AUERBACH'S WILDERNESS MEDICINE

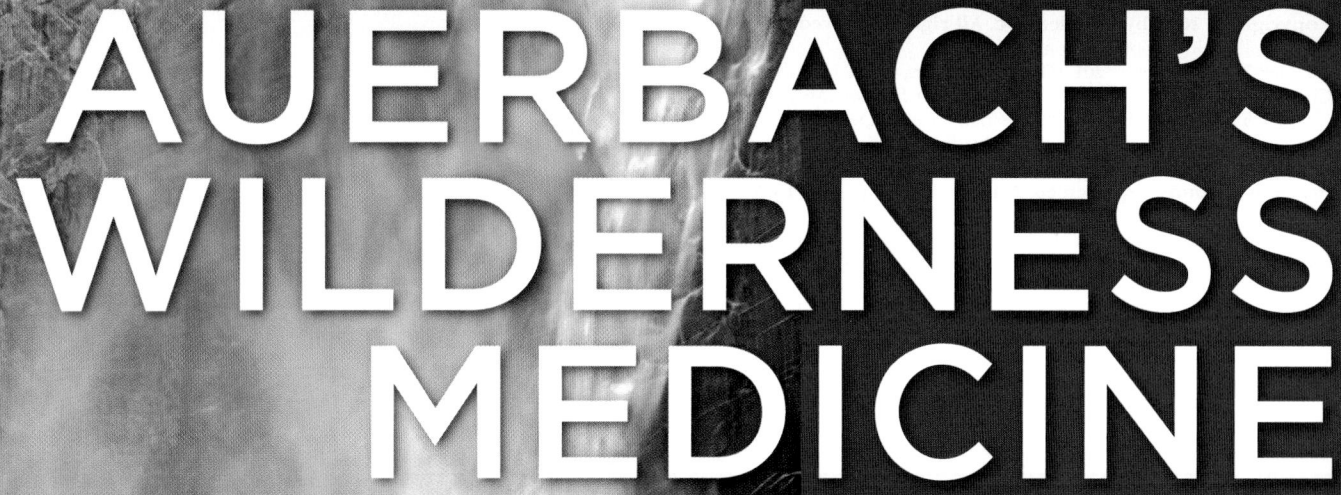

AUERBACH'S WILDERNESS MEDICINE

SEVENTH EDITION

EDITOR

PAUL S. AUERBACH
MD, MS, FACEP, MFAWM, FAAEM
Redlich Family Professor
Department of Emergency Medicine
Stanford University School of Medicine
Stanford, California

ASSOCIATE EDITORS

TRACY A. CUSHING, MD, MPH
Associate Professor
Department of Emergency Medicine
University of Colorado School of Medicine
Aurora, Colorado

N. STUART HARRIS, MD, MFA, FRCP (Edin)
Associate Professor of Emergency Medicine
Harvard Medical School
Chief, Division of Wilderness Medicine
Department of Emergency Medicine
Massachusetts General Hospital
Boston, Massachusetts

ELSEVIER

ELSEVIER

1600 John F. Kennedy Blvd.
Ste. 1800
Philadelphia, PA 19103-2899

Notices

International Standard Book Number: 978-0-323-35942-9

Executive Content Strategist: Kate Dimock
Content Development Manager: Lucia Gunzel
Publishing Services Manager: Patricia Tannian
Senior Project Manager: John Casey
Designer: Brian Salisbury

Printed in United States of America

Last digit is the print number: 9 8 7 6 5 4 3 2 1

Working together
to grow libraries in
developing countries

www.elsevier.com • www.bookaid.org

Contributors

Javier A. Adachi, MD, FACP, FIDSA
Associate Professor
Division of Internal Medicine
Department of Infectious Diseases, Infection Control and
    Employee Health
Adjunct Professor
Section of Infectious Diseases
Department of Medicine
Baylor College of Medicine
Adjunct Professor
Center for Infectious Diseases
The University of Texas Health Science Center at Houston
    School of Public Health
Houston, Texas

Norberto Navarrete Aldana, MD
Emergency Physician
Burns Intensive Care Unit
Hospital Simón Bolivar
Bogotá, Colombia

Martin E. Alexander, PhD, RPF
Adjunct Professor
Wildland Fire Science and Management
Department of Renewable Resources
Alberta School of Forest Science and Management
University of Alberta
Senior Fire Behavior Research Officer (Retired)
Canadian Forest Service, Northern Forestry Centre
Edmonton, Alberta, Canada

Susan Anderson, MD
Clinical Associate Professor
Division of Infectious Disease and Geographic Medicine
Center for Innovation and Global Health
Stanford, California;
Director of Travel Medicine
Palo Alto Medical Foundation
Palo Alto, California

Christopher J. Andrews, BE, MBBS, MEngSc,
**   PhD, JD, EDIC, GDLP, DipCSc, ACCAM**
Senior Lecturer, Medicine
University of Queensland
Brisbane, Queensland, Australia

E. Wayne Askew, PhD
Professor Emeritus
Department of Nutrition and Integrative Physiology
University of Utah
Salt Lake City, Utah

Dale Atkins, BA
President, American Avalanche Association
Vice President, Avalanche Rescue Commission
International Commission for Alpine Rescue, North America
    Training and Education Manager, RECCO, AB
Boulder, Colorado

Brian S.S. Auerbach, JD, MA, BE
Associate
Pepper Hamilton LLP
Philadelphia, Pennsylvania

Paul S. Auerbach, MD, MS, FACEP, MFAWM, FAAEM
Redlich Family Professor
Department of Emergency Medicine
Stanford University School of Medicine
Stanford, California;
Adjunct Professor
Department of Military and Emergency Medicine
F. Edward Hébert School of Medicine
Uniformed Services University of the Health Sciences
Bethesda, Maryland

Howard D. Backer, MD, MPH, FACEP, FAWM
Director
California Emergency Medical Services Authority
Sacramento, California

Aaron L. Baggish, MD
Assistant Professor
Cardiology Division
Department of Medicine
Associate Director
Cardiovascular Performance Center
Massachusetts General Hospital
Boston, Massachusetts

Buddha Basnyat, MD, MSc, FACP, FRCP (Edin)
Director
Oxford University Clinical Research Unit–Nepal
Medical Director
Nepal International Clinic and Himalayan Rescue Association
Kathmandu, Nepal

Pete Bettinger, PhD
Professor
School of Forestry and Natural Resources
University of Georgia
Athens, Georgia

Paul D. Biddinger, MD
Vice Chairman for Emergency Preparedness
Department of Emergency Medicine
Massachusetts General Hospital
Director
Emergency Preparedness Research, Evaluation and Practice
    Program
Harvard T.H. Chan School of Public Health
Boston, Massachusetts

Greta J. Binford, PhD
Associate Professor
Department of Biology
Lewis & Clark College
Portland, Oregon

Rebecca S. Blue, MD, MPH
Assistant Professor
Department of Preventive Medicine and Community Health
University of Texas Medical Branch at Galveston
Galveston, Texas

Ryan Blumenthal, MBChB (Pret), MMed (Forens) FC Path (SA), Dip Med (SA), PhD (Wits)
Senior Specialist
Department of Forensic Medicine
University of Pretoria
Pretoria, Gauteng, South Africa

Jolie Bookspan, PhD
Philadelphia, Pennsylvania

Ralph S. Bovard, MD, MPH, FACSM
Director
Occupational and Environmental Medicine Residency
Program
Midwest Center for Occupational Health and Safety
HealthPartners Medical Group
St. Paul, Minnesota

Warren D. Bowman Jr, MD
Clinical Associate Professor Emeritus
Department of Internal Medicine
University of Washington School of Medicine
Seattle, Washington

Leslie V. Boyer, MD
Associate Professor
Department of Pathology
Director
Venom Immunochemistry, Pharmacology, and Emergency
Response Institute
University of Arizona
Tucson, Arizona

Michael B. Brady, MA
Department of Geography
Rutgers University
Piscataway, New Jersey

Mark A. Brandenburg, MD
Medical Director
Bristow Medical Center
Bristow, Pennsylvania

Beau A. Briese, MD
Director
International Emergency Medicine
Department of Emergency Medicine
Houston Methodist Hospital
Houston, Texas

Millicent M. Briese, MA
Chief Executive Officer
Emergen International LLC
Houston, Texas

Calvin A. Brown III, MD
Department of Emergency Medicine
Brigham and Women's Hospital
Assistant Professor of Emergency Medicine
Harvard Medical School
Boston, Massachusetts

Colin M. Bucks, MD
Clinical Assistant Professor
Department of Emergency Medicine
Stanford University School of Medicine
Stanford, California

George H. Burgess, MSc
Director
Florida Program for Shark Research
Curator
International Shark Attack File
Florida Museum of Natural History
University of Florida
Gainesville, Florida

Sean P. Bush, MD, FACEP
Professor
Department of Emergency Medicine
Brody School of Medicine
East Carolina University
Greenville, North Carolina

Frank K. Butler Jr, MD
Chairman, Committee on Tactical Combat Casualty Care
Director, Prehospital Trauma Care
Joint Trauma System
San Antonio, Texas;
Adjunct Professor
Department of Military and Emergency Medicine
F. Edward Hébert School of Medicine
Uniformed Services University of the Health Sciences
Bethesda, Maryland

Dale J. Butterwick, MSc, CAT(C)
Associate Professor Emeritus
Faculty of Kinesiology
University of Calgary
Calgary, Alberta, Canada

Christopher R. Byron, DVM, MS, DACVS
Associate Professor of Large Animal Surgery
Large Animal Clinical Sciences
Virginia-Maryland College of Veterinary Medicine
Blacksburg, Virginia

Michael D. Cardwell, MS
Adjunct Faculty
Department of Biological Sciences
California State University
Sacramento, California

Steven C. Carleton, MD, PhD
Professor and W. Brian Gibler Chair of Emergency Medicine
Education
Department of Emergency Medicine
University of Cincinnati College of Medicine
Cincinnati, Ohio

Christopher R. Carpenter, MD, MSc, FACEP, FAAEM, AGSF
Associate Professor
Division of Emergency Medicine
Department of Medicine
Washington University in St. Louis School of Medicine
St. Louis, Missouri;
President, Academy for Geriatric Emergency Medicine
Chicago, Illinois

Scott P. Carroll, PhD
Research Associate
Department of Entomology and Nematology
University of California, Davis
Davis, California

John W. Castellani, PhD
Research Physiologist
Thermal and Mountain Medicine Division
US Army Research Institute of Environmental Medicine
Natick, Massachusetts

Michael J. Caudell, MD, FACEP, FAWM, DiMM
Professor
Department of Emergency Medicine and Hospitalist Services
Medical Director
Wilderness and Survival Medicine
Medical College of Georgia at Augusta University
Augusta, Georgia;
President
Appalachian Center for Wilderness Medicine
Morganton, North Carolina

Steven Chalfin, MD, FACS
Professor
Department of Ophthalmology
University of Texas Health Science Center at San Antonio
San Antonio, Texas

Nisha Charkoudian, PhD
Research Physiologist
Thermal and Mountain Medicine Division
US Army Research Institute of Environmental Medicine
Natick, Massachusetts

Samuel N. Cheuvront, PhD, RD
Research Physiologist
Thermal and Mountain Medicine
US Army Research Institute of Environmental Medicine
Natick, Massachusetts

Richard F. Clark, MD
Professor of Clinical Medicine
Division of Medical Toxicology
Department of Emergency Medicine
University of California, San Diego
San Diego, California

Kenneth S. Cohen, MA
Traditional Healer
Sacred Earth Circle
Nederland, Colorado

Richard W. Cole, MD, MPH, FACEP
Assistant Professor
Division of Aerospace Medicine
Department of Preventive Medicine and Community Health
University of Texas Medical Branch at Galveston
Galveston, Texas;
Clinical Instructor
Ultrasound Division
Department of Emergency Medicine
The University of Texas Health Science Center at Houston
Houston, Texas

Benjamin B. Constance, MD, FACEP, FAWM
Clinical Instructor
Department of Family Medicine
University of Washington School of Medicine
Chief and Medical Director
Tacoma Emergency Care Physicians
Tacoma General Hospital
Tacoma, Washington

Daniel G. Conway, DO, FACEP
Medical Corps
United States Army Medical Department
Department of Emergency Medicine
Fort Belvoir, Virginia

Donald C. Cooper, PhD, MBA
President and Chief Executive Officer
National Rescue Consultants, Inc.
Cuyahoga Falls, Ohio

Mary Ann Cooper, MD
Professor Emerita
University of Illinois at Chicago
Chicago, Illinois;
Founding Director
African Centres for Lightning and Electromagnetics
Kampala, Uganda

Kevin Coppock, MSc
Head of Mission—Myanmar
Médecins Sans Frontières (Doctors Without Borders)

Larry I. Crawshaw, PhD
Professor Emeritus
Biology Department
Portland State University
Professor Emeritus
Department of Behavioral Neuroscience
Oregon Health & Science University
Portland, Oregon

Gregory A. Cummins, DO, MS
Adjunct Instructor
Division of Primary Care
Department of Internal Medicine
Kansas City University of Medicine and Biosciences
Kansas City, Missouri

Tracy A. Cushing, MD, MPH
Associate Professor
Department of Emergency Medicine
University of Colorado School of Medicine
Aurora, Colorado

Jon Dallimore, MBBS, MSc
Specialty Doctor
Emergency Department
Bristol Royal Infirmary
Bristol, United Kingdom;
Co-Director, International Diploma in Expedition and
    Wilderness Medicine
Royal College of Physicians and Surgeons of Glasgow
Glasgow, United Kingdom;
General Practitioner
Vauxhall Practice
Chepstow, United Kingdom

Shawn D'Andrea, MD, MPH
Instructor of Emergency Medicine
Harvard Medical School
Boston, Massachusetts;
Chief
Emergency Medicine
Tsehootsooi Medical Center
Fort Defiance, Arizona

Daniel F. Danzl, MD
Professor and Chair
Department of Emergency Medicine
University of Louisville
Louisville, Kentucky

Kathleen M. Davis, BS, MS
Superintendent (Retired)
Montezuma Castle and Tuzigoot National Monument
National Park Service, Department of the Interior
Camp Verde, Arizona

Kevin Davison, ND, LAc
Director
Maui Regenerative Medicine
Haiku, Hawaii

Chad P. Dawson, MPS, PhD
Professor Emeritus
Department of Forest and Natural Resources Management
State University of New York College of Environmental Science
    and Forestry
Syracuse, New York

George R. Deeb, DDS, MD, FAWM
Associate Professor
Division of Oral and Maxillofacial Surgery
Department of Surgery
Virginia Commonwealth University
Richmond, Virginia

Janice A. Degan, RN, MS
Assistant Director of Research
Venom Immunochemistry, Pharmacology, and Emergency
    Response Institute
Arizona Health Sciences Center
University of Arizona
Tucson, Arizona

Thomas G. DeLoughery, MD, MACP, FAWM
Professor
Division of Hematology and Medical Oncology
Departments of Medicine, Pathology, and Pediatrics
Knight Cancer Institute
Oregon Health & Science University
Portland, Oregon

Arlene E. Dent, MD, PhD
Assistant Professor
Division of Pediatric Infectious Diseases and Rheumatology
Department of Pediatrics
Case Western Reserve University
Cleveland, Ohio

Alexandra E. DiTullio, MD
Attending Physician
Department of Emergency Medicine
The Queen's Medical Center
Honolulu, Hawaii

Katherine R. Dobbs, MD
Instructor
Division of Pediatric Infectious Diseases
Department of Pediatrics
Case Western Reserve University
Cleveland, Ohio

Eric L. Douglas, BA, EMT, DMT
Staff Instructor, Instructor Development Course
Emeritus Medic First Aid Master Trainer
Professional Association of Diving Instructors
Pinch, West Virginia

Jennifer Dow, MD
Medical Director
National Park Service—Alaska Region
Director
Emergency Department
Alaska Regional Hospital
Anchorage, Alaska

Herbert L. DuPont, MD, MACP
Mary W. Kelsey Distinguished Chair in Medical Sciences
Director, Center for Infectious Diseases
School of Public Health and McGovern Medical School
The University of Texas Health Science Center at Houston
Clinical Professor
Department of Medicine
Baylor College of Medicine
Houston, Texas

Thomas Eglin, MD
Assistant Professor of Family Medicine
Regional Assistant Dean
Pacific Northwest University of Health Sciences
Attending Physician
Emergency Department
Yakima Valley Memorial Hospital
Yakima, Washington

Timothy B. Erickson, MD, FACEP, FACMT, FAACT
Professor
Division of Toxicology
Department of Emergency Medicine
Director, UIC Center for Global Health
University of Illinois College of Medicine at Chicago
Chicago, Illinois

Thomas Evans, PhD
Chief Executive Officer
SAR3
Mountain View, California

Andrew J. Eyre, MD
Clinical Fellow
Harvard Medical School
Attending Physician
Department of Emergency Medicine
Brigham and Women's Hospital
Boston, Massachusetts

Joanne Feldman, MD, MS, UHM
Assistant Clinical Professor
Department of Emergency Medicine
University of California, Los Angeles
Los Angeles, California

D. Nelun Fernando, PhD
Hydrologist
Surface Water Resources
Water Science and Conservation
Texas Water Development Board
Austin, Texas

Paul G. Firth, MD
Assistant Professor
Harvard University
Pediatric Anesthesiologist
Department of Anesthesia, Critical Care, and Pain Medicine
Massachusetts General Hospital
Boston, Massachusetts

Mark S. Fradin, MD
Clinical Associate Professor
Department of Dermatology
University of North Carolina School of Medicine
Private Practice, Chapel Hill Dermatology, P.A.
Chapel Hill, North Carolina

Bryan L. Frank, MD, FAAMA, FAAPM, FAAARM
President
Global Mission Partners, Inc.
Yukon, Oklahoma

Esther E. Freeman, MD, PhD, FAAD
Assistant Professor
Department of Dermatology
Massachusetts General Hospital
Harvard Medical School
Boston, Massachusetts

CONTRIBUTORS

Luanne Freer, MD
Medical Director
Medcor at Yellowstone
Yellowstone National Park
Yellowstone, Wyoming;
Founder and Director
Everest ER
Himalayan Rescue Association
Mt Everest, Nepal

Tom Garrison, PhD
Professor Emeritus
Marine Science Department
Orange Coast College
Costa Mesa, California;
Adjunct Professor of Higher Education
Rossier School of Education
University of Southern California
Los Angeles, California

Alan Gianotti, MD, MS
Department of Emergency Medicine
Mills-Peninsula Medical Center
Burlingame, California;
Volunteer Physician
Himalayan Rescue Association Nepal
Kathmandu, Nepal

Robert V. Gibbons, MD, MPH
Task Area Manager
Battlefield Pain Management
United States Army Institute of Surgical Research
Joint Base San Antonio
Fort Sam Houston, Texas

Gordon G. Giesbrecht, PhD, FAsMA
Professor
Faculty of Kinesiology and Recreation Management;
    Department of Anesthesia
Director, Laboratory for Exercise and Environmental Medicine
Health, Leisure and Human Performance Research Institute
University of Manitoba
Winnipeg, Manitoba, Canada

Alina Goldenberg, MD, MAS
Department of Dermatology
University of California, San Diego
San Diego, California

Craig Goolsby, MD
Associate Professor
Department of Military and Emergency Medicine
F. Edward Hébert School of Medicine
Uniformed Services University of the Health Sciences
Bethesda, Maryland;
Director, Hybrid Simulation Lab
Val G. Hemming Simulation Center
Silver Spring, Maryland;
Attending Emergency Physician
Howard County General Hospital
Columbia, Maryland

Kimberlie A. Graeme, MD, FACMT
Clinical Associate Professor
Department of Emergency Medicine
University of Arizona College of Medicine
Medical Toxicologist
Department of Medical Toxicology
Banner—University Medical Center Phoenix
Phoenix, Arizona

Donald L. Grebner, PhD
Professor
Department of Forestry
Mississippi State University
Starksville, Mississippi

Colin K. Grissom, MD
Professor
Department of Internal Medicine
University of Utah School of Medicine
Salt Lake City, Utah;
Associate Medical Director
Shock Trauma Intensive Care Unit
Intermountain Medical Center
Murray, Utah

Peter H. Hackett, MD
Director, Institute for Altitude Medicine
Telluride, Colorado;
Clinical Professor
Department of Emergency Medicine
University of Colorado Denver School of Medicine
Aurora, Colorado

Charles Handford, MBChB (Hons), MRCS
General Duties Medical Officer
Royal Army Medical Corps
British Army

N. Stuart Harris, MD, MFA, FRCP (Edin)
Associate Professor of Emergency Medicine
Harvard Medical School
Chief, Division of Wilderness Medicine
Department of Emergency Medicine
Massachusetts General Hospital
Boston, Massachusetts

Seth C. Hawkins, MD, EMD
Assistant Professor
Department of Emergency Medicine
Wake Forest University
Winston-Salem, North Carolina

Charles G. Hawley, BS
Chairman
Safety at Sea Committee
United States Sailing Association
Portsmouth, Rhode Island

David M. Heimbach, MD, FACS
Professor Emeritus
Department of Surgery
University of Washington
Seattle, Washington

Carlton E. Heine, MD, PhD, FACEP, FAWM
Clinical Associate Professor
Elson S. Floyd College of Medicine
Washington State University
Spokane, Washington

Lawrence E. Heiskell, MD, FACEP, FAAFP
Emergency Physician
Founder and Director
International School of Tactical Medicine
Rancho Mirage, California

John C. Hendee, PhD
Professor Emeritus
Department of Conservation Social Sciences
College of Natural Resources
University of Idaho
Moscow, Idaho

Andrew A. Herring, MD
Director
Pain and Addiction Treatment
Department of Emergency Medicine
Highland Hospital
Oakland, California

Ronald L. Holle, MS
Meteorologist
Holle Meteorology and Photography
Oro Valley, Arizona

John R. Hovey, BS
Senior Instructor
Wilderness Medicine Institute
National Outdoor Leadership School
Lander, Wyoming

Martin R. Huecker, MD
Assistant Professor and Research Director
Department of Emergency Medicine
University of Louisville
Louisville, Kentucky

Christopher H. E. Imray, MB BS, DiMM, MSc, PhD, FRCS, FRCP, FRGS
Professor
Department of Vascular Surgery
University Hospital Coventry and Warwickshire NHS Trust
Warwick Medical School and Coventry University
Coventry, United Kingdom

Hillary R. Irons, MD, PhD
Assistant Professor
Department of Emergency Medicine
University of Massachusetts Medical School
UMass Memorial Medical Center
Worcester, Massachusetts

Kenneth V. Iserson, MD, MBA
Professor Emeritus
Department of Emergency Medicine
University of Arizona
Tucson, Arizona

Michael E. Jacobs, MD, MFAWM
Martha's Vineyard, Massachusetts

Ramin Jamshidi, MD, FACS
Assistant Professor
Department of Surgery
Department of Child Health
University of Arizona College of Medicine
Medical Director of Pediatric Trauma
Surgical Director of Pediatric Intensive Care
Maricopa Medical Center
Phoenix, Arizona

Joshua M. Jauregui, MD
Acting Assistant Professor
Division of Emergency Medicine
University of Washington School of Medicine
Seattle, Washington

James M. Jeffers, BA, LLB, LLM, MPhil, PhD
Senior Lecturer in Human Geography
College of Liberal Arts
Bath Spa University
Bath, United Kingdom

Amber M.H. Johnson, DO, DMD
Department of Oral and Maxillofacial Surgery
Virginia Commonwealth University
Richmond, Virginia

Kirsten N. Johnson, MD, MPH
Assistant Professor
Division of Emergency Medicine
Department of Family Medicine
McGill University
CEO, Humanitarian U
Montréal, Québec, Canada

Hemal K. Kanzaria, MD, MS
Assistant Professor
Department of Emergency Medicine
University of California, San Francisco
San Francisco, California

Misha R. Kassel, MD
Department of Emergency Medicine
Pali Momi Medical Center
Aiea, Hawaii

Stephanie Kayden, MD, MPH, CEDE
Assistant Professor
Harvard Medical School
Chief
Division of International Emergency Medicine and
    Humanitarian Programs
Department of Emergency Medicine
Brigham and Women's Hospital
Boston, Massachusetts

Katherine M. Kemen, MBA
Program Manager
Emergency Preparedness
Partners HealthCare
Boston, Massachusetts

Robert W. Kenefick, PhD
Research Physiologist
Thermal and Mountain Medicine Division
US Army Research Institute of Environmental Medicine
Natick, Massachusetts

Michael L. Kent, MD
Commander
Medical Corps, United States Navy
Assistant Professor
Department of Anesthesiology
F. Edward Hébert School of Medicine
Uniformed Services University of the Health Sciences
Staff Anesthesiologist
Bethesda, Maryland

Minjee Kim, MD
Assistant Professor
Division of Neurocritical Care
Ken and Ruth Davee Department of Neurology
Northwestern University Feinberg School of Medicine
Chicago, Illinois

Alexa B. Kimball, MD, MPH
Professor
Department of Dermatology
Harvard Medical School
Boston, Massachusetts

W. Taylor Kimberly, MD, PhD
Assistant Professor of Neurology
Harvard Medical School
Division of Neurocritical Care and Emergency Neurology
Department of Neurology
Massachusetts General Hospital
Boston, Massachusetts

Sean M. Kivlehan, MD, MPH
Clinical Instructor
Department of Emergency Medicine
Brigham and Women's Hospital
Harvard Medical School
Boston, Massachusetts

Judith R. Klein, MD
Assistant Clinical Professor
Department of Emergency Medicine
University of California, San Francisco
San Francisco General Hospital
San Francisco, California

Karyn Koller, MD, MPH
Associate Professor
Department of Emergency Medicine
Oklahoma University
Tulsa, Oklahoma

Brian J. Krabak, MD, MBA, FACSM
Clinical Professor
Department of Rehabilitation Medicine
Department of Orthopedics and Sports Medicine
University of Washington School of Medicine
Seattle, Washington

Andrew C. Krakowski, MD
Chief Medical Officer
DermOne, LLC
West Conshohocken, Pennsylvania

Michael J. Krzyzaniak, MD
Trauma, Critical Care, and Emergency Surgery
Department of Surgery
Naval Medical Center San Diego
San Diego, California

Peter Kummerfeldt, AD
Former Owner, OutdoorSafe Inc.
Former Survival Training Director
United States Air Force Academy
Colorado Springs, Colorado

Mark R. Lafave, PhD, CAT(C)
Professor and Athletic Therapy Program Coordinator
Department of Health and Physical Education
Mount Royal University
Calgary, Alberta, Canada

Ashley R. Laird, MD
Emergency Medicine
Asante Rogue Regional Medical Center
Medford, Oregon

Bruce Lampard, MD, FRCP, MIA
Lecturer
Division of Emergency Medicine
Department of Medicine
University of Toronto Faculty of Medicine
Toronto, Ontario, Canada

Michael A. Lang, BSc, DPhil
Assistant Adjunct Professor
Department of Emergency Medicine
Co-Director, San Diego Center of Excellence in Diving
University of California, San Diego
San Diego, California

Carolyn S. Langer, MD, JD, MPH
Associate Professor
Department of Family Medicine and Community Health
University of Massachusetts Medical School
Worcester, Massachusetts

Charlotte A. Lanteri, PhD
Deputy Director, Microbiology Section
Department of Pathology and Area Laboratory Services
Brooke Army Medical Center
San Antonio, Texas

Gordon L. Larsen, MD, FACEP, FAWM
Department of Emergency Medicine
Intermountain Health Care (IHC)
Dixie Regional Medical Center
St. George, Utah;
Medical Advisor
Zion National Park
Washington County, Utah

Justin S. Lawley, PhD
Instructor
Institute for Exercise and Environmental Medicine
Texas Health Presbyterian Hospital
University of Texas Southwestern Medical Center
Dallas, Texas

David J. Ledrick, MD, MEd
Associate Residency Director
Department of Emergency Medicine
Mercy Health—St. Vincent Medical Center
Toledo, Ohio

Jay Lemery, MD
Associate Professor
Department of Emergency Medicine
University of Colorado School of Medicine
Aurora, Colorado;
Fellow and Visiting Scientist
François-Xavier Bagnoud Center for Health and Human Rights
Harvard T.H. Chan School of Public Health
Boston, Massachusetts

Lisa R. Leon, PhD, FAPS
Research Physiologist
Thermal Mountain Medicine Division
US Army Research Institute of Environmental Medicine
Natick, Massachusetts

Benjamin D. Levine, MD, FACC, FAHA, FACSM
Professor
Division of Cardiology
Department of Internal Medicine
Distinguished Professor of Exercise Sciences
University of Texas Southwestern Medical Center
Director, Institute for Exercise and Environmental Medicine
Texas Health Presbyterian Hospital
Dallas, Texas

Matthew R. Lewin, MD, PhD
Director
Center for Exploration and Travel Health
California Academy of Sciences
San Francisco, California

James R. Liffrig, MD, MPH, FAAFP
Medical Director, FirstHealth Convenient Care
FirstHealth of the Carolinas Physicians Group
Pinehurst, North Carolina

Robin W. Lindsay, MD
Assistant Professor
Division of Facial Plastics and Reconstructive Surgery
Massachusetts Eye and Ear Infirmary
Department of Otolaryngology
Harvard Medical School
Boston, Massachusetts

CONTRIBUTORS

Grant S. Lipman, MD, FACEP, FAWM
Clinical Associate Professor
Department of Emergency Medicine
Stanford University School of Medicine
Stanford, California

Michael S. Lipnick, MD
Assistant Professor
Department of Anesthesia and Perioperative Care
University of California, San Francisco
Dive Medical Officer
California Academy of Sciences
San Francisco, California

Joanne Liu, MD, IMHL
International President
Médecins Sans Frontières (Doctors Without Borders)
Geneva, Switzerland

Andrew M. Luks, MD
Associate Professor
Division of Pulmonary and Critical Care Medicine
Department of Medicine
University of Washington School of Medicine
Seattle, Washington

Binh T. Ly, MD
Professor
Department of Emergency Medicine
University of California, San Diego
San Diego, California

Darryl J. Macias, MD
Professor
Department of Emergency Medicine
Medical Director
International Mountain Medicine Center
University of New Mexico
Albuquerque, New Mexico

Martin J. MacInnis, PhD
Postdoctoral Fellow
Exercise Metabolism Research Group
Department of Kinesiology
McMaster University
Hamilton, Ontario, Canada

Monika Brodmann Maeder, MD, MME
Senior Consultant
Department of Emergency Medicine
Bern University Hospital
Bern, Switzerland;
Senior Researcher
Institute of Mountain Emergency Medicine
European Academy of Bozen/Bolzano
Bolzano, South Tyrol, Italy

Edgar Maeyens Jr, MD
Private Practice
Dermatology
Coos Bay, Oregon

David S. Markenson, MD, MBA, FAAP, FACEP, FCCM, FACHE
Chief Medical Officer
Sky Ridge Medical Center
Lone Tree, Colorado;
National Chair
American Red Cross Scientific Advisory Council
Washington, DC

Armando Márquez Jr, MD
Assistant Clinical Professor
Department of Emergency Medicine
University of Illinois College of Medicine at Chicago
Chicago, Illinois

Thomas H. Marshburn, MD
Astronaut
National Aeronautics and Space Administration
Lyndon B. Johnson Space Center
Houston, Texas

Denise M. Martinez, MS, RD
Greenland, New Hampshire

Nicholas P. Mason, PhD, MB ChB
Consultant
Critical Care Medicine
Royal Gwent Hospital
Newport, United Kingdom

Michael J. Matteucci, MD
Assistant Professor
Department of Military and Emergency Medicine
F. Edward Hébert School of Medicine
Uniformed Services University of the Health Sciences
Bethesda, Maryland;
Emergency Medicine Department
Naval Medical Center San Diego
San Diego, California

Vicki Mazzorana, MD, FACEP, FAAEM, FAWM
Associate Professor
Emergency Medicine
Touro University Nevada College of Osteopathic Medicine
Las Vegas, Nevada

Loui H. McCurley
Chief Executive Officer
Pigeon Mountain Industries, Inc.
Lafayette, Georgia;
Technical Rescue Specialist
Alpine Rescue Team
Evergreen, Colorado

Henderson D. McGinnis, MD
Associate Professor
Department of Emergency Medicine
Wake Forest School of Medicine
Winston-Salem, North Carolina

Marilyn McHarg, O.Ont., MSc(A)
Private Consultant
Dundas, Ontario, Canada

Scott E. McIntosh, MD, MPH, FAWM, DiMM
Associate Professor
Division of Emergency Medicine
Department of Surgery
University of Utah School of Medicine
Salt Lake City, Utah

Carolyn Sierra Meyer, MD
Associate Physician
Emergency Medicine
Kaiser West Los Angeles Medical Center
Los Angeles, California

Richard S. Miller, MD
Professor of Surgery
Chief, Division of Trauma and Surgical Critical Care
Section of Surgical Sciences
Vanderbilt University Medical Center
Nashville, Tennessee

Michael G. Millin, MD, MPH, FACEP
Associate Professor
Division of Special Operations
Department of Emergency Medicine
Johns Hopkins University School of Medicine
Baltimore, Maryland;
Medical Director
Maryland Search and Rescue
State of Maryland

Alicia B. Minns, MD
Assistant Clinical Professor
Division of Medical Toxicology
Department of Emergency Medicine
Fellowship Director
Medical Toxicology Fellowship
University of California, San Diego
San Diego, California

John Mioduszewski, PhD
Center for Climatic Research
University of Wisconsin—Madison
Madison, Wisconsin

James K. Mitchell, PhD
Professor Emeritus
Department of Geography
Rutgers University
Piscataway, New Jersey

James Moore, BSc (Hons) Emergency Care
Director, Travel Health Consultancy
Exeter, Devon, United Kingdom;
Co-Director, International Diploma in Expedition and
    Wilderness Medicine
Royal College of Physicians and Surgeons of Glasgow
Glasgow, United Kingdom

Roger B. Mortimer, MD, FAAFP
Clinical Professor
Department of Family and Community Medicine
University of California, San Francisco
San Francisco, California;
Western Region Coordinator
National Cave Rescue Commission
Huntsville, Alabama

Michael J. Mosier, MD, FACS, FCCM
Associate Professor
Department of Surgery
Division of Trauma, Surgical Critical Care, and Burns
Loyola University Medical Center
Maywood, Illinois

Alice F. Murray, MB ChB
Instructor
Department of Emergency Medicine
Boston Medical Center
Boston, Massachusetts

Robert W. Mutch
Consultant
Fire Management Applications
Missoula, Montana

Ken Nguyen, PhD
Chief, Bacteriology Laboratory
Microbiology Section
Department of Pathology and Laboratory Services
Brooke Army Medical Center
San Antonio, Texas;
Company Commander
Troop Command, Brooke Army Medical Center
Joint Base San Antonio
Fort Sam Houston, Texas

Vicki E. Noble, MD
Associate Professor
Harvard Medical School
Director, Division of Emergency Ultrasound
Department of Emergency Medicine
Massachusetts General Hospital
Boston, Massachusetts

Robert L. Norris, MD, FACEP, FAAEM
Professor Emeritus
Department of Emergency Medicine
Stanford University School of Medicine
Stanford, California

Timothy C. Nunez, MD, FACS
Associate Professor
Division of Trauma and Surgical Critical Care
Section of Surgical Sciences
Vanderbilt University Medical Center
Tennessee Valley Veterans Administration Medical Center
Nashville, Tennessee

Karen K. O'Brien, MD
American Lake Division
Veterans Administration Puget Sound Healthcare System
Tacoma, Washington

Francis G. O'Connor, MD, MPH
Professor and Chair
Department of Military and Emergency Medicine
F. Edward Hébert School of Medicine
Uniformed Services University of the Health Sciences
Bethesda, Maryland

Terry O'Connor, MD
Emergency Physician
St Luke's Wood River Medical Center
Ketchum, Idaho

Lisa K. Oddy, MPH
Humanitarian U
Montréal, Québec, Canada

Bohdan T. Olesnicky, MD
CEO and President
SWAT Fuel, Inc.
Indian Wells, California

Edward J. Otten, MD, FACMT, FAWM
Professor
Departments of Emergency Medicine and Pediatrics
Director, Division of Toxicology
Department of Emergency Medicine
University of Cincinnati
Cincinnati, Ohio

Parveen K. Parmar, MD, MPH
Associate Professor
Director
Division of International Emergency Medicine
Department of Emergency Medicine
Keck School of Medicine
University of Southern California
Los Angeles, California

Sheral S. Patel, MD, FAAP, FASTMH
U.S. Food and Drug Administration
Silver Spring, Maryland

Ryan D. Paterson, MD, DiMM, DTM&H
Assistant Adjoint Professor
Section of Wilderness and Environmental Medicine
Department of Emergency Medicine
University of Colorado School of Medicine
Aurora, Colorado

Suchismita Paul, MD
Department of Dermatology & Cutaneous Surgery
University of Miami Miller School of Medicine
Miami, Florida

Lara L. Phillips, MD
Clinical Assistant Professor
Director
Wilderness Medicine
Department of Emergency Medicine
Thomas Jefferson University Hospital
Philadelphia, Pennsylvania

Justin T. Pitman, MD
Attending Physician
Department of Emergency Medicine
Mt. Auburn Hospital
Cambridge, Massachusetts;
Instructor of Emergency Medicine
Harvard Medical School
Boston, Massachusetts

Robert H. Quinn, MD
Professor and John J. Hinchey MD and Kathryn Hinchey Chair
Department of Orthopaedic Surgery
The University of Texas Health Science Center at San Antonio
San Antonio, Texas

Martin I. Radwin, MD
Chief of Gastrointestinal Endoscopy
Jordan Valley Medical Center
Salt Lake City, Utah

S. Christopher Ralphs, MS, DVM, DACVS
Staff Surgeon
Small Animal Surgery
Ocean State Veterinary Specialists
East Greenwich, Rhode Island

Wayne D. Ranney, MS
Adjunct Professor (Retired)
Department of Geology
Yavapai College
Prescott, Arizona;
President
Grand Canyon Historical Society
Flagstaff, Arizona

Mark A. Read, PhD, BSc
Manager
Operations Support
Great Barrier Reef Marine Park Authority
Townsville, Queensland, Australia

Sheila B. Reed, MS
Consultant
Disaster Risk Reduction and Development
Middleton, Wisconsin

Martin Rhodes, MBChB, DiMM
Medical Director
Antarctic Logistics & Expeditions LLC
Salt Lake City, Utah

Gates Richards, MEd, WEMT-I, FAWM
Special Programs Manager
Wilderness Medicine Institute
National Outdoor Leadership School
Lander, Wyoming

Robert C. Roach, PhD
Associate Professor
Director
Altitude Research Center
Department of Emergency Medicine
University of Colorado School of Medicine
Aurora, Colorado

George W. Rodway, PhD, APRN
Associate Clinical Professor
Betty Irene Moore School of Nursing
University of California, Davis
Sacramento, California

Nancy V. Rodway, MD, MPH
Medical Director
Lake County General Health District
Painesville, Ohio

Brent E. Ruoff, MD
Associate Professor and Chief
Division of Emergency Medicine
Washington University in St. Louis School of Medicine
St. Louis, Missouri

Renee N. Salas, MD, MPH
Division of Wilderness Medicine
Department of Emergency Medicine
Massachusetts General Hospital
Clinical Instructor
Department of Emergency Medicine
Harvard Medical School
Boston, Massachusetts

Richard S. Salkowe, DPM, PhD, FACFAS, FAWM
Medical/Training Officer
Florida Region 4 State Medical Response Team
Master Instructor–Leidos
Federal Emergency Management Agency Center for Domestic
    Preparedness
Research Associate
School of Public Affairs
University of South Florida
Tampa, Florida

Tod Schimelpfenig, WEMT-I, FAWM
Curriculum Director
Wilderness Medicine Institute
National Outdoor Leadership School
Lander, Wyoming

Andrew C. Schmidt, DO, MPH
Assistant Professor
Department of Emergency Medicine
University of Florida–Jacksonville
Jacksonville, Florida

CONTRIBUTORS

Sandra M. Schneider, MD, FACEP
Professor of Emergency Medicine
Hofstra Northwell School of Medicine
Hempstead, New York;
Attending Physician
John Peter Smith Hospital
Fort Worth, Texas

Robert B. Schoene, MD
Clinical Professor
Division of Pulmonary and Critical Care Medicine
Department of Medicine
University of Washington School of Medicine
Seattle, Washington;
Sound Physicians
The Intensivist Group
St. Mary's Medical Center
San Francisco, California

John Semple, MD, MSc, FRCSC, FACS
Head, Division of Plastic Surgery
Women's College Hospital
Professor
Department of Surgery
University of Toronto
Toronto, Ontario, Canada

Justin Sempsrott, MD, FAAEM
Executive Director
Lifeguards Without Borders
Jacksonville Beach, Florida

Jamie R. Shandro, MD, MPH
Associate Professor
Division of Emergency Medicine
Department of Medicine
University of Washington School of Medicine
Seattle, Washington

David Shaye, MD
Instructor
Division of Facial Plastic and Reconstructive Surgery
Massachusetts Eye and Ear Infirmary
Department of Otolaryngology
Harvard Medical School
Boston, Massachusetts

Susan B. Sheehy, PhD, RN, FAEN, FAAN
Associate Professor
Daniel K. Inouye Graduate School of Nursing
Uniformed Services University of the Health Sciences
Bethesda, Maryland

Robert L. Sheridan, MD, FAAP, FACS
Burn Service Medical Director
Boston Shriners Hospital for Children
Division of Burns
Massachusetts General Hospital
Professor of Surgery
Harvard Medical School
Boston, Massachusetts

Charles S. Shimanski, BA
Air Rescue Commission
International Commission for Alpine Rescue (ICAR)
Kloten, Switzerland;
Education Director
Mountain Rescue Association
San Diego, California

Joshua D. Shofner, MD
Dermatology Associates of Winchester
Winchester, Massachusetts

Tatum S. Simonson, PhD
Assistant Professor
Division of Physiology
Department of Medicine
University of California, San Diego
La Jolla, California

Eunice M. Singletary, MD, FACEP
Associate Professor
Department of Emergency Medicine
University of Virginia
Charlottesville, Virginia

William "Will" R. Smith, MD, FAWM
President and Medical Director
Wilderness and Emergency Medical Consulting, LLC
Jackson, Wyoming;
Medical Director
National Park Service
Washington, DC

Hans Christian Sørenson, MD, IMM
The Hospital, Tasiilaq
Tasiilaq, East Greenland

Susanne J. Spano, MD
Director
Wilderness Medicine Education
University of California, San Francisco Fresno
Fresno, California;
Assistant Clinical Professor
Department of Emergency Medicine
University of California, San Francisco
San Francisco, California

Matthew C. Spitzer, MD, DTMH
Past President, Board of Directors
Médecins Sans Frontières (Doctors Without Borders)—USA
Assistant Clinical Professor of Medicine
Center for Family and Community Medicine
College of Physicians and Surgeons
Columbia University
New York, New York

Brian Stafford, MD, MPH
Founder and Lead Guide
Wilderness Is Medicine
Ojai, California

Alan M. Steinman, MD, MPH
Rear Admiral (Retired)
United States Public Health Service
Director of Health and Safety
United States Coast Guard
Olympia, Washington

Giacomo Strapazzon, MD, PhD
Vice Head
Institute of Mountain Emergency Medicine
European Academy of Bozen/Bolzano
International Commission for Mountain Emergency Medicine
Bolzano, South Tyrol, Italy

Jeffrey R. Suchard, MD, FACEP, FACMT
Professor
Departments of Emergency Medicine and Pharmacology
University of California, Irvine School of Medicine
Irvine, California

CONTRIBUTORS

Julie A. Switzer, MD
Assistant Professor
Department of Orthopaedic Surgery
University of Minnesota
Minneapolis, Minnesota

Noushafarin Taleghani, MD, PhD, FAAEM
Clinical Associate Professor
Department of Emergency Medicine
Stanford University School of Medicine
Stanford, California

John Tanner, MD
Department of Emergency Medicine
Yakima Valley Memorial Hospital
Yakima, Washington

Shana L. Tarter, WEMT-I, FAWM
Assistant Director
Wilderness Medicine Institute
National Outdoor Leadership School
Lander, Wyoming

Owen D. Thomas, BMedSc (Phys), MBChB (Hons), DTM&H
Birmingham Medical Research Expeditionary Society
Birmingham, United Kingdom

Stephen H. Thomas, MD, MPH
Chairman
Emergency Department
Hamad General Hospital and Hamad Medical Corporation
Department of Medicine
Weill Cornell Medical College in Qatar
Doha, Qatar

Todd W. Thomsen, MD
Instructor in Medicine
Department of Emergency Medicine
Harvard Medical School
Boston, Massachusetts;
Attending Physician
Department of Emergency Medicine
Mount Auburn Hospital
Cambridge, Massachusetts

Robert I. Tilling, PhD
Volcanologist Emeritus
US Geological Survey
Menlo Park, California

David A. Townes, MD, MPH, DTM&H
Associate Professor
Division of Emergency Medicine
Department of Medicine
Adjunct Associate Professor
Department of Global Health
University of Washington School of Medicine
Seattle, Washington

Stephen J. Traub, MD, FACEP, FACMT
Associate Professor and Chair
Department of Emergency Medicine
Mayo Clinic Arizona
Phoenix, Arizona

Sydney J. Vail, MD, FACS
Associate Professor
Department of Surgery
University of Arizona College of Medicine—Phoenix
Chief, Division of Trauma and Surgical Critical Care
Director, Tactical Medicine Program
Vice Chairman
Department of Surgery
Maricopa Medical Center
Phoenix, Arizona

Karen B. Van Hoesen, MD
Clinical Professor
Department of Emergency Medicine
Co-Director, San Diego Center of Excellence in Diving
University of California, San Diego
San Diego, California

Michael VanRooyen, MD, MPH
Associate Professor of Emergency Medicine
Harvard Medical School
Chairman
Department of Emergency Medicine
Director
Division of International Health and Humanitarian Programs
Brigham and Women's Hospital
Boston, Massachusetts

Raghu Venugopal, MD, MPH, FRCPC
Assistant Professor
Division of Emergency Medicine
Department of Medicine
University of Toronto
Toronto, Ontario, Canada

Julian Villar, MD, MPH
Chief Fellow
Division of Critical Care Medicine
Department of Medicine
Stanford University School of Medicine
Stanford, California

Brandee L. Waite, MD
Associate Professor
Associate Director Sports Medicine Fellowship
Department of Physical Medicine and Rehabilitation
University of California, Davis School of Medicine
Sacramento, California

John B. Walden, MD, DTMH
Professor
Department of Family and Community Health
Director, International Health
Joan C. Edwards School of Medicine
Marshall University
Huntington, West Virginia

David A. Warrell, MA, DM, DSc, FRCP, FRCPE, FZS, FRGS, FMedSci
International Director
Royal College of Physicians
London, United Kingdom;
Emeritus Professor of Tropical Medicine
Nuffield Department of Clinical Medicine
University of Oxford
Oxford, United Kingdom

Ashley Kochanek Weisman, MD
Harvard Affiliated Emergency Medicine Residency
Brigham and Women's Hospital
Massachusetts General Hospital
Boston, Massachusetts

Timothy J. Wiegand, MD, FACMT, FAACT, FASAM
Associate Clinical Professor
Departments of Emergency Medicine and Public Health
  Sciences
Director of Toxicology
University of Rochester Medical Center
Rochester, New York

Stacie L. Wing-Gaia, PhD, RD, CSSD
Associate Professor
Department of Nutrition and Integrative Physiology
University of Utah
Salt Lake City, Utah

Sarah A. Wolfe, MD
Assistant Professor
Department of Dermatology
Duke University School of Medicine
Durham, North Carolina

Megann Young, MD, FACEP
Director
Wilderness Medicine Fellowship
University of California, San Francisco Fresno
Fresno, California;
Assistant Clinical Professor
Department of Emergency Medicine
University of California, San Francisco
San Francisco, California

Ken Zafren, MD, FAAEM, FACEP, FAWM
Clinical Professor
Department of Emergency Medicine
Stanford University Medical Center
Stanford, California;
Vice President
International Commission for Mountain Emergency Medicine
Associate Medical Director
Himalayan Rescue Association
Kathmandu, Nepal

Foreword

Before partaking of an urban existence, men, women, and children lived in austerity in the wilderness. So, the human race is not encountering wilderness medicine for the very first time. Before the advent of such wonders as antisepsis, randomized clinical trials, and emphasis on evidence, and therefore throughout most of the history of human existence and eventually, civilization, the practice of medicine was largely improvised and based on anecdotes and dogma, rather than evolving science. Given that humans had to make do with little or nothing before they had access to tests, drugs, and devices, the history of wilderness medicine might be considered to largely be the history of medicine itself. Advances in medicine have in general paralleled other sciences, with periodic insights into its essences, but there remain geographies and circumstances where wilderness medicine is uniquely essential.

We are in the midst of a scientific revolution, but recognize that optimal urban science is not necessarily applicable in austere environments. So, as we intentionally place ourselves in wild places isolated from cities and machines, wilderness medicine comes full circle and needs to remain different in certain ways from big city medicine. From this perspective, one might identify many potential starting points for our 21st century iteration of wilderness medicine. However, thoughtful reflection identifies two prominent threads. First, today's wilderness medicine "began" when urban, high-resource medicine became too sophisticated to practice in austere environments—when improvisation was required to replace more sophisticated methodology that was not available. Second, and very significant from a definition standpoint, wilderness medicine gained true identity when men and women began in earnest to explore environments that stressed normal human physiology to the point that unique pathophysiology was discovered. This phenomenon notably occurred with human endeavors at high altitude (mountaineering and aviation), under the ocean surface (diving), at extremes of temperature (cold and heat), and at the limits of endurance posed by natural disasters or forays into the ultimate frontier of space travel.

The history of wilderness medicine could be a textbook unto itself. The following paragraphs attempt to provide key examples of how the evolution of modern medicine simultaneously drew from and shaped the specialty.

Military medicine provides many examples of this interaction. For much of history, the greatest threats to soldiers were not battlefield combatants, but weather and infectious diseases. During the American Revolutionary War, 6,200 American soldiers were killed in action, while 10,000 died of disease. Typhus, smallpox, dysentery, diarrhea, and pneumonia were prevalent. The War of 1812 generated 2,200 American combat deaths and nearly 13,000 deaths from noncombat causes. Napoleon invaded Russia in 1812 with 680,000 soldiers, and retreated back to France five months later with 27,000. Most of the remainder had succumbed to hypothermia, frostbite, and typhus. It wasn't until World War II that the number of soldiers killed in combat outnumbered those who died from other causes, many of them environmental.

"*Medicine Under Sail,*" Zachary Friedenberg's history on the subject,[1] chronicles an oft-overlooked perspective of the early history of medicine. In the same vein, Homer made reference in book 4 of the *Iliad* to a medical naval incident in the Trojan War.[2] When Menelaus was wounded by a Trojan bowman, the fleet surgeon, Machaon (son of Aesculapius, god of medicine), was called to treat the wound:

> *Without delay he drew*
> *the arrow from the fairly fitted belt.*
> *The barbs were bent in drawing.*
> *Then he loosed the plate—the armorer's work—and carefully*
> *O'er looked the wound where fell the bitter shaft.*
> *Cleansed it from blood, and sprinkled over it*
> *with skill the soothing balsam of yore which*
> *the friendly Chiron to his father gave.*

Thomas Woodall (1569-1643) perhaps deserves the title "Father of Marine Medicine" because he was ahead of his time with observations of scurvy and views on the treatment of wounds, fractures, and amputations.[1] His extensive practical experience, astute observations, and cautious judgment persuaded him that the theories of oracles, such as Galen, often offered little in the way of useful medical knowledge. As stated in his 1655 book *The Surgeon's Mate*, Woodall divided wounds into three categories: (1) puncture wounds and lacerations, (2) gunshot wounds, and (3) bone fractures.[3] His treatment recommendations have a modern ring: "…remove unnatural things forced into the wound… which should be done with the least pain to the patient and avoiding arteries, nerves, and veins." The "unnatural things" to which he referred might include wood splinters from spars and masts, fragments from cannon fire, and other foreign objects embedded into people during commerce and conflict. Anesthesia was nonexistent in this era. In the case of removal being too difficult or painful, Woodall recommended "tarry if you may, while nature helps." His suggestions to ligate specific vessels that contributed to excessive bleeding and to place dressings soaked in wine over wounds were significant departures from the usual treatment of the day, which was wound cauterization with hot oil or a red-hot searing iron.

When limb wounds were severe, Woodall was not in a rush to amputate. This approach ran counter to the prevailing custom and for several hundred years afterward. Woodall reasoned that the need for amputation should be dictated by specific criteria: one-half or more of the limb should have been dismembered or irreparably damaged; a chronic suppurating wound be present; the patient's life be imminently in danger; or the remaining portion of the limb be unserviceable. His concepts were far more conservative and reasonable than those of military surgeons who practiced for the next two centuries, such as during the American Civil War, where immediate amputation of any limb with a gunshot wound was the customary practice. Woodall's conservative principles from three centuries past seem reasonable for modern physicians providing care for trauma patients in harsh or remote environments.

It was Admiral Horatio Nelson, a senior nonmedical officer in the British Royal Navy, who near the turn of the nineteenth century brought about a revolution in medicine, particularly in disease control, practiced on the high seas. Nelson's well-documented personal medical history provides a window into certain typical maladies and injuries for the ocean-going warrior or explorer of his era. As a midshipman, he sustained partial paralysis from an illness contracted at age 17, was stricken with malaria in the West Indies, contracted yellow fever in Nicaragua, suffered a laceration of his back and lost sight in his left eye during battles near Corsica, endured an abdominal wound during a military encounter at Cape St. Vincent, and had his right arm amputated below the shoulder after a severe injury from grapeshot during battle in the Canary Islands. His luck ran out in 1805 at Trafalgar, where a French sharpshooter's bullet delivered a fatal blow.

Largely as a result of Admiral Nelson's impressive understanding of the challenges of providing effective shipboard medical care, medical reforms in his and other navies became a reality. Much emphasis was directed at proper diet as it relates to disease prevention, a unique perspective at that time that is increasingly popular today. The success of this strategy is obvious from the historical record; the proportion of men sent sick to hospital from ships between the last decade of the 18th century and the first decade of the 19th century fell from a high of 38.4% (in 1793) to a low of 6.4% (in 1806).[4]

After the end of the American Civil War, the U.S. Army fought with many Native American tribes in the western states and territories. Military medical personnel and civilian practitioners became adept at extracting arrows and other primitive penetrating weapons. Instruments devised as early as 500 BC (such as the *belulcum*) for removing arrows became invaluable during the 1870s. These tools could dilate the point of entrance and widen the channel containing the arrow, to allow the head of the arrow to be grasped. North American Indian arrows were typically fired with great speed and force, and if not stopped by bone, could easily pass through a horse or bison. Not surprisingly, mortality from arrow wounds was high, with one 1871 report suggesting a fatality rate of approximately 30%.

The ensuing maturation of military medicine marked a turning point back to appreciation of wilderness medicine, or perhaps more appropriately, austere medicine. This occurred when the military began to move medicine to the front lines. Re-emergence of tourniquets applied in the field to extremities to control bleeding are illustrative. In the past two decades, bringing medicine to the point of action led to creation of tactical combat casualty care (TCCC)[5] and formation of the Special Operations Medical Association (SOMA), including collaboration with the Wilderness Medical Society (WMS). Soldiers with life-threatening injuries that previously would have been fatal are now stabilized on or near the battlefield before being evacuated to definitive trauma centers in their home countries.

Parallel to the contributions of military medicine were those of intrepid explorers. Many of the early "practitioners" of wilderness medicine were adventurers who accepted additional responsibilities. Although not a physician, Captain William Clark had sufficient medical knowledge to serve as the expedition doctor on the heralded Lewis and Clark expedition.[6] In the early days of exploration, expedition doctors were integral members of a dedicated team with expertise related to the logistics of the mission. The current expeditionary practice of retaining expert medical guests is a relatively recent phenomenon.

Infection from nonsterile surgical procedures and penetrating missiles was but one major challenge of this bygone era. Early explorers also had to contend with infectious diseases that could easily be passed between persons and that had the potential to bring any journey to a sudden halt. Throughout much of the course of its explorations, the Lewis and Clark expedition encountered indigenous tribes. These tribes had not been exposed to European-based diseases for many centuries, so were neither educationally nor immunologically capable of effective self-defense. The Americans learned of many settlements (especially along the Missouri River) that had been decimated by devastating epidemics of smallpox following contact with persons of European background. The concept of vaccination was gathering proponents at this time, and President Thomas Jefferson sent a sample of cowpox on the expedition with Lewis in hope that he could attempt to vaccinate the "natives."[7] Other infectious maladies of regular concern to Lewis and Clark included omnipresent venereal diseases, such as syphilis. Prior to 1800, mercury, already used as therapy for many infections and diseases, had

become the treatment of choice for syphilis. It was typically taken orally or used as a topical ointment in very liberal doses. Cures were few and far between, and the patient often succumbed to mercury poisoning before the syphilis entered its secondary or tertiary phase. During this era, cinchona for malaria was one of only a handful of medications that had the ability to produce an intended result. Thus, early physicians "were like hunters going into the field and shooting blanks."[8]

As exploration of the last great terrestrial and oceanic "blanks on the map" evolved into ever more sophisticated ventures in the 19th and early 20th centuries, wilderness medical care further evolved. "Physician/naturalists," trained physicians who could multitask as field biologists, began to accompany long, arduous explorations to the ends of the earth. While their medical training was certainly superior to that of William Clark and they could be considered more competent healers, these physicians still needed to be extremely skilled outdoorsmen to participate in these demanding adventures. To appreciate the extent of the sacrifices sometimes made by these physician-explorers, one need only recall the Englishman Edward Wilson—physician, polar explorer, natural historian, painter, and ornithologist. Wilson accompanied two of Robert Scott's exploratory Antarctic voyages in the early years of the 20th century, tragically perishing with his companions in March 1912 on the Antarctic plateau during the British team's return sledge journey from the South Pole. Edward Atkinson, research parasitologist and senior expedition surgeon for Scott's final, ill-fated 1910-1913 *Terra Nova* expedition, was part of the shore party that did not accompany Scott, Wilson, and their three companions during the final push to the Pole. By March 1912, Scott's party was clearly overdue and fear mounted that they had perished. That month, Atkinson, as senior officer in command of 13 men facing 4 months of darkness and intense cold, led a futile effort to locate Scott. In October of 1912, with the sun at last shedding some light and heat on the bleak Antarctic landscape, Atkinson once again set out with a search party. On November 12, they discovered the dead explorers within Scott's tent, which was partially buried in snow. Atkinson was first to enter the tent, where he read the diary entries of the polar party's final days of privation and suffering.[9]

During the 20th century, exploration of the limits of the human body and those of the earth's physical domain altered the manner in which people viewed the world and their place in it. While the pursuits of physical exploration and medicine may seem unlikely siblings, they deeply informed each other. Dr. Charles Houston, who served as an inspiration to many current wilderness medicine researchers and clinicians, embodied the modern adventurer-physician.[10] An accomplished mountaineer and Harvard-trained physician, Houston led two attempts to summit K2, included the ill-fated attempt in 1953 that claimed the life of one team member and nearly wiped out the entire team. While a naval flight surgeon during World War II, Houston conceived, and ultimately was one of the physician/scientists in charge of, Operation Everest in 1946. This study, sponsored by the U.S. Navy, was intended to benefit the aviation community by shedding light on human adaptation to and tolerance of extreme altitudes. Such research efforts were particularly timely because they occurred at a time when airplanes became capable of flying higher than humans could tolerate without support, such as from pressurized suits or cabins. Houston's high-altitude chamber research led to the first successful simulated "ascent" to the barometric pressure equivalent of the summit of Mt Everest, proving it could perhaps be reached in real life without supplemental oxygen. His research team's findings led to great advances in understanding the challenges of altitude and etiology of high-altitude illnesses. Houston later became a founding member of the WMS, and in doing so, drew attention to its mission and potential.

Houston's achievements were part of a blossoming of science exemplified by the discoveries of other legendary figures in altitude research and mountain medicine, including Drs. Herb Hultgren, John West, Robert Schoene, and Peter Hackett. While serving as a member of the American Medical Research Expedition to Everest in 1981, Hackett accomplished a successful summit of Mt Everest, climbing alone to the top from high camp, falling while traversing the Hillary step, and thereby fortunately uncovering a fixed rope that enabled him to self-rescue and live to tell the tale. He too became one of the founding members of the WMS. During this modern era, brave and high-spirited physician high-altitude adventurers Drs. Oswald Oelz, Charles Clarke, and Bruno Dürrer were pioneering by exploring, discovering, and innovating. There were and will be so many brilliant men and women who combine adventure with medicine.

One could write equally about the oceans that cover most of our planet, and about forests, rivers, canyonlands, or polar caps. There will hopefully always be mountains to climb, woods to wander, deserts to cross, and lagoons to explore. Each has its wilderness medicine history, from antiquity to modern times. There are lost people to find, victims of mishaps to rescue, and ever the need to make do with very little at the worst possible moments. We know more now about how to direct doctors, and how to facilitate location, stabilization, and transport of victims from remote and geographically challenging locales. Wilderness first responders are equipped with knowledge and training that allow for more advanced intervention that occurs with shorter transport times.[11] Search and rescue team training has become sophisticated and intense, in large measure because the wilderness medicine community has set the bar higher.

The logical evolution (and practical admixture) of wilderness medicine and wilderness search and rescue can be clearly seen in today's international Diploma in Mountain Medicine (DiMM). A cooperative idea initially developed in Europe in the late 1990s by the International Commission for Alpine Rescue, International Climbing and Mountaineering Federation, and International Society of Mountain Medicine, the extensive and comprehensive DiMM curriculum blends rigorous didactic and practical education in wilderness medicine with technical mountain rescue and self-sufficiency in the backcountry. Many mountain medicine organizations worldwide now offer the standard (or specialty module) DiMM curriculum, in the process bridging many nations and cultures.

The final linchpin in the modern enactment of wilderness medicine as a distinct entity is the selfless act of delivering medical care to the farthest reaches of the globe. Less fortunate people benefit from the emotionally taxing and sometimes courageous efforts of many wilderness medicine–trained volunteers who deliver medical support that ranges from immunizations during peaceful times to surgeries in the aftermath of natural disasters. Wilderness medicine breeds an ethos of service. Medical teams populated by wilderness medicine providers depart at a moment's notice to assist in humanitarian relief and disaster response. After many lessons learned from earlier treat-and-leave approaches, providers and organizations have embarked upon much more sustainable approaches to health care delivery, including vital education and training.

The modern history of wilderness medicine spawned the founding and maturation of important scientific societies dedicated to the discipline or one of its subspecialties. The WMS was formed in 1982; the International Society of Mountain Medicine in 1985; and the International Society of Travel Medicine in 1991. Phenomenal individuals who contributed to modern wilderness medicine have become too numerous to count. Modern wilderness medicine was conceptualized and organized by a dedicated and ambitious group of prime movers, and has become an enormous, growing community, reflected in part by the contributors to this textbook, some of whom have been involved in wilderness medicine for many decades. We admire the pioneers of the past, and have every confidence in the ability of today's leaders and innovators to carry us with great enthusiasm into the future.

Robert H. Quinn, MD
George W. Rodway, PhD

REFERENCES

1. Friedenberg ZB. Medicine Under Sail. Annapolis, MD: Naval Institute Press; 2002.
2. Homer. The Iliad and the Odyssey. London: John Ogilby; 1660.
3. Woodall T. The Surgeon's Mate. London: John League; 1655.
4. Allison RS. Sea Diseases: The Story of a Great Natural Experiment in Preventive Medicine in the Royal Navy. London: John Bale Medical Publications; 1943.
5. Butler FK, Hagmann J, Butler G. Tactical combat casualty care in special operations. Mil Med 1996;161(Suppl. 1):1–16.
6. Larsell O. Excerpts from: Medical aspects of the Lewis and Clark expedition (1804-1806). Wilderness Environ Med 2003;14:265–71.
7. Chuinard EP. Only One Man Died: The Medical Aspects of the Lewis and Clark Expedition. Fairfield, WA: Ye Galleon Press; 1999.
8. Paton BC. Adventuring with Boldness: The Triumph of the Explorers. Golden, CO: Fulcrum Publishing; 2006.
9. Campbell WC. Edward Leicester Atkinson: Physician, parasitologist, and adventurer. J Hist Med Allied Sci 1991;46:219–40.
10. McDonald B. Brotherhood of the Rope: the Biography of Charles Houston. Seattle, WA: The Mountaineers; 2007.
11. Backer HD. Editorial: what is wilderness medicine? Wilderness Environ Med 1995;6:3–10.

Preface

As the specialty of wilderness medicine matures, obligations grow. Education is the objective of this textbook and certainly essential, but to advance the field in all aspects, leadership and inspiration are required. In this seventh edition of *Wilderness Medicine*, the contributors are many of these leaders, and their writing and creativity are outstanding. Authors who are practitioners and researchers with an inestimable amount of experience share their knowledge and wisdom, and seek not only to teach, but to inspire those who will follow them. They have superbly pointed out not only what we already know, but also what we need to discover and learn, thereby directing a path toward observation, service, and experimentation, each of which is integral to the unique influence of wilderness medicine.

The breadth and depth of content of wilderness medicine have grown to the extent that two volumes of *Wilderness Medicine* are now required. The authors, assistant editors, and I are grateful to the publisher for using innovative techniques to create a comprehensive book with outstanding visual appeal, so that the blend of academia and art is at once logical and stimulating. In this edition, I am enormously grateful to the remarkable team at Elsevier, including Kate Dimock, Lucia Gunzel, Lauren Boyle, and Linda Belfus. My publishing family always sets the bar high and patiently helps me leap. My global academic family embraces this exciting specialty, and my biological family graciously allows me the time to pursue this endeavor.

Acquisition of new knowledge is exciting and challenging for academicians, practitioners, and students. Wilderness medicine draws not only from the timeless medical specialties of surgery, internal medicine, obstetrics and gynecology, pediatrics, and psychiatry, but from anywhere that medical science reaches out to improve the health and safety of patients. New chapters and deeper discussions within revised chapters introduce the reader to the trends that are most likely to become influential as we approach the next five years. Evidence-based medicine, genomics and personalization, and the imperative to translate all of this into how we live our lives and practice our craft in the field and hospital are new features of this edition. Other notable changes from the previous edition are a chapter on medical wilderness adventure races and expanded discussion of high-altitude medicine, improvisation, technical rescue, and wilderness medicine education, to name a few. We are proud to continue emphasis on how we approach the health of planet Earth. Wilderness conservation and preservation will remain in part the purview of wilderness medicine as we await a more concerted effort by the entire house of medicine to fulfill its obligation to play a leadership role in efforts to maintain the desired environment to support life on our planet.

The efforts of people and organizations engaged in all aspects of wilderness medicine are growing and increasingly collaborative. Wilderness medicine is firmly embedded in the activities of the military, and vice versa. As a responder to the 2015 earthquake disaster in Nepal, I witnessed once again that my remarkable colleagues in the wilderness medicine community are regularly at the front lines when calamity strikes. Whether it is an Ebola outbreak in West Africa, a typhoon in the Philippines, or a wildfire in Washington State, this book's contributors enthusiastically volunteer to serve. What I have learned since the last edition is that anywhere the ability to practice medicine in an austere setting is the task at hand, wilderness medicine knowledge and experience are essential.

In medical schools across the United States, and now in many other countries, wilderness medicine courses are taught and usually among the most popular electives. Wilderness experiences are used by undergraduate universities and medical schools to introduce students to one another early in their careers and facilitate collaborations. Competitive wilderness adventures in the cloaks of competitions and races are the backbone of reality entertainment. They all require medical planning and support. Wilderness recreation outpaces all other forms of time away from the urban work existence. Respite and renewal are inextricably linked to the wilderness. And when we seek to reach beyond ourselves, where do we go first to explore? The wilderness, of course.

At a time when humans are generally considered more of a burden to than saviors of the environment, we will more often be in the wilderness, learning its ways and hopefully not encroaching upon it. To impress upon others the need to preserve it, we will understand its offerings and document its beauty. To eliminate health care disparities, we will find a way to interact with indigenous people in a way that can preserve their surroundings and bring healing in the midst of horrific infectious diseases, violent conflicts, and post-disaster social and economic chaos. To fuel our existence, we will go beyond clear-cutting forests, pillaging oceans, and extracting fossil fuels that might never be replaced. If wilderness medicine helps make us aware that there is a wilderness and that without a concerted effort it will disappear, then that is a precious accomplishment by a noble specialty.

Judging by the quality of research, number of important publications, and attendance at educational gatherings, such as the combined sessions of the Wilderness Medical Society and International Society for Mountain Medicine, wilderness medicine is here to stay. For that, we are in great debt to those who came before us, who preached and practiced wilderness medicine long before anyone contemplated coalescing a specialty. One such visionary is Dr. Bruce Paton, whose artwork graces this Preface. We all have mentors and partners, and I have certainly had mine. Notable among them are Herb Hultgren and Charlie Houston in high-altitude medicine, Jeff Davis and Bruce Halstead in dive medicine, Warren Bowman in prehospital care, Bob Mutch in wildland fire management, Donald Trunkey in trauma care, Bruce Dixon in clinical diagnosis, Murray Fowler in veterinary medicine, Sherman Minton in envenomation, Bruno Dürrer in rescue, Steve French in bear behavior and attack, Cam Bangs and Alan Steinman in hypothermia, Joe Serra and Ed Geehr in humanism, Wongchu Sherpa in spirituality, and Ken Kizer in determination.

The spark has become a flame. I regularly see young people beam when they realize that medicine can be so enjoyable. There are hardcore science and service in wilderness medicine, but we are still "out there," away from electronic medical records, cost containment, and endless political debates about universal health care. We are in the field, responding because we are responsive, sticking our necks out to accept the adventure and risk, and then put something back. There is heroism in medicine, and wilderness medicine has its fair share, delightfully unsung. It is brave to document the wisdom of an indigenous healer, courageous to teach mountain safety to sherpas, and selfless to assist laypersons to fill the gaps in health care that cannot be provided during a humanitarian crisis. The settings in which we practice may sometimes be uncontrolled, but it is the domain of wilderness medicine experts to bring best practices to the unique bedsides posed on the side of a mountain, in a cave during a lightning storm, or on the beach of a faraway atoll. Wilderness medicine takes everything we have learned and then adds to it the spice of life. How much fun is that? Seven editions now, and I can't wait for the eighth.

Paul S. Auerbach

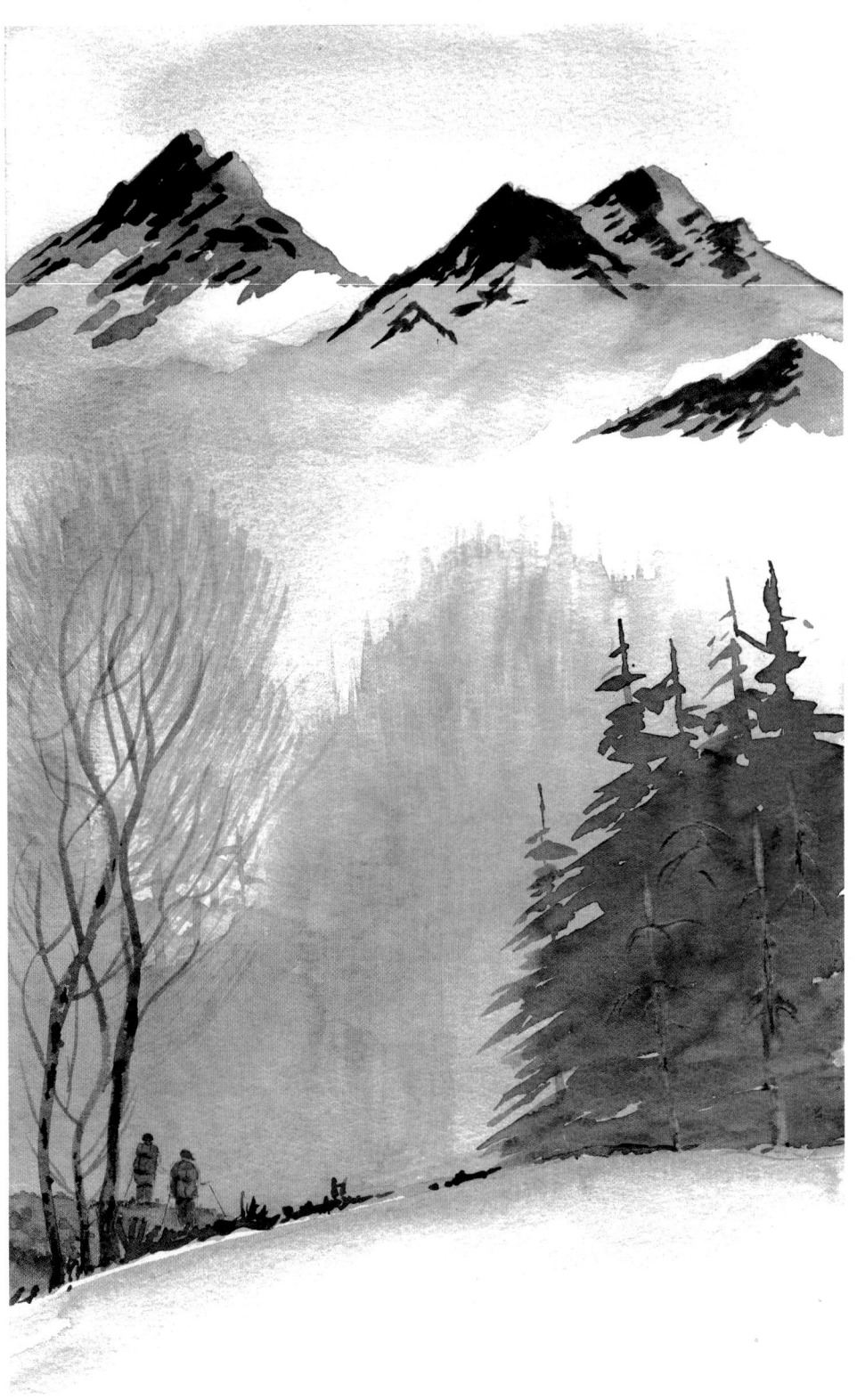

Aiming High
Bruce Paton

Contents

Video Contents

PHOTO CREDITS

Front and Back Cover, Spine, Part 17

Copyright 2016 Elizabeth Carmel

Parts 1 to 5, 9, 12, 14, 16

Courtesy Paul S. Auerbach

Part 6

Copyright iStockphoto.com/meikesen

Parts 7, 15

Copyright 2016 Mathias Schar

Part 8

Copyright iStockphoto.com/osmanpek

Part 10

Copyright 2016 Norbert Wu

Part 11

Copyright iStockphoto.com/Rumo

Part 13

Copyright iStockphoto.com/koldunova

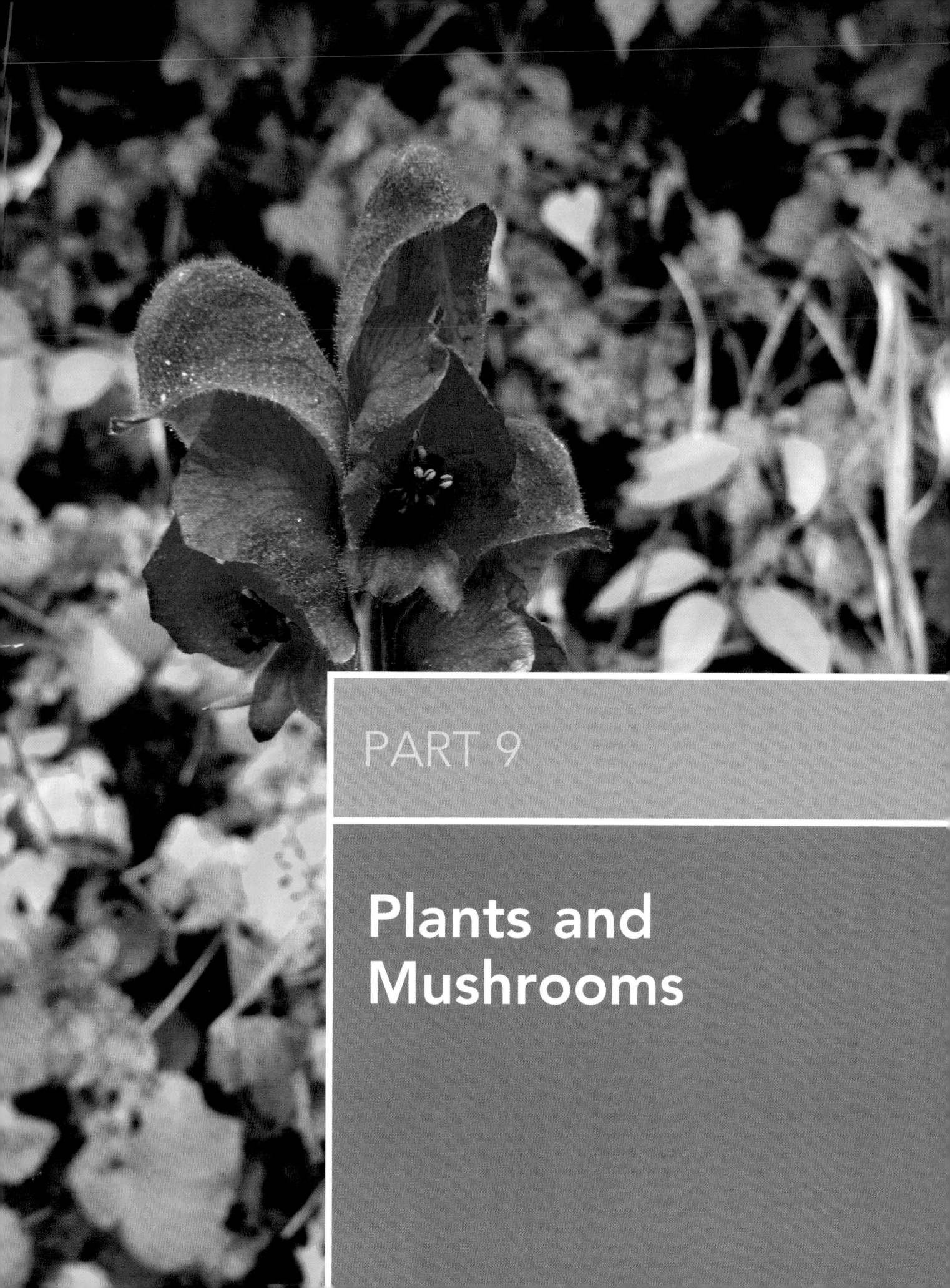

PART 9

Plants and Mushrooms

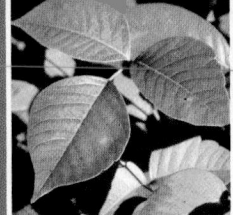

CHAPTER 64

Plant-Induced Dermatitis

ESTHER E. FREEMAN, SUCHISMITA PAUL, JOSHUA D. SHOFNER, AND ALEXA B. KIMBALL

Cutaneous exposure to plants may cause a wide array of skin problems. Plant-induced dermatitis can manifest in multiple ways, including weeping eczematous patches and plaques, vesicles and bullae, fine scaly patches, or any combination of these. Because the end result may be a generic response to injury, dermatitis is often an easy clinical diagnosis to make. However, determining the type of dermatitis affecting the patient can be difficult and frustrating. Acute care providers are often the first individuals to encounter and treat severe plant-induced dermatitis, so the ability to make a rapid and accurate diagnosis is crucial.

There are numerous subtypes of dermatitis: contact (irritant or allergic), photoallergic, nummular, asteatotic, stasis, seborrheic, atopic, and dyshidrotic. Dermatitis can manifest acutely with vesicles and bullae or in a chronic form with lichenification and hyperpigmentation. The acute nature of dermatitis is often itchy and uncomfortable, leading patients to seek emergency care. The history and physical examination are of the utmost importance in determining causality. A morphologic approach to the physical examination is a high-yield method for generating the appropriate differential diagnosis. Is the rash linear in nature? This often implies an external contactant. Is the rash in sun-exposed areas? This implies a photosensitive dermatitis.

In addition, the symptoms of the rash are important. Irritant reactions tend to decrescendo in severity, being the worst at presentation and gradually improving over time, whereas those that are allergic tend to crescendo, then decrescendo. They gradually build over 1 to 21 days to peak intensity, then slowly improve.

There are many clinical mimics of plant-induced dermatitis, including drug hypersensitivity reactions, connective tissue disease, superficial fungal infections, urticaria, and cutaneous T cell lymphoma. If a patient has persistent dermatitis that lasts longer than 1 month, a biopsy is often indicated to help differentiate possible mimickers. Pathology review of the biopsy specimen will help rule out other conditions and lead to appropriate therapy.

The subset of dermatitis discussed in this chapter is plant-induced dermatitis. Plant-induced dermatitis can be caused by contact with a wide variety of plants. Thousands of species of plants have been reported to cause dermatitis. The specific effects that each of these plants has on the skin have not been fully determined or described. The majority of medical literature regarding plant-induced dermatitis is anecdotal and has not been confirmed by independent observers. Few large-scale studies of the effects of plants have been performed. The exception is the *Toxicodendron* (poison ivy/oak/sumac) species of plants, because of their ubiquitous nature.

The most common injury to skin caused by plants is a simple scratch, laceration, or puncture wound. This can lead to bacterial or fungal infection. Plant-induced dermatitis reactions can be further subclassified. These include irritant contact dermatitis, allergic contact dermatitis, phototoxic dermatitis, and photoallergic dermatitis. Plants can also cause contact urticaria and foreign body reactions.

IRRITANT CONTACT DERMATITIS

A wide variety of plants cause irritant contact dermatitis, or nonallergic inflammation of the skin caused by direct contact with the offending plant. Most of these rashes are mild and self-limited, typically involving 1% to 2% body surface area (BSA). Irritant contact dermatitis causes transient redness and pruritus of the contacted skin. The spectrum of reactions ranges from linear scratch marks to weeping, ulcerated, red scaly plaques that may be difficult to link to the originating plant.

The most common cause of plant-induced contact dermatitis is irritant in nature. Irritant contact dermatitis can be further subdivided into traumatic (mechanical) and chemical causes. Most plants have the potential to cause traumatic skin injury. Some common plants in this category include rose thorns, cactus, orange trees, lemon trees, bougainvillea, and Euphorbiaceae.[37] Whether it is a thorn from a hawthorn tree, a cut from a sharp leaf edge, or scratches from briars, human skin is poorly prepared to protect itself from such insults (Figure 64-1).

Any foreign body embedded in the skin can cause a granulomatous reaction pattern. Some plants are more prone to causing this type of inflammatory reaction. Plants with thorns and barbs are the most likely culprits. Rose thorns and cactus spines are common offenders (Figure 64-2). Cacti are indigenous to the southwestern United States. They are popular as houseplants and can be grown indoors with proper care. Therefore, cactus injuries can be seen in a wide variety of locales.[116] The initial contact and acute injury may lead to chronic granulomatous inflammatory eruption, which typically takes 4 to 8 weeks to develop. It is the lag time that may make the diagnosis difficult. Clinically, the rash consists of erythematous and indurated papules, plaques, and nodules. The lesions are often grouped and localized, which is a clue to the diagnosis. Cactus spines may also penetrate so deeply into the skin that they cause pseudotumors of bone.[106]

The prickly pear (*Opuntia ficus-indica*) is found in North and Central America, as well as around the Mediterranean Sea. It is a member of the Cactaceae family. The fruit is covered with glochids. A unique example of mechanical trauma is from a glochid. Glochids are modified leaves that appear as tufts of barbed spines or hairs found on *Opuntia* species of cacti (Figure 64-3). They have sharp tips that penetrate skin and cause irritation by disrupting the epidermis. They are very loosely held to the cactus, release with the slightest touch, are quite irritating to skin, and cause variable amounts of discomfort and itching. They tend to break off from the cactus and work their way onto the skin, causing a granulomatous reaction that may resemble scabetic nodules.[106] They can also implant into the conjunctiva.[132] Glochids are present year-round and cause dermatitis in all seasons.

Similarly, penetrating injuries from a variety of cactus species, including *Echinopsis*, have been reported throughout the southwestern United States. Typical injuries manifest on the extremities as inflammatory papules. In rare cases, cactus spines can penetrate into bone and soft tissue spaces and cause inflammatory arthritis. Appropriate footwear and clothing, including gloves, are of utmost importance when encountering plants that can cause mechanical skin trauma. Treatment is to remove the spines from the skin. This is best done mechanically with a forceps under bright illumination and magnification if necessary[96,132] (Figure 64-4).

When biopsies are performed of the chronic (4 weeks after initial injury) inflammatory papules caused by cacti glochid implantation, a granulomatous reaction pattern is found.[79] Multiple multinucleated giant cells, histiocytes, granulomas, and organic plant material can be seen histologically under polarized light sources. Occasionally, a traumatic injury may implant one or more microbes. When performing a biopsy, one should also perform a tissue culture for bacteria, mycobacteria, and fungal species. This is especially true in cases with pustular morphologies.

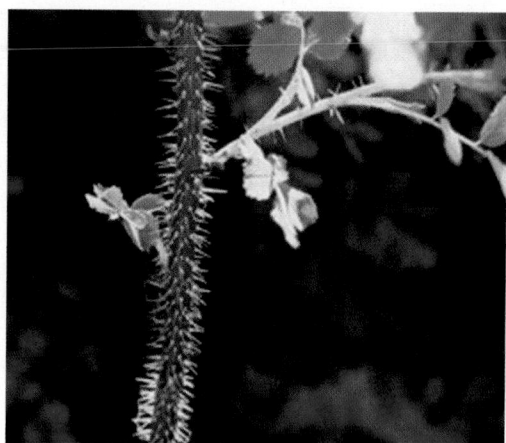

FIGURE 64-1 Spiny thorns of the rose bush. *(Courtesy USDA-NRCS PLANTS Database; Herman DE, et al: North Dakota tree handbook, USDA NRCS ND State Soil Conservation Committee, Bismarck, ND, 1996, NDSU Extension and Western Area Power Administration.)*

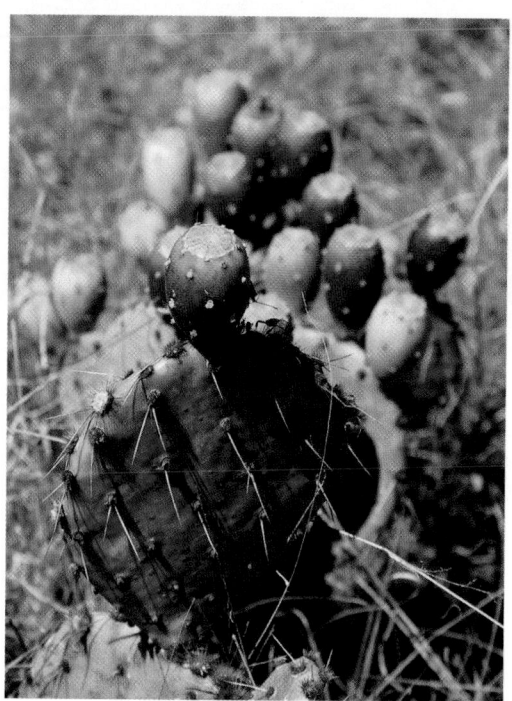

FIGURE 64-3 Prickly pear cactus. *(Courtesy Jon Sullivan.)*

Initial treatment should be prompt extraction of the cactus spines. The smaller the spine, the more difficult the removal.[79] This is a particular problem when encountering injuries from the beaver tail cactus (Figure 64-5), which has very small glochids that can be quite difficult to remove. Many methods of removal have been employed to remove the spines. Tweezers are often the first line of removal, and various gels, glue, tape, and facial masks have been tried.[86] The best method is mechanical removal with a small forceps or fine needle. Once removal is accomplished, a topical corticosteroid can be employed. A midpotency topical corticosteroid, such as triamcinolone acetonide (Aristocort, Kenalog) 0.1% cream or ointment, is often all that is needed. The general recommendation is to use topical corticosteroids for 2 weeks at a time to avoid skin atrophy; however, reports in the literature suggest use twice daily for up to 3 months for this indication.[116] Most granulomatous reactions resolve within 2 to 4 months.[36] Often, removal attempts are unsuccessful, and the glochids work their way to the surface over months to years. Supportive care with cool compresses with aluminum acetate solution 1:40 in water used as soak, compress, or wet dressing is very helpful. Administering pain medication and initiating prompt therapy for any coinfection are integral parts of the overall treatment plan.

Infections may also be inoculated into the skin from mechanical plant injury. The most well known is *Sporothrix schenckii* fungal infection occurring after a prick or puncture from a rose thorn. *S. schenckii* is a common dimorphic fungus found in organic material. The characteristic lymphangitic spread is easily recognized (Figure 64-6). Typically, an ulcerating nodule develops at the site of inoculation; then, over the next 3 weeks (range, 3 days to 12 weeks), nodules develop along the draining lymphatic channels. The nodules eventually ulcerate, and patients develop chronic lymphangitis. First-line therapy is itraconazole, 200 mg orally (PO) once daily for 2 to 4 weeks after all lesions have resolved, usually for a total of 3 to 6 months.[26,90] There are many other infections caused by traumatic implantation of bacteria, fungus, and algae into skin or underlying subcutaneous tissues (Box 64-1).

Another common problem is direct implantation of plant organic material into the skin. This implantation causes a foreign body reaction, such as that seen with a splinter. The goals of treatment are to remove the foreign material promptly and treat infections with the appropriate antimicrobial agent(s).

Wood dust can also cause an eczematous dermatitis of either the irritant or allergic type. The victims are nearly always woodworkers who have been repeatedly exposed. Allergic contact dermatitis occasionally develops. Rarely, an erythema multiforme–like configuration is noted.[50] Respiratory hypersensitivity, including asthma, to wood dusts is well documented.[118] Solid wood

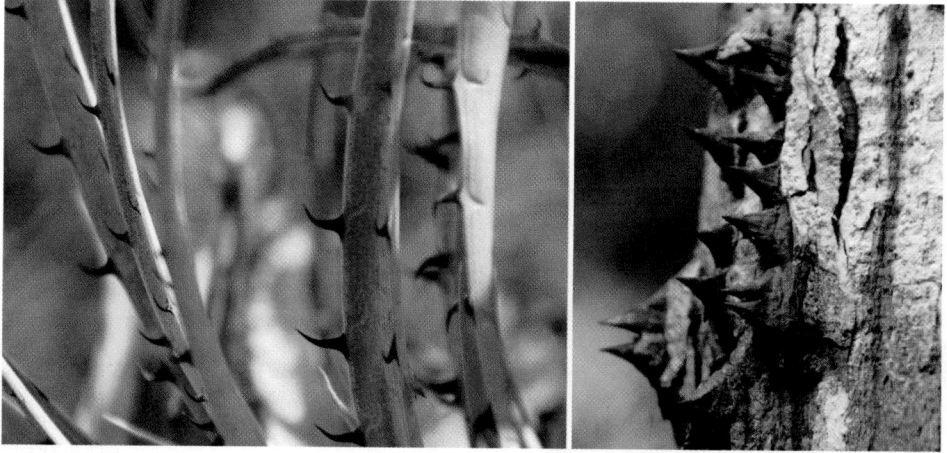

FIGURE 64-2 Many plants (including these from Peru) have evolved thorns and spines in self-defense. *(Courtesy Paul S. Auerbach.)*

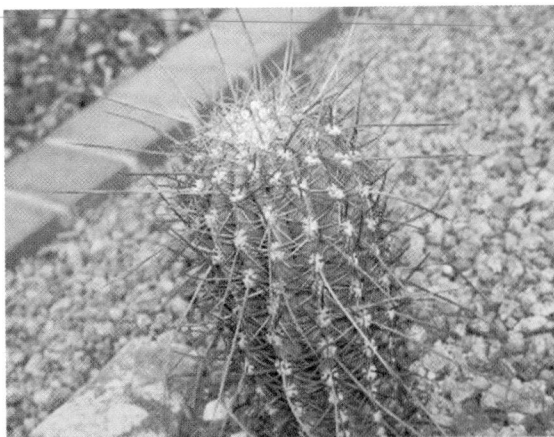

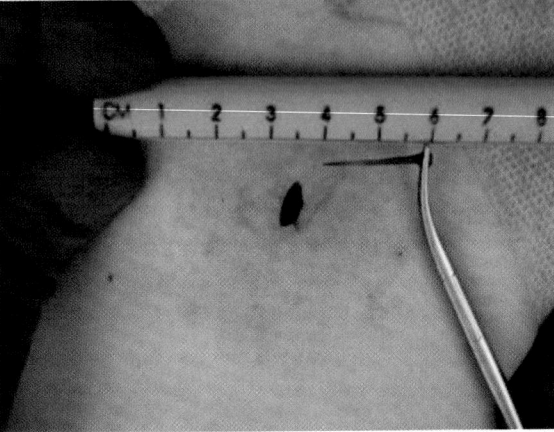

FIGURE 64-4 Penetrating cactus spine injury to mediastinum of a child. *(From O'Neill PJ, Sinha M, McArthur RA, et al: Penetrating cactus spine injury to the mediastinum of a child, J Pediatr Surg 43:e33, 2008.)*

has very rarely been reported to cause dermatitis.[123] Table 64-1 lists the most commonly reported woods that cause contact dermatitis. Dermatitis from woods is almost entirely seen in occupational settings. Treatment includes avoidance of the offending agents and use of ultrapotent topical corticosteroids, such as clobetasol 0.05% ointment twice daily to the affected areas for up to 2 weeks.

The most common form of plant-induced irritant contact dermatitis is from plant-derived chemicals. Acids, enzymes, isothiocyanates, phorbol esters, calcium oxalate, and alcohols cause these reactions. The chemicals are directly toxic to the skin and work by altering inherent pH balance, dissolving protective lipids of the stratum corneum, and denaturing skin proteins. These reactions require direct contact of the plant material with the

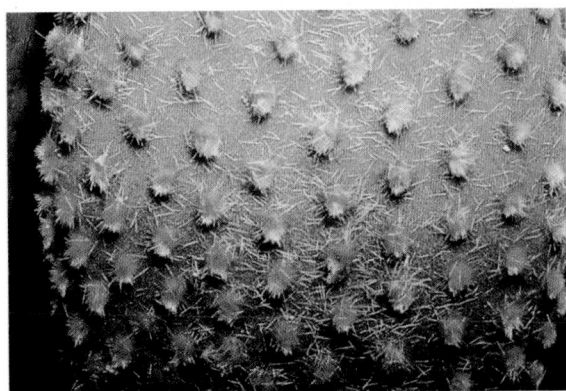

FIGURE 64-5 Beaver tail cactus. *(Courtesy Eric Lewis.)*

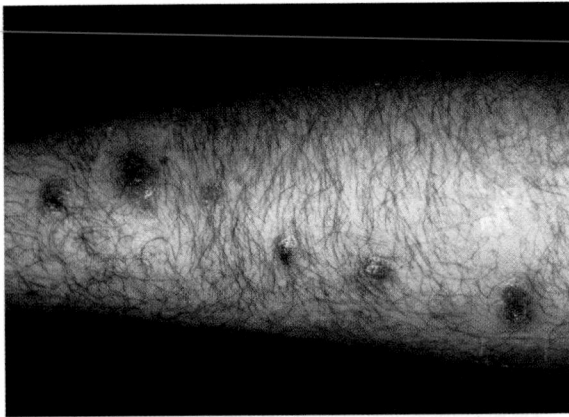

FIGURE 64-6 The characteristic red nodules that indicate lymphangitic spread of *Sporothrix schenckii.*

epidermis. Many factors can modify irritant reactions. The most important variables are duration of skin contact, concentration of the irritant, and underlying skin integrity and thickness.[8] Concentration of the irritant chemical in the plant will be at different levels in the stem, petals, roots, and leaves. Levels of the irritant also fluctuate at different times of the year, so someone could have a reaction in the summer months from contacting the leaves of an irritating plant and may not have the same reaction when touching the stem in winter.

Plants in the spurge (Euphorbiaceae) family exude a milky sap when traumatized. This sap contains a chemical mixture of irritating diterpenes and phorbol esters.[44] After skin contact, the reactions can vary from mild stinging and burning to erythema, vesiculation, and bulla formation. Blister formation typically occurs within 24 hours. Eczematous weeping plaques can also be seen in the first 24 hours. Reactions can last for 2 to 3 weeks. The spurge family is a large family of plants with more than 7000 described members. These plants are found predominantly in tropical climates; in the United States, they can be found mainly in Florida and the southwestern states. Some well-known members of the Euphorbiaceae family include the croton plant, wolfsmilk, manchineel tree, and snow-on-the-mountain (Figure 64-7 and Table 64-2).

Plants of the genus *Croton* are also members of the spurge family. These tropical plants are the source of croton oil. This oil had been used in the past as a purgative and for many medicinal remedies. The plants contain a mixture of phorbol esters and diterpenes in their leaves, stems, and seeds.[18] These

---

BOX 64-1 Infections Associated with Mechanical Plant Injury

Bacterial
Staphylococcus aureus
Clostridium tetani

Chromomycosis
Fonsecaea pedrosoi
Phialophora compacta
Phialophora verrucosa
Cladosporium carrionii
Rhinocladiella aquaspersa

Phaeohyphomycosis
Exophiala jeanselmei
Wangiella dermatitidis

Mycetoma
Madurella mycetomatis
Actinomadura madurae
Actinomadura pelletieri
Nocardia brasiliensis

Nocardia cavae
Nocardia asteroides
Streptomyces somaliensis
Madurella grisea
Leptosphaeria senegalensis
Petriellidium boydii
Aspergillus nidulans

Prototothecosis
Prototheca wickerhamii

Mycobacterial
Mycobacterium kansasii
Mycobacterium marinum
Mycobacterium ulcerans

Other Fungal
Blastomyces dermatitidis
Sporothrix schenckii
Histoplasma capsulatum

Data from references 71, 92, and 130.

TABLE 64-1 Sampling of Wood Trees That Cause Contact Dermatitis

Common Name	Botanical Name
African black walnut	*Mansonia altissima*
African blackwood	*Dalbergia melanoxylon*
Bolivian rosewood	*Machaerium acutifolium*
Brazilian box tree	*Aspidosperma* spp.
Cocobolo	*Dalbergia retusa*
Cordia	*Cordia goeldiana*
East Indian rosewood	*Dalbergia latifolia*
Ebony	*Diospyros celebica*
Honduran mahogany	*Swietenia macrophylla*
Iroko	*Chlorophora excelsa*
Litre	*Lithrea caustica*
Macassar ebony	*Diospyros celebica*
Mahogany	*Khaya* spp.
Milo wood	*Thespesia populnea*
Obeche	*Triplochiton scleroxylon*
Padauk	*Pterocarpus dalbergiodes*
Pao ferro	*Machaerium scleroxylum*
Perupok	*Lophopetalum dubicum*
Pine	*Pinus* spp.
Redwood	*Sequioa sempervirens*
Sapele wood	*Entandrophragma cylindricum*
Silky oak	*Grevillea robusta*
Sucupira	*Bowdichia nitida*
Tali wood	*Erythrophleum guineense*
Teak	*Tectona grandis*
Walnut	*Juglans nigra*
White ash	*Fraxinus americanus*
Zebrawood	*Astronium fraxinifolium*

Data from references 2, 3, 24, 25, 51, 52, 74, and 102.

TABLE 64-2 Common Members of the Euphorbiaceae Family

Common Name	Botanical Name
Poinsettia	*Euphorbia pulcherrima*
Candelabra cactus	*Euphorbia lactea*
Caper spurge	*Euphorbia lathyrus*
Chinese tallow	*Sapium sebiferum*
Crown-of-thorns	*Euphorbia splendens*
Cypress spurge	*Euphorbia cyparissias*
Manchineel tree	*Hippomane mancinella*
Pencil tree	*Euphorbia tirucalli*
Petty spurge	*Euphorbia peplus*
Sandbox tree	*Hura crepitans*
Snow-on-the-mountain	*Euphorbia marginata*
Sun spurge	*Euphorbia helioscopia*
Wolfsmilk	*Euphorbia purpurea*

Data from Asilian A, Faghihi G: Severe irritant contact dermatitis from cypress spurge, *Contact Dermatitis* 51:37, 2004; and Lovell CR: Irritant plants. In Lovell CR, editor: *Plants and the skin*, Oxford, 1993, Blackwell Scientific Publications, pp 42-95.

esters can cause immediate skin blistering, as well as a weeping eczematous eruption. These plants are found mostly in Central and South America, but approximately 40 species live in the southern United States. They typically appear as low-lying shrubs.

Some plants, such as those listed in Table 64-3, contain proteolytic enzymes, which cause skin irritation when contacted in sufficiently high concentrations. Plants such as *Mucuna pruriens* (cowhage) contain a proteolytic enzyme, mucunain, that causes intense itching immediately on contact. Its seed pods are covered with tiny stinging hairs called *trichomes*, which contain high concentrations of mucunain. This enzyme has been used for decades by practical jokers in its dried form as itch powder. Recently, medical researchers have made use of the irritant enzyme found in papaya. Papain is a proteolytic enzyme that is used in a number of commercial wound dressings to aid in degradation of necrotic tissue and to assist wound healing.[103]

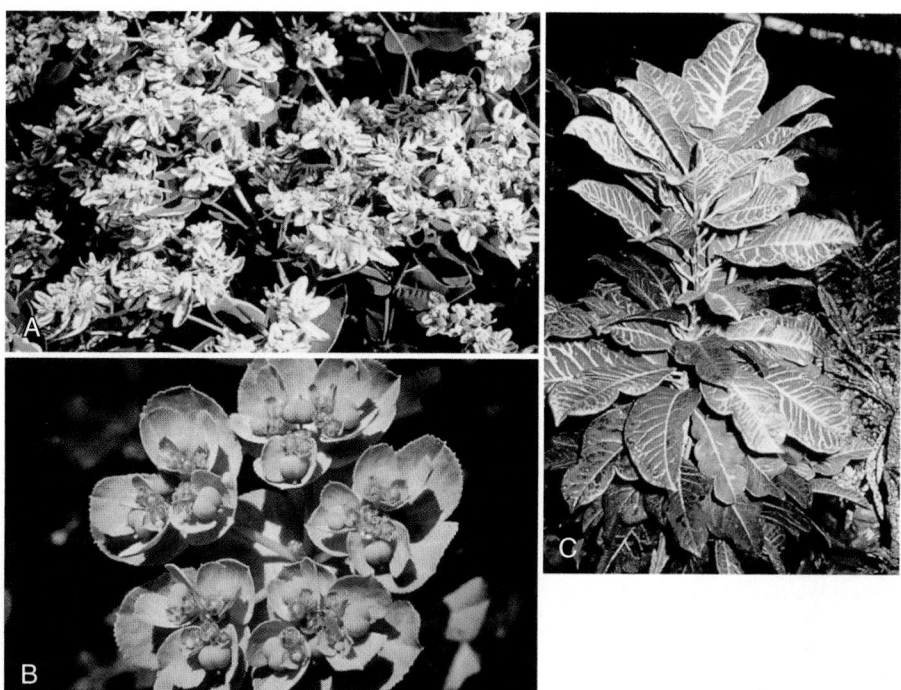

FIGURE 64-7 Common plants that induce irritant phytophotodermatitis. **A,** Snow-on-the-mountain. **B,** Wolfsmilk. **C,** Croton bush. (**C** *courtesy Yves Sell, Institute of Botany, Louis Pasteur University, Strasbourg, France.*)

TABLE 64-3 Common Plants with Irritant Enzymes

Common Name	Botanical Name	Proteolytic Enzyme
Cowhage	*Mucuna pruriens*	Mucunain
Crownflower	*Calotropis* spp.	Mudarin
Pineapple	*Ananas comosus*	Bromelin
Papaya	*Carica papaya*	Papain
Fig tree	*Ficus carica*	Ficin

Calcium oxalate is a common skin irritant. Calcium oxalate in plants is found in a crystalline needle-like form called *raphides*. It is present in irritating concentrations in many plants, including dumb cane, rhubarb, agave, daffodils, and hyacinths. Dumb cane (*Dieffenbachia* spp.) is a common houseplant well known to cause irritant skin and mucous membrane reactions (Figure 64-8).[30] The common name arises from the effect it has on persons who chew its leaves, which release calcium oxalate. Calcium oxalate causes irritation, swelling, salivation, pain, and blistering of mucous membranes. In an extreme case, the person is unable to speak normally.[133] When the sap of this plant contacts the eye, conjunctival swelling and corneal ulcers may occur.[87] Raphides are also found in *Agave* species. Irritant contact dermatitis has been reported in tequila distillery workers, who are in frequent contact with *Agave tequilana*.[110] Purpuric and irritant reactions have been reported after exposure to sap of *Agave americana*.[25,105] Immediate burning on exposure is characteristic of calcium oxalate toxicity.

Daffodils and hyacinths are among the many other species containing calcium oxalate, which is found in its highest concentration in the bulb.[121] Agricultural workers who gather these bulbs and flowers are at highest risk for irritant dermatitis, typically on the distal extremities where they came into contact with the plant.[62]

The family Solanaceae contains the peppers. These plant species contain several capsaicinoids, the most common of which is capsaicin. Capsaicin is a chemical compound that can cause skin and mucous membrane burning, itching, and in severe cases, vesiculation and bulla formation. Specialized cells of the plant's placenta produce capsaicin. Capsaicin binds to receptors on neurons and causes release of substance P from primary sensory neurons. With repeated applications, capsaicin causes depletion of substance P and desensitizes the neuron. This effect is used in clinical practice with topical application of capsaicin-containing compounds to skin in areas of chronic pain, such as for postherpetic neuralgia.

Brassicaceae (Cruciferae) is a large family of plants that causes irritant contact dermatitis. More than 3500 species live in temperate regions of the world.[32] Its members include horseradish (*Armoracia rusticana*), black mustard (*Brassica nigra*), and white mustard (*Sinapis alba*) (Figure 64-9). These plants contain glucosinolates, which are converted to isothiocyanate, which causes irritant dermatitis.[82] This reaction is catalyzed by the enzyme myrosinase. Substrate interacts with the enzyme after the plant is crushed, as in chewing.[32] Contact with these plants can cause a wide range of cutaneous reactions, including burning sensation, pain, red patches, and blister formation.

The Ranunculaceae family includes buttercups and Old Man's Beard (Figure 64-10). Table 64-4 lists a small sampling of plants in this family reported to cause irritant contact dermatitis. Protoanemonin is considered the primary irritant toxin in this group of plants. Reactions from these plants tend to be mild and rarely cause people to seek medical care. Table 64-5 includes plants and plant families that cause irritant phytocontact dermatitis and lists their primary irritant substance.[74,121]

It is currently believed that both irritation and contact sensitization are mediated by epidermally derived cytokines. Tumor necrosis factor-α (TNF-α), interferon-γ (IFN-γ), macrophage inflammatory protein-2 (MIP-2), and granulocyte-macrophage colony-stimulating factor (GM-CSF) are produced and secreted into tissue in response to both allergens and irritants. However, a number of other proteins are released only by allergenic stimulation.

In irritant contact dermatitis, the chemical irritant (which is usually an acid, alkali, surfactant, solvent, oxidant, enzyme, or toxin) damages keratinocytes. This damage is highly dependent on the concentration of the irritant. No sensitization or elicitation

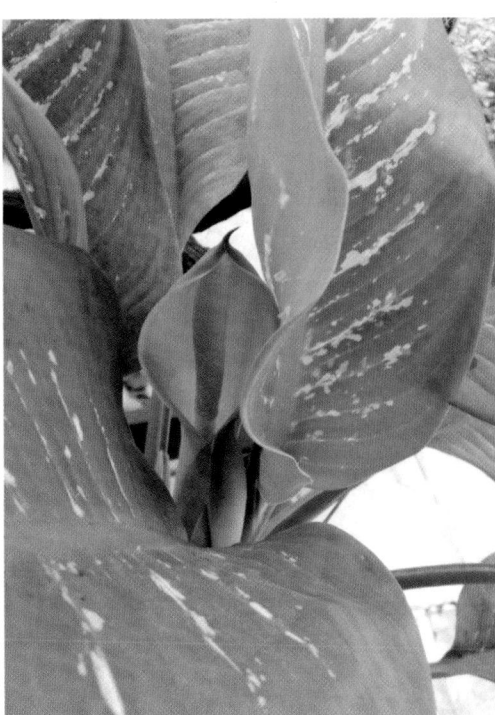

FIGURE 64-8 *Dieffenbachia* species.

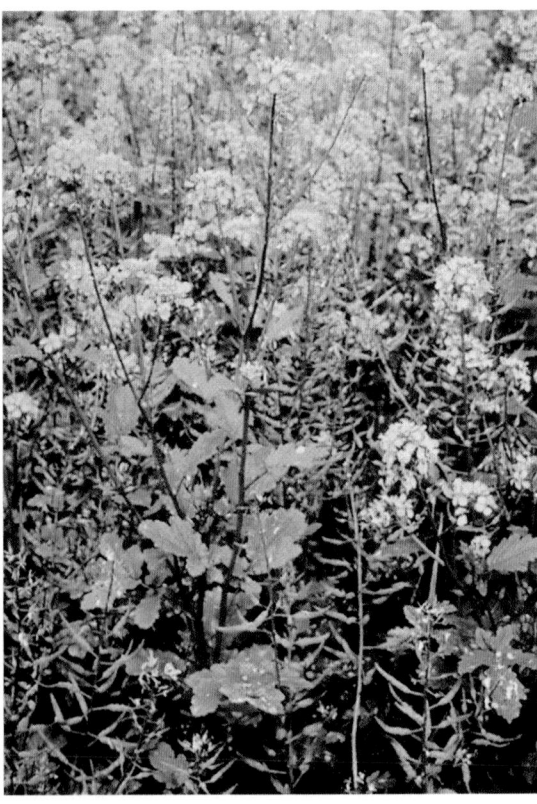

FIGURE 64-9 White mustard plant. *(Courtesy Yves Sell, Institute of Botany, Louis Pasteur University, Strasbourg, France.)*

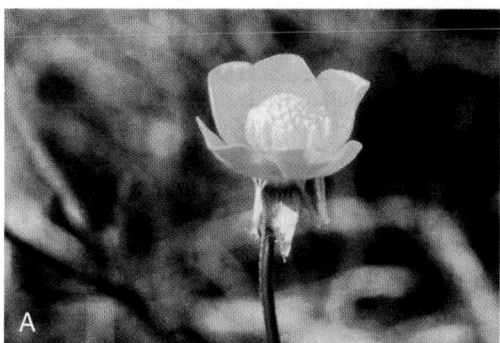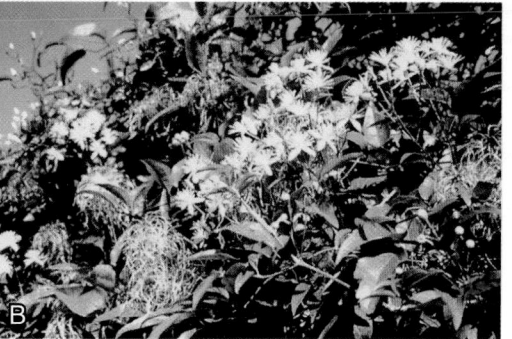

FIGURE 64-10 Plants of the family Ranunculaceae. **A,** Buttercup. **B,** Old Man's Beard. (*B courtesy Yves Sell, Institute of Botany, Louis Pasteur University, Strasbourg, France.*)

phase occurs, as is seen in allergic contact dermatitis, which is a key discerning feature between the two types of plant-induced contact dermatitis. The damaged keratinocyte activates phospholipase A$_2$. This in turn cleaves arachidonic acid and diacylglyceride (DAG) from the cell membrane. Arachidonic acid is converted into various prostaglandins and leukotrienes. Prostaglandins and leukotrienes cause endothelial cells to dilate and become leaky, resulting in edema. They also act on mast cells to release histamine and are chemoattractants for lymphocytes and neutrophils. Further recruitment of lymphocytes and neutrophils is facilitated by expression of intercellular adhesion molecule-1 (ICAM-1) by keratinocytes.[84] The DAG causes upregulation of genes for cytokines such as interleukin-1 (IL-1) and GM-CSF. These proteins then act to stimulate T cells and neutrophils. All these inflammatory cells combined with release of various cytokines and vasoactive substances lead to the clinical findings of irritant contact dermatitis. This is a continuing area of investigation.[107,134]

TREATMENT

Treatment of primary irritant dermatitis requires multiple steps. The victim must be removed from exposure to the irritant chemicals. Gentle cleansing of the wound with antibacterial soap, cool compresses, and watching for infection are essential. Antihistamines, such as hydroxyzine 10 to 25 mg PO four times daily, or diphenhydramine 25 mg PO two to four times daily, can help with itching. The sedating antihistamines tend to work better than the newer, nonsedating types (fexofenadine, loratadine, and desloratadine), although some patients respond well to the nonsedating forms. Topical medium-strength corticosteroids, such as triamcinolone 0.1% cream, may be applied twice daily to the affected areas for up to 2 weeks without risk for atrophy. Clobetasol 0.05% cream or ointment (an ultrapotent topical corticosteroid) can also be used in severe cases. In the case of topical medium-strength and ultrapotent topical corticosteroids, care should be taken to avoid application in the groin, axillae, and face. Typical application regimens are twice daily for 1 to 2

weeks. Cool compresses with aluminum acetate solution (Domeboro, Burow's solution) diluted 1:40 in water are very helpful for soothing pruritus and exudative skin irritation. Dermatitis generally heals in less than 7 days if no complications develop and if tissue damage is minimal. If the patient is unable to be removed from the source of irritation, no medicine, cream, or soak will alleviate the problem. People are sometimes forced to change occupations or hobbies, or at the very least modify their environment.

ALLERGIC CONTACT DERMATITIS

Allergic contact dermatitis is a type IV delayed hypersensitivity reaction. This form of contact allergy is much more common than is contact urticaria. The most common acute presentation is linearly arranged eczematous, edematous patches and plaques with

TABLE 64-4 Irritant Plants in the Family Ranunculaceae

Common Name	Botanical Name
American prairie crocus	*Pulsatilla patens*
Buttercup	*Ranunculus* spp.
Christmas rose	*Helleborus niger*
Meadow rue	*Thalictrum foliosum*
Pasque flower	*Pulsatilla vulgaris*
Pilewort	*Ranunculus ficaria*
Staves-acre	*Delphinium* spp.
Traveler's joy	*Clematis vitalba*
Windflower	*Anemone nemorosa*
Wolfsbane	*Aconitum napellus*

TABLE 64-5 Plants Causing Irritant Phytocontact Dermatitis and Their Primary Irritant Chemicals

Common Name	Botanical Name	Irritant Chemical
Agave	*Agave americana*	Calcium oxalate
Black mustard	*Brassica nigra*	Isothiocyanates
Buttercup	*Ranunculus bulbosus*	Protoanemonin
Coral plant	*Jatropha*	Thioglycoside
Cowhage	*Mucuna pruriens*	Proteolytic enzymes
Croton	*Croton tiglium*	Phorbol esters
Daffodils	Amaryllidaceae family	Calcium oxalate
Dumb cane	*Dieffenbachia* spp.	Calcium oxalate
Hyacinths	Liliaceae family	Calcium oxalate
Manchineel tree	*Hippomane mancinella*	Phorbol esters
May apple	*Podophyllium peltatum*	Podophyllin resin
Pencil tree	*Euphorbia tirucalli*	Triterpene alcohols
Prickly pear	*Opuntia* spp.	Spines
Spurges	Euphorbiaceae family	Shorbol and diterpene esters
Mustard, radish, etc.	Cruciferae (Brassicaceae) family	Isothiocyanates
Buttercups, pilewort	Ranunculaceae	Protoanemonin
Common caper	Capparidaceae family (e.g., *Capparis spinosa*)	Isothiocyanates
Peppers	Solanaceae family	Capsaicin
Spider plant	Cleomaceae family (e.g., *Cleome* species)	Isiothiocyanates

Data from High WA: Agave contact dermatitis, *Am J Contact Dermat* 14:213, 2003; and Ricks MR, Vogel PS, Elston DM, et al: Purpuric agave dermatitis, *J Am Acad Dermatol* 40:356, 1999.

TABLE 64-6 *Toxicodendron* Species

Common Name	Botanical Name
Western poison oak	*Toxicodendron diversilobum*
Eastern poison oak	*Toxicodendron quercifolium*
Poison ivy	*Toxicodendron radicans*
Rydberg's poison ivy	*Toxicodendron rydbergii*
Poison sumac	*Toxicodendron vernix*

varying amounts of vesiculation and bulla eruption. Occasionally, the eruption is widespread. If the face is involved, there can be severe eyelid swelling. Patients are quite distressed by their appearance. In severe cases, they can have systemic symptoms of fever, chills, fatigue, and lethargy. In its more chronic form, as is seen with the Compositae family, allergic contact dermatitis presents with lichenified eczematous plaques in exposed areas.

TOXICODENDRON (POISON IVY/OAK/SUMAC)

The most common cause of acute allergic contact dermatitis in the United States is from exposure to poison ivy, oak, and sumac plants (Table 64-6). In the past, allergic contact dermatitis caused by poison ivy, oak, or sumac was referred to as *Rhus* dermatitis. Recent botanical nomenclature places the poison ivy, oak, and sumac plants in the Anacardiaceae family in the genus *Toxicodendron*. The *Rhus* genus contains plants that are not known to cause allergic contact dermatitis. Therefore, the term "*Rhus* dermatitis" should be abandoned.

Toxicodendron weeds are fastidious. They do not grow in Alaska or Hawaii and do not survive well above 1500 m (5000 feet), in deserts, or in rain forests. They grow best along cool streams and lakes and luxuriate if it is also sunny and hot. They are found in every state of the continental United States. The plants have different configurations in different regions, but generally, poison ivy grows east of the Rockies, poison oak grows west of the Rockies, and poison sumac grows best in the southeastern United States. Because avoidance is the best prevention, it is important to learn what the plants look like in a given area (Figure 64-11). Once contaminated with the oil (resin), an average person has 1 to 4 hours to wash it off with soap and water to prevent dermatitis.

Poison ivy (*T. radicans*) grows in moist shady regions east of the Rockies. The plants thrive at sea level and do very poorly above 1500 m (5000 feet). Poison ivy is never found on the U.S. West Coast. The leaflets are 10 to 30 cm (4 to 12 inches) long and are found in groups of three. The shape of the leaves is often ovate or obtuse. The leaves can be shiny, smooth, and hairless, or they can be rough, hairy, and velvety[12,32] (Figure 64-12). Its characteristic shape has led to the adage, "Leaves of three, let them be" (Figure 64-13). It is a climbing shrub commonly found growing up the trunks of large trees, with aerial roots that are quite prominent.

Poison oak (*T. diversilobum*) is found in the west coastal states of North America and is given the designation *western poison oak*. It is a common shrub with multiple stems that form three leaflets. The leaves are larger on plants that grow in shade than on those grown in full or partial sunny conditions. It has many brown aerial roots and clusters of yellow flowers that bloom in the spring.[32] The flowers bear cream-colored berries. In the California hills, poison oak grows like a forest, but in cooler, dry climates, it remains isolated in small patches.

Poison sumac (*T. vernix*) is a fast-growing small tree or shrub. Some plants grow as tall as 12 m (40 feet), but the average height is about 4.5 m (15 feet). The plants are found in wet marshy regions of the United States. Its leaves are unique among *Toxicodendron* species. They are configured as 7 to 13 smooth oval leaflets attached along a central stem.[32] The plant forms pale-colored fruit. Nonpoisonous sumacs can be recognized by their jagged leaf margins and red berries.

All *Toxicodendron* plants have many interconnected channels that contain sap. When the plant is traumatized and a channel is broken open, the sap is extruded and hardens as a black resin

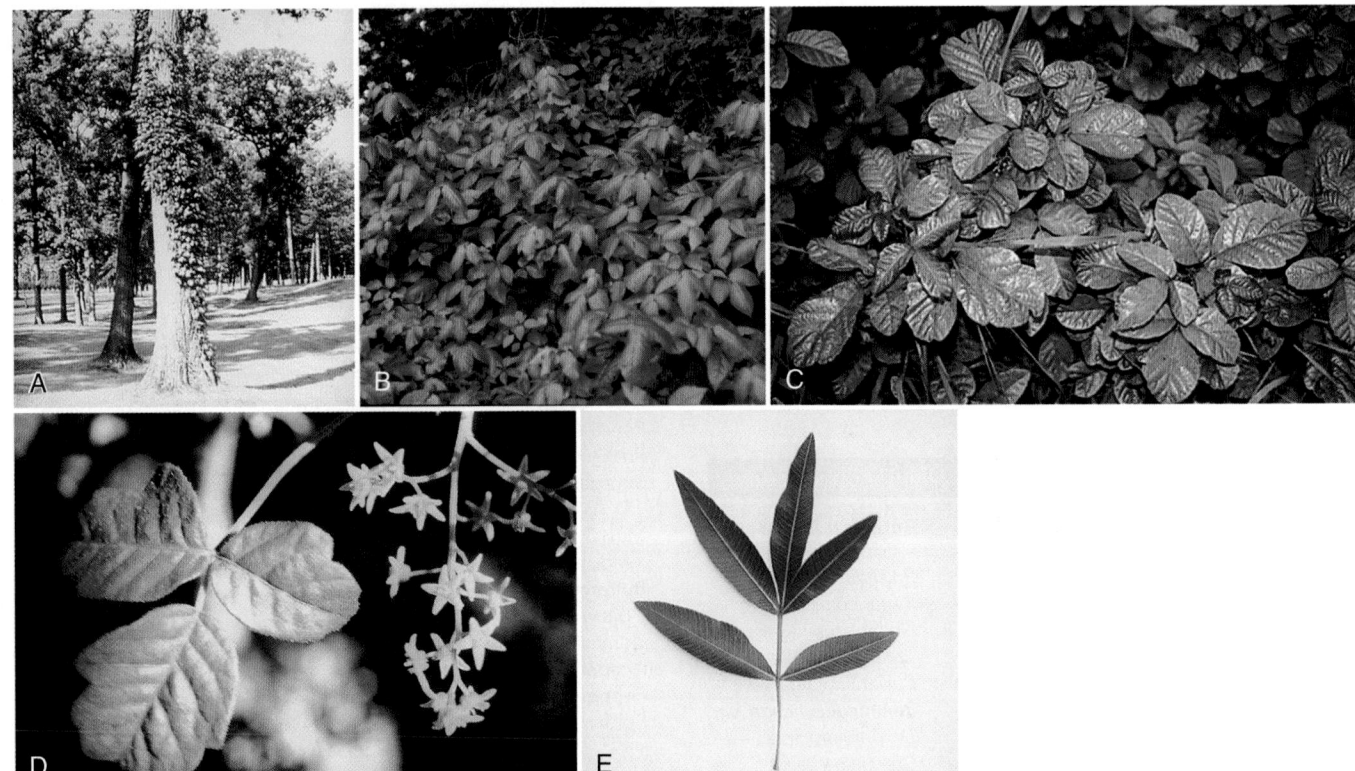

FIGURE 64-11 Plants in the *Toxicodendron* genus. **A,** Poison ivy. **B,** Poison ivy growing as a sea of vines. **C,** Poison oak. **D,** Poison oak, close-up. **E,** Poison sumac. (*C courtesy Paul S. Auerbach.*)

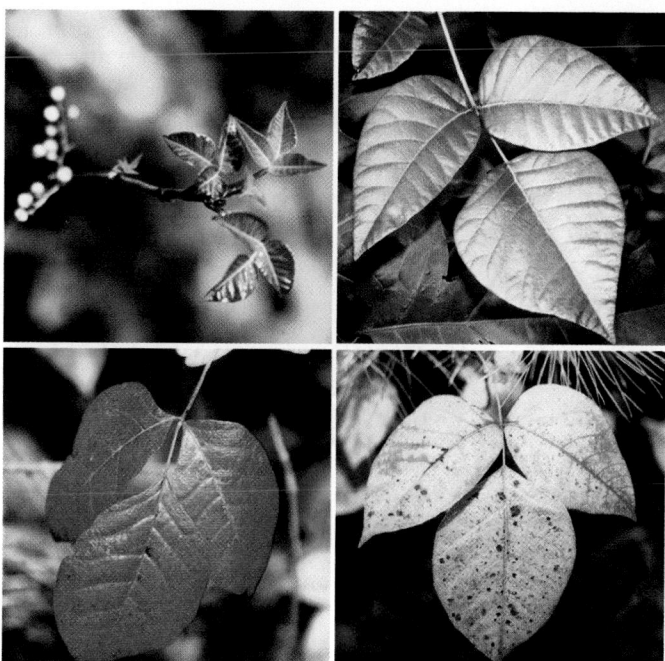

FIGURE 64-12 A to D, Poison ivy can have various appearances.

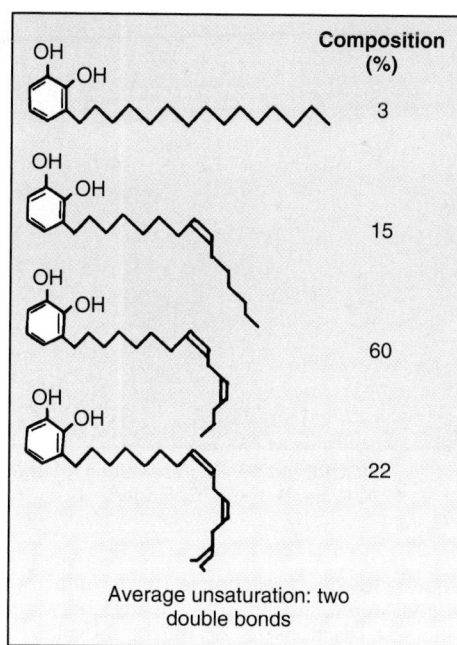

	Composition (%)
OH OH	3
OH OH	15
OH OH	60
OH OH	22

Average unsaturation: two double bonds

FIGURE 64-14 General structure and composition of poison ivy urushiol.

to seal off the damage. This sap is the material that contains the allergen urushiol.[32]

All parts of the plant contain the urushiol resin, which is a heavy, nonvolatile oil (Figure 64-14). In its natural state, the oil is colorless or slightly yellow. Because the oil is virtually invisible, many people fail to understand how they acquired the rash. It is not a vapor, because at 315° C (600° F) in a fire or oven, urushiol splatters like butter. In a camp or forest fire, it attaches to smoke particles and can be carried downwind. The oil also readily coats the fur of animals, which explains why people often contract the dermatitis from their outdoor pets. On exposure to air, the oil oxidizes, polymerizes, and turns black. This is a way to recognize the weeds, especially in autumn when the leaves fall off.

The amount of urushiol present in poison ivy and poison oak is roughly equal year-round, even when the plants are only sticks without leaves in the winter. As the leaves turn red and start to dry up in the fall, important nutrients, including urushiol, return to the stem and roots through subepidermal resin canals.[52] Therefore, dead leaves that fall to the ground are virtually devoid of urushiol.

Urushiol is exposed to skin when a plant that has been injured or bruised releases it to the surface of the leaf, petal, stem, or root. Clinical effects usually manifest 24 to 48 hours after contact in a previously sensitized individual[111] and 10 to 14 days after contact in a patient on first exposure. Typically, linear streaking of papulovesicles occurs; edema, weeping, and crusting are also often seen (Figure 64-15). A distinct linear nature is often a clue to the diagnosis of allergic contact dermatitis. On occasion, the eruption can appear to be urticarial in nature or can mimic cellulitis. Appearance of black dots on the skin in areas of involvement can be helpful in determining the etiology.[69] The black dots represent dried urushiol that has been oxidized by air (Figure 64-16). Severe itching leading to excoriations almost always accompanies the rash. This can lead to secondary infection.

The antigen is found in the milky sap, which is quickly absorbed into the skin. It is nearly impossible to wash off the sap quickly enough to prevent dermatitis. Once the sap touches the body, it is often spread by inadvertent transfer. This explains why patients often develop eruptions in sites distant from the initial contact with the plant. There are many unique urushiol chemicals. Collectively, they can be called *urushioids*. Each plant has a different urushioid concentration and composition. Urushioids have a structure that contains a benzene ring with a varying-length carbon side chain. Concentrations of the various urushioids of each plant depend on growing conditions and season, which also affect their antigenic properties. If the side chain is desaturated and longer, this increases the catechols' antigenicity. Conversely, if there is a substitution on the catechol ring, this reduces antigenicity.[84] Addition of an aliphatic side chain and presence of free phenolic groups also increase antigenicity.[121] Poison ivy contains predominantly urushiol III, poison oak contains mostly urushiol I, and poison sumac contains predominantly urushiol II.[32,84]

If the patient avoids repeat exposure, dermatitis resolves within 14 to 21 days in most cases. It is important to diagnose secondary impetiginization because this can lead to cellulitis if not treated with appropriate antibiotics. The most likely pathogens are *Staphylococcus aureus* and streptococcal species. Hyposensitization therapy has not proved practical or particularly effective and is rarely performed. Patients need to be informed to clean clothing thoroughly, through at least one complete automated hot-water wash and rinse cycle with detergent, and to clean any object that may have come in contact with the plant in order to avoid repeat exposure.

It is estimated that 50% to 70% of the population is sensitive to the causative antigen, urushiol. The amount of purified

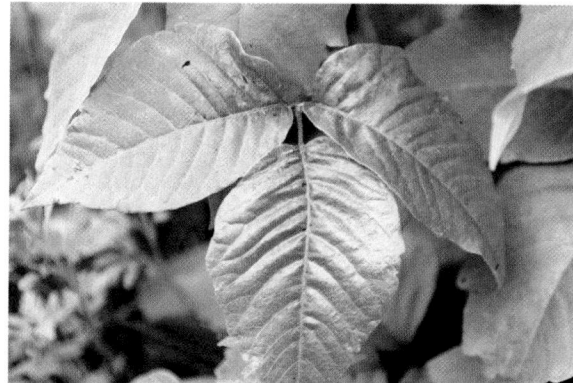

FIGURE 64-13 Close-up views of the characteristic three-leaf pattern of *Toxicodendron*. (*Courtesy Peter Schalock, Massachusetts General Hospital, Boston, Mass.*)

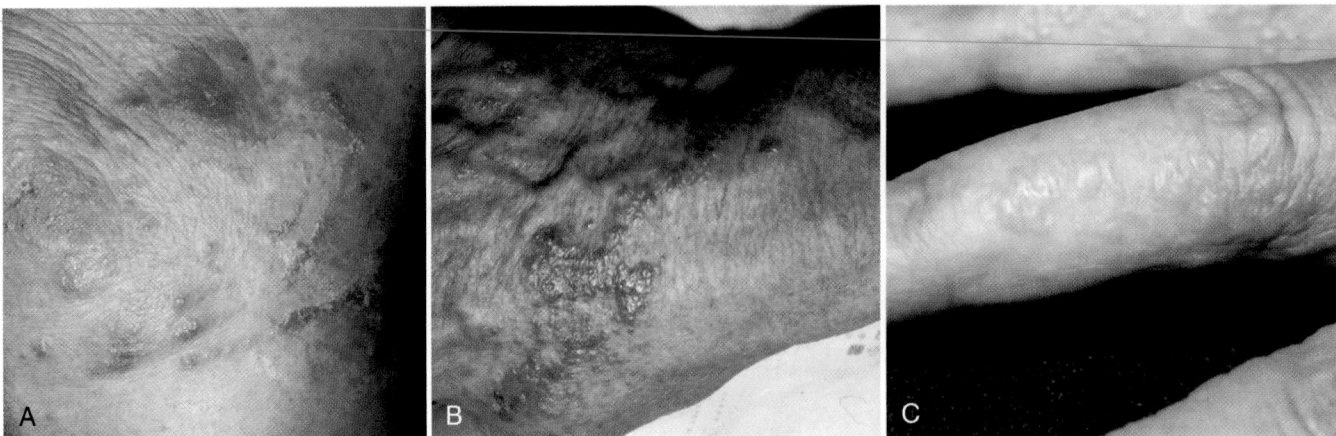

FIGURE 64-15 Representation of the linear nature of poison ivy–induced allergic contact dermatitis. A, Knee. B, Hand. C, Finger.

urushiol required to elicit a reaction is 2 to 2.5 mg.[47] Some people (~35%) are considered subclinically sensitive because they have negative skin test reactions to 2.5 mg of urushiol but react to higher concentrations, such as 5, 10, and 50 mg.[47] Clinically, this group is interesting because they invariably did not have poison ivy dermatitis as teenagers and often plucked the weeds with apparent impunity. However, usually in midlife after a bout of weed pulling, a rash spreads explosively. For unknown reasons, they have crossed the line into clinical sensitivity. If patch-tested with dilutions of urushiol, these individuals are often exquisitely sensitive and do not appear to lose their reactivity. The flare-up may last for several weeks, probably because of prior contamination of the home and workplace with urushiol oil. Treatment must be aggressive and more prolonged than usual.

A smaller group (10% to 15%) does not react to higher concentrations and cannot be sensitized by 1000 mg. This group was first detected and studied in passive transfer experiments in the 1950s.[48] These individuals are considered to be naturally tolerant, but it remains unclear whether they achieved that state by early antigenic exposure or by genetic luck. They have no inherent resistance to contact sensitization with other chemicals and otherwise appear healthy.[49] They may hold a clue to the molecular basis for immunologic tolerance.

From a practical standpoint, only 10% to 15% of Americans (up to 40 million people) can be categorized as exquisitely sensitive. Generally, these persons seek and need emergency medical care (Figure 64-17). They typically have had prior unpleasant experiences. Within 2 to 6 hours after exposure, swelling is accompanied by an erythematous, intensely pruritic, edematous, vesicular, and ultimately bullous eruption that can be associated with fever, malaise, and prostration (Figure 64-18). This true dermatologic emergency should be treated immediately and vigorously.

Extreme susceptibility tends to be familial; if one parent is supersensitive, children are likely to be as well. If both parents are sensitive, the chance of sensitive offspring is about 80%.[128] The level of individual sensitivity is not determined by severity of the initial bout of dermatitis, although almost one-half of patients admit to a memorable bout of dermatitis as a teenager. However, no more than 25% to 35% of patients at age 30 to 40 were stricken within the previous year.[42] When these patients are patch-tested with weak dilutions of urushiol, less than one-half react as might be expected from their history. An individual's level of reactivity does not change appreciably if he or she is tested monthly over a year; testing at less frequent intervals in very sensitive patients over 3 to 4 years has shown little or no change in the level of reactivity.[47] Repeated mild to moderate

FIGURE 64-16 Poison ivy–induced allergic contact dermatitis after a young woman accidentally pinched some poison ivy leaves behind her knee. Note the central black dots, which represent the dried urushiol.

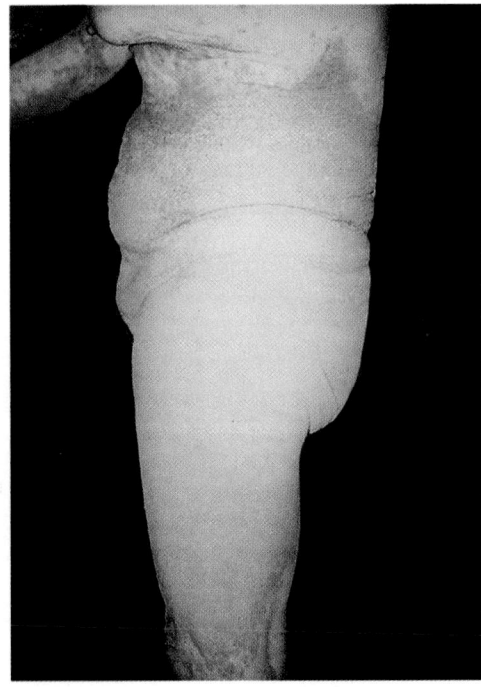

FIGURE 64-17 Generalized poison ivy dermatitis.

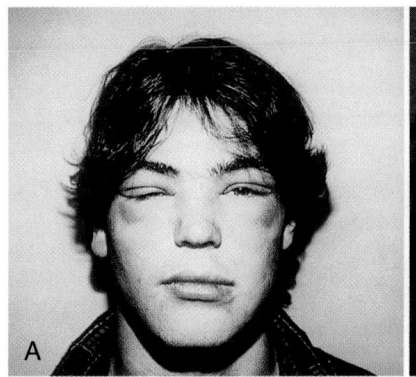 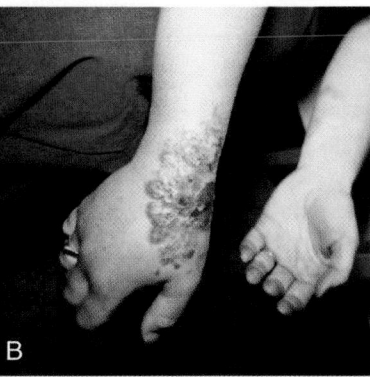 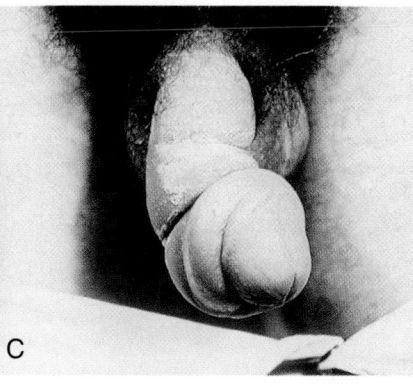

FIGURE 64-18 Severe acute poison oak dermatitis. **A,** Facial edema. **B,** Blisters. **C,** Penile edema. *(Courtesy Axel Hoke.)*

bouts of dermatitis maintain the sensitive state, whereas a single severe bout may produce a prolonged period of anergy or refractoriness, not unlike the clinical condition of "hardening" or unresponsiveness, which is well described in the industrial setting.[41,42,113]

The Anacardiaceae family accounts for most cases of allergic contact dermatitis in the United States. Table 64-7 catalogs the major members of this family and the plants most likely to cause dermatitis. Most individuals who spend a great deal of time outdoors know how to recognize these plants and appropriately avoid them. Figure 64-11 shows poison ivy, oak, and sumac. However, these are not the only plants that need to be considered. Table 64-8 lists some common plants causing allergic contact dermatitis.

In patients who have demonstrated allergic contact dermatitis to the *Toxicodendron* plants, there is a high risk of cross-reactivity with a number of other plants, including mango, oil from the cashew nut shell, fruit pulp from *Ginkgo biloba*, Japanese lacquer tree, and India marker ink tree. Mango dermatitis has been reported to be the leading cause of plant dermatitis in Hawaii.[121] (Figure 64-19). The allergens causing mango dermatitis are three resorcinol derivatives: heptadecadienylresorcinol, heptadecenylresorcinol, and pentadecylresorcinol.[95] Urushiol is found in the plant's leaves and stems and in its fruit's skin. Typically, people are exposed to the urushiol when they eat or manipulate the fruit that has yet to be peeled. Facial involvement, particularly of the lips, occurs after biting into a mango that still

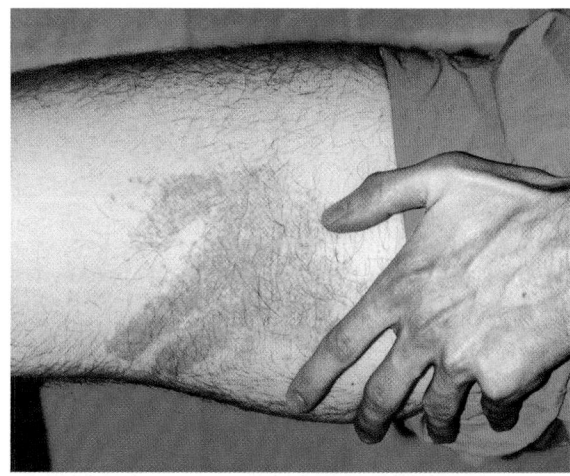

FIGURE 64-19 Pruritic and eczematous rash 3 days after onset. One week earlier, this 27-year-old man had peeled a mango, become distracted by a telephone call, and rested his left hand on his right leg. Three days later, contact dermatitis became apparent. When much younger, the patient had been sensitized to poison oak and poison ivy; the sap of the mango rind contains oleoresins that cross-react with the oleoresins of poison ivy. The rash resolved after 1 week of treatment with topical corticosteroids. *(From Tucker MO, Swan CR: Images in clinical medicine: The mango-poison ivy connection, N Engl J Med 339:235, 1998.)*

TABLE 64-7 Anacardiaceae Family

Common Name	Botanical Name
Brazilian pepper	*Schinus terebinthifolius*
Cashew	*Anacardium occidentale*
El litre tree	*Lithraea caustica*
Ginkgo tree	*Ginkgo biloba*
Indian marking nut	*Semecarpus anacardium*
Japanese lacquer	*Rhus vernicifera*
Korean lacquer tree	*Rhus vernicifera stokes*
Mango	*Mangifera indica*
Pepeo tree	*Mauria puberula*
Poison ivy	*Toxicodendron radicans* and *T. rydbergii*
Poison oak	*Toxicodendron diversilobum* and *T. toxicarium*
Poison sumac	*Toxicodendron vernix*
Poisonwood	*Metopium toxiferum*
Renges tree	*Anacardium melanorrhoea*

Data from Marks JG Jr, Elsner P, DeLeo VA: *Contact and occupational dermatology,* ed 3, St Louis, 2002, Mosby, pp 13-15.

TABLE 64-8 Plants Causing Allergic Contact Dermatitis

Common Name	Botanical Name
(Various)	*Alstromeria* spp.
(Various)	*Compositae* spp. (~20,000)
(Various)	*Grevilla* spp.
Lichen	*Cladonia, Evernia,* and *Primelia* spp.
Liverwort	*Frullania* spp.
Pine tree	*Pinus* spp.
Poison ivy	*Toxicodendron radicans*
Poison oak	*Toxicodendron diversilobum*
Poison sumac	*Toxicodendron vernix*
Primrose	*Primula obconica*
Ragweed	*Ambrosia* spp.
Tulip	*Tulipia* spp.

Data from Marks JG Jr, Elsner P, DeLeo VA: *Contact and occupational dermatology,* ed 3, St Louis, 2002, Mosby, pp 13-15.

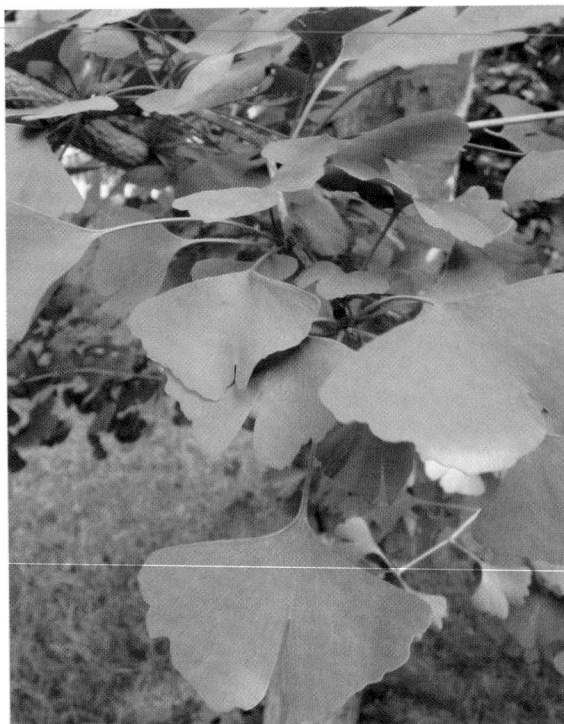

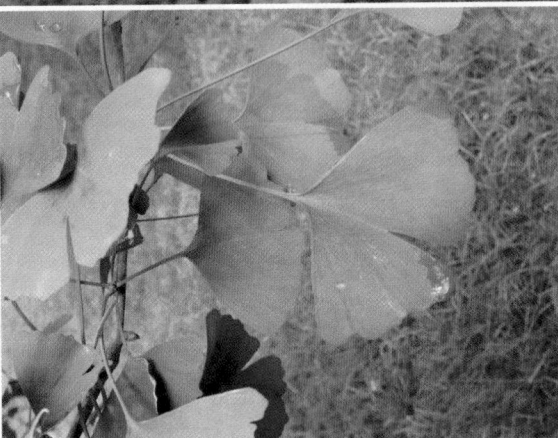

FIGURE 64-20 *Ginkgo biloba.*

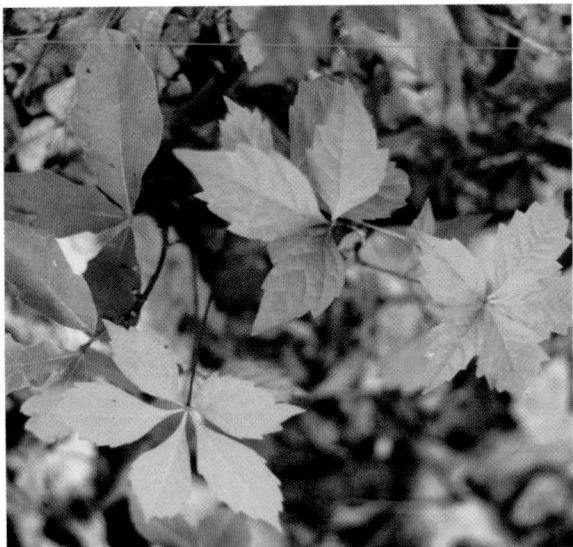

FIGURE 64-21 Poison ivy on the left, with three leaves, adjacent to the plant (Virginia creeper, with five leaves) for which it is commonly mistaken (*bottom* and *right*).

carries its outer peel. The other common area of involvement is the hand after individuals peel the fruit.[82] Once peeled, mangos are no longer allergenic. Cross-hypersensitivity between mango contact allergens and urushiol has been reported.[95]

The ginkgo tree, *Ginkgo biloba,* is commonly found in cities, where the trees thrive. Its characteristic split leaves are easily recognized (Figure 64-20). It has been reported to cause allergic contact dermatitis in joggers who run through debris on sidewalks and roadways containing ginkgo leaves, flowers, and fruit.

Multiple plants are similar in appearance to the poison ivy plant and need to be differentiated. Table 64-9 lists some of the

TABLE 64-9	Imposters of the Poison Ivy Plant
Common Name	**Botanical Name**
Boston ivy	*Parthenocissus tricuspidata*
English ivy	*Hedra helix*
Skunkbush sumac	*Rhus trilobata*
Virginia creeper	*Parthenocissus quinquefolia*

Data from McGovern TW, LaWarre SR, Brunette C: Is it or isn't it? Poison ivy look-a-likes, *Am J Contact Dermat* 11:104, 2000.

more common "imposters" for the poison ivy plant. The Virginia creeper, *Parthenocissus quinquefolia,* is frequently misidentified as poison ivy. Figure 64-21 shows poison ivy side by side with the Virginia creeper. English ivy, *Hedra helix,* is another plant that is often difficult to differentiate from poison ivy. *H. helix* has been reported to cause allergic contact dermatitis.[135]

IMMUNOLOGY OF POISON IVY AND POISON OAK DERMATITIS

The immunologic mechanism for allergic contact dermatitis is generally thought to be type IV cell-mediated delayed hypersensitivity.[43] An initial sensitization phase occurs, followed by an elicitation phase on subsequent exposure.

Allergic contact dermatitis is caused by haptens. Haptens are low-molecular-weight compounds, almost always 500 daltons or less, that exist as unprocessed antigen. They are lipid soluble, allowing them to pass into the stratum corneum.[77] Contact allergens are not immunogenic by themselves; they bind to epidermal proteins to generate new antigenic determinants.[66,76] Urushiol from poison ivy is a hapten. Percutaneous penetration of the hapten is followed by haptenization of self-proteins, which are then recognized by the innate immune system.[66] Sensing by Toll-like receptors (TLRs) and inflammasomes results in proinflammatory cytokines and chemokines that drive epidermal and dermal inflammation. Among these, TNF, IL-Iβ, and IL-18 are required for hapten-induced dendritic cell activation and migration from the skin to local lymph nodes.[66] Finally, antigen presentation by the skin dendritic cells at the lymph nodes to the naive and memory T cells leads to their activation and differentiation. These are the early immune events in the induction of allergic contact dermatitis.

Langerhans cells are the main antigen-presenting cells (APCs) in the skin. They are normally in a resting state, with minimal to no ability to stimulate T cells. In skin, keratinocytes are also part of the immune surveillance system. They respond quickly to every chemical insult, either irritant or allergenic, in antigen-dependent fashion, to produce a variety of cytokines. These function mainly to amplify future inflammatory responses.[10,93] Early on, they secrete TNF-α and ICAM.[1] Later, they release IL-1, IL-6, IL-8, and IL-10; still later, macrophage chemotactic factor and other cytokines are released.[9,55,56,93,100] These may in turn release acute-phase reactants from mast cells and endothelial cells, as seen in irritant responses.[10,93] Current research is attempting to identify which keratinocyte cytokines specify the allergic reaction, as distinct from simply injury. Nevertheless, it is known that the catechol molecules of poison oak and poison ivy enter the skin and bind through nucleophilic attack at benzene ring positions 4, 5, and 6 to surface proteins on APCs, which are primarily epidermal Langerhans cells. These cytokines from the keratinocytes cause Langerhans cells to mature and enter into an active state. Active Langerhans cells are then able to recognize and internalize antigens.

Langerhans cells are responsible for immunosurveillance. In the sensitization phase, when a hapten such as urushiol is applied to skin, it penetrates the stratum corneum. Urushiol then activates the skin's innate immune response, leading to upregulation of proinflammatory cytokines and eventual recognition of the antigen by activated APCs. These cells internalize the urushiol by pinocytosis. Proteolytic enzymes in lysosomes then process the urushiol. This processing consists of proteolytic degradation of the protein into smaller antigenic peptides. The antigenic peptides that have undergone chemical degradation associate with class II major histocompatibility complex (MHC) molecules and are expressed on the surface of the APCs.

The APCs then leave the epidermis and travel to regional lymph nodes, where they present processed antigen on the cell surface in context with a class I MHC molecule to the T cell receptor (TCR) complex on a CD8+ T cell, or in context with the class II MHC molecule to the TCR complex on a CD4+ T cell. Presence or absence of an urushiol-specific TCR is genetically determined. During early fetal development, the thymus interacts with various T cells. Through gene rearrangements, thousands of unique TCRs are produced that recognize unique antigens. If no T cell is present that recognizes the antigen complex on the APC, no reaction occurs, and the patient does not develop allergic contact dermatitis. To complete the sensitization signal, another surface protein (the B7 antigen) forms a co-stimulatory signal by binding to the CD28 ligand on the T cell. This then activates the T cell, which divides repeatedly to form a clone of urushiol-specific CD8+ and CD4+ cells. These subsequently expand into clones of circulating activated T effector and T memory lymphocytes.[65,81]

In the elicitation phase, with a new challenge by urushiol, the hapten enters the epidermis and again is internalized by Langerhans cells. It is processed and expressed by the MHC molecules, which then interact with the clone of T cells now specifically ready to interact with this MHC-antigen complex. This leads to the appearance of allergic contact dermatitis, typically within 24 to 72 hours of exposure. Langerhans cells in the skin that interact with T cells secrete IL-1, which stimulates the T cells to secrete IL-2 and express IL-2 receptors, which directly leads to activation, proliferation, and expansion of the T cell clone. Activated T cells will also secrete IFN-γ, which acts on keratinocytes to express ICAM-1, which allows them to interact directly with T cells.[84] Keratinocytes also secrete many cytokines that cause expansion and proliferation of these T cells. The CD8 lymphocytes elicit a cell-mediated cytotoxic immune response at the site of contact characterized by erythema, edema, and vesiculation resulting from destruction of epidermal cells and activation of the dermal vasculature. The clinical reaction is driven by the CD8 cytotoxic, effector T cells. This can be modified by CD4 T cells that may be either T helper type 1 (Th$_1$) or, more likely, Th$_2$ in nature.[65,81] In an individual patient, this determines the severity of dermatitis after exposure to the poisonous weeds. In addition, alternate pathways exist that account for the varying presentations of ACD. An acute eruption can begin within hours of initial exposure. Some have emphasized the presence of basophils in these hyperacute poison oak and poison ivy lesions and have proposed a role for basophil mediators in the pathogenesis of an early-onset acute reaction.[39] Others have proposed alternate hyperacute mechanisms involving mast cell degranulation, or a CD4 T cell–mediated induction of IgE reactivity.[64,67]

Suppressor pathways to decrease the extent of these pathways also exist. These mechanisms are poorly understood but include a number of specific pathways, such as elimination of primed dendritic cells by effector CD8 T cells, release of antiinflammatory cytokines, and activation of suppressor T cells.[128] These responses are generated to counterbalance or downregulate the type IV hypersensitivity reaction. It is the exposure to antigen through noncutaneous routes that leads to these suppressor pathways or, if there is a massive exposure, to antigen at the sensitization phase.[84] The final resulting skin reaction is a balance of sensitization and suppression of these antigen-specific reactions.

TREATMENT

Systemic corticosteroids are widely accepted as the first line of treatment for moderate to severe disease, especially given early and in large, therapeutic doses. In mild cases, ultrapotent topical steroids alone, such as clobetasol 0.05% ointment twice daily to the affected areas for 2 weeks, may suffice. If the reaction is of less than 2 hours' duration, intravenous (IV) hydrocortisone (adult dose 100 to 200 mg) or methylprednisolone (adult dose 500 mg to 1 g) can be curative. After a patient has suffered 4 to 6 hours with massive edema, erythema, and pruritus, IV therapy is highly effective, but it must be followed by more prolonged oral or intramuscular (IM) administration of corticosteroids. Most patients in this category seek help after 8 to 16 hours of discomfort, at which point IV therapy is less effective. In these circumstances, oral prednisone, 1 mg/kg/day for 3 to 4 days, followed by a slow taper over 2 to 3 weeks, helps many patients, but the danger lies in a sudden flare-up, which becomes poorly responsive to corticosteroids, at the end of therapy. This more often happens with rapid prednisone tapers. Whenever considering systemic corticosteroids for acute allergic contact dermatitis, the physician should evaluate the patient for active infection, vascular accident, endocrinopathy, or familial history of glaucoma. Side effects from oral corticosteroids include hypertension, increased risk for infection, adrenal insufficiency, glaucoma, cataracts, increased blood glucose, mood changes, osteoporosis, osteonecrosis, edema, weight gain, hypokalemia, peptic ulcer disease, bowel perforation, myopathy, Cushing's syndrome, adrenal suppression, and stunted growth in adolescents.

If dermatitis has been present for more than 24 hours, which is typically the case in clinical practice, the aggressive regimen is less successful. When the onset of dermatitis is delayed for several days and the eruption is mild or moderate, systemic therapy offers less benefit. In the situation of a mildly to moderately sensitive patient with delayed onset, topical corticosteroids are the mainstay of therapy. Typically, an ultrapotent topical steroid, such as clobetasol (Temovate), is used twice daily for no more than 14 days. Table 64-10 lists the most common topical corticosteroids and their classification. Prolonged use of ultrapotent corticosteroids may lead to skin atrophy. The face, axillae, and groin are highly susceptible to atrophy, so use of ultrapotent products should be avoided in these regions. In most mild cases of dermatitis, a medium- to high-potency topical corticosteroid and 15- to 30-minute cool compresses three or four times daily with a 1:40 dilution of aluminum acetate (Domeboro, Burow's solution) will suffice. A bath with 1 cup of Aveeno oatmeal per tub of water, in addition to therapy with antihistamines such as hydroxyzine or diphenhydramine, is helpful for the itching. Treatment is usually required for 1 to 2 weeks.

In more severe cases with the eyelids, hands, or more than 10% BSA involvement, a systemic corticosteroid, such as prednisone, in a tapering dose starting at 1 mg/kg, or triamcinolone (Kenalog), 40 mg IM, is employed, tapering slowly over a course of 2 to 3 weeks to avoid rebound. Antihistamines, such as hydroxyzine, 10 mg PO four times daily (up to 100 mg/day), or diphenhydramine, 25 mg PO two or three times daily, can be used to suppress itching. Calamine lotion and aluminum acetate compresses also help with the itching.

Topical immunomodulators, such as pimecrolimus (Elidel) 1% cream and tacrolimus (Protopic) 0.03% or 0.1% ointment, offer a noncorticosteroid treatment alternative. There is no risk of atrophy with these two agents. Studies show them to be helpful in alleviating allergic and irritant contact dermatitides, but expense is often a limiting factor.[5,6]

Most patients visit a pharmacy looking for over-the-counter (OTC) preparations; usually, they are disappointed. The eruption heals spontaneously in 7 to 10 days, so the most helpful option is an inexpensive agent, such as calamine lotion, which is comforting and helps form a crust. Aluminum acetate (Domeboro,

TABLE 64-10 Classification of Corticosteroids

Generic Name	Trade Name	Preparations Available
Ultrapotent		
Betamethasone dipropionate	Diprolene	0.05% cream or ointment
Clobetasol propionate	Temovate, Cormax	0.05% cream or ointment
Diflorasone diacetate	Psorcon	0.05% cream or ointment
Halobetasol propionate	Ultravate	0.05% cream or ointment
High Potency		
Amcinonide	Cyclocort	0.1% cream or ointment
Desoximetasone	Topicort	0.25% cream or ointment
Fluocinonide	Lidex	0.05% cream or ointment
Halcinonide	Halog	0.1% cream or ointment
Medium Potency		
Betamethasone valerate	Luxiq	0.1% cream or ointment, 0.12% foam
Fluocinolone acetonide	Synalar	0.025% cream or ointment
Fluticasone propionate	Cutivate	0.005% ointment or 0.05% cream
Hydrocortisone butyrate	Locoid	0.1% cream
Hydrocortisone valerate	Westcort	0.2% cream or ointment
Triamcinolone acetonide	Aristocort, Kenalog	0.1% cream or ointment
Low Potency		
Alclometasone dipropionate	Aclovate	0.05% cream or ointment
Clocortolone pivalate	Cloderm	0.1% cream
Desonide	DesOwen, Tridesilon	0.05% cream or ointment
Hydrocortisone acetate	Cortaid, Corticaine	0.5% cream or ointment

inadequate protection because urushiol is able to penetrate through rubber. Vinyl gloves are more protective, as are other plastic gloves. Leather gloves are acceptable. Many herbicides are available to kill the plants. Unfortunately, none is specific to *Toxicodendron* species. Proper cleaning of clothing is essential. Washing immediately with soap (detergent) and water has been shown to destroy urushiol. A lotion containing the organoclay quaternium-18 bentonite is very effective in preventing this type of dermatitis. If applied before contact with the urushiol resin, it has been proven to decrease poison ivy, oak, and sumac dermatitis by inactivating the resin.[85]

The best approaches to prophylaxis, based on an intimate understanding of the chemistry of urushiol and the biology of the weeds, are recognition and avoidance.[45] When this is not possible, protective clothing that is either disposable or washable should be worn. Wool is the best material to use as a protective barrier because it binds the allergen readily.[32] Clothing should be washed with detergent or, preferably, bleach to inactivate urushiol. Tools and other inanimate objects are best cleaned with a dilute solution of bleach. Bleach rapidly inactivates urushiol, and organic solvents such as alcohol, gasoline, and acetone can extract it from contaminated surfaces. For cleansing the skin after contact, a variety of products are available, some more useful than others. A commercially available OTC solvent is Tecnu, but this is merely an inexpensive petroleum solvent sold at a high price and should not be used for therapy. An excellent choice is rubbing (isopropyl) alcohol, which should be applied liberally for decontamination and followed by liberal use of water wash-off to avoid spreading the oil on the skin. Care should be taken to limit contact time with the skin, particularly with children, who may be susceptible to transcutaneous alcohol toxicity.

Use of soap is inferior to better solvents. The newer topical agent Zanfel has been shown to experimentally decrease urushiol-induced contact dermatitis. It is a mixture of alcohol solubles and anionic surfactants that binds to the urushiol antigen and renders it unable to induce an allergic reaction. If applied soon enough after exposure, it has the potential to decrease urushiol-induced allergic contact dermatitis.[35] The idea of using barrier preparations has become popular again, even though in the past, such creams and ointments proved disappointing.[97] The current favorite, an organoclay called IvyBlock, was developed to protect forestry workers against these weeds during national firefighting escapades.[46] This approach was confirmed in a multicenter

Burow's solution) 1 : 40 diluted in plain water and used as a soak, compress, or wet dressing is helpful, as is a 1% acetic acid wet dressing (white vinegar) in water. The soaks are performed for 15 to 30 minutes at a time and can be repeated as often as necessary. Regardless of the therapy chosen, time is required for healing.

Although field workers have mentioned that *Aloe vera* latex empirically improves wound healing, a major study in contact dermatitis showed that it was ineffective.[136] Topical lotions with anesthetics or antihistamines offer no additional benefit and may induce contact sensitization to the chemical additives. Allergic contact dermatitis is a self-healing disease if iatrogenic influences are avoided. Secondary superficial infections may occur in children, during hospitalization, or in cases with prolonged pruritus and scratching. Use of antibacterial soaps usually prevents this complication.

As the dermatitis heals and scales form after 10 to 14 days, the patient may note a resurgence of pruritus, which left untreated can lead to subacute lichenoid neurodermatitis (Figure 64-22). Judicious use of almost any corticosteroid cream or ointment, such as triamcinolone acetonide 0.025%, desonide 0.025%, or hydrocortisone 2.5%, helps alleviate symptoms.

PREVENTION

Prevention involves a combination of avoidance and destruction of plants. This can be done directly, by educating individuals at risk to recognize and avoid these plants, or indirectly, by wearing protective clothing and gloves when coming into contact with them. Rubber gloves that are the thickness of surgical gloves are

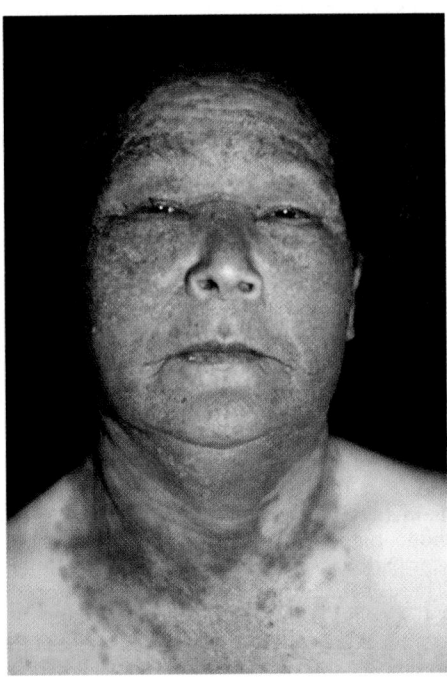

FIGURE 64-22 Resurgence of pruritus, leading to patch of subchronic lichenoid neurodermatitis.

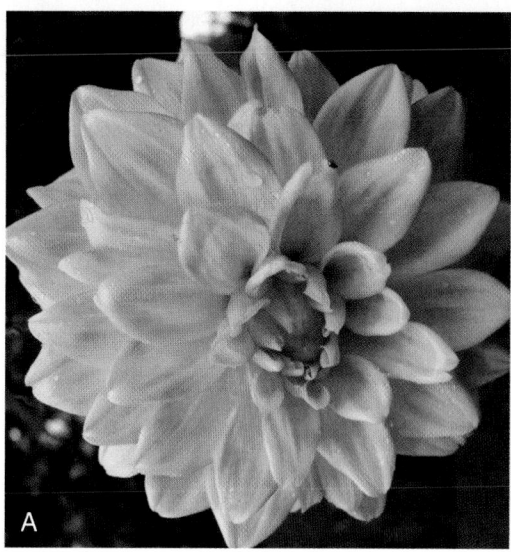
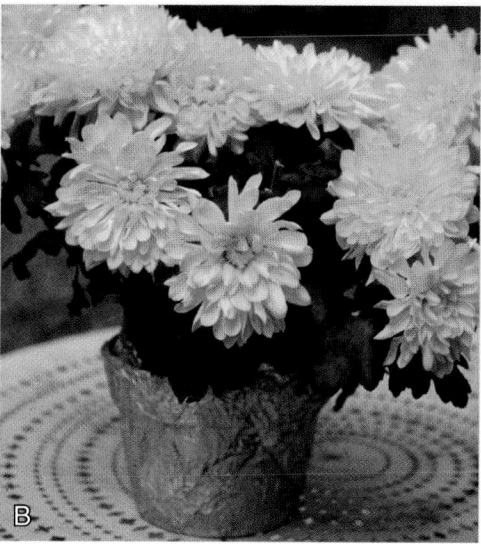
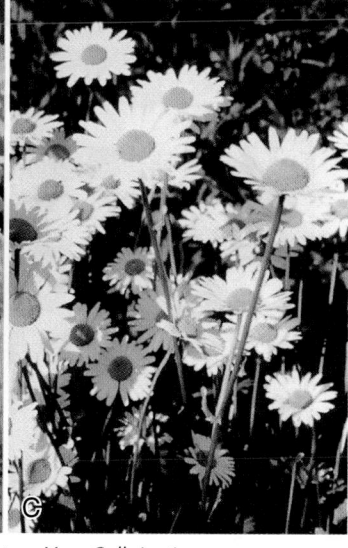

FIGURE 64-23 Compositae members. **A,** Dahlia. **B,** Chrysanthemum. **C,** Daisy. *(C courtesy Yves Sell, Institute of Botany, Louis Pasteur University, Strasbourg, France.)*

study.[85] The lotion can be obtained readily from a pharmacist or by major marketers. Oak-N-Ivy-Armor is a product marketed to be used as a preventive lotion. It actively binds urushiol and keeps it from contacting the skin. Similar topical preventive products include büji Block and Ongard. Stokogard outdoor cream, composed of a linoleic ester dimer, was removed from the market for lack of U.S. Food and Drug Administration (FDA) approval but is still available in industrial supply houses that are not regulated.[98] When the cream is first applied, it has a foul smell (like dead fish), resulting from release of the ester. The odor disappears in about 20 minutes, and the cream acts like a barrier to delay the penetration of urushiol oil. It must be washed off in 4 to 6 hours for protection.

COMPOSITAE FAMILY

There are more than 20,000 species of plants in the Compositae family. Box 64-2 provides a brief list of some of the more common members, and Figure 64-23 shows a few highly recognizable members. Compositae species have worldwide distribution. The allergens found in these plants are sesquiterpene lactones. More than 3000 individual sesquiterpene lactones have been identified.[33,54] The lactones are made in the trichomes found on the plant's surface. The allergen is not highly sensitizing; thus the individuals typically affected have repeated contact with the allergen and are usually involved in daily handling of plants: florists, nursery workers, horticulturists, and produce handlers.

Rarely, home gardeners or other people who spend long periods outdoors are affected. Allergenicity is increased by the presence of an α-methylene group attached to the lactone ring.[111] The dermatitis is fairly characteristic across the Compositae family. The clinical scenario is often a chronic lichenified eruption resembling photodermatitis.[84] Clues that this is not photodermatitis include involvement of the upper eyelids and submental region of the neck, areas that are classically spared in true photodermatitis. Definitive diagnosis can be made by patch-testing the patient to various portions of the actual leaf, stem, and petal against appropriate controls. A screening mixture of sesquiterpene lactones is available, but this mixture will miss some relevant allergies to Compositae plants. It is prudent to patch-test the patient with the actual plant that is suspected of causing the allergic reaction.

Ragweed (*Ambrosia* spp.) is a member of the Compositae family of plants; thus its allergen is a sesquiterpene lactone. Figure 64-24 shows a photo of common ragweed. Ragweed pollen likely contains two individual antigens, one that can cause respiratory ailments, such as asthma or allergic rhinitis, and another that contains sesquiterpene lactones and causes allergic

BOX 64-2 Familiar Compositae Plants

- Artichoke
- Black-eyed Susan
- Butterweed
- Chamomile
- Chicory
- Chrysanthemum
- Cornflower
- Daisy
- Dahlia
- Dandelion
- Endive
- Feverfew
- Goldenrod
- Ironweed
- Lettuce
- Marigold
- Mugwort
- Pyrethrum
- Ragweed
- Ragwort
- Sagebrush
- Sneezeweed
- Stinking mayweed
- Sunflower
- Tansy
- Tarragon
- Thistle
- Yarrow
- Zinnia

Data from Marks JG Jr, Elsner P, DeLeo VA: *Contact and occupational dermatology,* ed 3, St Louis, 2002, Mosby, pp 13-15.

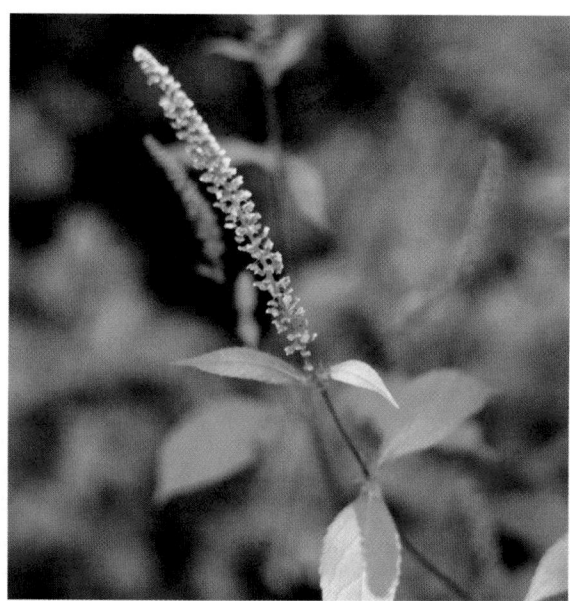

FIGURE 64-24 Ragweed, *Ambrosia* species.

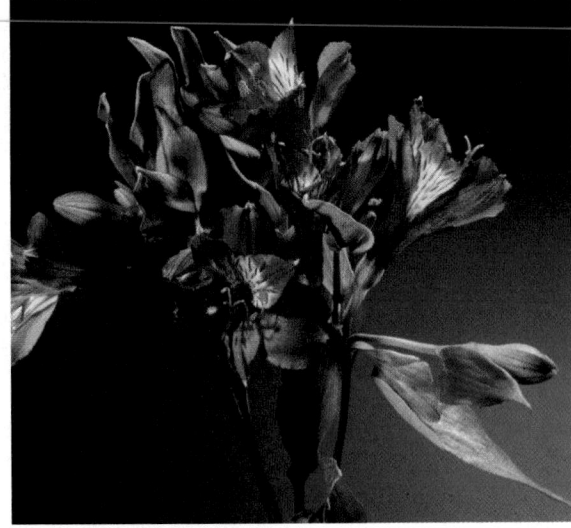

FIGURE 64-25 A familiar cut flower, Peruvian lily (*Alstroemeria* spp.).

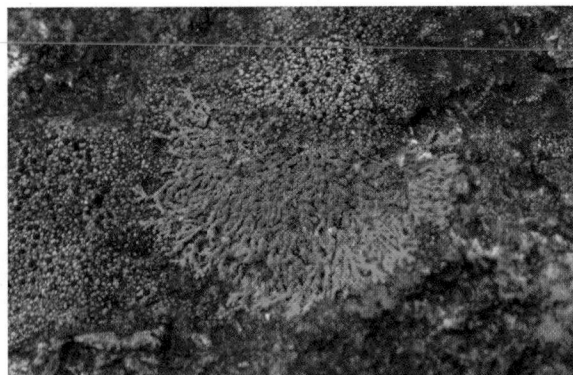

FIGURE 64-26 Close-up view of lichen. (*Courtesy Peter Schalock, Massachusetts General Hospital, Boston, Mass.*)

contact dermatitis. Clinically, patients show involvement of the head and neck region and other areas not covered with clothing. The dermatitis is chronic in nature and tends to mimic photo-contact dermatitis. In this case, the upper eyelid and submental regions may be involved, which is not the case in photocontact dermatitis. *Ambrosia deltoidea* is a weed in the Compositae family found in the southwestern United States that has also been reported to cause airborne allergic contact dermatitis. This plant bears little resemblance to common ragweed.[112]

Wild feverfew (*Parthenium hysterophorus*) is a weed in the Compositae family found throughout the western hemisphere. It is an acute cause of allergic contact dermatitis, although in clinical practice, it most often manifests as chronic lichenified dermatitis in areas chronically exposed to the allergen. Feverfew caused epidemic outbreaks of dermatitis in India after it was accidentally transplanted there. It is not a native plant to India and has thrived in its new environment. The epidemics have become so severe that it has been nicknamed the "scourge of India."[84]

Peruvian lily (*Alstroemeria* spp.) is a very popular cut flower. Its allergen is tuliposide A or α-methylene-γ-butyrolactone (Figure 64-25). Allergic contact dermatitis to this plant is the most common cause of allergic contact dermatitis in florists. Florists who repeatedly cut the flowers and stems are chronically exposed to the allergen. Consequently, they have the highest sensitization rate. It is a very rare cause of allergic contact dermatitis in individuals outside of the floral industry.

Liverworts (*Frullania* spp.) are members of the Jubulaceae family (related to mosses) that usually live on tree bark. They are small, reddish brown plants found most often in the Pacific Northwest. There are hundreds of species of *Frullania* plants. Similar to members of the Compositae family, this plant causes chronic lichenified dermatitis that is rarely seen in the acute phase. The allergen is sesquiterpene lactone. Allergic contact dermatitis caused by *Frullania* is a problem among lumberjacks and forest workers, but it may affect any individual who takes a walk in the woods.[84]

Grevillea banksii and *G. robusta* have been implicated as causing allergic contact dermatitis. These plants are native to Australia but have been transplanted around the globe. They grow as shrubs and are used in domestic landscaping. The allergen is a resorcinol. Similarly, *Dittrichia graveolens* (stinkwort) is a weed native to the Mediterranean but has become naturalized initially in Australia and now in the United States. It has recently been reported as a cause of allergic contact dermatitis in outdoor workers.[124]

Allergic contact dermatitis to lichens is seen most often in forestry workers and gardeners. Lichens live worldwide and grow just about anywhere (Figure 64-26). They are composed of algae and fungi that live in a symbiotic relationship. The allergens are usnic acid, atranorin, and evernic acid.[84] The clinical picture is very similar to that of Compositae dermatitis.[125]

The false heliotrope plant (*Phacelia crenulata*) is found in deserts of the southwestern United States. It causes acute allergic contact dermatitis in the direct areas of contact. A linear papulovesicular reaction, not unlike the reaction to *Toxicodendron*, is usually seen.

Two common, easily recognized plants that can cause allergic contact dermatitis are the tulip and primrose. The tulip (*Tulipia* spp.) is an early-spring flowering plant (Figure 64-27). Its allergen is tuliposide A, the same allergen found in *Alstroemeria* (Peruvian lily, discussed earlier). The allergen has its highest concentration in the epidermis of the bulb, from which originate the clinical findings of "tulip fingers," a chronic fissured and scaly eczematous rash of the fingertips in people who routinely handle the bulbs (Figure 64-28).[58] This is most common in commercial

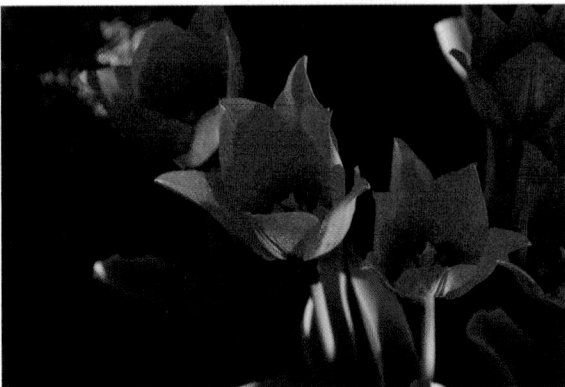

FIGURE 64-27 Tulip, *Tulipia* species.

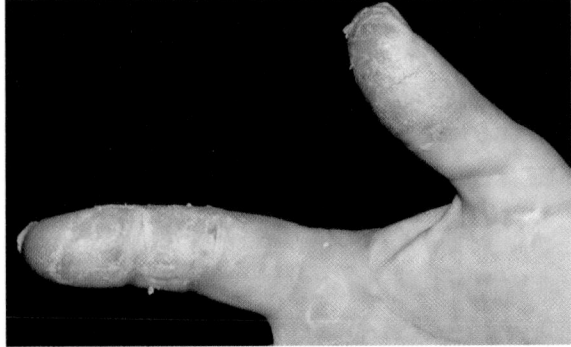

FIGURE 64-28 Eczematous scaly patches on the fingers of a floral worker.

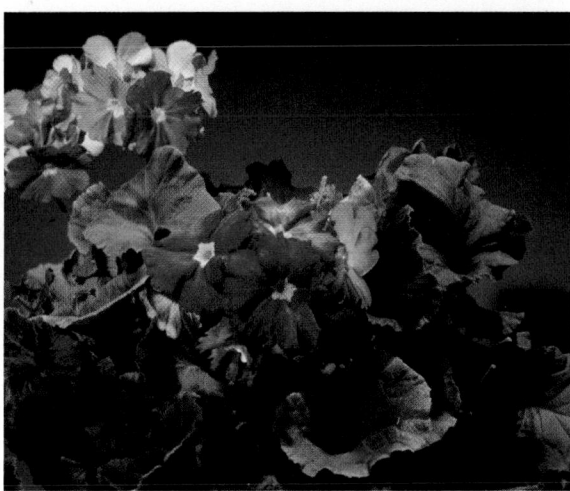

FIGURE 64-29 Primrose, a common houseplant.

gardeners; occasionally, an avid home gardener is affected. People who are allergic to tulips should avoid *Alstroemeria*.

Primrose (*Primula obconica*) is a common houseplant reported to cause allergic contact dermatitis in home gardeners (Figure 64-29). Its allergen is primin (2-methoxy-6-pentyl-1,4-benzoquinone). The allergen is found in the highest concentration in the trichomes of the stem and leaves. A genetically altered hybrid has been produced that does not make primin and thus has no potential to induce allergic contact dermatitis. This hybrid is likely responsible for the decrease noted in incidence of primin-induced allergic contact dermatitis.[28]

The creosote bush (*Larrea* spp.) is found throughout North and South America (Figure 64-30). It is a shrubby bush with leaves covered by a resinous substance. There are a few reports of this resin causing allergic contact dermatitis.[75]

The Hydrophyllaceae family of plants contains a class of chemicals called *phacelioids*.[104] These substances are related to urushiol and can be potent allergens. However, they do not cross-react with urushiol. The *Cineraria* hybrid has also been described as a cause of allergic contact dermatitis in the Compositae family.[29]

Not all cases of Compositae-induced dermatitis are allergic in nature. The glove artichoke (*Cynara solumus*) has been associated with an irritant vesicobullous reaction affecting the fingertips, although patch-test results have been negative.[101] Some patients have even presented with erythrodermic presentations, especially from the *Parthenium hysterophorus* (wild feverfew) species.[2]

Botanical extracts in cosmetics and topical medications can cause contact dermatitis.[61] This dermatitis is often irritant in

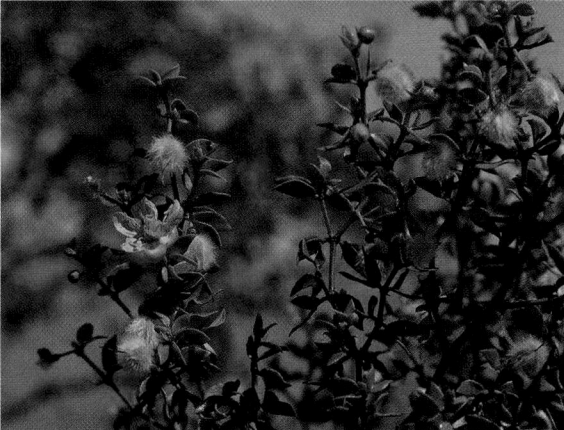

FIGURE 64-30 Leaves of the creosote bush are covered with a resinous substance. *(Courtesy Jon Sullivan.)*

nature, but allergic contact dermatitis has been reported in susceptible individuals. Plant products associated with cosmetic contact dermatitis include Compositae plants, tea tree oil, peppermint, lavender, lichens, and henna. In addition to the plant product, other allergens in these cosmetics include ingredients such as fragrance, preservative, dye, and sunscreen.[61]

Currently, resources are limited for patch-testing patients to plant irritants. The European and American baseline series includes sesquiterpene-lactone mix for Compositae and *Frullania*. Special plant series exist for testing Compositae, *Frullania,* Liliaceae, Alstroemeriaceae, Alliaceae, and the genus *Citrus.* However, testing for Anacardiaceae, Cruciferae, Capparaceae, Ginkgoaceae, Araliaceae, and Apiaceae is not currently available.[109]

CONTACT URTICARIA: IMMUNOLOGIC AND NONIMMUNOLOGIC SUBTYPES

Contact urticaria can be classified as immunologically or nonimmunologically induced. The immunologic subtype is caused by an immediate hypersensitivity reaction requiring antibody formation to a particular substance. These type I hypersensitivity reactions show a broad clinical spectrum, from mild skin hives to anaphylaxis. Prick testing and radioallergosorbent test (RAST) are of benefit in determining the cause in certain cases. The immunologic form of urticaria depends on the individual patient's immune activity or hyperactivity. There is no predictable manner to determine to which plants a person may develop a type I reaction. Food handlers and persons otherwise constantly exposed to plant products are likely to be more at risk. Many plant species have been reported to cause contact immunologic urticaria.[70,82] Patients typically present with urticarial wheals in areas of exposure within 1 to 2 hours of handling a particular plant. Occasionally, there is oral involvement with tongue and lip swelling. When there is prominent oral involvement, one must also consider consumed fruit as a cause. Box 64-3 provides a partial list of plants causing contact immunologic urticaria. Atopic individuals have been reported to be at higher risk for type I contact urticaria.[82]

Nonimmunologic plant contact dermatitis is caused by direct release of urticating substances onto or into the skin. There are four main families of plants contain stinging hairs or spines that can cause contact urticaria: Euphorbiaceae, Hydrophyllaceae, Loasaceae, and Urticaceae.[82] Most of these plants are found in the tropics, with the exception of stinging nettles, which have worldwide distribution and are found throughout the United States. Box 64-4 lists some of the more common nettle plants. The most common plant causing contact urticaria is the stinging nettle *Urtica dioica* (Figure 64-31). Within the *Urticaceae* family reside other plants capable of producing contact urticaria by means of the nonimmunologic route. Urticarial reactions are typically acute and resolve spontaneously, so the advice of a physician is rarely sought. Persistent paresthesias lasting hours have been reported.[88]

In the case of nonimmunologic urticaria, release of histamine from mast cells with vasodilation and leakage of fluid appears

BOX 64-3	Plants That Cause Immunologic Urticaria
Fruits	Mustard
Apple	Rapeseed
Carrot	
Celery	**Trees**
Parsley	Birch pollen
Potato	Western red cedar
Tomato	
	Vegetables
Plants	Chives
Tulip	Grains
	Lettuce
Spices	Onion
Cinnamon	
Garlic	

BOX 64-4 Plants in the Nettle Family

- *Urtica chamaedryoides*
- *Urtica dioica*
- *Urtica gracilis*
- *Urtica ferox*
- *Urtica membranacea*
- *Urtica urens*
- *Urtica pilulifera*
- *Urtica parviflora*

to be an early direct chemical change leading to clinical hives.[38,114] The molecular events in mast cell degranulation are thought to be similar to those described for immunogenic urticaria, with certain discrete differences. There is no evidence for a selective membrane receptor, such as the high-affinity immunoglobulin E (IgE) receptor that is now well characterized and required for immunologic degranulation of mast cells.[114,119] Instead, a receptor-independent mode of action occurs for all nonimmunologic histamine liberators, acting directly on a pertussis toxin–sensitive G protein to initiate a signal through phospholipase C activation, which degranulates mast cells of their histamine content.[91] There does not seem to be a requirement for methylation of the membrane phospholipids. Rather, a high intracellular calcium accumulation must occur, and the reaction is rapidly terminated without delayed mediator release.[108] Arachidonic acid metabolites are not formed in any amount.[14]

Figure 64-32, *A* and *B*, shows the stinging nettle plant and a close-up view of its spines. Contact with spines on the plant causes release of biologically active substances from the spines. These include histamine, acetylcholine, 5-hydroxytryptamine (serotonin), leukotriene B_4 (LTB$_4$), and leukotriene C_4 (LTC$_4$).[7,27,34,40] These chemicals lead directly to urticaria. There is no standardized therapy for stinging nettle dermatitis. Often the symptoms resolve in several hours. If pruritus is severe, treatment with diphenhydramine, 25 to 50 mg every 6 to 8 hours as needed, is indicated. Figure 64-32, *C*, illustrates the faint urticarial papules seen after contact with the stinging nettle plant.

Numerous plants have been associated with release of urticating substances. These include chili pepper (*Capsicum* spp.) and cowhage (*Mucuna pruriens*). In the case of chili pepper, the released chemical is capsaicin; with cowhage, it is mucanain.[84]

The pathogenesis of immunogenic contact urticaria is a variation of immediate type I hypersensitivity. The central cytologic reactor in skin is the mast cell, which has high-affinity IgE receptors in its membrane. An IgE molecule binds to the receptor by its Fc portion, exposing the Fab segments as recognition sites for circulating proteins. When a divalent protein antigen appropri-

ately bridges two IgE molecules, a series of biochemical events transpires that leads to mast cell degranulation. Initially, the plasma membrane is perturbed. Several lipids are phosphorylated and G proteins are activated, which in turn activate phospholipase C to hydrolyze phosphatidylinositol 4,5-bisphosphate (PIP$_2$) and yield two messengers: diacylglycerol (DG) and inositol triphosphate (IP$_3$).[20] IP$_3$ binds to its receptor on the endoplasmic reticulum, forming a calcium channel to release free calcium ions (Ca^{2+}) into the cytosol.[11,15,60,94] Simultaneously, DG activates protein kinase C in the plasma membrane, opening calcium channels and allowing entrance of extracellular Ca^{2+}, which further loads the cytosol with free Ca^{2+}, an important "messenger" in the stimulus secretion process.[78] G proteins interact with and release the nucleotide complexed to protein α-chains, some of which probably inhibit or stimulate cyclic adenosine phosphate and its actions as a second messenger.[20,122]

The result of the extensive alteration in intracellular milieu is activation of a serine proteinase and exocytosis of mast cell granule contents.[38,114] These come in three forms: preformed and rapidly released; preformed, bound to the granule matrix of heparin, and slowly released; and newly formed mediators. In addition, mast cells produce a variety of cytokines, including IL-1, IL-3, IL-4, IL-5, and IL-6; GM-CSF; and TNF-α.[120] These cytokines interact with cells and structures, such as endothelium in the skin, to amplify the various inflammatory responses.[38,114,120] In acute urticaria, the rapidly released preformed mediators account for most of the signs and symptoms. These mediators include histamine, chemotactic factors, and arylsulfatase. If the lesions persist or extend, other mediators, such as newly formed leukotrienes, heparin (or heparin fragments), cytokines, and a number of proteases, may be involved in the continuing tissue damage.

The sequence of inflammatory events leading to acute urticaria occurs most often in people with an atopic background, especially those with pollen allergies.[70] The patients with significant pollen allergies are also at risk for pollen-fruit allergy syndrome, described as a mucosal contact urticaria typically seen when these patients are exposed to *Betula pendula* (silver birch), *Artemisia vulgaris* (mugwort), or timothy grass (*Phleum pratense*).[68] Cross-reacting foods include apple, pear, carrot, celery, tomato, cherry, carrot, celery, aniseed, and peach. This group of people, mainly women and especially health care workers, have been found in recent years to be exquisitely sensitive to latex rubber gloves and sensitive to proteins in the natural latex from rubber trees in Asia.[22,73,83,115,126]

In the past decade, latex sensitivity has increasingly become a problem. More than 200 polypeptides are produced in natural latex rubber, many of them contact sensitizers, so that a single antigen is not likely to be identified for a given patient. In the clinical realm, IgE-mediated immediate-type hypersensitivity and thus the potential for anaphylaxis is a disastrous complication. In addition to the polypeptides appearing in natural rubber latex, many are found in a number of plants, particularly those consumed as food. One theory is that the cross-reacting allergens are "defense proteins" with a role to protect the plant from attack by pathogens.[72] Whether this is true requires further investigation, but it is also possible that by plant engineering, these allergens may be genetically removed from foods we consume.

In addition to fruit and nuts, mustard has been implicated in anaphylaxis.[99] In less severe cases, vesicular, eczematous rashes have been noted within hours of eating mustard or rapeseed, which is used widely in production of vegetable oils and margarine.[89] Recent reports also describe contact urticaria to raw potato, as well as the Solanaceae and Alliaceae families of plants, which include tomato, green bell pepper, jalapeño, chive, red leaf lettuce, serrano pepper, pasilla pepper, leek, red bell pepper, garlic, and yellow onion.

In contrast to urticarial reactions, erythema multiforme–like eruptions are well recognized after contact with bracelets and ornamental necklaces made of exotic woods, such as *Dalbergia nigra*.[50] Erythema multiforme has also been seen after exposure to more common plants, such as poison ivy, primula, and mugwort.[50,131] It is theorized that multiforme lesions result from vasculitis caused by deposition of immune complexes in or around the blood vessels.

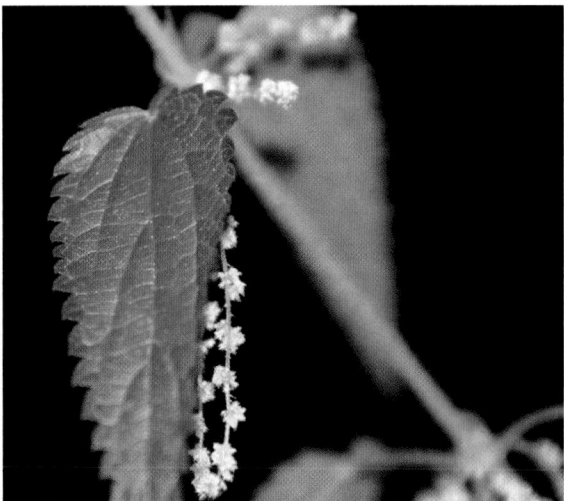

FIGURE 64-31 *Urtica dioica*, or stinging nettle. (*Courtesy Peter Schalock, Massachusetts General Hospital, Boston, Mass*).

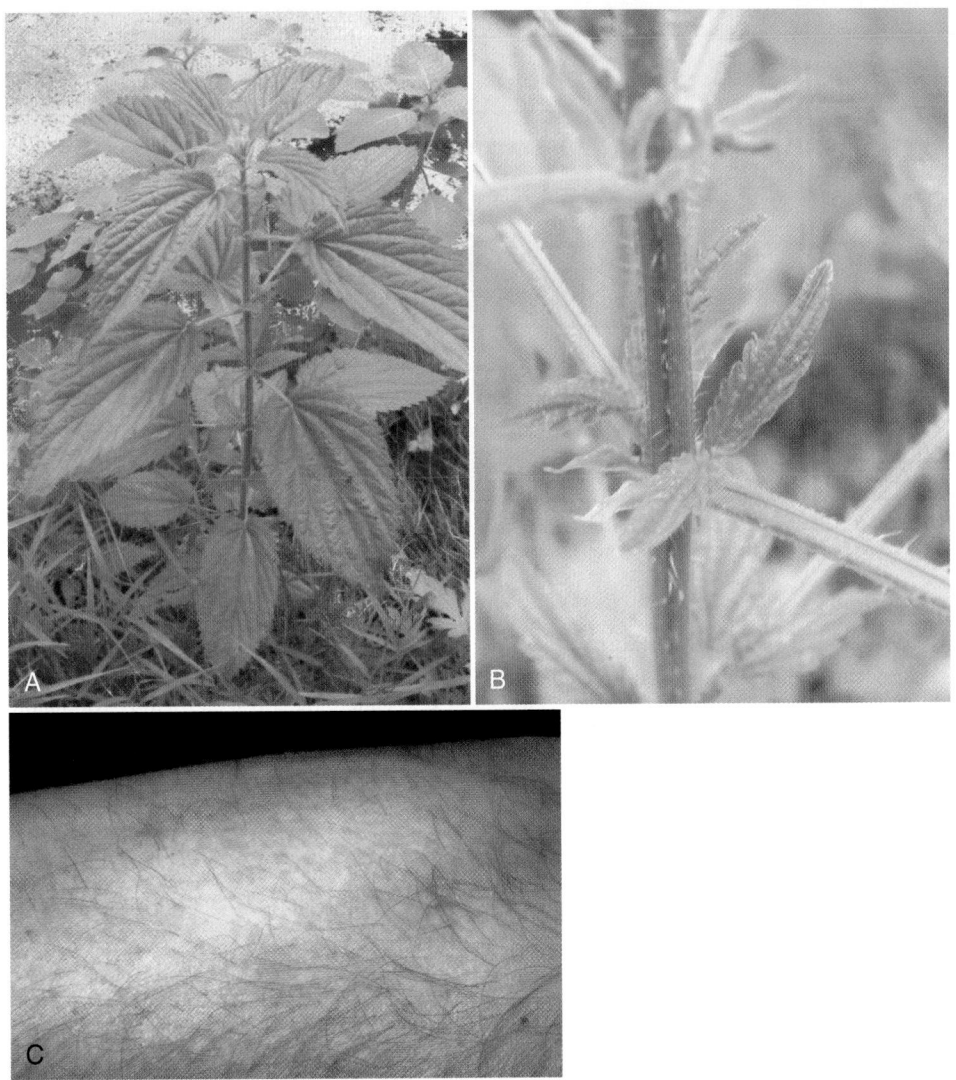

FIGURE 64-32 A, Stinging nettle. **B,** Close-up view of the stinging nettle spines. **C,** Urticarial papules induced after contact with the stinging nettle.

Diagnosis of immunogenic contact urticaria can be confirmed by simple tests. As a useful test, application of the suspected plant product to the antecubital fossa twice a day for several days may reproduce the wheal response. Open and closed patch tests, with examination of test sites in 2 to 6 hours, can be useful, as can more conventional prick, scratch, or scratch-chamber tests, in which the results are read in 15 to 20 minutes.[70] It is critical to determine whether urtication is immunologic or nonimmunologic, because this helps to quantify the risk for anaphylaxis.[53,70] For complete evaluation, an allergist obtains RASTs to quantify specific IgE in the patient's serum. More refined serologic tests include crossed radioimmunoelectrophoresis (CRIE) and CRIE inhibition.[23]

Patients with contact urticaria typically visit the emergency department when an eruption is extensive or extreme or if it is associated with stridor, wheezing, and collapse. Because mast cell degranulation is the central problem, epinephrine is the drug of choice because it stimulates cyclic adenosine monophosphate formation that opposes further degranulation. All patients at risk for severe urticaria should carry a method for epinephrine injection (e.g., EpiPen) with them at all times. Other supportive treatments for anaphylactic shock, such as albuterol, oxygen, or IV hydrocortisone, may be required. In less severe cases, antihistamines are valuable. IM or IV diphenhydramine in an adult dose of 25 to 50 mg usually stops progression of wheal formation and can be followed by oral hydroxyzine (10 to 25 mg three times daily) or cyproheptadine (4 mg three times daily) for 2 to 5 days.

Pure H$_1$ blockers, such as fexofenadine (60 mg twice daily), are also effective and do not depress the central nervous system, although the prescriber must be aware of any unique adverse reactions. It is important to make certain the patient is not inadvertently exposed to hidden parts of the plant on the body, in clothing, or in a towel, blanket, or knapsack. Recrudescence of the urticarial response usually can be traced to continuing unknown contact with the offending agent. In patients with high risk for urticarial eruptions and airway involvement, education regarding avoidance of the offending plant is crucial to maintenance of a symptom-free lifestyle.

PHYTOPHOTODERMATITIS

Plants and their components can interact with ultraviolet (UV) rays of the sun and produce a clinically distinct entity known as phytophotodermatitis. The two types of phytophotodermatitis are phototoxic and photoallergic. *Phototoxic* reactions, which appear clinically as an exaggerated sunburn, are analogous to irritant contact dermatitis. *Photoallergic* reactions, which appear eczematous, are analogous to allergic contact dermatitis. Phototoxic reactions are encountered more frequently and are often recognized by a clinician's knowledge of offending agents and the morphology of the exanthem. The reactions most frequently appear as linear red patches and plaques with or without edema, but also can be bullous in nature.[127] A characteristic finding is postinflammatory hyperpigmentation lasting for months to

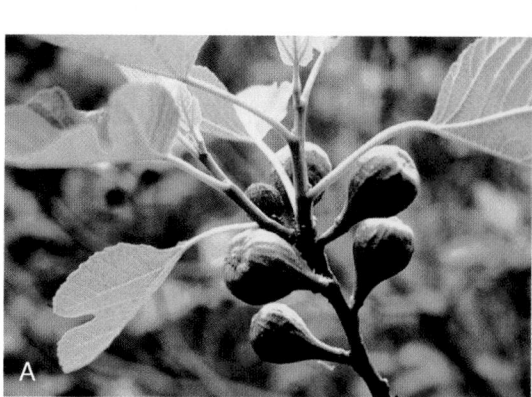
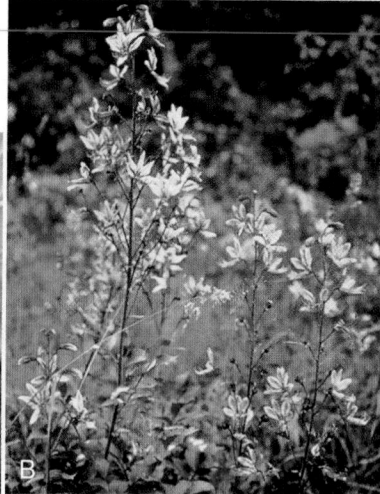

FIGURE 64-33 Phototoxic plants. **A,** Fig tree. **B,** Gas plant. (**B** *courtesy Yves Sell, Institute of Botany, Louis Pasteur University, Strasbourg, France.*)

years.[37] Most of these reactions are likely to go unreported or unrecognized, most often because of their mild nature, but also because it is often difficult to pinpoint the exact cause of the problem.

Phototoxic reactions are typically dose dependent and can occur in anyone if sufficient concentrations of UV light and the toxic plant material are achieved. In general, the wavelength of light needed to induce the most severe reactions is in the ultraviolet A (UVA) range, 320 to 400 nm.

For most phototoxic reactions, the plant toxin is a furocoumarin (psoralen). Furocoumarins intercalate into cellular DNA and cause formation of pyrimidine dimers, which interrupt DNA synthesis. This leads to cell damage and clinical effects. When UV light interacts with the psoralen molecule, it raises the energy level from the ground to an excited state. When the excited molecule returns to its ground state, energy is released that causes cross-linking of two strands of DNA. This interferes with DNA synthesis and ultimately cell division. This reaction is used to medical advantage in treatments such as PUVA (psoralen plus ultraviolet A) light therapy and in extracorporeal photopheresis. PUVA therapies are used for conditions ranging from vitiligo and psoriasis to cutaneous T cell lymphoma (CTCL). With extracorporeal photopheresis, a patient is connected by an IV line to a pheresis machine. Blood is drawn from the patient, and then leukocytes are isolated and exposed to a photoactive drug (psoralen), followed by exposure of blood to UVA light. This blood is then returned to the patient. This process causes cross-linking of DNA in the pathogenic T cells and death of these cells. This treatment is used almost exclusively for patients with CTCL and graft-versus-host disease (GVHD).

PHYTOPHOTOTOXIC CONTACT DERMATITIS

Furocoumarins include psoralen, 5-methoxy-psoralen (bergapten), 8-methoxy-psoralen (xanthotoxin), angelicin (isopsoralen), 5-hydroxy-psoralen (bergaptol), 8-hydroxy-psoralen (xanthotoxol), and limettin.[13,127] Psoralens are modified furocoumarins. Most of these chemicals are found in four plant families: Apiaceae, Rutaceae, Moraceae, and Leguminosae. Figure 64-33 shows a few examples of these plants. Figure 64-34 shows an example of the dermatitis that can result from exposure. Note the well-demarcated, angulated, hyperpigmented streaks that are characteristic of the disease.

Table 64-11 lists members of the families implicated in phytophototoxic contact dermatitis. Apiaceae, or Umbelliferae, is a well-recognized family that has an umbrella-like configuration to its flowers. In the United States, this family of plants is the most common cause of phytophototoxic dermatitis. The Moraceae and Leguminosae families are rare causes in the United States.[121]

So-called meadow dermatitis (dermatitis bullosa striata pratensis) occurs after exposure of wet human skin to psoralen-containing plants during daylight hours.[13] The most common offending plants are the yellow-flowered wild meadow parsnip and wild yellow flowered herb.[106] Bizarre linear configurations, such as an imprint, are often found on the lower extremities on bare skin after a walk through a field of a psoralen-containing weed.

Agriculture field work and grocery store work, in particular celery handling, have been the most frequently reported

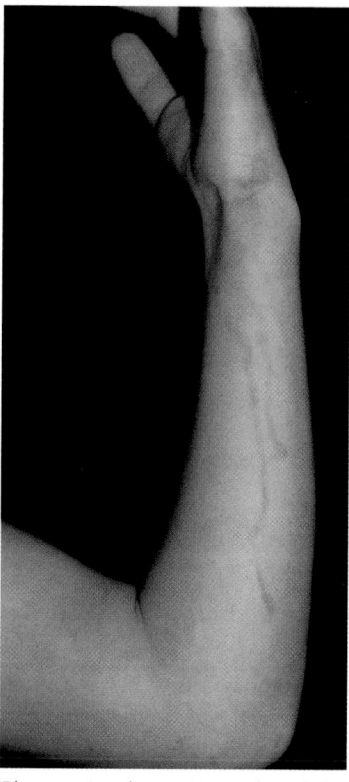

FIGURE 64-34 Phototoxic dermatitis induced by furocoumarins. (*Courtesy Richard A. Johnson, Massachusetts General Hospital, Boston, Mass.*)

TABLE 64-11 Common Members of the Umbelliferae, Rutaceae, Moraceae, and Leguminosae Families Found to Cause Phototoxic Contact Dermatitis

Common Name	Botanical Name
Umbelliferae (Apiaceae)	
Angelica	*Angelica gigas*
Celery	*Apium graveolens dulce*
Carrot	*Daucus carota*
Cow parsley	*Heracleum sphondylium*
Cow parsnip	*Heracleum lanatum*
Dill	*Anethum graveolus*
False bishop's weed	*Ammi majus*
Fennel	*Foenialum vulgare*
Giant hogweed	*Heracleum mantegazzianum*
Parsley	*Petroselinum crispum*
Parsnip	*Pastinaca sativa*
Queen Anne's lace	*Ammi majus*
Spring parsley	*Cymopterus watsonii*
Moraceae	
Fig	*Ficus carica*
Rutaceae	
Bergamot lime	*Citrus bergamia*
Berry rue	*Cneoridium dumosum*
Common rue	*Ruta graveolens*
Gas plant (burning bush)	*Dictamnus albus*
Grapefruit	*Citrus paradisi*
Lemon	*Citrus limon*
Lime	*Citrus aurantifolia*
Mexican lime	*Citrus aurantifolia*
Mokihana	*Pelea anisata*
Orange	*Citrus sinensis*
Zabon	*Citrus maxima*
Leguminosae	
Babchi (scurf-pea)	*Psoralea corylifolia*
Citrina	*Coronilla glauca*

Data from references 17, 19, 55, 59, 74, and 116.

BOX 64-5 Some Insecticides, Fungicides, and Herbicides That Cause Irritant Dermatitis (Pseudophytodermatitis)

- Captan
- Captofol
- Difolatan
- Dithiocarbamates
- Folpet
- Mancozeb (manganese and zinc ethylene-*bis*-dithiocarbamate)
- Maneb (manganese ethylene-*bis*-dithiocarbamate)
- Organophosphates
- Paraquat
- Phtahan
- Randox
- Sulfur

Data from Craigmill AL, editor: *Environmental Toxicology Newsletter*, University of California, Davis, 3:1, 1982; and Mark K, Brancaccio RR, Soter NA, et al: Allergic contact and photoallergic contact dermatitis to plants and pesticide allergens, *Arch Dermatol* 135:67, 1999.

primarily in field workers who are responsible for harvesting the celery plants.[121]

Pseudophytodermatitis has been used to describe dermatitis caused by arthropods that live on the plant or chemical agents that have been applied to plants.[121] One common arthropod causing dermatitis is the grain itch mite *Pediculoides ventricosus*, which can infest straw or hay. Numerous chemicals that are purposefully applied to plants can also cause contact dermatitis. Most often, these are insecticides, herbicides, or fungicides (Box 64-5). Waxes or azo dyes applied to various fruits and vegetables can also cause pseudophytodermatitis. Azo dyes are synthetic dyes containing the azo group (two connected nitrogen atoms) and are used in many industries, including the food industry.

PHYTOPHOTOALLERGIC CONTACT DERMATITIS

The phytophotoallergic reaction is exceedingly rare. Clinically, it manifests as an eczematous eruption localized to sun-exposed areas of the body that came into contact with the offending plant. It is likely underrecognized and underreported. Rare case reports are found throughout the literature. The plants reported to cause this reaction are tromso palm (*Heracleum laciniatum*), feverfew (*Parthenium hysterophorus*), garlic (*Allium sativum*), *Frullania*, and some coumarin (psoralen)–containing plants.[3,16,21,63,80,82] The clinical importance of these reactions is unknown. In the future, better screening methods may increase recognition of these reactions. Until then, only clinicians with access to extended patch-testing series or with sufficient suspicion and knowledge will recognize these reactions.

REFERENCES

Complete references used in this text are available online at expertconsult.inkling.com.

occupations associated with phytophototoxic dermatitis. Another occupation with reports of phytophototoxic dermatitis is bartending. Handling limes while mixing drinks, if combined with UV light, may cause this dermatitis.[4,31,50,57,117,129]

Berloque (pendant- or drop-like) dermatitis is perfume-induced phytophotodermatitis. Typically, a patient seeks care for hyperpigmented macules on the head and neck, with no obvious preexisting rash or dermatitis. Unfortunately, the hyperpigmentation can last for years. The original cause of this reaction was the oil of bergamot, which is derived from bergamot oranges and used in many perfumes. The oil contains a mixture of psoralens, including 5-methoxy-psoralen (5-MOP).

Pseudophytophotodermatitis is a reaction that has been reported to occur after prolonged human exposure to celery that has been infected with a psoralen-producing fungus (*Sclerotinia sclerotiorum*), more commonly known as "pink rot." This occurs

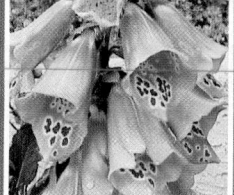

CHAPTER 65
Toxic Plant Ingestions

KIMBERLIE A. GRAEME

More than 46,000 plant exposures were reported to 57 American poison control centers (PCCs) in 2013, representing 2.25% of all human toxic exposures that year. This is likely an underrepresentation of plant exposures in the United States, because not all exposures are reported. The plant exposures most frequently reported to American PCCs were *Phytolacca americana* (American pokeweed), *Spathiphyllum* species (peace lily), *Prunus* spp. (cherry), *Ilex* spp. (holly), *Philodendron* spp., *Caladium* spp. (elephant ear), and *Malus* spp. (apple). Three deaths caused by plant poisoning were reported to PCCs in 2013.[226] The vast majority of reported plant exposures are accidental and occur in children. These exposures tend to produce mild symptoms. In fact, many exposures in children are to nontoxic or minimally toxic plants.

Worldwide, *Atropa belladonna* (deadly nightshade), *Datura* spp. (jimsonweed), *Brugmansia* spp. (angel's trumpet), *Hyoscyamus niger* (black henbane), *Conium maculatum* (poison hemlock), *Areca catechu* (betel nut), *Cascabela thevetia* (previously called *Thevetia peruviana*, or yellow oleander), *Nerium oleander* (common oleander), *Cerbera manghas* (sea mango), *Veratrum album* (hellebore), *Aconitum carmichaeli* (aconite), *Taxus* spp. (yew), *Chelidonium* spp. (greater celandine), *Colchicum autumnale* (autumn crocus), *Gloriosa superba* (glory lily), *Ricinus communis* (castor bean), *Atractylis gummifera* (bird-lime or blue thistle), and *Blighia sapida* (ackee fruit) cause significant morbidity and mortality.[101,108,111,145,203,209,338,354] The most serious poisonings generally occur in adults who have ingested the poisonous plants with intent for self-harm.[203,226,270] When plants are consumed with suicidal intent, the severity of symptoms is similar to other, nonplant, suicidal exposures.[270,304]

Serious poisoning can occur in wilderness exposure after persons consume meal-size portions of toxic plants that are mistaken for edible foods. These include hemlocks (*Conium maculatum* and *Cicuta maculata*) mistaken for wild carrots or parsnips, and autumn crocus (*Colchicum autumnale*) or death camas (*Zigadenus* spp.) mistaken for wild garlic or onion, respectively. War and famine can compel desperate, intentional, and prolonged ingestion of toxic plants. This may produce epidemics of chronic, devastating illnesses, such as Konzo from cassava (*Manihot esculenta*) and lathyrism from grass pea (*Lathyrus sativus*) consumption.

Although plants have been used for centuries as medications and mind-altering substances, there is a progressive trend of natural plant use as herbal medications (*Aconitum* spp., or aconitine) and to achieve legal intoxication (*Mitragyna speciosa*, or kratom, and *Argyreia nervosa*, or Hawaiian baby woodrose). Many medications prescribed by allopathic medical professionals have plant-based origins. Colchicine is derived from autumn crocus, a plant that was recommended for arthritis symptoms in *Des Materia Medica* in the first century AD. Furthermore, many popular drugs of abuse have plant-based origins. Ancient Incas used coca leaves (family Erythroxylaceae) medicinally. Cocaine was extracted from the leaves and abused recreationally. Bath salts, or synthetic cathinones, share a similar chemical structure to cathinone, found in khat (*Catha edulis*), a plant chewed socially in Arabia for millennia. Reasons for human exposure to toxic plants vary, but clinical presentations can be predicted if the plant species ingested is known. When identity of the ingested plant is unknown, general familiarity with toxic plant exposures and an organ system–based approach to evaluating patients may facilitate care.

GENERAL CONSIDERATIONS

Prompt and precise identification of the plant causing toxicity may not be feasible. Supportive care takes priority over plant identification. Airway, breathing, and circulation are assessed, including hydration status, end-organ perfusion, and urine output. Oral administration of activated charcoal (1 g/kg), up to 50 g, may aid gastrointestinal (GI) decontamination. However, recommendations on when to administer activated charcoal are challenging, because this has not been prospectively studied for most plant ingestions. If a patient is actively vomiting, activated charcoal likely will not contribute to decontamination. If the patient has depressed mental status or is likely to seize, administration of activated charcoal may result in pulmonary aspiration of charcoal and associated respiratory complications. Opinions on when to administer activated charcoal vary among toxicologists.

After emergency care is provided and the patient stabilized, a history should include time of ingestion, amount and part of plants ingested, initial symptoms, and time between ingestion and onset of symptoms. Method of preparation (e.g., drying, cooking, boiling) and number of persons who ate the same plant are important considerations. Plant identification may be aided by communication with PCC personnel and by Internet searches.[15,345,346]

Laboratory studies depend on clinical presentation and suspected plant exposure. Complications of poisoning include aspiration pneumonia, rhabdomyolysis, and deep vein thrombosis. Differential diagnosis is initially kept broad so that other illnesses, such as infection and trauma, are not missed. Table 65-1 provides signs and symptoms of toxic plant ingestions.

PLANT TOXINS

The discussion of plant toxins in this chapter is arranged on the basis of the organ systems primarily affected: central nervous, cardiovascular, gastrointestinal, hepatic, renal, hematopoietic, endocrine/metabolic, and reproductive system. Some plants contain toxins that injure many organ systems, especially if the toxins alter general cell functions, such as protein synthesis, production of adenosine triphosphate (ATP) in the mitochondria, or cell division. The discussion may note the chemical group to which the plants belong based on chemical structure. Most fall into one of the following categories: alkaloids, glycosides, resins, oxalates, or phytotoxins.

Alkaloids

Alkaloids are nitrogen-containing organic compounds that act as bases and form salts with acids. Plant alkaloids are soluble organic acid-alkaloid salts that contain nitrogen in a ring structure that is heterocyclic or aromatic, or both. Alkaloids are generally distributed throughout a given plant, so all ingested parts are toxic. Further subdivision into chemical groups is based on ring structure (Table 65-2).

TABLE 65-1 Effects of Toxic Plants on Organ Systems

System Involved	Syndrome	Common Name	Genus	Signs and Symptoms of Syndrome
Central nervous†	Anticholinergic*	Jimsonweed	*Datura*	See Box 65-1
		Angel's trumpet	*Brugmansia*	
		Deadly nightshade	*Atropa*	
		Black henbane	*Hyoscyamus*	
		Mandrake	*Mandrogora*	
	Nicotinic*	Tobacco	*Nicotiana*	See Box 65-2
		Poison hemlock	*Conium*	
		Betel nut	*Areca*	
		Blue cohosh	*Caulophyllum*	
		Golden chain tree	*Laburnum*	
		Kentucky coffee tree	*Gymnocladus*	
		Mescal bean bush	*Sophora*	
	Hallucinogenic*	Morning glory	*Ipomoea*	Hallucinations
		Nutmeg	*Myristica*	
		Marijuana	*Cannabis*	
		Peyote	*Lophophora*	
		Ibogaine	*Tabernanthe*	
		Khat	*Cathus*	
	Sedating†	Poppy	*Papaver*	Sedation
	Paralyzing‡	Yellow jessamine	*Gelsemium*	Weakness
	Epileptogenic*§	Strychnine	*Strychnos*	Twitching
		Water hemlock	*Cicuta*	Seizures
		Wild wisteria	*Securidacea*	Hyperreflexia
		Myrtle-leaved coriaria	*Coriaria*	GI distress
				Altered mental status
Cardiovascular†	Na⁺,K⁺ ATPase inhibitors	Foxglove	*Digitalis*	GI distress
		Common oleander	*Nerium*	Visual changes
		Yellow oleander	*Cascabela* (previously, *Thevetia*)	Altered mental status
		Squill	*Urginea*	Dysrhythmias
		Sea mango	*Cerbera*	Hypotension
		Lily of the valley	*Convallaria*	Hyperkalemia
		Ouabain	*Strophanthus*	
		King's crown	*Calotropis*	
	Sodium channel openers‡	Monkshood	*Aconitum*	GI distress
		Hellebore	*Veratrum*	Visual disturbances
		Death camas	*Zigadenus*	Paresthesias
		Rhododendron	*Rhododendron*	Altered mental status
		Azaleas	*Rhododendron*	Weakness/paralysis
				Dysrhythmias
				Hypotension
	Na⁺ and Ca⁺ transport inhibitors	Yew	*Taxus*	GI distress
				Altered mental status
				Dysrhythmias
				Widening of QRS
				Hypotension
Oral and gastrointestinal‖	Oral irritants	Philodendron	*Philodendron*	Hypersalivation
		Dumb cane	*Dieffenbachia*	Oropharyngeal edema
		Peace lily	*Spathiphyllum*	Vesicles
		Elephant's ear	*Colocasia*	Dysphagia
		Giant elephant's ear	*Alocasia*	Aphonia
				Airway compromise
	Gastrointestinal irritants	Chinaberry tree	*Melia*	GI distress
		Nightshade	*Solanum*	Neurologic symptoms
		Pokeweed¶	*Phytolacca*	Vomiting
				Foamy diarrhea
				Dehydration
				Altered mental status
				Plasmablasts
	Protein synthesis inhibitors	Castor bean	*Ricinus*	GI distress
		Rosary pea	*Abrus*	Dehydration
		Purging nut	*Jatropha*	Elevated liver enzymes
		Black locust	*Robinia*	Multiorgan failure

Continued

TABLE 65-1 Effects of Toxic Plants on Organ Systems—cont'd

System Involved	Syndrome	Common Name	Genus	Signs and Symptoms of Syndrome
	Hepatotoxins	Groundsel	*Senecio*	Venoocclusive disease
		Gordolobo	*Senecio*	Hepatomegaly
		Tansy ragwort	*Senecio*	Jaundice
		Comfrey	*Symphytum*	
		Mate	*Ilex*	
		Rattlebox	*Crotalaria*	
Renal	Oxalates	Rhubarb	*Rheum*	Hypocalcemia
		Sorrel	*Rumex*	Tetany
				Renal failure
	Other	Aloe	*Aloe*	Renal insufficiency
		Birthwart	*Aristolochia*	Renal failure
		Djenkol bean	*Pithecolobium*	
		Oduvan	*Cleistanthus*	
Hematopoietic	Anticoagulating	Yellow sweet clover	*Melilotus*	Bleeding
		Tonka bean	*Coumarouna*	
		Woodruff	*Galium*	
	Bone marrow inhibitors	Autumn crocus	*Colchicum*	GI distress
		Christmas bells	*Sandersonia*	Dehydration
		Glory lily	*Gloriosa*	Pancytopenia
		Podophyllum	*Podophyllum*	Weakness
	Hemolytic	Fava bean	*Vicia*	Hemolysis
				Hemoglobinuria
				Anemia
				Jaundice
Endocrine and metabolic	Hypoglycemia inducers§	Ackee fruit	*Blighia*	Vomiting
		Wild yams	*Dioscorea*	Seizures
		Cocklebur	*Xanthium*	Hypoglycemia
		Bird-lime	*Atractylis*	Metabolic acidosis
		Ox-eye daisy	*Callilepis*	Liver disease
	Mineralocorticoid inducers	Licorice	*Glycyrrhiza*	Hypertension
				Edema
				Weakness
				Rhabdomyolysis
				Hypokalemia
	Cyanogenic	Apple seed	*Malus*	GI distress
		Cherry pits	*Prunus*	Bitter almond breath
		Peach pits	*Prunus*	Agitation/seizures
		Plum pits	*Prunus*	Coma
		Apricot pits	*Prunus*	Metabolic acidosis
				Dysrhythmias

*Anticholinergic and nicotinic plants can be hallucinogenic and epileptogenic.
†Many plants that affect the central nervous system and cardiovascular system can result in sedation and seizures.
‡Cardiovascular agents that open sodium channels may also produce weakness or paralysis.
§Hypoglycemic agents are also epileptogenic.
‖The majority of toxic plants cause some gastrointestinal (GI) distress.
¶Also a hematopoietic poison.

Glycosides

Sugars in the form of acetals are called glycosides. In glycosides, a glycosyl group replaces an alcohol or a hydroxyl group. On hydrolysis, glycosides yield sugars (glycones) and aglycone compounds. The aglycone moiety accounts for most of the toxicity, although the sugar may enhance solubility and absorption. (Figure 65-1). Glycoside-producing plants include cardioactive, cyanogenic, saponin, anthraquinone, and coumarin glycoside compounds.

Resins

Resins are highly toxic compounds of diverse chemical and plant origin united by the physical characteristics of insolubility in water, absence of nitrogen, and solid or semisolid state on extraction at room temperature. Resins are usually mixed with other compounds, such as volatile or essential oils (oleoresins), gum (gum resins), and sugars (glycoresins).

Oxalates

Oxalates occur naturally in plants as soluble (sodium or potassium) or insoluble (calcium) oxalates or acid oxalates. Oxalates have corrosive effects and bind serum calcium, causing hypocalcemia.

Phytotoxins

Phytotoxins, or toxalbumins, are among the most toxic substances of plant origin. They are composed of large protein molecules that resemble bacterial toxins in structure and in their ability to act as antigens (Figure 65-2).

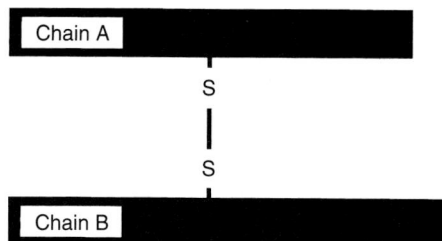

Amygdalin

↓ + Water

Aglycone

Mandelonitrile glucoside $+ C_6H_{12}O_6$

↓ + Water

Mandelonitrile $+ C_6H_{12}O_6$

↓

Benzaldehyde $+ HCN$

FIGURE 65-1 Hydrolysis of amygdalin, with its toxic aglycone group, yields hydrogen cyanide. The enzyme β-glucosidase, called emulsin, contained in plants can catalyze amygdalin hydrolysis.

Chain A
S
S
Chain B

FIGURE 65-2 The structures of ricin and abrin (phytotoxins isolated from the castor bean plant and the jequirity bean plant, respectively) are similar in structure to biologic toxins such as botulinum. These glycoproteins are composed of two peptide chains, designated A and B, connected by a disulfide bond.

CENTRAL NERVOUS SYSTEM TOXINS

ANTICHOLINERGIC PLANTS (TROPANE ALKALOIDS)

The plants discussed in this section produce an anticholinergic syndrome. Anticholinergic syndromes are more accurately termed *antimuscarinic syndromes*, because the syndrome is produced by antagonism of muscarinic receptors, with sparing of nicotinic receptors. However, the term *anticholinergic syndrome* is more frequently used and therefore is used here.

Plants contain tropane alkaloids (often called "belladonna alkaloids"), including atropine, hyoscyamine (the levorotatory isomer of atropine), and hyoscine (scopolamine).* Structures of the tropane alkaloids follow.

Tropane alkaloids are found in approximately 25 genera and 2000 species of plants. Plants causing human toxicity include

*References 51, 107, 166, 169, 209, 215, 217, 293, 324.

TABLE 65-2 Plant Alkaloids and Their Structures

Alkaloid Type	Alkaloid Structure	Examples
Indole		Ergonovine (ergots) Strychnine Physostigmine (calabar beans) Rauwolfia alkaloids (reserpine)
Isoquinoline		Opium alkaloids Emetine (ipecac)
Pyridine/ piperidine		Nicotine (tobacco) Arecoline (betel nut) Lobeline (Indian tobacco)
Purine		Caffeine Theobromine (cacao)
Quinoline		Cinchona alkaloids (quinidine)
Steroid		Veratrum alkaloids (false hellebore) Aconite (monkshood)
Tropane		Atropine (belladonna) Hyoscyamine Hyoscine (scopolamine)

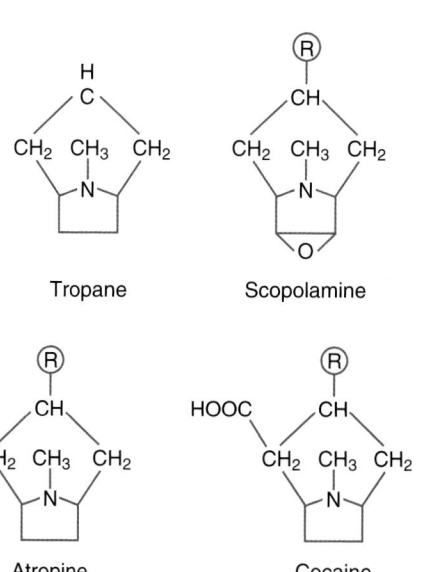

Tropane

Scopolamine

Atropine

Cocaine

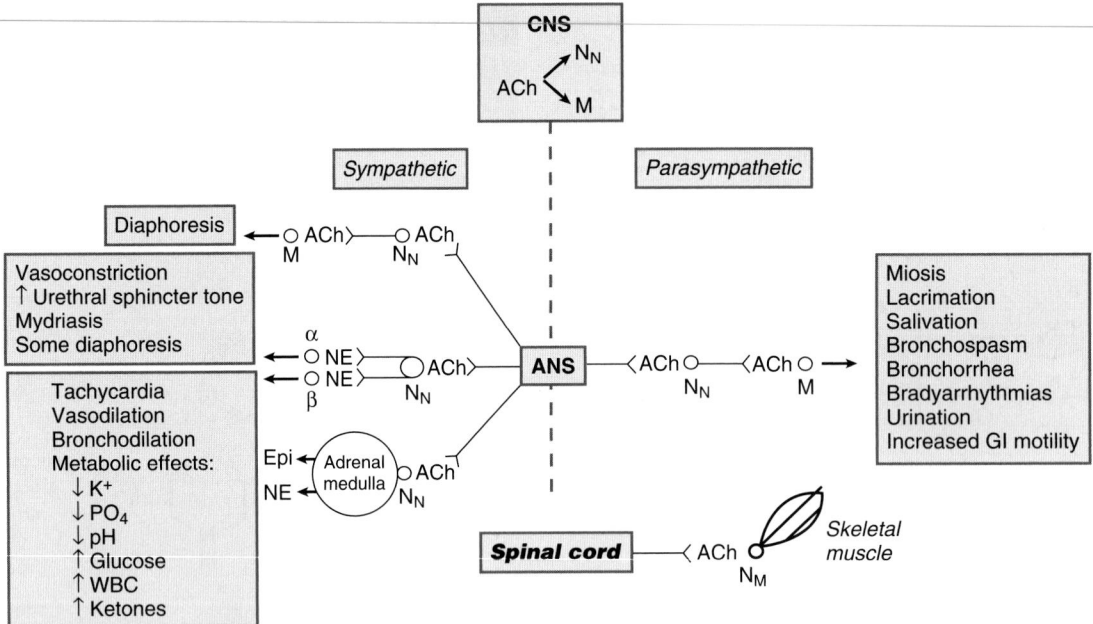

FIGURE 65-3 Nicotinic and muscarinic receptors of the central nervous system (*CNS*), autonomic nervous system (*ANS*), and peripheral skeletal muscles. Anticholinergic toxins (e.g., tropane alkaloids) antagonize muscarinic receptors, causing confusion, agitation, abnormal movements, hallucinations, and coma centrally, and mydriasis, anhidrosis, tachycardia, urinary retention, and ileus peripherally. Direct nicotinic agonists (e.g., arecoline, coniine, cytisine, lobeline, nicotine) stimulate nicotinic receptors; however, prolonged depolarization at the receptor causes eventual blockade of nicotinic receptors. *ACh,* Acetylcholine; *Epi,* epinephrine; *GI,* gastrointestinal; *M,* muscarinic receptor; *NE,* norepinephrine; N_M, nicotinic receptor at skeletal muscle; N_N, nicotinic receptor in nervous system.

Atropa belladonna (deadly nightshade), *Mandragora* spp. (mandrake), *Hyoscyamus niger* (black henbane), *Datura* spp. (jimsonweed), *Brugmansia* spp. (angel's trumpet), *Solanum* spp., and *Duboisia* spp. (corkwood tree).* The Solanaceae family includes *Solanum* and *Scopola carniolica,* sources of scopolamine.

Anticholinergic Syndrome

Toxicity may occur after ingesting or smoking plant parts. Tropane alkaloids competitively inhibit postsynaptic muscarinic receptors, producing the classic anticholinergic syndrome[58,125,136,257,266,293] (Figure 65-3 and Box 65-1). A useful clinical sign of anticholinergic toxicity is lack of perspiration in the axillae. Anticholinergic findings suggestive of poisoning may be remembered using the following mnemonic[266,307]:

*References 51, 136, 149, 166, 169, 209, 217, 257, 259, 265, 293, 308.

BOX 65-1 Anticholinergic Syndrome

Central
Central nervous sytem excitation
Agitation
Hallucinations
Lethargy
Coma
Respiratory depression
Mumbling speech
Muteness
Undressing behavior
Repetitive picking behavior

Peripheral
Tachycardia
Mydriasis
Blurred vision
Inability to accommodate (visually)
Flushed skin
Hyperthermia
Absent bowel sounds
Urinary retention
Dry mucous membranes

Hot as a hare (or Hot as Hades),
Blind as a bat,
Dry as a bone,
Red as a beet,
Mad as a hatter.

Jimsonweed

Datura species are generally known as jimsonweed or thorn apple, and *Brugmansia* species are generally known as angel's trumpet (Figure 65-4).[134,136,335] Young, thin, and tender stems of jimsonweed contain the highest concentration of tropane alkaloids.[217] However, the seeds also contain high concentrations of the alkaloids, and as little as one-half teaspoonful of seeds may cause death from cardiopulmonary arrest. The word "jimsonweed" is thought to be derived from Jamestown, Virginia, where British troops reportedly behaved bizarrely after consuming *Datura* in 1676. *D. stramonium* has reportedly been used in Haitian zombification rituals.[85,134,136] This plant is referenced in Homer's *Odyssey* and in the Shakespeare plays *Romeo and Juliet, Anthony and Cleopatra,* and *Hamlet.*[161] In cigarette form, jimsonweed has been used to treat asthma, heralding the current use of ipratropium bromide. *Datura* is still used as an herbal medicine, called Buah Kecubung, to treat allergic rhinitis in Malaysia.[219]

Reports of abuse of *Datura* and *Brugmansia* as hallucinogens continue to be reported in the United States and Europe.[136,215,276,324] Clusters of poisonings among adolescents are typical.[58,86,134,161,166,215,285,324] Frequently, a tea of the plant parts is brewed.[166] Smoking and ingesting various plant parts is described.[215] Report of toxicity after using a homemade *Datura* toothpaste has been reported.[260] Mass poisonings have occurred in Botswana and Slovenia after consumption of foods made with sorghum flour and buckwheat flour contaminated with seeds of *D. stramonium.*[245,261] Similar outbreaks have occurred elsewhere. In Athens, *Datura innoxia* was mistaken for blites (*Amaranthus blitum*) and consumed with vegetables, producing mass poisoning.[249]

Symptoms may appear within minutes and can last for days.[86,257,324] Tachycardia, dry mouth, nausea, vomiting, decreased GI motility with decreased bowel sounds, incoherence, disorientation, slurred speech, muteness, agitation, auditory and visual hallucinations, paranoia, mydriasis, hyperthermia, flushed skin, urinary retention, and hypertension have been

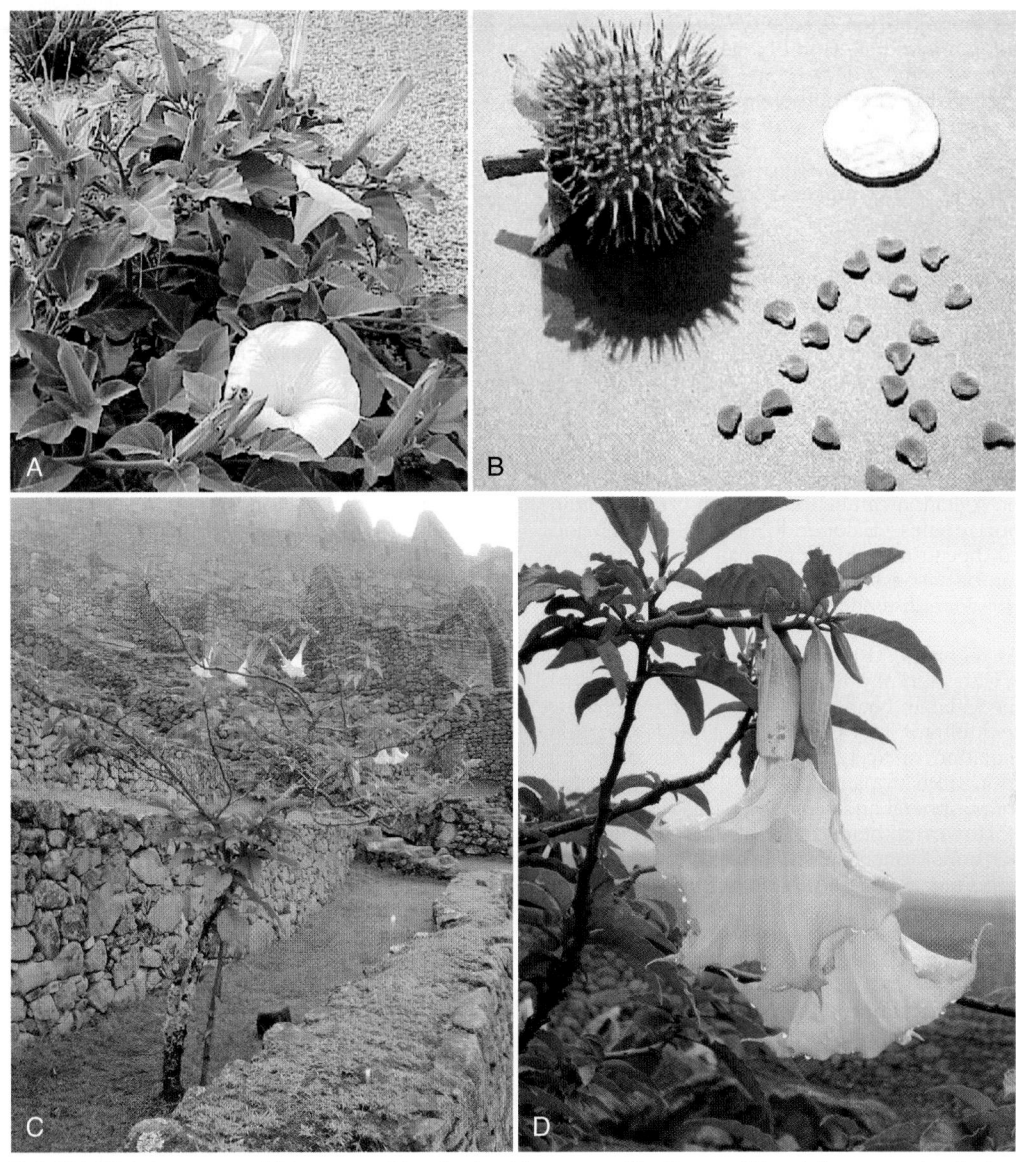

FIGURE 65-4 Jimsonweed (*Datura* spp.) is a bush with trumpet-like flowers **(A)** and thorny seedpods that contain numerous small, kidney-shaped seeds **(B)**. A nickel is shown for size comparison. Angel's trumpet (*Brugmansia* spp.) is a tree **(C)** with trumpet-like flowers **(D)**. *(Courtesy Kimberlie A. Graeme, MD, and Phillip Saba, MD.)*

reported.[86,166,215,257,266,285,324] Blurred vision and photophobia may be secondary to mydriasis. Isolated mydriasis and cycloplegia, including anisocoria, may be noted after topical contact to the eyes.[148,156,198,294,335] Anticholinergic poisoning should be suspected when patients are observed to communicate with imaginary friends with mumbling speech, while demonstrating repetitive picking behavior.[134,308] With severe toxicity, seizures, flaccid paralysis, and coma may ensue. Focal neurologic signs and posturing have been reported.[107,207,245,251,257,324] Users may be amnestic of events.[215] Studies may show leukocytosis, mild transient elevation of liver enzymes, elevated creatine phosphokinase (CPK) levels and other evidence of rhabdomyolysis, and changes on electrocardiogram (ECG) that are consistent with tachycardia and dysrhythmias.[86,107,136]

Death may result from behavioral changes, leading to trauma, drowning, or environmental exposure associated with hyperthermia or hypothermia.[166] Autopsy has revealed edema of the brain and lungs with focal hemorrhages within the alveoli, ischemic lesions and edema of the heart, and hyperemia of the sinusoidal tracts of the liver.[44]

Deadly Nightshade

Ingestion of *Atropa belladonna* (deadly nightshade) is less common than *Datura* or *Brugmansia* ingestion. All parts of deadly nightshade contain tropane alkaloids, but the highest concentrations are in the ripe fruit and green leaves; each berry may contain up to 2 mg of atropine. The berries may be mistaken for bilberries (hurtleberries) or blueberries. A family of eight had acute exposures to *A. belladonna* after eating both raw and cooked berries in a pie. The most severely poisoned patient had anticholinergic symptoms, with hypertonia, hyperthermia, respiratory failure, and coma, and required mechanical ventilation. Urine drug screens detected only atropine and not scopolamine, which is generally present in much smaller quantities.[221,293,308] A review of 49 children with acute deadly nightshade intoxication found that children most often demonstrated meaningless speech, tachycardia, mydriasis, and flushing; lethargy and coma were seen in the most severely poisoned children.[51] A patient with seasonal chronic ingestion presented with recurrent tachycardia, mydriasis, inability to concentrate, visual hallucinations, delusions, inappropriate laughter, dizziness, and headache.[169] The less frequently ingested velvet nightshade (*Solanum erianthum,* or potato tree) may produce anticholinergic syndromes.[162]

Mandrake

Mandragora officinarum (mandrake), which has a folklore history of being able to increase fertility, has recently been used as an aphrodisiac.[236] *Mandragora autumnalis* (autumn mandrake) has been mistaken for *Borago officinalis* (starflower or borage). Both autumn mandrake and borage grow in Mediterranean areas and have similar leaves and small, blue-violet flowers. Consumption of mandrake produces an anticholinergic syndrome.[265,266] All plant parts of the *Mandragora* spp. contain tropane alkaloids.[236]

Additional (Rare) Signs and Symptoms Seen with Anticholinergic Plants

Along with anticholinergic signs and symptoms, QT prolongation has been reported with some *Hyoscyamus reticulatus* exposures.[16] Polyneuropathies have been reported with angel's trumpet (*Brugmansia*) and *Hyoscyamus* spp. ingestions.[16,246,295,355]

Treatment

Treatment of anticholinergic plant exposure consists primarily of decontamination and supportive care, including airway protection, intravenous (IV) fluids, and vasopressors for hypotension resistant to IV fluids. Hyperthermia should be assessed and treated if significant. Agitation can be treated with careful administration of benzodiazepines. Haloperidol and phenothiazines should not be used, because these agents may worsen toxicity. Foley catheterization or nasogastric tube placement may be necessary if there is bladder distention or decreased gut motility, respectively.[125,166,169,251,293]

Some authorities recommend treating severe central anticholinergic syndrome with carefully titrated physostigmine, which is derived from the calabar bean of *Physostigma venenosum*. This cholinesterase inhibitor blocks acetylcholine degradation, resulting in accumulation of acetylcholine that overcomes the competitive inhibition from tropane alkaloids. Rapid, but often transient, reversal of peripheral and central nervous system (CNS) effects can ensue. However, bradycardia, asystole, ventricular arrhythmias, hypotension, bronchospasm, bronchorrhea, and seizures have been reported after rapid IV administration of physostigmine, limiting its use. Persons with cardiac conduction abnormalities are particularly susceptible to the cardiac complications. Use of physostigmine generally does not shorten hospital stay.[58,125,166,251,266,285,308,324]

Most patients with anticholinergic poisoning can be managed safely and effectively with supportive care alone.[307] If physostigmine is used, the patient should be on a cardiac monitor, with pulse oximetry, and a physician at the bedside should slowly administer graduated doses of the drug.[50,125,308]

NICOTINIC PLANTS (PYRIDINE AND PIPERIDINE ALKALOIDS)

The pyridine-piperidine group contains the major alkaloids nicotine, coniine, lobeline, arecoline, piperine, and isopelletierine. Structures of some pyridine/piperidine alkaloids follow:

Pyridine

Nicotine

Lobeline

Coniine

Plants containing nicotinic alkaloids include *Nicotiana* spp. (tobacco plants), *Conium maculatum* (poison hemlock), *Areca catechu* (areca palm, betel nut), *Caulophyllum thalictroides* (blue cohosh, squaw root), *Laburnum anagyroides* (golden chain tree), *Sophora secundiflora* (mescal bean bush, Texas mountain laurel), and *Sophora microphylla* (kowhai).[304]

Nicotinic Syndrome

Peripherally, acetylcholine is a neurotransmitter for autonomic and somatic motor fibers. It is stored in vesicles within the presynaptic neuron and released by calcium-dependent exocytosis into the synapse, where it binds to receptors and is eventually degraded by acetylcholinesterase. Acetylcholine can bind to two receptor types, nicotinic and muscarinic. Nicotinic receptors are located on postganglionic autonomic neurons (N_N receptors) and at skeletal neuromuscular junctions (N_M receptors). Plant toxins that are direct nicotinic agonists (e.g., arecoline, coniine, cytisine, lobeline, nicotine) prolong depolarization at these receptors and eventually cause blockade of nicotinic receptors. Clinical evidence of stimulation followed by blockade is apparent. Vomiting, diarrhea, abdominal pain, salivation, hypertension, tachycardia, bronchorrhea, tachypnea, muscle fasciculations, spasms, tremor, agitation, confusion, and convulsions (the stimulation) are followed by hypotension, bradyarrhythmias, asystole, respiratory failure, hyporeflexia, paralysis, and coma (the blockade). When it occurs, death is generally caused by respiratory paralysis[57,77,213,218,291,301,304] (Box 65-2; see also Figure 65-3).

Green tobacco sickness is a mild form of nicotine poisoning seen in tobacco-naive field workers with dermal exposure to leaves of green tobacco in wet environments. Nicotine, a water-soluble alkaloid, is absorbed dermally. The syndrome is characterized by weakness, salivation, nausea, vomiting, diarrhea, abdominal cramps, headache, dizziness, visual and hearing disturbances, respiratory depression, and occasionally fluctuations in blood pressure and heart rate. Neuromuscular blockade may result in death. A urinary nicotine metabolite, cotinine, may be helpful diagnostically.[20,213,291,313]

Tobacco Plants

Tobacco contains nicotine and related alkaloids with similar pharmacologic properties, such as anabasine, which is found in *Nicotiana glauca* (wild tree tobacco) (Figure 65-5). *N. glauca* has been mistaken for *Amaranthus hybridus* (marog) and eaten with porridge in South Africa. Ingestion of *N. glauca* is generally fatal. Anabasine, an isomer of nicotine that appears to be more toxic than nicotine, probably accounts for much of the toxicity of *N. glauca, N. debneyi,* and *N. rotundifolia*. Anabasine concentrations can be particularly high in the roots of the plants. Although there are more than 60 *Nicotiana* spp., some other, more common tobacco family members include *N. rustica* (Mapacho), *N.*

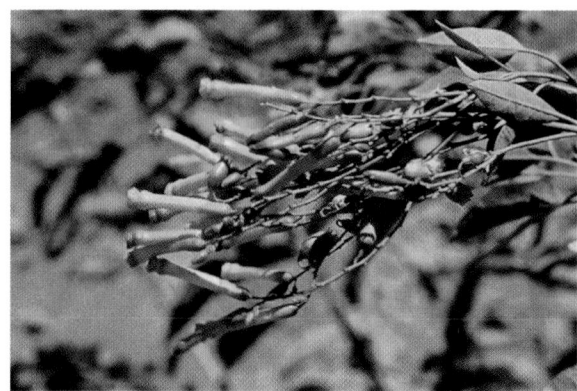

FIGURE 65-5 Tree tobacco (*Nicotiana glauca*).

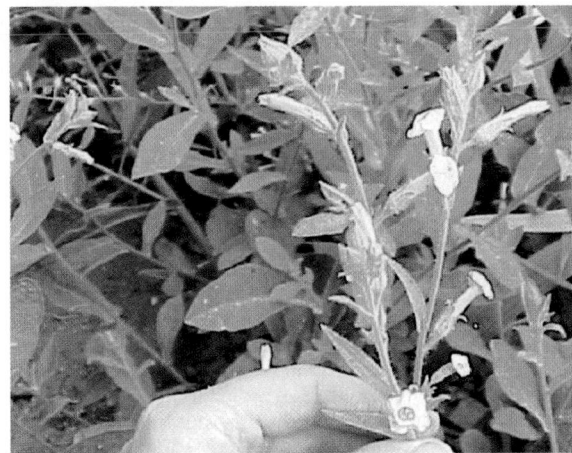

FIGURE 65-6 *Nicotiana trigonophylla* (desert tobacco) and other *Nicotiana* spp. are characterized by narrow, tube-like flowers. *(Courtesy Kimberlie A. Graeme, MD.)*

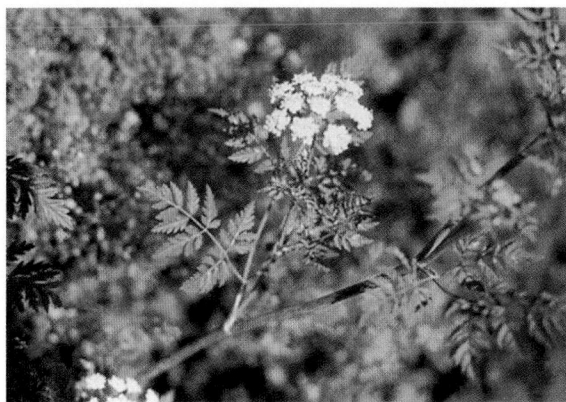

FIGURE 65-7 Poison hemlock (*Conium maculatum*).

tabacum (cultivated or common tobacco), *N. trigonophylla* (desert tobacco) (Figure 65-6), and *N. attenuata* (coyote tobacco). *N. tabacum* is the major source of commercial tobacco and contains 0.5% to 9% nicotine. *N. rustica* (Mapacho) tends to contain higher concentrations of nicotine than does *N. tabacum*. Lobeline, derived from the Indian tobacco plant *Lobelia inflata,* is a high-affinity nicotinic ligand. It can cause nicotine-like effects but is generally less toxic than is nicotine.[81]

Nicotine alkaloids are rapidly absorbed from the oral, GI, and respiratory tracts, as well as dermally. The kidneys excrete nicotine promptly after biotransformation in the liver and lungs. The half-life is 1 to 2 hours. Although the lethal dose of ingested nicotine is not well established, 2 to 5 mg may cause nausea, and 40 to 60 mg may be lethal in adult humans. In children, 1 mg/kg nicotine may produce significant toxicity. One to two cigarettes or less than 1 teaspoon of a nicotine solution used to refill electronic cigarettes could be lethal in a child if ingested and absorbed.[213,218,291,301,313]

Poison Hemlock

Conium maculatum, or poison hemlock, also known as spotted hemlock, California fern, Nebraska fern, stinkweed, fool's parsley, or carrot weed, is often mistaken for an edible plant, such as parsley, parsnip, or anise (Figure 65-7). However, it has a mousy odor, unpleasant bitter taste, and may irritate the mouth and throat. The stem is hollow with purplish to reddish brown spots. Its long taproot is solid and parsnip-like. Although all plant parts are poisonous, the unripe fruit is especially toxic. Poisonings are more common in the spring and summer. Poisoning may ensue after eating birds that have consumed poison hemlock. Coniine and γ-coniceine, the principal alkaloids in *C. maculatum,* are pyridine derivatives similar to nicotine. Coniine is more toxic than γ-coniceine. The alkaloid is volatile and susceptible to drying and heating.[37,291,338,346]

Conium maculatum was used in ancient times for capital punishment and murder. The primary action of the toxins is activation and then blockade of nicotinic acetylcholine receptors. Initially, stimulation causes sialorrhea, nausea, vomiting, diarrhea, abdominal cramping, hypertension, tachycardia, tremor, ataxia, confusion, and blurred vision, followed by dry mucosae, GI hypotonia, diminished cardiac contraction, hypotension, bradycardia, lethargy, and weakness, as with nicotinic syndrome. Muscles rapidly swell and stiffen, with multifocal necrosis of myocytes and associated muscle pain. Muscle fasciculations may be followed by flaccid paralysis, including respiratory paralysis. Rhabdomyolysis followed by acute tubular necrosis with renal failure may occur. Liver function tests (LFTs) and CPK and may be followed to assess rhabdomyolysis. Death is usually from respiratory failure. Autopsy may reveal congestion of the lungs and liver.[37,95,115,116,125,142,291,338,346]

Betel Nut

Areca catechu (areca palm) produces betel nut, a common masticatory drug in the Far East, Asia, India, and the South Pacific; it is shipped elsewhere (Figure 65-8). An estimated 10% to 25% of the world's population chews "betel quid." It is generally chewed with slaked lime paste (calcium hydroxide) wrapped in leaves of betel pepper (*Piper betel*), known as "quid," "punsupari," and "pan masala." Occasionally, tobacco is added. Quid is sucked in the lateral gingival pocket. Commercially, areca nut is marketed in the form of sweetened areca nut, known as "supari." *A. catechu* contains arecoline and guvacoline, which are hydrolyzed to arecaidine and guvacine, respectively. These are strong inhibitors of γ-aminobutyric acid (GABA) uptake. These arecal

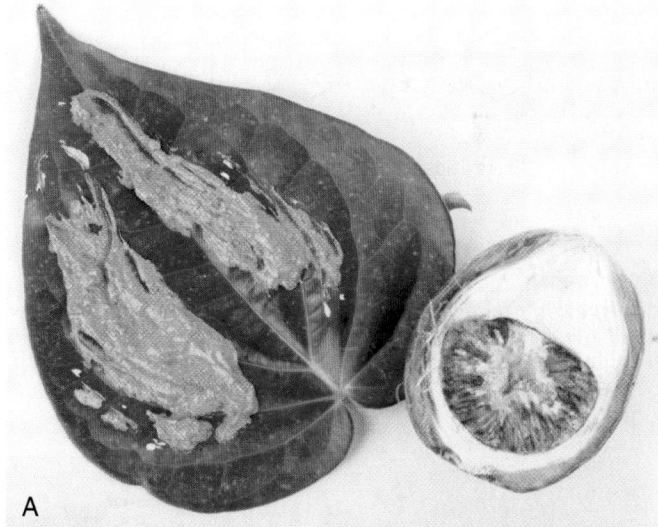

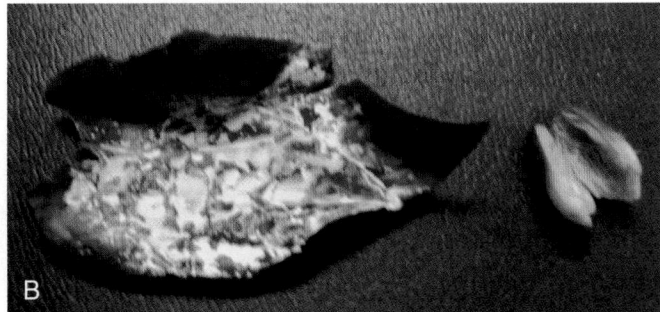

FIGURE 65-8 Betel nut (*Areca catechu*). (**A** copyright iStockphoto.com/nine_far; **B** courtesy Daniel Brooks, MD, and Tammy Tyree, NP.)

alkaloids are nicotinic and muscarinic. Betel pepper leaves contain betel oil, which contains psychoactive phenols and cadinene. These possess cocaine-like properties. Clinical effects resemble nicotinic syndrome, stimulant effects, and cholinergic toxicity, including CNS effects (dizziness, euphoria, subjective arousal, altered mental status, hallucinations, psychosis, convulsions), cardiac effects (tachycardia, hypertension, palpitations, arrhythmias, bradycardia, hypotension, chest discomfort, acute myocardial infarction in susceptible individuals), pulmonary effects (bronchospasm, tachypnea, dyspnea), GI effects (salivation, vomiting, diarrhea), urogenic effects (urinary incontinence), and musculoskeletal effects (weakness, paralysis). Use with calcium salts may result in hypercalcemia, hypokalemia, and metabolic acidosis with renal potassium wasting and renal insufficiency. Betel nut use is also associated with flushing, diaphoresis, warm sensations, red- or orange-stained lips, oral mucosa and saliva, and dark-brown– or black-stained teeth. Precancerous oral lesions may occur with chronic use. Areca nut chewing is associated with increased risk of oral and esophageal squamous cell carcinoma.[42,67,89,163,202, 203,232,297,315]

Golden Chain Tree

All parts of *Laburnum anagyroides* (golden chain tree) are toxic and contain the nicotinic alkaloids cytisine and *n*-methylcytisine. Cytisine is a quinolizidine alkaloid but is often classified with the pyridine and piperidine alkaloids. These alkaloids stimulate nicotinic ganglia. The toxins are concentrated in the seeds. Toxicity is generally only mild to moderate; however, an unusual fatality occurred in which 23 seedpods were found in the stomach of an adult at autopsy. Other plants that contain cytisine include Kentucky coffee tree (*Gymnocladus dioica*), necklace pod sophora (*Sophora tomentosa*), and mescal bean bush (*Sophora secundiflora*) (Figure 65-9) (see Hallucinogenic Plants, later). Structures follow[291]:

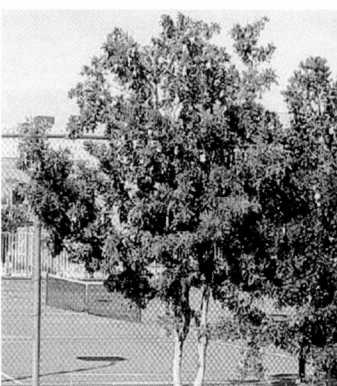

Quinolizidine   Cytisine

Blue Cohosh

Caulophyllum thalictroides is known as blue cohosh or squaw root. All parts of the plant contain the nicotinic alkaloid *n*-methylcytisine, which is much less potent than nicotine. Teas made from *C. thalictroides* have been used to induce labor and have reportedly resulted in newborn death and perinatal complications of stroke, congestive heart failure, respiratory failure, and circulatory collapse. The infant toxicity is thought to result from the toxic saponins, caulosaponin and caulophyllosaponin, rather than from the nicotinic alkaloids.[291]

Treatment

Treatment of nicotinic syndromes consists of supportive care with particular attention to airway protection and ventilation. Administration of activated charcoal has been used because it adsorbs nicotine in vitro. However, nicotine and related alkaloids are absorbed rapidly and often produce vomiting, which may limit usefulness of activated charcoal. These alkaloids may induce altered mental status, which can increase the risks associated with activated charcoal. Benzodiazepines and barbiturates are given for seizures. High urine output is maintained with aggressive IV fluids. Consider urine alkalinization. Treating initial excessive adrenergic stimulation with adrenergic antagonists is not advised, because this complicates the nicotinic blockade that typically follows. Symptomatic bradycardia may be treated with atropine. Atropine may also help to treat bronchorrhea. Hypotension can be treated with IV fluids and inotropic agents, if needed.[291,304]

OTHER NEUROMUSCULAR BLOCKING PLANTS

The nicotinic plants previously discussed produce a nondepolarizing neuromuscular blockade. Ingestion of yellow jasmine and exposure to the stinging nettle plant can produce weakness and paralysis.

Yellow Jasmine

Gelsemium sempervirens (Carolina or yellow jessamine) is a woody perennial evergreen vine with fragrant yellow flowers. It contains multiple indole alkaloids, including gelsemine, gelseminine, and gelsemoidin. Gelsemine binds to acetylcholine receptors at the neuromuscular junction (peripheral nicotinic acetylcholine receptors) and, to a lesser extent, at muscarinic receptors. A toddler who ate the blossoms of *G. sempervirens* experienced neuromuscular blockade with ataxia, dysarthria, facial weakness (including bilateral ptosis), extremity weakness, and transient coma. The child recovered without sequelae.[38]

Stinging Nettle

Urtica ferox is found in New Zealand. Dermal exposure most often produces pain, inflammation, urticaria, and allergic reactions (including anaphylactic reactions) when the leave tips break off and fine needles penetrate the skin. With large skin exposures, rapid onset of systemic symptoms may occur, including paresthesias, muscle weakness, paralysis, and respiratory failure. Peripheral neuropathy has been described. The toxin responsible for paralysis is not known.[304]

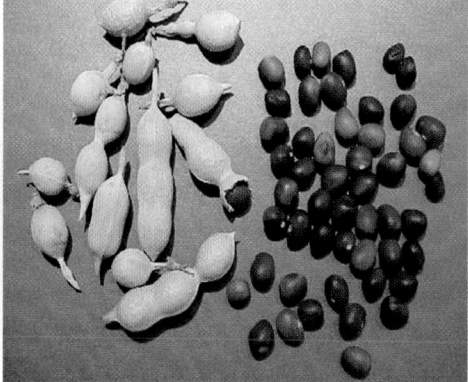
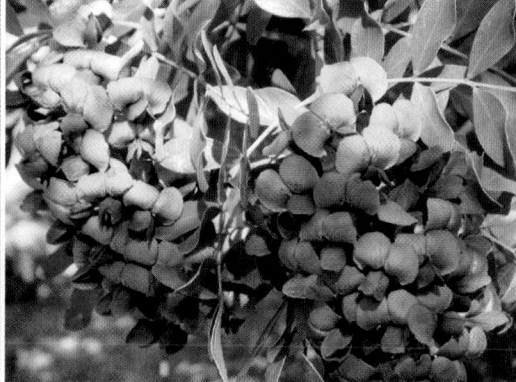

FIGURE 65-9 Mescal bean bush (*Sophora secundiflora*) **(A)** is characterized by bean pods that contain burnt-red seeds **(B)** and by purple blooms **(C)**. *(Courtesy Phillip Saba, MD, and Kimberlie A. Graeme, MD.)*

HALLUCINOGENIC PLANTS (INDOLES, PHENYLALKYLAMINES)

Many psychoactive plants are indole derivatives, which are among the most potent psychoactive compounds in nature and have the following structure:

Indole nucleus

Chemical relationships exist among serotonin, psilocybin (*Psilocybe* spp.), and D-lysergic acid diethylamide (LSD). Striking structural similarities exist between many potent psychoactive plant compounds and biochemically important neurotransmitters, as follows:

Serotonin

Psilocybin

Norepinephrine

Mescaline

Lysergic acid diethylamide

Tetrahydrocannabinol

Morning Glory

The active component of the naturally occurring hallucinogen found in the seeds of morning glory (*Ipomoea violacea*) (Figure 65-10) and Hawaiian baby woodrose (*Argyreia nervosa*) is ergine, or (+)-lysergic acid amide (LSA), an indole derivative.[134,253,254] Compared to LSD, LSA has a lower binding affinity for most serotonergic receptors, produces weaker psychedelic effects, and produces more sedation.[253] However, LSA may still produce psychosis through serotonergic and dopaminergic effects.[183,253] Hypertension has been reported.[183] Nonetheless, about 300 morning glory seeds, or enough to fill a cupped hand, are equivalent to 200 to 300 mg of LSD and have reportedly produced similar systemic and hallucinatory effects. Ingestion of Hawaiian baby woodrose seeds (*A. nervosa*), which also contain LSA, has similar effects.[124] *A. nervosa* is used in tribal medicine in parts of India.[253] Tutorials on the Internet provide instruction for ingestion of dried or fresh *A. nervosa* seeds and for preparation of aqueous

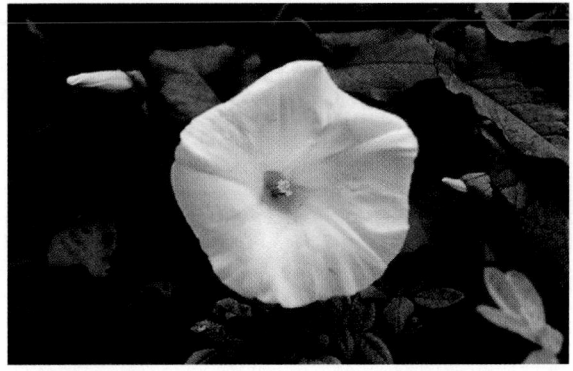

FIGURE 65-10 Morning glory (*Ipomoea violacea*).

and alcoholic extracts.[253,254] *Rivea corymbosa* (Ololiuhqui) also contains LSA. Some have postulated that fungal infection of these plants with ergoline alkaloid biosynthesis may be responsible for the LSA found in the hallucinogenic plants.[177]

Nutmeg

Myristica fragrans is used to make the spices nutmeg and mace (Figure 65-11). Mature rinds of the fruit split, revealing a bright-red, fringed, fleshy coating on the outside of its seed. The coating contains mace, and the seed contains nutmeg. Nutmeg contains myristicin, which is structurally similar to mescaline in peyote (*Lophophora williamsii*) and to kawain in kava (*Piper methysticum*), discussed later. Other alkylbenzene derivatives, such as safrole and elemicin, are also found in nutmeg. Nutmeg has been abused for its alleged hallucinogenic effects but may produce euphoria, lethargy, or obtundation. At very high doses, tachycardia, palpitations, anxiety, and anticholinergic-type signs are seen. Hallucinations and paranoid behavior can be observed at these higher doses. Nutmeg is most often abused by persons with limited access to more pleasant and more potent psychotomimetic agents. A person who ingested one grated nutmeg seed (7 g) had nausea, weakness, loss of coordination, vertigo, fainting, and paresthesias but no hallucinations.[26,303]

Cannabis

Cannabis preparations are largely derived from the female *Cannabis sativa* plant. The primary psychoactive component is δ-9-tetrahydrocannabinol (THC), which is most concentrated in the flowering tops. Marijuana generally contains 0.5% to 5% THC; however, sinsemilla and Netherwood varieties may contain up to 20% THC, and hashish and hashish oils have higher concentrations. Cannabinoids can be smoked or ingested. More recently, cannabis oils, or butter, with extremely high THC concentrations, have been promoted for "vaping," which involves using a vaporizer. A typical marijuana cigarette contains 0.5 to 1.0 g of cannabis, and the THC delivered varies from 20% to 70%, with bioavailability of 5% to 24%. As little as 2 mg of available THC produces effects in occasional users.[144]

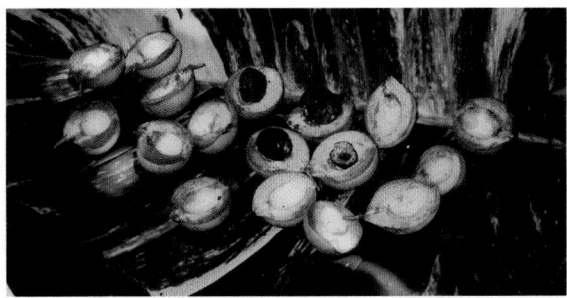

FIGURE 65-11 Nutmeg (*Myristica fragrans*). (*Courtesy Daniel Brooks, MD, and Tammy Tyree, NP.*)

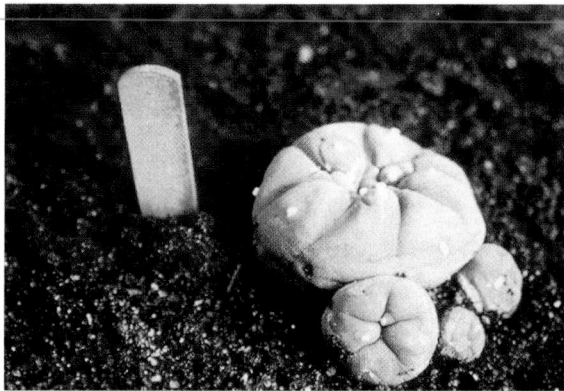

FIGURE 65-12 Peyote (*Lophophora williamsii*).

Cannabinoids bind to specific cannabinoid receptors in areas of the brain involved with cognition, memory reward, pain perception, and motor coordination. Cannabinoids act as neuromodulators in release and action of neurotransmitters (e.g., acetylcholine, glutamate).[93,144] Endogenous ligands for these receptors are endocannabinoids. The first endocannabinoid identified was anandamide, named after the Sanskrit word *ananda*, which means "bliss."

Desirable effects include mild mood-altering qualities, euphoria, altered perceptions, time distortion, and intensification of ordinary sensory experiences (e.g., gustatory, visual, and auditory sensations). Adverse effects include nausea, vomiting, anxiety, impairment of short-term memory and attention, mydriasis and slowly reactive pupils, and impairment of motor skills and reaction time. Psychotic symptoms have been reported in persons vulnerable to psychosis. Clinically, tachycardia may occur within minutes of THC exposure and last a few hours. Minor changes in blood pressure may occur. Exposed toddlers may present with lethargy, slurred speech, ataxia, and shaking.[39,144,340]

Peyote

Peyote use dates back to more than 5000 years ago.[54] The hallucinogenic peyote cactus *Lophophora williamsii* contains alkaloids that are phenylethylamines or isoquinolines, rather than indoles (Figure 65-12). Mescaline (3,4,5-trimethoxy-β-phenylethylamine), the primary psychoactive component of peyote, is structurally similar to the neurotransmitters norepinephrine and epinephrine and to hallucinogenic amphetamines. Pharmacologically, however, mescaline is similar to hallucinogenic indoles. Mescaline may affect the action of norepinephrine and serotonin, evidenced clinically by sympathomimetic effects, followed by marked visual hallucinations. Mescaline produces slight rises in blood pressure and heart rate, tachypnea, mydriasis, perspiration, flushing, nausea, salivation, hyperreflexia, ataxia, agitation, paranoia, psychosis, and urination. Type B botulism was associated with consumption of a ceremonial tea made from peyote that was stored in a jar by members of the Native American Church. Affected members had bilaterally symmetric, flaccid weakness in all extremities, dysphagia, nasal speech, and diplopia.[12,55,152]

San Pedro Cactus (*Echinopsis* or *Trichocereus* spp.)

Mescaline is also found in some *Trichocereus* spp. (or *Echinopsis* spp.), such as *T. pachanoi* (or *E. pachanoi*; the San Pedro cactus) and *E. peruviana* (Peruvian torch cactus). These cacti have been used medicinally by South American shamans.[242,55] The San Pedro cactus (*E. pachanoi* or *T. pachanoi*) also contains other psychoactive phenethylamines, including lophophine, homopiperonylamine, and lobivine, as does peyote.[47] *Trichocereus* spp. contain 3,4-dimethoxyphenethylamine, which has been isolated from these cacti and sold illicitly[250] (personal communication, Arizona police department).

Dona Ana Cactus

Coryphantha macromeris (Engelm) Br. and R. and its *runyonii* (Br. and R.) L. Benson variety contain methylated catecholamines, including the phenethylamine normacromerine (*N*-methyl-3,4-dimethoxy-β-hydroxyphenethylamine), which are believed to be psychoactive.[173]

MESCAL BEAN BUSH

The mescal bean bush or Texas mountain laurel (*Sophora secundiflora*) of the pea family (Fabaceae) produces dark-red hallucinogenic beans (mescal beans; see Figure 65-9). The beans contain the toxic alkaloid cytisine, which causes nausea, numbing sensations, hallucinations, unconsciousness, convulsions, and death through respiratory failure. The beans may be boiled in water and the mixture consumed, producing a delirium or "visionary trance." The origin of mescalism in modern peyote religion is debated. Mescal beans are worn during some peyote ceremonies.[12]

Iboga

Tabernanthe iboga (iboga or eboka) contains indole alkaloids, including ibogaine. The root of this plant is used in West Africa to communicate with ancestors, reportedly producing "visions" and "waking dreams." More recently, the roots have been ingested as a hallucinogenic substance of abuse. It produces altered states of consciousness, delusions, hallucinations, altered time perception, synesthesias (auditory, olfactory, and gustatory), mydriasis, tachycardia, tremor, and ataxia. Convulsions, paralysis, and lethal respiratory arrest have been reported. A man was found dead after ingesting a powdered root bark of *T. iboga* shrub mixed with sweet concentrated milk. Autopsy revealed pulmonary edema with hemorrhagic alveolitis and vascular congestion.[53,182,211]

Gifbol

Boophone disticha (gifbol, tumbleweed, veld fan, or windball) was historically used in Africa to poison arrow tips. It is now reportedly abused by teenagers for its hallucinogenic effects. In rats, it produces flaccid paralysis.[127]

Khat

The evergreen khat tree, *Catha edulis*, grows in East Africa and Arabia (Figure 65-13). Khat is also known as chat, qat, kat, kath, gat, eschat, miraa, murungu, qaad, and jaad. As early as 1237, khat was advocated in Arabic medical literature as a mood-elevating and hunger-suppressing agent. Khat leaves and bark continue to be chewed, with juice of the masticated plant being swallowed for stimulatory effects. Khat contains *cathinone* (2-amino-1-phenyl-1-propanone), cathine (norpseudoephedrine), and norephedrine. Cathinone, a phenylalkylamine, is the

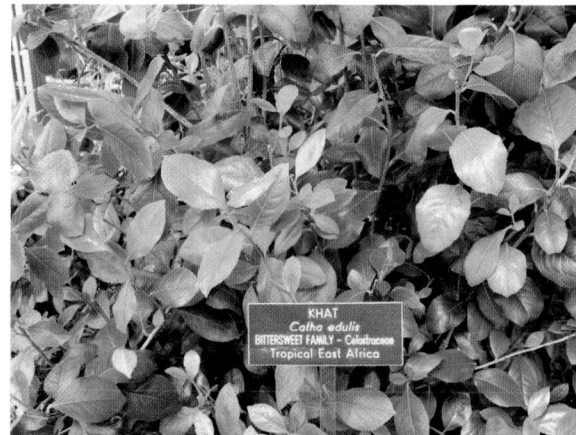

FIGURE 65-13 Khat (*Catha edulis*). *(Courtesy Daniel Brooks, MD, and Tammy Tyree, NP.)*

major psychoactive constituent. Structurally, cathinone is similar to amphetamines, and khat has been referred to as a "natural" amphetamine. Synthetic cathinones (known as "bath salts") have been manufactured and used illicitly. As with amphetamines, cathinone is an indirect sympathomimetic, inducing release of dopamine, serotonin, and norepinephrine.[4,6,9,53,56,154,235,240,252,327]

The structures of methcathinone, cathinone, and ephedrine follow:

Methcathinone

Cathinone

Ephedrine

Cathinone in fresh plant material must be extracted by masticating laboriously; this results in gradual absorption. As the leaf wilts, cathinone content decreases and the leaf loses its potency as a psychostimulant. Because only fresh leaves produce the desired stimulatory effects, in the past, khat use was generally limited to countries where khat was produced (e.g., North Yemen, Ethiopia, Kenya); however, khat is now air-freighted to Europe and the United States. Khat is transported damp, rolled in a banana leaf bundle called a marduff.

Desirable effects of khat include increased energy and alertness, feelings of increased endurance and self-esteem, enhanced imaginative ability, higher capacity to associate ideas, and euphoria. Cathinone has both positive chronotropic and inotropic effects. Tachycardia, increased blood pressure, tachypnea, and mydriasis are seen. Adverse effects include anorexia, hypomania, insomnia, delusions, paranoid psychosis, aggression, depression, anxiety, hyperthermia, stomatitis, oral lesions/cancers, gastritis, and endocrine disturbances. Khat use has been associated with vasoconstriction, acute myocardial infarction, leukoencephalopathy, and increased incidence of acute cerebral infarction. Khat is known to be habit forming and has been classified as a substance of abuse by the World Health Organization. Cathinone is a Schedule I controlled substance under federal regulations in the United States.*

ANTICHOLINERGIC PLANTS

Henbane (*Hyoscyamus niger*). jimsonweed (*Datura stramonium*), angel's trumpet (*Brugmansia* spp.) and mandrake (*Mandragora officinarum*) contain tropane alkaloids and can produce hallucinations, as discussed earlier.

Treatment

Treatment of patients exposed to hallucinogenic plants is generally supportive. First-line treatment for agitation is generally benzodiazepines.

SEDATING PLANTS

Poppy

Papaver somniferum flowers are large and white with purple stains at the base of each petal. They yield opium, a complex of more than 20 alkaloids, including morphine, codeine, and papaverine. Morphine was the first plant alkaloid isolated, by pharmacist Friederich Wilhelm Adam Serturner in 1806.[141] Seeds of *P. somniferum* are used in foods and beverages, including bagels, muffins, pastries, curry sauce, rice, and teas. Opiate toxicity from

poppy seed exposure occurred in a 6-month-old infant given 75 mL of strained milk made with 200 g of poppy seeds in 500 mL of milk, resulting in respiratory arrest requiring ventilation. Opiate toxicity has occurred after ingestion of a boiled poppy plant and after ingestion of spaghetti with poppy seeds. Poppy seed tea has been injected intravenously as a form of drug abuse, resulting in vomiting, hyperthermia, tachycardia, tachypnea, hypoxia, hypotension, myalgias, dyspnea, and rigors. Systemic reaction to foreign substances may account for much of the syndrome seen with injection. Poppy dependence has been described. Ingestion of poppy seeds can result in detectable levels of morphine and codeine by urine drug screen testing.[176,190,220,258,333]

PLANTS PRODUCING SPASTIC PARAPARESIS/ QUADRIPARESIS (NEUROTOXIC AMINO ACIDS)

Grass Pea

Lathyrus sativus (grass pea, chickling pea, vetchling, khasari, guaya, shan li dou, and pois carre), *Lathyrus cicero* L. (red pea), and *Lathyrus clymenum* L. contain the neuroexcitatory amino acid β-(*N*)-oxalyl-amino-L-alanine acid (BOAA), previously called β-*N*-oxalyl-L-2,3-diaminopropanoic acid (β-ODAP). Neuroexcitation is caused by BOAA being structurally similar to glutamate and acting as a glutamate receptor agonist. The toxic **BOAA** is thought to produce excessive and damaging neuroexcitation via glutaminergic pathways. Mitochondrial dysfunction is seen.

Chronic *L. sativus* (grass pea) ingestion may produce neurolathyrism, an upper motor neuron disease characterized by spastic lower-extremity paraplegia and occasionally quadriplegia. Mentation is generally unaffected. The illness was described in 46 BC by Hippocrates: "All men and women who continuously fed on the pulse were attacked by a weakness on the legs which remained permanent." Since that time, neurolathyrism epidemics have been reported during wartime, famine, and natural disasters. The most recent epidemics have been in Bangladesh, India, and Ethiopia. Toxicity is generally only seen when a person eats grass peas for 2 to 3 months and as 30% to 50% of their total dietary intake, or 400 to 500 g of seeds per day for several months. Despite chronic accumulation of toxin, the disease can appear to have a dramatically acute onset; however, detailed histories generally reveal some report of subacute weakness, myalgias, cramps, or stiffness.[25,349] Clinically, neurolathyrism appears similar to neurocassivism, or konzo (see Cyanogenic Plants, later).

CONVULSANT PLANTS (INDOLES, RESINS)

Strychnine

Strychnine, an indole found in seeds of the tree *Strychnos nux-vomica,* is a powerful CNS stimulant. Poisoning may occur after ingestion of rodent poisons containing strychnine, with use of illicit drugs contaminated with strychnine, or with use of herbal remedies contaminated with strychnine. Strychnine is especially concentrated in seeds and roots of the plant. The bark of *S. nux-vomica* also contains the alkaloid brucine, which is less potent than strychnine but produces similar toxicity when consumed. The *S. nux-vomica* tree has been confused with *Alstonia scholaris* (blackboard tree), resulting in fatal consumption of its bark due to brucine toxicity.[1]

Strychnine is a selective, competitive antagonist of glycine, a major inhibitory neurotransmitter, at its postsynaptic receptors in the spinal cord and brainstem. Poisoning produces an excitatory state, with hyperreflexia, hypersensitivity to stimuli, migratory rippling movements of muscles, twitching, rigidity, and spinal convulsions (generally, flexor spasm of upper limbs, extensor spasm of lower limbs, opisthotonic posturing, and jaw muscle spasms, all without loss of consciousness or postictal states). Minimal stimulation elicits diffuse muscle contractions. In between spasms, which last from 30 seconds to 2 minutes, muscles become completely relaxed. Respiratory and secondary cardiac failure may ensue during severe convulsions.

Treatment consists of supportive care, benzodiazepines, and barbiturates. Chemical paralysis with a nondepolarizing

---

*References 2, 4-6, 9, 19, 65, 90, 132, 154, 174, 208, 223, 235, 240, 252.

agent, endotracheal intubation, and mechanical ventilation may be required for severely poisoned patients. Hyperthermia, rhabdomyolysis, renal failure, and acidosis may occur secondary to convulsions. These complications often require treatment. Occasionally, death ensues despite aggressive treatment.[1,33,60,114,205,229,241,263,296,351]

Some *Strychnos* spp. in Africa contain alkaloids that produce curare-like effects. These alkaloids act through nondepolarizing and competitive mechanisms at the neuromuscular junction, competing with acetylcholine for the receptor and thus blocking nerve-to-muscle transmission. This results in paralysis; however, paralysis is not seen after ingestion of these species, because the toxic alkaloids are not absorbed from the GI tract.[263]

Wild Wisteria

The root of *Securidacea longepedunculata* (violet tree or wild wisteria) has been used as an intravaginal suicidal poison and abortifacient. The distilled oil of the root is primarily methyl salicylate; however, wild wisteria also contains the alkaloid securinine, a GABA-A receptor antagonist, which produces hyperreflexia, hypertonia, and seizures. Death can result within hours of placing the root intravaginally and is generally preceded by vomiting, diarrhea, and dehydration.

Water Hemlock

Water hemlock (*Cicuta maculata*) is one of the most toxic resin-containing plants. The resin of *C. maculata,* an unsaturated aliphatic alcohol called cicutoxin, has the following structure:

$$CH_2-CH_2-CH_2-(C\equiv C)_2-(CH\equiv CH)_3$$

with OH on the first carbon and CH(OH)–C₃H₇ grouping at the end:

$$\underset{OH}{CH_2}-CH_2-CH_2-(C\equiv C)_2-(CH\equiv CH)_3-\underset{\underset{C_3H_7}{CH(OH)}}{}$$

Cicutoxin

Species within the Umbelliferae (also called Apiaceae) family are divided into the *Cicuta* and *Oenanthe* genera. Nine subspecies of *Cicuta* are poisonous (Figure 65-14). *C. virosa* is common European water hemlock, whereas *C. maculata* and *C. douglasii* are found in North America. *Oenanthe crocata* (hemlock water dropwort) is found in Europe and North America. *Oenanthe* spp. contain oenanthotoxin.[118] Other common names for *Cicuta* spp. include cowbane, five-finger root, snake weed, snake root, wild carrot, dead man's fingers, death-of-man, poison parsnip, wild parsnip, beaver poison, children's bane, muskrat weed, spotted hemlock, spotted cowbane, musquash root, false parsley, fever root, mock-eel root, wild dill, spotted parsley, and carotte à Moreau. Roots have a parsnip- or carrot-like odor, and *Cicuta* spp. are often mistaken for edible plants, such as water parsnip, pignut, sweet flat, watercress, wild celery, wild ginseng, kvanne,

and wild carrots. The taste has been diversely described as unpleasant, resembling pine, or sweet tasting. Mature roots have air-filled chambers and extend from hollow stems. The plant is most toxic in the spring. All parts of the plant are toxic, but the roots contain the highest concentration of cicutoxin. Ingestion of as little as 2 to 3 cm of the root may be fatal to an adult. The severity of poisoning and latency to symptoms are proportional to the amount of plant ingested. The principal toxins, cicutoxin and oenanthotoxin, act as noncompetitive GABA antagonists in the CNS, resulting in unabated neuronal depolarization that manifests as seizures, including status epilepticus.[118,125,157,292]

Water hemlock poisoning should be considered in any patient who presents with cholinergic-like poisoning and abrupt onset of seizures. Early symptoms include muscarinic effects and involve primarily the GI tract: abdominal pain, nausea, vomiting, and diarrhea. Marked diaphoresis, salivation, and respiratory distress may be seen. Nicotinic effects are less prominent (see Figure 65-3). Tachycardia and hypertension or bradycardia and hypotension may be seen. Dysrhythmias may occur. Ataxia, paresthesias, muscle spasms, weakness, and coma have been reported. With severe poisoning, epileptiform seizure activity or spastic and tonic movements, including opisthotonos without electroencephalographic (EEG) seizure activity, may occur. Rhabdomyolysis and renal failure have been reported. Deaths may be associated with persistent seizures, cerebral edema, pulmonary edema, ventricular fibrillation, cardiopulmonary arrest, and disseminated intravascular coagulation. Survival beyond 8 hours generally indicates a good prognosis. Laboratory abnormalities include metabolic acidosis and elevated CPK and LFTs.

Treatment of water hemlock poisoning includes securing an airway, ventilation, and treating seizures with benzodiazepines and barbiturates. Phenytoin is contraindicated because it is ineffective for seizure control. Anticholinergic agents are not recommended because these agents do not reduce seizure activity. Continuous EEG monitoring may be helpful. Treatment of hypoxia, acidosis, hyperthermia, rhabdomyolysis, and cerebral edema should be provided. Hypotension can be treated with IV fluids and vasopressors. Recovery can take up to 4 days, and some patients never completely recover. Although survival has improved with aggressive supportive care, death may still ensue. Autopsies reveal pulmonary and cerebral edema, brain hemorrhages, and renal necrosis.[118,125,157,292]

Myrtle-Leaved Coriaria

Coriaria myrtifolia (myrtle-leaved coriaria, Currier's sumach, or Redoul sumach) grows in the western Mediterranean area. *C. myrtifolia* contains coriamyrtin, an analog of picrotoxin. The toxin is found in high concentrations in the berries, which resemble blackberries. Ingestion of only a few fruits can produce significant toxicity. The leaves are toxic. Rarely, individuals have become poisoned after eating snails acquired off the plant, after drinking the milk of goats that had been eating the plant, and

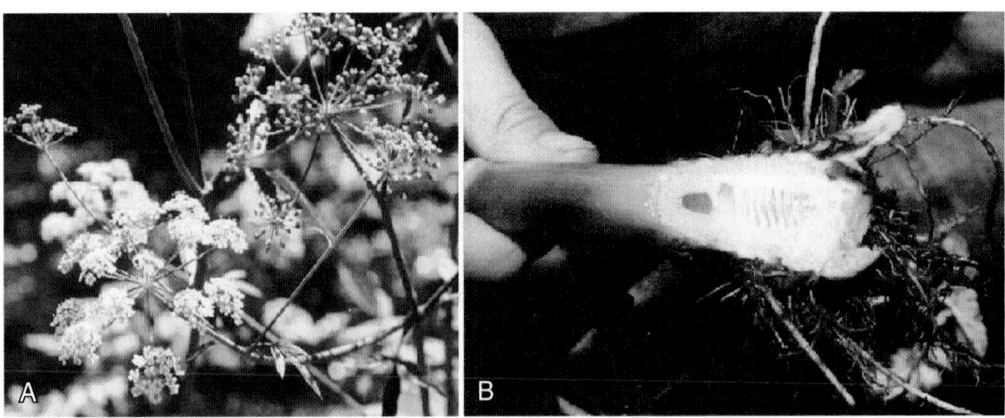

FIGURE 65-14 *Cicuta* species have characteristic flowering tops, typical of the Umbelliferae family **(A)**, and roots with air-filled chambers at the ends of hollow stems **(B)**. *(Courtesy Steven Curry, MD.)*

after consuming honey contaminated by its nectar. The leaves have been eaten when mistakenly thought to be the leaves of senna (*Cassia senna* L.). Initially, vomiting, abdominal pain, and drunken intoxication are seen. This may be followed by twitching, seizures (including status epilepticus), coma, and apnea. Death may occur. Treatment with benzodiazepines and barbiturates should be considered.[87]

Tutu

Tutu refers to the *Coriaria* spp. found in New Zealand, which include *C. angustissim*, *C. arborea*, *C. lurida*, *C. plumose*, *C. pteridoides*, and *C. sarmentosa*.[31] Although these plants are generally shrubs, *C. arborea* (tree tutu) may become an evergreen tree, reaching 6 m (20 feet) in height. The primary toxic is tutin, which is picrotoxin-like and produces GABA-A receptor suppression, resulting in anxiety and seizures. Some children who have eaten the attractive, seed-containing berries have died. The berries reportedly have a sweet, blueberry-like flavor. The whole plant is toxic, with the exception of the soft, black or purple petals, which are fleshy and called "berries."[31] Unfortunately, these "berries" contain highly toxic seeds that may be consumed with the berries. As described with other toxic plants, bees that have used tutu nectar have produced toxic, tutin-containing honey. The toxic derivative of tutin, hyenanchin (a hydroxytutin), may be present. Ingestion of the honey may produce vomiting, prolonged delirium, status epilepticus, and death. The seizures may present suddenly without warning. Ingestion of the plant may produce nausea, diarrhea, blurred vision, excitement, tremor, muscle spasms, weakness, incoordination, and coma. Nausea and vomiting may be delayed for 2 to 6 hours after consumption, followed by tonic-clonic seizures and respiratory compromise. The patient may report chest pain and rhonchi before respiratory arrest. If death occurs, it is generally within 24 hours. In survivors, the illness may last for several days, and patients may be amnesic on recovery. Practitioners in New Zealand recommend ECG, serum electrolytes, and a 12-hour observation period, with hospital admission if symptoms develop. There are no antidotes, and treatment is supportive. Benzodiazepines are often helpful and can be given prophylactically.[31]

Kratom

Kratom (*Mitragyna speciosa*) is a tree native to Southeast Asia; however, its plant parts are now popular as herbal drugs of abuse.[329] It contains the toxic alkaloids mitragynine, mitraphylline, and 7-hydroxymitragynine. Mitragynine is thought to have opioid effects, although stimulant effects are seen with ingestion of low doses of kratom. Other receptors besides opioid receptors are likely involved in toxicity. Toxicity is manifested as GI distress, palpations, nystagmus, tremor, altered mental status, and seizures. Psychosis may be seen with chronic abuse. A withdrawal syndrome featuring myalgias, insomnia, fatigue, and chest discomfort has been reported.[329]

Star Fruit

Patients with chronic renal disease are at risk of convulsions after ingesting star fruit (*Averrhoa carambola*). The proconvulsant toxin is caramboxin, a phenylalanine-like molecule with two carboxylic acid moieties. It is structurally similar to ibotenic acid, a toxin found in inebriating mushrooms. Caramboxin is able to activate NMDA glutamate (excitatory) neuroreceptors. Clinically, patients with kidney disease present with intractable hiccups, confusion, and status epilepticus. Toxicity occasionally progresses to death.[130]

Other Convulsants

Anticholinergic and nicotinic plants may produce seizures. Ingestion of plants that produce hypoglycemia, such as ackee (*Blighia sapida*), wild yam (*Dioscorea* spp.), cocklebur (*Xanthium* spp.), bird-lime (*Atractylis gummifera*), and ox-eye daisy (*Callilepis laureola*), are associated with seizures and discussed later. Ingestion of plants that produce multisystem organ failure, such as *Ricinus communis*, *Colchicinum autumnale*, *Poldophyllum* spp., and cyanogenic plants, may produce seizures. Plant-derived essential oils, such as eucalyptus oil, oil of wormwood (*Artemisia*

BOX 65-3 Cardiovascular Toxins Found in Plants

Alkaloids
Steroid (e.g., aconite, veratrum alkaloids)
Taxane (e.g., taxines)
Glycosides
Cardiac (e.g., lanatosides, oleandrin, thevetin)
Resins
Grayanotoxins (e.g., *o*-acetyl-andromedol)

absinthium), oil of wintergreen, and camphor, may produce seizures (see Table 65-4, later). Ingestion of plants that produce liver failure, such as *Chelidonium* (greater celandine), may produce seizures, as discussed later.

CARDIOVASCULAR TOXINS

Cardiovascular toxins found in plants are listed in Box 65-3.

CARDIOTOXINS THAT INHIBIT SODIUM/POTASSIUM ADENOSINE TRIPHOSPHATASE (CARDIAC GLYCOSIDES)

More than 200 naturally occurring cardiac glycosides have been identified. Plant cardiac glycosides are composed of a steroid backbone, an attached five-membered unsaturated lactone ring (six-membered for *Helleborus*), and either a carbohydrate or a sugar moiety in glycosidic linkage. The toxic aglycones are released by acid and enzymatic hydrolysis. The attached sugar moiety has no inherent cardiac action but may enhance solubility, absorption, and toxicity of the aglycone moiety. Cardiac glycosides bind to the membrane-bound enzyme sodium/potassium adenosine triphosphatase (Na^+/K^+ ATPase), increasing intracellular Na^+ and calcium ion (Ca^{2+}) levels and automaticity (Figure 65-15).[274] Cardiac glycosides are found in *Digitalis purpurea* (foxglove) (Figure 65-16), *Digitalis lanata*, *Nerium oleander*

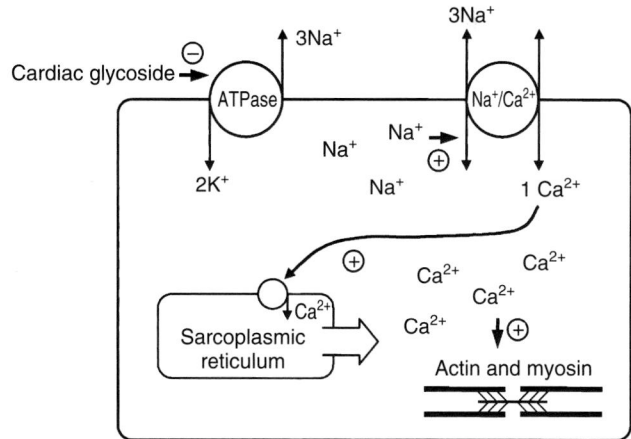

FIGURE 65-15 Cardiac glycosides bind to and inhibit the membrane-bound enzyme Na^+/K^+ ATPase in cardiac myocytes (shown), baroreceptor cells, and skeletal muscle cells. Inhibition of Na^+/K^+ ATPase in cardiac myocytes results in accumulation of intracellular Na^+, which results in accumulation of Ca^{2+} within myocytes via Na^+, Ca^{2+} exchangers. The resultant increase in intracellular Ca^{2+} stimulates further release of Ca^{2+} from the sarcoplasmic reticulum. The increased intracellular Ca^{2+} interacts with troponin C of the actin-myosin complex to cause increased contractions, seen as increased automaticity (e.g., premature ventricular contractions on electrocardiogram). Inhibition of membrane-bound enzyme Na^+/K^+ ATPase in baroreceptor cells and skeletal muscle cells contributes to increased vagal tone and hyperkalemia, respectively.

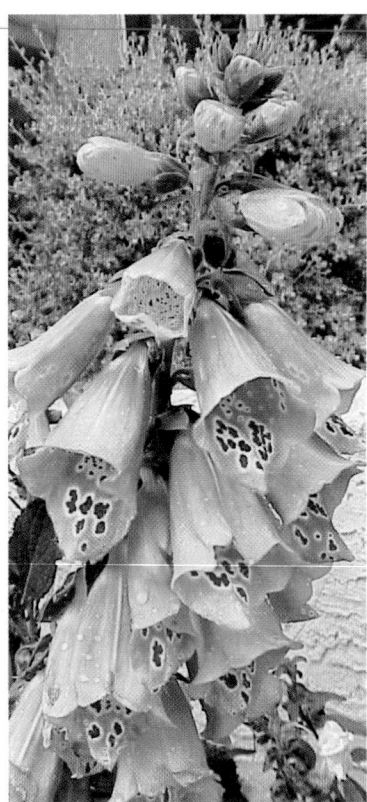

FIGURE 65-16 *Digitalis purpurea* (foxglove). *(Courtesy Kimberlie A. Graeme, MD.)*

(common oleander) (Figure 65-17), *Thevetia peruviana* (also called *Cascabela thevetia* and yellow oleander) (Figure 65-18), *Convallaria majalis* (lily of the valley) (Figure 65-19), *Urginea maritima* (squill or sea onion) (Figure 65-20), *U. indica, Cerbera manghas* (sea mango), *C. odollam* (pink-eyed cerbera), *Strophanthus* spp. (ouabain, poison rope), *Asclepias* spp. (balloon cotton, red-headed cotton-bush, and common milkweeds), *Calotropis procera* (king's crown), *Carissa spectabilis* (wintersweet), *C. acokanthera* (bushman's poison), *Plumeria rubra* (frangipani), *Cryptostegia grandifolia* (rubber vine), *Adenium multiflorum* (impala lily), *Euonymus europaeus* (spindle tree), *Cheiranthus, Erysimum* (wallflower), and *Helleborus niger* (henbane).* Cardiac glycosides are found in the African plant genera *Acokanthera, Boophone, Strophanthus, Adenium,* and *Catharanthus roseus* (Madagascar periwinkle). *C. roseus* contains vinca alkaloids that are antimitotic and produces metaphase arrest (as does colchicine from *Colchicum autumnale,* discussed later). *C. roseus* is the source of the antineoplastic drugs vincristine and vinblastine. *C. roseus* has hypoglycemic effects.[225,231]

Foxglove

Digitalis purpurea grows wild in parts of the United States and is cultivated as a garden ornamental plant. *D. purpurea* contains digitoxin, not digoxin. Withering reported medicinal use of extracts of *D. purpurea* based on a recipe for treating "dropsy."[155,239] The leaves have been consumed in a risotto when they were mistaken for borage (*Borago officinalis*) leaves, in a salad when mistaken for dandelion leaves, and in an herbal tea when mistaken for comfrey (*Symphytum officinale*).[52,204,234] Toxicity has been reported from consumption of contaminated field water with *Digitalis* plants growing nearby.[234] *D. lanata* (wooly foxglove or Grecian foxglove) was mistakenly substituted for plantain in herbal products, with resultant human cardiotoxicity.[305] *D. lanata* contains lanatosides A, B, and C, which yield digoxin and digitoxin. Intentional overdoses occur.[189,234]

---

*References 40, 98, 103, 125, 140, 142, 155, 193, 234, 300, 331, 334.

Oleander

All parts of *Nerium oleander* and *Thevetia peruviana* (*Cascabela thevetia*) are toxic, but the seeds contain more glycoside than do other parts of the plant. Yellow oleander (*T. peruviana* or *C. thevetia*), a native plant of tropical America, grows abundantly in the United States. Ingestion of a couple of seeds of yellow oleander, known as "lucky nuts," can result in death; however, the number of seeds ingested is a poor guide to the degree of poisoning. Yellow oleander contains the cardiac glycosides thevetin A and B, thevetoxin, neriifolin, peruvoside, ruvoside, and others. It is a popular suicide agent in Sri Lanka and India. Of patients admitted with yellow oleander poisoning in Sri Lanka, 43% had arrhythmias, many required temporary cardiac pacing, and 6% died shortly after admission. Common oleander (*N. oleander*), a native plant of the Mediterranean, grows abundantly in the United States. Common oleander contains the principal cardiac glycosides oleandrin and neriine, as well as folinerin and digitoxigenin. Severe toxicity has been reported after consumption of unprocessed common oleander leaves and prepared teas. Chronic toxicity has occurred with criminal intentional poisoning. Topical application of homemade *N. oleander* solutions onto psoriatic wounds has caused toxicity.[4,98,99,125,135,193,195,238,274,348]

Squill

Urginea maritima was used by ancient Egyptians and Romans as a diuretic, heart tonic, expectorant, emetic, and rat poison.

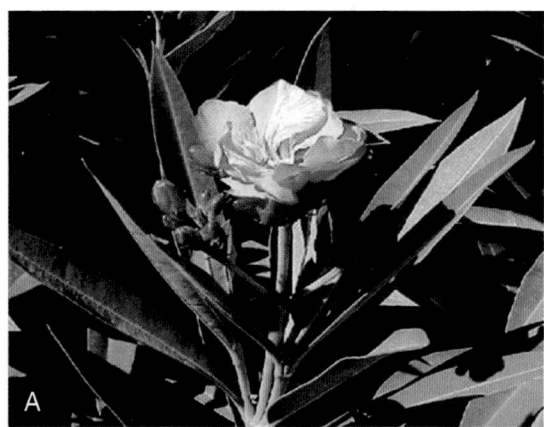

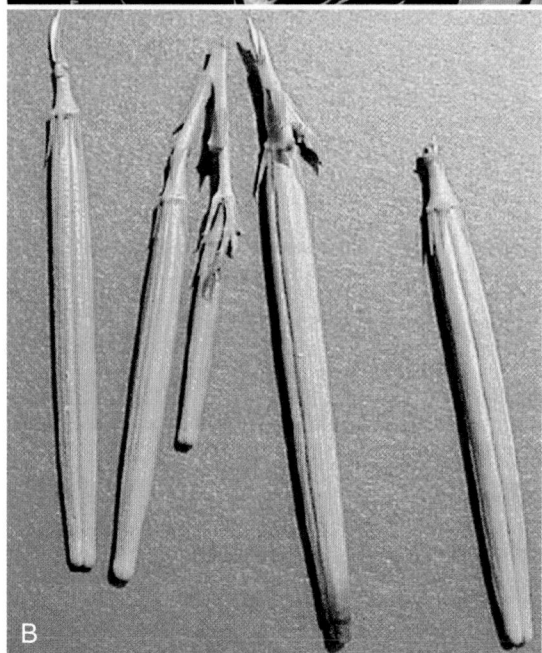

FIGURE 65-17 *Nerium oleander* (common oleander) plants have white or pink flowers **(A)** and long, narrow seedpods **(B).** *(Courtesy Kimberlie A. Graeme, MD.)*

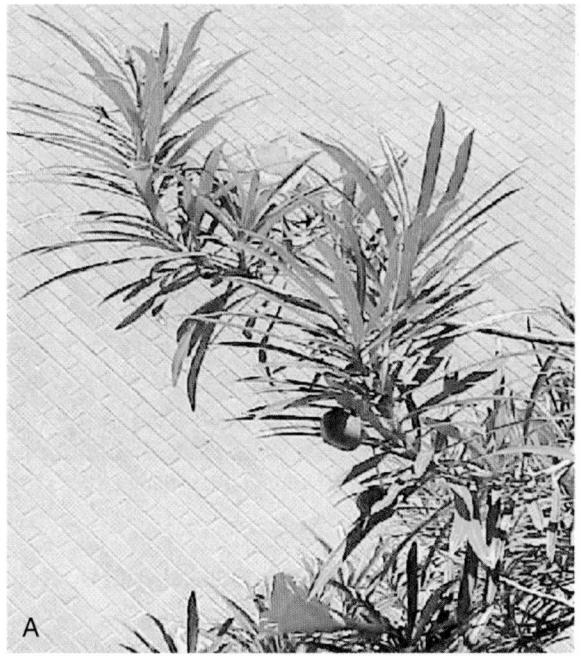

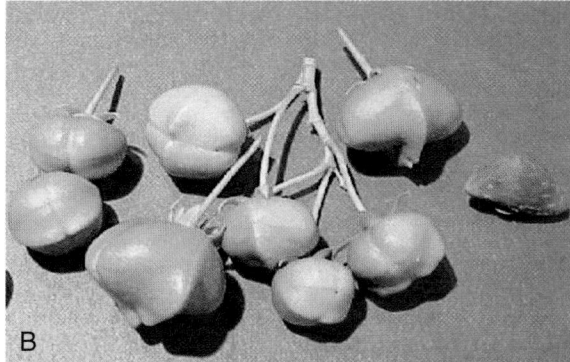

FIGURE 65-18 *Thevetia peruviana* (yellow oleander) has yellow flowers **(A)** with smooth seedpods, known as "lucky nuts," composed of green flesh surrounding a hard brown seed **(B)**. *(Courtesy Kimberlie A. Graeme, MD.)*

Squill contains several cardiac glycosides, including scillaren A, glucoscillaren A, scillaridin A, and scilliroside.[103,331,343]

Suicide Tree

Cerbera odollam (suicide tree, pong-pong tree, pink-eyed cerbera, yellow-eyed cerbera) contains cerberin, a cardiac glycoside. Ingestion of the seeds with suicidal and homicidal intent is reported in South Asia. Less often, suicidal ingestion occurs in

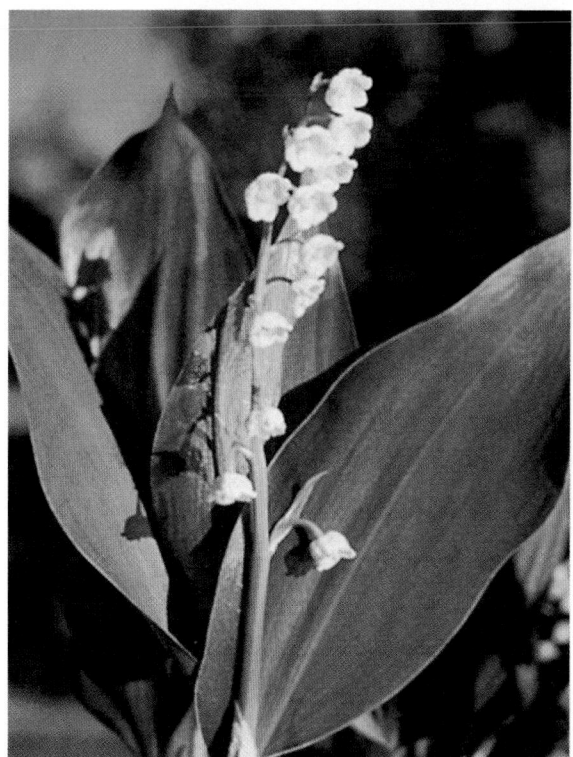

FIGURE 65-19 Lily of the valley (*Convallaria majalis*). *(Courtesy Donald Kunkel, MD.)*

the Western world, and has occurred after purchase of the seeds online. Anecdotal clinical improvement has been noted when toxicity is treated with digoxin-specific Fab fragments.[171]

Sea Mango

Cerbera manghas (sea mango) is similar to *C. odollam* (suicide tree). This tree grows in India, Vietnam, Cambodia, Sri Lanka, Myanmar (previously Burma), Madagascar, and Australia. The plant has large, white flowers that smell like jasmine. When the fruit is still green, it looks like a small mango. The inner fruit kernel is white, but on exposure to air turns violet, then dark gray, and then black. The crushed, white, fleshy kernel is often consumed as a suicide poison in India and Sri Lanka. The seeds are quite toxic. The leaves are less toxic. These plants contain the toxins cerberoside, cerberin, and odollin. After ingestion, death can occur within hours.[100,128,203,330]

Clinical Presentation

The onset of symptoms and duration of action are well known for certain glycoside preparations, such as digoxin, digitoxin, and

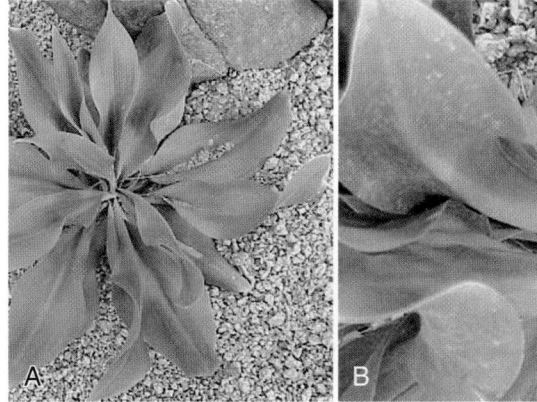

FIGURE 65-20 *Urginea* species (squill or sea onion) have broad leaves **(A)** and a red, underground bulb (some varieties have a white bulb) **(B)**. *(Courtesy Kimberlie A. Graeme, MD.)*

ouabain, but may vary considerably after plant ingestions. For example, oleandrin exhibits protracted binding times to cardiac myocardial tissues.[193] Generally, cardiac glycoside toxicity produces nausea, vomiting, diarrhea, abdominal tenderness, visual changes (appearance of yellow and green colors, "halos," geometric shapes, scintillations, photophobia), mydriasis, mental status changes (disorientation, psychosis, lethargy, stupor, dysarthria, weakness, dizziness, restlessness, seizures), cardiac disturbances (palpitations, premature ventricular beats, bradycardia, atrioventricular block, sinus node block, paroxysmal atrial tachycardia with block, junctional tachycardia, bidirectional ventricular tachycardia, ventricular arrhythmias, myocardial depression with cardiogenic shock, syncope), hyperkalemia, and death. When it occurs, death is generally caused by cardiotoxicity. The ECG may reveal nonspecific ST-segment and T-wave changes, similar to digoxin-induced changes.[96,135,195,204,234,274,305,34] [7] Serum digoxin levels may be elevated after exposure to plants containing cardiac glycosides, because antibody-based digoxin assays cross-react nonquantitatively with many cardiac glycosides. Digoxin immunoassays can only predict the presence of the glycoside, not the degree of toxicity.[99,140,193,331,204] Conversely, the degree of hyperkalemia often correlates with severity of toxicity.[99,128,204]

Treatment

Continuous cardiac monitoring for at least 24 hours is recommended because of the risk for arrhythmias. Cardiac glycoside toxicity from plant ingestions has been successfully treated with a single dose or multiple repeated doses of activated charcoal, cardiac pacing, antiarrhythmic agents, and digoxin-specific Fab fragments (e.g., Digibind, DigiFab). Maintenance of fluid and electrolyte balance is important. Potassium levels should be checked frequently. Correction of hyperkalemia with insulin and dextrose is recommended. Sodium polystyrene sulfonate resin is not recommended because total-body hypokalemia may ensue. Theoretically, administration of exogenous calcium could be harmful because of high intracellular calcium concentrations of poisoned myocytes. It is hypothesized that the heart may perform one final contraction without relaxation, a state termed *stone heart*. However, some have questioned the withholding of calcium, because some case reports and retrospective review suggest that calcium administration is generally not detrimental. Bradyarrhythmias have been managed with atropine and β-adrenergic agents. However, there is a theoretical risk for increasing tachyarrhythmias, which may be more difficult to treat. Some have advised against use of atropine and β-adrenergic agents unless bradycardia is life threatening. Some believe that cardiac pacing is a better alternative, although this may precipitate tachyarrhythmias as well. Ventricular tachycardia may persist despite electrical cardioversion, and electrical cardioversion can precipitate ventricular fibrillation or asystole. Therefore, electrical cardioversion is reserved for resistant cases.

For patients with tachyarrhythmias, lidocaine has been advocated. The role of magnesium is not known, although some have subjectively noted death after yellow oleander poisoning treated with IV magnesium. Amiodarone, quinidine, and calcium channel blockers are contraindicated because they may increase digitalis concentration; β-blockers are contraindicated because they may worsen heart block. Digoxin-specific Fab antibody fragments may couple to circulating cardiac glycosides and limit binding of cardiac glycosides to Na⁺/K⁺ ATPase. Administration of digoxin-specific Fab antibody fragments to reverse cardiotoxicity from plant glycosides has been successful in several animal and human studies. Clinical trials in Sri Lanka revealed that IV administration of 1200 mg of digoxin-specific antibody fragments reversed life-threatening cardiac arrhythmias and corrected hyperkalemia after yellow oleander poisoning. High doses of digoxin-specific Fab antibody fragments (e.g., 10 to 20 vials) may be needed. Animal studies indicate that fructose-1,6-diphosphate may be a beneficial treatment of cardiac glycoside poisoning. This is being studied in humans currently, but is not an established treatment.*

---

*References 74, 99, 100, 101, 128, 135, 171, 179, 193, 199, 204, 234, 274, 277, 279, 305.

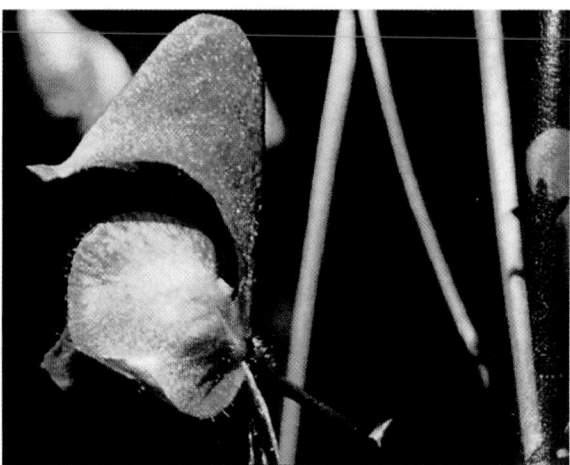

FIGURE 65-21 Monkshood (*Aconitum* spp.).

CARDIOTOXINS THAT OPEN SODIUM CHANNELS (STEROID ALKALOIDS, RESINS)

Steroid alkaloids form principal toxic components of several common cardiotoxic plants: *Aconitum* spp. (monkshood, wolfsbane, helmet flower), *Veratrum viride* (American hellebore, green hellebore), and *Zigadenus* spp. (death camas). Aconite is found in *Aconitum* spp., and veratrum alkaloids are found in *V. viride, V. nigrum* var. *japonicum* (false hellebore), *V. californicum* (skunk cabbage), *V. album* (white hellebore), *Z. paniculatus* (death camas), *Z. venenosus, Z. nuttallii,* and *Z. gramineus*.

Aconite

Aconite poisonings have become more common because of the use of *Aconitum* spp. (*A. napellus* [monkshood]; (Figure 65-21), *A. carmichaeli* (Chuanwa, Fuzi, Bushi), *A. brachypodium, A. vulparia,* and *A. kusnezoffii* (Caowu) in herbal products. *Delphinium* spp. (larkspur) demonstrate similar toxicity. All parts of these plants are toxic, with the roots being most toxic. *Aconitum* spp. contain diterpenoid-ester alkaloids, particularly aconitine, but also mesaconitine, hypaconitine, and yunaconitine, which are neurotoxins and cardiotoxins. Boiling these plants in water hydrolyzes aconite alkaloids to less toxic benzoylaconine and aconine derivatives. Soaking or boiling, termed *decoction,* is generally done when these plants are used as herbal medicines. The estimated lethal dose of wild plant is 1 g.[10,61-63,72, 120,125,200]

Aconite alkaloids activate voltage-sensitive sodium channels and affect excitable membranes of neural, cardiac, and muscle tissues. Aconite alkaloids bind to open voltage-gated sodium channels, producing a hyperpolarized state, with permanent activation of the channels. Hypaconitine affects sodium channels of the nerve membrane more selectively than aconitine and is more potent than aconitine and mesaconitine in producing neuromuscular block. These neurotoxins produce conduction block and paralysis through voltage-sensitive sodium channels in axons. In cardiac tissues, prolonged depolarization prevents repolarization of excitable membranes. Enhancement of the transmembrane inward sodium current during the plateau phase of the action potential prolongs repolarization in cardiac myocytes and induces delayed and early afterdepolarizations. Delayed afterdepolarizations result in increased automaticity, such as premature ventricular beats. Early afterdepolarizations produce lengthening of the QT interval. Hypotension and bradycardia may be induced by activation of the ventromedial nucleus of the hypothalamus.[10,62,61,72,120,125,200]

Symptoms begin within 3 minutes to 6 hours of aconite ingestion and may persist for several days. Nonspecific GI symptoms (nausea, vomiting, diarrhea) are accompanied by neurotoxicity and cardiotoxicity. Visual impairment, dizziness, vertigo, ataxia, paresthesias (e.g., numbness of mouth and extremities), hyporeflexia, weakness, paralysis, coma, restlessness, and convulsions may occur. Patients may present with chest pain, palpitations,

and syncope. Cardiac effects are clinically similar to cardiac glycoside toxicity, with enhanced vagal tone, bradycardia, heart
block, ectopic beats, supraventricular tachycardia, bundle branch
block, junctional escape rhythms, ventricular tachycardia, bifas-
cicular ventricular tachycardia, polymorphic ventricular tachycardia, torsades de pointes, ventricular fibrillation, asystole, and
hypotension. Bidirectional ventricular tachycardia, which is generally considered suggestive of cardiac glycoside toxicity, has
been reported with aconite poisoning. Elevated CPK and troponin levels, with or without evidence of myocardial infarction,
may occur. Myocardial necrosis and myocarditis have been
reported. Hypokalemia, metabolic or respiratory acidosis, respiratory alkalosis, and renal and hepatic impairment may be noted.
Occasionally, death ensues, generally from ventricular arrhythmias, such as refractory ventricular fibrillation. Respiratory paralysis may result in death.* A 17-year-old man ate immature
Delphinium root and developed seizures, ventricular fibrillation,
and cardiac arrest. He survived and later reported that he had
experienced a floating or flying sensation.[328]

Veratrum Alkaloids

Veratrum and Zigadenus spp. belong to the lily family. All parts
of these plants are toxic, with the rhizomes being more toxic
than the tops. Veratrum spp. have been found in sneezing
powders and have been accidentally ingested when mistaken for
Gentiana lutea (yellow gentian). Gentian wines are usually made
from G. lutea. When accidentally made from Veratrum spp.,
these wines can be toxic. V. viride has been mistaken for skunk
cabbage, ramps, and pokeweed (Phytolacca americana), producing toxicity after ingestion. Zigadenus spp. (foothill camas,
death camas, mountain camas) have been accidentally ingested
when mistaken for nontoxic wild onions (Allium macropetalum)
and sego lilies (Calochortus nuttallii). Amianthium muscitoxi-
cum (fly poison) and Schoenocaulon officinale (Sabadilla)
contain veratrum alkaloids. Veratrum alkaloids include protove-
ratrine, veratridine, cevadine, jervine, zygadenine, and zygacine,
which are found in the entire plant, although the bulb and flower
usually cause toxicity. These alkaloids are extremely toxic and
rapidly increase permeability of voltage-sensitive sodium channels in excitable cell membranes. This results in initial depolarization and then subsequent loss of membrane potential. Stimulation
of vagal fibers may result in bradycardia and hypotension.†

Symptoms generally occur within 30 minutes to 4 hours and
resolve within 24 to 48 hours, although symptoms may persist
for many days. Toxicity is characterized by headache, diaphoresis, salivation, nausea, vomiting, diarrhea, abdominal pain, hypotension, bradycardia, and shock. Syncope, respiratory depression,
scotomata, paresthesias, fasciculations, muscle spasticity, hyperreflexia, vertigo, ataxia, dizziness, coma, seizures, and death may
occur. ECG findings may mimic cardiac glycoside toxicity, including repolarization abnormalities (e.g., abnormal T waves and ST
segments), sinoatrial and atrioventricular blocks, and prolonged
QT intervals.[113,137,262,290,345,354]

Grayanotoxins

Resins called grayanotoxins are found in rhododendrons, mountain laurels, and azaleas. They produce toxicity similar to that
seen with the steroid alkaloids veratrum and aconite. They act
by binding to myocardial sodium channels and increasing their
permeability and by increasing vagal tone. Grayanotoxins inhibit
cardiac and respiratory actions within the CNS. Poisoning may
result from ingestion of leaves, flowers, or nectar. Grayanotoxin-
contaminated honey, termed "mad honey," is the most common
source. The nectar of Rhododendron spp. contains the grayano-
toxin o-acetyl-andromedol, formerly andromedotoxin, which is
transferred to humans through consumption of honey produced
by bees using the plant's nectar. "Mad honey" was reportedly
used as a biologic weapon against the Romans in 67 BC. Poisonings still occur in Asia Minor. "Mad honey" is sometimes taken
in hopes of enhancing sexual performance but may result in

toxicity. Symptoms include diaphoresis, hypersalivation, nausea,
vomiting, bradycardia, arrhythmias (atrioventricular blocks,
junctional rhythms), chest pain, hypotension, shock, dizziness,
syncope, circumoral and extremity paresthesias, incoordination,
and muscular weakness. A patient presented with acute myocardial infarction with normal coronary arteries after "mad honey"
ingestion.[168,302] Patients generally recover in 1 to 2 days. In Korea,
the blossoms of azaleas (R. mucronulatum) are used to make
wine, honeyed flower juice, and griddle cakes, with reported
toxicity.[3,69,71,88,168,180,191,196,339]

Treatment

Treatment of poisoning from cardiotoxins that open sodium
channels is supportive, with attention to fluid and electrolyte
balance. Atropine for bradycardia and vasopressors for fluid-
resistant hypotension are appropriate. Patients may require
mechanical ventilation and cardiopulmonary resuscitation. Magnesium may suppress early afterdepolarizations and polymorphic
ventricular tachycardia. Lidocaine, procainamide, flecainide, amiodarone, and hemoperfusion have been used to treat ventricular
arrhythmias secondary to aconite poisoning, as reported in
various case reports. Ventricular dysrhythmias may be resistant
to cardioversion and antiarrhythmic agents. Cardiopulmonary
bypass, extracorporeal membrane oxygenation, and ventricular
assist device placement have been used successfully for treatment
of aconite poisoning.*

OTHER CARDIOTOXINS

Taxine Alkaloids

Taxus spp. include T. baccata (English yew), T. brevifolia
(Western yew), T. cuspidata (Japanese yew), and T. sumatrana
(Sumatra or Chinese yew). The toxic alkaloids include taxines A
and B. Yew plants also contain nitriles, ephedrine, and irritant
oils. All parts of Taxus plants are toxic except the pulp, or aril,
which contains very little taxine. The seeds, which are surrounded by the aril, may be toxic if chewed sufficiently to allow
absorption of taxine. The plant is most toxic in the winter. Taxine
B, believed to be the primary cardiotoxic alkaloid, inhibits both
calcium and sodium transport across cell membranes.†

Most Taxus exposures occur in children, are accidental, and
are not associated with significant toxicity. However, serious
toxicity and death have occurred after intentional ingestions of
Taxus spp.. The lethal oral dose of yew leaves is 0.6 to 1.3 g/
kg body weight. GI toxicity is most common; dizziness, mydriasis, muscle weakness, altered mental status, and convulsions have
been reported. Severe toxicity is characterized by bradycardias,
heart blocks, ventricular tachycardia, ventricular fibrillation,
widened QRS complexes, hypotension, cardiac arrest, and death.
Brugada syndrome pattern has been noted on the ECG during
toxicity; it resolved with recovery. Hemolysis with multiorgan
failure has been reported.‡ Autopsies have revealed dilated
cardiac ventricles and congestion of the organs with pronounced
cerebral and pulmonary edema.[138] Plant parts are often found in
the stomach and small bowel on autopsy. 3,5-Dimethoxyphenol
demonstrated by gas chromatography–mass spectrometry of
blood or urine is a marker of Taxus poisoning.[119,138,268,270,344]

Reported yew-induced arrhythmias in humans are consistent
with arrhythmias induced by blockade of voltage-gated sodium
channels. These are described as bradycardia with wide QRS
complexes, despite normal electrolytes. Two patients who
ingested yew presented with severe cardiotoxicity and a wide
QRS complex, which appeared to respond favorably to administration of hypertonic sodium bicarbonate.[216,267,283] However,
sodium bicarbonate administration did not narrow the widened
QRS complex of Taxus-poisoned swine.[283] Because there is
minimal risk to administering sodium bicarbonate and possible
significant benefit, this treatment should be considered if widened

---

*References 61, 62, 72, 120, 125, 175, 200, 201, 203, 222, 243, 306, 353.
†References 113, 125, 129, 137, 158, 262, 271, 290, 345, 354.

*References 10, 61, 62, 69, 71, 97, 125, 129, 137, 196, 201, 222, 243, 262, 290, 306, 345, 353.
†References 119, 138, 185, 194, 203, 267, 268, 326, 336, 337, 347.
‡References 138, 185, 203, 216, 228, 267, 283, 326, 336, 337, 347.

QRS is noted. Lidocaine administration and cardiac pacing have been reportedly beneficial for treatment of humans poisoned with yew.[270,337]

ORAL AND GASTROINTESTINAL TOXINS

ORAL IRRITANTS (GLYCOSIDES, OXALATES)

Daphne

Coumarin glycosides may produce pronounced irritant effects. An example is daphne (*Daphne mezereum*), with its fragrant, succulent berries. The widely cultivated daphne presents a significant risk to curious children, for whom only a few ingested berries may be lethal. The fruits contain a coumarin glycoside and a diterpene that irritate mucous membranes, with swelling of the tongue and lips. Blisters form if berries are rubbed on the skin, and in the oral and GI tract if ingested. Severe gastroenteritis with GI bleeding may occur after ingestion. In addition, progressive weakness, paralysis, seizures, and coma may develop. Treatment is supportive.

Insoluble Oxalates

Plant exposures involving *Philodendron, Dieffenbachia* (dumb cane), *Spathiphyllum* spp. (peace lily) (Figure 65-22), *Colocasia* spp. (elephant's ear, common calla), and *Brassaia* (octopus tree, Queensland umbrella tree) are frequently reported.[184,206,256] *Alocasia macrorrhiza* (giant elephant's ear, taro), *Monstera deliciosa* (fruit salad plant, split-leaf philodendron), *Anum* spp. (dragon lily, voodoo lily), *Arisaema amurense* (cobra lily), and *Zantedeschia aethiopica* (calla lily, arum lily) can produce similar toxicity.[40,203,284] These plants contain insoluble oxalates arranged in numerous crystalline needles of calcium oxalate (raphides) contained in specialized cells (idioblasts). When stimulated, as by mastication, idioblasts forcefully release raphides that become embedded in exposed tissues, resulting in painful oropharyngeal edema, hypersalivation, vesicle formation, dysphagia, and aphonia. On occasion, airway obstruction occurs. These plants also contain trypsin-like proteases, histamine, and kinin-like substances that may contribute to toxicity.[206,284,320,342] In a mass foodborne illness in Chicago, patients presented with oral burning and facial edema after lunch in an office cafeteria serving a Chinese vegetable entrée found to contain raphides.[342]

Dieffenbachia is commonly known as "dumb cane" because of the person's inability to speak after chewing the plant. As with other plants containing insoluble oxalates, vesicle, bulla, and ulcer formation of the oral mucous membranes and epiglottis or esophageal erosions may occur after mastication and ingestion.[8] Respiratory obstruction resulting from edema and sudden death have been reported. Treatment is supportive, with special attention to maintaining a patent airway. Severe edema and potential for airway obstruction may warrant intensive care monitoring. After massive ingestions, hypocalcemia and its effects should be anticipated.[206,256,320,342]

GASTROINTESTINAL IRRITANTS (RESINS, ALKALOIDS)

Gastrointestinal toxins found in plants are listed in Box 65-4.

Chinaberry Trees

Melia azedarach plants are found throughout the southern United States and Hawaii (Figure 65-23). The chinaberry tree, also known as China tree, Texas umbrella tree, or white cedar tree, contains tetranortriterpenes (resins) identified as meliatoxins A_1, A_2, B_1, and B_2, which are enterotoxic and neurotoxic. The bark contains toosendanin. Gastroenteritis can occur after

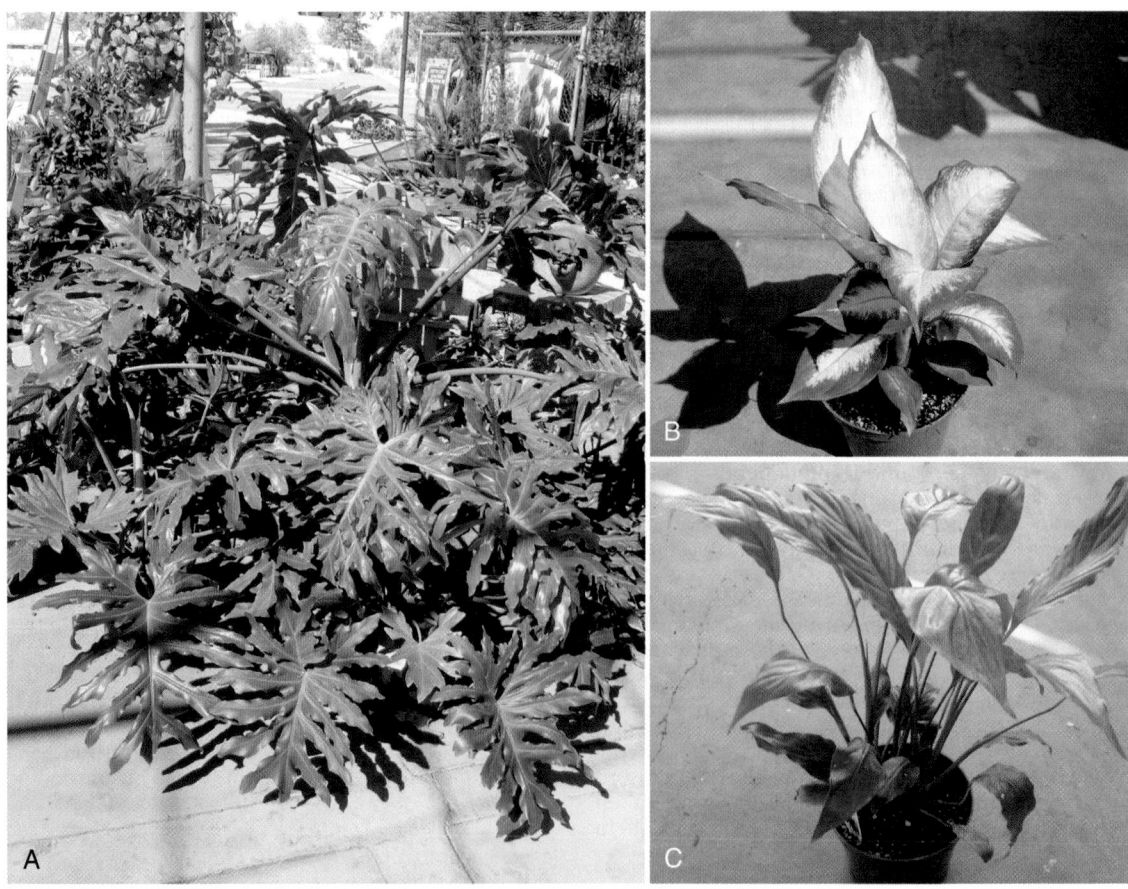

FIGURE 65-22 Plants that are oral irritants. *Philodendron* **(A)**, *Dieffenbachia* **(B)**, *Spathiphyllum* **(C)**. *(Courtesy Kimberlie A. Graeme, MD.)*

BOX 65-4 Gastrointestinal Toxins Found in Plants

Alkaloids
Amine (e.g., colchicine)
Isoquinoline and quinoline (e.g., emetine in ipecac)
Pyrrolizidine
Steroid (e.g., solanine)

Glycosides
Coumarin
Saponin (e.g., phytolaccatoxin)

Resins
Cicutoxin
Meliatoxins

Phytotoxins
Abrin
Curcin
Ricin

ingestion of any part of the plant, but typically occurs after berries are ingested by children. Immature berries are green but turn yellow and wrinkle with age. After ingestion of only one berry, severe gastroenteritis may ensue, often with bloody diarrhea. Symptoms may be rapid in onset or delayed by several hours after ingestion. In Chinese medicine, *M. azedarach* bark has been boiled and drank, with resultant nausea, vomiting, abdominal discomfort, diarrhea that can be bloody, dizziness, muscle soreness, weakness, ataxia, areflexia, coma, blurred vision, ptosis, numbness, and headache. Muscle tremors, convulsions, and death have been reported in children after ingestion of berries of the African variety of chinaberry tree. Fatalities are generally caused by respiratory arrest. Mild elevation of liver enzymes and CPK, as well as hypokalemia and acidosis, has been reported. Autopsy has revealed cerebral edema, midbrain necrosis, intracranial hemorrhage, pulmonary congestion, GI hemorrhage, yellow discoloration of the liver, and congestion of the kidneys. Treatment is supportive, with replacement of fluids and electrolytes. Patients with tachycardia and hypotension generally respond to IV fluids.[150,264]

Solanum

The genus *Solanum* makes up the largest group of steroid alkaloid–containing plants and includes *S. tuberosum* (potato), *S. gracile* (wild tomato), *S. carolinense* (horse nettle), *S. pseudocapsicum* (Jerusalem cherry), *S. dulcamara* (woody nightshade), *S. americanum* (black nightshade), and other nightshade plants. *Solanum* species are used medicinally in some countries. Solanine, a glycoalkaloid with a steroid-like moiety, has been isolated from more than 1700 different *Solanum* spp. It is found throughout the plants but is most concentrated in unripe fruits. Solanine generally produces gastroenteritis, but bradycardia, weakness, and CNS and respiratory depression may be seen. Treatment is supportive, with replacement of fluids and electrolytes. If hypotension ensues, patients generally respond to IV fluids. Atropine may be beneficial if bradycardia develops. Spontaneous recovery usually occurs in 1 to 3 days.[78,133]

Plants Containing Saponin Glycosides

Saponin glycosides are found throughout the plant kingdom, for example, in pokeweed (*Phytolacca americana*), English ivy (*Hedera helix*), tung tree (*Aleurites* spp.), ginseng (*Panax ginseng* or *P. quinquefolium*), and licorice (*Glycyrrhiza glabra*).[125] Saponins are GI irritants that facilitate their own intestinal absorption. Saponins may induce lysis of erythrocytes, causing hemolytic anemia. In addition, most saponins are found in combination with other toxins, resulting in diverse clinical syndromes.

Pokeweed. *Phytolacca americana*, or *P. decandra*, is most commonly known as pokeweed but is also called Virginia poke, inkberry, pocan, pigeonberry, American cancer-root, garget, red ink, American nightshade, scoke, jalap, and redwood. It may be mistaken for horseradish, parsnip, or Jerusalem artichoke. *P. americana* has green leaves with red stalks. Berries are green when immature and turn deep purple with maturity. Pokeberries typically leave a purple stain. The root is the most toxic part of the plant. *P. americana* is ingested intentionally in pokeweed salad and pokeberry teas. When prepared for ingestion, leaves should be parboiled, which entails boiling the leaves first in water that is discarded before boiling the leaves again and rinsing them with fresh water. However, parboiling does not necessarily offer complete protection against toxicity.[125]

The saponin glycosides phytolaccatoxin and phytolaccagenin account for the GI injury, which manifests as fulminant gastroenteritis, with vomiting and diarrhea 2 to 4 hours after ingestion. Diarrhea may appear foamy from the sudsing effect of saponin glycosides. Hypotension may follow significant GI fluid losses. Severe toxicity may include weakness, loss of consciousness, seizures, and respiratory depression.[125]

P. americana also contains mitogenic, hemagglutinating, and antiviral proteins. Pokeweed mitogen may induce morphologic changes in lymphocytes and plasma cells. An increased number of circulating plasmablasts and proplasmacytes, eosinophilia, and thrombocytopenia can be seen after ingestion or after handling *P. americana* with broken skin.

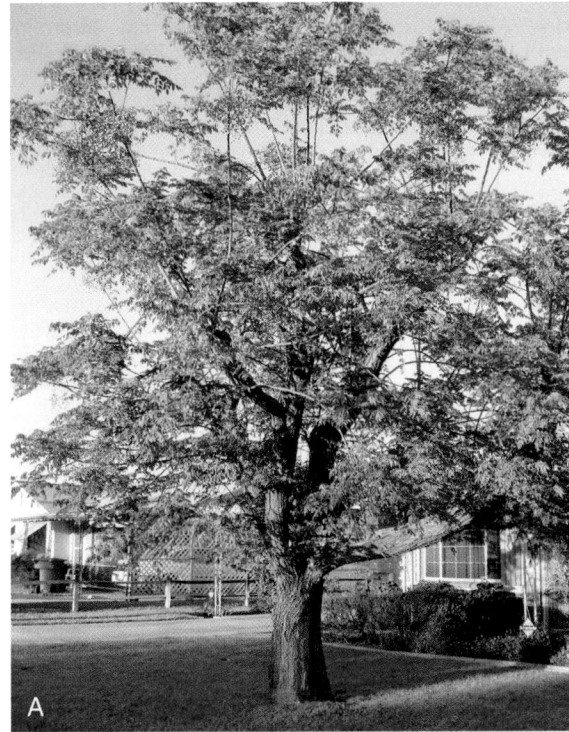
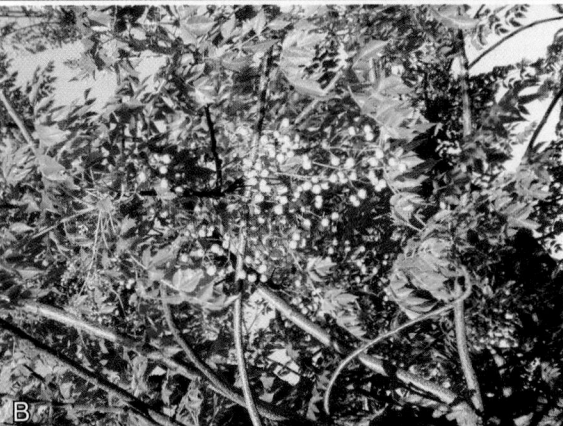

FIGURE 65-23 Chinaberry (*Melia azedarach*) tree **(A)** and berries **(B)**. *(Courtesy Kimberlie A. Graeme, MD.)*

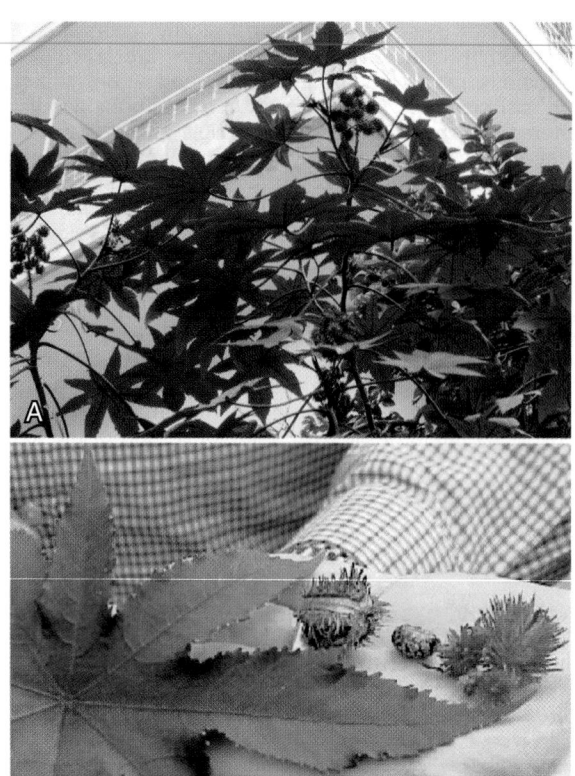

FIGURE 65-24 Castor bean plant (*Ricinus communis*) (A) contains ricin and is characterized by broad, serrated leaves, with fresh beans encased within a soft, thorny, red seedpod. With age, the seeds and their surrounding seedpod become brown, and the seeds develop hard shells that are difficult to penetrate (B). (*Courtesy Phillip Saba, MD, and Kimberlie A. Graeme, MD.*)

Treatment for acute toxicity includes fluid replacement for dehydration secondary to GI losses. Airway support may be needed. Seizures should be treated with benzodiazepines. Hematologic changes generally resolve within weeks.[125]

TOXINS THAT INHIBIT PROTEIN SYNTHESIS (PHYTOTOXINS)

Toxalbumins (Ricin, Abrin, Curcin, Robin, Phasin)

Toxalbumins are found in *Abrus precatorius* (jequirity bean, rosary pea, prayer bead; contains abrin), *Ricinus communis* (castor bean; contains ricin) (Figure 65-24, A), *Jatropha curcas* (purging nut) and *J. multifida*, which contain curcin, and *Robinia pseudoacacia* (black locust; contains robin and phasin). These toxins inhibit protein synthesis and cause cell death. The toxins are glycoproteins composed of two peptide chains, designated A and B, connected by a disulfide bond (see Figure 65-2). Chain B binds to the cell membrane. The toxin penetrates the cell by endocytosis. Chain A binds irreversibly and inactivates the ribosomes through glycosidase activity, which disrupts protein synthesis and results in cell death. Much of the toxicity is the result of endothelial cell damage, which causes increased capillary permeability, fluid and protein leakage, and edema.*

Ricin poisoning generally results from eating or chewing on the nut or seed; however, consumption of leaves may also produce toxicity.[270] Fresh, immature castor beans are encased within a soft, thorny, red seedpod. With age, the seeds and surrounding seedpod become brown, and the seeds develop hard

---

*References 7, 36, 45, 92, 94, 145, 164, 187, 247, 269.

shells that are difficult to penetrate, but can be punctured by teeth (Figure 65-24B). After a latent period of 1 to 6 hours, nausea, vomiting, diarrhea, hemorrhagic gastritis, abdominal pain, thirst, dehydration, hypotension, coma, hyporeflexia, seizures, respiratory compromise, and shock may occur. Liver disease, with elevated LFTs, is common. Death may occur from dehydration and electrolyte imbalances. Convulsions may precede death. Death on the third day or later is usually caused by multiorgan failure. Autopsy may reveal GI tract ulcerations, necrosis of the lymph nodes and liver, nephritis, and pulmonary edema.[45,92,94,145,187,247,269]

The oral lethal dose is estimated to be 1 mg/kg; theoretically, only one bean in a child and 8 to 10 beans in an adult could be fatal, although this rarely is the case. A discrepancy between the serious toxicity of isolated ricin exposure and the milder toxicity of ingested seeds of *Ricinus communis* is recognized. A young adult consumed 10 to 15 seeds of *R. communis* and experienced severe cramping abdominal pain and vomiting 4 hours after ingestion, without GI bleeding or abdominal guarding. He received IV fluids. By the third day, he had recovered completely. Other cases of oral ingestion of masticated seeds indicate that GI distress may be followed a few days later by elevated liver enzymes or hyperbilirubinemia, followed by complete recovery. In contrast, a Bulgarian broadcaster who was injected with isolated ricin died from severe gastroenteritis and multiorgan failure. Ingested *R. communis* is much less toxic than is parenteral ricin. The degree of mastication of castor beans may determine the degree of toxicity seen with oral ingestions. Fresh, soft seeds are likely to be more toxic than aged seeds that are enveloped by a hard coat. Although deaths have been reported with ingestions of a couple of seeds, toxicity is unlikely if mature seeds are swallowed intact. Furthermore, some of the toxin, which is a protein, is likely digested in the GI tract.[7,45,92,94,247]

Similarly, deaths have been reported after ingestion of fresh jequirity beans (*Abrus precatorius*) if the soft, immature bean is chewed or if the hard shell of the mature bean is adequately penetrated. The estimated human fatal dose of abrin is 0.1 to 1 mcg/kg. One-half a seed has been reported to cause toxicity in a child, and one chewed bean could be fatal. However, as with castor beans, the mature bean shell is often not penetrated; therefore significant toxicity is not often seen. For example, a 15-month-old child ingested more than 20 jequirity beans with only minor clinical toxicity, including mild hepatomegaly and mild elevation of aspartate aminotransferase/transaminase (AST).[92,112,269]

Symptoms generally begin within a few hours. Mild symptoms involve diarrhea alone. More severe symptoms include persistent vomiting, diarrhea, and abdominal pain, with associated hypovolemia and hypokalemia. Hemorrhagic gastritis with bloody diarrhea may ensue. Dehydration may be associated with shock and hepatorenal dysfunction. Severely ill patients may present with hyperthermia, mental status changes, and seizures. Systemic injury may appear in a delayed fashion as the cumulative effects of inhibition of protein synthesis mount. Delayed effects may occur 1 to 5 days after ingestion. Terminally, elevated serum LFTs and creatinine levels may be seen, indicating hepatorenal failure. If death occurs, it is generally 3 to 5 days after ingestion and is associated with seizures, tachycardia, GI distress, mucosal changes of the GI tract (including edema and hemorrhage of the Peyer's patches), focal necrosis and failure of the liver and kidneys, and retinal hemorrhage. Cerebral and pulmonary edema, hypertension, and pancreatitis have been observed.[7,92,112,269]

Jatropha species have attractive, sweet-flavored fruit that may entice children. Children may consume the seeds out of curiosity. Presentation of toxicity may be mistaken for organophosphate poisoning, with diaphoresis, vomiting, diarrhea, obtundation, and miosis reported in one case. Mydriasis has also been reported. Other cases have manifested with hemorrhagic gastroenteritis, hypotension, muscle spasm, and hyperpnea. Leukocytosis may be noted.[181,187]

Treatment

Treatment of toxalbumin poisoning is supportive, including fluid and electrolyte replacement. Patients who remain asymptomatic for 4 to 6 hours after ingestion of seeds may be discharged, with instructions to return if symptoms develop. Laboratory follow-up for delayed liver toxicity may be appropriate. Studies indicate that ricin antibody administered intravenously shortly after exposure could be beneficial. Animal studies indicate that vaccination with abrin and ricin toxoids may offer protection against subsequent abrin and ricin challenges, respectively. However, there does not appear to be cross-immunity between abrin and ricin toxoids. Toxoids and antibodies are not readily available. Detection kits for toxalbumins are being developed.[36,45,68,92,94,247,269]

HEPATOTOXIC AGENTS

Pyrrolizidine Alkaloids

It is estimated that 3% of the world's flowering plants contain toxic pyrrolizidine alkaloids.[281] Plants containing pyrrolizidine alkaloids include *Senecio vulgaris* (groundsel), *S. longilobus* (gordolobo), *S. jacobaea* (tansy ragwort), *S. latifolius* (Dan's cabbage or muti), *Symphytum officinale* (comfrey), *Gynura segetum*, *Ilex paraguanyensis* (mate), *Heliotropium* spp., *Crotalaria* spp. (rattlebox), *Amsinckia intermedia* (fiddle neck or tar weed), *Baccharius pteronoides*, *Astragulus lentiginosus*, *Gnaphalium*, *Cynoglossum*, *Echium*, *Tussilago farfara*, and *Adenotyles alliariae* (alpendost). These plants are consumed in herbal preparations, in breads made with grains that are contaminated with pyrrolizidine-containing weeds ("bread poisoning"), and in teas. For example, *Senecio* and *Crotalaria*, which are used to make "bush tea" in Jamaica, have been associated with hepatotoxicity. Less frequently, contaminated animal meat, milk, or honey from exposed animals or bees may be the source of exposure.

Pyrrolizidine alkaloids are heterocyclic compounds that act as alkylating agents and are activated in the liver. Activation by cytochrome P-450 and mixed-function oxidase systems forms reactive pyrrolic metabolites that alkylate proteins and DNA, thereby inhibiting protein and nucleic acid synthesis. The metabolites can also bind to glutathione, resulting in glutathione depletion. Toxicity results from a hepatic sinusoidal obstruction syndrome that presents as hepatic venoocclusive disease, hepatomegaly, cirrhosis, and Budd-Chiari syndrome, which is characterized by obstruction of the trunk or large branches of the hepatic vein.[49,122,275,278,281,309]

Young patients seem more susceptible than adults. Ingestion of 10 mg of pyrrolizidine alkaloid is probably enough to produce acute or chronic venoocclusive disease. Venoocclusive liver disease is characterized by nonthrombotic occlusion of the central veins of hepatic lobules. Histologic liver findings include central vein dilation, sinusoidal congestion, centrilobular necrosis, and fibrosis. Clinical evidence of intrahepatic portal hypertension may include painful hepatomegaly, ascites, weight gain, and jaundice. Hepatic failure and death may ensue. Neonatal death secondary to hepatotoxicity has been reported after intrauterine exposure to pyrrolizidine alkaloids from an herbal preparation. Neonatal ascites, skin edema, hepatomegaly, and anemia were noted. Elevated LFTs and bilirubin, as well as hyponatremia, may be seen. Occasionally, laparoscopic liver biopsy and hepatic and portal decompression are helpful in diagnosis and treatment, respectively. Treatment, including albumin infusions, diuretics, and therapeutic paracentesis, is supportive. *N*-acetylcysteine may reduce toxicity. Defibrotide, which has been used to treat venoocclusive liver disease of other etiology, may theoretically be useful. Cirrhosis and portal hypertension may be persistent.*

Kava Kava

Piper methysticum (kava kava) is used recreationally and medicinally in Polynesia and Micronesia. Traditionally, kava kava extracts are prepared from kava kava roots macerated with water or coconut milk. Kava kava is associated with yellowing of the skin and reddening of the eyes, termed *kava dermopathy*, and may be hepatotoxic.[49,121,207] More recent studies question the hepatotoxicity of kava kava. Some suggest that a contaminant, rather than *P. methysticum*, may be the culprit.[323]

---

*References 29, 49, 70, 122, 275, 278, 309, 310, 314, 356.

Greater Celandine

Chelidonium majus (greater celandine) is hepatotoxic. Patients are generally exposed through herbal use. Patients generally present with jaundice and elevated aminotransferases (transaminases), consistent with cholestatic hepatitis. Seizures may occur. The hepatotoxicity appears to be an idiosyncratic reaction.[49,270,321]

Black Cohosh

Cimicifuga racemosa (black cohosh), not to be confused with *Caulophyllum thalictroides* (blue cohosh), is hepatotoxic and produces an idiosyncratic hepatitis.[104] Exposure tends to be secondary to herbal use. It produces hepatonecrosis. Patients present with constitutional symptoms, jaundice, right-upper-quadrant abdominal pain, and elevated liver enzymes. Liver biopsy has revealed liver necrosis, with evidence of oxidative damage and protein adducts that may provoke an autoimmune response. Patients can make a full recovery.[104]

Coffee Senna

Cassia occidentalis (coffee senna, negro coffee, coffee weed, kasondi) ingestion is associated with hepatic failure, myopathy, and encephalopathy, with a high fatality rate. Young children may eat the beans and have fatal outcomes. Patients may present with fever, GI distress, lethargy, and abnormal behaviors (irritable, violent, self-mutilating). Physical examination may reveal hepatomegaly. Laboratory studies reveal elevated liver enzymes and coagulopathy. Histopathology may reveal myodegeneration of the skeletal muscle and fatty change with centrilobular necrosis of the liver.[237]

Other hepatotoxic plants include chaparral (*Larrea tridentate*, also known as the creosote bush or greasewood), aloe (*Aloe barbadenis miller*), germander (*Teucrium polium, T. chamaedrys*), senna, and mistletoe.[49,79,233,273,322] These are usually taken as herbal supplements. Chaparral contains the hepatotoxin nordihydroguaiaretic acid.[131] Plants that contain mitochondrial toxins (discussed later) may present with multiorgan failure, including liver failure.

RENAL TOXINS

SOLUBLE OXALATES

Soluble oxalates are found in rhubarb (*Rheum* spp., including *Rheum rhaponticum*) and sorrel (*Rumex* spp.) plants. Other plants containing oxalate include *Halogeton glomeratus* (saltlover), *Oxalis caerulea* (blue woodsorrel), *Oxalis corniculata* (creeping woodsorrel), *Portulaca oleracea* (common purslane), and *Tetragonia tetragonioides* (New Zealand spinach). Consumption of rhubarb leaves as a substitute for spinach resulted in several deaths in England during World War I. Soluble oxalates are rapidly absorbed by the GI tract. The oxalates may produce some corrosive effects on the GI tract, and mild toxicity may include only vomiting, diarrhea, and irritation of the oral and GI tracts. With more significant exposures, generalized disturbance of monovalent and divalent cation metabolism occurs. Serum ionized calcium levels may drop rapidly. Weakness, paresthesias, tetany, hyperreflexia, muscle twitches and cramps, hypotension, and seizures may develop. Acute renal failure may occur if calcium oxalate precipitates in urine and obstructs the renal tubules. Calcium oxalate crystals may be found in the myocardium and birefringent crystals in vascular walls.[27,110,288] The structures of oxalates follow:

$$
\begin{array}{ccc}
\text{COOH} & \text{COOK} & \text{COONa} \\
| & | & | \\
\text{COOH} & \text{COOH} & \text{COONa} \\
\text{Oxalic acid} & \text{Potassium oxalate} & \text{Sodium oxalate}
\end{array}
$$

Sodium bicarbonate lavage should be avoided because of the risk for sodium oxalate formation. IV calcium is recommended for tetany, prolonged QT interval, or low serum ionized calcium. Urine output should be maintained with generous fluid replacement to prevent deposition of calcium oxalate crystals in renal tubules. Of note, hemodialysis easily removes oxalate from the blood.[27]

OTHER NEPHROTOXINS

Aloe species contain aloins and aloinosides and can cause parenchymatous nephritis and acute renal failure. Initially, inflammation of the GI tract with bloody diarrhea is present, followed by fluid and electrolyte loss. Arthralgias and palpable purpura, followed by hematuria, proteinuria, renal failure, and death, were reported in a man who ingested juice extracted from four to five leaves of *Aloe vera* (*Aloe barbadenis*).[43,312]

Aristolocia clematitis (birthwart) contains aristolochic acid, which is nephrotoxic, producing interstitial nephropathy, called "aristolochic acid nephropathy." Recently, Balkan endemic nephropathy has been associated with *Aristolocia* seeds. Aristolochic acids are also carcinogenic. Wheat and other crops grown in close proximity to *Aristolocia* spp. are thought to take up aristolochic acids from the soil; there is concern of food crops becoming secondarily poisonous.[255,312]

Pithecolobium lobatum or *Archidendron jiringa* (djenkol bean, jering) has a sulfur-containing amino acid, djenkol acid. Djenkol beans resemble a flattened horse chestnut and are contained in large, dark-purple pods that grow on large trees. The beans are consumed intentionally as a delicacy in Indonesia, Malaysia, southern Thailand, and Myanmar. Poisoning is characterized by nausea, vomiting, spasmodic pain, hematuria, oliguria, and acute renal failure. A sulfurous odor may be noted on the breath and in the urine. Urine may contain needle-like crystals (djenkolic acid crystals). Animal studies and human renal biopsy results reveal acute tubular necrosis. Symptoms generally resolve with supportive care. Alkalinization of the urine may increase dissolution of djenkol crystals.[24,312]

Cleistanthus collinus (Vadisaaku, Oduvan, Oduvanthalai) is used as a suicidal and homicidal poison in India. All parts of the plant are toxic. Fresh leaves or extract of boiled leaves are generally consumed. *C. collinus* contains diphyllin glycosides, cleistanthins A and B, which are thought to be responsible for toxicity. The toxins inhibit proton pumps of the distal renal tubular cells. Toxicity is usually not evident until 3 to 4 days after ingestion. Distal renal tubular acidosis results, with urinary potassium wasting and metabolic acidosis. Renal failure may follow. The toxin antagonizes α-adrenergic receptors, causing hypotension. GI distress, altered mental status, dysrhythmias (bradycardia more often than tachycardia), hypotension, hypoxia, acute respiratory distress syndrome (ARDS), and muscle weakness are reported. Muscle weakness may manifest as dysarthria, dysphagia, ptosis, ocular palsies, and weak neck muscles leading to inability to hold up the head. Coagulopathy, elevated liver enzymes, elevated CPK, hypokalemia, hyponatremia, hyperchloremia, and urinary alkalosis are noted. Marked hypokalemia (<3 mEq/L) during hospitalization is associated with a worse prognosis. Treatment is supportive. Neostigmine and atropine have been advocated in case reports and animal studies. Animal studies indicate *N*-acetylcysteine may be beneficial. Mortality rates of 20% to 30% are reported, despite medical care. Death is usually caused by cardiac or respiratory failure.[21,32,80,230,317]

HEMATOPOIETIC TOXINS

PLANTS WITH ANTICOAGULANT PROPERTIES (LACTONE GLYCOSIDES)

Dipteryx odoratum (Dutch tonka bean) and *Coumarouna* (or *Dipteryx*) *oppositofolia* (English tonka bean) were among the first historically mentioned medical sources of coumarin. *Melilotus officinalis* (yellow sweet clover, yellow melilot, common melilot), *Asperula odorata,* and *Galium odoratum* (woodruff) contain significant quantities of coumarin. These coumarin-containing products have been consumed in teas. Yellow sweet clover poisoning is caused by dicumarol, a fungal metabolite produced from coumarin substrates in spoiling plants. Dicumarol interferes with synthesis of vitamin K–dependent coagulation factors, inducing coagulopathy. Generally, this has been a problem in livestock rather than humans.[186,272,278]

TOXINS THAT INHIBIT CELL DIVISION AND BONE MARROW

Colchicine

Colchicine toxicity can occur after ingestion of *Sandersonia aurantiaca* (Christmas-bells, Chinese lantern lily), *Gloriosa superba* (glory lily, flame lily), *Colchicum persicum*, and more often, *Colchicum autumnale*, all of the lily family. *C. autumnale* is commonly known as autumn crocus, wild saffron, meadow saffron, naked lady, naked boy, and son-before-the-father. It can be mistaken for an edible plant, such as leek, wild garlic, or bear's garlic (*Allium ursinum*). *C. autumnale* is found in Europe, North America, and Asia. All parts of the plant contain colchicine, an amine alkaloid, but the highest concentrations are found in the underground bulb. Colchicine binds selectively and reversibly to tubulin and prevents its polymerization into microtubules. This disrupts cell division, cell shape, mobility, and phagocytosis. Cells with the highest turnover rates, such as those of the GI mucosa and bone marrow, are affected most severely. Cell arrest in metaphase and abnormal nuclear morphology are seen at autopsy; the clumps of chromatin material seen in the nuclei are called colchicine bodies.[*]

Acute poisoning may occur after a latent period of several hours. Repeated ingestion of lower doses may have a latent period of days before onset of symptoms. Initial GI effects are severe abdominal pain, nausea, vomiting, diarrhea, and hemorrhagic gastroenteritis, which may result in electrolyte abnormalities, volume depletion, acidosis, shock, arrhythmias, and multiorgan failure. Muscular weakness and ascending paralysis may cause respiratory arrest, which may occur suddenly and with a clear sensorium. Respiratory arrest may be associated with pulmonary edema and cardiomegaly from hypertrophic myocytes. Patients may present comatose or convulsing. Myocardial toxicity, rhabdomyolysis, and pancreatitis have been reported. Initially, leukocytosis may be seen, but bone marrow depression with pancytopenia may follow, predisposing to hemorrhage and infection. Autopsy reveals hypocellular bone marrow. Autopsy may reveal diffuse vacuolization in the cytoplasma of hepatocytes and congestion of the liver, kidneys, spleen, lungs, and brain. Occasionally, hemorrhagic edema is seen. Isolated mitotic structures within the epithelium of the colon have been reported at autopsy. If a patient survives, it may take weeks to recover. Patients who survive severe toxicity may develop alopecia days to weeks after poisoning.[†]

Because of the severity of poisoning and frequent lethal outcomes after significant ingestion, aggressive decontamination should be considered. Colchicine-specific Fab antibody fragments have been used with success in France for management of acute poisoning with the drug form of colchicine, but this treatment is not commercially available. Therefore, treatment is symptomatic and supportive. Pulmonary function tests can be used to monitor respiration, assessing for fatigue and progressive ascending paralysis. Assisted ventilation is used as needed. Parenteral analgesics are given cautiously to relieve severe abdominal pain, because colchicine sensitizes patients to CNS depressants. Fluid and electrolyte replacement and occasionally blood component replacement and granulocyte colony-stimulating factor (G-CSF) may be necessary. Maintain adequate urine output and assess for infection.[11,17,46,48,101,126,151,165,350]

Podophyllum

Podophyllum peltatum is most commonly known as the mayapple but has also been called American mandrake. Because of this common name, it has been occasionally confused with true mandrake (*Mandragora officinarum*), an unrelated plant with anticholinergic properties. Toxicity from *P. peltatum* exposure is caused by the glucoside podophyllotoxin. *Dysosma pleiantha* also contains podophyllotoxin.[203] Acute toxicity after ingestion of *P. peltatum* may occur after a latent period of several hours, manifested by GI distress and associated hypovolemia. Nervous

---

*References 11, 46, 48, 82, 101, 123, 126, 172, 178, 203, 287, 312, 350.
†References 11, 46, 48, 82, 101, 109, 151, 165, 172, 178, 203, 287, 312, 350.

system effects (confusion, delirium, coma, peripheral neuropathy), bone marrow depression, and multiorgan failure may follow as a result of the antimitotic effect of podophyllotoxin. Treatment is similar to that for colchicine poisoning.[117]

PLANTS THAT INDUCE HEMOLYSIS

Fava Beans

Fava beans (*Vicia faba*) contain vicine and convicine, two metabolically inactive glycones that may be cleaved by β-glycosidase to produce toxins such as divicine and isouramil. Divicine, isouramil, and convicine are thought to be the primary toxins that account for the oxidative stress and hemolytic crisis seen in patients deficient in glucose-6-phosphate dehydrogenase (G6PD) who consume fava beans. Methemoglobinemia may occur. Favism has been reported in infants who ingest breast milk from mothers who have recently ingested fava beans and in fetuses of mothers who consumed fava beans. Clinically, favism is characterized by hemoglobinuria, anemia, and jaundice, secondary to hemolysis. Patients may present with fever, cyanosis, malaise, weakness, lethargy, nausea, vomiting, headache, and lumbar or abdominal pain. When methemoglobinemia occurs, cyanosis may be absent due to severe anemia from hemolysis. Levels of carboxyhemoglobin, a byproduct of hemolysis, may rise. Renal failure may ensue, secondary to hemolysis. With methemoglobinemia, patients with hypoxia, as determined by pulse oximetry, may appear unresponsive to supplemental oxygen. Methemoglobinemia causes unreliable and erroneous pulse oximeter readings. Arterial blood gas determination using multiwavelength co-oximetry is reliable and will generally reveal normal oxygen tension in the patient with methemoglobinemia. Supportive care is the mainstay of treatment. Occasionally, blood transfusions, exchange transfusions, and hemodialysis are needed. Remember that methylene blue treatment of methemoglobinemia may induce hemolysis in patients with G6PD deficiency; therefore, transfusion is preferable, when needed.[75,147,153,197]

ENDOCRINE AND METABOLIC TOXINS

PLANTS THAT INTERFERE WITH STEROID METABOLISM

Licorice

Licorice use predates the Babylonian and Egyptian empires. Its genus name, *Glycyrrhiza,* is derived from the Greek word for "sweet root." Adverse effects with chronic ingestion of *Glycyrrhiza glabra* (natural licorice) result from altered steroid metabolism. *G. glabra* contains glycyrrhizic acid, which is converted to 18-β-glycyrrhetinic acid in the GI tract. Both acids inhibit 11-β-hydroxysteroid dehydrogenase, an enzyme essential to in vivo conversion of cortisol to cortisone. Excessive local cortisol binds to and activates mineralocorticoid receptors in the kidneys, producing a hypermineralocorticoid syndrome, characterized by water and sodium retention with potassium excretion. Signs and symptoms of chronic ingestion include hypertension, edema, hypokalemia, metabolic alkalosis, headache, paresthesias, weakness, paralysis, tetany, and muscle cramps. Myopathy, myoglobinuria, and rarely thrombocytopenia have been reported. Heart failure, arrhythmias (e.g., torsades de pointes, ventricular fibrillation), and cardiac arrest have been attributed to licorice root ingestion.

Treatment consists of discontinuing exposure to licorice, maintaining good urine output, and alkalinizing the urine of patients with rhabdomyolysis. Occasionally, potassium-sparing diuretics (e.g., triamterene, spironolactone) are useful. Patients with torsades de pointes may respond to magnesium and potassium infusions.[30,59,105,109,139,167,214,312]

PLANTS WITH MITOCHONDRIAL TOXINS

Ackee Fruit

Blighia sapida trees, or ackee (akee) fruit trees, are indigenous to West Africa and prevalent in the West Indies, Central America, and southern Florida. Unripe ackee fruit has a closed yellow aril that is toxic. Ripe ackee fruit, with a spontaneously opened red aril, is

nontoxic. The seeds contain hypoglycin B and are toxic regardless of the maturation of the aril. Unripe ackee fruit contains hypoglycin A, or L(R,S)-2-amino-3-methylenecyclopropylproprionic acid, a water-soluble amino acid that is converted to methylenecyclopropylacetyl-coenzyme A in vivo. Both compounds are hypoglycemic agents; the second is a suicide inhibitor of β-oxidation of fatty acids. Inhibition of fatty acid metabolism results in microvesicular steatosis of the liver, hyperammonemia, metabolic acidosis, and hypoglycemia. Laboratory and histopathologic findings are indistinguishable from those of Reye's syndrome, but urine shows increased concentrations of glutaric and ethylmalonic acids after hypoglycin A exposure.[28,170,212,298]

Ackee fruit constitutes a traditional Jamaican breakfast and has been associated with Jamaican vomiting sickness. Ingestion of unripe ackee fruit caused an outbreak epidemic of fatal encephalopathy in West Africa, primarily affecting children ages 2 to 6 years, who experienced vomiting, hypotonia, convulsions, and coma. All children died within 48 hours of the onset of vomiting. Autopsy revealed massive liver steatosis and severe hypoglycemia. Urine concentrations of dicarboxylic acids were elevated. Similarly, an epidemic of more than 100 cases occurred in Haiti, associated with vomiting, abdominal pain, loss of consciousness, convulsions, and many deaths. Hypoglycemia was noted. The carnitine derivatives octanoylcarnitine and hexanoylcarnitine were noted in the urine, confirming exposure to hypoglycin. Fatal ackee fruit poisoning is more common in children than in adults. Adults are more likely to present with self-resolving cholestatic jaundice.[170,212,227,298,299]

Treatment is largely supportive and consists of securing an airway and administering IV fluids and dextrose. Before hypoglycemia was recognized, mortality rates of symptomatic unripe ackee fruit exposure approached 80%. Frequent glucose and electrolyte measurements with appropriate replacement are essential. Seizures are treated with benzodiazepines and barbiturates, remembering that serum glucose should be assessed and hypoglycemia treated in all seizing patients. Theoretically, riboflavin, clofibrate, glycine, methylene blue, and L-carnitine may be beneficial, although their efficacy is not established. Carnitine may facilitate transport of fatty acids into mitochondria and has been used for other toxins (e.g., valproate) that inhibit β-oxidation of fatty acids.[28,188,298,299]

Wild Yams

Dioscorea species contain dioscorines and dioscines. They are tuberous plants, commonly known as yams, used as a staple food in Africa and Asia. The tubers are usually detoxified in running water, soaking in salt water, boiling for several hours, squeezing out the juice, and roasting. The nondetoxified plant has been used in homicide, suicide, and hunting. CNS irritability with seizures, liver failure, and renal failure are seen. Hypoglycemia is reported.[312]

Cocklebur

Cocklebur (*Xanthium strumarium* and *X. spinosum*) has worldwide distribution and can be found along riverbanks, beaches, and lake shores. The stem is angled with red or black spots. The fruit is hard, brown, and woody; it contains two seeds that taste like sunflower seeds. The seeds and seedlings contain carboxyatractyloside, a sulfonated diterpenoid glycoside. This toxin inhibits oxidative phosphorylation and translocation of adenosine diphosphate (ADP) and ATP across mitochondrial membranes. Carboxyatractyloside is an analog of atractyloside, which is found in *Callilepis laureola* (ox-eye daisy) and *Atractylis gummifera* (bird-lime, blue thistle), discussed next. Drying of seeds does not diminish toxicity.

Patients present with acute abdominal pain, nausea, vomiting, diaphoresis, palpitations, drowsiness, and dyspnea, followed by respiratory depression. With severe poisoning, seizures, coma, and death may occur. Seizures may be repetitive, frequent, and difficult to treat. Patients may appear pale or with icterus and may be clammy, without pyrexia. Hepatomegaly and rhabdomyolysis may be noted. Laboratory findings may reveal elevated liver enzymes, elevated blood urea nitrogen and creatinine, hyponatremia, transient hyperglycemia followed by marked hypoglycemia, elevated CPK and CPK-MB, metabolic acidosis, and evidence of a consumption coagulopathy (diminished fibrinogen and prolonged prothrombin time). ECG may show ST-segment abnormalities. Death may occur within 2 days of ingestion. Autopsy findings include centrilobular hepatic necrosis, renal proximal tubular necrosis, microvascular hemorrhage of the cerebrum and cerebellum, and leukocytic infiltrates in the muscles, pancreas, lungs, and myocardium. Increased vascular permeability is suspected.

Treatment is supportive. Phenylbutazone, a nonsteroidal anti-inflammatory drug that is generally unavailable because of its toxicity, has been shown to reduce cytotoxic effects of carboxyatractyloside in rats.[311,332]

Bird-Lime/Blue Thistle

Atractylis gummifera (bird-lime, blue thistle) is found in North Africa and the Mediterranean region. It has a sugary taste and has been confused with edible wild artichoke. *A. gummifera* contains two poisonous glucosides: atractyloside and carboxyatractyloside. The glucosides inhibit oxidative phosphorylation, block transport of ADP at the mitochondrial membrane, and block conversion of ADP to ATP. The toxins inhibit the actions of P-450 and b_5 cytochromes. Clinically, headache, abdominal pain, vomiting, hematemesis, diarrhea, and dizziness are followed by liver failure, associated with jaundice and hepatitis. Seizures, coma, dysrhythmias, and renal failure may be seen. Laboratory studies reveal hypoglycemia, metabolic acidosis, uremia, and hyperkalemia. Death is generally from multiorgan system failure. Autopsy reveals lesions, necrosis, and congestion of the liver and kidneys.[145,146,311,312,332]

Ox-Eye Daisy

Callilepis laureola (ox-eye daisy, wildemagriet, impila) has been used as a medicinal plant in South Africa. It is administered to pregnant women to facilitate childbirth, but approximately 1500 deaths are reported each year from its use. In Natal, autopsies have shown hepatic and renal tubular necrosis. *C. laureola* contains the poisonous glucosides atractyloside and carboxyatractyloside.[40,341,231] Toxicity and treatment are similar to those for cocklebur and bird-lime exposure, as discussed earlier. Mortality has been reported at 90% by 5 days. *N*-acetylcysteine may be beneficial in treatment of plant toxicity from atractyloside and carboxyatractyloside.[49]

KARAKA

Corynocarpus laevigatus (karaka, New Zealand laurel) is a tall evergreen tree native to New Zealand. It contains the toxin karakin, which is hydrolyzed to 3-nitropropionic acid (3-NP), a toxic metabolite. *Astragalus mise* (timber milkvetch) also contains 3-NP, as does sugar cane infected by fungus. 3-NP is structurally similar to succinic acid, a substrate in the tricarboxylic acid (Krebs) cycle. 3-NP is an irreversible, competitive inhibitor of succinate dehydrogenase, the enzyme that converts succinic acid into fumarate. This results in inhibition of the Krebs cycle, which reduces ATP synthesis and interferes with energy production. Succinic acid and lactic acid accumulate. Excitotoxic and neurodegenerative effects are characterized by hypokinesia, dystonia, and chorea. It is thought that ingestion of one karaka kernel may produce toxicity. Initially, nausea, vomiting, diarrhea, and abdominal pain occur. Additionally, headache, altered mental status, nystagmus, tremor, and dizziness may be seen. With severe toxicity, coma, seizures, and respiratory failure occur. There may be delayed neurodegenerative disease that resembles Huntington's disease, with dystonia, choreoathetoid movements, and dyskinesia. Magnetic resonance imaging can reveal hypodensity of the basal ganglia (putamen and globus pallidus). Treatment is supportive, including benzodiazepines and barbiturates for seizures. Levodopa does not appear helpful for the neurodegenerative sequelae.[304]

GIFBLAAR

Dichapetalum cymosum (gifblaar) contains fluoracetate, which inhibits the Krebs cycle, reducing cellular respiration and often resulting in death. This is primarily a concern for cattle in Africa.[40]

CYANOGENIC PLANTS

Glycosides that yield hydrocyanic acid on hydrolysis are known as cyanogenic glycosides (see Figure 65-1). Cyanogenic glycosides include amygdalin, prunasin, linamarin, lotaustralin, and triglochinin.[64] Amygdalin (D-mandelonitrile-β-D-glucoside-6-β-glucoside), abundant in the Rosaceae family, is the cyanogenic compound found in seeds of *Malus* spp. (apples) and pits of *Prunus* spp., including cherries, peaches, plums, and apricots. Deaths have been reported after ingestion of apricot, apple, cherry, and other fruit seeds.[289] Black or wild cherries (*Prunus serotina*) are considered the most dangerous. Poisonings have resulted from milkshakes that contained apricot kernels and from apricot kernels sold in health food stores as snacks.[318] Linseeds (*Linum usitatissimum*) and cycad seeds (*Cycas* spp.) are also cyanogenic.[64,280]

Bamboo (*Dendrocalamus aspe, Bambusa nutans, B. mulfiplex, Thyrsostachys siamensis*) produces cyanogenic glycosides, including taxiphyllin (2-[β-D-glucopyranosyloxy]-2-[4-hydroxyphenyl] acetonitrile). When bamboo shoots are cut, a glycosidase enzyme in the shoot hydrolyzes the glycoside and produces hydrogen cyanide gas, which can be inhaled and has proved fatal. Ingestion of bamboo does not appear to produce cyanide toxicity.[286]

Cassava (*Manihot esculenta*) contains the cyanogenic glucoside linamarin, which is rapidly hydrolyzed to acetone cyanohydrin, which breaks down into hydrogen cyanide and acetone.[106,282] Both chronic and acute cyanide toxicity have been reported after ingestion of cassava. Chronic ingestion produces an upper motor neuron disease known as Konzo, or tropical spastic paraparesis. Konzo occurs after recurrent consumption of improperly prepared cassava during droughts in areas where cassava is a staple food, such as in Africa. To remove cyanogens, roots should be soaked; however, when water is scarce, this soaking process is limited.[22,23,106]

Cyanide combines with and inhibits many enzymes. It possesses great affinity for the ferric iron in cytochrome oxidase of the electron transport chain, accounting for most of its toxicity (Figure 65-25). By combining with cytochrome oxidase, cyanide prevents electron transport, thereby preventing ATP production by oxidative phosphorylation. Metabolic acidosis ensues. Humans detoxify cyanide by transferring sulfane sulfur to cyanide to form thiocyanate. Numerous sulfur sources are most likely acted on by various sulfurtransferases to form the sulfane sulfur needed to convert cyanide to thiocyanate. Administration of exogenous sulfane sulfur, such as sodium thiosulfate, can greatly facilitate detoxification.[76]

Clinically, GI distress, bitter almond breath, CNS changes (agitation, anxiety, excitement, weakness, numbness, hypotonia, spasticity, coma, seizures), respiratory changes (hyperpnea, dyspnea, apnea, cyanosis), cardiovascular changes (tachycardia and hypertension followed by bradycardia and hypotension, heart block, ventricular arrhythmias, asystole), and metabolic changes (anion gap metabolic acidosis) are seen. Skin color may be pink or cyanotic, and the partial pressure of oxygen may be normal in cyanide poisoning. ECG may reveal T-on-R phenomenon as a result of progressive shortening of the ST segment. Multiorgan failure and death may occur.[76,203,282]

Treatment

Red blood cell or plasma cyanide levels can be determined; however, treatment should be initiated promptly, without confirmation of exposure, in patients with evidence of toxicity. Patients with cyanogenic glycoside poisoning may respond to treatment with 100% oxygen and cyanide antidote kits. The traditional antidote kit contains sodium nitrite (3% solution given intravenously on the basis of hemoglobin and weight; generally, 300 mg in a nonanemic adult), and sodium thiosulfate (12.5 g in an adult). Traditional cyanide antidote kits are designed to induce methemoglobinemia through nitrite exposure. Cyanide binds preferentially to the ferric ion of methemoglobin rather than to that of cytochrome oxidase in the electron transport chain. Forming methemoglobin limits inhibition of electron transport by cyanide and restores cellular respiration. Sodium thiosulfate in

$$(1) \quad \text{Cyt-Fe}^{3+} + \text{HCN} \rightleftharpoons \text{Cyt-FeCN}$$

(Cytochrome oxidase)   (Hydrocyanic acid)   (Cytochrome oxidase-cyanide complex)

$$(2) \quad \text{Hb-Fe}^{2+} + \text{NaNO}_2 \rightleftharpoons \text{Hb-Fe}^{3+}$$

(Hemoglobin)   (Nitrites)   (Methemoglobin)

$$(3) \quad \text{Hb-Fe}^{3+} + \text{Cyt-FeCN} \rightleftharpoons \text{Hb-FeCN} + \text{Cyt-Fe}^{3+}$$

(Methemoglobin)   (Cytochrome oxidase–cyanide complex)   (Cyanomethemoglobin)   (Cytochrome oxidase)

$$(4) \quad \text{Na}_2\text{S}_2\text{O}_3 + \text{CN} \underset{\text{SCN}^- - \text{Oxidase}}{\overset{\text{Rhodanese}}{\rightleftharpoons}} \text{SCN}^- + \text{Na}_2\text{SO}_3$$

(Sodium thiosulfate)   (Cyanide)   (Thiocyanate)   (Sodium sulfate)

FIGURE 65-25 Principal steps in hydrocyanic acid poisoning and detoxification. *1*, Breakdown of cellular respiration resulting from the binding of cyanide to cytochrome oxidase. *2*, Conversion of the ferrous (Fe^{2+}) form of hemoglobin to the ferric (Fe^{3+}) form (methemoglobin) via nitrites. *3*, Preferential binding of cyanide to methemoglobin, liberating cytochrome oxidase and restoring cellular respiration. *4*, Providing exogenous thiosulfate to aid in formation of the less toxic thiocyanate via various sulfurtransferases, such as rhodanese. Thiocyanate is then excreted from the body. The reaction is slowly reversible via the enzyme thiocyanate oxidase, and rebound may occur.

the cyanide kit provides exogenous sulfane sulfur groups that bind to cyanide and form thiocyanate, which is much less toxic than cyanide. More recently available in the United States, hydroxocobalamin (Cyanokit) is also used to treat cyanide toxicity. Cyanide combines with hydroxocobalamin to form cyanocobalamin, which is excreted in the urine and bile. Sodium thiosulfate may be given with hydroxocobalamin, with theoretical synergistic therapeutic effects. Supportive care, including mechanical ventilation, IV fluids, and vasopressors, may also be used.[76,282,318]

REPRODUCTIVE TOXINS

Some plants that have been used as abortifacients are shown in Table 65-3.[34,73,101,224,231,352] Generally, a plant is not feticidal unless it produces severe toxicity or fatality in the mother.

Human teratogenesis from plant exposure is difficult to assess, because humans rarely chronically ingest toxic plants.

Discussion of teratogenesis in livestock can be found in other sources.[248]

OTHER TOXINS

OILS

Irritant oils, including various mustards (*Brassica* spp), horseradish (*Amoracia lapathifolia*), and protoanemonin from the buttercup family (Ranunculaceae), induce gastroenteritis. Essential oils, often found in combination with resins (oleoresins), are extracted commercially for use as rubefacients, salves, and liniments. Essential oils are summarized in Table 65-4.

ACKNOWLEDGMENT

I am grateful for having known Donald Kunkel, an exceptionally kind mentor, who guided me in the early editions of this chapter.

TABLE 65-3 Abortifacient Plants

Common Name	Genus	Species	Toxicity
Blue cohosh (or squaw root)	*Caulophyllum*	*thalictroides*	Nicotinic syndrome
Bryony	*Bryonia*	*dioica*	Nephrotoxic
Glory lily (or flame lily)	*Gloriosa*	*superba*	Toxins that inhibit cell division and bone marrow
Green hellebore	*Helleborus*	*viridis*	Cardiotoxic
Pennyroyal	*Mentha*	*pulegium*	Hepatotoxic
Nutmeg	*Myristica*	*fragrans*	Neurotoxic (hallucinogenic)
Potato tree	*Solanum*	*erianthum*	Neurotoxic (anticholinergic)
Ruda (or fringed rue)	*Ruta*	*chalepensis*	Multiorgan toxicity
Syrian rue (or espand)	*Peganum*	*harmala*	Neurotoxic (convulsant, paralytic, hallucinogenic)
Wild wisteria	*Securidaca*	*longepedunculata*	Neurotoxic (convulsant)
Yellow oleander	*Thevetia* or *Cascabela*	*peruviana* *thevetia*	Cardiotoxic

TABLE 65-4 Toxic Essential Oils

Common Name Of Oil	Genus and Species of Plant from Which Oil Is Derived	Toxin	Toxic Effect
Camphor[66]	*Cinnamomum camphora, Dryobalanops aromaticum, Ocotea usambarensis, Ocimum kilimandscharicum,* and others	Camphor	GI distress, headache, tremor, twitching, convulsions (including status epilepticus), delirium, coma, death
Clove[102]	*Syzygium aromaticum*	Eugenol	Hepatic failure
Eucalyptus[14,83,325]	*Eucalyptus globulus*	1,8-Cineole (eucalyptol)	Diaphoresis, CNS depression (hyporeflexia, weakness, ataxia, slurred speech, agitation, confusion, coma, respiratory depression, convulsions), GI upset (vomiting, diarrhea, abdominal pain), respiratory effects (bronchospasm, pneumonitis, pulmonary edema), metabolic acidosis, rhabdomyolysis, hypotension, death
Lavender[192]	*Lavandula* spp.	Linalool, linalyl acetate, lavandulyl acetate, terpinen-4-ol	CNS depression, confusion
Pennyroyal[13,18,319]	*Hedeoma pulegioides, Mentha pulegium*	Pulegone (oxidized to the toxic metabolite, menthofuran)	Hepatic failure, altered mental status, seizures, cerebral edema, multiorgan failure, shock, death
Pine[210]	*Pinus sylvestris* and other pine trees	1-α-Terpineol (damage also induced by lipophilic hydrocarbons)	Respiratory irritation (hemorrhagic and necrotic lungs), CNS depression
Sage[143]	*Salvia officinalis*	Thujone, camphor, cineole	Seizures
Wintergreen[41,159]	*Gaultheria procumbens*	Methyl salicylate	Salicylate poisoning (metabolic acidosis, respiratory alkalosis, CNS excitation, CNS depression, hyperthermia), laryngeal edema
Wormwood[35,91,160,244,316] (in the green liqueur, absinthe)	*Artemisia absinthium, A. pontica*	α- and β-Thujone	Psychoanaleptic effects, vomiting, neurotoxicity (vertigo, delirium, hallucinations, convulsions, coma), respiratory failure, death

CNS, Central nervous system; *GI,* gastrointestinal.

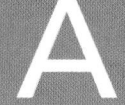

APPENDIX A

Common Toxic Plants

Common Name	Genus	Species	Toxin	Toxic Effect
Ackee (akee)	*Blighia*	*sapida*	Hypoglycin	Hypoglycemic
Aconite	*Aconitum*	spp.	Aconitine, mesaconitine, hypaconitine, yunaconitine	Cardiotoxic
Angel's trumpet	*Brugmansia*	*suaveolens*	Atropine, hyoscyamine, hyoscine	Anticholinergic
Apple seeds	*Malus*	spp.	Cyanogenic glycosides	Cyanogenic
Apricot pits	*Prunus*	spp.	Cyanogenic glycosides	Cyanogenic
Autumn crocus	*Colchium*	*autumnale*	Colchicine	Hematopoietic
Azalea (see Rhododendron)				
Belladonna (see Deadly nightshade)				
Bellyache bush	*Jatropha*	*gossypiifolia*	Curcin	Protein synthesis inhibition
Betel nut	*Areca*	*catechu*	Arecoline, arecaine	Nicotinic
Birthwart	*Aristolocia*	*clematitis*	Aristolochic acids	Nephrotoxic
Black cherry	*Prunus*	*serotina*	Cyanogenic glycoside	Cyanogenic

1460

Common Name	Genus	Species	Toxin	Toxic Effect
Black locust	*Robinia*	*pseudoacacia*	Robin, robitin (glycoside)	Protein synthesis inhibition
Black snake root (see Death camas)				
Blue cohosh	*Caulophyllum*	*thalictroides*	*n*-Methylcytisine, saponins	Nicotinic
Bushman poison bush (boesmansgif)	*Acokanthera*	*oppositifolia*	Cardenolides	Cardiotoxic
Carolina jessamine (aka yellow jessamine)	*Gelsemium*	*sempervirens*	Gelsemine, sempervirine	Psychoactive
Cassava (aka, manioc, tapioca)	*Manihot*	*esculenta*	Cyanogenic glycoside	Cyanogenic
Castor bean	*Ricinus*	*communis*	Ricin	Protein synthesis inhibition
Cherry	*Prunus*	spp.	Cyanogenic glycoside	Cyanogenic
Chinaberry tree	*Melia*	*azedarach*	Meliatoxin	GI irritant
Christmas rose	*Helleborus*	*niger*	Hellebrin, helleborin, helleborein	Cardiotoxic
Cobra lily	*Arisaema*	*amurense*	Calcium oxalate	Oral irritant
Coca	*Erythroxylon*	*coca*	Ecogonine	Psychoactive
Cocklebur	*Xanthium*	*strumarium*	Carboxyatractyloside	Metabolic toxin
Coral plant	*Jatropha*	*multifida*	Curcin	Protein synthesis inhibition
Corkwood tree	*Duboisia*	*myoporoides*	Tropane alkaloids	Anticholinergic
Daphne	*Daphne*	*mezereum*	Dihydroxycoumarin, diterpene mezerein	Coumarin glycosides
Day jessamine	*Cestrum*	*diurnum*	Tropane alkaloids	Anticholinergic
Deadly nightshade	*Atropa*	*belladonna*	Atropine	Anticholinergic
Death camas (aka black snakeroot)	*Zigadenus*	spp.	Zygacine, zygadenine	Cardiotoxic
Devil's trumpet (aka hairy thorn apple)	*Datura*	*metel*	Atropine, hyoscyamine, hyoscine	Anticholinergic
Dieffenbachia (aka dumb cane)	*Dieffenbachia*	spp.	Oxalate, asparagine	Oral irritant
Djenkol tree	*Archidendron* *Pithecolobium*	*jiringa* *lobatum*	Djenkol acid (amino acid)	Nephrotoxic
Elephant ear	*Colocasia*	*antiquorum*	Oxalates	Oral irritant
English bean (see Fava bean)				
False hellebore (aka Indian poke)	*Veratrum*	spp.	Veratrin	Cardiotoxic
Fava bean	*Vicia*	*faba*		Hemolytic anemia in patients with glucose-6-phosphate deficiency
Fishberry (or Levant nut)	*Anamirta*	*cocculus*	Picrotoxin	Convulsant
Foxglove	*Digitalis*	*purpurea*	Digitoxin, gitaloxin, gitoxin	Cardiotoxic
Glory lily	*Gloriosa*	*superba*	Colchicine-like alkaloids	Hematopoietic toxicity
Golden chain (aka golden rain)	*Laburnum*	*anagyroides*	Cytisine	Nicotinic
Horse bean (see Fava bean)				
Horse chestnut	*Aesculus*	spp.	Aesculin	Coumarin glycosides
Hyacinth bean	*Dolichos*	*lablab*	Cyanogenic glycosides	Cyanogenic
Hydrangea	*Hydrangea*	spp.	Cyanogenic glycosides	Cyanogenic
Inkberry (see Pokeweed)				
Jequirity pea (aka rosary pea, precatory bean)	*Abrus*	*precatorius*	Abrin	Protein synthesis inhibition
Jessamine (see Carolina jessamine)				
Jessamines	*Cestrum*	spp.	Tropane alkaloids	Anticholinergic
Jetbead	*Rhodotypos*	*tetrapetala*	Cyanogenic glycosides	Cyanogenic
Jimsonweed	*Datura*	*stramonium*	Atropine, hyoscyamine, hyoscine	Anticholinergic
Jonquil (see Daffodil)				
Kentucky coffee tree	*Gymnocladus*	*dioica*	Cytisine	Nicotinic
Larkspur	*Delphinium*	spp.	Aconitine-like (methyllycaconitine, lycoctonine)	Cardiotoxic Neurotoxic (curare-like in livestock)
Lily of the valley	*Convallaria*	*majalis*	Convallotoxin, convallarin, convallamarin	Cardiotoxic

Continued

Common Name	Genus	Species	Toxin	Toxic Effect
Lobelia (aka Indian tobacco)	Lobelia	spp.	Lobelamine, lobeline	Nicotinic
Mandrake (aka Satan's apple)	Mandragora	officinarum	Hyoscyamine, scopolamine	Anticholinergic
Marijuana	Cannabis	sativa	Tetrahydrocannabinol	Psychoactive
Mayapple	Podophyllum	peltatum	Podophyllotoxin	Hematopoietic
Mescal bean	Sophora	secundiflora	Cytisine	Psychoactive
(Common) Milkweed	Asclepias	syriaca	Asclepiadin	Cardiotoxic
Monkshood (aka aconite, wolfsbane)	Aconitum	spp.	Aconitine	Cardiotoxic and neurotoxic
Morning glory	Ipomoea	violacea	(+)-Lysergic acid amide	Psychoactive
Mountain laurel	Kalmia	latifolia	Andromedotoxin, arbutin, grayanotoxins	Cardiotoxic
Narcissus (see Jonquil)				
Night-blooming jasmine	Cestrum	spp.	Tropane alkaloids	Anticholinergic
Nutmeg	Myristica	fragrans	Myristicin	Psychoactive
Oleander	Nerium	oleander	Oleandrin, oleandroside, nevioside	Cardiotoxic
Oduvan(thalai)	Cleistanthus	collinus	Cleistanthin A and B	Nephrotoxic
Peach pits	Prunus	spp.	Cyanogenic glycosides	Cyanogenic
Peyote	Lophophora	williamsii	Mescaline, lophophorine	Psychoactive
Philodendron	Philodendron	spp.	Oxalate	Oral irritant
Physic nut (aka purging nut)	Jatropha	curcas	Curcin	Protein synthesis inhibition
Pigeonberry (see Pokeweed)				
Plum pit	Prunus	spp.	Cyanogenic glycosides	Cyanogenic
Poison hemlock	Conium	maculatum	Coniine, Coniceine	Nicotinic
Pokeweed	Phytolacca	americana	Triterpene saponins	GI irritant and hematopoietic
Potato tree	Solanum	erianthum	Tropane alkaloids	Anticholinergic
Purging nut (see Physic nut)				
Rattlepod (aka scarlet, wisteria tree)	Sesbania	spp.	Pyrrolizidine alkaloids	Hepatotoxic
Rhododendron (aka laurel, azalea)	Rhododendron	spp.	Grayanotoxins	Cardiotoxic
Rhubarb	Rheum	rhabarbarum	Oxalates	Nephrotoxic
San Pedro cactus	Trichocereus	pachanoi	Mescaline, lophophorine, and 3,4-dimethoxyphenethylamine	Psychoactive
Sea mango	Cerbera	manghas	Cerberoside, cerberin, and odollin	Cardiotoxic
Senecio (aka groundsel)	Senecio	longilobus	Pyrrolizidine alkaloids	Hepatotoxic
Squill	Urginea	maritima	Cardiac glycosides	Cardiotoxic
Star of Bethlehem	Ornithogalum	umbellatum	Cardiac glycosides, amine alkaloids	Cardiotoxic
Star fruit	Averrhoa	carambola	Caramboxin (phenylalanine-like)	Convulsant
Strawberry bush (see Burning bush)				
Suicide tree (or Pong-pong tree)	Cerbera	odollam	Cerberin	Cardiotoxic
Texas mountain laurel (see mescal bean)				
Tobacco	Nicotiana	tabacum	Nicotine	Nicotinic
Tree tobacco	Nicotiana	glauca	Anabasine	Nicotinic
Trumpet lily	Datura	arborea	Atropine, hyoscyamine, hyoscine	Anticholinergic
Tutu	Coriaria	arborea	Tutin (picrotoxin-like)	Convulsant
Water hemlock	Cicuta	maculata	Cicutoxin	Convulsant
Wild cherry (see Black cherry)				
Woody nightshade (see Nightshade)				
Yellow jessamine (see Carolina jessamine)				
Yellow oleander (aka be still tree, lucky nut tree)	Thevetia or Cascabela	peruviana thevetia	Thevetin, thevetoxin	Cardiotoxic
Yew	Taxus	spp.	Taxine	Cardiotoxic

APPENDIX B

Nontoxic Plants

African violet (*Saintpaulia ionantha*)
Air plant (*Kalanchoe pinnata*)
Aluminum plant (*Pilea cadierei*)
Aralia, false (*Dizygotheca elegantissima*)
Aralia, Japanese (*Fatsia japonica*)
Asparagus fern (*Asparagus plumosus*), berry
Baby's breath (*Gypsophilia paniculata*)
Baby's tears (*Helxine* [or *Soleirolia*] *soleirolii*)
Begonia (*Begonia rex*)
Bird of paradise* (*Strelitzia reginae*)
Bird's nest fern (*Asplenium nidus*)
Boston fern (*Nephrolepsis exaltata bostoniensis*)
Bromeliad family
California poppy (*Eschscholzia californica*)
Camellia (*Camellia japonica*)
Christmas cactus (*Schlumbergera bridgesii*)
Coffee tree (*Coffea arabica*)
Coleus
Coral berry* (*Aechamea fulgens, Ardisia crispa*)
Cornstalk plant (*Dracaena fragrans*)
Crape myrtle (*Lagerstromea indica*)
Creeping Charlie* (*Pilea nummularifolia*)
Crocus* (spring-blooming only)
Croton* (*Codiaeum variegatum*)
Dahlia
Dandelion (*Taraxacum officinale*)
Dogwood (*Cornus*)
Donkey's tail (*Sedum morganianum*)
Dragon tree (*Dracaena draco, Dracaena marginata*)
Easter cactus (*Schlumbergera bridgesii*)
Easter lily (*Lilium longiflorum*)
Echeveria: Mexican snowball, painted lady, plush plant
Emerald ripple (*Peperomia caperata*)
Fiddleleaf fig (*Ficus lyrata*)
Fig tree, weeping (*Ficus benjamina*)
Forget-me-not (*Myosotis alpestris, Myosotis sylvatica*)
Forsythia
Fuchsia
Gardenia
Geranium* (*Pelargonium*)
Gloxinia (*Sinningia speciosa*)
Grape ivy (*Cissus rhombifolia*)
Hawaiian ti plant (*Cordyline terminalis*)
Hawthorne (*Crataegus*), berry
Heavenly bamboo (*Nandina domestica*), berry
Hibiscus
Honeysuckle berry (*Lonicera*)
Ice plant
Impatiens walleriana
Jade plant (*Crassula argentea*)
Jasmine (*Jasminum rex*), Madagascar jasmine
Kalanchoe: maternity plant, monkey plant, panda bear plant
Lace plant, Madagascar (*Aponogeton senetralis*)
Lady, lady's slipper (*Cypripedium, Paphiopedilum*)
Lily of the Nile (*Agapanthus*)
Lipstick plant (*Aeschynanthus radicans*)
Maidenhair fern (*Adiantum*)
Marigold, African/American tall (*Tagetes*)
Moon cactus (*Gymnocalycium*)
Mother-in-law's tongue or snake plant (*Sansevieria trifasciata*)
Mother of pearls (*Grapetopetalum paraguayense*)
Nandina berry
Natal plum (*Carissa grandiflora*)
Norfolk Island pine (*Araucaria heterophylla*)
Old man cactus (*Cephalocereus senilis*)
Olive tree (*Olea europaea*)

Orchid (*Cattleya, Cymbidium, Oncidium*)
Oregon grape (*Mahonia aquifolium*)
Palm, bamboo (*Chamaedorea erumpeus*)
Pansy flower (*Viola*)
Paradise (*Howea* [or *Kentia*] *forsterana*)
Parlor (Chamaedorea [or Kentia] *elegans*)
Peanut cactus (*Chamaecereus sylvestri*)
Pellionia
Peony flower (*Paeonia*)
Peperomia
Petunia
Phlox
Piggyback plant (*Tolmiea menziesii*)
Pigmy date palm (*Phoenix roebelenii*)
Pocketbook (*Calceolaria herbeohybrida*)
Polka dot or freckle face plant (*Hypoestes sanguinolenta*)
Prayer plant (*Maranta leuconeura*)
Pussy willow (*Salix discolor*)
Pyracantha berry
Queen's tears (*Billbergia nutans*)
Rabbit's foot fern (*Davallia fejeensis*)
Rainbow plant (*Billbergia saundersii*)
Raphiolepsis
Rattlesnake plant (*Calathea insignis*)
Ribbon plant (*Dracaena sandriana*)
Rock rose (*Cistus*)
Rosary pearls (*Senecio rowleyanus*)
Rosary vine (*Ceropegia woodii*)
Roses (*Rosa*)
Rubber plant (*Ficus elastica*)
Schefflera plant (*Brassaia* [or *Schefflera*] *actinophylia*)
Sedum
Sensitive plant (*Mimosa pudica*)
Sentry (*Howea belmoreana*)
Silver heart (*Peperomia marmorata*)
Snake plant or mother-in-law's tongue (*Sansevieria trifasciata*)
Snapdragon (*Antirrhinum majus*)
Spider plant (*Anthericum, Chlorophytum comosum*)
Staghorn fern (*Platycerium bifurcatum*)
Starfish flower (*Stapelia*)
String of beads* (*Senecio rowleyanus, Senecio herreianus*)
String of hearts (*Ceropegia woodii*)
Swedish ivy (*Plectranthus australis*)
Sword fern (*Nephrolepsis cordifolia, Nephrolepsis exaltala*)
Tahitian bridal veil (*Gibasis geniculata, Tripogandra multiflora*)
Umbrella tree (*Schefflera actinophylla*)
Vagabond plant (*Vriesea*)
Velvet plant, purple (*Gynura aurantiaca*)
Venus fly trap (*Dionaea muscipula*)
Violet (*Viola*)
Wandering Jew (*Tradescantia albiflora*)
Wandering Jew—red and white (*Zebrina pendula*)
Wax plant (*Hoya exotica*)
Yucca
Zebra plant (*Aphelandre squarrosa*)
Zinnia

*This species has not been reported to cause illness, but other species may be toxic.

REFERENCES

Complete references used in this text are available online at expertconsult.inkling.com.

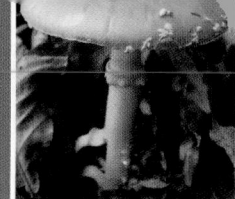

CHAPTER 66
Toxic Mushroom Ingestions

SANDRA M. SCHNEIDER AND TIMOTHY J. WIEGAND

> Had nature any outcast face? Could she a son condemn? Had nature an Iscariot?
> That mushroom—it is him. *Emily Dickinson*

Mushrooms are often considered the vermin of the vegetable world, likened to snakes, slugs, and worms. Some are regarded as mystical and others as delicacies. The locations of tasty morels are passed on from generation to generation, closely guarded from strangers. Each autumn and spring, foragers scour the woods for known delicacies and new ones untried. Some mushroom foragers search for "little brown mushrooms," not for their taste, but to evoke hallucinations.

Eating unidentified or misidentified species can be dangerous. In the vast majority of toxic ingestions (perhaps up to 95%), the mushroom was incorrectly identified. More than 40,000 species of fungi are currently described, with a few thousand new ones added each year. Only 100 species are toxic.[41]

The fungi kingdom contains molds, smuts, rusts, mildews, yeasts, and mushrooms, which are different from plants because they lack chlorophyll. *Yeasts* are single-cell organisms that divide using budding. *Mold* is any fungus that grows with thread-like connections and a fuzzy appearance. *Mildew, rust,* and *smut* are all fungi related to mushrooms and break down vegetable matter, leaving behind a white, red, or black powder, respectively. *Toadstool* is often used to describe toxic mushrooms. This chapter differentiates toxic mushrooms by their toxins and scientific names.

The body of a fungus is a dense network of branching filaments, or hyphae. The mushroom is the fruiting body of the fungus, containing the spores. The hyphae and mycelia generally occur in an underground network supporting the visible mushroom. Mushrooms often grow in large rings radiating from a central network of mycelia. In the past, these "fairy rings" were thought to have mystical influence (Figure 66-1). A fairy ring in northeast Oregon has been found to occupy an area over 10 km² (3.9 square miles). This ring is thought to be between 2000 and

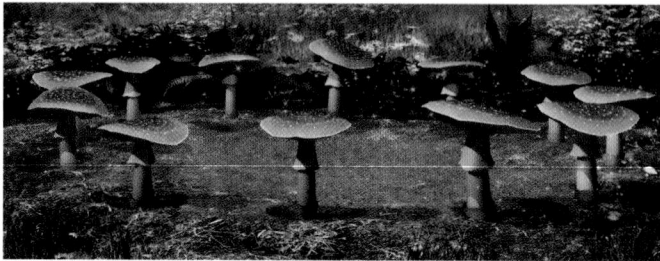

FIGURE 66-1 "Fairy ring" of mushrooms. (*Copyright iStockphoto.com/FairytaleDesign.*)

8000 years old, making it the oldest and largest single organism on the planet. Fungi are largely *saprophytic* (i.e., growing on decaying vegetable matter), involved with the decomposition of rotting materials, usually wood. They can also be *parasitic* (i.e., living on another living organism, injuring the host) or *symbiotic* (i.e., living together with each benefiting). Some emerge only after significant environmental changes, such as the large quantity of morels that may be found where a forest fire has recently occurred.

As a mushroom emerges from the ground, it is covered with a membrane or veil (Figure 66-2). As the mushroom grows (Figure 66-3), the membrane breaks, leaving residual marks known as *warts* on the cap of the mushroom (Figure 66-4). These warts may remain firmly attached to the mushroom or may remain as only residual spots, depending on the species of mushroom and environmental conditions. The emerging cap

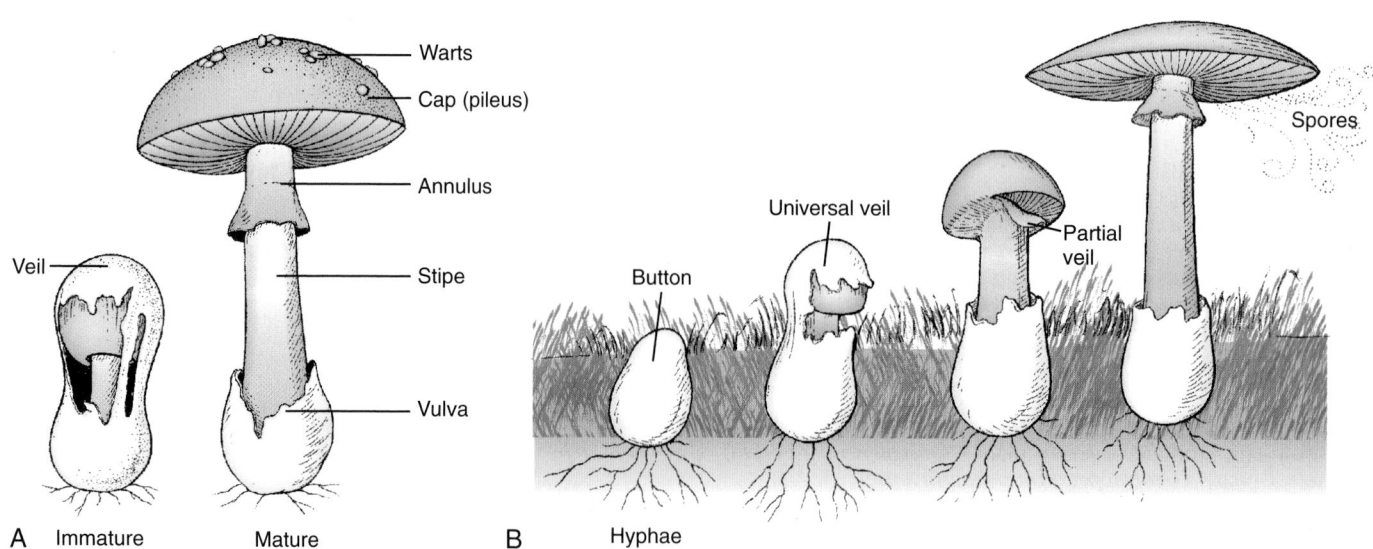

FIGURE 66-2 Structural characteristics (**A**) and life cycle (**B**) of mushrooms.

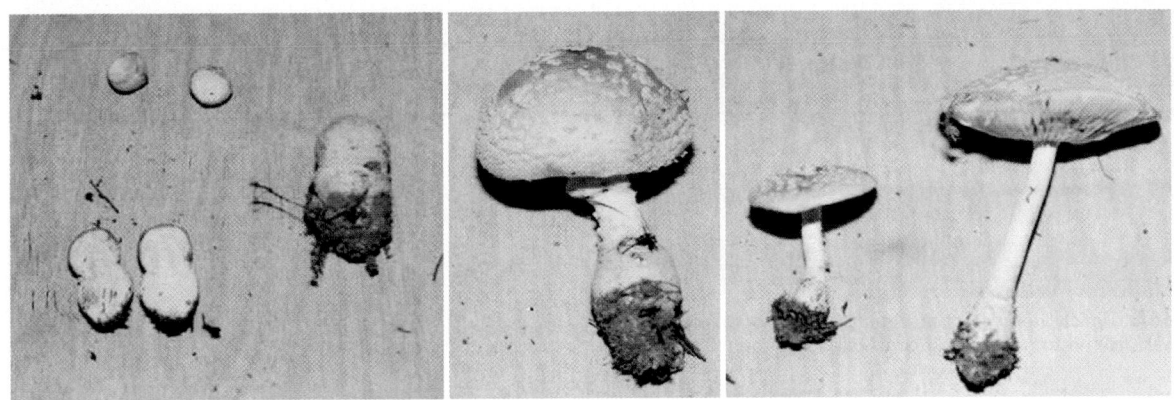

FIGURE 66-3 Growth of an *Amanita* species.

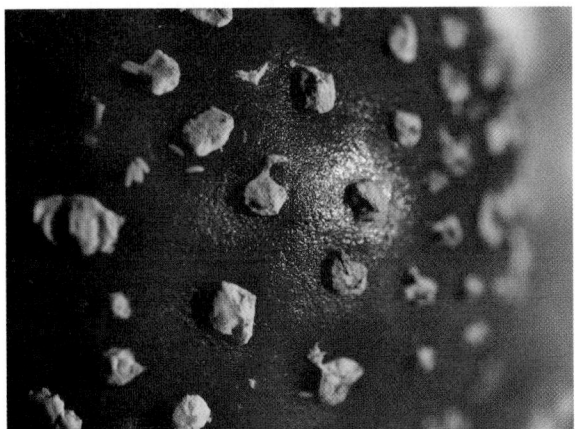

FIGURE 66-4 Warts on *Amanita muscaria*. (By Peter Rosbjerg from http://www.flickr.com. *Used with permission.*)

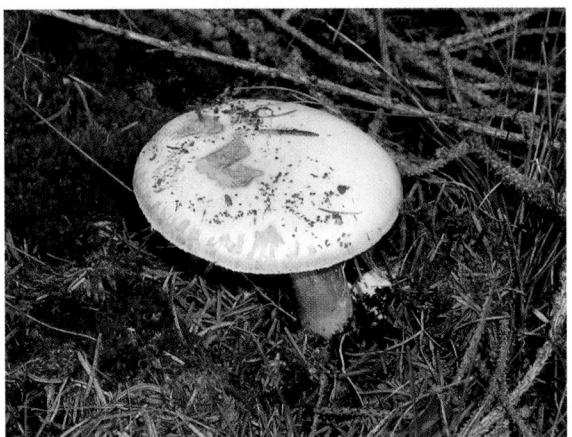

FIGURE 66-6 *Amanita phalloides*. (Grüner Knollenblätterpilz). (By Maja Dumat from http://www.flickr.com. *Used with permission.*)

takes on a shape consistent with the specific species, ranging from cylindrical to convex to funnel-shaped.

Gills located under the cap contain the spore-producing bodies. Some gills are covered with a second membrane or partial veil, which later pulls away to form an annulus, or ring, midway down the stalk of the mushroom. Gills may be attached firmly to the stalk, sometimes running down the stalk, or only to the cap itself (free gills) (Figure 66-5). Attachment of the gills is an important aid to identification of some poisonous mushrooms, such as *Amanita phalloides* (Figure 66-6).

The stalk (stipe) begins at the cap and ends either underground or in a cup (vulva) (Figure 66-7). A vulva at or just below ground level often is seen in a poisonous species. The stipe is generally located in the center of the cap and may or may not be tapered. The stipe of many poisonous species enlarges below the cap, ending in a bulb. The stipe may have a ringed membrane as evidence that the partial veil formerly protected the gills (Figure 66-8). Spores are produced by spore-forming bodies on the gills and expelled into the air after they mature.

Spores vary in size, color, and shape but are usually unicellular. They average 5 to 10 μm in diameter. Spores are useful in identifying mushroom species (Figure 66-9 and Box 66-1). They can be obtained by cutting the stipe of a fresh specimen close

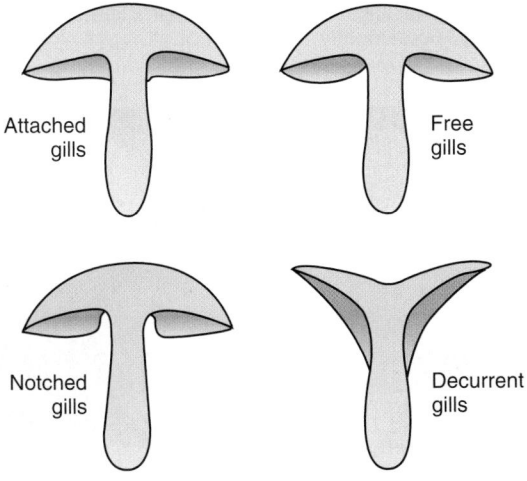

Attached gills

Free gills

Notched gills

Decurrent gills

FIGURE 66-5 Mushroom gill types.

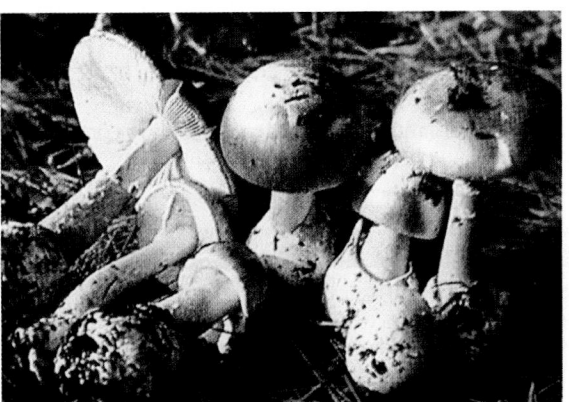

FIGURE 66-7 Death cap (*Amanita phalloides*).

1465

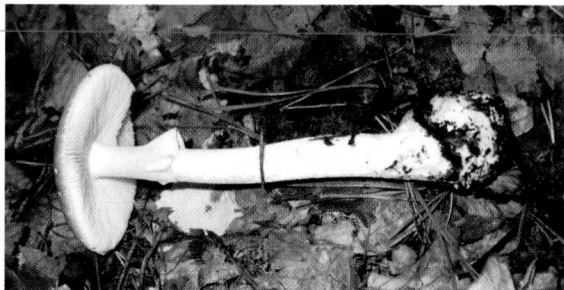

FIGURE 66-8 Typical features of an *Amanita* mushroom. *(By Tomasz Przechlewski from* http://www.flickr.com. *Used with permission.)*

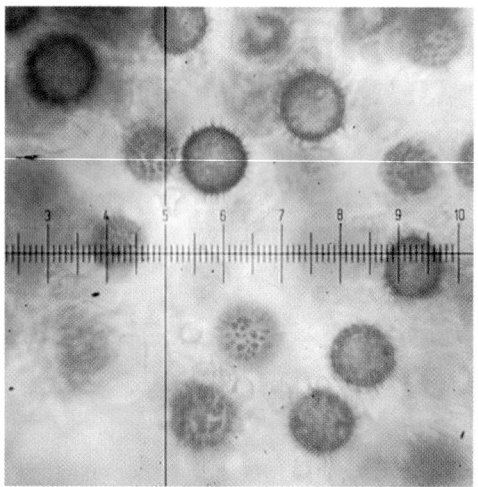

FIGURE 66-9 Spores from a mushroom. *(By Jason Hollinger from* http://www.flickr.com. *Used with permission.)*

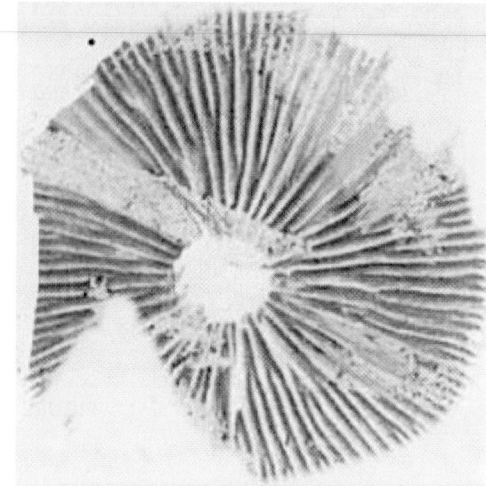

FIGURE 66-10 Spore print staining positive for amyloid.

to the gills, then laying the cap gill-side down on white paper for a few hours at room temperature. The initial color seen after removal of the gills is used for identification. With drying, the color may fade or change. Additional information about spores can be acquired by staining with Melzer's reagent (a solution of iodine and chloral hydrate). Spores that stain blue are called *amyloid,* indicating the presence of starch (Figure 66-10). This technique may be particularly useful in spore identification from gastric aspirates. Spores of *Amanita* species are amyloid. Thin-layer chromatography of spores available from a mycology laboratory, mushroom farm, or botany department is a more accurate aid to identification.

There are many species of mushrooms, including several that are hunted, that have no caps, gills, or stipe. They have developed alternative methods of releasing their spores. The "puffball" mushrooms are well known by the cloud of spores they release through a pore on the top surface of their spherical fruiting bodies (Figure 66-11). This spore release occurs when the spores are mature and may be initiated by a falling branch, errant placement of a deer's hoof, or the squeezing fingers of a curious child.

Mushrooms are composed of approximately 90% water, with 3% proteins and other nitrogen-containing compounds. The remainder is largely carbohydrate, fat, and a few vitamins. Some mushrooms may have high levels of minerals, such as selenium, iron, and potassium. Nutritionally unimpressive, mushrooms are consumed primarily for their taste and texture. Wild mushrooms have the additional allure of being free. This is changing in many parts of the northwestern United States, where some species of mushroom have become so profitable that pickers have had to buy commercial permits, and gun battles have erupted over territorial disputes.

Of the many varieties of wild mushrooms, few are deadly or cause serious illness. All mushrooms, including toxic ones, are safe to handle without gloves; however, handwashing after handling is strongly recommended. Many experts will even bite off and chew a small piece of mushroom to gather taste information before spitting it out. As in wine tasting, a thorough rinsing is recommended after each taste.

The American Association of Poison Control Centers (AAPCC) reports between 7000 and 9000 mushroom exposures annually, with most exposures occurring between June and October. Most of these occur in children younger than 6 years and are not serious or result only in mild gastroenteritis. These exposures are usually caused by ingestion of a small amount of mushroom growing in the backyard. More serious ingestions can occur when young adults or foragers confuse toxic mushrooms for edible or hallucinogenic species. More serious exposures with potentially life-threatening toxic effects occur in less than 1% of all cases reported to poison control centers.[59]

Many immigrants fail to realize that the nontoxic mushrooms from their native lands have toxic look-alikes in America. This is particularly true of Southeast Asian immigrants, who are attracted to the large *Amanita* species. Entire families have been poisoned, with many fatalities. The Russian roulette played by mushroom foragers is statistically safe. Some self-proclaimed experts are simply lucky; occasionally, they are not.

BOX 66-1 Obtaining Spore Prints

1. Obtain a fresh specimen.
2. Cut off stalk close to the gills.
3. Lay cap, gill side down, on white paper for several hours at room temperature.
4. Note color of spores on paper immediately after removal of cap. Drying may alter spore appearance.

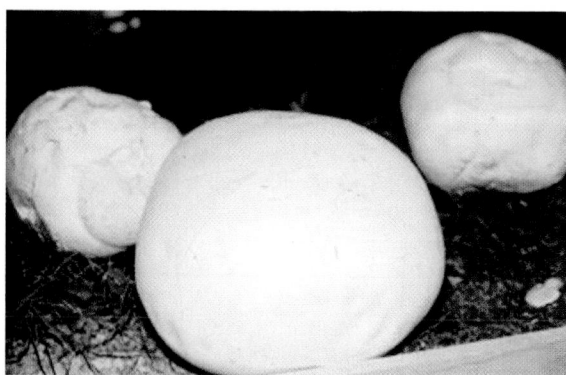

FIGURE 66-11 Puffball mushrooms (edible).

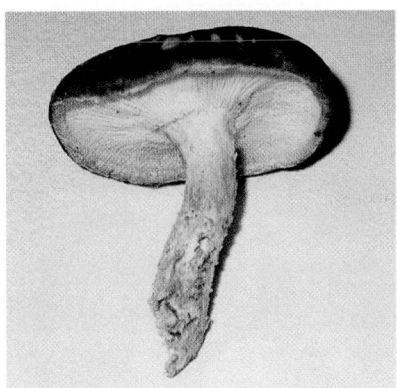

FIGURE 66-14 Shiitake mushroom.

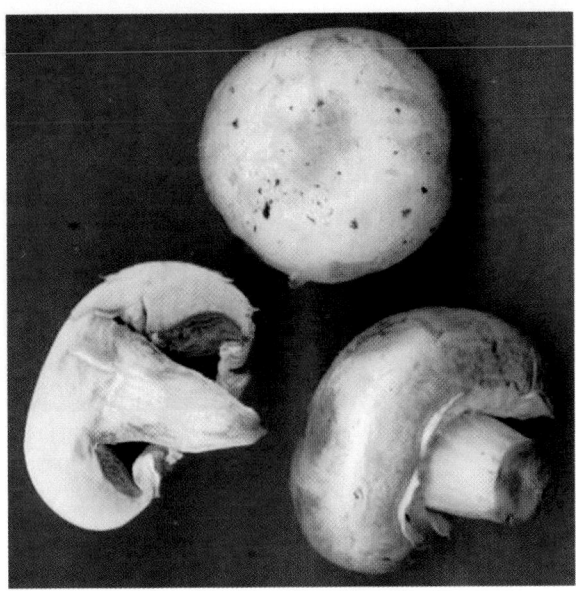

FIGURE 66-12 *Agaricus bisporus* (edible).

NONTOXIC MUSHROOMS

The most common commercially available mushroom in the United States is *Agaricus bisporus* (Figure 66-12). It is cultivated in abandoned mine shafts and caves. This small white mushroom with dark gills is often picked before the gills are fully exposed. Although the mushroom is considered nontoxic, hypersensitivity reactions and gastrointestinal (GI) symptoms have been reported. In some parts of the United States, close relatives of this common mushroom account for the largest percentage of toxic mushroom cases. Most often, *A. bisporus* causes GI disturbance. *Agaricus* species may be confused with the deadly *Amanita* species (Figure 66-13). The popular portobello mushroom is a type of *Agaricus bisporus. A. bisporus* can also be found in the wild.

Nontoxic mushrooms may carry environmental toxins, such as heavy metals and pesticides. Mushrooms with high lead concentrations have been gathered near highways.[36] High mercury concentrations are found in mushrooms from industrial sites.[98] Regular consumption of wild-grown edible mushrooms from areas surrounding former mercury mining sites in Slovakia led to concerning levels of heavy metals. Many mushrooms fruit among cultivated plants and may contain toxic levels of pesticides. Human toxicity has not been reported.

Fungi may cause allergic reactions. Molds that grow in damp locations in buildings have been suspected to cause a variety of patient complaints. They are one cause of the "sick building" syndrome that has resulted in some structures being vacated or demolished when the problem could not be remedied by conventional methods. Acute anaphylaxis from mushroom ingestion is rare, despite the presence of haptens capable of inciting an allergic response.[62] More often, symptoms develop from inhalation of spores.[84] Patients may present with anaphylaxis or, more frequently, with chronic hypersensitivity pneumonitis. Hypersensitivity reactions are described in workers exposed to cultivation of *A. bisporus* (the most popular commercially grown mushroom in America)[69] and shiitake (*Lentinus edodes*), the popular Japanese mushroom (Figure 66-14).[102] Asthma symptoms developed in almost 10% of shiitake-exposed workers. In one study, all workers had positive skin and inhalation challenge tests.[113] Spore counts correlate with asthma symptoms.

Gastroenteric symptoms after ingestion of mushrooms may not be caused by toxins. Bacterial food poisoning may occur in foods that coincidentally contain mushrooms. Small bowel obstruction occurred in a person who consumed 500 g of the edible mushroom *Cantharellus cibarius* (chanterelle) (Figures 66-15 and 66-16).[38] This was largely a result of poor mastication, because entire mushrooms were recovered from the patient's intestines. Improper preparation of edible mushrooms can result in severe toxicity. Staphylococcal food poisoning has been reported from improperly canned mushrooms.[66] Most wild mushrooms are nontoxic, and many are delicious. Morels (*Morchella esculenta* [Figure 66-17] or *M. deliciosa*) are highly prized delicacies. Chanterelles (*C. cibarius*) (see Figures 66-15 and 66-16) and several species of *Boletus* (Figures 66-18 and 66-19) are particularly tasty. The chicken mushroom (*Laetiporus sulphureus*) (Figures 66-20 and 66-21) is often used in place of chicken in Chinese dishes. Extracts of the shiitake mushroom, *L. edodes*, may have antimalarial properties.[136]

TYPES OF MUSHROOM TOXICITY

Mushroom toxicity can be classified into several types, which are summarized in Box 66-2. Detailed discussions of each type are presented in the sections that follow. Box 66-3 provides a method for identifying what type of mushroom may have caused a patient's illness.

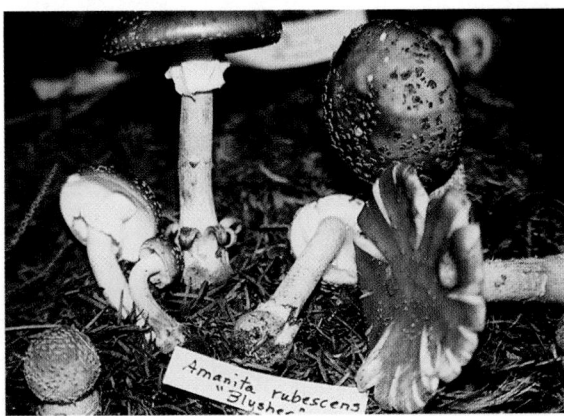

FIGURE 66-13 *Amanita rubescens.*

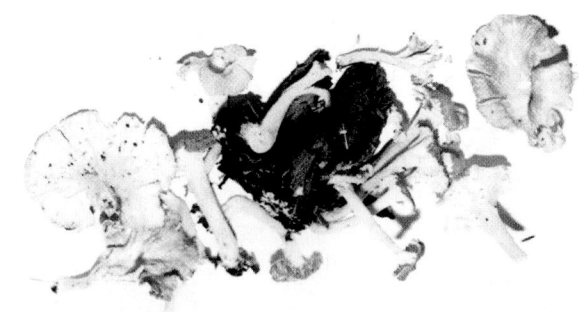

FIGURE 66-15 *Cantharellus cibarius* (edible).

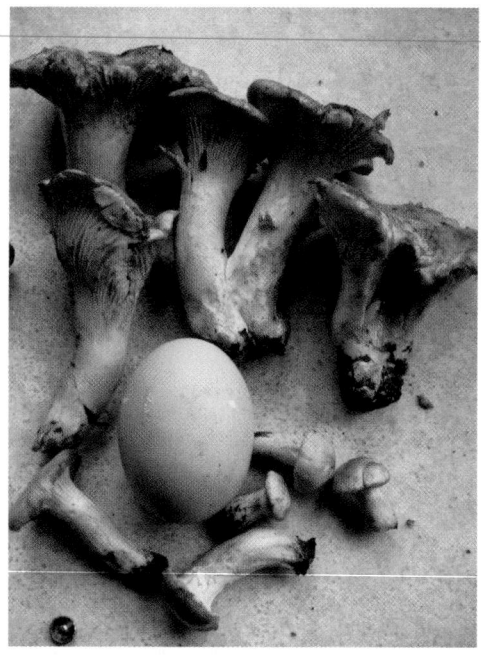

FIGURE 66-16 *Cantharellus cibarius* (chanterelles). *(By Tomasz Przechlewski from* http://www.flickr.com. *Used with permission.)*

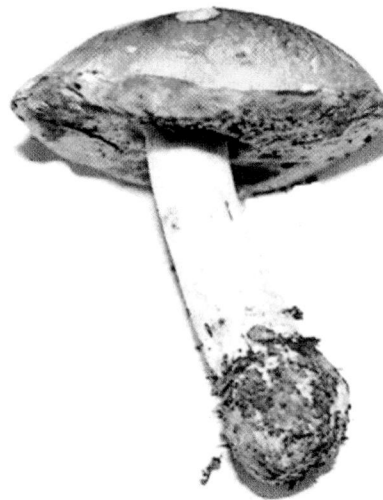

FIGURE 66-18 *Boletus edulis* (edible).

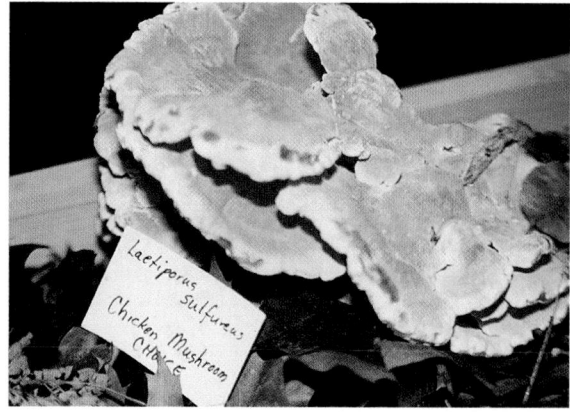

FIGURE 66-20 Chicken mushroom, *Laetiporus sulphureus* (edible).

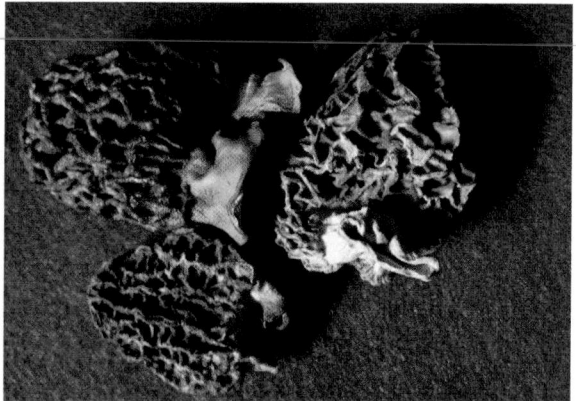

FIGURE 66-17 Morels (*Morchella esculenta*).

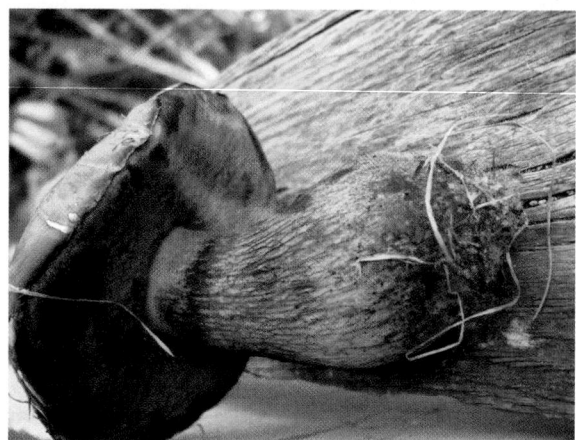

FIGURE 66-19 *Boletus luridus.* (By Tomasz Przechlewski from http://www.flickr.com. *Used with permission.)*

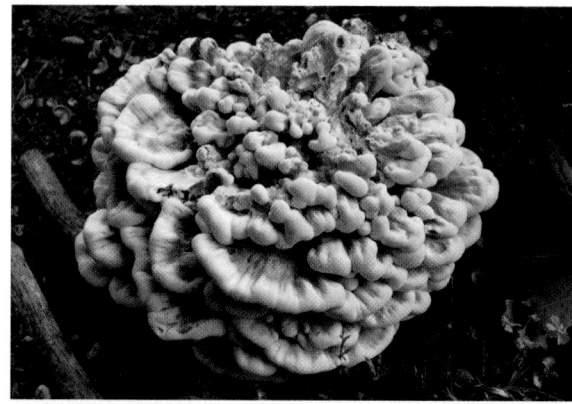

FIGURE 66-21 *Laetiporus sulphureus.* (By Carl Mueller from http://www.flickr.com. *Used with permission.)*

BOX 66-2   Types of Mushroom Toxicity

- Gastrointestinal irritants
- Disulfiram-like toxins
- Neurotoxins
  Muscarinic
  Isoxazole derivatives
  Psilocybin-hallucinogenic
- Protoplasmic
  Gyromitrin—hepatotoxic
  Amatoxin—hepatotoxic
  Orellanine—nephrotoxic

BOX 66-3 Guide to Mushroom Identification

1. Collect any specimens left at home—preferably uncooked.
2. Collect fresh specimens from gathering site(s).
3. Transport and store mushrooms in paper bags.
4. Spores can be recovered from gastrointestinal fluid.
5. Note initial toxicity and time since ingestion. Note symptoms or lack of symptoms among others ingesting mushrooms.
6. Contact a regional poison information center for assistance in locating an expert in identification.
7. When symptoms are not consistent with identified species, consider that the patient might have ingested another type of mushroom.

GASTROINTESTINAL TOXINS

Most toxic mushrooms fall into the group of GI irritants. This large, heterogeneous group of mushrooms causes GI distress, consisting of nausea, vomiting, and diarrhea, beginning 1 to 2 hours after ingestion and resolving in 6 to 12 hours. Even *A.*

bisporus, the common cultivated mushroom, may cause brief gastroenteritis in some individuals.[114] The mechanism is unknown.

CAUSATIVE MUSHROOMS

A large number of unrelated mushrooms cause GI symptoms with varying host responses (Box 66-4). *Chlorophyllum molybdites* (also known as *Lepiota morganii*) (Figure 66-22) is the most frequently ingested toxic mushroom in America. Most persons who ingest *C. molybdites* confuse it with *A. bisporus,* which it closely resembles. The common name for *C. molybdites,* green-spored parasol, describes the characteristics of this summer mushroom. The whitish cap is 10 to 40 cm (4 to 16 inches), initially smooth and round, and becomes convex with maturity. Tan or brown warts may be present. The gills are free from the stalk, initially white to yellow, and become green with maturity. The stalk is 5 to 25 cm (2 to 10 inches) long, smooth, and white. The ring is generally brown on the underside. Spores are green. The mushroom is common in most of eastern and southern North America and in California. In southern California, it is a common lawn mushroom.

Text continued on p. 1474

BOX 66-4 Mushrooms Reported to Cause Gastrointestinal Irritation

Agaricus
albolutescens
hondensis (Figure 66-23)
placomyces
silvaticus
silvicola
xanthodermus (Figure 66-24)

Amanita
brunnescens (Figure 66-25)
chlorinosma
flavoconia (Figure 66-26)
flavorubescens (Figure 66-27)
frostiana
parcivolvata
spissa
spreta
volvata

Boletus
luridus (see Figure 66-19)
pulcherrimus
satans
sensibilis

Chlorophyllum
molybdites (Lepiota morganii) (Figure 66-28)

Entoloma (Rhodophyllus)
lividum
nidorosum
rhodopolium
salmoneum (Figure 66-29)
strictius
vernum

Cantharellus (Figure 66-30)
bonari
floccosus
kauffmanii

Hebeloma
crustuliniforme
fastibile
mesophaeum
sinapizans

Lactarius
chrysorrheus (Figure 66-31)
glaucescens
helvus
representaneus
rufus (Figure 66-32)
scrobiculatus

torminosus (Figure 66-33)
uvidus

Lepiota
clypeolaria (Figure 66-34)
cristata (Figure 66-35)
lutea (Figures 66-36 and 66-37)
morganii
naucina

Lycoperdon
marginatum
subincarnatum

Morchella (Figures 66-38 and 66-39)
angusticeps
crassipes
deliciosa
esculenta (Figure 66-40)
semilibera (Figure 66-41)

Naematoloma (Hypholoma)
fasciculare

Omphalotus
olearius
illudens (Figure 66-42)
olivascens (Figure 66-43)

Paxillus
involutus

Ramaria (Clavaria)
formosa (Figure 66-44)
gelantinosa

Russula
emetica (Figure 66-45)

Scleroderma
aurantium
cepa (Figure 66-46)

Tricholoma
album
muscarium
pardinum
pessundatum
saponaceum
sejunctum
sulphureum
venenatum

Verpa
bohemica

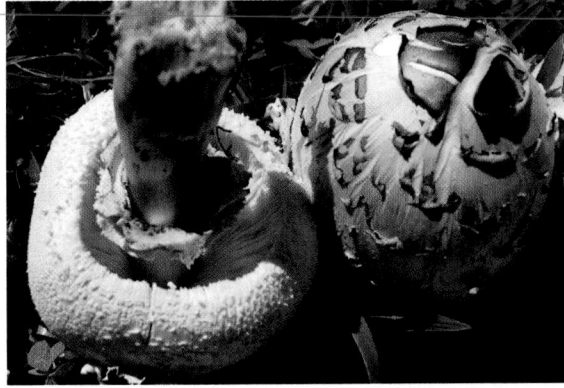

FIGURE 66-22 *Chlorophyllum molybdites* (also known as *Lepiota morganii*). *(By Jason Hollinger from http://www.flickr.com. Used with permission.)*

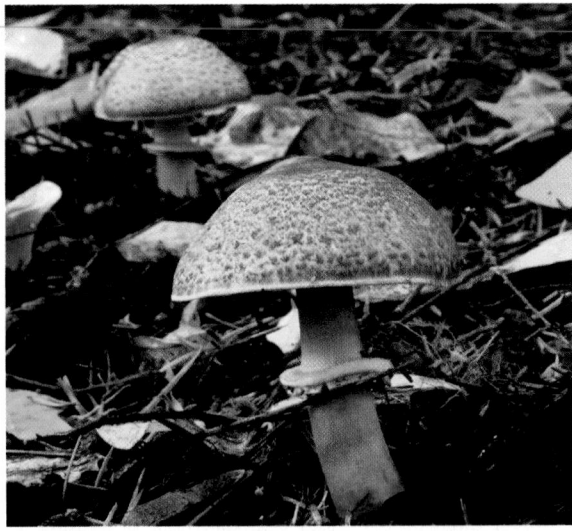

FIGURE 66-23 *Agaricus hondensis*. *(By Dan Bennett from http://www.flickr.com. Used with permission.)*

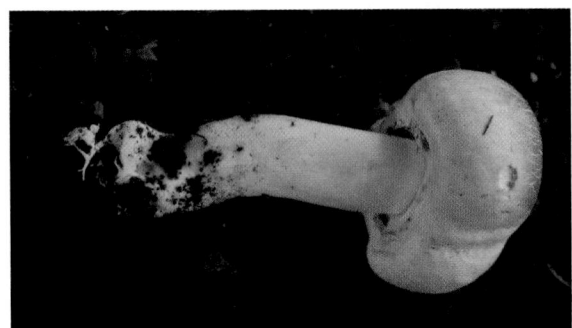

FIGURE 66-24 *Agaricus xanthodermus*. *(By Damon W. Smith from http://www.flickr.com. Used with permission.)*

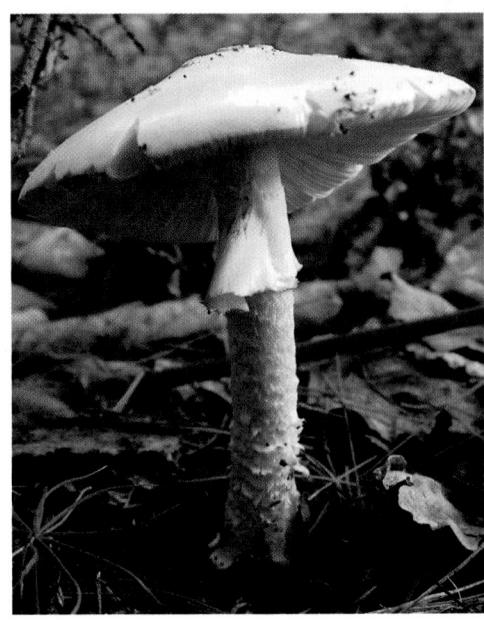

FIGURE 66-25 *Amanita brunnescens*. *(By Jason Hollinger from http://www.flickr.com. Used with permission.)*

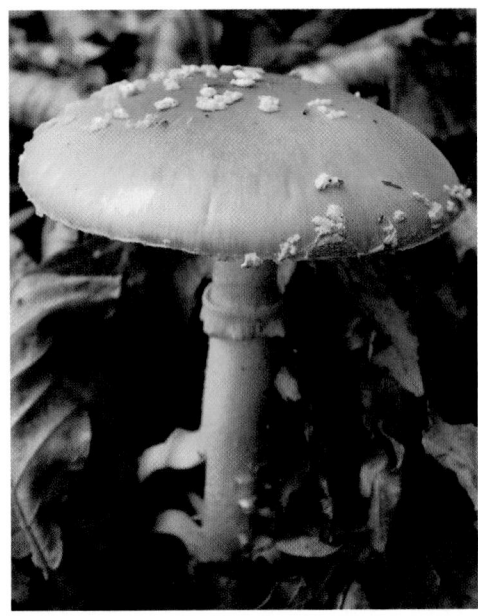

FIGURE 66-26 *Amanita flavoconia*. *(By Jason Hollinger from http://www.flickr.com. Used with permission.)*

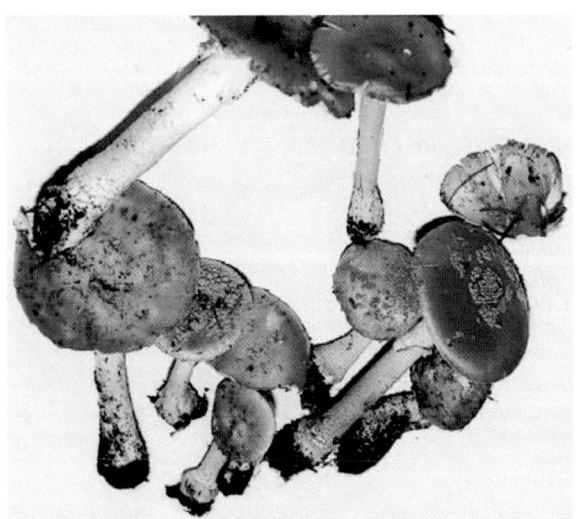

FIGURE 66-27 *Amanita flavorubescens*.

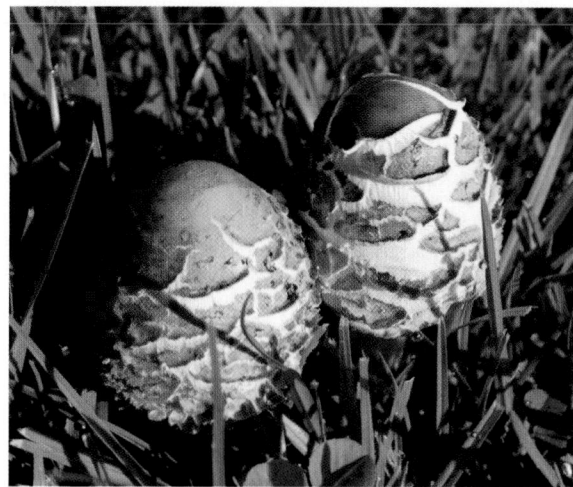

FIGURE 66-28 *Chlorophyllum molybdites (Lepiota morganii). (By Jason Hollinger from http://www.flickr.com. Used with permission.)*

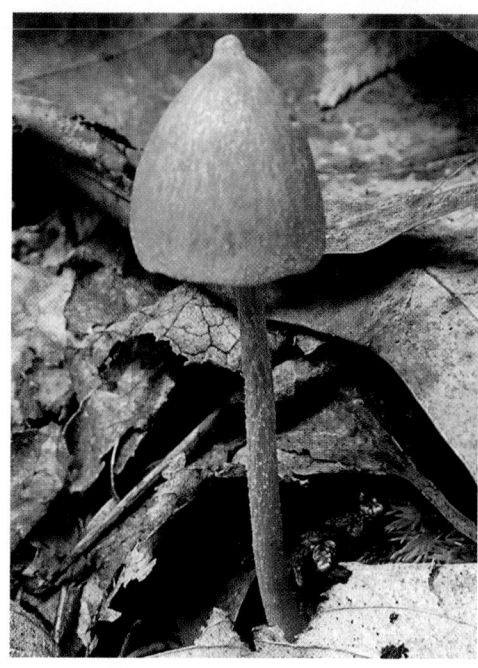

FIGURE 66-29 *Entoloma (Rhodophyllus) salmoneum. (By Jason Hollinger from http://www.flickr.com. Used with permission.)*

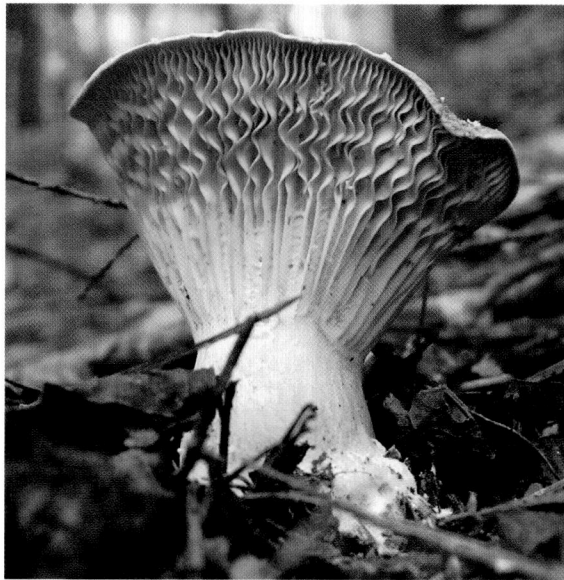

FIGURE 66-30 *Cantharellus mushroom. (By Jason Hollinger from http://www.flickr.com. Used with permission.)*

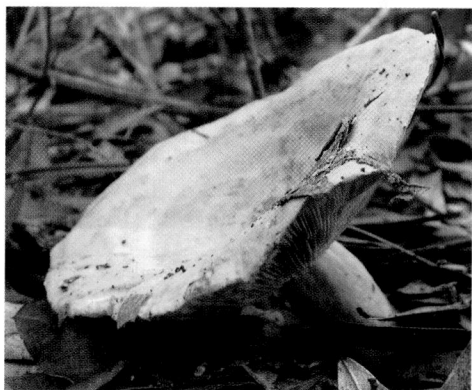

FIGURE 66-31 *Lactarius chrysorrheus. (By Jason Hollinger from http://www.flickr.com. Used with permission.)*

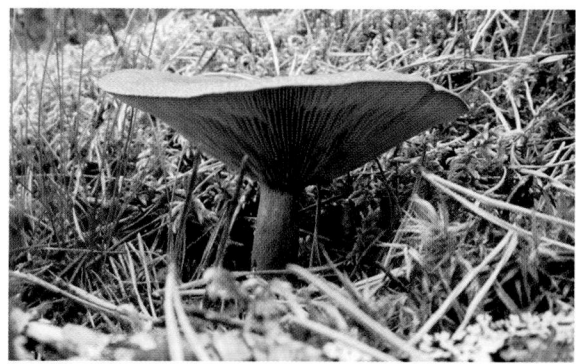

FIGURE 66-32 *Lactarius rufus. (By aSIMULAtor from http://www.flickr.com. Used with permission.)*

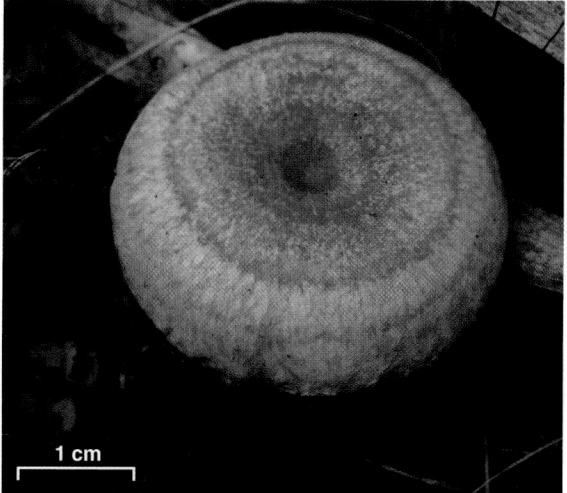

1 cm

FIGURE 66-33 *Lactarius torminosus. (By Jason Hollinger from http://www.flickr.com. Used with permission.)*

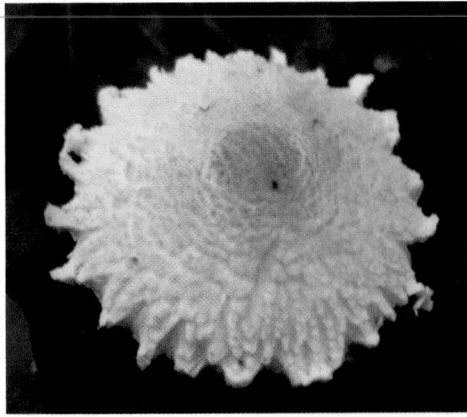

FIGURE 66-34 *Lepiota clypeolaria.* (By Tomasz Przechlewski from http://www.flickr.com. *Used with permission.*)

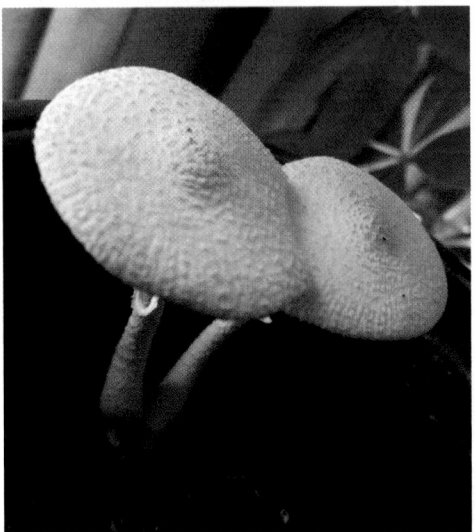

FIGURE 66-36 *Lepiota lutea.* (By Lara604 from http://www.flickr.com. *Used with permission.*)

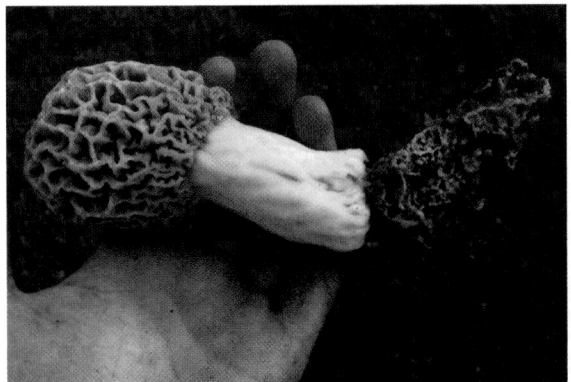

FIGURE 66-38 *Morchella sp.* (By Damon W. Smith from http://www.flickr.com. *Used with permission.*)

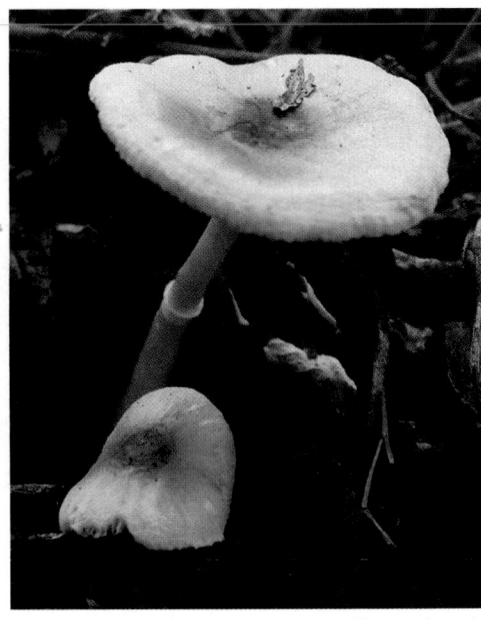

FIGURE 66-35 *Lepiota cristata.* (By Jason Hollinger from http://www.flickr.com. *Used with permission.*)

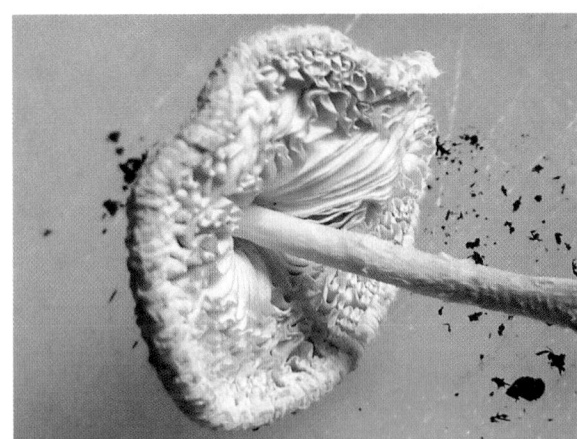

FIGURE 66-37 *Lepiota lutea.* (By Lara604 from http://www.flickr.com. *Used with permission.*)

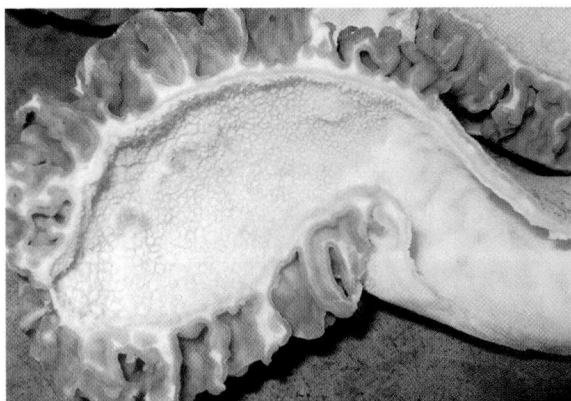

FIGURE 66-39 Inside of a *Morchella* mushroom. (By Damon W. Smith from http://www.flickr.com. *Used with permission.*)

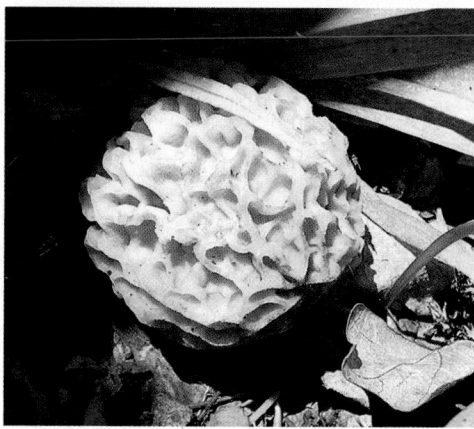

FIGURE 66-40 *Morchella esculenta.* (By Jason Sturner from http://www.flickr.com. *Used with permission.*)

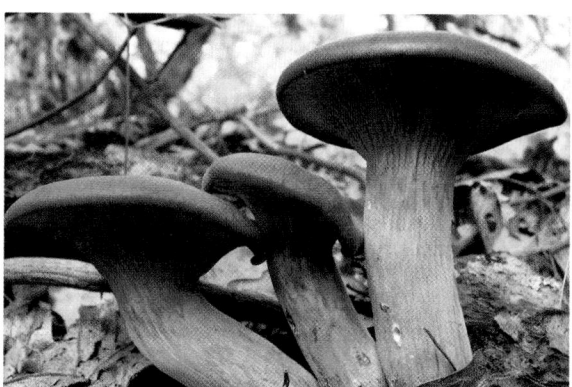

FIGURE 66-42 *Omphalotus illudens.* (By Jason Hollinger from http://www.flickr.com. *Used with permission.*)

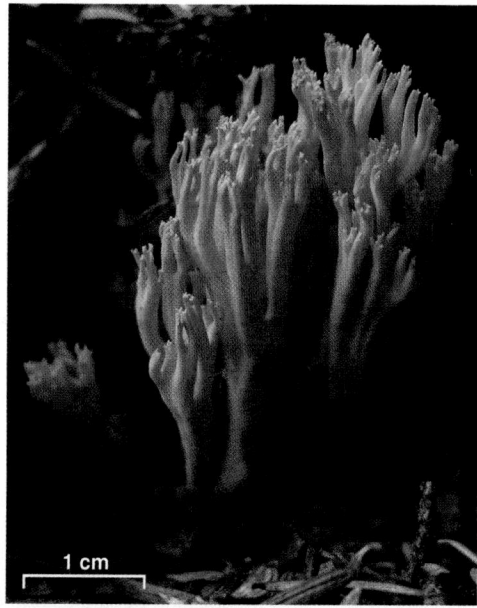

FIGURE 66-44 *Ramaria (Clavaria) formosa.* (By Jason Hollinger from http://www.flickr.com. *Used with permission.*)

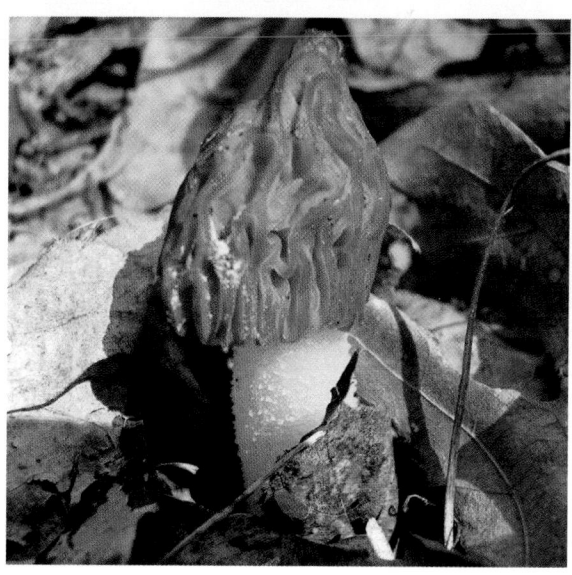

FIGURE 66-41 *Morchella semilibera.* (By Jason Sturner from http://www.flickr.com. *Used with permission.*)

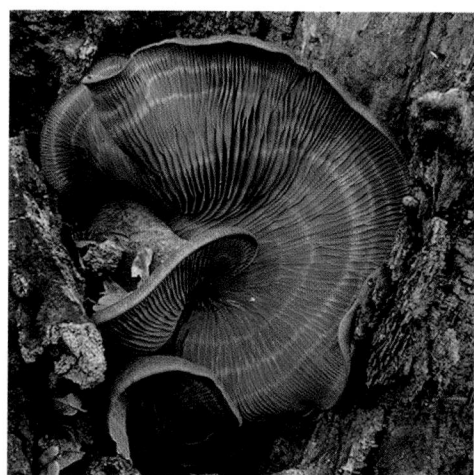

FIGURE 66-43 *Omphalotus olivascens.* (By Nathan Wilson from http://www.mushroomobserver.org/image/show_image/621 from http://www.flickr.com. *Used with permission.*)

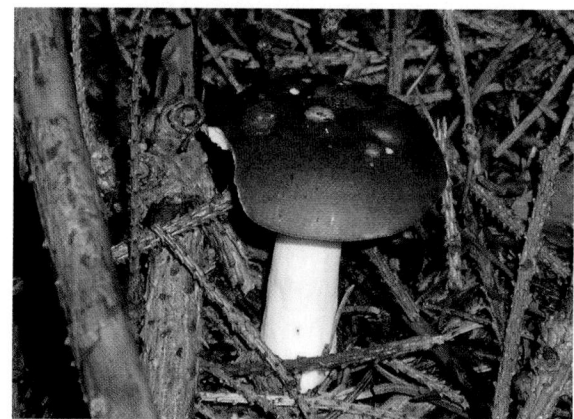

FIGURE 66-45 *Russula emetica.* (By Maja Dumat from http://www.flickr.com. *Used with permission.*)

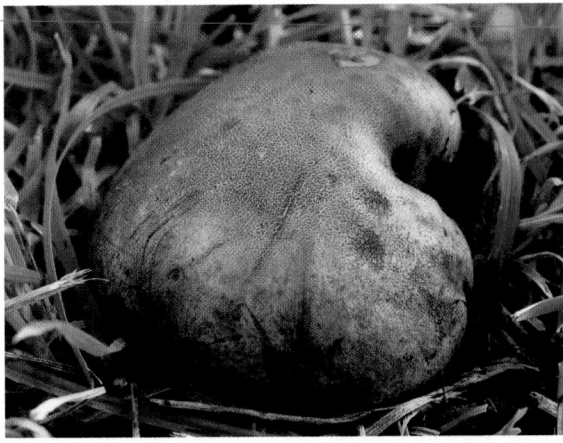

FIGURE 66-46 *Scleroderma cepa.* (By Jason Hollinger from http://www.flickr.com. Used with permission.)

Another common mushroom causing GI symptoms is the jack-o'-lantern. Its botanical classification is not completely settled. Most often, it is referred to as *Omphalotus illudens* (see Figure 66-42), *Omphalotus olearius*, or *Omphalotus olivascens* (see Figure 66-43). The mushroom is a bright orange-yellow mushroom with sharp-edged gills and often grows in clusters at the base of stumps or on buried roots of deciduous trees. The cap is 4 to 16 cm (1.6 to 6.3 inches) in diameter on a stalk that is 4 to 20 cm (1.6 to 8 inches) long. Gills are olive to orange, with white to yellow spores. The mushroom shows characteristic luminescence lasting 40 to 50 hours after collection. Members of this family are found in both eastern and western North America, generally in autumn and early spring. They may be mistaken for the edible species *C. cibarius* (see Figure 66-15). Some European reports have documented hepatic impairment and muscarinic effect following ingestion.[122] It is not clear whether the mushroom and its toxins are the same on both sides of the Atlantic.

Although the genus *Amanita* is most famous for its deadly member *A. phalloides* (see Figure 66-6), the genus also contains tasty nontoxic mushrooms (e.g., *Amanita caesarea* [Figure 66-47],

A. calyptrata, *A. velosa*). Several *Amanita* species cause GI symptoms indistinguishable from those caused by jack-o'-lantern mushrooms or *C. molybdites* (see Figure 66-28). *Amanita brunnescens* (see Figure 66-25) and *Amanita flavorubescens* (see Figure 66-27) are frequently listed as containing GI toxins, although they are occasionally listed as edible. Both have broad, yellowish to brown caps (3 to 15 cm [1.2 to 6 inches]) with loosely attached warts. The stalks are 3 to 18 cm (1.2 to 7.1 inches) long, enlarging toward the base with a superior ring. *A. brunnescens* stains reddish brown when bruised. As with most *Amanita*, these mushrooms are found in summer or fall associated with hardwoods or conifers.

Several members of the genus *Agaricus*, particularly *Agaricus albolutescens*, *A. silvaticus*, and *A. xanthodermus* (Figure 66-24), can cause GI symptoms. They resemble the cultivated mushrooms in grocery stores and are found in meadows and lawns in the summer and autumn. Table 66-1 lists the look-alike toxic and nontoxic mushrooms in this group.

TOXINS

A variety of toxins have been extracted from these mushrooms, although their structures are poorly described. Most are protein based and heat labile, although toxicity may not be completely eliminated with cooking. In some cases the toxin may be destroyed by heating (temperature and duration vary by species), parboiling, or even preserving in salt. Host response to a toxin varies; some persons can eat such mushrooms without harm, whereas others become quite ill. Some mushrooms also contain hemolysins and toxins that cause hemorrhage and hepatitis in animals.[63,118] Human hemolysis has not been reported.[63]

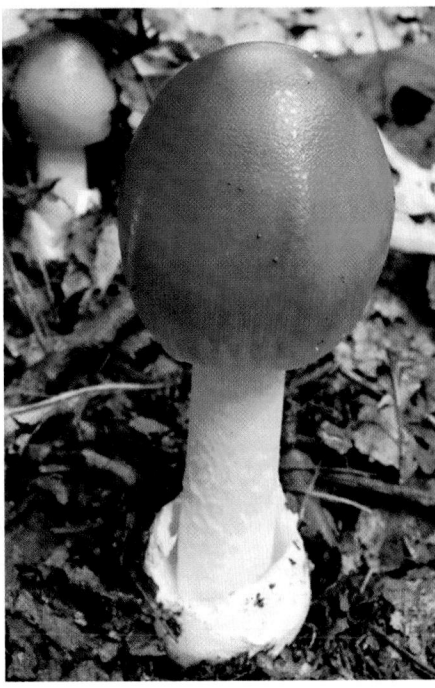

FIGURE 66-47 *Amanita caesarea.* (By Jason Hollinger from http://www.flickr.com. Used with permission.)

TABLE 66-1 Gastrointestinal Irritant Mushrooms Mistaken for Edible Species

Gastrointestinal Irritant	Edible Species
Agaricus albolutescens silvaticus xanthodermus (see Figure 66-24)	*Agaricus bisporus*
Amanita brunnescens (see Figure 66-25)	*Amanita flavorubescens* (see Figure 66-27)
	Amanita inaurata (Figure 66-48)
Chlorophyllum molybdites (see Figures 66-22 and 66-28)	*Lepiota* spp. (Figure 66-49)
	Agaricus bisporus (see Figure 66-12)
Entoloma spp. (see Figure 66-29)	*Pluteus cervinus*
	Entoloma abortivum
Hebeloma crustuliniforme	*Rozites caperata* (Figure 66-50)
Naematoloma fasciculare	*Armillaria mellea* (Figures 66-51 to 66-53)
	Naematoloma sublateritium
	Naematoloma capnoides
Paxillus involutus	*Lactarius* spp. (Figure 66-54)
Ramaria formosa (see Figure 66-44)	*Ramaria* spp.
Ramaria gelatinosa	
Scleroderma aurantium	*Lycoperdon perlatum* (Figure 66-55)
Tricholoma pessundatum	*Cantharellus cibarius* (see Figure 66-16)
Omphalotus olearius (see Figure 66-42)	*Laetiporus sulphureus* (see Figure 66-21)
	Armillaria mellea (see Figures 66-51 to 66-53)

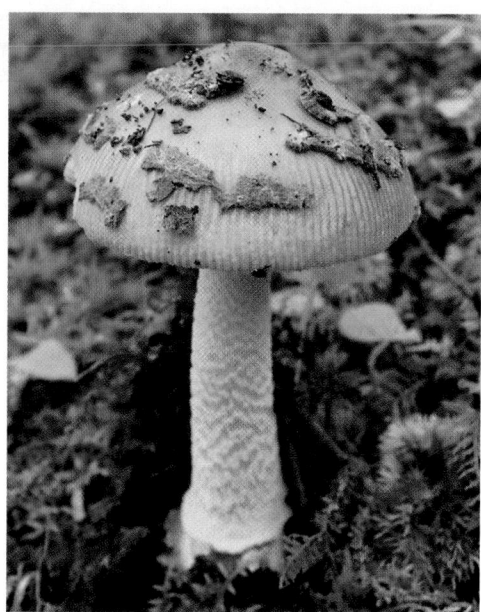

FIGURE 66-48 *Amanita inaurata.* (By Jason Hollinger from http://www.flickr.com. *Used with permission.*)

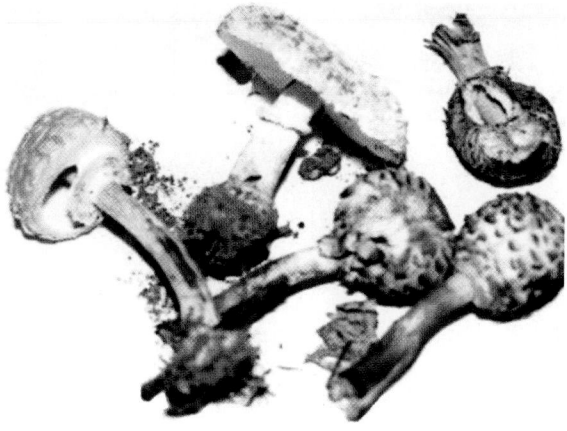

FIGURE 66-49 *Lepiota* species—some are toxic.

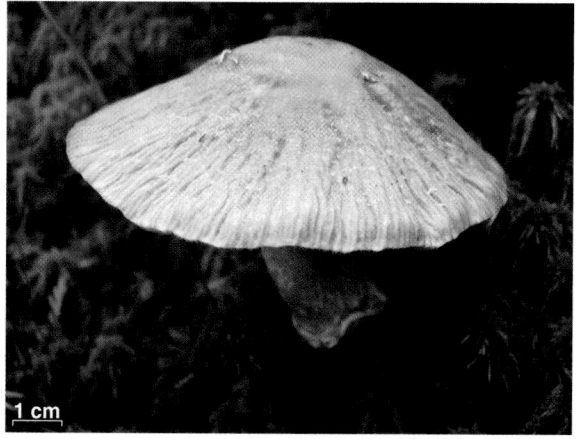

FIGURE 66-50 *Rozites caperata.* (By Jason Hollinger from http://www.flickr.com. *Used with permission.*)

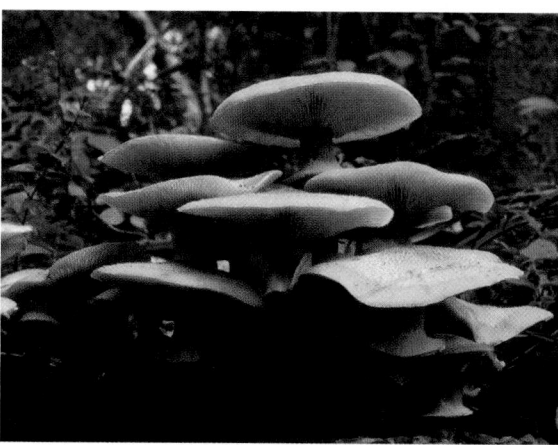

FIGURE 66-51 *Armillaria mellea.* (By Nathan Wilson from http://www.mushroomobserver.org/image/show_image/621 from http://www.flickr.com. *Used with permission.*)

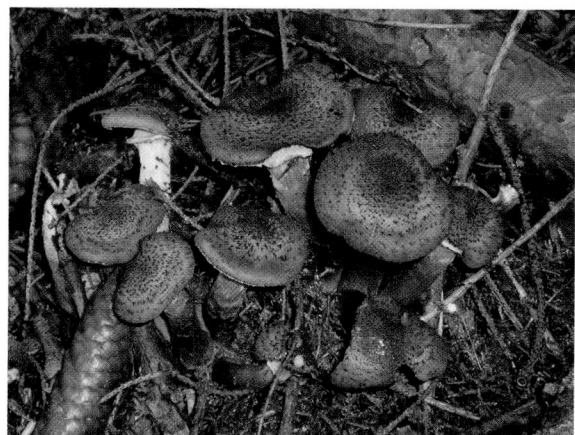

FIGURE 66-52 *Armillaria mellea.* (By Maja Dumat from http://www.flickr.com. *Used with permission.*)

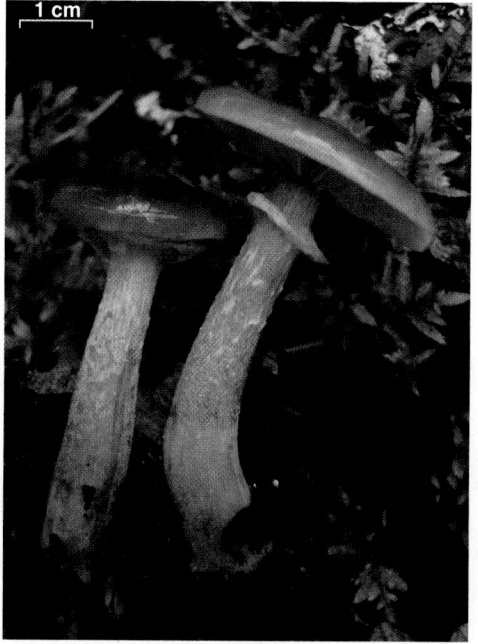

FIGURE 66-53 *Armillaria mellea.* (By Jason Hollinger from http://www.flickr.com. *Used with permission.*)

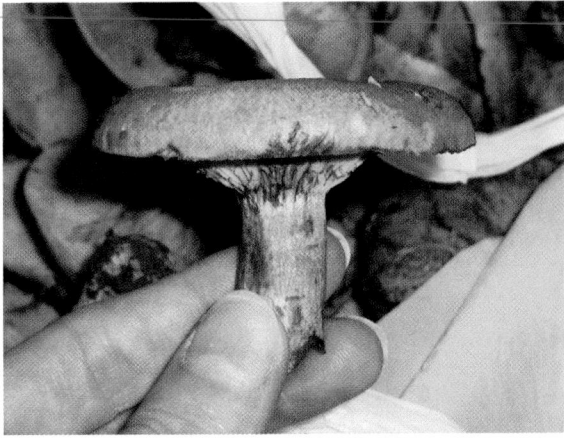

FIGURE 66-54 *Lactarius* sp. (*By Maja Dumat from* http://www.flickr.com. *Used with permission.*)

CLINICAL PRESENTATION

Within 1 to 2 hours of ingestion of these mushrooms, nausea, vomiting, intestinal cramping, and diarrhea develop. Stools are usually watery and occasionally bloody with fecal leukocytes. Chills, headaches, and myalgias may occur. Symptoms remit spontaneously in 6 to 12 hours. Most patients require only fluid and electrolytes replacement. A few serious cases reported in the literature have been associated with severe dehydration. In a review of 106 cases, all patients responded well to fluid and electrolyte replacement and occasional antiemetic or antidiarrheal medications.[23] Admitted patients were discharged in an average of 2 days. Persons whose symptoms are delayed (beginning 4 hours or more after ingestion) probably have ingested a more toxic mushroom, possibly *Amanita, Galerina, Lepiota,* or *Gyromitra.* Those who ingest these more toxic mushrooms present with very severe GI distress and may develop hepatic failure. Because nausea and vomiting are common symptoms seen with various types of mushroom exposures, careful attention to onset and timing of these symptoms is important in differentiating more severe, or even life-threatening, toxicity from relatively benign ingestions.

Recent reports of ingestion of jack-o'-lantern mushrooms describe mildly elevated liver transaminases.[122] Cases of metabolic acidosis and dehydration, and even death, are attributed to *C. molybdites*[15,116] (see Figure 66-22).

TREATMENT

Treatment is largely supportive and does not depend on the type of mushroom ingested (Box 66-5). Intravenous (IV) fluid and electrolytes replacement may be required. Although there is no

evidence, in a severe case, an antiemetic, such as ondansetron, 8 mg orally (PO/ODT) or intravenously (IV), or promethazine, 25 mg IV, may prevent further emesis. If a patient presents within 1 hour of ingestion and vomiting has not occurred, activated charcoal (1 g/kg) without cathartic is given PO or through nasogastric (NG) tube, although no evidence shows that its use decreases toxicity. Once vomiting starts, activated charcoal is likely useless. Most cases are self-limited.

Care should be taken not to dismiss early GI symptoms when several types of unknown mushrooms have been ingested. Individuals may ingest both GI irritant mushrooms and mushrooms containing serious toxins. Persons with prolonged gastroenteritis from unidentified mushrooms should be observed for 24 to 48 hours for development of delayed hepatic damage. Special efforts should be made in these cases to identify the ingested mushrooms.

DISULFIRAM-LIKE TOXINS

A fascinating toxicity is caused by some members of the *Coprinus* genus, known as "inky caps" (Figure 66-56). Individuals who ingest these mushrooms and subsequently ingest alcohol have symptoms similar to those of an alcohol-disulfiram (Antabuse) reaction.

CAUSATIVE MUSHROOMS

Several members of the *Coprinus* genus may contain disulfiram-like toxins (Box 66-6), but symptoms are most common with *Coprinus atramentarius.* The mushroom has a 2- to 8-cm (0.8- to 3.1-inch) cylindrical cap on a thin, 4- to 5-cm (1.6- to 2-inch) stalk. The cap is white or occasionally orange or yellow at the

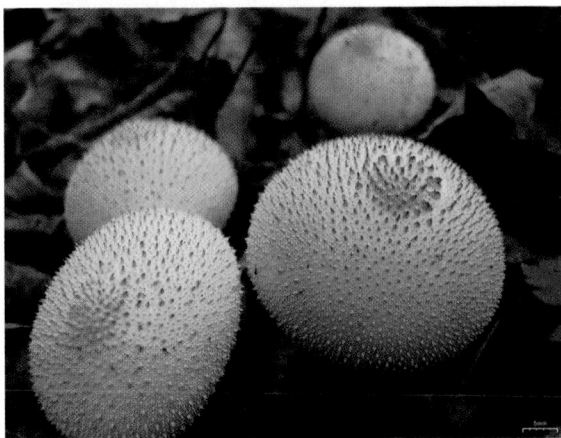

FIGURE 66-55 *Lycoperdon perlatum.* (*By Jason Hollinger from* http://www.flickr.com. *Used with permission.*)

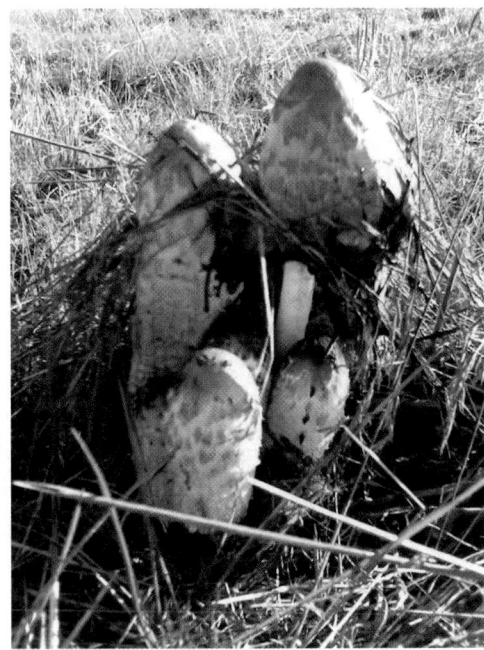

FIGURE 66-56 *Coprinus* sp. (*By Damon W. Smith from* http://www.flickr.com. *Used with permission.*)

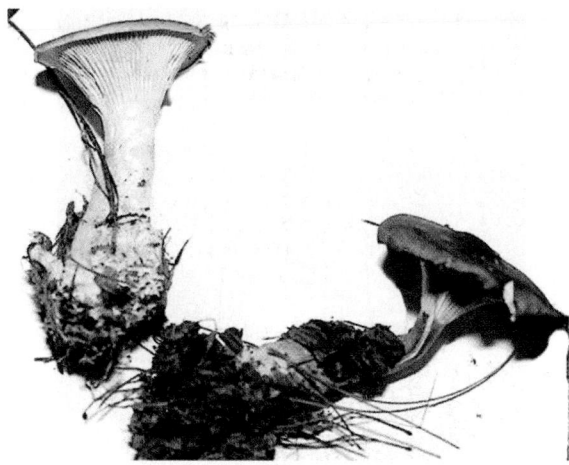

FIGURE 66-58 *Clitocybe* mushrooms—some are toxic.

top. The mature cap often develops cracks, which turn up at its margins. The cap blackens as it matures and then liquefies into the "inky cap." A ring may be present low on the stalk. Spores are black. *C. atramentarius* grows throughout North America in clusters of three or more in grass or wood debris. It often appears overnight after a rain. Several members of the *Coprinus* genus, including *C. atramentarius,* are edible if no alcohol is ingested for the next 72 hours. Other mushroom species contain coprine-like toxins. *Lepiota aspera* has caused disulfiram-like reactions in individuals who eat this mushroom and simultaneously consume ethanol.

TOXIN

Mushrooms causing a disulfiram reaction contain the toxin coprine, first isolated from the mushroom *C. atramentarius* in 1975.[46] Coprine is distinct from disulfiram and is most likely a derivative of glutamine. It probably is not present in the raw mushroom, but rather a hydrolyte created during cooking.[67]

Coprine (or its derivative L-aminocyclopropanol) inhibits acetaldehyde dehydrogenase, similar to the action of disulfiram. Acetaldehyde accumulates, leading to flushing, diaphoresis, headache, tachycardia, nausea, and vomiting. Some clinicians believe that coprine is a relatively poor inhibitor of acetaldehyde dehydrogenase and suggest that symptoms result from altered neurotransmitter levels.[86]

CLINICAL PRESENTATION

A history of wild mushroom ingestion within days before symptoms is rarely offered. Ingestion of the mushroom imparts sensitivity to alcohol, which begins 2 to 6 hours after ingestion and may last up to 72 hours. Within minutes of subsequent alcohol ingestion, the person experiences severe headache, flushing, and tachycardia. Hyperventilation, shortness of breath, and palpitations may occur. Chest pain and orthostatic hypotension occur in severe cases. Symptoms can be confused with an allergic reaction or acute myocardial infarction. Symptoms typically resolve spontaneously within 3 to 6 hours.

TREATMENT

Supportive and symptomatic treatments are suggested for patients with coprine toxicity (Box 66-7). Because these disulfiram-like symptoms may have other, more severe causes, baseline laboratory tests (blood urea nitrogen [BUN], creatinine, electrolytes, and glucose) should be drawn. Urine output should be monitored. IV fluids should be given to keep urine output at 50 mL/hr (children, 1 mL/kg/hr). Activated charcoal is not beneficial. Charcoal does not adsorb alcohol, and the coprine has already been absorbed by the time the reaction occurs. Hypotension generally responds to IV fluid administration. Severe hypotension refractory to fluid replacement should be treated with norepinephrine (initially 2 to 4 mcg/min; 0.05 to 0.1 mcg/kg/min in children and increased as necessary); norepinephrine stores are depleted in a true disulfiram reaction. Propranolol (0.5 to 3 mg IV; 0.01 to 0.02 mg/kg IV up to 1 mg in children) is used for severe symptomatic supraventricular tachycardia. Propranolol may be repeated as needed after 5 to 10 minutes.

NEUROLOGIC TOXINS

MUSCARINE

Muscarine was first isolated from the mushroom *Amanita muscaria* more than 150 years ago (Figures 66-59 and 66-60). A classic muscarinic reaction includes salivation, lacrimation, urination, diaphoresis, GI upset, and emesis (SLUDGE syndrome). Buddhist adepts may have used *A. muscaria* in the second to ninth centuries to achieve enlightenment.[43]

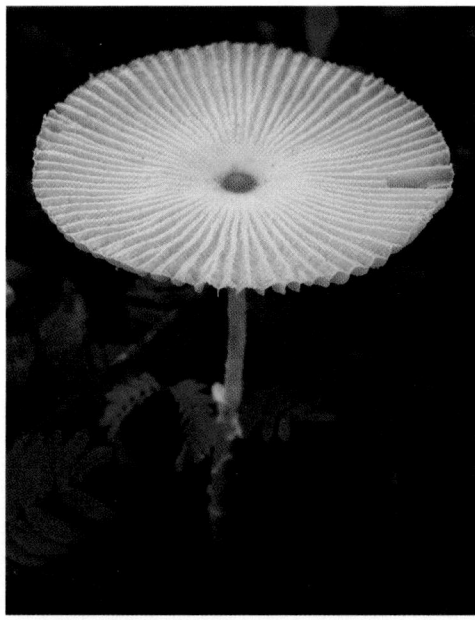

FIGURE 66-57 *Coprinus* sp. (*By Jason Hollinger from* http://www.flickr.com. *Used with permission.*)

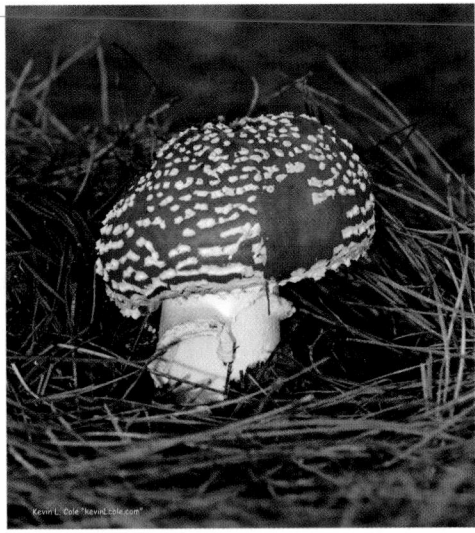

FIGURE 66-59 *Amanita muscaria. (By Kevin L. Cole from http://www .flickr.com. Used with permission.)*

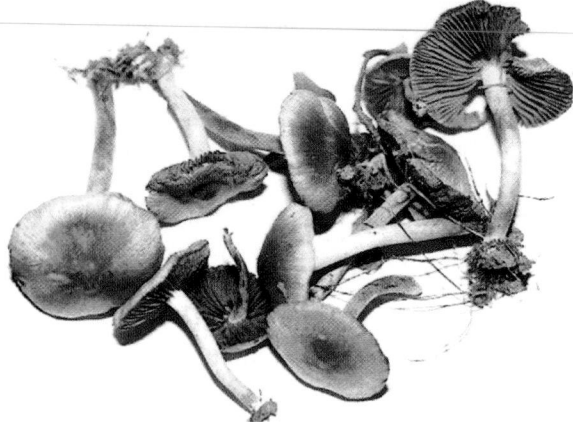

FIGURE 66-61 *Inocybe* mushrooms—some are toxic.

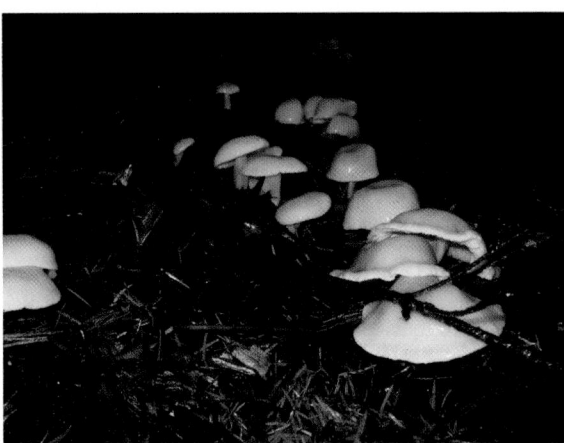

FIGURE 66-62 *Clitocybe* sp. *(By Damon W. Smith from http://www .flickr.com. Used with permission.)*

Causative Mushrooms

Amanita muscaria has a cap 5 to 30 cm (2 to 12 inches) in diameter that is scarlet red with white warts. The stalk tapers upward and is white, often hollow, and grows 15 to 20 cm (6 to 8 inches) in length. It has a prominent vulva and numerous rings. Gills are free and white, as are the spores. The mushrooms grow in eastern North America and throughout much of the western United States, often near *Boletus edulis.* They grow under hardwoods and conifers from summer to autumn.

Potentially toxic amounts of muscarine are found in some *Inocybe* (Figure 66-61) and *Clitocybe* mushrooms (Figure 66-62, Box 66-8, and Table 66-2; see also Figure 66-58). *Inocybe* mushrooms (see Figure 66-61) are small brown mushrooms with conical caps up to 6 cm (2.4 inches) in diameter. Stalks are 2 to 10 cm (0.8 to 4 inches) long, covered with fine, brown to white hairs. Gills are brown and notched; spores are brown. They are found typically under hardwoods and conifers in the summer and fall. All members of this family are considered poisonous.

In contrast, many *Clitocybe* mushrooms (see Figure 66-58) are edible, but except for *Clitocybe nuda* and its close relatives, they are not very tasty. A few contain muscarine. All *Clitocybe* mushrooms are whitish tan to gray mushrooms with caps 15 to 33 mm (0.6 to 1.3 inches) long on hairless stalks 1 to 5 cm (0.4 to 2 inches) long. Gills are decurrent (run down the stalk), and spores are white. They are usually single specimens (not clustered) found on lawns in the summer and fall.

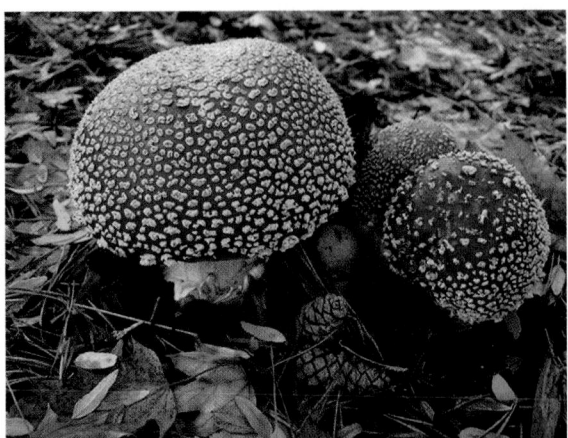

FIGURE 66-60 *Amanita muscaria. (By Damon W. Smith from http:// www.flickr.com. Used with permission.)*

BOX 66-8 Mushrooms Reported or Suspected of Containing Muscarine

Amanita
gemmata
muscaria (see Figures 66-59 and 66-60)
pantherina (Figure 66-63)
parcivolvata

Boletus
calopus
luridus
pulcherrimus
satanas

Clitocybe (see Figures 66-58 and 66-62)
aurantiaca
dealbata
nebularis

Hebeloma crustuliniforme
Inocybe (see Figure 66-61)
fastigiata
geophylla
nappies
patouillardii
pudica

Mycena pura (Figure 66-64)
Omphalotus (see Figure 66-42)
olivascens (see Figure 66-43)
olearius
illudens (see Figure 66-42)

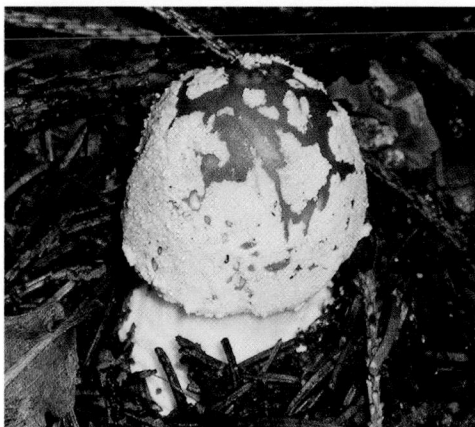

FIGURE 66-63 *Amanita pantherina. (By Maja Dumat from http://www.flickr.com. Used with permission.)*

Many *Inocybe* and *Clitocybe* mushrooms contain larger concentrations of muscarine than does *A. muscaria*. Other toxins (e.g., ibotenic acid) are present in *A. muscaria* and contribute to its toxicity.

Toxin

Muscarine is a quaternary trimethyl ammonium salt of 2-methyl-3-oxy-5-(amino) tetrahydrofuran. Muscarine stimulates postganglionic cholinergic receptors (muscarinic receptors), mimicking the action of acetylcholine. Muscarine stimulation of the GI tract leads to increased secretory activity, contraction amplitude, and peristalsis. Stimulation of the urinary tract leads to bladder contraction and increased peristalsis of the ureters. Stimulation of secretory tissue leads to salivation and lacrimation. Bronchoconstriction, flushing, and diaphoresis result from additional stimulation of bronchial and vascular tissues. Cardiac effects include reflex tachycardia or, more often, bradycardia and decreased atrioventricular conduction. Central nervous system (CNS) effects include headache, ataxia, and visual disturbances. The sensorium is generally not affected (except in ingestion of *A. muscaria*, which contains other CNS toxins).

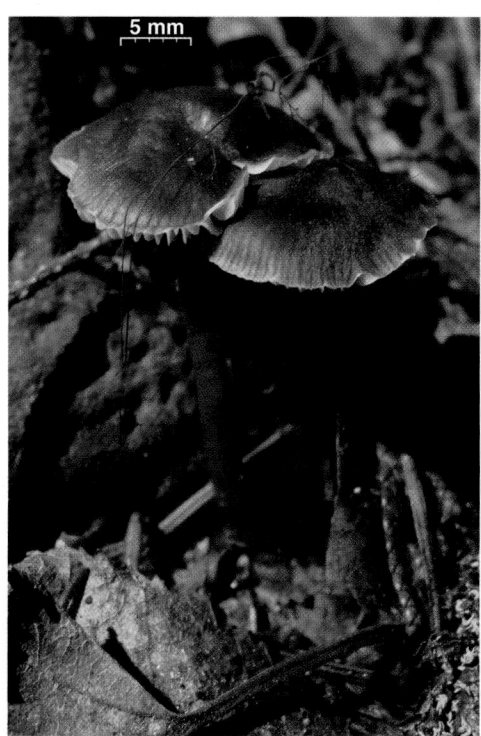

FIGURE 66-64 *Mycena pura. (By Jason Hollinger from http://www.flickr.com. Used with permission.)*

TABLE 66-2 Look-Alikes of Mushrooms Causing Muscarine Poisoning

Toxic Species	Edible Species
Clitocybe dealbata	*Marasmius oreades* (Figure 66-65)
Inocybe species (see Figure 66-61)	*Marasmius oreades*

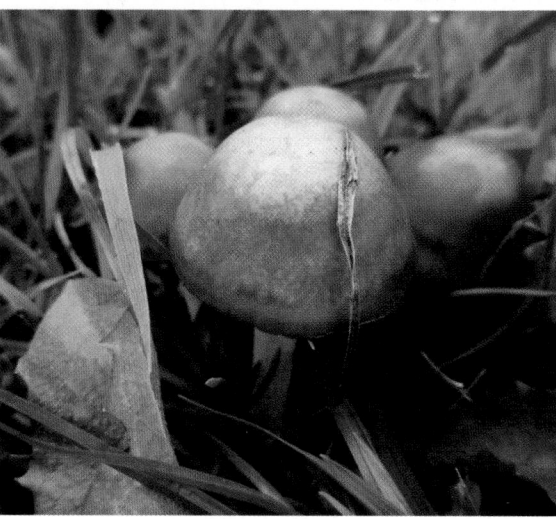

FIGURE 66-65 *Marasmius oreades. (By Becky Dewdney-York from http://www.flickr.com. Used with permission.)*

Clinical Presentation

Symptoms develop within 15 to 30 minutes after ingestion of muscarine-containing mushrooms. Typical symptoms include salivation, urination, lacrimation, diarrhea, diaphoresis, abdominal pain, nausea, and emesis. Bradycardia, bronchospasm, and constricted pupils are also noted. Copious bronchial secretions may cause respiratory failure requiring mechanical ventilation.

Symptoms remit spontaneously in 6 to 24 hours. In Europe, some deaths are reported from *Inocybe patouillardii*.[67] Although this mushroom is rarely eaten, ingestion carries a mortality rate of 6% to 12%, particularly among persons with preexisting pulmonary or cardiac disease. Most deaths occur within the first 12 hours as a result of respiratory failure or cardiovascular collapse.

Treatment

Treatment of muscarinic toxicity is outlined in Box 66-9. Many patients require supportive care with oxygen, suctioning, and IV fluid replacement. Activated charcoal and cathartics are rarely given because of the prominent emesis and diarrhea. Atropine is a muscarine antagonist but should be used only to control secretions or profound bradycardia. It should not be given prophylactically or for asymptomatic bradycardia because it may worsen the delirium, ataxia, and hallucinations induced by *A. muscaria*. Atropine is dosed at 0.01 mg/kg IV for children and 1 mg IV for adults. When secretions are life threatening, that

BOX 66-9 Treatment of Muscarinic Toxicity

1. Supportive care with oxygen, suctioning, and endotracheal intubation as needed.
2. Fluid and electrolyte replacement.
3. Atropine (if symptoms are life threatening) 0.01 mg/kg intravenously every 5 to 10 minutes until secretions are controlled. There is no upper limit to the dose if secretions are excessive. Atropine may worsen central nervous system effects of some mushrooms such as *Amanita muscaria*.

BOX 66-10   Mushrooms Reported or Suspected of Containing Ibotenic Acid, Muscimol, or Related Compounds

Amanita
cokeri
gemmata
muscaria (see Figures 66-59 and 66-60)
pantherina (see Figure 66-63)

Panaeolus campanulatus

Tricholoma muscarium

initial dose may be doubled on subsequent doses. There is no upper limit on the dose of atropine if secretions are severe and potentially life threatening. Symptoms resolve spontaneously within 24 hours.

ISOXAZOLE REACTIONS

The isoxazole derivatives ibotenic acid and muscimol produce CNS symptoms, including excitement and alteration in visual perception.

Causative Mushrooms

Several mushrooms contain ibotenic acid (Box 66-10 and Table 66-3). *A. muscaria* is described previously. *Amanita pantherina* (see Figure 66-63) is 5 to 15 cm (2 to 6 inches) long with a cap 5 to 15 cm in diameter. The cap is generally white to pink in the young specimen but becomes reddish brown or brown, often darker at the rim, with maturity. Fragments of the universal veil form warts on the cap but may be washed off by rain. The stalk has a distinct ring, with a vulva at the bottom. When the flesh is cut or injured (e.g., by insect larvae), it develops a pinkish tinge. Gills are free and produce white spores. The raw mushroom has minimal smell and tastes similar to a raw potato. It grows from June to November in woodlands throughout North America. *A. muscaria* and *A. pantherina* have been identified for sale in markets in Japan and elsewhere.

Toxin

Ibotenic acid is found in the bright-red cap of *A. muscaria* and undergoes decarboxylation during drying to form muscimol, which is more toxic than ibotenic acid. The potency of the cap remains high despite drying. Muscimol is a γ-aminobutyric acid (GABA) receptor agonist.[51] Muscimol increases CNS serotonin levels and decreases catecholamine levels. Ibotenic acid resembles GABA and in animals can act as GABA acts. Liquid chromatography (LC) can identify these compounds.[80,120] Ibotenic acid and muscimol are rapidly absorbed in the GI tract and excreted in urine. They can be identified by gas chromatography–mass spectometry (GC/MS) in the urine of patients that ingest *A. muscaria* or *A. pantherina*.[117]

Clinical Presentation

Ingestion of 10 mg of *A. muscaria* produces mild intoxication, dizziness, and ataxia. Ingestion of 15 mg leads to pronounced

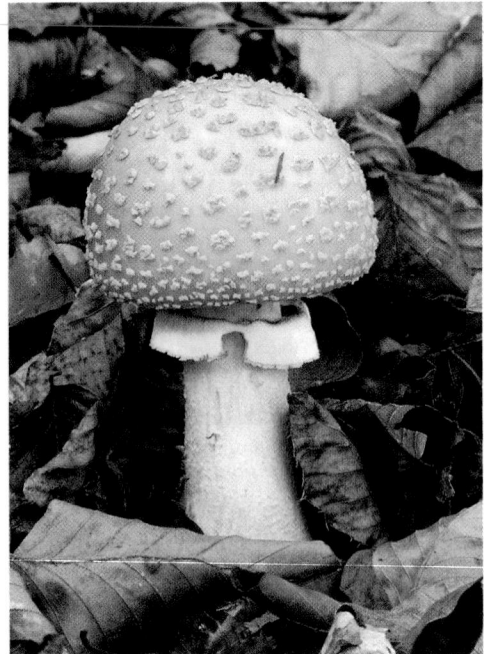

FIGURE 66-66 *Amanita rubescens.* (By Danel Solabarrieta from http://www.flickr.com. *Used with permission.*)

ataxia and visual disturbances.[39,78] Delirium or manic behavior may develop. Physical activity is accelerated, with inability to judge size. Visual hallucinations, seizures, and muscle twitching are common. Some patients complain of residual headache for up to 48 hours. Nausea, vomiting, hallucinations, restlessness, psychomotor agitation, and somnolence were common symptoms reported in a series of acute poisonings with fly agaric (*A. muscaria*) and panther cap (*A. pantherina*) ingestion.[71]

Symptoms begin within 30 minutes of ingestion and generally last 2 hours. Rare fatalities have been reported. Some people have ataxia and paralysis of ocular convergence.[39] In rare cases, symptoms last as long as 48 hours, depending on the dosage

TABLE 66-3   Look-Alikes of Mushrooms Containing Isoxazole Toxins

Toxic Species	Edible Species
Amanita muscaria (see Figures 66-59 and 66-60)	Amanita caesarea (see Figure 66-47)
	Amanita rubescens (see Figure 66-13)
	Armillaria mellea (see Figures 66-51 to 66-53)
Amanita gemmata	Russula spp. (see Figure 66-45)
Amanita pantherina (see Figure 66-63)	Amanita rubescens (Figures 66-66 and 66-67)

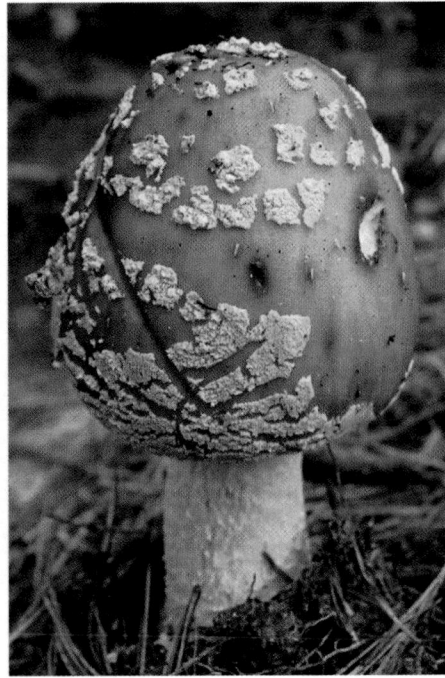

FIGURE 66-67 *Amanita rubescens.* (By Jason Hollinger from http://www.flickr.com. *Used with permission.*)

1. Supportive care.
2. Sedation as needed with benzodiazepine (diazepam, 2 to 5 mg IV every 10 minutes as needed) or phenobarbital (30 mg IV hourly).
3. If hyperpyrexia occurs (primarily seen in children), consider external cooling.

IV, Intravenously.

and individual host effect. There is a case report of psychosis lasting 5 days after ingestion of *A. muscaria*.[12] Ingestion of *A. pantherina* produces similar symptoms. In severe cases, seizures and CNS depression are observed[103] and rarely, death.[90]

Treatment

Treatment of patients with isoxazole reactions consists of supportive care (Box 66-11). Emesis caused by the toxin is unusual. Gastric emptying and activated charcoal administration are difficult because of CNS disturbances, have no proven effectiveness, and therefore are not recommended. Appropriate sedation with phenobarbital (30 mg IV hourly in adults, 0.5 mg/kg in children) or diazepam (2 to 5 mg IV repeated every 10 to 15 minutes in adults as needed, 0.1 to 0.3 mg/kg IV in children) is often necessary but requires caution. Phenobarbital or diazepam administered to treat *A. muscaria* ingestion may lead to unexpected apnea, flaccid paralysis, or both. Airway support and ventilatory assistance should be immediately available. Atropine may worsen the hallucinations, agitation, and delirium associated with isoxazole derivatives and should therefore be withheld unless the secretions or bradycardia are life threatening.

HALLUCINOGENIC MUSHROOMS

Perhaps the most sought-after mushrooms are "magic mushrooms," which are available as whole mushrooms in the wild and as spores (to grow your own) through mail-order catalogs. These mushrooms have been used for centuries for their hallucinogenic effects. Small, stone mushroom icons believed to be 3500 years old were found in Meso-American ruins.[67] Honey laced with *Psilocybe* can be purchased at Dutch coffee shops.

Causative Mushrooms

The most common hallucinogenic mushrooms are species of the *Psilocybe* genus (Box 66-12 and Table 66-4), which includes more than 100 species, not all of which cause hallucinations. These are "little brown mushrooms" (LBMs) (Figure 66-72). The cap is 0.5 to 4 cm (0.2 to 1.6 inches) in diameter (depending on the species), is usually smooth, and becomes sticky or slippery when wet. The stalk is slender and 4 to 15 cm (1.6 to 6 inches) long. Gills are gray to purple-gray; spores are dark, nearly black. The flesh of these mushrooms often turns blue or greenish when bruised or cut. The mushrooms are often mistaken for more poisonous species (e.g., *Galerina* [Figure 66-73] or *Inocybe* [see Figure 66-61]). These mushrooms also resemble *A. bisporus*. Regular grocery store mushrooms laced with lysergic acid diethylamide (LSD) or other hallucinogens are sold on the street as *Psilocybe*. Hallucinogenic mushrooms grow in a variety of habitats and are found throughout the world.

Other mushrooms, including members of the *Panaeolus* (see Figure 66-70) and *Gymnopilus* genera (see Figure 66-69), may contain psilocybin. *Panaeolus* mushrooms are also LBMs about the same size as *Psilocybe*. Gills are dark gray or black with black spores. They grow on dung throughout the tropics and subtropics of North America. Unlike *Psilocybe*, their caps do not become sticky or slippery when wet. The hallucinogenic effect and quantity of toxin varies among *Panaeolus* species.

Some *Gymnopilus* species (e.g., *Gymnopilus aeruginosus*) contain hallucinogens. These medium-sized mushrooms (cap, 5 to 15 cm [2 to 6 inches]; stalk, 5 to 12 cm [2 to 4.7 inches]) are variable in color (green, yellow, salmon, and red), with yellowish

Amanita
citrina (Figure 66-68)
porphyria

Conocybe
cyanopus
siligineoides
smithii

Gymnopilus (Figure 66-69)
aeruginosus
purpuratus
spectabilis
validipes

Naematoloma
popperianum

Panaeolus
campanulatus
castaneifolius
cyanescens
fimicola
foenisecii (Figure 66-70)

phalaenarum
semiovatus
sphinctrinus
subbalteatus

Psathyrella Sepulchralis
Psilocybe
baeocystis
caerulescens
caerulipes
cyanescens
cubensis
pelliculosa
semilanceata
strictipes
stuntzii

Stropharia
aeruginosa
coronilla
hornemannii
squamosal

TABLE 66-4 Look-Alikes of Mushrooms Containing Psilocybin or Psilocin

Toxic Species	Edible Species
Panaeolus foenisecii (see Figure 66-70)	*Psathyrella candolleana* (Figure 66-71) *Agrocybe pediades* *Marasmius oreades* (see Figure 66-65)
Panaeolus species (see Figure 66-70)	*Coprinus* spp. (see Figures 66-56 and 60-57)

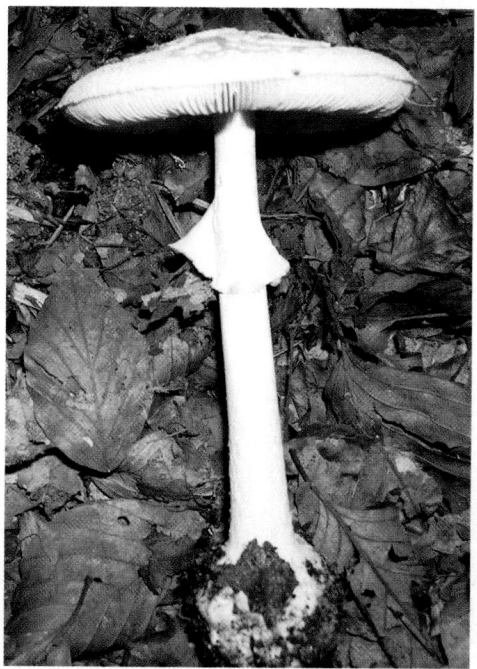

FIGURE 66-68 *Amanita citrina.* (By Tomasz Przechlewski from http://www.flickr.com. *Used with permission.*)

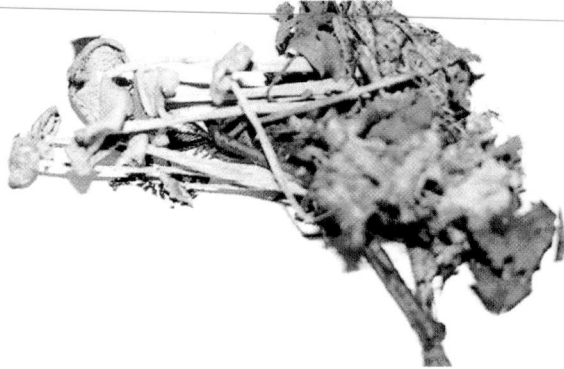

FIGURE 66-69 *Gymnopilus* mushroom—some are toxic.

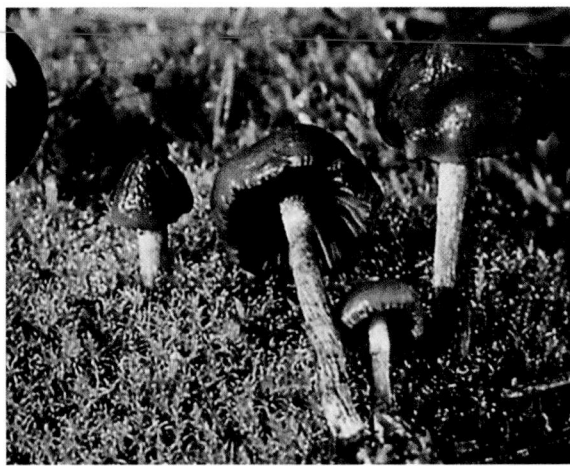

FIGURE 66-72 *Psilocybe caerulipes.*

gills and rusty spores. They grow on stumps or sawdust in the U.S. Pacific Northwest.

Visual hallucinations and ataxia were reported in a person ingesting *L. sulphureus* (see Figures 66-20 and 66-21), previously thought to be harmless.[3] It is not clear whether this mushroom contained hallucinogenic material or the individual ingested an additional mushroom.

Psilocybe sclerotia, or "magic truffles," have also been reported to contain psilocybin alkaloids. These have been a popular source of the psychoactive alkaloids because they had not typically been included in laws banning the sales of psilocybin-containing mushrooms.[92]

Toxin

Psilocybin and its somewhat unstable metabolite psilocin are indole compounds derived from tryptamine. These two toxins were first isolated by Albert Hofmann,[49] known as the father of LSD. Chemically, the toxins resemble 5-hydroxytryptamine (5-HT) and LSD and have similar effects. They maintain their potency in dried specimens.

Psilocybin, as well as LSD, inhibits the firing rate of serotonin-dependent neurons, particularly at the presynaptic receptors. It induces euphoria, hallucinations, and loss of time sensation. Many of these symptoms are similar to those seen with LSD. Some species contain phenylethylamine, which may be responsible for tachycardia and other adverse reactions.[5] In human volunteer studies, peak plasma levels were reached at 105 minutes.[45]

Clinical Presentation

Ingestion of 5 mg of psilocybin (10 mg of fresh *Psilocybe cubensis*) causes moderate euphoria. Ingestion of 10 mg leads to hallucinations and loss of time sensation. Heightened imagination occurs within 15 to 30 minutes of ingestion. Hallucinations may last for 4 to 6 hours. Serious side effects are rarely seen, but fever and seizures have been reported in children.[75] Up to 50% of patients have tachycardia and hypertension.[91] Ingestion resulting

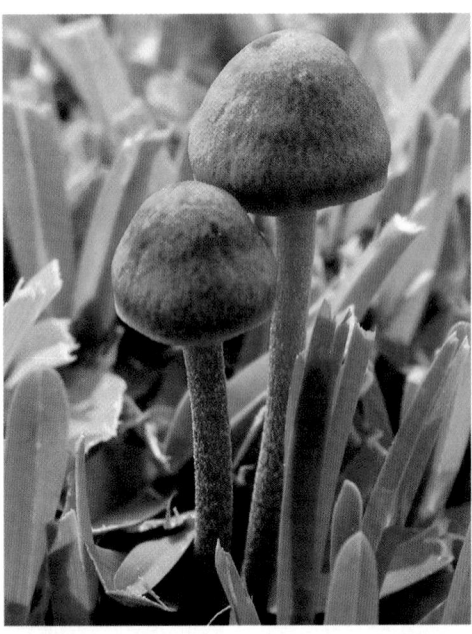

FIGURE 66-70 *Panaeolus foenisecii. (By Jason Hollinger from http://www.flickr.com. Used with permission.)*

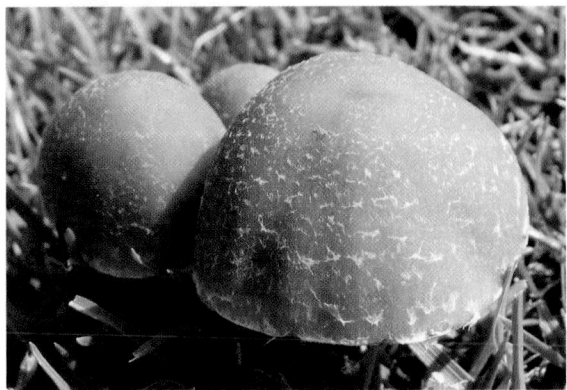

FIGURE 66-71 *Psathyrella candolleana. (By Jason Hollinger from http://www.flickr.com. Used with permission.)*

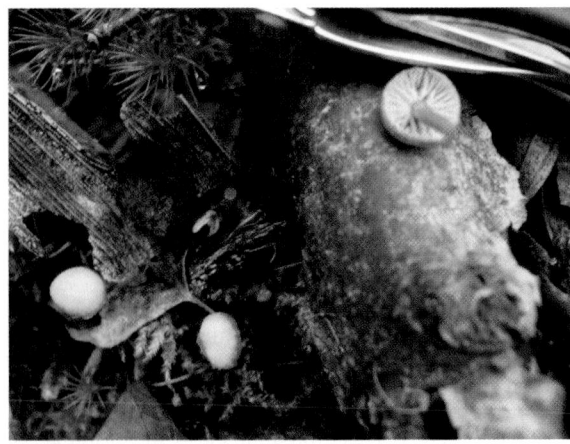

FIGURE 66-73 *Galerina marginata. (By Tomasz Przechlewski from http://www.flickr.com. Used with permission.)*

in myocardial infarction has been reported.[9] Flashbacks have been reported to occur in some persons for up to 4 months after ingestion.[7] Multifocal cerebral demyelination has been reported after ingestion of psilocybin-containing mushrooms.[115] Suicide while intoxicated with psilocybin-containing mushrooms has been reported in individuals with mental health or psychiatric disorders.[82]

Treatment

Recommendations for psilocybin toxicity are similar to those for isoxazole toxin (see Box 66-11). Initially, the patient should be placed in a quiet, supportive environment. Gastric emptying and activated charcoal administration are often impossible and may only enhance hallucinations. These modalities should be considered in patients with large ingestion who are brought early for treatment. Sedation can be accomplished when necessary with a benzodiazepine (e.g., diazepam, 0.1 mg/kg IV in children, or 2 to 5 mg IV in adults, repeated every 5 minutes as needed), phenobarbital (0.5 mg/kg IV in children, 30 mg IV in adults, repeated every 60 minutes as needed), chlorpromazine (50 to 100 mg intramuscularly [IM]), or haloperidol (5 mg IM). There is no evidence for the use of newer antipsychotic medications. Seizures can be controlled with diazepam in the doses just listed. Hyperpyrexia, seen primarily in children, is best treated with external cooling.

PROTOPLASMIC POISONS

GYROMITRA TOXIN

False morels (*Gyromitra esculenta* [Figure 66-74]) were once thought to be edible. During times of famine in Europe, ingestion of *Gyromitra* was encouraged.[44] Since 1793, these mushrooms have been suspected of causing toxicity, and since World War II, they have been known to cause hepatic failure, neurologic symptoms, and death. At present, they are collected, sold fresh, canned, and exported ("morschels") in Europe (Figure 66-75).[81] Symptoms appear 4 to 50 hours (usually 5 to 12 hours) after ingestion, with timing similar to that of *A. phalloides* poisoning. *Gyromitra* grows primarily in the spring and *A. phalloides* in the fall. Because of this difference in seasons and their distinct appearance, the identity of the two mushrooms is rarely confused.

Causative Mushrooms

Gyromitra esculenta (Figure 66-76) is approximately 5 to 16 cm (2 to 6.3 inches) in height with a reddish brown to dark-brown, irregularly shaped cap. The cap's surface is curved and folded, resembling a brain. The stalk is often as thick as the cap. The insides of the cap and stalk are hollow. This mushroom grows in the spring near pines and in sandy soil throughout North America. It is particularly common in Germany, Poland, and other eastern European countries. Mature species, particularly those with cap decay, may have increased toxicity. These mushrooms may be mistaken for morels, which are considered among the most delicious of wild mushrooms (Table 66-5).

Other members of the *Gyromitra* family contain gyromitrin. None of these mushrooms has been reported to cause toxicity in humans.

Toxin

Gyromitrin (*N*-methyl-*N*-formylhydrazone) was first isolated in 1967. This toxin is moderately volatile and heat sensitive. Cooking the mushrooms thoroughly and discarding the cooking liquid may decrease or eliminate the toxin. Symptoms have occurred despite proper cooking.

Once gyromitrin enters the stomach, hydrolysis yields *N*-methyl-*N*-formylhydrazine (MFH), which forms *N*-methylhydrazine or monomethylhydrazine (MH),[81] a component of rocket fuel. MH is a competitive inhibitor of pyridoxal phosphate, which interferes with enzyme systems (including decarboxylases, deaminases, and transaminases) requiring pyridoxine as a cofactor.[4] As a result, levels of GABA fall, interfering with neurotransmission.[61] It is believed that this decrease in GABA leads to altered mental status,

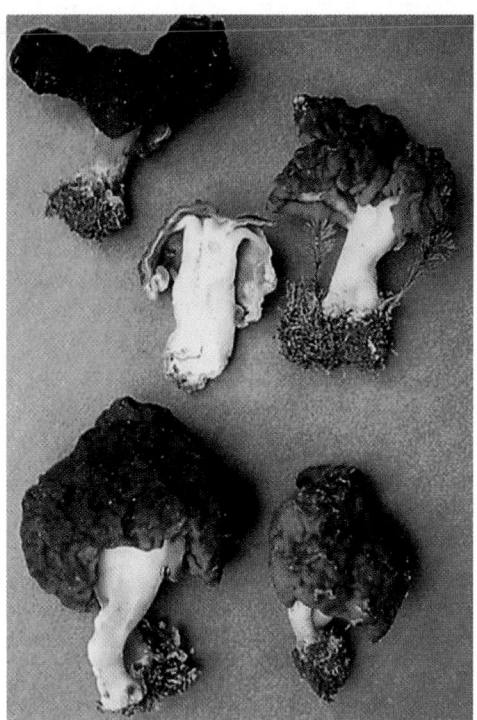

FIGURE 66-74 *Gyromitra esculenta*, which contains the hepatoxin gyromitrin. *(From Phillips R: Mushrooms of North America, Boston, 1991, Little, Brown.)*

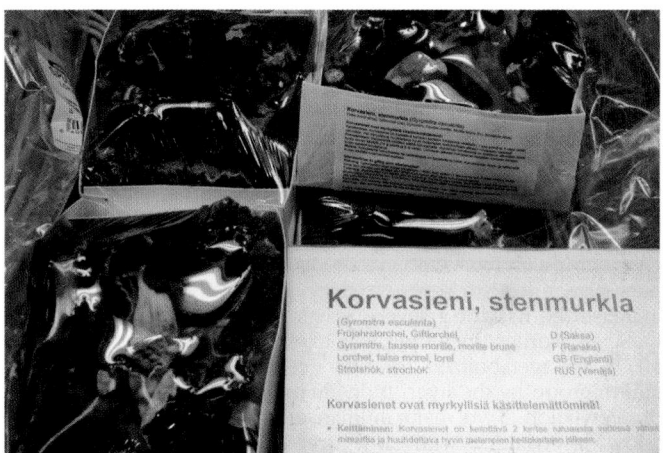

FIGURE 66-75 False morel fungi (*Gyromitra esculenta*) for sale at a department store in Helsinki. *(Courtesy Ilmari Karonen; Wikimedia Commons.)*

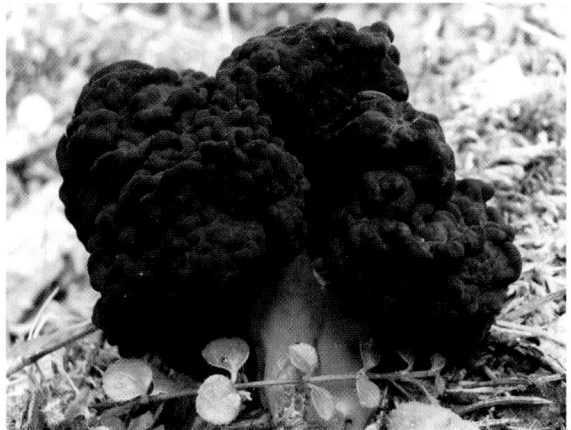

FIGURE 66-76 *Gyromitra esculenta*. *(By Jason Hollinger from http:// www.flickr.com. Used with permission.)*

TABLE 66-5 Look-Alike of Mushrooms Containing Gyromitrin

Toxic Species	Edible Species
Gyromitra esculenta (see Figure 66-76)	*Morchella esculenta* (see Figures 66-38 to 66-40)

seizures, or both. Recent questions have been raised about this widely accepted theory, because MH may cause seizures without a change in brain GABA levels.[74]

Both MFH and MH undergo oxidation in the liver into two highly reactive intermediates: a free methyl radical and an unstable diazonium compound.[81] These substances appear to produce local hepatic necrosis by blocking the activity of hepatic cytochrome enzyme systems, glutathione, and other hepatic biomolecules. There are significant concerns about long-term toxicity associated with repeated consumption of this mushroom. Each kilogram of fresh *G. esculenta* contains 3 to 100 mg gyromitrin. Fresh mushrooms contain 50 to 300 mg of MH per kilogram, and dried mushrooms up to 400 mg/kg. The human median lethal dose (LD_{50}) is suspected to be 20 to 50 mg/kg for adults and 10 to 30 mg/kg for children, or 0.4 to 1 kg of fresh mushrooms for an adult (average, 30 mushrooms) and 0.2 to 0.6 kg for a child.[81]

Clinical Presentation

Symptoms of gyromitrin toxicity are summarized in Box 66-13. They are generally delayed for 4 to 50 (average, 5 to 12) hours after ingestion. Initial symptoms include nausea, vomiting, and severe diarrhea. Some patients may have dizziness, weakness, muscle cramps, and loss of muscle coordination. In a severe ingestion, delirium, seizures, and coma are present. Hepatic failure develops over several days after ingestion, although hepatic damage is generally mild. Hypoglycemia, hypovolemia, severe hepatic failure, and death may occur.

Symptoms from gyromitrin toxin depend on amount consumed, toxin concentration, nature of the mushrooms, and other host factors. The variability of symptoms after ingestion of gyromitrin mushrooms is much greater than with other mushroom species. Some individuals can consume large quantities of *Gyromitra* with few or no symptoms. A second meal by the same person may lead to severe toxicity. Repeated consumption may increase the risk for a severe reaction.

Several drugs, including isoniazid, hydralazine, and probably MH,[18] are metabolized through acetylation of a hydrazine or amino group by the liver. Individuals vary greatly in the rapidity of acetylation. Two major human groups are termed "fast" and "slow" acetylators, with slow acetylation being an autosomal recessive trait. Slow acetylators in general have greater and more prolonged toxicity after ingestion of these drugs. Similar variation in toxicity in fast and slow acetylators is seen when *Gyromitra* mushrooms are ingested.

Treatment

Symptoms develop several hours after ingestion of *Gyromitra*. Treatment is summarized in Box 66-14. Activated charcoal (1 g/kg PO or via gastric tube) is of no value if given more than 1 hour after ingestion. At that time, most patients are asymptomatic and unaware that they have ingested a toxic mushroom. Pyridoxine has been useful in patients with neurologic disorders such as seizures and coma from MH toxicity and is of theoretical

BOX 66-13 Symptoms of Gyromitrin Toxicity

1. Onset of nausea, vomiting, and diarrhea within 4 to 50 (average, 5 to 12) hours.
2. Neurologic symptoms of dizziness, weakness, and loss of muscle coordination. Severe neurologic symptoms include coma, delirium, and seizures.
3. Hepatic failure begins 2 to 4 days after ingestion. Hepatic failure is often associated with hypoglycemia.

BOX 66-14 Treatment of Gyromitrin Toxicity

1. Activated charcoal if the patient presents within 1 hour of ingestion. Note that most of these patients will be asymptomatic.
2. Fluid and electrolyte replacement as needed.
3. Glucose replacement. Treat hypoglycemia with glucose infusion.
4. Pyridoxine, 25 mg/kg up to 20 g/day intravenously, to control seizures or coma.[6] If significant hepatic failure occurs, transfer patient to transplant facility.

benefit in those with gyromitrin toxicity. Persons who ingest *G. esculenta* and develop significant neurologic symptoms should receive pyridoxine (25 mg/kg IV initial dose, up to 20 g/day).[4,60,133] No evidence indicates that pyridoxine alters the course of hepatic disease. High-dose pyridoxine therapy may cause acute peripheral neuropathies.[2]

Baseline measurements of liver transaminases (alanine aminotransferase [ALT], aspartate aminotransferase [AST]), prothrombin time (PT), partial thromboplastin time (PTT), international normalized ratio (INR), BUN, creatinine, complete blood cell count (CBC), platelet count, glucose, and electrolytes should be performed. ALT, AST, PT, PTT, INR, BUN, and creatinine should be monitored at least daily for 3 to 4 days for the development of hepatic failure. Rapid deterioration of the liver (ALT or AST >2000 international units [IU], PTT >50 seconds) mandates immediate transfer to a tertiary center with liver transplantation capability. Persons with significant hepatic failure may require monitoring of blood glucose level every 2 to 4 hours and supplemental glucose administration for symptomatic hypoglycemia.

No specific antidote or treatment is available for the fulminant hepatic failure. The appropriate timing or necessity of liver transplantation is uncertain. In persons with fulminant hepatic failure from infectious causes, the presence of an abnormal PT (unresponsive to fresh-frozen plasma) and development of hepatorenal syndrome, grade II hepatic encephalopathy, hypoglycemia, and uncorrectable metabolic acidosis are used as signs that transplantation is needed on an emergent basis. Persons with fulminant hepatic failure from toxic ingestion, elevated bilirubin level, and young age are important indicators of a poor prognosis. As discussed later, the model for end-stage liver disease (MELD) score for assessing liver failure provides the best prognostic information. Mortality from gyromitrin poisoning is reported to be 15% to 35%.[32]

RENAL TOXICITY

Although originally thought to be an edible mushroom, *Cortinarius orellanus* was associated with 81 cases of renal toxicity in the 1950s.[42] This led to isolation of the toxin orellanine, which is found in the mushrooms *C. orellanus, Cortinarius speciosissimus,* and *Cortinarius gentilis.* Most cases occur in Europe and Japan.

Causative Mushrooms

Cortinarius orellanus has a small, smooth, brown to brownish red cap 30 to 80 cm (12 to 31 inches) in diameter. The stalk is somewhat yellow, often darker closer toward the soil. Gills are orange to rust with rust-colored spores. It grows in deciduous woods, most frequently in sandy soil underneath oaks and birches. It is ubiquitous throughout Europe. Some other species of *Cortinarius* are found in the United States and may be toxic (Figure 66-77 and Box 66-15). *Amanita smithiana,* which grows in the Pacific Northwest, has been associated with renal failure in the U.S. patients.[131] It may be mistaken for *Tricholoma magnivelare.*[129] *Amanita proxima* in France and *Amanita pseudoporphyria* in Japan have caused similar symptoms.[104]

Toxin

The two toxins isolated from *C. orellanus,* orellanine and orelline, are structurally related to paraquat and diquat. Their mechanism of action remains a mystery. These are heat-stable compounds,

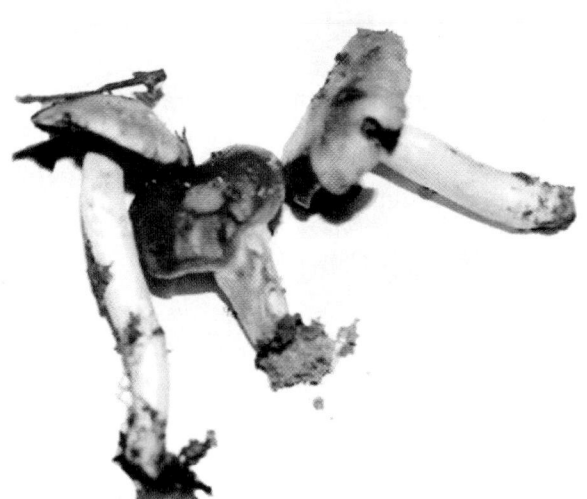

FIGURE 66-77 *Cortinarius* sp. (United States).

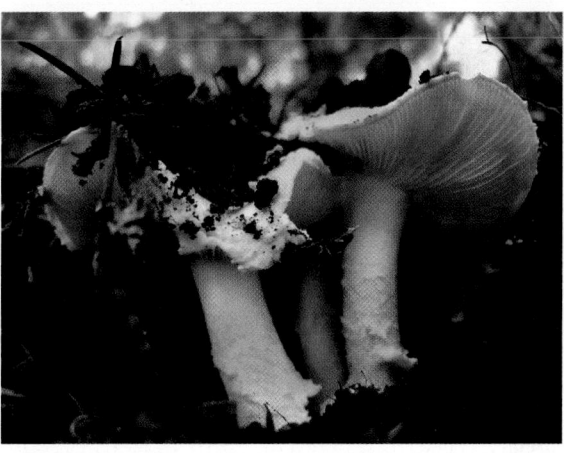

FIGURE 66-78 *Amanita smithiana*. *(By Heather Gardner-Madras from http://www.flickr.com. Used with permission.)*

unaffected by cooking. The toxin appears to cause intense interstitial nephritis with early fibrosis.[50] The toxin can be identified with thin-layer chromatography (TLC).[52] Orellanine is being evaluated as a potential chemotherapeutic agent for certain types of cancers, including metastatic renal cancer. High-performance liquid chromatography (HPLC) analysis is able to detect orellanine in urine and in extracts of Cortinaceae members.[47] *Amanita* species contain aminohexadrienoic acid,[104,129] which appears to be responsible for its renal toxicity.

Clinical Presentation

Persons who ingest these mushrooms are generally asymptomatic for 2 to 20 days. During this latent period, acute renal failure develops. Some persons develop neurologic changes, including paresthesias, taste impairment, and cognitive disorders.

Symptoms vary greatly. One case report described 26 soldiers who ate soup made of *C. orellanus* in nearly identical quantities.[11] Acute renal failure developed in 12 patients on or around day 11. Eight individuals later recovered normal renal function, whereas four required long-term dialysis or kidney transplantation. The other 14 soldiers showed no rise in BUN or creatinine levels but developed leukocyturia and hematuria that persisted for more than 1 month. Renal failure reportedly occurs in 30% to 46% of persons who ingest these mushrooms and become ill. Renal function returns in approximately 50% of affected patients.

Renal biopsy in patients with orellanine-induced renal failure shows changes in tubular epithelial cells and in actin filaments within their cytoplasm.[87] These biopsy changes may persist for up to 3 months.[11]

Treatment

In most persons who ingest nephrotoxic mushrooms, unexplained acute renal failure develops many days later. If a person presents within 1 hour after eating orellanine-containing mushrooms, gastric emptying and activated charcoal administration (1 g/kg PO or via gastric tube) is theoretically indicated to

prevent some absorption, decreasing the resultant toxicity. There is no evidence for its use. Early presentation is rare.

Once acute renal failure develops, baseline and repeated monitoring of BUN, creatinine, electrolytes, CBC, differential, and urinalysis should be performed to monitor renal function. Urine output should be monitored, and if it decreases, fluid administration should be used to achieve optimal hydration. Serum potassium, calcium, and magnesium should be monitored closely. If renal failure progresses, the patient should be transferred to a facility for hemodialysis and possible renal transplantation. Renal function may return to normal after months of dialysis dependency.

AMATOXINS

The mushrooms that contain amatoxins are responsible for more than 95% of fatalities caused by mushrooms (Box 66-16 and Table 66-6). *A. phalloides* is most common in central and eastern Europe; immigrants to the United States may have carried mushroom spores in wood products from eastern Europe. *Amanita verna* and *Amanita virosa* are more common in the United States. Toxicity has occurred from cooked or frozen mushrooms and even tea made from *Amanita* mushrooms.[94]

Causative Mushrooms

Mushrooms reported or suspected of containing amatoxins are listed in Box 66-16. The common names of *A. phalloides* (Figure 66-79; see also Figures 66-6 and 66-7) and its relatives, *A. verna* and *A. virosa* (Figures 66-80 and 66-81), are death cap, death angel, and destroying angel, reflecting their association with fatal outcome. *A. phalloides* has a white to greenish cap 4 to 16 cm (1.6 to 6.3 inches) in diameter, often with remnants of the veil as warts. The stalk is generally thick, 5 to 18 cm (2 to 7 inches) long, with a large bulb at the base, often with a vulva. A thin ring is usually present on the stalk. Gills are generally free and white to green in color; spores are white. The mushrooms grow under deciduous trees in the autumn.

Amanita virosa (see Figures 66-80 and 66-81) is more common in the United States. It resembles *A. phalloides*, but the cap is more yellow or white. *A. verna* is characteristically white. All grow in deciduous woods. Even mushroom experts have been tempted by the large white mushroom, which is tasty. The fatality rate is 35% in adults and 50% in children. Unfortunately, mushroom gatherers may mistake amatoxin-bearing *Amanita* species for edible mushrooms (see Table 66-6).

Some *Lepiota* mushrooms (see Figure 66-34), including *Lepiota castanea* and *Lepiota josserandii*, contain high concentrations of amatoxin. There have been two deaths attributed to *L. josserandii* in upstate New York.

Mushrooms that contain amatoxin may have a positive Meixner test. This test was first described by Wieland[132] in 1949 and popularized by Meixner.[77] A drop of liquid is expressed from a fresh mushroom onto print-free (ligand-free) newspaper and

---

BOX 66-15 Mushrooms Reported as Causing Renal Failure

Amanita
proxima
pseudoporphyria
smithiana (Figure 66-78)

Cortinarius
gentilis
orellanus

rellanus
rubellus
speciosissimus
splendens
venenosus

BOX 66-16 Mushrooms Reported or Suspected of Containing Amatoxins

Amanita
bisporigera
decipiens Jacquetant
hygroscopica Coker
ocreata
ocreata Peck
phalloides (see Figures 66-6, 66-7, and 66-80)
suballiacea Murr
tenuifolia Murr
verna
virosa (see Figures 66-80 and 66-81)

Conocybe
filaris

Galerina
autumnalis Smith and Singer (Figures 66-82 and 66-83)
badipes Kühn
beinrothil
fasciculata Hongo
helvoliceps
marginata
marginata Kühner (Figure 66-84)
sulciceps Boedjin
unicolor Sing
venenata AH Smith

Lepiota
brunneoincarnata Chodat and Martin
brunneolilacea Bon and Boiffard
castanea
castanea Quelet
citrophylla (Berk and Br.) Sacc.
clypeolaria (Bull.:Fr.) Kummer (see Figure 66-34)
clypeolarioides Rea
felina (Pers.:Fr) Karsten
fulvella Rea
fuscovinacea Moeller and Lange
griseovirens Maire
heimii Locq.
helveola
helveola Bres.
helveoloides Bon ex Bon and Andary
josserandii
josserandii Bon and Boiffard
kuehneri Huijsm. Ex Hora
langei Locq.
lilacea Bres.
locanensis Espinosa
ochraceofulva Orton
pseudohelveola Kühner ex Hora
pseudolilacea Huijsm.
rufescens Lange
subincarnata Lange
xanthophylla Orton

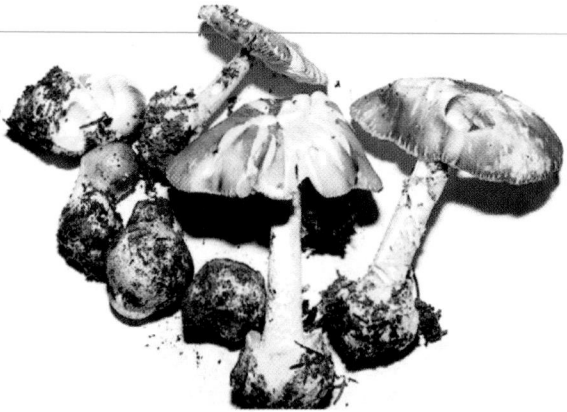

FIGURE 66-79 *Amanita phalloides*—toxic.

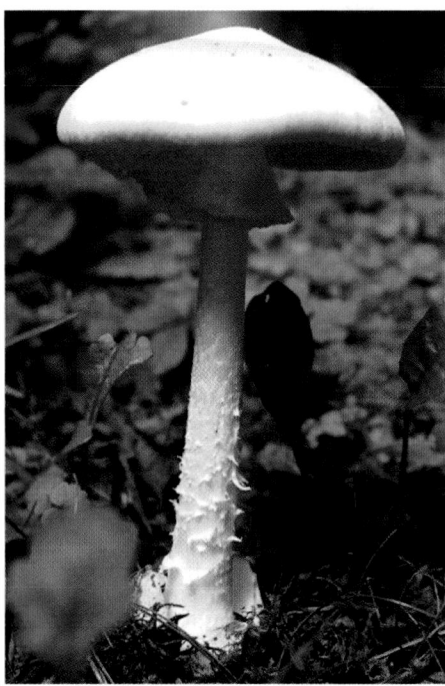

FIGURE 66-80 *Amanita virosa. (By Jason Hollinger from* http://www.flickr.com. *Used with permission.)*

TABLE 66-6 Look-Alikes of Mushrooms Containing Amatoxin

Toxic Species	Edible Species
Amanita phalloides (see Figures 66-6 and 66-7)	Amanita fulva (Figure 66-85)
Amanita verna	Lepiota flavovirens
Amanita virosa (see Figure 66-80)	Agaricus bisporus (see Figure 66-12)

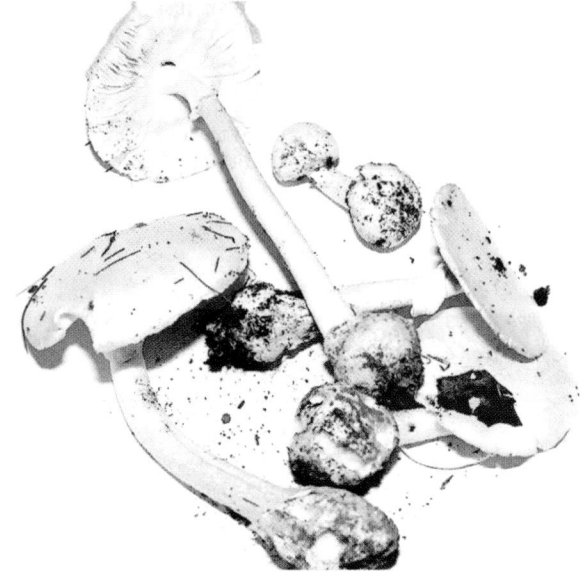

FIGURE 66-81 *Amanita virosa*—toxic.

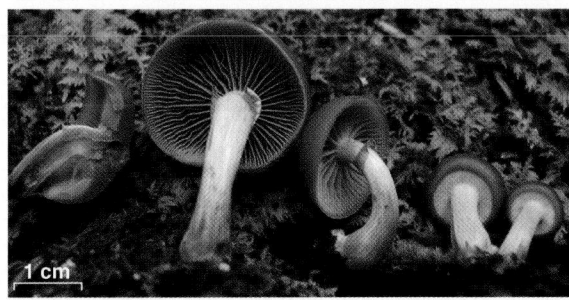

FIGURE 66-82 *Galerina autumnalis. (By Jason Hollinger from* http://www.flickr.com. *Used with permission.)*

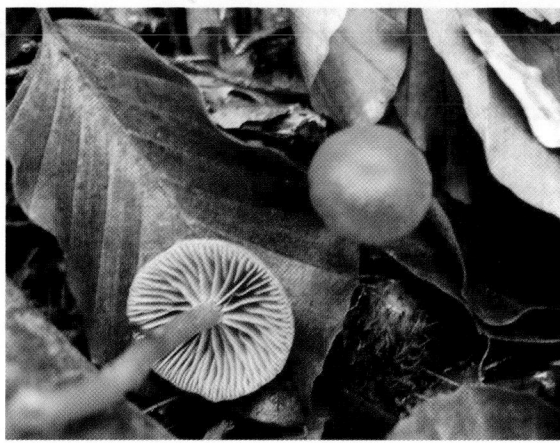

FIGURE 66-84 *Galerina marginata. (By Tomasz Przechlewski from* http://www.flickr.com. *Used with permission.)*

allowed to dry. A drop of concentrated (10 to 12 N) hydrochloric acid is added. A blue color develops within 1 to 2 minutes in the presence of amatoxins. Control tests on newspaper without mushroom juice and paper containing ligand should be conducted. False-positive results are common and can be elicited by excessive drying temperatures (>63°C [145.4°F]) or exposure to sunlight. The test can detect 2 mcg of α-amatoxin.[8] False-positive tests also occur from mushrooms containing psilocybin, terpenes, bufotenin, and other tryptamine compounds.[8] Almost 20% of gilled mushrooms that did not contain amatoxins tested positive in one study.[111] A positive test does not identify an amatoxin-containing mushroom, and further identification is necessary. TLC more accurately identifies the presence of amatoxin and can be done on mushroom liquid, human serum, or urine.[97] Radioimmunoassay (RIA), HPLC,[17] and a recently developed enzyme-linked immunosorbent assay (ELISA) test[89] can detect amatoxins in serum or urine.

Toxins

The mushroom *A. phalloides* contains two groups of toxins: amatoxins and phallotoxins. Each group contains several toxins. There are now eight identified amatoxins: α-amanitin, β-amanitin, γ-amanitin, ε-amanitin, amanin, amaninamide, amanullinic acid, and amanullin. Of these, α-amanitin is thought to be primarily responsible for human disease. α-Amanitin injected into animals produces hepatic toxicity characteristic of human ingestion of *A. phalloides.* In dogs, two phases of toxicity are seen. The first is cellular impairment with inhibition of protein and urea synthesis, followed by a second phase of hepatocellular changes, including condensation of nuclear chromatin and foaming of the cytoplasm.[73]

Phallotoxins include phalloidin, phalloin, phallisin, phallacidin, phallacin, phallisacin, and prophalloin. Phalloidin is the primary phallotoxin. Phallotoxins bind to F-actin, disrupting plasma membranes and causing massive efflux of calcium and potassium. Phallotoxins cause death in animals within 2 hours but are not

believed to play a role in human toxicity.[33] Humans may not even absorb these toxins, although they may be responsible for local gastric irritation. *A. virosa* contains amatoxins and virotoxins. Virotoxins resemble phallotoxin biochemically and also bind F-actin and cause death in animals within a few hours. Six different virotoxins have been isolated, but none is thought to play a role in human *Amanita* hepatotoxicity.

Amatoxins are heat stable and not destroyed by cooking, freezing, or drying. *A. phalloides* mushrooms stored in a freezer for 7 to 8 months have resulted in death.[48]

Amatoxins are concentrated in the cap, gills, ring, and stalk. Very small amounts have been detected in the spores, although much less than in the other tissues.[76] α-Amanitin has been detected in most *Amanita* species in concentrations ranging from 50 to 6000 ppm.[124] Phallotoxins are more concentrated in the bulb and vulva. The concentration of toxin in a given mushroom depends on environmental factors and the soil.[20] After ingestion, amatoxins are absorbed from the gut and actively transported into the liver through transport systems shared by bile acids and xenobiotics. Amatoxins do not appear to cross the placenta.[125] α-Amanitin is rapidly cleared from plasma.[55] Amatoxins are not protein bound. They bind to ribonucleic acid (RNA) polymerase II and inhibit formation of messenger RNA (mRNA).[23] This in turn inhibits transcription, because the reservoir of mRNA is depleted.

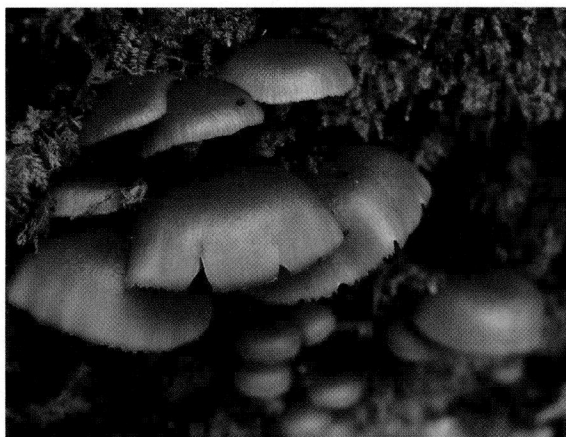

FIGURE 66-83 *Galerina autumnalis. (By Jason Hollinger from* http://www.flickr.com. *Used with permission.)*

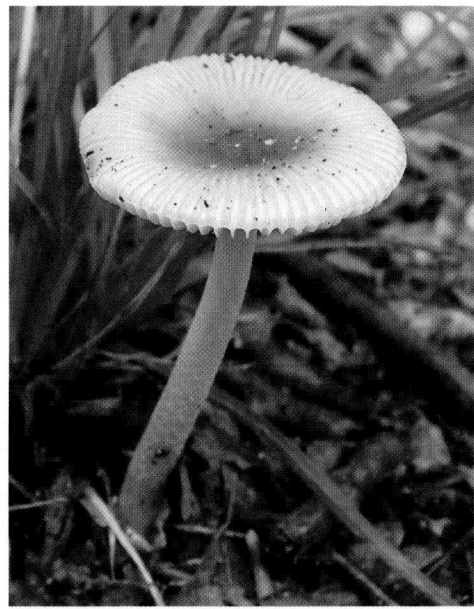

FIGURE 66-85 *Amanita fulva. (By Jason Hollinger from* http://www.flickr.com. *Used with permission.)*

Amatoxins are excreted into the bile, where they are reabsorbed and once again transported into the liver.[13] Interruption of this enterohepatic circulation could be a therapeutic tool. However, by the time clinical symptoms are present, enterohepatic circulation largely is complete, making its disruption ineffective.

Within the liver, α-amanitin may undergo some metabolism through the hepatic cytochrome system. Animal studies suggest that a more toxic metabolite may be produced through this metabolism, although this metabolite has never been isolated.[109,110] Nuclear fragmentation and condensation of chromosomal material have been observed within 15 hours of injection.[27] Glycogen is rapidly depleted, and fatty degeneration occurs within liver parenchymal cells. Mitochondria become swollen, and microvesicles appear throughout the cytoplasm.[27] Direct renal toxicity may occur.

Clinical Presentation

Symptoms of amatoxin poisoning are summarized in Box 66-17. People who ingest the mushroom *Amanita phalloides* feel well for 4 to 16 hours. Although nausea and vomiting are often reported with symptomatic mushroom exposures,[17] severe nausea, vomiting, abdominal cramps, and diarrhea follow this characteristic latent period with *A. phalloides* ingestion. Early complications include fluid and electrolyte imbalance (hypoglycemia, hypokalemia, and elevated BUN from dehydration). People in whom symptoms develop earlier (4 to 10 hours) are more likely to experience severe hepatotoxicity. Over the next 12 to 24 hours, the GI symptoms abate. The second latent period is followed by hepatic failure, which develops between 48 and 72 hours after ingestion in most patients. Hepatic failure may be of varying severity; it is frequently worse in children and depends minimally on the amount of mushroom ingested. Kidney failure can develop as a result of hepatic injury or possibly by direct renal toxicity to the kidneys.[37]

Children have greater toxicity and higher mortality, perhaps because of the relative quantity of mushrooms ingested or the varying metabolism in young children (differing levels of cytochrome enzymes). Previous experiments showed that ethanol concurrently ingested with *A. phalloides* decreased hepatotoxicity.[29] Therefore, decreased toxicity in adults could theoretically result from ingestion of ethanol with an *Amanita* mushroom dinner. More recently, however, ethanol failed to alter hepatotoxicity in an animal model poisoned with α-amanitin, which raises doubts about this explanation for increased toxicity in children.[108]

In addition to hepatic failure, endocrinopathies can develop, with hypocalcemia, decreased thyroid function, and elevated insulin levels in the presence of hypoglycemia.[58] Hypocalcemia may be caused in part by a loss of calcium through diarrhea or by a direct effect on osteoclasts. Renal failure may contribute to hypocalcemia. The thyroid abnormalities probably result from decreased hormone synthesis caused by overwhelming illness and blocked peripheral conversion of thyroxine (T_4) to triiodothyronine (T_3). Thyroid-stimulating hormone (TSH) depression may result from decreased synthesis caused by inhibition of RNA polymerase II by amatoxin. Hypothyroidism has not been clinically significant. Hypoglycemia is probably the result of several processes, including impaired hepatic gluconeogenesis, increased insulin release from the initial hyperglycemia, and tissue destruction of the pancreas.[30] Bone marrow toxicity with decreased neutrophils, lymphocytes, and platelets has been noted. Disseminated intravascular coagulation and coagulopathies secondary to hepatic dysfunction are common.[101] Pancreatitis occurs in up to

50% of patients.[30] Hypophosphatemia is particularly common in children, for unknown reasons. Myopathy has been associated with *Amanita* toxicity.[40]

Hepatic biopsy shows diffuse and severe steatosis with periportal inflammation and necrosis. Renal biopsy shows acute tubular necrosis with hyaline casts.[26] Extremely high levels of hepatic enzymes are seen. Level of liver transaminases are not helpful in predicting the patient's prognosis. A precipitous drop in liver transaminases, often to normal levels, may occur just before death. In addition to the biochemical factors (e.g., high transaminases) and coagulopathy, hypoglycemia and thrombocytopenia are associated with increased likelihood of mortality in amatoxin poisonings. High urea levels and hyponatremia, as well as certain clinical characteristics, including low mean arterial pressure, encephalopathy, mucosal hemorrhage, and oliguria/anuria, have also been shown to be indicative of prognosis.

Treatment

Attempts to treat *A. phalloides* poisoning have ranged from scientific to purely empirical (Box 66-18). Noting that rabbits were able to eat the *A. phalloides* mushroom with impunity, clinicians fed ground raw rabbit to patients with *Amanita* poisoning, without success.[121] Hemodialysis was long recommended but now has been shown to be ineffective, because the toxin is rapidly cleared from the plasma. Amatoxin is taken up in liver cells within 5 hours after IV administration.[25] In a retrospective study of 205 cases of amatoxin ingestion,[30] hemodialysis worsened the prognosis, and charcoal hemoperfusion did not improve outcome. Plasmapheresis has been used, but this appears to be ineffective because the toxin is largely intracellular and has caused cellular damage by the time symptoms appear.[93]

Despite this scientific evidence, the literature continues to report the use of dialysis/hemofiltration,[17] hemoperfusion, and plasmapheresis.[57] Antigen-binding fragment (Fab) monoclonal antibodies against amatoxin were developed and tested in mice. Although hepatic toxicity was greatly lessened, renal toxicity was 50 times greater than in control animals, possibly because of dissociation of the amatoxin-Fab molecule in the kidneys.[24]

Previously, thioctic acid and benzylpenicillin were recommended as treatments. Both these treatments are now questioned. In a retrospective study, thioctic acid was more frequently associated in humans with fatal outcome.[30] A more recent review of patients treated with a variety of antidotes showed benzylpenicillin was more effective than simple supportive care, but less effective than silymarin or antioxidant therapy;[21] the authors suggested abandoning the use of penicillin. However, because silymarin has not been easily available in the United States, some poison control centers may still recommend penicillin. If benzylpenicillin is used, the recommended dose is high: 300,000 to 1 million units/kg/day IV. Side effects are significant and include allergy, hyponatremia,[22] and granulocytopenia.[85]

Silymarin is the active component of the milk thistle *Silybum marianum*. It is an antioxidant that accumulates in the liver.[64] Silymarin binds tightly to the plasma membrane, stabilizing it,[95,96] and hinders amatoxin from penetrating the cell wall.[56,126,127] It is a free radical scavenger,[31,72,130] inhibits lipid peroxidation,[10,14,31,83] and stimulates RNA polymerase I.[130] In both retrospective studies, silymarin has shown promising reductions in mortality.[21,28] The IV form has recently become available in the United States as

IV, Intravenously.

Legalon. The IV dose of silybin dihemisuccinate is 5 mg/kg over 1 hour, followed by 20 mg/kg/day for 6 days or until liver transaminases normalize. There have been no controlled trials assessing IV silibinin, but review of uncontrolled trials and case reports suggest a lower mortality rate compared with other treatments, including penicillin and penicillin with silibinin.[35,79] The oral preparation (70-mg capsules) is less well studied; dosage recommendation is 1.4 to 4.2 g/day. Silymarin is most effective when started within 24 hours of ingestion.[35] Some poison control centers recommend obtaining milk thistle seed extract from a local nutrition or health food store if Legalon is not available. Milk thistle seed extract typically consists of 65% to 80% silymarin. Silymarin contains both silybin A and B, with silibinin being a 1:1 combination of silybin A and B.

Gastric decontamination (ipecac, gastric lavage, whole-bowel irrigation) may be useful in patients who can tolerate the procedure and have presented early.[1,128] Unfortunately, by the time patients with *Amanita* ingestions present to the hospital, the ingestion is many hours old, and intense nausea and vomiting may limit ability to administer activated charcoal. Although amatoxin has enterohepatic circulation, no data support any therapy designed to disrupt the enterohepatic circulation unless the ingestion is noted within the first few hours.[21] Likewise, there are no data to support forced diuresis.

The French have used hyperbaric oxygen as a treatment for *Amanita* toxicity.[65] Hyperbaric oxygen has been shown to have efficacy in animal models.

Recent animal work has suggested the use of antioxidants. Cimetidine has been shown to be effective in animals[109] and has been reportedly used in humans[21] (4 to 10 g/day IV for adults; pediatric dose not described). Vitamin C and *N*-acetylcysteine (NAC) have been used with some success.[21,123] NAC was not found to prevent *Amanita*-induced hepatoxicity in a mouse model. However, its free radical and reactive oxygen species scavenging properties may be beneficial.[128] Other reported treatments include aucubin and kutkin, both plant derivatives.[21]

Intravenous normal saline or Ringer's lactate is needed to replace GI fluid losses. Electrolyte losses (particularly potassium) may be significant. BUN, creatinine, CBC with differential, platelet count, electrolytes, glucose, calcium, phosphorus, magnesium, urinalysis, PT, PTT, INR, fibrinogen, amylase, protein, and albumin should be initially measured and repeated at least daily to monitor liver and renal function. Hyperglycemia is common on the first day, but insulin is generally not required. Hypoglycemia occurs after 24 hours and may be severe, requiring IV concentrated glucose. Therefore, bedside determinations of glucose level should be performed at least every 6 hours.

The patient with liver failure from *Amanita* will appear similar to a patient with any other type of advanced liver disease, with jaundice and asterixis. Hepatic encephalopathy can develop with elevated ammonia level and increased intracranial pressure. Tests of liver damage, including ALT, AST, alkaline phosphatase, ammonia, PT, and PTT, should be repeated at least daily and two or three times a day if hepatic failure develops. Transaminases that rise rapidly or are in excess of 2000 IU or PTT greater than 50 seconds signal severe toxicity and the need for referral to a transplant center.

Once liver failure begins, it is treated the same as any other fulminant hepatitis. Hypoglycemia is common. Supplemental glucose should be readily available. Dietary protein should be limited to 0.5 g/kg/day. There is no need to supply supplemental thiamin or multivitamins. Oral lactulose, 30 to 45 mL every 6 to 8 hours, may reduce hepatic encephalopathy. In patients who do not tolerate lactulose, neomycin (1 g PO three times daily) can be tried. PT, PTT, and INR should be measured at least twice daily once hepatic failure begins, and vitamin K (100 mg IM), fresh-frozen plasma (2 to 6 units initially), or both should be used to correct abnormalities in coagulation.

If hepatic failure progresses, a liver transplant may be required. The timing of the transplant is highly controversial. Criteria used for other causes of fulminant hepatic failure are often applied to amatoxin poisoning. Factors associated with poor prognosis in acetaminophen-induced hepatic damage include metabolic acidosis, PT greater than 50 seconds, and elevated serum creatinine (>2.0 mg/dL).[88] The largest study suggests that a person with ALT or AST level greater than 2000 IU, grade II hepatic encephalopathy, or PT greater than 50 seconds is at serious risk for death and should be considered for an emergency liver transplant.[23] Persons who met these criteria have survived without transplant.[70,99] The MELD score appears to be more effective than the King's College or Clichy's criteria for assessing the need for hepatic transplant. There are many online calculators for the MELD score, which uses bilirubin, INR, and creatinine levels.[134] Increased reparative enzymes may correlate with hepatic recovery.[53] These enzymes, including α-fetoprotein, retinal binding protein, γ-glutamyl transferase, and des-γ-carboxyprothrombin, are thought to be released during the healing phase of liver disease. Because hepatic failure develops rapidly, victims with toxicity due to mushrooms who have significant hepatic dysfunction must be transferred early to a transplantation site. Patients undergoing liver transplantation for fulminant hepatic failure (not caused by *A. phalloides*) have a 60% to 80% survival rate.[21] There are no statistics specifically for patients with mushroom poisoning. In Europe, an extracorporeal liver assistance device, the molecular adsorbent recirculating system (MARS), has been developed and used successfully in four patients.[19,54,68,112] MARS has been suggested as a bridge to liver transplantation[112] and in combination with therapeutic plasma exchange.[135] Early use may offer more benefit with regard to toxin removal. A temporary liver transplant was performed on a child and sustained her while her own liver recovered.[100]

Some persons who survive acute hepatic failure caused by *Amanita* without needing hepatic transplant may have persistent elevation in liver transaminases. In one study of 14 patients with severe *Amanita*-induced hepatotoxicity, eight showed persisted elevations in AST and ALT without normalization over a 1-year follow-up period.[23] All had biopsy evidence of chronic active hepatitis with positive anti–smooth muscle antibody and cryoglobulins. It is not known whether these persons will have an increased risk for hepatoma or will develop more serious complications of chronic active hepatitis.

Amatoxin ingestion during pregnancy does not appear to have serious consequences. Several reports now suggest that amatoxin does not cross the placenta.[107,119] In one study, 22 pregnant women poisoned during their pregnancy had similar outcomes to a control group; however, only five ingested mushrooms in their first trimester.[119]

MISCELLANEOUS REPORTS OF TOXICITY FROM MUSHROOMS

Occasional toxicity has been reported with other mushrooms. Erythromelalgia has been reported after ingestion of *Clitocybe amoenolens*.[34,106,105] The mushroom contains the toxin clitidine, which resembles nicotinic acid. *Tricholoma equestre* or *Russula subnigricans* ingestion is associated with rhabdomyolysis, respiratory failure, and hepatic and renal dysfunction.[6,16,104] Deaths from acute myocarditis and renal failure have been reported.[6]

APPROACH TO THE PATIENT WITH MUSHROOM POISONING

Four types of individuals develop mushroom toxicity: foragers, children, those seeking hallucinogenic "highs," and rarely, victims of attempted homicide. Most patients seek medical care only after symptoms develop. If small children are observed chewing on lawn mushrooms, caregivers should be advised to call the nearest regional poison information center.

Persons with agitation, altered perceptions, or frank hallucinations temporally related to mushroom ingestion are probably intoxicated with isoxazole or hallucinogenic mushrooms. Whether the mushrooms are picked accidentally or ingested intentionally, the treatment and clinical course are identical.

Persons who develop muscarinic symptoms (salivation, urination, diaphoresis, GI upset, emesis) present such a classic picture that it is rarely confused with any other presentation. Some drugs (e.g., bethanechol) may cause similar symptoms when taken in overdose. Patients with this variety of mushroom poisoning generally remain mentally clear and should be able to relate an appropriate history.

Patients with GI symptoms can be divided into those with early and those with delayed presentation. Those with early (within 2 hours of ingestion) GI symptoms generally have a benign course, except for persons with a mixed ingestion. Most guidebooks for mushroom hunters recommend eating only one variety of mushroom at a time, but more daring or foolish individuals mix multiple mushrooms and eat them frequently over the day. This makes diagnosis based on time of onset of symptoms difficult. Early onset of GI symptoms may mask more significant delayed symptoms. In these patients, identification of ingested mushrooms becomes essential to planning therapy.

Accurate botanical identification of the mushroom can be difficult. Only 800 of the 3000 species found in Europe can be identified without a microscope.[121] With the popularity of digital imaging, photos of suspicious mushrooms can be sent to poison control centers by e-mail and similarly can be forwarded to mycologists. This may save several hours of travel and may help initiate treatment, if needed, in a timelier manner. When multiple mushrooms are eaten together, the residual specimens brought from home may not be those causing toxicity. Cooking and refrigeration alter identifying features. Fresh mushroom specimens should be transported in a paper bag rather than in a plastic container to limit the effects of humidity. Finally, precise identification of even a good specimen can be difficult and should be done by an expert. Mycologists can be contacted through a poison control center, university, museum, or commercial mushroom grower.

In difficult cases, spores can be obtained from emesis or gastric-emptying procedures. Specimens should be refrigerated while awaiting analysis. More specific diagnosis can be made through TLC or RIA techniques. Botanical identification may not match the patient's symptoms. The patient should be treated according to time of onset of symptoms and condition when examined.

Patients with early-onset GI symptoms require supportive care with fluid and electrolyte replacement. For those with delayed GI symptoms or mixed ingestions containing amatoxin or gyromitrin mushrooms, treatment should begin as soon as possible. Toxic mushrooms can be differentiated by the season (spring: *Gyromitra*; autumn: *Amanita*).

Persons who have disulfiram-like reactions to alcohol should be questioned about prior mushroom ingestion. This situation is rarely correctly diagnosed because symptoms are thought to result from panic attacks, alcohol intoxication, or even an allergic reaction. Persons rarely relate their symptoms to the dinner of mushrooms eaten days earlier.

Any person with unexplained acute renal failure should be questioned about prior wild mushroom ingestion. Although *Cortinarius orellanus* is more common in Europe and Japan, it is found with increasing frequency in the United States. Because of the long delay before the onset of renal failure (1 to 2 weeks), the history of mushroom ingestion may be missed.

Mushroom poisoning cases remain relatively rare in the United States (they are still more common in parts of Europe and Asia), and until recently, up-to-date information was not accessible to the general public except through poison control centers. With the plethora of worldwide Internet connections, there are now mushroom experts readily available to answer questions about possible exposures within minutes to hours of contact. The active forager should use well-written field guides in addition to Internet sources and should cross-reference several sources before consuming any unknown mushrooms.

RECOMMENDED FIELD GUIDES

Arora D: *Mushrooms demystified,* Berkeley, Calif, 1986, Ten Speed Press.

Lincoff G: *The Audubon Society field guide to North American mushrooms,* New York, 1992, Knopf.

Lincoff G: *Simon & Schuster's guide to mushrooms,* New York, 1981, Simon & Schuster (European mushrooms).

Phillips R: *Mushrooms of North America,* Boston, 1991, Little, Brown.

Miller OK: *Mushrooms in North America,* New York, 2006, EP Dutton.

REFERENCES

Complete references used in this text are available online at expertconsult.inkling.com.

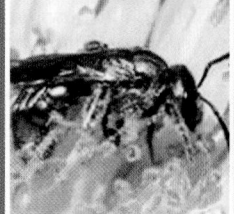

CHAPTER 67
Seasonal and Acute Allergic Reactions

JOHN TANNER AND THOMAS EGLIN

Allergic diseases are universal. Approximately 40% of people worldwide have one or more allergic diseases, and prevalence is increasing.[9,13,90] Allergic responses can range from annoying (e.g., allergic rhinitis) to life threatening (e.g., anaphylaxis).

Atopy is a predisposition to develop allergen-specific IgE hypersensitivity reactions (e.g., allergic rhinitis, bronchial asthma, atopic dermatitis, food allergy). It is often hereditary. Allergic rhinitis is the most common atopic disease and may be classified as seasonal (i.e., hay fever) or perennial. Aeroallergens (e.g., pollens) released from wind-pollinated plants (e.g., trees, grasses, weeds) cause seasonal allergic rhinitis. Perennial symptoms most often result from exposure to domestic allergens (e.g., dust mites, domestic pets, cockroaches, mold). In temperate climates,

patients with perennial allergic rhinitis may also have worsening symptoms during warmer months because of seasonal allergens.

Allergic reactions may present with skin and soft tissue manifestations of urticaria and angioedema. Urticaria is common, with a lifetime incidence of 20%. These superficial, erythematous, slightly raised, and pruritic lesions may occur anywhere on the skin. Typically acute, they may also be chronic. Angioedema results from swelling of dermis and subcutaneous tissues. If angioedema occurs in the upper airway, it can be life threatening. Angioedema and urticaria can be IgE-mediated hypersensitivity reactions or caused by other mechanisms (e.g., hereditary angioedema).

Anaphylaxis is the most severe form of allergic reaction and can be fatal if not treated promptly. Foods and medications are the most common causes of anaphylaxis. Anaphylaxis affects up to 2% of the worldwide population. Its incidence is increasing.[70,128] Anaphylactic reactions are likely underreported, particularly in cases of unexplained death. In one study, elevated tryptase levels (often found during acute anaphylaxis) were found in 13% of 68 cases of sudden unexpected death.[113]

ALLERGIC RHINITIS

Allergic rhinitis is an IgE-mediated inflammation of nasal mucosa characterized by nasal congestion, pruritus, rhinorrhea, and sneezing. It is the most common atopic disease and affects 10% to 30% of the global population.[90] For unclear reasons, prevalence of allergic rhinitis is increasing worldwide. Regional prevalence varies widely, from 5% in Tibet to greater than 40% in Australia.[29,30] Higher rates tend to occur in Western Europe, North America, and Australia. Lower rates are seen in Eastern Europe and south and central Asia.[21] Allergic rhinitis can lead to poor sleep, decreased school performance, decreased work productivity, and lower quality of life.[10,11,58,65,79,80,115]

EPIDEMIOLOGY AND RISK FACTORS

Allergic rhinitis typically first manifests in childhood or adolescence, then peaks in the second or third decade. Risk factors for allergic rhinitis are female gender, exposure to particulate air pollution, and history of maternal smoking during childhood.[21] The most important risk factor for development of allergic rhinitis is a family history of atopy, especially in cases with early onset. Risk is 30% greater if one parent or sibling is atopic and 50% or greater if both parents are affected.[85] Monozygous twins demonstrate a 45% to 60% concordance for allergic rhinitis.[32,34] Incomplete concordance for atopy in identical twins emphasizes the importance of environmental factors.[4] As with other atopic conditions (e.g., asthma, atopic dermatitis), allergic rhinitis tends to cluster in families. Multiple genes have been associated with allergic rhinitis.[24,35,100]

PATHOPHYSIOLOGY

Pathogenesis of allergic rhinitis consists of an acute allergic reaction and late inflammatory events. Acute clinical manifestations of allergic rhinitis are caused by a type I immediate hypersensitivity reaction. Late inflammatory events are mediated by cellular responses (i.e., by eosinophils, basophils, and T lymphocytes). Atopy is defined as the genetic predisposition to develop allergen-specific immunoglobulin E (IgE) antibodies. The underlying basis of immediate hypersensitivity is production of allergen-specific IgE (sensitization) antibodies. The sensitization process requires a cooperative effort between CD4 T lymphocytes and B lymphocytes (Figure 67-1). Sensitization begins with presentation by antigen-presenting cells (e.g., macrophages, dendritic cells) of an allergen to CD4 T lymphocytes in the context of a major histocompatibility complex. In response, CD4 T lymphocytes release cytokines, causing differentiation of B lymphocytes into immunoglobulin-secreting plasma cells; for example, release of the cytokine interleukin-4 (IL-4) or IL-13 from T lymphocytes promotes IgE switching.[27] Differentiation leads to isotype switching (i.e., production of specific antibody types) within the plasma cells. Once allergen-specific IgE antibodies are produced, allergens bind to mast cell surface IgE molecules in subsequent exposure, resulting in cross-linking of IgE molecules. Cross-linking causes mast cell or basophil degranulation that releases preformed and newly synthesized mediators. Histamine is the classic preformed mediator. Newly synthesized mediators include members of the arachidonic acid pathway (e.g., leukotrienes, prostaglandins, platelet-activating factor), neuropeptides (e.g., substance P), and cytokines (e.g., IL-4, IL-5).

Release of chemical mediators has various pathologic and clinical consequences. Stimulation of histamine receptors on sensory nerve endings causes sneezing and itching. Increased vascular permeability (produced by all the mediators) causes rhinorrhea. Leukotrienes and prostaglandins play major roles in nasal congestion.[132] Understanding of allergic rhinitis pathophysiology has been greatly enhanced by nasal challenge studies.[56] An allergic reaction consists of an early phase, characterized by mast cell or basophil degranulation, and a late phase, which occurs 4 to 6 hours after the early phase (see Figure 67-1).

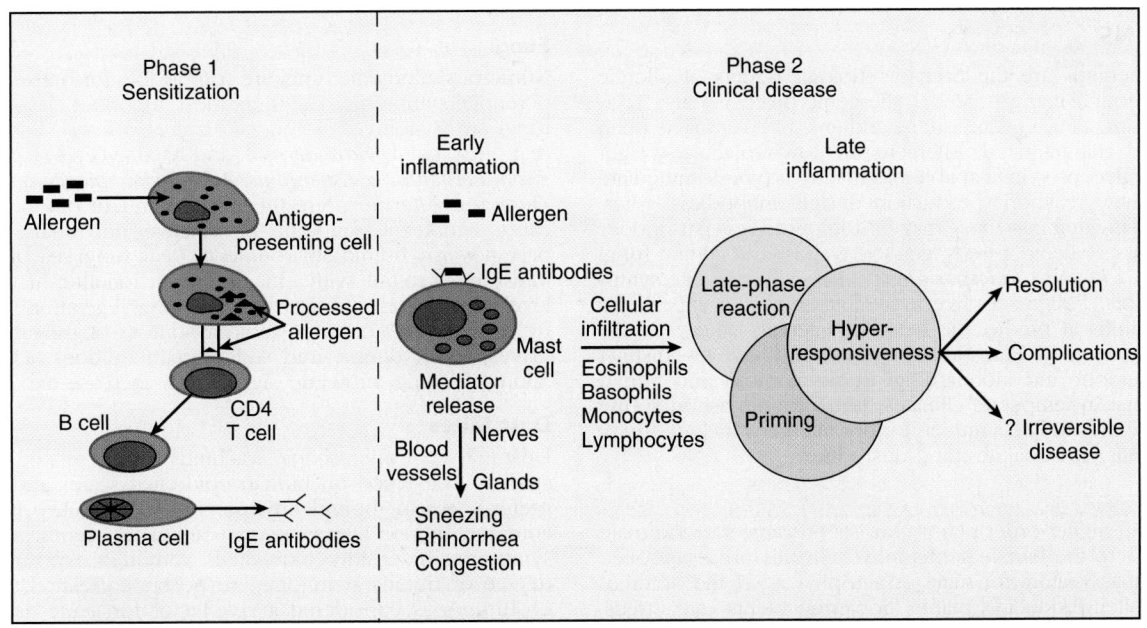

FIGURE 67-1 Natural history of allergic rhinitis (a simplified schematic). Individual becomes sensitized to an allergen in phase 1. Clinical disease develops in phase 2. Most individuals have an early response on reexposure to the allergen. Mast cell activation with mediator release dominates early response. After early response, individuals typically have cellular infiltration of nasal mucosa. This causes late inflammatory events, including spontaneous recurrence of mediator release (late-phase reaction), hyperresponsiveness to irritants, and increased allergen responsiveness (priming). *Circles* indicate heterogeneity of these late inflammatory events. Inflammation can resolve spontaneously, cause complications, or lead to an irreversible form of chronic rhinitis. *(From Naclerio R: Allergic rhinitis, N Engl J Med 325:860, 1991.)*

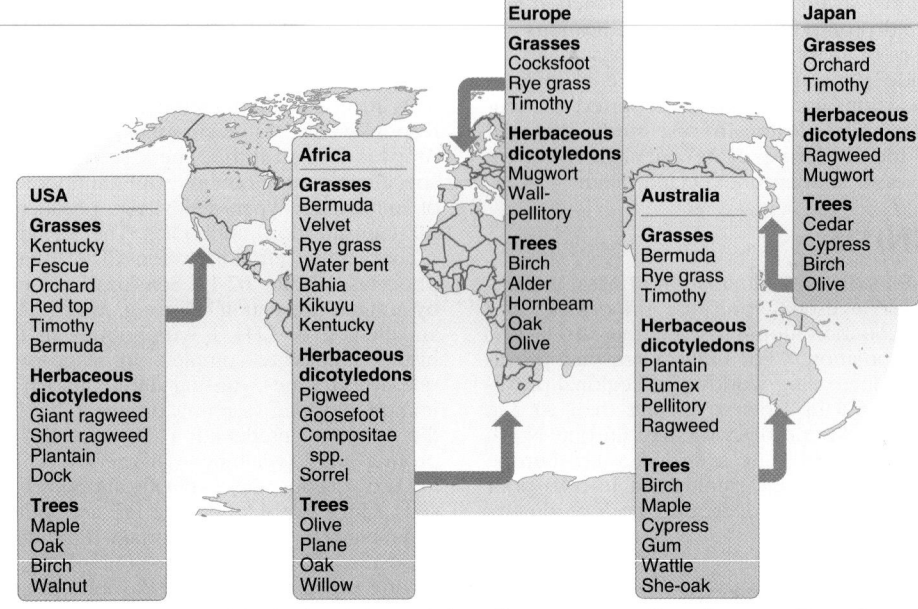

FIGURE 67-2 Selected worldwide distribution of clinically important pollen allergens. *(From Stewart GA, Peden DB, Thompson PJ, et al: Allergens and air pollutants. In Holgate ST, Church M, Broide D, et al, editors: Allergy, 4th ed, Edinburgh, 2012, Elsevier.)*

The hallmark of the late-phase reaction is an influx of inflammatory cells (e.g., eosinophils, basophils, T lymphocytes).[3] Basophils cause further histamine release. T lymphocytes release additional cytokines that enhance IgE production (via IL-4) and eosinophil activation (via IL-5). This cellular response leads to a recrudescence of symptoms many hours after initial allergen exposure. Leukotrienes, prostaglandins, and cytokines released in an early-phase reaction play an important role in recruiting late-phase cellular components to the inflammatory site. Although inhaled corticosteroids block both early- and late-phase reactions, systemic corticosteroids block only the late-phase reaction.

ALLERGENS

Airborne allergens are the primary etiologic agents of allergic rhinitis. Although many potential allergenic proteins exist, relatively few are clinically important and even fewer have been isolated and characterized. Allergens are low-molecular-weight proteins or glycoproteins capable of eliciting a type I immediate hypersensitivity reaction (production of IgE antibodies). Allergens can be divided into those that exist in outdoor versus indoor environments. Pollens of trees, grasses, weeds, and certain fungi (e.g., *Alternaria* and *Cladosporium* spp.) usually provoke symptoms outdoors. Pollen-sensitive individuals typically experience seasonal rhinitis at predictable seasonal intervals when specific allergens are released. Fungi are ubiquitous and have less distinct seasons. Outdoor and indoor fungi thrive in moist and humid environments. In temperate climates, fungi counts rise in spring and peak in mid- to late summer. Indoor allergens include fungi, furred animals, cockroaches, and dust mites.

Pollens

Pollination in higher-order plants consists of transfer of the male gametophyte to the female gametophyte. In this process, pollen grains serve as vectors for male gametophytes. Of the different types of pollen-producing plants, flowering plants (e.g., trees, grasses, weeds) are the most important allergens. Flowering plants can be divided into those that rely on animal vectors (e.g., insects, or entomophilous) or the wind (i.e., anemophilous) for pollination. Typically, only anemophilous plants (including trees, grasses, and weeds) cause allergic symptoms.[124] Pollens of entomophilous plants do not achieve high airborne concentrations. In temperate climates, anemophilous pollination occurs at predictable seasonal intervals. Awareness of relevant local botany

and pollination seasons allows prophylactic management of symptoms. Figures 67-2 and 67-3 list important pollen allergens and seasons.

In most temperate climates, tree pollination in spring marks the onset of allergy season. Grass pollen is a major cause of allergic rhinitis in sensitive individuals. In frost-free areas of the world, grass pollen may be present year-round. In temperate climates, grass pollination peaks in early summer. Unlike weed and tree pollen allergens, grass pollen allergens show extensive cross-reactivity among different species. Allergic individuals are typically sensitive to many species. In temperate climates, weeds typically generate pollen from end of summer through midfall.

Fungi

Numerous allergenic fungi are responsible for both seasonal and perennial symptoms. The three most important classes of allergic fungi are Zygomycetes (e.g., *Rhizopus, Mucor*), Basidiomycetes (e.g., rust, smut, *Ganoderma*), and Ascomycetes (e.g., *Cladosporium, Penicillium, Aspergillus, Alternaria, Epicoccum*). *Cladosporium* and *Alternaria* are the most abundant outdoor fungi and cause significant symptoms in sensitive individuals. Fungi grow best in warm, humid environments. Peak fungi season is typically midsummer to fall, with a marked reduction after first frost. Fungi levels may rise in spring, when decaying vegetation is uncovered by snow melt. Common outdoor sources of fungal growth are leaves, moist debris, and soil. Certain outdoor activities (e.g., raking, farming, mowing) significantly increase exposure.

Dust Mites

Dust mites are microscopic arachnids closely related to ticks and spiders. They feed on human epidermal scales and, like fungi, prefer a warm, humid environment. Dust mites are the most common indoor allergens and can cause significant perennial symptoms in sensitive individuals. Although exposure level and degree of rhinitis symptoms are poorly correlated, a dust level of 10 μg/g is considered a risk factor for acute asthma symptoms.[94] Common indoor sources of dust mite exposure include mattresses, pillows, blankets, upholstery, and stuffed toys. Dust mites can proliferate in sleeping bags stored in humid environments (e.g., damp basements).

Animals

Animals, especially cats, can be highly allergenic and in sensitized individuals can cause significant symptoms. Birds, rabbits,

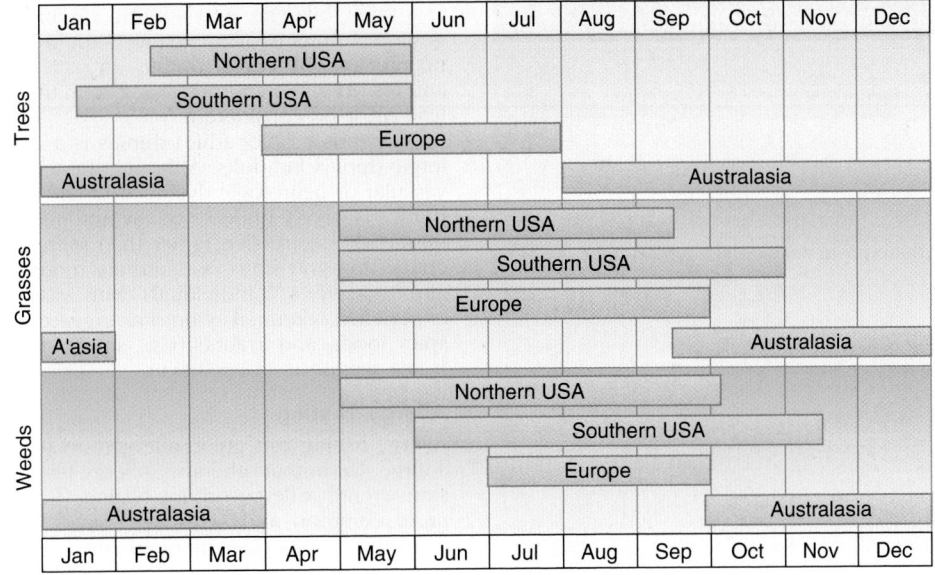

FIGURE 67-3 Pollen seasons in the United States, Europe, and Australasia. *(From Stewart GA, Peden DB, Thompson PJ, et al: Allergens and air pollutants. In Holgate ST, Church M, Broide D, editors: Allergy, 4th ed, Edinburgh, 2012, Elsevier. Modified from Sicherer SH, Eggleston PA: Environmental allergens. In Lieberman P, editor: Allergens in allergic diseases: Diagnosis and treatment, Totowa, NJ, 2000, Humana Press.)*

hamsters, guinea pigs, rats, and mice are other potentially allergenic pets. Feline and canine allergens include products of their salivary and sebaceous glands. Cat allergens can remain for months after cat removal. Cockroach allergens are frequently encountered in heavily infested, crowded, or multifamily dwellings.

Outdoors, inhalation of insect related allergens (e.g., moths, locusts, beetles, flies) may cause allergic symptoms.

FUNCTIONS OF THE NOSE

Function of the nose (i.e., to warm, humidify, and filter air) depends on turbulent airflow enhanced by three bilaterally symmetric turbinates (superior, middle, and inferior). The neurovascular system modulates nasal mucosa function. Nasal blood supply is via the ophthalmic (branch of the internal carotid) and internal maxillary (branch of the external carotid) arteries. Neural innervations include sensory (via the trigeminal nerve, responsible for the sneezing reflex) and autonomic (parasympathetic and sympathetic) nervous systems. Nasal congestion is related to blood pooling in the cavernous sinusoids (located within the turbinates) and mucosal edema. Sinusoid pooling is controlled by the autonomic nervous system. Parasympathetic stimulation causes vasodilation by opening capillaries and closing postcapillary venule sphincters, causing the sinusoid reservoirs to fill. Conversely, sympathetic stimulation contracts capillaries and relaxes postcapillary venule sphincters, allowing reservoirs to empty.

Asymmetric cyclic swelling and shrinking of turbinates between the two sides of the nose is common. This nasal cycle, occurring over 1 to 4 hours, results from alternating sympathetic discharge. It is responsible for the alternating unilateral nasal blockage experienced by allergic rhinitis sufferers.[51]

Olfaction is another major nasal function. Olfactory structures are on the roof of the nasal cavity above the middle turbinate. Significant turbinate edema can lead to poor ventilation and the associated hyposmia common to allergic rhinitis patients.

CLINICAL EVALUATION

Allergic rhinitis was described in 1929: "The three cardinal symptoms in nasal reactions occurring in allergy are sneezing, nasal obstruction and mucous discharge."[50] Allergic rhinitis symptoms range from intermittent and mild to incapacitating. The hallmark of allergic rhinitis is temporal correlation of symptoms with allergen exposure.[84] Common symptoms of allergic rhinitis (sneezing, nasal congestion, rhinorrhea, and pruritus of nose and eyes) are nonspecific. Itching and sneezing are the most distinctive complaints associated with allergic rhinitis.[85] Nasal congestion is more prominent in perennial than in seasonal rhinitis. In some patients, ocular symptoms predominate over nasal symptoms. Allergic rhinitis sufferers often experience priming effect (i.e., increased sensitivity to allergens after repeated exposure) and hyperresponsiveness to nonallergenic environmental stimuli (e.g., tobacco smoke, strong odors, pollutants, weather changes).[20]

Species-specific pollen production is predictable, so temporal correlation with symptoms is often helpful. Typically, tree pollen exposure causes symptoms in spring, grass and outdoor molds in summer, and weeds and outdoor molds in fall.[21] Ragweed sufferers characteristically start experiencing symptoms in late summer. In some regions, molds and pollens are perennial. In others, dust mites follow seasonal trends.[23,92] The terms *seasonal* and *perennial* may be inadequate to guide treatment decisions. The terms *intermittent* and *persistent* are more appropriate and better suited to guide diagnosis and treatment.[15]

In individuals with perennial rhinitis, it can be difficult to determine the responsible allergen(s). Upper respiratory tract diseases may mimic allergic rhinitis. Complications of allergic rhinitis include sinusitis, otitis media with effusion, and asthma flares.

Just as allergic symptoms may be vague, many physical signs are not exclusive to allergic rhinitis. Classically, nasal mucosa is pale blue and edematous, although this color is noted in only 60% of patients. Many individuals have erythematous mucosa.[51] In children, the "allergic salute" (upward nasal rubbing) and "allergic shiners" (dark, puffy circles under the eyes) may be present. Examine for septal deviation, polyps, and foreign bodies. Nasal discharge is usually clear to white. Discolored secretions are suggestive of chronic rhinosinusitis.[21] If congestion is profound, use of a topical decongestant (e.g., oxymetazoline) will improve visualization of the inside of the nose.

Allergic rhinitis is underdiagnosed and its severity underestimated.[81] Travel may unmask previously undiagnosed allergic rhinitis. Individuals may have acute worsening of symptoms during a wilderness sojourn (e.g., when traveling from winter to spring/summer) or can have marked improvement in symptoms (e.g., travel to high altitude, where offending allergens are decreased).

BOX 67-1   Differential Diagnosis of Rhinitis

Acute Rhinitis
Upper respiratory tract infection
Foreign body
Trauma
Chronic Rhinitis
Allergic
Nonallergic
   NARES (nonallergic rhinitis with eosinophilia syndrome)
   Chronic sinusitis
   Systemic diseases
     • Vasculitis
       — Wegener's granulomatosis
       — Churg-Strauss syndrome
     • Cystic fibrosis
     • Sarcoidosis
     • Hypothyroidism
Rhinitis medicamentosa
Medications
   Calcium channel clockers
   Angiotensin-converting enzyme (ACE) inhibitors
   β-Adrenergic blockers
Mechanical-anatomic obstruction
   Nasal polyps
   Foreign body
   Tumor
   Septal deviation
   Adenoid hypertrophy
Gustatory rhinitis
Atrophic rhinitis
Rhinitis of pregnancy
Cerebrospinal fluid leak
Vasomotor (idiopathic) rhinitis

Differential Diagnosis

To diagnose allergic rhinitis, the differential diagnosis of rhinitis must be considered (Box 67-1). Rhinitis can be classified as acute or chronic. The most common cause of acute rhinitis is a viral infection. Allergic rhinitis may be confused with viral rhinitis. Unlike the symptoms of allergic rhinitis, viral rhinitis symptoms typically persist less than 2 weeks, unless subsequent sinusitis develops. Nasal foreign body or trauma also can cause acute rhinitis. Unilateral symptoms suggest foreign body obstruction.

The differential diagnosis of chronic nonallergic rhinitis is broad. Nonallergic rhinitis with eosinophilia syndrome (NARES) is characterized by (1) symptoms similar to allergic rhinitis, (2) eosinophilia on nasal smear, and (3) a negative skin test.[57] Chronic rhinosinusitis, a potential complication of allergic rhinitis, typically causes nasal congestion, sinus pressure, postnasal drip, cough, and diminished senses of smell and taste. Symptoms of chronic rhinosinusitis are subtle and may require radiologic evaluation (e.g., computed tomography). Systemic diseases (e.g., vasculitis, cystic fibrosis) may cause chronic rhinitis. Rhinitis medicamentosa, usually secondary to overuse of topical α-adrenergic vasoconstrictors (e.g., oxymetazoline), is associated with profound nasal congestion due to rebound effects on withdrawal of the decongestant after prolonged (i.e., 5 to 7 days) topical use. Medications implicated in chronic rhinitis include nonsteroidal antiinflammatory drugs (NSAIDs), angiotensin-converting enzyme (ACE) inhibitors, and β-adrenergic blockers.

Examine for mechanical and anatomic abnormalities. Nasal polyps have a pearly, smooth, peeled-grape–like appearance and are often bilateral. Nasal polyps may be associated with chronic sinusitis, asthma, and aspirin sensitivity.[114] Unilateral symptoms should always heighten suspicion for a foreign body or tumor. Some degree of septal deviation is common, and unless symptoms are severe, treatment is unnecessary. In children, adenoid hypertrophy must be considered.

Gustatory rhinitis symptoms are caused by a cholinergic response to stimuli (e.g., eating, running, exposure to cold air). Atrophic rhinitis is a rare condition that manifests in older adults

as a thick, bilateral, and odorous discharge with little nasal congestion.[43] Rhinitis of pregnancy should be considered if there is no previous history of rhinitis. In patients with clear rhinorrhea and history of central nervous system trauma, cerebrospinal fluid leak must be considered.

Vasomotor (idiopathic) rhinitis is a common cause of nonallergic rhinitis in adults. Although the term implies an etiology of vascular or neurologic dysfunction, the mechanism of vasomotor rhinitis is poorly understood. Symptoms of vasomotor rhinitis are frequently obstructive rather than secretory. Symptoms of nasal congestion and sinus pressure are more common than sneezing and rhinorrhea.[73] Individuals with vasomotor rhinitis typically experience perennial symptoms triggered by changes in weather, spicy foods, and irritants (e.g., smoke, strong scents, chemicals). It is a diagnosis of exclusion.

Allergy Testing

Allergy testing can guide allergen avoidance as well as provide a target for immunotherapy. Allergy testing can be performed by skin or radioallergosorbent testing (RAST). Skin testing is the more common and sensitive assay.[60] For skin testing, minute quantities of specific allergens are injected into the dermis. A positive response depends on allergen-specific release of histamine. In RAST, evidence of allergen-specific IgE is detected from patients' serum. Given its lesser sensitivity, greater cost, and longer turnaround time for results, RAST is typically reserved for patients whose skin tests might be difficult to interpret (e.g., patients with severe eczema or dermatographism).

TREATMENT

Treatment of allergic rhinitis begins with attempting to avoid offending allergens. Avoidance is often difficult. Allergens can be ubiquitous outdoors, as well as indoors if patients are unable to part from a beloved pet. Pharmacologic intervention is often necessary. Treatment should be individualized on the basis of symptoms, seasonal patterns, and presence of possible comorbid conditions. The best therapeutic agent effectively addresses both early- and late-phase reactions.[125] Medications available for allergic rhinitis treatment include histamine-1 (H_1-) antihistamines, decongestants, intranasal or oral glucocorticoids, anticholinergics, cromolyn sodium, and leukotriene receptor antagonists (LTRAs). Immunotherapy may be considered in moderately to highly sensitive individuals.

Avoidance

Although it may be difficult to avoid pollen, certain common-sense measures can decrease exposure. Outdoor activities should be limited or avoided on days when pollen counts are high. Pollen counts typically peak in late morning to midafternoon.[134] Limiting high-risk activities (e.g., leaf raking, lawn mowing, farming) can reduce exposure to outdoor fungi. Important indoor fungal control measures include dehumidification, proper ventilation, fungicide use in contaminated areas, and removal of substrate for fungal growth. Reduce dust mite exposure by covering mattresses and pillows with allergen-proof encasings, frequent washing of bedding in hot water, and removal (or treatment) of carpeting. A limited approach (e.g., using allergen-proof encasings without additional measures) may not be effective.[126] For symptoms related to animal allergens, remove the animal from the indoor environment. This option is often not exercised. If the pet stays in the home, bath it at regular intervals and keep it out of sleeping areas. High-efficiency particulate air (HEPA) filters remove animal allergens from the environment[25] but do not improve symptoms.[135]

Antihistamines and Decongestants

H_1-antihistamines are first-line therapy for treatment of allergic rhinitis.[99] They are most effective against seasonal rhinitis, in which sneezing, itching, rhinorrhea, and watery eyes are the most prominent symptoms. Only 33% to 50% of seasonal allergic rhinitis sufferers obtain complete relief with H_1-antihistamine therapy alone.[12] H_1-antihistamines have little effect on nasal congestion because histamine plays only a minor role in the pathophysiology

TABLE 67-1 Newer-Generation Antihistamines

Chemical Name	Trade Name	Dosage		Minimum Age
		Adult	Children (<12 Years)	
Cetirizine	Zyrtec	10 mg daily	2.5-10 mg daily	6 mo
Levocetirizine	Xyzal	5 mg daily	1.25-2.5 mg daily	6 mo
Loratadine	Claritin	10 mg daily	2.5-10 mg daily	2 yr
Desloratadine	Clarinex	5 mg daily	1.0-2.5 mg daily	6 mo
Fexofenadine	Allegra	60 mg bid to 180 mg daily	30 mg bid	2 yr
Azelastine	Astepro	2 sprays per nostril bid	1 spray per nostril bid	6 yr
Olopatadine	Patanase	2 sprays per nostril bid	1 spray per nostril bid	6 yr

bid, Twice daily.

of congestion. H_1-antihistamines are usually inadequate for treatment of perennial rhinitis, in which nasal congestion is often a predominant symptom.

H_1-antihistamines occupy H_1 receptors on cells and block histamine binding. Older- and newer-generation H_1-antihistamines are equally effective, but newer-generation (second- and third-generation) H_1-antihistamines are much less sedating and have fewer anticholinergic side effects. First-generation H_1-antihistamines (e.g., chlorpheniramine, diphenhydramine, brompheniramine, clemastine, hydroxyzine) are generally available over the counter (OTC), and although safe, can effect cognition[78] and impair driving performance.[88]

Newer-generation H_1-antihistamines are safe, effective, and well tolerated and do not have anticholinergic or anti–α-adrenergic activity[59] (Table 67-1). Most are given once daily. All are approved for use in children, and some (e.g., cetirizine, levocetirizine, desloratadine) are approved for patients as young as 6 months. Azelastine and olopatadine are safe and effective in relieving most allergic rhinitis symptoms and are the only H_1 receptor antagonists available as nasal spray formulations.[7,64] Although H_1-antihistamines have a relatively rapid onset of action, they are most effective if taken before exposure (e.g., before pollen season begins) or if used on a regular basis.

Given H_1-antihistamines' limited effect on nasal congestion, using a decongestant may be helpful. Decongestants act by stimulating α-adrenergic receptors and reduce blood flow to the sinusoids. Most oral formulations are short acting (4 to 6 hours) and available OTC. Pseudoephedrine is often used but of questionable efficacy.[53] Insomnia and irritability are the most common side effects. Individuals with hypertension, glaucoma, or cardiac arrhythmias should use oral decongestants only under a physician's supervision. Topical decongestants (e.g., oxymetazoline) have a prompt onset of action (within minutes) and provide rapid relief of symptoms. To decrease risk of rhinitis medicamentosa, topical decongestant use should be limited to no more than 3 to 5 days.

Intranasal Corticosteroids

Intranasal corticosteroids are the gold standard of treatment for allergic rhinitis. Intranasal corticosteroids are more effective than H_1-antihistamines and LTRAs,[131,133] control all symptoms of allergic rhinitis, and may improve allergic ocular symptoms.[8] Intranasal corticosteroids can be used as first-line therapy for patients with perennial rhinitis. Corticosteroids control protein synthesis by influencing gene transcription within the cell.[63] Corticosteroids have an inhibitory effect on late-phase reactions. Unlike their oral counterparts, intranasal corticosteroids also inhibit the early-phase reaction.[1]

Several preparations of intranasal corticosteroids are available (Table 67-2). Fluticasone and mometasone are potent and have negligible systemic effects.[110] Maximal benefit of nasal corticosteroids may not be realized until 1 to 3 weeks after initiation of therapy. For patients with seasonal rhinitis, start nasal corticosteroid therapy shortly before onset of pollen season. There is no role for regular use of oral corticosteroids in the treatment of allergic rhinitis. When symptoms are severe (e.g., during peak pollen season), a short course (3 to 5 days, without a rapid taper) of oral corticosteroids may be appropriate[21] and may facilitate delivery of nasal corticosteroids to nasal mucosa.

The most common side effects of intranasal corticosteroids are local irritation (10%) and bleeding (4% to 8%).[21] Side effects are higher during winter months because of drier conditions. Although rare, nasal septal perforation has been reported with use of intranasal corticosteroids.[112] If septal ulceration and crust formation are noted, treatment with saline spray should be instituted and corticosteroid therapy should be discontinued until the nasal mucosa has healed. Long-term studies have shown no evidence of mucosal atrophy associated with the use of intranasal corticosteroids.[18] Nasal corticosteroids are rapidly metabolized. Although hypothalamic-pituitary-adrenal axis suppression is rare, it is prudent to monitor growth of pediatric patients receiving intranasal corticosteroids.

Leukotriene Receptor Antagonists

Previously indicated only for asthma, LTRAs are now approved for use in allergic rhinitis. Cysteinyl leukotrienes are products of the arachidonic acid pathway and important mediators of allergic inflammatory effects. Leukotrienes cause vasodilation and nasal congestion. As antagonists, LTRAs can significantly reduce nasal congestion.[62] In addition, leukotrienes encourage mucus

TABLE 67-2 Intranasal Corticosteroids*

Generic Name	Trade Name	Recommended Dose (Each Nostril)	Amount Per Spray (mcg)	Minimum Age (Years)
Beclomethasone	Beconase AQ	1-2 sprays bid	42	6
Budesonide	Rhinocort Aqua	1-4 sprays daily	32	6
Flunisolide	Nasarel	2 sprays bid	29	6
Fluticasone propionate	Flonase	1-2 sprays daily	50	4
Fluticasone furoate	Veramyst	1-2 sprays daily	27.5	2
Mometasone	Nasonex	1-2 sprays daily	50	2
Triamcinolone	Nasacort AQ	1-2 sprays daily	55	2
Ciclesonide	Omnaris	1-2 sprays daily	50	6

bid, Twice daily.
*All preparations are aqueous based.

production, leading to rhinorrhea. Nasal lavage leukotriene levels are increased in patients with seasonal and perennial allergic rhinitis.[122] LTRAs block binding of cysteinyl leukotrienes to respiratory tract CYS-LT1 receptors.

Montelukast (LTRA) and loratadine (antihistamine) are equally effective in alleviating nasal symptoms.[91] Montelukast was significantly less effective than the nasal corticosteroid fluticasone propionate in relieving nasal symptoms.[74] The effectiveness of combining LTRAs and H₁-antihistamines is unclear. One study found that the combination of montelukast with loratadine was more effective than either agent alone. Other studies have refuted this finding.[82,86] For treatment of allergic rhinitis, LTRAs perform as well as H₁-antihistamines, but not as well as nasal corticosteroids.

Oral LTRAs include montelukast, pranlukast, zafirlukast, and zileuton. Only montelukast is approved for use in both allergic rhinitis and asthma. The recommended dosage of montelukast for adults and adolescents (≥15 years) is 10 mg at bedtime. Pediatric dosing is age dependent: 4 mg (6 months to 5 years) and 5 mg (6 to 14 years). Both are given at bedtime. LTRAs appear to be well tolerated. Liver toxicity has been reported with zafirlukast[103] and zileuton but not with montelukast.

Other Medications

Cromolyn sodium and nasal anticholinergic drugs are other treatments for allergic rhinitis. Cromolyn is believed to inhibit mast cell degranulation. It is much less potent than nasal corticosteroids but is very safe. As with H₁-antihistamines, cromolyn sodium is effective for relief of sneezing, itching, and rhinorrhea, but less so for nasal congestion.[21] For optimal effect, it requires regular use and frequent dosing (three to four times daily). Cromolyn may be used as a prophylactic treatment before exposure to a known allergen (e.g., visiting a person with a cat). In a similar circumstance, if rhinorrhea is the predominant allergic symptom, use of a nasal anticholinergic (e.g., ipratropium) may be beneficial and can reduce postnasal drip. The recommended dosage of ipratropium is 1 to 2 sprays in each nostril two to four times a day. Nasal dryness is the primary side effect of intranasal ipratropium.

Immunotherapy

Allergen immunotherapy seeks to achieve tolerance in a sensitized person by exposing the person to gradually increasing amounts of allergen. Traditionally administered subcutaneously, many allergen extract preparations can now be administered sublingually. Although the precise mechanism is unclear, immunotherapy leads to induction of allergen-specific IgG "blocking antibodies," decreases in allergen-specific IgE, modulation of mast cell or basophil function, and increases in suppressor T cells (CD8).[39]

In patients with allergic rhinitis, efficacy of immunotherapy has been well established.[33,76] Most individuals obtain a degree of relief and thus have better symptom control with less medication. Immunotherapy should be considered in patients who respond poorly to medical therapy, who experience significant medication side effects, or in whom allergen avoidance is not possible. Immunotherapy involves weekly exposure of allergens at escalating doses until a maintenance dose is reached, typically within 4 to 6 months. Maintenance can consist of one or more therapeutic exposures per month and can be influenced by the number of allergen sensitivities. Optimal duration of immunotherapy is not clear; recommendations are from 3 to 5 years.[22]

Approach to Treatment

Treatment of allergic rhinitis should be based on duration and severity of symptoms.[14] Mild or intermittent symptoms may be treated with oral H₁-antihistamine, intranasal H₁ blocker and/or decongestant, or LTRA. More severe or persistent symptoms may require treatment with intranasal glucocorticoids. Patients using intranasal glucocorticoids derive no additional benefit from oral antihistamines.[101,28] In contrast, if symptoms are inadequately controlled using intranasal glucocorticoids, adding intranasal H₁-antihistamines or ocular H₁-antihistamines (for ocular symptoms) can improve symptom relief.[49,66] Patients with severe symptoms

may also benefit from a short course of systemic glucocorticoids. Ipratropium may be given for persistent rhinorrhea and an intranasal H₁-antihistamine for residual nasal congestion.[21] Immunotherapy should be considered in patients who fail to respond to the previous measures.

PREVENTION

Individuals with significant allergic rhinitis should obtain adequate supplies of appropriate medications (i.e., intranasal H₁-antihistamines, LTRAs, or intranasal glucocorticoids) before travel. If an unprepared traveler develops significant allergic rhinitis symptoms in the field, many general medical kits will only contain medications with less efficacy and more side effects (e.g., oral H₁-antihistamines and corticosteroids).

URTICARIA AND ANGIOEDEMA

Angioedema and urticaria often occur together, share a number of common etiologies, and have similar pathophysiology. Urticaria (i.e., hives) are intensely pruritic, erythematous, and plaquelike lesions caused by release of inflammatory mediators (e.g., histamine) by mast cells and basophils in the superficial dermis. Individual lesions resolve within 24 hours. Angioedema is caused by leakage of fluid in the deeper layers of the dermis and subcutaneous tissues. Angioedema presents as less well-defined, localized swelling in nondependent portions of the body. Angioedema and urticaria may be triggered through IgE-mediated allergic reactions or occur via nonallergenic pathways.

URTICARIA

Acute urticaria is defined as urticaria of less than 6 weeks' duration. Lesions vary in size from less than 1 cm (0.4 inch) to several centimeters. In severe reactions, the lesions may become confluent (Figure 67-4). The lifetime incidence of urticaria is about 20%. Urticaria may occur alone, with angioedema, or as part of an anaphylactic reaction. Common causes can include IgE-mediated allergic reactions to drugs or foods, infections, or direct activation of mast cells. Studies in children with acute urticaria have documented a high rate of infections as well as the concurrent use of antibiotics.[6]

IgE-mediated type I hypersensitivity reactions are the most common cause of acute urticaria and anaphylactic responses.

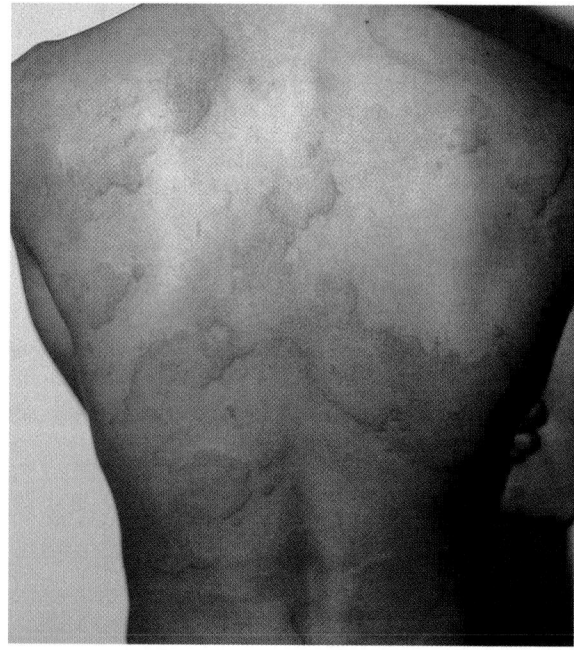

FIGURE 67-4 Urticaria. *(From Grattan CEH: Urticaria and angioedema. In Bolognia JL, Jorizzo JL, Schaffeer JV, editors: Dermatology, 3rd ed, London, 2012, Saunders.)*

Type I reactions occur when an antigen binds to specific IgE antibodies attached to high-affinity IgE receptors on mast cells. Antigen binding causes cross-linking of adjacent IgE antibodies and leads to mast cell degranulation and histamine release. In children, foods such as peanuts, tree nuts, milk, soy, and eggs are common triggers. In adults, latex, shellfish, and fish are also culprits.[6,138] Insect envenomations (e.g., bee, wasp, hornet, fire ants) are a common environmental source. Urticarial reactions have been reported with most antibiotics; β-lactam antibiotics (e.g., penicillin, cephalosporins) are most common. Drug hypersensitivity reactions may be responsible for up to 20% of fatalities from anaphylaxis. IgG autoantibodies and immune complexes can also elicit non-IgE immune-related mast cell histamine release and present with urticaria. Plant-induced dermatitis is discussed in Chapter 64.

Urticaria can also result from direct mast cell degranulation induced by drugs, foods, contact allergens, or physical stimuli. Narcotics (e.g., morphine) often cause a reaction at the site of injection. Radiocontrast medium can cause nonallergic anaphylaxis (previously called anaphylactoid reactions) by a similar mechanism, with rash, hypotension, and respiratory compromise. Vancomycin is known for the generalized flushing called "red man syndrome," also mediated by direct mast cell stimulation.

Some foods and drugs can cause urticaria by IgE-mediated mast cell activation or through nonallergenic pathways. Children are more sensitive to nonallergic foods (e.g., tomatoes, strawberries). Nonselective NSAIDs are cyclooxygenase (COX)-1 inhibitors and may cause a reaction involving altered leukotriene metabolism. Even in NSAID-sensitive patients, selective COX-2 inhibitors typically do not induce urticaria.[138]

Reactions and skin lesions may also be caused by interaction of IgG antibodies with antigens such as drugs, viruses (e.g., infectious mononucleosis, hepatitis B), and bacteria to form complexes. These complexes aggregate in blood vessels and activate the complement cascade, generating anaphylatoxins that cause mast cells to degranulate and release histamine. Immune complex–mediated skin lesions may include purpura and urticarial vasculitis.[93] Lesions that resemble urticaria, but are painful and leave residual bruising, may be manifestations of urticarial vasculitis.

Physical urticaria is induced by mechanical stimuli, temperature alterations, or photoreactions. Dermographism is caused by mast cell histamine release induced by firm stroking of skin. Cholinergic urticaria results in fine, intensely pruritic lesions caused by heat exposure (e.g., exercise, warm temperature, hot bath). Cold-induced urticaria usually affects exposed skin but may cause dramatic anaphylaxis in susceptible individuals who dive into cold water. Urticaria of skin exposed to the sun has a broad differential diagnosis, including porphyria or photodermatitis caused by oral medications or topical contact.

Urticarial rashes can widely vary in severity, from acute, isolated pruritic rash to skin manifestation of life-threatening anaphylaxis. Angioedema can occur simultaneously and can be life threatening if it involves the airway.

Diagnosis of acute urticaria is based on history and physical examination. Routine laboratory work is not typically indicated unless other diagnoses are being considered. Acute generalized urticaria after exposure to a known or likely allergen may herald onset of anaphylaxis. Urticaria accompanied by signs or symptoms of involvement of other organ systems (e.g., hypotension, respiratory or gastrointestinal [GI] symptoms) is consistent with anaphylaxis. Immediate treatment with epinephrine is indicated. Patients with persistent urticaria, GI symptoms, and eosinophilia should be evaluated for parasitic GI infection. In a young child with an upper respiratory infection, acute urticaria is likely caused by an infectious stimulus. Unintentional weight loss and chronic urticaria not responsive to antihistamine therapy may be evidence of lymphoproliferative disease. Chronic urticaria in a patient with weight gain or other symptoms of thyroid suppression may indicate the need to test for antithyroid antibodies.

Treatment

Urticaria typically responds well to oral antihistamines. A short course of prednisone has been shown to decrease duration of

symptoms.[93] High incidence of concurrent infection has resulted in less frequent glucocorticoid use in children. Treatment guidelines recommend a nonsedating (newer-generation) H_1-antihistamine in standard or double dose. A sedating H_1-antihistamine (e.g., diphenhydramine or hydroxyzine) may be used at bedtime to help with sleep. Some studies have shown additional improvement by adding an H_2-antihistamine (e.g., ranitidine or cimetidine).[72] Oral prednisone, 20 mg twice daily for 4 days, may be considered for adults with severe pruritus.[93] Box 67-2 lists treatment guidelines. Patients presenting with urticaria associated with anaphylaxis require treatment with epinephrine and intravenous (IV) fluids and careful observation for at least 6 hours. H_1-antihistamines and glucocorticoids are typically given to reduce the possibility of delayed or biphasic reactions, although only a benefit for skin manifestations has been proved.

ANGIOEDEMA

Angioedema shares similar pathologic features with urticaria, but the postcapillary leakage in angioedema occurs in deeper layers of dermis and subcutaneous tissues, leading to swelling of face, lips, tongue, extremities, or genitalia (Figure 67-5).[102] Angioedema can be caused by mast cell release of mediators of vascular permeability (e.g., histamine, leukotrienes, prostaglandins). Familial, acquired, and ACE inhibitor–related angioedema are bradykinin mediated. Some episodes of angioedema are idiopathic.

Similar allergic and nonallergic factors that trigger mast cell–mediated urticaria can cause angioedema. Mast cell–mediated angioedema almost always presents with urticaria.[106] Direct mast

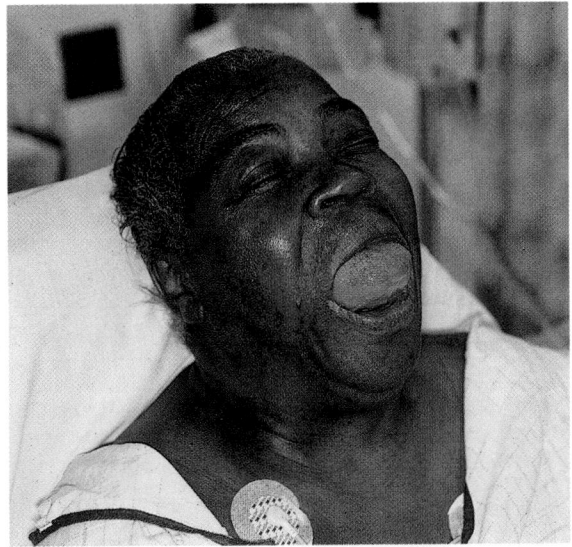

FIGURE 67-5 Angiotensin-converting enzyme (ACE) inhibitor–induced angioedema. *(From Roberts JR, Custalow CB, Thomsen TW, editors: Roberts and Hedges' clinical procedures in emergency medicine, 6th ed, Philadelphia, 2014, Elsevier.)*

1. If symptoms are mild and do not involve the airway:
   • Administer antihistamines such as diphenhydramine, 50 mg every 6 hours (other antihistamines acceptable).
   • Administer glucocorticoids such as prednisone, 20 to 40 mg twice daily for 5 to 7 days (dosing not established by trials).
2. Severe symptoms mandate treatment according to guidelines for anaphylaxis (see Boxes 67-6 and 67-7).

cell activation (e.g., by opiates or radiocontrast media) can cause angioedema. NSAIDs can precipitate urticaria and angioedema by various pathways involving prostaglandins and arachidonic acid metabolism.

In bradykinin-mediated angioedema, increased bradykinin levels cause increased vascular permeability. Patients may report a burning sensation. Pruritus and urticaria are usually absent. Hereditary angioedema (HAE) and acquired angioedema result from decreased levels of functional C1 esterase inhibitor, which increases bradykinin production. Onset of hereditary angioedema is usually during childhood. Late-onset acquired angioedema is associated with lymphoproliferative disorders. ACE inhibitors interfere with breakdown of bradykinin. ACE inhibitor angioedema accounts for 20% to 30% of angioedema. It typically affects soft tissues of the face and oral cavity (e.g., lips, tongue, soft palate, glottic structures). It can cause rapid onset of stridor, loss of airway patency, and death. Angioedema can also cause intestinal edema, with episodes of colicky pain, diarrhea, and vomiting.

Treatment

Identification of underlying etiology has therapeutic implications. Angioedema with urticaria is likely mast cell mediated and should be treated with antihistamines and glucocorticoids (Box 67-3). If there is any evidence of anaphylaxis (e.g., stridor, hoarseness, upper airway involvement, hypotension), epinephrine is indicated. Continuous airway monitoring is mandatory. In patients with airway edema, early endotracheal intubation is preferred. It may be a difficult intubation because airway anatomy can change rapidly and may be distorted by swelling.

Angioedema caused by excessive bradykinin is usually thought not to be responsive to antihistamines, glucocorticoids, and epinephrine. However, several small studies have shown benefit. Box 67-4 lists treatment recommendations. In one study, patients treated with antihistamines were extubated significantly sooner than were controls.[44] In angioedema with airway involvement, treatment with these medicines poses minimal risk and should be considered. Icatibant is a synthetic bradykinin B_2 receptor antagonist approved for treatment of HAE. A small case series of patients with ACE inhibitor–related angioedema treated with icatibant showed dramatic reduction in time to resolution of symptoms (4.4 vs. 33 hours) compared with a historical control group.[2] Icatibant should be considered for ACE inhibitor–related angioedema involving the airway. Availability may be limited because of cost (U.S. $8000 per dose). Fresh-frozen plasma contains ACE

1. Discontinue drug if patient is taking an ACE inhibitor.
2. Initiate early airway management if patient has stridor or airway compromise.
3. Often, treat with corticosteroids and antihistamines because of concern about possible allergic etiology (doses as in Box 67-3).
4. If the airway is involved:
   • Consider treatment with icatibant, 30 mg subcutaneously, if available (off-label treatment supported by case series).
   • Consider treatment with fresh-frozen plasma as a second-line therapy (usual dose, 15 mL/kg).
5. Nebulized epinephrine (0.5 to 1.0 mL of 1 : 1000) may be considered to help relieve swelling in the oral and upper airway regions.

and is widely available; rapid improvement in symptoms after its administration is reported.[52] Patients with HAE should have a well-delineated plan of treatment for acute episodes. This may include home administration of medications and rapid transport to an emergency department for airway management and further medical treatment.

WILDERNESS CONSIDERATIONS

Potential for allergic reactions is not limited by geography. An expedition health care provider can prepare by reviewing medical histories and allergy lists to ensure medications are available in the field. Group medical kits typically include antihistamines, corticosteroids, and epinephrine to treat serious reactions. Patients with airway angioedema require close monitoring. The decision to evacuate a patient with angioedema to a higher level of care depends on acuity and severity of symptoms, medical provider experience, available resources, and options for timely evacuation under medical supervision. Physicians treating angioedema should anticipate the need for advanced airway management.

ANAPHYLAXIS

Anaphylaxis is a systemic, life-threatening allergic reaction that follows exposure to an allergen.[109] It is the most severe form of hypersensitivity reaction and involves multiple organ systems. Clinical manifestations may occur in skin, upper respiratory tract, lower respiratory tract, GI tract, and cardiovascular system. Anaphylaxis was first described in canine experiments involving sea anemone venom. Canine subjects experienced no ill effect from initial immunization, but died when later exposed to nonlethal doses of venom.[95]

Anaphylactic reactions should be described as either allergic or nonallergic. Allergic anaphylaxis describes reactions mediated by an immunologic mechanism (e.g., IgE, IgG, or immune complex complement related). Nonallergic anaphylaxis describes anaphylaxis from any nonimmunologic cause. "Anaphylactoid" has been used to describe severe, non–IgE-mediated allergic reactions. The term is no longer recommended;[17,116] *IgE-mediated allergic anaphylaxis* may be used when appropriate. Idiopathic anaphylaxis describes reactions in which no trigger can be identified[45,118] (Box 67-5).

ETIOLOGY

Foods are the most frequent cause of anaphylaxis.[136] Egg, cow's milk, wheat, soybean, peanut, tree nuts (e.g., hazelnut, walnut,

IgE-Mediated Allergic Anaphylaxis
Food
Drugs (penicillin, cephalosporins, insulin, sometimes aspirin and other NSAIDs)
Insect stings and bites
Exercise (food dependent)
Other (exposure to antivenom or aquatic proteins)

Allergic Anaphylaxis (Not IgE Mediated)
Radiologic contrast material
Disturbances in arachidonic acid metabolism
   Aspirin and other NSAIDs
Complement activation
   Transfusion reactions
Other causes

Nonallergic Anaphylaxis
Direct stimulation of mast cells
   Drugs (opiates, vancomycin)
   Physical stimuli (e.g., heat or cold)
Exercise
Other causes

Idiopathic Anaphylaxis

IgE, Immunoglobulin E; *NSAIDs,* nonsteroidal antiinflammatory drugs.

cashew, almond), fish, and shellfish (e.g., shrimp, lobster, crab) account for more than 90% of all food-related anaphylactic reactions. In children, peanuts are the most frequent cause of food-induced anaphylaxis.[108] Individuals may accidentally ingest allergenic food when it is disguised by misleading labeling or contaminated during food preparation.

Drugs (e.g., antibiotics) may cause allergic and nonallergic anaphylaxis. Penicillin and its derivatives are most often implicated, with reactions occurring in one to five patients per 10,000 courses of treatment.[55] Opiates and vancomycin can directly degranulate mast cells and basophils. These reactions do not require prior sensitization. Aspirin and other NSAIDs can provoke IgE-mediated and non–IgE-mediated allergic reactions; they inhibit the COX pathway, increasing synthesis of lipoxygenase pathway products[68] (e.g., leukotrienes) that are important mediators of inflammation. In patients with asthma and chronic urticaria, this is the predominant mechanism for anaphylaxis.

Common outdoor causes of anaphylaxis are envenomation (e.g., Hymenoptera, i.e., bee sting), contact with aquatic proteins, and antivenom therapy (e.g., for snakebite). Estimated incidence of insect sting anaphylaxis is 0.3% to 3%.[104] Hymenoptera-related anaphylactic reactions are common in individuals younger than 20. These reactions are more likely to be fatal in older adults. Typically, children's reactions are milder (e.g., urticaria only) than those of adults. Individuals who experience a sting-related anaphylactic reaction have a 50% to 60% risk of anaphylaxis after subsequent insect stings.[104] Offending insects vary by geographic location. In the United States, yellow jackets cause most allergic reactions, whereas in Europe, honeybees and wasps cause the majority of insect sting–related reactions. Although rare, anaphylaxis can result from bites by certain insects, such as the kissing bug *Triatoma protracta*, the deerfly *Chrysops discalis*,[54] and ticks.[16]

Physical stimuli may provoke nonallergic anaphylactic reactions. In exercise-induced reactions, symptoms typically begin after 5 minutes of moderate to heavy exercise and resolve within 30 minutes to 4 hours after exercise cessation.[129] Approximately 50% of affected individuals are atopic, and most engage in regular vigorous exercise. A coinciding factor, such as ingestion of an allergenic food (e.g., shellfish)[75,89] or NSAID, may be necessary to induce this type of reaction. In cold-induced reactions, symptoms occur after exposure to a cold stimulus, such as being outside on a cold day, holding a cold object, or eating a cold food.

Recurrent anaphylaxis without identifiable cause is known as idiopathic anaphylaxis. Idiopathic anaphylaxis most often results in urticaria and/or angioedema, although all organ systems may be affected. Diagnosis of idiopathic anaphylaxis is one of exclusion. Patients who have frequent episodes are less likely to undergo remission. Acute treatment is identical to that for other forms of anaphylaxis. Long-term treatment may require regular use of oral corticosteroids.

In anaphylactic reactions caused by transfusion of blood products and immunoglobulins, complement activation plays a key role. Transfusion of incompatible blood type can cause cytotoxic anaphylactic reactions if complement-fixing antibodies to formed elements of blood (e.g., red cells, white cells, platelets) are present. In γ-globulin–related anaphylactic reactions, immune complex aggregation occurs when antigen-antibody complexes activate complement.

EPIDEMIOLOGY AND RISK FACTORS

Anaphylaxis affects 0.05% to 2% of the population, and its incidence is increasing.[70,128] Asthma is a risk factor for anaphylaxis.[42] Risk factors for death from anaphylaxis include severe asthma, cardiovascular disease, mastocytosis, and certain medications (e.g., β-blockers, ACE inhibitors).[98] Food, insect stings, and medications are the most common triggers for anaphylaxis. Frequently, no trigger is identified.[118,130]

Anaphylaxis is an infrequent occurrence in the outdoor setting. The National Outdoor Leadership School (NOLS) database recorded two cases of anaphylaxis and 149 cases of acute allergic reaction over 20 years (2.5 million participant-days).[111] There were no deaths.

PATHOPHYSIOLOGY

In anaphylaxis, clinical consequences of hypersensitivity are systemic. The primary event underlying anaphylactic episodes is degranulation of mast cells and basophils.[71] Histamine is the most important mediator and responsible for most of clinical manifestations. Important effects of histamine include vasodilation, increased vascular permeability, smooth muscle contraction, stimulation of nerve endings, and glandular secretion. Arachidonic acid metabolites (e.g., prostaglandins, thromboxane A_2, platelet-activating factor) are also released from mast cells and basophils, causing airway smooth muscle contraction, increased vascular permeability, goblet and mucosal gland secretion, and peripheral vasodilation. Platelet-activating factor also contracts smooth muscle and enhances vascular permeability. A late-phase reaction may occur many hours to days after the initial event.

CLINICAL PRESENTATION

Clinical manifestations of anaphylaxis may occur in various organs, including the skin (urticaria, angioedema, flushing), upper respiratory tract (rhinitis, stridor, hoarseness), lower respiratory tract (wheezing, bronchospasm, cough), GI tract (abdominal pain, diarrhea, vomiting), and cardiovascular system (tachycardia, hypotension, shock). Urticaria and angioedema are the most common manifestations, occurring in 83% to 90% of individuals with anaphylaxis.[61] The second most common manifestations are respiratory tract symptoms, followed by dizziness or syncope and GI symptoms. Cardiovascular collapse with shock can occur rapidly and without other antecedent symptoms. Table 67-3 presents the frequency of different signs and symptoms of anaphylaxis.

No single sign or symptom can be used to diagnose anaphylaxis. A standard definition of anaphylaxis has only recently been established. In 2005 an international symposium was convened by the U.S. National Institutes of Health (Allergy and Infectious Disease) and the Food Allergy and Anaphylaxis Network. This meeting created criteria to diagnose anaphylaxis (Box 67-6).[109]

Most anaphylactic reactions occur soon (within 5 minutes to 2 hours) after exposure to an inciting agent, but other patterns are possible. Protracted anaphylaxis can begin suddenly or gradually, but the clinical manifestations are prolonged, sometimes requiring hours or even days of resuscitation. Typically, abrupt

TABLE 67-3 Frequency of Signs and Symptoms in Patients with Anaphylaxis

Signs and Symptoms	Percentage of Cases
Cutaneous	>90
Urticaria (hives) and angioedema (localized swellings beneath the skin, most often on the lips and eyes)	85-90
Flush	45-55
Pruritus (itch) without rash	2-5
Respiratory	40-60
Dyspnea (shortness of breath), wheeze, cough	45-50
Upper airway angioedema (e.g., swelling in throat)	50-60
Rhinitis (runny nose, nasal congestion)	15-20
Dizziness, Syncope (Loss of Consciousness), Hypotension (Low Blood Pressure)	30-35
Abdominal	25-30
Nausea, vomiting, diarrhea, cramping pain	
Miscellaneous	
Headache	5-8
Substernal pain	4-6
Seizure	1-2

Based on a compilation of 1784 patients, reviewed in Lieberman P: Anaphylaxis and anaphylactoid reactions. In Middleton E et al, editors. *Allergy: Principles and practice*, 5th ed, St Louis, 1998, Mosby–Year Book, pp 1079-1092.

BOX 67-6 Clinical Criteria for Diagnosing Anaphylaxis

Anaphylaxis is highly likely when any one of the following three criteria is fulfilled:

1. Acute onset of an illness (minutes to several hours) with involvement of skin, mucosal tissue, or both (e.g., generalized hives, pruritus or flushing, swollen lips-tongue-uvula), and at least one of the following:
   a. Respiratory compromise (e.g., dyspnea, wheeze-bronchospasm, stridor, reduced PEF, hypoxemia)
   b. Reduced BP or associated symptoms of end-organ dysfunction (e.g., hypotonia [collapse], syncope, incontinence)
2. Two or more of the following that occur rapidly after exposure to a likely allergen for that patient (minutes to several hours):
   a. Involvement of the skin-mucosal tissue (e.g., generalized hives, itch-flush, swollen lips-tongue-uvula)
   b. Respiratory compromise (e.g., dyspnea, wheeze-bronchospasm, stridor, reduced PEF, hypoxemia)
   c. Reduced BP or associated symptoms (e.g., hypotonia [collapse], syncope, incontinence)
   d. Persistent gastrointestinal symptoms (e.g., crampy abdominal pain, vomiting)
3. Reduced BP after exposure to known allergen for that patient (minutes to several hours):
   a. Infants and children: low systolic BP (age specific) or greater than 30% decrease in systolic BP*
   b. Adults: systolic BP of less than 90 mm Hg or greater than 30% decrease from that person's baseline

From Sampson HA et al: Second symposium on the definition and management of anaphylaxis, *J Allergy Clin Immunol* 117:391-397, 2006.
PEF, Peak expiratory flow; *BP*, blood pressure.
*Low systolic blood pressure for children is defined as less than 70 mm Hg (1 month to 1 year old), less than 70 mm Hg + (2 × age) (1 to 10 years old), and less than 90 mm Hg (11 to 17 years old).

symptom onset is associated with increased symptom severity. Fatalities usually result from airway obstruction or cardiovascular collapse.[17]

DIAGNOSTIC TESTS

Plasma histamine and serum tryptase can help diagnose anaphylaxis. Both may be elevated during an acute episode. For best results, measure plasma histamine 10 to 60 minutes and serum tryptase 1 to 2 hours after symptom onset.[67]

TREATMENT

Anaphylaxis is a medical emergency. Treatment depends on severity and organ system(s) involved. For a mild allergic reaction limited to the skin (e.g., urticaria without anaphylaxis), antihistamines alone may be effective. Individuals with cutaneous reactions should be monitored closely for signs of respiratory or cardiovascular compromise. Clinical evidence of additional organ system involvement may require more aggressive measures (e.g., administration of fluids, bronchodilators, and epinephrine). Box 67-7 details acute management of anaphylaxis.

Epinephrine

Treatment for anaphylaxis is epinephrine. Epinephrine treats the primary symptoms of anaphylaxis: upper airway obstruction, lower airway obstruction, urticaria, angioedema, hypotension, and shock.[118] No randomized controlled trials of epinephrine in anaphylaxis have been published. Given that available evidence is compelling, it is unlikely a randomized controlled trial will ever be performed.[77,117] International evidence-based guidelines strongly recommend that epinephrine be given for anaphylaxis.[119]

Most fatalities result from delayed treatment.[36,96] If indicated, prompt administration of epinephrine is key. Intramuscular (IM) injection of epinephrine into the anterolateral thigh is preferred. This site provides faster absorption and higher plasma epinephrine levels than does subcutaneous administration or deltoid injection.[120,121] If reactions are life threatening or patients do not

respond to IM epinephrine, IV epinephrine may be administered. IV epinephrine should be used with caution in persons older than 35 or with known coronary artery disease. Continuous epinephrine infusion is preferred to an IV bolus of epinephrine.[38,83] Bolus dosing of IV epinephrine should only be performed if the patient is in cardiac arrest.

Aerosolized aqueous epinephrine can prevent upper airway edema but is inadequate to abort systemic anaphylaxis.[26] Use of OTC epinephrine inhalation aerosol bronchodilators (e.g., Primatene Mist) is generally not recommended because they lack adrenergic specificity (i.e., are non–β_2 selective) and have extremely short half-life. These agents should also be used with caution in individuals with a history of coronary artery disease and arrhythmias.

BOX 67-7 Management of Anaphylaxis

General Measures

1. Place individual in supine position with feet elevated.
2. Establish and maintain airway.
3. Administer oxygen.
4. Place a venous tourniquet above the reaction site (e.g., insect sting or drug administration site) to decrease systemic absorption of antigen.
5. Obtain IV access and infuse normal saline (20 mL/kg over 10 minutes). Repeat as needed to achieve a systolic blood pressure of 90 mm Hg in an adult.

Epinephrine Use and Treatment of Hypotension

1. Administer aqueous epinephrine, 1:1000, 0.3 to 0.5 mL (0.3 to 0.5 mg) IM in the anterolateral thigh. Epinephrine dosage for children is 0.01 mL/kg. Repeat once or twice as necessary at 5- to 15-minute intervals to control signs and symptoms.
2. If the reaction is life threatening or if patient does not respond to IM epinephrine, administer epinephrine IV. Mix 0.1 mL (0.1 mg) of 1:1000 aqueous epinephrine in 10 mL of normal saline (final dilution, 1:100,000) and infuse over 10 minutes (10 mcg/min). If hypotension persists, a continuous epinephrine infusion may be started by adding 1 mL (1 mg) of 1:1000 epinephrine to 250 mL of normal saline, creating a concentration of 4 mcg/mL. Infuse this solution at a rate of 1 mcg/min (15 minidrops/min or 4 macrodrops/min, depending on the infusion set being used). Rate of infusion can be increased to 4 to 5 mcg/min if clinical response is inadequate. In children and infants, starting dosage is 0.1 mcg/kg/min, up to maximum of 1.5 mcg/kg/min.
3. If epinephrine and fluids are ineffective, an IV dopamine infusion should be initiated.
4. Norepinephrine, a potent vasopressor, can be used to treat severe hypotension that is unresponsive to administration of epinephrine, fluids, and dopamine.
5. Individuals taking a β-blocker medication may require treatment with glucagon (1 to 5 mg IV over 2 minutes). Continuous infusion of glucagon may be necessary.

Treatment of Bronchospasm

1. Administer a β_2-adrenergic agonist (e.g., albuterol, metaproterenol, pirbuterol, or terbutaline) via nebulization as required for bronchospasm that is not relieved by epinephrine.
2. Continuous nebulization may be required if bronchospasm persists.
3. Treatment with an anticholinergic (ipratropium) may be beneficial.

Antihistamines and Corticosteroids

1. Administer diphenhydramine, 25 to 50 mg (1 mg/kg in children), or chlorpheniramine, 10 to 20 mg (2.5 to 5 mg in children), IV over 3 minutes; IM or PO when the reaction is not severe. Addition of cimetidine, 300 mg, or ranitidine, 50 mg, IV over 5 minutes may be beneficial.
2. Most authorities advocate use of glucocorticoids to decrease likelihood of a late-phase reaction. Standard therapy includes hydrocortisone 200 to 300 mg or 125 to 250 mg methylprednisolone IV, or in milder cases, prednisone 30 to 60 mg orally.

IM, Intramuscular(ly); *IV*, intravenous(ly); *PO*, orally.

Epinephrine autoinjectors (e.g., EpiPen) are popular for their ease of use. Carrying epinephrine in ampule form with syringes and needles offers the benefit of multiple dosing. Smaller syringes, such as tuberculin or insulin syringes, can be used to avoid accidental overdose. Needle length should be sufficient to allow IM administration.[37]

Treatment of Hypotension

Place the patient in supine position to improve venous return. Sitting the patient upright may lead to death from decreased vascular tone.[97] If the supine position cannot be tolerated (e.g., because of respiratory distress or vomiting), the patient should be placed in semirecumbent or lateral decubitus position.

Patients with hypotension not rapidly responsive to epinephrine should be treated with IV fluids. Normal saline should be given in bolus doses of 20 mL/kg (1 to 2 L for an adult) over 10 minutes and repeated as necessary. Vasopressor drugs may be needed to treat hypotension if response to epinephrine and fluids is inadequate. Dopamine is often the initial drug of choice. Norepinephrine, a potent vasopressor, can be used to treat severe hypotension that is unresponsive to epinephrine, dopamine, and fluids. Glucagon may be necessary to treat refractory hypotension (e.g., patients taking β-adrenergic blockers) that is resistant to standard therapeutic regimens.[40,137] Atropine can be used to treat hypotension associated with bradycardia. Medical antishock trousers have been used successfully to treat refractory hypotension associated with anaphylaxis.[87]

β₂-Adrenergic Agonists

To treat severe wheezing, an aerosolized β₂-adrenergic agonist (e.g., albuterol) is recommended. Place in a nebulizer and administer as guided by symptom severity (intermittently or continuously). Nebulized anticholinergic agents (e.g., ipratropium) can also be used for treatment of bronchospasm.

Glucocorticoids

Limited evidence supports use of glucocorticoids in anaphylaxis. In a Cochrane Database systematic review, no studies met inclusion criteria for the review. Authors were unable to make recommendations for the use of glucocorticoids in the treatment of anaphylaxis.[19] Most authorities recommend glucocorticoids to decrease the likelihood of a late-phase reaction.[69]

Antihistamines

Limited evidence supports use of antihistamines in anaphylaxis. After treatment with epinephrine, antihistamines may be used to relieve itching and urticaria. Combining an H₁-antihistamine and an H₂-antihistamine may be more effective than administering an H₁-antihistamine alone.[72,107] Transient hypotension, bradycardia, and arrhythmias have been reported after rapid IV administration of cimetidine.

Biphasic Reactions

Recurrence of anaphylaxis after initial symptom resolution is known as a biphasic reaction. Biphasic reactions occur in up to 20% of patients, typically in the first 8 hours, but may occur several days later.[127] Prolonged monitoring has been recommended to monitor for biphasic anaphylactic reactions. Two large reviews of anaphylaxis found that less than 5% of patients had biphasic allergic reactions, of which 1% to 2.3% were deemed clinically important.[105] No deaths were reported.[46]

Medical Evacuation

The decision to transport patients to a higher level of care depends on skill and experience of medical providers, as well as available resources. If adequate supplies are available and care can be provided by a physician with experience in the management of anaphylaxis, patients with rapid and thorough response to initial treatment may not require evacuation. Local resources should include the ability to provide advanced airway management, IV access, and additional doses of medications, especially epinephrine and IV fluids. Every case of anaphylaxis deserves serious consideration of evacuation to a higher level of care. Special consideration should be given in cases of severe reaction, asthmatic patients, ingested allergen with possible continued absorption, and individuals with a previous history of biphasic reaction.[123] The Wilderness Medical Society's guidelines on use of epinephrine in wilderness settings state that "because of the life-threatening nature of anaphylaxis, as well as the possibility of a biphasic reaction, field victims of anaphylaxis should be evacuated if possible to definitive or hospital-based care."[37]

Sequelae and Aftercare

After resolution of symptoms, patients should continue a short course of oral antihistamines and glucocorticoids. Patients should be referred to an allergist or similarly qualified expert to identify precipitating agents so that preventive measures can be taken. Individuals with a history of anaphylaxis should carry at all times a device allowing self-injection of epinephrine. A medical information bracelet should be worn. Epinephrine autoinjectors, including multidose versions, require a prescription. Patients should obtain this immediately.

PREVENTION

Patients with drug allergies should avoid using new medicines in a wilderness setting. For instance, persons with a previous history of sulfa allergy should not start acetazolamide in the field to prevent acute mountain sickness. Although risk of cross-reactivity is low, it is prudent first to use this medicine in a suitable setting before moving to a remote high-altitude environment.[47]

Travelers with food allergies should be especially cautious with regard to food preparations. Individuals with peanut allergy need to consider regional differences in food preparation and the possibility of food contaminated with peanut-based products.

Medical providers should use latex-free gloves in anticipation of the possibility that they will be caring for persons with latex allergy.

Evaluation and treatment by an allergist or other appropriately trained medical provider is critical in patients with a history of allergic anaphylaxis. Immunotherapy can lead to substantial reductions in future episodes of anaphylaxis.[41,48]

ACKNOWLEDGMENT

We would like to thank the previous author, Dr. Naresh Patel, for his contribution to this chapter.

REFERENCES

Complete references used in this text are available online at expertconsult.inkling.com.

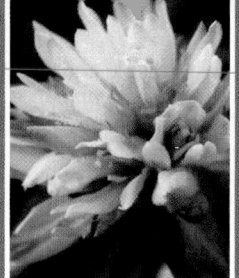

CHAPTER 68

Ethnobotany: Plant-Derived Medical Therapy

KEVIN DAVISON AND BRYAN L. FRANK

The history of ethnobotany begins before the advent of written records. In all ancient civilizations, plants served as important elements of food, shelter, dyes, ornamentation, religious rituals, and medicines. The term *ethnobotany* refers to an individual culture's use of specific plants. Medicinal use of the plant kingdom has been termed *herbalism, plant medicine,* and *natural-based medicine* and is called *phytomedicine* in its current application. The word *herb* is broadly defined as a nonwoody plant that dies down to the ground after flowering. The most commonly used interpretation, however, is any plant used for medicinal therapy, nutritional value, food seasoning, or dyeing another substance.

The history of the discovery of the medicinal uses of plants by humans remains conjectural. Many scenarios probably occurred. Perhaps, in a prehistoric jungle of South America, a pool of water containing fallen plant material leached out some of the precious medicinal constituents of leaves, flowers, stems, and bark. Tannins, glycosides, sugars, and alkaloids from the bark were infused into the waters. Because of burning fever and severe dehydration, an extremely ill native drank from the pool, and his fever miraculously disappeared. The pond became known for its magical healing powers. If the water held bark from the cinchona tree, the native may have serendipitously discovered quinine.

Archaeologic evidence shows that prehistoric humans used plants extensively to treat physical ailments. Instinct and trial and error led to the realization that, for example, cinchona bark controlled intermittent fevers, animals fed ergotized grain aborted their fetuses, and the latex sap from the opium poppy could be eaten to alleviate pain. Innumerable medicinal plant traditions, some originating as far back as 2700 BC, remain intact. Ethnobotanically, the use of plant-based medicines in a particular culture represented much more than an individual's efforts to survive. Analyzing the methods and degrees of use of indigenous medicines reveals information about cultural philosophy, ingenuity, and sophistication. The Chinese developed an extensive and elaborate system for prescribing, classifying, and processing herbs that dates back to the third millennium BC. The formulas identified the specific effect of each herb and interactions with other herbs. Less tolerable herbs were blended with those that would counteract undesirable effects. Formulas were custom-blended, taking into account a victim's constitution and the stage of the disease. Some of the ancient knowledge from these writings is being used in contemporary herbal preparations commercially sold as "patent" (readily available in pill form) medicines.

Many native tribes of New Guinea, Indonesia, and the Amazon use single-herb formulations to treat almost all medical conditions, as they did thousands of years ago. In the West, written records dating to the Sumerians accurately describe medicinal uses of specific plants.[120] In the same period of about 3000 years ago, the first Asian written record, the Ben Tsao Gan Mu, was compiled by the Chinese. It listed more than 360 medicinal plants and their classifications, uses, contraindications, and methods of action as perceived at that time. Roman and Greek herbal remedies were described in the writings of Hippocrates and later in those of Galen, providing a pattern for development of the Western medical tradition. Hippocrates was an advocate of using a few simple plant preparations, along with fresh air, rest, and proper diet, to help the body's own "life force" eliminate problems. In contrast, Galen promoted use of direct intervention to correct the imbalances that cause disease, employing large doses of complicated mixtures that included animal, plant, and mineral ingredients.[134]

The earliest European compendium that listed the uses and properties of medicinal plants, *De Materia Medica,* was written by the Greek physician Dioscorides in the first century AD. He described about 600 plants, and his work remained the authoritative herbal medicinal resource into the 17th century.[45]

Herbalism was practiced in many different ways during and after the Middle Ages. There were learned traditional herbalists and lay practitioners, as well as wandering herbalists, who professed pagan animism or Christian superstitions that often were more influential in healing than were the herbs' properties. Little was added to the knowledge of herbalism during this period. After the Middle Ages and invention of the printing press in the 1400s, hundreds of herbal publications were compiled. Most early works were available only in Latin or Greek; it was not until the 15th through 17th centuries that the great age of herbalism was appreciated in English.[120]

Tides changed in European herbalism when a Swiss pharmacist-physician named Theophrastus Bombastus Von Hohenheim, better known as Paracelsus (1490 to 1541), introduced a new dimension. He advocated chemistry and chemical processing and used mineral salts, acids, and other preparations in medicinal therapies. This was a departure from the plant-based medicinal methods of the past. During the latter part of the 17th century, the predominance of plant medicines slowly eroded. In 1806, Freidrich Serturner, a small-town German pharmacist, became known for his efforts to isolate organic acids from plants in an attempt to find the active ingredient in opium. He discovered organic alkaloids, which became known as the first set of active plant constituents.[169] Because of their physiologic activity, the search for plant alkaloids continued into the 20th century.

Discoveries quickly followed. The bronchodilator and antitussive ephedrine, from the herb *Ephedra sinica,* was often used in Chinese medicinal formulas for bronchial asthma. Discovery of morphine led to creation of all the narcotic analgesics. The bark of the cinchona tree was found to contain quinine in 1819, which led to development of antimalarial drugs.

The traditional herbal extract from rhubarb (*Rheum* spp.) has several active compounds. These compounds mediate many of the pharmacologic effects, such as its purgative action (from sennosides); antibacterial, antifungal, and antitumor activities (from anthraquinones); antiinflammatory and analgesic activities; and improvements of lipid metabolism (from stilbenes). Treatment of leukemias from an extract of Madagascar periwinkle (*Catharanthus roseus*), known as vincristine, has been highly effective.[46]

Discoveries in the 19th and 20th centuries included atropine (from belladonna leaves, *Atropa belladonna*) in 1831, cocaine (from coca leaves, *Erythroxylum coca*) in 1860, ergotamine (from *Claviceps purpurea*) in 1918, and tubocurarine in 1935.[134]

European settlers brought herbal knowledge and their medicinal methods to the Americas. Because of the abundance and wide use of plants on the new continents, they also learned much from indigenous peoples. The colonists found that conditions afflicting them, such as malaria and scurvy, were treated effectively with herbs by the Native Americans.[136] In the 1700s, herbal medicine continued to have popular applications in lay circles, but was also investigated by the new medical establishment. Although creation of a small, elite group of learned professionals was thought to violate political and constitutional concepts of the early American democratic movement, the practice of medicine was carried over from England and Scotland during pre-Revolutionary days. Before a professional medical class was established, most illness in America was treated within the family or extended-family network.

Many concepts were modified in the colonies between 1765, when the first medical school opened, and 1850, when more than 42 schools of medicine had been recognized. Inquiry into *Digitalis purpurea* (foxglove) by William Withering exemplified the change in perspective from anecdotal folk medicine to a critical examination for specific uses of botanicals from a biochemical point of view. During the early 1800s, the trend was to look at the efficacy of botanicals and their intrinsic value from a more scientific perspective.

Several developments delayed appreciation of herbalism by physicians in the colonies. For instance, Samuel Thomson promoted a system of herbal medicine by proselytizing about his patented method of herbal prescribing, which used many Native American herbs. A central theme in his approach was advocacy of self-prescribing based on the philosophies and herbal prescriptions found in his book, *New Guide to Health*. The right to sell "family franchises" for use of the Thomsonian method of healing was the basis of a widespread lay movement between 1822 and Thomson's death in 1843. Thomson adamantly believed that no professional medical class should exist and that democratic medicine was best practiced by laypersons within a Thomsonian "family unit."[43] Although his methods were considered crude and unscientific, he had more than 3 million faithful followers in 1839. Founded on ignorance, prejudice, and dogma, the Thomsonian school did little to help physicians accept European and American herbal medicines. European physicians in the Thomsonian movement wanted to separate themselves from lay practitioners by creating requirements and standards for the practice of Thomsonian medicine. Thomson was adamantly against this, but a decade after his death, the Thomsonian physicians formed the Eclectic School of Medicine, which attempted to unite "professional physicians," Thomsonianism, and traditional herbal medicine. Establishment of several Eclectic medical schools was a step toward validating herbal medicine, but failed to bring herbalism into the mainstream medical establishment. The founding of the American Medical Association and the Flexner Report on medical education in 1910 thoroughly established the modern pharmaceutical industry in the medical education system.[43]

Because of the availability of pure, active constituents from plant drugs and synthetic drugs that began to appear on the market toward the end of the 19th century, the prescribing habits of physicians began to change. The sensibility and predictability of administering exact doses were appealing. For example, the pure alkaloid of quinine, rather than a foul-tasting extract of cinchona bark containing variable percentages of quinine and other alkaloids with different physiologic properties, could be prescribed for malaria.

Many "crude drugs" were standardized for therapeutic activity. Digitalis, which still retains its status in the *United States Pharmacopeia* (USP), is one example. Of the 200 plant drugs officially listed in the USP in 1936, about 19% are still official today.[169] An estimated 25% of all prescriptions dispensed in community pharmacies between 1959 and 1980 contained ingredients extracted from higher plants. For a significant number of synthetic drugs, natural drug products continue to serve as either models or starting points for synthesis.

EVOLUTION OF PHYTOPHARMACEUTICALS

The drive toward patenting and ownership in the pharmaceutical industry has been a strong incentive to research and develop plant-based products. Because a plant cannot be patented, however, little U.S. effort has gone into developing herbal medicines during the past century. The principal active constituents of botanicals are investigated for their biologic activity, but in many cases, these are less effective than is the whole crude extract of an herb.[134]

One problem in development of the U.S. botanical pharmaceutical industry has been quality control. In addition, lack of standardization plagues plant-based products. Quality control and standardization of crude plant extracts for herbal medicines were virtually nonexistent until recently,[134] or we might be using more botanical medicines for common ailments. In Europe and Asia, where pharmaceutical firms have been producing standardized phytopharmaceuticals (plant-based standardized extracts) for decades, research and development have demonstrated that they make economic and medical sense. Europeans use phytopharmaceuticals as part of their mainstream medical practice. In hospitals, they are used primarily as adjuvant therapies. More than 70% of general practitioners in Germany prescribe phytopharmaceuticals, and the public health insurance system pays for most of these prescriptions. The total annual market for phytopharmaceuticals in Germany is $1.7 billion. Beginning in 1993, the licensing procedure for German physicians required knowledge of phytotherapy.[152]

Production and evaluation of botanical medicines have improved significantly in the past six decades. In crude plant evaluation, modern laboratory analysis can determine the percentage of active constituents, as well as solubility, specific gravity, melting point, optical rotation, and water content. Scientists detect resins, alkaloids, flavonoids, enzymes, essential oils, fats, carbohydrates, and protein content. They can precisely assay using liquid, high-pressure liquid, paper, and thin-layer chromatographies; spectrophotometry; atomic absorption; and magnetic resonance imaging. These methods improve predictability and therapeutic effectiveness of standardized crude botanical medicines, which are then evaluated for their efficacy in animal studies to determine pharmacologic potency, activity, and toxicity. U.S. and European companies have set strict quality control guidelines to ensure optimal yields of pharmacoactive constituents, with acceptable levels of impurities, pesticides, residual solvents, and heavy metals, and acceptable bacterial counts.

Specific cultivation and harvesting techniques affect the therapeutic value of a given herb, which is related to the amount of active constituents in a specific medicinal plant. Methods of packaging, storage, and transport can dramatically affect stability of active compounds. Extracts and concentrates are obtained by adding appropriate solvents to raw herbs, which draws out the active constituents. The most common method is *infusion,* which is analogous to a tea bag being steeped in hot water to make tea; in this case, water is the solvent. When the water is slowly evaporated, the concentrate contains the active constituents.

Pure ethanol is a solvent that is often used to concentrate active herbal constituents. Immersing a high-quality bulk or raw herb in pure ethanol for hours or days, depending on the herb and the part used, and then pressing the solids out, yields an herbal *tincture.* The alcoholic tincture is diluted with water to yield a 20% alcohol tincture. In another method, a 20% alcohol mixture is the solvent. *Fluid extracts* can be made by vacuum-distilling off some of the alcohol; this avoids elevating the temperature, which may affect some of the active constituents. Another concentration process, *solid extraction,* yields a solid or semisolid product that can then be powdered or granulated for administration.

Once an extract is produced, qualitative and quantitative analyses can be performed to assist in standardization. The percentage of known active constituents is assayed, to obtain predictable clinical results.

An herbal infusion is generally a better source of active compounds than is an air-dried or a sun-dried powdered herb (Figure 68-1), but its action may not be as strong as those of concentrates, such as tinctures, solid extracts, and fluid extracts. Potency of an extract can be defined by (1) percentage of active constituents or (2) concentration. Herbalists express concentration as an equivalency: a four-to-one extract is equivalent to or derived from four parts of the crude herb to yield one part extract. This is usually written as "4:1 solid extract." Longer shelf life, greater effectiveness, and higher concentration of active constituents make a more standardized (thus better) product than is the raw powdered herb; however, efficacy is difficult to compare.

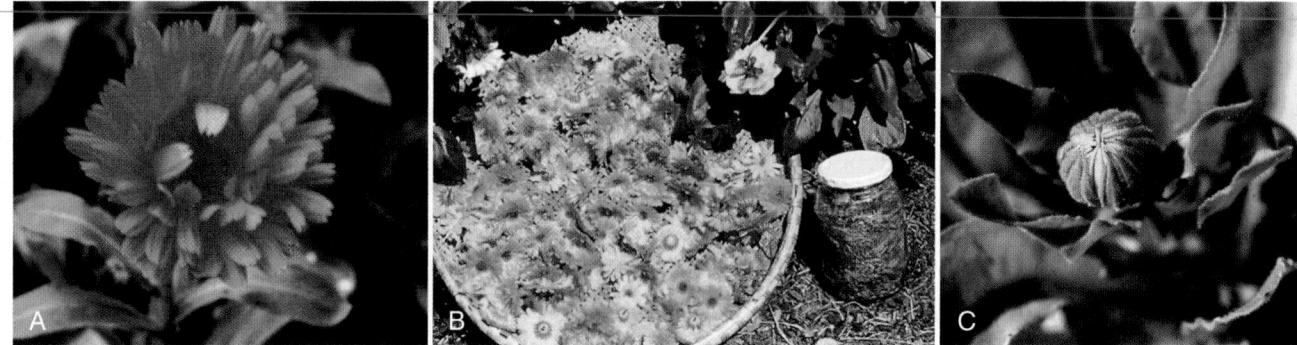

FIGURE 68-1 A, *Calendula officinalis.* **B,** Calendula drying and dried in a jar. **C,** Calendula flower bud. (**A** and **B** *courtesy Cascade Anderson Geller;* **C** *courtesy Jill Stansbury.*)

An example of a product that is standardized by the percentage concentration of pharmacoactive glycosides is *Ginkgo biloba* extract, marketed in Europe under the trade names Tanakan, Rokan, and Tebonin. It is typically standardized as 24% flavonoid glycoside. In experimental models, *G. biloba* extract has been shown to prevent metabolic and neuronal disturbances of cerebral ischemia and hypoxia.[101,115]

Quality control is addressed for many herbal products when the known clinical effectiveness can be attributed to a specific active constituent. Improved analytic methods and use of high-quality herbs (i.e., high in active constituents) help ensure standardization. In Europe, dosage is expressed in milligrams of active constituents, a system that favors consistency. The main difference between the infusion or extraction method, and chemical isolation or synthesis, is that the extracts still contain all the synergistic cofactors that enhance function of the active ingredient. This important aspect of herbal medicine is lost once the active constituent is removed from the whole plant.

HERBAL PREPARATIONS FOR CLINICAL AND WILDERNESS USE

Botanical preparations can be readily and accurately prescribed for travelers and wilderness enthusiasts who need medical help. Throughout the ages, botanicals have been useful adjunctive therapeutic agents. Knowing which preparations from the natural pharmacopeia can be used and how to use them engenders a sense of integration with the natural environment. Indigenous peoples who depend on the botanical world hold a vast amount of untapped knowledge. Wilderness enthusiasts should help preserve this understanding of the natural world and do what they can to save natural habitats. Further investigation into the plant kingdom for useful medicinal agents will aid in these efforts.

As for allopathic medicine, a word of caution is appropriate. Naturopathic remedies are sometimes offered as substitutes for more accepted Western medical remedies. The practitioner should always use the best and most proven remedy available. An example is treatment for spider bite, which is discussed from an allopathic perspective in Chapter 43, and mentioned briefly later in the discussion on a potential use for an activated charcoal poultice. The practitioner who selects any less commonly supported therapy should be aware of the science supporting the choice of therapy.

Herbal medicines can be prepared by decoction or infusion of bulk or raw herbs or by making an extract, a concentrate, or a tincture.

Infusions are prepared like a standard tea. The soft parts of plants—flowers, stems, and leaves—are placed in a warmed pot. Boiling water is poured over the herb, and the pot is covered to prevent beneficial essential oils from evaporating. The mixture infuses for approximately 10 minutes and then is strained. The supernatant can be used immediately or refrigerated in an airtight container for as long as 2 days. A standard adult dose of an herbal preparation is 28.3 g (1 oz) of dried herb in 473.2 mL (1 pint) of water, or 1 tbsp per cup. The amount is doubled if the herb is fresh.

Generally, it is best to take infusions hot by the cupful, three times daily for a chronic problem and up to every 1 or 2 hours during an acute illness. To make infusions palatable, many herbalists add licorice, aniseed, or honey. The hard or woody parts of plants, such as bark, seeds, roots, rhizomes, and nuts, have tough cell walls that must be broken down by longer heating before they impart their constituents to water. The herbs can be first broken into small pieces by chopping, crushing, or hammering.

Traditionally, a *decoction* was prepared in an earthen crock reserved especially for making herbal preparations. In the past, herbalists believed that some quality of the medicine was affected by the type of vessel or container in which the brew was prepared. Contemporary practitioners generally recommend use of stainless steel, ceramic, or enamel, and specifically discourage use of aluminum or other alloyed-metal pots. The herb is placed in the container and covered with cold water. The mixture is brought to a boil, covered, and simmered for 10 to 45 minutes, depending on the type and part of the herb being used. A decoction can be strained, flavored, or sweetened like an infusion and is consumed while hot.

Modern practitioners use the most efficient and predictable forms of specific herbal medicines. *Concentrates* in capsule form are most effective and easiest to administer. The standard herbal concentrate found in the marketplace is in a ratio of 4:1. Ease of administration and dosing and predictability of clinical effects have made this the industry standard. Herbal *tinctures* are extracted into a specific percentage of alcohol and can be mixed easily to make formulas tailored to personal circumstances. Formula prescribing is an art; a combination may be many times more effective than a single herb. Classic formulas for common ailments have been cataloged since the first herbal compendiums were recorded centuries ago. In this chapter, however, the focus is on single herbs and their specific uses, identification, and preparation.

HOMEOPATHIC USE OF BOTANICALS

Medical pioneer Samuel Hahnemann developed a radically different system of medicine nearly 200 years ago. Homeopathy is derived from the Greek words *homoios,* which means "similar," and *pathos,* which means "disease" or "suffering." The law of similars states that a substance that causes a set of symptoms in pharmacologic doses can be used as a cure for similar symptoms (even if the etiologic agent is different) if that substance is given in a homeopathic dilution. Most homeopathic remedies are prepared from plant, mineral, and animal products. In homeopathic medicine, there is a perfectly matched simillimum (the most effective medicine) if the predominant symptoms of a disease or illness match the symptoms produced when the substance is taken in large doses by a healthy individual. For example, the herb *Atropa belladonna,* which contains atropine, is poisonous.

In excessive doses, the herb causes death; in moderate doses, it creates hot, feverish states; and in tiny (homeopathic) doses, it can effectively treat certain types of fevers, viral syndromes, and inflammatory states.

A homeopathic dilution is created by taking a prepared tincture ("mother tincture") of a botanical or an extract from nonplant sources and diluting it in a sequential or serial method. The difference in a homeopathic dilution is in its methodology. To be effective, a homeopathic medicine must be succussed (shaken or agitated) mechanically or manually a prescribed number of times between the serial dilutions. The succussion method originally discovered by Hahnemann is said to "dynamize" the medicine. The succussion method is purported to affect the water molecules, creating a "memory" that the water molecules store in a lattice formation. This is similar to the storage of information on a magnetic disk or tape, except the signature resonance pattern is created from interaction of the original tincture within the water's lattice structure. The dilution can range from a 1× potency, which is a decimal dilution of a given ingredient (one part mother tincture per nine parts solute), to a 1 cup (one part mother tincture to 99 parts solute), to an extremely dilute 200c (one part mother tincture per 99 parts solute, then serially diluted 200 times with one part of the subsequent solution, then diluted with 99 parts solute each of 200 times; thus, a 1:99 dilution each of 200 times). A high-potency dilution (serially diluted more than 30 times in the × [1:9 dilution each time] potencies and more than 12 times in c [1:99 dilution each time] potencies) would be taken much less frequently than would be a low-potency dilution.

To make a 30× homeopathic preparation of *Arnica montana,* 1 drop of the plant tincture is added to 9 drops of pure water, and the mixture is succussed 50 to 100 times. Next, 1 drop from that solution would be added to 9 drops of pure water and again succussed 50 to 100 times. This is repeated 30 times to yield the desired 30× homeopathic remedy. The number refers to the number of succussions and the letter to the ratio of the mother tincture to pure water. Thus, a 30× remedy is a 1:9 dilution repeated 30 times.

The mechanisms by which homeopathy works have yet to be elucidated, even though it has been practiced effectively for several hundred years. In 1900, an estimated 15% of U.S. physicians were prescribing homeopathic remedies.[124] Recent studies have shown effective results in clinical trials using homeopathic medicines.[34,95,110] Mechanisms of action for many common pharmaceuticals also remain unknown. Many theories in medicine are still based largely on empirical observations rather than on theoretical understanding.

One herbal folk remedy for bruises, sprains, strains, and rheumatism in European and Native American medicine is topical application of the plant *Arnica montana* (leopard's bane). Consistent with the homeopathic principle, toxic quantities of the whole-plant extract of arnica produce the same set of symptoms that it is intended to cure when administered internally in a homeopathic dose or when the tincture or oil is applied topically to the affected area.

Arnica is contained in herbal and homeopathic doses in numerous ointments, salves, and poultices for the treatment of trauma resulting from localized sprains, strains, or contusions. Controlled studies in Germany have shown that effective products for sprains from athletic activity use an ointment that contains homeopathic arnica.[182]

TOPICAL APPLICATION

The earliest method of plant administration was topical application. Although many plants contain generalized moisture-enhancing properties, some were found to be particularly effective in ameliorating specific acute conditions when applied topically. Two methods are used to apply remedies to the skin. The *endermatic* method applies medicine on the skin without friction, as when applying a compress to the dermis and epidermis after an abrasion or laceration. The *epidermatic* method uses friction and is most effective with botanical oils, liniments, ointments, and medicated warm and cold friction rubs, primarily for subdermal contusions and trauma, to effect circulatory changes.[59]

Topical application of medicinal plants is useful for many conditions, including abrasions, lacerations, burns, insect bites, infections, rashes, and dermatoses. Other applications include contusions, varicosities, joint pain, inflammation, and musculotendinous aches, strains, and sprains.

Topical herbal remedies are applied with a poultice, compress, fomentation, or ointment. Probably the most common, the *poultice* is used to apply a remedy to a skin area with moist heat. A poultice is prepared by bruising or crushing the medicinal parts of the plant to a pulpy mass, then applying this to the affected area and covering it all with a moist heat source. If dried plants are used (or fresh plants if necessary), the materials are moistened by mixing with a hot, soft, adhesive substance such as moist flour or corn meal. A good way to apply a poultice is to spread the paste or pulp on a hot, wet cloth, which is wrapped around the affected area to help retain moisture and heat. The cloth is moistened with hot water as necessary. With irritant plants, such as those used in a mustard plaster, the paste is kept between two pieces of cloth to prevent direct contact with the skin. After the poultice is removed, the area is washed well with water to remove any residue. A poultice can be used to soothe, to irritate, or to draw impurities from the affected area, depending on which plants are applied.

A *fomentation* is a hot cloth soaked with an herbal infusion or decoction. Fomentations are generally less active than poultices. A cold compress is used for conditions that require an antiinflammatory cure. A cold, infusion- or decoction-soaked cloth is applied to an area and then removed when the body's circulation has warmed the cloth to body temperature. The botanicals' active constituents determine what actions the external applications will impart. For example, a poultice with an astringent herb, such as *Hamamelis* (witch hazel), has an entirely different effect from one made with a strong vasodilator and rubefacient, such as capsicum (cayenne pepper).

Ointments are another method of topical administration. Most ointments are made in a base of petroleum jelly, stable vegetable oils, beeswax, or a combination of these. The extract from the desired botanical is suspended within the base to create a stable solid product. Topical botanical products have the same function as do topical pharmaceutical ointments and are used to treat lacerations, abrasions, infections, and insect bites. Other uses for botanical topicals include hemostatic, antiinflammatory, antihistamine, rubefacient, analgesic, emollient, and circulatory stimulant actions. Herbal poultices, compresses, and ointments deliver their active compounds transdermally, as do pharmaceutical topical agents.

The first uses of most medicinal plants were probably topical. In contemporary herbology, many of these plants are also used internally. Whole plants containing more than one ingredient with biologic activity generally invoke synergistic action of several components to produce the therapeutic action. Thus, most botanicals have multiple applications for therapeutic purposes. Herbalists and homeopaths treat trauma of the skin, muscles, tendons, ligaments, and joint tissue with a topical agent in ointment or poultice form and give the same medicine internally in minute (homeopathic) doses to enhance the activity, as with concurrent use of arnica ointment and homeopathic arnica.

The major precaution in medical botany is to identify *toxicity*. Some of the most effective topical agents can be toxic if ingested. Most of these plants found in the wild could not be taken in sufficient doses to be fatal before causing gastrointestinal (GI) upset. A tincture, herbal concentrate, or powdered version of the plant, however, could have deadly potential and bypass obvious GI manifestations.

USE OF HERBAL MEDICINE IN THE WILDERNESS

Travelers in the wilderness can choose preprocessed herbal preparations or naturally available plants in the immediate vicinity. A surprisingly large number of minor medical conditions encountered in an outdoor setting can be treated with plants in that location. North American recreational areas are home to medicinal plants that have been used by Native Americans for centuries. Recreationists in desert, alpine, and river environments can find medicinal plants in abundance. Almost all plants encountered during an alpine trek in North America have some medicinal property, as do many in tropical and subtropical regions.

Considerations for using herbal products in the wilderness are availability, ease of application, incidence of side effects, toxicity, spectrum of applicability, affordability, and effectiveness.

AVAILABILITY AND APPLICATION

If a condition can be improved by application of a local botanical growing in the immediate vicinity, the pharmacy is immediately available. Plants may be in season, plentiful, and easily harvested. Finding the appropriate plants can be challenging, however, depending on the location, the season, the traveler's familiarity with botanicals, and the type of medical condition. During mild seasons and at elevations conducive to plant growth in the continental United States, the chances of finding common plants are good. Otherwise, standardized commercial preparations of these herbs can be carried. These are packaged for long storage life, sanitary and convenient application, and standardization of active ingredients.

Hundreds of plants can be applied topically for a variety of conditions. Most of the readily available plants, even if properly identified, require some form of processing for the active constituents to be used fully. Furthermore, expertise in the field requires years of training by a knowledgeable botanist and herbalist. It also requires knowledge of plants' seasonal variations, ecologic niches, and precise identifications. However, a person who is neither a botanist nor a herbalist can gain basic understanding of a few plant medicines that have a wide spectrum of applicability and broad range of geographic distribution.

SIDE EFFECTS AND TOXICITY

The American Association of Poison Control Centers annually reports plant ingestion as a significant category of accidental poisoning. In 1997, 5.6% of U.S. poisonings came from plants and mushrooms. Of the substances that were involved in pediatric poisonings, plants were responsible for 7.4% of exposures.

Side effects or toxic reactions from botanicals are rare. Among the botanicals covered in this chapter, toxicity is not a major consideration, although anything can be toxic when used excessively or indiscriminately. Many toxic plants produce GI distress, vomiting, or diarrhea before they cause any severe neurologic or cardiorespiratory derangement. Often, toxic side effects are caused by one substance in a plant. When isolated, minute amounts of an alkaloid may be potentially dangerous, but when ingested in a form modified by other constituents, the altered drug effect allows tolerance of larger amounts of the toxic substance or substances.

As is true for any medication, medicinal plants should be applied appropriately, and doses for internal use should not exceed recommendations. Pregnancy and nursing may be contraindications. Doses for almost any herb can be found in numerous references.[134] Felter[59] stated that "as a rule, doses usually administered are far in excess of necessity and it is better to err on the side of insufficient dose and trust to nature, than to overdose to the present or future harm or danger of the patient." In general, for the self-harvested herbs presented in this chapter, the dry, crushed, herbal adult dose should be 1 tsp per cup or 8 oz of water; when the fresh herb is used, the amount should be twice that. Although no absolute law exists for administering medicines to children, Cowling's rule takes the child's age at the next birthday and divides by 24 to determine what fraction of the adult dose should be given.[59]

SPECTRUM OF APPLICABILITY

Most herbal medicines that have been catalogued and used historically are specifically indicated for one condition, although additional therapeutic effects have been noted over time. All the botanicals covered here have multiple uses. Comfrey (*Symphytum officinale*) may be used as a topical antiinflammatory agent; it also has constituents that are effective for GI conditions when taken internally. *Aloe vera* gel is an excellent topical agent for abrasions and burns; taken internally, the latex portion serves as an effective laxative. *Calendula officinalis* has antimicrobial properties that make it an effective topical dressing for mild infectious conditions, whereas internally it has antipyretic effects.[120]

AFFORDABILITY

If the herbalist collects plants and processes them personally, the cost is minimal. The purchase price of botanicals depends on the rarity and origin. Some exotic and rare botanicals from Asia and the Amazon rain forest demand a high price on the world market. *Panax ginseng* has long been regarded by Asian peoples as a prized herbal tonic and can cost hundreds of dollars per root, depending on the size, origin, and age. *Panax quinquefolius* (American ginseng), can cost as much as $52 per pound and was valued at $62 million as a cash crop in 1992.[19] Many exotic herbal and animal-derived medicines from China have prices as high as those of precious metals.

Most of the herbs produced in the continental United States and used for common ailments average 20¢ to 30¢ per dose (equivalent to 1 tsp of herbal tincture). Prices are not yet standardized. Quality control for production and supply and demand seem to dictate the cost of the mass-marketed herbal products. The best way to obtain a standardized product with a good quality-to-price ratio is to acquire the product from a botanical company that has been in business for at least 10 years and sells only to licensed health care practitioners.

NORTH AMERICAN PLANT MEDICINES

EPHEDRA (*Ephedra* species)

Description and Habitat

Common names for ephedra include Brigham Young weed, desert herb, Mormon tea, squaw tea, and teamsters' tea.

Ephedra spp. are shrubs with erect, straw-like branches found in desert or arid regions throughout the world and in the southwestern U.S. deserts. The Chinese ephedra called Ma Huang, *Ephedra sinica,* is found throughout Asia; *Ephedra distacha* is found throughout Europe; *Ephedra trifurca* or *Ephedra viridis* (desert tea) (Figure 68-2), *Ephedra nevadensis* (Mormon tea), and *Ephedra americana* (American ephedra) (Figure 68-3) are found in North America; and *Ephedra gerardiana* (Pakistani ephedra)

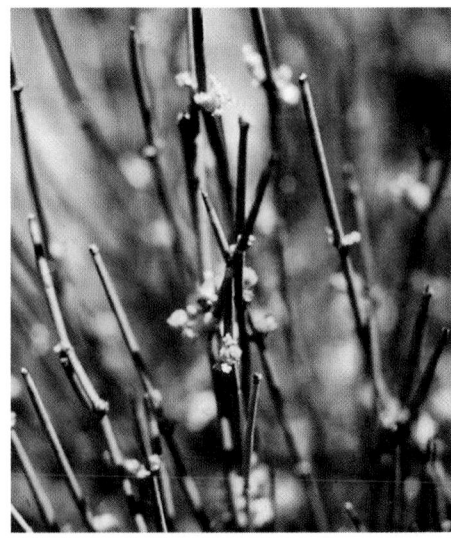

FIGURE 68-2 *Ephedra viridis. (Courtesy Cascade Anderson Geller.)*

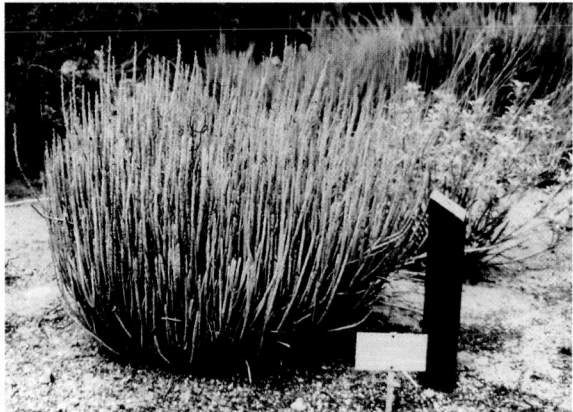

FIGURE 68-3 *Ephedra americana. (Courtesy Jill Stansbury.)*

is found in Pakistan and India. The 0.6- to 2.1-m (2- to 7-foot) shrubs grow on dry, rocky, or sandy soils. The broom-like shrub has many jointed green stems with two or three small, scale-like leaves that grow at the joint of stems and branches (Figure 68-4).

Pharmacology

Ephedra is generally used for its alkaloid content, which tends to consist of ephedrine, pseudoephedrine, and norpseudoephedrine. The various species vary significantly in both alkaloid type and alkaloid content. In *E. sinica,* the total alkaloid content can be from 3.3% to 20%, with 40% to 90% being ephedrine and the remainder pseudoephedrine.[52] The North American varieties, such as Mormon tea (*E. nevadensis*), are reported to contain no ephedrine.

Ephedra's pharmacology centers on the actions of ephedrine. Ephedrine and pseudoephedrine are used widely in prescription and over-the-counter (OTC) drugs to treat asthma, hay fever, and rhinitis.[68]

The central nervous system (CNS) effects of ephedrine are similar to those of epinephrine but are much milder, and the duration of action is much longer. The cardiovascular effects are increased blood pressure, cardiac output, and heart rate. In addition, ephedrine increases brain, heart, and muscle blood flow while decreasing renal and intestinal circulation. Relaxation of bronchial, airway, and uterine smooth muscles also occurs.[68]

Pseudoephedrine has weaker CNS and cardiovascular system actions but has bronchial smooth muscle relaxation effects. Because it has fewer side effects, it is used more often than ephedrine for asthma.[68] Pseudoephedrine also demonstrates significant antiinflammatory activity.[81,102] Per 100 g, the dry leaf of ephedra is reported to contain 5 g protein, 5810 mg calcium, and 500 mg potassium.[52]

Native American and European Medicinal Uses

Ephedra has been used extensively in the West and in Asia for upper respiratory conditions such as asthma, bronchitis, and hay

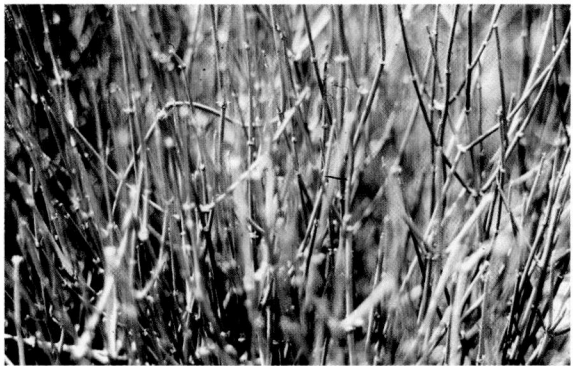

FIGURE 68-4 Ephedra. *(Courtesy Jill Stansbury.)*

fever. It has also been used to treat edema, arthritis, fever, hypotension, and urticaria.[38] It is said to be valuable as a diuretic, febrifuge, and tonic.[120]

Navajo Indians applied the dried, crushed, long leaf of ephedra to syphilitic sores, and Hopi Indians drank a tea from the branches and twigs of a related species for the same condition.[176] Other tribes used the ground and roasted root for making bread.[52]

Mormon tea is a folk remedy for colds, gonorrhea, headache, nephritis, and syphilis. Mexicans mix the leaves with tobacco and smoke them for headaches.[52]

Modern Clinical and Wilderness Applications

Ephedra has proved to be an effective bronchodilator for treating mild to moderate asthma and hay fever. The common preparations include other herbs, such as licorice (*Glycyrrhiza glabra*) and grindelia (*Grindelia camporium*), that have antitussive and expectorant effects.

Ephedrine promotes weight loss.[134] Appetite suppression plays a role, but increased metabolic rate of adipose tissue is the main mechanism.[8] The weight reduction effects can be enhanced by up to 60% with addition of methylxanthine.[54]

In response to accumulating evidence of adverse effects related to *Ephedra,* the U.S. Food and Drug Administration (FDA) banned the sale of *Ephedra*-containing supplements on the retail market.

In the wilderness, specifically the desert, Mormon tea from the raw herb *E. nevadensis* or *E. viridis* can be useful for hay fever, mild asthma, bronchitis, or upper respiratory infection (URI). These species contain minimal amounts of ephedrine and principally contain pseudoephedrine; thus, they can be used without some of the unpleasant side effects of the Asian species. They can also be used for mild fevers associated with influenza or URI.

The shrubs are typically found growing on dry, rocky, or sandy slopes. The leaves can be picked fresh or sun-dried for 6 to 8 hours and can be prepared as a steeped tea or an infusion. Generally, the dose should be the equivalent volume of 1 tsp of dried, crushed stems per 8 oz of water, steeped for 10 minutes. The patient should not exceed a dose of this amount given six times daily. Once harvested, the leaves can be kept for an indefinite period for later use if stored in an airtight container.

Toxicity

According to Duke,[52] an infusion of ephedra produced "prompt and extensive contraction of uterine muscle when applied to smooth muscle strips of virgin guinea pig uteri." Ephedra may also elevate blood pressure. Frequent use may result in nervousness and restlessness. It should be used with caution if the patient has hypertension, heart disease, thyrotoxism, diabetes, or benign prostatic hypertrophy. Ephedra should not be used with antihypertensive or antidepressant medications.

GOLDENSEAL (*Hydrastis canadensis*)

Description and Habitat

Hydrastis has a perennial root or rhizome that is tortuous, knotty, and creeping (Figure 68-5). The internal color is bright yellow, with numerous long fibers. The stem is erect, simple, herbaceous, and rounded, from 15 to 30 cm (6 to 12 inches) in height, becoming purplish and bearing two unequal terminal leaves. The leaves are alternately palmate with three to five lobes, hairy, dark green, and cordate at the base. The flowers, which are evident in early spring, are solitary, terminal, small, and white or rose colored.

The plant is a native of eastern North America and cultivated in Oregon and Washington. The parts used are the dried rhizome and roots.

Pharmacology

The alkaloids derived from *Hydrastis* are hydrastine (1.5% to 4%), berberine (0.5% to 6%), berberastine (2% to 3%), canadine, hydrastinine, and related compounds. Other constituents include meconin, chlorogenic acid, phytosterins, and resins.[134]

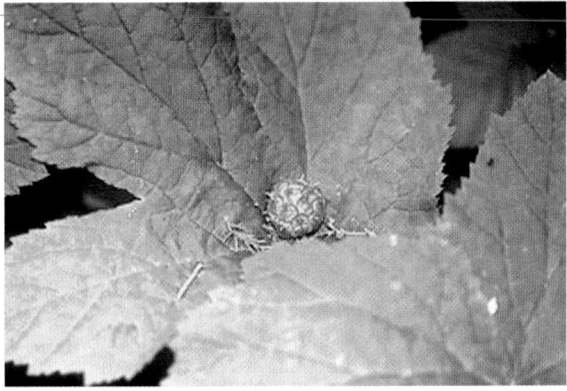

FIGURE 68-5 Goldenseal (*Hydrastis canadensis*).

Native American and European Medicinal Uses and Folklore

Native Americans used *Hydrastis* extensively as an herbal medicine and clothing dye. The Cherokee Indians used the roots as a wash for local inflammations, as a decoction for general debility and dyspepsia, and to improve appetite. The Iroquois Indians used a decoction of the root for whooping cough, diarrhea, liver trouble, fever, sour stomach, flatulence, pneumonia, and heart trouble.[129]

Early European uses date back to 1793. In *Collections for an Essay Towards a Materia Medica of the United States,* Benjamin Smith Barton noted that *Hydrastis* was useful as an eyewash for conjunctival inflammation and as a bitter tonic. In the pharmacy of the 19th century (1830), goldenseal was listed among the official remedies in the first revision of the New York edition of the USP. It was listed in the USP until 1926 and recognized in the *National Formulary* until 1955.[82]

Modern Clinical and Wilderness Applications

Goldenseal is among the top sellers in the American herbal medicine market. It is used as an antiseptic, hemostatic, diuretic, laxative, tonic, and antiinflammatory for inflammation of the mucous membranes. It has also been recommended for hemorrhoids, nasal congestion, sore mouth and gums, conjunctivitis, external wounds, sores, acne, and ringworm.[117]

Modern research into the active ingredients berberine and hydrastine has shown why some of the folk applications are effective. The most widely studied component is *berberine*. This isoquinoline alkaloid has demonstrated antibiotic, immunostimulatory, anticonvulsant, sedative, febrifugal, hypotensive, uterotonic, choleretic, and carminative (promoting elimination of intestinal gas) activities.[134] Berberine has broad-spectrum antibiotic activity. The antimicrobial activity has been demonstrated on protozoa, fungi, and bacteria, both in vitro and in vivo. Antimicrobial action has been noted against *Staphylococcus, Streptococcus, Chlamydia, Corynebacterium diphtheriae, Escherichia coli, Salmonella typhi, Vibrio cholerae, Pseudomonas, Shigella dysenteriae, Entamoeba histolytica, Trichomonas vaginalis, Neisseria gonorrhoeae, Neisseria meningitidis, Treponema pallidum, Giardia lamblia, Leishmania donovani,* and *Candida albicans.*[134] Berberine inhibits adherence of bacteria to host cells.[161]

Active ingredients in the crude botanical may be responsible for the wide-spectrum effectiveness of *Hydrastis.* The antifungal properties, for example, prevent overgrowth of *Candida,* which frequently occurs with use of other antibiotic therapies.

Other studies have shown the immunostimulatory activity of berberine-containing plants. Berberine increases blood flow through the spleen; improved circulation may augment immune function of this lymphoid organ.[147] Berberine also activates macrophages.[109] Historically, berberine-containing plants have been used as febrifuges, and in rat studies they have an antipyretic effect three times as potent as that of aspirin.[134]

Plants such as goldenseal are very effective in treating acute GI infections. In several clinical studies, berberine has successfully treated acute diarrhea caused by *E. coli, S. dysenteriae,*

Salmonella, Klebsiella, Giardia, and *V. cholerae.*[14,41,49,75,100,148,153] Berberine-containing plants, in addition to having antimicrobial properties, influence the enterotoxins produced by offending pathogens.[28,162,163]

Gastrointestinal illness is a major concern of travelers to areas with questionable sanitation. Both waterborne and food-borne bacterial and protozoal infections are concerns for persons in wilderness and Third World environments. Some experts recommend using a berberine-containing botanical source prophylactically at least 1 week before a visit to questionable areas and for 1 week after return.[134]

Various eye complaints involving the conjunctivae and surrounding mucous membranes have been effectively treated with forms of berberine extract. Studies point to the effectiveness of berberine in treating infection caused by *Chlamydia trachomatis.* Clinical trials found that a 2% berberine solution compared favorably with sulfacetamide. Although the symptoms resolved more slowly with the berberine extract, the rate of relapse was much lower in the berberine-treated group.[10,130]

A standardized form of *H. canadensis* is beneficial for generalized digestive disorders (acute dysentery, gastritis) and for infective, congestive, and inflammatory states (sinusitis, pharyngitis, stomatitis) of mucous membranes. A typical dose depends on the source and method of the extract. For the previous conditions, the following doses, three times a day, are recommended: dried root or as infusion, 2 to 4 g; tincture (1:5), 6 to 12 mL (1.5 to 3 tsp); or solid extract (4:1 or 10% alkaloid content), 250 to 500 mg. *Hydrastis* can also be used as a wash or rinse for conjunctivitis, sinusitis, and pharyngitis. Eye drops, nasal lavage, and gargle are applied in a 5% preparation of a 1:5 tincture, or 1 to 2 tsp of powdered herb in 8 oz of water to create an infusion for application to inflamed mucous membranes. This can be repeated three times daily.

Toxicity

Berberine and berberine-containing plants are generally nontoxic. In recommended doses, berberine-containing plants have not been shown to be toxic in clinical trials. The median lethal dose (LD_{50}) of berberine sulfate in mice is approximately 25 mg/kg, and in dogs, intravenous (IV) doses up to 45 mg/kg do not produce lethal or gross toxic effects.[147] *Hydrastis* should not be used during pregnancy, and long-term ingestion may interfere with metabolism of B vitamins.

ARNICA (*Arnica montana*)

Description and Habitat

Arnica is a perennial plant generally found in mountainous areas of Canada, the northern United States, and Europe. The plant reaches a height of 30 to 60 cm (12 to 24 inches) and generally contains from one to nine large, daisy-like flower heads, which bloom during summer months (Figures 68-6 to 68-8).

Pharmacology

The flower is used both internally and externally for medicinal effects. The rootstock is used to make commercial preparations

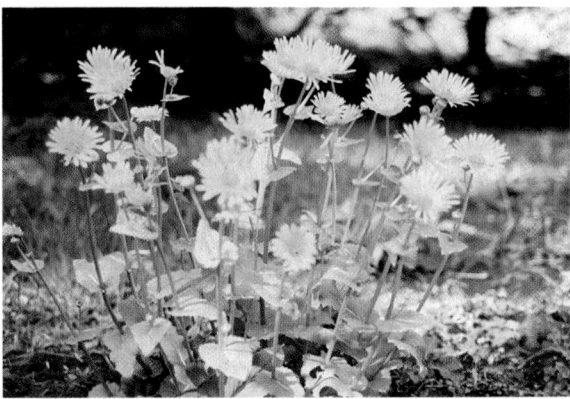

FIGURE 68-6 *Arnica montana.* (Courtesy Jill Stansbury.)

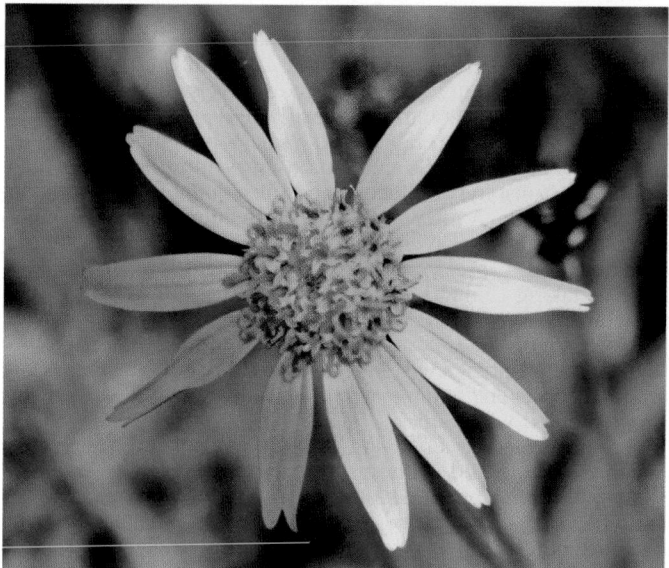

FIGURE 68-7 *Arnica latifolia. (Copyright iStockphoto.com/SnowOwl Moon.)*

for tinctures and oils that are applied topically. The active constituents of the plant drug are flavonoids, volatile oils, and plant pigments (carotenoids).[177] Specific constituents include arnicine, formic acid, thymohydroquinone, lobelamine, and lobeline (piperidine alkaloid).[34]

Native American and European Medicinal Uses and Folklore

Catawba Indians administered the tea of arnica roots to treat back pain. In Europe, the flower heads have been used since the 16th

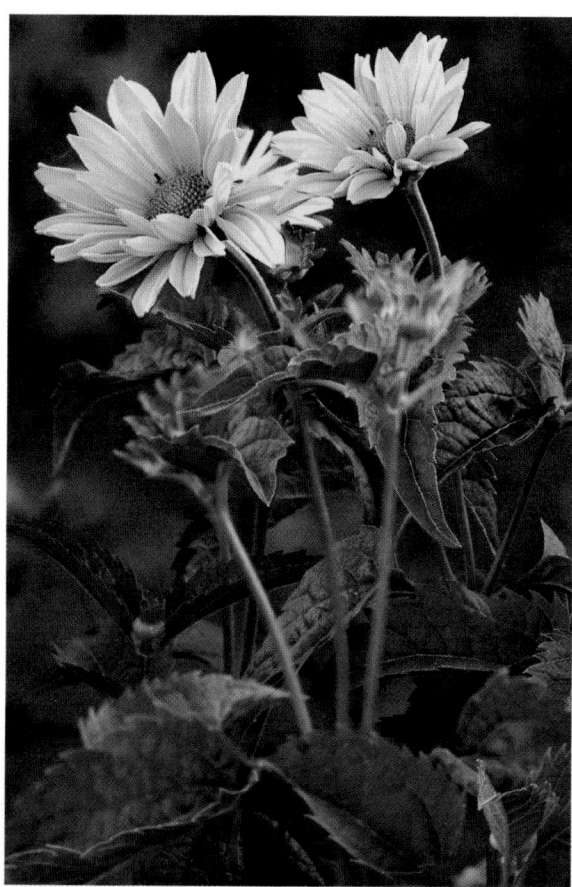

FIGURE 68-8 *Arnica montana. (Copyright iStockphoto.com/AGE photography.)*

century as an application for bruises and strains.[175] European arnica was included in the USP from the early 1800s until 1960 and recognized for its effects on the healing of bruises and sprains.

Specific instructions given in the *American Dispensory* in 1922 listed arnica as effective for "muscular soreness and pain from strain or overexertion; advanced stage of disease, with marked enfeeblement, weak circulation, and impaired spinal innervation; … tensive backache, as if bruised or strained; [and] … headache with tensive, bruised feeling and pain on movement."[59] Arnica in concentrated tincture form has been a popular, but not necessarily safe, medicine to treat inflammatory swellings and to relieve the soreness of myalgia and effects of bruises and contusions. Doses above the therapeutic range cause vagal inhibition when ingested and may cause toxicity if the concentrated tincture is applied topically. Therefore, the most common use has been fomentation of the flowers for topical application in the treatment of strains and sprains.

Modern Clinical and Wilderness Applications

Contemporary use of *A. montana* is generally limited to topical commercially prepared ointments and salves, in conjunction with internal homeopathic (low dose) use for the same indications. Although its alkaloid (arnicine) and volatile oil (thymohydroquinone) are both relatively toxic, the actions of these constituents are extremely useful in resolving contusions and soft tissue injuries. Most ointments are found to contain a 1× homeopathic dilution of arnica tincture, which is about 4% by volume. Oral dosage is given in homeopathic potencies of 6× to 200c, depending on severity of the condition.

For application in the wilderness, most naturopathic first-aid kits include both ointment and the oral homeopathic forms of arnica. For direct use of the plant in treating minor sprains and strains, 2 tsp of the dried flower tops can be steeped in 1 cup of water for 10 minutes, and the infusion applied in a cold compress to the affected area. This should be repeated every 2 hours in addition to standard first-aid procedures. The infusion lasts 1 day if refrigerated and a few hours if not; therefore it is best to use a fresh infusion whenever possible. In addition, if available, the oral homeopathic preparation (30× to 200c) should be taken three times daily until swelling is reduced significantly. A topical ointment can be applied every 2 to 3 hours for this condition instead of the compress.

According to Weiss,[176] arnica is safe and effective for topical contusions and for stimulating granulation and epithelialization. A tablespoon of tincture is added to 500 mL of water, and the gauze compress is then placed on the wound. This stimulates local circulation and acts on peripheral vasculature. After granulation has occurred, ointments may be applied.

Toxicity

Arnica tincture or infusion can be toxic if the concentration is too high. Undiluted tincture should not be used internally or in compress form over an open wound. Vagus nerve inhibition is the primary toxic effect; GI irritation is also noted. Toxic reactions include gastric burning; nausea; vomiting; headache; decreased temperature; dyspnea; cardiovascular collapse; convulsions; motor, sensory, and vagal paralysis; and death.[34]

GARLIC (*Allium sativum*)

Description and Habitat

Garlic is a member of the lily family. It is a perennial plant cultivated worldwide (Figure 68-9). The garlic bulb is composed of individual cloves enclosed in a white skin. The medicinal herb is found in the bulb and is used either fresh or dehydrated. Garlic oil, which also has medicinal value, is obtained by steamed distillation of the crushed fresh bulbs.[117]

Pharmacology

The medicinal compounds in garlic generally contain sulfur and have been the subject of most research on garlic. Two primary compounds are an odorless chemical called alliin and the enzyme allinase, which begins a cascade of chemical reactions when the

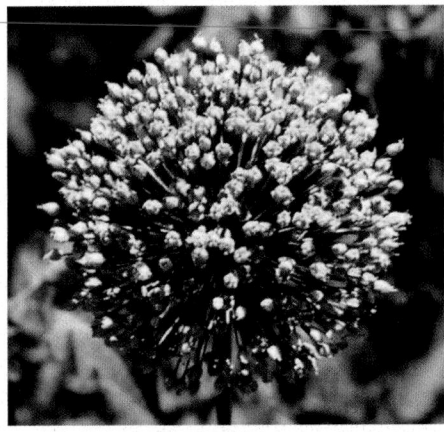

FIGURE 68-9 Garlic blossom (*Allium* sp.). *(Courtesy Cascade Anderson Geller.)*

garlic clove is cut, crushed, or bruised. Alliin is converted to allicin, which is responsible for the characteristic odor of garlic. Allicin is strongly antibacterial and considered to be the major source of the antimicrobial effects of garlic. Breakdown products of allicin include diallyl sulfide, disulfide, and trisulfide. Heat speeds up the reaction, so cooked garlic and steamed distilled garlic oil contain little or no allicin. About 0.1% to 0.36% of the volatile oils in garlic is composed of sulfur-containing compounds (e.g., allicin, diallyl sulfide, diallyl trisulfide). These volatile oils are thought to be responsible for most of the pharmacologic properties of garlic. Other constituents of garlic include S-methyl-L-cysteine sulfoxide, protein (16.8% by dry weight), a high concentration of trace minerals (particularly selenium and germanium), vitamins, glucosinolates, and the enzymes allinase, peroxidase, and myrosinase.[134,142]

Native American and European Medicinal Uses and Folklore

Throughout history, garlic has played an important part in medicinal herbology. Clay garlic bulbs dating back to 3750 BC were found in Egypt. Preserved garlic bulbs were discovered in the tomb of Tutankhamen. An entire basket of these bulbs from the tomb of Kha at Thebes is in the Turin Egyptian museum. The Greek historian Herodotus recorded that an enormous amount of money was spent on garlic for the builders of the great pyramids. One of the earliest Sanskrit manuscripts, the Bower manuscript, devotes its entire first section to garlic, describing its legendary origins. It states that garlic keeps in order the three fluids and can cure thinness, weakness of digestion, lassitude, coughs, inflammation of the skin, piles, glandular swellings in the abdomen, splenic enlargement, indigestion, constipation, excessive urination, worms, wind in the body (rheumatism), leprosy, epilepsy, and paralysis.

Within the traditional medical circles of Greece and Rome, medieval Europe, and the Far East, similar claims may be found. Galen, Dioscorides, and Aristotle extolled garlic as an excellent medicine. Hippocrates recommended garlic as a diuretic; to regulate digestion; to treat bowel pains, inflammations, and infections; and to regulate menstruation. Early Chinese and European herbalists used garlic as a heating and drying agent, and therefore to prevent and cure diseases arising from cold, poisons, excesses of diet and drink, and sluggish metabolism.

In 1858, Pasteur noted garlic's antimicrobial properties. Albert Schweitzer used garlic in Africa to treat amebic dysentery. Garlic was also used as an antiseptic to prevent gangrene during both world wars.

Modern Clinical and Wilderness Applications

The pharmacologic effects of garlic are based on its activity as a hypoglycemic and hypolipemic regulating agent,* anticoagulant,†

---

*References 7, 9, 15, 23, 25, 29-31, 39, 40, 76, 89, 90, 93-95, 98, 99, 106, 107, 137.
†References 6, 22, 27, 28, 32, 66, 92, 121, 135, 149, 158.

---

antihypertensive,[122,143] antimicrobial,[1,4,5,36,62,111,121,136,168] detoxifier of heavy metals,[3] and immune system modulator.[97]

Animal and human studies have substantiated that garlic lowers serum cholesterol and triglyceride levels and increases the amount of high-density lipoproteins. Dietary atherosclerosis was significantly reduced in rabbits fed garlic consistently for weeks; also, an extract of garlic and onions was more effective than clofibrate against hyperlipidemia and subsequent lipid deposition within the aorta.[24] After 4 months of feeding rabbits a high-cholesterol diet, the average lipid content in the aorta of the control animals rose from 5.95 to 13.75 mg/100 g dry weight. Animals taking clofibrate for 4 months had 7.95 mg, and garlic-fed animals 6.23 mg/100 g dry weight of lipid content in the aorta.[24] Other studies of experimental atherosclerosis in rabbits support these findings.[91,106] Decreased atheromatous lesions seem to be a consistent finding in rabbits fed high-cholesterol diets supplemented with garlic.

Of various sulfur-containing amino acids isolated from garlic, S-methylcysteine and S-allylcysteine exert the greatest antilipidemic effects.[89] Components of garlic can combine with the sulfhydryl group, the functional part of coenzyme A that is necessary for biosynthesis of fatty acids, cholesterol, triglycerides, and phospholipids. The lipid-lowering effect may best be attributed to inactivation of the sulfhydryl group.[9] In vitro and in vivo tests show reduced conversion of acetate into cholesterol by liver tissues.[39] Because sulfhydryl groups are involved at all levels of metabolic activity, the impact of garlic could be more extensive. Studies suggest that garlic may lower blood pressure by acting the same way as prostaglandin E_1, by decreasing peripheral vascular resistance.[138]

As a nutritional supplement, garlic is composed of magnesium, iron, copper, zinc, selenium, calcium, potassium chloride, germanium, sulfur compounds, amino acids, and vitamins A, B_1, and C. Garlic increases the body's capacity to assimilate thiamine by enhancing its absorption. Thiamine is a key part of the cocarboxylase enzyme system, which has beneficial effects on liver cells; this may explain why garlic offers prophylaxis against liver and gallbladder damage. In one study, garlic was shown to protect hepatocytes in tissue culture from the damage of carbon tetrachloride.[138]

Antioxidant activity has been attributed to garlic and garlic derivatives. The free radical scavenger action of garlic may be explained by its germanium, glutathione, selenium, and zinc content. The last three are key components of the antioxidant enzyme superoxide dismutase and glutathione peroxidase. Animal studies show that feeding garlic oil enhanced physical endurance in normal rats and also reduced the decrease in endurance induced by isoproterenol, a synthetic catecholamine that induces myocardial necrosis.[151]

Garlic inhibits platelet aggregation in animals; similar effects can be demonstrated in vitro and in vivo in humans.[47,157] Ajoene, an antiplatelet extract of garlic, was found to potentiate the antithrombotic effect of antiinflammatory drugs. Under fasting conditions, inhibition of platelet aggregation by garlic or its extracts is dose related.[159]

The garlic effect may be linked to inhibition of thromboxane synthesis or to altered properties of the plasma membrane. Methyl (2-propenyl) trisulfide, another component of garlic, is 10 times more potent as an inhibitor of platelet aggregation than is diallyl disulfide or trisulfide.[6] Thrombocyte aggregation inhibition is enhanced by two other compounds, 2-vinyl-1,3-dithiene and allyl-1,5-hexidienyl-trisulfide.[18]

Garlic and its juice or oil also enhance fibrinolysis.[26] In a double-blind, placebo-controlled trial, cycloallin, a component of garlic, was given to volunteers and patients after myocardial infarction and significantly increased fibrinolysis 1.5 hours later.[57] Chutani and Bordia[42] observed that the increase took place 6.5 to 12 hours after garlic intake. Daily garlic ingestion for 1 month generated a 72% to 85% increase in fibrinolysis in patients with ischemic heart disease.[146]

The pharmacologic versatility of garlic is best reflected by its antiviral, antifungal, antiprotozoan, antiparasitic, and antibacterial activities.[4,5,36,62,137,164,181] Laymen are credited with being the first to describe the scientific basis for medicinal use of garlic extract.[179]

Huddleson and colleagues[85] and Cavallito and Bailey[37] demonstrated in 1944 that garlic juice and allicin at low concentrations inhibited growth of *Staphylococcus, Streptococcus, Bacillus, Brucella,* and *Vibrio* species. Recent studies using serial dilutions and filter paper disk techniques have shown that fresh garlic, powdered garlic, and vacuum-dried preparations were effective antibiotic agents against many bacteria, including *Staphylococcus aureus,* α- and β-hemolytic *Streptococcus, E. coli, Proteus vulgaris, Salmonella enteritidis, Citrobacter,* and *Klebsiella pneumoniae.*[134] These studies compared the antimicrobial effects of antibiotics, including penicillin, streptomycin, chloramphenicol, erythromycin, and tetracycline, with those of garlic. Beside confirming garlic's well-known antibacterial effects, studies demonstrated its effectiveness in inhibiting growth of certain antibiotic-resistant bacteria.[1,56,154]

Garlic has also demonstrated significant antifungal activity against a wide range of fungi.[2,4,86,128,131,141,150,169] From a wilderness perspective, inhibition of fungi that can affect the skin (*Microsporum, Trichophyton, Epidermophyton,* and *Candida albicans*) can be significant. Garlic juice applied topically is an effective alternative in treating fungal skin diseases.[4] Garlic compares well with nystatin, gentian violet, and six other reputed antifungal agents used to treat *C. albicans.*[2,131,141,150]

Garlic has long been associated with prophylaxis against influenza virus. In vivo studies with mice revealed that garlic administration protected mice against intranasal inoculation with influenza viruses and enhanced reproduction of neutralizing antibodies after vaccine administration.[136] In vitro studies showed that garlic has antiviral activity against influenza B virus and herpes simplex virus type 1.[166] Preliminary studies revealed significant enhancement of natural killer (NK) cell activity in humans administered raw or cold, aged whole-clove garlic preparations daily for 3 weeks.[97] Antiviral activity of garlic in humans may result from the direct toxic effect on viruses and enhanced NK cell activity that destroys virus-infected cells.

Wilderness Medical Applications

Uses of garlic in the outdoor setting can be extensive. Its use as a food should be encouraged despite its odor, particularly in people with elevated cholesterol levels, heart disease, hypertension, diabetes, asthma, fungal infections, respiratory infections, and GI disorders (intestinal parasites, dysentery). A macerated garlic poultice and garlic slices serve as topical agents for fungal infections, ulcerated wounds, pyoderma, and other skin infections. The poultice can be used directly on the dermatologic problem, and as a suppository it can be used to treat vaginitis, particularly infections caused by *C. albicans.* For this application, one to two fresh-chopped cloves can be made into a poultice. This should be kept on the affected site for several hours and changed at least once every 6 hours with a fresh preparation. If the garlic causes epidermal irritation, its use is discontinued.

Prophylactic use during the flu season can reduce incidence of infection. Within the first 48 hours of onset of a flu or URI, one or two cloves can be consumed with a carbohydrate source to prevent stomach irritation. Alternatively, two or three oil-of-garlic capsules can be taken. For persons concerned about the social-segregating aspect, extracts that preserve the allicin content but remain odorless can be used.

Toxicity

For the vast majority of individuals, garlic is nontoxic at usual doses. However, some people develop allergic contact dermatitis or irritation of the digestive tract. Apparently, they are unable to detoxify allicin and other sulfur-containing components. Prolonged consumption of large amounts of raw garlic by rats results in anemia, weight loss, and failure to grow.[137]

GINGER (*Zingiber officinale*)

Description and Habitat

Ginger is an upright perennial herb with tuberous rhizomes, from which an aerial stem grows to 1.5 m (5 feet) in height. It is native to southern Asia, although it is cultivated in the tropics. Extracts

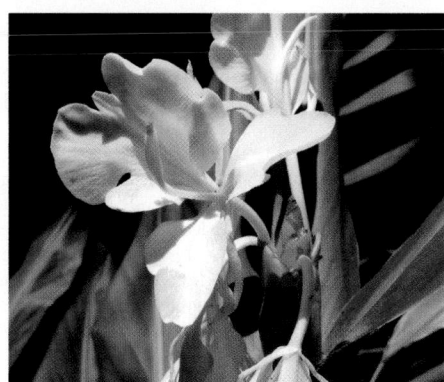

FIGURE 68-10 Ginger (*Zingiber officinale*) flower. (*Courtesy Kevin Davison.*)

and dried ginger are produced from dried unpeeled ginger; peeled ginger loses much of its essential oil content.[171]

Pharmacology

Ginger is composed of a rich variety of nutrients and enzymes. The general composition is starch (50%); protein (9%); lipid (6% to 8%) composed of phosphatidic acid, lecithin, free fatty acids, and triglycerides; protease (up to 2.26%); volatile oils (1% to 4%), the principal components of which are three sesquiterpenes (bisabolene, zingiberene, zingiberol); vitamins, especially niacin and vitamin A; and resins.[171]

Native American and European Medicinal Use

Zingiber officinale is native to southern Asia and tropical Africa (Figures 68-10 and 68-11). Therefore, it did not have a role in the early herbal preparations of European and Native American herbal medicine.

Modern Clinical and Wilderness Applications

Clinical use of ginger for antiinflammatory action, cholesterol-lowering effects, and relief of dizziness and motion sickness is

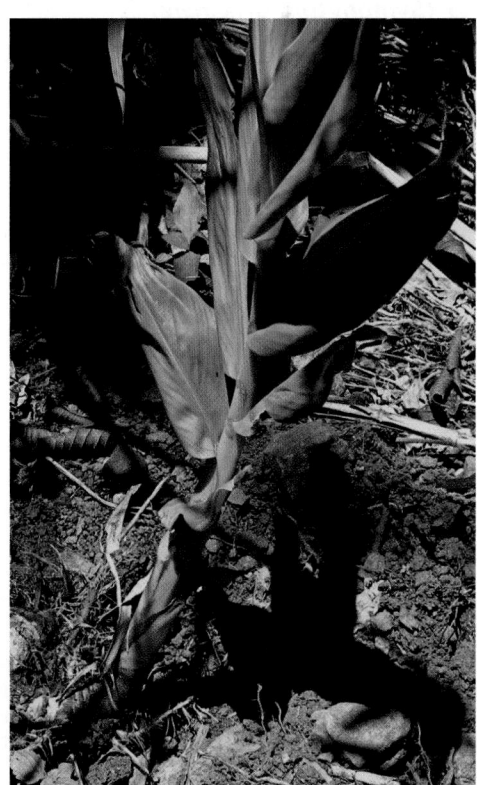

FIGURE 68-11 Ginger plant with rootstock. (*Courtesy Kevin Davison.*)

A choleretic effect (promotion of bile flow to the gallbladder and small intestine) and conversion of cholesterol into bile acids are enhanced by ginger ingestion and may be responsible for its overall cholesterol-lowering effect.

An early Eclectic medical text listed ginger as a local stimulant, sialogogue, diaphoretic, and carminative.[59] Powdered ginger in a large quantity of cold water taken before sleep frequently "breaks up" a severe cold, and a hot infusion of ginger tea is a popular remedy for similar use to mitigate the pains of dysmenorrhea.[59] Ginger may relieve painful spasmodic contractions of the stomach and intestine. The antiinflammatory action of ginger is thought to be caused by potent inhibition of inflammatory compounds, such as prostaglandins and thromboxanes.[108] Ginger is also known to contain strong plant proteases such as bromelain, ficaine, and papain, which may explain some of its antiinflammatory action.[171]

Ginger has been used historically for major GI complaints. It is generally regarded as an excellent carminative (promoting elimination of intestinal gas) and intestinal spasmolytic.[134] One of the most noted uses of ginger in contemporary herbal medicine that applies to wilderness medicine is its action on the symptoms of motion sickness and seasickness.[72,73,133] Ginger is also a significant antiemetic. It has long been used for treatment of nausea and vomiting associated with pregnancy. The efficacy of ginger has been confirmed in hyperemesis gravidarum, a severe form of nausea and vomiting during pregnancy. Ginger root powder at a dose of 250 mg four times a day brought a significant reduction in both severity of nausea and number of attacks of vomiting during pregnancy.[61] To treat motion sickness and vertigo, two 500-mg capsules of powdered ginger root are eaten 20 to 30 minutes before the precipitating event. The same dose is used for the nausea of pregnancy during the acute attack. The raw ginger root can be grated using 1 tsp in 4 oz of water, steeped for 10 minutes, and taken every 30 minutes until the symptoms of motion sickness abate.

Toxicity

There appears to be no toxicity associated with ginger root ingestion.

COMFREY (*Symphytum officinale*)

Description and Habitat

Comfrey is a perennial herb with a stout spreading root that is divisible for propagation (Figure 68-12). Comfrey grows about 1 m (3.3 feet) high and has coarse, bristly, oblong, lanceolate leaves. The tubular flower can be purplish, blue, white, red, or yellow (see Figure 68-12, *A*). About 25 *Symphytum* species are described; they are indigenous to countries around the Mediterranean Sea and in northern Asia. Comfrey is typically found in moist meadows and other wet places in the United States and Europe.

Pharmacology

The chemical constituents of *S. officinale* roots include carbohydrate, predominantly sucrose; the amino acids serine and asparagine; the phenolic acids chlorogenic acid, caffeic acid, and *p*-coumaric acid; the alkaloids choline and allantoin; and the pyrrolizidine alkaloids viridiflorine, echinatine, heliosupine, symphytine, echimidine, and lasiocarpine.[172] The most concentrated (0.88% to 1.71%) alkaloid, allantoin, is generally credited with comfrey's beneficial effects.

Native American and European Medicinal Uses and Folklore

In Europe, comfrey is a common perennial grown in the garden for animal fodder. Russian comfrey is often promoted as a medicinal herb for use as a tonic. Comfrey is also cultivated in Japan as a green vegetable. A tonic made from comfrey has been used in American herbal medicine for hundreds of years.[113]

Comfrey has long been known as an external agent for rehabilitation of musculoskeletal and orthopedic injuries. Its former name, "bone knit," derives from the external use of poultices of

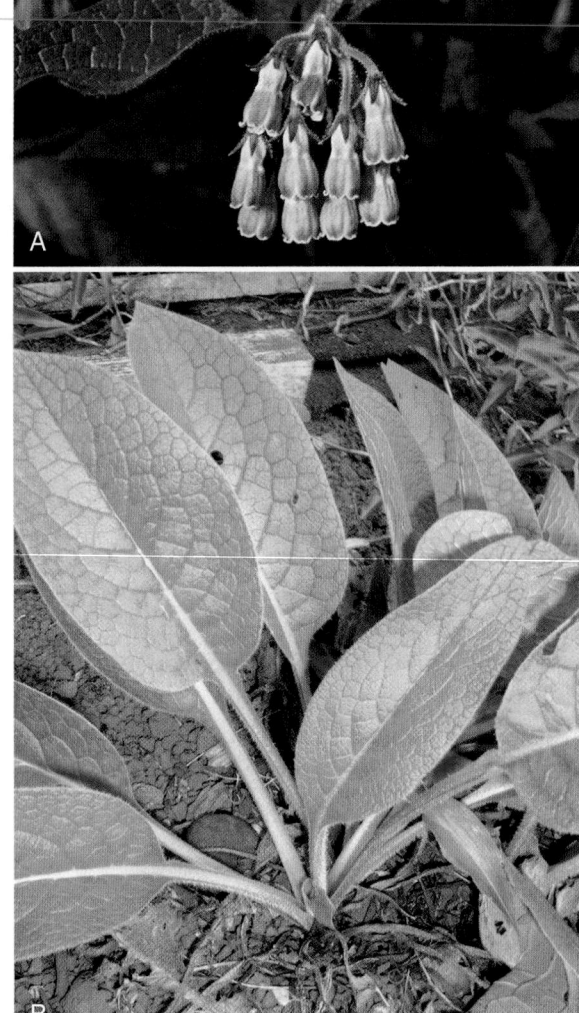

FIGURE 68-12 A, Comfrey (*Symphytum officinale*) flower. **B,** Comfrey (*Symphytum officinale*) leaf. (**A** *courtesy Cascade Anderson Geller.*)

leaves and roots, which were believed to help heal burns, sprains, swellings, and bruises. Comfrey has been claimed to heal gastric ulcers and hemorrhoids, suppress bleeding, and relieve bronchial congestion and inflammation.[16] The healing action of a poultice derived from the roots and leaves is probably related to the presence of allantoin, an agent that promotes cell proliferation. The underground parts contain 0.6% to 1.3% allantoin and 4% to 6.5% tannin.[35,127] Comfrey extracts applied topically have been reported to heal wounds and bones in about one-half the normal time. In herbology, a general rule is that "if anything is broken, use comfrey."[180] Herbalists have also found that the allantoin concentration from a fluid extract of comfrey can increase the rate of wound healing of lacerations sufficiently to avoid the use of sutures.[178]

In European folklore, comfrey was regarded as an herb having unsurpassed ability to heal any injured or broken tissue. The mucilage (gelatinous mucopolysaccharide) of the comfrey root was named "the great cell proliferator," helping new flesh and bones to grow. Comfrey was one of the main herbs found in any poultice or fomentation. European herbalists considered comfrey exceptional for coughs and soothing inflamed tissues. Comfrey is effective for treating upper respiratory inflammation and has been used successfully to treat hemorrhagic conditions of the lungs.

Modern Clinical and Wilderness Applications

Comfrey lotions and salves containing 0.5% to 2.5% allantoin have been used for sprains, strains, and contusions. In the 1980s, comfrey became controversial because of potential hepatotoxicity. Members of the family Boraginaceae (*Heliotropium,*

Symphytum) contain a variety of related pyrrolizidine alkaloids reported to cause hepatotoxicity in animals. Although no hepatotoxic episodes from ingestion of comfrey have been reported in humans, the potential exists, so caution is advised when using comfrey for internal consumption.[113] Topical use of comfrey products as yet poses no concern for toxicity.

As a topical agent after acute trauma, such as musculoskeletal injuries, strains and sprains, or contusions, comfrey is an exceptional medicine.[17] A prepared gel of comfrey with a standardized allantoin concentration should be carried during travel or camping expeditions in the wilderness.

The raw herb can be used if the plant is nearby. The herb is readily identifiable, but should not be confused with foxglove (*Digitalis purpurea*), and should be used with caution when taken internally in its raw state. For use in a poultice or compress, the leaves may be picked damp, macerated, and applied topically for up to 24 hours.

Toxicity

Comfrey is not recommended for routine internal ingestion. Animal studies indicate that hepatic damage is an eventual outcome if the herb is consumed over a long period.

ALOE (*Aloe vera*)

Description and Habitat

The aloe is a perennial plant native to South and East Africa and is also cultivated in the West Indies and other tropical and temperate areas. The leaves, which emerge from a central rosette produced by a central fibrous root, are 30 to 60 cm (12 to 24 inches) long, narrow, fleshy, and light green with spiny teeth on the margins (Figure 68-13). Aloe is easily cultivated as a houseplant and can be grown in a sunny, warm spot with good drainage.

The genus *Aloe* comprises more than 300 species, which are members of the Liliaceae (lily) family. *Aloe* spp. are perennial succulents native to Africa. They are not cacti and should not be confused with American aloe, the century plant.

Pharmacology

Two important products are derived from aloe: a gel and latex. Aloe gel is a clear gelatinous material extracted from the mucilaginous cells found in the inner tissue of the leaf (see Figure 68-13). It is obtained by crushing the leaves and straining the mass repeatedly to remove cellular debris. The result is a clear gel, which is the product most frequently used in the health food and cosmetic industries. It is generally devoid of anthraquinone glycosides. A variety of compounds have been identified in *Aloe* spp., including polysaccharides, tannins, organic acids, enzymes, vitamins, minerals, saponins, and steroids.[113]

The bitter yellow latex of aloe contains cathartic anthraquinone glycosides, mostly barbaloin, as the active constituents. The concentrations of the glycosides vary with the type of aloe, ranging from 4% to 25% of aloe in concentration. The water-soluble fraction of aloe is called aloin and is a mixture of active

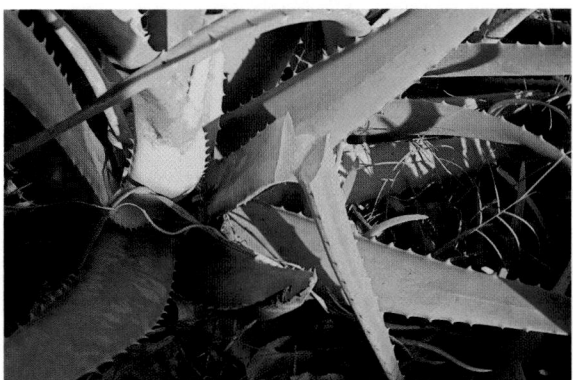

FIGURE 68-13 *Aloe vera* with exposed latex gel. (*Courtesy Kevin Davison.*)

glycosides. Cathartics have been derived from extracts of the latex and can create strong purgative effects by stimulating the large intestine.

Native American and European Medicinal Uses and Folklore

Fresh *Aloe vera* gel is well known for its domestic medicinal values.[69,116,132,139] It has been dubbed the burn plant, first-aid plant, and medicine plant. When fresh, the gel relieves thermal burns and sunburns and promotes wound healing. It also has moisturizing and emollient properties. Because of these effects, aloe is widely used as a home remedy.

Aloin and other anthraquinone derivatives of aloe are extensively used as active ingredients in laxative preparations. Aloin is also used as an antiobesity preparation.[117] Aloe or aloin extracts are used in sunscreens and other cosmetic preparations, as well as in drugs for moisturizing, emollient, or wound-healing purposes.

In folk medicine, aloe is used for condylomas, warts, abnormal skin growths, and cancers of the lip, anus, breast, larynx, liver, nose, stomach, and uterus.[52] Folklore suggests that parts of the plants should be chewed to purify the blood. The pulp is said to possess wound-healing hormonal activities and "biogenic stimulators," and is used for intestinal ailments, sore throat, and ulcers. In India, aloe is used to treat piles and rectal fissures. Slukari hunters in Africa's Congo basin rubbed their bodies with the gel to eliminate the human scent, making them less likely to disturb prey. During epidemics of influenza, Lesotho natives take a public bath in an infusion of *Aloe latifolia*.[52]

Modern Clinical and Wilderness Applications

Although numerous claims have been made for aloe gel, its most common lay use is in the treatment of minor burns and skin irritations. In 1935, a report described the use of aloe in the treatment of radiation-induced dermatitis.[44] This study followed a 5-week course of topical applications of either the whole leaf or the leaf macerated into gel, resulting in complete wound healing after 4 months. In 1937, studies used a calamine- and lanolin-based aloe preparation to treat skin irritations resulting from burns, pruritus vulvae, and poison ivy. The results suggested that aloe stimulated tissue granulation and accelerated wound healing.[113]

Barnes[12] evaluated the effect of 5% aloe ointment on sandpaper-abraded fingertips and found the wound-healing rate was two to three times that of controls, as measured by decreased electrical potential of the wound. Other studies measured tensile strength of the healed surgical wounds of mice. Healing occurred within 9 days, an improvement over the results in control mice.[70]

Studies of antibacterial activity of aloe extracts have been attempted several times, yielding mixed results. In 1963, studies of the antibacterial effect of macerated *Aloe vera* gel found no activity against *Staphylococcus aureus* and *Escherichia coli*.[63] Other studies have determined that *Aloe chinensis* is effective against *S. aureus, E. coli,* and *Mycobacterium tuberculosis,* although *Aloe vera* showed no inhibitory effect.[71] The latex possesses in vitro activity against several pathogenic strains of bacteria, although the whole leaf minus the latex from the leaf epidermis and mesophyll of aloe showed no activity.[118] Two commercial preparations of aloe gel were found to exert antimicrobial activity against gram-negative and gram-positive bacteria and *C. albicans* when used in concentrations greater than 90%.[78]

The moisturizing effect of aloe may be beneficial for treatment of burns. The healing process may be related to mucopolysaccharides along with sulfur derivatives and nitrogen compounds in the gel, but this has not been well substantiated.[112] In attempts to document the antiinflammatory effects of aloe, a 1976 study found that *Aloe vera* had bradykinase activity in vitro, but this was not confirmed in vivo.[65]

Evidence for the internal use of aloe has been limited to studies involving mucous membrane tissue repair. Corneal ulcers treated with aloe extracts had more healing, less cellular reaction, and fewer signs of irritation than did control groups.[113] Topical application of *Aloe vera* gel after periodontal flap surgery reduced postoperative pain more than did the saline control, and swelling of the treated tissue was less marked than with the control.[80]

Because of easy recognition and administration, use of the aloe plant in the wilderness environment is practical. The wild plant can yield an excellent preparation for dermal abrasions, cuts, and superficial wounds. A leaf cut from the base of a healthy plant can be conveniently carried. This allows the gel to remain intact, protected by the outer skin of the leaf. It can be squeezed from the inside through the cut portion directly onto superficial wounds with or without a gauze dressing. A standardized preparation of *Aloe vera* may be used as an antibacterial agent and emollient for superficial wounds or dermatitis.

In the event of constipation, the mixture of aloe gel and latex can be scraped or squeezed from the leaf cortex and ingested, 1 tbsp three times daily, or until a mild laxative effect is noted. A gel and latex mixture produces less cathartic effect than does latex alone. Because of the bitterness of the gel and latex, the mixture should be taken with food or a flavored beverage.

Toxicity

Because of its cathartic effects, oral aloe is not advised if gripping pain is associated with constipation. Aloe taken orally is contraindicated in pregnancy. Otherwise, aloe has no reported toxicity.

PLANTAIN (*Plantago major*)

Description and Habitat

The common broadleaf plantain is a familiar perennial "weed" found along roadsides and in meadowlands (Figure 68-14). Plantain belongs to the family Plantaginaceae, which contains more than 200 species, 25 to 30 of which have domestic use (Figures 68-14 to 68-16). *Plantago major* is a small weed with a rosette of ribbed leaves and small, projecting seed stalks. Its seeds, known as "psyllium seeds" in North America, resemble those of another species, *Plantago psyllium*. The leaves contain 84% water, 2.5% protein, 0.2% fat, and 14% carbohydrate; trace amounts of calcium, phosphorus, iron, sodium, and potassium; and beta-carotene, riboflavin, niacin, and ascorbic acid. Biochemically identified compounds include allantoin, adenine, baicalein, baicalin, benzoic acid, chlorogenic acid, choline, cinnamic acid, ferulic acid, L-fructose, fumaric acid, gentisic acid, D-glucose, *p*-hydroxybenzoic acid, indican, lignoceric acid, neochlorogenic acid, oleanolic acid, plantagonine, planteose, saccharose, salicylic acid, scutellarein, sitosterol, sorbitol, stachyose, syringic acid, tyrosol, ursolic acid, vanillic acid, and D-xylose.[52]

Native American and European Medicinal Uses and Folklore

Historically, plantain has long been used for stings, bites, and irritations from venomous insects and reptiles. Folk medicine of the eastern United States suggests using crushed plantain leaves to stop the itching of poison ivy. It has also been reported to

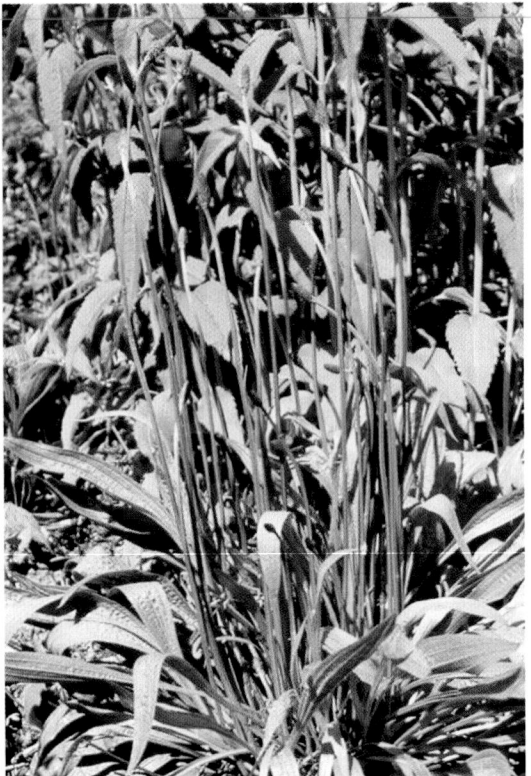

FIGURE 68-15 *Plantago laycedota. (Courtesy Jill Stansbury.)*

help relieve toothache. Ancient herbalists maintained that plantain had "refrigerant" (imparting a cooling sensation to the mucosa and allaying thirst), diuretic, and astringent properties. When the leaves are applied to a bleeding surface wound, hemorrhage lessens. In the highlands of Scotland, plantain is still called *slan-lus*, or "plant of healing."

In the United States, plantain has been known as "snake weed," from the belief that it is effective for bites from venomous creatures. Felter[59] noted that "the crushed leaves were very effective for the distressing symptoms caused by puncture by the horny appendages of larvae of *Lepidoptera* and the irritation produced by certain caterpillars, as well as the stings of insects and bites of spiders." In Native American folklore, the plant was

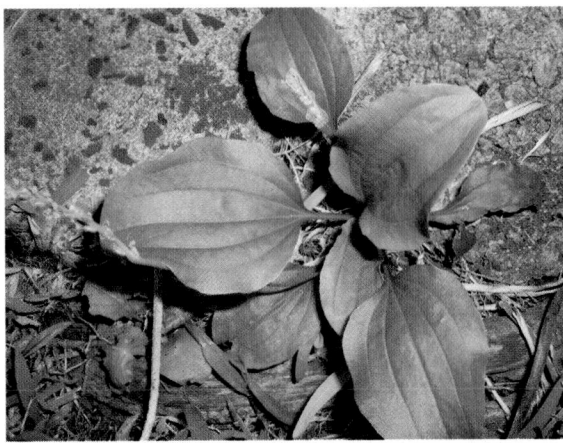

FIGURE 68-14 Plantain (*Plantago major*). (*Courtesy Cascade Anderson Geller.*)

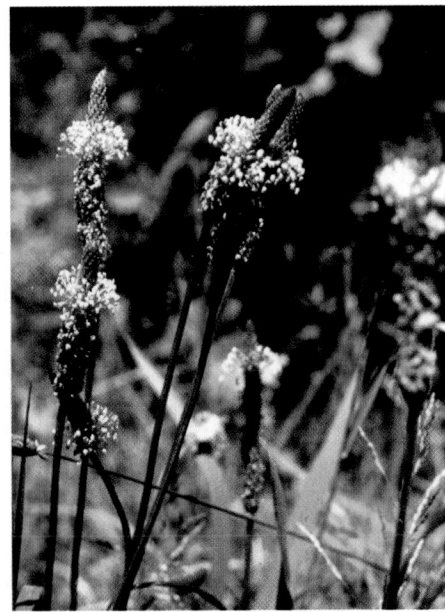

FIGURE 68-16 *Plantago*—flowering plantain. (*Courtesy Jill Stansbury.*)

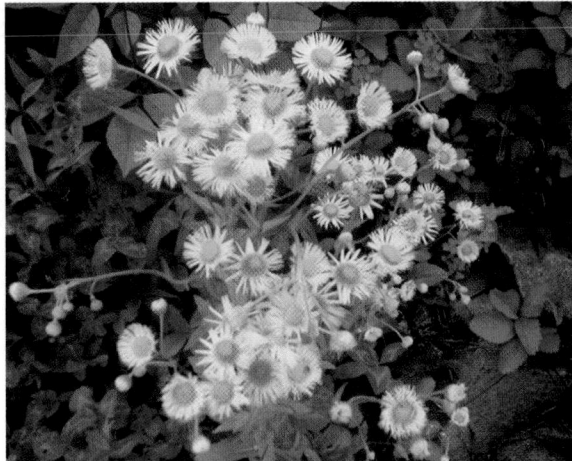

FIGURE 68-17 Chamomile (*Matricaria chamomilla*).

known as "white man's foot," in reference to its trait of growing in the settlements of white people. The Shoshoni Indians heated the leaves and applied them in a wet dressing for wounds.[177]

Modern Clinical and Wilderness Applications

Plantain is readily available in recreational areas of North America. This plant is extremely useful for various superficial wounds, abrasions, stings, and bites of mildly venomous insects. The constituents in the crushed leaves have an antihistaminic effect and anesthetic quality. In the event of a tooth fracture, a compress or poultice of 0.5 tsp of fresh leaves may be used on the tooth's exposed nerve root. Seeds of the plantago plant are useful for spastic colon, an effect that appears to be related to their mucilaginous properties. Psyllium seeds, known on the Asian continent as "flea seed husk," are often used as a bulk laxative. The seeds are collected from the stalk, and 2 tsp of fresh seeds in 4 oz of water are taken twice a day for mild constipation. Water should be ingested throughout the day to alleviate the condition and assist the laxative effect.

Because of its astringent quality, an infusion of the leaves is recommended to treat diarrhea. The preparer pours 1 pint of boiling water on 1 oz of the herb and leaves it in a warm place for 20 minutes. After straining and cooling, 0.5 cup is ingested three or four times a day.

Toxicity

No known toxicities are attributed to *Plantago*.

CHAMOMILE (*Matricaria chamomilla*)

Description and Habitat

Chamomile is a low-growing perennial with a hairy, prostrate branching stem (Figure 68-17). It blooms late in July through September and is found growing throughout North America and Europe. The name *chamomile* is derived from the Greek *chamos* (ground) and *melos* (apple), which refer to the plant's low growth and the apple-like scent of its fresh blooms.[156] The flower head is about 2.5 cm (1 inch) in diameter, has a conical receptacle, and is covered by yellow disk-like flowers surrounded by 10 or 20 white, down-curving ray flowers.

Pharmacology

The most important chemicals associated with chamomile are the volatile oils containing tiglic acid esters, chamazulene, farnesene, and α-bisabolol oxide. These volatile oils are destroyed if the herb is boiled.[157]

Native American and European Medicinal Uses and Folklore

A distinction should be made between the German and Roman species of chamomile, although they have been used interchangeably for centuries. German chamomile is preferred on the European continent, whereas Roman chamomile has been used widely in Great Britain. In the United States, German chamomile is much more widely consumed.[123]

German chamomile has a long tradition as a folk or domestic remedy. It has been used as an external compress or fomentation for gout, sciatica, inflammations, lumbago, rheumatism, and skin ailments. Infusions, decoctions, and tinctures have long been used internally to treat colic, convulsions, croup, diarrhea, fever, indigestion, insomnia, teething, toothaches, and bleeding or swollen gums. Historically, Roman chamomile was used similarly.[52,117] Chamomile is also a folk remedy for cancer.

Modern Clinical and Wilderness Applications

The principal biochemical constituent of chamomile is *chamazulene*. It is found in both species of chamomile and is reported to have antihistaminic properties.[58] Both histamine release and inhibition of histamine discharge have been considered mechanisms for the potential antiallergic action of chamazulene.

In Germany, chamomile products include tinctures, extracts, teas, and salves, widely used as antiinflammatory, antibacterial, antispasmodic, and sedative agents.[123] Studies have shown that chamazulene and α-bisabolol have antiinflammatory activity. Chamazulene may constitute as much as 5% of the essential oil. Other studies have shown that α-bisabolol has a protective effect against peptic ulcer, as well as antibacterial and antifungal effects. α-Bisabolol has reduced fever and shortened the healing time of skin burns in laboratory animals.[48] Most commercial European chamomile preparations have been standardized with regard to chamazulene and α-bisabolol content.[169]

According to Rudolph Weiss,[176] one action of chamomile is to reduce gastric motility and secretions, which would alleviate colic and painful spasm. About 20 flavones and flavonols, such as apigenin, are found in the aqueous portion of the distillation process. These are three times as effective at spasmolytic activity as is the opium alkaloid papaverine. Chamomile also has a significant calming effect and has traditionally had application as a mild sedative.

Chamomile is a good botanical to have on hand when traveling or camping. For infants experiencing restlessness and discomfort from teething, one-third of the adult dose may provide relief. For treatment of conditions (intestinal gas, colic, peptic ulcers) that may arise from excessive nervous tension, 2 tsp (or one standard teabag) of the flower tops can be added to a cup of boiling water and infused for 5 to 10 minutes; 2 to 3 cups may be taken over 30 minutes for acute intestinal colic.

ECHINACEA (*Echinacea* species)

Description and Habitat

Echinacea is a perennial herb native to the midwestern region of North America, from Saskatchewan to Texas (Figures 68-18 and 68-19). Species include *Echinacea angustifolia* and *Echinacea purpurea*. The plant produces a characteristic large, pale-purple flower and thick, hairy leaves and grows 60 to 90 cm (2 to 3 feet) high. The dried root is typically used for medicinal purposes.

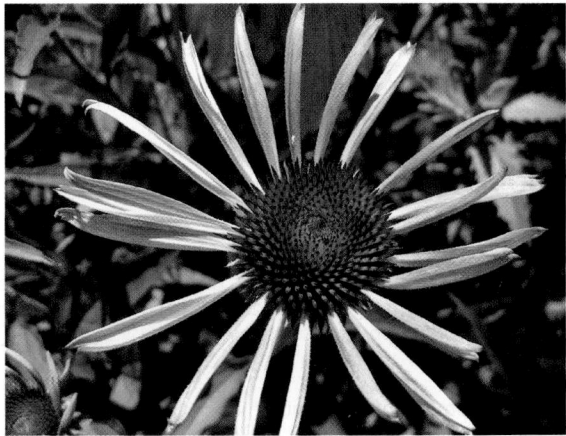

FIGURE 68-18 Echinacea flower. (*Courtesy Jill Stansbury.*)

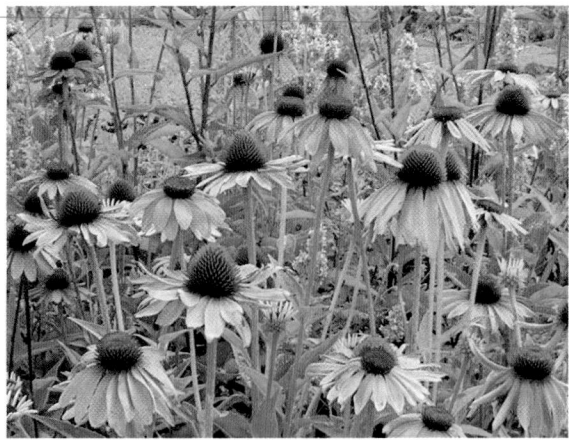

FIGURE 68-19 Echinacea (*Echinacea purpurea*).

Pharmacology

The compounds currently identified from *Echinacea* spp. are inulin, glucose, fructose, betaine, echinacin, echinacoside, 3-(*m*-trihydroxyphenyl) propionic acid, and nonspecific resins.[170]

Native American and European Medicinal Uses

This medicinal herb came to the attention of American herbalists in the late 1800s. Echinacea was originally used by the Indian tribes of Nebraska and the Sioux for treatment of snakebite and as an antiseptic and analgesic. Eclectic practitioners used it externally for the same purposes but used it internally to treat "bad blood" or any condition that manifested signs of local or systemic infection, whether bacterial or viral.

Modern Clinical and Wilderness Applications

Echinacea is probably the most common botanical used and known by the public, especially in relation to its immunomodulating effects. Many have empirically found that it can reduce symptoms and derail the onset of URIs and minor influenza episodes. However, an evaluation of *E. angustifolia* in experimental rhinovirus infections concluded that extracts of this plant's root, either alone or in combination, did not have clinically significant effects on infection with the virus or on the clinical illness that results from it.[167]

Echinacea is also a good systemic adjunct for treatment of any contusion or laceration. The polysaccharide component echinacin can maintain structure and integrity of the collagen matrix in connective tissue and ground substance, and it can accelerate wound healing experimentally.[134] Echinacin also has a cortisone-like effect, with intermediate stabilization of inflammation reactions. Inulin, a major component of echinacea, is a powerful activator of the immune system's alternative complement pathway. It may increase host defense mechanisms for neutralization of viruses, destruction of bacteria, and increased action of white blood cells (lymphocytes, neutrophils, monocytes, eosinophils) within areas of infection. Extracts of the root have been shown to possess interferon-like properties. As an immune stimulant early in infection, and for post-trauma rehabilitation, doses are taken orally three times daily: tincture (1:5), 30 to 60 drops, or solid extract (dry powdered extract, 6:1), 250 to 500 mg.

CALENDULA (*Calendula officinalis*)

Description and Habitat

Calendula, a member of the daisy and dandelion family, is found throughout Asia, North America, and Europe (see Figure 68-1). It is most often known as the pot marigold. The flower is generally used for production of a tincture.

Pharmacology

Calendula's chemical constituents include flavonoids, carotenes, saponin, resin, and volatile oils. The volatile oil content is responsible for localized increase in blood circulation and diaphoresis.

The resin content is responsible for antimicrobial and antiinflammatory action of the topical application.

Native American and European Medicinal Uses

Native Americans apparently did not use calendula extensively; early European literature mentions only its medicinal role. Calendula, however, is one of the best topical applications for treatment and prevention of infection and skin irritation. Early American surgeons highly regarded its ability to treat and prevent postsurgical infections.

Modern Clinical and Wilderness Applications

A fluid or water extraction, or an oil infusion (prepared as a tincture but using vegetable oil instead of alcohol) of calendula should be used in the initial treatment of lacerations, abrasions, and scalds; immediately after any required debridement and cleaning of a wound; and for generalized inflammation of mucous membranes. It has shown its usefulness in dermatitis and in vaginal, sinus, ophthalmic, and middle and external ear infections. The choice of application mode (ointment, tincture, or fluid extract) depends on the wound. The succus (fluid extract) of the flower should be applied for irrigation of wounds and for ophthalmic uses.

GENTIAN, BITTER GENTIAN, YELLOW GENTIAN (*Gentiana* L. species)

Description and Habitat

More than 300 species of gentian are found throughout the world (Figure 68-20). It is especially common in mountainous regions of southern and central Europe, Eurasia, and western North America. All parts are used, but it is primarily the roots and rhizomes that are medicinal. Because of concern that overharvesting may endanger this genus, partial root/rhizome collection or leaf-only preparations are recommended.

Pharmacology

The yellow gentian is native to Europe and has been used as a digestive bitter, antiinflammatory, and aid to treating infection. Secoiridoids, γ-pyrones, and triterpenoids are among the most notable studied constituents. The bitter secoiridoid gentiopicroside (2% to 4% of the root) is known to have antibacterial and smooth muscle–relaxing effects consistent with gentian's traditional use as a digestive bitter, antibacterial, and antiarthralgic.[109,145]

Native American and European Medicinal Uses

Gentian has been used since ancient times. The genus is named after King Gentius, the king of Illyria (180 to 167 BC), and it was described by Dioscorides in *De Materia Medica*. Although gentian is native to Europe, it is generally considered one of the best stomach tonics worldwide. In Germany, it is approved by the Commission E for digestive disorders (loss of appetite, fullness, flatulence)

Traditionally, gentian has been used for chronic dyspepsia, indigestion, and poor digestive function. The root, rhizome, or cut herb is steeped and drunk 15 to 30 minutes before eating,

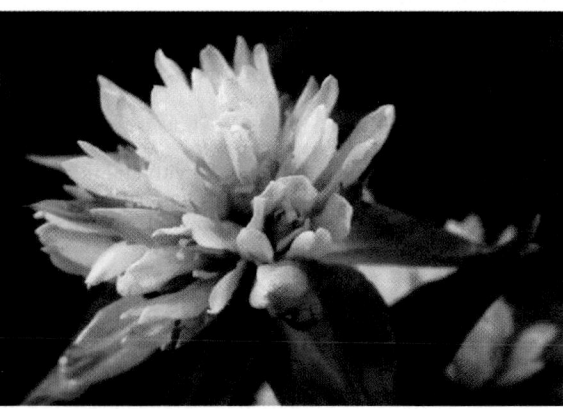

FIGURE 68-20 Gentian (*Gentiana lutea*).

especially in the evening. It stimulates appetite and disperses the "full" and "not hungry" sensation. It is very bitter.

Modern Clinical and Wilderness Applications

A tea of the leaf, root, or rhizome is most convenient and readily available in many areas at altitude or below tree line. Gentian can be very helpful for indigestion and digestive dysfunction brought about by poor food quality, weakness, and overexertion that impairs appetite. This tea can also be very helpful for fever or joint inflammation from infection, fatigue, and overuse. In Chinese herbal medicine, gentian is an essential component of Long dan xie gan wan, an excellent herbal formula for fever, viral infection, headache, iritis, cystitis, urethritis, genital herpes, and liver dysfunction.

DESERT PARSLEY, FERN-LEAFED LOMATIUM (*Lomatium dissectum*, Nutt.)

Description and Habitat

Lomatium, a perennial herb, is native to the western United States and grows predominantly at low to middle elevation in temperate to arid regions (Figure 68-21). The genus *Lomatium* contains more than 80 species, used more or less interchangeably. It is found on wooded or brushy rocky slopes, alpine meadow steppes, or dry hillsides. The root is drunk as an infusion, chewed, or pounded for topical application.

Pharmacology

The root extract has been shown to inhibit completely the cytopathic effects of rotaviruses in vitro.[126] The active constituent from *Lomatium suksdorfii*, suksdorfin, is related to coumarin and has been shown to strongly inhibit human immunodeficiency virus (HIV)-1.[114] This finding is consistent with its use as an antiinfective. Flavonoids and ichthyotoxic (fish-killing) tetronic acids have also been identified.[174]

Native American and European Medicinal Uses

Lomatium was highly revered by Native Americans and used for a wide variety of problems. It gained legendary status in the U.S. Southwest when Native Americans used it during the influenza pandemic of 1917. The Paiutes of Nevada treated sore throats with a decoction of the root. Many Native American groups considered *Lomatium* important for treatment of tuberculosis, asthma, and other lung diseases. It was also used internally and topically for venereal disease. Naturopathic physicians in the western United States have popularized use of *Lomatium* as an antiviral when the root extract is taken internally, for vaginitis when used as a douche, or as an oral rinse to treat periodontal disease.[13]

Modern Clinical and Wilderness Applications

Because of unconfirmed toxicity, it is probably best to avoid the tops of *Lomatium,* but the root is very helpful for URIs, viral illnesses, sore throats, mouth infections, and topical local

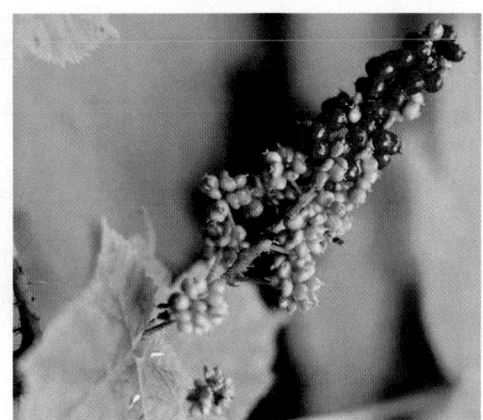

FIGURE 68-22 Devil's club flower (*Oplopanax horridus*). (*Courtesy Jill Stansbury.*)

infections. In the clinic, specific root isolates (with resins removed) are used; in naturopathic medicine, these are considered specific for herpes infections. These isolates are also thought to reduce the incidence of a benign hive-like rash that appears in individuals sensitive to *Lomatium*. A pioneer in naturopathic medicine, John Bastyr, said the appearance of the rash is a sign to decrease the dose, not discontinue the medicine.[13]

In the wilderness, *Lomatium* may be a significant aid in treating and preventing a wide variety of microbial and viral infections. It is easily prepared from fresh or recently dried root as a decoction.

DEVIL'S CLUB (*Oplopanax horridus*)

Description and Habitat

Native to North America, *Oplopanax* is an erect, slightly spreading deciduous shrub present in moist but well-drained forested and riverbank ecosystems (Figures 68-22 and 68-23), from coastal Alaska to central Oregon, east to Idaho, Montana, northwestern Alberta, southwestern Yukon, and the Canadian Rockies, with a few populations near northern Lake Superior, the upper peninsula of Michigan, and Ontario. The stems, leaves, and petioles have a dense armor of needle-like yellow spines that can cause injury and irritation. Flowers are small, whitish, and numerous in compact terminal pyramidal clusters. Notably, *Oplopanax* is a member of Araliacea, which includes *Panax ginseng* (Asian ginseng), *Panax quinquefolius* (American ginseng), and *Aralia nudicauli* (sarsaparilla).

Pharmacology

The best-known constituents of devil's club include saponin triterpenoid glycosides, which have been described primarily in Japanese and Russian *Oplopanax*. There has been much discussion as to whether these saponins are similar to the ginsenosides

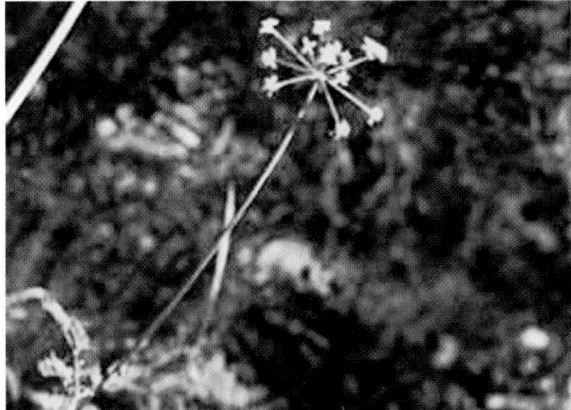

FIGURE 68-21 Desert parsley or fern-leafed lomatium (*Lomatium dissectum,* Nutt).

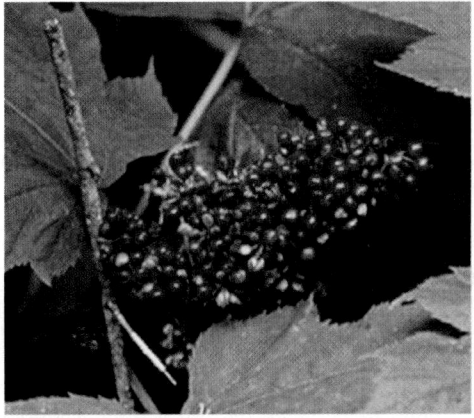

FIGURE 68-23 Devil's club (*Oplopanax horridus*). (*Courtesy Jill Stansbury.*)

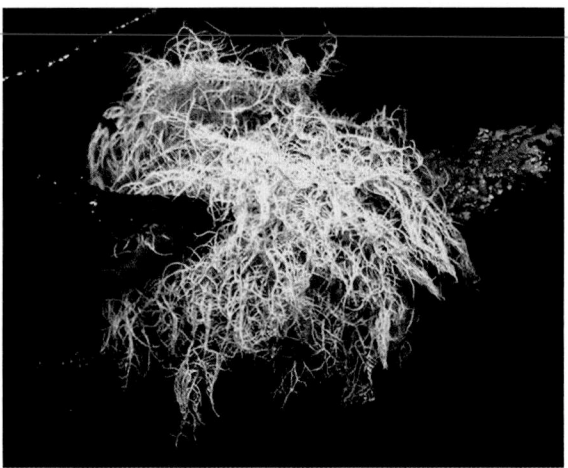

FIGURE 68-24 Old man's beard (*Usnea* sp.).

in *Panax* spp., consistent with devil's club traditional use among Native Americans as a tonic. Sterols, sesquiterpenes, and polyenes have been shown to have significant action against mycobacteria, fungi, and common bacteria such as *S. aureus, Bacillus subtilis, Pseudomonas aeruginosa, E. coli, and C. albicans.*[105] These findings are consistent with the primary historical use of devil's club internally and topically for all varieties of infection, including tuberculosis.

Native American and European Medicinal Uses

It is difficult to overstate the importance of this herb to the native peoples of North America. Devil's club is of extreme significance as a spiritual and shamanic herb, including purification and healing, protection against evil spirits, and gaining of supernatural powers, and as an emetic and purgative. Its primary uses as medicinal herb are for infections, fever, arthritis, respiratory ailments, bleeding after childbirth, pain, broken bones, digestive ailments, stomach complaints, and even dandruff and lice.

European medicinal use of *Oplopanax* is mostly in formulas for joint pain, arthritis (especially autoimmune arthritis), and rheumatism. The root is considered to be an effective expectorant and respiratory stimulant. Marketers have played up the adaptogenic potential of *Oplopanax*, calling it "Alaskan ginseng" or "Pacific ginseng." Commercial products also emphasize the root, whereas traditional uses and much of the research have focused on the inner bark of the stem.

Modern Clinical and Wilderness Uses

Modern clinical use is focused primarily on joint pain, osteoarthritis, and inflammatory arthritides. Devil's club is used in various formulas or as a single herb. It is often found as an antiinfective combination in combination with devil's claw (*Harpagophytum*), cat's claw (*Uncaria* spp.), or one of its western companions, chaparral (*Larrea tridentata*) and Oregon grape (*Berberis aquifolium*). Decoction of the inner bark of the stem is the primary method of preparation, but other parts, such as the inner bark (burned, and the ash used topically), whole stems, berries, leaves, and root, have all been used. In the wilderness, an infusion or decoction of the stem's inner bark is easily prepared and may help allay fatigue, ease joint or headache pain, or serve as an expectorant. In the practice of traditional medicine, devil's club appears to be "good for everything."

OLD MAN'S BEARD (*Usnea* species)

Description and Habitat

Usnea species are lichens (composed of fungi and algae in a stable symbiotic relationship) that are ubiquitous in old-growth forests of the U.S. Northwest (Figures 68-24 and 68-25). They can be seen hanging from shrubs or conifers, often lightly tethered to the tree bark, or lying on the forest floor, especially after a storm. It is difficult for anyone but an expert to distinguish between species of usneas, but they typically have a long, single,

unbranched (or sparsely branched) central cord colored from white to yellow with an outer portion that is gray to pale green.

Native American and European Medicinal Uses

This plant has been used since ancient times in the Americas, Europe, and China. Native Americans saw *Usnea* as representing the male gender and the northerly direction and maintaining the "respiratory" system of the planet (namely the trees); they saw its human uses as secondary to this crucial function.[88] *Usnea* appears in the ancient Chinese herbal, the *Shennong Ben Cao Jing* (*Divine Farmer's Materia Medica*, ~200 BC), and it is classified as a phlegm-resolving herb. Among northwestern Native Americans, it has been used as bedding, as sanitary napkins, and to wipe slime when cleaning salmon. Most significantly, however, it is used as a wound dressing and bandage material,[173] because of not only its wispy soft form, but also its antibacterial properties. In Europe, it has been used predominantly as a topical medication, employing the active constituent usnic acid, present in many lichens, and as an antibiotic, antiinflammatory, and analgesic substance.[83] Since its isolation in 1844, usnic acid has been the most studied of lichen constituents and one of the few to be commercially available. In addition to bacterial inhibition of staphylococci, streptococci, pneumococci, and mycobacteria, usnic acid has been shown to have antiviral, antiprotozoal, and antiproliferative effects consistent with its traditional use.[87] Also present in *Usnea*, but less well studied than usnic acid, are the organic acids usnaric, thamnolic, lobaric, and stictinic.

Modern Clinical and Wilderness Uses

Although pure usnic acid has been used for weight loss in recent times, this use cannot be considered safe and has been associated with liver failure.[55] *Usnea* has been used in several formulas in modern-day China, usually paired with the seaweed *Laminaria* or *Sargassum* (or both) for treatment of thyroid cancer,[84] and in the treatment of bronchitis with profuse sputum.[50] Other current uses include lozenges for oral inflammation and many different salves and creams with antimicrobial and antiinflammatory action.

In the wilderness, *Usnea* is readily available in the regions mentioned earlier. It makes excellent bandages for wounds, superficial infections, and contact dermatitis. Most herbalists recommend collection from the ground so as not to disturb growth on shrubs or trees. Soft and wispy *Usnea* is applied directly to

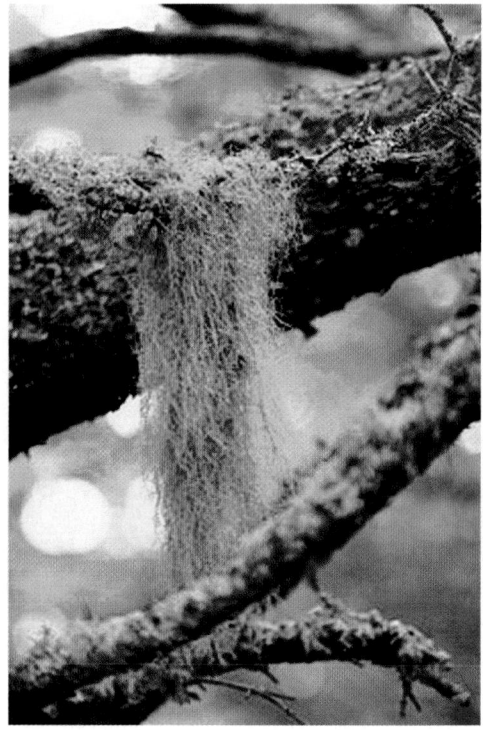

FIGURE 68-25 *Usnea* sp. *(Courtesy Jill Stansbury.)*

the affected area and held in place by whatever means are available. Alternatively, dry *Usnea* may be powdered and sprinkled directly on wounds, affording antimicrobial wound protection.

FIRST-AID KIT OF NATURAL PRODUCTS

A natural products first-aid kit should contain a variety of products that are easy to obtain and replace and that have a wide spectrum of use, including herbs (Box 68-1), homeopathic preparations, and vitamin and enzyme supplements (Table 68-1).

HOMEOPATHIC MEDICINES

Homeopathy can be an excellent source of relief and treatment for emergencies and general first-aid situations. Homeopathic preparations include powders, tablets, tinctures, lotions, ointments, creams, and sprays. Advantages of homeopathy are ease of administration, lack of toxicity, rapid action, and small volume of material. Disadvantages are the degree of understanding and competence required to become an effective prescriber and the lack of readily available sources of each medicine at most North American pharmacies.

A kit made exclusively of homeopathic medicines can cover most first-aid emergency situations. For the acute, straightforward injury or malady without a complex set of symptoms, the correct simillimum and rapid amelioration of symptoms are not difficult to achieve. This section discusses a few indications for use of homeopathic medicines and the preparation most often used. Unless otherwise noted, a 6× to 12× potency in lactose pellet form should be given every 15 to 30 minutes immediately after the injury until noticeable improvement occurs. If no effect is noted after the first two doses, the medicine selection should be reconsidered.

The personal experience of one of the authors (KJD) exemplifies the relief that can be obtained from an acute injury with the appropriate homeopathic medicine:

I was bitten on the lip by a small centipede while sleeping. I instantly experienced swelling and intense burning pain. Local application of ice provided no relief. I chose the homeopathic medicine *Apis mellifica* in a 6c potency because the wound was shiny and felt hot, and the swelling was increasing. After sublingual ingestion of two pellets, I waited 1 to 2 minutes, still in excruciating pain with no change in symptoms. My next selection was cantharis in a 6c potency, because a key symptom for this remedy is extreme red and hot burning pain of the face. Less than 30 seconds after administration, the pain was almost undetectable. Total relief was obtained within a few minutes after being bitten. As an unintended control, I have had no homeopathic kit available after other centipede bites, and the pain generally lasted for hours and the residual swelling for days. Reactions from different centipedes can cause different sensations and symptoms, however, so cantharis may not work for all bites.

Proper selection of the simillimum or indicated homeopathic medicine requires the ability to note the subtle differences in the ways the patient responds to apparently similar traumatic or toxicologic influences. An appropriate homeopathic field guide that lists specific indications and differentiations for each homeopathic remedy should accompany any first-aid kit. It is essential to understand the specific homeopathic indications for each of the remedies (simillima) on hand. Otherwise, the chance of obtaining a successful outcome is small.

Practitioners and the homeopathic industry have realized the difficulty of single-remedy prescribing, which involves understanding and memorizing indications for every homeopathic medicine. Therefore, medicines have been developed that combine remedies to cover a large number of the symptoms and symptom characteristics that typically accompany most ailments. These medicines, known as *complex* or *combination* homeopathic preparations, can be very helpful for the new user.

SINGLE PREPARATIONS AND THEIR INDICATIONS

Aconite

Tincture of the whole plant with its root is derived when monkshood or wolfsbane (*Aconitum napellus*) begins to flower. Aconite is indicated for acute states of emotional disturbance, including anxiety and intense fear or pain. This is one of the key remedies that should be administered after an acute injury that has dazed, shocked, or frightened the patient. Persons who are fearful or restless, cannot tolerate being touched, and have pain followed by numbness and tingling sensations are most responsive to aconite. Those with sudden onset of fever, nausea, and vomiting and who exhibit symptoms of fear, restlessness, and anxiety may also benefit.

Apis

The original tincture is manufactured from the whole honeybee and from dilutions of its venom (*Apis mellifica*). Apis is used for insect stings, particularly from bees and related insects, when the wound is swollen, shiny, and hot to the touch. Treatable symptoms from other conditions are histamine reactions (resulting in facial flushing; puffiness or swelling around the mouth, face, and eyes), sunburn, hives, burns, and early stages of abscesses and frostbite. If symptoms include a stinging, burning, or swelling quality and subside by applying cold rather than heat, apis is the indicated remedy.[144]

Arnica

Tincture comes from the whole fresh plant, flowers, and dried roots of leopard's bane or Fallkraut (*Arnica montana*). Arnica is indicated for blunt traumatic wounds (resulting in both deep and superficial hematomas), contusions, swelling, and localized tenderness. It is also effective for sore muscles, as well as sprains, fractures, dislocations, and internal bleeding. We recommend taking a 6× to 30× potency every 15 minutes to 3 hours for the first few days after a severe injury. The more severe the injury, the more frequently the dose is taken for the first day. As symptom severity decreases, the medicine is taken less often. Arnica can be helpful in decreasing severity of symptoms and recovery time.

Arsenicum

Derived from arsenic trioxide, arsenicum is used for skin rashes (those that feel warm but are relieved by hot applications), hay fever, asthma (especially when accompanied by notable anxiety), diarrhea, vomiting, and gastroenteritis (especially from foodborne microbes).

Belladonna

Belladonna (*Atropa belladonna*, deadly nightshade) is a perennial herbaceous plant native to Europe, North Africa, western Asia, and some parts of Canada and the United States. The foliage and berries are extremely toxic, containing the tropane alkaloids scopolamine and hyoscyamine, which are used as pharmaceutical anticholinergics, including the drug atropine. Belladonna has been used throughout history as a poison administered orally or by arrow tips. Used in eye drops by women in the past to dilate their pupils and appear seductive, the name is translated as "beautiful woman." As a homeopathic preparation, belladonna

---

BOX 68-1 Herbal Medicines Recommended for a First-Aid Kit

Aloe gel and powder capsules
Arnica ointment
Calendula gel, ointment, and tincture
Chamomile tincture
Comfrey gel or ointment
Echinacea tincture or freeze-dried powder capsules
Ephedra freeze-dried powder capsules
Goldenseal tincture or ointment
Hypericum ointment or tincture
Plantain tincture
Witch hazel fluid extract or tincture

TABLE 68-1 Uses for Phytopharmaceuticals

Plant Medicines	Analgesic	Antibiotic	Antifungal	Antiinflammatory	Astringent	Antiseptic	Decongestant	Sedative
Aconitum napellus	—	—	—	—	—	—	—	Homeopathic internal
Apis mellifica	—	—	—	Homeopathic topical, internal	—	—	—	—
Arnica montana	Homeopathic internal Botanical topical	—	—	Homeopathic topical, internal	—	—	—	—
Arsenicum album	—	—	—	—	—	—	—	Homeopathic internal
Bromelain	—	—	—	Botanical internal	—	—	—	—
Calendula	—	—	Botanical internal, topical	Botanical topical	Botanical topical	Botanical topical	—	—
Chamomile	Botanical internal, topical	Botanical internal, topical	—	Botanical internal, topical	—	Botanical topical	Botanical internal	Botanical homeopathic internal
Comfrey	—	—	—	Botanical topical	—	—	—	—
Echinacea	Botanical internal, topical	Botanical internal, topical	Botanical internal, topical	Botanical internal	—	Botanic homeopathic topical	—	—
Ephedra	—	—	—	—	—	—	Botanical internal	—
Goldenseal	—	Botanical internal, topical	Botanical internal, topical	Botanical topical	Botanical internal, topical	Botanical topical	—	—
Hypericum	—	—	—	—	—	Homeopathic topical, internal	—	Homeopathic internal
Peppermint	—	—	—	—	—	—	Botanical internal, topical	—
Plantain	—	—	—	Homeopathic topical, internal	Botanical topical	Botanical topical	—	—
Rhus toxicodendron	—	—	—	—	Botanical topical	—	—	—
Witch hazel	—	—	—	—	Botanical topical	—	—	—

has a long history of use to treat various conditions, including motion sickness, headache, seizures, vertigo, pharyngitis, bronchitis, influenza, tonsillitis, sinusitis, epistaxis (nosebleed), inflammations, constipation, and cystitis.

Cockle

Indian cockle (*Cocculus indica*) is used to treat motion sickness, vertigo, nausea, and jet lag and to restore normal sleep cycle.

Hypericum

The tincture comes from the whole fresh plant and flowers of St John's wort (*Hypericum perforatum*). Indications include any pain that affects the peripheral or central nervous system and exhibits shooting pains that travel in a dermatomal pattern (e.g., sciatica). Wounds that affect nerve endings, such as injuries to fingers, toes, or teeth, are improved by hypericum. Pain from dental surgery, toothache, injury to the coccyx, and first- and second-degree dermal burns are other indications.

Ledum

Ledum is made from leaves and stems of the whole fresh plant of wild rosemary (*Ledum palustre*). Homeopathic indications include puncture wounds from small, sharp objects (e.g., nails, needles) and some mosquito bites when the injured area feels cold, swollen, and numb and the pain would be relieved by application of cold.

Poison Nut

From the seeds, blossoms, and bark of *Strychnos nux-vomica* (nux vomica, poison nut) come the highly poisonous, intensely bitter alkaloids strychnine and brucine. As a homeopathic preparation, nux vomica may be the most diversely useful remedy for common diseases. It should be considered during bouts of influenza and with associated GI symptoms of vomiting and diarrhea. Nux vomica is probably the most helpful remedy for hangover from ingestion of alcohol. Other indications include nausea, heartburn, headache, vertigo, GI cramping, colic, constipation, upset stomach, cystitis, allergic rhinitis, cough, asthma, sinusitis, pain, and stiffness.[20,21,60,104,140]

Rhus

The homeopathic preparation of *Rhus* comes from leaves and stems of the whole fresh plant of poison ivy. This is the remedy of choice for the urticaria caused by poison ivy exposure and is also helpful for some cases of poison oak. Other skin rashes that are red, weeping, blistered, and swollen with itching can be treated with *Rhus*. It is also effective for treatment of connective tissue irritations with swelling, stiffness, and tightness. *Rhus* is often used for overuse injuries (e.g., fasciitis, tendinitis) and some forms of arthritis, especially when the injured area feels better with warm applications and movement. Note that the name of this preparation may change, because *Toxicodendron* is now the correct name of the genus.

COMBINATION PREPARATIONS FOR ACUTE SPRAINS AND STRAINS

Homeopathy companies have created combination remedies for the general public that can be used without the need for in-depth understanding of homeopathic prescribing. These remedies are designed to cover a broad range of symptoms associated with acute ailments and trauma-induced medical conditions. They are sometimes touted to be effective for many disorders on the basis of empirical observations, rather than on the basis of randomized, blinded studies. Practitioners are advised to be aware of the possibility for unsubstantiated claims of clinical efficacy for these and any other medications marketed for profit.

Traumeel is a combination homeopathic formula that is effective for treatment of trauma and inflammatory changes affecting skin, connective tissue, and muscle.[67] The preparation comes in liquid, tablet, and ointment form. Traumeel includes remedies indicated for traumatic injuries (sprains, strains, contusions) and resulting pain, swelling, and ecchymoses. Many German studies have demonstrated its effectiveness.[33] Traumeel may be the

primary homeopathic medicine chosen for the first-aid kit because of its wide range of applications and multiple delivery systems.

Inflamyar ointment is a uniquely formulated homeopathic medicine that combines eight ingredients to provide treatment of traumatic sports-related injuries, such as sprains, bruises, and muscle strains. This formula developed from a long tradition of German homeopathic salves also is available as a homeopathic tincture. It has been used with great success for immediate relief and resolution of bursitis, sciatica, and acute and chronic inflammation, as well as pain of rheumatic and arthritic conditions. After strenuous exercise, massaging Inflamyar into tender points will help prevent soreness the next day. Routine self-massage with Inflamyar into tender points has been shown to restore flexibility and elasticity to muscles, tendons, and ligaments.

Herbal Combination Formulas

In the tradition of Chinese herbal medicine, many formulas have been developed over the centuries to treat acute ailments. Many of these formulas were kept secret and reserved for the nobility and ruling class. As the field of Chinese herbology has become more accessible to the general population, some of the secret formulas have been mass-produced into convenient pill form, known as "patent medicines." Many are extremely useful for acute conditions.

Zheng Gu Shui ("Rectify Bones Liquid") trauma lotion is used for sprains, strains, and bruises. It is also indicated for back pain and arthritis pain. The herbs of which it is composed invigorate circulation, relieve pain, induce a pleasant warming feeling, and accelerate healing. This formula has long been a mainstay of martial artists, massage therapists, and Chinese herbalists. It should be applied to affected areas two to three times daily, keeping the liquid away from mucous membranes and open cuts. It accelerates resolution of bruises and connective tissue injuries, reducing swelling, pain, and inflammation. It is produced by Guangxi Yulin Pharmaceutical Factory, which is well known in China and has been honored with awards for quality and effectiveness. This product can be ordered through the Institute for Traditional Medicine (ITM; see Appendix at the end of this chapter) and from most Chinese herbal pharmacies.

NUTRITIONAL SUPPLEMENTS

For immune system support, antiinflammatory action, and pain relief, many natural products in the nutritional supplement category have proved to be effective agents.

Bromelain

Bromelain is a naturally occurring proteolytic enzyme found in pineapple that is used to reduce pain and swelling after sprains and strains of soft tissues. Ingested on an empty stomach, the complex proteases in bromelain are absorbed intact and have significant antiedema, antiinflammatory, and coagulation-inhibiting effects. Bromelain exhibits fibrinolytic activity and acts to inhibit fibrinogen synthesis, decreasing kininogen and bradykinins.[119] For treatment of injuries and postsurgical recovery, 125 to 400 mg is ingested three times daily at 30 minutes before or 90 minutes after a meal. Bromelain is nontoxic even at high doses and is generally prepared as 100-mg tablets.

Papain

As with bromelain, papain is a naturally occurring plant enzyme (from papaya fruit) that exhibits proteolytic activity. Papain is generally used externally to neutralize bee, ant, or wasp venom. It is available as commercial meat tenderizer (e.g., Adolph's) or in tablet form. After removal of the stinger, a thick paste is prepared from water and tenderizer (or five or six crushed tablets) and applied to the area as soon as possible.

A convenient form that contains bromelain, papain, and pancreas-derived proteolytic enzymes is the product Wobenzym. This product has had decades of use in addition to clinical trials to back its claims as an effective proteolytic antiinflammatory. Suggested use is three tablets three times a day or as directed by the practitioner. Wobenzym N is taken on an empty stomach at least 45 minutes before meals.

Vitamin C

Ascorbic acid has both wound-healing and antiinflammatory effects. Vitamin C is required for hydroxylation of proline and subsequently for synthesis of effective collagen. Studies have shown that the stress associated with injury and wound healing results in an increased need for vitamin C.[125] For acute trauma and acute upper respiratory allergy, vitamin C in larger doses (2 to 5 g/day in divided doses) has been claimed to reduce anaphylactic reactions and recovery time.[77] Therefore, for any traumatic event, high-dose vitamin C should be administered as part of the treatment.

Vitamin D$_3$

Classically known in deficiency to cause rickets, vitamin D$_3$ has demonstrated profound impact on the immune system. It has been stated that no other single nutrient supplement could save more health costs and provide more prevention. Vitamin D$_3$ is available in capsule or liquid form. Daily doses of 1000 to 5000 international units (IU) are recognized to support health and wellness, decrease susceptibility to multiple cancers, and enhance the glucose-insulin response, among other benefits. During travel, increased dosing may offer protection from communicable infections or may help clear upper respiratory conditions more quickly.

FOR ACUTE GASTROENTERITIS

Pill Curing (Kang Ning Wan, "Healthy Quiet Pill"), botanically called Coix Formula, consists of 16 herbal medicines that are collectively effective for relieving disturbances caused by motion sickness, food poisoning, overeating, excessive alcohol consumption (nausea, headache, vomiting), difficulty passing stool, loose stools, and GI cramping and pain. Coix Formula is currently produced in a convenient globule form. One or two capfuls of globules are swallowed with warm water every hour until symptoms improve. Relief should occur within 4 hours of administration. Pill Curing (or Culing) is also available as a Chinese patent (or prepared) medicine from ITM or from a Chinese herbal pharmacy. The package includes 10 vials; the usual dose is 1 to 2 vials, each containing multiple small pilules to be swallowed all at once. Relief is generally within hours. This is an all-purpose remedy claimed to be useful for everything from traveler's diarrhea, to hangover, to the common cold. Coix Formula is well known to provide relief from motion sickness, food poisoning, excessive eating, drinking alcohol, nausea, headache, vomiting, diarrhea, constipation, GI cramping, and generalized pain.

Diarrhea

While using botanicals or any other remedy for diarrhea, it is critical to continue to maintain adequate hydration through oral and IV means as necessary. The primary medical risk of common diarrhea still remains dehydration.

Travelers may use a pharmaceutical, such as loperamide, to limit or stop diarrhea. Botanicals may help to quiet the intestinal tract, although typically not as aggressively as do pharmaceutical agents. Most botanicals that help to relieve diarrhea contain the compounds tannin, pectin, and mucilage. Tannins have astringent action that decreases intestinal inflammation. Pectin is a soluble fiber that adds bulk to the stool and soothes the gut. Pectin is the "pectate" in the OTC antidiarrheal medicine Kaopectate. Mucilage soothes the digestive tract and adds bulk to the stool by absorbing water and decreasing swelling.

Agrimony (*Agrimonia eupatoria*) contains high amounts of tannin and is endorsed by the German Commission E for common diarrhea. Apple (*Malus domestica*) pulp is high in pectin, which is amphoteric, acting as a remedy for diarrhea and helping with constipation because of its action as a stool softener. Bilberry and blueberry (*Vaccinium* spp.) are rich in both pectin and tannins and thus offer relief for common diarrhea. Blackberry and raspberry (*Rubus* spp.) are also both high in tannins and may be effective in the treatment of diarrhea. Carob (*Ceratonia siliqua*) powder has been shown to reduce diarrhea duration by as much as 50% in children with bacterial or viral diarrhea.

Cooked carrots (*Daucus carota*) are good choices for adults or infants with diarrhea. Carrots soothe the digestive tract, decrease diarrhea, and provide vitamins and minerals often lost during sickness. Fenugreek (*Trigonella foenum-graecum*) seeds contain up to 50% mucilage. They swell in the gut to relieve diarrhea and also soften the stool, having amphoteric action like apple. Portions should be limited to avoid gut irritability that may be experienced with too large a dose.

Oak (*Quercus* spp.) in the form of a tea made from 2 tsp of dried oak bark is recommended by the German Commission E for treating diarrhea. Psyllium (*Plantago ovata*) is known for its use in relieving constipation; it also has a high mucilage content that makes it useful for treating diarrhea (amphoteric). Caution is advised with this botanical, as for many others; if allergic symptoms arise after its use, it should not be further used.

FOR ACUTE HEMORRHAGIC CONDITIONS

The product Yunnan Bai Yao ("Yunnan white medicine"), produced in the western Chinese province of Yunnan, has been used for centuries as a first-line approach to trauma that results in internal or external bleeding. It is prescribed in China for excessive menstrual cramps and bleeding, bleeding ulcers, trauma-induced swelling, bleeding wounds, and allergic reactions to insect bites. It comes in powder (4 g per bottle) and capsule (packets of 20) form and contains one red pellet that is to be ingested only for serious bleeding conditions. Dose is 1 to 2 capsules four times daily. The powder can be applied externally after the wound has been properly cleaned. This product is exclusively produced in China from a proprietary formula and can be obtained from most Chinese herbal pharmacies. Other botanicals recognized for anticoagulant properties include clove (*Syzygium aromaticum*) and helichrysum (*Helichrysum italicum*).[103] Each of these also is reported to offer antiseptic activity.

FOR DERMATOLOGIC CONDITIONS

SssstingStop Gel

The Boericke and Tafel SssstingStop gel is for temporary relief of itch, pain, and redness of nonpoisonous insect bites and stings from insects, including mosquitoes, bees, and wasps. It also soothes fever blisters and cold sores. According to Boericke and Tafel, the London School of Hygiene and Tropical Medicine conducted two clinical studies using mosquitoes not fed for 24 hours and human volunteers and reportedly proved that the medicines in SssstingStop provide dependable, effective relief.

SssstingStop combines three natural homeopathic medicines prepared from botanical sources and listed in the *Homeopathic Pharmacopoeia of the United States* (HPUS). It contains no hydrocortisone or other steroids, antihistamines, "-caine" anesthetics, or any synthetic medicines. It is applied to the affected skin area, with applications repeated as needed. Ingredients are *Echinacea angustifolia* (1×, 10%), *Ledum palustre* (1×, 10%), *Urtica dioica* (1×, 10%), and citronella and eucalyptus oils in a water-gel base.

Ching Wang Hun (or Jing Wan Hong) Burn Ointment

This rapid-acting analgesic and burn-healing salve is a remarkable herbal medicine. It is effective for chemical, thermal, electrical, radiation, and solar burns. It can also be used to decrease inflammation and stimulate regeneration of the skin and is used for contact dermatitis (poison oak, ivy, sumac), hemorrhoids, and infected skin. The ointment is applied liberally to the affected areas. Ideally, it is covered with a dressing to prevent accumulation of dirt and grime and to reduce the red stain that occurs if the ointment contacts clothing. It should be reapplied and the dressing changed once or twice a day. This ointment is made by one of the best-known manufacturers in China and can be ordered through ITM (see Appendix) and from most Chinese herbal pharmacies.

Other Skin Therapies

Other botanicals with applications for skin conditions should be considered for inclusion in the travel first-aid kit. As previously noted, aloe (*Aloe vera*) has been used since ancient times to treat burns and other wounds and trauma. Arnica (*Arnica montana*) is well recognized for its efficacy to treat trauma, bruises, swelling, and other wounds. Comfrey (*Symphytum officinale*) has been used since ancient Greece for skin problems. Activated charcoal is indicated for a wide variety of poisonous plant and other topical dermatological conditions. In these cases, activated charcoal poultices may be applied topically.

FOR GENERAL HEALTH AND WELLNESS

It is always advisable to begin travel in a healthy condition, which should include pretravel preparations. Certain botanicals are useful to enhance the immune system and act as a general tonic. Teas, capsules, and powdered preparations that promote general health and wellness are available with multiple botanicals combined. These typically may include gingko biloba, American or Asian ginseng (*Panax quinquefolius* or *P. ginseng*), echinacea (*Echinacea* spp.), evening primrose (*Oenothera biennis*), garlic (*Allium sativum*), gotu kola (*Centella asiatica*), milk thistle (*Silybum marianum*), peppermint (*Mentha piperita*), purslane (*Portulaca oleracea*), thyme (*Thymus vulgaris*), chamomile (*Matricaria recutita*), and horsetail (*Equisetum arvense*). These and other botanical combinations provide antioxidant, antiaging, and antiinflammatory effects and may help promote better energy, clearer thinking, better mood, emotional stability, desirable enhanced hormone levels, and general immune support.

JET LAG AND TRAVEL FATIGUE[64]

St John's wort (*Hypericum perforatum*) is a common OTC remedy that is one of the most widely used botanicals in Europe. It contains the compound hypericum, which shows significant improvement for anxiety, depression, and feelings of worthlessness in clinical studies. Some studies have also shown beneficial effects to improve sleep quality. Once thought to be caused primarily by a monoamine oxidase (MAO) inhibitor effect, studies now indicate that additional influencing compounds are present, and that their combination yields the clinical result without side effects. *St John's wort is not advised during pregnancy.*

Lemon balm or Melissa (*Melissa officinalis*) is recommended by the German Commission E as a sedative and to soothe the stomach. Active compounds include terpenes, which are also found in juniper, ginger, basil, and clove, although none has a reputation as a bedtime herb comparable to lemon balm. Valerian root (*Valerian officinalis*), another botanical endorsed by the German Commission E for promotion of sleep, is usually taken as a tea, although capsules may be easier for travel. It has also been recommended for anxiety, restlessness, and nervousness. More than 80 OTC sleeping aids in the United Kingdom (UK) contain valerian root. The common hangover feeling often associated with prescription anxiety and sleep medications is not prevalent with this plant remedy.

Lavender (*Lavandula* spp.) is typically used in massage oil or diffused into the air to promote relaxation and rest, as well as to reduce irritability. Be aware, however, that some species of lavender, notably Spanish lavender, are actually stimulants. Passionflower (*Passiflora incarnata*) is a mild sedative and is included in more than 40 OTC sleep preparations in the UK. Despite extensive use worldwide for centuries to treat nervous tension, anxiety, and insomnia, the FDA has not approved this botanical remedy. Chamomile (*Matricaria recutita*) tea has been used as a bedtime beverage for centuries. The constituent chemical apigenin is one of the most effective sedative botanical compounds. Rooibos (*Aspalathus linearis*) is a shrubby African legume that is a favorite for bedtime tea among many South Africans. Its popularity has spread to the United States. In addition to promoting sleep, it is used to calm the digestive tract and reduce nervous tension.[53] Homeopathically, *Cocculus indicus* may be very useful for jet lag and to help restore the normal sleep/wake cycles in the new destination.

MOTION SICKNESS AND SEASICKNESS

Cocculus indicus and tabacum are two leading homeopathic remedies for motion sickness and seasickness. Ginger has been used traditionally for acute motion sickness as well as other causes of simple dyspepsia. As a quick and easy travel method, take $\frac{1}{2}$ tsp of fresh ginger, finely dice it, and swallow it whole.

COUGH, COLD, AND FLU

The Great Plains Indians chewed echinacea, the mountain daisy or coneflower, for centuries to treat colds, flu, and other ailments (see earlier discussion). Naturopathic and integrative medical physicians encourage using echinacea for general immune support. Echinacea increases a chemical in the body called properdin, which activates the immune system[53] and is responsible for increasing defense against viruses and bacteria. Echinacea extracts have demonstrated antiviral activity against influenza, herpes, and other viruses.

Garlic (*Allium sativum*) contains the chemical allicin, one of the plant kingdom's most potent, broad-spectrum antibiotics. Ginger (*Zingiber officinale*) contains nearly a dozen antiviral compounds, including sesquiterpenes that have specific action against rhinoviruses. Other compounds include gingerols and shogaols, known to relieve pain and fever, suppress cough, and mildly sedate to encourage rest. Onion (*Allium cepa*) is closely related to garlic and has similar antiviral activities. Citrus fruits and other plants containing vitamin C are important as a part of the diet or as a supplement to reduce severity and duration of cold symptoms.[79] Amazonian fruit camu camu (*Myrciaria dubia*) has the world's highest vitamin C content, and other good sources include acerola, bell peppers, cantaloupe, and pineapple.

Elderberry (*Sambucus nigra*) is a herb containing two compounds that are active against influenza viruses. It also prevents the virus from invading respiratory tract cells. The patented drug Sambucol contains elderberry and has demonstrated antiviral activity in preliminary trials against Epstein-Barr virus, herpesvirus, and HIV. Forsythia (*Forsythia suspensa*) and honeysuckle (*Lonicera japonica*) are common Chinese traditional approaches to treating colds and influenza. Anise (*Pimpinella anisum*) is recognized by the German Commission E as an expectorant. In larger doses, anise has antiviral properties. Ephedra (*Ephedra sinica*) is known as Ma Huang in traditional Chinese medicine and has long been used as a potent decongestant. Ephedra's chemicals, ephedrine and pseudoephedrine, dilate bronchial airways. Caution is important because the compounds in ephedra may also lead to elevated blood pressure, insomnia, and agitation. The FDA has placed restrictions on their distribution because of occasional deaths, especially with overuse.

PAIN AND TRAUMA[64]

It is critically important that a competent health care provider provide a proper evaluation for the patient who presents with pain. A number of botanicals should be considered for treating pain.

As previously mentioned, aloe (*Aloe vera*) has been used since ancient times to treat burns and other wounds and trauma. Arnica (*Arnica montana*), or coneflower, is well recognized for its efficacy to treat trauma, bruises, swelling, and other wounds. Calendula (*Calendula officinalis*) reduces inflammation and promotes wound healing. Clove (*Syzygium aromaticus*) has been recognized for its usefulness for dental pain. Clove oil is applied directly to the gum and tooth involved. Evening primrose (*Oenothera biennis*) is rich in the amino acid tryptophan. Studies have demonstrated that tryptophan supplements are effective in relieving pain of acute and chronic conditions. Although the oil has been often recommended by some, much of the tryptophan is lost in the oil extraction process, so powdered seeds should be a better choice. Ginger (*Zingiber officinale*) is a highly effective pain reliever. Furthermore, ginger may be applied to painful areas topically, such as with hot ginger compresses for abdominal cramps, headache, or joint pain. Kava kava (*Piper methysticum*) is a tropical herb that has demonstrated analgesic effectiveness comparable to aspirin. Chewing the leaves leads to mouth numbness, and therefore kava kava can be useful for dental pain, canker sores, and sore throat.

Peppermint (*Mentha piperita*) contains menthol, which has anesthetic effects. Because peppermint oil is typically very concentrated, mix a few drops in a tablespoon of coconut or olive oil to decrease the potential to irritate the skin. Never drink peppermint oil, because a small amount can be toxic. Red pepper (*Capsicum* spp.) has become a popular natural choice for pain therapy, both in OTC and pharmaceutical preparations. Pain-relieving compounds called salicylates, similar to salicins, are the botanical equivalent of aspirin. Additionally, the red peppers contain capsaicin, a compound that stimulates the body's natural endorphins and depletes the pain transmitter substance P. One should wash hands thoroughly after applying capsaicin-containing cream so as not to rub it accidentally into the eyes. It is best first to use a small portion on a limited skin area to determine that it will be tolerated and to be able to discontinue use promptly if it leads to skin irritation.

Turmeric (*Curcuma longa*) is found in curries and has long been a staple of South Asian cuisine. It has some of the most potent botanical antiinflammatory properties known. Turmeric has recently gained recognition and popularity. Willow bark (*Salix* spp.) contains salicin, from which aspirin was derived approximately 100 years ago. Willow may provide relief for a wide variety of pains. It should be avoided by persons who are allergic to aspirin compounds. Do not give willow or similar products to young children who have a viral syndrome, because of the risk of inducing Reye's syndrome.

FROSTBITE, HEAT EXHAUSTION, AND HEATSTROKE[64]

Ginkgo biloba should be considered as a botanical approach to managing frostbite or chilblains. Containing numerous compounds that include terpenes, flavones, proanthocyanidins, and ginkgolides, *Ginkgo* can improve arterial and venous circulation, especially in the brain, eyes, ears, and limbs. It may scavenge free radicals, perhaps the mechanism for its protective effect on vasculature. Common dosing is 50 mg up to three times daily.

Aloe (*Aloe vera*) is indicated for frostbite. Common oak (*Quercus rubor*) has astringent properties. It can be applied topically as a poultice of the leaves, bark, and acorns or as a tea or capsule. Lungwort (*Pulmonaria officinalis*), commonly known in French as "the cardia herb," has been recognized as being of benefit for frostbite. Black walnut (*Juglans nigra*) has been mentioned as a remedy for frostbite.

Sunstroke (heatstroke) and overheating may be addressed with a variety of botanicals to cool the body and help dispel excess heat. American ginseng (*Panax quinquefolius*) and Siberian ginseng (*Eleutherococcus senticosus*), both prepared as a tea, are noted for efficacy in heat exhaustion. Peppermint (*Mentha piperita*) should be considered as a cool forehead compress or used orally. Black mulberry (*Morus nigra*) may be beneficial, prepared as a tea. Passionflower (*Passiflora incarnata*) is also noted for clinical benefits to treat heatstroke and heat exhaustion.

ACTIVATED CHARCOAL FOR TRAVEL[64]*

Activated charcoal is an exciting natural remedy from the botanical world that is deceptively ordinary at first appearance. It possesses extraordinary properties that may help to clear toxins, fight microbial infections, and offer other significant health-producing effects.

Charcoal is the blackened residual of burning wood and other products, before complete consumption. For the purpose of medicinal care, hardwoods, coconut shells, and bones are the most common starting materials, and commercial medical- or

*NOTE: Consultation with a competent health care professional is appropriate for all infectious illnesses. *Do not delay consultation* if you are using activated charcoal.

food-grade charcoal is called *activated charcoal*. Activated charcoal is further processed by exposing the source material to gas or to oxygen or steam at extremely high temperatures, resulting in a carbonization or oxidation process that renders the material to be microporous, with pores measuring 1 micron in high-quality activated charcoal. Because of this microporosity, 1 g (1/4 tbsp) has a surface area of 500 to 1500+ m^2, as determined by gas adsorption.

Activated charcoal is listed by the FDA as a Class I "safe and effective" agent to treat acute poisoning. It adsorbs gases, liquid, and dissolved solids by having them adhere within the microporous structure. This occurs due to the structural framework and resultant van der Waals forces.

Medicinal activated charcoal is available in powder, tablet, capsule, and even toothpaste form and can be used internally and topically for a diverse set of clinical conditions. In addition to adsorbing certain toxins, it can also adsorb and thereby inactivate bacteria, viruses, fungi, and parasites. Charcoal filters are used in many portable and industrial water-treatment devices and are readily available in lightweight, portable containers.

Plant and Other Poisons or Medications Neutralized by Activated Charcoal

Plant poisonings may be neutralized by activated charcoal (Box 68-2). Activated charcoal poultices may be applied topically for poison ivy or stinging nettle skin reactions or internally when these plants are internally consumed.[165a]

When the amount of poison consumed is unknown, a general rule is to administer 1 g of activated charcoal per kilogram of body weight, or about 0.5 g of activated charcoal per pound of body weight.

How to Make an Activated Charcoal Poultice

Activated charcoal poultices are easy to make and may provide benefit for many topical illnesses. For its simplest application, pure charcoal powder may be sprinkled on wounds, including skin ulcers, abrasions, lacerations, and decubitus ulcers. Activated charcoal may be applied with a gauze, muslin cloth, or paper towel underneath to provide a barrier between the activated charcoal powder and the topical surface. Using this technique, the poultice may also be applied over the closed eyelids for eye infections, on the ears for otitis, in the nose for hemostasis of epistaxis, and on the skin for ant bites, bee/wasp stings, scorpion stings, or spider bites,[21a,51] and for topical eruptions such as from poison ivy, oak, or sumac. In any circumstance where a practitioner uses a naturopathic remedy instead of or in addition to an accepted allopathic remedy for a potentially life-threatening situation, it must be done in full recognition of the quality of the science supporting the remedy.

It is imperative that the activated charcoal poultice be sufficiently moistened that the dressing remains moist for 10 to 12 hours. A dry poultice will not adsorb and neutralize the intended target. An excellent poultice may be made from equal parts of powdered or blended activated charcoal and ground flaxseed, or

---

BOX 68-2 Botanical Poisons Neutralized by Activated Charcoal

Alder	Lily of the valley
Autumn crocus	Mistletoe
Azalea	Monkshood
Black nightshade	Oleander
Bryony	Poison ivy
Buckthorn berry	Poison oak
Christmas rose	Poison sumac
Daphne	Privet berry
Deadly nightshade	Rhododendron
Foxglove	Savin juniper
Hemlock	Spindle tree berry
Holly berry	Thorn apple
Honeysuckle berry	Woody nightshade
Jerusalem cherry	Yew
Laburnum	

with therapeutic clay such as bentonite or zeolite. After changing the poultice, discard the used poultice.

Although a tattooing effect when applying charcoal on open wounds may be a concern, this does not generally seem to be an issue and should be minimized if the charcoal is placed with a barrier (e.g., moist gauze, muslin cloth, paper towel) against the wound surface.

ESSENTIAL OIL REMEDIES FOR TRAVEL[64]

Essential oils are natural aromatic compounds found in the seeds, bark, stems, roots, flowers, and other parts of plants. Potent and widely used botanical products, they are extracted through steam distillation and cold pressing. Essential oils provide many opportunities for maintaining health and wellness during travel. Highly fragrant, the aromatherapeutic uses are only a part of essential oil–rich benefits. Essential oils typically deliver quick and potent clinical effects because the oils are much more powerful and effective than the dry herbal products. Essential oils may be diffused, inhaled, placed in baths, applied topically, or taken internally for a variety of ailments. Essential oils are well absorbed but do not build up in the body; they are excreted after yielding their benefits.

Historically, cinnamon, frankincense, myrrh, and sandalwood were considered very valuable and at times were exchanged for gold along the ancient trade routes. French chemist René-Maurice Gattefossé is credited with rediscovering the benefits of essential oils in modern times, having treated a severely burned hand with pure lavender oil in 1937.* Dr. Jean Valnet, a contemporary of Gattefossé, successfully treated injured soldiers during World War II using therapeutic-grade essential oils. He continued his work with essential oils and became a renowned world leader in development of aromatherapy practices.

Manufacture of essential oils is a highly specialized process and requires large amounts of raw materials for distillation of the oils. For example, as many as 12,000 rose blossoms are required to distill 5 mL of essential rose oil; 100 pounds of plant material is required to produce 1 pound of lavender essential oil. Certain citrus oils are extracted by compression and others by using solvents, which are later removed from the final product.

Essential oils are thought to activate the brain's limbic system.† The odor of fragrant essences also stimulates various hormones and other metabolic processes. Olfactory responses to various fragrances have been documented extensively. The oils may be used individually or in complex blends, depending on user experience and desired benefits.

Many essential oils have antibacterial, antifungal, and antiviral properties. Essential oils that are best for cleaning include lemon, grapefruit, eucalyptus, peppermint, tea tree, lavender, and rosemary.

Thieves blend essential oil was developed based on the ingredients found in the "Four Thieves Vinegar" or "Marseilles Vinegar," which was used to protect against the plague in the 15th century; this essential oil blend was prepared by thieves and grave robbers who wanted protection from the plague and other ailments.[165] Diffusing Thieves blend of cinnamon, clove, eucalyptus, lemon, and rosemary oils can kill 99% of airborne bacteria in 12 minutes. This makes Thieves blend a consideration for airline and other similar crowded travel (Box 68-3).

Use of Essential Oils during Travel

Essential oils typically come as single or blended combinations in small bottles of 5 to 15 mL. Based on the particular clinical need, as highlighted next, one is able to choose an essential oil collection and use the drops in a diffuser or directly from the bottle to inhale, placed on the palmar wrists and areas of distress and rubbed in topically, or taken orally as a drop or in water. It is very important *only* to use the essential oils "neat" (no dilution) when so indicated and only to take those essential oils internally

---

*www.vanderbilt.edu/AnS/psychology/health_psychology/what_is_aromathery.html.

†www.yalescientific.org/2011/11/aromatherapy-exploring-olfaction/.

BOX 68-3   Thieves Blend Essential Oil Properties

Cinnamon bark (*Cinnamonum verum*): Antiseptic, antiviral, antibacterial, antifungal, COX inhibitor (antiinflammatory), a strong oxygenator

Clove (*Syzygium aromaticum*): Antiseptic, antiviral, antifungal, COX inhibitor (antiinflammatory), one of the highest ORAC (Oxygen Radical Absorbance Capacity) values of any plant in the world*

Eucalyptus (*Eucalyptus radiata*): Antiinflammatory, antiseptic, antiviral, antibacterial, antifungal, supports respiratory system

Lemon (*Citrus limon*): Antiseptic, immune stimulating, purifying and uplifting

Rosemary (*Rosmarius officinalis*, CT cineol): Antiseptic, antiinfectious, reduces mental fatigue, eases anxiety

*www.orac-info-portal.de/download/ORAC_R2.pdf.

---

that are approved for this use. Some essential oils need to be diluted for either topical or oral use. The recommended amount of essential oil remedies and acceptable methods of use should be listed on the package or container.

Aromatic Uses. When diffused into the air, essential oils can be either stimulating or calming and soothing. Beyond their emotional benefits, diffusing essential oil can rid air of unwanted odors and some airborne pathogens. Oil diffusers with low or no heat are recommended to minimize any change in the chemical structure of the oil. Rosemary, lavender, peppermint, grapefruit, chamomile, lemon, and ylang ylang essential oils have been shown to calm the mind and emotions, as well as enhance memory and test performance. Clary sage oil helps with premenstrual syndrome (PMS). It should not be overused for this or any other purpose.

Topical Uses. Essential oils may be easily absorbed by the skin and may be safely applied topically to unbroken surfaces because of their microparticle composition. Essential oils often yield a prompt local benefit to the treated area. Chamomile specifically has been shown to decrease hives. Highly favored for massage and beauty therapies, essential oils have calming as well as restorative properties; furthermore, some are natural disinfectants. Topical essential oils should usually be blended with other oils, waxes, or alcohols. Citrus essential oils should not be applied when there will be direct sunlight exposure.

Essential oils that are generally regarded as safe to use undiluted on the skin include lavender, German chamomile, tea tree, sandalwood, and rose geranium. It is especially important only to use half-strength (or more dilute) oils on children and infants. Box 68-4 lists essential oils that are generally considered safe for infants and children.

BOX 68-4   Essential Oils Generally Safe for Infants and Children

Bergamot (*Citrus bergamia*)*
Cedarwood (*Cedrus atlantica*)*
Chamomile, Roman (*Chamaemelum nobile*)
Cypress (*Cupressus sempervirens*)
Frankincense (*Boswellia carteri*)
Geranium (*Pelargonium graveolens*)
Ginger (*Zingiber officinale*)
Lavender (*Lavandula angustifolia*)
Lemon (*Citrus limon*)*
Mandarin (*Citrus reticulata*)*
Marjoram (*Origanum majorana*)
Melaleuca (tea tree) (*Melaleuca alternifolia*)
Orange (*Citrus aurantium*)*
Rose Otto (*Rosa damascena*)
Rosemary (*Rosmarinus officinalis*)*
Rosewood (*Aniba rosaeodora*)
Sandalwood (*Santalum album*)
Thyme (*Thumus vulgaris*, CT linalol)
Ylang ylang (*Cananga odorata*)

From www.abundanthealth4u.com/Essential_Oils_Care_for_Babies_and_Children_s/40.htm.
*Always use these in diluted form for infants and children.

Internal Uses. Because of their microparticle composition, essential oils may be absorbed into the bloodstream from the skin for internal benefits. When used as dietary supplements, some essential oils have been shown to have powerful antioxidant properties, whereas others help support healthy antiinflammatory responses.[11] Although many essential oils are commonly regarded as safe for internal use, others should not be taken internally. *Only use essential oils internally if they have the appropriate dietary supplement facts on the label.*

It is highly recommended that only 100%-pure, therapeutic-grade essential oils be used in any manner, and all label warnings and instructions must be followed. CPTG (Certified Pure Therapeutic Grade) is the accepted standard for pure essential oils; the essential oils that carry this designation are guaranteed to be pure, natural, and free of synthetic compounds or contaminants. Essential oils should be stored in dark-colored bottles. Most remain potent for 5 to 10 years, whereas citrus essential oils retain potency for 1 to 2 years.

Common Essential Oil Remedies during Travel

Prevention. Using essential oils is a sound approach to maintaining health before and during travel. Because the oils are concentrated, the containers are small enough that a well-stocked travel kit does not require much space or weight in packing. Some of the most common essential oils to consider include lemon, grapefruit, eucalyptus, peppermint, tea tree (*Melaleuca*), lavender, and rosemary. One of the best essential oil combinations is the Thieves blend.[96]

Frankincense offers muscle relaxation and sedative support that may be very helpful to gain rest during travel. Likewise, lemon, orange, and valerian may be calming. Lemongrass is said to be a revitalizer. Patchouli is reported to be both a relaxant and a stimulant, as is ylang ylang. Other essential oils specifically reported as beneficial for jet lag and travel fatigue include eucalyptus, geranium, grapefruit, lavender, and peppermint.

Motion Sickness and Seasickness. Essential oils to consider for motion sickness include ginger, lavender, patchouli, and peppermint. With a few drops placed over the mastoid, at the base of the skull behind the ears, and also on the navel, relief may be quite rapid. When possible, a warm compress may be placed over the abdomen after applying the essential oil for further comfort. In addition, one may inhale the oils for 15 to 20 minutes or even place 1 to 2 drops on the tongue.

Cough, Cold, and Flu. Cough, colds, and flulike illnesses may often be cleared with the administration of essential oils by diffusion, orally, or topically. Many essential oils are antimicrobial and immune stimulants. Some also are mucolytic and anticatarrhal, reducing nasal congestion and thick mucus that often accompanying these ailments. Thieves blend can be used for all these conditions. Individual oils with antimicrobial benefits include blue tansy, citronella, clove, eucalyptus, frankincense, lemon, lemongrass, myrtle, patchouli, peppermint, rosemary, rosewood, and tea tree essential oils. Eucalyptus offers mucolytic and expectorant benefits, as do helichrysum, lemon, and myrtle.

Diarrhea, Dysentery, and Vomiting. Various essential oils calm the GI tract and may offer relief for episodes of diarrhea and vomiting, including fennel, lavender, nutmeg, patchouli, and peppermint. Nausea is covered in the section on motion sickness. Clove is known to protect the stomach. Lavender and valerian are antispasmodic and vermifuges (anthelmintics). Orange is an antispasmodic. Patchouli, peppermint, and rosemary are digestive aids. Essential oils should be considered for food poisoning; patchouli, peppermint, rosemary, tarragon, and the Thieves blend may be helpful. These may be taken as a few drops on the tongue or diluted in a small amount of water.

Pain and Trauma. Essential oils that have disinfectant properties include hyssop, oregano, tea tree, thyme, and Thieves blend. Helichrysum, rose otto, and geranium are known to help reduce bleeding, and clove, elemi, and myrrh should be considered for infected wounds. Essential oils that promote healing include Canadian hemlock, dorado azul, lavender, and tea tree. These may be used singly or blended and applied topically two to five times per day, diluting as indicated per essential oil used. Box 68-5 provides a recommended natural first-aid spray.

BOX 68-5 Essential Oils Natural First-Aid Spray

2 drops cypress
2 drops lavender
3 drops tea tree
Blend essential oils with ½ tsp of salt.
Add this blend to 8 oz of distilled water in a spray bottle.
Shake until dissolved.
Spray topically as indicated.

More than 60 different essential oils have been shown to have analgesic properties. Wintergreen essential oil contains 85% to 99% methyl salicylate. Peppermint, clove, and helichrysum should be considered to treat muscle pain. Dental pain may be treated with black pepper, clove, Idaho tansy, tea tree, and wintergreen. With these, one may apply the oil diluted 50:50 with water directly to the tooth and gum.

Box 68-6 lists essential oils that may be applied to insect bites and stings. Apply 1 to 2 drops directly on each bite or sting three to four times daily. In addition, various essential oils are excellent natural mosquito repellents (Box 68-6).

Frostbite. Conventional medical care is recommended, with integrative care to further promote healing. Essential oils may increase blood flow and provide gentle warming to frostbitten tissues. Essential oils to consider include helichrysum, peppermint, cypress, lavender, and marjoram. Apply 1 to 2 drops of the essential oil or blend topically to the affected areas and *very gently* massage the extremities to increase circulation and soothe the affected areas, followed by a mildly warm compress. Helichrysum is also known for nerve healing and regeneration. This approach may be repeated for a total of two or three treatments daily, even after the extremities are warmed, to provide relief and promote healing.

Heat Exhaustion and Heatstroke. After sunburn, lavender essential oil may be applied directly or in a 50:50 blend with water to promote a cooling sensation and healing of skin.

For heat exhaustion, remove clothing (if possible) and apply a cool, moist washcloth to the skin, adding peppermint essential oil for cooling sensation. Peppermint essential oil increases blood flow to the skin, perhaps helping the body to release heat more quickly and return to normal body temperature. Consider using peppermint mist in a spray bottle by adding 25 drops of peppermint essential oil to a 6-oz water bottle, and spray when feeling overheated.

Contraindications to Essential Oils on Travel

Essential oils should only be used during pregnancy under a competent physician's orders and care. Essential oils are *not* indicated for use in the eyes, ear canal, or open wounds. One may apply any natural oil, such as extra virgin, cold-pressed coconut oil or olive oil, to the affected area if redness or irritation develops while using essential oils topically.

BOX 68-6 Essential Oils for Insect Bites and Mosquito Repellent

Insect Bites/Stings	Clove
Basil	Dorado azul
Eucalyptus	*Eucalyptus globulus*
Lavender	*Eucalyptus radiata*
Peppermint	Geranium
Rosemary	Idaho tansy
Tea tree	Lavender
	Lemon
Natural Mosquito Repellents	Lemongrass
Basil	Peppermint
Blue cypress	Thyme

INDICATIONS FOR BOTANICAL AND ESSENTIAL OIL REMEDIES

Boxes 68-7 and 68-8 list indications for botanical remedies and essential oil remedies, as used in the first-aid kit of natural products.

BOX 68-7 Botanical Remedies for Travel: Indications

Aloe vera gel, liquid, powder capsules: Promotes healing; burns, sunburn, abrasions, cuts, hives, frostbite, gastrointestinal distress, constipation

Anise: Mucolytic, expectorant, antiviral

Arnica ointment, capsules, tea, tincture: Disinfecting; wound healing; sprains, strains, bruises, dislocations, muscle pain, joint pain, bites, stings, sunburn

Calendula gel, ointment, tincture: Cuts, bruises, antiinflammatory, bites, stings, sunburn, antibacterial, antiviral, antifungal

Chamomile tincture: Relaxant, somnolent, antibacterial, antiviral, immune support, stings

Echinacea tincture or capsules: Immune support, cough, colds, flu, antibacterial, antiviral, antifungal, wound repair

Gingko biloba extracts, tinctures, capsules: Enhanced circulation, arrhythmias, altitude sickness, hangover, headache, frostbite, antioxidant, free radical scavenger, immune support

Hypericum* (St John's wort) capsule, ointment, tincture, tea: Jet lag, sedative, anxiolytic, antidepressant, bites, stings, scabies, bruises, cuts, burns, sunburn

Plantago capsule, tincture, tea: Diarrhea, constipation, burns, sunburn, bites, stings, poison ivy, laryngitis, pharyngitis, antibacterial, astringent

Valerian capsules, tincture, tea: Jet lag, sedative, antianxiety, arrhythmias, palpitations, improves circulation, lowers high blood pressure, improves cardiac output, gastrointestinal spasm

Coix Formula: Motion sickness, food poisoning, excessive eating and alcohol, nausea, headache, vomiting, diarrhea or constipation, gastrointestinal cramping, generalized pain

Zheng Gu Shui: Sprains, strains, bruises, muscle pain, arthritis pain

*Avoid in pregnancy, and use caution with sunlight.

BOX 68-8 Essential Oils: Indications*

Clove (*Syzygium aromaticum*): Antiinflammatory, antiseptic, antiviral, antibacterial, antifungal, antiinfectious, antiparasitic, antiaging, antioxidant, analgesic, anticoagulant, immune stimulant, anticonvulsant, disinfectant, stomach protectant, warming

Eucalyptus (*Eucalyptus globulus*): Antiviral, antibacterial, antifungal, antiaging, antiinfectious, antiinflammatory, antirheumatic, antiseptic, deodorant, insecticidal, mucolytic, expectorant

Frankincense (*Boswellia carterii*): Anticatarrhal, antidepressant, antiinfectious, antiseptic, expectorant, immune stimulant, muscle relaxant, sedative

Helichrysum (*Helichrysum italicum*): Antiviral, antiinflammatory, antispasmodic, expectorant, mucolytic, anesthetic, anticoagulant, anticatarrhal, antioxidant, liver stimulant/detoxifier, skin and nerve regenerator

Lavender (*Lavandula angustifolia*): Antifungal, analgesic, antiseptic, anticonvulsant, vasodilator, antispasmodic, antiinflammatory, vermifuge (anthelmintic)

Orange (*Citrus sinensis*): Antiseptic, antidepressant, antispasmodic, digestive aid, circulatory stimulant, sedative, tonic

Patchouli (*Pogostemon cablin*): Antiinflammatory, antifungal, antimicrobial, antiseptic, antitoxic, astringent, decongestant, deodorant, diuretic, insecticidal, stimulant, relaxant, digestive aid, tonic

Peppermint (*Mentha piperita*): Antiinflammatory, antiviral, antiparasitic, antibacterial, gallbladder, digestive stimulant, pain reliever, analgesic, antispasmodic

Rosemary (*Rosmarinus officinalis*): Antifungal, antibacterial, antiviral, antiparasitic, liver protecting, cardiotonic, digestive, detoxicant, anxiolytic

Tea tree (*Melaleuca alternifolia*): Antiviral, antibacterial, antifungal, antiparasitic, antiseptic, antiinflammatory, antioxidant, decongestant, immune stimulant, insecticidal, tissue regenerator

Ylang ylang (*Cananga odorata*): Antiinflammatory, antispasmodic, antiseptic, antidepressant, vasodilator, regulates heartbeat, antidiabetic, tonic, sedative

*For blended essential oils (Thieves blend), see Box 68-3.

Appendix

COMPANIES

BOIRON

Natural Home Health Care LeKit contains 36 single-remedy medicines in distinctive blue tubes, including the commercial flu remedy Oscillococcinum. The home kit also contains four external remedies: tinctures of calendula and hypericum, and ointments of arnica and calendula. Travel LeKit is a more compact collection of single remedies (22 multidose and 16 one-dose tubes) plus the flu remedy.

BIOLOGICAL HOMEOPATHIC INDUSTRIES (BHI)

BHI is the U.S. distributor of the German line of complex homeopathic remedies manufactured by Heel:
http://www.heel.com

BIORESOURCE INC.

BioResource Inc. is the U.S. distributor of quality German botanical and homeopathic medications such as Inflamyar ointment.
http://www.bioresourceinc.com

INSTITUTE FOR TRADITIONAL MEDICINE (ITM)

http://www.itmonline.org
ITM is a nonprofit resource for Chinese herbal medicines, patent formulas (prepared medicines), and professional herbal formulas for practitioners. Jintu is the nonprescription resource for the products listed here:
http://www.itmonline.org/jintu.

Website to access Wobenzym N and other products that are generally sold only to health care practitioners:
http://www.pureprescriptions.com

BOOKS

NATURAL HEALTH AND MEDICINE

Frank B: *Travel well, naturally: an essential guide to staying healthy on personal, business or mission travel.* Yukon, OK, 2014, ReGenesis Health.

Lust J, Tierra M: *The natural remedy bible,* New York, 1990, Pocket Books.

Murray M, Pizzorno J: *Encyclopedia of natural medicine,* Rocklin, Calif, 1991, Prima.

Weil A: *Health and healing: Understanding conventional and alternative medicine,* Boston, 1983, Houghton Mifflin.

HERBS AND HERBALISM

Murray M: *The healing power of herbs,* Rocklin, Calif, 1991, Prima.

Weiss RF: *Herbal medicine,* Beaconsfield, UK, 1988, Beaconsfield.

HOMEOPATHY BOOKS

Boericke W, Boericke O: *Boericke's materia medica with repertory,* New Delhi, 1991, B Jain.

Kruzel T: *The homeopathic emergency guide,* Berkeley, Calif, 1992, North Atlantic Books/Homeopathic Education Services.

Reckeweg HH: *Homotoxicology: Illness and healing through antihomotoxic therapy,* ed 2, Albuquerque, 1984, Menaco.

Subotnick S: *Sports and exercise injuries: Conventional, homeopathic, and alternative treatments,* Berkeley, Calif, 1991, North Atlantic Books.

PRACTITIONERS

AMERICAN ASSOCIATION OF NATUROPATHIC PHYSICIANS

4435 Wisconsin Ave, NW, Suite 403
Washington, DC 20016
202-237-8150 telephone
866-538-2267 toll-free
202-237-8152 fax
http://www.naturopathic.org

HERBAL MEDICINES

HERB RESEARCH FOUNDATION

http://www.herbs.org

NUTRITIONAL PRODUCTS

CRANE HERB COMPANY

745 Falmouth Rd
Mashpee, MA 02649
800-227-4118
http://www.craneherb.com (registration required)

THORNE RESEARCH

25820 Highway 2 W
PO Box 25
Dover, ID 83825
800-228-1966
http://www.thorne.com

METAGENICS

100 Avenida La Pata
San Clemente, CA 92673
800-692-9400
http://www.metagenics.com

MOUNTAIN PEAK NUTRITIONALS

3310 SW Vista Dr
Portland, OR 97225
877-686-7325

VITAL NUTRIENTS

45 Kenneth Dooley Dr
Middletown, CT 06457
888-328-9992
http://www.vitalnutrients.net

REFERENCES

Complete references used in this text are available online at expertconsult.inkling.com.

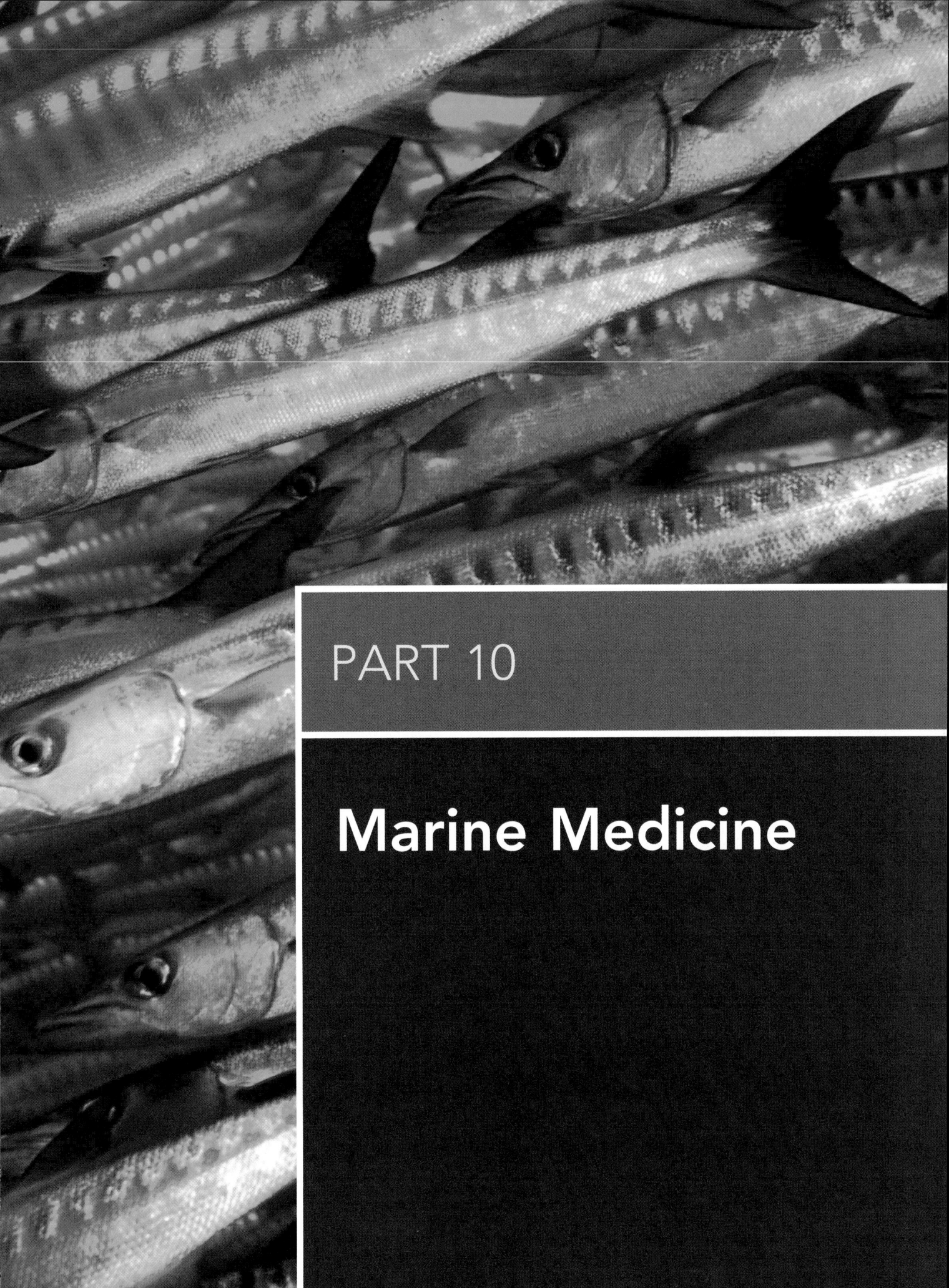

PART 10

Marine Medicine

JUSTIN SEMPSROTT, ANDREW C. SCHMIDT, SETH C. HAWKINS, AND TRACY A. CUSHING

> *To have faith is to trust yourself to the water. When you swim you don't grab hold of the water, because if you do you will sink and drown. Instead you relax, and float.* A. Watts[247]
>
> *A lack of oxygen does not simply involve stoppage of the engine, but total ruin of what we took to be the machinery.* J.S. Haldane[91]

Humankind is surrounded by water; it covers 75% of Earth's surface, and is integral to our survival and development. Water can be dangerous, responsible for hundreds of thousands of drowning deaths per year. The earliest recorded drowning resuscitation is from Syria in 1237 BC, when two soldiers rescued the king of Aleppo from the Orontes River. The king is shown being held upside down as part of an inversion technique used for thousands of years in attempts to revive drowning patients. During the late 16th century, several societies were founded in Europe in response to increasing numbers of deaths on commercial waterways, where boating and shipping were the primary mechanisms of transportation. Drowning became a substantial public health issue, and in response, several national societies were formed. With proliferation of swimming pools and rapid expansion of recreational water activities, drowning became not only an occupational hazard but also a significant recreational hazard. This chapter reviews classification, pathophysiology, clinical presentation, treatment, and prevention of drowning, and emphasizes the importance of safety and injury prevention.

CLASSIFICATION AND TYPES OF SUBMERSION INJURIES AND DROWNING SCENARIOS

Drowning is an international public health problem that has been complicated by lack of a uniform definition, proliferation of confusing subdefinitions, inadequate epidemiologic studies, and conflicting clinical management paradigms. In response to dialogue at the 2002 World Conference on Drowning, a consensus panel and the World Health Organization adopted the following definition: "Drowning is the process of experiencing respiratory impairment from submersion/immersion in liquid."[238] According to this new classification system, drowning outcomes should be classified as drowning death, drowning with morbidity, and drowning without morbidity. Drowning is now considered a process and not an outcome. Other water-related conditions that do not primarily involve the airway and respiratory system are submersion injuries rather than drowning. For example, this definition of drowning specifically excludes water rescues during which submersion does not involve the respiratory system; if the rescued person maintains his or her airway above water throughout the event, it would be considered a submersion injury rather than a drowning.[237]

The consensus panel of 2002 also concluded that the terms *wet drowning, dry drowning, active drowning, passive drowning, silent drowning, near-drowning,* and *secondary drowning* should no longer be used in drowning terminology.[238] However, because these terms are still widely in use by medical professionals and laypersons, it is important to be familiar with them.

One of the most common previous classification systems divided drowning into two possible outcomes: drowning and near-drowning. This system was problematic because the term *near-drowning* had 20 different published and often conflicting definitions. The preferred nomenclature is *nonfatal* drowning. Data on nonfatal incidents were often excluded from epidemiologic and research studies of drowning because the victim had

survived. This was a detriment because information about survival of drowning can have a major impact on public health initiatives and optimization of treatment protocols.[163,238] Excluding nonfatal drowning incidents from statistics on drowning meant that such incidents were often underreported; excluding information about survivors of a life-threatening event from epidemiologic data is rare in medicine. The term near-drowning should no longer be used in drowning terminology; it should be replaced by the terms preferred since 2002 for the subsets of drowning: *drowning death, drowning with morbidity,* and *drowning without morbidity.*[237,253]

Another common previous classification system differentiated drowning incidents by presumed physiologic mechanism: wet or dry. Wet drowning, a term that described aspiration of water during the drowning process, was thought to occur in 80% to 90% of drowning deaths, with the remaining individuals experiencing dry drowning, in which no water is found in the lungs, presumably due to laryngospasm. Reanalysis of the original autopsy studies leading to these distinctions has brought this classification into question. The actual existence of dry drowning has not been proven; additionally, if laryngospasm does occur, it likely relaxes with progressing hypoxemia. Existence of such a reflex holds no prognostic or treatment significance. The terms wet drowning and dry drowning should not be used.

Other classifications that describe the mechanism of drowning include *active drowning, passive drowning,* and *shallow water syncope* or *shallow water blackout. Active drowning* and *passive drowning* are historical terms that most likely represented witnessed and unwitnessed drowning incidents, respectively.[238] The terms have no usefulness for epidemiologic or clinical understanding of drowning. *Shallow water syncope* is a syndrome that occurs primarily among competitive swimmers, free-divers, and spearfishers who attempt to stay underwater for long periods without the need to breathe. Individuals hyperventilate before submersion, resulting in hypocapnic respiratory alkalosis. By artificially reducing the proportion of carbon dioxide in arterial blood, the time until a person needs to breathe is prolonged; at the same time, the body's consumption of oxygen may lead to such a low level of blood oxygen that the person becomes unconscious. Because the compulsion to breathe from hypoxemia is less potent than the drive from acidosis or hypercapnia, a person may become unconscious from hypoxemia before the carbon dioxide level rises adequately to stimulate breathing, which leads to drowning.

INCIDENCE AND EPIDEMIOLOGY

The World Health Organization Global Burden of Disease Update estimated that 372,000 people drowned worldwide in 2012; this represented 7% of all injury-related deaths.[253] Statistical data likely underestimate the true incidence of drowning. This is largely due to underreporting, particularly in middle- and low-income countries, where many drowning victims never make it to a hospital. It is estimated that for every reported drowning death, another four go unreported.[101] Codes from the *International Classification of Diseases 10th edition* (ICD-10) have recently been altered to improve drowning and subtype categorizations, but many

DROWNING AS A LEADING CAUSE OF DEATH AMONG 1-14 YEAR OLDS, SELECTED COUNTRIES

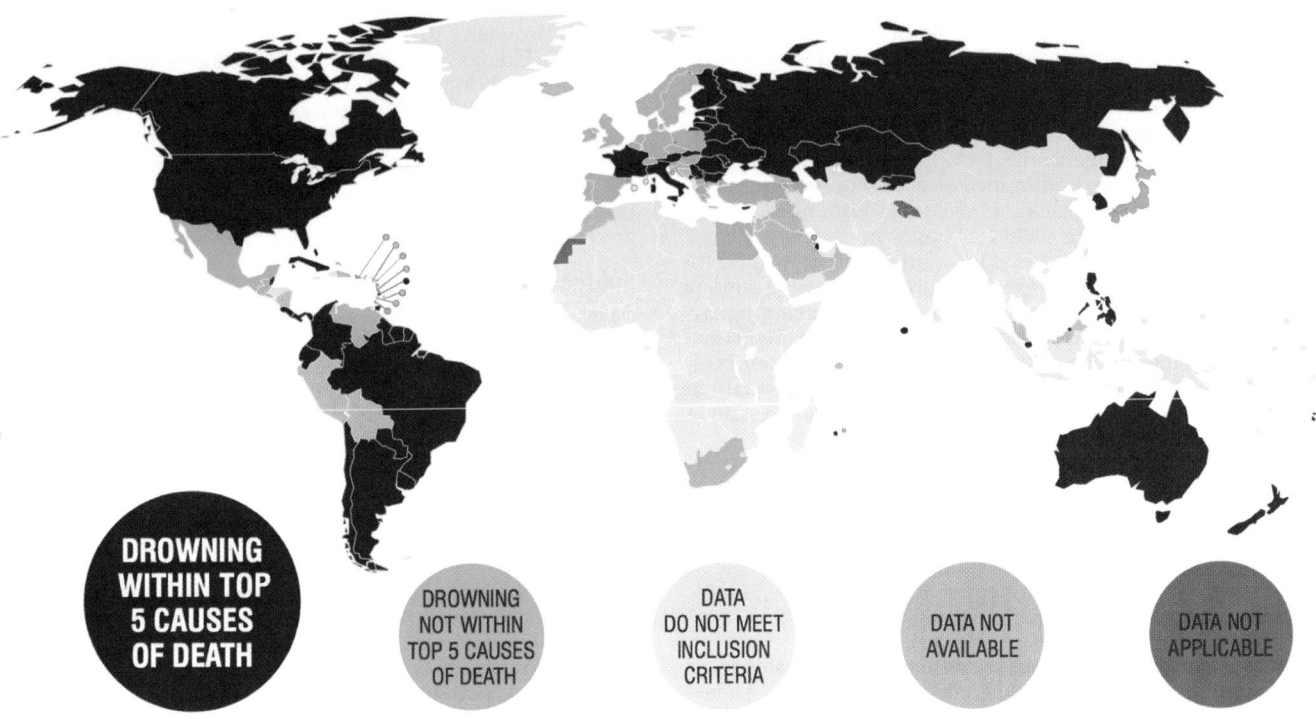

DROWNING WITHIN TOP 5 CAUSES OF DEATH

DROWNING NOT WITHIN TOP 5 CAUSES OF DEATH

DATA DO NOT MEET INCLUSION CRITERIA

DATA NOT AVAILABLE

DATA NOT APPLICABLE

FIGURE 69-1 According to the World Health Organization, drowning is a leading cause of death among those 1 to 14 years of age worldwide. *(From WHO. Global report on drowning: preventing a leading killer. 2014. http://www.who.int/violence_injury_prevention/global_report_drowning/en/.)*

countries still fail to report sufficiently specific codes to the World Health Organization with regard to data on drowning deaths.[136] A further complication is that drowning deaths caused by floods and natural disasters are not reflected in these numbers; such events include the great tsunami of December 2004, which resulted in more than 100,000 deaths by drowning, and Hurricane Katrina in New Orleans in 2005. Drowning deaths resulting from assaults, suicides, and boating accidents are not typically classified as drowning, because they are usually classified based on the primary cause of death, and secondary diagnoses (e.g., drowning) are not captured.

Worldwide, drowning occurs overwhelmingly (>91%) in low- and middle-income countries. Drowning is the third leading cause of accidental injury death worldwide. India and China both have particularly high drowning mortality rates,[139] together contributing 43% of all drowning deaths worldwide and 41% of the total disability-adjusted life years attributed to drowning worldwide. In China in 2001, drowning was the leading cause of injury death among children between 1 and 14 years of age.[252] The global burden of drowning in 2002 is shown in Figure 69-1; territories are sized in proportion to the absolute number of people who died from drowning that year.

In the United States, the National Center for Injury and Prevention Control reported 4308 fatal unintentional drowning deaths in 2012, or 1.37 deaths per 100,000 people.[41] Boating-related incidents accounted for an additional 651 deaths, with 71% of those attributed to drowning.[41] Drowning ranks as the 10th leading cause of injury death overall in the United States, but it overwhelmingly affects younger age groups: Drowning is the leading cause of death by unintentional injury among children between the ages of 1 and 4 years, and ranks second among children between the ages of 5 and 9 years; it is the sixth leading cause of injury death for those between the ages of 15 and 24 years.[40] California, Florida, and Texas reported the highest numbers of drowning deaths in 2006.[38] It is estimated that for every pediatric drowning death, an additional four children are hospitalized for nonfatal drowning; many of these children require prolonged intensive care and may suffer permanent neurologic disability.[40,136]

The economic costs of drowning are among the highest of any injury group, largely because the most severe complications and most deaths occur in individuals between the ages of 0 and 15 years. At this young age, there is a large impact on future economic productivity. An estimated 1 million disability-adjusted life years were lost as a result of premature death or disability from drowning worldwide in 2004.[196,252] A single nonfatal drowning survivor with severe neurologic impairment can accrue more than $4.5 million in medical treatment costs over a lifetime.[40]

RISK FACTORS

Drowning tends to involve specific populations, age groups, and locations (Box 69-1). Understanding risk factors is important to implementing prevention and public health programs to decrease the incidence of drowning.

AGE

Young people have the highest likelihood of drowning. A bimodal age distribution characterizes childhood drowning, with

---

BOX 69-1 Factors Common to Drowning Incidents

Age: toddlers, teenage boys
Location: home swimming pools, bathtubs, buckets
Gender: males more often than females
Race: black children are at higher risk than other groups
Drugs: particularly alcohol
Trauma: secondary to diving, falls

children less than 4 years old and adolescent males accounting for the peaks. There is an additional smaller peak later in life among persons over 65 years of age.[192] In 2005, of all children between the ages of 1 and 4 years who died in the United States, 31% died from drowning.[40] Children are at high risk of drowning because many cannot swim or swim well, they have a large head-to-body ratio (increasing the risk of head submersion), there is a lack of barriers around pools and bathtubs, and there are lapses in supervision. Toddlers are especially at risk because they are able to move about independently but are unable to recognize water hazards or to effect self-rescue. Despite the American Academy of Pediatrics (AAP) recommendation never to leave a child unsupervised in the bathtub, one study reported that nearly 33% of parents leave children unattended in this setting.[214] Children bathing with a sibling who was less than 2 years old who were unsupervised for a brief time accounted for 22% to 58% of bathtub drowning deaths.[34] Drowning among adolescents and teenagers is often seen with risk-taking behaviors, lack of supervision, and drug and alcohol intake. The scene of drowning in this age group is most commonly a natural body of water, such as a lake, pond, or river. Incidents often occur far from medical assistance and may take place where rescue is challenging; however, these events are often witnessed.[7,32,45,192,193] Among people who are more than 65 years old, deaths are evenly divided between open-water drowning and bathtub-related drowning, often from falls or exacerbations of concomitant illnesses (e.g., cardiac arrhythmias), which may not be recognized at autopsy.[192]

GENDER

In 2012, males were three times more likely than females in all age groups to die from unintentional drowning in the United States.[38] The incidence of drowning in females peaks at 1 year of age and declines throughout the rest of life. This trend is thought to be due to increased risk-taking behavior and greater alcohol consumption among males as compared with females. Worldwide, males have a higher mortality rate from drowning as compared with females in all age groups and regions.[184]

RACE

In the United States between 1999 and 2010, the rate of fatal drowning for blacks was 1.4 times higher than that of whites.[41] The rate was twice as high for Alaska natives and Native Americans as for whites.[40] In Alaska, drowning rates are twice as high among Native American children as compared with white and black children.[6] In the 10- to 14-year-old age group, the fatal drowning rate for blacks is 3.7 times that of white children of the same age, and is 2.6 times higher for Alaska native and Native American children.[38,79] This pattern is reflected in the military, where black soldiers drown 62% more often than white soldiers.[15] The reasons behind racial differences in drowning rates are unclear, but suspected factors are decreased routine access to swimming pools, less emphasis on swimming lessons, and less participation in recreational water-related activities.[161] If, overall, minorities participate in fewer water-related activities, their drowning rates per exposure may be even higher than reported.[27]

LOCATION

Familiar or Unfamiliar Places

Any body of water, no matter how shallow or small, can be the site of drowning. Oceans, seas, and rivers account for fewer drownings than do backyard pools, recreational lakes, bathtubs, and buckets of water. In the United States, drownings involving young children occur primarily in fresh water; children less than 1 year of age most often drown in bathtubs, buckets, or toilets, whereas those between 1 and 4 years of age most often drown in residential pools.[5,14,23,32,45,161,192] Despite these statistics, only a small proportion of home pools are properly protected, and most are easily accessible by ambulatory toddlers and curious children.[204,218] One study found that most young children who drowned in residential pools had been out of sight of adults for

less than 5 minutes, and were in the care of one or both parents at the time.[188] Among individuals between the age of 5 and 64 years, drowning typically occurs in open-water recreational settings such as lakes, rivers, and oceans.[32,185] Persons over age 65 have the highest rates of bathtub drowning per age group.[192]

Visitors to domestic and international locations are at a higher risk for drowning than natives in the same region. After motor vehicle accidents and homicide, drowning is the leading cause of injury death among U.S. citizens traveling abroad.[231] In island locations, it is the leading cause of injury death; it accounts for 63% of traveler deaths by injury as compared with 3.5% for native citizens of the respective countries.[88,231] Lack of familiarity with the environment,[133] lack of understanding of local hydrology, overestimation of abilities, and use of alcohol while vacationing are likely contributors to drowning rates among travelers.

Submerged Vehicle Incidents

Some studies suggest that approximately 10% of all drownings occur via a submerged vehicle. During natural disasters, drowning in a submerged vehicle occurs in as many as 10% of all motor vehicle accident deaths.[216,256] A more recent study[219] demonstrated that, of 83 drowning deaths in vehicles, more than 92% of victims had insignificant traumatic injuries, suggesting that the primary source of death in submerged vehicles is drowning rather than trauma.

Many suggestions in the popular media about how to manage entrapment in a submerged or submerging vehicle are incorrect and can paradoxically lead to increased risk of death. These poor suggestions include allowing the passenger compartment to fill with water so it will be easier to open doors, waiting until the vehicle hits the bottom to maintain orientation, relying on kicking out the windshield or opening the door to exit, and relying on breathing trapped air in the passenger compartment.

One series of Canadian studies looked at ways to deal with a submerging vehicle situation and possible ways to reduce fatality rates. These data demonstrated that a vehicle floats for 30 seconds to 2 minutes prior to sinking. In this phase, windows can be easily opened and used for exit, assuming that the risk outside the vehicle (e.g., swift water or a nonswimmer exiting into deep water) is not greater than the risk inside the vehicle. In one trial, three adults were able to release a child mannequin from a rear child seat and exit the vehicle within 51 seconds. During the sinking phase (after 2 minutes), occupants can breathe as water rises inside the vehicle but chances for escape and survival decrease considerably because rising water pressure makes it more difficult to exit through doors and windows. In the third, submerged phase, the vehicle is full of water and no air pockets exist, so the chance of survival is negligible. The following escape procedure is recommended: Immediately unfasten all seat belts and then open all the windows. If children are present, they should be released from restraints and held by an adult. Once all passengers are free of restraints, children should be assisted out of the open windows first, followed by adults (Box 69-2).[97]

Scuba Diving Accidents

The Divers Alert Network reported 138 deaths internationally in 2006 from scuba diving accidents.[58] Fifty-one of these were in the United States, with Florida having the highest incidence, followed by California. The cause of death was reported in 58 cases (77% of the total); of those, 86% were attributed to

---

BOX 69-2 Submerged Vehicle Escape Procedure

Seat belts: unfastened
Windows: open
Children: if present, released from restraints and brought close to an adult who can assist in their escape
Out: children should be pushed out of the window first, and followed immediately

From McDonald GK, Giesbrecht GG: Vehicle submersion: a review of the problem, associated risks, and survival information. *Aviat Space Environ Med* 84:498-510, 2013.

drowning, by far the most common cause of death in this series. Several patients had known preexisting medical conditions, including cardiovascular disease, which may have contributed to drowning.

Water Birthing Incidents

Water birth (i.e., labor and delivery while immersed in water) may be a risk factor for drowning. Documented adverse neonatal outcomes from underwater birth include unexplained death, drowning, asphyxiation, water intoxication, hyponatremia with seizures, water aspiration leading to respiratory distress and failure, pulmonary edema, hypoxic-ischemic encephalopathy, and pneumonia and other infections, including *Pseudomonas* and *Legionella* infection.[70,76,169,180] Other observational series have shown similar Apgar scores, rates of neonatal resuscitation, and complications for both regular births and water births.[78,169] There has been a vigorous debate in the pediatrics and obstetrics community regarding the safety of this birth modality, but what is undisputed is that there are few reliable data demonstrating the safety of water birthing.[207] In 2014, the AAP and American College of Obstetricians and Gynecologists (ACOG) issued a joint position paper stating that "the practice of immersion in the second stage of labor (underwater delivery) should be considered an experimental procedure that only should be performed within the context of an appropriately designed clinical trial with informed consent." However, the authors[102] of this position paper have been criticized for nearly exclusive reliance on low-level evidence in case studies, while failing to cite or review higher-level evidence in prospective studies; using an outdated literature review; and misrepresentation of studies that were reviewed (evidencebasedbirth.com/waterbirth/). It should be noted that, in contrast to the AAP-ACOG position paper, the American College of Nurse Midwives,[6b] the American Association of Birth Centers,[6a] and the Royal College of Midwives[203a] all released counterstatements declaring evidence-based support for the safety of water births, and specifically the low drowning risk for neonates during these deliveries.

ABILITY TO SWIM

Although popular, swimming programs for young children do not fully protect against drowning; children should always be supervised while swimming. There is some evidence that children ages 1 to 4 years with some formal swim instruction were less likely than matched controls (3% versus 26%, respectively) to die by drowning.[31] The latest recommendation from the AAP is that children as young as 1 year old can be enrolled in formal swimming courses. This does not replace the need for direct supervision and use of pool barriers and alarms. Swimming lessons are recommended for nearly all children after the age of 4 years. Prevention focuses on supervision, restricting access to home pools, and reducing use of drugs and alcohol among teenagers around water.[4-6]

Highly experienced swimmers are not immune from drowning; competitive swimmers and breath-hold divers sometimes engage in intentional hyperventilation and die as a result of shallow water syncope. Breath-hold diving is defined as in-water activity without self-contained or surface-supplied breathing gas. Breath-hold activities include snorkeling, spearfishing, and free-diving, from which there were 34 fatal drowning cases reported worldwide by the Divers Alert Network in 2006.[58] More than half occurred in the United States, primarily in Florida, Hawaii, California, and Texas; this may be the result of higher rates of reporting in the United States than other countries and suggests that safety and prevention strategies should be a focus in specific geographic regions. Twelve cases were associated with blackout due to hypoxemic loss of consciousness, likely as a result of intentional hyperventilation to prolong breath-holding time.

According to the International Swimming Federation, open-water swimming is defined as any competition that takes place in a lake, river, or ocean. Several studies have demonstrated a risk for hypothermia during open-water swimming competitions, but the amount of risk varied depending on the modality of temperature measurement used and remains unclear.[28,36]

ALCOHOL AND DRUGS CONTRIBUTING TO DROWNING INCIDENTS

Alcohol has been implicated as a contributing factor in 25% to 50% of recreational water-related deaths and in 20% of boating-related fatalities.[33,60,131,133,159] Studies have demonstrated blood alcohol levels of 100 mg/dL or more as a factor in 25% of boating-related fatalities,[33] in 25% of teen drowning deaths,[193] and in 33% of drowning deaths of young adults between the ages of 20 and 34 years. In Australia, 21% of people who drowned during a 5-year period had measurable blood alcohol levels.[69] Despite federal laws that prohibit alcohol use during recreation on open water, a survey of adults in the United States showed that 31% of 597 respondents reported operating a motorboat while under the influence of alcohol; these operators were overwhelmingly males between 25 and 34 years of age.[134] Impaired judgment caused by intoxicants can lead to accidents as well as loss of body heat, decreased laryngeal reflexes, higher risk of aspiration, decreased supervision of children, and decreased use of safety devices, such as personal flotation devices (PFDs).[192,260] Illicit recreational drug use with and without alcohol has been reported as a factor in water-related deaths.[33] All types of drugs that affect judgment can result in watercraft overcrowding, speeding, and inattentive or reckless handling, and in failure to wear PFDs.

PREEXISTING DISEASE

Risk of submersion injury or death in water increases significantly when medical conditions compromise the chance for self-rescue and survival. Situations are particularly dangerous for unpredictable medical conditions, such as cardiac and neurologic conditions. Individuals with relevant preexisting conditions should never be alone in the water and must optimize treatment for the underlying condition before engaging in water-related activities.

Seizure disorders increase the risk of drowning among adults and children in both natural bodies of water and in homes.[16,18,29] Drowning is the most common cause of death by unintentional injury among patients with seizure disorders.[190] One study found the risk of drowning among people with epilepsy to be 15 to 19 times greater than that of the general population.[16] It is when a patient is alone that the risk of death increases drastically. Other neurologic conditions (e.g., cerebrovascular accident, arteriovenous malformation) that manifest as seizure have also been associated with drowning.[81]

Cardiac disorders associated with dysrhythmias may manifest while a person is submerged in water; however, the exact mechanism for rhythm disturbance as a result of submersion remains unclear.[2,25] Prolonged QT syndrome, a conduction disorder associated with sudden death, has been linked by forensic molecular screening to some drowning deaths, indicating a theoretically possible gene-specific dysrhythmogenic presentation of prolonged QT syndrome triggered by swimming.[3,137] Adverse events, such as unstable tachycardia or loss of consciousness from myocardial infarction, may lead to drowning deaths.

CHILD ABUSE, HOMICIDE, AND SUICIDE

Abuse or neglect should be investigated in any suspicious fatal or nonfatal pediatric drowning; thorough social service and legal investigation is needed. One series found abuse or neglect to account for 19% of bathtub drowning deaths among patients less than 5 years old.[193] In the adult population, homicide by drowning is relatively uncommon. The postmortem determination of death by drowning (as opposed to body disposal in water after another mechanism of homicide) is very difficult to make. Drowning by suicide is relatively uncommon.[175,240,251] An Australian study of 123 suicides by drowning found women to more commonly choose a bathtub or the ocean for drowning, whereas men selected rivers, ditches, and lakes.[35]

BOATING-RELATED DROWNING

Recreational and commercial boating accidents are among the leading causes of unintentional drowning. Deaths result from capsized vessels or falls overboard. The risk of drowning is determined by the water depth and temperature, distance from shore, and currents, including hydraulics at the bases of dams or spillways. Alcohol use, lack of personal protective equipment, and unsafe boating practices are involved in many boat-related drowning incidents.[33,131] In 2013, the U.S. Coast Guard reported 2620 injuries and 560 deaths as a result of recreational boating accidents;[236] Of these deaths, 431 were the result of drowning; 362 (84%) of these victims were not wearing PFDs or lifejackets. Studies suggest there is significant underuse of PFDs among recreational boaters.[115,191] In the United States in 2013, alcohol was the leading contributing factor in 16% of fatal boating accidents, followed by operator inexperience and careless or reckless operation. Most fatal accidents occurred with open motorboats, followed by canoes and kayaks. States with the highest death rates (i.e., > 10 per 100,000 registered boats) were Alaska, Hawaii, Montana, Idaho, Utah, Texas, Louisiana, and Vermont.[236]

The international commercial fishing industry also contributes to boating-related drowning deaths. The International Labor Organization estimated that 45 million people worldwide were employed in aquaculture industries in 2007[103]; most are located in Asia and Africa. Death rates among commercially employed fisherman are among the highest of any occupation.[132,199] In the United States, death rates of fishermen are 16 times higher than those of police and firefighters and 8 times higher than those of persons who drive motor vehicles for a living.[235]

Another population affected by water transport and drowning is that of refugees seeking asylum, who are often in rough weather and poorly equipped, overcrowded boats without life-jackets. A 2004 study reported that 4000 asylum seekers are estimated to drown annually at sea.[61,189] The 2014 crisis of refugees fleeing war-torn Middle Eastern countries has resulted in numerous drowning deaths. According to the United Nations High Council on Refugees (UNHCR), there were 410 documented drowning deaths in the first 6 weeks of 2015 among 80,000 people crossing the eastern Mediterranean, which is a 35-fold increase from 2015.[233a]

PATHOPHYSIOLOGY

The pathophysiology of submersion has been extensively studied in animal models, yet there remain ambiguities with regard to the exact sequence of events and mechanisms of drowning in humans. The effect of submersion on mammals was initially reported in scientific literature during the late 1800s, and most early research involved animal models. In a classic monograph from 1965, Greene noted that "inundation of the upper airway, the bronchial tree and segments of the alveolar spaces blocks gas exchange in the lung and produces asphyxia. Thus drowning involves the rapid development of hypoxemia, hypercapnia, and acidosis with the associated sequence of hypertension, bradycardia, apnea, and terminal gasping."[86] Although these observations remain largely accurate for humans, they were based on mammalian experiments designed to simulate drowning.[100,135,170] Early animal research examined the hemodynamic and electrolyte effects of drownings that occurred in water types of different osmolality (i.e., saltwater versus freshwater drowning). Although some models indicated a pathophysiologic difference between the two, this has proved to be of limited applicability in humans. Early canine experiments showing hypervolemia in freshwater aspiration and hypovolemia and hypernatremia in saltwater aspiration[157] have not been reproduced, and human research has failed to replicate the course observed in animals.[205] Hypervolemia has not been observed in human freshwater aspiration, and most humans have total fluid aspiration of less than 4 mL/kg.[141,153] More than twice that amount is required to effect the changes in blood volume seen experimentally. Similarly, an aspirated amount of 22 mL/kg is required before systemic electrolyte changes result[152]; therefore, the distinction between saltwater and freshwater drowning is of limited utility for humans. Most authorities recommend discontinuation of this distinction so the focus can be on the common pathway of hypoxemia, acidosis, pulmonary injury, and multiorgan system failure that remain the hallmarks of drowning pathophysiology.[8,81,127,149,178,181,182,238]

THE HUMAN BODY AND WATER

The degree to which a body floats (i.e., its buoyancy) depends on the amount of air in the lungs, body fat, and type and distribution of clothing. When the lungs are maximally filled with air (close to total lung capacity), the body has approximately 2.5 kg (5.5 lb) of flotation. It has greater buoyancy during inspiration as the lungs fill with air, and lesser buoyancy during expiration. Clothing can affect both heat conservation and buoyancy, and can be integral to survival in the wilderness water environment. PFDs are specifically designed to increase buoyancy (Figure 69-2).[168] The percentage of body fat is a factor in the ability to conserve body heat during prolonged immersion.

THE INITIAL EVENT

Drowning begins when the patient's airway is below the surface of a liquid medium, usually water, and the patient must breathe but cannot surface to do so. There is typically an initial period of struggle with attempted breath-holding. This struggle may not occur during trauma-associated submersion, when the patient may have been unconscious before or upon entry into water.[127,178] After gasping occurs, the initial struggle may be followed by laryngospasm to protect the lower airways from liquid in the upper airways, although the prevalence and relevance of this distinction to the ultimate pathophysiology is controversial.[127,177,205] It is now believed that all drowning patients likely aspirate at least a small amount (< 30 mL) of liquid. Particularly during cold-water submersion, the initial event is accompanied by a drive to hyperventilate caused by stimulation of thermal skin receptors, in addition to increasing hypoxemia. During this initial time, patients often swallow large amounts of water to avoid aspiration.[153] Eventually, the outcomes of breath-holding are hypoventilation, hypercapnia, respiratory acidosis, and hypoxemia. Loss of consciousness ensues and cardiopulmonary arrest follows (Figure 69-3).

The duration of tissue hypoxemia, timing of rescue, and institution of effective cardiopulmonary resuscitation (CPR) and field resuscitation are significant factors that affect whether the initial submersion injury is survivable. The duration of submersion, water temperature, and tissue susceptibility to hypoxemia determine the effects of submersion on different organ systems and likelihood of survival.

PULMONARY SYSTEM

Aspiration of water of any type and volume immediately affects alveolar ventilation, gas exchange, and mechanical characteristics of the lung.[56,74,178] Hypoxemia is the hallmark of pulmonary pathophysiology during drowning. Breath-holding and apnea lead to a rise in partial pressure of carbon dioxide and a fall in partial pressure of oxygen in both the alveolar and arterial blood. In addition, inhalation of any liquid causes surfactant disruption and alveolar collapse, resulting in areas of ventilation/perfusion ($\dot{V}/\dot{Q}$) mismatch, shunting, and further worsening of hypoxemia. Pulmonary sequelae may range from asymptomatic to acute respiratory distress syndrome (ARDS), depending on the amount of water aspirated and duration of submersion. Usually, symptoms of pulmonary involvement are present immediately; however, there are reports of delayed ARDS after an initially normal chest radiograph.[56]

Volumes of aspirated liquid of as little as 1 to 3 mL/kg are sufficient to cause disruptions in alveolar gas exchange and thus hypoxemia. Diminished pulmonary gas exchange occurs in part due to surfactant disruption as a result of aspiration. Surfactant is produced by type 2 pneumocytes, pulmonary epithelial cells responsible for maintaining alveolar surface tension, increasing pulmonary compliance, and preventing atelectasis. Disruption of surfactant leads to malfunctioning of the alveolar epithelial lining and increased $\dot{V}/\dot{Q}$ mismatch. Interstitial and microvascular damage ensues in response to alveolar-capillary basement membrane disruption, releasing an inflammatory cascade that results in pulmonary edema caused by extravasation of fluid into the alveolar space, bronchospasm, worsening $\dot{V}/\dot{Q}$ mismatch,

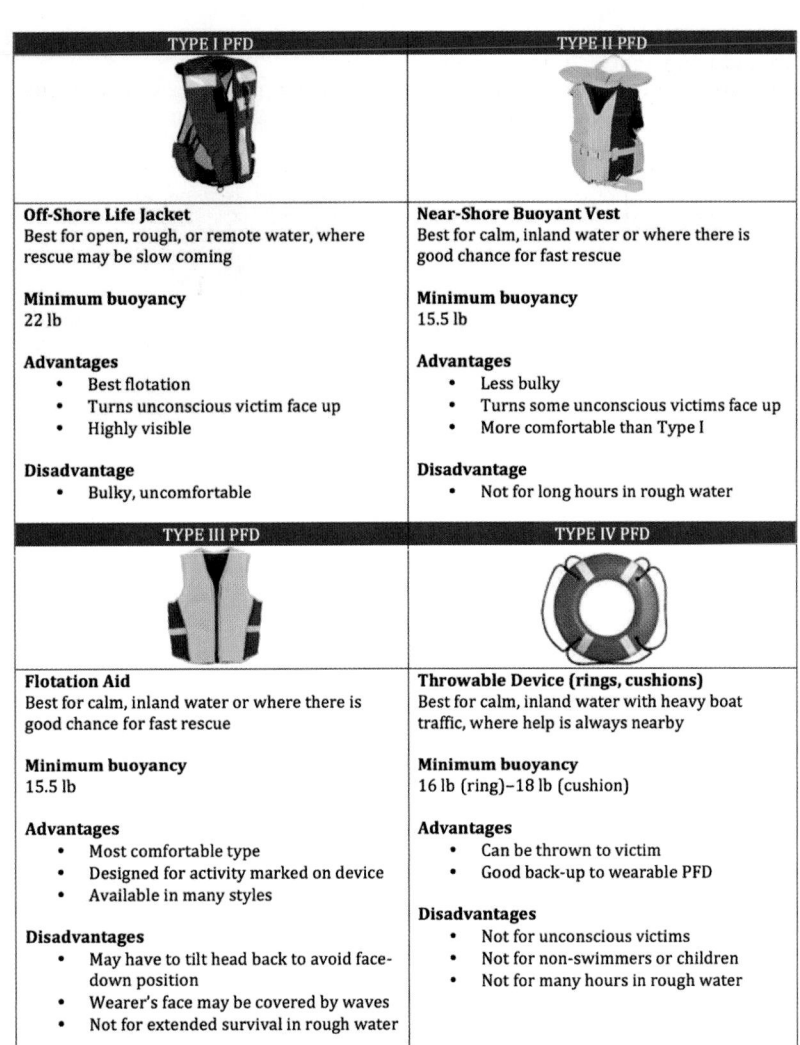

TYPE I PFD	TYPE II PFD
Off-Shore Life Jacket Best for open, rough, or remote water, where rescue may be slow coming **Minimum buoyancy** 22 lb **Advantages** • Best flotation • Turns unconscious victim face up • Highly visible **Disadvantage** • Bulky, uncomfortable	**Near-Shore Buoyant Vest** Best for calm, inland water or where there is good chance for fast rescue **Minimum buoyancy** 15.5 lb **Advantages** • Less bulky • Turns some unconscious victims face up • More comfortable than Type I **Disadvantage** • Not for long hours in rough water
TYPE III PFD	TYPE IV PFD
Flotation Aid Best for calm, inland water or where there is good chance for fast rescue **Minimum buoyancy** 15.5 lb **Advantages** • Most comfortable type • Designed for activity marked on device • Available in many styles **Disadvantages** • May have to tilt head back to avoid face-down position • Wearer's face may be covered by waves • Not for extended survival in rough water	**Throwable Device (rings, cushions)** Best for calm, inland water with heavy boat traffic, where help is always nearby **Minimum buoyancy** 16 lb (ring)–18 lb (cushion) **Advantages** • Can be thrown to victim • Good back-up to wearable PFD **Disadvantages** • Not for unconscious victims • Not for non-swimmers or children • Not for many hours in rough water

FIGURE 69-2 Current classification of the types of personal flotation devices.[104] *(Courtesy Justin Sempsrott, MD; adapted from Personal Flotation Device Manufacturers Association: pfdma.org/choosing/types.aspx.)*

and hypoxemia.[127] Areas of hypoxic pulmonary vasoconstriction further worsen shunting and increase pulmonary hypertension, leading to increased pressure across the alveolar-capillary basement membrane and further extravasation of fluid into the alveoli. In severe cases, patients present with ARDS, profound hypoxemia, noncardiogenic pulmonary edema, and a significant alveolar-arterial oxygen gradient. In profoundly ill patients, intubation and artificial ventilation may be required, increasing the risk of subsequent ventilator-associated lung injury and ventilator-associated pneumonia. With adequate resuscitation and treatment of patients without significant neurologic compromise, pulmonary dysfunction may initially be severe, but ultimate recovery of baseline lung function after drowning is the rule rather than the exception.[87,153]

Contamination by debris from petroleum products, sewage, sand, and organic matter is more common in saltwater and brackish water. Such debris accentuates the possibility of further inflammation and lung injury, which increases mortality rates. Inhalation of mud, sand, and other particulates may require fiberoptic bronchoalveolar lavage to cleanse the airways. Aspiration of microbes and related potential infections are discussed later. Figures 69-4 to 69-6 show examples of foreign body and contaminant aspiration after drowning.

Swimming-Induced Pulmonary Edema

Swimming-induced pulmonary edema has been described in several case reports as affecting scuba divers, Navy SEALS, and individuals (e.g., triathletes) who engage in strenuous surface swimming. The pathophysiology of this disorder is unclear, but proposed mechanisms include central blood pooling related to immersion and strenuous swimming resulting in elevated pulmonary artery pressure and diastolic dysfunction. Experimental equine data demonstrate increases in right ventricular and pulmonary arterial pressures with varying degrees of submersion in water, presumably resulting in capillary fracture. The case definition of swimming-induced pulmonary edema consists of acute hypoxemia during or immediately after a swimming event, a demonstrable chest radiograph abnormality with resolution within 48 hours in the absence of evidence of underlying pulmonary infection, and aspiration of water or attempted breathing against a closed glottis. The significance of this clinical entity is unclear, and it appears to be relatively uncommon.[147,209]

CENTRAL NERVOUS SYSTEM

The central nervous system (CNS) is highly sensitive to even brief periods of hypoxemia and is the organ system most susceptible to the negative effects of drowning. The major determinant of survival and long-term morbidity from drowning is the extent of CNS injury. Most submersion patients suffer a brief period of unconsciousness caused by cerebral hypoxia. Full neurologic recovery rarely occurs after 10 minutes of anoxia in normothermic conditions; hypothermia under controlled circumstances can prolong this to more than 40 minutes.[254] In most cases, prolonged

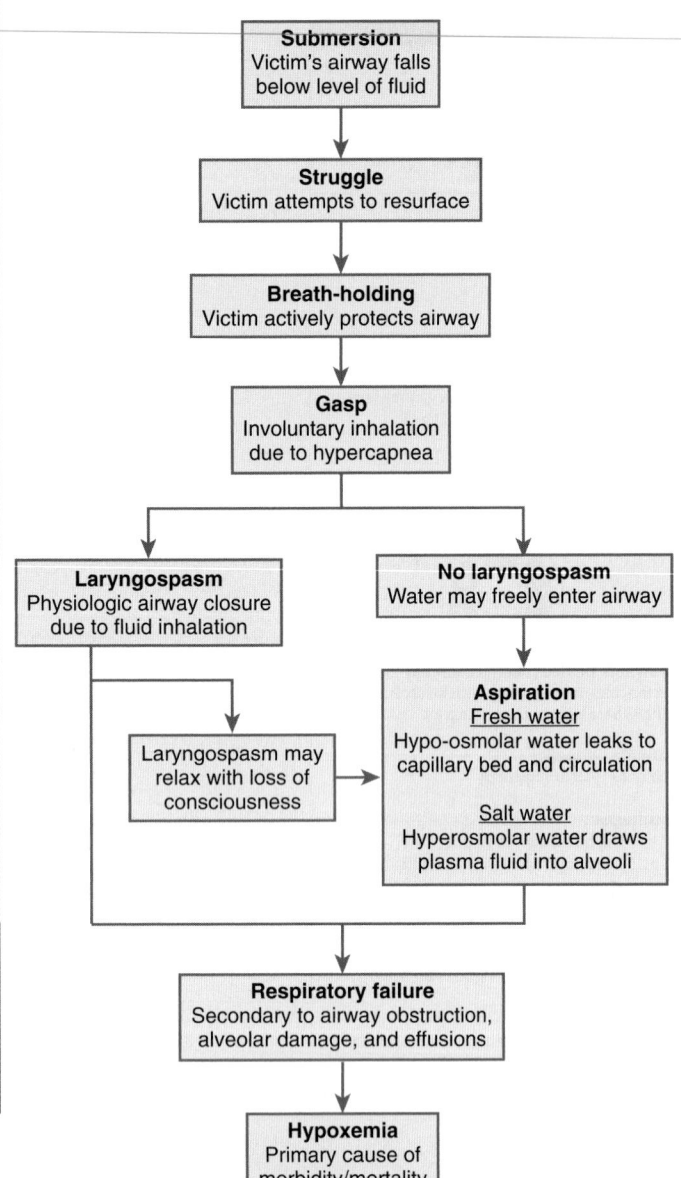

Submersion
Victim's airway falls below level of fluid

↓

Struggle
Victim attempts to resurface

↓

Breath-holding
Victim actively protects airway

↓

Gasp
Involuntary inhalation due to hypercapnea

↓

Laryngospasm
Physiologic airway closure due to fluid inhalation

No laryngospasm
Water may freely enter airway

Laryngospasm may relax with loss of consciousness

Aspiration
Fresh water
Hypo-osmolar water leaks to capillary bed and circulation

Salt water
Hyperosmolar water draws plasma fluid into alveoli

↓

Respiratory failure
Secondary to airway obstruction, alveolar damage, and effusions

↓

Hypoxemia
Primary cause of morbidity/mortality

FIGURE 69-3 Pathophysiologic events of the drowning process. *(Courtesy Andrew Schmidt, DO, MPH.)*

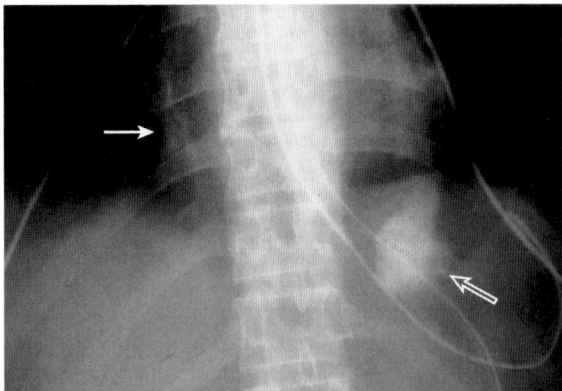

FIGURE 69-4 Chest radiograph taken in the emergency department, showing sand bronchograms in the right lower lobe *(solid arrow)*. Note sand within the gastric fundus *(open arrow)*. (From Dunagan DP, Cox JE, Chang MC, et al: Sand aspiration with near-drowning: radiographic and bronchoscopic findings, Am J Respir Crit Care Med 156:292, 1997.)

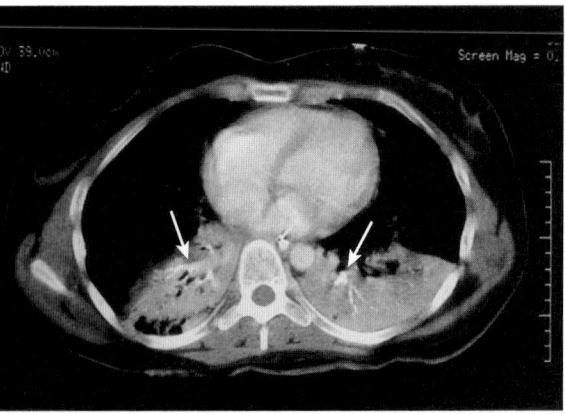

FIGURE 69-5 Chest CT scan showing bilateral sand bronchograms within the lower lobes *(arrows)* as well as significant air space opacification. *(From Dunagan DP, Cox JE, Chang MC, Haponik EF: Sand aspiration with near-drowning: radiographic and bronchoscopic findings, Am J Respir Crit Care Med 156:292, 1997.)*

submersion leads to death from neurologic asphyxia. Even with aggressive CPR and return of spontaneous circulation, drowning is associated with significant neurologic morbidity. Patients who present either awake or with blunted mental status have a better prognosis than those who present in a coma; the mortality rate in one study was as high as 34% among patients who were comatose on arrival at the hospital.[52,151] Of surviving patients, 10% to 23% demonstrated severe and persistent neurologic sequelae.[52,151] Prolonged hypoxemia and acidosis lead to neuronal cell death and demyelination.[26,110,143] Thus, the longer the submersion time, the more CNS damage suffered. Areas of high metabolic activity in the brain that are most susceptible to damage from hypoxemia include gray matter (more than white), vascular end zones, cerebral cortex, thalamus, basal ganglia, and hippocampus. Initial computed tomography (CT) scanning of the brain after submersion that shows any abnormalities of edema, loss of differentiation between gray and white matter, or focal infarct is highly predictive of a poor outcome. Conversely, a normal initial CT scan of the brain is of little prognostic value.[195,201]

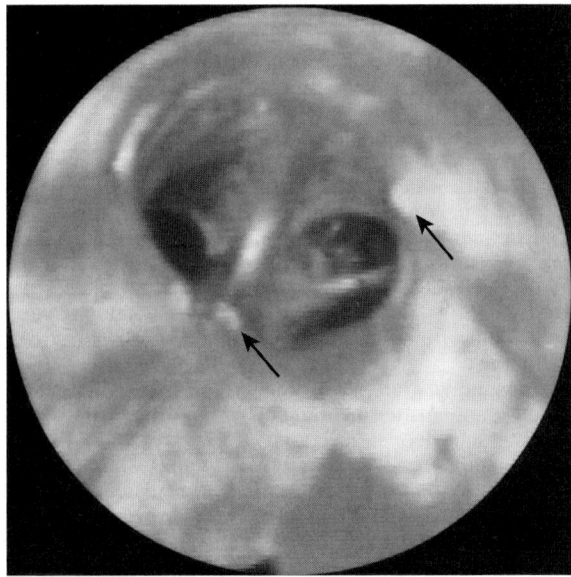

FIGURE 69-6 Fiberoptic bronchoscopy, demonstrating pieces of sand *(arrows)*, significant airway erythema, and inflammation following drowning and sand aspiration. *(From Dunagan DP, Cox JE, Chang MC, et al: Sand aspiration with near-drowning: Radiographic and bronchoscopic findings, Am J Respir Crit Care Med 156:292, 1997.)*

After the initial hypoxic event, subsequent reperfusion of damaged neurons can result in cell lysis, as well as interstitial and cerebral edema that are further worsened by systemic acidosis, hypotension, hyperglycemia, and, if present, seizure activity.[181] Hypothermia can increase cerebral tolerance of ischemia and hypoxemia. There are multiple case reports of survival with good neurologic outcomes after prolonged submersion, particularly among children. This is thought to result from decreased cerebral oxygen demand in the setting of hypothermia.[21,51,205,206,211,225] This requires rapidly induced hypothermia before the onset of anoxic damage, which occurs with sudden submersion into very cold water. Therapeutic hypothermia (TH) in cases of cardiac arrest has resulted in an improved neurologic outcome, and there are several case reports of complete neurologic recovery after TH in drowning patients.[13,245,250] Drowning patients often arrive hypothermic at temperatures below the 32° to 34°C (90° to 93°F) goal of TH. This is an area of active research, and in the absence of randomized control trials of TH in non–ventricular fibrillation cardiac arrest, the decision to initiate TH is based on expert consensus and theoretical benefit. This is discussed further in the hypothermia section.

CARDIOVASCULAR SYSTEM

Cardiac rhythm, output, and function are affected by hypoxemia and acidosis, with more severe manifestations in prolonged submersion.[162] Dysrhythmias may occur as a result of acidosis and hypoxemia. Decreased cardiac output may result from direct effects of hypoxemia on the myocardium. Pulmonary hypertension caused by aspirated fluid can result in right ventricular overload, and further decrease cardiac output. Patients with underlying cardiac disease may be more susceptible to the effects of hypoxemia on myocardial function. A sudden cardiac dysrhythmia may precipitate submersion and drowning in patients with preexisting cardiac disease, although during postmortem analysis, this can be difficult to discern from submersion-related injury.

HEMATOLOGIC AND ELECTROLYTE DISTURBANCES

Prior data supporting the notion of systemic electrolyte disturbances from aspiration of saltwater are of little practicality for treatment of human drowning patients, because such derangements are rarely seen. Massive (i.e., > 22 mL/kg) instillation of saltwater in animal models resulted in disturbances in serum sodium, chloride, magnesium, and calcium,[46,255,260] presumably as a result of osmotic gradients across the alveolar epithelium. Humans who die by drowning aspirate less than 4 mL/kg of fluid volume.[149,152,156] Similarly, canine models have demonstrated gross hemolysis, resulting in hyperkalemia and disseminated intravascular coagulation after large-volume aspiration; however, clinically relevant changes in hematocrit and hemoglobin levels are rarely seen in human drowning patients.[153] Therefore, routine observation and laboratory analysis with treatment for measured abnormalities are all that are indicated in the hospital setting.

HYPOTHERMIA

For patients who do not drown immediately upon entering cold water, subsequent fatal or nonfatal drowning may result from hypothermia.[48,100] Water at 91.4°F (33°C) is thermally neutral, where heat loss equals heat production for a swimmer without clothes; water any colder than this leads to ongoing heat loss. The thermal conductivity of cold water is 25 to 30 times that of air.[100,130] Even in only moderately cold water, hypothermia may ensue rapidly and lead to a loss of consciousness and subsequent drowning. This is particularly true in children, who have less subcutaneous fat and relatively greater body surface area compared with adults.[21,49,84,94] Survival is unlikely after 60 minutes in water that is cooler than 32°F (0°C); however, people who have not submerged can survive for up to 6 hours at a water temperature of 59°F (15°C) (Table 69-1).[47]

TABLE 69-1 Estimated Survival Times in Cold Water

Water Temperature	Exhaustion or Unconsciousness in	Expected Survival Time
21-27°C (70-80°F)	3-12 hr	3 hr to indefinitely
16-21°C (60-70°F)	2-7 hr	2-40 hr
10-16°C (50-60°F)	1-2 hr	1-6 hr
4-10°C (40-50°F)	30-60 min	1-3 hr
0-4°C (32.5-40°F)	15-30 min	30-90 min
<0°C (<32°F)	<15 min	<15-45 min

Courtesy U.S. Search and Rescue Task Force: ussartf.org/cold_water_survival.htm.

There are many factors that affect an individual's response to cold-water immersion. Dramatic recoveries after prolonged hypothermia have been documented in children and adults.[186,211,225,259] These case reports of increased survival are associated with ice cold (< 6°C) water that rapidly induces the protective effects of the mammalian diving reflex. *Gradual* onset of hypothermia while drowning worsens outcomes. Therapeutic hypothermia (TH) is an area of active research in post cardiac arrest, where it has been shown to decrease cerebral metabolic demand and improve neurologic outcomes.[109] Protocols for TH were adopted by the American Heart Association in 2002 and by the European Resuscitation Council in 2003 for out-of-hospital cardiac arrest patients. Case reports of survival after submersion in cold water with profound hypothermia have provoked questions as to whether this would provide the same physiologic effect of neuroprotection for drowning patients who become rapidly hypothermic, and might warrant maintenance of a low core temperature in comatose drowning patients.[127,241] A panel of experts during the World Congress on Drowning in 2002 concluded that "drowning victims with restoration of adequate spontaneous circulation who remain comatose should not be actively rewarmed to temperature values above 32° to 34°C (90° to 93°F). If core temperature exceeds 34°C (93.2°F), hypothermia at 32° to 34°C (90° to 93°F) should be achieved as soon as possible and sustained for 12 to 24 hours."[245] There are several cases of full neurologic recovery after submersion with subsequent TH.[155,242] Optimal temperature management for submersion patients remains an area of active discussion.

The pathophysiologic response to hypothermia ranges from shivering that contributes to increasing the metabolic rate, to coma, massive metabolic acidosis, and spontaneous ventricular fibrillation. Patients progress from mild hypothermia, characterized by shivering, increased metabolic rate, and tachycardia, to profound hypothermia at varying rates, depending on surrounding water temperature, protection and clothing, duration of exposure, and position in the water (Figure 69-7).

Though not specifically drowning or hypothermia, in some cases, patients suffer from immersion syndrome, which involves sudden death from bradycardia, tachycardia, or ventricular fibrillation and cardiac arrest from cold-water exposure before onset of systemic hypothermia.[178] Immersion in cold water (< 5°C [< 41°F]) produces a rapid fall in core body temperature. Heat loss through convection and conduction is further compounded by increased muscle activity during swimming and struggling.

The "diving reflex" in diving mammals is a vestigial but inducible reflex in humans that may contribute to survival in cases of prolonged submersion and subsequent hypothermia.[49,84,95,141] The reflex is activated by vagal stimulation from cutaneous receptors that respond to cold by shunting blood to the brain and cardiac muscles and away from the skin, extremities, and splanchnic vascular beds, along with bradycardia and a decreased metabolic rate. Bradycardia and vasoconstriction in all vascular beds (except those serving the heart and brain) result in the preserved mean arterial pressure for those organs and overall decreased cardiac output. The reflex may be inducible in only 15% to 30% of humans,[22] but may be a contributing factor for persons who survive drowning.[64,84,121] However, some discount its role.

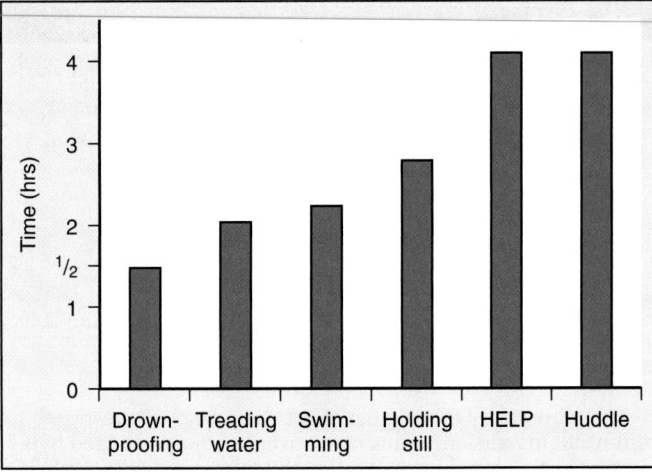

FIGURE 69-7 Survival times in cool (10° C [50° F]) water using various techniques in several situations. HELP, heat escape lessening posture. *(Data from Collis ML: Survival behaviour in cold water immersion. In Proceedings of the Cold Water Symposium, Toronto, Royal Life-Saving Society of Canada, 1976.)*

Although the mechanism is not completely understood, there are researchers that propose "autonomic conflict" as an additional mechanism of death during immersion in cold water. During submersion in cold water with breath-holding, the sympathetic nervous system is activated during the cold shock response, and the parasympathetic nervous system is activated through the diving reflex. This simultaneous activation of both limbs of the nervous system has triggered dysrhythmias in healthy human volunteers, which has been extrapolated as a mechanism of death through fatal dysrhythmias in drowning patients.[19a,53,146,229,230]

Immersion hypothermia occurs as the core temperature falls. It is discussed in detail in Chapter 8.

MANAGEMENT: THE ELEMENT OF TIME

Time plays a significant role in determining the ultimate outcome of rescue of a drowning patient. The duration of anoxic time may be unknown or unreliable for a variety of reasons, including an unwitnessed event or unrecognized call for help (e.g., the waving of hands or thrashing about may be confused with play activity). Witnesses may exhibit panic and frantic behaviors, further impairing effective rescue.

Time is of the essence. The published world record for conscious breath-holding while underwater is 17 minutes and 4 seconds,[228] and it should be noted that this feat was achieved after months of training under highly controlled circumstances, which included extensive pre-oxygenation. Most humans are unable to stay conscious underwater or avoid aspiration after a few minutes. Irreversible neurologic deficits are common after 4 to 5 minutes.[51] The longest documented period of submersion time in an unconscious patient with survival is 66 minutes[24] (a pediatric patient in cold water). Hypothermia may offer a protective benefit and prolong the time during which resuscitation can still be successful. There are case reports in which patients survived after 40 minutes of submersion in cold water with complete or nearly complete recovery.[211,225,259] The lowest recorded temperature in a human with subsequent survival and neurologic recovery was taken from a Norwegian skier trapped in a frigid river, who had a core body temperature of 13.7° C (56.6° F) when extricated.[77] Table 69-1 describes time parameters surrounding expected survival at various water temperatures.

An extremely rapid response is required in some cases, whereas no immediate response or body recovery is required in others. This decision depends on the characteristics of the patient, presumed length of submersion, possible associated traumatic injuries, and water temperature. It is unnecessary to put rescuers at risk to retrieve a drowned patient whose survival would defy physiologic reality. The initial evaluation and total time of submersion should help clinicians determine the appropriate duration of resuscitative efforts on a drowned patient with potentially significant morbidity or brain death.

CLINICAL PRESENTATION: A CASE HISTORY

This case demonstrates many of the clinical features of drowning patients. The patient was a 52-year-old previously healthy male who worked the night shift on a barge in the brackish waters of the Duwamish Slough near Puget Sound. One night, he tripped on an uncoiled rope on the deck and fell 20 feet into the water. Despite struggling to swim, he lost his orientation and drifted under the barge. Another worker saw him fall and drift under the boat, so he astutely threw his flashlight into the water away from the side of the boat. The patient saw the light, desperately swam to it, and was subsequently pulled from the water by coworkers. His total submersion time was approximately 2 minutes.

Emergency personnel transported the patient to Harborview Medical Center. In the emergency department, he was anxious but alert and oriented, and mildly short of breath with a cough. His vital signs were as follows: respiratory rate, 24 breaths/min; pulse, 115 beats/min; blood pressure, 145/100 mm Hg; and temperature, 36° C (96.5° F). The remainder of his examination was normal except for diffuse rhonchi throughout both lung fields. Arterial blood gas levels were as follows: pH, 7.48; arterial partial pressure of carbon dioxide ($PaCO_2$), 32 mm Hg; and arterial partial pressure of oxygen (PaO_2), 58 mm Hg on a face mask with high-flow oxygen. A chest radiograph showed a normal cardiac silhouette with diffuse bilateral patchy opacities. He was admitted to the intensive care unit for observation.

Within the first hour, his gas exchange worsened despite adequate alveolar ventilation. He was endotracheally intubated and placed on mechanical ventilation in the volume ventilation mode. Despite high concentrations of oxygen, his gas exchange capabilities further deteriorated, and he was given a trial of positive end-expiratory pressure (PEEP). At 15 cm H_2O pressure, the patient's blood pressure fell to 76/52 mm Hg. Volume resuscitation was increased. A pulmonary artery catheter was placed to monitor cardiac function. During the initial PEEP trial, pulmonary capillary wedge pressures were low (i.e., < 10 mm Hg). The cardiac index fell from 2.8 to 1.8 L/min/m² body surface area after the PEEP was increased from 10 to 15 cm H_2O. PEEP was therefore reduced to 10 cm H_2O and more vigorous volume resuscitation was instituted, after which the cardiac index and blood pressure improved so that PEEP could safely be increased, which was necessary to maintain adequate oxygenation.

Over the next 6 days, the patient's lung compliance initially decreased and then increased; his chest radiograph worsened and then slowly improved; and his gas exchange improved so that he was extubated on hospital day 10. It was another 2 months before he was able to be physically active, and he had dyspnea on exertion for approximately 6 months after his accident. At hospital discharge, pulmonary function tests showed a moderate decrease in both vital capacity and total lung capacity, mild obstruction of airflow, and severely decreased diffusion capacity for carbon monoxide. Over the next 6 months, the patient's vital capacity and total lung capacity returned to normal, but his diffusion capacity remained mildly decreased.

This case demonstrates a number of important features of drowning with aspiration and respiratory failure. First, the patient was extremely lucky that his fall was witnessed and subsequent rescue was rapid, limiting exposure and submersion times. He arrived at the hospital conscious and alert, one of the best prognostic signs, and had no comorbid conditions. His clinical course was consistent with acute lung injury from aspiration of brackish water, and the initial worsening and subsequent improvement of lung mechanics and gas exchange were typical of ARDS. Fortunately, he had no other organ failure, and his recovery was unremarkable.

There is a spectrum of types of morbidity from drowning, ranging from asymptomatic to unresponsive, apneic, and pulseless. Classification systems based on observations from first-aid providers assist with determination of which patients require hospitalization.[221]

ON-SCENE MANAGEMENT

The scene at drowning incidents is often chaotic. Patients are not usually found flailing in the water; rather, they are more commonly found floating on or motionless underneath the surface. Rescue attempts must always take into consideration the safety of rescuers to avoid creating additional victims. Safety devices should be used to tow the patient, or life preservers should be thrown to people in trouble before a human lifesaver enters the water. Persons without current training in water-rescue techniques specific to the conditions (e.g., open water, swift water, ice) should never enter the water to rescue a drowning patient. Well-intentioned but ill-advised heroic efforts can create additional victims and compound the tragedy.[68]

Upon arrival at the scene, accurate timing and documentation of the course of events, including vital signs, clinical state, and environmental conditions, should begin.[19] The scene description, estimation of time of submersion, type and temperature of the water and air, and events during transport to the hospital may be critical information. If multiple patients or rescuers are present, the accident scene may be disorganized, so it is imperative that someone assume a leadership role. After the patient is out of the water, basic life support should be instituted. Evaluation for concomitant trauma and associated injuries should be assessed once the patient is out of the water. Findings and circumstances consistent with child abuse, seizures, cardiac arrhythmias, trauma, and other medical issues should be ascertained.

Hypoxemia is the most significant consequence of submersion, so immediate attention to the airway and oxygenation is of paramount importance to the outcome. Appropriate resuscitative measures should be instituted immediately after extrication from the water and continued by rescuers at the scene. Although there are various products and training techniques designed to promote rescue breathing in the water, this is difficult in the best of circumstances, and is generally discouraged except when performed by trained rescuers (Figure 69-8). Rapid extrication from the water is the priority to ensure that CPR and rescue breathing are adequate. In-water rescue breathing should only be instituted when rapid extrication is not feasible. Transport to an emergency facility with ongoing CPR should take place unless resuscitation is determined to be futile or successful.[8] Concomitant hypothermia sometimes makes clinical determination in the field difficult at best.

THE ASYMPTOMATIC PATIENT: GRADES 0 AND 1

Patients with no other comorbid conditions who have been rescued from the water and who are alert, with a clear chest examination on auscultation, no respiratory distress, and with or without coughing, may not need further medical care but still present a dilemma. Although there are published reports of delayed complications in drowning patients who were initially minimally symptomatic, these case reports have recently come under scrutiny. More recent studies show that patients may have minimal symptoms that become progressively worse over the next 5 to 8 hours, but patients who are truly asymptomatic do not show delayed complications. Minimally symptomatic patients should be advised to seek care if they develop worsening symptoms over the ensuing 8 hours.*

Hypothermia is often difficult to ascertain at the scene, so it may be prudent to have the person evaluated, even if only briefly, at a medical facility.[8] Conscious and cooperative patients should be protected against hypothermia with passive warming techniques, protected from wind, and offered dry clothes and blankets. If the person remains asymptomatic with normal vital signs and stable arterial oxygen saturation (if testing is available) on ambient air for 10 to 15 minutes, then it is not likely that the person will require further medical care.

THE SYMPTOMATIC PATIENT: GRADES 2, 3, AND 4

All submersion patients requiring on-scene intervention or resuscitation, or showing signs of distress (e.g., anxiety, tachypnea, dyspnea, syncope, persistent cough, presence of foam in the mouth or nose, changes in vital signs), should be evacuated or transported to a hospital for evaluation.

Protection of the airway to ensure oxygenation and ventilation is the first priority. Maintaining perfusion to reverse the metabolic consequences of acidosis comes next. The airway should be protected from aspiration by placing the patient in a lateral recumbent (i.e., recovery) position if possible. Vomiting is common with submersion, and aspiration can worsen lung injury. Measures should be taken to prevent hypothermia and shivering. Rescuers must maintain vigilance and treat cardiac dysrhythmias that may arise as a result of hypoxemia. The management actions listed in Table 69-2 can then be considered. Routine cervical spine immobilization is unnecessary and should be reserved for patients with a known or suspected significant mechanism of injury, or worrisome clinical examination (see Cervical Spine Injury, later).[246]

THE PATIENT IN RESPIRATORY OR CARDIOPULMONARY ARREST: GRADES 5 AND 6

Approximately half of drowning resuscitations involve bystander CPR.[19,192] Initiation of immediate ventilatory support and early CPR, if indicated, results in a better prognosis and outcomes.[19,50,64,81,94,181,185,216] In an 11-year study of pediatric drowning incidents in Houston, Texas, the biggest predictor of survival was prompt CPR by lay responders.[249] Initiation of chest compressions while the patient remains in the water is ineffective, delays extrication, and may further endanger the patient and rescuer. Effective CPR cannot realistically be started until the patient is out of the water and on a solid surface. Alternatively, rescue breathing should be initiated as soon as the patient's airway can be opened, even if in the water; this intervention improved survival rates threefold in one series of cases[222] (see Figure 69-8). The success of this intervention often depends on a well-trained and skilled rescuer, but is very useful in the appropriate setting. An example would be a child who is being pulled unconscious toward a boat or land in calm water. The extra few seconds taken to provide rescue breaths can provide critical oxygenation that may delay otherwise imminent cardiac arrest caused by hypoxemia.

When the individual is out of the water, either mouth-to-mouth or mouth-to-nose ventilation can be used.[8] If it is available at the scene, supplemental oxygen should be initiated as soon as possible. If the patient is spontaneously breathing, a face mask with a reservoir bag of approximately 2.5 L can be used. If a

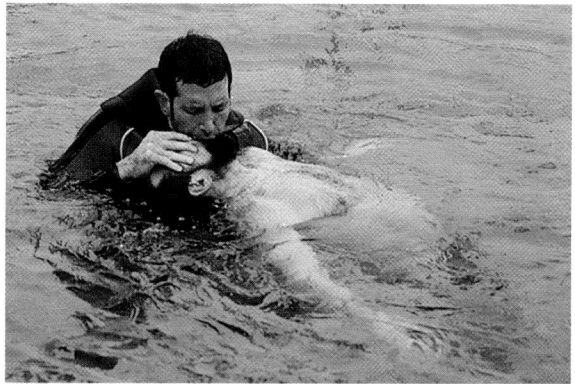

FIGURE 69-8 Mouth-to-mouth ventilation in the water is difficult in the best of circumstances. *(Courtesy Alan Steinman, MD.)*

*References 42a, 87, 111, 134a, 148a, 171a, 178a, 181a, 187a, 198a, 206a, 221.

TABLE 69-2 Prehospital Management and Classification of Drowning Patients

Grade	The Asymptomatic Patient		The Symptomatic Patient			The Patient in Respiratory or Cardiopulmonary Arrest	
	0	**1**	**2**	**3**	**4**	**5**	**6**
Mortality (%)	0	0	0.6	5.2	19	44	93
Pulmonary Examination	No cough or dyspnea	Normal auscultation with cough	Rales, small amount of foam	Acute pulmonary edema	Acute pulmonary edema	Respiratory arrest	Cardiopulmonary arrest
Cardiovascular Findings	Radial pulses	Radial pulses	Radial pulses	Radial pulses	Hypotension	Hypotension	
On-scene Management	Release at scene with education	Rest, rewarm, reassure, and release	Oxygen via nasal cannula; observe for 6-24 hr	Oxygen via nonrebreathing mask; advanced cardiac life support	Oxygen via nonrebreathing mask; advanced cardiac life support	Load and go	
Transport	No	No	Transport or observation	Yes	Rapid	Rapid	
En Route Management			Vital signs	Vital signs	Possible endotracheal tube and manage pressure	Advanced cardiac life support	
Hospital Management			Emergency department or overnight observation	Admission for observation	Intensive care unit	Intensive care unit	Intensive care unit

Courtesy Justin Sempsrott, MD. Adapted from Szpilman D: Near-drowning and drowning classification: a proposal to stratify morality based on the analysis of 1,831 cases, *Chest* 112:660, 1997.

nonrebreathing mask, portable positive end-expiratory pressure (PEEP) valve, or portable continuous positive airway pressure (CPAP) device is available, oxygen should be delivered at a high flow rate (i.e., 10 to 15 L/min). Using CPAP and PEEP in the field remains an area of controversy. Multiple emergency medical services (EMS) systems have successfully used this modality for management of acute pulmonary edema in congestive heart failure.[227,245] To date, there are no randomized controlled studies of the application of either prehospital PEEP or CPAP for drowning patients, and only several case reports of CPAP application for drowning.[59] A CPAP mask should be used cautiously if there is any concern about vomiting or loss of airway protective reflexes.

Draining water from the lungs of submersion patients dates back to the 17th and 18th centuries, but is no longer recommended. The Dutch method consisted of rolling subjects over a barrel; another method involved flinging subjects over a horse, which was then made to trot. In 1975, the Heimlich maneuver was introduced for victims of choking, which was subsequently recommended as a treatment for drowning patients. This maneuver is no longer recommended for drowning.[202] For patients who have swallowed large amounts of water, gastric distention can interfere with ventilation by increasing intraabdominal pressure. In such instances, gastric decompression by nasogastric tube is recommended.[7,198,202] Digital or visual examination for foreign bodies should be done, and if one is present, it should be removed with a swipe or grasp of the fingers. Foreign bodies (e.g., sand, beach flotsam, seaweed) were reported in up to 54% of cases in one series of surf beach-related submersions.[140]

Vomiting during resuscitation has been reported in 86% of cases involving drowning patients receiving CPR.[140] If vomiting occurs, the patient should be rolled onto the side or have the head turned to the side and vomitus removed with a cloth or finger-sweep maneuver.[181] If spinal injury is of concern, the patient should be logrolled, maintaining linear integrity of the head, neck, and torso.[8] The risk of aspiration from vomiting may be reduced by application of cricoid pressure during endotracheal intubation.[178] Because most beaches, riverbanks, boat ramps, and other waterway access points are sloped, patients should be placed perpendicular to the incline so that the head and feet are at the same level.[20]

When the patient is out of the water and the airway and breathing have been addressed, the presence or absence of adequate circulation should be ascertained. In cases of hypothermia or hypotension, a pulse may be difficult to identify. If ventilation or cardiac function is impaired, chest compressions should be initiated as soon as the patient is removed from the water. For patients who are more than 1 year old, an automated external defibrillator (AED) may be used to evaluate the heart rhythm. AED electrode pads with pediatric attenuation should be used for children who are between 1 and 8 years old.[8] However, some believe that there is no major role for an AED in this setting[19,192] because ventricular fibrillation is rare after drowning in an otherwise healthy patient, and a priority should be placed on oxygenation and ventilation over defibrillation.[19] If the field rescue team is capable of advanced life support (ALS), then cardiac monitoring, intravenous or intraosseous access, fluids, and medications should be administered according to ALS protocols. Basic life support or advanced cardiac life support should continue until the patient's core body temperature is more than 30°C (86°F).[8] Table 69-2 shows a classification scheme for drowning field assessment and management.

CERVICAL SPINE INJURY

Cervical spine injury is rare in drowning except in high-impact accidents, such as high-speed boating accidents, surf-related injuries, and diving accidents.[107,246] Evaluation of the breathing pattern and breath sounds is critical, because abnormal respiratory patterns can indicate cervical spine injury unrelated to direct pulmonary injury from submersion. Unless a focal neurologic deficit, significant mechanism of injury, altered mental status/unreliable examination, or midline neck or back tenderness (or a distracting injury preventing patient identification of such tenderness) is present, routine spine immobilization is unnecessary and may

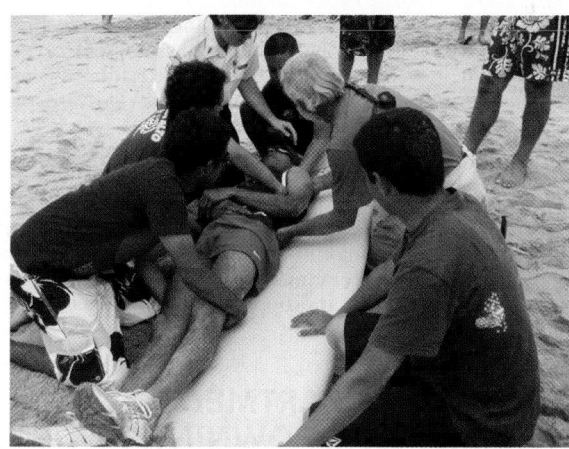

FIGURE 69-9 Surfboards can be used for spinal immobilization. *(Courtesy Lifeguards Without Borders.)*

delay lifesaving resuscitation measures.[107,246] In cases in which neck injury is likely based on the mechanism of injury or suggested by physical examination, appropriate immobilization should be considered.[246] In the wilderness water setting, surfboards, paddles, or small watercraft may be used to immobilize and transport the patient (Figure 69-9). Evaluation for additional fractures or internal or intracranial injuries should be considered for any patient with a cervical spine injury.[64,95,181]

THE OBVIOUSLY DEAD OR STILL-SUBMERGED PATIENT

Some persons may appear to be dead when they are retrieved from the water. They are unresponsive with a normal temperature, demonstrate postmortem lividity, and may be asystolic and apneic. If CPR has been in progress for more than 25 to 30 minutes with no return of vital signs, persons who are retrieved from warm water may be considered dead at the scene.[45,67,194] However, because of case reports of neurologically intact survival after submersion for more than 60 minutes in icy cold (< 6°C) water,[43,63,75,105] rescue crews must start and continue life support measures for all persons who are not obviously dead or who are hypothermic. After 1 hour of submersion in warm water, scene rescue efforts should transition to body recovery efforts.[168] Many drowning deaths become medical examiner cases, because the possibility of foul play must be investigated, and appropriate local authorities should be contacted.

TERMINATING RESUSCITATION EFFORTS

The decision to end CPR in drowning cases is an emotionally charged issue. In remote wilderness settings, it may become necessary to terminate resuscitation efforts on scene; this decision should be based on the distance to definitive care, time the patient has been submerged, and condition of the patient. The standard of care in the field is to terminate resuscitation efforts if there is no return of spontaneous circulation after 25 to 30 minutes of chest compressions or if the patient was submerged for more than 1 hour[67,168] (see Prognosis and Termination of Resuscitation, later).

EN ROUTE TO DEFINITIVE CARE

During transport, the goal is optimization of oxygenation, ventilation, and perfusion. Supplemental oxygen should be delivered by a simple or nonrebreathing face mask or nasal cannula. A pulse oximeter should be used to monitor arterial oxygen saturation, but rescuers should recognize that pulse oximetry might be inaccurate as a result of hypothermia and peripheral vasoconstriction. Body heat loss should be minimized by keeping the patient dry, out of the wind, and covered with blankets. Although shivering is a good prognostic sign, it increases tissue oxygen demand and caloric expenditure, and should be avoided by warming the patient, removing wet clothing, and protecting the patient from wind and weather. Detailed assessment of neurologic status with attention to fluctuations in the patient's Glasgow Coma Scale score should be made repeatedly. The use of ALS medications should follow standard protocols. The core body temperature and acid-base status of the patient may not be known in the field, making effects and metabolism of drugs unpredictable. Drugs should be used only when absolutely necessary, preferably in a hospital setting. If active rewarming techniques using cardiopulmonary bypass or extracorporeal membrane oxygenation are anticipated, EMS protocols dictating transport of the patient to appropriately equipped facilities are recommended.

EMERGENCY DEPARTMENT TREATMENT OF DROWNING PATIENTS

Upon arrival at the medical facility, the patient's airway, breathing, circulation, and mental status should be reassessed. Patients who initially presented with minimal symptoms may develop worsening pulmonary function over the next several hours.

Box 69-3 outlines the emergency department care of drowning patients. Rapid correction of hypoxemia and acidosis are the most important priorities. Although severe drowning cases are true medical emergencies, if patients reach the emergency department before cardiac arrest and are given timely and effective treatment, nearly all will recover without significant neurologic or pulmonary sequelae.[50,117,212,213]

Because of the potential delay in symptom manifestations, even asymptomatic patients should be observed for a minimum of 4 hours. For asymptomatic patients, if there is a history of significant or prolonged submersion, clinicians may choose to

---

BOX 69-3 Emergency Department Management of Drowning Patients

Check Airway/Ventilation
Adequate ventilation
  Supplemental oxygen: nonrebreathing mask at 12-15 L/min or via demand valve
Inadequate ventilation
  Borderline patients: consider CPAP
  Comatose patients or those with PaO_2 < 90 mm Hg on 15 L/min nonrebreathing mask or $PaCO_2$ > 45 mm Hg: endotracheal intubation with PEEP as needed

Diagnostics
Arterial blood gas studies for mechanically ventilated patients, SpO_2 monitor for spontaneously breathing patients
Chest radiograph
Cardiac monitor
Cervical spine radiograph/trauma evaluation if indicated by mechanism
Assess for hypothermia, hypoglycemia, electrolyte abnormalities

Further Interventions
Intravenous access, hydration
Nasogastric tube if significant aspiration/ingestion of water

Disposition
Admit
  All patients with abnormal vital signs, abnormal radiologic findings, respiratory symptoms, or abnormal findings on blood gas measurements
  ICU admission preferred for all patients not being admitted for simple observation
  Rehydration and ventilatory stabilization should be underway prior to ICU admission
Criteria for discharge in 4-6 hours
  Asymptomatic (no cough or respiratory complaints)
  No vital sign or examination aberrancies (in particular, normal SpO_2 on room air, normal lung auscultation, normal Glasgow Coma Scale score)
  No diagnostic abnormalities (normal chest x-ray)

---

obtain arterial blood gas measurements to look for a widened alveolar-arterial gradient, or they may obtain chest radiographs to inspect for occult injury.[121,150,177,183] A patient with a normal chest radiograph taken on admission may have a markedly abnormal radiograph several hours later[143]; regardless of the patient's clinical appearance, a baseline chest radiograph should be obtained.[121] Asymptomatic patients may be safely discharged from the emergency department if they have a normal Glasgow Coma Scale score, respiratory effort, chest radiograph, and oxygen saturation on room air after 4 to 8 hours of observation.*

Patients may present with a range of respiratory symptoms, from mild cough to profound hypoxemia and respiratory distress. Symptomatic patients may complain of cough, sore throat, chest tightness, and/or shortness of breath. The first and most important step is to evaluate the airway and breathing to address hypoxemia and acidosis. Even if the patient is adequately breathing with spontaneous and unassisted ventilations, the patient should still be provided with supplemental oxygen.

If the patient is unable to maintain effective spontaneous breathing (to prevent hypoxemia) and ventilation, CPAP or endotracheal intubation should be considered. Severe hypoxemia and intubation are not unusual with drowning; in one series, 53% of drowning patients had severe hypoxemia, and 36% required mechanical ventilation.[153] Serial arterial blood gas measurements may be helpful to determine the degree of hypoxemia and whether patients are improving without advanced airway management. Arterial blood gas measurements will determine (1) alveolar ventilation (i.e., acceptable $PaCO_2$ and pH); (2) gas exchange (i.e., PaO_2 > 60 mmHg on supplemental oxygen); and (3) perfusion (i.e., no metabolic acidosis). CPAP can be used in a brief trial before proceeding to endotracheal intubation in awake patients with low PaO_2 levels despite administration of high-flow oxygen. If arterial blood gas parameters cannot be maintained and the patient is not improving with less invasive measures, including CPAP, mechanical ventilation should be initiated using the volume-ventilation mode and a high level of supplemental oxygen. Other criteria for endotracheal intubation include a patient who is unable to handle his or her secretions or who has a seriously altered mental status. After advanced airway management, consider nasogastric or orogastric tube placement to prevent aspiration of gastric contents. The core temperature should be monitored. All patients with abnormal vital signs, hypoxemia, abnormal chest radiographs, or any respiratory distress should be admitted to the hospital for, at a minimum, observation.

IN-HOSPITAL TREATMENT OF DROWNING

Although the complexity of patient management is as variable as the condition of the patient, clinicians facing complex management decisions should keep in mind that nearly all successful clinical interventions focus on correction of acidosis, hypoxemia, and hypoperfusion. The following paragraphs present a systems-based discussion of in-hospital management of drowning.

From an epidemiologic and medical systems standpoint, the 2002 First World Congress on Drowning in Amsterdam made the following recommendations regarding in-hospital treatment of drowning[73]:

- Registration of drowning patients and collection of clinical data regarding in-hospital resuscitation and treatment of complications of drowning are recommended.
- Development of a uniform reporting system to register and collect these data (similar to the Utstein-style set of guidelines established for the uniform reporting of cardiac arrest) is desirable. Lack of standard definition and outcome criteria hinder the exchange of data across medical and basic science specialties. In 1990, a group of researchers studying

---

*References 37, 42a, 87, 111, 134a, 148a, 171a, 178a, 181a, 187a, 198a, 206a, 213, 221.

out-of-hospital cardiac arrest met at the Utstein Abbey in Norway and set forth consensus criteria for uniform reporting of data related to cardiac arrest. A similar consensus was reached at the 2002 World Congress on Drowning, which set forth the criteria for reporting drowning data and recommended that only three outcomes be recognized: death, no morbidity, and morbidity (this was further categorized as moderately disabled, severely disabled, vegetative state/coma, and brain death).[111]

- Hospital treatment of severe drowning patients should be concentrated in specialized centers.

PULMONARY MANAGEMENT

Therapy usually begins in the field with oxygen given by nasal cannula or face mask. Progression to a nonrebreathing mask or to noninvasive positive-pressure ventilation is determined by the initial response to oxygen therapy, respiratory symptoms, arterial oxygen saturation, and arterial blood gas analysis. When the decision has been made to begin mechanical ventilation, low tidal volumes (i.e., 6 mL/kg) should be used initially, and PEEP started at a low level (i.e., 5 to 10 cm H_2O) if a PaO_2 of more than 60 mm Hg cannot be maintained with a fraction of inspired oxygen of 0.6. Positive-pressure strategies such as PEEP should be used judiciously, because higher intrathoracic pressure may impair venous return and result in hypotension, decreased cardiac output, and further compromise of systemic oxygen delivery. Caution should be used if there is any concern about vomiting before applying a CPAP mask. However, at appropriate levels and when needed, PEEP can be remarkably effective for recruiting edematous or collapsed alveoli, and can thus improve gas exchange and oxygenation in patients with atelectasis, substantial aspiration, and pulmonary edema. Volume ventilation is preferred to ensure that adequate alveolar ventilation (i.e., approximately 10 L/min in adults) is delivered, reflected by acceptable pH and $PaCO_2$ levels.

A feature of drowning is cough and respiratory irritation caused by inhaled water and particles in the tracheobronchial tree. Cough and bronchospasm can impair airflow, resulting in $\dot{V}/\dot{Q}$ mismatch and hypoxemia. Aerosolized albuterol, which is a relatively selective β_2-adrenergic agonist, is the initial treatment of choice for bronchospasm. It can be administered to spontaneously breathing patients via face mask or to intubated patients using a T-piece adaptor. Ipratropium via nebulizer may be added to decrease bronchial smooth muscle spasm.[17,172,200]

Discontinuation of ventilatory support should follow standard principles. The timing may be influenced by surfactant regeneration, which is a situation uncommon in other mechanically ventilated patients. Surfactant washout or functional inactivation caused by drowning requires 2 to 4 days of CPAP and PEEP to allow adequate surfactant regeneration.[73] There has been interest in administration of exogenous surfactant for drowning patients with acute respiratory failure.[244] Theoretical benefits include more rapid improvement in pulmonary function and decreased required duration of mechanical ventilation,[89] as well as reduced infection rates because of surfactant's role in pulmonary immune function.[90] Although published case reports generally suggest a benefit,[82,124,217,220] multipatient studies have shown more variable results.[9,118,243,248] Prophylactic antibiotics to prevent pneumonia after drowning are not recommended (see Infectious Diseases, later). Most patients without underlying pulmonary disease or prolonged resuscitation or mechanical ventilation times recover full pulmonary function, as shown in Figures 69-10 and 69-11.

CARDIOVASCULAR SYSTEM AND HEMODYNAMICS

Avoidance of hypoxemia and acidosis requires monitoring and support of cardiac output and peripheral perfusion. From a hemodynamic perspective, drowning patients are likely to have mild intravascular dehydration.[197] Mechanical ventilation can reduce the circulating blood volume through increased intrathoracic pressure and decreased central venous return. Controlled studies have shown that hydration and adequate systemic blood

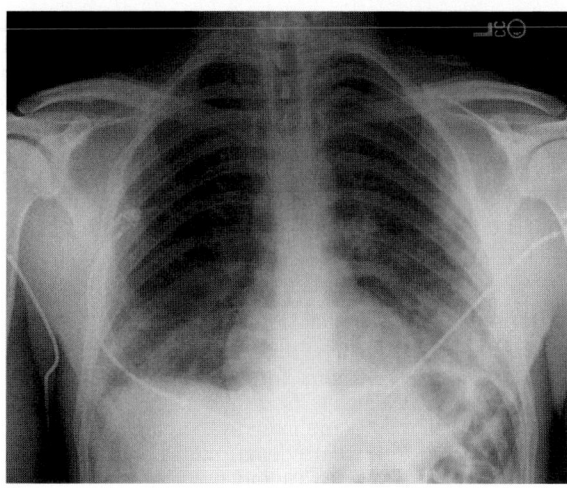

FIGURE 69-10 Submersion-related pulmonary edema. *(Courtesy U.S. Navy.)*

pressure are critical to successful resuscitation; without adequate volume resuscitation, neither inotropic support nor mechanical ventilation alone results in adequate tissue oxygenation or survival.[197,223]

Dysrhythmias seen during resuscitation after drowning most likely result from hypoxemia, acidosis, and hypothermia rather than from a primary cardiovascular abnormality. Correction of the acid-base status and oxygenation may be the only treatments required. The dysrhythmias observed in controlled animal models of drowning and in human drownings include bradycardia, tachycardia, absent or decreased P waves, a widened PR interval, a widened QRS wave, ST segment elevation or depression, inverted or peaked T waves, atrioventricular dissociation, atrial fibrillation, premature ventricular contractions, and ventricular fibrillation.[158] The cause of dysrhythmias is variable, and parameters (e.g., comorbidity, ingestions, trauma, electrolyte disturbances, primary cardiac pathology [ischemia, heart failure]) other than any immediate drowning pathophysiology should be considered.

After initial cardiopulmonary and hemodynamic stabilization, further invasive monitoring should be considered to help guide therapy. An arterial catheter can be used to monitor the blood pressure and arterial blood gases. A pulmonary artery catheter may be useful for hemodynamically unstable patients or those requiring PEEP of 15 cm H_2O pressure or more to maintain oxygenation. Pulmonary capillary wedge pressure and cardiac output determinations allow a quantitative approach to fluid management in the hypotensive patient. Vasopressor agents (e.g.,

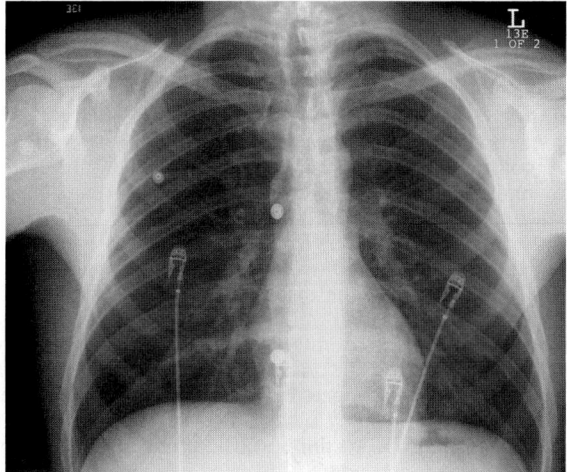

FIGURE 69-11 Resolution of the edema seen in Figure 69-10. *(Courtesy U.S. Navy.)*

dopamine, dobutamine, norepinephrine) may be required to maintain the mean arterial pressure adequate for tissue perfusion, but there is no evidence to suggest they improve the final outcome.[158] An ongoing need for vasopressors after the initial resuscitation and stabilization phases should prompt consideration of other causes of circulatory compromise, such as ongoing volume loss, cardiac failure or ischemia, traumatic injuries, or septic shock. Significant hypothermia can compromise cardiac function, cause dysrhythmias, and decrease the efficacy of electrical and pharmacologic interventions.[232,233]

CENTRAL NERVOUS SYSTEM

Global hypoxemia and hypoperfusion can result in cerebral anoxic injury with consequent focal or generalized neurologic deficits. Inflammatory damage from hypoxemia and reperfusion leads to loss of cell membrane integrity, resulting in extracellular fluid movement and cerebral edema, ultimately producing elevated intracranial pressure (ICP) and possible uncal herniation. The best preventive measure against this cascade of neurologic injury is correction of hypoxemia and hypoperfusion.

Accurate assessment of the neurologic status upon presentation is crucial to predicting the outcome. Serial neurologic examinations, brain imaging, and physiologic testing during the initial 24 to 72 hours of therapy may be helpful for assessing the patient's neurologic progress and projected outcome.[110] Measurements of ICP and cerebral oxygenation have been used as monitoring parameters, but a consensus recommendation from the Brain Resuscitation Task Force of the 2002 World Congress on Drowning states there is insufficient evidence that routine ICP monitoring and management alter outcomes.[245]

Certain neuroimaging modalities may be helpful for diagnosing conditions of particular concern, but routine imaging is rarely helpful for the drowning patient. CT scanning may detect severe brain injury if the scan is abnormal early during the patient's presentation[195]; however, in most cases, unless traumatic injury is suspected, the initial scan is normal and has limited usefulness.[201,224] Magnetic resonance imaging (MRI) and spectroscopy may each be more helpful than CT for showing early signs of injury and cerebral metabolic changes.[62] There is insufficient evidence to support the use of other neurologic diagnostic tools (e.g., brainstem auditory evoked potential response, somatosensory evoked potentials).[110]

Neurologic conditions of concern include seizures, metabolic disorders, and CNS infections. Seizures may occur as a result of cerebral edema or meningitis and should be treated appropriately. An electroencephalogram (EEG) may be helpful for detecting occult seizures; however, if seizures are not suspected, an EEG is of limited usefulness.[21,245] Diuretics and mannitol have been recommended if there is evidence of cerebral edema, but no studies have documented that osmotic diuretics improve the neurologic outcome of drowning patients. Critically ill and ventilated intensive care unit patients have shown improved outcomes if glucose levels are maintained in the range of 80 to 140 mg/dL. Although this study did not address drowning specifically, this should be considered part of the metabolic treatment of ventilated drowning patients.[239] Hyperglycemia has been linked to worse outcomes from acute brain injury.[11] Hypoglycemia should be prevented and can be seen in conjunction with hypothermia and alcohol use (both of which are common in drowning), and can cause direct brain damage and impaired cerebral functioning.[14,19,112]

In the past, controlled hyperventilation to a PaCO$_2$ of 30 mm Hg was advocated as a neuroprotective measure to prevent elevated ICP in the setting of trauma. It was believed that by decreasing cerebral PaCO$_2$, the resultant cerebral vasoconstriction would decrease the ICP. However, active hyperventilation is only indicated for brief periods of established elevated ICP, and metaanalyses suggest the evidence for this intervention is not as strong as for many other ICP interventions.[72,145] Hyperventilation for neuroprotection or ICP reduction in drowning patients is not recommended.

Corticosteroids for lung or cerebral injury were previously advocated for treatment of drowning. There is scant evidence to suggest a benefit to their administration. Steroids are not currently recommended because of their potential deleterious side effects (e.g., hyperglycemia, adrenal suppression, compromised immunity), which may complicate the clinical picture.[14,83,143,153]

As advancements are made in out-of-hospital resuscitation and EMS, patients increasingly survive incidents that would previously have been fatal. However, although cardiovascular functioning may be preserved, neurologic deficits may be profound and immediately call into question the benefit of "survival," or may be insidious and affect the quality of life in more subtle ways. Despite normal MRI and CT studies, longitudinal psychological monitoring may uncover deficits that are not apparent after initial imaging or presentation, because neuropsychiatric sequelae can develop many years after drowning. The importance of understanding these parameters to develop improvements for patients' future quality of life cannot be understated.[106]

HYPOTHERMIA

Hypothermia in the field can be metabolically and neurologically protective; there have been remarkable cases of survival after prolonged submersion and low body temperatures. Unless other obvious signs of death are present, patients should be rewarmed while resuscitation continues and until the body temperature reaches 30° to 35° C (86° to 95° F).[192] Resuscitation can be terminated if at that temperature there is no cardiac activity.[19] There are currently no formal guidelines beyond the recommendations of the 2002 World Congress regarding use of TH in drowning patients, so the current standard of care is rewarming. Guidelines of the American Heart Association and the European Resuscitation Council currently call for TH in comatose patients with return of spontaneous circulation after cardiac arrest.[171] Inducing mild hypothermia (32° to 34° C [90° to 93° F]) or only rewarming to that level and sustaining these temperatures for 12 to 24 hours may result in better neurologic outcomes for drowning patients with or without preceding cardiac arrest.[19,119,171] Drowning patients often arrive hypothermic at temperatures below the 32° to 34° C (90° to 93° F) range of TH. This is an area of active research, and in the absence of randomized control trials of TH in non–ventricular fibrillation cardiopulmonary arrest, the decision to initiate TH is based on expert consensus and theoretical benefit. Drowning patients with restoration of adequate spontaneous circulation who remain comatose should not be actively rewarmed to temperature values above 32° to 34° C (90° to 93° F). If the core temperature exceeds 34° C (93.2° F), hypothermia at 32° to 34° C (90° to 93° F) should be achieved as soon as possible and sustained for 12 to 24 hours. A more complete discussion of hypothermia and its management can be found in Chapters 7 and 8.

RENAL SYSTEM

Acute tubular necrosis and renal failure can result from hypoperfusion, acidosis, and hypoxemia. Hemolysis and myoglobulinuria may follow muscle trauma.[100,121] Creatine phosphokinase and urine myoglobin levels and urine output should be followed. Dialysis may be necessary in severe cases to correct volume overload from oliguria, hyperkalemia, or profound acidosis. With appropriate resuscitation with crystalloid fluids, rhabdomyolysis and acute tubular necrosis can be successfully treated.[100]

DECOMPRESSION ILLNESS

Posthypoxic encephalopathy and hypothermia may cloud the diagnosis of decompression sickness in a drowned scuba diver. If the clinical scenario suggests that decompression sickness is likely, hyperbaric oxygen therapy should be considered (see Chapter 71).

INFECTIOUS DISEASES

Infections from submersion, most often pulmonary in nature, are difficult to predict, and there is no evidence to support the use of prophylactic antibiotics.[83,174] When infections occur, the mortality rate may be as high as 60%.[65] Bacterial, fungal, and amebic pathogens have been implicated. The primary sites of infection are the lungs and CNS, both of which create potential for systemic spread and septic shock.

Aspirated lake, pond, or canal water is more likely to be contaminated than swimming pool and hot tub water. Infections from *Pseudomonas* and *Vibrio* species occur from ocean water aspiration. Leptospirosis may result from aspiration of sewage or water contaminated by rats.[95] Vomiting with subsequent aspiration of gastric contents may lead to infection with gastrointestinal and oropharyngeal microorganisms. *Streptococcus pneumoniae* and *Staphylococcus aureus,* as well as aerobic gram-positive bacteria from the patient's oropharynx, have been found in submersion pulmonary infections, and gram-negative bacteria have been reported to be virulent pathogens following drowning.[19] *Aeromonas hydrophila* is a facultative, anaerobic, gram-negative bacteria found in both fresh water and saltwater, and has been reported to cause fatal pneumonia.[148]

Fungal infections after drowning are quite rare but can be overwhelming, even in immunocompetent individuals. They are often fatal, perhaps because of a delay in diagnosis. Infections from *Pseudallescheria boydii* and its anamorph *Scedosporium apiospermum,* found in water polluted with soil and sewage, have been reported weeks to months after drowning incidents.[19,120] CNS invasion and brain abscesses have been reported with these organisms,[116,120,144] and most reported cases have been fatal. Current treatment is with voriconazole, which has greater CNS penetration than do other antifungal medications. Other fungal infections include invasive *Aspergillus* species, resulting in invasive CNS infection subsequent to pulmonary aspiration pneumonia, particularly in warm climates with drowning in stagnant water. Severe cases should be treated with a combination of voriconazole and caspofungin.[129]

Amebic infection is a rare but potentially fatal complication of drowning. Primary amebic meningoencephalitis (PAM), an infection with a high mortality rate, is caused by *Naegleria fowleri,* a thermophilic ameba found in standing fresh water, such as lakes and ponds. One study in the southwestern United States found *Naegleria* in five out of six wells sampled and in 26.6% of groundwater samples near the location of two drowning deaths from primary amebic meningoencephalitis. The organism is prevalent particularly in warm climates.[126] It usually enters humans through the nasopharynx, with subsequent infection of the olfactory nerve and then the CNS. About 235 PAM cases worldwide have been described in the medical literature, with only a few reported cases of survival (the PAM mortality rate is approximately 95%).[55,99] Most cases have been reported in subtropical or temperate zones; underreporting in tropical regions has been suggested.[55] In the Americas, PAM has been reported in Venezuela, Brazil, Cuba, Mexico, and the United States.[1] Cases occur primarily during summer months (July to September) in southern and southwestern states, with the majority occurring in Texas and Florida.[258] Clinical features are similar to bacterial and viral meningitis and include fever, headache, neck stiffness, anorexia, vomiting, and altered mental status. Primary amebic meningoencephalitis is rapidly progressive, and death typically occurs within 3 to 7 days. The primary treatment is intravenous and intrathecal amphotericin B. Additional drugs reported to be helpful in combination with amphotericin B include rifampin, azithromycin, and the azole drugs.[39,92]

Despite the risks of infection associated with drowning, prophylactic antibiotics are not recommended.[83,174] Monitoring of temperature, tracheal aspirates (with Gram staining and culture), respiratory status, and chest radiographs should guide the clinician's use of antibiotics for established pneumonia. Mental status changes, headache, and fever without evidence of pulmonary infection should prompt consideration of CNS infection. The severity and high mortality rates of fungal and amebic infections are partly the result of the prolonged time for organisms to be grown and identified in culture in combination with the aggressiveness of the pathogens. The location and duration of submersion, water type and temperature, duration of hospital stay, and immune status of the patient help guide the infectious disease

workup and direct initial antibiotic coverage until the regimen can be narrowed to organism-specific drugs.

PROGNOSIS AND TERMINATION OF RESUSCITATION

One of the most difficult tasks faced by physicians involves end-of-life decisions and counseling. These include declaration of a resuscitation as futile, and discussions regarding prognosis with families of comatose patients.

Declaring a patient dead as a result of drowning is complicated by the fact that many of the most dramatic and physiologically unexpected recoveries from cardiac arrest have been in young patients after cold-water drowning.[24,226] Because of this particular consideration with drowning and hypothermia patients, the duration of submersion, water temperature, patient core body temperature, and cardiac electrical or echocardiographic activity should be considered before declaration of death. If there is any uncertainty, resuscitation should be continued until the patient is rewarmed to 30° to 35° C (86° to 95° F).[192] Functional recovery with minimal neurologic impairment and the ability to independently perform activities of daily living occurs in approximately 17% of patients who require resuscitation in the emergency department.[194]

Similarly challenging are neurologically devastated patients who have survived emergency resuscitation. Because hypoxemia is the initial and primary insult with drowning and because the brain is one of the most sensitive organs to hypoxemia, this unfortunate scenario is not unusual. As one wilderness medicine specialist states, "It is clear that we are limited in our medical ability to 'treat' the global hypoxic-ischemic insult sustained by the victim of a significant submersion accident ... preservation of patients in persistently vegetative states is a tragedy of our time."[57]

Factors known to be useful for predicting outcomes in drowning are listed in Box 69-4. In the absence of profound hypothermia, the neurologic status of a patient on admission to the emergency department is of paramount importance for predicting survival with intact neurologic function. Persons who are alert when admitted seldom die.[51,54,114,154,176] Age is included in many prognostic recommendations, but its significance has been contested. Some authorities consider an age of 3 years or younger as a favorable prognostic factor,[57,128,165] whereas others view it as unfavorable.[176,178,210] Prognostic indicators in pediatric patients include the Glasgow Coma Scale score[54] and the presence of spontaneous breathing.[62,85,114,122]

It is difficult to predict the ultimate outcome based on initial presentation, but several different classification systems help clinicians address questions regarding the potential for recovery.[45,50,114,123] Some persons have expressed concern that these systems may miss potential survivors. An ABC classification of patients based on presenting neurologic examination was established and refined by Modell, Conn, and Barker[50,151] (Table 69-3). This system categorizes patients on the basis of their condition within 1 hour of emergency department presentation and whether they were at that time A, *a*lert; B, *b*lunted in consciousness; or

---

BOX 69-4 Prognostic Signs in Submersion Incidents

Positive Signs
Alert on admission
Brief submersion time
On-scene basic or advanced life support
Good response to initial resuscitation measures

Negative Signs
Fixed, dilated pupils in emergency department
Submerged longer than 5 minutes
No resuscitation attempts for more than 10 minutes
Preexisting chronic disease
Arterial pH < 7.10
Coma on admission to emergency department

TABLE 69-3 Classification of Drowning Patients

Category	Description
A	Awake—fully oriented
B	Blunted—arousable; purposeful response to pain
C	Comatose—not arousable; abnormal response to pain
C_1	Flexor response to pain
C_2	Extensor response to pain
C_3	Flaccid
C_4	Arrested

C, comatose. Comatose patients were further categorized according to abnormal neurologic responses: C_1, flexor response; C_2, extensor response; C_3, flaccid; and C_4, cardiac arrest. In their series on children, Conn and coworkers[51,52] reported that all patients in category A survived and were neurologically normal, and all but one patient in category B survived. Patients in category C showed variable responses, with increasingly poor outcomes from C_1 to C_4. In another pediatric study, 37% of subjects who presented in the C_3 stage (i.e., no response to pain, fixed and dilated pupils, absence of spontaneous respiration, hypotension, and poor perfusion) had complete recovery despite predicted poor outcomes.[173] The classification system is therefore highly specific for predicting patients with good outcomes, but shows a significant amount of variability with regard to outcomes among patients with category C presentations.

Graf and colleagues[85] developed a prediction rule based on variables that predicted vegetative state or death: history of CPR, CPR longer than 25 minutes, hyperglycemia on arrival, or absence of pupillary light reflex on arrival. Those variables, plus male gender and an initial blood glucose level of more than 200 mg/dL, had the strongest associations with unfavorable outcomes in comatose children. Other studies have shown similar results, suggesting that poor outcomes are the rule rather than the exception in cases of cardiopulmonary arrest after drowning.[221]

Of special consideration with drowning patients is that most prediction rules, although good for predicting unfavorable outcomes, are not sufficiently sensitive to reliably predict favorable outcomes. As previously emphasized, there are multiple case reports of neurologically intact survival after prolonged resuscitation from drowning. It is therefore recommended that drowning patients be treated aggressively for 48 hours to determine if meaningful recovery is possible.[45,192] Withdrawing therapy from survivors who show no clinical improvement after 48 hours can then be considered.

Emergency care providers should understand that drowning incidents may be psychologically devastating for families. One study showed that 24% of parents separated after a drowning incident involving their child.[57] Siblings present during a pediatric drowning may suffer survivor's guilt. Families who have experienced a drowning incident have demonstrated posttraumatic stress syndrome, sometimes for years, and developed otherwise unexpected substance abuse patterns and sleep disturbances.[57] Counseling services should be offered to families of patients involved in a serious drowning incident or death.

DROWNING PREVENTION AND SURVIVAL

Prevention is a plausible strategy for reducing the incidence of permanent injury and death as a result of drowning. It can take the form of preimmersion interventions or postimmersion actions taken by individuals and groups to prevent complications and deaths related to drowning.

PREIMMERSION INTERVENTIONS

Drowning represents a serious public health problem worldwide, yet the majority of incidents are likely preventable.[19,141] Prevention strategies appear to be successful in avoiding fatal drownings,[81,98,138,167,216,257] and countries that have implemented prevention programs have reduced their drowning death rates.[164] Some authorities suggest that certain measures (e.g., fencing, lifeguard training, water safety training at a young age) shown to be helpful in high-income countries may not be relevant to curtailing drowning deaths in low- and middle-income countries because of geographic, social, cultural, and behavioral factors. They note a striking absence of adequate data regarding incidence rates, risk factors, intervention effectiveness, and cost-effectiveness in these settings.[108]

Preimmersion Interventions by Age

Strategies are broken down into four distinct age groups (Figure 69-12). For children who are 4 years old and younger, prevention is based on increased supervision. Children should swim only with "touch" supervision (i.e., within an arm's reach of an adult), and need to be protected from or closely supervised at all times around any bodies of water, including those as small as bathtubs, toilets, and buckets.[6,71,125,214] Children between the ages of 1 and 4 years may be enrolled in survival swimming courses. For children between the ages of 5 and 15 years, swim instruction and awareness of hazards have been shown to decrease mortality rates.[44,196] Even after swimming lessons, children of all ages

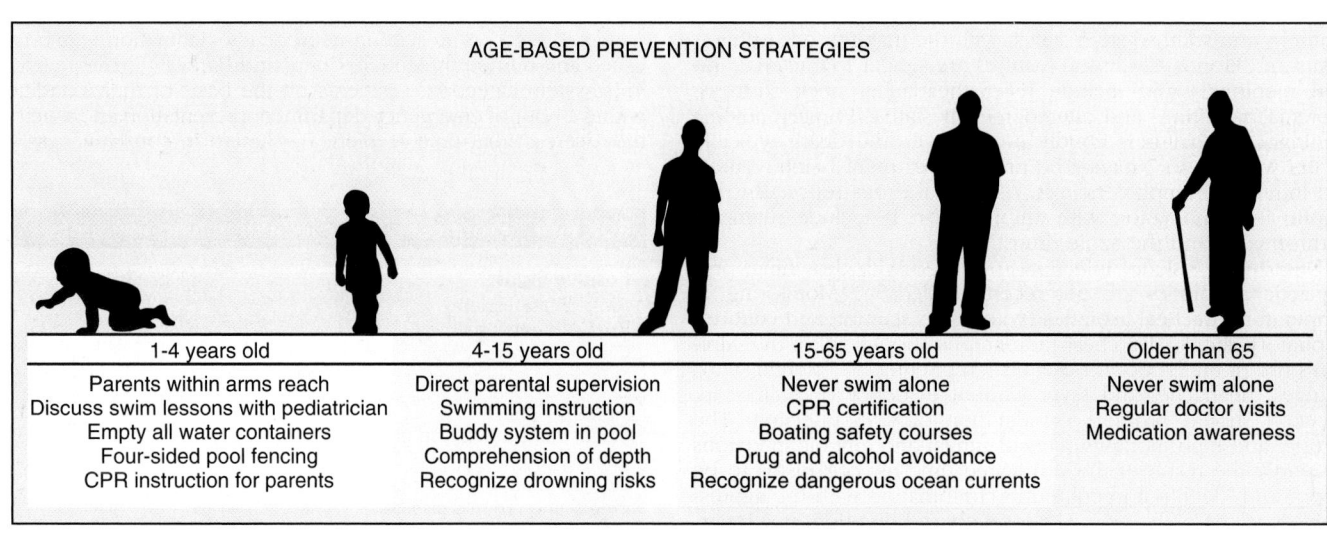

AGE-BASED PREVENTION STRATEGIES

1-4 years old	4-15 years old	15-65 years old	Older than 65
Parents within arms reach	Direct parental supervision	Never swim alone	Never swim alone
Discuss swim lessons with pediatrician	Swimming instruction	CPR certification	Regular doctor visits
Empty all water containers	Buddy system in pool	Boating safety courses	Medication awareness
Four-sided pool fencing	Comprehension of depth	Drug and alcohol avoidance	
CPR instruction for parents	Recognize drowning risks	Recognize dangerous ocean currents	

FIGURE 69-12 Age-based prevention strategies for drowning prevention. (*Courtesy Andrew Schmidt, DO, MPH.*)

BOX 69-5 Recommendations for Water Safety from the American Academy of Pediatrics

Infants and Children
Careful supervision
Empty all water containers, such as buckets and child pools
Do not allow swimming lessons to provide a false sense of security
Install four-sided fences around swimming pools
CPR instruction and 9-1-1 phone access
Use of flotation devices

Children 1-4 Years Old
Swimming instruction
Buddy swimming with supervision/lifeguard
Personal flotation devices
Knowing the depth of the water prior to entry
Recognizing drowning risks, such as skating on thin ice

Adolescents
Avoidance of alcohol and drug use
CPR instruction
Prohibiting alcohol use during boat operation
Proper training in scuba diving and water-sporting activities
Recognizing rip currents and other dangerous water situations

should wear PFDs as recommended during water sports and around aquatic environments.[6,71] For individuals who are 15 to 65 years old (especially toward the younger end), prevention strategies include risk-taking behavior reduction (especially use of alcohol and other performance-impairing drugs during aquatic activities) and increased understanding of potential hazards and mechanisms for survival and self-rescue should an incident occur. Adolescents in particular may benefit from counseling regarding swimming in remote locations or in areas not designated as approved for swimming.[71] Swimmers who are more than 65 years old may have comorbid conditions or be using medications that can affect their cognitive or physical abilities in the water, so they should be aware of potential medication effects before engaging in water activities. Water entry should be feet first any time the depth of water is unknown.[71] Box 69-5 outlines the formal recommendations for water safety from the AAP[4]; other agencies have developed similar formal guidelines.[38]

Swimming Pool Safety

Prevention involving swimming pools has been particularly successful. Legislation regarding residential pools and fences has been shown to reduce by 50% or more the incidence of drowning in communities with large numbers of swimming pools.[193,208] Inadequate enforcement of local ordinances and inadequate operation or maintenance of barrier equipment are contributing factors to childhood drowning.[161] Absence of fencing around pools increases the risk of drowning fourfold.[187] Studies have shown that pool fencing should be four-sided, with a minimum height of 1.5 m (5 feet) and a self-locking gate.[33,133] Proper gate closure should be emphasized, because a fence alone does not prevent drowning.[23] Even when locks are present, they are often nonfunctional or in an unlocked position; barrier equipment may be inadequately maintained or operated.[161,203] Ground pools should be filled so that the water level is as close as possible to the surrounding external ground, making self-extrication easier for a struggling person who reaches the side of the pool and does not have sufficient physical strength to pull up to gain exit from the water. Pool alarms and rigid pool covers may provide additional protection and should be used in addition to, not in place of, fencing.[30] Fish and garden ponds should be eliminated or fenced if small children can be near them.[133]

Supervision and Lifeguards

In almost 90% of drowning incidents, there is no supervising individual, or the individual is absent at the time of the incident.[193] This has been further validated in developing nations, such as Bangladesh, where one-third of children who die by drowning are unaccompanied. Of the remaining two-thirds, more than 40% are accompanied only by a child who is 10 years old

or younger.[44,196] Young children should never be left alone, even momentarily, where there is accessible water.[5,34,98,214]

Figure 69-1 shows international drowning rates with territories sized in proportion to the absolute number of people who died from drowning over the course of 1 year. It is informative to compare results in regions that have long-standing traditions of lifeguarding, such as England, North America, and Australia, with regions that do not. Using its own surveillance data, the United States Lifesaving Association has calculated the chance that a person will drown while attending a beach protected by United States Lifesaving Association–affiliated lifeguards at 1 in 18 million (0.0000055%).[234] Other studies found that the presence of a lifeguard positively affects the outcome of drowning.[81,216] Observation by pool lifeguards is also associated with decreased rule violations.[93] Lifeguards not only perform actual drowning rescues, but are also active in swimming education and drowning prevention. CPR training and competency are not mandated for lifeguards in all international areas, so this remains a target for intervention.[193] Case fatality rates can be as high as 42% for individuals under the supervision of lifeguards, suggesting that in some regions, there is an opportunity to improve lifeguard efficacy.[193] International organizations such as the International Life Saving Federation (ilsf.org) and national affiliates such as the United States Lifesaving Association (usla.org) promote modern open-water and pool lifeguarding principles worldwide. A number of groups are involved with exporting lifeguard training and practice to countries with high drowning rates and low or nonexistent lifeguard and drowning prevention programs. These agencies (e.g., Nile Swimmers [NileSwimmers.org], International Surf Lifesaving Association [ISLASurf.org], Lifeguards Without Borders [lifeguardswithoutborders.org]) also provide oversight to private lifeguarding agencies; they offer preventive education and promote lifeguarding techniques in areas where such activities are absent. Other private-sector agencies have developed unique courses and curricula for water safety and supervision. One example is Landmark Learning, a wilderness medicine school in the southeastern United States that developed a Wilderness Starguard program in cooperation with the Starfish Aquatics Institute and the American Safety and Health Institute (landmarklearning.edu/courses/starfish-aquatics-institute/wilderness-starguard). This certification course trains students to serve as lifeguards and water safety personnel in wilderness settings.

Training for Out-of-Hospital Personnel

On-scene resuscitation is associated with improved outcomes. Persons designated to attend the scene of drowning incidents should have specialized training and triage ability to deliver the patient to the appropriate medical center.[98] Lifeguard agencies should conduct routine interagency training sessions with EMS workers, firefighters, and other personnel who may respond to drowning or rescue incidents to discuss management and extrication strategies. Specific training is available for open-water and swift-water rescuers, and personnel should seek certification appropriate to the aquatic environments in which they participate. In the United States, the *National Fire Protection Association 1670 Standard on Operations and Training for Technical Rescue*[166] regulates the components of swift-water rescue training, including operational and technical training.

Swimming Lessons and Boating Instruction

One possible intervention to prevent drowning is to promote swimming lessons. Although this seems intuitively sensible, some studies suggest there is no solid evidence that swimming lessons are an effective public health measure to reduce drowning.[216] Potential explanations for this finding are that swimming ability or lessons may lead to overconfidence in a water setting, swimming in hazardous situations, increased exposure to water, or reduced parental vigilance.[6,10,12,160,215] Others debate the validity of positions that argue against swimming lessons.[80,142] More recent studies suggest that lessons may reduce the incidence of drowning in young children,[257] and emerging data from developing nations show that swim instruction may have a lifelong protective effect and decrease mortality rates.[44] Swimming instruction may improve survival ability in water, but should not be seen as a guarantee against drowning. Even in studies showing a protective benefit from swimming lessons, many persons in the drowning cohort were relatively skilled swimmers.[31]

The optimal time to begin swimming education remains controversial. Prehospital trauma life support (an expert consensus certification course) workers and other authors recommend swimming education for children who are younger than 3 years old.[165,178] Commercial training programs, such as Child Drowning Prevention and Infant Swimming Resources, offer specific floating training to children in this age group.[42,113] Multiple studies show that swimming skills can be taught and retained at a young age.[10,66,179] Two case-control studies suggest that participation in formal swimming education prevents 40% to 88% of drowning incidents among children who are 1 to 4 years old.[31,257] Based on recent research showing that drowning victims between the ages of 1 and 4 years were less likely to have had formal swimming instruction,[31,257] the AAP updated its recommendations to allow formal survival swimming lessons as early as 1 year of age.[5] Unless there is a cause for exception, all children who are 4 years of age or older should be enrolled in formal swim instruction. No level of swim training or instruction should replace direct, uninterrupted, and competent supervision of children in and around the aquatic environment. Some suggest that educational efforts to explain high-risk situations and avoidance activities may be more beneficial than actual swimming instruction.[6,98,216] Formal training in boating skills and self-rescue can prevent drowning and help boaters and paddlers manage the consequences if they enter the water.

Personal Flotation Devices

All individuals involved in water sports should be familiar with PFDs and particular devices that may be recommended or required for their specific activities. In 2013, 84% of persons who died by drowning aboard boats were not wearing PFDs. Air-filled swimming aids (e.g., water wings, floaties) should not replace PFDs.[30] The AAP further states that water wings and floaties are detrimental to safety and can allow a child to reach water beyond his or her depth and then easily fall off or be removed, resulting in drowning. Drowning survival, prevention, and self-rescue hinge on correct PFD selection. PFDs are categorized based on the amount of buoyancy they provide and type of activity in which they will be used (see Figure 69-2). As of September 22, 2014, the U.S. Coast Guard issued a ruling that it would abandon the "type" classification as presented in Figure 69-2. No new terminology has yet been approved or disseminated, and many manufacturers still use the type classification.[104]

Preventive Equipment

By selecting safety equipment appropriate to the conditions, many hazards can be controlled by individuals in the water setting. This includes activity-specific helmets, wetsuits or thermal protection, PFDs, and survival suits. Newer-generation white-water helmets feature multilayer impact shells with specially designed retention systems to keep the helmets in place during water sports. Wetsuits or drysuits can be lifesaving in cold-water environments by preventing cognitive, motor, and other adverse physiologic consequences of hypothermia. Whistles that are lightweight, operate without a pea, and can be carried in pockets or attached to survival gear greatly increase the chance of a wet individual being located if he or she is lost. Beacon locator systems and other boating safety technology can reduce open-water boating-related fatal drownings by allowing rescuers to locate persons in a timely manner. Using boats that are correctly configured and equipped for the chosen environment is critical for all paddling sports.

Education About Alcohol and Drugs

Despite similar pathophysiology and injury patterns between motorized water- and land-based vehicular injuries, there is greater legal and societal acceptance of alcohol use during motorized water sports. There is also widespread social acceptance of alcohol ingestion while recreating in and around water, and a plethora of advertisements promote its appeal. Strategies similar to those used to curtail alcohol drinking while driving

may have a similar effect on alcohol drinking while boating.[134] In addition to impaired cognition that may result in a collision while operating a vessel, impairment from drugs or alcohol can significantly hinder an individual's ability to self-rescue. Decreased situational awareness and/or physical stamina required for self-rescue and peer rescue in an aquatic environment are risky and should be discouraged.[33,98,192,216] This is an area amenable to law enforcement.

POSTIMMERSION ACTIONS

Individuals venturing into remote settings that include water exposure should be mentally and physically trained and prepared to act if an accident occurs. Preparation, education, and proper equipment are crucial factors for the prevention of and response to a drowning event. Ideally, all activities involving water exposure should include safety personnel either in or beside the water who have predetermined roles if a victim gets into trouble. This is not necessarily a formal lifeguard; many drowning rescues have been accomplished as a result of the astute situational awareness of bystanders. Rescuer safety should always be considered; there are numerous case reports of well-intentioned rescuers dying while attempting to perform rescues. One Australian study examined cases over a 6-year period where adults attempting to rescue children died by drowning. In 93% of cases when the adult died, the child they were attempting to rescue survived.[68] Having safety personnel in place can be as simple as having one team member downstream on the shore before everyone else runs a rapid, or as complex as rigging a safety line before making a stream crossing. It is critical that rescuers never exceed their level of training or abilities.

A key educational intervention is the principle of "reach, throw, row, go" (Figure 69-13). First, attempt to reach the victim with a rope, branch, oar, paddle, or other object while safely remaining on shore or in a boat. Second, throw any floating object to the victim; ideally, this is a buoy or PFD; improvised items include something like a soccer ball, empty cooler, or dry bag full of air. Third, row or paddle to the victim in a boat, kayak, canoe, surfboard, or any other large watercraft capable of safely simultaneously floating both the rescuer and victim. The final option, "go," should be reserved as a last resort for professional rescuers. An uncertified would-be rescuer has a high risk of becoming a second drowning victim, either by succumbing to the same environmental dangers as the original victim or by being dragged underwater by the panicked victim. If it becomes necessary for an untrained rescuer to enter the water to effect a rescue, it is critically important to never physically engage an actively drowning person. The rescuer should swim toward the victim while wearing a PFD and carrying an additional PFD for the victim. Stop a safe distance (i.e., greater than two arms' lengths) and throw or push the second PFD to the victim, avoiding direct contact. When the victim is wearing the given PFD and no longer is in a state of panic, he or she can be safely assisted to shore or a boat.

The person who is suddenly thrown into water must remain calm and make a plan based on the situation. For example, if a person wearing a backpack falls into moving water while crossing a stream, the backpack must be removed before the person attempts to swim, to avoid being pulled underwater by the pack. If a person falls into a calm lake or ocean, the person should attempt to float on the back and discard any items that might be weighing the person down. For rip currents (i.e., surface ocean currents that form as the result of channeled water returning seaward), a person should relax and swim parallel to shore instead of struggling against the current. All of these situations can be compounded by cold-water or prolonged immersion. The person must stay relaxed, remember to turn the head to breathe, and remain in the HELP position (Figures 69-14 and 69-15) while not swimming. Rhythmically turning the head to breathe as the face-down body bobs to the surface helps to promote controlled breathing, especially in open water or surf. Achieving adequate respiration with this maneuver becomes very difficult in rough water, currents, and tides or if there is concurrent injury; however, the chances for successful survival increase with practice.

RECOMMENDED RESCUE TECHNIQUES			
Reach	Throw	Row	Go
Lowest risk to rescuer	→ → → → → → → → →		Highest risk to rescuer
Weak/injured victim, unable to swim, close to shore	Weak/injured victim, unable to swim, far from shore	Long distance, victims unable to grasp rope	Should be reserved for trained rescuers, swim floatable object to victim, never contact active victim
Branches, poles, paddles, clothing	Rope bags, ring buoys, coolers, soccer ball, PFD, air-filled dry bag	Kayak, canoe, surfboard	PFD, rescue buoy, ring buoy, cooler, soccer ball, air-filled dry bag

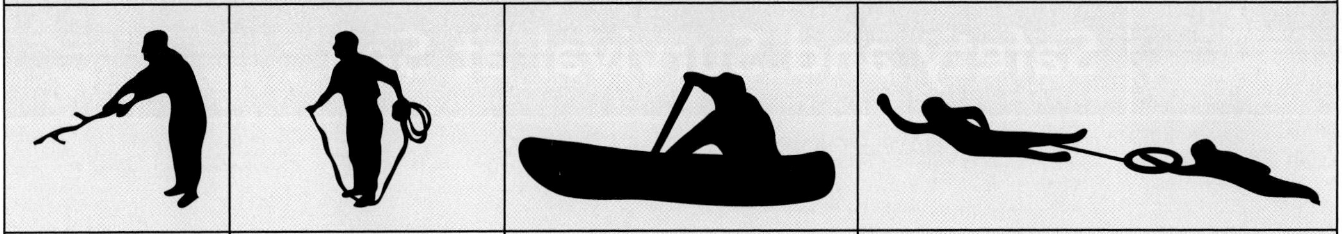

FIGURE 69-13 Reach, throw, row, go: recommended rescue techniques in submersion incidents. *(Courtesy Andrew Schmidt, DO, MPH.)*

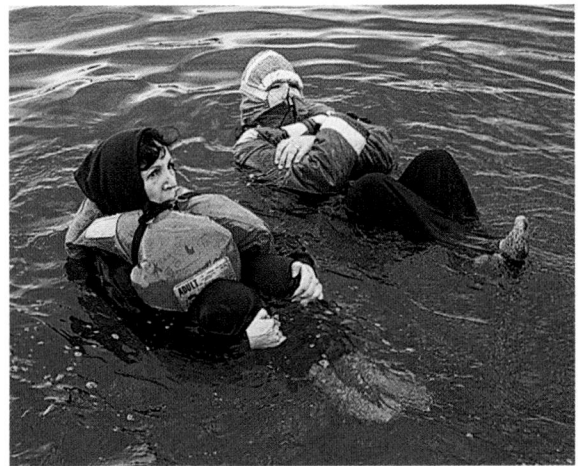

FIGURE 69-14 Heat escape lessening posture (HELP). *(Courtesy Alan Steinman, MD.)*

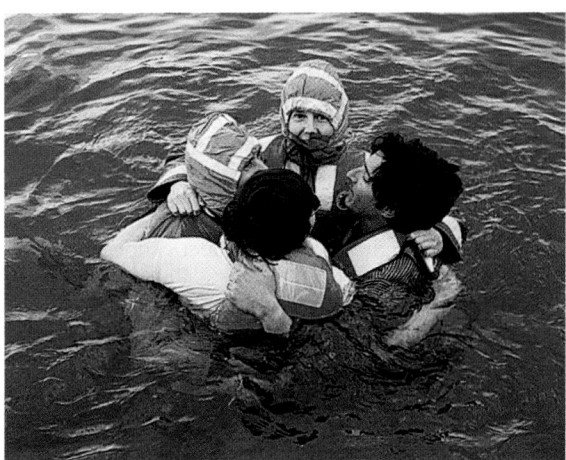

FIGURE 69-15 Huddle technique. *(Courtesy Alan Steinman, MD.)*

If rescue is not immediate, a decision must be made by the victim as to whether swimming to safety or staying in place is the best course of action. Trying to swim a great distance in hope of rescue increases exposure of the body's surface area to cold water and thus heat loss by convection. It also increases loss of energy that might be better spent keeping the head above the water surface for a longer time. Decisions such as this are made easier by preventive planning before and during activities in and around water. Individuals anticipating recreation in a water environment should have a premeditated plan that includes appropriate equipment, as well as practiced swimming, rescue, lifesaving, and resuscitation skills. Boats, canoes, kayaks, and rafts should meet accepted standards and be kept in good condi-

tion. All boats and vessels should be equipped with U.S. Coast Guard–approved PFDs or other flotation devices in sufficient numbers to equip all participants. Courses on boating safety, rescue, and navigation are offered by the U.S. Coast Guard in most waterways and by numerous private companies for various boating sports.

REFERENCES

Complete references used in this text are available online at expertconsult.inkling.com.

It is difficult for us to grasp the idea that parts of our planet remain in an almost primordial state of wildness and isolation. There are only a few places left on Earth where merely getting across them is an achievement: Antarctica...the Sahara...the Southern Ocean...the wilderness of ice or sand or water or terrible places where nature retains power over humans to terrify and diminish.
Derek Lundy, Godforsaken Sea

The greatest wilderness on Earth is the sea. Water covers two-thirds of the planet and, except for the sun, has the greatest influence on global weather patterns. Although it may take hours or days to succumb to exposure in most environments, death at sea can happen in under a minute. Compared with desert heat, high-altitude hypoxia, and polar subzero temperatures, water is the most hostile and life-threatening natural environment for inadequately equipped survivors.

The 1979 Fastnet Race distinguished itself as the worst disaster in the long history of ocean yachting. A surprise storm crossed the Irish Sea between southwest England and southern Ireland, and exploded without warning in the midst of the Fastnet racing fleet. Suddenly, 2700 men and women in 303 ocean-sailing yachts unwittingly became participants in hundreds of incidents of survival at sea. Winds of force 10 (55 knots) with much stronger gusts, and seas as high as 15 m (50 feet) knocked down 48% of the fleet until their masts paralleled the water; 33% of the fleet experienced knockdowns substantially beyond horizontal, including total inversions and full 360-degree rolls for at least 26 yachts. Despite a massive response of rescue personnel and equipment, 24 yachts were abandoned and 5 vessels sank. Fifteen sailors died and 136 were rescued from disabled yachts or the water. The official Fastnet Race Inquiry noted, "The common link among all 15 deaths was the violence of the sea, an unremitting danger faced by all who sail." It concluded, "The sea showed that it can be a deadly enemy and that those who go to sea for pleasure must do so in the full knowledge that they may encounter dangers of the highest order."[5] The Fastnet storm had two positive results. First, boats, safety gear, and safety procedures were improved dramatically. Second, sailors began to talk realistically about the risks of sailing and came to regard safety as a necessary component of their craft. The first public Safety at Sea Seminars were held in Annapolis and New York after the Fastnet shock. Since then, hundreds of safety and seamanship seminars have been held across the United States and other sailing locales (Figure 70-1).

Twenty years later, on the edge of the Southern Ocean, the Sydney to Hobart race between the southeast coast of Australia and the island of Tasmania became a terrifying ordeal for 115 yachts. Within a day of leaving harbor, an explosive low-pressure cell, a "southerly buster," formed over the fleet as it entered Bass Strait. In its aftermath, 6 men died, 55 men were rescued, and 12 boats either sank or were abandoned. One hundred participants were seriously injured and five drowned. Fractured ribs, lacerations, and head trauma were the most common injuries. The 330-page investigative report recommended strict guidelines for improved safety gear, life rafts, and communication equipment. In 2012, five sailors perished while participating in the Full Crew Farallones Race out of San Francisco. An independent review panel of experts under the auspices of the U.S. Sailing Association (often known as U.S. Sailing) subsequently issued a full and detailed report of this disaster. This report can be read in its entirety, together with other safety reports and reviews of sailing accidents, on the U.S. Sailing website.[11]

HOW DO PEOPLE DIE IN RECREATIONAL BOATING ACCIDENTS?

For ocean racing sailors and voyaging seafarers, most emergencies and accidents occur during extreme weather conditions created by violent ocean storms (Figure 70-2). In contrast, most recreational boating accidents in the United States occur in fair weather, with flat to 30-cm (1-foot) seas, light (0- to 10-km/hr [0- to 6-mph]) winds, and good daytime visibility. Most of these accidents happen close to home, on inland lakes, ponds, rivers, and coastal bays, which are the most common areas used for pleasure boating.

The most recent U.S. recreational boating statistics available from the Coast Guard from their annual report "Recreational Boating Statistics 2014"[8] indicate there were 610 boating fatalities (14% decrease from 2012 to 2013; 9% increase from 2013 to 2014). This Boating Accident Reporting Database (BARD) report is a compilation of accident data from individual states and trust territories, and it recounts the fascinating, if macabre, stories of how people die while boating. Capsizing and falls overboard from open motorboats, rowboats, canoes, and kayaks account for more than half of fatalities. Vessels involved in accidents with the greatest number of casualties are open motorboats (47%), personal watercraft (17%), cabin motorboats (15%), canoes (13%), and kayaks (10%). Eight of every 10 boaters who drown were in vessels less than 21 feet in length. The BARD reports an average of 5000 recreational boating accidents annually. Sixty percent of all accidents involve operator and passenger controllable factors, and 25% involve boat or environmental factors. Operator inattention, improper lookout, operator inexperience, excessive speed, and machinery failure rank as the top five primary contributing factors in accidents. Alcohol use is the leading known contributing factor in fatal boating accidents; where the primary cause is known, alcohol use is the leading factor in 21% of deaths.

Eighty percent of deaths occurred on boats where the operator received no boating safety instruction. However, this statistic is misleading, because the overall number of boaters who have received boating safety training is unknown. Collision with another vessel is the most common type of accident, followed by flooding/swamping, collision with a fixed object, grounding, and water-skier mishaps, accounting for 30% of fatalities. Open motorboats less than 8 m (26 feet) in length and personal watercraft make up two-thirds of the watercraft involved in collisions. Drowning is the cause of death in 63% (178 of 282) of open powerboat fatalities, but it is the cause of death in only 35% (12 of 34) of personal watercraft fatalities; this discrepancy suggests

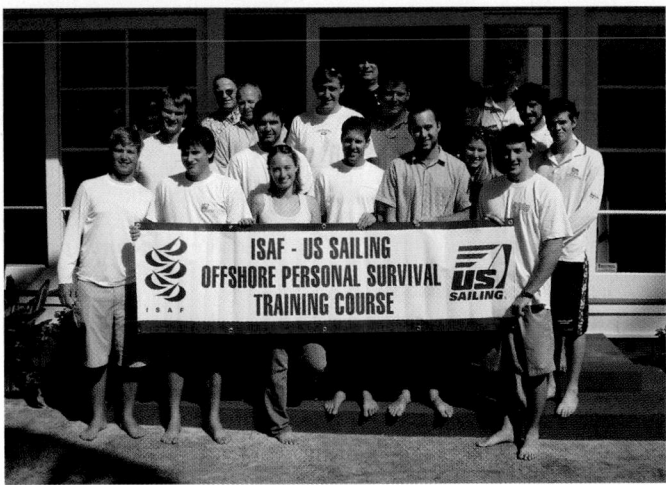

FIGURE 70-1 U.S. Sailing Safety at Sea courses offered around the country are a great way to be exposed to expert opinions and hands-on training with safety gear.

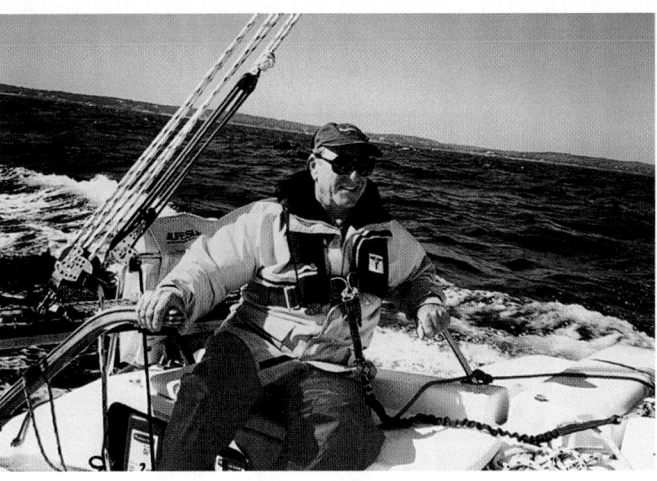

FIGURE 70-3 Protection from sun, wind, and water, eye protection, and a harness and inflatable life jacket are just some of the "kit" for offshore sailors.

that use of life jackets (sometimes called personal flotation devices [PFDs]) on personal watercraft has a significant impact on mortality rates.

These statistics indicate that one of the greatest threats to a boater's safety in "home waters" is an inexperienced, inattentive operator motoring at excessive speed, unaware that another vessel or individual may be nearby. Constant vigilance is necessary in order to take evasive action and avoid collision. Sixty-nine percent of all fatalities in accidents on recreational boats described in the BARD report are from drowning, and 84% of victims were not wearing a life jacket. The full report may be reviewed at the website of the U.S. Coast Guard's Boating Safety Resource Center, along with the annual JSI study of life jacket wear rates.[9]

Fractures, lacerations, contusions, head injuries, and low back sprains are the most frequent injuries in boating. Burns, hypothermia, amputations, carbon monoxide poisoning, and dislocations are among the next most common problems. Open motorboats and personal watercraft are the vessels most frequently involved in passenger injuries from trauma, while canoes and rowboats account for 33% of boaters affected by hypothermia. Explosions from propane stoves and carbon monoxide poisoning from bad exhaust systems accounted for only two fatalities in 2014, or less than 1% of all deaths.

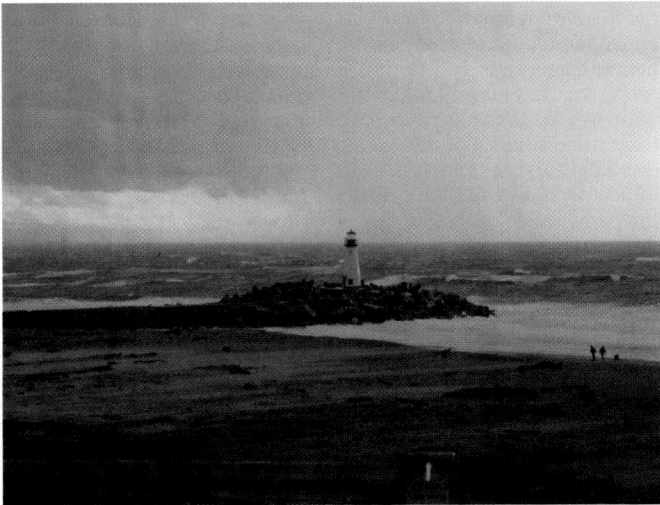

FIGURE 70-2 Sailors need to be able to "weather the storm they cannot avoid"; breaking entrances may force them to wait out the gale until a channel can be safely navigated.

PERSONAL SAFETY GEAR

LIFE JACKETS

Annual Coast Guard recreational boating fatality statistics reemphasize that boaters should wear life jackets. In 2014, for example, 418 (69%) of 610 recreational boating fatalities where the cause of death is known were due to drowning. Of drowning victims where the life jacket status is known, 84% were not wearing a life jacket.

The vast majority of these drowning victims were in boats under 7 m (21 feet), including open motorboats (43%), canoes (17%), and kayaks (12%). Each annual Coast Guard report estimates that at least 85% to 90% of small vessel drowning deaths could have been prevented if a life jacket had been worn. The most common causes of drowning include capsizing of a vessel, falls overboard, flooding/swamping, and collision with a fixed object. Life jackets help prevent drowning in water at any temperature and are crucial in combating the lethal effects of cold water. When boating in cold waters (< 70°F [21°C]), the cold shock response (see Chapter 8) is the primary cause of drowning. A high-buoyancy life jacket (Figures 70-3 and 70-4) is essential to survival; it keeps the head above water and maximizes the airway freeboard (distance from the water to the mouth), which prevents aspiration immediately following sudden immersion. Some states require everyone in boats 21 feet long or less to wear a life jacket between November 1 and May 1. Few boaters routinely wear life jackets, and delay in donning them until facing storm conditions, losing protection during both collisions and falls overboard. During the Dauphin Island Race in Mobile Bay, Louisiana, a fleet of 118 sailboats was overtaken by a fast-moving (but widely predicted) line of squalls. Videos and testimony from the sailors in that race indicate that many delayed putting on life jackets despite the ominous front that approached the fleet. Six sailors drowned in that race (some of whom were wearing low-buoyancy life jackets). The 2014 National Life Jacket Wear Rate Observational Study reported that from 2006 to 2014, usage rates for adults in open motorboats varied from 4.5% to 5.8%, with a 2013 figure of 5.8%.

Nonswimmers, children, and inexperienced crew should wear life jackets at all times whenever on deck or in an open boat. Everyone on deck should wear a life jacket in heavy weather, at night, when visibility is reduced, when the boat is traveling quickly, or while traversing cold waters. In warm waters, experienced boaters who are strong swimmers implicitly acknowledge a degree of risk by not wearing a life jacket.

When boating in cold weather, a foam-lined float coat can be worn either with or in lieu of a life jacket, although the combination of float coat and life jacket is demonstrably safer. In addition to providing 7 kg (15.5 lb) or more of flotation, the coat offers

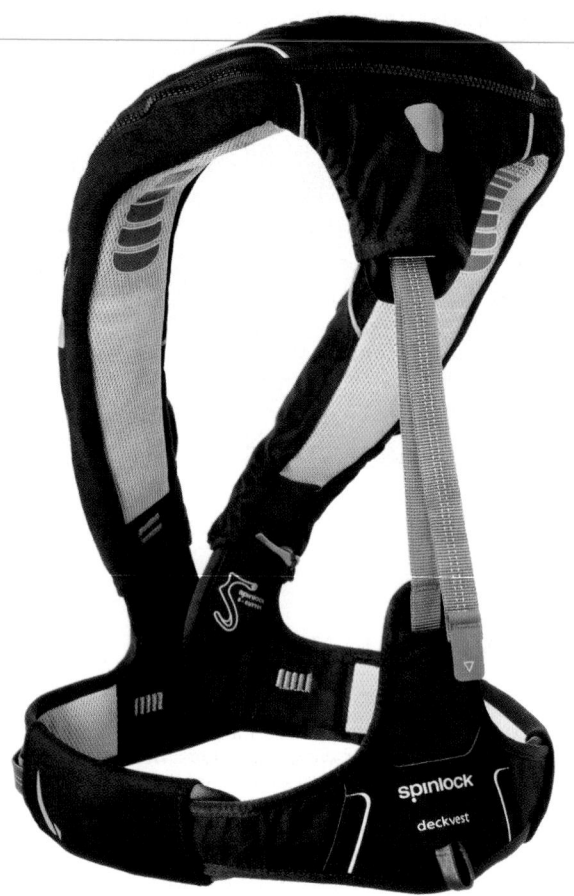

FIGURE 70-4 Modern life jacket-harness combinations combine some features of climbing gear with personal flotation. While not approved by the U.S. Coast Guard, this model from Spinlock meets ISO standards for life jackets and is approved in much of the rest of the world.

excellent protection against hypothermia and cushions the ribs and thorax from injury during a fall on deck. Most models are approved as type III* flotation devices (for calm, inland waters, or where fast rescue is likely). For additional flotation or hypothermia protection, many float coats can be combined with bib overalls. Use of these gear items in tandem has the added benefit of extended survival time in very cold water.

The primary reasons cited by veteran sailors for not wearing life jackets include discomfort and inconvenience. Virtually all inherently buoyant (foam or kapok-filled) type I offshore life jackets and type II near-shore life buoyant vests are bulky, uncomfortable, awkward to wear, too warm in summer, and limit mobility. The common type III flotation aid and many type V

---

*In the fall of 2014, the U.S. Coast Guard announced that life jackets would no longer be classified by type as part of the process of harmonization with ISO (international) life jacket standards. A new North American standard, UL 12402, was in the process of being approved as this book went to print. This standard is based on the ISO 12402 standard and will use different levels to denote the lifesaving potential of the devices. Proposed levels are roughly equivalent to the buoyancy of the life jacket in Newtons, and will be level 50, 70, 100, 150, or 275. The new standard includes dramatically different labels that show the conditions under which the life jackets are to be used and, in some cases, not used, as well as the righting ability of the device and sizing recommendations. As of January 2016, two sections of UL 12402 were approved: -5 and -9. These cover the Level 50 and Level 70 devices (-5), and the means to test life jackets (-9). Life jackets made to this standard will be legal in both the United States and Canada, which will preclude the need to have separate products for each country. Level 150 (-3) and Level 100 (-4) portions of the standard were being worked on by the Standards Technical Panel as of the date of this writing (summer 2016). Boaters are advised to rely on the label instructions found inside every life jacket to assess the conditions for appropriate use of a given product.

vests are comfortable and wearable, but have significant limitations, including low total buoyancy (generally 70 N or 15.5 lbf), poor reserve buoyancy (as the wearer is immersed, buoyancy does not increase, because the life jacket is already immersed), low freeboard, inability to turn the unconscious victim face up (righting ability), and inability to support the head (and thus maintain an airway). These type III and V life vests are suitable only for calm water and should be worn in situations where a quick rescue is assured. Life jackets should be selected according to comfort and practicality in order to maximize compliance.

The Inflatable Advantage

Inflatable vests have a low profile and lightweight design that allow them to lie flush against the body so they do not restrict movement, resulting in ease of wear and superb flotation. For offshore sailors, vests provide 150 N (33.7 lbf) of buoyancy, compared with 100 N (22.5 lbf) in foam type I and 70 N (15.5 lbf) in foam types II and III. Incremental buoyancy enables a person to float high in the water, easing inspiration and expiration, and reduces risk of seawater aspiration in rough seas (see Figures 70-3 and 70-4). Avoiding mouth immersion is vital to prevent drowning. When possible, victims should face downwind and away from oncoming waves to avoid splash-over of water into the airway, although a natural tendency is to assume a face-into-the-waves attitude. By keeping the head, neck, and chest higher out of the water, it is easier to adopt the heat escape lessening position (HELP) (see Figure 69-14). With buoyancy high on the chest, there is also superior righting ability and head support. Inflatables with 150 N of buoyancy can be purchased with an integral safety harness, and all vests can be equipped with strobe or LED safety lights, whistles, crew overboard (COB) beacons, and other attention-attracting gear (see discussions of safety harnesses, as well as other equipment, below) (see Figure 70-3).

The U.S. Coast Guard has approved a wide variety of inflatable life jackets with varying buoyancies (70, 100, 150, and 275 N [16, 24, 35, and 60 lbf]). Water-activated inflatable vests should be worn at all times by nonswimmers because they might panic after falling overboard and not deploy their manual inflation ripcord; children must be older than 16 years and weigh more than 36 kg (80 lb) to have these types of vests count in a vessel's inventory. Even strong swimmers should consider wearing a water-activated model. Head injury from a surprise fall or an inadvertent head injury from the boom might render a person unconscious or stunned and leave the person face down in the sea with a deflated manual inflation vest. More importantly, any sudden, unexpected immersion can be very disorienting, especially when compounded by a cold shock response and reduced swimming ability due to clothing, footwear, and gear. When interviewed, survivors of boat accidents involving quick, unanticipated immersion consistently report that they might not have been able to find the "ripcord" and activate it, because of the disorientation that occurs with cold-water immersion. Wearing an inflatable vest that automatically responds to immersion negates having to locate the "jerk to inflate" lanyard.

Newer models of inflatable vests have 1F (water-activated) and 3F (manually activated) inflators that have a single point indicator to show if the vest is armed with an unused carbon dioxide (CO_2) cylinder, so-called cylinder seal indication. The indicator allows the user to determine whether the life jacket is properly armed and ready for use. Newer inflators will not deploy unless the wearer is immersed in water, and are highly resistant to incidental water contact, such as sea spray or rain. Older models suffered from premature and undesired inflation. All automatic vests have a manual backup ripcord for inflation, plus a backup oral inflation tube that can also be used to deflate the bladder routinely and in an emergency.

Like all mechanical systems on-board ship, inflatable vests require regular inspection and maintenance according to the manufacturer's instructions. Prior to each use, the CO_2 cylinder must be in place and unused. With newer 1F and 3F models, this can be verified by looking for the green indicator. Older models may require investigation under the protective shroud and unscrewing of the cylinder. Users should note whether the life jacket has a water-activated inflator. Every season, the CO_2 cylinder should be removed and the vest orally inflated as much as possible and left to stand for at least several hours to assess for leaks. If the vest becomes soft, it should be established that the oral inflation tube valve is seated. If the oral inflation tube is not the leak source, the vest should be destroyed or returned to the manufacturer for further analysis. The water-soluble bobbins should be inspected and replaced as scheduled (generally every 2 years). One must know how to rearm, deflate, and repack any inflatable vest according to instructions. A life jacket should be maintained as though one's life depends on it, because it certainly does.

Boaters who resist wearing any type of vest may tolerate an inflatable vest packed in a compact belt pack. This vest is carried in a belt pack around the waist, and is the least cumbersome of any flotation device. After inflation in water, the horseshoe-shaped device must be pulled over the head and secured with straps to the chest (similar to a regular inflatable life vest) while the swimmer works to stay afloat; it offers 100 N to 150 N (22 to 35 lbf) of buoyancy. This device is not suitable for nonswimmers or children. It is becoming more common due to the increasing popularity of stand-up paddleboards because of lack of interference when paddling.

An additional option is one of the increasingly lightweight, stole-type vests that fit close to the chest but do not look like the original suspenders-appearing vests (see Figure 70-4). They are more like athletic equipment, and are available as water-activated models that can be converted to manual-only operation when desired.

Testing a Life Jacket

One should test and wear any new vest in a pond or pool and practice the HELP position. The wearer should float in a slightly reclining position with 3 to 4 inches of freeboard. Life jackets should be close fitting with small arm holes, or at least grip the torso so that they stay in place. Life jackets that ride up on the wearer's chest allow the wearer to sink lower in the water, reducing the airway freeboard.

Children require a properly fitted model with leg straps to prevent the vest from sliding up over the arms and head (this is also effective for adults). Common size ranges for children's life jackets are 0 to 30 lb, 30 to 50 lb, and 50 to 90 lb. The best life jackets for children under 23 kg (50 lb) should have a bifold head support to right a face-down child and keep the child face-up in water. An additional option is to have children wear safety harnesses to keep them on deck. It is dangerous to buy a life jacket that is too large for a child (in anticipation of future growth); incorrect sizing of a life jacket compromises its usefulness and may have tragic consequences. The PFD should fit snugly with zippers closed and straps tightened. Test the fit by having the child raise his or her arms over the head while an adult lifts the PFD by the shoulder straps. If the PFD slips upward or slides up to touch the child's nose, further adjustment is necessary. Adults can also perform this test by jumping into the water wearing the PFD to see if it slips upward, or have someone pull forcefully on the shoulder straps from above. Falling overboard with the PFD rising up and covering the face and head is an alarming and life-threatening situation.

For young sailors, there are many styles, rated buoyancies, designs, and constructions. These were reviewed in the June 2013 issue of *Practical Sailor;* the following month's issue reviewed some newer designs for "active" adult sailors (racers) and kayakers.

IMMERSION (SURVIVAL) SUITS

Immersion (survival) suits are the ultimate protection from hypothermia and drowning. An immersion suit combines properties of a life raft, life jacket, and dry suit. Most models include a watertight full-length zipper, watertight hood, face seal for wind and water protection, detachable mitts, neoprene wrist seals, integral boots, inflatable head pillow for optimum flotation angle, integrated lifting harness, water-activated safety light (strobe or LED), whistle, and buddy line. Their general bulkiness (one size fits a 50- to 136-kg [110- to 300-lb] person) and built-in gloves make them impractical for continued wear while actively working aboard ship. The Coast Guard now requires personnel onboard

their vessels to wear a dry suit (not an immersion suit) when the ocean water temperature is less than 50°F (10°C), and a less bulky antiexposure suit with insulating underwear and clothing when temperatures are between 50° and 59°F (10° and 15°C). A type III life jacket is still necessary to provide adequate flotation if the head pillow and flotation are not integral to the suit.

One potential disadvantage of survival suits (as with high-buoyancy life jackets) is that their buoyancy may impede escape from an overturned craft. The person may become trapped in the cabin, under the cockpit, or under the trampoline of a multihull. "When the trampoline is on top of you, buoyancy is your enemy," said one multihull sailor, who barely survived after capsizing his vessel while wearing his survival suit. One should always don the suit topside (never below decks or in the wheelhouse) and move away quickly from a rolling, unstable craft. In high latitudes (over 40 degrees), many experts recommend that a survival suit be carried for each person onboard, although the bulk and expense make this somewhat impractical for recreational boaters. Crew should read instructions for suit use because there is a specific technique and sequence for donning the suit, pulling the hood over the head, zipping, and closing the face flap. In practice, the suit should be closed and made watertight in less than 60 seconds. Suits should be inspected regularly for tears or deterioration, and zippers lubricated with Zipper-Ease or other lubricant. A partially closed immersion suit serves only to keep the victim afloat and alive until the victim dies of the cold shock response, immersion hypothermia, or drowning; there are cases of professional fishermen who died from these causes while wearing immersion suits when forced to abandon ship in cold waters.

Water-activated inflatable life vests also may lead to entrapment. In the 2012 Chicago-Mackinac race, two sailors drowned when their sailboat capsized in a powerful squall; they were unable to free themselves from underwater entanglement (see ussailing.org/racing/offshore-big-boats/big-boat-safety-at-sea/safety-incident-reports/ for incident reports regarding recent sailboat accidents).[1] In the incident report, survivors describe how inflated life jackets and attached tethers impeded their escape. Required skills for any sailor include safety equipment familiarity, PFD deflation and air bleeding, use of a quick-release clip on a tether, PFD, and underwater knife use and deployment.

If one has to enter cold water voluntarily (e.g., to free a fouled propeller) without protection of a specialized suit, one must acclimate gradually to frigid water in anticipation of the cold shock response. Upon entering, one must control one's breathing while wearing a safety harness with the tether held by an alert crew member. Once breathing is controlled, the person may proceed.

SAFETY HARNESSES

Safety harnesses (see Figure 70-4) are made from 50-cm (2-inch) nylon webbing or are integrated into inflatable life jackets, with a breaking strength exceeding 1450 kg (3300 lb), and attach the wearer to the vessel. Harnesses are worn when sailing in rough weather, at night, when on deck alone or out of sight of crew, or when both hands are occupied. In heavy weather, a harness should be worn at all times, even in the cockpit. A harness should fit snugly around the chest, 2 inches below the armpits. Tethers connect the harness to through-bolted deck fittings or dedicated jacklines, and are made from uncoated stainless steel wire, HMPE rope, or webbing running fore and aft to a through-bolted pad eye or cleat. Cockpit pad eyes or jacklines should be established within reach of the companionway, so crew can clip on before entering the cockpit. Many newly-awakened sailors, groggy with sleep and unaware of sea conditions, have been lost overboard transitioning from cabin to cockpit during a change of watch. Jacklines should be continuous, allowing crew to roam without having to unclip. Low-stretch webbing is preferable to wire and rope because webbing tends to lie flat on deck and does not roll underfoot. Wire jacklines should be inspected for broken strands, and webbing and rope for ultraviolet (UV) damage and weakening. Recently manufactured tethers have colored threads that will break if the tether has been overtensioned and stretched (also called an overload indicator or overstress indicator). Tethers should be no more than 2 m (6.6 feet) long with an elastic core to keep them from dragging underfoot; a second tether 1 m (3.3 feet) long helps triangulate support and ensures continuous contact with the ship while changing positions. Tethers are best used in confined places, such as the cockpit and at the helm. Ideally, the tether should be attached to the boat such that it will not allow the wearer to be dragged in the water alongside or behind the boat. However, this may not be possible; sailors have drowned while being dragged alongside the vessel by their harness and tethers. The chest shackle should be a quick-release snap shackle that can be released under load if the wearer is trapped under a capsized boat or feels he or she might drown due to being dragged. The ship's end should have a locking snap hook, not one that will accidentally self-release from a pad eye. It should be possible to accomplish the clip on/off process with one hand, and never require a sailor to use both hands to connect or loosen the hook at the end of the harness tether. A double-action carabiner only opens when squeezed "between one hand" (between fingers and palm), and eliminates the possibility of accidental opening. Another option is the double-action locking safety hook, which can be opened with one hand.

The harness should be donned before leaving the cabin, and tether secured before leaving the companionway. While underway, crew should hook the tether onto the windward (uphill, upwind) jackline whenever possible; a crew person is more likely to fall to leeward, and the shorter tether length will keep a person on deck instead of dragging the person through the water. Women should not adjust the chest strap below their bust line, because breast injury may occur from upward force placed on the harness under sudden tension; there are female-specific harness designs. Inflatable life jackets are available with an integral safety harness; this convenient combination may be the most important piece of personal safety gear at sea. A harness keeps the crewmember aboard, prevents separation from the vessel if and when a crewmember falls overboard, and can guide escape from an overturned craft, especially when someone is disoriented.

CREW OVERBOARD

REMAINING ABOARD

Falling overboard (most often from collision) with subsequent drowning is the most common cause of a marine fatality in recreational boating and commercial shipping. In stormy weather, the safest location is inside the cabin. Following these rules can prevent virtually all crew-overboard (COB) incidents:

  Remain sober, especially if you expect to go on deck for any reason.
  Wear nonskid footwear that grips well on a rolling and wet deck, and have nonskid paint or pads in critical work areas.
  Walk in a crouched position with a low center of gravity and wide-based stance when the boat is rolling, heeling, or pitching.
  If the boat's motion is too violent for a person to stand, then crawl or slide along the deck.
  Use a safety harness and tether as a "third hand," secured to a strong attachment point.
  Use a safety harness whenever going aloft in the rigging or climbing any superstructure.
  Avoid leaning overboard with all your weight on a lifeline or stanchion, and use a strong adjustable boat hook to pick up a mooring and dock lines or extend to a COB.
  Know the location of secure handholds and grab rails so you can find them at night.
  Know safe routes to avoid tripping on deck hardware, vents, and hatches, especially at night; use spreader lights if necessary to illuminate the deck. Be aware, the helmsperson will lose night vision temporarily (Figure 70-5).
  Do not urinate from the afterdeck in rough weather unless you are kneeling and attached with a safety harness. In really rough weather, consider urinating into cockpit scuppers.
  Wear a safety harness whenever seasick; vomit into a bucket rather than leaning overboard.

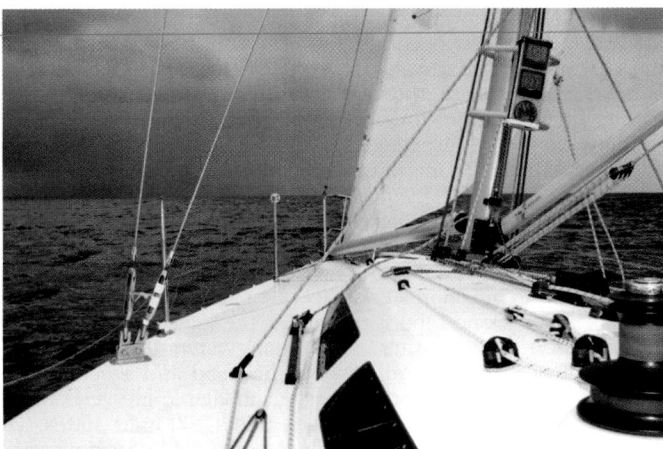

FIGURE 70-5 Clean side decks on this ocean racer provide fewer trip hazards, but not a great deal to hold on to. Toe rails on modern boats may only extend aft from the stem to abeam of the mast. Using jacklines would make going to the foredeck dramatically safer.

  In heavy weather, sleep in the harness and be ready to attach the tether to a cockpit pad eye before coming on deck.
  Check the integrity of pulpits, stern rails, handrails, stanchions, lifelines, and jacklines. Look for cracks on welds, corrosion of fittings at terminals, and telltale rust streaks on plastic coating. Current standards for lifelines do not allow vinyl coating, because it can hide corrosion. Inspect for broken strands on lifelines. Check for sun damage, chafe, and stretching on jacklines, and keep these lines taut with minimal slack.
  Clip on when sailing alone, when sailing short-handed, at night from dawn to dusk, in conditions with poor visibility, when reefed, and in heavy weather.
  Practice "boom awareness" and know the boom's position relative to your head and body while walking on deck, and while tacking and jibing. Walk forward facing the boom, and keep low when returning on the opposite side, with the boom always in sight. Offshore, use a boom preventer at all times, in all conditions, and on all points of sail (not just running downwind) to prevent being knocked overboard. A vessel's boom might be thought of as a deck-sweeping club designed to knock overboard anyone not paying close attention, with the added complication that he or she will probably be unconscious.
  Crew should maintain physical fitness, agility, and balance. This may involve extra time exercising and balance exercises in a gym, prior to a trip.

There is some debate in the Safety at Sea "world" about whether to have the engine on when rescuing a COB. Much of what we know about COBs came from studies done by the Sailing Foundation in Seattle. The researchers found that many victims became injured from propeller strikes, especially if visual contact with the victim was lost as the vessel approached. The conclusion was to maneuver under sail to avoid injuring the victim with the vessel's propeller. Other studies conducted by the Sailing Squadron at the Naval Academy in Annapolis, Maryland, were done with the engine on as a backup to sails.

If used, the engine can be started and left in neutral, ready to be used if needed in the final approach. Rescuers must ensure that all lines are aboard before engaging the engine, to avoid fouling the propeller. It is advisable to return to neutral when close to the victim. The main danger to the victim is being sucked under the stern while the propeller is turning and the boat is moving forward under power

RECOVERY OF CREW OVERBOARD

Time is the critical factor in recovering a crew overboard (COB). (We prefer the gender-neutral term *crew overboard [COB]*, which is gaining popularity in the United States, but some product

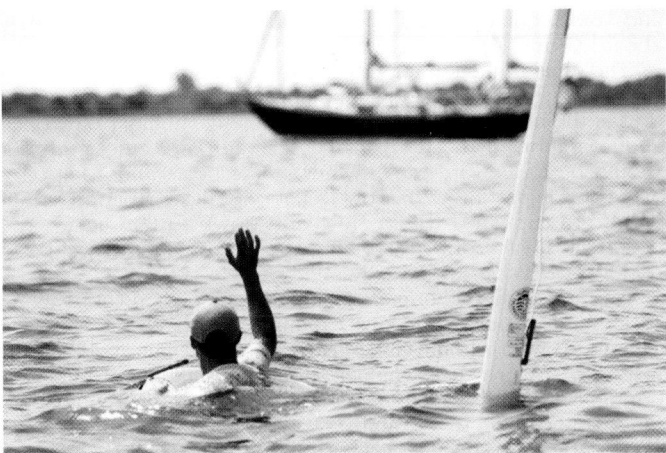

FIGURE 70-6 This crew overboard module consists of an inflatable horseshoe-shaped buoyant device, 1.8-m (6-foot) inflatable locator pylon with a light, and self-opening sea anchor.

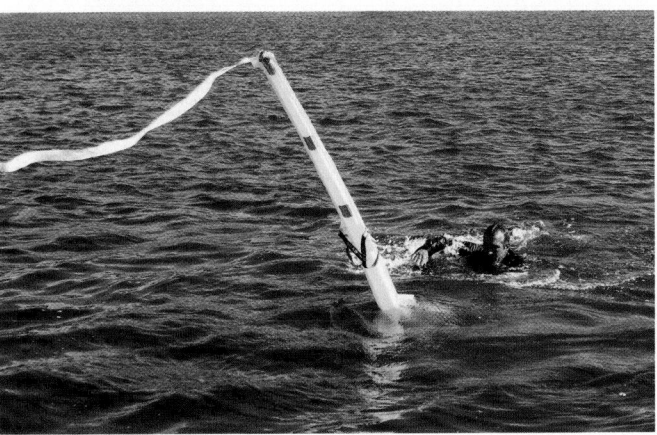

FIGURE 70-7 The MOB Dan Buoy is a ballasted, inflatable pylon with a light at the top, very visible streamer, drogue, and enough buoyancy to float the victim.

names, as well as global positioning system [GPS] functions, still use the term *man overboard [MOB]*.) A well-rehearsed rescue under competent leadership with clear communication during rescue maneuvers is most likely to succeed. When someone is observed falling overboard, shout "crew overboard." The crew should then initiate the COB function to create a COB waypoint. Most GPS receivers will store a waypoint named COB, and will also make this the GOTO waypoint, thus providing guidance back to the geographic position of the victim at the time of the accident. A pan-pan should be broadcast on the very high frequency (VHF) radio to alert vessels in the area. Heavy winds, large seas, and strong currents decrease the relevance of the GPS waypoint in marking the COB, because the person may drift downwind and especially down-current while the boat returns to the scene; however, it is still better to have a last known point for a starting position than no position at all. One or more crew should be tasked with spotting and pointing at the victim continuously without losing sight of the victim. Floating objects should be thrown overboard, including buoyant cushions, horseshoe buoys, ring buoys, and extra life jackets, to "litter" the water surrounding the victim. Gear may provide extra flotation to the victim and provides visual cues for the spotter. Unfortunately, most of these objects will drift faster than a person can swim in winds over 10 knots, so the COB cannot be expected to retrieve a thrown life jacket after falling overboard.

Special equipment designed for locating and retrieving a COB should be deployed immediately. This gear should be ready for easy deployment and instant release. Too often, gear is protected against accidental loss by extra wraps of line to the stern pulpit or rigging, and a delay in releasing COB gear will leave it too far from the victim. A COB pole is a 4- to 5-m (12- to 15-foot) floating flagpole that is ballasted to remain upright in rough seas. Without a small drogue (a cone-shaped device to slow a vessel's drift downwind), it will quickly drift away from the designated area. When released from its canister, a crew overboard module (Figure 70-6) automatically deploys a CO_2-activated horseshoe buoy and a 2-m (6-foot) inflatable locator pylon equipped with a drogue and water-activated, lithium-powered light. The SOS Dan Buoy is a throwable pylon that inflates to 6 feet high, with 150 N (35 lbf) of buoyancy and a light on top. The swimmer can grab the pylon handles for support (Figure 70-7).

A variety of lights have been developed to serve as rescue beacons worn by the COB or thrown overboard. An overboard marker strobe marks the site, illuminates the scene for rescuers, and automatically activates when thrown into water. Waterproof personal rescue strobe lights attached to a life jacket can flash for 8 hours at 1-second intervals and are visible a mile away. A strobe light together with a proper whistle (with a special flat design to prevent the whistle body from holding water and dampening sound) should be attached to every life jacket.

In the last decade, a number of personal COB beacons have become available, which is fortuitous because the speed of

offshore sailboats has greatly increased during the same period; faster sailboat speeds imply longer distances between a sailboat and the COB. There are several variations on a theme in current models:

A beacon transmits a signal (commonly on the retired EPIRB frequency 121.5 Mhz) when immersed in water or activated; remaining crew uses a radio direction finder or automatic direction finder to home in on the victim.

A device worn by all crew members ceases transmitting to an onboard base station when the wearer goes overboard. The station then sounds an alarm and stores a waypoint on a GPS so that the victim's initial location is known (Figure 70-8).

A radio allows the victim to communicate by voice with the mother ship, using a small VHF transceiver, possibly equipped with a GPS and digital selective calling (DSC) capabilities.

A personal locator beacon (PLB) may be carried and activated. It is designed to communicate with the Search and Rescue Satellite-Aided Tracking (SARSAT) system, a rescue coordination center, and rescue agencies (Figure 70-9). This system works reliably and worldwide, but it could take too long for the U.S. Coast Guard to arrive at the position. A

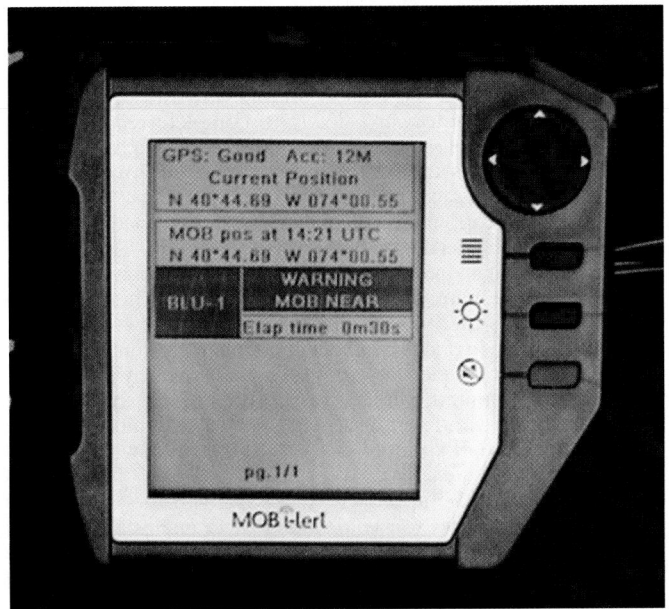

FIGURE 70-8 Cessation-of-transmission crew overboard devices alert the helmsman when a particular crewmember's pendant loses contact with the base station. The device stores a waypoint for immediate navigation back to the "swimmer."

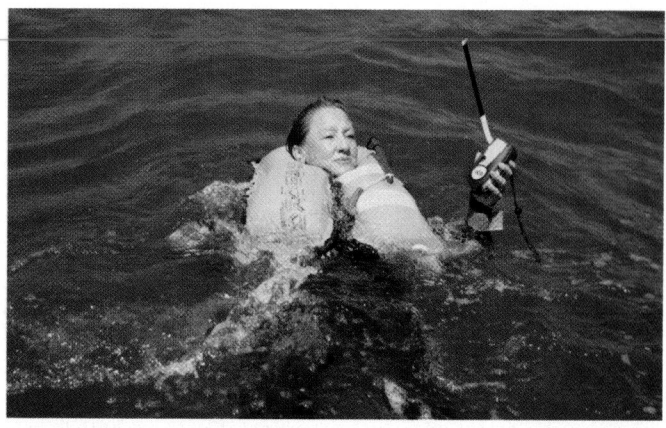

FIGURE 70-9 A personal locator beacon (PLB) may be an excellent link back to the Coast Guard, but if you are too far offshore, you may not survive until the Coast Guard arrives. Consider a MOB beacon that alerts the crew on the mother ship, or better yet, both methods.

PLB broadcasts little information of use to the rescuing crew on the vessel or the fleet in which it is sailing.

The beacon contains a GPS and ability to transmit on automatic identification system (AIS) frequencies or both AIS and DSC frequencies, so the mother ship can determine both the position of the victim and that the victim is overboard. This requires that the mother ship have the ability to receive AIS and DSC signals; several modern VHF transceivers have this capability. Ideally, they are with a chart plotter so that the victim's position can be constantly plotted relative to the rescuing vessel.

With these new systems, it is essential that all components integrate seamlessly, because they function together to locate and retrieve the COB.

Crew Overboard Maneuvers

The goal in overboard recovery is to return as quickly as possible to the COB using the simplest maneuver. A boat traveling at a speed of 8 knots moves away from the COB at about 3.9 m (13 feet)/second or 244 m (800 feet)/minute. At that rate, one-half mile is traversed in 3 minutes. Motorboats should reduce speed, return in a simple circle, and approach the victim heading upwind, with the victim about 6 m (20 feet) to one side. Sailboats under power alone can return by simply circling back and approaching the COB in the same manner. Contact should be established with the COB by using a rescue throw rope (i.e., a floating polypropylene line in an easily throwable, high-visibility, nylon storage bag). If the boat is drifting downwind, the vessel should be advanced forward slowly to complete recovery over the leeward side. Sailboats under sail should approach on a close reach, which allows the vessel to speed up or slow down as needed by changing course or luffing the mainsail.

The "quick stop" recovery maneuver is designed for rapid COB recovery, especially with short-handed crews. This method enables the boat to reduce speed immediately by turning into the wind and allowing the headsail (jib) to back. Thereafter, the helmsman keeps the boat turning through the eye of the wind, until headed downwind. The jibe will be relatively gentle because the main is kept sheeted in during the maneuver. After passing abeam of the victim, the jib is dropped (or furled), and the boat heads up to the wind (on a close reach) to stop alongside the victim at an angle of about 60 degrees to the wind with the sails luffing.

The COB must be approached slowly, with the boat under good control, in order to avoid hitting or dragging the COB as soon as the COB is contacted and attached to a retrieval device. By sailing the final approach to the COB on a close reach, the sails can be fully luffing or trimmed to maintain forward movement if short of the mark. The technique is similar to picking up a mooring under sail. Communication with the victim is essential, providing instructions on the rescue plan, what is required of the victim, and reassuring the victim that recovery will occur. Eye and voice contact should be maintained until the COB is safely aboard (Box 70-1).

The final direction of approach used by the rescue boat involves factors that include conditions of the sea, wind strength, drift of the boat relative to the COB, maneuverability of the boat, and condition of the COB. If the seas are large, the approach should be to leeward (downwind) so the boat cannot fall off a wave and injure the COB. Low to flat seas allow an approach to windward (upwind) with a slow drift down to the victim. The boat will always drift faster than the person in the water, so retrieval gear should be ready at all times.

An injured, hypothermic, or unconscious person (not waving or looking at the rescue boat) requires assistance by a rescue swimmer, who should take steps to avoid the cold shock response. The rescue swimmer should be tethered to the boat during recovery, trained in water rescue and lifesaving techniques, and able to recognize warning signs of panic as the swimmer approaches the victim. If the COB is unconscious, possible head and neck injury should be considered; the cervical spine should be stabilized before hoisting the victim out of the water if injury is suspected. The life jacket itself may be used to control the head and neck if it is tightened in the upper chest area.

Recovering an unconscious person from the water is extremely difficult and puts a second person (at least) in a very precarious position. Unless the water is very calm, it is nearly impossible for the victim to avoid aspirating water, causing drowning if the head injury has not been fatal in the first place. The decision to risk a second life in recovering a body must be carefully considered.

Bringing the Victim Aboard

The goal is to bring the COB onboard as quickly as possible. Different rescue techniques should be practiced with the planned boat and crew prior to deciding which methods and modifications work best. The Lifesling pack was developed to enable a single individual to retrieve a person overboard. Stanchion-mounted, the Lifesling[11] pack contains a pliable center section horseshoe, 120 feet of three-eighths-inch floating polypropylene line, and an optional water-activated personal marker light. The flexible floating horseshoe collar can be used as a hoisting sling (Figure 70-10). The collar should be deployed from the stern pulpit and delivered by repeatedly circling the victim, just as a ski boat maneuvers to deliver the towrope to a fallen water-skier. After securing the horseshoe over the head and under the arms, pull the victim back to the boat and make the retrieval line fast to a cleat in the cockpit. At this point, the pace of rescue can be slowed, because the victim cannot be lost and is not likely to drown. The Lifesling can be used with a long halyard, capable of reaching to the bight of line at the Lifesling, or it can be used

---

BOX 70-1   Engine On or Engine Off?

There's some debate in the Safety at Sea "world" about whether to have the engine on when rescuing a crewmember overboard. Much of what we know about crewmembers overboard came from studies done by the Sailing Foundation in Seattle. The research found that many victims became injured due to propeller strikes, especially if visual contact with the victim was lost as the vessel approached. Their conclusion was to maneuver under sail to avoid injuring the victim with the vessel's propeller. Other studies conducted by the Sailing Squadron at the Naval Academy in Annapolis, Maryland, were done with the engine on as a backup to sails.

If used, the engine can be started and left in neutral, ready to be used if needed in the final approach. Rescuers must ensure all lines are aboard before engaging the engine, to avoid fouling the propeller. It is advisable to return to neutral when close to the victim. The main danger to the victim is being sucked under the stern while the propeller is turning and the boat is moving forward under power. Other experienced sailors have pointed out that sailing a boat back to the victim in light winds may be slow compared with firing up the engine and powering directly into the wind.

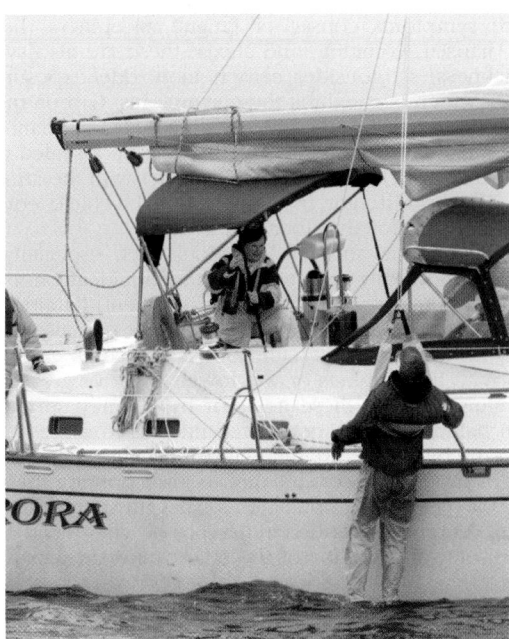

FIGURE 70-10 Getting the person in the water back onboard is not a simple task. The Lifesling provides flotation, connects the victim to the vessel, and serves as a lifting sling.

with a 3:1 tackle with 65 feet of line. On smaller sailboats (< 30-foot length overall) that have smaller winches, the 3:1 tackle reduces tension on the fall of the tackle and makes winch operation easier. Note that in Lifesling demonstrations and clinics, students frequently improvise the lifting tackle rigging and end up with suboptimal results. As with all rescue methods, practice with the planned boat and crew to increase familiarity with rescue systems and concomitant likelihood of success.

Lifelines are an obstacle to bringing the COB back on deck, but are an important source of protection for remaining crew. Lifelines may be secured at the stern (or transom) with lashing, rather than shackles or pins, so they can be easily cut and released in a recovery.

The most important factors for a successful rescue are the crew's familiarity with the boat and COB equipment, leadership of the captain, and expert teamwork developed during practice of rescue maneuvers. In 2005, a Crew Overboard Rescue Symposium[4] was conducted on San Francisco Bay during which hundreds of rescues were performed. The resulting publication reviews challenges for a successful recovery, required crew skills, preferred recovery maneuvers, and helpful equipment for locating and retrieving the victim. It is a must-read for every boater. It is also available in a slightly different format on the U.S. Sailing website.[12]

EMERGENCIES AT SEA

FIRE AT SEA

Causes

Uncontrolled fire is a disaster aboard ship. Fires aboard wood and fiberglass boats can double in size every 10 seconds. Approximately 7500 pleasure boat fires and explosions occur annually; of the boats affected, 10% are declared total losses. More than one-half of the 2700 fire-related injuries incurred each year occur on small, open motorboats. According to statistics compiled by Boat U.S. Marine Insurance claims investigations,[3] the leading causes of fires on boats (55%) are alternating current (AC) and direct current (DC) wiring faults. The most common electrical problem is related to chafed wires creating short circuits. Many fires are started by battery cables, bilge pump wires, or instrument wires chafing on hard objects, such as vibrating engines or sharp-edged bulkheads. The DC voltage regulator is responsible for 25% of electrical fires. Eleven percent of fires are started by

the boat's AC system, frequently at the shore power inlet box. AC heaters and other household appliances that have been brought onboard cause a small number of fires. Twenty-four percent of fires are started by overheated propulsion systems. Frequently, an intake or exhaust cooling water passage is obstructed, causing the engine to overheat and melt down hoses and impellers. These fires tend to be less serious, but because of the amount of smoke and in areas with flammable fuels, they appear more threatening. Often the fires are simply smoldering rubber, until the engine compartment is opened, allowing fresh air to enter. In Florida, lightning is a major cause of boat fires in marinas. Box 70-2 lists ways to prevent fires aboard ship.

Fire from Fuels, Liquids, and Gases

The explosive potential of fuel depends on its chemical properties and where vapors accumulate in enclosed, unventilated spaces. Hazardous liquids are classified according to flash point, the lowest temperature at which a liquid releases sufficient vapor to sustain burning. "Flammable liquids," such as gasoline,

---

BOX 70-2 Fire Prevention at Sea

1. Sniff the engine compartment before starting a gasoline engine and before starting the electric bilge blower. Bilge blowers are ignition-protected, but it is still a good idea. Run the bilge blower for at least 4 minutes before starting the engine.
2. Use appropriately sized marine-grade wire. Periodically inspect the wiring for cracks, charring, and deteriorating insulation. Wiring connectors and terminals should be tightly set and periodically inspected for looseness. Each electrical circuit should have fuses or circuit breakers according to American Boat and Yacht Council Standard E-11.
3. Battery compartments must not be completely enclosed, and must allow hydrogen gas to escape through the lids of the battery boxes. Even sealed AGM (absorbed glass mat) and gel batteries can generate hydrogen gas if overcharged.
4. Consult a professional to develop an appropriate ship's grounding system. See westmarine.com/WestAdvisor/Marine-Grounding-Systems for the best article on the complicated topic of vessel grounding.
5. Observe all precautions when taking on fuel. Close all hatches and ports before filling the tanks, and extinguish all flames. Ventilate the boat after fueling.
6. Never leave the stove unattended while in use.
7. Store extra fuel on deck in approved plastic containers, or in a locker that is sealed from the main cabin and drains overboard.
8. Store outboard motor and fuel tank on deck in approved fuel containers.
9. Transfer gasoline and other flammable liquids from one container to another on deck or off the boat, not below decks.
10. Inboard engines require meticulous inspection and maintenance. Perform a routine visual inspection of any operating engine and the exhaust system. Keep seawater strainers for the engine cooling system clean. Become an expert in examining and repairing all components of the fuel system. On vessels with an engine room, consider having a mirror-finished piece of stainless steel that will make it obvious if you have a fine spray of fuel or other liquids in the air.
11. Install a heat-activated automatic fire-extinguishing system in the engine compartment, together with smoke and flame detectors.
12. Properly store fuels, solvents, paints, brushes, and combustibles in a deck storage locker. Keep all rags in metal containers with the lid tightly closed. Do not keep oily rags below decks or in the engine compartment.
13. Place fire extinguishers away from the intended area of use so that they are accessible, and have them inspected and maintained on a scheduled basis.
14. Read the extinguishers' instructions periodically, and practice on a controlled fire away from the boat.
15. Remove extinguishers from their brackets and invert them several times to ensure that the agent inside is loose and flowing.

turpentine, lacquer thinner, and acetone, have flash points below 38°C (100.4°F), meaning they release enough vapor at warm temperatures to form burnable and explosive mixtures. "Combustible liquids," such as diesel oil, kerosene, and hydraulic fluid, have flash points above 38°C (100.4°F).

Gasoline is the most hazardous fuel, causing 60% of fuel-related fires. Typical problem areas are fuel lines, engine connections, and leaking fuel tanks. The first warning sign is frequently the odor of leaking gasoline. Vapors can ignite from heat in the engine compartment and from liquid spills over hot engine parts. Five mL (1 tsp) of gasoline can vaporize and cause an explosion, and 237 mL (1 cup) of gasoline has the explosive potential of several sticks of dynamite. Vaporized gasoline is heavier than air, so it accumulates in the lowest part of any enclosed space, generally the bilge. It is therefore critical to run the bilge blower for at least 4 minutes before starting the engine. Diesel fuel is much less explosive than gasoline. However, pressurized diesel fuel spurting from a burst fuel line will ignite and burn when it strikes something hot, such as the exhaust manifold. Charging batteries generate hydrogen, which accumulates in the battery compartment or the compartment overhead; the gas is lighter than air, highly flammable, and potentially explosive. Sparks from a nearby electric motor may set off an explosion from excess hydrogen produced by overcharging batteries.

A popular galley stove fuel is liquefied petroleum gas (LPG), either propane or butane. Both are highly explosive, heavier than air, and may accumulate in the bilge. Like gasoline, free propane in the bilge is potentially explosive. Proper LPG tank installation requires a completely self-contained vapor-tight locker that opens only above decks. A drain should be located at least 51 cm (20 inches) from any opening to the boat's interior, and should not be submerged while the boat is underway. A pressure gauge connected to the LPG cylinder valve helps indicate a leak somewhere in the system. It is not, as many believe, intended to show the quantity of LPG in the tank. A regulator to reduce pressure in the gas line to the stove and an electric solenoid valve complete the delivery. Safety standards recommended by the American Boat and Yacht Council require an LPG sniffer in the system to continually monitor the air for LPG. The sniffer should be installed at a low point where gas is likely to accumulate; if any is detected, an alarm sounds, and the sensor shuts off the solenoid and gas flow to appliances. Newer LPG stoves have a built-in thermosensor to shut off the gas supply if a burner flame is accidentally extinguished by a draft or wind. The safest practice is to never leave any lighted galley stove unattended. Expert professional assistance is recommended when installing a complete fuel supply system. As of April 2002, propane cylinders must be equipped with an overfill protection valve, because overfilled cylinders may explode after overheating. If a LPG leak is suspected, the propane tank should be shut off using the manual valve, and the main battery switch should be used to kill electrical power to all electrical devices. All hatches and ports should be opened to ventilate the boat, and the ignition-protected bilge or engine room exhaust blower should be activated to remove any leaked gas.

The system should be periodically pressure-tested for leaks, especially after rough weather, or repairs or maintenance to the system using the LPG sniffer. In order to check for a leak properly, the cylinder valve should be opened with the solenoid switched on and all appliance valves closed, and the pressure gauge reading recorded. The cylinder hand valve should be closed in order to assess the pressure drop over intervals of 3 to 5 minutes; if the pressure drops, there is a leak. Soapy water may be used to look for the leak source, because leaking gas will generate bubbles.

To avoid accidents after cooking, switch off the solenoid first, leave the burner ignited until the line is cleared of gas, and then turn the burner off. When appliances are not in use or the boat is unattended, the cylinder valve must be closed. Most importantly, a stove should never be used as a cabin heater; open combustion and flames can deplete a cabin of oxygen and release carbon monoxide, asphyxiating the sleeping crew. Carbon monoxide is a colorless and odorless gaseous byproduct of incomplete combustion; severe exposure can be lethal. Early

exposure symptoms consist of fatigue, sleepiness, headache, malaise, nausea, vomiting, and ataxia; these are also symptoms of seasickness, so consider carbon monoxide exposure when several crewmembers exhibit these symptoms. Carbon monoxide detectors should be installed below decks. LPG appliances, such as cabin heaters, manufactured for boats have a sealed combustion chamber, which is not in direct contact with the atmosphere aboard. This is different from recreational vehicle equipment, which is not safe for use aboard a boat.

Stove alcohol is another hazardous fuel, especially if one burner is accidentally extinguished and liquid alcohol used in priming the burner pours onto an adjacent flaming burner, causing a flare-up. A nonpressurized burner can also reignite if refilled with alcohol while still hot. Alcohol fires can be extinguished with fire blankets or wet towels. A stove grease fire can be extinguished with these items or by liberally sprinkling the fire with baking soda. A good precaution is to place a kettle of water on the burner before lighting it; this helps contain any high flames arising from excess alcohol used in priming the burner.

Charcoal grills are popular on boats; however, they should not be used on boats berthed in marinas or when wind can blow hot ashes onto the surface of the boat or a nearby craft.

FIGHTING FIRES

The best way to manage a fire in the engine compartment is to install a properly sized, automatic discharging extinguisher system, which interrupts combustion with chemical materials or gases. Fire-suppressing alternatives to Halon gas (now banned because it breaks down atmospheric ozone) are fluoropropane and fluoroethane (FM-200 for occupied spaces, and FE-241 for unoccupied spaces, respectively). These fire suppressants can be automatically discharged from extinguishers by devices that sense ultraviolet radiation or temperature above 79°C (174.2°F). Automatic systems should also have a manual trigger for activation. Portable fire extinguishers should be discharged into the engine compartment through fire ports (Figure 70-11), which minimize the amount of fresh air allowed into the compartment with fire. Shut down the engine either automatically or manually when fighting a fire in the compartment. Automatic shutoff for diesel engines, generators, and engine room blowers is now required in the event of an extinguisher discharge. Diesel engines consume large volumes of air when running and can quickly deplete the extinguishing agent. The area should be allowed to cool before opening hatches or inspection ports, because fresh air may rekindle the fire, either by diluting the concentration of extinguishing agent or by introducing oxygen.

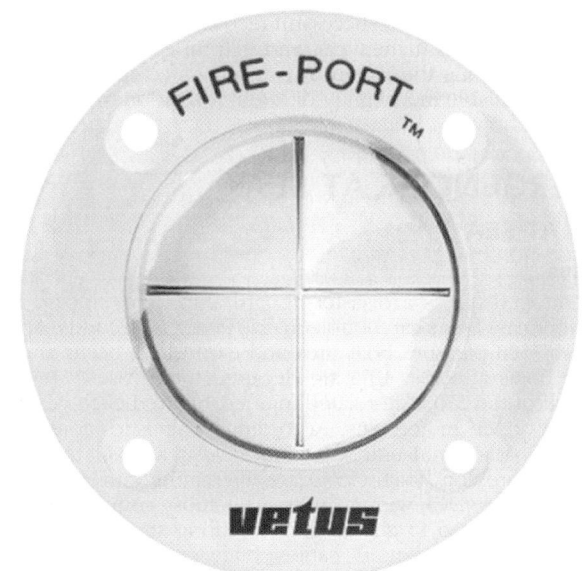

FIGURE 70-11 Portable fire extinguishers should be discharged into the engine compartment through fire ports.

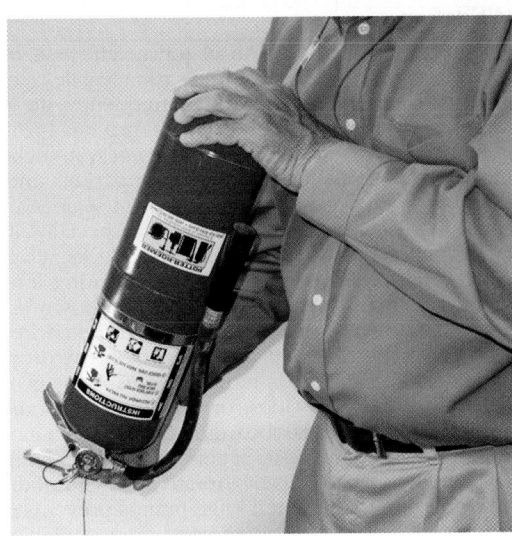

FIGURE 70-12 Dry chemical fire extinguishers should be inspected to ensure the pressure gauge indicates a full charge, and should be inverted regularly to unpack the extinguishing agent.

In the United States, fires are categorized by letter designations. Class A fires involve common combustible products such as wood, canvas, and plastic (items that leave an Ash). Class B fires are flammable liquids such as kerosene, diesel, gasoline, and alcohol (items that Boil). Class C fires result from an electrical fault, but generally involve class A or B materials once the circuit is deenergized (think of electrical Charge). Class D fires involve burning metals such as lithium batteries or possible flare contents (think of Don't, because these fires are extremely difficult to deal with). Fire classes in countries using ISO standards will find that the letter designations are slightly different, but are defined on the extinguisher's label.

The Coast Guard requires all recreational vessels to have portable fire extinguishers (Figure 70-12). Because many boaters have never used a fire extinguisher, it is important to read instructions and become familiar with use before a fire extinguisher is actually required. The standard multipurpose dry chemical extinguisher (filled with monoammonium phosphate) and newer dry chemicals can be used on all types of fires. Dry chemical fire extinguishers work by preventing access to oxygen and interrupting the chemical reaction of fire. ABC dry chemical extinguishers are painted red. The chief disadvantage of ABC extinguishers is that the monoammonium phosphate powder is difficult to clean up and damages electronic equipment. Halotron 1 is a relatively new, clean, "no residue" agent for portable extinguishers (also painted red) that discharges as a rapidly evaporating liquid. It is safe for electronics and computers, and is a good alternative to older dry chemical powders. A major drawback of all portable extinguishers is the extremely brief window of opportunity provided to put out the fire. The common B-1 extinguisher discharges completely in just 10 to 13 seconds. Units with greater capacity simply deliver more chemical over the same period. Because of a short discharge time, more than one fire extinguisher should be available to cope with a large blaze.

The acronym "PASS" is used to remind users of how to use a portable extinguisher. P stands for Pull; the pin on the extinguisher's head must be pulled for activation. A is for Aim, because there is a limited amount of discharge time. S stands for Squeeze; release the extinguishing agent. Finally, S stands for Sweep; the most effective use of the agent is to sweep across the base of the flames. Fires extinguished with dry chemicals should be considered hazardous until cooled to room temperature. A single portable extinguisher should be dedicated to the engine compartment, a second to the galley (where it should be reachable even if the stove is on fire), a third to the area under the fore hatch, and the fourth (and largest size practical to stow) in a cockpit locker. It is also recommended to have one in each stateroom. The crew should know all locations. One should

never have to walk more than half the boat's length to reach an extinguisher. The ideal location for a portable extinguisher in a closed compartment is next to the exit door. Fires involving common combustible solid material can be brought under control by cooling with large amounts of water. Fires involving flammable or combustible liquids can be smothered to remove oxygen by using a fire blanket (required for many ocean races on sailboats). Electrical fires can be difficult to extinguish because the heat source (a shorted wire) can reignite fire even after a fire extinguisher has been used. Deenergizing the electrical circuit can often control electrical fires, especially when a short circuit is generating sufficient heat to cause other materials to combust. Every boat must have a main battery switch and/or AC breaker to turn off the entire electrical system. Water does not extinguish electrical fires, but may be effective on the resulting class A fire after the electrical circuit has been disconnected. See Box 70-3 for fire-fighting guidelines.

FLOODING

Flooding, with potential for sinking, is a threat to every boater. Boat U.S. Marine Insurance examined 50 claims[2] from recreational boats that sank while underway, ranging from a tiny personal watercraft to a 16.5-m (54-foot) ocean-going sailboat. Thirty-four percent of boats sank because of leaks at through-hull fittings, outdrive boots, or raw water cooling system/exhaust. The single most critical reason that small motorboats flood in open water relates to transom height. Engine transom cutouts may be only inches above the waves, and the motor well may not protect the cockpit. Often, weight distribution of passengers and gear to the stern contributes to the problem. Weight distribution problems may be exacerbated by heavier four-stroke outboards when used with boats that are not designed for the incremental weight.

Flooding may occur from system failure or construction (6% of boats sank after coming down hard off of waves and then splitting open), or structural damage from collision and extreme

---

BOX 70-3 Guidelines for Fighting Fire at Sea

1. Attack fire immediately at the source. Detection and reaction time must be immediate, before the fire burns out of control. Prepare a plan that has been shared with the crew so that everyone knows their responsibilities and the location of equipment.
2. Initiate a MAYDAY call immediately. The purpose is to alert ships in the area in which the crew may have to abandon ship. Always state your position clearly.
3. When fire is discovered, all crew should report on deck as quickly as possible with life jackets and fire extinguishers in hand. Ensure that the life raft is away from the fire. This is another good reason to store life rafts on deck or in a deck-accessible locker.
4. Slow the boat to reduce relative wind, and steer to keep smoke and flames clear of the crew and vessel. Keep the fire on the downwind side of the ship, exposing the smallest amount of the boat's structure to the flames.
5. Crew should always have a clear escape route when fighting a fire.
6. Cut off the source(s) of the fire (e.g., fuel supply, electric current, and ventilation system). Turn off blowers, and stop the engine if fire is in engine compartment.
7. Shut off the air supply to the fire. Close hatches, doors, and vents to all compartments free of people.
8. If you must open a hatch to discharge a portable extinguisher, beware of burning your hands or face. As fresh air enters the compartment, the fire will rise to the air source and flare up. The safest way to open a hatch is to wear gloves and stand on the hinged side of the hatch while it is opened. A "fire port" that allows a fire extinguisher to be discharged without opening an engine compartment can easily be retrofitted to a boat.
9. If the fire is too large or out of control, abandon ship before the fuel tanks explode.
10. Check the engine compartment frequently to detect smoke/fire.

BOX 70-4 Sources of Flooding

Failure of through-hull fittings involving the following systems: head, galley, wash basins, shower sump, bilge pumps, centerboard pins and cables, engine exhaust, engine cooling, deck and cockpit drains, bait box, drain plugs (for small boats), knot meter sensor, depth sounder sensor, propeller shaft stuffing box, shaft struts, shaft log, rudder post, and keel bolts

Failure of hose connections, clamps, pipes, and fittings

Open hatches, companionways, portholes, and ventilators

Siphoning of seawater back into the boat because of poor system design or failure of a check valve

Collision with large floating or submerged objects (e.g., vessel, container, whale, rock, reef)

Structural failure in hull, deck, or rigging

Punctured hull from overboard broken spars (e.g., after dismasting)

Clogged scuppers or cockpit drains

Waves entering the cockpit of an outboard-powered motorboat through the transom engine cutout

BOX 70-5 Damage Control Kit

Assorted hose clamps and tools to adjust them

Conical wood or foam plugs, preferably secured at each through-the-hull opening, and spares

3M Fast Cure 5200 cartridges, or epoxy putty sticks

Caulking gun, extra cartridges

Triangular collision mat, spare plywood for patches

Water-activated fiberglass repair fabric (Syntho-Glass)

Pruning saw with spare blades, bolt, and rigging cutters

Drifts matching the size of clevis pins

Duct tape, electrical tape, and self-amalgamating tape

Self-tapping stainless steel screws, threaded rod, bolts, nuts, and large washers

Extra buckets

weather (Box 70-4). Before abandoning ship, quickly assess damage; time is the limiting factor. Proper tools and repair supplies (Figure 70-13) must be stocked in a damage control kit (Box 70-5), and the crew must know how to use them effectively. Before departure, specific duties are assigned to crewmembers in case of emergency, so they know what to do in the event of flooding, COB, fire, grounding, and dismasting. Duties include damage control, radio transmission of a MAYDAY message (which can be cancelled later if necessary), and preparation to abandon ship.

Flood Mitigation

Early detection of flooding is crucial for an effective response. Visual inspections of the bilge, engine room, galley, and head while underway should be performed frequently, to maintain watertight integrity at all times. Port lights, hatches for the main companionway, engine room, lazarettes, cockpit lockers, fish holds, and other potential breaches require gaskets and proper dogging (locking) devices to ensure watertight seals. All of these seals should be closed while underway, especially in heavy weather, no matter the temperature below decks. Place storm boards over large windows to protect them during long ocean crossings. Flooding may occur either from top down or bottom up. After a knockdown or wave breaking over the cockpit, water may go straight below decks if the companionway drop boards are not in place. These boards require a means to secure them that is operable from both sides, or a lanyard that can be tied securely to keep trapezoidal boards from upward movement. Severe flooding, with damage to batteries, electronics, navigation station, and engine, usually results from top-down flooding. Loss of electrical and engine-mounted bilge pumps prevents dewatering the ship and reduces the amount of time available for the crew to identify the source and stem the flow.

Discharge plumbing requires seacocks. Regularly inspect through-hull fittings, the engine drive shaft stuffing box, clamps, and hoses. Avoid polyvinyl chloride pipes or any other domestic plastic plumbing fittings for through-hull fittings below waterline; these materials are prone to fracture if struck by shifting stores. Preferred materials are Marelon (reinforced noncorrosive plastic) or silicon bronze, together with two stainless steel hose clamps over hose barbs. Post a diagram showing locations of all through-hull fittings and routes of connecting hoses in the cabin. Seacocks should be readily accessible and unobstructed, and easy to find even in conditions of darkness or reduced visibility. Install U-shaped antisiphon loops above the highest waterline, because the waterline changes as the boat heels in. Without these loops, water can siphon back through the hose and into the bilge.

Reliable manual bilge pumps may mitigate mild flooding (Figure 70-14). A high-capacity pump or multiple pumps can buy time for locating and plugging the leak. However, no pump can keep up with even a modest-sized hull breach. If a boat is equipped with an automatic bilge pump(s), install a cycle counter on the pump and an "on" light to alert crew when the pump is activated. A second emergency pump mounted above the first, using a separate float switch, can provide added pumping capability if the first pump cannot keep up with the leak. In this case, an alarm installed in the circuit will alert crew to flooding in excess of what the first pump can handle.

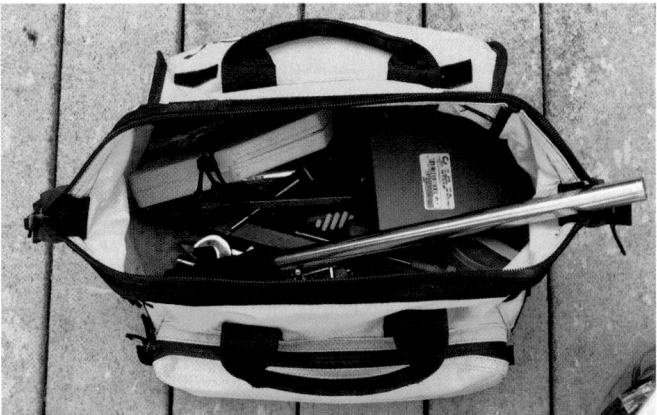

FIGURE 70-13 Damage control kits are not suitable for making fine furniture; in fact, one may have to remove the furniture in the vessel's saloon to get to the source of the leak. Saws, hammers, rivet tools, Band-It tools, and a rechargeable drill are just some of the items one needs to carry.

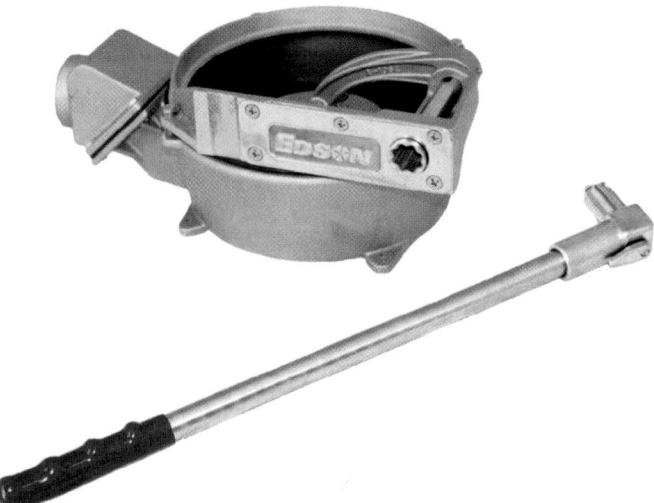

FIGURE 70-14 To be effective, a manual bilge pump has to allow the user to operate it for an extended period of time. A long handle and convenient location, along with a high-capacity pump, make a tremendous difference.

Bilges should be kept clean and free of debris to avoid clogging the pump strainer. New boats frequently have debris (sawdust, masking tape, wire ties) remaining from construction that can clog pumps. Regular inspection and maintenance of the entire pumping system is strongly recommended. Aluminum-body bilge pumps may corrode from the inside out, especially while retaining saltwater. They may appear to be in perfect condition, when in fact they may be useless. Hoses crack with age, rubber components become dry and brittle, valves jam, and moving parts deteriorate through wear and corrosion. To guarantee reliability, manual bilge pumps should annually be disassembled, inspected, and cleaned. Bilge pump handles should be easily accessible and secured with a lanyard near the pump to avoid loss after a knockdown or rollover. Offshore boats require at least two manual bilge pumps, one operable from above decks and one from below decks. A captain should have thorough knowledge of the capacities of a boat's compartments and a means to pump them out if flooded. Test the pump's capabilities by intentionally flooding the bilges (preferably with fresh water) and timing how long it takes to pump out the water.

The volume of water entering through a defect in the boat's hull depends on the breach size and its depth below waterline. A hose that is 2.5 cm (1 inch) in diameter disconnected from a seacock 30 cm (1 foot) below waterline allows 75 L (20 gal) of seawater per minute into the cabin, which is about as much as the best manual bilge pump and a fit operator can handle. A disconnected open seacock of the same diameter just 60 cm (2 feet) below waterline admits three times that amount of water. A boat equipped with the largest manual diaphragm bilge pump can pump a maximum of 1 gallon per stroke if fitted with a 2-inch hose together with an able and inexhaustible crew member; such a pump is rated at 30 gpm based upon a 30-stroke per minute rate. It is therefore critically important to locate and stop the leak, rather than fight what is likely a losing battle by pumping to prevent sinking. There are, however, emergency large-capacity hydraulic bilge pumps capable of pumping hundreds of gallons per minute. Large-capacity pumps may be installed on larger boats with sizeable engine rooms and are capable of saving vessels when pumping large amounts of water is required. Engine-driven front-mounted/clutched centrifugal pumps are the best solution if there is room for the installation and hoses. An alternative is to use one or more high-capacity DC centrifugal pumps.

As water rises in the cabin, a leak becomes more difficult to locate. The inflow rate decreases as the depth of water inside increases, because the pressure gradient is reduced. At a critical level of flooding, the inflow rate may slow sufficiently to allow pumps to handle the volume, so one is best advised to keep pumping. A point of zero net flooding may be reached from inherent buoyancy of the boat as it settles in the water, which is another reason the ship should not be abandoned unless it continues to flood. Many small wood and fiberglass boats float when fully flooded or swamped. Boats less than 6 m (20 feet) in length constructed in the United States after July 1972 are required to have sufficient built-in flotation to remain afloat when swamped. Small boats (e.g., day sailors, small open motorboats) can obtain additional buoyancy by lashing down unused life jackets, cushions, and fenders.

A tapered, soft, and dry wood plug sized to fit a leaking through-hull fitting (including propeller shaft) can serve indefinitely as an emergency seal; the plug will absorb water and swell to seal the fitting or any small puncture in the hull (Figure 70-15). Plugs should be removed from the damage control kit at the beginning of the voyage and attached to their respective through-hull fittings with lanyards; this makes them instantly available and helps crew find them in the dark. Forespar's Sta-Plug is a new damage control product. It is a tapered circular cone-shaped plug about 23 cm (9 inches) tall and 12 cm (4.75 inches) across at the base, made of soft foam that is a spongy but firm cellular material, coated with a flexible sealer that adds strength and color. The TruPlug can be used as a temporary or emergency plug in boating applications where water would enter a circular, oval, or irregular hole caused by mechanical failure or hull breach due to impact.

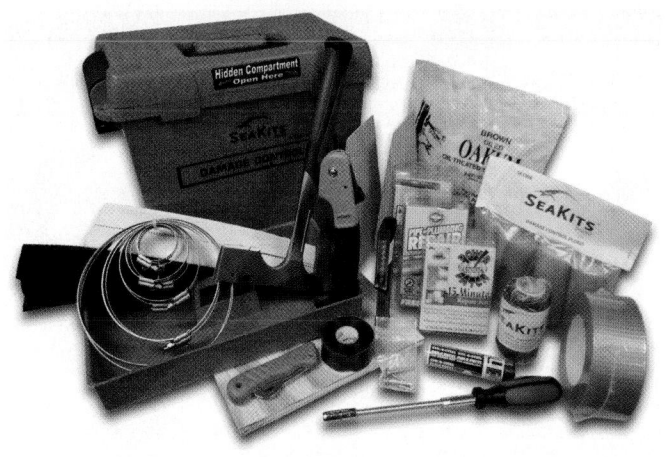

FIGURE 70-15 A damage control kit focused on flooding. Tapered wooden (or foam) plugs, underwater epoxy, saws, and hose clamps provide a variety of tools to stem the flow. *(Courtesy WheelHouse Technologies, Inc, Hudson, MA.)*

Large holes can be overlaid with a collision mat (Figure 70-16) placed outside the hull to supplement a temporary interior patch. The mat is a triangular-shaped piece of heavy canvas or vinyl-coated fabric with grommets and lines that enable it to be positioned and secured on the exterior surface. The mat is held in place by water pressure and lines. Collision mats can be purchased or improvised by using a small sail or awning material, although it is a mistake to make the mat too large; generally 1.2 m (4 feet) on an edge of the triangular shape is adequate. Water pressure automatically spreads the patch over the hole to form an effective seal and holds it in place. A commercial hull repair kit features flexible oval concave sheet metal plates with rubber gaskets. A bolt is welded to the intended exterior piece. The exterior oval plate is passed through the hull breach; the second plate is used to reinforce it from the inside. Finally, the plates are tightened together with a thumbscrew.

In the absence of specialized repair equipment, any soft, pliable material, such as a life jacket, mattress, blanket, or foam pad, can be used to slow water rushing through a break in the hull. When placed against the exterior hull, the suction effect created by flow and hydrostatic pressure will generally provide clamping pressure to the plug or patch. If a plug is positioned from inside the cabin, it should be shored up with a board and braced with a metal or wood pole (e.g., oar, mop handle, boat hook, whisker pole, strut, bunk rail). The eventual solution to a hull repair may start with a crude internal patch to slow the flow of water, followed by an external patch, followed by an improved internal patch with plywood and bracing. The vessel's pumps may then be able to handle the remaining leaks.

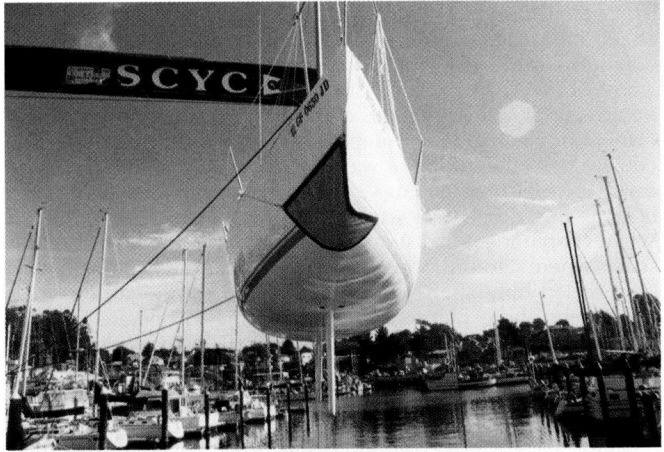

FIGURE 70-16 A collision mat consists of a triangular piece of fabric that is held in place with lines attached to each corner. Water pressure and the lines hold it in place.

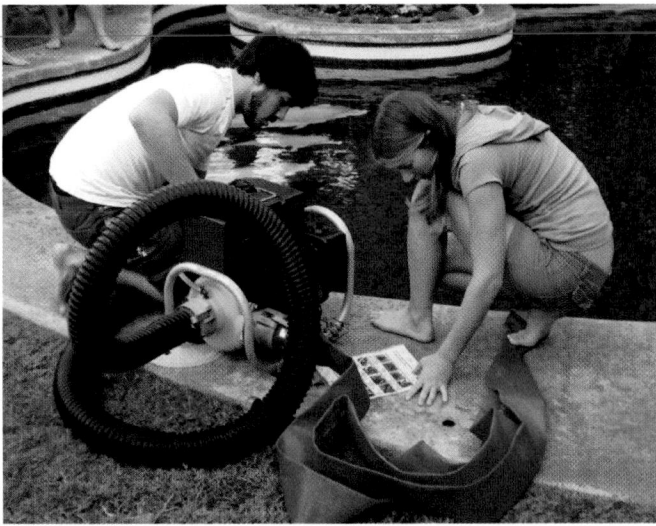

FIGURE 70-17 Coast Guard gasoline-powered dewatering pumps are extremely effective, but are also a bit cryptic in their use. Note that she is reading the waterproof instructions, while he ponders the controls. Some are self-priming, while others may have a hand pump to draw water into the pump body.

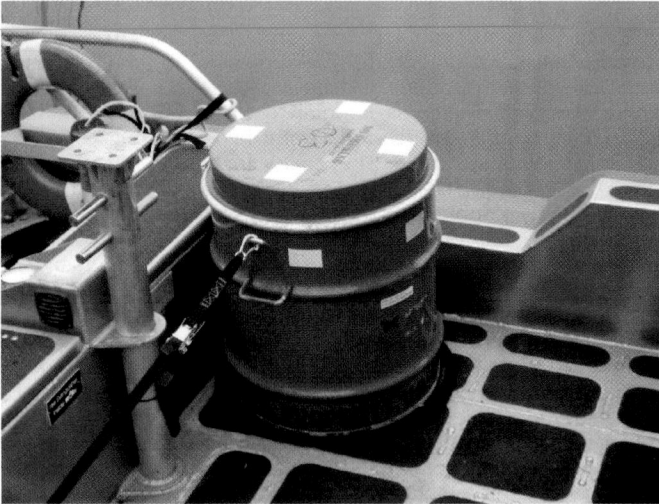

FIGURE 70-18 Larger P-6 pump carried on a Coast Guard 29-foot response boat.

Underwater patching compounds can be used to bond a solid plate over the hole or to impregnate expandable material or packing to serve as plugging material. Patching compounds vary in cure speed, ease of mixing, mixed viscosity, and adhesiveness. Some products work only on specific hull materials (e.g., wood, fiberglass, or aluminum). Direct repairs should be supplemented with additional measures to help slow water inflow. The vessel should be heeled away from the area of damage to decrease hydrostatic water pressure. This is relatively easy to accomplish under sail. Crews of powerboats should shift items to the side opposite the leak and slow the forward speed if water is entering a hole in the bow.

When ingenuity and improvisation fail to stop flooding, the U.S. Coast Guard can supply a portable gasoline-powered dewatering pump to assist a sinking vessel. The unit is simple to operate and comes in a waterproof barrel with hoses, gasoline, and illustrated operating instructions (Figure 70-17). When dropped from an aircraft into the sea, a retrieving line will be dropped to the deck crew. Two people are required to lift the pump from the sea onto the deck. The standard CG P-1B dewatering pump can pump 450 Lpm (120 gpm) at 3 m (10 feet) lift, and is capable of running 4 to 5 hours on a tank of gas. The P-1B pump, known as the drop pump, is carried by helicopter and by any of the Coast Guard rescue craft. A larger pump, the CG P-6 (classified as a dewatering/fire-fighting pump) is carried by Coast Guard search and rescue (SAR) ships and is placed either onboard or passed via lines, depending on weather conditions (Figure 70-18). Pump capacity is 950 Lpm (250 gpm) at 3.6 m (12 feet) lift; it runs 4 to 5 hours on a tank of gas. Both pumps are dramatically more effective than even the most robust manual or electric bilge pump. However, 950 Lpm (250 gpm) is equivalent to the inflow of water from a 3-inch hole (a relatively small breach) only 60 cm (2 feet) below waterline; any larger hole at this depth will exceed the capacity of even the P-6. Whatever pump is used should be run outside, not in an enclosed space where carbon monoxide may accumulate. Pumps should be refueled only after the engine is stopped. As with all safety equipment, these pumps can be confusing to operate for non-professionals, especially at night while a ship is swamping or sinking. Attendance at a safety at sea seminar or other survival training is highly recommended to become familiar with infrequently used and new safety gear.

Some oceangoing cruising vessels are built with watertight compartments to confine flooding to a limited area. Crew should know locations of watertight doors and have knowledge of their operation. If flooding and sinking are inevitable, the captain should consider running the boat onto shore.

COLLISIONS WITH OTHER VESSELS

International regulations for preventing collisions at sea are referred to as COLREGS. They define the responsibility of ships when collision is possible between two boats, as when crossing each other, overtaking, or meeting head on. Although the *stand on* vessel, which has the right of way over the *give way* vessel, is permitted to hold course and speed, rules require that both ships take any actions necessary to avoid an imminent collision. In the presence of large ships, small boats must be especially vigilant. All tow vessels or large craft, such as freighters or tankers operating on inshore waters, should be considered restricted in maneuverability. Rules 3 and 18 of the Inland Navigational Rules make it clear that a sailing vessel does *not* have the right of way over these vessels. In commercial traffic areas, a deck watch must be maintained at all times, and approaching ships should be hailed on VHF channel 13 (the vessel's pilothouse), or channel 16 if no response, if the ship's course or intentions are uncertain. If two vessels are in a crossing situation and the bearing (angle) between them remains constant, collision is inevitable. Visibility from the pilothouse of a large vessel may be partially obstructed by containers, fishing gear, or other items on deck; small craft may not be seen by the ship's lookout or pilot, show up on radar (Figure 70-19), or be granted the right of way. Reduced visibility

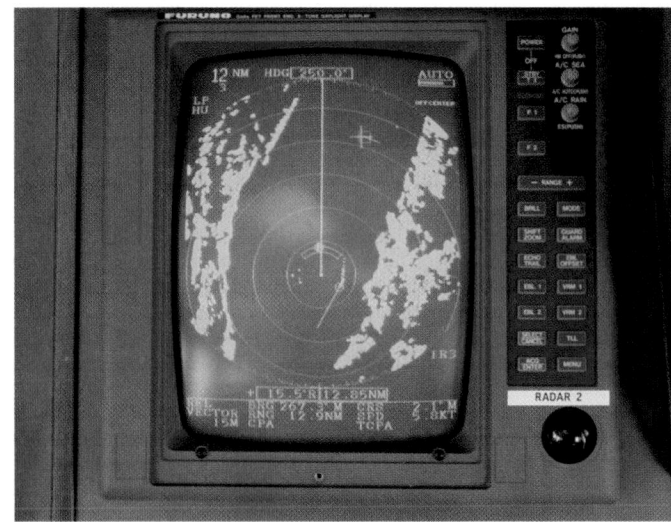

FIGURE 70-19 Although radar reflectors make a vessel incrementally more visible on a ship's radar, it is a lot easier for you to see them than vice versa. Keeping a radar watch in shipping channels makes sense, as it does here in the Strait of Juan de Fuca.

is a major cause of collisions along shipping lanes for commercial and recreational small craft. Every crew should be prepared for defensive action.

Automatic Identification System

Although radar, visual observations, and plotting are the anticollision tools for most mariners, a relatively new tool for avoiding collisions is the automatic identification system (AIS), which is required on a variety of commercial vessels and is also available for use by smaller craft. AIS transceivers consist of automated VHF radios that transmit information about the vessel's position, speed, and course, as well as name, classification, call sign, and maritime mobile service identity (MMSI) number, while also receiving the same information from similarly equipped vessels. The transceivers have a dedicated GPS to obtain position data, and use two VHF channels to send and receive data. Three categories of AIS transceivers are in use:

Large ship AIS receivers are class A (for commercial ships), which transmit more information, more frequently, and with more transmission power.

Class B transceivers are used on vessels not rated as Safety of Life at Sea (SOLAS) vessels and on recreational boats; they transmit fewer data fields, less frequently, and at lower power.

Receive-only models "eavesdrop" on transmissions of other vessels but do not send out information about the vessel on which they are installed.

The two transmitting systems are compatible, but the class A system is more robust. As of 2014, some domestic commercial vessels, including self-propelled vessels of 20 m (65 feet) or more in length and those engaged in commercial service, are required to have onboard a properly installed, operational, Coast Guard type–approved AIS.

All AIS class A transceivers and some class B models incorporate a display that allows other vessels to be plotted and provides a list of vessels and their threat potential, or provides this information to a chart plotter, network display, or radar. Alarms can be set to warn if another vessel will pass within a certain distance, so that vessels posing the greatest threat are highlighted.

Comparisons between benefits of radar and AIS are common, but the best solution is to have and use both technologies. Radar can detect large vessels, buoys, non-AIS vessels, shorelines, harbor configurations, and rocks. Radar requires training and experience to operate and interpret. AIS provides critical information about vessels and aids navigation on vessels equipped with transceivers, but no information about other threats.

Using Radar to Avoid Collisions

Radar is invaluable in conditions of poor visibility (Figure 70-20). At night or in fog, radar can be used to identify other ships, hazards to navigation, squalls, and other local weather that may endanger a vessel.

Small, affordable radar units are available for recreational boaters. Most are simple to operate, but require practice and patience for mastery. The radar horizon is a function of radar antenna height and target height; the higher each is located above sea level, the better the range of visibility. Modern units integrate a variety of data, including electronic bearing lines, rings that give a fast reference point to a target, and the variable range mark, which marks the range to a target at a particular time. These data are invaluable for avoiding collision with another vessel. Many units can be integrated with electronic chart displays and interfaced with computers for precision course plotting and tracking during navigation in narrow and complicated passages. A big advance in collision avoidance is the automatic radar plotting aid (ARPA), which works in conjunction with the main radar and is required (under COLREGS rule 7) to be used whenever a risk of collision exists. ARPA provides automated long-range scanning, sounds an alarm when a vessel comes within a predetermined distance, calculates the speed and bearing of other vessels, and automatically calculates course alternatives to avoid collision. Radar's interface with AIS provides the most comprehensive data set for collision avoidance.

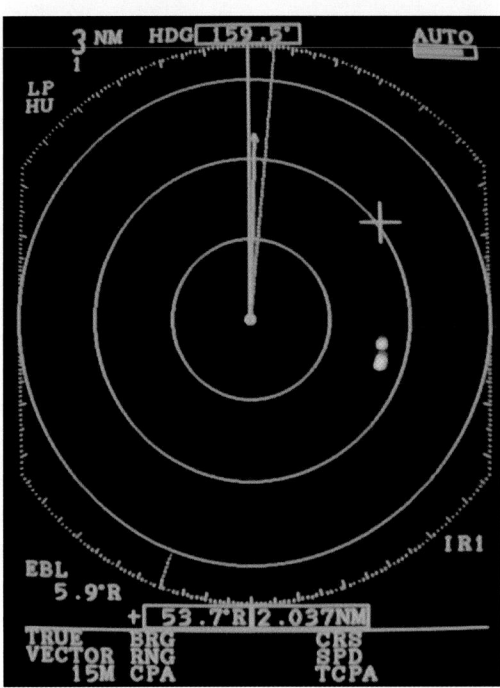

FIGURE 70-20 Plotting aids, such as ARPA and MARPA, remove much of the doubt about whether or not the other vessel is going to pass safely.

One problem common to radar units on small boats is that during storm conditions, large commercial ships and yachts may be lost on the radar screen because of echoes from nearby tall waves. Intense reflection of radar signals from the sea is called *sea clutter*. Fiberglass and wooden boats with wood spars are nearly invisible to radar. Regardless of construction, all boats should have a radar reflector mounted at all times while in shipping lanes, on the open sea, or under conditions of reduced visibility.

Search and rescue transponders (SARTs) render the object to which the SART is mounted significantly more conspicuous on a nearby vessel's radar screen. The radar-SART is used to locate a survival craft or distressed vessel by creating a series of dots on a rescuing ship's radar display. Essentially, it functions as an active radar reflector. SART is an excellent aid for life rafts and boats in distress, which usually do not return noticeable radar reflections on their own. A SART will only respond when interrogated by 9 GHz X-band (3 cm wavelength) radar, which is standard on all SAR craft but not on all commercial craft, which often use 3 GHz S band radar. New SARTs respond to both bands.

An important function of radar is the ability to maintain an electronic guard zone. The radar scans this zone, preset as the circle formed by a given radius, and sounds an alarm when a new target enters the guard zone for a certain number of sweeps. Unfortunately, commercial ships and solo ocean racers may rely too much on radar while they run on autopilot, and fail to post a lookout on deck. This is a clear violation of rule 5 of the COLREGS: "Every vessel shall at all times maintain a proper lookout by sight and hearing."

Visual Means of Avoiding Collisions

For collision avoidance, many cruising sailboats install a masthead strobe light. Although these are highly visible, masthead strobes are not accepted internationally as legal running lights, and the Coast Guard does not recommend them. A flashing strobe light may be interpreted as a distress signal, paradoxically inviting an unwelcome convergence of ships. Shining a powerful spotlight on the mainsail, turning on spreader lights, or igniting a white "anticollision" flare can be an effective alternative means of alerting a ship to the danger of collision. It is recommended that cruising sailboats have a masthead tricolor light for coastal and offshore cruising when sailing (to extend the range of visibility), in addition to deck-level lights for meeting, powering, crossing, and passing maneuvers when vessels are nearby. The LED tricolor masthead light combines sidelights, sternlight, and all-round white light (for anchoring) and is notable for its energy efficiency, durability, longevity, and brightness. The U.S. Coast Guard Navigation Rules,[10] International-Inland, specifies light requirements for every description of watercraft.

Mariners should recognize the different patterns of lights displayed by commercial ships. Beyond U.S. coastal waters, many ships do not always show appropriate lights, and the risk of collision is increased. Box 70-6 reviews tips to prevent collisions at sea.

Sailors crossing the North Atlantic in summer along a great circle route to Europe need to beware of colliding with icebergs. Every year from February to July, more than 10,000 icebergs are separated from Greenland glaciers. Global warming has had a profound effect on the number of icebergs; it increases local production of icebergs because ice shelves fragment in warming coastal waters. In August 2010, a giant ice sheet measuring 260 km^2 (100 mi^2) broke off from the floating portion of Peter-

mann Glacier. By 2012, splintered fragments had drifted southwest, and on July 15, 2012, a 130-km^2 (50-mi^2) piece calved from the northern tip of the glacier and drifted into Baffin Bay. At least 1000 icebergs drift in the Labrador Current south and east of Newfoundland and are a hazard to mariners above 41 degrees north latitude. Navigation around icebergs is complicated by dense fog often present over the Grand Banks region, and the difficulty of detecting icebergs with radar. U.S. and Canadian Coast Guards broadcast iceberg reports twice daily. The International Ice Patrol[7] broadcast times and frequencies can be obtained from the International Ice Patrol in New London, Connecticut.

HEALTH MAINTENANCE AT SEA

THE FEARSOME FIVE

The "Fearsome Five" are health issues that must be addressed to maintain optimal physical and mental performance: food (calorie depletion), fluid (dehydration), Fahrenheit (hypothermia), fatigue (sleep deprivation), and fitness (injury, illness, infection).

Food

To keep the crew well fed, meals on a long sea voyage should be simple, high calorie, and easy to digest. Some meals should be prepared in advance to minimize the risk of seasickness for the cook, who would otherwise be required to spend extended periods below decks. Snacks should be readily available. Energy bars, trail mix, crackers, and fresh or dried fruit are good choices. Sips of water help speed absorption and digestion of snacks. The goal is to avoid hypoglycemia with depletion of reserve muscle and liver glycogen stores.

Fluid

Common causes of dehydration include excessive sweating from fever or vigorous exercise (especially in hot weather), profuse/protracted diarrhea/vomiting, and restricted use of potable water. Seasickness and gastroenteritis may cause dehydration. Fluid loss at rest in a thermoneutral environment ($28°$ to $30°C$ [$82°$ to $86°F$] and 50% relative humidity) is via skin, lungs, and kidneys. Each of these organs has an obligatory daily fluid loss of approximately 500 mL (1 pint). Minimal daily body water loss is therefore 1500 mL (1.6 quarts). Headache, nausea, lethargy, apathy, lightheadedness, and hypotension can develop with a deficit of 1 to 2 L (2 to 4 pints; 3% to 5% of total body water); these symptoms can mimic those of seasickness and heat exhaustion. Boaters often fail to appreciate both heat absorption and the drying effects of warm breeze on skin. Continuous evaporation of sweat removes the visible reminder of fluid loss, and quick-drying fabrics accentuate this invisible evaporative loss. Signs of overheating also may be less obvious if the body absorbs radiant heat from the sun while a breeze cools the skin. Exposure to sunny, hot, breezy, and dry conditions promotes increased fluid loss from the lungs, because the air we inhale and exhale is humidified in the nose and bronchial tree, increasing "insensible loss." Boaters are more susceptible to dehydration during this "ideal boating weather." On an average summer day, sailors should consume a minimum of approximately 2 quarts of fluid. Feeling thirsty is not always a reliable early sign of dehydration. However, the sensation of thirst should not be ignored, and one should drink fluids until thirst is satisfied. A good way to determine the hydration level is to monitor the color of urine. Clear to pale-yellow urine indicates sufficient fluid consumption. Dark yellow or tan-colored urine indicates dehydration.

There are a variety of causes of and remedies for limited fluid intake onboard. Poor taste of a boat's tank water can reduce voluntary fluid intake; powdered drink mixes or fresh citrus fruits can counteract bad-tasting water. Seasick sailors often suffer from dehydration because of recurrent nausea and vomiting. When rehydrating seasick crew, frequent sips of small volumes of water are often more effective than drinking large volumes at a single sitting. Self-imposed water restriction is sometimes practiced to reduce urinary frequency, especially in rough weather, when it is often difficult for crew to go below to use the head. In these circumstances, having the helmsman make a brief change of

---

BOX 70-6 Preventing Collisions at Sea

1. Post a lookout with a 360-degree view of the horizon.
2. Know the rules of the road and right of way.
3. Use radar (if available) and running lights. A tricolor masthead light is most visible and cannot be obstructed by sails or other gear when sailing in the open ocean.
4. An automatic information system (AIS) allows one to plot large vessels on the chart plotter or AIS display, and helps prevent collisions at night and in busy traffic lanes.
5. Mount radar reflectors at least 4 m (13 feet) above the waterline.
6. Do not assume that other boats have operational or unobstructed running lights. Be aware that outside of U.S. waters, navigation lights on foreign ships may not match standard configurations.
7. Observe Rule 7 of the COLREGS: "When a vessel has any doubt as to whether a risk of collision exists, she shall assume it does and avoid it." Be prepared to change course and speed.
8. Ask yourself, "Can I be seen?" If you cannot see the wheelhouse windows of a ship, they probably cannot see you. Deck cargo, cranes, and containers can make it impossible for watchkeepers on a ship to see you up to 3 miles in front of the vessel. Do not assume you are seen, even in daylight.
9. If you hear a foghorn, stop and let the other ship steer around you.
10. If a collision threatens, sound the danger signal (five or more short blasts on the horn), and take whatever actions are necessary to save your boat.
11. Maintain radio contact with other ships in the area. VHF channel 13 is the bridge-to-bridge channel. Use VHF channel 16 if there is no response.
12. Avoid congested shipping routes if possible, and avoid navigating in the harbor's incoming and outgoing traffic separation lanes designated for commercial traffic. If you have to cross the traffic lanes, do so at right angles and remain in them for the shortest possible amount of time.
13. When your boat is in the way of another vessel, the right of way does not automatically grant you safe passage. Regardless of the COLREGS, be prepared to take evasive action. Caution is the primary rule of the sea to avoid collision.
14. To avoid collision with another vessel, make early and obvious changes in course and/or speed. Port-to-port is a good rule for most head-on passing situations (sound one whistle). In overtaking situations, sounding one whistle means you are overtaking on the starboard side of the overtaken vessel, and sounding two whistles means the port side.
15. Give large ships a wide berth. Whenever possible, avoid meeting or overtaking tugboats towing vessels or barges near river bends, bridges, and narrow channels.
16. Observe the bearing of an approaching vessel (the direction relative to you). If the bearing does not change, and if the distance between the two boats is decreasing, you are on a collision course.

course allows the crew to safely go below decks. Men suffering from prostate enlargement may also voluntarily restrict fluids in order to urinate less frequently. Some drugs for seasickness accentuate urinary retention in men with enlarged prostates; these medications should be tried before going to sea to evaluate for potential side effects.

Fahrenheit

Hypothermia (see Chapters 7 and 8) may develop acutely when crew falls overboard and remains immersed in cold water (< 25°C [77°F]) or over a period of hours to days during prolonged exposure to the elements, as when wind, rain, and seawater inundate the crew on deck in cold ambient temperatures. For sailors, staying warm requires staying dry. Good foul-weather gear (including sea boots, hat, and waterproof gloves), combined with insulating layers of clothing made with modern synthetic fabrics (highly breathable, moisture-wicking, and fast drying), are essential. Mild hypothermia, defined as a core temperature above 32°C (90°F), is the only level of hypothermia that can be treated onboard. More severe hypothermia requires evacuation to a medical facility. Sustained uncontrollable shivering is the most reliable and earliest sign of drop in core temperature, and usually begins in earnest at 35°C (95°F). Other clues are alterations in motor skills and changes in mental status. As blood is diverted from muscles and nerves, there is loss of manual dexterity, large muscle coordination, and strength. Clumsiness occurs while performing simple tasks, such as adjusting binoculars or using navigational instruments. Walking safely on deck and working with lines and gear become hazardous. Subtle changes in mental status cause impaired judgment, confusion, and disorientation. Initial treatment of a conscious and shivering mildly hypothermic person (core temperature above 32°C [90°F]) is to prevent further cooling and heat loss. This person is capable of rewarming himself or herself and does not require evacuation. The victim should be sheltered from wind and water, and wet clothing replaced with multiple layers of dry insulating garments after the skin is completely dried. If dry clothing is not available, an external vapor barrier should be added with additional foul weather gear. A windproof layer minimizes convective and evaporative heat loss. When practical, the victim should be wrapped in blankets, a sleeping bag, sails, or sail bags. Provide calories with simple carbohydrate foods and sugar-based liquid drinks, and allow vigorous shivering to generate rewarming heat. Warm liquids are psychologically beneficial but do not significantly increase rewarming rates.

Avoid warming skin directly because this inhibits shivering. Warm showers will not warm the core; instead, they may cause vasodilation and severe hypotension (circumrescue collapse).

Fatigue

Sleep deprivation and fatigue impair physical and mental performance, and foster cognitive errors, poor judgment, mood changes, and even hallucinations. Sailors often have irregular sleep schedules, prolonged watches, and difficult sleeping conditions. The crew should sleep in secure sea berths that are narrow with lee cloths, so they do not roll around, fall out, or battle to stay in their berths. The challenge is to improve sleep efficiency. Sleep cycles have light and deep stages of rest. A 1-hour nap can quickly bring about deeper restorative sleep. Regular watch and sleep schedules, and napping to reduce fatigue are recommended. Sleep deprivation increases susceptibility to seasickness, and many medications for seasickness cause drowsiness, which may further disrupt regular sleep schedules and patterns.

Fitness

Seasickness, sunburn, and dehydration are the most frequent ailments, and together with infections, are the most common illnesses for otherwise healthy cruising sailors. Sailors are constantly exposed to solar radiation (see Chapter 16). Sunlight is reflected off water, especially from choppy seas; reflected rays can burn eyes and undersides of the mouth, nose, and chin. Overcast days afford little relief, because most radiation is transmitted and scattered through haze and high clouds. Boaters especially suffer from sunburn on cloudy days, because they neglect to take measures for sun protection, such as using sunscreen or wearing protective clothing, hats, and sunglasses. Certain medications increase the skin's sensitivity to sun exposure; medications should be reviewed for this possibility and extra precautions taken.

Soft tissue extremity injuries are common, usually caused by trips and falls during sailing maneuvers, especially in heavy weather. Being caught in lines or struck by objects, including sheets, blocks, lines, and hardware, contributes to most injuries. Typical injuries are contusions, lacerations (most often on hands), sprains, and strains. Severe injuries, such as fractures, concussions, and dislocations, are not common. Most injuries occur in the cockpit or on the foredeck.

In the enclosed and tight quarters of a boat, upper respiratory infections are easily spread by crew coughing and sneezing airborne droplets; advise ill crew to sneeze/cough into the crook of the arm to avoid contaminating hands and surrounding surfaces. Viral and bacterial gastroenteritis can quickly spread by improper hand washing before leaving the head and prior to food preparation and eating. Poor hand washing facilitates spread of intestinal disease by contaminating cookware, dishes, utensils, and food. All crew should wash hands carefully with soap and water, followed by application of an alcohol-based hand sanitizer and air-drying the hands.

SEASICKNESS

Seasickness is the most prevalent medical illness for mariners at sea, and causes a significant number of maritime rescue operations, putting crew and rescue personnel at unnecessary risk. During stormy weather, mariners frequently consider seasickness a medical emergency and justification for medical evacuation. Each year, seaworthy yachts are abandoned because their exhausted and despondent crews have lost the collective will to persevere. In the words of a professional mariner, "They are wet, seasick, scared, and want to go home."

Anyone can develop seasickness with sufficient stimuli; however, individual susceptibility is variable. Only persons without a functioning vestibular system are fully immune. Pregnant women are highly susceptible, especially in the first trimester.

Seasickness involves a conflict of sensory input processed by the brain to orient the body's position. Someone positioned in the cabin of a heeling or rolling boat is inviting seasickness. Below decks, eyes oriented to cabin sole and ceiling detect no tilt from vertical, while fluid in the inner ear's vestibular system (semicircular canals and otolith organs) constantly shifts, sending neural messages that the head and body are not vertical. Position sensors (proprioceptors) in the neck, muscles, and joints send additional signals, depending on how a person shifts and secures himself or herself from falling. This mix of sensory data from eyes, inner ear, and position sensors arrives in complex and conflicting combinations, creating a "sensory conflict" that activates the emetic center in the brainstem. According to Dr. Charles Oman, Director of the Man Vehicle Laboratory at the Massachusetts Institute of Technology and an authority on motion sickness, the sensory conflict is also a sensory cue and "expectancy conflict." The expectancy conflict occurs when signals from the inner ear do not match expectations based on one's commanded self-movement, or concurrent visual or proprioceptive cues. When the motor cortex generates motor signals for movement, it also generates predicted sensory feedback of our motion. If there is a conflict in expected sensory input with actual movement (e.g., the effect of a rolling boat on our motion), an expectancy conflict develops that activates the autonomic and emetic centers, and symptoms of seasickness develop. If one eliminates these conflicts, one can prevent seasickness: if the eyes are seeing what the ears are feeling and what the brain is expecting, one has a good chance of experiencing a great day at sea.

Seasickness often presents with nausea and vomiting. Another facet of seasickness not often recognized is the *sopite syndrome*, which refers to profound drowsiness and persistent fatigue following provocative motion stimulation. Yawning has been shown to be a behavioral marker of the sopite syndrome; additional signs include boredom, sighing, pallor, dry mouth or salivating, headache, dizziness, and lethargy. With sustained exposure to the stimulus, gastric emptying is inhibited. Subsequently, the hands and face sweat, becoming cold and clammy; belching, salivation, nausea, retching, and vomiting ensue. Some people experience headache, apathy, and depression. Moreover, seasickness impairs cognitive function. Sailors often lose the ability to multitask, making it difficult to analyze and integrate complex data, leading to poor reasoning, impaired judgment, and faulty decisions. Cognitive failure may also present as short-term memory loss. As seasickness becomes more severe, symptoms worsen, and include rapid mental, emotional, and physical deterioration marked by progressive dehydration, loss of manual dexterity, and ataxia.

Preventing and Treating Seasickness

Medication is more effective in preventing symptoms than in reversing them. Therefore, antiseasickness medication should be taken well in advance, before leaving port, or the night prior to departure. See discussion of medications below.

All voyagers should begin their journey well hydrated, well rested, and free of aftereffects of alcohol, which impairs vestibular function by sensitizing the vestibular apparatus to motion. Bland foods, such as crackers, fruit, trail mix, and popcorn, should be eaten throughout the day, even if one is not hungry, to maintain energy levels until meals are regularly tolerated. Drink small amounts of fluid frequently to avoid dehydration. Many sailors believe drinks with high amounts of vitamin C prevent seasickness; however, there are no clinical data to support this notion. Ginger is available in 250-mg capsules and sold in marine stores as Sailors' Secret. The suggested dose is 1 g every 4 to 6 hours. Foods containing lower concentrations of ginger, such as gingersnap cookies, ginger ale or tea, and candied ginger may be helpful. However, ginger may cause heartburn and even biliary colic in the setting of gallstones.

Both field and laboratory experiments have documented efficacy of acupressure in preventing seasickness. However, some experts consider acupressure no better than placebo. One sea trial showed that acustimulation suppressed symptoms of motion sickness. Pressure is applied on the Neiguan P6 acupuncture point on the forearm over the median nerve, found two to three fingerbreadths proximal to the wrist joint between the two prominent finger flexor tendons. There are commercially available elastic wrist straps with plastic studs that create pressure over the P6 point. The ReliefBand is an electric stimulator that operates under the same principle.

After departure, one can mitigate the symptoms of seasickness using the following multifaceted approach. Limit time below decks while underway to minimize sensory conflict. Stay on deck amidships (center) or aft (toward the stern), where motion is less severe. Maintain a broad view of the horizon, using both direct and peripheral vision; this provides a stable and level point of reference. Avoid close-focused visual tasks, such as prolonged reading and writing. Exposure to fumes (especially diesel) and odors may stimulate nausea. Sleep deprivation also increases susceptibility to seasickness. Take seasickness medication at the suggested intervals, and taper the dose after the first or second day.

At the first sign of seasickness, a direct remedy for many is to take the helm and steer, standing and feeling the waves, using clouds, the horizon, and distant marks as references, anticipating the boat's motion by "riding" the waves. "Wave riding" synchronizes sensory input and expectations of motion. One should keep the head, shoulders, and hips aligned to stay in balance and gracefully gain postural control. Sitting in the cockpit, one can still ride the waves and watch the horizon. "Postural anticipation of the boat's motion is the natural cure for seasickness," states Chuck Oman, who developed the concept of wave riding.

Seasick crew can easily fall or be washed overboard. They should always wear a safety harness on deck and be closely monitored. Seasick crew should not be allowed to move to lifelines to vomit overboard; a bucket should be readily available. In storm conditions, or if symptoms progress, the safest place to be secured is in the cabin, resting in a well-ventilated bunk, face-up with eyes closed and head still.

The antihistamines meclizine (Bonine) and dimenhydrate (Dramamine) are available over the counter (OTC) without prescription. They are effective for preventing seasickness, as are the other prescription medications listed in Table 70-1. The popular antihistamine cinnarizine (Stugeron) is not sold in the United States but is available OTC in Europe, Bermuda, Mexico, and Canada (and can be obtained legally from online Canadian pharmacies). Many sailors favor it because it is less sedating than other antihistamines and has fewer reported side effects (described below).

Side effects of OTC antihistamines include drowsiness, dry mouth, blurred vision, irritability, urinary retention, dizziness, and headache. Meclizine (Bonine) causes less drowsiness and confusion. Antihistamines cause thickened bronchial secretions, and should be used cautiously in people with asthma and chronic obstructive pulmonary disease. An effective nonprescription drug for drowsiness is the decongestant pseudoephedrine, which is available in doses of 30 to 100 mg (immediate release, adult: 30-60 mg; sustained release, adult: 120 mg; maximum, 240 mg/day); caffeine 200 mg is also useful. Newer-generation nonsedating antihistamines are ineffective at preventing seasickness.

Parenteral antinausea medications include the phenothiazine-derivative promethazine hydrochloride (Phenergan). Promethazine is useful for prophylactic and active treatment of seasickness and can be administered as a suppository, by intramuscular injection, and orally as a tablet or syrup. Anticholinergic side effects include constipation, xerostomia, blurred vision, and urinary retention. Promethazine should be used with caution in persons with decreased gastrointestinal motility, urinary retention or obstruction, benign prostatic hypertrophy, xerostomia, or visual problems. Rare but serious adverse effects of promethazine include extrapyramidal reactions. The oral disintegrating tablet ondansetron (Zofran) is extremely effective for vomiting; however, it does not treat or prevent other symptoms of seasickness. Transdermal scopolamine hydrobromide (Transderm Scōp patch) is the most popular anticholinergic agent used for motion sickness prevention. Scopolamine prevents motion-induced nausea by inhibiting vestibular input to the central nervous system, inhibiting the vomiting reflex. The drug is delivered via an adhesive patch placed behind the ear at least 4 hours before departure; the patch will last for up to 3 days, often with minimal side effects. The scopolamine disk's integrity should be maintained, and not be cut or torn. Apply only one patch at a time. The administering person should be sure to wash his/her hands

TABLE 70-1	Medications for Seasickness	
Medication	**Dose**	**Interval**
Diphenhydramine (Benadryl) (OTC)	25- or 50-mg tablet	6 to 8 hr
Dimenhydrinate (Dramamine) (OTC)	50- or 100-mg tablet (maximum 400 mg/day)	4 to 6 hr
Meclizine (OTC)	12.5- or 25-mg tablet (maximum 100 mg/day)	6 to 8 hr
Bonine (Meclizine) (OTC)	25-mg chewable tablet	6 to 8 hr
Cinnarizine (Stugeron)	15-mg tablet (maximum 100 mg/day)	6 to 12 hr
Scopolamine (Transderm Scōp)	1.5-mg skin patch	72 hr
Promethazine (Phenergan)	12.5-, 25-, or 50-mg tablet, suppository, deep intramuscular injection	Variable intervals, depending on dose/preparation

thoroughly after application; there may be temporary blurring of vision and pupillary dilation if drug residuum on hands contacts the eyes. The most common adverse effects of anticholinergic medications are dry mouth (66%) and drowsiness (17%). Other undesirable side effects include blurred vision (which may persist for weeks), dry mucous membranes, and short-term memory loss. Scopolamine is contraindicated in children, men with prostatic hypertrophy, and people with narrow-angle glaucoma; remove the patch immediately if a patient complains of the sudden onset of eye pain. Long-term use may produce withdrawal symptoms such as nausea, dizziness, headache, and equilibrium disturbances. Scopolamine in pill form (Scopace) is no longer available in the United States or Canada.

All therapies are subject to placebo effect, and there are no well-controlled trials comparing and evaluating different treatments for seasickness. It is not uncommon for one drug in a category (e.g., antihistamine) to be effective and a related drug to provide no benefit; the same is true for side effects. Medication side effects should be evaluated by trying different drugs while on shore. If all else fails, follow Samuel Johnson's 18th-century advice: "To cure seasickness, find a good big oak tree and wrap your arms around it."

MARINE WEATHER

THUNDERSTORMS AND SQUALL LINES

A single thunderstorm generally encompasses an area less than 3 km (2 mi) in diameter. The storm typically lasts approximately 30 minutes, with marked fluctuations in wind, temperature, and barometric pressure. The National Weather Service (NWS) considers a thunderstorm severe if it produces hail at least 2 cm (0.75 inch) in diameter, winds 93 km/hr (58 mph) or stronger, or a tornado. Of the estimated 100,000 thunderstorms that occur on inland and coastal areas in the United States, 10% are classified as severe. Eighteen hundred thunderstorms occur at any moment around the world, totaling 16 million a year. A squall line is a fast-moving row of violent thunderstorms, often more than 160 km (100 mi) long. An intense cold front 64 to 483 km (40 to 300 mi) behind the squall line contains most of the gusting winds and rain normally found in the front. A squall line is visible on both radar and to the naked eye, where it appears as a wall of boiling black clouds arising from the water.

Rapid growth of cumulus clouds is the primary indicator of a forming thunderstorm. The faster the clouds build, the more violent the resulting storm, because steep pressure gradients within the cloud generate high winds. Within the thunderhead are columns of rapidly sinking air called downdrafts. Downdrafts along the leading edge of the thunderstorm form the gust front. This zone of advancing cold air is characterized by a sudden increase in wind speed. Strong and highly localized downdrafts are called downbursts, the smallest of which are microbursts. Airplane pilots refer to these as wind shear. Downbursts are extremely intense concentrations of sinking air. On reaching the surface, they fan out radially in all directions, often generating winds at the gust front in excess of 150 knots. They are short-lived, typically lasting less than 15 minutes. A single thunderstorm can produce a series of downdrafts affecting an area several miles long, and persist an hour or more. Blowing spray under or slightly ahead of the storm may be the only indicator of its presence. A gust front often precedes a microburst. The combination of these two extremely strong and shifting wind systems can blow equipment and personnel off the deck and can easily capsize small craft and large sailboats.

In the United States, squalls occur predominantly during spring and summer in association with thunderstorms generated by towering cumulus clouds. The larger the cloud's size (and radar echo), the more wind potential within the cloud; the taller the cloud (especially above 6096 m [20,000 feet]), the more energy potential for stronger winds. Most squall formations occur at night when cloud tops radiate heat back into space, enhancing their ability to grow. Squall-generated winds rarely strike without warning. A rapid fall in temperature is the precursor of a local storm. The bigger the drop, the stronger the winds. Rain preced-

ing wind suggests that stronger winds are coming. Occasionally, thunderstorms may form with the building of the cumulus cloud and not be associated with typical rain, thunder, and lightning. These violent winds are called white squalls. The only warning may be the sudden appearance of a cold, shifting wind with an increase in velocity.[2]

The inquiry into the 2011 Chicago Yacht Club Race to Mackinac reviewed the impact of a thunderstorm with powerful winds on the capsize of the 35-foot, ultralight, low-stability sailing vessel *WingNuts*. (The full report is available at ussailing.org/racing/offshore-big-boats/big-boat-safety-at-sea/safety-incident-reports/). When the *WingNuts* encountered a "wall of wind" with a speed of over 50 knots, it was blown over, capsized, and turtled. Six of the crew members, including one who was below decks at the time, were able to free themselves from the vessel; two who were unable to do so died as a result of head injuries and drowning. Weather and the boat's design were the dominant factors. The report issued the following weather description: "As they ran north at speeds in the high teens, the *WingNuts* team tracked the weather with several tools, including NOAA weather radio forecasts and WX weather overlays on the boat's GPS and radar. The forecast for Northern Lake Michigan area degraded throughout Sunday. A Severe Thunderstorm Watch was established at 1925 CDT, and subsequently the National Weather Service at Gaylord, MI, issued ever more urgent warnings." In a report produced after the race at the request of the Independent Review Panel, the Gaylord office described the developments this way: "During the late evening of July 17, a disorganized cluster of thunderstorms over Wisconsin and Upper Michigan moved into Lake Michigan and eventually evolved into a line of thunderstorms that crossed northern Lower Michigan. From a radar perspective, the storms were initially somewhat disorganized and marginally severe. As the cluster of storms progressed into Lake Michigan, however, one particular cell rapidly developed and intensified just prior to midnight EDT [2300 CDT]." During this intense thunderstorm, 37 other boats were knocked down but recovered upright.

Large sailboats, such as the clipper topsail schooner *The Pride of Baltimore,* have also been knocked down and sunk by these unexpected powerful winds. In May 1986, a sudden storm rumbled across the Atlantic and unleashed its strength over a small patch of the Bermuda Triangle. With furious precision, its 70-knot winds overwhelmed the 97-ton, 34-m (110-foot) clipper ship heading home from Europe; survivors reported that the ship immediately barrel-rolled in the heavy wind and sank. Daniel S. Parrott's book *Tall Ships Down* provides more information on the loss of *The Pride of Baltimore,* as well as four other traditionally rigged vessels, the *Pamir, Albatross, Marques,* and *Maria Asumpta.*

Sources of Marine Weather Information

To avoid or prepare for a thunderstorm, sailors must monitor local weather conditions. The National Oceanographic and Atmospheric Administration (NOAA) transmits on VHF-FM radio recorded messages, which are repeated every 4 to 6 minutes, and updated every 2 to 3 hours with the latest local information. Broadcasts usually can be received 20 to 60 miles from transmitting antennas. Stations are identified on the radio channel display as WX-1, WX-2, and WX-3. Nationwide, more than 860 transmitters provide coverage to all 50 states and adjacent marine areas. In many areas, the Coast Guard broadcasts weather information on VHF channel 22. Listings of schedules and frequencies for coastal and offshore weather broadcasts are available in a number of publications, including the *Admiralty List of Radio Signals,* volume III, and *Reeds Nautical Almanac.* Box 70-7 lists the definitions of storm warnings.

Many newer VHF radios have a weather-alert function known as Weather Watch. When the radio receives a warning signal from NOAA, it sounds a special alerting tone, signifying an urgent NOAA weather forecast. Some radios automatically tune to the active weather channel, whereas others require manual tuning. NOAA improved their severe weather warnings by encoding both the area affected by severe weather and the nature of the severe weather (e.g., hurricane, winter storm, high wind, severe

BOX 70-7 Storm Warnings

1. Small craft advisory: generally associated with sustained winds of 18 to 33 knots (30.5 to 61.2 km/hr [19 to 38 mph]) and/or sea conditions dangerous to small boats.
2. Gale warning: sustained winds of 34 to 47 knots (62.8 to 86.9 km/hr [39 to 54 mph])
3. Storm warning: sustained winds of over 48 knots (88.5 km/hr [55 mph]). If winds are associated with a tropical cyclone, the storm warning display indicates forecast winds of 48 to 63 knots (88.5 to 117.5 km/hr [55 to 73 mph]).
4. Hurricane warning: sustained winds of 64 knots (119.1 km/hr [74 mph]) and greater as the result of a tropical cyclone
5. Special marine warning: winds of 35 knots or more generally lasting less than 2 hours. These are usually associated with an individual thunderstorm or an organized series of thunderstorms, as in a squall line.

---

thunderstorm). Called Specific Area Message Encoding, this feature is intended to make weather warnings more customized so that users will not tune out possibly lifesaving warnings. Offshore sailors can receive a variety of high-seas marine weather broadcasts with single-sideband (SSB) high-frequency (HF) radios. The U.S. Coast Guard broadcasts NWS high-seas forecasts and storm warnings from each coast. All broadcasts are upper single-sideband HF, with additional broadcasts on medium frequency (MF). The time schedules and frequencies for these transmissions can be found in the National Geospatial-Intelligence Agency (NGA) Publication 117, titled *Radio Navigation Aids*. A less comprehensive list for specific locations can also be found in *Reeds Nautical Almanac*. For schedules and much more information on NWS marine products, visit NOAA's National Weather Service Marine Forecasts at web page nws .noaa.gov.

The U.S. Coast Guard sends a facsimile of a weather chart (weatherfax) from their East, Gulf, and West Coast communication centers. These marine weather charts are updated every 6 hours and available within 3.5 hours of the valid update time. Weatherfaxes contain graphic charts and forecasts compiled by the NWS; they are broadcast on HF radio bands between 3.5 and 30.0 MHz. Lists of transmitters, frequencies, and times can be found in *Reeds Nautical Almanac* or online at NOAA's page listed above. This site contains text forecasts, ocean current and surface analysis charts, wave charts, buoy reports, and prognosis charts (500-millibar [mb] charts) for weather outlooks of 12, 24, 36, 48, and 96 hours.

Software can integrate weather forecasting with optimal routing for safety and sailing performance. Weather files (called GRIB files) can be downloaded and overlaid onto an electronic chart, and routing formulas can then be applied incorporating the boat's known performance characteristics. Mariners can obtain sea state and weather data directly from NOAA buoys moored offshore by using the Internet. The National Data Buoy Center website is ndbc.noaa.gov; the website lists more than 1200 buoys around the world that one can find on the site's world map to obtain real-time observation of weather conditions.

NAVTEX is a worldwide land-based radio navigation warning service, transmitting text-only messages (in English) to a dedicated onboard receiver. The unit can be programmed to receive both specific stations and message categories; it can print out area weather forecasts, gale warnings, navigation warnings, ice warnings, and relayed distress messages on the assigned frequency of 518 kHz. Vital messages (e.g., gale warnings, SAR information) activate an alarm in the receiver as the message is being printed.

Traditional Weather Forecasting Methods

Even without expensive electronic equipment, mariners can predict changes in local weather by using their own observations. All crewmembers should learn the cloud types or augment their knowledge base through use of a photo atlas of cloud formations, to identify the variety of clouds and their significance. During the day, a sailor can learn to recognize a squall line, growth of a cumulus to a cumulonimbus cloud with its characteristic anvil head on the downwind side (a thunderhead), and the cloud sequence and wind changes of an approaching cold and warm front. "Mare's tails and mackerel scales; soon it's time to shorten sails," refers to cirrus and cirrocumulus formations (long puffy clouds at high level, commonly known as a mackerel sky). This cloud formation signifies unsettled weather, with the approach of a warm front. Two weather concepts can be helpful for predicting changes in weather: the crossed-winds rule, popularized by the meteorologist Alan Watts, and Buys Ballot's law. The crossed-winds rule states that whenever the upper-level wind flow (determined by observing the direction of the cirrus clouds at 6096 to 9144 m [20,000 to 30,000 feet]) and lower-level surface winds are crossed, the weather is going to change. Buys Ballot's law states that in the Northern Hemisphere, if you stand with the wind blowing at your back, a high pressure will be at 90 degrees to your right, and a low pressure 90 degrees to your left (remember "low-left"). If application of the crossed-winds rule and Buy Ballot's law indicates a low is approaching, the weather will certainly deteriorate into a warm front, with increasing winds and rain. Once past, a cold front follows. If the upper-level flow either matches or directly opposes the surface wind, weather is likely to remain stable for a while.

During daylight, a band of low, dark, and smooth tubular roll clouds can often be seen at the leading edge of a squall, preceding a cold front. The faster a roll cloud approaches, the stronger the wind is likely to be, and the more agitated the sea appears under it. When the sea is observed beneath the roll cloud, the cloud is about 2 miles away; because clouds typically move at about 40 km/hr (25 mph), the face will arrive in about 5 minutes.

A barometer is one of the most important weather instruments onboard a small boat. By 1 to 4 hours before an approaching thunderstorm, there is a sharp drop in barometric pressure of about 1.5 mb. If the atmospheric pressure is fluctuating very little, it means weather is likely to remain stable. A pronounced rise in pressure heralds fair weather.

The sea state is a valuable clue to approaching weather patterns. Large ocean swells precede a heavy weather system, whereas chop without swells often reflects a local, more isolated, and temporary disturbance. An alert observer can calculate the distance between a vessel and a thunderstorm within earshot. The distance of lightning from an observer can be determined by noting the time between the flash and the bang of associated thunder. For each 5-second count from flash to bang, lightning is 1.6 km (1 mi) away. Lightning is discussed in more detail in the following section and Chapter 5.

In order to meet the challenge of finding the most reliable, accurate weather information and mastering the art and science of weather forecasting, a sailor departing on an extended coastal cruise or ocean passage anywhere in the world can contract with a professional weather routing company; these services provide assistance in determining a favorable weather window for departure, and continued support for weather forecasting and routing during passage. Such consultation provides an invaluable additional layer of safety and confidence.

LIGHTNING

Lightning is one of nature's most destructive phenomena (see Chapter 5). Boating, fishing, and swimming rank second only to playing sports on an open field as the most dangerous activities associated with lightning strike. A cruising sailor in Florida, the lightning capital of America, can expect at least one strike to his or her boat in its lifetime.

Lightning protection systems do not prevent lightning strikes. They may, in fact, increase the possibility of the boat being struck. The purpose of lightning protection is to reduce the damage to the boat and the possibility of injuries or death to crew from lightning.

Tall and narrow objects, with highly charged and focused electric fields, are likely to attract lightning. Metal itself does not attract lightning. A sailboat mast, radio antenna, fishing outrigger, fishing rod, and even crew standing on deck are all good targets.

In a marina or anchorage, the boat with the tallest mast is usually the most vulnerable to a strike.

The most critical factor initiating the lightning streamer emanating from the boat is not only the mast height but also its electric potential. The crackling bluish-green light sometimes seen in a ship's rigging at night during thunderstorms is not lighting but a type of electrical discharge (corona discharge) called St Elmo's fire. It may even appear like a stream of fire as it trails from the mast. Magellan's storm-battered crew regarded the "fire" as a sign of divine protection by St Elmo, the patron saint of mariners. Captain Ahab saw St Elmo's fire and reassured his ill-fated crew aboard the whaler *Pequod*, "The white flame but marks the way to the white whale."

St Elmo's fire occurs when there is a large difference in electrical charge between the mast and surrounding air. This causes air molecules to be split apart by the voltage streaming off the mast, and resulting gas begins to glow. Do not climb the rigging for closer inspection, because there are 30,000 volts per centimeter of space surrounding the masthead.

Lightning is too erratic and unpredictable for full protection to be possible. Many experts advocate providing an adequate conductive path from the masthead through to the water by the shortest, most direct route possible, using an elaborate bonding system. All wire rigging and large metal objects should also be connected to an underwater ground plate. This is especially important for boats constructed from wood, composites, and fiberglass; these nonconductive hulls impede the passage of electrical charge to the water. Steel and aluminum hulls with traditional aluminum spars are excellent conductors of electricity and can easily carry electrical charges to the ground. The objective of bonding is to prevent injury to the crew, catastrophic damage to the boat, and severe damage to electrical systems and electronic equipment. Even with the best system, this is not always accomplished. Without grounding, a bolt of lightning will find its way to the sea from the base of the mast, usually through some part of the hull.

Mitigating the Damage from Lightning

The best advice on preventing and mitigating lightning strikes is to follow the practices recommended by the American Boat and Yacht Council for both lightning protection and grounding. At a minimum, the mast should be fitted with an air terminal. This consists of a solid 0.375-inch copper or 0.5-inch aluminum rod attached to the top of and extending at least 6 inches above the vessel's mast. Its skyward tip should be rounded. The path to the ground must be a highly conductive material of low resistance so that current passing through will not create heat sufficient to melt the conductor. The bonding system must be complete. Half measures may invite massive electrical charges into the boat and then fail to provide a safe path to the water; it would be preferable to remove the half measures and sail without a bonding system (other than one exclusively for electronics). Copper wire with a minimum of 4 American wire gauge (AWG), not 8 AWG as previously suggested, is required in saltwater, and a ground plate (with sharp rather than round edges), ideally made of solid copper or bronze with a dimension of at least 930 cm² (1 foot²), is recommended. The ground plate should be located as close to the mast as possible on the bottom exterior of the underwater hull.

Lead keels on sailboats make excellent ground plates only when properly connected to the base of the mast and only if not encapsulated with fiberglass. Some motor and auxiliary sailboats use the exposed surface of the engine prop and shaft as a ground plate. With engine grounding, damage may occur from the heat generated by a powerful strike. All masts constructed of wood or other nonconductive materials (e.g., carbon fiber with epoxy resins) require wire or a solid copper strap from the masthead to the ground plate.

Lightning can also generate a side flash, which is the secondary flow of current from the charged area to some object near the path of the strike to the water, especially dangerous to crew who are accidentally nearby. Simple grounding of the mast to the ground plate prevents major hull damage but does not prevent side flashes. As current follows a designated path to the ground, another electric potential is created between the ground system and the objects surrounding it. The entire boat becomes high voltage, and the secondary electric current, called the side flash, is created.

The oft-quoted wisdom that a 45-degree cone-shaped zone of protection is created under the mast is false. Lightning has been known to directly penetrate this supposed area of safety, and a person can still be electrocuted by voltage along the deck surface or by side flash if the mast is struck. The key to preventing secondary current flows is to equalize the voltage of all metallic objects onboard by establishing a common electrical ground for the entire boat, that is, a complete bonding system. Any area capable of collecting a large static charge, including each piece of metal equipment onboard, all electronic instruments, and radio equipment, must be bonded to the same discharge system used to protect the boat from effects of the initial lightning strike. This is accomplished by connecting No. 6-gauge copper cable from all metal objects to the common ground. This includes shrouds, stays, tanks, the rudder, engine blocks, electric winches, pulpits, pedestals, arches, radar masts, and seacocks. Switching off or disconnecting electronic equipment is advised, but will not necessarily protect it. Portable electronics, computers, handheld GPS units, and radios can be placed in the galley oven, which acts like a Faraday cage, or in a designated grounded metallic box. Everything electronic that uses modern microprocessors is vulnerable in an electrical storm. A new way of bonding the boat recommends grounding the mast at deck level to a continuous loop outside the cabin, connected to multiple cables down to the grounding plate and supplemental electrodes near the water line to further disperse electrical charge. This method is still in early stages of development.

Crewmembers may become part of the current path if they are in contact with, or come between, two different metal objects that are not connected (e.g., by grasping the stanchion or rigging while holding an aluminum steering wheel). The best protection in the event of a direct lightning strike, even if the boat is grounded and bonded, is to remain low in the boat (preferably in a cabin and dry) and away from shrouds, the mast and other metal objects, wiring, and electric conductors. Crew should refrain from using all electrical equipment (Box 70-8).

OTHER WEATHER PHENOMENA AT SEA

Waterspouts

Waterspouts are maritime tornadoes. Although less common than lightning and downbursts, they are generated by the same dynamic forces found in the squall line at the leading edge of an advancing cold front or in a rapidly building summer afternoon thunderstorm. The danger of a waterspout lies in the powerful revolving winds, which may exceed 400 km/hr (250 mph), and the very low pressure at its center, which may cause tightly enclosed spaces to explode. Waterspouts are visible during the day, when most of them occur, and can also be located and tracked by radar. The average forward speed is 50 km/hr (30 mph) but may vary from nearly stationary to 120 km/hr (70 mph). An area of turbulent water in the distance is the earliest visible sign of a waterspout; as it approaches, spray rises upward and joins the funnel cloud with its characteristic snakelike, gyrating appendage. Waterspouts usually last only 30 to 60 minutes. Preparation of the boat and crew is similar to that for a thunderstorm. Because a waterspout is relatively narrow, steering a course perpendicular to its projected path (the direction the clouds are going) is a logical avoidance maneuver.

Hurricanes and Cyclones

A hurricane is a type of tropical cyclone—an organized rotating weather system that develops in the tropics (see Chapter 107). Tropical cyclones are classified as a:
- Tropical depression: an organized system of thunderstorms with closed low-level circulation and maximum sustained winds of 33 knots (38 mph) or less.
- Tropical storm: an organized system of strong thunderstorms with well-defined circulation and maximum sustained winds of 34 to 63 knots (39 to 73 mph).

BOX 70-8   Protecting Crew from Lightning Injury

1. Get out of the water. If possible, get off the water and away from the water.
2. Get off the beach. If stranded, squat down and place legs and ankles together. Keep the surface area of the body in contact with the ground to a minimum. Spread people out to maximize the possibility that some will survive a lightning strike.
3. If possible, get off the boat, including a boat at anchor or in a marina.
4. Remove wetsuits and other wet clothing. Put on dry clothing and foul weather gear, hat, boots, and a personal flotation device. Wet bodies make good electrical conductors, but wet foul weather gear may provide protection by lowering surface resistance and guiding the current around the body.
5. Remove all metal articles, especially jewelry, scuba tanks, and weight belts.
6. Avoid direct contact with all metal objects, including handrails, engine, stove, rigging, and spars.
7. Do not touch any of the boat's installed electrical equipment, including navigation instruments and radios. Use a handheld VHF radio for emergency communications during the storm.
8. Do not simultaneously touch two metal objects, such as the engine throttle and spotlight handle.
9. Stay away from the mast, stays, shrouds, and wet sails.
10. Stay out of areas where bridging between two highly charged areas, or side flashes, may occur. These areas include the foredeck, between the mast and the head stay, or a seat between an outboard engine and the portable metal fuel tank or steering wheel.
11. If caught in a storm while on a sailboard, lower the sail and mast and sit down on the board.
12. If fishing or trawling, stop and lay the rods and trawls horizontal in the boat.
13. Put nonessential crew and passengers below decks, in the center of the cabin. Stay out of the companionway, engine room, and head. If there is no cabin, stay low in the boat.
14. If possible, put the boat on autopilot to minimize contact with a metal wheel.

• Hurricane: an intense tropical weather system with well-defined circulation and sustained winds of 64 knots (74 mph) or higher.

The Saffir-Simpson Hurricane Wind Scale is a 1 to 5 rating based on the hurricane's intensity. Category 1 has sustained winds up to 153 km/hr (95 mph), and category 5, sustained winds in excess of 250 km/hr (155 mph). In the western North Pacific Ocean, hurricanes are called *typhoons* (super typhoons have sustained winds exceeding 241 km/hr [150 mph]) and in the Indian Ocean, *cyclones*. On average each year, 10 tropical storms, 6 of which become hurricanes, develop in the Atlantic Ocean, Caribbean Sea, or Gulf of Mexico.

The center (eye) of a hurricane is relatively calm. The most violent winds and rainfall are found in the eye wall, a ring of thunderstorms 15,240 m (50,000 feet) high. Coastal sailors seeking harbors of refuge from the destructive wind and sea still have to prepare for the greater threat of the storm surge; this is a large dome of water, often 80 to 160 km (50 to 100 mi) wide, that sweeps across the coastline where the hurricane makes landfall. The surge of high water, topped by huge waves, is devastating. In August 2005, Hurricane Katrina flooded and destroyed cities of the Gulf Coast with its 6-m (20-foot) storm surge. In October 2012, Hurricane Sandy became the largest Atlantic hurricane on record (as measured by diameter, with winds spanning 1800 km (1100 miles). Its storm surge hit New York City on October 29, flooding streets, tunnels, and subway lines and cutting power in and around the city.

When given the choice, some sailors head out to sea, risking their lives to save their boats. This may be a reasonable strategy for a battleship but is rarely a prudent decision for an offshore sailing craft. The best tactic for dealing with the fury of hurricanes at sea is to avoid them. The HMS *Bounty* (originally built for the 1962 film *Mutiny on the Bounty*) sank in the Atlantic Ocean off the coast of North Carolina after attempting to outrun or navigate around a massive hurricane. The vessel had started taking on water, its engines failed, and the crew of the stately historic craft had to abandon ship as it went down in the immense seas. The captain and one crewmember perished, and the remaining crew were rescued from life rafts by helicopters. The ship left New England just prior to the arrival of the storm. Ironically, one of the last posted messages on Facebook said: "Rest assured that the *Bounty* is safe and in very capable hands. *Bounty*'s current voyage is a calculated decision … NOT AT ALL … irresponsible or with a lack of foresight as some have suggested. The fact of the matter is … A SHIP IS SAFER AT SEA THAN IN PORT!"

In the Northern Hemisphere, wind blows counterclockwise around the eye of a hurricane. Facing into the wind and stretching the right arm back 120 degrees will point at the eye. In the Southern Hemisphere, wind blows clockwise around the eye. Facing into the wind and stretching the left arm back 120 degrees will point to the eye. In the Northern Hemisphere, the strongest winds are to the right side of the hurricane's path, where the forward speed over the water adds to the local wind speed; this is the more dangerous semicircle. In the Southern Hemisphere, the strongest winds are on the left side of the path. Although recommendations include placing the boat in the so-called safe or navigable semicircle and avoiding the strongest winds surrounding the eye of the hurricane, the safest course is to stay out of its path entirely.

Hurricane track forecasting has acknowledged limits and errors, and the U.S. National Hurricane Center is not infallible. Hurricanes are inherently unpredictable, even when the best computer models are used to predict the path. In October 1998, when category 5 Hurricane Mitch (the fourth-strongest Atlantic basin hurricane in recorded history) slammed into Honduras, the 82-m (286-foot), four-masted, steel-hulled *Fantome* was doomed. Despite every evasive action taken by the experienced captain (based on the updated forecast track), the massive hurricane swirled menacingly into his path and eventually sank the cruise ship with loss of the entire crew. The plots of the ship's daily locations off the coast of Central America and those of the hurricane exactly overlap each other, as though Mitch were actively chasing the ship before finally devouring it.

The expected track error for a hurricane is 160 km (100 mi) on either side of the predicted track for each 24-hour forecast period. For a 72-hour forecast, an error of 480 km (300 mi) to the left or right of the predicted forecast track can be expected, and for a 96-hour forecast, 650 km (400 mi) to either side is applied. That would make the storm's potential swath for destruction 800 miles wide, a considerable area to avoid if a vessel can only travel at 6 to 7 knots in storm conditions. In order to take meaningful evasive action, a hurricane needs to be monitored at least every 6 hours, the official forecast interval for the NOAA/NWS Storm Prediction Center. The National Hurricane Center in Miami, Florida, provides advisory updates on developing tropical storms and hurricanes 24 hours a day online at the National Hurricane Center website: nhc.noaa.gov.

SEA CONDITIONS AND BREAKING SEAS

The U.S. Sailing Farallones Panel Report of *Low Speed Chase* Capsize issued in July 2012 explores the danger of sea conditions in shoal waters (Figure 70-21) (see ussailing.org/racing/offshore-big-boats/big-boat-safety-at-sea/safety-incident-reports/ for the *Low Speed Chase* reports and other incident reports involving sailboats). "On April 14, 2012, at 14:36:40 PDT, while racing in the Full Crew Farallones Race out of San Francisco, CA, the sailing vessel *Low Speed Chase*, with eight crew aboard, encountered breaking waves when rounding Maintop Island, the northwest point of SE Farallon Island. The vessel, a Sydney 38, was less than 0.2 nautical miles (400 yards) from the point, crossing a 4-fathom shoal at near-low tide in a 25-knot northwest wind on a heading of approximately 235° magnetic. The morning forecast predicted 'wind waves 3 to 7 feet, NW swell 12 to 15 feet at 13 seconds.' A set of larger than average waves capsized

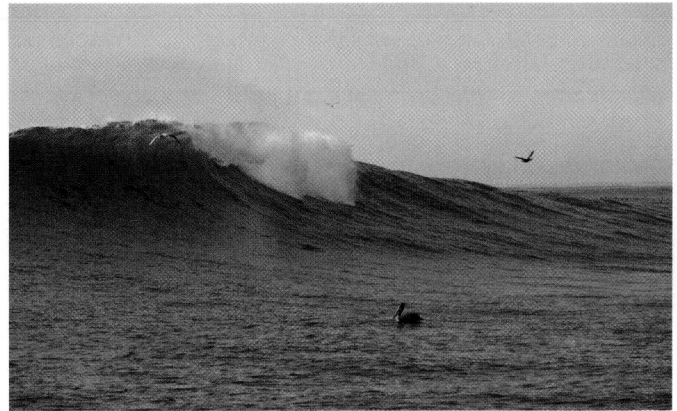

FIGURE 70-21 Breaking seas can occur when the depth of the water is less than 2.5 times the significant wave height. Waves may break very infrequently, lulling skippers into a false sense of security. Know wave heights and depths.

BOX 70-9 Visual and Sound Distress Signals at Sea

1. If other vessels are in sight, stand in an unobstructed area and slowly and repeatedly raise and lower outstretched arms as though you are flapping wings.
2. Sound a foghorn (SOS: 3 short blasts, then 3 long, then 3 short), ring a ship's bell, or blow a whistle continuously.
3. At night, point a flashlight at another boat and flash SOS (dot dot dot, dash dash dash, dot dot dot) repeatedly.
4. Fly the ship's ensign upside down, or fly the recognized distress flag: an orange flag with a black square under a black ball. Any square flag with a ball shape above or below is also a recognized distress signal.
5. Wave any brightly colored clothing or foul weather gear attached to a paddle or pole.

the boat and drove it onto the rocky shore. Seven of the eight crew members were thrown into the water. Two of those in the water made it to shore and survived, but five did not. One of the survivors rode the boat to shore. Whether or not a wave will break in shallow water depends on the size and steepness of the wave, water depth, and shape of the bottom contour. Wavelength and period are related, and the wavelength (L) of a wave with a 14-second period is 1000 feet. Depths over half of that (L/2 or 500 feet) are considered "deep water," and depths of less than L/20 (50 feet) are considered "shallow water" for wave dynamics.

Waves slow down as they reach shallow water and "feel the bottom," but the period is unchanged, so the kinetic energy is converted into the potential energy of a slower, taller wave. This increases as the depth decreases until the wave becomes unstable and breaks. If this process happens gradually (e.g., a gently sloping beach), then the waves will form "spilling" breakers, with the water tumbling down the sloping face of the wave. If the breaker forms quickly (e.g.., a faster-moving wave and a more steeply sloping shoreline), then a "plunging" breaker forms, with the face becoming vertical, curling, and then collapsing into the trough.

In storm-tossed seas, expect larger, more dangerous waves; the height varies, and some can be double the height of average waves in a given area. Strong tidal currents, common near inter-island passages, inlets, canal exits, and river mouths, can interact with wind-driven waves to produce high waves and perilous conditions. The same concept applies to adverse currents. When a current's speed approaches or exceeds 25% of the speed of oncoming wind-driven waves, the current stops the wave energy from moving forward; the wave energy builds vertically until the steep waves begin to break, endangering small craft. Current and tide tables should be checked in the regional *Nautical Almanac* in order to calculate the optimal time for safe passage by coordinating local weather with the predicted currents. Sailing parallel (beam-to) to high breaking seas (see Figure 70-21) should be avoided; the curl of a plunging breaker can easily capsize a boat. Capsizing may occur in seas that are not exceptionally high. On December 21, 2004, the 23-m (75-foot) *Northern Edge,* with six fishermen aboard, capsized off the New England coast in a snow squall with 5-m (15-foot) seas and 56-km/hr (35-mph) winds (an average North Atlantic winter storm). The lone survivor said, "We were dredging (for scallops) … then came a wave and the boat was hit broadside, and it just flipped." The bodies of the other five fishermen were never recovered from the 4°C (39°F) water after the U.S. Coast Guard searched a 4791-km² (1850-mi²) area for more than 40 hours. None of the fishermen was wearing a survival suit. According to a preliminary investigation, the water-tight door to the engine room and forward compartment was open, but scuppers to the main deck (openings along the deck that allow water to escape) were closed.

EMERGENCY COMMUNICATIONS AND DISTRESS SIGNALS
VISUAL AND SOUND DISTRESS SIGNALS

The simplest signaling strategies and devices are often overlooked. Box 70-9 lists some simple signaling techniques. Pyrotechnic distress signals have a replacement interval of 42 months from date of manufacture and are labeled with the expiration date. Expired flares can be kept onboard as spares, but will not be counted in the vessel's required inventory if boarded. The U.S. Coast Guard requires all boats over 16 feet on U.S. waters to carry three visual distress signals for day use and three for night use.

Handheld flares have varying effectiveness for attracting attention during daylight (Figure 70-22). Luminosity ratings range from 500 to 15,000 candlepower. The lowest-rated flares are virtually invisible in daylight at 0.4 km (0.25 mi), and the highest-rated flares are only slightly more visible. For daytime use, orange smoke devices are the most effective way to attract attention. SOLAS-graded smoke canisters are superior to handheld smoke flares. They float and emit orange smoke for 3 to 4 minutes. Immediately after ignition, the canister should be hurled in the water downwind of the craft. All orange smoke devices have a few seconds of delay in activation; direct inspection of the pyrotechnic device should never be performed after ignition. Smoke signals have a visible range of 1.6 to 5 km (1 to 3 mi) in daylight, depending on wind. Helicopter pilots find smoke signals readily visible, and in addition, smoke often conveys the strength and direction of the wind at sea level (Figure 70-23).

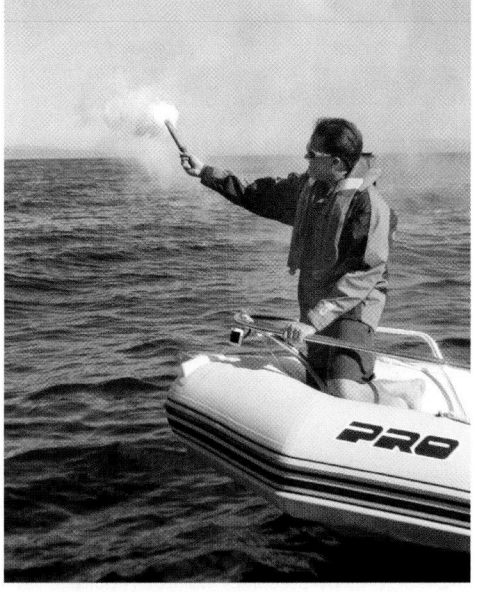

FIGURE 70-22 SOLAS red hand flare during the day. The smoke may attract more attention, but at night the red light is unmistakable.

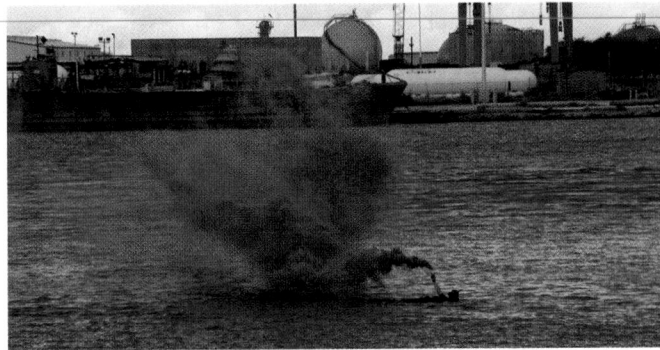

FIGURE 70-23 Coast Guard rescue swimmer with a small handheld smoke flare. This instantly shows the helicopter crew the wind direction.

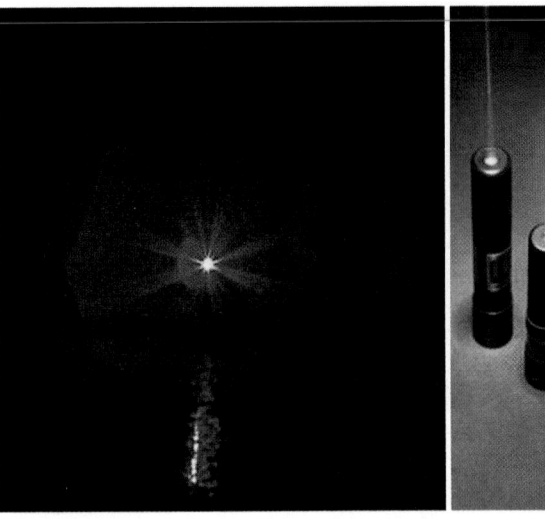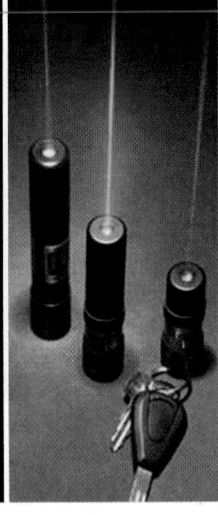

FIGURE 70-25 Although using a laser is exceedingly effective, Coast Guard members will abort a mission if they determine that their pilots have been "illuminated" by a laser. This is a shame, because laser flares are compact and have an exceedingly long range. However, it is not worth the risk to pilots if they are "targeted" with a laser.

After sunset, a flare's luminosity, burn time, and attained altitude are all considerations relevant to use. An aerial flare (meteor or parachute) should be used to attract attention or alert a ship or an aircraft at night, followed by a handheld flare to guide rescue craft to the distressed boat's location (Figure 70-24). Because of the curvature of the Earth, sighting distances are limited. A high-altitude flare can alert a ship over the horizon from the crippled vessel. The greater the height, the longer and farther the signal can be seen by a distant viewer. A parachute flare at 305 m (1000 feet) is seen as a brief flash of light on the horizon from 64 km (40 mi) away, but from 32 km (20 mi), it appears to be 152 m (500 feet) above the horizon and is visible longer. Luminosity and burn time are more important than altitude in helping craft to home in on the ship's location. The rated visible range assumes a ship in the area has an alert lookout standing on the bridge watching for and anticipating the signal, on a clear night with calm seas.

Whenever possible, flares should be chosen that meet SOLAS (International Convention for Safety of Life at Sea) standards. There are three SOLAS pyrotechnic types: a red hand flare that burns for 60 seconds at 15,000 candela (Figure 70-25); a red rocket parachute flare that soars to 305 m (1000 feet) and lasts for 40 seconds at 30,000 candela; and a 4-minute smoke canister

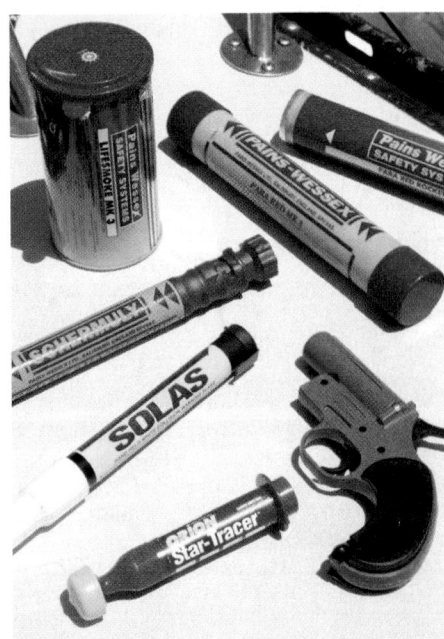

FIGURE 70-24 SOLAS pyrotechnics do not require a launcher, but some recreational flares do. Do not drop it overboard, or it could render the rest of your signals irrelevant.

(see Figure 70-23). All three are self-contained, waterproof, and found on commercial ships and life rafts, as well as on racing sailboats participating in offshore races.

All pyrotechnics are hazardous, capable of melting life-raft rubber and burning skin. Handheld red flares may drip considerable ash and slag, and should be held high, at arm's length, away from the raft or boat deck, and over the water. Crewmembers should be in a stable position when igniting a flare. All adhesive fastenings and covers on the flare should be removed and the device properly oriented after identifying the rocket or flare exit end. Some flares are activated by pulling a lanyard from the "business" end, while others are activated by pulling a lanyard from the "handle" end. After the signal is activated, shield the user's eyes. If a rocket or flare fails to ignite immediately, it may not ignite at all or there may be a lag time before firing. The flare should be held in a safe position for 60 seconds; if there is still no ignition, the flare should be thrown into the sea. Once activated, the flare should be treated as a live explosive, and should not be visually inspected or put back into the raft.

Red rocket parachute flares are designed to attract attention of potential rescuers out of sight over the horizon. They are the brightest, longest-burning aerial distress signals. For practical purposes, a parachute flare has a useful range of about 16 km (10 mi), regardless of its rated range or altitude. These flares drop slowly beneath a nonflammable parachute and burn for 40 seconds. The SOLAS models burn four times brighter and up to 50% longer than Coast Guard–approved models. Red is the standard distress signal, but a white parachute flare provides far more illumination than does a red one, especially if a collision is imminent. The main body of the rocket is contained within the launch tube. After the firing mechanism is activated, the flare tube should be held in both hands using gloves or a cloth to prevent the tube from slipping because of its powerful recoil.

Red meteor (aerial) hand-launched or pistol-launched flares (see Figure 70-23) should also be launched downwind approximately 80 degrees above the horizon. These flares are less effective than parachute flares because the burn time is only 5 to 9 seconds, and they are best used by firing in sequence. The first flare is fired to attract attention and the second about 10 seconds later to confirm distress and general position. Because of their lower altitude and brightness, visibility is limited to 5 to 8 km (3 to 5 mi) at night, and with these limitations, these flares are best suited for guiding nearby rescuers to the boat after it has already been spotted, or in inland waters where the distances are shorter.

NONPYROTECHNIC SIGNALS

The fullest effort should be made to use inexhaustible signal resources, such as signal mirrors, flashlights, or kites, before using flares. Rescue lights are no longer recommended because of hazard to airline pilots and rescue personal. The bright beam of the laser light (see Figure 70-25) may force a pilot to head back to base, unable to finish the search, and poses a potential hazard to injuring the pilot's eyes and vision. Pilots and aircrew require an eye examination before returning to duty after laser exposure. This is unfortunate because laser "flares" are visible over a long distance, have excellent duration, and are very compact. Pyrotechnic flares should not be fired in the direction of high-flying commercial aircraft; pilots and crew cannot see low-altitude flares and other signals when they are flying at 9144 m (30,000 feet). Flares should be used sparingly, and not all expended in an attempt to signal the first passing ship or low-flying aircraft, which might pass close by without seeing the signals.

Signal mirrors are inexhaustible devices and more effective than flares in daylight. Mirrors are especially useful when trying to attract the attention of aircraft, even those flying at high altitudes. The signal should be directed at the airplane when it is still in the distance and approaching the vessel. Signal mirror flash can be seen at a distance of up to 64 km (40 mi) from the air on a clear day. Mirror signaling should start as soon as a plane is audible, because flashing light may be visible to passing aircraft before a plane comes into view. Mirrors are also useful at night, where they can be used to increase vessel conspicuity by reflecting back a ship's searchlight, making the raft or ship easier to locate in the dark. Improvised reflective surfaces can be fashioned from materials such as compact discs, foil space blankets, jewelry, eating utensils, fishing lures, and credit cards. See Box 70-9 for other signals.

Coast Guard rules state that every boat must carry a device capable of producing a 4-second blast audible from 800 m (0.5 mi). This requirement can be met with chemical propellant–powered horns, lung-powered horns, or whistles. Plastic horns threaded into a metal canister often malfunction; spare parts and propellant should be kept onboard. Most handheld horns are barely audible at half a mile, and are inaudible at three-quarters of a mile. The same is true for lung-powered horns and whistles, which are barely audible at 400 m (0.25 mi). In the absence of a working sound device aboard ship, percussion of metal objects such as a spoon or winch handle against a pot can be used to sustain a continuous, albeit crude, bell-like sound.

Rescue ships and aircraft use radar to locate a life raft or vessel in distress. Commercial life rafts and lifeboats increase their visibility on the radar screen by using an electronic radar reflector known as a search and rescue transponder (SART). Once activated by an incoming radar signal (the interrogating radar), the SART is capable of sending back an enhanced electronic signal to any commercial radar located on a ship within a 16-km (10-mi) radius and up to 80 km (50 mi) on the radar screen of an aircraft flying at 914 m (3000 feet). It is much more effective than a simple radar reflector. Carbon sails also make excellent radar targets for planes and rescue craft, and should be left up at least partially, or deeply reefed, for as long as possible.

Commercially available yacht radar reflectors have variable performance.* Sailors have tales of having been seen at great distances when using their favorite radar reflector, but it is more likely that a small vessel with radar will see a ship than that a ship will see a small vessel with a radar reflector. The effectiveness of many radar reflectors varies with the fourth power of their radius, so larger reflectors are dramatically more effective. Small aerodynamic radar reflectors have virtually no effectiveness, even if mounted near the masthead.

Fluorescent dye marker can be seen by airplanes and has a daytime visibility of 3 to 8 km (2 to 5 mi). In moderate weather, dye lasts for approximately 30 minutes. It dissipates far more quickly in rough seas. The ideal time for using dye is just prior to an anticipated aircraft arrival or in a known flight path. A sea anchor will keep the drift rate of the boat similar to that of the dye.

Handheld waterproof personal safety lights offer portable, compact signaling and can flash for hours on a single replaceable battery. New LED models last far longer on a set of AA batteries and are less expensive than the xenon strobes they have replaced. Although not an internationally recognized distress signal, they are effective when supplemented with other recognized distress signals.

CELLULAR TELEPHONES

According to the U.S. Coast Guard, sailors use cellular phones more often than marine radios to call for assistance simply because more boaters carry cellular phones than VHF radios aboard their craft. Although sailors should be prepared to use any form of communication in an emergency, a cellular phone has several disadvantages associated with its use that make a marine VHF radio a better choice in many circumstances.

- Currently, 16 to 32 km (10 to 20 mi) offshore is the average effective range of cellular phones; range is determined by line of sight to the cellular antenna. Therefore, use is restricted to populated areas where there is coastal cellular coverage. Gaps in coverage make them unreliable, even for coastal use.
- Cellular communication is "narrowcast" between two parties, in contrast to the more public "broadcast" over VHF radio; this excludes potential assistance from boats that might be in the immediate vicinity.
- Cellular phone reliance excludes the possibility of avoiding a collision with a large ship because of inability to contact the pilothouse of the ship by cellular phone, as one could with a VHF radio (Table 70-2).
- In SAR operations, no practical way exists to maintain continuous communication with a number of rescue craft via cellular phone.
- The Coast Guard is unable to use radio direction-finding equipment to locate the vessel in distress if the vessel is

---

*See the 1995 radar reflector study performed by Stan Honey, Jim Corenman, and Chuck Hawley at SRI Labs in Menlo Park, California: ussailing.org/racing/offshore-big-boats/big-boat-safety-at-sea/safety-incident-reports

TABLE 70-2	Useful Marine Channels (VHF Radio)
06	Intership safety communications. Frequently used by boats engaged in towing.
09	Boater calling. Use to initiate contact with other boats, and ship to shore (hailing channel). Commercial and noncommercial.
12	Port operations, traffic advisories.
13	Intership navigation safety (bridge to bridge). Use this channel to contact a ship when there is danger of collision, or other emergencies near to both vessels.
14	Port operations and some Coast Guard shore stations. Used by Vessel Traffic Service in some harbors.
16	International distress, safety, and calling
22A	Working Coast Guard ships and shore stations, Coast Guard marine information broadcasts. Switch to 22A after contacting the Coast Guard on 16.
68, 69, 71	Noncommercial intership and ship to coast.
70	Digital selective calling (voice communications not allowed).
72	Noncommercial intership only.
78A	Noncommercial intership and ship to coast.
87A, B	Reserved for AIS digital communications.
WX 1 to 9	NOAA (National Oceanic and Atmospheric Administration) weather radio broadcasts on 162 MHz.

using a cellular phone, as it can with the VHF-FM signal. (New features of Rescue 21 may allow cellular triangulation in the future, but so far the cellular providers generally provide the positional information to the Coast Guard.)

- A cellular telephone has limited battery power and longevity, and cellular telephones in general have poor durability and water resistance.

If a cellular phone is the only communications link onboard, it can be made more robust as a communications tool with a 12V charger and waterproof case. A comprehensive list of emergency phone numbers should include local hospitals and physicians, regional Coast Guard rescue coordination centers, harbormasters, and maritime towing services.

SATELLITE PHONES

Portable satellite telephones are a versatile and useful tool for offshore sailors. Depending on the carrier, they can provide either coastal or worldwide voice and data communications for a reasonable initial, per-minute, and per-megabyte cost. (Prices are subject to change; few areas of consumer electronics change faster than the options available for satellite communications; both voice and data options are expanding continuously, and prices for both hardware and airtime are falling precipitously.) Service resellers can also rent phones or data terminals on a weekly or monthly basis, which may make sense for a single voyage or a summer of sailing. Due to the high cost of data, traditional web browsing is impractical, especially given slow data transfer rates. Generally, an email-forwarding service, such as Sailmail, will be used to strip away undesired images and spam. For small data files, such as GRIB weather charts, the cost is not excessive and speed not prohibitively slow. (The excellent, informative website sailmail.com has a variety of services for long-distance communication, including an SSB-based network of stations providing email service around the world.)

Satellite telephones require a clear view of the sky to operate, because the antenna must be directly visible to the satellite, or they may be used with a docking station and remote external antenna (which in turn can see the sky/satellite). Satellite phones are the primary high-seas communication alternative to SSB transceivers, although SSB transceivers have distinct advantages. When the mast comes down and antennas for the SSB and VHF are lost, a satellite phone may be lifesaving, especially when help is out of range of the handheld VHF radio. A satellite phone is an invaluable addition to the abandon-ship bag. When not in use, the satellite phone should be stored in a waterproof container together with a list of the critical phone numbers of the rescue coordination centers and Coast Guard communications centers in the area. Newer models can be preprogramed in the SOS function. A push of a button alerts the rescue service of choice and helps establish two-way communications to assist in their response. These models also are GPS enabled, which allows users to text message their location. Distress alerts and position data continue to transmit every 5 minutes until the user cancels the SOS; a fully charged battery will transmit for 26 hours in this mode.

Iridium is a popular phone providing reliable worldwide voice coverage without gaps. These portable phones can be used for text messages, voice transmissions, sending and receiving email and Internet communications, and serving as a WiFi connection. The Iridium communication system uses low earth–orbiting satellite constellations (see information on pricing, above).

Globalstar offers portable phones under the SPOT Global Phone and the Globalstar brands. Coverage for the Globalstar system is largely continental land areas and coastal waters out to about 200 miles. For many voyagers, this provides necessary coverage. The voice quality is very good, and data speeds are better than with Iridium.

Inmarsat, known for large ship terminals, offers the IsatPhone Pro and ruggedized IsatPhone 2, which uses geostationary satellites and provides nearly worldwide coverage (except at very high latitudes). The Fleet One system has been designed for small recreational and fishing boats, and provides global coverage for voice transmission, data transmission, Internet access, and text

messages. Fleet One also supports Inmarsat's free 505 safety service, which in an emergency directs a call straight through to a Maritime Rescue Co-ordination Centre.

Each of these companies offers a wide array of payment plans for voice, short message service, and data. Each service offers the ability to call virtually any phone number in the world to get weather routing, medical advice, or miscellaneous information.

GLOBAL MARITIME DISTRESS AND SAFETY SYSTEM AND DIGITAL SELECTIVE CALLING

Until the new Global Maritime Distress and Safety System (GMDSS) is fully implemented, the Coast Guard and many recreational and commercial ships continue a radio watch on VHF channel 16. The GMDSS is a worldwide infrastructure, controlled from a shore-based communications center, to coordinate assistance to vessels in distress. This fully automated system uses satellite and digital communication techniques that require upgraded radio equipment and communication protocols. GMDSS simplifies routine communications at sea and facilitates regular weather forecasts, navigation warnings, and distress relays in the form of maritime safety information. Digital selective calling (DSC) technology permits a VHF radio (with DSC capability) to call another radio selectively using digital messages, similar to the modem on a computer. As with a direct-dial telephone call on land, only the vessel called receives the initial message. Every vessel has its own unique MMSI number. The radio must therefore be registered in order to be properly identified in an emergency or to be called directly by another boat using a DSC radio.* The vessel's MMSI and information about the boat are registered in the Coast Guard's national distress database. For VHF radios, channel 70 (156.525 MHz) is used exclusively for digital distress alerts, safety announcements, and calling using DSC techniques. No other uses are permitted. Distress messages can be sent automatically with DSC radios. The vessel's identity is permanently coded into the unit, and its position can be determined from the data output of a GPS receiver linked to the radio. On a DSC-equipped radio, the receiver sounds an alarm if it receives an "all ships call" (distress or otherwise), group call, or call specifically to that vessel.

A distress alert (equivalent to MAYDAY) can be sent to a shore-based rescue coordination center covering the area. Once the alert is sent, the radio will automatically repeat the call at intervals of between 3 and 4 minutes until the center acknowledges receipt of the message on channel 70. Subsequent communication should continue on channel 16 or another selected frequency for voice transmission. A verbal MAYDAY can also be sent immediately on channel 16 after the first alert. Most DSC-equipped transceivers can monitor channel 70 for DSC and channel 16 or other channels for voice transmission.

VHF-FM MARINE RADIOS

The VHF-FM radio transceiver is among the most popular marine communication systems, because it is a user-friendly, inexpensive, and reliable form of communication. It allows communication with those in the marine community of greatest utility: the U.S. Coast Guard, bridge tenders, fuel docks, yacht clubs, race committees, recreational boats, and even large ships. VHF radios specialize in ship-to-ship and ship-to-shore communication. VHF may also be used to check weather reports. Best of all, marine VHF radios are easy to use, even for crew with minimal experience.

The VHF signal range is limited to the line of sight and therefore depends on the height of transmitting and receiving antennas. A transmission range of 25 to 50 km (15 to 30 mi), and frequently farther when communicating to the Coast Guard, can be expected between boats having masthead-mounted antennas.

---

*To obtain and register a MMSI number, see the Boat U.S. website at http://www.boatus.com/mmsi, or the SeaTow website at http://www.seatow.com/boating_safety/mmsi.

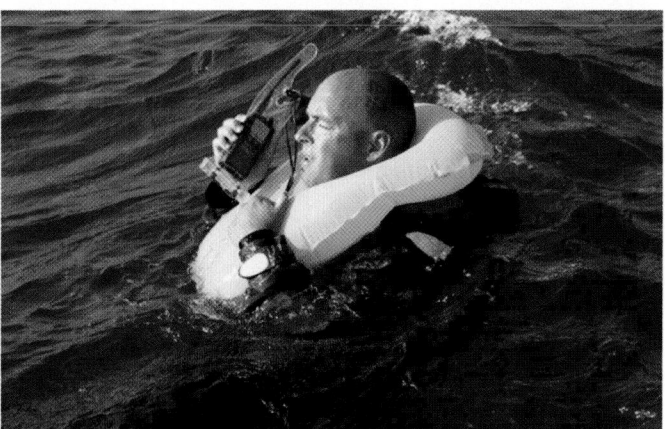

FIGURE 70-26 A waterproof handheld VHF radio allows a person to call not only his boat but other boats in the fleet, should he go over the side. The low height-of-eye requires that one call early and often before the receiving party is over the horizon.

Communication is not private, which is a distinct advantage in maritime emergencies and SAR operations. VHF is the open party line connecting all vessels within range of the signal. Should a vessel broadcast a MAYDAY call, all boats in the area monitoring distress channel 16 will likely receive the call.

Offshore boats should have both a fixed mount radio, wired to the ship's electrical system with a masthead sailboat antenna, as well as a portable handheld VHF radio (Figure 70-26). Fixed mount radios not only have a higher antenna but also transmit at 25 W, and can therefore be heard for longer distances and over weaker signals. During an emergency, use the fixed mount radio for the initial distress call. The vessel should carry a spare antenna that can be substituted for the masthead antenna in the event of the boat being dismasted; this applies to owners of powerboats as well, because the antenna itself can be broken. In an emergency, a VHF antenna may be improvised by extracting 17.9 inches of center conductor from a piece of coaxial cable, while leaving the shield to one side.

After a knockdown or capsize, a handheld radio can operate independently of the ship's radio antenna (the mast may have been lost or antenna damaged), and can operate if the electrical system of the mother ship has been compromised, which is a common occurrence during a variety of emergencies at sea (e.g., flooding, fire). Consequently, the handheld radio is virtually indispensable during SAR operations and helicopter evacuation, when one is required to be mobile and on deck. Handheld radios can also be used to communicate with the mother ship from a dinghy, and are essential for communicating with rescue personnel from a life raft.

The range of handheld units is up to 5 km (3 mi), or further if communicating with a Coast Guard shore station. Transmit power is limited to 6 W, and all radios have the option to transmit at 1 W. Transmitting uses 15 times more battery power than does receiving; to maximize battery life, transmission should be used sparingly and initial contact should always be attempted first using lower 1-W transmit power. Higher transmission powers should be used only if contact cannot be established at lower power. Although the range of handheld radios is less than that of high-powered fixed-installation VHF radios, reliable communication can generally be established with any visible aircraft or vessel. When quoted, battery life is based on the 90/5/5 standard, meaning that the radio is on standby (no noise) for 90% of the time, receiving (audible signals) for 5% of the time, and transmitting for 5% of the time.

Digital selective calling (DSC) has affected handheld VHF and fixed mount radios. Several manufacturers offer handheld radios with built-in GPS receivers and ability to send the same DSC distress calls that a fixed mount radio can send. The combination of GPS and VHF radio simplifies their use considerably. An MMSI number should be requested* and assigned to the handheld radio–GPS unit so that it can function properly.

The most important VHF channel is channel 16, the distress and safety frequency (156.8 MHz). This frequency is used to initiate contact between two vessels and is the only frequency continuously monitored by the Coast Guard. When a radio is not active on another channel, it should be left monitoring channel 16, eavesdropping for distress and hailing calls. This can be accomplished by using the DualWatch or TriWatch functions on the radio (the radio switches quickly between channel 16 and one or two other channels), or by using a programmable scan feature. Table 70-2 lists other VHF-FM channels often used by pleasure craft.

A VHF radio is one of the best ways to summon help from the Coast Guard and other vessels. Prior to DSC, emergency procedure words were used to indicate the severity of distress:

MAYDAY: when there is a likelihood of losing the vessel or someone's life; distress.

Pan-Pan: when the vessel has a breakdown or there is a medical issue, but it is not life-threatening; urgency.

Sécurité: when there is an important message for other ships, such as describing a floating hazard or a buoy that is out of position; safety.

These words are still effective when requesting assistance. An example of a MAYDAY call is as follows:

"MAYDAY, MAYDAY, MAYDAY. This is the vessel Surprise, Surprise, Surprise." (Urgency word and vessel name three times.)

"We are located at 36 degrees 52.2 minutes north, 122 degrees, 19.7 minutes west." (Location from either the GPS or any display that shows position.)

"Surprise is a 38-foot yawl with a blue hull and a tan deck." (Description of vessel.)

"We are taking on water, and we cannot find the leak. We request immediate assistance." (Nature of the emergency.)

"There are six souls onboard. We have a life raft, and EPIRB, and life jackets." (Number of crew and information on safety equipment.)

"This is the vessel Surprise standing by on channel 16." (Complete the call and let potential responders know that you are standing by.)

DSC and the completion of the Rescue 21 network have made many of these techniques and terms less important, although sailors should continue to know procedure words and how to broadcast a MAYDAY. If the ship's radio has DSC capability (all radios sold for more than a decade have DSC built in), the process of transmitting a MAYDAY consists of lifting a small red distress flap and pressing the uncovered red button. This sends the digital equivalent of a MAYDAY, with the unique vessel ID (MMSI number) and precise position of the signaling vessel. This information will be displayed and stored on any vessel within range that has a DSC radio, as well as by the Coast Guard's Rescue 21 network. On many boats, the transmitted position will be transferred to a chart plotter as well. In this situation, the voice transmission of the VHF serves as a complement, allowing the crew in distress to add details to the distress call on channel 16 or whatever channel has been used, as directed by the Coast Guard.

Unfortunately, the Federal Communications Commission (FCC) and Coast Guard report that around 50% of the radios in use are not set up to use DSC and Rescue 21, because the radios predate the DSC requirement, the radio is not connected to an operating GPS, or the owner has not programmed the MMSI number into the VHF. An older noncompliant radio should be upgraded to one with DSC capability in order to take advantage

---

*You can request an MMSI number from the Federal Communications Commission (fcc.com), SeaTow (seatow.com/boating_safety/mmsi), or BoatU.S. (boatus.com/mmsi). For international use, the FCC is the best choice. However, for use within the United States, BoatU.S. has a free service and an easy-to-use online form. Remember to jot down your user name and password so that you can update your MMSI registration information if your situation changes or you sell your boat.

of one of the best and least expensive ways to get help in an emergency.

SSB-HF RADIOS

For communication offshore beyond VHF range, a more powerful and elaborate single-sideband (SSB) radio transmitter is required. The SSB's clear advantage over the satellite phone is that a transmitted distress message (voice and via DSC) will be heard by anyone who is listening or monitoring SSB frequencies, which are part of the internationally adopted Global Maritime Distress Safety System (GMDSS). All commercial ships operating under GMDSS are required to monitor marine SSB frequencies while at sea. Satellite phones cannot provide ship-to-ship safety communications or communications with rescue vessels or aircraft because the phone numbers of those craft are unknown. An SSB radio allows an unlimited number of people to listen in on a transmission. Other nearby commercial and recreational vessels that are monitoring the airwaves could lend a hand or communicate directly to offer advice, act as relay, or help in other ways. SSB is also the only way to participate in various regional safety and cruising nets, such as the Bahamas Air Sea Rescue Association (BASRA) Weather, Safety, and Traffic Net; Cruiseheimers Net; or Chris Parker's popular Marine Weather Center. Many cruising events, such as the Atlantic Rally for Cruisers' Caribbean 1500, require participants to have an SSB radio onboard, so that they can stay in contact and share important safety and weather bulletins. Until recently, all offshore sailboat races required SSB equipment, including daily check-ins to report positions.

Medium-frequency/high-frequency marine radio-telephone equipment operates between 2 and 23 MHz. This equipment can also be used to receive high seas weather broadcasts and, in combination with a laptop computer and special HF modem, can provide an easy and relatively inexpensive way to send and receive email. The five principal SSB email system providers for the recreational market are CruiseEmail, MarineNet, SailMail, WinLink, and SeaWave. Each provider uses a different software package with the Pactor-2 or Pactor-3 modem. Email is not just for social exchanges; it offers cruising boats a safety advantage for communicating safety-related data to boats around the world. Depending on the radiofrequency band and atmospheric conditions, the communication range may be several thousand miles.

As of August 1, 2013, the U.S. Coast Guard terminated its radio guard of the international distress and calling frequency 2182 kHz, and the international DSC distress and safety frequency 2187.5 kHz. On HF bands, the frequencies 4125 kHz (channel 450), 6215.5 kHz (channel 650), 8291.0 kHz (channel 850), 12,290.0 kHz (channel 1250), and 16,420 kHz (channel 1650) have all been designated for distress and safety calls. The HF transceivers can call and receive voice and digital communications to and from anywhere in the world on land and sea. As with a VHF radio, DSC (see below) can be used with the SSB radio when it is interfaced with GPS and has its own registered MMSI. All U.S.-flagged vessels require a Ship Radio Station License from the FCC to get an MMSI number. This number will be coded for international waters and registrations entered into the international SAR database. The Coast Guard transmits voice and weather information on various marine HF frequencies. The transmitters cover the Atlantic and Pacific Oceans, Caribbean, Gulf of Alaska, and Gulf of Mexico.*

The best way to select an optimum emergency frequency is to listen to the quality of a radio broadcast. Any station that is received loudly and clearly will also provide good reception for an emergency broadcast when needed. SSB is an excellent receiver for voice weather and weatherfax broadcasts. Optimal use of a marine SSB radio requires instruction and practice. Mobile Marine Radio (ShipCom) in Mobile, Alabama, is the sole

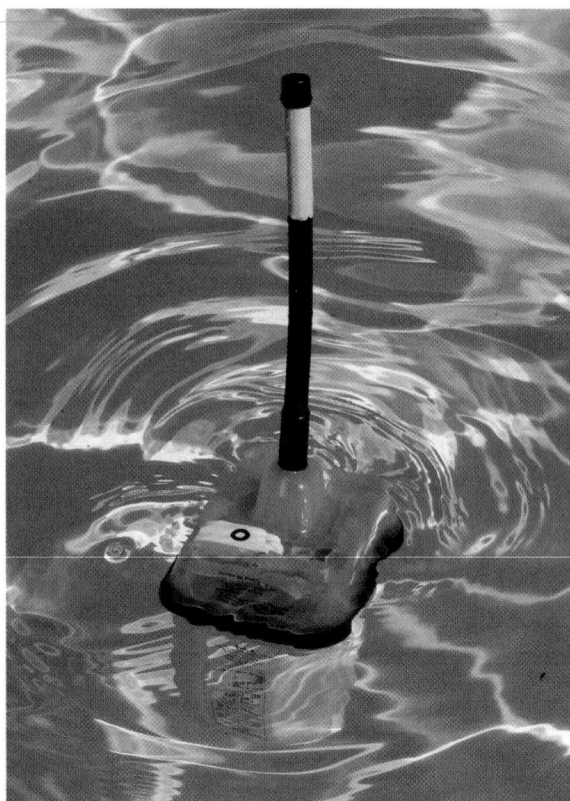

FIGURE 70-27 EPIRBs float upright and can transmit while bobbing in the water next to a life raft or damaged vessel. They include a tether that must be attached to the vessel or raft so that the EPIRB does not drift away.

provider of worldwide ship-to-shore HF SSB (and VHF in some locations) radiotelephone service in the United States.†

EMERGENCY BEACONS

Emergency position-indicating radio beacons (EPIRBs) are hand-held portable radio transmitters that can transmit signals interpreted as MAYDAY calls (Figure 70-27). These signals are the satellite-linked equivalent of a 9-1-1 call for mariners in distress. In the absence of a marine radio, or when out of range of coastal VHF stations, an EPIRB is the most important piece of signaling equipment. An EPIRB should be used when there is a life-threatening emergency; activation should be considered the equivalent of a MAYDAY call on VHF or SSB. The EPIRB should be located in a readily accessible location.

EPIRB signals are transmitted on established distress frequencies of 406/121.5 MHz. Signals are monitored by the global COPAS-SARSAT (search and rescue satellite-aided tracking) satellite system, coordinated by the United States, Canada, France, and Russia. This system (Figure 70-28) is a constellation of polar orbiting and geostationary satellites fitted with transponders to receive the distress signal and locate the beacon. Polar satellites orbit 966 km (600 mi) above the earth and have an orbit time of 105 minutes.

First-generation class A and class B beacons are no longer in use, having been replaced by the superior categories 1 and 2 EPIRBs and PLBs (personal locator beacons). The 406-MHz EPIRB provides the most reliable worldwide coverage. Satellites with 406-MHz transponders can store the signal in memory until a ground station is in view and then can retransmit the signal. The distress signal is quickly relayed to a ground station called

---

*Up-to-date schedules and frequencies used are online at nws.noaa.gov/om/marine/hfvoice.htm and weather.gov/om/marine/hfvprod.htm.

†Complete information regarding these radiotelephone channels can be obtained by calling 251-666-5110 or found online at shipcom.com/services.

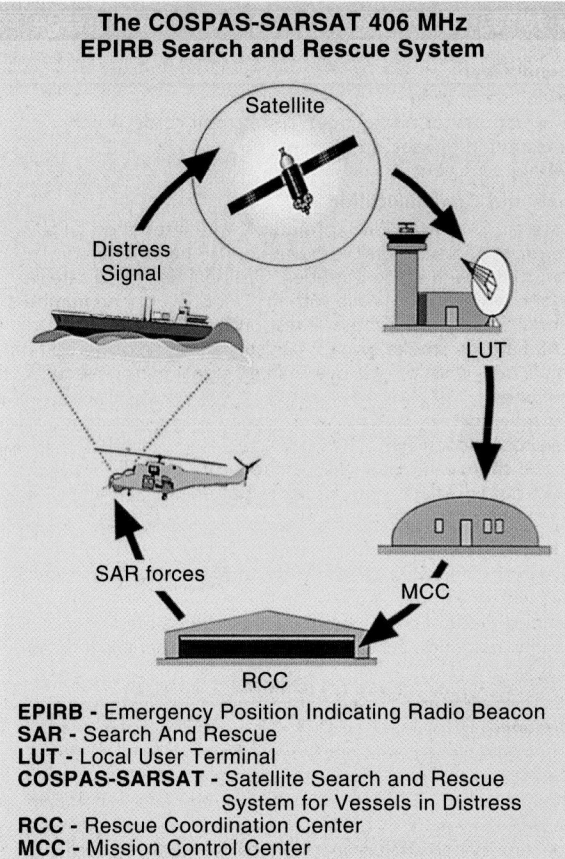

The COSPAS-SARSAT 406 MHz EPIRB Search and Rescue System

Satellite

Distress Signal

LUT

SAR forces

MCC

RCC

EPIRB - Emergency Position Indicating Radio Beacon
SAR - Search And Rescue
LUT - Local User Terminal
COSPAS-SARSAT - Satellite Search and Rescue System for Vessels in Distress
RCC - Rescue Coordination Center
MCC - Mission Control Center

FIGURE 70-28 With an EPIRB or a PLB, one is able to transmit to a worldwide network that listens for distress signals, and then forwards them to the correct agency. Register the EPIRB!

a local user terminal, passed on to the mission control center, and relayed to the appropriate maritime rescue coordination center. Satellites are able to compute the beacon position to within 2 km (1.24 mi). The 406-MHz EPIRB transmits a digital signal with a unique identification code, which can be instantly identified through a NOAA-encoded transmission program. If the unit is properly registered with NOAA, vital information regarding the vessel can be passed on to SAR units. All registered EPIRBs are issued a dated decal that provides proof of registration and includes a unique 15-character hexadecimal code, registration expiration date, and the vessel's eight-digit registration code. Every owner who registers an EPIRB receives a sticker from NOAA printed with the beacon's registration number. This number should be verified to match the ID number on the beacon before it is attached to the unit. If the numbers do not match, the beacon is not properly registered. According to NOAA, 30% of beacons are not registered by their owners (registration can be done online at beaconregistration.noaa.gov/).

Another reason to register an EPIRB is to prevent unnecessary SAR operations. According to the Coast Guard, 96% of all EPIRB distress signals are false alarms resulting from faulty or accidental activation. If the rescue coordination center is able to phone the contacts listed on the beacon's registration form, they can in the majority of cases validate legitimacy of the distress signal.

The newest generation of EPIRB is the 406-MHz unit with a GPS interface or a built-in GPS receiver. The GPS-enabled beacon (also called a self-locating beacon) transmits its exact location within 100 m (328 feet), using GPS-derived latitude and longitude coordinates, along with the EPIRB signal. GEOSAR satellites receive the signal as soon as the beacon is activated. Position information is continually updated and stored every 20 minutes in the unit as long as it maintains a direct connection to the GPS receiver.

All EPIRBs have a homing signal at 121.5 MHz. This is the homing frequency used by SAR vessels and aircraft equipped with radio direction-finding equipment to locate the craft in distress. Once activated, the EPIRB should be left on until the emergency is over; to update position, it must broadcast continuously. EPIRB radio signals cannot penetrate water, wood, metal, or fiberglass (the unit must be outside the cabin), but signals will be received when transmitted from inside a life raft, on deck, or on the water's surface. All category 1 and 2 EPIRBs will transmit for at least 48 hours at −40° C (−40° F). PLBs will transmit for at least 24 hours, and some transmit for more than 40 hours.

Many cruising sailors believe a 406 EPIRB alert will bring rescuers in a matter of hours, or at most a couple of days. These expectations are unrealistic in many parts of the world. Although the SARSAT system and rescue coordination centers that support 406 EPIRBs save more than 1000 lives each year, the system is far from perfect. Some nations responsible for rescue coordination centers covering specific areas have failed to ratify the Search and Rescue Convention of 1979, and even after signing, lack resources to meet their obligations under the guidelines. These rescue coordination centers are not equipped to carry out effective SAR operations in their designated areas; moreover, SAR may not be a top priority for the planet's poorest countries. For example, when the 10-m (32-foot) Down East cutter *Leviathan* went down in a storm off the island nation of Madagascar, a 6-hour EPIRB signal was not picked up by the rescue coordination center in Madagascar, because the center is not available on a 24-hour basis. Rescue ships and planes were not immediately diverted to the beacon's location, and 10 days passed before an air search was launched in the Western Indian Ocean. By then, the task was futile; the cruising couple and lifeboat were never found.

Potential delays justify carrying a second 406-MHz EPIRB when cruising in remote areas and far offshore. While the EPIRB is activated, continue signaling by all other methods available. EPIRBs with lithium batteries have a shelf life of 10 years (although the recommended battery replacement interval is 5 years), making it feasible to store the second one in the life raft. If a single EPIRB is carried on a vessel, it should be packed into an abandon-ship bag or other storage area for safety gear, or it should be mounted in a special bracket for automatic activation and deployment (category I).

SEND DEVICES

Satellite emergency notification devices (SENDs) allow brief messages to be sent either one way (to shore) or two ways, either from continental and coastal waters or worldwide. A variety of devices are available, and this is an area of rapid technological development. A feature common to all devices is the ability to send an emergency message to a private firm that can then forward the message to the appropriate rescue agency. A second common feature is the ability to leave a "bread crumb trail" of locations that track one's vessel or personal movements, which can in turn be followed by selected individuals.

Although many consider a SEND to be a second-tier safety product compared with an EPIRB or a PLB, it has been instrumental in many rescues and extremely helpful in instances where the track function has helped document events aboard a vessel prior to an accident. Safety experts generally recommend that an EPIRB or a PLB be the first choice in alerting rescue agencies, but a SEND device can also provide useful information to friends and family, as well as to rescue agencies.

ABANDON SHIP AND LIFE RAFTS
DECISION TO ABANDON SHIP

There are many reasons to abandon ship.[6] Flooding, fire, or collision damage will generally sink a vessel if not controlled quickly. Crew should only abandon ship when the vessel is about to sink or is burning out of control. The adage "always step up to the life raft" means it is best to abandon the vessel no sooner than when the decks are awash. All options should be considered. Abandoning ship prematurely puts crew at greater risk than remaining with a disabled craft. With rare exceptions, a floating disabled vessel is always the best lifeboat. The mother ship provides a stronger and more visible rescue platform than does a life raft. It is better stocked with provisions and equipment for communication and survival; conditions will always be more harsh in a life raft.

LIFE RAFT CLASSIFICATIONS

The three classes of life rafts (ocean, offshore, and coastal) refer to regions where the ship will be sailing and reflect differences in size, design, construction, quantity of survival stores, and packed equipment. For vessels cruising on a small boat near land, an inshore rescue platform, such as ResQpod, affords an adequate level of protection. Such platforms are not a substitute for a coastal life raft, and are suitable for use only on protected bays, sounds, and inland waters, especially in warm waters. A stable inflatable or rigid dinghy can also support the crew on inland waters and very near shore when abandoning ship. Coastal rafts are rated for open water, mostly protected or within 20 miles of shoreline; they have one or two buoyancy tubes and a manually or automatically erected canopy. This is ideal for offshore fishermen and coastal cruisers who need a light, compact raft, but its equipment must be augmented with a well-stocked abandon-ship bag (as with all rafts; see below). Offshore rafts are designed to ISO 9650 specifications, and are most appropriate for boats encountering offshore conditions for a relatively short duration but that are not taking a transoceanic voyage (Figure 70-29). SOLAS A Transoceanic Life Rafts are intended for the toughest conditions, with water temperatures below 5°C (41°F). These rafts include the greatest array of equipment and are the most sturdily constructed, to maximize self-sufficiency and permit survival for extended periods of time.

Regardless of the raft selected, the gear supplied will seem woefully inadequate, or at least that is the frequent lament from those who have abandoned ship. Due to the low likelihood that a life raft will ever be used, severely limited space available for survival gear, and desire to limit the amount of perishable items in the raft, it becomes incumbent on the raft owner to add incremental gear in the form of a grab bag, ditch bag, or abandon-ship bag. Regardless of its name, this bag contains incremental gear to improve the chances of rescue, and comfort and safety of the crew while awaiting rescue. See Box 70-10 for a comprehensive list of gear, but focus on having an EPIRB and a source of water before other items.

The life raft should be serviced according to the manufacturer's recommended interval by an authorized service facility. Owner and/or crew can request to be present when the raft is unpacked and repacked. The owner has a deep personal interest in seeing how well the job is done, and the raft's service appointment is an invaluable opportunity to become familiar with all components. Sailors should be intimately familiar with boarding

methods, equipment onboard, expiration dates of supplies (e.g., flares, batteries), and inflation methods.*

HOW TO ABANDON SHIP

All crew should don personal flotation equipment prior to entering the life raft. Excess layers of quick-drying clothing are recommended. One crewperson should broadcast a MAYDAY message on all available radios. A satellite telephone should be used to notify appropriate contacts of the crew's condition and coordinates of the ship's location. A 406-MHz EPIRB should be activated, and the life raft should be launched after locating the abandon-ship bag. Duplicates of essential communication equipment should be in this bag; if such equipment is not in the bag because it is in everyday use while sailing, a laminated list should be made of equipment to be loaded into the bag before

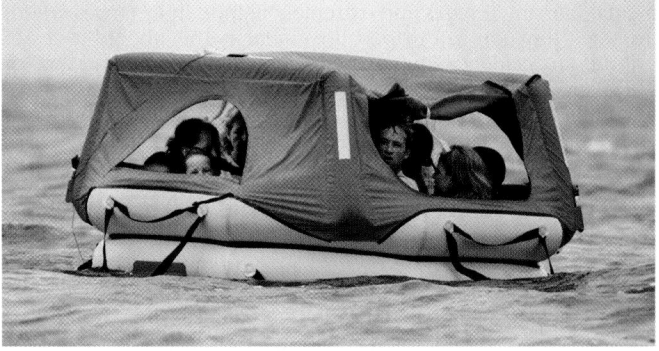

FIGURE 70-29 Example of a modern offshore life raft. There are lots of options for adjusting visibility and ventilation, excellent ballasting, and redundant buoyancy.

*An excellent way to become more familiar with life raft designs, features, and survival techniques is to take a U.S. Sailing Safety at Sea course, or a Sea Survival course outside of the United States. These courses combine lectures on a wide variety of safety topics, as well as demonstrations and hands-on interactions. See ussailing.org/seminars.

abandoning ship. It is recommended to augment the modest amount of survival gear found in most life rafts by having select items packed inside the raft container at its annual repack (include VHF radio, EPIRB, food, water maker, medical kit, signal pack, sharp knives). However, it is not recommended to put those items in the raft if they might be needed independently. These items may be packed into a waterproof bag securely attached by a short line to the raft.

For extended offshore and ocean trips, each crew member should have an easily accessible prepacked waterproof bag containing extra dry clothing, personal medications, passport, prescription glasses and sunglasses, personal strobe, safety harness and tether, wallet, and any other personal valuables and necessities. If the vessel's abandon-ship bag has been properly stocked, little else is needed from the sinking ship except synthetic blankets, jerry jugs of freshwater, extra food, and navigation tools; freshwater containers should be filled no more than two-thirds full so that they float. Additional communication and signaling equipment should be collected from the stricken vessel, even if emergency equipment has already been placed in the bag or raft, because it might become essential for backup if other equipment fails. This includes an EPIRB, SART, PLB(s), and a waterproof handheld VHF radio. In a life raft, one can never have too many EPIRBs, radios, flares, and fishhooks (see Box 70-10).

Life Raft Storage

Store the raft securely, either on deck with hardware capable of withstanding shearing forces due to capsize, or in the cabin. The life raft must be rapidly deployable in all conditions (offshore racing rules require 15 seconds or less) to maximize the chance of successful use.

If storing the raft on deck, a hard canister version is recommended, designed to withstand the rigors of a wet, salty environment (Figure 70-30). Rafts enclosed in a fabric valise that are stored on deck are much less waterproof than the canister models, and often end up with water vapor, rainwater, or seawater trapped inside, which can cause deterioration of seams and result in leaks. Some manufacturers now use a vacuum-bagging process to protect the raft from water intrusion while stored. Deck-mounted canister models have a hydrostatic release, which releases the raft from its cradle and allows it to float to the surface if the crew cannot manually launch it before the boat sinks. If the raft is stored below decks, make sure it too can be brought above decks and launched within 15 seconds. For offshore racers, rafts stowed below cannot be heavier than 40 kg (88 lb).

Launching the Raft

Before launching the raft, firmly secure the line coming out of the canister or valise to a strong point on the vessel. The canister

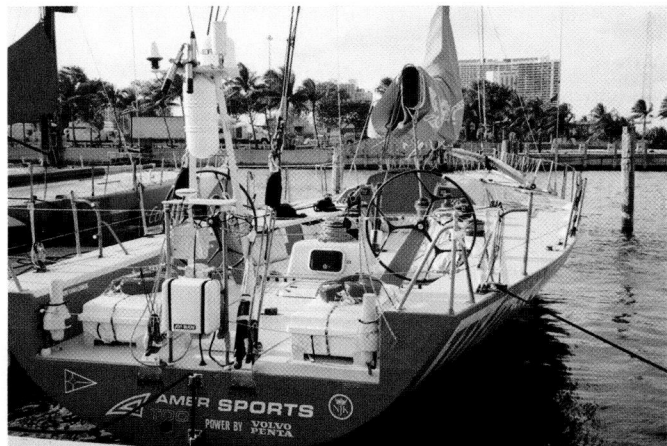

FIGURE 70-30 On the round-the-world racing Volvo 60s, 70s, and 65s, safety gear is stored where it can be reached quickly in an emergency. Redundancy and the highest-quality gear give sailors the best possible chances in inhospitable oceans.

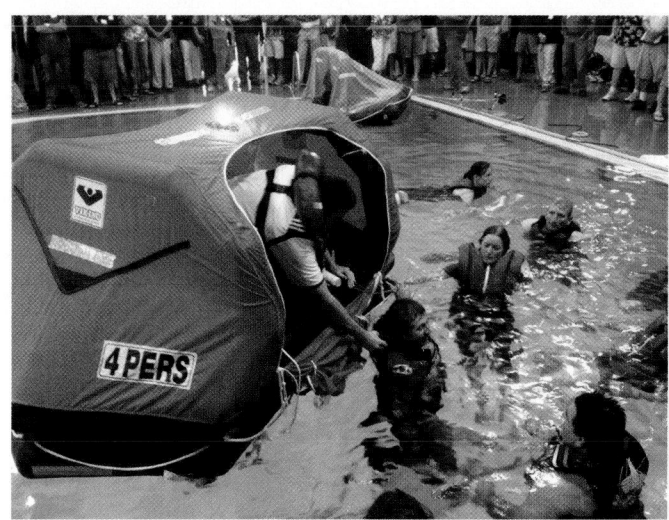

FIGURE 70-31 Keeping dry is advised when boarding a life raft, but it is not easily done. Safety at Sea Seminars allow sailors to practice launching, boarding, and righting a capsized raft.

should be thrown overboard on the downwind (leeward) side of the boat before inflation. Inflating the raft while it is still onboard is dangerous because it may become wedged in the rigging of the sinking ship or be punctured accidentally. A sharp jerk on the outstretched painter triggers the nitrogen/CO_2 cylinder and inflates the raft. Full inflation normally takes less than 30 seconds; care should be taken that the canopy arches inflate completely before boarding. The hissing sound heard after inflation does not signify a leaking or defective raft. The relief valve is simply releasing excess gas pressure. If the raft fails to inflate in the water, it should be brought onboard and manually inflated with the hand pump.

The first crew into the raft should be strong and free of seasickness; the abandon-ship bag should be handed directly to that person. If possible, the abandon-ship bag should be firmly attached to the painter so that it cannot be lost during transfer. The first aboard then helps remaining crew to board, while trying to keep water out of the raft (Figure 70-31). When possible, the crew should remain as dry as possible and enter the raft directly from the sinking boat, rather than from the water. If immersion is unavoidable, ease into the water slowly to avoid the cold shock response. Rafts are intentionally stable and drift slowly, and are therefore hard to maneuver to a person in the water. Therefore, the first person into the raft should throw the heaving line to those who might have drifted away. The line has a rubber doughnut-shaped quoit attached to the end, which allows a person to hold on firmly. Be sure to protect the airways of unconscious crew once they are in the raft, to avoid drowning. If rescuers must enter the water to rescue additional crew, they should be secured to the raft with a safety line.

LIFE IN THE RAFT: EXTENDING SURVIVAL TIME AND ANTICIPATING RESCUE

After successfully abandoning ship and securing both crew and equipment in the life raft, begin preparations for rescue. Panic, fear, and hopelessness can easily defeat the best-equipped and most experienced crew; an optimistic crew is more likely to survive. If the EPIRB is activated and the raft is near busy shipping lanes, the probability of rescue in a few days is high.

After everyone is aboard, the painter line should be payed out quickly and evenly to separate the raft from the sinking vessel. A safety knife is located in a pocket by the entrance of the raft to cut the painter should the ship begin to sink irreversibly. If the ship remains afloat, the raft should be attached to the wreckage with a quick release line; wreckage is easier to spot than a small life raft during rescue, and the main vessel remains a source of additional food and supplies. Because of the

CO_2/nitrogen mixture in the raft's interior space, the life raft should be ventilated periodically and thoroughly. The floor should be inflated separately with the manual pump to provide stability and insulation from the cold sea. With recovery of each crewperson from the sea, a significant volume of water enters the raft, adding to what may enter through wave action. Bail the raft as dry as possible, wring out all clothing, and bail again. All equipment should be inventoried and then secured. The EPIRB should be activated and left on until rescue is completed.

The first medical action should be distribution of seasickness medication. In a life raft (sometimes referred to as "an inflatable vomitorium"), everyone is susceptible to seasickness, especially in the first 24 hours. The raft should be made as dry as possible, and every effort should be made to maintain and conserve body heat, strength, and morale, in order to prepare for rescue.

No immediate danger exists if the raft capsizes with the crew inside, because there is sufficient air available in the space under the canopy. It is frequently necessary to enter the water in order to right the raft, unfortunately, because it is unlikely to right itself unless rolled again by successive waves. With the raft empty, pulling on the righting strap at the bottom can right it. One or more crew should kneel on the downwind side with feet braced on the CO_2 cylinder, and lean back (Figure 70-32). The raft will right easily when caught by the wind. It may also be possible to right the raft from inside.

To avoid recurrent capsizes in heavy wind and seas, take additional measures. Every raft is equipped with a cone-shaped sea anchor; this device is essential in rough weather. It provides stability in high winds, helps prevent capsizing, aids in directional control, and helps reduce drift. The benefit of reducing drift in storm conditions is controversial, because the raft may become sluggish with the sea anchor deployed. If sea room is sufficient, occupants may be more comfortable and the raft less likely to capsize if it is allowed to drift at the same rate as the waves. Weight distribution is also critical to avoid capsizing. Most of the crew should be positioned on the windward side, the side from which the sea anchor is deployed, to act as ballast. Weight on the windward side reduces the chance of the raft being lifted and flipped over by the wind. In seas with high wave crests, the crew must be prepared to maintain the raft's balance and quickly shift as needed to prevent capsize in the opposite direction.

Signals and Watch Schedules

Each type of distress signal should be reviewed, with inventory of signaling devices available, and an agreed-upon order of use. The most important duty aboard the raft is to maintain a continuous and effective lookout for land, ships, rescue boats, and airplanes. A watch schedule should be created to rotate duties every

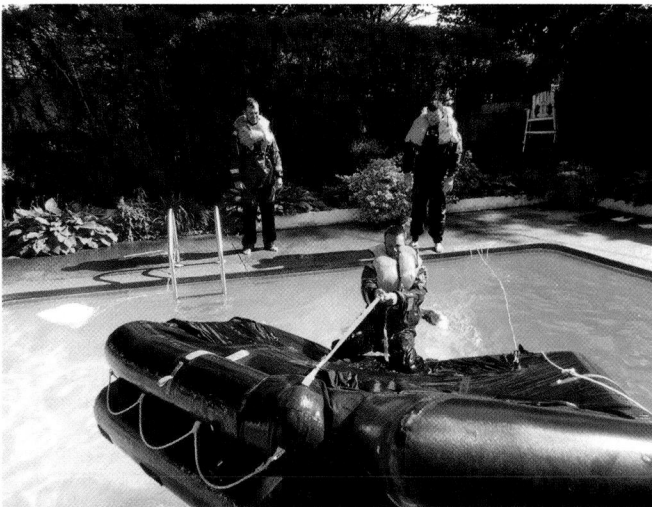

FIGURE 70-32 Righting a life raft is not difficult, but remember to keep the inflation bottle (cylinder) close to the feet so that it does not strike one on the head.

2 hours. In calm seas, intermittent observations should be performed while standing up in the raft. The visible horizon is 2.6 nautical miles if the observer's eye is at 1.5 m (5 feet); raising the eye to 3 m (10 feet) (standing up in the raft as it rides on a swell) adds another mile.

Raft Maintenance

The raft is subject to tears, punctures, and chafe, which may cause air chambers to leak and lose air-holding integrity. As the temperature drops at night, the raft should be topped off with the manual pump to keep chambers taut with no apparent folds, which will provide the fabric floor with greater rigidity and support. The raft's pressure relief valves will prevent overinflation, but they must be operational (not plugged with provided emergency valve caps) during daytime to release heated expanding air. The raft should be protected against sharp, pointed, and abrasive objects, such as knives, tools, or angular debris.

Internal and/or external dome lights are attached to the canopy. These lights help survivors find the raft at night when abandoning ship and provide interior lighting; they are not intended to be rescue lights. Occupants should determine if the light(s) can be turned off for energy conservation if not needed.

Health Issues and Hypothermia

If sea conditions permit, the raft door should be left open to permit the crew to view the horizon and allow circulation of fresh air. After seasickness, no other condition is more debilitating than chronic sleep deprivation. Sleep deprivation causes decreased alertness with blackouts of attention, which become increasingly prolonged and frequent. A groggy, inattentive lookout can easily miss the opportunity to observe and signal a passing ship. Conversely, the person may begin to hallucinate and see ships and planes. Inability to make quick decisions may further jeopardize the rescue. Crew should rest, and be encouraged to stretch and relax muscles that are constantly working to keep the body stable in the raft. Each person's recumbent body should be insulated against heat loss, especially from the cold raft floor. Hypothermia, rather than exposure to severe weather, is the greatest threat to survival in most abandon-ship scenarios. A Mylar blanket reduces body heat loss by 80% to 90%; however, the major heat loss in raft survivors is by conduction through the raft floor, against which a foil blanket affords little protection. The raft floor should be lined with sails, tarps, and extra clothing. The double-layer floor also protects against the bumps of sharks, dorado, and other fish. In tropical climates, spraying salt water directly on skin or clothing to cool the body by evaporation is not recommended. Salt-encrusted skin is more likely to break down and become infected. Dry clothing protects skin from painful saltwater boils and other bacterial infections. Apply emollient creams to knees, hands, elbows, and buttocks to decrease skin abrasion and wear. Any area of skin breakdown should be treated with antiseptic or antibiotic cream and covered with a dry dressing.

Water

It is imperative to drink water at regular intervals to avoid dehydration and heat-related illness. In tropical climates, keep clothing on to help reduce fluid losses; long-sleeved shirts, trousers, and a hat are more effective than shorts and T-shirts in prolonging the cooling effects of evaporative fluid loss, as well as offering superior sun protection.

Body water losses in excess of 8% to 10% of body weight cause significant deterioration in mental and physical performance. Hallucinations and delirium from hypernatremia (high serum sodium levels) are common with progressive dehydration; death occurs with acute dehydration when water loss approaches 15% to 20% of body weight. By contrast, complete starvation leads to death in 40 to 60 days provided there is enough fresh water to drink. Decrements in physical and cognitive performance do not begin in well-hydrated individuals until they acutely lose 10% or more of body weight. Fit and healthy individuals are able to maintain a normal work capacity during short periods (< 10 days) on severely restricted diets. Reducing activity to a minimum decreases food and water requirements.

Water requirement changes dramatically with exercise, sweating, diet, and ambient conditions. Evaporative loss from sunlight in an open boat in the tropics is estimated at 2.4 L (5 pints) per day if the body is at rest.

Life rafts may be equipped with 500 mL (1 pint) to 1 L (2 pints) per person in 125-mL sachets; it is recommended that castaways should restrict water intake to about 600 mL (1.25 pints) daily, unless supplies are plentiful. Analysis of protracted voyages in life rafts during World War II found that the critical amount of potable water for survival was 120 to 240 mL (4 to 8 oz) per day.

Hand-operated, portable reverse-osmosis desalination units contain a semipermeable membrane that allows only fresh water to pass. The water makers weigh 2.5 pounds, and produce 250 mL (1 cup) of water in 15 minutes, or 1 L (2 pints) per hour by hand pumping, which is enough for the occupants in a 4-to 12-person offshore life raft. As an added benefit, the units remove bacteria, viruses, protozoa, and other contaminants.

Rainwater can be collected with the life raft canopy. An exterior gutter collects and routes the water to a large container for storage. Daily canopy washing with seawater, whenever practical, can help remove the buildup of salt deposits. In a heavy sustained downpour, rain should be allowed to rinse the canopy before water is collected.

Fish and other sea creatures contain water with extremely low salt content in their eyes, flesh, and cerebrospinal fluid. Fish blood has a high salt concentration and is not recommended. Juices can be pressed out of the flesh by twisting pieces of fish in a cloth. The blood from sea birds and turtles is a source of hydration for castaways.

Seawater is not potable. After continuous exposure to harsh elements, intolerable thirst may drive castaways to drink seawater. Succumbing to this powerful temptation is a major cause of death and hastens dying. Seawater is approximately four times saltier than blood. Drinking seawater usually causes immediate vomiting. If ingested and absorbed, seawater triggers a process of osmosis in which free water is shifted from the intracellular space into the blood and other extracellular fluids to restore equilibrium. The fluid shift dehydrates every cell in the body, including brain cells, which contributes to the reported madness in persons who have drunk large quantities of seawater.

At high latitudes, old sea ice is a good source of water. Sea ice loses its salt content after one year. The ice is brittle, bluish in color, and has round edges. New sea ice is gray, salty, opaque, and hard. Melting the ice allows tasting and judging of salinity. If the temperature drops to freezing, seawater can be collected in a can and allowed to freeze. Fresh water freezes first. Therefore, the salt concentrates in the center, forming slush surrounded by ice containing very little salt. Sea ice should not be confused with ice from an iceberg. Water from melted iceberg chunks is glacial fresh water. As a last resort, chewing a piece of gum or cloth will help moisten the mouth and reduce thirst.

Unless survivors are assured of an early rescue or have a reverse-osmosis water maker, they should consume no water in the first 24 hours, and use the body's reserves; thereafter, survivors should restrict intake to about 500 mL (1 pint) a day. If water is plentiful, drink up to 1 L (1 quart) daily.

Food

Nutrition is the last priority for survival. If rescue is expected to take many days or weeks, the crew should eat little or nothing for the first 24 hours; thereafter, lifeboat rations of carbohydrates should be eaten. Some rations should be saved until rescue is imminent, when extra energy will be needed. Rations should be regarded as more of a medicine to extend survival time, rather than as a meal. Dried food should not be consumed unless water is available, and protein intake should be limited to conserve the body's water. When 2 or more quarts of fresh water are available per day, normal eating patterns may be resumed.

Fish are usually the mainstay of a diet at sea once survival routine and water consumption have been established. The raft casts a dark shadow beneath the surface, which appears as a safe haven for a variety of fish, especially dorado (school dolphin). With practice and patience, fish can be taken near the sea surface with a harpoon, gaff, or spear gun. Care must be taken not to puncture the raft with these devices. At night, fish are attracted to bright lights. Instead of a flashlight, a signal mirror or any other shiny surface may be used to reflect moonlight onto the water.

When bringing a fish aboard the raft, the creature should be wrapped in a piece of cloth or canvas, because both dolphin and wahoo have serrated teeth and tend to thrash wildly when they come out of the water. Wounds from fish-induced bites, punctures, and scrapes heal poorly and easily become infected. A cutting board should be ready to kill the fish quickly by cutting the spine right behind the head. A large fish can be stunned with a blow to the top of the head at eye level. Simply covering its eyes will calm it down sufficiently to position for a quick kill.

Certain fish are inherently poisonous (see Chapter 77); these are usually located around shoals and reefs in shallow waters. These include pufferfish, porcupine fish, and ocean sunfish (Mola). Any fish with spines or bristles instead of scales should not be eaten.

As a general rule, a fish that smells bad after storage should not be eaten. If there is uncertainty about the safety of a fish, it should be tested for edibility. If the flesh burns, stings, or tastes bad on the tip of the tongue, it should not be consumed. If it has an acceptable taste, a small piece should be eaten every hour for 3 to 4 hours initially, and if there are no ill effects after 12 hours, edibility and nontoxicity may be inferred. If there is excess fish after eating, the flesh may be cut into thin strips about an inch wide and one-half inch thick, and spread out to dry in the sun on a flat surface. If the flesh is cut with the muscular fibers running the long way, the strips can be hung on a piece of string and allowed to dry in the open air under the raft canopy. Fish spoils within hours in the heat, so the drying process should be started immediately after the fish is caught. Fresh-caught fish (except tuna), as well as dried turtle and bird meat, are good for days when the heat and humidity are not too high. Most ocean fish can safely be eaten raw. Freshwater fish should not be eaten raw because they harbor parasites.

Seaweed is valuable in two ways. As a floating nest, it can harbor a variety of small edible creatures, including small fish, barnacles, crabs, and other crustaceans. All kelp and almost all brown and green seaweed are edible, although of limited nutritive value. Red seaweed is highly toxic, and any seaweed that tastes bitter may be one of the rare poisonous varieties.

Many sea creatures follow a raft. Dolphins and whales may accompany the boat, but are not likely to harm the survivors in a raft. Sharks can be a menace as they swim about the raft for days or even weeks, and drive away other potentially edible fish. The shark's habit of frequently bumping a raft with its abrasive skin causes wear on the flotation chambers. Blood and offal should be disposed of at night to avoid attracting sharks and other carrion feeders, preferably when the raft is moving. Contamination of the waters around the raft, resulting in a waste trail for sharks to follow, should be avoided, and hooked or speared fish should be brought aboard as quickly as possible.

RESCUE AND EVACUATION OF THE SICK AND INJURED

Transferring personnel from a boat or a life raft to a rescue ship or helicopter entails risk for everyone; this may well be the most dangerous aspect of the survival ordeal.

AUTOMATED MERCHANT VESSEL REPORTING PROGRAM

AMVER, the Automated Merchant VEssel Reporting program[1] (formerly named the Automated Mutual-Assistance Vessel Rescue System) provides resources to help any vessel in distress on the high seas. AMVER is sponsored by the U.S. Coast Guard, and uses a unique, computer-based, global ship reporting system to assist worldwide maritime SAR authorities. Although reporting is voluntary for ships from many countries, AMVER participation is mandatory for U.S.-flag shipping. With the advent of the GMDSS, the role of AMVER complements the emerging technology. Today, more than 22,000 ships from over a hundred nations participate in AMVER. An average of 4000 ships are on the AMVER plot each day, and this number continues to increase. These merchant ships are not specifically designed for SAR and their crews may not be trained for recovering survivors from small boats or life rafts under storm conditions. Offshore, however, they may be the only rescue option.

In ship-to-ship rescue, collision between vessels is the greatest risk. The typical scenario is of a large merchant ship with limited maneuverability approaching a smaller vessel in distress with almost no maneuverability. Bringing a small boat alongside a commercial ship in a gale is a skill that cannot effectively be practiced; "Even under ideal circumstances, it is a highly danger-ous, heart in the throat, adrenaline-fueled action," a transpacific racing sailor once said who had abandoned ship and was aided by a huge container ship. Unless the rescue craft is designed for rescue work, the captain and crew experienced, and the seas relatively calm, it is much safer for boats and crew to use a smaller craft to transfer personnel between the boats. Options include a rigid-hull inflatable boat, lifeboat, or even a life raft. In rough seas, a boat or survival raft should never be secured to the rescue vessel. The constant battering of the two hulls is likely to damage the smaller craft, and may sink it. Whether to approach the rescue vessel upwind or downwind depends on wind, sea, and size and relative drift of the two vessels. Becoming pinned and capsizing are risks when sitting in the lee (downwind) side of a large, rolling ship.

The transfer of personnel between ships is also hazardous if sick, injured, or exhausted crewmen are required to climb a cargo net or pilot ladder; climbing out can be a difficult task even for a healthy crewman.

A large rescue ship most often approaches upwind of the survival craft unless the ship's rate of drift is much greater than that of the craft. This provides a calmer sea in the lee of the rescue vessel as it slowly drifts to the survivors' craft. If a sea anchor is deployed, it should be pulled in to prevent entangle-ment in the rescue vessel's propeller. Communication should be established with the rescue craft on channel 16 to coordinate the rescue. If the raft is to be lifted aboard with injured survivors, the floor must be fully inflated. Lifting lines should be attached firmly to the towing bridles on both sides of the raft, along with two steadying lines to each side.

The dangerous climb up a net, pilot ladder, or Jacob's ladder during a rescue should not be attempted without a safety line. When boarding a rescue ladder, the climb out of the life raft should be initiated when the raft is on the crest of a wave; at that moment, transfer to the ladder should be attempted. Sub-sequently the survival craft will drop down while the crewmem-ber is ascending and in theory reduces the danger of the craft rising up on a wave and crushing the climber. The safest proce-dure is to be hoisted up to the deck in a harness by a deck cargo crane.

HELICOPTER EVACUATION

Helicopter emergency evacuation and rescue have become rela-tively common within 483 km (300 mi) of coastline. A detailed briefing is radioed to the crew when the helicopter is en route to the vessel in distress. A crewmember should be assigned to monitor the radio and listen for the pilot's radio briefing on channel 16 VHF radio, or 2182 or 4125 kHz on SSB radio; radio contact should be maintained with the pilot until the evacuation is completed (Figure 70-33).

All loose gear onboard must be well secured, including cockpit cushions, coils of line, winch handles, dive gear, hats, and clothing. Any gear not secured on deck will become a flying missile in the 161-km/hr (100-mph) downdraft generated by the helicopter. This debris may be sucked into the intake of the helicopter's engine or become tangled in the rotor blades.

All crew should wear life jackets, with extra layers of clothing to protect against the chilling downdraft. Avoid shining flashlights and laser lights on the helicopter. Flares should not be fired in the vicinity of a helicopter.

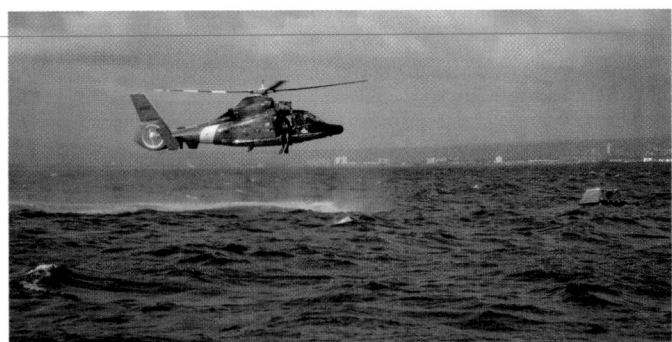

FIGURE 70-33 Coast Guard MH-65 helicopter off of Pearl Harbor, Hawaii. With a duration of about 3 hours, the MH-65 is used within 100 miles of the coast.

The transfer device is either a rescue basket or a Stokes litter (Figure 70-34). Selection depends on the victim's medical condi-tion and whether it is necessary to remain horizontal during the hoist. The horizontal position is particularly important for persons with suspected spine injuries or severe hypothermia. A basket is the preferred device for lifting; baskets are easy to enter, espe-cially in rough weather, and have positive flotation. The basket will settle on the sea surface, enabling someone in the water to float into it.

A horse collar sling (Figure 70-35) is a padded loop placed over the body, around the back, and underneath the armpits. The hoist is made with the line in front of the face. Always wear a PFD when entering the basket or hoist, and follow directions for securing safety straps.

The helicopter builds up static electricity traveling to the rescue scene, and the charge is transferred down the cable to the basket. The basket should touch the deck or the water first to discharge any static electricity. Failure to follow this procedure will deliver a strong, but nonlethal, electric shock to the victim. The orange steadying line, which is lowered first, is safe to handle and will not produce any shock.

The hoist cable or steadying line should never be attached to any part of the vessel or life raft, even temporarily. The winch operator will react immediately, and move to sever the cable from the hauling winch to prevent disaster.

If a Coast Guard helicopter picks up survivors from a life raft, survivors may be instructed to sit on the roof and on the inflated support arch to help stabilize the raft from capsize and decrease the amount of surface exposed to downdraft. A rescue swimmer

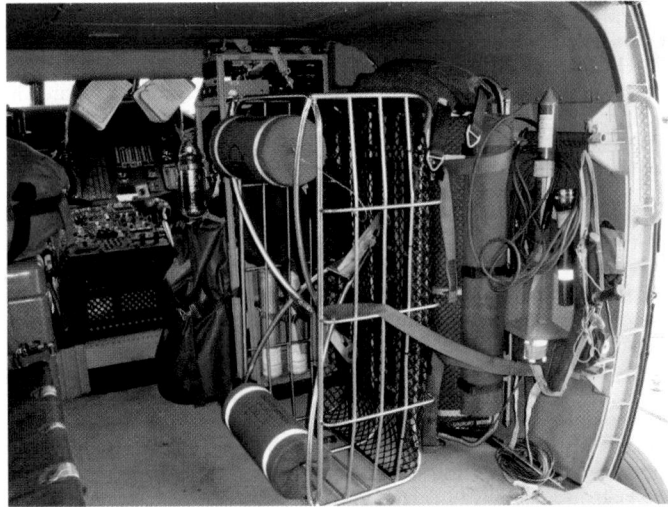

FIGURE 70-34 The interior of an MH-60 Jayhawk is crowded, even before the survivors are taken onboard. The basket, rafts, and pumps can be seen in the photo. This gear can be jettisoned if room is needed for rescued mariners.

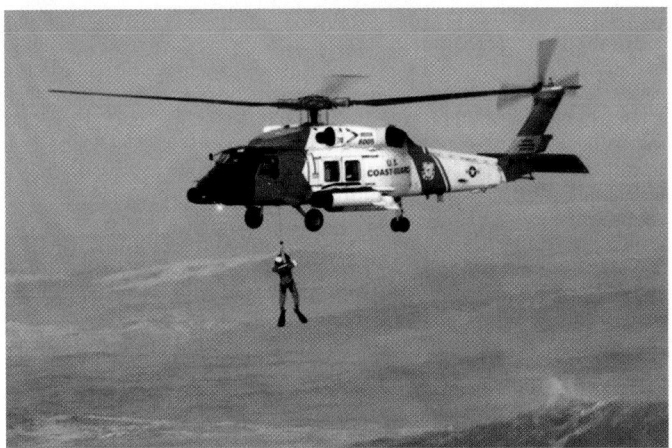

FIGURE 70-35 Rescue swimmer being hoisted by an MH-60 Jayhawk with a lifting sling.

TABLE 70-3 Coast Guard Search and Rescue Helicopters

Model	MH-60T Jayhawk	MH-65D Dolphin
Crew	Pilot, copilot, rescue swimmer, flight mechanic	
Maximum takeoff weight	9926 kg (21,884 lb)	4300 kg (9480 lb)
Maximum speed	180 knots	175 knots
Range	700 NM	375 NM
Duration	6 hours	3 hours
Capacity (additional people [passengers])	4+6	4+5

from the helicopter crew will assist in transfer, and when crew are required to jump into the water in order to be hoisted aloft. The raft may also be used as an intermediate rescue platform between the distressed vessel and the helicopter.

The helicopter is a versatile, effective and powerful means of transportation and rescue, with multiple applications for safe and effective SAR.*[3] The U.S. Coast Guard operates two types of helicopters (Table 70-3).

The C-130 Hercules is the largest of the U.S. Coast Guard SAR fleet, with a range in excess of 1609 km (1000 mi). It can air drop an enormous amount of lifesaving equipment, including dewatering pumps, life rafts, and survival and signaling equipment. A new twin-engine turboprop, the HC144 Ocean Sentry Medium Range Surveillance Aircraft, has joined the Coast Guard's air wing. Although it is smaller than the Hercules, the Ocean Sentry has similar systems, allowing it to carry out a wide range of Coast Guard surveillance, SAR, and transport missions. It can be outfitted with mission system pallets, a roll-on, roll-off suite of electronic equipment that enables the air crew to compile data from the aircraft's multiple integrated sensors to transmit and receive both classified and unclassified information from other assets, including other aircraft, surface vessels, and shore facilities (uscg.mil/acquisition/mrs). It can cruise at 215 knots and has a range of 2100 nautical miles.

REFERENCES

Complete references used in this text are available online at expertconsult.inkling.com.

___
*To view an excellent instructional video for recreational boaters on helicopter rescue, see the Cruising Club of America website: cruisingclub.org/seamanship/seamanship_safety_heli.htm.

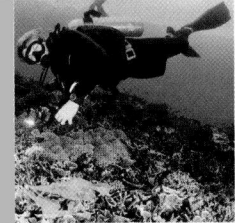

CHAPTER 71
Diving Medicine

KAREN B. VAN HOESEN AND MICHAEL A. LANG

There are five generally recognized global diving communities, each with its own set of medical, operational, training, and regulatory frameworks: recreational (including diving that is technical in nature), public safety, scientific, commercial, and military.

Recreational scuba diving is an adventurous and comparatively safe activity for a cross section of the general public. It is practiced by individuals of all ages who prior to training complete a medical history form (e.g., as provided by the Recreational Scuba Training Council). If there are any potential contraindications, the participant is referred to a physician (preferably one trained in diving medicine) for further evaluation. The diving depth window for recreational divers breathing from an open-circuit scuba system with compressed air or an enriched air mixture of nitrogen and oxygen (nitrox) is generally limited to 40 m (130 feet). Technical diving often far exceeds recreational diving in depths and times, may use mixed gases, and commonly incurs obligatory decompression stops. Using advanced equipment (such as multiple cylinders and gases or closed-circuit rebreathers [RBs]) mandates an advanced level of training and an in-depth knowledge of decompression techniques and equipment.

Public safety diving is an activity practiced by lifeguards, law enforcement officers, firefighters, U.S. Coast Guard personnel, Environmental Protection Agency workers, Department of Homeland Security personnel, and others. This type of diving is performed as a function of search and rescue attempts, crime scene investigations or body recoveries, or hazardous material recoveries. The public safety diving community consists of employees from various jurisdictions but also has a large contingent of volunteer divers who participate in the search and rescue teams of sheriff, police, or fire departments. The public safety diver's exposure to contaminants in the water column or sediments is of acute and chronic medical concern, yet can be largely mitigated by using encapsulated diving equipment and appropriate decontamination procedures following a dive. Radiologic, chemical, and microbiologic hazards can trigger a number of serious systemic or dermatologic signs and symptoms. Often, the connection is not made between the diving exposure and the clinical presentation, which emphasizes the need for further medical and operational education of public safety divers.

Scientific diving is performed by scientists whose sole purpose for diving is to use their expertise in making underwater observations and gathering data to advance knowledge. Medical, training, and operational standards are consensually promulgated by the American Academy of Underwater Sciences (AAUS; aaus.org), a professional society recognized by the U.S. Department of Labor Occupational Safety and Health Administration (OSHA). Due to the international and interdisciplinary nature of marine science, international organizations are increasingly adhering to AAUS standards. This facilitates the conduct of collaborative, multiinstitutional, international diving research projects. Many of these research projects are conducted at remote sites such as under polar ice, at South Pacific atolls and coral reefs, and from research vessels at otherwise inaccessible dive sites adjacent to third-world countries. As such, diving safety risk assessment and mitigation are carefully planned in consideration of emergency evacuation, hyperbaric chamber location, method of transport, and emergency oxygen supplies.

Commercial diving activities involve underwater construction, troubleshooting for and inspections of underwater structures, oil field work, and ship's husbandry, among other tasks. Like scientific diving, commercial diving is governed by OSHA (29CFR1910 Subpart T, Commercial Diving Operations). The Association of Diving Contractors International sets standards for commercial diving, collects exposure data, and creates educational and training tools for the commercial diving community.

Most military diving procedures are under the auspices of the U.S. Navy. Several Department of Defense sections manage diving operations, but by and large, the Navy tables and Navy-specified dive computers are the standard; the Navy's *Diving Manual* is the reference source, and its dive school curriculum is often the baseline for training. Of the five diving communities, the military and commercial diving sectors are best equipped from a resource and training perspective to manage diving emergencies, such as decompression sickness (DCS) and gas embolism.

The diving communities recognize that DCS is a risk of diving, but the incidence rates are acceptable; in fact, DCS occurs infrequently. Nonetheless, scuba diving can be a physically demanding activity because of intrinsic hazards of the aquatic environment and the physiologic effects of breathing compressed gas at depth.

The hazards of diving include the generic problems found in other aquatic activities, such as drowning, immersion pulmonary edema, hypothermia, skin and ear, nose, and throat disorders, water-borne infectious diseases, and interactions with hazardous marine life, as well as unique problems related to the increased pressure gradients underwater and effects of increased partial pressures of gases on human physiology.

There are many millions of recreational, public safety, scientific, commercial, and military divers worldwide; hundreds of thousands of new recreational divers are trained each year. The U.S. recreational diver population is estimated at 2.7 to 3.5 million divers based on the Diving Equipment and Marketing Association Certification Census and the Professional Association of Diving Instructors entry-level diver certification history.[145] Diving is conducted in every imaginable aquatic setting, including the open ocean and along the shores of oceans, fresh water, and confined environments such as aquariums. Despite the extent of activity, diving-related fatalities and serious injuries are rare. For recreational divers, the average death rate (based on data derived from case claims of insured divers) is 16.4 deaths (range 12.1 to 22.9) per 100,000 divers per year.[82] The fatality rate per dive is a better measure of exposure risk.[283] Training dive logs have reported a mean annual fatality rate of 0.48 deaths per 100,000 student dives per year.[243] The chance of suffering DCS during any single recreational dive is approximately 4 in 10,000 in warm water and 59 in 10,000 in cold water.[281]

The most up-to-date information about recreational diving accidents is compiled by the Divers Alert Network (DAN), a not-for-profit diving safety medical organization supported by clinical and academic affiliations, including the University of California at San Diego and a network of referral diving physicians. Established in 1980, DAN provides diving medical assistance to recreational, public safety, and scientific diving communities all over the world. Services include dissemination of medical information online (DAN.org) and through a medical hotline (919-684-9111), research results from studies and workshops, educational courses, and insurance products. DAN is a member-supported organization with more than 250,000 American members and an additional 175,000 international (IDAN) members.

The number of diving-related accidents in North America reported by DAN has been relatively stable over the past three decades. DAN's research department analyzes these observational data to eliminate reporting bias and for completeness of information about the frequency and type of diving performed. Diving medical safety continues to be DAN's primary mission-oriented focus. One of DAN's key roles in the diving industry is management of recreational diving fatality and accident data. Diving-associated fatalities peaked in the mid-1970s, with annual rates as high as 150, and have been stable since that time, with an average of 84 (range 77 to 91) fatalities per year.[82] In a recent effort to further define the scope of diving fatalities and overcome the perennial problem of uncertain total numbers (denominators), DAN researchers used claims data from 2000 to 2006 from insured members. Over that 7-year period, there were 187 death claims among 1,141,367 insured member-years, for which the mean annual fatality rate was 16.4 (range 12.1 to 22.9) deaths per 100,000 persons.[82] Fatality data from the British Sub-Aqua Club are similar for the same period, with 14.4 deaths per 100,000 divers.

DAN hosted a 2010 workshop on Recreational Diving Fatalities[283] to address industry concerns about root-cause analysis (trigger, disabling agent/action, disabling injury, and cause of death) of diving accidents and to solicit input from industry leaders about possible intervention strategies. Denoble and colleagues stated, "The most common disabling injuries associated with death were asphyxia, arterial gas embolism (AGE), and acute cardiac related events. The most common root causes were gas supply problems, emergency ascent, cardiac health issues, entrapment/entanglement, and buoyancy trouble. The risk for death while diving increased with age, starting in the early-thirties years of life. This is likely due to the naturally increased prevalence of cardiac disease with age, but an increased association of AGE and asphyxia were also associated with aging."[81]

Since scuba diving made its debut in the United States in 1951, the nature of the diving population has substantially changed. Scuba divers of the 1950s and 1960s were generally "water people" who were well-trained, strong swimmers; experienced in breath-hold diving; and mostly male. For these individuals, donning a scuba tank and regulator was a natural extension of a familiar activity. These early scuba divers seldom encountered problems that required attention from the general medical community. However, as scuba diving equipment became more available, adventure-minded persons from all walks of life became attracted to the sport. Popularization of recreational scuba diving in recent years has attracted participants who are poorly conditioned, have little or no experience in aquatic or other sports, are of advanced age, have significant underlying medical conditions, or are sometimes severely disabled. Because of the hostile and unforgiving nature of the aquatic environment and the time-sensitive nature of underwater emergencies, such persons may be at increased risk for a diving-related injury or illness. Certain medical conditions may constitute temporary or absolute contraindications to diving.

In the past two decades, recreational divers have increasingly sought out more technically complicated, and often more remote, diving activities in efforts to increase the amount of time or depth attained underwater. Although these advanced diving techniques (e.g., using an RB apparatus or mixed gas) have long been used in scientific, commercial, and military diving programs under controlled and supervised conditions, there are significant concerns about the safety of "technical" diving in the typically less-controlled recreational setting.

All primary care physicians should be prepared to answer basic questions about fitness for diving and to initially manage diving-related medical emergencies. Every emergency medical treatment facility should be prepared to evaluate a dive accident victim, provide emergency care, and if needed, arrange appropriate transport to a hyperbaric treatment facility if a diver is suspected to be suffering from DCS or AGE. The DAN emergency hotline (919-684-9111) is available for consultation with diving medical experts.

This chapter focuses primarily on the pressure-related diving syndromes collectively known as dysbarism; additional conditions relevant to diving are discussed in other chapters (e.g., immersion hypothermia in Chapter 8, submersion incidents in Chapter 69, hyperbaric oxygen therapy in Chapter 72, and hazardous marine life in Chapters 73 to 75).

HISTORICAL PERSPECTIVE

Humans did not evolve for an aquatic existence and are not well adapted for functioning in the aquatic environment. Nonetheless, for thousands of years, humans have been breath-hold diving to gather food and other natural resources from the oceans. There is archaeologic evidence that Neanderthal man breath-hold dived for shellfish 40,000 years ago. The Ama of the Izu Peninsula of Japan and the Haenyeo of the South Korean Island of Jeju (in both cases women) have been breath-hold diving to collect shellfish, lobster, sea urchins, octopus, and seaweed for at least 6000 years. Women of the Yahgan, Alakaluf, and other nomadic sea-going female Fuegian peoples of southern Patagonia engaged in similar diving practices for probably 5000 years before these primitive Native Americans became extinct in the late 19th and early 20th centuries. The fires that these divers built to warm themselves along the shores of what is now known as the Straits of Magellan inspired Ferdinand Magellan to name the area Tierra del Fuego (land of fire).

Written records of diving for salvage and military purposes date back to around 500 BC, when the Greek historian Herodotus recorded the feats of Scyllis and his daughter Cyana as they dived in the Mediterranean Sea for the Persian king Xerxes during the 50-year war between Greece and Persia. Many early cultures around the Mediterranean Sea made use of divers in military operations, usually to cut the anchor cables of ships, bore holes in the hulls of enemy vessels, and build harbor defenses. In 360 BC, Aristotle described the use of diving bells (basically, upside-down buckets) to supply air to sponge fishermen, and in 332 BC, Alexander the Great is reported to have gone underwater in a specially constructed glass diving bell (Colimpha) to observe his divers removing defensive obstructions from the besieged harbor of Tyre.

Colorful accounts of military and salvage divers dot the history of Roman and other early cultures. By 100 BC, diving operations around the major shipping ports of the eastern Mediterranean were so well organized that there were legally binding payment schedules, which recognized that the risk to the diver increased with depth underwater.

Although written records of diving in the Americas were not discovered until after European explorers arrived in the New World in the 16th century, Peruvian artifacts dating to AD 200 show divers wearing goggles and holding fish, so it is reasonable to assume that breath-hold diving had been practiced long before the Europeans arrived. Spanish explorers are reported to have enslaved native divers and forced them to dive for pearls in the Caribbean. These explorers also made extensive use of divers to salvage galleons wrecked in the Caribbean and along the coast of Florida.

Human underwater exploits remained limited to breath-hold diving until approximately 300 years ago, when a series of technological developments began to expand human underwater activity. These developments principally involved the use of different types of external air supplies to prolong submergence.

In the 17th century, primitive bells containing air were carried from the surface, allowing Swedish divers to stay underwater longer than a single breath and to salvage cannons from Stockholm's harbor.[228] In 1690, Sir Edmund Halley devised a leather tube to carry surface air to barrels, which resupplied air to manned bells at a depth of 18 m seawater (msw) (60 feet seawater [fsw]). These barrels were submerged, and the air they contained was compressed.[73]

The first practical diving suit was fabricated by Augustus Siebe in 1837.[5,73,228] Atmospheric air was supplied to the diver as compressed air from a manually powered pump on the surface. By 1841, French engineers had developed the technique of using compressed air to keep water and mud out of caissons sunk to the bottom of riverbeds for bridge footings and tunnels. Soon thereafter, it was noted that people working in a compressed-air environment sometimes suffered joint pains, paralysis, and other medical problems soon after leaving the caisson. This poorly understood condition was called caisson's disease, and was the first recognition of what is now known as decompression sickness (DCS).[236]

Underwater diving remained an esoteric activity having limited commercial and military utility until the 1930s. By that time, and increasingly during World War II, the military importance of submarines and other undersea activities became evident to navies around the globe. With the development of submarine forces came the need to train men to escape from submarines that became disabled at depth (an all-too-frequent occurrence in the early days of submarines). Given the shallow operational depths of these early boats, it was usually possible to escape by simply exiting the vessel and ascending to the surface. It was noted early that failure to exhale while ascending through the water column led to pulmonary overpressurization accidents and a new and dramatic syndrome that we now know to be AGE.

In 1865, the French engineers Rouquayrol and Denayrouze developed a device that could supply air on demand at increased ambient pressures relative to the 1 atmosphere of pressure found at sea level. These inventors were able to supply air on demand at appropriate breathing pressure to persons underwater with a "demand regulator," (versus a free-flowing breathing apparatus). This device originally required a surface air supply connection.[5] The demand valve regulator was later modified to supply auxiliary oxygen for pilots operating at high altitude. In 1943, while working with the French resistance against Nazi Germany, Jacques-Yves Cousteau and Emile Gagnon combined a demand valve regulator with a compressed-air tank, giving rise to what they called a self-contained underwater breathing apparatus, or *scuba*.

The potential military usefulness of scuba was immediately recognized and led to a considerable amount of investigation during World War II. As initially configured, scuba was used in an open-circuit mode in which exhaled air was simply vented into the water. This was wasteful of the compressed-air supply and had other disadvantages for military uses. Further work led to refinement of RB devices (both closed-circuit and semiclosed-circuit systems), such as Christian Lambertsen's amphibious respiratory unit.[13] These RB systems conserved the breathing gas by using a carbon dioxide scrubber and recirculating all or part of each exhalation (see Rebreather Diving, later). These specialized scuba systems were useful for military purposes because they allowed longer submergence times and could be used in clandestine operations or when disarming pressure-sensitive explosive devices. However, they had a greater frequency of mishap, so RB systems were not widely used until the 1970s for science. In the 1990s, there began a resurgence of interest in RBs by technical recreational divers.

After World War II, development and marketing of open-circuit scuba equipment to the general public made the underwater world accessible to growing numbers of people. The first civilian scientific diving course was taught at the Scripps Institution of Oceanography in 1951 by Conrad Limbaugh and Andreas Rechnitzer. This was the precursor curriculum to the Los Angeles County Parks and Recreation Scuba Program pioneered in 1954 by Al Tillman and Bev Morgan, the first recreational diving training association in the United States. In the last six decades, scuba diving has opened the underwater world to millions of divers and hundreds of millions of film and photography observers. Scuba is now used as a basic tool with myriad commercial, military, scientific, public safety, and recreational applications (Box 71-1).[10]

BOX 71-1   Types of Diving

Commercial Diving
  Harvest of Natural Resources
    Oil and natural gas
    Minerals (e.g., gold)
    Fish and shellfish
    Pearls, corals, and shells
    Algae
    Wood (e.g., underwater logging)
    Aquaculture
  Salvage and Recovery Operations
    Maintenance and Construction
      Ship hulls
      Nuclear power plants
      Bridges and tunnels
      Piers and jetties
      Aquariums
      Water treatment plants
      Sewers
      Dams
    Underwater Photography and Motion Picture Productions
  Scientific Diving
    Marine Studies
      Biology
      Geology
      Archeology
      Other sciences
    Polar Ice Diving
  Public Safety Diving
    Rescue Operations
  Recreational Diving
    Sport-Diving Instructors and Tour Guides

TYPES OF DIVING AND DIVING EQUIPMENT

There are several general types of diving, each using different equipment and having different logistical support needs. From the least to the most sophisticated equipment used, the types of diving are breath-hold diving, open-circuit scuba diving, RB diving (closed-circuit and semiclosed-circuit diving), and surface-supplied (tethered) diving. Mixed gas and technical diving, saturation diving, and one-atmosphere diving are also discussed later.

BREATH-HOLD DIVING

Breath-hold diving is the simplest and oldest form of underwater activity, dating back thousands of years. In breath-hold diving, no supplemental air source or underwater breathing device is used, so submergence is limited to the length of time the diver can hold the breath. There are several types of breath-hold diving, each characterized by activity and equipment.

Snorkeling is the most common form of breath-hold diving. Snorkelers typically use a face mask to facilitate underwater vision, fins for propulsion, a snorkel to breathe air while swimming facedown on the water's surface, attire for environmental protection (e.g., a neoprene wetsuit or full-body spandex [Lycra] suit), and sometimes lead weights to counterbalance the positive buoyancy of a wetsuit or one's innate positive buoyancy. Snorkelers remain mostly on the surface, breathing through the snorkel with face submerged, with little actual diving under the surface. Snorkeling is widely practiced at tropical resorts to introduce people to the beauty of coral reefs.

Freediving generally refers to one of several types of competitive breath-hold diving. Freediving is classified as an "extreme sport," and many consider it to be the original extreme sport. Competitive freediving dates back to at least the early 1900s, with

perhaps the best recorded account involving the Greek sponge diver Giorgios Haggi Statti. In 1913, he was offered a few dollars to dive more than 61 msw (200 fsw) underwater to retrieve the anchor of the Italian ship *Regina Margherita* that had become stuck in the Aegean Sea at a depth of 70 msw (230 fsw). He freed the anchor after three consecutive dives of between 1.5 and 3.5 minutes' duration, diving as deep as 80 msw (263 fsw). He did not consider this an especially taxing feat, saying that he had dived as deep as 110 msw (361 fsw) and stayed underwater for as long as 7 minutes on other occasions. Some consider Haggi Statti to be the "father of freediving." However, it was not until Jacques Mayol of France dived to 101 msw (331 fsw) in 1976, considered a stunning feat at the time, that freediving really began to grow in popularity as an extreme sport. In 1988, the film *The Big Blue* portrayed the lives of Jacques Mayol and Italian Enzo Maiorca as competitive freedivers and further popularized the sport. Extreme no limits freediver record holders, known as the world's deepest man and woman, are Herbert Nitsch (253.2 msw; 831.8 fsw) and Tanya Streeter (160 msw; 525 fsw).

Competitive freediving attracts athletes from around the world and is regularly featured on sports television channels. The sport is governed by the Association Internationale pour le Développement de l'Apnée (also known as the International Association for the Development of Apnea [AIDA; aida-international.org/]) or the International Association for the Development of Freediving. Since 1992, AIDA has been the officiating body for freediving, setting standards and recognizing records. AIDA recognizes eight types of freediving and breath holding; descriptions of these disciplines and the world records for each can be found in Table 71-1.

Medical Problems of Breath-Hold Diving

The major medical concern of breath-hold diving is development of hypoxia leading to loss of consciousness and drowning, especially if submergence is preceded by hyperventilation (see Hyperventilation and Shallow Water Blackout, later). Breath-hold divers also may become hypothermic, become entangled in underwater debris (e.g., fishing line, ropes, and cables) or vegetation, be harmed by marine animals, or be injured by boats or other watercraft. Divers are also subject to barotrauma of the ears, sinuses, and lungs, as described later. Although it is a very rare occurrence, breath-hold divers also can suffer from DCS (see Decompression Sickness, later).

SCUBA DIVING

Scuba diving uses a cylinder fitted with a single-hose, two-stage regulator that supplies compressed air to the diver at a pressure equal to ambient water pressure. Dive cylinders are available in a range of sizes and are predominantly made of aluminum or steel. Common volumes are 80 cubic feet of filtered, oil-free compressed air pressurized to approximately 3000 pounds per square inch gauge (psig; 250 bar). Compressed air in a full cylinder weighs approximately 6 pounds, which affects the buoyancy of the cylinder toward the end of the dive. High-pressure steel cylinders are pumped to 3500 psi and are heavier than their aluminum counterparts of similar volume.

The regulator reduces pressure in two stages. The first stage is attached to the cylinder and makes an initial reduction in pressure from high (3000 psi) to intermediate pressure (145 psi) delivered to the lower-pressure second stage attached to the diver's mouthpiece.

Like the snorkeler, the scuba diver wears a face mask covering the eyes and nose. Full-face masks cover the entire face to allow underwater vision and communication. Fins are donned for propulsion; a thermal protection suit, weight belt, and buoyancy compensator combine to adjust buoyancy underwater and for surface flotation in case of an emergency. Dive computers that track time and depth underwater have largely replaced wristwatches and depth gauges. A compass and dive light may be worn as auxiliary equipment, but a submersible pressure gauge is required to monitor air consumption. Because of the higher thermal conductivity of water, divers typically wear neoprene wetsuits to stay warm (as well as to provide protection from

TABLE 71-1 AIDA Competitive Freediving World Records (as of July 2016)

Discipline	Description	World Record: Male	World Record: Female
Pool			
Static apnea	Resting, immersed breath holding in controlled water (pool)	Stephane Mifsud 11 min 35 sec 06/2009	Natalia Molchanova 9 min 02 sec 06/2013
Dynamic apnea, without fins	Horizontal swim in controlled water	Mateusz Malina 226 m 11/2014	Natalia Molchanova 182 m 06/2013
Dynamic apnea, with fins	Horizontal swim in controlled water	Mateusz Malina 285 m 05/2016	Natalia Molchanova 237 m 09/2014
Ocean			
Constant weight, without fins	Vertical self-propelled swimming to a maximum depth and back to the surface without a line	William Trubridge 101 m 12/2010	Sayuri Kinoshita 72 m 04/2016
Constant weight, with fins	Vertical self-propelled swimming to a maximum depth and back to the surface without a line	Alexey Molchanov 128 m 09/2013	Natalia Molchanova 101 m 09/2011
Free immersion	Vertical excursion propelled by pulling on the line during descent and ascent; no fins	William Trubridge 121 m 04/2011	Natalia Molchanova 91 m 09/2013
Variable weight	Vertical descent to a maximum depth on weighted sled; ascent by pulling up the line with kicking	Stavros Kastrinakis 146 m 11/2015	Nanja Van Den Broek 130 m 10/2015
No limits	Vertical descent to a maximum depth on a weighted sled; ascent with a lift bag deployed by the diver	Herbert Nitsch 214 m 06/2007	Tanya Streeter 160 m 08/2002

AIDA, Association Internationale pour le Développement de l'Apnée.

sunburn, scrapes, and stinging marine life), even in relatively warm tropical oceans. These suits maintain a layer of water warmed by body heat between the skin and suit. The suits are typically 7 mm in thickness when diving in temperate water, and 2 to 3 mm (or Lycra) when diving in warm tropical water. An impermeable drysuit and undergarments are usually worn when diving in water colder than 10° C (50° F). Drygloves attached to the drysuit provide increased thermal protection for the hands, which is an important safety consideration in polar diving. Increasingly, electrically heated undergarments (e.g., BlueHeat by Diving Unlimited International) worn underneath drysuits are available to use as adjuncts to passive thermal protection. In addition to the preceding basic equipment, additional equipment (e.g., dive knife, camera, spear gun, and/or game bags) may be needed for safety, navigation, communication, or other purposes.

REBREATHER DIVING

Although the first self-contained underwater dive is thought to have been as a scuba dive, it was actually first done with the assistance of a RB in the 1880s. RB devices for diving were perfected over the years, but with the advent of scuba in the 1940s, RBs were relegated primarily to military operations. In the 1970s, scientific diving research using RBs was successfully performed from saturation habitats, such as by the nationally sponsored Scientist-in-the-Sea programs TEKTITE I and II.[65] Beginning in the 1990s, use of RBs started to increase in technical recreational diving (especially for underwater photography and cave diving).

RBs are used in recreational, technical, and military diving activities and have a place in the scientific diving community's underwater research toolbox. Current RBs mandate continuous attention and monitoring of equipment life-support functions that may detract from the purpose of diving missions. The amount of time invested in training, maintaining equipment before and after a dive, and keeping up the skill level requirements of advanced

RBs is generally not realistic for broad application within the recreational and scientific diving communities. Furthermore, the commercial industry rarely uses this technology. More recently, the diving industry has recognized that although there will always be a limited universe of technical RB divers, nontechnical RB divers are needed to meet the needs of the scientific diving community. RBs have in some cases been demonstrated to be a powerful tool for extended range and technical diving. There also exists an extraordinary potential to extend bottom times and diving activities in depths less than 30 msw (99 fsw), coupled with a reduced logistical footprint for remote site diving.

Rebreather Devices

A brown paper bag can be considered the simplest form of RB. Inhaling from, and exhaling into, a bag allows two things to occur, neither of which is physiologically advantageous: (1) Carbon dioxide accumulates, and (2) the air becomes hypoxic. A RB is an underwater life-support system that consists of one-way valves to ensure unidirectional gas flow, a counterlung, and the ability to remove carbon dioxide through a scrubber (soda lime) and replace it with oxygen. There is a finite absorbing capacity of scrubbers, requiring periodic replacement. Scrubbers are prone to installation and packing errors, although new models exist as prepacked canisters.

Some publications comprehensively discuss the types of RBs currently available for recreational, technical, commercial, scientific, and military diving; the history of RBs; the applicable physics, physiology, and theory of RB diving; operational predive, dive, and postdive procedures; and RB maintenance.[243,278]

Oxygen Rebreather. The oxygen RB supplies pure oxygen via a demand valve that feeds into the whole breathing loop. There is depth- and time-dependent potential for oxygen toxicity. Generally, a maximum partial pressure of oxygen (PO_2) of 1.6 ATA is not to be exceeded due to increased potential for oxygen toxicity to result in a seizure. The maximum operating depth for breathing 100% oxygen would be 6 msw (19 fsw) for a single exposure of 45 minutes (per NOAA limits).

Semiclosed-Circuit Rebreather. A semiclosed-circuit RB uses a nitrox mix supplied via a constant mass flow regulator and demand valve. A quantity of gas is periodically bled into the water column. The PO_2 can be variable and uncertain, and can change with the workload and depth.

Manual Closed-Circuit Rebreather. The manual closed-circuit RB consists of a source of diluent gas and oxygen supplied via a constant mass flow regulator; it can be adjusted manually as well. Triple-redundant oxygen sensors with a PO_2 display warrant careful attention because the cells are prone to failure. No gas escapes into the water column. Normal operation of this relatively simple life-support system relies on diligence of the diver.

Electronic Closed-Circuit Rebreather. The electronic closed-circuit RB system consists of a source of diluent gas, oxygen source, and battery-powered microprocessor. Triple-redundant oxygen sensors monitor PO_2 in the loop. From these data the microprocessor sends information to a solenoid valve, triggering when to open to add more oxygen into the system. Normal operation requires little diver input, but this is a complicated, electronically managed system that can foster complacency and has many failure points.

Open-Circuit Scuba System versus Rebreather Approach

Several helpful presentations comparing open-circuit scuba systems with RBs were made at the Rebreather Forum 3 in Orlando, Florida, on May 18 to 20, 2012; Lang and Steller have summarized the presentations discussed here in their report on the AAUS Rebreather Colloquium in Monterey, California, in September of that year.[175a] Simon Mitchell of the University of Auckland discussed a 90-msw/20-minute dive.[198a]

Open-Circuit Air Approach. The narcotic effect of nitrogen would incapacitate the diver at this depth of 10 ATA, so that work could not be accomplished with compressed air. The inspired PO_2 at depth would be 2.1 ATA (1.3 ATA is the generally accepted advisable maximum for technical diving) with the concomitant risk of oxygen toxicity. The gas density would be quite high at 13 g/L (8 g/L is often considered the advisable maximum), rendering the work of breathing very high. Further, decompression on air is known to be very inefficient. For the bottom depth of this profile, one would ideally use a helium-based mix (trimix 13:47, where 13% O_2 gives a PO_2 of 1.3 ATA, 40% N_2 gives an equivalent narcosis level as an air dive to 40 m, and the 47% balance will be He). Decompression would ideally consist of EAN_{36} (36% O_2 and the balance N_2) from 27 m, and 100% O_2 from 6 m. The total run time for this open-circuit dive would be 131 minutes and 18 seconds. Gas volumes required for such a dive are calculated by multiplying the ambient pressure by the time by the surface air consumption rate for each of the depth levels, and then adding the totals and including a 1.3 safety factor. For a 90-m/20-minute profile with the decompression as described, a dive would require 7852 L of trimix (expensive He), 1365 L of EAN_{36}, and 991 L of O_2. The big problem with the open-circuit scuba system for this dive profile is that it takes longer to decompress because the optimal PO_2 (1.3 ATA) is not breathed at each stage of decompression on ascent.[175a]

Rebreather Approach. Using a RB eliminates the need to carry multiple bottles for various stages of the dive profile. No bubbles are emitted from the unit, warm humidified gas is breathed, there is minimal gas consumption (which is important on deeper dives), the optimal mix is always available during descent and ascent of a dive, and the RB allows for constantly optimal PO_2 diving. The logistical aspects of a 90-msw/20-minute RB dive are more complex than those for an open-circuit dive. Besides the dive platform and topside support, bailout gas requirements must be planned as they would be for open-circuit diving. Checklists are imperative; they outline a step-by-step procedure for preparing a RB before a dive to ensure the unit will perform for the planned dive. Going through the checklists demands no rushing, no shortcuts, and no distractions, and there must be methodical, meticulous attention to detail. The carbon dioxide scrubber needs to be packed and installed, and the following items checked: one-way valves, general assembly of the unit, positive and negative pressure, diluent and oxygen pressures, and sensor calibrations.

When discussing the procedures for the four phases of an RB dive, Simon Mitchell also observed that the diver must perform the final RB check and ensure that the cylinders are open; the set point for oxygen is appropriate for the surface and the descent; the mouthpiece is closed when it is out of the mouth; a leak check is done; and a minimal loop volume is maintained (poor buoyancy is exhibited with a high loop volume); if the loop is open, it can be flooded and buoyancy lost. On descent, one must ensure that the ears are cleared, buoyancy adjustments are made, situational awareness is maintained, PO_2 and diluent are checked to maintain the loop volume, and the set point is changed at some time during the dive. Once on the bottom, one must ensure that the bailout is checked and working, set point is changed to a bottom mix, and PO_2 is checked. On ascent, one must ensure that PO_2 is frequently checked, given that the diver's life depends on it; minimal loop volume is maintained; buoyancy is monitored; situational awareness is maintained; oxygen is manually added as needed; and the mouthpiece is shut off before removing the unit at the surface.[175a]

Andrew Fock of the Alfred Hospital Hyperbaric Service in Melbourne presented the results of his survey on RB fatalities at the forum.[113a] Data were taken from the Internet, and in some cases, the information was incomplete and/or unconfirmed. Actual numbers of fatalities and accidents are unknown because of lack of reporting, and there is also uncertainty about numbers of RB divers worldwide, RB dives logged per year, and numbers of RB units currently being used. Data therefore are estimates taken from the Rebreather World website, a Dutch RB survey, a Diver Mole survey, and a British Slovakia Club survey. For the time frame of 1998 to 2010, the following observations were provided:

1. The increased potential for RB diving accidents includes high-risk behavior and RB unit cleaning and assembling procedures.
2. Approximately 20 RB deaths per year were reported worldwide from 2005 to 2010, with the top three causes identified as hypoxia, carbon dioxide intoxication, and oxygen-induced seizure.
3. Consideration of the relative safety of manual and electronic RB units acknowledges that manual units have no electronic failure potential because they are human operated. However, divers are required to know the PO_2 at all times. Electronic units monitor PO_2 without distraction, which allows divers to become complacent and not worry about PO_2. It is an accepted fact that both systems have the potential to fail.
4. The number of deaths involving manual and electronic units appear to be proportional to the current market share of each type of unit. No one brand of RB is more dangerous than another.
5. Proper training and understanding of physics and physiology will make RB diving safer. It is clear that progress is being made toward a simpler, more robust RB.[175a]

William Stone of Stone Aerospace in Austin, Texas, shared his views of three truths about RBs[266a]:

1. Sensors are the "eyeballs" of any autonomous system; if you cannot see what is going on, you are headed for trouble. This translates to RB reliability and user safety. Being aware of the PO_2 and autocalibration are essential.
2. Redundancy paths must exist for all critical systems. There must be a clear and simple abort mechanism to a safe haven with no accumulation of a need for decompression.
3. The industry should mine data and learn more about the RB to better assess the nature of the triggers.[175a]

Finally, Thalmann remarked, "A scuba regulator is the steam engine of diving gear. It has been around for a long time. It has been honed to a fine art and is incredibly reliable. By comparison, a rebreather is like a space shuttle."[269a] RBs are a form of reemerging technology for the scientific, recreational, and technical diving communities, first used extensively for underwater research in TEKTITE II.[65] Notwithstanding this early RB use, the vast majority of the experience of the scientific and recreational diving communities is with no-decompression, open-circuit scuba systems.[193a]

Disappointment about the failure to replace standard open-circuit scuba systems with RBs since 1970 has been expressed by many. RBs appear to be more expensive, but one must ask whether they truly are, because with them, one can accomplish twice the work in a given unit of time and carry out investigations or missions that take more bottom time than one has with open-circuit scuba systems.

Mechanical failure is more likely with RBs than with open-circuit scuba systems, but the risk is mitigated because RBs have an extra underwater breathing apparatus. RB diving is more dangerous by an order of magnitude than is open-circuit diving. RBs have facilitated many fabulous dives for research and discovery; however, RBs are very complex and being used by fallible humans in a hostile nonrespiratory environment that has the potential to create many problems. Most mishaps are preventable; this fact emphasizes the importance of following proper procedures, including those for assembly and maintenance of equipment, and using checklists.[175a]

SURFACE-SUPPLIED (TETHERED) DIVING

Surface-supplied (tethered) diving uses several different technologic systems; in all of them, the diver breathes gas (compressed air or mixed gas) supplied by a hose from a surface source or a diving bell at a pressure equal to the ambient water pressure.

The best-known form of surface-supplied diving is classic hardhat diving, which is sometimes called mud diving or blackwater diving because it is often done in harbors with a muddy bottom and in dirty water with almost no visibility. In this type of diving, which was portrayed in the 2000 movie *Men of Honor,* the diver wears a large bronze helmet with glass faceplates, canvas suit, weight belt and weighted shoes, and other gear. Altogether, the traditional hardhat diver's gear weighs 87 kg (192 lb). Although traditional hardhat gear is still used in a variety of settings, most surface-supplied divers use modern gear that is not as heavy or cumbersome as traditional gear has communication capabilities, and can keep the diver warm.

Surface-supplied diving is most often used in commercial or military settings and can be combined with hot-water suits. It is frequently performed in arduous circumstances. The diver often operates in total darkness in cold water or in clear offshore waters where oil platforms are located. Working against a current or surge and performing tasks primarily by feel are commonplace.

The diving techniques of surface-supplied diving are quite different from those of scuba diving, and are not further discussed here; however, most of the physiologic and medical problems of surface-supplied divers are identical to those encountered in scuba diving.

MIXED-GAS DIVING

Diving can be done using either compressed air or mixed gas. Compressed air is most commonly used, especially with scuba systems, but there are a number of settings where mixed gas is needed or preferred.

In mixed-gas diving, a breathing mixture other than compressed air (e.g., a mixture in which the concentrations of nitrogen and oxygen have been changed or in which a different inert gas such as helium is substituted for nitrogen) is used. Mixed-gas diving can be used in surface-supplied, saturation, RB, or scuba diving modes, although historically it has been used most often in surface-supplied or saturation diving operations.

Mixed-gas diving has been used for many decades, but because of the greater logistical support required and associated greater expense and hazards, it has been used primarily in commercial, scientific, and military diving operations. This has changed in the past 15 years as technical divers have sought to go deeper and stay down longer. Increasing numbers of recreational divers now use mixed gas, especially nitrox.

Enriched Air Nitrox

Nitrox is a breathing gas mixture containing oxygen and nitrogen in concentrations different from those found in air. Nitrox was popularized when Dick Rutkowski began in 1985 to transfer this methodology from the scientific diving community to the recreational diving world after his retirement from the NOAA Diving Program. Nitrox use was the initial core training curriculum of the International Association of Nitrox and Technical Divers. More than a dozen different such mixtures have been used by recreational and scientific divers, all of which are lumped under the term *nitrox,* but the two most commonly used are the ones labeled by NOAA as nitrox I (containing 32% oxygen and 68% nitrogen, denoted as EAN_{32}) and nitrox II (containing 36% oxygen and 64% nitrogen, denoted as EAN_{36}). Each nitrox mixture, or blend, requires its own decompression parameters, bottom time limits, and maximum operating depth. Most modern-day dive computers are easily programmable in their settings for the oxygen content of a nitrox mix. Nitrox tables are used as infrequently as are air tables; most scuba training agencies have abandoned their teaching and use in favor of dive computers.

Of note, the term *nitrox* historically was used to refer to gas mixtures having less than 21% oxygen. These mixtures were used in diving habitats or other saturation diving situations in which the diver wanted to avoid, or at least lessen, the risk for oxygen toxicity. Technically, if the oxygen percentage is adjusted to greater than 21%, the mixture is called *enriched air nitrox* (EAN) or *oxygen-enriched air* (OEA), although *EAN* and *nitrox* are used interchangeably in the common parlance of divers.[133]

Beginning in the 1980s, an increasing number of recreational divers began using EAN to extend bottom time (compared with what was possible using compressed air) and reduce the risk for DCS. Many thousands of recreational EAN divers have been certified in recent years, and EAN has become the norm on many live-aboard charter dive boats.

EAN diving enthusiasts typically claim that nitrox is safer than compressed air because it carries less risk for DCS for equivalent bottom times. At relatively shallow depths, EAN diving allows considerably increased bottom times before decompression is required, when compared with compressed air diving. For instance, at 18 msw (60 fsw), EAN diving allows an extra 45 minutes (60 minutes with air, 105 minutes with EAN). However, this advantage diminishes greatly at depths beyond 30 msw (100 fsw). At 30 msw (100 fsw), EAN diving provides for only 8 extra minutes.[171]

Although diving with nitrox may lessen the risk for DCS compared with diving with compressed air, it definitely does not eliminate all risk, and EAN has risks of its own. The main concern is with central nervous system (CNS) oxygen toxicity, which usually manifests suddenly (with few, if any, prodromal symptoms) by loss of consciousness and seizures. Because of the risk for CNS oxygen toxicity at a maximum PO_2 of 1.6 ATA, EAN_{32} must not be used below 40 msw (130 fsw) and EAN_{36} is limited to a maximum operating depth of 34 msw (110 fsw).

A diver can still suffer DCS diving with EAN if he or she stays down too long, surfaces too fast, bypasses a required decompression stop, or uses the wrong nitrox decompression table or dive computer oxygen setting for the particular breathing medium. Furthermore, although nitrox may increase a diver's allowable no-decompression bottom time, this is often irrelevant because a bottom time is as much a function of gas supply as it is of the decompression limit (i.e., most scuba divers will exhaust their gas supply before reaching the no-decompression limit).

Nitrox use for recreational diving purposes is now a mainstream practice and readily available at the majority of live-aboard and dive store operations.[171] EAN has advantages and disadvantages (Box 71-2), with the advantages most likely realized in a setting that ensures adherence to safety.

Heliox

Other than nitrox, the most commonly used mixed gas is heliox, or oxy-helium, a mixture of helium and oxygen. Helium is used as the inert gas, replacing nitrogen (and thus eliminating the risk for nitrogen narcosis). With heliox, the oxygen level is reduced to prevent oxygen toxicity. Like nitrox, heliox is a generic term that applies to a number of different blends or mixtures of helium and oxygen.

BOX 71-2   Advantages and Disadvantages of Enriched Oxygen Nitrox Diving Compared with Compressed Air at Depths Between 15 and 40 msw (50 and 130 fsw)

Advantages

Decreased risk for decompression sickness
Decreased occurrence of nitrogen narcosis
Reduced residual nitrogen time
Shorter surface interval times
Reduced decompression times if maximum bottom time limits are
  exceeded
Reduced surface intervals between diving and flying

Disadvantages

Requires special training
Requires equipment dedicated for use with nitrox only
Increased oxidation of scuba cylinders
Possible increased rate of deterioration of equipment
Increased fire hazards
Potential for nitrox mixing and filling problems
Risk for central nervous system oxygen toxicity

Because it causes negligible, if any, narcosis and is easier to breathe at greater depths (because of reduced density), heliox is the preferred gas for commercial diving at depths beyond 40 msw (130 fsw). The major problems with helium are its expense (which precludes its widespread use in recreational or scientific diving), greater thermal conductivity, and hindrance of speech. In commercial and military settings, helium speech unscramblers are typically used. However, at depths beyond 183 msw (600 fsw), and especially with rapid descent, helium causes a poorly understood condition known as *high-pressure nervous syndrome* (HPNS). HPNS is characterized by dizziness, nausea, vomiting, postural and intention tremors, fatigue, somnolence, myoclonic jerking, stomach cramps, numbness, and sleep disturbances.[17] HPNS is a major barrier to prolonged manned undersea activity at depths beyond 183 msw (600 fsw).

Trimix

Trimix is a generic term referring to mixtures of helium, nitrogen, and oxygen. This breathing medium was pioneered by military and commercial diving interests for operations at depths greater than those possible by diving with compressed air. Helium replaces some of both the nitrogen and oxygen in an effort to eliminate or minimize nitrogen narcosis and to prevent CNS oxygen toxicity. The precise concentrations of helium, nitrogen, and oxygen used in trimix vary according to the specific depth profile of the dive. Obviously, in deep-diving operations, the percentages of both nitrogen and oxygen will be much less than those present in air, which means that a "travel" gas mixture is needed for breathing in shallower depths that must be traversed to get to the depth at which the trimix will be used. Currently, the U.S. Navy specifies the use of trimix for diving at depths greater than 58 msw (190 fsw), and trimix is typically used in extreme-depth (> 183 msw [600 fsw]) commercial diving because the addition of small amounts of nitrogen partially mitigates the occurrence of HPNS.

A spin-off of trimix that has begun to be used in recreational diving is an oxygen-enriched trimix, or *helitrox*. A trimix blend commonly used in this setting is 26% oxygen, 17% helium, and 57% nitrogen (trimix 26/17). Helitrox advocates promote its use for diving to depths of up to 46 msw (150 fsw), either using helitrox to decompress or switching to pure oxygen at the 6-msw (20-fsw) decompression stop.

A new world record for open-circuit scuba diving using trimix was set by the South African Nuno Gomes in June 2005 when he dived to 318.25 msw (1044 fsw) in the Red Sea. It took 20 minutes to descend to depth, incurring more than 12 hours of decompression on ascent. A total of nine different gas mixes were used for the dive (4 trimix, 3 nitrox, 1 air, and 1 oxygen). Also in June 2005, Pascal Bernabé of France dived to 330 msw (1100 fsw) off Propriano, Corsica, using an open-circuit scuba system (an event unwitnessed by Guinness). His descent time

was only 10 minutes, requiring decompression of 9 hours. On 19 September 2014, Ahmed Gabr, a 41-year-old Egyptian special forces officer and technical diving instructor, recorded a Guinness World Record open-circuit scuba dive of 332.35 msw (1,090 fsw) off Dahab, Egypt. His descent time took 12 minutes to maximum depth, incurring nearly 13 hours and 35 minutes of decompression on ascent.

A high incidence of fatalities among divers using trimix has limited its use in recreational diving, but interest in its use remains high, and the recent emergence of trimix dive computers for RBs portends a much greater future use of trimix.

TECHNICAL DIVING

Beginning in the late 1980s, a small but rapidly growing number of recreational divers began to use mixed-gas systems, RBs, and other technical systems previously used only by military and commercial divers to dive deeper and stay down longer than was possible with conventional scuba systems. Technical diving (a term coined in 1990) is employed by wreck, cave, and deep decompression divers.

Technical diving represents the leading edge of underwater discovery and challenge. Its technology and techniques are at the forefront of diving developments. This type of diving is inherently more hazardous than typical recreational diving because diving deep is more hazardous, has a smaller margin for error, and relies on technology more extensively. Mitigation of these hazards has improved through training of divers and advances in equipment design.

Despite its hazards, technical diving has markedly increased in global popularity, as witnessed by establishment of the International Association of Nitrox and Technical Divers, Technical Diving International, and other technical diving associations. Technical diving conferences drawing thousands of divers have proliferated in the United States, Europe, and Asia, as have manufacturers of equipment that cater specifically to needs of the technical diving community.

SATURATION DIVING

The physiology and pathophysiology of saturation diving have been thoroughly reviewed.[38] Under pressure, the diver begins to absorb increased amounts of nitrogen or other inert gas, depending on the breathing medium, until a new equilibrium is established according to the pressure of the depth of submergence. In most deep-diving scenarios, the time needed to "off-gas," or *decompress,* inert gas upon returning to normal atmospheric pressure may be much greater than the time spent at depth. The need to minimize prolonged decompression after deep diving led to development of saturation diving. In the late 1950s, experiments by Navy diving medical officers George Bond and Robert Workman coincided with those of Jacques-Yves Cousteau and Edwin Link in the commercial sector, all of whom were working on ways to stay underwater at great depths long enough to perform useful work.[5]

The basic concept of saturation diving is that after approximately 24 hours at any given depth, the diver's tissues establish equilibrium with the gases in the breathing mixture. From that point forward, if the diver can be kept at pressure for a prolonged period, the decompression obligation remains essentially the same no matter how long the diver remains at that depth. Modern saturation complexes allow divers to live for days in large chambers at the pressure of a given work site and to be transported to the underwater site by locking into a personnel transfer capsule or sealed diving bell. When the desired depth is reached, the water pressure equals the gas pressure within the capsule and divers may exit the personnel transfer capsule into the water while breathing gas is supplied by umbilical hoses. To maintain the diver's thermal balance in the cold water found at great depths, heated water through an umbilical is circulated in a hot-water suit.

Medical considerations include the prolonged time the diver spends in isolation in a saturation chamber, exposure to potentially toxic gases and bacteria, and bubble formation during decompression. Hyperoxia may lead to production of reactive oxygen species that interact with cell structures, causing damage to proteins, lipids, and nucleic acid. Hyperoxia and vascular gas bubble formation may lead to endothelial dysfunction.[38] Saturation diving in commercial and military applications has proven to be a safe and controlled method for working underwater, obviating the need for multiple decompressions and ascents as utilized with surface diving. To date, no long-term impact on health attributable to saturation diving has been documented.

Another application of saturation diving, used primarily for scientific purposes, uses underwater habitats. These are steel chambers situated at a given depth of water and pressurized with a compressed-gas atmosphere at the same pressure as the surrounding water. Divers may live for days or weeks in the habitat, leaving the chamber with scuba equipment (excursions) to perform studies or observe marine life in its natural state. In this specialized type of diving, rigorous precautions are taken to avoid inadvertent surfacing, thermal stress, and skin and ear infections during prolonged stays in the continuously moist environment of the habitat. Prolonged saturation decompression schedules, often taking several days, are required to return divers safely to sea level pressure upon completion of the underwater mission.

POLAR DIVING

Approximately four decades ago, scientists were first able to enter the undersea polar environment to make biologic observations for a nominal period of time. The conduct of underwater research in extreme environments, such as under ice, requires special consideration of diving physiology, equipment design, diver training, and operational procedures. Since the days when the first ice dives were made in wetsuits and double-hose regulators without buoyancy compensators or submersible pressure gauges, novel ice-diving techniques have expanded the working envelope based on the scientific need to include the use of dive computers, oxygen-enriched air, RB units, blue-water diving, and drysuit systems. The 2007 International Polar Diving Workshop in Svalbard, Norway, drew together polar diving scientists, equipment manufacturers, physiologists, decompression experts, and diving safety officers, who coordinated their expertise to form recommendations for diving in extreme conditions.[175] The polar diving environment has unique hazards associated with marine life, types of emergencies that may develop, and physiologic considerations, as discussed below.

Marine Life Hazards

Few polar animal species are considered dangerous to the diver. Southern elephant seals (Mirounga leonina) and Antarctic fur seals (Arctocephalus gazella) may become aggressive during the late spring/early summer breeding season. Crabeater seals (Lobodon carcinophagus) have demonstrated curiosity about divers and aggression toward humans on the surface. Leopard seals (Hydrurga leptonyx) have been known to attack humans on the surface and have threatened divers in the water. There is a single known in-water fatality caused by a leopard seal.[211] Should an aggressive seal approach a diver in the water, the diver's response is similar to that for a shark. Polar bears (Ursus maritimus) and walruses (Odobenus rosmarus) in the Arctic are considered predatory mammals against which diving personnel must be safeguarded. Encounters with all of the aforementioned mammals are usually restricted to areas of open water, ice edges, or pack ice. Divers in the fast ice around McMurdo Station, Antarctica, may encounter Weddell seals (Leptonychotes weddellii) in the water. Occasionally, a Weddell seal returning from a dive may surface to breathe in a dive hole to replenish its oxygen stores after a hypoxic diving exposure.[167] Usually, the seal will vacate the hole after it has taken a few breaths, particularly if divers are approaching from below and preparing to surface. Divers must approach such a seal with caution because an oxygen-starved seal may aggressively protect its air supply. Weddell seals protecting their surface access will often assume a head-down, tail-up posture to watch for rivals. Divers entering or exiting the water are particularly vulnerable to aggressive male

Weddell seals, which tend to bite each other in the flipper and genital regions. There are no recorded incidents of killer whale (Orcinus orca) attacks on divers.

Polar Diving Emergencies

The best method for mitigating scuba diving emergencies is prevention. Divers must halt operations any time they become unduly stressed because of cold, fatigue, nervousness, or other physiologic reasons. Diving is also terminated if there are equipment difficulties, such as free-flowing regulators, tether-system entanglements, leaking drysuits, or buoyancy problems. Emergency situations and accidents rarely have a single major cause; more often, they result from accumulation of several minor problems. Maintaining the ability to not panic and to think clearly is the best preparation for the unexpected.

Most emergencies can be mitigated by assistance from a dive buddy; contact between two comparably equipped divers in the water is, therefore, important. Loss of contact with the dive hole may require a diver to retrace his or her path. Scanning the water column for the downline is done slowly and deliberately because the strobe light flash rate may be reduced in cold water. If the hole cannot be found, an alternate access to the surface may need to be located. There will often be open cracks at the point where fast ice touches a shoreline. Lost divers need to constantly balance a desirable lower air consumption rate in shallow water with the need for the wider field of vision available from deeper water. Maintaining safe proximity to the surface access point has made losing the dive hole an unlikely occurrence. Loss of the tether on a fast-ice dive that requires its use is one of the most serious polar diving emergencies. Lost diver search procedures are initiated immediately (i.e., assumption of a vertical position under the ice where the tethered buddy will swim a circular search pattern just under the ceiling to catch the untethered diver). The danger associated with loss of a tether in low visibility is mitigated if the divers have previously deployed a series of benthic lines. If a diver becomes disconnected from the tether downcurrent under fast ice, it may be necessary to crawl along the bottom to the downline. To clearly mark the access hole, divers deploy a well-marked downline; establish recognizable "landmarks" (such as specific ice formations) under the hole at the outset of the dive; leave a strobe light, flag, or other highly visible object on the substrate just below the hole; or shovel surface snow off the ice in a radiating spoke pattern that points the way to the dive hole.

The under-ice platelet layer can be several meters thick and become a safety concern if positively buoyant divers are trapped within this layer, become disoriented, and experience difficulty extricating themselves. The most obvious solution is to exhaust air from the drysuit to achieve negative buoyancy. If this is not possible and the platelet layer is not too thick, the diver may stand upside-down on the hard undersurface of the ice so that the head is out of the platelet ice to orient to the position of the dive hole and buddy. Another concern is that abundant platelet ice dislodged by divers will float up and plug a dive hole.

Fire is one of the greatest hazards for any operation in polar environments. Low humidity ultimately renders any wooden structure susceptible to combustion, and once a fire has started, it spreads quickly. Dive teams must exercise utmost care when using heat or open flame in a dive hut. If divers recognize during the dive that the dive hut is burning, they must terminate the dive and ascend to a safety hole or to the undersurface of the ice next to the hole (but not below it) in order to conserve air.

Physiologic Considerations in Polar Diving

Cold Water. A cold ambient temperature is the overriding limiting factor on dive operations, especially for the thermal protection and dexterity of hands. Dives are terminated before the hands become too cold to effectively operate gear or grasp a downline. Loss of dexterity can occur quickly (in 5 to 10 minutes if hands are inadequately protected). Grasping a camera, net, or other apparatus increases the rate at which a hand becomes cold. Switching the object from hand to hand or attaching it to the downline may allow the hands to rewarm. Dryglove systems and, more recently, electrically heated gloves and socks have greatly improved thermal protection of the hands and feet. The cold environment can also cause chilling of the diver, resulting in reduced cognitive ability with progressive cooling. To avoid life-threatening hypothermia, it is important to monitor progression of the following symptoms: cold hands or feet, shivering, increased air consumption, fatigue, confusion, inability to think clearly or perform simple tasks, memory loss, reduced strength, shivering cessation while still cold, and finally, hypothermia. Heat loss occurs because of inadequate insulation, exposure of areas such as the head when a hood is inadequate, and breathing cold air. Scuba cylinder air is initially at ambient temperature and chills from expansion as it passes through the regulator. Air consumption increases as the diver cools, resulting in additional cooling with increased ventilation. Significant chilling also occurs during safety stops while the diver is not moving.

Polar diving requires greater thermal insulation, which results in decreased general mobility and increased potential for buoyancy problems. Fatigue results from increased drag, increased swimming effort, and the need to don and doff equipment.

Surface Cold Exposure. Dive teams are aware that the weather can change quickly in polar environments. While they are in the field, all divers and tenders have in their possession sufficient cold-weather clothing for protection under any circumstance. Possible circumstances include loss of vehicle power or loss of a fish hut caused by fire. Boat motor failure may strand dive teams away from the base station. Supervisors and tenders on dives conducted outdoors must also be prepared for the cooling effects of inactivity while waiting for divers to surface. In addition, food and water are part of every dive team's basic equipment. Besides serving as emergency rations, water is important for diver rehydration after the dive.

Hydration. In addition to the dehydrating effect of breathing filtered, dry, compressed air on a dive, the low humidity of the Antarctic and Arctic regions can lead rapidly and insidiously to dehydration. Continuous effort is advised to stay hydrated and maintain proper fluid balance. Urine should be copious and light colored, and diuretics (e.g., coffee, tea, and alcohol) should be avoided before a dive.

Decompression. Mueller[210] reviewed the effect of cold on decompression stress. The relative contributions of tissue nitrogen solubility and tissue perfusion to the cause of DCS are not completely resolved. Overwarming of divers, especially active warming of cold divers following a dive, may induce DCS. Therefore, divers in polar environments should avoid becoming cold during decompression and/or after the dive, and if they feel hypothermic, should wait before taking a hot shower until they have rewarmed themselves, for example, by walking. The effect of cold on bubble grades (as measured by Doppler scores) may be the same for a diver who is only slightly cold as for one who is severely hypothermic. Long-term health effects for divers with a high proportion of cold water dives is amenable to investigation.

A 2007 research report from the Navy Experimental Diving Unit entitled "The influence of thermal exposure on diver susceptibility to decompression sickness"[125] is misinterpreted by some divers to think they should be cold during the dive if they want to reduce decompression risk. This misinterpretation of the results of an exemplary study may be causing divers to unnecessarily endure uncomfortable diving conditions. There is no substitute for comfort and safety on a dive. Gerth and associates[125] questioned the conventional wisdom that cold at depth increases the risk of DCS. After conducting a carefully designed experiment, they were surprised to find that exactly the opposite was true. Some degree of cooling was beneficial, as long as the diver was warm during ascent. The temperature regimes used for their experiment were hardly reflective of operational diving conditions, and therefore extrapolation of the results is questionable in practice.

Dive computers were examined for use by scientific and recreational divers[174] and have now been effectively used in diving programs for more than three decades in lieu of U.S. Navy or other dive tables. Battery changes may be needed more frequently because of higher discharge rates in extreme cold. Advantages of dive computers over tables include their display

of ascent rates, no-decompression time remaining at depth, and dive profile downloading function. Future dive computer functions should provide for additional safety and functional features.[172] Safety stops of 3 to 5 minutes between the depths of 3.3 to 10 msw (10 to 30 fsw) are required for all dives.[173]

ONE-ATMOSPHERE DIVING

Clearly, humans cannot reliably or safely function at the greatly elevated pressure of deep water, and the human factor aspects of diving have become the limiting factors in manned exploration of the ocean depths. This has led to numerous developments in one-atmosphere diving systems. In the 15th century, Leonardo da Vinci drafted schematic drawings of systems that look similar to modern one-atmosphere diving systems, but these systems had to await late 20th-century advances in metallurgy, engineering, and communications before they could become functional.

One-atmosphere absolute (ATA) diving systems are, in essence, small submarines with various types of propulsion systems and manipulators that allow the operator to work at great depth. The interior of the unit is maintained with environmental control systems to retain safe physiologic parameters. These systems range from one-person ATA suits (e.g., Exosuit by Nuytco research; nuytco.com), in which a diver can walk or "fly" through the water (Figure 71-1), to submersibles that accommodate two or more occupants (e.g., Curasub by Nuytco Research).

DIVING PHYSICS

Divers encounter many challenging environmental conditions underwater. These include cold, changes in light transmission and sound conduction, lack of air to breathe, increased density of the surrounding environment, and increased atmospheric pressure. Not surprisingly, diverse medical problems are related to diving (Box 71-3).

Of the various environmental factors affecting divers, pressure is by far the most important because it contributes either directly or indirectly to the majority of serious diving-related medical problems. Therefore, knowing the basic physics and physiologic

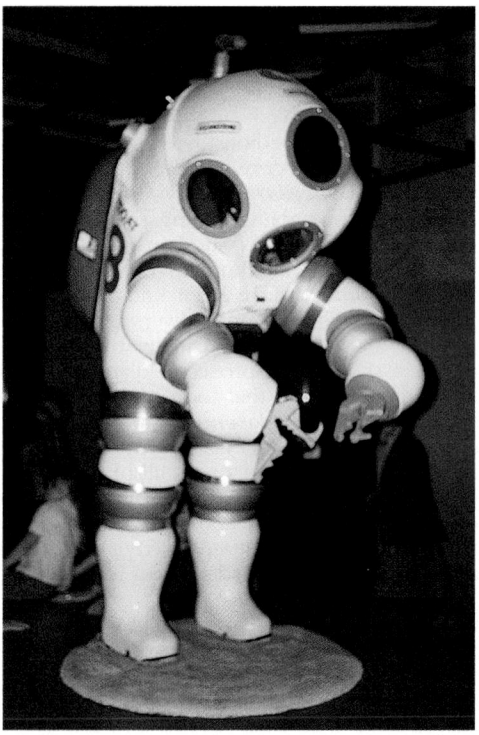

FIGURE 71-1 JIM diving suit. The diver remains at sea level pressure inside the suit and can work for prolonged periods of time at extreme depths underwater. (*Courtesy Kenneth W. Kizer, MD.*)

BOX 71-3 Medical Problems of Divers

Problems Related to Environmental Exposure

Motion sickness
Near drowning
Hypothermia
Heat illness
Sunburn
Phototoxic and photoallergic reactions
Irritant and other dermatitis
Infectious diseases
Mechanical trauma

Disorders Related to Diving

Barotrauma
Arterial gas embolism
Decompression sickness
Dysbaric osteonecrosis
Dysbaric retinopathy
Immersion pulmonary edema
Shallow water blackout

Problems Related to Breathing Gas

Inert gas narcosis
Hypoxia
Oxygen toxicity
Hypercapnia
Carbon monoxide poisoning
Lipoid pneumonitis

Problems Related to Hazardous Marine Life

Miscellaneous Problems

Hyperventilation
Hearing loss
Carotid-related blackout
Panic and other psychological problems

effects of pressure is essential to understanding and treating pressure-related disorders.

Diving-related disorders most often develop acutely because of problems caused by the mechanical effects of pressure on closed air spaces (barotrauma) or problems, such as nitrogen narcosis or DCS, caused by breathing gases at elevated partial pressure. Less often, clinical effects are delayed for months or years, as in the case of dysbaric osteonecrosis, the pathophysiology of which is not well understood.[254]

Pressure is defined as the force per unit of area. *Atmospheric pressure* is the pressure exerted by the air above the earth's surface and varies with altitude. At sea level, atmospheric pressure is 760 mm of mercury (mm Hg), or 14.7 lb per square inch (psi). *Barometric pressure* at sea level is generally referred to as 1 atmosphere (atm). *Absolute pressure* is the total barometric pressure at any point. With pressure gauges calibrated to read zero at sea level, gauge pressure is the amount of pressure greater than atmospheric pressure. In general, gauge pressure is 1 atm less than absolute atmospheric pressure. It is necessary to specify whether pressure is expressed in terms of *gauge* (psig) or *absolute pressure* (psia). Except in situations requiring laboratory precision, the following units are commonly used to express water pressure:

Feet of seawater (fsw)
Feet of fresh water (ffw)
Meters of seawater (msw)
Meters of fresh water (mfw)
Atmospheres absolute (ATA)
Pounds per square inch gauge (psig)
Pounds per square inch absolute (psia)

As a diver descends underwater, absolute pressure increases much faster than in air. Each foot (0.3048 m) of seawater exerts a force of 0.445 psig. Therefore, if the 14.7 psi pressure of 1 atm is divided by 0.445 psi per foot of seawater, the absolute pressure will have doubled at 33 fsw. In the ocean, each 33 feet of depth adds one additional atmosphere of pressure. The gauge pressure at 33 fsw is 14.7 psig (in excess of atmospheric pressure), and the absolute pressure is 29.4 psia. Because of the weight of

solutes in seawater, seawater is slightly heavier (64 lb/ft³) than is fresh water (62.4 lb/ft³). In fresh water, 10.4 msw (34 fsw) equals one additional atmosphere of pressure.

The pressure change with increasing depth is linear, although the greatest relative change in pressure per unit of depth change occurs nearest the surface, where it doubles in the first 33 fsw. Table 71-2 lists commonly used units of pressure measurement in seawater.

When a diver submerges, the force of the tremendous weight of the water above is exerted over the entire body. Except for spaces that contain air, such as the lungs, sinuses, intestines, and middle ears, the body behaves as a liquid. The law that describes the behavior of pressure in liquids is named for the 17th-century scientist Blaise Pascal. Pascal's law states that pressure applied to any part of a fluid is transmitted equally throughout the fluid. Thus, when a diver reaches 10 msw (33 fsw), pressure on the surface of the skin and throughout the body tissues is 29.4 psia or 1520 mm Hg (Figure 71-2). The diver's body is generally unaware of this pressure, except in spaces of the body that contain air. The gases in these spaces obey Boyle's law (Figure 71-3), which states that the pressure of a given quantity of gas at constant temperature varies inversely with its volume. Thus, air in the middle ear, sinuses, lungs, and gastrointestinal tract is reduced in volume during compression or descent underwater. Inability to maintain gas pressure in these body spaces equal to the surrounding water pressure leads to various untoward mechanical effects, which are discussed below.

Because of the weight of the water exerting pressure over the chest wall, humans can breathe surface air through a snorkel or tube connected to the surface typically only to a depth of 1 to 2 feet. Attempts to breathe at greater depths through the tube are not only impossible but are dangerous, because the respiratory effort greatly augments the already physiologic negative-pressure breathing. In other words, when the respiratory muscles are relaxed at sea level, alveolar pressure is equal to surrounding air pressure. At a depth of 1 foot, the total water pressure on the chest wall is nearly 91 kg (200 lb). Because of loss of normal chest expansion and pressurization of intraalveolar air, the diver has to use forceful negative-pressure breathing to draw surface air into the lungs through the tube. Even at a depth of 1 foot, the great respiratory effort required is rapidly fatiguing, and respiration becomes impossible at further depths of only a few inches. Forced negative-pressure breathing can ultimately result in pulmonary capillary damage, with intraalveolar edema or hemorrhage. Symptoms include dyspnea and hemoptysis. Should this occur, there is no specific treatment; therapy is purely supportive.

BAROTRAUMA

Gas pressure in the various air-filled spaces of the body is normally in equilibrium with the surrounding environment. However,

TABLE 71-2 Commonly Used Units of Pressure in the Underwater Environment

Depth (fsw)	Depth (msw)	psig	psia	ATA	mm Hg (absolute)
Sea level		0.0	14.7	1	760
33	10	14.7	29.4	2	1520
66	20	29.4	44.1	3	2280
99	30	44.1	58.8	4	3040
132	40	58.8	73.5	5	3800
165	50	73.5	88.2	6	4560
198	60	88.2	102.9	7	5320
231	70	102.9	117.6	8	6080
264	81	117.6	132.3	9	6840
297	91	132.2	147.0	10	7600

ATA, atmospheres absolute; fsw, feet of seawater; msw, meters of seawater; psia, pounds per square inch absolute; psig, pounds per square inch gauge.

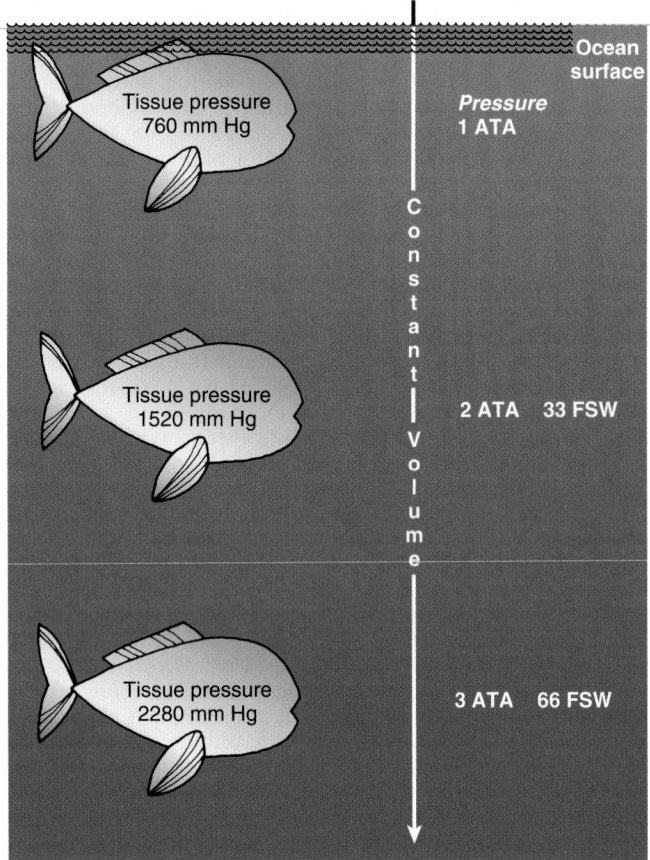

FIGURE 71-2 Pascal's law. Pressure applied to any part of a fluid is transmitted equally throughout the fluid.

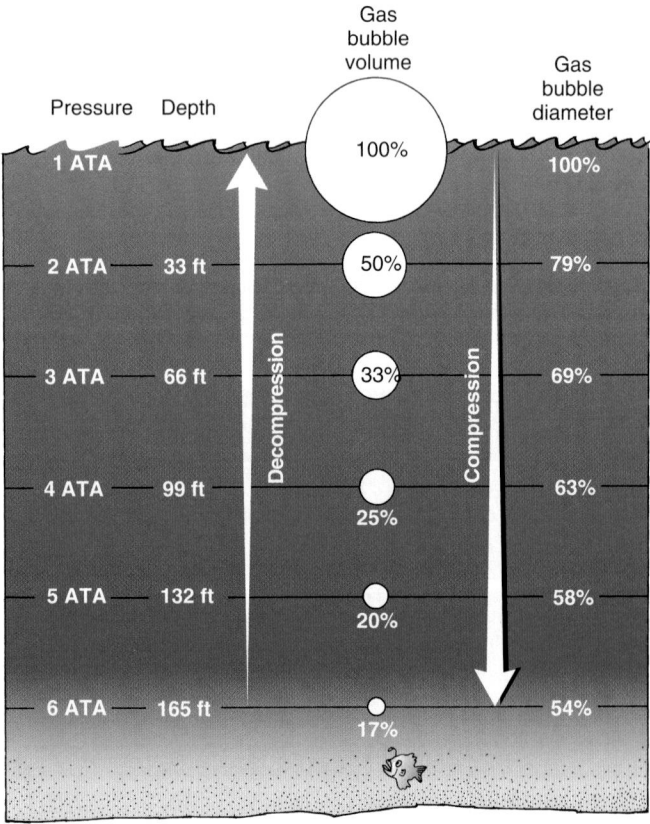

FIGURE 71-3 Boyle's law. The volume of a given quantity of gas at constant temperature varies inversely with pressure: $P_1V_1 = P_2V_2$.

if anything obstructs the passageways of gas exchange for these spaces and a change in ambient pressure occurs, pressure disequilibrium develops. The tissue damage resulting from such pressure imbalance is known as barotrauma and commonly referred to as a *squeeze*.

Overall, barotrauma is the most common medical problem in scuba diving, potentially involving any structure or combination of structures that leads to entrapment of gas in a closed space. This includes the ears, sinuses, lungs, gastrointestinal tract, teeth, portion of the face under a face mask, and skin trapped under a fold in a drysuit.

BAROTRAUMA OF DESCENT

Mask Barotrauma

For humans to see underwater, an air space must be present between the eyes and water. In scuba diving, this is created using a face mask consisting of tempered safety glass in a soft malleable mask that seals across the forehead, on the sides of the face, and under the nose to allow nasal exhalations into the mask space to maintain air pressure inside the mask. As a diver descends in the water, the ambient pressure increases; thus, the volume within the mask decreases. The diver must add air to the gas inside the face mask to equalize the water pressure. If inexperience or inattention causes the diver to forget to maintain this balance, negative pressure in the mask can be sufficient to rupture capillaries, causing petechiae, skin ecchymosis, subconjunctival hemorrhage, lid edema, and, rarely, hyphema. This unusual condition is known as *mask barotrauma* or *squeeze* (Figure 71-4; see also Figure 48-20). Most divers with mask barotrauma are asymptomatic. The condition usually resolves over a few days to a week without any intervention, but can be treated with cold compresses and analgesics if needed. Face mask barotrauma is easily prevented simply by exhaling through the nose during descent.

In recent years, full-face masks, which are standard issue for commercial, military, and public safety divers, have become more popular with recreational divers as more models have become available (e.g., Ocean Reef, Ocean Technology Systems, Scubapro), but they are still not commonly used. A full discussion of the advantages and disadvantages of full-face masks is beyond the scope of this chapter, but these masks should be remembered as a potentially good alternative for persons who have trouble with face mask fit, face mask flooding, or feelings of claustrophobia.

Orbital hemorrhage and subperiosteal orbital hematoma from face mask barotrauma are unusual complications and can be

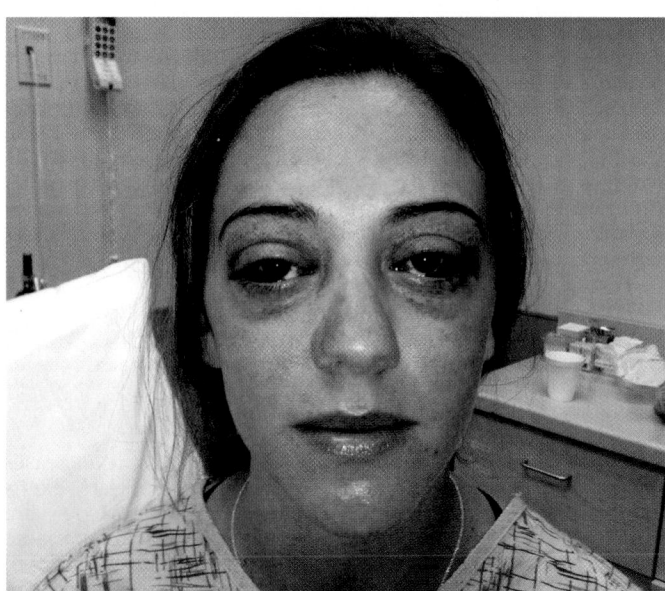

FIGURE 71-4 Mask barotrauma. A novice diver with mask barotrauma, showing subconjunctival hemorrhages, petechiae, and edema.

associated with diplopia, proptosis, and visual loss.[3,44,176,245,302] Although such neurologic findings after scuba diving may suggest AGE or neurologic DCS, the presence of the unmistakable stigmata of mask squeeze and a consistent history should prompt consideration of orbital hemorrhage. Under these circumstances, instead of immediate referral to a hyperbaric facility, the diver should be referred for immediate orbital CT scanning or magnetic resonance imaging (MRI) and ophthalmology consultation, because of the possibility of permanent vision loss caused by compression of the optic nerve or elevated intraocular pressure. In rare cases, surgical intervention may be necessary.[245] Recompression is contraindicated for orbital hemorrhage unless the diver also suffers from AGE or DCS.

Sinus Barotrauma

The four paired paranasal sinuses (frontal, maxillary, ethmoid, and sphenoid) have narrow connections to the nasal cavity via the sinus ostia. If there is inability to maintain the air pressure in any sinus during descent, a relative vacuum develops in the sinus cavity. This negative pressure causes congestion of the mucosal lining with subsequent edema and intramucosal bleeding and possible hematoma, hemorrhagic bullae, and bleeding into the sinus (Figure 71-5). In cases of sinus barotrauma, the diver usually experiences increasingly severe pain over the affected sinus during descent, which often causes the diver to abort the dive and return to the surface. On ascent, the remaining gas in the sinus expands and may force mucus and blood into the nose and mask.

The frontal sinus, followed by the maxillary sinus, is most commonly affected by barotrauma,. With maxillary sinus involvement, the diver often experiences pain in the maxillary teeth caused by compression of the posterior superior branch of the fifth cranial nerve, which runs along the base of the maxillary sinus. Additionally, maxillary sinus barotrauma can cause compression or ischemic neurapraxia of the infraorbital branch of the fifth cranial nerve, causing tingling and numbness of the cheek and upper lip.[43,220] Other complications include sinusitis from infection of the intrasinus fluid, or periorbital emphysema from air dissecting through the lamina papyracea from the ethmoid sinus into the orbits.[234] Unilateral optic neuropathy and a case of

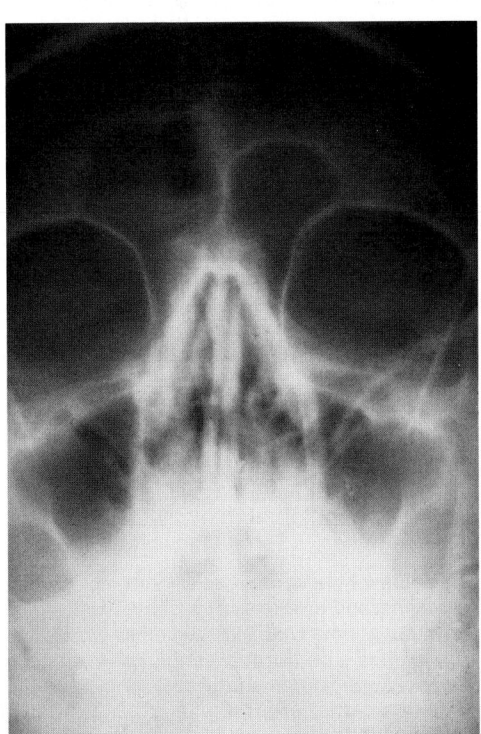

FIGURE 71-5 Frontal sinus barotrauma that first occurred 3 days earlier. Note the persistent air-fluid level. *(Courtesy Kenneth W. Kizer, MD.)*

transient vision loss at depth from possible sphenoidal sinus barotrauma have been reported.[130,139]

Treatment of sinus barotrauma involves use of systemic (e.g., pseudoephedrine) and topical (e.g., phenylephrine or oxymetazoline) vasoconstrictors, analgesics, abstinence from diving until resolved, and antihistamines if needed. Antibiotics are indicated only if signs of sinusitis, including fever or purulent nasal drainage, are present. In the field, a 3- to 5-day course of corticosteroids may hasten recovery and allow an otherwise healthy diver to return to diving. On rare occasions, drainage of the affected sinus by an otolaryngologist is required for persistent pain.

Sinus barotrauma usually occurs in the setting of a diver who has an upper respiratory infection or severe allergies, or who has an anatomic deformity such as nasal polyps or a deviated septum. Divers with a history of sinusitis or middle-ear barotrauma may be more prone to sinus barotrauma.[279] Consequently, prevention of sinus barotrauma includes avoidance of diving when suffering from an upper respiratory infection, while symptomatic from allergic rhinitis, and when sinusitis, nasal polyps, or any other condition is present that impairs free flow of air from the sinus cavity to the nose. Significant nasal deformity may predispose to sinus barotrauma and warrant surgical correction to allow one to continue diving.

External Auditory Canal Barotrauma. A tight-fitting wetsuit hood or drysuit hood can trap air in the external auditory canal and potentially lead to painful external ear squeeze during descent as the volume of air is reduced according to Boyle's law. External ear canal barotrauma can occur if cerumen, exostoses, or foreign objects, such as earplugs, block the canal.

Symptoms and signs of external ear canal barotrauma include pain, swelling, erythema, petechiae, and/or hemorrhagic blebs of the ear canal wall, and possible bleeding when the diver's hood is removed. Bullae may be present in the canal and on the tympanic membrane. In very severe (and very rare) cases, the tympanic membrane can rupture from negative pressure in the ear canal. The diver, feeling pain in the canal, may believe there is inadequate equalization of the middle ear and attempt a forceful Valsalva maneuver, which increases pressure on the tympanic membrane, leading to rupture. If this occurs, further diving is contraindicated until the tympanic membrane has healed.

Treatment of ear canal barotrauma includes washing the canal with lukewarm water. Bullae should not be incised. Antibiotic drops, such as a fluoroquinolone preparation combined with hydrocortisone, should be used to prevent infection due to contamination with seawater and should always be prescribed for tympanic membrane perforation.

Ear canal barotrauma can be prevented by remembering to break the seal of the wetsuit hood to allow water to fill the external ear canal before descent. Earplugs should never be worn when scuba diving, with perhaps the exception of vented, flexible, fitted earplugs often used by freedivers to prevent ear infections (e.g., Doc's Proplugs).

Middle Ear Barotrauma. Middle ear barotrauma is the most common medical problem in scuba diving, probably affecting more than 40% of divers at one time or another.[128] The problem can be explained by direct application of Boyle's law (Figure 71-6), potentially compounded by the structure of the eustachian tube.

Boyle's law describes the inverse relationship of pressure and volume in an enclosed air space and explains why the greatest relative volume change for a given depth change occurs near the surface, where the greatest risk for middle ear squeeze occurs. As the diver descends, hydrostatic water pressure forces the tympanic membrane inward, and the volume within the middle ear cavity is reduced. The diver can add air into the middle ear through the eustachian tube, equalizing the pressure in the middle ear cavity with the external ambient pressure.

Because each foot of seawater exerts a pressure of approximately 23 mm Hg, a diver who descends 76 cm (2.5 feet) and does not equalize pressure in the middle ear will develop a relative vacuum in the middle ear because of contraction of air volume. If middle ear pressure cannot be equalized on descent, the diver should ascend several feet to minimize the pressure

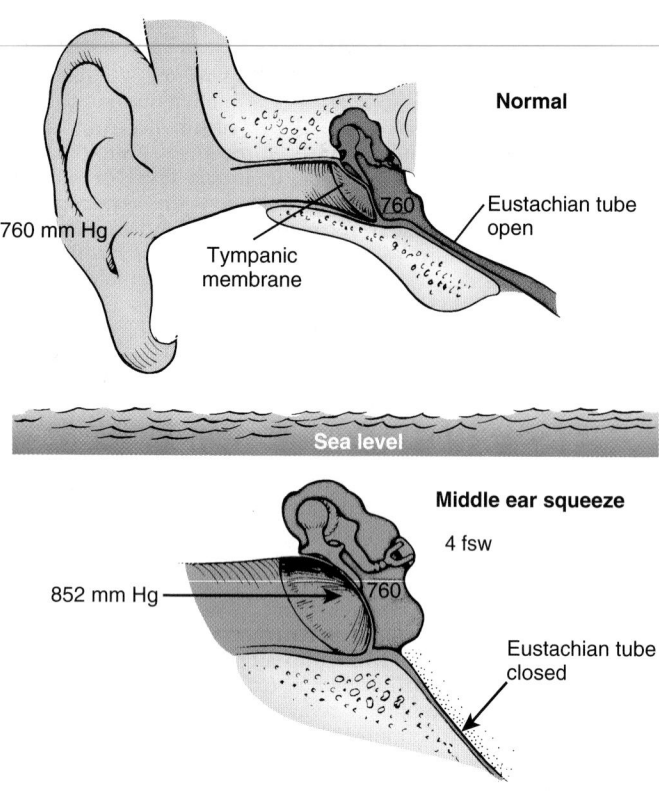

FIGURE 71-6 Middle ear barotrauma. Symptoms include fullness and pain caused by stretching of the tympanic membrane.

imbalance while attempting to equalize. Typically, the diver notices slight pain at a pressure differential of 60 mm Hg between air in the middle ear and ambient water pressure. This pressure differential causes the tympanic membrane to stretch and bulge inward, causing increasing discomfort and, eventually, severe pain. Additionally, when the tissues lining the middle ear cavity are exposed to this vacuum, vasodilation, edema, transudation, and vascular rupture occur, causing bleeding into the mucosa and middle ear cavity.

At a depth of 1.2 msw (4 fsw), a pressure differential of 90 mm Hg is generated, and the unsupported, flutter-valve, medial one-third of the eustachian tube collapses and becomes obstructed. At this point, attempts to autoinflate the middle ear by the Valsalva or Frenzel maneuver may be unsuccessful. The diver must ascend to equalize middle ear pressure with ambient environmental pressure.

If a diver does not heed the initial symptoms of middle ear barotrauma and allows the pressure differential to reach 100 to 400 mm Hg (i.e., at depths of 1.3 to 5.3 msw [4.3 to 17.4 fsw]), the pressure imbalance may lead to rupture of the tympanic membrane.[111] Symptoms of middle ear barotrauma include ear pain during descent, sensation of fullness, and reduced hearing in the affected ear. There may be mild tinnitus or vertigo. With tympanic membrane rupture, pain is relieved, but cold caloric stimulation created by seawater entering the middle ear cavity causes severe vertigo with nausea, vomiting, and disorientation underwater. The vertigo may resolve after a few minutes or continue for hours after surfacing.

The otoscopic appearance of the tympanic membrane in cases of middle ear barotrauma varies with the severity of injury. A commonly used grading scheme is the TEED classification, which grades severity according to the amount of hemorrhage in the tympanic membrane (Table 71-3).[102] Each higher grade tends to be more painful than the preceding one, except for grade 5, which may be relatively painless. With grade 5, cessation of pain corresponds with the membrane tearing, which immediately equalizes pressure in the middle ear with the external environment. Use of this grading scheme facilitates communication when describing these injuries.

In addition to having an abnormal-appearing tympanic membrane, persons with middle ear barotrauma occasionally have a small amount of bloody drainage around the nose or mouth. Audiometry usually reveals conductive hearing loss.

Middle ear barotrauma should be treated with decongestants and analgesics, although most cases clear spontaneously in 3 to 7 days without complication. Antihistamines may be used if the eustachian tube dysfunction has an allergic component. Divers should abstain from diving until the condition has resolved. Combining an oral decongestant with a long-acting topical nasal spray (such as 0.5% oxymetazoline or phenylephrine) for the first few days is usually most effective. Repeated gentle autoinflation of the middle ear by using the Frenzel maneuver also can help to displace any collection of middle ear fluid through the eustachian tube. If the tympanic membrane has ruptured, antibiotic drops, such as a fluoroquinolone preparation combined with hydrocortisone, should be used to prevent infection due to contamination with seawater. The diver should refrain from diving until the tympanic membrane is fully healed. The majority of tympanic membrane perforations from diving heal spontaneously without complications in 1 to 3 months. Surgical repair can be considered if healing has not occurred by 1 month.

Prevention is key for middle ear barotrauma. Training must emphasize the importance of early and frequent pressure equalization techniques. The diver should start equalizing immediately upon descending below the surface. Without equalization, the eustachian tube may become "locked" by 1.2 msw (4 fsw), as described earlier.

There are several maneuvers for equalizing pressure in the middle ear. The *Valsalva maneuver* involves blowing with an open glottis against closed lips and nostrils to increase pressure in the nasopharynx to inflate the middle ear through the eustachian tube. This may force open a collapsed eustachian tube. The *Toynbee maneuver* is performed by swallowing with a closed glottis while the lips are closed and nostrils pinched. The *Frenzel maneuver* is performed by pinching the nose, closing the glottis, and keeping the mouth closed while moving the jaw forward and down. This moves the pharyngeal muscles, which open the eustachian tube. This does not increase intracranial pressure. Descending feet first underwater also makes it easier to equalize pressure in the middle ear.

Divers who understand the pathophysiology of middle ear barotrauma generally take steps to inflate the middle ear immediately while submerging and thereby prevent the problem as they descend in the water. If middle ear pressure is kept equal to or greater than water pressure, no problem should occur. However, if the diver forgets to inflate the middle ear or suffers from eustachian tube dysfunction (caused by mucosal congestion due to upper respiratory infection, allergies, smoking, mucosal polyps, excessively vigorous autoinflation maneuvers, or previous maxillofacial trauma), middle ear barotrauma may occur. This most often happens just after the diver leaves the surface, with the diver complaining of ear fullness or pain. Generally, the pain rapidly becomes so severe that the diver either corrects the problem or aborts the dive.

Topical and oral decongestants are often used before diving to facilitate clearing the ears.[227] Pseudoephedrine has been

TABLE 71-3 TEED Grading System for Middle Ear Barotrauma

Grade	Description
0	Symptoms without otologic findings
1	Erythema and mild retraction of the tympanic membrane
2	Erythema of the tympanic membrane with mild or spotty hemorrhage within the membrane
3	Gross hemorrhage throughout the tympanic membrane
4	Grade 3 changes plus gross hemorrhage within the middle ear (hemotympanum)
5	Free blood in the middle ear plus perforation of the tympanic membrane

reported to reduce the incidence and severity of middle ear barotrauma in novice divers.[36] Using intranasal surfactant has been suggested to improve eustachian tube function to prevent middle ear barotrauma during repetitive diving.[97] Divers are sometimes taught not to use decongestants before diving because of theoretical concern about the medication wearing off while diving and causing problems during ascent; however, no data support this concern, and judicious use of oral or nasal decongestants can facilitate pressure equalization.

Inner Ear Barotrauma. A serious but relatively unusual form of aural barotrauma is inner ear barotrauma in the form of labyrinthine window rupture. This is the most serious form of aural barotrauma because of possible injury to the cochleovestibular system, which may lead to permanent deafness or vestibular dysfunction.[100,110]

Inner ear barotrauma results from rapid development of markedly different pressures between the middle and inner ear, as may occur from an overly forceful Valsalva maneuver or an exceptionally rapid descent, during which middle ear pressure is not adequately equalized. During descent, the tympanic membrane is pressed inward, pushing the stapes against the oval window. Perilymph and endolymph are not compressible; the resulting increased pressure causes the round window to bulge outward. The diver may attempt a forceful Valsalva maneuver to equalize the middle ear. This raises intracranial pressure, which is propagated through the perilymphatic duct to the inner ear, causing the round or oval window to rupture. This pressure dysequilibrium may cause several types of injury to the cochleovestibular apparatus, including hemorrhage within the inner ear; rupture of Reissner's membrane, leading to mixing of endolymph and perilymph; fistulation of the oval or round window, with development of a perilymph leak; or a mixed injury involving any or all of these conditions.[226] During ascent, the expanding middle ear gas may be forced through the perilymph fistula and enter either into the scala tympani or scala vestibule, which may damage cochlear or vestibular structures, leading to permanent hearing loss.

The classic triad of symptoms indicating inner ear barotrauma is roaring tinnitus, vertigo, and hearing loss. In addition, a feeling of fullness or "blockage" of the affected ear, nausea, vomiting, nystagmus, pallor, diaphoresis, disorientation, and/or ataxia may be present in varying degrees. Symptoms of inner ear barotrauma may develop immediately after the injury or be delayed for hours, depending on the specific damage and the diver's activities during and after the dive. Vigorous isometric exercise after a dive may complete an incipient or partial membrane rupture. Findings on physical examination may be normal or reveal signs of middle ear barotrauma or vestibular dysfunction. Audiometry may demonstrate mild to severe high-frequency sensorineural hearing loss or severe loss of all frequencies. Symptoms usually improve with time. Tinnitus tends to decline over time, and vestibular injury is centrally compensated. The diver may be left with high-pitch tone and high-frequency hearing loss.

Persons with inner ear barotrauma should be treated with bed rest (head elevated to 30 degrees), avoidance of strenuous activity or straining that can lead to increased intracranial pressure, and symptomatic measures as needed. There is a good prognosis for full recovery of hearing in 3 to 12 weeks. Labyrinthine window fistulas usually heal spontaneously, and data support initial conservative treatment.[226] Deterioration of hearing, worsening vestibular symptoms, or persistent significant vestibular symptoms after a few days heralds the need for detailed otolaryngologic evaluation and possible surgical exploration and fistula closure. No consensus exists as to how long to wait before surgical intervention. If a perilymph fistula is suspected, one recommendation is to explore the ear surgically as soon as possible or if symptomatic after 24 hours.[29] Patients with a tear in Reissner's membrane have manifestations similar to those with inner ear hemorrhage, although there will be persistent localized sensorineural hearing loss commensurate with the area of membrane tear. Management is the same.

Prevention of this condition is aimed at avoiding sudden, dramatic increases in middle ear pressure. Special emphasis during diver training and education should be placed on gentle pressure equalization. Upper respiratory tract infections and allergies reduce eustachian tube function and may precede inner ear barotrauma.

A diagnostic dilemma exists whenever a diver complains of vertigo, tinnitus, and hearing loss after diving. These symptoms are classic for labyrinthine rupture, in which case recompression is contraindicated because of the potential for further barotrauma to worsen the injury. Conversely, these symptoms may indicate a diagnosis of inner ear DCS, which requires expeditious treatment in a hyperbaric chamber. In such cases, the most important differential feature for diagnostic use on a dive boat or other diving site is a careful history as to time of onset and dive activities preceding the onset of symptoms. If symptom onset was during descent and ear clearing was difficult or impossible, requiring forcible Valsalva maneuvers, perilymph fistula is more likely. If the onset was during or after a decompression dive, DCS must be assumed and hyperbaric chamber treatment sought. In some cases, however, it simply is not possible to rule out DCS or rarely, AGE, and a "trial of pressure" in the hyperbaric chamber may be necessary.

Suit Barotrauma

If an area of the diver's skin becomes trapped under a fold or wrinkle of a drysuit, causing a closed air space, the pressure-induced contraction of air under the fold and resulting partial vacuum can cause transudation of blood through the skin. This is unusual and generally benign, although the resultant skin ecchymosis may have a dramatic appearance. Thick thermal undergarments (e.g., 400-g Thinsulate jumpsuit) worn under the drysuit in extremely cold water allow for significant squeeze prior to symptoms. Suit squeeze requires no treatment and resolves in a few days to a few weeks.

Dental Barotrauma

Dental barotrauma, or barodontalgia (tooth squeeze), is an infrequent yet dramatic type of barotrauma. This painful condition, sometimes called aerodontalgia, is caused by entrapped gas in the interior of a tooth or in the structures surrounding a tooth. The confined gas develops either positive or negative pressure relative to ambient pressure, which exerts force on surrounding sensitive dental structures and causes pain.

Barodontalgia may be caused by an array of dental conditions, including caries, defective restorations, oral tissue lacerations, recent extractions, periodontal abscesses, pulpal or apical lesions or cysts, and endodontal (root canal) therapy.[233] If a pocket of trapped air remains at sea level pressure while ambient pressure increases during descent, the tooth can implode or empty cavity fill with blood. Conversely, air that is forced into a tooth during descent can expand during ascent, causing the tooth to explode. To prevent barodontalgia, a diver should wait at least 24 hours after dental treatment (including fillings) before diving. Approximately 5% of French military divers reported dental barotrauma (fracture or loss of dental restoration) at the time of medical examination.[129]

Other causes of tooth pain associated with pressure changes are less well understood. Pulpitis or other dental infections can produce pain during a dive. Upper tooth pain associated with pressure changes should raise suspicion for a pathologic condition in the maxillary sinus.

Lung Barotrauma

Lung barotrauma, or lung squeeze, is a very unusual form of barotrauma that has been observed with breath-hold diving. Persons having this syndrome complain of shortness of breath and dyspnea after surfacing from a deep (> 30.5 msw [100 fsw]) breath-hold dive. The diver may cough up frothy blood, and a chest radiograph may show pulmonary edema. The condition is treated with supplemental oxygen and respiratory support as needed. Symptoms typically resolve within a few days; however, breath-hold fatalities have been linked to lung squeeze.

The classic understanding of lung squeeze is that it occurs when a diver descends to a depth at which the total lung volume is reduced to less than the residual volume. At this point, transpulmonic pressure exceeds intraalveolar pressure, causing transudation of fluid or frank blood (from rupture of pulmonary capillaries) and overt manifestations of pulmonary edema and hypoxemia. According to this scenario, a breath-hold diver with a total lung volume of 6000 mL and a residual volume of 1200 mL could dive to only 6000/1200 or 5 ATA (equal to 40.2 msw [132 fsw]) before lung squeeze would occur. However, breath-hold divers have dived much deeper without apparent problems.

In 1968, Schaefer and associates reported that breath-hold divers pool their blood centrally, accumulating a central volume increase of as much as 1047 mL at 27.4 msw (90 fsw).[252] If it is assumed that this adjustment in pulmonary blood volume reduces the residual volume, then theoretically, it should be possible for the diver with a total lung volume of 6000 mL to breath-hold to 6000/(1200 − 1047 = 153 mL), or almost 40 ATA. Although deep breath-hold dives seem to support the beneficial effect of central pooling of blood, cases of lung squeeze continue to occur at much shallower depths. The exact pathophysiology of this condition remains unclear.[182]

Underwater Blast Injury

Barotrauma can be caused by underwater explosions. Shock waves from a blast are propagated farther in the dense medium of water than in air.[62] Underwater explosions may result from ordnance or ignition of explosive gases during cutting or welding operations.

Underwater blasts can cause serious injuries to divers. Body cavities that contain air, such as the lungs, intestines, ears, and sinuses, are most vulnerable. Pneumothorax, pneumomediastinum, and air embolism may result from laceration of the lungs and pleura.[146] There may be intestinal perforation, subserosal hemorrhage, and subsequent peritonitis. Subarachnoid hemorrhage and rupture of the aorta and left ventricle have been reported in diving-related fatalities caused by underwater explosions.[235] The occurrence of blast-related air embolism at depth, which worsens with ascent to the surface, requires hyperbaric treatment. Otherwise, management of underwater blast injuries is the same as for terrestrial blast injury.

BAROTRAUMA OF ASCENT

Reverse Sinus or Ear Barotrauma (Reverse Squeeze)

The sinuses and ears are subject to barotrauma during ascent as well as descent. As the ambient pressure drops, the volume of the gas within the sinus or ear cavities expands, causing pain and tissue damage if not released. Gas pressure can exceed intravascular pressure in adjacent tissue, causing local ischemia. In the sinuses, a cyst or polyp can act as a one-way valve; air enters the sinus as the diver descends but cannot escape as the diver ascends. Fainting underwater as a result of frontal sinus pain has been reported.[112]

Pain can develop in the ear during ascent because of expanding gas pressure in the middle ear that is not released through the eustachian tube. If a diver makes frequent descents and ascents during a dive or multiple short dives back-to-back (bounce diving), the mucosal lining of the eustachian tube can become inflamed, making equalization of pressure in the ears difficult. The eustachian tube may not allow air to escape fast enough, and the pressure rises in the middle ear during ascent. This results in pain and often tinnitus and vertigo, and may lead to outward rupture of the tympanic membrane.

Alternobaric Vertigo

An unusual type of aural barotrauma is alternobaric vertigo. This usually occurs with ascent and is caused by sudden development of unequal (between the two ears) middle ear pressure, which causes asymmetric vestibular stimulation and resultant pronounced vertigo.[186] Vertigo, nausea, and vomiting may occur as the diver ascends. Although usually only transient and requiring no treatment, alternobaric vertigo may precipitate a panic response, leading to drowning or pulmonary barotrauma with resultant air embolism. The incidence of diving injuries due to alternobaric vertigo is unknown. The condition can be mitigated underwater by holding onto the ascent line and/or assistance from the dive buddy. Rarely, alternobaric vertigo lasts for several

hours or days, in which case it should be treated symptomatically after excluding inner ear barotrauma. Diving should be avoided when middle ear equalization is compromised.

Facial Baroparesis (Alternobaric Facial Palsy)

The seventh cranial nerve courses through the middle ear and mastoid process via a bony channel. Parts of the nerve may be directly exposed to middle ear pressures through a defect in the canal wall. During ascent, if the eustachian tube mucosa is swollen due to irritation, infection, or allergy, middle ear pressure may exceed the capillary pressure of the facial nerve and cause ischemic neuropraxia.[99,148,149,152,207] The diver may complain of ear fullness and pain after surfacing, along with facial palsy symptoms. The diver is unable to close the eye on the affected side, and the mouth may be affected. Otoscopy reveals a bulging tympanic membrane.

The diver can try the Toynbee maneuver, as described above, to release middle ear overpressure. Oral and topical decongestants should be used. The middle ear gas is eventually absorbed; this reduces the pressure. However, permanent damage of the nerve can occur if the pressure is elevated for too long. Myringotomy is the preferred treatment to remove air from the middle ear cavity.[152] Recompressing the diver to 1 msw (3 fsw) can also restore capillary circulation to the nerve. The diver's diving profile and lack of other neurologic symptoms and signs help exclude the diagnosis of AGE or DCS.

Gastrointestinal Barotrauma

Because the intestines are pliable, contraction of intraluminal bowel gas during descent does not cause barotrauma. In unusual situations, however, expanding gas can become trapped in the gastrointestinal tract during ascent and cause gastrointestinal barotrauma, which is also known as aerogastralgia.[68,185] This infrequent condition has been noted most often in novice divers, who are more prone to aerophagia; in divers who repeatedly perform the Valsalva maneuver in the head-down position, which may force air into the stomach; in those who chew gum while diving; and in divers who consume large quantities of carbonated beverages or legumes shortly before diving.

Divers with gastrointestinal barotrauma typically complain of abdominal fullness, colicky abdominal pain, belching, and flatulence. Rarely, syncope has been reported and is presumed to result from a combination of decreased venous return and vagal reflex. Most often, gas accumulates in the gastric antrum.

The physical examination of a diver having symptoms of gastrointestinal barotrauma is usually normal because the condition typically resolves by the time medical care is obtained. However, abdominal distention, tympany, and abdominal tenderness may be found. In an extreme case, there may be signs of cardiovascular compromise as a result of obstruction of venous return.[101]

Gastric rupture is uncommon and normally occurs with blunt abdominal trauma. Gastric rupture secondary to barotrauma is very rare, with only 15 cases reported in the literature.[39,146a,206,274] Air that is swallowed during the dive expands rapidly during an uncontrolled ascent, causing gastric rupture and pneumoperitoneum.[168,206] Abdominal compartment syndrome from tension pneumoperitoneum has been reported in a diver.[39] Pneumoperitoneum from gastric rupture should be treated with needle decompression prior to surgery. Pneumoperitoneum has also been reported after pulmonary barotrauma; air escaping from alveolar rupture enters the mediastinum and can progress to the abdomen through either the esophageal or aortic hiatus.[168] This can lead to a diagnostic dilemma (see section below). Gastrointestinal barotrauma is most often self-remedied by elimination of the excess gas. Hyperbaric treatment may be necessary in very rare, severe cases.

Pulmonary Barotrauma

The most serious type of barotrauma is pulmonary barotrauma of ascent, which results from expansion of gas trapped in the lungs. If a diver does not allow the expanding gas to escape, a pressure differential develops between the intrapulmonary air space and ambient pressure. The combination of overdistention of alveoli and overpressurization causes the alveoli to rupture, producing a spectrum of injuries collectively referred to as pulmonary barotrauma.

Divers suffering pulmonary overpressurization usually report a history of rapid and uncontrolled ascent to the surface before the onset of symptoms (typically as a result of running out of air, panic, or sudden development of uncontrolled positive buoyancy, as may occur when a diver drops his or her weight belt or inadvertently inflates his or her buoyancy compensator). However, pulmonary barotrauma may occur in divers who ascend slowly with no discernible cause. In these cases, there is presumed to be localized overinflation of the lung in these cases. Underlying lung pathology could theoretically lead to air trapping. One published case reports a 25-year-old male with coccidioidomycosis who suffered AGE after a normal ascent and was found to have a right upper lobe cavitary lesion on chest CT.[106] Pulmonary barotrauma has also been reported during normal ascent in divers with bullous disease.[196]

Localized overinflation of the lungs from focally increased elastic recoil may occur in divers who ascend at a proper rate.[63,64] Theoretically, if there are focal areas of decreased compliance in the lungs, adjacent areas of normal compliance would be subjected to greater forces, leading to barotrauma.[114] With immersion in diving, central pooling of blood causes an increase in intrapulmonary blood volume, and the lungs become stiffer. This decreased compliance may increase the risk for pulmonary barotrauma.

If a given intrapulmonary gas volume is trapped by forcible breath-holding or a closed glottis, or, even in a small portion of the lung, by bronchospasm during ascent, intrapulmonary volume increases (according to Boyle's law) until the elastic limit of the chest wall is reached. After that, intrapulmonary pressure rises until, at a positive differential pressure of about 80 mm Hg, air is forced across the pulmonary capillary membrane. This air usually enters either the pulmonary interstitial spaces or pulmonary capillaries.

It is important to remember that there is significant change in barometric pressure in shallow water. Boyle's law dictates greater volume changes for a given change in depth near the surface than at greater depths. Thus, shallow depths are the most danger-ous for breath-holding ascents. A pressure differential of only 80 mm Hg (alveolar air) above ambient water pressure on the chest wall, or about 1 to 1.3 msw (3 to 4 fsw) of depth underwater, is adequate to force air bubbles across the alveolar-capillary membrane. Fatal pulmonary barotrauma has occurred from breath-holding during an ascent from a depth as shallow as 1.3 msw (4 fsw).[20]

The diagnosis of pulmonary barotrauma is based on development of characteristic symptoms after diving. Actual clinical manifestations may take several forms, depending on the course traveled by the extraalveolar air. Once alveoli rupture, air can remain in the interstitium, causing localized pulmonary injury and alveolar hemorrhage. Air can travel along perivascular sheaths and dissect into the mediastinum. This air can track superiorly to the neck, resulting in subcutaneous emphysema, and can dissect inferiorly and posteriorly, causing pneumoperitoneum. Air may dissect to the visceral pleura, causing a pneumothorax. If air enters the pulmonary vasculature, it can travel to the heart and embolize systemically, causing AGE (Figure 71-7).

Clinical Manifestations of Pulmonary Barotrauma. The specific clinical manifestations of pulmonary barotrauma depend on the location and amount of air that escapes into an extraalveolar location.

Local Pulmonary Injury. Air can rupture alveoli, causing localized pulmonary injury and capillary bleeding without other signs of pulmonary barotrauma, such as pneumomediastinum or AGE. Diffuse alveolar hemorrhage has been described as a rare manifestation of pulmonary barotrauma.[8] The diver may complain of chest pain, cough, and hemoptysis without any neurologic findings. Intraparenchymal lung injury and bleeding may be seen on chest x-ray. A diver with local pulmonary injury without any evidence of AGE does not require recompression and should be treated with supportive care. However, a complete history and neurologic evaluation must be performed to be certain the diver did not have a transient episode of neurologic dysfunction immediately after the event that could herald an AGE. Subtle parietal lobe dysfunction may be the only abnormality detected by the time the diver reaches the emergency department or hyperbaric chamber.[218]

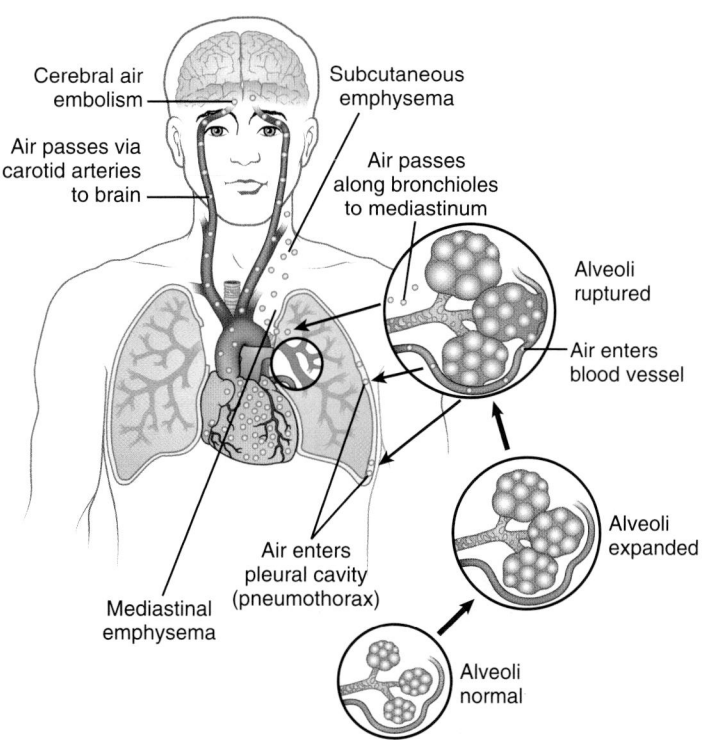

Cerebral air embolism
Subcutaneous emphysema
Air passes via carotid arteries to brain
Air passes along bronchioles to mediastinum
Alveoli ruptured
Air enters blood vessel
Alveoli expanded
Air enters pleural cavity (pneumothorax)
Mediastinal emphysema
Alveoli normal

FIGURE 71-7 Pulmonary barotrauma. Diagram of different manifestations of pulmonary barotrauma, including mediastinal emphysema, subcutaneous emphysema, pneumothorax, and arterial gas embolism.

Pneumomediastinum, or mediastinal emphysema, is the most common form of pulmonary barotrauma, resulting from pulmonary interstitial air dissecting along bronchi to the mediastinum. The diver may be asymptomatic or complain of substernal chest pain. Respiratory distress is typically not present. If air dissects from the mediastinum up to the neck, the diver may experience hoarseness and neck fullness. Subcutaneous emphysema may be present and palpated as crepitance under the skin of the neck and anterior chest. In severe cases, the diver may complain of marked chest pain, dyspnea, and dysphagia. *Hamman's sign* (also known as Hamman's murmur or Hamman's crunch) is a crunching, rasping sound, synchronous with each heartbeat and heard over the precordium during auscultation of the chest. It may rarely be heard when air is present in the mediastinum around the heart. Radiographs may show extraalveolar air in the neck or mediastinum, or both, although radiographs are rarely necessary to make the diagnosis. The presence of air on a radiograph may be very subtle and is often best visualized along the pulmonary artery and aorta, and along the edge of the heart.

Treatment of pneumomediastinum is conservative, consisting of rest, avoidance of further pressure exposure (including flying in commercial aircraft), and observation. Supplemental oxygen administration may be useful in severe cases. Hyperbaric treatment is indicated only in cases associated with AGE. As mentioned above, any transient neurologic symptom in the presence of pneumomediastinum suggests AGE.

Pneumothorax is an infrequent manifestation of diving-related pulmonary barotrauma, because it requires that air be vented through the visceral pleura, a path generally having greater resistance than does air tracking through the interstitium. Although pneumothorax has been reported to occur in 5% to 10% of cases of AGE,[231] in the authors' experience its occurrence is much less frequent. Despite being infrequent, pneumothorax must be considered and excluded whenever pulmonary barotrauma or AGE is suspected, because a simple pneumothorax can become a tension pneumothorax during ascent in a hyperbaric chamber.

In cases of diving-related pneumothorax, the diver usually complains of pleuritic chest pain, breathlessness, and dyspnea, just as with pneumothorax from any other cause. Radiographs may confirm the diagnosis. Because the majority of diving-related pneumothoraces are small, treatment may consist simply of supplemental oxygen and close observation, repeating the chest x-ray at intervals to ensure resolution. Tube thoracostomy is usually reserved for a larger pneumothorax or if the diver is to undergo hyperbaric treatment. A chest tube is necessary if the diver is recompressed, because the expanding intrapleural gas of the pneumothorax cannot otherwise be vented to the environment during depressurization from hyperbaric treatment, and it may convert to a lethal tension pneumothorax.

Tension pneumothorax is one of a very few diving-specific disorders that can quickly kill a diver at the dive site (or in a hyperbaric chamber), but is curable if recognized. Although pneumothorax may result from pulmonary barotrauma, it is also associated with severe blunt chest trauma (e.g., from an underwater blast, landslide, or cave-in or from collision with a boat) or may develop spontaneously, as has been observed with other outdoor sports.[163]

Divers developing a pneumothorax underwater will almost always develop shortness of breath, dyspnea, and pleuritic chest pain, although these symptoms may not be recognized or their significance may not be recognized at the time. Shortness of breath always worsens during ascent, although the chest pain often improves during ascent as the pneumothorax enlarges and the lung no longer touches the chest wall. Breath sounds will be noted to be diminished when the chest is auscultated.

Treatment of tension pneumothorax in divers is with closed chest thoracostomy.

ARTERIAL GAS EMBOLISM

Arterial gas embolism (AGE) is the most feared complication of pulmonary barotrauma. It is one of the most dramatic and serious injuries associated with compressed-air diving and is a major cause of death and disability among recreational divers.[160] Many diver deaths officially listed as drowning probably have been cases of AGE. Unfortunately, the accident investigation and postmortem evaluation of many diving accident victims are insufficient to establish the precise cause of death. Autopsies of diving accident victims should be performed according to special procedures.[50,51,75]

PATHOPHYSIOLOGY

AGE results from air bubbles entering the pulmonary venous circulation from ruptured alveoli. When air is introduced into the pulmonary capillary blood, gas bubbles are showered into the left atrium; from the atrium, the bubbles move to the left ventricle and subsequently the aorta. From the aorta, they are distributed throughout the arterial vasculature. Bubbles may enter the coronary arteries and produce electrocardiogram (ECG) changes and elevation of cardiac enzymes, but rarely myocardial injury.[262] Myocardial dysfunction resulting from ischemia and stunning caused by gas bubbles in the coronary arteries after diving has been reported in a patient who developed acute pulmonary edema while diving.[251] Gas embolization to the coronary arteries also may induce arrhythmias.[156]

Most of the bubbles entering the aorta pass into the systemic circulation, lodging in small- and medium-sized arteries and occluding the more distal circulation. Bubbles travel up the carotid or vertebral arteries to embolize the brain, causing a combination of mechanical and reactive sequelae. Most bubbles pass through the cerebral vasculature after varying amounts of delay.[127] Occlusive bubbles lodge most frequently in small arterioles with a diameter of 30 to 60 μm, which are found at the junction between the white and gray matter.[83] Vascular occlusion causes distal ischemia, which is compounded by damage to the vascular endothelium and disruption of the blood-brain barrier, with resultant cerebral edema. Systemic hypertension occurs, cerebrospinal fluid pressure rises, and there is reactive hyperemia causing loss of autoregulation of cerebral perfusion. Cerebral blood flow now reflects changes in systemic blood flow.[109]

Bubbles damage the vascular endothelium, causing release of vasoactive substances both in the brain and lungs,[141] and adversely affect nitric oxide–mediated endothelial cell function.[37] These mechanisms explain the delayed effects of air embolization on circulatory dynamics.

Depending on the site or sites of circulatory occlusion, AGE produces myriad and often disastrous consequences. The neurologic pattern may be confusing as showers of bubbles randomly embolize the brain's circulation, producing ischemia and infarction of diverse brain regions. Combined carotid and vertebral artery embolization may produce severe, diffuse brain injury (Figure 71-8).[160]

AGE typically develops during ascent or immediately after the diver surfaces, at which time the high intrapulmonary pressure resulting from lung overpressurization is relieved, allowing bubble-laden pulmonary venous blood to return to the heart and pass into the systemic circulation. It is axiomatic that symptoms of AGE develop within 10 minutes of surfacing from a dive, although most often they are clearly evident within the first 2 minutes. Sudden loss of consciousness during ascent or upon surfacing from a dive should be considered to represent air embolism until proven otherwise.

In a pulmonary overpressure accident, as soon as normal breathing resumes at the surface of the water, the pressure differential that drives air bubbles into the pulmonary capillaries is equalized. From this point on, usually no further intraarterial air is introduced.

ARTERIAL GAS EMBOLISM AND SUDDEN DEATH

Approximately 4% of divers who suffer an AGE die immediately, presenting with sudden loss of consciousness, pulselessness, and apnea. These victims are not responsive to immediate cardiopulmonary resuscitation or recompression. It was previously thought that sudden death from AGE was caused either by reflex arrhythmias from brainstem embolization or by myocardial ischemia and

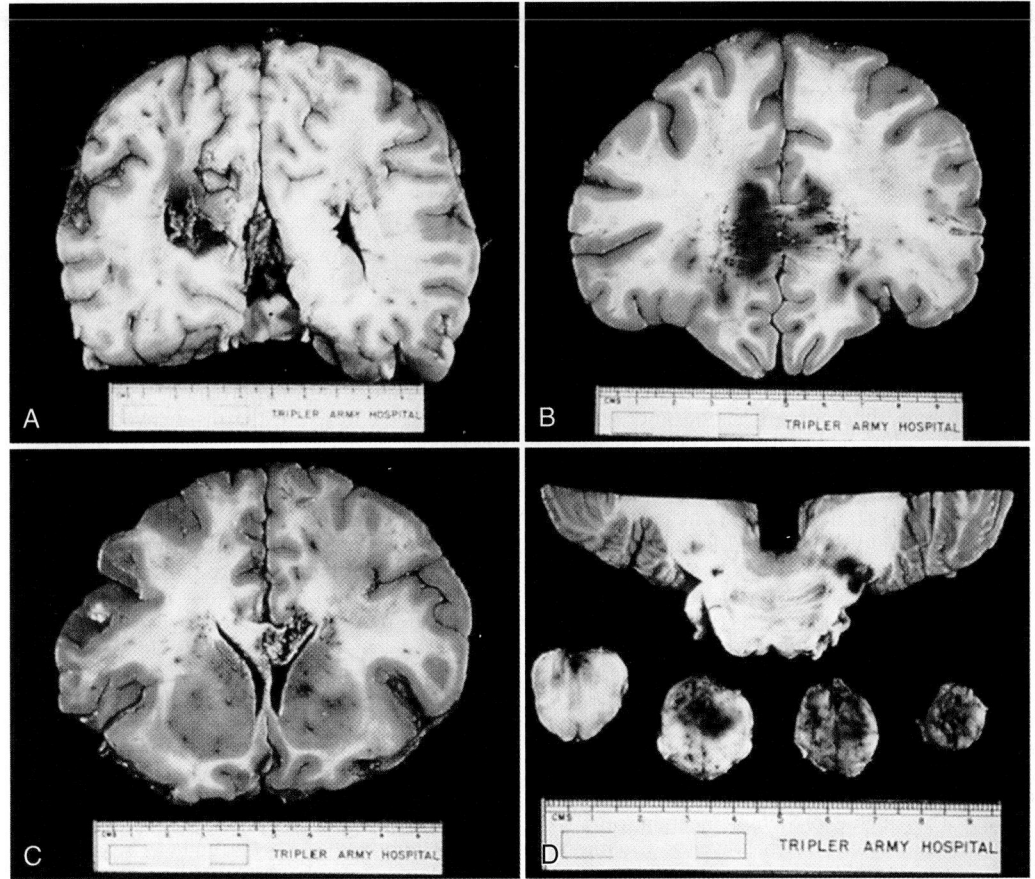

FIGURE 71-8 A to **D,** Cross sections of the brain of a 31-year-old male sport diver who suffered an arterial gas embolism, dying 4 days after the accident and after receiving extended hyperbaric oxygen therapy. Bubble-induced infarcts are found throughout the brain in the distribution of both the carotid and vertebral arteries. *(Courtesy Kenneth W. Kizer, MD.)*

death due to coronary artery embolization and occlusion.[48,109] However, these mechanisms do not explain what is seen in animal models or clinically in humans. Accidental injection of air into the coronary arteries of humans during cardiac catheterization does not result in sudden death. There is only one case report of myocardial infarction associated with an AGE,[66] and biochemical evidence for myocardial ischemia in cases of AGE has not been found.[262]

In sudden death from AGE, there is complete filling of the central vascular bed with air.[215] Radiographs of fatal cases of AGE demonstrate massive amounts of air in the central vasculature (Figure 71-9).[219] Autopsies typically reveal large amounts of air in the central vascular bed, particularly in the pulmonary arteries and right ventricle. Currently, it is believed that the primary mechanism of cardiac arrest in most cases of AGE is vascular obstruction caused by air, leading to pulseless electrical activity.[215,219]

CLINICAL MANIFESTATIONS

Clinical manifestations of cerebral air embolism are sudden, dramatic, and often life-threatening. Approximately 4% of victims of AGE suffer immediate cardiac respiratory arrest and die. Another 5% die in the hospital from consequences of the AGE or drowning that can accompany AGE. More than one-half of the remaining victims of AGE have complete functional recovery.

Victims of AGE present with varied neurologic and systemic signs and symptoms depending on the amount and distribution of air. Neurologic manifestations of AGE are typical of an acute stroke, although hemiplegia and other purely unilateral brain syndromes are infrequent. Loss of consciousness, monoplegia or asymmetric multiplegia, focal paralysis, paresthesias or other sensory disturbances, convulsions, aphasia, confusion, blindness

or visual field defects, vertigo, dizziness, or headache is most often observed (Table 71-4).[84,109,160,197,218]

The physical findings of AGE are extremely variable and depend on the specific site or sites of vascular occlusion. Neurologic findings generally dominate the clinical picture because of the frequency of cerebral involvement. All patients with

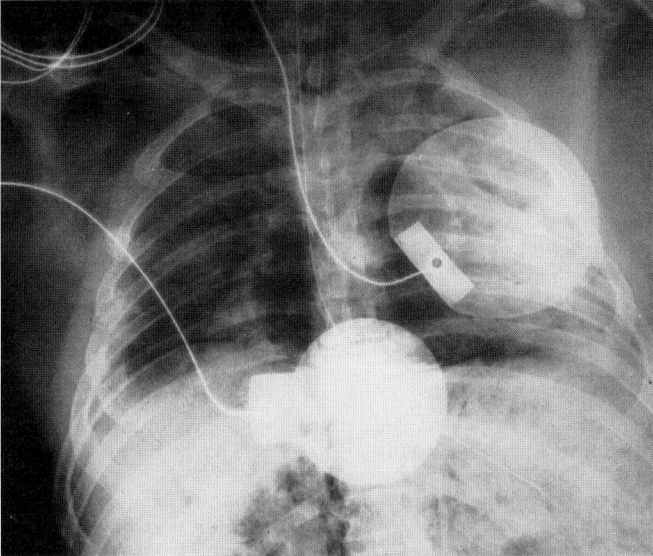

FIGURE 71-9 Chest radiograph of a diver who died suddenly from an arterial gas embolism, showing complete filling of the central vascular bed with air. Note the air in the heart and carotid arteries.

Condition	Symptoms	Signs
Arterial gas embolism	Seizure (focal or general), unconsciousness, confusion, headache, visual disturbances, bloody sputum (rare)	Hemiplegia, monoplegia, altered level of consciousness, blindness, visual motor deficit, focal motor or sensory loss
Mediastinal-subcutaneous emphysema	Substernal pain, hoarse voice, neck swelling, dyspnea	Subcutaneous crepitus, gas patterns on radiographs of the mediastinum and neck
Pneumothorax	Chest pain, dyspnea	Loss of breath sounds, hyperresonant chest percussion, tracheal shift

suspected AGE should be carefully examined for neurologic deficits. Often, the neurologic findings are subtle and require detailed examinations, including cognitive function testing.[218] Such testing is rarely possible at the dive site, so divers who have a history suggestive of AGE (e.g., loss of consciousness after ascending from a dive) but who do not manifest any gross symptoms or signs of neurologic injury in the field should be given the benefit of the doubt and transported to the nearest emergency department for initial stabilization and referral to a hyperbaric treatment facility. Specific manifestations of pulmonary barotrauma (such as subcutaneous or mediastinal emphysema) should be carefully sought.

Persons suffering an AGE may present with various hematologic and biochemical abnormalities. Gas bubbles distribute systemically and are thought to cause direct organ injury or injury to the vascular endothelium, or both. AGE patients usually present with hemoconcentration due to plasma extravasation from endothelial injury. The degree of hemoconcentration correlates with the neurologic outcome of the diver.[264] Creatinine kinase (CK) is elevated in nearly all cases of AGE and correlates with eventual neurologic outcome of the diver.[262] The more elevated the CK, the less likely is full functional recovery. The majority of elevated CK is from skeletal muscle (the MM component). CK-MB (derived from cardiac muscle) is elevated in some cases, and nonspecific ECG changes can occur; however, true myocardial infarction due to AGE is extremely rare.[34] Even in cases of AGE with elevated CK-MB, functional studies of the heart show no evidence of wall motion abnormalities following recovery.[251,262] Bubbles cause injury to other organs. Elevated serum glutamic oxaloacetic transaminase, serum glutamic pyruvic transaminase, and lactate dehydrogenase can be found in victims of AGE.[263] Despite elevations of these enzymes, organ function usually does not decline.

AGE can lead to loss of consciousness upon surfacing; hence, it is not unexpected to find evidence of aspiration and drowning clinically and on chest x-ray. Radiographic findings consistent with aspiration can be found in more than 50% of chest x-rays of victims with AGE.[135] However, many of the same radiographic findings may be seen with venous gas embolism.[162]

Rarely, air bubbles may be visualized in the retinal arteries, or sharply circumscribed areas of glossal pallor (Liebermeister's sign) may be noted, but these findings cannot be relied upon to make the diagnosis. The diagnosis of AGE is clinical and based on the diving history and symptoms. Any diver who loses consciousness or presents with symptoms or signs of serious neurologic injury within 10 minutes of surfacing from a dive must be considered to have suffered an AGE.

TREATMENT

All cases of suspected AGE must be referred for hyperbaric oxygen treatment as rapidly as possible. This is the primary and essential treatment for the condition.[98]

As noted earlier, initial neurologic manifestations of AGE may resolve by the time the diver reaches a medical facility. Regardless, all patients should be referred for hyperbaric consultation if the history is suggestive of AGE, because neurologic impairment is difficult to exclude in the acute setting and subtle neurologic injuries may progress and become irreversible. Although

early treatment with hyperbaric oxygen therapy (HBOT) is more likely to be efficacious than is delayed treatment, there are many reports of divers improving with HBOT after delays longer than 6 hours.[189]

DAN has a diving medicine physician available 24 hours a day, 7 days a week, who can help with diagnosis and immediate care of an injured diver and provide the location of the nearest hyperbaric treatment facility. DAN can assist with arrangement of transport and treatment for all diving injuries. In the United States, the DAN hotline number is 919-684-9111.

Prehospital Care

The affected diver should be given supplemental oxygen at a high flow rate (15 L/min by nonrebreather facemask) as soon as possible starting on the dive boat or in the field and continued during transport, emergency department evaluation, and transfer to the hyperbaric treatment facility. Supplemental oxygen enhances the rate of resolution of inert gas bubbles and treats arterial hypoxemia.

AGE patients should be maintained in the supine position, both in the field and during transport to an emergency medical treatment facility or hyperbaric chamber. Historically, much attention was directed toward keeping the AGE patient in the Trendelenburg position in the field. This was based on anecdotal reports and limited experimental data.[127,169,280] The rationale for keeping the patient with AGE in the head-down position was the belief that the weight of the column of blood would force bubbles through the cerebral capillary bed, that the buoyancy of the bubbles would keep them in the aorta or heart, and that the weight of the spinal fluid might compress bubbles in the spinal cord. These benefits were never well demonstrated or experimentally confirmed. More recent studies showed that the Trendelenburg position did not keep bubbles from being distributed to the systemic circulation.[47] Additionally, it is more difficult to oxygenate patients in a head-down position, and if someone is maintained in this position for longer than 30 to 60 minutes, it may cause or worsen cerebral edema.

Because the AGE event so often occurs while the victim is in the water, he or she frequently suffers concomitant drowning. The rescuer must be prepared to provide cardiopulmonary resuscitation and to protect the airway from aspiration of gastric contents secondary to vomiting.

While life support measures are being instituted, a member of the diving or rescue team should contact the nearest civilian or military hyperbaric treatment facility and contact an air ambulance if air evacuation is required. Aircraft selection is crucial because the stricken diver should not be exposed to a significantly lower atmospheric pressure in the aircraft. Ideally, the diver should be transported by aircraft pressurized to sea level so that any intraarterial bubbles do not further expand. In the case of helicopter evacuation or in the event that an unpressurized aircraft is required, the flight altitude must be maintained as low as possible, not to exceed 305 m (1000 feet) above sea level, if possible.

Intravenous fluid resuscitation should be started for divers with AGE. As mentioned earlier, victims of AGE present with hemoconcentration from plasma extravasation due to endothelial injury from gas bubbles. It is important to maintain adequate intravascular volume because inert gas cannot be effectively eliminated from tissues or from intravascular bubbles at the arteriolar-capillary level without sufficient capillary perfusion. Additionally, autoregulation of blood flow in the brain is lost following AGE, and cerebral perfusion passively follows the systemic blood pressure. Hypotension should be avoided in cases of AGE. Intravenous infusion of isotonic solution should be started, and urine output maintained at 1 to 2 mL/kg/hr.[74]

The AGE-affected diver should be transported to a hyperbaric treatment facility as quickly as possible. Delay prolongs cerebral ischemia and cellular hypoxia, resulting in significant cerebral edema, which typically leads to a more difficult course of therapy. Transport should still be undertaken even if delay is unavoidable. Remarkable improvement has been seen in cases in which treatment was delayed for more than 24 hours after the onset of neurologic manifestations.[157]

If the AGE-stricken diver is first seen at a hospital emergency department or clinic, baseline laboratory tests, including hemoglobin and creatine phosphokinase, chest radiograph, and other diagnostic tests (such as an ECG) should be obtained while transport to a hyperbaric treatment facility is being arranged. CT or MRI of the brain should be deferred until after initial hyperbaric treatment unless intracranial hemorrhage, carotid artery dissection,[212] or other nondiving injury is strongly suspected. Diagnostic imaging has low sensitivity and should not delay initiation of hyperbaric oxygen therapy.

Hyperbaric Oxygen Therapy

Hyperbaric oxygen therapy (HBOT) consists of rapidly increasing ambient pressure to reduce intravascular bubble volume and restore tissue perfusion. Oxygen-enriched breathing mixtures enhance bubble resolution and deliver oxygen to hypoxic nervous tissue, followed by slow decompression to avoid bubble re-formation.[33,74,76] Additional details regarding HBOT tables used for treating AGE are provided in Chapter 72. Although patients with AGE have successfully been treated in a monoplace hyperbaric chamber,[290] it is better for these patients to be treated in multiplace hyperbaric chambers (Figure 71-10) capable of being pressurized to 6 ATA and in which both air and oxygen can be administered to the patient. There is growing evidence that HBOT to 2.8 ATA with 100% oxygen may be more effective treatment than initial pressurization to 6 ATA for divers with AGE because of the typical several-hour delay in bringing the patient to a chamber and, thus, less need for the higher pressure to resolubilize bubbles (and perhaps a greater immediate need for tissue oxygenation).[85,86,159,160,179,180]

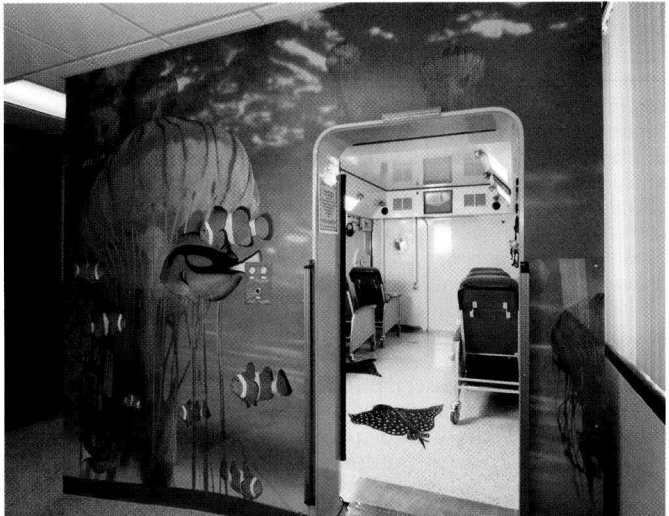

FIGURE 71-10 Example of a large modern hyperbaric chamber. A hyperbaric chamber for treating decompression sickness or arterial gas emboli should preferably have a pressure capability of at least 6 ATA (165 fsw) and should have space for an attendant to provide ongoing hands-on care and repeated neurologic examinations. It must have provisions for supplying 100% oxygen and other gases for treating the stricken diver.

Although the majority of victims with AGE have neurologic deficits when examined, initial manifestations may spontaneously resolve by the time the victim is seen by medical personnel. Occasionally, a person has symptoms but no reproducible neurologic deficits on physical examination.[160,178] Nonetheless, all patients must be referred for diving medicine consultation and hyperbaric treatment if the history is suggestive of AGE, because neurologic impairment is impossible to exclude in the acute care setting, and waiting to complete definitive diagnostic studies may allow subtle neurologic injuries to become irreversible.[218] Additionally, patients with AGE who show clinical improvement or recovery may deteriorate a few hours later.[232] Therefore, early HBOT is recommended even for patients who have spontaneous recovery.

Adjunctive Treatment

Over the years, numerous medications (e.g., heparin, low-molecular-weight dextran, aspirin, corticosteroids) have been proposed as adjuncts to recompression and hyperbaric oxygen for treatment of AGE and DCS; however, experimental and clinical data do not support the use of any of these for AGE.

Lidocaine had been proposed as an adjuvant to HBOT for treatment of AGE. Limited experimental data support its use. Lidocaine is a class IB antiarrhythmic agent and a local anesthetic that crosses the blood-brain barrier and may have cerebroprotective effects by modulation of inflammatory mediators, preservation of cerebral blood flow, reduction in cerebral metabolism, and deceleration of ischemic ion fluxes. In animal models of AGE and brain ischemia, lidocaine acts to preserve blood flow in the brain, reduce brain edema and intracranial pressure, and preserve neuroelectrical function.[199,205] When given prophylactically, lidocaine reduces brain dysfunction after AGE in cats[108] and improves recovery of brain function in cats and dogs with AGE when given therapeutically.[98,107] Human data are less impressive because many of the case studies contain patients with both AGE and DCS.[61,90,291] Although earlier studies reported significantly less neurocognitive deficit in patients when lidocaine was used prophylactically during left heart valve surgery,[205] follow-up studies have not shown any neuroprotective effect of lidocaine during adult cardiac surgery.[192,204] Overall, the evidence does not support the use of lidocaine as an adjunct to recompression for treatment of AGE.

PREVENTION OF PULMONARY BAROTRAUMA AND ARTERIAL GAS EMBOLISM

In view of the potentially catastrophic consequences of AGE, one of the key goals of scuba diving training is to prevent pulmonary overpressure accidents. Divers must be warned of the potentially great intrathoracic volume changes that can occur at shallow depths and be trained to keep an open airway during ascent, particularly through the last 3 msw (10 fsw) to the surface. If equipment malfunction or depletion of air supply at depth makes this impossible, the diver must make every attempt to exhale continuously during an "emergency swimming ascent" in order to vent the increasing volume of air from within the lungs. With a satisfactory air supply, the diver should simply breathe normally on ascent to the surface, taking care to ascend slowly near the surface.

INDIRECT EFFECTS OF PRESSURE

Several diving-related problems may develop as a result of breathing gases at higher-than-normal atmospheric pressures. Chief among these are nitrogen narcosis, oxygen toxicity, and DCS.

DALTON'S LAW OF PARTIAL PRESSURES

Dalton's law of partial pressures states that the total pressure exerted by a mixture of gases is the sum of the pressures that would be exerted by each of the gases if it alone occupied the total volume. The partial pressure of a gas in a mixture is the pressure exerted by that gas alone. The symbols for partial

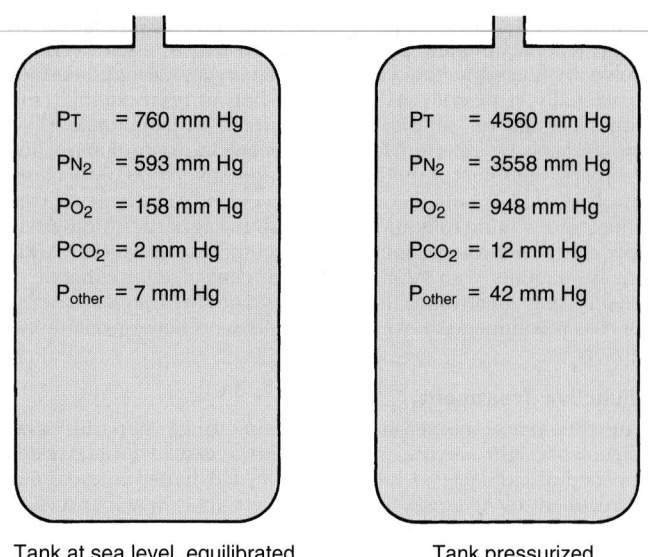

PT = 760 mm Hg	PT = 4560 mm Hg
PN2 = 593 mm Hg	PN2 = 3558 mm Hg
PO2 = 158 mm Hg	PO2 = 948 mm Hg
PCO2 = 2 mm Hg	PCO2 = 12 mm Hg
Pother = 7 mm Hg	Pother = 42 mm Hg
Tank at sea level, equilibrated with ambient air pressure	Tank pressurized with compressed air to 6 ATA (165 fsw)

FIGURE 71-11 Dalton's law of partial pressures. The total pressure exerted by a mixture of gases is the sum of the pressures that would be expected of each of the gases if it alone were present and occupied the total volume.

pressure of oxygen, nitrogen, carbon dioxide, and water vapor are P_{O_2}, P_{N_2}, P_{CO_2}, and P_{H_2O}, respectively. Dalton's law states that in an air mixture, the total pressure (PT) = P_{N_2} + P_{O_2} + P_{H_2O} + P_{other}. The partial pressure of each gas in the mixture is found by multiplying the percentage of that gas present by the total pressure. In Figure 71-11, in a mixture of air, nitrogen is assumed to be present in a proportion of 78%, oxygen at 21%, and carbon dioxide at 0.03%, and the balance composed of water vapor and other trace gases.

The partial pressures of inspired gases in a gas mixture, not their percentages, are of prime importance in diving. For example, it has been shown that in hyperbaric chamber treatment of DCS, 100% oxygen can be safely used at depths to 2.8 ATA (60 fsw) for 20-minute periods with the subject at rest in the dry chamber. On the other hand, with 21% oxygen in a helium-oxygen mixture at 20 ATA (600 fsw), the diver would breathe 0.21 × 20 ATA, or 4.2 ATA of oxygen, which would rapidly produce CNS oxygen poisoning. This type of problem is avoided in deep diving by reducing the oxygen percentage in the gas mixture to between 0.35 and 0.50 ATA, so that the P_{O_2} will be between 266 and 380 mm Hg.

The scuba diver who uses open-circuit compressed air is subject to the effects of the component gases in the air according to their partial pressures. Thus, even though the gas mixture is simply air with normal percentages of oxygen and nitrogen, the increases in partial pressures of these gases and those of the trace contaminants at sea level create numerous potential problems related to the breathing medium. Most notable among these for scuba divers is the problem of nitrogen narcosis.

NITROGEN NARCOSIS

Nitrogen narcosis, also known as rapture of the deep or inert gas narcosis, is development of intoxication due to increased partial pressure of nitrogen in compressed air at increased depth. Nitrogen narcosis is important to divers because it causes anesthetic-like euphoria, overconfidence, and deterioration in judgment and cognition, all of which can lead to serious errors in diving techniques, accidents, and drowning. Many divers have died as a consequence of nitrogen narcosis.

During the 1930s, Behnke and associates[13,14] first suggested that mood changes described by divers breathing compressed air at 200 fsw were caused by a high inspired P_{N_2}. Much has been learned since that time, and in-depth analysis of inert gas narcosis

has been provided by Bennett[16-18] and recently reviewed by Clark.[58]

Although the exact mechanism of inert gas narcosis is not known, the intoxicating effect of nitrogen is believed to be similar to the effects of gaseous anesthetics. According to currently accepted theory, alteration in electrical properties of cellular membranes is affected by absorption of gas molecules into their lipid component. The theory is supported by the observation that the greater the lipid solubility of a given gas, the greater is its narcotic potency. Thus, higher partial pressures of pure nitrogen are required to produce an anesthetic effect than is the case with nitrous oxide, the effects of which can be achieved by much lower partial pressures; nitrous oxide is much more soluble in lipid than is nitrogen. The lack of narcotic effect of helium is in accord with its low lipid solubility. Indeed, substitution of helium for nitrogen as the inert gas in the diver's breathing gas prevents nitrogen narcosis and is the main reason helium-oxygen mixtures are used for deep diving. In experimental rats, the activities of interneuronal $GABA_A$ receptors are desensitized during exposure to high partial pressures of nitrogen.[177] The actual mechanism of nitrogen narcosis is probably multifactorial.

Typically, a scuba diver breathing compressed air develops symptoms of nitrogen narcosis at depths between 21 and 31 msw (70 and 100 fsw). These symptoms include light-headedness, loss of fine sensory discrimination, giddiness, and euphoria. Symptoms progressively worsen at deeper depths. At depths over 46 msw (150 fsw), a diver becomes severely intoxicated, presenting with increasingly poor judgment and impaired reasoning, overconfidence, and slowed reflexes. At depths of 76 to 91 msw (250 to 300 fsw), auditory and visual hallucinations may occur, along with feelings of impending blackout. Most divers lose consciousness when they reach a depth of 122 msw (400 fsw).

Of note, individual and diurnal variability occur in the depth of onset and severity of symptoms in nitrogen narcosis. Oceanographic parameters, such as visibility and light penetration, can affect the onset or severity of narcosis. Also, some degree of acclimatization allows experienced divers to work more safely at greater depths than can inexperienced divers. Nonetheless, nitrogen narcosis is a major problem for all compressed-air divers at depths greater than 31 msw (100 fsw). This is one of the reasons why it is recommended that recreational divers not dive deeper than 39 msw (130 fsw).

Treatment of nitrogen narcosis simply requires ascent to a shallower depth (usually < 21 to 31 msw [70 to 100 fsw]), where symptoms promptly clear. Of course, the condition is prevented by avoiding deep dives. In commercial diving, where there may be good reasons to dive deeper than 31 msw (100 fsw), the problem is prevented by using heliox. In general, the effects of inert gas narcosis resolve by decreasing the partial pressure of the inert gas. However, there is evidence to indicate that some of the symptoms of nitrogen narcosis can be persistent. Measures of critical flicker fusion frequency (a measure of visual acuity) remained significantly altered 30 minutes after a single dive to 30 msw (97 fsw).[7] Symptoms were reversed by treatment with 100% oxygen, suggesting that some of the neurologic alterations caused by nitrogen narcosis may persist in a manner similar to delayed recovery from anesthetics.

OXYGEN TOXICITY

Although oxygen is essential for most life on Earth, it becomes a poison at elevated partial pressures. Oxygen toxicity in divers can affect either the CNS or pulmonary system. Understanding oxygen effects is necessary for safe diving operations. A complete discussion of the complex pathophysiology of oxygen toxicity is beyond the scope of this chapter. Thorough reviews of oxygen under pressure for diving and hyperbaric exposures are available.[38,57]

Inspired high P_{O_2} occurs in diving in two ways. Breathing 100% oxygen underwater or in a hyperbaric chamber is one. The second results from Dalton's law of partial pressures. If a normal 21% oxygen gas mixture is breathed at 10 ATA (300 fsw), an inspired P_{O_2} of 2.1 ATA is generated, which is equivalent to breathing 100% oxygen at 36 fsw. Again, it is the partial pressure of a gas that determines its biologic effects.

Pulmonary Oxygen Toxicity

Retrolental fibroplasia in premature infants and pulmonary oxygen toxicity in adults are well-known problems associated with use of therapeutic oxygen. Pulmonary oxygen toxicity is induced by breathing above-normal, but relatively low, Po_2 for prolonged periods. The limit for indefinite exposure without demonstrable lung damage is generally considered to be a Po_2 of approximately 0.5 ATA. On a time-dose curve, it is generally considered safe to breathe 100% oxygen at 1 ATA for up to about 20 hours, or at 2 ATA for up to 6 hours. This time can be lengthened significantly by using intermittent exposures, such as interspersing a 5-minute air break between every 20 minutes of oxygen breathing.[138] At 2.8 to 3 ATA (60 to 66 fsw), at which depth 100% oxygen is used to treat DCS and gas gangrene, pulmonary oxygen toxicity is rarely a problem, because CNS manifestations usually intervene before sufficient time elapses to induce pulmonary damage. Pulmonary oxygen toxicity and its relationship to professional diving have been reviewed.[284] Using hyperbaric oxygen according to U.S. Navy Treatment Table 6 (used to treat DCS; see Chapter 72, Figure 72-11) does not produce clinical manifestations of pulmonary oxygen toxicity. However, animal studies involving more extreme oxygen exposures have shown a pathologic sequence of alveolar capillary endothelial damage, with increased permeability leading to pulmonary edema and hemorrhage. Variations in susceptibility are seen among species, but interruption of exposure usually results in reversal of pathologic changes.[59]

The most common clinical manifestation of pulmonary oxygen toxicity is substernal discomfort on inhalation. If exposure continues, this can progress to severe burning substernal pain and persistent cough. Reduction of inspired Po_2 to 0.21 to 0.5 ATA usually results in prompt relief. Severe cases of pulmonary oxygen toxicity may require endotracheal intubation and positive end-expiratory pressure ventilation to achieve adequate arterial oxygenation at the required lower partial pressures of inspired oxygen.

Central Nervous System Oxygen Toxicity

During the 1880s, the French physiologist Paul Bert described convulsions in animals breathing 100% oxygen at elevated chamber pressures. Behnke and others observed the same phenomenon in humans in the 1930s. Donald's classic observations on divers were published in 1947 and provide much of the current knowledge on predisposing factors and clinical manifestations of CNS oxygen toxicity.[87,88]

In brief, Donald found that at a given duration and pressure of oxygen, a diver in the water was more susceptible to oxygen-induced seizures than was the same diver in a warm, dry hyperbaric chamber. Based on this observation, a limit of 7.6 msw (25 fsw) was imposed for military special operations dives using 100% oxygen. Donald found a wide variation in oxygen tolerance among subjects exposed to the same conditions, as well as variability in oxygen tolerance in the same diver from day to day. Most people can tolerate breathing 100% oxygen for 30 minutes at rest at 2.8 ATA in a dry chamber, although some present with toxicity at this exposure.

Common symptoms and signs of CNS poisoning are shown in Box 71-4. Unfortunately, some people may have no warning symptoms, and the first manifestation of CNS oxygen toxicity may be a generalized seizure. If an oxygen-induced seizure occurs underwater, there is a high risk for drowning and death. With increased use of RBs and mixed-gas technical diving, oxygen toxicity is a serious consideration. Apart from physical injury or drowning, an oxygen seizure does not produce harmful or residual effects. CNS oxygen toxicity due to HBOT is discussed in Chapter 72.

CONTAMINATED BREATHING GAS (CARBON MONOXIDE POISONING, HYPERCARBIA)

As breathing-gas cylinders are pressurized or filled, the sea level partial pressure of each gaseous component is multiplied.

BOX 71-4 Typical Manifestations of Central Nervous System Oxygen Poisoning

Apprehension
Feeling of air hunger
Sweating
Nausea
Focal muscle twitching
Isolated jerking of a limb
Auditory changes (such as "hearing bells ringing")
Tunnel vision
Diaphragmatic flutter
Convulsion

Therefore, any contaminant in the air source can potentially become dangerous to the diver at the elevated pressure found underwater. Compressor motors must be free of oil that could be pumped into tanks; otherwise, oil mist in the air may cause the diver to suffer lipoid pneumonitis.[161]

Compressed-air inlets should always be situated so that they avoid engine exhaust from the compressor, parking lots, or other combustion sources that produce carbon monoxide. Because carbon monoxide is colorless, odorless, and tasteless, the diver cannot detect it unless it is accompanied by other contaminants. The first warning of carbon monoxide poisoning may be headache, nausea, or dizziness during the dive. Examination at the surface may show lethargy, mental dullness, and nonspecific neurologic deficits, which may be confused with those accompanying DCS or air embolism. The cherry red skin color often mentioned in standard medical texts is rarely observed in carbon monoxide poisoning. Holt and Weaver[143a] reported a case of carbon monoxide poisoning in a commercial diver who was initially diagnosed and treated for presumed AGE. Fortunately, the treatment of choice for serious acute carbon monoxide poisoning, DCS, and air embolism is HBOT.

Another potential breathing gas problem involves carbon dioxide. Alveolar partial pressure of carbon dioxide ($PaCO_2$) reflects the arterial PCO_2; therefore, even as ambient pressure increases at depth, the $PaCO_2$ remains constant at approximately 40 mm Hg unless environmental or physiologic changes occur. Hypercapnia can occur because of increased PCO_2 in the breathing gas or decreased pulmonary ventilation. Unless there is regulator malfunction or contaminated breathing gas, hypercapnia is exceptionally rare in open-circuit scuba diving. Hypercapnia can occur in helmet or chamber diving if these closed spaces are inadequately ventilated or the breathing gas becomes contaminated by carbon dioxide, and in closed-circuit scuba diving (i.e., using an RB) if there is failure of the carbon dioxide–absorbent (scrubbing) material. It is believed that hypercarbia was the primary cause of David Shaw's death at Boesmansgat cave in South Africa in January 2005.[201] Shaw was attempting to recover the remains of 20-year-old Deon Dreyer, who had drowned in the cave on Mount Carmel farm more than 10 years earlier, from a depth of 276 m (905 feet).

At sea level, a concentration of 5% to 6% inspired carbon dioxide leads to dyspnea, increased respiratory rate, and mental confusion. At 10% inspired carbon dioxide, pulse rate and blood pressure may fall to the point that unconsciousness occurs. With prolonged exposure to 12% to 14% inspired carbon dioxide, such that the $PaCO_2$ exceeds 150 mm Hg, central respiratory and cardiac depression can be fatal.

HYPERVENTILATION AND SHALLOW WATER BLACKOUT

Hypocapnia can result from hyperventilation during or before diving. The well-known symptoms of hyperventilation, dizziness, and paresthesias around the mouth and in the distal extremities have been postulated to cause unconsciousness among divers, but whether this actually occurs is unclear. In contrast, unconsciousness associated with hyperventilation before a breath-hold dive is caused by hypoxia, rather than hypocapnia.

BOX 71-5 Causes of Unconsciousness in Divers

Breath-Hold Divers
Underwater hypoxemia after hyperventilation before the dive (shallow water blackout)
Near drowning

Divers Using Compressed-Gas Equipment
Hypoxic breathing gas
Contaminated breathing gas (such as carbon monoxide)
Equipment failure or exhaustion of breathing gas
Near drowning
Inert gas narcosis
Oxygen toxicity
Pulmonary barotrauma with arterial gas embolism

Divers Using Rebreathing Equipment
Carbon dioxide toxicity
Oxygen toxicity
Hypoxia

In what is commonly described as *shallow water blackout,* a diver hyperventilates before a dive, lowering alveolar PCO_2 to 20 to 30 mm Hg. However, because hemoglobin is nearly saturated with oxygen during normal respiration, there is little gain in arterial PO_2 by hyperventilating. In an underwater swim, even in a shallow swimming pool, exercise-induced hypoxia sufficient to cause unconsciousness may occur before arterial PCO_2 reaccumulates to provide sufficient stimulus to breathe.[12]

In a deep breath-hold dive, the problem is compounded by the effect of increased pressure. In addition to the initial depression of arterial PCO_2 secondary to hyperventilation, elevations occur in alveolar and arterial PO_2. During the dive, these serve to suppress the respiratory response to hypercarbia. During descent in the water, $PaCO_2$ increases from the increased pressure, but after oxygen consumption at depth, depressurization on return to the surface causes a dramatic drop in alveolar and arterial PCO_2. Even if $PaCO_2$ rises to the stimulatory breakpoint during ascent, hypoxemia may cause unconsciousness and near drowning. An expansion of Edmonds' most common causes of unconsciousness in divers is presented in Box 71-5.[101] Breath-hold diving fatalities average 3 per 10,000 divers annually.[191]

DECOMPRESSION SICKNESS

In the mid19th century, tunnel and bridge workers who labored in caissons pressurized with compressed air were sometimes observed to suffer joint pains, paralysis, and other medical problems after leaving the high-pressure caissons. The condition was not understood and became dubbed caisson disease or compressed-air illness.[236] Of course, these early high-pressure workers were experiencing the same symptoms that were later observed in divers and aviators, and that we now know to be decompression sickness (DCS).

For many decades, caisson disease remained a medical curiosity, but because of its occurrence in increasingly important areas of activity in the 20th century, considerable research has been directed to better understanding its causes and finding effective treatment.

DCS is caused by formation of bubbles of inert gas (e.g., nitrogen) within both intravascular and extravascular spaces after reductions in ambient pressure. This may occur in divers during or after decompression from being underwater; in persons in a caisson or hyperbaric chamber in which pressures are greater than at sea level; or in aviators, astronauts, or hypobaric (high-altitude) chamber workers who travel rapidly from sea level to pressures less than 0.5 ATA. DCS is also a major concern in commercial divers who breathe heliox and then switch breathing gases to nitrox; bubbles can form in the absence of a decrease in ambient pressure because of local tissue supersaturation due to a change in breathing gas.

CAUSE

Although DCS is a topic of considerable research and discussion among divers and diving medicine practitioners, it is fortunately rare. Based on DAN's Project Dive Exploration data, a DCS incidence summary based on 137,451 dive profiles collected from 1995 to 2008 resulted in a diagnosis of 41 cases.[95] Profiles were collected from various diving environments. Deep-wreck divers in the North Atlantic had a DCS incidence of 0.181%, whereas the incidence among warm-water live-aboard divers was 0.006%.[96]

To understand the cause of DCS, one must appreciate the temporal relationship between inert gas uptake and elimination. Earth's atmosphere is composed of 78% nitrogen and 21% oxygen; it is the presence of this inert nitrogen that forms the crux of the DCS problem. If it were safe for a diver to breathe 100% oxygen while underwater, one could prevent DCS because oxygen is rapidly metabolized by the body, and for all practical purposes does not contribute to bubble formation on ascent. Unfortunately, breathing pure oxygen at increased atmospheric pressure causes CNS toxicity. To prevent this, divers breathe an inert gas diluent (e.g., nitrogen) and thus must be concerned with inert gas (nitrogen) absorption and potential bubble formation during decompression.

The partial pressures of inspired gases increase as a diver descends. At 4 ATA (99 fsw), the absolute pressure is 3040 mm Hg (see Table 71-2), 79% of which is nitrogen (2400 mm Hg, as compared with 600 mm Hg PN_2 at sea level). Accounting for water vapor and carbon dioxide, the resulting alveolar partial pressure of nitrogen (PAN_2) at this depth is approximately 2360 mm Hg. This PAN_2 is rapidly reflected across the alveolar-capillary membrane to the arterial blood, where (according to Henry's law) nitrogen becomes physically dissolved in the blood. Henry's law states that the amount of gas dissolved in a liquid at any given temperature is a function of the partial pressure of the gas in contact with the liquid. Thus, the amount of nitrogen absorbed by tissues during a dive is a function of depth (pressure) and time.

PATHOPHYSIOLOGY

DCS is a multisystem disorder caused by the separation of gas bubbles in the body's tissues as a result of inadequate decompression time, leading to an excessive degree of gas formation. Rapid decompression, due to either a rapid decrease in ambient atmospheric pressure from rapid ascent or omission of decompression stops, causes inert gas (nitrogen) to come out of solution and form bubbles in tissue and venous blood. Conceptually, DCS is the same illness whether it occurs in high-altitude aviators or deep-sea divers, although there are some differences in the symptoms of the disease, depending on whether it is caused by hyperbaric or hypobaric exposure.

Paul Bert first described bubbles in the bloodstream in experimental animals after decompression in 1878.[21] Bubbles form within tissues in which the inert gas partial pressure exceeds the pressure within the tissue. It is believed that bubble formation is initiated at sites of stable gas micronuclei.[282] The physiologic sequelae of bubble formation in tissue and venous blood are myriad. These effects include cellular distention and rupture; mechanical stretching of tendons or ligaments, producing pain; and intravascular or intralymphatic occlusion, resulting in congestive ischemia and infarction, or lymphedema. Boycott and colleagues[35] described a method for prevention of compressed-air illness in divers when a pressure reduction ratio not exceeding 2:1 is observed.

Venous Gas Emboli

The presence of bubbles in tissues or venous circulation does not imply DCS. Venous gas emboli (VGEs) probably originate in extravascular tissue and enter the bloodstream, where they enlarge. These bubbles travel to the right heart and are trapped by the pulmonary capillaries when the gas diffuses into alveoli. VGEs can be observed in the veins or right heart after diving using ultrasound or echocardiography.[94,266] VGEs can be found in varying quantities in some divers with no symptoms of DCS. There is no direct correlation of bubbles with DCS; however, their presence is thought by some researchers to be a marker of decompression stress.[118,183] Recent data suggest that there are some individuals who are more prone to developing VGEs after diving, leading to the concept of "bubble-prone" and

TABLE 71-5 Common Symptoms and Signs of Decompression Sickness

Condition	Symptoms	Signs
Musculoskeletal decompression sickness, limb bends	Severe joint pain, single joint or multiple joints involved, paresthesia or dysesthesia around the joint, lymphedema (uncommon)	Tenderness, which may be temporarily relieved by local pressure with a blood pressure cuff; pain worsened by movement of the joint
Neurologic decompression sickness		
Spinal cord	Back pain, girdling abdominal pain, extremity heaviness or weakness, paralysis, paresthesia of extremities, fecal incontinence, urine retention	Hyperesthesia or hypoesthesia, paresis, anal sphincter weakness, loss of bulbocavernosus reflex, urinary bladder distention
Brain	Visual loss, scotomata, headache, dysphasia, confusion	Visual field deficit, spotty motor or sensory deficits, disorientation or mental dullness
Fatigue	Profound generalized heaviness or fatigue	May precede signs of other forms
Cutaneous manifestations	Intense pruritus	No visible signs, mottling, local or generalized hyperemia or marbled skin (cutis marmorata)
Chokes	Dyspnea, substernal pain that is worsened on deep inhalation, nonproductive cough	Cyanosis, tachypnea, tachycardia
Vasomotor decompression sickness (decompression shock)	Weakness, sweating, unconsciousness	Hypotension, tachycardia, pallor, mottling, hemoconcentration, decreased urine output
Inner ear (vestibular) decompression sickness	Tinnitus, vertigo, nausea, vomiting	Ataxia, possible nystagmus and positive Romberg's test, acute sensorineural hearing loss

"bubble-resistant" individuals.[55,56,118] Because VGEs occur much more frequently than does DCS and are easily detected even in safe dives, Doppler bubble detection is used to develop models of DCS, for evaluating safe diving profiles, and for diving medicine research.

In some circumstances, VGEs can enter the arterial circulation through a right-to-left shunt, such as a patent foramen ovale (PFO), atrial septal defect, or intrapulmonary arteriovenous anastomoses,[187] or by overwhelming the pulmonary capillary filtration system. Arterialized VGEs can produce symptoms of AGE and may play a role in certain types of DCS, particularly involving the skin, inner ear, and CNS.[202,208,277,297] Further research on PFO and diving is discussed below.

Biochemical Effects of Bubbles

Intravascular bubbles cause multiple biophysical effects at the blood-bubble surface interface because bubbles are viewed by the immune system as foreign matter and incite an inflammatory reaction. One step in the process is activation of the Hageman factor, which in turn activates intrinsic clotting, kinin, and complement systems, producing platelet activation, cellular clumping, lipid embolization, increased vascular permeability, interstitial edema, and microvascular sludging. The overall effects are decreased tissue perfusion and ischemia.

The pathophysiologic changes associated with scuba diving and DCS have been extensively studied but remain poorly understood. More recent attention focuses on the roles played by cellular and biochemical changes involved in inflammation, oxidative stress, and vascular endothelial cell activation. Scuba diving without DCS results in physiologic consequences that include increased oxidative stress, impaired endothelial function, platelet activation, neutrophil activation, and increase in microparticles.[222,239,267,271,272] How these factors contribute to DCS is unclear. Gas bubbles are associated with platelet aggregation.[6] Complement activation by bubbles has been reported in vitro and in vivo in animals and proposed as a mechanism for DCS in humans.[142,287,288] Bubbles cause endothelial disruption, leading to extravasation of plasma into the interstitium, causing an increase in hematocrit level.[31,221] Leukocytes adhere to bubbles and denuded endothelium. Microparticle increase and production may play a role in neutrophil activation, resulting in vascular leak and DCS in mice and humans.[270,273,303] Nitric oxide is now thought to play a role in bubble formation.[300] Endothelial nitric oxide, an important vasodilator with antiatherogenic properties, can attenuate bubble formation and DCS incidence, most likely by reducing gaseous nuclei from which bubbles form. Activation of heat shock proteins may lead to protection from bubble-induced injury during decompression.[24,113,194]

Clinical Manifestations

The clinical manifestations of DCS are protean (Table 71-5), with neurologic and musculoskeletal systems most often affected. Symptoms and signs of DCS include joint pain, cutaneous rashes, neurologic dysfunction, pulmonary edema (chokes), and shock; death may follow. DCS is often categorized as type I and type II, with type I referring to the mild forms of DCS (cutaneous, lymphatic, and musculoskeletal) and type II including the neurologic and other serious forms (pulmonary chokes and inner ear DCS). Some investigators have advocated using type III DCS to refer to combined AGE and DCS with neurologic symptoms.[216] However, this term should not be used; *biphasic decompression illness* accurately describes the presentation of AGE and DCS occurring together.

Although categorization of DCS as types I and II is firmly entrenched in the literature, its use is not advocated. It is clinically more meaningful to refer to the body systems affected when discussing patients with DCS, especially in light of the growing awareness that all cases of DCS must be considered serious and treated vigorously.

Musculoskeletal Decompression Sickness

Musculoskeletal DCS, or *the bends*, is development of pain in and around major joints after diving or other hyperbaric or hypobaric exposures. It is the most common manifestation of DCS, occurring in approximately 70% of patients.[193,236,244] This form of DCS is often referred to as limb bends, joint bends, or pain-only bends.

The term *bends* originated at the beginning of the 20th century, when caisson workers on the Brooklyn Bridge who were suffering from DCS of the hips were noted to walk stiffly, bending forward at the hips.[236] Coworkers would describe the stricken men as walking as if they were trying to do the *Grecian bend*, a term for the forward-bending, stiff-at-the-hips way that stylish women of the day would walk because of their tight corsets. Over time, the term became shortened to just bends.

The shoulders and elbows are the joints most often affected by DCS in scuba divers, but any joint may be involved. Hips and knees are most commonly affected in saturation divers, caisson workers, and aviators. The reason for the different anatomic predilection is not known.

The pain of joint bends is usually described as "boring" or a dull ache deep within the joint, although it may also be characterized as sharp or throbbing. It is sometimes described as "tearing" or feeling like tendinitis or bursitis. It may radiate to surrounding areas. Movement of the joint can worsen the pain, so the joint is usually held immobile. An area of vague numbness or dysesthesia may surround the affected joint, but this typically does not conform to any anatomic distribution and should not be confused with neurologic involvement. There also may be erythema around the joint, and the joint may be mildly swollen. The joint may also be tender to touch.

Sometimes divers will complain of having a "niggle" after a dive. *Niggle* is a British colloquialism referring to mild pain in a single joint that improves 10 to 15 minutes after the onset of pain and then disappears without treatment. Whether niggles should be treated with recompression is controversial, but the safest approach is to treat them with at least the protocol in U.S. Navy Treatment Table 5.

Differentiating between limb bends and trauma or other causes of joint pain may be aided by inflation of a sphygmomanometer cuff placed around the joint to 150 to 250 mm Hg.[247] If the pain is due to DCS, inflation of the cuff may immediately relieve the pain by reducing the gas volume in tendons and ligaments. This relief suggests that the mechanism of pain is gas expansion (bubbles) in tendons and ligaments, which stretches nerve endings. The pain of limb bends recurs when the cuff is deflated. The test is helpful when it is positive, but lack of a response cannot be used to rule out the presence of DCS; this must be done with a "test of pressure" in a hyperbaric chamber. Importantly, most often there may be neither abnormal physical signs (other than splinting or stiffness from pain) nor abnormal radiographic findings.

Limb bends pain alone is not immediately threatening to life or function, but indicates that bubbling may be occurring in venous blood. Often, patients who begin with musculoskeletal DCS and are not treated progress to more serious forms of DCS. In addition, it is impossible to completely exclude subtle neurologic signs in a field setting. Likewise, as discussed later, untreated DCS may lead to osteonecrosis of major joints.

Fatigue

Profound fatigue that is out of proportion to the activity performed underwater, or otherwise while under increased atmospheric pressure, may be an early manifestation of DCS. Although its cause is unknown, a feeling of severe fatigue after diving demands careful evaluation for other manifestations of DCS.

Cutaneous Decompression Sickness (Skin Bends)

DCS may present with a variety of cutaneous manifestations, including scarlatiniform, erysipeloid, or mottled rashes; pruritus; and formication. Occasionally, localized swelling or peau d'orange may result from lymphatic obstruction, and rarely, an entire limb may become edematous.

Skin manifestations are relatively uncommon and, in and of themselves, are usually not serious. However, mottling or marbling of the skin *(cutis marmorata)* is often a harbinger of more severe DCS (Figure 71-12). The exact physiologic basis of the mottled skin lesion is unknown. Skin bends should be easily distinguished from cutaneous barotrauma, "wetsuit dermati-

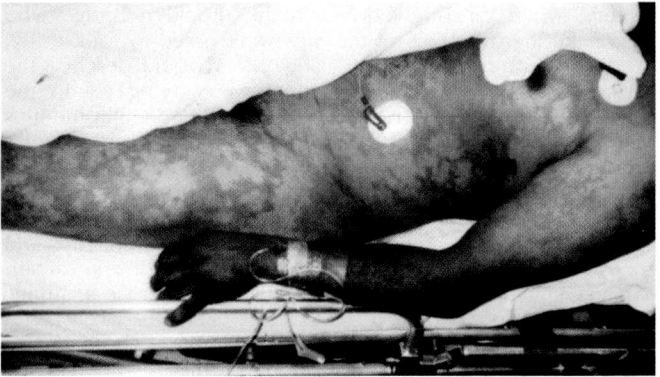

FIGURE 71-12 Cutis marmorata is mottling of the skin seen in severe cases of decompression sickness.

tis,"[170,250] marine envenomation, or other skin rashes often seen in divers.

Itches, or "the creeps," is a type of skin bends seen during decompression in hyperbaric chamber workers when the skin is exposed to the high PN_2 in compressed air. This is a highly pruritic skin reaction most intensely felt on body parts exposed to the compressed air. The sensation is often described as feeling like ants crawling over one's body.

In hyperbaric chambers, inert gas from the external environment is absorbed directly into skin, and itches represent bubble formation in the skin during decompression. The concentrations of dissolved gases in ocean water are essentially constant at all depths, so the skin is not exposed to elevated partial pressures of inert gases underwater.

Pulmonary Decompression Sickness (Chokes)

The chokes is an unusual but very serious form of DCS characterized by burning substernal pain (especially on inhalation), cyanosis, dyspnea, and nonproductive cough. Animal studies have demonstrated gas bubbles or foam in the pulmonary arteries, right atrium, and right ventricle after unsafe decompression. The chokes probably represents massive pulmonary gas embolism with mechanical obstruction of the pulmonary vascular bed by bubbles. Typically, symptoms of pulmonary venous air embolization begin when 10% or more of the pulmonary vascular bed is obstructed. Patients with the chokes can progress rapidly to profound shock or neurologic DCS. The specific clinical and radiographic manifestations of the chokes are similar to those seen with VGEs from other causes.[162]

Symptoms of VGEs include air hunger, dyspnea, cough, and chest pain. Findings may include pallor, diaphoresis, tachypnea, tachycardia, hypotension, cyanosis, expiratory wheezing, neurologic signs, and a mill-wheel heart murmur. Victims may also exhibit increased central venous or pulmonary artery pressure, electrocardiographic changes of ischemia or cor pulmonale, decreased end-tidal carbon dioxide fraction, and precordial Doppler sounds of circulating gas bubbles. Echocardiography may show gas bubbles in the right atrium and ventricle. Rarely, air may be visualized in the main pulmonary artery on chest radiographs; this is pathognomonic for pulmonary air embolism.[146,162,219]

Neurologic Decompression Sickness

Neurologic impairment may occur as the sole manifestation of DCS or as part of a larger dysbaric syndrome. Neurologic DCS is manifested by myriad symptoms and signs because of the random nature by which DCS affects the nervous system. Although any level of the CNS may be affected, the most commonly involved site in divers is the spinal cord, specifically the lower thoracic and lumbar regions. Although much less frequently affected than the CNS, the peripheral nervous system also may be involved.[150]

Based on military experience, neurologic DCS was believed to occur in only 10% to 20% of DCS cases,[244] but neurologic manifestations of DCS have been found in 50% to 60% of scuba diving casualties treated in Hawaii[105,153] and have been reported in similarly high frequencies in other populations of sport divers.[74,84]

Classically, dysbaric spinal cord injury occurs in the lower thoracic, lumbar, and sacral portions of the cord, producing low back pain, subjective "heaviness" in the legs, paraplegia or paraparesis, lower extremity paresthesia or dysesthesia, and sometimes bladder or anal sphincter dysfunction. General malaise or fatigue is often noted as well. Involvement of the cervical and thoracic cord may cause chest or abdominal pain and weakness or sensory disturbances in the upper extremities. Absence of the bulbocavernosus reflex, elicited by gently squeezing and pulling the glans penis to seek reflex contraction of the anal sphincter, often foretells a poor prognosis, as does absence of the superficial anal reflex, which can be elicited in the male or female by stroking the perianal region.

The mechanism of spinal cord DCS is multifactorial, involving autochthonous inert gas bubble formation in the cord[116,225] and in the epidural vertebral venous plexus (Batson's plexus), with resulting congestive infarction of the spinal cord.[132] There are other mechanisms that are not well understood.[140,225]

DCS of the brain produces a variety of symptoms, most of which are indistinguishable from AGE. These include dizziness, vertigo, altered mentation or level of consciousness, generalized weakness, and visual deficits (e.g., diplopia, scotoma, visual field defects, and blindness). Involvement of the cerebellum or inner ear may produce ataxia and loss of balance.

Inner Ear or Vestibular Decompression Sickness

The *staggers* is another classic DCS syndrome. In this case, the inner ear is primarily affected; the name derives from the unsteady gait that results from vestibular damage. Manifestations include dizziness, vertigo, nystagmus, tinnitus, nausea, and vomiting. In contrast to inner ear barotrauma, which generally has a favorable prognosis, inner ear DCS carries a high risk for residual inner ear damage despite appropriate treatment.

Inner ear DCS has been most often seen in saturation divers, when there is a rapid ascent on heliox, or when switching gases on ascent during very deep dives. However, there are increasing reports of inner ear DCS in technical and sport divers. A PFO has been associated with inner ear DCS, suggesting that shunted VGEs may play a role in inner ear injury.[202,277]

Vasomotor Decompression Sickness

Vasomotor DCS, or *decompression shock,* is a rare, life-threatening form of DCS. The pathogenesis of this shock syndrome is not completely understood. It is believed to be caused by a rapid shift of fluid from intravascular to extravascular spaces secondary to diffuse bubble embolization, ischemia, and hypoxia.[54] Hypotension may also result from massive venous air embolization of the lungs.

Despite vigorous intravenous fluid replacement, the hypotension of decompression shock may not respond until recompression is undertaken. Unfortunately, the condition is highly lethal, and most patients do not survive long enough to undergo recompression unless a hyperbaric chamber is immediately available.

LONG-TERM SEQUELAE OF DECOMPRESSION SICKNESS

Although DCS is the most overt manifestation of inadequate decompression after diving, it has now been clearly established that there may be long-term sequelae of diving related to inadequate decompression, even if the diver never manifests overt DCS. The most described problem is dysbaric osteonecrosis.

Dysbaric Osteonecrosis

Dysbaric osteonecrosis is a form of avascular or aseptic necrosis of bone associated with pressure changes. The major joints (shoulders, elbows, hips, and knees) are most often affected, although any bone can be involved.[53,104,195]

Dysbaric osteonecrosis was first recognized in compressed-air workers in the early 1900s.[224] Since then, its incidence in professional divers has been found to range from less than 1% to more than 80%, depending on the age of the diver and type of diving. Its occurrence correlates well with deep diving, decompression diving, occurrence of DCS, and missed decompression.[77,104,147,195,286] Most diving medicine experts consider dysbaric osteonecrosis a long-term sequela of inadequate decompression.

Fossil evidence of avascular necrosis has been found in marine mosasaurs and plesiosaurs of the Cretaceous period, suggesting that at least some of these extinct giant marine lizards dived deeply.[246] Likewise, although modern marine mammals were previously thought to be immune to DCS, it has been recently found that sperm whales, which dive to depths exceeding 3048 msw (10,000 fsw) and stay underwater for as long as an hour, also suffer from dysbaric osteonecrosis.

Dysbaric Retinopathy

Infrequently, DCS affects the eyes, producing a wide array of acute ophthalmic effects, including homonymous hemianopsia,

cortical blindness, central retinal artery occlusion, retinal hemorrhage, nystagmus, convergence insufficiency, and optic neuropathy.[41,42] Long-term ophthalmic findings in divers have been observed.

A retinal fluorescein angiography survey of asymptomatic divers found a higher incidence of retinal pigment epithelium than in nondivers, and various capillary changes at the fovea.[237] The significance of these abnormalities is unclear because none of the divers had visual loss. Similarly, the cause of such changes is unclear, although they are postulated to be the result of small bubble microembolization.

DIAGNOSIS

As with AGE, diagnosis of DCS is clinical and based on history of exposure to increased atmospheric pressure and subsequent development of characteristic symptoms and signs. The majority of patients with DCS become symptomatic in the first hour after surfacing from a dive, with most of the remainder noticing symptoms within 3 hours after diving. The majority of all symptoms manifest within 24 hours after diving, unless they appear as a result of further decompression, such as high-altitude exposure.

A variety of laboratory abnormalities may be demonstrated in DCS, but most have little or no usefulness in the immediate management of patients. However, two tests that may be useful are urine specific gravity and hematocrit; intravascular volume depletion and hemoconcentration are common in serious DCS because of increased vascular permeability caused by endothelial damage and release of kinins. The results of these tests can help guide replacement fluid therapy. The hematocrit percentage is commonly in the high 50s or 60s in serious DCS. Low serum albumin is reported in cases of neurologic DCS due to increased vascular permeability; however, sensitivity of hypoalbuminemia as a predictor of DCS is very low.[120]

As with laboratory tests, radiographic evaluation of patients with suspected DCS may yield various findings, but the radiographs are rarely useful in acute management of the patient. Bone radiographs of patients with acute joint bends do not show abnormalities. Months to years later, they may demonstrate findings of dysbaric osteonecrosis. Noncardiogenic pulmonary edema may be seen on chest radiographs of persons with pulmonary or vasomotor DCS.

Both CT and MRI have been used to evaluate neurologic DCS injury, although conventional CT has poor sensitivity for early lesions and is unable to image spinal cord lesions.[143,155] Limited clinical data support the feasibility and efficacy of MRI in these conditions,[119,181,265,289] especially when intracranial injury is suspected, although the urgency of obtaining HBOT makes these modalities useful primarily for postrecompression evaluation of residual deficits. Neither imaging nor laboratory data should be used to confirm the diagnosis of DCS or to decide if a diver with suspected DCS needs HBOT.

TREATMENT

All persons with suspected DCS should be referred to a hyperbaric treatment facility as quickly as possible because HBOT is the primary and essential treatment for this condition. The physician must have a high index of suspicion when diagnosing DCS, because the often-diverse manifestations of DCS may present a very confusing clinical picture. The history of the dive profile is helpful if the diver knowingly violated decompression procedures, but DCS may occur on dives that should be safe according to current decompression schedules.[1] In addition, the reported depth and time of the dive are often not accurate.

Management of DCS must begin as soon as the condition is suspected.[74] Divers may be far from a hyperbaric chamber when their symptoms develop, so treatment is often initiated in the field or at a general acute care facility. Supplemental oxygen at a high flow rate (10 L/min by nonrebreather face mask) should be administered as soon as possible, beginning on the dive boat or otherwise in the field and continued during transport, emergency department evaluation, and transfer to a hyperbaric

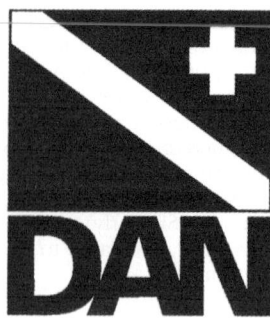

FIGURE 71-13 Logo for the Divers Alert Network. *(Courtesy Divers Alert Network.)*

treatment facility. Supplemental oxygen enhances the rate of resolution of inert gas bubbles and treats hypoxemia. Of equal importance is maintenance of intravascular volume to ensure capillary perfusion for elimination of microvascular inert gas bubbles and tissue oxygenation. Intravenous infusion of isotonic solution should be started and run at a flow rate sufficient to maintain urine output at 1 to 2 mL/kg/hr. If there is spinal cord involvement, an indwelling urinary catheter may be needed because of sacral nerve root dysfunction and urinary retention. Intractable vomiting or vertigo should be treated with appropriate parenteral agents. Diazepam has been quite effective in providing relief from the vertigo associated with inner ear DCS. Advanced life support measures should be undertaken appropriate to the patient's clinical condition.

Arrangements must be made for transfer to the nearest hyperbaric chamber. Because of the large number and frequently changing status of hyperbaric chambers, no list is provided here. To locate an active chamber, the reader is referred to the Divers Alert Network (DAN) (Figure 71-13).

Before a patient is transferred to the hyperbaric treatment facility, it is imperative to contact the chamber to determine its availability. The chamber may be out of service or already being used to treat another patient. The physician should never send a patient without first discussing the transfer with hyperbaric treatment personnel.

If airborne evacuation is required, it is critical to obtain an aircraft that can maintain sea level cabin pressurization during flight. Examples of such aircraft are the military C9 and C-130 Hercules, Learjet, and Cessna Citation. In the case of helicopters (which cannot be pressurized), the crew must maintain the lowest possible flight altitude, preferably never greater than 305 m (1000 feet) above the starting elevation. This is always problematic in evacuations from mountain lakes. All resuscitative measures must be maintained in flight.

At the hyperbaric treatment facility, one of several standard hyperbaric treatment protocols is followed. In a multilock compressed-air chamber, the patient and an attendant can be pressurized with compressed air, and the patient given 100% oxygen by face mask.

As with AGE, hyperbaric treatment of DCS has undergone significant evolution over the past two decades and is discussed in more detail in Chapter 72.

HBOT is most often successful, but the likelihood of success is difficult to predict for any given diver. In general, the sooner after the onset of symptoms that treatment begins, the better the outcome,[9] although treatment after delays of many hours, or even days, often results in full functional recovery. In one series of 92 sport scuba divers treated after a significant delay between the offending dive and start of hyperbaric treatment, 85% had good results when standard U.S. Navy treatment tables were followed.[74] Similar results were achieved in another series of 50 patients.[158] Even despite a delay of 48 hours or longer for HBOT, 76% of divers with DCS had full recovery.[131] Such treatment is usually given according to U.S. Navy Tables 5 and 6 (Figure 71-14). Any patient with neurologic or pulmonary DCS requires treatment with U.S. Navy Table 6 (see Figure 71-14B), with extension of

the hyperbaric oxygen periods, depending on how the patient responds.

Monoplace hyperbaric chambers are used to treat DCS and air embolism,[136,159] although the conventional wisdom is to use a multiplace chamber whenever possible because of the free access to the patient that is possible in these larger chambers and greater flexibility in possible treatment regimens.

U.S. Navy Treatment Table 7 is an option for serious DCS cases; however, this treatment table should be reserved for patients with major deficits because of its length and commitment of resources. The diver and attendant are held at 2.8 ATA for at least 12 hours, and longer if needed, with the patient breathing oxygen in 30-minute periods as tolerated. A final, slow, 32-hour decompression follows, regardless of the time spent at 2.8 ATA. Details of Table 7 are found in the *U.S. Navy Diving Manual.*[278]

Patients with DCS who have residual symptoms after their initial HBOT should receive repetitive treatments until symptoms have completely resolved or the patient shows no further improvement in response to two consecutive treatments. Most individuals need no more than 5 to 10 treatments. Treatments can be given daily or twice daily as shown in U.S. Navy Table 5, 6, or 9 (2-hour treatment at 2.4 ATA). A small number of patients have residual neurologic deficits that may either be permanent or improve gradually over 6 to 12 months.

Another potentially useful recommendation for dealing with recurrence of neurologic symptoms and signs after apparently successful HBOT of neurologic DCS has been advanced by Edmonds.[101] Frequent postrecompression recurrences of neurologic manifestations led him to institute multiple 30-minute,

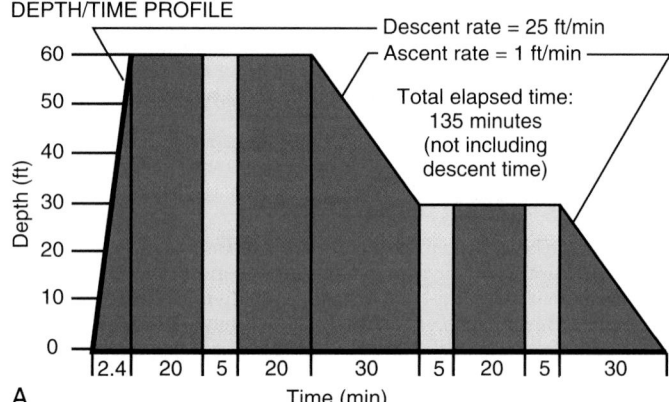

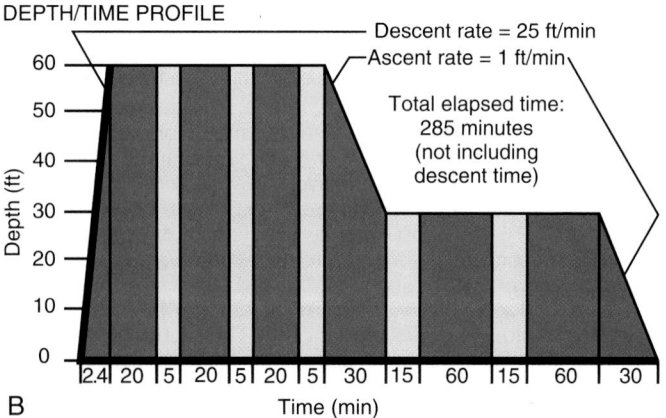

FIGURE 71-14 Examples of U.S. Navy decompression tables. *Dark shading* represents oxygen breathing; *light shading* represents air breathing. A, U.S. Navy Treatment Table 5, oxygen treatment of type 1 decompression sickness. B, U.S. Navy Treatment Table 6, oxygen treatment of type 2 decompression sickness. *(Modified from Department of the Navy: U.S. Navy diving manual, vol 2, rRv 2, Flagstaff, Arizona, 1988, Best Publishing.)*

sea-level, oxygen-breathing periods with 30-minute air breaks for 6 to 8 hours following treatment and observation in the hospital, rechecking the vital capacity frequently to detect and prevent pulmonary oxygen toxicity.

Remote treatment of DCS when access or transport to a recompression facility is not possible is controversial. Mild DCS (limp pain or rash) with no neurologic manifestations can be treated without recompression if HBOT is not possible. A consensus guideline for management of mild DCS in remote locations has been published.[203] In-water recompression has been used successfully for severe neurologic DCS in remote locations; however, in-water recompression carries a significant risk of drowning, hypothermia, hyperoxia, and dehydration. In-water recompression requires special training and equipment, and is beyond the scope of this chapter.[26-28,240,241,278]

Adjunctive Treatment

Corticosteroids. Although experimental proof of their efficacy is lacking, high-dose parenteral corticosteroids were widely used in the past as an adjunct to recompression treatment of both neurologic DCS and AGE. Anecdotal data suggesting that steroids were beneficial in combination with HBOT have been reported,[74,154,178] but there have been no published clinical series or controlled trials demonstrating their efficacy. In contrast, controlled studies of high-dose parenteral dexamethasone and methylprednisolone in DCS-affected dogs and pigs showed that use of glucocorticoids as an adjunct to conventional HBOT produced no benefit, and even suggested that the animals treated with steroids had inferior outcomes.[91,115]

Anticoagulants and Nonsteroidal Antiinflammatory Drugs. Because intravenous bubbles can induce platelet adherence, antiplatelet agents, such as aspirin and nonsteroidal antiinflammatory drugs (NSAIDs), have been tried prophylactically and therapeutically, but without success. Although use of tenoxicam has been shown to decrease the total number of treatments required for DCS, the outcomes of the divers in the control and treatment groups were unchanged.[19] Therefore, NSAIDs and aspirin are not routinely recommended as adjuncts for treatment of DCS. Of note, divers who are paralyzed from DCS should be treated (e.g., with subcutaneous low-molecular-weight heparin) to prevent thromboembolic disease.

PREVENTION

Ever since DCS was first recognized, efforts have been directed at prevention. Such efforts have used all manner of interventions, but to date the only proved way to prevent DCS is to limit the time a diver spends at increased pressure (depth) and to ensure that decompression from increased pressure is sufficiently slow, or staged, so that the body's burden of excess inert gas is eliminated without forming bubbles. Such depth/time ascent schedules have given rise to a variety of decompression tables.

A number of preconditioning techniques, such as exercise, vibration, antioxidants, and time spent in a heated sauna, have been investigated as protective measures against stress and DCS. Studies suggest that a single bout of moderately intense aerobic exercise 2 to 24 hours prior to diving significantly decreased the bubbles detected by ultrasound in the pulmonary artery after diving.[25,52,92] As discussed above, the presence of VGEs does not predict DCS but may be a marker of decompression stress. Other benefits of exercise may include activation of heat shock protein and increased nitric oxide production, resulting in protection of endothelial function..[93,194] Madden and colleagues[188] demonstrated that high-intensity cycling before diving decreased VGEs, circulating microparticles, and neutrophil response. They suggested that exercise may decrease preexisting gas micronuclei before the dive, resulting in decreased VGEs after diving.

Predive vibration[124] and predive sauna treatment[24] both show a decrease in VGEs. Predive antioxidants have been reported to decrease brachial artery flow–mediated dilation, suggesting that antioxidants may reduce endothelial dysfunction in divers.[223] The proposed mechanism behind these preconditioning methods remains unclear.

DECOMPRESSION SICKNESS IN BREATH-HOLD DIVERS

Conventional wisdom has always held that DCS does not occur in breath-hold divers, because they do not breathe air at an increased atmospheric pressure. However, it appears that neurologic DCS occurs among professional breath-hold divers in some settings.

A condition known as *taravana* was first described among pearl divers in the Tuamotu Islands of the South Pacific in the early 1960s.[69,70] These breath-hold divers make 40 to 60 dives per day to depths of 24 to 30 msw (80 to 100 fsw), spending about 2 minutes underwater each dive and remaining on the surface for 3 to 4 minutes between dives. These divers often complain of vertigo, nausea, euphoria, numbness, and partial or complete paralysis of the extremities after several hours of diving. In some cases, the diver loses consciousness for seconds to minutes after noting symptoms. Many of these divers have died either suddenly or after developing other symptoms. Nonfatal symptoms are usually transient, resolving in minutes to a few weeks. The symptoms immediately resolve with recompression.[229]

The symptoms of the taravana diving syndrome are similar to what has been more recently reported as occurring among some Japanese Ama divers, who have been reported to suffer dizziness, nausea, euphoria, numbness and weakness of extremities, dysarthria, and loss of consciousness after several hours of making 20 to 40 dives per hour to depths of 9 to 27 msw (30 to 90 fsw).[164,166]

With both the Tuamotu pearl divers and Japanese Ama, as well as in one instance of a U.S. Navy diver making repetitive breath-hold dives to depths of over 100 fsw in a submarine escape tank training tower, only neurologic symptoms have been observed. Joint pain and skin signs that are often seen in DCS have not been observed.

The mechanism of CNS damage after repetitive breath-hold diving is poorly understood. Venous gas bubbles were described in an Ama diver who had made 30 dives to 45 to 50 fsw in less than an hour.[242] It is possible that inert gas accumulates in the peripheral tissues of these divers consequent to the repeated back-to-back exposure to elevated atmospheric pressures. Gas bubbles are then released from peripheral fatty tissues, bypass the usual lung-filtering mechanism via pulmonary arteriovenous or cardiac intraatrial shunts, enter the systemic circulation, and cause cerebral embolization. Nothing has been reported about the prevalence of PFO in these populations, but there is no reason to believe that it is less than in other populations where it has been studied (i.e., about 25% of people). It is also possible that intravascular microbubbles (i.e., bubbles < 21 μm in diameter) that would pass through the lungs[45,46] could impair the blood-brain barrier transiently,[141] although this alone seems unlikely to explain the cerebral lesions that have been demonstrated by MRI.[166] Whatever the mechanism, symptoms and neurologic lesions that these divers suffer after repetitive breath-hold dives are now well documented.[165,301]

LONG-TERM HEALTH EFFECTS OF DIVING

Long-term untoward health effects related to diving may result from CNS injury as a result of AGE or DCS. These effects may include motor paresis or paralysis; paresthesias and other sensory disturbances; bladder, bowel, and sexual dysfunction; seizures; hearing loss; vertigo, tinnitus, and balance disorders from inner ear injury; dysbaric osteonecrosis; dysbaric retinopathy; hearing loss; and possible personality changes and loss of intellect.

A number of informal observations have been made over the years suggesting that long-time divers suffer some loss of intellect and may experience significant changes in personality, although confounding variables (e.g., use of alcohol) have always complicated such observations. There is now increasing evidence that divers may suffer subclinical CNS injury from paradoxic gas embolization and, possibly, other mechanisms.[297] For example, in MRI studies, long-time divers have been found to have more subcortical cerebral lesions than did controls. Studies in professional divers report decreased cognitive abilities, such as decreased mental flexibility, as well as lower verbal memory intelligence and sustained attention in divers reporting memory and concentration loss[67,268]; recreational divers do not show evidence of deficiencies of general higher cognitive function.[137] Overall, there is growing evidence that long-time divers suffer untoward health effects related to repeated exposures to a hyperbaric environment and breathing compressed gas.

UNUSUAL CONDITIONS OF UNCERTAIN ORIGIN FOLLOWING DIVES

IMMERSION PULMONARY EDEMA

Acute immersion pulmonary edema has been associated with both scuba diving and swimming. Numerous case reports describe scuba divers developing pulmonary edema while at depth during a dive.[134,238,258,299] In the majority of these cases, the divers were healthy with no predisposing factors for development of pulmonary edema (e.g., no evidence of cardiac disease or hypertension). Other reports describe pulmonary edema associated with heavy exertion in surface swimmers.[184,190,256,292] Many of these reports are of healthy males in military fitness training programs who presented with dyspnea, cough, tachypnea, hypoxemia, and hemoptysis after a strenuous swim. Immersion pulmonary edema is now recognized in triathlon swimmers.[49,198]

The exact mechanism for stress failure of the pulmonary capillaries is unknown. Racehorses are known to develop extremely high pulmonary vascular pressures, leading to stress failure of capillaries.[293] Physiologic changes that occur with immersion most likely contribute to the overall pathophysiology. Immersion causes central pooling of blood, which increases preload. Decreased core body temperature from cold water causes redistribution of blood flow to thoracic vessels and vasoconstriction. Increased sympathetic outflow also leads to vasoconstriction. Hence, immersion causes increased cardiac output and increased pulmonary vascular resistance. Reduction in functional residual capacity and vital capacity occurs by blood displacement into the lungs; there is also reduction in lung compliance.

Increased pulmonary blood flow and vascular pressure most likely cause stress failure of pulmonary capillaries. In scuba divers, use of a regulator with high inspiratory resistance could lead to negative-pressure pulmonary edema.

Radiographic findings include Kerley B lines, cephalization of flow, air-space consolidation, and normal cardiac size (Figure 71-15). Treatment is conservative because hypoxemia usually resolves within 12 hours. Treatment includes supplemental oxygen and inhaled β_2-adrenergic agonists for symptomatic relief. Diuretics are often given; however, most patients improve dramatically within the first 12 hours without their use. Older divers with cardiac risk factors need to be evaluated for a cardiac event that may have precipitated acute pulmonary edema. Reversible myocardial dysfunction has been reported in 28% of a group of divers with immersion pulmonary edema and associated with age over 50 years and hypertension.[122]

There is no way to predict whether or not a scuba diver will develop acute pulmonary edema; however, low lung volumes, pulmonary hypertension, and underlying cardiopulmonary disease, particularly occult hypertension, may be common predisposing factors for immersion pulmonary edema.[121,230,256] Many divers in the case reports have returned to diving without any recurrence of symptoms; however, divers must be cautioned about recurrence. Rare fatalities are reported from immersion pulmonary edema.[60,261]

INTERNAL CAROTID ARTERY DISSECTION

Dissection of the internal carotid artery and associated thromboembolic stroke have been reported (rarely) after scuba diving. These have been initially incorrectly diagnosed as AGE.[11,126,212]

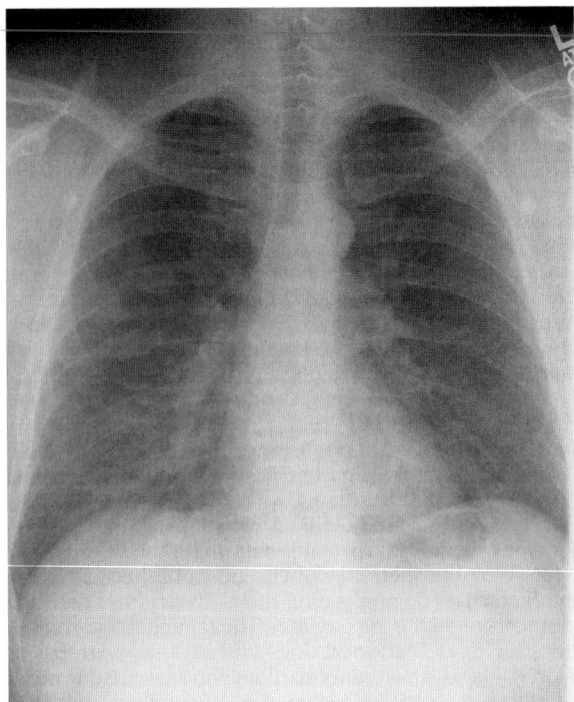

FIGURE 71-15 Chest radiograph of a diver with immersion pulmonary edema, showing bilateral patchy opacities consistent with pulmonary edema after an uneventful dive.

Although conceivably related to intravascular bubble-induced endothelial injury, the cause is a mystery.

Internal carotid artery dissection has been reported after a variety of situations involving neck trauma, hyperextension of the neck in athletic activities, and invasive diagnostic procedures, as well as spontaneously in persons having connective tissue disorders (e.g., Marfan's syndrome, fibromuscular dysplasia, and cystic medial necrosis), although its cause is unknown in most cases.

Symptoms of internal carotid artery dissection include unilateral headache, with or without ipsilateral neck pain, and other neurologic symptoms of intracranial origin. In all published cases involving divers, the condition was diagnosed after hyperbaric treatment for presumed AGE; HBOT produced no improvement in symptoms, or the condition worsened after HBOT. The preferred diagnostic modality is magnetic resonance or arteriography; ultrasound may be helpful.

Primary treatment of this condition entails anticoagulation aimed at preventing further thromboembolic complications. Most patients regain full function if appropriately treated.

MEDICAL FITNESS FOR DIVING
GENERAL CONSIDERATIONS

Although diving is an enjoyable sport that is safer than many other activities, the risks associated with diving are increased by certain physical conditions. Persons who intend to take up scuba diving should first be medically cleared. The diving examination should focus on conditions that may put the diver at increased risk for DCS, pulmonary barotrauma, and any conditions that could invoke Boyle's law or lead to loss of consciousness in the water. Special attention must be paid to the pulmonary, otolaryngologic, cardiac, and neurologic systems, as well as the person's psychological stability. The diver must be able to withstand cold stress and the physiologic effects of immersion and have sufficient exercise capacity to deal with possible stressful situations and emergencies. An increasing number of fatalities in diving are associated with cardiovascular disease, so particular attention should be directed to whether the diver can be expected to meet the performance requirements likely to be encountered in diving.

In general, contraindications for diving fall into five general categories:

1. Persons who are unable to equalize pressure in one or more of the body's air spaces and are thus at increased risk for barotrauma.
2. Persons who have a medical or psychiatric condition that may become manifest underwater or at a remote diving site and endanger the diver's life because of the condition itself, because it occurs in the water, or because inadequate medical help is available.
3. Persons who have impaired tissue perfusion or diffusion of inert gases and thus increased risk for DCS.
4. Persons who are in poor physical condition and thus at increased risk for exertion-related medical problems (the factors compromising the physical condition may be physiologic or pharmacologic).
5. Women who are pregnant, because the fetus may be at increased risk for dysbaric injury.

MEDICAL CLEARANCE FOR DIVING

Different medical standards are in place for the various diving communities: recreational, scientific, commercial, and military. The most common questionnaire used by recreational divers is the Recreational SCUBA Training Council Medical Statement, which can be downloaded at wrstc.com/standards-downloads/. Medical standards for scientific divers fall under the auspices of AAUS and can be downloaded at aaus.org/diving_standards. The Association of Diving Contractors International, Inc. lists medical standards for commercial diving that can be downloaded at adc-int.org.

Medical clearance guidelines divide the risks of diving into severe risk, relative risk, and temporary risk. *Severe risk* includes conditions that are absolute contraindications to diving, as well as conditions that put the diver at significant risk for injury or drowning. A potential diver with any of these conditions should be discouraged from diving. *Relative risk* refers to conditions that might represent a moderately increased risk that may be acceptable to the diver. The physician must base his or her judgment on assessment of the individual patient in each of these cases. *Temporary risk* may preclude diving while a condition is being treated. The diver may dive safely once the condition has resolved.

Table 71-6 lists the general guidelines for medical clearance for diving. Physicians and medical personnel of the Divers Alert Network (DAN) are available for consultation by telephone during normal business hours (919-684-2948) for all issues related to fitness for diving.

SPECIFIC CONDITIONS OF CONCERN WITH REGARD TO DIVING

Neurologic Disorders

Any neurologic abnormality that affects a diver's exercise capacity, leads to unconsciousness underwater, or has waxing and waning neurologic symptoms that can be difficult to distinguish from neurologic DCS must be strongly considered to be a contraindication to diving. Persons with spinal cord or brain abnormalities in which perfusion is impaired may have a theoretically increased risk for DCS.

Seizures. A history of epilepsy or other seizure disorder has traditionally been an absolute contraindication for diving. Seizures occurring underwater almost always lead to fatal drowning. Even if seizures are well controlled with medication, the individual should be disqualified from diving. Factors involved with diving (stress, exercise, hyperventilation, hypothermia, hypercapnia, and sensory deprivation) may lower the seizure threshold. Elevated oxygen partial pressures are suggested to increase the likelihood of a seizure in a diver with epilepsy; however, there are no data to support this notion.[2] Investigators have proposed that individuals with well-controlled seizures may be allowed to dive only if wearing a full-face mask. If a seizure occurs

underwater, it is conjectured that it is unlikely the diver will drown.[2,259]

Once an individual has discontinued antiepileptic medication for 5 years and has a normal neurologic workup (including an electroencephalogram [EEG]), the person may return to diving because the risk for having another seizure is the same as for the general population. A history of febrile seizures in childhood, seizures due to sepsis or drug ingestion, or posttraumatic seizures of childhood are not disqualifying for diving, as long as there is no ongoing seizure problem.

Head Injury. Any significant head injury that increases the risk for delayed seizures is a contraindication to diving. Such injuries include significant brain contusion, subdural hematoma, skull fracture, or loss of consciousness or amnesia for more than 24 hours. In a case of minor head injury that does not have any associated symptoms and that does not require anticonvulsant medication, scuba diving can be considered after 6 asymptomatic weeks.[4]

Unexplained Syncope. Unexplained loss of consciousness should be viewed as a contraindication to diving, for the same reasons as for seizures.

Migraine Headaches. Scintillating scotomata, paresthesias, weakness, and other neurologic symptoms associated with migraines and other types of vascular headaches may be confused with symptoms of AGE or DCS if they occur soon after diving. If such symptoms are misinterpreted, it may lead to unnecessary medical evacuation and HBOT. Depending on the specific situation, migraine headaches may be a relative contraindication to diving.

Cardiovascular Disorders

Immersion in water causes redistribution of blood from the periphery to the core. Increased cardiac preload during immersion can precipitate pulmonary edema in patients with impaired left ventricular function, increased pulmonary artery pressure, or significant valvular disease. Because an increasing proportion of scuba diving fatalities are due to coronary artery disease, individuals over 40 years of age should undergo risk assessment for coronary artery disease prior to diving.

Atrial Septal Defect. An atrial septal defect allows right-to-left intracardiac shunting of blood and increases the risk for paradoxic embolization of bubbles[298]; hence, the presence of an atrial septal defect is an absolute contraindication for diving. A ventricular septal defect does not allow right-to-left shunting and is not a contraindication for diving.

Patent Foramen Ovale. Patent foramen ovale (PFO) and diving has gained a lot of attention in the last few years. A PFO has the potential for a right-to-left shunt, and several studies suggest that a PFO may increase the risk for serious DCS.[72,123,208,253,276,285,296,297] However, the overall risk for DCS in divers with a PFO is very small, and routine screening for a PFO is not indicated.[32] It is reasonable to look for a PFO in cases of neurologic DCS, because the risk for right-to-left shunting increases with the size of the PFO, and some data suggest a significantly higher risk for recurrent serious DCS in persons having a larger (grade 2 or 3) PFO.[276]

If a PFO is identified, a diver may consider closure of a PFO to continue diving. However, this remains controversial. Honek and associates reported on 47 divers found to have a large PFO on medical screening.[144] Twenty divers who had suffered "unprovoked" decompression illness underwent transcatheter closure, and 27 divers (who either had not suffered decompression illness despite the presence of the PFO or who declined closure) were not closed. Not surprisingly, PFO closure reduces arterialization of venous inert gas bubbles after chamber dives; however, there was no difference in clinical outcomes. Billinger and colleagues[22] demonstrated reduction in decompression illness after PFO closure. Over a 5-year follow-up, the incidence of neurologic decompression illness per 10,000 dives in the closed and unclosed groups was 0.5 and 35 cases, respectively, which barely reached statistical significance because there were only five cases of decompression illness (one in the closure group and four in the nonclosure group). Closing a PFO may reduce the risk of neurologic decompression illness, but the procedure carries risks and

TABLE 71-6   Guidelines for Medical Clearance for Recreational Diving

System	Severe Risk Conditions	Relative Risk Conditions	Temporary Risk Conditions
Neurologic	Seizures Transient ischemic attack or cerebrovascular accident Serious decompression sickness with residual deficits	Complicated migraine Head injury with sequelae Herniated disk Peripheral neuropathy Multiple sclerosis Spinal cord or brain injury Intracranial tumor or aneurysm	Arterial gas embolism without residual, in which pulmonary air trapping has been excluded and the probability of recurrence is low
Cardiovascular	Intracardiac right-to-left shunt (atrial septal defect) Hypertrophic cardiomyopathy Valvular stenosis	Coronary artery bypass grafting Percutaneous transluminal coronary angioplasty or coronary artery disease History of myocardial infarction Congestive heart failure Hypertension Dysrhythmias Valvular regurgitation	Pacemaker: if the problem necessitating pacing does not preclude diving; pacemakers must be certified by the manufacturer to withstand pressure
Pulmonary	Spontaneous pneumothorax Impaired exercise performance due to respiratory disease	Asthma or reactive airway disease Exercise-induced bronchospasm Solid, cystic, or cavitating lesions Pneumothorax caused by surgery, trauma, or previous overinflation Immersion pulmonary edema Interstitial lung disease	
Gastrointestinal	Gastric outlet obstruction Chronic or recurrent small bowel obstruction Severe gastroesophageal reflux disease Paraesophageal hernia	Inflammatory bowel disease Functional bowel disorders	Unrepaired hernias of the abdominal wall Peptic ulcer disease associated with obstruction or severe reflux
Metabolic and endocrine	Pregnancy	Insulin-dependent diabetes mellitus Non–insulin-dependent diabetes mellitus	
Otolaryngologic	Open tympanic membrane perforation Tube myringotomy Middle ear or inner ear surgery Tracheostomy	Recurrent otitis externa, otitis media or sinusitis Eustachian tube dysfunction History of tympanic membrane perforation, tympanoplasty or mastoidectomy Significant conductive or sensorineural hearing loss History of round or oval window rupture	Acute upper respiratory infection Acute sinusitis Acute otitis media
Orthopedic		Amputation Scoliosis with impact on respiratory performance Aseptic necrosis	Back pain
Hematologic		Sickle cell disease Leukemia Hemophilia Polycythemia vera	
Behavioral health	Inappropriate motivation to dive Claustrophobia Acute psychosis Untreated panic disorder	Use of psychotropic medications Previous psychotic episodes	

Modified from Recreational SCUBA Training Council (RSTC) Medical Statement: wrstc.com.

should be carefully considered on a case-by-case basis. Commercial and technical divers who perform dives that are considered provocative might be appropriate candidates. Other divers may choose to adopt more conservative dive profiles.

The South Pacific Underwater Medicine Society (SPUMS) and United Kingdom Sports Diving Medical Committee (UKSDMC) have published a joint position statement on persistent foramen ovale and diving.[260] In 2015, the Undersea and Hyperbaric Medical Society (UHMS) and DAN held a 1-day workshop to establish consensus guidelines from the joint position statement on PFO and diving. Workshop proceedings are available at diversalertnetwork.org.[79a] Box 71-6 summarizes the guidelines on PFO and diving.

Coronary Artery Disease.   As scuba diving has become more popular, older divers are pursuing the activity and more deaths from coronary artery disease are occurring among scuba

divers in the water. In recreational divers, cardiac events are associated with approximately a quarter of diving fatalities.[80] In addition to the need for cardiac reserve during an in-water emergency, carrying tanks, donning equipment, and swimming against water currents entail significant physical stresses. Symptomatic coronary artery disease is a contraindication for diving. However, a history of myocardial infarction is not a disqualification for sport diving per se, particularly after revascularization or comparable procedures, and if the diving candidate is able to achieve 6 metabolic equivalents during an exercise stress test.[200]

Dysrhythmias.   Benign dysrhythmias that do not interfere with exercise tolerance are not disqualifying. Individuals with well-controlled atrial fibrillation who are taking anticoagulation medications should be able to scuba dive without undue risk.

Hypertension.   Whether a hypertensive person may safely dive is based largely on the therapy required for blood pressure

BOX 71-6 Position Statement on Patent Foramen Ovale (PFO) and Diving by the Undersea Hyperbaric Medicine Society (UHMS) and the Divers Alert Network (DAN)

Statement 1

Routine screening for patent foramen ovale (PFO) at the time of dive medical fitness assessment (either initial or periodic) is not indicated

Statement 2

Consideration should be given to testing for PFO under the following circumstance:

- A history of more than one episode of decompression sickness (DCS) with cerebral, spinal, vestibulocochlear or cutaneous manifestations. Noncutaneous manifestations of mild DCS and headache as an isolated symptom after diving are not indications for PFO investigation.

Statement 3

If testing for PFO is performed, then the following is recommended:

- That testing is undertaken by centers well practiced in the technique
- The testing must include bubble contrast, ideally combined with transthoracic echocardiogram (TTE), because this best facilitates cooperation with provocation maneuvers. Use of two-dimensional and color-flow echocardiography without bubble contrast is not adequate.
- The testing must include the use of provocation maneuvers to promote right-to-left shunting, including Valsalva release and sniffing as described in the supporting references (both undertaken when the right atrium is densely opacified by bubble contrast).

Statement 4

Interpreting a positive PFO screening result:

- A spontaneous shunt without provocation or a large, provoked shunt following diving when venous gas emboli are present is recognized as a risk factor for those forms of DCS listed in Statement 2.
- Smaller shunts are associated with a lower but poorly defined risk of DCS. The significance of minor degrees of shunting needs to be interpreted in the clinical setting that led to testing.

Statement 5

Following diagnosis of a PFO considered likely to be associated with increased DCS risk, the diver may consider the following options in consultation with a diving physician:

- Stop diving
- Dive more conservatively: There are various strategies that might be employed to reduce the risk of significant venous bubble formation after diving, or the subsequent right-to-left shunting of such bubbles across a PFO. The appropriateness of this approach, and the strategies chosen, need to be considered on an individual basis, and in discussion with a diving medicine expert. Examples include: reducing dive times to well inside accepted no-stop limits; performing only one dive per day; use of nitrox with air dive planning tools; intentional lengthening of a safety stop or decompression time at shallow stops; avoidance of heavy exercise and unnecessary lifting or straining for at least 3 hours after diving
- Close the PFO. It is emphasized, however, that closing a PFO after an episode of DCS cannot be considered to provide assurance that DCS will not occur again.

Statement 6

The options outlined in Statement 5 require careful consideration of the risks and benefits and the clinical setting that led to screening.

Statement 7

Following closure of a PFO and before returning to diving, the diver requires a repeat bubble contrast echocardiogram demonstrating shunt closure, a minimum of 3 months after the closure.

Statement 8

Diving should not be resumed until satisfactory closure of the PFO is confirmed, and the diver has ceased potent antiplatelet medication (aspirin is acceptable)

Statement 9

Venous bubbles can also enter the systemic circulation through intrapulmonary shunts, although the role of this pathway in the pathogenesis of DCS is not as well established as PFO. These shunts are normally closed at rest. They tend to open with exercise, hypoxia, and beta-adrenergic stimulation, and close with hyperoxia. It is therefore plausible that exercise, hypoxia, and adrenergic stimulation after a dive could precipitate DCS when it might not otherwise have occurred, while supplemental oxygen is likely to minimize this effect.

From Denoble PJ, Holm JR, eds. Patent foramen ovale and fitness to dive consensus workshop proceedings. Durham, NC, Divers Alert Network, 2015.

---

control and the presence of any other contraindications that are often associated with hypertension (e.g., coronary artery disease or diabetes). Diving has little effect on blood pressure, and when a regimen of weight control, diet, and antihypertensive medication is successful, diving usually can be allowed. Occult hypertension is thought to be a risk factor for immersion pulmonary edema.[121]

Pulmonary Disorders

Any lesion or disease that impedes airflow from the lungs increases the risk for pulmonary barotrauma and the possibility of AGE. Additionally, respiratory disease due to either structural disorders of the lungs or chest wall may impair exercise performance and is exacerbated by the effects of immersion and increased gas density while diving.

Spontaneous Pneumothorax. A history of a spontaneous pneumothorax is an absolute contraindication for diving. Individuals with a history of spontaneous pneumothorax are often found to have small blebs on the surface of the lungs that may be at increased risk for rupture while diving, causing pulmonary barotrauma and AGE. A history of previous spontaneous pneumothorax carries a significant incidence of recurrence, even after many years, and the candidate must be advised against compressed-gas diving. A pneumothorax that occurs while the diver is underwater or in a hyperbaric chamber can rapidly progress to become a life-threatening tension pneumothorax as the pleural cavity air expands (per Boyle's law) during ascent. Surgical procedures designed to prevent recurrence (such as pleurodesis or apical pleurectomy) do not correct the underlying lung abnormality.

A history of a traumatic or iatrogenic pneumothorax is not a contraindication to diving. In these cases, inspiratory/expiratory high-resolution chest CT scanning can rule out significant air trapping.

Asthma. In the past, asthma was considered an absolute contraindication for diving because of the person's increased risk for air trapping and pulmonary overinflation while diving. However, many persons with asthma dive with no apparent increased risk for pulmonary barotrauma.[217] Criteria for clearing a person with a history of asthma to dive include:

1. Asymptomatic adult with a past history of childhood asthma
2. Well-controlled asthma with known triggers with normal pulmonary function tests (with or without medication) with a reduction of less than 20% in peak mid-expiratory flow after exercise
3. No evidence of cold-induced wheezing or exercise-induced bronchospasm

A more complete discussion of the issues relating to asthma and diving can be found in the article by Van Hoesen and Neuman.[283a]

Bullous Lung Disease. Pulmonary blebs or cysts can trap air and lead to local pulmonary overpressure accidents during decompression. If a ball-valve or flutter-valve effect allows such a bleb or cyst to equalize with the elevated breathing pressure during compression or descent, but blocks escape of air during decompression, rupture could cause pulmonary barotrauma and air embolism. Similarly, individuals with significant obstructive lung disease should be disqualified from diving.

Diabetes

Like asthma, insulin-dependent diabetes mellitus (IDDM; also known as type 1 diabetes mellitus) was formerly considered a contraindication for diving because of the risk for a hypoglycemic reaction underwater that would lead to incapacitation, unconsciousness, and drowning. Hypoglycemic reactions may result from sudden bursts of energy expenditure, as may occur in dealing with emergencies. Underwater incapacitation due to hypoglycemia not only endangers the life of the diver but may also risk the lives of other persons during rescue attempts, and can lead to drowning. However, many patients with IDDM have been diving safely for years, and guidelines for divers with IDDM exist through the American Diabetes Association and the YMCA. Persons with diabetes who are well controlled on insulin, accustomed to vigorous physical exercise, knowledgeable about their condition, and who dive with prepared buddies usually can be cleared for diving. Guidelines for recreational diving with diabetes can be found on the DAN website.

Pregnancy

There is near unanimity that a woman who is pregnant, or who may be pregnant, should suspend compressed-air diving until after delivery. Animal studies have produced conflicting results in different species and laboratories, but the possibility of bubble formation in fetal or placental tissues leading to fetal demise or malformation is a concern, even during a dive that is safe for the mother.

Ear, Nose, and Throat Disorders

Any condition that inhibits or precludes the ability to clear the ears or sinuses may be disqualifying for diving. Likewise, any condition that impairs eustachian tube function may preclude an individual from diving; such conditions include frequent ear infections, mastoiditis, and cholesteatoma; a history of surgery for a middle ear disorder may also be a factor in precluding diving. A chronic perforated tympanic membrane is a contraindication for diving. A healed or repaired tympanic membrane perforation is usually not a problem for diving. Persons who have had a stapedectomy or stapedotomy should not dive, because of increased risk for oval window fistula and inner ear barotrauma. Chronic sinus disease or polyps, allergic rhinitis, or nasal septal deviation may make clearing the sinuses difficult. Individuals with inner ear disease, such as Ménière's disease, with recurrent vertigo should not dive.

Sickle-Cell Disease or Trait

The chances that a sport diver will breathe a hypoxic gas mixture are remote, but possible. Other concerns are heavy exertion in cold water or local compromise of microvascular blood flow by bubble evolution during decompression, which could lead to sickling and a vicious cycle of hypoxia, leading to further sickling.

Panic Disorders

A person prone to panic attacks may have such an attack underwater, prompting the diver to make a rapid uncontrolled ascent that may precipitate pulmonary barotrauma and AGE. The majority of dive accidents usually result from human error, not medical problems. Any condition that can lead to poor judgment and panic underwater should be disqualifying for diving.

Abdominal Hernias

There is a rare but potential risk for trapping expanding gas in a herniated loop of bowel during ascent. In general, diving should be suspended until surgical repair is completed.

Poor Physical Condition

Sport scuba diving may seem deceptively easy until an emergency occurs that requires swimming against a current, rescue of a buddy diver, or other vigorous activity. The diver should be capable of performing sudden strenuous activity before entering the water. Regular swimming or other exercise programs to ensure cardiovascular fitness are encouraged.

MEDICATIONS AND DIVING

In a survey of 531 divers, more than 50% reported taking over-the-counter medications within 6 hours of diving and 23% reported taking prescription medications (10% reported taking cardiovascular medication).[89] Many recreational divers today have underlying medical conditions that require chronic medication use. Lack of prospective experimental data on the impacts of increased pressure or a gas mixture on medication metabolism poses a challenge to physicians who desire data-driven answers. However, most diving and hyperbaric physicians approach the question of medical fitness to dive less from a medication perspective (i.e., the possible influences of depth or a gas mixture on a particular medication's actions) and more from consideration of the tangible influences of the patient's underlying medical conditions. As an example, persons with heart failure are poor candidates for diving because of their underlying heart disease, not because they take medications to control blood pressure. The critical caveat to this approach is that any medication that alters consciousness, impairs judgment, or decreases response time must be scrutinized. Although it is possible that the effect of such medications is increased secondary to the narcotic effects of nitrogen, the fact that these effects exist at all should warrant caution and second thoughts before initiating a dive.

An unusual situation in this regard, but one that is certainly plausible in today's scuba diving population, involves persons who have been treated with bleomycin (e.g., for testicular cancer). The concern is that bleomycin sensitizes the lungs to oxygen toxicity. Scuba divers who dive to depths of 18 to 36 msw (60 to 120 fsw) on compressed air would be exposed to the equivalent of 0.63 to 1.05 ATA oxygen, an amount sufficient to cause concern, because there is no known minimal safe oxygen exposure in bleomycin-treated patients.[151,304] A recent review of patients with a history of bleomycin use treated with HBOT did not demonstrate significant pulmonary complications. Although the clinical setting of HBOT exposes people to oxygen partial pressures of 2 to 3 ATA, these patients require close observation and usually undergo regular pulmonary function testing. As such, there is generalized caution among diving physicians when determining the suitability of diving for patients who have taken this medication.[275]

Another area of concern involves medications whose side effects may create diagnostic confusion in the case of DCS. An example of such a medication is mefloquine (Larium), used for malaria prophylaxis. Among its known potential side effects are vertigo, nausea, dizziness, anxiety, hallucinations, mania, sleep disturbances, and seizures. Depending on the specific circumstances, the side effects of the drug could be confused with DCS or AGE.

The side effects of some drugs may be especially problematic for divers because of the environment of diving. For example, divers in tropical locations may be exposed to intense sunlight, increasing the risk for a phototoxic reaction, which is a recognized side effect of many commonly prescribed medications. A few drugs have been studied under hyperbaric conditions and found to be at least relatively safe for divers; these include pseudoephedrine,[36,269] transdermal scopolamine,[23,294] and the antihistamine clemastine.[257] Other drugs that appear to be safe by virtue of their extensive use by divers and absence of reported untoward effects include aspirin, acetaminophen, warfarin, chlorpheniramine, and oxymetazoline.

Given the unknowns about the behavior of most medications in the diving environment, the following precautions are appropriate:

1. Whenever possible, avoid all drugs when diving.
2. Any medication that impairs mental judgment or physical capacity should be very carefully considered before being used when diving. If the medication is used, the expected benefits of its use should outweigh its risks.
3. Never take a drug for the first time before diving.
4. Always consider whether the reason for taking a drug is reason itself not to dive.
5. Always consider the known side effects of a drug and whether those would be a problem when diving.

DIVING WITH DISABILITIES

In recent years, many persons with limb amputations or other serious orthopedic impairment, spinal cord injury, cerebral palsy, or similar physical condition have sought to participate in scuba diving. Some of these persons were accomplished athletes or divers before an accident changed their physical status. For others, scuba diving is a completely new experience, offered as part of a rehabilitation program. Whatever the case, it is clear that persons having "disabilities" can enjoy diving as much as anyone else if they are properly trained, understand their condition and the limitations it causes them, and make appropriate adjustments, when necessary, for their condition.[78] When done in this context, scuba diving can open exciting new vistas for some disabled persons. Williamson and coworkers[295] demonstrated significant improvements in self-concept and body image among a group of young people with disabilities, including brain damage following head injury, congenital deafness, blindness, spinal cord dysfunction, and major limb amputations. These individuals were examined according to standard diving medicine practice regarding pulmonary and ear, nose, and throat status, and detailed psychological testing. Motivation proved to be an important predictor of success. The subjects were given extensive scuba diving training with a minimum of one-on-one instructor attention.

In any of these situations, the diver and buddy need to fully understand the concerns attendant to the condition (e.g., autonomic dysreflexia, skin breakdown, personal hygiene, and a possible increased risk for DCS) and the wisdom of taking a conservative no-decompression approach to diving.

FLYING AFTER DIVING

Diving is often done at remote destinations, and many divers travel considerable distances after packing in as many dives as possible. The question of when it is safe to fly after diving comes up often. Flying too soon after diving can seriously jeopardize decompression safety, leading to development of DCS during or after the flight because of the reduced atmospheric pressure present in most commercial aircraft.

The normal commercial aircraft cabin pressure is equivalent to an altitude exposure of approximately 1500 to 2500 m (5000 to 8000 feet), which is sufficient pressure reduction to cause dissolved nitrogen to come out of solution and form intravascular bubbles. Based on published DAN data gathered from 1987 to 1999, 17% (382/2222) of divers in the DAN injury database had their first symptom during or after flying.[117]

With continued growth of the dive-travel industry, the issue of when it is safe to fly after diving is important. Based on years of experimental work done by DAN in collaboration with Duke University, the following guidelines for flying in commercial aircraft after recreational diving have been established[255]:

1. For single no-decompression dives, a minimum preflight surface interval of 12 hours is suggested.
2. For multiple dives per day or multiple days of diving, a minimum preflight surface interval of 18 hours is suggested.
3. For dives requiring decompression stops, there is insufficient experimental or published evidence on which to base a recommendation. However, it would seem prudent that such divers should exercise caution, and a preflight surface interval substantially longer than 18 hours seems warranted. The longer the interval between diving and flying, the lower the DCS risk.

Two recent studies have looked at in-flight echocardiography in divers returning from a week of diving and found that a small percentage of divers develop venous bubbles during flight despite a preflight surface interval of 24 hours. The majority of bubbles occurred in individuals who also developed bubbles after diving.[55,56] None of these divers developed DCS.

Despite these guidelines, it is important to emphasize that no rule about flying after diving can be guaranteed to prevent DCS. These recommendations simply represent the best estimate of a safe surface interval for the majority of sport divers.

SAFE SCUBA DIVING

Sport scuba divers are fortunate that the most colorful marine life and abundant natural light exist at shallow depths. This obviates the need to dive deep. Indeed, 130 fsw should be considered a deep dive for sport diving and, for all intents and purposes, the maximum depth for recreational diving.

Recreational diving is usually done hours to days away from the nearest hyperbaric chamber, so the occurrence of DCS or AGE usually necessitates a major effort to evacuate an afflicted diver to the chamber. This often requires the use of special aircraft. Unfortunately, the delay between symptom onset and treatment may cause the damage to be poorly responsive to hyperbaric treatment. Therefore, divers should do their utmost to avoid developing AGE or DCS.

The need to take a conservative approach to depth and time is even more compelling when one considers that individual variability in DCS susceptibility, workload during the dive, water temperature, and exercise or altitude exposure following a dive may confound any set of decompression tables or dive computers. Indeed, the potentially devastating consequences of DCS, even with the most vigorous hyperbaric treatment, mandate that divers always dive with the prevention of this disease foremost in their minds.

Based on common trends seen in diving accidents and fatalities, the following suggestions for safe diving are recommended[213]:

- Ensure physical fitness to dive: train for your sport and be sure that you exercise regularly and follow a healthy diet.
- Use the buddy system.
- Follow your training: check your gauges often, respect depth and time restrictions, and do not dive beyond your training limits.
- Weight yourself properly and remember to dump your weights when appropriate.
- Ensure that your skill level and familiarity are appropriate for conditions.
- Have equipment serviced and maintained regularly.
- Account for all divers (a physical, individual response should be received from every diver before entering and after exiting the water).
- Avoid overhead environments (e.g., caves and tunnels) unless you are properly trained and equipped.
- Breath-hold divers should remember to use the buddy system and be aware of the dangers of shallow water blackout.

Diving in mountain lakes requires significant adjustments in decompression tables to account for decreased atmospheric pressure at the surface of the lake. Dive computers must be calibrated for altitude. Boni and associates[30] pointed out that for the same depth bottom time of a dive, surfacing at a lower ambient air pressure than sea level necessitates longer decompression time. Several decompression tables for altitude diving have been calculated and tested in the field.[15,71,209] The U.S. Navy Standard Decompression Tables can be used up to an altitude of 701 m (2300 feet).

Even when safe diving practices are followed, unexplained DCS cases sometimes occur.[1] Two mechanisms are postulated to account for these cases. After an otherwise safe dive, one well within the specified decompression procedure, elevated inert gas tensions exist in tissues and venous blood, and some individuals may develop VGEs. If a physiologic PFO allows intermittent retrograde flow from the right to left atrium, VGEs can become AGEs. The potential for this type of paradoxic gas embolism has been demonstrated in recent years for both PFO and other types of intracardiac and pulmonary shunts, as discussed above.

Another plausible explanation for DCS occurring after safe diving postulates that focal pulmonary barotrauma, or inadvertent breath holding during ascent, produces local air trapping during ascent and releases microbubbles into the systemic circulation. These microscopic "seed" bubbles in arterialized blood pass through the capillary bed to become bubble nuclei in venous blood, precipitating overt bubble formation and the classic manifestations of DCS.

DIVE ACCIDENT INVESTIGATION

When investigating a dive accident, whether for treatment purposes or as part of a forensic evaluation in the event of a fatal accident, the investigator begins by taking a detailed dive accident history. A number of specific details must be determined about the patient's diving activities, time of symptom onset, and nature and progression of symptoms, in addition to the medical history and other information that should be obtained for any patient. The history related to diving should specifically solicit information in the following areas[214]:

1. Type of dive and equipment used. Inquire specifically as to whether a decompression computer, diving watch, and depth gauge were used. Was compressed air or mixed gas used, and what was the source of the gas? Was an RB used?

2. Number of dives; depth, bottom, or total dive times; and surface interval or intervals between dives for all dives in the 72 hours preceding symptom onset. This information will be needed by the diving medicine consultant because it allows calculation of any omitted decompression and thus helps decide the likelihood of the patient having DCS or other problems. Unfortunately, the diver's interpretation of whether required decompression was omitted cannot be the sole source of data; this is notoriously unreliable. If a dive computer was used, it should be checked for information about any omitted decompression times; one should also ascertain whether the computer was worn on all dives.

3. Whether and how much in-water recompression was attempted. This is relevant to the likelihood of the diver having DCS. If a dive computer was used, the diver should be asked whether the specified decompression profile was followed.

4. Site of diving (e.g., ocean, lake, or quarry) and the environmental conditions (e.g., water temperature or presence of current or surge) associated with the dive. These factors enter into the differential diagnosis and may raise the possibility of the symptoms being caused by something other than a bubble-related problem. For example, DCS is more common after diving in cold water (other things being equal), and motion sickness may develop in a diver swimming back to shore on a choppy sea, even if there was no problem with seasickness before or during the dive.

5. Presence of predisposing factors for DCS. A number of factors have been associated with increased risk for DCS. These include dehydration, vigorous exercise underwater, advanced age, obesity, poor physical conditioning, local physical injury, and multiple repetitive dives in individuals who have not been acclimatized.

6. Whether the dive was complicated by running out of air, an untoward marine animal encounter, trauma, or other unexpected event. For example, low back pain suggestive of DCS may be caused by muscle strain from lifting a scuba tank or climbing into the dive boat, and tingling or numbness in an extremity may be caused by jellyfish envenomation.

7. Whether the patient flew in an airplane, went jogging, or engaged in any other particular activity after diving but before the onset of symptoms. If so, the effect of the activity on the symptoms should be ascertained. Some activities (e.g., flying in an unpressurized aircraft or vigorously exercising immediately after diving) may precipitate DCS in someone who might otherwise not be affected, and trivial dysbaric symptoms may become severe after similar activities.

8. Time of symptom onset. Symptoms that began soon after getting in the water (e.g., nausea from motion sickness), even if they worsen afterward, are not likely to be from DCS. Pulmonary symptoms that develop at depth are much more consistent with immersion pulmonary edema than with AGE.

INVESTIGATION OF DIVING FATALITIES

In the event of a fatal diving accident, information gathered from the diving accident history should be supplemented with an appropriate diving accident autopsy, thorough evaluation of the diving equipment used, and a detailed environmental history.[75] Guidelines for scuba diver death investigations have been published.[40,50,51,214,283] An excellent symposium on investigation of diving fatalities for medical examiners and diving physicians in 2014 was sponsored by the UHMS and DAN.[79] Environmental factors, such as weather, currents, wave action, visibility, water temperature, potential for entanglement, and dangerous marine life, must be considered. The diving equipment should be carefully studied for proper function and the amount of compressed air in the tanks, and the air should be analyzed for contaminants. The diver's medical and psychological histories should be sought because they may contain clues to a coincidental medical event that led to the diver's death but was unrelated to the dive. Aside from obvious psychosocial risk factors, such as alcoholism, drug abuse, or panic disorder, use of a scuba dive for suicide or homicide must be considered.

Unique aspects of the diving victim autopsy should include careful search for subcutaneous emphysema or other physical signs of pulmonary barotrauma and search for signs of marine envenomation. For example, before the surface of the body is washed, it should be examined for evidence of nematocysts from coelenterate stings. In addition, in contrast to the thoracic incision being made first, the calvarium should be opened before other incisions are made in order to prevent accidental introduction of air into the intracranial circulation. A finding of gas bubbles in intracranial vessels may result from AGE or DCS. Postmortem introduction of gas into the cerebral veins can be avoided if the calvarium is opened underwater.[75] Likewise, the initial thoracic incision must be made with care to determine whether pneumothorax is present. A careful search should be made for gas bubbles in the major blood vessels and heart. The middle ear should be examined for the presence of blood, and tympanic membranes and sinuses examined for evidence of barotrauma.

In many scuba fatalities, the pathologist may ascribe the death to drowning when there is no evidence of a diving-related malady, such as air embolism or evidence of equipment malfunction. Sudden cardiac death due to underlying cardiac disease should also be considered because these cases should be reported as natural death and not drowning.[248]

Meticulous investigation of dive accidents is important to find equipment, procedural, or medical causes that could be useful for improving the safety of diving and to gather information for legal procedures that often follow diving accidents. A unique approach to diving fatality investigation exists in the San Diego Diver Death Review Committee, which consists of personnel from the San Diego Lifeguards, San Diego Police Department, Medical Examiner's Office, Scripps Institution of Oceanography, University of California San Diego Hyperbaric Center, U.S. Coast Guard, and San Diego State University Diving Safety. The committee represents a multiagency dive team for scene investigation, equipment analysis, autopsy by the medical examiner, and input from diving medicine specialists. Representatives from all these groups review each diver death in San Diego to determine the cause and manner of death. The committee provides related information to agencies and the public for prevention and education to promote safety for the local diving community.[249]

REFERENCES

Complete references used in this text are available online at expertconsult.inkling.com.

Hyperbaric oxygen therapy (HBOT) is a method of treating both acute life-threatening and chronic conditions by delivering oxygen at partial pressures greater than the normal sea level barometric pressure of 760 mm Hg. The patient breaths 100% oxygen intermittently or continuously while inside a chamber that is pressurized to at least 1.4 times the atmospheric pressure at sea level. The field of hyperbaric medicine has shown increasing applicability in the past 60 years. An estimated 2000 hospitals offer HBOT, and another 500 to 700 non–hospital-based programs also offer HBOT. HBOT is useful for treating diving injuries, acute carbon monoxide poisoning, necrotizing fasciitis, crush injuries, problem wounds, and radiation injuries.

Portable hyperbaric chambers are available for use in remote wilderness settings; however, their use is currently limited to diving injuries and altitude illness. HBOT has been proposed for other applications related to wilderness medicine, such as frostbite, brown recluse spider bites, and heatstroke (Box 72-1). However, few data exist to support routine use of HBOT for these. Additionally, HBOT has been suggested as an adjunct to field management of combat trauma in remote settings.

One-year accredited training fellowships in diving and hyperbaric medicine, recognized by the Accreditation Council for Graduate Medical Education, are available throughout the United States. The American Board of Preventive Medicine and the American Board of Emergency Medicine offer subspecialty board certification in undersea and hyperbaric medicine for individuals who have completed fellowship training.

HISTORY OF HYPERBARIC MEDICINE

Treatment with compressed-air therapy dates to 1662, when the British clergyman Henshaw treated acute medical disorders with increased pressures and treated chronic disorders with decreased pressures.[197] Compressed air was used to treat caisson disease, or decompression sickness (DCS), in the late 1800s. Medical use of hyperbaric oxygen (HBO) began in the 1930s with the first systematic studies on the physiologic effects of oxygen.[13] Extensive research on oxygen toxicity and safe oxygen limits was conducted during the 1940s, when oxygen was incorporated into the treatment tables of the U.S. Navy for diving injuries.

True clinical hyperbaric medicine began in the 1950s and 1960s, with the use of HBOT for anaerobic infections, including gas gangrene and clostridial infections, and for carbon monoxide poisoning.[32,198] During the 1970s, HBOT was used widely to treat a variety of conditions with little scientific basis. In 1976, the Undersea Medical Society established a multidisciplinary committee to review research and clinical data on the uses of HBOT. Every 3 years, the committee publishes a critical review of approved indications for HBOT (Table 72-1).[246] In 1986, the Undersea Medical Society changed its name to the Undersea and Hyperbaric Medical Society to incorporate the expanding field of hyperbaric medicine.

MECHANISMS OF HYPERBARIC OXYGEN

HBOT is inhalation of oxygen at a pressure greater than atmospheric pressure measured at sea level, which is 1 atmosphere (atm). An individual is placed inside a hyperbaric chamber that is pressurized with air or oxygen. The atmospheres absolute (ATA) is the sum of the atmospheric pressure and the hydrostatic pressure as measured in the chamber. For every increase of 10 meters of seawater (msw; equivalent to 33 feet of seawater [fsw]), a pressure increase of 1 atm (760 mm Hg) is present. At 20 msw (66 fsw), the absolute pressure in the chamber is 3 ATA. Increasing the atmospheric pressure in the hyperbaric environment causes both mechanical reduction in bubble size and increased partial pressure of oxygen in tissues.

EFFECTS OF HYPERBARIC OXYGEN ON OXYGEN CONTENT

The oxygen content of blood is the sum of oxygen carried by hemoglobin and oxygen dissolved in the blood plasma. At 1 atm at sea level, 98% of the oxygen content of normal blood is bound to hemoglobin. The oxygen content of blood plasma is determined by the solubility of oxygen in plasma at 37° C (98.6° F), which at a partial pressure of oxygen (PO_2) of 100 mm Hg results in oxygen in solution of only 0.31 mL/dL. Once hemoglobin is fully saturated, further increases in PO_2 can only increase the amount of oxygen physically dissolved in the plasma. As PO_2 increases in inspired air, the amount of oxygen dissolved in plasma increases linearly (Figure 72-1). For every atmosphere of pressure increase, 1.8 mL/dL of oxygen is dissolved in plasma. At 3 ATA, approximately 6.8 mL/dL of oxygen can be dissolved in plasma. Because normal oxygen extraction at the tissue level is 5 mL/dL (at normal cardiac output), plasma alone can carry enough oxygen to meet the metabolic needs of tissues. In addition, this increase in oxygen-carrying capacity dramatically increases the driving force for oxygen diffusion.

EFFECTS OF AN ELEVATED PARTIAL PRESSURE OF OXYGEN

The increase in tissue oxygen concentration has important physiologic and biochemical effects in both normal and diseased tissue. HBO causes vasoconstriction and edema reduction; inhibits neutrophil adhesion; inhibits infection; upregulates growth factors and growth factor receptors; modulates inflammation; increases neovascularization, angiogenesis, and osteogenesis; and reduces ischemia-reperfusion injury. Recent studies show that HBO stimulates vasculogenic stem cell growth and release of stem cells derived from bone marrow[148,217] (Box 72-2).

Recent work by Thom[217] shows that breathing oxygen at pressures greater than 1 ATA increases production of reactive oxygen species and reactive nitrogen species, which elicit signaling molecules in transduction pathways that then generate a variety of growth factors, hormones, hypoxia-inducible factor, stem and progenitor cells, and cytokines. Through these activation pathways, HBO improves neovascularization and improves postischemia tissue survival.

Vasoconstriction

Hyperoxia-induced vasoconstriction occurs in both the arterial and venous vasculature and has been demonstrated in cerebral, retinal, renal, muscular, and myocardial circulations. Despite reduction in blood flow from vasoconstriction, cellular metabolism is not compromised by increased tissue oxygen partial pressures and increased oxygen diffusion pressure.[65] Reduced edema occurs because filtration of capillary fluid is decreased, whereas vascular outflow and improved oxygen delivery are maintained. This vasoconstriction can be beneficial in peripheral edema and intracerebral edema, and decreases edema

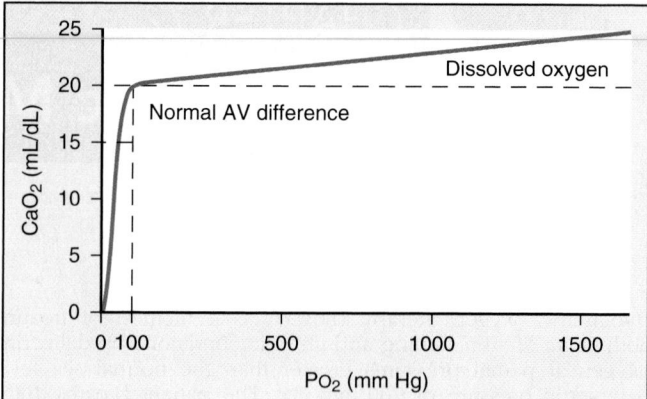

FIGURE 72-1 Effects of hyperbaric oxygen on the oxygen content of arterial blood. The blood oxygen content (CaO_2) under normal conditions is approximately 20 mL/dL and carried almost exclusively by hemoglobin. The normal oxygen extraction (arterial-venous [AV] difference) is approximately 5 mL/dL, or about one-quarter of total CaO_2. During hyperbaric oxygen therapy, dissolved oxygen in plasma can be increased to provide the entire AV difference without unloading oxygen from hemoglobin.

in burns and postischemic tissues.[22,161,166,167] Blood flow in the microcirculation is improved through decreased interstitial fluid pressures from edema reduction. This effect is important for treatment of brain injuries from carbon monoxide poisoning or arterial gas embolism, spinal cord DCS, and crush injuries.

Bacteriostatic and Bactericidal Effects of Hyperbaric Oxygen

HBO has been shown to have a potent inhibitory effect on the growth of various microorganisms. HBO causes a direct bactericidal effect on anaerobic bacteria through production of toxic radicals in the absence of free radical degrading enzymes, such as superoxide dismutase, catalases, and peroxidases.[98] HBO also has a bacteriostatic effect on selected facultative and aerobic organisms.[110,260] A tissue PO_2 of 30 to 40 mm Hg is necessary for oxidative killing of microorganisms by neutrophils. Increased PO_2 in infected and hypoxic tissue enhances neutrophil function and return of antimicrobial activity. A single 90-minute exposure increases the respiratory burst activity of neutrophil-like cells after exposure and an increase in the phagocytosis of *Staphylococcus aureus*.[3] HBO also augments the bactericidal action of aminoglycosides and potentiates the effect of certain sulfonamides.[80,103] Aminoglycoside and cephalosporin antibiotic transport across the bacterial cell wall requires tissue oxygen tensions above 30 mm Hg. Overall, HBO enhances antibiotic transport and augments efficacy.

Angiogenesis

HBO influences angiogenesis and vasculogenesis, the two processes that cause neovascularization. Angiogenesis is growth of new blood vessels from local endothelial cells. Vasculogenesis is recruitment and differentiation of circulating stem and progenitor

cells to form new blood vessels. HBO mobilizes circulating stem and progenitor cells in both humans and mice by stimulating bone marrow endothelial nitric oxide synthase.[68,72,220] HBO also stimulates stem cell growth factor production through augmented synthesis of hypoxia-inducible factor.[93,148] Some of the mobilized cells will migrate to peripheral sites, where they function as de novo endothelial progenitor cells and contribute to wound vasculogenesis.

Wound Healing

The relationship between tissue wound hypoxia and wound healing has been well documented.[94,95] Tissue hypoxia decreases fibroblast replication, collagen deposition, angiogenesis, resistance to infection, and intracellular leukocyte bacterial killing, which are all oxygen-sensitive responses essential to normal wound healing. Intermittent elevation of tissue PO_2 reverses local tissue hypoxia and corrects the pathophysiology related to oxygen deficiency and impaired wound healing. HBO enhances collagen synthesis, stimulates angiogenesis, improves leukocyte function of bacterial killing, and blunts systemic inflammatory responses.[92,95,127] In addition, HBO stimulates vascular endothelial growth factor release and induces platelet-derived growth factor receptor appearance.[24,195,208] The net result of serial increased PO_2 from HBOT is improved local host immune responses, clearance of infection, enhanced tissue growth, angiogenesis with progressive improvement in local tissue oxygenation, and epithelialization of hypoxic wounds.

Ischemia-Reperfusion Injury

Ischemia-reperfusion injury is tissue damage that occurs after reperfusion of ischemic tissue. Ischemia-reperfusion injury is mediated by oxygen-derived free radicals, such as superoxide and hydroxyl free radicals, which are produced during prolonged periods of ischemia followed by reperfusion. These oxyradicals can lead to cell death by lipid peroxidation and generation of further free radicals. Oxyradicals are generated from xanthine oxidase and neutrophils. Neutrophil endothelial adhesion and subsequent release of free radicals play an important role in endothelial and microcirculatory damage.[107,184] Tissue reperfusion is inhibited by adherence of circulating neutrophils to vascular endothelium by beta$_2$ integrins.

HBO protects tissues from reperfusion injury. HBO provides additional oxygen so that reperfused tissues can generate scavengers such as superoxide dismutase, catalase, peroxidase, and glutathione, which detoxify destructive oxygen radicals before they damage tissues.[60] HBO antagonizes the beta$_2$ integrin system, which initiates adherence of neutrophils to postcapillary venule endothelium.[216,222] Reperfusion injury may be inhibited by HBO

TABLE 72-1 Approved Indications for Hyperbaric Oxygen Therapy

Indication	HBO Mechanism	Treatment Profile	Number of Treatments
Air or gas embolism	Bubble reduction Inert gas washout Modulation of ischemia-reperfusion injury and inflammation Treats ischemia	U.S. Navy Table 6 or 6A Repeat treatment with U.S. Navy Table 5 or 6, or 2.4 ATA	1-10 or to clinical plateau
Decompression sickness	Bubble reduction Inert gas washout Modulation of ischemia-reperfusion injury and inflammation Treats ischemia	U.S. Navy Table 6 Repeat treatment with U.S. Navy Table 5 or 6, or 2.4 ATA	1-10
Arterial insufficiencies Central retinal artery occlusion	Modulation of ischemia-reperfusion injury	2-2.8 ATA BID to clinical plateau Consider U.S. Navy Table 6 if no improvement	6
Enhancement of healing in select problem wounds	Treats ischemia Modulation of ischemia-reperfusion injury and inflammation Upregulation of growth factors, growth factor receptors, and circulation stem cells Inhibition of infection Angiogenesis	2-2.5 ATA	10-30
Carbon monoxide poisoning	Carbon monoxide washout Treats ischemia Modulation of ischemia-reperfusion injury and inflammation	2.4-3 ATA	1-3
Clostridial myositis and myonecrosis (gas gangrene)	Inhibition of toxins Suppresses organism growth Treats ischemia	3 ATA TID in first 24 hr, then BID for 2-5 days	3-10
Compromised grafts and flaps	Treats ischemia Angiogenesis Upregulation of growth factors, growth factor receptors	2-2.5 ATA BID initially until graft/flap appears stable	10-20
Crush injury, compartment syndrome, and acute ischemia	Treats ischemia Limits edema Modulation of ischemia-reperfusion injury and inflammation	2-2.5 ATA	2-14
Delayed radiation injury and soft tissue and bony necrosis	Treats ischemia Angiogenesis Upregulation of growth factors, growth factor receptors	2-2.5 ATA For prophylaxis: 20 sessions before surgery in radiated field 10 sessions after surgery	30-60
Idiopathic sudden sensorineural hearing loss	Supraphysiologic levels of oxygen in tissue	2-2.5 ATA	10-20
Intracranial abscess	Inhibition of infection Cerebral vasoconstriction and edema reduction Modulation of inflammation	2-2.5 ATA 1-2 times per day	10-20
Necrotizing soft tissue infection	Inhibition of infection Treats ischemia Modulation of inflammation	2-3 ATA BID until stabilization	5-30
Refractory osteomyelitis	Treats ischemia Inhibition of infection Stimulates osteoclasts	2-2.5 ATA	20-40
Severe anemia	Treats ischemia	2.4-3 ATA 3-4 times per day until replacement or red blood cells by regeneration or transfusion	1-20
Thermal burn injury	Inflammation modulation Upregulation of growth factors, growth factor receptors, and circulation stem cells Inhibition of infection	2-2.5 ATA TID in first 24 hours, then BID	20-30

ATA, atmospheres absolute; BID, twice a day; TID, three times a day.

through decreased leukocyte venular endothelial adherence, release of toxic oxygen species, and arteriolar vasoconstriction; hence, progressive arteriolar vasoconstriction is inhibited.[259] HBO inhibits intracellular adhesion molecule 1 expression, which plays a role in neutrophil adhesion and ischemia-reperfusion injury.[35] Additionally, HBO upregulates transforming growth factor beta₁, which decreases reperfusion injury by upregulating bcl-2 and inhibiting tumor necrosis factor alpha.[78] Nitric oxide plays an important role in ischemia-reperfusion injury, regulating vascular tone and neutrophil adhesion. HBO appears to increase nitric oxide production by inducing nitric oxide synthase production.[10,35,221] It is possible that the beneficial effect of HBO in ischemia-reperfusion injury is primarily mediated by nitric oxide.[34]

HBO increases the ischemic tolerance of multiple organs in animal models by induction of antioxidant enzymes and antiinflammatory proteins. HBO has been shown to be beneficial in almost all animal models of ischemia-reperfusion injury, and results in increased microvascular perfusion in skeletal muscle and improved skin flap survival.[116,252,259,261] It may be an important adjunct for treatment of tissue at risk for reperfusion injury that can accompany crush injury, limb replantation, compartment syndrome, arterial gas embolism (AGE), and DCS. New data suggest a role of HBO in preventing ischemia-reperfusion injury associated with myocardial infarction and cerebral ischemia.

TYPES OF HYPERBARIC CHAMBERS

MONOPLACE HYPERBARIC CHAMBERS

Monoplace, or single-person, chambers account for the majority of hyperbaric chambers in the United States. They accommodate a single patient, and the chamber is pressurized either with 100% oxygen or with air while the patient breathes oxygen through a mask or hood. Monoplace chambers are easier to maintain, require less space, and are less expensive than are multiplace chambers. They can be configured with noninvasive and invasive monitoring. Specially adapted ventilators and monitoring systems in some monoplace chambers allow for treatment of critically ill patients. During treatment, there is no direct access to the patient. Therefore, the chamber must be decompressed for an emergency, which can limit its use in some critically ill patients (Figure 72-2). Most monoplace chambers cannot exceed a treatment depth of 3 ATA.

MULTIPLACE HYPERBARIC CHAMBERS

Multiplace chambers hold two or more people and allow more than one patient to be treated at a given time, accompanied by

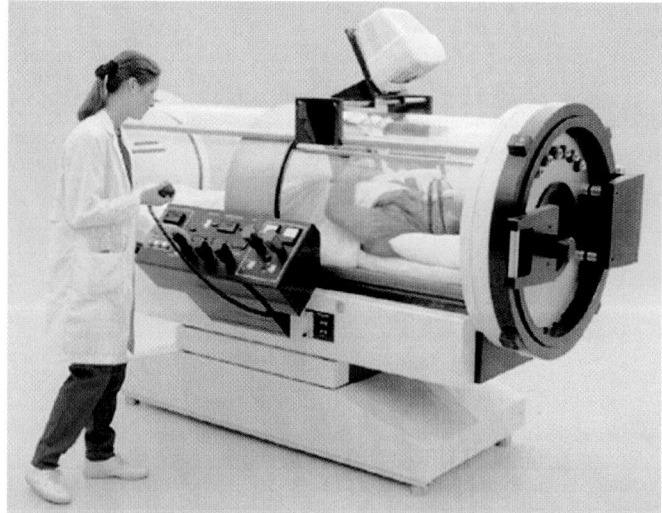

FIGURE 72-2 Monoplace hyperbaric chamber. Monoplace chambers hold a single patient, usually in an environment of pure oxygen. Attendants remain outside the chamber during treatment.

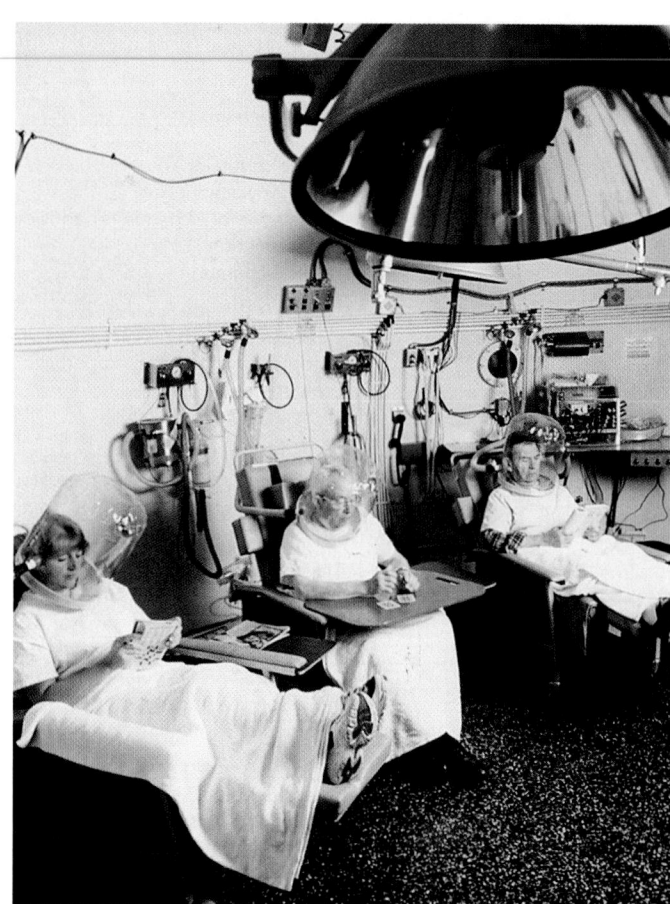

FIGURE 72-3 Multiplace hyperbaric chamber. Multiplace chambers allow more than one patient at a time to receive HBO. Attendants may accompany the patients during treatments. *(Courtesy Duke University Photography, Les Todd.)*

attendants, including technicians, nurses, and respiratory therapists (Figure 72-3). The chamber is pressurized with air; 100% oxygen is delivered by face mask, using a head tent, or through an endotracheal tube. Multiplace chambers allow for intensive care–level monitoring, mechanical ventilators, vascular pressure monitoring, intravenous (IV) infusion pumps, blood gas analysis, and medication administration. Multiplace chambers can maintain a treatment pressure of 6 ATA and are ideal for treatment of diving injuries, particularly DCS and AGE. General anesthesia, surgery, chest tube placement, and cardiopulmonary resuscitation have been performed inside multiplace chambers. They have the disadvantage of a risk for DCS to attendants during long treatments.

PORTABLE RECOMPRESSION CHAMBERS

Portable monoplace recompression chambers have been developed for use in remote areas for treatment of both diving injuries and high-altitude illnesses.

HYPERBARIC CHAMBERS FOR ALTITUDE ILLNESS

Several portable hyperbaric chambers are available for emergency treatment of severe acute mountain sickness, high-altitude pulmonary edema, and high-altitude cerebral edema, particularly when descent is not feasible or while awaiting evacuation (Figures 72-4 to 72-6). They are constructed of relatively lightweight fabrics and require no use of portable oxygen. The portable chambers are pressurized with ambient air using manual foot pumps or hand pumps, and can simulate a descent of 1500 to 2500 m (5000 to 8200 feet). Hyperbaric treatment should only be used as an emergency measure and is not a substitute for descent or evacuation.

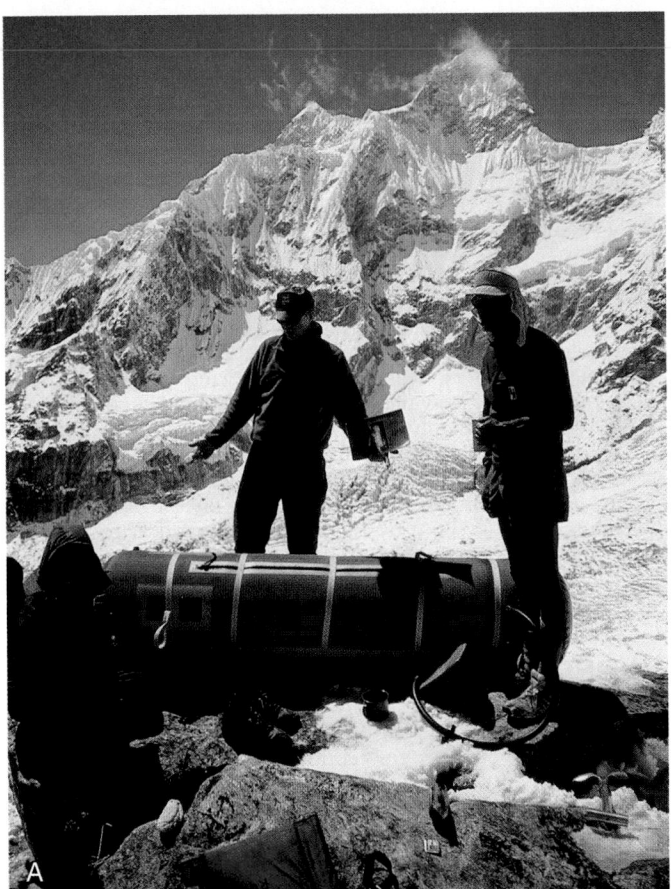

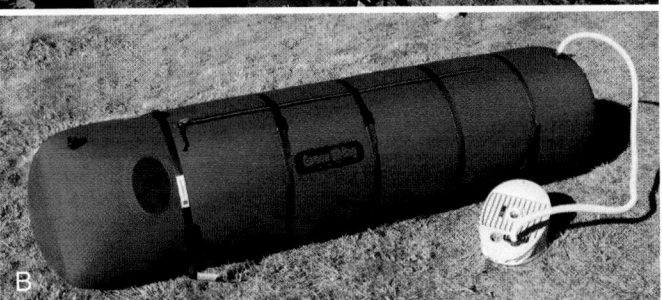

FIGURE 72-4 Chinook Medical Gear's Gamow portable altitude chamber. **A,** In the field. **B,** Close up. *(Courtesy Chinook Medical Gear, Inc.)*

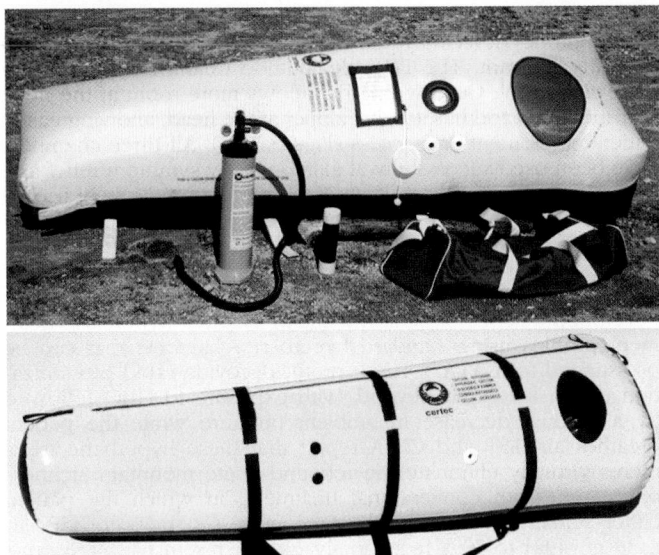

FIGURE 72-5 Certec chamber. *(Courtesy Certec Company.)*

weight (the bag, pump, and carrying day pack weigh approximately 7 kg [15 lb]), and easy to use. It measures 2.5 × 0.6 m (8 × 2 feet) and can maintain an internal pressure of 2 psi (104 mm Hg or 0.13 atm). The Certec hyperbaric chamber has two bags: an outside envelope made to withstand tension and provide stability and an inside envelope of polyurethane that allows for more durability of the chamber (Figure 72-5). The Certec chamber weighs 4.8 kg (10.5 lb) and measures 2.2 × 0.65 m (7 × 2 feet); it can be pressurized to a slightly higher inflation pressure (internal pressure of 165 mm Hg or 0.22 atm or 3.2 psi) than can the Gamow bag. Compared with the Gamow

The patient should be told to breathe normally and instructed on equalizing his or her ears by swallowing or by the Valsalva maneuver. The patient is placed inside the portable chamber, zipper pulled shut, and bag inflated with the foot pump to 2 psi (104 mm Hg) above ambient pressure. Two pop-off pressure values are set at 2 psi and prevent overpressurization of the bag. All portable chamber bags must be pumped continually 8 to 12 times per minute in order to flush air through the chamber to prevent carbon dioxide buildup. Patients should be treated for approximately 1 hour and then removed from the bag and reassessed. Additional cycles of descent and reassessment are continued until the patient improves and is able to descend or evacuation is available. Patients with severe high-altitude pulmonary edema may not be able to lie flat; hence, one end of the chamber can be propped up 30 to 40 cm (12 to 16 inches). In severe cases, a patient can breathe oxygen at 4 to 6 L/min during treatment by placing an oxygen bottle inside the chamber.

Different brands of portable chambers are available for use at high altitude. The Gamow bag (Figure 72-4) was invented by Dr. Igor Gamow at the University of Colorado. It is cylindrical, light-

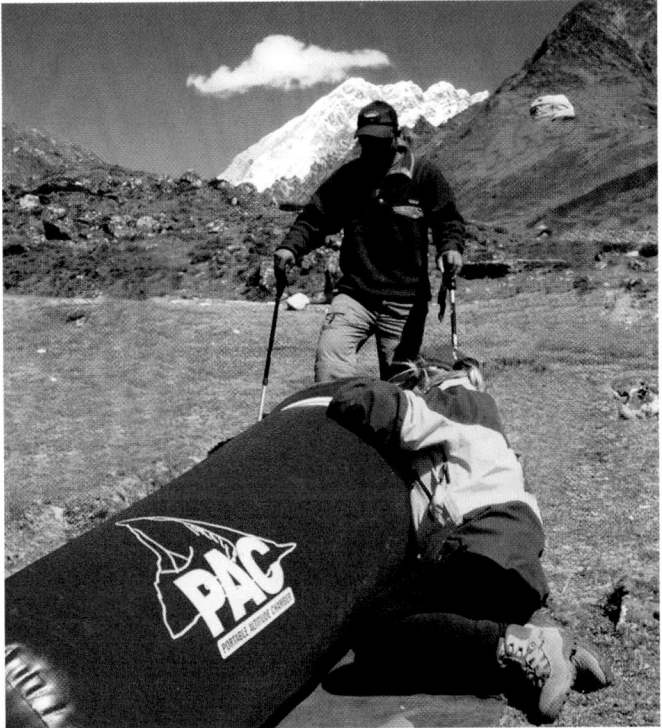

FIGURE 72-6 Treksafe Portable Altitude Chamber. *(Courtesy Treksafe Company.)*

bag, this is equivalent to about 800 m (2625 feet) more of simulated altitude descent; however, it is unclear whether this is clinically relevant. The Portable Altitude Chamber is about the same size as the Gamow bag but allows more room at the head and shoulders and has a radial zipper at the head, allowing easier patient assessment and access (Figure 72-6). All three chambers have been used successfully at altitude; early symptom relief and improvement in peripheral oxygen saturation and cerebral oxygenation have been reported.[7,96] These chambers have no utility for treatment of diving injuries.

The Life Support Technology (LST) Group and the Center for Investigation of Altitude Medicine (CIMA) in Cusco, Peru, have developed a series of acute mountain sickness hyperbaric treatment profiles using standard hyperbaric chambers that can be pressurized to 3 ATA.[37] These profiles provide rapid pressurization to sea level and beyond, with exposure to HBO followed by a gradual decrease in ambient pressure while the patient breathes air. LST and CIMA report that these hyperbaric treatments virtually eliminate the rebound acute mountain sickness often seen with conventional treatment, in which the patient either remains at altitude or is recompressed back to 1500 to 2438 m (4921 to 7999 feet) briefly, and then returns to the same altitude where symptoms were first manifested. These are proposed protocols and are not the standard of care in treating acute mountain sickness.

HYPERBARIC CHAMBERS FOR DIVING INJURIES

Sturdier portable chambers exist for treatment of diving-related injuries. Although there are a number of hard, small recompression chambers used in commercial diving operations, these chambers are not collapsible or easily portable. Two collapsible chambers, used primarily by the U.S. Navy and commercial diving operations, are pressurized with air from a scuba cylinder while the patient breathes 100% oxygen from a face mask. The patient can be transported within the portable chamber to a large recompression facility and moved under pressure into a large multiplace chamber. Unlike the lightweight portable chambers used for treatment of altitude illnesses, these have a working pressure of 3.3 ATA or 48 psi (equivalent of 75 fsw).

The SOS Hyperlite Hyperbaric Stretcher is the most widely used collapsible chamber for treatment and transportation under pressure of a patient suffering from DCS or AGE to a permanent recompression chamber (Figure 72-7). The chamber is made of seamless Vectran-braided tube with coated nylon bladder, has two removable endplates with a communication system, and can deliver 100% oxygen to the patient. It is capable of a standard treatment depth of 3.3 ATA and weighs approximately 50 kg (110 lb). Also called the Emergency Evacuation Hyperbaric

Stretcher, or Hyperlite 1, it is certified for use within the U.S. Department of Defense and is currently in use by the U.S. Coast Guard, all four branches of the U.S. military, the National Aeronautics and Space Administration, and the Russian navy. SOS Group is currently developing larger multioccupant collapsible chambers with maximum operating pressures up to 6 ATA.

Another collapsible, portable hyperbaric chamber is the Italian-made GSE chamber. A smaller version, the Hyperbaric Backpack, is also available. This chamber is 76 cm (30 inches) in diameter, 2 m (7 feet) long, and weighs 42 kg (92 lb). It is a double bag of translucent composite polyester and specified for 6 ATA. Another chamber, the Chamberlite 15, is probably the simplest unit on the market and one of the lightest in weight. It is capable of providing 100% oxygen at 2 to 2.4 ATA pressure with special adapters. This unit is constructed of foldable polyurethane, has 10 viewing ports, and weighs less than 18 kg (40 lb), making it highly portable by standard stretcher or two-person carry. The depth of treatment is limited, however, because treatment of diving injuries requires a minimum treatment depth of 2.82 ATA. It has been used in studies on carbon monoxide poisoning and may be a useful tool for emergency treatment of carbon monoxide poisoning in the field.[196]

CONTRAINDICATIONS TO HYPERBARIC OXYGEN THERAPY

ABSOLUTE CONTRAINDICATIONS

HBOT is safe, with very few contraindications. Untreated *pneumothorax* is an absolute contraindication to treatment, because it may progress to a tension pneumothorax during decompression. Once a chest tube has been placed, the patient can safely undergo HBOT. Treatment with bleomycin, disulfiram, and doxorubicin may enhance toxic effects when used concurrently with HBOT; patients taking one of these medications must be reviewed individually for the risks and benefits of HBOT.[109]

RELATIVE CONTRAINDICATIONS

Any condition that interferes with pressure equalization in the sinuses, ears, or lungs (e.g., acute or chronic sinusitis, otitis media, upper respiratory infection) is considered a relative contraindication. Nasal and oral decongestants can be used before treatment; myringotomy or placement of tympanoplasty tubes can facilitate treatment in certain situations. Use of bronchodilators and slow ascent rates can allow individuals with chronic obstructive pulmonary disease to undergo HBOT.

COMPLICATIONS OF HYPERBARIC OXYGEN THERAPY

OXYGEN TOXICITY

In 1878, Bert described seizures and death in animals exposed to 3 to 4 ATA. This central nervous system (CNS) manifestation of oxygen toxicity became known as the *Paul Bert effect*.[19] In 1899, pulmonary oxygen toxicity was described after prolonged exposures to 0.74 to 1.3 atm of oxygen.[125] Tissue injury from oxygen is mediated by reactive oxygen species that are produced by chemical reactions involving single electron transfers to molecular oxygen or its metabolites. These reactive oxygen species include superoxide anions, hydroxyl radials, and hydrogen peroxide.

Under normal oxygen conditions, cells have adequate antioxidant defenses. These defenses include antioxidant enzymes such as superoxide dismutase and catalase, and low-molecular-weight scavengers such as glutathione and vitamin E. As PO_2 increases, these defenses are overwhelmed and reactive oxygen species cause lipid peroxidation, protein oxidation, sulfhydryl depletion, and oxidation of pyridine nucleotides, leading to cell membrane disruption, cell injury, and death.[61]

Clark has written a thorough review of the pathophysiology of oxygen toxicity during hyperbaric exposures.[45a]

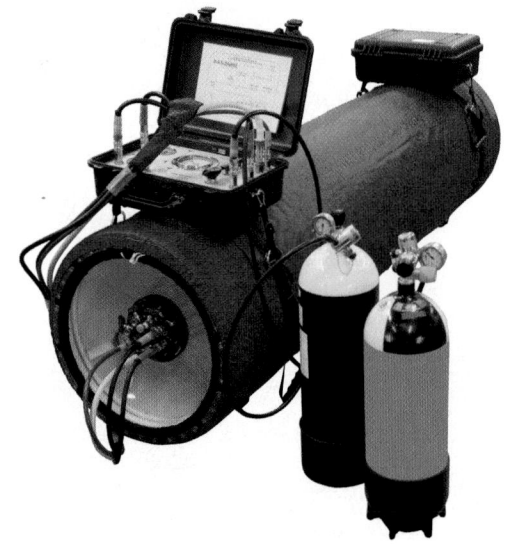

FIGURE 72-7 The Hyperlite by SOS Limited is pressurized with air from a scuba cylinder. The injured diver breathes 100% oxygen from a separate oxygen bottle. (*Courtesy SOS Group.*)

BOX 72-3 Signs and Symptoms of Central Nervous System Oxygen Toxicity

Diaphoresis	Tinnitus
Bradycardia	Nausea
Palpitations	Vomiting
Euphoria	Vertigo
Apprehension	Lip or facial twitching
Visual fields constriction	Seizures

Central Nervous System Oxygen Toxicity

CNS toxicity occurs during oxygen exposures of 1.4 atm or greater. Symptoms may include dizziness, irritability, facial twitching, tunnel vision, tinnitus, nausea, and seizures (Box 72-3). The incidence of oxygen-induced seizures is 1 to 3/10,000 patients treated at 2 to 2.5 ATA. Susceptibility to oxygen-induced seizures varies among individuals and in any single individual from day to day. Factors that increase susceptibility include exertion, increased partial pressure of carbon dioxide (PCO_2), increased metabolic rate from fever, thyrotoxicosis, adrenal stress, and acute cerebral injury. Catecholamines can lower the seizure threshold and increase the risk for CNS oxygen toxicity. Oxygen-induced seizures are self-limited and resolve quickly after oxygen has been discontinued. No permanent neurologic sequelae have been reported from HBO-induced seizures, and anticonvulsants are not indicated. Intermittent exposure to brief periods of air during HBOT significantly extends the oxygen tolerance and prevents oxygen toxicity. Individuals with a history of seizures or who are taking medications that can lower the seizure threshold can still receive HBOT; oxygen breathing periods are reduced from 30 minutes to 20 minutes as a precaution.

Remove oxygen at the first sign of CNS toxicity (e.g., when feelings of apprehension are noted or when sweating, nausea, or twitching is observed). After all symptoms have resolved, oxygen therapy can be resumed. Shortening the duration of oxygen exposure can prevent the recurrence of symptoms. Treatment for an oxygen-induced seizure involves removing the oxygen mask, maintaining the airway, and preventing self-injury by the patient. Of note, the chamber pressure should be kept constant until the seizure activity ceases to prevent possible pulmonary barotrauma. There is no reason for a person who has had an oxygen-induced seizure not to receive normobaric 100% oxygen if it is medically indicated.

Pulmonary Oxygen Toxicity

Retrolental fibroplasia in premature infants and pulmonary oxygen toxicity in adults are well-known problems associated with the use of therapeutic oxygen. Pulmonary oxygen toxicity is induced by breathing an above-normal but relatively low PO_2 for prolonged periods. The limit for indefinite exposure without demonstrable lung damage is considered to be a PO_2 of approximately 0.5 ATA. On a time-dose curve, it is considered safe to breathe 100% oxygen at 1 ATA for up to about 20 hours, or at 2 ATA for up to 6 hours. This time can be lengthened significantly by using intermittent exposures, such as interspersing a 5-minute air break between every 20 minutes of oxygen breathing

Symptoms of early pulmonary oxygen toxicity include substernal burning, slight cough, mild dyspnea, and chest tightness, and can be seen in patients treated for DCS, air embolism, and gas gangrene when treatments are prolonged. These symptoms resolve after discontinuing therapy. Pulmonary oxygen toxicity is rare using current treatment tables. Patients do not experience significant alteration in pulmonary gas exchange when treated with standard HBOT protocols.[37a,248]

BAROTRAUMA

The most common side effect of HBOT is middle ear barotrauma caused by inadequate equalization of pressure in the middle ear. This may result from an upper respiratory infection, eustachian tube dysfunction, or inadequate techniques of equalization.

Middle ear barotrauma typically occurs during compression, causing pain and hemorrhage within the middle ear, rarely leading to tympanic membrane rupture. It can be prevented by slow compression rates with frequent stops, proper autoinflation techniques, and use of decongestants. For individuals who have significant difficulty clearing their ears, bilateral tympanotomies can be placed. In an emergency, myringotomies can be performed. Sinus barotrauma results from blockage of the sinus ostia due to upper respiratory infection, or allergic sinusitis or rhinitis. Symptoms include pain in the maxillary or frontal sinus. Oral or nasal decongestants before treatment may allow the patient to proceed with HBOT.

CLAUSTROPHOBIA

Some patients may experience claustrophobia or confinement anxiety in both monoplace and multiplace chambers. Benzodiazepines can be given before treatment to help relieve anxiety.

VISUAL REFRACTIVE CHANGES

Patients who undergo more than 20 HBOT treatments often develop progressive myopia that is temporary and reverses completely within a few weeks after discontinuing HBOT. The exact mechanism is not known but appears to be lenticular in origin.[41,128,170] Treatment with HBOT beyond 150 treatments is associated with an increased risk for irreversible refractive changes or development of new cataracts. In the United States, HBOT treatments rarely exceed 60 in number.

PRACTICAL ASPECTS OF HYPERBARIC TREATMENT

EVALUATION OF THE PATIENT FOR HYPERBARIC OXYGEN THERAPY

For elective treatments, patients are assessed for appropriateness of HBOT and contraindications to treatment. Patients should be screened for a history of seizures, pulmonary disease including asthma or chronic obstructive pulmonary disease, implanted devices such as cardiac pacemakers or intrathecal pumps, and claustrophobia. Eustachian tube function and ability to clear the ears can be assessed by examining the tympanic membrane with an otoscope and asking the patient to hold his or her nose and swallow or perform a simple Valsalva maneuver. If the tympanic membrane moves with either maneuver, the eustachian tube is patent.

In emergency situations, patients may be unconscious and thus cannot be screened for contraindications to HBOT. If the patient is not alert, it may be necessary to endotracheally intubate for airway protection; it is safer to sedate combative or semicomatose patients and mechanically ventilate them than to restrain and attempt to control an agitated patient in the chamber. Patients who are sedated and intubated generally do not need myringotomies, because passive inflation of the middle ear space during hyperbaric compression will occur. If necessary, an emergency myringotomy can be performed. Under direct visualization of the tympanic membrane, a perforation is made in the anterior-inferior quadrant of the tympanic membrane with a 21-gauge spinal needle. Patients with diving injuries and carbon monoxide poisoning should be maintained on 100% oxygen by face mask at 10 to 15 L until treatment is initiated in the hyperbaric chamber.

PREPARATION FOR HYPERBARIC TREATMENT

Preparation of a hyperbaric patient requires strict attention to certain safety issues and protocols. For fire safety reasons, patients must wear hospital-supplied clothing of either 100% cotton or a blend of 50/50 polyester-cotton. Undergarments must be 100% cotton. Silk, wool, waffle weave, and nylon and other synthetic materials are prohibited. Watches must be inspected for pressure compatibility. Excessive cosmetics, lotions, and perfumes should be removed. Patients must be inspected for matches, lighters,

BOX 72-4 Guidelines for Equipment Use in Hyperbaric Chambers

Equipment Not Allowed to Be Used in Chamber
Telemetry device
Defibrillator
Brush-driven motor (noninvasive blood pressure machines)
Laser printer (electrocardiogram strips)
Pneumatic stockings
Patient-controlled anesthesia pump
Non–pressure-tested intravenous pump
Transport ventilator
Unnecessary equipment, such as pulse oximetry device
Off-gassing batteries and equipment supplied by > 12 volts
48-watt power source

Equipment Allowed Inside Chamber
Electrocardiogram monitor
Bard Harvard pump
HBO-approved intravenous pump
HBO-approved ventilator
Doppler device
Permanent pacemakers (check with manufacturer for whether they have been pressure tested)
Swan-Ganz and arterial line
Pressure bag
Drains, Foley catheter, nasogastric tube, endotracheal tube cuff
Glass bottles inspected by HBO staff and vented if necessary

HBO, hyperbaric oxygen.

and smoking materials, all of which are prohibited. The hyperbaric staff should follow established protocols at their facility. In general, staff must (1) ensure eustachian tube patency, (2) remove all medical devices not required during hyperbaric treatment, (3) cap all IV catheters that are not in use, (4) empty a Foley bag or have the patient void before chamber entry, (5) have labeled medications available, (6) confirm a good signal on all monitors and check that monitors and IV pumps are fully charged, and (7) ensure that the ventilator is functioning correctly on the surface. A list of equipment that is prohibited and allowed inside a hyperbaric chamber is presented in Box 72-4.

PEDIATRIC CONSIDERATIONS

Generally, indications for HBOT in the pediatric population are similar to those in adult patients. Critically ill pediatric patients can safely receive HBOT when attended by experienced personnel.[104] Accidental carbon monoxide poisoning and serious burns are common afflictions in pediatric age groups. Invasive procedures can result in iatrogenic cerebral gas embolism in children. Figure 72-8 shows a 7-day-old infant with clostridial omphalitis from an umbilical vein catheter that developed into gas gangrene of the abdominal wall. The child was treated successfully with HBOT at the University of California, San Diego, Hyperbaric Center.[179] This center has also successfully treated a child with acute hepatic artery thrombosis after liver transplantation (Figure 72-9).[77]

Special attention must be paid to reduce evaporative, conductive, and convective heat losses in the chamber, because children have an increased risk for hypothermia. An oxygen hood can be used for most children older than 3 to 4 years. In younger children, the neckdam can be pulled down to waist level, which allows the child's hands to be free inside the hood (Figure 72-10). Although there are no studies on the safe limits of exposure to HBO for children, in practical experience there is no increased risk for developing pulmonary or neurologic oxygen toxicity. Additionally, there are no significant differences in side effects or morbidity rates with HBOT for children compared with adults.[186] One theoretical problem with HBOT exists for the child with a ductus arteriosus–dependent congenital heart disorder. The increased PO_2 could result in ductal constriction, limiting cardiac output, so this must be considered when treating an infant with congenital heart disease.[234]

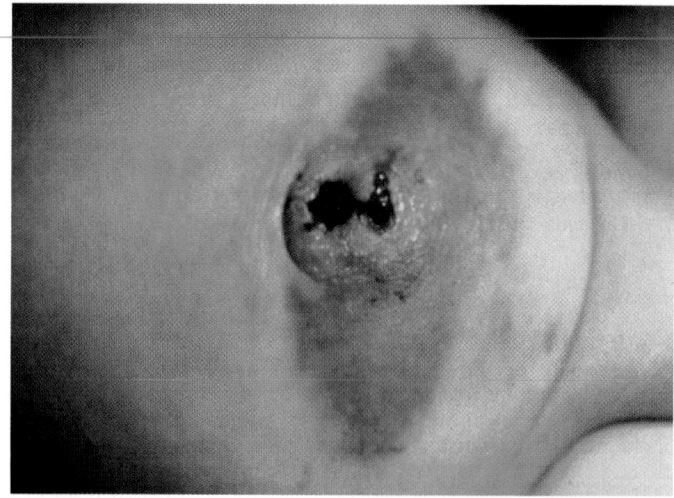

FIGURE 72-8 A 7-day-old infant with gas gangrene of the abdominal wall due to *Clostridium perfringens* treated with HBOT with a good outcome.

APPROVED CLINICAL APPLICATIONS OF HYPERBARIC OXYGEN THERAPY

ARTERIAL GAS EMBOLISM

AGE can result from pulmonary barotrauma while diving (see Chapter 71). Pulmonary barotrauma typically occurs when a diver ascends rapidly while holding the breath because of panic or running out of air. Rapid expansion of gas causes pulmonary overdistention and disruption of the alveolar capillary membrane. Air enters the pulmonary veins, travels to the heart, and enters the systemic circulation. Air embolism may result from causes other than diving, many of which are iatrogenic. Pulmonary barotrauma can occur from blast injuries, mechanical ventilation, penetrating chest trauma, and bronchoscopy. As discussed in Chapter 71, venous gas embolism occurs after scuba diving and in large volumes can enter the arterial circulation via a patent foramen ovale, atrial septal defect, or intrapulmonary arteriovenous anastomosis, or by overwhelming the pulmonary capillary network.

Box 72-5 summarizes the surgical and invasive procedures and nonsurgical causes of gas embolism.[235] Documented AGE, presumably from venous gas embolism, has occurred during

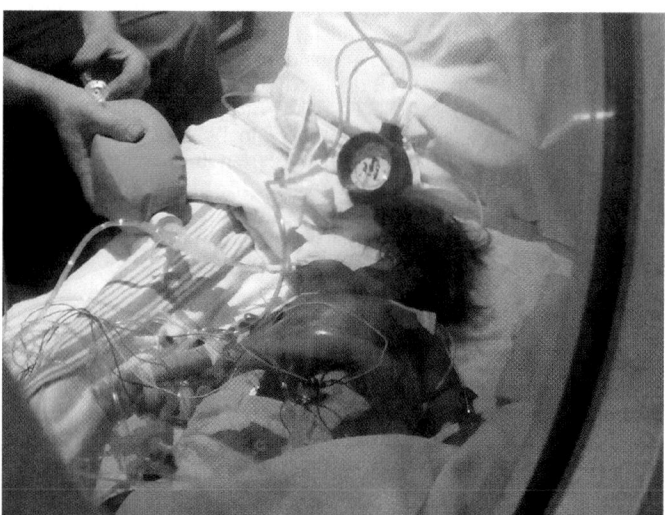

FIGURE 72-9 An 11-month-old boy undergoing HBOT for acute hepatic artery thrombosis after liver transplantation.

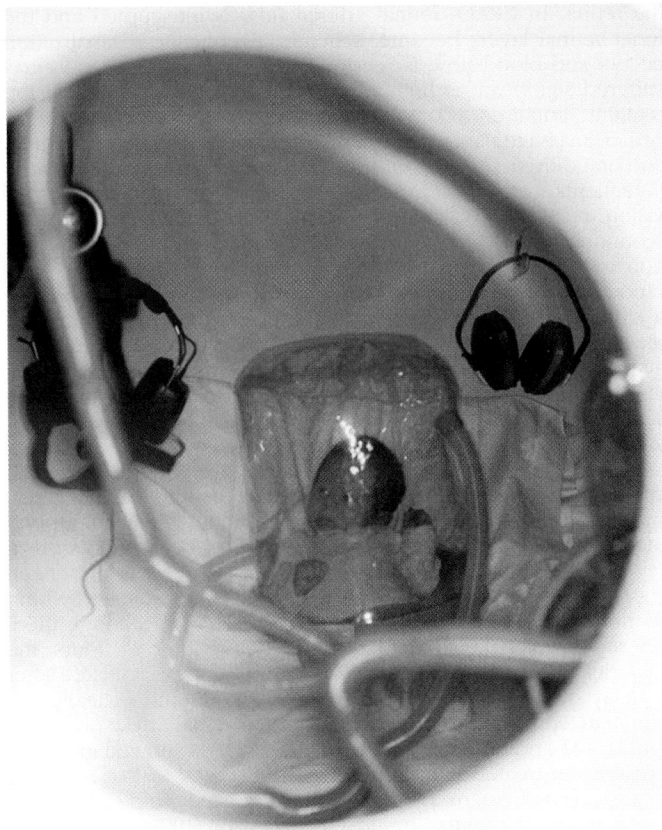

FIGURE 72-10 Child being treated in a hyperbaric chamber with the neckdam of the oxygen hood around his waist.

central venous catheterization, mechanical ventilation, cardiopulmonary bypass, angioplasty, lung biopsy, percutaneous hepatic puncture, liver transplant, hemodialysis, gastrointestinal endoscopy, hydrogen peroxide irrigation and ingestion, spine surgery, oral sex, sexual intercourse after childbirth, transurethral prostatectomy, laparoscopy, arthroscopy, hysteroscopy, and cesarean delivery.* Abnormal neurologic findings after cardiovascular or neurologic surgery or dialysis should make one consider AGE.

*References 8, 9, 18, 46, 49, 57, 89, 101, 108, 141, 152, 155, 226, 231, 233, 240, 250.

AGE manifests with a sudden alteration in consciousness, confusion, focal neurologic deficits, cardiac arrhythmias, and death. AGE requires immediate recompression. HBOT reduces the volume of gas bubbles, thereby restoring the blood flow, and improves oxygen delivery to ischemic, hypoperfused tissues. HBOT reduces cerebral edema and decreases ischemia-reperfusion injury. Treatment for AGE had traditionally been done according to U.S. Navy Table 6A, with an initial excursion to 165 feet (6 ATA) for 30 minutes to enhance bubble compression (Figure 72-11). Animal studies showed no additional benefit from compression to 6 ATA compared with 2.82 ATA.[120] Current recommendations include initial recompression to 2.82 ATA

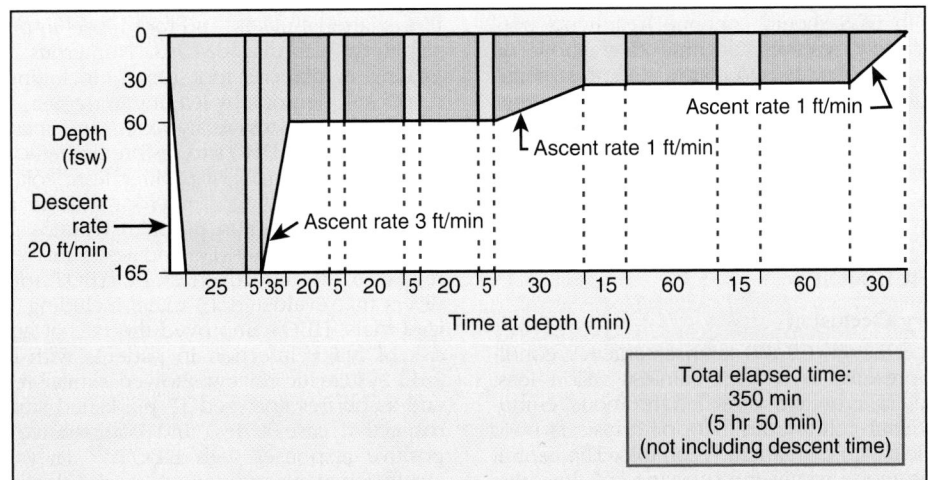

FIGURE 72-11 U.S. Navy Treatment Table 6A. fsw, feet of seawater. (*Redrawn from* U.S. Navy Diving Manual.)

while breathing 100% oxygen. If there is no improvement or clinical deterioration, deeper recompression to 6 ATA can be instituted. The diver breathes a mixture of 50% nitrogen and 50% oxygen below 2.82 ATA. Repetitive treatments are recommended until there is no further stepwise improvement.[149]

The Divers Alert Network has an on-call diving physician available 24 hours a day, 7 days a week, who can assist in triage and arrangement of transport and treatment for all diving injuries. In the United States, the network can be reached at 919-684-9111.

DECOMPRESSION SICKNESS

Decompression sickness (DCS) results from generation of bubbles of inert gas in the tissues and blood that interfere with organ function by occluding blood flow and other biochemical events (see Chapter 71). DCS may result from rapid ascent from diving, flying after diving, ascent in an unpressurized aircraft, or exposure in a hyperbaric or hypobaric chamber. Definitive treatment of DCS is immediate recompression and HBOT. HBOT causes immediate reduction in bubble volume, increase in the diffusion gradient for inert gas from the bubble into surrounding tissues, oxygenation of ischemic tissue, and reduction in cerebral edema. Other beneficial effects of HBOT that probably play a role in treating DCS are reduction in neutrophil adhesion to the capillary endothelium and prevention of ischemia-reperfusion injury.[131]

Various hyperbaric treatment regimens for DCS have been described. However, there are no human prospective, randomized studies for treatment of DCS. In general, U.S. Navy Table 6 has become the standard of treatment for pain-only and neurologic DCS.[214] Occasionally, U.S. Navy Table 5 is still used for pain-only DCS, but many diving physicians have discontinued its use.[75] U.S. Navy Tables 5 and 6 are shown in Chapter 71, Figure 71-14. These tables consist of compression to 60 fsw (2.8 ATA), initially with intermittent oxygen breathing. Theoretical advantages of using helium and oxygen in the Comex 30 table have been reported.[111] Longer oxygen treatment tables exist that feature extended decompression profiles for refractory cases of DCS involving the CNS.

The choice of treatment table and number of treatments required depend on the clinical severity of illness, response to treatment, and residual symptoms after initial recompression. If the delay to treatment is not excessive, the majority of patients with DCS have complete resolution of symptoms after a single hyperbaric treatment. Patients with severe DCS involving the spinal cord or a prolonged delay to recompression may have incomplete resolution of symptoms and often require repetitive treatments. Although delay to treatment worsens the outcome for severely injured divers, currently available data have not established a maximum time after which recompression is ineffective.[4,53] In one series of 76 divers, even despite a delay of 48 hours or longer for HBOT, 76% of divers with DCS had full recovery.[79] Patients with DCS should continue treatments until symptoms have completely resolved or until they show no further improvement in response to two consecutive treatments. Most individuals need no more than 5 to 10 repetitive treatments. Repetitive treatments can be given daily or twice daily as described in U.S. Navy Table 5, 6, or 9 (2-hour treatment at 2.4 ATA). A small number of patients have residual neurologic deficits that may either be permanent or improve gradually over 6 to 12 months.

ARTERIAL INSUFFICIENCIES

Central Retinal Artery Occlusion

Central retinal artery occlusion (CRAO) is an emergency condition of the eye that presents as sudden painless vision loss. Causes of CRAO include atherosclerosis-related thrombus, embolism, vasospasm, and giant cell arteritis. The prognosis is poor and patients are often left with permanent vision loss. The central retinal artery enters the globe within the substance of the optic nerve and serves the inner layers of the retina. The long posterior ciliary arteries supply blood to the choroid and outer layers of the retina. In CRAO, retinal arterial flow is interrupted and the inner retinal layers become ischemic. Eventually, recanalization occurs and blood flow is reestablished. The retina typically has suffered significant ischemia and cell death, however, so vision remains impaired. Conventional therapy for CRAO includes ocular massage, anterior chamber paracentesis, pentoxifylline, and oral diuretics; however, these modalities rarely restore vision.

Patients with CRAO present with sudden painless loss of vision, resulting in a clinical assessment of "light perception" to "counting fingers." Complete loss of vision with no light perception is more indicative of ophthalmic artery occlusion, with no blood flow in the choroidal vessels. In 15% to 30% of individuals, a cilioretinal artery is present that supplies the area around the macula; hence, central vision may be preserved in these individuals with CRAO. Ocular findings in patients with CRAO may include an afferent papillary defect and "boxcarring" of arterioles. The retina typically appears pale yellow or white due to ischemia; a cherry red spot may develop in the macula.

In cases of elevated partial pressures of oxygen, the choroidal circulation may supply enough oxygen to the inner retinal layers by diffusion to maintain viability of the inner retina.[121] Supplemental oxygen at normobaric pressures has been successful at reversing retinal ischemia in CRAO.[36,56,204] HBO has also been successful in restoring vision in cases of CRAO if initiated within 24 hours or less of onset of vision loss.[14,121,145,175] Although there are reports of patients responding to HBOT after 24 hours, the majority do not have return of vision if therapy is initiated after a delay of 24 or more hours. Murphy-Lavoie and colleagues[157] summarized 29 studies in the literature of retinal artery occlusion and HBOT and found that overall, 65% of cases showed improvement when treated with HBO.

Patients with signs and symptoms consistent with CRAO with onset within 24 hours should be placed on 100% oxygen at 1 ATA immediately. If vision improves significantly with normobaric oxygen within 15 minutes, the patient should be admitted and given intermittent normobaric oxygen for 15 minutes every hour. If there is no response within 15 minutes, HBOT should be initiated. Adjunctive therapies to lower intraocular pressure or cause retinal vasodilation can be started while HBOT is being arranged. Recommended protocols for HBOT range from 2 to 2.8 ATA for 90 minutes twice daily for a minimum of 3 days.[156] U.S. Navy Table 6 has also been considered for treatment if there is no improvement at 2.8 ATA after 20 minutes. HBOT should be continued twice daily until there is no further visual improvement after 3 consecutive days. If a patient has return of vision during HBOT, inpatient monitoring and intermittent supplemental oxygen should be considered.[157]

Enhancement of Healing in Selected Problem Wounds

Problem or chronic wounds are usually present in a compromised host and fail to respond to medical and surgical management. The incidence and prevalence of these wounds are increasing. Such wounds include venous leg ulcers, pressure ulcers, arterial ulcers, and foot ulcers in patients with diabetes or significant vascular disease. Numerous factors impair wound healing in diabetic foot ulcers, including impaired autonomic responses, neuropathy leading to trauma, impaired microvascular perfusion, local tissue hypoxia, and increased rates of wound infection. Using HBOT to restore tissue PO_2 into the normal range can stimulate fibroblast proliferation, collagen synthesis, neutrophil oxidative killing of microorganisms, and angiogenesis.

The most common problem wounds treated with HBOT are diabetic foot wounds. Liu and associates[124] published a systematic review of the effectiveness of HBOT for chronic diabetic foot ulcers that evaluated 13 trials, including 7 prospective randomized trials. HBOT improved the rate of healing and lowered the risk of major infection in patients with diabetic foot ulcers. A 2012 systematic review showed similar results.[69] In 2014, Worth and associates analyzed 17 published studies (clinical trials, retrospective case series, and comparative case series) showing positive responses with HBOT.[253] They also reviewed arterial insufficiency ulcers, venous stasis ulcers, and pressure ulcers. HBOT is not indicated in routine pressure ulcer management or for primary management of venous stasis ulcers. Primary treatment of arterial insufficiency ulcers is to improve blood flow using angioplasty, surgical revascularization, or other interventional techniques.

Other treatments to hasten recovery include negative pressure wound therapy (wound vacuum-assisted closure), bioengineered tissue grafts, topical debriding agents, platelet-derived growth factor, and surgical closure in combination with HBOT. Not all wounds should be treated with HBOT. For example, HBOT is not a substitute for surgical revascularization in arterial insufficiency, for which a comprehensive, multidisciplinary approach is advised.

HBOT is administered at 2 to 2.5 ATA for 90 to 120 minutes once or twice daily. Patients hospitalized with limb-threatening infections or significant peripheral arterial occlusive disease may require twice-daily treatments until stabilized. Many of these wounds are slow to respond and may require 30 to 60 HBO treatments. Appropriate wound care is extremely important to facilitate healing, and many hyperbaric chambers are associated with wound care centers.

Figure 72-12 shows a 58-year-old diabetic man with Wagner grade 3 plantar foot wound with necrosis and cellulitis. He refused amputation and was treated with 30 hyperbaric treatments. He responded with granulation of the wound tissues and eventual epithelialization and closure.

CARBON MONOXIDE AND CYANIDE POISONING

Carbon monoxide poisoning is a significant health problem in the United States, accounting for more than 50,000 emergency department visits annually. Poisonings occur primarily from fire smoke, exhaust from internal combustion engines, and inhalation of fumes from faulty gas furnaces. Carbon monoxide poisoning has also occurred in recreational boaters and campers who use internal combustion engines and fossil fuel heaters in enclosed spaces.

Carbon monoxide toxicity is mediated by a number of mechanisms that lead to hypoxic stress. Carbon monoxide binds to hemoglobin with an affinity 200 times that of oxygen, resulting in a shift of the hemoglobin-oxygen dissociation curve to the left and tissue hypoxia. Additionally, carbon monoxide binds to myoglobin and cytochrome oxidase, interfering with intracellular respiration and increasing oxidative stress, both of which contribute to cell death. Carbon monoxide causes the production of reactive oxygen species, leading to neuronal necrosis and apoptosis.[177] In addition to hypoxic stress, carbon monoxide poisoning leads to a complex cascade of biochemical events involving inflammatory and immunologic processes.[215,216,218,219,222] A poor correlation exists between tissue hypoxia and blood carboxyhemoglobin levels.

The most common signs and symptoms of carbon monoxide poisoning are headache, nausea, vomiting, dizziness, malaise, and confusion. Chest pain and shortness of breath may occur. Severe exposures result in loss of consciousness and death.[82,245] Carbon monoxide poisoning can result in delayed neurologic sequelae, characterized by deterioration in cognitive and motor function that appears days to weeks after the initial insult. Delayed neurologic sequelae are reported in up to 46% of acute carbon monoxide poisoning victims.[223,247]

Supplemental oxygen is the standard treatment for carbon monoxide poisoning. Oxygen hastens dissociation of carbon monoxide from hemoglobin and provides enhanced tissue oxygenation. Use of HBOT for treatment of carbon monoxide poisoning is based on the following mechanisms:

- HBOT accelerates the rate of carbon monoxide dissociation from hemoglobin; the carboxyhemoglobin half-life is decreased from 5.5 hours breathing air to 23 minutes breathing 100% oxygen at 3 ATA.[29,169]
- HBOT accelerates dissociation of carbon monoxide from cytochrome oxidase, thereby improving oxidative phosphorylation at 3 ATA.[31]
- HBOT prevents carbon monoxide–mediated brain lipid peroxidation and leukocyte-mediated inflammatory changes in the brain by inhibition of leukocyte beta$_2$ interferons.[215,216]
- HBOT reduces brain inflammation and improves mitochondrial oxidative processes.[218]
- HBOT decreases cerebral edema and maintains adequate cerebral oxygen delivery.
- HBOT reduces necrosis and protects against accelerated apoptosis.[33]

Animal models of carbon monoxide poisoning and HBOT demonstrate more rapid improvement in cardiovascular status, lower mortality rates, and a lower incidence of neurologic sequelae.[100,171,227]

HBOT is recommended for patients with a carboxyhemoglobin level greater than 25% or with signs of serious carbon monoxide poisoning, including prolonged unconsciousness, neurologic symptoms, cardiovascular dysfunction, or severe acidosis, irrespective of the carboxyhemoglobin level. HBOT should be used more liberally in pregnant patients because of enhanced fetal vulnerability to carbon monoxide and hypoxia.[234] Controversy exists surrounding HBOT for mild to moderate cases of carbon monoxide poisoning and whether HBOT can prevent delayed neurologic sequelae. Six randomized, controlled clinical trials during acute carbon monoxide poisoning had conflicting results; however, the studies varied in quality, study design, and outcomes. The studies that showed no benefit from HBOT had long treatment delays and poor follow-up.[55,135,180,189,223,247] The largest randomized clinical trial with the best study design and follow-up demonstrated a significant benefit of HBOT in decreasing the incidence of delayed neurologic sequelae.[247] A recent review article by Hampson and colleagues[84] discusses practice recommendations in acute carbon monoxide poisoning, including recommendations for HBOT. The recommended treatment protocol for carbon monoxide poisoning is 2.4 to 3 ATA for 90

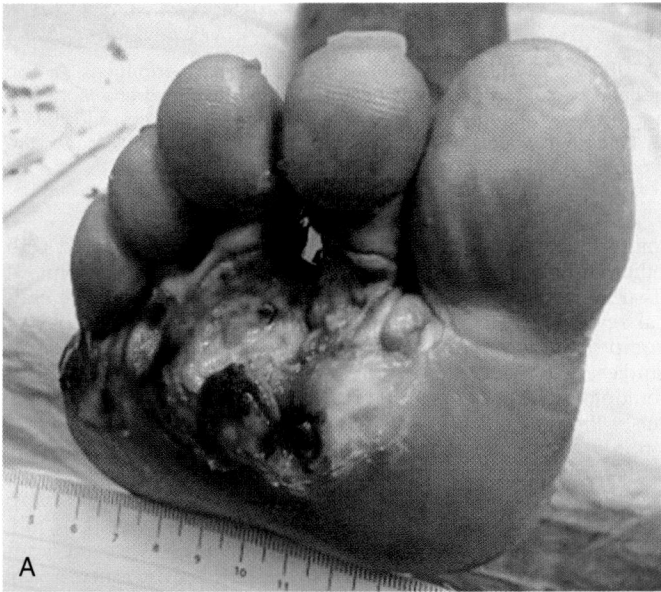
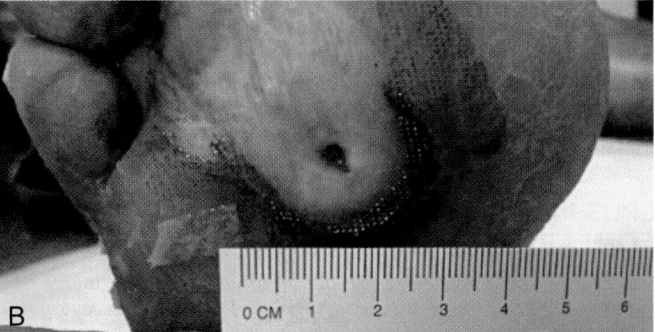

FIGURE 72-12 Diabetic foot wound. **A,** A 58-year-old diabetic man with Wagner grade 3 plantar foot wound. **B,** After 30 HBO treatments, he had almost complete closure of his wound, eliminating the need for amputation. (*Courtesy of Caesar Anderson, MD*).

to 120 minutes[247] for a total of three treatments at 6- to 12-hour intervals.[83]

Using HBOT to treat cyanide poisoning is less clear. Hydrogen cyanide often accompanies carbon monoxide poisoning; the toxic effects of cyanide and carbon monoxide are synergistic.[165] Treatment for hydrogen cyanide poisoning includes hydroxocobalamin with or without sodium thiosulfate. Amyl nitrite and sodium nitrite induce methemoglobin to bind hydrogen cyanide, which can further impair the oxygen-carrying capacity in the presence of carbon monoxide. HBO may directly reduce the toxicity of cyanide and maintain adequate oxygen delivery to the brain during the peak insult from hydrogen cyanide. In recent work in animal models after cyanide poisoning, HBO was beneficial in increasing cerebral tissue oxygen partial pressures and in reducing respiratory distress and cyanosis.[118] There are no controlled clinical trials of HBOT for pure cyanide poisoning or carbon monoxide poisoning complicated by cyanide. The use of HBOT is supported only by anecdotal cases; the clinical literature is limited.[25,71,117,123,190]

CLOSTRIDIAL MYONECROSIS (GAS GANGRENE)

Invasive clostridial infection usually results from injury or contamination of wounds. Clostridial myositis accompanied by myonecrosis (gas gangrene) is an acute, rapidly progressive invasive infection of muscles characterized by toxemia, edema, tissue death, and gas production. *Clostridium* is an anaerobic, spore-forming, gram-positive encapsulated bacillus. The most common species isolated is *C. perfringens* (isolated in 80% to 90% of wounds); others include *C. novyi*, *C. septicum*, and *C. histolyticum*. *C. perfringens* is a facultative anaerobe that can multiply freely in tissues with an oxygen tension of 30 mm Hg and demonstrates restricted growth at oxygen tensions of 70 mm Hg. Although more than 20 toxins are produced, the most prevalent and lethal is alpha-toxin, which causes hemolysis and tissue necrosis. HBOT does not kill clostridial organisms; it has a bacteriostatic effect and at oxygen tensions of 250 mm Hg inhibits alpha-toxin production.[237]

Treatment for clostridial infections consists of surgical debridement, antibiotics, and HBOT as soon as possible to stop alpha-toxin production and to save potentially viable tissue. Multiple retrospective clinical studies report improved overall survival rates and a decreased rate of amputation. The lowest rates of morbidity and mortality are achieved with initial conservative surgery and rapid initiation of HBOT.[5,73,90,112,173,181]* This approach not only saves lives but also saves limbs and tissues because no major amputations or excisions are done prematurely and demarcation of dead tissue is allowed.

HBOT for gas gangrene should be given at 3 ATA every 8 hours for the first 24 hours and then twice per day at 2.4 to 3 ATA for 2 to 5 days. When daily assessment reveals no further evidence of ongoing tissue necrosis, HBOT can be stopped. Figure 72-13 shows a young female who fell while riding her horse and sustained gas gangrene due to *C. perfringens*. After aggressive surgical debridement, antibiotics, and HBOT, a graft was placed to cover her wound, and she made an excellent recovery.

COMPROMISED GRAFTS AND FLAPS

HBOT is extremely useful in flap salvage when tissue is compromised by decreased perfusion, irradiation, or hypoxia. HBOT can help maximize viability of compromised grafts and flaps by improving tissue oxygenation and increasing flap capillary density. HBOT enhances graft and flap survival by decreasing the hypoxic insult, enhancing fibroblast function and collagen synthesis, stimulating angiogenesis, and inhibiting ischemia-reperfusion injury. Since 1966, experimental animal studies have shown improved skin flap survival in animals treated with HBOT compared with controls.[11,142,160,191] In an ischemic flap model in rats, HBOT increased microvascular blood flow during reperfusion, compared with untreated ischemic controls, by reducing neutrophil endothelial adherence in venules and blocking progressive arteriolar vasoconstriction associated with reperfusion

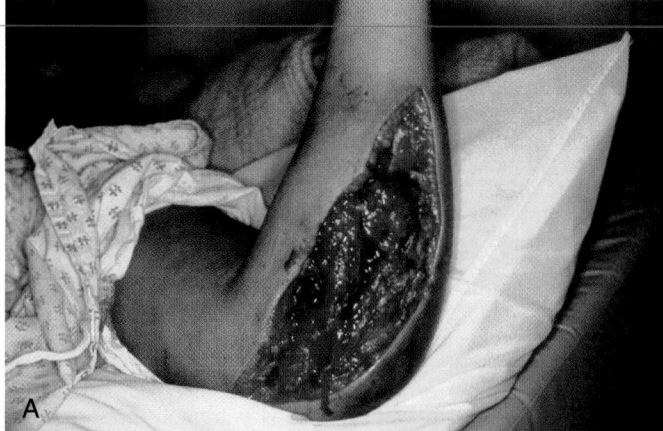

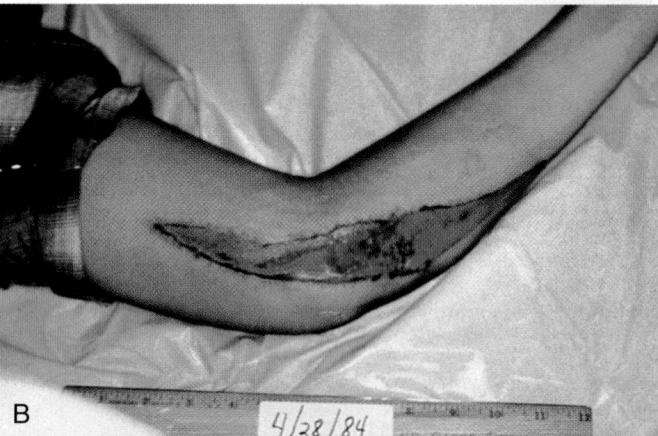

FIGURE 72-13 Gas gangrene due to *Clostridium perfringens*. **A,** The patient presented with myonecrosis from gas gangrene and was aggressively treated with surgical debridement, antibiotics, and HBOT. **B,** Once her wound was stabilized, a graft was placed to cover the wound.

injury.[259] Flap survival with HBOT averaged 90%, compared with other studies with failure rates as high as 67% in compromised tissues.[27,172,244] Baynosa and Zamboni[11,12] published extensive critical reviews of HBOT and its applications to different types of compromised flaps and grafts in both animal and clinical human studies that demonstrates the benefit of adjunctive HBOT for multiple types of grafts and flaps with various causes of compromise. Prompt initiation of HBOT as soon as flap or graft compromise is identified maximizes tissue viability and ultimately graft or flap salvage.

HBOT is most effective when started as soon as signs of flap compromise appear. Initial treatments should be twice daily at a pressure of 2 to 2.5 ATA for 90 to 120 minutes. Once the graft or flap appears more viable, HBOT can be given once a day until the flap appears stable. The average number of treatments varies from 10 to 20. In patients who have had previous graft or flap failure, 20 treatments prior to flap placement can prepare the site with granulation tissue, followed by 10 to 20 treatments after flap or graft placement to ensure tissue survival. Figure 72-14 shows a dusky, ischemic flap after surgery; it improved dramatically with a single HBOT treatment.

CRUSH INJURIES AND SKELETAL MUSCLE COMPARTMENT SYNDROMES

HBOT is a therapeutic adjunct to treatment of crush injury and skeletal muscle compartment syndrome. Posttraumatic cytogenic and vasogenic edema reduce tissue oxygenation, contributing to hypoxia and ischemia. There may be secondary tissue destruction caused by reperfusion injury. HBOT (1) increases tissue oxygen tension in hypoxic tissue during the early postinjury period when oxygen demand is greatest; (2) causes vasoconstriction

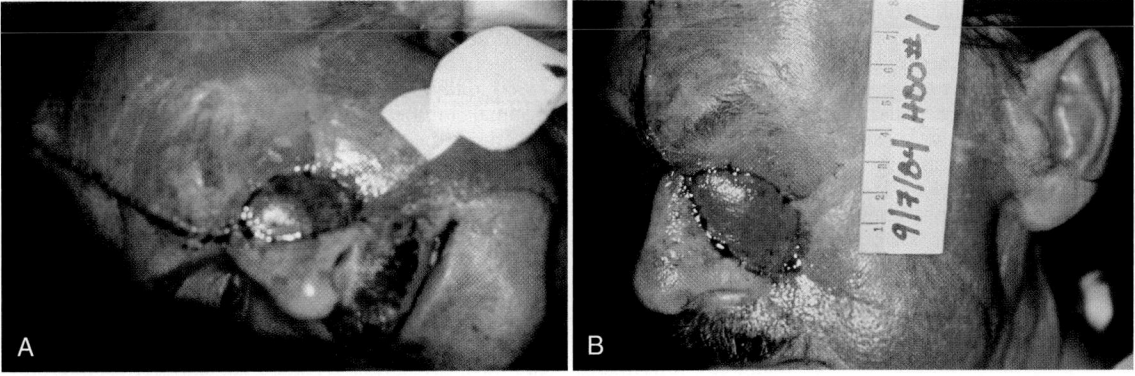

FIGURE 72-14 HBOT and compromised flap. **A,** Shortly after surgery, the flap appeared dusky and ischemic. **B,** The patient was treated with one round of HBOT and had immediate improvement in color and blood flow to the wound.

and edema reduction while maintaining hyperoxygenation; (3) improves blood flow in the microcirculation by decreasing interstitial fluid pressures attributed to edema reduction; and (4) mitigates reperfusion injury that accompanies crush injuries and skeletal muscle compartment syndrome.

Numerous animal studies and clinical series support use of HBOT for crush injuries and compartment syndrome.[51,70,166,207,208,259] A randomized, double-blinded clinical trial in crush injuries showed a statistically significant 94% healing rate in the HBOT group compared with 59% in controls.[26] A complete summary of the supporting literature and an evidence-based review is provided by Strauss.[206]

Early initiation of HBOT within 4 to 6 hours of injury or ischemia is essential. HBOT is administered at 2 to 3 ATA for 90 to 120 minutes. The number of treatments depends on the pathophysiology. Patients with crush injuries require HBOT three times a day for the first 2 days, two times a day for the next 2 days, and daily for an additional 2 days. Suspected reperfusion injuries after reimplantations, placement of free flaps, or transient ischemia only require one or two treatments. Signs of impending compartment syndrome include increasing pain, particularly with passive stretch, a tense compartment, and hyperesthesia or weakness in the distal extremity. If compartment pressures indicate that fasciotomy is not required, HBOT should be given three times within 24 hours. If clinical indications and compartment pressure measurements dictate immediate fasciotomy, HBOT can be used after surgery to reduce morbidity from residual injury due to swelling and ischemia.

DELAYED RADIATION INJURIES (SOFT TISSUE AND BONY NECROSIS)

Radiation kills normal tissue and causes loss of vascularity and cellularity. Delayed radiation complications are seen after a latent period of 6 months or more and may develop many years after exposure. Radiation leads to progressive obliterative endarteritis with resultant tissue ischemia and fibrosis. Dental extractions and other surgical procedures are associated with high complication rates when performed on heavily irradiated tissues.

HBOT stimulates fibroplasia, angiogenesis, and increased cellularity in radiated tissue by mechanisms similar to those described above for wound healing.[150] HBO can correct diminished stem and progenitor cell mobilization caused by irradiation and chemotherapy.[72] HBOT has been used prophylactically before oral surgery in a radiated tissue field and to treat delayed radiation tissue injury. HBOT has been used successfully for many years in treatment and prevention of mandibular osteoradionecrosis.

From randomized, prospective trials of bone grafts to irradiated tissue in humans, a standard protocol has been developed for use of HBOT when surgery is performed in irradiated tissue.[132,133] This protocol of 20 to 30 preoperative HBOT treatments followed by 10 postoperative treatments has been shown to be effective for head and neck therapy after radiation surgery, including bone graft reconstruction, soft tissue vascular flaps, and tooth extraction. In a recent review by Hampson and associates,[82] 73% of 43 patients treated for mandibular necrosis showed complete resolution and 21% had significant improvement. HBOT is also beneficial for prophylaxis of osteoradionecrosis. Figure 72-15 demonstrates improvement in osteoradionecrosis with use of HBOT.

This clinical success has led scientists to apply HBOT to radiation injuries at other sites. HBOT has been shown to be beneficial in other forms of soft tissue radionecrosis, including radiation proctitis, enteritis, and cystitis.[20,28,40,59,84] Additionally, HBOT is useful in treatment of laryngeal and tracheal radionecrosis, and for soft tissue necrosis of the head, neck, and chest wall, the latter particularly after mastectomy.[38,62] A more recent application has been use of HBOT to treat neurologic injuries secondary to radiation, including transverse myelitis, brain necrosis, optic neuritis, and brachial and sacral plexopathy.[58] Although evidence of

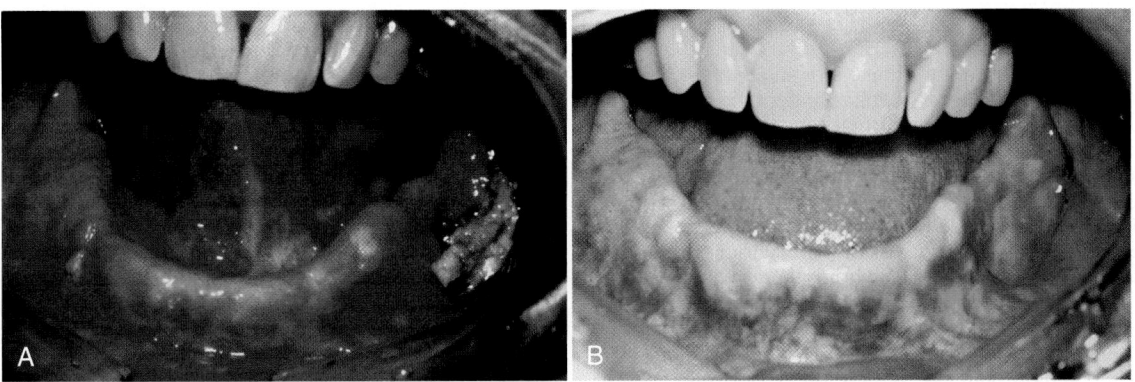

FIGURE 72-15 Patient with osteoradionecrosis of the mandible before **(A)** and after **(B)** HBOT.

beneficial HBOT for radiation-induced neurologic injuries is anecdotal, because of the severe consequences of injury to the CNS, HBOT should be given serious consideration.

HBOT for radiation injury is administered at 2 to 2.5 ATA daily for 20 to 40 treatments. Some patients benefit from additional treatments, so utilization review should occur at 60 treatments. To prevent osteoradionecrosis in patients who require extraction of teeth in previously irradiated jaws, the patients should receive 20 treatments before extraction, followed by 10 treatments after extraction. If osteoradionecrosis is already present, the treatment protocol changes to 30 preextraction treatments, or surgical resection followed by 10 postresection treatments.

A frequent concern of practitioners referring patients for HBOT with radiation injury is the fear that HBOT will accelerate malignant cancer growth or cause a dormant malignant tumor to be reactivated. Feldmeier[58] extensively reviewed this subject and found that both clinical reports and animal studies show no enhancement of cancer growth or recurrence rates.

IDIOPATHIC SUDDEN SENSORINEURAL HEARING LOSS

Idiopathic sudden sensorineural hearing loss is loss of at least 30 dB over at least three contiguous frequencies within 3 days. In addition to sudden unilateral hearing loss, individuals present with tinnitus, vertigo, and a sensation of aural fullness. Although the cause of this type of hearing loss is unclear, possible pathophysiologic mechanisms include vascular occlusion, cochlear membrane damage, ischemia, viral infections, labyrinthine membrane breaks, diseases associated with immunity, and trauma. Perilymph oxygen tension decreases significantly with sudden sensorineural hearing loss. HBOT increases the perilymph PO_2 by 9.4-fold.[114] Additional benefits of HBOT in the treatment of idiopathic sudden sensorineural hearing loss may include antiinflammatory effects, blunting of ischemia-reperfusion injury, and edema reduction.

Murphy-Lavoie and colleagues[158] and Piper and associates[178] have published the most comprehensive reviews of HBOT treatment efficacy for idiopathic sudden sensorineural hearing loss. There are more than 100 publications evaluating the use of HBOT for the condition, including 8 randomized controlled trials. The majority of these studies have shown that HBOT has significant efficacy as an adjunct to medical therapy.

The recommended treatment is 100% oxygen at 2 to 2.5 ATA for 90 minutes daily for 10 to 20 treatments. The best outcomes occur by combining oral corticosteroids with HBOT, particularly in patients with profound hearing loss treated within 2 weeks from symptom onset.

INTRACRANIAL ABSCESS

HBOT is an adjunct to treatment for intracranial abscess. The overall mortality rate for intracranial abscess is 2.7% to 25% in patients with underlying immune deficiency or neoplasm.[254] In certain patients with complications or in patients who pose therapeutic problems, HBOT has been beneficial when used as an adjunct. Over 109 cases of intracranial abscess treated with adjunctive HBO have been reported in the literature, with an overall mortality rate of 0% to 3.4%.[115,136,211]

Proposed mechanisms of HBOT in intracranial abscess include reduction in brain swelling, inhibition of anaerobic organisms found in the abscess, enhancement of neutrophil-mediated phagocytosis of infecting organisms, and treatment of concomitant skull osteomyelitis. HBOT has been recommended as a complement to currently accepted standard procedures in patients with multiple abscesses or abscesses in a deep or dominant location; in a compromised host with an abscess; in patients who are poor surgical candidates or for whom surgery is contraindicated; or in patients in whom there has been no response to standard surgical and antibiotic treatment or who have deteriorated further after undergoing standard treatment.[6] Because of significant mortality rates and long-term sequelae, it is unlikely that a rigid, human, double-blind controlled study can be done.

For the treatment of intracranial abscess, HBOT is administered at 2 to 2.5 ATA, with 60 to 90 minutes of oxygen administration per treatment. Initially, HBOT should be administered twice daily depending on the condition of the patient. The optimal number of treatments is unknown; treatments should be based on the patient's clinical response and radiologic findings. In reported series, the average number of HBOT sessions was 14. Utilization review is recommended after 20 treatments.

NECROTIZING SOFT TISSUE INFECTIONS

HBOT is recommended as an adjunct to surgical debridements, antibiotic treatment, and goal-directed critical care therapy for necrotizing soft tissue infections (including crepitant anaerobic cellulitis, progressive bacterial gangrene, necrotizing fasciitis, Fournier's gangrene, nonclostridial myonecrosis, and zygomycotic gangrenous cellulitis), particularly for compromised hosts when the mortality rate is expected to be high. Detailed descriptions of each of these infections are beyond the scope of this chapter, but can be found in a recent summary.[97] These infections are typically mixed aerobic-anaerobic infections of subcutaneous tissues, fascia, and muscle. HBOT adversely affects anaerobic bacterial growth and improves neutrophil function. The hyperoxygenated tissue zone surrounding the infected area may be of significance in preventing extension of invading microorganisms.

Studies continue to demonstrate the beneficial effect of HBOT in management of necrotizing soft tissue infections. Patients treated with HBOT show a statistically significant lower mortality rate, decreased incidence of amputation, and improved long-term outcome.[47,97,112,181,183,194,200,249] There are no randomized, double-blinded, controlled clinical trials comparing the outcomes of patients treated with HBOT with patients not treated with it, because it would be unethical to perform such trials when morbidity and mortality rates have improved in patients treated with HBOT compared with those not treated with HBOT before it became available. HBOT can be both cost-effective and saving of life and limb, particularly for the sickest patients.

HBOT for necrotizing fasciitis is given at 2.4 to 3 ATA for 90 to 120 minutes twice daily until the patient has stabilized and infection is controlled. If the infection is severe, the recommendation is to give 3 ATA three times in the first 24 hours, followed by twice-daily treatments for up to 30 treatments.

REFRACTORY OSTEOMYELITIS

Refractory osteomyelitis recurs or persists after standard therapy with aggressive surgical debridement and antibiotics. HBOT can elevate tissue oxygen tension in infected bone to normal or above-normal levels.[130] Osteoclast function of removing necrotic bone is an oxygen-dependent process; osteoclasts do not function properly in hypoxic bone. HBOT has a stimulatory effect on osteoclast function.[144,150] Experimental animal models have demonstrated the benefit of HBO for refractory cases of osteomyelitis.[144,229] No prospective, randomized clinical human trial examining the effect of HBOT on refractory osteomyelitis exists, however. The overwhelming majority of published animal data, human case series, and prospective trials support using HBOT as a beneficial adjunct for management of refractory osteomyelitis.[87] The highest reported cure rates were obtained when HBOT was combined with culture-directed antibiotics and concurrent surgical debridement. Of patients who failed to respond to repetitive surgery and antibiotic care, 63% to 86% have had infections successfully arrested with addition of HBOT.[2,39,138] HBOT is indicated in patients who fail to respond to surgical debridement and appropriate antibiotics, or in whom osteomyelitis recurs after appropriate management.

In addition to long-bone osteomyelitis, specific cases of refractory osteomyelitis deserve special consideration because of their potential for life-threatening infections or their central neuraxial locations. HBOT has been recommended for mandibular, sternal, vertebral, and cranial osteomyelitis and for malignant external otitis. In one circumstance, it was used to treat progressive and potentially fatal *Pseudomonas aeruginosa* osteomyelitis involving

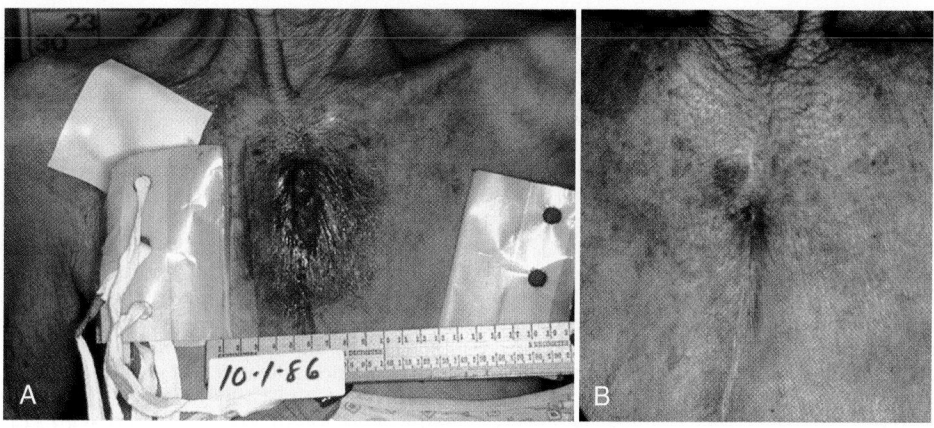

FIGURE 72-16 A, Woman with sternal osteomyelitis following coronary artery bypass graft that failed repeated debridements and two 6-week courses of IV antibiotics. **B,** After 40 sessions of HBOT, she had complete closure of the wound and resolution of osteomyelitis.

the external auditory meatus with osteomyelitis of the temporal bone.[1,48,159,174,187,258]

HBOT is used as an adjunct to standard surgical and antibiotic treatment for refractory osteomyelitis. Figure 72-16 shows a woman who developed sternal osteomyelitis after coronary artery bypass grafting. She was treated with two debridements and two separate 6-week courses of IV antibiotics. There was no improvement in her wound, and she was eventually referred for HBOT. After 40 treatments, she had complete resolution of her sternal infection and closure of the wound. HBOT is administered at 2 to 2.5 ATA for 90 to 120 minutes once per day, for an average of 20 to 40 treatments.

SEVERE ANEMIA

Severe anemia occurs when sufficient red cell mass is lost to compromise tissue oxygenation in a patient who, for medical, personal, or religious reasons, cannot or will not receive a blood transfusion. HBOT can dissolve enough oxygen to meet the oxygen requirements of tissues in the severely anemic patient until the bone marrow restores hemoglobin and red cell mass. Animal studies demonstrate the beneficial effect of HBOT in hemorrhagic shock models.[23,134,255] HBOT has been used successfully to correct accumulating oxygen debt in untransfusible patients and to reverse organ dysfunction in severe anemia associated with hemorrhagic shock.[74,76,143] The best published series of use of HBOT for treatment of exceptional anemia is reported by Hart; 26 patients with severe, exceptional blood loss anemia, defined as class IV hemorrhage, demonstrated a 70% survival rate.[88] Van Meter published a systematic review of HBOT for treatment of severe anemia.[236] HBOT may be used concurrently with erythropoietin, fluorocarbons, or stroma-free polymerized hemoglobin.

THERMAL BURNS

HBOT is used as an adjunct for treatment of thermal burns and has been shown to improve morbidity and mortality rates, reduce the length of the hospital stay, and decrease the need for surgery. The rationale for use of HBOT is to minimize edema, enhance host defenses, preserve marginally viable tissue, reduce ischemia-reperfusion injury, enhance leukocyte killing, preserve adenosine triphosphate (ATP), stimulate angiogenesis, and improve wound healing. Experimental data in animals have shown that HBOT reduces generalized edema and wound size.[102,167] Additionally, HBOT has a beneficial effect on angiogenesis and epithelial regeneration.[21] Biopsies of control animals showed progression to full-thickness injury, and biopsies of animals treated with HBOT showed preservation of dermal elements and capillary patency.[203]

Clinical experience in human burn patients suggests improved wound healing, reduction in mortality rates, decrease in the need

for surgical procedures and resuscitative fluid requirements, and reduced hospital stay attributed to adjunctive HBOT.[42-44,81] In a prospective, randomized, controlled, double-blind trial comparing HBOT with sham controls in a human burn model, Niezgoda and colleagues[161] demonstrated significant reductions of wound size, hyperemia, and wound exudates in the HBOT group. Current recommendations include serious burns greater than 20% of the total body surface area or involving the hands, face, feet, or perineum that are deep partial- or full-thickness injuries. Although use of HBOT for burn treatment is approved by the Undersea and Hyperbaric Medical Society, some burn centers around the country do not use HBOT except for carbon monoxide poisoning. A 2004 Cochrane Review found insufficient evidence to support or refute use of HBOT in the management of thermal burns.[241] In a recent evidence-based review, Cianci and colleagues[45] analyzed 22 clinical series; 20 of these reports demonstrated benefit of the use of HBOT in thermal injury.

HBOT should be initiated as soon as possible after injury. Initially, three treatments at 2 to 2.5 ATA for 90 minutes of oxygen delivery within the first 24 hours are recommended, and then twice-daily treatments for 10 to 14 days for 20 to 30 treatments. Further treatments are often used to optimize graft uptake. Patients rarely need more than 50 treatments. Careful attention to fluid management is critical, because initial fluid requirements of burn patients can be several liters per hour. Ambient temperature in the chamber should be comfortable because thermal instability can be problematic, particularly within 1 to 2 hours of burn wound dressing changes. In cases of concurrent inhalation injury, patients can be maintained on ventilator support during treatment.

TRENDS IN HYPERBARIC OXYGEN THERAPY RESEARCH

ACUTE MYOCARDIAL ISCHEMIA

In animal studies, HBOT reduces the ischemic effect of coronary artery occlusion.[202,224] Thomas and coworkers demonstrated that a combination of thrombolytic therapy and HBOT is more effective in reducing the size of a myocardial infarction than either treatment alone.[224] In a rabbit model of aortic atherosclerosis, HBOT not only halted the progression of the disease but also accelerated the regression of atherosclerotic lesions.[113] HBOT decreased the size of necrosis in rat myocardium after irreversible occlusion of the left coronary artery.[52] HBOT may lessen or inhibit reperfusion injury by protecting oxidative metabolism in reperfusion-stunned myocardium. The Hyperbaric Oxygen and Thrombolysis in Myocardial Infarction study showed that treatment with HBO in combination with thrombolysis resulted in attenuated creatine phosphokinase rise, more rapid resolution of pain, and improved ejection fraction.[201]

Dekleva and colleagues[50] demonstrated that HBOT in conjunction with streptokinase in acute myocardial infarction reduced left ventricular volumes with associated increases in ejection fraction. In a controlled trial, patients who underwent percutaneous coronary intervention for acute myocardial infarction or unstable angina and received HBOT in the early peri-PCI period had lower clinical restenosis rate and less frequent development of late anginal symptoms.[193] The authors postulate that HBOT may induce expression of antioxidant enzymes that offer protection against atherosclerosis and reduce oxidation products in high-density lipoproteins. Additionally, fibrinolysis derived from endothelial cells and blood flow are enhanced by HBOT, which could result in reduction in recurrent thrombosis.[225] The results are provocative; larger randomized trials are indicated.

Bennett and colleagues compared all studies of acute coronary syndrome treatments that included HBOT; this metaanalysis consisted of six trials with 665 patients.[15] They found a significant decrease in mortality rates with HBOT ($P = .02$). There was evidence from individual trials of reduction in the risk for major adverse coronary events ($P = .03$) and certain dysrhythmias ($P = .01$) following HBOT. The review also showed that HBOT following acute coronary syndrome reduced the amount of time until pain relief following the onset of angina ($P < .0001$). Evidence from these few trials suggests that HBOT is associated with reduction in risk of death, volume of damaged muscle, risk of major adverse coronary events, and time to relief from ischemic pain. However, because of study flaws, low numbers of patients, and inconsistency of timing of HBOT for myocardial injury, the authors caution that the results be carefully interpreted. Further studies are required to define the mechanistic role of HBOT in myocardial ischemia.

ACUTE CEREBRAL ISCHEMIA

The effectiveness of HBOT in cerebral ischemia is controversial. It is difficult to compare studies because of different stroke models in different species with different HBOT protocols. Recent work demonstrates that HBOT appears to be protective in various models of focal cerebral ischemia.[199,210,256] In three recent reports using magnetic resonance imaging in an animal model, HBOT given 40 minutes to 6 hours after stroke onset was neuroprotective; HBOT improved infarct volume reduction and neurologic outcome.[126,188,238] Early HBOT may stop the process of ischemic infarct growth by rapidly restoring oxygen and energy to ischemic but still viable brain tissue. Other proposed mechanisms of HBOT include reduction of extracellular dopamine and inhibition of cyclooxygenase-2 overexpression in the cerebral cortex,[256,257] as well as effects on antiinflammatory and antiapoptotic responses.

Although animal studies suggest a possible role of HBOT in treating acute cerebral ischemia, clinical studies of humans have failed to show significant benefit from HBO, probably in part due to the long time window between symptom onset and HBOT.[17,162,185] Bennett and colleagues[17] reviewed 11 randomized controlled trials involving 705 patients and found no difference in case fatality rates at 6 months in those receiving HBOT or controls. Although some measures of disability and functional performance indicated improvement following HBOT, the authors found no good evidence that HBOT improved clinical outcomes.

TRAUMATIC BRAIN INJURY

Traumatic brain injury (TBI) can result in short- or long-term problems with memory, equilibrium, vision, headaches, decision making, judgment, fatigue, sleep, irritability, and emotional lability. TBI is one of the defining injuries of modern military conflict; an estimated 10% to 20% of U.S. service members suffer mild TBI from wars in the Middle East. TBI also occurs in nonmilitary activities that include motor vehicle accidents and sport and recreational accidents (e.g., bicycling, skiing). Incident rates vary widely; a rate of 130/100,000 individuals per year is a conservative estimate. HBOT has been proposed as a treatment for patients with TBI. Possible mechanisms by which HBOT may have

a beneficial effect include modulation of ischemia-reperfusion; reduction of brain inflammation and edema; improvement of oxygen availability to idling, but viable, neurons in the brain; and increase in metabolic performance of chronically impaired neurons leading to improved integrative plasticity.[141a]

There are multiple case reports of off-label use of HBOT for TBI that describe improvement in cognitive function; however, these reports have been criticized because they are not controlled trials. Randomized controlled trials report conflicting outcomes. In a 2012 Cochrane Review, Bennett and associates[16] reviewed seven studies involving 571 people (285 receiving HBOT); none of the studies were blinded. Although a few studies showed that HBOT might reduce the risk of death, there was little evidence that HBOT improved outcomes.

Wolf and colleagues[251] studied 50 U.S. Air Force personnel diagnosed with TBI in a double-blinded, randomized controlled study and found that compared with controls, HBOT did not reduce symptoms following concussion or symptoms of posttraumatic stress disorder. In a multicenter, double-blinded, sham-controlled clinical trial of 72 military service members with mild TBI, HBOT showed no benefit compared with sham compressions, although both groups improved compared with those who received care for postconcussive symptoms alone.[147] HBOT is currently not the standard of care for patients with TBI.

ORGAN TRANSPLANTATION

HBOT has been suggested to limit the ischemia-reperfusion injury that can complicate organ transplantation.[34,153] In animal studies, use of HBOT in transplantation has shown a positive response. HBOT influences ischemia-reperfusion injury and consequent acute cellular rejection. Several clinical studies have been published on using HBOT with liver transplantation. All such studies relate either to its use in the posttransplantation period for management of hepatic artery thrombosis[54,77,140] or its use in acute liver failure prior to transplantation. One major potential advantage of HBOT is that it affects the processes of ischemia-reperfusion injury and acute cellular rejection through numerous cellular and molecular mechanisms. HBOT has been shown to stimulate hepatocyte proliferation after liver resection in animal and human studies.[209,228] In addition, it may play a role as a liver support adjunct for fulminant hepatic failure, posttransplantation graft dysfunction, and acute hepatic artery thrombosis. More research is required on the influence of HBOT in liver transplantation, specifically its effect on the immune response.

APPLICATIONS FOR HYPERBARIC OXYGEN THERAPY IN WILDERNESS MEDICINE

HBOT plays a significant role in wilderness medicine for treatment of diving-related illnesses and altitude illness. HBOT has been investigated in other wilderness-related entities, such as frostbite, brown recluse spider bite, and, more recently, heatstroke. HBOT has also been successful in treating necrotizing soft tissue infection from a stingray puncture and *Vibrio vulnificus* septicemia and cellulitis from eating raw fish.[182,243] HBOT has been tried in an experimental rat model of sea nettle envenomation. Although it had no effect on mortality rate, HBOT protected against venom-induced decreases in brain blood flow and maintained oxygenation in envenomed animals.[151]

FROSTBITE

The first case of HBOT use with cold injury was reported by Ledingham in 1963, followed by a number of reports for its use in the 1970s. Numerous case reports are available, but controlled trial data are lacking. Initial experiments in rabbits showed that HBOT had no effect on tissue loss and variation of injury.[66,67,85] However, other studies have shown benefit. If HBOT was administered immediately after rewarming, the mean tissue loss was decreased in rabbits. This benefit was significantly reduced by delays in treatment, particularly beyond 24 hours.[67,168] Research into the pathophysiology of frostbite has revealed marked similarities to inflammatory processes seen in thermal burns, ischemia-reperfusion injury, and crush injury.[154] Hence, HBOT has theoretical advantages as an adjunct in the treatment of frostbite. An 11-year-old boy who suffered deep frostbite on six fingers was treated with HBOT and had complete recovery after 14 days.[242] In another report, HBOT was shown to improve skin microcirculation by increasing the number of nutrient capillaries in frostbitten areas on the toes.[63] A young female who suffered frostbite to her fingers and was treated with HBOT had complete return of function, with superficial tissue loss to one finger only.[64] A case of frostbite due to contact with liquid helium gas was successfully treated with HBOT with good recovery.[192] Kemper and associates[105] reported a case of deep frostbite of the toes treated with HBOT after a 21-day delay with good outcome. They reviewed 17 human case reports of frostbite treated with HBOT, all showing positive effects with no amputations.

The ideal time to initiate HBOT for frostbite is during the rewarming period because of the reperfusion aspect of the injury. Although there is no standard protocol, HBOT can be given at 2 to 2.5 ATA for 90 to 120 minutes three times in the first 24 hours, followed by twice-daily treatments until there is no longer threatened tissue loss. If a frostbitten limb has already been rewarmed and is at risk for significant tissue loss, HBOT is still indicated to help hasten demarcation, decrease the risk for infection, enhance the survival of the damaged tissue in the gradient of injury, and improve flap survival.

BROWN RECLUSE SPIDER BITE

The brown recluse spider (Loxosceles reclusa) is known to cause necrotic skin lesions in humans. Most bites resolve spontaneously, but a few progress to severe local necrosis and tissue loss (see Chapter 43). Treatment of brown recluse spider bites with HBOT remains controversial. HBOT has been proposed to directly inhibit neutrophil adherence to the endothelium and to decrease venom-induced ischemia-reperfusion injury, as well as perhaps inactivate sphingomyelinase or other components of the venom.[146] HBOT may minimize the wound size by increasing oxygen tension within the wound and thereby increasing angiogenesis and fibroblast proliferation.

Animal models show conflicting data. In experimental models using rabbits, there was neither reduction in lesion size nor histologic improvement from HBOT.[176] Similarly, there was no decrease in lesion size in a swine model.[91] Two reports have shown benefit in controlled animal studies. One showed histologic improvement in a rabbit model, but found no difference in lesion size.[205] A randomized, controlled trial using rabbits demonstrated that HBOT reduced the size of lesions, even when treatment was delayed by 2 days.[139] A single treatment given immediately was as effective as were multiple treatments.

Several case studies in humans suggest that HBOT may be beneficial in managing dermatonecrosis associated with L. reclusa. Svendsen first described the use of HBOT for treatment of brown recluse spider bites.[212] He treated six patients who had clinically deteriorating lesions with HBOT 2 to 6 days after the bite with twice-daily treatments for 3 days. All lesions healed well without surgery, skin sloughing, or significant scarring. Kendall and Caniglia reported 47 cases with good outcomes; only 1 of 48 patients required skin grafting.[106] Maynor and colleagues treated 14 patients, all of whom healed without scarring, disability, or a need for skin grafting.[137] Two cases of potentially devastating bites, one to the glans penis and another to the periorbital region on a child's face, were both treated with HBOT and had good outcomes.[30,99]

Tutrone and colleagues published a review of the treatment of brown recluse spider bites with HBOT[232] and found it may be effective at reducing scarring and complications. However, there are no randomized, controlled trials of HBOT in human cases of Loxosceles envenomation and no standardized HBOT protocols.

HBOT can be given at 2 to 2.5 ATA for 90 to 120 minutes on a daily basis for 2 to 10 treatments. Systemic symptoms, size of the dermatonecrotic lesion, and area of surrounding erythema should be assessed on a daily basis.

HEATSTROKE

Heatstroke is characterized by significant hyperthermia, altered mental status, and varying degrees of multiple-organ failure. In rodents, heatstroke causes vasoplegic shock, intracranial hypertension, and cerebral ischemia and injury.[122] In experimental studies on rats, HBOT was beneficial in resuscitating rats with experimental heatstroke. HBOT reduced heatstroke-induced arterial hypotension, hypoxia, plasma tumor necrosis factor-alpha overproduction, and cerebral ischemia. HBOT improved survival rates during heatstroke by augmenting mean arterial pressure and local cerebral blood flow and by decreasing multiple-organ dysfunction.[164,230] In a diabetic rat model of heatstroke, HBOT increased survival times by reducing heat-induced activated inflammation and ischemic and oxidative damage in the hypothalamus and other brain regions.[119] In another rat model for heatstroke, activated protein C or HBOT was equally effective in reducing heat-induced inflammation, a hypercoagulable state, and multiple-organ injury. Combined activated protein C and HBOT reduced these heatstroke reactions better than did activated protein C or HBO alone.[213]

Additionally, HBOT has been used to successfully treat a heatstroke patient with multiple-organ dysfunction.[163] HBOT is not standard therapy for heatstroke, however. Further work is needed to support its use as an adjunct to conventional treatment options in severe cases.

FIELD TREATMENT OF COMBAT TRAUMA

Because the indications for HBOT closely overlap those preset in combat casualties, HBOT has been increasingly used by U.S. and NATO forces for treatment of combat-related trauma.[86,129,239] Hart reviewed preliminary wound statistics from Operation Iraqi Freedom.[86] Approximately 70% of injured soldiers sustained extremity trauma. Of 560 surgical procedures performed, 31% were complicated by persistent tissue necrosis, wound infection, graft failure, or delayed wound healing. HBOT is effective in correcting tissue ischemia and hypoxia, as an adjunctive treatment for compartment syndrome, and for controlling wound infections and augmenting healing. Field use of HBOT for combat injuries could limit the extent of surgical debridements, improve tissue flap and graft survival rates, decrease wound infection rates, and improve healing rates for complex wounds. HBOT could be used as a temporizing measure pending operating room availability.

Several portable hyperbaric chambers have been suggested for use in field treatment. The Hyperlite Hyperbaric Chamber or Emergency Evacuation Hyperbaric Stretcher is ideal for remote locations without hospital support. The U.S. Navy's Transportable Recompression Chamber System is a multiplace chamber designed for treatment and evacuation of injured divers, but can be used for any emergency hyperbaric treatment and moved to almost any location. The Fly Away Recompression Chamber is a much larger system (61 m³ [200 feet³]), consisting of a double-lock recompression chamber capable of treating divers or any patient in need of HBOT. A multiplace hyperbaric chamber could be put aboard a designated hospital ship for treatment of combat wounds.

REFERENCES

Complete references used in this text are available online at expertconsult.inkling.com.

PAUL S. AUERBACH, GEORGE H. BURGESS, AND ALEXANDRA E. DiTULLIO

The expanses of oceans, estuaries, and fresh waters that cover the earth are the greatest wilderness. Seventy-one percent (or 362 million km^2 [139,768,981 miles^2]) of the earth's surface is composed of ocean, the volume of which exceeds 523 km^3 (325 million miles^3). Underneath the surface lie huge mountain ranges, deep valleys, and many active volcanoes. Nearly one-half of the sea floor is composed of an abyssal plain, which lies at an average depth of 4 km (2.5 miles) and is largely devoid of life forms. Within the undersea realm exist four-fifths of all living organisms. Hundreds of thousands of marine species have been taxonomically described and thousands are as yet undiscovered.

The opportunity for direct encounters with aquatic organisms continues to increase because of enhanced recreational, industrial, scientific, and military oceanic and freshwater activities related to ever-rising human populations. The most common cause of injuries is handling of animals that bite and sting in self-defense, followed by provoked encounters and then unprovoked encounters.

Nearly 80% of the world's population resides in coastal regions. In the United States, 50% of the population lives within 80 km (50 miles) of a coastline. It is estimated that 127 million U.S. citizens live along the coasts. A significant proportion of this population is directly involved as entrants into the aquatic world. Therefore, it is imperative that clinicians be familiar with hazards unique to the aquatic environment.

Although noxious marine organisms are concentrated predominantly in warm temperate and tropical seas, particularly in the Indo-Pacific region, hazardous animals may be found as far north as 50 degrees latitude. Saltwater aquariums in private homes and public settings, intercontinental seafood shipping, and increasing accessibility of air travel to aquatic recreationists, most notably scuba/skin divers and surfers, contribute to the risks.

Like the rainforest, the ocean depths have the potential to reveal virtually limitless active pharmaceutical agents, including antihelmintic, anticoagulant, antifungal, antimalarial, antiprotozoal, antituberculosis, antiinflammatory, and antiviral compounds.[129] Genetically engineered reproduction of the adhesive protein of the popularly consumed marine mussel *Mytilus edulis* has created a tissue adhesive agent that may one day prove superior to cyanoacrylic compounds. The annelid sandcastle worm *(Phragmatopoma californica)* manufactures a glue used to construct a protective home of sand and shell fragments. This is being investigated as a tissue adhesive for fragmented human bones. Toxins isolated from ascidians (tunicates, or sea squirts) include cyclic peptides, some of which (ecteinascidin-743, aplidine) have undergone evaluation for cancer chemotherapy; others (e.g., thiocoraline and kahalalide F) may follow. Investigative techniques continue to improve. In pursuit of anatomic information that can elucidate the biology and ecology of fish, evolution, cellular physiology, and aquatic models of human disease, nuclear radiologists have performed in vivo nuclear magnetic resonance imaging (MRI) and spectroscopy of anesthetized (tricaine methanesulfonate [MS222]) aquatic organisms.[26] Most marine organisms rely on antimicrobial components of their innate immune defenses to combat pathogens. From this unique perspective, scientists seek to identify novel antimicrobials, among which the most promising are marine cationic antimicrobial peptides, defined as small (10 to 40 amino acids) peptides containing a prevalence of positively charged residues (lysine and arginine).[147] As examples, these have been found in teleost fishes (pardaxin, pleurocidin, hepcidin), tunicates (styelin, clavanin), chelicerates (big defensin, tachyplesin), crustaceans (callinectin), gastropods (dolabellanin), and mollusks (mytilin). Their activities include synergy to induce cell lysis, modulating the host immune response, chemotaxis, macrophage development, production or inhibition of cytokines, and so forth. Sponges (phylum Porifera) and sharks (order Selachii) have become particular foci of biomedical screening over the past three decades.

Despite the wondrous nature of the deep, danger exists. The ubiquity of hazardous creatures and their propensity to appear at inopportune times make it imperative to be aware of them, to respect their territorial rights, and to avoid unpleasant contact with them.

DIVISIONS AND DEFINITIONS

Dangerous aquatic animals are divided into four groups: (1) those that bite, rip, puncture, or deliver an electric shock without envenomation; (2) those that sting (envenom),[173] discussed in Chapters 74 and 75; (3) those that are poisonous on ingestion (see Chapter 77); and (4) those that induce allergies (see Chapter 78). Aquatic skin disorders are discussed in Chapter 76.

IN DEFENSE OF THE FISH

As in all nature (except for humans), indiscriminate aggression is rarely involved when injuries are inflicted by aquatic animals. Most injuries result from gestures of warning or self-defense; aquatic creatures rarely attack humans without provocation. Attacks are made in defense of young, in territorial dispute when mating activities are interrupted, or during active procurement of food. *Caution* is the key word when dealing with potentially injurious aquatic creatures.

GENERAL PRINCIPLES OF FIRST AID

The physician must adhere to fundamental principles of medical rescue. Although many injuries and envenomations have unique clinical presentations, the cornerstone of therapy is immediate attention to the airway, breathing, and circulation. Along with specific interventions directed against a particular venom or poison, the rescuer must simultaneously be certain that the victim maintains a patent airway, breathes spontaneously or with assistance, and is supported by an adequate blood pressure. Because marine attacks and envenomations often affect swimmers and divers, the rescuer should anticipate drowning (see Chapter 69), immersion hypothermia (see Chapter 8), and decompression sickness or arterial air embolism (see Chapters 71 and 72). Any victim rescued from the ocean should be thoroughly examined for signs of a bite, puncture, or sting if such is a possibility.

WOUND MANAGEMENT

Whether the injury is a bite, abrasion, or puncture, meticulous attention to basic wound management is necessary to facilitate healing and minimize posttraumatic infection.

WOUND IRRIGATION

All wounds acquired in the natural aquatic environment should be vigorously irrigated with sterile diluent, preferably normal saline (0.9% sodium chloride) solution. Seawater is not recommended as an irrigant, because it carries a hypothetical infection risk. Sterile water or hypotonic saline is acceptable. Tap water (preferably disinfected) is a suitable alternate irrigant if a sterile solution cannot be obtained in a timely manner.[5] Irrigation should be performed before and after debridement. A 19-gauge needle or 18-gauge plastic intravenous (IV) catheter attached to a syringe that delivers a pressure of 7031 to 14,061 kg/m[2] (10 to 20 psi) will dislodge most bacteria without forcing irrigation fluid into tissue along the wound edges or deeper along dissecting tissue planes. Convenient ring-handle syringes with blunt irrigation tips and IV tubing that connects to standard IV bags are useful. At least 100 to 250 mL of irrigant should be flushed through each wound. If a laceration is from a stingray, proteinaceous (and possibly) heat-labile venom may be present in the wound. Therefore, if the wound is still painful at the time of irrigation, the irrigant may be warmed to a maximum temperature of 45°C (113°F).[9]

Antiseptic may be added to the irrigant if the wound appears to be highly contaminated. Povidone-iodine solution in a concentration of 1% to 5% may be used with a contact time of 1 to 5 minutes.[199] When antiseptic irrigation is completed, the wound should be thoroughly irrigated with normal saline or tap water to minimize tissue toxicity from the antiseptic. Antiseptics that are particularly harmful to tissues include full-strength hydrogen peroxide, povidone-iodine scrub solution, hexachlorophene detergent, and silver nitrate.

Scrubbing should be used to remove debris that cannot be irrigated from the wound. Sharp surgical debridement is preferable to sponge scrubbing, which may increase infection rates, particularly when applied with harsh antiseptic solutions. Poloxamer 188 (Pluronic F-68), a nontoxic, nonionic surfactant skin wound cleanser (found in Shur-Clens 20%), does not offer any significant advantage over traditional sterile saline irrigation.

WOUND DEBRIDEMENT

Debridement is more effective than irrigation at removing bacteria and debris. Crushed or devitalized tissue should be removed with sharp dissection to provide clean wound edges and encourage brisk healing with minimal infection risk. The limitations are those imposed by anatomy, specifically skin tautness or the presence of vital structures. Anesthesia of wound edges may be attained by regional nerve block or local infiltration with lidocaine or bupivacaine, which do not damage local tissue defenses. A topical anesthetic mixture containing epinephrine may be less desirable because of the vasoconstrictive effects and theoretical infection-potentiating effects. Definitive wound exploration, debridement, and repair should be undertaken in an appropriate sterile environment. It is often impractical to explore complex wounds in the emergency department, and some wounds may necessitate surgical exploration in the operating room. Operating loupes can be used as needed to inspect the wound for residual foreign material, such as sand, seaweed, tooth or spine fragments, or integumentary sheath shards. Standard radiographs, static soft tissue techniques, computed tomography, ultrasound, MRI, or fluoroscopy should be used preoperatively or perioperatively to localize spines or teeth.

WOUND CLOSURE

The decision to close a wound must weigh the risk of infection. The incidence of infection is high in wounds acquired in natural bodies of water because such wounds may be contaminated with venom or potentially virulent microorganisms, or both; because early adequate irrigation and debridement are often unavailable; and because definitive care is often delayed. Tight wound closure restricts drainage and promotes bacterial proliferation, particularly from anaerobes, which are common contaminants. Wounds at high risk in this regard include those on the hands, wrists, or feet; punctures and crush injuries; wounds into areas of fat with poor vascularity; and wounds to victims who are immunosuppressed. Whenever possible, the use of sutures to close dead space in contaminated wounds should be minimized because the absorbable sutures act as foreign bodies.

PROPHYLAXIS AGAINST TETANUS

Any wound that disrupts the skin can become contaminated with *Clostridium tetani*. Anaerobic bacteria, predominantly of the genus *Clostridium*, have been isolated in shark tissue and as part of the oral flora of alligators and crocodiles. Proper immunization with tetanus toxoid virtually eliminates the risk of disease. Although it was previously accepted that the protective level of toxin-neutralizing antibody is 0.01 antitoxin unit/mL, it appears that clinical tetanus can develop despite an antibody level many times that amount. Therefore, it is imperative to provide an early and adequate booster injection. If the victim is older than age 50 years, is from an underdeveloped country, or cannot provide a definite history of tetanus immunization, it is likely that circulating toxin-neutralizing antibody will be suboptimal. Prophylaxis should be provided according to the scheme shown in Chapter 21 in Table 21-6. Tdap (tetanus, reduced diphtheria, and acellular pertussis vaccine) should be used instead of Td for routine tetanus boosters and wound management in adolescents and adults.

BACTERIOLOGY OF THE AQUATIC ENVIRONMENT

Wounds acquired in the aquatic environment are soaked in natural source water and sometimes contaminated with sediment. Penetration of the skin by the spines or teeth of animals, the razor edges of coral or shellfish, or mechanical objects such as the blades of a boat propeller may inoculate pathogenic organisms into a wound. Sports activities, such as surfing, snorkeling, diving, and fishing, lead to ubiquitous abrasions and minor lacerations that heal slowly and with marked soft tissue inflammation. Fishing boats, bearing decks and other structures that seldom are adequately cleaned, are particularly rich sources of pathogens. Wounds acquired in the aquatic environment tend to become infected and may be refractory to standard antimicrobial therapy. Not infrequently, indolent or extensive soft tissue infections develop in the normal or immunocompromised host.[15,151] A clinician faced with a serious infection caused by an aquatic injury frequently needs to administer broad-spectrum antibiotics to a patient before definitive laboratory identification of pathogenic organisms has been obtained.

MARINE BACTERIOLOGY

Marine Environment

Ocean water provides a saline milieu for microbes. The salt dissolved in ocean water (3.2% to 3.5%) is 78% sodium chloride (sodium 10.752 g/kg; chlorine 19.345 g/kg). Other constituents include sulfate (2.791 g/kg), magnesium (1.295 g/kg), potassium (0.39 g/kg), bicarbonate (0.145 g/kg), bromine (0.066 g/kg), boric acid (0.027 g/kg), strontium (0.013 g/kg), and fluorine (0.0013 g/kg). The temperature of the surface waters varies with latitude, currents, and seasons. Tropical waters are warmer and maintain a more constant temperature than do temperate and subtropical waters, which are subject to substantial meteorologic variation. Shallow and turbulent coastal waters are generally richer in nutrients than is the open ocean, which is reflected in the diversity of life that can be identified in the intertidal zone. Although the greatest number and diversity of bacteria are found near the ocean surface, diverse bacteria and fungi are found in marine silts, sediments, and sand and within the oral cavities of marine organisms. In ocean waters having marked differences in salinity/density, the greatest concentration of bacteria is noted at the thermocline, where changes in both temperature and salinity are usually found.[159] Marked vertical salinity stratification is the norm in estuaries where freshwater inflow "floats" over the top of a denser wedge of marine waters. This effect is less active in other coastal waters, where tide- and wind-driven perturbations may create a more even distribution of sediments, microbes, salinity, and temperature. Microbes are most abundant in areas that have the greatest numbers of higher life forms. Growth requirements are species specific with respect to the use of organic carbon and nitrogen sources, requirements for various amino acids, vitamins and cofactors, sodium, potassium, magnesium, phosphate, sulfate, chloride, and calcium. Most marine bacteria are facultative anaerobes, which can thrive in oxygen-rich and oxygen-poor environments. Few are obligatory aerobes or anaerobes. Some marine bacteria are highly proteolytic, and the proportion of proteolytic bacteria seems to be greater in the oceans than on land or in freshwater habitats.[159] It has been observed that sharks may harbor bacteria that are resistant to many drugs; this phenomenon could be a result of natural immunity, or it may be that some of these animals have encountered synthetic drugs that found their way into the sea via effluents.

Diversity of Organisms

Unique conditions of nutrient and inorganic mineral supply, temperature, and pressure have allowed evolution of unique, highly adapted marine microbes.[215,216] In addition, numerous other bacteria, microalgae, protozoa, fungi, yeasts, and viruses have been identified in or cultured from seawater, marine sediments, marine life, and marine-acquired or marine-contaminated infected wounds or body fluids of septic victims. In their natural environment, the bacteria serve to scavenge and transform organic matter in the intricate cycles of the food and growth chains. Some of these bacteria are listed in Box 73-1.[157] Enteric pathogenic bacteria have been isolated from sharks.[76] A shark attack victim in South Africa who sustained serious injuries to his lower extremities was reported to have developed a fulminant infection attributed to *Bacillus cereus* shown to be sensitive to fluoroquinolones, amikacin, clindamycin, vancomycin, and tetracyclines and resistant to penicillin and cephalosporins (including third-generation cephalosporins). In another report, one shark

---

BOX 73-1 Bacteria and Fungus Isolated from Marine Water, Sediments, Marine Animals, and Marine-Acquired Wounds

Achromobacter	*Micrococcus sedentarius*
Acinetobacter lwoffii	*Moraxella lacunata*
Actinomyces	*Mycobacterium marinum*
Aerobacter aerogenes	*Neisseria catarrhalis*
Aeromonas hydrophila	*Pasteurella multocida*
Aeromonas salmonicida	*Photobacterium (Vibrio)*
Aeromonas sobria	*damsela*
Alcaligenes faecalis	*Propionibacterium acnes*
Alteromonas espejiana	*Proteus mirabilis*
Alteromonas haloplanktis	*Proteus vulgaris*
Alteromonas macleodii	*Providencia stuartii*
Alteromonas undina	*Pseudomonas aeruginosa*
Bacillus cereus	*Pseudomonas cepacia*
Bacillus subtilis	*Pseudomonas maltophilia*
Bacteroides fragilis	*Pseudomonas putrefaciens*
Branhamella catarrhalis	*Pseudomonas stutzeri*
Chromobacterium violaceum	*Salmonella enteritidis*
Citrobacter	*Serratia*
Clostridium botulinum	*Staphylococcus aureus*
Clostridium perfringens	*Staphylococcus epidermidis*
Clostridium tetani	*Streptococcus*
Corynebacterium	*Vibrio alginolyticus*
Edwardsiella tarda	*Vibrio carchariae*
Enterobacter aerogenes	*Vibrio cholerae*
Erysipelothrix rhusiopathiae	*Vibrio fluvialis*
Escherichia coli	*Vibrio furnissii*
Flavobacterium	*Vibrio harveyi*
Fusarium solani	*Vibrio mimicus*
Grimontia (Vibrio) hollisae	*Vibrio parahaemolyticus*
Klebsiella pneumoniae	*Vibrio splendidus I*
Legionella pneumophila	*Vibrio vulnificus*
Micrococcus luteus	

---

attack victim in Australia grew both *Vibrio parahaemolyticus* and *Aeromonas caviae* from his wounds, whereas another grew *Vibrio alginolyticus* and *Aeromonas hydrophila* from his wounds.[162] It is now fairly well known that *Vibrio* species and *Aeromonas* species are potential pathogens residing in ocean water and fresh water.

Marine bacteria are generally halophilic (thrive in saline conditions), heterotrophic (require exogenous carbon and nitrogen-containing organic supplements), motile, and gram-negative rod forms. *Halomonas venusta,* a halophilic, nonfermentative, gram-negative rod, was reported as a human pathogen in a wound that originated from a fish bite.[200] Previous opinions that enteric pathogens (associated with the intestines of warm-blooded animals) deposited into marine environments ultimately succumb to sedimentation, predation, parasitism, sunlight, temperature, osmotic stress, toxic chemicals, or high salt concentrations may be untrue.[75] Pathogens may accumulate in surface water in association with lipoidal particulates, from which they are rapidly dispersed toward the shore by wave and wind activity. In addition, dredging, storms, upwellings, and other benthic disturbances may churn enteric organisms into the path of wastewater nutrients. In the United States, coastal and Great Lakes beaches regularly have bacteria counts above the Environmental Protection Agency's threshold values for safety. Sewage spills and intentional industrial effluent release contribute to harmful contamination, notably including enteric bacteria.

WOUND INFECTIONS CAUSED BY *VIBRIO* SPECIES

Vibrio organisms can cause gastroenteric disease (gastroenteric *Vibrio* infections are discussed in Chapter 82) and soft tissue infections, particularly in immunocompromised hosts. Extraintestinal infections may be associated with bacteremia and death. *Vibrio* species are the most potentially virulent halophilic organisms that flourish in the marine environment. The teeth of a great white shark were swabbed and yielded *V. alginolyticus, V. fluvialis,* and *V. parahaemolyticus.*[30] Mako shark tooth culture has yielded *V. damsela, V. furnissii,* and *V. splendidus I.*[6] *V. parahaemolyticus* has also been identified in freshwater habitats.[10] Water that is brackish (salinity of 15 to 25 parts per thousand [ppt]) allows growth of *Vibrio* species if appropriate nutrients are present; *V. vulnificus* infection has been documented after exposure to waters with salinities of 2 and 4 ppt. The optimal season for exposure appears to be summer, when water temperatures encourage bacterial proliferation. In most studies reported, infections seem to cluster during summer months; this may be related to increased numbers of people at the seashore.[63] This has been corroborated to some degree by the observation that *V. parahaemolyticus* cultured from marine mammals was recovered only in warmer months of the year in the northeastern United States or in animals from subtropical regions. Sharks appear to develop some immunity to autochthonous *Vibrio* species, as suggested by detection of a binding protein similar to the immunoglobulin M (IgM) subclass of immunoglobulin. Allochthonous (for the shark) *Vibrio* species, such as *V. carchariae,* may be the agents of elasmobranch disease when the animal is under stress. Other species, such as *V. anguillarum* and *V. tapetis,* are pathogens of aquatic vertebrates or invertebrates.[12]

Vibrio species are halophilic, gram-negative rods that are facultative anaerobes capable of using D-glucose as their sole or principal source of carbon and energy.[51] These organisms are part of the normal flora of coastal waters not only in the United States but also in many exotic locations frequented by recreational and industrial divers and seafarers. *Vibrio* species are mesophilic organisms and grow best at temperatures of 24° to 40°C (75.2° to 104°F), with essentially no growth below 8° to 10°C (46.4° to 50°F). Certain other "marine bacteria" are facultative psychrophiles (thrive in cold temperatures) or barophiles (thrive in high pressures), or both. *Vibrio* species seem to require less sodium for maximal growth than do other more fastidious marine organisms, a factor that explains their presence in estuarine waters and allows explosive reproduction in the 0.9% saline environment of the human body. At least 11 of the 34 recognized

Vibrio species have been associated with human disease.[51] Wound infections have been documented to yield *V. cholerae* O group 1 and non-O1, *V. parahaemolyticus, V. vulnificus, V. alginolyticus,* and *V. damsela.* Septicemia, with or without an obvious source, has been attributed to infections with *V. cholerae* non-O1, *V. parahaemolyticus, V. alginolyticus, V. vulnificus,* and *V. metschnikovii. Vibrio* may infect fish, causing significant mortality rates in fish culture facilities. The affliction manifests with lethargy, loss of appetite, skin sores, exophthalmia, and gastrointestinal hemorrhage.

Vibrio parahaemolyticus

Vibrio parahaemolyticus is a halophilic gram-negative rod. The organisms are found in waters along the entire coastline of the United States. Generally, the incidence of clinical disease is greatest in warm summer months when the organism is commonly found in zooplankton. *V. parahaemolyticus* absorbs onto chitin and to minute crustacean copepods that feed on sediment. It has been postulated that unusual warm coastal currents (such as El Niño) may contribute to increased proliferation of *Vibrio* species. The optimal growth temperature of *V. parahaemolyticus* is 35° to 37°C (95° to 98.6°F); under ideal conditions, the generation time has been estimated at less than 10 minutes, with explosive population growth from 10 to 10^6 organisms in 3 to 4 hours.

Extraintestinal wound infections are most common in persons who suffer chronic liver disease or immunosuppression. Although more than 95% of *V. parahaemolyticus* strains associated with human illness are positive for the Kanagawa reaction (production of a cell-free, heat-stable hemolysin on high-salt-mannitol [Wagatsuma] agar), the relationship of this reaction to pathogenicity is not yet clear. Furthermore, most marine strains are not Kanagawa positive. Virulence factors include proteases, beta-hemolysins (thermostable direct hemolysin [tdh] and tdh-related hemolysin [trh]), adhesins, and the expression of virulence genes, including the toxR operons.[12,174] Some primary soft tissue infections previously attributed to *V. parahaemolyticus* may theoretically be attributed to misidentified *V. vulnificus.*

Vibrio vulnificus

Vibrio vulnificus (formerly known as a "lactose [fermenting]-positive" vibrio) is a halophilic gram-negative bacillus. *V. vulnificus* (Latin for "wounding") is found in virtually all U.S. coastal waters and has been reported to cause infection worldwide.[11] It prefers salinity of 0.7% to 1.6%; and although it prefers a habitat of warm (at least 20°C [68°F]) seawater, it can be found in much colder water. It does not appear to be associated with fecal contamination of seawater. It has been shown to exist in Chesapeake Bay with bacterial counts comparable to those reported from the Gulf of Mexico.[213]

V. vulnificus may or may not have an acidic polysaccharide capsule (opaque colony), which confers protection against bactericidal activity of human serum and phagocytosis and thus renders the organism more virulent in animals. At extremely low frequency, some strains can shift between unencapsulated (avirulent; translucent colony) and capsulated (virulent) serotypes. The encapsulated isolates show exquisite (positive) sensitivity to iron. Virulent isolates can use 100% but not 30% saturated (normal for humans) transferrin as an iron source, as well as iron in hemoglobin and hemoglobin-haptoglobin complexes. *V. vulnificus* exhibits enhanced growth and virulence in the presence of increased serum iron concentration or saturated transferrin-binding sites.[2] *V. vulnificus* is classified into three biotypes: biotype 1 is pathogenic for humans and biotype 2 is pathogenic for fish.[51,53] Biotype 3 causes soft tissue infections and septicemia following contact with fish from freshwater ponds; it was first noted in Israel. Within biotype 1, various genetically distinct subgroups identified by randomly amplified polymorphic deoxyribonucleic acid (DNA) polymerase chain reaction (PCR) appear to be especially virulent.[8] Furthermore, complete genomic sequencing of *V. vulnificus* YJ016, a biotype 1 strain, reveals gene clusters related to pathogenicity (cell adhesion, colonization, cytotoxicity, and tissue destruction), including capsular polysaccharide, siderophore biosynthesis and transport, and heme receptor and transport.[53] In vivo antigen technology can

identify virulence genes produced and expressed in humans.[102] The ability of biotype 1 to multiply and produce a toxic metalloprotease in human serum may be a prominent virulence factor.[206]

Infection worsens rapidly after the initiation of symptoms and has been noted most frequently in men older than age 40 years with preexisting hepatic dysfunction (particularly cirrhosis), end-stage renal impairment, leukopenia, or impaired immunity (malignancy, leukemia, hypogammaglobulinemia, human immunodeficiency virus [HIV] infection, diabetes, bone marrow suppression, long-term corticosteroids), although it has been reported in young, previously healthy individuals.[22,94,107,109,134] One case followed application of fish blood by a healer as a traditional remedy to a chronic leg ulcer in an obese patient suffering from recurrent erysipelas.[184] Preexisting liver disease is a predictor of death, with 50% of such individuals in one series succumbing to the illness.[87] Persons with high serum iron levels (from chronic cirrhosis, hepatitis, thalassemia major, hemochromatosis, multiple transfusions [such as are given for aplastic anemia]) or achlorhydria (low gastric acid; may be iatrogenically induced with H_2 blockers) may be at greater risk for fulminant bacteremia.[2,178,193] This has been attributed in part to the protective effect of gastric acid, the iron requirement of the organism, and the effects of liver disease (decreased polymorphonuclear leukocyte and macrophage activity, flawed opsonization, and shunting of portal blood around the liver). It has been proposed that an effective host response against *V. vulnificus* and similar iron-sensitive pathogens (e.g., *Listeria monocytogenes, Klebsiella* spp., and *Yersinia* spp.) is in part augmented by hepcidin, a cysteine-rich cationic antimicrobial peptide central to iron metabolism.[8,204] *V. vulnificus* produces a siderophore *(vulnibactin)* and a protease that may enhance pathogenicity.[2] Other pathogenicity factors may be the polysaccharide capsule, hemolysin, type IV pili and other proteases, including a serine protease and a 45-kDa metalloprotease regulated through quorum sensing at a lower temperature than core body temperature.[134,205]

The syndrome consists of flu-like malaise, fever, vomiting, diarrhea, chills, hypotension, and early skin vesiculation that evolve into necrotizing dermatitis and fasciitis, with vasculitis and myositis (Figures 73-1 and 73-2).[214] Hematogenous seeding of vibrios to secondary cutaneous lesions is probable. Primary wound infections (≈ 30% of cases) rapidly show marked edema, with erythema, vesicles, and hemorrhagic or contused-appearing bullae, progressing to necrosis.[63] This may require radical surgical debridement or amputation. Up to 25% of these victims may have sepsis. When *V. vulnificus* is recovered from the blood of a victim with sepsis attributable to a wound infection, the case fatality rate may exceed 30%.[87] Necrotizing fasciitis from this bacteria has also been described to produce a fatal toxic shock–like syndrome.[63] Extracellular elastin-lysing proteases elaborated by the organism, as well as a potent collagenase, probably contribute

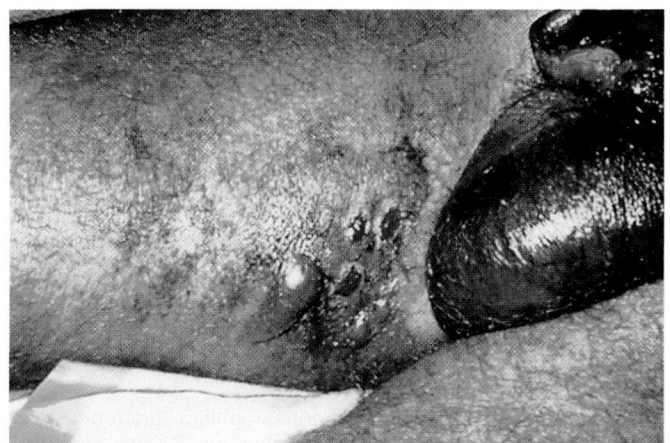

FIGURE 73-1 Ecthyma gangrenosum associated with *Vibrio vulnificus* sepsis. *(Courtesy Edward J. Bottone, MD, Department of Microbiology, Mt Sinai Hospital, New York.)*

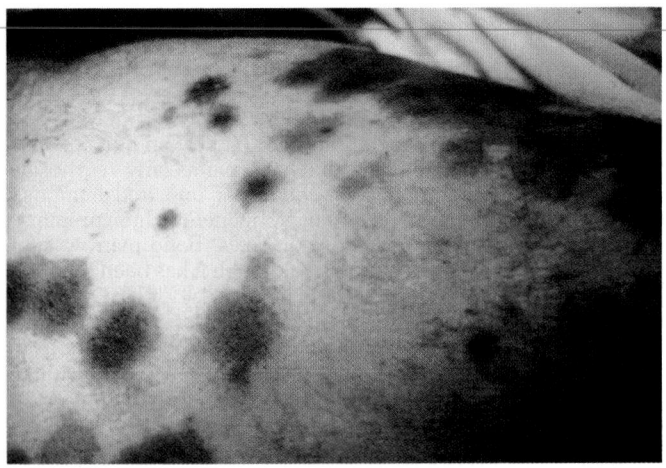

FIGURE 73-2 Torso of a victim with *Vibrio vulnificus* sepsis.

to rapid invasion of healthy tissue. *V. vulnificus* also produces a cytotoxin-hemolysin and phospholipases. Cytolysin produced by most pathogenic strains of *V. vulnificus* is extremely toxic to mice when injected intravenously and results in severe perivascular edema and neutrophil infiltration in lung tissues.[98,145] The precise roles of these and other factors (pili, mucinase, chondroitinase, hyaluronidase) in the in vivo pathogenicity of the organism have yet to be determined. Bleeding complications (which may include gastrointestinal hemorrhage and disseminated intravascular coagulation) are common and may be attributed in part to thrombocytopenia. Gastroenteritis is more common (15% to 20%) with the septicemic presentation than with primary wound infection and may exist as an isolated entity (≈ 10% of cases), although it is debated that illness has been erroneously attributed to the asymptomatically carried organism. *Vibrio vulnificus* endometritis has been reported after an episode of intercourse in the waters of Galveston Bay, Texas.[188] Another series of nine cases of *Vibrio* infections, in most cases the species being *vulnificus,* was reported associated with finning injuries of the hands.[50] Other presentations of *V. vulnificus* infections have included meningitis, necrotizing fasciitis following lightning strike in a windsurfer, spontaneous bacterial peritonitis, corneal ulcers, epiglottitis, and infections of the testes, spleen, and heart valves.[195]

The explosive nature of the syndrome can lead to gram-negative sepsis and death, reportedly in up to 50% of cases. The mortality rate may be as high as 90% in victims who become hypotensive within 12 hours of initial examination by a physician. For wound infections from all *Vibrio* species, the organism may only be recovered from blood specimens in less than 20% of victims.[87] Appropriate antibiotics should be administered as soon as the infection is suspected (see later). In one report, *V. vulnificus* sepsis was treated with antibiotic therapy, debridement of necrotic tissues, and direct hemoperfusion using polymyxin B immobilized fiber, which served as an artificial reticuloendothelial system and removed endotoxin from the circulating blood.[163] In an immunocompetent victim who acquired a *V. vulnificus* hand infection from peeling shrimp, treatment with oral ciprofloxacin was successful. In a series of seven patients treated for primary skin and soft tissue infections secondary to *V. vulnificus,* prompt operative exploration and debridement were correlated with a decrease in the intensive care unit and hospital length of stay, particularly if the surgery occurred within 72 hours from the time of infection.[83] The authors noted that all patients had necrosis of underlying subcutaneous tissue, whereas some did not demonstrate skin necrosis.

Vibrio mimicus

Vibrio mimicus is a motile, nonhalophilic, gram-negative, oxidase-positive rod with a single flagellum. It can be distinguished from *V. cholerae* by its inability to ferment sucrose, inability to metabolize acetylmethyl carbonyl, sensitivity to polymyxin, and negative lipase test. An ear infection may follow

exposure to ocean water. Isolates are sensitive to tetracycline. Physicians who collect stool samples for culture to identify suspected *V. mimicus* must alert the laboratory to use appropriate culture media (thiosulfate-citrate–bile salts–sucrose [TCBS] agar).

Vibrio alginolyticus

Vibrio alginolyticus, found in seawater, has been implicated in soft tissue infections (e.g., those caused by coral cuts or surfing scrapes), sinusitis, and otitis, particularly after previous ear infections or a tympanic membrane perforation. Although bacteremia has been reported in immunosuppressed patients and patients with burns, *V. alginolyticus* does not generally carry the virulent potential of *V. vulnificus.*[128] Typical symptoms include cellulitis, with seropurulent exudate. Its distinguishing microbiologic features are stated to be sucrose and lactose fermentation, growth in 1% tryptone broth plus 10% NaCL, positive Voges-Proskauer reaction, negative urease reaction, and susceptibility to vibriostatic compound O/129. However, because these indices may vary, identification may be difficult. Antibiotic resistance may be a feature of *V. alginolyticus* infection.

Photobacterium damsela

Photobacterium (formerly *Vibrio* or *Listonella*) *damsela,* formerly enteric group EF-5 and so-named because it is pathogenic for the damselfish, causes wound infections similar to those attributed to vibrios. Rapidly progressive infection leading to muscle necrosis and fasciitis or to sepsis and death may transpire in an immunosuppressed victim or person with normal immunity.[72,74,185] This may be related to an extracellular cytolysin (damselysin) or other unidentified enzymes or virulence factors.

Vibrio cholerae

Vibrio cholerae is associated with severe gastroenteritis (see Chapter 82). With regard to tissue infection, a case of necrotizing fasciitis and septic shock caused by *V. cholerae* non-O1 (not agglutinated in cholera polyvalent O1 antiserum) acquired in San Diego, California, has been described.[202] The victim suffered from preexisting diabetes mellitus complicated by chronic plantar ulceration of the affected limb. *V. cholerae* may cause severe disease signs in Japanese sweetfish (ko-ayu or *Plecoglossus altivelis*), certain shrimp (e.g., *Penaeus monodon*), and ornamental fish in India.[13,82,182]

Growth in Culture

Although plating on standard clinical laboratory media may detect only 0.1% to 1% of the total number of microorganisms found in seawater or marine sediment, most marine bacteria that are pathogenic to humans can be readily recovered on standard media. Although pathogenic *Vibrio* species can grow on conventional blood agar media, other marine bacteria may require saline-supplemented media and incubation at 25°C (77°F) instead of the standard 35° to 37°C (95° to 98.6°F). In culture, marine bacteria may grow at a slower rate than terrestrial bacteria, which delays identification. Pleomorphism in culture may be attributed to adaptation to small concentrations of nutrients in seawater. Most organisms require sodium, potassium, magnesium, phosphate, and sulfate for growth; a few require calcium or chloride.

All *Vibrio* species grow in routine blood culture mediums and on nonselective mediums, such as blood agar. TCBS agar is selective and recommended for detection of marine *Vibrio* organisms, although cellobiose–polymyxin B–colistin (CPC) agar may be as good or better.[20,120] An alternative is Monsur taurocholate-tellurite-gelatin agar. A large clinical laboratory near the ocean might consider routinely using TCBS or CPC agar. Pathogenic vibrios generally grow on MacConkey agar. All species except *V. cholerae* and *V. mimicus* require sodium chloride for growth. Enrichment broth (alkaline peptone water with 1% NaCl) is recommended for isolation of vibrios from convalescent and treated patients. Another enrichment broth that may be more effective is 5% peptone, 1% NaCl, and 0.08% cellobiose (PNC) at pH 8.0.[91] A comparison of strategies for detection and recovery of *V. vulnificus* from marine samples of the western Mediterranean coast determined that the best strategy consisted of the combination of culture-based methods (3-hour enrichment in alkaline-saline peptone water at 40°C [104°F], followed by culture on CPC agar) and DNA-based procedures (specific PCR amplification of the presumptive colonies with primers Dvu 9V and Dvu 45R).[6]

Key characteristics that aid in separation of *Vibrio* species from other medically significant bacteria (Enterobacteriaceae, *Pseudomonas, Aeromonas, Plesiomonas*) are motility by polar flagella, production of oxidase, fermentative metabolism, requirement of sodium chloride for growth, and susceptibility to the O/129 vibriostatic compound. *V. vulnificus* can be cultured from blood, wounds (bullae), and stool. The laboratory must be cautioned to use selective culture media with a high salt content (3% NaCl) for prompt identification. Suggestive features include positive fermentation of glucose, positive catalase and oxidase tests, positive indole test, positive reaction for both lysine and ornithine decarboxylase, positive o-nitrophenyl-β-D-galactopyranoside, and inability to ferment sucrose. A useful identification scheme for pathogenic *Vibrio* species is found in the chapter on *Vibrio* in the most recent edition of the American Society for Microbiology's *Manual of Clinical Microbiology.*

Because growth of *V. vulnificus* in culture generally requires 48 hours, current research is directed at a more rapid diagnostic test. Direct identification of *V. vulnificus* in clinical specimens by nested PCR has been accomplished using serum specimens and bulla aspirates from septicemic patients, as well as from fish, sediments, and water.[7,115] Simultaneous detection of five marine fish pathogens (*V. vulnificus, Listonella anguillarum, Photobacterium damsela, Aeromonas salmonicida,* and *V. parahaemolyticus*) has been accomplished using multiplex PCR and a DNA microarray.[73] This technique has not yet been applied to diagnosis of pathogens afflicting humans.

Mycobacteria must be cultured in media such as Middlebrook 7H10 or 7H11 agar or Lowenstein-Jensen medium; fungi require a medium such as Sabouraud dextrose or brain-heart infusion/Sabhi agar. Antibiotic susceptibility testing can be performed using established procedures, except for addition of NaCl 2.3% to the Mueller-Hinton broth or agar used for disk diffusion. Certain commercial test kits may not accurately identify marine organisms. In the setting of wound infection or sepsis, the clinician should alert the laboratory that a marine-acquired organism may be present. If a laboratory does not have time or resources to perform a complete identification, the bacteria may be sent to a reference laboratory. Marine bacteria are kept in the American Type Culture Collection. Because of the diversity of species, complete agreement has not yet been reached on comprehensive taxonomic criteria for identification.

Antibiotic Therapy

The objectives for management of infections from marine microorganisms are to recognize the clinical condition, culture the organism, and provide antimicrobial therapy. Management of marine-acquired infections should include therapy against *Vibrio* species. Antibiotic selection should be guided by the most current recommendations. Historically, third-generation cephalosporins (cefoperazone, cefotaxime, or ceftazidime) provide variable coverage in vitro; first- and second-generation products (cefazolin, cephalothin, cephapirin, cefamandole, cefonicid, ceforanide, or cefoxitin) appear to be less effective in vitro. The organism has been reported in some cases to be resistant in vitro to third-generation cephalosporins, mezlocillin, aztreonam, and piperacillin.[149] A combination of cefotaxime and minocycline seems to be synergistic and extremely effective against *V. vulnificus* in vitro.[56] Oral cultures taken from two captive moray eels at the John G. Shedd Aquarium in Chicago demonstrated *V. fluvialis, Photobacterium damsela, V. vulnificus,* and *Pseudomonas putrefaciens* to be sensitive to cefuroxime, ciprofloxacin, tetracycline, and trimethoprim-sulfamethoxazole.[69] Imipenem-cilastatin is generally efficacious against gram-negative marine bacteria, as are trimethoprim-sulfamethoxazole and tetracycline. Gentamicin, tobramycin, and chloramphenicol have tested favorably against *P. putrefaciens* and *Vibrio* strains. Nonfermentative bacteria (such as *Alteromonas, Pseudomonas,* and *Deleya* species) appear to be sensitive to most antibiotics. In a mouse model, combination

therapy with minocycline and cefotaxime was more effective than either drug alone.[55]

Quantitative wound culture has no advantage before the appearance of a wound infection. Pending a prospective evaluation of prophylactic antibiotics in the management of marine wounds, the following recommendations are based on the indolent nature and malignant potential of soft tissue infections caused by *Vibrio* species:

Minor abrasions or lacerations (such as coral cuts or superficial sea urchin puncture wounds) do not require prophylactic antibiotics in the host with normal immunity. Persons who are chronically ill (as with diabetes, hemophilia, or thalassemia) or immunologically impaired (as with leukemia or acquired immunodeficiency syndrome [AIDS], or undergoing chemotherapy or prolonged corticosteroid therapy), or who suffer from serious liver disease (such as hepatitis, cirrhosis, or hemochromatosis), particularly those with elevated serum iron levels, should be placed immediately after the injury on a regimen of oral ciprofloxacin, trimethoprim-sulfamethoxazole, or tetracycline (or doxycycline), because these persons appear to have an increased risk of serious wound infection and bacteremia. Cefuroxime may be a useful alternative. Penicillin, ampicillin, and erythromycin are not acceptable alternatives.[135,137] Norfloxacin may be less efficacious against certain vibrios.[136,153] Other quinolones (ofloxacin, enoxacin, pefloxacin, fleroxacin, lomefloxacin) have not been extensively tested against *Vibrio;* they may be useful alternatives, but this awaits definitive evaluation. Appearance of an infection indicates the need for prompt debridement and antibiotic therapy. If an infection develops, antibiotic coverage should be chosen that will also be efficacious against *Staphylococcus* and *Streptococcus,* because these are still quite common perpetrators of infection. In general, the fluoroquinolones, which are particularly effective for treating gram-negative bacillary infections, may become less and less useful against resistant staphylococci.[192] If *Staphylococcus* is a β-lactamase–producing strain, a semisynthetic penicillin (nafcillin or oxacillin) should be chosen, with a cephalosporin such as cefazolin or cephalothin used if there is a history of delayed-type penicillin allergy. Vancomycin is recommended in the event of methicillin resistance.[122]

Serious injuries (from an infection perspective) include large lacerations, serious burns, deep puncture wounds, or a retained foreign body. Examples are shark or barracuda bites, stingray spine wounds, deep sea urchin punctures, scorpaenid (scorpionfish) spine envenomations that enter a joint space, and full-thickness coral cuts. If the victim requires hospitalization and surgery for standard wound management, recommended antibiotics include gentamicin, tobramycin, amikacin, ciprofloxacin, or trimethoprim-sulfamethoxazole. Cefoperazone and cefotaxime may or may not be effective. There is a recommendation in the literature advocating use of ceftazidime in combination with tetracycline (or doxycycline).[108] Chloramphenicol is an alternative agent less commonly used because of hematologic side effects. Imipenem-cilastatin or meropenem may be used in a circumstance of sepsis or treatment failure. Meropenem has shown excellent in vitro activity against the Vibrionaceae and may be useful for eradicating infections produced by these organisms.[57] Patients who simultaneously receive imipenem or ciprofloxacin and theophylline may have an increased tendency to seizures.[165] If the victim is managed as an outpatient, the drugs of choice to cover *Vibrio* are ciprofloxacin, trimethoprim-sulfamethoxazole, or tetracycline. Cefuroxime is an alternative. It is a clinical decision whether oral therapy should be preceded by a single IV or intramuscular (IM) loading dose of a similar or different antibiotic, commonly an aminoglycoside.

Infected wounds should be cultured for aerobes and anaerobes. Pending culture and sensitivity results, the patient should be managed with antibiotics as described previously. In a person who has been wounded in a marine environment and has rapidly progressive cellulitis or myositis, *V. parahaemolyticus* or *V. vulnificus* infection should be suspected, particularly in the presence of chronic liver disease. If a wound infection is minor and has the appearance of a classic erysipeloid reaction (*Erysipelothrix rhusiopathiae*), penicillin, cephalexin, or ciprofloxacin should be administered (see Chapter 76). *E. rhusiopathiae* attributed to a pet goldfish has been reported to cause necrotizing fasciitis in a diabetic patient.[168] It is also cultured in episodes of infective endocarditis, although the origins of the infections are often not identified.[117,196]

If sepsis is severe, additional aggressive measures beyond surgery and antibiotics, such as administration of recombinant human activated protein C, may be required.[4] Hyperbaric oxygen therapy has been used as adjunctive therapy in *V. vulnificus* septicemia and cellulitis, but there is no standard recommendation for this modality for this indication.[203]

FRESHWATER BACTERIOLOGY

Diversity of Organisms

The natural freshwater environment of ponds, lakes, streams, rivers, lagoons, harbors, estuaries, and artificial bodies of water is probably as hazardous as the ocean from a microbiologic standpoint. Waterskiing accidents, propeller wounds, fishhook punctures, lacerations from broken glass and sharp rocks, fish fin punctures, and crush injuries during white-water expeditions are commonplace. A large number of bacteria have been identified in fresh water and associated sediments and animals. In fringe areas of the ocean that carry brackish water (NaCl content < 3%), marine bacteria, salt-tolerant freshwater bacteria, and brackish-specific bacteria, such as *Agrobacterium sanguineum*, are noted. The combined effects of human and animal traffic and waste disposal increase the risk for coliform contamination. In Great Britain, antibiotic-resistant *Escherichia coli* have been documented in rivers and coastal waters.[170] Coxsackievirus A16 has been isolated from children stricken ill after bathing in contaminated lake water.[64] Of particular note is the presence of virulent species, such as *Chromobacterium violaceum*, *V. parahaemolyticus*, and *A. hydrophila*, associated with serious and indolent wound infections.[201] The last can be cultured from natural bodies of water, as well as from the mouths of domesticated aquarium fish, such as the piranha.[158] Biologic control agents, such as guppy fish bred in wells to control mosquito proliferation, can carry bacterial pathogens, such as *Pseudomonas*.[49]

One investigation sampled water, inanimate objects, and animals from freshwater environments in California, Tennessee, and Florida.[10] Bacteria isolated were predominantly gram-negative and included *A. hydrophila*, *Flavobacterium breve*, *Pseudomonas* species, *V. parahaemolyticus*, *Serratia* species, *Enterobacter* species, *Plesiomonas shigelloides*, *Bacillus* species, *Acinetobacter calcoaceticus*, and *Alcaligenes denitrificans*.

Primary amebic meningoencephalitis is caused by infection with *Naegleria fowleri*, a thermophilic, free-living ameba found in freshwater environments. The infection is associated with human activities that allow entry of water into the nose, from where the ameba migrate to the brain via the olfactory nerve.

Wound Infections Caused by *Aeromonas* Species

Aeromonas hydrophila (Latin for "gas producing" and "water loving") is a gram-negative, facultatively anaerobic, polarly flagellated, non–spore-forming, motile rod and member of the family Vibrionaceae that commonly inhabits soil, freshwater streams, and lakes.[3,14,112,198] *Aeromonas* species are widely distributed and found at wide ranges of temperature and pH. Five species *(A. hydrophila, A. sobria, A. schubertii, A. veronii,* and *A. caviae)* of the nine that have been recovered from clinical material have been linked with human disease; there are 13 or more distinct genotypes.[1] *A. hydrophila* is pathogenic to amphibians, reptiles, and fish. Soft tissue and gastroenteric infections predominate in humans. Virulence factors elaborated by *Aeromonas* species include hemolysin, cytotoxin, enterotoxin, cholera toxin–like factor, and hemagglutinins.[27,197] *Aeromonas* species are sometimes misidentified as members of the genus *Vibrio* by commonly used screening tests.[1]

A wound, particularly of the puncture variety, immersed in contaminated water may become cellulitic within 24 hours, with erythema, edema, and a purulent discharge.[166,211] The lower extremity is most frequently involved. This usually occurs from stepping on a foreign object or being punctured underwater. The appearance may be indistinguishable from typical streptococcal cellulitis, with localized pain, lymphangitis, fever, and chills. Untreated or managed with antibiotics to which the organism is not susceptible, this may rarely progress to a severe gas-forming soft tissue reaction, bulla formation, necrotizing myositis, or osteomyelitis. An appearance similar to ecthyma gangrenosum caused by *Pseudomonas aeruginosa* has been reported in *Aeromonas* septicemia.

Fever, hypotension, jaundice, and chills are common manifestations of septicemia.[105] Additional clinical manifestations include abdominal pain or tenderness, altered consciousness, acute renal failure, bacteremic pneumonia, and coagulopathy.[99] In a manner analogous to the pathogenicity of virulent *Vibrio* species, the chronically ill or immunocompromised host (e.g., chronic liver disease, neoplasm, diabetes, uremia, corticosteroid therapy, extensive burns) is probably at greater risk of a severe infection or complication, such as meningitis, endocarditis, or septicemia.[96] Freshwater aspiration may result in *A. hydrophila* pneumonitis and bacteremia.

There are numerous case reports of infections linked to *Aeromonas* species. Infection has been reported following the bite of an alligator. A 15-year-old boy suffered an *A. hydrophila* wound infection after a bite from his pet piranha. For unknown reasons, there is a marked preponderance of male victims. This may represent the phenotypic variation of critical bacterial adhesins or more likely may simply reflect activity patterns of male humans. Corneal ulcer caused by *A. sobria* was reported after abrasion by a freshwater reed.[47] Medicinal leeches can harbor *Aeromonas* in their gut flora; soft tissue infections related to this phenomenon have been reported.[175] The genus *Plesiomonas* also belongs to the family Vibrionaceae; it has been linked to aquarium-associated infection complicated by watery diarrhea and fever.

Because of the microbiologic similarity of *Aeromonas* on biochemical testing to members of the Enterobacteriaceae, such as *E. coli* or *Serratia* species, it is important to alert the laboratory to the clinical setting. In the microbiology laboratory, *Aeromonas* species may be identified on the basis of positive oxidase reaction, no growth on TCBS agar, growth on MacConkey agar, and resistance to the vibriostatic compound O/129.[105]

Gram's stain of the purulent discharge may demonstrate gram-negative bacilli, singly, paired, or in short chains. Given the appropriate clinical setting (after a wound acquired in the freshwater environment), this should not be casually attributed to contamination.[98] *A. hydrophila* is generally sensitive to chloramphenicol, aztreonam, gentamicin, amikacin, tobramycin, trimethoprim-sulfamethoxazole, cefotaxime, cefuroxime, moxalactam, imipenem, ceftazidime, ciprofloxacin, and norfloxacin. For a severe infection, initial therapy that includes an aminoglycoside provides coverage against concomitant *Pseudomonas* or *Serratia* infection. As has been demonstrated with *Vibrio* species, first-generation cephalosporins, penicillin, ampicillin, and ampicillin-sulbactam are not efficacious, perhaps because of production of β-lactamase by the organism. *Aeromonas* species are capable of producing chromosomally encoded β-lactamases induced by β-lactam antibiotics. This leads to resistance to penicillins, cephalosporins, and monobactams. The β-lactamase inhibitors, such as clavulanate, are not effective against these β-lactamases, so that amoxicillin-clavulanate may not kill *Aeromonas*.[146] The optimal therapy for invasive infections caused by cefotaxime-resistant *A. hydrophila* is not known, but a recent study of in vitro and in vivo (mice) activities of fluoroquinolones suggest that ciprofloxacin may be as effective as cefotaxime–minocycline.[104] In this study, ciprofloxacin and levofloxacin showed greater activity than did gatifloxacin, moxifloxacin, and lomefloxacin.

Initial therapy of a severe soft tissue infection related to *Aeromonas* should include aggressive wound debridement to mitigate the potentially invasive nature of the organism. In one case of severe cellulitis unresponsive to debridement, fasciotomy, and antibiotic therapy, treatment with hyperbaric oxygen was felt to contribute to successful infection control.[127]

Infections Caused by a Fish Pathogen, *Streptococcus iniae*

Streptococcus iniae is a pathogen of fish, noted to cause subcutaneous abscesses in Amazon freshwater dolphins (Mammalia:

Inia geoffrensis) kept in captivity.[207] Epizootic fatal meningoencephalitis in fish species caused by streptococci has been observed in outbreaks affecting tilapia, yellowtail, rainbow trout, and coho salmon. *S. iniae* has emerged as a serious pathogen of farmed barramundi in Australia.[29] Persons who handle these fish are at risk for bacteremic illness, which can manifest as cellulitis or sepsis. Endocarditis, meningitis, and arthritis have been noted to accompany *S. iniae* infection.

The tilapia (*Oreochromis* and *Tilapia* species) are also known as St Peter's fish or Hawaiian sunfish. The surfaces of these commonly aquacultured fishes may be colonized with *S. iniae*. Persons of Asian descent have been identified as prone to infection, probably because they often prepare this fish with the intent to dine. Typically, the victim recalls puncturing the skin of the hand with a fin, bone, or implement of preparation. Cellulitis with lymphangitis and fever is common, without skin necrosis or bulla formation.[207]

In culture, *S. iniae* shows β-hemolysis. However, it may appear to be α-hemolytic because the narrow zone of β-hemolysis is ringed by a more prominent zone of α-hemolysis. Therefore, it may be misidentified as a *viridans* streptococcus and thus considered a contaminant. A reasonable approach to antibiotic therapy includes penicillin, cefazolin, ceftriaxone, erythromycin, clindamycin, or trimethoprim-sulfamethoxazole. In one series, ciprofloxacin showed slightly less efficacy in vitro.

Infection Caused by *Desmodesmus armatus*

Two cases of soft tissue infection cause by the chlorophyll-containing alga *Desmodesmus armatus* were reported.[110a] In immunocompetent adults sustaining a deep puncture wound to the foot in one case and open fracture-dislocation of the knee in the other case, infection investigated by fungal cultures of the soft tissues revealed green colonies consistent with a chlorophyllic organism that was identified as *D. armatus*. Both patients underwent surgical debridement and healed without recurrence. In these cases, no antifungal drug therapy was administered.

A General Approach to Antibiotic Therapy

Management of infections acquired in fresh water should include therapy against *Aeromonas* species. First-generation cephalosporins provide inadequate coverage against growth of fresh water bacteria. Third-generation cephalosporins provide excellent coverage, whereas second-generation products are less effective. Ceftriaxone may not be efficacious against *Aeromonas* species. Ciprofloxacin, imipenem, ceftazidime, gentamicin, and trimethoprim-sulfamethoxazole are reasonable antibiotics against gram-negative microorganisms. Trimethoprim or ampicillin alone may be inefficacious.

Whether to begin antimicrobial therapy before establishment of a wound infection is controversial. Pending prospective evaluation of prophylactic antibiotics in wounds acquired in fresh water, the following recommendations are based on the potentially serious nature of soft tissue infections caused by *Aeromonas* species:

Minor abrasions or lacerations do not require the administration of prophylactic antibiotics in the host with normal immunity. Persons who have chronic illness, immunologic impairment, or serious liver disease, particularly those with elevated serum iron levels, should be placed immediately on a regimen of oral ciprofloxacin or norfloxacin (first choice), trimethoprim-sulfamethoxazole (second choice), or doxycycline-tetracycline (third choice; use only in the setting of allergy to the first two choices, because resistance has been observed), because these persons appear to have an increased risk of serious wound infection and bacteremia. Penicillin, ampicillin, erythromycin, and trimethoprim do not appear to be acceptable alternatives. The appearance of an infection indicates the need for prompt debridement and antibiotic therapy. If an infection develops, antibiotic coverage that will also be efficacious against *Staphylococcus* and *Streptococcus* should be chosen, because these are likely the most common perpetrators of infection.

If the victim requires surgery and hospitalization for wound management, recommended antibiotics include ciprofloxacin, gentamicin, or trimethoprim-sulfamethoxazole. Imipenem-cilastatin is an extremely powerful antibiotic that should be used in a circumstance of sepsis or treatment failure. If the victim is to be managed as an outpatient, the oral drug of choice is norfloxacin (or ciprofloxacin), trimethoprim-sulfamethoxazole, or tetracycline or doxycycline. It is a clinical decision whether oral therapy should be preceded by a single IV or IM loading dose of a similar or different antibiotic, commonly an aminoglycoside.

Infected wounds should be cultured. Pending culture and sensitivity results, the patient should be managed with antibiotics as outlined previously. If fever or rapidly progressive cellulitis characterized by bullae and large areas of necrosis develops, *A. hydrophila* infection should be suspected. Less rapidly progressive *Aeromonas* infections may have the appearance of streptococcal cellulitis.[100]

SHARKS

Myth and folklore surround sharks, the most feared of sea creatures. Although dreaded, sharks are among the most graceful and magnificent denizens of the deep (Figures 73-3 and 73-4). Sharks may be found in all seas but the Southern Ocean and occur in some tropical rivers and riverine lakes. Sharks range in size from the dwarf and cylindrical dogfishes *Etmopterus perryi* and *E. carteri* (21 cm [8.3 inches]) to the plankton-feeding whale shark *Rhincodon typus* (17-21 m [56-69 feet] and 22,700 kg [50,000 lb]) (Figures 73-5 and 73-6).

Attacks by these occasionally savage animals have always held enormous fascination for scientists, adventurers, and clinicians. The problem was highlighted for the U.S. military in 1945 during World War II, when crew members from the USS *Indianapolis* perished in shark-inhabited waters. On July 30, the heavy cruiser was sunk by a Japanese torpedo, resulting in hundreds of deaths plus reports of an estimated additional 60 to 80 shark attack fatalities of survivors left adrift for 5 days. This estimate is certainly a high figure inflated by historical misinterpretation of scavenge bites on already dead servicemen and some exaggeration, but nevertheless, the approximately two dozen bites on live and dying seamen involved in this tragedy represents the largest documented incidence of mass shark attacks (GHB interviews with survivors).

The bull shark *Carcharhinus leucas* (Figure 73-7) is a frequent visitor and occasional resident of tropical and warm-temperate rivers and a regular denizen of reefs and other nearshore marine habitats. It commonly penetrates 161 km (100 miles) or more up freshwater rivers, such as the Ganges, Nile, and Zambezi, and

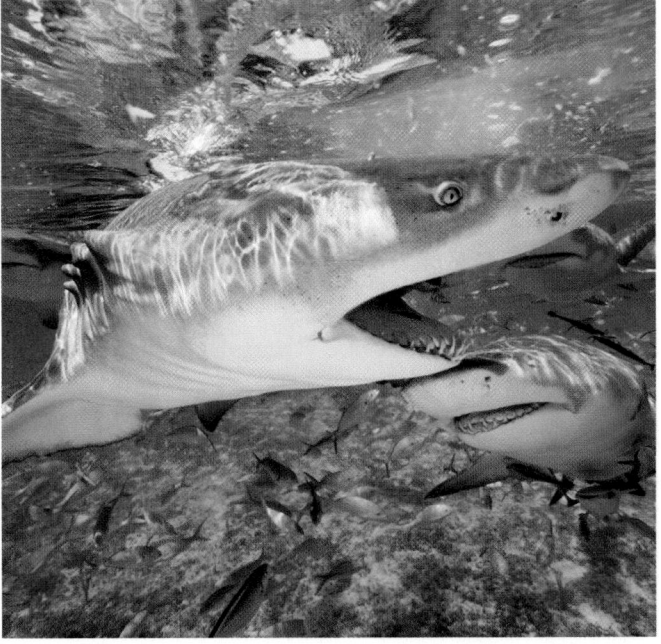

FIGURE 73-3 Schooling sharks. *(Copyright Stephen Frink.)*

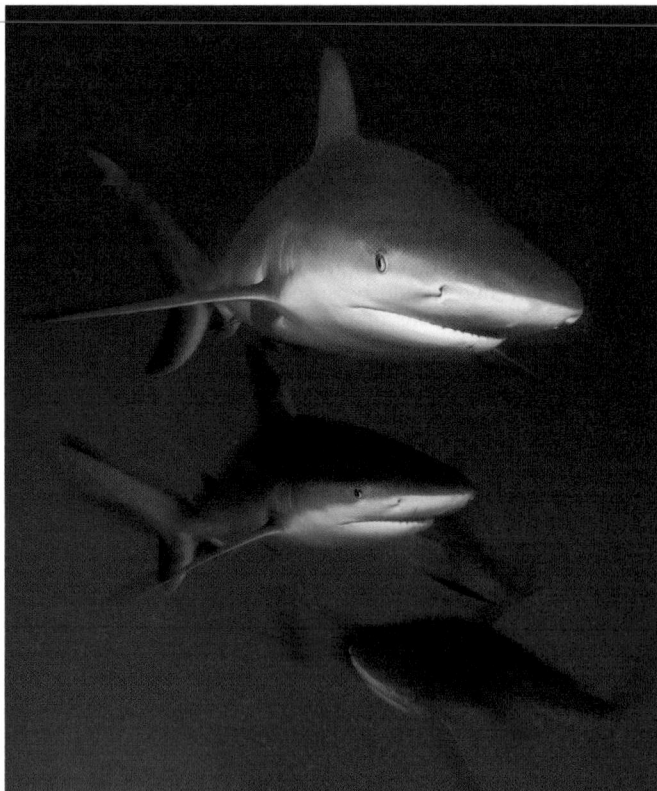

FIGURE 73-4 Caribbean reef sharks. *(Courtesy Jennifer Hayes.)*

has been seen in the Amazon River at Iquitos, Peru, 4000 km from the Atlantic Ocean, and as far inland as Illinois in the Mississippi River.[140,187] These sharks also live in Lake Nicaragua and have had their aggressive behavior attributed in part to high levels of testosterone. During the summer of 2001, the "Summer

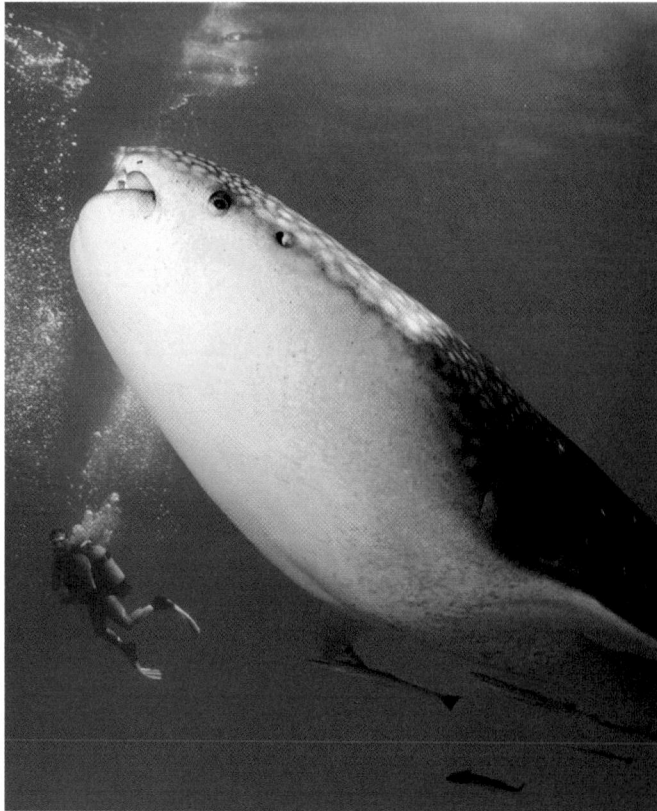

FIGURE 73-5 Whale shark. *(Copyright Stephen Frink.)*

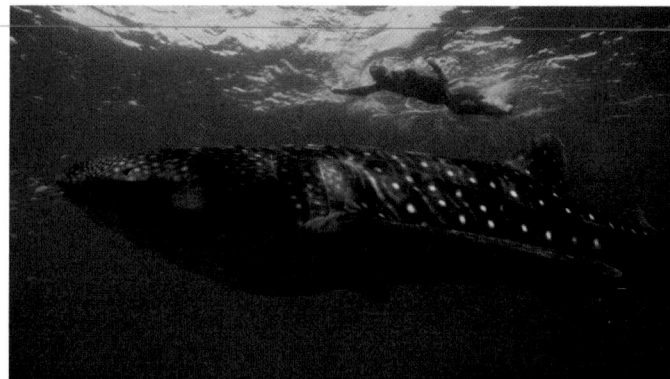

FIGURE 73-6 Snorkeler soars above a whale shark. *(Copyright Carl Roessler.)*

of the Shark" in the U.S. media, a bull shark was believed to have attacked an 8-year-old child off the Gulf Coast of Florida.

The International Shark Attack File (ISAF) has its origin from the Shark Research Panel created by the Office of Naval Research (ONR) in 1958. The File was initiated by Perry W. Gilbert and Leonard P. Schultz in 1958 for the Smithsonian Institution, American Institute of Biological Sciences, Cornell University, and the ONR. In 1967, the data were sent to Mote Marine Laboratory in Sarasota, Florida, where H. David Baldridge analyzed 1165 reported attacks and case histories and prepared a special technical report, "Shark Attack Against Man," for the U.S. Navy Bureau of Medicine and Surgery in 1973. After a period of maintenance at the National Underwater Accident Data Center at the University of Rhode Island, in 1988 the Shark Attack File moved to the University of Florida at Gainesville, where it is maintained by the Florida Museum of Natural History under the direction of George H. Burgess.[36] It remains an authoritative collection of analyzed data, containing a series of more than 6000 individual investigations from the mid-1500s to the present. Smaller regional scientific records of shark attacks are maintained by the Taronga Zoo (Australia), California Department of Fish and Game, Hawaii Department of Land and Natural Resources, Natal Sharks Board (South Africa), and University of Sao Pãulo (Brazil). All of these organizations serve as cooperators with ISAF, feeding results of regional investigations into the ISAF database. Hundreds of cooperating scientific observers located throughout the world act in a similar capacity, ensuring broad international coverage.

The world's shark populations are in danger from overfishing, particularly in light of their slow growth rate, late sexual maturation, relatively lengthy gestation periods, and low number of offspring. Each year, 26 to 73 million sharks representing 1.21 to 2.29 million metric tons (2.7 to 5 billion pounds), or about 10 million sharks for each shark-related human fatality, are killed in

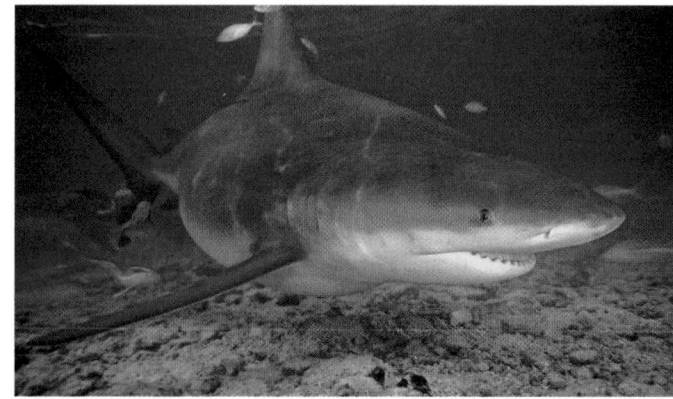

FIGURE 73-7 Bull shark. *(Courtesy Marty Snyderman.)*

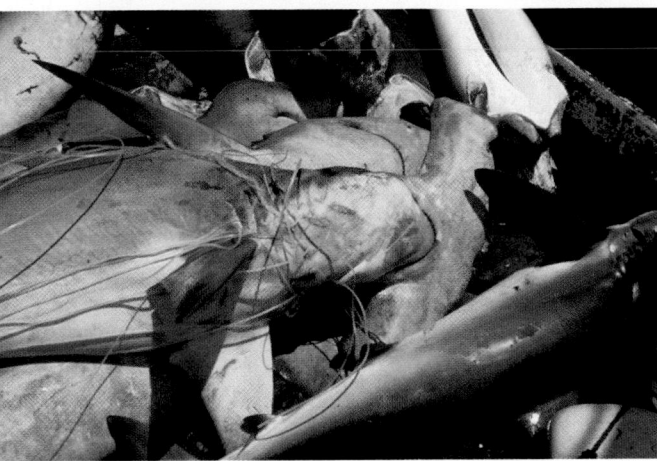

FIGURE 73-8 Shark slaughter. *(Copyright Stephen Frink.)*

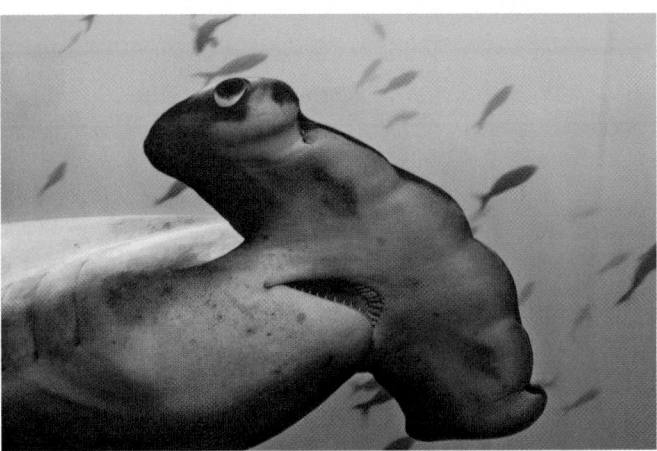

FIGURE 73-10 Hammerhead shark. *(Copyright Stephen Frink.)*

fisheries.[59] One-half of this total represents incidental bycatch (nontargeted captures in fishing nets or on longlines fishing for other species).[23] The National Marine Fisheries Service estimates that 20 million metric tons of marine wildlife are killed and thrown back into the sea as bycatch (Figure 73-8). Such nonlanded bycatch likely increase the above estimate of shark deaths, which was calculated using East Asian shark fin–trade landings. Sharks killed by commercial fishing in U.S. waters average 20,000 metric tons (44,092,000 lb) per year. Great declines in shark populations along the eastern coast of the United States occurred over the last two decades of the 20th century (now moderated through U.S. fishery regulation), but declines continue through much of the (unregulated) world. Some commercially targeted species declined by as much as 80%; the most dramatic declines were seen in dusky sharks. The flesh of most sharks is deemed of low value in American markets, and innumerable animals were ground into fertilizer or simply discarded at sea.

The fishery interest in sharks centers on the fins, including those of the blue, hammerhead (Figures 73-9 to 73-11), silky (Figure 73-12), mako, and thresher sharks. These are of great value in Eastern Asia, where they are made into shark fin soup, a traditional dish that signifies high economic status and is reputed to be an aphrodisiac. Interest in fins has also spawned the heinous and wasteful practice of finning, in which a shark is captured, its fins are sliced off (Figures 73-13 to 73-15), and then it is returned to the water (Figure 73-16).[124] Shark fin soup, which dates back from the Chinese Sung Dynasty in 960 AD, is sold for upward of $150 per bowl. The prepared fins themselves may sell for more than $800 per pound. It has been estimated that 350 tons of shark fins may be consumed each year. The

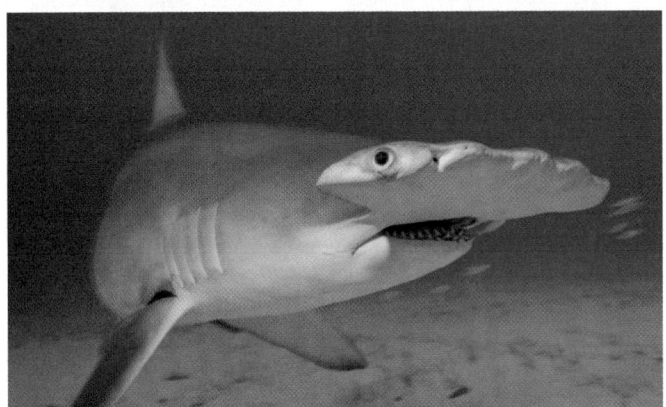

FIGURE 73-11 Hammerhead shark. *(Copyright Stephen Frink.)*

International Commission for the Conservation of Atlantic Tunas (ICCAT) created a ban on shark finning in November 2004, to join the United States, which banned shark finning in the Atlantic Ocean in 1993 and in the Pacific Ocean in 2002, in such a prohibition. Shark flesh is a major food source in both developed countries (commonly the fish in European "fish and chips") and undeveloped countries (artisanal fisheries). Mako shark flesh is similar to that of swordfish and often serves as a more than adequate culinary substitute. Sharks do not routinely appear to carry ciguatera toxin, except in the liver; however, serious poisoning from shark ingestion has been reported (see Chapter 77).[28]

In Tahiti and some other Polynesian locations, sharks are occasionally mercilessly killed simply to acquire their teeth for jewelry manufacture. The great white shark has been declared a protected species in South Africa, Australia, the Maldives, California, and the Atlantic waters of the United States. In 1991, the South African government declared the great white shark (Figures 73-17 to 73-20) a protected species within 322 km (200 miles) of

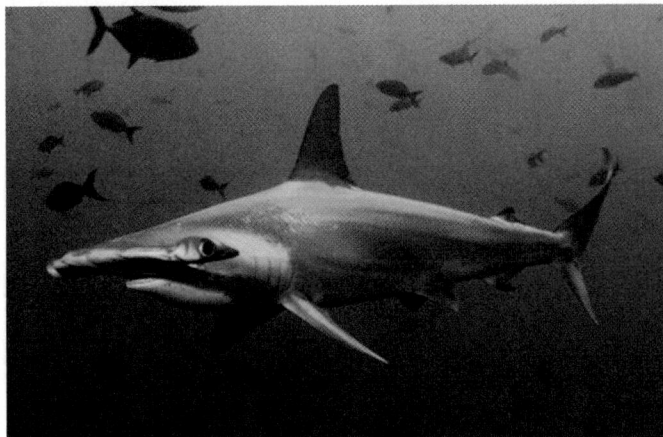

FIGURE 73-9 Hammerhead shark in Cocos Island. *(Copyright Carl Roessler.)*

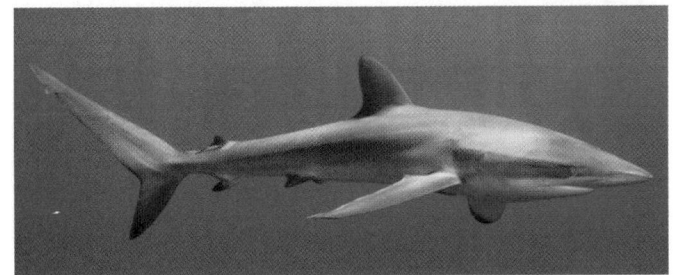

FIGURE 73-12 Silky shark. *(Courtesy Marty Snyderman.)*

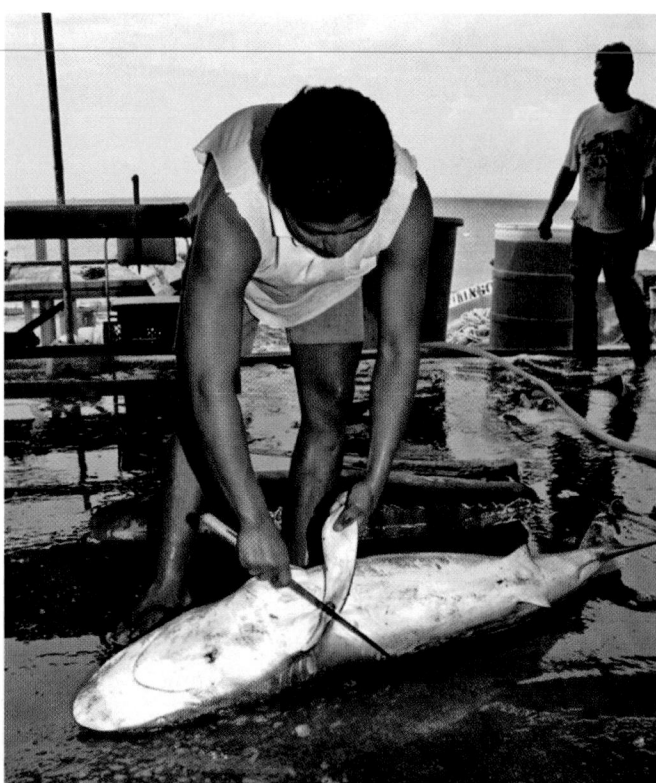

FIGURE 73-13 Finning a shark. (Courtesy Marty Snyderman.)

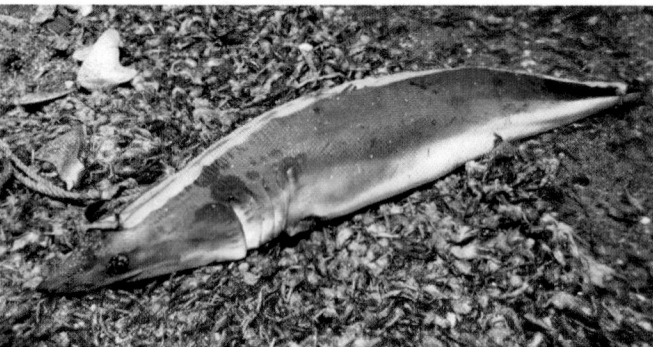

FIGURE 73-15 Shark that has been finned and discarded. (Copyright Nobert Wu: norbertwu.com.)

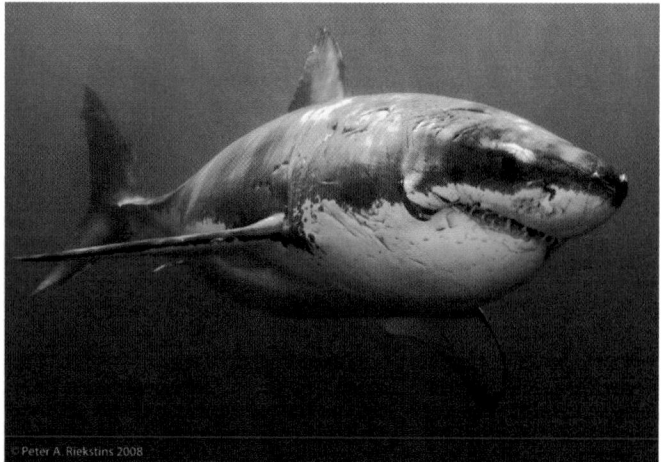

FIGURE 73-17 Great white shark shows its battle scars. (Copyright Peter Riekstens.)

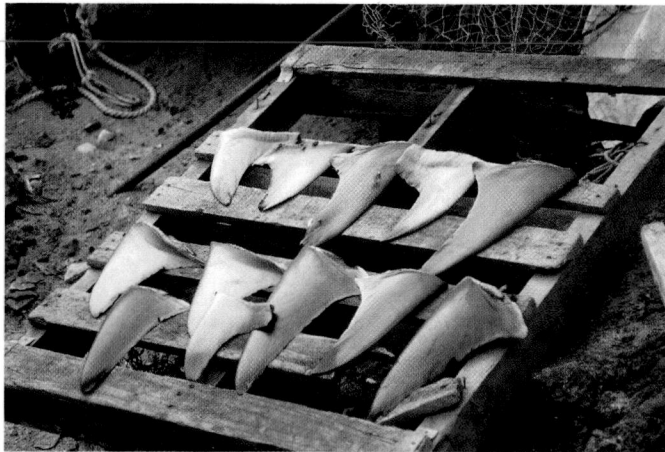

FIGURE 73-14 Shark finning. (Copyright Howard Hall.)

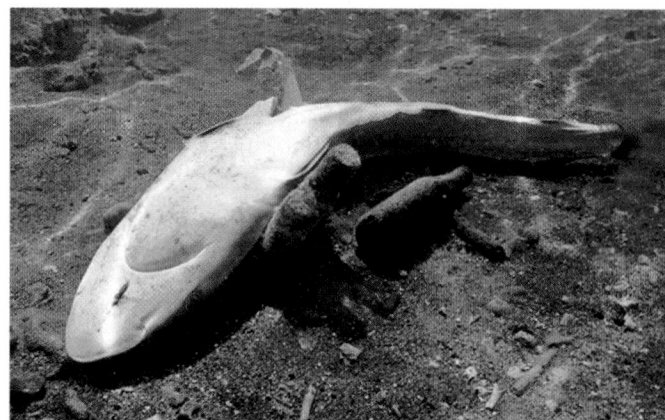

FIGURE 73-16 This dead shark is a victim of finning. (Courtesy Marty Snyderman.)

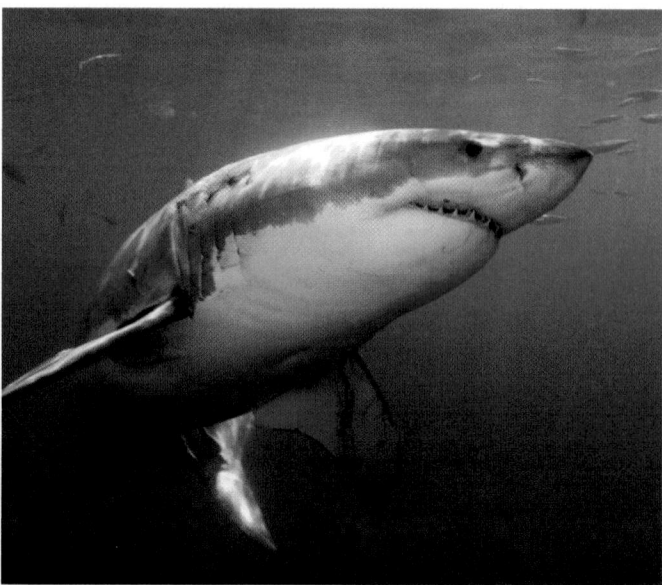

FIGURE 73-18 Great white shark. (Copyright Stephen Frink.)

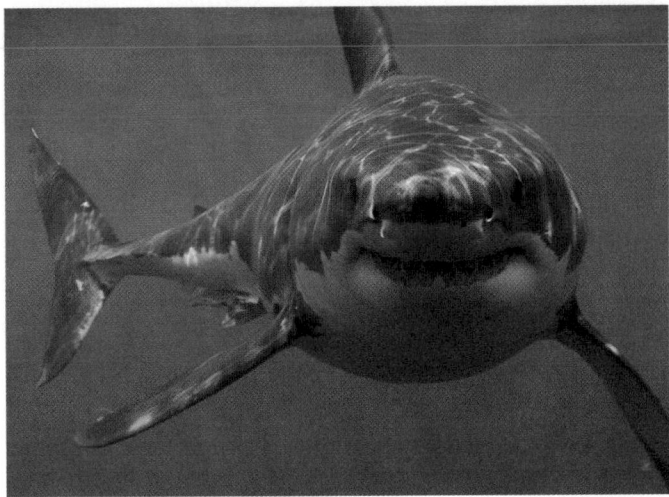

FIGURE 73-19 Great white shark approaches. *(Courtesy Paul S. Auerbach, MD.)*

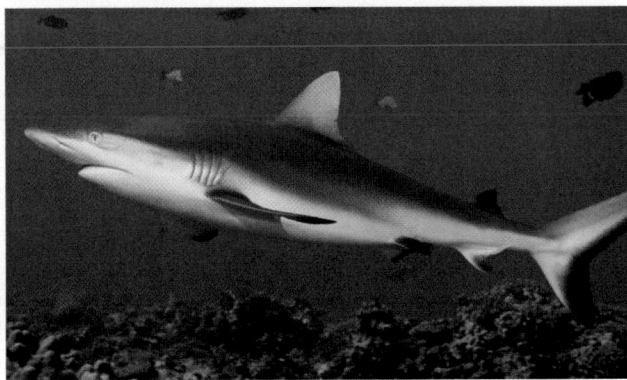

FIGURE 73-21 Grey reef shark. *(Copyright Stephen Frink.)*

its coast. The U.S. government has lowered allowable shark fishing quotas in Atlantic waters, and Australia closely monitors its shark fisheries. In October 2004, a global wildlife treaty by the Convention on International Trade in Endangered Species (CITES) offered new protection to great white sharks. In other areas, however, sharks and their relatives are largely unregulated and populations are in serious decline. Some species, especially those that enter rivers, are potentially at risk of extinction.

Of note is the failure of designation of "no-take" areas within marine coral reef ecosystems to demonstrably diminish the depletion of reef shark species, such as the whitetip reef shark and grey reef shark (Figure 73-21) in Australia, as opposed to no-entry zones. The latter are aerially surveyed and strictly enforced exclusion areas. Anything less appears to allow widespread predation by humans upon sharks.[161] Poaching and underreporting of catches are rampant.

LIFE AND HABITS

Sharks (from *xoc,* pronounced "shock," a Yucatee word from the Mayan language and a glyph for "fish") have inhabited the oceans for at least 400 million years.[24] They appeared on the planet during the Devonian period, approximately 200 million years before the dinosaurs. Indeed, many living species of sharks belong to the same genera as species from the Cretaceous period, one hundred million years ago.[177] Ancestral sharks may have been enormous; *Carcharocles megalodon,* which inhabited the

seas between 20 million and 1.5 million years ago, probably grew to a length of more than 15 m (49 feet), with teeth longer than 15.2 cm (6 inches). This was a predator of astronomic proportions that apparently largely fed on whales and manatees.

Shark attack is perhaps first depicted on a vase dated circa 725 BC from the Island of Ischia west of modern-day Naples, and it is recorded in early Greek literature. Some 35 of about 375 species of sharks have been implicated in the 75 shark attacks on humans that currently occur annually worldwide (on-average, 65 attacks per year were recorded by the ISAF in the first decade of the 21st century), and another 35 to 40 species are considered potentially dangerous.[86] It is often opined that shark attacks may be underestimated, largely because of failure to report.[189] Even if this is the case in a world made increasingly smaller by mobile phones, the Internet, and social media, it is unlikely that a completely accurate estimation would change the epidemiologic significance, compared with other causes of water-related deaths.

U.S. coastal waters typically are the setting for one-third or more of the annual number of shark attacks. The great American colonial painter John Singleton Copley's 1778 painting *Watson and the Shark* (Figure 73-22), which depicts an encounter between the Englishman Brook Watson (1735-1807) and a shark that bit off his right foot in Havana Harbor in 1749, is one of the earliest authenticated records of a shark attack.[24] ISAF has records of attacks going back into the mid-1500s. ISAF data document an average of six deaths per year during the past decade, with a long-term trend of a declining number of fatalities over the last 11 decades. Of the 72 unprovoked shark attacks worldwide in 2014 (dropping from 75 in 2013 and 83 in 2012), 63% of those attacks occurred in North American waters but none of the three worldwide fatalities occurred in the region.[33] The worldwide

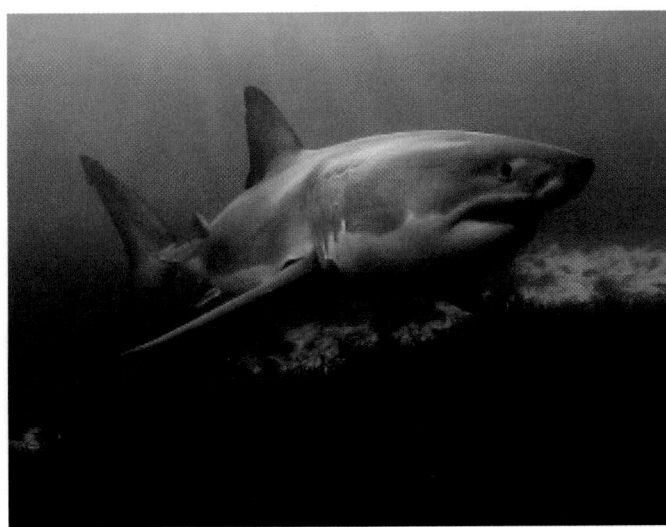

FIGURE 73-20 Great white shark. *(Copyright Howard Hall.)*

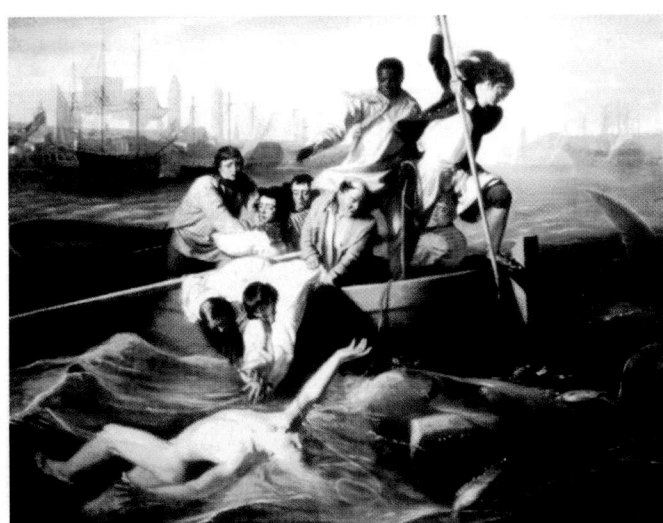

FIGURE 73-22 *Watson and the Shark,* by John Singleton Copley, 1778. *(Copyright 2005 Museum of Fine Arts, Boston.)*

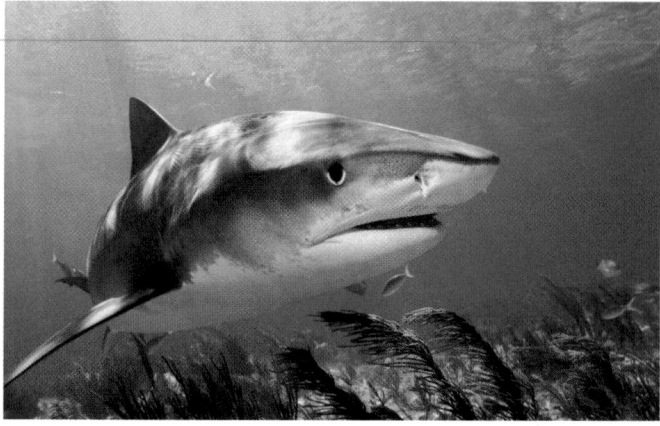

FIGURE 73-23 Tiger shark. (Copyright Stephen Frink.)

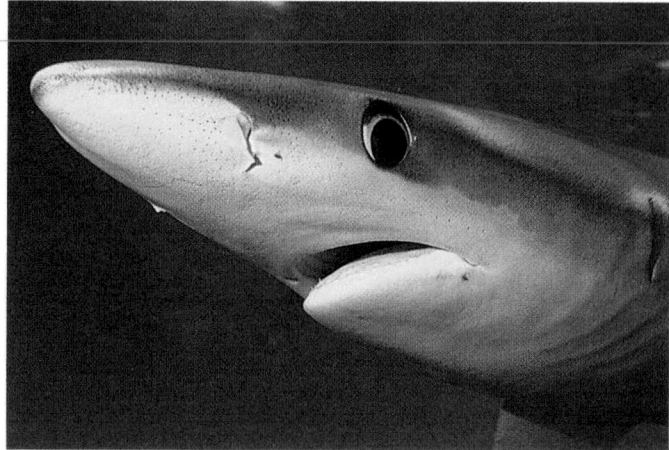

FIGURE 73-25 Blue shark, considered a dangerous species. (Courtesy Marty Snyderman.)

shark attack fatality rates have declined from over 50% in the early 20th century to 7% in the first decade of this century, largely reflective of advances in medical and first-responder capabilities and beach safety practices.[86] Greater institutional capacity in the United States results in significantly lower mortality rates than those in other areas of the world.

The most frequently documented offenders are three larger animals: the great white, bull, and tiger (*Galeocerdo cuvier*) (Figure 73-23) sharks. All three reach large sizes, routinely seek larger prey items, and have broadly serrated teeth that facilitate shearing. Bull sharks are perhaps the species of greatest concern owing to their habitat preference (inshore waters, including estuaries and rivers, which places them close to human activity) and tenacious mode of attack.[38,46,61] The species is certainly underrepresented in attribution statistics because its distributional range overlaps those of many species similar in appearance. An outbreak of shark attacks off Pernambuco, Brazil, largely involved this species.[85] However, blacktip (*Carcharhinus limbatus*) and possibly spinner (*Carcharhinus brevipinna*) sharks, which are thought to be involved in most of Florida's numerous (15 to 20 per year) minor bites, may be involved in even more incidents.[36] Identification of attacking species is a difficult task because victims seldom see the attacker well enough to make an accurate identification and because identification of most shark species, especially requiem sharks of the family Carcharhinidae, is notoriously difficult, even for trained scientists. Definitive identification can be made by examining tooth fragments left behind in a wound, but this is an infrequent occurrence. Thus, easily identified species, such as white, tiger, and nurse sharks, sit high on documented attacker lists, whereas most requiem shark incidents are grossly underreported. Less commonly reported attackers include the sand tiger (ragged tooth) (Figure 73-24), blue (Figure 73-25), blacktip reef (Figure 73-26), bronze whaler, lemon

(Figures 73-27 to 73-29), shortfin mako (Figure 73-30), grey reef (Figure 73-31), oceanic whitetip (Figures 73-32 and 73-33), sandbar, sevengill, Caribbean reef, and dusky sharks (ISAF data). Hammerhead (Figure 73-34), Galápagos, and nurse (Figure 73-35) shark attacks are rarely reported. The famous series of attacks along the New Jersey shore in the summer of 1916 are thought to be attributable to a single great white shark. Tiger sharks are the most commonly identified attackers in the Hawaiian Islands and other tropical regions. Most attacks are reported from North America, with Florida (and its central east coast)

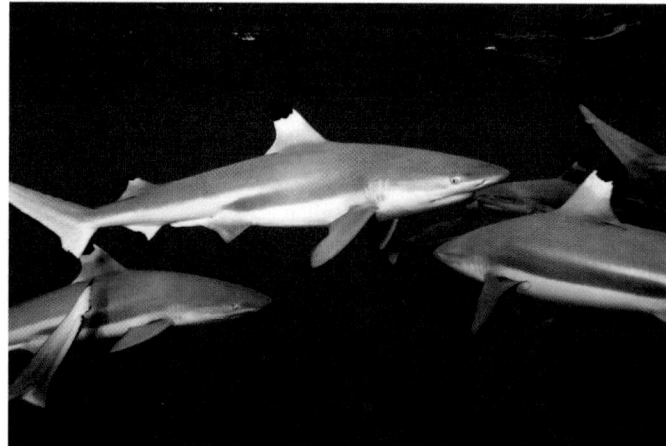

FIGURE 73-26 Blacktip reef shark. (Copyright Stephen Frink.)

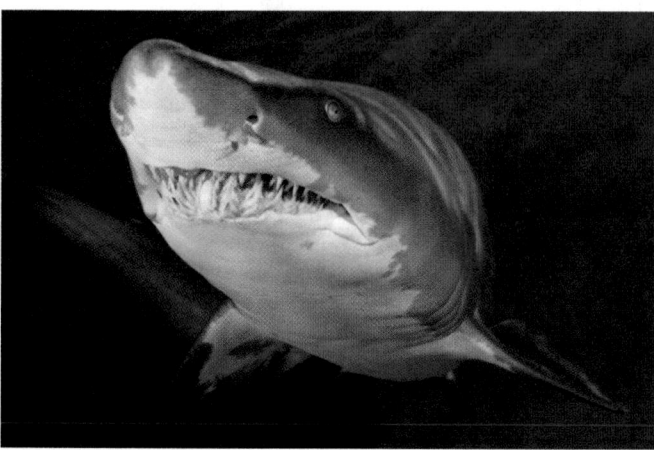

FIGURE 73-24 Sand tiger shark. (Copyright 2011 Norbert Wu: norbertwu.com.)

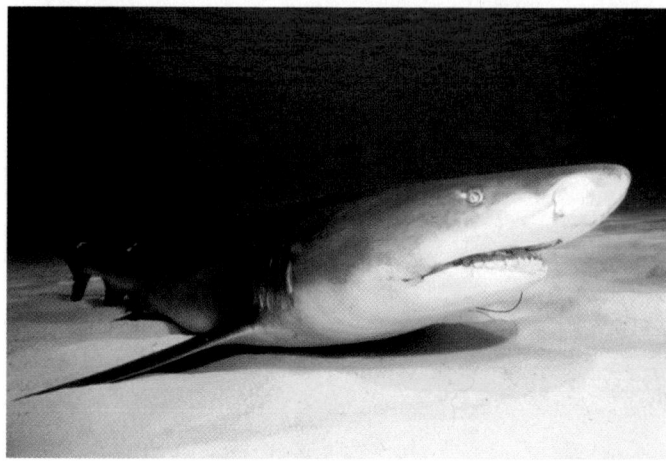

FIGURE 73-27 Lemon shark. (Courtesy Howard Hall.)

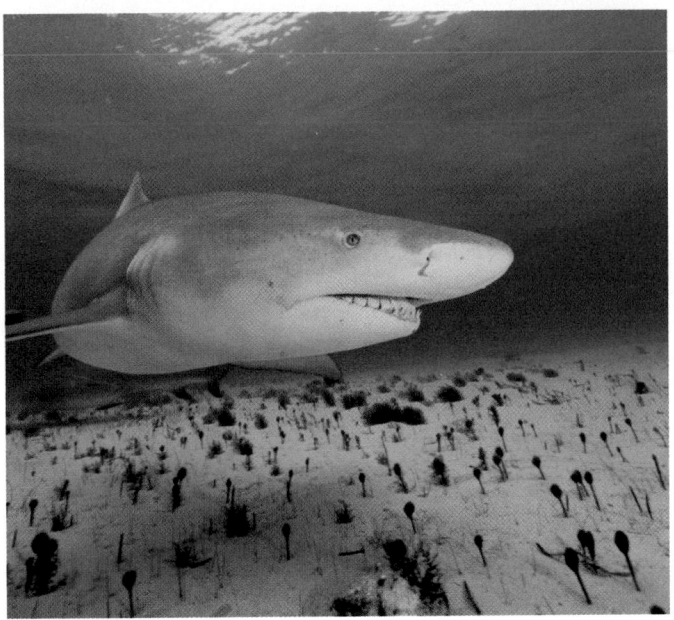

FIGURE 73-28 Lemon shark. (*Copyright Stephen Frink.*)

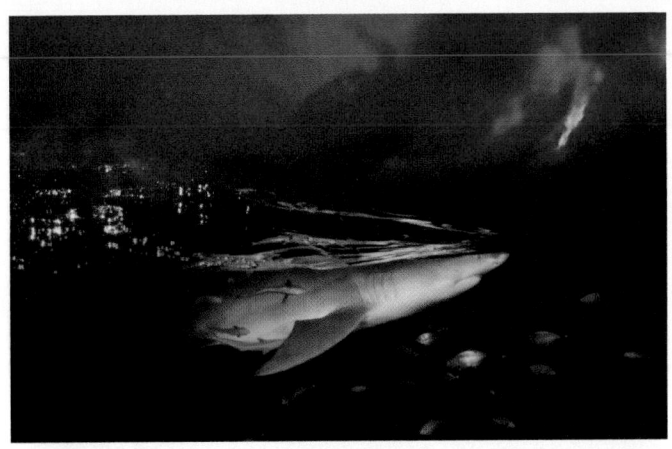

FIGURE 73-29 Lemon shark at dusk. (*Copyright David Doubilet.*)

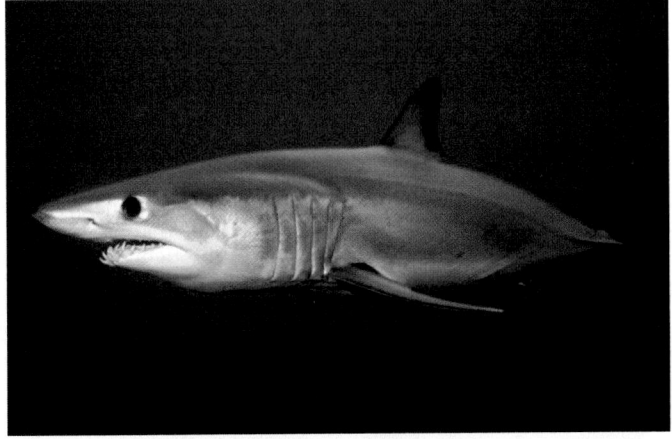

FIGURE 73-30 Mako shark. (*Courtesy Marty Snyderman.*)

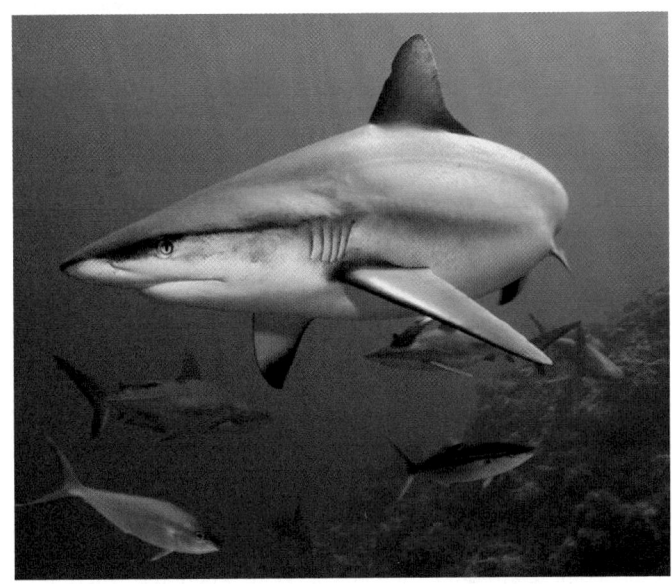

FIGURE 73-31 Grey reef shark. (*Copyright Stephen Frink.*)

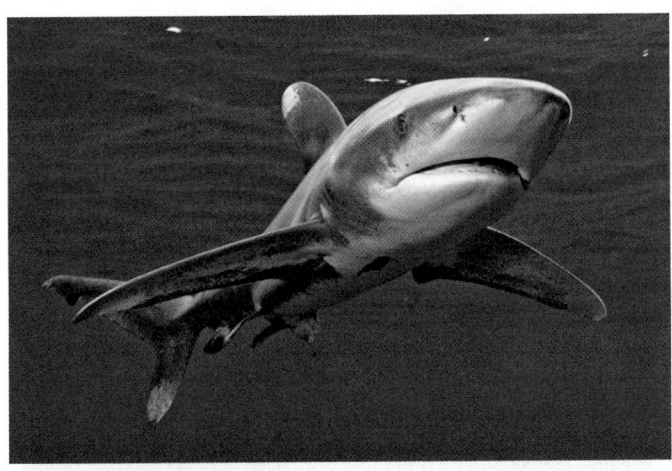

FIGURE 73-32 Oceanic whitetip shark, *Carcharhinus longimanus.* (*Copyright 2000 Norbert Wu: norbertwu.com.*)

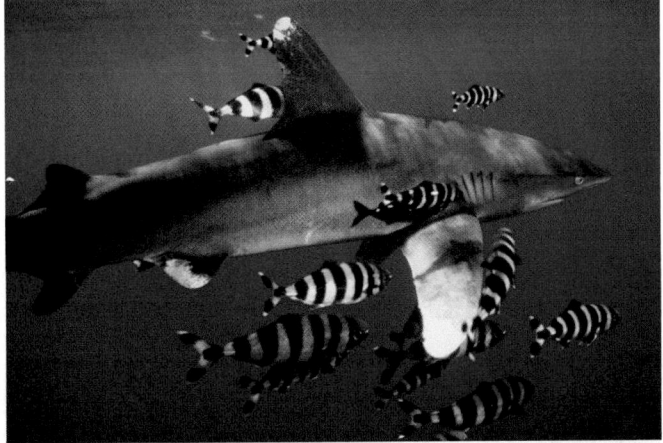

FIGURE 73-33 Oceanic whitetip shark. (*Copyright Carl Roessler.*)

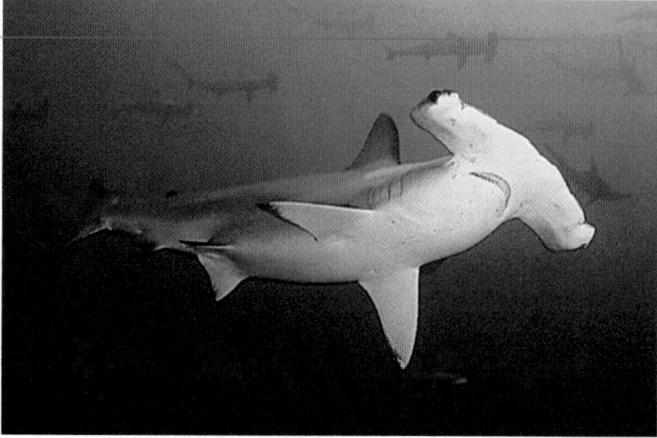

FIGURE 73-34 Hammerhead sharks, schooling off Cocos Island. The positioning of the eyes is reputed to increase the peripheral vision of these apex predators. (*Courtesy Howard Hall.*)

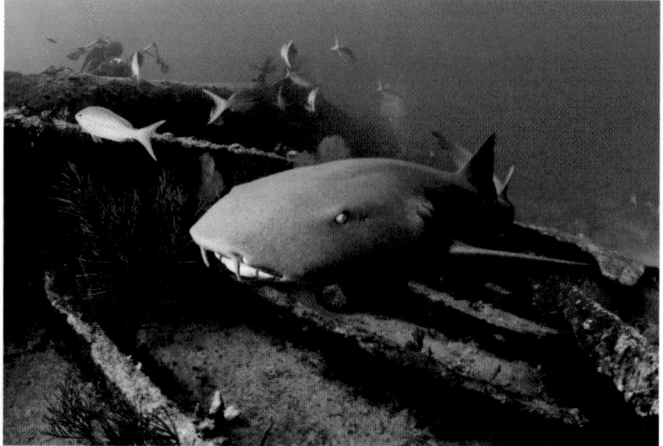

FIGURE 73-35 Nurse shark. (*Copyright Stephen Frink.*)

leading the list. A "leveling off" of annual shark attack numbers during the past decade suggests that it is possible that people are becoming a bit more intelligent about when and where they enter the water.

Sharks are carnivorous; many are apex predators. Their danger to humans results from the combination of size and dentition. Some species are also aggressive. The three largest sharks, the whale shark (Figure 73-36) (the largest fish at 15.2 m [50 feet] in

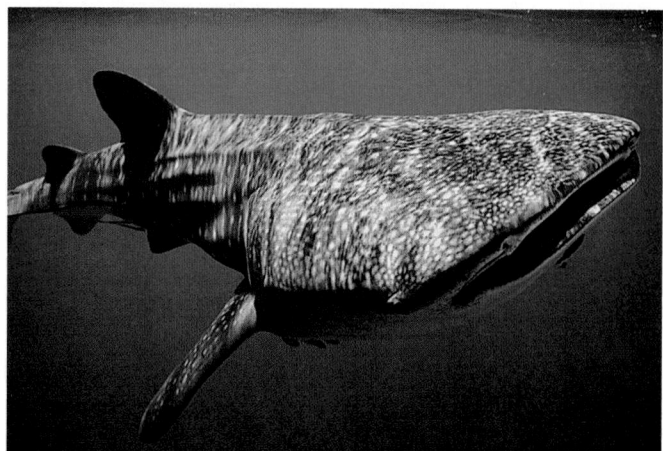

FIGURE 73-36 Whale shark (*Rhincodon typus*), the largest fish in the sea, is fortunately a plankton eater. (*Copyright 2000 Norbert Wu: norbertwu.com.*)

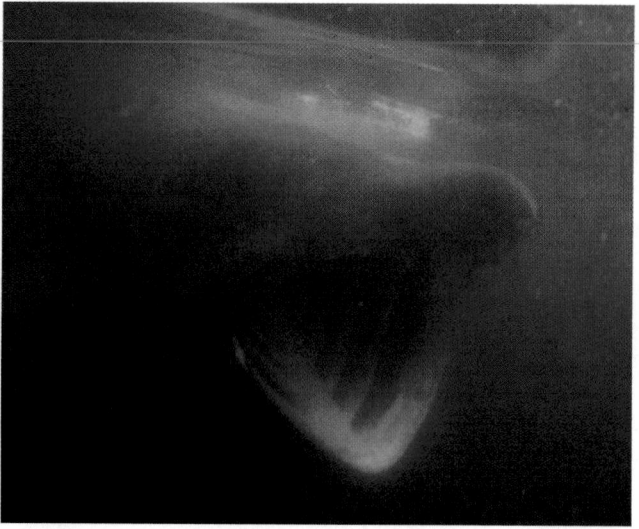

FIGURE 73-37 Basking shark. (*Copyright 2011 Norbert Wu: norbertwu.com.*)

length and more than 18,181 kg [40,000 lb]), basking shark (Figure 73-37), and megamouth shark, eat plankton and use their gill rakers as filters. Even small sharks may have powerful jaws and sharp teeth. Any species reaching a length of 2 m (6.5 feet) must be considered potentially dangerous because its dentition and jaw strength at that size can inflict serious injury on a human. White shark attacks are most common in the waters of southern Australia, the south coast of South Africa, the middle Atlantic coast of North America, and the American Pacific coast north of Point Conception, California. Attacks by great white sharks, which reach a length of nearly 6 m (20 feet) (making it the largest predatory shark), off the coast of northern California have led to the designation of a "red [or bloody] triangle" bordered on the north by Point Reyes and Tomales Bay, through the Farallon Islands to the west, and down south to Año Nuevo and Point Sur facing the Monterey Bay. This is a breeding area for elephant seals *(Mirounga angustirostris)* (Figure 73-38), which yield 91-kg (200-lb) pups, perfect food for the immense predators. In an

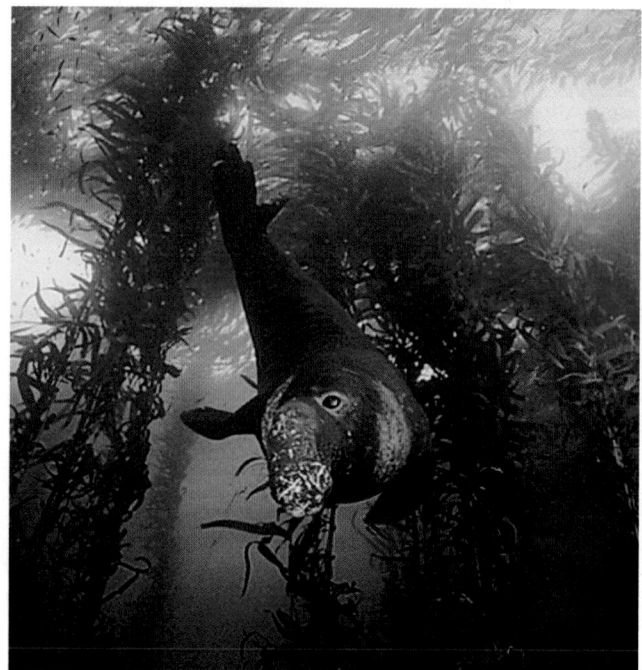

FIGURE 73-38 The elephant seal, shown here swimming through a kelp bed, is a favorite food for the great white shark. (*Courtesy Howard Hall.*)

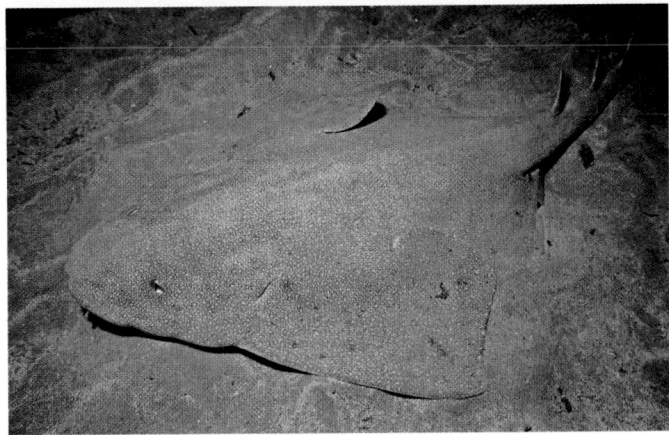

FIGURE 73-39 Angel shark. *(Courtesy Marty Snyderman.)*

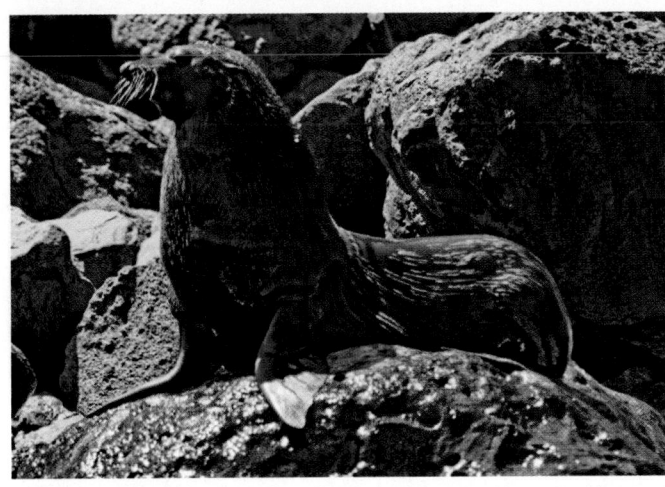

FIGURE 73-41 Bull Guadalupe fur seal. *(Courtesy Marty Snyderman.)*

analysis of California attacks, Miller and Collier attributed unprovoked attacks north of San Miguel Island to white sharks, whereas those south of this area involved members of the families Carcharhinidae (requiem sharks), Sphyrnidae (hammerheads, which can grow to more than 5.5 m [18 feet] in length), and possibly Squatinidae (angel sharks) (Figure 73-39).[133] Great white sharks follow established migration patterns and so are seen with regularity in certain locations, such as Guadalupe Island, 232 km (145 miles) off the coast of Mexico's Baja peninsula (Figure 73-40). In this instance, they have followed schools of tuna and reside from September to December with Guadalupe fur seals *(Arctocephalus townsendi)* (Figure 73-41), northern elephant seals, and California sea lions *(Zalophus californianus)*.

The white, tiger *(Galeocerdo cuvier)* (≤ 5.5 m [18 feet] and 909 kg [2000 lb]) (Figure 73-42), and bull *(C. leucas)* (3.5 m [11.5 feet]; 364 kg [800 lb]) sharks are considered the most dangerous with regard to attacks on humans. The great hammerhead *(Sphyrna mokarran)* (Figure 73-43) shark has a reputation as an attacker in equatorial waters, but its reputation is overstated, probably because of its appearance. The hammerhead has ampullae scattered over its entire undersurface that are sensitive to electromagnetic fields, which in combination with its highly developed sense of smell, lateral eye placement (Figure 73-44), and maneuverability gained by its cephalofoil head shape make this shark a superior predator. In the pelagic realm, the oceanic whitetip shark is to be respected because of its aggressive nature. This species was implicated in many of the attacks and scavenge bites on survivors of the USS *Indianapolis* and in 2010 was involved in a pair (possibly trio) of severe Red Sea attacks, including a fatality.

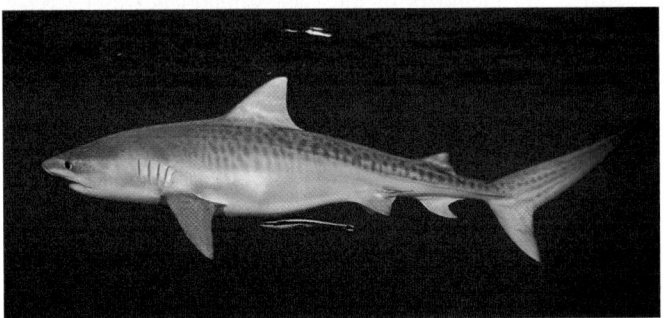

FIGURE 73-42 Tiger shark. *(Courtesy Marty Snyderman.)*

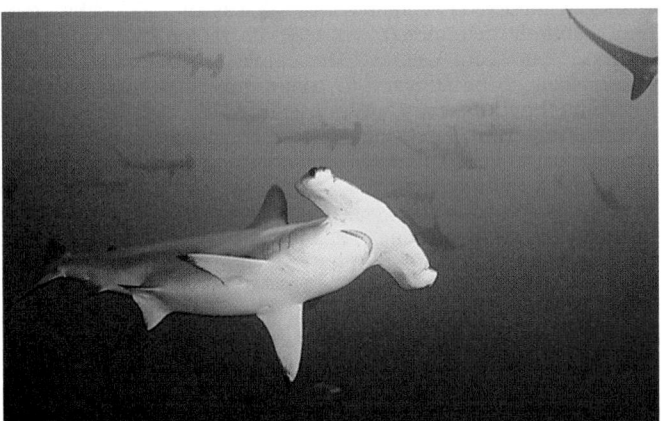

FIGURE 73-43 The great hammerhead *(Sphyrna mokarran)*.

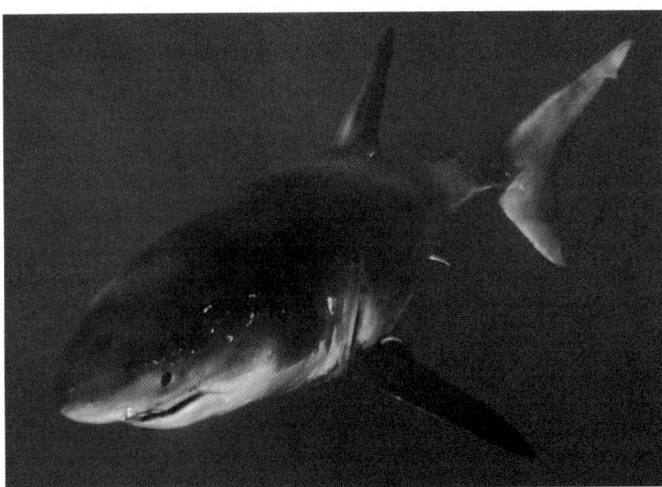

FIGURE 73-40 A massive great white shark photographed near Guadalupe Island, Mexico. *(Copyright Peter Riekstens.)*

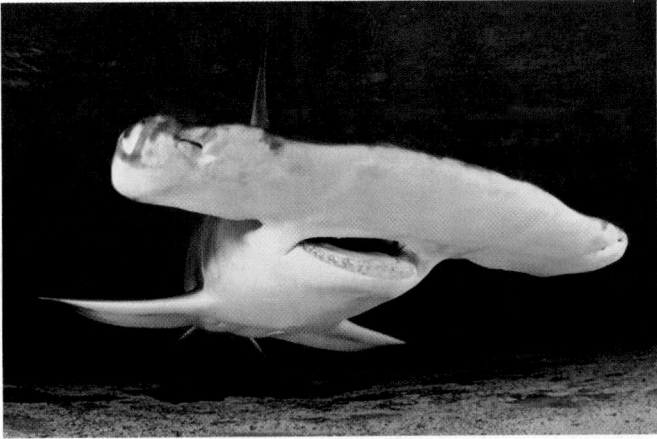

FIGURE 73-44 Lateral eye placement of the hammerhead shark. *(Courtesy Marty Snyderman.)*

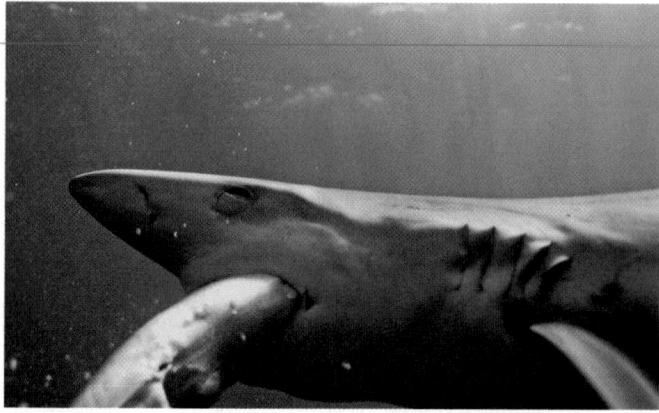

FIGURE 73-45 Blue shark bites a mackerel, demonstrating the nictitating membrane that protects the eyes. *(Courtesy Marty Snyderman.)*

Sharks are members of the class Chondrichthyes (subclass Elasmobranchii), or cartilaginous (skeleton) fishes, which also includes skates, rays, and chimaeras.[48] Unlike many bony fish, sharks do not possess swim bladders for flotation, so in most species the large liver, which contains the oil squalene, contributes to their limited buoyancy. Thus, most sharks must stay in nearly constant motion to keep from sinking and to drive oxygenated water past the gills. Only a few groups of bottom-dwelling species rest for extended periods of time. Although sharks are not highly intelligent, they are endowed with remarkable sensory systems and well-developed sensory lobes of the brain. These systems allow the shark to locate struggling fish, swimmers, or divers. Their color vision is poor but well compensated for by the acute perception of motion and contrast; the eye musculature is adapted for fixation with any body motion. Whether or not sharks are attracted to certain colors, such as international orange, is not entirely determined, but research biologists refer to this color as "yum-yum yellow." The empirical observation is that sharks seem to be attracted to contrasting colors. The tapetum lucidum ("bright tapestry," responsible for the eye shine seen at night) is a series of reflecting plates containing silver guanine crystals in the choroidal layer behind the retina, which reflects light from a photoreceptor back along the same optical path to restimulate the rods and cones and thereby increase sensitivity of the eye. This is present in sharks that are active in low-light environments.[186] The tapetum also functions to shield the retina from bright light near the surface by manipulating pigment granules. The eyes of many species are protected by upper and lower eyelids and the nictitating membrane (Figures 73-45 and 73-46). The great white shark, which does not have the membrane, rotates its eyes in the sockets to avoid injury. Keen olfactory and gustatory chemoreceptors permit taste and the recognition of blood, urine, or peritoneal fluid in the water (in some cases, one

part blood in 100 million parts of water, or concentrations of fish flesh in dilutions of one part in 10 billion parts of seawater). Sharks are most sensitive to chemicals that are similar to those produced by normal prey, such as amino acids, amines, and small fatty acids.[138] The nostrils are located on the underside of the snout just in front of the mouth. They open into sacs lined with folds of tissue containing cells used to detect smells. The odor-detecting system is constantly bathed by currents of water in both the resting and moving states.

Sharks have relatively large brains for their body size. Up to two-thirds of the shark brain can be devoted to smell. The nostrils are the openings of the olfactory organs and do not take part in breathing, which is accomplished by oxygen extraction from the water passing over gill filaments, exiting through a series of 10 to 14 gill slits (five to seven per side). Additionally, sharks possess skin chemoreceptors that detect chemical irritants. The lateral line organs are small openings along the sides of the shark's body that register motion in the water. The lateral line system extending from the back along the side to the tail responds to sonic vibrations or pulsed low-frequency (20 to 60 cycles/sec; < 800 Hz) sound waves.[48] Perhaps the most ornate series of telereceptors is located about the head, within the jelly-filled ampullae of Lorenzini, which are extremely sensitive to electrical voltage gradients (generated by the muscle contractions of fish; detection down to a $1/10^6$ volt applied across a centimeter of seawater). Continuing research is directed at delineating the piscine ability to recognize electric fields. The common smooth dogfish (*Mustelus canis*) can detect an electrical voltage gradient of 5/1000 of a microvolt, whereas the brains of certain sharks can discern 15-billionths of a volt.[71] Sharks also have extremely sensitive hearing, which may detect prey underwater from a distance of 914 m (3000 feet). Hammerhead sharks have a laterally expanded skull (cephalofoil), which spreads sensory receptors over a wider area and perhaps provides anterior lift during swimming.

Shark skin (*shagreen*) is composed in part by placoid scales (dermal denticles). These microscopic appendages have the same origin as teeth, with a pulp cavity, dentine, and vitreodentine (enameloid) covering. The denticles are embedded in the skin and mouths of sharks and rays, and protect them from predators and parasites, reduce mechanical abrasion to the animal, accommodate sensory organs, and minimize swimming-induced drag.[176] Some sharks can alter their coloration because melanin in the skin darkens near the ocean surface and lightens at depth distant from sunlight. Scale-rasping behavior has been demonstrated in the juvenile lesser spotted dogfish (*Scyliorhinus canicula*), which uses this body armor to anchor food items near its tail in order to allow bite-sized pieces to be torn away by rapid jaw and head movements.

Research has been conducted on isolation of potential antineoplastic agents from shark cartilage, organs, and body fluids.[54,116,148,150] For instance, sphyrnastatins have been isolated from the hammerhead shark *Sphyrna lewini*.[150] Squalamine, produced by the spiny dogfish, is a low-molecular-weight aminosterol as well as a broad-based antibiotic with antibacterial, antifungal, and antitumor properties. Squalene derived from shark liver boosted the immune system in experimental mice with sarcoma. Shark cartilage (which despite marketing claims does not appear to have significant antineoplastic activity) is used in creation of artificial skin for humans and is an ingredient in cosmetics, and shark blood and liver oil are being investigated for hematologic and immunologic properties.[86] The latter is used in preparations to shrink hemorrhoids. Angiogenesis inhibitors (U-995 from the blue shark *Prionace glauca* and water-soluble neovastat [AE-941]) have been derived from shark cartilage.[54,65] Shark cartilage may also affect lymphocyte migration into murine tumors.[70]

SHARK FEEDING AND ATTACK

As previously noted, sharks are well equipped in the sensory aspects of feeding. They seem particularly able to avoid detection by potential prey, by virtue of coloration and a stealthy approach.[31] Sharks feed in two basic patterns: (1) normal or subdued, with

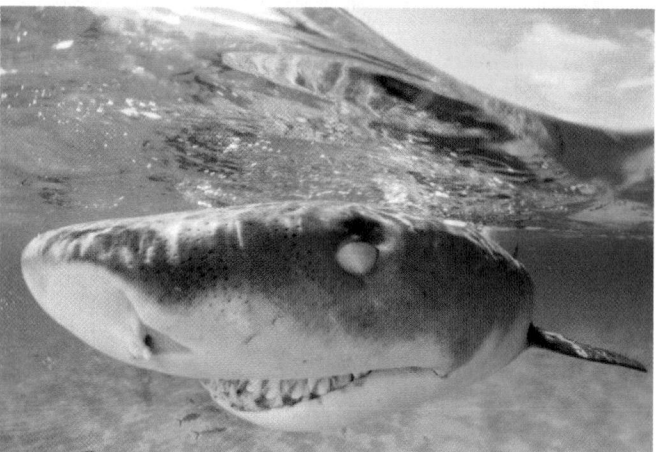

FIGURE 73-46 Shark protects its eyes. *(Copyright Stephen Frink.)*

slow, purposeful group movements; and (2) frenzied or mob, as the result of an inciting event. The latter is precipitated by sudden presentation of commotion or food or blood in the water. Frenzied behavior is enhanced by the proximity of other sharks in large numbers. In a frenzy, sharks become fearless and savage, snapping at anything and everything, including each other. Shark feeding frenzies are rare in nature, but may occur in association with major aviation or maritime disasters. Most reports of feeding frenzies have been the result of humans providing food to induce the event.

Threat displays in sharks include pointing the pectoral fins downward (most common threat sign), a "hunch" posture (nose up, pectoral fins down, back hunched), body shiver (shark hesitates or stalls in the water and appears to shudder—seen in silvertip sharks), jaw gape, sideways turn (flank exposure with slow swimming), tail "popping" (noise from exaggerated tail beats), laterally exaggerated swimming, rapid approach and retreat, and gill cavity billowing. After a shark decides to attack, the "posture" may involve a combination of swimming erratically with elevated snout, hunched back, pectoral fin depression, stiff lateral bending of the body, and rapid tail motion, in contrast to its normal sinuous and graceful swimming style.[43,97] In bursts of speed, a shark can use its powerful caudal fin muscles, and some species may attain speeds in the water of 32 to 64 km/hr (20 to 40 mph). Lamnid sharks, which include mako and white sharks, swim with a lunate tail sweep similar to that employed by tuna, facilitated by interposition of aerobic, fatigue-resistant red muscle and anaerobic, rapidly fatiguing white muscle.[180] Because sharks do not possess a swim bladder, they can ascend rapidly in pursuit of prey without incurring barotrauma.[177] As the carchariniform shark prepares to strike, it rapidly opens and closes its jaws up to three times each second, depresses the pectoral fins (from horizontal to as much as 60 degrees downward) in a braking action, and elevates the head. During a bite of a large prey item, the shark shakes its head and forebody in an effort to tear flesh from its prey. If the object of such a bite is human, there may be gouge marks left on bones or teeth shattered and embedded in the human skeleton. The white shark often bites and releases its prey prior to returning to consume the weakened creature. Large sharks swallow food whole without chewing it. Some smaller sharks or juveniles, perhaps because they are gape-limited with respect to feeding, may repeatedly suck and spit prey into and out of the mouth in order to reduce food in size.[125,139] Analysis of human remains recovered from a tiger shark indicate that the human victim was dismembered and then swallowed and digested.[95]

It is difficult to postulate hunger as the sole attack motive, because more than 70% of victims are bitten only once or twice. "Hit-and-run" attacks, in which the shark bites, then releases and leaves the area, are most common. Usually the spike-like lower teeth are used first in feeding; these anchor the victim to allow the serrated upper teeth to carve through the flesh. Solitary upper tooth slashes might indicate attacks unrelated to feeding. Up to 60% of wounds involve only the upper teeth. To aid in cutting, the shark shakes or rolls its head. At the moment of the strike, the shark rolls its eyes back in the sockets and uses the ampullae of Lorenzini to home in on the victim.

Like all predators, sharks commonly attack young, old, injured, or sick prey.[34] They are selective feeders with clear dietary preferences. Sea turtles, penguins, seals, and stingrays are consumed by certain large shark species; fish, squid, and shrimp are commonly taken by moderate- and small-sized species. Humans are not preferred food items because they are not normal inhabitants of the sea. Sharks often eat other sharks. The great white shark cruises along the bottom of the ocean preparing to launch an attack on an unsuspecting surface animal. It can strike with enough force to lift the animal out of the water and breach itself (Figure 73-47), tearing a 50-lb chunk of flesh from its victim or even decapitating the animal (Figure 73-48). The cookie-cutter (or cigar) sharks *Isistius brasiliensis* (Figure 73-49A) and *Isistius plutodus* (see Figure 73-49B) create circular crater-like wounds approximately 5 to 6 cm (2 to 2.4 inches) in diameter when they attack pinnipeds, tunas, billfishes, and other large fish. Postmortem bites on humans have been documented; recently a Hawaiian swimmer suffered a nonlethal bite.[89] Sharks have short intestines, seem to be able to selectively digest ingested foodstuffs, and may be able to keep portions of what they ingest intact for prolonged periods of time, perhaps as a method to regulate nourishment. Relatively intact human limb segments have been removed from shark stomachs many days after ingestion.[39]

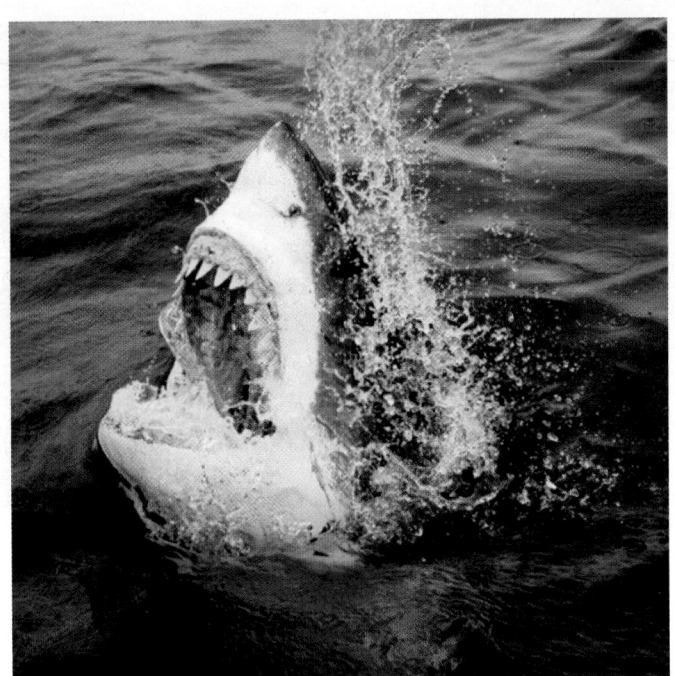

FIGURE 73-47 Great white shark begins to breech. (*Copyright Stephen Frink.*)

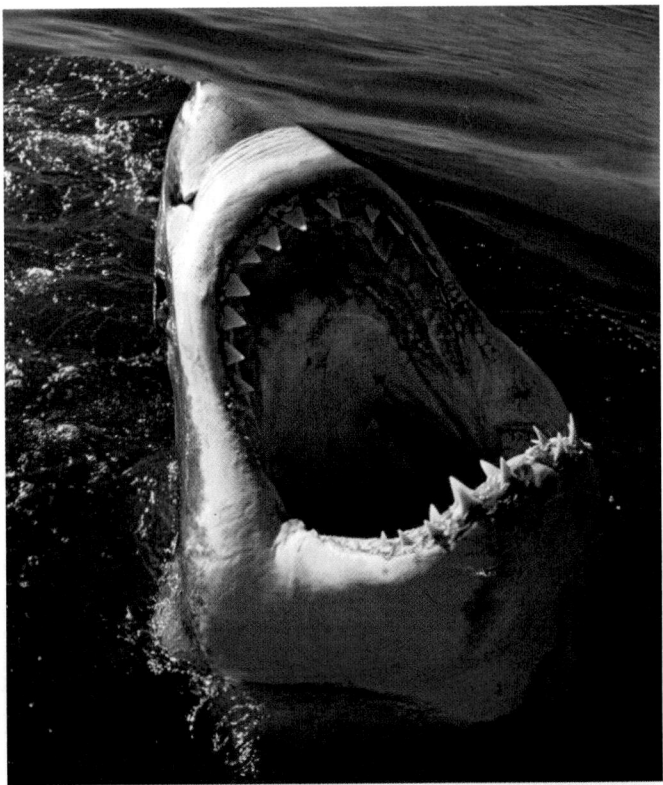

FIGURE 73-48 Great white shark (*Carcharodon carcharias*) with open jaws on surface, Neptune Islands, South Australia. Protected species. (*Copyright Gary Bell: oceanwideimages.com.*)

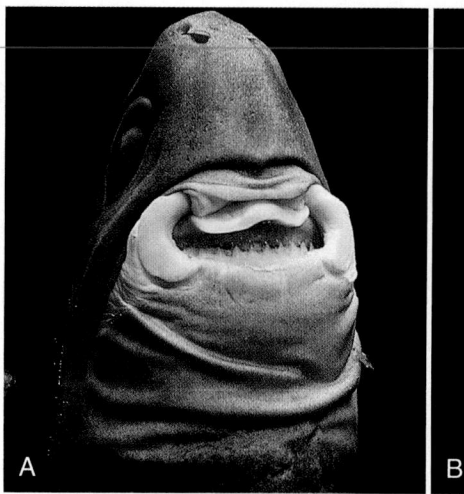
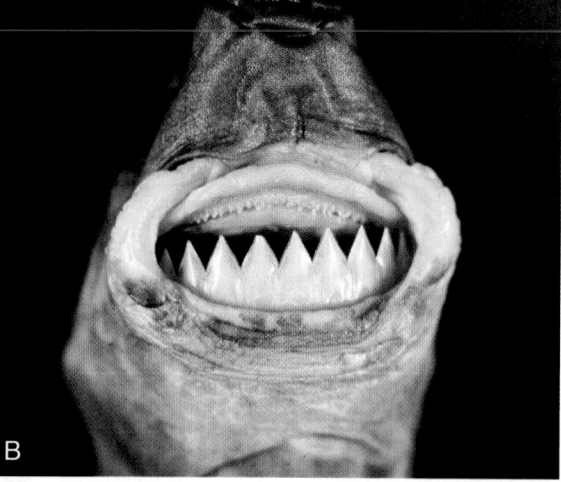

FIGURE 73-49 The cookie-cutter sharks *Isistius brasiliensis* **(A)** and *Isistius plutodus* **(B)** cut pieces of flesh off their prey with their unusual tooth configuration. (**A** *courtesy George H. Burgess;* **B** *copyright 2000 Norbert Wu: norbertwu.com.*)

It is difficult to generalize about shark attacks on humans. Most attacks likely occur as cases of mistaken identity in which the shark misinterprets the splashing of humans at or near the water surface as the activity of normal prey items. Less commonly, attacks may be direct feeding events in which large sharks simply perceive the human as appropriate sized and demonstrating appropriate behavior patterns. Finally, overt agonist behavior related to territoriality or personal space may contribute to some attacks, especially in the reef environment. Current explanations suggest that frightened persons engaged in erratic escape activity are more likely to incite attack. This has been demonstrated in the case of the grey reef shark, *Carcharhinus amblyrhynchos*. Aggression may be aggravated by purely anomalous behavior, violation of courtship patterns, or territorial invasion. More docile behavior tends to be the rule with other reef sharks, such as the silvertip *(Carcharhinus albimarginatus)* (Figure 73-50), blackfin *(C. melanopterus),* or whitetip *(Triaenodon obesus)* (Figures 73-51 and 73-52). A variety of environmental cues, including lunar periodicity, likely influence the presence of sharks and/or propensity to attack.[37]

The great white shark *(Carcharodon carcharias)* has been captured off Cuba at a length of 5.9 m (19.5 feet) and an estimated weight of 2045 kg (4500 lb); it is claimed, but not proved, that it can attain a length of 7.6 m (25 feet) and a weight of

2500 kg (5500 lb). It attains maturity at a length of approximately 4 m (13 feet). It is a man-attacker, but not always a man-eater. This statement reflects the observation that this highly feared animal usually releases its victim following a single "inquisitory" bite, a behavior it also employs on floating pieces of Styrofoam, surfboards, and marine mammals it does not consume, such as sea otters. Humans may survive and avoid consumption by having the ability to retreat to boats or surfboards prior to return of the shark, a luxury unavailable to the white shark's normal prey. This is small consolation to the unfortunate victim, who

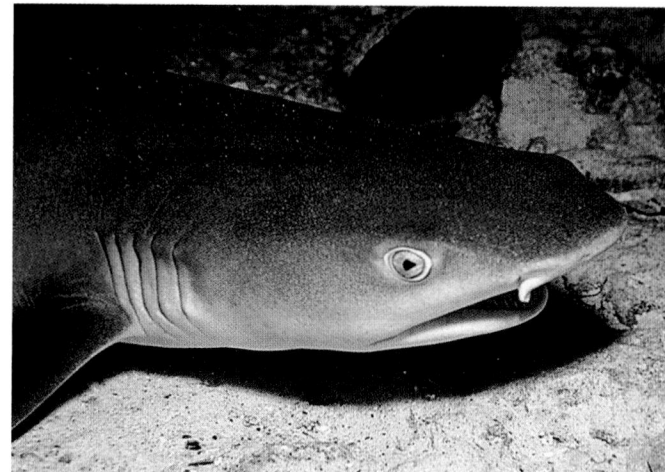

FIGURE 73-51 Whitetip reef shark. This species tends to be fairly docile. (*Courtesy Paul S. Auerbach, MD.*)

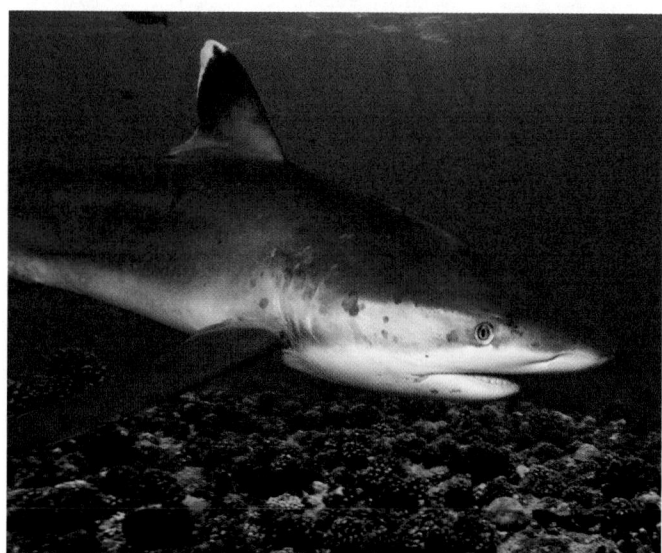

FIGURE 73-50 Silvertip reef shark. (*Copyright Stephen Frink.*)

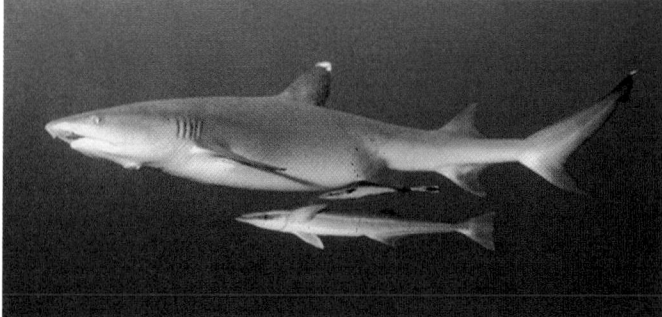

FIGURE 73-52 Whitetip reef shark with remora. (*Copyright Carl Roessler.*)

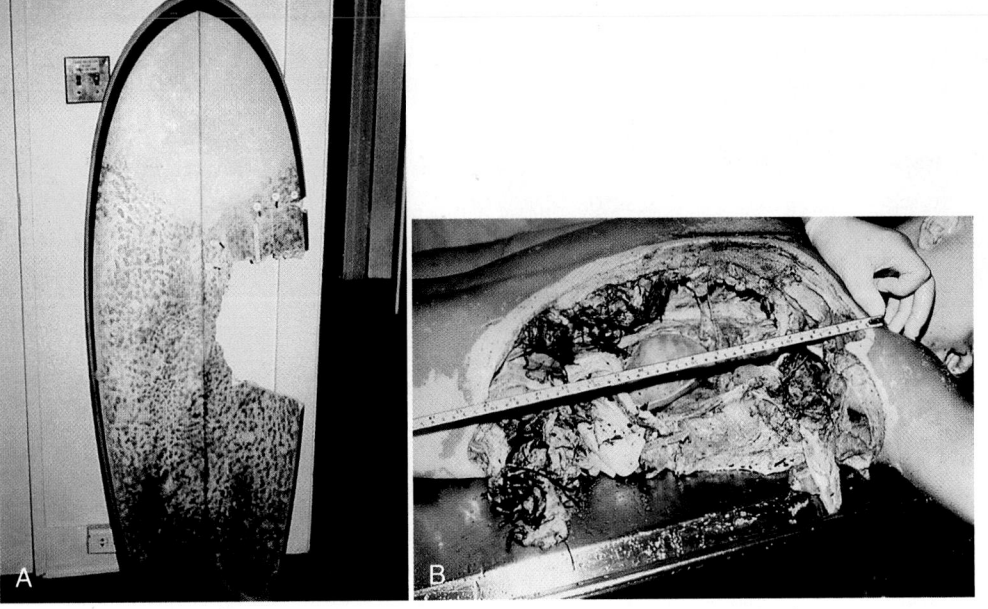

FIGURE 73-53 Victim of great white shark attack. **A,** Damaged surfboard ridden by the victim. **B,** Massive thoracic injury after a single bite. It was estimated that the shark was 6 m (20 feet) long. *(Courtesy P. Crossman, Coroner's Division, Salinas, California.)*

may have an entire hemithorax or limb removed (Figure 73-53). The great white shark has only recently been closely observed in the wild and is thus the subject of much speculation about predation strategies.[131] The feared trait of great white sharks is that they initiate contact with humans.[67] Their unpredictable nature ranges from a seemingly docile approach to a research boat to a powerful attack on a surface sea lion. Because adults feed largely on pinnipeds, the "bite-and-spit" behavior is considered a means of avoiding injury from struggling prey (Figure 73-54) while allowing the prey to weaken from exsanguination. However, it has also been observed that white sharks will sometimes chase and seize wounded prey, holding onto them during exsanguination, so there is no absolute feeding pattern.[103] It has been offered that a shark may release the victim to avoid self-drowning, because of the need to take water into its mouth in order to oxygenate gill tissues.[18] Another possibility is that it might be necessary for a shark to initiate the bite from a wide-opened jaw position.

One theory is that a shark that largely consumes a human victim does so because the victim was solitary in the water.[68] Breath-hold diver behavior and the similarity of the silhouette of a contemporary surfboard to that of a surface seal may be responsible for white shark attacks on humans. Most attacks on humans occur at or near the water's surface because this is where humans most often are found. One fatal attack in 1989 with two victims was on sea kayakers off the coast of southern California. From 1900 to 2014, there were 2777 unprovoked white shark attacks on humans, resulting in 497 fatalities worldwide (unpublished ISAF data). In 2014, there were 72 unprovoked attacks and 3 fatalities. The most recent attack statistics can be obtained from the ISAF at flmnh.ufl.edu/fish/sharks/isaf/isaf.htm.

Shark attacks have occurred from the Atlantic waters of Canada to southern New Zealand, with most between latitudes 46 degrees N and 47 degrees S, because of the increased presence of humans and sharks in warmer waters. The odds of being attacked by a shark along the North American coastline are approximately 1 in 11.5 million (ISAF data). From a worldwide perspective, danger is greater during summer months (more people in the water, expanded shark ranges), in recreational areas (splashing, noise), from dusk to dawn (preferred feeding time for many sharks), and in murky, warm (> 20° C [68° F]) water. By contrast, white sharks prefer cooler water, and attacks have occurred in waters as cold as 10° C [50° F]).[194] Attacks in northern California occur more frequently in clearer water at temperatures of less than 16° C [60° F].[133] Shark attacks in Hawaiian waters are infrequent but, as in most areas of the world, on the rise.[208] Tiger shark attack increases in Hawaii may be due in part to attraction to seagoing green turtles that come close to land, but most likely are simply reflective of rising human recreational utilization (especially surfing) of coastal waters.

Although most attacks occur within 30.5 m (100 feet) of shore, this is an artifact of the high human density in this region rather than a reflection on shark distribution. Other areas, such as mouths of rivers and inlets, edges of channels and drop-offs, and reefs and other hard-bottom relief features, are areas of shark abundance. Because of their ability to detect contrasts, sharks have a predilection to attack bright, contrasting, or reflective objects. Movement is an added attraction to sharks, which have been known to bite surfboards, boats, propellers, float bags, fishing bags, crab traps, and buoys. Because there does not appear to be any pattern of shapes, colors, or sizes to the biting behavior of white sharks on inanimate objects, it is possible that these sharks strike unfamiliar objects to determine potential food value or to protect territory.[60] Some shark attacks in northern California coastal waters have involved swimmers on surfboards (black on white), who entered migratory elephant seal (white

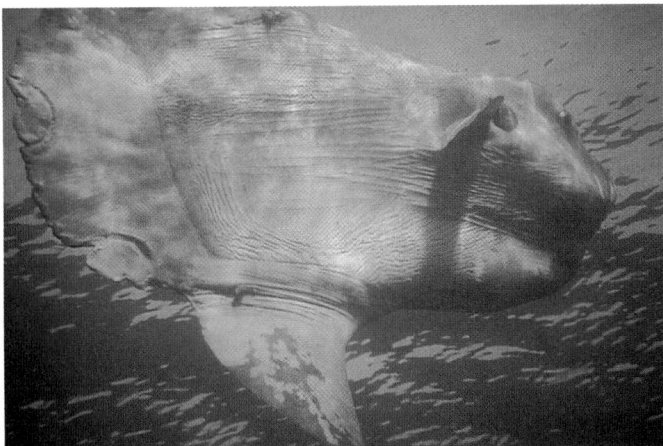

FIGURE 73-54 Giant sunfish *(Mola mola)*. Note the shark bites on the posterior end of the fish. *(Courtesy Paul S. Auerbach, MD.)*

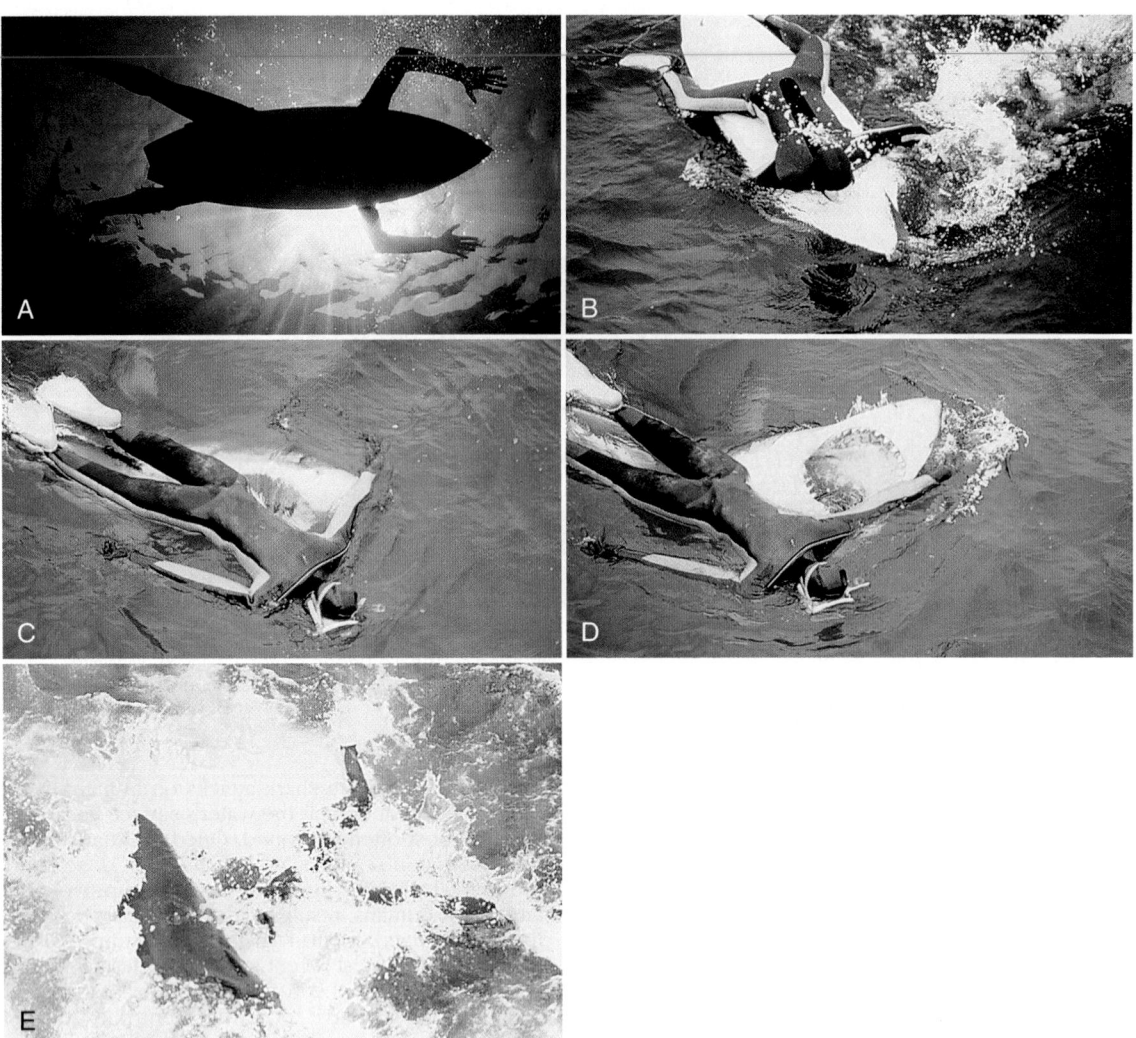

FIGURE 73-55 A, Silhouette of diver on surfboard to demonstrate similarity in shadow and contour to a sea lion at the surface. **B,** A great white shark passes underneath a dummy on a surfboard before making an attack. **C,** The shark begins to elevate its head from the water. **D,** With jaws wide, the shark attacks the dummy. **E,** With great commotion, the dummy and surfboard are dragged beneath the surface. *(Courtesy Images Unlimited, Inc. A courtesy Al Giddings; B courtesy Rosemary Chastney; C to E courtesy Walt Clayton.)*

shark food) habitats (Figure 73-55). The color black may encourage great white shark interest, perhaps resembling the dark coloration of certain marine mammals.[37] Great white sharks congregate in autumn in the waters around the rocky Farallon Islands, 43.5 km (27 miles) off the Golden Gate Bridge near San Francisco, where they actively pursue seals. They also congregate, seasonally and predictably, in other locations, such as around Guadalupe Island off the coast of Mexico. Great white sharks have been observed to use hunting strategies involving anchor points or lairs, rather than random attacks. The attack locations possibly are selected by a balance between prey detection, competition with other sharks, and water conditions that allow a swift vertical attack.[126] In a study of the behavior of great white sharks and their pinniped prey during predatory attacks, it was noted that white sharks feed on phocids (elephant seals) more frequently than on otariids (sea lions). It was also noted that certain prey might be deemed less palatable after initial sampling on the basis of perceived low energy value.[103]

Most shark attack victims are bitten by a single shark, violently and without warning. In the majority of attacks, the victim does not see the shark before the attack. Attacks occur predominately from below or from the side. The most common (80%) attack type is hit and run, in which the victim is seized and released, or slashed on an extremity.[32,90] This frequently occurs in shallow water and has been attributed to (1) mistaken identity of potential

prey, (2) juvenile sharks with poor predatory ability, or (3) situational provocation.[19,36] Another type is a "sneak" attack on a diver or swimmer in deeper water, whereby a shark attacks without being seen. Finally, "bump-and-bite" attacks have the shark make contact with the victim prior to actually biting. This may be an attempt by the shark to determine the defensive abilities of its prey or to wound the victim before the definitive strike. A shark may circle a victim prior to bumping. Severe skin abrasions (Figures 73-56 and 73-57) and bruising from the shark skin can be produced in this manner. The sneak and bump-and-bite attacks generally are perpetrated by larger animals and are thought to be part of intentional feeding behavior.

CLINICAL ASPECTS

The jaws of the major carnivorous sharks are crescent-shaped and contain up to five or six rows or series of sharp ripsaw triangular teeth, which are replaced every few weeks by advancing inner rows (Figure 73-58). The teeth of sharks are not attached directly to the jaw cartilage, but are held in place by a collagenous membrane in a shallow depression known as the tooth bed.[138] Each species has distinctively shaped teeth.[186] However, teeth of the great white shark reveal no consistent pattern of size or arrangement of the marginal serrations that are sufficiently characteristic within an individual shark to serve as a

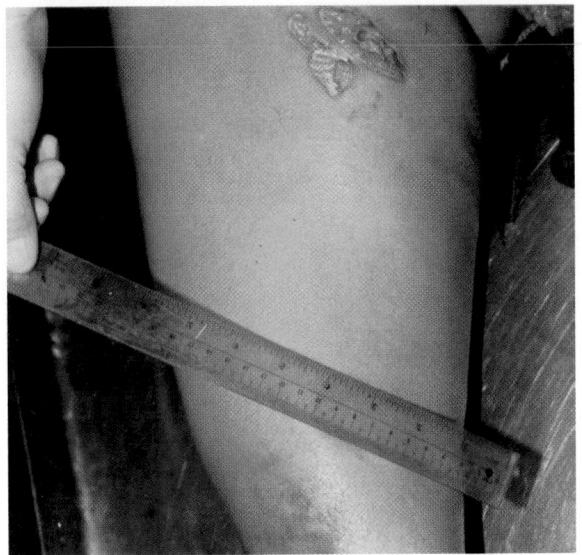

FIGURE 73-56 Skin abrasion and bruise from shark denticles. (Courtesy George H. Burgess.)

reliable index of identification of a tooth as originating from that particular shark. Tooth shape and size are useful in determining its place in the jaw, and serrations are sufficiently distinctive to enable the potential identification of an individual tooth as having been the cause of a particular bite mark.[143] The size of a shark can be determined from forensic analysis of bite damage and the two evolutionary lineages of sharks most often involved in attacks, the carcharhinoids and lamnoids, are discernable by dental characteristics.[121] A nomogram has been developed that can be used to estimate the body length of a great white shark from measurements of the tooth or bite mark morphology.[142] Although normal tooth replacement takes 7 to 14 days, in some species a lost tooth can be replaced within 24 hours. Sharks are born with a full set of teeth (covered by a protective ectodermal sheath), and in some cases have up to 15 rows of replacement teeth available. Amazingly, some sharks produce up to 25,000 teeth in a lifetime, as teeth are shed frequently (Figure 73-59);

FIGURE 73-57 Skin abrasions from shark denticles. (Courtesy George H. Burgess.)

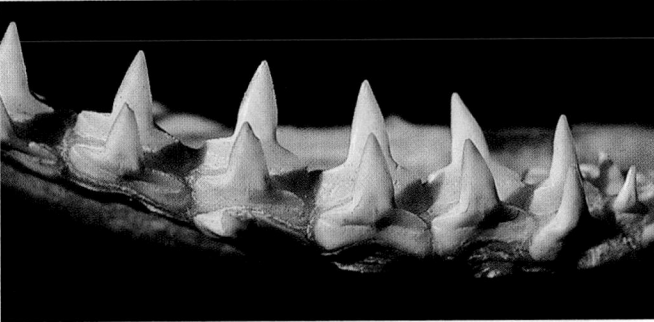

FIGURE 73-58 Teeth of bull shark (Carcharhinus leucas). (Copyright 2000 Norbert Wu: norbertwu.com.)

this explains the abundance of fossil shark teeth in paleontologic excavations. The upper jaws generally have larger cutting teeth, whereas the sharp lower teeth are designed to fasten onto and hold prey during capture.[77] The bamboo shark (Chiloscyllium plagiosum), which dines largely on crustaceans, is able to fold its teeth inward on a flexible broad ligament in order to crush and consume its normal prey.[167]

Shark teeth are cartilaginous, strengthened by the deposition of calcium phosphate crystals (apatite) in a protein matrix, all covered by an enameloid substance. They are considered to be as hard as granite and as strong as steel. In a large great white shark, the largest serrated triangular teeth can grow to 6.4 cm (2.5 inches), with 26 upper and 24 lower teeth exposed in the front row. The height of the enamel of the largest tooth in the upper jaw is proportional to the animal's length, so a body length of up to 7.6 m (25 feet) may be possible based on recovered teeth. Teeth and fragments embedded in clothing or the victim may assist in identification of the biting species. The upper jaw is advanced forward and protruded to allow its participation in the biting action (Figure 73-60). The biting force of tiger (Figure 73-61) and dusky sharks is estimated at as high as 21 tons per square inch across the tooth tips. By comparison, humans have been estimated to bite with a force of 15 tons per square inch. Severe shark bites result acutely in massive tissue loss, hemorrhage, shock, and death. Even a smaller animal, such as a young lemon shark, can bite with bone-crushing force.[79] The potential for destruction is enormous, in parallel with other predators, such as tigers, lions, and bears.

Lentz and colleagues reviewed the mortality rates and management of 96 shark attacks and developed the Shark-Induced Trauma (SIT) Scale.[118] Arms and especially lower legs are the most common trauma regions in shark attacks on humans (Figure 73-62). Sharks most often attack from below and behind. Therefore, the legs and buttocks are most frequently bitten (Figures 73-63 and 73-64), perhaps an indication of leg movement and the available body mass of buttocks and thighs. This is followed in frequency by the hand(s) and arm(s), as the victim attempts to fend off the shark (Figures 73-65 to 73-67).[39] Because sharks

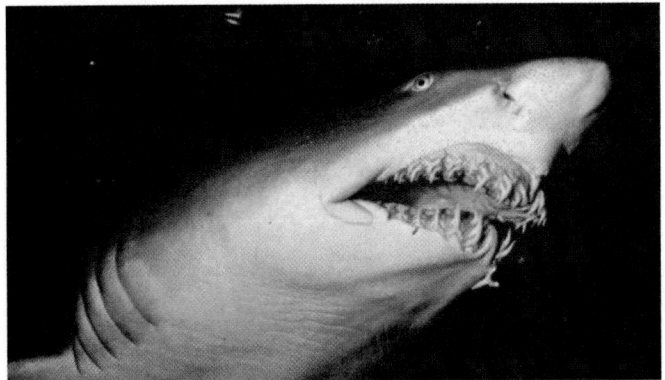

FIGURE 73-59 Shark shedding tooth. (Copyright Lynn Funkhouser.)

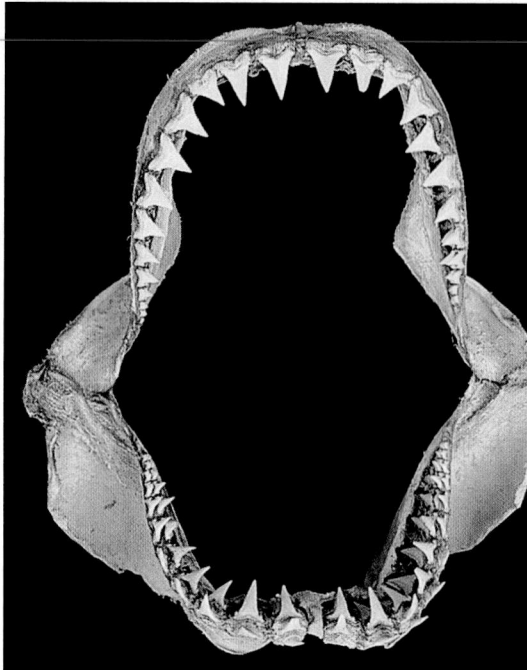

FIGURE 73-60 Jaw of a great white shark. (Copyright 2000 Norbert Wu: norbertwu.com.)

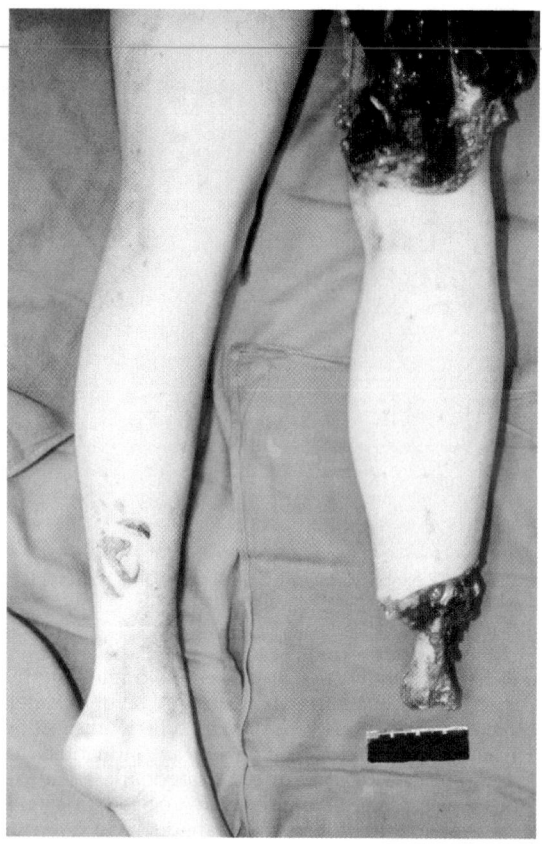

FIGURE 73-62 Tiger shark spin and pull. (Courtesy George H. Burgess.)

do not chew their food, their method of biting and rolling or thrashing allows flesh to be stripped from the victim. Teeth may be embedded in prey (Figure 73-68), but fractured bones are surprisingly rare.[95] Degloving injuries occur when a victim attempts to pull an extremity from the mouth of a biting shark, raking soft tissue across sharp teeth (Figure 73-69). Skin lacerations may display tooth patterns (Figure 73-70). Proximal femoral artery disruption carries a poor prognosis because of torrential hemorrhage (Figure 73-71). Although fractures are not common, broken ribs often accompany intrathoracic, intraperitoneal, and retroperitoneal injuries. Spiral gouges or crescent-shaped grooves horizontal to the shaft on bones indicate the bite and roll activity of an attacking shark.[95] In 2007, an Australian abalone diver claimed to have been partly swallowed head first by a great white shark, which released him when the man fought his way free.

Because the victim is generally far from medical assistance, blood loss may be profound. The wounds have historically been fatal in 15% to 25% of attacks, but have averaged under 10% over the past decade, with major causes of death listed as hemorrhage and drowning. Rapid response and prehospital care are undoubtedly improving this statistic, as have advances in major trauma treatment gained in part from lessons learned in 20th-century wars.

In a retrospective review of 12 corpses recovered from Okinawa, Japan, with shark-induced, mostly postmortem injuries, the characteristic injury features were felt to be sharp incision without abrasion, wound with a serrated edge, triangular or rectangular flap of skin, regular arrangement of marks that correspond to shark teeth, gouge marks on bone, and severance of the body part at the joints without a fracture.[93] Postmortem bites from sharks and other marine creatures, such as sea lice, can

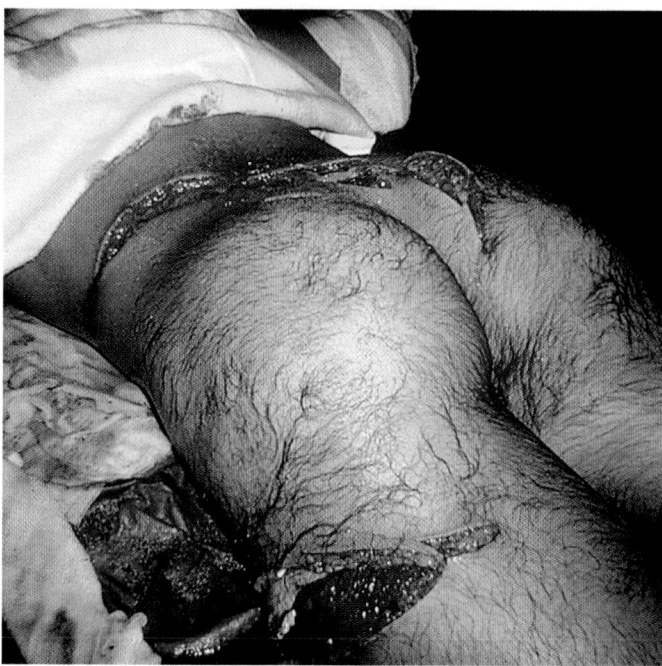

FIGURE 73-63 Shark bite of the buttocks and thigh. (Courtesy T. Hattori, MD.)

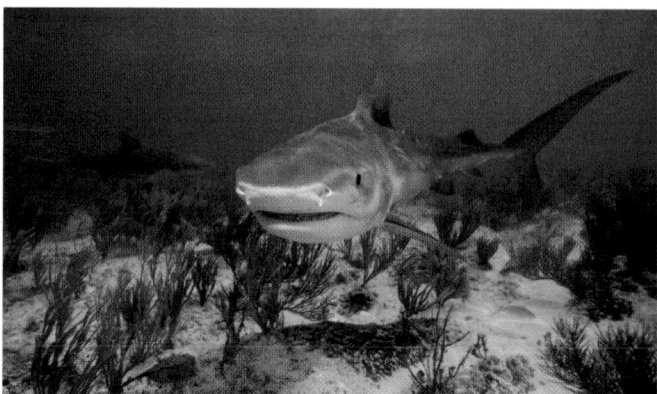

FIGURE 73-61 Tiger shark on a reef. (Copyright Stephen Frink.)

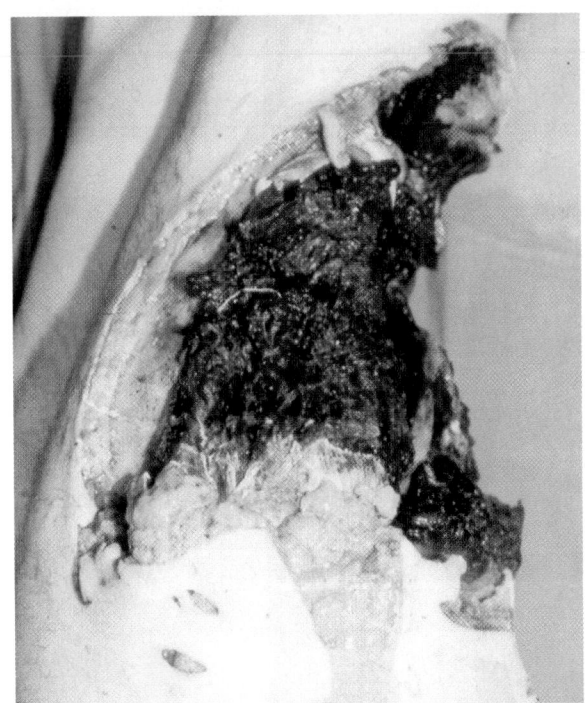

FIGURE 73-64 Typical thigh wound from shark bite. (Courtesy George H. Burgess.)

create the appearance of inflicted injury and obscure the true cause of death.[40] It therefore becomes important to differentiate postmortem artifacts from injuries that may have been inflicted while the victim was alive. For instance, the drowned victim may be bitten by sharks. If the wounds do not penetrate blood vessels or vital structures, they should be suspected of being noncontributory to the fatal event. However, when only part of a body is recovered, it is difficult to determine if a shark bite was the

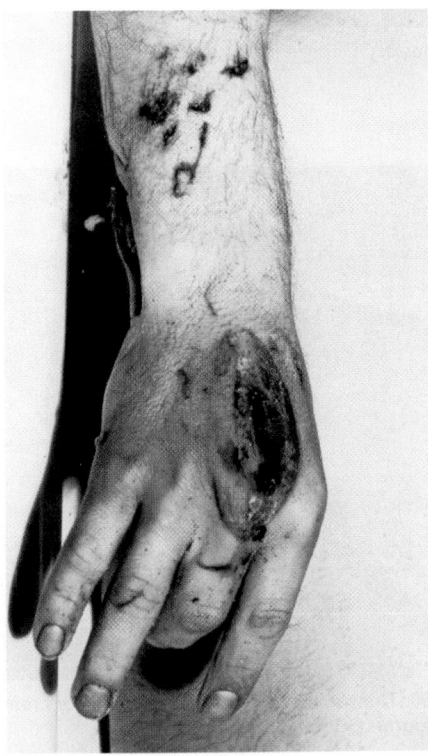

FIGURE 73-65 Defensive wound of the hand from shark bite. (Courtesy George H. Burgess.)

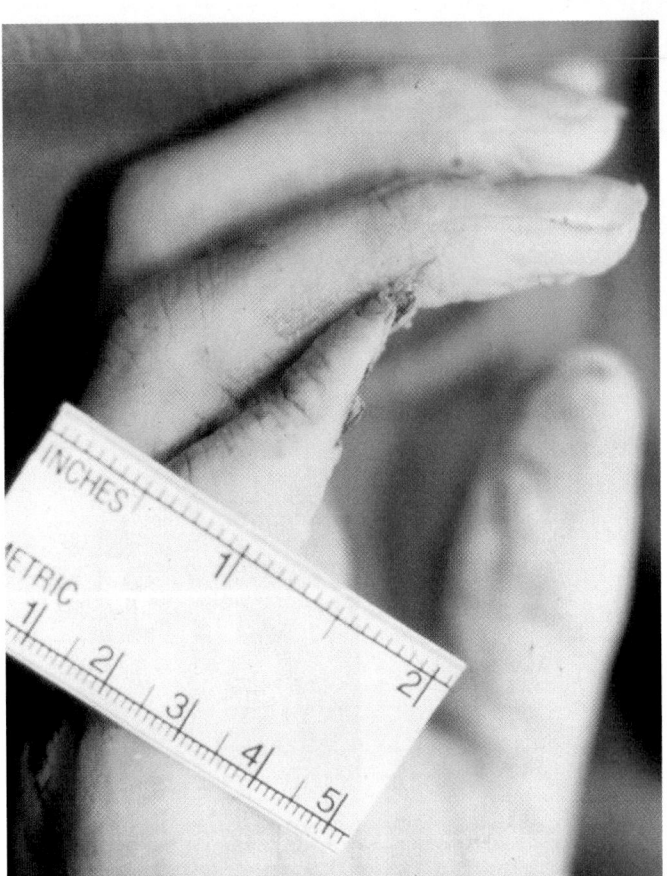

FIGURE 73-66 Defensive wound of the finger from shark bite. (Courtesy George H. Burgess.)

inciting event. Furthermore, sharks are capable of maintaining tissues within their stomachs for weeks at a time without digestion occurring, which may further obscure determination of time of death.[123] Bite configurations may be pathognomonic for some species, but species identification is difficult in most cases. The circular and C-shaped injuries inflicted by the cookie-cutter shark (I. brasiliensis, I. plutodus) are made by small erect teeth in the upper jaw and triangular teeth in the lower jaw, resulting in the distinctive carving of a plug of flesh (Figure 73-72).[212] Cookie-cutter sharks have been implicated in bites on live and dead humans[89,93,123] (Figure 73-73). Two cases of fatal great white shark attack were reported where the only tissues recovered were lung fragments.[41] The authors concluded that the only tissue to escape being consumed or lost in fatal shark attacks associated with dismemberment may be lung. Aerated lung tissue from a recently killed victim may rise to the surface, as opposed to fluid-filled lung tissue that would be characteristic of a drowning.

Sharks can grow to be quite large and are strong creatures. Fishermen are injured by thrashing animals on boat decks and in fishing nets. In one unusual incident reported to the author (PSA) by Dr. Edward Paget, the captain of a fishing ship jumped into the ocean in order to free a whale shark caught in a net. The enormous animal bumped him against the ship. The captain suffered mild abdominal pain, which worsened to the extent that he sought care in a hospital at Majuro in the Marshall Islands. He was transferred 300 miles by airplane to Dr. Paget, who observed signs of blood loss and localized peritonitis. At surgery, the victim was found to have 3400 mL of intraperitoneal blood with clots and a gangrenous 2-inch segment of sigmoid colon that necessitated a diverting colostomy.

TREATMENT

In most cases, the immediate threat to life is hypovolemic shock. In one series compiled by the South African Natal Sharks Board,

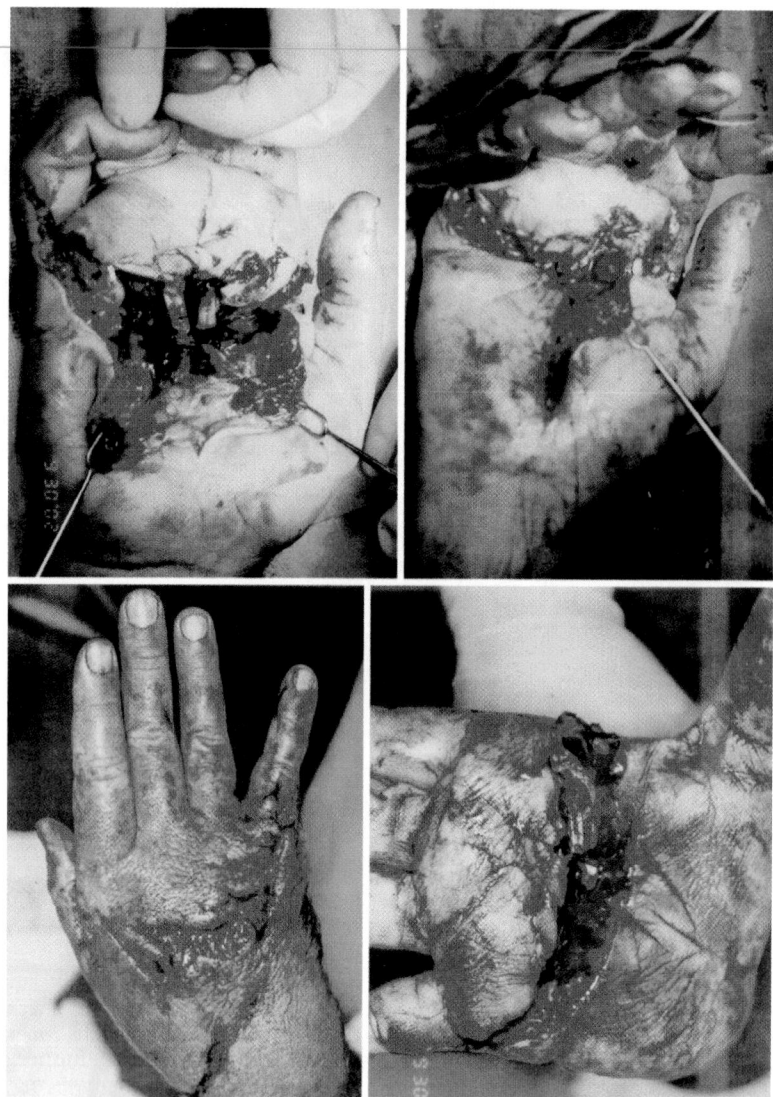

FIGURE 73-67 Nondefensive shark bite of the hand. *(Courtesy George H. Burgess.)*

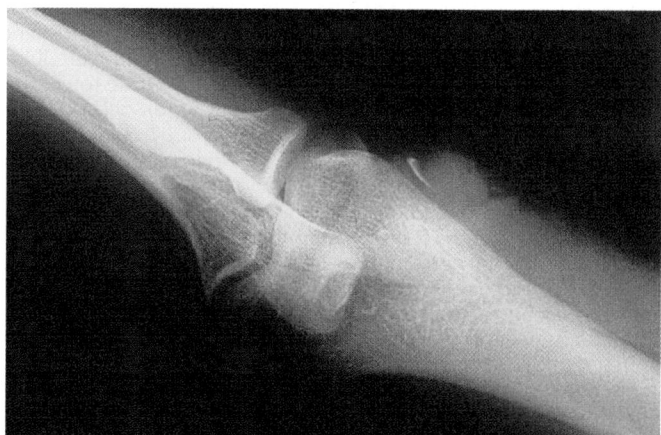

FIGURE 73-68 The presence of a shark tooth in the arm is revealed by x-ray examination.

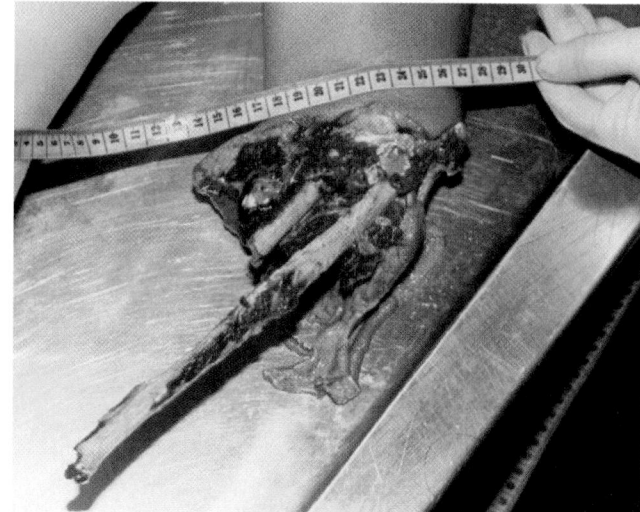

FIGURE 73-69 Tiger shark "bite and spin" behavior creates a degloving injury. *(Courtesy George H. Burgess.)*

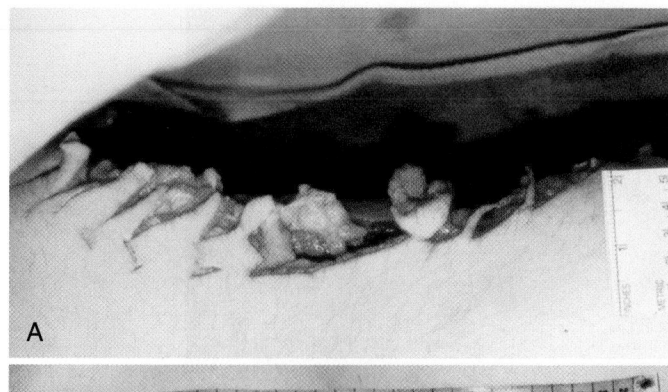

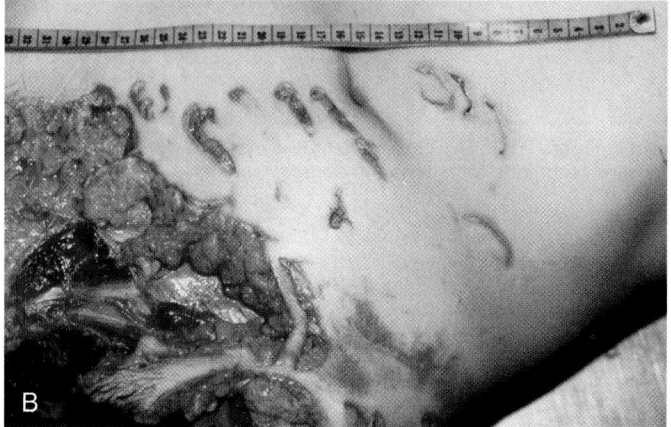

FIGURE 73-70 A, Shark bite creates wound edge that displays tooth pattern. **B,** Tooth pattern and wounds created by bite of a tiger shark. *(Courtesy George H. Burgess.)*

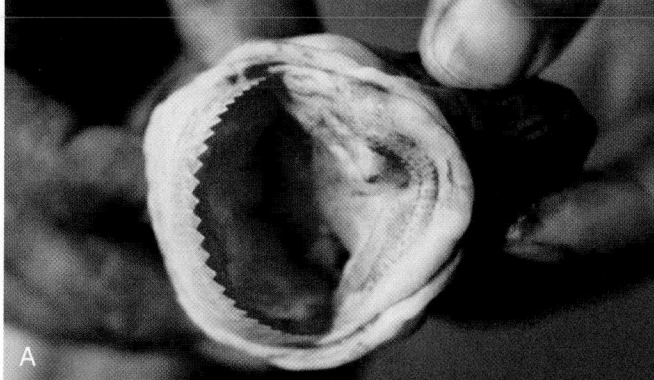

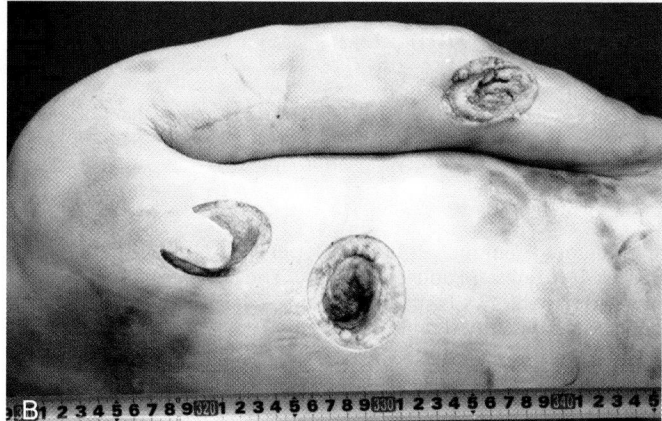

FIGURE 73-72 A, Jaws of the cookie-cutter shark. **B,** Postmortem wounds created by cookie-cutter shark bites. *(Photos courtesy Y. Makino.)*

death occurred most frequently as a result of exsanguinating hemorrhage from a limb vascular injury. Thus, it is occasionally necessary to compress wounds or manually constrict arterial bleeding while the victim is in the water. As soon as the victim is out of the water, all means available must be used to ligate large, disrupted arteries or to apply compression dressings. In one incident, dental floss was used by a fast-thinking companion of the victim to ligate a severed vessel while in the field, likely saving the victim's life. If necessary, judicious use of pressure points or tourniquets should be entertained, taking care to avoid excessive ischemia time in treated tissue. If intravascular volume must be replaced in large quantities, at least two large-bore IV lines should be inserted into the uninvolved extremities to deliver crystalloid (lactated Ringer's solution, normal saline, or hyper-

tonic saline), colloid, or blood products.[141,191] If prolonged transport is necessary, central IV access may be helpful.[154]

The victim should be kept well oxygenated and warm while being transported to a facility equipped to handle major trauma. Blood losses should be replaced with whole blood or packed red blood cells and fresh-frozen plasma.[190] The precise ratio of crystalloid to blood products and proper mean arterial blood pressure end point of primary resuscitation in the presence of a major vascular injury are the subjects of ongoing investigations.[179] The victim should be thoroughly examined for evidence of cervical, intrathoracic, and intraabdominal injuries. Because *Clostridium* can be cultured from ocean water, tetanus toxoid 0.5 mL IM

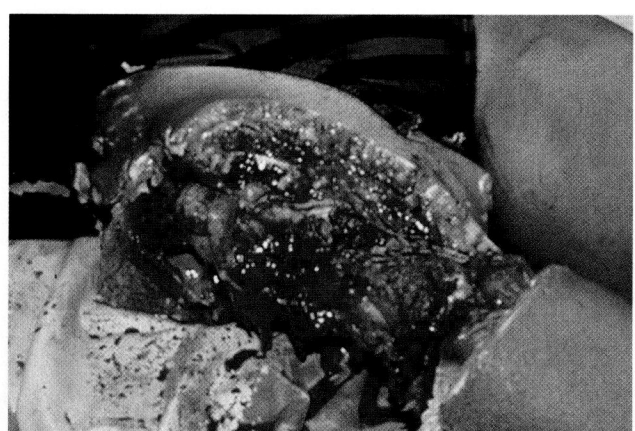

FIGURE 73-71 Shark bite of the proximal thigh. This unfortunate victim exsanguinated from a disrupted femoral artery. *(Courtesy Kenneth W. Kizer, MD.)*

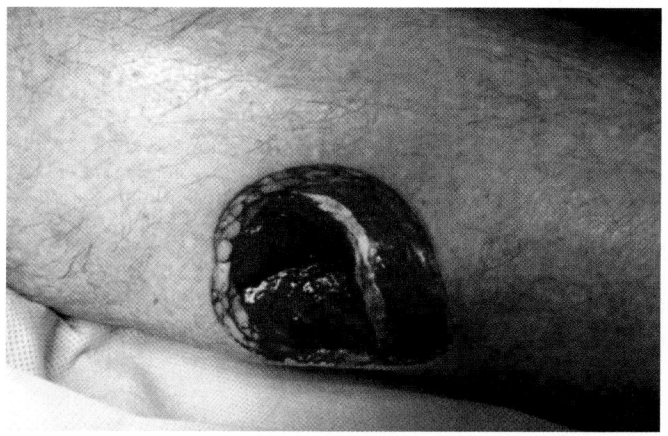

FIGURE 73-73 Cookie-cutter shark bite on a live human. *(Photo courtesy Peter Galpin.)*

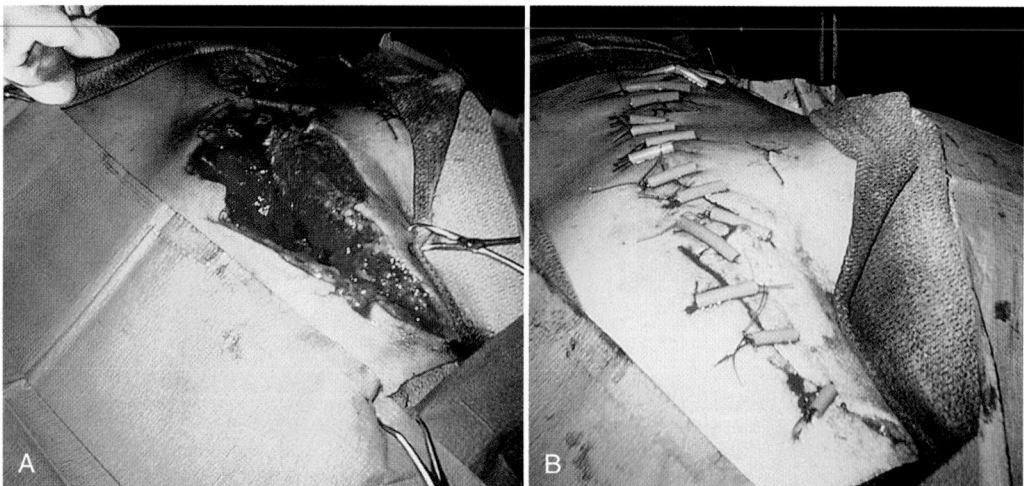

FIGURE 73-74 Operative repair of shark bite wound shown in Figure 73-53. **A,** Debridement and exploration of the wound in the operating room. **B,** Proper closure technique with tension-releasing sutures. (*Courtesy T. Hattori, MD.*)

and tetanus immune globulin (HyperTET, Grifiols, Barcelona) 250 to 500 units IM must be given. The administration of prophylactic antibiotics is more controversial. The victim of a shark bite should be treated with an IV third-generation cephalosporin, trimethoprim-sulfamethoxazole, an aminoglycoside, ciprofloxacin, or some reasonable combination of these agents. Imipenem-cilastatin or meropenem should be reserved for established wound infections or early indications of septicemia, particularly in the setting of immunosuppression. The rationale for prophylactic antibiotics is that shark wounds are prone to heavy contamination with seawater, sand, plant debris, shark teeth, and shark mouth flora. After a clinical infection is recognized, wounds should be cultured for aerobes and anaerobes by insertion of sterile swabs deeply into available lesions.

Proper operative intervention is mandatory.[35,52] It is inappropriate to attempt emergency department exploration of what often prove to be extensive and complicated wounds. In the operating room, devitalized tissue should be widely debrided and the wound irrigated copiously to remove all foreign material (Figure 73-74). An x-ray may reveal one or more shark teeth in the wound (see Figure 73-68). Shark teeth and fragments should be identified and removed to avoid infection initiated by a contaminated foreign body. Vascular repair should be completed when necessary.[212] Unless it is absolutely necessary to achieve tight closure, the wound should be carefully undermined and closed loosely around multiple drains (preferably closed systems) or packed open to await delayed primary closure. Although there is debate about whether to use internal or external fixation of grossly open and contaminated fractures, it seems logical to recommend surgical stabilization to facilitate vascular and soft tissue repair. In the pediatric population, damage to the physis and future limb length discrepancy should be anticipated.[79]

The abrasion associated with a shark bumping should be managed like a second-degree burn, with daily debridement and application of antiseptic ointment.

Postoperative management may be prolonged and complicated by acute renal failure attributed to hypovolemia and shock, massive blood transfusion, myoglobinuria, and administration of nephrotoxic antibiotics. Rehabilitation may include creation of prosthetic devices.

A reasonable "shark pack" should be available in emergency facilities and rescue vehicles near shark-inhabited waters. This must be portable and should include items necessary to control hemorrhage and initiate IV therapy.

Shark phobia is a real entity that causes the victim to be unwilling to enter the ocean. In one case, it has been treated successfully by a self-administered systematic desensitization program that followed a hierarchical progression of entry into the ocean combined with deep muscle relaxation technique.[106]

PREVENTION

Every precaution should be taken to avoid shark attack, beginning with an intimate knowledge of the local waters. The following is precautionary advice and a list of alternatives for action in the event of a confrontation:

Avoid shark-inhabited water, particularly at dawn, dusk, and at night. Do not swim through schools of bait fish in the presence of sharks. Do not enter waters posted with shark warnings. Surfers are generally at greater risk than divers. Do not disguise yourself as a pinniped (seal). Do not swim with animals (such as dogs or horses) in shark waters. Shark behavior can be unpredictable, so it is best not to remain in the water with sharks, particularly if you are fearful. Although some persons believe that sharks can be domesticated, there is no such thing as a friendly shark. Photograph hazardous sharks from within the confines of a protective cage (Figures 73-75 and 73-76), rather than from an unprotected position.

Swimmers should remain in groups. Isolation creates a primary target, eliminates companion surveillance, and removes the opportunity for postattack assistance. When diving, maintain constant vigilance. Do not wander far from shore, particularly if you are a solitary swimmer.

Turbid water, drop-offs, deep channels, inlets, mouths of rivers, and sanitation waste outlets are areas frequented by sharks and should be avoided. Water clarity is cited as turbid in 64% of all attack incidents, so it appears that sharks attack at least one-third of the time in clear water. Humans are most often attacked

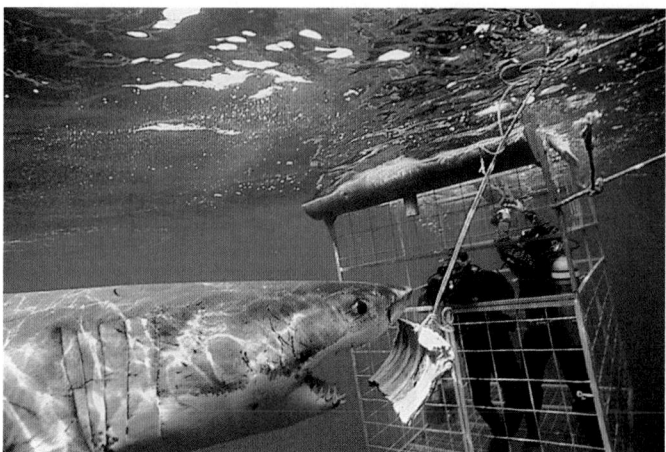

FIGURE 73-75 Caged divers view an inquisitive great white shark. (*Courtesy Carl Roessler.*)

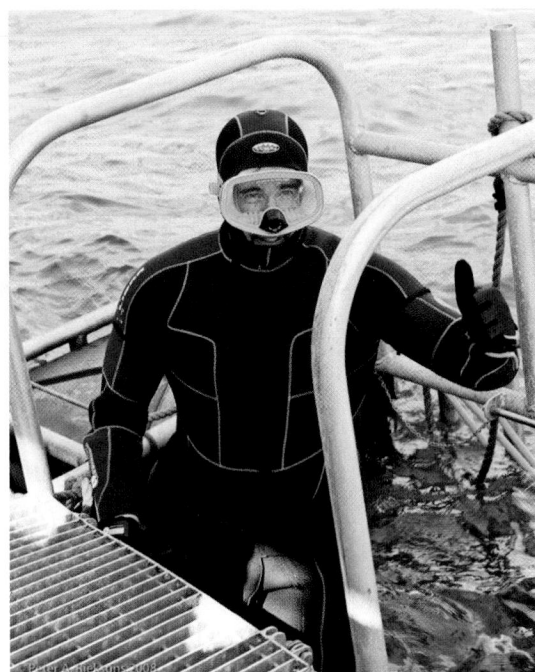

FIGURE 73-76 The author descends in a cage to photograph great white sharks. (*Copyright Peter Riekstens.*)

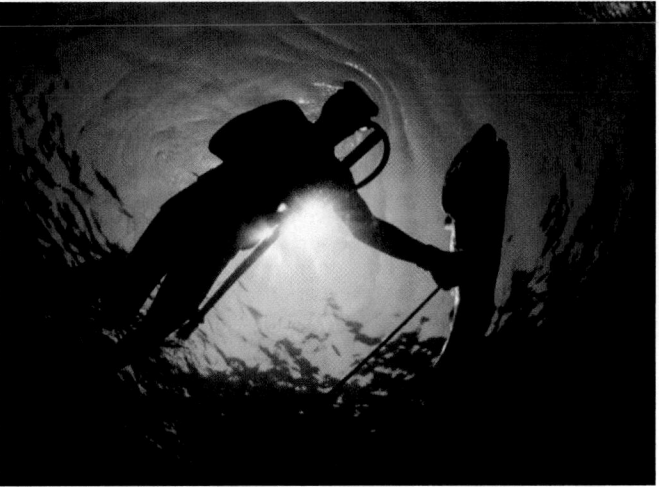

FIGURE 73-77 Blue water hunter with white sea bass off Catalina Island, California. (*Copyright 2000 Norbert Wu: norbertwu.com.*)

in shallow water or beyond the breakers. Do not swim in waters frequented by recreational or commercial fishers. Do not swim in water that has been recently churned up by a storm. Be alert when crossing the troughs between sandbars.

Blood and other body fluids (including peritoneal fluid) attract sharks. No person should be in shark waters with an open wound. Women have historically been advised to avoid diving during menstruation, although there are no data to support attraction of sharks to the discharge of menstruation. Given the shark's well-documented acute sense of smell, it seems possible that menstrual blood is attractive.

Brightly reflective swimwear or diving equipment and shiny snorkeling gear attract certain sharks. Bright (international) orange and other contrasting colors appear to be particularly attractive to sharks. Flat black is probably the least attractive color, except in the instance of the great white shark, which may be preferentially attracted to this color. There is scant evidence that sharks are more attracted to light-skinned bathers, but differential tanning and base skin color producing lighter palms of the hands and soles of the feet may contribute to bites to these appendages, especially when movement is involved.

Captured fish must be tethered at a distance from any divers. There is no greater chemical attractant for a shark than fish blood, and the thrashing of a speared fish is greatly attractive. Do not dive or swim in the presence of spear fishermen (Figure 73-77). Divers who harvest abalone should be aware that the banging and prying noise of an "abalone iron" might attract sharks.

The presence of porpoises in the water does not preclude the presence of sharks (it is not uncommon for both to be pursuing the same prey items). Be alert for the presence of a shark whenever schools of fish behave in an erratic manner or when pods of porpoises cluster more tightly or head toward shore.

Do not tease or corner a shark. This is particularly true with captive animals. Do not pull on a shark's tail. Do not chase after a shark. If a shark begins to act in an erratic manner, do not photograph it at close range using a strobe flash apparatus. There is now evidence that shark feeding, as perpetrated by shark diving operators, may be followed by shark attack upon humans.

If a shark appears in shallow water, swimmers should leave the water with slow, purposeful movements, facing the shark if possible and avoiding erratic behavior that could be interpreted as distress. If a shark approaches in deep water, the diver should remain submerged, rather than wildly swim to the surface to

escape. The diver should move to defensive terrain with posterior protection to fend off, as best as possible, a frontal attack. It is inadvisable to trap a shark in a position from which it must attack to obtain freedom. Fighting sharks is difficult; they are best repulsed with blunt blows to the snout or probing of the eyes or gills. If possible, the bare hand should not be used, to avoid severe abrasions or lacerations. A stream of air bubbles from a scuba regulator directed into the face of a shark may serve as an initial deterrent, but this does not work most of the time. Although spears, knives, shotgun shell- or 30.06-loaded power-heads (bang sticks) (Figure 73-78), strychnine-filled spears, and carbon dioxide darts can kill small sharks, they can worsen the situation if they are misapplied or their application promotes frenzy in a school of sharks.

Do not splash on the surface or create a commotion in a manner that might cause a shark to interpret your behavior as that of a struggling fish. Surface activity, including the sound of marine engines and perhaps the sounds created by helicopter rotor wash, attracts sharks. During a helicopter rescue, exit the water as soon as possible.

Although there is no question that shark avoidance is the most reliable maneuver, shark defense techniques and repellents are constantly evolving. In response to shark attacks on downed airmen and sailors during World War II, copper acetate (20%) blended with a water-soluble wax and nigrosine-type black dye (80%) was packaged as a slowly dissolving (3 to 4 hours) 6-oz waxy cake for deployment as "shark chaser" by the Office of

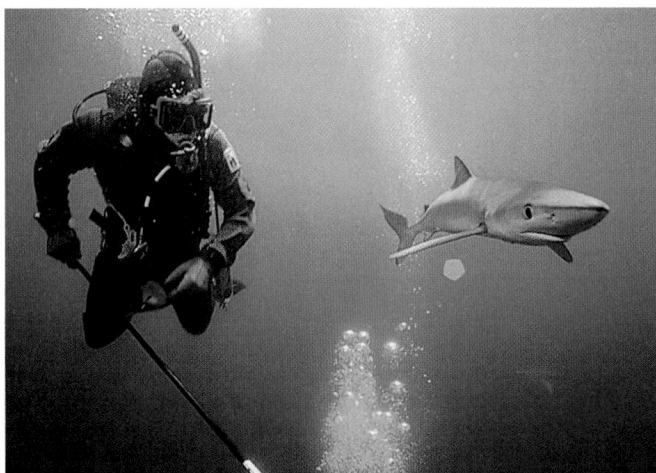

FIGURE 73-78 Diver carrying a bang stick in the presence of a blue shark. (*Courtesy Howard Hall.*)

Naval Research of the U.S. Navy.[17] It was theorized that the dye released as a dark (often black or purple) cloud similar to defensive mollusk secretions, and that the copper acetate both inhibited feeding and resembled the decaying carcasses of sharks, so that sharks would thus be repelled. Unfortunately, although a morale booster, this was not a reliable deterrent. Its use was discontinued by the Navy in 1976. Limited progress has been made since that time. Recreational beaches in Australia and South Africa are protected with extensive gill net systems (meshing) to kill animals seeking to enter the surf zone. These work by reducing population sizes over time, thereby minimizing shark-human interactions. This type of prevention measure is increasingly under attack by biologists and conservationists because of its highly negative impact on populations of threatened sharks, sea turtles, sea birds, and sea mammals. Exclusion nets (large-mesh nets intended to prevent interaction between humans and sharks) have been employed in a limited number of locales. Logistic and economic considerations preclude widespread utility. Electric shark barriers (cable device) using 0.8-msec pulses 15 times per second to create a field of 4 volts per meter seem to generate a fright response in sharks longer than 1.2 m (4 feet) and are being investigated.[44,171] Their benefits include repulsion rather than shark capture or destruction. However, some sharks respond weakly to these stimuli. Abalone divers in South Australia work from one-person, self-propelled shark cages.

Experimental devices for individuals include chain-mesh diving suits (Figures 73-79 and 73-80), inflatable dull-colored plastic protective bags (yellow is easy for aircraft to spot, but most attractive to sharks), acoustic and handheld electrical field transmitters, surfactants and other chemical repellents (e.g., firefly and the Red Sea and western Indian Ocean Moses sole, *Pardachirus marmoratus* [Figure 73-81] glandular extract [pardaxin]).[58] Pardaxin is an excitatory polypeptide neurotoxin that forms voltage-gated pores and triggers neurotransmitter release.[113] The ichthyotoxic secretion from the fish, which appears as a milky substance from a series of glands located along the dorsal and anal fins, also contains shark-repellent lipophilic constituents that appear to be steroid monoglycosides.[152,183] Another sole, *Pardachirus pavoninus,* which lives in the tropical regions of the western Pacific and eastern Indian Oceans, secretes pavoninins 1 through 6. These shark-repelling substances are ichthyotoxic steroids, N-acetyl-glucosaminides.[209] It appears that in sharks, the gills or pharyngeal cavity is the target organ(s) for the repellent action. For the exudate from the Moses sole, concentrations of 10 to 25 g/m³ are needed to elicit an immediate indication of repellency. However, it has been estimated that about 24 kg (53 lb) of any effective drug would have to be contained within an enveloping "drug cloud" in the volume of water through which a slowly approaching shark might swim in its final 10 seconds of approach as it attacked a human in the ocean.[17]

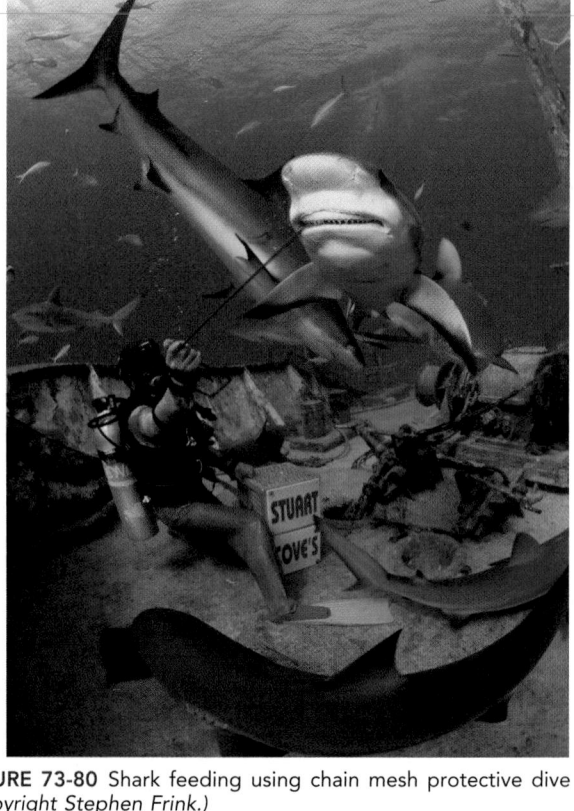

FIGURE 73-80 Shark feeding using chain mesh protective dive suit. *(Copyright Stephen Frink.)*

Studies have indicated that shark-repellent efficacy of alkyl sulfate surfactants is due to their hydrophobic nature.[169] In tests conducted on juvenile swell sharks *(Cephaloscyllium ventriosum),* the aversive response of sharks to these surfactants increased with carbon chain length from octyl (8) to dodecyl (12), decreased with the addition of ethylene oxide groups, and was not affected by counterions (e.g., magnesium for sodium). Still, for the most effective synthetic detergent repellent (e.g., sodium dodecyl sulfate [SDS]), the concentration needed in the water is 800 g/m³. These findings show that a chemical carried in a life jacket cannot be reliably useful against sharks, because to meet the Navy's potency requirement for a nondirectional surrounding-cloud–type repellent, it would have to be instantaneously effective at a concentration of no less than 100 parts per

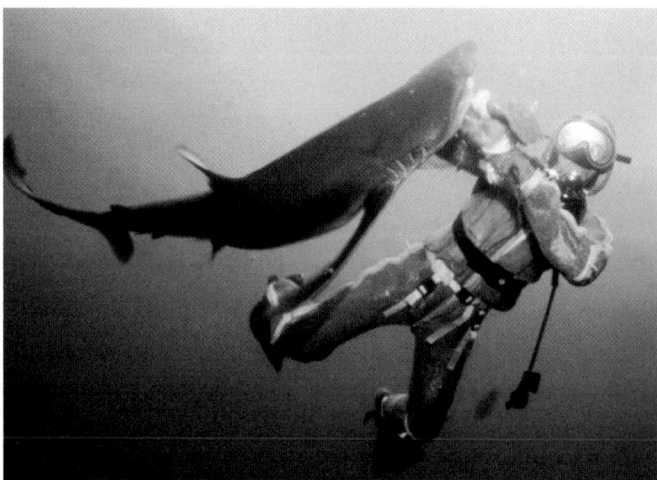

FIGURE 73-79 Diver wearing chain mesh metal suit for shark protection. *(Courtesy Howard Hall.)*

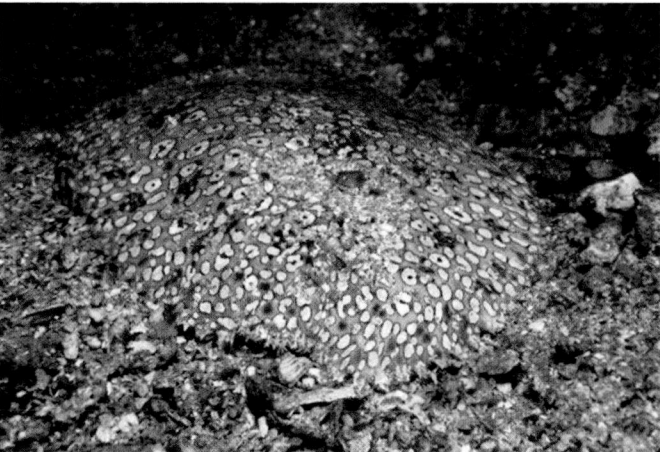

FIGURE 73-81 Moses sole, *Pardachirus marmoratus,* Thailand. *(Copyright 2000 Norbert Wu: norbertwu.com.)*

billion (0.1 μg/mL). Most tests have been performed on bait-attracted blue sharks *(Prionace glauca)*. In chemical repellent tests on white sharks, using an air-powered syringe gun to deliver 250 mL of a 10% seawater solution of SDS, it was demonstrated that large white sharks could be effectively repelled if a substantial dose reached the mouth cavity and remained there long enough to stimulate the relevant receptors. However, this has not proved practical in a field situation.[144] Future direction of chemical shark repellent research include delineation of the morphologic target sites of chemical and natural shark repellents, investigation of natural bioactive toxins as repellents, and identification and purification of semiochemicals (e.g., exudates or body secretions of predators that act as alarm pheromones) to be used as repellents.[169]

The Shark Shield series of shark-deterrent devices are distributed by Shark Shield Pty Ltd (sharkshield.com) in South Australia, based on the original technology that led to development of the SharkPOD (which is now discontinued). The Shark Shield produces an electrical field that is detected by sharks through the ampullae of Lorenzini and that is believed to cause discomfort and muscle spasms in the animals. The Shark Shield unit incorporates electrodes that project the field from the unit to create an invisible protective shield that surrounds the user. The electrodes must be immersed in the water in order to give protection to the wearer. One electrode is encased in a short antenna, which trails out from the ankle, secured with a neoprene cuff. The second electrode is a pad designed to be worn on the scuba cylinder. This pad electrode attaches to the cylinder by means of a special quick-release fastening device. Under no circumstances should the two electrodes be placed any closer to one another than 900 mm (35.43 inches), as this will reduce the deterrent effect. A full-length wetsuit or drysuit must be worn when using the Shark Shield Scuba unit to reduce the skin stimulation effect caused by the configuration of the two electrodes. The unit is strapped to the thigh or can be placed in the buoyancy compensator pocket. In tests, the unit has deterred sharks at distances of up to 8 m (26 feet), but with an average distance of 4 to 5 m (13 to 16 feet) from the unit. More recent studies on the Shark Shield as a deterrent to white sharks showed conflicting data. In a first trial of attaching the deterrent to static bait, the proportion of baits taken was not affected by the electrical field; however, it took an increased amount of time for the sharks to take the bait with the electrical field in place.[92] In a second experiment, using a towed seal decoy, the electrical field significantly decreased the number of shark strikes and interactions with the decoy.[92] These studies may indicate that shark response to the electrical field is contextually specific.

As for any shark-deterrent strategy, it cannot be assumed to provide perfect protection, because the animals are unpredictable, and it is impossible to state with assurance that they will always be deterred. A fatal attack by a great white shark upon a SharkPOD-equipped diver in 2002 has been attributed to the device not being used in accordance with the manufacturer's specifications, but the device produced sufficient current to deter human rescue attempts. Regardless of assignment of fault, it emphasizes that no device should be assumed 100% effective in all circumstances. The reader is advised to check on the availability and status of warranties and representations prior to committing to any particular purchase.

BARRACUDA

To many divers, the barracuda appears more sinister than the shark and is more highly feared. Barracuda are distributed from Brazil north to Florida, and in the Indo-Pacific from the Red Sea to the Hawaiian Islands. Of the 22 species of barracuda, only the great barracuda *(Sphyraena barracuda)* has been implicated in human attacks. Smaller species of barracuda may be found in large schools.

LIFE AND HABITS

The great barracuda is encountered in all tropical seas and is reputed to grow to 2.5 m (8.2 feet) and 50 kg (110 lb) but is

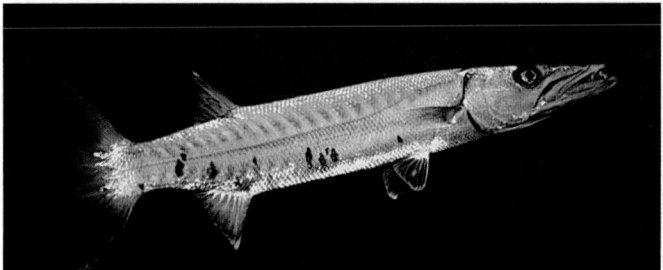

FIGURE 73-82 Great barracuda *(Sphyraena barracuda)*. *(Courtesy Paul S. Auerbach, MD.)*

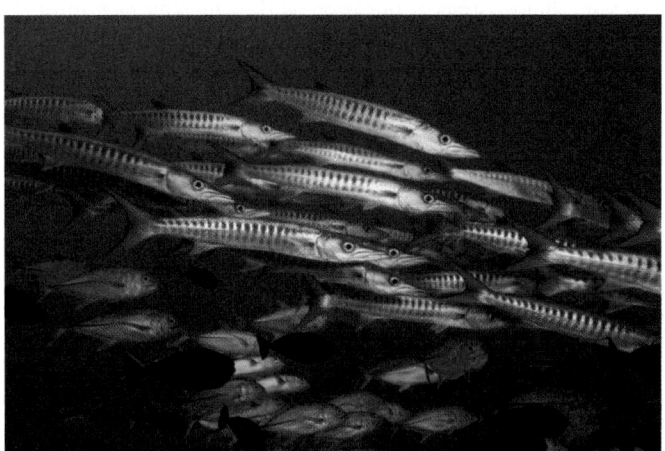

FIGURE 73-83 Schooling barracuda. *(Copyright Stephen Frink.)*

rarely sighted at a length greater than 1.5 m (5 feet) (Figures 73-82 and 73-83). The world record weight of a captured barracuda is approximately 102 lb, from 2013 International Game Fish Association (IGFA) data. A solitary swimmer, the fish is extremely swift and has the disconcerting habit of hovering near divers, opening and closing its toothy mouth as part of the respiratory process. The barracuda possesses an elongated narrow mouth filled with nearly parallel rows of large knife-like cutting teeth, similar in appearance to those of canines (Figure 73-84).

Barracuda capture fish with a swift and voracious feeding strike. They can attack fish larger than the gape of their powerful jaws and often sever prey into pieces. In an evaluation of the functional morphology of bite mechanics in the great barracuda, it was observed that prey are impacted at the corner of the mouth

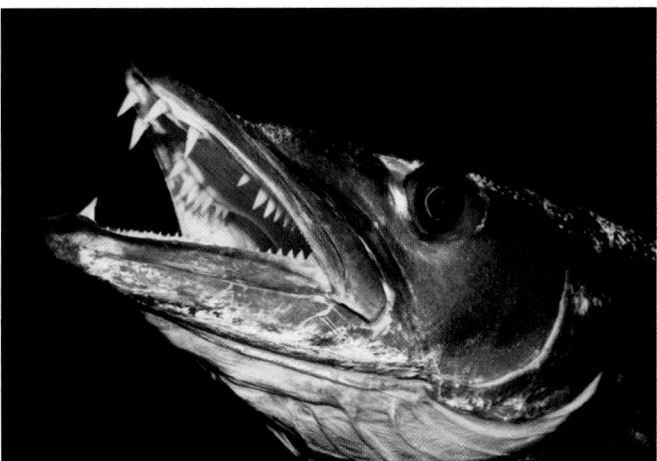

FIGURE 73-84 Jaws of the great barracuda, with canine-type teeth. *(Copyright Stephen Frink.)*

during capture in an orthogonal (right-angle) position; rapid repeated bites and short lateral head-shakes cut the prey into pieces. A palatine bone embedded with dagger-like teeth opposes the mandible at the rear of the jaws and provides for a scissor-like bite capable of shearing flesh and bone.[78]

Although great barracuda seldom attack divers, when they do it is rapidly and fiercely, often out of confusion in murky waters. More commonly the fish charges through shallow water to bite the dangling legs of a boater, particularly if a shiny anklet or toe ring (which resembles a fishing lure) is worn. Persons have been bitten on the scalp while wearing a barrette or on the face when trying to feed a barracuda by holding dead fish bait in their mouths. Wounds to the hand are commonly incurred during removal of hooks. Barracudas normally feed with sudden and rapid bursts of speed. They often slice a natural prey item in two with almost surgical precision as they literally race through the prey.

The great barracuda is a well-known leaper, frequently leaving the water when hooked or (apparently) when chasing prey. With an increase in boating traffic in barracuda-inhabited Florida waters, incidents of accidental contact between barracudas and "speeding" vessels have become more commonplace. Concurrently, incidents involving leaping sturgeons and boat-based humans have become a regular source of injury in Florida waters.[210] The resulting collision between heavy, large-toothed fishes and humans at great speed can be catastrophic.

Considering the great frequency with which barracuda are encountered and the low number of reported attacks, they do not pose nearly the hazard of sharks.

CLINICAL ASPECTS

Barracuda bites produce straight or V-shaped lacerations, in contradistinction to the crescent-shaped bite of the shark. Except for this difference and the magnitude of injury, the surgical problems generated by the barracuda do not differ from those of the shark. The clinician encounters tissue loss, moderate hemorrhage, and wound infections.

TREATMENT

Barracuda bites are treated identically to shark bites. If a barracuda is captured, it should not be eaten in ciguatera toxin–endemic regions (see Chapter 77).

PREVENTION

Barracuda are attracted to underwater commotion, irregular motion, surface splashing, and shiny objects. These should all be avoided. It is unwise to dangle a body part adorned with reflective jewelry in front of the jaws of a barracuda. In general, divers should avoid wearing rings, exposed watches (the glass or plastic face plate is attractive when reflecting light), necklaces, earrings, and bracelets, because these are contributors to attacks by both barracudas and sharks. Like sharks, barracudas are highly attracted to speared fishes and owing to their predilection to remain close to divers, often make lightning-quick dashes to poach such captures. Speared fishes should always remain on the spear tip and the spear held at length away from the spear fisher until it is deposited in the support boat.

MORAY EELS

LIFE AND HABITS

Moray eels (Figures 73-85 to 73-90) are found in tropical, subtropical, and some temperate waters. Members of the order Anguilliformes, family Muraenidae, some individuals of the larger species may attain lengths of 3.0 m (9.84 feet), diameters of more than 35 cm (13.78 inches), and weights in excess of 34 kg (75 lb). Morays are muscular and powerful bottom dwellers, residing in holes or crevices or under rock and coral (Figure 73-91). They have a snake-like appearance and usually lack scales or pectoral fins. Distinguishing features of the morays

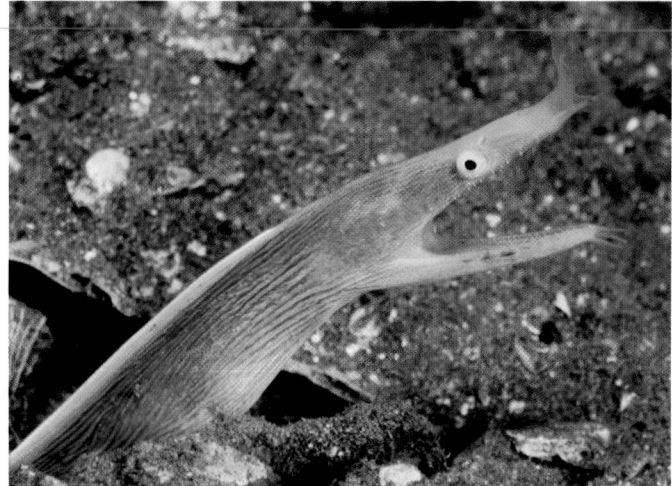

FIGURE 73-85 Moray eel. *(Copyright Stephen Frink.)*

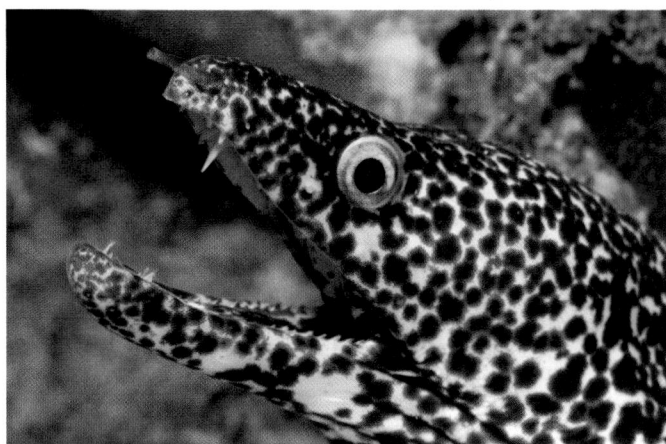

FIGURE 73-86 Spotted moray eel. *(Copyright Stephen Frink.)*

include the small, round gill openings and robust dentition. The skin of moray eels is rubbery to leathery and mucus coated (to protect from infection). They typically have poor eyesight and rely on their sense of smell to locate prey. Moray eels exhibit three different types of reproductive ability: gonorchist (dedicated male or female, without the ability to change gender), simultaneous hermaphrodite (both sex organs, able to mate with either gender), or protogynous hermaphrodite (can be born as a female or male; female can change to male if need be).

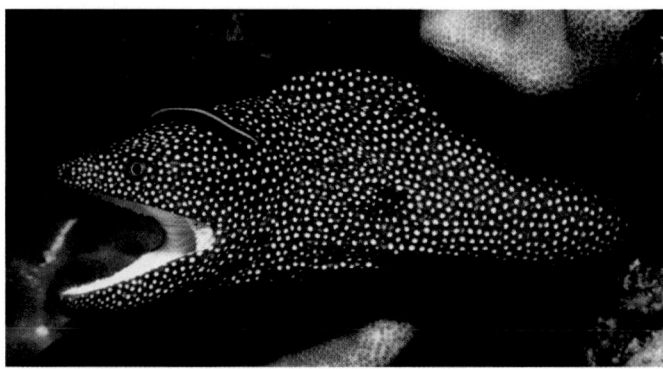

FIGURE 73-87 Blue-striped cleaner wrasse on moray eel in the Coral Sea. *(Copyright Carl Roessler.)*

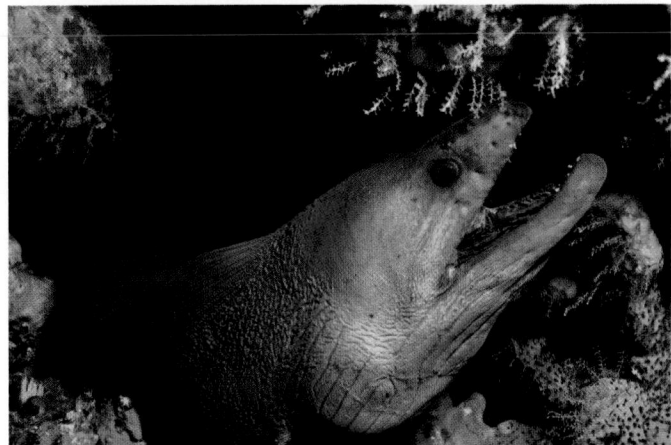

FIGURE 73-88 Large green moray eel. (Copyright Stephen Frink.)

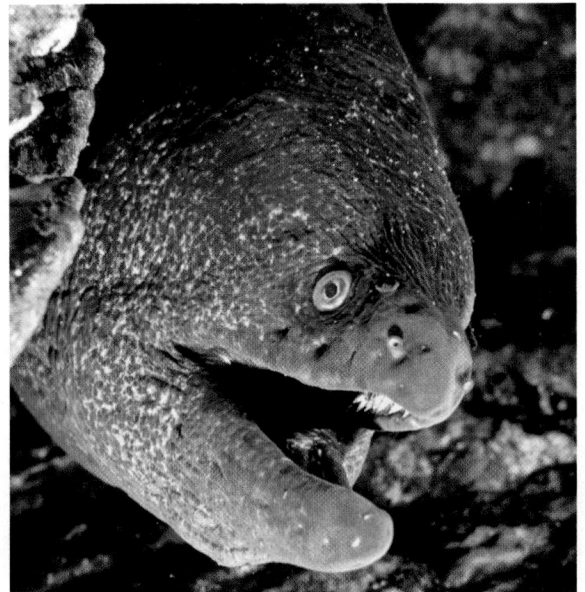

FIGURE 73-89 Large moray eel. (Courtesy by Marty Snyderman.)

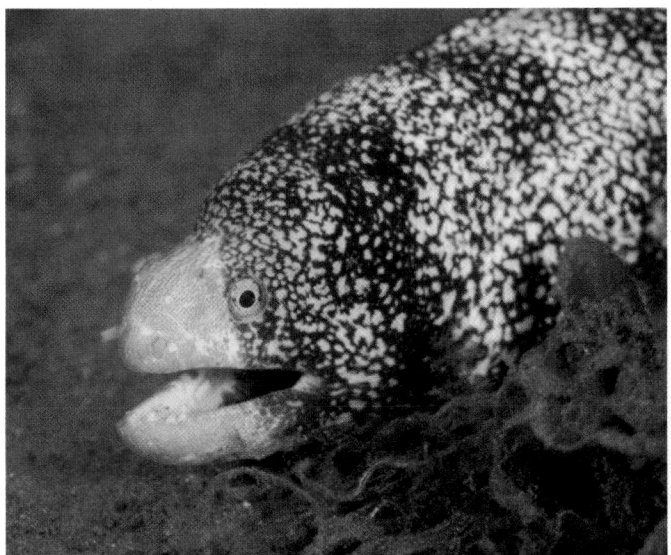

FIGURE 73-90 Moray eel. (Copyright Lynn Funkhouser.)

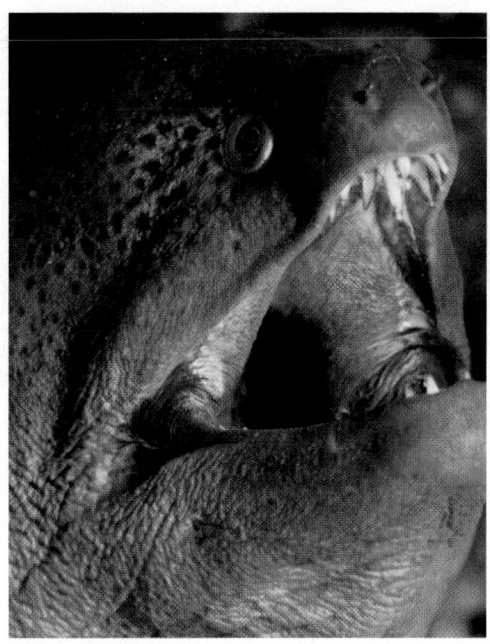

FIGURE 73-91 Moray eel. (Copyright Stephen Frink.)

Fortunately, eels usually evade confrontation unless cornered or provoked. Bites typically occur when a diver intentionally probes into a coral bed or cave, or a fisher reaches into a net and offers a hand to an aggravated eel. Aquarium-housed morays may strike when handled improperly. Most moray eels are easily intimidated; however, an aggressive eel may strike out in competition for prey. Elderly, vision-impaired eels or seemingly docile animals may attack without specific provocation, especially at night. In U.S. coastal waters, the species most often observed are the California, green, and spotted morays.

CLINICAL ASPECTS

Morays are forceful and vicious biters that can inflict severe puncture wounds with their narrow and viselike jaws, which are equipped with long, sharp, retrorse, and fanglike teeth. Normal eel prey includes fish, crustaceans, octopi, and other small marine animals. Molar-type teeth are present in some species; these species typically consume crustaceans. A moray eel has the tenacity of a bulldog and will hold on to a victim rather than strike and release. Multiple small puncture wounds are common after the bite of smaller eels, with the hand most commonly involved. Large avulsion injuries may occur (Figure 73-92).[160] If the eel is ripped forcefully from the victim, the resulting lacerations may be even more extensive.

TREATMENT

Moray bites are treated in a manner analogous to that of shark bites. If the eel remains attached to the victim, the jaws may need to be broken or the animal decapitated to effect release. The primary wound should be irrigated copiously and explored to locate any retained teeth. The risk of infection is high, particularly in bites to the hand, because the symbiotic flora associated with the moray's oral cavity is apparently unusually rich. Uncomplicated small puncture wounds generated by individual teeth should be left unsutured to allow drainage and the victim given appropriate prophylactic antibiotics. If the wound is extensive and more linear in configuration (resembling a dog bite), the wound edges may be debrided and loosely approximated with nonabsorbable sutures or staples, in which case antibiotics should be administered. If the wound is severe, vital structures should be assessed in routine operative fashion. In all cases, it is prudent to inspect the wound at 24 and 48 hours to detect the onset of infection. If not appropriately treated initially, infections may persist for months, even years.

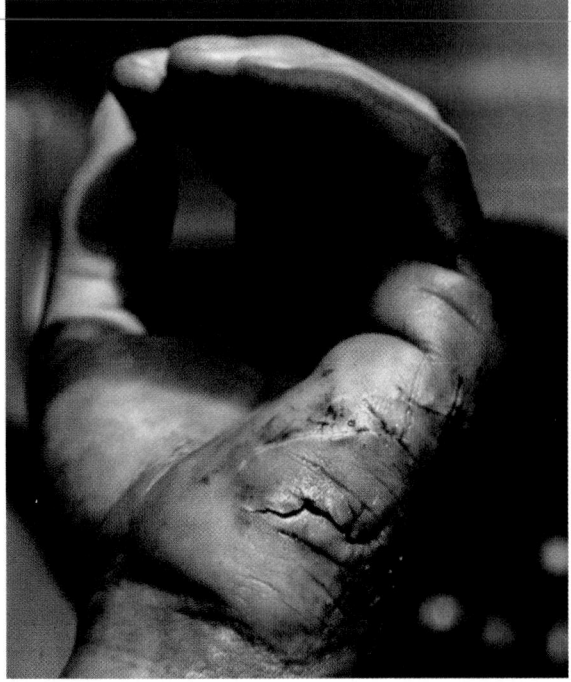

FIGURE 73-92 Moray eel bite. *(Photo by Marty Snyderman.)*

PREVENTION

It is unwise for a snorkeler or diver to place a hand underneath unexplored coral or rock unless it has been probed or otherwise disturbed specifically in search of an eel. Divers seeking lobsters should be aware that the objects of their hunt commonly share the same microhabitat with morays. All fishing nets should be handled carefully. A dive guide who feeds moray eels (Figure 73-93) by holding a loaf of bread or bait fish in his mouth is foolishly offering his nose and mouth as a target for an unpredictable eel.

GIANT GROUPERS

Some of the larger species of sea basses or groupers (family Serranidae) may grow to exceed 3.6 m (11.8 feet) and 227 kg (500 lb) (Figures 73-94 to 73-96). Distributed in both tropical and temperate seas, they are curious, occasionally pugnacious, and voracious feeders. Although not aggressive like a shark, a giant grouper should be respected for its fearlessness, bulk, and

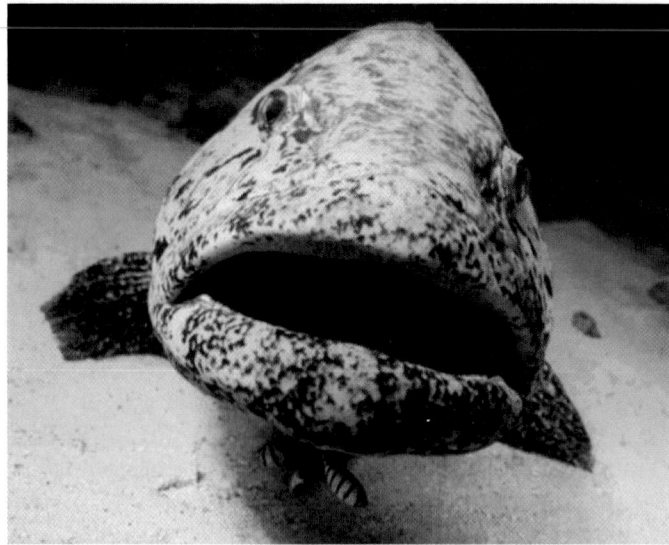

FIGURE 73-94 Giant grouper or potato cod, Great Barrier Reef, Australia. *(Copyright 2000 Norbert Wu: norbertwu.com.)*

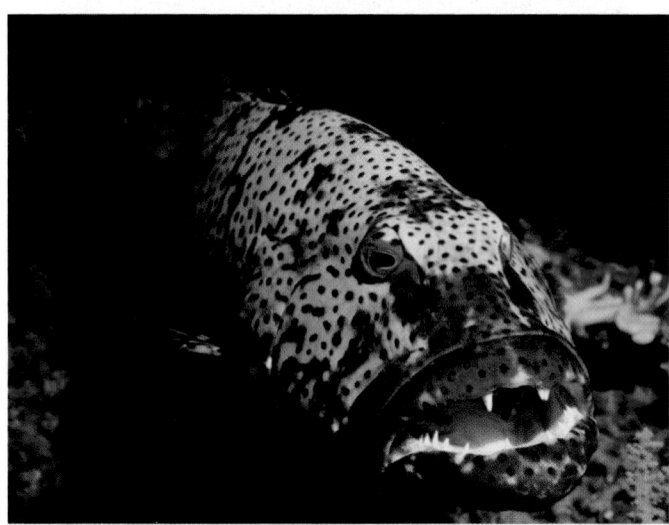

FIGURE 73-95 Grouper in the Red Sea. *(Copyright Carl Roessler.)*

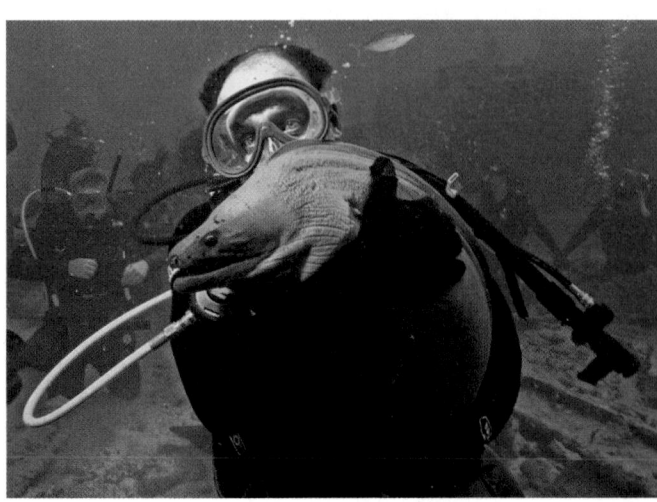

FIGURE 73-93 Diver handling large moray eel. *(Courtesy Marty Snyderman.)*

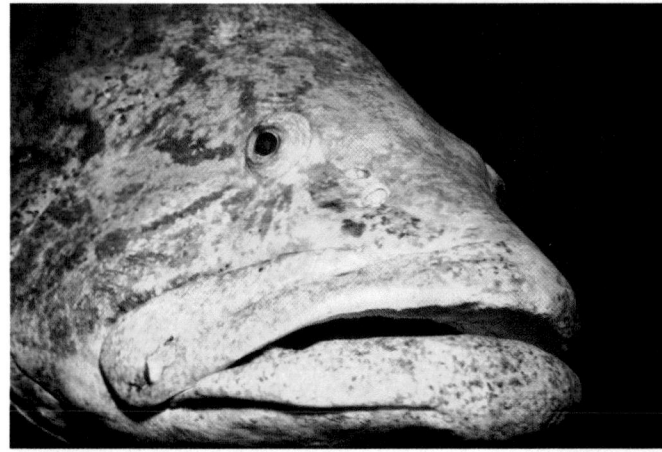

FIGURE 73-96 Face of large potato cod in the Coral Sea. *(Copyright Carl Roessler.)*

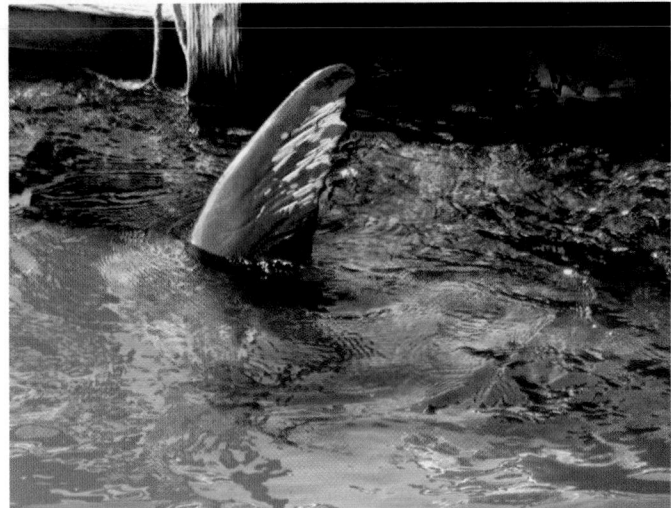

FIGURE 73-97 Sea lion playfully lifts a fin in the water. *(Courtesy Paul S. Auerbach, MD.)*

cavernous mouth. Groupers can be found frequenting ship-wrecks; swimming in caves, caverns, and holes; and lurking behind large rocks and coral outcroppings. They are territorial and may become aggressive while protecting their domain. Bite wounds may be ragged with extensive maceration and are treated the same as shark bites. Large groupers should not be eaten in ciguatera toxin–endemic regions. It is always wise to visually survey an underwater cave before entering or exiting. The diver should not block the exit if a grouper is attempting to escape and should not carry speared fish. Many scare tactics used against sharks are of no avail with groupers. In a freak accident in 2006, a Florida free-diver was reported to have drowned after he shot a large grouper with a spear gun. The wounded grouper wedged itself into a hole and the man became entangled around his wrist in the line attached to the spear.

SEA LIONS AND SEALS

Sea lions (family Otariidae) and seals (family Phocidae) are mild-mannered mammals (Fig. 73-97) except during the mating season, when the males may become aggressive, and during the breeding season, when both genders attack in defense of their newborn pups (Figure 73-98). Divers have been seriously bitten and there-fore should avoid ill-tempered and abnormally aggressive animals. There is nothing unique about the clinical aspects of these inju-ries, except for the posttraumatic infections. The bites are treated the same as shark bites.

"Seal finger" (spekk finger, blubber finger) (see Chapter 76) follows a bite wound from a seal or from contact of even a minor skin wound with a seal's mouth or pelt. It has traditionally been an occupational hazard of seal hunters, but has now been noted in persons trying to save seals and aquarium workers. One case was attributed to a polar bear bite (which may or may not have eaten a seal). The affliction is characterized by an incubation period of 1 to 15 (typically 4) days, followed by painful swelling of the digit, with or without destructive articular involvement. Severe pain may precede appearance of the initial furuncle, stiffness, or swelling. As the lesion worsens, the skin becomes taut and shiny, and the entire hand may swell and take on a brownish violet hue. It is quite possible to have involvement of adjacent fingers. Tenosynovitis and arthritis have been noted, which may progress to joint destruction and arthrosis. There may be painless, nonsuppurative lymphadenopathy. It is common for the affliction to run a protracted course.[84] Current thinking focuses on *Mycoplasma* species (such as *M. phocidae* or *M. phocacerebrale*) as the inciting pathogens, which is consistent with their cytopathogenic potential.[16] Therefore, microbiologic evaluation of a lesion should include culture for mycoplasmas in addition to standard aerobes and anaerobes. Infection with *E. rhusiopathiae* is in the differential diagnosis, but usually is

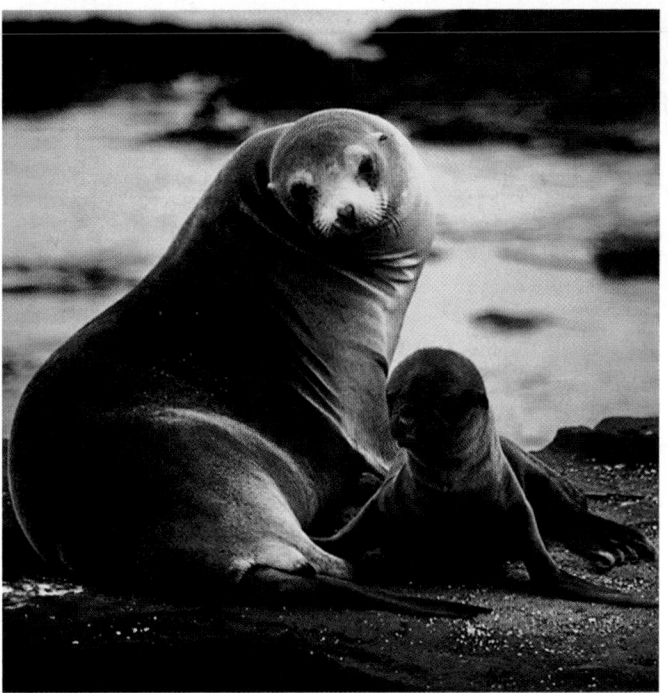

FIGURE 73-98 Sea lion and pup. Parents of both genders aggressively protect their young. *(Courtesy Paul S. Auerbach, MD.)*

characterized by a more erythematous and bordered rash spread among multiple fingers. There have been case reports of *Bis-gaardia hudsonensis,* a member of the family Pasteurellaceae, causing seal finger.[181]

The recommended therapy is tetracycline 1.5 g initially, fol-lowed by 500 mg four times a day for 4 to 6 weeks.[42] β-Lactam antibiotics, cephalosporins, and erythromycin are not efficacious. Fluoroquinolone or macrolide antibiotics may be useful if tetra-cycline is not available. Early (in the first week) incision to relieve elevated tissue pressure may be efficacious, but delayed joint debridement has not proved useful. Early antibiotic therapy is key to successful treatment. Preventive measures include wearing gloves and washing all wounds vigorously with soap and water, perhaps followed by an isopropyl alcohol rinse.

NEEDLEFISH

Marine needlefish (family Belonidae) are slender, tubular, elon-gate, silver, and lightning-quick surface swimmers found in tem-perate and tropical seas (Figure 73-99). They resemble, but are

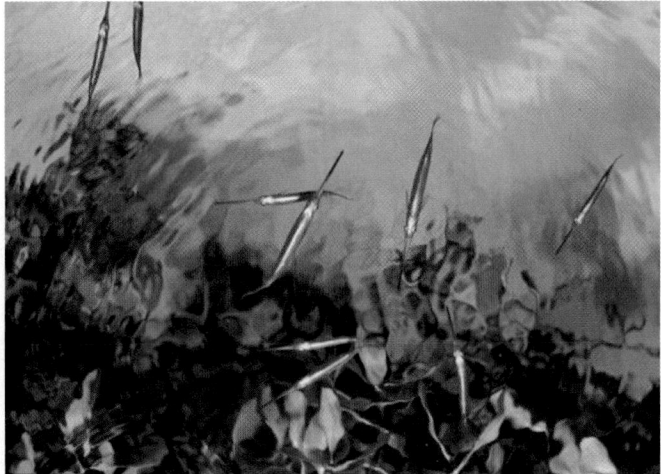

FIGURE 73-99 Needlefish in mangrove swamp, Solomon Islands. *(Copyright 2000 Norbert Wu: norbertwu.com.)*

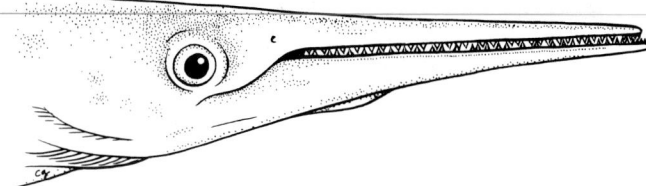

FIGURE 73-100 Needlefish beak, capable of causing a penetrating injury.

not related to, the freshwater gar and may attain streamlined lengths of up to 1.35 m (4 feet). Possessed of an elongated pointed snout, which forms one-quarter the length of the fish and contains numerous small pointed teeth (Figure 73-100), the fish moves rapidly, often leaping out of the water in fear or when attracted to lights or windsurfers. It has been hypothesized that a needlefish can exit the water at a speed of approximately 64 km/hr (40 mph), which approximates the speed of a flying fish. The needlefish, or garfish, is an occupational hazard for persons who fish from small canoes at night in tropical Indo-Pacific ocean waters.[21] On occasion, they have flown into people, spearing them in the chest, abdomen, extremities, head, and neck. In one reported case, a fish caused brain injury by creating an internal carotid-cavernous sinus fistula after orbitocranial perforation.[130] In another case, the calcified elongated jaws of a needlefish embedded in a woman's neck were retained for more than a month before removal.[25] In others, penetration of the knee by *Tylosurus crocodilus* (little sea crocodile) occurred in an ocean surface swimmer in New Caledonia and of the chest of a spear fisher in Hawaii.[110,155] Exsanguination from a neck wound has been anecdotally reported from Papua New Guinea. A penetrating leg injury from a needlefish, with major vascular injury (popliteal vein, anterior tibial and peroneal arteries), occurred in the leg of a windsurfer off the coast of the Outer Banks of North Carolina.[119] A chest wound can be accompanied by a pneumothorax. Death may occur from chest or abdominal penetration. The depth of penetration of the animal may be augmented by the speed at which the victim approaches the piscine projectile. Treatment is according to the nature of the injury. All wounds should be debrided and irrigated, followed by a search for foreign material. Radiographs appropriate to identify foreign bodies should be obtained. Two semiparallel lines of opacity representing the jaws of the fish are pathognomonic of a needlefish beak.[101,110,119] A small superficial wound may cause the physician to underestimate an internal injury. The major risk is wound infection, attributed to bacteria in the carnivorous fish teeth. Injury prevention is difficult, although it has been suggested that canoes be positioned in a circle to allow spearing of fish in a central pool of light. "Flying fishes" (Exocoetidae) pose less risk, because they have blunt heads.

LARGE LEAPING FISH

Many fish leap from the water, but injuries are extremely uncommon. A case of a wahoo (150 cm, 22.5 kg [5 feet, 50 lb]), family Scombridae, leaping from the water and biting a victim on the upper extremity has been reported.[88] The sharp teeth generated extensor tendon lacerations on the dorsal hand and forearm that required surgical repair. A careless fisherman can easily be cut by a wahoo or other large mackerels of the genus *Scomberomorus,* including the king mackerel *Scomberomorus cavalla,* when extracting a fishing lure. The latter also is a well-documented jumper. Although bluefish *(Pomatomus saltatrix)* are not leapers, they have sharp, conical mackerel-like teeth and most bites occur as the fish are handled out of the water. The fish is quick to bite while on deck (earning the nickname "choppers") and can grow to 1.2 m (4 feet) and more than 12 kg (26.4 lb). They occur in schools and often feed in a frenzied fashion, but in-water attacks on humans are largely theoretical.[111] During a World War II beach landing along the North African coast, bluefishes were reported to attack wading soldiers. As previously described, barracuda frequently exit the water in pursuit of fishing lures, jewelry, or shiny metallic objects that resemble lures, as well as when chasing bait fishes, and regularly are involved in aerial accidents with humans.

The sailfish, which can approach speeds in the water of 113 km/hr (70 mph), sports an elongated bill. Although not considered a predator, a sailfish has on at least a few occasions driven its bill into a human victim (Figure 73-101), in one case causing a colon perforation in a snorkeler. Other istiophorid species, including blue, black, and white marlin, exhibit similar speed and jumping ability (Figure 73-102).

The swordfish *(Xiphias gladius)* is a billfish usually found in deep waters (Figure 73-103). In one case, a male victim was attacked three times by a swordfish in shallow water near the

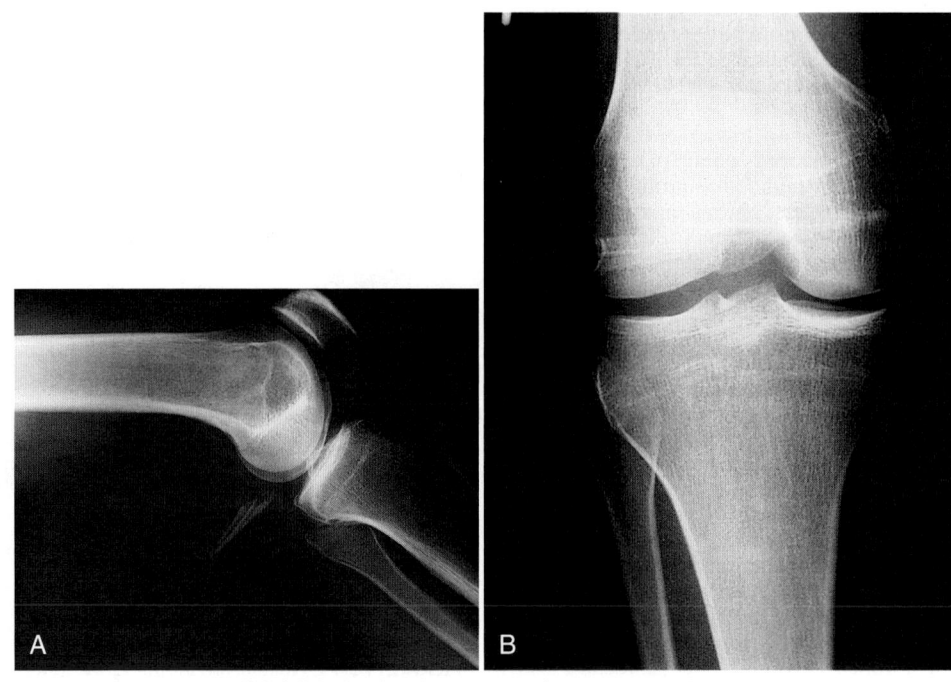

FIGURE 73-101 Sailfish bill lodged in the posterior knee. **A,** Lateral view. **B,** Anterior view.

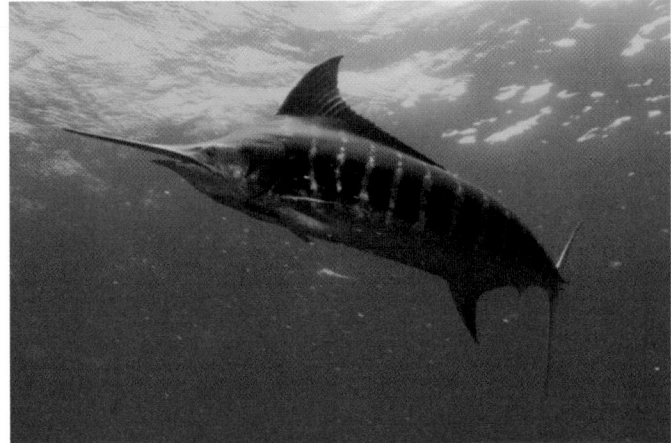

FIGURE 73-102 Black marlin. *(Copyright Norbert Wu: norbertwu .com.)*

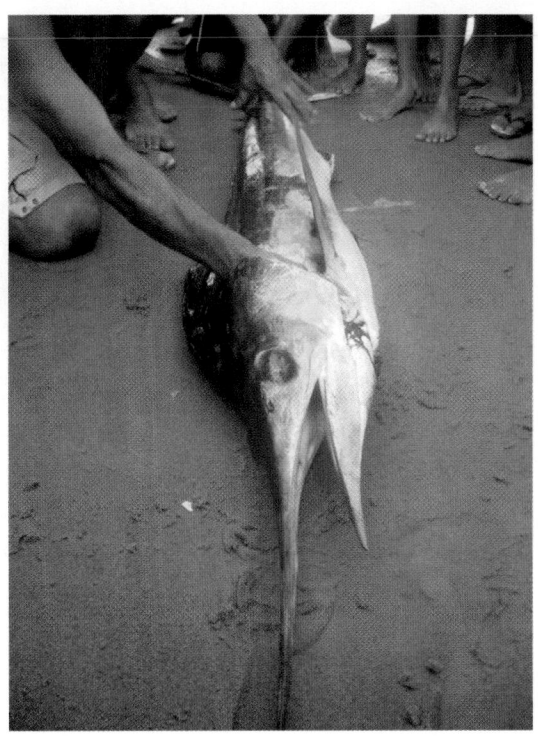

FIGURE 73-104 Swordfish that speared the posterior knee of a human victim. *(Courtesy Vidal Haddad, Jr.)*

beach, sustaining multiple punctures to the leg (Figure 73-104).[80] In another case, a young man had the left upper lobe of his lung pierced by the tip of a swordfish, requiring left upper lobe segmentectomy.[45]

Many persons have been knocked unconscious or otherwise injured by leaping sturgeons on the Suwannee River in Florida.[210] One was reported severely injured with a ruptured spleen. Sturgeon weigh up to 200 pounds and attain lengths of up to 8 feet.

KILLER WHALES

The killer whale, *Orcinus orca,* is not a ferocious killer of humans in the wild. The largest of the living mammalian dolphins, these magnificent animals (Figure 73-105) grow to 10 m (33 feet) and 9090 kg (10 tons) and are found in all oceans. They usually travel in pods of up to 40 individuals. Swift, smart, and enormously powerful creatures, they feed on squid, fish, birds, seals, walruses, and other whales. Their powerful jaws are equipped with cone-shaped teeth directed back into the throat, designed to grasp and hold food. The killer whale can generate enough crushing power to bite a seal or porpoise in two with a single snap. Nonetheless, although killer whales are believed not to prey on humans, they should be regarded with respect and kept at a distance in their natural habitat. Mistaken for a sea lion, a human would be a nice snack for a killer whale.

In captivity, killer whales are playful creatures and seem intelligent, without the primal behavior of sharks. However, they have been documented in several incidents involving handlers in North American public aquaria. In two highly publicized events, captive killer whales appeared to pursue their handlers, in one case attempting to cause injury by repetitive battering, and in the other case grabbing a female handler by the hair, killing her. The

behavioral dynamics of such a large predator maintained in confined space and subjected to intense conditioning warrant review.

Other whale species, such as the finback, have rammed boats, theoretically in defense of their young. Similarly, the unrelated but similarly sized planktivorous whale shark *(R. typus)* also has rammed ships. Territorial behavior should be anticipated and respected.

GIANT CLAMS

Although many adventure stories describe divers being caught in the clamp of a giant clam (family Tridacnidae), there are no verifiable reports of such a calamity resulting in a major injury. *Tridacna gigas* can attain a length of 1 m (3.3 feet) (Figure 73-106) and weigh as much as 300 kg (660 lb). The mantles may be quite colorful (Figures 73-107 and 73-108). The hazard to divers is hypothetical.

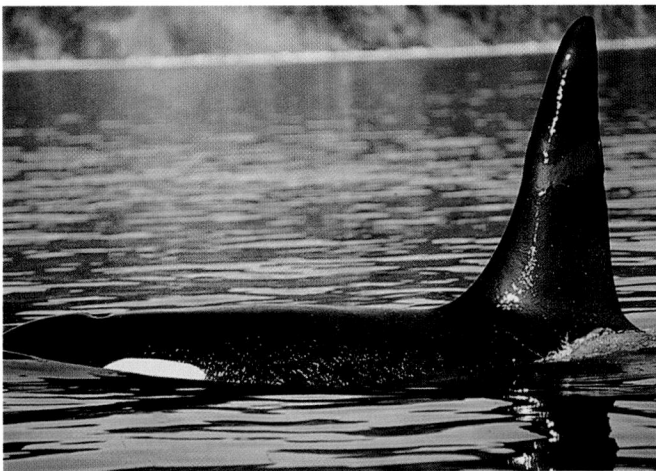

FIGURE 73-105 Distinctive markings of a killer whale near the San Juan Islands, Washington State. *(Copyright 2000 Norbert Wu: norbertwu.com.)*

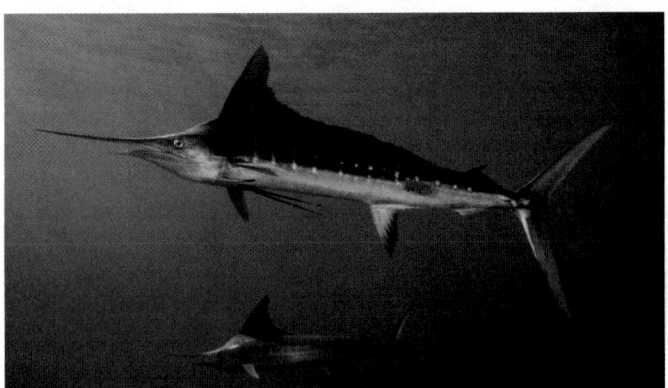

FIGURE 73-103 Swordfish. *(Copyright Howard Hall.)*

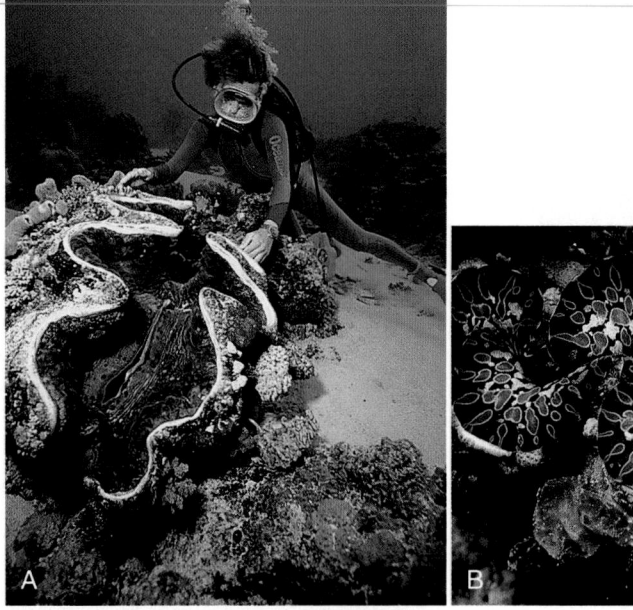

FIGURE 73-106 Giant clams. **A,** Giant clam with diver. **B,** Giant clam mantle (*Tridacna* sp.) obtains its coloration from algae used for photosynthesis. (*A courtesy Howard Hall; **B** copyright 2000 Norbert Wu: norbertwu.com.*)

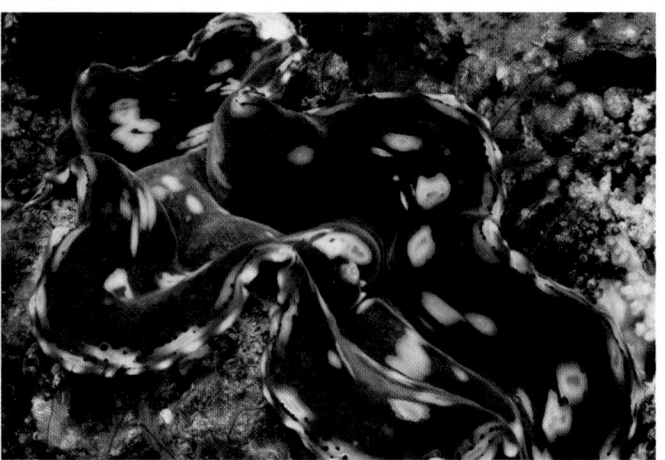

FIGURE 73-107 Mantle of the giant clam. (*Copyright Stephen Frink.*)

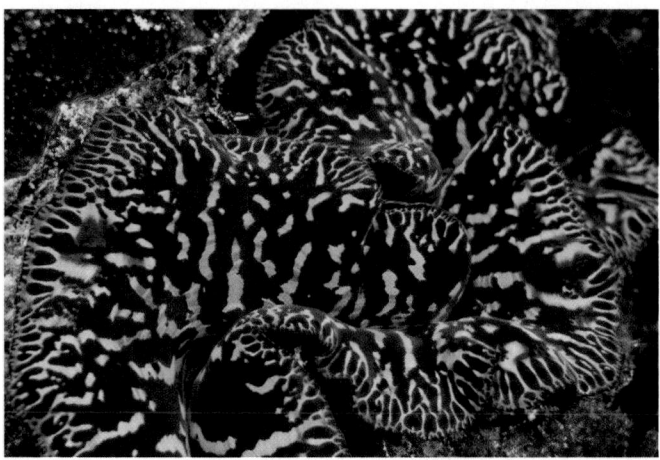

FIGURE 73-108 Colorful mantle of the giant clam. (*Copyright Stephen Frink.*)

GIANT SQUID

The giant ("colossal") squid (possibly *Mesonychoteuthis hamiltoni*), a cephalopod (10 arms), grows to a length in excess of 17.4 m (57 feet) and weight of 909 kg (2000 lb), with long (10-m [32.8-feet]) menacing tentacles, eyes with a diameter of nearly 35 cm (13.7 inches, the size of a dinner plate), and a razor-sharp beak that it uses to eat prey. *Architeuthis dux*, the "giant squid," may have a mantle that does not exceed 2.25 m (7.4 feet). It has been filmed underwater by Japanese scientists at an overall estimated length of 8 m (25 feet). The tentacles are armed with chitinous serrated rings equipped with teeth on each of the suckers. The suckers are approximately 4 cm (1.5 inches) in diameter. The giant Humboldt squid (Figures 73-109 to 73-111) demonstrates typical giant squid features. Sperm whales have been examined with sucker wounds with a diameter of 46 cm (18 inches), which would extrapolate to a truly monstrous squid,

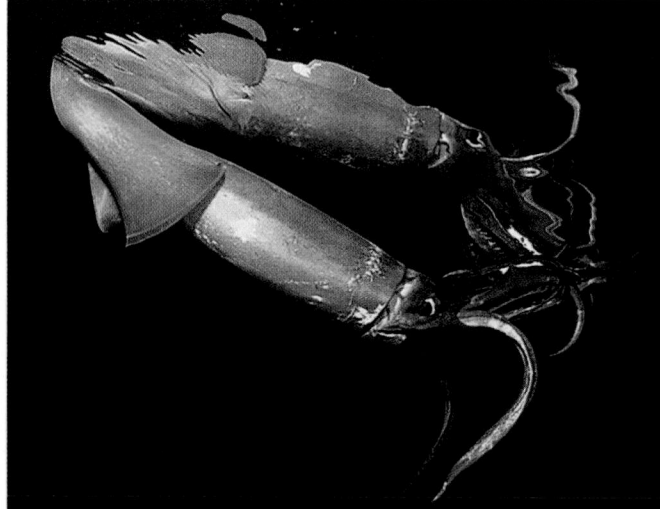

FIGURE 73-109 Giant Humboldt squid (*Dosidicus gigas*) attains a length of 15 feet and weight of 50 pounds. It is a voracious carnivore. (*Copyright 2000 Norbert Wu: norbertwu.com.*)

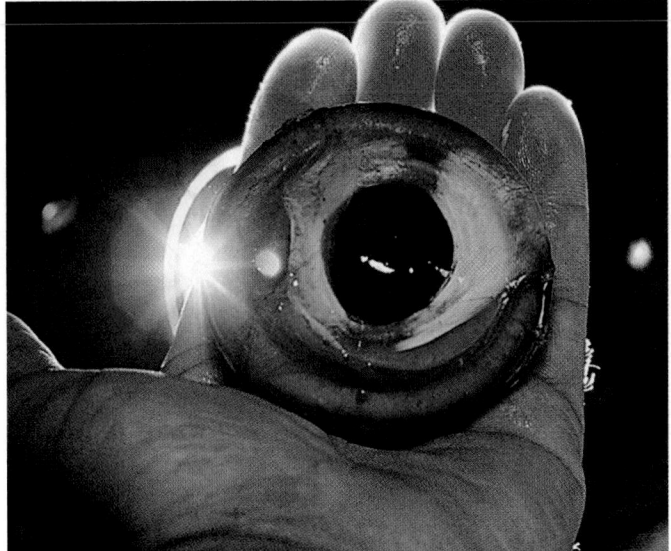

FIGURE 73-110 Eyeball of a giant Humboldt squid cut up by local fishermen. *(Copyright 2000 Norbert Wu: norbertwu.com.)*

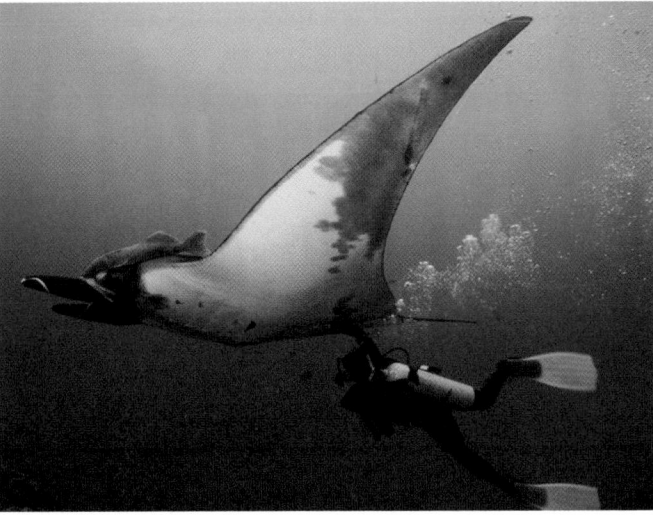

FIGURE 73-112 Diver strokes the belly of a manta ray. *(Copyright Carl Roessler.)*

estimated at 60 m (197 feet) in length. However, sucker scars expand in size as a whale grows, casting doubt on these projections. The battles between sperm whales and colossal squid are legendary, but humans are unlikely to encounter this awesome animal, which is found at depths far beyond the range of a sport scuba diver.[66] With increased deep-sea exploration by small submersibles, we may learn more about this fascinating creature. It is possible that a hungry colossal squid might ingest a human, but this has not yet been observed and is not likely to occur.

GIANT OCTOPUS

The Pacific giant octopus *Octopus dofleini* is a predator that has been captured at 272 kg (598 lb) with an arm span of more than 9.1 m (30 feet). It ranges off the western North American coast from northern California to Alaska and off Eastern Asia southward to Japan. This cephalopod is armed with suckers on eight arms and a parrot-like chitinous mouth located centrally underneath the head. Although it exhibits curiosity, it does not exhibit aggression directed against humans. However, it possesses the strength and agility to easily overwhelm a human. The animals have been reported to remove a dive mask or pull a regulator from divers. In open water, it is capable of squirting a large cloud of ink, which it sheds as evasive strategy. Folklore from the South Pacific tells of native breath-hold divers being subdued and drowned by angered captive octopuses.

GIANT MANTA RAY

The giant manta ray *Manta birostris* can have a wingspan of more than 6 m (19.7 feet) and a weight of 1600 kg (3520 lb) (Figure 73-112). The caudal appendage carries a vestigial stinger that poses no threat to humans. However, the coarse dermal denticles can create severe abrasions, which generally occur when intrusive divers attempt to ride these gentle and accommodating creatures. Similar abrasions can occur from attempts to ride whale sharks, *R. typus,* which also have large caudal fins that can readily shed an offending diver during regular swimming locomotion. In addition to potential injury, riding of large marine animals is behaviorally altering and illegal in many areas.

MANTIS SHRIMP

The mantis shrimp (Crustacea: Stomatopoda, "foot-mouth") (Figure 73-113) is not a true shrimp but resembles a large flattened shrimp or miniature lobster (≤ 36 cm [14.2 inches]) equipped with a pair of legs that serve as specialized jackknife claws (Figure 73-114). The tail carries numerous sharp spines that may project beyond the edge of the sturdy tail fin. Lacerations may be induced by either the front raptorial (prey-acquiring) claws or the tail, particularly when the mantis shrimp attacks an unwary victim. The strike from the paired claws may be

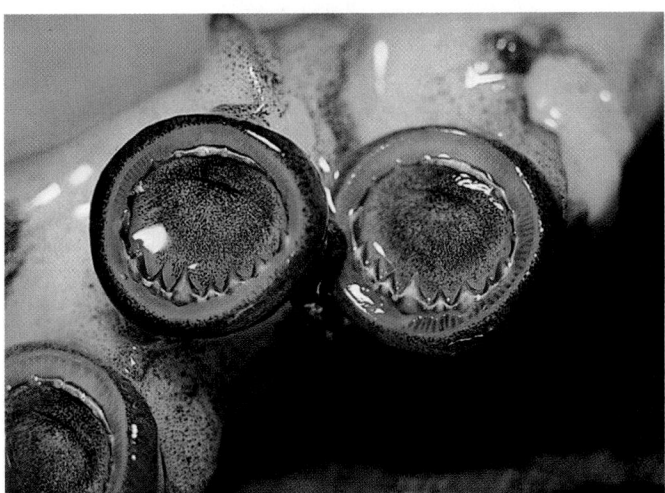

FIGURE 73-111 Suckers of the giant Humboldt squid are lined with razor-sharp teeth. *(Copyright 2000 Norbert Wu: norbertwu.com.)*

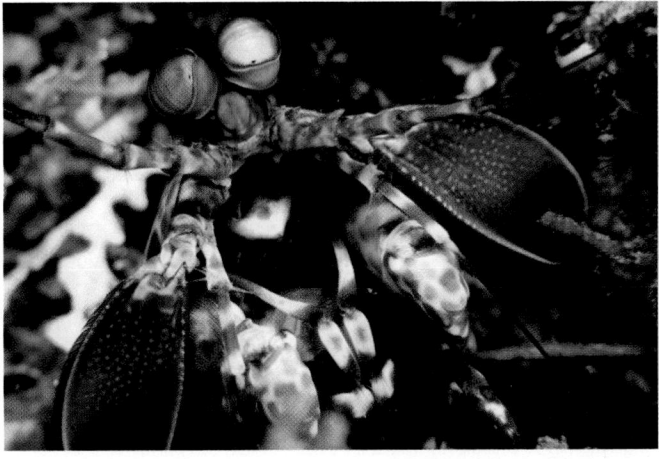

FIGURE 73-113 Mantis shrimp. *(Copyright Stephen Frink.)*

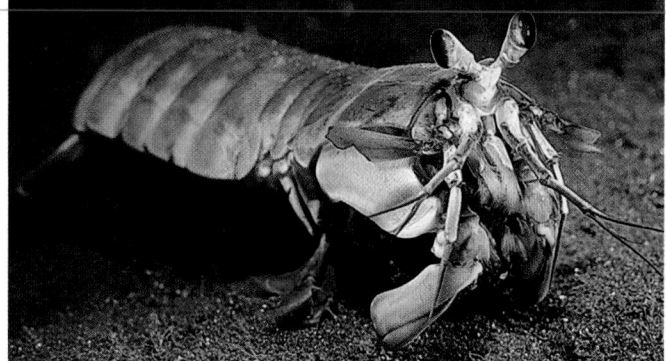

FIGURE 73-114 Mantis shrimp, ready to strike with its claws. *(Copyright 2000 Norbert Wu: norbertwu.com.)*

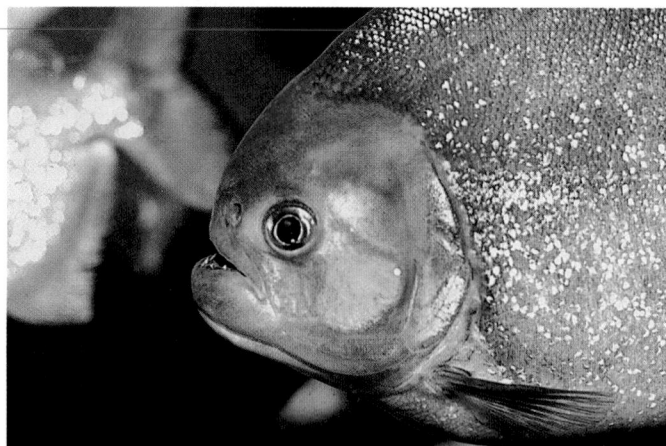

FIGURE 73-116 Piranha. *(Copyright 2000 Norbert Wu: norbertwu.com.)*

completed in a few milliseconds and is considered one of the fastest actions in the animal kingdom. It has been claimed that an attacking mantis shrimp struck with enough force to crack a diver's face mask and it is said that aquarium-held creatures have broken aquarium glass. Certain species use a spearing action, whereas others use a smashing technique. In the Caribbean, the mantis shrimp is known as "thumb splitter." The peacock mantis shrimp *Odontodactylus scyllarus* from the Indo-Pacific (Figure 73-115) can be afflicted with a disease that digests areas of its dorsal cuticle and eventually is lethal. This may explain one anecdotal report of a human finger wound (which led to amputation) characterized by cartilage destruction and from which no pathogenic organism could be cultured. The mantis shrimp is a superb predator, in part because it has the most highly developed eyes of any crustacean. One species, *Lysioquillina glabriuscula,* when faced with a rival male or a predator, adopts a position that accentuates fluorescent markings on its antennae and carapace, to make the creature more visible to an approaching enemy.

PIRANHA

South American freshwater characins include the piranha *Serrasalmus nattereri* (Figure 73-116), equipped with a formidable set of razor-sharp teeth (Figures 73-117 and 73-118). They are attracted by blood or commotion. Piranhas are widespread in rivers and lakes, and number approximately 30 species of the genera *Pygocentrus* and *Serrasalmus.*[81] These small fish may attack in schools of several hundred, although this reputation is largely borne of folklore rather than of documentation. Its reputation as an attacker of humans, like that of the barracuda, is greatly overstated. Natives living near piranha-inhabited waters express much more concern over freshwater stingrays (genus *Potamotrygon*) than about piranhas. Although an overwhelmed

human could theoretically be reduced to a shiny skeleton in short order, most attacks on humans are caused by a single fish biting only once, resulting in a single, circular, crater-like wound (Figure 73-119). Bathers are injured most often in dammed waters because of fish proliferation, spawning, and parental-care

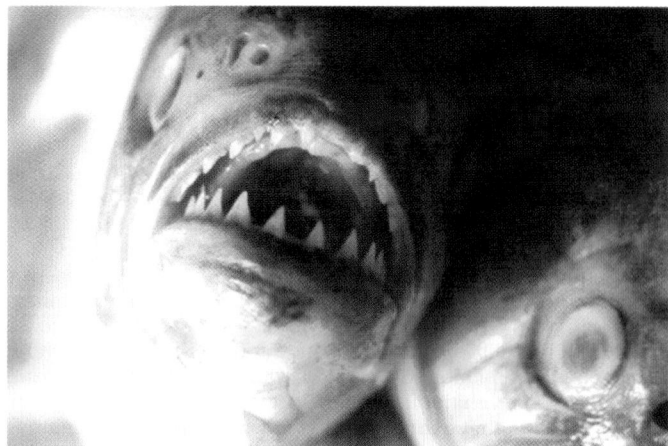

FIGURE 73-117 Teeth of the piranha. *(Courtesy V. Haddad, Jr.)*

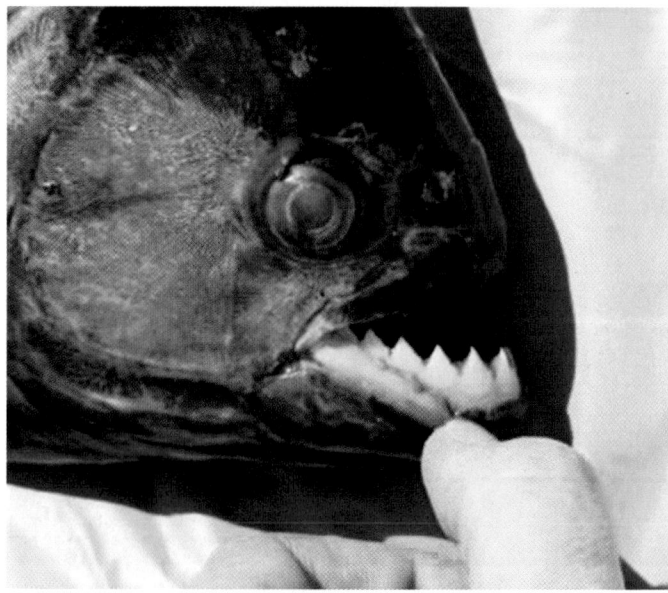

FIGURE 73-118 Piranha teeth. *(Courtesy George Hertner, MD.)*

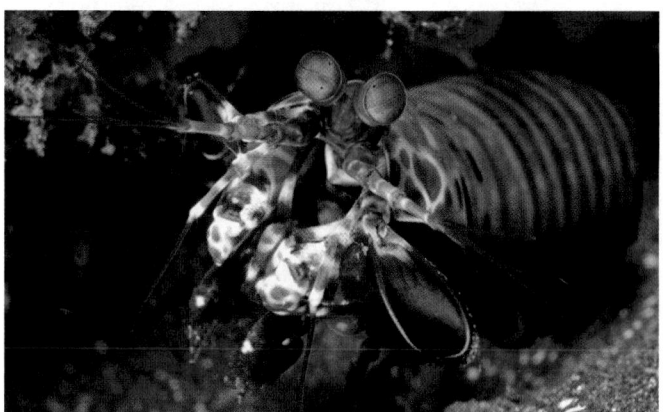

FIGURE 73-115 Peacock mantis shrimp. *(Courtesy Marty Snyderman.)*

MARINE MEDICINE

PART 10

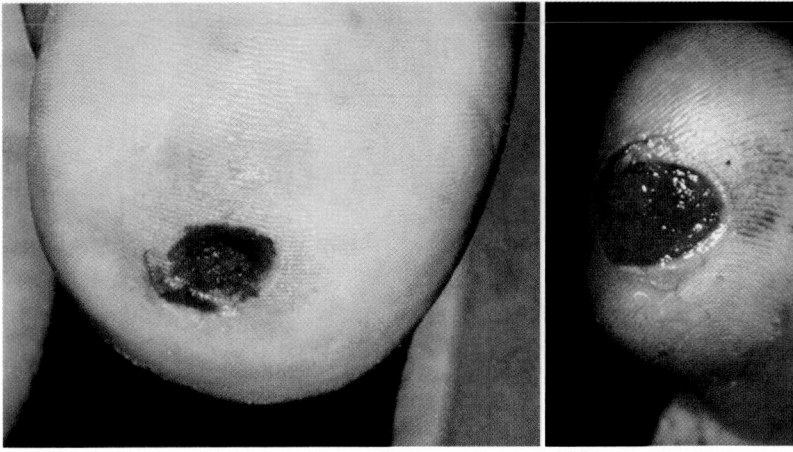

FIGURE 73-119 Crateriform bite wounds caused by piranhas. (Courtesy Vidal Haddad, Jr.)

behavior.[114,164,194] In one series of attacks by speckled piranhas (*Serrasalmus spilopleura*), it was noted that most bites occurred on the lower extremities, particularly on the heel. One bite was sufficient to amputate a toe.[81] Prevention measures might include clearance of waterweeds at bathing sites or placement of net enclosures around bathing areas. Other characid freshwater fish with fearsome teeth include the South American dogfish (Figure 73-120).

SNAPPING TURTLE

Snapping turtles (family Chelydridae) may bite humans when they are provoked on land; bites are not initiated while the animals are in the water. The biting speed is quite rapid and powerful, as evidenced by the aggression of the common snapper *Chelydra serpentina*. The larger alligator snapper *Macroclemys temminckii* is less aggressive.[36] The Florida snapping turtle *Chelydra osceola* is found only in Florida. Softshell turtles (Trionychidae) readily bite if harassed.

TRIGGERFISH

Triggerfish (named for its fin apparatus) (Figures 73-121 and 73-122) of the family Balistidae may be gregarious or unimposing, but during mating season the females of at least two species (*Pseudobalistes fuscus* and the larger titan triggerfish *Balistoides viridescens*) can become extremely territorial in guarding their nests and eggs during certain parts of the lunar cycle and thus aggressive, inflicting painful bites. The former can grow to 55 cm

(22 inches) and the latter to 75 cm (30 inches). The strong jaws each carry eight long, protruding, and chisel-like teeth (Figure 73-123) in an outer row, backed by an inner row of six teeth.[156] Usually the fish "bites and runs," commonly on the legs (Figure 73-124), hands, or head of the human victim, but the orange-striped triggerfish *Balistoides undulatus* has been reported to bite and not release. It is common to have to strike the fish in some manner to get it to release. In the Gilbert Islands, a release technique is to bite the fish on the top of the head. If attacked by a triggerfish, one should retreat from the area of the nest by swimming laterally away, rather than straight up, to leave the cylinder of water above the nest. Care should be exercised when reaching into fishing nets in areas inhabited by triggerfishes; coauthor

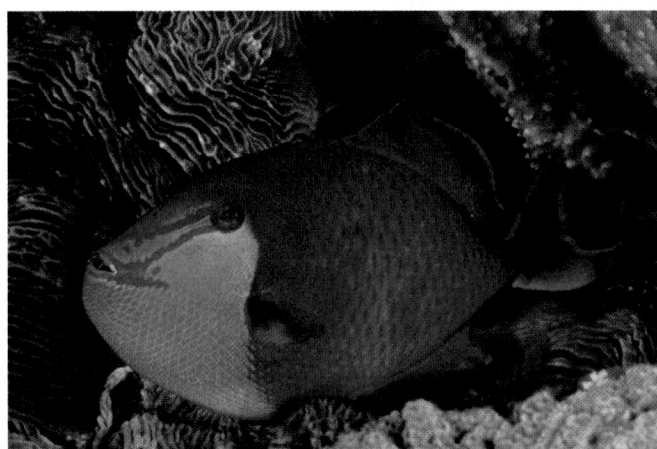

FIGURE 73-121 Triggerfish. (Copyright Lynn Funkhouser.)

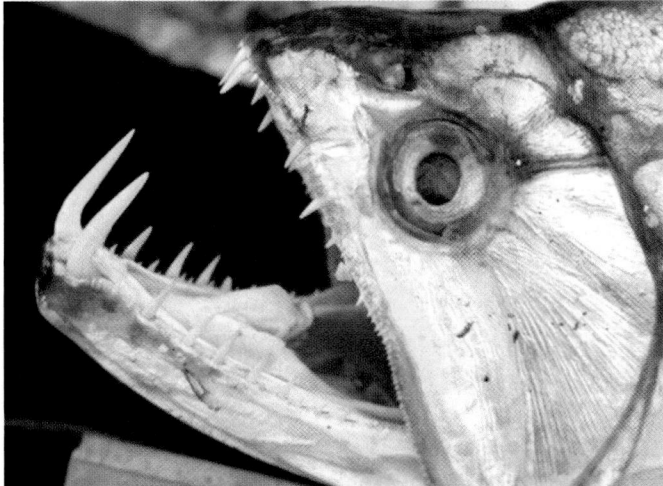

FIGURE 73-120 South American freshwater characid dogfish. (Courtesy Vidal Haddad, Jr.)

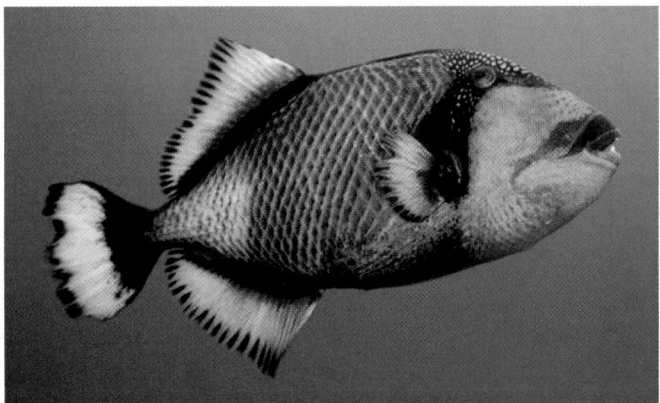

FIGURE 73-122 Titan triggerfish. (Copyright Stephen Frink.)

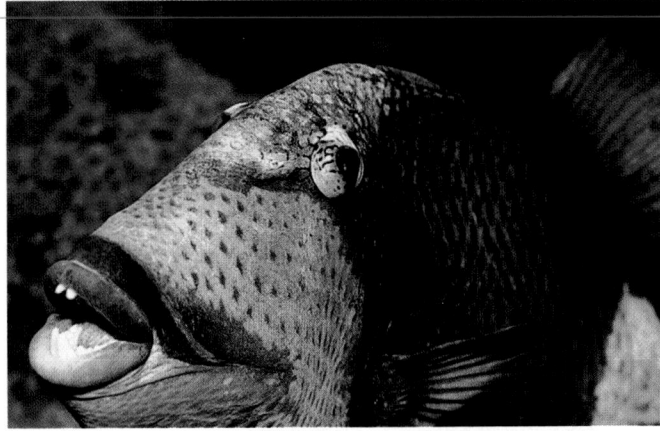

FIGURE 73-123 Triggerfish. *(Courtesy John Randall.)*

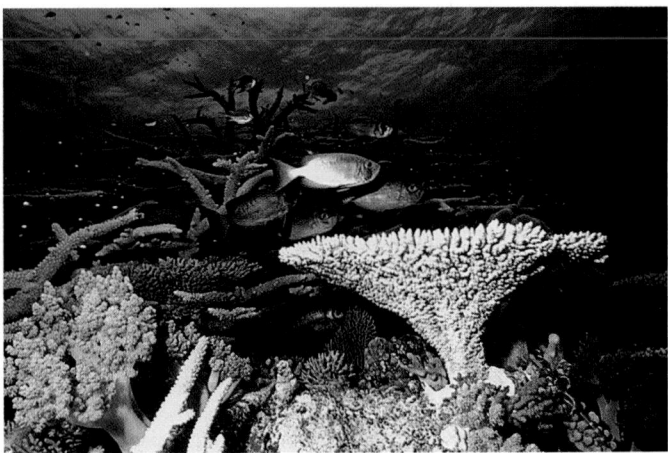

FIGURE 73-125 Coral garden. *(Courtesy Paul S. Auerbach, MD.)*

GHB received a painful bite to the first web space of the hand from a cryptic subadult grey triggerfish *(Balistes capriscus)* when sorting a trawl catch off the Florida Everglades.

SAWFISHES

Cartilaginous fishes that reach shark-like sizes (to 7 m), sawfishes are actually rays of the family Pristidae. Five species inhabit tropical waters worldwide. All species are highly endangered due to their habitat choices (shallow nearshore waters, including estuaries and lower stretches of rivers) and the presence of a peculiar elongated, toothed rostrum (the "saw"); humans frequent, modify, and fish in the waters in which sawfishes are found. Sawfish rostra are easily entangled in nets, and the animals readily take a baited hook.

There are no documented cases of sawfish-diver interactions, but fishery-caught sawfishes are very dangerous to handle when brought up to the boat, dock, or beach. They rapidly shake their heads from side to side defensively, and the combination of great size and power and sharp rostral teeth makes live release a difficult task. It is best to simply cut the fishing line, leaving the hook in the mouth (as is best done with live sharks). The hook will eventually rust and be dislodged, and these tough creatures hopefully do not suffer from the inconvenience. A net-caught sawfish is a bigger problem and must be cut out of the net.

Recommended medical treatment is the same as measures applied for shark attack. The complications can also be similar, including retained foreign bodies and wound infections.

STONY CORALS
LIFE AND HABITS

The anthozoan Madreporaria, or true (stony) corals, exist in colonies that possess calcareous outer skeletons (the origin of calcium carbonate, or limestone) with pointed horns or razor-sharp edges, or both (Figure 73-125). There are nearly 1000 species of corals. Reef-forming corals live in waters at temperatures of 20°C (68°F) or higher, generally at depths of up to 20 fathoms (120 feet), although they are seen at depths of up to 83 fathoms (500 feet). A "coral head" is actually a colony of individual polyps. Certain coral species, such as *Plexaura homomalla,* have been investigated as sources of prostaglandins and other pharmaceutical precursors to treat conditions as diverse as asthma, leukemia, and infections. Pieces of coral have been evaluated for use as bone grafts.

Coral reefs are under pressure worldwide from climatic changes, human-induced sedimentation and salinity modification, chemical poisons (e.g., cyanide used for fishing, pollution), natural predators (e.g., crown-of-thorns sea star), and mechanical destruction (e.g., ship anchors, diver contact, and explosives).

CLINICAL ASPECTS

Snorkelers and divers, particularly photographers and spear fishermen, frequently handle or brush against these living reefs, resulting in superficial cuts and abrasions on the extremities (Figure 73-126) while simultaneously injuring the corals. Coral cuts are probably the most common injuries sustained underwater. The initial reaction to a coral cut is stinging pain, erythema, and pruritus, most commonly on the forearms, elbows, and

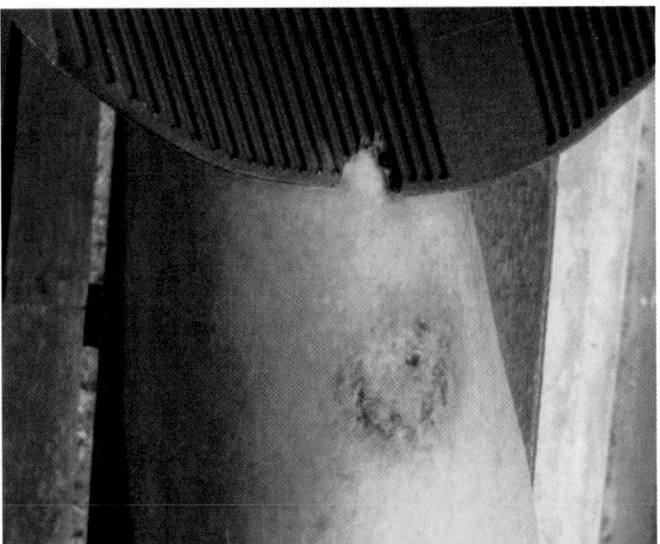

FIGURE 73-124 Leg and dive fin bitten by *Pseudobalistes flavimarginatus* triggerfish. *(Copyright Corinne Paollilo.)*

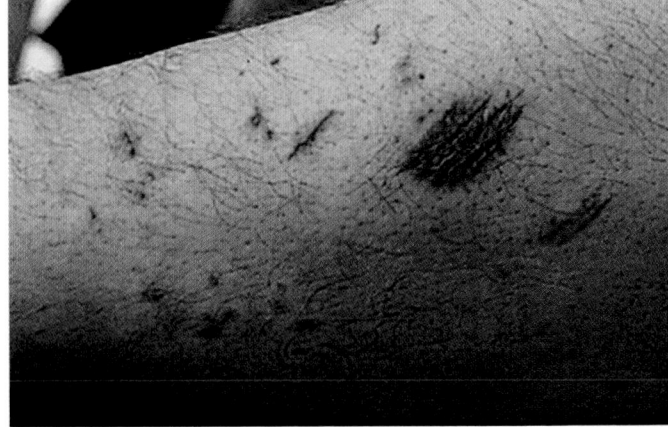

FIGURE 73-126 Abrasions of the leg from bumping against sharp coral. *(Courtesy Paul S. Auerbach, MD.)*

knees. Divers without gloves frequently receive cuts to the hands. A break in the skin may be surrounded within minutes by an erythematous wheal, which fades over 1 to 2 hours. The red, raised welts and local pruritus are called *coral poisoning*. Low-grade fever may be present and does not necessarily indicate an infection. Blistering may occur. With or without prompt treatment, the wound may progress to cellulitis with ulceration and tissue sloughing. These wounds heal slowly (3 to 6 weeks) and result in prolonged morbidity. There may be a stage of subacute fleshy granulomatous dermatitis, followed by chronic lichenoid dermatitis, in which the lesions harden, become smaller, and take on a shiny, lichenoid appearance.[62] In an extreme case, the victim develops cellulitis with lymphangitis, reactive bursitis, local ulceration, and wound necrosis. Chronic dermal granulomata following a coral scrape or cut should invoke suspicion for *Mycobacterium* infection, including species *marinum* or *haemophilum*.[172]

TREATMENT

Coral cuts should be promptly and vigorously scrubbed with soap and water and then irrigated copiously with a forceful stream of fresh water or normal saline to remove all foreign particles. Using medicinal hydrogen peroxide to bubble out "coral dust" is occasionally helpful. Any fragments that remain can become embedded and increase the risk for an indolent infection or foreign body granuloma. If stinging is a major symptom, there may be an element of envenomation by nematocysts (see Chapter 74). A brief rinse with diluted acetic acid (vinegar), lidocaine, or nonscalding hot water may diminish the discomfort (after the initial pain from contact with the open wound). Topical decontamination should be followed by a normal saline or tap water rinse. If a coral-induced laceration is severe, it should be closed with adhesive strips rather than sutures if possible; preferably it should be debrided for 3 to 4 consecutive days and closed in a delayed fashion.

A number of approaches can be taken with regard to subsequent wound care. One method is to apply twice-daily sterile wet-to-dry dressings, using saline or a dilute antiseptic (povidone-iodine 1% to 5%) solution. Alternatively, a nontoxic topical antiseptic or antibiotic ointment (mupirocin, bacitracin, or polymyxin B–bacitracin-neomycin) may be used sparingly and covered with a nonadherent dressing (e.g., Telfa). Secondary infections are dealt with as they arise. A final approach is to apply full-strength antiseptic solution, followed by a powdered topical antibiotic, such as tetracycline. No method has been supported by any prospective trial.

Despite the best efforts at primary irrigation and decontamination, the wound may heal slowly, with moderate-to-severe soft tissue inflammation and ulcer formation (Figure 73-127). All devitalized tissue should be debrided regularly using sharp dissection. This should be continued until a bed of healthy granulation tissue is formed. Wounds that appear infected should be cultured and treated with antibiotics as previously discussed. Lichenoid papules, which may be flat or dome shaped, may respond to treatment with betamethasone dipropionate 0.05% cream applied twice daily for 2 weeks under occlusive dressings.[45] Residual postinflammatory hyperpigmentation is possible.

The victim who demonstrates malaise, nausea, and low-grade fever may have a systemic form of coral poisoning or be manifesting early signs of a wound infection. It is prudent at this point to search for a localized infection, procure wound cultures or biopsy specimens as indicated, and initiate antibiotics pending confirmation of organisms. If the victim is started on an antibiotic and does not improve, a supplemental trial of a systemic glucocorticoid (prednisone 80 mg tapered over 2 weeks) is not unreasonable. In the absence of an overt infection, the natural course of the wound is to improve spontaneously over a 4- to 15-week period.

A hypertrophic scar may form following coral abrasion. First-line therapy is silicone sheets and gels applied to the scar. Intralesional corticosteroid injection is second-line therapy. One therapeutic regimen is triamcinolone acetonide in concentrations of 10 to 40 g/mL injected every 4 to 6 weeks. This is felt to

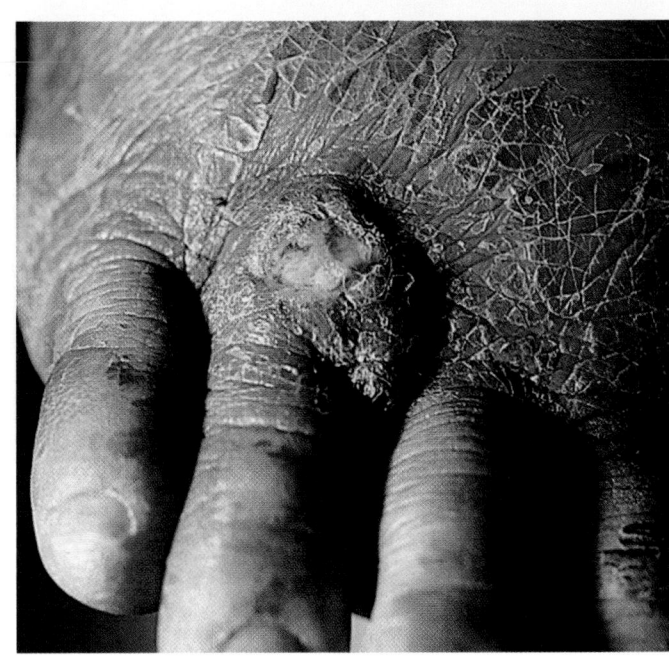

FIGURE 73-127 Poorly healing wound following coral cut. *(Courtesy Paul S. Auerbach, MD.)*

alter collagen and glucosaminoglycan synthesis and reduce inflammation and fibroblast proliferation. Another approach is compression therapy to thin the skin by reducing the cohesiveness of collagen fibers in hypertrophic scars. Select newer therapies to treat hypertrophic scars include intralesional interferon, 5-fluorouracil, or bleomycin; application of topical retinoic acid, imiquimod, or tacrolimus; cryotherapy; excision; and laser therapy.[132]

PREVENTION

Divers exploring near coral reefs must take every care to avoid coral cuts. Protective clothing and gloves should be impenetrable. Snorkelers and underwater photographers in shallow water should wear adequate hand, elbow, and knee protection.

ELECTRIC FISH AND RAYS

Only two groups of electric fish are marine; the remainder are freshwater animals. They rarely pose a health hazard but rather are curious creatures surrounded by superstition and folklore. The marine electric fish include stargazers *(Astroscopus)* (Figure 73-128), electric rays *(Torpedo* and *Narcine),* and skates (Rajidae). The electric eel (Figure 73-129) is a freshwater Amazonian animal (see below).

Electric rays are found in temperate and tropical oceans. Of the class Chondrichthyes, they are round-bodied, with short tails and thick bodies (compared with stingrays). In California, *Torpedo californica* (Figure 73-130) attains a length of 1.2 m (4 feet) and weight of 36 to 41 kg (80 to 90 lb). It swims slowly and sluggishly and is usually found partially buried in bottom mud and sand. Well camouflaged, its dorsal surface is multicolored and the ventral surface creamy white. The externally visible electric organs are located on each side of the anterior part of the disk between the anterior extension of the pectoral fin and the head, extending from above the level of the eye backward past the gill region onto the ventral surface. The electric organs are composed of a honeycomb network of modified muscles organized into columnar prism-like structures and connective tissue, which generate an electrical charge by neuromuscular activity. The muscle cells (electroplaques) are stacked 500 to 1000 deep, creating up to 500 cm² of surface area. The electroplaques depolarize in series and in parallel simultaneously, producing amperage sufficient to stun prey. Species in the tropical eastern Pacific include

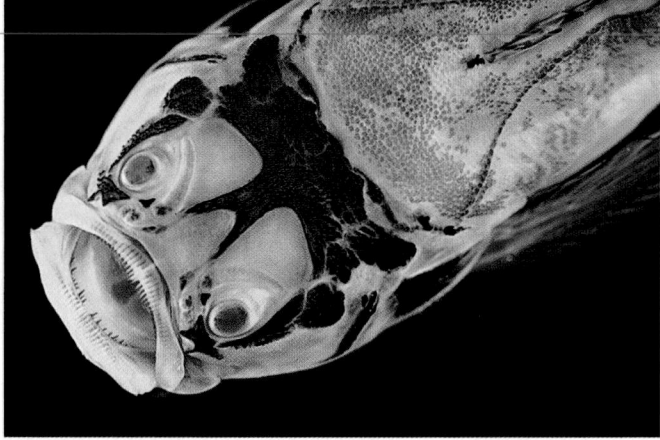

FIGURE 73-128 Stargazer (*Astroscopus zephyreus*) with electric plates above each eye. *(Copyright 2000 Norbert Wu: norbertwu.com.)*

the smaller-bodied lesser ray *Narcine entemedor* and the bulls-eye ray *Diplobatis ommata* (Figure 73-131).

Generally the ventral surface of the ray is negative and the dorsal side is positive. An electrical discharge is reflexively produced on contact, often in a series exhaustive for the fish. This necessitates a period of recharging. Electricity is delivered in doses of 8 to 220 volts. The Atlantic *Torpedo nobiliana* produces 180 to 220 volts. Although the shock is of low amperage, it is sufficient to stun a grown man and might induce drowning. Recovery from the shock has been reported anecdotally to usually be uneventful. An electric ray should not be handled. The energy generated by skates is considerably less, measured in millivolts to 1 to 2 volts.

The electric eel, *Electrophorus electricus,* is a freshwater fish (not related to true eels) that is a member of the knifefishes. Electric eels reside in the Amazon and Orinoco Rivers and other related bodies of water in South American basins. This species generates the potential to electrically shock victims by manipulating the sodium ion concentration in specialized cells called electrocytes. The current generated has been estimated to attain a maximum of 500 to 650 volts in the adult animal, with lesser amounts in juvenile animals. This is of a severity that may incapacitate a human. Because the creatures may deliver repeated

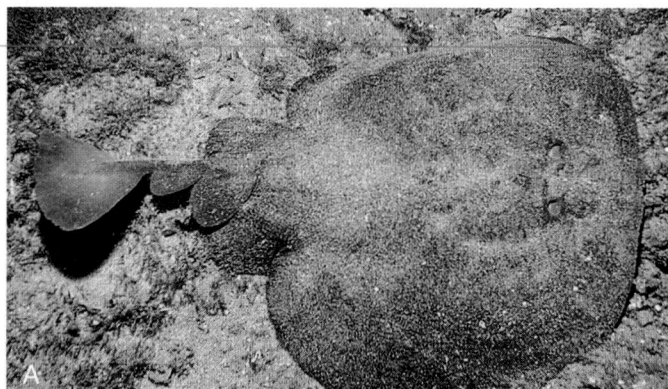
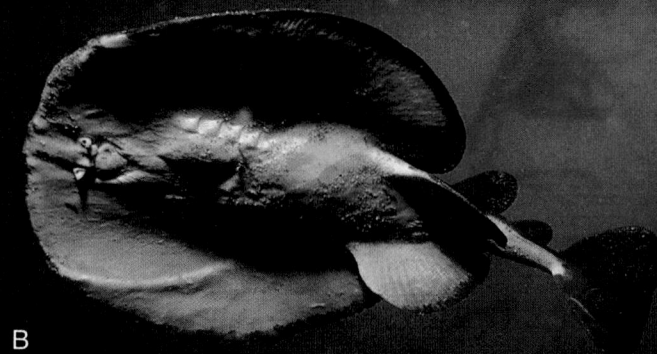

FIGURE 73-130 Electric ray *(Torpedo californica)*. **A,** Dorsal view. **B,** Ventral view. *(Copyright 2000 Norbert Wu: norbertwu.com.)*

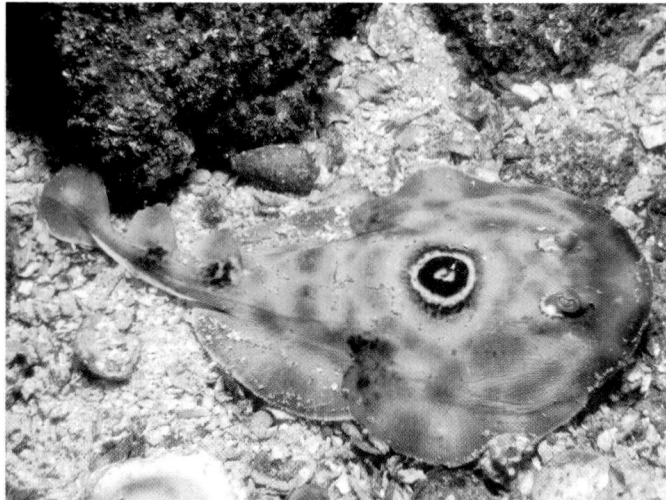

FIGURE 73-131 Bull's-eye electric ray. *(Courtesy Paul S. Auerbach, MD.)*

shocks, they should be given wide berth and not be handled. The mechanism of electricity generation is sufficiently unique to warrant study for application to development of a new type of battery.

REFERENCES

Complete references used in this text are available online at expertconsult.inkling.com.

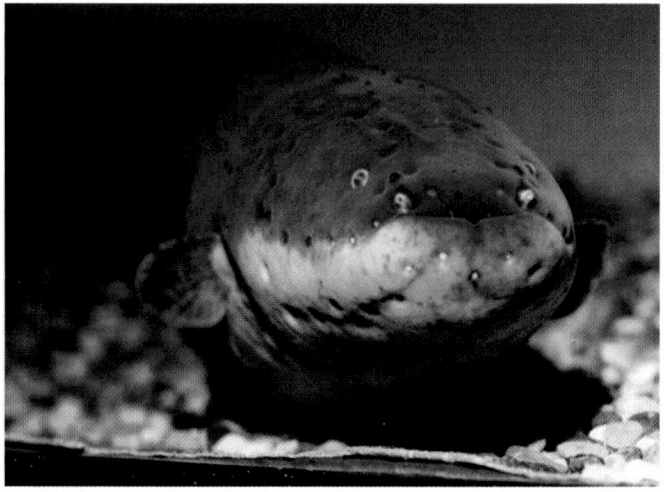

FIGURE 73-129 Electric eel, Steinhart Aquarium. *(Copyright 2000 Norbert Wu: norbertwu.com.)*

PAUL S. AUERBACH AND ALEXANDRA E. DiTULLIO

Stinging aquatic animals pose a hazard for swimmers and divers. They constitute a large collection of marine organisms that include invertebrates and vertebrates, and that range from primitive to extremely sophisticated organisms. This chapter discusses envenomation by aquatic invertebrate life-forms. Chapter 75 discusses envenomation by aquatic vertebrate life-forms. Chapter 73 discusses infections associated with aquatic wounds and the relevant antimicrobial therapies. Standard wound care measures, such as antitetanus immunization, should be undertaken whenever there is penetration of the skin.

The science of poisons, biotoxicology, is divided into plant poisons, or phytotoxicology, and animal poisons, or zootoxicology. *Toxinology* connotes the science of toxic substances produced by or accumulated in living organisms, their properties, and their biologic significance for the organisms involved.[139] Animals in which a definite venom apparatus is present are sometimes called phanerotoxic, whereas animals whose body tissues are toxic are termed cryptotoxic.[173] Naturally occurring aquatic zootoxins may be designated as oral toxins (which are poisonous to eat and include bacterial poisons and products of decomposition), parenteral toxins (venom produced in specialized glands and injected mechanically [by spine, needle, fang, fin, or dart]), and crinotoxins (venom produced in specialized glands and administered as slime, mucus, or gastric secretion). Within these three subdivisions, further classifications are by phylogeny, chemical structure, and clinical syndrome.

Although all venoms are poisons, not all poisons are venoms. Venoms can be released in varying amounts and have evolved for conquest and defense. It is theorized that offensive (prey capture and digestion) venoms are generally perioral (mouth, fang, or tentacle) and that defensive venoms are aboral (tail and sting) or dermal (barb and secretion). In the evolutionary scheme, it appears that many venomous fish seek a specific form of self-defense, whereas poisonous fish are noxious in a nonspecific manner.[7] A brief comparison of the features of venoms and poisons shows that, generally, poisons produced in skin, muscle, blood, or organs are heat stable (46° to 49°C [115° to 120°F]) and gastric acid stable and carry seasonal toxicity. They are not "released," and may lack a well-defined biologic function. Venoms are more commonly heat labile, gastric acid labile, and nonseasonal in toxicity.

In snakes, the latency, toxicity, and duration of venom effects are related to the route of envenomation. Intravascular injection is significantly more lethal than intraperitoneal or transcutaneous injection, as determined by the dose that produces 50% lethality in a group (LD_{50}). This principle is not commonly applied to marine venoms because few encounters involve direct intravascular injection.

Most venoms are high-molecular-weight amalgams of vasoactive amines, proteolytic enzymes, and other biogenic compounds. These substances denature membranes, catabolize cyclic 3′,5′-adenosine monophosphate, degranulate mast cells, provoke histamine release, initiate arachidonate metabolism, accelerate coagulopathy, interfere with cellular transport mechanisms, disrupt metabolic pathways, impede neuronal transmission, and evoke anaphylaxis and shock. Toxin-containing venoms from marine and other creatures include components, such as incretin mimetics, sarafotoxins, antiarrhythmics, and bradykinin-potentiating and natriuretic peptides, that may be applicable to cardiovascular drug discovery.[90] Although many marine venoms are composed of protein and polypeptide subunits, they lack sufficient immunogenicity to allow development of antitoxins or antivenoms. Poisons represent metabolic by-products and are usually of lower molecular weights.

The taxonomy of marine animals can sometimes be confusing. The hierarchy, in descending order, is kingdom, phylum, class, order, family, genus, and species.

Treatment recommendations are constantly evolving in response to acquisition of data, clinical observations, and preferences of expert rescuers and physicians.

ALLERGIC REACTIONS

ANAPHYLAXIS

An envenomation or the administration of antivenom can elicit an allergic reaction. In the previously sensitized individual, the antigen (venom, aquatic protein, or animal serum) forms a complex with immunoglobulin E (IgE) and perhaps with IgG homocytotropic antibodies or activated complement cleavage products attached to the membranes of mast cells and basophils. This induces membrane permeability, which allows degranulation or membrane production of histamine, serotonin, kinins, prostaglandins, platelet-activating factor, eosinophil and neutrophil chemotactic factors, leukotrienes, and other bioactive chemical mediators.[9]

The signs and symptoms of anaphylaxis may occur within minutes of exposure. They include hypotension, bronchospasm, tongue and lip swelling, laryngeal edema, pulmonary edema, seizures, cardiac arrhythmia, pruritus, urticaria, angioedema, rhinitis, conjunctivitis, nausea, vomiting, diarrhea, abdominal pain, gastrointestinal bleeding, and syncope. Most severe allergic reactions occur within 15 to 30 minutes of envenomation, and nearly all occur within 6 hours. Fatalities are often related to airway obstruction or hypotension. Acute elevated pulmonary vascular resistance may contribute to hypotension that results from generalized arterial vasodilation.[10,12]

Treatment

Decisive treatment should be instituted at the first indication of hypersensitivity. Specific treatment recommendations for anaphylaxis are found in Box 67-7.

ANTIVENOM ADMINISTRATION

A number of marine envenomations, such as those by the box-jellyfish and certain sea snakes, may provoke administration of specific antivenom by the treating clinician. Marine antivenoms are raised in horses or sheep and therefore may be antigenic in humans, inducing both immediate and delayed hypersensitivity. Most authorities recommend that a skin test be performed for sensitivity to horse serum, if the clinical situation permits, after a sea snake envenomation. A skin test should be done only after deciding to administer antivenom; it is *not* done to determine whether antivenom is necessary. The purpose of sensitivity testing is to allow adequate prophylaxis against anaphylaxis. The skin test is performed with an intradermal injection into the upper extremity of 0.02 mL of a 1 : 10 dilution of horse serum test material in saline, with 0.02 mL saline in the opposite extremity as a control. Erythema and a wheal with pseudopodia appear in 15 to 30 minutes in a positive response. Because antivenom contains many times the protein content of horse serum used for skin testing, the use of antivenom for skin testing may increase the risk of anaphylactic reaction. If the skin test is positive, the antivenom intended for intravenous (IV) infusion should be diluted in sterile water to a 1:100 concentration for administration. Successive vials should be less dilute if the allergic reaction is minimal (controlled by antihistamines and epinephrine). A negative skin test does not preclude the possibility of an anaphylactic response to antivenom administration.

The rationale for administering antivenom is to provide early and adequate neutralization of the toxin at the tissue site of entry before it gains systemic dominance. Except for stonefish antivenom, the product is preferentially administered intravenously, taking care to provide adequate doses for children and older adults, who have a decreased volume of distribution and increased sensitivity to venom effects. The antivenom intended for IV administration should always be diluted with normal saline, Ringer's lactate, or dextrose 5% in water.

Marine antivenoms are produced and distributed in the Indo-Pacific regions. They include the following:

Chironex fleckeri (box-jellyfish) antivenom, from Commonwealth Serum Laboratories (CSL), Parkville, Victoria, Australia. This hyperimmune sheep globulin preparation may be used to neutralize the stings of *C. fleckeri* and *Chiropsalmus* species. It may not be as efficacious as commonly believed.

Enhydrina schistosa (beaked sea snake) antivenom, from CSL. This hyperimmune horse globulin preparation may be used to neutralize the bites of most sea snakes. It is prepared by immunizing horses with venom from *E. schistosa* and the Australian tiger snake *Notechis scutatus*.

Notechis scutatus (tiger snake) antivenom, from CSL, has traditionally been recommended as the antivenom of second choice against the bites of most sea snakes. However, it has been written that tiger snake antivenom is not effective against sea snake bites, and so it should not be relied upon for clinical efficacy in humans.[228]

Synanceja trachynis (stonefish) antivenom, from CSL. This hyperimmune horse globulin preparation may be used to neutralize the stings of stonefish and more virulent scorpionfish species, although it is rarely used for the latter.

A person who is known to be sensitive to horse or sheep serum, has a positive skin test, or develops signs of an allergic reaction or anaphylaxis during antivenom therapy requires aggressive medical management. A recipient of antivenom should be pretreated with 50 to 100 mg of IV diphenhydramine (1 mg/kg in children). After this, the initial dose of antivenom is administered at a rate no faster than one vial each 5 minutes. If no allergic manifestation ensues, the antivenom can be administered at a more rapid rate. If signs of anaphylaxis develop, usually heralded by an urticarial eruption or pruritus, 0.1- to 0.2-mL aliquots of antivenom should be alternated with 3- to 10-mL (0.03- to 0.1-mg) IV doses of aqueous epinephrine 1:100,000 (infused over 5 to 10 minutes). Alternatively, an epinephrine drip may be prepared as discussed in Chapter 67. The victim should be managed in an intensive care unit, with electrocardiographic and blood pressure monitoring. The dose of epinephrine should not elevate the pulse rate to greater than 150 beats/min. The administration of IV epinephrine may cause transient hypokalemia as potassium is driven intracellularly; cessation of the epinephrine infusion may create transient hyperkalemia as the potassium regains entry into the extracellular space. If a victim is highly allergic to antivenom, serious consideration should be given to supportive therapy (including hemodialysis) without antivenom administration.

In one series, stonefish antivenom was administered to 24 victims in a dose of one or two ampules by the intramuscular (IM) route, without any "immediate reactions" reported.[198] In this same report, six victims received box-jellyfish antivenom by the IV route without immediate or delayed reactions. Anecdotal reports indicate that box-jellyfish antivenom has been administered by the IM route in the field more than 90 times to date without any episode of anaphylaxis.

SERUM SICKNESS

The formation of IgG antibodies in response to antigens present in antivenom (prepared in heterologous serum) results in the deposition of immune complexes in many tissue sites, notably in the walls of blood vessels. These complexes induce vascular permeability, activate the complement cascade and chemotactic factors, degranulate mast cells, and trigger the release of proteolytic enzymes. Decreased levels of C_3 and C_4 are accompanied by increased C_{3a}/C_{3a} des-arginine, a split product C_3.[74,112] Although immune complexes can be measured by various tests (Raji cell IgG assay and C_{1q}-binding assay), levels of immune complexes may not correlate with the clinical presentation.[74,147] Cutaneous venulitis may precede vasculitis. Dermal biopsy of lesional skin may reveal leukocytoclastic vasculitis.

Symptoms are generally present within 8 to 24 days and include fever, arthralgias, malaise, urticaria, lymphadenopathy, urticarial and morbilliform skin rashes, peripheral neuritis, and swollen joints. It is not uncommon for the primary urticarial lesion to be noted at the injection site. Serum sickness is managed with administration of corticosteroids. An initial loading dose of prednisone (40 to 60 mg for adults, and 2 to 5 mg/kg, not to exceed 50 mg, for children) should be administered and maintained daily until symptoms markedly resolve. The corticosteroid should be tapered over a 2- to 3-week course to avoid induction of adrenal insufficiency. Aspirin or other nonsteroidal antiinflammatory agents are rarely helpful and may be contraindicated because of circulating immune complex–induced platelet dysfunction.

PHYLUM PORIFERA
SPONGES
Life and Habits

There are approximately 5000 species of sponges (phylum Porifera, predominantly of class Demospongiae), which are supported by horny, but elastic, internal collagenous skeletons of spongin, some forms of which we use as bath sponges. Sponges are without digestive, excretory, respiratory, endocrine, circulatory, and nervous systems. Embedded in the connective tissue matrices and skeletons are spicules of silicon dioxide (silica) or calcium carbonate (calcite), by which some sponges can be definitively identified. In general, sponges are stationary acellular animals that attach to the sea floor or coral beds and may be colonized by other sponges, hydrozoans, mollusks, cnidarians, annelids, crustaceans, echinoderms, fish, and algae. These secondary cnidarian inhabitants are responsible for the dermatitis and local necrotic skin reaction termed *sponge diver's disease (maladie des plongeurs)*.[192] In recognition of a medicinal property, the ancient Greeks burned sea sponges and inhaled the vapors for prophylaxis against goiter.[49] Sponges harbor various biodynamic substances, with possible antineoplastic, antibacterial, growth-stimulating, antihypertensive, neuropharmacologic, psychopharmacologic, and antifungal properties. A number of sponges produce crinotoxins that may be direct dermal irritants, such as subcritine, halitoxin (*Haliclona* species), *p*-hydroxybenzaldehyde, and okadaic acid. These may be present in surface or internal secretions. Murine monoclonal antibodies against okadaic acid intended for use in an assay system for the detection of diarrhetic shellfish poisoning have been prepared from the sponge *Halichondria okadai*.[209] The causative agent of Dogger Bank itch, (2-hydroxyethyl) dimethylsulfoxonium chloride, has been isolated from the marine sponge *Theonella aff. mirabilis*.[215]

Clinical Aspects

Two general syndromes, with variations, are induced by contact with sponges. The first is a pruritic dermatitis similar to plant-induced allergic dermatitis, although the dermatopathic agent has not been identified. Rarely, erythema multiforme or an anaphylactoid reaction may be present. A typical offender is the friable Hawaiian (Figure 74-1) or West Indian fire sponge (*Tedania ignis*), a brilliant yellow-vermilion-orange (Figure 74-2) or reddish-brown organism with a crumb-of-bread appearance

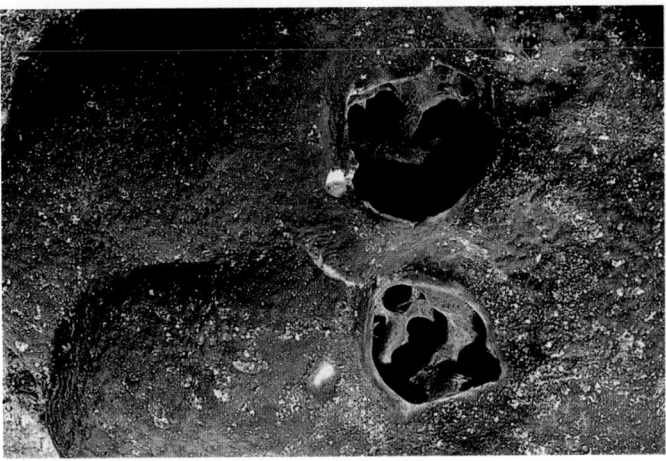

FIGURE 74-1 Pacific fire sponge. *(From Norbert Wu, with permission: norbertwu.com.)*

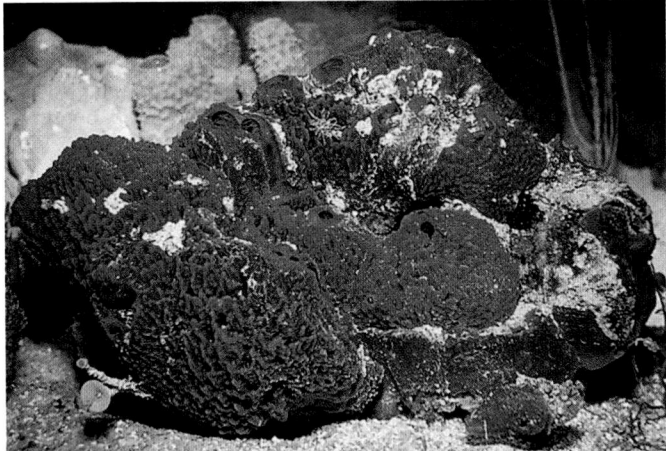

FIGURE 74-2 Atlantic fire sponge. *(Courtesy Dee Scarr.)*

found off the Hawaiian Islands and the Florida Keys.[180,189] Other "fire sponges" have a similar appearance (Figure 74-3). This sponge grows in thick branches, which extend from a larger base and are easily broken off. Other culprits include *Fibula* (or *Neofibularia*) *nolitangere,* the poison bun sponge (Figure 74-4) (and the related sponge *Neofibularia mordens*), and *Microciona*

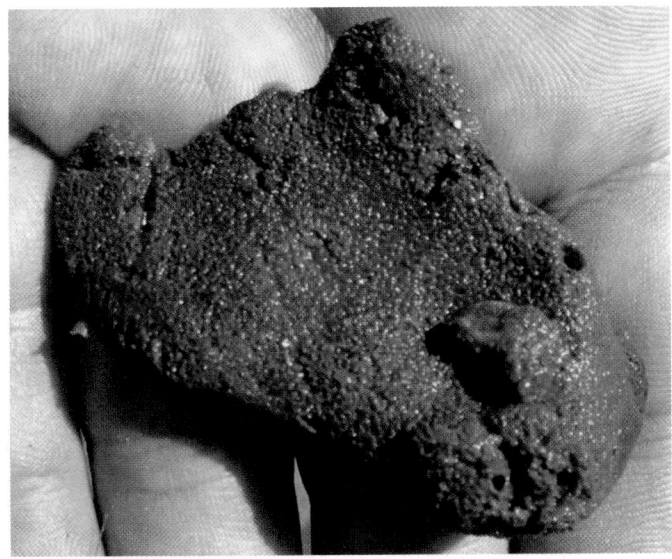

FIGURE 74-3 Fire sponge. *(Courtesy Vidal Haddad, Jr.)*

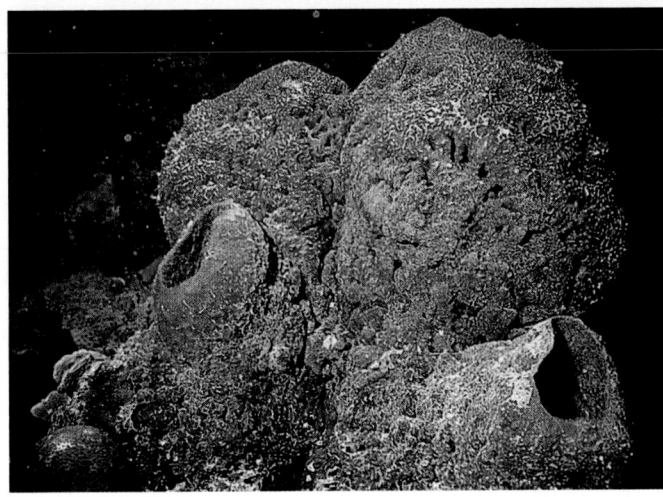

FIGURE 74-4 Poison bun sponge *Neofibularia nolitangere. (Courtesy Dee Scarr.)*

prolifera, the red moss sponge (found in the northeastern United States).[104] *F. nolitangere* is found in deeper water and grows in clusters, with holes (oscula) large enough to admit a diver's finger. It is brown (Figure 74-5) and bready in texture, so it may crumble in the hands.

Within a few hours after skin contact, but sometimes within 10 to 20 minutes, the reactions appear. They are characterized by itching and burning, which may progress to local joint swelling, soft tissue edema, vesiculation, and stiffness, particularly if small pieces of broken sponge are retained in the skin near the interphalangeal or metacarpophalangeal joint. Most victims of sponge-induced dermatitis have hand involvement, because they handled the sponges without proper gloves. In addition, abraded skin, such as that which has been scraped on stony coral, may allow more rapid or greater absorption of toxins.[173] When the sponge is penetrated, torn, or crumbled, the skin is exposed to the toxic substances. Untreated, mild reactions subside within 3 to 7 days. When large skin areas are involved, the victim may complain of fever, chills, malaise, dizziness, nausea, muscle cramps, and formication. Bullae induced by contact with *M. prolifera* may become purulent. Systemic erythema multiforme, dyshidrotic eczema, or an anaphylactoid reaction may develop 1 to 2 weeks after a severe exposure.[237] The skin may become mottled or purpuric, occasionally after a delay of up to 10 days.[189]

The second syndrome is irritant dermatitis and follows penetration of small spicules of silica or calcium carbonate into the skin. Most sponges have spicules; toxic sponges may possess crinotoxins that enter microtraumatic lesions caused by the spicules.

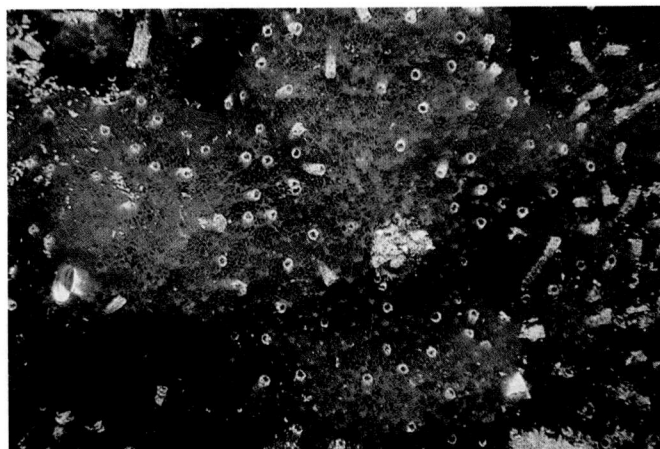

FIGURE 74-5 Crumb-of-bread appearance of poison bun sponge. *(Courtesy Dee Scarr.)*

In severe cases, surface desquamation of the skin may follow in 10 days to 2 months. No medical intervention can retard this process. Recurrent eczema and persistent arthralgias are rare complications.

Treatment

Because distinguishing clinically between the allergic and spicule-induced reactions is usually impossible, it is reasonable to treat for both. The skin should be gently dried. Spicules should be removed, if possible, using adhesive tape, a thin layer of rubber cement, or a facial peel. As soon as possible, dilute (5%) acetic acid (vinegar) soaks for 10 to 30 minutes 3 or 4 times a day should be applied to all affected areas.[189,193,236] Isopropyl alcohol (40% to 70%) is a reasonable second choice. Although topical steroid preparations may help relieve the secondary inflammation, they are of no value as an initial decontaminant. If they precede the vinegar soak, they may worsen the primary reaction. Delayed primary therapy or inadequate decontamination can result in the persistence of bullae, which may become purulent and require months to heal.

Erythema multiforme or dyshidrotic eczema may require administration of a systemic glucocorticoid, beginning with a moderately high dose (prednisone, 60 to 100 mg) tapered over 2 to 3 weeks. Anecdotal remedies for management of sponge envenomation that have been suggested without demonstration of efficacy include antiseptic dressings, broad-spectrum antibiotics, methdilazine, tripelennamine, phenobarbital, diphenhydramine, promethazine, and topical carbolic oil or zinc oxide cream.[189]

After the initial decontamination, a mild emollient cream or steroid preparation may be applied to the skin. If the allergic component is severe, particularly if there is weeping, crusting, and vesiculation, a systemic glucocorticoid (prednisone, 60 to 100 mg, tapered over 2 weeks) may be beneficial, as might a potent topical steroid preparation. Severe itching may be controlled with an antihistamine.

Clostridium tetani has been cultured from sea sponges, so proper antitetanus immunization should be part of sponge dermatitis therapy. Frequent follow-up wound checks are important because significant infections sometimes develop.[105] Infected wounds should be cultured and managed with antibiotics (see Chapter 73). Because of infection risk, sponges should not be used to pack wounds. If sponge poisoning induces an anaphylactoid reaction, standard resuscitation using epinephrine, bronchodilators, corticosteroids, and antihistamines should be undertaken.[237]

As mentioned previously, sponge diver's disease is not caused by any toxin produced by the sponge, but rather, is a stinging syndrome related to contact with the tentacles of the small anemone *Sagartia rosea* (family Sagartiidae) or anemones from the genus *Actinia* (family Actiniidae) that attach to the base of the sponge. Treatment should include that for cnidarian envenomation (see below).

Prevention

All divers and net handlers should wear proper gloves. Sponges should not be broken, crumbled, or crushed with bare hands. If the victim brings a specimen, the physician should take care to document its appearance. Dried sponges may remain toxic.

PHYLUM CNIDARIA

The phylum Cnidaria (previously called coelenterates [hollow gut]) contains an enormous group of approximately 10,000 species, at least 100 of which are dangerous to humans. Only members of the phylum Cnidaria (sometimes referred to as cnidarians) produce the capsule commonly called a cnida (also called cnidocyst).[55] The word *cnida* is derived from the Greek word κνίδη, which means "nettle." For practical purposes the cnidarians can be divided into four main groups: (1) hydrozoans, including hydroids, fire corals, and creatures such as the Portuguese man-of-war; (2) scyphozoans, such as true jellyfish; (3) anthozoans, such as soft corals (alcyonarians), stony corals, sea pens, and anemones; and (4) cubozoans, such as box-jellies.

Gorgonians (order Gorgonacea, class Anthozoa, subclass Alcyonaria) secrete mucinous exudates having toxic effects in experimental animals that can be characterized as hemolytic, proteolytic, cholinergic, histaminergic, serotonergic, and adrenergic.[71] Fenner divides jellyfish into three main classes: scyphozoans (true jellyfish), with tentacles arising at regular intervals around the bell; cubozoans (e.g., box-jellyfish), with tentacles arising only from the corners (and these may be further divided into carybdeids [e.g., Irukandji jellyfish], with only one tentacle [except in rare cases] arising from each lower corner of the bell, and chirodropids, which have more than one tentacle in each corner of the bell); and other jellyfish, such as members of the hydrozoans (e.g., *Physalia* species).

MORPHOLOGY, VENOM, AND VENOM APPARATUS

Cnidarians are carnivorous predators that feed on other fish, crustaceans, and mollusks. They are radially symmetric animals of simple structure (95% water) and exist in two predominant life forms—either sedentary, asexual polyps (hydroids) or free-swimming and sexual medusae. They are the lowest form of life organized into different layers.[173] Generally, the polyps are sac-like creatures attached to the substrate at the caudal (aboral) end, with a single orifice or mouth at the upper end surrounded by stinging tentacles (dactylozooids). This form predominates in the hydrozoans and anthozoans. The medusa is a bell-shaped creature, with a floating gelatinous umbrella from which hang an elongated tubular mouth and marginal nematocyst-bearing tentacles. This form predominates in the scyphozoans and is also found in the hydrozoans.

Cnidocytes (include nematocytes, spirocytes, and ptychocytes) are mature living cells that encapsulate the nonliving intracytoplasmic capsules called cnidae (or cnidocysts: include nematocysts, spirocysts, and ptychocysts), within which are found the stinging apparatus. Cnidae are secreted by the Golgi apparatus of cells (cnidoblasts: include nematoblasts, spiroblasts, and pychoblasts) specialized for this function. Nematocysts are initially found in differentiating clusters. After differentiation into the different types of capsules, the clusters break up to allow single nematocytes to migrate to tentacles, where they become mounted in specialized tentacle epithelial cells, called battery cells.[200] The nematocytes are located on the outer epithelial surfaces of the tentacles (Figure 74-6) or near the mouth and are triggered by contact with the victim's body surface. The nematocyst is contained within the cnidoblast, to which is attached a single pointed "trigger," or cnidocil. The undischarged nematocyst (3 to 100 μm in diameter) varies in shape and is under high osmotic pressure created during capsule morphogenesis by synthesis of poly-γ-glutamate in the capsule matrix. Minicollagen networks determine the structure of the nematocyst wall.[46] The nematocyst contains a hollow, sharply pointed, coiled, or folded "thread" tubule (nema) (Figure 74-7). This tubule may attain

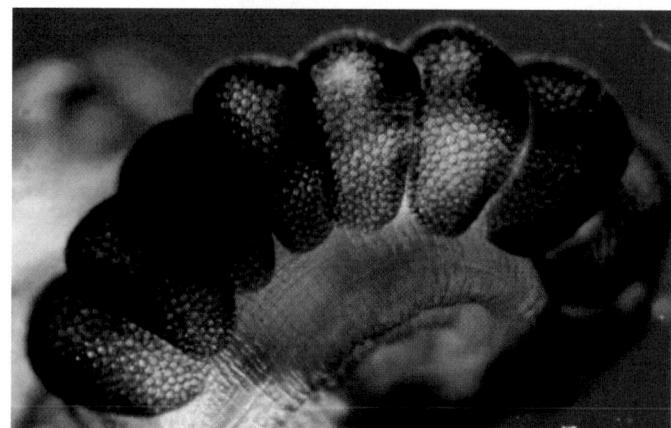

FIGURE 74-6 Unfired nematocysts on a *Physalia* tentacle. *(Courtesy Peter Parks.)*

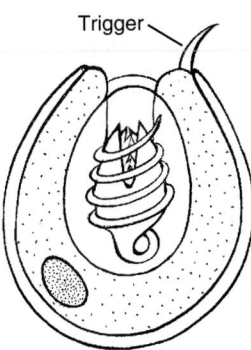

FIGURE 74-7 Nematocyst before discharge.

lengths of 200 to 850 μm and is sufficiently hardy to penetrate a surgical glove. The tubule is initially formed outside the capsule and then invaginates within the wall, so that in the undischarged state, the toxin is located in the folds and invaginations of the tubule's membrane. This membrane hardens via disulfide bond isomerization to form bridges between minicollagen peptides as the capsule attains its final size.[200]

The tubule is lined with hollow barbs, which help it penetrate and anchor into the victim. In the undischarged state, the barbs occupy the lumen of the twisted and folded tubule. When the cnidocil is stimulated, either by physical contact or by a chemoreceptor mechanism, it causes the opening of a trapdoor (operculum) in the cnidoblast, and the venom-bearing tubule is everted (Figure 74-8) within 3 μsec. This exocytosis has been hypothesized to occur because of osmotic swelling of the capsular matrix caused by high concentration of poly-γ-glutamate, influx of water (leading to a hydrostatic pressure of up to 150 atm), release of intrinsic tensile forces (up to 375 MPa on the inner capsule wall), or deformation of the wall-induced internal pressure.[91,92,200] The sharp tip of the thread tube enters the victim's skin (Figures 74-9 and 74-10), and envenomation occurs as toxin is translocated by hydrostatic forces from the surface of the everted and extended tubule through the now helically arranged (Figure 74-11) and extended hollow barbs.[121,122] It has been estimated that the velocity of ejection attains 2 m/sec, which corresponds to an acceleration of 40,000 g, with an estimated skin striking force of 2 to 5 psi.[53] This is one of the most rapid mechanical events found in nature. A human encounter with a large Portuguese man-of-war could conceivably trigger the release of several million stinging cells (Figure 74-12). It has been estimated that more than

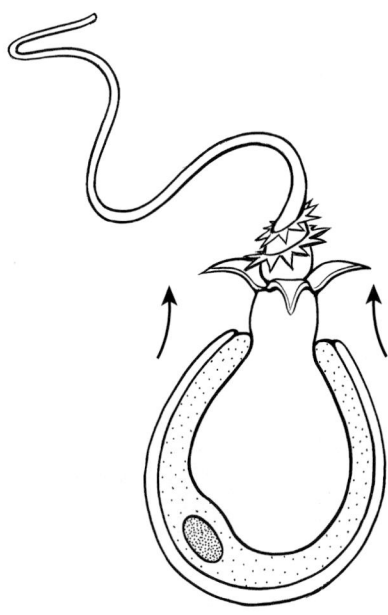

FIGURE 74-8 Nematocyst after discharge.

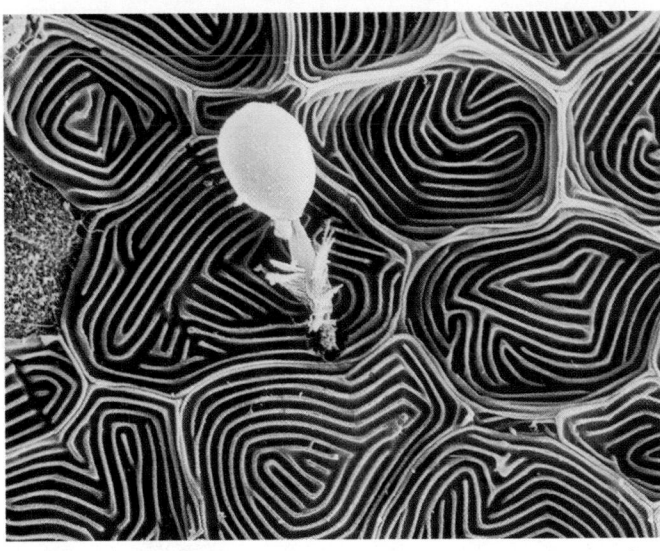

FIGURE 74-9 Discharged nematocyst that penetrated human skin. *(Scanning electron micrograph by Thomas Heeger, MD.)*

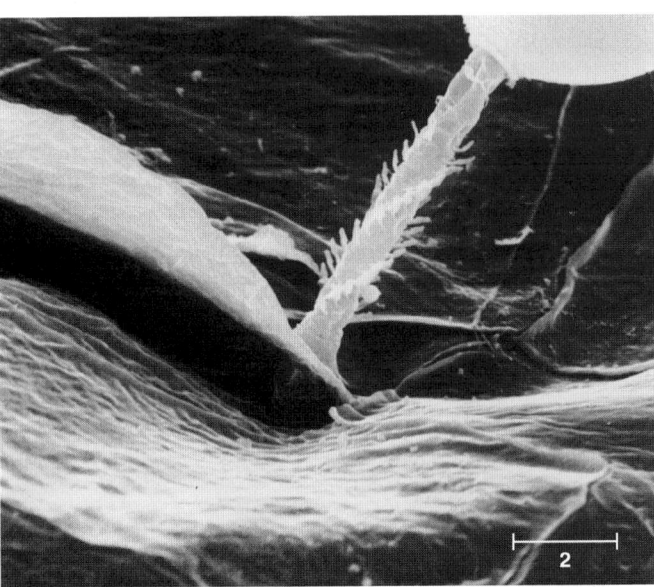

FIGURE 74-10 An everted tubule of a nematocyst from a lion's mane jellyfish *(Cyanea capillata)* has entered the skin and has lifted an epithelial cell. *(Scanning electron micrograph by Thomas Heeger, MD.)*

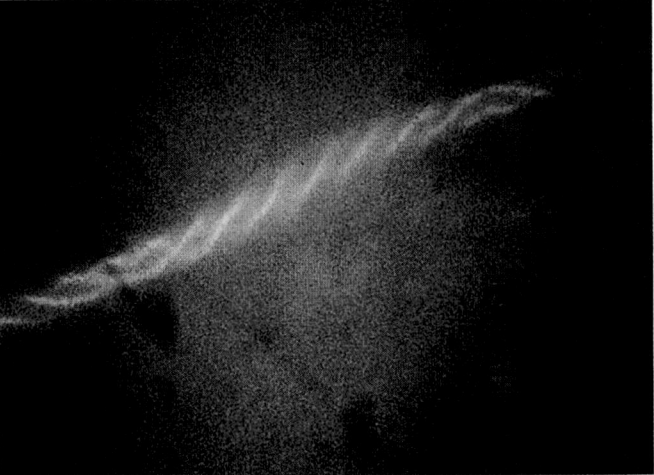

FIGURE 74-11 Helical arrangement of barbs on the tubule of a nematocyst. *(Courtesy Amit Lotan.)*

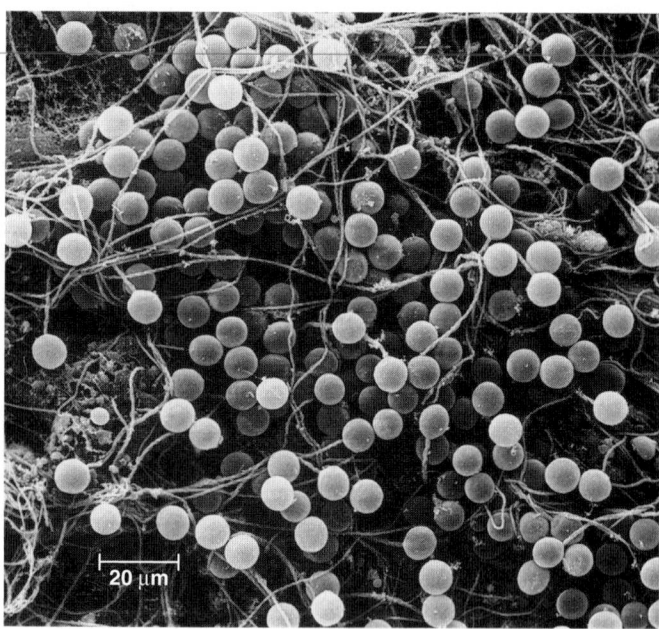

FIGURE 74-12 Nematocysts of a jellyfish (*Versuriga anadyomene*, Philippines), mostly discharged as seen by everted tubules. *(Scanning electron micrograph by Thomas Heeger, MD.)*

In the case of the Indo-Pacific box-jellyfish *C. fleckeri*, which may carry up to 59 tentacles bearing millions of nematocysts, it is the cigar-shaped microbasic p-mastigophores that are most important in human envenomation (Figure 74-13). The capsule of the structure holds a hollow coiled tube and granular matrix. The thread tube has a thick butt end that is attached to the operculum. The tube contains three rows of helically arranged spines. When the nematocyst fires into the human victim, the tube everts through the opercular end of the nematocyst, with the butt anchoring first to keep the nematocyst adherent to the victim. The thread then everts through the hollow butt and uncoils, presenting the spines and accompanying toxins to the living tissue. Although the major toxic fractions appear to be present in the nematocysts, there appears to be toxic material present in tentacles denuded of such organelles.[23] The largest nematocysts of *C. fleckeri* can penetrate human skin to a depth of 0.9 mm.[139]

Cnidarian venoms are viscous mixtures of proteins, carbohydrates, and other nonproteinaceous components. Although they are heat labile in vitro, this does not seem to apply in the clinical setting. To date, they have been difficult to fractionate. The primary difficulties encountered in jellyfish venom purification have been lack of stability and tendency of active toxins to adhere to each other and to support matrices.[156] Lyophilized crude venom can be prepared in water by homogenization, sonication, and rapid freeze-thawing. A second technique consists of grinding samples with a glass mortar and pestle and using phosphate-buffered saline. This has been done to prepare crude venom from isolated nematocysts of the box-jellyfish, the bells of Irukandji jellyfish, and the oral lobes of blubber jellyfish.[227] Analyses of Western blot tests showed that box-jellyfish antivenom reacted specifically with the venom of each jellyfish, but there is not yet any clinical significance to this observation. Because toxicity was found in the Irukandji jellyfish venom derived by the mortar-and-pestle method, but not by the lyophilization method, the former was deemed the more efficacious method. Within box-jellyfish venom are protein components ranging from 18 to more than 106 kDa.

2000 sting penetrations can occur within a single square millimeter of skin. The threads penetrate the epidermis and upper dermis, where the venom diffuses into the general circulation. The agitated victim moves about and assists the venom's distribution by the muscle-pump mechanism. On the basis of mouse studies, it appears that the rapid death of a victim is related to the venom that is discharged directly into capillaries, as opposed to that which must diffuse from the dermis into the bloodstream.

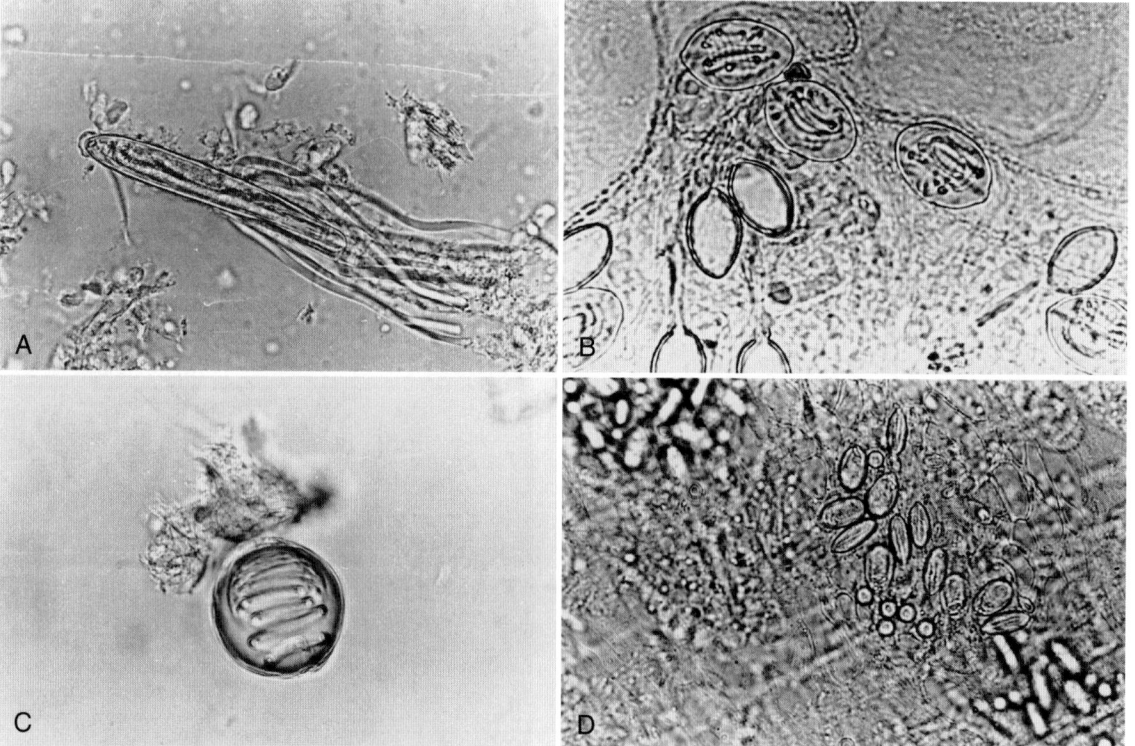

FIGURE 74-13 Nematocyst identification guide. **A,** Microbasic p-mastigophore (undischarged) of *Chironex fleckeri.* Capsule length, 75 µm. **B,** Same (discharged and undischarged) of Irukandji. **C,** Isorhiza (undischarged) of bluebottle (*Physalia physalis*). **D,** Clustered isorhizas and euryteles on tentacle of "hair jelly" (*Cyanea*). *(Courtesy Bob Hartwick.)*

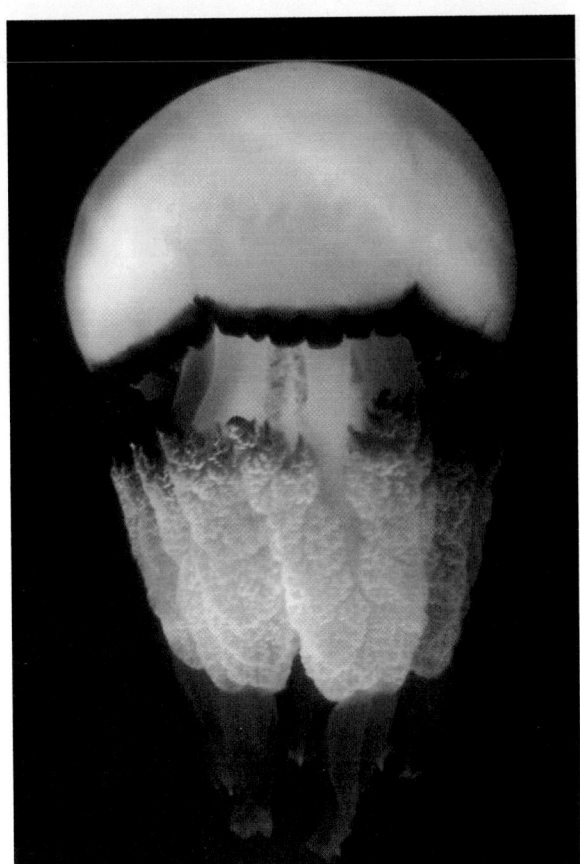

FIGURE 74-14 Rhizostome medusa, *Rhizostoma pulmo* (Mediterranean Sea). *(Courtesy Thomas Heeger, MD.)*

Cytolytic toxins have been characterized from *Physalia physalis*, *Rhizostoma pulmo* (Figure 74-14), *C. fleckeri,* and *Carybdea marsupialis*. Hemolytic activity, phospholipase A$_2$, and α-chymotrypsin–like serine protease activity have been noted in the venom of *Rhopilema nomadica*.[80] Many jellyfish and marine animal venoms generate autonomic neurotoxicity.[36] This may be a result of their ability to affect ion transport (sodium and calcium in particular), induce channels or pores in nerve and muscle cell membranes, alter membrane configurations, and release mediators of inflammation. Cnidarian venoms can target the myocardium, Purkinje fibers, atrioventricular node, and aortic ring, as well as injure the hepatic P-450 enzyme family.

Freshwater jellyfish, such as the Appalachian mountain jellyfish *Craspedacusta sowerbyi,* do not appear to pose a hazard to humans.

CNIDARIAN SYNDROME

Clinical Aspects

For clinical purposes, a considerable phylogenetic relationship exists among all stinging species, so that the clinical features of the cnidarian syndrome are fairly constant, with a spectrum of severity. The severity is related to the season and species (venom potency and configuration of the nematocyst), number of nematocysts triggered and size of the animal (venom inoculum), size and age of the victim (the very young and old and the smaller person tend to be more severely affected), location and surface area of the sting, and health of the victim. The wise clinician suspects a cnidarian envenomation in all unexplained cases of collapse in the surf, diving accidents, and near-drownings. Any victim in distress pulled from marine waters should be carefully examined for one or more cutaneous lesions that may provide the clue to a cnidarian envenomation.

Mild envenomation may result in only an annoying dermatitis, whereas severe envenomation can progress rapidly to involve virtually every organ system, resulting in significant rates of morbidity and mortality. Clinical envenomation is described here by severity, with the understanding that there is a fair amount of overlap. In the following paragraphs, syndromes associated with specific classes of creatures are discussed in greater detail.

Mild Envenomation. The stings caused by the hydroids and hydroid corals, along with lesser envenomations by *Physalia, Velella velella* (Figure 74-15), *Drymonema dalmatinum* (stinging cauliflower), *Olindias sambaquiensis* (Figure 74-16) (known as *relojinho* in Portuguese; endemic to the Blanca Bay area south of Buenos Aires province and found on the southeastern Brazilian coast) (Figure 74-17), scyphozoans, and anemones, result predominantly in skin irritation.[82,106] *Nemopilema nomurai (echizen kurage)* is a large stinging jellyfish, with a maximum bell size of 2 m and weight of 200 kg, that blooms in the orient.[98] There is usually an immediate pricking or stinging sensation, accompanied by pruritus, paresthesias, burning, throbbing, and radiation of the pain centrally from the extremities to the groin, abdomen, and axillae. The area involved by the nematocysts becomes red-brown-purple, often in a linear whiplike fashion, corresponding to tentacle prints (Figures 74-18 and 74-19). Other features are blistering, local edema, angioedema, and wheal formation (Figures 74-20 to 74-23), as well as violaceous petechial hemorrhages. Dyspnea due to upper airway obstruction associated with severe facial swelling is possible.[5] The papular inflammatory skin rash is strictly confined to areas of contact and may persist for up to 10 days. Areas of body hair appear to be somewhat more protected from contact than hairless areas. If envenomation is slightly more severe, the aforementioned symptoms, which are evident in the first few hours, can progress over a course of days to local necrosis, skin ulceration, and secondary infection. This is particularly true of stings from certain anemone (*Sagartia, Actinia, Anemonia, Actinodendron,* and *Triactis*). A painless "jellyfish sting," in which there is a pattern of hyperpigmented linear streaks, might represent phytophotodermatitis (e.g., from citrus juice spilled on skin and later exposed to light).[21]

Untreated, the minor to moderate skin disorder resolves over 1 to 2 weeks, with occasional residual hyperpigmentation for 1 to 2 months. Rubbing can cause lichenification. Local hyperhidrosis, fat atrophy, and contracture may occur.[27] Mondor's disease of the breast has been reported following jellyfish stings.[94] Facial swelling with sterile abscess formation has been reported.[201] Permanent scarring or keloids may result. Persistent papules or plaques at the sites of contact may demonstrate a predominantly mononuclear cell inflammatory infiltrate, which may represent a delayed hypersensitivity response to an antigenic component of the cnidarian nematocyst or venom. This may be accompanied by localized arthritis and joint effusion. It has been suggested that sensitization may occur without a definite history of a previous sting, because cnidarians may release antigenic and allergenic venom components into the water. Granuloma annulare, which is usually both a sporadic and familial inflammatory

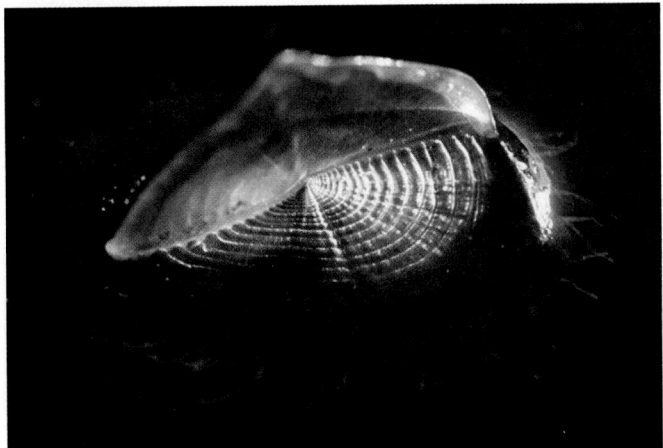

FIGURE 74-15 By-the-wind sailor, *Velella velella. (From Norbert Wu, with permission: norbertwu.com.)*

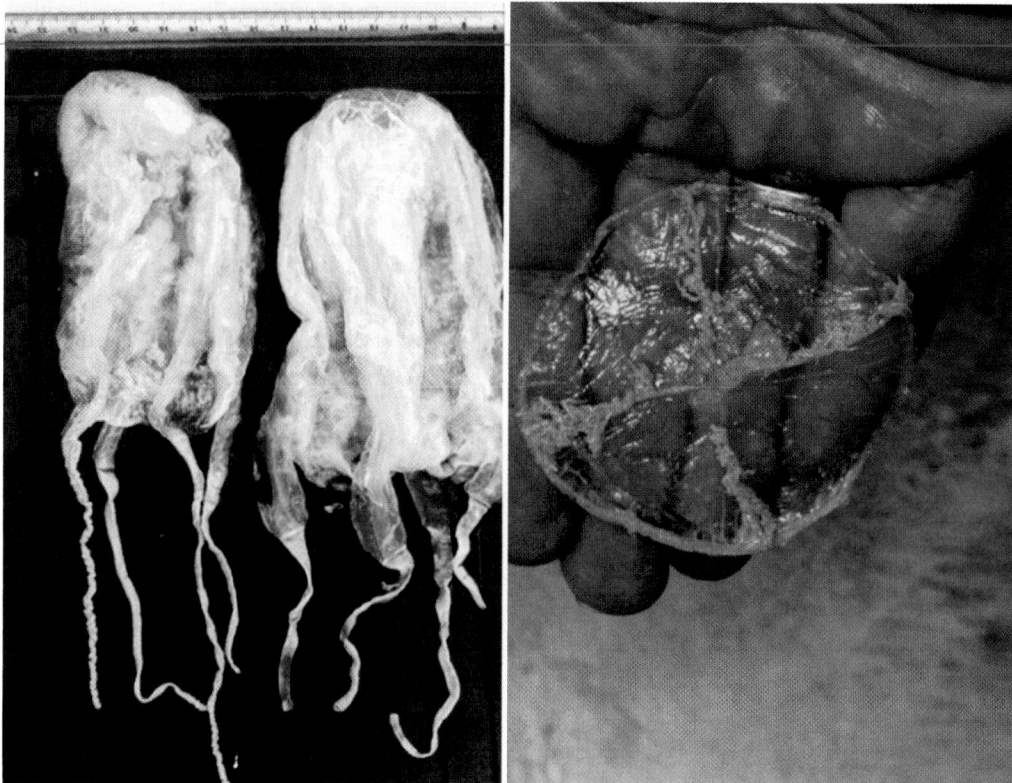

FIGURE 74-16 *Tamoya* and *Olindias* species jellyfishes. *(Courtesy Vidal Haddad, Jr.)*

dermatosis, has been associated with *Physalia utriculus* envenomation.[128] Gangrene has been observed.

Moderate and Severe Envenomation. The prime offenders in this group are the anemones, *Physalia* species, and scyphozoans. The skin manifestations are similar or intensified (as with *Chironex*) and compounded by the onset of systemic symptoms, which may appear immediately or be delayed by several hours:

Neurologic: Malaise, headache, aphonia, diminished touch and temperature sensation, vertigo, ataxia, spastic or flaccid paralysis, mononeuritis multiplex, Guillain-Barré syndrome, parasympathetic dysautonomia, plexopathy, radial-ulnar-median nerve palsies, brainstem infarction (not a confirmed relationship), delirium, loss of consciousness, convulsions, coma, and death[28,39,65,140,160]

Cardiovascular: Anaphylaxis, hemolysis, hypotension, small artery spasm, bradyarrhythmias (including electromechanical dissociation and asystole), tachyarrhythmias, elevated serum troponin I level in the absence of myocardial injury, vascular spasm, deep venous thrombosis, thrombophlebitis, acute myocardial infarction, congestive heart failure, and ventricular fibrillation[87,133,176]

Respiratory: Rhinitis, bronchospasm, laryngeal edema, dyspnea, cyanosis, pulmonary edema, and respiratory failure

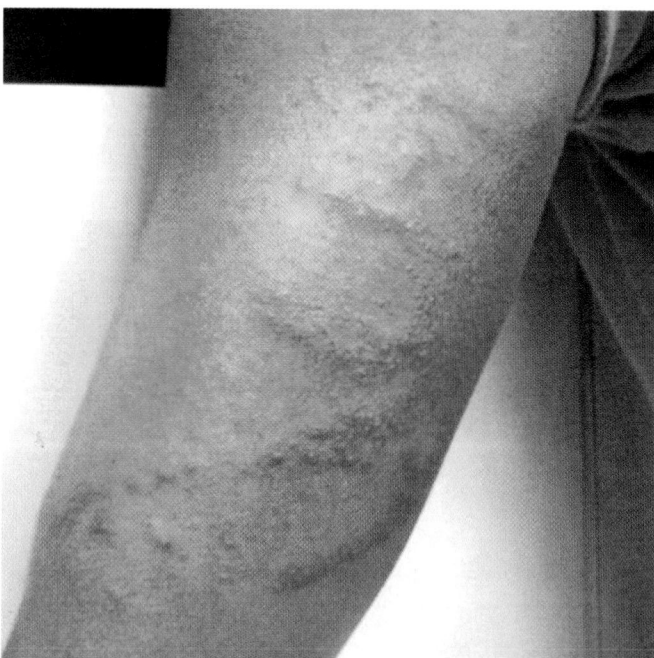

FIGURE 74-17 Skin irritation from sting of *Olindias* species. *(Courtesy Vidal Haddad, Jr.)*

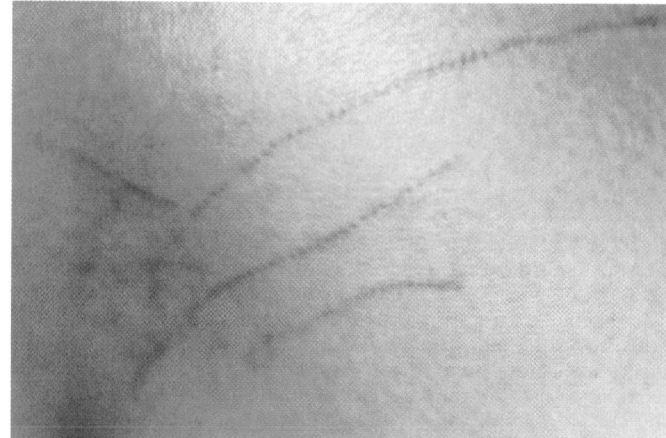

FIGURE 74-18 Telltale *Physalia* species sting pattern. *(Courtesy Vidal Haddad, Jr.)*

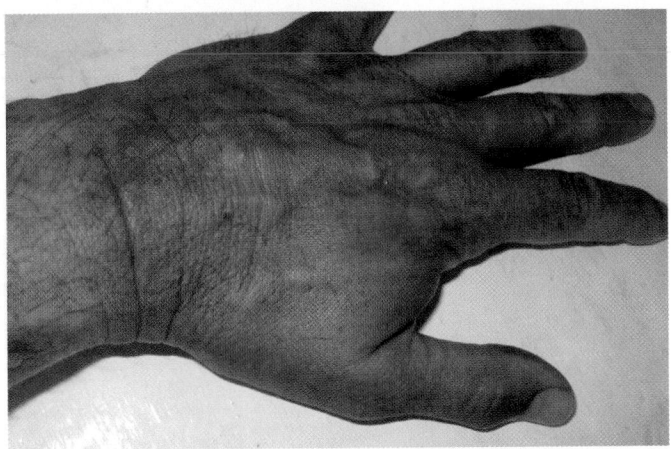

FIGURE 74-19 Man-of-war sting. *(Courtesy Paul S. Auerbach, MD.)*

Musculoskeletal or rheumatologic: Abdominal rigidity, diffuse myalgia and muscle cramps, muscle spasm, fat atrophy, arthralgias, reactive arthritis (seronegative symmetric synovitis with pitting edema),[217] and thoracolumbar pain

Gastrointestinal: Nausea, vomiting, diarrhea, paralytic ileus,[163] dysphagia, hypersalivation, and thirst

Ocular: Conjunctivitis, chemosis, corneal ulcers, corneal epithelial edema, keratitis, iridocyclitis, elevated intraocular pressure, synechiae, iris depigmentation, chronic unilateral glaucoma, and lacrimation[75,76,229]

Other: Acute renal failure, lymphadenopathy, chills, fever, and nightmares

The extreme example of envenomation occurs with *C. fleckeri*, the dreaded box-jellyfish. *Physalia* and anemone stings, although extremely painful, are rarely fatal. Death after *Physalia* stings has been attributed to primary respiratory failure or cardiac arrhythmia, which may have reflected an element of anaphylaxis.[32,194] Confirmed deaths after cnidaria envenomation have been attributed to *C. fleckeri, Chiropsalmus quadrigatus,* and *Chiropsalmus quadrumanus* (Figure 74-24).[139] *Stomolophus nomurai* (the sand jellyfish) has caused at least eight deaths in the South China Sea.[56] Although there have been other deaths, the animals have not been definitively identified.

Clinical reports and studies on the serologic response to jellyfish envenomation suggest that allergic reactions may play a significant pathophysiologic role in humans. When crude or

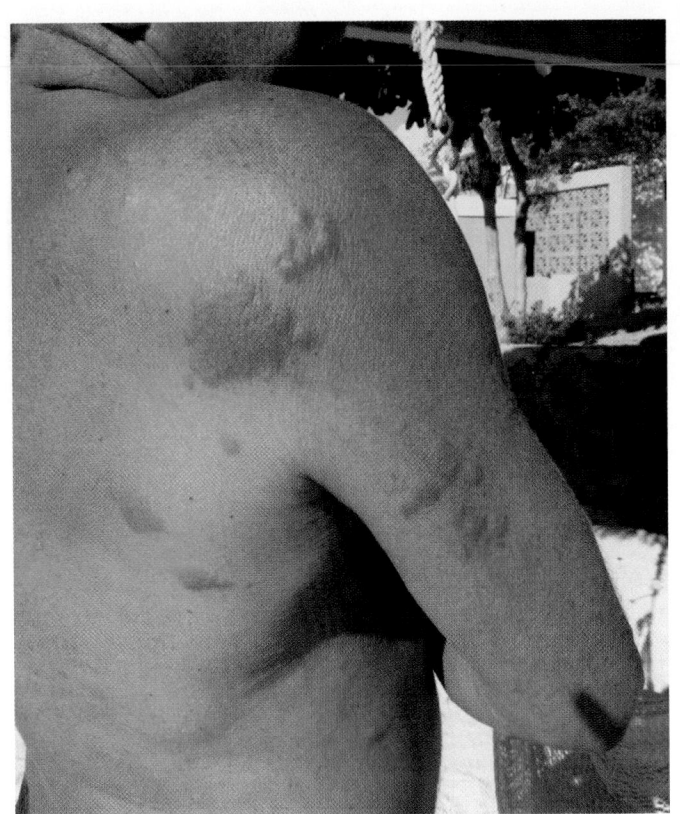

FIGURE 74-21 Jellyfish sting. *(Courtesy Paul S. Auerbach, MD.)*

partially purified nematocyst venom and an antigen are used in an enzyme-linked immunosorbent assay (ELISA), both IgG and IgE can be detected.[74,174] Elevated specific anti–jellyfish IgG and IgE may persist for several years, recurrence of the clinical cutaneous reaction to jellyfish stings may occur within a few weeks

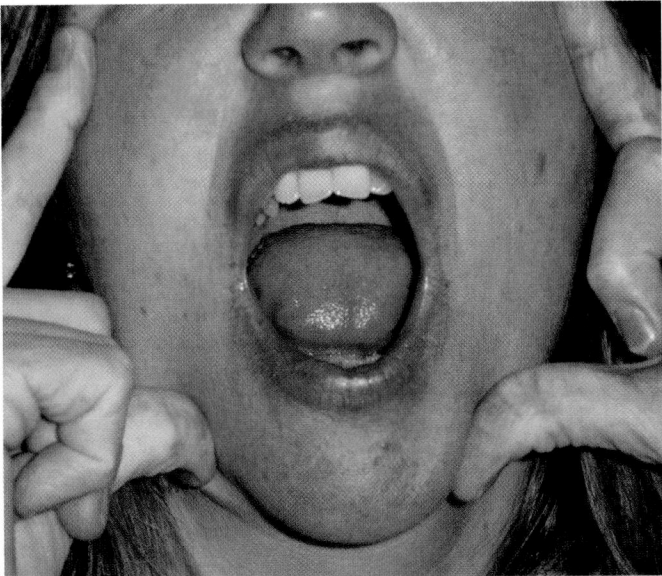

FIGURE 74-20 Jellyfish sting around the lips.

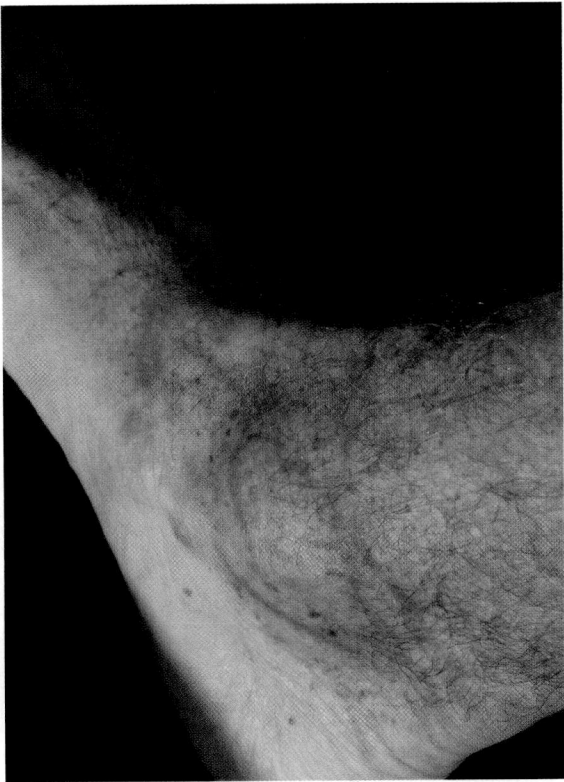

FIGURE 74-22 Jellyfish sting of the ankle. *(Copyright Stephen Frink.)*

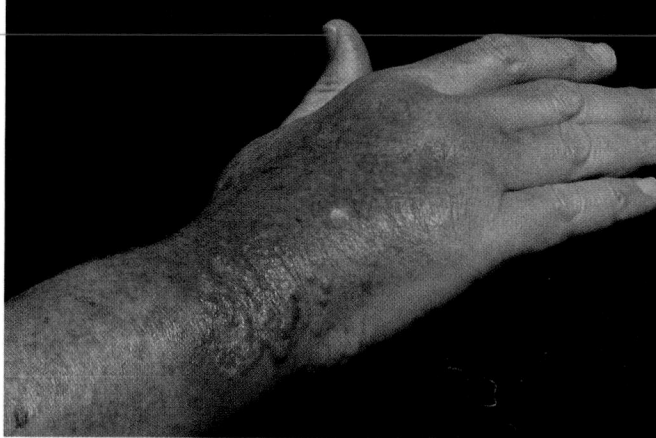

FIGURE 74-23 Severe jellyfish sting of the wrist. (Copyright Stephen Frink.)

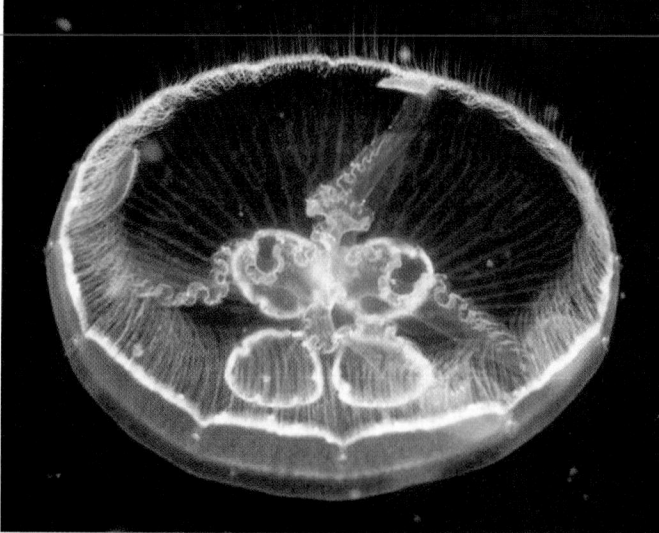

FIGURE 74-25 Moon jellyfish, *Aurelia aurita*. (From Norbert Wu, with permission: norbertwu.com.)

without additional contact with the tentacles, and serologic cross-reactivity occurs between the sea nettle (*Chrysaora quinquecirrha*) and *P. physalis*. In a case of significant envenomation by the moon jellyfish *Aurelia aurita* (Figure 74-25), the victim developed significant cross-reacting antibodies to *C. quinquecirrha* antigens.[31]

Persons with extracutaneous or anaphylactoid responses to a cnidarian sting have been noted to have higher specific IgG and IgE antibody levels.[174] However, elevated persistent specific anti–jellyfish serum IgG concentrations are not protective against the cutaneous pain resulting from a natural sting.[30] A false-positive ELISA serologic test to venom may occur, as demonstrated by negative skin testing.

A person stung by *P. physalis* may have recurrent cutaneous eruptions for 2 to 3 weeks after the initial episode, without repeated exposure to the animal. This may take the forms of lichenification, hyperhidrosis, angioedema, vesicles, large bullae, nodules that resemble erythema nodosum, granuloma annulare, or a more classic linear urticarial eruption.[8,29,129] Recurrent eruptions have also followed a solitary envenomation by the cnidarian *Stomolophus meleagris*.[26] In a histologic study of delayed reaction to a Mediterranean Sea cnidarian, skin biopsy demonstrated grouping of human leukocyte antigen–DR-positive cells with Langerhans cells and helper/inducer T lymphocytes, which indicates the possibility of a type IV immunoreaction.[162]

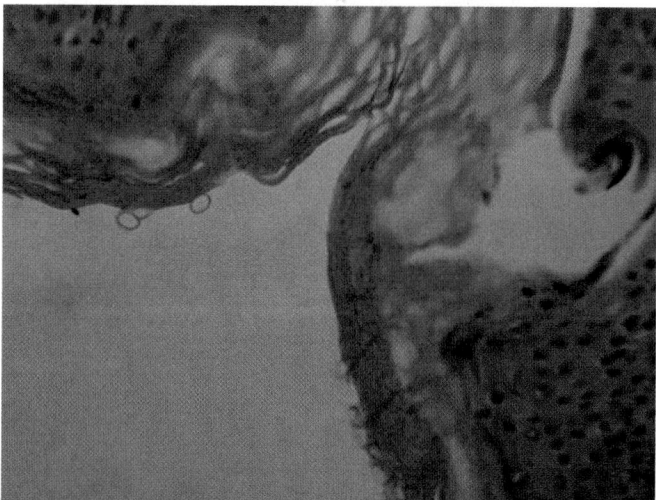

FIGURE 74-24 Skin biopsy from a child after fatal sting from *Chironex fleckeri*. Nematocysts are seen on the skin. (Courtesy Jamie Seymour, MD.)

Venom-specific IgG antibodies appear to persist for longer periods than IgM antibodies. The binding of brown recluse spider venom and purified cholera toxin to anti-*Chrysaora* and anti-*Physalia* monoclonal antibodies indicates that there may be a common or cross-reacting antigenic site or sites between these toxic substances and certain cnidarian venoms.[154]

Acute regional vascular insufficiency of the upper extremity has been reported after jellyfish envenomation. It can be manifested by acral ischemia, signs and symptoms of compartment syndrome, and massive edema.[222]

Treatment

Therapy is directed at stabilizing major systemic decompensation, opposing the venom's multiple effects, and alleviating pain. The following is a generalized overview; treatment related to the specific class of organism is discussed in detail in later paragraphs.

Systemic Envenomation. Generally, only severe *Physalia* or Cubomedusae stings result in rapid decompensation. In both cases, supportive care is based on the signs and symptoms. Hypotension should be managed with prompt IV administration of crystalloid, such as lactated Ringer's solution or normal saline. This must be done in concert with detoxification of any nematocysts (particularly those of *Chironex* or *Chiropsalmus*) that are still attached to the victim, to limit perpetuation of envenomation. Hypotension is usually limited to very young or older adult victims who suffer severe and multiple stings, the effects of which are worsened by fluid depletion that accompanies protracted vomiting. Hypertension is an occasional side effect of a cubomedusan envenomation, such as that of the Irukandji *Carukia barnesi*. Excessive catecholamine stimulation is one putative cause, which has prompted clinical intervention with benzodiazepines, magnesium, and phentolamine, an α-adrenergic blocking agent (5 mg intravenously as an initial dose, followed by an infusion of up to 10 mg/hr). Bronchospasm may be managed as an allergic component. If the victim is in respiratory distress with wheezing, shortness of breath, or heart failure, supplemental oxygen administration will be necessary by face mask or a continuous positive airway pressure/bilevel positive airway pressure (CPAP/BiPAP) circuit. Arterial blood gas measurement may be used to guide oxygen therapy. Seizures are generally self-limited but should be managed with IV diazepam for 24 to 48 hours, after which time they rarely recur.

Any victim with a systemic component should be observed for a period of at least 6 to 8 hours, because rebound phenomena after successful treatment are not uncommon. All older adult victims should undergo electrocardiography and be observed on a cardiac monitor, with frequent checks for arrhythmias. Urinalysis demonstrates the presence or absence of hemoglobinuria, indicating hemolysis after the putative attachment of *Physalia* venom to red blood cell membrane glycoprotein sites.[79] If this is the case, the victim's urine should be alkalinized with bicarbonate to prevent precipitation of pigment in the renal tubules, while moderate diuresis (30 to 50 mL/hr) is maintained with a loop diuretic (such as furosemide or bumetanide) or mannitol (0.25 g/kg intravenously every 8 to 12 hours). In rare instances of acute progressive renal failure, peritoneal dialysis or hemodialysis may be necessary.

If there are signs of distal ischemia or an impending compartment syndrome, standard diagnostic and therapeutic measures apply. These include Doppler ultrasound or angiography, or both, for diagnosis; regional thrombolysis for acutely occluded blood vessels; measurement of intracompartmental tissue pressures to guide fasciotomy; and so forth. Reversible regional sympathetic blockade may be efficacious if vasospasm is a dominant clinical feature. However, vasospasm associated with a jellyfish envenomation may be severe, prolonged, and refractory to regional sympathectomy and intraarterial reserpine or pentoxifylline.[1]

A small child may pick up tentacle fragments on the beach and place them into his or her mouth, resulting in rapid intraoral swelling and potential airway obstruction, particularly in the presence of exceptional hypersensitivity. In such cases, an endotracheal tube should be placed before edema precludes visualization of the vocal cords. In no case should any liquid be placed in the mouth if the airway is not protected. In 1999, a lifeguard in Cairns, Australia, drank from a container containing 4-day-old *C. fleckeri* tentacles. He fortunately suffered only a sore throat and transient shortness of breath.

C. fleckeri, the box-jellyfish, produces the only cnidarian venom for which a specific antidote exists (see below). To date, the venoms of *Physalia* and *Chrysaora* species have not been sufficiently purified as antigens to permit the production of an antitoxin. Antivenom administration should accompany the first-aid protocol previously described.

Pain Control. Often, mild pain can be controlled by treating the dermatitis. However, if pain is severe and there is no contraindication (such as head injury, altered mental status, respiratory depression, allergy, or profound hypotension), administration of a narcotic (fentanyl 50 to 100 mcg intravenously; morphine sulfate 2 to 10 mg intravenously; hydromorphone 1 to 2 mg intravenously) will be appreciated by the victim. Severe muscle spasm has been empirically noted to respond to 10% calcium gluconate (5 to 10 mL intravenously by slow push), diazepam (5 to 10 mg intravenously), or methocarbamol (1 g, no faster than 100 mg/min through a widely patent IV line).

Treatment of Dermatitis. If a person is stung by a cnidarian, the following steps should be taken:

Immediately rinse the wound with seawater, not with freshwater. Do not rub the wound with a towel or with clothing to remove adherent tentacles. Nonforceful rinsing with fresh water or a rubbing variety of abrasion (the latter in the absence of simultaneous application of a decontaminant such as papain or vinegar) is felt to stimulate any nematocysts that have not already fired. Surf lifesavers (lifeguards) in the United States and Hawaii have reported that a hot shower applied with a forceful stream may decrease the pain of an envenomation. If this is successful, theoretical explanations are that the mechanical effect of the water stream (which dislodges tentacle fragments and stinging cells) supersedes the deleterious (sting-stimulating) effect of the hypotonic water, or that the heat has a beneficial effect. Remove any gross tentacles with a forceps or a well-gloved hand. In an emergency, the keratinized palm of the hand can be used because it is relatively protected, but care must be taken to avoid becoming envenomed.

Acetic acid 5% (vinegar) is the treatment of choice to inactivate *C. fleckeri* toxin. Vinegar does not always alleviate the pain from a *Chironex* sting, but it interrupts the envenomation. It may not be extremely effective against *Chrysaora* or *Cyanea*. The detoxicant should be applied continuously for at least 30 minutes or until the pain is relieved. Then the tentacles should be removed.

A sting from the Australian *P. physalis,* a relatively recently differentiated species, should not be doused with vinegar, because this may cause discharge of up to 30% of nematocysts.[63]

For stings from other species, there are substances that may be more specific and therefore more effective (see below). Alternatively, nonspecific substances may be effective. Depending on the species, the most popular remedies include lidocaine (4% to 15%), isopropyl alcohol (40% to 70%), dilute ammonium hydroxide (which may prove to be caustic), sodium bicarbonate (particularly for stings of the sea nettle *C. quinquecirrha*), olive oil, sugar, urine, and papain (papaya latex [juice] or unseasoned meat tenderizer [powdered or in solution]). The last is supposed to work by cleaving active polypeptides into nontoxic amino acids. Lime or lemon juice has been observed on occasion to be effective. Ammonia has been noted to be relatively ineffective for stings of *Carybdea marsupialis* in the Adriatic Sea.[159] There is some evidence that alcohol may stimulate the discharge of nematocysts in vitro; the clinical significance is as yet undetermined. The rescuer must remember that pain relief may not equate with nematocyst inhibition.[139] A commercial aqueous solution of aluminum sulfate (20%) and 1.1% anionic surfactant in aqueous solution (Stingose) has been mentioned in the past as effective on the basis that the aluminum ion interacts with proteins and long-chain polysaccharide components to denature and inactivate venom. Prior treatment with topical alcohol or methylated spirits reduces effectiveness of the aluminum sulfate solution. This product has essentially fallen out of favor with clinician jellyfish experts in Australia.

Perfume, aftershave lotion, and high-proof liquor are not particularly efficacious and may be detrimental. Other substances mentioned to be effective at one time or another, but that are to be condemned on the basis of inefficacy and toxicity, are organic solvents such as formalin, ether, and gasoline. Household ammonia has been recommended, but may be caustic.

Immersing the area in hot water is increasingly recommended, despite the premise that a hypotonic solution is felt to cause nematocysts to discharge. One study compared hot (40° to 41°C [104° to 105.8°F]) water immersion to papain meat tenderizer or vinegar for treatment of a single-tentacle *Carybdea alata* (Hawaiian box-jellyfish; also known as *Alatina alata*) sting to the forearm, and the hot water immersion was found to be the most efficacious.[150] In a crayfish model of envenomation, exposure to heat reduced the lethality of extracted *C. fleckeri* venom.[38] At temperatures of 43°C (109.4°F) and greater, venom lost its lethality more rapidly the longer the exposure time. Because of the speed of onset of symptoms after *C. fleckeri* envenomation, this approach may be of limited clinical usefulness, and until human clinical confirmation against other species is obtained, hot water application should not automatically be extrapolated to other species.

Once the wound has been soaked with a decontaminant (e.g., vinegar), remaining (and often essentially invisible) nematocysts must be removed. The easiest way to do this is to apply shaving cream or a paste of baking soda, flour, or talc and to shave the area with a razor or similar tool. If sophisticated facilities are not available, the nematocysts should be removed by making a sand or mud paste with seawater and using this to help scrape the victim's skin with a sharp-edged shell or piece of wood. The rescuer must take care not to become envenomed; bare hands must be rinsed frequently. If a scrub brush or pad has been used to treat the envenomation, this step may not result in much, if any, clinical improvement.

No systemic drugs (other than antivenom for a *Chironex* envenomation) are of verifiable use. Ephedrine, atropine, calcium, methysergide, and hydrocortisone have all been touted at one time or another, but no proof exists that they help. Antihistamines may be useful if there is a significant allergic component. Administration of epinephrine is appropriate only in the setting of anaphylaxis.

It is not recommended to use the pressure-immobilization technique for venom containment because this may discharge more nematocysts. A venolymphatic proximal (to the injury) occlusive tourniquet should be considered only if a topical detoxicant is unavailable, the victim suffers from a severe systemic reaction, and transport to definitive care is delayed.

A topical anesthetic ointment (lidocaine 2.5%) or spray (benzocaine 14%), antihistaminic cream (diphenhydramine or tripelennamine), or mild steroid lotion (hydrocortisone 1%) may be soothing. These are used after the toxin is inactivated. Paradoxic reactions to benzocaine are rarely noted.

Victims should receive standard antitetanus prophylaxis.

Prophylactic antibiotics are not automatically indicated. Each wound should be checked at 3 and 7 days after injury for infection. Any ulcerating lesion should be cleaned three times a day and covered with a thin layer of nonsensitizing antiseptic ointment, such as mupirocin. A jellyfish sting to the cornea may cause a foreign body sensation, photophobia, and decreased or hazy vision. Ophthalmologic examination reveals hyperemic sclera, chemosis, and irregularity of the corneal epithelium with stromal edema. Depending on the extent of the wound, the anterior chamber may demonstrate the inflammatory response of iridocyclitis (flare with or without cells).[233] The victim should be referred to an ophthalmologist, who may prescribe steroid-containing eye medications, such as prednisolone acetate 1% with hyoscine 0.25%. Applying a traditional skin detoxicant directly to the cornea is not recommended, because it is likely to worsen the tissue injury. Cycloplegia achieved with topical cyclopentolate (0.5% to 1%) may prove useful to achieve pain relief.[229]

It is worth commenting on the perpetual discussions about the efficacy of topical decontaminants. It has been observed that certain substances that have been used to diminish the pain of a jellyfish sting, such as isopropyl alcohol, when tested in vitro (e.g., with tentacle preparations) may cause the nematocysts that reside on the tentacles of a jellyfish to discharge their contents. These observations have provoked some persons to advise against the use of the substances as remedies for jellyfish stings, sometimes stating that it would be dangerous to use them. However, what is observed under the microscope does not always match up with the observed beneficial clinical effect. Clearly, more research needs to be done to determine which decontaminants are clinically beneficial and which are detrimental, and the meaning of the various forms and activities of nematocysts under different conditions, including exposure to topical first-aid remedies.

Delayed Reaction. A delayed reaction, similar in appearance to erythema nodosum, may be noted in areas of skin contact and may be accompanied by fever, weakness, arthralgias, painful joint swelling, and effusions. This may recur multiple times over the course of 1 to 2 months. The treatment is a 10- to 14-day tapered course of prednisone, starting with 50 to 100 mg. Prednisone administration may need to be prolonged or repeated with each flare of the reaction.

Persistent Hyperpigmentation. Postinflammatory hyperpigmentation is common after the stings of many jellyfish and other lesser cnidarians. A solution of 1.8% hydroquinone in a glycol and alcohol base (70% ethyl alcohol and propylene glycol mixed at a 3:2 ratio), twice a day as a topical agent for 3 to 5 weeks, has been used successfully to treat hyperpigmentation after a *Pelagia noctiluca* sting.

Persistent Cutaneous Hypersensitivity. Persistent local dermal hypersensitivity may occur after a jellyfish sting, such as that from the Hawaiian box-jellyfish *C. alata*.[203] This is characterized by erythematous papulonodular lesions in the pattern of the original sting, which may persist for months. Treatment, which may be unsatisfactory, consists of topical and intralesional steroids.

Prevention

A topical jellyfish sting inhibitor has been commercialized. Safe Sea ("jellyfish-safe sunblock") by Nidaria Technology, Ltd, Zemah, Jordan Valley, Israel (nidaria.com) was compared in a blinded fashion with conventional sunscreen for protection against *Chrysaora fuscescens* (sea nettle) and *Chiropsalmus quadrumanus* jellyfish. Subjects were stung with jellyfish tentacles on each forearm for up to 60 seconds, and erythema and pain were assessed at 15-minute intervals over a 2-hour period. The jellyfish sting inhibitor prevented sting symptoms of *C. fuscescens* in 10 of 12 subjects and diminished the pain of the jellyfish sting in the remaining two subjects.[103] It was equally impressive with *C.*

quadrumanus. Another author performed a double-blind, randomized, placebo-controlled field trial using Safe Sea in an ocean setting, with participants snorkeling in the Gulf of Mexico and Caribbean. This study showed a relative risk reduction of 82% when Safe Sea was used to prevent jellyfish stings as compared with placebo (sunscreen), where notable common species encountered were *C. quinquecirrha* (sea nettle), *C. quadrumanus*, and *Linuche unguiculata* (thimble jellyfish).[19] The inhibitor is formulated to inactivate jellyfish stinging in several ways: (1) it is hydrophobic and thus prevents tentacles from making sufficient skin contact to induce a sting; (2) glycosaminoglycans in the inhibitor mimic the same compounds found in the jellyfish bell, thus causing self-recognition; (3) the inhibitor contains a competitive antagonist to nonselective receptors on the jellyfish that bind to amino acids and sugar secretions from prey; and (4) calcium and magnesium within the inhibitor block transmembrane signaling channels of the jellyfish, thereby altering the osmotic forces required to generate the firing pressure within the nematocyst capsule[103] The product has not yet been tested prospectively against *Physalia*, *Carukia*, or *Chironex* species.

Derma Shield is a topical formulation that contains lanolin, aloe vera, and vitamin E. According to the manufacturer, this chemically inert (1-vinyl-2-pyrrolidone) barrier protectant is hydrophobic (dimethicone and stearic acid) and does not wash off but is shed as the epithelium sloughs naturally. It has been reported anecdotally by ocean bathers to protect against the agents of seabather's eruption.

Smerbeck and coworkers were assigned a U.S. patent in 1999 for a method and composition of polymeric quaternary ammonium salts for protecting the skin from jellyfish stings.

A protocol has been developed to establish the effectiveness of topical agents to block the firing of nematocysts.[35] Unreliable topical barriers include petrolatum, mineral oil, silicone ointment, cocoa butter, and mechanic's grease.

If jellyfish are sighted, they should be given a wide berth because the tentacles may trail great distances from the body. All swimmers and divers in hazardous areas should be on constant alert. Persons should not dive headfirst into jellyfish-infested waters; it is far safer to walk in. Bathers should wear protective clothing in infested areas. This includes Lycra stinger suits or a double thickness of pantyhose. In hot weather, it is possible to cause human heat storage while stinger suits are being worn during beach activities, so one should be cognizant of the potential for heat-related illness when out of the water.[190] If stinger enclosures are present, bathers should stay within the netted barriers, although it should be noted that the small (2-cm) Irukandji jellyfish will pass with ease through the mesh of a stinger net. Many bathers suffering from Irukandji envenomations in northern Queensland, Australia, were swimming in a stinger enclosure at the time of their envenomation.

Divers concerned about jellyfish tentacles dangling from the surface or congregations of creatures at the surface should remain deeper than 20 feet and should always check snorkel and regulator mouthpieces for tentacle fragments before entering the water in endemic areas. In areas inhabited by anemones and hydroid corals, protective gloves should be worn when handling specimens. Beached dead jellyfish or tentacle fragments washed up after a storm can still inflict serious stings. Any person stung by a jellyfish should leave or be assisted from the water because of the risk of drowning.

CLASS HYDROZOA

The hydrozoans range in configuration from the feather hydroids and sedentary *Millepora* hydroid coral to the free-floating siphonophore *Physalia* (Portuguese man-of-war).

Hydroids

Hydroids are the most numerous of the hydrozoans. The feather hydroids of the order Leptomedusae, typified by *Lytocarpus philippinus* (fire weed or fire fern), are feather-like or plumelike (Figure 74-26) animals that sting the victim who brushes against or handles them.[169] After a storm, the branches may be fragmented and dispersed through the water, so that merely diving

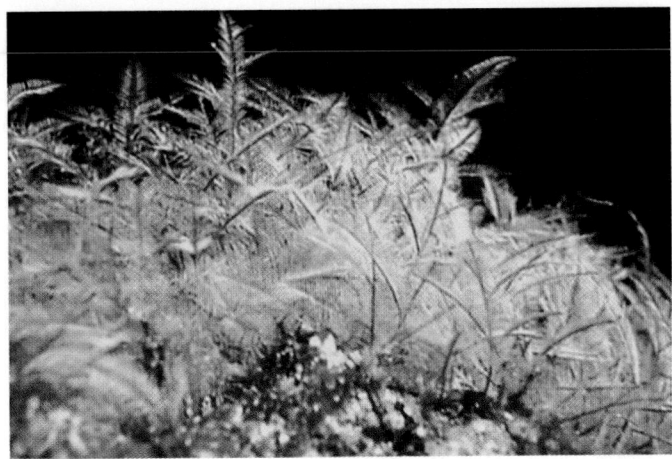

FIGURE 74-26 Cnidarian hydroid. *(Courtesy Paul S. Auerbach, MD.)*

or swimming in the vicinity causes itching and may induce visible skin irritation.

Clinical Aspects. Contact with the nematocysts of a feather hydroid induces a mild reaction, which consists of instantaneous burning, itching, and urticaria. If the exposure is brief, the skin rash may not be noticeable or may consist of a faint erythematous and miliary irritation (Figure 74-27). A second variety of envenomation consists of a delayed papular, hemorrhagic, or zosteriform reaction (Figure 74-28) with onset 4 to 12 hours after contact. Rarely, erythema multiforme or a desquamative eruption may develop. In turbulent waters or in a strong current, fragments may be washed into a diver's mask or regulator mouthpiece; this will be evident as a burning sensation in the conjunctivae or oral mucous membranes. Systemic manifestations (such as abdominal pain, nausea, vomiting, diarrhea, muscle cramps, and fever) are rarely reported and are associated with large areas of surface involvement. Allergic sensitization and subsequent anaphylaxis have been proposed.

Treatment. The skin should be rinsed with seawater and gently dried without abrasive activity. Application of freshwater and brisk rubbing are strictly prohibited because they encourage any nematocysts remaining on the skin to discharge and thus worsen envenomation. An application of 5% acetic acid (vinegar) or isopropyl alcohol (40% to 70%) to the skin for 15 to 30 minutes has traditionally been recommended to relieve the cutaneous reaction. In an in vitro evaluation, vinegar and urine caused discharge of a few nematocysts in 10% to 15% of defensive tentacle polyps; methylated spirits were found to cause gross discharge of microbasic mastigophores in all defensive polyps.[169] Fresh water did not cause discharge. On the basis of this study, the authors recommended that irrigation with fresh water and

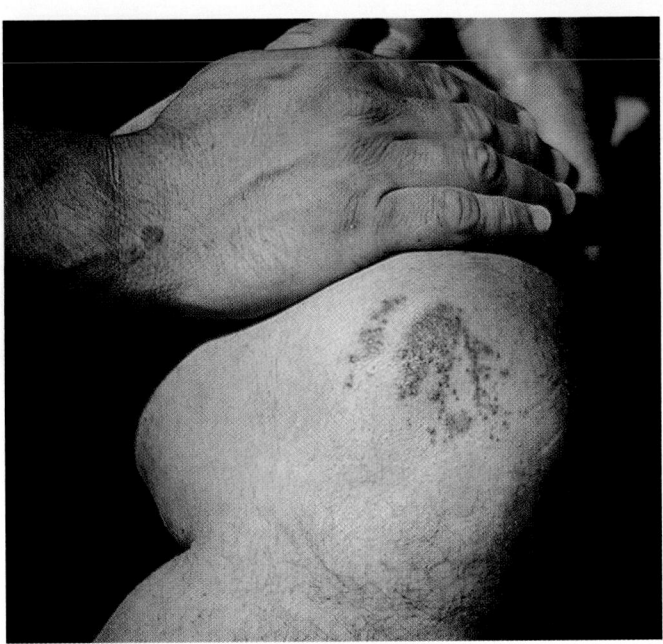

FIGURE 74-28 Fernlike hydroid print on the knee of a diver. *(Courtesy Paul S. Auerbach, MD.)*

the application of ice be used to treat acute stings. However, the clinical correlation remains to be described.

Alternative topical agents are addressed in the larger discussion on therapy for cnidarian stings. After pain relief is achieved, a mild steroid cream (hydrocortisone 1%) or moisturizing lotion may be applied.

Fire Coral

The stony, hydroid, and coral-like *Millepora* species (e.g., *Millepora alcicornis*), or fire corals, are not true corals. They are widely distributed in shallow tropical waters. Sessile creatures, they are found attached to the bottom in depths of up to 1000 m (3281 feet). They are often mistaken for seaweed because they attach to pilings, rocks, shells, or coral. Although smaller segments resemble Christmas trees or bushes 7.6 to 10.2 cm (3 to 4 inches) in height, they may attain heights of 2 m (6.6 feet). The color ranges from white to yellow-green, with pale yellow (Figure 74-29) most common. Rare purple fire corals exist. Fire coral is structured on a razor-sharp calcium carbonate (calcic limestone) exoskeleton, which is an important component in the development of coral reefs. The outcroppings assume upright, clavate, blade-like, honeycomb, or branching calcareous growth

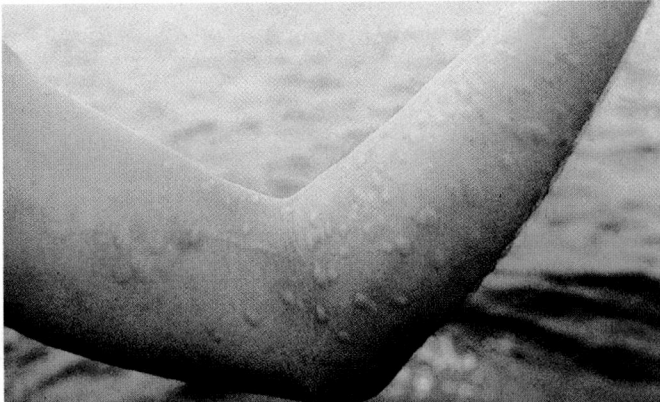

FIGURE 74-27 Hydroid sting on the arm of a diver. *(Courtesy Neville Coleman.)*

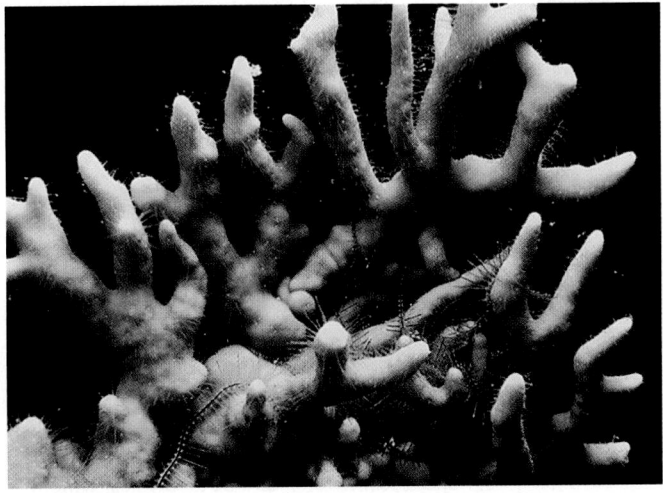

FIGURE 74-29 Fire coral. *(Courtesy Paul S. Auerbach, MD.)*

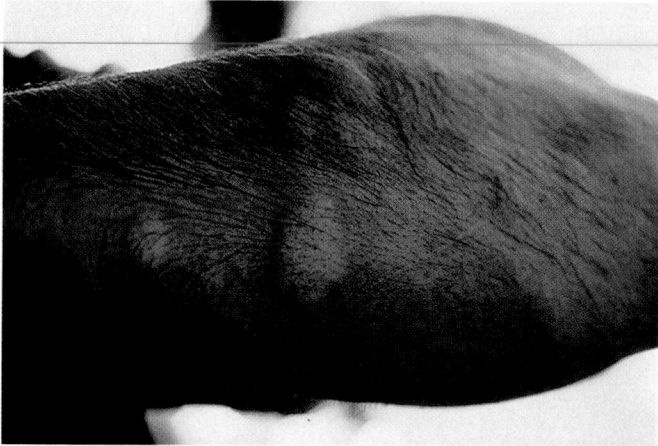

FIGURE 74-30 Fire coral sting of the author. *(Courtesy Kenneth Kizer, MD.)*

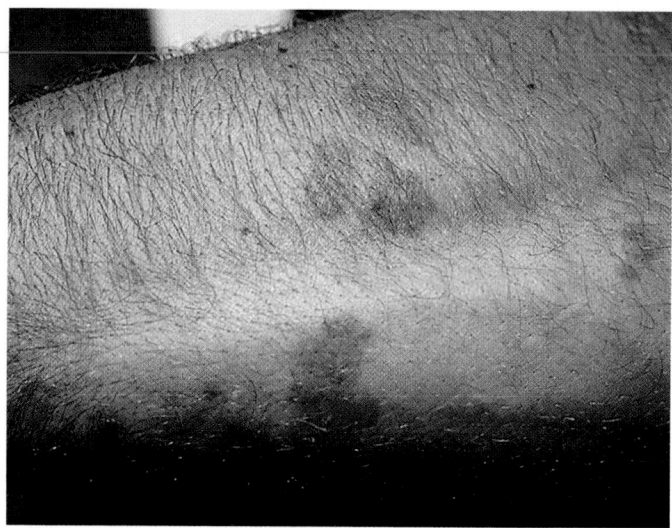

FIGURE 74-31 Hyperpigmentation of forearm depicted in Figure 74-24 after a fire coral sting. *(Courtesy Kenneth Kizer, MD.)*

structures that form encrustations over coral and objects such as sunken vessels. From numerous minute surface gastropores protrude tiny nematocyst-bearing tentacles, wherein lies the stinging apparatus. *M. alcicornis* probably accounts for more cnidarian envenomations than any other species. Unprotected and unwary recreational scuba enthusiasts handle, kneel on, or lean on this marine stinger.

Clinical Aspects. Immediately after contact with fire coral, the victim suffers burning or stinging pain, rarely with central radiation. Intense and painful pruritus follows within seconds, which frequently induces the victim to rub the affected area vigorously, worsening the envenomation. Over the course of 5 to 30 minutes, urticarial wheals develop, marked by redness, warmth, and pruritus (Figure 74-30). The wheals become moderately edematous and reach a maximal size in 30 to 60 minutes. Untreated, they flatten over 14 to 24 hours and resolve entirely over 3 to 7 days, occasionally leaving an area of hyperpigmentation (Figure 74-31) that may require 4 to 8 weeks to disappear. The pain generally resolves without treatment in 30 to 90 minutes.

A hemorrhagic or ulcerative lesion(s) may occur acutely. In the case of multiple stings, regional lymph nodes may become inflamed and painful. This does not necessarily indicate a secondary infection. The skin may take on the appearance of leukocytoclastic vasculitis.[157] Long thoracic mononeuritis with serratus anterior muscle paralysis has been described after *Millepora* sting, confirmed by demonstrated presence of immune-specific IgG.[142] Delayed skin reaction after Red Sea fire coral injury was characterized by superficial granulomas and atypical CD30+ lymphocytes (Figure 74-32).[141] In another series, contact with fire coral resulted in a typical pruritic urticarial lesion and blister formation, followed by a lichenoid stage that developed 3 weeks after the initial injury; resolution, with residual hyperpigmented macules, required 15 weeks.[2] A persistent cutaneous reaction characterized by eczematous dermatitis lasting more than 18 months is possible.[157] Grouped or linear papulonodular lesions, round or oval

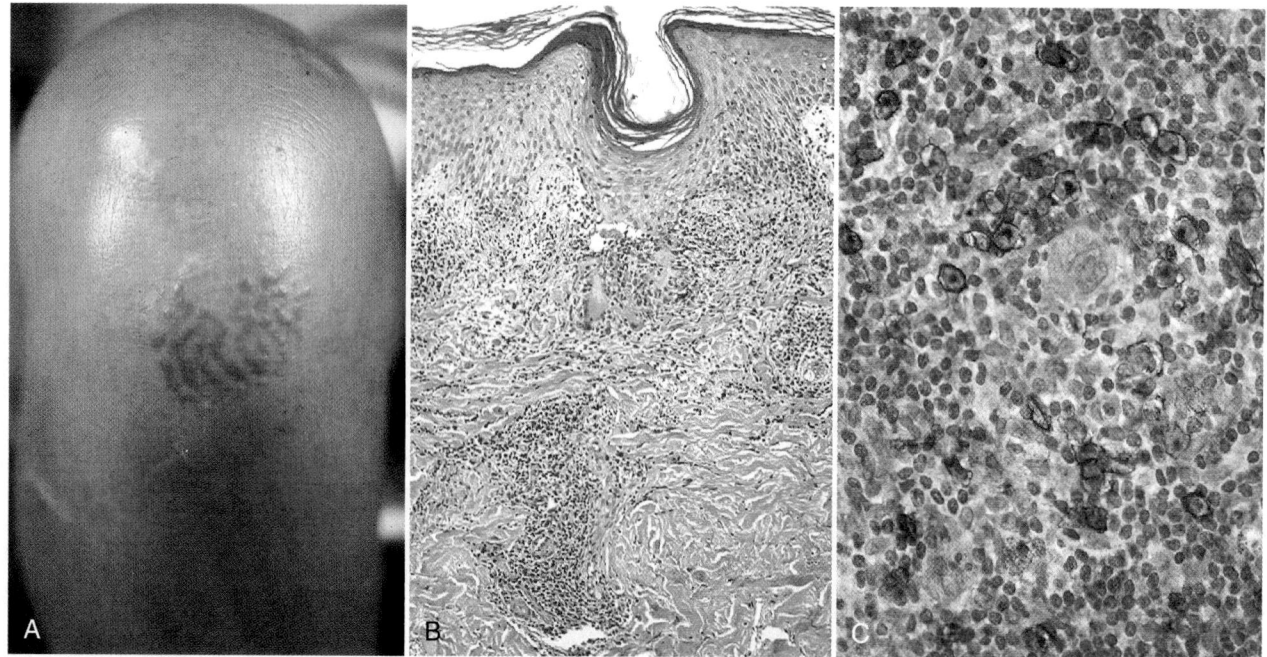

FIGURE 74-32 A, Streaks of red papules on the knee of a victim stung by a Red Sea fire coral. **B,** Wedge-shaped inflammatory infiltrate with edema of the papillary dermis and an epithelioid granuloma (hematoxylin and eosin, ×100). **C,** CD30+ atypical lymphoid cells (alkaline phosphatase–antialkaline phosphatase, ×400). *(Courtesy Dr. Clelia Miracco.)*

in shape, may follow as a delayed reaction to a jellyfish sting.[211] In a rare case, a full-thickness skin burn may occur.[175]

Renal minimal change disease (nephrotic syndrome, renal failure) responsive to corticosteroid therapy has been associated with fire coral exposure.[164]

Treatment. The skin should be rinsed liberally with seawater and then immediately soaked with acetic acid 5% (vinegar) or isopropyl alcohol (40% to 70%) until pain is relieved. Alternative topical agents are discussed in the larger cnidarian treatment section, earlier. Residual dermatitis is generally not very severe and can be managed in a fashion similar to that used after a feather hydroid sting. If the rash becomes eczematous and indolent, it may respond to a course of systemic corticosteroids (prednisone, 60 to 100 mg, tapered over 2 weeks). Divers should avoid touching with bare skin anything resembling coral. For example, the underwater statue of Jesus at John Pennycamp Park in Key Largo, Florida, is encrusted with fire coral, so posing divers have been envenomed.

Physalia (Man-of-War)

The Atlantic Portuguese man-of-war *(Physalia physalis)* of the phylum Cnidaria, order Siphonophorae, is a pelagic (open sea) polymorphic colonial siphonophore that inhabits the surface of the ocean. It is constructed of a blue or pink-violet and iridescent floating sail (pneumatophore) that is filled with nitrogen and carbon monoxide and up to 30 cm (11.8 inches) in length, from which are suspended multiple nematocyst-bearing tentacles, which may measure up to 30 m (98 feet) in length (Figures 74-33 and 74-34). It has been reported that an Australian version of *P. physalis* is present in northern Australian waters.[64] This jellyfish is characterized by float lengths of up to 15 cm (5.9 inches), up to five thick, dark blue "main" tentacles, and up to 10 other long,

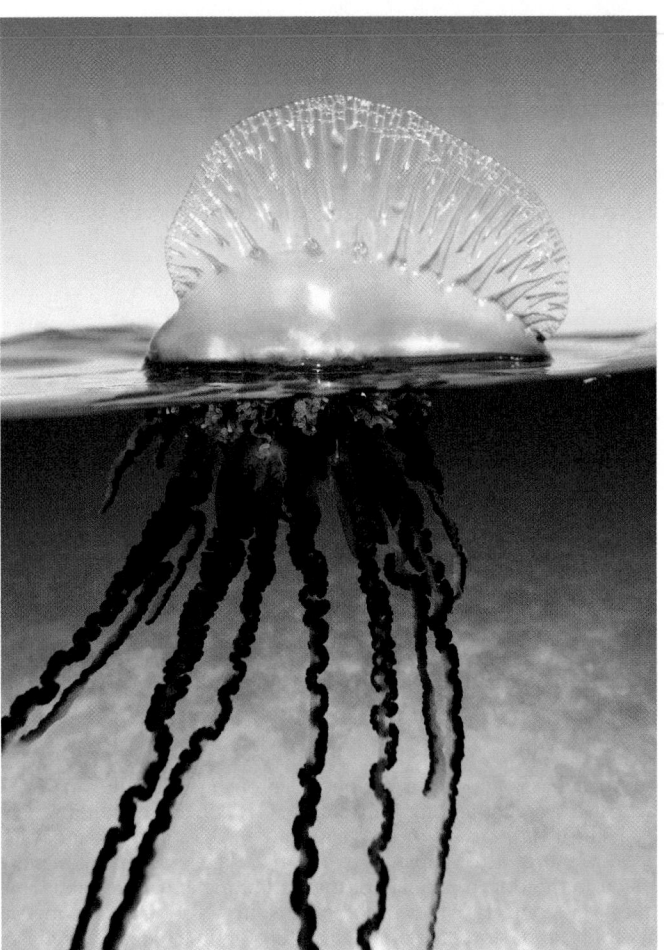

FIGURE 74-34 Portuguese man-of-war. *(Copyright Stephen Frink.)*

thin, and pale-colored tentacles. The smaller Pacific bluebottle *(Physalia utriculus)* usually has a single fishing tentacle, which attains lengths of up to 15 m (49.2 feet) (Figure 74-35). In some species, the sail can be deflated to allow the animal to submerge in rough weather.

The physaliae depend on the winds, currents, and tides for movement, traveling as individuals or in floating colonies that resemble flotillas. They are widely distributed but seem to abound in tropical waters and in the semitropical Atlantic Ocean, particularly off the coast of Florida and in the Gulf of Mexico. Envenoming has been reported as far south as the coast of Brazil.[47] Their arrival at surf's edge can transform a halcyon vacation into a stinging nightmare. Unfortunately, the peak appearance time for both the man-of-war and sea nettle is July through September, which is prime beach season.

As is the case for icebergs, much of the story is below the water surface. Because the tentacles are nearly transparent, they pose a hazard to the unwary (Figure 74-36). As the animal moves in the ocean, the tentacles rhythmically contract, sampling the water for potential prey. If the tentacle strikes a foreign object, the nematocysts are stimulated and discharge their contents into the victim. Each tentacle in a larger specimen may carry more than 750,000 nematocysts. To increase the intensity of the "attack," the remainder of the tentacle shortens in such a way as to create loops and folds, presenting a greater surface area and greater number of nematocysts for offensive action in "stinging batteries" (Figure 74-37).

Detached moistened tentacles, often found by the thousands fragmented on the beach, carry live nematocysts capable of discharging for months. Air-dried nematocysts may retain considerable potency, even after weeks (Figure 74-38). The loggerhead turtle *(Caretta caretta)* (Figure 74-39) feeds on *Physalia*. Like the clownfish with the sea anemone, the brightly colored fish *Nomeus*

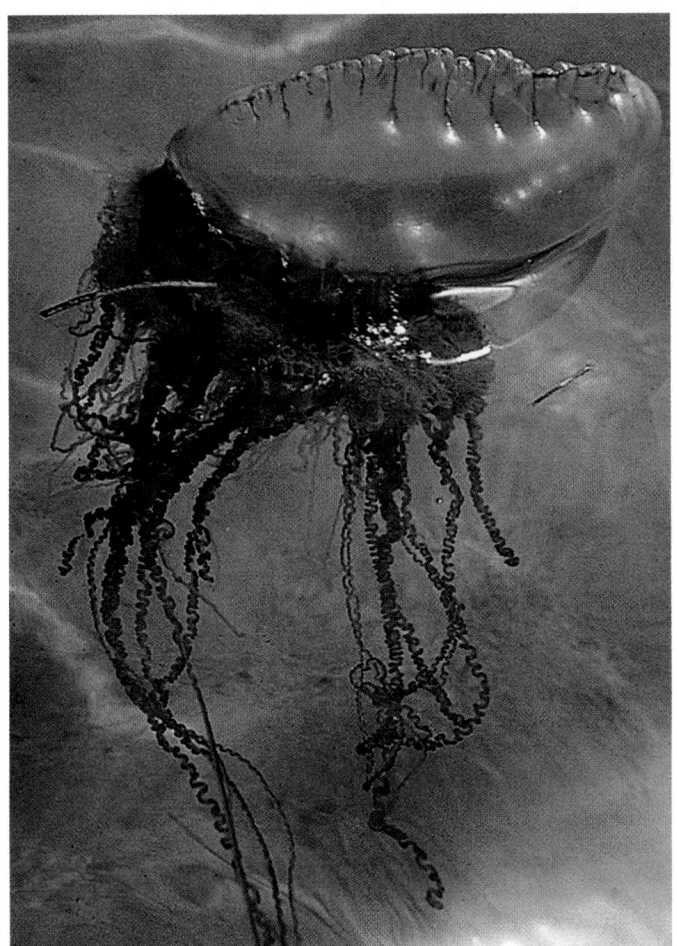

FIGURE 74-33 Atlantic Portuguese man-of-war. *(From Norbert Wu, with permission: norbertwu.com.)*

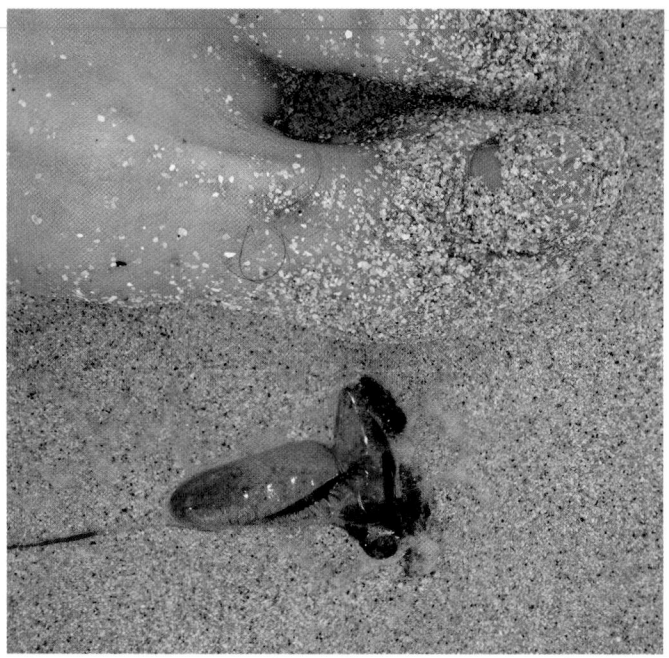

FIGURE 74-35 Tiny stinging jellyfish on the beach in Hawaii. (Courtesy Paul S. Auerbach, MD.)

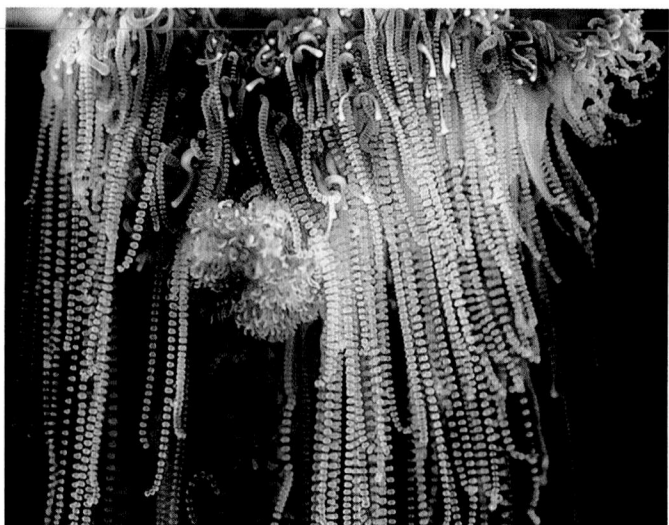

FIGURE 74-37 Tentacles of the Atlantic Portuguese man-of-war. Nematocysts may number in the hundreds of thousands on tentacles coiled into "stinging batteries." (Courtesy Larry Madin, Woods Hole Oceanographic Institution.)

gronovii has a unique symbiotic relationship with the man-of-war, living freely among the tentacles. A species of nudibranch (sea slug), *Glaucus atlanticus*, eats the tentacles and nematocysts of *P. physalis*. The nematocysts are not digested and ultimately reside in the dorsal papillae of the nudibranchs, where they may sting on contact. Other nudibranchs are also able to ingest hydroids and store their stinging cells in the cerata, or flesh appendages. Dermatitis can also result from contact with water containing venom that has already been released from stimulated nematocysts. The Mediterranean octopus *Tremoctopus violaceous* stores intact dactylozooid segments in its suckers for later use.[29]

Clinical Aspects. *Physalia* envenomations can be quite painful. *P. utriculus* usually causes only local pain and dermatitis, or rarely, minor systemic symptoms, but *P. physalis* can potentially cause major systemic symptoms, as discussed previously. The most common presentation is immediate local stinging/searing/sharp pain from the sting followed by an erythematous maculopapular linear rash that can later show vesicles or even skin necrosis. Pain usually improves in the first few hours, and local symptoms resolve in 72 hours.[206] More severe systemic symptoms, which generally only occur with stings from *P.*

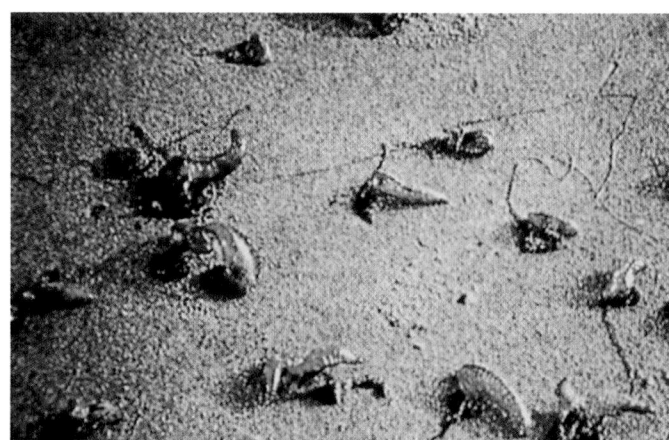

FIGURE 74-38 Pacific man-of-war washed ashore may retain stinging potency for weeks. (Courtesy John Williamson, MD.)

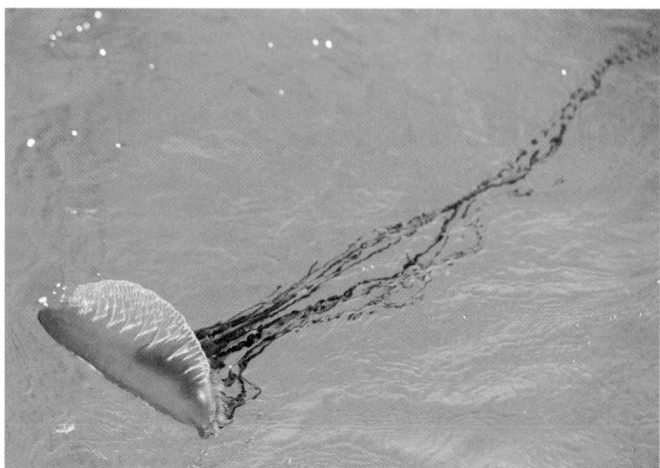

FIGURE 74-36 Stinging tentacles of Portuguese man-of-war trail in the water. (Copyright Stephen Frink.)

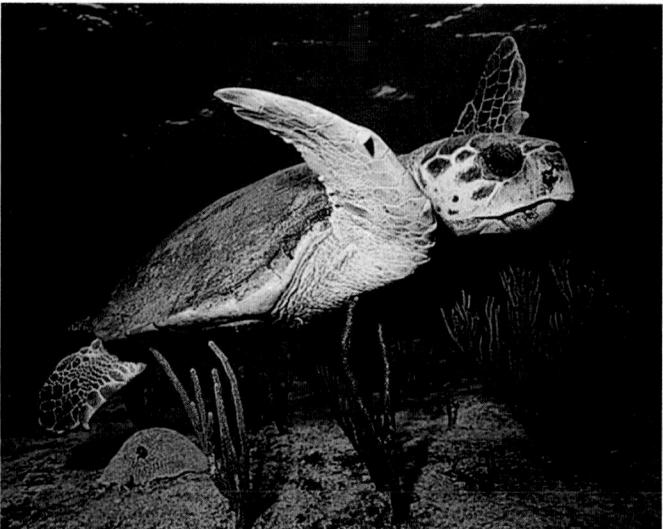

FIGURE 74-39 The loggerhead turtle sometimes dines on jellyfish tentacles. (Courtesy Howard Hall.)

physalis, include nausea, vomiting, muscle cramps, dyspnea, anxiety, abdominal pain, and headache; rarely, death occurs.[109]

Treatment. Treatment of *Physalia* envenomations is still controversial. As discussed earlier, if a specific decontaminant is not immediately available, washing with seawater and removal of any adherent tentacles is primary field treatment. Commercial (chemical) cold or ice packs applied over a thin dry cloth or plastic membrane have been shown to be effective when applied to mild or moderate *P. utriculus* (or bluebottle) stings.[53] Whether the melted water from ice applied directly to the skin can stimulate the discharge of nematocysts has not been determined. However, a recent randomized controlled trial of hot water (45°C [113°F]) immersion versus ice packs for pain relief for bluebottle stings showed hot water to be the favored treatment, with statistically significant reduction in reported pain.[123] To support this approach, it has been observed by physicians in Australia that hot packs and hot showers (45°C [113°F]) are efficacious for relieving pain of bluebottle stings. As stated previously, application of vinegar may increase nematocyst discharge in vitro and is not yet a universally accepted treatment. Other treatments that may be effective for pain relief include lidocaine, Stingose (20% $MgSO_4$), baking soda, and papain.

Seabather's Eruption

Seabather's eruption, commonly termed sea lice (pika-pika around the Belize barrier reef; sea poisoning, sea critters, and ocean itch are other names), refers to a dermatitis that results from contact with ocean water.[95] It has become a seasonal problem afflicting oceangoers in southern Florida and across the Caribbean; it has been reported in Brazil and Papua New Guinea.[81,210] It predominantly involves covered areas of the body and is commonly caused by pinhead-sized (0.5 mm) greenish brown to black larvae of the thimble jellyfish *Linuche unguiculata* (Figure 74-40), which breeds in Caribbean waters throughout the summer, with a peak in May.[208] *L. unguiculata* exists in three swimming stages during its life cycle: planula (free-swimming larva), ephyra (immature medusa), and adult medusa. It is likely that all three swimming stages initiate the eruption.[165,181] Another culprit off Long Island, New York, has been the planula larval form (visible at 2 to 3 mm) of the sea anemone *Edwardsiella lineata,* which carries hundreds of nematocysts.[66,67] Given the number of cnidarians that inhabit the oceans of the world and the cross-reactivity of antigens, it is likely that etiologic organisms are numerous.

Clinical Aspects. A swimmer who encounters the stinging forms usually complains of cutaneous discomfort (stinging, tingling, or a pins-and-needles sensation) after contact, often while in the water or soon after exiting. Application of freshwater may intensify the sting. The eruption occurs a few minutes to 12 hours after bathing and consists of erythematous and intensely pruritic

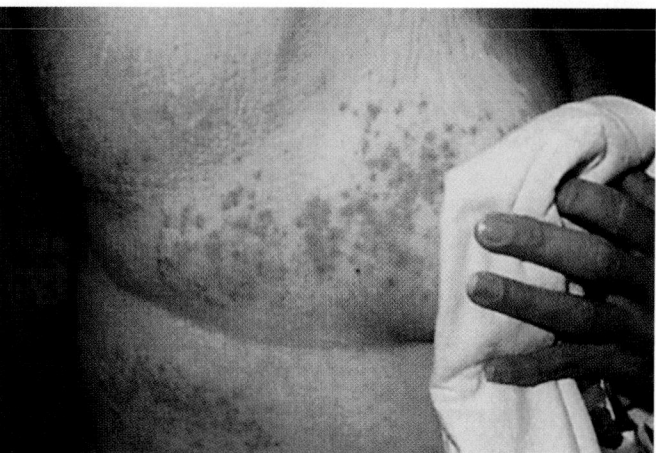

FIGURE 74-41 Seabather's eruption. *(From Wong DE, Meinking TL, Rosen LB, et al: Seabather's eruption,* J Am Acad Dermatol *30:399, 1994.)*

wheals, vesicles, or papules that persist for 2 to 14 days and then involute spontaneously. When a bathing suit has been worn by a woman, the areas commonly involved include the buttocks, genital region, and breasts (Figure 74-41). A person at the water's surface (commonly a person who surfaces after a dive) may suffer stings to the exposed neck (Figure 74-42), particularly if there has been recent motorboat activity in the vicinity, which may disturb and fragment the causative jellyfish. Nematocysts adherent to scalp hair may sting the neck as the hair hangs down. Individual lesions resemble insect bites. Coalescence indicates a large inoculum (Figure 74-43). Surfers develop lesions on areas that contact the surfboard (chest and anterior abdomen). The rash may also be seen under bathing caps and swim fins or along the edge of the cuffs of wetsuits, T-shirts, or stinger suits (Figure 74-44).[208] In children with extensive eruptions, fever is common. Low-grade fever may be noted in adults.[210] Other symptoms may include headache, chills, fatigue and malaise, vomiting,

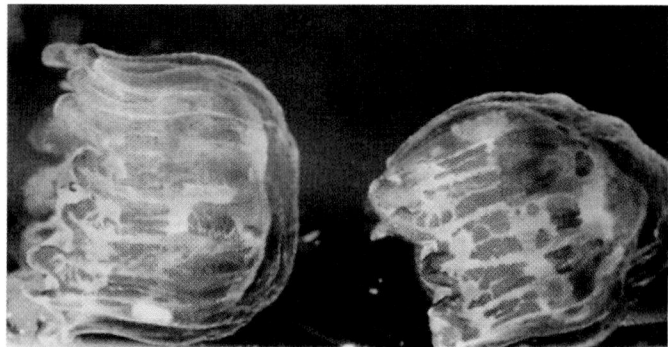

FIGURE 74-40 Mature *Linuche unguiculata,* the causative agents of seabather's eruption. The planula or larvae of these cnidarians were collected from plankton tows and grown to maturity at the University of Miami. Slightly smaller than their brethren found in the open ocean, these specimens are approximately 2 cm in diameter when open and 1 cm when contracted. *(Courtesy David Taplin and Terri L. Meinking.)*

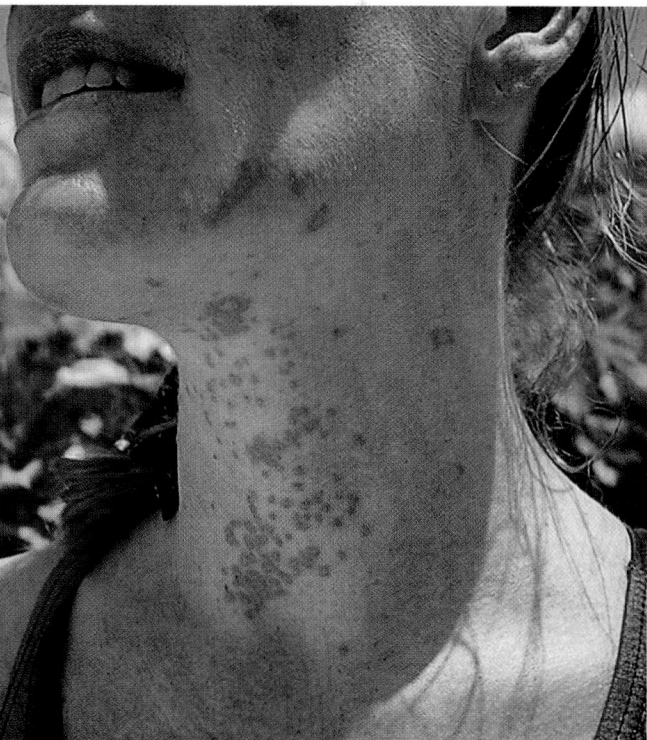

FIGURE 74-42 Seabather's eruption on the neck of a diver in Cozumel, Mexico. *(Courtesy Paul S. Auerbach, MD.)*

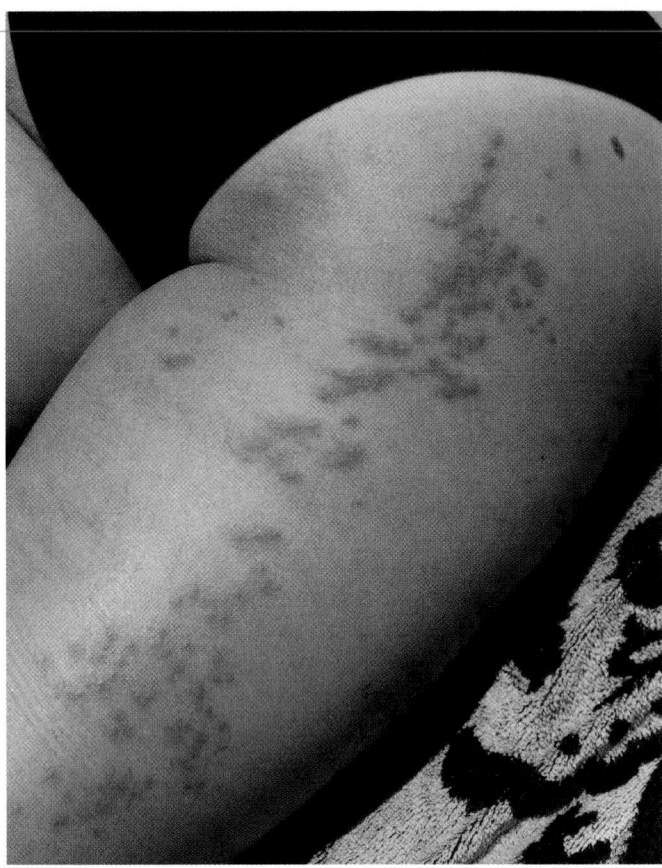

FIGURE 74-43 Seabather's eruption. *(Copyright Stephen Frink.)*

conjunctivitis, and urethritis. Itching is often pronounced at night and awakens the victim from sleep. Burnett and Burnett[22] reported blurred vision and left arm weakness in a teenager stung by an adult *Linuche*. People who note a stinging sensation during the primary contact while still in the water may have a higher incidence of previous sensitization to the antigen or antigens. Persons who wear clothing that has been contaminated with the larvae may suffer recurrent reactions. Prior sensitization may precede prolonged (≤ 6 weeks) reactions (rash and pruritus).

Elevated IgG levels specific for *L. unguiculata* can be measured by ELISA in the sera of victims who have suffered from seabather's eruption. The extent of the cutaneous eruption or sting severity appears to correlate with the antibody titer.[33] In an evaluation of southeastern Florida victims envenomed by *L. unguiculata*, histopathologic examination of inflammatory papules demonstrated superficial and deep perivascular and

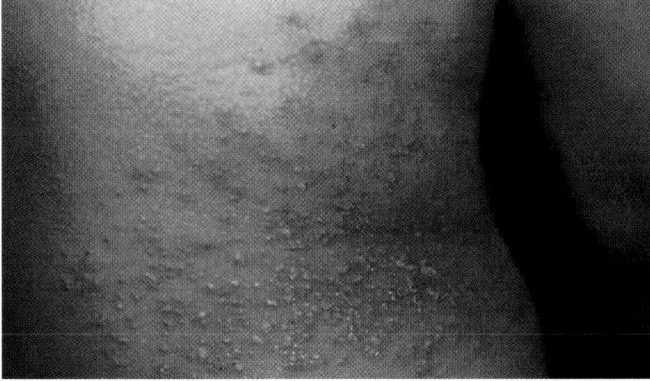

FIGURE 74-44 Seabather's eruption in an area under the weight belt. *(Courtesy Doug Wong, MD.)*

interstitial infiltrate consisting of lymphocytes, neutrophils, and eosinophils.[234]

Treatment. Field management is identical to that for any cnidarian sting (see earlier), with the empirical observation that topical papain may be slightly more effective as an initial decontaminant than vinegar, isopropyl alcohol, or other substances. Papain application may be more effective if undertaken with a mildly abrasive scrub pad. Whether the pain relief is due to nematocyst inactivation or counterirritation is not yet known. Substances that are believed to be ineffective include hydrogen peroxide, garlic, antifungal spray, anti–head lice medication, petroleum distillates, fingernail polish, and citrus juice.

The skin eruption is self-limited and usually remits within 10 days. However, in a severe envenomation, the rash may persist for up to 4 weeks and leave atrophic scars.[125] Further treatment is palliative and consists of calamine lotion with 1% menthol. Because the lesions rarely extend into the dermis, a potent topical corticosteroid may be helpful in mild cases, but benefit is not invariably attained. In a more severe case, an oral or parenteral antihistamine or systemic corticosteroid may be used. A thorough soap and water scrub (not a casual rinse) on leaving the water provides partial prophylaxis. Avoidance logically includes advice to ocean bathe in abbreviated swimwear (which may, however, expose a person to other stings), to maintain tightly occlusive cuffs on dive skins and wetsuits, to change swimwear as soon as possible after leaving the water, and to use caution during high season for *L. unguiculata* (April to July off southern Florida) or *E. lineata* (August to November off Long Island) and when there are strong onshore winds. Swimwear worn and suspected to be contaminated with nematocysts should be washed in detergent and fresh water and dried before wearing.[180]

True sea lice are parasites on marine creatures and do not cause this disorder.

Gonionemus Species

These small hydrozoans are distributed worldwide but have been reported as causing severe envenomation only in the Sea of Japan near Vladivostok, Russia, and at the northwestern shores of Honshu Island, Japan.[56] It is a small creature of 5 to 15 mm in diameter across the bell, with a symmetric, right-angled cross visible in the transparent part.

When the reaction is painful, the victim suffers muscle, joint, chest, and pelvic pain for up to 3 days. There may be muscle fasciculations. In a respiratory presentation, the victims suffer rhinitis, tearing, hoarseness, cough, and shortness of breath. In addition, there may be a combination of symptoms, such as sore throat, tachycardia, vomiting, and mild hypertension. Psychiatric depression and hallucinations may occur.[152]

It has been noted that envenomation may occur under a bathing suit. In addition, a similar syndrome was reported after ingestion of raw seaweed, to which was presumably attached the jellyfish.[56]

CLASSES CUBOZOA AND SCYPHOZOA

The classes Cubozoa and Scyphozoa contain the larger medusae or jellyfish, including the deadly box-jellyfish and variably injurious species (e.g., *Chironex, Cyanea, Chiropsalmus,* and *Chiropsella,* which were formerly classified as *Chiropsalmus* spp.). These creatures are armed with some of the most potent venoms in existence. Jellyfish are mostly free-swimming pelagic creatures; however, some can be found at depths of more than 2000 fathoms. They may be transparent or multicolored and range in size from a few millimeters to more than 2 m (6.5 feet) in width across the bell, with tentacles up to 40 m (131 feet) in length. Like physaliae, the scyphozoans depend on wind, currents, and tides for transport and are widely distributed (Figure 74-45). Some vertical motion may be produced by rhythmic contractions of the gelatinous bell, from which originate the feeding tentacles.

Some jellyfish contain less than 5% solid organic matter. Regardless, they can withstand remarkable temperature and salinity variations, although they do not fare well with violent activity and thus may descend to great depths during stormy surface weather. Some scyphozoans avoid sunlight; others follow an

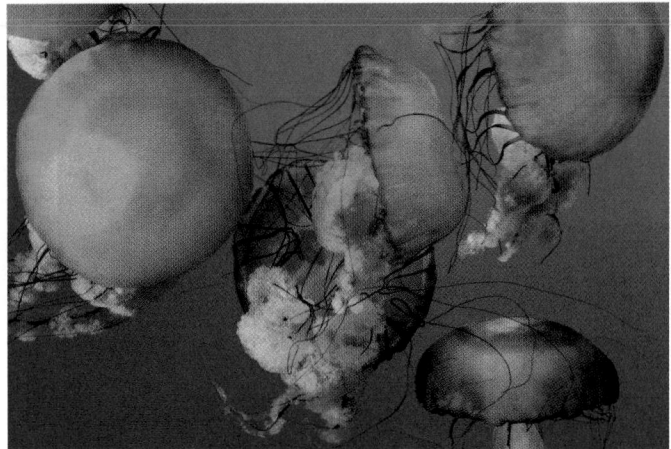

FIGURE 74-45 Schooling jellyfish. *(Copyright iStockphoto.com/Gary Adams.)*

opposite pattern. Certain jellyfish have adapted to local nutrient (largely algal) supply and have lost their ability to sting humans (Figure 74-46).

In eastern coastal waters of the North American continent, the creatures appear to grow larger as they progress north (Figure 74-47), so that true giant jellyfish, typified by *Cyanea capillata* (lion's mane), are found in Arctic waters (Figure 74-48). Tentacles (which may number up to 1200) of larger specimens may exceed 30 m (100 feet) in length.[29] *Pelagia* species (purple-striped or mauve stingers) are commonly found in large numbers off the California coast and appear in the Mediterranean Sea in abundance every 10 to 12 years.[166] *P. noctiluca* (Figure 74-49) phosphoresces at night, hence its name.[139] *Olindias sambaquiensis* is a jellyfish that stings bathers in South American coastal waters. *R. nomadica* is a tropical jellyfish that has invaded the eastern Mediterranean.[61,120,121] As another example, stings from *S. nomurai* in the Bohai waters of China produce severe pulmonary edema, coma, convulsions, psychoses, and death. Australian jellyfish include the blubber jellyfish (*Catostylus* species), hair jellyfish (*Cyanea* species), little mauve stinger (*P. noctiluca*), and the cuboid-shaped jellyfish (*C. fleckeri* and *Chiropsalmus* species). A number of cubomedusan (box-shaped jellyfish) scyphozoans of a highly toxic nature inhabit Indo-Pacific and, less frequently, Caribbean waters. These include *Carybdea rastoni* (jimble) (Figure 74-50) and *Carybdea marsupialis* (sea wasp), *Chiropsella bronzi, Chiropsalmus quadrigatus* and *Chiropsalmus quadrumanus,* and *Chironex fleckeri.*[172] The carybdeids of the order Carybdeida have four tentacles only, whereas the chirodropids of the order Chirodropidae may have up to 60 tentacles. All are frequently called box-jellyfish.

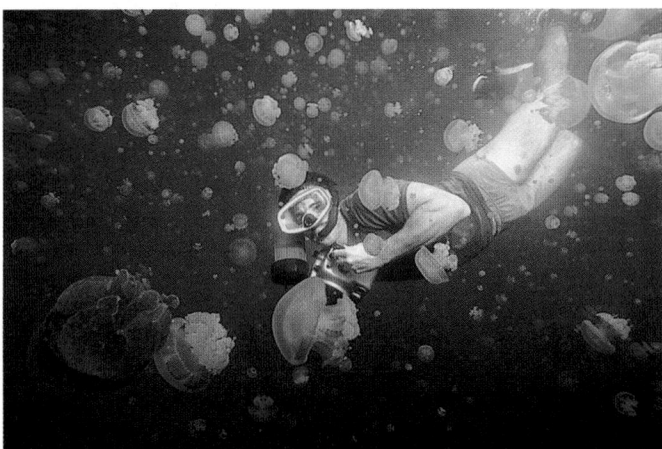

FIGURE 74-46 The author snorkels in Jellyfish Lake in Palau, Micronesia. The jellyfish have evolved to subsist on algae and thus no longer pose a stinging hazard to humans. *(Courtesy Avi Klapfer.)*

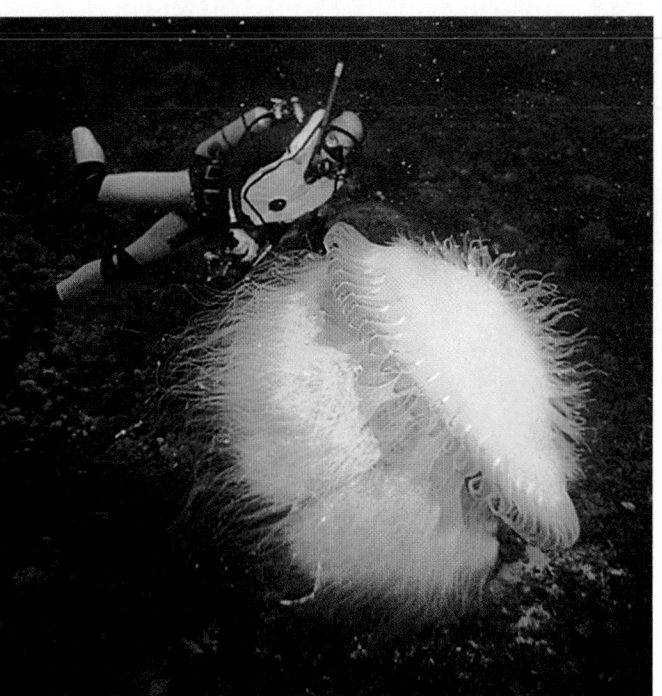

FIGURE 74-47 Lion's mane jellyfish *(Cyanea capillata). (Courtesy Carl Roessler.)*

Chironex (Box-Jellyfish)

The dreaded chirodropid box-jellyfish (*C. fleckeri* Southcott), often misnamed the sea wasp, is a venomous sea creature that can induce death in less than 60 seconds with its potent sting. Like all other scyphozoans, it is a carnivore, adapted to deal rapidly with prey. A member of the group of Cubomedusae jellyfish, it ranges in size from 2 to 30 cm across the bell. Although these creatures seem to prefer quiet, protected, and shallow areas, chiefly in the waters off northern Queensland, Australia, they can be found in the open ocean. A seasonal alternation of polypoid and medusoid generations from winter to summer, respectively, appears to account for the shift in preferred habitat from tidal estuaries to the open eulittoral zone.[86] Stinger season

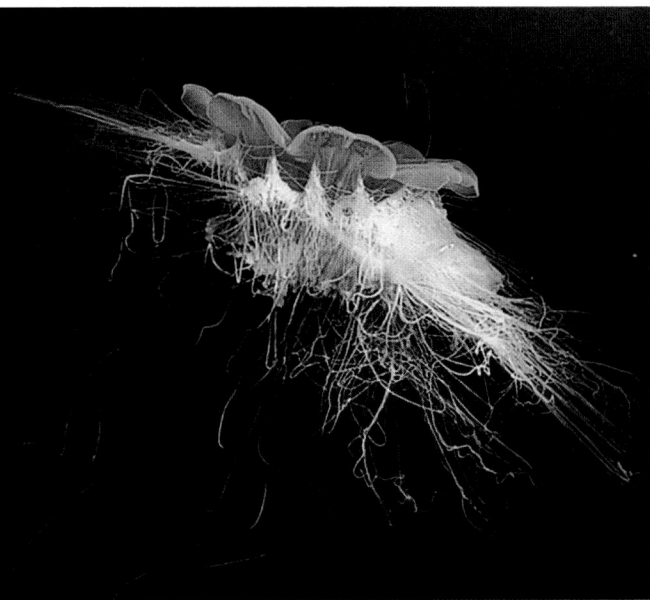

FIGURE 74-48 Lion's mane jellyfish *(Cyanea capillata)* can reach 3 m (10 feet) in diameter in Arctic waters. *(From Norbert Wu, with permission: norbertwu.com.)*

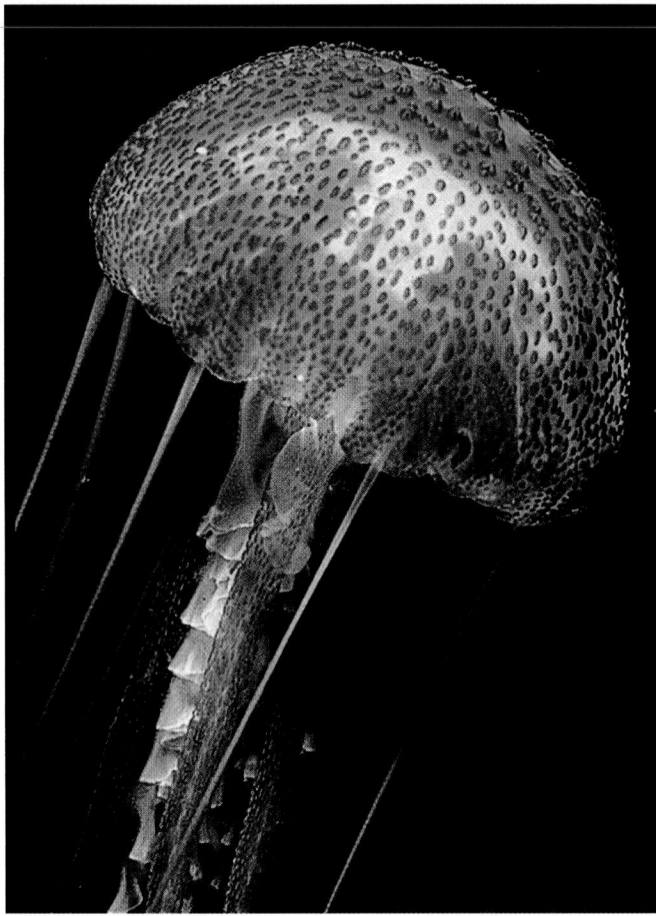

FIGURE 74-49 Mauve stinger *(Pelagia noctiluca)*. *(Courtesy Larry Madin, Woods Hole Oceanographic Institution.)*

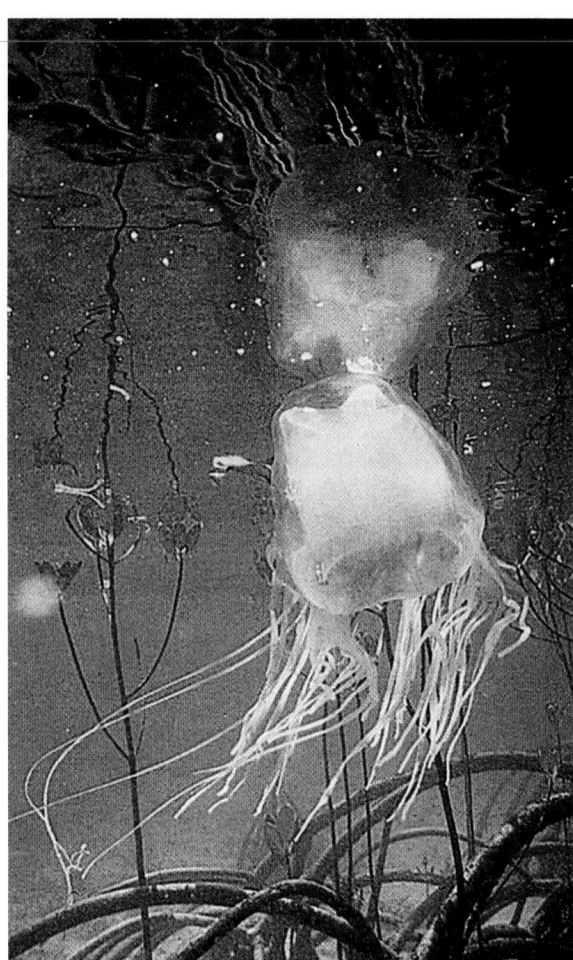

FIGURE 74-51 Box-jellyfish *(Chironex fleckeri)*, swimming just beneath the surface of the water. *(Courtesy John Williamson, MD.)*

in the Northern Territory of Australia is from October 1 to May 31.[42] Swimming and bathing are precluded in the littoral and estuarine waters of Indonesia, Malaysia, and Northern Australia during this season, which coincides with the hottest tropical months in the Southern Hemisphere.[158] However, it is likely that *Chironex* ("the assassin's hand") may be present year-round in the Northern Territory.[59] *Chironex* are fragile and photosensitive and thus are found submerged during bright sunlight hours (Figure 74-51), seeking the surface in the early morning and late afternoon and evening. The visual system of the box-jellyfish has 24 eyes of different types (eyes with spheric lenses, pigment pit eyes, and pigment slit eyes), which may possibly be used for an avoidance response or attraction to light.[72] Box-jellyfish are swift and graceful travelers, capable of sailing along at a steady 2 knots.

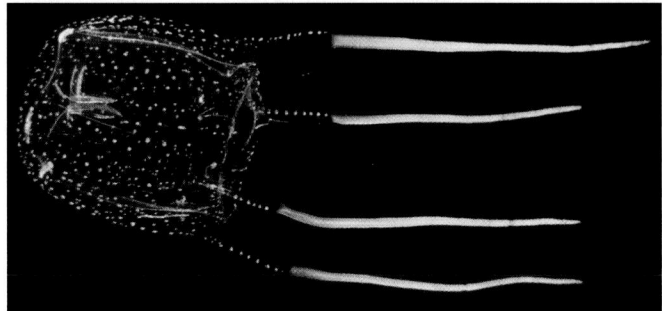

FIGURE 74-50 Jimble box-jellyfish or southern sea wasp *(Carybdea rastoni)* in Southern Australia. *(From Gary Bell: oceanwideimages.com.)*

An adult *Chironex* carries up to 15 broad tentacles (Figure 74-52) in each corner (pedalium, or foot) of its bell (up to 60 tentacles total, each with a length of up to 3 m [10 feet]) and has enough venom (> 10 mL) to kill three adults.[44,196] As *Chironex* grows in size, the ratio of mastigophores (nematocysts believed to hold the lethal venom component for prey) to less injurious organelles increases.[37] Two fractions have been isolated from the venom: a "lethal" fraction of molecular weight 150,000, and a lethal-hemolytic-dermatonecrotic fraction of molecular weight 79,000. At least 72 fatalities have been verified in Australian and Southeast Asian waters, with greater numbers probably lacking official documentation. Thus, the box-jellyfish is a much greater true hazard than the more fearsome shark. Other jellyfish, such as *C. rastoni* and *P. noctiluca*, infrequently cause severe prolonged reactions and have rarely been reported to lead to death, but are capable of causing dramatic immediate reactions (Figure 74-53).

Sudden death in a child has followed envenomation by *Chiropsalmus quadrumanus* (also sometimes described as a box-jellyfish) in the Gulf of Mexico at Crystal Beach, Texas.[14] Death was attributed to acute arrhythmia after a catecholamine surge, followed by cardiogenic shock and pulmonary edema.

Clinical Aspects. The extreme example of envenomation occurs with *C. fleckeri* (after Dr. Hugo Flecker) (Figure 74-54).[158] Death is attributed to hypotension, profound muscle spasm, muscular and respiratory paralysis, and subsequent cardiac arrest. Recent evidence suggests that *C. fleckeri* toxin has direct effects on the myocardium and may be cardiotoxic.[40,93] The overall mortality rate after box-jellyfish stings may approach 15% to 20% in select locales. Most commonly, bathers, frequently aboriginal children, are stung in shallow and remote coastal waters. The

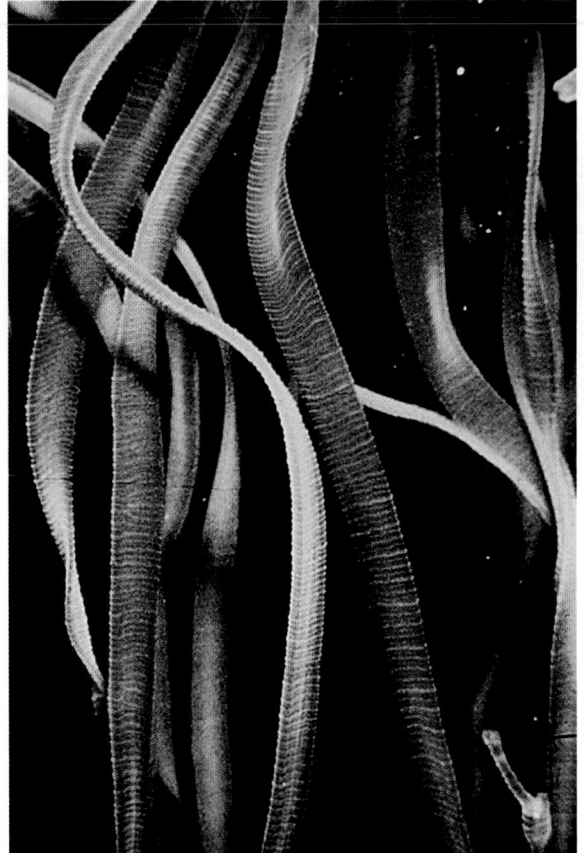

FIGURE 74-52 Close-up of the tentacle mass of an adult box-jellyfish *(Chironex fleckeri)*. *(Courtesy Bob Hartwick.)*

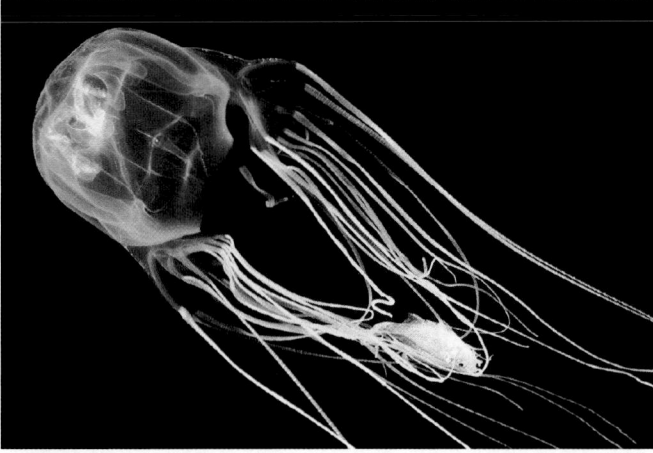

FIGURE 74-54 Box-jellyfish with prey in Australia. *(Copyright David Doubilet.)*

victims do not recognize the small, semitransparent, and submerged creature, which may approach as a member of a small armada. Most stings are minor; severe reaction or death follows skin contact with tentacles longer than 6 to 7 m (20 to 23 feet), although 10 cm of tentacle is capable of delivering a lethal dose of venom.[158,197] The sting is immediately excruciatingly painful, and the victim usually struggles purposefully for only a minute or two before collapse. The toxic skin reaction may be intense, with rapid formation of wheals, vesicles, and a darkened reddish brown or purple whiplike flare pattern with stripes 8 to 10 mm in width (Figures 74-55 and 74-56). With major stings, skin blistering occurs within 6 hours, with superficial necrosis in 12 to

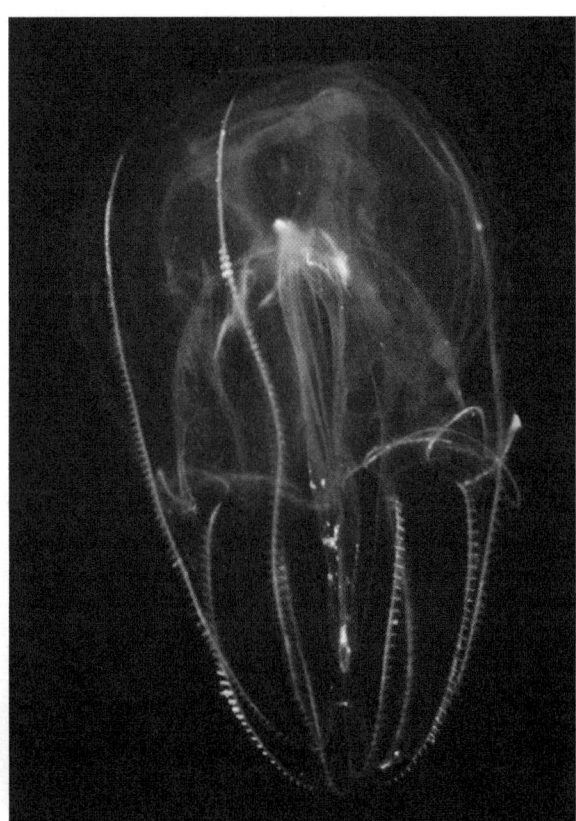

FIGURE 74-53 Box-type jellyfish in open water in Tonga. *(Copyright Carl Roessler.)*

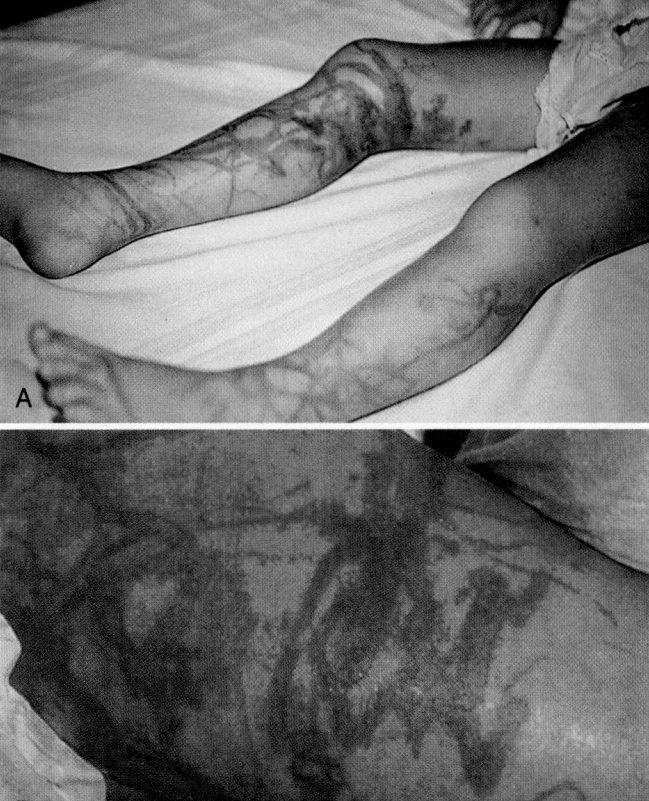

FIGURE 74-55 Intense necrosis (here, at 48 hours) is typical of a severe box-jellyfish *(Chironex fleckeri)* sting. **A,** Involvement of nearly an entire limb. **B,** Skin darkening can be rapid with cellular death. *(Courtesy John Williamson, MD.)*

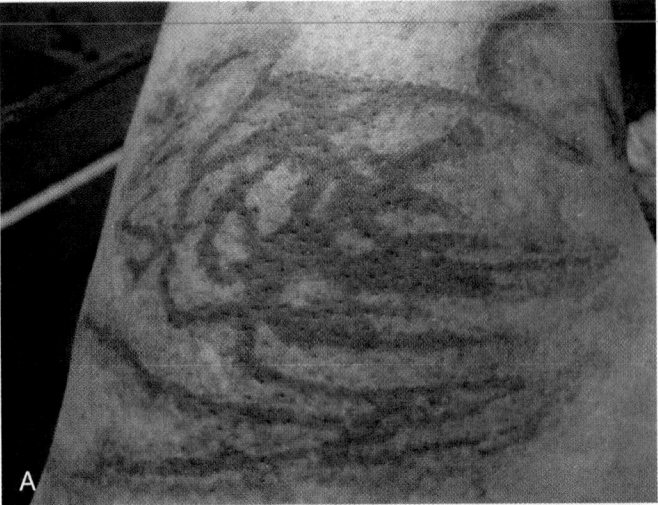

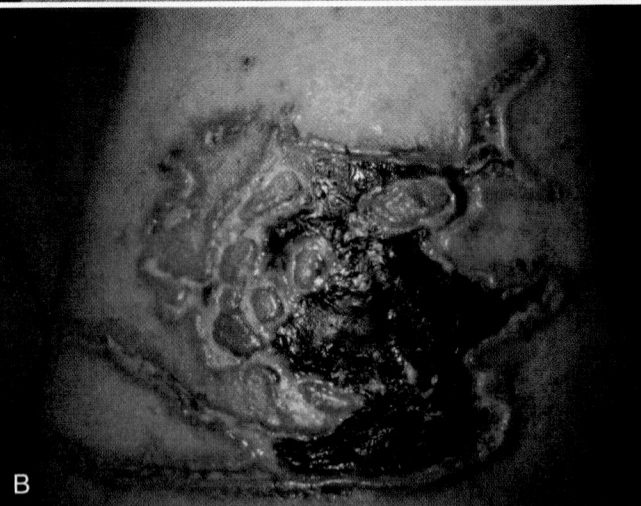

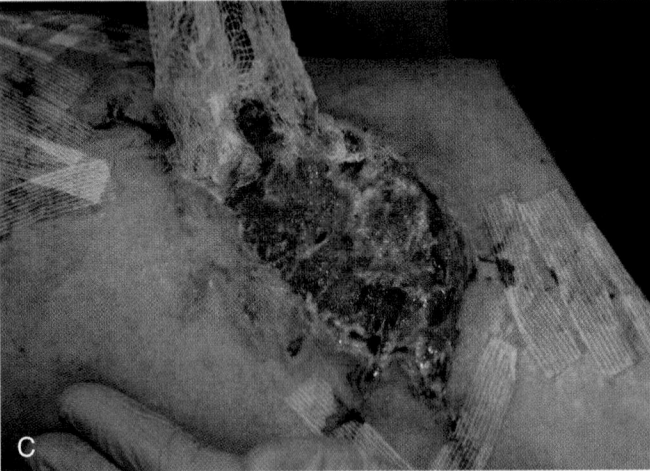

FIGURE 74-56 Progression of a severe jellyfish sting. **A,** Soon after the sting. **B,** Within a few weeks, severe necrosis is evident. **C,** Treatment required excision and skin grafting. *(Courtesy Stefan Caporale.)*

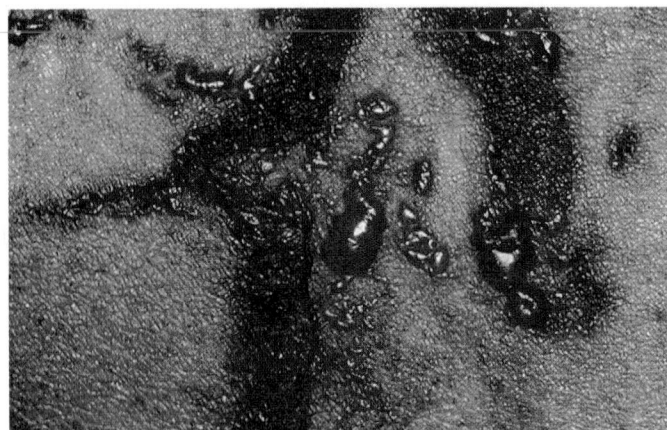

FIGURE 74-57 Incipient necrosis and blistering within 24 hours of box-jellyfish *(Chironex fleckeri)* envenomation. *(Courtesy John Williamson, MD.)*

One case of *Chironex* envenomation in a pregnant woman has been reported.[111,223] A 20-year-old woman in the 34th week of pregnancy suffered apparent respiratory arrest but was successfully revived with rescue breathing at the scene. The victim received antivenom in the hospital and delivered a healthy child at term by cesarean section. It is interesting to note that one rescuer was 37 weeks pregnant and received a sting from tentacles adherent to the victim, but she also delivered uneventfully.

Identification of *Chironex* envenomation is sometimes possible by nematocyst recovery from the skin. This can be done by scraping with a scalpel or by applying sticky tape. In the former technique, the skin is firmly scraped with a sterile scalpel blade, which is then placed in a container. Five to 10 mL of distilled water is added, and the container is sonicated for 5 minutes to remove any nematocysts adherent to the blade. The solution is syringed through a 13-mm Millipore filter, which leaves the nematocysts, debris, and skin cells on the paper. A 0.5% eosin stain is syringed through the filter paper, which is allowed to dry, after which it is placed on a glass slide, fixed, and mounted with a cover slip. In the sticky tape technique, transparent household sticky tape is applied to the sting site, stroked several times to ensure adherence, and then removed and placed sticky side up on a glass slide, with the ends secured to the slide with additional tape.[45]

Treatment. In the case of a known or suspected box-jellyfish envenomation, the victim must be assessed rapidly for adequacy of breathing and supported with an airway and

18 hours (Figure 74-57). The skin defects that result from a severe envenomation can be profound (Figure 74-58). On occasion, a pathognomonic frosted appearance with a transverse cross-hatched pattern has been observed (Figure 74-59). This appearance may be primarily the result of the application of aluminum salts used for decontamination. More severe reactions and increased mortality rates in women and small children have been attributed to their greater hairless body surface area and smaller body mass.

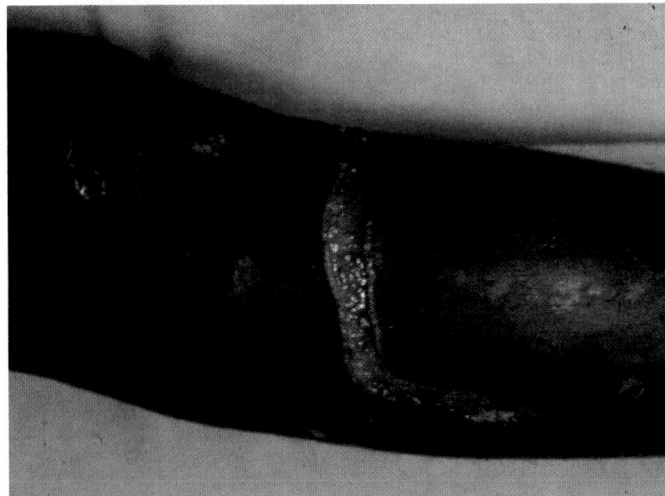

FIGURE 74-58 Skin destruction 3 weeks after an untreated box-jellyfish *(Chironex fleckeri)* envenomation. *(Courtesy John Williamson, MD.)*

return. Such a bandage should be loosened for 90 seconds every 10 minutes and should be completely removed after 1 hour. In no case should an arterial tourniquet be applied. Use of a proximal constriction band has not been proved to be helpful.

Up until recently, it has been recommended that *Chironex* antivenom be administered intravenously as soon as possible. Following the "antivenom approach," the IM route is less preferred, because peak blood levels may not be obtained for 48 hours after administration by this route. One author has recommended consideration of intraosseous administration if the IV route is not available.[44] The antivenom is supplied in vials (1.5 to 4 mL of liquid) containing 20,000 units by CSL (Figure 74-61). The initial dose is one vial (diluted 1:5 to 1:10 in isotonic crystalloid; dilution with water is not recommended) administered intravenously over 5 minutes, or three vials into three different sites (generally on the thigh) intramuscularly. IM antivenom has been administered successfully over the years by members of the Queensland Surf Life-Saving Association and the Queensland Ambulance Transport Brigade.[62] Although the antivenom is prepared by hyperimmunizing sheep and adverse reactions reported have been rare and mild, the prudent physician is always prepared to treat anaphylaxis or serum sickness.[42] It has been stated that it cannot be overemphasized that timely administration of antivenom might be lifesaving, particularly in light of the fact that most deaths from *Chironex* stings occur in the first 5 to 20 minutes.[223] In addition to its lifesaving properties, early administration of antivenom is felt to markedly reduce pain and decrease

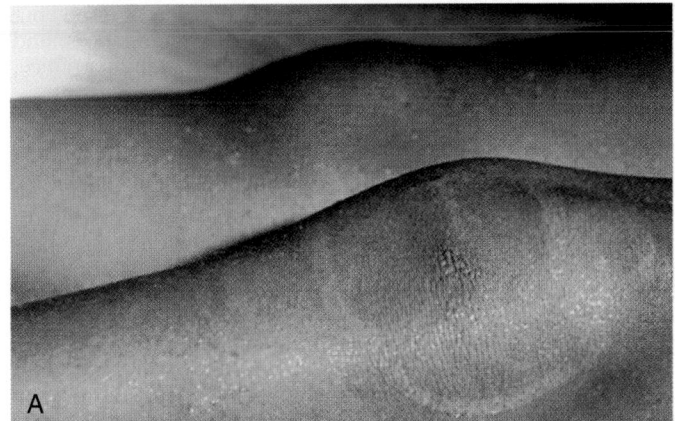
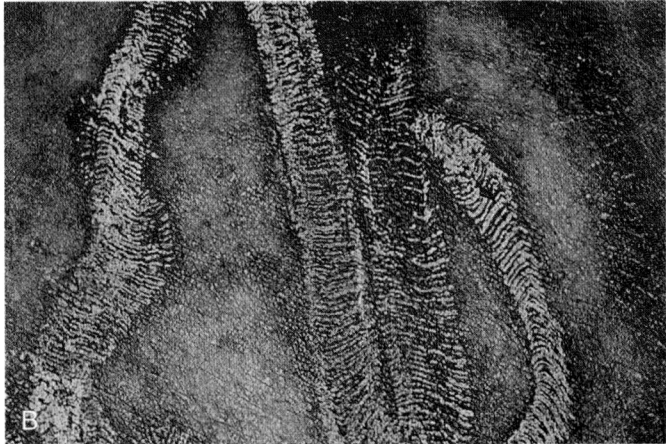

FIGURE 74-59 Frosted cross-hatched pattern pathognomonic for a box-jellyfish envenomation. **A,** The victim of this sting expired rapidly. **B,** The enhanced frosted appearance is a result of application of a spray of aluminum sulfate. *(Courtesy John Williamson, MD.)*

artificial ventilation if necessary. The victim should be moved as little as possible. It is essential to immediately and liberally flood, for a minimum of 30 seconds, the skin surrounding any adherent tentacles with 5% acetic acid (vinegar) before any attempt is made to remove them; this paralyzes the nematocysts and avoids worsening the envenomation (Figure 74-60). Significant pain relief should not be expected from this maneuver, which may actually worsen the pain briefly.[13,218] Although most nematocysts cannot penetrate the thickened skin of the human palm, the rescuer should pay particular attention to his or her own skin protection. If acetic acid is not available, aluminum sulfate surfactant (Stingose) may be substituted, although its efficacy has not been well demonstrated for a *Chironex* envenomation. A number of experts recommend that isopropyl alcohol *not* be used as a topical decontaminant for a box-jellyfish envenomation, based on in vitro observations of inefficacy and nematocyst discharge after application of this detoxicant.[86,197] Clinical confirmation of this recommendation has not been published.

Pressure-immobilization is no longer recommended to prevent absorption of *Chironex* venom.[4,115] Certain experts have questioned its efficacy and noted that large affected skin surfaces cannot be effectively bandaged. Others have noted that application of pressure might promote nematocyst discharge, which is believed to be more harmful than foregoing any attempt to devascularize the area immediately below the bandage in order to prevent distribution of venom into the general circulation.[8,161,182,196,225,226] In any event, it is reasonable to splint or otherwise immobilize the limb to prevent motion.

In the absence of antivenom (see below) and facing a prolonged transport prior to supportive intensive care, a rescuer might apply a constriction bandage proximal to the site of an extremity sting, to impede lymphatic and superficial venous

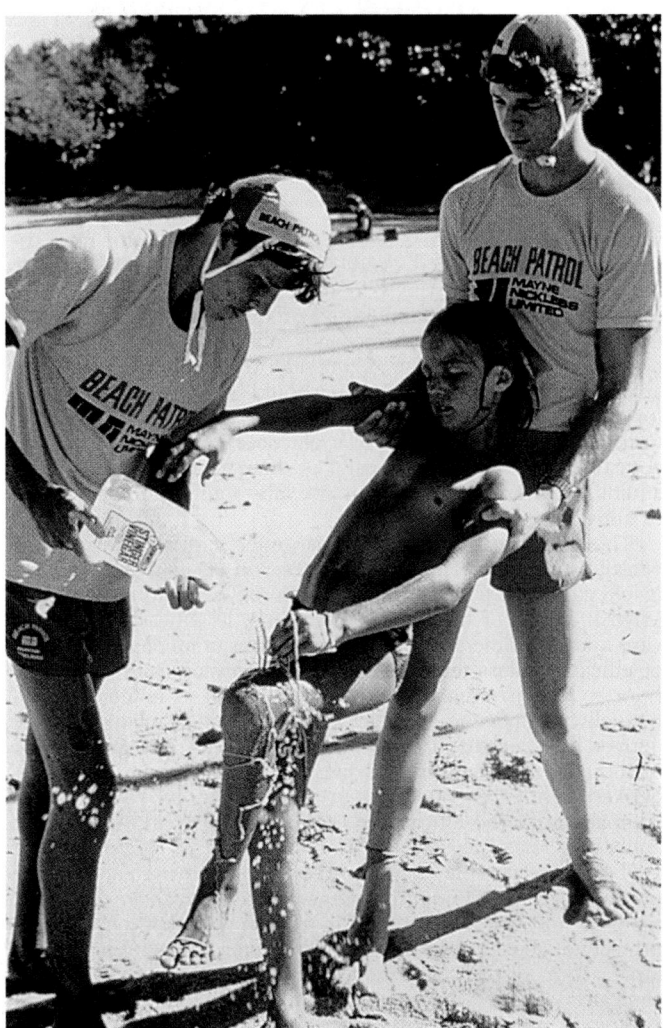

FIGURE 74-60 Surf lifeguards pour vinegar on the leg of a simulated box-jellyfish envenomation. Note how they restrain the victim's arms to prevent him from handling the harmful tentacles. *(Courtesy John Williamson, MD.)*

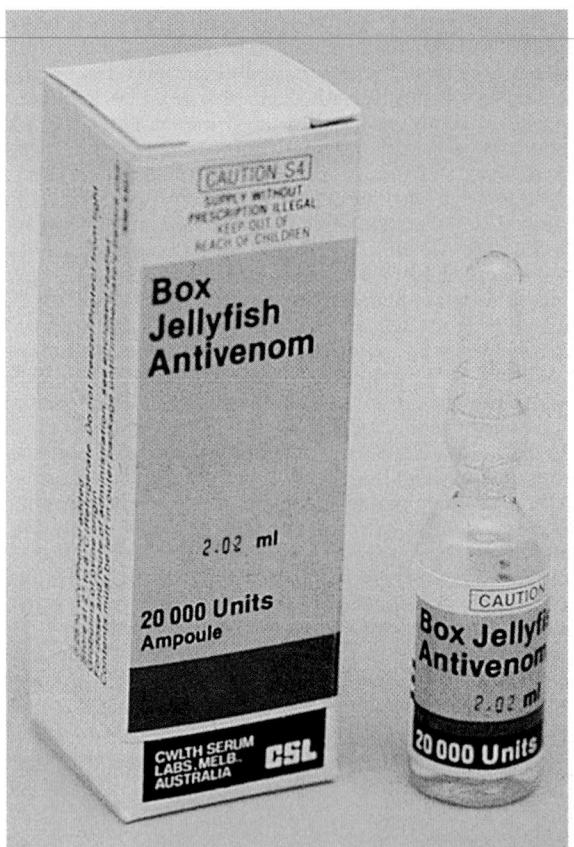

FIGURE 74-61 Box-jellyfish antivenom. *(Courtesy John Williamson, MD.)*

subsequent skin scarring.[224] Antivenom administration may be repeated once or twice every 2 to 4 hours until there is no further worsening of the skin discoloration, pain, or systemic effects. A large sting in an adult may require initial IV administration of up to three vials. The antivenom may also be used to neutralize the effects of a *Chiropsella* (formerly *Chiropsalmus*) envenomation.[167,196,230] Antivenom should be stored in a refrigerator at 2° to 10° C (35.6° to 50° F) and must not be frozen.[29] Concomitant administration of a glucocorticoid (such as hydrocortisone 200 mg intravenously) is often recommended for its antiinflammatory activity but is no substitute for administration of antivenom.

The usefulness of antivenom is under scrutiny and not universally supported. There is not 100% consensus that antivenom is effective for treatment of human envenomations by box-jellyfish. Some of the arguments against its efficacy include in vitro and experimental animal observations of incomplete or lack of efficacy, unless the antivenom is administered for protection prior to venom administration.[51,231] Some have noted that CSL box-jellyfish antivenom, which is raised against "milked" venom derived from electrical stimulation of tentacles stretched over a membrane, may not have complete efficacy against tentacle-derived venom encountered in vivo. In an in vivo (rodent) comparison of the efficacy of CSL box-jellyfish antivenom with antibodies raised against nematocyst-derived *C. fleckeri* venom, antibodies were able to neutralize the cardiovascular collapse produced by the venom, but large amounts of antivenom were required and needed to be preincubated with the venom to be protective. The authors interpreted these results to indicate a very rapid action of the toxins and that antivenom is unlikely to be clinically effective because it cannot be administered early enough.[231] The effectiveness of the antivenom remains the subject of debate, because no controlled trials or observational studies exist to support its effectiveness.[43] Furthermore, administration of antivenom in the actual field situation is often delayed and suboptimal, and deaths have occurred despite its administration.

None of these observations mandates that it not be used, but they do call into question whether, in what circumstances, and to what degree antivenom might be effective. Until further notice, its use is still widely recommended.

Another line of inquiry seeks to understand whether there is any benefit to adjunctive therapy if antivenom is used. In an investigation that sought to quantify the in vivo cardiovascular effects of box-jellyfish venom in rats, efficacy of pretreatment with antivenom, verapamil, and magnesium sulfate was undertaken. Box-jellyfish venom was injected intravenously and produced a transient hypertensive response followed by hypotension and cardiovascular collapse. Pretreatment with antivenom did not have any effect on the venom-induced pressor response but prevented cardiovascular collapse in some of the animals. Administration of verapamil alone or in combination with antivenom did not have any beneficial effect; however, verapamil negated the protective effects of antivenom. Magnesium sulfate administration alone was not beneficial; however, combined with antivenom, it prevented cardiovascular collapse in all animals. In a different study in which a cell-based assay for screening of antidotes to and antivenom against *C. fleckeri* venom was deployed, it was determined that box-jellyfish antivenom could neutralize certain effects of the venom only if added prior to administration of the venom, and that felodipine and MgSO₄ potentiated detrimental effects of the venom. The extrapolation of these animal data to humans treated with antivenom is theoretical.[168]

Burnett and Calton[17,25,34] discovered that verapamil can prolong the lives of mice challenged with box-jellyfish, sea nettle, or Portuguese man-of-war venom. Verapamil was considered to be inactive or deleterious in anesthetized laboratory pigs envenomed with box-jellyfish venom.[207] Extrapolation of these data to humans is as yet untested. Although there is logic to using verapamil from a theoretical pharmacologic perspective (venom affects calcium influx through voltage-dependent channels; elevated calcium levels may represent cell death), the suitability of using verapamil as an adjunct to therapy in humans has been questioned because of the perceived problem of administering a hypotensive agent during an episode of cardiac decompensation.[89] In a cell-based assay to evaluate antidotes to box-jellyfish venom, verapamil had no effect and felodipine was detrimental.[107] Calcium channel–blocker drug use is currently not recommended for any form of jellyfish sting.

If a sting is mild (not life-threatening), one may use nonmoist ice packs for initial pain relief, along with a parenteral analgesic. Even with successful treatment, skin irritation may persist for months, marked by discolored striae, intermittent desquamation, and pruritus. Type IV hypersensitivity reactions with *Chironex* stings may occur more commonly than previously thought; they may be attributable to retained foreign material.[155]

Irukandji Jellyfish

Carukia barnesi, the carybdeid jellyfish known as Irukandji, is a small (1 to 2.5 cm across the bell) translucent jellyfish with four thin nematocyst-covered tentacles (5 to 7 cm in length at rest, and up to 70 cm [27.5 inches] extended) found off the coast of northern Australia in both inshore and open waters.[11,116,143,191] Barnes demonstrated that *C. barnesi* causes Irukandji syndrome.[11] With this species, most stings occur near shore and during the afternoon.[158] Because the jellyfish tend to aggregate, victims often present in clusters. Furthermore, victims can be stung inside stinger-resistant enclosures, even when the mesh is as small as 2 cm diagonally.[57]

It has been reported that additional species of jellyfish can cause Irukandji syndrome. These include *Alatina mordens, C. alata, Malo maxima, Carybdea xaymacana,* and perhaps others.[118,119,232] Other carybdeid medusae that envenom with varying severity include the jimble (*C. rastoni*) and fire jelly (*Tamoya haplonema*). The morbakka is a stinging creature that resembles the Irukandji but is larger. Its bell, which measures up to 12 by 16 cm, is covered with clumps of nematocysts and may be as dangerous to handle as the meter-long tentacles. This animal may have been previously misidentified as *Tamoya*. An Irukandji-like syndrome has been reported in South Florida divers, but the jellyfish species was not identified.[77]

Clinical Aspects. The immediate skin reaction is characterized by stinging pain that is often not severe, followed by erythema at the sting site. Within minutes, irregularly spaced papules of 2 mm in diameter may develop. The venom may then induce a more severe reaction of restlessness, muscle pain and spasm, severe lumbosacral back pain, lower leg pain, priapism, abdominal pain, pancreatitis, parasympathetic dysautonomia, respiratory difficulty (including painful breathing), headache, shivering, tremor, nausea, and vomiting, which progress to profound weakness and collapse. Localized piloerection and sweating have been reported to occur commonly. Generally, the discomfort remits in 6 to 24 hours; however, it occasionally recurs. The *Irukandji syndrome* (named by Hugo Flecker for an Aboriginal tribe in the Cairns region of Australia) presupposes massive catecholamine release, with abdominal and chest pain, a sensation of chest tightness, pallor or peripheral cyanosis, vomiting, diaphoresis, hypertension (diastolic blood pressure to 140 mm Hg), oliguria, tachycardia, ventricular tachycardia, cardiomyopathy, severe pulmonary edema, cerebral edema, troponin leak, and hypokinetic heart failure.[44,63,130,148,177] This resembles what might be seen with a pheochromocytoma. Papilledema and coma in a child have been described.[60] Although the systemic syndrome can be quite distinctive, there may be minimal cutaneous signs of envenomation.[83,148] Two deaths have been reported, both attributed to intracerebral hemorrhage associated with hypertension.[58]

It is interesting to note that many Irukandji-like stings occur inside stinger enclosures (bathing nets) designed to exclude *C. fleckeri*. Although residents of Irukandji-endemic areas are often aware that stinger-resistant enclosures do not prevent entry of the smaller jellyfish, many tourists, particularly those from countries other than Australia, are not aware.[85,148]

Treatment. It is not determined whether or not there is a suitable topical decontaminant for an Irukandji sting, and it has been noted that the skin manifestations may be comparatively innocuous, so rapid field therapy may not be undertaken. In addition to the standard cnidarian measures and supportive therapy, IV phentolamine (5 mg initially, followed by 5- to 10-mg doses as needed) may be administered to control high blood pressure. However, because acute cardiac failure may be a feature of envenomation, administration of an α-adrenergic blocking drug should be undertaken with close cardiovascular monitoring and perhaps preliminary echocardiography, supplemented as needed in a case of severe or rapidly progressive illness.[117] Administration of box-jellyfish antivenom does not significantly relieve symptoms. Propranolol or other β-adrenergic blockers should not be used to control tremor, as these might precipitate catastrophic hypotension, or might contribute to unopposed α-adrenergic stimulation predisposing to myocardial ischemia.[57] Fentanyl has been suggested for pain relief because it does not cause cardiac depression.[117] One report noted resolution of agitation and sympathetic features, and significant resolution of pain, in a victim of Irukandji syndrome treated with magnesium sulfate (loading dose 10 mmol [≈ 2.5 g or 20 mEq], followed by an infusion of 5 mmol/hr).[41]

Chrysaora (Sea Nettles)

Sea nettles (such as *C. quinquecirrha* and *C. capillata*) are considerably less lethal animals and can be found in both temperate and tropical waters, particularly in the Chesapeake Bay, where they are found in seasonal plague proportions.[139] Not as dangerous as the Indo-Pacific box-jellyfish, they are still capable of inducing a moderately severe sting. *C. quinquecirrha* and similar species carry a proteinaceous venom that contains at least seven enzymes, with at least one antigenic and thermolabile component that is cardiotoxic, neurotoxic, and dermatonecrotic.[73] The venom also contains histamine, histamine releasers, prostaglandins, serotonin, and kinin-like factors (kinin-like factors have also been found in venoms of *C. fleckeri* and *P. physalis*).[23] Large intradermal injections of crude sea nettle venom in normal saline produced immunosuppression (T cells) for several days, with a homologous reaction against the same cnidarian antigen and a heterologous reaction against antigens contained within vaccinia and herpes simplex viruses and tetanus bacillus.[212]

Clinical Aspects. The clinical presentation of a sea nettle envenomation is similar to that of *Physalia* species, with perhaps a greater incidence of systemic complications. Death is exceedingly rare. Elevated levels of serum anti–sea nettle venom IgM, IgG, and IgE may persist for years in victims who suffer exaggerated reactions to *C. quinquecirrha* stings. These antibodies cross-react with *Physalia* venom and have been postulated to be of value in identifying victims at risk for a severe reaction.[24] This technique is not widely available or frequently used, and its reliability and reproducibility require further verification.

The reaction after a sting by the blubber jellyfish (*Catostylus* species) is relatively mild, with the formation of wheals, erythema, and pruritus limited to the areas of contact. Systemic effects are exceedingly rare. *Cyanea* species carry long thin tentacles that induce a similar effect, with occasional muscle aching, nausea, and drowsiness, particularly in small children. *Pelagia* species also induce wheals, which are more circinate or irregularly shaped and may not follow a linear pattern. The venom is sufficiently toxic to cause a severe generalized allergy, with bronchospasm and pruritus.

Treatment. Treatment for a sea nettle envenomation is similar to that for the sting of *Physalia* species. Baking soda may be the most effective commonly available initial detoxicant, followed by papain and Stingose. One study found that ammonia, ethanol, and vinegar may increase the sensation of pain from sea nettle envenomation and cause discharge of nematocysts.[16] Topical lidocaine is the anesthetic of choice if a patient presents with painful lesions. Monoclonal antibodies to jellyfish venoms have been developed that demonstrate cross-reactivity among venoms of a variety of cnidarians, which may allow development of a single protective antivenom or vaccine.

CLASS ANTHOZOA

The class Anthozoa includes sea anemones, stony (true) corals (subclass Zoantharia), and soft corals (subclass Alcyonaria). Anemones are considered here because they envenom.

Actinaria (Anemones)

Actinarians (sea anemones) are abundant (1000 species) multicolored animals with sessile habits and a flower-like appearance (Figures 74-62 and 74-63). They are composed of stalked, finger-like projections capable of stinging and paralyzing passing fish. Their sizes range from a few millimeters to more than 0.5 m (1.7 feet); they are found at depths of up to 5303 m (2900 fathoms). The insides of some anemones can be eaten after they are dried.

Anemones can be colorful creatures and may be found in tidal pools, where the unwary brush up against them or inquisitively

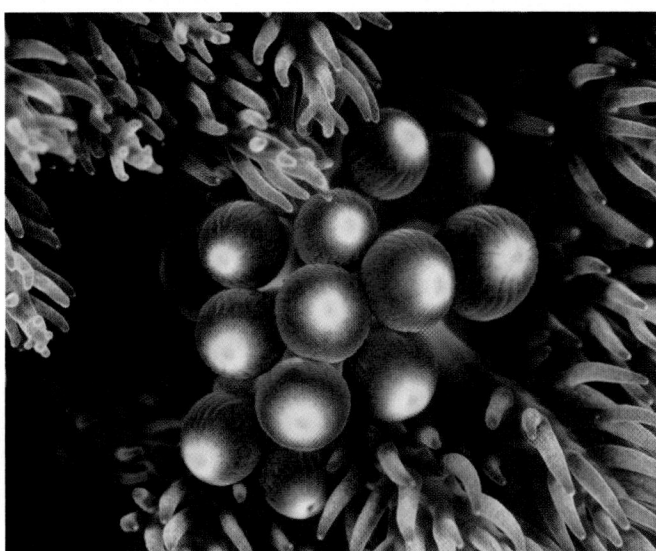

FIGURE 74-62 Detail of grape-like vesicles of sea anemone (*Actinaria* species). (*From Gary Bell: oceanwideimages.com.*)

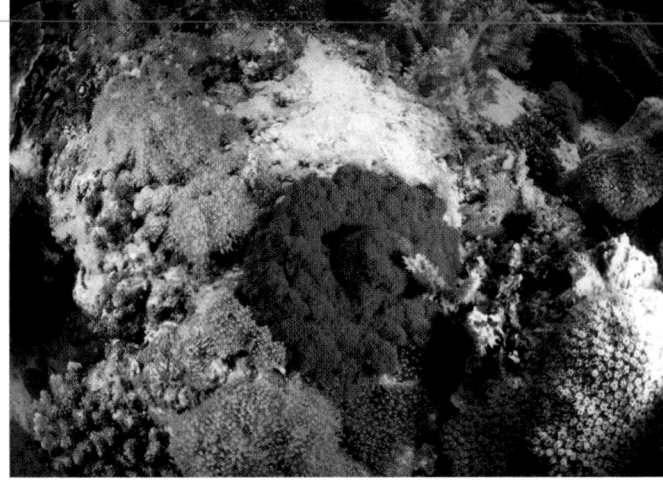

FIGURE 74-63 Orange stinging anemone. (Copyright Lynn Funkhouser.)

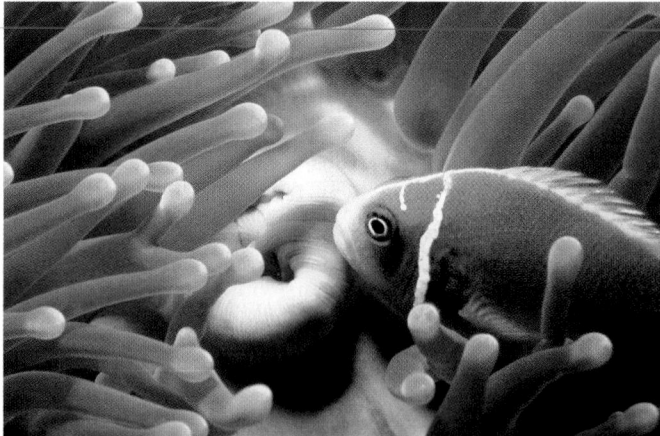

FIGURE 74-65 Clownfish in peaceful coexistence with a sea anemone. (Courtesy Paul Auerbach, MD.)

touch them. Other anemones burrow into bottom mud or sand. Like other cnidarians, they possess tentacles loaded with one of two variations of the nematocyst, either the sporocyst or the basitrichous isorhiza (basitrich). These wreak havoc once stimulated by an unfortunate victim. Some sporocysts are adhesive and act to hold and envenom prey. To present a greater number of nematocysts to the victim, an exposed anemone inflates the tentacles by filling them with water. Many anemones also secrete mucus, which covers the anemone's body and may contain cytolytic and hemolytic protein toxins. These may serve to repel potential predators.

Although a number of sea animals, such as clownfish (anemonefish) of the genera *Amphiprion* and *Premnas*, live in symbiosis with certain anemones (*Heteractis* species, *Stichodactyla* species, *Macrodactyla doreensis*, *Entacmaea quadricolor*, and *Cryptodendrum adhaesivum*), humans are not so fortunate and are frequently stung when attempting to handle these not so delicate "flowers." The clownfish have evolved resistance to the anemone's sting by repeated contact and development of a mucous coat (Figures 74-64 and 74-65), and perhaps by immunity.[137]

Sea anemones contain biologically active substances, including neurotoxins (sodium channel inactivation, stabilizing the open state conformations), cardiotoxins, hemolysins (for erythrocytes and platelets), and proteinase inhibitors.[138,186] A ubiquitous and well-studied class of sea anemone toxins is composed of cytolytic polypeptides of four known groups based on differing molecular properties and modes of action.[195] Cytolytic toxins

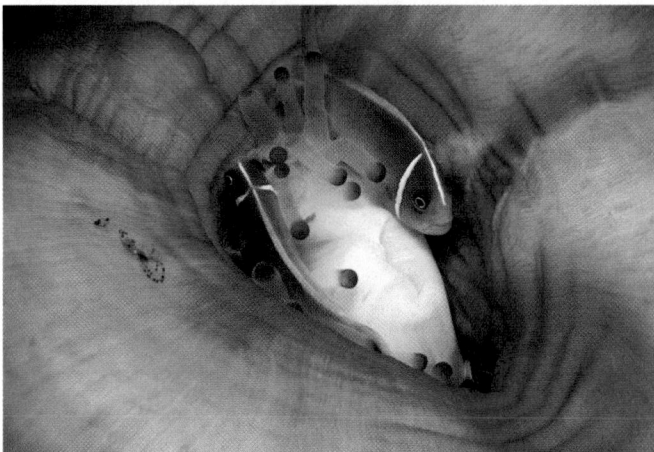

FIGURE 74-64 Clownfish nestled in anemone. (Copyright 2011 Norbert Wu: norbertwu.com.)

elaborated by anemones include cytolysins, which are thought to exert their effect by damaging membranes via pore or channel formation. A cytolytic toxin has been isolated from the Indo-Pacific sea anemone *Stoichactis kenti*.[15] The anemone *Actinia equina* elaborates cytolytic polypeptide toxins known as equinatoxins, which may induce hemolysis and cardiorespiratory arrest in animals, attributed by some to coronary vasospasm.[124] Tenebrosin-C from the anemone *Actinia tenebrosa* is a positive inotrope that can be inhibited by the cyclooxygenase blockers indomethacin and aspirin, a lipooxygenase blocker and leukotriene antagonist, and mepacrine (a phospholipase A_2 inhibitor).[69] Potassium channel toxins have been isolated from the sea anemones *Bunodosoma granulifera* and *Stichodactyla helianthus*.[88,151] Palytoxin has been found in the sea anemone *Radianthus macrodactylus*.[126] Granulitoxin is a lethal neurotoxic peptide isolated from *B. granulifera*.[178]

Clinical Aspects. Most victims are stung when they handle or accidentally brush against an anemone in shallow water. Nudists may acquire genital injuries; small children may accidentally or intentionally ingest tentacles. The dermatitis caused by contact with an anemone is similar in all regards to that from fire coral or a small man-of-war; it is often likened to a bee sting. The variation in skin reaction is related to the specific toxicity of the venom, so that while *Actinia* species produce painful urticarial lesions, *Anemonia* species induce paresthesias, edema, and erythema. Most commonly, the initial skin lesion is centrally pale with a halo of erythema and petechial hemorrhage. This is soon followed by edema and diffuse ecchymosis. If the envenomation is severe, intense local hemorrhage, vesiculation, necrosis, skin ulceration, and secondary infection may occur, particularly after the stings of certain species (*Sagartia*, *Actinia*, *Anemonia*, *Actinodendron*, and *Triactis*). In Floridian waters, the turtle grass anemone *Viatrix globulifera*, translucent-white and less than 2.5 cm (1 inch) in diameter, is very hazardous, particularly for fishermen wading on grass flats. The Hell's fire sea anemone (*Actinodendron plumosum*) is aptly named. Systemic reactions are less likely after the sting of an anemone than after that of a man-of-war; reactions include fever, chills, somnolence, malaise, weakness, nausea, vomiting, and syncope. Fulminant fatal hepatic failure 3 days after a sea anemone sting of approximately 3 cm (just greater than 1 inch) in diameter on the scapula and complicated by coma, severe coagulopathy, and renal failure has been attributed to *Condylactis* (Figure 74-66) (commonly found in reefs and lagoons of south Florida, the Bahamas, and the Caribbean) on the basis of a positive serum test of IgG by ELISA at a dilution of 1:450.[70]

In most cases, mild envenomations resolve within 48 hours. More severe reactions, characterized by discoloration and vesicle formation, may become indolent, with eschar leading to residual hyperpigmentation, hypopigmentation, or keloid formation.

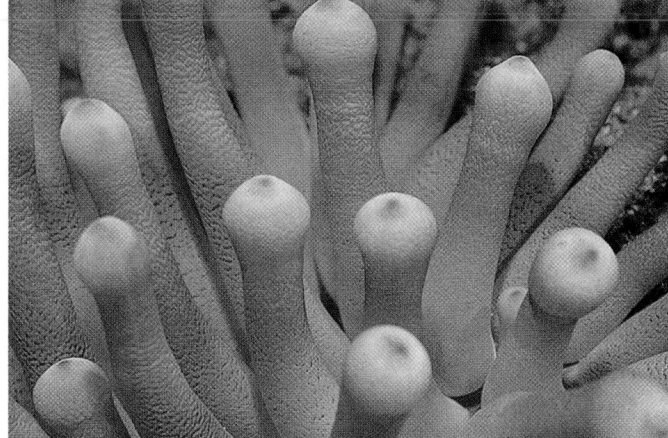

FIGURE 74-66 Giant anemone *(Condylactis gigantea). (From Norbert Wu, with permission: norbertwu.com.)*

Sponge fisherman's (diver's) disease is caused by contact with an anemone *(Sagartia* or *Actinia)* that attaches itself symbiotically to the base of a sponge. A few minutes after contact with the sponge, the victim's skin begins to itch and burn, with development of erythema and small vesicles. As described previously, this transforms to a darkened purple appearance, with frequent systemic components (headache, nausea, vomiting, fever, chills, and muscle spasm).

Treatment. Treatment for an anemone envenomation is similar to that for the sting of *Physalia* species. The dermatitis is frequently more severe and may require prolonged wound care consisting of debridement and antibiotic therapy for secondary infection. The healing process is generally slower after an anemone sting than after a man-of-war envenomation.

PHYLUM ECHINODERMATA

The phylum Echinodermata ("spiny skin") has five classes: sea lilies, brittle stars, starfish, sea urchins, and sea cucumbers. Only the last three are of medical interest in humans, although some brittle stars carry toxins capable of causing paralysis and death in small animals.

STARFISH

Life and Habits

Starfish are simple, free-living, stellate echinoderms covered with thorny spines of calcium carbonate crystals held erect by muscle tissue. The creatures move on the ocean floor by means of tube feet located under the arms (rays). They eat other echinoderms, mollusks, coral, worms, and poisonous shellfish. Starfish proliferation and the destruction of coral beds within the Great Barrier Reef off the coast of Australia is a conservation issue of international concern. The starfish everts its membranous stomach through its mouth and secretes digestive enzymes that destroy coral polyps. Only the stark white coral skeleton remains. The crown-of-thorns starfish *(Acanthaster planci)* is found in the coral reef communities of the Great Barrier Reef, throughout the Pacific and Indian Oceans, in the Red Sea, and in the Gulf of California.

Venom and Venom Apparatus

Glandular tissue interspersed in or lying underneath the epidermis (integument) produces a slimy venomous substance. The carnivorous *A. planci* is a particularly venomous species, normally 25 to 35 cm (10 to 14 inches) in diameter but up to 70 cm (27.5 inches) in diameter, with 7 to 23 arms (Figure 74-67). The sharp, rigid, and venomous aboral spines of this animal may grow to 4 to 6 cm (1.6 to 2.4 inches) (Figure 74-68). Potentially toxic saponins and histamine-like compounds have been isolated from the spine surfaces; crude venom extracts demonstrate hemolytic, capillary permeability–increasing, myotoxic (via

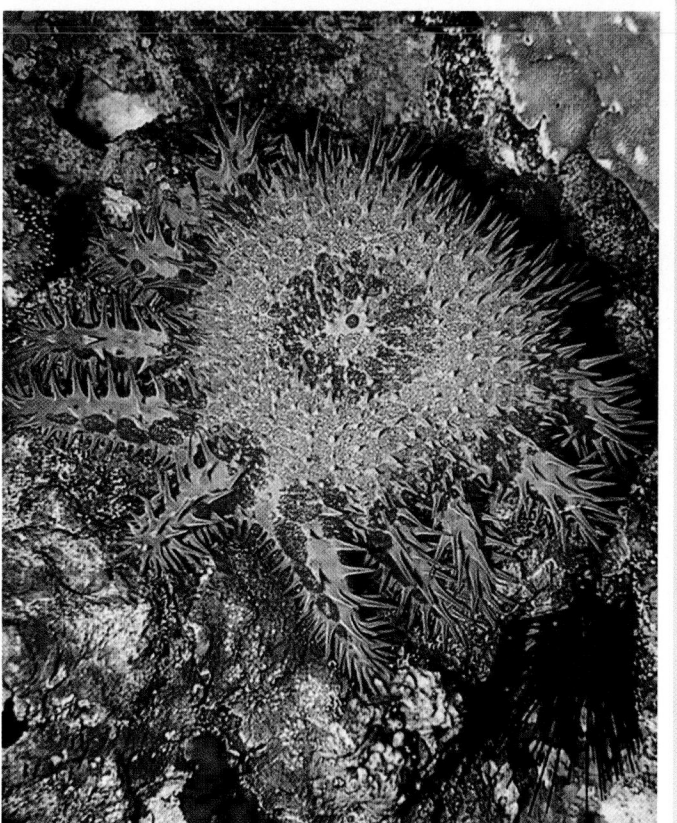

FIGURE 74-67 Crown-of-thorns starfish *(Acanthaster planci). (Courtesy Paul S. Auerbach, MD.)*

phospholipases A_2-I and -II), myonecrotic, and anticoagulant effects. The *A. planci* lethal factor is a potent hepatotoxin in laboratory animals.[185,187] A case report described abnormal liver function after *A. planci* envenomation of a 19-year-old.[113] Plancinin is an anticoagulant purified from the crown-of-thorns starfish. This peptide shows activity in mice that suggests a longer duration of action than heparin.[100] Severe systemic hypotension, thrombocytopenia, and leukopenia were induced by *A. planci* venom in dogs.[188] Indomethacin, a cyclooxygenase inhibitor, suppressed the hypotension. *A. planci* venom caused smooth (uterine) muscle contraction in rats, which was blocked by inhibitors of prostaglandin synthesis but not by atropine.[101]

Other starfish that might envenom humans are those of the genus *Echinaster*. The slime (cushion) star *Pteraster tessalatus*, which inhabits Pacific coastal waters from Puget Sound to Alaska,

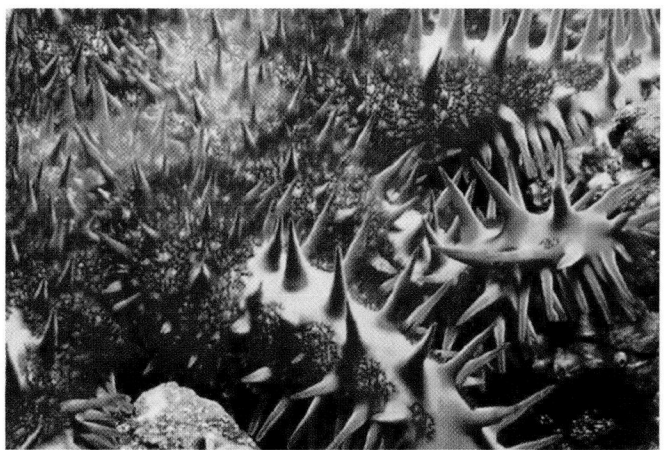

FIGURE 74-68 Spines of the crown-of-thorns starfish *(Acanthaster planci). (Courtesy Paul S. Auerbach, MD.)*

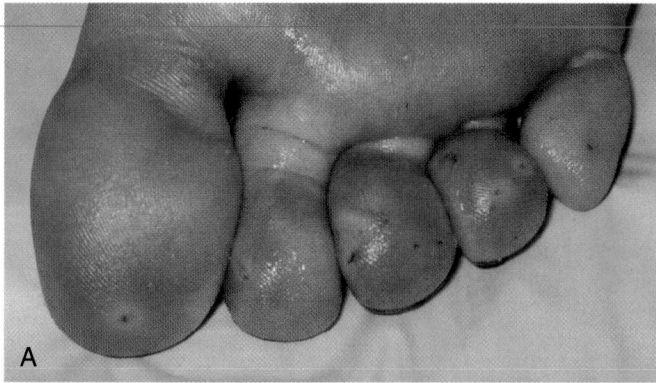

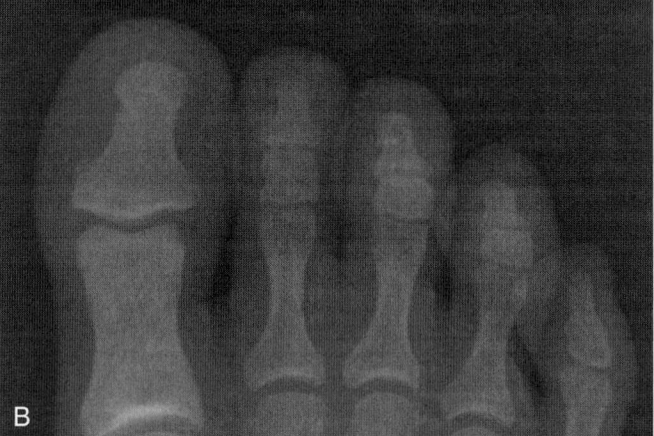

FIGURE 74-69 A, Crown-of-thorns starfish spine punctures to the toes. **B,** X-ray of foot of the same patient demonstrates retained spine fragments. *(Courtesy Brian Lin, MD.)*

generates the unique defense of copious gelatinous or rubbery, poisonous mucus to repel natural enemies. No human injuries have been reported to date.

Clinical Aspects

The ice pick–like spine of *A. planci* can penetrate the hardiest of diving gloves. Most spines are composed of porous crystalline magnesium calcite, articulated at the base and extremely sharp, with three raised cutting edges at the tips. As the spine enters the skin, it carries venom into the wound, with immediate pain, copious bleeding, and mild edema. The pain is generally moderate and self-limited, with remission over a period of 30 minutes to 3 hours. However, it may be of a severity to require narcotic analgesia (Figure 74-69). The wound may become dusky or discolored. Multiple puncture wounds may result in acute systemic reactions, including paresthesias, nausea, vomiting, lymphadenopathy, and muscular paralysis. If a spine fragment is retained, a granulomatous lesion may develop akin to that seen after a sea urchin puncture wound. A previously sensitized victim may suffer a prolonged reaction lasting for weeks or even months and consisting of local edema and pruritus. Tenosynovitis may affect multiple fingers simultaneously after a single puncture wound.[3] Contact with other, less injurious starfish may induce a pruritic papulourticarial eruption (irritant contact dermatitis).

Treatment

Immersion therapy may provide some relief from the pain. The wound should immediately be immersed into nonscalding hot water to tolerance (45°C [113°F]) for 30 to 90 minutes or until there is significant pain relief. The pain is occasionally severe enough to require local anesthetic infiltration. The puncture wound should be irrigated and explored to remove all foreign material. Because of the stout nature of the spines, retainment of a fragment is rarer than with sea urchin puncture. However, if a victim steps on a starfish and creates a shearing motion, the tips of spines may remain in the wound(s). If any question of a foreign body exists, a soft tissue radiograph often identifies the fractured spine. Not infrequently, the victim suffers an indolent contact dermatitis from handling a starfish such as Solaster papposus, the sun (Figure 74-70) or rose star. The dermatitis may be managed in standard fashion with topical solutions, such as calamine with 0.5% menthol, or a corticosteroid preparation. Systemic therapy is supportive. Granulomas from retained spine fragments may require excision. Starfish that have ingested poisonous shellfish are themselves toxic on ingestion.

SEA URCHINS

Life and Habits

Sea urchins are free-living echinoderms that have an egg-shaped, globular, or flattened body. A hard skeleton (test) composed of fused calcareous plates surrounds the viscera and is covered by regularly arranged spines and triple-jawed (pincerlike) pedicellariae. These pedicellariae (globiferous, or glandular) are sometimes used for defense (Figure 74-71). Urchins are nocturnal and omnivorous (mostly in pursuit of algae) eaters, yet are shy, nonaggressive, and slow-moving animals found on rocky bottoms or burrowed in sand and crevices (Figure 74-72). Their bathymetric range extends from the intertidal zone to great depths. The raw or cooked gonads of several species are eaten as a great delicacy by humans.

Venom and Venom Apparatus

Of the approximately 600 species of sea urchins, roughly 80 may be venomous to humans.[114] The venom apparatuses of sea urchins consist of the hollow, venom-filled spines and the triple-jawed globiferous pedicellariae. Venom may also be released from within a thin integumentary sheath on the external surface of the spines of certain urchins.

The spines of sea urchins, formed by calcification of a cylindric projection of subepidermal connective tissue, may be non–venom bearing, with solid blunt and rounded tips (Figure 74-73), or venom bearing (as in the families Echinothuridae and Diadematidae [Figure 74-74]), with hollow, long, slender, and sharp needles (Figure 74-75). These are extremely dangerous to handle. The spines, which are attached to the shell with a modified ball-and-socket joint, are brittle and break off easily in the flesh, lodging deeply, and removal is difficult. They are keen enough to penetrate rubber gloves and fins. *Diadema setosum* (black sea urchin) spines may exceed 1 foot in length. *Echinothrix* species also carry lengthy spines. The purple sea urchin *Strongylocentrotus purpuratus* (Figure 74-76) of California has much shorter spines. The genera *Asthenosoma* (Figures 74-77 and 74-78) and *Aerosoma* have special venom organs (sacs) on the sharp tips of the aboral spines (Figure 74-79), which introduce the potent venom.

Pedicellariae are small, delicate seizing organs attached to the stalks scattered among the spines. These are considered to be

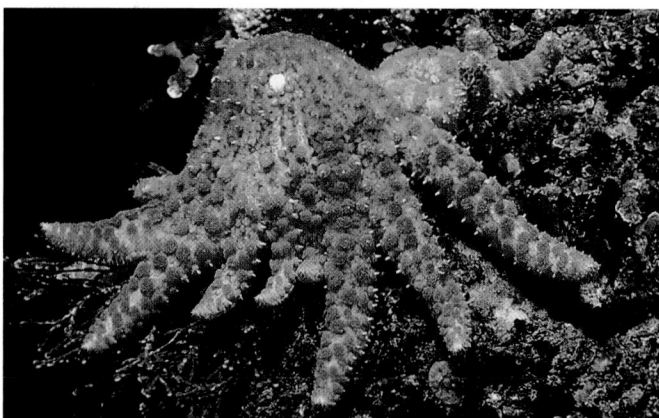

FIGURE 74-70 Sun starfish *(Solaster)*. *(From Norbert Wu, with permission: norbertwu.com.)*

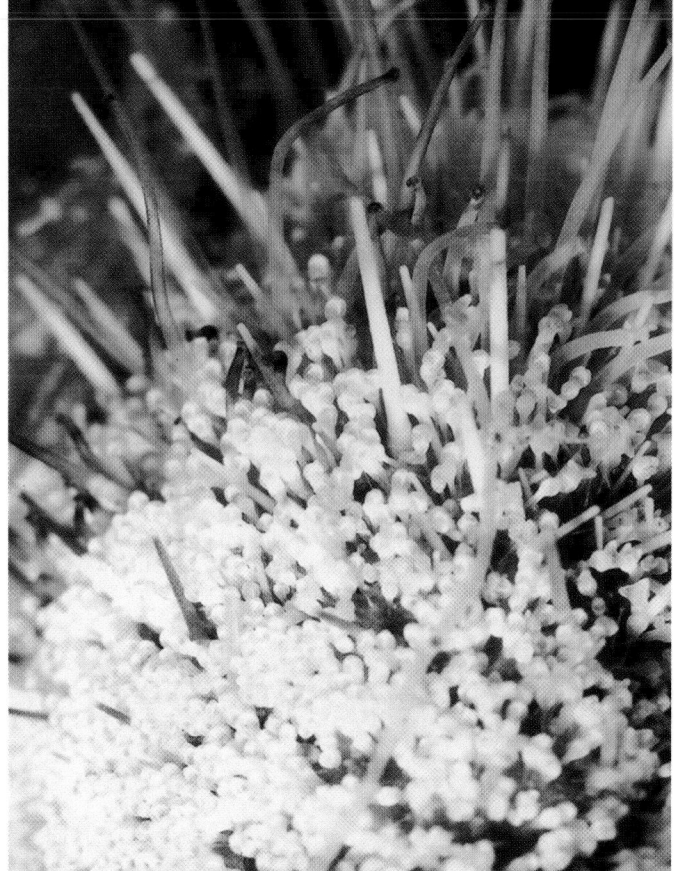

FIGURE 74-71 Globiferous pedicellariae are equipped with venom glands. *(Courtesy Dietrich Mebs.)*

modified spines with flexible heads.[173] Globiferous pedicellariae, typified by those found in *Toxopneustes pileolus* (flower urchin) (Figure 74-80) and *Tripneustes* species, have globe-shaped heads that contain the venom organs (Figure 74-81). The terminal head, with its calcareous pincer jaws (two to four, but usually three), is attached by the stalk to the shell plates of the sea urchin. The outer surface of each opened "jaw" is covered by a large venom gland, which is triggered to contract with the jaw on contact. When the sea urchin is at rest in the water, the jaws are extended, slowly moving about (Figure 74-82). Anything that

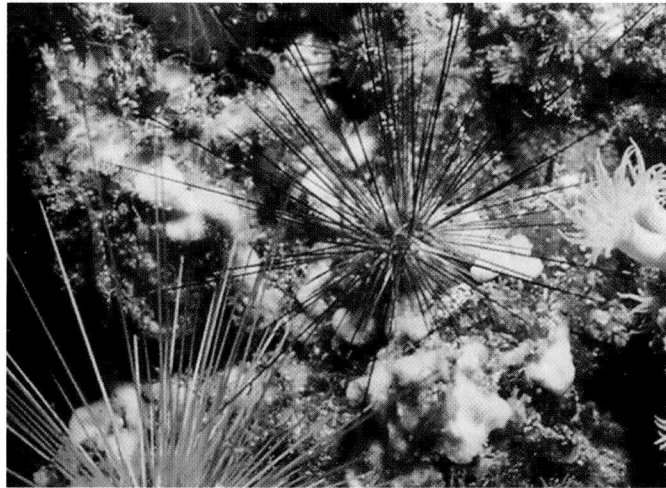

FIGURE 74-72 Needle-like spines of sea urchins in their natural habitat. *(Courtesy Kenneth Kizer, MD.)*

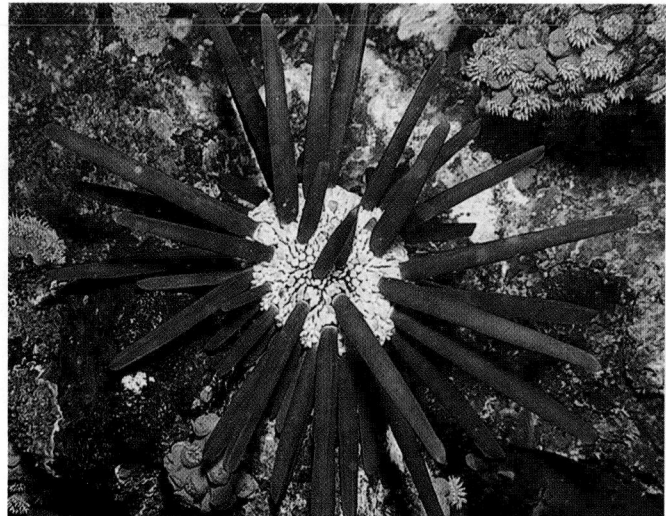

FIGURE 74-73 Nontoxic "pencil" urchin with blunt, rounded tips. *(Courtesy Paul S. Auerbach, MD.)*

touches them is seized. As long as the object is moving, the pedicellariae continue to bite and envenom. Once a pedicellaria attaches to a victim, it will be torn from the shell rather than let go. Detached pedicellariae may remain active for several hours. The *Toxopneustes* sea urchin also has solid spines, but these are nonvenomous.

The venom of sea urchins contains various toxic fractions, including steroid glycosides, hemolysins, proteases, serotonin,

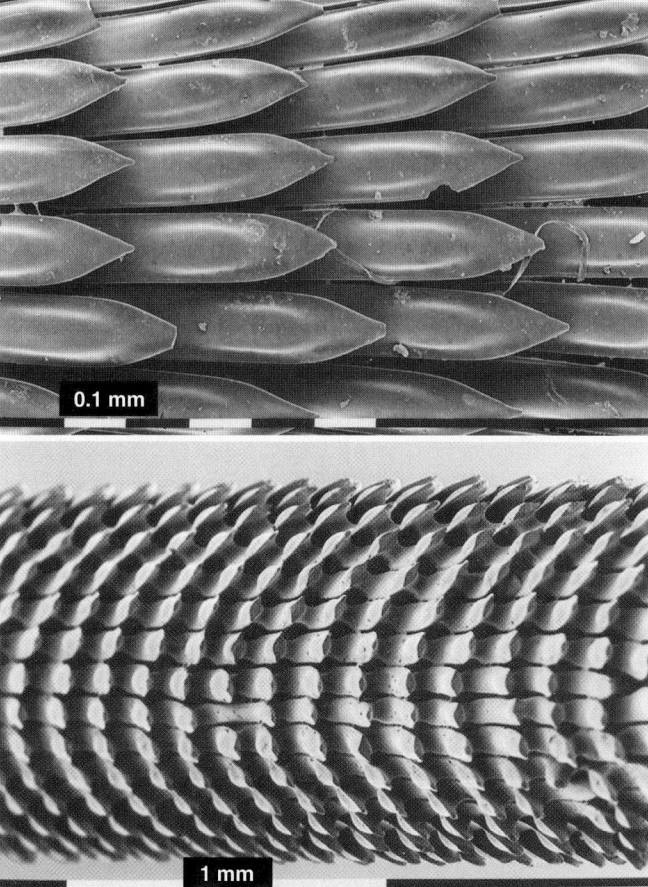

FIGURE 74-74 The spines of the diadematid sea urchin (*Diadema* species) are covered with small, tilelike structures. *(From Meier J, White J: Handbook of clinical toxicology of animal venoms and poisons, Boca Raton, Florida, 1995, CRC Press. Courtesy Dr. J. Meier.)*

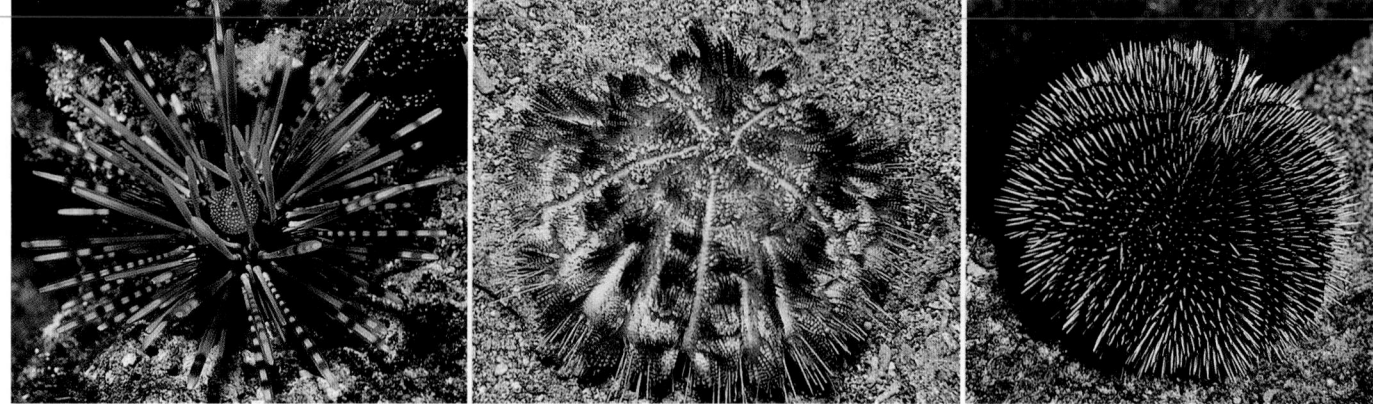

FIGURE 74-75 Three examples of sharp-spined (venomous) sea urchins. (Courtesy Paul S. Auerbach, MD.)

and cholinergic substances. The Pacific *Tripneustes* urchin carries a neurotoxin with a predilection for facial and cranial nerves. A toxic substance from the sea urchin *T. pileolus* induces histamine release from rat peritoneal mast cells.[202] Contractin A (a mannose-containing glycoprotein) from the pedicellariae of the same species causes contraction of isolated guinea pig tracheal smooth muscle.[145] Other substances that have been identified from sea urchin spines or pedicellariae include D-galactose–binding lectins and heparin-binding and hemolytic lectins.[144]

Clinical Aspects

Most victims are envenomed when they step on, handle, or brush up against a sea urchin.[54] Because the creatures tend to be nocturnal, divers are most commonly injured in dark waters during night diving activities, particularly in small caves or shallow turbulent waters. Young inquisitive children who explore tide pools frequently handle urchins incorrectly and may be injured. If a diver moves a hand slowly toward a spiny (venomous) sea urchin, the spines may align to offer the greatest defense.

Venomous spines inflict immediate and intensely painful stings.[110] The pain is initially characterized by burning, which

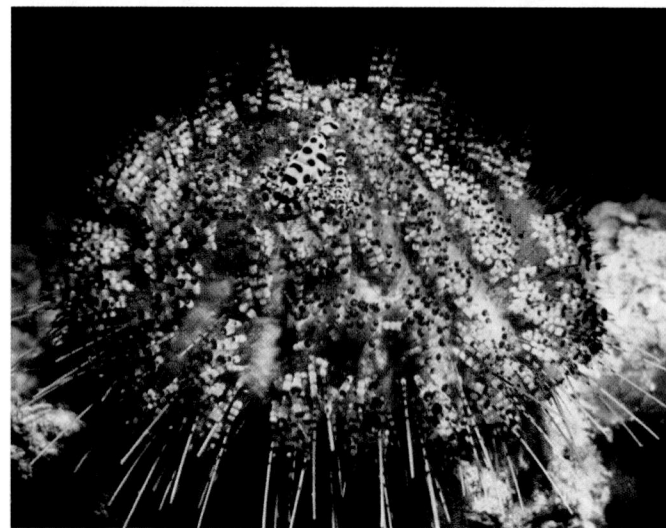

FIGURE 74-77 Pair of shrimp on an *Asthenosoma* anemone. (Copyright Carl Roessler.)

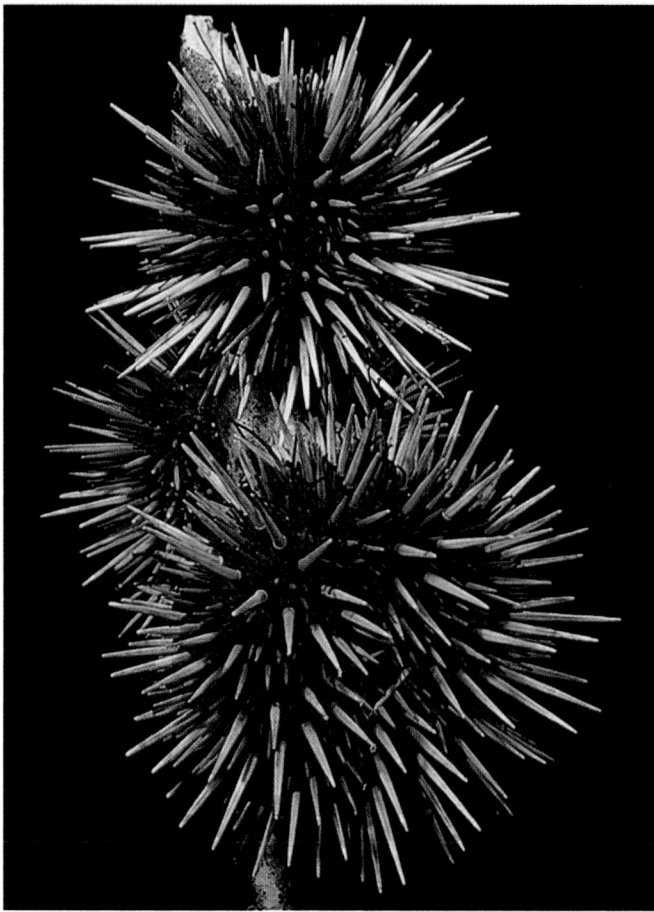

FIGURE 74-76 Purple sea urchins. (Courtesy Howard Hall.)

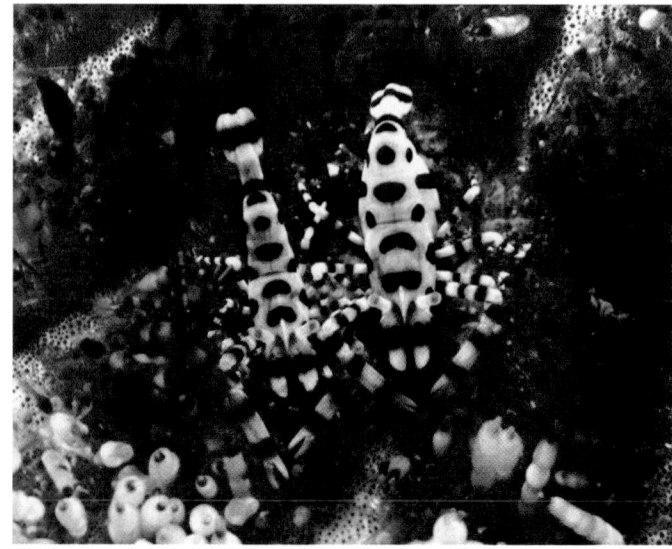

FIGURE 74-78 Porcelain shrimp in fire urchin. (Courtesy Paul S. Auerbach, MD.)

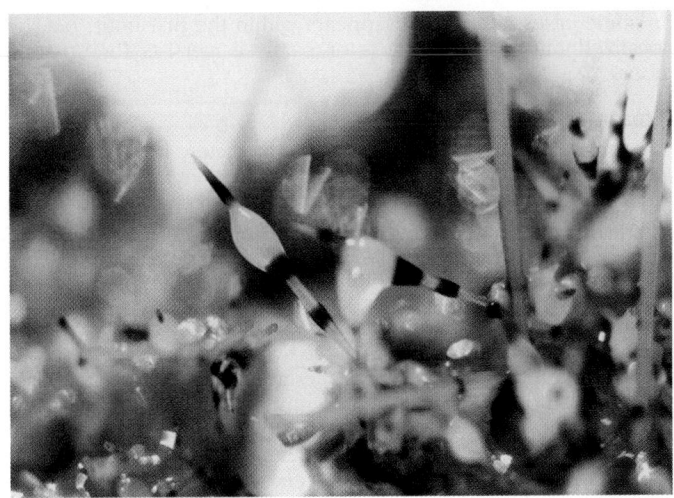

FIGURE 74-79 The tips of the short spines of the leather urchin (e.g., *Asthenosoma* from the Indo-Pacific) are encased by a venom gland. (*Courtesy Dietrich Mebs.*)

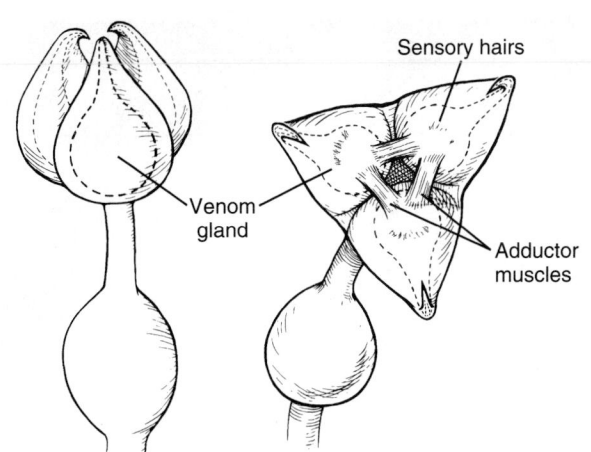

FIGURE 74-81 Globiferous pedicellaria of a sea urchin, used to hold and envenom prey.

rapidly evolves into severe local muscle aching with visible erythema and swelling of the skin surrounding the puncture site or sites (Figure 74-83). Frequently, a spine breaks off and lodges in the victim. Some sea urchin spines (such as those of *D. setosum* or *S. purpuratus*) contain black-purplish dye, which may give a false impression of spines left in the skin (Figures 74-84 to 74-86). Soft tissue density x-ray techniques, ultrasound, computed tomography (CT), or magnetic resonance imaging (MRI) may reveal a radiopaque foreign body. If a spine enters a joint, it may rapidly induce severe synovitis. Over time, if the spine remains embedded in or near the joint, this may progress to arthritis.[114] There may be a symptom-free period of 1 to 2 months between the initial injury and the onset of fusiform swelling, limited motion, and pain of the affected joint, which reflect joint effusion and soft tissue thickening, followed by osteolysis, sharply demarcated bone erosion, and periosteal reaction. Radiography may not reveal a visible spine but may show soft tissue swelling and osteolysis.[213] Gadolinium-enhanced MRI may be useful to identify subtle changes, such as synovial proliferation.[114] If multiple spines have penetrated the skin, particularly if they are deeply embedded, systemic symptoms that may rapidly develop include nausea, vomiting, paresthesias, numbness and muscular paralysis, abdominal pain, syncope, hypotension, and respiratory distress. The presence of a frank neuropathy may indicate that the spine has lodged in contact with a peripheral nerve. The pain

from multiple stings may be sufficient to cause delirium. Secondary infections and indolent ulceration are common. A delayed hypersensitivity–type reaction (flare-up) at the sites of the punctures has been described, in which the victim demonstrates erythema and pruritus in a delayed fashion, 7 to 10 days after primary resolution from the initial envenomation.[6] The sensitizing antigen in such cases has yet to be identified. Hepatic transaminasemia after a relatively minor puncture has been reported, which may have been caused by the envenomation or by therapy with cephradine and mefenamic acid.[235] Eosinophilic pneumonia has been associated with, but not proved to be related to, foot injury from a sea urchin.[108]

Three separate unusual cases have been reported to the lead author since 1993 by neurologists. In each case, the victim sustained multiple punctures from one or several black sea urchins in Hawaiian waters. The immediate clinical reaction was typical, but it was followed in 6 to 10 days by severe bulbar polyneuritis with respiratory insufficiency. In two cases, the victims were hyporeflexic and appeared to suffer a Guillain-Barré variation with elevated protein levels in the cerebrospinal fluid. In the other case, the victim manifested meningoencephalitis documented by MRI. The temporal relationship to the urchin stings suggests an autoimmune phenomenon.

A spine that enters a finger in proximity to the nail apparatus may cause a subungual or periungual granulomatous nodular lesion. Excision may cause permanent nail plate dystrophy. Small, firm, and erythematous chronic inflammatory cutaneous nodules (granulomas) of the palms, dorsa of the hands, elbows, knees, and other areas of skin contact may be persistent.[97]

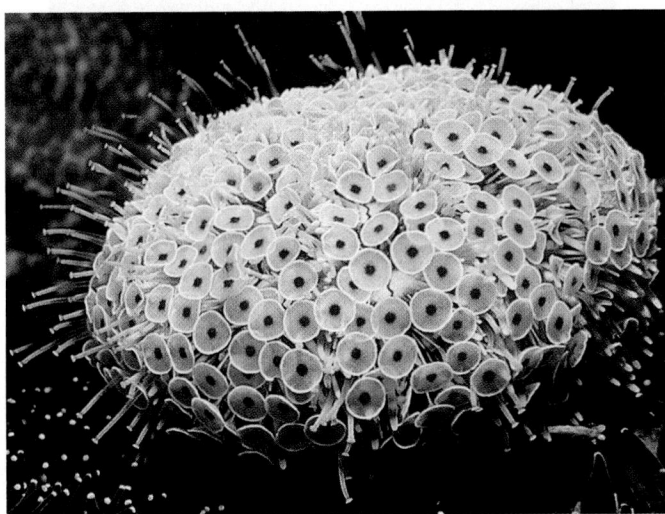

FIGURE 74-80 Flower urchin (*Toxopneustes pileolus*). (*Courtesy Ken Kizer, MD.*)

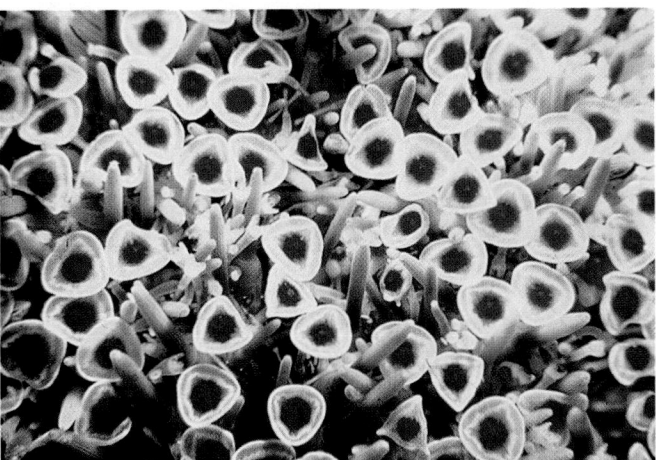

FIGURE 74-82 Close-up of opened flower urchin (*Toxopneustes pileolus*) pedicellariae seeking prey. (*Courtesy Ken Kizer, MD.*)

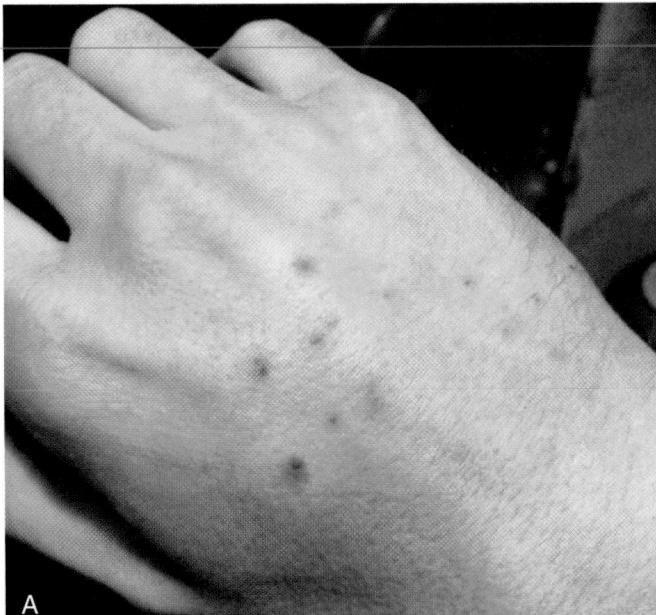

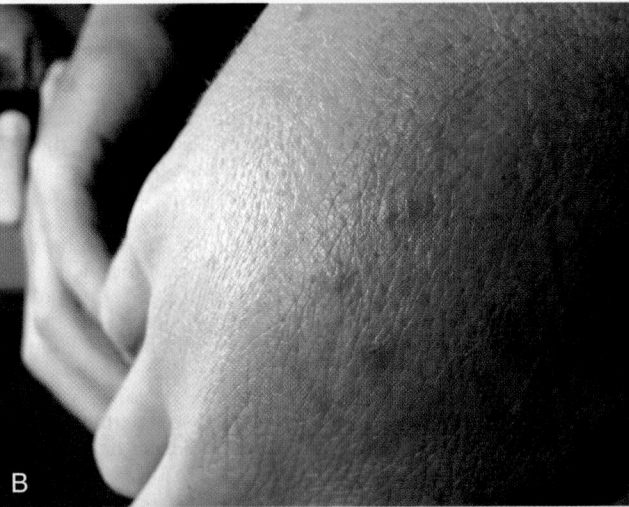

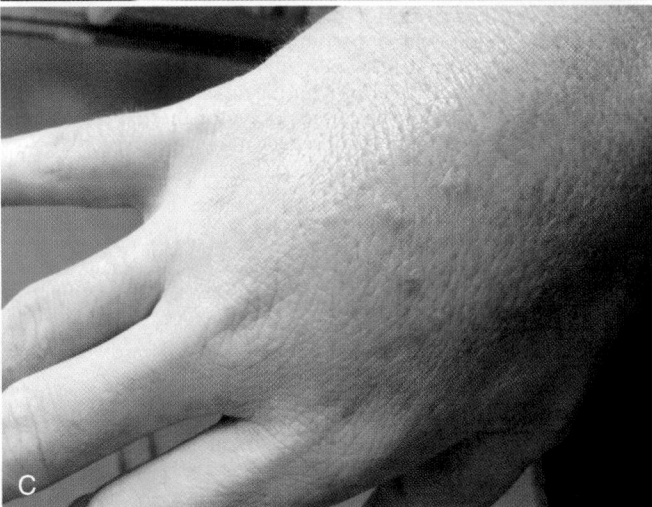

FIGURE 74-83 Swelling of the hand associated with sea urchin punctures. **A,** Soon after the injury. **B,** 24 hours after the injury. **C,** Resolving swelling. *(Courtesy John Martin.)*

The stings of pedicellariae are often of greater magnitude, causing immediate intense radiating pain, local edema and hemorrhage, malaise, weakness, paresthesias, hypesthesia, arthralgias, aphonia, dizziness, syncope, generalized muscular paralysis, respiratory distress, and hypotension; death is a rare occurrence.

In some cases, the pain disappears within the first hour, but the localized muscular weakness or paralysis persists for up to 6 hours.

Treatment

The envenomed body part should immediately be immersed in nonscalding hot water to tolerance (upper limit, 45°C [113°F]) for 30 to 90 minutes in an attempt to relieve pain. Hot candle wax application has been used successfully. Any pedicellariae still attached to the skin must be removed or envenomation will continue. This may be accomplished by applying shaving foam and gently scraping with a razor. Embedded spines should be removed with care because they easily fracture. Black or purplish discoloration surrounding the wound after spine removal is often merely spine dye and therefore may be of no consequence. Although some thin venomous spines may be absorbed within 24 hours to 3 weeks, it is best to remove those that are easily reached. All thick spines (calcium carbonate, magnesium carbonate, and silica) should be removed because of the risk of infection, foreign body encaseation granuloma, or dermoid inclusion cyst.

Although some persons recommend crushing embedded spines in situ, external percussion to achieve fragmentation may prove disastrous if a chronic inflammatory process is initiated in sensitive tissue of the hand or foot. If the spines have acutely entered joints or are closely aligned to neurovascular structures, the surgeon should take advantage of an operating microscope in an appropriate setting to remove all spine fragments. The extraction should be performed as soon as possible after the injury. If the spine has entered an interphalangeal joint, the finger should be splinted until the spine is removed to limit fragmentation and further penetration. This also may control the fusiform finger swelling (Figure 74-87) commonly noted after a puncture in the vicinity of the middle or proximal interphalangeal joint. It is inappropriate to rummage about in a hand wound in the emergency department, virtually looking for a needle in a haystack. After a spine has been embedded in soft tissue for 24 to 48 hours, the spine dye may be absorbed, and the spine becomes flesh colored and very difficult to locate. If the spine is lodged

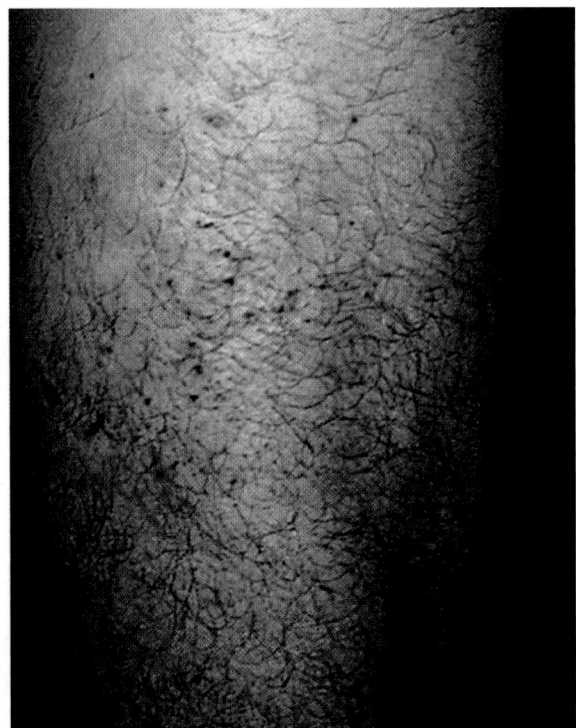

FIGURE 74-84 Thigh of the author demonstrating multiple sea urchin punctures from black sea urchins *(Diadema)*. Within 24 hours, the black markings were absent, indicative of spine dye without residual spines. *(Courtesy Ken Kizer, MD.)*

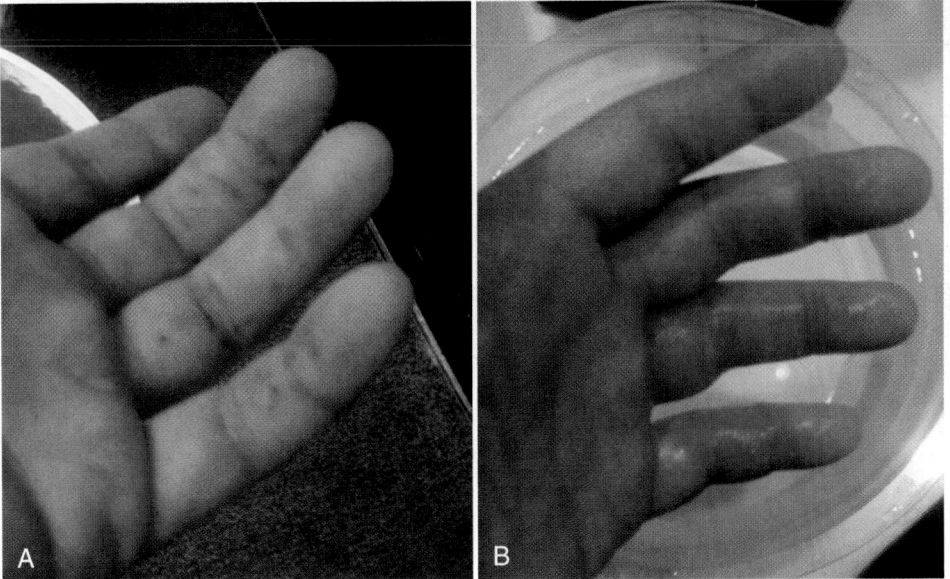

FIGURE 74-85 A, Multiple sea urchin punctures to hand soon after injury and following a soak in hot water. **B,** Same hand after 6 days without intervening therapy other than soaking. Lack of discoloration indicates absorption of dye from sea urchin spines and probable absence of retained fragments.

in avascular tendon or ligament, the spine dye may persist for a longer period, allowing easier identification of the foreign body. If surgery is undertaken to remove a spine, particularly of the hand, an elliptical skin incision may allow better visualization with magnification to aid in complete spine removal.[146]

If the presence of a spine is in question, soft tissue density radiographic techniques for a radiopaque foreign body may be diagnostic. CT or MRI (Figure 74-88) may be quite useful to locate spine fragments. Although the calcium carbonate is relatively inert, it is accompanied by slime, bacteria, and organic epidermal debris. Therefore, secondary infections are common (Figure 74-89), and deep puncture wounds are an indication for prophylactic antibiotics.

Some sea urchin spines are phagocytosed in the soft tissues and ultimately dissolve. The granulomas caused by retained sea urchin spine fragments have sarcoidal histologic features and

generally appear as flesh- or dye-colored surface or subcuticular nodules 2 to 12 months after the initial injury (Figure 74-90).[171] In thin-skinned areas, these nodules are erythematous and rubbery, painless, and infrequently umbilicated. In thicker-skinned areas (palms, soles, and knees) that are frequently abraded, they have a keratinized appearance. Although necrosis and microabscess formation may be evident microscopically, suppuration is unusual. Rarely, the destructive nature of the inflammatory process may be severe enough to necessitate amputation of a digit. If a spine cannot be removed and becomes a nidus for cyst or granuloma formation, the lesion may be removed surgically. Intralesional injection with a corticosteroid (triamcinolone hexacetonide, 5 mg/mL) is less efficacious but may be successful. Erbium-YAG laser (emission wavelength 2940 nm) ablation has been used to destroy multiple sea urchin spines in the sole of the foot, with resulting circumscribed crater

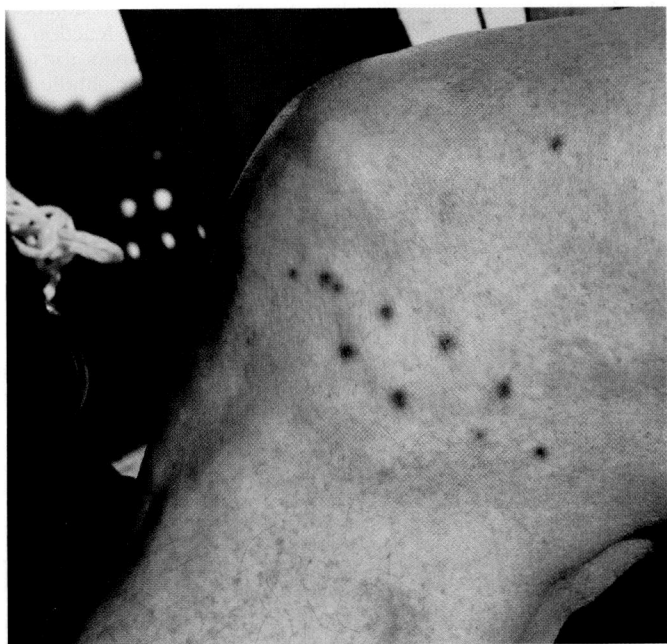

FIGURE 74-86 Sea urchin spines that have punctured the knee. *(Copyright Stephen Frink.)*

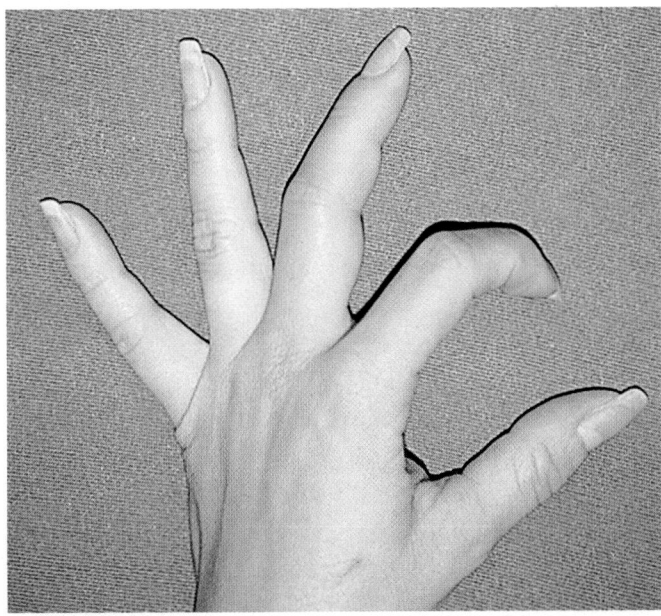

FIGURE 74-87 Finger swelling from sea urchin puncture. A single spine entered the palm over the mid–third metacarpal bone. Swelling was severe in the second and third digits. *(Courtesy Paul S. Auerbach, MD.)*

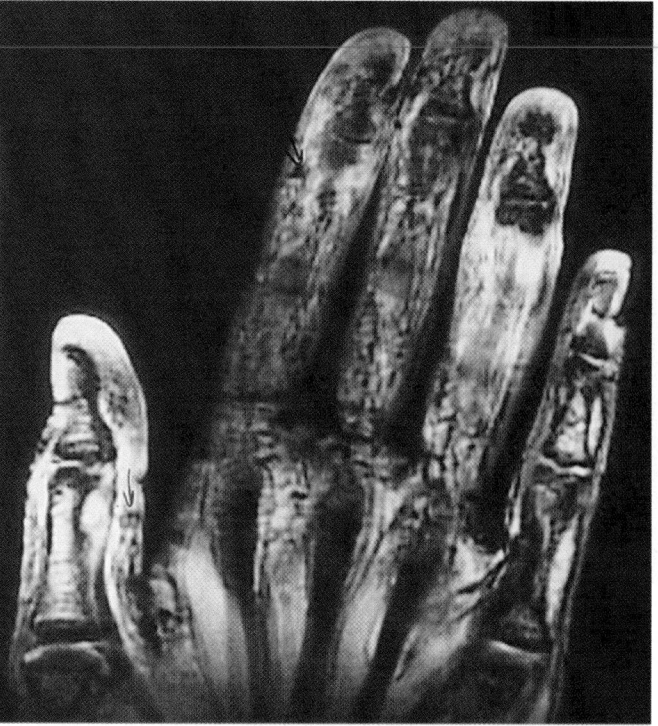

FIGURE 74-88 Magnetic resonance imaging of the hand of a victim of multiple sea urchin spine punctures, demonstrating the presence of spine fragments in the soft tissues. *(Courtesy Paul S. Auerbach, MD.)*

lesions with tiny pinpoint areas of bleeding and scattered focal hyperkeratosis without scarring but with some delayed (2 years) granulomatous reactions.[183] Systemic antiinflammatory drugs may be minimally helpful but are not substitutes for removal of the spine. A diffuse delayed reaction, consisting of cyanotic induration, fusiform swelling in the digits, and focal phalangeal bony erosion, may be treated with a systemic corticosteroid and

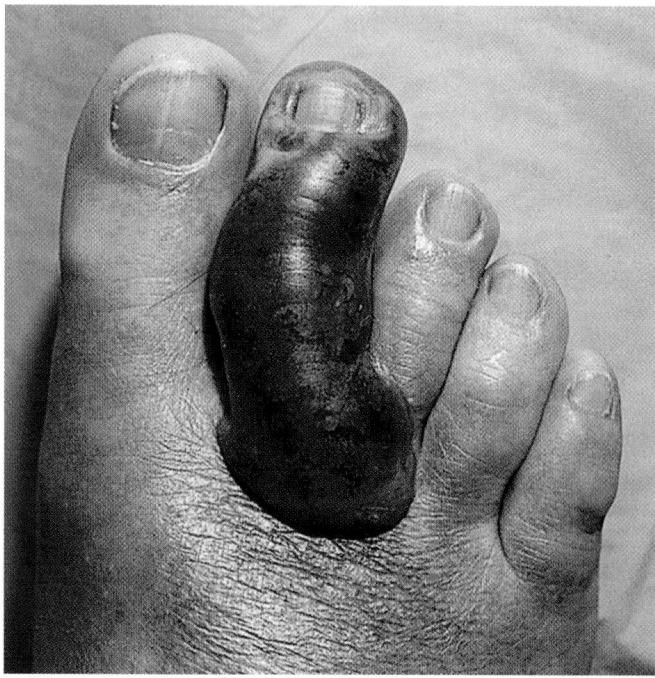

FIGURE 74-89 Infection after sea urchin puncture. The rapid-onset, gas-containing hemorrhagic blister and severe cellulitis with sepsis are common features of infection with *Vibrio* species. *(Courtesy Paul S. Auerbach, MD.)*

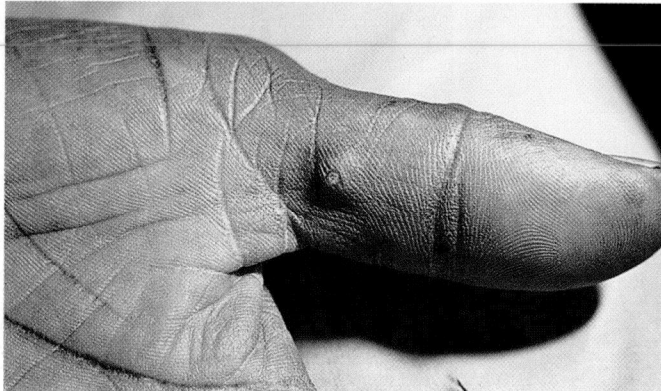

FIGURE 74-90 Subcuticular nodule after sea urchin puncture. *(Courtesy Paul S. Auerbach, MD.)*

antibiotics. Sea urchin spine arthritis of the hand in the proximal interphalangeal joint not responsive to antibiotics or nonsteroidal antiinflammatory agents has been successfully treated with synovectomy of the joint combined with removal of granulation tissue around the joint.[213]

SEA CUCUMBERS

Life and Habits

Sea cucumbers are free-living worm- or sausage-shaped bottom feeders of diverse external patterns and coloration (Figure 74-91) that are essentially scavengers. They are cosmopolitan in distribution, found in both shallow and deep waters. Cucumbers are harvested as a food (trepang, bêche-de-mer) in the South Pacific.

Venom and Venom Apparatus

Cucumbers produce in their body walls a visceral cantharidin-like liquid toxin (holothurin). Holothurin is concentrated in the tentacular organs of Cuvier, which can be projected and extended anally when the animal mounts a defense (Figure 74-92). Toxic genera include *Actinopyga*, *Stichopus*, and *Holothuria*. Some cucumbers dine on nematocysts and thus can secrete cnidarian venom as well.

Clinical Aspects

Holothurin may induce contact dermatitis when the tentacular organs directly contact the skin. Generally, the substance is diluted in the surrounding ocean water and the reaction is minimal; however, persons who dissect sea cucumbers topside in the preparation of food products may inadvertently handle the toxin and develop papular skin irritation. The major risk for

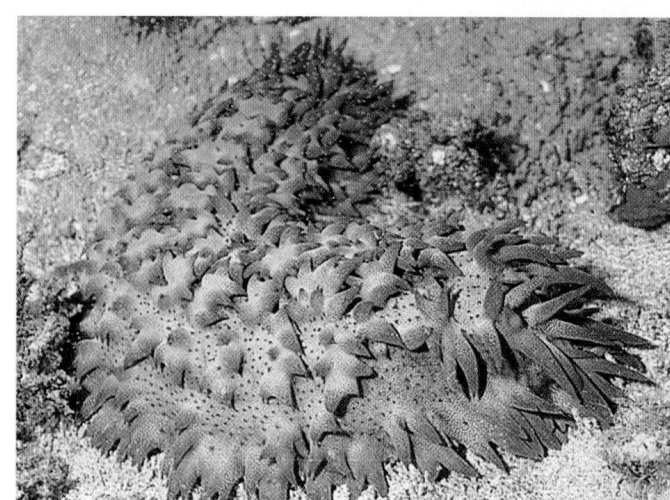

FIGURE 74-91 Sea cucumber. *(Courtesy Paul S. Auerbach, MD.)*

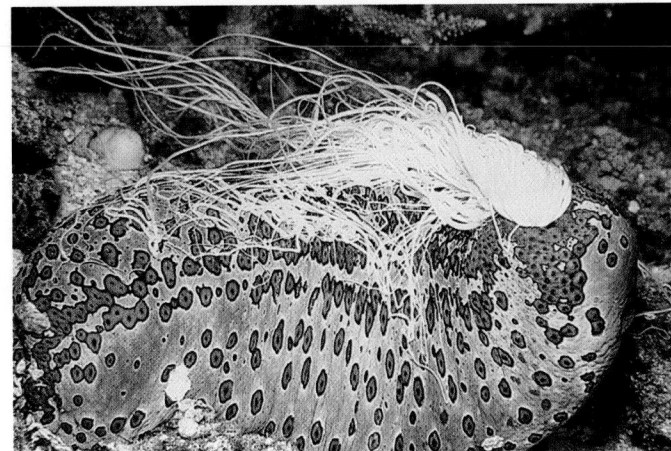

FIGURE 74-92 Extruded tentacular organs of Cuvier from within a sea cucumber. *(Courtesy Paul S. Auerbach, MD.)*

divers is to the corneas and conjunctivae, which may become intensely inflamed if directly contacted by tentacular fragments or high concentrations of the toxin. This may occur if the mask is cleared in the immediate vicinity of recent sea cucumber manipulation. A severe reaction may lead to blindness. Holothurin is a potent cardiac glycoside and may cause severe illness or death on ingestion.

Treatment

The management of holothurin-induced contact dermatitis is similar to that for starfish dermatitis. A topical or systemic corticosteroid may be necessary to manage a severe reaction. Because cucumbers that dine on nematocysts may secrete cnidarian venom, the initial skin detoxification should include topical application of 5% acetic acid (vinegar), papain, or 40% to 70% isopropyl alcohol. If an eye is involved, it should be anesthetized with 1 or 2 drops of 0.5% proparacaine and then irrigated with 100 to 250 mL of normal saline to remove any residual foreign matter. The cornea should be stained with fluorescein to identify corneal defects. A proper slit-lamp examination is optimal to determine whether inflammation extends into the anterior chamber or involves the iris. If there is no sign of infection, a moderate approach to the inflammatory keratitis includes regular instillation of cycloplegic, mydriatic, and corticosteroid ophthalmic solutions. Prompt referral to an ophthalmologist is essential.

PHYLUM ANNELIDA

ANNELID WORMS

Life and Habits

There are 6200 species of segmented marine worms (phylum Annelida, class Polychaeta), either free-moving or sedentary. Some free-moving members are considered toxic and may attain 30 cm (1 foot) in length. The worms are predominantly carnivorous and exist in the tidal zone to depths of 5000 m (16,405 feet), mostly as bottom feeders. Each segment of the worm possesses paddle-like appendages (parapodia) for locomotion. From these project numerous silky or bristle-like setae, which are capable of puncturing the victim (Figures 74-93 to 74-97).

The chitinous urticating bristles are arranged in soft rows about the body. When a worm is stimulated, its body contracts and the bristles are erected. There are no associated venom-producing cells. Easily detached, the bristles penetrate skin like cactus spines and are difficult to remove. The ubiquitous bottom-dwelling bristleworm *Hermodice carunculata* is frequently handled in Floridian and Caribbean waters by snorkelers and divers. This worm can attain a length of one foot and a width of 2.54 cm (1 inch). It is found on coral, under rocks, and moving among sponges. The body is green or reddish with tufts of white bristles. *Chloeia flava* is found along the Malayan coast, *Chloeia*

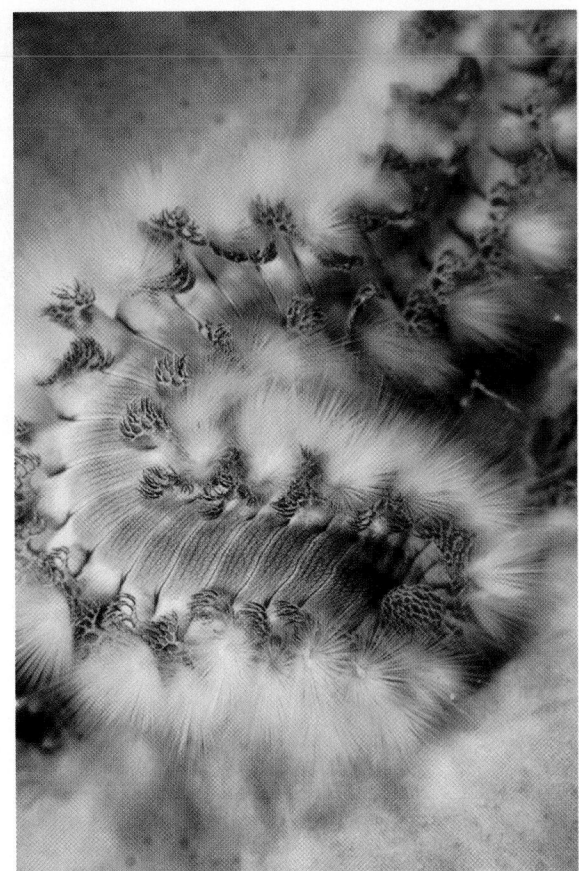

FIGURE 74-93 The chitinous spines of a bristleworm are easily dislodged into the skin of an unwary diver. *(Copyright Stephen Frink.)*

viridis in the West Indies, Gulf of California, and Gulf of Mexico south to Panama, and *Eurythoe complanata* in Australia and other tropical seas. Other worms, such as *Chloeia euglochis,* are free swimming. Some marine worms possess strong chitinous jaws with pharyngeal teeth and can inflict painful bites.

Clinical Aspects

The bite or sting of an annelid worm may induce intense inflammation typified by a burning sensation with a raised, erythematous, and urticarial rash, most frequently on the hands and fingers (Figure 74-98). Edema and papules ensue, with rare necrosis. The setae are easily fractured into the skin and are generally not visible on external inspection, although the victim may report a

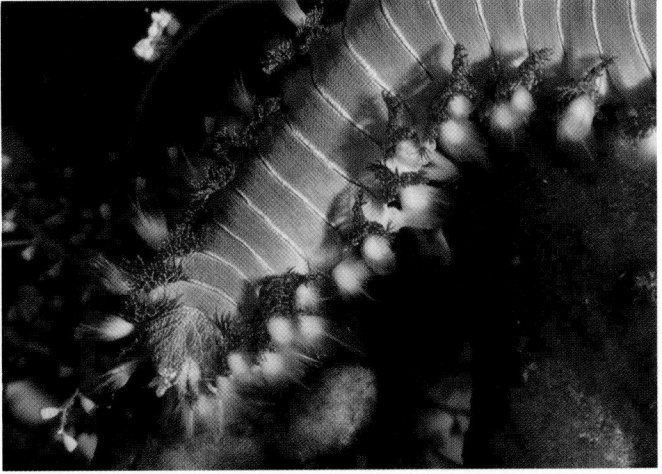

FIGURE 74-94 Bristleworm I. *(Copyright Stephen Frink.)*

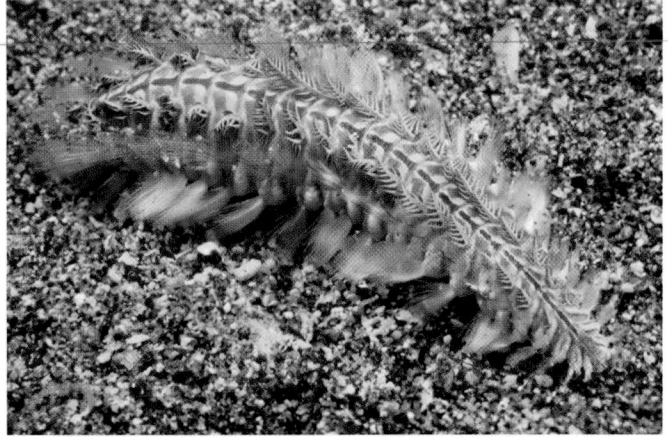

FIGURE 74-95 Bristleworm. *(Copyright Stephen Frink.)*

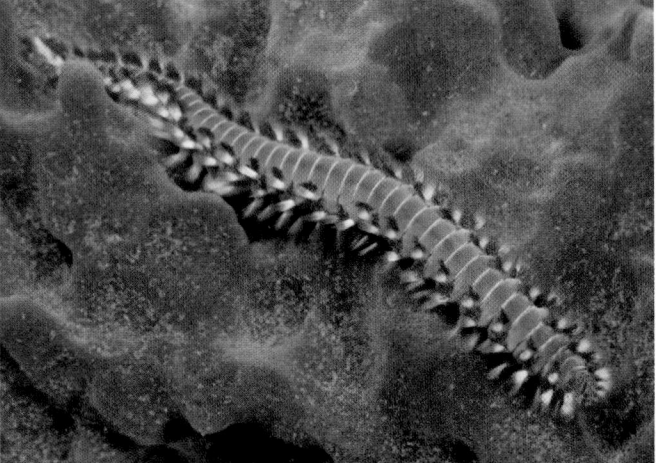

FIGURE 74-96 Bristleworm. *(Copyright Stephen Frink.)*

sensation of pricking or abrasion. Untreated, the pain is generally self-limited over the course of a few hours, but the inflammatory component of erythema and urticaria may last for 2 to 3 days, with total resolution of the skin discoloration over 7 to 10 days. With multiple stings, marked local soft tissue edema and pruritus may develop. Secondary infections and cellulitis may occur if the eczematous component is severe.

Treatment

All large visible bristles should be removed with forceps. The skin should be dried (without scraping, to avoid breaking or

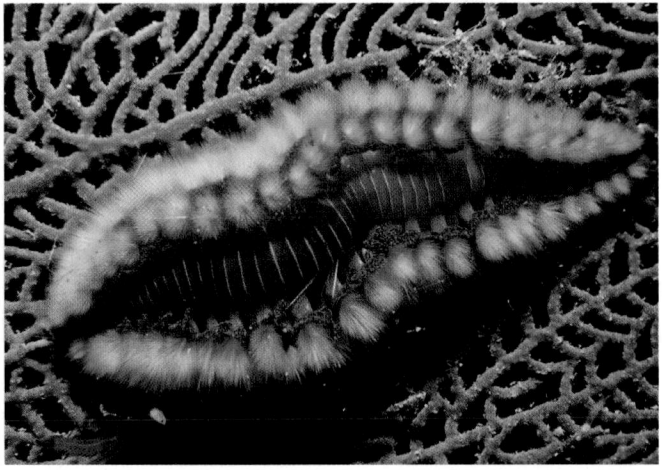

FIGURE 74-97 Bristleworm. *(Courtesy Marty Snyderman.)*

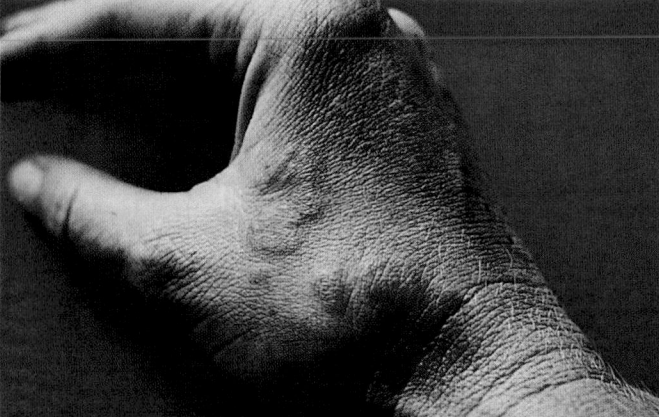

FIGURE 74-98 Skin rash caused by a bristleworm. *(Courtesy Paul S. Auerbach, MD.)*

embedding the spines further into the skin) so that a layer of adhesive tape may be applied to remove the remaining smaller spines, which are too tiny for individual extraction. Application of tape may force spines into the tissue, causing pain. Alternatively, a facial "peel" or thin layer of rubber cement may be applied and removed. After this maneuver, 5% acetic acid (vinegar), 40% to 70% isopropyl alcohol, or a paste or solution of unseasoned meat tenderizer (papain) or application of a papain-impregnated scrub brush may provide some pain relief. If the inflammatory reaction becomes severe, the victim may benefit from administration of a topical or systemic corticosteroid.

PHYLUM MOLLUSCA
MOLLUSKS

The phylum Mollusca (45,000 species) encompasses a group of unsegmented, soft-bodied invertebrates, many of which secrete calcareous shells. Generally, a muscular foot is present with various modifications. Of the five main classes, three predominate in their hazard to humans: the pelecypods (such as scallops, oysters, clams, and mussels), the gastropods (such as snails and slugs), and the cephalopods (such as squids, octopuses, and cuttlefish [Figures 74-99 and 74-100]). Mollusks are often implicated as the transvectors in poisonous ingestions.

CONE SNAILS (CONE SHELLS)
Life and Habits

There are approximately 500 species of these circumtropical, beautiful, yet potentially lethal, univalve and cone-shaped shelled

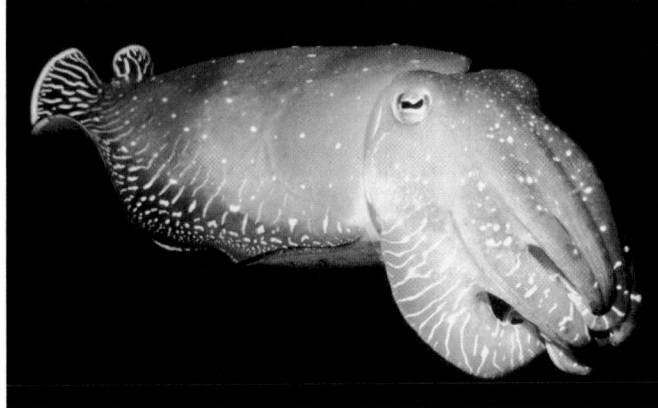

FIGURE 74-99 Giant cuttlefish in the Coral Sea. *(Copyright Carl Roessler.)*

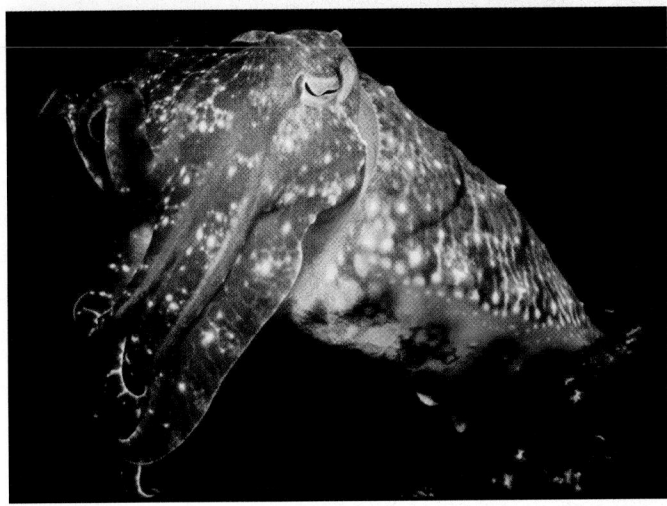

FIGURE 74-100 Curious cuttlefish in Papua, New Guinea. *(Copyright Carl Roessler.)*

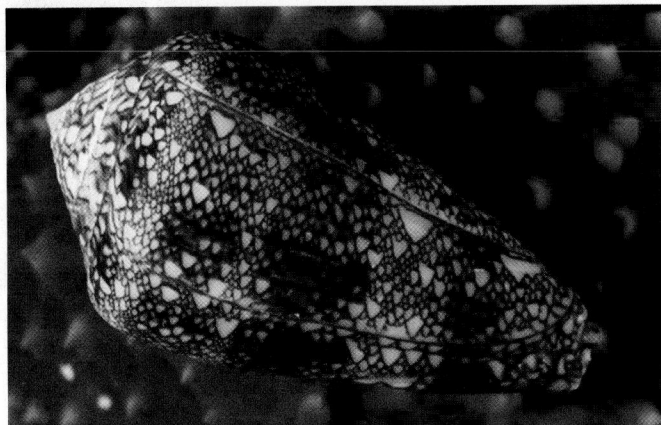

FIGURE 74-102 *Conus dalli*, in the Sea of Cortez. *(From Norbert Wu, with permission: norbertwu.com.)*

mollusks of the class Gastropoda, family Conidae, genus *Conus* (Figures 74-101 and 74-102).[136] Most of these carnivores carry a highly developed venom apparatus, and at least 18 species have been implicated in human envenomations, with occasional fatalities (≈ 16 to 30 have been recorded).[78] These include *Conus aulicus* (court), *Conus geographus* (geographer), *Conus gloriamaris* (glory of the sea), *Conus marmoreus* (marbled), *Conus omaria* (pearled), *Conus striatus* (striated) (Figure 74-103), *Conus textile* (textile) (Figure 74-104), and *Conus tulipa* (tulip).

Most harmful cone snails (cones) are creatures of shallow Indo-Pacific waters; variance in feeding habits and venom production accounts for varying toxicity. Atlantic species, such as *Conus ermineus* (turtle) are less toxic. *Conus regius* (crown or queen) and *Conus spurius* (Chinese alphabet) are found in Florida waters. Apparently, cones that feed on fish or mollusks are the most dangerous. Less toxic stings are attributed to cones that feed on marine worms. Predominantly nocturnal creatures, cones burrow in the sand and coral during the daytime, emerging at night to feed. They have two eye stalks, but vision is poor, so chemosensory prowess is required to identify and approach prey.[204]

Venom and Venom Apparatus

Cone snails are predators that feed by injecting rapid-acting venom by means of a detachable, dartlike radular tooth (or radula) (Figure 74-105). To do this, the head of the animal must extend out of the shell. The venom apparatus is composed of a set of minute, harpoon-like, chitinous, and hollow radular teeth associated with a venom bulb, a long convoluted duct, and a radular sheath (Figure 74-106).[139] The barbed teeth, which may attain a length of 1 cm (0.34 inch), are housed within the radular sheath. The act of envenomation is performed by release of a radular tooth from the sheath into the pharynx, where it is "charged" with venom from the venom duct and then transferred to the extensible proboscis. This appendage, which may extend in some species as far back as the spire of the shell, grasps the venom-impregnated and barbed tooth and thrusts it into the flesh of the victim. In normal small fish prey, the cone snails may deploy a hunting method of initial rigid paralysis with fin tetanus to tether the prey to the radular tooth, and then flaccid paralysis to allow consumption. This has been observed in the fish-hunting snail *C. purpurascens*.[205] Remarkably, cone snails can switch rapidly between venom distinct for predation (high in prey-specific toxins) and venom for defense (high in paralytic toxins).[50]

The venom is composed of biologically active peptides (> 100 conotoxins have been identified) of 13 to 35 amino acids in length.[153] The majority of the unique *Conus* peptides appear to be derived from a few gene superfamilies (A, M, and O), which results in the biologically active venom components.[52] Peptide families in the A-superfamily include the α-conotoxins and the αA-conotoxins, which antagonize the nicotinic acetylcholine receptor, as well as the κA-conotoxins, which may act by blocking voltage-gated potassium channels. The μ-conotoxins, in the M-superfamily, block voltage-gated sodium channels. The ψ-conotoxins are noncompetitive antagonists of the nicotinic

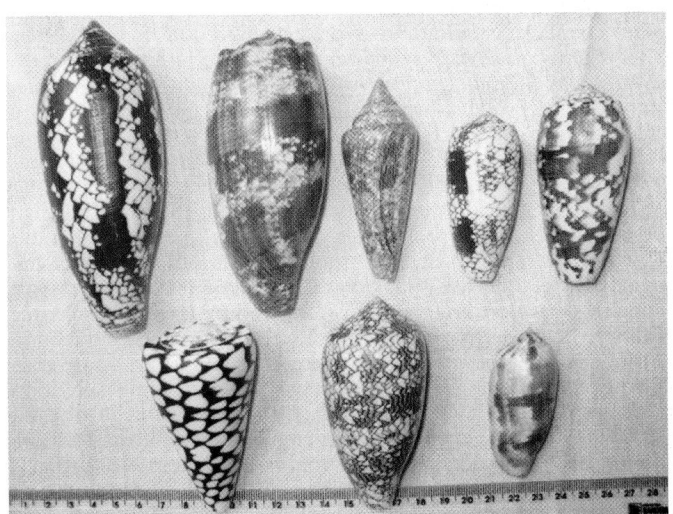

FIGURE 74-101 Assorted cone snails. *(Courtesy Vidal Haddad, Jr.)*

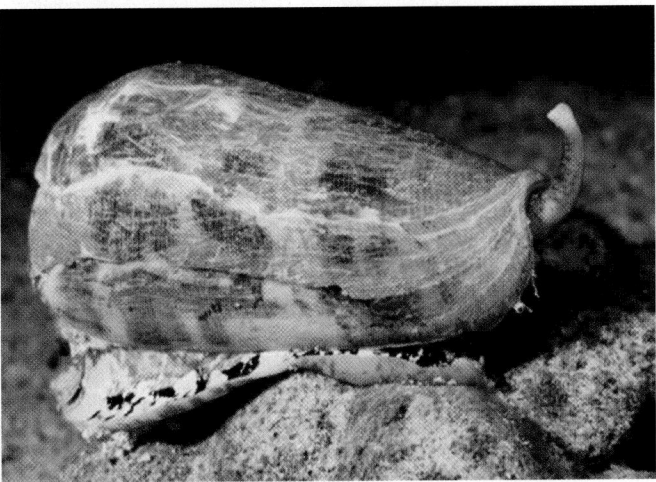

FIGURE 74-103 Conus striatus. *(From Norbert Wu, with permission: norbertwu.com.)*

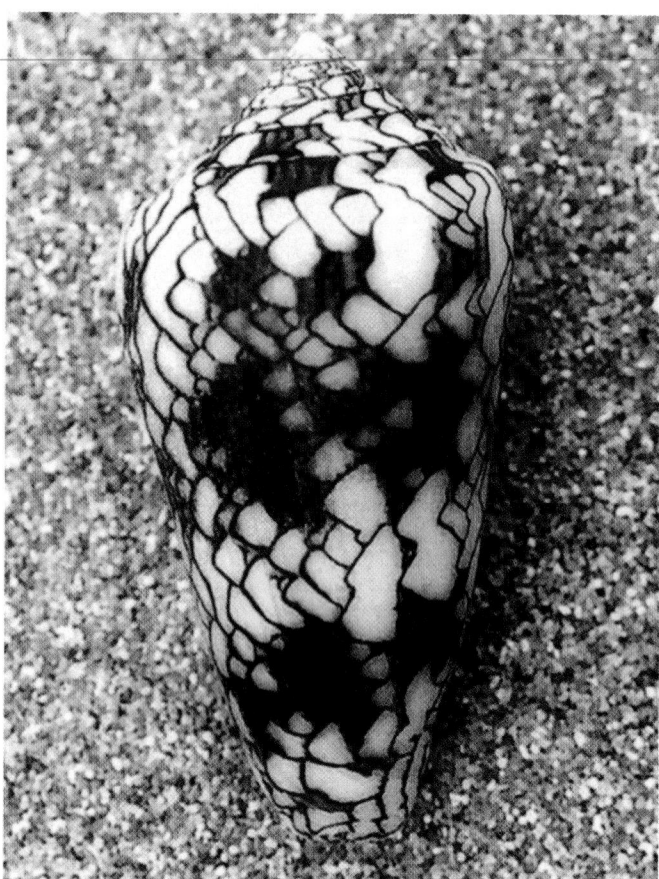

FIGURE 74-104 Cone snail, *Conus textile,* from the Red Sea. (*Courtesy Dietrich Mebs.*)

acetylcholine receptor. In the O-superfamily are the ω-conotoxins, which block voltage-sensitive calcium channels; δ-conotoxins, which delay inactivation of voltage-sensitive sodium channels; μO-conotoxins, which block voltage-gated sodium channels; and κ-conotoxins, which block voltage-gated potassium channels.[136]

Smaller peptides are probably strategic from an evolutionary perspective because of the speed of diffusion through a poisoned

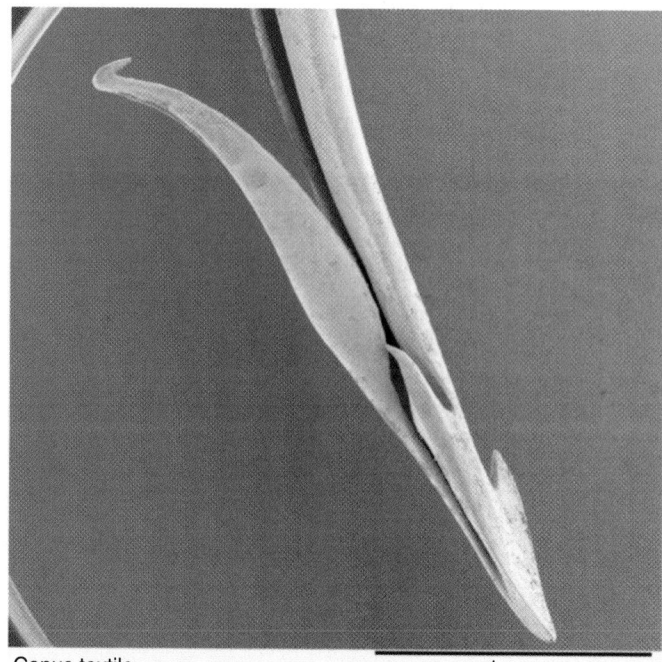

Conus textile   1 mm
FIGURE 74-105 Radula of *Conus textile.* (*Courtesy Dietrich Mebs.*)

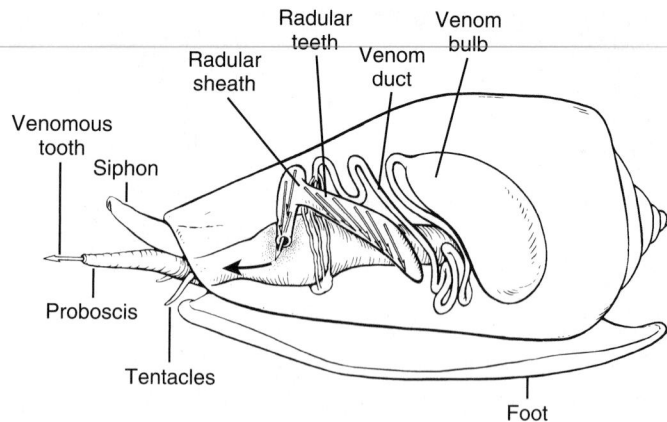

FIGURE 74-106 Venom apparatus of the cone snail.

fish. The venom targets are neuromuscular transmission and ion channels. Because there is a redundancy of sites of action at the neuromuscular junction, presynaptically and postsynaptically, minute amounts of conotoxins effect neuromuscular blockade.[216]

At the same site as tetrodotoxin and saxitoxin, μ-conotoxins bind and modify muscle sodium channels.[84] Voltage-dependent calcium uptake at the presynaptic cleft, and cholinergic transmission in avian and mammalian neuromuscular junctions are inhibited by ω-conotoxins, such as that from *C. geographus.*[48] These ω-conotoxins bind to neuronal (N-type) rather than the cardiac (L-type) calcium channels, which prevents the calcium influx necessary for neurotransmitter release. N-type calcium channels are expressed almost exclusively on neurons, and they are implicated in synaptic release of neurotransmitters such as substance P and calcitonin gene–related peptide within nociceptive sensory neurons. Ziconatide, a synthetic form of the ω-conopeptide MVIIa, is a potent analgesic intended for human application directly to the spinal cord and to prevent cell death in the brain after head trauma and ischemic events.[216] The α-conotoxins block the nicotinic acetylcholine receptor.[78,145] A subset of the α-conotoxins known as α-conotoxins RgIA and Vc1.1 produces both acute and long-lasting analgesia, and accelerates recovery of function after nerve injury, perhaps through immune-mediated mechanisms.[134] A sleeper peptide in *C. geographus* venom causes test animals to enter a deep sleeplike state.[78] Conantokins G and T, which are selective inhibitors of certain subtypes of the *N*-methyl-D-aspartate (NMDA) receptor, exhibit potent antinociceptive effects in several models of injury-induced pain, which holds promise as a novel therapeutic approach for the control of pain.[127] Furthermore, if conotoxins targeting NMDA receptors can be translated into effective drugs, this may lead to another approach to the treatment of epilepsy.[96] A novel conotoxin isolated from *Conus virgo* inhibits vertebrate voltage-sensitive potassium channels.[102] Serotonin is present in venom from the cone snail *Conus imperialis,* which is a worm feeder.[135] In the act of envenomation, milky venom from the venom duct is transformed into a clear product, which may indicate conversion from an ineffective to an effective toxin.

Clinical Aspects

Most stings occur on the fingers and hand, as the unknowledgeable fossicker (i.e., a prospector, or collector) incorrectly handles a hazardous specimen. Mild stings are puncture wounds that resemble bee or wasp stings, with associated burning or a sharp stinging sensation. Initial pain is followed by localized ischemia, cyanosis, and numbness in the area surrounding the wound. Numbness may occur without preceding pain, or in a rare case, the envenomation may be without any specific dermal sensation. More serious envenomations induce paresthesias at the wound site, which rapidly encompass the limb and then become perioral before becoming generalized. Partial paralysis transitions to generalized muscular paralysis, causing diaphragmatic dysfunction and respiratory failure; bronchospastic respiratory distress is not commonly seen. Coma has been observed, and death is attributed to diaphragmatic paralysis or cardiac failure. Other symptoms include dysphagia, syncope, weakness, failing coordination, areflexia, aphonia, dysarthria, diplopia, ptosis, absent gag reflex, blurred vision, and pruritus. The sting of *C. geographus* may be rapidly toxic, with progression to cerebral edema, coma, respiratory arrest, and cardiac failure within a few hours, perhaps even 1 hour. Although mild stings may cause symptoms of nausea, blurred vision, malaise, and weakness for only a few hours, severe envenomation may induce symptoms that require 2 to 3 weeks to achieve total resolution. *C. textile* and *C. marmoreus* have been reported to kill humans. A fatality has been attributed to *C. gloriamaris,* but this has not been confirmed.[139]

Treatment

No antivenom is available for cone shell envenomation. Numerous therapies have been recommended, including the pressure-immobilization technique (see Figure 35-30 in Chapter 35), application of a proximal lymphatic–venous occlusive bandage, incision and suction, soaking in nonscalding hot water to tolerance (upper limit, 45° C [113° F]) until pain is relieved, injection of a local anesthetic (1% to 2% lidocaine without epinephrine), and local excision. The pressure-immobilization technique makes sense and should be applied.

Cardiovascular and respiratory support are the usual priorities after severe envenomation. The wound should be inspected for the presence of a foreign body (the radula). Edrophonium (10 mg intravenously for an adult) has been suggested as empirical therapy for paralysis. A rational approach would be to administer an edrophonium (Tensilon) test to determine effectiveness. The clinician should choose a weak muscle group for which strength can be objectively measured, then inject edrophonium (2 mg intravenously). If there is improvement, this is followed by edrophonium (8 mg intravenously). Adverse reactions to edrophonium (an anticholinesterase inhibitor) include salivation, nausea, diarrhea, and muscle fasciculations. These can be ameliorated with atropine, 0.6 mg intravenously.

Cone shells should be handled only when wearing proper gloves; if the proboscis protrudes, the cone should be dropped. If the animal must be carried, it should always be lifted by the large posterior end of the shell, although this does not afford complete protection. A collector should never carry a live cone inside a wetsuit, clothing pocket, or buoyancy compensator pocket.

OCTOPUSES

Life and Habits

Octopuses and cuttlefish are cephalopods that are usually harmless and retiring. On occasion, they are noted to manifest "curiosity" or "play behavior," by navigating mazes or manipulating objects without intent to feed or create a habitat. True octopuses are inhabitants of warmer waters with little tolerance for extremes in salinity. They prefer rocky bottoms and rock pools in the intertidal zones. The entertainment media have created the image of a giant creature that envelops its victim in a maze of tentacles and suction cups. However, most dangerous (envenoming) creatures are smaller than 10 to 20 cm (4 to 8 inches) and do not squeeze their victims at all. On the other hand, there are reports in the South Pacific of breath-hold spearfishermen drowned while hunting octopuses. The method used to kill the animals was to allow an octopus to cling to a diver, who would bite the animal between the eyes as the combatants surfaced. Apparently, the octopuses were large enough (4-m [13-foot] tentacle span) to resist the technique. *Octopus apollyon* can be pugnacious and may bite, in one case causing an immediate reaction of bradycardia and hypotension.[20]

Octopus bites are rare but can result in severe envenomations. Fatalities have been reported from the bites of the Australian blue-ringed (or "spotted") octopuses, *Octopus (Hapalochlaena) maculosa* and *Octopus (Hapalochlaena) lunulata.* These small creatures, which rarely exceed 20 cm (8 inches) in length with tentacles extended, are found throughout the Indo-Pacific (Australia, New Zealand, New Guinea, Japan) in rock pools, under discarded objects and shells, and in shallow waters,

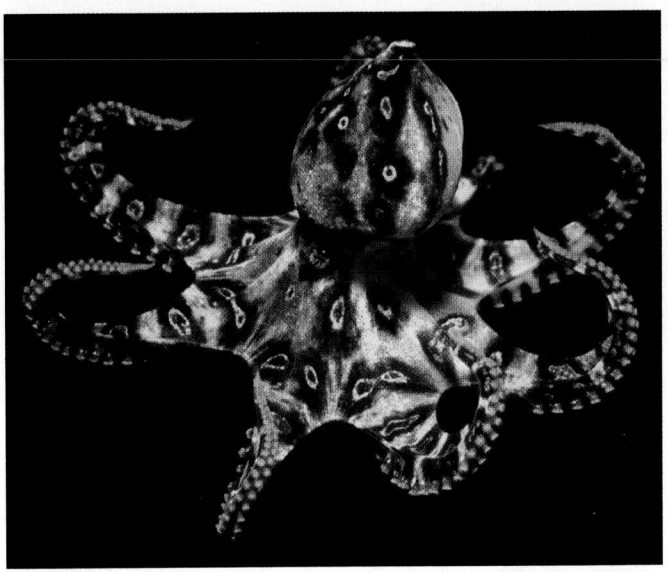

FIGURE 74-107 Extremely venomous temperate blue-ringed octopus (*Hapalochlaena maculosa*), in Southern Australia. *(From Gary Bell:* oceanwideimages.com.)

posing a threat to curious children, tidepoolers, fossickers, and unwary divers.[199] Divers rarely spot them in water deeper than 3 m (10 feet). The bodies are oblong and pyriform, with a pointed tail and conspicuous excrescences on the upper surface.[18] In Australian waters, *H. maculosa,* the southern species, is smaller and yellow. *H. lunulata* is found in the north; larger, darker, and predominantly brownish, it favors the warmer tropical water. A third species, the blue-lined octopus (*Hapalochlaena fasciata*) has been described along the east coast (New South Wales) of Australia.[149] It has blue lines on the body and blue rings on the arms. When any of these animals is at rest, it is covered with dark brown to yellow-ochre bands over the body and arms, with superimposed blue patches or rings.[196] When the animal is excited or angered, the entire body darkens and the blue circles or stripes glow iridescent peacock blue, a trait shared by other animals, such as the peacock flounder (*Bothus lunatus).* The colorful appearance is attractive to small children, who can easily handle the 25- to 90-g animal (Figure 74-107). The smallish *Octopus joubini* of the Caribbean, which lives in small shells and empty containers, such as submerged bottles, is dangerous to a lesser degree; envenomation causes pain followed by numbness, fever, and nausea. The large common octopus, *Octopus vulgaris,* is nontoxic (Figure 74-108). Many octopuses can release inky fluid into the water, which is used to confuse attackers, but this mechanism is not present in the blue-ringed octopus. The chameleon-like changing of colors to match the surroundings is accomplished with pigment cells (chromatophores) (Figures 74-109 to 74-112).

Venom and Venom Apparatus

The venom apparatus of the blue-ringed octopus consists of the salivary glands (anterior and posterior), salivary ducts, buccal mass, and beak. The mouth is located ventrally and centrally at the base of the tentacles and is surrounded by a circular lip fringed with finger-like papillae, leading into a muscular pharyngeal cavity. This anatomic complex (buccal mass), concealed by the tentacles, is fronted by two parrot-like, powerful, and chitinous jaws (the beak), which bite and tear with great force at food held by the suckers. The salivary glands, particularly the posterior ones, secrete toxin (sometimes called maculotoxin or cephalotoxin)–containing venom via the salivary ducts into the pharynx. This venom, normally released into the water to subdue crabs, may be injected into the victim with great force through the dermis down to the muscle fascia.[199] The venom of *H. maculosa* has been extensively studied. The toxin, maculotoxin (molecular weight less than 5000), contains at least one fraction identical to

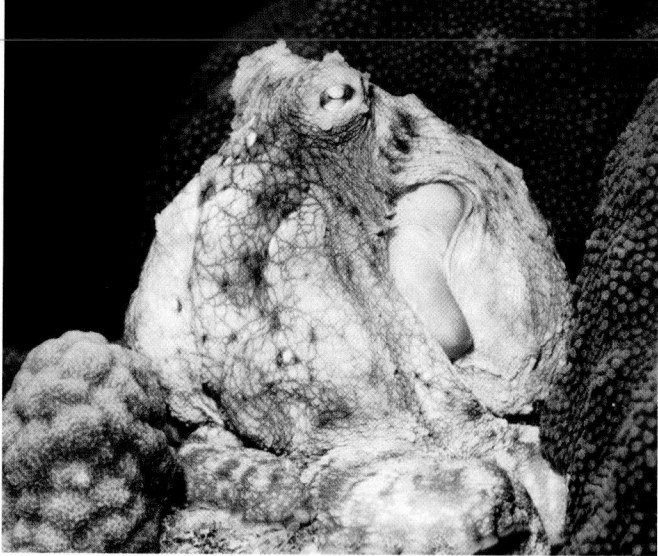

FIGURE 74-108 *Octopus vulgaris. (Copyright Stephen Frink.)*

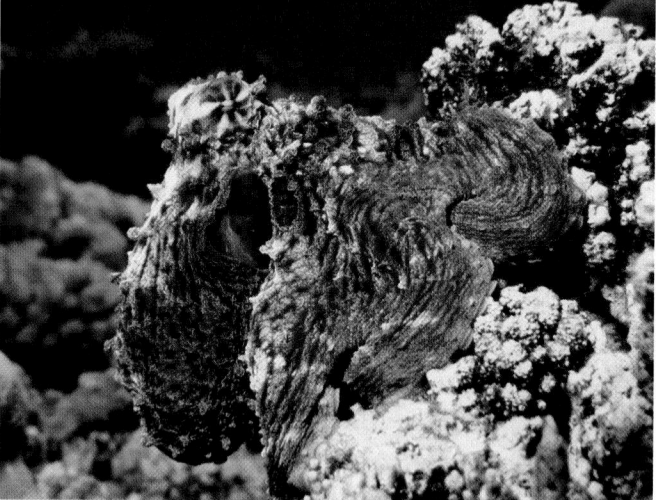

FIGURE 74-109 *Octopus posed atop coral in the Coral Sea. (Copyright Carl Roessler.)*

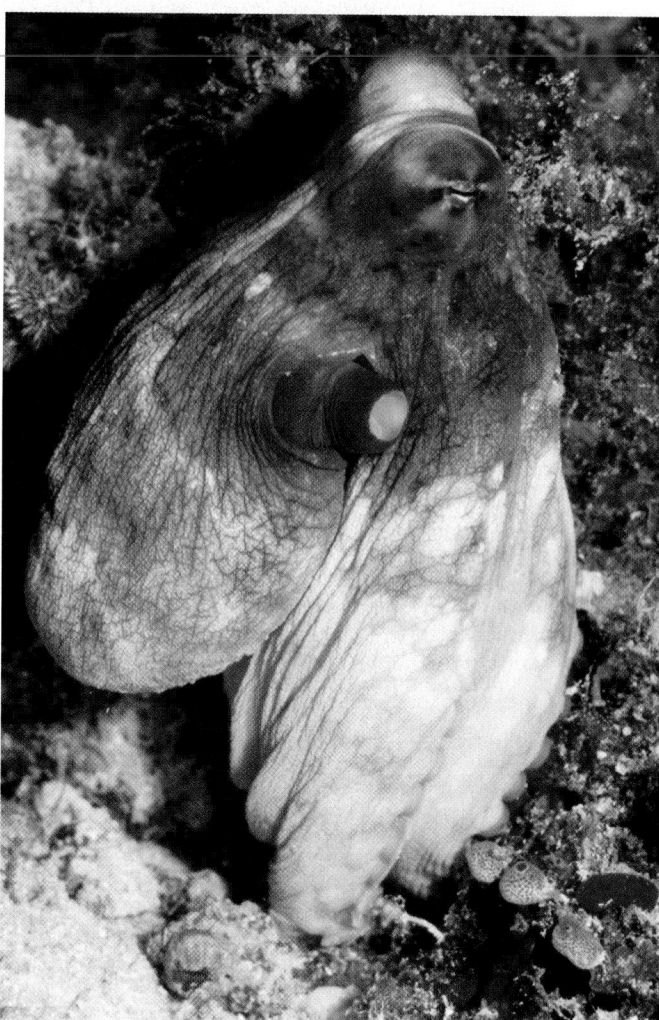

FIGURE 74-111 *Octopus vulgaris. (Copyright Stephen Frink.)*

tetrodotoxin (TTX, with the chemical formula $C_{11}H_{17}O_8N_3$) of molecular weight 319.3, which blocks peripheral nerve conduction by interfering with sodium conductance in excitable membranes by blocking voltage-gated sodium channels.[99,184] The toxin, as well as the tetrodotoxin precursor anhydrotetrodotoxin, is produced by bacteria of the Vibrionaceae family, and is passed along the food chain to the octopus.[216] In a study of the intraorganismal distribution of tetrodotoxin in two species of blueringed octopuses (*H. fasciata* from New South Wales, Australia, and *H. lunulata* from Indonesia), TTX was detected in posterior salivary gland, arm, mantle, anterior salivary glands, digestive gland, testes contents, brachial heart, nephridia, gill, and oviductal gland of *H. fasciata*, but only in the posterior salivary gland, mantle tissue, and ink of *H. lunulata*. The highest concentrations of TTX reside in the posterior salivary gland. The distributional data suggest both offensive and defensive functions of TTX.[219]

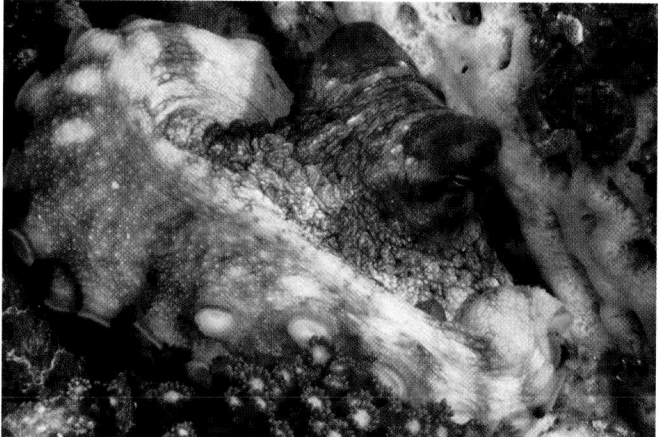

FIGURE 74-110 *Octopus vulgaris. (Copyright Stephen Frink.)*

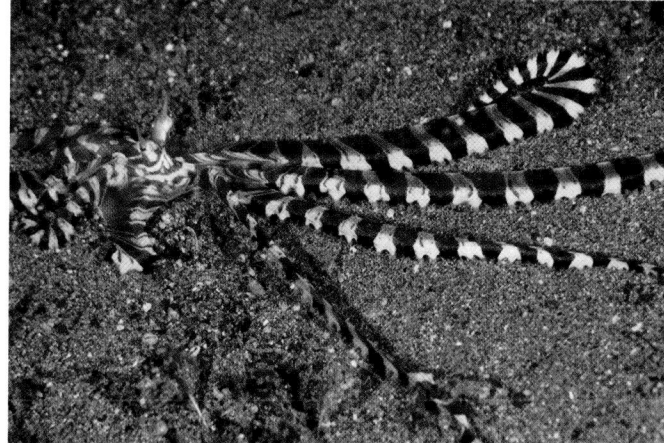

FIGURE 74-112 Mimic octopus. *(Copyright Lynn Funkhouser.)*

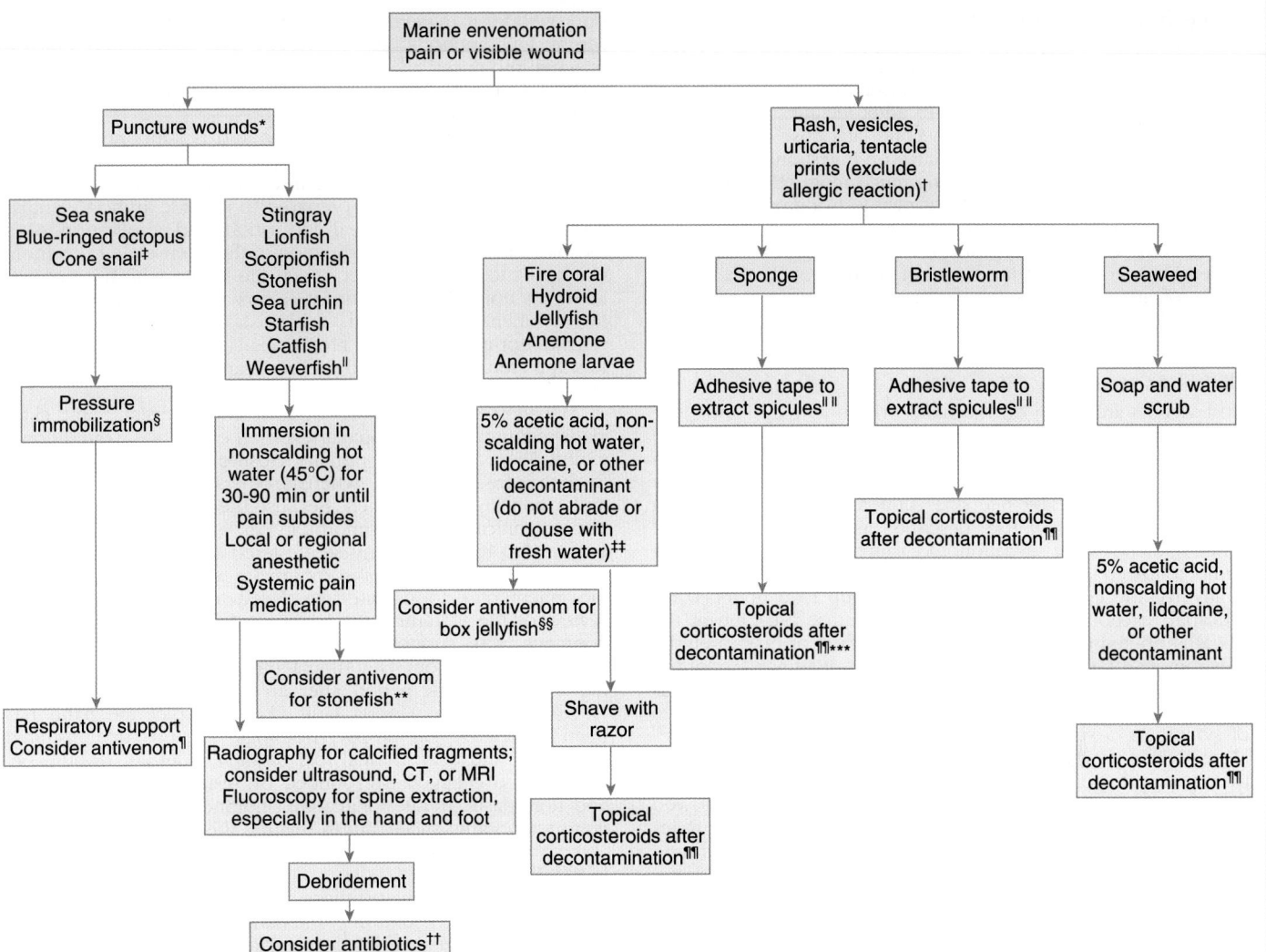

FIGURE 74-113 Algorithmic approach to marine envenomation. *A gaping laceration, particularly of the lower extremity, with cyanotic edges suggests a stingray wound. Multiple punctures in an erratic pattern with or without purple discoloration or retained fragments are typical of a sea urchin sting. One to eight (usually two) fang marks are usually present after a sea snake bite. A single ischemic puncture wound with an erythematous halo and rapid swelling suggests scorpionfish envenomation. Blisters often accompany a lionfish sting. Painless punctures with paralysis suggest the bite of a blue-ringed octopus; the site of a cone shell sting is punctate, painful, and ischemic in appearance. †Wheal-and-flare reactions are nonspecific. Rapid onset (within 24 hours) of skin necrosis suggests an anemone sting. Broad "tentacle prints" with cross-hatching or a frosted appearance after application of aluminum-based salts suggests a box-jellyfish (*Chironex fleckeri*) envenomation. Ocular or intraoral lesions may be caused by fragmented hydroids or cnidarian tentacles. An allergic reaction must be treated promptly. ‡Sea snake venom causes weakness, respiratory paralysis, myoglobinuria, myalgias, blurred vision, vomiting, and dysphagia. The blue-ringed octopus injects tetrodotoxin, which causes rapid neuromuscular paralysis. §As soon as possible, venom should be sequestered locally with a proximal venous-lymphatic occlusive band of constriction or (preferably) the pressure-immobilization technique, in which a cloth pad is compressed directly over the wound by an elastic wrap that should encompass the entire extremity at a pressure of 70 mm Hg or less. Incision and suction are not recommended. ¶Early ventilatory support has the greatest influence on outcome. The minimal initial dose of sea snake antivenom is 1 to 3 vials; up to 10 vials may be required. ‖The wounds range from large lacerations (stingrays) to minute punctures (stonefish). Persistent pain after immersion in hot water suggests a stonefish sting or a retained fragment of spine. The puncture site can be identified by forcefully injecting 1% to 2% lidocaine or another local anesthetic agent without epinephrine near the wound and observing the egress of fluid. Do not attempt to crush the spines of sea urchins if they are present in the wound. Spine dye from sea urchin spines that have already been extracted will disappear (be absorbed) in 24 to 36 hours. **The initial dose of stonefish antivenom is one vial per two puncture wounds. ††The antibiotics chosen should cover *Staphylococcus, Streptococcus,* and microbes of marine origin, such as *Vibrio.* ‡‡Acetic acid 5% (vinegar) is a good all-purpose decontaminant and mandated for the sting from a box-jellyfish. Alternatives, depending on the geographic region and indigenous jellyfish species, include isopropyl alcohol, bicarbonate (baking soda), lidocaine, papain, and preparations containing these agents. Application of water heated to 45°C may be effective for relieving pain. §§The initial dose of box-jellyfish antivenom is one ampule intravenously or three ampules intramuscularly. ¶¶If inflammation is severe, steroids should be given systemically (beginning with at least 60 to 100 mg of prednisone or its equivalent), and the dose should be tapered over a period of 10 to 14 days. ‖‖An alternative is to apply and remove commercial facial peel materials. ***An alternative is to apply and remove commercial facial peel materials followed by topical soaks of 30 mL of 5% acetic acid (vinegar) diluted in 1 L of water for 15 to 30 minutes, several times a day, until the lesions begin to resolve. Anticipate surface desquamation in 3 to 6 weeks.

This paralytic agent rapidly produces neuromuscular blockade, notably of the phrenic nerve supply to the diaphragm, without any apparent direct cardiotoxicity. It has been estimated that enough venom (25 g) may be present in one adult octopus to paralyze 750 kg of rabbits or 10 adult victims.[196,199] An adult blue-ringed octopus can inject a second fatal dose of toxin after a 1-hour interval. The venom is active on ingestion or by parenteral administration, the latter being much more effective. Other components of the venom, which include hyaluronidase, histamine, 5-hydroxytryptamine, tyramine, serotonin, and hapalotoxin (believed to derive from tyrosine, but still not confirmed as being present), are not believed to be major contributors to the clinical effects of an octopus bite.[179] Because most venoms and toxins with molecular weights less than 30,000 are poor antigens, octopus venom elicits no good antivenom.[199]

Clinical Aspects

Most victims are bitten on the hand or arm as they handle the creature or "give it a ride." No blue-ringed octopus bites have yet been reported from an animal in the water.[221] An octopus bite usually consists of two small puncture wounds produced by the chitinous jaws. The bite goes unnoticed or causes only a small amount of discomfort, described as a minor ache, slight stinging, or pulsating sensation. Occasionally, the site is initially numb, followed in 5 to 10 minutes by discomfort that may spread to involve the entire limb, persisting for up to 6 hours. Local urticarial reactions occur variably, and profuse bleeding at the site is attributed to a local anticoagulant effect or may rarely be a harbinger of coagulation abnormalities. Within 30 minutes, considerable erythema, swelling, tenderness, heat, and pruritus develop. By far the most common local tissue reaction is absence of symptoms, a small spot of blood, or a tiny blanched area.[220] More serious symptoms are related predominantly to the neurotoxic properties of the venom. Within 10 to 15 minutes of the bite, the victim notices oral and facial numbness, rapidly followed by systemic progression.[221] Voluntary and involuntary muscles are involved, and the illness may rapidly progress to total flaccid paralysis and respiratory failure. Other symptoms include perioral and intraoral anesthesia (classically, numbness of the lips and tongue), diplopia, blurred vision, aphonia, dysphagia, ataxia, dizziness, myoclonus, weakness, sense of detachment, nausea, vomiting, peripheral neuropathy, absent deep tendon reflexes, flaccid muscular paralysis, sensation of chest tightness, and respiratory failure, which may lead to death. Ataxia of cerebellar configuration may occur after envenomation that does not progress to frank paralysis. Jerking limbs have been mentioned, as have poorly reactive or unreactive pupils. The victim may collapse from weakness and remain awake, so long as oxygenation can be maintained. When breathing is disturbed, respiratory assistance may allow the victim to remain mentally alert despite being paralyzed. Cardiac arrest is probably a complication of the anoxic episode.[214] Although tetrodotoxin is a potent vascular smooth muscle depressant, it does not appear to often produce significant hypotension in humans; however, hypotensive crisis has been mentioned in the literature as a complicating factor.

Treatment

First aid at the scene might include the pressure-immobilization technique (see Fig. 35-30, Chapter 35), although this is as yet unproved for management of octopus bites. A monoclonal rabbit serum IgG antibody has been effective against tetrodotoxin injected into mice.[131,135,170] This raises the possibility of the practical use of passive immunotherapy in the event of tetrodotoxin poisoning.

Treatment is based on symptoms and is supportive. Prompt mechanical respiratory assistance has by far the greatest influence on the outcome. Respiratory demise should be anticipated early, and the rescuer should be prepared to provide artificial ventilation, including endotracheal intubation and application of a mechanical ventilator. The duration of the intense clinical venom effect is 4 to 10 hours, after which the victim who has not suffered an episode of significant hypoxia shows rapid signs of improvement. If no period of hypoxia occurs, mentation may remain normal. Complete recovery may require 2 to 4 days. Residua are uncommon and related to anoxia rather than venom effects.

Management of the bite wound is controversial. Some clinicians recommend wide circular excision of the bite wound down to the deep fascia, with primary closure or an immediate full-thickness free skin graft, whereas others advocate observation and a nonsurgical approach. Because the local tissue reaction is not a significant cause of morbidity, excision is presumably recommended to remove any sequestered venom. Kinetic studies of radiolabeled venom absorption are necessary to track the movement of octopus bite–introduced tetrodotoxin. Based on review of the literature, this author would favor a nonsurgical approach with supportive therapy. As previously mentioned, there is no antivenom. Granuloma annulare of the hand developing over a 2-week period after an octopus (presumed to be *O. vulgaris* of the Florida Gulf Coast) bite of the hand has been reported.[68] On biopsy, histologic sections demonstrated superficial and deep dermal foci of altered dermis, presumably degenerated collagen, surrounded by histiocytes, lymphocytes, and fibroblasts. Intralesional triamcinolone acetonide injections were temporarily successful in treating the primary lesion.[132]

Prevention

All octopuses, particularly those less than 20 cm (8 inches) in length (including *O. joubini* of the Caribbean), should be handled with gloves. Divers need to be familiar with the lethal creatures in their domain. Giving an octopus a ride on one's back, shoulder, or arm is not recommended.

SUMMARY

A summary algorithmic approach to marine envenomation (Figure 74-113) can be followed when the causative agent cannot be definitively identified.

REFERENCES

Complete references used in this text are available online at expertconsult.inkling.com.

See Chapter 74 for a discussion of infections associated with aquatic wounds and the relevant antimicrobial therapy. An analysis that compared DNA sequences from 233 fish species was used to create a family tree for spiny-rayed fishes. This indicates that previous estimates of approximately 200 venomous fishes should be revised to suspect at least 1200 fishes in 12 clades (a group of biologic taxa or species that share features inherited from a common ancestor) as perhaps venomous.[97]

A common clinical question is how best to image embedded spines, such as those from stingrays, scorpionfishes, or sea urchins. Some prove to be radiopaque and some are not. One limited study evaluated intraarticular foreign bodies using sea urchin spines and chicken thigh-leg combinations.[61] Pending further evidence, computed tomography (CT) and magnetic resonance imaging (MRI) appear to be more reliable modalities for imaging than plain radiography, ultrasonography, or fluoroscopy. However, for reasons of limiting radiation exposure or expense, one of the latter three may be chosen as the initial imaging technique.

STINGRAYS

Stingrays are the most commonly incriminated group of fish involved in human envenomations. They have been recognized as venomous since ancient times, known as "demons of the deep" and "devil fish." Aristotle (384 to 322 BC) made reference to their stinging ability. Stingray spines were used in certain Mayan bloodletting procedures and rituals.[55]

Stingrays are members of the class Chondrichthyes (cartilaginous fish), subclass Elasmobranchii (plates and gills; with sharks and chimaeras), order Rajiformes (which contains stingrays [Dasyatidae], guitarfish [Rhinobatidae], skates [Rajidae], electric rays [Torpedinidae], eagle rays [Myliobatidae], mantas [Mobulidae], and freshwater rays [Potamotrygonidae]). Twenty-two species of stingrays are found in U.S. coastal waters, 14 in the Atlantic and 8 in the Pacific. The family Dasyatidae includes most of the species that cause human envenomation. It is likely that at least 2000 stingray injuries take place each year in the United States. On the west coast of the United States, the round stingray (*Urolophus* [or *Urobatis*] *halleri*) is a frequent stinger; along the southeastern coast, it is the southern stingray (*Dasyatis americana*). Most attacks occur during the summer and autumn months as vacationers venture into surf that may be laden with congregating (for spawning purposes) rays. Freshwater species do not inhabit U.S. waters. They are found in South America, Africa, and Southeast Asia. Skates are related to rays and look similar, but do not carry a sting, so are harmless to humans.

LIFE AND HABITS

Stingrays are cartilaginous fish that are usually found in tropical, subtropical, and warm temperate oceans, generally in shallow (intertidal) water areas, such as sheltered bays (Figure 75-1), shoal lagoons, river mouths, and sandy areas between patch reefs (Figure 75-2).[76] Although rays are generally found above moderate depths, at least one deep-sea species has been discovered. Rays can enter brackish and freshwaters as well. For instance, freshwater stingrays are common in rivers and tributaries in South America (Figure 75-3).[52]

Rays are small (several inches) to large (up to 4 m × 2 m [12 feet × 6 feet]) creatures observed lying on top of the sand and mud or partially submerged, with only the dorsally placed eyes and spiracles and part of the tail exposed (Figure 75-4). Their dorsoventrally flattened bodies are round-, diamond-, or kite-shaped, with wide pectoral fins that look like wings (Figure 75-5). The large fleshy cephalic lobes that appear to extend from the front of the head in manta rays are continuations of modified and enlarged pectoral fins. Rays are nonaggressive scavengers and bottom feeders that burrow into the sand or mud to feed on worms, mollusks, and crustaceans. The mouth and gill plates are located on the ventral surface of the animal (Figure 75-6). The flattened shape is largely configured by the modified pectoral fins, or "wings," of the animal. These wings ripple or flap to propel the animal through the water (Figure 75-7).

VENOM AND VENOM APPARATUS

The venom organ of stingrays consists of one to four venomous stings on the dorsum of an elongate, whip-like caudal appendage. Anatomic types of stingray venom organs, and thus stinging ability, are differentiated into four groups based on their adaptability as a defense organ (Figure 75-8): (1) the gymnurid type (butterfly rays, or Gymnuridae), with a poorly developed sting of up to 2.5 cm (1 inch) placed at the base of a short tail; (2) the myliobatid type (eagle and bat rays, or Myliobatidae), with a sting of up to 12 cm (4.7 inches) placed at the base of a cylindrical caudal appendage that terminates in a long whip-like tail; (3) the dasyatid type (stingrays and whip rays, or Dasyatidae), with a sting of up to 37 cm (14.5 inches) placed at the base or further out on the caudal appendage that terminates in a long whip-like tail; and (4) the urolophid type (round stingrays, or Urolophidae), with a sting of up to 4 cm (1.5 inches) located at the base of a short, muscular, and well-developed caudal appendage. The efficiency of the apparatus is related to the length and musculature of the tail and to the location and length of the sting. Eagle rays and some mantas (Atlantic *Mobula mobular* and Pacific *Mobula japanica*) have a stinging apparatus, but it is less of a threat because the spine is located at the base of the tail and is not well adapted as a striking organ. Although the Pacific manta (*Manta birostris*) may grow to a width ("wingspan") of 6 m (20 feet) and weight of 1800 kg (4000 lb), it dines on small fish, crustaceans, and microorganisms (Figures 75-9 and 75-10). There is some DNA evidence and a prevailing opinion that all mantas may be of the same species (*M. birostris*), which will in time render other Latin names and some common names obsolete. Many divers have "hitched" a ride on the wings of a manta; there are no reports of envenomation. However, manta skin is rough and can abrade unprotected human skin. A stingray "hickey" is a mouth-bite created by powerful grinding plates that produces superficial erosions and ecchymosis in an oral pattern. People who hand-feed stingrays may incur this type of injury.[37] The suction force generated by a stingray is sufficient to pull in a large amount of soft tissue, for example, from an obese thigh. This may result in a large and painful contusion or hematoma.

In all cases, the venom apparatus of stingrays consists of a bilaterally retroserrate spine or spines and the enveloping integumentary sheath or sheaths. The elongate and tapered vasodentine (modified dentin permeated by blood and capillaries) spine is

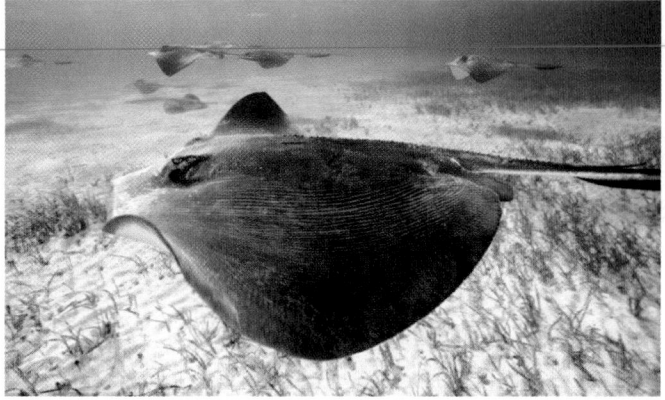

FIGURE 75-1 Stingrays gliding in shallow reef waters. (Copyright Stephen Frink.)

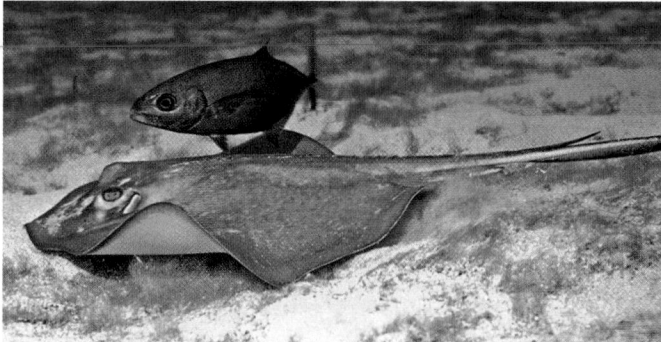

FIGURE 75-2 Stingray glides along the sandy ocean bottom. (Courtesy Marty Snyderman.)

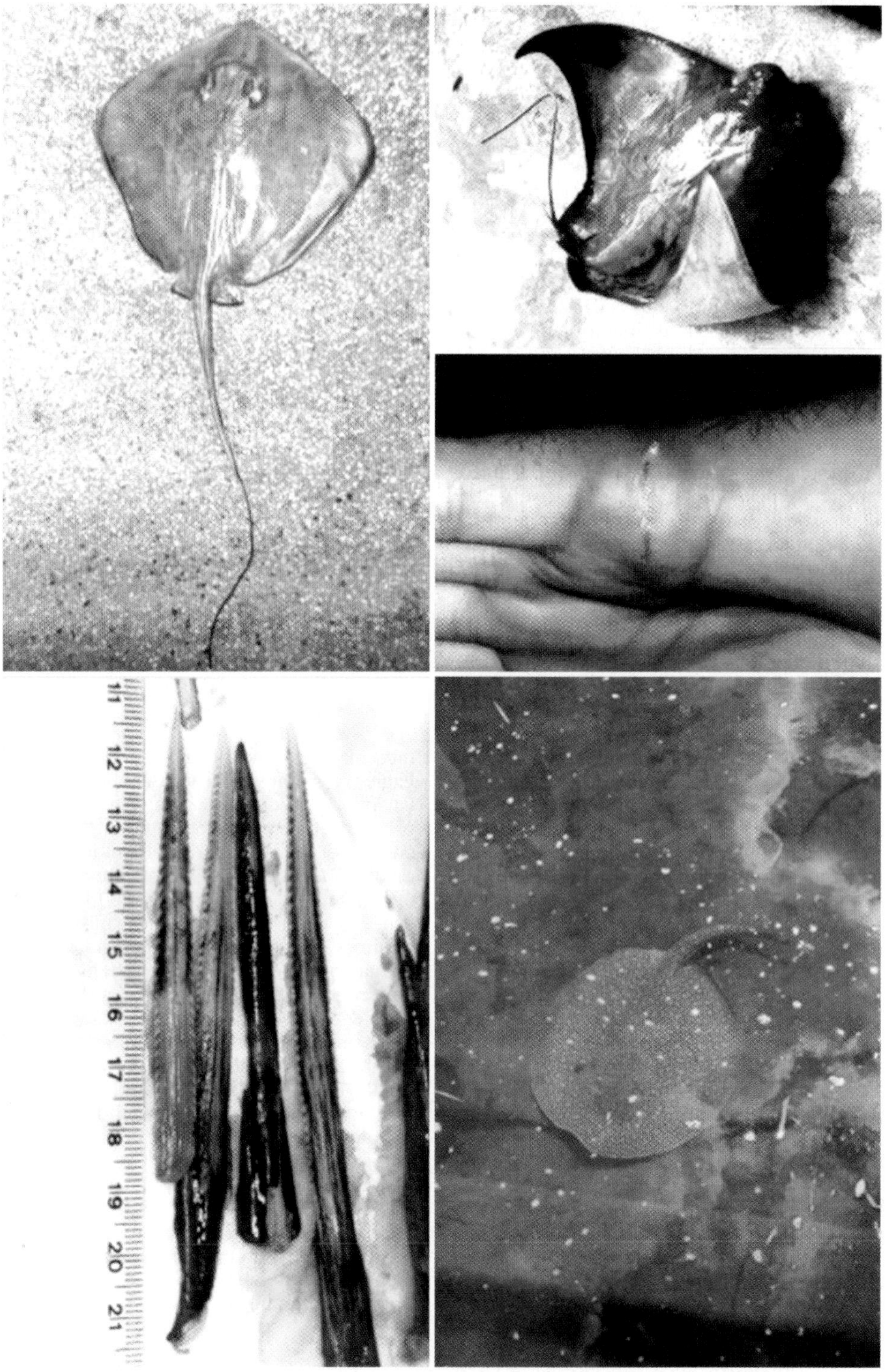

FIGURE 75-3 Freshwater stingray features and injury. (Courtesy Vidal Haddad, Jr.)

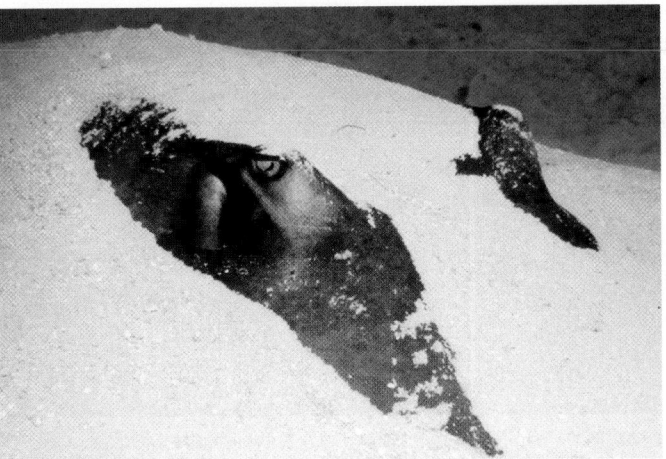

FIGURE 75-4 Stingray nestled in the sand. Only the eyes and spiracles are visible. *(Copyright Stephen Frink.)*

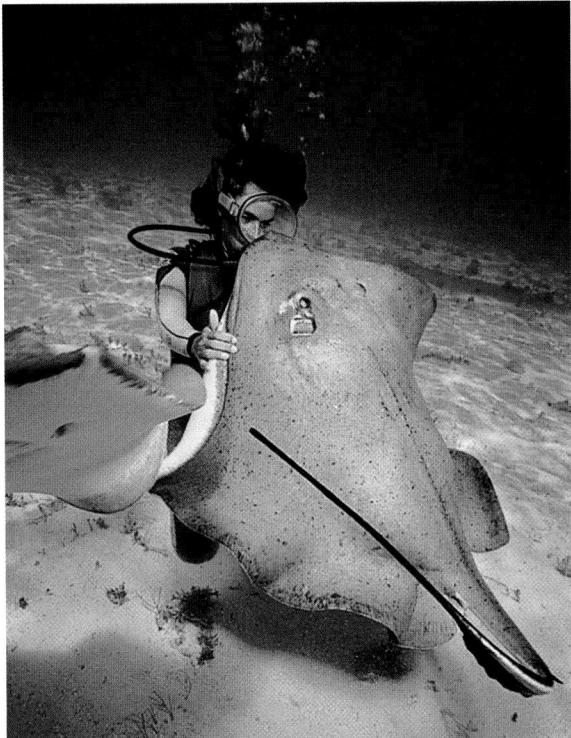

FIGURE 75-5 Diver cavorting with a large stingray. *(Courtesy Howard Hall.)*

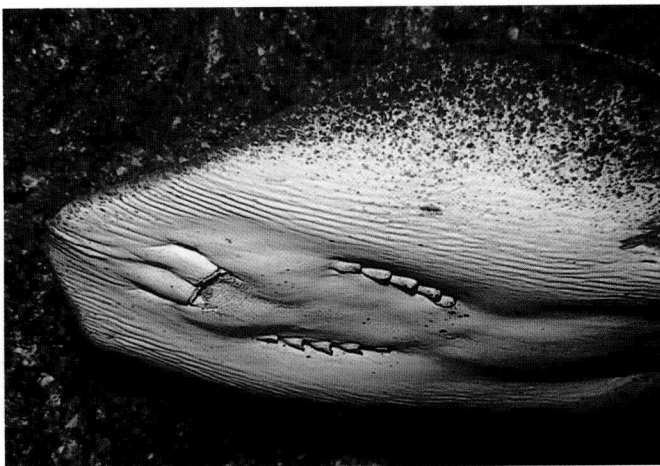

FIGURE 75-6 Ventral surface of a stingray, demonstrating mouth and gill plates. *(Courtesy Paul S. Auerbach, MD.)*

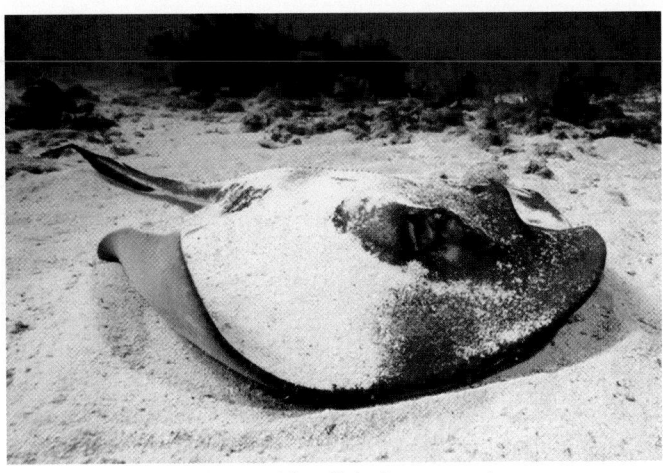

FIGURE 75-7 Large stingray lifts off the bottom and prepares to move away. *(Copyright Stephen Frink.)*

firmly attached to the dorsum of the tail (whip) by dense collagenous tissue and is edged on either side by a series of sharp retrorse teeth. Along either edge on the underside of the spine are the two ventrolateral grooves, which house the soft venom glands. The entire spine is encased by the integumentary sheath, which also contains some glandular cells. The sting is often covered with a film of venom and mucus. The spine is replaced if detached.

The venom contains various toxic fractions, including serotonin, 5′-nucleotidase, and phosphodiesterase. Russell and others have investigated the pharmacologic properties of stingray venoms.[33,90] In animal studies, they demonstrated significant

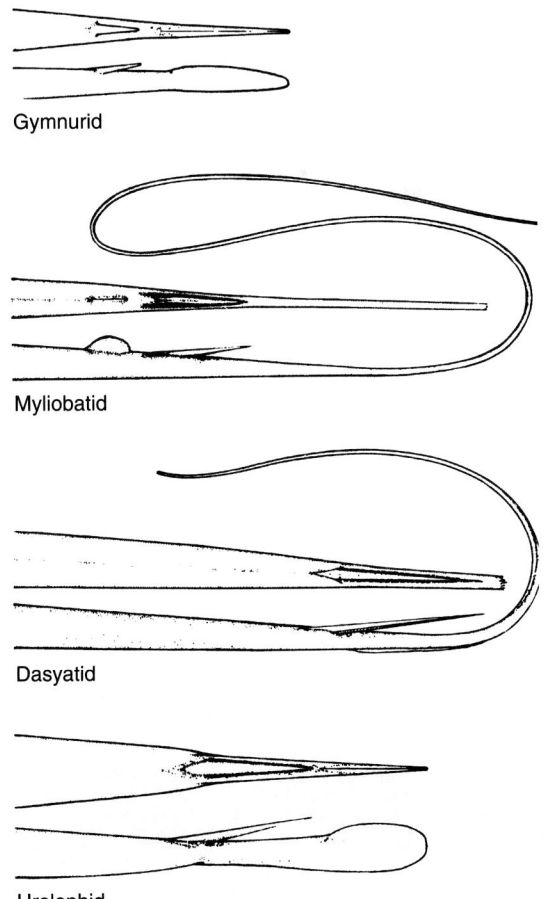

Gymnurid

Myliobatid

Dasyatid

Urolophid

FIGURE 75-8 Four anatomic types of stingray venom organs.

1723

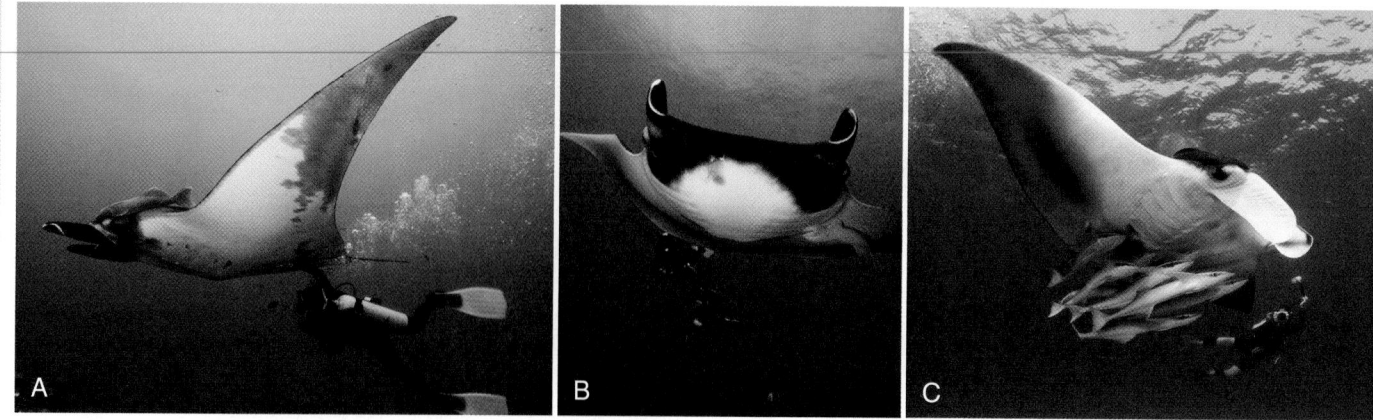

FIGURE 75-9 Manta rays. **A,** Diver strokes the belly of a manta ray. **B,** Pacific manta ray. **C,** Atlantic manta ray. (**A** copyright Carl Roessler; **B** and **C** copyright Stephen Frink.)

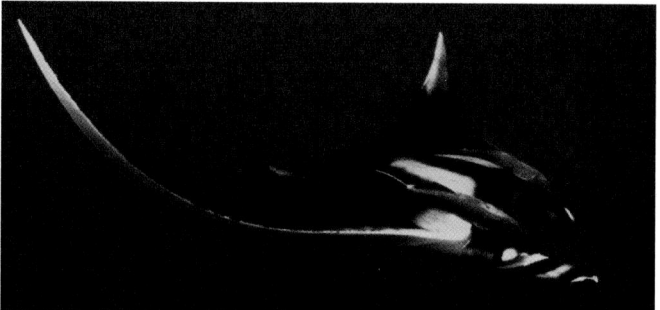

FIGURE 75-10 Manta ray. (Copyright 2011 Norbert Wu: norbertwu.com.)

venom-induced peripheral vasoconstriction, bradycardia, tachycardia, atrioventricular block, ischemic Q and ST-T wave abnormalities, asystole, central respiratory depression, seizure activity, ataxia, coma, and death. The venom did not appear to be a paralytic neuromuscular agent. Research on stingray venom from the 1950s observed that heating the venom to a temperature above 50°C (122°F) diminished some biologic effects. Haddad analyzed proteins from freshwater stingray *(Potamotrygon falkneri)* venom using SDS-polyacrylamide gel electrophoresis and identified components with gelatinolytic, caseinolytic, and hyaluronidase activities.[52] Others have identified hyaluronidase from the freshwater stingray *Potamotrygon motoro* and fibrinolytic activity from the venom of *Dasyatis sephen* and *Aetobatus narinari*.[77,70] A novel bioactive peptide, Porflan, from the stingray *Potamotrygon gr. orbignyi* induces leukocyte rolling and adherent cells, and is proinflammatory in mice.[29]

Electric rays are discussed in Chapter 73.

CLINICAL ASPECTS

Stingray "attacks" are purely defensive gestures that occur when an unwary human wading in shallow waters handles, corners, or steps on a camouflaged creature (Figure 75-11). A frequently cited estimate of annual stingray injuries incurred in U.S. coastal waters is 750 to 1500, although there is no reliable reporting system for these injuries. Estimates are higher in tropical regions. The tail of the ray reflexively whips upward and accurately thrusts the caudal spine or spines into the victim, producing a puncture wound or jagged laceration (Figure 75-12). The integumentary sheath covering the spine is ruptured and venom is released into the wound, along with mucus, pieces of the sheath, and fragments of the spine. On occasion, the entire spine tip is broken off and remains in the wound (Figure 75-13).[91] "Domesticated" stingrays, such as those that congregate at "Stingray City" in the waters off Grand Cayman Island (Figures 75-14 to 75-16), are habituated to the presence of humans and apparently pose less hazard for a spine puncture, but may still be induced to bite. It has been observed that there are hematologic differences between stingrays at tourist and nonvisited sites that reflect suboptimal stingray health in response to stress.[94]

A stingray wound from a spine puncture is both a traumatic injury and an envenomation. The former involves the physical damage caused by the sting itself. Because of the retrorse serrated teeth and powerful strikes, significant lacerations can result. Secondary bacterial infection is common. Osteomyelitis may occur if the bone is penetrated. Most injuries occur when the victim steps on a ray; another common cause is handling a ray during its extraction from a fishing net or hook.[35] The lower extremities, particularly the ankle and foot, are involved most often, followed by the upper extremities, abdomen, and thorax. In a rare case, the heart may be directly injured.[88] The tragic death in September 2006 of 44-year-old naturalist Stephen Irwin

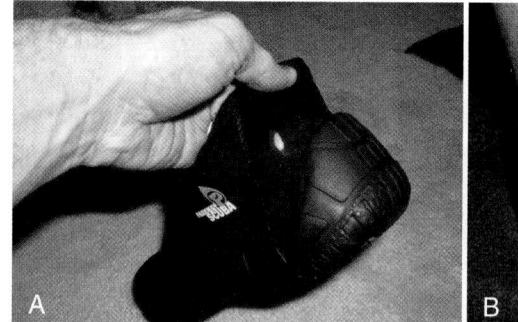
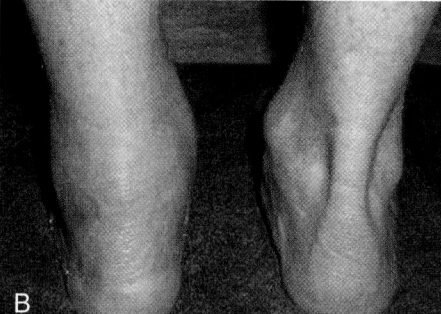
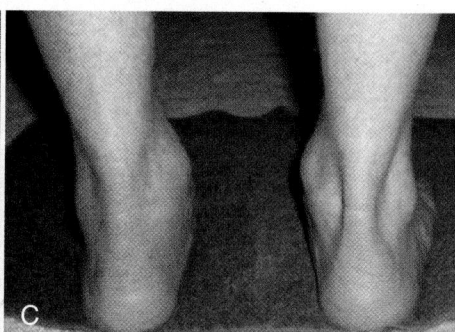

FIGURE 75-11 Stingray puncture wound. **A,** Puncture through neoprene boot in a typical location near the Achilles tendon. **B,** Stingray wound compared with normal foot 2 months following injury. **C,** Stingray wound compared with normal foot 6 months following injury. (Courtesy Bob Luce.)

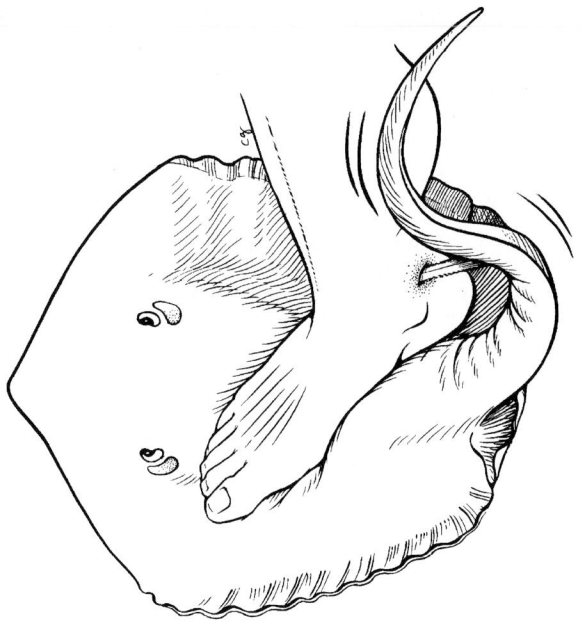

FIGURE 75-12 The stingray lashes its tail upward into the leg and generates a deep puncture wound.

occurred at Batt Reef off the remote coast of northeastern Queensland, Australia, when he swam directly over a stingray that thrust a stingray spine into his chest. Death was attributed to a direct heart puncture. He was filming a documentary titled *Ocean's Deadliest.* Fatalities have occurred after abdominal penetration and from exsanguination from the femoral artery. There have been reported cases of survival following cardiac injury, including one from the sting of a blue-spotted stingray *(Dasyatis kuhlii;* now *Neotrygon kuhlii)* that leaped into the boat of a 75-year-old man.[84] Pseudoaneurysms of the superficial femoral artery and posterior tibial artery caused by stingray envenomation have been reported.[18,57] One death has been attributed to tetanus

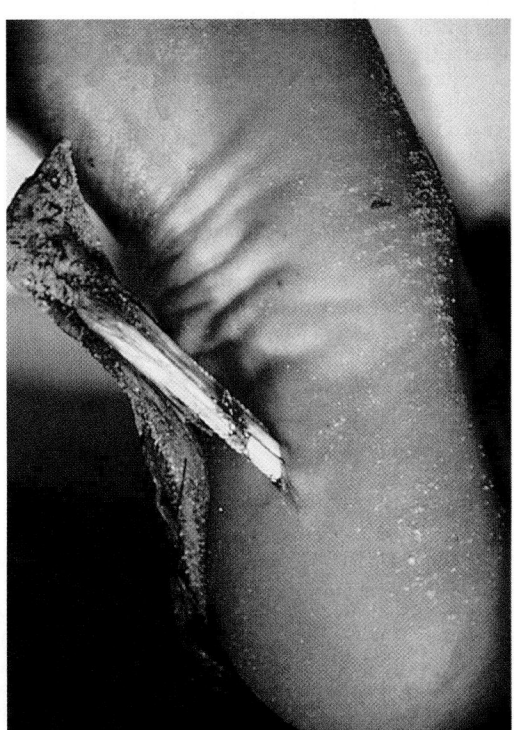

FIGURE 75-13 Stingray spine tip broken off into the heel of a victim. *(Courtesy Robert D. Hayes.)*

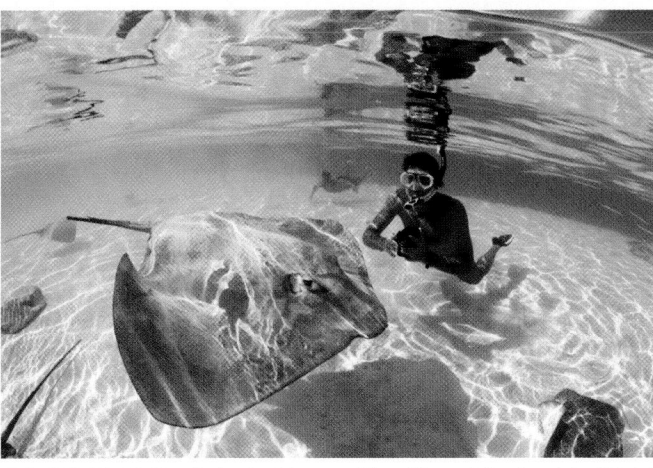

FIGURE 75-14 Snorkeler in Stingray City. *(Copyright Stephen Frink.)*

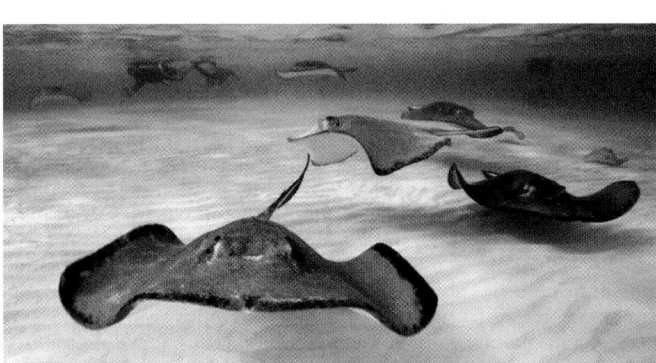

FIGURE 75-15 Stingrays in Stingray City. *(Copyright Stephen Frink.)*

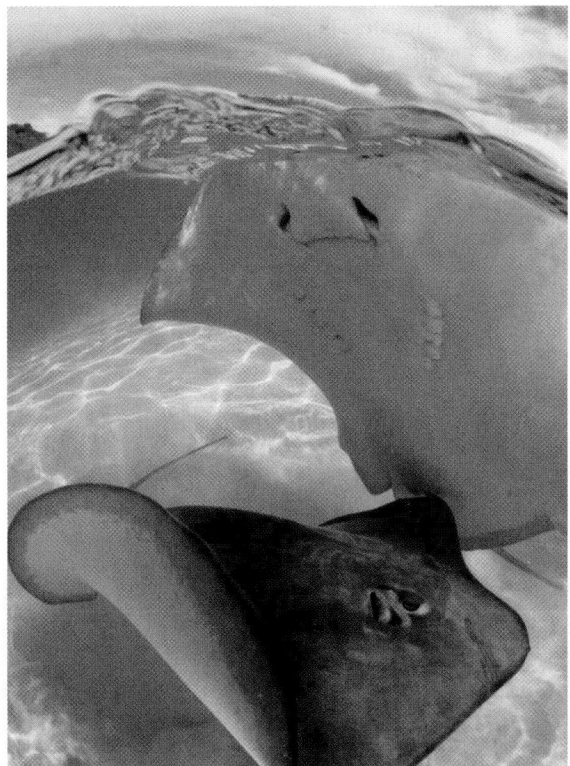

FIGURE 75-16 Paired stingrays in Stingray City. *(Copyright Stephen Frink.)*

complicating a leg wound. In one rare case, a women experienced vocal cord paralysis while eating raw stingray after ingesting a barb that lodged in her arytenoid.[71] A spine partially or totally denuded of its sheath and venom glands may not cause an envenomation.[38] A detached stingray spine may be used as a weapon. A man stabbed between the shoulder blades with stingray spine suffered a direct spinal cord injury at the level of T7-T8. He was extremely fortunate to make nearly a complete recovery after delayed operative removal.[49]

The envenomation classically causes immediate local intense pain, edema, and variable bleeding. The pain may radiate centrally, peaks at 30 to 60 minutes, and may last for up to 48 hours. The wound is initially dusky or cyanotic and rapidly progresses to erythema and hemorrhagic discoloration, with rapid fat and muscle hemorrhage and necrosis.[11,62] Although the mechanisms causing pain, edema, and necrosis are not definitively determined, it is possible that the mucus covering the animal might contribute to the injury.[70] If discoloration around the wound edge is not immediately apparent, within 2 hours it often extends several centimeters from the wound. Hemorrhagic blisters resembling a severe thermal burn or frostbite may occur and may be worsened by overzealous therapeutic hot-water immersion.[93,103] Minor stings may simulate bacterial cellulitis. Delayed healing seen following stingray injuries is usually attributed to direct venom toxicity and infections. One analysis of the tissue surrounding a necrotic center 96 hours after envenomation revealed a perivascular and interstitial mononuclear cell infiltrate with numerous eosinophils and rare neutrophils. The phenotype of the lymphoid population was predominately CD3[+] T cells that coexpressed CD4[+] and contained T cell–restricted intracellular antigen (TIA[+]) granules corresponding to the NK1.1 subpopulation of CD4[+] T cells. Abundant eosinophils in the vicinity of a stingray soft tissue wound have been noted.[87] All of these findings indicate a possible immunologic reaction, which, if present, might contribute to delayed healing of stingray injuries.[45]

Systemic manifestations include weakness, nausea, vomiting, diarrhea, diaphoresis, vertigo, tachycardia, headache, syncope, seizures, inguinal or axillary pain, muscle cramps, fasciculations, generalized edema (with truncal wounds), paralysis, hypotension, arrhythmias, and death.[48,60] The paralysis may represent spastic muscle contractures induced by pain, which are a tremendous hazard for a diver or swimmer. The clinical syndrome associated with freshwater stingray envenomation may in general be more severe than that associated with marine stingray envenomation.[9]

When handled, a stingray may place its underside adjacent to a human limb or even wrap itself around a leg. The stingray may then bite the victim with a powerful crushing force sufficient to sever a digit or to create a substantial hematoma (Figure 75-17). A lesser wound may amount to a "stingray hickey."[36,37] Rays will

sometimes soar ("fly") out of the water, particularly in the vicinity of a motorized boat. This behavior is attributed to a defensive maneuver, although rays will also jump in the act of birth and to dislodge parasites. In 2008, a woman in a boat was killed from head injuries from the blunt impact of a spotted eagle ray that landed in the boat.

TREATMENT

The success of therapy is largely related to the rapidity with which it is undertaken. Treatment is directed at combating the effects of the venom, alleviating pain, and preventing infection. As soon as possible, the wound should be soaked in nonscalding hot water to tolerance (upper limit 45°C [113°F]) for 30 to 90 minutes. This might attenuate some of the thermolabile components of the protein venom (although this has never been proved in vivo) or interrupt nerve impulse transmission, and, in some envenomations, it relieves pain.[31] Hot water immersion likely has minimal or no effect on the ultimate degree of soft tissue necrosis. If hot water for immersion and irrigation (see below) is not immediately available, the wound should be irrigated immediately with nonheated water or saline. If sterile saline or water is not available, tap water may be used. This removes some venom and mucus and may provide minimal pain relief.

There is no indication for addition of ammonia, magnesium sulfate, potassium permanganate, or formalin to the soaking solution. Under these circumstances, they are toxic to tissue and may obscure visualization of the wound. During the hot water soak (or at any time, if soaking is not an option), the wound should be explored and debrided of any readily visible pieces of the spine or its integumentary sheath, which would continue to envenom the victim. Although the standard recommendation is to remove the spine and fragments as soon as possible (to limit the extent of envenomation and pain), if a spine is seen to be lodged in the victim and has acted as a dagger deeply into the chest, abdomen, or neck (this is extremely rare) and may have penetrated a critical blood vessel or the heart, it should be managed as would be a weapon of impalement (e.g., a knife). In this case, the spine should be left in place (if possible) and secured from motion until the victim is brought to a controlled operating room environment where emergency surgery can be performed to guide its extraction and control bleeding that may occur upon its removal.[84]

Cryotherapy may be disastrous by causing or exacerbating local tissue damage, and no data yet support the use of antihistamines or steroids. One local remedy, application of the cut surface of one-half a bulb of onion directly to the wound, has been reported to decrease the pain and perhaps inhibit infection after a sting from the blue-spotted stingray *N. kuhlii* (Figure 75-18).[104] The author noted that this approach is used in the Northern Territory of Australia for other fish spine stings, and that the medicinal use of the Liliaceae plant family has been recorded in many cultures. No other folk remedy, including application of macerated cockroaches, cactus juice, "mile-a-minute" leaves, fresh human urine, or tobacco juice, has been proved effective.[80]

Local suction, if applied in the first 15 to 30 minutes, has been suggested by some clinicians to be of potential value (this is controversial), as may a proximal constriction band (also controversial) that occludes only superficial venous and lymphatic return. If a constriction band is deployed, it should be released for 90 seconds every 10 minutes to prevent ischemia.

Pain control should be initiated during the first debridement or soaking period. Narcotics may be necessary. Local infiltration of the wound with 1% to 2% lidocaine (Xylocaine) or bupivacaine 0.25% (not to exceed 3 to 4 mg/kg total dose in adults; not approved for children under the age of 12 years) without epinephrine may be useful. A regional nerve block may be necessary.

After the soaking procedure, the wound should be x-rayed (Figures 75-19 and 75-20) or otherwise imaged, then prepared in a sterile fashion, reexplored, and thoroughly debrided, particularly of hemorrhagic fat and obviously necrotic tissue. Wounds may be packed open for delayed primary closure or sutured

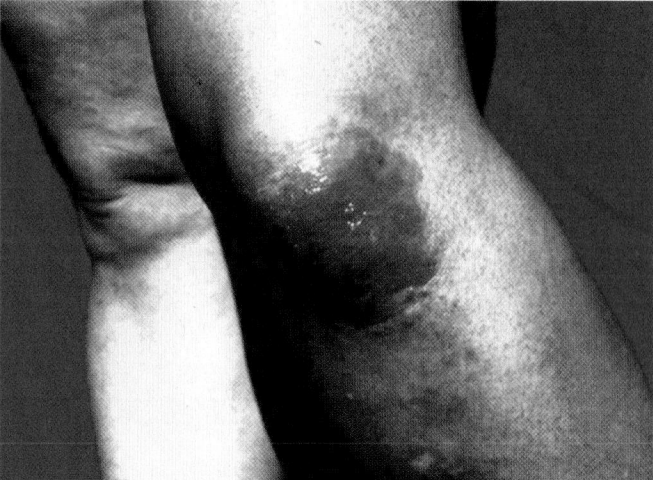

FIGURE 75-17 Stingray suction bite incurred at Stingray City, Grand Cayman Island.

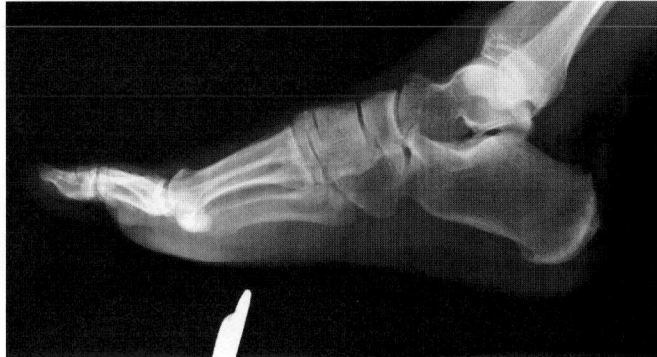

FIGURE 75-20 X-ray of a foot shows tiny fragment of stingray spine that caused inflammatory response. *(Photo courtesy Mathias Schar.)*

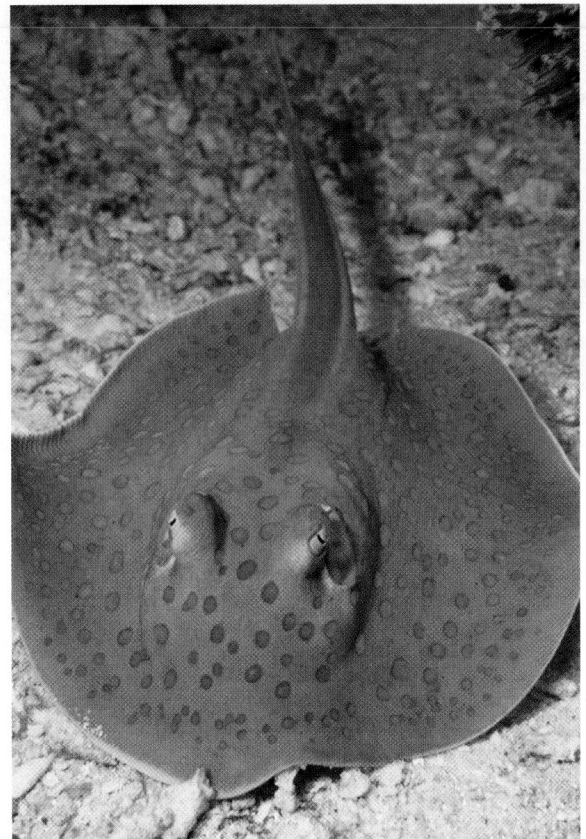

FIGURE 75-18 Blue-spotted stingray. *(Copyright Stephen Frink.)*

loosely around adequate drainage in preference to tight closure, which might increase the likelihood of wound infection. Another approach that has been mentioned is wound excision followed by packing with an alginate-based wick dressing.[39,80] Prophylactic antibiotics are recommended because of the high incidence of ulceration, necrosis, and secondary infection. Necrotizing fasciitis

caused by *Vibrio alginolyticus* has followed stingray injury in a victim with preexisting hepatic cirrhosis.[59] It has also been attributed to *Photobacterium damsela* (formerly *Vibrio damsela*) in a person with normal immunity punctured by a stingray in the tibialis anterior muscle.[10] If the abdominal cavity is penetrated, the victim should receive cefoxitin, clindamycin-gentamicin, or another intravenous regimen intended to cover bowel flora in addition to any antibiotic(s) chosen to cover marine microbes.

If the treatment plan is to treat and release, the victim should be observed for at least 3 to 4 hours for systemic side effects. Properly treated wounds may require a few months to fully heal with complete resolution of local tissue swelling (Figure 75-21). Wounds that are not properly debrided or explored and cleansed of foreign material may fester for weeks or months.[41] Such wounds may appear infected, but what really exists is a chronic draining ulcer initiated by persistent retained organic matter. Within the first few weeks after an envenomation, a foreign body can sometimes be observed by soft tissue radiograph, ultrasound, CT, or MRI. After a few weeks, exploration may reveal erosion or necrosis of adjacent soft tissue structures, synovitis, and/or the formation of an epidermal inclusion cyst or other related foreign body reaction.[12,101] As with other marine-acquired wounds, indolent infection should prompt a search for unusual microorganisms. A case of invasive fusariosis *(Fusarium solani)* after stingray

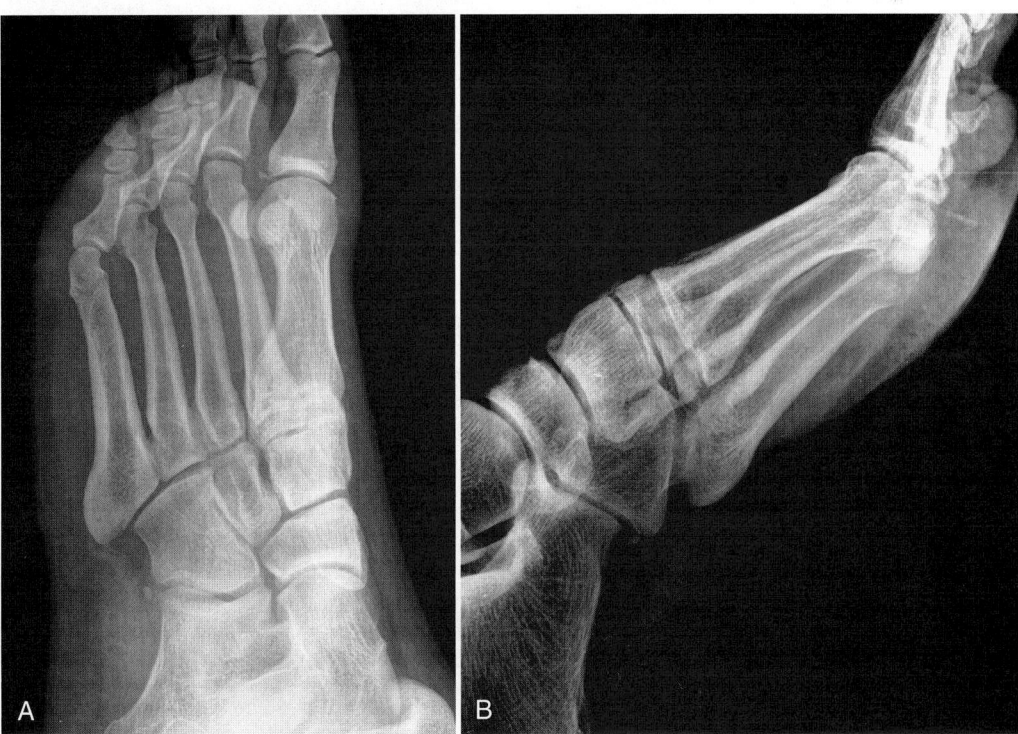

FIGURE 75-19 Radiographs demonstrating stingray spine tip at level of the first metatarsophalangeal joint. **A**, Oblique view. **B**, Lateral view. *(Courtesy Chris Fee.)*

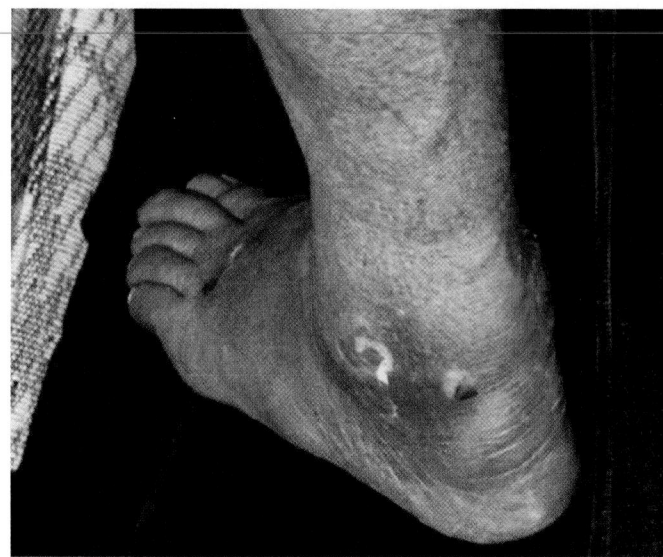

FIGURE 75-21 Initial severe inflammatory response from stingray puncture near the Achilles tendon. This injury required many weeks to heal. *(Courtesy Bob Luce.)*

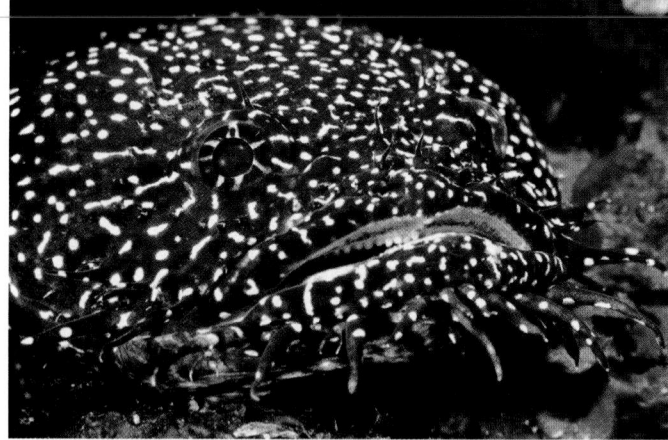

FIGURE 75-22 Toadfish. *(Courtesy Marty Snyderman.)*

envenomation responsive to sequential debridement and keto-conazole (the latter of indeterminate effect) has been reported.[58] Necrotizing fasciitis due to *Photobacterium (Vibrio) damsela* followed a leg laceration caused by a stingray. Notably, the patient had the wound sutured primarily and was not prescribed an antibiotic at the time of the repair.[10] Hyperbaric oxygen therapy has been cited to contribute to wound healing in a refractory case of stingray-induced soft tissue necrosis and postulated infection.[87] Another treatment to accelerate wound healing in a refractory case is topical recombinant human platelet-derived growth factor-BB (becaplermin gel 0.01%) every 12 hours underneath a moist dressing.[7]

PREVENTION

A stingray spine can penetrate a wetsuit, leather or rubber boot, and even the side of a wooden boat; therefore, a wetsuit or pair of athletic sneakers is not adequate protection. People walking through shallow waters known to be frequented by stingrays should shuffle along and create enough disturbance to frighten off any nearby stingrays. The same precautions hold true when one is accompanied by animals such as horses.[86]

SCORPIONFISH AND SIMILAR VENOMOUS FISH

Scorpionfish are members of the family Scorpaenidae and follow stingrays as perpetrators of piscine vertebrate stings. Distributed in tropical and less commonly in temperate oceans, several hundred species are divided into three groups typified by different genera on the basis of venom organ structure: (1) *Pterois* (zebrafish, lionfish, and butterfly cod), (2) *Scorpaena* (scorpionfish, bullrout, and sculpin), and (3) *Synanceja* (stonefish). All have a bony plate (stay), which extends across the cheek from the eye to the gill cover. Each group contains a number of different genera and species; at least 80 species of the family Scorpaenidae have been implicated in human injuries or studied anatomically, biochemically, or physiopharmacologically.

Other venomous fish that sting in a manner similar to scorpionfish include the Atlantic toadfish (family Batrachoididae, genus *Thalassophryne*) (Figure 75-22), with two venomous dorsal fin spines and venomous spines on the gill covers, and the Pacific ratfish *(Hydrolagus colliei)* (Figure 75-23) and European ratfish *(Chimaera monstrosa)*, both with a single dorsal venomous spine.[51] Toadfish hide in crevices and burrows, under rocks and debris, or in seaweed, sand, or mud. They may change coloration

rapidly and remain superbly camouflaged. Rabbitfish (family Siganidae) (Figure 75-24) and leather jacks (leather backs or leather jackets, family Carangidae) carry venomous spines or fins and pose additional risks. Stargazers (family Uranoscopidae) have spines but do not appear to be venomous (Figures 75-25 and 75-26).

LIFE AND HABITS

Zebrafish (lionfish, firefish, or turkeyfish) are beautiful, graceful, and ornate coral reef fish generally found as single or paired free

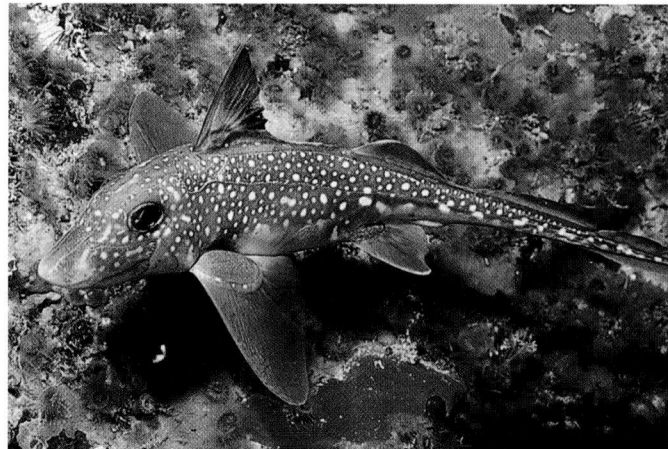

FIGURE 75-23 Ratfish *(Hydrolagus colliei).* *(Courtesy Howard Hall.)*

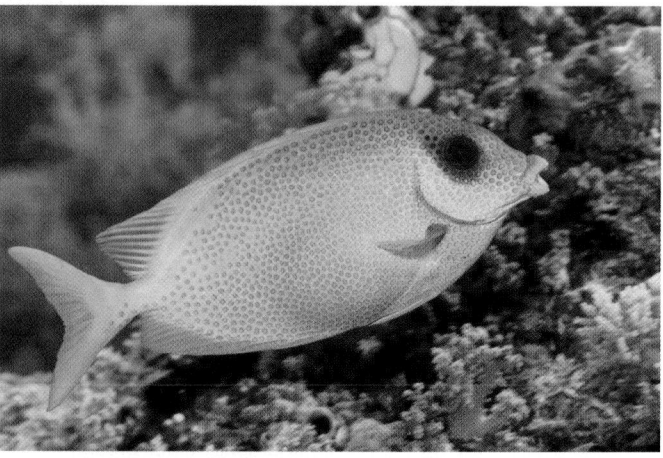

FIGURE 75-24 Rabbitfish. *(Courtesy Marty Snyderman.)*

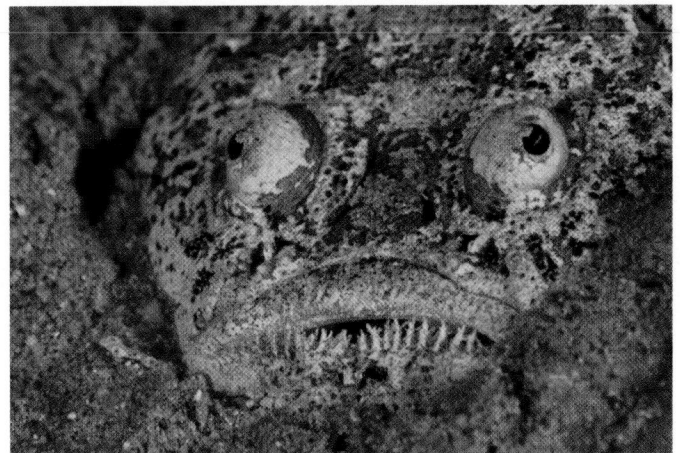

FIGURE 75-25 Stargazer. *(Copyright Lynn Funkhouser.)*

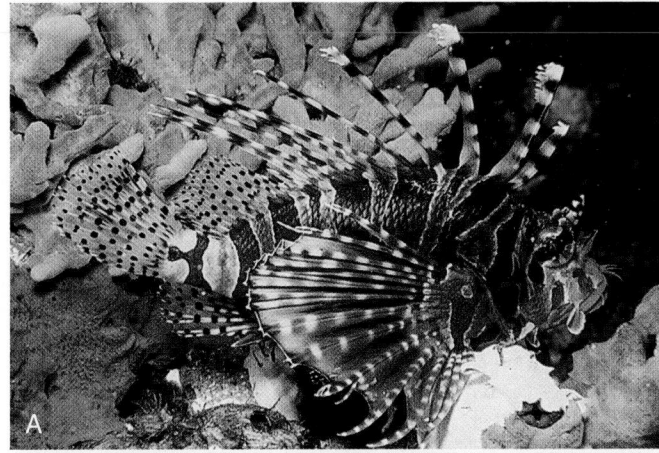

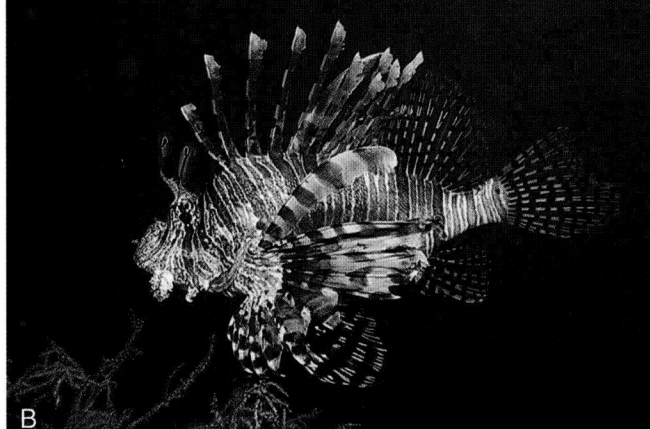

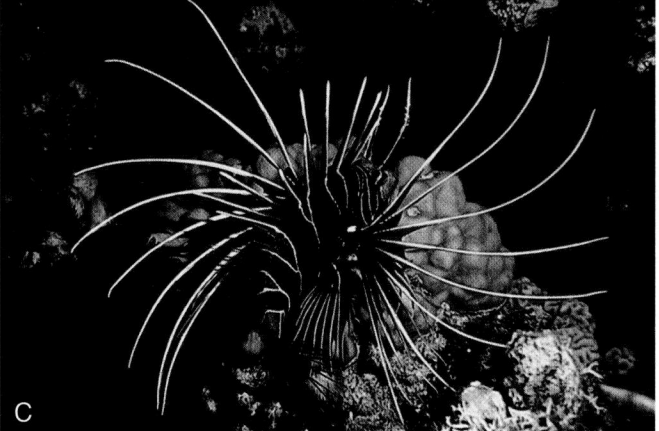

FIGURE 75-27 Three examples of lionfish. **A,** Juvenile lionfish from Sulawesi, Indonesia. **B,** Adult lionfish. **C,** Lionfish from the Red Sea. *(Courtesy Paul S. Auerbach, MD.)*

swimmers or hovering in shallow water (Figure 75-27). They are increasingly popular as aquarium pets and are imported illegally as part of the "underground zoo." They have relatively recently been introduced to the Atlantic Ocean, perhaps released from aquaria, and have been spotted from North Carolina to South Florida.[4] They are proliferating in areas such as the Bahamas (Figure 75-28). To date, introduction of "exotic" (sometimes referred to as alien, nonnative, nonindigenous, or introduced) species of fishes has not resulted in the extinction of native species in marine habitats, but this has been mentioned as a concern because of the feeding behavior of zebrafish. The western red lionfish *Pterois volitans* is a recently introduced species.[89]

Scorpionfish proper *(Scorpaena)* dwell on the bottom in shallow water, bays, coral reefs and along rocky coastlines to a depth of 50 fathoms. Their shape and coloration provide excellent camouflage, allowing them to blend in with the ambient debris, rocks, and seaweed (Figures 75-29 to 75-33). They can be captured by hook and line and serve as important food fish in many areas. The protective coloration and concealment in bottom structures make scorpionfish difficult to visualize. Some species bury themselves in the sand, and most dangerous types lie motionless on the bottom. In the United States, they are found in greatest concentration around the Florida Keys and in the Gulf of Mexico, off the coast of southern California, and in Hawaii.

Stonefish live in shallow waters, often in tide pools and among reefs (Figures 75-34 to 75-35). They frequently pose motionless and absolutely fearless under rocks, in coral crevices or holes, or buried in the sand or mud. The fish use their pectoral fins to dredge sand or mud from beneath themselves, so that they can settle with only the mouth and eyes exposed.[63] They are so sedentary that algae frequently take root on their skin (Figures 75-36 and 75-37). They are usually 15 to 20 cm (6 to 8 inches) in length, but can grow to 30 cm (12 inches). Stonefish are not indigenous to North American coastal waters.

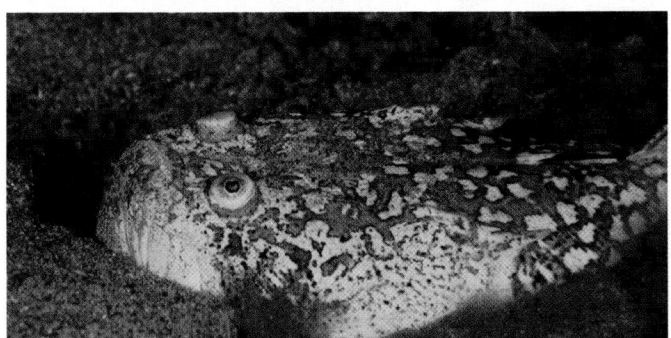

FIGURE 75-26 Stargazer. *(Copyright Lynn Funkhouser.)*

VENOM AND VENOM APPARATUS

The venom organs are the 12 or 13 (of 18) dorsal (Figure 75-38), 2 pelvic, and 3 anal spines, with associated venom glands. Although they are frequently large, plume-like, and ornate, the pectoral spines are not associated with venom glands. Each spine is covered with an integumentary sheath, under which venom filters along grooves in the anterolateral region of the spine from the paired glands situated at the base or in the midportion of the spine. It is estimated that the two venom glands of each dorsal stonefish spine carry 5 to 10 mg of venom, closely associated with antigenic proteins of high molecular weight (between 50,000 and 800,000).[22] Scorpionfish venom contains multiple toxic fractions and, in the case of stonefish venom, has been likened in potency to cobra venom. It contains a mixture

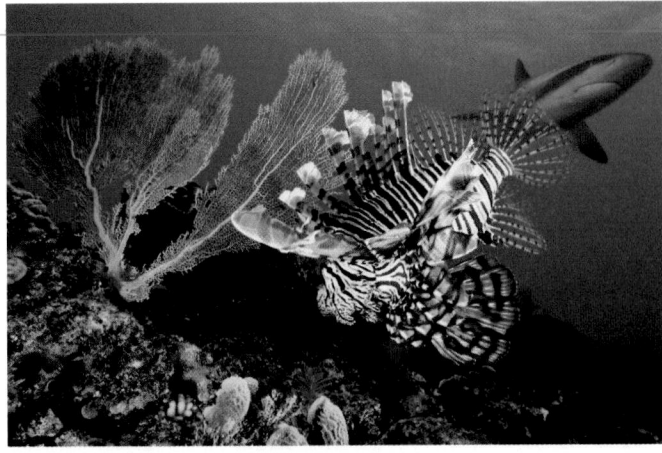

FIGURE 75-28 Invasive lionfish with Caribbean reef shark in the Bahamas. *(Copyright David Doubilet.)*

production of nitrous oxide and activation of potassium channels.[99] The nondialyzable opalescent venom retains full potency for at least 24 to 48 hours after the death of a scorpionfish.[67] Extrapolating from the LD$_{50}$ of 0.36 mcg/g in mice, it is estimated that 18 mg relayed by six intact spines might cause death in a 60-kg (132-lb) human.[65]

Pterois species carry long, slender spines with small venom glands covered by a thin integumentary sheath. An extract of lionfish spine tissue contains acetylcholine and a toxin that affects neuromuscular transmission.[28] *Scorpaena* species carry longer heavy spines with moderate-sized venom glands covered by a thicker integumentary sheath. *Synanceja* species carry short, thick spines with large, well-developed venom glands covered by an extremely thick integumentary sheath (Figures 75-39 and

of proteins containing several enzymes, including hyaluronidase.[63] Hyaluronidase is a spreading factor in venoms because it degrades hyaluronate, which helps structure connective tissue. The major toxic component of *Synanceja* venom (stonustoxin) is a protein of molecular weight 148,000 (comprising alpha and beta subunits of molecular weights 71,000 and 79,000, respectively) that is both antigenic and heat labile. Similar purified toxins from other species are trachynilysin from *Synanceja trachynis* (Australian estuarine stonefish) and verrucotoxin (a glycoprotein) from *Synanceja verrucosa* (reef stonefish).[92] The principal action of stonefish venom appears to be direct muscle toxicity, resulting in paralysis of cardiac, involuntary, and skeletal muscles.[46] In an analysis of biologic activity, stonefish (*Synanceja horrida,* the Indian stonefish) venom exhibited edema-inducing, hemolytic, hyaluronidase, thrombin-like, alkaline phosphomonoesterase, 5'-nucleotidase, acetylcholinesterase, phosphodiesterase, arginine esterase, and arginine amidase activities.[65] In a recent evaluation, chromatographic analysis with electrochemical detection showed the presence of substances comigrating with norepinephrine, dopamine, and tryptophan. Serotonin (5-hydroxytryptamine) was not detected.[44] Crude venom of the stonefish *S. verrucosa* possesses numerous enzymatic properties, including hyaluronidase, 8 esterases, and 10 aminopeptidases.[43] Intracellular Ca^{2+} levels are increased by venoms of the soldierfish *(Gymnapistes marmoratus),* lionfish *(P. volitans),* and stonefish *(S. trachynis),* possibly via formation of pores in the cellular membrane, which, under certain conditions in experimental animals, may lead to necrosis.[27] In addition, trachynilysin activity on the heart, often noted as negative inotropy, may also be a function of Ca^{2+} influx.[92] The hemolytic activity of stonustoxin may in some part depend on surface tryptophan residues.[106] The cardiovascular effects of stonefish venom have been attributed in part to its activity at muscarinic receptors and adrenoceptors, and pain effects perhaps to its activity at bradykinin receptors.[23] Similar receptor activity, neutralized by stonefish antivenom, has been noted with lionfish venom.[25] The pain-causing protein in bullrout *(Notesthes robusta)* venom is an algesic protein (169.8 to 174.5 kDa) called nocitoxin.[54]

Stonefish venom causes pulmonary edema in laboratory animals, which may reflect general vascular permeability.[65,68] It also causes species-restricted (nonhuman) hemolysis and platelet aggregation.[64] Scorpionfish venom also causes acute inflammatory lung injury in mice, with hemorrhage and alveolar macrophage activation.[13] Profound endothelial relaxation may contribute directly to hypotension.[73] The neuromuscular toxicity appears to be a consequence of the venom's dose-dependent presynaptic and postsynaptic actions at the myoneural junction, which include release and depletion of neurotransmitter from the nerve terminal, followed by irreversible depolarization of muscle cells and microscopically observable muscle and nerve damage.[69] Hypotension observed in envenomed laboratory animals may be due in part to binding to receptors on endothelial cells, causing

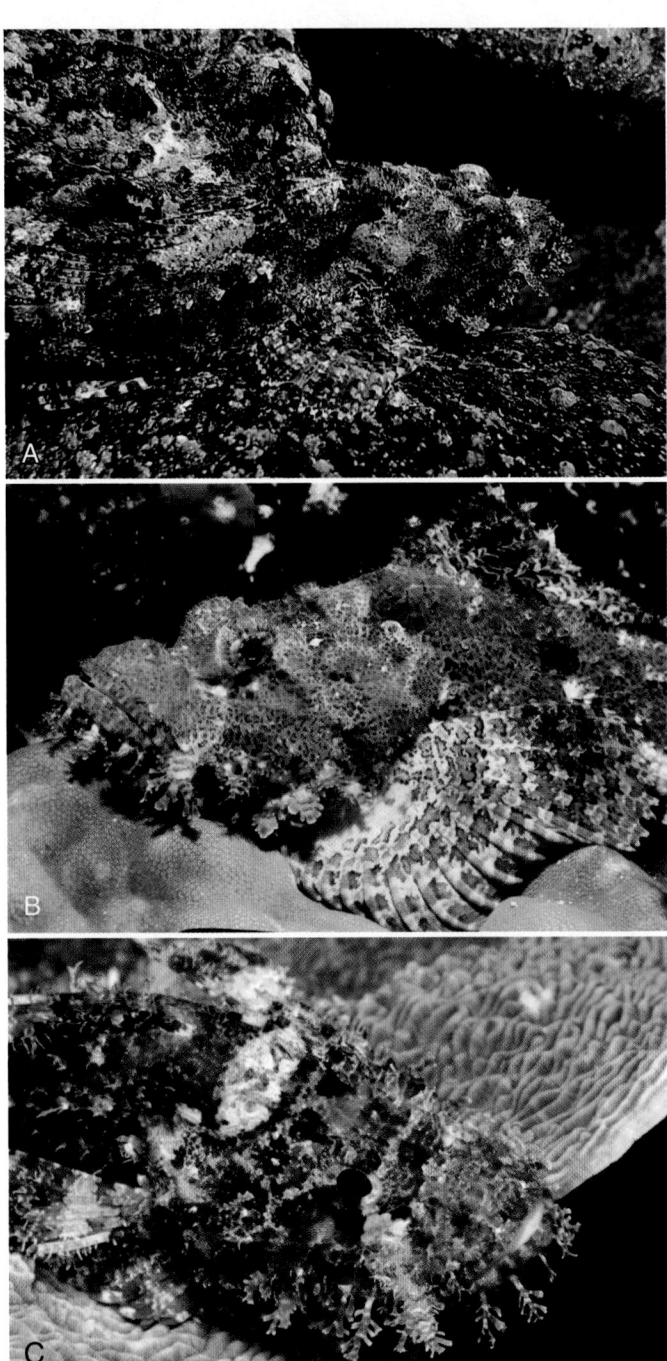

FIGURE 75-29 Three examples of scorpionfish. **A,** Scorpionfish assuming the coloration of its surroundings. **B,** Scorpionfish in the Red Sea. **C,** Scorpionfish. (**A** *courtesy Paul S. Auerbach, MD;* **B** *copyright Carl Roessler;* **C** *copyright Stephen Frink.)*

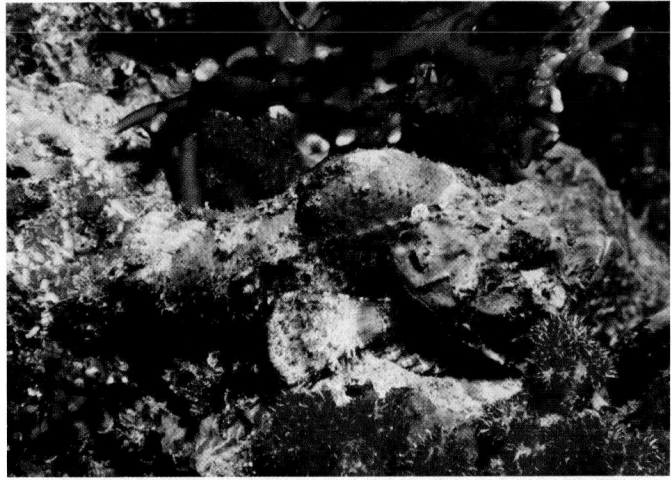

FIGURE 75-30 Scorpionfish camouflaged like debris in Fiji. *(Copyright Carl Roessler.)*

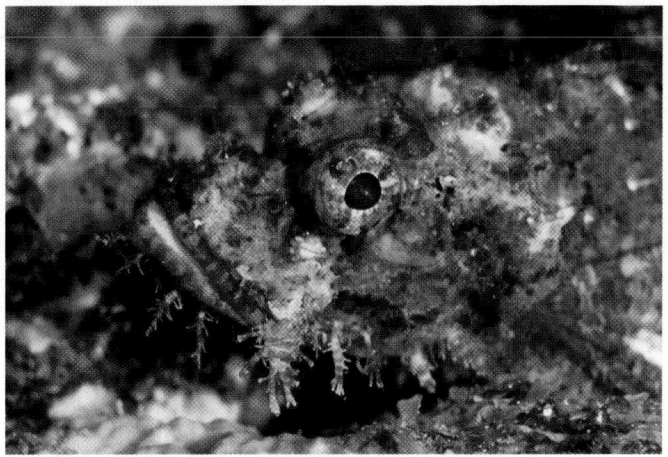

FIGURE 75-33 Raggy scorpionfish. *(Copyright 2011 Norbert Wu: norbertwu.com.)*

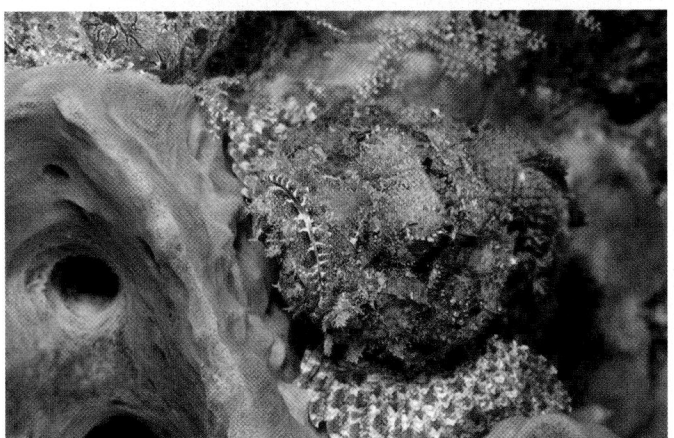

FIGURE 75-31 Scorpionfish nestled on a sponge. *(Copyright Stephen Frink.)*

spiny dorsal fin and flares out the armed gill covers and pectoral and anal fins. If provoked while still in the water, it actually attacks. The venom is injected by a direct puncture wound through the skin, which tears the sheath and may fracture the spine, in a manner analogous to that of a stingray envenomation. Fishermen are commonly injured, particularly when emptying nets or extracting hooks from captured fishes.[50]

CLINICAL ASPECTS

Native residents of the Indo-Pacific islands have great fear of a sting from the dreaded venomous stonefish, such as the "ikan hantu" (devil fish), Tahitian "nohu" ("nofu" or "no'u," the waiting one) or the Australian "warty ghoul." The presentation of the injury is similar to that of stingray envenomation in that the unwary diver or fisherman steps on or handles the fish. In the United States, marine aquarists and beneficiaries of illegal importation of tropical animals are increasingly envenomed as they unknowledgeably handle *P. volitans, Pterois radiata,* or *Scorpaena guttata.* In Indo-Pacific waters, envenomations of the foot and lower extremity are more commonly caused by the stonefish, such as *S. horrida, S. trachynis,* or *S. verrucosa.* Scorpionfish stings vary according to the species, with a progression in severity from the lionfish (mild) through the scorpionfish (moderate to severe) to the stonefish (severe to life threatening). The severity of envenomation depends on the number and type of stings, species, amount of venom released, and age and underlying health of the victim. Pain is immediate and intense, with

75-40). However, the skin over the venom gland is loosely attached, so when a human treads on the fish, the skin is pushed down the spine and the venom gland is compressed by the crumpled sheath. The pressure forces the venom gland to empty up the paired narrow ducts so that venom and glandular tissue spurt into the wound.[47]

When any of these fish is removed from the water, handled, stepped on, or otherwise threatened, it reflexively erects the

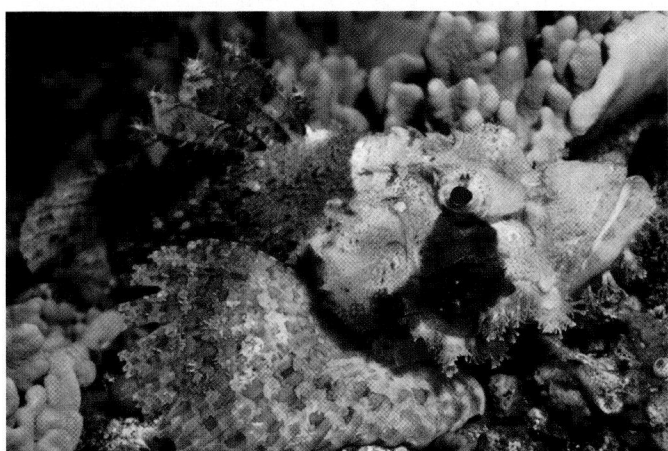

FIGURE 75-32 Scorpionfish. *(Copyright Stephen Frink.)*

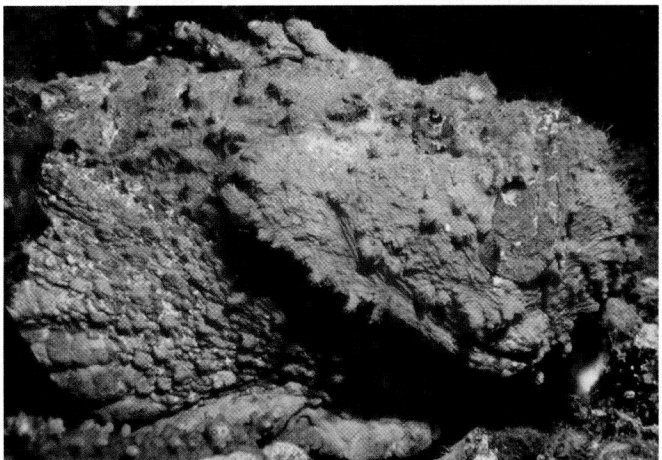

FIGURE 75-34 Stonefish in Papua New Guinea. *(Copyright Carl Roessler.)*

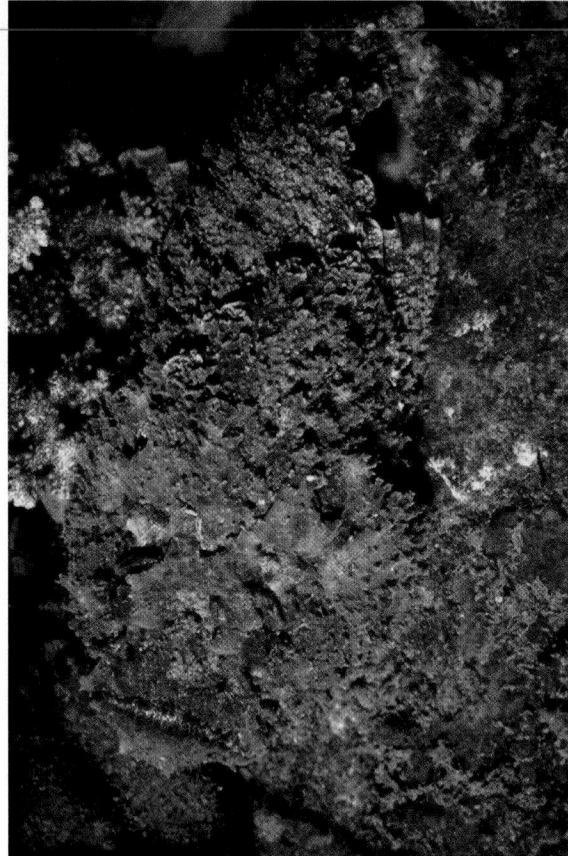

FIGURE 75-35 Stonefish. *(Copyright Lynn Funkhouser.)*

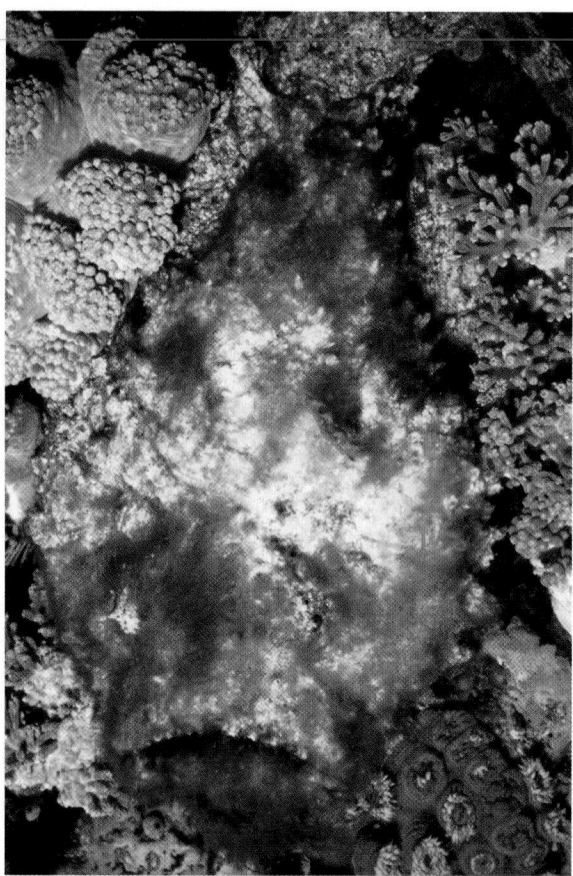

FIGURE 75-37 Stonefish. *(Copyright Lynn Funkhouser.)*

radiation centrally. Untreated, pain peaks at 60 to 90 minutes and persists for 6 to 12 hours. With a scorpionfish or stonefish envenomation, pain may be severe enough to cause hallucinations or delirium and may persist at high levels for hours (scorpionfish) or days (stonefish).[50] The wound and surrounding area are initially ischemic and then cyanotic (Figure 75-41), with more broadly surrounding areas of erythema, edema, and warmth. Vesicles may form (Figure 75-42). Human (hand) vesicle fluid after the sting of the lionfish *P. volitans* was analyzed for mediators of inflammation and demonstrated an appreciable quantity of prostaglandin $F_{2\alpha}$; thromboxane B_2, prostaglandin E_2, and 6-keto-prostaglandin $F_{1\alpha}$ were present in negligible quantities. Whether or not residual venom is present in blister fluid is a matter of conjecture. Rapid tissue sloughing and close surrounding areas of cellulitis, with anesthesia adjacent to peripheral hyperesthesia, may be present within 48 hours. Necrotic

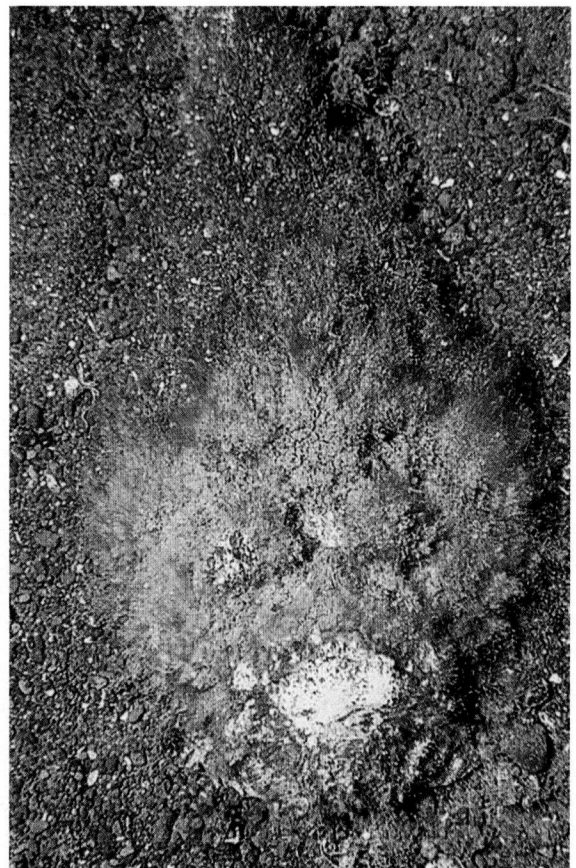

FIGURE 75-36 Some stonefish are so sedentary that algae grow on their skin. *(Courtesy Paul S. Auerbach, MD.)*

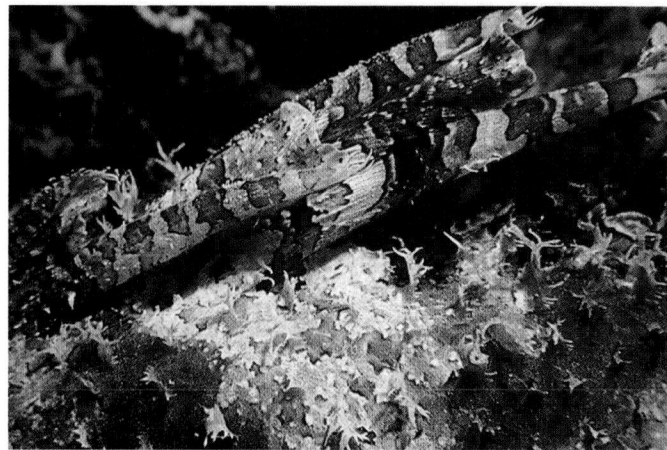

FIGURE 75-38 Scorpionfish spines. *(Courtesy Kenneth Kizer, MD.)*

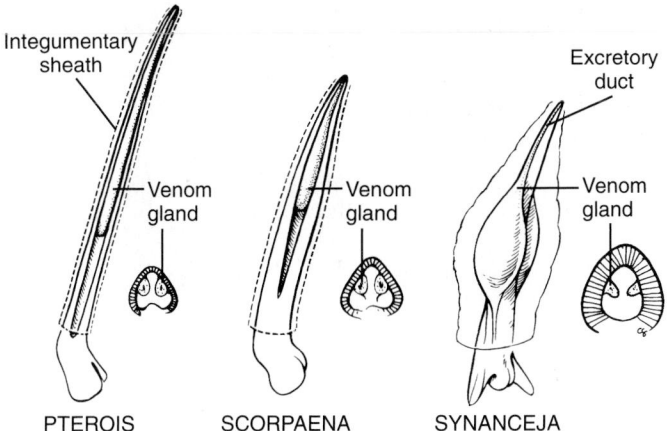

FIGURE 75-39 Lionfish (*Pterois*), scorpionfish (*Scorpaena*), and stonefish (*Synanceja*) spines with associated venom glands.

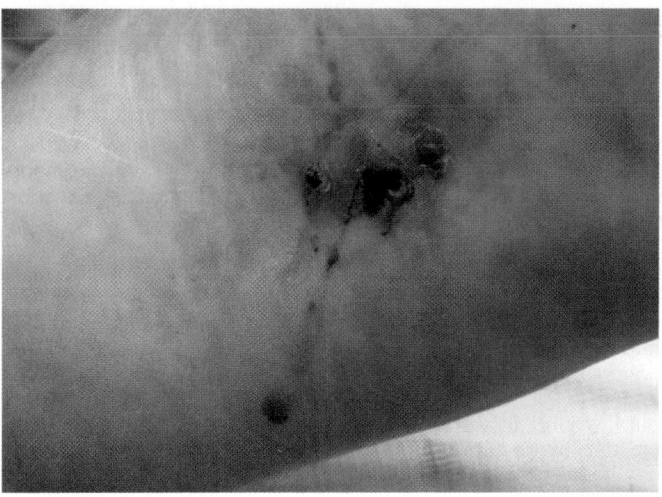

FIGURE 75-41 Stonefish puncture wound. (*Courtesy Richard Lyon, MD.*)

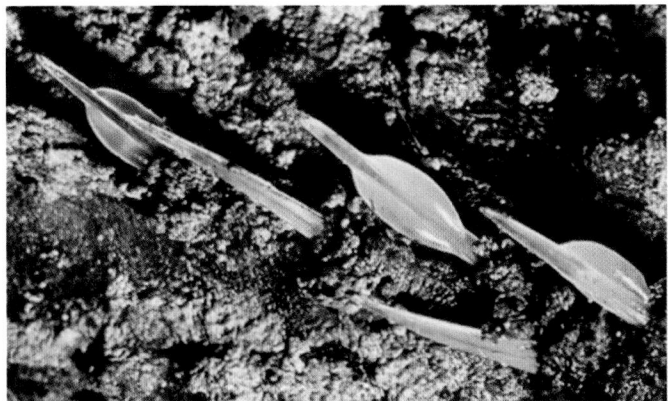

FIGURE 75-40 Spines of the venomous stonefish, demonstrating venom glands. (*Courtesy John Williamson, MD.*)

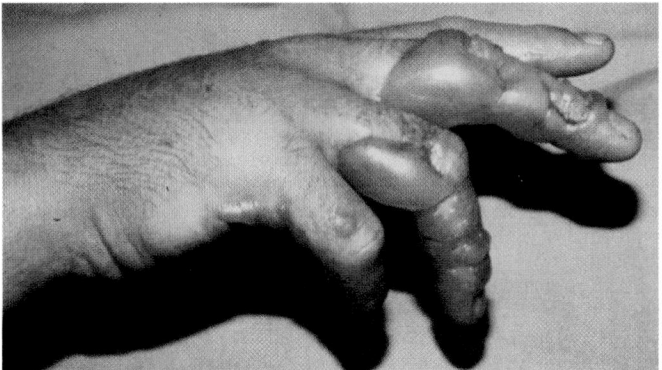

FIGURE 75-42 Vesiculation of the hand 48 hours after the sting of a lionfish. (*Courtesy Howard McKinney.*)

ulceration is rare but may occur after a lionfish envenomation (Figure 75-43).[85] Severe local tissue reaction is more common after the sting of a scorpionfish or stonefish.

Systemic effects include anxiety, headache, tremors, maculopapular skin rash, nausea, vomiting, diarrhea, abdominal pain, diaphoresis, pallor, restlessness, delirium, seizures, limb paralysis, peripheral neuritis or neuropathy, lymphangitis, eosinophilia, arthritis, fever, hypertension, respiratory distress, bradycardia, tachycardia, atrioventricular block, ventricular fibrillation, congestive heart failure, pulmonary edema, pericarditis, hypotension, syncope, and death.[16,72] Pulmonary edema is a bona fide sequela.[72] Death in humans, which is extremely rare, usually occurs within the first 6 to 8 hours. The wound is indolent and may require months to heal, only to leave a cutaneous granuloma or marked

tissue defect, particularly after a secondary infection or deep abscess. Mild pain may persist for days to weeks. Lionfish envenomation has been used as a fabricated chief complaint to seek a prescription for narcotic drugs.[98] After successful therapy, paresthesias or numbness in the affected extremity may persist for a few weeks.

TREATMENT

As soon as possible, the wound or wounds should be immersed in nonscalding hot (upper limit 45° C [113° F]) water to tolerance. This may inactivate at least one of the thermolabile components of the protein venom that might otherwise induce a severe

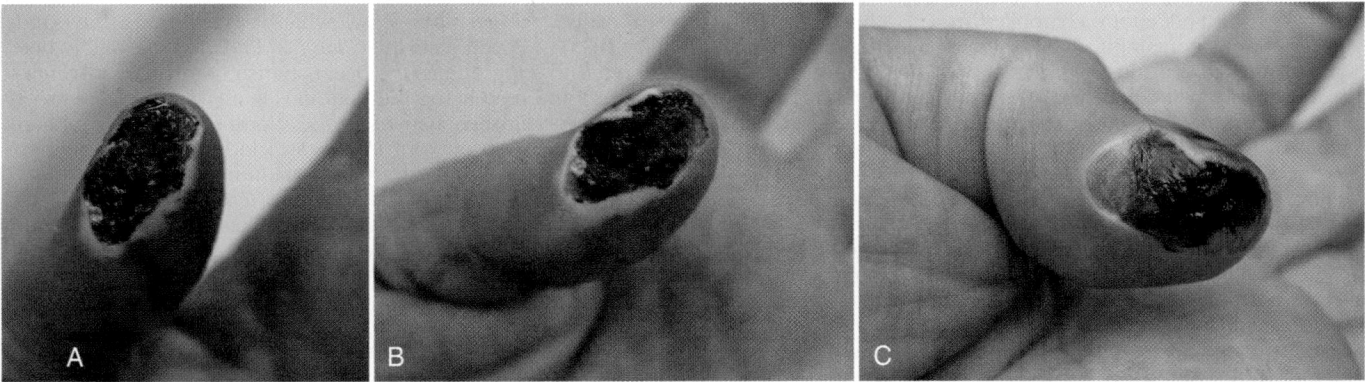

FIGURE 75-43 Necrotic ulceration following a lionfish sting at 5 (**A**), 7 (**B**), and 11 (**C**) days. (*Photos courtesy Elly Wray.*)

systemic reaction. Platelet aggregation in blister fluid is inhibited by heat treatment, which suggests that the venom or some other active component may be neutralized. The soak should be maintained for a minimum of 30 minutes and may continue for up to 90 minutes. Recurrent pain that develops after an interval of 1 to 2 hours may respond to a repeat hot water treatment. As soon as is practical, all obvious pieces of spine and sheath fragments should be gently removed from the wound. Vigorous irrigation should be performed with warmed sterile saline to remove any integument or slime. If pain is severe or inadequately controlled (in terms of degree or rapidity of relief) by hot water immersion, local tissue infiltration with 1% to 2% lidocaine without epinephrine or regional nerve block with an anesthetic, such as 0.25% bupivacaine, may be necessary. After injection with a local or regional anesthetic, the hot water immersion should be discontinued or closely observed, to avoid inadvertent creation of a burn wound in the now insensate body part. Infiltration with emetine hydrochloride, potassium permanganate, or Congo red has been abandoned, despite reports of favorable experiences with acidic emetine. The biochemical bases for the success of folk remedies, such as application of meat tenderizer, mangrove sap, or green papaya (papain), have yet to be confirmed. The effectiveness of alternative remedies may be related to the protein behavior of the venom, which is inactivated by heat, extremes of pH (it is partially inactivated at pH of greater than 8.6 and completely at a pH of less than 4), hydrogen peroxide, iodine, and potassium permanganate (which is, unfortunately, tissue toxic). One health care provider has recommended using vitreous humor from the black rock cod *Epinephelus daemelii* as a topical pain relief preparation for a sting from this species. Currently, no data are available to support topical administration of empirical remedies, such as mineral spirits, organic dye, ground liver, or formalin. Cryotherapy is absolutely contraindicated, to avoid an iatrogenous cold-induced injury.

Although the spine rarely breaks off into the skin, the wound should be explored to remove any spine fragments, which will otherwise continue to envenom and act as foreign bodies, perpetuating an infection risk and poorly healing wound. If the spine has penetrated deeply into the sole of the foot, surgical exploration should be performed in the operating room with magnification. Vigorous warmed saline irrigation should be performed. Wide excision and debridement are unnecessary. Because of the nature of the puncture wound, tight suture or surgical tape closure should not be undertaken; rather, the wound should be allowed to heal open with provision for adequate drainage. If the puncture wound is high risk (deep, into the hand or foot, or both), prophylactic antibiotic(s) should be administered. It is wise to remove blister fluid using aseptic technique.

Stonefish envenomation may cause profound tissue necrosis. This may be of a severity to require debridement, including amputations of soft tissues and bone.

A stonefish antivenom is manufactured by the Commonwealth Serum Laboratories (CSL Limited, Parkville, Victoria, Australia) (Figure 75-44). In cases of severe systemic reactions from stings of *Synanceja* species, perhaps from soldierfish (*G. marmoratus*) or bullrout (*N. robusta*), and rarely from other scorpionfish, it is administered intramuscularly or diluted for intravenous administration.[24,32] The antivenom is supplied in vials containing 1.5 to 3 mL of liquid containing 2000 units of hyperimmune F(ab')$_2$ horse serum active against *S. trachynis*, with 1000 units (one-half a vial) capable of neutralizing 10 mg of dried venom.[30] F(ab')$_2$ preparations are obtained by pepsin treatment of IgG at pH 2, whereas Fab fragments are produced by papain treatment at pH 7 to 8.[100] The former product is believed to be easier to standardize than the latter, and better in its plasma distribution and venom neutralization. After skin testing to estimate the risk for an anaphylactic reaction to equine sera, the antivenom should be given. If skin testing is omitted, anticipate and be prepared to treat an allergic reaction. As a rough estimate, one vial of antivenom should neutralize one or two significant stings (punctures). For one or two puncture wounds, administer one vial; for three or four puncture wounds, two vials; for more than four puncture wounds, administer three vials. One or more additional vials may be necessary if there is recurrent severe pain. When not in use, the antivenom should be protected from light and stored at 2° to 8°C (35.6° to 46.4°F), and never frozen. Unused portions should be discarded.

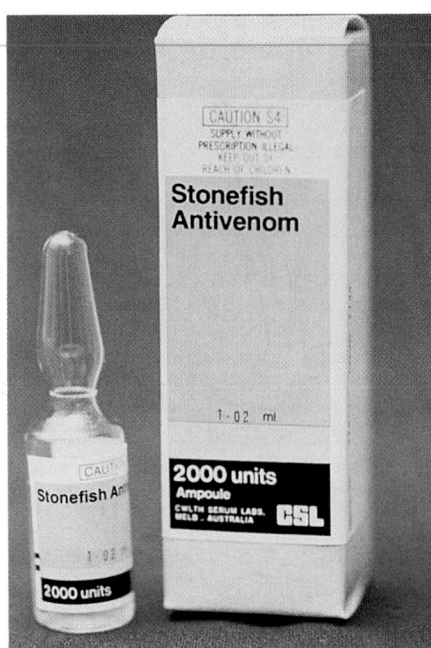

FIGURE 75-44 Stonefish antivenom. *(Courtesy John Williamson, MD.)*

The fact that stonefish antivenom cross-reacts with most piscine venoms suggests that piscine venoms may possess structural similarities in addition to their functional similarities, which include induction of profound cardiovascular changes, release of nitric oxide from endothelial cells, smooth muscle contraction, depolarizing action on nerve and muscle cells, and potent cytolytic activity.[26]

PREVENTION

The most effective way to prevent envenomation is to avoid handling or setting down upon a scorpionfish. A diver should make a careful inspection before contacting the ocean floor or a rocky ledge. Amateur aquarists should be exceedingly cautious when handling exotic tropical fish. Seemingly dead fish may yield an unpleasant surprise for the unwary.

CATFISH

LIFE AND HABITS

Approximately 1000 species of catfish inhabit both freshwaters and saltwaters; many of these are capable of inflicting serious stings. Marine animals include the Oriental catfish (*Plotosus lineatus*), which lurks in tall seaweed and can inflict extremely painful stings, the larger sailcat (*Bagre marinus*), and the common sea catfish (*Galeichthys felis*), which hovers along the sandy bottom. The coral catfish (*Plotatus lineatus*) has also been reported to sting humans.[95] Ocean catfish, particularly juveniles, "swarm" and feed along the bottom (Figure 75-45). There are 39 species of catfishes native to the North American continent. Freshwater catfish of North America include the brown bullhead (*Ameiurus nebulosus*), Carolina madtom (*Noturus furiosus*), channel (*Ictalurus punctatus*), blue (*Ictalurus furcatus*), and white (*Ameiurus catus*) catfish. Some of the catfish of South America can grow to a very large size (Figures 75-46 and 75-47).

The catfish derives its name from the well-developed sensory barbels ("whiskers") surrounding the mouth. The barbels of catfish carry well-developed sensory organs that are used to transmit both touch and taste. All catfishes are adapted to foraging in muddy and dark waters, where feeding by senses is essential.

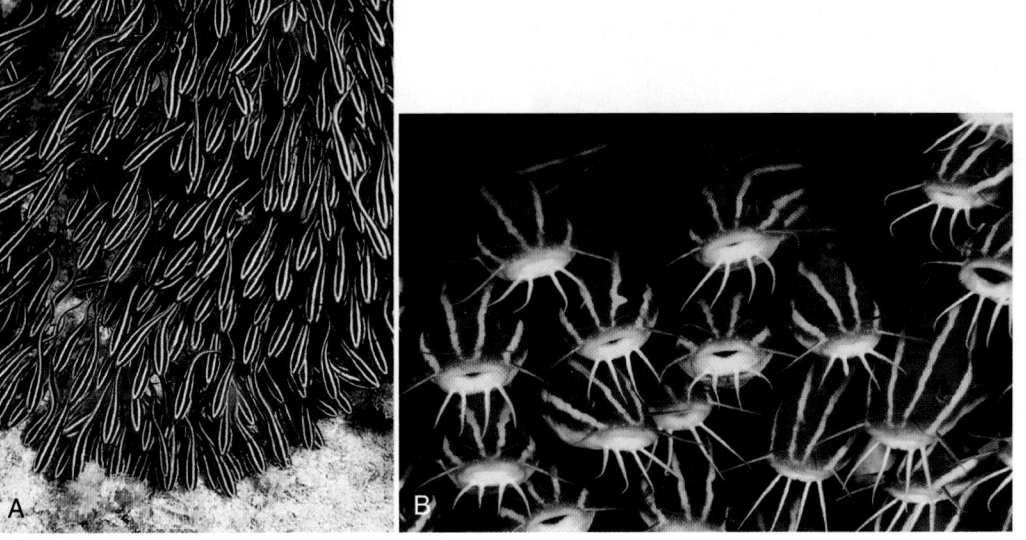

FIGURE 75-45 Marine catfish. **A,** Juvenile ocean catfish. **B,** Marine catfish. (**A** copyright 2006 Norbert Wu: norbertwu.com; **B** copyright Lynn Funkhouser.)

Catfish possess a slimy skin without any true scales. Marine catfish, unlike freshwater catfish, frequently travel in large schools. Most freshwater catfish are bottom feeders noted for their junkyard diet. They are poor swimmers and not very evasive.

The South American astroblepids have flattened suctorial lips that allow them to scale cliffs. Tiny South American (Amazonian) catfish of the genus *Vandellia* (species *cirrhosa, balzanii, plazaii, sanguinea,* and *beccarii*) are known as "urethra fish" in English, *candirú* by Brazilians, and *canero* by Spanish speakers.[15]

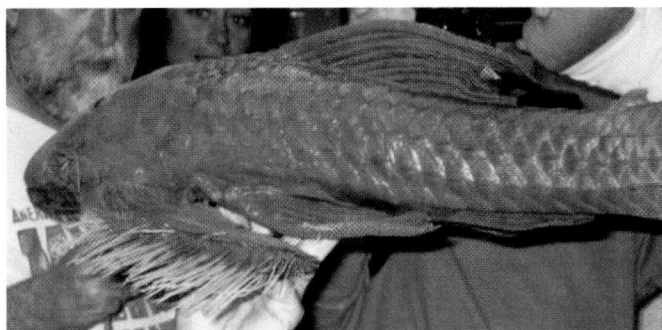

FIGURE 75-46 Amazonian catfish with pectoral fin spines. (*Courtesy George Hertner, MD.*)

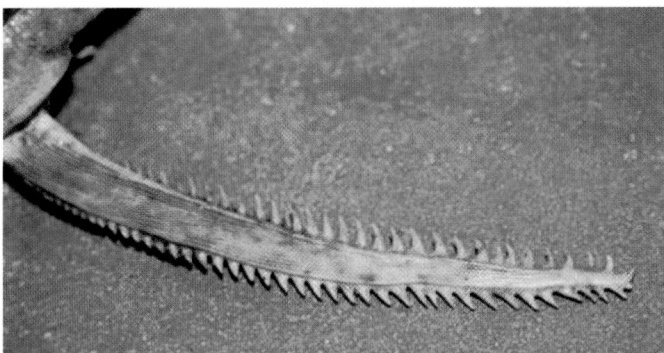

FIGURE 75-47 Amazonian catfish pectoral spine. (*Courtesy George Hertner, MD.*)

Approximately 2.5 to 7.5 cm (1 to 3 inches) long, they carry short spines on their gill covers (Figure 75-48). This "vampire fish" is predominately a bottom-feeding "junkfish" found in murky or muddy waters in the Amazon and Orinoco Rivers and perhaps select tributaries and is putatively attracted to urine (water motion, warmth). It can swim into the gills of a larger fish, or reputedly up the human urethra or other urogenital apertures, where it extends the spiny gill covers and thus becomes embedded, preventing removal by pulling on the fish's tail. Within the gills of a fish, it anchors itself with its spines and rasps with teeth to obtain a blood meal. Within the human urethra, it causes extreme pain and inflammation. Because the animal normally seeks the outflow stream from a larger fish's gills (where it may enter and parasitize the host fish), perhaps it is not urinophilic, but merely swimming into a stream. Others theorize that it is attracted to ammonia. Natives wear pudendal shields when urinating in natural bodies of water. A tight-fitting bathing suit is certainly prudent.

At best, extraction is painful (Figure 75-49). Amputation of the penis by natives has been described in the older literature. Ingestion of the green fruit of the jagua (xagua or xaqua) tree or buitach apple *(Genipa americana)* as a concoction (tea) apparently works to dispel the urethra-lodged candirú by the action of a large quantity of citric acid (megadose vitamin C), which softens calcium spines. Other references cite placement of either or both plants (or their extracts) within the urethra (or other invaded body orifice) in order to dispatch and dissolve the fish. Typically, removal is performed mechanically while the victim is anesthetized. The veracity of the threat of the candirú to humans has been called into question.[11a]

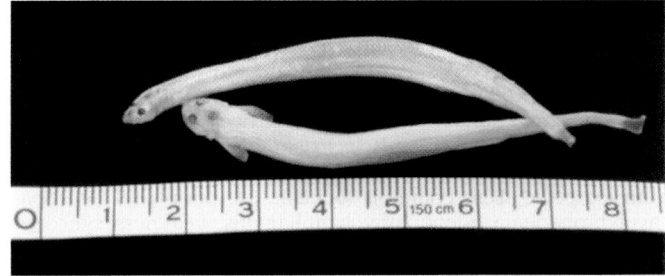

FIGURE 75-48 Amazonian catfish (candirú), which can enter the human urethra. (*Courtesy Vidal Haddad, Jr.*)

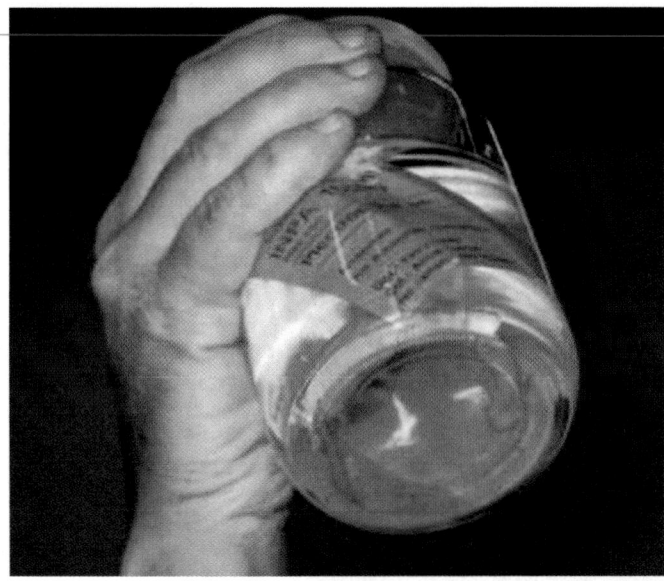

FIGURE 75-49 Candirú extracted from human urethra. *(Courtesy George Hertner, MD.)*

VENOM AND VENOM APPARATUS

The venom apparatus of the catfish consists of the single dorsal and two pectoral fin spines ("stings") and the axillary venom glands. Both the dorsal and pectoral spines are exquisitely sharp and can be locked into an extended position by the fish when it is handled or becomes excited. The spines are enveloped by glandular tissue within an integumentary sheath; some spines are barbed or have sharp retrorse teeth. Scattered reports note envenomation in persons who handled only the tail of the fish, such as the Arabian Gulf catfish (*Arius thalassinus),* which suggests the presence of a toxic skin secretion (crinotoxin). Other observers note that toxin released from epidermal skin cells can cause throbbing pain, tissue necrosis, and perhaps muscle fasciculations.[42] Oriental catfish toxin, which is poorly antigenic, contains vasoconstrictive, hemolytic, edema-forming, dermatonecrotic, and other biogenic fractions.[96] It behaves in vivo much like a milder version of stingray venom. In contrast, the crinotoxin of the Arabian Gulf catfish contracts smooth muscle and stimulates release of prostaglandins; pretreatment with atropine and indomethacin attenuates the response.[3,95] Furthermore, wound healing responses are accelerated by repeated local application of preparations from the epidermal secretions of another Arabian gulf catfish (*Arius bilineatus,* Valenciennes).[2]

Clinical Aspects

Most stings are incurred when a fish is handled, which creates an injury out of proportion to the mechanical laceration. Other injuries occur when the animal is accidentally or intentionally stepped upon or kicked (Figure 75-50). When the spine penetrates the skin, the integumentary sheath is damaged, and the venom gland exposed. Catfish stings are described as instantaneously stinging, throbbing, or scalding, with central radiation up the affected limb. Normally the pain subsides within 30 to 60 minutes, but in severe cases it can last for 48 hours. The area around the wound quickly appears ischemic, with central pallor that gradually becomes cyanotic before the onset of erythema and edema. Swelling can be severe, and secondary infections are frequent; gangrenous complications have been reported. Common side effects include local muscle spasm, diaphoresis, and fasciculations. Bleeding from the puncture wounds may be more severe than expected. Less common sequelae are peripheral neuropathy, lymphedema, adenopathy, lymphangitis, weakness, syncope, hypotension, and respiratory distress. Death is extremely rare. A marine catfish (*Genidens genidens*) sting caused a fatal heart perforation in a fisherman, who fell upon a net carrying several catfish.[53] "Finning" occurs when a person is punctured by a fin

while handling a fin. This often occurs when removing a hook from a fish or a fish from a net. In one instance of catfish finning, in addition to the immediate typical immediate toxic reaction, the victim suffered recurrent episodes of pain and swelling on the dorsum of the hand over the course of 6 months, which eventually led to spontaneous skin rupture and blood-tinged fluid drainage.[1] Plain radiography revealed two catfish spines embedded in the soft tissues between the third and fourth metacarpal bones. Thirteen months after the initial injury, one spine was removed easily with local exploration; more extensive surgery did not lead to successful localization of the second spine, but revealed extensive edematous tenosynovitis. Because of the clinical course, the patient was treated presumptively for *Mycobacterium marinum* infection. Development of a necrotizing fasciitis-like reaction of the hand requiring extensive debridement was noted in a case report describing catfish spine envenomation.[20] In another case, the radial artery was lacerated by a spine that became embedded in the volar-radial aspect of the nondominant wrist (Figure 75-51).[40] This was repaired by lateral arteriorrhaphy rather than segmental resection and reanastomosis (Figure 75-52).

The sting of the marine catfish is usually more severe than that of its freshwater counterparts and may have a propensity to more local hemorrhage.[79] Infection risk is similar to that for any aquatic-acquired wound, in that *Vibrio* and *Aeromonas* species may be pathogens and the infection may be polymicrobial.[81,82] Other organisms that have been reported to be associated with marine or freshwater catfish-related injuries include *Edwardsiella tarda, Citrobacter freundii, Fusobacterium mortiferum, Morganella morganii, Providencia rettgeri, Enterococcus faecalis, Pseudomonas aeruginosa, Mycobacterium terrae,* and *Enterobacter cloacae.*[82] *E. tarda* is a gram-negative bacillus of the family Enterobacteriaceae that is mainly associated with aquatic environments and the animals that inhabit them, particularly catfish and other cold-blooded animals.[5,8] It may be a pathogen for eels and catfish. If *E. tarda* infection is determined, it is sensitive in vitro to ampicillin, aminoglycosides, β-lactamase stable

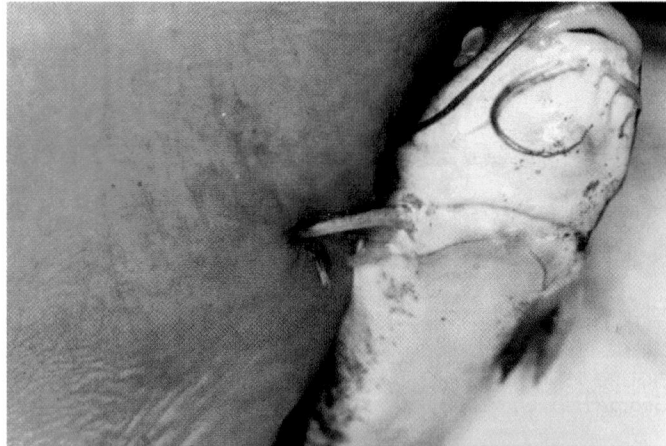

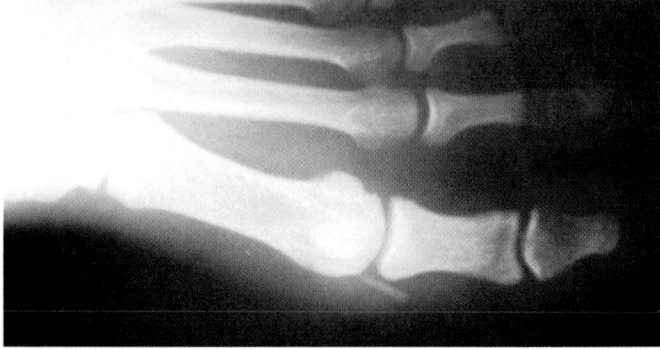

FIGURE 75-50 Catfish spine broken off into foot. *(Courtesy Vidal Haddad, Jr.)*

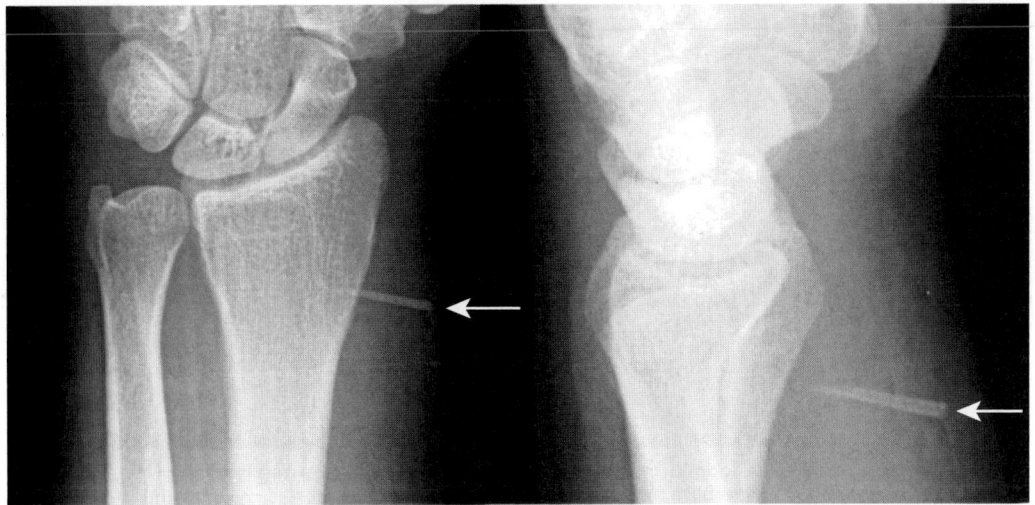

FIGURE 75-51 Plain films with a catfish fin in the volar wrist. *(Courtesy Ekkehard Bonatz.)*

cephalosporins, quinolones, tetracycline, and trimethoprim-sulfamethoxazole.[8]

TREATMENT

There are no specific antidotes. As with stingray and scorpionfish envenomations, the success of therapy is related to the rapidity with which it is undertaken. With catfish envenomations, in contrast to those of stingrays, constriction bandages have never been recommended for first aid. The wound should be immediately immersed in nonscalding hot water to tolerance (upper limit 45°C [113°F]) for 30 to 90 minutes or until there is significant pain relief. This may inactivate heat-labile components of the venom and perhaps helps to reverse local toxin-induced vasospasm. There is no evidence that adding mineral salts, solvents, antiseptics, or other chemicals to the water is of additional benefit. Cryotherapy is not efficacious. A popular and unstudied local (U.S. rural) remedy is to rub the sting with skin mucus (slime) from the catfish. If the hot water soak is not sufficient to control pain, local infiltration of the wound with buffered (alkalinized) bupivacaine or lidocaine without epinephrine or a regional nerve block may be necessary. It has been theorized that the pH alteration offered by the alkalinized local anesthetic may neutralize venom.[75] The wound should be explored surgically to remove all spine and sheath fragments. Standard radiographs or soft tissue exposures may locate a radiopaque foreign body (Figure 75-53). Advanced imaging may be necessary. The wound should be left unsutured to heal, to allow adequate drainage and minimize the risk of infection. All wounds must be carefully observed for infection until healed. If the puncture wound is of high infection risk (i.e., deep or into the hand or foot), a prophylactic antibiotic(s) should be administered.

PREVENTION

Catfish should be handled without grabbing the dorsal or pectoral fins, preferably by using a mechanical instrument or gaff. If possible, *Plotosus lineatus* should not be handled at all.

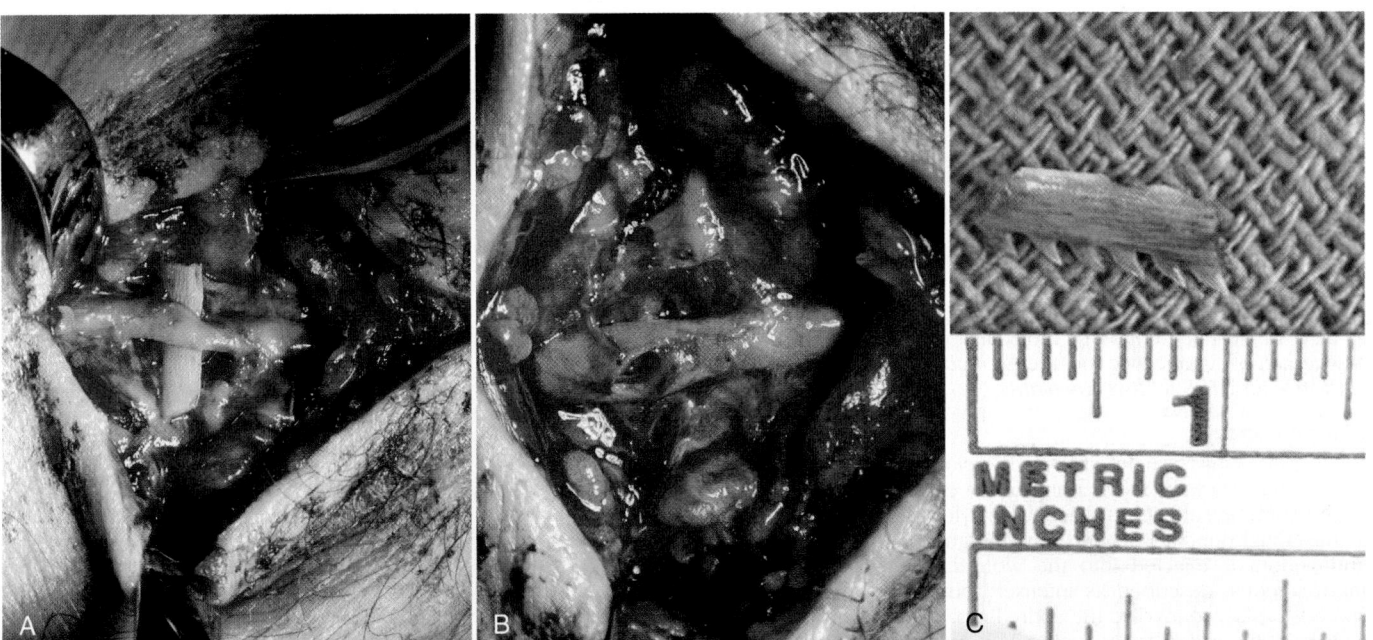

FIGURE 75-52 **A,** Catfish spine piercing the radial artery. **B,** Radial artery with residual holes from catfish spine, which has been removed. **C,** The retrobarbed structure of the catfish spine is apparent. *(Courtesy Ekkehard Bonatz.)*

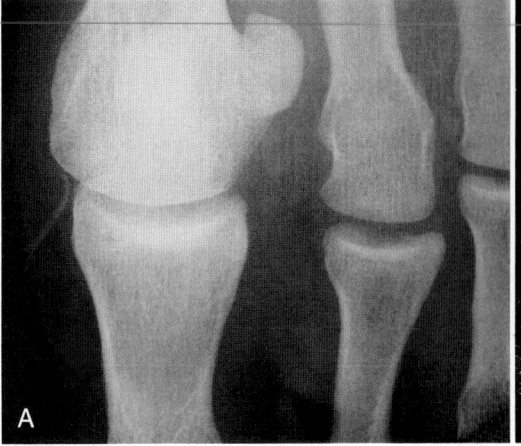
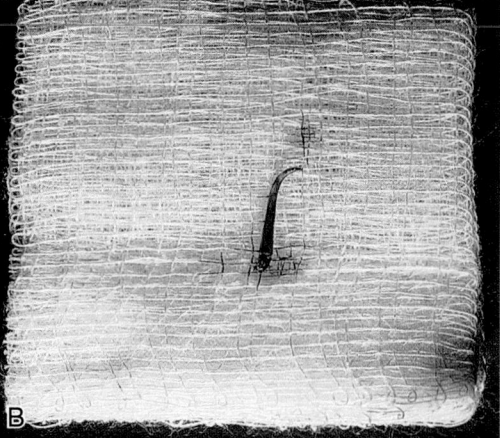

FIGURE 75-53 Catfish spine lodged in the foot. **A,** Radiograph shows a foreign body. **B,** The spine removed. *(Courtesy Paul S. Auerbach, MD.)*

WEEVERFISH

LIFE AND HABITS

The weeverfish (*Echiichthys* species, formerly named *Trachinus*) (Figure 75-54) is the most venomous fish of the temperate zone. It is found in the Black Sea, Mediterranean Sea, eastern Atlantic Ocean, North Sea, and European coastal areas. Common names for the weeverfish include adder-pike, sea dragon, sea cat, and stang. Weeverfish are small (10 to 53 cm [4 to 21 inches]) marine creatures that inhabit flat sandy or muddy bays, usually burying themselves in the soft bottom with only the head partially exposed. They lead sedentary lives but when provoked can strike out with unerring accuracy. "Weevers" are terrors to fishermen working in shallow sandy areas.

VENOM AND VENOM APPARATUS

The venom apparatus consists of four to eight elongate (up to 4.5 cm [1.75 inches] in length) and needle-sharp dorsal and two opercular and dagger-like dentinal spines, associated holocrine glandular tissue, and a thin, enveloping stratified squamous epithelium integumentary sheath. When excited, the fish extends the dorsal fin and expands the operculum, projecting the opercular spine out at a 35- to 40-degree angle from the longitudinal axis of the body. Weeverfish survive for hours out of the water, and the toxin remains potent for hours in dead animals, particularly when they are well refrigerated. Although incompletely characterized, the unstable (heat-labile) protein venom (ichthyoacanthotoxin) contains several peptides, at least one protein of high molecular weight (324,000), and possibly 5-hydroxytryptamine, epinephrine, norepinephrine, histamine, and mucopolysaccharide components. To date, serotonin has not been identified in weeverfish venom. The greater weeverfish (*Echiichthys draco*) releases a protein venom, dracotoxin, which has membrane-depolarizing and hemolytic activities. It appears to be a single polypeptide of molecular weight 105,000.[21] Other weeverfish of significance include *Echiichthys vipera*, *Echiichthys radiatus*, and *Echiichthys lineolatus*.

Clinical Aspects

Weeverfish stings usually afflict professional fishermen or vacationers who wade or swim along sandy coastal areas. The thrust of the spine is sufficient to penetrate a leather boot and creates a substantial puncture wound. The integumentary sheath is torn, and venom is injected into the wound. The onset of pain is instantaneous, described as intensely burning or crushing, and spreads rapidly to involve the entire limb. The pain usually peaks at 30 minutes and subsides within 24 hours, but can last for days. Its intensity can induce irrational behavior and syncope; even narcotics are poorly effective. An account dating from 1782 informs that a fisherman amputated his own finger to alleviate the pain caused by a weeverfish sting.[17] If an upper extremity is envenomed, the pain may radiate into the thorax and mimic the symptoms of myocardial ischemia.[56] The puncture wound bleeds little and often appears pale and edematous initially. The sting of *E. vipera* may bleed freely. Over the course of 6 to 12 hours, the wound becomes erythematous, ecchymotic, and warm. The edema may increase for 7 to 10 days, causing the entire limb to become markedly swollen. Secondary bacterial infections are common, and gangrene has been reported. The indolent wound may require months to heal, depending on the nature of the sting and underlying health of the victim. Raynaud's phenomenon in an envenomed digit occurring a few weeks after a weeverfish sting has been reported.[19] This may develop in a delayed fashion and persist for months after envenomation.[78] Persistent edema has been noted to last for more than 1 year.

Systemic symptoms associated with weeverfish envenomation include headache, delirium, aphonia, fever, chills, dyspnea, diaphoresis, cyanosis, nausea, vomiting, seizures, syncope, hypotension, and cardiac arrhythmias. Death has been reported, perhaps attributable to direct intravascular injection of venom.[14]

TREATMENT

The wound should be immersed immediately in nonscalding hot water to tolerance (upper limit 45° C [113° F]) for 30 to 90 minutes or until there is significant pain relief. This may inactivate heat-labile components of the venom and perhaps helps reverse local vasospasm that might contribute to local sequestration of venom and inhibition of free bleeding. Addition of mineral salts, ammonia, vinegar, urine, or other substances to the water is of no proved value. Immersion in hot water is often a less successful therapy for a weeverfish sting than for that of a scorpionfish. When the heat inactivation method is inadequate to control pain,

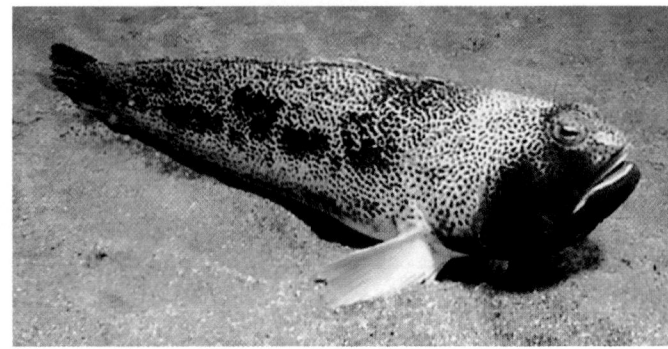

FIGURE 75-54 Greater weeverfish (*Echiichthys draco*), Mediterranean Sea. *(Courtesy H. Göthel.)*

it is necessary to infiltrate the wound with a local anesthetic (1% to 2% lidocaine without epinephrine) or perform a regional nerve block. The liberal use of narcotics is often required. Prolonged immersion cryotherapy is contraindicated. However, a practice known as "thermic shock" has been touted by practitioners along the French Mediterranean coast. This consists of application of intense local temperature variation (heat for 2 to 10 minutes, followed by application for 10 to 30 minutes of an ice cube insulated within a tissue or thin cloth).

Rarely, a spine breaks off into the skin. The wound should be explored gently, all fragments of sheath should be removed, and the wound should be irrigated vigorously with warmed saline. Wide excision and debridement are unnecessary. Because of the nature of the puncture wound, tight suture or surgical tape closure should not be undertaken; rather, the wound should be allowed to heal open with provision for adequate drainage. If the puncture wound is high risk (i.e., deep or into the hand or foot), prophylactic antibiotic(s) should be administered. No commercial antivenom is currently available.

PREVENTION

Weeverfish hide in bottom sand and mud; thus, people must shuffle along with adequate footwear. These fish are easily provoked and should be avoided by scuba divers. They should never be handled alive and must be treated with extreme caution even when dead. Weeverfish survive for hours out of the water, and careless handling of a seemingly dead fish may result in an envenomation.

VENOMOUS (HORNED) SHARKS

LIFE AND HABITS

Horned sharks are species that possess dorsal fin spines. In the United States, the group is essentially limited to the spiny dogfish *(Squalus acanthias)* (Figure 75-55). These and similar animals are distributed throughout sub-Arctic, temperate, tropical, and sub-Antarctic seas. The Port Jackson shark *Heterodontus portusjacksoni* (Figure 75-56) is particularly dangerous.

The fish are sluggish and prefer cooler water and shallow protected bays. They are erratic in their migration and may be found singly or in schools. Voracious feeders, they eat other fish, coelenterates, mollusks, crustaceans, and worms.

The venom apparatus consists of a spine anterior to each of two dorsal fins and the associated venom glands.

CLINICAL ASPECTS

As with other vertebrate stings, there is immediate intense stabbing pain that may last for hours and is accompanied by erythema and edema. Although systemic side effects are rare, fatalities are possible.

TREATMENT

Treatment is the same as for stingray envenomation.

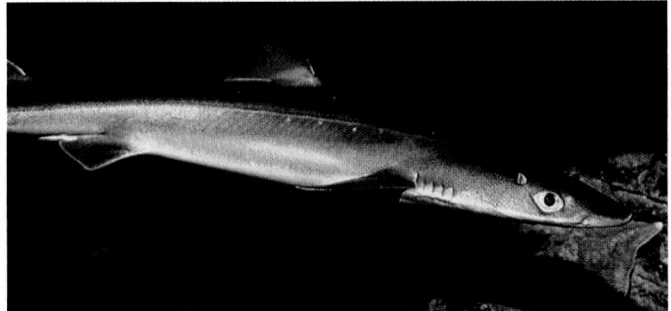

FIGURE 75-55 Spiny dogfish *(Squalus acanthias)*. *(Copyright 2006 Norbert Wu: norbertwu.com.)*

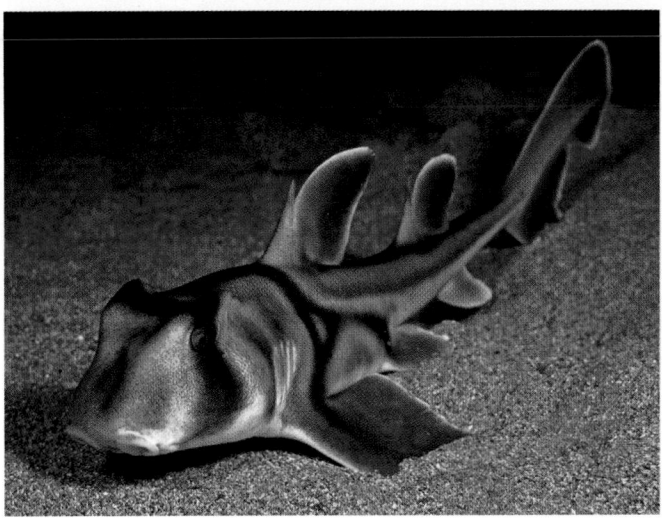

FIGURE 75-56 Port Jackson shark. *(Courtesy Marty Snyderman.)*

SURGEONFISH

LIFE AND HABITS

The surgeonfish (doctorfish or tang) is a tropical reef fish of the family Acanthuridae that carries one or more retractable jackknife-like epidermal appendages ("blades") on either side of the tail (Figure 75-57). When the fish is threatened, the blade may be extended out at a forward angle, where it serves to inflict a laceration. There does not appear to be any associated envenomation.

CLINICAL ASPECTS

A victim cut by a surgeonfish notes a laceration or deep puncture wound that is immediately painful; it usually bleeds freely. The pain is moderate to severe and of a burning nature. Systemic reactions are infrequent and consist of nausea, local muscle aching, and apprehension.

TREATMENT

The wound should be irrigated and then soaked in nonscalding hot water to tolerance (upper limit 45° C [113° F]) for 30 to 90 minutes or until pain is relieved, although this may be of variable efficacy. It should be scrubbed vigorously to remove all foreign material and watched closely for development of a secondary infection. Unless absolutely necessary for hemostasis, sutures should not be used to close the wound.

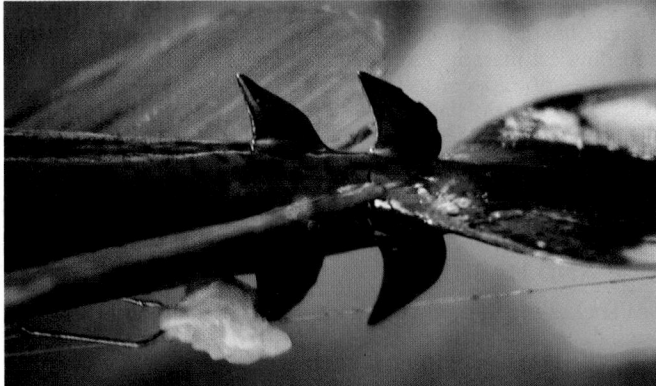

FIGURE 75-57 Surgeonfish "blades." *(Courtesy Paul S. Auerbach, MD.)*

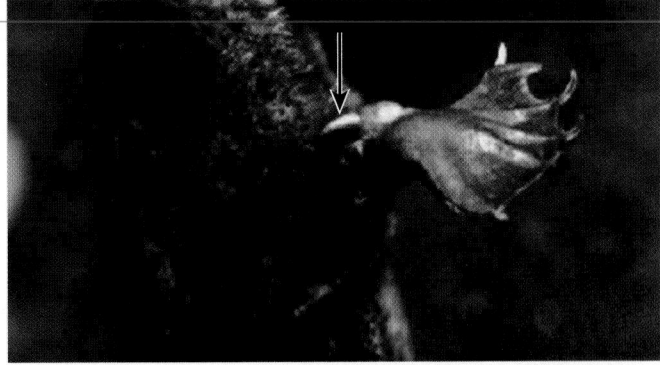

FIGURE 75-58 The poison-delivering spur (*arrow*) is found only on the male platypus's hind limbs. *Ornithorhynchus anatinus.* (*Used with permission via the GNU Free Documentation License; copyright 1995 E. Lonnon.*)

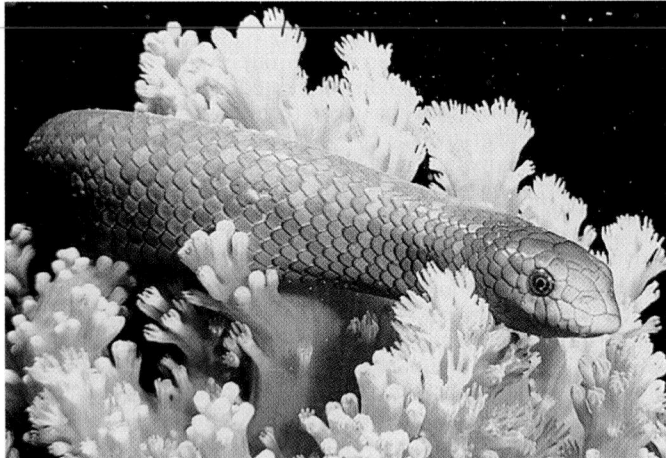

FIGURE 75-59 Olive sea snake. (*Courtesy Michele Hall.*)

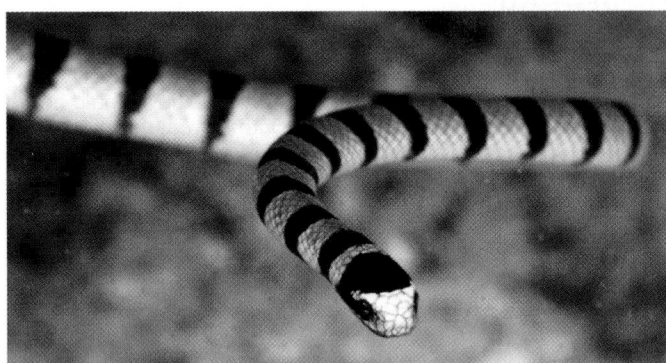

FIGURE 75-60 Sea snake. (*Copyright Lynn Funkhouser.*)

PLATYPUS

VENOM AND VENOM APPARATUS

The platypus *Ornithorhynchus anatinus* (Figure 75-58) is a furry venomous mammal that inhabits riverine systems of eastern Australia between northern Queensland and southern Tasmania.[34] These strange, fat animals have bills like a duck, webbed feet, a paddlelike tail, and claws on the feet. The male animal has an erectile keratinous spur on each hind limb linked via a distensible duct to a venom gland. There is a duct on each side that connects the spur to a venom gland situated under the thigh muscles. The venom appears to have components that mediate a type I hypersensitivity reaction with mast cell degranulation, which is consistent with the clinical presentation of soft tissue edema. Other venom fractions include a natriuretic peptide, proteases, and hyaluronidase. Venom-induced local edema in laboratory rats is attenuated by ketanserin and, to a lesser degree, by cimetidine, which may indicate a role of 5-hydroxytryptamine and histamine in the pathogenesis of the envenomation.

CLINICAL ASPECTS

Normally, the platypus is a shy creature; however, when provoked, it grasps its opponent with the hind legs and thrusts a spur or spurs into the victim, when 2 to 4 mL of venom may be released. When a human is envenomed, symptoms include immediate severe pain, tissue edema, and prolonged local sensitivity to painful stimuli. Movement, even remote (such as coughing), worsens the pain. The pain and hyperesthesia may generalize for several days before the pain recedes back to the envenomed limb. The pain may last for weeks, and in a severe case, muscle mass may be lost.

TREATMENT

Therapy is supportive and includes pain medication, wound care, and physical therapy after the acute episode. Hot water immersion does not appear to be of benefit acutely. Short-term corticosteroid therapy has been suggested to diminish pain and mitigate swelling, but there is no proof that antiinflammatory agents are definitively useful.

SEA SNAKES

LIFE AND HABITS

Sea snakes (Figures 75-59 to 75-62) of the family Hydrophiidae (subfamilies Hydrophiinae [genera *Hydrophis, Hydrelaps, Kerilia, Thalasophina, Enhydrina, Acalyptophis, Thalassophis, Kolpophis, Lapemis, Astrotia, Pelamis,* and *Microcephalophis*] and Laticaudinae [genera *Laticauda, Aipysurus,* and *Emydocephalus*]) are probably the most abundant reptiles on Earth. There are at least 52 species, all venomous. Species implicated in serious envenomations or human fatalities include *Astrotia stokesii, Enhydrina schistosa, Hydrophis ornatus, Hydrophis cyanocinctus, Lapemis hardwickii, Pelamis platura,* and *Thalassophis viperina.*

The snakes are distributed in the tropical and warm temperate Pacific and Indian Oceans, with the highest number of

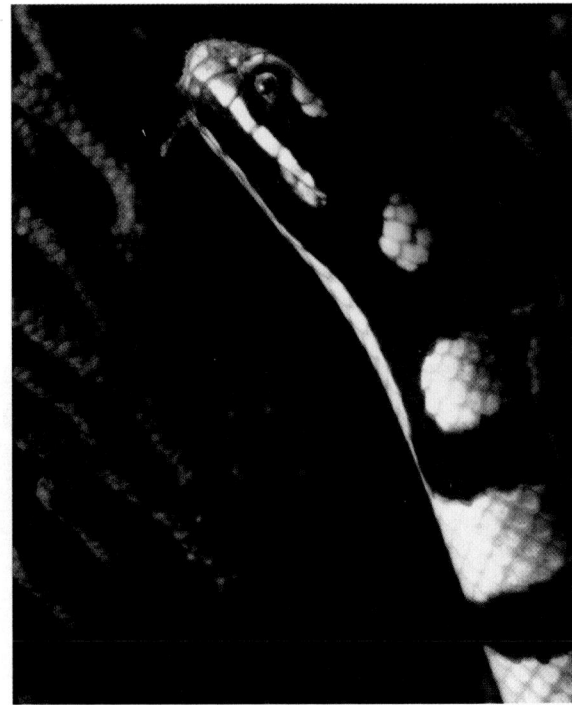

FIGURE 75-61 Sea snake. (*Copyright Lynn Funkhouser.*)

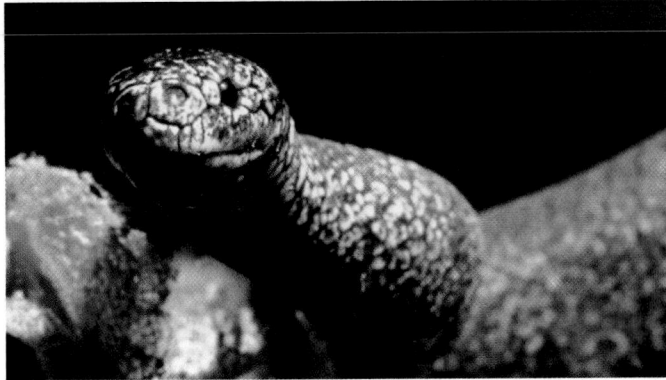

FIGURE 75-62 Olive sea snake in the Coral Sea. (Copyright Carl Roessler.)

envenomations occurring along the coast of Southeast Asia, in the Persian Gulf, and in the Malay Archipelago. No sea snakes live in the Atlantic Ocean or in the Caribbean Sea. Hawaii is the only U.S. state that has sea snakes (predominantly *P. platura*). The Pacific snakes usually inhabit sheltered coastal or coral reef waters and congregate about river mouths, and only on rare occasion do they venture into the open ocean. *P. platura*, the most widely distributed sea snake, is pelagic and may be found in the Pacific coastal waters of Central and South America. It does not migrate to the Caribbean, because of the freshwater barrier of Gatun Lake in the center of the Panama Canal.

Although sea snakes have the general appearance of land snakes, true sea snakes and sea kraits have valve-like nostril flaps and rudimentary ventral plates, without gills, limbs, ear openings, sternum, or urinary bladder. Most species of sea snakes are 0.9 to 1.2 m (3 to 4 feet) long, but some attain lengths of up to 2.7 m (9 feet). They are sinuous scaled creatures whose bodies are compressed posteriorly into a flat, paddle-shaped tail designed for marine locomotion (Figure 75-63). They swim in an undulating fashion and can move backward or forward in the water with equal speed. On land, however, they are awkward and do not survive readily. They may be brightly colored, such as the yellow-bellied sea snake, *P. platura*. With a single lung, the sea snake is capable of diving to 100 m (328 feet) and remaining submerged for 2 hours. The sea snake is an air breather and must surface periodically. The sea snake can be distinguished from a sea eel (Figure 75-64) by the presence of scales and absence of gills and fins.

Sea snakes use an air retention mechanism in the lungs to control buoyancy. Their food, small fish swallowed whole, is captured underwater, usually around bottom rocks and coral.

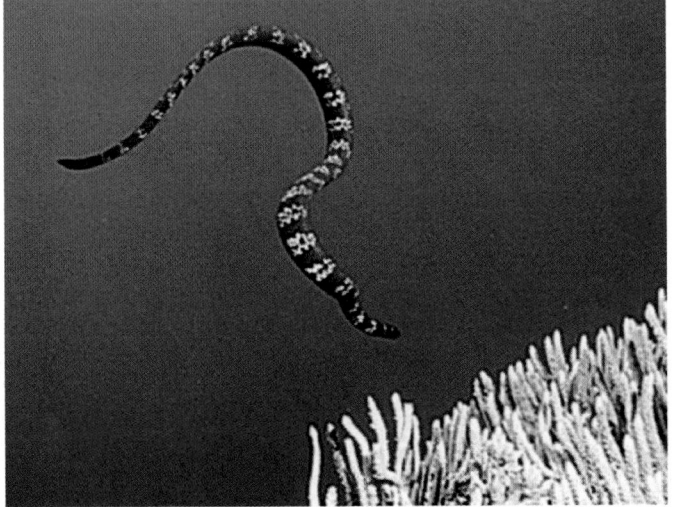

FIGURE 75-63 Sea snake in the Coral Sea. (Courtesy Carl Roessler.)

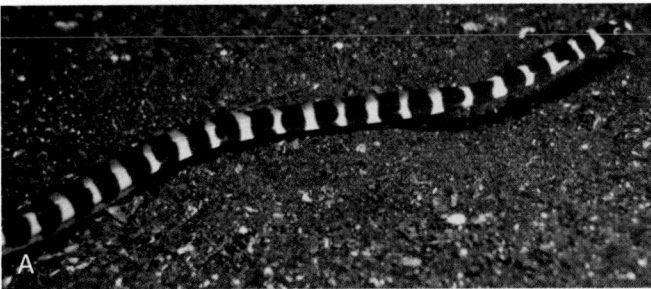

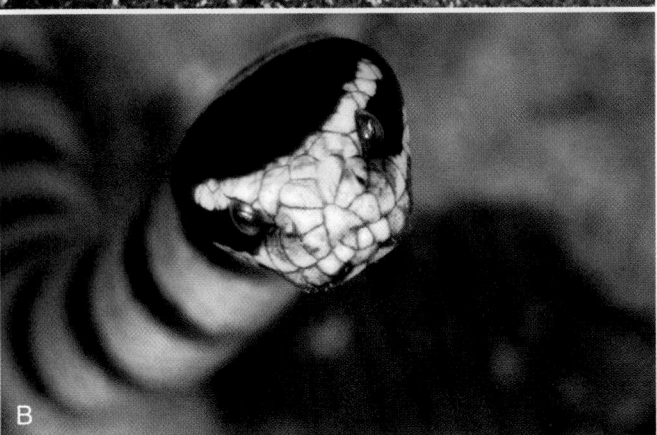

FIGURE 75-64 Harmless snake eel (A) mimics venous sea snake (B), Sulawesi Island, Indonesia. (A copyright 2006 Norbert Wu: norbertwu .com; B copyright Lynn Funkhouser.)

In general, sea snakes are docile creatures and flee when approached. However, when cornered or handled, they may become aggressive and strike out. During the reproductive season, some males adopt more irritable attitudes. The banded sea snake (sea krait) *Laticauda semifasciata* is served as a food (raw, smoked, or cooked) in certain Asian countries, notably Japan and the Philippines.

VENOM AND VENOM APPARATUS

The well-developed venom apparatus consists of two to four hollow maxillary fangs and a pair of associated venom glands. Fortunately, because the fangs are short and easily dislodged from their sockets, most bites (≈80%) do not result in significant systemic envenomation. Most fangs, except for those of *A. stokesii* and *Aipysurus laevis*, are not long enough to penetrate a wetsuit. The venom yield of sea snakes varies with species and is largely related to the size of the venom glands. An average-sized snake can produce 10 to 15 mg of venom, which is approximately 10 times the lethal dose in humans.

The protein venom is highly toxic and includes stable peripheral neurotoxins more potent than those of terrestrial snakes. Neuromuscular transmission is blocked predominantly at the postsynaptic membrane and caused by attachment of toxin to the alpha subunit of the acetylcholine receptor. Presynaptic toxin in sea snake venom has been less well studied but appears to be related to inhibition of transmitter release by blocking resynthesis of acetylcholine from choline. It seems probable that the action of *L. semifasciata* venom on excitable membranes is to alter ionic permeability, particularly that of sodium and chloride, without effect on Na^+,K^+-dependent adenosine triphosphatase activity. Calcium transport abnormalities are currently under investigation. Among other fractions of the venom are phospholipases, nerve growth factors, capillary permeability factor, anticomplement-active factor, enzymes (including acetylcholinesterase, hyaluronidase, leucine aminopeptidase, 5′-nucleotidase, phosphomonoesterase, and phosphodiesterase), and hemolytic and myotoxic compounds, which result in skeletal muscle necrosis, intravascular hemolysis, and renal tubular damage. Myonecrosis is related to phospholipase A, which may inhibit calcium

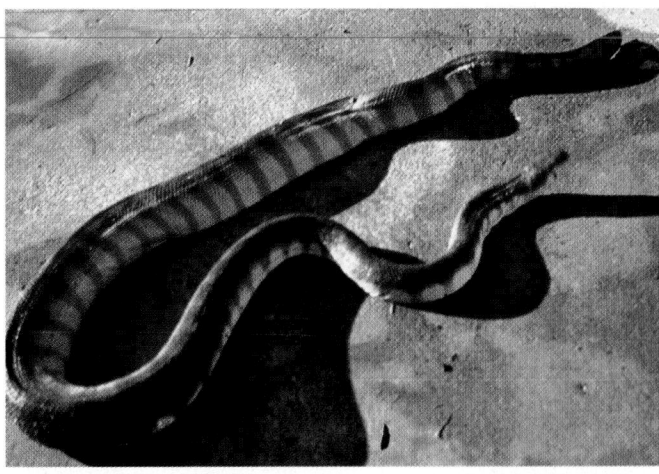

FIGURE 75-65 Beaked sea snake (*Enhydrina schistosa*). A common sea snake of Southeast Asia, the average length is about 1 m (3 feet). This creature inflicts a high proportion of the sea snake bites recorded in Asian coastal waters. *(Courtesy Sherman Minton, MD.)*

uptake into the sarcoplasmic reticulum. Neurotoxins are believed to exert their toxicity by binding in a nondepolarizing fashion to the nicotinic acetylcholine receptor and blocking neuromuscular transmission.[83]

The venoms of sea snakes are similar, as reflected in positive reactions during immunodiffusion, immunoelectrophoresis, and cross-neutralization by antivenom against heterologous venoms, and amino acid composition and sequences of neurotoxins. This is a reflection of phylogenetic relationships and is a logistic aid in preparation of effective antivenom.

Although large venom yields have been obtained from *A. stokesii*, *E. schistosa* is considered the most dangerous sea snake (Figure 75-65). *E. schistosa* is the most widely distributed sea snake in the Arabian sea. *Aipysurus duboisii* and *Acalyptophis peronii* from the Coral Sea have recently be shown to carry venoms of high human lethality potential. In an evaluation of poisonous land and sea snakes representative of those encountered in Saudi Arabia, sea snakes were noted to have an average lethal dose in dogs of 0.05 mg/kg, in comparison with the average lethal dose of vipers (1.13 mg/kg) and elapids (0.69 mg/kg).[102] Deaths were attributed to respiratory paralysis and failure.

CLINICAL ASPECTS

Bites are usually the result of accidental handling of snakes snared in the nets of fishermen or of accidentally stepping on a snake while wading. Most sea snake poisonings occur in remote fishing villages and in boats engaged in fishing. Nearly all bites involve the extremities.

The diagnosis of sea snake bite is based on the following:

Location. A person usually must have been in the water or handling a fishing net containing a sea snake to have been bitten. Some snakes may foray briefly onto land, particularly in areas of heavy mangrove growth, but it is quite unusual for a bite to occur out of the water. Because snakes may inhabit sheltered coastal waters and frequently congregate near river mouths, a bite can occur in an estuarine setting, up to 5 km (3 miles) inland.

Absence of pain. Initially, a sea snake bite does not cause great pain and may resemble no more than a pinprick.

Fang marks. These are multiple pinhead-sized, hypodermic-like puncture wounds, usually 1 to 4, but potentially up to 20. If the skin is not broken, envenomation cannot occur. In some cases, particularly with a superficial injury through the arm or leg of a neoprene wetsuit, the fang marks may be difficult to visualize because of lack of a localized reaction.

Identification of the snake. If excellent digital photographs of the snake can be taken, these should be used for identification by an expert. If the decision is made to capture or kill the snake, this should be done very carefully. The snake may be killed with a nonmacerating blow behind the head.

Development of characteristic symptoms. These include painful muscle movement, lower extremity paralysis, arthralgias, trismus, blurred vision, dysphagia, drowsiness, vomiting, and ptosis. Neurotoxic symptoms are rapid in onset and usually appear within 2 to 3 hours. If symptoms do not develop within 6 to 8 hours, there has almost certainly not been a clinically significant envenomation.

Envenomation by a sea snake characteristically shows an evolution of symptoms over a period of hours, with the latent period being a function of venom volume and victim sensitivity. The onset of symptoms can be as rapid as 5 minutes or as long as 8 hours. There is no appreciable local reaction to a sea snake bite other than the initial pricking sensation. The first complaint may be euphoria, malaise, or anxiety. Over 30 to 60 minutes, classic muscle aching and stiffness (particularly of the bitten extremity and neck muscles) develop, along with a "thick tongue" and sialorrhea, indicative of speech and swallowing dysfunction. Within 3 to 6 hours, moderate to severe pain is noted with passive movements of the neck, trunk, and limbs. There may be a brief period of spastic muscular and neurologic reflex hyperreactivity. Ascending flaccid or spastic paralysis follows shortly, beginning in the lower extremities, and deep tendon reflexes diminish and may disappear. Nausea, vomiting, myoclonus, muscle spasm, ophthalmoplegia, ptosis, dilated and poorly reactive pupils, facial paralysis, trismus, and pulmonary aspiration of gastric contents are frequent complications. Occasionally, bilateral painless swelling of the parotid glands develops.

Severe envenomations are marked by progressively intense symptoms within the first 2 hours of symptoms. Victims become cool and cyanotic, begin to lose vision, and may lapse into coma. Failing vision is reported to be a preterminal symptom. If peripheral paralysis predominates, the victim may remain conscious if hypoxia is avoided. Leukocytosis may exceed 20,000 white blood cells per milliliter; elevated plasma creatine kinase is variable. Elevated glutamic oxaloacetic transaminase reflects hepatic injury. Pathognomonic myoglobinuria becomes evident about 3 to 6 hours after the bite and may be accompanied by albuminuria and hemoglobinuria. Cerebrospinal fluid is normal. Respiratory distress and bulbar paralysis, pulmonary aspiration–related hypoxia, electrolyte disturbances (predominantly hyperkalemia), and acute renal failure (attributed in part to myonecrosis and pigment load) all contribute to the ultimate demise, which can occur hours to days after the untreated bite. Preterminal hypertension may occur. The mortality rate is 25% in victims who do not receive antivenom and 3% overall.

It is interesting to note the effects of sea snake (*A. laevis*) venom on prey fish.[107] The prey are subdued in six stages, which correlate roughly to certain aspects of a human envenomation: stage 1, increased ventilatory rate; stage 2, loss of mouth control, fin control, coordination, and buoyancy; stage 3, depressed ventilation, weakness, and ineffective swimming; stage 4, apnea; stage 5, near paralysis and body color darkening; and stage 6, death.

TREATMENT

If possible, the offending snake should be identified (see above), taking care not to increase the number of victims. The therapy for bites by snakes of the family Hydrophiidae is similar to that for terrestrial snakes of the family Elapidae. The affected limb should be immobilized and maintained in a dependent position while the victim is kept as quiet as possible. The pressure-immobilization technique for venom sequestration (see Figure 35-30) should be applied. If the bite is on a digit where a compression bandage cannot be applied, a loose constriction bandage that constricts only the superficial venous and lymphatic flow may be applied proximal to the wound. This should be released for 90 seconds every 10 minutes and should be completely removed after 4 to 6 hours. If the bite is older than 30 minutes, neither technique may be very effective.

There is no clinical enthusiasm for incision and suction therapy, which has been universally relegated to therapeutic history.

The victim must be kept warm and as still as possible. As with terrestrial snakebite, cryotherapy (immersion into ice water) is inefficacious and potentially harmful.

With any evidence of envenomation, sea snake antivenom (an equine pepsin-digested immunoglobulin from CSL Limited) prepared against the venoms of *E. schistosa* and the Australian tiger snake *Notechis scutatus* should be administered intravenously after appropriate skin testing for equine serum hypersensitivity. If skin testing is omitted, anticipate and be prepared to treat an allergic reaction. Tiger snake *(N. scutatus)* antivenom was formerly recommended for use if sea snake antivenom is unavailable, but this is no longer recommended, because tiger snake antivenom does not appear to be efficacious against sea snake bites in humans.[105] However, it is still commented in product literature that one vial of CSL sea snake antivenom is equivalent to 2 to 4 vials of CSL tiger snake antivenom. Sea snake antivenom is specific and absolutely indicated in cases of envenomation. Supportive measures, although critical in management, are no substitute. Administration of antivenom should begin as soon as possible and is most effective if initiated within 8 hours of the bite. Each vial of sea snake antivenom contains 1000 units of antivenom in 15 to 35 mL of liquid. The minimum effective adult dosage is one vial (1000 units), which neutralizes 10 mg of *E. schistosa* venom. The victim may require 3000 to 10,000 units (3 to 10 vials), depending on the severity of the envenomation. The proper administration of antivenom is clearly described on the antivenom package insert. Antivenom should be protected from light and stored refrigerated at 2° to 8°C (35.6° to 46.4°F). It must not be frozen.

Commercial Thai cobra *(Naja kaouthia)* antivenom was found to be effective in neutralizing sea snake *(L. hardwickii)* venom in mice. The application of this finding to humans is as yet undetermined.[66]

Sea snake envenomation may induce severe physiologic derangements that require intensive medical management. Urine output and measured renal function should be closely monitored, because hemolysis and rhabdomyolysis release hemoglobin and myoglobin pigments into the circulation, which precipitates acute renal failure. If hemoglobinuria or myoglobinuria is detected, urine should be alkalinized with sodium bicarbonate and diuresis promoted with a loop diuretic (furosemide or bumetanide) or mannitol, to avoid progressive nephropathy. Acute renal failure may necessitate a period of peritoneal dialysis or hemodialysis. Hemodialysis offers an alternative therapy that may be successful if antivenom is not available.

Respiratory failure should be anticipated as paralysis overwhelms the victim. Endotracheal intubation and mechanical ventilation may be required until antivenom adequately neutralizes the venom effects. Serum electrolytes should be measured regularly to guide administration of fluids and electrolyte supplements. Hyperkalemia related to rhabdomyolysis and renal dysfunction must be promptly recognized and treated.

As previously mentioned, symptoms usually occur within 2 to 3 hours after envenomation. If there is no early evidence of envenomation, the victim should be observed for 8 hours before discharge from the hospital.

SUMMARY

A summary algorithmic approach to marine envenomation can be followed when the causative agent cannot be positively identified (see Figure 74-113).[6] Once the physician has made a commitment to a course of treatment based on a presumption of what creature has caused the injury, the subtleties of therapy can be deployed.

REFERENCES

Complete references used in this text are available online at expertconsult.inkling.com.

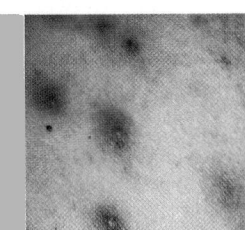

CHAPTER 76
Aquatic Skin Disorders

EDGAR MAEYENS JR AND SARAH A. WOLFE

Human interaction with marine and freshwater aquatic environments is becoming more frequent. People travel to remote and exotic areas to participate in aquatic activities. When in these areas, be they for vacation or adventure, contact with aquatic animals, plants, and microbes is responsible for allergic reactions, trauma, infections, and envenomations. The dermatologic manifestations of many of these disorders are presented in this chapter.

PHYTOPLANKTON DERMATOSES

This category of aquatic dermatoses includes diseases caused by algae, cyanobacteria, and dinoflagellates. Each of these organisms produces predictable disorders in aquatic life forms and humans. When phytoplanktons are "blooming," they are able to cause a variety of dermatoses. Terminology defining these disorders can be ambiguous and misleading. Current taxonomy and genetic techniques are redefining and clarifying the exact nature and origins of these organisms, thus allowing more accuracy, less ambiguity, and better comprehension of disease states produced by phytoplankton.

The following vignettes attempt to differentiate organisms. Absolute separation of species is not possible, because chimerism is prevalent and gene sharing occurs.

CYANOBACTERIA

Cyanobacteria are true gram-negative bacteria, although they are often erroneously referred to as "blue-green algae." Their habitats include almost every conceivable environment, from soil to freshwater lakes and oceans. Some are endosymbionts in plants, sponges, slime molds, and protozoans, for whom they provide energy. Cyanobacteria do not possess a nucleus (prokaryotic) or membrane-bound organelles. Most species are autotrophic.

Aquatic cyanobacteria can form "blooms" (massive reproduction in an area) in both marine and freshwater environments, giving the appearance of blue-green paint or scum on the water surface. If these blooms are created by toxin-producing cyanobacteria, they can be harmful to both animals and humans and thus become "harmful blooms." These toxins can be hepatotoxins, cytotoxins, neurotoxins, and endotoxins. Because of the ability to produce harmful blooms, cyanobacteria are confused with dinoflagellates, which also produce harmful blooms. Examples of cyanobacteria toxin–related diseases are paralytic shellfish poisoning, neurotoxic shellfish poisoning, diarrheic shellfish poisoning, amnestic shellfish poisoning, and ciguatera fish poisoning. Common to all blooms are lipopolysaccharides, which are a cause of skin irritation. Cyanobacteria toxins are not absorbed through the skin but only via ingestion or inhalation. All of these toxins are resistant to boiling.

DINOFLAGELLATES

Dinoflagellates are organisms common to all types of aquatic ecosystems. Approximately one-half of the species are photosynthetic[63]; the remainder are heterotrophic and feed by phagotrophy and osmotrophy. Dinoflagellates are prominent members of the zooplankton and phytoplankton marine and freshwater ecosystems. Of the 2000 living species, more than 1700 are found in oceans and 220 in freshwater.[171] These organisms are frequently and erroneously referred to as "algae," because most are eukaryotic and derive energy by photosynthesis. Dinoflagellates exist as biflagellate unicells, plasmodia (i.e., multinucleated organisms), and coccoid stages.

Dinoflagellates are at their greatest concentration in temperate coastal waters, where they bloom in middle to late summer when sunshine and vertical stability allow aggregations to develop.[171] In tropical waters and nutrient-poor temperate regions, all types of phytoplankton are generally scant. In polar waters, diatoms predominate over dinoflagellates.

About 75% to 80% of toxic phytoplankton species are dinoflagellates.[33] When dinoflagellates bloom, *red tides* are produced and frequently kill fish and/or shellfish, either directly via toxin production or by clogging fish gills, depleting oxygen, or other means.[165] Colors of red tides vary from red to red-brown to brown. Anthropogenic and natural factors contribute to their development. Dinoflagellate toxins are some of the most potent biotoxins known. Accumulation in fish or shellfish produces diseases in humans like neurotoxic shellfish poisoning, paralytic shellfish poisoning, diarrheic shellfish poisoning, and ciguatera fish poisoning. Blooms, when aerosolized, produce cutaneous disorders in humans, such as dermatitis and urticaria (Figure 76-1).

ALGAE

The derivation of the term *alga* is from the Latin word for "seaweed." Algae are a very large and diverse group of autotrophic, unicellular (microscopic), or multicellular (macroscopic)

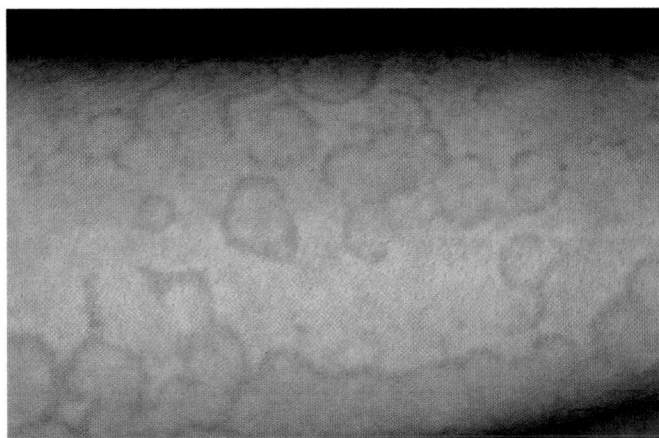

FIGURE 76-1 Red tide dermatitis. Petaloid pattern of urticaria following swimming in red tide–contaminated water. *(Courtesy Edgar Maeyens, Jr., MD.)*

TABLE 76-1 Potency Ranking of Topical Steroids*

Potency	Generic	Sizes
High potency (not for use on face, groin, or axillae)	Clobetasol propionate 0.05% cream/ointment	15, 30, 45, 60 g
	Fluocinonide 0.05% cream/ointment	15, 30, 60 g
Medium potency (not for use on face, groin, or axillae)	Triamcinolone 0.1% cream/ointment	15, 80, 454 g
	Betamethasone valerate 0.1% cream/ointment	15, 45 g
Low potency (safe for face, groin, or axillae)	Hydrocortisone 2.5% cream/ointment	30 g
	Desonide 0.05% cream/ointment	15, 60 g

*These topical steroids must be applied once or twice daily. Larger volumes or multiple tubes may be needed for greater surface area involvement.

organisms. They are eukaryotic and therefore possess a nucleus enclosed within a membrane and membrane-bound chloroplasts (photosynthetic machinery derived from cyanobacteria).[4] Phylogenetically, chloroplasts are membrane-bound organelles containing DNA similar to that of cyanobacteria. It is presumed that chloroplasts represent reduced cyanobacteria endosymbionts.[4] Traditional terminology has used the terms *algae* and *cyanobacteria* synonymously and is currently regarded as outdated.[4]

The exact number of algae species is estimated to be 1 to 10 million and most are microalgae.[14] They are found in all waters (both fresh and marine), the atmosphere, and soil. Microscopic forms suspended in the water column are designated phytoplankton. When conditions are present that facilitate proliferation, overgrowth occurs, resulting in "algal blooms." Waters containing algal blooms become discolored, asphyxiate or poison surrounding aquatic life forms, and threaten the health of humans. Algae have been compared with plants but differ in many ways. For instance, algae are devoid of certain structures found in land plants, such as roots, leaves, stems, and vascular tissues.[13] Plants and algae are photosynthetic. Algal photosynthetic pathways vary among different groups, some deriving energy from photosynthesis and uptake of organic carbon and others utilizing photoautotrophism.

Sargassum algae Dermatitis

Definition. *Sargassum* is a brown macroalgae distributed throughout tropical and temperate oceans. The name is derived from the Sargasso Sea, which is home to several species of *Sargassum*. Their habitat is coral reefs and shallow water. Although these species are normally benthic, they can exist in planktonic and pelagic forms.

Physiology. Certain species of these algae grow to lengths of several meters. They are brown or deep green in color. To keep afloat, the algae possess air vesicles or bulb-like gas-filled bladders. When detached from their moorings, *Sargassum* become beach drift. *Sargassum* in quantity usually appear as a large, tangled mass. Many fishes use these algae as habitat.

Clinical Presentation. Contact with skin can result in an exuberant erythematous, urticarial-like dermatitis (Figure 76-2).[28]

Treatment. Symptomatic treatment with oral antihistamines and topical corticosteroids is usually adequate (Tables 76-1 and 76-2).

Prevention. Avoid contact with these algae, not only when they are part of beach drift, but also when they are floating mats.

Lyngbya Dermatitis

Lyngbya majuscula is an alga that produces tissue-damaging toxins. Direct contact with *Lyngbya* can result in serious skin reactions and tissue necrosis.

Definition. *L. majuscula* (also known as *Microcoleus lyngbyaceus*) is finely filamentous and dark green or olive in color. It grows in hairlike masses in clumps at depths of up to 30 m

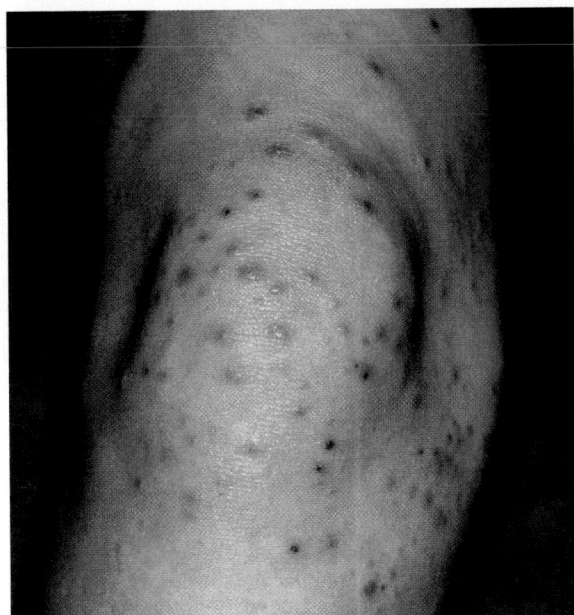

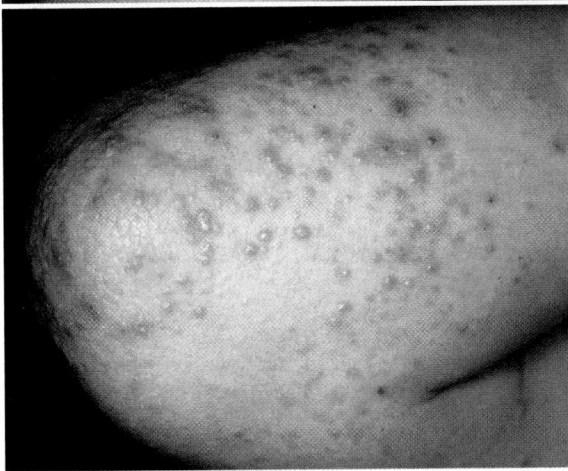

FIGURE 76-2 An urticaria-like papular eczematous dermatitis from contact with *Sargassum algae*.

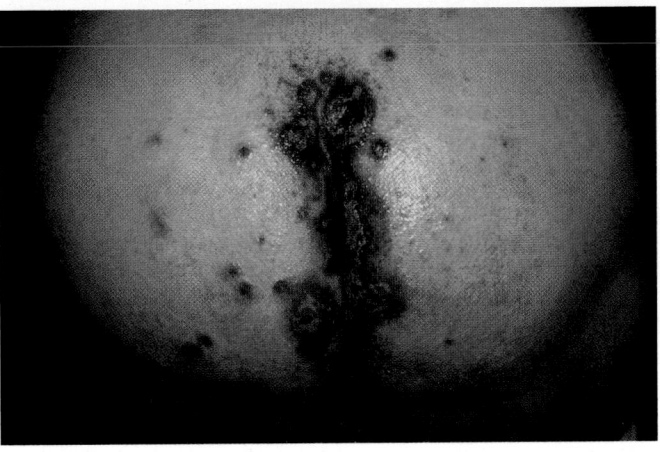

FIGURE 76-3 Rare and extreme example of superficial necrosis and inflammation secondary to dermonecrotic toxins of *Microcoleus lyngbyaceus*. *(Courtesy Edgar Maeyens, Jr., MD.)*

(100 feet) and is often found entangled with other algae in tide pools and reef flats.[162]

Epidemiology and Risk Factors. *Lyngbya* is found throughout the Pacific and Indian Oceans and the Caribbean Sea. Strong currents and winds dislodge the alga from its normal habitat, fragment it, and carry it to the surf line. Dermatitis occurs only when the alga or its fragmented components are trapped beneath swimwear. On exiting the water, algae fragments are either washed off or dry out, rendering them harmless.

Pathophysiology. *L. majuscula* produces the dermatonecrotic toxins lyngbyatoxin A and debromoaplysiatoxin. Toxicity varies depending on season, type, and location of the algae.[133] Not every strain of *Lyngbya* is toxic. It is the potency and/or concentration of these toxins against the skin that determines the degree of cutaneous damage.

Clinical Presentation. Within minutes to hours of contact, pruritus, burning sensations, and erythematous dermatitis develop in a swimsuit-patterned distribution. This is followed by varying degrees of blister formation, which ultimately may progress to epidermal and dermal necrosis (Figures 76-3 and 76-4). Additional symptoms can include periorbital edema, irritation of nasal mucosa, conjunctivitis, headache, and fatigue.[81] Symptoms last a few hours to days. Skin necrosis takes weeks to resolve. Anatomic locations typically are the genital, perineal, and perianal regions.

Differential Diagnosis. Differentiating *Lyngbya* dermatitis from "seabather's eruption" and "swimmer's itch" can be difficult when there is limited contact with the algae.

Treatment. Treatment consists of prompt cleansing with copious amounts of soapy water to remove residual algal fragments. This is followed with two to three sequential isopropyl alcohol rinses and then application of a topical corticosteroid ointment (Table 76-1). Severe dermatitis may require oral corticosteroids. If necrosis is present, any of a variety of agents and techniques may be used to facilitate wound healing and prevent

TABLE 76-2 Topical Antipruritics and Oral Antihistamines		
Product (Brand Name)	**Chemical Name**	**Adult Doses [Children <12 Years Doses]**
Topical Antipruritics		
Camphor/menthol (Sarna)	Camphor 0.5%/menthol 0.5%	Apply up to 4 times a day
Pramoxine (Sarna Sensitive, Gold Bond Anti-Itch)	Pramoxine HCl 1%	Apply up to 4 times a day
Neutrogena Norwegian Formula Soothing Relief Anti-Itch Moisturizer	Camphor 0.1%/lidocaine HCl 2%	Apply up to 4 times a day
Pramosone cream, ointment, lotion	Hydrocortisone acetate 1% or 2.5% with pramoxine HCl 1%	Apply up to 4 times a day
Aveeno Oatmeal Bath	Colloidal oatmeal	Daily as needed
Oral Antihistamines		
Allegra	Fexofenadine	180 mg daily [30 mg twice a day; minimum age 2 years]
Claritin	Loratidine	10 mg daily [2.5-10 mg daily; minimum age 6 months]
Zyrtec	Cetirizine	10 mg daily [2.5-10 mg daily; minimum age 6 months]
Benadryl	Diphenhydramine	25-50 mg every 6 hours [12.5-25 mg every 6 hours; minimum age 2 years]

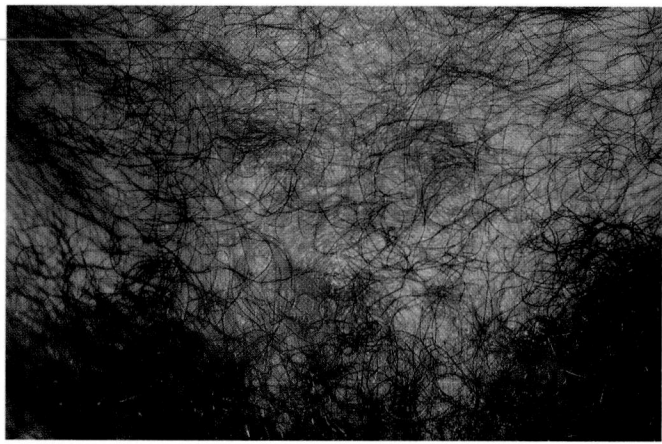

FIGURE 76-4 Folliculitis in the bathing trunk area caused by *Microcoleus lyngbyaceus*. (*Courtesy Edgar Maeyens, Jr., MD.*)

infection. Choices are predicated upon the severity of the process and the care provider's preferences. Methods range from sterile saline cleanses followed by white petroleum jelly to Hydrofera Blue bacteriostatic wound dressings (Hydrofera LLC, Willimantic, Connecticut). Difficulty with breathing may indicate a systemic allergic response causing bronchospasm or early signs of anaphylaxis, requiring epinephrine and antihistamines.

Sequelae. If the condition is diagnosed and treated promptly, no adverse sequelae occur. If diagnosis and therapy are delayed, skin necrosis will occur, resulting in possible secondary infection with severe scarring.

Prevention. Remove swimsuits and shower with soap on exiting the water. Avoid waters where algae densities are high or algae blooms exist. Swimsuits and swim gear must be machine washed to remove any residual algae fragments.

Ciguatera Dermatitis

Definition. Ciguatera fish poisoning is the name given to a food-borne illness caused by consumption of fish contaminated with ciguatoxins (see Chapter 77). Dermatoses can occasionally be a feature of the illness. Ciguatera dermatitis is not diagnostic of ciguatera fish poisoning, because it is nonspecific and manifests with a wide range of clinical presentations.

Epidemiology and Risk Factors. Ciguatoxin accumulates in predator fish, such as grouper, snappers, amberjacks, and barracudas. Ciguatoxin is produced by dinoflagellates, such as *Gambierdiscus toxicus*.[188] The toxin is heat resistant, so it cannot be destroyed by cooking. Ciguatoxin-producing dinoflagellates are localized to tropical waters of the Caribbean and Pacific. Ciguatoxin is found in hundreds of species of reef fish.

Pathophysiology. The precise pathophysiology of ciguatoxin dermatitis is unknown.

Clinical Presentation. Dermatologic manifestations of ciguatera fish poisoning include intense generalized pruritus associated with a diffuse, maculopapular eruption that can progress to bullae or desquamation (Figure 76-5). Other manifestations that have been reported include hair and nail loss, intense diaphoresis leading to dehydration, cyanosis, and urticaria.

Diagnostic Tests. No routine test exists to diagnose ciguatera dermatitis.

Treatment. There is neither a specific therapy nor an antidote for ciguatera fish poisoning. Treatment of cutaneous manifestations, as well as systemic ciguatera fish poisoning, is symptomatic and supportive.

Sequelae. No long-term cutaneous adverse effects have been reported.

Prevention. Avoid ingestion of fish likely to be ciguatoxic.

Prototheca Dermatitis

Prototheca spp. are unicellular algae lacking chlorophyll. *Prototheca* spp. are often preliminarily misidentified as fungi in tissue and cultures. They are infrequent causes of cutaneous and systemic infections.

Definition. The genus *Prototheca* consists of nonpigmented algae from the family Chlorellaceae. Human and animal infections have been caused by an achlorophyllic mutant of the green algae *Chlorella pyrenoidosa*. Three species of *Prototheca* are recognized: *Prototheca stagnora, P. wickerhamii,* and *P. zopfii. P. wickerhamii* and *P. zopfii* are the pathogens most commonly implicated in human prototothecosis.[24,53,95,181]

Epidemiology and Risk Factors. *Prototheca* spp. occur globally on every continent except Antarctica.[101] *Prototheca* have been isolated from fresh and marine water, streams, lakes, sewage treatment systems, tree slime, and soil. Infections usually occur after inoculation into skin following exposure to contaminated water or soil. The incubation period for the onset of symptoms is not well known.[190] Periods of weeks to months have been reported.[38,173] Most people do not recall the moment of trauma and thus the duration of incubation. Preexisting skin wounds facilitate entry of *Prototheca*. Person-to-person transmission has not been reported. The organism is of low virulence. Immunosuppressed persons or persons taking immunosuppressive medications are at increased risk of acquiring prototothecosis.[91,101,181] The infection is usually localized in healthy individuals, but can disseminate in the immunocompromised.

Pathophysiology. *Prototheca* species are unicellular, aerobic, and spherical organisms without chlorophyll that have hyalin sporangia that reproduce asexually. They are unable to produce energy from photosynthesis and therefore exist as saprophytes.[24] *Prototheca* species are distinct from fungi and bacteria in size, morphology, and method of reproduction.

Histologically, organisms can be found within giant cells or lying freely in the dermis. *Prototheca* cells are round; each cell, or sporangium, contains two to eight tightly packed endospores (Figure 76-6). Sporangia are described as being frambesiform (raspberry-like). The organism stains well with Grocott-Gomori methenamine silver nitrate, colloidal iron, and periodic acid–Schiff.[18,70]

Clinical Presentation. Clinical features of human prototothecosis include:

1. Superficial Cutaneous Lesions. These manifest as papulonodules or verrucous plaques with or without ulcerations[47] (Figure 76-7). Bullous lesions may occur, with subsequent rupture, drainage, and crusting.[18,70] Rarely, eczematous and cellulitis-like lesions occur.

2. Olecranon Bursitis. The elbow is swollen and erythematous and, on occasion, drains spontaneously. This is not accompanied by fever or chills. The presentation is similar to other causes of bursal inflammation. A history of preceding trauma should suggest prototothecosis.[18,47,70]

3. Systemic Infection. Immunosuppressed patients, such as those undergoing chemotherapy or infected with human immunodeficiency virus (HIV), are more predisposed to disseminated infection than are immunocompetent persons. At least

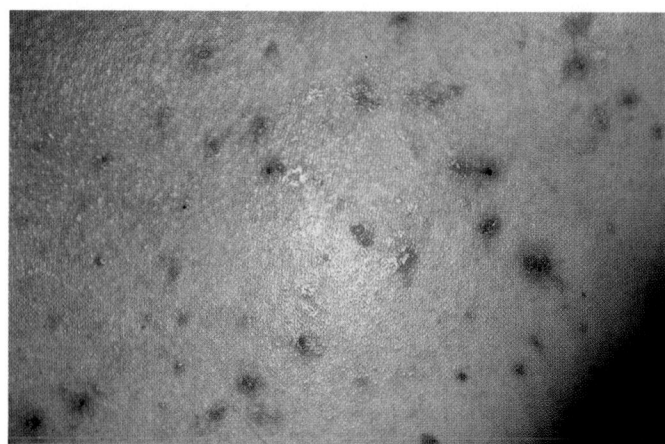

FIGURE 76-5 Ciguatera dermatitis. Thirty-year-old man's posterior hemithorax showing papules and rare blisters as a cutaneous manifestation of his ciguatera intoxication. (*Courtesy Edgar Maeyens, Jr., MD.*)

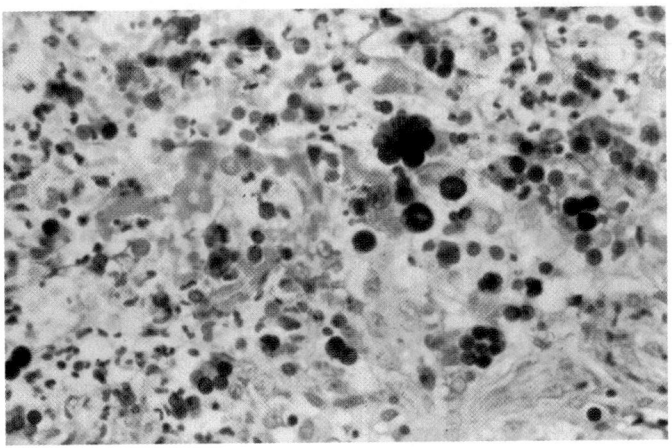

FIGURE 76-6 Protothecosis histology. (*Courtesy Edgar Maeyens, Jr., MD.*)

50% of reported individuals with cutaneous protothecosis are immunosuppressed.[31,136]

Mucosal Protothecosis. Lacoviello and colleagues reported a case of protothecosis of the esophagus complicating prolonged endotracheal intubation.[100]

In cases associated with a traumatic episode, the initial lesion is a tender, red papule or an asymptomatic nodule that enlarges, becomes pustular, and ulcerates. Purulent, malodorous, and blood-tinged discharge may be present. Satellite lesions surrounding the primary lesion develop and frequently become confluent. Lesions can become verrucous and resemble chromomycosis. Regional lymph nodes may develop metastatic granulomas. Lesions extend centrifugally and occasionally disseminate. In the olecranon bursitis form, infection develops several weeks after an elbow injury and is localized to the bursa. Overlying sinus tracts may develop.[129]

Differential Diagnosis. The differential diagnosis includes the following diseases: atypical *Mycobacterium* infection, chromoblastomycosis, pyoderma gangrenosum, deep fungal infection, blastomycosis-like pyoderma, and Majocchi's granuloma.

Diagnostic Tests. Diagnosis of protothecosis can be made either by tissue biopsy or tissue culture. If uncertainty exists as to the exact nature of the organism, electron microscopy reveals a double-layered cell wall and no chloroplasts. These are features differentiating *Prototheca* from other algae.

Treatment. There is no defined pharmacologic protocol for eradication of *Prototheca*. Protothecosis shows no tendency to self-heal. It is a chronic and progressive disease.[85] Cutaneous lesions are cured with surgical excision. Amphotericin B has been used successfully.[31] Prolonged treatments with the algaecidal agents ketoconazole, itraconazole, fluconazole, and voriconazole[60] have been reported effective.[92,118,170]

Human Pythiosis Dermatitis

The aquatic fungus-like organism *Pythium insidiosum* is a zoosporic plant pathogen and newly emerging human pathogen. It is phylogenetically more closely related to algae than to true fungi.[62] *P. insidiosum* is a long-recognized plant pathogen causing seed decay and root rot of seedlings.[58] The disease in humans and animals is called *pythiosis*.

Definition. Pythiosis is a cutaneous/subcutaneous disease of humans and animals. Although primarily a cutaneous and intestinal disease of animals (horses, cats, dogs, and cattle), it is now an emerging human pathogen that presents as a localized or systemic/vascular form.[58]

Epidemiology and Risk Factors. The organism is found in tropical, subtropical, and temperate areas of the world. Preferential ecologic niches are swampy environments, where the organism produces mobile biflagellate zoospores that are attracted chemotactically to traumatized human and animal tissues.[86] The disease has been identified in the United States, Australia, Asia, South and Central America, and New Zealand. Individuals with hemoglobinopathies are especially susceptible to developing systemic disease.[182]

Pathophysiology. The chemoattractants keratin and collagen from wounded skin attract *P. insidiosum* sporangia, which release biflagellated, mobile zoospores. Zoospores are attracted to hair and lacerated skin, where they encyst on contact. At the time of encystment in tissue, the flagellae detach and the zoospores become globose, forming germ tubes in 24 hours. Once attached, encysted zoospores secrete an amorphous material that acts as an adhesive substance.[122] *Pythium* species produce pectic and cellulolytic enzymes, macerating enzymes, and phytotic fungal products.[58] The role of these enzymes in production of the granulomatous response seen in human tissue is unknown.

Clinical Presentation. Cutaneous pythiosis typically begins as a pustule at the site of inoculation. The inflammatory response to the organism mimics cellulitis and eventuates in suppurative necrosis. Prototypically, the lower extremities are most frequently involved, but any cutaneous surface is vulnerable (Figures 76-8 and 76-9). Pythiosis can also progress to a systemic disease involving the vascular system, where it causes arterial occlusion.[21]

Differential Diagnosis. Although not a true fungus, *P. insidiosum* has some morphologic characteristics in common with the order Zygomycetes. These similarities are best appreciated histologically by their resemblance to the Zygomycetes *Aspergillus* and *Mucor*. Zygomycetes fungi are ubiquitous in nature, found in soil and decaying vegetation.

Hyphae of *P. insidiosum* species are broad, branched at right angles, usually nonseptate, and irregularly shaped. They are

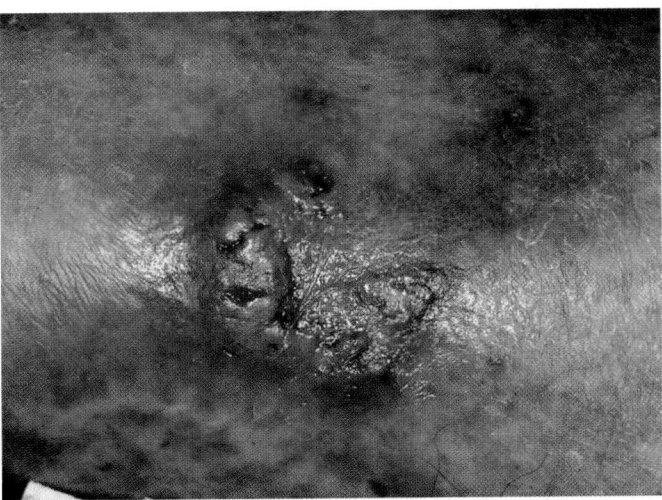

FIGURE 76-7 Protothecosis of anterior leg. (*Courtesy Edgar Maeyens, Jr., MD.*)

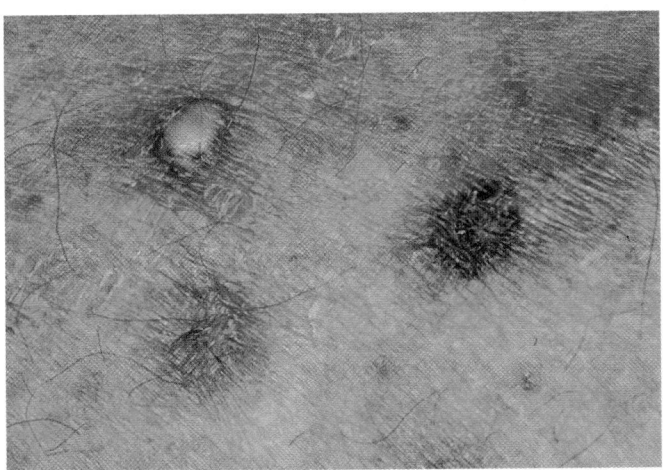

FIGURE 76-8 Human pythiosis. A pustule at the site of inoculation of *Pythium insidiosum*.

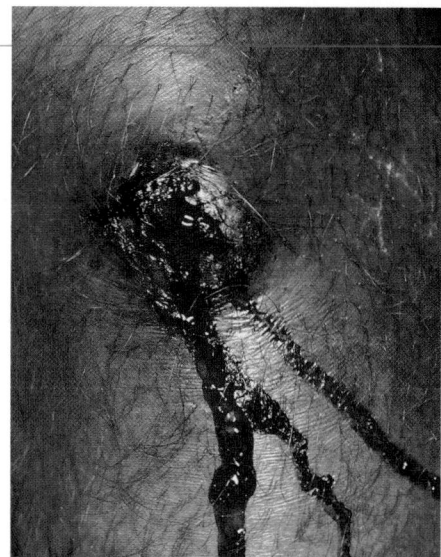

FIGURE 76-9 Human pythiosis. Suppurative necrotizing cellulitis of *Pythium insidiosum* infection.

described as ribbon-like (Figure 76-10).[7] Fungi of the class Zygomycetes (e.g., *Mucor, Rhizopus,* and *Absidia*) are etiologic agents of a variety of infections in humans. Diseases caused by this group of fungi were formerly termed mucormycoses but are now called zygomycoses.

The spectrum of zygomycoses includes cutaneous, gastrointestinal, renal, central nervous system, pulmonary, and rhinocerebral infections.[7] Cutaneous zygomycosis has been associated with burns, traumatic wounds, surgical wound infections, contaminated dressings, and intramuscular injections.[7] Cutaneous zygomycosis begins with erythema and induration, gradually evolving into a necrotic ulcer virtually identical to pythiosis. It is believed that many cases of pythiosis have been misdiagnosed as therapeutically nonresponsive zygomycosis.

Diagnostic Tests. It is possible to culture pus, lesion exudate, or biopsy material on Sabouraud glucose or brain heart infusion agar. In 24 to 48 hours at 28° to 37°C (82.4° to 98.6°F), there appears a flat or submerged, colorless or white growth with short or no apparent aerial hyphae.[86] Cotton blue dye–assisted microscopic examination shows broad, nonseptate, and/or sparsely septate hyaline hyphae.

Histopathologic examination of lesional tissue reveals broad, branched, and nonseptate or sparsely septate hyphae. The organism is best visualized with Gomori methenamine silver (GMS) or periodic acid–Schiff (PAS) stains. Microscopically, *P. insidiosum* resembles the hyphae of Zygomycetes (Figure 76-11).[86]

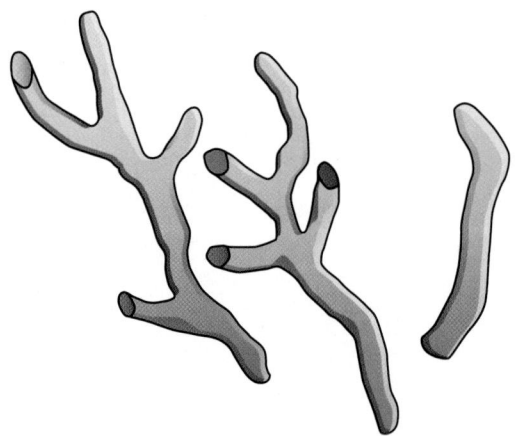

FIGURE 76-10 *Pythium insidiosum.* Illustrations of *Pythium insidiosum* with right-angled branching, broad, nonseptate hyphae. These are microscopically similar to the Zygomycetes. *(Courtesy Jan Mucklestone.)*

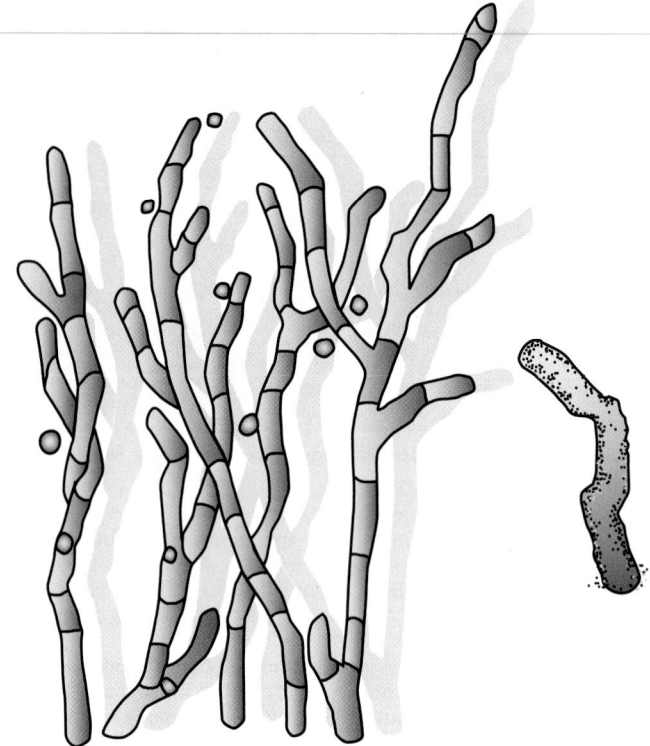

FIGURE 76-11 *Pythium insidiosum.* Illustration of *Aspergillus niger* showing its septated branching hyphae contrasted with the nonseptated hyphal elements of *Pythium insidiosum. (Courtesy Jan Mucklestone.)*

Fluorescein-labeled *P. insidiosum* antiglobulin and immunoperoxide procedures are specific for the organism in tissues.

Serologic tests, such as enzyme-linked immunosorbent assay (ELISA) or immunodiffusion, are also diagnostic.[20] In the absence of a positive culture, polymerase chain reaction and a species-specific DNA probe from ribosomal DNA complex have proven useful in identifying *P. insidiosum.*

Treatment. Little information exists on the efficacy of therapy. Whether a single agent or combination of antimycotic agents can be curative has not been clearly established. Medical treatment alone for vascular and systemic involvement is ineffective.[89] Most patients require both extensive surgical treatment and medical treatment. Treatment results with conventional antimycotic medications, such as amphotericin B, have been contradictory. *Pythium sp.* do not possess ergosterol in their cytoplasmic membranes, so do not respond to medications directed against ergosterol. In vitro studies have recently identified minocycline and tigecycline as potentially effective therapies.[108,113] There are isolated case reports of successful treatment with itraconazole and terbinafine for 1 year.[158] Immunotherapy with *P. insidiosum*–antigen injection has been effective for complete or partial remission[182] following uncleared systemic infection treated with surgery or antimycotics.

Prevention. Given that pythiosis occurs in animals and humans that frequent aquatic habitats harboring *P. insidiosum,* awareness of the potential for infection should prompt avoidance of aquatic environs such as ponds, marshes, and bodies of water rich in plants or decaying organic material. Cleansing of lacerations or abrasions acquired in such environments should be prompt and thorough. If a cutaneous wound exists prior to entry into a body of water, protective covering is recommended.

BACTERIAL INFECTIONS

AEROMONAS HYDROPHILA INFECTIONS

The Aeromonads are inhabitants of brackish and freshwater. Currently, the four main species of *Aeromonas* are *A. hydrophila,*

A. caviae, A. salmonicida, and *A. sobria.* The spectrum of disease ranges from soft tissue infection to sepsis, and increasingly, diarrheal disease.

Definition

Aeromonas organisms are gram-negative, nonsporulating, facultative anaerobic bacilli. Formerly of the family Vibrionaceae, they have been reclassified as members of their own family, Aeromonadaceae. *A. hydrophila* have polar flagella.

Epidemiology and Risk Factors

These Aeromonads have a ubiquitous presence and can be found in a wide variety of aquatic environs, including brackish, fresh, bottled, chlorinated, well, and polluted waters. Entrance into soft tissue is gained through open wounds. Immunocompromised people more commonly develop serious complications, such as septicemia, meningitis, gastroenteritis, and pneumonia.[3]

Pathophysiology

A. hydrophila is the cause of most *Aeromonas* soft tissue infections. Pathogenicity results from production of the virulence factors cytotoxic enterotoxin (Act), heat-stable cytotoxic enterotoxin (Ast), and heat-labile cytotoxic enterotoxin (Alt). Hemolysins, aerolysins, and serine proteases are also present.[46]

Clinical Presentation

Cellulitis develops within 8 to 48 hours and may progress to focal, superficial, and cutaneous necrosis with purulent discharge (Figure 76-12), ecthyma gangrenosum–like cutaneous necrosis, fasciitis, myonecrosis, and osteomyelitis. On occasion, infections may be associated with gas production. Ecthyma gangrenosum and myonecrosis are uncommon and tend to occur in immunocompromised individuals.

Differential Diagnosis

A. hydrophila cutaneous infections must be differentiated from streptococcal or *Pseudomonas aeruginosa* cellulitis, abscesses, and septicemia with ecthyma gangrenosum. *Vibrio* and *Serratia* species mimic both environmental exposures and cutaneous manifestations of *Aeromonas* infections. Presented with an individual who has cellulitis secondary to a water-related injury, one must consider *Aeromonas* and *Vibrio* species infections. In the rare gas-producing infections, evaluate for other gas-producing organisms, such as *Clostridium* species.

Diagnostic Tests

Culture exudates and purulent material from wounds. Surgical samples of myonecrotic tissue should be cultured. Differentiation

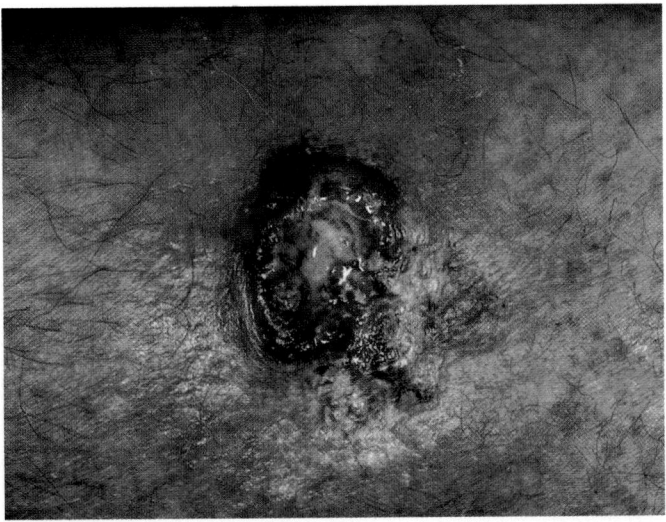

FIGURE 76-12 Trauma-induced necrotic ulcer of the anterior leg of a fisherman caused by *Aeromonas hydrophila*. *(Courtesy Edgar Maeyens, Jr., MD.)*

of *Aeromonas* from other gram-negative rods can be readily facilitated by culturing on blood agar containing ampicillin 10 or 30 μg/mL in a selective growth media or in cefsulodin-Irgasan-novobiocin agar.[82]

Treatment

Wounds should be drained and debrided as needed. *Aeromonas* species are all usually sensitive to third-generation cephalosporins, carbapenems, and aztreonam. Fluoroquinolones are highly active against *Aeromonas*.[179] Pertinent disease-producing *Aeromonas* species are resistant to early-generation penicillins and cephalosporins, such as amoxicillin-clavulanate and cephalexin, but are typically sensitive to piperacillin-tazobactam.[5] Resistance to trimethoprim-sulfamethoxazole, aminoglycosides, and tetracycline are increasingly being reported.[96]

Prevention

Do not enter any body of water with an open wound or abrasion. If skin trauma occurs while in fresh or brackish water, perform meticulous wound cleansing upon exiting. A prophylactic course of fluoroquinolones should be considered if there appear early signs of infection, such as erythema, purulence, or increasing pain.

CHROMOBACTERIUM VIOLACEUM INFECTIONS

The bacterium *Chromobacterium violaceum* rarely causes human disease, but can result in life-threatening sepsis with multiple metastatic abscesses. *C. violaceum* septicemia is clinically similar to melioidosis, the causative agent of which is *Burkholderia pseudomallei*.[80] Microscopically, *C. violaceum* can be confused with vibrios.

Definition

C. violaceum is found in water and soil. It is capable of producing skin abscesses, sepsis, and metastatic abscesses, and carries a mortality rate of greater than 50%. The mortality rate increases up to 75% to 80% for persons with septicemia or sepsis.[111,156,164]

Epidemiology and Risk Factors

C. violaceum is found in water and soil. It is abundantly present in the tropics and subtropics. More than three dozen cases have been reported in the United States, almost all from the southeast, primarily Florida.[137,164] Infections occur primarily in the summer months. Cases have been reported from Africa, India, South America, and Australia.[55,116] *C. violaceum* infects humans through exposure of nonintact skin to contaminated water and soil or after ingesting contaminated food or water.

Physiology

C. violaceum is a facultative, anaerobic, elongated, gram-negative bacillus that is slightly curved and therefore resembles the vibrios. It produces purple pigment (violacein), from which it derives its name. Violacein protects the microorganism's cell membrane from oxidation and peroxidation.[125] *C. violaceum* adapts well to either aerobic or anaerobic conditions because it has an efficient and flexible energy-generating metabolism. *C. violaceum* is also a reporter strain in quorum sensing.[110]

Clinical Presentation

The initial symptom is inflammation of soft tissue with or without adenopathy. Clinically, this manifests as cellulitis. As the infection progresses, there is focal abscess formation. Untreated, cellulitis rapidly progresses to sepsis and metastatic abscesses (Figures 76-13 and 76-14). The entire infectious process can occur suddenly, leading to a life-threatening situation. It is not unusual for *C. violaceum* infection to present as sepsis with fever, pneumonia, and spleen, liver, and lung abscesses.[116]

Differential Diagnosis

The initial stages of infection may resemble staphylococcal or streptococcal cellulitis. Cutaneous ulcerations are similar to those found in the diseases of leishmaniasis, melioidosis, and ulceroglandular tularemia and superficial infections caused by

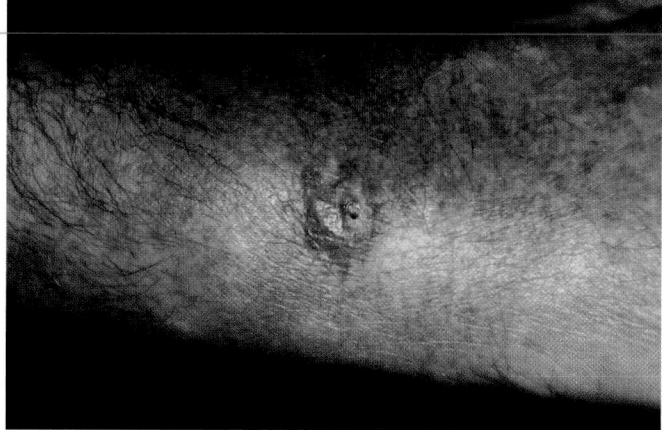

FIGURE 76-13 A minor abrasion while snorkeling led to this forearm infection with *Chromobacterium violaceum*. (*Courtesy Edgar Maeyens, Jr., MD.*)

Aeromonas and *Pseudomonas*. Systemic infection with *C. violaceum* must be differentiated from melioidosis.

Treatment

Although the optimal antibiotic therapy is not known, *C. violaceum* is typically susceptible to fluoroquinolones, tetracycline, imipenem, and trimethoprim-sulfamethoxazole.[102,157,195] It is resistant to penicillin and first-generation cephalosporins, and its susceptibility to third-generation cephalosporins is variable. Aztreonam (Azactam), a product of *C. violaceum*, is a monobactam antibiotic active against gram-negative bacteria and most strains of chromobacterium.[56]

Prevention

Avoid exposure to soil and/or stagnant or potentially contaminated water if there has been even a minor injury to the skin. If this is the situation, seek prompt medical attention at the first sign of cutaneous inflammation or purulence.

PSEUDOMONAS AERUGINOSA INFECTIONS

In 1850, Sèdillot noted blue-green discharges on infected surgical dressings. In 1925, Osler defined the organism as an opportunistic or secondary invader of damaged tissue. The name *aeruginosa* derived from cultured organisms having the color of verdigris, that is, the rust of copper or brass. *Pseudomonas aeruginosa* is one of the most serious sources of nosocomial bacterial infections.

Definition

P. aeruginosa is a ubiquitous, motile, nonfermentative, primarily aerobic, gram-negative rod.[1,77] Ultrastructurally, *P. aeruginosa* possesses a polar flagellum and many surface pili. Virtually all

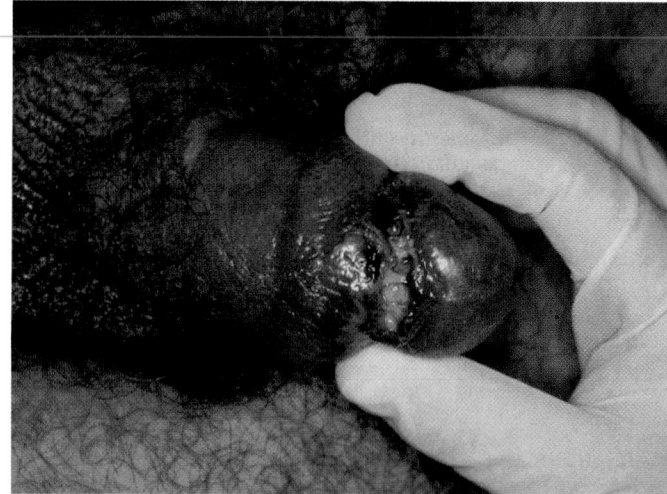

FIGURE 76-15 *Pseudomonas aeruginosa*. Primary infection of the penis in a young man with atopic dermatitis following hot tubbing. (*Courtesy Edgar Maeyens, Jr., MD.*)

strains produce an extracellular polysaccharide matrix necessary for biofilm formation.[149,172] It is a fastidious organism that survives extremes of temperature, under hostile conditions and with minimal nutritional support. It infects humans, other vertebrates, animals, and plants. The infection is often associated with moist conditions or environs. *Pseudomonas* skin infections can follow exposure to hot tubs, swimming pools, and whirlpools (Figures 76-15 and 76-16). *P. aeruginosa* is the most common cause of skin disorders in occupational saturation divers and can occur after recreational use of diving suits. Skin infection manifestations in these divers include folliculitis, abscesses (primarily of the head and neck), and otitis externa[1,99]

Epidemiology

P. aeruginosa, although primarily a nosocomial pathogen, grows in a wide variety of environments with minimal nutritional components.[127] It is commonly found in soil, water, and plants, but healthy humans and animals can be colonized. Up to 7% of healthy humans carry *P. aeruginosa* on their skin and in their nasal mucosa and throat. A rate of fecal carriage as high as 24% has been reported.[127]

Pathogenesis

Healthy humans are resistant to *Pseudomonas* skin infection. It is only when barrier functions of the skin are disrupted that *P. aeruginosa* organisms become invasive. *Pseudomonas* contains

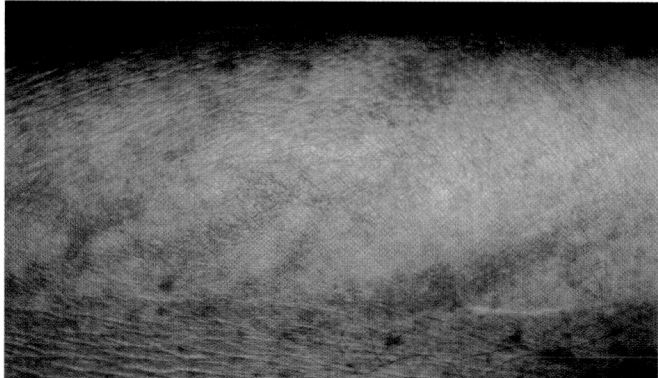

FIGURE 76-14 *Chromobacterium violaceum*. Lymphangitis of the forearm. (*Courtesy Edgar Maeyens, Jr., MD.*)

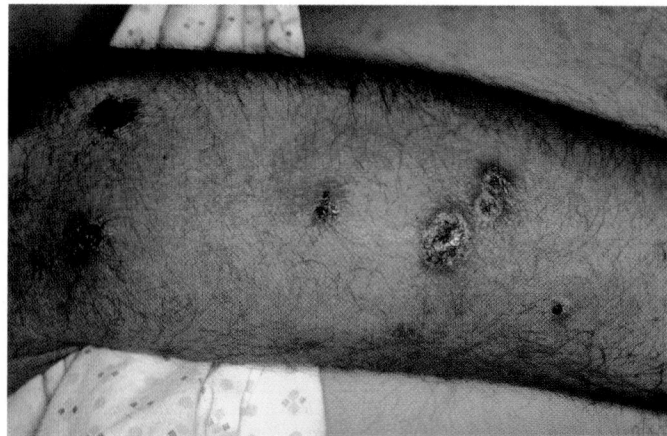

FIGURE 76-16 *Pseudomonas aeruginosa*. Primary infection of the forearm of a young man with atopic dermatitis following hot tubbing. (*Courtesy Edgar Maeyens, Jr., MD.*)

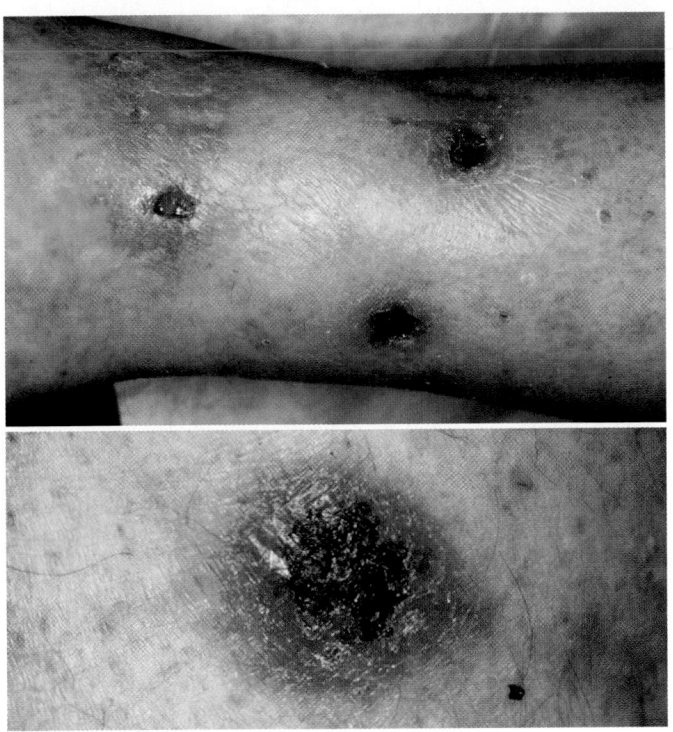

FIGURE 76-17 *Pseudomonas aeruginosa.* Discrete foci of necrotizing vasculitis (ecthyma gangrenosum) caused by *P. aeruginosa.*

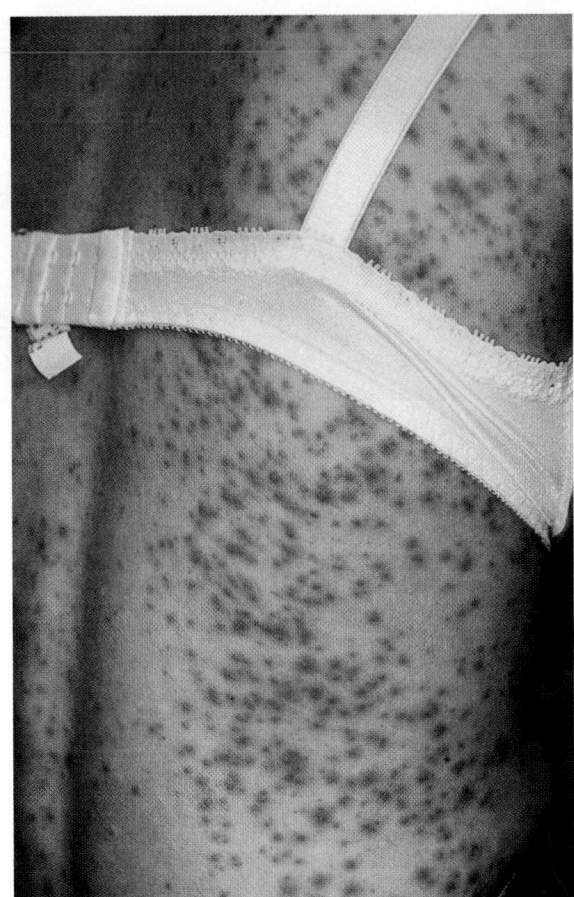

FIGURE 76-18 Hot tub folliculitis. *(Courtesy Edgar Maeyens, Jr., MD.)*

virtually all major classes of bacterial virulence systems and can potentially infect any site in the body. The virulence is in part determined by the status of the host resistance, such as the site of infection, comorbid conditions, and immune function. An example is ecthyma gangrenosum, which is cutaneous necrotizing vasculitis seen in persons with *P. aeruginosa* bacteremia (Figure 76-17).

Hot Tub Folliculitis

Definition. One of the more common types of cutaneous *Pseudomonas* infections is hot tub folliculitis, which is infection of the infundibuli of hair follicles by *P. aeruginosa.*

Epidemiology. This infection is seen most often following immersion in inadequately chlorinated whirlpools or hot tubs, but can occur following swimming or scuba diving, both of which produce hyperhydration and maceration of the epidermis that predispose to *Pseudomonas* colonization and invasion. Numerous cases of "hot tub" or "whirlpool" dermatitis have been described.[34,150,184] Eruptions can also occur after use of heated recreational water sources, such as swimming pools, water slides, and communal bathtubs. Contaminated bath toys, loofah sponges, moisturizing creams, and diving suits have been implicated as fomites in cases of *Pseudomonas* folliculitis.[23,59,61,77]

Pathophysiology. Histologically, an inflammatory response, primarily composed of polymorphonuclear leukocytes, surrounds and infiltrates the follicular epithelium. Clinically, this manifests as a pustule surmounting an erythematous papulonodule. Depending on the stage of evolution of this infection, purulence may or may not be present, and only inflammatory papulonodules may be evident (Figures 76-18 and 76-19). Histopathologically and microbiologically, this folliculitis rarely demonstrates the bacterium.

Clinical Presentation. The eruption is perifollicular in distribution and appears within 48 hours of exposure. It is most pronounced in the skin folds, trunk, buttocks, and proximal extremities, whereas the head and neck are typically spared.[154,198] The extent and severity of the eruption depend on the concentration of bacteria in the water source, duration of exposure time, presence or absence of preexisting skin disease, water temperature, and individual susceptibility. Pruritus and mild pain are common associated symptoms. Other symptoms include external

otitis, conjunctivitis, tender breasts, enlarged and tender lymph nodes, fever, and malaise.[77,151] Serious infections arise in immunocompromised and debilitated individuals. Rapid progression to severe systemic disease, as manifested by hemorrhagic bullae, pneumonia, or septicemia, suggests immunosuppression.[57,66,148]

Diagnostic Tests. Bacterial culture from a pustule helps to confirm the diagnosis, although clinical presentation is often sufficient.

Treatment. Hot tub folliculitis usually resolves spontaneously without therapy in 7 to 14 days. Keeping the skin dry and cool expedites resolution without formal therapy. Systemic infection may be treated with a fluoroquinolone (ciprofloxacin or levofloxacin), an antipseudomonal penicillin, antipseudomonal cephalosporin, carbapenems, or monobactams (e.g., aztreonam)

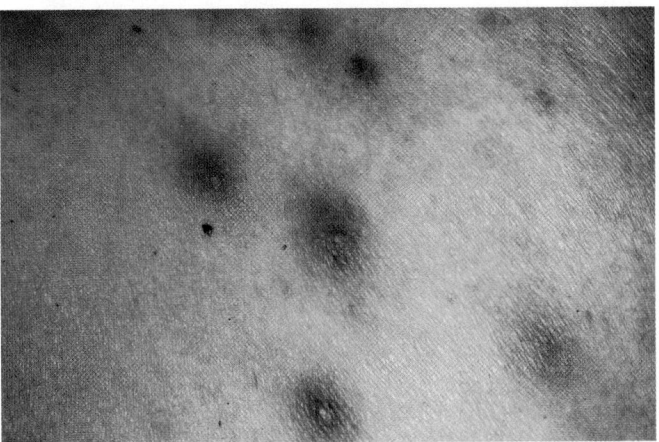

FIGURE 76-19 Hot tub folliculitis. *(Courtesy Edgar Maeyens, Jr., MD.)*

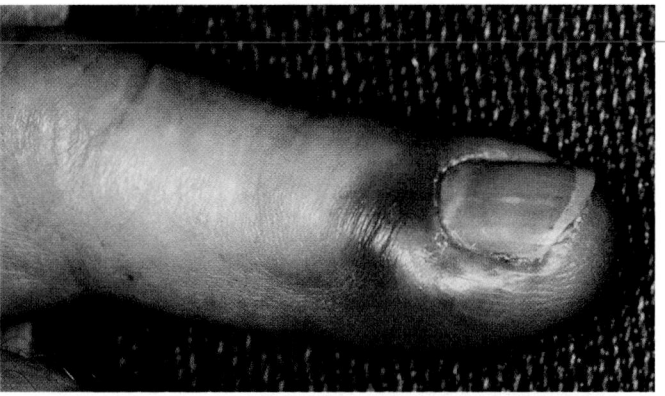

FIGURE 76-20 Green nail syndrome. Acute purulent *Pseudomonas aeruginosa* paronychia with early pigment formation.

as single agents. Aminogylcosides must be given in combination with another antibacterial agent for systemic infection.

Prevention. Prevention of *P. aeruginosa* infection requires either use of adequate disinfectant or avoidance of recreational closed-water systems and disinfection of reservoirs that are vehicles of transmission. Prompt drying of skin when exposed to wet, environmental conditions can prevent or at least minimize the degree of infection. Once colonization occurs, showering does not appear to prevent the disorder.[151]

Green Nail Syndrome

Definition. Green nail syndrome is defined as greenish-black discoloration of the nail plate secondary to the combination of pigments, pyocyanin, and pyoverdin synthesized by the bacterium *P. aeruginosa*.

Pathophysiology. Hydration of paronychial skin, usually with entry into the epidermal barrier, predisposes to colonization with *P. aeruginosa*. Infection follows, producing erythema, edema, pain, and discoloration of the adjoining nail plate. If the course of infection is prolonged, the infection extends into the hyponychium, at which point onycholysis occurs.

Among the many virulent factors of *P. aeruginosa* are pyocyanin. Pyocyanin damages cells by producing hydrogen peroxide and superoxide. These substances impart pigment to the nail plate and hyponychium. The typical discoloration of the nail plate seen in green nail syndrome is bluish-green and is the end point of the combination of two different pyocyanins (Figures 76-20 and 76-21). With loss of the epidermal barrier function in onycholysis, a polymicrobial infection may ensue.

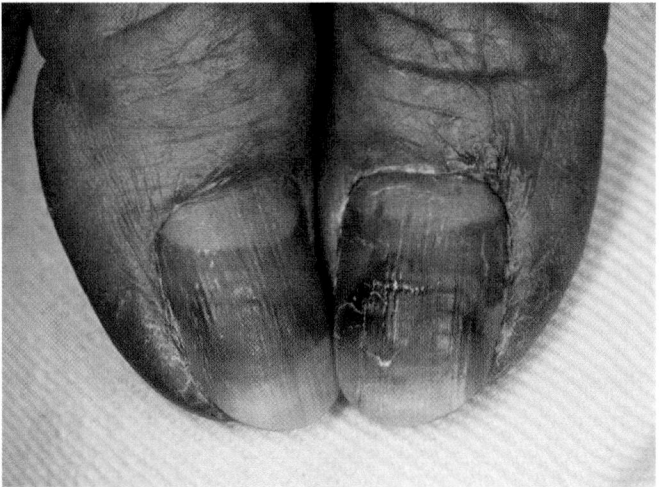

FIGURE 76-21 Green nail syndrome. Greenish-black discoloration of *Pseudomonas onychia*.

Risk Factors. Prolonged or frequent exposure to water, such as water sports, tending bar, and housecleaning, predisposes individuals to *Pseudomonas* paronychia, especially if the nails and the cuticles are poorly manicured.

Clinical Presentation. Infection is characterized by onycholysis and bluish-green discoloration of the nail plate with or without paronychia.[9] With paronychia, pain and swelling of nail fold tissue is the initial presentation. Occasionally, foci of purulence develop. If infection is not promptly treated, pigmentary changes within the nail plate appear and infection of the nail bed and matrix follow.

Differential Diagnosis. Without the pigmentary changes of the nail plate, diagnosis of *P. aeruginosa* as an etiologic agent is not clinically possible. Pseudomonal infection should be suspected if the patient has a history of abundant water exposure. Otherwise, consider *Staphylococcus* species, nonpseudomonal gram-negative organisms, or polymicrobial species as causes.

Diagnostic Tests. Culture purulence if present. No additional tests are needed once the pigmentary changes occur.

Treatment. Cessation of water exposure, debridement of the affected nail plate and subungual debris, and topical antibiosis effect resolution. Twice-a-day topical application of the antibiotics tobramycin ophthalmic solution or nadifloxacin cream, or soaks with antiseptics such as diluted acetic acid solution or 0.1% octenidine dihydrochloride solution are therapeutic options. To reduce swelling and erythema of the paronychium, application of a topical corticosteroid cream or ointment, such as clobetasol, is beneficial[10,140,146] (see Table 76-1).

Otitis Externa

Definition. Otitis externa is a general term that includes more than one inflammatory or infectious disease process of the external auditory canal or ear itself. Etiologically, it is rarely unifactorial. Contributing causes include inflammatory dermatoses such as seborrheic dermatitis and psoriasis; physical factors of trauma, heat, humidity, and moisture; and microbial exposure.[119] *Pseudomonas* is the most common causative microorganism.[183] Malignant otitis externa is an infection involving the external ear and skull base that can be life-threatening.

Epidemiology and Risk Factors. Any of the common causes of otitis externa are potentially worsened in an aquatic environment. For example, moisture, humidity, and heat are important predisposing factors for "swimmer's ear," which is characterized by erythema, edema, and pronounced dermatitis. Water encourages epidermal maceration, predisposing to secondary bacterial or fungal infection. According to Springer, freshwater is particularly prone to producing swimmer's ear.[168] Otitis externa does not appear to be associated with bacterial indicators of recreational water quality, such as fecal coliform bacteria or *Enterococcus* or *Pseudomonas* organisms.[30]

Diabetes mellitus and immunosuppression facilitate development of malignant otitis externa.[71]

Pathophysiology. The epidermis of the adult pinna and ear canal is normally as resistant to infection as is skin elsewhere. The adult ear canal is a cul-de-sac approximately 5 mm (0.2 inches) in diameter and 25 mm (1 inch) in length lined by stratified squamous epithelium.[183] The outer one-third of the canal produces cerumen, an acidic-waxy mantle mixed with sloughed epithelial cells. Cerumen is a physiologic barrier to infection. However, this barrier is not present to the same degree in the more delicate epithelium of the inner two-thirds of the ear canal. In addition, darkness and inaccessibility to air flow create an excellent milieu for certain microbial growth.

Interaction of moisture retention, moderate to high temperatures, and bacterial colonization predispose an individual to otitis externa (Figure 76-22). Other predisposing factors include canal occlusion by exostoses, cerumen plugs, ear plugs, and entrapped particles of sand; trauma related to mechanical attempts to clean the canal; intrinsic dermatoses; cerumen degradation; and pH variation above the normal pH of 4 to 5. Bacterial otitis externa is most often caused by *P. aeruginosa,* other gram-negative bacteria, and *Staphylococcus* species.

Clinical Presentation. Initial symptoms of otitis externa are pruritus of the ear canal, a sense of pressure or fullness within

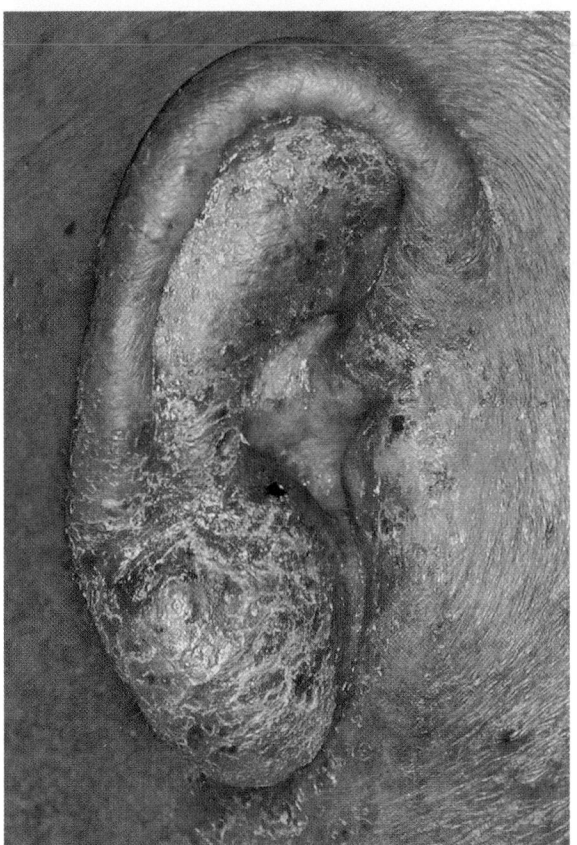

FIGURE 76-22 Otitis externa. The entire pinna is erythematous, edematous, scaly, and colonized by *Staphylococcus aureus*.

the canal, and diminished hearing. As inflammation progresses, the pain intensifies. Pain is elicited by applying pressure to the external auditory meatus or the tragus or by pulling on the lobule. Initially, there is a dermatitis, which if left untreated, is followed by progressive inflammation, edema, superficial fissures, serous exudate, and microbial overgrowth. Secondarily infected otitis externa may be associated with or progress to otitis media, canal occlusion, cervical lymphadenopathy, headache, nausea, fever, cellulitis, associated purulent discharge, and toxemia. Infection can extend to periauricular soft tissues, the parotid gland, and the temporomandibular joint. A condition called infectious eczematous dermatitis occurs when exudate from the infected ear canal discharges onto the surrounding skin of the neck or face, producing secondary infection or dermatitis of those areas.

Malignant otitis externa (Figure 76-23) usually manifests with severe pain and purulent discharge. Otologic examination reveals excessive granulation tissue at the junction of the cartilaginous and osseous components of the external auditory canal.[71] Infection penetrates the cartilage surrounding the external auditory canal and extends into the middle ear, mastoid air cells, and temporal bone. This is a severe and dangerous infection that could extend into the brain, producing thromboses of the venous sinuses and carotid artery, resulting in cerebral infarction.

Differential Diagnosis. Cholesteatomas are able to produce a thick, malodorous discharge that can be confused with infected otitis externa. Although *P. aeruginosa* and *S. aureus* are the predominant organisms producing infection, other bacteria and fungi can produce identical clinical presentations. These organisms include *Proteus mirabilis, Enterococcus faecalis, Bacteroides fragilis, Acinetobacter calcoaceticus, Aspergillus,* and *Candida*.[49,73,191,194]

Diagnostic Tests. Bacterial swab culture can help to identify causative bacteria; however, tissue biopsy culture may be indicated if swab culture–directed therapy is not diagnostic.

Treatment. The guiding principal of treatment of uncomplicated otitis externa is to treat with a topical anti-septic or antibiotic formulation and to combine this with a topical steroid to hasten reduction of associated itch or pain. Although numerous effective antimicrobial combinations will result in resolution in 1 to 2 weeks, common options include acetic acid (vinegar) in a 1:1 mixture with rubbing alcohol, Cortisporin Otic (generic form: neomycin/polymyxin B/hydrocortisone 1%) or 0.3% ofloxacin otic.[87,152] Note that patients should apply enough medicine to coat the ear canal and remain with their head in side tilt for 3 to 5 minutes. If the canal is edematous to the point of occlusion, a gauze wick soaked with the topical antibiotic ofloxacin otic should be inserted and kept in place for 24 to 72 hours. Systemic antibiotic use with a quinolone antibiotic, such as ciprofloxacin or ofloxacin, is only indicated when complications of cellulitis, adenopathy, fever, or profuse, purulent discharge are present. Antibiotics should be continued for at least 7 to 10 days in addition to topical therapy. Intravenous antibiotics are indicated when the infection worsens or does not respond to therapy within 48 hours.

For symptomatic control, analgesics are required for pain control, and short courses of systemic corticosteroids can reduce edema and any associated dermatitis. Before institution of corticosteroids, antibiotics must be started. For example, prednisone 40 mg daily for 4 days may be given simultaneously with the antibiotic.

Treatment of malignant otitis externa consists of debridement of all necrotic tissue, including cartilage and bone, plus administration of antipseudomonal antibiotics. The treatment of choice is IV ciprofloxacin, switched to oral ciprofloxacin, for 2 to 8 months once clinical markers improve.

An antipseudomonal beta-lactam antibiotic (piperacillin, piperacillin-tazobactam, ceftazidime, cefepime) may be indicated if ciprofloxacin resistance is present.[17]

Sequelae. Acquired atresia of the external auditory canal may rarely be a consequence of chronic otitis externa.

Prevention. Resolution of all existing dermatoses prior to water activities is recommended. One must thoroughly dry both the pinnae and ear canals after completion of aquatic activities. Seeking low-humidity environs will allow for continued epidermal water evaporation and drying. Rubbing alcohol applied directly to the ear canal facilitates water evaporation. Dilute acetic acid (vinegar 1 part to 3 parts water) ear rinses lower the pH of the auditory canal and discourage bacterial proliferation. When

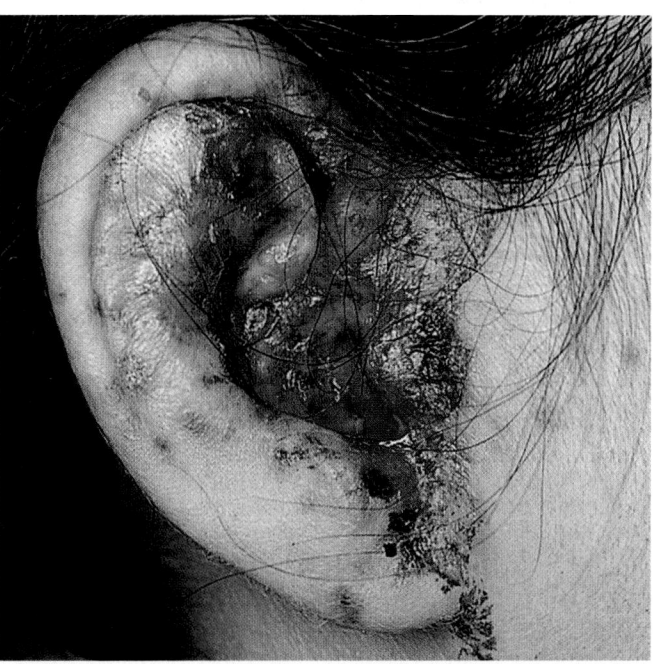

FIGURE 76-23 Malignant otitis externa. *(Courtesy Edgar Maeyens, Jr., MD.)*

available, blow-drying the canals with a hair dryer is very effective.

VIBRIO VULNIFICUS INFECTIONS

The bacteria *Vibrio vulnificus* is a part of normal marine flora and a recognized virulent pathogen. The organism has been isolated in warm (20°C [68°F] or warmer) coastal waters and in waters with salinity of 0.7% to 1.6%.[131] It is also found in brackish inland waters. *V. vulnificus* is detectable at high concentrations in filter-feeding sea life, such as aquatic animals, oysters, mussels, clams, scallops, and crabs, and also fish inhabiting coral reefs.[169]

Definition

V. vulnificus is a curved, flagellated, and gram-negative rod. The genus *Vibrio* is classified in the family Vibrionaceae, along with the genera *Photobacterium, Aeromonas,* and *Plesiomonas.* Infection with *V. vulnificus* can be localized to skin or be systemic.

Epidemiology and Risk Factors

Individuals develop cutaneous infection following contamination of a preexisting wound or as a result of an injury acquired while a person is exposed to warm, coastal waters. Primary bacteremia occurs following ingestion of raw or undercooked seafood, particularly oysters, without direct skin injury. Individuals who are especially at risk include those with liver disease and hemochromatosis, or chronic diseases, including diabetes mellitus and persons who are immunocompromised.[106]

Clinical Presentation

The course of the initial wound infection is erythema, edema, and pain that rapidly progresses to cellulitis with characteristic hemorrhagic bullae.[18] Primary bacteremia can result in metastatic cutaneous lesions that evolve into hemorrhagic bullae and necrotic ulcers.[48] Septicemia is virtually inevitable in the presence of fasciitis.

Pathophysiology and Histology

Skin lesions caused by *V. vulnificus* may, in part, be attributed to the destructive capabilities of enzymes released during infection. These enzymes are proteolytic, collagenolytic, and elastolytic. In the latter stages of cutaneous infection, there is intercellular edema and necrosis of the epidermis, dermis, and subcutaneous fat (Figure 76-24). The histopathologic features are infiltration of the dermis and subcutaneous tissues by a mixed inflammatory cell infiltrate composed of neutrophils, lymphocytes, and histiocytes, with areas of necrosis.

Differential Diagnosis

Staphylococcal and streptococcal infections induce identical patterns of cellulitis. Skin infections with *P. aeruginosa* and *Aeromonas* species mimic the hemorrhagic and necrotic lesions occurring in the later stages of *Vibrio* infection.

Diagnostic Tests

Culturing wound or bulla fluid is recommended. One should obtain blood cultures if the patient is febrile, has hemorrhagic bullae, or is septic.

Treatment

Because of the severity and rapid progression of *V. vulnificus* wound infections, prompt diagnosis plus antimicrobial therapy and early surgical debridement of necrotic tissue are recommended.[84] Fasciotomies are necessary to control infection in the presence of necrotizing fasciitis.[81] Despite prompt diagnosis and treatment, the mortality rate remains high, especially in people who are chronically ill, are immunologically compromised, or have liver disease. Favored treatment for serious skin infections or septicemia includes the use of a tetracycline analog and a third-generation cephalosporin antibiotic. Specific treatment options include combining doxycycline or minocycline (both 100 mg orally twice daily) with either IV ceftriaxone (1 g a day) or IV cefotaxime (2 g three times a day).[106] Alternately, levofloxacin 500 mg daily, intravenously or orally, may be

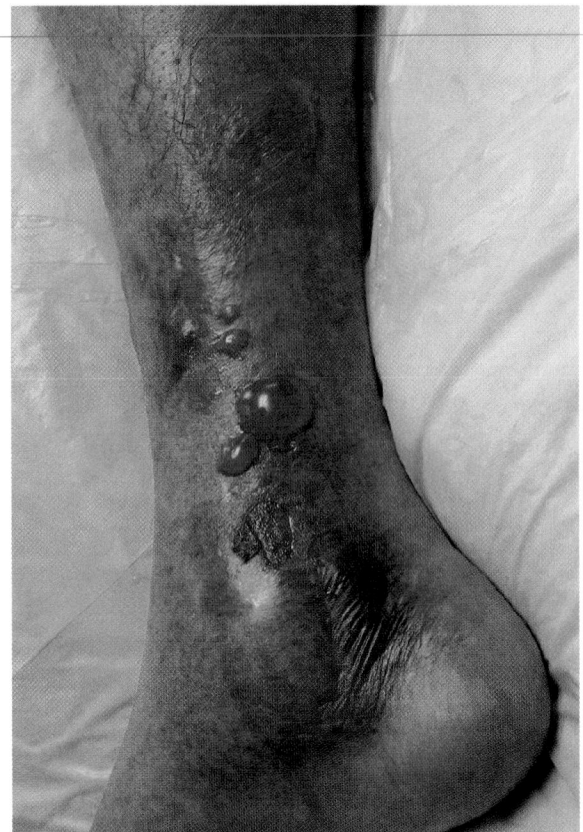

FIGURE 76-24 *Vibrio vulnificus* infection. Cellulitis with bullae and hemorrhage. *(Courtesy Sarah A. Wolfe, MD.)*

given.[42] For minor, localized wound infections, oral treatment with a tetracycline or fluoroquinolone is sufficient.

Prevention

Avoid entering warm coastal waters with a preexisting skin wound. Promptly attend to any injury acquired in an aquatic environment with meticulous wound care. Persons with known risk factors should avoid eating undercooked seafood, especially oysters.

SHEWANELLA PUTREFACIENS INFECTIONS

The taxon *Shewanella* species contains, among others, two bacteria known to be human pathogens. These are *Shewanella algae* and *Shewanella putrefaciens.* Key characteristics of these gram-negative, mobile rods are production of hydrogen sulfide gas on triple sugar iron (TSI) slants, positive catalase and oxidase reactions, and release of trimethylamine as it participates in the decay of rotting fish.[90]

Definition

S. putrefaciens is a member of the family Vibrionaceae. It is most frequently recovered from aquatic reservoirs (freshwater, marine water, and sewage), fish, and aquatic animals, but can also be found in poultry, beef, dairy products, soil, oil emulsions, natural gas, and oil fields.[155] *S. algae* is a tetrodotoxin-producing isolate recovered from red algae.[160] This group of bacteria infrequently is the cause of cutaneous and systemic disease in humans.

Pathophysiology

S. putrefaciens produces the extracellular enzymes DNAase, lipase, and lecithinase.[160] Other enzymatic activities detected among select *Shewanella* isolates include tyrosine alkyl sulfatase, elastase, and chitinase.[90] The exact role of these enzymes in human disease can at best be inferred. Chen suggests possible exotoxin involvement in *S. putrefaciens* cellulitis.[41] *S. putrefaciens* is frequently found in association with other bacterial pathogens, rendering its pathogenic role unclear.[43,90] This bacterium produces trimethylamine as it participates in the decay of rotting fish; hence, the name putrefaciens, meaning putrid.[121]

Clinical Presentation

Skin and soft tissue manifestations include wound infections, cellulitis, dacryocystitis, and otitis externa.

Risk Factors

Persons with underlying diseases, such as hepatobiliary disease, malignancy, or renal failure, or those who are immunocompromised are at risk for bacteremia and fulminant illness. The course of localized skin infections is believed to proceed from colonization to invasion, especially in individuals with open wounds.[197] Tissues with compromised circulation are predisposed to infection with *Shewanella* species.

Differential Diagnosis

Clinically, there is nothing unique about cutaneous infections with *S. putrefaciens* or *S. algae*. They often manifest as necrotic areas with marked inflammation and necrosis not dissimilar to other gram-negative soft tissue infections. Therefore, deciphering these organisms from other gram-negative infections is necessary for proper treatment. *Vibrio vulnificus* and *Aeromonas* species should be considered with a rapidly progressive soft tissue infection. *Pseudomonas* species are the organisms most frequently mistaken for *Shewanella* using routine bacterial culture techniques.

Diagnostic Tests

Obtain routine specimens for Gram's stain, culture, and sensitivity. Colonies in culture have a pink water-soluble pigment or reddish-tan color. However, specific microbiologic laboratory testing is necessary for differentiation of *Shewanella* species. Automated identification systems are unable to differentiate between *S. putrefaciens* and *S. algae,* because *S. algae* is not included in these systems' databases. Retrospectively, it has become apparent that most *Shewanella* infections that had been previously attributed to *S. putrefaciens* were actually caused by *S. algae.* Species differentiation of *S. algae* and *S. putrefaciens* can be obtained with extensive phenotypic characterization.[78] Use of 16S rRNA gene sequence analysis correctly identifies the species.[22]

Treatment

Shewanella species are usually susceptible to levofloxacin, aminoglycosides, most third- and fourth-generation cephalosporins, and piperacillin.[174]

Prevention

If a person is immunocompromised, exposure to aquatic environments presents a potential for infection. Open wounds should be protected from exposure to freshwater lakes and oceans.

MYCOBACTERIUM MARINUM INFECTIONS

Mycobacterium marinum is a nontuberculous mycobacterium commonly recognized as the etiologic agent of "fish tank" or "swimming pool granuloma."[26] Most infections manifest 2 to 3 weeks after contact with contaminated water. Infections are localized primarily to skin.

Definition

M. marinum is found in freshwater and saltwater environs. It is an acid-fast, rod-shaped bacillus of Runyon group 1 and is a photochromogen producing yellow pigment when cultured and exposed to light. In contradistinction to *Mycobacterium tuberculosis,* which cannot multiply outside of the host, *M. marinum* is a free-living soil and water saprophyte. It is an infrequent human pathogen.

Epidemiology and Risk Factors

Persons at risk for infection with *M. marinum* are those who incur trauma while in contact with fresh or marine water, marine

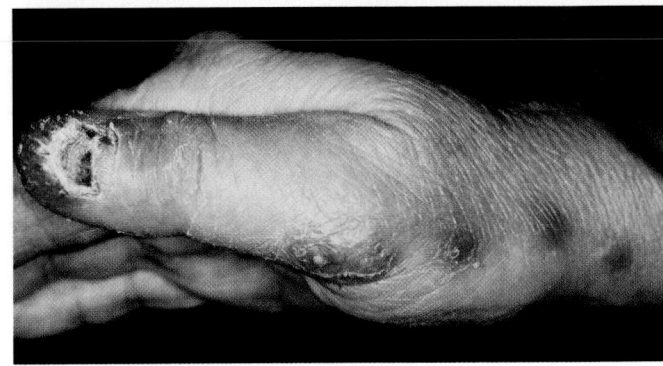

FIGURE 76-25 *Mycobacterium marinum* nodular lymphangitis.

animals, or aquariums. Tap water is considered to be a reservoir for most nontuberculous mycobacteria, where they may be present as a biofilm.[64] Immunosuppression predisposes an individual to a more aggressive cutaneous infection and systemic dissemination.

Pathophysiology

Because the optimal temperature range for growth in tissues is 31° to 32°C (87.8° to 89.6°F), cooler extremities are infected more often than are warmer body sites. *M. marinum* is capable of growing at temperatures as high as 37°C. An example of this is their ability to cause systemic infection in persons who are immunocompromised.[88] At the time of inoculation, *Mycobacteria* are phagocytized by macrophages. The organisms are either destroyed by macrophages or escape extracellularly to spread cell to cell. Cytokines, such as tumor necrosis factor (TNF), facilitate destruction of the bacterium. In the absence of TNF, *Mycobacteria* are engulfed by macrophages but not destroyed.[50]

Clinical Presentation

Within 2 to 3 weeks of inoculation into skin, a papule, nodule, or shallow ulceration develops. The upper extremities are the most commonly involved sites. Lesional pain and induration are common. As the inflammatory process progresses, nodules predominate over ulcerations. There may be progression of nodules along lymphatics in up to 50% of infections. Lymphatic distribution of nodules is called "sporotrichoid" because of the resemblance to sporotrichosis (Figures 76-25 to 76-29). Lymphadenopathy is inconsistent in its occurrence. Extracutaneous infections include septic arthritis, bursitis, osteomyelitis, and tenosynovitis. Dissemination to viscera or bone marrow is rare. Immunocompromised individuals are those most at risk for development of disseminated infection with fever and lymphadenopathy.

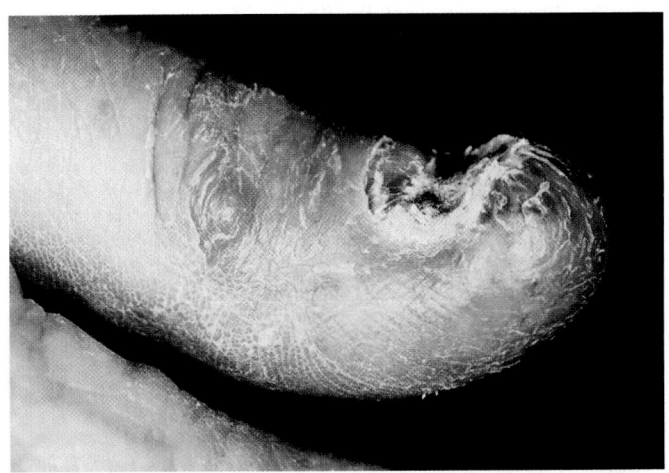

FIGURE 76-26 Dermatitis-like initial infection with *M. marinum*.

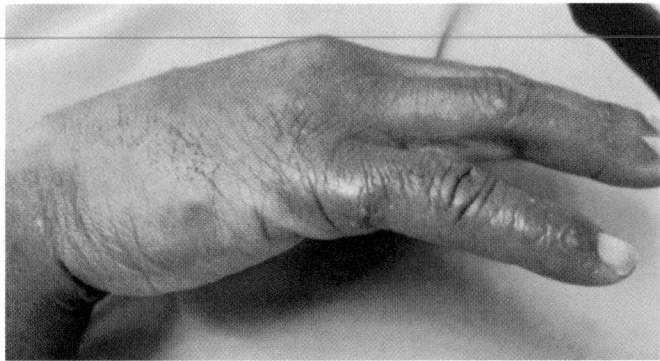

FIGURE 76-27 The granulomatous nodules of *M. marinum* lymphangitis following infection of the fingertip. *(Courtesy Sarah A. Wolfe, MD.)*

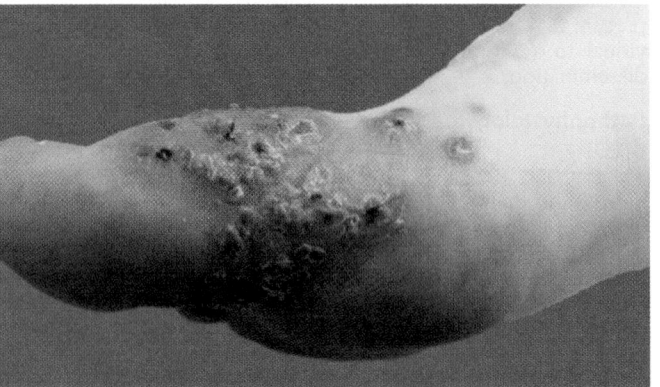

FIGURE 76-28 Vesicular eruption at site of inoculation with *Mycobacterium marinum*. *(Courtesy Jessica Kim So, MD.)*

Differential Diagnosis

The following diseases share morphologic similarities to cutaneous *M. marinum* infections: sporotrichosis, sarcoidosis, nocardiosis, tularemia, cutaneous protothecosis, leprosy, leishmaniasis, cowpox, verrucae vulgaris, iododerma, bromoderma, chronic pyogenic infections, and other cutaneous mycobacterioses.

Diagnostic Tests

Diagnosis of *M. marinum* infection is confirmed by tissue biopsy culture grown on standard *Mycobacterium* culture medium (Lowenstein-Jensen) at 30° to 32°C (86° to 89.6°F), or more rapidly by polymerase chain reaction where testing is available.[52,139] Histopathologically, acid-fast bacilli are visualized in only 10% to 13% of biopsies. Approximately 70% to 80% of tissue cultures are positive (Figure 76-30). Skin tests show cross-reactivity between *M. marinum* and *M. tuberculosis*.

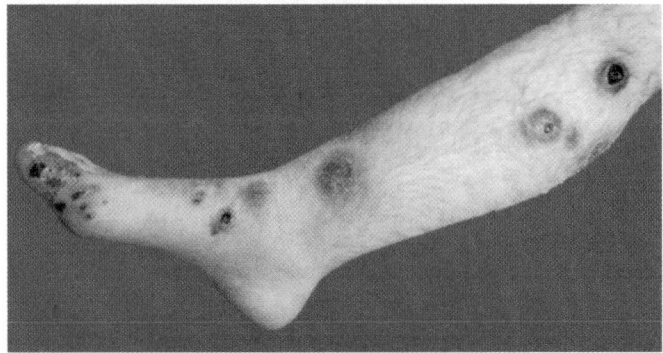

FIGURE 76-29 Lymphocutaneous (sporotrichoid) spread of *Mycobacterium marinum*. *(Courtesy Jessica Kim So, MD.)*

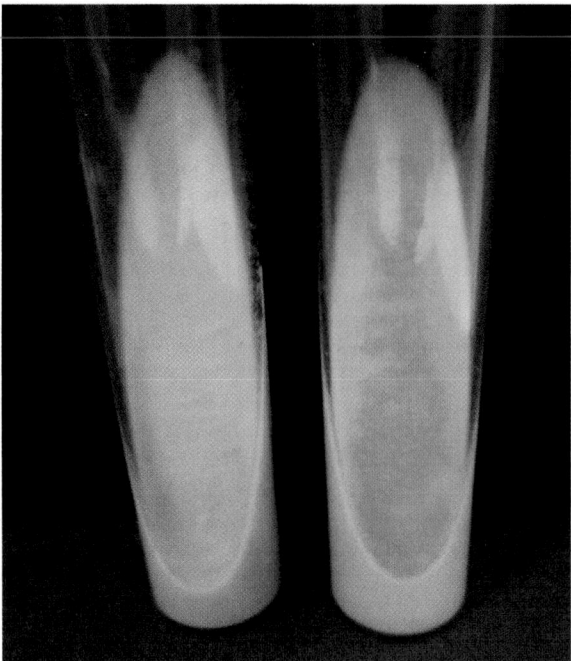

FIGURE 76-30 Tissue cultures grew smooth photochromogenic colonies supportive of a diagnosis of *Mycobacterium marinum*. **A**, photoprotected cultures grew buff-colored colonies. **B**, cultures exposed to light grew colonies producing yellow pigment. *(Courtesy Jessica Kim So, MD.)*

Treatment

There is no consensus on treatment, and *M. marinum* has a natural pattern of multidrug resistance.[6] Most cases of *M. marinum* are treated empirically because routine antibiotic susceptibility testing is not available in most laboratories. Testing may be necessary, however, following months of treatment failures. Successful monotherapy for focal soft tissue infections includes clarithromycin, minocycline, doxycycline, amikacin, and sulfamethoxazole.[6,192] For treatment failure or more extensive infection, combination treatment may be warranted.[139] Options include clarithromycin plus ethambutol, ethambutol plus rifampin, or a combination that includes a tetracycline. High resistance to doxycycline has been reported in Taiwan.[192] Treatment is recommended for 1 to 2 months beyond clinical clearance; for most, this equates to 3 to 4 months total. Involvement of deeper structures, such as joints, tendons, or bone, may require months longer. Surgical debridement may be beneficial in cases of treatment failure or when closed spaces of the hand are involved, although appropriateness of this modality has not been well studied.

Prevention

Cognizance of the potential for *M. marinum* infection in aquatic environments, avoidance of entry into such environments when skin wounds are present, and prompt attention/hygiene to wounds sustained while in an aquatic environment will help avoid infection.

MELIOIDOSIS

Melioidosis, also called Whitmore's disease, was first described by the pathologist Alfred Whitmore as a "glander-like" disease among drug addicts in Rangoon, Burma.[140] This name is derived from the Greek *Melis* (distemper of asses) and *Eidos* (resemblance).[130] Once solely perceived as an esoteric tropical disease, melioidosis is now increasingly recognized as an important public health problem worldwide. *Burkholderia pseudomallei* is the causative agent.

Definition

B. pseudomallei are small, gram-negative, oxidase-positive, aerobic, and mobile bacilli that reside in soil and water. The entry

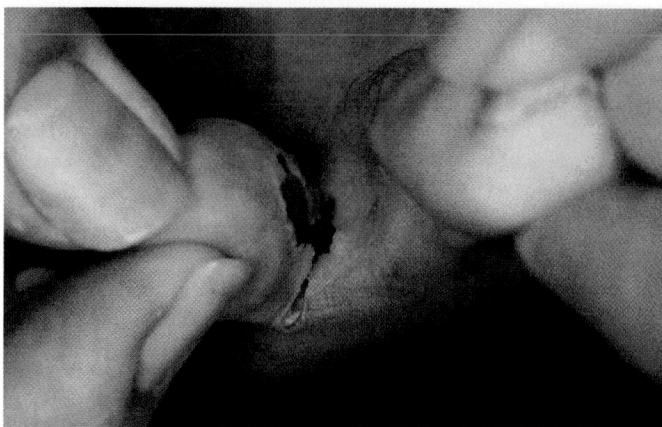

FIGURE 76-31 Melioidosis. Foot web space infection with *Burkholderia pseudomallei*.

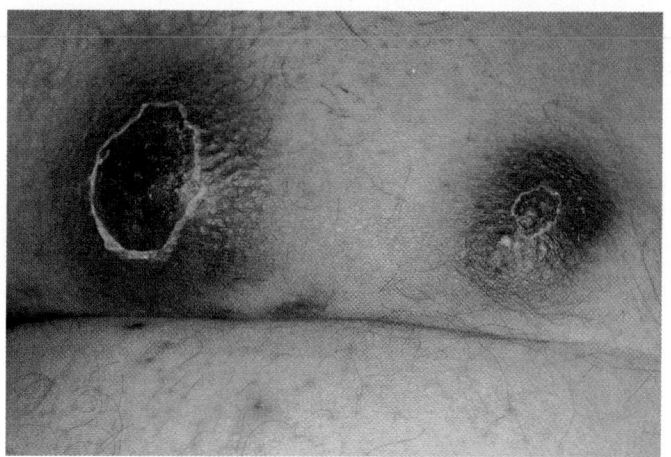

FIGURE 76-33 Melioidosis. Cutaneous abscesses in an individual with chronic melioidosis.

sites for infection are primarily percutaneous and via inhalation. Common disease manifestations include pneumonia and cutaneous disease, but infection may extend to multiple organs, including the central nervous system. The mortality rate is as high as 40% in endemic areas.[186] This section focuses on cutaneous disease.

Epidemiology and Risk Factors

Although northern Australia and Southeast Asia are recognized as highly endemic, cases have also been reported in the Indian subcontinent, China and Taiwan, the Indian Ocean islands, the Americas, and Africa.[104,186] Risk factors for infection include diabetes, heavy alcohol use, chronic lung disease, chronic kidney disease, and, less frequently, thalassemia, glucocorticoid therapy, and cancer.[52,105] Infection is more common in adults than children; however, children are more likely than adults to develop primary cutaneous melioidosis.[120]

Localized Form. *B. pseudomallei* enter the skin through any type of breach in the epidermal barrier or via a laceration. Mucous membranes may occasionally be a site of entry. After entry into the skin, acute inflammation is followed by cellulitis and then abscess formation, ulceration, and lymphadenitis (Figure 76-31). Rarely, superficial soft tissue infection can progress to necrotizing fasciitis or a cutaneous granulomatous reaction mimicking mucormycosis[189] (Figure 76-32).

Chronic Form. Chronic melioidosis characteristically presents as multiple abscesses widely disseminated to organ systems that include the spleen, liver, muscles, or skin (Figure 76-33). This form of the disease can reactivate many years after the primary infection. Draining sinuses from lymph nodes or bones may develop.

Differential Diagnosis

Cutaneous lesions must be differentiated from those of *Staphylococcus* species, *Streptococcus* species, *Pseudomonas* species, varicella-zoster virus, *Bacillus anthracis* bacteria (the cause of anthrax), and variola virus.

Diagnostic Tests

Gram's staining of skin abscesses and sputum show small, gram-negative bacilli; the bacilli look like bipolar safety pins when stained with Wright or methylene blue stains. Culture is the gold standard for diagnosis. The medium used for culture is Ashdown agar, but *B. cepacia* selective agar is an effective substitute if the Ashdown agar is not available.[135] Other tests include polymerase chain reaction assays, direct immunofluorescence microscopy, and enzyme immunoassays, but each is less sensitive than culture.[79,123,193]

Treatment

Treatment requires an initial intensive therapy with IV antibiotics for at least 10 days followed by oral eradication therapy for 3 months at a minimum. The intensive therapies of choice are ceftazidime, meropenem, or imipenem.[39,44,161] The addition of trimethoprim-sulfamethoxazole during treatment with ceftazidime may be beneficial for severe disease.[167] Trimethoprim-sulfamethoxazole is the best antibiotic for eradication therapy.[51] In pediatric cases verified to have localized skin infection, oral treatment alone with high-dose trimethoprim-sulfamethoxazole plus folic acid for 3 months has resulted in clearance.[120]

Prevention

There is no vaccine for melioidosis. Individuals with skin lesions, diabetes mellitus, renal failure, immune deficiencies, and chronic lung disease should avoid contact with soil or standing water, especially in endemic disease areas. In health care settings, use blood and body fluid precautions.

ERYSIPELOTHRIX RHUSIOPATHIAE (ERYSIPELOID)

Erysipelothrix rhusiopathiae, formerly known as *Erysipelothrix insidiosa*, is a gram-positive bacterium that causes an infection of skin known as erysipeloid. In 1909, Rosenbach isolated the organism from a patient with a cutaneous lesion.[143] Rosenbach labeled the infection erysipeloid to differentiate it from erysipelas, a cellulitis caused by group A streptococci.[142]

Definition

E. rhusiopathiae is an aerobic or facultatively anaerobic, nonmobile, non–spore-forming, and gram-positive bacillus. It is found worldwide as a commensal or pathogen in many invertebrate and vertebrate species.[143] The primary terrestrial reservoir is domestic swine.[143]

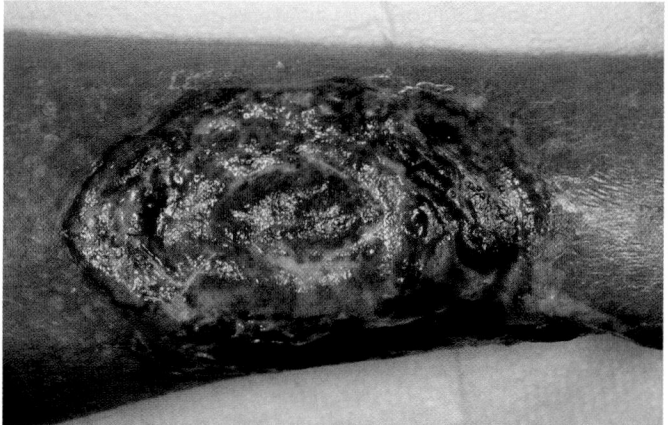

FIGURE 76-32 Melioidosis. An exuberant granulomatous infection caused by *Burkholderia pseudomallei* clinically mimicking mucormycosis.

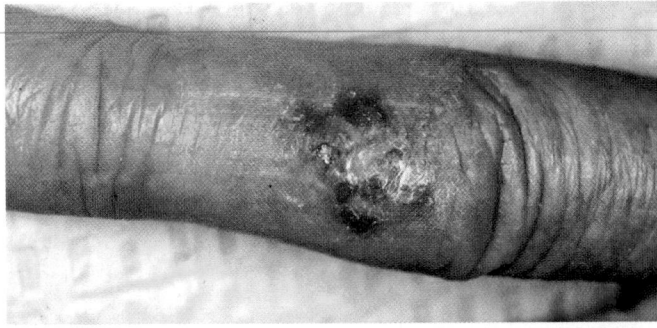

FIGURE 76-34 *Erysipelothrix rhusiopathiae.* Early skin lesion of *E. rhusiopathiae* with central pallor and raised, marginated, erythematous borders.

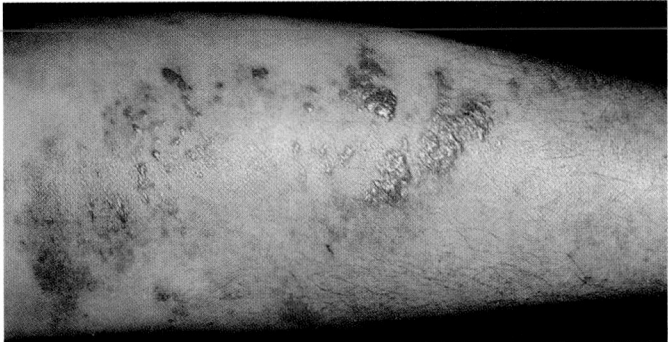

FIGURE 76-36 *Erysipelothrix rhusiopathiae* infection. *(Courtesy Edgar Maeyens, Jr., MD.)*

Epidemiology

In the aquatic environment, *E. rhusiopathiae* inhabits the exterior mucoid slime of fish and can be cultured from the skin of mammals, such as whales. Direct contact with marine animals is one source of infection. Persons at greatest risk are fisherman, fish handlers, butchers, slaughterhouse workers, and so forth.[142] *E. rhusiopathiae* can survive 12 days in sunlight, 4 months in putrefied flesh, and 9 months in buried carcasses.

Pathophysiology

E. rhusiopathiae gains entrance into the skin via abrasions or puncture wounds. Hyaluronidase, neuraminidase, and surface proteins are its virulence factors.[159] Having an ability to evade phagocytosis and to replicate intracellularly facilitates *E. rhusiopathiae* pathogenicity.[67]

Clinical Presentation

Erysipeloid has three clinical presentations in humans: localized cutaneous, diffuse cutaneous, and generalized or systemic.

In the localized cutaneous (erysipeloid) form, *E. rhusiopathiae* enters the skin through a puncture wound or abrasion, usually of the finger or hand. One to 7 days later, the lesion begins as a minor, purple-red irritation or infected paronychia with edema and a small amount of purulent discharge. Characteristically, the peripheral edge of the lesion spreads slowly with central fading (clearing), resulting in a well-demarcated, erythematous or violaceous ring[93] (Figure 76-34). The infected site is typically warm and edematous with associated pruritus and pain. There is often proximal progression along the dorsal edge of the finger into the web space and then distally along the adjoining finger. Suppuration is absent. Infection seldom occurs on the palm. Although the infection is generally limited to the hand (Figure 76-35), it may spread to the wrist and forearm.[94] Regional, painful

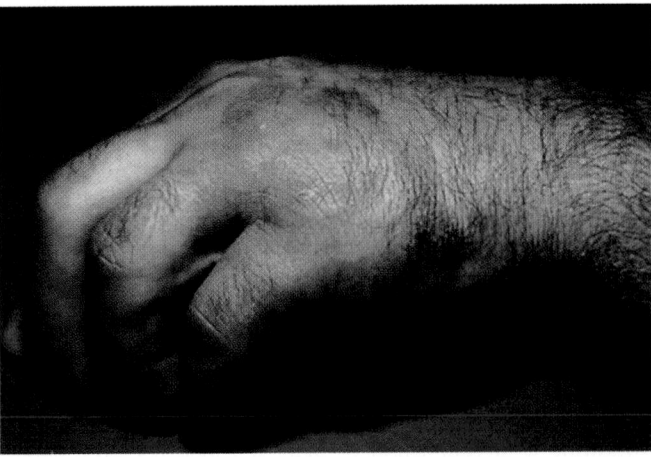

FIGURE 76-35 Typical appearance of *Erysipelothrix* skin infection. *(Courtesy Paul S. Auerbach, MD.)*

lymphadenopathy is present in a third of patients; low-grade fever and arthralgias are less common.[130]

In the diffuse cutaneous form, the infection progresses proximally from the initial site to involve remote areas of the body or multiple areas regionally[69] (Figure 76-36). Fever and adenopathy are common, blood cultures are negative, and the course is more protracted than the localized form.

Systemic involvement with *E. rhusiopathiae* infection is rare. Endocarditis is the most common sequela of systemic erysipeloid and carries a mortality risk approaching 40%.[67] In systemic *E. rhusiopathiae* infection, characteristic skin lesions may be present in 40% of patients.

Differential Diagnosis

Staphylococcal or streptococcal cellulitis is the most frequent simulator. Vibrios and *Shewanella putrefaciens* also cause cellulitis.

Diagnostic Tests

For a definitive diagnosis of infection with *Erysipelothrix*, isolation of the organism is required. Biopsy specimens of infected tissues and/or blood cultures enable isolation of *E. rhusiopathiae* by routine culture techniques. No serologic tests are available.

Treatment

Although erysipeloid usually is self-limited and runs its course within 3 weeks, resolution is facilitated by antibiotic therapy. Most strains are susceptible to penicillins, cephalosporins, ciprofloxacin, clindamycin, and imipenem.[177] For isolated skin involvement, the first-line treatment is with penicillin V 500 mg orally every 6 hours or cephalexin 500 mg orally four times a day for 7 days. Alternatively, ciprofloxacin 250 mg orally twice a day for 7 days is rapidly effective.[12] *E. rhusiopathiae* is resistant to vancomycin, aminoglycosides, chloramphenicol, erythromycin, and trimethoprim-sulfamethoxazole. If arthritis, septicemia, or endocarditis is present, aqueous penicillin G should be administered in a dose of 2 to 4 million units intravenously every 4 hours for 4 to 6 weeks,[138] although oral therapy may be initiated after 2 weeks in patients who do not have endocarditis.

Prevention

Wearing protective clothing and gloves is recommended whenever handling marine mammal skin or body parts. Handle fish with care so as not to be punctured by their spines or lacerated by their scales.

MYCOPLASMA INFECTIONS

Seal Finger

Mycoplasma species are the smallest free-living organisms colonizing animal, plant, and insect kingdoms.[141] They are prokaryocytes lacking cell walls. *Mycoplasma* devolved from gram-positive bacteria through reductive evolution.[141] When initially discovered, they were believed to be viruses.

Definition. Seal finger is the sobriquet given to a unique infection, usually of a digit, acquired by exposure to pinnipeds

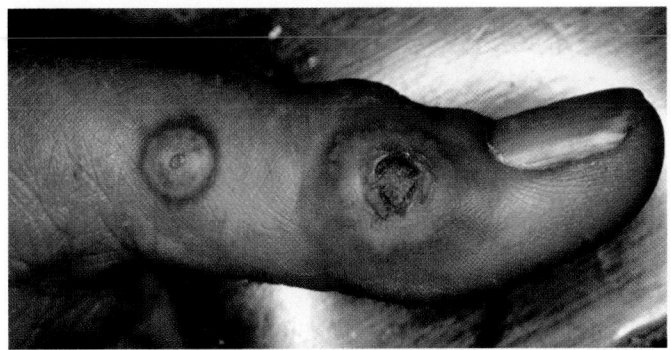

FIGURE 76-37 Seal finger secondary to *Mycoplasma*. *(Courtesy Edgar Maeyens, Jr., MD.)*

(seals, walruses, and sea lions).[180] It is believed that *Mycoplasma* inoculation occurs following direct contact with the skin or mucous membranes of one of these animals. Infection sites, most frequently the digits, become swollen and very painful. If the soft tissue infection is not treated promptly, tenosynovitis, bone marrow edema, periarticular osteoporosis, and interphalangeal effusion may occur.[115]

Pathophysiology. The disorder is believed to be secondary to infection with *Mycoplasma* strains *Mycoplasma phocacerebrale* and *Mycoplasma phocarhinis,* which were initially isolated from seals.[180] These strains are new species of *Mycoplasma* unique to seals and possibly other pinnipeds.[72] Some believe that these *Mycoplasma* species may be part of the normal flora of seals.[72] Several species of *Mycoplasma* are commensals in the animal's genitourinary tract and in the human oral cavity and genital mucosa.[15] Toll-like receptors interact with *Mycoplasma,* provoking an inflammatory response.[112] Antigen-antibody reactions or inflammatory cytokines result in cytolysis.

Clinical Presentation. Clinical manifestations begin after an incubation period of a few hours to 3 to 4 days, although some report an incubation period of 1 to 15 days.[11] Initially, an inflammatory papule rapidly develops into a nodule with swelling, slight purulence, and severe pain (Figure 76-37). Edema and stiffness of the digit are common sequelae.[54,117] If joint involvement occurs, it is usually in the joint nearest the site of entry of the organism.[72] Untreated, atrophy of cartilage, bone resorption, and, ultimately, arthrosis develop.[117] Secondary bacterial infection may occur in skin lesions, producing purulence and lymphangitis. Fever and leukocytosis may accompany the infection. Seal finger can resolve spontaneously with few or no sequelae or can last for several months. No immunity is conferred.[117]

Differential Diagnosis. Presentation can be with edema and erythema, both local and diffuse, resembling erysipeloid or cellulitis as seen with infection by *V. vulnificus.* The edema of erysipeloid is more pronounced than that of seal finger. Atypical mycobacterial infection may mimic seal finger, but produces much less pain in the initial inflammatory phase.

Parapoxvirus infection most closely resembles seal finger. Viruses within this group include the orf and paravaccinia viruses. Both of these viruses produce pustulovesicular lesions.

Orf virus infection is acquired from sheep (orf), whereas the paravaccinia virus is acquired from cows (milker's nodules). Tanapox virus, a monkey virus, can cause solitary nodules similar to those seen with seal finger. Herpetic whitlow not only resembles seal finger morphologically but is as painful. Bacterial furunculosis and an inflammatory response to foreign bodies must be considered.

Risk Factors. Frequent or prolonged exposure to marine mammals, direct contact with live marine mammals, and contact with secretions, excretions, blood, or tissue will increase the opportunity for trauma and infection.

Diagnostic Tests. Because of its small size, *Mycoplasma* cannot be visualized with routine microscopy. One can acquire material for culture, but the organism has very fastidious growth requirements and is very difficult to grow in a cell-free medium.

Specimens for culture should not be allowed to desiccate. If culture material cannot be transported to a diagnostic laboratory immediately on collection, it should be frozen at −70° C (−94° F).[180] If available, molecular-based systems, such as polymerase chain reaction and enzyme-linked immunosorbent assays, can identify *Mycoplasma.*

Treatment. After contact with marine animals or bites from handling marine animals, especially pinnipeds, cleanse the wounds thoroughly with soap and water. If signs of infection occur, treat with tetracycline. Tetracycline is given orally at 500 mg four times a day for 4 to 6 weeks.[72] The sooner that therapy is begun, the greater the chance for resolution of infection and prevention of joint involvement.

Prevention. Be aware of the potential for infection when handling pinnipeds or their by-products. Practice good hygiene by wearing gloves, and washing with soap and water after each exposure. If the skin is damaged while handling pinnipeds, seek immediate medical attention and start empirical treatment with tetracycline.

PARASITES

ANISAKIDOSIS

Definition

Anisakidosis, formerly known as anisakiasis, is caused by accidental ingestion of larval nematodes of the family Anisakidae, which include *Anisakis* and *Pseudoterranova* in raw fish and cephalopods.[98]

Epidemiology and Risk Factors

Anisakis simplex is a parasitic nematode of several marine organisms. Accidental ingestion by humans eating raw fish, cephalopods, or undercooked fish can lead to infestation.[35]

Pathophysiology and Clinical Presentation

Adult stages of *A. simplex* and *Pseudoterranova decipiens* reside in the mucosa of stomachs of marine mammals. It is from here that unembryonated eggs produced by adult females pass into the feces of their hosts. In the water, eggs become free-swimming larvae. Larvae ingested by crustaceans morph a third time, becoming infective to predators. Humans ingesting these fishes and manifesting symptoms will often have larvae infiltrating the mucosal linings of their stomachs. Larvae rarely actually then develop in humans. Instead, once embedded in the gastric or intestinal mucosa they die by means of proteolytic enzymes.[75]

Sensitization to *Anisakis* larvae may cause an acute allergic reaction, such as urticaria, angioedema, or anaphylaxis. If a person has been previously sensitized to *Anisakis* antigens, allergic reactions are faster in onset and much more severe. The wide spectrum of allergic reactions to *A. simplex* include, in addition to the aforementioned, rhinitis, conjunctivitis, asthma, and allergic contact dermatitis (Figure 76-38). Consumption of raw and smoked fish may increase sensitization to Anisakidae (Figure 76-39).

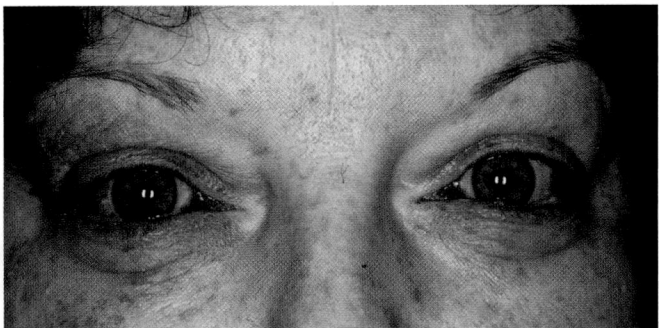

FIGURE 76-38 Anisakidosis. Conjunctivitis from an allergic response to *Anisakis simplex.*

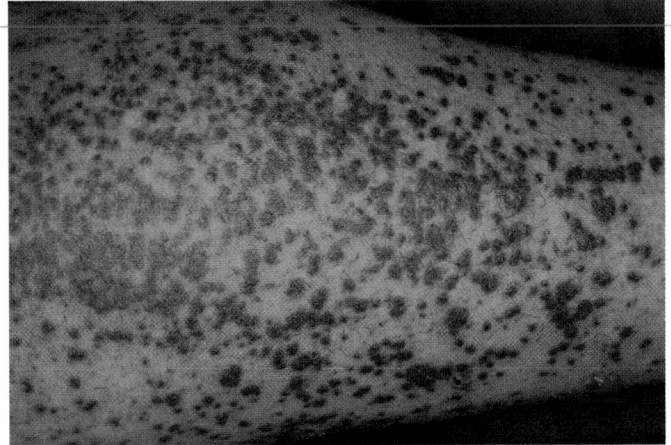

FIGURE 76-39 Cutaneous manifestations of a severe allergic response to *Anisakis simplex* antigens after ingestion of smoked salmon (same person with conjunctivitis).

Differential Diagnosis

Allergic reactions to seafood are the primary differential diagnoses. Most purported seafood allergies are actually reactions to *A. simplex* or the marine larval nematode *Pseudoterranova*.

Treatment

In the majority of persons, symptoms fade spontaneously. Endoscopic removal of worms results in a prompt cure. Treatment of allergic responses is with symptomatic and supportive therapies. Although not approved by the Food and Drug Administration, albendazole 400 mg orally twice daily for 6 to 21 days was successful in cases.[126]

Prevention

Thoroughly cooking seafood for at least 10 minutes over 65°C (149°F) or freezing it at −28.9°C (−20°F) for 24 hours is necessary to destroy all larvae. Adequate cooking or freezing does not destroy larval antigens and therefore will not prevent allergic reactions.

SCHISTOSOME CERCARIAL DERMATITIS

Definition

Schistosome cercarial dermatitis, known as swimmer's itch, is an inflammatory response to cutaneous infestation with any of several blood flukes (schistosomes) of the genera *Trichobilharzia, Ornithobilharzia, Gigantobilharzia, Orientobilharzia, Austrobilharzia, Bilharziella, Heterobilharzia,* and some species of the *Schistosoma* genus.[76] The particular flukes discussed here are animal pathogens that do not parasitize humans beyond the skin to cause systemic infection. The geographic distribution of these dermatoses is worldwide, occurring in Arctic, temperate, and tropical zones. Swimmer's itch is most commonly seen after exposure to cercariae-laden fresh or brackish water or, less often, saltwater.[107] This process is nearly exclusively cutaneous with only localized pruritus. Rarely, there may be fever, lymphadenopathy, and edema, particularly in those with repeated exposures.

Epidemiology

The definitive hosts of these nonhuman schistosomes are aquatic birds, such as ducks, gulls, and geese, in addition to mammals, such as beaver, mice, muskrats, and ungulates. The life cycle begins when eggs of the adult schistosomes are eliminated via feces of infested hosts. When eggs are deposited in water, they hatch and release small swimming larvae (miracidia). On finding their specific intermediate hosts (snails), miracidia penetrate the snails' soft flesh and metamorphose into forked-tail cercariae. Mature cercariae exit the snail in search of a definitive avian or mammalian host to complete their life cycle (Figure 76-40).[16]

The probability of infection is highest in the morning hours when cercarial emergence is greatest[166,178] and increased when more time is spent in the water. Prevalence is higher in warmer summer months when both human water activities and emergence of the cercariae peak. Shallow waters where snail populations are most numerous are sites of the highest infection risk, though infection can still occur at deeper water depths.

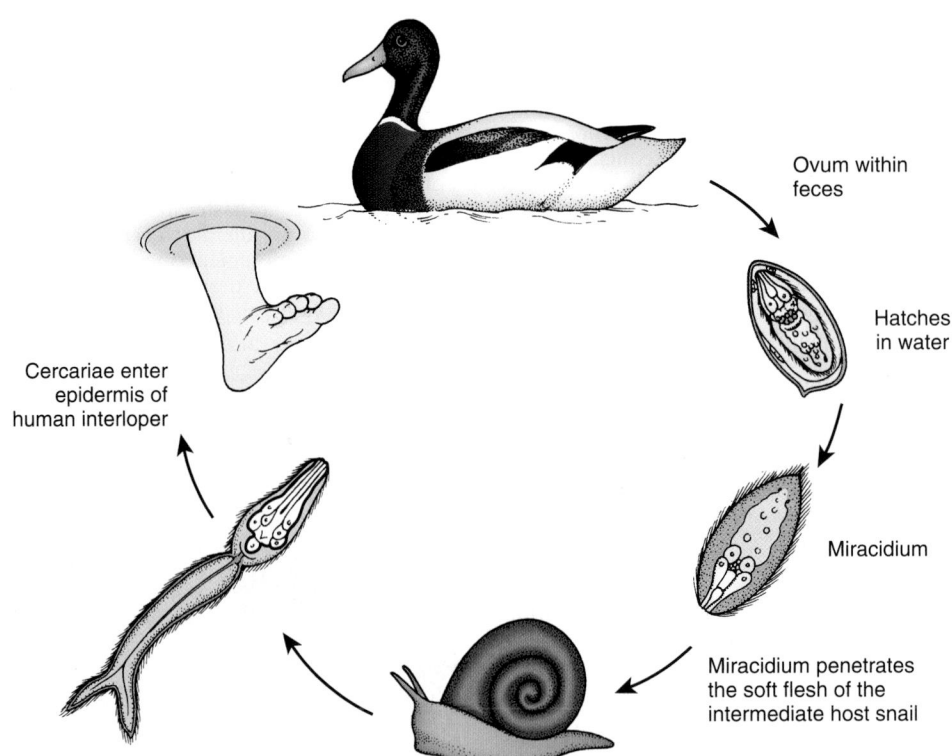

Ovum within feces

Hatches in water

Miracidium

Miracidium penetrates the soft flesh of the intermediate host snail

Cercariae enter epidermis of human interloper

FIGURE 76-40 Schistosome cercarial life cycle. *(Courtesy Edgar Maeyens, Jr., MD.)*

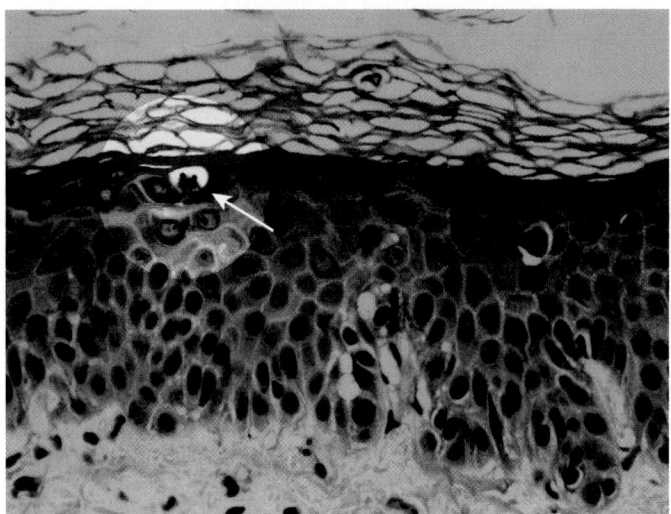

FIGURE 76-41 Schistosomiasis. Schistosome cercaria beneath the stratum corneum of the epidermis (H&E, original magnification ×10). *(Courtesy Ronald Rapini, MD.)*

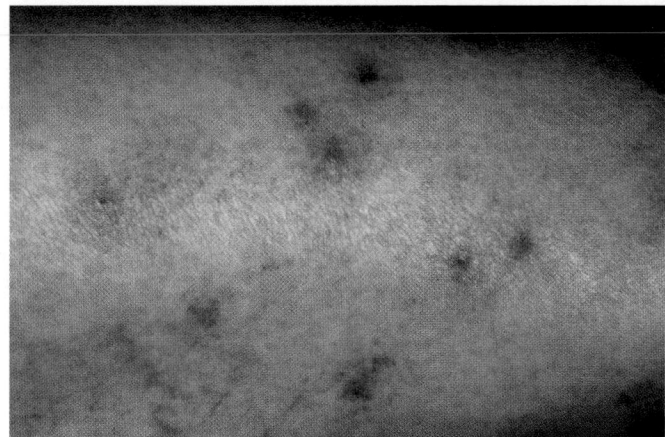

FIGURE 76-43 Schistosome cercarial dermatitis: Multiple papulovesicles in a sensitized individual following clam digging. *(Courtesy Edgar Maeyens, Jr., MD.)*

Pathophysiology

Penetration of human skin by cercariae induces a localized inflammatory response. The immunologic response is IgE-mediated histamine release. The degree of inflammation varies depending on previous exposure to and the numbers of penetrating cercariae. A primary exposure results in development of pruritic macules and papules within 1 to 2 days of infection, whereas infection in a previously sensitized individual results in transient eruption of macules inside of 20 minutes, followed by a papular and then vesicular eruption associated with intense pruritus in the following hours to days.[97] Once in human skin, these nonhuman cercariae are unable to develop further and are destroyed by the inflammatory infiltrate.

Histopathologically, the epidermis shows varying degrees of spongiosis. Extremely rarely, cercariae are found on histopathologic examination. Cercariae are located in the epidermis (Figure 76-41). There is edema of the upper dermis and superficial perivascular inflammatory infiltrate composed of lymphocytes, histiocytes, and eosinophils.[25] Histopathologically, swimmer's itch resembles arthropod assaults and seabather's eruption.

Clinical Presentation

Within minutes of cercarial penetration, tingling, burning, and itching appear. Initially, an erythematous macule develops, which promptly evolves into a papule. When the allergic response is severe, papules vesiculate (Figures 76-40 to 76-43). Without

therapy, the eruption disappears in 7 to 14 days.[76] Exposed body surfaces are the primary areas of involvement, helping to differentiate this from seabather's eruption; however, covered surfaces may also be involved. Pruritus with scratching can lead to secondary infection. *Staphylococcus aureus* and *Streptococcus* species are the most common bacteria associated with secondary infection.

Differential Diagnosis

The differential diagnosis includes papular urticaria, arthropod assaults, nettle dermatitis, and *Toxicodendron* (poison ivy, poison oak, and poison sumac) contact dermatitis.

Diagnostic Tests

The complete blood count may show mild eosinophilia; otherwise, there are no specific diagnostic tests.

Treatment

Because the inflammatory response is self-limited, therapy need only be symptomatic. The use of over-the-counter antihistamines plus antipruritic lotions or creams (Table 76-2) is usually all that is needed. If moderate to severe dermatitis occurs, topical corticosteroid creams (see Table 76-1) in conjunction with oral corticosteroids (Table 76-3) may be indicated.[36] Secondary bacterial infection, depending on the degree and extent, is treated with topical antiseptic (mupirocin or bacitracin) ointment or cream or systemic antibiotics. An empirical trial of oral cephalexin or clindamycin may be indicated if secondary infection is severe.

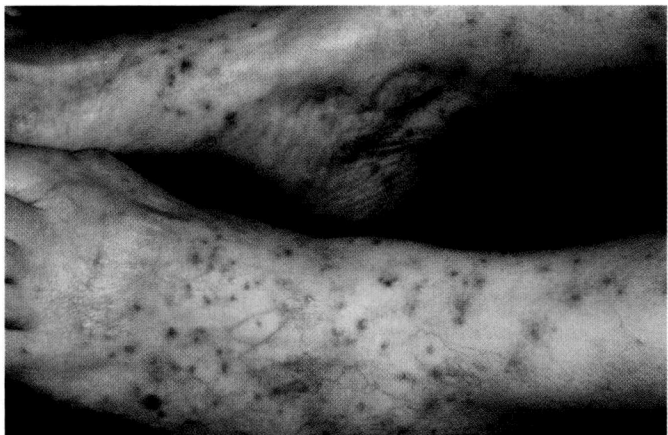

FIGURE 76-42 Schistosome cercarial dermatitis of the feet and ankles. *(Courtesy Edgar Maeyens, Jr., MD.)*

TABLE 76-3	Systemic Steroids
Steroid	**Dose**
Oral Steroid	
Prednisone	Dosing schedule A: 40 mg orally every morning for 7 days
	Dosing schedule B: 2-week tapering course starting at 35 mg orally every morning for 2 days; then decrease by 5 mg every 2 days
Intramuscular Steroid	
Kenalog (Triamcinolone)	40-60 mg deep intramuscularly into a large muscle mass (gluteus maximus)

Prevention

Methods to reduce the risk of cercarial dermatitis include the following[36,37]:

Avoid wading or swimming in marshy areas and areas with dense vegetation, or other areas where snails are plentiful.

Swim as far away from shore as safety allows, thereby minimizing exposure to vegetation and snails.

Obey posted signs that indicate that water is unsafe.

Use of waterproof sunscreens has been reported to prevent infestation.

CUTANEOUS LARVA MIGRANS

Definition

Cutaneous larva migrans (creeping eruption) is a superficial infestation of skin caused by the dog and cat hookworms *Ancylostoma braziliense, Ancylostoma caninum, Uncinaria stenocephala,* and *Bunostomum phlebotomum.*[74,145] Rarely, the human hookworms *Gnathostoma spinigerum* and *Strongyloides stercoralis* can cause similar findings. Although not directly related to water environs, this infestation may be acquired by humans while participating in water-related activities.

Epidemiology and Risk Factors

Ancylostoma braziliense larvae reside in the intestinal tract of dogs and cats. Second-stage, noninfectious larvae are excreted in feces and then mature in soil. Mature, third-stage infectious larvae are able to survive in sand or soil when adequate conditions prevail. Larvae penetrate the skin of humans who come in direct contact with such soil. The condition is more common among children living in warm, humid climates. Cutaneous larva migrans is the most common dermatologic disorder affecting vacationers to tropical countries.[83]

Pathophysiology

On percutaneous penetration, larvae migrate within the superficial dermis, causing a strong inflammatory reaction along the course of migration. Migration is random, forming curvilinear lines of edema and erythema. The leading edge is frequently vesicular. Larvae are rarely found on histopathologic examination, because they are usually 1 to 2 cm (0.4 to 0.8 inches) beyond the vesicle. Larvae are able to advance several centimeters a day (Figure 76-44). The inflammatory response is intensely pruritic.

Clinical Presentation

Larval penetration of the skin causes a tingling sensation, followed by pruritus, inflammation, and vesicle formation. As the larvae migrate, they leave in their wake a serpiginous, inflamed, and edematous tract. Common locations include the feet, buttocks, and back.[153] There may be a single tract or multiple tracts, or a folliculitis-like presentation. The folliculitis-like presentation

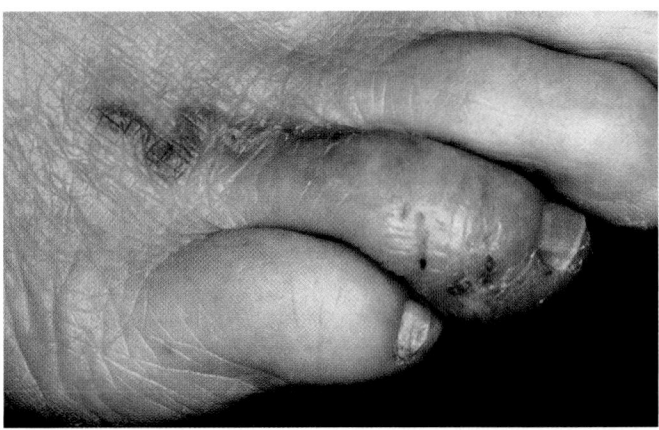

FIGURE 76-44 Cutaneous larva migrans. *(Courtesy Edgar Maeyens, Jr., MD.)*

occurs when multiple larvae penetrate the skin simultaneously in a localized area, such as the back of a person who had been lying on infested sand. Previously sensitized individuals develop an exaggerated allergic response with accentuation of all symptoms. Animal hookworm larvae do not survive in human skin and die in a few weeks, at which time there is spontaneous clearing of signs and symptoms.

Diagnostic Tests

Skin biopsies are nondiagnostic because larvae are virtually never found. Rarely, peripheral eosinophilia is present with a massive infestation or in a severely allergic person infested with numerous larvae.

Differential Diagnosis

The differential diagnosis of migratory skin lesions is either infectious or inflammatory. Infectious migratory diseases include: strongyloidiasis, myiasis, hookworm, gnathostomiasis, dracunculiasis, fascioliasis, sparganosis, erythema chronicum migrans, and dermatophytosis. Inflammatory dermatoses include photodermatitis and phytophotodermatitis.

Treatment

This is a self-limited infection; however, symptoms may persist for months if the infection is not treated early. Therapy for cutaneous larva migrans includes ivermectin 12 mg as a single dose, albendazole 400 mg daily for 5 to 7 days, or topical 10% thiabendazole (two 0.5-g tablets crushed and mixed with 10 g of petrolatum) twice a day until clear.[19,32,109,147,175] Antibiotics may be needed if secondary infection occurs.

Prevention

In sandy areas frequented by dogs and cats, do not sit or lie on damp sand or soil, especially during rainy season. Wear footgear in similar situations. Cover the ground with an impenetrable material before sitting or lying down.

LEECHES

Leeches are annelids of the class Hirudinea. Approximately 600 species have been identified. Many are blood-sucking endoparasites and ectoparasites that attach themselves to vertebrae hosts and suck blood.

Definition

Leeches vary in shape and color. They are typically cylindrical and elongated, but can be broadly ovoid. The ventral surface is flat and dorsal surface is convex. Leeches possess suckers at both anterior and posterior ends of their body. Sizes range from 5 mm to 45 cm (0.2 to 18.0 inches) in length. Colors vary from dark brown to black to brightly colored or mottled. The crop (stomach) of the leech can store up to five times its body size in blood. They are hermaphroditic or protandrous (at first male, than later female).[124]

Epidemiology and Risk Factors

Worldwide, there are many different types of leeches. They can be divided into freshwater, marine, and land leeches. The typical freshwater leeches attach themselves to humans and animals entering ponds or muddy-bottomed rivers. At the time of attachment, leeches secrete an adhesive mucoid substance enhancing suction power. They possess blade-like jaws having 60 to 100 small teeth. Land leeches live in the tropical rain forests of South America and southeast Asia on shrubs and under stones. Marine leeches live on and feed on fish.

The one leech known as an internal leech, *Limnatis nilotica,* is found in western Asia, northern Africa, and southern Europe. *L. nilotica* attaches to mucous membranes of the nasal pharynx and esophagus when ingested via contaminated water.

Pathophysiology

After attachment and beginning of feeding, leeches secrete at least three anticoagulants: seratin, hirudins, and ornatins.

Hirudins block collagen-mediated platelet activation. They are antithrombotic agents secreted from buccal glands. Seratin inhibits platelet-collagen interactions, and ornatins are glycoprotein IIb-IIIa antagonists and platelet aggregation inhibitors. Feeding is painless, as leeches secrete an analgesic substance currently not identified.[68,163] Spontaneous detachment occurs on engorgement, usually within an hour or less, leaving behind bleeding attachment sites. The anticoagulant effect lasts for up to 12 hours before spontaneous cessation of bleeding occurs.

Clinical Presentation

The telltale sign of having been parasitized by a leech is a puncture wound oozing blood. Puncture sites may become painful, erythematous, edematous, and pruritic.[114] Bacteria and viruses from prior blood feedings can survive within a leech and be transmitted to humans, thereby causing secondary infectious diseases.[128]

Treatment

Mechanical removal is the treatment. Remove the leeches carefully so as not to leave behind pieces of teeth in the skin. Leeches have very sensitive taste and smell receptors. The key to successful removal is breaking suction of the leech at each attachment site with little or no trauma to the organism. Too aggressive removal can cause regurgitation of crop contents and resultant infection. A drop of any essential oil near the mouthpart causes rapid release by the leech. Overzealous use of essential oils may cause the leech to regurgitate and potentially contaminate the attachment site. If without essential oils, use a fingernail or sharp object to break the sucker seals and cause the leech to release its jaws. Do not apply caustic chemicals, such as alcohol, or a lit cigarette to the leech, as these techniques can also result in regurgitation of stomach contents.[125] Do not forcibly pull off the leech, as this also may result in regurgitation. Cleanse puncture sites thoroughly with soap and water and observe for signs of infection. If oozing is continuous, apply a hemostatic dressing, such as QuikClot gauze, under pressure for 15 minutes.

Prevention

Protect skin from leech attachment by wearing or adjusting clothing when in leech-infested environs. "Leech socks" (any long, light-colored socks pulled over pant legs to allow visualization of leeches and prevent their attachment to skin) should be worn when walking in infested areas. These are light colored to allow visualization of ascending leeches.

Sequelae

Some individuals experience severe allergic reactions or even anaphylaxis from leech bites. Allergic reactions manifest locally as swelling and itching at the attachment sites or as generalized urticaria.

YEAST

PITYROSPORUM FOLLICULITIS

Definition

Pityrosporum folliculitis is a condition most commonly occurring in young or middle-aged adults characterized by follicular papulopustules involving the upper torso.[8] The condition is the result of overgrowth of normal skin yeast of the genus *Pityrosporum*. Two species commonly associated with *Pityrosporum* folliculitis are *Pityrosporum ovale* and *Pityrosporum orbiculare*. Together they are classified as *Malassezia furfur*, of which there are other group members making up the *M. furfur* complex.[103]

Pathophysiology

M. furfur is a lipophilic, dimorphic, gram-positive, double-walled, and saprophytic budding yeast.[8] Growth and proliferation occur in an environment rich in free fatty acids. Sebaceous glands produce triglycerides, which break down into free fatty acids. Any condition creating an increase in free fatty acids encourages proliferation of *M. furfur*.

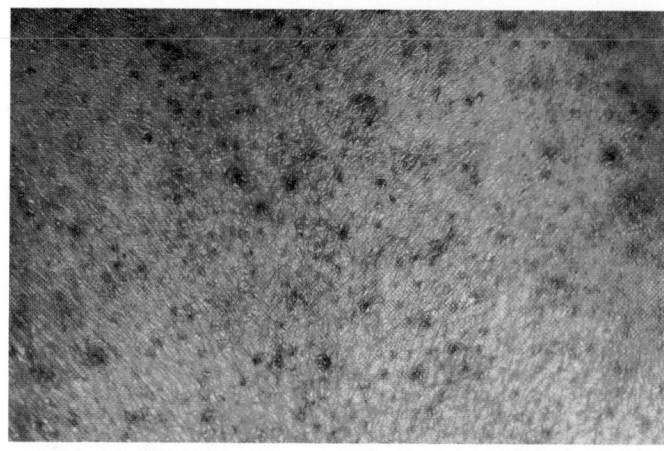

FIGURE 76-45 *Pityrosporum* folliculitis. Follicular papulopustules on the back of a scuba diver after his wetsuit had been removed. (*Courtesy Edgar Maeyens, Jr., MD.*)

Epidemiology and Risk Factors

The surface of normal skin is colonized by *Pityrosporum* in 90% to 100% of humans. Individuals living in humid and hot climates experience increased incidence of *Pityrosporum* folliculitis.[8] Conditions or agents facilitating overgrowth of these yeasts include cosmetics, sunscreens, body lotions, occlusive clothing, and having hot, moist skin from wearing wetsuits.[8]

Medical disorders that can predispose a person to *Pityrosporum* folliculitis include diabetes, leukemia, lymphoma, and immunodeficiency states.[27] Medications known to be associated with the occurrence of *Pityrosporum* folliculitis include antibiotics, anticonvulsants, immunosuppressants, and systemic steroids.[27] All of these medications tend to alter normal skin flora, thereby favoring yeast proliferation.

Clinical Presentation

Pityrosporum folliculitis manifests clinically as an acneiform eruption. The distribution is usually on the upper torso, and infrequently on the neck and face. The lesions are typically dome-shaped papules of 2 to 4 mm in diameter. Some papules are topped by tiny pustules. Pruritus is common (Figure 76-45).

Differential Diagnosis

Pityrosporum folliculitis closely resembles acne, but is unresponsive to acne therapy. *Pseudomonas* and *Staphylococcus* folliculitis are simulators.

Diagnostic Tests

Gram's stain of purulence from the follicular ostia reveals numerous yeast forms, and potassium hydroxide (KOH) preparation from a skin scraping may show a characteristic "spaghetti and meatball" appearance of the hyphae and spores. Skin biopsies stained with hematoxylin and eosin show numerous yeasts within the follicular ostia. Conventional culture techniques rarely detect *M. furfur* because the organism requires free fatty acids for growth.

Treatment

Treatment is with a topical antifungal or systemic antifungal, or both. Ketoconazole 2% cream or miconazole cream twice daily for a month, as well as twice weekly application of selenium sulfide shampoo, may be effective. For disease not responsive to topicals, oral itraconazole 200 mg daily for 7 days is effective.[134] Alternately, fluconazole prescribed either as 100 mg daily for up to 3 weeks may result in clearance.[144]

Prevention

When in hot and humid climates, wear light, loose-fitting clothing and avoid occlusive sunscreens and body lotions. After diving, remove wetsuits promptly, dry the skin thoroughly, and stay cool and dry.

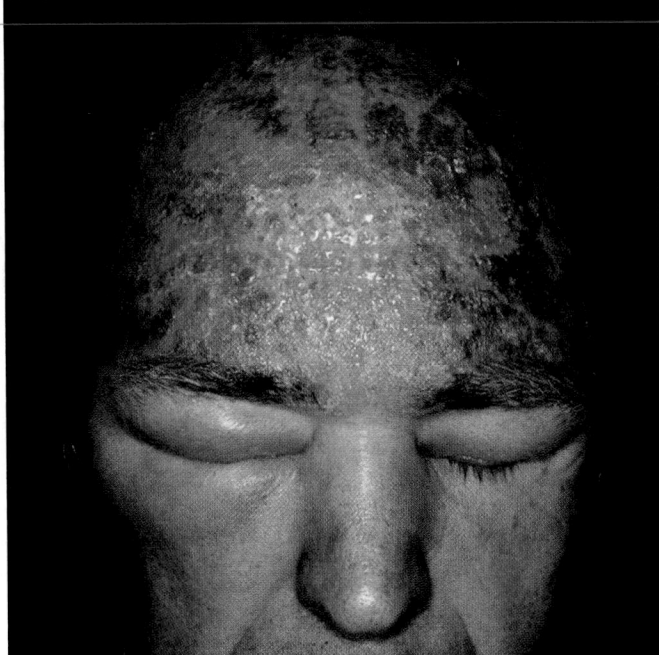

FIGURE 76-46 Severe allergic contact dermatitis secondary to a neoprene hood. *(Courtesy Edgar Maeyens, Jr., MD.)*

DERMATOSES RELATED TO DIVING
ALLERGIC CONTACT DERMATITIS

The use of wetsuits, masks, rubber mouthpieces, and swim gear predisposes a person to development of allergic contact dermatitis. Clinically, the majority of these allergic reactions manifest as clearly delineated areas of dermatitis of the body surfaces in contact with diving gear.

Definition

Allergic contact dermatitis related to diving gear is due to allergies to one of several chemicals used in the development and processing of rubber (Figure 76-46). Dermatitis associated with wetsuits can also be nonallergic, for example, intertrigo, maceration, and folliculitis.

Pathophysiology

Rubber is an organic substance obtained from plants or is artificially synthesized. More than 99% of the world's natural rubber is extracted from the *Hevea brasiliensis* tree. There are many types of natural and synthetic rubber, each with its unique processing technique and chemical content. Many chemical additives are potent allergens. Rubber itself does not cause allergic contact dermatitis. It is the chemical additives used to cure rubber that are the antigenic components of rubber products. Local heat, maceration, and perspiration enhance the potential for developing allergic contact dermatitis. Sensitivity is acquired most easily if the allergen is applied to damaged skin.

Clinical Presentation

Rubber allergic contact dermatitis is a cell-mediated immune response by T lymphocytes to the presence of inciting antigens. The onset of dermatitis becomes apparent hours after antigen exposure. Depending on an individual's previous antigen exposure and the degree of his or her rubber sensitivity, clinical manifestations will be more or less acute.

The acute phase of rubber dermatitis manifests as erythema, edema, pruritus, and vesiculation. In the context of neoprene diving suits, goggles, and so forth, dermatitis is clearly confined to areas of contact with rubber. Chronic allergic dermatitis is characterized by inflammation, pruritus, and cutaneous lichenification. Edema seen in chronic contact dermatitis is usually less than that of acute dermatitis and appears as diffuse thickening and accentuation of skin tension lines (Figures 76-46 to 76-48).

Differential Diagnosis

Irritant contact dermatitis due to direct chemical damage is the primary differential diagnosis. However, it has a different clinical spectrum than does allergic contact dermatitis. Acute irritant dermatitis can present in a spectrum from mild erythema and irritation to florid dermatitis with marked inflammation, edema, pain, and vesiculation. Onset of irritant contact dermatitis is rapid without delay, versus the relatively slow onset of allergic contact dermatitis.

Treatment

Basic methods of treatment apply regardless of whether the dermatitis is secondary to diving masks, goggles, mouthpieces, or wetsuits. Reversal of the T-cell–driven response is the objective. Whether inflammation is mucosal or cutaneous, the mainstay of therapy is removal or elimination of the inciting chemicals and suppression of the inflammatory response. For mild allergic reactions, topical corticosteroids are effective (see Table 76-1). Systemic corticosteroids, such as prednisone, are used to treat severe allergic reactions (see Table 76-3). Mucosal reactions, if with ulceration, respond to application of triamcinolone acetonide 0.1% in dental paste (Kenalog in Orabase) three times a day and at bedtime for 5 to 7 days, in addition to 10 to 20 mg oral prednisone for 2 to 3 days. Triamcinolone acetonide 40 to 60 mg deep intramuscularly may be needed for extensive blistering reactions. Systemic antihistamines provide symptomatic relief from pruritus (see Table 76-2). Secondary infection presents as purulence, pain, or lymphangitis.

Prevention

Avoidance of known allergen(s) is the only prevention.

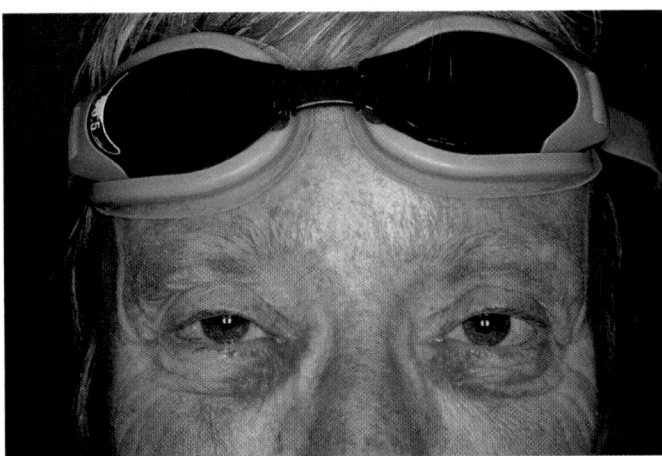

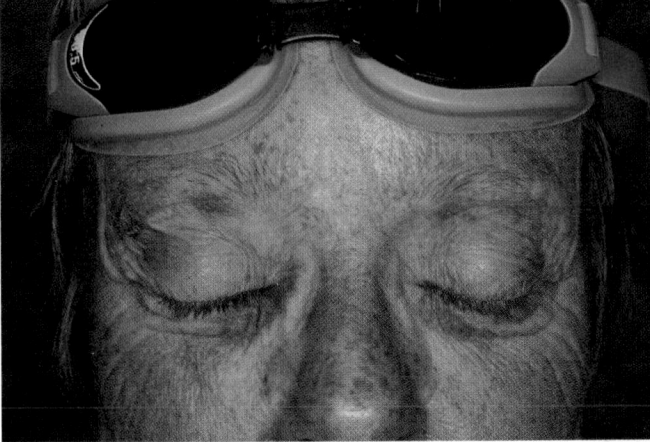

FIGURE 76-47 Allergic dermatitis. Periorbital allergic contact dermatitis from rubber goggles.

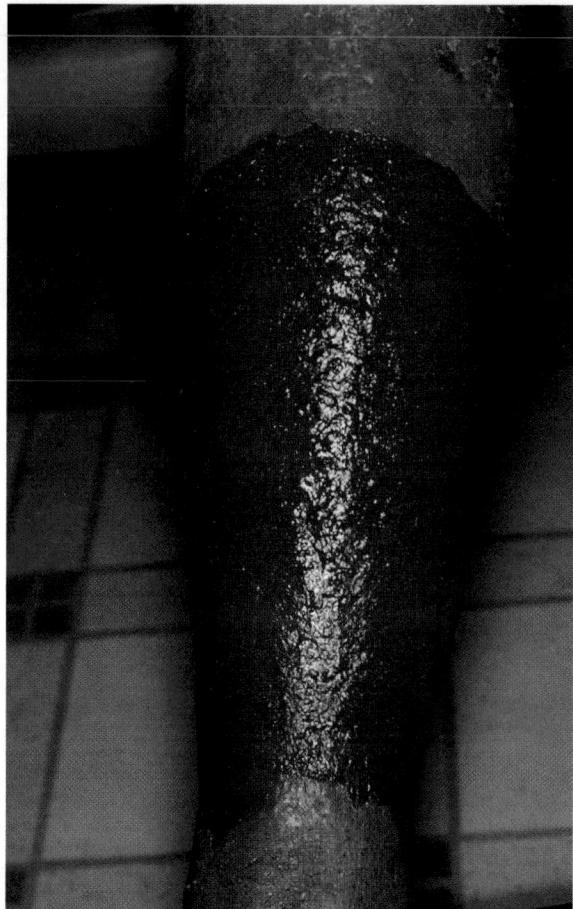

FIGURE 76-48 Allergic dermatitis. Allergic contact dermatitis of a leg caused by an elastic wrap. Notice the clear cut-off distribution of the dermatitis, differentiating this from a diffuse cellulitis.

CUTANEOUS DECOMPRESSION SICKNESS: AN OVERVIEW

Definition

Cutaneous decompression sickness (CDS) is defined as a disorder of the skin occurring in scuba divers or caisson workers as a consequence of depressurization. This results in bubbles forming in the skin from dissolved gases coming out of solution. CDS may occur as an isolated occurrence or in conjunction with other organ system "bubble diseases," such as decompression sickness with or without associated arterial gas embolism. Thermal cooling is also a contributory factor. Excessive skin gas pressure over ambient pressure (called gaseous supersaturation) is critical in development of bubbles occurring during or after ascent from depth. Once bubbles form, they may initiate the release of inflammatory mediators, obstruct vascular or lymphatic vessels, or directly or indirectly stimulate the release of neurotransmitters.

Epidemiology and Risk Factors

Although there is little written about the rates of CDS, in a study of more than 5000 patients treated at a Chinese hyperbaric unit, cutaneous abnormalities were the most common symptom of decompression sickness.[194] Additionally, a majority of divers who suffer from CDS also have a right-to-left cardiac shunt, typically as a patent foramen ovale, although some have pulmonary shunts.[187]

Pathophysiology

Tissue solubility of compressed gases varies. Nitrogen is highly lipid soluble. After a person dives while breathing nitrogen, the greatest amounts of this dissolved gas are deposited in lipid-rich tissues, which become supersaturated. The rash of CDS clinically favors body areas with larger amounts of subcutaneous fat, such as the trunk, thighs, abdomen, arms, and buttocks. The

FIGURE 76-49 Cutis marmorata. *(Courtesy Edgar Maeyens, Jr., MD.)*

precise pathophysiology of CDS remains unverified. In one proposed scenario, for individuals with a right-to-left cardiac shunt, the mechanism may be due to venous microbubble emboli entering the arterial circulation. Upon entering the circulatory system, bubbles are absorbed into tissues and/or amplified peripherally, becoming emboli. Buttolph and colleagues used a swine model to study CDS, and were able to demonstrate vascular congestion on tissue histology as the most common finding.[27] They also described neutrophil adhesion to vessel walls and vascular occlusion. They demonstrated a perturbation of the endothelium or neutrophils, or both. These authors concluded that "the marbling or cutis marmorata forms of cutaneous presentations in CDS are principally vascular congestion, possibly as a result of inflammation."[27]

Clinical Presentation

Clinically this condition presents as a broad, purple marbled, or mottled appearance of the skin and is usually confined to parts of the body with larger amounts of subcutaneous fat, in particular the trunk and thighs. If the diver experiences CDS in future dives, the same sites are typically involved.[187] Clinical manifestations include itching and varying degrees of pain. The term cutis marmorata is often used erroneously to describe CDS. True cutis marmorata presents as a reddish-blue reticulated vascular pattern surrounding central pale areas. The cause of this process involves cooling of the skin and subcutaneous fat with subsequent vasodilation of the deep dermal venous plexus and contraction of superficial arterioles and venules, not gas emboli. This is a transient, asymptomatic normal physiologic process that occurs with drops in ambient temperatures (Figures 76-49 and 76-50). In contrast, CDS almost universally demonstrates an erythematous, blotchy appearance. Depending on the location of the bubbles, cutaneous manifestations vary. For example, when bubbles are present in larger vessels of the deep dermis or subcutaneous

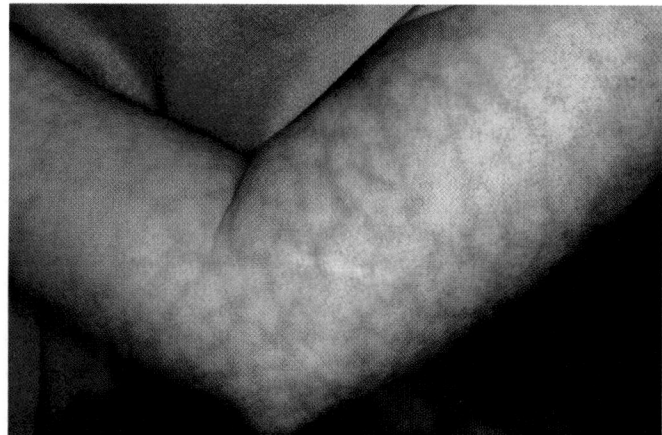

FIGURE 76-50 Cutis marmorata. *(Courtesy Edgar Maeyens, Jr., MD.)*

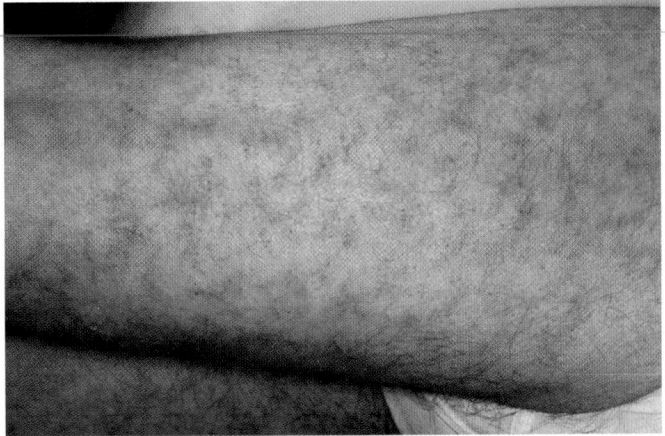

FIGURE 76-51 Marbling of the thigh in cutaneous decompression sickness. (*Courtesy Edgar Maeyens, Jr., MD.*)

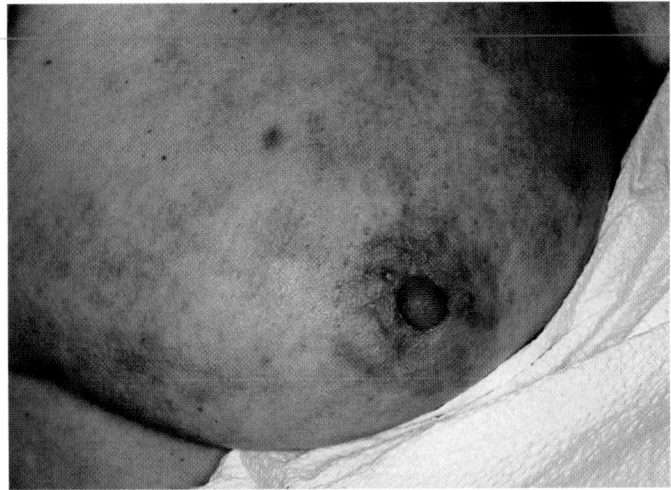

FIGURE 76-52 Blotchy erythema of the breast in cutaneous decompression sickness. (*Courtesy Edgar Maeyens, Jr., MD.*)

tissue, the clinical presentation is that of marbling (Figure 76-51). If the capillaries or venules of the superficial plexus are affected, the skin develops blotchy erythema (Figure 76-52).

Treatment

The initial response is first-aid treatment by having the diver breathe 100% oxygen. Definitive therapy is recompression to increased pressure while the diver breathes 100% oxygen[176] (see Chapter 71).

REFERENCES

Complete references used in this text are available online at expertconsult.inkling.com.

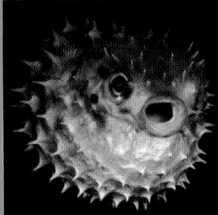

CHAPTER 77
Seafood Toxidromes

ALICIA B. MINNS, MICHAEL J. MATTEUCCI, BINH T. LY, AND RICHARD F. CLARK

At least three-quarters of the world's population live within 10 miles (16 km) of a coast. One of many reasons why populations congregate near the sea is the abundance of food beneath the ocean's surface. Seafood provides a significant percentage of the protein in the diets of many cultures. Presently, 200 to 240 million tons of fish are harvested each year, with 50% of the total coming from coastal regions. Per capita fish consumption has increased in recent decades. Americans consume 7.3 kg (16.4 lb) of fish per person per year.[190] The ocean is one of our last plentiful food resources. International trade has dramatically increased year-round availability of assorted seafoods, many of which come from distant geographic locations.[446]

Throughout time, humans have recognized that toxic seafood is associated with seasons of the year, phases of the moon, water temperature, weather conditions, waterfowl deaths, the color of waves that wash onto shore, and many other circumstances. Unfortunately, none of these factors has proven entirely reliable in predicting when seafood poisoning occurs.

Marine creatures whose consumption can lead to poisoning include dinoflagellates, coelenterates, mollusks, echinoderms, crustaceans, fishes, turtles, and mammals. Most marine biotoxins are naturally occurring poisons derived directly from marine organisms, including phytotoxins (plant poisons) and zootoxins (animal poisons). Ingestible toxins may be classified by specific toxin or by the donor organ of origin ingested by the victim. *Ichthyosarcotoxin* is a general term for poison derived from the fresh flesh (muscle, viscera, skin, or slime) of any fish. The geographic location, dietary and clinical histories, and appropriate index of suspicion figure prominently in diagnosis and treatment of fish poisoning.

Data on food-borne disease outbreaks in the United States show that fish are the vehicle of transmission in 19% of cases, mollusks in 7%, and crustaceans in 4%.[81] Some 90% of outbreaks of seafood-related illnesses and 75% of individual cases come from contaminated raw molluscan seafood (e.g., oysters, clams), histamine poisoning (scombroid), and ciguatoxin found in reef fish species.[349] In general, marine toxins are heat stable and largely unaffected by cooking. Marine poisoning causes mostly gastrointestinal and neurologic symptoms. Many marine toxins target voltage-gated sodium channels in myelinated and unmyelinated nerves, resulting in a range of peripheral neurologic effects.[226]

MONITORING MARINE ALGAE THAT PRODUCE PHYTOTOXINS AND SEAFOOD THAT MAY CAUSE POISONING

Despite the increasing risk of human poisoning from contaminated seafood, standards and methods of screening and law enforcement vary worldwide.[497] According to the U.S. Department of Agriculture, imports account for more than 55% of total U.S. seafood consumption. The largest sources of seafood imported into the United States are Canada, Asia, and Latin America. The U.S. Food and Drug Administration (FDA) has been criticized for inadequate inspection of all food imports.[349] In 1995, the FDA switched to a new program for seafood safety known as the Hazard Analysis and Critical Control Point (HACCP) system. This program became mandatory for the seafood industry on December 18, 1997.[155] The HACCP focuses on the following: (1) identification of sources and points of contamination; (2) levels of the hazard(s) of concern, transmission rate, and transport of microorganisms; and (3) possibility of exposure of the consumer to the contaminant. The HACCP concentrates on preventing hazards rather than relying on spot checks and random sampling of products. The most effective control strategies can then be implemented. For shellfish- and virus-associated diseases, data suggest that harvesting from unapproved sources is associated with more than 30% of outbreaks.[301] Among imports, the biggest risks relate to histamines and scombroid poisoning, mainly from tuna and mahi-mahi imported from Argentina, Taiwan, and Ecuador. For foods traveling great distances, refrigeration is the most critical aspect of controlling illness. Although there has been progress in improving standards for imported seafood in the United States, only 5% to 7% of the 8500 firms importing seafood in the country during 2002 and 2003 were inspected by regulators.[114]

The United States is the second largest importer of shrimp worldwide. Shrimp aquaculture currently accounts for approximately 30% of the world's supply. The FDA has amended the food additive regulations to provide for the safe use of ionizing radiation for control of food-borne pathogens in fresh or frozen molluscan shellfish.[156]

Molluscan poisoning is mainly a problem with domestic seafood. In 1991, California was the first state to require restaurants that serve or sell Gulf Coast oysters to warn prospective customers about possible deleterious effects from *Vibrio* contamination, particularly *Vibrio vulnificus*.[389] Other states have since adopted these warning regulations. In addition, fishermen are now required to refrigerate oysters within 6 hours after harvesting from the Gulf of Mexico. Regulations require oyster lot tagging, labeling, and record retention to facilitate trace-back investigations of outbreaks. The United States and Canada allow the sale of oysters if there are less than 10,000 colony-forming units per gram (CFU/g) of *Vibrio parahaemolyticus*. However, in outbreaks in the Pacific Northwest in 1997 and New York in 1998, oysters had less than 200 *V. parahaemolyticus* CFU/g of oyster meat, suggesting that human illness can occur at lower levels.[77]

Approximately one-third of U.S. shellfish beds carry bans or limitations on harvesting because of high levels of fecal coliform bacteria. The fecal indicator system for shellfish-harvesting waters has been effective in protecting consumers against general types of bacteria in fecal contamination. However, several pathogenic bacteria are not predicted by the system. The efficacy of methods for virus recovery may range from 2% to 47%.[517] The most promising of the new detection methods are based on molecular techniques. Deoxyribonucleic acid (DNA) hybridization and polymerase chain reaction (PCR) have the advantages of specificity for particular pathogens, sensitivity, and speed (most assays are completed within a few hours). The PCR has been used in shellfish to detect *Salmonella*, *Vibrio* species, and viruses, including hepatitis A virus and norovirus. High-performance liquid chromatography (HPLC) has also been used to detect and quantify many shellfish toxins.[18,23,105,289,375,418] Phytotoxin-producing marine algae are responsible for the syndromes of paralytic, neurotoxic, and diarrhetic shellfish poisoning. Closure of fisheries (product harvest areas) depends on the density of algae. In some cases, the decision to close a fishery is based on the toxicity level in shellfish; in others, algae in the water and toxin in shellfish must both be found. In Florida, more than 5000 cells/L of *Ptychodiscus brevis* must be detected before fisheries are closed. The quarantine level of saxitoxin (a neurotoxin found in marine dinoflagellates) varies between countries and ranges from 40 to 80 mg of toxin per 100 g (3.5 oz) of seafood, as determined through mouse bioassay.[21] The higher number is used in the United States and is monitored by the Interstate Shellfish Sanitation Conference and the FDA.

The maximal acceptable concentration of diarrhetic shellfish toxin (okadaic acid) also varies between countries because of lack of precise analytic methods for quantification. Countries with established regulations apply 4 to 5 mouse units or 20 to 25 mg equivalents of okadaic acid as an acceptance limit. In the United Kingdom, the Ministry of Agriculture, Fisheries, and Food shellfish surveillance program tests harvested shellfish weekly from April to October and sporadically during the winter for the presence of toxins.[421] The United States, Canada, and Portugal monitor for domoic acid (the cause of amnesic shellfish poisoning) and use 2 mg/100 g of seafood as the threshold. Ciguatoxins are monitored infrequently because of difficulties associated with the assay. In French Polynesia, ciguatoxin at 0.06 ng/g of seafood as determined by mosquito bioassay is considered toxic; in the United States (Florida, Hawaii), detection of the toxin at any level by immunoassay renders the fish unmarketable. Two primary features render toxin surveillance difficult: performance problems of the assays and impracticality of surveying every fish.

SUSTAINABLE AND SAFE SEAFOOD INITIATIVES

Recently, there have been numerous initiatives by private nonprofit organizations to promote practices that will result in sustainable fisheries, restoration of marine ecosystems, and safer seafood arriving to markets. These initiatives include the industry-centric FishWise (fishwise.org), which encourages sustainable use of fisheries by educational and certification programs primarily directed toward producers/harvesters, distributors, and retailers in the industry. In addition, FishWise periodically publishes an updated list of fish containing a low level of mercury that is useful for both consumers and industry (Box 77-1). Other initiatives, such as those by the Blue Ocean Institute (blueocean.

BOX 77-1 Fish Containing a Low Level of Mercury*

Abalone (United States farmed)
Arctic char†* (farmed)
Catfish (farmed)
Clams
Cod, black/sablefish,† Pacific† (United States and Canada)
Crab, Dungeness/king/Tanner/snow (United States and Canada)
Crawfish (United States farmed)
Flounder, arrowtooth/starry (United States and British Columbia, Canada)
Haddock (United States handline)
Hake (United States Atlantic)
Halibut (Pacific†)
Herring (United States Atlantic)
Lobster, American (United States and Canada)
Lobster, spiny (United States, Mexico [Pacific], and Bahamas)
Mackerel (United States Atlantic)
Mahi-Mahi (United States and international handline)
Mussels, blue† (farmed)
Oysters (Pacific, Eastern-wild†)
Pollock† (United States)
Salmon (Alaska-wild† and British Columbia, Canada†)
Sardines (Pacific†)
Scallops (United States wild and farmed)
Sea bass, black† (north of North Carolina)
Shrimp† (United States and Canada)
Sole (English†)
Squid†
Tilapia† (United States, South and Central America farmed)
Trout (United States farmed, Rainbow†)
Tuna, albacore (United States and Canada [Pacific], international handline)
Tuna, skipjack (United States and international handline)
Tuna, tongol (Malaysian and international handline)
Tuna, yellowfin (Handline)

*See fishwise.org for further information.
†These fish are also low in polychlorinated biphenyls.

BOX 77-2   Representative Ichthyocrinotoxic Fish Hazardous to Humans

Phylum Chordata
Class Agnatha
Order Myxiniformes: hagfishes, lampreys
  Family Myxinidae
    Myxine glutinosa: Atlantic hagfish
    Petromyzon marinus: sea lamprey, large nine-eyes
Class Osteichthyes
Order Anguilliformes: eels
  Family Muraenidae
    Muraena helena: moray eel
Order Perciformes: perch-like fishes
  Family Serranidae
    Grammistes sexlineatus: golden striped bass
    Rypticus saponaceus: soapfish
Order Tetraodontiformes: triggerfishes, puffers, trunkfishes
  Family Canthigasteridae
    Canthigaster jactator: sharp-nosed puffer
  Family Diodontidae
    Diodon hystrix: porcupinefish
  Family Ostraciontidae
    Lactoria diaphana: trunkfish
    Lactoria fornasini: trunkfish, boxfish
  Family Tetraodontidae
    Arothron hispidus: puffer, toadfish, blowfish, rabbitfish
    Fugu xanthopterus: puffer
Order Batrachoidiformes: toadfishes
  Family Batrachoididae
    Opsanus tau: oyster toadfish
    Thalassophryne maculosa: toadfish

org), include a more consumer-based focus with educational outreach that includes smartphone applications that provide instant, color-coded guides to sustainable seafood.

ICHTHYOSARCOTOXISM

The term *ichthyosarcotoxism* describes a variety of conditions arising as the result of poisoning by fish flesh. Many toxins are generally not destroyed by heat or gastric acid. Various toxins are found in the musculature, viscera, blood, skin, or mucous secretions of the fish. Further classification is based on the specific organ system poisoned, for example, ichthyocrinotoxins (glandular secretions), ichthyohemotoxins (blood), ichthyohepatotoxins (liver), ichthyootoxins (gonads), ichthyoallyeinotoxins (hallucinatory), and gempylotoxins (purgative).

ICHTHYOCRINOTOXICATION

Ichthyocrinotoxic fish poisoning is induced by ingestion of glandular secretions not associated with a specific venom apparatus; this usually involves skin secretions, poisonous foams, or slimes. Examples of these toxic fish are certain filefish, pufferfish, porcupinefish, trunkfish, boxfish, cowfish, lampreys, moray eels, and toadfish (Box 77-2). Cyclostome poisoning results from ingestion of the slime and flesh of certain lampreys and hagfishes. Pahutoxin and homopahutoxin have been isolated from secretions of the Japanese boxfish *Ostracion immaculatus*.[163]

Ichthyotoxic skin secretions may cause a bitter taste.[183] Ingestion of ichthyocrinotoxins causes gastrointestinal symptoms within a few hours of ingestion, characterized by nausea, vomiting, dysenteric diarrhea, tenesmus, abdominal pain, and weakness. Most victims recover within 24 hours; however, some individuals have symptoms for up to 3 days. Therapy is supportive and based on symptoms. Additionally, some slime, such as "grammistin" from the soapfish (*Rypticus saponaceus* of the family Grammistidae), can cause contact irritant dermatitis.[209] This dermatitis is managed with cool compresses of aluminum sulfate and calcium acetate (Domeboro). All suspect fish should be washed carefully with water or brine solution and skinned before being eaten.

ICHTHYOHEMOTOXICATION

Ichthyohemotoxic fish are perfused with "poisonous blood," the toxicity of which is usually inactivated by heat and gastric juice. Examples are various eels, such as morays, anguilliforms, and congers. The syndrome is predominantly gastrointestinal and should be treated according to symptoms. Hematologic complications are rare. Risk of intoxication is increased by ingestion of raw or undercooked fish.

ICHTHYOHEPATOTOXICATION

Ichthyohepatotoxic fish carry toxin predominantly in the liver. The remainder of the fish may be nontoxic. Fish that are always toxic fall into two basic groups: (1) Japanese perch–like fish (e.g., mackerel, sea bass, porgy, sandfish) and (2) tropical sharks (e.g., requiem fish, sleeperfish, cowfish, great white shark, catfish, hammerhead, angelfish, Greenland fish, dogfish).[371] Some skates and rays, whose phylogeny is similar to that of sharks, harbor ichthyohepatotoxins.

Ingestion of the Japanese perch–like fish group causes an onset of symptoms within the first hour, with maximal intensity over the ensuing 6 hours.[445] Symptoms include nausea, vomiting, headache, flushing, rash, fever, and tachycardia. No fatalities have been reported.

Ingestion of tropical shark liver (and occasionally of the musculature), such as that of the Greenland shark *(Somniosus microcephalus)*, results in "elasmobranch poisoning" (Box 77-3).[25] Symptoms are noted within 30 minutes of ingestion and include nausea, vomiting, diarrhea, abdominal pain, malaise, diaphoresis, headache, stomatitis, esophagitis, muscle cramps, arthralgias, paresthesias, hiccups, trismus, hyporeflexia, ataxia, incontinence, blurred vision, blepharospasm, delirium, respiratory distress, and coma; death may ensue. Recovery varies from several days to weeks. If only the flesh is eaten, the symptoms are mild and gastroenteric, with spontaneous resolution.

In 1993, 200 people in Madagascar were poisoned after ingesting a single shark identified as *Carcharhinus leucas*. They all experienced symptoms, and 30% died. Two lipophilic toxins were isolated from the shark liver and named carchatoxin-A and carchatoxin-B.[47] Trimethylamine oxide, found in shark liver and

BOX 77-3   Representative Poisonous Sharks (Elasmobranchs) Hazardous to Humans

Phylum Chordata
Class Chondrichthyes
Order Squaliformes: sharks
  Family Carcharhinidae
    Carcharhinus melanopterus: blacktip reef shark
    Carcharhinus menisorrah: gray reef shark
    Galeocerdo cuvier: tiger shark
    Prionace glauca: blue shark
  Family Dalatiidae
    Somniosus microcephalus: Greenland shark, sleeper shark, nurse shark
  Family Hexanchidae
    Hexanchus griseus: cow shark, gray shark, mud shark
  Family Isuridae
    Carcharodon carcharias: white shark
  Family Scyliorhinidae
    Scyliorhinus canicula: dogfish, lesser-spotted cat shark
  Family Sphyrnidae
    Sphyrna diplana: hammerhead shark
  Family Squatinidae
    Squatina dumeril: monkfish, angel shark
  Family Triakidae
    Triaenodon obesus: white-tip houndshark

flesh, has also been implicated in shark poisoning.[14] A similar syndrome has occurred in sled dogs that ingest large quantities of shark flesh.

Therapy is supportive and based on symptoms. If the victim is treated within 60 minutes of ingestion of the shark liver or other viscera, gastrointestinal decontamination with activated charcoal (50 to 100 g [1.8 to 3.6 oz]) may be of value. Fish liver or any shark viscera should not be eaten. However, drying the flesh properly may minimize toxicity.

ICHTHYOOTOXICATION

Ichthyootoxic fish possess toxic gonads that may vary in toxicity with the reproductive cycle. The musculature is generally nontoxic. Examples are sturgeon, alligator gar, salmon, pike, minnow, carp, catfish, killifish, perch, and sculpin. Sea urchins may be toxic during the reproductive period.[25] This toxicity is exemplified by *Paracentrotus lividus* (Europe), *Tripneustes ventricosus* (West Africa), and *Diadema antillarum* (West Indies). Heat does not inactivate the toxin.

Symptoms begin within an hour of ingestion and include nausea, vomiting, diarrhea, headache, dizziness, fever, thirst, xerostomia, bitter taste, tachycardia, seizures, paralysis, and hypotension; death occasionally occurs. Treatment is supportive and based on symptoms. The roe of any fish should not be eaten during the reproductive season.

ICHTHYOALLYEINOTOXICATION

Ichthyoallyeinotoxic fish induce hallucinatory fish poisoning. These are predominantly reef fish of the tropical Pacific and Indian reefs; they carry these heat-stable toxins mainly in the head, brain, and spinal cord and in lesser amounts in the musculature. Typical species include surgeonfish, chub, mullet, unicornfish, goatfish, sergeant major fish, grouper, rabbitfish, rock cod, drumfish, rudderfish, and damselfish. Hallucinatory mullet poisoning has been described as a seasonal condition that occurs only during the summer months in restricted areas on the Hawaiian islands of Kauai and Molokai.[211] Symptoms can develop within 5 to 90 minutes of ingestion and include dizziness, circumoral paresthesias, diaphoresis, weakness, incoordination, auditory and visual hallucinations, nightmares, depression, dyspnea, bronchospasm, brief paralysis, and pharyngitis.[25] No fatalities have been reported. Various toxins, including indoles akin to lysergic acid diethylamide, have been implicated, the sources being algae and plankton eaten by the fish.[438] Heating the fish does not appear to lessen the severity of poisoning.

Therapy for ichthyoallyeinotoxic fish poisoning is supportive and based on symptoms. Haloperidol or benzodiazepines may be administered if the victim is agitated, psychotic, or violent. The victim should be observed until normal mental status is regained. The head, brain, or spinal cord of any tropical fish should not be eaten.

GEMPYLOTOXICATION

Gempylotoxic fishes are pelagic mackerels that produce an oil with a pronounced purgative effect. The "toxin" is contained in both the musculature and bones. No particular characteristic distinguishes a gempylotoxic fish from a nontoxic fish of the same species. The castor oil fish *(Ruvettus pretiosus)* is named for its purgative properties.

The victim suffers from abdominal cramping, bloating, mild nausea, and diarrhea, usually within 30 to 60 minutes of ingestion. The disorder is self-limited and resolves in 12 to 18 hours. Diarrhea often occurs without concomitant systemic effects. Fever, bloody or foul-smelling stools, or protracted vomiting suggest infectious gastroenteritis. No specific antidote is available. If the victim cannot tolerate oral fluids because of nausea or severe abdominal cramping, administration of intravenous fluid and antiemetics may be indicated. Antimotility agents are not recommended unless the diarrhea is debilitating because inhibition of peristalsis prolongs transit time of the toxin through the gut and may increase the duration of the disorder.

SPECIFIC TOXIC SYNDROMES RELATED TO SEAFOOD CONSUMPTION

Three specific toxic syndromes related to fish consumption are scombroid poisoning, tetrodotoxin (puffer fish) poisoning (both described in Table 77-1) and grass carp gallbladder poisoning.

SCOMBROID POISONING

Scombroid, the most commonly reported seafood poisoning in the United States, occurs after eating fish with high levels of accumulated histamine or other biogenic amines. The first report of scombroid poisoning was published in 1830 and involved five sailors who consumed bonito fish, a member of the Scombridae family; hence the name of the syndrome.[285] Other members of the family Scombridae include albacore, bluefin and yellowfin tuna, mackerel, saury, needlefish, wahoo, and skipjack. Fish not from the Scombridae family that can produce scombroid include mahi-mahi (dolphinfish), kahawai, sardine, black marlin, pilchard, anchovy, herring, amberjack (yellowtail or kahala), and the Australian ocean salmon *Arripis truttaceus*.[322,428,443,471] Most of these fish species are rich in free histidine in their muscle tissues.[222] Scombroid poisoning accounts for 3% of food-related outbreaks reported to the Centers for Disease Control and Prevention (CDC) in Atlanta.[79] Underreporting is likely because of the short duration of illness and its resemblance to an allergic reaction. Because greater numbers of fish that were previously considered not to be a risk for scombroid poisoning are now recognized as potentially "scombrotoxic," it has been suggested that the syndrome be more appropriately called *pseudoallergic fish poisoning*.[388]

Pathophysiology

During conditions of inadequate preservation or refrigeration, the musculature of dark-fleshed or red-muscled fish undergoes bacterial decomposition.[33,371] The normal surface bacteria *Proteus morganii, Klebsiella pneumoniae, Aerobacter aerogenes, Escherichia coli, Alcaligenes metalcaligenes,* and others have been implicated in the putrefactive process, which includes decarboxylation of the amino acid L-histidine to histamine and saurine (a phosphate salt of histamine).[471,551] This most often occurs when fish is held at ambient or high temperatures for several hours.[114] The term *saurine* originated because of association of scombrotoxism with saury, a Japanese dried fish delicacy.[220] Because of this process, the "scombrotoxin" was initially thought to be histamine, which is commonly found in large amounts in the flesh of the fish usually implicated. Evidence initially suggesting that histamine may be the causative toxin of scombroid fish poisoning was presented in an investigation of a small outbreak.[336] The urinary excretion of histamine and its metabolite, *N*-methylhistamine, was measured in three persons who had scombrotoxism after ingestion of marlin. There was no increase in the principal metabolite of prostaglandin D_2 (a mast cell secretory product considered to indicate release of histamine from mast cells), supporting the hypothesis that the excess histamine was from the fish rather than endogenously produced in the victims. Histamine levels greater than 20 to 50 mg/100 g are frequently noted in scombrotoxic fish, and it is not unusual to record levels in excess of 400 mg/100 g.[428] However, it is possible that some other compound may be responsible for scombroid symptoms, because the syndrome cannot be reproduced solely by administration of equal or even massive doses of histamine by the oral route. Histamine is rapidly inactivated by enzymes in the gastrointestinal tract and on first pass through the liver, with very little reaching the systemic circulation. Other compounds, such as cadaverine, putrescine, or *cis*-urocanic acid, may be present in the decomposed fish flesh and may either facilitate absorption or inhibit gastrointestinal or hepatic degradation of histamine.[43,407,471] Whatever the causative toxin, it is heat stable and not destroyed by cooking. Affected fish typically have a sharply metallic or peppery taste but may be normal in appearance and color. Not all persons who eat a scombrotoxin- or histamine-contaminated fish become

TABLE 77-1   Seafood Toxidromes

Toxidrome	Seafoods	Regions	Causative Organisms	Toxins Produced	Mechanisms of Action	Clinical Manifestations	Time of Symptom Onset After Ingestion	Duration of Illness	Treatment
Fish-Related Toxic Syndromes									
Scombroid	Albacore, tuna, wahoo, mackerel, skipjack, bonito, mahi-mahi	Worldwide	Presumably, bacteria within the fish transform histidine to histamine	Histamine, saurine	Histamine response	Diffuse erythema, flushing, nausea, vomiting, pruritus, headache, urticaria, bronchospasm	Minutes	Resolves in 8-12 hr	Histamine-1 and -2 blockers, antiemetics
Tetrodotoxin	Puffer fish (fugu), porcupinefish, sunfish	Tropical and subtropical	*Pseudomonas* species	Tetrodotoxin	Na⁺ channel blocker, blocks axonal transmission	Paresthesias of lips and tongue, hypersalivation, weakness, ataxia, tremor, dysphagia, seizure, bronchospasm, hypotension, nausea, vomiting, diarrhea, death	10 min to 4 hr	Hours to days	Supportive, aggressive airway management, intravenous fluids, inotropic agents, ? anticholinesterase agent
Algal Bloom–Related Toxic Syndromes									
Ciguatera	Tropical and semitropical reef fish such as barracuda, grouper, snapper, jack	Worldwide, most common in Indian Ocean, South Pacific, Caribbean	*Gambierdiscus toxicus* and other species	Ciguatoxin, maitotoxin, GT1-4, palytoxin	Na⁺ channel blocker	Gastroenteritis followed by neurologic symptoms: dysesthesias, hot/cold reversal, weakness, respiratory paralysis	2-6 hr	Days to months	Supportive, ? intravenous mannitol
Clupeotoxin	Herring, sardines, anchovies, tarpons, bonefish	Caribbean, Indo-Pacific, Africa	*Ostreopis siamensis*	Palytoxin	Inhibits Na⁺K⁺-ATPase	Metallic taste, nausea, vomiting, diarrhea, paresthesias, hypotension, death	30-60 min	Days	Supportive, ? early gastric emptying
Paralytic shellfish poisoning	Shellfish	Northeast and northwest coasts of United States, Philippines, Alaska, North Sea	*Protogonyaulax, Alexandrium catarella, Pyrodinium, Saxidomus, Gonyaulax*	Saxitoxin, neosaxitoxins, gonyautoxins	Na⁺ channel blocker, may suppress atrioventricular nodal conduction	Paresthesias of face and extremities, numbness, dysphonia, dysphagia, ataxia, weakness, paralysis, death from respiratory failure	30-60 min	Weeks	Supportive, activated charcoal, ventilatory support

Syndrome	Source	Organism	Toxin	Mechanism	Clinical Manifestations	Onset	Duration	Treatment
Neurotoxic shellfish poisoning	Shellfish	Ptychodiscus brevis	Brevetoxins	Modulate Na$^+$ channel	Circumoral paresthesias, ataxia, gastrointestinal symptoms; if aerosolized, may cause conjunctivitis, bronchospasm	Minutes to hours	Several hours to a few days	Supportive
Diarrhetic shellfish poisoning	Shellfish	Dinophysis, Prorocentrum	Okadaic acid and others	Phosphatase A$_1$ and A$_2$ inhibitors	Acute gastroenteritis	30 min-2 hr	2-3 days	Supportive
Amnestic shellfish poisoning	Shellfish	Nitzschia pungens, Pseudonitzschia australis	Domoic acid	Glutamate antagonist	Gastroenteritis, seizures, coma, anterograde memory disorder	1-24 hr	24 hr-12 wk	Supportive, benzodiazepines for seizures
Possible estuary-associated syndrome	Estuarine fish	Pfiesteria piscicida	Unidentified	Unknown	Headache, skin lesions, eye irritation, respiratory irritation, learning and memory deficits, cognitive impairment	Within 2 wk of exposure	Improves within 3-6 mo	No treatment; cholestyramine for persistent symptoms
Haff disease	Buffalo fish	? Blue-green algae	Unknown	Unknown	Severe muscle pain, rhabdomyolysis, weakness, tachycardia, hypotension	6-12 hr	Days	Supportive, intravenous fluids, ? diuretics
Azaspiracid poisoning	Shellfish	Azadinium spinosum	Azaspiracid	Cytotoxic	Nausea, vomiting, diarrhea	Within hours	2-3 days	Supportive, intravenous fluids
Yessotoxin	Shellfish	Protoceratium reticulatum, Lingulodinium polyedrum, Gonyaulax spinifera	Yessotoxin	Unknown	Restlessness, dyspnea, shivering, cramps	Within hours		Supportive, intravenous fluids

ATPase, adenosine triphosphatase.

ill, possibly because of uneven distribution of decay within the fish.

Clinical Presentation

The effects of scombroid fish poisoning occur within minutes after consumption of the fish. Symptoms are similar to an allergic reaction (which it is not) and typically include headache, diffuse erythema, a sense of warmth without elevation in core temperature, nausea, vomiting, diarrhea, abdominal cramps, conjunctival injection, pruritus, dizziness, and a burning sensation in the mouth and oropharynx.[30,254,322] Flushing of the head, neck, and upper torso is characteristic. Severe effects, such as bronchospasm, generalized urticaria, hypotension, palpitations, and dysrhythmias, have been reported but are not frequent.[176,119,220,548,] In most healthy victims, the syndrome is self-limited, resolving within 6 to 12 hours. In rare cases, symptoms can persist beyond 24 hours.[222] In patients with preexisting respiratory or cardiac disease, effects of the poisoning can precipitate more severe illness.[50,322] Scombroid reactions may be markedly more severe in patients taking isoniazid because of this compound's blockade of gastrointestinal tract histaminase.[495] Death has never been reported after scombroid poisoning. Assays of histamine and its metabolite in urine samples of scombroid-poisoned patients demonstrated elevated levels compared with controls, although histamine measurement is neither common in clinical practice nor recommended. Histamine levels poorly correlate with clinical manifestations and do not affect management decisions.

Treatment

Gastric decontamination for scombroid poisoning is not indicated, because symptoms occur rapidly and vomiting can be a primary effect of the toxin. Symptoms can be lessened or controlled with administration of histamine-1 (H_1) receptor antagonists, such as diphenhydramine or hydroxyzine, administered initially in doses of 25 to 50 mg orally or intravenously. Histamine-2 (H_2) receptor antagonists (e.g., ranitidine, famotidine) have also been shown to relieve most of the symptoms; a combination of H_1 and H_2 receptor antagonists may be most effective.[45,193] Vomiting is usually controlled by an antihistamine, but occasionally requires addition of a specific antiemetic, such as ondansetron. The persistent headache of scombroid poisoning may respond to famotidine or a similar drug if standard analgesics are not effective.[19] Intravenous fluids and inhaled bronchodilators should be used as needed. Vasopressors are rarely necessary because hypotension is usually mild and responds to intravenous fluid administration. Corticosteroids are generally not indicated.

Prevention

The only effective method for prevention of scombroid fish poisoning is consistent temperature control at less than 40° F (4.4° C) at all times between catching and consumption.[114] It has been difficult to reduce the occurrence of scombroid poisoning in the United States; recreational catches likely play a major role.[222] No fish should be consumed if it has been handled improperly or has the smell of ammonia. Fresh fish generally has a sheen or oily rainbow appearance; "dull" packaged fish should be avoided. If an episode of scombroid poisoning is recognized, it is important to report it promptly to local public health authorities to prevent additional exposures, particularly if the food was served in a public eating establishment.[221]

TETRODOTOXIN POISONING

Tetrodotoxin (TTX) is a potent neurotoxin found in a variety of creatures and has been isolated from animals of four different phyla, including puffer fish, California newt, blue-ringed octopus, poison dart frogs, ivory shell, and trumpet shell. TTX is characteristic of the order Tetraodontiformes.[458] The suborder Tetraodontoidei contains three families of fish (Tetraodontidae, Diodontidae, and Canthigasteridae), including puffer fish (toadfish, blowfish, globefish, swellfish, balloonfish, toado) and porcupinefish. Sunfish (*Mola* species) are members of the suborder Moloidei. Tetrodotoxin was named around 1911 after searching for the active ingredient in fugu ovaries.[160] Isolation of the chemical was achieved in the 1950s. In the 1970s, the major toxin in certain poison dart frogs was identified as TTX. Crystalline TTX was isolated in 1978. The puffer fish, sometimes called a globefish, is one of the better-recognized species that contains TTX. These fish can be found in both freshwater and saltwater and can inflate their bodies to a nearly spherical shape using air or seawater.[198] Human TTX poisonings have also occurred after consumption of gastropod mollusks.[534] Envenomation from the blue-ringed octopus is rare, but poisonings have occurred from their consumption.[154,531]

Puffer fish poisoning has been recognized for millennia. Ancient Asian literature documents the dangers of eating puffer fish.[198] There are references to puffer fish in hieroglyphics of the ancient Egyptian dynasty of 2700 BC. Scholars suggest this fish was known to be poisonous during Egyptian times. Mosaic sanitary laws against eating fish without fins and scales may have been derived to avoid fish containing TTX; the TTX-containing fish in the region inhabited by the Israelites were scaleless.[198]

Captain James Cook, the British explorer, recorded in 1774 his experience after eating a piece of liver from a puffer fish purchased from a native fisherman during his voyages in the Pacific Ocean.[505] Before preparing the fish for eating, it was described and drawn. Cook tasted the liver and wrote of a vivid feeling of extraordinary weakness and numbness.[198] There has been some contention that TTX (also known as puffer powder) was used as a component of the Haitian voodoo potion in the zombie ritual.[484] This has been challenged on grounds, among others, that under the usual conditions of extreme alkaline storage, any TTX in a "zombie potion" would be decomposed irreversibly into pharmacologically inactive products.[251,537]

In humans, the most common exposure to TTX is through the ingestion of fugu, a special preparation of puffer fish.[73] Sporadic cases have been reported in the United States.[85] In Japan, chefs must undergo a rigorous certification process before they are allowed to prepare fugu. The fillet of the puffer fish contains very small concentrations of TTX. Fugu is served raw with paper-thin slices placed into an ornate configuration. The presence of small quantities of TTX gives the desired effect of slight oral tingling. Importation of fugu into the United States is illegal, but smuggling has resulted in cases of poisoning. At least 50 of the more than 100 species of these fish have been involved in poisonings of humans or may be intermittently toxic.[406] Many species other than fish also contain TTX (Box 77-4).

Many years ago, when TTX was believed to be present exclusively in puffer fish, it was controversial whether TTX was endogenous. It is now known that TTX is accumulated through the food chain, in a several-step process starting with marine bacteria as the primary source.[351] TTX may be produced by *Pseudomonas* species that live on skin of the puffer fish.[544] This would explain the transmittal of toxicity between toxic and nontoxic fish through skin contact. Other investigators have found that *Vibrio* and other species isolated from intestines of puffer fish produce TTX.[512] The exact origin of TTX in the food chain, however, remains unknown. Distribution of TTX in the body of a puffer fish appears to be species-specific. In general, the liver and ovaries have the highest toxicity, followed by intestines and skin.[351] Female fish are considered more toxic than are males because there are especially high concentrations of TTX in ovaries. The musculature is less toxic but still may contain a significant amount of TTX. The toxin is heat stable and not inactivated by freezing. There occurs seasonal variation of TTX concentration, with peak levels during spawning season. TTX is likely accumulated as a biologic defense agent.[351]

Pathophysiology

TTX blocks the action potentials in nerves by binding to the pores of voltage-gated, fast sodium channels in nerve cell membranes. TTX has a unique nonprotein structure and is widely used as a research tool to study sodium channels. Mouse bioassays demonstrate that the minimal lethal dose of TTX by intraperitoneal injection is 8 to 20 mg/kg.[337] Interaction of TTX with the sodium channel is thought to be stoichiometric, with each TTX molecule interfering with one channel. TTX affects the

BOX 77-4 Non-Tetraodontiformes Containing Tetrodotoxin

Phylum Chordata

Order Caudata

Family Salamandridae
Taricha granulosa: rough-skinned newt
Notophthalmus viridescens: eastern newt
Triturus: European newts
Pleurodeles: ribbed newts
Cynops: fire belly newts
Paramesotriton: warty newts
Tylototriton: crocodile newts

Order Anura

Family Bufonidae
Atelopus: stubfoot toad

Phylum Mollusca

Order Caenogastropoda

Family Buccinidae
Babylonia japonica: ivory shell
Family Naticidae
Natica lineata: lined moon shell
Natica vitellus: calf moon shell
Polinices didyma: bladder moon shell
Family Ranellidae
Charonia sauliae: trumpet shell

Order Octopoda

Family Octopodidae
Hapalochlaena maculosa: Australian blue-ringed octopus

Phylum Echinodermata

Order Paxillosida

Family Astropectinidae
Astropecten polyacanthus: starfish

Phylum Nemertea

Order Paleonemertea

Family Cephalothricidae
Cephalohrix linearis: ribbon worm

Phylum Platyhelminthes

Order Polycladida

Family Planoceridae
Planocera multitentaculata: flat worm

Phylum Arthropoda

Order Decapoda

Family Xanthidae
Atergatis floridus: xanthid crab

Order Xiphosura

Family Limulidae
Carcinoscorpius rotundicauda: mangrove horseshoe crab

Data from Dunn J: Algae kills dialysis patients in Brazil, BMJ 312:1183, 1996; Edwards C, Beattei KA, Scrimgeour CM, et al: Identification of anatoxin-A in benthic cyanobacteria (blue-green algae) and in associated dog poisonings at Loch Insh, Scotland, Toxicon 30:1165, 1992; Gessner BD, Middaugh JP: Paralytic shellfish poisoning in Alaska: A 20-year retrospective analysis, Am J Epidemiol 141:766, 1995; Rosen L, Loison G, Laigret J, et al: Studies on eosinophilic meningitis. 3. Epidemiologic and clinical observations on Pacific Islands and the possible etiologic role of Angiostrongylus cantonensis, Am J Epidemiol 85:17, 1967; and Tatsumi M, Kajiwara A, Yasumoto T, et al: Potent excitatory effect of scaritoxin on the guinea-pig vas deferens, taenia caeci and ileum, J Pharmacol Exp Ther 235:783, 1985.

spike-generating process of sodium channels, not the resting or steady-state voltage.[249]

TTX interferes with both central and peripheral neuromuscular transmission. Although it is not a depolarizing agent, in animals it causes depression of the medullary respiratory mechanism, intracardiac conduction, and myocardial and skeletal muscle contractility. At the microcellular level, the mechanism of action of TTX is linked to the axon rather than to the nerve end plate. TTX blocks axonal transmission by interfering with sodium conductance within the depolarized regions of the cell membrane, perhaps by acting at a metal cation binding site in the sodium channel, without affecting presynaptic release of acetylcholine or its effects on the neuromuscular junction.[4,212] There is no apparent effect on potassium permeability.[404] Saxitoxin, implicated in paralytic shellfish poisoning, has essentially the same action as does TTX on the nerve membrane, although it is believed to have a discrete receptor.[254] The poison in freshwater puffers may be composed of TTX or saxitoxin, the predominant toxin depending on the species. The lethal dose (LD_{50}) for mice is 10 mg/kg when TTX is administered by intraperitoneal, intravenous, or subcutaneous routes.[482]

Animal studies suggest that TTX has a peripheral effect that results in vasodilation independent of α- or β-adrenergic receptors.[233,250,301] Further studies suggest a dose-dependent action. At low doses, systemic blood pressure is lowered, although perfusion pressure is initially maintained. Higher doses of TTX result in a profound fall in blood pressure.[249] Experiments with animal models using TTX from blue-ringed octopi demonstrate a similar profound hypotension. Agonists (norepinephrine or phenylephrine) have been the most effective agents in raising blood pressure in models of TTX poisoning.[154]

Clinical Presentation

Clinical manifestations typically develop within 30 minutes of ingestion but may be delayed by up to 4 hours. In a 2002 outbreak in Bangladesh of 37 people (from eight families) who were poisoned from inadequately prepared puffer fish, 31 victims developed symptoms within 2 hours and 8 died.[2] Death has been recorded within 17 minutes of exposure. The extent and type of symptoms vary according to the individual and amount of TTX ingested. Usually, paresthesias of the lips and tongue are followed by several signs; they may be as mild as diaphoresis or as life-threatening as hypotension, respiratory failure, and coma.[85] Other commonly described symptoms include weakness, headache, body paresthesias, and gastrointestinal symptoms such as nausea, vomiting, and abdominal pain. Hypersalivation, ataxia, cyanosis, dysphagia, aphonia, dyspnea, blurred vision, bronchorrhea, and bronchospasm have been described.[2,85,94,101] Early miosis may progress to mydriasis with poor pupillary light reflex.[482] A disseminated intravascular coagulation—like syndrome is heralded by petechial skin hemorrhages that can progress to bullous desquamation and diffuse stigmata of prolonged coagulation. Hypotension can be profound and may be refractory to treatment. Bradycardia and atrioventricular node conduction abnormalities may be present. Complete cardiovascular collapse with respiratory paralysis precedes death. Normal consciousness may be maintained until shortly before death.[160,482] In some older reports, 60% of victims died, most within the first 6 hours. Survival past 24 hours is a good prognostic sign.

Treatment

Treatment of TTX is primarily supportive, with aggressive airway management and assisted ventilation.[439] Decontamination may be considered with 1 g/kg of activated charcoal given as soon as practical following presentation if no contraindications (such as vomiting or altered mental status) are present. Atropine may be used to treat bradycardia in conjunction with adequate oxygenation ($SaO_2 > 92\%$). Intravenous fluid resuscitation should be initiated for hypotension; however, use of vasopressors may be required to maintain perfusion. α-Agonists, such as phenylephrine or norepinephrine, are more likely to be effective. No antidote is currently available to treat TTX poisoning.

Cholinesterase inhibitors, such as edrophonium and neostigmine, have been used to treat victims of TTX poisoning, with mixed results. Some case reports suggested subjective improvement in neurologic symptoms after administration of cholinesterase inhibitors.[91,482] A recent case series suggested that neostigmine may help overcome respiratory muscle paralysis, which is the predominant cause of death.[91] Other case reports noted no improvement after infusion of these compounds.[2,310,479] Antihistamines and steroids have also been used without clear benefit.[310]

A minor intoxication with TTX may be limited to paresthesias and mild dysphagia. In such a case, the victim should be observed in the emergency department or intensive care unit for at least 8 hours to monitor for deterioration, particularly in respiratory function. The victim should not be discharged until symptoms are clearly improving. Although it is water soluble, TTX is very difficult to remove from fish, even by cooking. It is prudent to avoid all puffers, even when prepared by an expert.

GRASS CARP GALLBLADDER POISONING

Fish gallbladder has long been used as a folk remedy in China and Southeast Asia. In a case series of 17 patients from Vietnam, the most common reason for ingestion was for symptoms of arthritis.[533] The toxin is found in the bile of freshwater fish of the family Cyprinidae. Grass carp (Ctenopharyngodon idellus) accounts for 80% of freshwater fish gallbladder poisonings in China.[276] Serious illness is attributed to the nephrotoxic and hepatotoxic properties of a toxin in bile.[88] The toxic ingredient is 5-α-cyprinol sulfate, a 27-carbon salt, which is heat stable and not destroyed by ethanol.[19,272] Most cases have occurred in Hong Kong, Taiwan, and South Korea. Two cases were reported in the United States in immigrants who ate raw gallbladders from carp caught in Maryland.[70] One of the patients required hemodialysis for acute renal failure.

Several hours after ingestion, abdominal pain, nausea, vomiting, and watery diarrhea develop. This can be accompanied by marked elevations in concentrations of liver enzymes (aspartate and alanine aminotransferases).[121] The hepatitis is usually self-limited, although fulminant liver failure and death have been reported.[253,533] Nephrotoxicity occurs in moderate to severe poisonings and may be profound, leading to oliguric or nonoliguric renal failure within 48 to 72 hours after ingestion.[409,533] Renal and liver biopsies demonstrate acute tubular necrosis and hepatocellular injury. With appropriate supportive care, including dialysis, patients typically recover. Acute renal failure accounts for more than 80% of deaths, although the mortality rate has declined, likely due to advances in intensive care and renal salvage therapy.[276]

POISONINGS ASSOCIATED WITH ALGAL BLOOMS

Although there are thousands of species of microalgae that form the base of the food chain, fewer than 60 species are toxic or harmful. These toxic species may cause significant rates of death in fish and shellfish, seabirds, and marine mammals, as well as human illnesses and death. Algal toxins have resulted in more than 500,000 incidents per year, with an overall mortality rate of 1.5% on a global basis.[510] In the United States, harmful algal blooms now threaten virtually every coastal state, and the number of toxic species is increasing. Algae can reproduce rapidly, even to the point of discoloring the sea, producing "red tides."[446] Several distinct clinical syndromes exist: ciguatera fish poisoning, clupeotoxic fish poisoning, paralytic shellfish poisoning, neurotoxic shellfish poisoning, diarrhetic shellfish poisoning, amnestic shellfish poisoning, possible estuary-associated syndrome, and Haff disease (see Table 77-1). Besides these more familiar syndromes, several newer syndromes have been characterized recently, including illness due to azaspiracid toxins, yessotoxin, and palytoxin.

Most dinoflagellate toxins are neurotoxins, causing toxicity via their interaction with voltage-sensitive ion channels or specific receptors associated with neurotransmitter release. Some block the channel pore physically and prevent ion conductance (hydrophilic low-molecular-mass toxins and large polypeptide toxins). Others alter voltage-dependent gating through binding to intramembranous receptor sites (alkaloid toxins and related lipid-soluble toxins) or intracellular sites (polypeptide toxins).[510]

CIGUATERA POISONING

The word ciguatera is derived from the Spanish name cigua for the sea snail Turbo pica found in the Caribbean Spanish Antilles.[26,475] Ciguatera poisoning, a neurotoxic syndrome, has been recognized throughout history, with one of the earliest cases reported in the 4th century when Alexander the Great refused to allow his soldiers to eat fish, and another during the Tang Dynasty in China.[452] One of the earliest written records of suspected ciguatera poisoning is from the journal of Captain William Bligh, who described symptoms consistent with ciguatera in 1789 after eating mahi-mahi.[452] In addition, it was also quite possibly ciguatera that was illustrated by Captain James Cook while sailing on the Resolution in the South Pacific in 1774.[368]

Ciguatera fish poisoning is an important cause of food-borne disease and is endemic throughout subtropical and tropical regions of the Indo-Pacific and Caribbean. More than 400 species of fish have been implicated to cause ciguatera fish poisoning. In the United States, it is a prominent nonbacterial type of food poisoning associated with fish, second only to scombroid, with cases having been reported in many states.[79,171,215,332,507] Outbreaks of ciguatera are most common between the months of April and August. In endemic areas, the incidence is estimated to be between 500 and 600 cases per 10,000 people.[278] Worldwide, ciguatera may affect more than 50,000 persons each year. Most cases in the United States occur in Hawaii and Florida, with the incidence in Florida estimated to be five cases per 10,000 people.[142] The true incidence of ciguatera fish poisoning is difficult to ascertain because of underreporting. It is believed that only 2% to 10% of cases are reported to health authorities.[159] Outbreaks of ciguatera have been associated with ingestion of warm-water, reef-dwelling fish caught in the zone between the latitudes of approximately 30 and 35 degrees.[29,199] In addition, the advent of flash-freezing and shipping of fish around the world has accounted for several cases of ciguatera in nonendemic areas.[215]

The most frequently implicated reef fishes are listed in Box 77-5. Of reported cases, 75% (except in Hawaii) involve barracuda, snapper, jack, or grouper. Hawaiian carriers of the toxin include parrot-beaked bottom feeders and surgeonfishes, particularly those inhabiting waters with high dinoflagellate populations, such as those with disturbed coral reefs.[232] Other fish that have been reported as ciguatoxic are listed in Box 77-6. Ciguatera has also been reported after ingestion of farm-raised salmon.[130] There is one report of ciguatera from consumption of jellyfish.[550]

Pathophysiology

The blue-green and free algal dinoflagellate Gambierdiscus toxicus is thought to be responsible for producing ciguatoxins.[452] G. toxicus adheres to dead coral surfaces and marine algae that are consumed by smaller herbivorous fish.[182,278] Although G. toxicus is very likely responsible for the majority of ciguatoxins encountered in fish, the cyanobacterium Trichodesmium erythraeum can produce water- and lipid-soluble precursors to the

---

BOX 77-5 Reef Fish Frequently Implicated in Ciguatera Poisoning

Phylum Chordata
Order Anguilliformes
Family Muraenidae: moray eels

Order Mugiliformes
Family Mugilidae: mullets

Order Perciformes
Family Acanthuridae: surgeonfishes
Family Carangidae: jacks
Family Labridae: wrasses
Family Lethrinidae: emperor fish
Family Lutjanidae: snappers
Family Scaridae: parrotfishes
Family Serranidae: groupers
Family Sparidae: porgies
Family Sphyraenidae: barracuda

Order Tetraodontiformes
Family Balistidae: triggerfishes

From Gilbert DN, Moellering RC, Sande MA: The Sanford guide to antimicrobial therapy, ed 34, 2007, Sperryville, Virginia, Antimicrobial Therapy, Inc., pp 98-99.

BOX 77-6 Some Fish Other Than Those in Box 77-5 That Are Known to Be Ciguatoxic

Albulidae (ladyfishes)
Chanidae (milkfishes)
Clupeidae (herrings)
Elopidae (tarpons)
Engraulidae (anchovies)
Synodontidae (lizardfishes)
Congridae (true eels)
Ophichthidae (snake eels)
Belonidae (needlefishes)
Exocoetidae (flying fishes)
Hemiramphidae (halfbeaks)
Aulostomidae (trumpetfishes)
Syngnathidae (seahorses)
Holocentridae (squirrelfishes)
Apogonidae (cardinalfishes)
Arripidae (sea perches)
Chaetodontidae (butterfly fishes)
Cirrhitidae (hawkfishes)
Coryphaenidae (dolphins)
Gempylidae (oilfishes)
Gerridae (silverfishes)
Gobiidae (gobies)
Istiophoridae (sailfishes)
Kuhliidae (bass)
Kyphosidae (rudderfishes)
Mullidae (goatfishes)
Pempheridae (sweeperfishes)
Pomacentridae (damselfishes)
Pomadasyidae (grunts)
Priacanthidae (snapper)
Scatophagidae (spade fishes)
Sciaenidae (croakers)
Scombridae (tunas)
Scorpaenidae (scorpionfish)
Siganidae (rabbitfishes)
Xiphiidae (swordfishes)
Zanclidae (idol)
Bothidae (flounders)
Aluteridae and Monacanthidae (filefishes)
Ostraciontidae (trunkfishes)
Batrachoididae (toadfishes)
Antennariidae (sargassumfish)
Lophiidae (goosefish)
Ogcocephalidae (longnose batfish)

toxins that may generate ciguatera syndrome.[141] Other dinoflagellates, such as *Prorocentrum concavum, Prorocentrum mexicanum, Prorocentrum rhathymum, Gymnodinium sanguineum,* and *Gonyaulax polyedra,* may generate toxins that play a role in ciguatera syndrome.[383,480]

Larger reef fish eat the contaminated smaller fish, thereby becoming vectors as ciguatoxin is bioconcentrated up the food chain. It has long been assumed that smaller fish within a given species are safer to eat than the larger ones. However, a recent study sampling different species from French Polynesia found no relationship between toxicity of the fish and size.[164,209,220,371] Although the entire fish is toxic, viscera (particularly the liver) and roe are considered to carry the highest concentrations of toxin.[28] No plankton feeders have so far been reported to be ciguatoxic.

It has been suggested that proliferation of toxic algae may be triggered by contamination of water from a number of sources, including industrial wastes, golf course runoff, metallic compounds, ship wreckage, or other pollutants.[199] In the Marshall Islands (Micronesia), consequent to nuclear testing, the incidence of toxin-producing plankton has tripled.[393] Similar observations have been made with respect to various military activities (dumping and explosives) in the Line Islands and Gilbert Islands (Kiribati, Central Pacific), Hao Atoll (Tuamotu Archipelago, French Polynesia), Gambier Islands (French Polynesia), and

others.[403] Yet another cause of toxic dinoflagellate proliferation may be transfer and dumping of ballast water from large ocean-going vessels.

Ciguatera is associated with more than five toxins, including fat-soluble quaternary ammonium compounds (ciguatoxins), a water-soluble component (maitotoxin, from the Tahitian vernacular name *maito* for the striated surgeonfish *Ctenochaetus striatus*), a maitotoxin-associated hemolysin (lysophosphatidylcholine, or lysolecithin), and a ciguatoxin-associated adenine triphosphatase (ATPase) inhibitor.[202,290,296,413] Scaritoxin (isolated from *Scarus gibbus*) is similar to the fat-soluble component and is specific to parrotfishes.[86] Lipid-extracted toxins from *G. toxicus* have been designated GT-1, GT-2, and GT-3; a water-soluble toxin is designated GT-4.[126,327] Chemical analysis of ciguatoxins demonstrates that they closely resemble brevetoxin C (from *P. brevis*) and okadaic acid, isolated from marine sponges and the dinoflagellate *Prorocentrum lima*.[152,339] Identification of okadaic acid from the Caribbean dinoflagellate *P. concavum* lends support to the notion that this toxin may be more significant in ciguatera poisoning than previously thought. Another compound, named prorocentrolide, has also been found in reef-dwelling fish with okadaic acid and has been implicated in diarrhetic shellfish poisoning, another common fish-borne illness.[152,219]

Three major ciguatoxins (CTX-1, CTX-2, and CTX-3) are usually found in the flesh and viscera of ciguateric fishes. Each is found in variable concentrations; this may account for the inconsistency of reported clinical signs and symptoms.[296] CTX-2 is a diastereomer of CTX-3.[295] Ciguatoxins may result from oxidation of gambiertoxins, possibly through the cytochrome system in fish liver.[297] The lipid components have been characterized as crystalline, colorless, heat-stable compounds with a molecular weight of approximately 1100 daltons, with functional hydroxyl and quaternary nitrogen groups.

Ciguatoxins are potent Na^+ channel toxins and exert their effects by activating voltage-sensitive Na^+ channels. The Na^+ channels open at resting membrane potentials, leading to spontaneous firing of neurons, giving rise to neurologic signs and symptoms of ciguatera.[226] One mechanism of their action may be that they falsely occupy calcium receptor sites that modulate sodium pore permeability in neural, muscle, and myocardial membranes.[35] This effect could allow increased membrane permeability to sodium and cause sustained depolarization. Electrophysiologic studies of the sural and common peroneal nerves in humans with ciguatera, demonstrating reduced light touch, pain, and vibratory sensation in the extremities, showed prolongation of the absolute refractory, relative refractory, and supernormal periods. These findings indirectly suggest that ciguatoxin may abnormally prolong sodium channel opening in nerve membranes.[62] This influx of sodium is antagonized by the presence of TTX.[40]

In vitro studies have also shown that scaritoxin causes release of norepinephrine and acetylcholine and increases sodium channel permeability.[469] Maitotoxin as well may trigger release of norepinephrine and stimulate cellular uptake of calcium and has been hypothesized to stimulate cholinergic receptors by inhibiting acetylcholinesterase.[40,438] However, evidence suggests that highly purified ciguatoxin preparations may not have anticholinesterase effects in vivo.[288]

Hypertension occurring with ciguatera can be suppressed in animal models with phentolamine (an α-antagonist), suggesting α-adrenergic receptor activity. Although purified ciguatoxin appears to have cardiac stimulatory effects (increasing heart rate and output), maitotoxin is a myocardial depressant in vitro, which may explain variation in clinical presentation. Isolated human atrial trabeculae show concentration-dependent positive inotropy with CTX-1 that is not reversed with mannitol.[294] Cardiac calcium conduction effects have been implicated in the activity of maitotoxin, because its action is inhibited in the presence of verapamil, magnesium ions, or low-calcium-concentration solutions. In mice, injection of maitotoxin can induce a marked increase in the total calcium content of the adrenal glands and a rise in the plasma cortisol concentration.[473] When injected into mice, ciguatoxin targets the heart, adrenal glands, and autonomic nervous system.[475] Ciguatoxin and CTX-4c (a derivative), administered in repeated doses, cause the mouse heart to suffer septal and ventricular interstitial fibrosis, accompanied by bilateral ventricular hypertrophy.[477] Ciguatoxin is a potent substance, with an LD_{50} in mice of 0.45 mg/kg in purified form. Maitotoxin is even more potent, with an LD_{50} of 0.13 mg/kg in mice. It is interesting to note that ciguatoxins can become toxic to fish in higher concentrations, thus potentially limiting levels of these compounds carried by a fish.[293] However, the toxin or toxins may reside in skeletal muscle or other tissues of the fish in association with proteins that may be protective of the carrier.[195]

All identified toxins associated with ciguatera are unaffected by freeze-drying, heat, cold, and gastric acid and do not affect the odor, color, or taste of the fish. There is some evidence that cooking methods can alter the relative concentrations of the various toxins. For example, boiling fish flesh will remove water-soluble toxins, but frying or grilling the flesh may increase toxicity of lipid-soluble toxins as a result of releasing lipid-soluble components from the cellular compounds to which they are normally bound.[140]

Clinical Presentation

Ciguatera fish poisoning is associated with gastrointestinal, cardiovascular, neurologic, and neuropsychiatric symptoms and signs. The meal containing ciguatoxins is generally unremarkable in taste and smell. Symptoms may develop within minutes of ingestion, although they generally occur within 2 to 6 hours after the meal. Almost all victims develop symptoms by 24 hours.[26,142] The severity of symptoms seems to follow a dose-dependent pattern, with victims who eat larger portions of ciguatoxic fish experiencing more severe symptoms (Box 77-7). In addition, there are variable concentrations of ciguatoxin within a fish, depending on the fish size, age, and part consumed, with higher concentrations in the viscera, especially the liver, spleen, gonads, and roe.[266,282]

The most common initial symptoms reported in cases of ciguatera include acute gastroenteritis, with abdominal cramps, nausea, vomiting, and diarrhea.[26] These symptoms rarely persist for longer than 24 hours but may require fluid resuscitation.[142] Myriad other symptoms reported in ciguatoxic patients are listed in Box 77-7. Headache is a common symptom, and victims often complain of experiencing a metallic taste. In a well-described clinical outbreak affecting a group of scuba divers who consumed coral trout (Cephalopholis miniata), the most common symptoms were weakness, cold sensitivity, paresthesias, a taste sensation of carbonation, and myalgias.[2] Two men suffering from ciguatera poisoning had painful ejaculation with urethritis, which in turn may have induced dyspareunia (pelvic and vaginal burning) in their female partners after intercourse.[280] In a North Carolina outbreak in 2007, six of the seven sexually active patients reported onset of painful intercourse beginning in the first few days after onset of illness. Although sexual transmission of ciguatoxin has been documented, painful intercourse as a consequence of ciguatera fish poisoning is not commonly described.[282] Neurologic symptoms seem to develop after initial gastrointestinal symptoms. Paresthesias and myalgias are typically seen within the first 24 hours and usually resolve by 48 to 72 hours after ingestion of ciguatoxins, although there have been reports of neurologic symptoms persisting for weeks to months.[27,286,372,282]

Many case reports of ciguatera describe symptoms of a sensory perception of "hot and cold reversal," and loose, painful teeth. Although the presence of these symptoms is suggestive of ciguatera, their absence does not exclude the possibility of the disease.[27] Although there have been reports of a paradoxic reversal of temperature perception, resulting in cold feeling hot rather than hot feeling cold, other reports demonstrated that gross temperature discernment remains intact and the description of paradoxic heat perception may be misleading.[61] These authors describe the symptoms as intense, painful tingling or "electric shock" rather than true reversal of hot and cold perception.[61] This peculiar symptom may have a delayed onset of 2 to 5 days, may last for months after ingestion, and is otherwise seen only with neurotoxic shellfish poisoning (brevetoxins), caulerpicin (from the green alga Caulerpa) toxicity, or turban shell poison-

BOX 77-7   Signs and Symptoms Associated With Ciguatera Poisoning

Abdominal pain
Nausea
Vomiting
Diarrhea
Chills
Paresthesias (particularly of the extremities and circumoral region)
Pruritus (particularly of the palms and soles)
Tongue and throat numbness or burning
A sensation of "carbonation" during swallowing
Odontalgia or dental dysesthesias
Dysphagia
Dysuria
Dyspnea
Weakness
Fatigue
Tremor
Fasciculations
Athetosis
Meningismus
Aphonia
Ataxia
Vertigo
Pain and weakness in the lower extremities
Visual blurring
Transient blindness
Hyporeflexia
Seizures
Nasal congestion and dryness
Conjunctivitis
Maculopapular rash (erythematous, with occasional desquamation)
Skin vesiculations
Dermatographia
Sialorrhea
Diaphoresis
Headache
Arthralgias
Myalgias (particularly in the lower back and thighs)
Insomnia
Bradycardia
Hypotension
Central respiratory failure
Coma

ing.[132,536] These symptoms are commonly associated with polyneuropathy, predominantly affecting sensory small fibers.[414] Pruritus is another vague but often described sensation in victims of ciguatera. The onset of pruritus may be delayed for more than 24 hours but is rarely, if ever, seen in the absence of other symptoms.[152,286] Pruritus may persist for weeks and be exacerbated by any activity that increases skin temperature (blood flow), such as exercise or alcohol consumption.[286] Ciguatera-associated pruritus may occasionally become severe and may improve after treatment with histamine receptor antagonists. Delayed symptoms also include hiccups.

Tachycardia and hypertension are often described in ciguatera poisoning, in some cases after transient bradycardia and hypotension, which can be severe.[87] Hallucinations, flushing, flaccid paralysis, and fever occur but are uncommon. More severe reactions tend to occur in persons previously stricken with the disease. Severely affected persons may report intermittent symptoms for up to 6 months, with gradual diminution in frequency and intensity. There may be regional variability to the symptoms of presentation.[27,334] Reappearance or worsening of symptoms after alcohol consumption has been described.[282] Other foods and behaviors associated with symptom recurrence include nuts, caffeine, port wine, chicken, other fish, and physical activity/exertion.[159] Persons who have ingested parrotfish (scaritoxin) have been reported to suffer from classic ciguatera poisoning, as well as a second phase of toxicity 5 to 10 days after the initial onset, consisting of ataxia, dysmetria, and resting or kinetic tremor.[95] Although both gastrointestinal and neurologic effects are the hallmarks of ciguatera intoxication, there are regionally dependent differences in clinical presentation. Neurologic effects predominate in the Indo-Pacific region, whereas gastrointestinal symptoms predominate in the Caribbean.[226] Consumption of Indian Ocean fish has led to a further syndrome characterized by hallucinations, incoordination, loss of equilibrium, depression, and nightmares. Sensitization with repeated exposure has been described, leading to more rapid onset of effects.[226]

Whether ciguatoxin crosses the placenta is not known, but exposures during pregnancy have resulted in normal fetal outcomes.[424] Transmission via breast milk has been reported.[257] In small children, symptoms of ciguatera poisoning may be no more specific than irritability, sleep disturbance, nausea, and vomiting.[518] Other reported symptoms include carpopedal spasm, ptosis, and inconsolability.

An overall death rate of 0.1% to 12% has been reported with ciguatera, but the lower percentage seems more likely with modern supportive care. Death is usually attributed to respiratory paralysis.[244]

Diagnosis

Diagnosis of ciguatera poisoning is based on clinical symptoms. The differential diagnosis includes paralytic shellfish poisoning, eosinophilic meningitis, type E botulism, organophosphate insecticide poisoning, TTX poisoning, and psychogenic hyperventilation.[27,402] Temperature-related dysesthesia has also been reported in neurotoxic shellfish poisoning from consumption of shellfish contaminated with brevetoxin. Therefore, neurotoxic shellfish poisoning should be considered in the differential diagnosis. Unreliable folklore used in the past to aid in predicting ciguatoxic seafood includes the advice that a lone fish (separated from the school) should not be eaten. Other myths include that ants and turtles refuse to eat ciguatoxic fish, that a thin slice of ciguatoxic fish does not show a rainbow effect when held up to the sun, and that a silver spoon tarnishes in a cooking pot with ciguatoxic fish.[102] Ciguatoxin may be detected in the flesh of fish by two immunoassay techniques, a mouse bioassay where a sample of the fish is injected intraperitoneally into a mouse, and a rapid IgG assay.[215] Rapid immunoassays have largely replaced using mice and other archaic tests (e.g., feeding fish to a mongoose or cat to observe for neurologic symptoms or death). HPLC is also available for ciguatoxins and okadaic acid. Unfortunately, tests for ciguatoxin are still of limited clinical benefit because most institutions do not have the equipment needed for their performance. Multiple individuals presenting with the same symptoms that are consistent with ciguatera fish poisoning after consuming the same fish strongly supports the diagnosis.

Treatment

If possible, a piece of the implicated fish should be obtained in the event that analysis for ciguatoxins can be performed. Treatment of ciguatera poisoning is primarily supportive. Intravenous hydration with crystalloid and electrolyte replacement may be necessary for dehydration. Severe or refractory hypotension may require a vasopressor. Antiemetics such as ondansetron may be beneficial. Atropine has been shown to be effective in patients with symptomatic bradycardia or excess cholinergic stimulation.[152] Gastric decontamination is rarely indicated, because presentation is usually delayed and gastroenteritis has already occurred. Activated charcoal may bind some of the toxin in the gastrointestinal tract, but this is not useful when presentation is more than 1 to 2 hours after exposure.

Many traditional remedies have been used for centuries to treat ciguatera. Edrophonium, neostigmine, corticosteroids, pralidoxime, ascorbic acid, pyridoxine (vitamin B_6), salicylic acid, colchicine, and vitamin B complex have all been tried with variable success; however, there is no current clinical support for these modalities.[334] Local anesthetics (e.g., lidocaine, tocainide) have also been administered for treatment of ciguatera.[63,279] These agents are effective blockers of sodium influx and may antagonize the sodium channel effects of ciguatoxin. In addition, amitriptyline has been used for its sodium channel–blocking effects, as well as its potent antimuscarinic effects.[55,60,115] Nifedipine has been used to counteract cellular uptake of calcium caused by

maitotoxin, and to relieve headache.[60] Although there is limited experience with most of these therapies, they may be beneficial in cases refractory to supportive care alone.

Mannitol has become the most widely applied therapy in severe cases of ciguatera poisoning.[53,453] Most reports of its success are based on limited data with small numbers of patients.[135,364,369,519] One series described successful treatment with mannitol in 24 victims of ciguatera poisoning. Each was infused with up to 1 g/kg of a 20% mannitol solution intravenously over 30 minutes. None of the victims received more than 250 mL.[364] The mechanism by which mannitol might be effective in abating the neurologic symptoms from ciguatera poisoning is unknown, but suggested theories have included acting as a free radical scavenger, acting as a competitive inhibitor of ciguatoxin at the cell membrane, and promoting a decrease in Schwann cell edema.[369,519] It is also possible that the osmotic action of mannitol may render ciguatoxin inert.[364,369] Curiously, mannitol therapy seems to have no beneficial effect on mice administered a sublethal intraperitoneal dose of ciguatoxin (CTX-1).[298] A more recent double-blinded, randomized study of mannitol therapy found no difference in resolution of symptoms when compared with saline.[414] Of note, therapy was not initiated until an average of 19 hours after exposure in the mannitol group and 40 hours after exposure in the saline group. In humans, the empirical observation is that mannitol has greater benefit if administered early in the course of illness, so the delay may have diminished the effect in this study. One concern with administration of mannitol in the setting of ciguatera is that patients may present dehydrated. In these cases, patients should be adequately rehydrated before administration of mannitol. During recovery from ciguatera, it is recommended that victims exclude fish, shellfish, alcoholic beverages, and nuts and nut oils from their diet, as these could result in exacerbation of the syndrome.[437] Gabapentin has been used successfully for treatment of chronic symptoms after ciguatera poisoning, but symptoms seem to recur after cession of therapy in some patients.[372]

Prevention

For travelers, common sense dictates avoiding any fish that local fishermen and residents do not eat, or fish caught in areas known to be endemic for ciguatera. Any level of Caribbean ciguatoxin of 0.1 ppb or more of fish tissue is thought to be a health risk.[282] Because of the accumulation of toxin, all oversized fish of any predacious reef species (such as jack, snapper, barracuda, grouper, or parrot-beaked bottom feeder) should be suspected to be toxic. Moray eels should never be consumed. Internal organs of implicated fish seem to concentrate the toxin and should therefore be avoided. Natural events, such as hurricanes and earthquakes, have been associated with an increased incidence of ciguatera, presumably because of reef disturbance. El Niño storms may also affect the incidence of ciguatera in the Pacific.[29]

CLUPEOTOXIC FISH POISONING

Clupeotoxic fish poisoning involves plankton-feeding fish that ingest blue-green algae and dinoflagellates. This poisoning is distinguished from ciguatera on the basis of the severity and high fatality rate of clupeotoxic fish poisoning and identification of the implicated clupeoid fish. These fish of the order Clupeiformes are found in tropical Caribbean, Indo-Pacific, and African coastal waters. Toxicity is reported to increase during warm summer months. Viscera are considered to be highly toxic. Previously, the toxin was poorly characterized as a result of infrequency of the syndrome and rare access to toxic animals. The first case to shed light on clupeotoxism was reported in a Madagascar woman who died after eating a sardine, *Herklotsichthys quadrimaculatus*.[362] This same sardine has been implicated in clupeotoxism in Fiji and the Philippines.[540,539] The causative toxin was identified as palytoxin or its analog, which distinctly differed from ciguatoxin. Palytoxin is an extremely poisonous nonprotein agent of low molecular weight that has been isolated from various zoanthid soft corals of the genus *Palythoa,* and subsequently from many other organisms such as seaweed and shellfish.[194,510]

Palytoxin was found in the dinoflagellate *Ostreopsis siamensis*, which caused blooms along the coast of Europe, resulting in extensive death of edible mollusks and echinoderms, and human illness.[510] Since the structure of palytoxin was reported in 1981, numerous palytoxin-like substances have been described from various marine organisms.[117] Palytoxin has been found in mackerel (*Decapterus macrosoma*), filefish (*Altera scripta*), freshwater puffer fish (*Tetraodon* sp.), triggerfish (*Melichthys vidua*), and several species of crab (*Demania reynaudii, Demania alcalai, Lophozozymus pictor*).[6,117,161,267] Palytoxin poisoning was recently suspected after cowfish (*Lactoria diaphana*) ingestion.[431] Other examples include the families Clupeidae (herrings and sardines), Engraulidae (anchovies), Elopidae (tarpons), Albulidae (bonefishes), and Pterothrissidae (deep-sea slickheads).[25,325]

Pathophysiology

The benthic dinoflagellate *O. siamensis* is the most probable toxin source.[362,535] As with ciguatoxin, the poison typically does not impart any unusual appearance, odor, or flavor to the fish. The exact mechanism of palytoxin effects remains to be elucidated. However, in vitro studies have demonstrated multiple effects. Palytoxin appears to increase cell permeability to sodium in neuronal cells by converting the sodium-potassium ATPase pump to a permeable channel to monovalent cations, allowing potassium efflux and sodium influx. The subsequent membrane depolarization may open voltage-dependent calcium channels in synaptic nerve terminals, cardiac cells, and smooth muscle cells. In addition, there is increased intracellular calcium concentration through the sodium-calcium exchanger. Ultimately, the increase in intracellular calcium stimulates release of neurotransmitters from nerve terminals, histamine from mast cells, and vasoactive agents from the vascular endothelium.[353,510] Palytoxin may also increase cytosolic hydrogen concentration.[510]

Clinical Presentation

Symptoms of palytoxin exposure vary greatly, depending on the route of exposure. This was originally described using several animal species and various routes of exposure.[516] Deaths have occurred due to palytoxin injection in animals and ingestion in humans. Additional symptoms have been observed to be caused by dermal, ocular, and inhalational exposure in humans. Ingestion in humans reportedly causes abdominal cramps, nausea, diarrhea, limb paresthesias, muscle spasm, and respiratory distress. Of this cluster of symptoms, the predominant physical findings appear to be respiratory distress and extreme tonic muscle contractions. Severe debility leading to death may occur within 15 minutes of the onset of symptoms.[199] A case definition for human poisonings was offered by Tubaro and colleagues.[489] Mortality rates have been reported to be as high as 45%. One of the most commonly reported complications appears to be rhabdomyolysis, with peak creatine kinase levels typically occurring 24 to 36 hours after symptom onset.[117,359] A recent case series of confirmed palytoxin poisoning from Taiwan included a patient that had a fatal dysrhythmia attributable to hyperkalemia following ingestion of *Herklotsichthys quadrimaculatus* (goldspot herring).[532] Surviving family members of this outbreak reported persistent myalgias as well as axonal sensorimotor polyneuropathy. A postmortem examination in one case after ingestion of *Sardinella marquesensis* (Marquesan sardine) flesh and viscera demonstrated enterocolitis and the sequelae of hypotension and acute heart failure.[325]

Inhalational exposure has also been described. In the summer of 2005, a massive proliferation of the tropical microalga *Ostreopsis* spp. broke out along the Mediterranean coastline of Liguria, near Genoa, Italy. Approximately 200 people experienced fever, conjunctivitis, and respiratory distress after exposure to this marine aerosol. Palytoxin and a new analog, ovatoxin-A, were later identified.[96] Dermal exposures have also been described, specifically with handling of marine zoanthids containing palytoxin sold in the home aquarium trade.[216,353] There is a great deal of conflicting information regarding the risks of palytoxin exposure from store-bought aquarium zoanthids. Numerous unconfirmed anecdotal stories can be found by affected individuals online at coral reef hobbyist forums. Palytoxins are not found in all commercially available zoanthid species, but they clearly occur in potentially dangerous concentrations in a select few.[117]

Treatment

Therapy is supportive and based on symptoms, with a focus on aggressive hydration to prevent renal failure associated with rhabdomyolysis. Because of the severe nature of this intoxication, early gastric emptying is desirable; however, the disease is so unusual and so rarely suspected that gastric emptying is not often considered. Patients should be monitored for development of hyperkalemia and life-threatening dysrhythmias during the course of treatment. Aggressive management and early intensive care are essential.

Prevention

Clupeotoxic fish should be avoided, especially during summer months. These fish are indigenous to Caribbean, African coastal, and Indo-Pacific waters. The viscera of suspicious fish can be fed to experimental animals to see if illness is generated. Because a rapid and sensitive hemolysis neutralization assay for palytoxin is available, the toxin's presence in seafood should become easier to determine.[41] Persons handling zoanthid coral should wear protective gloves to decrease the risk of local and systemic toxicity.

PARALYTIC SHELLFISH POISONING

Shellfish have been implicated in poisonings for centuries, if not millennia. Epidemics of shellfish toxicity have been linked to proliferation of dinoflagellates and other small marine organisms responsible for red tides or blooms in oceans around the world. The Bible refers to red tides in Exodus 7:20-21, where "the waters that were in the rivers were turned into blood, and the fish that was in the rivers died; and the river stank." The Red Sea was so named by ancient Greeks for its red appearance in certain seasons when red tides occurred. Red tides are described in the *Iliad* and were first recognized by North American Indians as luminescence or "flickering" of ocean waves.[68]

Perhaps the first published description in the Western world of a patient with clinical findings suggestive of paralytic shellfish toxicity dates back to 1689. An article from a French journal named *Ephemeredes des Curieux de la Nature* described a young woman who had ingested mussels.[90,197] The description notes that her symptoms included fever, chest pain, respiratory insufficiency, nausea, seizures, and tachycardia. She had emesis induced, bringing up the mussels, and eventually recovered. For years after this report, the incidence and cause of paralytic shellfish toxicity were undocumented throughout the world, but epidemics were known to occur in certain seasons and under certain conditions. Improvements in monitoring and public health reporting have demonstrated patterns of occurrence. Gessner and Middaugh[173] described 54 outbreaks of paralytic shellfish poisoning in Alaska occurring in 117 individuals between 1973 and 1992. The California Paralytic Shellfish Poisoning Prevention Program has been so successful that it has been a model of surveillance for many other countries.[379] Paralytic shellfish poisoning has been a reportable condition in California since 1927, with more than 500 cases and 30 deaths reported since that time. In California, there is an annual 6-month quarantine (May through October) on locally harvested mussels, clams, and oysters.

Of the several types of neurologic diseases occurring after ingestion of shellfish, PSP is one of the most common. This syndrome is most frequently reported during summer months when water temperature is highest, but has also been recorded from May to November.[184,197] Some authors suggest that the toxin responsible for PSP may be present in significant concentration in some shellfish, such as the Alaskan butter clam, in certain areas year round, and that shellfish harvested from untested waters of these regions never be consumed.[172] The most commonly implicated varieties of shellfish include mussels, clams, oysters, and scallops.[173,197,252] Lobster hepatopancreas toxicity has also been noted.[144] Although almost all outbreaks have been described from shellfish consumption, 13 cases of paralytic shellfish poisoning were diagnosed in Florida in 2002 after ingestion of puffer fish containing saxitoxin, rather than TTX.[78] To distinguish the puffer fish poisonings from those caused by TTX, the puffer fish syndrome is becoming known in the literature as *saxitoxin puffer fish poisoning*.[144]

Pathophysiology

The major toxin sources of paralytic shellfish poisoning include marine dinoflagellates of the genera *Alexandrium* (formerly *Gonyaulax*), *Gymnodinium*, and *Pyrodinium*. Bacterial origins of the toxin have also been proposed.[144]

Dinoflagellates produce a number of toxins, the most commonly identified of which is saxitoxin. If a single organism predominates, it can discolor the water, creating a black, blue, pink, red, yellow, brown, or luminescent "tide."[97] Organisms can multiply rapidly from a concentration of 20,000/L to more than 20 million/L. These plankton can release massive amounts of toxic metabolites into the water, at times leading to enormous mortality rates in various bird and marine populations, including large mammals such as dolphins and even whales. Large numbers of dead animals on the beach suggest a colored tide. The trend toward increased numbers and magnitude of blooms is attributable to many factors, including coastal development, dumping of sewage, fertilizer runoff, and ocean warming. Kills by the dinoflagellate *Karenia* (formerly *Gymnodinium breve* and *Ptychodiscus brevis*) *brevis* are estimated at 100 tons of fish per day. The problem is markedly increasing in Europe.[498]

A limited number of the approximately 1200 species of dinoflagellates has been implicated in human toxic syndromes.[412] Paralytic shellfish poisoning has been linked to the dinoflagellate *Protogonyaulax*, species *catanella* (U.S. Pacific coast), species *tamarensis* var. *excavata* (U.S. Atlantic coast and Europe), and *Gymnodinium catenatum* (northwestern Spain).[321,470] These creatures are relatively fastidious and prefer to bloom in warm, sunlit water of low salinity. Some algal organisms may release their toxin in the form of microscopic cysts, which can hibernate at the sediment-water interface. In mollusks, the greatest concentration of toxin is found in the digestive organs (e.g., the dark hepatopancreas), gills, and siphon.[426] Toxic benthic dinoflagellate cysts may be transported by dredging operations, potentially introducing a dinoflagellate population into a new region.[541]

Although the origin of paralytic shellfish toxins is assumed to be dinoflagellates, the toxins have been isolated in both marine and freshwater bivalves that are not associated with dinoflagellates. It has not been determined how this has occurred.[356] The bacterium *Moraxella* isolated from *Protogonyaulax tamarensis* has been shown to produce paralytic shellfish toxins in culture. Toxin production can increase in nutritionally deficient environments.[268]

The paralytic shellfish toxins identified to date are 18 related tetrahydropurine compounds produced mainly by dinoflagellates of the genus *Alexandrium*. These include saxitoxin, neosaxitoxin, and the gonyautoxins (GTX1, GTX2, GTX3, GTX4, GTX5), with the best characterized being saxitoxin.[167] Saxitoxin ($C_{10}H_{17}N_7O_4$) takes its name from *Saxidomus giganteus*, the Alaskan butter clam. *P. brevis* is a toxic dinoflagellate that produces a milder toxin. Other dinoflagellates considered poisonous to animals or humans include *Gonyaulax catenella*, *Pyrodinium phoneus*, *Pyrodinium bahamense* var. *compressa*, *Gonyaulax monilata*, *Gonyaulax polyhedra*, *Gymnodinium veneficum*, and *Exuviaella maria-lebouriae*.[363] *S. giganteus* and the Washington clam (*Saxidomus nuttalli*) may carry the toxin in their neck parts for up to 2 years; however, no physical characteristic distinguishes a carrier animal.

Unfortunately, a direct human serum assay to identify the toxin responsible for paralytic shellfish poisoning is not readily available to clinicians. Paralytic shellfish poisoning is assessed in foodstuff using a mouse bioassay, in which a 20-g mouse is injected with 1 mL of an acid extract of the shellfish, and the time taken for the animal to die is recorded. One mouse unit (mu), or 0.18 mg, is the amount of injected saxitoxin that kills a test mouse in 15 minutes.[498] In most countries, the action level for closure of a fishery is 400 mu/100 g shellfish. Polyclonal enzyme-linked immunosorbent assays (ELISAs) that measure saxitoxin, neosaxitoxin, and gonyautoxins 1 and 3 may be rea-

sonable screening techniques. Other testing methods under investigation include a sodium channel–blocking assay, spectrometry, thin-layer chromatography, and fluorometric HPLC.[167,309] An automated tissue culture (neuroblastoma cell) bioassay may become a valid alternative to live animal testing.[240]

Saxitoxin and related compounds are water soluble and heat and acid stable. At least 24 saxitoxin-like congeners have been identified, with an array of hydroxyl, carbamyl, and sulfate substitutions on the backbone structure, and also with large variation in potency.[196,144] Like TTX, they can be destroyed to a certain extent in an alkaline medium but not by ordinary cooking. Saxitoxins are chemically distinct from TTX, but both act on site 1 of the voltage-dependent sodium channel, blocking influx of sodium into excitable cells and restricting signal transmission along nerve and muscle membranes.[277] Although the threshold levels for causing illness in humans are not definitively known, it has been suggested that ingestion of 200 to 500 mg would cause at least mild symptoms; 500 to 2000 mg, moderate illness; and more than 2000 mg, serious or fatal illness. However, serious symptoms have been reported after ingestion of less than 100 mg of saxitoxin in adults. During peak red tide seasons, each mussel may accumulate up to 50,000 mu of saxitoxin. Mussel concentrations of saxitoxin have been determined to be too high for consumption when seawater dinoflagellate counts are as low as 200/mL.[426] A saxitoxin concentration of greater than 75 to 80 mcg/100 g foodstuff is considered hazardous to humans. In the 1972 New England red tide, the concentration of saxitoxin in blue mussels exceeded 9000 mg/100 g foodstuff. In cases of paralytic shellfish poisoning in Massachusetts, saxitoxin concentrations of 24,400 mg/100 g were recorded in raw mussels. With oral ingestion of saxitoxin, the LD_{50} for mice is 263 mg/kg. It has been estimated that as little as 0.5 to 1 mg of saxitoxin can be fatal in humans.[426]

Neither steaming nor cooking affects potency of the toxin. Commercial processing of shellfish does not eliminate the toxin or potential for toxicity; therefore, public health agencies in the United States and Canada strictly monitor these canning industries.

Clinical Presentation

Onset of symptoms of paralytic shellfish poisoning is rapid. Within 30 to 60 minutes of ingestion, victims complain of paresthesias, numbness, vertigo, and tingling of the face, tongue, and lips. Cranial nerve dysfunction, including dysarthria, dysphonia, dysphagia, and even blindness, can occur.[173,197,220,321] Other early symptoms include light-headedness, floating sensation, ataxia, weakness, hyperreflexia, incoherence, sialorrhea, thirst, abdominal pain, nystagmus, dysmetria, headache, diaphoresis, sensation of loose teeth, chest pain, high blood pressure, and tachycardia. Neurologic symptoms progress to involve the extremities and trunk over the first 1 to 2 hours. Limb weakness may begin any time after sensory changes, and gradually progresses to ataxia, and finally paralysis. Reflexes are frequently normal throughout progression of the disease, and patients remain awake and alert. Death results from respiratory failure with diaphragmatic and chest wall muscle paralysis.

Although some victims have nausea, vomiting, or diarrhea, lack of gastroenteritis and thus early self-decontamination may in part explain why the mortality rate from paralytic shellfish poisoning approaches 25% in some older series.[26,515] More recent reports cite a lower incidence of fatalities, probably because of improvements in supportive care. Hypotension can result from direct action of the toxin on vascular smooth muscle, although both diastolic and systolic hypertension have been reported.[249,172] Toxicity is generally not delayed more than 10 to 12 hours, with a median onset of 3 hours. The prognosis is good for individuals surviving past 12 hours, but weakness can persist for weeks. Children seem to be more sensitive to saxitoxin than are adults. In milder cases, alcohol ingestion appears to increase toxicity. Saxitoxin is structurally similar to TTX and shares a common mechanism of action. Intoxication causes superimposable symptoms; these two syndromes can only be differentiated by their area of distribution or by isolation and identification of the specific toxin.[149]

Treatment

No antidote is currently available for saxitoxin or paralytic shellfish poisoning. The victim should be closely observed in the hospital for at least 24 hours for respiratory insufficiency. Airway patency and respiratory support are of utmost importance, because even patients with severe symptoms of poisoning often do well if expeditiously supported with mechanical ventilation. Although gastric emptying has been advocated by some authors when shellfish suspected of containing saxitoxin are ingested, airway collapse can be rapid and induction of emesis should not be attempted.[220] These toxins bind well to charcoal, so an oral dose of charcoal should be administered if this can be done safely.[88] Some clinicians suggest that atropine administration may worsen symptoms of paralytic shellfish poisoning and should be avoided, because saxitoxin and its derivatives may have antimuscarinic effects.[425] Several studies have suggested that acidity may enhance the potency of saxitoxin, leading some authors to speculate that serum alkalinization might be of benefit to victims, although the efficacy of this practice has yet to be established.[11,208,316,366]

At least one human case report and some animal data have implied that dialysis or hemoperfusion may benefit some victims of severe PSP.[26,388] Other reports are less optimistic, because in vitro trials have demonstrated that dialysis is not effective in removing saxitoxin.[136,208] Some clinicians have suggested enhancing renal clearance with diuresis, but no study supports this practice. Maintaining normal urine output should suffice in most cases.

Prevention

The most important aspect of managing paralytic shellfish poisoning is prevention. It has been said that one should not eat shellfish in the Northern Hemisphere in months that contain the letter *r*. It has become more apparent with changing ocean conditions that shellfish in many parts of the world may be contaminated throughout the year because of high water concentrations of *Gonyaulax*. Most coastal agencies monitor dinoflagellate concentrations off the shores of developed countries and restrict shellfish harvesting during high-risk periods. Despite aggressive public health monitoring in a known endemic region, a recent outbreak in Washington State was described following noncommercial harvesting in mid-September because posted signs restricting collection of shellfish were not visible in the darkness.[223] In addition, harvesting management strategies, such as harvesting parts of the organisms known to be safe and discarding the parts of the organism that may pose a threat, are in place.[144] Many outbreaks of this illness have occurred on isolated islands where public health monitoring is infrequent and intensive care medicine resources scarce. Saxitoxin found in southern puffer fish off the coast of Florida is much more concentrated within the muscle than in the liver; therefore, even careful preparation of these puffer fish fillets would not prevent intoxication to consumers.[277]

NEUROTOXIC SHELLFISH POISONING

Neurotoxic shellfish poisoning, often described clinically as a milder version of paralytic shellfish poisoning, results from consumption of molluscan shellfish contaminated with brevetoxins produced by the dinoflagellate *Kareni brevi, which* creates a colorful tide when it blooms and is considered endemic to the Gulf of Mexico. Brevetoxins are potent ichthyotoxins associated with large numbers of dead birds, fish, and mammals. In 1996, 149 manatees died along the southwest Florida coast; brevetoxin was implicated as the primary cause of the epizootic.[51] Signs and symptoms of intoxication in fish include violent twisting and corkscrew swimming, defecation and regurgitation, pectoral fin paralysis, caudal fin curvature, loss of equilibrium, quiescence, vasodilation, convulsions, and fatal respiratory failure.[24]

Pathophysiology

K. brevis produces a group of at least 10 toxins, known as brevetoxins.[24] These toxins are designated PbTx-1 to PbTx-10 and are potent, lipid-soluble, cyclic polyether compounds that bind to and modulate voltage-gated sodium channel activity.[116] Brevetoxins produce acute neuronal injury and death in rat cerebellar neurons.[38] In a canine model, brevetoxins produce depolarization of tracheal and bronchial smooth muscle.[394] Intratracheal brevetoxin instillation in rats resulted in systemic distribution of brevetoxin, which suggests that initial respiratory irritation and bronchoconstriction may be only part of the toxicologic syndrome with brevetoxin inhalation.[34]

Although a human assay to detect the presence of brevetoxins is not readily available to clinicians, a number of distinct methods, in addition of the traditional mouse bioassay, have been developed using ELISA, HPLC, or liquid chromatography paired with mass spectrophotometry, receptor binding assay, and radioimmunoassay to detect the presence of brevetoxins in environmental and biologic samples.[493]

Clinical Presentation

Ingestion of shellfish contaminated with brevetoxin can induce neurotoxic shellfish poisoning. The condition resembles ciguatera toxin poisoning in symptoms but does not have a major paralytic component. Death has not been reported in humans. Symptoms include circumoral and limb paresthesias, dizziness, ataxia, muscle aches, and gastrointestinal symptoms. The median incubation time for this illness is 3 to 4 hours, and it lasts several hours to a few days.[333] Most neurotoxic shellfish poisoning outbreaks have occurred along the Gulf of Mexico or on the west coast of Florida, in coastal Texas, in North Carolina, and in New Zealand.[333]

Unlike other shellfish poisoning syndromes, neurotoxic shellfish poisoning can cause a respiratory irritation syndrome. When large blooms of *K. brevis* occur near the shoreline, wind and wave action can aerosolize the toxin; if sea breezes blow the aerosolized toxin onshore, rapidly reversible conjunctivitis, rhinorrhea, and bronchospasm with nonproductive cough can occur in sensitive individuals.[220] Severe respiratory distress is uncommon, but asthmatics may have respiratory effects that may persist for days following just 1 hour of brevetoxin exposure.[259]

Treatment

As with paralytic shellfish poisoning, there are no antidotes available for treatment of neurotoxic shellfish poisoning. Management consists mainly of supportive and symptomatic care. Although death has not been reported, patients should be monitored for respiratory deterioration. Because patients with asthma are at particular risk for more prolonged and perhaps more severe respiratory symptoms, additional precautions to address respiratory dysfunction are advisable in this population.

Prevention

Avoiding consumption of contaminated shellfish in known endemic areas, such as the coastline of the Gulf of Mexico, adjacent areas of the United States, and New Zealand, during warning periods is key. Although neurotoxic shellfish poisoning is mainly a result of consuming contaminated shellfish, certain healthy omnivorous and planktivorous finfish may accumulate and retain high levels of brevetoxins in their muscles and viscera.[334] There are no guidelines warning against consumption of muscle meat from finfish that are harvested during or after red tides, but there are some cultural communities that engage in whole fish consumption. Because the highest levels of brevetoxins found in healthy finfish were detected in the liver and stomach, consuming these parts may place persons consuming whole fish at higher risk for neurotoxic shellfish poisoning.

DIARRHETIC SHELLFISH ILLNESS

Diarrhetic shellfish poisoning is a rapid-onset illness with gastrointestinal symptoms, which although typically severe, are self-limited. Ingestion of shellfish contaminated with dinoflagellates belonging to the genus *Dinophysis* (*Dinophysis fortii, D. acuminata, D. norvegica,* and *D. acuta*) or *Prorocentrum* (*P. lima* and *P. minimum*) causes diarrhetic shellfish poisoning. Lipid-soluble toxins accumulate in shellfish fatty tissues and the hepatopancreas of mussels. They exert their effects mainly on the human small intestine, leading to diarrhea and degenerative changes of the absorptive epithelium.[318,498] Symptoms include rapid onset (30 minutes to 2 hours) of diarrhea, nausea, vomiting, abdominal pain, and chills. Rarely, symptoms are delayed up to 12 hours. The syndrome is self-limited and resolves after 2 to 3 days. From 1976 to 1982, diarrhetic shellfish poisoning was diagnosed in at least 1300 persons in Japan. The period of greatest toxicity appears to be May to August. In 1981, more than 5000 cases were reported in Spain.[538] Other outbreaks have occurred in The Netherlands and Chile.[201] In 1993, a particularly severe episode occurred in Spain with unusual symptoms; analyses revealed a complex toxin profile, with both paralytic and diarrhetic shellfish toxins present.[166]

DSP toxins include okadaic acid, okadaic acid diolester, dinophysistoxins (DTX-1 to DTX-4), and pectenotoxins.[3,315,496,521,538] Okadaic acid was first isolated from a sponge (Halichondria okadai) in the Pacific.[461] It is a specific and potent inhibitor of protein synthesis and inhibits phosphatases A_1 and A_2 in vitro. Okadaic acid induces diarrhea because it increases phosphorylation of proteins, which either controls sodium secretion of intestinal cells or influences permeability of cell membranes.[100,124] It is a potent tumor promoter in mouse cells and can act as a genotoxin.[150] Other diarrhetic shellfish toxins exert various effects in experimental animals: pectenotoxins induce liver necrosis, and yessotoxins (from the Japanese scallop Patinopecten yessoensis) induce intracytoplasmic edema in cardiac muscle.[474,476] Minimal doses of okadaic acid and DTX-1 necessary to cause diarrhetic shellfish poisoning symptoms are 40 mg and 36 mg, respectively.[203] Metals (e.g., aluminum, copper, lead, mercury, cadmium) in concentration at or below acceptable levels in mussels synergistically increase cytotoxicity of low concentrations of okadaic acid in cultured cells.[485]

Increasing incidents of phytoplankton blooms with a danger of toxin release have necessitated searching for new diagnostic methods that can detect toxin quickly and reliably. A variety of techniques, including radioimmunoassay using antibodies raised in rabbits, competitive ELISA, idiotypic antiidiotypic competitive immunoassay, rapid tissue culture assays, and cytotoxicity assays, can identify the presence of okadaic acid.[92,104,292,429,491] A unified bioscreen for detection of diarrhetic shellfish toxins and microcystins (as from blooms of the cyanobacteria Microcystis aeruginosa) uses capillary electrophoresis coupled with a liquid chromatography–linked protein phosphatase bioassay.[48] A protein phosphatase A_2 inhibition assay has been shown to be rapid, accurate, and reproducible; it can detect concentrations as low as 0.063 ng/mL in aqueous solutions and 2 ng/g in mussel digestive glands.[490] The Japanese quarantine standard is 200 ng of okadaic acid per gram of shellfish tissue. Four times this amount of toxin has been identified in northeastern Pacific Ocean mussels. Okadaic acid and related toxins are potent tumor-growth promotors and immunosuppressants in animals, but the effect of exposure in humans is unknown.[110]

AMNESTIC SHELLFISH POISONING

Domoic acid is produced in nature by the phytoplankton algae Pseudonitzschia species, which are widely distributed across the world.[275] Domoic acid, the toxin responsible for amnestic shellfish poisoning, is an excitatory neurotransmitter first described in Japan in 1958 and isolated from the red algae Chondria armata.[466] The first documented human outbreak of poisoning with this compound was in 1987 from Prince Edward Island, Canada, when more than 150 people became ill after ingesting cultured blue mussels, Mytilus edulis, later found to be contaminated with domoic acid.[239,373,472,530] Four of these individuals died, and the clinical description of persistent memory impairment in many survivors prompted the nickname of amnestic shellfish poisoning.[153] The source of the toxin in these cases was found to be Nitzschia pungens, a diatom that had been ingested by the mussels before humans ate them.[30,456] The toxin is concentrated in the mussels' hepatopancreas.

Epidemics of domoic acid poisoning have been prominent in other marine life, especially sea birds.[49,514,527] A large number of dead and distressed pelicans and cormorants were noted in

Monterey Bay, California in September 1991.[527,528] Autopsies performed on dead birds demonstrated they had consumed large quantities of anchovies from the bay. Subsequent testing showed the anchovies contained high levels of domoic acid. This was the first report documenting the presence of domoic acid in the United States. Water samples taken in the area identified significant quantities of the diatom Pseudonitzschia australis, which were able to produce domoic acid when grown in a laboratory environment.[169,527] Three species of Pseudonitzschia are now known to produce domoic acid.

Undefined mortality events with signs of neurologic poisoning of California sea lions (Zalophus californianus) have been reported over multiple years, with domoic acid identified as a causative agent in 1998. That year, 400 sea lions were found stranded on shore from Monterey Bay to San Diego. The poisoning was correlated with a late spring bloom of the diatom P. australis, generating anchovies contaminated with domoic acid. Clinical signs in sea lions included ataxia, head weaving, seizures, or coma. Seizures varied in severity but were continuous during the period of toxicosis, lasting about 1 week, followed by treatment-aided recovery or death.[386]

Domoic acid has also been detected in Gulf shellfish (Gulf Coast oyster, Crassostrea virginica) and phytoplankton in the Gulf of Mexico, although no outbreaks of amnestic shellfish poisoning have been recorded in this region. The toxic N. pungens forma multiseries has also been confirmed in Korea, Japan, Oslofjord, Scandinavia, the northeastern and northwestern United States, eastern and western Canada, and eastern South America.[127]

In the fall of 1991, the latest reported epidemic of domoic acid poisoning occurred in Washington State.[260] More than 20 people who consumed razor clams were affected. Subsequent testing confirmed the presence of domoic acid in razor clams along the coasts of both Washington and Oregon, although mussels tested in these areas were virtually free of toxin. Dungeness crabs collected from these waters were also found contaminated with domoic acid. Many contaminated filter-feeding marine organisms, such as shellfish and finfish, have been identified as domoic acid vectors. However, in terms of human health risks, species such as market squid, scallops, mussels, and razor clams are of most concern because of their demand by the seafood-consuming public.

Pathophysiology

Domoic acid was first isolated in 1958 following investigations on the antihelmintic and insecticidal activity of seaweed extracts. After the 1987 epidemic of neurotoxic illness on Prince Edward Island, Canada, significant evaluation of the surviving victims was undertaken. Chemical analysis at various laboratories ruled out all other known toxic causes of the symptoms displayed by patients.[530] Intraperitoneal injection of extracts of implicated mussels into mice produced a syndrome characterized by reproducible scratching followed eventually by death.[373,472] The toxin was finally identified as domoic acid.

Domoic acid is a water-soluble, excitatory neurotransmitter and a glutamate receptor agonist. It is structurally related to kainic acid, a potent neurotoxic amino acid.[361,419,472,530] This group of compounds is excitatory and acts on three types of receptors in the central nervous system (CNS), with those in the hippocampus being the most sensitive. Domoic acid seems to work by activating kainate receptors in the brain more potently than does kainic acid itself. The result of this stimulation is extensive damage to the hippocampus, as well as less severe injury to portions of the thalamic and forebrain regions.[321,398,472] There may also be mechanisms mediated by non-N-methyl-D-aspartate (NMDA).[468]

It was estimated that the mussels implicated in the Canadian outbreak of amnestic shellfish poisoning contained a total amount of domoic acid in excess of 6 kg, with most being concentrated in the digestive glands.[184,530] Other organisms known to produce domoic acid include the phytoplankton Alsidium corallinum and C. armata. Subsequent research suggests that other phytoplankton, such as Amphora coffeaeformis, can also produce domoic acid. Scientists continue to monitor shellfish and marine microorganisms to determine the presence of other sources. There are 10 isomers of domoic acid identified to date; however, some of these have a significantly lower amount of toxicity than does the parent compound.[287] Domoic acid is relatively stable and does not degrade at room temperature. Also, cooking will not increase the safety of the shellfish product if it is contaminated with domoic acid.[320] There is wide variation in tissue distribution and retention of domoic acid; for example, razor clams have been shown to retain domoic acid for up to a year and contain domoic acid throughout all tissues, whereas most of the toxin is confined to the viscera in mussels and fish.[287]

Clinical Presentation

As a result of the Prince Edward Island event, numerous laboratory-based toxicity studies were performed in order to characterize the toxicity of domoic acid. Multiple regimens that have been investigated include intraperitoneal, intravenous, intra-arterial, intrauterine, and oral dosing and direct brain injections, making a direct comparison of domoic acid toxicity between species difficult. Studies have been performed in monkeys, mice, rats, birds, and fish. The most notable clinical signs of toxicity include scratching and seizures in rodents, vomiting in monkeys, spiral-swimming in fish, and tremors and scratching behavior in birds.[287,373,344]

Humans involved in the Canadian epidemic of amnestic shellfish poisoning had initial symptoms of nausea, vomiting, abdominal cramps, and diarrhea 1 to 24 hours after ingestion.[373,472] Neurologic symptoms initiated with memory loss began within 48 hours after ingestion and progressed in some victims to seizures, hemiparesis, ophthalmoplegia, and coma. Some victims displayed purposeless grimacing and chewing. Follow-up neuropsychological testing on affected patients displayed predominantly an anterograde memory disorder, with most other cognitive functions preserved.[373] The most severely affected individuals also had retrograde amnesia. Labile blood pressure and cardiac dysrhythmias were recorded in a few individuals, suggesting that domoic acid may be cardiotoxic.[381] Elevations in blood urea nitrogen and creatine phosphokinase were also noted in many victims and have been recorded in animals suffering domoic acid poisoning, possibly resulting from exertional myopathies or tremors.[373,528]

The onset of symptoms in victims of the Prince Edward Island epidemic ranged from 15 minutes to 38 hours, with the average approaching 5 hours.[373,472] Increased age was identified as a risk factor for both severity of illness and memory loss. Males were found to be more susceptible.[381] Most fatalities occurred in the oldest victims, with postmortem findings suggesting neuronal loss or necrosis, accompanied by astrocytosis.[373] The most severe damage was to the hippocampus and amygdala, which are brain areas known to participate in memory function. Lesions were also noted in the claustrum and the septal and olfactory regions. Retinal lesions have also been reported.[381] No lesions were found in the motor nuclei of the brainstem. Hippocampal lesions in victims at autopsy resembled those seen in the brains of animals injected with kainic acid.[373,321,442] A follow-up study on patients from the Montreal area suggested that bronchial secretions became so profuse in the hours after mussel ingestion that one-half of the severely affected individuals required endotracheal intubation.[373] Pupillary dilation or constriction, and piloerection were also common findings. Approximately 10% of involved patients demonstrated persistent memory loss or other neuropathies. Of patients exhibiting neurologic toxicity, maximal effects were noted within the first 3 days after mussel ingestion, and maximal improvement in neurotoxicity occurred in 24 hours to 12 weeks after ingestion. At 4 and 6 months following exposure, several patients had distal atrophy, with weakness of the extremities and hyporeflexia. Electromyography findings were consistent with an acute nonprogressive neuronopathy involving anterior horn cells or diffuse axonopathy predominantly affecting motor axons.[381] Another clinical syndrome, called *domoic acid epileptic disease,* is characterized by spontaneous recurrent seizures weeks to months after domoic acid poisoning and atypical behaviors in animals. There is at least one human who had persistent seizures 1 year after his initial poisoning.[386]

Treatment

As with most other shellfish toxins, no antidote exists for amnestic shellfish poisoning. Based on the alleged mechanism of action of both domoic and kainic acid, it is possible that benzodiazepines may be beneficial in controlling some of the excessive hippocampal activity and seizures.[361,528] Animal studies have suggested a lowered mortality rate in groups in which benzodiazepines are used after domoic acid exposure. There may also be a role for NMDA antagonists.[37]

Prevention

Many regulatory agencies worldwide have established biotoxin monitoring programs. Although monitoring programs have been effective at preventing human toxicity, chronic domoic acid toxicity has been characterized in other mammalian species, such as sea lions.[287] To protect seafood consumers, authorities have established an action limit of 20 mcg of domoic acid per gram of shellfish tissue. This is based on retrospective estimations of concentrations of 200 mcg of domoic acid per gram of mussel tissue, which caused illness during the amnestic shellfish poisoning outbreak and incorporates a safety factor of 10. This regulatory limit has been adopted by the United States, the European Union, New Zealand, and Australia. Levels exceeding this limit trigger closure of the affected beaches and shellfish harvesting areas.[287]

POSSIBLE ESTUARY-ASSOCIATED SYNDROME

Pfiesteria piscicida is a toxic dinoflagellate that inhabits estuarine and coastal waters of the eastern United States and has been associated with fish kills and a human illness that has been labeled possible estuary-associated syndrome. Since 1991, *P. piscicida* and other *Pfiesteria*-like species have been implicated in massive fish kills in estuaries of North Carolina, Maryland, and the Chesapeake Bay.[181,186,433] *P. piscicida* is responsible for a fish disease formally known as ulcerative mycosis. *Pfiesteria* is primarily a benthic organism, but can exist in at least 24 different life stages. Fish swimming into an area with *Pfiesteria* may be exposed to a toxin that is produced by the dinoflagellate. These fish develop characteristic ulcerative lesions and erratic swimming behavior. *Pfiesteria* have now been found in coastal waterways extending from Delaware to the Gulf Coast of Alabama.

Although it is not associated with seafood ingestion, possible estuary-associated syndrome is associated with seafood contact. The first report of adverse health effects in humans was described after an accidental laboratory exposure; investigators working with *Pfiesteria* developed respiratory and eye irritation, skin rashes, and cognitive and personality changes.[181] During the 1990s, commercial fishermen who were exposed to waterways with *Pfiesteria* species reported similar symptoms.[186,188,188,433] The route of exposure is unknown, although it is thought to be either by prolonged direct skin contact with toxin-laden water or via aerosols after breathing the air over areas where fish are dying from toxic *Pfiesteria*.

Individuals with high exposure complain of headache, skin lesions, skin burning on contact with water, eye irritation, upper respiratory tract irritation, muscle cramps, and neuropsychological symptoms, including increased forgetfulness and difficulties with learning and higher cognitive function.[188] No consistent physical findings or laboratory abnormalities have been found. When skin lesions appear, they are erythematous, edematous papules on the trunk or extremities that resolve within a few days to a week after exposure. Thorough neuropsychological testing has documented deficits in higher cognitive function and learning and functional memory.[188] The severity of cognitive dysfunction was directly related to the degree of exposure. The exact nature of the neurocognitive deficit is unknown; however, rats exposed to water containing *Pfiesteria* toxins have shown significant learning impairments.[290,291] Deficits may be expected to improve within 3 to 6 months after cessation of exposure to affected waters.[460] The natural history of the syndrome is improvement in most symptoms without treatment; however, cholestyramine has been successfully used in patients with persistent symptoms.[434] The clinical improvement seen in cases treated with cholestyramine may be due to interruption of enterohepatic circulation of the toxin, although this hypothesis has not been confirmed.[435]

Diagnosis of the syndrome is difficult because the specific causal toxins have not yet been identified and a biomarker of exposure has not been developed. Current recommendations for diagnosis include (1) development of symptoms within 2 weeks after exposure to estuarine water, (2) memory loss or confusion of any duration, or three or more symptoms from the complex as described in the preceding paragraph, and (3) no other cause for symptoms identified.[76] A multiplex PCR assay is being developed for rapid identification of *P. piscicida* and other toxic *Pfiesteria* species.[331] Possible estuary-associated syndrome is not infectious and has not been associated with eating fish or shellfish caught in waters where *P. piscicida* has been found. Brief, direct water contact, including swimming, has not been associated with symptoms. No deaths have been associated with exposure to *Pfiesteria* species. People should avoid areas with large numbers of diseased, dying, or dead fish.

HAFF DISEASE

Haff disease is a syndrome characterized by severe muscle pain and rhabdomyolysis after consuming fish. It was first described in 1924 around the shores of Königsberg Haff, a bay on the Baltic Sea.[551] Further outbreaks have occurred in Sweden, Russia, and Brazil.[36,131,436,444] Twenty-three cases in total have been reported in the United States, most associated with eating buffalo fish (*Ictiobus cyprinellus*) or crawfish, bottom-feeding species found in the Mississippi River and its tributaries. Two cases have been associated with ingestion of a salmon meal.[281] Haff disease is most likely the result of a heat-stable toxin in blue-green algae that is eaten by fish; however, the toxin is currently unidentified.[75]

Haff disease manifests as generalized muscle pain and tenderness, rigidity, weakness, and rhabdomyolysis. Chest and back pain are common complaints.[213,549] Tachycardia, hypertension, tachypnea, and drop in temperature can also occur. Elevated serum creatine kinase occurs with leukocytosis, myoglobinuria, and elevation of lactate dehydrogenase and other muscle enzymes. Symptoms appear approximately 18 hours after eating fish (range, 6 to 21 hours).[75] Pathologically, there is neuromyodystrophy with necrosis in motor neurons of the brain and spine, coagulation necrosis of muscle, and myoglobinuric nephrosis. Treatment includes large volumes of intravenous fluids and diuretics to prevent renal failure from myoglobin toxicity. The diagnosis is based on the clinical presentation, laboratory data, and food history.

BLUE-GREEN ALGAE BLOOMS

Blue-green algae are worldwide freshwater cyanobacteria that proliferate rapidly in a bloom, discoloring the surface of the water and spoiling its odor and taste. Cyanobacteria in terrestrial water, freshwater, brackish water, and seawater produce toxins that are acute and chronic hazards to human and animal health and are responsible for isolated, sporadic animal fatalities each year. Typical algal species include *M. aeruginosa, Anabaena flos-aquae, Nodularia spumigena, Nostoc, Oscillatoria agardhii,* and *Aphanizomenon flos-aquae*.[99,143,345,405]

During conditions of a bloom (warm stagnant water, frequently enhanced by phosphorus and nitrogen fertilizers), the toxins are concentrated enough to become a significant hazard to wild and domestic animals and have been responsible for the deaths of livestock and dogs.[99,139,207,347,499] In most species of toxic cyanobacteria, the toxins are cyclic heptapeptides called microcystins, or cyanoginosins. More than 60 cyanobacterial toxins have been isolated from blue-green algae.[99,440] The toxins are of multiple configurations and include alkaloids, polypeptides, and lipopolysaccharides (endotoxins).[450]

Anatoxin-a and homoanatoxin-a are potent nicotinic agonists that act as postsynaptic, depolarizing neuromuscular blocking agents. Along with saxitoxin, these toxins cause animals to collapse quickly from neuromuscular paralysis, with features of staggering, muscle fasciculations, gasping, and convulsions.[206] Anatoxin-a(s) ("second" anatoxin-a) is an anticholinesterase that causes demonstrable cholinergic toxicity in animals.[67,206] Anatoxin-a and anatoxin-a(s) are both derived from *Anabaena flos-aquae*. Nodularins and microcystins cause hepatotoxicosis. Cylindrospermopsin is a protein synthesis inhibitor that induces necrotic tissue injury of multiple organs. Cyanobacterial lipopolysaccharide endotoxins are responsible for gastroenteritis and skin irritations.[99] In mice, administration of microcystin-LR causes rapid hepatocellular necrosis with hemorrhagic shock.[108,478]

Human exposure to blue-green algae blooms has resulted in allergic reactions, skin irritations, gastroenteritis, pulmonary consolidation, and liver damage.[99,374] A person who swims through a bloom may suffer local effects, such as conjunctivitis, facial swelling, or papulovesicular dermatitis. Ingestion of contaminated water causes dysenteric diarrhea, with green slimy stools. This may be associated with elevation of γ-glutamyl-transpeptidase and alanine aminotransferase levels. Inhalation of toxins is a probable exposure route; microcystin-LR and anatoxin-a cause significant toxicity in mice via intranasal aerosol exposure.[153] In 1996, more than 50 people with associated liver damage died at a hemodialysis clinic in Brazil. Microcystins are thought to have been present in the water used for hemodialysis.[99,134]

Treatment is supportive in humans and animals. Cyclosporine A has been shown to inhibit the fatal effects of microcystins administered to mice. In humans, no specific treatment is recommended other than fluid and electrolyte supplementation as needed, because all sequelae appear to be self-limited.

AZASPIRACID SHELLFISH POISONING

Azaspiracid poisoning was first described in 1995 in the Netherlands after an outbreak of severe vomiting and diarrhea from ingestion of mussels from Ireland. Although the symptoms were typical of diarrhetic shellfish poisoning, concentrations of the toxins associated with diarrhetic shellfish poisoning were very low in these shellfish. Therefore, an alternate, and in this case novel, causative agent was sought.[494] The toxin was originally named "Killary-toxin" based on the origin of these shellfish from Killary Harbour, Ireland. This unique toxin was later renamed azaspiracid toxin based on its chemical structure. Over the last decade, several analogs of this structurally distinct, heat-stable marine toxin have been identified. Shellfish contaminated with azaspiracids have been documented in several European countries and recently in the UnitedStates.[264]

Pathophysiology

The producing organism was originally thought to be *Protoperidinium crassipes*. However, it is now known to be produced by the small dinoflagellate *Azadinium spinosum*.[246] Limited availability of the pure toxins has impeded necessary investigations of azaspiracid poisoning. Initially, AZA1 toxin was isolated from the Killary mussels. Investigations have shown that AZA1 is cytotoxic to many cell types, including the liver, lung, pancreas, thymus, spleen, and especially small intestine. These effects are time and concentration dependent.[494] Several analogs of AZA have been identified. Some studies indicate that AZAs might have different targets. For example, AZA4 inhibits plasma membrane calcium channels.[162]

Clinical Presentation

The symptoms of azaspiracid poisoning appear within hours of ingestion and include nausea, vomiting, severe diarrhea, and stomach cramps. The illness persists for 2 to 3 days. To date, no long-term effects have been reported.[494] Most information regarding AZA toxicology has been obtained from in vitro and in vivo experiments. Mice injected with low doses of AZA developed slowly progressive paralysis, difficulty breathing, and listlessness. Large oral doses in mice demonstrated widespread organ damage, particularly necrosis in the lamina propria within the small intestine.[162] Azaspiracid poisoning remains a rare illness, although underreporting is probably likely because of the short duration and benign course of the illness.

Diagnosis

Levels of AZA vary significantly among mussels harvested from a given region. The European Commission regulatory limit is 0.16 mg/kg shellfish. Previous reports have determined the presence of AZA by liquid chromatography–mass spectrometry/mass spectrometry.[264] Other detection methods, such as ELISA, have been developed for AZA but are not commercially available.[494]

Treatment

At present, there is no specific treatment for azaspiracid poisoning. Treatment is primarily supportive, with a focus on preventing dehydration, and antiemetics for nausea and vomiting.

Prevention

Several incidents of human intoxication were the impetus for implementation of a national surveillance program that monitors levels of AZA in shellfish from all production areas in Ireland weekly. There have since been no further reports of azaspiracid poisoning incidents associated with Irish shellfish. In 2008, an outbreak occurred in France and Ireland following accidental dispatch to consumers of AZA-contaminated shellfish; the shellfish were held in quarantine following AZA confirmation.[162]

YESSOTOXIN POISONING

Yessotoxins (YTXs) were first isolated in 1986 from the Japanese scallop *P. yessoensis* and Norwegian mussels. They have since been observed in several countries, including New Zealand, Chile, Italy, Spain, the United Kingdom, and Canada.[8] Recently, YTX has been identified in French shellfish originating from the Mediterranean.[8] Yessotoxin and its analogs are produced by the dinoflagellates *Protoceratium reticulatum, Lingulodinium polyedrum,* and *Gonyaulax spinifera.*[488,492] YTX and its analogs were initially included in the group of toxins causing diarrhetic shellfish poisoning. However, they have recently been classified and regulated separately, because they do not share the same mechanism of action and only have been shown to be toxic to mice by intraperitoneal injection.[488,492] Similar to other marine toxins, the principal vectors for YTXs are scallops and mussels, which can accumulate large quantities of YTX, particularly in the hepatopancreas, because of their filter feeding nature.

More than 100 YTX analogs have been reported from shellfish and microalgae, although the structures of only about 40 of them have been identified. Although no reports of human poisoning induced by YTX have been recorded, YTX-contaminated shellfish have been reported worldwide.[367] In a mouse model, intraperitoneal injection of lethal doses of YTX or homoYTX caused symptoms similar to those of paralytic shellfish poisoning, with restlessness, dyspnea, shivering, jumping, and/or cramps.[22] Several studies have demonstrated a range of median LD_{50} values of from 80 to 750 mcg/mL.[488] The target organ of YTX appears to be cardiac muscle, where ultrastructural changes in mitochondria and myofibrils have been demonstrated.[488] Other YTX analogs cause fatty degeneration of the liver and pancreas. Oral administration in mice does not seem to cause behavioral changes or death. However, changes in the cardiac muscle were observed with repeated oral dosing. These changes resolved by 90 days.[492] Although the mechanism of action of YTX remains to be elucidated, it appears to exert a modest indirect effect on calcium channels.[488]

Due to the high number of existing analogs of YTX, methods of detection and quantification are complex. Mouse bioassay is the official method accepted to detect YTXs. However, it is time consuming and expensive, and lacks specificity.[367] Several other methods of detection are available and include functional assays, structural assays, and chemical methods. However, some of these methods have not been validated, and the gold standard for detection has yet to be determined.

OTHER TYPES OF SHELLFISH AND INVERTEBRATE POISONING

Callistin Shellfish Poisoning

The Japanese *Callista* clam (*Callista brevisiphonata*) is toxic during the spawning months of May to September, at which time cholinergic compounds in the ovaries are increased. Intoxication resembles cholinergic crisis, with both muscarinic and nicotinic components. Within an hour of ingestion of the heat-stable toxin, patients may experience generalized pruritus, urticaria, erythema, facial numbness and paralysis, hypersalivation, diaphoresis, fever, chills, nausea, vomiting, diarrhea, bronchorrhea, and bronchospasm.[25] Therapy is supportive, and recovery is usually complete within 2 days. In severe cases of cholinergic crisis, particularly with marked bradycardia, atropine (0.5 mg or more intravenously every 5 minutes, titrated to dry secretions, with adequate ventilation) may be administered.

Venerupin Shellfish Poisoning

The Japanese lake-harvested oyster (*Crassostrea gigas*) and clam (*Tapes semidecussatus*) occasionally feed on toxic dinoflagellate species of the genus *Prorocentrum,* posing the greatest risk during the months of December through April.[25,200] The heat-stable toxin induces rapid onset of gastrointestinal distress, headache, and nervousness, followed at 48 hours by hepatic dysfunction, manifested by elevation of liver enzymes, leukocytosis, jaundice, and profound coagulation defects. Delirium and coma may ensue, and death occurs in 33% of victims. Therapy is supportive. Any victim who shows early symptoms of gastroenteritis should be monitored for 48 to 72 hours for signs of liver failure. There is not yet clinical experience with exchange transfusion, chemotherapy, hemoperfusion, or liver transplantation in management of profound liver failure associated with this disorder.

Tridacna Clam Poisoning

Giant clams of the species *Tridacna maxima* are eaten in French Polynesia.[25] This species can cause poisoning characterized by nausea, vomiting, diarrhea, paresthesias, tremor, and ataxia. Severe cases can be fatal. The toxin appears to be concentrated in the mantle and viscera of the clam. Therapy is supportive.

Whelk Poisoning

In Japan, poisoning has followed ingestion of mollusks of the genera *Neptunea, Buccinum,* and *Fusitriton* (whelks, or ivory shells). The toxin is located in the salivary glands and has been characterized as tetramine.[13] Tetramine (trimethylammonium) is a naturally occurring quaternary ammonium compound that has been identified in anemones, gorgonians, jellyfishes, and mollusks.[12] Symptoms include headache, dizziness, nausea, vomiting, blurred vision, and dry mouth. No fatalities have been reported. Therapy is supportive.[25]

Ivory Shell Poisoning

Human poisonings have followed consumption of the ivory shell *Babylonia japonica,* which is widely distributed along the coastline of Japan. The toxin, surugatoxin, is located in the midgut of the animal and reputed to be produced by a gram-negative bacterium on which the snail feeds. Surugatoxin and ivory shell toxins appear to have autonomic ganglionic blocking action. Symptoms include abdominal pain, diarrhea, nausea, vomiting, oral paresthesias, syncope, and seizures.[201] TTX has also been identified in *B. japonica.*

Abalone Poisoning

Abalone poisoning follows ingestion of the viscera of certain Japanese abalone (tsunowata, or tochiri), particularly from the Island of Hokkaido, where *Haliotis discus* and *Haliotis sieboldi* are found. Symptoms include severe urticaria, erythema, pruritus, edema, and skin ulceration. The reaction appears to be of a photosensitive nature, as the lesions are confined to areas of ultraviolet exposure. The toxin may be derived from chlorophyll contained in the seaweeds on which the abalone feed.[25] Therapy is supportive.

Cephalopod Poisoning

In certain areas of Japan, intoxications have resulted from ingestion of squid and octopus. Symptoms develop within 10 to 20 hours and consist of nausea, vomiting, diarrhea, abdominal pain, headache, weakness, paralysis, and seizures. Although most victims recover within 48 hours, deaths have occurred.[25] Therapy is supportive.

Sea Cucumber Poisoning

Sea cucumbers are eaten throughout Asia and in some Pacific islands, where they are known as trepang, sea slugs, cucumbers, erico, or hai shen. Gastroenteritis is induced by saponins of the triterpinoid variety, such as holothurin. The typically self-limited disorder consists chiefly of abdominal pain, nausea, and diarrhea.

Sea Hare Poisoning

Sea hares are marine gastropod mollusks prevalent in certain South Pacific waters, including Fiji. *Aplysia* species have been considered to be toxic since Roman times. *Aplysia juliana* secretes an antibacterial and antineoplastic protein found in the water-soluble fraction of a fetid secretion lethal to crabs. Human poisoning has been reported after ingestion of *Dolabella auricularia* (known as *veata* in Fiji).[410,448] The symptoms begin approximately 30 minutes after eating and include prickling skin sensations, vomiting, diarrhea, shaking, tremors, fasciculations, arthralgias, dyspnea, visual disorientation, altered sensorium, and fever. The course of illness may exceed a week. It has been suggested that sea hare poisoning in humans might be a form of subacute organobromine intoxication.

Ingestion of the sea hare *Aplysia kurodai* was associated with acute liver damage with sustained elevations of aminotransferases. Microscopic findings in a liver biopsy specimen revealed characteristic apoptotic hepatocytes accompanied by mitotic hepatocytes. Bioactive substances in the sea hare might induce such apoptosis of hepatocytes in the liver.[411]

Anemone Poisoning

In the South Pacific, ingestion of the green or brown anemones *Radianthus paumotensis* or *Rhodactis howesii* (mata-malu samasama) has been associated with severe illness and death. Accidental deaths generally involve small children, whereas adults may be the unfortunate recipients of improperly cooked anemone or may be intentionally stricken in acts of suicide. The toxic substances are found in the nematocysts and the tentacles. Anemones have been used for criminal purposes in the South Pacific.[25] *Physiobranchia douglasi* is poisonous if eaten raw but is reputedly safe if cooked.[201]

Ingestion of the raw anemone induces an altered mental status within 30 minutes, often immediately after ingestion. The victim becomes agitated or confused, delirious, and then comatose. Other symptoms include fever, seizures, myalgias, abdominal pain, respiratory failure, and hypotension; death may follow. Contact with the skin, particularly mucous membranes, is extremely painful, with rapid inflammation and vesiculation.

Treatment is symptomatic and supportive. Because of the rapid onset of symptoms, the rescuer must be prepared to provide advanced life support within the first hour after ingestion.

A toxic protein has been isolated from the sea anemone *Urticina piscivora*. It is a potent cardiac stimulatory protein and potent hemolysin on erythrocytes of the rat, guinea pig, dog, pig, and human, causing toxicity at concentrations as low as 10^{-10} M.[98]

Crab Poisoning

Human intoxications have followed ingestion of crabs in many Indo-Pacific islands. Most of the toxic crab species are members of the family Xanthidae and include the genera *Demania, Carpilius, Atergatis, Platypodia, Zosimus, Lophozozymus,* and *Eriphia*. Clinical symptoms develop 15 minutes to several hours after ingestion and include nausea, vomiting, diarrhea, perioral and extremity paresthesias, ataxia, aphasia, respiratory distress, altered mental status, coma, and rapid death.

A number of toxins have been isolated from crab species, and there is marked similarity to paralytic and TTX shellfish poisonings. Saxitoxin, neosaxitoxin, and gonyautoxins have been isolated from crab species in Okinawa and from *Eriphia sebana* and *Atergatis floridus* from Australian coral reefs.[302-305] TTX and palytoxin have also been characterized from poisonous crabs.[6] In Thailand, TTX was responsible for an epidemic involving 71 persons (2 died) who ate toxic eggs from the horseshoe crab *Carcinoscorpius rotundicauda*.[248] The poisonous mosaic crab *L. pictor* from the Indo–West Pacific region has caused several fatalities in the Philippines and Singapore. The toxins were concentrated in the gut and hepatopancreas, whereas the muscle was less toxic. Captive crabs lose toxicity almost completely by 24 days.

Coconut crab (*Birgus latro*) poisoning is manifested as nausea, vomiting, headache, chills, myalgias, and exhaustion, with occasional deaths. Asiatic horseshoe crabs (*C. rotundicauda*) are eaten in Thailand, where they cause *mimi* poisoning. Symptoms include nausea, vomiting, diarrhea, abdominal cramps, dizziness, palpitations, weakness, lower extremity paresthesias, aphonia, perioral burning, pharyngitis, sialorrhea, syncope, paralysis, and death. Again, the toxin appears highly similar to saxitoxin.[89]

Crab lung has followed aspiration of tiny fragments of North American blue crab shells into the lung, necessitating removal with fiberoptic bronchoscopy. The diagnosis of occult aspiration should be considered in anyone with an unexplained cough who has recently consumed cracked crab, particularly while intoxicated.

Freshwater crabs are a potential source of human paragonimiasis, a parasitic disease that was prevalent in Asia until the 1960s.[93] Paragonimiasis usually causes pulmonary disease with productive cough and bloody sputum. CNS involvement has also been reported.[382] The disease is contracted by eating raw crab infected with the metacercariae of *Paragonimus* species. Areas known to be endemic are Vietnam, China, Japan, Korea, Ecuador, and Liberia.[5,93,106,346,382,408,504]

BACTERIAL AND VIRAL PATHOGENS IN SEAFOOD

Shellfish, particularly bivalve mollusks, contaminated with bacteria or viruses are implicated more than any other marine animal in seafood-related human illness.[301,376] As filter feeders, bivalve mollusks filter large quantities of water unselectively to gather plankton and extract oxygen, which allows concentration of bacteria and viruses (along with biologic toxins, pesticides, industrial chemicals, radioactive wastes, toxic metals, and hydrocarbons). They are sessile invertebrates that generally inhabit shallow waters close to shore and pollution sources. Standard purification (with ultraviolet light or ozone) for 48 to 72 hours may not significantly reduce these contaminants, or effectively remove viruses.[242,418] Viruses and naturally occurring bacteria that cause disease and death are of great concern because they are so common. The greatest risk of death from consumption of raw shellfish is among people with underlying health conditions.

BACTERIA ASSOCIATED WITH FECAL CONTAMINATION

Bacterial pathogens associated with fecal contamination have accounted for only 4% of the shellfish-associated gastroenteritis outbreaks in the United States.[397] In the early 1900s, most reported illnesses in the United States were associated with bacterial pathogens from fecal contamination; the primary causative agent was *Salmonella*. Since the institution of the National Shellfish Sanitation Program in the 1920s, illnesses from typhoid fever have drastically declined.[122,397,520] *Salmonella typhi* is still responsible for outbreaks of illness in other countries.[454,455] Nontyphoidal *Salmonella* species, including *Salmonella paratyphi* and *Salmonella enteritidis*, have been detected in shrimp and bivalves. Eight *Salmonella* shellfish infections were reported in the United States between 1984 and 1993, and *S. enteritidis* phage type 19 was responsible for an outbreak of infections from cockles in the United Kingdom.[189,522]

Other important bacteria include *Shigella, Campylobacter, Yersinia, Listeria, Clostridium, Staphylococcus,* and *Escherichia coli*.[230] *Shigella* was responsible for 111 cases of shellfish illness and four outbreaks in the United States.[397] *Shigella* has a low infectious dose and a long survival time in clams and oysters.

Campylobacter species have been isolated from shellfish, but their role in seafood infections is not known.[520] *Listeria monocytogenes* has been identified in high rates in isolates from fresh and processed fish and shellfish.[228] *Listeria* seafood-borne infections are probably underreported in the United States. *Yersinia enterocolitica* has also been identified in fish and shellfish; however, most *Yersinia* infections are not associated with seafood.[230,397] *E. coli* has not been an important source of seafood-related illness, although *E. coli* is found in shellfish.[59]

Another potential nidus for infection includes fish bone ingestions. A recent case report describes a 37-year-old previously healthy male who presented with fever and abdominal pain from *Streptococcus constellatus* bacteremia. He developed hepatic abscesses and thrombosis of the superior mesenteric vein, and was ultimately found to have ingested a fish bone that perforated his duodenum, pancreas, and superior mesenteric vein. Other similar cases are reported where patients, who unknowingly ingest fish bones, develop hepatic abscesses from perforation and subsequent infection with *S. constellatus*. *S. constellatus* is part of the normal flora of the human oral cavity; however, it can cause abscess formation in deeper tissue spaces. In the setting of bacteremia, abscess formation may occur in distant areas, such as the lung, brain, liver, and kidney.[174]

Vibrio Poisoning and Septicemia

Over the past few decades, naturally occurring bacteria, particularly those belonging to the family Vibrionaceae, are becoming a more important cause of shellfish illness.[234] Three *Vibrio* species, *V. cholerae*, *V. parahaemolyticus*, and *V. vulnificus*, are the most important vibrios associated with human illness.[122] *Vibrio* organisms can cause gastroenteric disease and soft tissue infections after consumption of raw shellfish. This can lead to bacteremia and death, particularly in immunocompromised hosts. Between 1988 and 1996, 422 infections from *V. vulnificus* were reported to the CDC and 43% of patients presented with primary septicemia.[427] In 2002, 452 patients were reported to the CDC with noncholera *Vibrio* infections. Of these, 45% were hospitalized and 11% died.[509] *V. parahaemolyticus* was found in 35% of the victims, and *V. vulnificus* was found in 73% of the patients who died.[509]

Vibrio species may be the most virulent halophilic organisms that flourish in the marine environment. In general, they are not associated with fecal contamination, so surveillance methods mentioned earlier for bacteria and viruses do not correlate with the presence of *Vibrio*. *Vibrio* species proliferate in warmer water. Infections seem to cluster during summer months, which may be related to increased numbers of people at the seashore.[329] *Vibrio* species grow best at moderate temperatures of 24° to 40°C (75.2° to 104°F), with essentially no growth below 8° to 10°C (46.4° to 50°F).[59] They can grow in brackish waters and require less sodium for maximal growth than do other, more fastidious marine organisms, a factor that allows explosive reproduction in the saline environment of the human body. *V. parahaemolyticus* has also been identified in freshwater habitats.[20]

Gastrointestinal illness has been associated with toxigenic O group 1 (O1) *V. cholerae*, non-O1 *V. cholerae*, *V. parahaemolyticus*, *V. fluvialis*, *V. mimicus*, *V. hollisae*, *V. furnissii*, *V. alginolyticus*, and *V. vulnificus*.[61,187,385,390,427,464,522] Septicemia, with or without an obvious source, has been attributed to infections with non-O1 *V. cholerae*, *V. parahaemolyticus*, *V. alginolyticus*, *V. vulnificus*, *V. hollisae*, and *V. metschnikovii*.[1,46,86,187,236,263,265,274,307,427]

Whenever a *Vibrio* species is suspected, the microbiology laboratory must be alerted to use an appropriate selective culture medium for stool cultures, such as thiosulfate-citrate-bile salts-sucrose (TCBS) agar or Monsur taurocholate-tellurite-gelatin agar.[308,335] Pathogenic *Vibrio* species generally grow on MacConkey agar. The stool specimen should be collected if possible within the first 24 hours of illness and before administration of antibiotics; specimens should not be allowed to dry. The specimen may be transported in the semisolid transport medium of Cary and Blair; buffered glycerol-saline is not satisfactory, because glycerol is toxic to vibrios. Tellurite-taurocholate-peptone broth is adequate. All *Vibrio* species grow in routine blood culture media and on nonselective media, such as blood agar. New,

rapid PCR tests are available for detection of *V. vulnificus* at the point of harvest.[64,365]

Key characteristics that aid in separation of *Vibrio* species from other medically significant bacteria (*Enterobacteriaceae*, *Pseudomonas*, *Aeromonas*, *Plesiomonas*) include production of oxidase, fermentative metabolism, requirement of sodium chloride for growth, and susceptibility to the 0/129 vibriostatic compound.[247] Species that cannot be identified in the hospital microbiology laboratory may be referred to a state laboratory or the CDC. Many sensitive and reliable PCR methods are now used to detect various strains of *Vibrio* species in oyster tissue and water samples.[34,290,503]

***Vibrio vulnificus* Infection.** Illnesses due to *V. vulnificus* are the leading cause of mortality associated with seafood consumption in the United States. The organism accounts for an estimated 100 food-borne cases per year, with nearly all cases being sporadic and linked to consumption of raw oysters harvested on the Gulf Coast during summer months.[122] *V. vulnificus* is a free-living, motile, halophilic, gram-negative bacillus. It is naturally present in marine environments, has a worldwide distribution, and is found throughout the United States.[397,471]

The growth of *V. vulnificus* is favored in waters with intermediate salinity. The optimal temperature for its growth (doubling time 15 minutes) is 35°C (95°F).[338] Below 10°C (50°F), it enters a nonculturable state and is viable but ceases to replicate.[360] The *V. vulnificus* count in the marine environment and in shellfish increases and peaks during summer months, as does the incidence of *V. vulnificus* infections.[217]

V. vulnificus may appear as one of two colonial morphotypes: opaque and virulent, or translucent and less virulent. The opacity of the colony of the virulent morphotype is caused by an acidic mucopolysaccharide capsule. This capsule increases resistance of the organism to bactericidal activity of human serum and to phagocytosis, and thus renders the organism more virulent. At extremely low frequency, some strains can shift between unencapsulated and capsulated serotypes.[542]

Growth of encapsulated isolates is improved in the presence of iron, but these are unable to use transferrin-bound iron. In patients with iron overload and transferrin saturation greater than 75%, free iron is available for use. Additionally, virulent isolates can use the iron in hemoglobin and hemoglobin-haptoglobin complexes.[56,58,547] *V. vulnificus* can bind specifically to human intestinal cells and quickly induce cytotoxic effects.[273] In vivo studies show that 4 hours after inoculation into the duodenum, the organism is found in the systemic circulation via bacterial translocation.[241]

Clinical Presentation. There are two clinical syndromes of *V. vulnificus* infection: primary septicemia and wound infection. The wound infection syndrome consists of flu-like malaise, fever, vomiting, diarrhea, chills, hypotension, and early skin vesiculation that evolves into necrotizing dermatitis, with vasculitis and myositis. Primary septicemia occurs when *V. vulnificus* is acquired through the gastrointestinal tract. Blood cultures are positive for the organism in 97% of patients. Septic shock, disseminated intravascular coagulation, and death may occur.[508] Infections occur 12 hours to 7 days after ingestion of contaminated raw or undercooked seafood, particularly raw oysters. The mortality rate of patients with primary septicemia is 56% and increases to 92% when there is septic shock.[214]

Gastroenteritis was previously thought to exist as an isolated entity in 10% of cases. However, it is more likely that other enteric pathogens are the causal agents and that *V. vulnificus* illness has been erroneously attributed to the asymptomatically carried organism.[233]

V. vulnificus is also implicated in other infectious presentations, including meningitis, spontaneous bacterial peritonitis, corneal ulcers, epiglottitis, osteomyelitis, rhabdomyolysis, endocarditis, and infections of the testes and spleen.[128,148,255,324,486,501,508,526] Necrotizing fasciitis and myositis have been reported after *V. vulnificus*-contaminated seafood ingestion.[162] *V. vulnificus* endometritis has been reported after an episode of sexual intercourse in the water of Galveston Bay, Texas.[481]

The severity of *V. vulnificus* infections is related to both bacterial characteristics and host factors. In patients with liver disease, such as cirrhosis and alcoholism, portal hypertension allows shunting of the organism around the liver. These patients also have impaired immune systems, thus promoting virulence of *V. vulnificus*.[384] Persons with high serum iron levels (from cirrhosis, hepatitis, thalassemia major, or hemochromatosis) are at increased risk for infection.[58,274,508] Any individual with impaired immunity (e.g., malignancy, human immunodeficiency virus [HIV] infection, diabetes, long-term corticosteroid use) is at greater risk for fulminant bacteremia.[463]

Treatment. Early recognition of *V. vulnificus* infection is essential for effective treatment. Blood and wound cultures should precede immediate and aggressive antibiotic and supportive treatment. Current recommendations include doxycycline (100 mg intravenously every 12 hours) combined with ceftazidime (2 g intravenously every 8 hours) or ciprofloxacin (400 mg intravenously every 12 hours).[178] Other antibiotics that have been suggested include imipenem/cilastatin, meropenem, trimethoprim-sulfamethoxazole, carbenicillin, tobramycin, gentamicin, and many third-generation cephalosporins. Supportive care includes crystalloid and vasopressor agents for hypotension.

***Vibrio parabaemolyticus* Infection.** *V. parabaemolyticus* is a gram-negative rod that can cause mild to moderate gastroenteritis when consumed in raw or partially cooked seafood. It is more widely distributed than is *V. cholerae* or *V. vulnificus*, because it occurs in cooler and more saline waters. It has been reported in temperate, subtropical, and tropical coastal regions.[32,77,205,319] The organisms are found in marine and estuarine waters along the entire coastline of the United States. In the largest reported outbreak in North America of culture-confirmed *V. parabaemolyticus* infections, during July and August 1997 in the Pacific Northwest, 209 persons became ill and 1 person died after eating raw or undercooked oysters.[77] *V. parabaemolyticus* has been recovered at frequencies up to 25% in frozen peeled shrimp.[525] In the past decade, *V. parabaemolyticus* has become the leading cause of bacterial gastroenteritis associated with seafood consumption in the United States.[122] During 2012, a Pacific Northwest strain of *V. parabaemolyticus* was responsible for several outbreaks along the Atlantic Coast. Six percent of patients were hospitalized; none died. The number of food-borne *V. parabaemolyticus* cases traced to Atlantic Coast shellfish was threefold greater in 2012-2013 compared with the annual average number reported during 2007-2011.[350]

Ingestion of raw or partially cooked seafood contaminated with *V. parabaemolyticus* (shrimp, oysters, crab, or fish) is followed in 6 to 76 hours by explosive diarrhea, nausea, vomiting, headache, abdominal pain, fever, chills, and weakness. In immunocompetent persons, *V. parabaemolyticus* causes mild to moderate gastroenteritis with a mean duration of illness of 3 days. Serious illness and death can occur in persons with underlying disease (preexisting liver disease, diabetes, iron overload states, or a compromised immune system).[263] The stools may contain blood and classically demonstrate leukocytes on methylene blue staining. The syndrome generally resolves spontaneously in 24 to 72 hours but may cause significant fluid and electrolyte depletion. Stool cultures should be obtained before initiation of antibiotic therapy. Panophthalmitis with this organism requiring enucleation occurred in a man who suffered a corneal laceration.[462] A course of oral ciprofloxacin, trimethoprim-sulfamethoxazole, or tetracycline may shorten the duration of the severe gastroenteritis.

***Vibrio mimicus* Infection.** *V. mimicus* is a motile, nonhalophilic, gram-negative, oxidase-positive rod with a single flagellum. It can be distinguished from *V. cholerae* by its inability to ferment sucrose, inability to metabolize acetylmethyl carbonyl, sensitivity to polymyxin, and negative lipase test.[113] Multiple toxins are produced by *V. mimicus*, including cholera-like toxin, enterotoxin, and hemolysin.[385,430,523] *V. mimicus* causes a syndrome of gastroenteritis (diarrhea, nausea, vomiting, abdominal cramps, fever, and headache) after ingestion of raw oysters, crawfish, crab, or shrimp. It was identified by PCR in 11 individuals with gastroenteritis from eating raw turtle eggs.[65] Nonfatal bacteremia resulting from *V. mimicus* has been reported.[265] The median incubation period is 24 hours, with delayed diarrhea noted up to 3 days after ingestion of contaminated seafood. Isolates are sensitive to tetracycline, ciprofloxacin, and norfloxacin.[329]

***Vibrio alginolyticus* Infection.** *V. alginolyticus* can cause gastroenteritis in immunocompetent individuals and bacteremia in immunosuppressed patients.[307,390] More commonly, it is implicated in soft tissue infections (such as those caused by coral cuts or surfing scrapes), sinusitis, and otitis media and externa.[168,307,391,487]

***Vibrio cholerae* Infection.** In developing countries, cholera caused by toxigenic *V. cholerae* is a major public health problem. The last several cholera pandemics were caused by consumption of fecally contaminated water.[529] *V. cholerae* is commonly linked to ingestion of raw or inadequately cooked mollusks and crustaceans and is responsible for the third highest number of shellfish-related illnesses, behind other noncholera *Vibrio* species and Norwalk virus.[247,522] Toxigenic O group 1 *V. cholerae* infections are associated with secretory, profuse watery diarrhea, nausea, and vomiting. Because the stool is virtually isotonic, large amounts of fluid and electrolytes are lost, leading to rapid dehydration, shock, acidosis, and renal failure. Treatment consists of aggressive intravenous and oral fluid replacement. In an outbreak in Italy, all strains were resistant to tetracycline, but patients responded to ciprofloxacin.[311] Untreated, the disease remits in 3 to 8 days.

Nontoxigenic, non-O1 *V. cholerae* strains cause gastroenteritis and septicemia.[217] Self-limited (24 to 48 hours) nausea, vomiting, abdominal cramping, and invasive diarrhea with blood and fecal leukocytes are typical. Spontaneous non-O1 *V. cholerae* bacteremia and peritonitis have been reported in patients with cirrhosis after eating raw oysters.[300,377,399] Meningitis and death have also been associated with non-O1 *V. cholerae*.[77,263]

Other Vibrios. *V. metschnikovii* caused bacteremia in a patient with cholecystitis; the authors postulated that it may have been associated with long-term carriage after seafood ingestion.[236] *Vibrio cincinnatiensis* caused meningitis; a relationship to foreign travel, seawater exposure, or seafood ingestion has not been established.[46] *V. fluvialis*, previously designated as enteric group EF-6 or group F, is common in the marine environment. It causes diarrheal disease associated with vomiting, abdominal pain, dehydration, and fever.[464] Fatal gastroenteritis has been reported.[265] This bacterium can be mistaken in the microbiology laboratory for *Aeromonas hydrophila*, from which it can be distinguished by growth in 60 to 70 parts per thousand sodium chloride solution. *V. hollisae* and *V. furnissii* have both been linked to gastroenteritis after seafood ingestion, and *V. hollisae* has been associated with septicemia.[1,181]

Prevention of *Vibrio* Infection. The Interstate Shellfish Sanitation Conference, a shellfish-industry group, has sought to decrease the number of contamination-related illnesses by public education, limiting harvesting to certain periods, facilitating rapid refrigeration of shellfish after harvest, and studying postharvest treatments to prevent bacterial growth.[103] Recently, postharvest high-pressure processing of oysters has demonstrated significant reductions in *V. vulnificus* levels but variable results with other *Vibrio* species; further studies are ongoing.[103] Persons who are immunosuppressed or chronically ill, particularly those with hepatic insufficiency, should not eat raw or partially cooked shellfish. All seafood should be cooked thoroughly, protected from cross-contamination after cooking, and eaten promptly or stored at temperatures above 60°C (140°F) or below 4°C (39.2°F) to prevent proliferation of *Vibrio* species.

VIRUSES ASSOCIATED WITH FECAL CONTAMINATION

Most infections associated with consumption of shellfish are viral in origin. More than 120 enteric viruses can be found in human sewage. These viruses can produce a variety of symptoms, including gastroenteritis, meningitis, paralysis, myocarditis, and hepatitis. Compared with other food-borne illnesses, those caused by viruses are less severe and seldom fatal. Norovirus (previously Norwalk virus) is the leading cause of nonbacterial illnesses in shellfish consumers.[122] Norovirus illnesses occur more frequently during the late fall through winter because of increased stability of the virus at lower temperatures, reduced solar inactivation, and bioaccumulation of the pathogen by shellfish.[122] Other viruses that have been isolated from seafood include hepatitis viruses (A, non-A, and non-B), enteroviruses (echovirus, poliovirus, coxsackievirus A and B), adenoviruses, rotaviruses, and, most commonly, small round viruses (norovirus, calicivirus, Snow Mountain agent, and small rounded structured viruses).[376]

Harvest areas are surveyed and closed for fecal contamination. However, the relative absence of fecal coliform bacteria in areas of shellfish harvesting does not indicate freedom from viral contamination. Outbreaks of norovirus and calicivirus have been caused by oyster harvesters discharging sewage overboard.[74] In addition, shellfish depuration processes that eliminate bacteria do not necessarily remove viral contaminants.[418] Steamed clams probably pose a significant risk because household cooking techniques are often insufficient to kill viruses. Although it takes 4 to 6 minutes of pressure-cooker steaming for the internal temperature of soft-shell clams ("steamers") to reach 100° to 106°C (212° to 222.8°F), it requires only 60 seconds for the shells to open, at which point they may appear cooked.[258] Poliovirus can survive (7% to 13%) in oysters that are steamed, fried, baked, or stewed.[129]

Methods using PCR amplification of target viral genomes provide a rapid, specific, and sensitive test for detection of viruses.[16,17] Amplification of viral ribonucleic acid (RNA), DNA, and complementary DNA (cDNA) has shown a high prevalence of human viruses that would not be detected by use of classic techniques.[375] PCR has been used to detect the presence of hepatitis A virus in oysters and scallops during an outbreak, and small rounded structured viruses, adenoviruses, enteroviruses, and noroviruses in shellfish.[16,17,20,105,289,375,418]

Hepatitis Viruses

Oysters, mussels, and clams harvested from waters contaminated with raw sewage are the most frequent cause of food-borne viral hepatitis A. Often, there is a long incubation period of 2 to 8 weeks, so it is common for hepatitis A to occur 3 to 4 weeks after gastroenteritis attributed to consumption of shellfish.[397] Symptoms include fever, jaundice, nausea, and abdominal pain; diarrhea is rare. Treatment is supportive.[42]

Enteroviruses

Enteroviruses are commonly isolated from marine water and shellfish. In the United States, up to 63% of shellfish in areas closed for harvesting and up to 40% of shellfish in areas open for harvesting were positive for enteroviruses.[401] In contaminated waters in Venezuela, 40% of harvested shrimp contained enteroviruses.[52] Enterovirus outbreaks have not been characterized, and the impact of enteroviruses on public health is not fully appreciated.[301]

Small Round Viruses

Small round viruses include norovirus, calicivirus, Snow Mountain agent, and small rounded structured viruses. These viruses are a major cause of shellfish-associated gastroenteritis.[74,84,133,270,451,456] Caliciviruses are small, single-stranded RNA viruses and have been responsible for a number of oyster-related gastroenteritis outbreaks in Louisiana.[74,84] Reverse transcription PCR (RT-PCR) assay can easily detect norovirus in contaminated water, shellfish, and stool from infected people.[270,418] The virus may be excreted in the feces of food handlers and harvesters for 48 hours after recovery from infection.[44] Symptoms, including nausea, vomiting, fever, abdominal cramps, and nonbloody diarrhea, appear 24 to 48 hours after ingesting contaminated shellfish and resolve over 1 to 2 days. Antibodies to norovirus have been measured in the serum of patients with gastroenteritis, and electron microscopy or RT-PCR can detect virus in stool.[270] Treatment is supportive and complications are rare.

BOTULISM

Botulism is a paralytic disease caused by the potent natural toxin of *Clostridium botulinum*. Toxins A to G have been identified, but only A, B, E, F, and G cause human illness.[395,447] Seafood-related botulism can be caused by raw, parboiled, salt-cured, or fermented meats from marine mammals (seal, walrus, whale) or fish products (particularly salmon and salmon roe).[210] Toxin type E spores are found in mud and sediment in northern coastal areas and inland lakes, accounting for the prevalence of type E toxin in fish-borne botulism (although types A and B may also be involved). Improperly preserved (smoked, dried, or canned) foods are at high risk for *C. botulinum* toxin proliferation. The technique of hanging meat for decomposition (flavor and texture improvement) supports growth of the nonproteolytic, psychrotolerant forms of *C. botulinum,* which may grow at temperatures as low as 4°C (39.2°F).[210]

In the last four decades in the United States, more than 10% of outbreaks of food-borne botulism have been related to the consumption of fish. Using quantitative PCR analysis, the prevalence of the *C. botulinum* type E gene was 10% to 40% in raw fish samples and 4% to 14% in fish roe samples in Finland.[225] In 1991, 91 patients were hospitalized in Cairo with botulism intoxication associated with eating *faseikh* (uneviscerated salted mullet fish); *C. botulinum* type E was isolated.[513] In 2002, eight individuals from an Alaskan village on the Bering Sea contracted botulism type E from eating fluke from a Beluga whale that had washed up on shore several weeks before.[326]

C. botulinum spores germinate in an environment of appropriate pH (>4.6), warm temperature (> 10°C [50°F]), sufficient moisture, and an anaerobic environment. The toxins are proteins of an approximate molecular weight of 150,000 Da and are absorbed in the proximal gastrointestinal tract.

Clinical Presentation

The toxin affects the presynaptic cholinergic neuromuscular junction, where it blocks release of acetylcholine and causes flaccid paralysis.[28] Signs and symptoms develop within 12 to 36 hours of ingestion and include nausea, vomiting, abdominal pain, and diarrhea, followed by dry mouth, dysphonia (hoarseness), difficulty swallowing, facial weakness, ptosis, nonreactive or sluggishly reactive pupils (third cranial nerve), mydriasis, blurred or double vision (sixth cranial nerve), descending symmetric muscular weakness leading to paralysis, and bulbar and respiratory paralysis. With adequate ventilatory support, mentation frequently remains normal. Death occurs in 10% to 50% of cases, depending on availability of antitoxin and appropriate intensive care facilities.

If botulism is suspected, a careful food history should be obtained and suspected food items collected. Laboratory confirmation of botulism is achieved when botulinum toxin or viable *C. botulinum* is detected in food, toxin is demonstrated in the victim's serum or stool, or the organism is cultured from stool. Toxin types are distinguished using type-specific antitoxin.[28] The standard test is a bioassay involving intraperitoneal injection of toxin into mice and monitoring for development of botulism-specific symptoms. The test is performed in a limited number of public health laboratories, and final results may not be available for up to 48 hours.[446] To determine the clinical need for botulism antitoxin, a number of tests may be helpful. Electromyography should be performed using repetitive stimulation at 40 Hz or greater; a positive test shows diminished amplitude of the muscle action potential with a single supramaximal stimulus, and facilitation of action potentials using paired or repetitive stimuli.[28] Cerebrospinal fluid (CSF) may be examined for white blood cells and protein (to rule out infectious causes), and an edrophonium (Tensilon) challenge test may be performed to rule out myasthenia gravis. The vital capacity should be monitored as a sensitive indicator of clinical deterioration.

Treatment

Ventilatory support should be provided at the first sign of respiratory inadequacy. As of March 13, 2010, heptavalent botulinum antitoxin (HBAT, Emergent BioSolutions) became the only botulinum antitoxin available in the United States for naturally occurring noninfant botulism. HBAT contains equine-derived antibody to the seven known botulinum toxin types with the following potency values: 7500 U anti-A, 5500 U anti-B, 5000 U anti-C, 1000 U anti-D, 8500 U anti-E, 5000 U anti-F, and 1000 U anti-G. HBAT is composed of less than 2% intact immunoglobulin G

(IgG) and 90% or more Fab and F(ab)$_2$ immunoglobulin fragments. BabyBIG (botulism immune globulin) remains available for infant botulism through the California Infant Botulism Treatment and Prevention Program.[80] A physician who seeks antitoxin should first contact the state health department. If this is unsatisfactory, the CDC may be telephoned at 770-488-7100 (24 hours a day). Before administration, the victim should be skin tested for hypersensitivity to horse serum. If horse serum test material is not available, 0.1 mL of a 1:10 dilution of antitoxin in saline may be used. The antitoxin should not be stored at a temperature greater than 37° C (98.6° F).

An adjunct to therapy in type B is administration of guanidine, which increases release of acetylcholine from nerve endings, although use is limited by hemopoietic and renal toxicity, and it has not been well studied after increased availability and use of antitoxin. The dose is 15 to 35 mg/kg/day orally in four divided doses.

Prevention

Prophylaxis with antitoxin is not currently recommended; neither is general pentavalent (A to E) toxoid immunization.[10,380] The best prevention is public health education with respect to food preparation and avoidance of improperly stored food products. Because the spores are frequently detected in fish intestines, it is important to clean fish properly and to avoid consumption of the viscera, even in salt-cured products. To eliminate spores in food, heat or irradiation may be used. Types A and B may survive boiling for several hours (particularly at the lower temperatures associated with higher altitude) and generally require pressure heating at 120° C (248° F) for 30 minutes; type E spores are killed at 80° C (176° F) after 30 minutes. Preformed toxin is inactivated after heating for 20 minutes at 80° C (176° F) or 10 minutes at 90° C (194° F). Germination is inhibited by acidification, refrigeration, freezing, drying, or the addition of salt, sugar, or sodium nitrate; however, heating remains the most reliable technique.[28]

PARASITES IN SEAFOOD

Most parasites of marine animals are of little public health concern to humans. However, there are at least 50 species of helminths found worldwide in fishes, crabs, crayfishes, and bivalves that can cause human infections. With increasing consumption of raw seafood such as sushi and sashimi, the number of documented human infections is increasing. The overall risk of human infection is small.

FISH TAPEWORM

In the United States, consumption of raw fish (sushi) has led to more frequent recognition of infestation with the fish tapeworm, *Diphyllobothrium latum*. Salmon appears to be a popular culprit.[107,138,224,483] Diphyllobothriasis is also reported from eating raw flesh of redlip mullet.[95] The fish tapeworm has a complex life cycle, in which a gravid egg released into freshwater releases a ciliated coracidium, which is eaten by a crustacean intermediate host. The coracidium penetrates the intestinal wall of the crustacean and then develops into a procercoid larva. A fish eats the small crustacean, and the procercoid larva migrates through the intestinal wall of the fish into fish muscle, where it changes into a plerocercoid larva. It is this final larval stage that is ingested by a human and that subsequently attaches to the intestine, where it grows into a mature tapeworm.

Classic symptoms include subacute abdominal pain, nausea, vomiting, diarrhea, and weight loss. Proglottids may be passed in the stool. Chronic *D. latum* infestation may induce megaloblastic anemia, as the tapeworm splits the vitamin B$_{12}$ intrinsic factor complex and prevents absorption of the vitamin.[185] The diagnosis can be made by examination of the stool for typical proglottids or operculate egg forms, which measure 60 to 75 mm in length. Proper identification of the eggs is important to differentiate them from the ova of trematodes, such as *Paragonimus westermani*, endemic in southeast Asia, which may be carried by immigrants to the United States.[1] For documented *D. latum* infestation, praziquantel (5 to 10 mg/kg in one dose for adults or children) is the recommended treatment.[180,358,357] Magnesium sulfate as a purgative has been used to help expel the worm.[483] Niclosamide, 2 g orally as a single dose, can also be used for treatment.[370] Because a worm may not be identifiable if expulsion is delayed or follows a purge, stool analysis should be repeated at 3 months to confirm successful therapy.

Fish tapeworm infection can be avoided by cooking fish until the parts for consumption reach a temperature of at least 56° C (133° F) for 5 minutes, or by freezing the fish to −18° C (0° F) for 24 hours or −10° C (14° F) for 72 hours.[524]

TREMATODES

Humans can acquire intestinal infection from the trematode *Nanophyetus salmincola*, which infests salmonid fishes such as steelhead trout or salmon.[137] Canine infection with this fluke is a well-known phenomenon in the Pacific Northwest of the United States. Humans ingest the flesh of fish infested with the metacercariae, which excyst in the host and attach to the upper small bowel. The worms release eggs that are detected in the stool approximately 1 week after ingestion of infected fish.

Symptoms of nanophyetiasis include diarrhea, eosinophilia, abdominal discomfort, bloating, nausea, vomiting, weight loss, and fatigue. Although symptoms may resolve spontaneously over a period of months, antihelmintic treatment is recommended. Praziquantel (25 mg/kg orally three times a day for 1 day) is the first-line treatment. Other regimens have included bithionol (50 mg/kg orally for two doses), niclosamide (2 g orally for three doses), or mebendazole (100 mg orally twice a day for 3 days).[137]

Numerous other trematode infections cause enormous morbidity worldwide via liver and intestinal flukes. For instance, in Southeast Asia, opisthorchosis caused by the liver fluke *Opisthorchis viverrini* is quite serious. The cercariae are ubiquitous in cyprinid fish.[175] Clonorchiasis occurs when humans eat raw or undercooked freshwater fish harboring the metacercariae of *Clonorchis sinensis*.[422]

NEMATODES

Anisakiasis

Thousands of restaurants serve sushi in the United States, and many do so without specific knowledge of the various parasites that can infest their fare. For instance, many serve raw salmon, squid, shrimp, and mackerel.

The first report of acute gastric anisakiasis caused by penetration of the *Anisakis* larvae through the gastric mucosa was by Van Thiel in 1960.[500] It is a rare problem in the United States, but is increasingly noted in Japan, where raw fish is more commonly eaten.[261,457] In a Japanese series, the fish consumed included predominantly mackerel; less common perpetrators included horse mackerel, bream, squid, sardines, and bonito.[457] In the United States, anisakine nematodes are present in many commercial fish intended for raw or semiraw consumption, such as Pacific herring (thus, herring worm disease), sablefish, Pacific cod (thus, codworm disease), arrowtooth flounder, petrale sole, coho salmon, Pacific ocean perch, silvergray rockfish, yellowtail rockfish, and bocaccio.[345] In rare cases, the anisakine worm can be present in tuna or yellowtail. Preservation of marine mammals along the western coast of the United States has been linked to greater worm burdens in fishes associated with these mammals, such as Pacific rockfish, red snapper, and salmon.[323]

Life and Habits. Anisakine nematodes, members of the order Ascarida (suborder Ascaridae), are found in great numbers in the viscera and muscles of fish.[341] There are 30 genera in the family Anisakidae, including *Anisakis* and *Pseudoterranova* (or *Phocanema*). Adult worms infest the stomachs of marine mammals, burrowing in clusters into the mucosal surface. Eggs passed in the stool embryonate and hatch in seawater to produce second-stage larvae, which are ingested by crustaceans, which are in turn eaten by squid or fish. In these hosts, larvae migrate through the gut wall and encyst in the viscera or musculature.[366] The fish may then pass the parasite to other fish, humans, or back to another marine mammal. The coiled *Anisakis* larva grows to approximately 2.5 to 3 cm (1 to 1.2 inches) in length and 0.5 to 1 mm in diameter. Fish are usually the intermediate (transport) host for larval anisakines.

The definitive host for *Phocanema decipiens* is the seal; *Anisakis* larvae grow to maturity in the whale. Shellfish are not infested. Only four genera of anisakine nematodes have been implicated in human anisakiasis: *Anisakis, Phocanema, Porrocaecum,* and *Contracaecum.* In the United States, all cases are related to larval stages of *Anisakis simplex* and *Phocanema decipiens.*[323]

Clinical Presentation. Symptoms from ingestion of *Anisakis* may begin within 1 hour of ingestion of raw fish and include severe epigastric pain, nausea, and vomiting. The presentation may mimic an acute abdomen. Asymptomatic gastroduodenal anisakiasis has also been a cause of acute urticaria and severe anaphylaxis in sensitized patients.[111,158,165] If the anisakine worms (such as *Phocanema*) do not implant and the infection is luminal without tissue penetration, the worms may be coughed up, vomited, or defecated, generally within 48 hours of the meal.[109] If the worm is felt in the oropharynx or proximal esophagus, the "tingling throat syndrome" is described.[323] An anisakine worm was documented in the tonsil of a 6-year-old girl with recurrent tonsillitis.[39]

Intestinal anisakiasis is more often delayed in onset (≤ 7 days after ingestion) and marked by abdominal pain, nausea, vomiting, diarrhea, fever, eosinophilia (particularly with gastric anisakiasis), and occult blood in the stool.[109] This may be easily confused with appendicitis, regional enteritis, gastric ulcer, colonic or other gastrointestinal carcinoma, or, most commonly, other causes of small bowel inflammation with partial obstruction.[54,243,432,465] In one study, 29% of patients with Crohn's disease had detectable specific total immunoglobulin (IgG), IgM, and IgA antibodies against *A. simplex.*[192] Anisakiasis has also manifested as small bowel obstruction requiring surgical resection.[416]

Diagnosis and Treatment. Definitive diagnosis of anisakiasis is usually made on the basis of morphologic characteristics of the whole worm when the creature is expelled by the patient or removed from the stomach after endoscopic examination.[411] Contrast-enhanced radiographs of the gastrointestinal tract may reveal threadlike gastric filling defects approximately 30 mm (1.2 inches) in length, which are typical, with a circular or ring-like shape.[54,457] Mucosal edema and pseudotumor formation are also seen. Ultrasonography can be useful in identifying intestinal anisakiasis.[227] However, once the worms have migrated to extragastric sites, the diagnosis can be difficult.

Early fiberoptic gastroscopy is recommended for patients in whom acute gastric anisakiasis is suspected and for those who have eaten raw fish within 6 to 12 hours before the onset of gastric symptoms. The *Anisakis* worm is usually found in the greater curvature of the stomach, often associated with severe mucosal edema.[245] Worms may also penetrate the intestinal wall.

The larvae of *Anisakis* can be visualized on endoscopy and removed with biopsy forceps. Fourth-stage larvae of *A. simplex* and *Pseudoterranova (Phocanema) decipiens* are found in the intestine and stomach of humans.[262] The larva is visible in the mucosa or buried within the submucosa, surrounded by an intense inflammatory granulomatous response.

When laparotomy is performed for presumed appendicitis, the diagnosis is based on identification of the worm in an inflamed segment of appendix, cecum, small intestine, mesentery, or omentum.[66,118] The only effective therapy for inflamed bowel is resection.

Antibodies to the ileal worm have been detected by radioallergosorbent test (RAST), ELISA, and immunofluorescent antibody assay, but these laboratory methods are not widely available.[192] Physical removal by endoscopy or surgery is the treatment of choice. The use of albendazole (400 mg orally, twice daily for 6 to 21 days) is of questionable efficacy.[180]

Prevention. The larvae are extremely difficult to identify in fish flesh, because they are colorless and normally tightly coiled in a spiral of approximately 3 mm. Only cooked (above 60°C [140°F]) or previously frozen (to −20°C [−4°F] for 24 hours) fish should be eaten. Smoking (kippering), marinating, pickling, brining, and salting may not kill the worms.[109] Candling is an inadequate method of surveillance, particularly in dark-fleshed fish infested with *Anisakis* larvae. Fish should be gutted as soon as possible after they are caught to limit migration of worms from viscera into muscle.

Irradiation of fish to limit their infectivity is controversial because of potential generation of long-lived free radicals within the fish, as well as germination of spores of *Clostridium botulinum.*[523] To date, this practice is not legal for seafood in the United States, although it is used in other countries.

Eustrongylides

Eustrongylides is a genus of roundworms that can invade fish in its larval form and thus be consumed by humans in their quest for sushi and sashimi. *Eustrongylides* may also parasitize bait minnows, which are sometimes swallowed whole by fishermen. The worms are released into the human gastrointestinal tract, where they attain lengths of 15 to 30 cm (6 to 12 inches) and penetrate the intestinal wall to enter the peritoneal cavity. Symptoms include unexplained abdominal pain, peritonitis, and fever in a live-bait fisherman. Surgical intervention may be required in pursuit of the acute abdomen, at which time the characteristically bright red worm is identified.[524]

Gnathostoma

Approximately 12 *Gnathostoma* species are responsible for gnathostomiasis, also known as larva migrans profundus or nodular migratory eosinophilic panniculitis. This systemic infection is caused by tissue destruction by migrating larvae.

Gnathostomiasis was first described in humans in 1889 in Thailand and has been endemic in Southeast Asia.[147] However, with advent of increased international travel, reports of gnathostomiasis are becoming more common in other regions of the world. Often, this is the result of travelers becoming infected in Southeast Asia and returning to other countries, as with 16 cases reported in London in 2003.[330] There also appear to be newly endemic regions such as Central and South America. Mexico's first case was reported in 1970, but gnathostomiasis is now endemic in many regions of that country.[125,299] *Gnathostoma* larvae are acquired by ingestion of raw or undercooked freshwater snakes and fish, particularly *Monopterus albus* (swamp eel), *Fluta alba* (eel), *Clarias batrachus* (catfish), or *Channa striatus* (snake-headed fish).[299] In Mexico, gnathostomiasis is particularly related to ingestion of ceviche (a dish made of raw fish marinated in lime juice).[355,400]

Life and Habits. There are 12 known species of *Gnathostoma,* all having similar life cycles. The definitive hosts are dogs, felines, and wild mammals.[299] The first intermediate hosts are crustaceans, which are ingested by the second intermediate hosts, fish. Humans then ingest the larvae found in these second intermediate hosts, leading to gnathostomiasis.

Clinical Presentation. Symptoms, which begin within 24 to 48 hours after ingestion of larvae, are nonspecific: fever, arthralgias, myalgias, malaise, anorexia, vomiting, diarrhea, and abdominal pain.[299] Cutaneous gnathostomiasis manifests as migratory swelling and inflammation, most often affecting the trunk, that appears 1 to 20 weeks after ingestion.[83,299] Visceral gnathostomiasis occurs when larvae migrate through internal organ systems such as the lungs, gastrointestinal tract, genitourinary tract, or CNS. CNS infections may manifest with radiculomyelitis with severe radicular pain followed by paralysis.[49] Eosinophilia is a common but nonspecific finding.

Diagnosis and Treatment. Definitive diagnosis is by isolation of the larvae from lesion biopsies.[83] ELISA has been used with a sensitivity of 93% and specificity of 96.7% in one study.[83] A clinical diagnosis may be made in a patient with a history of ingesting raw or partially cooked fish, migratory swelling, and eosinophilia.[354] The standard treatment for gnathostomiasis is albendazole (400 mg twice daily for 21 days), which results in a cure rate of 92%. Single-dose ivermectin (200 mg/kg) results in a 76% cure rate.[272]

Prevention. Adequate cooking of food is preventive, as is freezing to −20°C (−4°F) for 3 to 5 days. Lime juice is not effective at killing *Gnathostoma.*[299]

OTHER TYPES OF POISONING RELATED TO SEAFOOD

POISONING BY ENVIRONMENTAL CONTAMINATION

In the process of concentrating fish proteins as a food source, a variety of protein-bound, non–water-soluble, or non–alcohol-soluble toxic compounds may be preserved. These include organic mercurials, hydrocarbons, dioxins, polychlorinated dibenzofurans, chlorinated pesticides, and heavy metals (e.g., antimony, arsenic, cadmium, chromium, cobalt, lead, phosphorus, mercury, nickel, and zinc).[23,102,459] The overall public health risk for environmental contamination is concerning; however, the true risk of exposure is unknown.

Higher concentrations of polychlorinated biphenyls and dioxin-like compounds are found in Inuit people in the Arctic because of their traditional diet, which includes large quantities of sea mammal fat.[23] Data suggest that there may be an elevated risk of multiple myeloma in groups with high consumption of dioxin-contaminated fish from the Baltic Sea and Alaska, and accidental exposure in Italy.[420] Dioxin has been found in Dungeness crabs in Humboldt Bay, California.

In Taiwan, high levels of copper, zinc, and arsenic were found in oysters. The long-term exposure to metals from seafood consumption is potentially dangerous, although the real risk is unknown.[204] Urine arsenic levels have been shown to increase twofold to sevenfold after consumption of certain types of seafood (mackerel, herring, crab, and tuna).[15] Consumption of fish rich in amines has been shown to increase excretion of N-nitrosodimethylamine in the urine, because of increased formation of carcinogenic N-nitrosamines.[502]

Mercury is found in marine organisms in the form of methylmercury (MeHg) and is concentrated in the food chain. Increased fish consumption is associated with higher blood levels of mercury.[312] MeHg is neurotoxic and crosses the placenta and blood-brain barrier. Prenatal poisoning causes mental retardation and cerebral palsy. The risk of this from seafood is unclear. High blood and hair concentrations of mercury have been found in fishermen of coastal villages, and adverse effects have been reported.[342,392] Controversy exists over fetal risk from exposure to low-dose MeHg from maternal consumption of fish.[23] A study of children exposed to MeHg from seafood in a Madeira fishing community did not show mercury-associated deficits.[340] A longitudinal cohort study of children showed no adverse outcome with either prenatal or postnatal MeHg exposure.[112]

In the past several years, benefits of seafood containing long-chain omega-3 fatty acids have become popularized. This is partially responsible for increased seafood consumption. These fatty acids have been shown to decrease the risk of cardiac sudden death and coronary artery disease in both men and women.[6,218] However, small amounts of mercury are commonly found in the same fish, and studies have shown increased mercury levels in persons with increased seafood ingestion.[191,543] These same studies have shown conflicting data on whether elevated levels of mercury diminish the cardioprotective effect of omega-3 fatty acids. More study is needed. Omega-3 fish oil supplements have not been shown to contain elevated levels of mercury.[157]

Spills of toxic chemicals and petroleum by-products will certainly continue to expand the list of carcinogens to which humans are exposed through the marine environment. Although radiation exposure is not known to induce production of new marine poisons, ingestion of radioactive fish poses a potential radiation hazard. Divers are exposed to a variety of environmental contaminants while exploring polluted waters. These hazards include solvents, nuclear wastes, herbicides, chemical effluents, and sewage.

RED SEAWEED POISONING

Seaweed is a common component in the diet of individuals living in the Pacific Islands and the Pacific Rim. It can be eaten raw or cooked. Most *Gracilaria* species are nontoxic and edible, but a number of poisonings and deaths have been reported in Japan, Guam, and Hawaii. Ingestion of the red seaweeds *Gracilaria verrucosa* (ogonori) and *Gracilaria chorda* (tsurushiramo) is associated with a toxic syndrome, including gastroenteritis and death.[352] It is commonly referred to as *Japanese ogonori poisoning.*

In 1991 in Guam, 13 individuals became ill and 3 died after ingesting the red alga *Polycavernosa tsudae* (formerly *Gracilaria tsudae* or *edulis*).[201] Symptoms consisted of diarrhea, abdominal cramping, vomiting, generalized numbness, perioral and extremity paresthesias, numbness of the fingertips, diaphoresis, jaw aching, muscle spasms, tremors, and hypotension. *Gracilaria lemanaeformis* may have been responsible for three illnesses in California in 1992.[71] In Japan, two people became ill with nausea, vomiting, and hypotension and one died after ingestion of *G. verrucosa.* Prostaglandin E$_2$ is suggested as the toxic component of *G. verrucosa,* and polycavernosides, which are glycosidic macrolides, are the probable toxins in *G. tsudae.*[352,545,546]

An outbreak of acute gastroenteritis from ingestion of the red alga *Gracilaria coronopifolia* occurred in Hawaii in 1994, in which seven individuals reported symptoms of diarrhea, nausea, vomiting, and a burning sensation in the mouth and throat.[71] Aplysiatoxin and debromoaplysiatoxin have been isolated as the causative agents.[343] These toxins are probably produced by blue-green algae that are found on the surface of *G. coronopifolia* and are known to cause contact dermatitis in swimmers in Hawaii. Aplysiatoxin and debromoaplysiatoxin experimentally cause edema and bleeding of the small intestine, leading to hemorrhagic shock.[231]

SEA TURTLE POISONING (CHELONINTOXICATION)

Various tropical Pacific, particularly Japanese, marine turtles are toxic when ingested (Box 77-8).[449] The term *chelonintoxication* comes from the order Chelonii. All portions of the turtle are toxic and the freshness of the meat is irrelevant. In Madagascar, 60 people became ill after eating sea turtle in 1994. The mortality rate was 7.7%.[387] Lyngbyatoxin A has been isolated from meat of a green turtle, *Chelonia mydas,* that was involved in a fatal intoxication.[535] The source of the toxin was suspected to be blue-green algae belonging to the genus *Lyngbya.* The sea turtle may feed on sea grass contaminated with this alga.

Symptoms develop from 1 to 48 hours after ingestion and include ulcerative glossitis and stomatitis, pharyngitis, diaphoresis, hypersalivation, nausea, vomiting, diarrhea, abdominal pain, vertigo, icterus, desquamative dermatitis, hepatosplenomegaly, centrilobular hepatic necrosis with fatty degeneration, renal failure, somnolence, and hypotension. The mortality rate can be as high as 28% to 44%. Therapy is supportive and based on symptoms.

Various *Salmonella* serotypes have been isolated from pet turtles (*Pseudemys* [or *Chrysemys*] *scripta elegans*) imported into and from the United States.[123,269,313] Pet-associated salmonellosis was a significant problem in the 1970s. In 1975, Canada banned importation of turtles, and the FDA prohibited sale of small turtles in the United States the same year. However, the popularity of iguanas and other reptiles is increasing; these reptiles can also

---

BOX 77-8 Representative Marine Turtles Hazardous to Humans

Phylum Chordata
Class Reptilia
Order Chelonia: turtles
  Family Cheloniidae
    Caretta caretta gigas: Pacific loggerhead turtle
    Chelonia mydas: green turtle
    Eretmochelys imbricata: hawksbill turtle
  Family Dermochelyidae
    Dermochelys coriacea: leathery turtle
  Family Trionychidae
    Pelochelys bibroni: soft shell turtle

transmit *Salmonella* to humans. Reptile-associated salmonellosis causes febrile gastroenteritis, septicemia, and meningitis; one death has been reported from myocarditis from *Salmonella virchow* in a small child.[72,123,348]

LIVER POISONING: HYPERVITAMINOSIS A

Hypervitaminosis A can occur with ingestion of the liver of certain polar bears, seals, sea lions, whales, dolphins, walruses, husky dogs, and Pacific sharks. The vitamin A content of shark liver can reach 100,000 IU/g. A typical ingestion involves exposure to more than 1 million (and occasionally 3 to 8 million) IU of vitamin A. The recommended daily allowance is 4000 to 5000 IU. Symptoms of hypervitaminosis A include formication, headache, apathy, drowsiness, giddiness, irritability, photophobia, nausea, vomiting, diarrhea, polyarthralgia, seizures, desquamative dermatitis, ophthalmoplegia, and elevated CSF pressure with an idiopathic intracranial hypertension type of presentation (acute or chronic, the latter with headache, lip fissuring, papilledema, decreased visual acuity, and tinnitus).[145,328] Elevated levels of serum glutamic oxaloacetic transaminase and serum vitamin A (markedly in excess of 70 mg/dL) may be measured. A normal serum beta-carotene level excludes the possibility of a plant source (e.g., carrots or mangoes) for the vitamin.[328] The syndrome is rarely fatal and resolves in 2 to 8 weeks.

AMEBIC INFECTIONS

Free-living, amphizoic amebas belonging to the genera *Naegleria*, *Acanthamoeba*, and *Balamuthia* can cause significant CNS pathology in human beings. Approximately 350 cases of human infection have been reported to date.[317,397] These amebas are ubiquitous in nature; they are found in soil, lakes, ponds, swimming pools, hot springs, and warm water around the world. Human infection caused by amebas has significantly increased over the past 10 years.[317]

Free-living amebas are responsible for three disease entities: (1) primary amebic meningoencephalitis produced by *Naegleria fowleri*, (2) granulomatous amebic encephalitis caused by *Acanthamoeba* species and *Balamuthia mandrillaris,* and (3) *Acanthamoeba* keratitis caused by *Acanthamoeba* species.

PRIMARY AMEBIC MENINGOENCEPHALITIS

Primary amebic meningoencephalitis (PAM) is a fulminant, rapidly progressive CNS infection produced by *N. fowleri*. It was first described in 1965 by Malcolm Fowler and Rodney Carter in four human cases of meningoencephalitis from *N. fowleri*.[142] Worldwide, approximately 180 cases of PAM have been reported, with more than 80 cases in the United States alone.[69,120,283,304,398,506] *N. fowleri* multiplies and grows between 40° and 45°C (104° and 113°F). In response to adverse environmental conditions, such as cold temperature, the ameba encysts and remains in the sediment in the bottoms of lakes, rivers, and pools.

Infections occur in healthy children and adults who contact the ameba while swimming in polluted water in manmade lakes, ponds, and swimming pools, or the ameba may be inhaled with dust from air.[317] Infection is more common during summer months. Amebas enter the CNS through the nasal mucosa and olfactory neuroepithelium. Amebic trophozoites travel up the unmyelinated fila olfactoria of the olfactory nerves and through the cribriform plate to the subarachnoid space.[241] They proliferate and penetrate into the CNS, causing edema and necrosis. The incubation period is from 1 to 15 days. Symptoms include severe headache, fever, nausea, vomiting, and stiff neck. Rapid neurologic deterioration, accompanied by signs of fulminant meningitis with seizures, coma, and death, follows within 2 to 3 days.

Diagnosis is made by direct visualization of trophozoites in the CSF, along with polymorphonuclear pleocytosis, elevated protein, and low glucose. *Naegleria* trophozoites typically measure 8 to 12 mm (0.3 to 0.5 inches) in diameter with indistinct cytoplasm, round nucleus, and perinucleolar halo.[317] *N. fowleri* causes acute leptomeningitis and hemorrhagic necrosis of the orbitofrontal cortex, olfactory bulbs, and base of the brain, with edema of the cerebral hemispheres and cerebellum. Computed tomographic (CT) scan of the brain shows nonspecific cerebral edema.[256,415] Early detection and treatment are essential because this disease carries a very poor prognosis, with mortality rate of 98%. To date, there are six cases of successful treatment of PAM in individuals who were treated very early in the clinical course.[57,378,423,511] Treatment includes high-dose intravenous (1 to 1.5 mg/kg/day) and intrathecal (1 to 1.5 mg/day) amphotericin B.[179] Oral ketoconazole (200 to 400 mg/day) and rifampicin (10 mg/kg/day; maximum 600 mg/day) have been used in addition to amphotericin B.[378]

PAM should be suspected in any previously healthy individual who has been exposed to fresh warm water within 7 days of the onset of illness and who has clinical findings of bacterial meningitis with a basilar distribution of exudate by head CT.[69]

GRANULOMATOUS AMEBIC ENCEPHALITIS

Several species of *Acanthamoeba* and *B. mandrillaris* are pathogenic opportunistic amebas that cause granulomatous amebic encephalitis (GAE), mainly in victims who are immunocompromised, debilitated, diabetic, or alcoholic. GAE has been reported in patients with systemic lupus erythematosus, acquired immunodeficiency syndrome (AIDS), or bone marrow transplantation.[9,146,271,467] However, two cases of GAE caused by *B. mandrillaris* occurred in apparently immunocompetent individuals.[398] Approximately 170 cases of GAE have been reported worldwide.[317]

Acanthamoeba species are ubiquitous in nature; they have been found in ocean water, ponds, sewage, rivers, air-conditioner filters, cooling towers, eye-wash stations, and dust. Some of the *Acanthamoeba* opportunistic species include *A. castellanii, A. hatchetti, A. culbertsoni, A. astronyxis, A. polyphaga, A. rhysodes,* and *A. mauritaniensis.*[317] *B. mandrillaris* has not been isolated from the environment, although, like *Acanthamoeba*, it probably exists in cyst form. Trophozoites and cysts can enter through the lungs and ulcerations in the skin. Olfactory neuroepithelium may also act as a portal of entry.[235,317] The incubation period is unknown but is probably weeks.

Both *Acanthamoeba* species and *B. mandrillaris* produce chronic granulomatous encephalitis. The clinical presentation may mimic tuberculous meningitis or viral encephalitis. Symptoms include headache, fever, seizures, personality changes, cranial nerve palsies, hemiparesis, and coma. There may be skin ulcerations. The amebas cause hemorrhagic necrosis and foci of encephalomalacia in occipital, parietal, temporal, and frontal lobes. The lesions are multifocal and most numerous in the basal ganglia, midbrain, brainstem, and cerebral hemispheres.[317] Vasculitis can occur, and trophozoites are often found invading vascular walls.[396] The amebas multiply and can disseminate throughout the body. Other organs involved (at the time of autopsy) include the liver, lungs, kidneys, adrenals, pancreas, lymph nodes, and heart.[9,467]

Magnetic resonance imaging (MRI) and CT scans have shown multiple enhancing lesions in the cerebral hemispheres and cerebellum, but the scans are nondiagnostic.[256,396,415] Diagnosis is difficult, because amebas are rarely observed in the CSF. Examination of the CSF shows a moderate mononuclear pleocytosis, elevated protein, and low glucose. Definitive diagnosis is made by direct visualization of amebic trophozoites and cysts within brain tissue. Unfortunately, there is no effective treatment for GAE, and the mortality rate is 100% in immunocompromised patients.[317] Although pentamidine isethionate, propamidine, sulfadiazine, and ketoconazole are effective in vitro, these drugs do not appear to be useful because of the underlying immunosuppression of most of these patients.[317] Based on tissue-culture studies, pentamidine isethionate appears to be the best choice for treatment of *B. mandrillaris* encephalitis.[417] One case of widespread granulomatous skin lesions in an immunocompromised patient resulting from *A. rhysodes* was successfully treated with intravenous pentamidine isethionate for 4 weeks, topical chlorhexidine gluconate, and ketoconazole cream, followed by oral itraconazole.[441] Miltefosine is a drug that has shown in vitro activity against free-living amebas, but as an investigational drug.

It is not readily available in the United States. However, with CDC assistance, miltefosine has been administered since 2009 for amebic infections as single-patient emergency use with permission from the FDA. Although the number of *B. mandrillaris* and *Acanthamoeba* species infections treated with a miltefosine-containing regimen is small, it appears that a miltefosine-containing treatment regimen does offer a survival advantage for patients with these often fatal infections. The CDC now has an expanded access investigational new drug protocol in effect with the FDA to make miltefosine available directly from the CDC for treatment in the United States.[82]

ACANTHAMOEBA KERATITIS

Acanthamoeba keratitis is caused by *Acanthamoeba*, a genus containing at least 24 species of free-living amebic protozoa.[317] It is ubiquitous in nature, existing both in soil and in nearly all water sources and supplies, and has been found in seawater, lakes, rivers, and streams, and is commonly found in water supplies, such as tap and bottled water, drinking fountains, eye-wash stations, dental units, and dialysis machines. Despite its near universal presence, *Acanthamoeba* infection in humans is relatively uncommon. The combination of corneal epithelium barrier disruption, whether from trauma or from contact lens wear, and exposure to a sufficient inoculum of *Acanthamoeba* substantially increases the risk of keratitis.

Acanthamoeba enters the corneal stroma through minor trauma or abrasion, causing chronic corneal inflammation, which can impair vision and lead to vascularized corneal scarring, perforation, and loss of the eye. Poor lens hygiene and overnight wear are the dominant risk factors for development of keratitis. The incidence of *Acanthamoeba* keratitis is estimated at 0.33 to 1.0 per 10,000 hydrogel contact lens wearers per year.[7]

Symptoms include severe eye pain, photophobia, conjunctival inflammation, and blurred vision. Diagnosis is made by identification of the trophozoites or cysts by corneal scrapings or biopsies. The treatment of choice for *Acanthamoeba* keratitis is 0.02% polyhexamethylene biguanide or propamidine (0.1%) with topical polymyxin B, gramicidin, or neomycin.[177,284] Other topical drugs that have been used for the treatment of this form of keratitis include antibiotics (e.g., aminoglycoside, neomycin) and antifungals (e.g., azole, itraconazole, metronidazole, voriconazole). Oral itraconazole has been used in severe cases to prevent potential spread of trophozoites into adjacent tissues. Penetrating keratoplasty and corneal grafting have been performed.[151] Contact lens wearers should use sterile solutions for lenses and should consider not wearing contact lenses while engaging in water sports.[229]

DISEASES CAUSED BY OCCUPATIONAL EXPOSURE TO SEAFOOD

The number of fishers and fish farmers has been growing at an average rate of 3.5% per year since 1990.[237,238] There is great variation in work activities for the different types of seafood, including working aboard fish trawlers, aquaculture production, working inland as capture fishers or in processing, food preparation activities, laboratory technicians and researchers, pet food production, shell grinders, and jewelry polishers. Adverse respiratory reactions are mainly the result of biologic and chemical agents associated with processing, preserving, storage, and transport of seafood. Several types of seafood cause occupational respiratory allergy, although shellfish are some of the most allergenic species of seafood. Agents with the potential to cause respiratory disease include high-molecular-weight seafood proteins, microbes containing "fish juice," biogenic amines, degradation compounds, and digestive enzymes.[238] Additional contaminants not associated with seafood, such as parasites, protochordates, marine toxins, bacterial toxins, chemical additives, spices, and gasses produced by anaerobic decomposition (hydrogen sulfide), have been reported to cause toxicity.[237,238]

PATHOPHYSIOLOGY

Adverse reactions to seafood can be immune mediated or nonimmune mediated.[306] A number of seafood allergens have been characterized, including shellfish muscle protein, tropomyosin, and other crustacean allergens, including arginine kinase, myosin light-chain kinase, and sarcoplasmatic calcium-binding protein.[306] These proteins can cause typical IgE-mediated symptoms in individuals who have been sensitized through ingestion. By contrast, aerosolized seafood proteins responsible for asthmatic reactions encountered in occupational environments have not been well described.

CLINICAL PRESENTATION

Occupational asthma is the most frequent work-related respiratory disease reported in the seafood industry. The prevalence varies from 2% to 36%, with differences in prevalence partly due to inconsistent definitions of occupational asthma.[237] A higher prevalence is associated with exposure to crab and shrimp. Symptoms may develop from weeks to years after exposure, and are more severe at work, with improvement noted on weekends. Rhinitis, conjunctivitis, and skin rashes on exposed portions of the body accompany or precede respiratory symptoms. The prognosis of occupational asthma is variable and depends on several factors, including duration of exposure, pulmonary function testing at the time of diagnosis, and type of agent involved.

Approximately 75% of workers with occupational asthma are left with permanent hyperresponsiveness, even after removal from the exposure, although the magnitude of their symptoms is generally mild. In patients who remain exposed, asthma is likely to worsen.[314]

TREATMENT

A definitive diagnostic test for occupational asthma does not exist.[31] Questionnaires are very sensitive but not very specific. The specific inhalation challenge test is considered the reference standard. However, it is not widely available and false-negative results occur. Other objective tests include the prick skin test or specific IgE to the offending allergens, or documentation of increased nonallergenic bronchial responsiveness. These tests have positive predictive values of 76% to 89%. Therefore, a negative test does not exclude the diagnosis, whereas a positive test is not confirmatory.[31,237] Monitoring of peak expiratory flow is inexpensive and easily available; however, performance is effort dependent and often poorly performed.[170] Diagnosing occupational asthma should be performed in a stepwise manner, incorporating the compatible clinical history and objective testing. Once the diagnosis of occupational asthma is made, the worker must be removed from the exposure. Inhaled steroids can hasten improvement.

PREVENTION

Atopy is the most important host factor associated with development of sensitization to high-molecular-weight allergens and for development of occupational asthma, although there is a general consensus that there is no place for prescreening and exclusion from employment of atopic individuals.[170] Smoking has also been associated with sensitization to snow crab.[170] Potential primary prevention measures include engineering controls to improve ventilation, administrative controls to reduce the number of workers exposed or duration of exposure, and use of personal protective equipment. There are currently no regulatory exposure standards for seafood allergens.

REFERENCES

Complete references used in this text are available online at expertconsult.inkling.com.

Seafood, including all edible fish and shellfish, has been a mainstay of diets throughout the world for centuries, playing a key role in the nutrition and economy of nations around the globe. In the United States, fish and shellfish consumption has increased in recent decades, perhaps because of its increasingly recognized nutritional benefits, such as providing low-fat, high-quality protein as well as omega-3 fatty acids essential for heart and brain health. In 2012, the United States was ranked the third largest consumer of seafood in the world, behind China and Japan, consuming a total of 4.5 billion pounds of fish and shellfish.[143] This equated to 14.4 pounds of fish and shellfish per person in 2012, up from 11.8 pounds in 1970. Table 78-1 illustrates trends in per capita seafood consumption in the United States since 1970. Since 2001, shrimp has continued to rank as the most consumed seafood in the United States, with 3.8 pounds of shrimp consumed per person in 2012, down from a record of 4.4 pounds in 2006.[142] Table 78-2 lists the most frequently consumed seafood in the United States in 2012.

Given this trend toward increased fish and shellfish consumption, there has been growing recognition and appreciation of seafood allergies, which can range from mild cutaneous reactions to life-threatening anaphylaxis and death. It is important that clinicians be prepared to recognize, treat, and prevent fish and shellfish allergies. Understanding the epidemiology, pathophysiology, biologic classification, and spectrum of cross-reactivity of seafood with other potential allergens is instrumental in achieving this goal.

EPIDEMIOLOGY

Food allergies pose a significant threat to human health. Bock and coworkers estimate that food allergies are the leading identifiable cause of anaphylactic reactions presenting to emergency departments in the United States. Overall, there are approximately 29,000 anaphylactic reactions per year, resulting in 150 deaths annually.[23] The actual incidence of anaphylaxis due to food allergies depends on the diagnostic criteria used. One study reported a 13% incidence among a sample of patients presenting with food-related allergic reactions,[165] whereas another reported an incidence of 51%.[39] In a study of patients presenting with food allergies to an allergy center in Singapore, 66% had a history of anaphylactic reaction to a food allergen.[193]

Food allergies are common. It is estimated that 4% to 5% of adults and 5% of children under the age of 3 years in the United States have a food allergy.[181] Seafood allergy is the most common food allergy in adults, with as much as 2.3% of the general population reporting a seafood allergy.[180] Unlike many food allergies, seafood allergies appear to be more common in adults than in children. Similar to the situation with peanut allergy, individuals with fish and shellfish allergies generally remain clinically reactive lifelong. A 2002 telephone survey conducted in the United States determined that fish allergies afflicted 0.1% and 0.4% of children and adults, respectively, whereas 0.1% of children and 2% of adults reported a shellfish allergy. Shellfish rank as the leading cause of IgE-mediated food allergies in the U.S. adult population, as well as the leading cause of visits related to a food allergy to an emergency department.[39,180] Another analysis estimated that shellfish are the number one cause of food allergies among individuals older than age 6 years presenting to EDs in the United States with food allergies.[165]

Although the specific causes of food allergies vary in different countries according to regional dietary patterns, seafood allergies appear to be one of the leading causes of food allergies worldwide. In Korea, where whelk is commonly eaten, allergy to this mollusk has been reported.[99] Similarly, barnacle allergy has been identified in the Portuguese population.[121] In a study of patients with food allergies in Singapore, crustacea accounted for 34%, mollusks 19%, and fish 4% of food allergies.[193] A telephone survey in Canada reported a probable prevalence of fish and shellfish allergies to be 0.48% and 1.42%, respectively,[19] similar to the allergy patterns reported in the U.S. population. In a survey of food allergies in schoolchildren in Asia, a high prevalence of shellfish allergy was seen, with rates of 5.23% and 5.12% in 14- to 16-year-olds in Singapore and the Philippines, respectively. This was in comparison to similar groups of children born in Western countries, where peanut and tree nut allergies were found to be much more prevalent,[176] possibly reflecting differences in patterns of seafood consumption in Asian and Western countries.

BIOLOGIC CLASSIFICATION OF SEAFOOD

Seafood can be classified mainly into four categories of organisms: fish, crustacea, mollusks, and echinoderms, with each belonging to a different phylum. Because most individuals with a seafood allergy are not allergic to all types of seafood, basic understanding of the biologic classification of fish and shellfish can be helpful to guide patients regarding selective avoidance diets. Table 78-3 provides an overview of the taxonomic relationships among seafoods.

Fish belong to the phylum Chordata, with most edible fish belonging to the class of bony, ray-finned fish, Actinopterygii (superclass Osteichthyes). Sharks (including dogfish), rays, and skates are the exception, belonging to the Chondrichthyes class of cartilaginous fish. The most frequently consumed fish in the United States fall into several orders: Salmoniformes (salmon, trout, whitefish), Siluriformes (catfish), Pleuronectiformes (flounder, halibut, sole, flatfish), Perciformes (bass, perch, snapper, tuna, mackerel, tilapia, swordfish), Gadiformes (codfish, pollock), and Clupeiformes (herring, sardines, anchovies).[139] Table 78-4 describes the taxonomic relationships among edible fish species.

Shellfish can be broken down into two distinct phyla. Crustacea, which include shrimp, prawns, crab, lobster, barnacles, krill, and crayfish, are classified as arthropods, sharing the Arthropoda phylum with spiders, centipedes, and insects. The Mollusca phylum includes eight classes, three of which are important for human consumption: Gastropoda (snails, abalone), Bivalvia (mussels, oysters, scallops, clams), and Cephalopoda (squid, octopus, cuttlefish).[139,191]

Sea cucumbers and sea urchins and their products, including *uni*, or sea urchin coral, and *roe*, or sea urchin ovaries, make up a very small percentage of marine organisms consumed by humans. Sea urchins and sea cucumbers belong to the phylum Echinodermata, with sea urchins belonging to the class Echinoidea, and sea cucumbers belonging to the class Holothuroidea.[139]

IMMUNOLOGIC MECHANISMS OF SEAFOOD ALLERGIES

Although nonimmunologic reactions to fish and shellfish occur, true seafood allergies are reactions mediated by immunoglobulin E (IgE) that represent a failure of the body's oral tolerance

TABLE 78-1 U.S. Seafood Consumption for Selected Years from 1970 to 2012 (Pounds per Capita)

Seafood	1970	1980	1990	1995	2000	2005	2007	2009	2010	2011	2012
Total	11.8	12.5	15.0	15.0	15.2	16.2	16.3	16.0	15.8	15.0	14.4
Fresh/frozen	6.9	7.9	9.6	10.0	10.2	11.6	12.1	12.0	11.6	10.9	10.5
Canned	4.5	4.3	5.1	4.7	4.7	4.3	3.9	3.7	3.9	3.8	3.6
Cured	0.4	0.3	0.3	0.3	0.3	0.3	0.3	0.3	0.3	0.3	0.3

From National Oceanic and Atmospheric Administration: Fisheries of the United States: noaa.gov.

TABLE 78-2 Top Ten Most Frequently Consumed Seafoods in the United States in 2012

Seafood	Weight (lb/capita)
1. Shrimp	3.800
2. Canned tuna	2.400
3. Salmon	2.020
4. Tilapia	1.476
5. Pollock	1.167
6. Pangasius	0.726
7. Crab	0.523
8. Cod	0.521
9. Catfish	0.500
10. Clams	0.347
Total	14.6

Data from National Marine Fisheries Service: Top 10 U.S. consumption by species chart, calculated by Howard Johnson, H.M. Johnson & Associates for NFI: aboutseafood.com/about/about-seafood/Top-10-Consumed-Seafoods.

TABLE 78-3 Taxonomic Relationships Among Seafoods

Phylum	Class	Common Name Representatives
Chordata	Actinopterygii	Bony, ray-finned fish (see Table 78-4)
	Chondrichthyes	Cartilaginous fish (sharks, rays, skates)
Arthropoda	Crustacea	Shrimp, crab, lobster, barnacles, crayfish, krill
Mollusca	Gastropoda	Snails, abalone, whelk
	Bivalvia	Mussels, oysters, scallops, clams, cockles
	Cephalopoda	Squid, octopus, cuttlefish
Echinodermata	Echinoidea	Sea urchin
	Holothuroidea	Sea cucumber

Data from Myers P, Espinosa R, Parr CS, et al: The animal diversity web, 2008: animaldiversity.org.

TABLE 78-4 Taxonomic Relationships Among the Edible Fishes

Class	Order (Suborder)	Common Name
Chondrichthyes	Elasmobranchii	Sharks
Actinopterygii	Acipenseriformes	Sturgeons, paddlefish
	Anguilliformes	Common eels, morays
	Atheriniformes	Silversides, jacksmelts, grunions
	Beloniformes	Sauries, needlefish, flying fish
	Clupeiformes	Herring, sardines, alewives, shad, menhaden, anchovies
	Cypriniformes	Minnows, carp, suckers
	Elopiformes	Tarpons, ten-pounders
	Esociformes	Pike, pickerel, muskellunge
	Gadiformes	Codfish, ling cod, pollock, haddock, tomcod, hake, codling, whiting
	Gonorynchiformes	Awa, milkfish
	Lampridiformes	Opah
	Lophiiformes	Monkfish, goosefish
	Mugiliformes	Mullets
	Osmeriformes	Smelts, eulachon, capelin
	Perciformes (Ammodytoidei)	Sand lances
Actinopterygii (cont.)	Perciformes (Labroidei)	Cichlids (tilapia), tautogs, wrasses, surf perch
	Perciformes (Percodei)	Bass, crappies, bluegills, sea bass, sunfish, perch, bluefish, jacks, pompanos, dolphin fish, snapper, groupers, scups, grunts, porgies, pomfrets, sheepsheads, snooks, robalos, bigeyes, catalufas, croakers, butterfly fish, goatfish, mojarras, rudderfish, weakfish, drums, sauger, threadfins, walleye
	Perciformes (Scombroidei)	Mackerel, tuna, cutlassfish, albacore, bonitos, kingfish, swordfish, sailfish, barracuda, billfish, marlin, spearfish, tenggiri fish
	Perciformes (Stromateoidei)	Butterfish
	Perciformes (Zoarcoidei)	Wolffish
	Percopsiformes	Trout-perch, sand rollers
	Pleuronectiformes	Flounders, halibut, sole, dabs, turbots, flatfish
	Salmoniformes	Trout, salmon, whitefish, graylings, lake herring
	Scorpaeniformes	Rockfish, scorpionfish, greenlings
	Siluriformes	Catfish
	Tetraodontiformes	Pufferfish, boxfish, trunkfish

From Myers P, Espinosa R, Parr CS, et al: The animal diversity web, 2008: animaldiversity.org.

mechanisms. Oral tolerance can be defined as "an active nonresponse to antigens delivered via the oral route."[123] It involves both prevention of uptake of allergenic proteins from the gut into the bloodstream and suppression of the immune system's allergenic response to such proteins once they enter the system.

Under physiologic conditions, luminal barriers within the gastrointestinal tract prevent the uptake of the majority of potential food allergens that enter the gut. Potentially allergenic proteins are degraded into nonimmunogenic forms by gastric acid and digestive enzymes, whereas IgA antibodies secreted by B cells in the gut bind foreign proteins and prevent their uptake. However, even under physiologic conditions, approximately 2% of ingested proteins cross the protective epithelium of the gastrointestinal tract intact and are absorbed into the bloodstream as immunologically active antigens.[80] Usually these antigens do not elicit allergic reactions because of the body's innate mechanisms that suppress the immune response to food allergens. This process of immune suppression begins when an intact antigen escapes the protective barriers of the gut and is taken up and presented by antigen-presenting cells (APCs), including B cells, dendritic cells, and macrophages. APCs then activate regulatory and suppressor T cells, which secrete suppressive cytokines, transforming growth factor β and interleukin-10 (IL-10). Through this series of steps, a state of oral tolerance is achieved whereby the immune system essentially "ignores" the food antigen. In the case of high-dose oral antigen exposure, tolerance is mediated by a different mechanism, specifically, lymphocyte clonal anergy and/or deletion.[29,34]

When oral tolerance mechanisms fail to inhibit the body's immune response to ingested food antigens, food allergies can develop. True seafood allergies are type I immediate hypersensitivity IgE-mediated reactions that result from a chain of molecular and cellular interactions involving APCs, T cells, and B cells (Figure 78-1). Production of allergen-specific IgE (sensitization) antibodies forms the underlying basis of immediate hypersensitivity; atopy is defined as the genetic predisposition to developing allergen-specific IgE antibodies. The sensitization process requires a cooperative effort between CD4 T lymphocytes and B lympho-

cytes. It begins with presentation of an allergen to CD4 T lymphocytes by APCs in the context of a major histocompatibility complex. Cytokines released from CD4 T lymphocytes as a result of this interaction cause differentiation of B lymphocytes into immunoglobulin-secreting plasma cells. This differentiation leads to isotype switching (production of specific antibody types) within plasma cells. For example, release of cytokines IL-4 or IL-13 from T lymphocytes promotes IgE switching.[50] Once allergen-specific IgE antibodies are produced, subsequent exposure and binding of the allergens to IgE molecules on the surface of mast cells results in cross-linking of the IgE molecules. Consequently, mast cells or basophils degranulate and release both preformed and newly synthesized mediators. The prototype preformed mediator is histamine, and the newly synthesized mediators include those of the arachidonic acid pathway (leukotrienes, prostaglandins, and platelet-activating factor), neuropeptides (e.g., substance P), and cytokines (e.g., IL-4, IL-5).

Release of chemical mediators has various pathologic consequences that can cause both local and systemic clinical manifestations. Histamine causes vasodilation and increased vascular permeability, smooth muscle contraction, stimulation of sensory nerve endings, and glandular secretions, with clinical effects including nasal congestion, rhinorrhea, urticaria, angioedema, laryngospasm, cough, wheezing, and shock. Products of the arachidonic acid pathway have similar effects.

Allergic reactions consist of an early phase characterized by mast cell or basophil degranulation, and a late phase, which occurs 4 to 6 hours after the early phase. The hallmark of the late-phase reaction is influx of inflammatory cells, such as eosinophils, basophils, and T lymphocytes. For example, basophils cause further histamine release, and T lymphocytes release additional cytokines that enhance IgE production (via IL-4) and eosinophil activation (via IL-5). As a result of further inflammatory activity by these cells, there is recrudescence of symptoms many hours after the initial allergen exposure. Leukotrienes, prostaglandins, and cytokines released in the early-phase reaction play an important role in recruiting the late-phase cellular components to the inflammatory site.

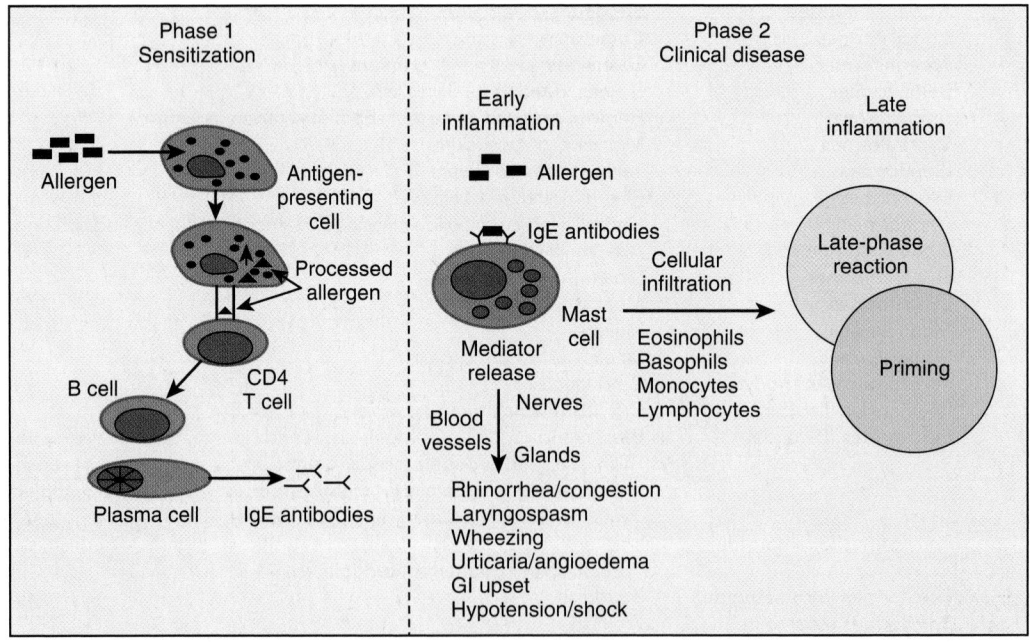

FIGURE 78-1 The natural history of IgE-mediated allergic reaction (simplified schematic). During phase 1, the individual becomes sensitized to an allergen. During phase 2, clinical disease develops. An overwhelming majority of individuals have an early response on reexposure to the allergen. Activation of mast cells and release of mediators dominate the early response. After the early response, most individuals have an influx of inflammatory cells, causing late inflammatory events, including spontaneous recurrence of release of mediators (late-phase reaction) and increased responsiveness to the allergen on reexposure (priming). *Circles* indicate the heterogeneity of these late inflammatory events. (*Modified from Naclerio R: Allergic rhinitis,* N Engl J Med *325:860, 1991.*)

In theory, prior exposure and sensitization to a food allergen must occur before development of a clinically significant allergic reaction. The exposure may occur through cutaneous or inhalation routes, cross-sensitization via similar antigens, placental transfer, or as a result of hidden ingredients or contaminants in other foods. Risk factors for development of food allergies include early age of antigen exposure, extensive delay of oral exposure (possibly causing sensitization by topical exposure rather than inducing tolerance via oral exposure), family history of atopy, presence of asthma or other atopic disease, and medications (e.g., antacids) or medical conditions that reduce acidity within the gut and allow more potential allergens to escape the natural protective barriers of the gastrointestinal tract.[29,181,197] In one study, more than half of patients with food allergy had concomitant allergic rhinitis, asthma, and/or atopic dermatitis.[193] In another study, codfish-allergic individuals were orally challenged with fish digested with gastric enzymes at pH 2.0 and 3.0. Patients experienced allergic symptoms sooner or at a lower dose when the codfish was predigested at pH 3.0 compared with pH 2.0, underscoring the role of gastric digestion in the process of food allergen tolerance.[197]

CLINICAL MANIFESTATIONS

Clinical manifestations of fish and shellfish allergies are similar to those of other IgE-mediated food allergy reactions, ranging from mild urticaria to life-threatening anaphylaxis. In the U.S. telephone survey cited earlier, 55% of finfish reactions and 40% of shellfish reactions were severe enough to cause the sufferers to seek evaluation by a physician.[180] IgE-mediated reactions generally have a rapid onset, with allergic symptoms developing within minutes to an hour of exposure and most reactions occurring within 30 minutes.[1,30,46,74] However, a delayed onset (3 to 24 hours after exposure) of symptoms may occur and has been noted with, among other seafoods, dogfish,[163] cuttlefish,[177] abalone,[119] and limpets.[134] A biphasic reaction may occur, whereby the individual appears to recover and then experiences a late-phase reaction with recrudescence of symptoms after an asymptomatic period. In one pediatric study, a biphasic reaction was seen in 6% of anaphylaxis patients.[98]

Symptoms of seafood allergy are often, but not always, related to the route of exposure and can occur after ingestion, cutaneous contact, and inhalation. Following ingestion of an offending seafood, the most commonly reported signs and symptoms include generalized itching and urticaria; angioedema, particularly swelling of the lips and tongue; pulmonary manifestations, including dyspnea, wheezing, and chest tightness; gastrointestinal complaints, including nausea, vomiting, diarrhea, and abdominal cramping; and shock.[101,180] It is direct contact of the allergenic food with the oral mucosa that causes pruritus and angioedema of the lips, tongue, throat, and palate—a constellation of symptoms known as oral allergy syndrome.[37,52] In patients with underlying atopic disease, exposure to fish and shellfish allergens can cause exacerbations of eczema[169] and, less commonly, asthma symptoms.[84] Because ongoing exposure to a food allergen may cause chronic urticaria, the presence of an undiagnosed food allergy should be sought in patients with chronic urticaria.[52]

In general, ingestion of the allergic seafood leads to gastrointestinal symptoms, urticaria, and possible vascular compromise, whereas skin contact results in mainly dermatologic symptoms. Exposure by inhalation typically causes respiratory symptoms. For example, there are documented cases of patients allergic to fish presenting with skin reactions after handling raw fish,[136,157] as well as symptoms of asthma in fish-allergic children after inhalation of aerosolized fish.[161] However, this is by no means the absolute rule; systemic reactions after cutaneous and inhalational exposure may occur. In one case study, a 2-year-old fish-allergic child experienced facial urticaria and angioedema after her grandfather, who had eaten fish 2 hours earlier, kissed her.[131] In another report, a shellfish-allergic patient experienced anaphylaxis after kissing her boyfriend, who had recently ingested shrimp.[185] In one survey, 8.6% of fish-allergic and 10% of shellfish-allergic individuals experienced more severe reactions following inhalational or dermal, rather than ingestion, exposure. These

allergic individuals were able to consume the offending antigen without significant sequelae.[180]

Vascular involvement is not uncommon in patients with seafood allergies. In one review of patients with seafood allergies, 8% of patients with fish allergy and 13% of patients with shrimp allergy developed anaphylactic shock after seafood challenge.[101] Manifestations of vascular involvement may include hypotension, a subjective "sense of doom," respiratory distress progressing to asphyxia, dysrhythmias, and myocardial infarction. Near-fatal and fatal reactions may begin with only mild symptoms, such as oral allergy syndrome, before rapidly progressing to cardiovascular collapse. Risk factors for severe anaphylactic reactions are the presence of other atopic disease(s), inadvertent ingestion of the offending food, rapid onset of symptoms, failure to promptly treat with epinephrine, and a history of prior anaphylaxis to the causative food.[52]

One form of anaphylaxis that occurs in the setting of seafood allergy is *food-associated, exercise-induced anaphylaxis.* Affected patients develop anaphylaxis if they exercise within 2 to 6 hours of ingesting an allergenic food, but remain asymptomatic if the same food is ingested without exercise. Although the mechanism is poorly understood, shellfish and wheat flour are the most common causes of food-associated, exercise-induced anaphylaxis.[18,211]

OCCUPATIONAL SEAFOOD ALLERGIES

Hypersensitivity reactions to fish and shellfish in the seafood processing industry due to occupational exposure are increasingly recognized. Rather than ingestion, most reactions are associated with direct contact or inhalational exposure during cutting, cleaning, cooking, or drying of seafood.[100] Occupational reactions have been reported in a variety of seafood workers, including fishermen, seafood-processing workers, canners, restaurant cooks, delivery persons, and other workers associated with the seafood industry.[31,49,105,174] Occupational seafood allergy can manifest as rhinitis, conjunctivitis, asthma, urticaria, contact dermatitis, or oral allergy syndrome.[4,86] Studies performed on snow crab workers demonstrated a 33% incidence of asthma, 24% incidence of skin rash, and 18% rate of rhinitis or conjunctivitis related to inhalational exposure or skin contact with snow crab meat or by-products.[31] In a survey of occupational allergies in seafood workers in Australia and South Africa, skin reactions accounted for 78% to 81% of reported problems, followed by asthmatic symptoms (7% to 10%) and nonspecific allergic symptoms (9% to 15%).[117] Although rare, vascular involvement related to occupational seafood exposure has been reported.[174]

In most studies, occupational asthma appears to be the most prominent clinical presentation of seafood allergy, with a reported prevalence of 7% to 36%.[86] Seafood implicated in occupational asthma include all the major seafood groupings: oysters,[141] clams,[49] shrimp,[49,105] prawns,[61] fish,[42,51] snow and king crabs,[31,151] lobsters,[105,154] sea squirts,[89] abalone,[40] powdered marine sponges,[16] cuttlefish,[194] and clam liver extract.[91] In one case study, shark cartilage powder was reported to have caused a fatal occupational asthma attack.[153] Hypersensitivity pneumonitis may result from occupational exposure to seafood allergens and has been documented secondary to mollusk shell dust inhalation.[152] Clinical manifestations of hypersensitivity pneumonitis include dyspnea, fever, chills, cough, and malaise. With chronic low-level allergen exposure, fever and chills may be absent, with symptoms of exertional dyspnea, fatigue, and weight loss predominating.[104]

Dermatologic occupational seafood allergy has been less well studied but generally takes the forms of contact urticaria and a chronic recurrent dermatitis known as protein contact dermatitis.[4,78,138] The estimated prevalence of occupational protein contact dermatitis ranges from 3% to 11%.[86] The most frequent clinical presentation is chronic or recurrent eczema that may be limited to the fingertips or extend to the wrists and arms. Initial manifestations include itchy, erythematous, and vesicular lesions, which usually progress to chronic eczema, with episodic acute exacerbations after repeated contact with the culprit allergen.[4,78] Some cases of chronic paronychia (after handling the allergenic food) may also be a variant of protein contact dermatitis, with redness and swelling of the proximal nail fold.[196] In some cases, percutaneous sensitization to seafood allergens may occur via direct skin contact in the workplace, as may occur with seafood packers or delivery persons. If ongoing exposure occurs, the individual may develop allergic symptoms and even anaphylaxis following ingestion of the offending seafood.[174] Risk factors for sensitization and clinical allergy in seafood workers include the presence of atopy, as well as the duration and intensity of exposure to the potential allergen.[90,182]

DIFFERENTIAL DIAGNOSIS

Diagnosing a seafood allergy can range from a simple to an extremely complex process. There are a number of hidden allergens in foods, as well as seafood allergy mimics (such as seafood toxins and allergens present in seafood parasites), that can easily go unrecognized. When evaluating a patient with a suspected seafood allergy or a patient with an apparent allergic reaction to an unknown allergen, it is important to obtain a careful history and consider a broad differential diagnosis.

Many nonseafood products contain fish and shellfish, often unbeknownst to the consumer. For example, imitation crab meat is usually made of pollock or monkfish. Surimi, which is processed fish meat usually derived from Alaskan pollock in the United States, is commonly used for seafood-flavored snacks, sauces, flavors, "meatless" hot dogs, sausages, pepperoni sticks, imitation crab, and pizza toppings.[205] Anchovies are a routine ingredient in Caesar salad dressing and Worcestershire sauce. Fish gelatin is a common stabilizing and gelling agent in foods, often used in marshmallows, gummy candies, and other desserts. Many pills and medications contain chitin, a component of the outer skeleton of crustacea and other arthropods. Additionally, many products may be unintentionally contaminated with seafood because they are processed in a facility that also handles seafood. Although the allergenic potential of some of these products has not been well studied, it is important to consider them as potential sources in patients presenting with allergic symptoms. A thorough history may help to identify these accidental ingestions, especially in patients with a known seafood allergy who present with an allergic reaction of unknown cause.

Apparent seafood allergies can also be caused by seafood parasites, rather than the particular fish or shellfish consumed. The parasite *Anisakis simplex* can be a cause of allergic reactions in individuals after consuming parasitized seafood.[10,11,92] *A. simplex* is a nematode that infects fish worldwide and can cause health issues in humans via transient infection after consuming raw or undercooked flesh of infected fish, or via allergy. The allergic reaction is a typical IgE-mediated reaction, presenting as acute urticaria, angioedema, or anaphylaxis following ingestion of infected fish.[11] To date, 13 different *Anisakis* allergens have been characterized.[3] One of the responsible allergens, Ani s 3, is the invertebrate panallergen tropomyosin, capable of cross-reacting with shellfish tropomyosins, adding to the diagnostic dilemma when faced with a patient with a potential seafood allergy.[8,11,68,122,204] Another *Anisakis* allergen, the secretor allergen Ani s 1, has been identified as the major allergen for diagnosing *Anisakis* allergy, with sensitivity and specificity values in vivo and in vitro approaching 100%.[63]

Evidence also suggests that *Anisakis* allergy contributes to occupational respiratory and skin allergies in seafood workers. Armentia and colleagues found *A. simplex* to be the cause of occupational asthma in two seafood workers.[5] In a case report by Scala and coworkers, *Anisakis* was found to be the allergen responsible for contact urticaria and inhalational asthma in a seafood factory worker.[173] In one study looking at the prevalence of *Anisakis* sensitization and related symptoms in fish-processing factories, the prevalence of sensitization to *Anisakis* was found to be higher than that for the fish being processed and was associated with a higher risk of allergic reactions.[145] These findings underscore the importance of considering *Anisakis* allergy in patients presenting with first-time allergic symptoms following consumption of seafood, especially if that seafood has been tolerated in the past. Unfortunately, studies suggest that ingestion of

frozen or cooked seafood, which is recommended for anisakidosis prophylaxis, does not prevent IgE-mediated allergic reactions to *Anisakis*. Given the prevalence of parasitism of fish and shellfish by *Anisakis,* for patients diagnosed with *Anisakis* allergy, a seafood-free diet is recommended.[132]

A common mimicker of IgE-mediated seafood allergy is scombroid poisoning (see Chapter 77). Scombroid intoxication results from ingestion of dark-meat fish (tuna, salmon, marlin, mahi-mahi, bluefish, mackerel, and others) containing high levels of free histamine produced by bacteria in the fish flesh during spoilage.[33] Usually within 10 to 30 minutes of ingestion, the histamine produces symptoms that mimic IgE-mediated allergy, including perioral tingling and burning sensations, flushing, urticaria, and gastrointestinal complaints, and may progress to bronchospasm, tachycardia, and hypotension. Symptoms that suggest scombroid intoxication include headache, dizziness, and perioral tingling and burning, as well as a history of consuming fish that tasted peppery or bitter.[33]

Other types of seafood poisoning (ciguatoxin, fish or diarrheic shellfish poisoning, and others) may result in a variety of physical complaints, but these are usually clinically distinct from IgE-mediated allergic reactions. Similarly, seafood-associated illness may occur secondary to bacterial and viral causes, such as poisoning due to toxins (botulism, *Staphylococcus*) or gastroenteritis from bacterial or viral infection.[33] These illnesses also tend to be clinically distinct from IgE-mediated reactions.

DIAGNOSIS

A critical step in diagnosing seafood allergy, or any other food allergy, is obtaining a thorough and accurate history, including specific symptoms, food(s) ingested around the time of symptom onset, timing of the reaction, prior history of similar reactions, presence of known food allergies, and any exacerbating factors, such as exercise. Patients should also be questioned about possible contaminants or hidden allergenic ingredients in ingested food(s), particularly if the inciting allergen is unknown. Although taking a good history is of utmost importance, research suggests that medical history alone is insufficient in diagnosing food allergy. In one study of children with a self-reported food allergy, the allergic reaction was reproducible in only 40% by double-blind, placebo-controlled food challenge.[22]

Contributing to the challenge of diagnosing food allergies are several confounding factors. Preparation and processing methods, as well as the part of seafood ingested, may all contribute to the allergenicity of any particular seafood. In one study, pomfret and hilsa fish lost their allergenicity significantly when they were boiled and fried compared with raw extracts, and bhetki and mackerel remained strongly, if not more, reactive once cooked.[32] Another study found that patients with salmon and tuna allergies had negative reactions to canned salmon and tuna challenges, suggesting that the major antigen(s) in these fish may be considerably heat labile.[21] Finally, Kobayashi and colleagues demonstrated less allergenicity in fish dark muscle compared with white muscle, suggesting that the part of the fish ingested may lead to variable allergic responses.[95]

In patients with suspected seafood allergy, skin prick tests (SPTs) are a relatively safe, inexpensive, and useful screening tool. Commercial extracts are not available for every seafood species; therefore, mixed extracts are often used. Additionally, actual raw or cooked food itself can be used for skin testing. SPTs may be contraindicated in patients with a history of a severe anaphylactic reaction to the seafood being tested or in patients with significant skin disease. Given the fact that SPTs measure sensitization to a particular allergen, and sensitization is not equivalent to allergic disease, caution must be taken in interpreting SPT results. Multiple studies comparing SPTs with double-blind, placebo-controlled food challenges have found that a positive SPT does not always correlate with symptomatic seafood allergy.[20,22,73] Thus, SPTs have high sensitivity and excellent negative predictive value, but low specificity and poor positive predictive value.[52] Specifically, patients with positive results on SPT may not necessarily have clinically significant allergic disease. However, a study using mean wheal diameters to predict positive food challenges with shrimp suggested that skin testing for seafood allergy may not be as problematic as was once thought.[88] Mean wheal diameter of 30 mm (1.2 inches) after an SPT provided 80% and 95% predictive probability for positive food challenge in subjects with allergies to black tiger prawn and giant freshwater prawn, respectively. This study suggested that the predictive probability of SPTs can be helpful in cases where food challenge cannot be performed.[88]

In vitro diagnostic methods, such as serum immunoassays to determine food-specific IgE antibodies, can also be useful screening tools, particularly for patients in whom skin testing is contraindicated. Serum immunoassays are fraught with the same diagnostic dilemmas as is skin testing, in that in vitro reactivity, like cutaneous sensitization, does not necessarily correlate with clinical allergy.[130] Thus, many patients with positive serum immunoassay testing may not have allergic disease when exposed to the allergen in question.[20,73] Studies by Sampson and colleagues, however, suggest that quantitative measurement of food-specific IgE antibodies may be a useful predictive tool in identifying patients with clinical reactivity.[170,171] In one study, diagnostic levels of IgE, called "decision points," were established that could predict clinical reactivity with greater than 95% certainty to a variety of allergenic foods, including fish, eggs, peanuts, and milk. Diagnostic IgE levels were identified at 20 kU (A)/L or greater for fish allergy.[171] The predictive value of using diagnostic IgE levels to substantiate clinical reactivity was confirmed in a prospective study in which more than 95% of clinical food allergies, including fish allergy, were correctly identified using quantitative serum food-specific IgE concentrations.[170] These findings suggest that serum immunoassay testing may be a safe alternative to oral challenge in patients suspected of having IgE-mediated food allergy.

Atopy patch tests (APTs) have been evaluated as useful tools for diagnosis of food allergy. In the classic patch test, the suspected allergen is applied to a piece of cloth or paper, which is placed on intact skin and covered with an impermeable barrier for 24 to 48 hours. The patch is then removed and the skin examined.[104] However, recent studies have found that APTs add little predictive value to standard SPT and IgE measurements in the diagnostic workup of suspected food allergies and thus cannot be routinely recommended.[125]

The gold standard test in verifying a particular food allergen is the double-blind, placebo-controlled food challenge.[24] This should not be performed in persons who have experienced life-threatening reactions and should be undertaken only under close physician supervision. Dried or freeze-dried foods are encapsulated in opaque, dye-free capsules; alternatively, the food of interest can be hidden in a food vehicle. Appropriate identical placebo-controls are prepared. Although such testing is time consuming and labor intensive, it permits precise diagnosis.

When a certain type of seafood is suspected of producing symptoms, a diagnostic elimination diet can support the diagnosis. Once the offending allergen is eliminated from the diet, the allergic reactions should not occur. The food is then reintroduced to determine if the allergic reaction is reelicited. Diagnostic elimination diets should only be used in persons who have experienced mild allergic symptoms.

Although the methods described previously are useful in diagnosing food allergies, the diagnosis of occupational allergies often requires a different approach, especially in the case of occupational asthma due to inhalation of a seafood allergen. If the allergic individual notes the onset of asthma symptoms related to work exposure, and there is improvement during weekends or vacation, occupational asthma should be suspected. Asthma is verified by appropriate pulmonary function tests, such as spirometry with and without bronchodilators. If the history of asthma is suspected but not corroborated by physical examination or spirometry, it may be necessary to perform a provocation test with inhaled methacholine or histamine to document airway hyperreactivity. The diagnosis depends ultimately on provocation of symptoms by bronchial inhalation challenge with the suspected allergen to simulate industrial exposure.[104] Such evaluation can be performed at the workplace or in a controlled laboratory environment. If a workplace challenge is performed,

the subject's lung function is monitored during the workday with the idea that lung function will decline during the work period because of workplace exposure to the offending allergen. Laboratory challenge is the diagnostic method of choice for diagnosis of occupational asthma, because it allows for identification of a specific etiologic agent (unlike a workplace challenge, where many different allergens may confound the test).[104] Because of inherent dangers of exposing an allergic individual to high doses of allergen, laboratory challenge should occur under close observation in a hospital setting.

Occupational allergic contact dermatitis may also require a specialized approach. Approximately 90% of occupational dermatitis involves the hands, usually the palm and back of the wrist[104]; therefore, dermatitis in a different distribution should raise doubt about the diagnosis. Additionally, location of the dermatitis and location of exposure to the allergen must be matched. Although routine atopy patch testing is not recommended as part of the diagnostic workup of food allergy, in the case of suspected occupational skin disease, patch testing may be useful in demonstrating allergic contact dermatitis to a suspected allergen.[104]

MANAGEMENT

Treatment of acute allergic reaction due to seafood is the same as for any other allergic reaction and depends on the severity and specific symptoms of the reaction. Treatment should begin with assessment and management of the ABCs. For mild cutaneous reactions, antihistamines alone may be sufficient. In patients with severe reactions, epinephrine should be promptly administered intramuscularly or, in refractory cases, intravenously. Intravenous fluids and vasopressors should be used to manage hypotension refractory to epinephrine. Respiratory symptoms, such as wheezing, can be treated with an aerosolized β_2-agonist. To decrease the risk of a delayed, or late-phase, reaction, systemic glucocorticoids should also be given. Because of the risk of a recurrence of symptoms after initial recovery, patients should be observed for a period of several hours up to 24 hours, depending on the severity of the allergic reaction. If severe respiratory or cardiac compromise is present, the patient should be hospitalized.

AFTERCARE

All individuals at risk for anaphylaxis should carry a device for self-injection of epinephrine and carry a medical information card or wear a medical information bracelet. Patients should be referred to an allergist for evaluation and testing to help determine the nature and extent of the seafood allergy.

Avoidance is the only treatment for seafood allergy. Because the allergens present in fish and shellfish are molecularly different (see Molecular Biology section), patients with an allergy to fish generally do not need to avoid shellfish, and vice versa. Allergists typically recommend removing all edible fish from the diet when the patient has a demonstrated history of severe allergic reaction to any fish and/or if there is a positive skin test or serum immunoassay to a fish extract. Similarly, an individual who previously had a severe allergic reaction to a shellfish would be advised to avoid all shellfish. In patients with a history of severe anaphylactic reaction or allergic reactions to many types of seafood, avoidance of all fish and shellfish may be the safest strategy.

In patients with a history of less severe allergic reaction to a particular seafood, research suggests that selective avoidance diets may be reasonable. Studies using double-blind, placebo-controlled fish challenges[20,73] and other tests[48] in fish-allergic children have shown that individuals are not uniformly sensitive to all fish species; hence, sensitivity to one species does not automatically warrant dietary elimination of all seafood. Studies of fish challenges are often negative in children with negative skin tests.[20] Therefore, it seems reasonable to recommend dietary elimination of any seafood species for which there has been a demonstrated allergic reaction or a positive SPT or in vitro test. If a patient tests positive by SPT or in vitro testing to a particular seafood item, but has no history of clinical allergy to that seafood

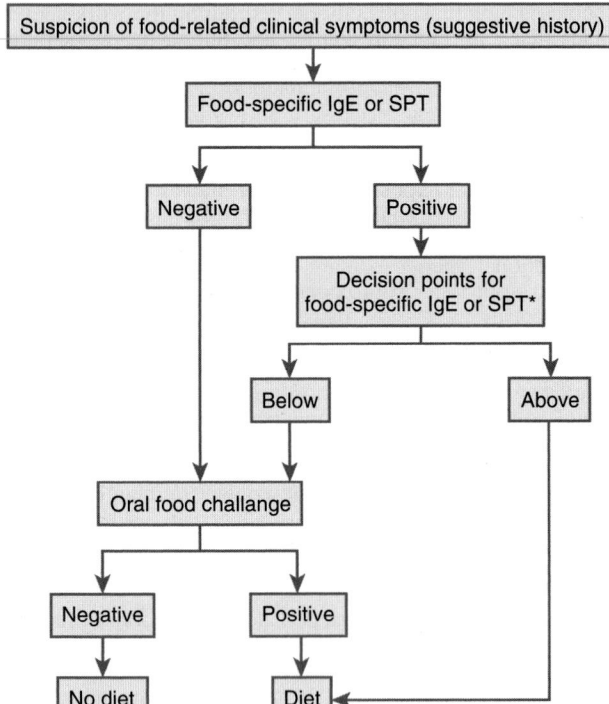

FIGURE 78-2 An algorithmic approach to diagnosing food allergies, including seafood allergies, proceeding from suspicion of food-related symptoms to final recommendations on a specific elimination diet. *Diagnostic decision points appear to be population, age, and allergen dependent. SPT, skin prick test. *(From Niggemann B, Beyer K: Diagnosis of food allergy in children: Toward a standardization of food challenge, J Pediatr Gastroenterol Nutr 45:400, 2007.)*

species, a double-blind, placebo-controlled food challenge can be performed to determine whether true clinical allergy exists. Given the high negative predictive value of SPTs, seafood species for which patients have no history of allergic reaction and have tested negative by a SPT could be permitted in the diet after oral challenge. In the setting of a newly diagnosed seafood allergy to a particular fish or shellfish species, it is reasonable to allow patients to consume other seafood items that have not previously caused allergic symptoms.

Niggemann and colleagues have proposed an algorithmic approach to diagnosing food allergies, including seafood allergies (Figure 78-2).[146] In this algorithm, all patients with a suspected food allergy should undergo food-specific IgE or SPT. If negative, an oral challenge can be conducted. If the initial IgE or SPT is positive, previously established food-specific IgE or SPT "decision points" should be evaluated. If the patient's quantitative IgE or SPT wheal diameter is above the previously established decision point, the food should be eliminated from the diet, but if it falls below the decision point, oral challenge can be conducted.[146]

Education is crucial following an allergic reaction to seafood. Patients should be counseled to read all food labels for the possibility of hidden or unexpected allergenic ingredients or allergic contaminants. Since passage of the United States Food Allergen Labeling and Consumer Protection Act of 2004, food labels have been required to clearly state the presence of eight specified food allergens, including fish and crustacean shellfish. However, mollusks are not included in this labeling mandate.[60] Patients should be informed about the potential for allergic reaction after aerosolization of the offending allergen, as may occur during cooking of seafood, either at home or in fish markets. Finally, patients should be cautioned about the potential for exposure to seafood allergens via inadvertent cross-contact, as in restaurants where equipment is shared for seafood and nonseafood cooking, or during contact with contaminated saliva during kissing or utensil sharing.[131,185]

MOLECULAR BIOLOGY OF SEAFOOD ALLERGIES

The major allergens responsible for IgE-mediated allergic reactions due to fish and shellfish are the parvalbumin and tropomyosin proteins, respectively.[47,53,54,110,175] Since the original characterization of these allergens in codfish and shrimp models, researchers have continued to characterize these proteins and confirm their allergenicity in a wide variety of species of fish and shellfish, as well as identify new classes of proteins also implicated in the development of seafood allergies. Tables 78-5 and 78-6 list the allergens characterized in fish and shellfish to date.

FISH ALLERGENS

Of the seafood allergens that have been isolated and purified, the best characterized is the major allergen of the codfish, Gad c 1, which belongs to the group of muscle tissue proteins called parvalbumins and was first identified in the Baltic cod *(Gadus callarias)*.[54] Parvalbumins are small (12-kD) calcium-binding proteins responsible for mediating the concentration of calcium in white muscle of lower vertebrates and skeletal muscle of higher vertebrates. Parvalbumins exist in two different isoforms, alpha and beta. In fish, parvalbumin beta appears to be a cross-reactive panallergen. Parvalbumins resist heat and enzymatic degradation,[205] making them ideally suited food allergens capable of withstanding extreme temperatures during cooking and proteolytic breakdown in the digestive tract.

Since the original characterization of parvalbumin in codfish, parvalbumins have been identified as allergens in numerous other fish species. Lindstrom and coworkers identified a parvalbumin, designated Sal s 1, as the major allergen in Atlantic salmon *(Salmo salar)*.[116] A second parvalbumin, Gad m 1, has been characterized in the Atlantic cod *(Gadus morhua)* and was found to have greater homology with Sal s 1 than with Gad c 1 (75% with Sal s 1 compared with 62.3% with Gad c 1).[45,119] Parvalbumin antigens have also been identified as major allergens in three species of mackerel (Sco j 1, Sco a 1, Sco s 1), carp (Cyp c 1.01, Cyp c 1.02), Alaska pollock (The c 1), pilchard (Sar sa 1.0101), threadfin, Indian anchovy, pomfret, tenggiri, and Indian scad.[17,71,113,128, 189,200] Studies performed on red and golden snapper revealed a 51-kD protein as a major allergen that is hypothesized to be a parvalbumin tetramer.[164] Interestingly, the 12-kD protein isolate believed to be fish parvalbumin was only found to be a minor allergen in both species of snapper.[164] Studies on tuna have produced inconclusive results. Bugajska-Schretter and associates demonstrated IgE reactivity to tuna parvalbumins in sera from fish-allergic patients,[27] and another study reported identification of parvalbumin as a major allergen in bigeye tuna (Thu o 1).[178] Other studies have failed to detect allergenicity to tuna parvalbumins, suggesting that tuna fish allergy may be caused by an allergen other than parvalbumin.[198,209]

In addition to parvalbumin proteins, other antigens are also emerging as major fish allergens. A second codfish allergen, p41, has been identified that is a 41-kD IgE-reactive protein homologous to an aldehyde phosphate dehydrogenase.[44,62] The purified p41 protein binds specifically to reaginic IgE from cod-allergic individuals. The p41 protein was also found to bind to monoclonal antibodies specific for the first calcium-binding site of parvalbumins, suggesting that p41 may have a calcium-binding site corresponding to an IgE epitope similar to that of Gad c 1.[62] Fish enolase and aldolase have also been identified as significant fish allergens in cod, salmon, and tuna.[97]

Type 1 collagen, a component of muscle and skin in several fish species, was recently identified as a potential major allergen. Hamada and colleagues identified a high-molecular-weight allergen recognized by one fish-allergic serum sample in surimi made from walleye pollock.[69] IgE immunoblotting and amino acid analysis identified the allergen as collagen. In another study, Sakaguchi and coworkers demonstrated IgE antibodies to fish gelatin (type 1 collagen) in fish-allergic children.[168] Anaphylaxis following ingestion of marshmallows containing fish gelatin has been reported.[96] In a study by Hamada and colleagues, five of eight serum samples obtained from fish-allergic individuals

TABLE 78-5 Allergens Characterized in Fish

Protein	Species	Allergen	Reference
Parvalbumin	Baltic cod (Gadus callarias)	Gad c 1	54
	Atlantic cod (Gadus morhua)	Gad m 1	44, 199
	Atlantic salmon (Salmo salar)	Sal s 1	116
	Mackerel (Scomber japonicus, Scomber australasicus, Scomber scombrus)	Sco j 1, Sco a 1, Sco s 1	71
	Alaska pollock (Theragra chalcogramma)	The c 1	200
	Carp (Cyprinus carpio)	Cyp c 1.01, Cyp c 1.02	188
	Pacific pilchard (Sardinops sagax)	Sar sa 1.0101	17
	Indian anchovy (Stolephorus indicus)		113
	Pomfret (Pampus chinensis)		113
	Tenggiri papan (Scomberomorus guttatus)		113
	Threadfin (Polynemus indicus)		113
	Indian scad (Decapterus russelli)		128
	Bigeye tuna (Thunnus obesus)	Thu o 1	178
	Red snapper (Lutjanus argentimaculatus)		164
	Gold snapper (Lutjanus johnii)		164
Collagen, type 1	Bigeye tuna (Thunnus obesus)		70
	Alaska pollock (Theragra chalcogramma)		69
Aldehyde phosphate dehydrogenase homologue	Cod	p41	44, 62
Vitellogenin	Trout caviar		58
	Beluga fish caviar	Hus h 1	156
Alpha S1-casein-like protein	Kingfish caviar		35
Aldolase	Cod		97
	Salmon		97
	Tuna		97
Enolase	Cod		97
	Salmon		97
	Tuna		97

TABLE 78-6 Allergens Characterized in Crustacea and Mollusks

Protein	Species	Allergen	Reference
Tropomyosin (Crustacea)	Brown shrimp (Penaeus aztecus)	Pen a 1	47
	Indian white shrimp (Penaeus indicus)	Pen i 1	175
	Neptune rose shrimp (Parapenaeus fissurus)	Par f 1	114
	Sand shrimp (Metapenaeus ensis)	Met e 1	110
	Tiger prawn (Penaeus monodon)		167
	King prawn (Penaeus latisulcatus)		167
	Chinese spiny lobster (Panulirus stimpsoni)	Pan s 1	107
	American lobster (Homarus americanus)	Hom a 1	107
	Red crab (Charybdis feriatus)	Cha f 1	106
	Krill (Euphausia superba)	Eup s 1	140
	Krill (Euphausia pacifica)	Eup p 1	140
	Amphipods (Gammarus and Caprella spp.)		135
	Acorn barnacle (Balanus rostratus)	Bal r 1	186
	Goose barnacle (Capitulum mitella)	Cap m 1	186
Tropomyosin (Mollusks)	Pacific flying squid (Todarodes pacificus)	Tod p 1	129
	Octopus (Octopus vulgaris)	Oct v 1	83
	Pacific oyster (Crassostrea gigas)	Cra g 1, Cra g 2	82
	Razor clam (Ensis macha)	Ens m 1	87
	Mussel (Perna viridis)	Per v 1	38
	Scallop (Chlamys nobilis)	Chl n 1	38
	Abalone (Haliotis midae, Haliotis discus, Haliotis rufescens)	Hal m 2, Hal d 1, Hal r 1	36, 38, 119
	Turban shell (Turbo cornutus)	Tur c 1	81
	Common whelk (Buccinum undatum)	Buc u 1	99
	Fan shell (Pinna atropurpurea)	Pin a 1	109
	Brown garden snail (Helix aspersa)	Hel as 1	7
Arginine kinase	Tiger prawn (Penaeus monodon)	Pen m 2	210, 167
	King prawn (Penaeus latisulcatus)		167
	White shrimp (Litopenaeus vannamei)	Lit v 2	64
Myosin light chain	White shrimp (Litopenaeus vannamei)	Lit v 3	12
Sarcoplasmic calcium-binding protein	Tiger shrimp (Penaeus monodon)		179
	White shrimp (Litopenaeus vannamei)	Lit v 4	13

reacted to bigeye tuna collagen.[70] Furthermore, studies of allergens in red and golden snapper revealed a heat-stable high-molecular-weight protein believed to be collagen as a minor allergen in both snapper species.[164]

Fish allergy may result from allergy to protamine sulfate, a protein found in the sperm of salmon, trout, herring, and other species belonging to the families Salmonidae and Clupeidae. Protamine sulfate is a low-molecular-weight protein used as a heparin antagonist. Because of case reports of fish-allergic patients experiencing anaphylaxis after administration of protamine sulfate, extreme caution or use of alternative therapies in fish-allergic patients is advised by some experts.[41,94,158]

Allergic reactions, including anaphylaxis, have also been reported after ingestion of fish roe and caviar. In several case reports, the allergic individuals experienced a reaction after eating Beluga caviar, trout roe, or whitefish roe but had no allergy to fish or other types of roe.[58,120,156] In another case, a woman experienced an allergic reaction after consuming rainbow trout roe, and serum analysis demonstrated cross-reactivity with other types of fish roe.[120] A 118-kD protein, Hus h 1, has been identified as the culprit allergen in Beluga caviar allergy.[156] This is the hormone vitellogenin, found in fish eggs, and has also been proposed as the causative allergen in trout roe allergies.[58,156] A 33-kD alpha S1-casein–like allergen, a well-known major allergen in cow's milk, was identified as the culprit allergen in a subject who experienced anaphylactic shock after consuming kingfish caviar.[35] Although sea urchins fall into a different phylum from fish, it is worth mentioning sea urchin roe allergy, as several case reports have reported anaphylactic reactions following consumption of sea urchin roe.[75,162]

CRUSTACEAN ALLERGENS

The crustacea family includes shrimp, prawns, crabs, lobsters, crayfish, krill, and barnacles, and is a commonly reported cause of food allergy. The major allergen in crustacea has been identified as tropomyosin, an essential protein for muscle contraction found in vertebrates and invertebrates. Tropomyosin was originally identified as the major allergen in shrimp.[47,110,175] Subsequent studies have identified tropomyosin as the major allergen in other crustacean species, as well as in mollusk species. Although tropomyosins are major allergens in shellfish, arachnids (mites), and insects (cockroaches, midges), the tropomyosins of vertebrates such as cattle and chicken are considered nonallergenic, possibly because of their greater susceptibility to breakdown by digestive enzymes, as compared with shellfish, arachnid, and insect tropomyosins.[126] Invertebrate tropomyosins share a high (up to 100%) amino acid sequence homology with other invertebrates and a much lesser (50% to 60%) homology with vertebrate tropomyosins, supporting their role as the panallergen responsible for cross-reactivity across crustacea, insects, arachnids, and mollusks. This also helps explain the lack of allergenicity of vertebrate tropomyosins (see Cross-Reactivity section).[14,67,108]

Convincing evidence for the role of tropomyosin as a major shrimp allergen originated with studies by Daul and coworkers.[47] Using the brown shrimp (Penaeus aztecus) model, a 36-kD tropomyosin protein named Pen a 1 was identified and shown to react with the sera of 82% of shrimp-allergic individuals.[47] Similar tropomyosins were also identified as the major allergens in other shrimp species, including Pen i 1 in Indian white shrimp (Penaeus indicus), Met e 1 in sand shrimp (Metapenaeus ensis), and Par f 1 in Neptune rose shrimp (Parapenaeus fissurus).[110,114,175] A study of the black tiger prawn (Penaeus monodon) and king prawn (Penaeus latisulcatus) identified several major antigens in both species, with one thought to represent tropomyosin and another arginine kinase.[167] Studies of other crustacea have identified tropomyosin as the major allergen in American and Chinese spiny lobsters (Homarus americanus and Panulirus stimpsoni), designated Hom a 1 and Pan s 1, respectively, and red crab (Charybdis feriatus), named Cha f 1.[106,107] Two major IgE-binding proteins of 35- to 37-kD and 97-kD were demonstrated in extracts of lobster in pooled sera from subjects with respiratory symptoms caused by Norwegian lobster (Nephrops norvegicus).[206] The 35- to 37-kD allergen likely represented tropomyosin, but made up only 0.02% to 1% of the total protein. The 97-kD allergen made up 7% to 15% of the total protein, suggesting the presence of another major allergen in addition to tropomyosin in Norwegian lobster.

Tropomyosin proteins have also been identified as the major allergens in two species of krill, designated Eup s 1 in Euphausia superba and Eup p 1 in Euphausia pacifica, with the krill tropomyosins showing high IgE-binding epitope sequence homology to shrimp tropomyosin Pen a 1.[140] Tropomyosins were found to be the major allergens in gammaridean and caprellid amphipods.[135] Amphipods can be accidentally collected with seaweed during seaweed harvest and therefore become part of nori (dried laver) sheets used in sushi making and as condiments in other foods, raising concerns about the safety of nori sheets in individuals with shellfish allergies. Finally, tropomyosins have been identified as major allergens in two species of barnacle, Bal r 1 in the Acorn barnacle (Balanus rostratus) and Cap m 1 in the Goose barnacle (Capitulum mitella).[186] These tropomyosins shared higher sequence identity with mollusk tropomyosins compared with other crustacean tropomyosins, suggesting that barnacle tropomyosin is evolutionarily more closely related to the molluscan tropomyosin family.[186]

In addition to tropomyosins, other major allergens have been identified and characterized in crustacea, particularly shrimp. A 356–amino acid protein designated Pen m 2 has been found in tiger shrimp (P. monodon). This protein showed homology to arginine kinase from other crustacea and was found to react with serum IgE from shrimp-allergic individuals.[210] A similar 40-kD protein was isolated from white Pacific shrimp (Litopenaeus vannamei) and identified as arginine kinase.[64] Designated Lit v 2, this new protein was recognized by IgE in serum from shrimp-allergic individuals and had 96% identity to Pen m 2.[64] Arginine kinase has also been identified as a major allergen in king prawns.[167] Another new shrimp allergen, a myosin light-chain protein in white Pacific shrimp, is named Lit v 3.[12] Lit v 3 demonstrated IgE binding in 55% of white Pacific shrimp-allergic individuals.[12] A 20-kD allergen was purified from the abdominal muscle of black tiger shrimp and identified as a sarcoplasmic calcium-binding protein (SCP).[179] Of sera from 16 crustacea-allergic individuals, eight reacted to SCP, whereas 13 reacted to tropomyosin, supporting SCP as a crustacean allergen.[179] An SCP in white Pacific shrimp (L. vannamei), named Lit v 4, has been identified as a major allergen, particularly in the pediatric population.[13]

MOLLUSK ALLERGENS

Molluscan shellfish allergy has been ascribed to nearly all of the commonly consumed types of mollusks, including terrestrial and marine snails, whelk, limpet, and abalone among the gastropods; oyster, clam, scallop, mussel, and cockle among the bivalves; and squid, octopus, and cuttlefish among the cephalopods. Tropomyosins appear to be the major allergens in mollusks, and specific tropomyosin allergens have been characterized in all classes of mollusks.[191]

In the cephalopod class, the tropomyosin Tod p 1 was found to be the major allergen in the Pacific flying squid (Todarodes pacificus).[129] In studies on the common octopus (Octopus vulgaris), the tropomyosin protein Oct v 1 was designated as the major octopus allergen, including identification of several IgE-binding epitopes with sequence similarities to IgE-binding epitopes of other molluscan shellfish and crustacea.[83] Amino acid sequence analysis demonstrates 64% homology between Oct v 1 and shrimp tropomyosin Pen a 1, and 63% homology between Tod p 1 and Pen a 1.[191]

In the bivalve class of mollusks, tropomyosin allergens have been characterized in the Pacific oyster (Cassostrea gigas), razor clam (Ensis macha), mussel (Perna viridis), and scallop (Chlamys nobilis).[38,82,87] Cra g 1 and Cra g 2 were isolated from the oyster, with Cra g 1 having 76% sequence homology with mussel tropomyosin, 74% with abalone tropomyosin, and 58% with M. ensis (shrimp) tropomyosin.[82] Studies on razor clam allergens isolated three major allergens between 30 and 45 kD in size that demonstrated IgE binding with serum from a razor clam–allergic patient. One allergen, designated Ens m 1, is likely clam tropomyosin.[87] Other studies identified tropomyosin as the major allergen in the scallop, designated Chl n 1, and the mussel, named Per v 1, and confirmed their reactivity to IgE antibodies from shellfish-allergic subjects.[38]

Among the gastropods, tropomyosins have been demonstrated to be major allergens in the abalone (Hal m 2, Hal d 1, Hal r 1), turban shell (Tur c 1), common whelk (Buc u 1), and fan shell (Pin a 1).[36,38,81,99,109,119] There are at least two major allergens in the abalone, *Haliotis midae*.[119] The first, a 38-kD IgE-binding protein designated Hal m 2, is likely tropomyosin.[119] Another study identified tropomyosin as the major allergen of *Turbo cornutus*, a horned turban mollusk and popular food item in Japan. The major allergen, named Tur c 1, was found to be 35 kD in size and identified as tropomyosin, but it was found to have an IgE-binding epitope dissimilar to those in oyster and shrimp tropomyosins.[81] Studies identifying the major allergens in common whelk revealed three IgE-binding proteins. One, with a molecular weight of 40 kD, was presumed to be tropomyosin (Buc u 1).[99] A study of snail tropomyosin found that brown garden snail (*Helix aspersa*) tropomyosin, named Hel as 1, shared high homology with other edible mollusk tropomyosins (69% to 84% identity). However, tropomyosin reacted with only 18% of the sera from snail-allergic patients, suggesting that tropomyosin may be only a minor allergen in snails.[7]

In addition to tropomyosins, many studies have identified nontropomyosin allergens in numerous mollusk species, including snails, whelk, pen shell, fan shell, abalone, and limpet in the gastropod family; oyster, scallop, and razor clam in the bivalves; and squid, octopus, and cuttlefish in the cephalopod family.[191] Most of these nontropomyosin allergens remain to be identified, although research suggests that some of them may be hemocyanin, myosin heavy chain, and amylase.[191]

CROSS-REACTIVITY

Cross-reactivity may be defined as "the recognition of distinct antigens by the same IgE antibody, demonstrable by in vivo and in vitro tests, which clinically manifests as reactions caused by antigens that are homologous to different species."[205] Individuals may demonstrate sensitization by positive allergy testing to multiple species of fish and/or shellfish without demonstrating overt symptoms after consumption of that particular seafood, although the clinical significance of this observation is unclear. As discussed previously, the major allergens responsible for allergies due to fish and shellfish are parvalbumins and tropomyosins, respectively. The homology of the epitopes of these proteins across different types of seafood is thought to produce cross-reactivity.

When looking at cross-reactivity within the class of bony fish, it is estimated that approximately 50% of individuals allergic to a particular fish species will be allergic to another fish species.[195] Among crustacea, cross-reactivity appears to be even higher, with approximately 75% of individuals allergic to a crustacean species being allergic to another type of crustacea, likely because of the greater degree of similarity among tropomyosins compared with parvalbumins.[195] Both clinical and serologic cross-reactivity among fish and shellfish have been well documented. However, some studies have produced conflicting results, suggesting that the mechanisms of cross-reactivity and responsible allergens have not been completely elucidated. Furthermore, most studies have only looked at in vitro and serologic cross-reactivity, with few studies testing for actual clinical cross-reactivity.

Although some degree of cross-reactivity is common, species-specific allergies have been reported to sole, swordfish, tuna, and shrimp.[6,85,93,133] In studies on monospecific fish allergies, subjects with allergies to multiple fish species showed IgE binding to 12- to 13-kD bands (parvalbumins), whereas monosensitive subjects showed IgE binding to unique bands at 40 kD in tuna,[85] 25 kD in swordfish,[93] and 6 to 7 kD and 40 kD in tropical sole.[6] Such monospecific reactions are thought to be secondary to IgE antibodies to minor, species-specific antigens rather than to the major allergenic proteins, parvalbumins and tropomyosins.

It is noteworthy that because different antigens are responsible for causing allergic reactions to fish and shellfish, cross-reactivity between fish and shellfish does not occur. Allergy to both fish and shellfish in a single individual may occur, but it is not due to cross-reactivity. Nonetheless, in the American telephone survey previously discussed, it was estimated that 10% of individuals with a seafood allergy have an allergy to both fish and shellfish,[180] perhaps reflecting an atopic predisposition in this population.

FISH CROSS-REACTIVITY

Both serologic and clinical cross-reactivity across different fish species have been demonstrated and are hypothesized to be secondary to the major fish allergen parvalbumin. In adults with clinical sensitivity to cod, positive skin prick reactions were reported to mackerel, herring, and plaice, and sera from the same individuals demonstrated IgE binding to a protein in the 11- to 14-kD region of mackerel, herring, and plaice extracts, likely representing parvalbumin.[72] Mackerel, herring, and plaice inhibited codfish immunoassays and demonstrated at least the presence of serologic cross-reactivity to different fish species.[72] Cross-reactivity among IgE epitopes for six different fish species, including cod, tuna, salmon, perch, carp, and eel, was demonstrated by IgE-immunoblot inhibition experiments.[27] In another study, when sera from fish-allergic individuals were incubated with recombinant carp parvalbumin, IgE-reactivity to cod, tuna, and salmon was lost, suggesting the presence of common epitopes across these fish species.[189] In a study of children with codfish allergy, skin testing was most frequently positive with eel (85%), bass, dentex, sole, and tuna (55%), whereas it was least frequently seen with dogfish (10%).[48] This suggests the presence of common epitopes, but also supports the presence of significant variation within these common epitopes. Cross-reactivity across nine commonly consumed fish in Norway was studied. Cod, salmon, pollock, herring, and wolffish had the most potent cross-reactive allergens, whereas halibut, tuna, flounder, and mackerel were the least allergenic, suggesting that cross-reactivity among IgE epitopes is highest in the setting of close phylogenetic relationships between fish species.[198]

Other studies have demonstrated similar variable cross-reactivity among different fish species. In one case study, a 4-year-old boy experienced anaphylactic reactions on contact with many different types of fish, including cod, tuna, salmon, trout, and eel, among others.[115] In other studies of individuals with fish allergy confirmed by skin test and immunoassay reactivity, the majority of subjects reacted to only one type of fish, whereas a much smaller proportion of individuals reacted to two or more species of fish on oral challenge.[20,73] These studies demonstrate that while clinically significant cross-reactivity exists, it varies across allergic individuals, and that sensitization as indicated by positive allergy testing cannot always predict clinically significant allergic reactions. Similarly, up to 40% of patients sensitized to fish (positive allergy testing) do not present with symptoms on consumption of other fish species,[195] supporting the observation that subclinical sensitization is not always predictive of clinical hypersensitivity.

As a whole, the fish parvalbumins share amino acid homologies ranging from 60% to 80%, which both supports the role of parvalbumin as a major fish allergen and helps to account for the variable clinical cross-reactivity seen in fish-allergic individuals.[118] Variable clinical cross-reactivity and monospecific fish allergies can also be explained by the presence of nonparvalbumin and species-specific fish allergens. Thus, it seems that parvalbumin is a panallergen in most or all fish species, whereas some species contain additional species-specific allergens.[192]

Cross-reactivity with nonfish parvalbumins may exist. One case report documented a patient who experienced anaphylaxis following consumption of frog legs, with subsequent protein microsequencing implicating the alpha isoform of frog parvalbumin as the causative allergen.[76] Subsequent studies have demonstrated in vitro cross-reactivity between frog and fish beta-parvalbumins, suggesting that parvalbumins may be a new family of cross-reactive allergens.[77]

SHELLFISH CROSS-REACTIVITY

Cross-reactivity among shellfish is more extensive than fish cross-reactivity. It is due to the panallergen tropomyosin, which has significant sequence homology throughout crustacea and mollusks, as well as in other invertebrates, such as arachnids and insects.[160] In the American telephone survey discussed previously, 38% of individuals reported an allergy to more than one type of crustacea, 49% had an allergy to more than one type of mollusk, and 14% reported an allergy to both crustacea and mollusks.[180] Studies have demonstrated marked homology between shrimp, crab, and lobster tropomyosins, as well as likely cross-reactivity between shrimp and crab, and shrimp and lobster as evidenced by IgE inhibition assays.[106,107] In addition, studies on krill have used immunoblot to demonstrate in vitro cross-reactivity between krill, shrimp, lobster, and crab tropomyosin.[140] A study found that 81% of atopic shrimp-allergic individuals demonstrated cross-reactivity to crab, crayfish, and lobster by SPT.[46] Cross-reactivity has been demonstrated among shrimp, crab, crayfish, and lobster by positive skin testing.[203]

Studies of cross-reactivity among mollusks using laboratory analysis and SPT have demonstrated cross-reactivity among abalone, snail, white mussel, black mussel, oyster, and squid.[119] Laboratory methods have been used to demonstrate cross-reactivity of abalone, scallop, and mussel tropomyosins.[38] These studies establish subclinical cross-reactivity, but because oral challenges were not performed, the clinical significance of these observations remains to be investigated.

In addition to cross-reactivity within the crustacea and mollusk phyla, cross-reactivity between crustacea and mollusks has been widely reported. Inhibition experiments were used to demonstrate cross-reactivity between oyster and crustacean, and between squid and shrimp.[30,103] One group of researchers was able to demonstrate in vitro cross-reactivity between squid and shrimp tropomyosin allergens, but not between squid and octopus or squid and other mollusks.[129] In a study of patients with a history of shrimp anaphylaxis, 100% of patients' sera reacted with tropomyosins from 13 different crustacea and mollusks, although because oral challenges were not conducted, the clinical importance is uncertain.[108]

Shellfish cross-reactivity has been reported in circumstances of occupational seafood allergy and food-dependent, exercise-induced anaphylaxis. In one case, a seafood restaurant worker presented with occupational asthma and urticaria after contact with shrimp and scallops, with laboratory analysis confirming cross-reactivity between shrimp and scallops.[66] A 14-year-old girl with a recurrent history of oral swelling and discomfort after ingesting shrimp, crab, squid, and octopus presented with similar symptoms after scallop ingestion followed by intensive exercise.[211] Laboratory investigation demonstrated that her serum IgE reacted to multiple types of crustacean and mollusk tropomyosins, with the level of IgE-reactivity and species-specific IgE scores correlating directly with the degree of sequence homology between each seafood tropomyosin and shrimp tropomyosin. In the case of scallops, the patient's scallop-specific IgE score was not as high as for shrimp and other shellfish, consistent with the lesser homology in the amino acid sequence of scallop tropomyosin with shrimp tropomyosin and consistent with the observation that other immunologic mechanisms, specifically food-dependent, exercise-induced anaphylaxis, was necessary for clinical reactivity.[211]

SHELLFISH CROSS-REACTIVITY WITH INSECTS AND ARACHNIDS

Invertebrate tropomyosin is also found in nonmarine allergenic organisms, including cockroaches, dust mites, and other insects and arachnids, and has been demonstrated to be a major allergen in dust mites and cockroaches via inhalational exposure.[2,9,172] Between shrimp and fruit fly, shrimp and cockroach, and shrimp and house-dust mite, tropomyosin sequence identities share 87%, 90%, and 89% homologies, respectively, supporting the role of tropomyosin as an invertebrate panallergen.[160] A growing body of evidence suggests that this highly conserved tropomyosin protein is responsible for causing cross-reactivity between shell-fish and inedible arthropoda and insects.[43,57,108,122,207] For example, inhibition experiments demonstrated cross-reactivity between shrimp and nonbiting midges (chironomids).[57] In other studies, cross-reactivity was demonstrated between crustacean, chironomid, and cockroach tropomyosins.[207] Immunoblot and inhibition studies demonstrated in vitro cross-reactivity between Atlantic shrimp and German cockroaches.[43] Sera from shrimp-allergic subjects demonstrated IgE reactivity against grasshopper, cockroach, and fruit fly tropomyosins.[108] Tropomyosin IgE from shrimp-allergic individuals demonstrated cross-reactivity to mite, cockroach, and lobster tropomyosins.[14] In a study of five patients with barnacle allergy, two patients demonstrated in vitro cross-reactivity to house-dust mites, although the responsible cross-reactive allergen was not identified.[121]

Skin prick studies demonstrated cross-reactivity between shellfish and other arachnids and insects. For example, there are significant correlations between positive SPT with chironomid extract and various crustacea.[57] In a study of patients attending an allergy clinic in Hong Kong, Wu and colleagues found that 90% of patients with shellfish allergy demonstrated house-dust mite cross-reactivity by SPT.[208] In one unique study, Orthodox Jews with dust mite/cockroach hypersensitivity were found to have positive SPTs and IgE reactivity to shrimp. Because they had never been exposed to shellfish due to religious dietary prohibitions, it is hypothesized that sensitization to shrimp tropomyosin occurred via cross-reactivity to house-dust mite or cockroach tropomyosin.[59]

The previously discussed studies support the presence of in vitro and serologic cross-reactivity between shellfish and nonmarine allergenic organisms. Accumulating data suggest that this cross-reactivity also has important clinical implications. In one study, a series of individuals developed both laboratory and clinical evidence of shrimp allergy over the course of immunotherapy for house-dust mite allergy, suggesting that dust mite allergen served as the sensitizing agent in causing the shrimp allergy.[202] In a series of patients with asthma induced by snail consumption, house-dust mite sensitization was likely the causal event, although tropomyosin was thought to play only a minor role as a cross-reactive allergen.[201] Clinical cross-reactivity was demonstrated in a study in which asthmatic subjects sensitized to house-dust mite showed laboratory and clinical allergy to limpets.[15]

FUTURE DIRECTIONS

The current standard of care for managing seafood allergies is avoidance diets and provision of a self-injectable epinephrine device. Much research is under way to develop new strategies for treating and preventing seafood allergies. Some of the therapeutic modalities currently under investigation include sublingual and oral immunotherapy, anti-IgE therapy, peptide immunotherapy, traditional Chinese medicine, DNA immunization, and development of hypoallergenic seafood for human consumption.[28,55]

Although traditional allergen-specific immunotherapy was discovered nearly a century ago and has been used successfully in the treatment of peanut allergy, it is currently not recommended because of an unacceptably high incidence of dangerous systemic allergic reactions during the treatment course.[144,150] Additionally, there appears to be a potential for developing hypersensitivity to cross-reacting food allergens, such as shrimp, as described in subjects undergoing house-dust mite immunotherapy.[202] Given the high incidence of adverse reactions using traditional immunotherapy, alternatives are currently under investigation and promising new methods are being developed. For example, sublingual immunotherapy, originally developed to treat allergic rhinoconjunctivitis and asthma, was used successfully and safely to treat hazelnut food allergy in hazelnut-allergic patients.[56] Studies looking at the efficacy of specific oral tolerance induction or oral immunotherapy in inducing desensitization to food allergens have yielded promising results, although the long-term effects of such therapy have not been rigorously investigated.[26,28,124,147,155] In one study including patients with fish allergy, a standardized oral immunotherapy protocol induced desensitization, as evidenced by conversion from skin test positive to skin test negative, following treatment in 78% of subjects who completed the oral immunotherapy protocol.[155]

Another promising modality currently in clinical trials is recombinant humanized monoclonal anti-IgE antibodies. These IgG antibodies directed against the IgE molecule bind to freely circulating IgE, creating antigen-antibody complexes that are then cleared from the circulation. Use of anti-IgE appears to decrease levels of circulating free IgE, inhibit early- and late-phase responses to allergens, suppress inflammation, and improve control of allergic diseases.[55,127] A clinical trial using anti-IgE in the treatment of peanut allergy found that a large number of patients had a significant decrease in clinical symptoms in response to peanut challenge following treatment.[111]

Peptide immunotherapy is a therapy currently under investigation that uses peptide fragments containing reactive epitopes rather than the complete protein allergen, the hypothesis being that these peptide fragments are immunogenic but are theoretically unable to cross-link IgE molecules, activate mast cells, and cause clinical allergic symptoms.[25,28] Use of these peptide fragments for immunotherapy would thus render T cells unresponsive to subsequent allergen exposure without causing dangerous systemic allergic reactions during the course of therapy. Thus far, clinical studies using peptide immunotherapy for bee venom sensitivity and cat allergy have demonstrated promising results, with subjects experiencing a significant decrease in allergic symptoms after allergen exposure following therapy.[25,137,148,149,190] Studies using peanut allergen peptides suggest that peptide immunotherapy may have a future role in treatment of food allergies, including seafood allergy.[65,79]

Traditional Chinese medicine and use of herbal remedies have gained attention as potential modalities for treating allergic diseases, including food allergies. In studies on peanut allergy using murine models, the food allergy herbal formula-1 and the simplified food allergy herbal formula-2 significantly reduced IgE levels and blocked anaphylactic reactions to peanuts for up to 5 weeks following therapy.[112,184] Although Chinese herbal remedies hold promise and have shown efficacy in murine models, human studies are only currently under way, and the active ingredients and mechanism of action of these remedies remain to be delineated.[181]

A new approach for treatment of food allergy is DNA immunization.[183] With this strategy, a plasmid DNA (pDNA) vector encoding a specific food allergenic protein would be injected subcutaneously or delivered orally. The pDNA sequence would be taken up by APCs, the DNA transcribed and translated, and the allergenic protein then presented on the surface of the APC as an endogenously produced protein. This endogenous protein would induce a Th1 response (rather than Th2 as occurs in allergic disease) with suppression of allergen-specific IgE production, thus producing desensitization to the specific food allergen.[28,166] Although promising in murine models, allergen DNA immunization is likely years away from practical use.

Genetic alteration of epitopes on food allergens to suppress their allergenicity is currently under investigation as a method for producing safer allergens for immunotherapy. Hypoallergenic foods could be developed for consumption by individuals with food allergies. For example, studies on shrimp tropomyosin (Pen a 1) have demonstrated that substitution of critical amino acids in Pen a 1 epitopes results in significant reduction of IgE binding while still preserving immunogenicity.[102] Such a mutated molecule could be used safely and effectively for immunotherapy without the risk of allergic reaction during treatment, or the mutant could be incorporated into the genome to create a hypoallergenic organism.[102] A recombinant hypoallergenic carp parvalbumin mutant has been constructed that has 95% reduced IgE reactivity and diminished allergenicity as demonstrated by in vitro assays and in vivo SPT, but retains immunogenicity, making it a candidate for immunotherapy.[187] Studies using genetic transformation technology to modify the allergic structure in shrimp are under way,[37,159] with the eventual goal of producing nonallergenic transgenic seafood that is safe for consumption by individuals with seafood allergy.

REFERENCES

Complete references used in this text are available online at expertconsult.inkling.com.

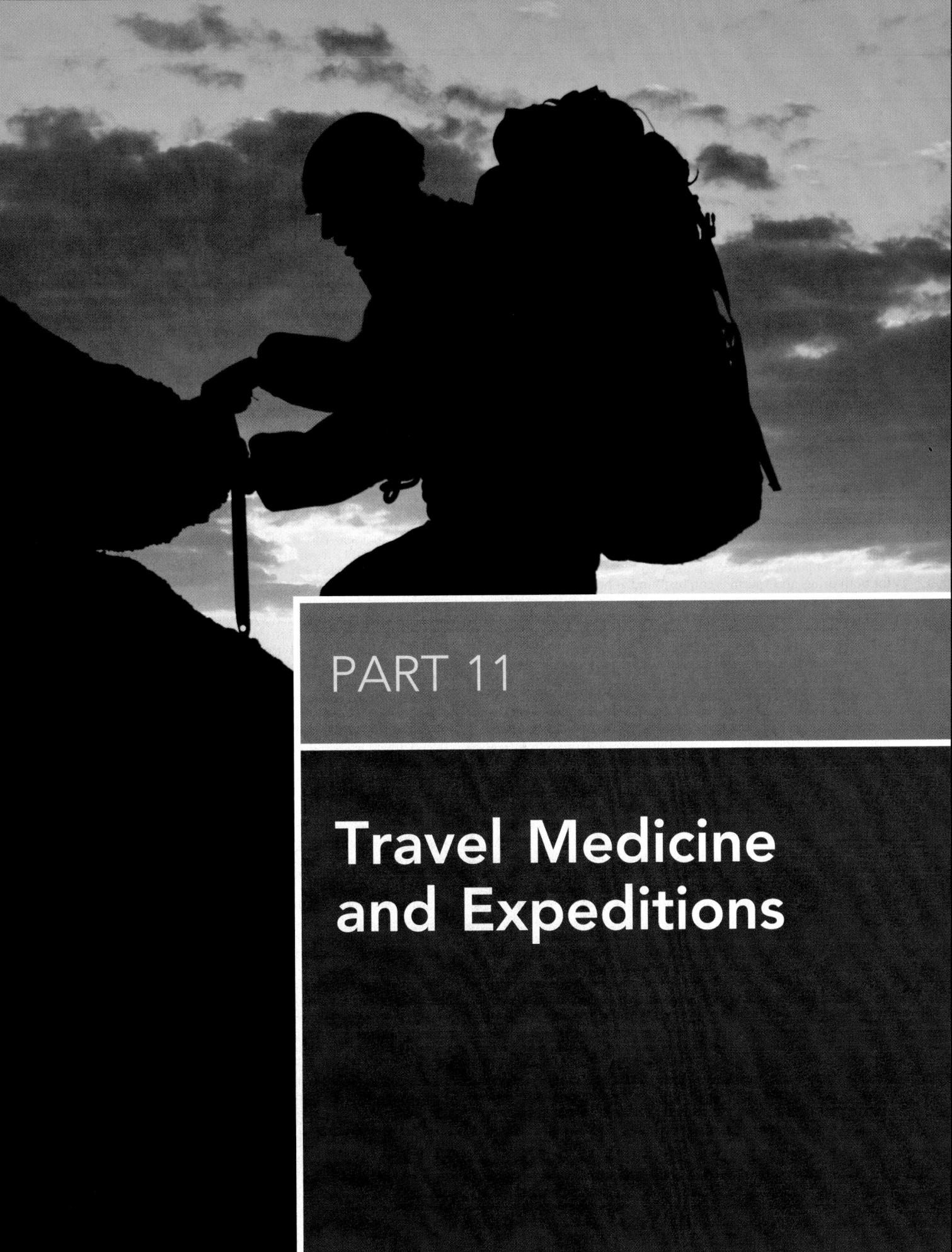

PART 11

Travel Medicine and Expeditions

International travelers, particularly those participating in wilderness and outdoors activities, have unique health needs based largely on their underlying health and specific geographic destination.[64] Exposure to unfamiliar cultures, poor sanitation, and harsh environments may have a deleterious effect on health and interfere with the purpose and enjoyment of the trip.

The multidisciplinary specialty of travel medicine shares principles with the fields of public health, infectious diseases, tropical medicine, environmental medicine, and wilderness medicine. Travel medicine integrates features of these disciplines with geographic and chronologic data to formulate an approach to health risk assessment for a given journey.[67]

SOURCES OF INFORMATION

As a basic introduction to travel medicine, this chapter focuses on advice for the healthy adult traveler from the United States. Closely related topics are covered extensively in other chapters. Children and unhealthy travelers are beyond the scope of this chapter. Excellent information about travel medicine–related vaccines for children has been published,[72,88] and reference tables for both drugs and vaccines can be found at http://www.istm.org. A published review on the approach to travelers with underlying medical conditions is available in the *International Journal of Antimicrobial Agents*.[44]

The U.S. Centers for Disease Control and Prevention (CDC) publishes several authoritative sources of information on travel medicine. *Health Information for International Travel,* commonly called the "Yellow Book," is updated annually. Two other periodicals, the weekly *Morbidity and Mortality Weekly Report* (or *MMWR*) and *Summary of Health Information for International Travel* (the "Blue Sheet," published biweekly), provide updated information on the status of immunization recommendations, worldwide disease outbreaks, and changes in health conditions.

A reliable way to obtain current travel health information, including vaccine requirements, malaria chemoprophylaxis, and disease outbreaks for various regions of the world, is to consult the CDC Database of Health Information for International Travel website (http://www.cdc.gov/travel/yb/index.htm). For nonmedical information of interest to the traveler, the U.S. Department of State can be accessed at http://travel.state.gov/. (See Resources for Travel Medicine Information, later.)

If an extended stay in a given country is planned, American travelers should register with the U.S. Smart Traveler Enrollment Program (STEP) before arriving in the foreign country. This will allow the traveler to receive important information from the embassy regarding safety conditions in the destination country, such as travel warnings and severe weather updates. It will also allow the U.S. embassy, family, and friends to contact a traveler in the event of an emergency. American travelers abroad who experience any emergency should contact the nearest U.S. consulate or embassy or call the U.S. Department of State, which can help provide additional assistance, information regarding logistics, and emergency planning.

Several months before departure, travelers should ascertain whether their health insurance policies cover the costs of hospitalization, treatment, and emergency evacuation back to the United States for illness or injuries occurring abroad. Travelers should obtain such a policy, particularly if their travel involves remote locations where medical care is marginal or nonexistent.

For example, when trekking in the Himalayas, insurance that covers helicopter rescue evacuation is important. Air ambulance repatriation back to the United States for life-threatening emergencies may require a separate insurance policy. Depending on the insurer, chronic medical conditions may be excluded or covered only if they are certified to be under control for a period of time before departure. Elderly travelers may find it more difficult to obtain this type of medical insurance. Medicare generally only covers health care expenses arising in the United States and its territories. Some credit card services provide worldwide medical referrals and arrangements for emergency transportation for their cardholders, but do not actually cover the costs incurred. What the traveler needs is a short-term health insurance policy that specifically covers medical expenses and medical evacuation during foreign travel.

TRAVEL HEALTH RISK ASSESSMENT

Pretravel medical preparation should be individualized through review of the (1) geographic destination, duration, and purpose of the trip; (2) style of travel, including information about sanitation and environmental hazards; (3) underlying health of the traveler; and (4) available access to medical care during the trip (Box 79-1). Risk assessments should also include special considerations for environmental exposures, such as whether the traveler might be exposed to extreme weather conditions, high altitude, or aquatic activities.

In addition, discussions on immunizations, prevention of malaria, self-treatment of traveler's diarrhea, and prevention and treatment of common ailments, such as jet lag, motion sickness, sun exposure, altitude illness, and insect and animal bites, should be reviewed with the traveler when these issues are applicable. Some attention, at least in the form of patient education, should be given to address personal safety, sexually transmitted diseases, prevention of vehicular trauma, and emergency medical evacuation.

PRETRAVEL PREPARATIONS

Trips with multiple destinations and travel lasting longer than a few weeks increase the complexity of pretravel medical preparation. Extensive travel often mandates carrying travel medical kits that are more extensive, given that a traveler is more likely to become ill as time and number of destinations increase. Travelers who camp or live in small villages often have greater exposure to vectors of disease than do those staying in urban, air-conditioned hotels or resorts. If accommodations are deemed to be high risk for exposure to disease vectors, travelers should plan to take appropriate precautions. For example, portable bed nets and permethrin-containing sprays help protect against mosquitoes and other biting insects.

Teachers, students, missionaries, relief workers, agricultural consultants, field biologists, and adventure travelers are often considered high risk for exposure to endemic infectious diseases, such as hepatitis B, tuberculosis, and meningitis; insect-borne diseases, such as malaria, yellow fever, leishmaniasis, filariasis, plague, and typhus; and diseases associated with animal exposures, such as rabies, leptospirosis, and anthrax.

All travelers should be cautioned about blood-borne infections, such as those contracted through using contaminated needles, syringes, and other medical or dental devices or during

BOX 79-1 History for Travel Risk Assessment

Travel Details

Geographic itinerary
    Sequence of countries visited
    Urban versus rural travel
Duration and season of travel
Style of travel and accommodations
    Airline and resort hotel versus bus and camping
Reason for travel and planned activities
    Packaged tour versus business versus adventure
Access to competent medical care during travel

General and Special Personal Health Issues

General Health Status

Age and weight
Pregnant or lactating
History of routine immunizations
Allergies to drugs and vaccines
Medications taken on a regular basis

Special Medical Issues

History of travel immunizations
Impaired immunity from disease or treatment
- Human immunodeficiency virus (HIV)
- Transplantation
- Malignancy and its treatment
- Immunoglobulin A (IgA) deficiency
- Asplenia
- Use of immunocompromising drugs (e.g., corticosteroids)
Underlying medical or physical conditions
- Diabetes mellitus
- End-stage renal disease requiring dialysis
- Chronic obstructive pulmonary disease requiring oxygen therapy
- Heart disease, including recent myocardial infarction
- Gastrointestinal diseases, including cirrhosis
- Disability requiring special transport or accommodations

emergency medical or dental care, injections, tattoos, and transfusions. Travelers should be cautioned about sexually transmitted infections contracted during unprotected sexual encounters with new partners, especially with commercial sex workers. Gonorrhea and *Chlamydia* infection, common in the industrialized world, have worldwide distribution, including remote locations. Human immunodeficiency virus (HIV) infection, syphilis, chancroid, and lymphogranuloma venereum are more prevalent in the developing world.

Most international travelers should begin pretravel medical preparations 4 to 6 weeks before the date of departure so that multidose immunization schedules can be completed, protective immunity developed, and necessary medications and special supplies obtained. Medical preparations for an international trip that includes many tourist destinations are often uncomplicated for people in good health. However, advance planning and consultation with a travel medicine expert is recommended for people with allergies, special health needs (e.g., pregnancy, infancy, advanced age, disabilities), or chronic underlying health conditions (e.g., cardiovascular or respiratory disease, compromised immune system, diabetes, psychiatric disorder, renal failure, organ transplant, seizure disorder).

People who participate in global relief operations in regions affected by political unrest, war, terrorist activity, famine, or natural disaster should ideally prepare broadly for travel to any part of the world well in advance of possible deployment. These people often face unique exposures to diseases, in part because of impaired infrastructure at the destination. Health care workers traveling to West Africa to assist in caring for patients, such as those with Ebola virus disease, must plan to arrive with sufficient personal protective equipment to practice appropriate infection control precautions. Too frequently, volunteers anxious to help in the aftermath of a disaster, leave their home country poorly prepared to protect their own health.

Vaccine-preventable diseases (e.g., diphtheria, measles, polio, hepatitis, typhoid fever) and exotic infectious diseases (e.g., malaria, schistosomiasis, leishmaniasis, trichinosis) are important.[26,56] However, cardiovascular diseases and trauma account for more morbidity and mortality among American travelers and expatriates than do infectious diseases. This underscores the importance of not only addressing travel-specific health needs, but also seriously considering preparations to handle chronic illnesses.

Accident prevention is essential because injuries are the leading cause of preventable death among travelers. Road traffic accidents account for the majority of injury-related deaths.[122,123] If travelers consider driving an automobile while abroad, they must be aware of the possible differences in vehicle safety features, road conditions, and behavior of local drivers. Driving in even a developed country can be hazardous when signs cannot be read or the traffic patterns are reversed. If the traveler rides bicycles, mopeds, or motorcycles, he or she should wear a helmet. The traveler should avoid driving any vehicle at night and should never drink alcohol and drive. In addition to road traffic accidents, important causes of travel-related morbidity are injuries from falls, drowning, animal bites, fires, and poisonings.

Travelers should remain vigilant at all times to help guarantee personal safety. Even if statistical numbers are available for the incidence of certain illnesses or accidents during travel, it may be impossible to determine if the risk is high or low, because this may depend on the personal perception of the traveler.[56] People should consciously avoid risky situations that could lead to traumatic events such as sexual assault or kidnapping. Women traveling alone or under difficult circumstances must consider the possibility of sexual assault and plan to carry emergency contraception.[96] Up-to-date information on personal risk at specific destinations can be obtained from the U.S. Department of State website (http://www.state.gov).

Finally, travel advisers need to understand that culture shock generated by travel to remote areas might lead to psychological breakdown, especially if a person is traveling alone or with a person who has a psychiatric disorder.[56] Importantly, if travelers (before the trip) are made aware of the potential differences or absence of medical resources in a country, they may be more accepting, and they or their caregivers might cope more easily with the psychological impact of a medical emergency.

HAZARDS OF AIR TRAVEL

Changes in barometric pressure cause the majority of health-related problems during air travel. Although the cabin is pressurized to an altitude of approximately 1524 m (5000 feet), pilots can be authorized to climb to avoid threatening weather, resulting in an increase in cabin altitude to 2438 m (8000 feet). At this altitude, everyone is mildly hypoxic; however, a patient with underlying lung disease, such as chronic obstructive pulmonary disease (COPD), can become dangerously hypoxic. Pretravel assessments and trial exposures to lower fraction of inspired oxygen can help determine whether supplemental oxygen might be necessary during a flight. If that is the case, planning is needed because airlines often need several days to arrange supplemental O_2, and not all flights offer it. After a myocardial infarction, travelers are advised not to travel for at least 3 weeks.[44,101] Flying less than 12 to 18 hours after scuba diving may increase the risk of decompression sickness.[56]

Transmission of respiratory pathogens, such as *Mycobacterium tuberculosis*, is possible. However, because of the use of high-efficiency particulate air (HEPA) filters in passenger aircraft, the immediate risk is largely to travelers seated close to an infected person. Arthropods, such as mosquitoes, can transmit diseases such as malaria, dengue fever, and chikungunya virus infection during passenger airline travel, but such concerns are mitigated by disinfection practices followed by many airlines traveling in high-risk locations. Modern passenger airplanes are exposed to measurable cosmic radiation, which has been shown to pose a negligible risk to occasional travelers, but a potential risk to long-haul pilots and crew.[25]

JET LAG

Symptoms of fatigue, impaired concentration, performance, and sleep may occur when normal circadian rhythm is disrupted by travel across multiple (usually five or more) time zones.[25,128] In most people, more symptoms occur, and a longer period of adaptation is required, following eastward travel than with westward travel. The typical adjustment time is 1 day per hour of time zone change without intervention. Short-acting hypnotic medication, timed exposure to bright light, and melatonin have been used to shorten the period of adjustment.[25,128]

To avoid possible periods of amnesia associated with hypnotic agents,[85] these are best avoided during flight and should only be used when the traveler can schedule uninterrupted sleep during the time the drug is active. Any hypnotic, including benzodiazepines and the nonbenzodiazepine drugs zolpidem, zaleplon, and eszopiclone, should be used in the lowest effective dose. Such medications should probably be tried before travel to ensure tolerance. If desired, hypnotics should be taken for the first several nights after arrival in the new time zone and after return to the original time zone. Alcohol ingestion should be avoided because it interferes with rapid eye movement (REM) sleep.

Exposure to bright light on arrival to a new destination helps to "reset" the timing of melatonin production because the light suppresses melatonin production by the pineal gland. The specific recommendation is to seek exposure to bright sunlight in the evening after westward travel and in the morning after eastward travel. The recommendations become more complicated when travel exceeds eight time zones. Exposure too early to light might actually inhibit adaptation.[25,128]

To facilitate adaptation, melatonin may be taken at the new bedtime after eastward travel (and in the second half of the night after westward travel) in a dose as low as 0.5 mg until one becomes adapted to the new time.[57,107] In the United States, melatonin is a dietary supplement and may be contaminated with impurities, so its potency is not guaranteed.[103]

Based on a review of jet lag,[107] a summary of recommendations follows, depending on whether a person is traveling westward or eastward.

Before Travel

1. For a westward journey, shift the timing of sleep to 1 to 2 hours later for a few days before the trip; seek exposure to bright light in the evening.
2. For traveling eastward, shift the timing of sleep to 1 to 2 hours earlier for a few days before the trip; seek exposure to bright light in the morning.
3. Try to get an adequate amount of sleep.

In Flight

1. Try to be comfortable.
2. Drink plenty of water to stay hydrated.
3. Do not drink caffeine if you want to sleep.
4. Consider a short-acting sleep medication. Do not take sleep medication combined with alcohol, or if there is a risk for deep vein thrombosis.

On Arrival

1. Expect to have trouble sleeping until you become adjusted to local time.
2. If you are sleep deprived, take a nap after arrival. Continue to take daytime naps if you are sleepy, but keep them as short as possible to avoid ruining nighttime sleep.
3. Consider using sleep medication at bedtime for a few nights until you are adjusted to local time.
4. Melatonin may be taken at the new bedtime after eastward travel (and in the second half of the night after westward travel) in a dose as low as 0.5 mg until one becomes adapted to the new time.
5. Seek exposure to bright light in the evening if traveling westward. Seek exposure to bright light in the morning if traveling eastward.
   a. However, after westward travel across more than eight time zones, for the first 2 days after arrival, avoid bright light for 2 to 3 hours before dusk. Starting on the third day, seek exposure to bright light in the evening.
   b. After eastward travel exceeding eight time zones, for the first 2 days after arrival, avoid bright light for the first 2 to 3 hours after dawn, then starting on the third day, seek exposure to bright light in the morning.
6. Avoid caffeine after midday because it may interfere with sleep at night.

DEEP VEIN THROMBOSIS

Deep vein thrombosis (DVT) and its associated risk for pulmonary embolism are recognized as potential complications of flights that last for 6 or more hours.[111,112] DVT occurs more often in persons using oral contraceptives and in those with cardiovascular risk factors, active malignancy, or recent surgery.[20,51,79,81] Pulmonary embolism occurs in only 1 to 2 travelers per 1 million long-haul flights.[68] On the other hand, up to 10% of travelers who were not using support stockings sustained asymptomatic DVT in the calf after a flight of 8 hours or longer.[112]

As safety permits during long-haul flights, travelers should be encouraged to move frequently about the cabin. If this is not possible, isometric exercise is recommended. Using below-the-knee support stockings is encouraged; low-molecular-weight heparin may be used in high-risk travelers under the guidance of the traveler's primary care physician. Aspirin is not recommended because it does not appear to reduce the risk of DVT.[32]

IMMUNIZATIONS FOR TRAVEL

Immunizations may be divided into three categories: required, recommended, and routine. Table 79-1 details vaccine schedules and booster intervals for adult travelers who are assumed to have received the primary series of routine vaccines as children.[22,87,99] Vaccinations for traveling children can be found in tables referenced in Resources for Travel Medicine Information (see later). The international traveler should have all current immunizations recorded in a World Health Organization (WHO) International Certificate of Vaccination. This yellow document is recognized

---

TABLE 79-1 Vaccines and Immunoglobulin for Adult Travelers Who Completed Childhood Immunizations

Vaccine	Route (Dose)	Schedule	Side Effects, Precautions, and Contraindications*	Comments
Hepatitis A (Havrix and Vaqta)	IM (1.0 mL)	Primary: 2 doses Additional booster doses: not recommended	Local reactions: <56% Fever: <5% Headache: 16%	Prevaccine hepatitis A serology may be cost-effective for some travelers (see text).
Hepatitis B (Recombivax HB and Engerix-B)	IM (adult and pediatric formulations)	Primary: 1 dose at 0, 1, and 6 months Booster: not routinely recommended Accelerated schedules (see text)	Local reaction: 3%-29% Fever: 1%-6%	

TABLE 79-1 Vaccines and Immunoglobulin for Adult Travelers Who Completed Childhood Immunizations—cont'd

Vaccine	Route (Dose)	Schedule	Side Effects, Precautions, and Contraindications*	Comments
Hepatitis A and B antigens combined (Twinrix)	IM (1.0 mL)	Primary: 1 dose at 0, 1, and 6 months Booster: not routinely recommended Accelerated schedules (see text)	Local reactions: approximately 56% Systemic reactions: similar to single-antigen products	Give at least 2 doses of vaccine before departure to provide protection against hepatitis A.
Influenza	IM (0.5 mL)	One dose of current vaccine annually	Local reactions: <33% Systemic reactions: occasional Allergic reaction: rare Avoid in those with history of anaphylaxis to eggs.	
Influenza (FluMist)	Intranasal (0.5 mL)	Primary: 1 dose per season	Mild upper respiratory tract symptoms: occasional Avoid in those with history of anaphylaxis to eggs, Guillain-Barré syndrome, or immunosuppression.	Approved for persons 5 to 49 years old
Japanese B encephalitis (Ixiaro)	IM (0.5 mL) 2 months to 3 years: 0.25 mL >3 years: 0.5 mL	Primary: 1 dose at 0 and 28 days Booster: >1 year following primary series, booster if continued risk		Ixiaro is a Vero cell culture–derived formulation. A single booster >1 year after completion of primary series if ongoing risk
Measles (monovalent or combined with rubella and mumps, MMR)	SC (0.5 mL)	Primary: 2 doses separated by at least 1 year Booster: none (Unless born prior to 1956; then see CDC recommendation.)	Fever, 5-21 days after vaccination: 5%-15% Transient rash: 5% Local reaction among those who received killed vaccine (1963-1967): 4%-55% Severe allergic reactions, CNS complications, thrombocytopenia (MMR): rare Avoid in pregnancy, immunocompromised hosts, and those with history of anaphylaxis to eggs or neomycin.	Do not give immune globulin within 3 months of vaccine dose. If MMR and yellow fever vaccine are not given simultaneously, separate by 28 days or longer.
Meningococcal polysaccharide-protein conjugate quadrivalent vaccine (Menactra)	IM (0.5 mL)	Primary: single dose Booster: not recommended for routine use; every 5 years recommended for ongoing risk	Local reactions: 10%-60% Systemic reactions: occasional fever, headache, and malaise	Replaces quadrivalent polysaccharide vaccine (Menomune)
Mumps	SC (0.5 mL)	Primary: 1 dose (usually as MMR) Booster: none	Mild allergic reactions: uncommon Parotitis: rare Avoid in pregnancy, immunocompromised hosts, and those with history of anaphylaxis to eggs or neomycin.	Do not give immune globulin within 3 months of vaccine dose. If MMR and yellow fever vaccine are not given simultaneously, separate by 28 days or longer.
Pneumococcal polysaccharide Conjugate vaccine (PCV 13)	SC or IM (0.5 mL)	Primary: single dose at age 65 or age 60 if high risk Booster: high-risk patients after 5 years from initial dose	Mild local reactions: approximately 50% Systemic symptoms: <1% Arthus-like reaction with booster doses occurs. Avoid in those with moderate to severe acute illness.	Opportunity to update routine vaccination in older travelers
Poliomyelitis	SC or IM (0.5 mL)	Booster: one adult dose	Local reactions: occasional	Additional boosters not recommended. Access CDC or WHO databases for current regions with polio transmission.

Continued

Vaccine	Route (Dose)	Schedule	Side Effects, Precautions, and Contraindications*	Comments
Rabies Human diploid cell vaccine (HDCV); purified chick embryo cell (PCEC); rabies vaccine adsorbed (RVA)	IM (1.0 mL)	Preexposure: 1 dose at 0, 7, and 21 or 28 days Booster doses depend on ongoing risk and results of serology (see text)	Mild local or systemic reactions: occasional Immune complex–like reactions after booster dose of HDCV (2-21 days after vaccination): 6%	Target children in endemic areas who might not tell parents about bites.
Rubella	SC (0.5 mL)	Primary: 1 dose (usually as MMR) Booster: none	Transient arthralgias in adult women beginning 3-25 days after vaccination: up to 25% Arthritis: <2% Avoid in pregnancy, immunocompromised hosts, and those with history of anaphylaxis to neomycin.	Do not give immune globulin within 3 months of vaccine dose. If MMR and yellow fever vaccine are not given simultaneously, separate by 28 days or longer.
Tetanus- diphtheria (Td)	IM (0.5 mL)	Booster dose every 10 years	Local reactions: common Systemic symptoms: occasional Anaphylaxis: rare Arthus-like reactions possible after multiple previous boosters Avoid if Guillain-Barré syndrome occurs 6 weeks or earlier after previous dose.	Consider booster at 5 years for travelers to remote areas or regions without adequate health care facilities when sustaining punctures or other significant wounds is possible.
Tetanus-diphtheria with acellular pertussis (Tdap)	IM (0.5 mL)	One-time dose (wait at least 2 years since last Td), then resume Td every 10 years.	Similar to Td	Do not confuse Tdap with the pediatric formulation (TDaP), which can cause adverse reactions in adults.
Typhoid Ty21a	Oral capsules	Primary: 1 capsule every other day for 4 doses Booster: every 5 years if ongoing risk	Gastrointestinal upset or rash: infrequent Avoid in pregnancy and in persons with febrile illness, taking antibiotics, or in immunocompromised state.	Refrigerate capsules. If already taking mefloquine, separate doses by 24 hours.
Typhoid Vi polysaccharide	IM (0.5 mL)	Primary: single dose Booster: every 2 years if ongoing risk	Local reaction: 7% Headache: 16% Fever: <1%	
Varicella	SC (0.5 mL)	Primary: 2 doses at 4-week interval or longer. No booster	Local reactions: 20% Fever: 15% Localized or mild systemic varicella rash: 6% Avoid in immunocompromised hosts, if severe allergic reactions to gelatin or neomycin, or if serum immune globulin within 5 months.	Rare transmission of vaccine strain to susceptible hosts; therefore, avoid if close contacts are immunosuppressed.
Varicella-zoster virus (VZV) vaccine	SC (0.5 mL)	One dose		Recommended for all adults over 60 years old, including those with previous history of zoster Decreases the incidence of postherpetic neuralgia
Yellow fever	SC (0.5 mL)	Primary: single dose Booster: every 10 years	Mild headache, myalgia, fever (5-10 days after vaccination): 25% Immediate hypersensitivity: rare Viscerotropic syndrome or neurotropic disease: rare (see text) Avoid if allergic to eggs. Contraindicated in immunocompromised hosts	If person can eat eggs without a reaction, person can take vaccine.

Modified from information in Centers for Disease Control and Prevention (CDC): *Health information for international travel*, 2014 (http://wwwnc.cdc.gov/travel/page/yellowbook-home-2014); and Hill DR, Ericsson CD, Pearson RD et al: Guidelines for the practice of travel medicine, *Clin Infect Dis* 43:1499, 2006.

IM, Intramuscularly; *SC*, subcutaneously.

*Moderate or severe acute illness with or without fever or a serious reaction to a previous dose is a contraindication to all vaccines.

BOX 79-2 Vaccination in HIV-Positive Adults

Generally Avoid
- Varicella-zoster virus (VZV) vaccine
- Bacille Calmette-Guérin (BCG) vaccine
- Oral polio vaccine
- Oral typhoid vaccine

Avoid if CD4+ Cells <200
- Yellow fever vaccine
- Measles vaccine

Give Routinely
- Tetanus/diphtheria (or Tdap) vaccine
- Hepatitis B vaccine
- *Streptococcus pneumoniae* vaccine
- *Haemophilus influenzae* type b (Hib) vaccine
- Influenza vaccine, yearly
- Hepatitis A vaccine

Give if Indicated for Travel
- Typhoid Vi vaccine
- Meningococcal vaccine
- Polio, IPV vaccine
- Rabies vaccine
- Japanese encephalitis
- Tick-borne encephalitis (JE) vaccine

worldwide and has a dedicated page for documentation of the yellow fever vaccine. Recent copies of the document do not contain a separate page for the cholera vaccine validation because the WHO officially removed cholera vaccination from the International Health Regulations in 1973. If given, cholera vaccination can be recorded in the space provided for "Other Vaccinations" in the newer booklets.

Contraindications to vaccinations are often overstated. In general, live-virus vaccines and attenuated bacterial vaccines are contraindicated during pregnancy and in persons with impaired immune systems due to medical conditions (e.g., HIV, asplenia, congenital immune deficiencies) or medical therapy (e.g., corticosteroids, cancer chemotherapy, radiation therapy, or immune suppression therapy in the organ transplant patient). Comprehensive review of contraindications to immunizations by underlying host deficiency is beyond the scope of this chapter; reviews are available.[44] Box 79-2 outlines vaccination practices for the patient with HIV, which is a reasonable approach to vaccination in most immunocompromised hosts, in whom live-virus and live-attenuated bacterial vaccines should generally be avoided.

REQUIRED TRAVEL VACCINES

"Required" immunizations are not only those regulated by WHO, but also those required by some countries. For example, yellow fever vaccine may be required for entry into some WHO member countries, whereas smallpox and cholera vaccinations are no longer required for international travel according to WHO regulations. However, some countries continue to "require" cholera vaccination in practice. Meningococcal vaccine is not required by WHO but is by certain countries; for example, Saudi Arabia requires meningococcal vaccination for persons arriving for the Hajj or Umrah pilgrimages.

Yellow Fever Vaccine

Yellow fever (YF) is a viral infection transmitted by mosquitoes in equatorial South America and Africa (Figure 79-1). YF vaccine is a live-attenuated viral vaccine that is highly protective.[83,131] It is given as a single dose for primary immunization; the booster interval is 10 years. According to WHO, a single dose of the vaccine is sufficient to confer lifelong immunity, but more data are needed documenting duration of immunity after vaccination. Because of age-related risk of encephalitis after immunization, most authorities agree that the YF vaccine is contraindicated in infants less than 6 months of age, and immunization should usually be delayed until the infant is 9 months or older.[33] The vaccine is generally not recommended for persons older than 60

years, immunocompromised, or pregnant. If the pregnant traveler cannot avoid or postpone travel to a highly endemic area, risk of the disease should be greater than the theoretical risk of adverse effects from the vaccine. A small case series demonstrated significant increase in relapse rates among travelers with multiple sclerosis (MS) who received YF vaccine, so unless there is a significant risk for YF, MS patients should not receive the vaccine.[45]

Three types of reactions to YF vaccine have been described. The most common is a general hypersensitivity or anaphylactic reaction to components of the vaccine. The vaccine includes proteins from chickens and eggs, because the virus is cultured in eggs. The vaccine is therefore contraindicated in persons with a history of anaphylactic reaction to chickens or eggs. If able to eat eggs without a reaction, the person can receive YF vaccine.

Vaccine-associated neurologic disease (YEL-AND) manifests as several distinct neurologic syndromes. These syndromes are caused either by virus entering the central nervous system (CNS) and causing infection, thereby resulting in neurotropic disease (i.e., meningoencephalitis), or by autoimmune damage to neuronal tissues causing syndromes such as Guillain-Barré or acute disseminated encephalomyelitis (ADEM).[116]

Vaccine-associated viscerotropic disease (YEL-AVD) has been reported in a small number of first-time recipients of YF vaccine.[29,116] This is a severe reaction that mimics fulminant YF infection, resulting in multiorgan failure and death. The disease is thought to be infection by the attenuated vaccine strain facilitated by an altered host response, rather than by a change in virulence of the vaccine strain. Persons who have successfully received a first dose of YF vaccine are unlikely to be at risk with a booster dose if they have remained immunocompetent hosts. Two potential risk factors for YEL-AVD are previous thymectomy and older age. Thymectomy was documented in four of the first 23 cases, but as of 2010 had not been documented in any subsequent case. The incidence of YEL-AVD in persons older than 60 is estimated at 1.4 to 1.8 cases per 100,000 doses, which is significantly higher than the estimated 0.3 to 0.4 cases per 100,000 doses in the general population.[116] Despite these two purported risks, the small number of cases makes accurate risk factor assessment difficult.[10,116]

Although complications from YF vaccine are rare, the potential lethality of YEL-AVD prompts careful risk assessment, especially when considering first-time vaccination in older travelers. Some countries may be listed as endemic for YF, but certain locations within the country may pose no risk. If a person for whom the vaccine is contraindicated (or not advised because the person is not truly at risk) must travel to a country where a YF vaccine is required for entry, then according to WHO regulations, a signed statement indicating that the YF vaccine could not be given because of medical contraindications should be acceptable in lieu of documented vaccination. The statement should be written on letterhead stationery and accompanied by authoritative stamps or seals. Contacting the embassy or consulate of the country may be necessary to help guarantee that the letter of waiver will be accepted.

Cholera Vaccine

Cholera is an intestinal infection caused by *Vibrio cholerae* that involves profuse secretory diarrhea. The injectable cholera vaccine is not very efficacious, even when the primary series of two doses given 1 week or more apart is received.[105] WHO no longer endorses a requirement for this vaccine before entry into any country. For countries that still require cholera vaccination for travelers arriving from cholera-endemic areas, recording a single cholera dose in the traveler's International Certificate of Vaccination should suffice to meet this regulation.

Travelers going to areas endemic or epidemic for cholera are encouraged to strictly follow food and water precautions intended to prevent all forms of travel-associated diarrhea. Oral killed and live-attenuated vaccines[97] are available in some countries, but at present, there are no standardized recommendations for use of cholera vaccines, although health care workers and relief workers traveling to higher-risk areas might be suitable candidates. Likewise, travelers to cholera-endemic areas who are achlorhydric or have had a partial gastrectomy are logical candidates for the vaccine. Two oral, whole-cell killed vaccines are available. Dukoral (Crucell, The Netherlands), licensed in many European countries and Canada, is administered in two doses 1 to 6 weeks apart (three doses in children 2 to 6 years old). Shanchol (Shantha Biotechnics, India) is administered in two doses 2 weeks apart to persons more than 1 year old.[34]

Smallpox Vaccine

The requirement for smallpox vaccine for international travel was removed from WHO regulations in 1982. The CDC has embarked on an initiative to immunize health care providers, first responders, and others involved in bioterrorism preparedness, but the vaccine is not otherwise available, and travel is not considered a sufficient reason for vaccination.[113]

RECOMMENDED TRAVEL VACCINES

"Recommended" vaccines are those that are not routinely given during childhood in the United States but are advised for travelers based on the travel health risk assessment. Vaccines in this category include those for hepatitis A and B, typhoid fever, meningococcal meningitis, Japanese encephalitis virus, rabies, tick-borne encephalitis, varicella-zoster virus (VZV), influenza, and bacille Calmette-Guérin (BCG). The VZV vaccine is supposed to be used routinely in the United States, but for many adult U.S. travelers, it remains a vaccine that must be added. The influenza vaccine is often but not routinely used in children; it is recommended for many travelers. Although BCG vaccination is used in children

in the developing world, it is not used in U.S. children. Some vaccines are now routinely recommended for children. These include hepatitis B (since 1991), hepatitis A (more recently in United States),[27] and meningococcal vaccine, which is recommended for all 11- to 12-year-olds and young adults before starting higher education. Because of these practices, in the future, more travelers will likely have been vaccinated with recommended vaccines.

Hepatitis A Vaccine

Hepatitis A is the second most common vaccine-preventable travel-associated infectious disease, after influenza, and hepatitis A virus (HAV) is the most common cause of viral hepatitis. In the absence of vaccination, HAV infection occurs in 6 to 30 persons per 100,000 travelers per month who visit high- and medium-endemic destinations.[132] Risk is high even among those residing in "first-class" accommodations. Adventure travelers who venture off usual tourist routes may be at increased risk compared with other groups of travelers. Although HAV infection is asymptomatic in young children and self-limited in most adults, it causes greater than 2% mortality in infected adults older than 40, considerable morbidity during travel, and lost productivity after travel. Vaccination against HAV should be considered for all travelers to regions with moderate to high endemicity.

Individuals who have a history of jaundice, who were born before 1950, or who were born or resided for lengthy periods in endemic regions are likely to have natural immunity to HAV.[120] They should be screened for immunoglobulin G (IgG) antibodies

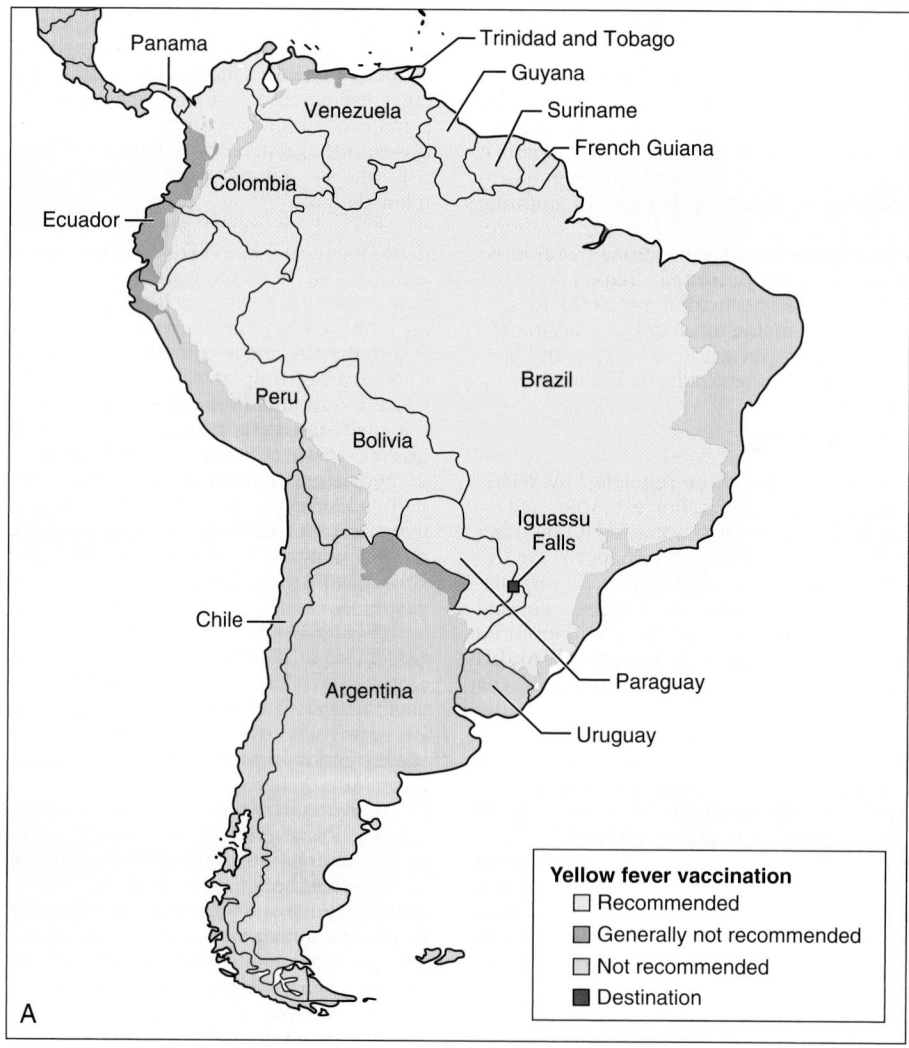

FIGURE 79-1 A, Yellow fever vaccination recommendations in South America.

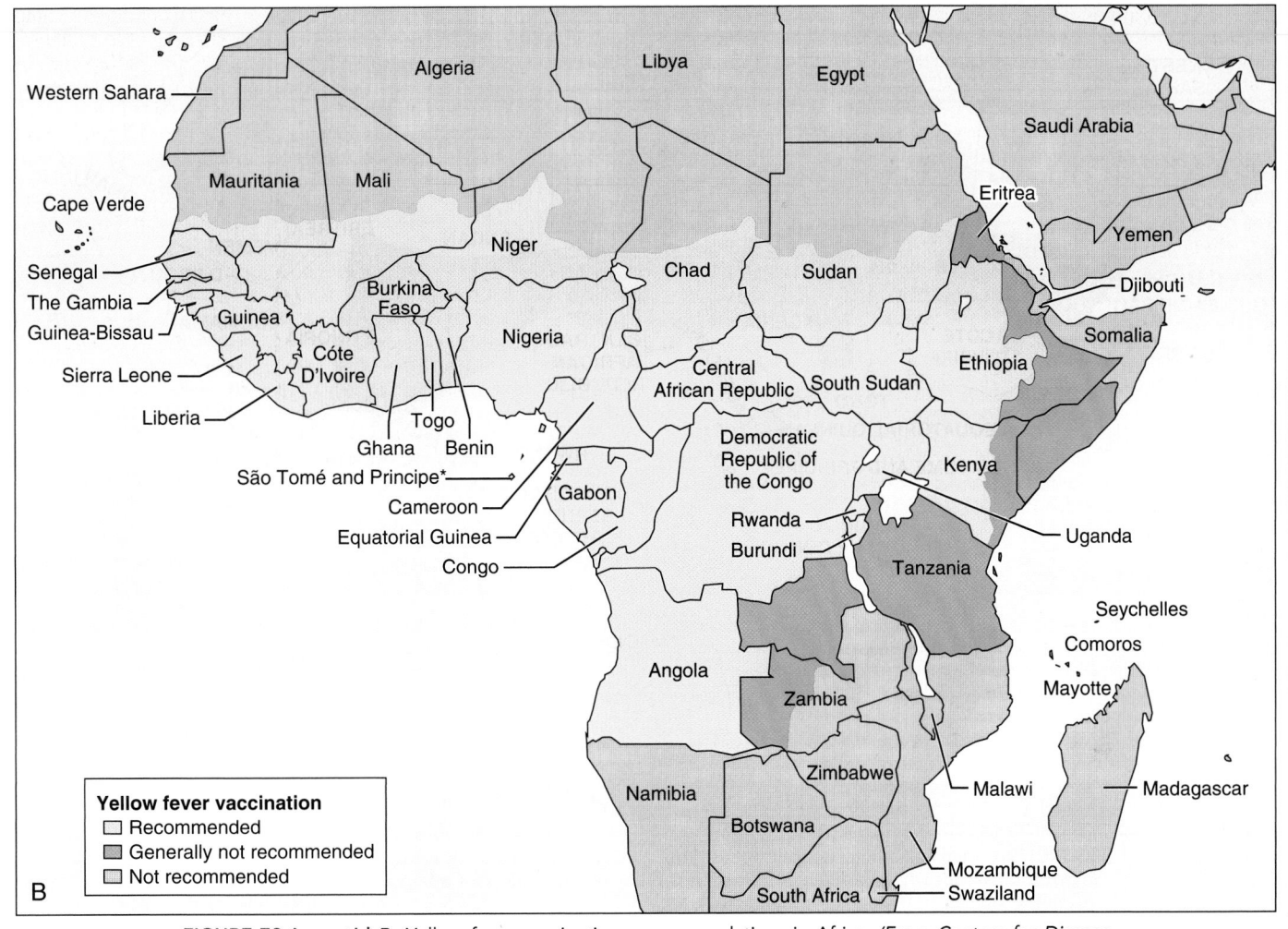

FIGURE 79-1, cont'd B, Yellow fever vaccination recommendations in Africa. (*From Centers for Disease Control and Prevention:* Health information for international travel, *2014. http://wwwnc.cdc.gov/travel/ yellowbook/2014/chapter-3-infectious-diseases-related-to-travel/yellow-fever.)*

against HAV, because if these are present, it is possible to avoid the cost of vaccination, which is usually more expensive than serologic testing. However, because vaccination of HAV-immune persons is not associated with adverse consequences, a traveler who does not have time before departure to be tested should be vaccinated.

A single dose of monovalent hepatitis A vaccine leads to seroconversion of 80% by 2 weeks and 99% after 1 month following vaccination.[38,126,132] For most healthy people, one dose of the monovalent HAV vaccine administered at any time before departure should provide adequate protection. Immune globulin is seldom indicated, except in older individuals, in whom HAV infection is more life threatening, and persons who are immunocompromised and therefore might not respond to the vaccine.[38,132] Postexposure prophylaxis with immune globulin is recommended for nonimmunized persons who are exposed to HAV.[132]

The HAV vaccine products are thought to be interchangeable. After two full doses separated by 6 to 12 months, protection is likely lifelong, so booster doses are not recommended in immunocompetent travelers.[126] Travelers who fail to receive their second dose of HAV vaccine within 6 to 12 months should attempt to complete the series; however, protective antibody levels have been produced even when the second dose was given 8 years after the initial dose.[60]

Hepatitis B Vaccine

Hepatitis B vaccine was added to the list of vaccines recommended for routine immunization of U.S. children in 1991, and consideration should be given to vaccinating all U.S. adults

regardless of travel. Risk to short-term travelers is low; however, travelers should be vaccinated when contact with body fluids or blood is possible (e.g., through sex or medical work), when it is anticipated that medical care might be received in a developing country, or if the person is a frequent short-term traveler. Long-term travelers and expatriates should be vaccinated.[58]

Two recombinant vaccines (Engerix-B and Recombivax HB) are thought to be interchangeable. A series started with one hepatitis B vaccine may be completed with another. The standard regimen for both vaccines is one dose at each of 0, 1, and 6 months. After any of the hepatitis B vaccination regimens, additional boosters are not recommended for normal hosts. Engerix-B is approved by the U.S. Food and Drug Administration (FDA) for an accelerated dosage schedule of 0, 1, and 2 months, with a booster dose at 12 months for long-lasting protection. Although a highly accelerated 3-week schedule is not FDA approved, literature supports dosing at 0, 7, and 21 days, with a 12-month booster with either licensed vaccine.[63,65] This regimen affords 65% protection at the end of 1 month and 100% seroconversion at 13 months. This is an attractive option for at-risk travelers who plan to depart in the next 3 to 4 weeks. An interrupted series can be completed without being restarted if the series cannot be completed before travel.

A combined hepatitis A and hepatitis B vaccine is dosed at 0, 1, and 6 months. Because a smaller dose of HAV antigen is used in this preparation, travelers must receive their second dose before travel for reliable protection. Literature supports a highly accelerated 3-week dosing regimen, with a 12-month booster using the combination vaccine.[89]

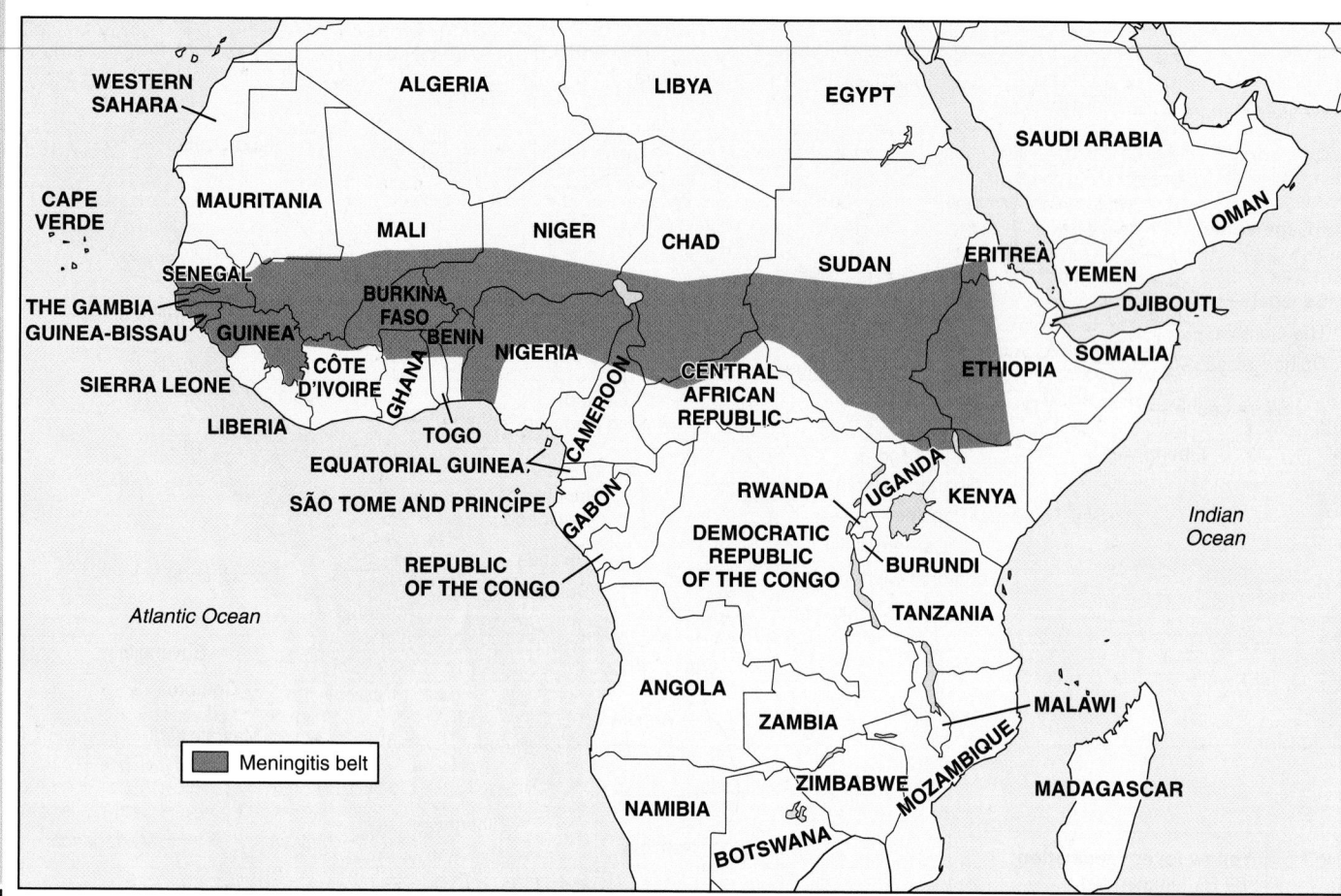

FIGURE 79-2 Meningitis belt. Consult details in the CDC Yellow Book for locations within each country where, and seasons when, pretravel vaccination is recommended. *(From Centers for Disease Control and Prevention:* Health information for international travel, *2014.* http://wwwnc.cdc.gov/travel/yellowbook/2014/chapter-3-infectious-diseases-related-to-travel/meningococcal-disease#3972.)

Typhoid Fever Vaccine

Typhoid is an insidious febrile illness caused by *Salmonella enterica* serotype Typhi. The incidence of typhoid fever among American travelers is estimated at 1 to 10 cases per 100,000 travelers.[95] Among reported cases in the United States., the majority were acquired during international travel.[71,75] The risk to travelers is highest among visitors to the Indian subcontinent, where the incidence is estimated at more than 100 cases per 100,000 native persons.[95] Travelers most at risk are those visiting friends and relatives (VFR). Visitors to Central and South America, Africa, and Asia should be considered for typhoid vaccination when they might be exposed to conditions of poor sanitation and hygiene, even for short periods.[23,118]

Increasing antibiotic resistance among *S. enterica* serotype Typhi infections is another reason to be vaccinated.[1,13] However, the current vaccines afford only 50% to 80% protection, and emergence of *S. enterica* serotype Paratyphi, against which protection is not afforded by current vaccines, underscores the importance of food and beverage hygiene among travelers.[75]

The two vaccines currently available offer a similar degree of protection. The parenteral purified Vi polysaccharide typhoid vaccine is administered as a single injection, with a booster recommended every 2 years. The oral Ty21a typhoid vaccine uses a live-attenuated strain of *S. enterica* serotype Typhi. One capsule is taken every other day for four doses (a three-dose regimen is recommended in Europe).[17] A booster regimen is recommended every 5 years.

Meningococcal Vaccine

Vaccine protection against meningococcal meningitis is recommended for long-term travelers to the sub-Saharan "meningitis belt"[27,36,100] (Figure 79-2). Short-term travelers to this region should receive vaccine if they will travel during the dry season (December to June) or have extensive contact with local people. The quadrivalent meningococcal vaccine is required for travel to Saudi Arabia for Umrah or the annual Hajj religious pilgrimages. Regardless of travel, the classic recommendation has been that young adults who will live in school dormitories and persons with complement deficiencies who will have prolonged contact with a local population, such as in a refugee camp, or with surgical or functional asplenia should be vaccinated. Travelers to regions where outbreaks are occurring should be vaccinated. Practitioners who do not subscribe to commercial information services that are routinely updated should check the CDC website (http://www.cdc.gov/travel) periodically to determine where epidemic disease of any causation is occurring.

Quadrivalent meningococcal polysaccharide vaccine induces immunity against serogroups A, C, Y, and W-135. A single dose appears to provide immunity for 5 years. However, a single-dose quadrivalent meningococcal polysaccharide-protein conjugate vaccine is the preferred vaccine for those older than 2 years, with a booster recommended every 5 years for ongoing risk.[37] Travelers who had previously been vaccinated with polysaccharide vaccine and need revaccination should receive a conjugate vaccine. However, neither the polysaccharide nor the conjugate vaccine provides immunity against serogroup B. The FDA recently approved a vaccine (Trumenba) active against four *Neisseria meningitidis* serogroup B strains prevalent in the United States, for use in adolescents and young adults age 10 to 25 years. It has not been recommended for travelers because *N. meningitides* serogroup B infections are rare in sub-Saharan Africa.[125]

Japanese Encephalitis Virus Vaccine

Japanese encephalitis (JE) is an arboviral infection transmitted by mosquitoes in Asia and Southeast Asia. Transmission is year-round in tropical and subtropical areas and during the late spring, summer, and early fall in temperate climates. JE virus is not considered a risk for short-term travelers visiting usual tourist destinations in urban and developed resort areas.[47]

Personal protective measures to prevent mosquito bites can greatly reduce risk of infection. The overall incidence of JE among people from nonendemic countries traveling to Asia is estimated at less than 1 case per 1 million travelers. However, travelers who stay for prolonged periods (including expatriates) in rural areas with active JE virus transmission are likely to be at a risk similar to that of the susceptible resident population (~5 to 50 cases per 100,000 children per year). Persons on short trips may be at risk if they are staying in rural areas or have high mosquito exposure.[47] Thus, vaccination should be offered to both long- and short-term visitors to rural areas when travel will occur during transmission season, particularly when mosquito exposure might be high and significant time will be spent outdoors.

Two vaccines (JE-Vax, Ixiaro) are FDA approved, but only Ixiaro, a Vero cell culture–derived formulation, is available. Previously recommended only for use in persons 17 years or older, Ixiaro is now approved by the FDA for use in children 2 months or older. A single dose of Ixiaro has been shown to effectively boost antibody levels in persons previously vaccinated with JE-Vax, but the duration of protection is unknown. The primary immunization schedule for Ixiaro is two doses, on days 0 and 28, with therapy completed 1 week or longer before travel. In patients receiving JE-Vax, fewer than 1% of patients reported redness, swelling, tenderness, and pain after injection.[47] Systemic adverse events reported included headache (26%), myalgias (21%), influenza-like illness (13%), and fatigue (13%).

The single-dose, live-attenuated SA 14-14-2 JE vaccine manufactured in Chengdu, China (available in destination countries such as Nepal) has been effectively used extensively in South and Southeast Asia for decades with an acceptable safety profile.

Rabies Vaccine

Rabies is an acute, progressive encephalomyelitis caused by neurotropic viruses in the family Rhabdoviridae[56] (see Chapter 31). Although rabies is endemic in much of the world, the risk of rabies for most travelers is very low.[55] Avoidance of dog bites eliminates much of the risk.[77] Other animal species important for transmission of rabies to travelers include monkeys, mongooses, bats, and foxes. Preexposure rabies immunization should be considered for rural travelers, particularly adventure travelers who go to remote areas, persons with occupational (veterinarians) or recreational (spelunkers) exposure, and expatriate workers, missionaries, and their families living in countries where rabies is a recognized risk. Children should be targeted for pre-exposure vaccination in high-risk regions, because they may not tell their parents when they have been bitten or exposed to rabies virus.

Any of the three tissue culture–derived inactivated virus rabies vaccines can be administered intramuscularly in the deltoid (not gluteal) muscle in a pre-exposure schedule of 0, 7, and 21 (or 28) days.[77] For persons who continue to be at risk of exposure, a booster can be given every 2 years, or less frequently based on annual serology testing. For persons engaging in high-risk activities (veterinarians, cavers, adventure travelers to Asia and Africa), serologic testing every 2 years and booster vaccine, if necessary, are recommended.

In the event of an exposure, the vaccinated traveler must understand how to clean the wound thoroughly and immediately seek two additional doses of vaccine. Pre-exposure vaccination obviates the need for postexposure administration of rabies immune globulin (RIG), which is an important consideration because RIG may be very difficult to obtain abroad.[77] Persons who are exposed without having had pre-exposure rabies vaccination require both RIG and a four-dose course of rabies vaccine given over 14 days, as recommended by the U.S. Advisory Committee on Immunization Practices.[104] Persons with immunosuppression should still receive five doses of the vaccine.[77]

Mild local reactions (pain at the injection site, redness, swelling, and induration) to rabies vaccine occur in 60% to 89% of persons receiving human diploid cell vaccine (HDCV) and 11% to 57% of persons receiving purified chick embryo cell vaccine (PCECV). Adverse reactions are self-limited, lasting a few days.[77] For persons receiving HDCV and PCECV, 6.8% to 55.6% and 0% to 31% of recipients, respectively, developed mild systemic symptoms that included low-grade fever, myalgia, headache, dizziness, and gastrointestinal (GI) upset. Systemic hypersensitivity reactions, characterized by urticarial rash, angioedema, and respiratory symptoms, occurred much less frequently in patients receiving HDCV and PCECV vaccination types. A serum sickness–like syndrome is possible after HDCV; sudden death and encephalomyelitis are very rare.[77]

Tick-Borne Encephalitis Vaccine

Tick-borne encephalitis (TBE) is a viral illness transmitted predominantly by bites of *Ixodes* ticks during spring and summer months in rural forested areas of central and eastern Europe, Scandinavia, Siberia, and northern Japan. Infection can lead to central nervous system (CNS) effects of meningitis, encephalitis, or meningoencephalitis in about 20% to 30% of infected persons.[56] Infection can occur after ingestion of unpasteurized dairy products from infected cows, goats, or sheep.[54]

There are no licensed vaccines for TBE in the United States.[6,46] The standard dosing regimen is three doses given over 1 year. Accelerated schedules exist, but doses would likely need to be administered in the destination country. Whereas expatriates can consider obtaining vaccine at their new location, it is much more practical for most travelers to at-risk areas to use stringent tick bite precautions (e.g., repellents and insecticides, protective clothing, frequent tick surveillance) and to avoid unpasteurized dairy products.

Bacille Calmette-Guérin Vaccine

The BCG vaccine is intended to prevent tuberculosis (TB). The vaccine is currently not recommended for most U.S. travelers, including expatriates. This is because it is believed to be of varying efficacy in preventing adult forms of TB.[56] Persons taking short trips for tourism or business to developing countries where TB is common among the indigenous population are not at great risk for contracting TB. However, expatriates or travelers who will live among foreign residents or work in foreign orphanages, schools, hospitals, or similar facilities are at significant risk of exposure to TB infection.[35] Such travelers should be tested with a purified protein derivative (PPD) skin test before the trip, and if the test is negative, they should be retested 3 months after their return to a developed country and yearly thereafter. In the setting of travel and exposure, persons who convert from a negative to a positive PPD skin test should be treated with isoniazid for 9 months, regardless of age. Interferon-γ release assays (IGRAs) are blood tests that measure host cell–mediated immune response to *Mycobacterium tuberculosis* antigen. IGRAs appear to have high specificity but variable sensitivity compared with the TB skin test. IGRAs may be most useful in BCG-vaccinated patients and in persons unlikely to return for reading of a skin test.[56]

Varicella-Zoster Virus (Chickenpox) Vaccine

Varicella-zoster virus (VZV) infections are common throughout the world. Primary infection with VZV is known as chickenpox. After primary infection with VZV, the virus often stays dormant. It can reemerge as shingles later in life.[56] A traveler with a history of chickenpox can be considered immune. Many adults have had exposure to VZV, so if time permits, serum immunity should be documented before considering vaccination. If a person is not immune, two doses of single-antigen varicella vaccine should be given 4 to 8 weeks apart.[78]

Influenza Vaccine

Each year, the influenza vaccine antigen composition is based on projections of winter influenza activity in North America (or South America). The vaccine differs depending on the hemisphere in which one lives, and therefore may not protect against the precise influenza strains circulating elsewhere in the world. As a result of when the projections are made, the vaccination may not be available for at-risk travelers from the United States during late spring through early autumn.[21]

Travelers from the United States may be exposed to influenza when traveling during winter months in the northern hemisphere; between April and September in the southern hemisphere; and year-round in the tropics. Travelers from diverse locations may be brought together during cruises, resulting in an outbreak of influenza during periods when influenza transmission might otherwise not frequently occur.[124] Risk for acquiring influenza during long-haul flights exists if a person infected with influenza is seated close to a susceptible individual. For these reasons, influenza should be considered a travel-related infection, and influenza vaccine should be recommended to travelers.[21]

Other Vaccines

According to the CDC, anthrax vaccine is not recommended for travelers. A killed bacterial vaccine for plague exists, but the dosing schedule is long and protection is uncertain. An alternative for select persons at risk (e.g., field biologists) for plague is a daily 100-mg dose of doxycycline, which can double as protection against malaria. The protective efficacy of this regimen against plague is inferred from treatment recommendations.[56]

ROUTINE VACCINES

"Routine" immunizations are those customarily given in childhood and then updated in adult life, regardless of travel.[87] Visits to travel medicine clinics afford opportunities to update immunizations through booster doses of routine vaccines.

The routine vaccines currently recommended in childhood include those against tetanus, diphtheria, pertussis, measles, mumps, rubella, varicella, polio, *Haemophilus influenzae* type b (Hib), hepatitis A/B, pneumococcus (PCV), and rotavirus. Routine immunization schedules for children, including nuanced changes in routine schedules for traveling children, can be found in the CDC's Yellow Book.[56]

Diphtheria, Tetanus, and Pertussis Vaccine

Primary immunization in young children is accomplished with five doses of a combination vaccine containing full doses of tetanus/diphtheria toxoid combined with acellular pertussis antigen (DTaP). The diphtheria/tetanus vaccine (Td) classically used for booster doses in older children and adults has no pertussis component and a lower dose of diphtheria antigen. Absence of a pertussis booster for adults has led to waning immunity and susceptibility to the disease.[2,22] Therefore, adolescents (11 to 18 years) and adults (>19 years) should receive a single dose of tetanus/diphtheria with acellular pertussis (Tdap). The Td vaccine should then be used every 10 years or after an exposure to tetanus to maintain tetanus immunity.[87] Travelers to remote locations who might sustain open wounds and be unable to safely obtain a tetanus booster should be given a Td booster if it has been 5 or more years since the prior booster. This should particularly be considered when a person plans travel to areas of the world where diphtheria remains a risk (e.g., most countries of Africa, Asia, South Pacific, Middle East, eastern Europe, South America, Haiti, Dominican Republic.).

Poliomyelitis Vaccine

All traveling adults should have received a primary course of polio vaccine. Vaccination campaigns worldwide have been largely successful in making some regions (e.g., western hemisphere, Europe, western Pacific) polio-free.[31] However, some regions continue to have circulating wild poliovirus (WPV). This is often caused by political instability that interferes with vaccination programs, or because of regional reimportation of polio virus, or because the live oral polio vaccine (OPV) has replicated and regained some properties of WPVs, which leads to small outbreaks of vaccine-derived poliovirus (VDPV) infection that are clinically indistinguishable from WPV infection.[28,30] Travel medicine practitioners should routinely check the CDC or WHO websites for the latest information regarding recommendations

for polio prevention. Adult travelers to at-risk regions should receive a one-time booster dose of inactivated polio vaccine (IPV).[56]

Measles, Mumps, and Rubella Vaccine

Measles is endemic in large portions of the world.[56] Travelers to developing countries are at risk for acquiring measles. Measles cases in the United States are largely caused by importation of measles from other countries, with the largest proportion of cases occurring in unvaccinated individuals.[50] If travelers have received two doses of a measles-containing vaccine, usually given in childhood as the measles, mumps, and rubella (MMR) vaccine or the MMR plus varicella vaccine (MMRV), they should be protected. Adults born after 1956 who have not received two doses of live measles vaccine and who do not have a physician-documented history of infection or laboratory evidence of immunity should receive two doses of MMR vaccine separated by at least 28 days.[80] The measles component of the combination vaccines distributed in the United States contains a live-attenuated virus. Measles-containing vaccines are therefore contraindicated in pregnancy and in all immunocompromised persons (except persons with HIV and CD4 counts ≥ 200 cells/μL, for whom measles vaccination is recommended).[80]

Haemophilus Influenzae Type B (Hib) Vaccine

The risk for *H. influenzae* type b disease is the same in traveling children as it is in children who reside in developed countries. Traveling children should be kept up to date according to standard pediatric vaccination schedules.

Pneumococcal Vaccine

The pneumococcal polysaccharide vaccines (PCV13 and PPSV23) should be offered routinely, regardless of travel, to people 65 and older and those 19 and older with significant comorbidities, as recommended by the CDC. Many older travelers as well as high-risk individuals may not have been vaccinated, so a visit to the travel clinic is an ideal opportunity to bring these people up to date.[121]

MALARIA

Malaria is a mosquito-transmitted, blood-borne, parasitic infection present throughout tropical and developing areas of the world (Figure 79-3) (see Chapters 39 and 40). In the United States, 1500 to 2000 cases of malaria are reported annually to the CDC. Almost all of these cases are in returning travelers. Although the risk to travelers is relatively low compared with other medical problems (e.g., diarrhea, respiratory problems), malaria is the most common preventable infectious cause of death among travelers and one of the most common causes of fever in the returning traveler. Most travelers who develop malaria have not used chemoprophylaxis, were prescribed inappropriate chemoprophylaxis, or were not compliant with their medication regimen.[52,110]

Travelers often fail to use appropriate personal protective measures (PPMs). Visitors to friends and relatives (VFR) are now recognized as a group that disproportionally accounts for malaria occurring among travelers.[4] These persons typically grow up in a malaria-endemic region, immigrate to a malaria nonendemic region (subsequently losing much of their protective immunity), and then return to a malaria-endemic region to visit friends and relatives. This population needs to be counseled to practice the same PPMs and chemoprophylaxis as should other travelers to malaria-endemic regions. Although newer medications for malaria chemoprophylaxis have been introduced, rising drug resistance, breakdown in malaria control, and continuing reports of real or perceived adverse effects from antimalarial medications contribute to difficulties in protecting travelers against malaria.

MALARIA RISK ASSESSMENT

Assessment of risk for malaria requires knowing the details of a traveler's itinerary, including specifics of travel within a country. For instance, a geographic area may be listed as endemic for malaria, whereas urban travel may represent no appreciable risk,

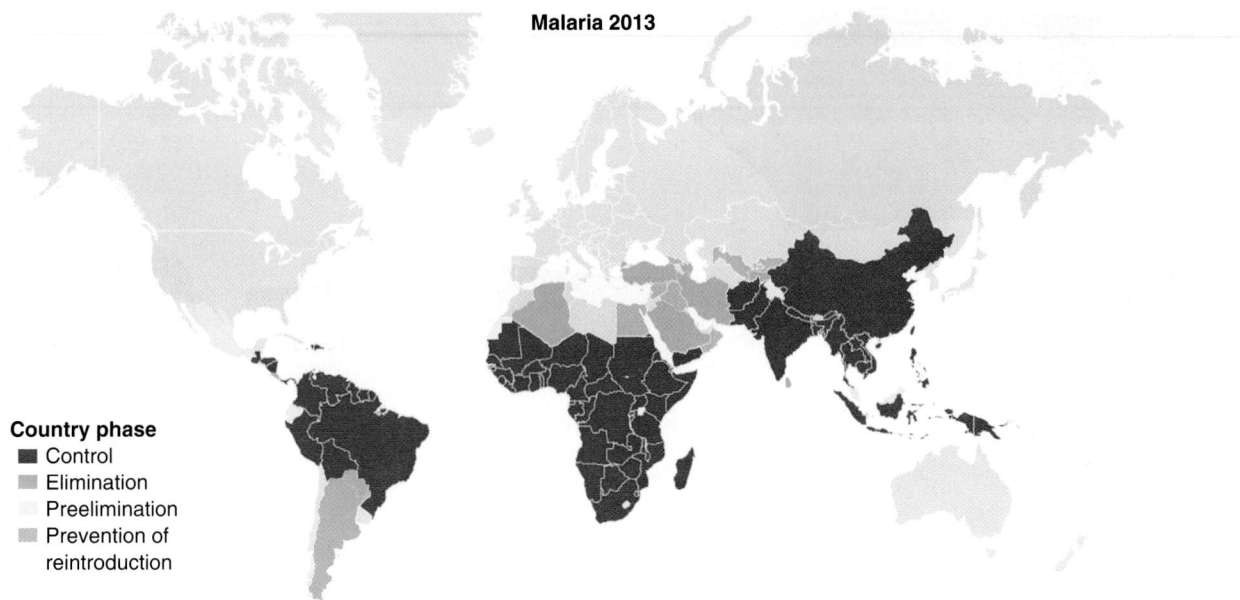

Malaria 2013

Country phase
- ■ Control
- ■ Elimination
- ■ Preelimination
- ■ Prevention of reintroduction

FIGURE 79-3 Worldwide distribution of malaria based on data from the WHO 2013 World Malaria Report. (*From* http://worldmalariareport.org.)

so chemoprophylaxis might be delayed until rural travel begins. When health facilities in the area are reliable, the traveler might need only to practice PPMs and perhaps take along standby therapy if duration of travel exceeds the minimum incubation time (~1 week) for malaria.

Season of travel (dry vs. rainy) and elevation of a destination influence risk, although climate change is altering our general understanding of these patterns.[84] Type of accommodation (e.g., camping vs. sleeping in air-conditioned well-screened room) influences whether to recommend permethrin-coated products such as bed nets. Location and duration of stay impact the amount and type of chemoprophylaxis (e.g., weekly mefloquine vs. daily doxycycline or atovaquone/proguanil for long-term travel) providers should recommend. A medical history must address the possibility of known intolerance of an antimalarial medication, drug-drug interactions, and contraindications (e.g., mefloquine and depression).

Any traveler determined to be at risk for malaria should be educated about the serious nature of malaria; risks posed by itineraries; how to avoid mosquito bites; antimalarial drug compliance; and how to seek medical care expeditiously in the event that fever occurs during or after travel. Up to 20% of cases of *Plasmodium vivax* malaria in travelers may have onset more than 6 months after travel. A helpful pneumonic for travelers is the ABCD of malaria prevention: awareness of risk, bite avoidance, compliance with drugs, and diagnose promptly.

Health departments in other countries may offer differing recommendations regarding malaria prophylaxis, thereby confusing the traveler. The advising provider must take the traveler's medical history, itinerary, and individual risk into account to create an individualized plan based on relevant information.

PRECAUTIONS AGAINST INSECTS
(see Chapter 45)

No drug completely prevents malaria. Many chemoprophylactic regimens do not absolutely prevent the liver phase of *P. vivax* infection. At the outset, travelers should be told to practice PPMs against malaria in addition to taking prophylactic medication.[49] Only perfect avoidance of mosquito bites can successfully prevent mosquito-borne diseases, such as malaria, chikungunya virus infection, or dengue fever.[48,59] Resistance to antimalarial compounds is increasing in some malaria-endemic regions.

The female *Anopheles* mosquito transmits malaria parasites. Depending on the species of mosquito, bites most frequently occur between dusk and dawn, during which travelers should take appropriate precautions or limit time outdoors. At-risk persons should wear protective clothing and apply insect repellents to exposed areas of skin. They should sleep in well-screened or air-conditioned rooms or within bed nets, the protective efficacy of which can be increased by application of insecticide (e.g., permethrin). Treated bed nets and clothing retain residual insecticide activity for weeks (sprayed) to months (soaked).[84] In addition to repelling mosquitoes, permethrin insecticides are effective against gnats, ticks, chiggers, bedbugs, scorpions, centipedes, beetles, and flies. Permethrin is a chemical derivative of alkaloids (pyrethrums) naturally occurring in the chrysanthemum plant family. When permethrin is allowed to air-dry before treated items are used, it is relatively nontoxic and suitable for treatment of external clothing and mosquito nets (Figure 79-4). It is not recommended for direct skin application, because skin hypersensitivity reactions may occur.[84]

The three most highly recommended repellents for disease prevention are the synthetic repellent N,N-dimethyl-*m*-toluamide (DEET); the plant-derived terpene repellent *p*-menthane-3,8-diol (PMD) from lemon eucalyptus; and the piperidine icaridin (also known as picaridin).[84] Picaridin appears to be better tolerated on skin than DEET and should not damage fabric or plastics.

In the United States, according to the Environmental Protection Agency (EPA), DEET-containing repellents are the most commonly used. Concentrations of DEET that afford a reasonable duration of protection are in the range of 30% to 40%. Higher concentrations of DEET do not protect better; rather, protection lasts longer. Particularly in concentrations of less than 30%, DEET appears to be safe for use on infants and children older than 2 months. DEET repels not only mosquitoes but also ticks, chiggers, fleas, gnats, and flies. Care should be taken in its application to avoid applying it to the eyes or mouth. When sunscreen and insect repellent need to be used simultaneously, the sunscreen should be applied first to avoid increasing absorption of DEET.[84]

MALARIA CHEMOPROPHYLAXIS
(see Chapter 40)

Selection of a malaria chemoprophylaxis agent is determined by the geographic destination and pattern of drug resistance among malaria strains transmitted at the destination. As shown in Table 79-2, chloroquine is still appropriate for chemoprophylaxis in some regions of the world (Caribbean, Central America west of Panama Canal, some Middle East countries). For much of the

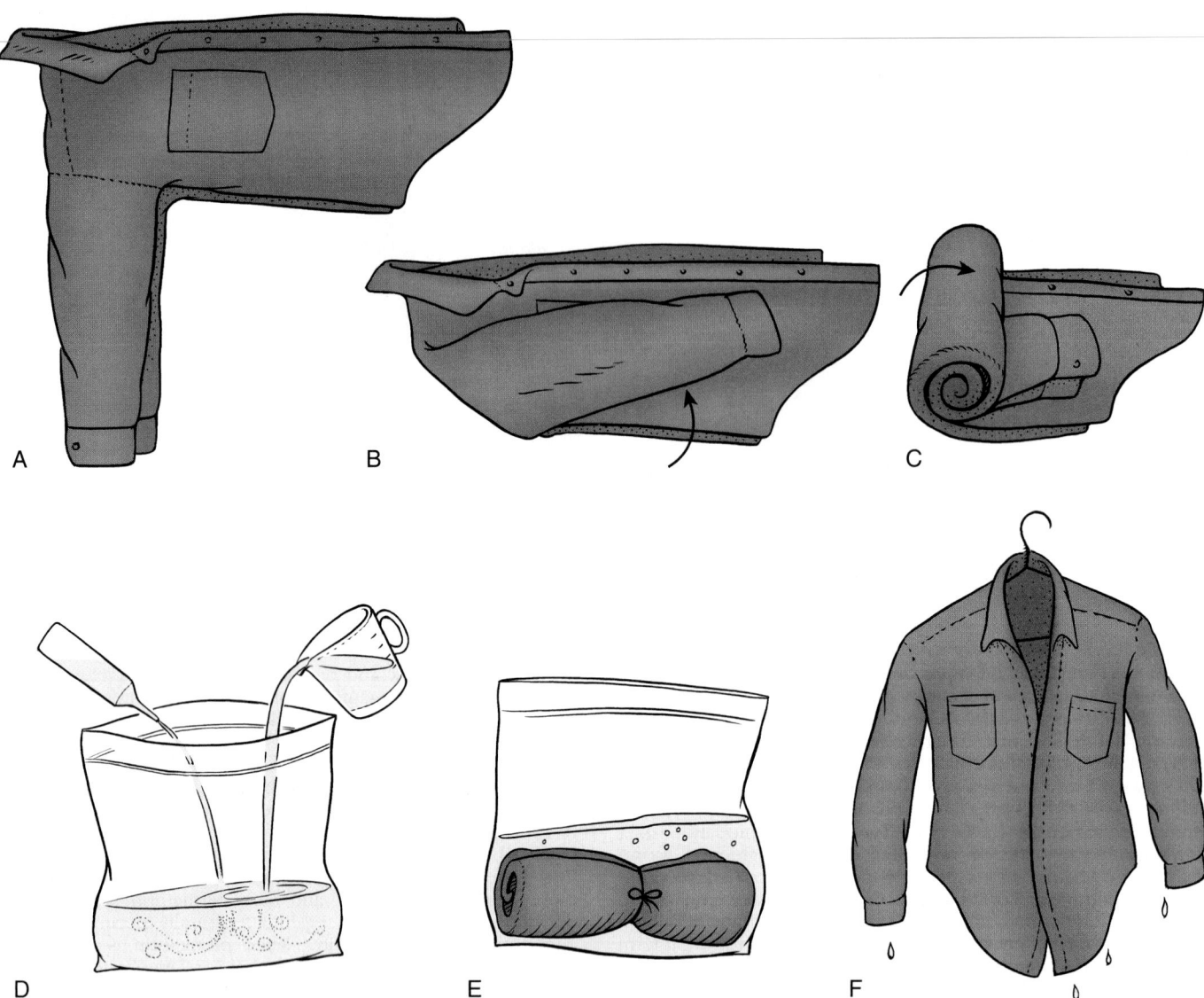

FIGURE 79-4 Technique for impregnating clothing or mosquito netting with permethrin solution. **A** to **C,** Lay jacket flat and fold it shoulder to shoulder. Fold sleeves to inside, roll tightly, and tie middle with string. For mosquito net, roll tightly and tie. **D,** Pour 60 mL (2 oz) of permethrin into plastic bag. Add 1 L (1 quart) water. Mix. Solution will turn milky white. **E,** Place garment or mosquito netting in bag. Shut or tie tightly. Let rest 10 minutes. **F,** Hang garment or netting for 2 to 3 hours to dry. Fabric can also be laid on a clean surface to dry. *(Redrawn from Rose S:* International travel health guide, *North Hampton, Mass, 1993, Travel Medicine, with permission.)*

TABLE 79-2	Chemoprophylaxis Drugs by Regions of Drug Resistance		
		Drugs	
Malaria Drug Resistance	**Country or Region**	**Preferred**	**Alternatives**
Chloroquine-sensitive	Central America (west of Panama); parts of Mexico; Haiti/Dominican Republic; most of the Middle East; states of the former Soviet Union; northern Africa; Argentina and Paraguay; parts of China	Chloroquine	Atovaquone/proguanil Doxycycline Mefloquine Primaquine Hydroxychloroquine
Chloroquine-resistant	Most of malarious South America, including Panama, west of the former Panama Canal Zone; most of Asia and Southeast Asia; sub-Saharan Africa; Oceania; parts of Iran, Oman, Saudi Arabia, and Yemen	Atovaquone/proguanil Doxycycline Mefloquine	Primaquine
Chloroquine-, mefloquine-, and sulfonamide-resistant	Thailand borders with Myanmar and Cambodia	Doxycycline Atovaquone/proguanil	

TABLE 79-3 Malaria Chemoprophylaxis Drug Regimens for Adults

Drug	Dose	Regimen	Comments and Adverse Effects
Chloroquine	500 mg/wk	Begin 1-2 weeks before arrival in malarious area; continue drug weekly while in, and for 4 weeks after leaving, the malarious area.	May exacerbate psoriasis Pruritus (persons of African descent), headache, bitter taste: common Transient visual blurring, partial alopecia skin eruptions, reversible corneal opacity: occasional
Hydroxychloroquine	200 mg/wk	As with chloroquine	As with chloroquine
Mefloquine	250 mg/wk	As with chloroquine	Take with food. Avoid concurrent alcohol. Avoid if history of depression, psychosis, seizures, or cardiac conduction abnormality. Dizziness, nausea, diarrhea, nightmares, insomnia, mood alteration, headache: common
Doxycycline	100 mg daily	Begin 1-2 days before arrival in malarious area; continue drug daily while in, and for 4 weeks after leaving, the malarious area.	Use sunscreen. Stains teeth (fetuses and children age <8 yr) GI upset, photosensitivity, *Candida* vaginitis: common
Atovaquone/proguanil	250 mg/100 mg daily	Begin 1-2 days before arrival in malarious area; continue drug daily while in, and for 7 days after leaving, the malarious area.	Take with food. Avoid if CLcr <30 mL/min. Nausea, abdominal pain, headache: common Transient increase in transaminases: occasional
Primaquine	30 mg base daily	Begin 1-2 days before arrival in malarious area; continue drug daily while in, and for 2 days after leaving, the malarious area.	Take with food. Avoid if G6PD deficiency. GI upset: common

CLcr, Creatinine clearance; *GI*, gastrointestinal; *G6PD*, Glucose-6-phosphate dehydrogenase.

malaria-endemic world, chloroquine-resistant *Plasmodium falciparum* malaria (CRPF) dictates the drug of choice. In a limited area of the world, chloroquine-, mefloquine-, and sulfonamide-resistant malaria is a concern. Where chloroquine-resistant *P. vivax* (CRPV) is a concern, recommendations for CRPF, which is also present in these regions, suffices for CRPV as well. Table 79-3 provides doses and schedules for drugs typically used in malaria chemoprophylaxis.[56]

Travelers should start taking drugs with a weekly dosing regimen (chloroquine or mefloquine[56]) 1 to 2 weeks before departure. This allows time for familiarity with the side effects of the drug while the drug attains steady-state levels in the body, enables the traveler to habituate to the timing of doses, and gives the traveler time, while at home, to switch to an alternative drug in the event of intolerable side effects. Antimalarial drugs with a daily dosing schedule (doxycycline, atovaquone/proguanil, or primaquine phosphate[5,52]) are started 1 to 2 days before entering the malaria-endemic area.[56] Doxycycline, chloroquine, and mefloquine chemoprophylactic regimens should be continued for 4 weeks after the traveler leaves a malaria endemic area to prevent malaria in the immediate post-travel period. Atovaquone/proguanil should be continued for 7 days, and primaquine for 2 days, after leaving a malaria endemic area.[56] Travelers should be warned not to stop or switch the antimalarial regimen during the trip without the advice of a knowledgeable health care provider.

In addition to geographic considerations, convenience of dosing regimen, cost, and adverse effect profile of the malaria chemoprophylaxis agents combine to play an important role in choice and traveler compliance when taking the medication. Although inexpensive, doxycycline is associated with sun sensitivity rash.[56] Mefloquine has the greatest purported neuropsychiatric side effects.[56,109] Studies indicate that doxycycline and atovaquone/proguanil have relatively advantageous side effect profiles, are well tolerated, and are therefore often the most popular agents.[109]

Some travelers may not be able to take an optimal chemoprophylactic regimen. During pregnancy, doxycycline (category D), atovaquone/proguanil (category C), and primaquine (potential risk of hemolysis in the fetus) are contraindicated. The most recent data suggest that mefloquine (category B as of 2011) is probably safe for use during pregnancy.[56] Doxycycline is contraindicated in children younger than 8 years.

STANDBY SELF-DIAGNOSIS AND DRUG TREATMENT

For travelers who spend prolonged time in very-low-risk areas, where risks of chemoprophylaxis might exceed the risk of malaria, the approach of self-diagnosis[61,90,129] and self-treatment,[93] instead of malaria chemoprophylaxis, is an option. This may also be appropriate for persons taking suboptimal chemoprophylaxis or for those taking appropriate chemoprophylaxis who travel to remote areas where the risk of breakthrough clinical illness due to resistant malaria is high. This approach mandates that the traveler who develops a febrile illness and begins antimalarial treatment also seeks rapid, definitive medical care.

Self-diagnosis of malaria using rapid diagnostic tests (RDTs) by travelers in the field can be accompanied by a high false-negative rate depending on the test, species of malaria, and presence of other infectious agents.[76] When travelers who develop a febrile illness elect to self-treat and are subsequently evaluated medically, they often are found not to have had malaria. Recent expert consensus concludes that self-diagnosis and self-treatment cannot routinely be recommended and should be considered only after expert consultation.[56] In the United States, the currently preferred recommendation for self-treatment of suspected malaria is either atovaquone/proguanil (four 250-mg tablets taken as a single daily dose for 3 days) or artemether/lumefantrine (3-day treatment based on weight).[56]

In addition to malaria, enteric fever, scrub typhus, leptospirosis, and dengue are common causes of undifferentiated febrile illness that travelers may acquire in the tropics. If empirical drug self-treatment is started for presumed malaria and then malaria is ruled out, empirical antibiotic therapy for another presumed cause may need to be started. Oral azithromycin may be an option for the empirical treatment of enteric fever, scrub typhus, and leptospirosis while the medical workup is underway.[12,95,98]

TRAVELER'S DIARRHEA
(see Chapter 82)

The term *traveler's diarrhea* (TD) usually refers to abrupt onset of loose stools accompanied by abdominal cramps. Other symptoms often include nausea, vomiting, fever, and malaise. Tenesmus and bloody stools are uncommon features. According to the

CDC, it is estimated that 30% to 70% of international travelers develop travel-related diarrhea, depending on the destination and season of travel.[56] Most cases of TD are self-limited and resolve within 1 to 2 days; 90% of cases resolve by 7 days.[56] Despite this, a substantial percentage of travelers change activities because of symptoms, which can severely impact a trip. Current evidence indicates that 4% to 32% of patients with bacterial gastroenteritis may develop postinfectious irritable bowel syndrome (IBS), leading to chronic, episodic symptoms of IBS.[41]

Diarrhea associated with travel can result from multiple causes, including a change in normal diet, food poisoning (toxins), viral infections (e.g., rotavirus, norovirus), and parasites (e.g., *Giardia lamblia*, *Entamoeba histolytica*, *Cryptosporidium*). However, bacteria such as enterotoxigenic (ETEC) and enteroaggregative (EAEC) *Escherichia coli*, *Shigella*, *Campylobacter*, *Aeromonas*, *Salmonella*, noncholera *Vibrio*, and *Plesiomonas* account for the majority of cases.[39,66] The major causal role of bacteria explains the benefits of antimicrobial agents for treatment and prevention of the syndrome.[39]

The world can be divided into high-, intermediate-, and low-risk regions for TD[66,127] (Figure 79-5). The risk of TD is highest during the first week of travel. The style of travel may confer increased risk of disease (e.g., backpacking seems to carry a higher risk for TD than staying at resorts).[66] Although strict adherence to food hygiene when traveling is still recommended, the advice to "cook it, peel it, boil it, or forget it" has been shown to have marginal benefit in preventing TD.[66] Nevertheless, thoroughly cooked food, dry food, and fruits and vegetables that can be peeled by the traveler are generally considered safe, whereas tap water, ice cubes, fruit juices, fresh salads, unpasteurized dairy products, cold sauces and toppings, open buffets, and undercooked or incompletely reheated foods should be avoided.

TABLE 79-4 Recommended Agents for Traveler's Diarrhea Chemoprophylaxis

Agent	Dosage	Comments and Adverse Effects
Bismuth subsalicylate (Pepto-Bismol)	Two tablets chewed four times daily	Avoid in persons who should not take aspirin or who are taking anticoagulants. Black stool and tongue may occur.
Fluoroquinolones*		Occasional
Norfloxacin	400 mg PO daily	gastrointestinal
Ciprofloxacin	500 mg PO daily	upset, rash, and allergic reaction
Rifaximin	200 mg PO daily	Well tolerated because rifaximin is not absorbed

*Other fluoroquinolones can be predicted to be effective but have not been studied in prophylaxis; *PO*, orally.

CHEMOPROPHYLAXIS

Bismuth subsalicylate (BSS)–containing compounds and antimicrobial agents are successful for prevention of TD (Table 79-4).[66] Antimicrobial prophylaxis for TD is not recommended for most travelers.[56] Antimicrobial prophylaxis might be a reasonable strategy for a traveler who is taking a brief trip to a high-risk area and cannot afford even a brief illness. According to current

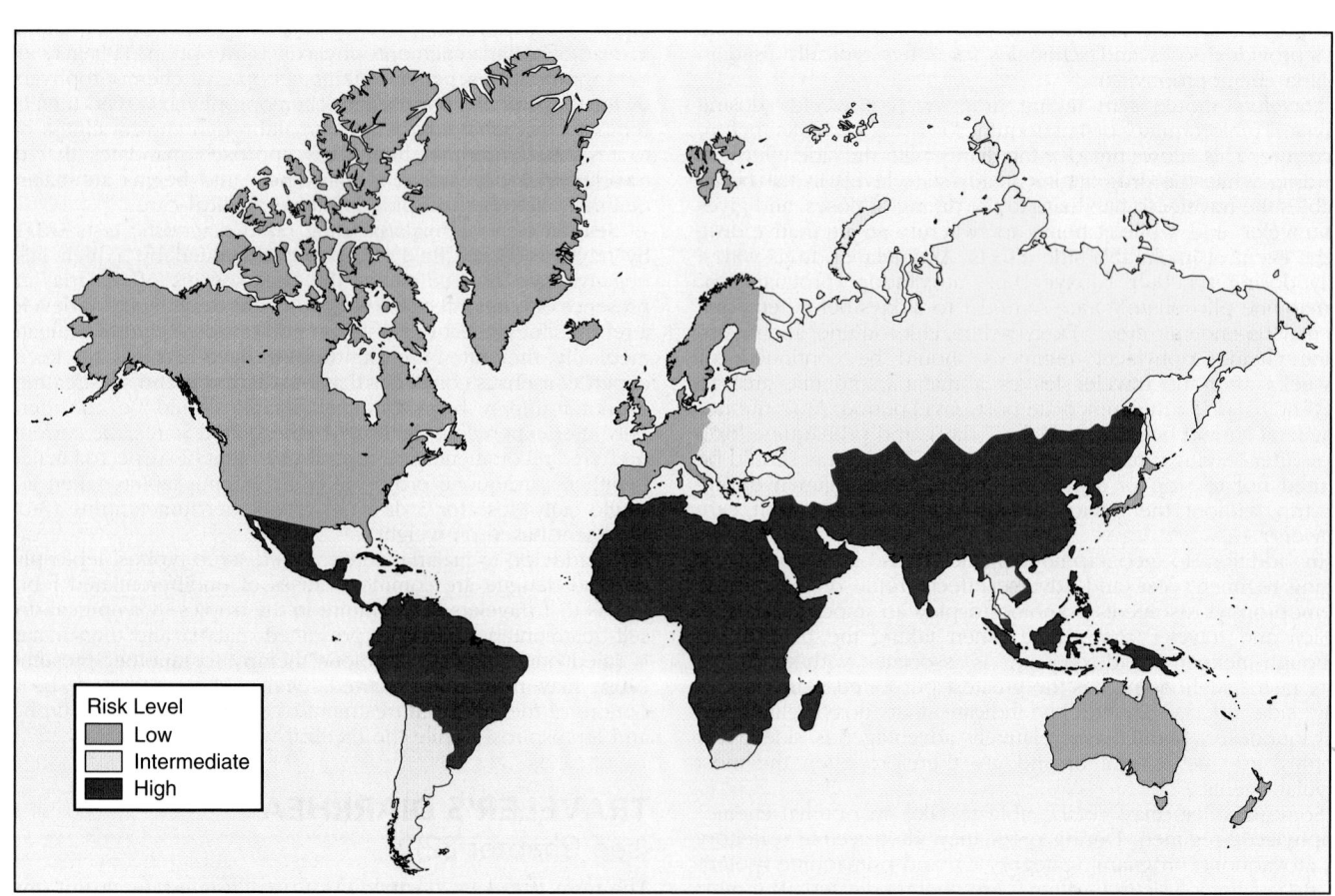

FIGURE 79-5 Risk areas for traveler's diarrhea: low risk, less than 4%; intermediate risk, approximately 8% to 15%; high risk, approximately 40%. Thailand has recently been reclassified as intermediate risk, based on data from Bangkok, Phuket, and Chiang Mai. *(Courtesy R. Steffen, MD.)*

Risk Level
- Low
- Intermediate
- High

guidelines, travelers who are competitive athletes, politicians, on essential business, or going to special events or who have significant underlying comorbidities can be considered for antimicrobial prophylaxis. Confirmation that between 4% and 32% of patients with bacterial gastroenteritis may develop postinfectious IBS[41] and the availability of rifaximin[66] have rekindled interest in chemoprophylaxis of TD.

Using probiotics to prevent TD cannot be recommended at this time because of inconclusive evidence.[56,66] *Lactobacillus* GC, *Saccharomyces boulardii*, and other combination probiotics have been studied with inconclusive results regarding prevention of TD.[66] Anecdotal reports exist favoring use of probiotics for prevention of TD, but direct evidence is lacking.

Bismuth subsalicylate, which is active in large part because of its antimicrobial properties, can successfully prevent approximately 65% of cases of traveler's diarrhea.[66] Disadvantages include cost and dosing regimen, risk of salicylate toxicity, and adverse effects of tongue and stool blackening.

Trimethoprim-sulfamethoxazole (TMP-SMX) and doxycycline are no longer recommended for prevention of TD because of increasing worldwide bacterial resistance. Fluoroquinolones successfully prevent up to 90% of TD cases.[66] Rifaximin is a nonabsorbed antimicrobial agent with an excellent safety profile and usefulness only in the management of enteric diseases. A daily dose of rifaximin may prevent 58% to 70% of cases of TD,[43,66] but it should only be offered as prophylaxis in patients deemed high risk by current guidelines.

SYMPTOMATIC TREATMENT

Fluid replacement has long been the cornerstone of therapy for TD. Dehydration and decreased oral intake are the greatest risks to health in patients with TD. However, when loperamide is used to treat TD, addition of oral rehydration solution (ORS) has not been demonstrated to add to the clinical benefit of loperamide alone.[24] Despite this, dilute fruit juices or flavored mineral water are typically adequate when used for oral rehydration during most episodes of TD. Packets of oral rehydration salts, which can be reconstituted with clean water to make ORS, are available in pharmacies globally.

Table 79-5 lists medications and their doses for symptomatic relief of TD. Agents that offer insufficient or no relief include anticholinergics, adsorbents such as kaolin-pectin preparations, and probiotics (e.g., *Lactobacillus*). Because of insufficient information or lack of availability, calmodulin and enkephalinase inhibitors (zaldaride and racecadotril, respectively) cannot be recommended.

Bismuth subsalicylate reduces the number of stools passed in traveler's diarrhea by approximately 50%.[66] Although BSS can be recommended for mild diarrhea, for moderate to severe disease, loperamide works better and with a faster onset of action.[62] Opiates and diphenoxylate are effective, but CNS and other side effects, plus poor tolerance among elderly persons, limit their usefulness.[66] Because it is safe and efficacious, loperamide has become the symptomatic treatment agent of choice.[66]

The combination of loperamide and an antimicrobial agent is the treatment of choice for TD.[3,66] Loperamide appears to be safe,[24] even in children, as long as doses are kept in the recommended range and the drug is stopped if diarrhea persists despite several days of treatment. Most experts prefer, however, to avoid using loperamide in children under 6 years of age.[56] Although the combination of loperamide and an antibiotic was more efficacious than an antibiotic alone in the treatment of *Shigella* dysentery,[86] most experts prefer not to use loperamide when the patient has high fever or grossly bloody stools, which are usually not present in TD[56] (Figure 79-6).[66]

Traveler's diarrhea can also be treated with empirical antibiotic therapy. An antibiotic with concurrent use of loperamide often leads to relief in a few hours. A fluoroquinolone is the empirical antimicrobial of choice for the treatment of TD for travelers in most parts of the world. Because of increased resistance, specifically found in *Campylobacter jejuni* and *Shigella* strains from patient with TD in South and Southeast Asia, the preferred agent for empirical treatment of TD in these areas is azithromycin. In addition, azithromycin can be used in pregnant women and children (10 mg/kg/day for 3 days) and in patients who do not respond to a fluoroquinolone within 48 hours.[3,27,66] Given resistance patterns worldwide,[66,127] TMP-SMX can no longer be recommended for empirical treatment of TD.[66]

Rifaximin, a nonabsorbed antimicrobial agent with broad activity against enteric pathogens, is effective in treatment of TD in regions of the world where enterotoxigenic *E. coli* is the predominant pathogen.[42,66,117] Rifaximin is not recommended for treating bloody diarrhea or when an invasive pathogen is suspected, limiting its usefulness as a therapeutic agent.

Either a fluoroquinolone or azithromycin can be used for treatment of TD that occurs despite prophylaxis. Table 79-6 provides recommended dosages of antimicrobial agents. A 3-day treatment course has been shown to be as effective as a single dose for the treatment of TD.[66] Travelers who do not respond to empirical antibiotic treatment or who have persistent diarrhea for more than 1 week should seek medical attention.

In the wilderness, *Giardia lamblia* can be an important cause of ongoing diarrhea that is unresponsive to antibiotics. Metronidazole (250 mg three times daily for 5 days), tinidazole (2 g once), or nitazoxanide (500 mg twice daily for 3 days) can be used for empirical treatment of infection with *Giardia*.[56,94]

HIGH-ALTITUDE ILLNESS
(see Chapter 2)

High-altitude illness is generally considered to exist as one of three syndromes: acute mountain sickness (AMS),[19] high-altitude cerebral edema (HACE),[130] or high-altitude pulmonary edema (HAPE).[119] High-altitude illness can occur when travelers ascend rapidly to altitudes greater than 3000 m (9850 feet), particularly if the traveler fails to acclimatize as higher altitudes are reached.[19,69] Of persons who ascend rapidly to moderate altitude (1900 to 3000 m [6250 to 9850 feet]), approximately 25% develop at least mild AMS. Symptoms of AMS are usually experienced within 6 to 12 hours of arrival at altitude and are characterized by headache, fatigue, sleep disturbance, dizziness, and anorexia.[7,18,53,69] These symptoms typically resolve spontaneously over 1 to 3 days, as long as the traveler does not ascend further. The risk of AMS in the individual traveler is uncertain, although travelers with preexisting medical conditions, such as lung disease, kidney disease, hypertension, eye problems, epilepsy, and coronary artery disease, benefit from consulting an altitude medicine expert before travel.[70,73,82]

TABLE 79-5	Recommended Agents for Symptomatic Treatment of Traveler's Diarrhea	
Agent*	**Dosage**	**Comments and Adverse Effects**
Bismuth subsalicylate (Pepto-Bismol)	1 oz PO every 30 minutes for 8 doses	Delayed onset of action. Avoid in persons who should not take aspirin or who are taking anticoagulants. May interfere with absorption of other antimicrobials, notably fluoroquinolones and doxycycline. Black stools and tongue may occur.
Loperamide (Imodium)	4 mg PO, then 2 mg after each loose stool, not to exceed 8 mg daily	Rapid onset of action. Best results occur with loperamide plus an antimicrobial agent. Very well tolerated.

*See text for discussion of other agents; *PO,* orally.

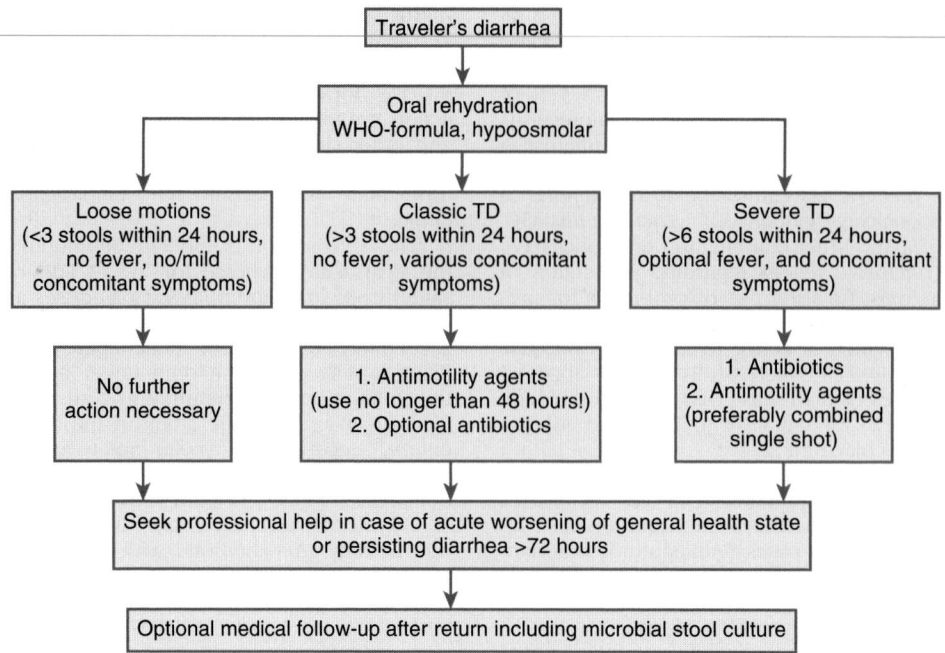

FIGURE 79-6 Management of acute traveler's diarrhea. *WHO*, World Health Organization. *(Modified from Kollaritsch H, Paulke-Korinek M: Durchfallerkrankungen. In Löscher T, Burchard GD, editors:* Tropenmedizin in Klinik und Praxis mit Reise- und Migrationsmedizin, *4th ed, New York, Stuttgart, 2010, Georg Thieme Verlag.)*

Acclimatization is the best way to prevent altitude illness. Gradual ascent is critical. Ideally, travelers should spend a few days ascending to 3000 m (9850 feet), then gradually ascend above 3000 m so that the elevation at which they sleep does not increase more than 300 to 500 m (990 to 1640 feet) per night.[69] The carbonic anhydrase inhibitor acetazolamide (Diamox) hastens acclimatization by increasing ventilation, bicarbonate diuresis, and arterial oxygen levels.[40] A dose of 125 mg twice daily can be taken 1 day before ascent and continued for at least 2 days once the highest altitude is reached.[16,69] Acetazolamide is contraindicated in persons who have had a life-threatening reaction to sulfa drugs. Extremity and circumoral paresthesias occur in 35% to 90% of persons taking acetazolamide, which can be very bothersome for some people, so the trekker should be warned about this potential side effect.[9]

Although dexamethasone has been used for prevention of all three major syndromes of high-altitude illness, it does not hasten acclimatization. Given the potential adverse effects of dexamethasone, which include glucocorticoid toxicity and adrenal suppression, it should only be used for prevention of altitude illness if the patient cannot take another agent.[9,53,69] However, dexamethasone should be used for treatment of AMS/HACE in conjunction with descent.[69]

For climbers who have previously developed HAPE and want prophylaxis for subsequent travel to altitude, nifedipine, 30 mg (extended-release preparation) every 12 hours, can be prescribed.[8,69] Although acetazolamide speeds acclimatization, no data support its role specifically in HAPE prevention.[69] In accordance with Wilderness Medical Society practice guidelines, salmeterol (125 mcg inhaled twice daily),[108] tadalafil (10 mg twice daily), and dexamethasone (8 mg twice daily) are also effective for prevention of HAPE.[69,74] Oxygen and nifedipine are used as adjuncts combined with descent for treatment of HAPE.[92,119]

If AMS symptoms do not resolve or symptoms worsen with evidence of HACE or HAPE, descent is imperative. Descending only 500 to 1000 m (1640 to 3280 feet) can be lifesaving. Acetazolamide (250 mg twice daily) can also be added for treatment of AMS.[69]

Treatment of the symptoms of AMS is also important. Antiemetics such as ondansetron, a serotonin antagonist, can be

TABLE 79-6	Recommended Antimicrobial Agents for the Treatment of Traveler's Diarrhea	
Agent	**Dosage**	**Comments**
Fluoroquinolones		
Norfloxacin	400 mg PO bid for 3 days	Occasional gastrointestinal upset, rash, and allergic reactions. After 24 hours, patients
Ciprofloxacin	500 mg PO bid for 3 days	can reevaluate themselves before taking next dose. If diarrhea persists, or if fever or
Ofloxacin	200 mg PO bid for 3 days*	passage of bloody stools was present, finish 3 days of therapy.
Levofloxacin	500 mg PO qd for 3 days*	
Azithromycin	1000 mg PO once, *or*	A single 500-mg dose suffices when *Escherichia coli* is the predominant enteropathogen;
	500 mg daily for 3 days	agent of choice for diarrhea occurring in Southeast Asia.
Rifaximin	200 mg PO tid for 3 days†	Should not be used to treat persons with fever, grossly bloody stools or in whom an invasive enteropathogen is otherwise suspected.

PO, Orally; *bid,* twice daily; *qd,* once daily; *tid,* three times daily.
*Single doses of ofloxacin and levofloxacin have been studied and appear equivalent to 3-day regimens. A single dose of any fluoroquinolone likely will suffice.
†400 mg PO bid for 3 days was also efficacious in one study.

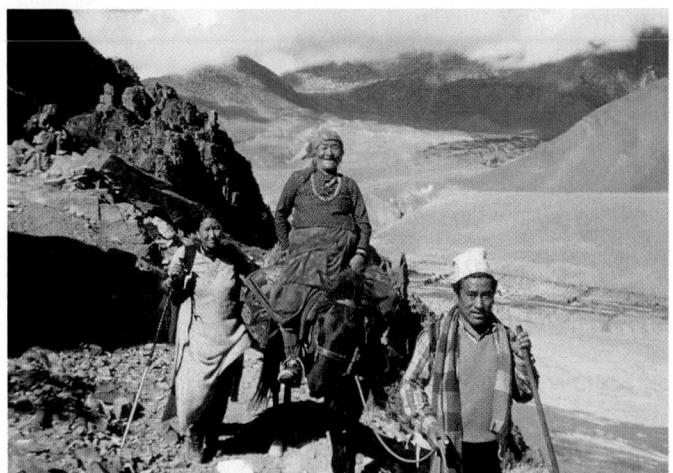

FIGURE 79-7 Pilgrims going to Muktinath sacred temple at approximately 3700 m (12,139 feet) in the Mustang region of Nepal.

effective to treat nausea caused by AMS.[69] Another beneficial effect of acetazolamide (125 mg taken before dinner) is stabilization of periodic breathing, which leads to hypoxemia during sleep. It is important to note that because not all medical problems at high altitude are caused by altitude-related illness, a differential diagnosis must be formulated.[15]

Older travelers and other groups, such as pilgrims traveling to remote, sacred areas at high altitude, may have comorbidities that require prior attention[11,14] (Figure 79-7). Porters may be sojourning to high altitude without adequate clothing or equipment, predisposing them, for example, to hypothermia and frostbite. Trekkers and travelers could check with the trekking agency to ensure that the porters who will accompany them on their wilderness trip are adequately equipped.

RADIATION FROM THE SUN
(see Chapter 16)

Sunscreens should be applied in sufficient quantities to achieve protection from solar radiation.[102] At least 1 oz is required to adequately protect an adult who is average size and wearing a small bathing suit. Sunscreen should be applied at least 20 minutes before sun exposure (or as directed by the manufacturer). Care must be taken to apply sunscreen under the chin and to other skin that might be burned because of reflected ultraviolet (UV) rays. A sun protection factor (SPF) of at least 15 is preferred, but SPF relates mainly to protection against ultraviolet B (UVB) rays. Ultraviolet A (UVA) radiation is also deleterious to skin. Only sunscreens with specific added ingredients offer protection against UVA rays. The consumer should purchase "broad-spectrum" sunscreens with UVA/UVB protection. Although products vary somewhat in their ability to withstand water exposure, any sunscreen should be reapplied at regular intervals after swimming, profuse sweating, or ongoing exposure to the sun. Sunblocks containing emulsified titanium dioxide are useful to protect especially sensitive skin or to block UV exposure in persons taking doxycycline for malaria prophylaxis.[102]

MOTION SICKNESS

Oral scopolamine preparations to prevent motion sickness are convenient for short-duration travel.[114] For longer-duration travel (e.g., cruises, prolonged or frequent automobile or bus trips), transdermal sustained-release scopolamine may be employed. Scopolamine is contraindicated in persons with urinary tract obstruction or glaucoma and can cause dry mucous membranes and drowsiness.[114] Other medications for motion sickness prevention are meclizine and dimenhydrinate, but sedation can be a limiting factor because both cause sleepiness.

TRAVEL MEDICAL KIT

Travelers are advised to prepare a travel medicine kit appropriate for their itinerary. Such a kit should contain adequate supplies of all prescription medications normally taken, medications for malaria and diarrhea, and remedies for common problems such as headache, musculoskeletal pain, allergies, nasal and sinus congestion, cough, jet lag, and constipation. Travelers should be instructed to carry prescription medications in their handheld luggage and copies of their prescriptions, because finding exact replacements for medications can be very difficult in certain parts of the world. A second supply of critically necessary medications might be placed in checked luggage to guard against loss in the event that hand luggage is stolen or misplaced.

Depending on the individual and itinerary, insect repellent, sunscreen, topical antiseptic ointment, antifungal cream or powder, and medications for motion sickness, allergic reactions, and high-altitude illness should be included. Female travelers should be reminded to carry personal sanitary supplies, because disposable tampons and pads may be difficult to obtain in developing countries. Sexually active travelers of both genders should take along a supply of high-quality latex condoms. Kits carried by medical professionals on trips to remote areas (e.g., trekking and climbing expeditions in the Andes or Himalayas) should include equipment for a wider variety of injuries, infections, and medical conditions.

POST-TRAVEL MEDICAL CARE AND SCREENING

Although travel medicine practitioners generally focus on pretravel advice, prevention, and self-treatment of disease, they may be called for advice by returned travelers who are ill. They should be generally familiar with common and life-threatening conditions after travel and how to triage post-travel complaints.[115] Particularly when a traveler presents only with constitutional symptoms, the differential diagnosis may be broad. It can often be narrowed by considering incubation time, geographic area of disease acquisition, immunizations, malaria chemoprophylaxis, dietary habits, insect and rodent exposure, animal bites, and intimate or sexual contact with foreign residents or fellow travelers.

The approach to post-travel illness has been extensively reviewed.[91,106,115] In a traveler who develops high fever weeks, months, or even years after travel in a malarious area, malaria should be actively sought and treated. Many physicians practicing in developed countries are unfamiliar with the clinical presentation of malaria and may fail to include malaria in the differential diagnosis. This holds true for typhoid, typhus, dengue, leptospirosis, and other causes of febrile illness in the traveler recently returned from a developing country. When empirical treatment needs to be started for a returned traveler for a febrile illness without any particular focus and malaria is ruled out, ceftriaxone (for enteric fever) and doxycycline (for rickettsial illnesses and leptospirosis) are good choices.

Diarrhea that develops within approximately the first week after travel can be assumed to be TD and treated empirically. Persistent or remittent diarrhea should prompt a diagnostic workup. Antibiotic-resistant bacterial enteropathogens, intestinal parasites, or even hepatitis may account for prolonged symptoms. TD may unmask inflammatory bowel disease; persistent symptoms raise concern for coincidental biliary tract disease or even intestinal malignancy.

Returned travelers may complain of unusual skin lesions or rashes. Tropical infections that might present with cutaneous manifestations include cutaneous myiasis, cutaneous larva migrans, larva currens, and cutaneous or mucocutaneous leishmaniasis. Because secondary bacterial infection can occur with these conditions, the skin lesion may initially improve with therapy for bacterial skin infections. If the lesion fails to resolve completely, however, consultation with a tropical medicine specialist is recommended.

Many parasitic infections may have unfamiliar signs and symptoms. Eosinophilia may be a clue to some parasitic diseases.

Nonspecific symptoms in a recently returned traveler, in whom common, non–travel-related illness has been excluded, probably should be referred for expert evaluation.

RESOURCES FOR TRAVEL MEDICINE INFORMATION

Telephone Information

Centers for Disease Control and Prevention (CDC) Traveler's Health Hotline: +1-800 CDC-INFO (+1-800-232-4636).

U.S. Department of State Overseas Citizens' Services: U.S.-based telephone number, 888-407-4747, and from overseas, +1-202-501-4444.

Official References

Centers for Disease Control and Prevention (CDC): *Health information for international travel,* New York, 2015, Oxford University Press (revised annually).

Morbidity and Mortality Weekly Report, Centers for Disease Control and Prevention, 1600 Clifton Rd, MS E-90. Atlanta, GA 30333. Telephone: +1-404-498-1150. Subscriptions are available at the website: http://www.cdc.gov.

World Health Organization (WHO): *International travel and health, vaccination requirements and health advice,* 2012, World Health Organization Publications Center USA, 49 Sheridan Avenue, Albany, NY 12215 (revised frequently).

Pretravel Clinic Directories

American Society of Tropical Medicine and Hygiene: http://www.astmh.org.

International Society of Travel Medicine: http://www.istm.org.

Travelers' Clinic Directory

English-Speaking Physicians: International Association for Medical Assistance to Travelers (IAMAT): https://www.iamat.org.

Locations:

1623 Military Rd #279, Niagara Falls, NY, USA, 14304-1745. Telephone: 716-754-4883.

67 Mowat Ave, Suite 036, Toronto, Ontario, M3K 3E3 Canada. Telephone: 416-652 0137.

ACKNOWLEDGMENT

The authors extend special thanks to Charles D. Ericsson for his previous contributions to this chapter.

REFERENCES

Complete references used in this text are available online at expertconsult.inkling.com.

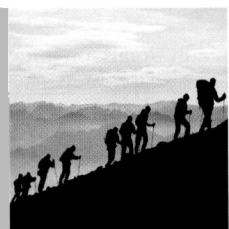

CHAPTER 80

Expedition Medicine

JON DALLIMORE, NICHOLAS P. MASON, AND JAMES MOORE

HISTORICAL BACKGROUND

The desire for exploration runs deep in the human spirit. "The Journey" appears as a recurring theme in historical, religious, and literary records of numerous societies. It is used as a vehicle to describe and understand the mystery of human existence: the Exodus of the Israelites from Egypt and their wandering in the wilderness for 40 years, recorded in the Pentateuch books of the Old Testament; Homer's *Odyssey,* describing the journey of Odysseus home from the Trojan Wars; and the voyage of Marlow along an African river in Conrad's *Heart of Darkness.*

The *Oxford English Dictionary* defines an expedition as "a journey undertaken by a group of people with a particular purpose, especially that of exploration, research or war."[55]

A history of expeditions is beyond the scope of this chapter. Readers are referred to excellent works published on this topic.[1,19] The first clearly documented expeditions are those of Harkhuf, who was the governor of Upper Egypt during the 23rd century BC and whose three explorations along the Nile are recorded on his tomb at Aswan. In modern times, the golden age of expeditions and exploration stretches from the middle of the 19th century to the middle of the 20th century, although it has been mentioned that many of those who occupy a prominent place in the Western imagination were merely recorders of preexisting civilizations, rather than genuine explorers of untrodden ground.[1] Despite this observation, many expeditions that took place during this period illustrate both the varied environments and the recurring controversies that surrounded expeditions then and continue to do so today:

- The jungle explorations of David Livingstone during his 6-year search for the origin of the Nile and the subsequent search for Livingstone by the journalist Henry Stanley[63] were sponsored by the *New York Herald* to further boost the newspaper's circulation.
- The disputed claims of Robert Cook and of the celebrity-obsessed Robert Peary as to who, if either, may have reached the North Pole.[32]
- The ill-fated journey of Robert Falcon Scott to the South Pole, who discovered that he had been beaten by Roald Amundsen by 5 weeks, and then died with the rest of his team on the return journey only 11 miles from the food cache that might have saved them.[20]
- Charles Darwin's scientific voyages[14] to the southern hemisphere in *The Beagle,* which revolutionized our understanding of humans' place on the planet.
- Sven Hedin's expeditions[30] to the deserts of Central Asia.
- Early British attempts on the north side of Mt Everest during the 1920s and 1930s;[67] Charles Houston's expeditions to K2;[37] the first ascent of an 8000-m (26,247-foot) peak by Maurice Herzog;[33] and the ascent of Mt Everest by Sir Edmund Hillary and Tenzing Norgay.[39]

EXPEDITION DEMOGRAPHICS

In the six decades since Hillary and Tenzing stood on the summit of Mt Everest, the demographics of expeditions, particularly mountaineering expeditions to the Great Ranges, have changed dramatically. Although audacious, groundbreaking ascents continue to be made,[11,23] mountains that were once the domain of only an elite group of climbers, who served long apprenticeships to gain the skills necessary to survive in hostile surroundings, now are frequently attempted by less experienced mountaineers.

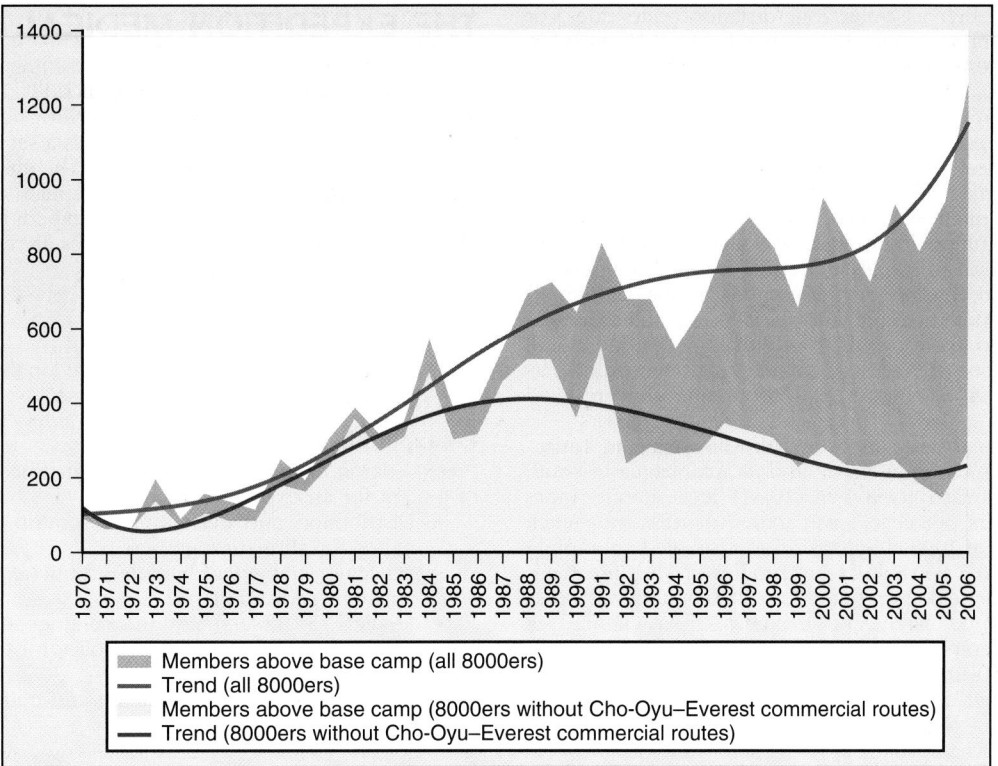

FIGURE 80-1 Climbing activity (members above base camp) for all 8000-m (26,247-foot) peaks between 1970 and 2006, with the Mt Everest and Mt Cho Oyu commercial routes shown separately. (*Data from Salisbury R, Hawley E: The Himalaya by the Numbers, Golden, CO, 2007, The American Alpine Club.*)

Where once expedition members were chosen for their experience and ability to function autonomously, many now utilize the infrastructure of a commercial expedition and purchase the services of highly experienced guides to fulfill their summit dreams. There has also been an explosion in charity treks over the last 20 years, which has contributed to large numbers of unfit wilderness- and altitude-naive individuals being led into an environment for which they may be totally unprepared.

Many accounts from leaders, guides, physicians, and a growing number of books recount expeditions in the commercial era in an unfavorable light.[7,15,31,45,46,61] Figure 80-1, from the Himalayan Database, shows climbing activity on all the 8000-m (26,247-foot) peaks between 1970 and 2006, separating out the commercial routes on Mt Everest and Mt Cho Oyu. This demonstrates the large increase in the number of people attempting these routes. The increased popularity of the highest peaks has been mirrored on lower peaks and by nonclimbing trekkers. Figure 80-2 illustrates the numbers of climbers with permits issued for the 18 Nepalese group B climbing peaks, which includes the most popular peaks below 7000 m (22,966 feet), formerly known as "trekking peaks," between 1996 and 2009. The number of visitors to Sagarmatha National Park of Nepal has increased massively over the last 35 years. Between 1972 and 1973 there were approximately 1400 visitors; 7492 persons visited in 1989 and 25,925 in 2001. Visitor numbers fell during the recent civil unrest but were reported at more than 20,000 in 2004, increased to 30,599 in 2008, and exceeded 37,000 in 2014.[58]

The increase in popularity and accessibility of expeditions has, in all likelihood, been accompanied by a decrease in the experience and wilderness skills of expedition participants. There is certainly a need for data to substantiate the anecdotal accounts of the guides and medical professionals who provide medical cover for these trips or who work at high-altitude rescue posts in Nepal. Increasing familiarity of the general public with wilderness environments and "extreme sports" via the media has resulted in an exponential growth in adventure tourism. The better commercial companies vet participants for appropriate

experience. However, many do not. Strangers, whose primary motivation is completing a trek or climb, are often grouped together. Individuals acclimatize to their environments at differing rates, which presents significant challenges for group leaders adhering to tight schedules. Members are frequently unaccustomed to adapting goals to weather, terrain, or the needs of other team members.

Recently, many countries have seen development of the "charity trek" business, in which supporters of charities attempt

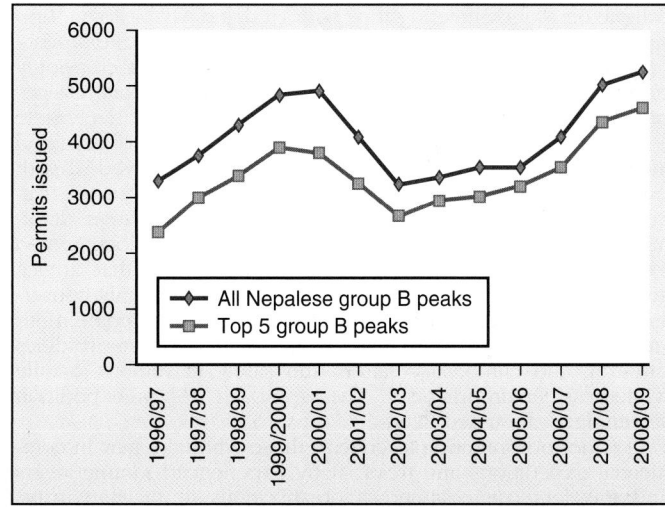

FIGURE 80-2 Permits issued by the Nepal Mountaineering Association for the 18 Nepalese group B climbing peaks, formerly known as "trekking peaks," between 1996 and 2009. The five most popular peaks—Mera, Island Peak (Imja Tse), Pharchamo, Lobuche, and Pokhalde—are grouped separately. (*From Nepal Mountaineering Association.*)

endurance events such as treks, long-distance cycle rides, or summit climbs to raise money through individual sponsorship of these efforts. These have been further popularized by widely publicized "celebrity treks" that make light of the risks.[41,43] Inexperienced participants entirely depend for their safety on the advice, guidance, and care provided by the trek organizers. When this guidance is misplaced, the results can be catastrophic, as the tragic events on the Thorung La in October 2014 illustrate. Despite a well-recognized weather pattern in the Bay of Bengal resulting in unseasonably high snowfalls over the Annapurna region of Nepal, the rapidly deteriorating conditions were ignored, and poorly equipped groups lacking in mountaineering experience and knowledge were led from the safety of shelter to their deaths. More than 50 people died, although the number of Nepalese trekking staff who died has never been finalized, and more than 500 people were rescued by helicopter.[16]

Three very popular destinations are Mt Kilimanjaro in Tanzania, Mt Everest Base Camp in Nepal, and Mt Aconcagua in South America. Mt Kilimanjaro at 5895 m (19,341 feet) attracts more than 50,000 climbers per year, fewer than 70% of whom reach the summit. Between 1996 and 2003, 25 tourists died attempting to reach the summit.[29] Sensible ascent profiles of Mt Kilimanjaro would suggest that trekkers require 7 to 9 days above 2500 m (8202 feet) to ascend safely and maximize their chances of summit success. A comparative study of commercial charity treks found that 15 of 20 treks planned only 4 nights above 2500 m (8202 feet).[38,53] There are many reasons for this. The Tanzanian government levies a charge in excess of $70 per day for each day tourists spend in the national park, and as a result, in an attempt to maximize profits, trekkers are encouraged to climb the mountain as quickly as possible, thereby putting lives at risk. None of the charity groups surveyed offered the option of an acclimatization ascent of Mt Meru (4566 m [14,980 feet]) before attempting Kilimanjaro.

Tourists may choose to ignore sensible ascent profiles, but this is not the case for their employed porters, without whom they would be unable to make an attempt on the mountain. No formal statistics are available, but porters die as a result of altitude illness or from hypothermia when guides push on in bad weather.[44] The difficulties faced by mountain porters are discussed in more detail later.

PREEXISTING MEDICAL CONDITIONS

More participants with complex medical problems are attempting expeditions. There is once again need for international data. The medical advisor to a major British commercial expedition company has described his experience of clients who successfully completed mountaineering trips with Hodgkin's lymphoma; epilepsy; insulin-dependent diabetes; a cardiac pacemaker; post–coronary angioplasty, or post–renal transplant.[35] It is increasingly common for prospective clients to have a history of depression, anxiety, hypertension, asthma, or diabetes.[36] Comparatively little is known about the effects of altitude on the majority of common medical problems.[27] Most published recommendations deal with cardiopulmonary pathologic conditions at altitude but are frequently based on theoretical considerations rather than documented experience.[10,34,47,52,56] The result of this lack of documented experience with preexisting medical conditions is that advice given to potential expedition participants may be unduly conservative and prohibitive. It is apparent that, with appropriate motivation, care, and planning, people with significant comorbidities can trek and climb successfully and safely in remote, hostile wilderness environments.[35] The approach to preexpedition screening is discussed later.

It is not our intention to criticize those who take part in commercial expeditions and treks. Many experienced mountaineers and travelers use commercial organizations to facilitate trips. However, the days of the ad hoc expedition physician, who often learned his or her trade extemporaneously while caring for friends while climbing, are receding. It is in the context of these demographic changes that the 21st-century expedition medical officer (EMO) is expected to operate.

THE EXPEDITION MEDICAL OFFICER

Providing health care in an expedition setting is a specialist area of practice, requiring not only medical skills, but also the ability to live and work in a potentially austere or hostile environment. This distinctive area of practice demands a set of skills and qualities seldom found in other disciplines. The attributes of an experienced EMO may be divided into three main categories that will be required simultaneously during an expedition, but not necessarily in equal measure. These categories are clinical skills, expedition skills, and personal skills.

CLINICAL SKILLS

An EMO's clinical skills can be considered in three further categories, depending on the expedition phase.

Preexpedition Phase

Preexpedition clinical skills are crucial to successful preparation of a team for an expedition:

- Distribution and evaluation of pretrip medical questionnaires for all team members
- Advice on travel vaccinations and, when appropriate, antimalarial medication
- Medical risk assessment and contingency planning
- Developing the expedition's policy for treating indigenous peoples
- Preexpedition medical briefing and training
- Medical kit preparation

Expedition Phase

The EMO needs to have broad-based clinical skills. As in nonexpedition clinical practice, the EMO typically has a specialist interest, such as tropical medicine, envenomation, or high-altitude medicine. However, other than for the situation of the high-altitude environment, this is unlikely to provide the majority of the expedition medical caseload, which will generally consist of common, usually minor, ailments, most frequently gastrointestinal (GI) illnesses, followed by minor orthopedic and trauma problems, respiratory conditions, and other minor medical and surgical problems.[3,13,57] The required clinical skills of the EMO will also be influenced by the location, environment, expedition goals, and preexisting medical conditions.

Location. Remoteness of the expedition location will determine the level of clinical autonomy required. An EMO working in an isolated environment where evacuation is likely to take days or weeks, or with poor communications, would be expected to manage complex and difficult cases that elsewhere would be evacuated. In contrast, a team equipped with good communications and reliable and rapid access to definitive care might be confident working with a much lower level of medical support.

Environment. The expedition environment also influences the medical skills that are required of the EMO. A medic operating above 3000 m (9843 feet) requires familiarity with high-altitude conditions and frequently with cold injuries. This skill set is quite different from that required when operating in a jungle environment, where the likely injuries and illnesses include those resulting from local flora and fauna. Dive, cave, and maritime expeditions each require familiarity with the environment and activity-specific medical problems.

Goals. There is a long tradition within medical and scientific expeditions for the EMO also to be part of the research team to offer specific scientific skills in addition to providing medical care. More often, the EMO may provide medical support for a building project in a developing country, where traumatic injuries are likely to form a significant part of the EMO's workload. Personal development expeditions usually include a mixture of local project work with adventurous activities. Program participants, particularly on youth expeditions, may have psychological problems, so strong personal communication and counseling skills may be advantageous for the EMO. Other expedition types may include working with media production teams or film crews. The scope, duration, and workload encountered on such expeditions vary enormously and have the potential to stress not only one's clinical skills, but also ethical and professional boundaries (see later).

Preexisting Medical Conditions. As previously discussed, increasing numbers of people with complex medical problems are successfully taking part in expeditions. EMOs should be fully familiar and able to deal with many conditions that lie outside their normal area of practice.

The EMO will often be required to possess nursing skills not normally required in the EMO's routine practice. EMOs typically need to record regular vital signs, dress wounds, clean and change soiled patients, and reposition patients to prevent pressure ulcers while awaiting rescue or evacuation. These skills are crucial to delivery of good remote-environment medical care.

Postexpedition Phase

In this phase the EMO will be responsible for the following:
- The expedition medical report
- Postexpedition medical advice for expedition members, including referral to specialists
- Follow-up where appropriate

EXPEDITION SKILLS

Expedition medicine is frequently practiced in challenging and hostile environments. A successful EMO must be capable of functioning autonomously and confidently in such environments and must possess appropriate expedition skills to permit the EMO to work effectively, without jeopardizing the safety of the expedition members. Such skills should be commensurate with the environment where the EMO is required to practice and might include the following:
- Basic camp craft: erecting a tent or hammock efficiently, cooking on a stove, and living safely and comfortably in the expedition environment
- Survival skills appropriate to the type of expedition
- Navigation: a vital skill to enable the EMO to operate safely and independently, and essential for locating casualties and organizing evacuations
- Radio communication skills: proficiency in the use of radios and satellite telephones
- Rope work and mountaineering skills

PERSONAL SKILLS

Desirable personal qualities of the EMO include self-awareness, good communication skills, empathy and compassion, adaptability, a sense of humor, and skills to facilitate conflict resolution.

Self-Awareness

An EMO should have a realistic understanding of his or her strengths and weaknesses and how the EMO interacts with the expedition team. The close proximity of expedition living heightens even minor tensions. The EMO is required to care for any team member who becomes ill or is injured, regardless of personal feelings toward the individual.

Communication Skills

Good communication skills are crucial to effectively eliciting a patient's problems and concerns. This includes communicating information and discussing treatment options and providing psychological and emotional support.[48] These communication skills are not only useful while practicing medicine, but also when working as an arbitrator in times of team conflict. This is discussed in greater detail later.

In the event of a death or serious injury, it may fall to the EMO to deal with the media (see later).

Empathy and Compassion

Emotional support of expedition members forms an important part of the EMO's responsibility. It is not unusual for individuals to place considerable emotional significance on their participation in an expedition. It may be the holiday of a lifetime or may be undertaken as affirmation after bereavement, divorce, or illness. With such psychological weight placed on the expedition, an injury or illness in an alien and threatening environment can result in an emotional response that is far greater than for a comparable problem at home, where the individual has readily available familiar support mechanisms. Increased availability of satellite telephones can actually worsen the situation. When things go wrong, the first reaction of a person is often to want to speak to family or friends. This can heighten the person's natural feeling of homesickness and further compound the emotional response. That said, reassurance that all is well at home can be very comforting when operating in remote areas.

Adaptability

A key quality of any EMO is the ability to adapt practice to the surrounding environment or conditions. Having the expectation that things may not go as planned is the first step in making allowances for these eventualities and preparing accordingly. One practical expression of this is planning a medical kit so that drugs and equipment can be used for more than one problem. The ability to think imaginatively and dynamically in changing circumstances is a crucial attribute of any EMO.

Sense of Humor

A great asset is a good sense of humor, and this is especially true of the EMO. Self-deprecating humor aids humility, promotes courage, and can diffuse tense and difficult situations. This sense of humor must be combined with sensitivity, patience, and compassion; always having a cheerful countenance can be viewed as being flippant or dismissive.

Skills of Conflict Resolution

There will be times of increased stress or pressure. The pressure has the potential to spill into professional conflict. Much that has been written on the art of conflict resolution[28] can probably be summarized in one word—*communication*. The EMO might be in the position of arbitrator during times of expedition conflict. The key to avoiding most issues of conflict is first to examine and resolve them during the expedition planning stage rather than to refrain from discussing them. Clear dialogue should highlight and resolve any issues in the following three categories:
- Decision making and hierarchy
- Expectations
- Purpose, morals, and ethics

Examine all areas that might cause a problem, and work through the issues. It is useful to consider worst-case scenarios and examine resolution strategies.

Honesty and integrity are two key aspects. There is often the temptation to skip uncomfortable issues, with the assumption that they can be addressed in a time of need during the expedition. All expedition team members should be encouraged to discuss uncomfortable issues ahead of time.

Decision Making and Hierarchy. Expedition medics are part of the expedition leadership team. Their decisions may inevitably affect members of the team, and occasionally the entire group. Therefore, it is important that persons making such decisions do so with good judgment and authority. During the planning stages, typical questions that should be asked are the following:
- Who is in overall charge of the expedition?
- What authority does the expedition medic have over factors that may influence the expedition timetable, particularly where safety is concerned?
- If an issue arises between the medic and expedition leader that cannot be solved, who can act as a mediator?

If there is an expedition medical team, establishing clarity of roles, responsibilities, and command hierarchy within this team is vitally important. By having a clear understanding of the skills, knowledge, and background of the medical team members, the lead medical officer will be able to make more informed decisions and avoid professional disagreements. This exercise should be completed at an early stage of the expedition (preferably in the planning stages) to avoid later difficulties.

Expectations. Team members may have differing expectations of the role of the expedition medic. This depends on their individual knowledge and experience and their confidence in caring for themselves. Expedition medics also vary in how much they expect individuals to look after themselves. Initially running daily clinics, where medical issues can be addressed in a more controlled environment, will enable the medical officer to decide on appropriate levels of input.

It is unlikely that the expedition medic will practice at the same intensity as in normal hospital environment, which some individuals might find frustrating. However, periods of intense activity may be required at any stage of the expedition with little or no warning. For many clinicians, this "rapid response" may be unfamiliar unless they are specialists in prehospital or emergency care.

There may be expectations surrounding the level of involvement the medic is expected to have in nonmedical expedition activities. Medical officers who opt out of nonmedical expedition work are likely to cause resentment among other hard-working team members. There must be a balance so that medic involvement in expedition activities and ensuing tiredness does not affect the ability to provide medical care in the event of an emergency.

Medics may find themselves in the position of having to provide medical care for indigenous populations. This remains a contentious subject. There is a requirement to balance help for persons in distress against the potential to undermine local health care systems. Medical officers working on expeditions in or near poor communities will be surrounded by health care problems that in their normal practice could be improved with simple interventions. There is no easy solution, and all team members are likely to find it difficult not to intervene at varying levels. The approach to providing medical care for local populations should be part of preexpedition planning and should be appropriately resourced, because use of expedition medical supplies to treat local populations might put the health of the expedition team at risk.

Another area of expectation to consider is health care and communication equipment. Members should have a clear understanding of access to medical and communication equipment while on expedition.

Conflict Stemming From Expedition Purpose, Ethics, and Morals. All team members also must have a clear understanding of the purpose of the expedition. This is equally important for the EMO. One can easily agree to take part in an expedition based on the location and work, without necessarily taking into consideration ethical or moral issues behind the trip, as in the following examples:
- Commercial adventure/charity expeditions
- TV/film production work—often in exciting locations, but sometimes with potentially questionable ethics
- Impact of the expedition on local people
- Disaster medicine and humanitarian aid work—may be motivated by good intentions, but with the potential to be carried out inappropriately
- Environmental issues associated with the expedition

Ethical considerations permeate every part of an expedition, from the expedition purpose or goal, through delivery of care to expedition members and affiliates, to the impact on host cultures and countries. The four principles of ethical debate and behavior[6] that can be appropriately applied to the individuals and expedition as a whole[2] are as follows:
1. Autonomy—the rights of individuals to decide for themselves to accept or refuse treatment, ideally based on an informed decision-making process
2. Doing of good—beneficence—making sure individuals are working for the benefit of others, through preparation, appropriate training, and delivery of care
3. Avoidance of harm—nonmaleficence—choosing when and when not to intervene and having awareness of the consequences of one's actions (physical, verbal, or emotional) on all parties, including the expedition team members, local communities, and the host country
4. Justice, equity, and fairness

WHO IS QUALIFIED TO BE THE EXPEDITION MEDICAL OFFICER?

The first EMOs were physicians who frequently combined providing medical care with their role as climbers or as physiologic or other scientific researchers.[37,39,62,64,68,71] Skills and knowledge were generally passed on to aspiring EMOs in an informal manner. With growth of commercial expeditions, many physicians with little or no experience or understanding of expedition medicine accepted the offer of a reduced-price place on an expedition. This provided the pretense of medical cover to the group, sometimes with disastrous consequences. The EMO does not necessarily need to be a physician. Emergency medical care on expeditions has been provided safely by registered nurses or paramedics with appropriate training and experience similar to civilian and military prehospital caregivers. There is no information as to how care provided by a nonphysician EMO compares with that provided by a physician; however, UK emergency nurse practitioners have demonstrated equally competent levels of skill and knowledge compared with traditionally trained medical colleagues.[5,59] No established medical specialty encompasses all the skills and knowledge required for the safe practice of expedition medicine.

If expeditions do not have a formal EMO, the preexpedition and postexpedition and expedition phases may be performed by different people. Preexpedition medical screening and planning and provision of training and medical kits may be provided by a corporate (company) EMO, whereas care in the field is delivered by the expedition leader or guide. Nonmedical veterans of many expeditions may be more experienced than the EMO, so, along with appropriately trained expedition leaders, they can provide a high standard of emergency care to expedition members. Box 80-1 gives an example of the lifesaving care provided by an expedition leader to a Nepalese porter during an expedition to Baruntse. The role of telemedicine in providing expert medical support to expeditions without an EMO and the legal responsibility of non–medically qualified leaders providing medical care to members of their group are discussed later. One unique model of care is the Everest Base Camp Medical Clinic (Everest ER), founded in 2003 by Dr. Luanne Freer to address the problems of expeditions on Mt Everest. The temporary clinic offers medical care to all expeditions on the Nepalese side of Mt Everest during the spring climbing season.[18,22]

Paralleling the explosive growth in commercial expeditions and increased formalization of all aspects of medical training are many courses around the world offering some form of wilderness, expedition, or mountain medical training. In August 1997, the medical commissions of the International Mountaineering and Climbing Federation (UIAA), International Committee on Alpine Rescue (ICAR), and International Society for Mountain Medicine (ISMM) established minimal requirements for courses in mountain medicine. These standards, last updated in 2010, have been adopted across many countries. There are now 17 UIAA-ICAR-ISMM–approved basic diploma courses in mountain medicine available worldwide. Courses are offered in France, Germany, Italy, United Kingdom, Norway, Canada, United States, Japan, and Nepal with supplementary courses in expedition medicine and rescue available in several countries.[54] With growing concern about possible litigation from expedition clients (see Legal and Ethical Considerations, later), there should be consensus among expedition medical providers about the core knowledge and clinical competencies required to practice expedition medicine in each of its major environments. Table 80-1 provides details of the UIAA-ICAR-ISMM syllabus for the Diploma in Mountain Medicine.

Satellite expeditions medically coordinated from a single, central base camp allow utilization of broader skill sets and abilities, with the most qualified or experienced medic able to provide advice or support from a central location (Figure 80-3). The numerous variations based on this theme might include having the senior EMO based with the group deemed at highest medical risk, with outpost medical support provided from that location.

BOX 80-1   Nepali Porter with Severe HACE and HAPE

A 50-year-old Nepali porter working for a commercial expedition that did not have a medical officer was taken ill at Makalu Base Camp (5450 m [17,881 feet]) in Nepal. The following is a summary of the excellent contemporaneous notes made by the expedition leader outlining the lifesaving treatment he gave to the porter:

08:20: Porter found to be semiconscious, vomiting, and to have frothy, blood-stained fluid around his mouth.

08:30: According to expedition medical protocols, the porter was given 8 mg of dexamethasone IM. He was unable to cooperate to swallow nifedipine. Shortly afterwards, the porter fitted and lost consciousness. His breathing became labored, irregular, and noisy. He was placed in a hyperbaric bag and monitored.

08:45: Contacted Kathmandu office of expedition company and confirmed need for urgent helicopter evacuation.

09:00: Regained consciousness but became distressed and disorientated. He was removed from the hyperbaric bag but seized again and once again rapidly lost consciousness.

09:10: The porter was placed back in the hyperbaric bag at 30° and monitored.

10:30: Intermittently regained consciousness but now appears unconscious. Unresponsive to sound. Respiratory rate 20 breaths/min.

11:15: Removed from hyperbaric bag. Had vomited and been incontinent of urine. Slurred speech and unable to stand. Still unable to take nifedipine. Rapidly deteriorated and put back in hyperbaric bag after it had been cleaned and his clothes changed.

14:00: Conscious and alert. Removed from hyperbaric bag. Complaining of headache. Began to become increasingly drowsy so placed back in hyperbaric bag.

14:30: Conscious and alert. Given further 4 mg dexamethasone IM. Able to take 20 mg nifedipine orally. Remained conscious and alert.

17:00: Remains out of hyperbaric bag, sleeping but rousable. Paracetamol 1 g.

20:30: Given further 4 mg dexamethasone IM and 20 mg oral nifedipine. Headache easing.

The porter was monitored overnight by his brother making observations every hour. He continued to receive regular dexamethasone and nifedipine. The following morning, when he was evacuated by helicopter to Kathmandu, his condition was much improved, although he remained very ataxic. He was cared for at the Kathmandu offices of the expedition company, where he was also reviewed by a Western physician, and made a complete recovery.

From Paul Donovan, expedition leader with Jagged Globe.
HACE, High-altitude cerebral edema; *HAPE,* high-altitude pulmonary edema; *IM,* intramuscularly.

TABLE 80-1   UIAA-Approved Basic Syllabus for the Diploma in Mountain Medicine

Basics of	Minimal Time (hr)	Instructors	Training
Altitude	3	High altitude experienced doctor	Theory
Hypothermia	4	Experienced doctor	Theory
Avalanche	4	Experienced doctor + mountain guide or avalanche/ski patroller	Theory + practical
Frostbite	2	Experienced doctor	Theory
Submersion and immersion in water	1	Experienced doctor	Theory
Heat and solar radiation	1	Experienced doctor	Theory
Survival in the mountains/exhaustion	4	Experienced doctor	Theory + workshop
Children and mountains	1	Experienced doctor (pediatrician)	Theory
Practical traumatology	4	Experienced doctor	Workshop
Weather	1	Mountain guide or meteorologist	Theory
Rescue techniques (introduction)	1	Experienced mountain rescue doctor, team member and/or mountain guide	Theory
Rescue techniques (practical)	2	Experienced mountain rescue doctor, team member and/or mountain guide	Practical
Mountaineering techniques in summer and winter, and personal mountaineering equipment	18	Mountain guides	Practical
Information About			
Nutrition	1	Experienced doctor or nutritionist	Theory
Exercise physiology	1	Physiologist or experienced doctor	Theory
Travel medicine	1	Experienced doctor	Theory
Navigation in the mountains	4	Mountain guide	Workshop + practical
Personal first-aid kit	1	Experienced doctor	Theory
Legal aspects	0.5	Experienced lawyer or doctor with medico-legal experience	Theory
Stress management	1	Experienced doctor	Theory
Preexisting clinical conditions	3	Experienced doctor	Theory
Analgesia in the field	1	Experienced doctor	Theory
International mountaineering organizations	0.5		Theory
Additional subjects selected by the course organizer	40		Theory, workshop + practical
Total	**100 hr**		

From http://www.theuiaa.org/upload_area/files/1/DIMMreg_20101-3.pdf.
UIAA, International Mountaineering and Climbing Federation.

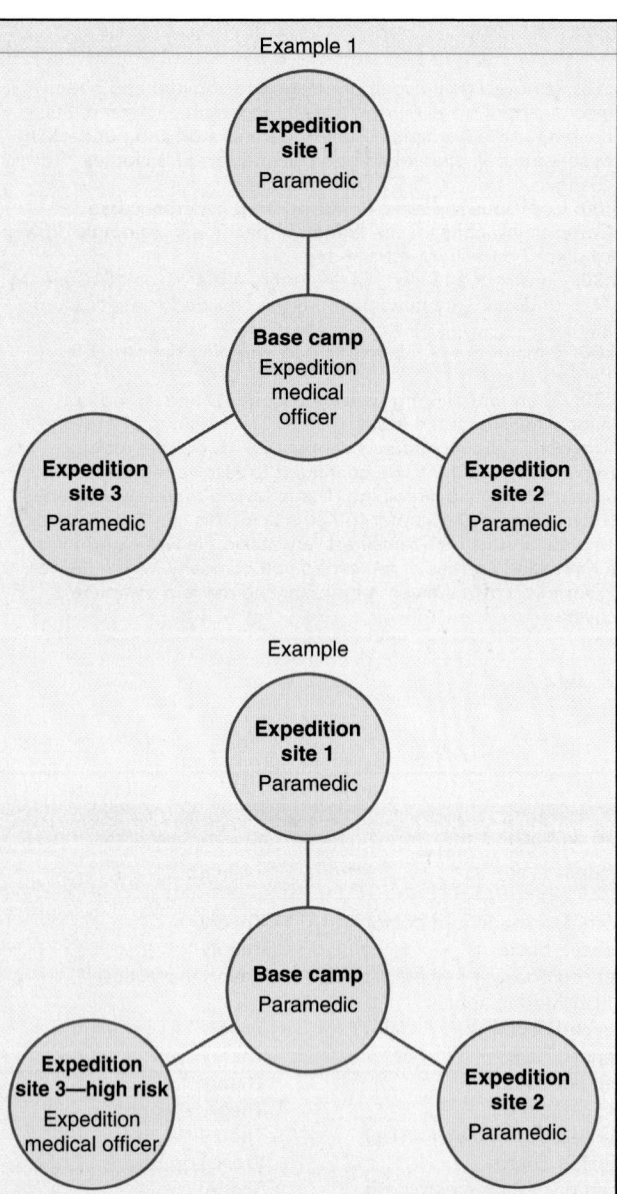

Example 1

Expedition site 1
Paramedic

Base camp
Expedition medical officer

Expedition site 3
Paramedic

Expedition site 2
Paramedic

Example

Expedition site 1
Paramedic

Base camp
Paramedic

Expedition site 3—high risk
Expedition medical officer

Expedition site 2
Paramedic

FIGURE 80-3 Allocation of medical staff according to level of risk and skills required at each expedition site. In Example 1 the expedition medical officer (EMO) with the highest level of skill and competency is based centrally with equal access to each expedition site. In Example 2 the EMO with the highest level of skill and competency has been allocated to the expedition site with the highest risk.

EXPEDITION MEDICAL PLANNING

The EMO should aim to prevent illness and injury and to treat as quickly and appropriately as possible persons who sustain injuries or become unwell. The chance of successfully achieving these aims is greatly increased by careful preexpedition planning, which should include medical screening of all expedition members and risk assessment and management. Other team members should also receive preexpedition medical training. Box 80-2 provides an expedition medical planning checklist.

MEDICAL SCREENING

Persons with special health care needs should be involved with careful preexpedition planning to aim for a safe and successful trip. Certain chronic illnesses and disabilities mean that some individuals will be unable to participate fully, but with forethought, they can still enjoy a worthwhile challenge or experience. The stresses and strains of expedition life may exacerbate

BOX 80-2   Expedition Medical Planning Checklist

☐ Advise and brief the team on medical issues (general and specific to expedition environment).
☐ Undertake medical screening of all expedition members.
☐ Encourage all participants to have a preexpedition dental checkup.
☐ Provide advice on immunizations and malaria prophylaxis.
☐ Organize appropriate first-aid training for all expedition members.
☐ Obtain, pack, and transport medical supplies and kits.
☐ Undertake a risk assessment, and prepare associated documents.
☐ Investigate local health services and medical facilities.
☐ Anticipate and plan evacuation of a severely ill or injured person from each part of the expedition.
☐ Consider the effects of weather and natural disasters such as tsunami, volcanic eruption, and earthquake.
☐ Prepare a communication network in case of evacuation.
☐ Organize medical insurance with full emergency evacuation coverage.
☐ Confirm that professional indemnity insurance will cover expedition medical officer role.

underlying joint problems, inflammatory bowel disease, respiratory illnesses, angina, and other long-standing health issues. The main concerns are that if conditions worsen, definitive medical care may be very remote and evacuation times prolonged.

Before a decision can be made regarding an expedition team member's suitability for the proposed trip, it is essential to consider all risks that may lead to serious illness, or even death. For some persons, a different trip with less demanding objectives may be more suitable.

All participants should complete a detailed health questionnaire (Box 80-3). The information may prompt a request for further details from the patient, family physician, or specialist. Undeclared medical conditions may mean that the EMO is not in a position to give comprehensive medical care because of inadequate knowledge or lack of appropriate medications. It is important to determine the severity of the condition and whether the disease is stable, worsening, or improving. One useful predictor of future performance is the individual's prior ability to cope with wilderness travel in other isolated or remote areas. The individual may need to be involved in the final decision and take into consideration expedition duration and environment, presence of medical support, field communications, remoteness of location, and evacuation options.

All team members should be fully financially insured. Incomplete medical disclosure may invalidate insurance coverage.

GENERIC PREEXPEDITION ADVICE FOR PERSONS WITH PREEXISTING MEDICAL CONDITIONS

Any illness should be stable and well controlled before departure, and the individual, family physician or specialist, and EMO must

BOX 80-3   Health Questionnaire for Preexisting Medical Conditions

• Do you have a history of convulsions, asthma, or diabetes?
• Do you have any allergies?
• Have you ever had any heart problems?
• Have you experienced recurring back or joint problems?
• Please give details of any psychological or psychiatric illness, including eating disorders, deliberate self-harm, overdoses, depression, anxiety, or psychosis.
• Do you have any objections to any form of treatment, including blood transfusions or immunizations?
• Do you have any disabilities or ongoing medical problems?
• Do you take any medications?
• Any other medical conditions including surgical operations?

agree on a self-management plan. For example, in the case of a person with diabetes, a summary of the condition and recent test results, such as serial blood glucose levels, electrocardiogram, hemoglobin A_{1c}, and medications, are important data points for anyone who assumes care of the individual. Additional items of medical equipment may be required, so the EMO may need to acquire familiarity with uncommon medications and new equipment. During the expedition, support and advice will be readily available from the EMO. Where sufficient communications exist, it may be possible to obtain advice from an individual's physicians at home, but this should not be relied on. Potential risks and possible difficulties obtaining further medical help should be discussed openly beforehand.

Where appropriate, with conditions such as diabetes or epilepsy, other team members should have an understanding of the individual's condition and should be able to give emergency treatment if required, such as for management of hypoglycemia or convulsions. Explicit guidelines about actions to be taken with any warning signs of a worsening condition should be documented in advance. An action plan for asthmatic patients can be downloaded at http://www.asthma.org.uk/advice-asthma-action-plan.

It is important that, where appropriate, all participants are aware of and prepared to accept the risks that an individual's preexisting medical condition can bring to an expedition, such as the need for evacuation. The individual must be physically and psychologically prepared for the planned expedition. Training in a similar environment will enable an assessment to be made of how an individual will cope during the expedition.

If there have been problems during a trip, prompt reassessment should be advised on return to the home country. It is important to send a report of any significant problems to the patient's physician.

VACCINATIONS, MALARIA CHEMOPROPHYLAXIS, AND PERSONAL MEDICATION

Vaccinations

The EMO should ensure that all expedition participants have received complete proper childhood vaccinations schedule. Many communities visited by expedition teams will be vaccine naive, having never had the opportunity to receive immunizations. Ensuring childhood vaccinations reduces the chance of contracting vaccine preventable disease and, more importantly, not introducing it into local populations. Certain vaccinations recommended for travel will not be part of the childhood schedule. Expert advice should be sought as to which vaccines are appropriate for the expedition, based on location, expedition activities, and access to definitive and reasonable health care. Some countries may demand certification of vaccination, such as for yellow fever. Information about appropriate travel vaccinations can be found at http://www.cdc.gov/vaccines/schedules/index.html or www.nathnac.org.

Malaria Chemoprophylaxis

People undertaking expeditions to the tropics should obtain accurate advice regarding malaria chemoprophylaxis (see Chapter 40). One must ensure the following:
- Take the malaria chemoprophylaxis appropriate for the area to be visited.
- Take tablets as prescribed, and remember to take them for the recommended time after leaving the malaria risk area.
- Malaria chemoprophylaxis is never 100% reliable

Personal Medication

Individuals taking personal medication should ensure that:
- They have sufficient quantities for the duration of the trip, plus extra in case of emergency or delays.
- Medication can be stored appropriately.
- Medication does not contravene any international border restrictions (see www.incb.org for more accurate information about transporting medications across borders).
- Medication is not likely to interact with travel vaccinations or malaria chemoprophylaxis.

BOX 80-4 Formal Risk Assessment

- [ ] Hazard
- [ ] Risk
- [ ] Risk level
- [ ] Control measures
- [ ] Additional action
- [ ] Review mechanism

Potential Hazards
- Physical
- Biologic
- Chemical
- Human-made
- Personal safety
- Environmental impact

Personal medication should be carried in hand luggage to help prevent it from becoming lost.

Medication should be accompanied by an official letter detailing its intended use and the prescribing authority. This should be signed by the prescriber, with an official stamp, and, where possible, the needed language translations. Individuals should consider the possibility of resupplying medicine in country.

RISK MANAGEMENT

Potential risks to expedition members should be systematically identified and control measures instituted to reduce the risk.[4] This easily neglected exercise is an important part of expedition planning. The EMO should work closely with the expedition leader to formulate a formal risk assessment (Box 80-4). All team members must be fully informed before departure of the risks to which they are likely to be exposed and the means of hazard control, and they must understand that it is not possible to eliminate all risk completely (Box 80-5). With this information, they can make an informed decision about their participation in the expedition.
- A *hazard* is anything that may cause harm. Examples are fall from a height, rockfall, motor vehicle crash, and high environmental temperature.
- The *risk* is the chance that somebody could be harmed by a hazard. The chance may be very low, but there may be very serious consequences.

Risk assessments should periodically be reviewed during the expedition because hazards change. For example, while ascending Mt Kilimanjaro in Tanzania (5895 m [19,341 feet]), the hazards change from those of a tropical environment to those of a high-altitude environment.

BOX 80-5 Briefing the Expedition Team

Topics to Cover for Hazard Control and Risk Reduction
- [ ] The importance of clean water and hygienically prepared food
- [ ] Dangers of the sun—sunburn, dehydration, and heat illnesses
- [ ] The need for good personal hygiene to prevent skin and other infections
- [ ] Promoting sexual health by avoiding risky sexual activity
- [ ] Awareness of emotional problems such as isolation, homesickness, and conflict within the group
- [ ] Drug-taking behavior must be avoided, and alcohol should be used only in moderation
- [ ] Avoiding bites and stings, use of insect repellents, and dangers of walking barefoot
- [ ] Special risks for some activities, such as high-altitude mountaineering, scuba diving, kayaking, and sailing
- [ ] Appropriate preexpedition immunizations and choice of suitable antimalarials
- [ ] Preexpedition fitness, including a dental checkup
- [ ] Preparation of a suitable personal first-aid kit and first-aid training tailored to the environment and activities planned

The most serious risks while traveling are falls and other injuries; drowning; road traffic collisions; altitude illness and heatstroke; serious infections (malaria, blood borne viruses), and homicide.[4] Although the list is not exhaustive, Table 80-2 highlights the environment-specific hazards and risks that should be systematically evaluated during risk assessment.

Country-Specific Risks

Detailed information about safety and security, local laws and customs, entry requirements, and health risks for all countries can be obtained through the following websites:

- Australia: http://www.dfat.gov.au
- Canada: http://www.voyage.gc.ca
- United Kingdom: http://www.gov.uk/foreign-travel-advice
- United States: http://www.travel.state.gov
- U.S. Centers for Disease Control and Prevention: http://www.cdc.gov/travel
- World Health Organization: http://www.who.int

Before departure, or shortly after arrival on location, local medical facilities, local and regional hospitals, clinics, and pharmacies should be identified and, if possible, inspected. Embassies often provide useful information regarding good-quality medical

TABLE 80-2 Expedition Risks and Hazards: General and Specific to Environment

Setting/Cause	Hazard/Risk
Hazards Common to Most Expedition Environments	
Solar radiation	Sunburn
High or low ambient temperatures	Heat and cold injuries
Hot, dry environments	Dehydration and heat exhaustion
Poor water and food quality	Gastrointestinal illnesses
Isolation	Unfavorable psychological reactions
Overcrowding	Upper respiratory and other infections
Attitudes and behavior	Sexually transmitted infections, injuries
Wildlife Hazards	
Dogs	Infected bite wounds and rabies
Leeches	Wound infections
Snakes	Envenomation
Ticks	Typhus and other tick-borne diseases
Hippos	Animal attacks, capsizing of boats
Parasites	Infestations
Bears	Multiple injuries
Local Conditions	
Lack of shelter	Hypothermia
Dangerous roads	Road traffic collisions
Open fires and stoves	Burns and scalds
Endemic diseases	Malaria, schistosomiasis, dengue fever, encephalitis, blood borne viruses
Human factors	Assault, kidnapping, terrorism, conflict
Environment-Specific Hazards	
High Altitude	
Altitude	Altitude-related illness (acute mountain sickness [AMS], high-altitude cerebral edema [HACE], high-altitude pulmonary edema [HAPE], altitude-related cough)
Solar radiation	Sunburn and ultraviolet (UV) keratitis (snowblindness)
Cold	Hypothermia and tissue cold injury
Avalanche and rockfall	Traumatic injury
Blizzard	Becoming lost and hypothermic
Lightning	Lightning injuries
Climbing	Falls and traumatic injury
Snow holing	Carbon monoxide poisoning
	Asphyxiation
Desert	
Solar radiation and extreme heat	Sunburn and heat illnesses
Lack of water	Dehydration, collapse
Snakes and scorpions	Envenomation
Jungle	
Heat/high humidity	Heat exhaustion, syncope, prickly heat
River crossing	Drowning and being swept downstream
Deadfall	Injuries
Plant life	Skin reactions, anaphylaxis
Animal and insect	Snakebite, infected bites, arbovirus infections
Maritime	
Sun and wind	Sunburn/windburn and UV keratitis
Cold and heat	Thermal injuries
Saltwater	Saltwater boils
High waves	Seasickness, drowning
Ropes and pulleys	Hand trauma
High rigging	Falls and traumatic injury
Isolation	Interpersonal conflict, adverse psychological reactions

services; some insurance companies list approved hospitals or local physicians. In some parts of the world, emergency assistance may be obtained from the military. This includes search and rescue support using helicopters, inflatable rafts, and all-terrain vehicles. National parks staff and nongovernmental organizations (NGOs) may offer support in certain circumstances. In some parts of the world, there is risk from natural disasters. For further information, see http://www.preventionweb.net/english/hazards/.

EXPEDITION MEDICAL TRAINING

When operating in wilderness areas, it is common to provide medical care in remote hostile environmental conditions. The EMO will usually carry out his or her role independently with finite medical supplies, sometimes with limited communications and unreliable casualty evacuation facilities. Patient evacuation may be delayed for many reasons. When the EMO is required to look after more than one patient or casualty, resources will be stretched to the limit. It is therefore important that expedition team members be trained to give first aid and second aid. The exact nature of medical training for expeditions to wilderness areas should be tailored to suit the environment. For example, it may need to include training in tropical illnesses, malaria, cold injury, and high-altitude illness. Many of these subjects are not covered in "standard" first-aid courses. Advanced techniques that should be taught include use of select prescription medications, use of specialized rescue equipment, and reduction of simple fractures and dislocations.[12] All team members should have completed basic first-aid training. Essential topics for persons who operate in wilderness areas are the following:

- Safe approach to the injured casualty, including scene assessment
- Basic life support, including management of cardiac arrest and choking
- Understanding the causes of shock and its field treatment, especially control of bleeding
- Care of the unconscious patient, including potential causes of loss of consciousness in the expedition's environment
- Management of acute medical problems (e.g., asthma, hypoglycemia, convulsions)
- Packaging and moving patients, including stretchers and logrolling
- Patient medical reports

There is no clear consensus in the United States regarding "industry standards" for wilderness first aid.[69] In the United Kingdom, British Standard 8848 was established in April 2007 and revised in 2014. This simply states, "The venture provider shall check the first aid qualifications of the leadership team and ensure that they are commensurate with the needs of the venture."[9] Boxes 80-6 and 80-7 list common expedition complaints and recommended training courses for wilderness first aid.

EXPEDITION MEDICAL KIT PREPARATION

Choosing, assembling, and packing an expedition medical kit takes time and effort. Factors dictating the composition of medical kits are as follows:

- Number of expedition team members, including local staff
- Duration of the expedition
- Distance from medical help
- Presence of endemic diseases or environmental hazards, such as high altitude and extreme cold
- Type of activities, such as diving, rock climbing, vehicle-based travel, sailing, or caving
- Medical skills of the team
- Preexisting medical problems of the group members
- Cost, weight, and bulk

It is not possible to prepare for every possible eventuality, and there is always a balance between being underprepared and having too much in a kit.[40] For detailed recommendations regarding medical kit contents, see Appendix to this chapter.

BOX 80-6 Common Injuries and Illnesses during Wilderness Expeditions

Common Expedition Complaints
- Blisters
- Orthopedic injuries, including fractures and dislocations
- Splinters and other foreign bodies

Common Expedition Medical Conditions
- Infections, such as diarrhea, upper respiratory, and urinary
- Asthma
- Convulsions
- Fainting
- Headaches

Serious Medical Problems
- Anaphylaxis
- Chest pain
- Abdominal pain
- Cough and shortness of breath

Important Injuries
- Head and spinal injuries
- Chest injuries
- Abdominal trauma
- Pelvic injuries

Environmental Injuries
- Altitude-related illness
- Heat illnesses—heat exhaustion and heatstroke
- Cold injuries—frostbite and hypothermia
- Diving injuries
- Venomous bites and stings

Patient Handling
- Moving, lifting, and straightening of injured casualties
- Patient transportation, including improvised stretchers

Diagnostic Equipment

This should include simple diagnostic apparatus such as stethoscope, sphygmomanometer, otoscope, urine testing strips, lightweight pulse oximeter, near-patient malaria testing kits, and low-reading thermometer.

Medical Kit Packaging

Containers should be lightweight, robust, and allow easy identification of the contents. Depending on the environment, the containers should protect from impact, crush, dust, moisture, and other contamination. Medications may need to be protected from extremes of hot and cold (see Appendix: Drug Stability in the Wilderness).

In general, liquid medicines are best avoided because of weight and bulk. Tablets should be in blister packs to protect from damage during transport. Glass ampules are less robust than plastic ampules; both need to be protected from extremes of cold and heat. For insulin, snakebite serum, and other medications that must be kept cold, specialized pouches are available, such as those produced by Frio (http://www.friouk.com). Food vacuum flasks have been used to protect medication from desert heat and Arctic cold.

When preparing the medical kit, related items should be packed together. For example, dressing materials should be in one box, tablets in another. This means that many different boxes do not have to be opened to deal with one clinical problem. It

BOX 80-7 Recommendations for Comprehensive Training Courses for Wilderness Medicine

Basic First Aid
- Cardiopulmonary resuscitation (CPR) and choking management
- Control of bleeding
- Wound and burn management
- Bone and joint medicine
- Treatment of the unconscious casualty

is helpful to mark clearly the contents on the lid of each box, so that the boxes do not need to be opened to determine the contents.

Problems of Transporting Controlled Drugs

Morphine and other controlled drugs should be taken on overseas expeditions only under strict supervision. Some countries impose stringent laws,[26] including the death penalty, for possession of opiates. In the United Kingdom, a Home Office license is required to export controlled drugs, but this does not protect the individual from applicable laws in other countries.[25] If controlled drugs are dispensed, this should be recorded in a controlled drugs register.

A valuable source of information on carrying medications can be found through the International Narcotics Control Board.[42] Information is heavily weighted toward narcotics and drugs that affect the central nervous system, such as benzodiazepines, and the website contains information only for countries willing to submit data. Nevertheless, it is a valuable resource for the EMO. The EMO should pay particular attention to any medications that affect the central nervous system, any that can be abused (e.g., steroids), injectables, and large quantities of certain medications. As with personal medication, the medical kit and medication should be accompanied by an official letter, detailing the kit's intended use, the person for whom it is intended, and the prescribing authority. This should be signed by the prescriber, with an official stamp, and where possible, needed language translations.

Treating Infections

Antibiotics and antimicrobials are frequently used on expeditions to treat or prevent GI illness, wound and skin infections, respiratory infections, and important tropical illnesses such as malaria, typhus, and leptospirosis. A range of familiar antibiotics should be carried to cover common, important infections. The chosen antimicrobials should be tailored to local resistance patterns, where known, and should cater to persons who may have antibiotic allergies.

Analgesia

Many injuries and illnesses are painful, so a comprehensive range of analgesics should be available. Analgesia should be offered regularly to control pain. Ketamine may be considered by experienced practitioners for its analgesic and anesthetic properties.

Other Essential Drugs

Regardless of whether there is an asthmatic team member, all expedition medical kits should include a salbutamol inhaler and medications to treat anaphylaxis: injectable chlorphenamine, epinephrine, and prednisone or hydrocortisone. Both motion sickness and GI illness can cause incapacitating nausea and vomiting. Suitable antiemetics include ondansetron (Zofran), cyclizine (Marezine, Marzine, and Emoquil in U.S.), and prochlorperazine (Compazine, Stemzine, Buccastem, Stemetil, and Phenotil). The latter may be given intramuscularly or via the buccal route. Other injectable drugs to consider include local anesthetic agents, parenteral antibiotics, and intravenous (IV) fluids.

Creams and Ointments

Antiseptic creams, antibiotic ointment for conjunctivitis, antifungal preparations, a mild corticosteroid ointment, and antimicrobial cream or ointment for burns should be included in all kits.

Emergency Equipment

Depending on the expedition, the EMO may consider advanced airway equipment if the provider is competent in its use, and if rapid evacuation is possible in the event of using such a device, or the condition requiring such a device can be managed, unsupported, for a prolonged period. Similar consideration should be given to the appropriateness of oxygen therapy. Transporting oxygen in useful quantities presents major logistical challenges that will be beyond the scope of many expeditions.

For persons operating in areas where they may encounter severe trauma, a combat application tourniquet and QuikClot

may be required for treatment of torrential hemorrhage. It is important to base the decision to carry such equipment on a realistic assessment of the likelihood of a safe and rapid evacuation of any casualty requiring such interventions. Many different emergency splints are available to manage orthopedic injuries. Improvisation is always an option.

Obtaining Medical Supplies

Purchasing medical supplies for expedition medical kits can be quite expensive. Some pharmaceutical companies may donate drugs, particularly if there is recognition of sponsorship. Hospitals and pharmacists may provide drugs at their cost. Many drugs can be purchased less expensively in destination countries, but there are important concerns regarding efficacy and counterfeit drugs.

Base Camp and Satellite Medical Kits

A comprehensive medical kit should be kept at base camp.[25] Satellite camps should have smaller kits tailored to the size of the group, medical training of team members, and likelihood of serious illness or injury. In addition, each team member should carry personal medication, with some spares (Box 80-8). For more prolonged expeditions or remote field stations, mechanisms must be in place to resupply medical kits.

Medical Kits for Special Environments

The same basic medical kit can be used in many different theaters of operation; however, modifications will be required, depending on activities and environment[60]:

- *Tropical regions:* The kit should include spare antimalarial drugs and near-patient testing kits, snakebite antivenom (controversial), and larger quantities of antibiotics for wound and skin infections. It is worth considering IV fluids for treatment of dehydration and heat illness.
- *Mountaineering expeditions:* Trips above 4000 m (13,123 feet) must include acetazolamide, dexamethasone, and nifedipine. Larger groups may consider bringing a portable hyperbaric chamber and oxygen cylinders. Chemical oxygen generators (e.g., emOx) are available in some countries.
- *Maritime and diving trips:* Seasickness medication, ear drops for otitis externa, and treatments for marine envenomation should be considered.

COMMUNICATIONS TECHNOLOGY

Expedition communication technology consisting of two-way radios (AM, high-band FM, or UHF), mobile telephones, or satellite telephones is increasingly financially accessible to even small and lightweight expeditions. Many companies now offer ready-to-use expedition communication packages complete with web hosting.

If satellite communications are part of the expedition kit, ensure that the correct documentation and visa paperwork is in place. Some countries (e.g., India) will not allow personal satellite phones into the country without appropriate documentation. Arriving without this is likely to result in a fine or even imprisonment.

Communications operate at different levels:

- *Internal communications* between expedition members to facilitate expedition logistics, information exchange, and

---

> ### BOX 80-8 Team Members' Medical Kit
>
> - ☐ Blister kit
> - ☐ Adhesive plasters and dressings
> - ☐ Antiseptic wipes
> - ☐ Simple analgesic—acetaminophen or preferred painkiller
> - ☐ Antihistamine tablets
> - ☐ Hydrocortisone 1% cream—chlorphenamine tablets
> - ☐ Antiemetic and oral rehydration sachets
> - ☐ Personal medication, including antimalarials if appropriate
> - ☐ Insect repellent and sunblock

BOX 80-9 Principles of Good Radio Procedure for Expeditions

Good radio procedure is marked by the following:
- *Clarity:* Always identify yourself and whom (you think) you are addressing. Speak slowly and clearly.
- *Accuracy:* Use the NATO phonetic alphabet to spell difficult or unusual words.
- *Brevity:* Be brief. Think about what you are going to say before transmission. If in doubt, write it down.

End each message with "Over."

Send message "Understood, over" or "Roger that, over" to acknowledge a received message.

Send message "Standing by" if you are continuing to monitor the frequency.

End message with your identity and "Out" if you have finished transmitting.

Use the mnemonic ETHANE to facilitate accurate transmission of casualty information:
- **E**xact location
- **T**ype of incident
- **H**azards
- **A**ccess
- **N**umber of casualties
- **E**mergency services on scene or required

NATO, North Atlantic Treaty Organization.

BOX 80-10 Telemedicine Saves Climber's Frostbitten Toes

A 48-year-old male and one companion set out on an attempt to cross Antarctica.

The team utilized kites to harness wind power and propel themselves across the ice while on skis. They averaged 47.5 km (28.5 miles) per day for 81 days and covered a total of 3854 km (2312 miles) in that time. Temperatures ranged between −30° and −45°C (−22° to −49°F). With wind chill and at higher elevations, temperatures likely were as low as −60°C (−76°F). The expedition spent much of the time between 2896 m (9500 ft.) and 3658 m (12,000 ft.).

On day 22 of the expedition, the man injured his right big toe. His toenail broke, and the distal toe subsequently became swollen and developed a friction blister. The fluid underwent repeated freezing and thawing, which contributed to cold injury. Initial care involved ibuprofen, 800 mg twice daily, and dressing the toe with both antibiotic ointment (fucidin and polysporin) and medical tape each morning and evening. On day 38, the patient sought medical advice via satellite phone from the physician based at the Union Glacier Camp (Figure 80-4). An additional opinion was requested from a UK expert in frostbite injuries; Internet communication was established, and he confirmed the diagnosis of frostbite.

On completion of the expedition, the great toe improved. After several weeks of recovery, the toe sloughed necrotic tissue, and no bone involvement was suspected. Additional consultation at the Intermountain Burn Center confirmed that both toes would likely recover without surgical debridement or amputation. The toes eventually healed as predicted.

Contributed by Professor Chris Imray.

medical care. This may be over considerable distances for large expeditions with several sites. It is crucial that expedition members be familiar with radio procedures to facilitate accurate transmission of information (Box 80-9).
- *Communication with local agencies,* such as national park authorities, the military, embassies, or rescue services. It is important to ensure that one knows before departure correct telephone numbers and radio frequencies used by these agencies.
- *Communication with the expedition home country* for contact with the expedition head office, sponsors, or the media, and for expedition members to remain in touch with their families.
- *Telemedicine* is facilitation of health care delivery by exchange of health care information across distances. This can range from simple telephone advice to transmission of complex diagnostic images or data for remote analysis.[72] Telemedicine clearly has significant potential to deliver diagnostic services and expert advice into remote areas. The French Institut de Formation et de Recherche en Medecine de Montagne (Ifremmont), based in Chamonix, offers a subscription service for expedition trip leaders, guides, and EMOs that can help in expedition medical preparation. It provides 24-hour telephone access to expert medical advice in French or English in the event of a medical problem.

Box 80-10 outlines the story of a British climber who sustained frostbitten toes on Mt Aconcagua and avoided amputation through consultation with the UK Frostbite Advice Service. This service has existed since 2005 and helped approximately 150 climbers with a combination of remote service advice, often using digital imaging, and rapid follow-up consultation on return to the United Kingdom. Contact details for both Ifremmont and the UK Frostbite Advice Service are given in the Resources section at the end of this chapter.

When using communications of any type to discuss confidential patient details, remember that there is always the possibility that someone unintended may be listening.

LEGAL AND ETHICAL CONSIDERATIONS OF EXPEDITION MEDICINE

Most people who venture into wilderness areas are willing to help sick or injured travelers in their own party or strangers whom they may encounter. In some countries, such as France, laws exist that make it an offense to not provide assistance to somebody in peril. These are sometimes referred to as Good Samaritan laws. In other parts of the world, offering assistance remains only an ethical and not a legal obligation.

DUTY OF CARE

Each person has a duty of care not to injure others; however, this duty is different in certain circumstances. Leaders or members of a group have a clear duty of care to the other members of their group. Moral and ethical duties may exist to rescue another person, but these must be distinguished from legal duties. Common law does not impose a legal duty on an individual to rescue another person; however, a legal duty may be imposed on certain people in certain circumstances. A physician is under a legal duty to render emergency care to his or her own patient,

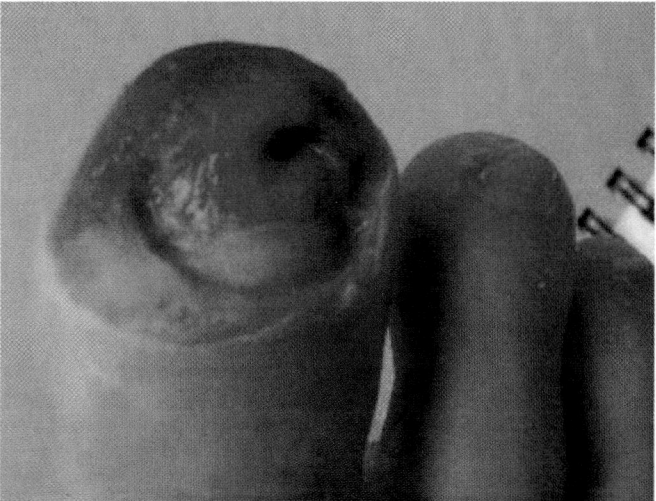

FIGURE 80-4 Initial photograph of patient's frostbite on day 38 (December 12, 2011) of the expedition. *(From Russell KW, Imray CH, McIntosh SE, et al: Kite skier's toe: an unusual case of frostbite. Wilderness Environ Med 24(2):136-140, 2013.)*

although professional bodies such as the UK General Medical Council expect physicians to provide emergency assistance even when off duty: "In an emergency, wherever it may arise, you must offer anyone at risk the assistance you could reasonably be expected to provide."[24] Whether a physician is treating a patient, advising a patient, or advising an expedition company, a clear duty of care exists in law. All who provide medical care or advice, whether physicians, nurses, paramedics, or laypersons, must do so reasonably and carefully.

A parent is under a legal duty to rescue his or her child. Police and fire service personnel are under a legal duty to rescue people in distress. Once a person undertakes the rescue, there is a legal duty to do everything possible to complete the rescue without causing personal injury. The law does not expect any rescuer to lose his or her life, even when circumstances mean that there is a legal duty to rescue. In a court of law, assessment of whether an individual has met the duty of care expected of that individual would is judged according to the principles discussed next.

Level of Control and Age/Experience of the Ill or Injured Person

Supervision of any wilderness activity must be appropriate to the age and experience of the participants. This is particularly important when working with children or youths, who cannot be expected to have the same degree of knowledge in wilderness situations as would an older, more experienced adult. For commercial groups with inexperienced adults, suitable guidance should be given by persons who are familiar with the environment and management of common problems. Appropriate staff-to-participant ratios should be determined to ensure adequate supervision.

Comparison with Peers

The courts will compare the provided standard of care with that expected from a person with similar experience and training acting in the same or similar circumstances. In effect from April 2007, British Standard 8848 describes recommended safety standards for expeditions and other adventure travel. This standard was revised in 2014.[69]

Likelihood of an Incident Occurring

In law, if an accident has happened before in similar circumstances, it could do so again, and precautions should be put in place to prevent recurrence.

Maintenance of Equipment and Cost of Precautions

It is essential that medical, safety, and rescue equipment be appropriate for the wilderness area to be visited. Procedures must be in place to guarantee that equipment is fit for purpose and correctly stored and packaged to prevent damage when being transported into the theater of operation. Adequate funds must be invested in providing adequate medical kits and supplies, but a court might understand that cost of excessive precautions might preclude the activity in the first place.

Emergency Situations

In the case of an emergency, the court will take into account the specific circumstances, such as the need to act with speed in a hazardous situation, in determining whether a practitioner has acted with reasonable care. Courts recognize that medicine is practiced in remote areas and that medical resources are limited.

Standard of Care

In UK law, the case of *Bolam v Friern Hospital Management Committee* (1957) produced the following definition of what is reasonable: "The test is the standard of the ordinary skilled man exercising and professing to have that special skill. A man need not possess the highest expert skill at the risk of being found negligent. It is sufficient if he exercises the skill of an ordinary man exercising that particular art." This definition is supported and clarified by the case of *Bolitho v City and Hackney Health Authority* (1993), where the House of Lords ruled that any decision must have a logical basis.[8]

Courts have indicated that they are not prepared to allow inexperience as a defense in actions of professional negligence. If a physician is unable to exercise reasonable care in carrying out a particular task, the physician should not undertake that task. If a practitioner professes to be an expedition physician (and as such, having a "specialist" skill), the provider's actions are judged against what might reasonably be expected of a competent expedition physician, even if this is the first time the practitioner has ever taken on such a role.

Confidentiality

All persons who are ill or injured must be confident that sensitive medical information will be kept confidential. For example, such information will not be made known to the rest of the expedition team or other individuals who are not directly involved in medical treatment or nursing care. However, in the United Kingdom, the General Medical Council has made it clear that physicians also have a duty to the public at large. Rare circumstances can arise where confidentiality needs to be broken so that the health and safety of other expedition members are not jeopardized. The expedition leader may need to be informed that an individual is concealing an illness or refusing treatment. Box 80-11 gives an example of a situation where a patient's withholding information about his past medical history engendered significant consequences for himself and the expedition.

Consent

Before starting treatment, the recipient must give consent. This means explaining what treatment is planned and ensuring that the patient is aware of the rescuer's level of training and experience. There must also be agreement to continue treatment. Consent may be implied from the circumstances. Voluntary submission to treatment usually indicates consent. In the expedition or wilderness setting, verbal consent must often be sufficient. In situations where treatment carries considerable risk, or is controversial, informed consent should be obtained, documented, and ideally witnessed by an observer.

The concept of consent is governed by the law of battery. Without consent, treatment is assault. The law usually presumes

---

BOX 80-11 Urinary Retention at Concordia

A 68-year-old man was taking part in a commercial trek to K2 Base Camp at Concordia in Pakistan and over the Ghondokoro La (5585 m [18,323 feet]). As part of preparation for the trip, he had been required to complete a comprehensive medical questionnaire that was screened by the company medical officer, a physician with long-standing experience in mountain and wilderness medicine. The trekker declared no significant health problems.

Having arrived at Concordia, the group leader was woken at around midnight by one of the trekkers to say that his tent mate, the 68-year-old man, was unable to pass urine and was in considerable discomfort. He was well hydrated and had suffered no trauma. He again denied any significant past medical history. A satellite telephone call was made to the company's medical officer, but the connection was poor and a detailed discussion of the case was not possible.

Simple measures, including diazepam administration and sitting the man in a large bowl of warm water, produced no result. The man was now in considerable pain. An inquiry was made of all the other groups camping at Concordia that night, but none had a urinary catheter. Eventually, an intravenous administration set was found, from which was improvised a urinary catheter. The man was successfully catheterized by the group leader, who had previously trained as a radiographer. This produced 1.5 L of heavily blood-stained urine.

After a considerable wait due to bad weather, the man was evacuated by helicopter to the District Headquarters Hospital at Skardu, where it became apparent that he had a history of prostatism and had been previously taking finasteride. Because of his failure to declare his history of prostatic problems, the man's insurance was void and he was required to finance his evacuation and treatment in Pakistan.

consent in an emergency situation when immediate action is necessary for protection of the patient's life. The law presumes that most reasonable persons under the same or similar circumstances would want their lives saved, if at all possible. Competent patients have the right to refuse treatment, even if, in the rescuer's opinion, this will not be in their best interest.

Competence and Capacity

A competent person has the right to refuse treatment if the person understands the consequences of such a refusal; however, a competent adult may lack the capacity to consent as a result of a comatose state. Intoxicated adults, however, have been deemed by some courts to have the capacity to consent. Severe intoxication that substantially impairs understanding is a "gray zone."

The only person who can give consent to treatment for someone age 16 or older is that person himself. Consent to treatment for a child younger than 16 years is given by a parent or guardian, although the child should be given information relevant to his or her age and understanding, and the child's consent also should be sought. Children under 16 years can consent to medical treatment themselves if, in the opinion of the physician, they are capable of understanding the nature and consequences of that treatment. When taking children under age 16 on an expedition, it is wise to gain written permission from the parent or guardian that medical care can be given if it is thought to be in the child's best interest.

Negligence

To prove negligence and sue for damages, the plaintiff must establish a usual standard of care, then prove a breach of that standard of care and that as a result of that breach, there is demonstrable injury. It must also be proved that the breach of duty was the logical and legal cause of the claimed injury (causation).

Contributory negligence is a factor that reduces liability. For example, a novice expedition member may forget to pack essential survival items, despite being informed that these items were required. Any settlement for negligence related to not having the items might then be reduced.

How Much Should Laypersons be Taught About Medicine?

In the United Kingdom, the law does not prohibit any person from practicing medicine or dentistry; however, it is an offense for any person to pretend to be or imply that he or she is a physician. Thus, the essence of what treatment should be provided by laypeople is largely a matter of patient consent and understanding.

Persons who participate in hazardous activities may, in many circumstances, be held to consent to the risks and rigors dictated by such a circumstance. In other words, if you become injured or ill, you have accepted that medical care may be of a less satisfactory nature than in a modern emergency department. It is very important that group members are involved in the risk assessment process and are aware of the level of medical care that can be provided.

Laypeople should be taught sufficiently to enable any expedition to be safe insofar as that can be achieved. There exists a duty of care to exercise skills consistent with training, experience, and procedures. The duty of care will obviously vary. Care rendered by a completely untrained "Good Samaritan" providing urgent assistance in extreme or remote circumstances can easily be distinguished from the setting of a simple bony fracture by a trained first-aider acting at the direction of medical personnel providing advice by telephone or radio. The duty of care is defined in each individual circumstance.[17]

Legal Position of a Physician Advising Care to be Administered by a Layperson

Persons accepting responsibility to provide medical, nursing, or paramedical help must be judged according to the state of their knowledge and experience and the extent to which they follow directions or advice given to them by more highly or appropriately qualified personnel removed from the accident scene. The higher the degree of training provided and greater the detail of medical support in place, the greater is the expectation of the patient to be properly treated and rigor with which the duty of care is interpreted by lawyers.

Liability on Commercial Expeditions

Medical indemnity is discussed in detail later (see Professional Indemnity Insurance). Most medical indemnity organizations provide Good Samaritan coverage for physicians acting in any part of the world. The British Medical Defence Union (MDU) defines a Good Samaritan act as "The provision of clinical services related to a clinical emergency, accident or disaster when you are not present in your professional capacity but as a bystander," and states that "MDU members who have a current Professional Indemnity Policy are covered for claims arising from Good Samaritan acts anywhere in the world."[51] However, in an expedition setting, this would apply only where a team member just *happens* to be a physician. It would certainly not cover a physician receiving any form of inducement (e.g., a discount in the trip fee or sponsorship in kind) that implies the physician has an official medical role on the expedition.

Expedition companies have a responsibility in common law to ensure that any EMO they choose to employ is suitably experienced. In the event of a claim for negligence, the claim would normally be made against the expedition company. A liability disclaimer signed by a patient before receiving treatment is unlikely to carry much weight before a court. However, a "letter of understanding" detailing the risks and the individual's acceptance of these risks would make it clear to a judge that the participant was fully aware of the expedition environment and medical care available.

Expeditions Departing Without an EMO

Many smaller expeditions do not have the resources to be able to take an EMO into the field; however, the team still needs medical advice and suitable medical pack. In these cases, an EMO may:

- Provide advice on travel medicine, such as required vaccinations or recommended antimalarial chemoprophylaxis.
- Supply private prescriptions for an expedition. It should be kept in mind that drugs may be used for treatment of trip members previously unknown to the EMO. In these situations, the EMO (who retains a duty of care) should provide clear written guidelines, which should include indications, contraindications, doses, and side effects. It would also be prudent for the EMO to seek written assurance from the person to whom prescriptions are supplied that the medication prescribed will be used only for immediate treatment of expedition members in wilderness areas and not as a substitute for seeking professional medical advice when such is readily available.
- Delegate responsibility for initiating treatment to a trip leader.

Medical Records

Brief, accurate, and contemporaneous medical records should be made for all clinical encounters. In serious illness or injury, this is essential so that detailed clinical information can be given to those who deliver definitive care to the patient. This principle applies to both medical and nonmedical expedition staff providing medical care; Box 80-1 is an example of excellent record keeping by a nonmedical expedition leader. Whenever a patient is evacuated or referred to a formal medical facility, the person should be accompanied by clear notes outlining the history and treatment. If there are later concerns about the standards of care given in a wilderness setting, comprehensive clinical notes will help to defend actions if legal activities occur. Examples of suitable medical records for use in the field can be found at http://medex.org.uk/diploma/resources.php.

PROFESSIONAL INDEMNITY INSURANCE

Professional indemnity insurance is an increasingly contentious issue and with considerable international variation. In the United

Kingdom, professional indemnity insurance is provided by four national organizations: the Medical and Dental Defence Union of Scotland, the MDU, the Medical Protection Society, and the Royal College of Nursing. Each organization generally provides discretionary indemnity to its members for a period of volunteer or charity work, such as accompanying an expedition or trek, or being based in a mountain or wilderness clinic. Importantly, "This is dependent on the doctor confirming he or she is suitably trained and equipped to undertake that work."[51] There are a number of countries where indemnity insurance is not available, including Australia, the United States, and Canada and their dependent territories. Work for which the physician receives financial remuneration will be considered for indemnity coverage, but is likely to be charged on a pro rata basis of up to $6500 per year (as of April 2010). In the United States, medical professional liability insurance is provided by private insurance companies at considerable cost. Any American EMO needs to discuss indemnity with his or her insurance company on an individual basis.

Canadian physicians obtain indemnity insurance through the Canadian Medical Protective Association (CMPA). Fees vary from province to province. The CMPA will indemnify its members only for treating Canadian citizens in the province where they work. The CMPA does not provide indemnity insurance for overseas expedition work, so this must therefore be obtained privately. Private medical indemnity insurance can be very difficult to obtain and prohibitively expensive.

In Australia, the situation is more complex, particularly since the financial collapse in 2002 of one of the major providers of medical indemnity insurance. A variety of medical defense organizations provide cover, depending on whether the physician is self-employed or works in public hospitals. It would appear that the majority of organizations might consider providing indemnity cover for their members carrying out volunteer work in a similar manner, and with similar conditions, to the British organizations discussed earlier.

Many EMOs practice expedition medicine with inadequate indemnity insurance. We are unaware of any indemnity claim that has been brought against an EMO, but regrettably, in the current litigation climate and with the changing attitude and demographics of expedition members, it seems only a matter of time before such legal proceedings occur. It is crucial that anybody considering undertaking expedition medical work is competent to undertake the work and has a full discussion with his or her medical defense organization. With the risk for litigation and number of commercial expeditions offering medical professionals the chance to practice expedition medicine, it seems wise for anybody considering EMO activities to obtain a suitable and robust qualification, such as the Diploma in Mountain Medicine.

Nurses and paramedics acting as EMOs should inform their respective professional indemnity carriers about the potential extended scope of practice. The scope of professional indemnity insurance provided varies among national professional bodies. In the United Kingdom, nurses are assumed to work within a skill set commensurate with their level of knowledge and training and in the event of a claim would be held accountable for straying from a suitable level of competency.[66]

Some organizations requiring a medic will dictate the level of professional indemnity (PI) and personal liability (PL) coverage required. For example, the British Broadcasting Corporation (BBC) requires medics to demonstrate that they have £5 million PI and PL coverage. Currently, the RCN will provide coverage up to £2 million, necessitating the need for a separate policy.

ETHICAL CONSIDERATIONS OF INTERACTING WITH LOCAL POPULATIONS

A frequent problem confronting an expedition is the extent to which medical treatment should be provided for a local population. When an expedition arrives in a new village, particularly if it is known that there is an EMO on the expedition, a queue of local people often forms to seek consultation and treatment. There are no absolute ethical guidelines for this situation. Each

---

BOX 80-12   Interacting with Local Healers

The left hand of a young Sherpa boy who presented to the Community Action Nepal–International Porter Protection Group Rescue Post at Machermo in the Gokyo Valley of Nepal with a gangrenous accessory digit (Figure 80-5). His mother had been advised by a local shaman to tie a piece of the child's hair around the accessory digit. The boy was referred to the Hillary Trust Hospital at Khunde, where he underwent amputation of the digit under ketamine anesthesia without complications.

expedition must decide the policy it will adopt. The factors discussed next should be taken into consideration.

Preexpedition Planning

A decision should be made at the planning stage of the expedition as to the degree the expedition will offer medical care to local people. This decision is influenced by two major factors:
- Expedition resources and budget
- Preexisting medical facilities in the area being visited

The location of local health care facilities should be researched before the expedition. It is crucial that when local health care facilities exist, however basic, the expedition does not undermine them. Local clinics continue to provide care long after an expedition has departed and are not helped in their task if an expedition falsely raises the expectations of local communities. If an expedition intends to provide treatment for local people, as in a region that lacks local health care facilities, it is important that this is anticipated and budgeted, and that extra resources are allocated.

During the Expedition

During the expedition walk-in, it is important to visit local health care facilities and to meet the staff. Such visits can provide encouragement for the local staff and inspiration for the visiting EMO, because the work carried out in such posts, often with minimal resources, is frequently impressive. It offers the opportunity to discuss with local staff the best ways in which the expedition should interact with the community. It is also useful to discuss the existence of any indigenous healers in the area and to be guided by the local health staff in which way to interact with them (Box 80-12). The visit should also be used to determine the best ways to evacuate sick expedition members if direct air evacuation is not available.

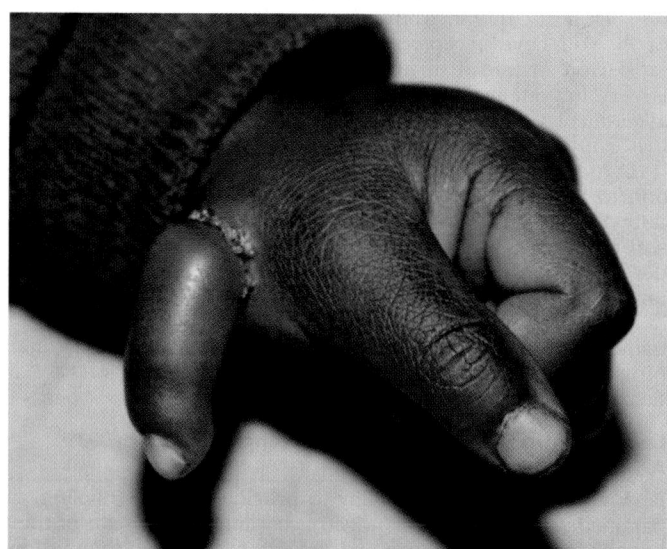

FIGURE 80-5 The left hand of a young Sherpa boy with a gangrenous accessory digit.

If local people are treated, only acute problems should be addressed. Any patient requiring ongoing treatment or follow-up should be referred to the local health care facility with a formal letter of referral. On the walk-out, it is courteous and helpful to leave any unused drugs and items of equipment that might be useful with the local health care facilities. It is essential that those receiving the donated medical items are aware of the proper use of drugs and equipment, because trade names (and sometimes generic names) differ in various countries.

Treating Local Staff

Although the extent to which expeditions should treat members of local populations is open to debate, the manner in which local staff working for the expedition should be treated is not. They should receive the same medical care as do other members of the expedition. George Finch,[21] a member of the 1922 Mt Everest expedition, wrote at the time:

There is only one form of transportation for this cumbersome, and at times dangerous, work: the native mountain people. The natives of the Himalayas, like all mountain people, are very tough and healthy as can be; they are resolute and brave, yet always of friendly and cheerful disposition, and are excellent porters if they are treated right. But they have to be cared for properly, that is, they must be clothed appropriately and supplied with ample provisions to keep them in peak performance.

Unfortunately, this self-evident sentiment is not the experience of many local staff, who are regularly required to work without adequate clothing or shelter and too frequently abandoned and left to fend for themselves when they fall ill. This abuse of local staff, and in particular portering staff, is one of the most shameful features of modern expeditions.[49,50] Box 80-13 tells the typical story of a sick porter abandoned by his expedition. Box 80-14 gives a Nepalese porter's perspective of his work.

The International Porter Protection Group offers the following guidelines for the care of local staff[65]:

1. Clothing appropriate to season and altitude must be provided to porters for protection from cold, rain and snow. This may mean: windproof jacket and trousers, fleece jacket, long johns, suitable footwear (boots in snow), socks, hat, gloves and sunglasses.
2. Above the tree line porters should have a dedicated shelter, either a room in a lodge or a tent (the trekkers' mess tent is no good as it is not available till late evening), a sleeping mat and a decent blanket or sleeping bag. They should be provided with food and warm drinks, or cooking equipment and fuel.
3. Porters should be provided with life insurance and the same standard of medical care as you would expect for yourself.
4. Porters should not be paid off because of illness/injury without the leader or the trekkers assessing their condition carefully. The person in charge of the porters (sirdar) must let their trek leader or the trekkers know if a sick porter is about to be paid off. Failure to do this has resulted in many deaths. Sick/injured porters should never be sent down alone, but with someone who speaks their language and understands their problem, along with a letter describing their complaint. Sufficient funds should be provided to cover cost of rescue and treatment.
5. No porter should be asked to carry a load that is too heavy for their physical abilities (maximum: 20 kg (44.1 lb.) on Kilimanjaro, 25 kg (55.1 lb.) in Peru and Pakistan, 30 kg (66.1 lb.) in Nepal). Weight limits may need to be adjusted for altitude, trail and weather conditions; experience is needed to make this decision. Child porters should not be employed.

BOX 80-14 Porter Poetry

Porter
by Laxman Tamang

I am a porter, a small man.
I carry luggage for the rich
and the foreigners.
I eat worse food than they do,
Wear tattered clothes,
Get a meagre salary,
Walk faster than them.
What can I do?
Such is my fate.
I pass my days this way.
I forget my agonies this way.

From *On a donkey's back—Poetry of the Nepalese mountain porters*, Vineland, NJ, 2008, Yileen Press.

BOX 80-13 Another Nepalese Porter with HAPE and HACE

A 22-year-old Nepalese porter from the foothills of Nepal was portering for a commercial Swiss trek. Shortly after arrival at Gokyo (4750 m [15,584 feet]), which he had previously visited without problems, he began to feel unwell. As the evening progressed, he developed a headache and went to bed. He awoke in the night with severe dyspnea and orthopnea. By morning his condition had worsened. It is unlikely that the Swiss leader was aware that one of his porters was sick or that the group's sirdar had paid him off at 250 Nepalese rupees (just over $3) per day and left him to descend alone.

The porter was found collapsed at the side of the trail, about an hour's walk from Gokyo, semiconscious and vomiting, by Dutch and British trekkers. The British group's Sherpa guide carried the porter 5 km (3.1 miles) to the Community Action Nepal–International Porter Protection Group Rescue Post at Machermo (4400 m [14,436 feet]), where he was diagnosed as having severe HAPE and HACE. This proved refractory to treatment with oxygen, nifedipine, dexamethasone, tadalafil, and inhaled β_2-agonists, and it was feared that the porter would die. Thanks to the generosity of trekkers staying in the village, who between them donated the $4500 cost of the rescue flight, the porter was flown by helicopter the following day to Khunde Hospital (3800 m [12,467 feet]), where he made a full recovery and was able to leave the hospital unaided 24 hours later.

HACE, High-altitude cerebral edema; *HAPE*, high-altitude pulmonary edema.

BIOMEDICAL RESEARCH

There is a long-standing tradition of physiologic and medical research on expeditions, particularly at high altitude, where such work has made major contributions to understanding cardiorespiratory physiology at sea level as well as at altitude.[70] It is crucial that any research on human participants during an expedition meet the same ethical criteria as if it were carried out at home, namely:

- The project must have received ethics approval at the home institution and, wherever possible, from a comparable institution in the country where the research is to be carried out. This is particularly important if the research involves local populations.
- Informed consent must be obtained from all participants, who have the right to withdraw from the research at any point.
- The participants' rights to confidentiality must be respected and every step taken to ensure that data are collected and stored securely.

DEALING WITH THE MEDIA

Because of the inherent nature of expeditions, serious accidents, injury, and deaths can occur. On such occasions, it may fall to the EMO to talk to the media. This can be a very stressful experience. The manner in which such incidents are reported can have a significant effect on the public's and the legal profession's long-term interpretation of events. Box 80-15 gives guidelines on the best ways in which to interact with journalists and reporters.

BOX 80-15 The Media-Savvy Mountain Medic

Journalists want a good story, but this may conflict with your medical responsibilities and ethics. Your job is to lower the temperature, not to add fuel.

- **Never speculate, embroider, or blame**—your insurers won't like it and the true cause of an accident or a death may be unexpected. Stick to the medical facts.
- **Never name victims**—this is a job for embassies and the police. Even if next-of-kin know, they need time to tell other family members and close friends. They should not learn of a serious accident or death via a TV or radio bulletin.
- **Never say "no comment"**—you'll sound guilty. Just give a few simple facts to help a journalist. But if you say too little, unscrupulous hacks will make it up anyway. Scrupulous reporters will just speculate.
- **Always offer appropriate sympathy**—it's only human in the case of death or serious injury but it's often forgotten. Try not to over-state the case—death is a "tragedy" but calling off an expedition because the entire team has diarrhea is merely "unfortunate" or "careless."
- **Always keep promises to journalists**—it's wise to keep them on your side. Broadcasters, in particular, work to very tight deadlines, so failing to deliver information on time may well attract negative coverage or speculation.
- **Always tell the truth**—even if you can't tell the full story. A "quick bleed" is often a good policy if there's been a mistake, but insurers don't like it so don't say too much.

You should always try to prevent a crisis turning into a media disaster and feeding frenzy. And remember, inquests and other court cases can turn on public perception rather than legal argument.

RESOURCES

Institut de Formation et de Recherche en Medecine de Montagne (Ifremmont), Remote Mountain Medicine Consultation Service, Chamonix, France
   http://www.ifremmont.com/en/contacts
   Telephone: +33-826-14-8000
   E-mail: contact@ifremmont.com
UK Frostbite Advice Service
   For e-mail or telephone advice on frostbite from anywhere in the world, contact:
   http://www.christopherimray.co.uk/highaltitudemedicine/frostbite.htm
   or
   http://www.thebmc.co.uk/how-to-get-expert-frostbite-advice
Dr. David Hillebrandt
   Telephone: +44-1409-253814
   E-mail: dh@hillebrandt.org.uk
Dr. Paul Richards
   Telephone: +44-1268-568240
   E-mail: paul@medex.org.uk
International Porter Protection Group
   http://www.ippg.net

APPENDIX Recommended Medical Kit

Quantities are for a group of 10 persons on a 6-week high-altitude mountaineering expedition. The list may be useful as a checklist when preparing kits for other types of expeditions.

ANTIMICROBIALS

Ceftriaxone powder for injection	4 g	5 ampules
Chloramphenicol 1% ointment	4 g	3 tubes
Clarithromycin	250 mg	40 tablets
Ciprofloxacin	500 mg	50 tablets
Amoxicillin/clavulanic acid	250/125 mg	84 tablets
Doxycycline	100 mg	80 tablets
Mebendazole	100 mg	20 tablets
Metronidazole	400 mg	100 tablets
Metronidazole suppositories	1 g	10 suppositories
Quinine sulfate	200 mg	50 tablets
Rabies vaccine	1 mL	5 vials

PAINKILLERS, LOCAL ANESTHETICS/SEDATIVES

Aspirin	325 mg	32 tablets
Bupivacaine 0.25% for injection	10 mL	5 vials
Acetaminophen/codeine	30/300 mg	80 tablets
Diclofenac	50 mg	100 tablets
Ibuprofen	400 mg	80 tablets
Ketamine solution for injection	10 mg/mL	2 vials
Ketorolac solution for injection	30 mg/mL	5 vials
Lidocaine 1% for injection	5 mL	10 ampules
Lidocaine 2% gel	30 mL	2 tubes
Lorazepam solution for injection	2 mg/mL	5 vials
Midazolam solution for injection	5 mg/5 mL	5 vials
Acetaminophen	500 mg	100 tablets
Tetracaine 0.5% eye drops	15 mL	6 bottles
Eszopiclone	7.5 mg	20 tablets

GASTROINTESTINAL

Bisacodyl	5 mg	20 tablets
Antacid tablets		100 tablets
Oral rehydration solution sachets		100 sachets
Loperamide	2 mg	50 capsules
Prochlorperazine	5 mg	56 tablets
Prochlorperazine solution for injection	12.5 mg/mL	5 vials
Prochlorperazine suppositories	25 mg	10 suppositories

CARDIOVASCULAR

Bisoprolol	2.5 mg	20 tablets
Atropine solution for injection	600 mcg/ 1 mL	5 vials
Enoxaparin for injection	80 mg/ 0.8 mL	10 prefilled syringes
Nitroglycerin sublingual spray	400 mcg/ spray	1 bottle

RESPIRATORY/ALLERGY

Epinephrine 1:1000 solution for injection	1 mL	10 ampules
Beclometasone for inhalation	200 mcg	2 canisters
Chlorphenamine	4 mg	60 tablets
Chlorphenamine solution for injection (UK)	10 mg/mL	5 vials
Diphenhydramine solution for injection (U.S.)	25-50 mg	5 vials
Hydrocortisone powder for injection	100 mg/ 2 mL	5 vials
Prednisone	5 mg	100 tablets
Albuterol for inhalation	90 mcg	2 canisters

ALTITUDE

Acetazolamide	250 mg	250 tablets
Dexamethasone	2 mg	40 tablets
Nifedipine	20 mg	20 capsules
Portable altitude chamber and/or oxygen cylinders		1

OTHER MEDICATION

Multivitamins with minerals		500 tablets
Dimenhydrinate	50 mg	40 tablets

CREAMS AND OINTMENTS

Acyclovir cream 5%	2 g	6 tubes
Hemorrhoidal cream		1 tube
Mupirocin cream	15 g	6 tubes
Betamethasone sodium phosphate 0.1%; neomycin sulfate 0.5%	10 mL	4 bottles
Clotrimazole 1% cream	20 g	6 tubes
Aqueous cream	50 g	1 tube
Fluconazole	150 mg	4 tablets
Hydrocortisone 1% cream	15 g	6 tubes
Sunblock SPF 25+		4 tubes

DRESSINGS

Adhesive plasters		50 assorted
Alcohol swabs	100	2 boxes
Cotton wool		4 packets
Crepe bandages	7.5 cm	4 units
Medium wound dressing		2 units
Eye dressing		4 units
Fluorescein eye test strips/ minims		10 strips/ minims
Gauze swabs	5 × 5 cm	100 swabs
Nonadherent dressing	10 cm²	5 dressings
Nonadherent dressing	5 × 5 cm²	5 dressings
Hypoallergenic tape	2.5 cm	2 rolls
Adhesive strips, assorted		4 packets
Triangular bandages		8 bandages
Petrolatum gauze	10 cm²	10 rolls
Zinc oxide roll plaster		2 rolls

INJECTION EQUIPMENT AND INTRAVENOUS (IV) FLUIDS

2-mL, 5-mL, 10-mL syringes		20 of each
25-, 23-, and 21-gauge hypodermic needles		20 of each
IV cannulas, 14 gauge, 18 gauge		10 of each
Giving sets		5 units
Normal saline	1 L	6 bottles
Hartmann's solution	500 mL	8 bottles
Dextrose 5%	500 mL	4 bottles

AIRWAY CARE

Oropharyngeal airways (sizes 2, 3, 4)	2 of each
No. 6 nasopharyngeal airway	2 units
Bag-valve-mask device	1 unit
Minitracheostomy set	1 unit
Endotracheal tubes, 7 mm, 9 mm	2 of each
Laryngeal mask airway sizes 3, 4	2 of each
I-gel supraglottic airway sizes 3, 4	1 of each
Catheter mounts for above	2 units
Laryngoscope	1 unit
Oxygen tubing	1 unit
Oxygen cylinder	1 unit
Handheld suction unit	1 unit

MAJOR TRAUMA

Nonsterile examination gloves	100 pair
Tuff cut scissors	1 unit
Chest drain 32 Fr	2 units
Heimlich valve	2 units
Kendrick Traction Device	1 unit
SAM Splint	2 units
Adjustable cervical collar (Stifneck Select)	2 units
Urinary catheter 14 Fr	2 units
Catheter bag and tubing	2 units
Bladder syringe, 50 mL	2 units
Nasogastric tube 12 Fr	2 units
Disposable scalpels	2 units
Gloves sterile (medium)	10 pair
Sutures:	
2/0 silk straight	4 units
4/0 nonabsorbable suture	5 units
5/0 nonabsorbable suture	5 units
Staples and remover	1 unit
Needle holder	1 unit
Toothed forceps	1 unit
Dressing scissors (straight/ straight 5-inch)	1 unit
Spencer Wells forceps	2 units
Tissue/super glue (e.g., LiquiBand)	5 units
Dental first-aid kit	1 unit
Low-reading thermometer	1 unit
Thermometer (digital)	1 unit

EXAMINATION

Pen flashlight	3 units
Stethoscope	1 unit
Aneroid sphygmomanometer	1 unit
Ophthalmoscope/auriscope	1 unit

Travelers to tropical and subtropical areas of the world, where hygiene conditions are poor and ecologic conditions are permissive, may encounter infectious agents that are no longer endemic or have never existed in temperate regions of the world. Although economic development and industrialization of developing countries of the tropics have resulted in a decreased health burden of many tropical infectious diseases, it is important to realize that there is still a risk for exposure for the traveler who is unaware of appropriate measures to prevent or treat such conditions. The most important consideration in the management of this problem, which is increasing as international travel expands, is appropriate preventive measures through counsel with a travel medicine specialist and prophylaxis using safe drugs and vaccines. This topic has been reviewed in several excellent publications.[11,52,70,81]

This chapter discusses infectious diseases that are uncommon or do not exist in North America and thus may be less familiar to most health professionals there. Other chapters give specific details relevant to malaria (Chapter 40), tick-borne diseases (Chapter 42), infectious diarrheas (Chapter 82), and travel medicine (Chapter 79). The infectious diseases discussed in this chapter should not be considered a complete listing. This is especially important to keep in mind in an era when diseases once thought to be eliminated or nonexistent in North America are emerging or reemerging at the same time as large-scale movements of human and vector populations.

MAJOR VIRAL INFECTIONS

This section describes certain viral infections that may be acquired outside North America. Emphasis is placed on viral infections that have recently been recognized as highly pathogenic and endemic in select tropical areas, such as those caused by filoviruses, and those for which effective preventive or therapeutic measures exist, such as viral hemorrhagic fever caused by the yellow fever virus, some types of viral hepatitis, and Japanese B encephalitis.

MAJOR VIRAL HEMORRHAGIC FEVERS

A diverse group of ribonucleic acid (RNA) viruses can produce the hemorrhagic fever syndrome. Fever, headache, myalgia, and malaise generally characterize the early phase of the clinical presentation of all these infections, which develops over several hours to 3 to 4 days. In the full-blown hemorrhagic fever syndrome, nonspecific clinical symptoms are followed by hemorrhagic signs, including petechiae and bleeding from the gums and gastrointestinal (GI) tract. Loss of plasma volume and a capillary leak syndrome may ensue, manifested in some individuals as increased hematocrit with hypotension and shock. Elevated blood urea nitrogen and creatinine levels indicative of renal dysfunction may develop. Death is caused by a combination of intractable hypotension, bleeding, electrolyte imbalances, and renal failure. There are many viral causes of this syndrome (e.g., Rift Valley fever), but not all of these are discussed here. In general, the management principles are the same and consist primarily of supportive therapy.

YELLOW FEVER

European physicians did not recognize the clinical syndrome now known as yellow fever (YF) until the late 1490s. Initially described by Columbus in the West Indies, large-scale epidemics were later observed throughout the Americas and tropical Africa in the 1700s and 1800s. After epidemic YF in Texas, Louisiana, and Tennessee caused 20,000 deaths in the 1880s, the Yellow Fever Commission was organized to study the problem. Identification of the mosquito vector, *Aedes aegypti*, and definitive studies conducted by the U.S. military under the leadership of Walter Reed were followed by massive campaigns to eradicate mosquito breeding sites. This led to virtual elimination of urban YF from the Americas. The last case of YF acquired in the continental United States was reported in 1911. Because it is difficult if not impossible to eliminate jungle reservoirs, cases continue to be reported annually from South America and tropical Africa.[68]

Virology and Pathophysiology

Yellow fever is a single-stranded RNA flavivirus. Strain differences are of little clinical relevance, although they may be of use in epidemiologic studies. The pathophysiologic mechanisms operating in viral hemorrhagic fevers are not well defined. In general, viral replication occurs at the site of inoculation. After the virus spreads to lymph nodes and monocyte-rich organs, further reproduction results in massive viremia.

The liver is the principal target organ. Pathology studies show coagulative necrosis of hepatocytes and appearance of various markers of cell involvement (e.g., Councilman and Torres bodies). The degree of physiologic derangement is usually much more severe than expected for the extent of hepatic damage seen on pathology examination. Perivascular edema and occasional focal bleeding occur in the kidneys, heart, and brain, but these changes are less severe than expected for the degree of clinical disease.

Ecology and Epidemiology

In the Americas, primates in the forest canopy serve as hosts for the YF virus. Mosquitoes of the genus *Haemagogus* transmit infection. Because this vector does not travel far from the forest, jungle YF occurs when humans enter jungle areas or the forest border zones. Urban YF involves a different vector, *Aedes*, that is highly anthropophilic, lives in and around human habitations, and prefers domestic water storage containers for breeding. In Africa, *Aedes* species serve as the main vectors.[67,91]

Currently, both the Americas and Africa have a constant low level of jungle YF because of inability to control either the monkey reservoir or the mosquito vector. Estimates from the 1990s placed the burden of disease at about 200,000 cases per year, resulting in approximately 30,000 deaths, primarily in sub-Saharan Africa.[77] Some suggest that these rates are underestimated by at least 10-fold. After mass YF vaccine campaigns in Africa beginning in 2006, current estimates of YF disease burden in Africa for 2013 were 130,000 cases and 78,000 deaths.[47]

Clinical Presentation and Diagnosis

Although YF may appear as an undifferentiated viral syndrome in patients who have only mild disease, classic disease is characterized by a triphasic pattern. The infection phase begins with sudden onset of headache, fever, and malaise, often accompanied by bradycardia and conjunctival suffusion. After about 3 to 4 days, patients often experience brief remission. Within 24 hours, the intoxication phase develops, characterized by jaundice, recrudescent fever, prostration, and in severe cases, hypotension, shock, oliguria, and obtundation. Hemorrhage usually manifests as hematemesis; bleeding from multiple sites may occur. Signs of poor prognosis include early onset of the intoxication phase, hypotension, severe hemorrhage with disseminated intravascular coagulation (DIC), renal failure, shock, and coma. Death occurs in 20% to 50% of cases.

Diagnosis is difficult in the infection phase. With development of the classic syndrome, the differential diagnosis narrows somewhat, but still includes malaria, leptospirosis, typhoid fever, typhus, Q fever, viral hepatitis, and other viral hemorrhagic fevers. Laboratory diagnosis is confirmed by detection of virus-specific immunoglobulin M (IgM) and IgG antibodies in acute and convalescent serologic assays, available through the U.S. Centers for Disease Control and Prevention (CDC). It is important to obtain a YF vaccination history, because IgM antibodies to YF vaccine virus can persist for several years after vaccination. Serologic cross-reactions occur with other viruses, so positive results should be confirmed with a more specific test (e.g., plaque-reduction neutralization test). Early in the illness, YF virus or YF virus RNA can often be detected in the serum by virus isolation or nucleic acid amplification testing (e.g., reverse-transcriptase polymerase chain reaction [RT-PCR]). However, by the time overt symptoms are recognized, the virus or viral RNA is usually undetectable.

Management

Appropriate management of viral hemorrhagic fevers requires awareness of the geographic distribution of disease and travel history of the patient. In the first several days of infection, differentiation of a viral hemorrhagic fever from other infectious diseases is almost impossible. However, occurrence of an undifferentiated febrile syndrome in a traveler from a YF-endemic area warrants a careful physical examination, thick and thin blood smears to rule out malaria, and blood cultures for bacterial pathogens (e.g., *Salmonella typhi*). In recently returned travelers, dengue serologic tests should be considered. Progression to the intoxication phase or any sign of volume disturbance, renal failure, or hemorrhage mandates immediate admission to an intensive care unit (ICU). There is no effective antiviral therapy for YF. Intensive supportive care and management of end-organ failure are paramount. Severe disease carries a mortality rate of 50%.

Prevention

Avoidance of this potentially fatal infection is possible through use of YF vaccine. The vaccine strain 17D is a live-attenuated virus grown in chicken embryos. More than 95% of vaccinated persons achieve significant antibody levels within 10 days. Repeat vaccinations were previously recommended every 10 years, but in 2013 the World Health Organization (WHO) recommended that a single dose of YF vaccine confers lifelong protection against YF disease. However, countries with vulnerable populations and susceptible vector species may define their own YF vaccine entry requirements. WHO also recommended that all endemic countries introduce YF vaccine to their routine infant immunization programs.[59,96] YF vaccine is generally well tolerated, with headache or malaise occurring in less than 10% of vaccinated persons. Rare allergic side effects occur primarily in persons with hypersensitivity to eggs. Other serious adverse events, including death, have been reported, with the greater risk being associated with age greater than 60 years.[59,68] Vaccination is not recommended during the first 6 months of life or in other situations where live-virus vaccines are contraindicated. Although pregnant women have received the vaccine without adverse effect to themselves or their infants, it is not recommended for use in this group because of possible teratogenic effects. Other means of reducing the risk for YF (and any mosquito-borne infectious disease) include liberal use of mosquito repellent and netting in endemic areas. Outbreak control in endemic countries is primarily through focused vaccination campaigns.

DENGUE

Dengue has been reported since the late 1700s. Since World War II, increased attention has focused on the dengue virus, largely as a result of recognition of dengue hemorrhagic fever (DHF) and dengue shock syndrome (DSS). Dengue is the most common insect-borne viral infection worldwide. The infection has been reported in more than 100 countries, with a recent estimate of 390 million dengue infections per year, of which 96 million are symptomatic.[15,50]

Virology and Pathophysiology

The etiologic agent is a single-stranded RNA flavivirus, which may be one of four serotypes, denoted DEN-1 through DEN-4. As with YF, local viral replication is followed by dissemination to lymphocyte- and macrophage-rich areas, where most of the reproductive activity occurs. Infection with one virus serotype provides long-lasting immune protection against that type only. After infection with one serotype, a subsequent infection with a heterologous serotype may result in a more severe clinical course. Non-neutralizing antibodies produced in response to the primary infection are thought to facilitate entrance of the heterologous virus into host macrophages. Although cases of DHF and DSS may result from this "immune enhancement," severe DHF and DSS also occur with other serotypes in the absence of previous infection with a heterologous dengue virus serotype.[42,50] Pathology studies of DHF and DSS show hemorrhage, congestion, and perivascular edema of multiple organs. The liver may show areas of focal necrosis. As with YF, the extent of pathologic findings does not correspond to severity of the clinical course.

Ecology and Epidemiology

Aedes aegypti is the principal vector for dengue. In the Americas and Asia, viral transmission is maintained through a mosquito-human cycle without a major animal reservoir. Monkey carriers have been identified in Africa and Asia, but their importance in transmission is unclear. *Aedes albopictus*, an anthropophilic dengue vector from Southeast Asia, has also been recognized in the western hemisphere. Both these mosquitoes are capable of large-scale transmission to humans in endemic areas. Currently, dengue is endemic in tropical and subtropical Asia, Africa, South America, and the Caribbean basin.

Clinical Presentation

Most dengue infections appear after an incubation period of 2 to 14 days, either as an undifferentiated viral syndrome with fever and mild respiratory or GI symptoms or as dengue ("breakbone") fever (DF) with bone pain, generalized myalgia, severe headache, and retro-orbital pain. Febrile illnesses that appear more than 2 weeks after putative exposure to dengue virus are unlikely to be caused by this virus. After 1 to 3 days, a quiescent period may ensue. There may be a subsequent second episode of fever accompanied by a patchy maculopapular or morbilliform rash that spreads outward from the chest and ultimately desquamates. Lymphadenopathy and leukopenia occur during this phase of the illness. The distinct severe forms of dengue disease referred to as either DHF or DSS may occur around the usual time of recovery. These are caused by development of capillary leak syndrome with associated hemorrhagic manifestations (Figure 81-1).

In 2009, WHO changed the classification of DF/DHF/DSS to dengue and severe dengue (D/SD).[57] Warning signs (WS) have been established to help clinicians identify symptomatic patients who should be hospitalized and closely monitored (D+WS).[56] "Dengue without warning signs" (previously DF) is defined as laboratory-confirmed dengue, fever, and at least two of the following: nausea, vomiting, rash, leukopenia, arthralgia, myalgia, and a positive tourniquet test. "Dengue with warning signs" (D+WS, previously DHF) includes the previous features plus any of the following warning signs: abdominal pain or tenderness, persistent emesis, volume overload (edema), mucosal bleeding, lethargy, hepatomegaly, or hemoconcentration. "Severe dengue" (previously DSS) includes laboratory-confirmed dengue and shock, significant volume overload with respiratory distress, severe clinical bleeding, or organ failure.[57,93] Most studies have noted SD primarily in infants and young children, usually with a history or serologic evidence of previous heterologous dengue infection.

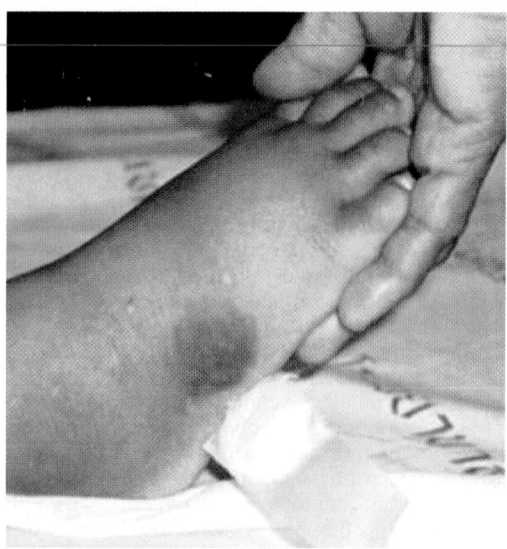

FIGURE 81-1 A Thai child with dengue hemorrhagic fever and hemorrhagic sequelae.

Prevention and Management

There is currently no vaccine to protect against dengue infection or disease, although several encouraging candidates are in development with clinical trials.[50]

Awareness of the local epidemiology of severe dengue, especially the occurrence of other cases, is important in establishing the diagnosis. The diagnosis may be confirmed by a fourfold change in antibody titer between acute and convalescent sera or by presence of antidengue IgM antibodies. In the United States, isolation of the virus from serum can be arranged through state health departments. Management is symptomatic. Hydration should be vigorously maintained. Acetaminophen may be given for fever and myalgia, but salicylates should not be used. The WHO guidelines state that patients diagnosed with dengue plus warning signs should be hospitalized for close monitoring and interventions. Infants diagnosed with dengue without warning signs should probably be admitted, whereas older patients diagnosed with dengue without warning signs may be managed as outpatients. Outpatient care requires careful monitoring of hematocrit, platelets, and electrolytes. If warning signs develop, hospitalization is appropriate for rapid and continuous assessment. Progression to severe dengue is a medical emergency and requires immediate hospitalization. There is no specific antiviral chemotherapy. Supportive measures with careful monitoring are appropriate.

LASSA FEVER

Four viral hemorrhagic fevers—Lassa, Marburg, Ebola, and Crimean-Congo—have been associated with outbreaks of fatal person-to-person spread. Although the overall number of clinical cases in travelers caused by these viruses is small, they represent potentially significant threats as emerging diseases. They have also achieved notoriety as a group as a result of media interest and their potential use as agents of bioterrorism.

Lassa fever was first recognized in 1969, when several nurses caring for febrile patients at a mission hospital in Lassa, Nigeria, became ill. Since that time, seroepidemiologic studies have established a large area of endemicity and broad spectrum of clinical manifestations of infection.

Epidemiology

The principal animal host for this virus is the rat, *Mastomys natalensis,* which prefers living in and around human dwellings. The rodents become chronically infected, secreting viral particles for long periods. Natural infection in humans occurs after rodent contamination of food and drink, inhalation of aerosolized rodent secretions, or contact with rodent material through skin abrasions. Lassa fever has been reported in several areas of sub-Saharan West Africa, with outbreaks noted in Nigeria, Sierra Leone, Guinea, and Liberia. Recent evidence indicates an expanded region of endemicity, including Mali, Burkina Faso, Côte d'Ivoire (Ivory Coast), and Ghana.[82] It affects up to 500,000 people, with 5000 deaths annually.[43] Secondary human infection (nosocomial) has been reported and may occur after contact with infected secretions.[46]

Virology and Pathophysiology

Lassa virus is a single-stranded RNA arenavirus. Proliferation and dissemination presumably occur after initial replication at the inoculation site. As with the flaviviral diseases, the extent of end-organ involvement noted at autopsy does not account for the rapid death of infected patients. Platelet dysfunction and endothelial permeability are probably induced by host factors.[79,100] DIC, believed to be a major cause of bleeding and death in patients with other viral hemorrhagic fevers, appears to play a relatively minor role in arenavirus infections. The liver is most consistently the organ in which pathologic changes are observed at autopsy.

Clinical Presentation

Most (80%) Lassa virus infections are asymptomatic. The incubation period is 3 to 21 days. Patients hospitalized with Lassa fever show a distinct clinical syndrome. Fever, malaise, and purulent pharyngitis often develop after insidious onset of headache. Retrosternal chest pain, possibly a result of pharyngitis and esophagitis, suggests the diagnosis. The combined presence of retrosternal chest pain, fever, pharyngitis, and proteinuria is the best predictor of Lassa fever. Hemorrhagic complications (hematemesis, vaginal bleeding, hematuria, lower GI bleeding, and epistaxis) were seen in fewer than 25% of patients with Lassa fever. Nonfatal disease usually begins to resolve in 8 to 10 days. The combined presence of fever, sore throat, and vomiting was associated with a poor prognosis (relative risk for death, 5.5). Terminal stages of fatal disease were accompanied by hypotension, encephalopathy, and respiratory distress caused by stridor (presumably secondary to laryngeal edema). The most common complication after recovery from Lassa fever is sensorineural hearing loss, presumably caused by host immune response reactions against elements of the inner ear.[36]

Diagnosis

Establishing an accurate diagnosis is extremely difficult during the early phase of the infection. As the classic clinical syndrome develops, differentiation from other viral hemorrhagic fevers depends on serologic confirmation. Serologic diagnosis is made by indirect fluorescent antibody (IFA) analysis of acute and convalescent sera or detection of Lassa-specific IgM antibody. Clotted whole blood may be sent to the CDC for viral culture if handled appropriately. If the diagnosis is suspected, the CDC should be contacted immediately for assistance in diagnosis, isolation, and management.

Management

Ribavirin has been used with success in patients with Lassa fever. It is most effective if started early in the course of the illness. For adults, a 2-g loading dose, followed by 1 g every 6 hours for 4 days, then 0.5 g every 8 hours for 6 days, is recommended. Additional supportive care, with maintenance of appropriate fluid and electrolytes, ventilation and blood pressure support, and treatment with broad-spectrum antibiotics for concomitant bacterial superinfections, is often necessary.

Lassa fever has been associated with outbreaks of fatal person-to-person spread. Secondary infection (nosocomial) occurs through direct contact with infected persons or their secretions.[46] The role of aerosols in person-to-person spread is unclear. Blood and body fluids should be considered infectious. In light of the potentially fatal outcome of Lassa fever and the relative ease of transmission, the CDC has published specific recommendations for management of possible or confirmed cases. If a person has (1) a compatible clinical syndrome (especially pharyngitis, vomiting, conjunctivitis, diarrhea, and hemorrhage or shock); (2) relevant travel history, including time spent in an endemic area; and (3) prior contact within 3 weeks of presentation with a person or animal from an endemic area suspected of having a viral hemorrhagic fever, the person should be isolated and local, state, and federal health officials contacted. Ideally, an isolation unit with negative air pressure vented outside the hospital should be used. However, lack of a negative-pressure room alone is not a reason for transfer to another medical care facility.

Transmission of Lassa fever virus to medical staff can be reduced by routine blood and body fluid precautions as well as strict barrier nursing. Barrier nursing includes wearing gloves, gown, mask, shoe covers, and, if there is risk for splashing fluids, goggles whenever entering the patient's room. Decontamination of solid articles and rooms may be accomplished with 0.5% sodium hypochlorite solution. Recommendations for management of patients with viral hemorrhagic fever have been published.[18,23]

No vaccine is available for Lassa virus. Prevention is through avoidance of contact with rodents, especially in geographic areas where outbreaks occur.

EBOLA AND MARBURG VIRUSES

Ebola and Marburg viruses are closely related, large RNA viruses known as filoviruses. They cause severe viral hemorrhagic fever syndromes with some of the highest case fatality rates (~90%) of any known infectious disease. Both are endemic in focal areas of central and southern Africa.

Ebola virus seropositivity has been noted in Sudan, Democratic Republic of the Congo, the Central African Republic, Côte d'Ivoire, and Kenya. In 2014, the largest Ebola epidemic in Western Africa was reported. The first cases of Ebola were identified in Liberia in March 2014 near the Guinean border. During the epidemic, inadequate health infrastructure, lack of training and supplies, poor transportation and communication, and public fear contributed to continued transmission. As of March 2016, a total of 28,610 Ebola cases with 11,308 deaths had been reported in Sierra Leone, Liberia, and Guinea.[99a] The majority of cases and deaths occurred between August and December 2014. Contact cases were also detected in Italy, Mali, Nigeria, Senegal, Spain, United Kingdom, and United States.[10,37,58,99a]

Marburg disease is found in South Africa, Zimbabwe, and Kenya. In 2005, there was an outbreak that caused over 300 deaths in Angola.[24] Since then, sporadic cases have been observed, especially in Uganda.[31]

Although there is no definitive evidence indicating the animal reservoir that maintains these filoviruses in nature, current evidence strongly suggests that bats are involved.[66] Person-to-person transmission has been well documented, primarily through contaminated needles and contact with the secretions of infected individuals.[12,87]

Pathophysiology and Clinical Presentation

Ebola and Marburg viruses are presumed to act through similar pathophysiologic mechanisms that involve initial infection of monocytes, macrophages, and dendritic cells, which are then distributed through the circulation to many organs and cell types. The viruses suppress both innate and adaptive host immune responses, leading to overwhelming infection and wide release of proinflammatory cytokines and chemokines, causing fever, vascular instability, hypotension, and shock, followed by multiorgan failure and death.[12,31,37]

Patients present after an incubation period of 4 to 10 days with fever, headache, and myalgias. Diarrhea and abdominal pain are common. In many patients, rash, conjunctivitis, sore throat, and chest pain appear early in the disease. As in other hemorrhagic fevers, hemorrhage, hypotension, shock, and electrolyte abnormalities mark fatal courses. The high mortality reported in various outbreaks and transmission to health care workers caring for patients emphasizes the importance of intensive supportive care and precautions that limit contact with body secretions of infected individuals.

Diagnosis and Treatment

If these diseases are suspected, strict isolation procedures should be instituted and the local health authorities and the CDC notified immediately. Diagnosis may be made on a serologic basis or by polymerase chain reaction (PCR). There appears to be no serologic cross-reactivity between the two viruses.

While there are no licensed vaccines against Ebola or treatments with proven efficacy in humans (as of October 2015), the 2014 Ebola epidemic triggered rapid scale-up in research and development efforts. Three vaccine candidates have shown encouraging preclinical results and are undergoing Phase 2 and 3 clinical trials, and several other candidates are in Phase 1 trials. Blood or plasma from convalescent patients may be beneficial. Humanized monoclonal antibodies (ZMapp, Mapp Biopharmaceutical, San Diego) targeted at Ebola proteins is currently being studied in human safety and efficacy trials. Other medications in expedited clinical trials include antivirals and small interfering RNAs.[12,17,49,99b,101]

CRIMEAN-CONGO HEMORRHAGIC FEVER

Virology and Epidemiology

The etiologic agent of Crimean-Congo hemorrhagic fever (CCHF) is a bunyavirus. Ixodid ticks serve as both reservoirs and vectors of the virus. Infection in humans results from tick bites or direct contact with infected secretions from crushed ticks, animals, or humans. Most cases occur in individuals with occupations or living conditions that bring them in contact with domestic goats, sheep, or cattle on which ticks feed.[65] The disease has been observed in southeastern Europe, south-central Asia, the Middle East, and much of Africa.[13] Nosocomial transmission through contact with infected body fluids has been well documented.[65]

Pathophysiology and Clinical Presentation

Pathophysiologic mechanisms of CCHF are presumably similar to those of other hemorrhagic fevers.[30] One in five infections results in clinical disease, with case fatality rate ranging from 30% to 50%. The incubation period is approximately 1 week, with initial symptoms of fever, severe headache, myalgias, vomiting, and diarrhea. Various forms of hemorrhage, including petechiae, large ecchymoses, melena, and hematemesis, are more pronounced in CCHF than in other hemorrhagic viral diseases. Severe cases progress rapidly to DIC, shock, and death.

Diagnosis

The diagnosis of CCHF virus infection can be confirmed with acute and convalescent serologic evaluation for a fourfold rise in IgG antibody titers. The virus can be detected by PCR or cultured from whole blood if it is drawn during the first week of symptoms and kept on dry ice (or at −70°C [−94°F]) during shipment to the CDC.[92]

Management

Initial management of CCHF is similar to that for Lassa, Marburg, and Ebola virus infections, with strict patient isolation and notification of health authorities. The primary treatment is supportive therapy, with attention to fluid balance and electrolytes, oxygenation, and hemodynamic support. Although not confirmed in clinical trials, ribavirin has good activity in vitro against CCHF virus. The CDC recommends that patients believed to have CCHF receive intravenous (IV) ribavirin in the doses suggested for treatment of Lassa fever.[40] Persons in contact with CCHF patients should receive prophylactic ribavirin as suggested for Lassa fever contacts. To date, almost all therapy has used the oral form of ribavirin.

HEMORRHAGIC FEVER WITH RENAL SYNDROME AND HANTAVIRUS CARDIOPULMONARY SYNDROME

Hantaviruses, when transmitted from rodent reservoirs, cause two significant human diseases: hemorrhagic fever with renal syndrome (HFRS) in Asia and Europe and hantavirus cardiopulmonary syndrome (HCPS) in the Americas. HFRS first came to the attention of Western medical science during the Korean conflict, when febrile illness accompanied by bleeding and renal failure developed in 3000 United Nations troops and was ultimately found to be caused by the *Hantavirus* species Hantaan virus.[51] Mortality ranged from 5% to 10%. A similar, less severe syndrome (nephropathia epidemica) had been recognized in Scandinavia since the 1930s. HCPS was first recognized in a cluster of deaths in the southwestern United States in 1993, but was brought to public attention in 2012 with an outbreak of 10 cases of HCPS, three of which were fatal, in Yosemite National Park.[27] A non-specific febrile illness is followed by shock and alveolar pulmonary edema caused by the Hantavirus Sin Nombre virus.

Epidemiology

Hantaviruses cause chronic, nondebilitating infections of various rodent species. Human infection is initiated by contact with rodent secretions or inhalation of aerosolized rodent material. The disease occurs most commonly in rural areas, although occasional urban outbreaks occur, presumably with the common house rat as vector. Cases have been described most often from Asia, including China, Korea, Japan, and the Soviet Union, but the disease also occurs in Eastern Europe.[64] The Sin Nombre virus appears to cause chronic infection of the deer mouse, *Peromyscus maniculatus,* which is the main reservoir of the virus in the United States. Since the initial outbreak, additional cases have been described across the United States and South America. The risk for infection is likely related to rodent exposure, but transmission is infrequent.

Virology and Pathophysiology

Members of the genus *Hantavirus* (family Bunyaviridae) are enveloped single-stranded RNA viruses that form one of the largest viral families, with more than 300 species. The most common virus associated with HFRS in Asia is the Hantaan virus. The most common European Hantavirus is Puumala virus, which causes a mild form of HFRS termed *nephropathia epidemica.* Severe HFRS cases in Europe have been caused by the Hantavirus Dobrava-Belgrade virus. Sin Nombre virus is one cause of HCPS in the United States. Hantaviruses enter host endothelial cells and spread rapidly.[83]

Clinical Presentation

Hantaviruses cause a vascular leak syndrome. As with most viral hemorrhagic fevers, infection may be asymptomatic or accompanied by mild nonspecific illness. In the classic severe form, an initial febrile phase is associated with petechiae, proteinuria, and abdominal pain. After 3 to 5 days, a hypotensive phase occurs, with decreased platelet count and more severe hemorrhagic phenomena. An oliguric phase follows with concomitant electrolyte abnormalities. A diuretic phase usually commences 10 days after the onset of illness. Death occurs from hemorrhage, hypotension, and pulmonary edema, presumably secondary to fluid overload and renal failure. With modern management, the case fatality rate of classic HFRS is about 5%. The more benign nephropathia epidemica syndrome has a case fatality rate of less than 1%. In this disease, hypotension, shock, and hemorrhagic manifestations are rare. With HCPS, there is usually a prodromal illness with fever and mild respiratory or GI symptoms, followed by shock and pulmonary edema. The tempo of the disease at this stage may be rapid and may require respiratory and circulatory support in an ICU. HCPS has a case fatality rate of 50%.[54]

Diagnosis

The diagnosis of HFRS, nephropathia epidemica, and HCPS is confirmed by IFA or enzyme-linked immunosorbent assay (ELISA) for antibodies in acute and convalescent sera. IgM antibody determination may also be helpful. Virus isolation is difficult, but PCR and immunohistochemical staining may be useful when applied to affected tissues.

Management

Care of patients with HFRS is supportive. With HFRS, renal dysfunction occurs early, and patients require institution of dialysis soon after diagnosis to prevent fluid overload and correct electrolyte disturbances. Patients' secretions should be handled with care, and enteric precautions (but not strict isolation) are prudent. It is not clear whether person-to-person transmission of the virus through direct inoculation occurs. For the Hantaviruses, viremia recedes and antibody levels rise as the clinical phase appears.

Accordingly, nosocomial transmission or hematogenous transmission with *Hantavirus* infections has not been frequently documented, although presumed nosocomial transmission has been reported. No vaccine is available.

JAPANESE B ENCEPHALITIS

Japanese B encephalitis (JE) is only one of several arthropod-borne viruses that may cause encephalitis in different areas of the world. Others include Murray Valley encephalitis in Australia; tick-borne encephalitis in Europe, for which a vaccine exists; and La Crosse, West Nile, and St. Louis encephalitis in the United States. JE has been recognized in Japan since the 19th century. It is the only arboviral encephalitis for which an effective inactivated vaccine has been developed. Vaccine use in Japan and elsewhere since the 1960s has resulted in a significant decrease in the disease rate; however, the inactivated mouse brain–derived JE vaccine (JE-VAX) is no longer being produced because it was associated with adverse reactions, usually with the third dose. An inactivated Vero cell–derived JE vaccine (Ixiaro) has been licensed for use in adult travelers and just recently in children as young as 2 months.[29] This vaccine is recommended if traveling to an endemic region for longer than 30 days.

Epidemiology

In Asia, JE is the most common cause of encephalitis. Of the estimated 35,000 to 50,000 cases annually, 20% to 30% of infected individuals die, and of those who recover, 30% to 50% have neurologic sequelae.[29] Transmission correlates with monsoon rains in the tropics and with the summer and fall seasons in temperate regions. Rice field–breeding and other culicine mosquitoes serve as vectors. In addition to humans, birds and pigs can be infected. Pigs play an important role as amplifying hosts because they develop high-grade viremia from which large numbers of mosquitoes may become infected.[62] Most infections in endemic areas occur in children, whereas all age groups of previously unexposed populations are at risk. Transmission of JE currently occurs in India, Southeast Asia, China, Korea, Indonesia, and the Western Pacific region.[22] Routine use of JE vaccine in Japan has been eliminated because of low risk in this country.

Virology and Pathophysiology

Transmitted by mosquitoes, JE is caused by a neurotropic flavivirus that is phylogenetically related to West Nile and dengue viruses. After initial replication near the mosquito bite, viremia occurs, which if prolonged may seed infection to the brain. The cytopathologic effect of the flavivirus is believed to cause nerve cell destruction and necrosis.

Clinical Presentation

Incubation period is typically 2 to 15 days. Most infections do not cause clinical illness. Many patients recall a mild, undifferentiated febrile illness, which probably coincides with the viremic phase of infection. Patients with encephalitis often report a similar prodrome. The encephalitis syndrome is not easily distinguished from other arboviral encephalitides. The patient usually complains of headache, lethargy, fever, and confusion and may display tremors or seizures. One clinical series suggested that the presence on admission of (1) unresponsiveness to pain, (2) low level of anti–Japanese B encephalitis virus IgG or IgM antibodies in serum or cerebrospinal fluid (CSF), or (3) virus in CSF culture was associated with death. Of the 16 patients with fatal disease, all died within 7 days of hospitalization.[20]

Diagnosis

Acute and convalescent sera for antibody determination (virus neutralization or hemagglutination inhibition assays) provide the only reliable method of diagnosis of JE. Paired sera should be sent for these assays through state health departments. Sensitive assays for determinations of IgG and IgM antibodies in serum and CSF have been developed but are not yet widely available. Because most patients seek treatment long after the viremic phase, blood cultures are rarely positive for the virus, and CSF cultures are often positive only in patients with a poor prognosis.

Management

There is no specific therapy for JE. The main interventions are prophylactic: vaccination and reduced arthropod exposure. Supportive care may require an ICU. Because the virus is present in body fluids, especially CSF, blood and body fluid precautions should be considered.

NAMED HEPATITIS VIRUSES

Although infectious hepatitis has been a well-known clinical entity for hundreds of years, it is only in the last few decades that identification of specific viral pathogens has been possible. The causes of hepatitis may be divided into two groups. First, the "named," or more accurately, *lettered,* viruses now include hepatitis A to G. These are associated with defined clinical syndromes and elevated liver function tests. Second, other organisms that cause hepatitis as part of a more systemic infection include Epstein-Barr virus, cytomegalovirus, toxoplasmosis, and leptospirosis.

Hepatitis A

Epidemiology. Hepatitis A virus (HAV) is transmitted by the fecal-oral route through either person-to-person contact or ingestion of contaminated food or water. Food items typically associated with outbreaks are raw or undercooked clams and shellfish. Risk factors include contact with a HAV-infected person, international travel, household or personal contact with a child who attends a child care center, food-borne outbreaks, male homosexual activity, and use of illegal drugs.[7,45] Occasional cases are associated with exposure to nonhuman primates. Transmission by blood transfusion has been reported, but this is an uncommon source of infection. Hepatitis A is endemic worldwide, but underdeveloped nations have a higher prevalence than those in North America. Most persons in these areas show serologic evidence of past infection with HAV. Hepatitis A is a common viral infection occurring in travelers, but rates are declining with increased use of hepatitis A vaccine.

Virology and Pathophysiology. HAV is a picornavirus with a single-stranded RNA genome. Although the pathophysiologic mechanism has not been delineated, most infections begin with introduction of viral particles into the proximal GI tract. Brief viremia precedes seeding of hepatocytes, where viral replication has been documented. With replication, hepatocellular necrosis is accompanied by lymphocytic infiltration. In the majority of cases, hepatic regeneration occurs after acute disease, and no significant sequelae are observed. Chronic infection does not occur with hepatitis A.

Clinical Manifestations. The incubation period for HAV ranges from 2 to 7 weeks. The infection may be asymptomatic or mild, especially in children, but also in a minority of adults. The classic syndrome includes anorexia followed by nausea, vomiting, fever, and abdominal pain. These symptoms may be accompanied by hepatosplenomegaly. Aspartate transaminase (AST) and alanine transaminase (ALT) levels rise within a few days of the onset of symptoms. In children, AST and ALT return to normal levels in 2 to 3 weeks, whereas in adults, resolution of elevated serum transaminase levels may take several months. Bilirubin level rises shortly after AST and ALT elevations. Jaundice usually follows GI symptoms by several days to a few weeks. Resolution of jaundice may take another 3 to 4 weeks. The syndrome is occasionally preceded by arthralgias and rash, but these prodromal symptoms are uncommon. Resolution of acute disease is permanent in most patients, but rare cases of relapse have been noted. Pregnant women have a higher risk for severe illness than the general adult population. Anti-HAV antibody (primarily IgG) is detectable in the blood for many years after infection. Presence of the antibody confers immunity. Accordingly, reinfection with HAV is not believed to occur.

Diagnosis. The clinical presentation of hepatitis A is usually milder than that of other types of viral hepatitis. Consequently, the symptoms are not distinctive enough to allow a firm diagnosis, which requires detection of hepatitis A antigen in the stool or serologic evaluation for HAV-specific IgM or total anti-HAV antibody. Stool hepatitis A antigen is maximal before the onset of symptoms but may be detected as long as 2 weeks after the onset of disease. A more practical test is measurement of HAV-specific IgM antibody, which is usually present by the time symptoms are recognized and generally absent 6 months later. Measurement of anti-HAV antibodies may be helpful in evaluating possible causes of past icteric episodes or for seroepidemiologic studies, but their presence does not differentiate recent from past infection.

Management. No specific therapy exists for hepatitis A. Affected persons are usually managed as outpatients and should be instructed on enteric precautions to avoid transmission to others. Although infectivity drops sharply soon after the onset of jaundice, it is prudent to maintain enteric and blood-drawing precautions for about 2 weeks after jaundice appears. Nosocomial transmission has also been documented, but most spread probably occurs before jaundice and diagnosis.

Prevention. Active immunization with hepatitis A vaccine is recommended for most travelers to at-risk areas.[4] In addition, hepatitis A vaccine is now recommended as part of routine U.S. infant/child immunization programs, for postexposure prophylaxis, and for close contacts of newly arriving international adoptees.[3,4,25]

Hepatitis B

The spread of hepatitis by parenteral means was noted in 1885. Recognition in the 1960s of specific viral particles (the Australia antigen) in the serum of hepatitis patients led to identification of the responsible agent.

Epidemiology. With widespread use of serologic markers for hepatitis B disease, it became apparent that spread occurs through exchange of blood, semen, or rarely, saliva of infected people. Although spread is possible from persons with acute disease, the primary sources of viral particles are chronic carriers. Persons are defined as "carriers" if blood samples obtained 6 months apart both contain hepatitis B surface antigen particles (HBsAg). The carrier state follows acute infection in up to 90% of infected infants and 10% of adults. Risk factors for acquisition of hepatitis B infection in the United States include IV drug use, homosexual activity, and working in health care. In the United States, most patients are adults, and the carrier rate in the general population is less than 0.5%. In many areas of the developing world, most infections occur in infancy or childhood, and chronic carriers may constitute as much as 10% to 20% of the total population; thus, travelers are more likely to be exposed to carriers than is the nontraveling population. The risk is higher in persons regularly exposed to body fluids, including medical personnel and persons with many sexual partners.[103]

Virology and Pathophysiology. Hepatitis B virus (HBV) is a DNA virus unrelated to the agent responsible for hepatitis A. Infection occurs naturally in humans and can be induced easily in some nonhuman primates. Most HBV infections are subclinical. In those resulting in clinical disease, entry of the virus into the liver is followed by viral replication and hepatocellular necrosis. HBsAg, a viral particle, appears in the bloodstream within 3 months of infection. In most cases, IgM antibody to the hepatitis B core antigen (HBcAg) appears first, followed by anti-HBsAg (surface) antibody. Antibody to a third hepatitis antigen, the e antigen (HBeAg), is present for variable periods. The course of the disease varies widely, depending on a number of factors that are not well defined. In brief, most cases are self-limited and resolve in 4 to 6 months. In these patients, anti-HBsAg or anti-HBcAg IgG antibodies can be detected for years after the episode of hepatitis. Chronic carriers do not develop anti-HBsAg antibody, but rather maintain measurable levels of HBsAg. Similarly, carriers with persistent HBeAg detectable in blood samples appear to be more infectious than carriers without circulating HBeAg. The intricate network of antibody-antigen relationships in hepatitis B is believed to play a role not only in development of acute and chronic hepatitis, but also in the many extrahepatic syndromes associated with hepatitis B. Immune complex formation has been suggested as etiologic in hepatitis B–associated arthritis, rash, arteritis, and renal disease.[21]

Clinical Presentation. The incubation period for hepatitis B ranges from 7 to 22 weeks; however, the patient may be antigenemic for a large portion of that time. Manifestations of HBV infection are similar to those of hepatitis A and include fever, anorexia, nausea, vomiting, and abdominal pain. In addition, a prodrome of rash, arthralgia or arthritis, and fever is seen in up to 20% of hepatitis B patients, compared with its rarity in hepatitis A. Glomerulonephritis is occasionally seen. Jaundice usually appears a short time after the onset of GI symptoms. In the self-limited form of disease, recovery is complete by 6 months. Some HBV infections follow a fulminant course; case fatality rates are 2% or less in most series. In addition to complete resolution or death, three other sequelae are possible with acute hepatitis B. First, a person may become an asymptomatic chronic carrier and remain HBsAg positive but have no detectable active hepatitis. Second, a person may have *chronic persistent hepatitis,* a term used to describe persistent, but not progressive, hepatic inflammation (usually monitored by serum transaminase levels), often with HBsAg in the serum. Third, persons with chronic active hepatitis may be HBsAg positive and have progressive hepatitis, which may result in cirrhosis and death directly related to liver disease. Any of these three conditions results in the presence of HBV particles in the blood.[61]

Diagnosis. A variety of antigen and antibody tests have been developed for diagnosis and monitoring of HBV disease. The most practical and widely available test for diagnosis of acute disease is the assay for HBsAg. Antigen is usually present before the onset of symptoms and persists during symptomatic disease. Occasionally, HBsAg may be undetectable in patients with clinical disease caused by hepatitis B. In these cases, antibody to HBcAg is often present. Later, antibody to HBsAg will appear, but this is often long after the episode of clinical hepatitis.

Management. Management is similar to that of hepatitis A. Prolonged viremia makes blood and body fluid precautions necessary until the absence of HBsAg antigen and presence of antibody to HBsAg are established. For patients with chronic infection, therapy with interferon-α and an antiviral (lamivudine, tenofovir, entecavir, adefovir, or telbivudine, depending on individual clinical characteristics) is recommended.[63] Even in individuals with good prognostic indicators, the response rate in terms of long-term clearance of virus and seroconversion only approaches 30%.

Prevention. Universal immunization of U.S. infants beginning at birth and catch-up immunization of children and adolescents are the current recommendations. Vaccination for at-risk adults is also advised. Travelers to highly endemic areas who stay for 6 or more months or have close contact with inhabitants should be vaccinated. Available vaccines are discussed in Chapter 79.

Delta Hepatitis (Hepatitis D)

Hepatitis with the delta agent was first suspected in 1977, when cases of severe hepatitis B disease and exacerbations of hepatitis were being evaluated.

Epidemiology. Delta virus infection is found only in patients concomitantly or previously infected with hepatitis B. Transmission follows a pattern similar to HBV infection. In the United States, affected populations are IV drug abusers and multiply transfused hemophiliac patients. Serologic evidence of delta virus disease has been documented in the Mediterranean basin, West Africa, and parts of South America.[94]

Virology and Pathophysiology. The delta agent has been termed a *defective virus* because it requires HBV activity for its own replication.[76] The agent is a single-stranded RNA enclosed in a protein coat of HBsAg. The delta agent infects cells at approximately the same time as HBV (coinfection), or it may be introduced later in the course of persistent HBV infection (superinfection). In coinfected patients, the clinical picture may not differ from hepatitis B, but a higher percentage of such patients develop severe disease than do those with hepatitis B alone. Patients superinfected with the delta agent develop flare-ups of hepatitis, which may become fulminant. After the acute infection, the delta agent can cause progressive disease in previously stable hepatitis B patients. In general, infection with the delta agent worsens the prognosis of HBV disease. The diagnosis can be made by detection of antibody to the delta antigen in the serum.[76]

All HBV-infected individuals should be tested for anti–hepatitis D virus (HDV) IgG antibodies at least once.

Management and Prevention. Management of acute hepatitis consists of supportive care. Only interferon-α has proven antiviral activity against HDV and is associated with clearance in approximately 20% of infected patients.[2,94] Precautions against transmission are the same as for hepatitis B. There is no specific vaccine or immunoglobulin for the delta agent. The best preventive measure is to be vaccinated for hepatitis B, because delta agent infection cannot occur in the absence of the former virus.

Hepatitis C

As serologic methods for the diagnosis of hepatitis A, hepatitis B, and delta agent were developed, it became apparent that there was a group of persons with hepatitis for which no etiologic agent had been identified. This syndrome, previously termed "non-A, non-B" (NANB) hepatitis, was thought to be caused by a heterogeneous group of etiologies. It is now clear that a majority of such cases were caused by hepatitis C.[90]

Epidemiology. Risk factors for hepatitis C include IV drug use and, before routine testing, transfusion of blood products. Nonparenteral routes of infection are less important for hepatitis C than for hepatitis B. Hepatitis C is a global problem. Approximately 80% of exposed individuals develop chronic infection, which may lead to cirrhosis in 20% of patients and hepatocellular carcinoma in up to 5% of this patient subset. Rates of infection vary from 1% to 5% in most Western countries to 20% in parts of the Middle East, such as Egypt.

Virology and Clinical Manifestations. Hepatitis C virus (HCV) is a single-stranded RNA virus of the Flaviviridae family. Acute disease is indistinguishable from HAV or HBV infections. Most infections are asymptomatic, with jaundice occurring in fewer than 20% of infected individuals. Transition to chronic hepatitis after an insidious asymptomatic infection is the usual pattern. Chronic hepatitis may be asymptomatic or associated with nonspecific symptoms, such as lethargy, nausea, and abdominal discomfort. The patterns of cirrhosis and hepatocellular carcinoma, when these occur, do not differ significantly from those of other conditions. Extrahepatic syndromes associated with HCV infection include porphyria cutanea tarda, membranous glomerulonephritis, and mixed cryoglobulinemia.

Diagnosis. Two types of tests are available for diagnosis: serologic assays and RNA detection tests. Serologic testing detects only IgG antibodies, and assays for IgM or early/acute infection are not available. False-negative results may occur early in the course of acute infection. Within 15 weeks of exposure, the majority of HCV-infected patients will seroconvert. Standard immunoassay testing is used by clinical laboratories to detect antibodies to HCV. In addition, several rapid tests for HCV antibodies have been developed for point-of-care testing, including an over-the-counter testing kit that has been approved by the U.S. Food and Drug Administration (FDA). These rapid tests have sensitivities and specificities equivalent to standard immunoassays and can be performed on various patient specimens, including finger-stick blood, serum, plasma, and saliva.[60] Viral RNA can be detected in blood 1 to 2 weeks after exposure and before IgG detection. Assays for detection of HCV RNA are used to detect infection in infants born to HCV-infected mothers, for monitoring patients receiving antiviral therapy, and to identify seropositive patients who have persistent HCV infection. RNA tests can give false-positive and false-negative results. Viral RNA can also be shed intermittently, making a single negative assay inconclusive.

Management and Prevention. Prevention of hepatitis C largely depends on risk reduction, especially with respect to IV drug use. Pooled immunoglobulin has been used after exposure, but this should be procured from donors screened for hepatitis C; however, it is not generally recommended. Unlike hepatitis B, protective antibody responses have not been demonstrated. Treatment of acute hepatitis C is supportive. People with chronic HCV infection are at risk for developing cirrhosis and primary hepatocellular carcinoma. Treatment of chronic infection is rapidly improving with development of direct-acting oral agents. Oral antiviral regimens offer the potential of a cure to more patients than had been seen with previous interferon-α–based regimens, with significantly improved tolerability and safety profiles. The Infectious Diseases Society of America and American Association for the Study of Liver Diseases provide frequently updated recommendations on the management of chronic hepatitis C infection at http://www.hcvguidelines.org.[1]

The goal of HCV therapy is sustained virologic response, a marker for cure of the infection, defined by continued absence of detectable HCV RNA at least 12 weeks after completion of therapy. Treatment is recommended for all HCV-infected persons, except those with limited life expectancy (<12 months). The highest priority for immediate treatment is for patients with advanced fibrosis, compensated cirrhosis, severe extrahepatic disease, and liver transplant recipients. Regimen selection is based on the HCV genotype, with specific considerations for patients with cirrhosis, HIV coinfection, post–liver transplant infection, and severe renal impairment. In general, treatment-naive patients without cirrhosis are treated for 12 weeks, whereas those with cirrhosis are treated with longer courses (typically 24 weeks). Regimens based on oral direct-acting antiviral agents are highly efficacious, with cure rates greater than 90% in treatment-naive patients infected with HCV genotypes 1, 2, 3, and 4. Limited data are available regarding patients infected with the less common HCV genotypes 5 and 6.

Hepatitis E

Hepatitis E is an RNA virus provisionally placed in the Caliciviridae family. It is the second most common cause of viral hepatitis transmitted via the enteric route. The epidemiologic characteristics are similar to hepatitis A. However, hepatitis E has animals (pigs and deer) as its reservoir.[88] This group of infections is especially important in the Indian subcontinent, Middle East, and Africa. The incubation period is 2 to 6 weeks. The disease is usually self-limited but may be associated with severe illness in pregnant women. Diagnosis in travelers from endemic areas can be made on the basis of IgM antibody to hepatitis E in serum or testing of stool for viral antigen. PCR for hepatitis E may be available in some centers. In the United States, testing for hepatitis E is best undertaken in returned travelers with clinical hepatitis, although a more severe illness may occur in persons with underlying liver disease. Prophylaxis is appropriate advice for travelers and involves counseling on precautions regarding ingestion of food and water in endemic areas. In 2011, China licensed the first vaccine to prevent hepatitis E infection; it is not yet available globally.[102]

Hepatitis F and Hepatitis G

Hepatitis F is a putative hepatitis virus of uncertain significance, first described in France. Hepatitis G is a member of the Flaviviridae family with limited homology to hepatitis C. Its significance as a cause of hepatitis is also unclear.

MAJOR BACTERIAL INFECTIONS

This section reviews several bacterial diseases of relevance to the overseas traveler, including typhoid fever, meningococcal disease, pertussis, diphtheria, and tetanus. Other chapters deal with bacterial causes of gastroenteritis and diarrhea (Chapter 82), tick-borne diseases (Chapter 42), and zoonoses (Chapter 34).

TYPHOID AND PARATYPHOID FEVER

Typhoid fever was recognized as a clinical entity in the 1800s and was first associated with transmission by the fecal-oral route in the 1870s. Although effective treatment with chloramphenicol became possible in 1948, the disease continues to be a major cause of morbidity and mortality in the developing world.

Epidemiology

Enteric fever (typhoid or paratyphoid) occurs worldwide, but its prevalence and attack rates are much higher in underdeveloped countries. Humans are the only host for *Salmonella enterica* serotype Typhi (*S.* Typhi), the most common cause of the enteric fever syndrome. Almost all cases are contracted through ingestion of contaminated food or water. Transmission occurs through a variety of mechanisms, most often contact with a chronic carrier of the organism, especially food handlers, and ingestion of untreated waste material or sewage. Improved sewage and tracking of chronic carriers have greatly reduced the incidence in developed countries, although several hundred cases a year are reported to the CDC. Enteric fever is estimated to cause 26 million illnesses and 200,000 deaths per year.[34] This may be underestimated because diagnosis can be difficult (especially in children) and because enteric fever is not a reportable disease in most countries. Travel to Asia and especially India is associated with the highest risk for contracting enteric fever.[39]

Bacteriology and Pathophysiology

Salmonella species are gram-negative enteric bacilli. Enteric fever is primarily caused by *S.* Typhi and *S. enterica* serotypes Paratyphi A, B, and C. Increasing incidence of disease caused by *S.* Paratyphi A has been seen in some highly endemic areas of Asia.[35] *Salmonella* species are easily grown on routine bacterial culture plates, but if multiple organisms are present, media with selective growth inhibitors may be needed for optimal sensitivity. After ingestion of food or water containing the pathogen, organisms are subjected to the acid stomach environment, which results in significant bacterial killing. If the organisms pass through the small intestine, several processes may occur. The bacteria may simply pass through, causing few clinical symptoms. If the bacteria multiply and invade the mucosa, a gastroenteritis-like syndrome will result. Typhoid fever requires penetration of the intestinal mucosa and intestinal lymphatics, where intracellular replication of *S.* Typhi occurs. Soon thereafter, bacteria seed the bloodstream and are transported to reticuloendothelial cells throughout the body, where further intracellular replication can take place. After the acute episode of infection is over, *Salmonella* species may remain and asymptomatically reproduce in scarred or chronically inflamed tissues. Persons may shed organisms from such foci for years and serve as a source of outbreaks while they themselves are asymptomatic. The most common site for such colonization is the chronically diseased gallbladder.

Clinical Presentation

After exposure to the pathogen, 10 to 14 days usually pass before the onset of clinical illness. Some patients may experience gastroenteritis early in the course of disease, and abdominal pain or diarrhea may be present when the classic typhoid fever picture develops. Fever is usually the first sign of disease. Fever increases slowly over several days and may remain constant for 2 to 3 weeks, after which defervescence begins. With antibiotic therapy, fever resolves more rapidly, often within 3 to 4 days. Relative bradycardia may accompany fever. Most patients also report headache, malaise, and anorexia. Rose spots (2- to 4-mm maculopapular blanching lesions) are classically described on the trunk, although they are not seen in the majority of patients. Hepatomegaly and splenomegaly have been reported in a large number of patients.[16] Laboratory investigations early in the course may show a high white blood cell (WBC) count, anemia, and mild elevations of serum hepatic enzyme levels, including AST, lactate dehydrogenase, and alkaline phosphatase. Later in the disease course, leukopenia (WBCs <3500/mm^3) develops. Uncomplicated and untreated typhoid fever resolves in 3 to 4 weeks. Several complications may herald or contribute to death. Intestinal perforation, presumably secondary to necrosis of lymphoid areas of the bowel wall, may lead to peritonitis and death. Significant GI hemorrhage may occur but rarely is fatal. Secondary pneumonia is common. A subgroup of patients has more severe disease, which may include myocardial involvement, mental status changes, hyperpyrexia, and multisystem failure. Data on case fatality rates are limited; the global mortality rate is estimated to be 1%.[34]

Diagnosis

Culture of a bacterial species associated with the syndrome (most likely *S.* Typhi) from a normally sterile fluid is the gold standard; however, it is expensive and requires expertise that many developing countries cannot afford. Multiple studies have evaluated usefulness of various diagnostic tests. In general, bone marrow culture is the most sensitive method, detecting up to 90% of cases; blood cultures are less sensitive. Both methods are most useful in the first week of disease. Stool cultures and string test cultures may be positive later in the disease course but provide only circumstantial evidence of the causative agent. Other sero-diagnostic methods in development have not yet proved useful.[8]

Management

Chloramphenicol had been the mainstay of treatment for typhoid fever since the late 1940s. Ampicillin and trimethoprim-sulfamethoxazole (TMP-SMX) were the traditional alternatives. Multidrug resistance to traditional first-line agents is now widespread, so ciprofloxacin is the current first-line antibiotic. Unfortunately, increasing resistance to quinolones has been observed, especially from the Indian subcontinent. In cases of quinolone resistance, either laboratory or clinical, ceftriaxone or other third-generation cephalosporins are indicated.[9] Azithromycin is another useful alternative for treatment of uncomplicated enteric fever.[38] Other treatment modalities include fluid support and adequate nutrition. Corticosteroids have been used empirically for many years. A single randomized double-blind study showed that administration of high-dose dexamethasone (3 mg/kg for the first dose, followed by 1 mg/kg every 6 hours for eight more doses) with chloramphenicol resulted in significantly lower mortality in patients with severe typhoid fever than in those treated with chloramphenicol alone.[55] Severe typhoid fever was defined in this study by the presence of obtundation, delirium, stupor, coma, or shock. High-dose corticosteroids are not recommended for patients with less severe disease and should be used cautiously in those with severe disease.[33]

Prevention

Even when vaccines are given before travel, it is important to observe routine hygiene, preparation, and handling precautions for ingestion of food and water to prevent enteric fever and acquisition of other pathogens by the fecal-oral route. Currently, two vaccines are available in the United States for prophylaxis. The live-attenuated oral vaccine containing the Ty21a strain of *S.* Typhi is given as a four-dose series, with 1 day between each dose. Immunosuppression, antibiotic use, and gastroenteritis are contraindications to the use of this vaccine. It is licensed for use in those 6 years and older, and a booster is recommended every 5 years. The parenteral vaccine contains the Vi (virulence) polysaccharide of *S.* Typhi purified from formalin-killed bacteria. It is administered as a single intramuscular (IM) injection and is therefore most useful when vaccination is required on short notice. It is licensed for persons 2 years and older, and a booster is required every 2 years. *S.* Paratyphi lacks the Vi antigen, so the Vi-based vaccine offers no cross-protection against paratyphoid fever. There is limited evidence that Ty21a vaccine may provide cross-protection against *S.* Paratyphi A and B, although there are currently no licensed vaccines against *S.* Paratyphi.[95]

MENINGOCOCCAL DISEASE

Classically, meningococcal meningitis attacks children and young adults and is often seen in epidemic form. Although the advent of effective antibiotic therapy and useful vaccines has greatly improved the ability to manage this disease, it remains a major problem in many parts of the world.

Epidemiology

Cases of meningococcal disease occur sporadically worldwide, with epidemic disease generally limited to developing nations. The five predominant strains of meningococcal infections are A, B, C, Y, and W-135. The epidemiology of meningococcal disease is highly dynamic with considerable fluctuations and frequent outbreaks and epidemics. Serogroup A (and less so serogroup C) is most frequently associated with epidemics in sub-Saharan Africa. Increasingly, serogroup W-135 has emerged in Saudi Arabia (associated with the Hajj pilgrimage) and West Africa.[97] Epidemic situations clearly pose the greater health problem to both travelers and resident populations. The "meningitis belt" in

sub-Saharan Africa, a region that extends from Ethiopia in the east to Senegal in the west, experiences 100 to 800 cases per 100,000 population per year. In contrast, the United States and Europe experience approximately 1 case/100,000/yr.[53]

Particularly in sub-Saharan Africa and China, the disease demonstrates yearly incidence peaks and periodic massive outbreaks, the exact determinants of which are unknown. Transmission of the organism occurs by exchange of respiratory secretions; contact is believed to be important in the spread of disease. Asymptomatic transient nasopharyngeal carriage of the meningococcus, occurring with a baseline prevalence of 5% to 10%, may increase during epidemic periods and in close contacts of cases. The secondary attack rate among household contacts of patients with sporadic disease is 2:1000 to 4:1000, whereas that in epidemics ranges from 11:1000 to 45:1000 household contacts.

Bacteriology and Pathogenesis

Neisseria meningitidis is a gram-negative diplococcus that grows easily on several common media, including chocolate and blood agar. The organism is characterized further on the basis of serologic analysis of capsular antigens. The most common serogroups are A, B, C, Y, and W-135. In the United States, the current serogroup distribution is 23% serogroup B, 31% serogroup C, 35% serogroup Y, and the remainder serogroup W-135 and other serogroups.[53] Asymptomatic persons may carry various serotypes of *N. meningitidis* in the nasopharynx for short periods. An antibody response is often generated to these strains during asymptomatic carriage. The conditions that cause one person to become clinically ill with invasive disease while another carrier remains healthy are not well understood. The route of entrance of the organism to the bloodstream and central nervous system (CNS) is presumably through the nasopharynx or respiratory tract.

Clinical Presentation

Meningococcal disease may appear in a variety of forms, including but not limited to bacteremia with septic shock; meningitis, often accompanied by bacteremia; and pneumonia. Sustained meningococcemia may lead to severe toxemia with hypotension, fever, and DIC. In the fulminant presentation, adrenal hemorrhage may lead to Waterhouse-Friderichsen syndrome, and death may follow intractable shock. In the United States, the case fatality rate for sustained meningococcemia is generally higher than for meningococcal meningitis. There is also a clinical syndrome of chronic meningococcemia with a much more insidious onset.

Meningitis caused by *N. meningitidis* classically begins with fever, headache, and a stiff neck. It may also be accompanied by bacteremia and any of several skin manifestations, including petechiae, pustules, or maculopapular rash. In either meningitis or bacteremia, progression of petechiae to broad ecchymoses is a poor prognostic sign. As with septic meningococcemia, severe meningitis may progress with mental status deterioration, hypotension, congestive heart failure, DIC, and death. The case fatality rate of meningococcal meningitis with or without bacteremia is estimated to be about 10%.[48] In classic cases of meningitis or bacteremia with sepsis, the peripheral WBC count is elevated, with polymorphonuclear neutrophil (PMN) cell predominance. CSF is typically purulent, usually with more than 500 PMNs/mm^3. There may be a more heterogeneous cell population and fewer cells if CSF is obtained early in the course or if the patient has been treated with antibiotics. The CSF glucose level is usually low and protein high, as in other bacterial meningitides. Gram stain of CSF may show gram-negative diplococci.

Meningococcal pneumonia is a well-known but less common clinical entity described in military recruit populations involving serogroup Y organisms.

Diagnosis

The presumptive diagnosis in an epidemic can be made on the basis of clinical presentation and purulent CSF. The presence of characteristic bacterial forms on Gram stain is also suggestive. A definitive diagnosis requires culture of the organism from CSF or a normally sterile fluid (usually peripheral blood). This may be impossible in the case of a patient who was previously treated with antibiotics before CSF culture. Several commercial kits for measuring meningococcal antigen are now available for use on CSF or blood samples; they have variable sensitivity and specificity.

Management

Treatment of meningococcal meningitis or sepsis is a medical emergency. Fortunately, the organism remains sensitive to a large number of antibiotics. In developed countries, patients are treated with pencillin G alone or a third-generation cephalosporin. Typical duration of therapy is 7 to 10 days, although 3 to 4 days of IV therapy has been effective without increased risk of relapse. During epidemics in developing countries, a single IM injection of long-acting chloramphenicol or ceftriaxone can be sufficient treatment for meningitis.[84] Antibiotic treatment before culture or hospital referral is recommended in clinically suspected cases. Supportive care should include close monitoring for hypotension and cardiac failure. Development of DIC is an ominous sign. Although focal bleeding and adrenal necrosis may lead to acute adrenal insufficiency, the role of replacement steroids in the treatment of Waterhouse-Friderichsen syndrome is unclear.

Because the infectious agent has been found in household contacts and in persons exposed to oral secretions, contacts should receive prophylaxis to eradicate the organism. Rifampin, 600 mg orally every 12 hours for four doses, is standard adult prophylaxis. Children should receive 10 mg/kg of rifampin every 12 hours for four doses if older than 1 month and 5 mg/kg every 12 hours for four doses if younger than 1 month. More recently, alternate regimens using ceftriaxone and ciprofloxacin have also been proved to be efficacious, although rifampin remains the standard.

Ceftriaxone is given intramuscularly as a single dose (125 mg for children <15 years and 250 mg for people >15 years). Ciprofloxacin is given at 20 mg/kg (maximum 500 mg) orally as a single dose.

Prevention

Several meningococcal vaccines are available and include a quadrivalent meningococcal polysaccharide vaccine (MPSV4) and quadrivalent meningococcal polysaccharide vaccines conjugated to diphtheria toxins (MCV4). These quadrivalent vaccines contain serogroups A, C, Y, and W-135. Vaccination with MCV4 is recommended for all adolescents age 11 to 18 years. In addition, meningococcal vaccination is recommended for younger and older individuals with increased risk for invasive meningococcal disease, such as those with asplenia, complement deficiencies, military recruits, college students living in dormitories, and travelers to countries where meningococcal disease is hyperendemic or epidemic.[6,32] In 2014 the FDA approved a meningococcal serogroup B vaccine for use in individuals age 10 to 25 years. The serogroup B vaccine is now recommended for routine use in infants in the United Kingdom although it is not yet recommended for routine vaccination in the United States.[73]

PERTUSSIS

Pertussis, or whooping cough, was first recognized as a major threat in the 1500s. After introduction of a vaccine in the 1940s, the incidence of pertussis dropped sharply among immunized populations; however, neither natural infection nor immunization results in lifelong immunity. Older siblings and adults with mild or unrecognized disease are important sources of pertussis. Humans are the only known reservoir.

Epidemiology

Pertussis is found throughout the world. The incidence is highest in undeveloped countries, where immunization rates are low and socioeconomic conditions predispose to many communicable diseases. Pertussis is highly infectious, with attack rates of greater than 90% in unvaccinated household contacts. Untreated individuals remain infectious for more than 6 weeks. In the United States, the most severe disease occurs in children under 5 years old and particularly in young infants. Transmission is by airborne particles from respiratory secretions of infected persons.

Bacteriology and Pathophysiology

Bordetella pertussis is a gram-negative coccobacillus. The organism produces several toxins when present in the respiratory tract. Pertussigen stimulates lymphocytosis and hemagglutination. Dermonecrotic toxin and tracheal cytotoxins damage respiratory epithelium. In addition, endotoxin is produced. During the course of the somewhat protracted disease, complications can occur that may cause death. The most serious of these are secondary pneumonia and encephalopathy. In addition, fits of coughing often result in pneumothorax, hemorrhage (facial, conjunctival, CNS), and aspiration.

Clinical Presentation

Classic pertussis develops after an incubation period of 7 to 10 days. The disease appears in three stages: catarrhal, paroxysmal, and convalescent. The catarrhal stage lasts 1 to 2 weeks and resembles an undifferentiated upper respiratory tract infection with cough and mild fever. Progression of the cough to yield the classic whoop (which results when the patient gasps for breath after a prolonged coughing episode) marks the paroxysmal stage, which again can last as long as 2 weeks. During this stage, the WBC count may show marked lymphocytosis. Finally, cough resolves during the convalescent stage. Death may occur from pertussis alone or from complications such as aspiration pneumonia. Recent case fatality rates for Americans were 0.4% for all persons and 1% for patients younger than 1 year. The disease in adults is often milder, although it may show a severe classic pattern. Some investigators believe mild or atypical disease in adults may serve as a reservoir for infection of susceptible children.

Diagnosis

Laboratory tests for the diagnosis of pertussis include culture, PCR, and serology, which must be used in conjunction with clinical and epidemiologic data. Culture is considered the gold standard because it is the only method with 100% specificity, and it is best done from nasopharyngeal (NP) specimens collected during the first 2 weeks of cough. PCR on NP specimens has excellent sensitivity and turnaround time, although the high sensitivity of PCR increases the risk for false-positives. PCR is best done on samples obtained within 4 weeks of cough onset. Pertussis serologic tests are generally more useful for diagnosis in adults and in the later stages of disease.[72]

Management

Treatment with antibiotics, unless begun in the incubation or catarrhal period, has little effect on the course of the disease. Antibiotics can reduce subsequent transmission to contacts, however, and should be instituted as soon as the diagnosis is made. Macrolides are the drugs of choice, with azithromycin, erythromycin, or clarithromycin all appropriate choices for first-line treatment and prophylaxis. For infants from birth to age 5 months, azithromycin is given at 10 mg/kg as a single oral dose for 5 days. For older infants, children, and adults, azithromycin is given at 10 mg/kg (maximum 500 mg) as a single oral dose on day 1, then 5 mg/kg (maximum 250 mg) as a single oral dose on days 2 through 5. Other useful agents include doxycycline, TMP-SMX, and chloramphenicol. In infants with severe disease, corticosteroids may provide some improvement. Perhaps more important than specific antibiotics is supportive care, including hydration, nutrition, care to maintain adequate ventilation, and supplemental oxygen. In addition, external stimuli, which seem to exacerbate symptoms, should be kept to a minimum.

Prevention

Universal immunization of children younger than 7 years, as well as boosters for adolescents (age 11 to 18 years) and adults, is recommended. In addition, it is recommended that women receive a booster with each pregnancy.[26,28] In the United States, acellular pertussis vaccines are currently used. The pertussis vaccine is combined with diphtheria and tetanus toxoids (pediatric DTaP formulation and adolescent/adult Tdap formulations). The Tdap replaces Td to boost waning pertussis immunity in the adult population, where the majority of pertussis infections are perpetuated. In cases of pertussis exposure, immunization of unimmunized or underimmunized individuals should be initiated. In addition, chemoprophylaxis (with azithromycin, erythromycin, or clarithromycin) should be started for all household contacts and other close contacts regardless of age and immunization status. If 21 days has elapsed since exposure, chemoprophylaxis is of limited value.[89]

DIPHTHERIA

Diphtheria, once a highly feared cause of morbidity and mortality in young people, can be controlled with appropriate vaccination. However, according to some surveys, waning immunity has left many adults (18 years of age or older) with inadequate circulating levels of antitoxin against diphtheria. Newer vaccine recommendations are aimed at ameliorating waning immunity.

Epidemiology

Humans are the natural host for *Corynebacterium diphtheriae*. Person-to-person spread occurs through contact with respiratory secretions or diphtheritic skin lesions. A carrier state exists in which people who have either been immunized or previously infected can harbor the organism and asymptomatically transmit it to others. Evidence suggests that diphtheria can be transmitted through food or water, but this is not a major route of transmission.

Bacteriology and Pathogenesis

C. diphtheriae is a gram-positive, club-shaped bacillus. On Gram stain, the clustered bacteria have the characteristic "Chinese letter" configuration. The organisms grow on standard media, but to avoid overgrowth of other oral flora, selective media (Loffler's culture medium or cysteine-tellurite agar) are suggested. The presence of a lysogenic bacteriophage in some *C. diphtheriae* organisms induces production of diphtheria toxin. The toxin is produced as a single molecule with two subunits, fragments A and B. Fragment B facilitates attachment to the cell membrane of host cells, and after attachment, fragment A enters the cell. Cell death results from large-scale disruption of protein synthesis capabilities.

Clinical Presentation

The most important manifestation of diphtheria is respiratory tract infection. Illness begins after an incubation period of approximately 1 week with nonspecific symptoms of malaise, fatigue, mild sore throat, and slight fever. The classic lesion is exudative pharyngitis progressing to a greenish gray membrane that is difficult to dislodge. This membrane may spread over the posterior pharynx, tonsils, and uvula and down the respiratory tree to involve the larynx and trachea. Any one of these areas may be involved selectively, and the severity of illness is to some extent related to the area grossly involved. In severe disease, swollen tissues may result in a bull-neck appearance. Major complications include obstruction of the respiratory tract, which may result from direct parapharyngeal swelling or laryngeal involvement in young children, and sloughing of the tracheobronchial membrane in older patients. In addition to respiratory tract damage, toxin directly injures myocardial and neural tissue. Endocarditis occurs in some patients. Early signs in the first week of disease include ST-segment–T-wave depression and atrioventricular conduction abnormalities on the electrocardiogram (ECG). Congestive heart failure and cardiac enlargement may develop. Neurologic deficits usually begin with pharyngeal and cranial nerve paralysis. Cranial nerve paralysis may progress to bilateral motor paralysis, which generally resolves over 3 to 6 months. In the tropics, cutaneous diphtheria is seen frequently. The skin lesions are not consistent in appearance, and range from very superficial impetigo-like lesions to deep ulcers. In most cases of cutaneous disease, absorption of toxin is not great enough to cause the multisystem involvement seen in respiratory tract disease. The prevalence of skin lesions increases the overall likelihood of coming in contact with toxigenic *C. diphtheriae*.

Diagnosis

Reliable isolation of the organism requires a selective medium and several days of culture. Treatment should be started as soon as the patient is evaluated and is guided by clinical manifestations.

Management

Because the toxin and not the organism per se mediates life-threatening clinical manifestations of diphtheria, neutralization of absorbed toxin is crucial. A horse-derived antitoxin is available from the CDC and should be administered as soon as the diagnosis is seriously considered. A 0.1-mL test dose of intradermal antitoxin diluted to a 1:1000 concentration (with a saline control) is observed for 20 minutes. If no reaction occurs, full doses can be given intravenously. Antitoxin should be diluted to 1:20 in saline and given no faster than 1 mL/min. The dose depends on the location and severity of disease. A dose of 20,000 to 40,000 units is recommended for pharyngeal/laryngeal disease of less than 48 hours' duration, 40,000 to 60,000 units for moderate cases with nasopharyngeal disease, and 80,000 to 120,000 units for severely ill patients with diffuse neck swelling or illness of more than 3 days' duration.[5] Erythromycin or penicillin G may be given to eradicate the carrier state, although their use has no effect on the clinical course of disease. Close observation is crucial to evaluate the need for respiratory support, especially in young children. Serial ECGs and neurologic evaluation establish the onset of complications. If significant conduction abnormalities are present, continuous heart monitoring should be undertaken. Strict bed rest is recommended for all patients for 2 to 3 weeks. Immunization should be given during convalescence, because disease survival does not necessarily confer immunity.

Prevention

Close contacts of patients with respiratory diphtheria should receive diphtheria vaccine if they have not received at least three doses previously or if 5 or more years have elapsed since the last dose. In addition, unimmunized or partially immunized contacts should receive either IM benzathine penicillin (600,000 units if younger than 6 years, 1.2 million units if older than 6 years) or 7 to 10 days of erythromycin (40 mg/kg/day for children or 1 g/day for adults, in four divided doses). Antitoxin is not recommended for contacts. The most important way to prevent diphtheria in adults, however, is to ensure that all adults receive a booster dose of Tdap every 10 years.

TETANUS

Tetanus was recognized by the early Greeks and remains a cause of infant and adult mortality. The current mortality rate approaches 90% and 40% for untreated infants and adults, respectively. Tetanus toxoid immunization has drastically reduced the incidence of disease in populations with high coverage rates.

Epidemiology

The tetanus bacterium and its spores are ubiquitous. Approximately 10% of the general population carries *Clostridium tetani* in fecal flora. Person-to-person spread is not an important cause of this disease. Disease occurs when the organism is introduced into an environment suitable for its growth, specifically wound sites with an anaerobic environment. In the developing world, the vast majority of cases are in neonates as a result of umbilical stump infections.

Bacteriology and Pathophysiology

C. tetani is a gram-positive, anaerobic, spore-forming rod. The spores are hardy and can occasionally survive boiling for short periods. After proliferating in an appropriate anaerobic environment, *C. tetani* releases the toxin tetanospasmin, which in generalized disease reaches the spinal column and CNS by hematogenous spread. The toxin is taken up by inhibitory neurons, where it interferes with release of inhibitory neurotransmitters, resulting in disinhibition of motor groups. Disinhibition of sympathetic nervous system neurons occurs through a similar mechanism. The result is muscular spasm of varying severity and signs of sympathetic nervous system hyperactivity, including tachycardia, sweating, arrhythmias, and high blood pressure.

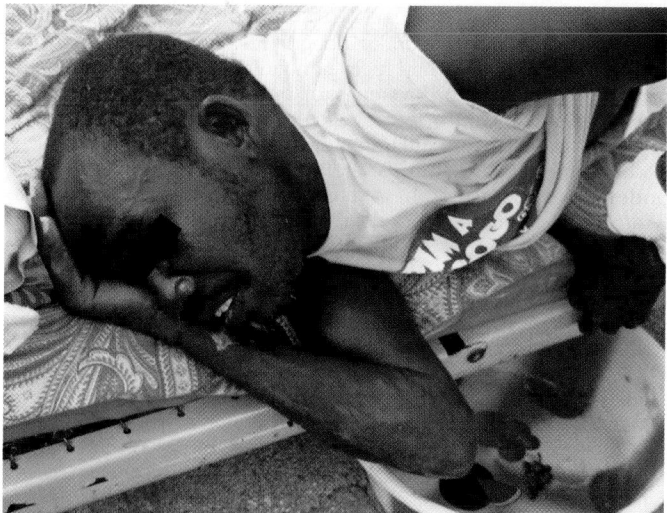

FIGURE 81-2 Patient with tetanus following a leg wound suffered during the 2010 earthquake in Haiti. Note difficulty with handling of oral secretions. *(Courtesy Paul S. Auerbach, MD.)*

Clinical Presentation

A tetanus-prone wound precedes most adult disease, which may not be evident at presentation. Localized tetanus, with spasm of a focal set of muscle groups, may occur and remain localized for weeks, then slowly resolve. This form of tetanus is much less common than is the generalized form, which often begins with trismus, or spasm of the masticator muscle group (Figure 81-2). Gradual onset of spasm of other muscle groups usually involves the trunk and extremities. Because the posterior muscles are stronger during spasms, the patient exhibits lumbar lordosis, with the neck and legs extended and arms flexed at the elbows (opisthotonos). Spasms seem to be exacerbated by external stimuli, such as sudden sound or light. The primary danger is loss of ability to breathe, especially during prolonged spasms. Respiratory failure is the main cause of death. The clinical picture in neonatal tetanus is similar but begins with restlessness and failure to nurse, with progression to tetany and sympathetic overactivity (Figure 81-3). There is no definitive laboratory test to confirm the diagnosis of tetanus, but the clinical picture is adequate in the majority of cases.

Management

Emergency medical treatment of tetanus patients should include (1) excision of the wound, (2) administration of human tetanus immunoglobulin (TIG; 3000 to 6000 units in a single dose), and (3) administration of an antibiotic effective against *C. tetani*, such as penicillin or metronidazole for 10 to 14 days.[41] Depending on the severity of disease, different levels of supportive care and sedation may be appropriate. Benzodiazepines may be given to mildly affected patients for sedation. Patients should be evaluated carefully for dysphagia. If dysphagia is present or other respiratory difficulties arise, endotracheal intubation or a tracheostomy should be performed. With prolonged spasms, hypoxia and cyanosis may occur, and mechanical ventilation with pharmacologic paralysis is appropriate. At the same time, attention must be given to fluid balance and nutrition. Enteral feeding by a nasogastric tube is the least invasive way to supply both. β-Adrenergic blockers have been suggested to relieve symptoms of autonomic overactivity, such as tachycardia and hypertension, but their prophylactic use has no proven benefit. Sources of sensory stimulation should be reduced when the spasms are uncontrolled.

Prevention

Although rare cases of tetanus have occurred in previously immunized persons, immunization is considered at least 99.9% effective. Several vaccine formulations are available in the United States. Children younger than 7 years may receive either DTaP

or DT (diphtheria and tetanus toxoid only) vaccine. A third vaccine, Tdap, is manufactured for use in persons at least 7 years old and consists of tetanus toxoid and a smaller amount of diphtheria toxoid and pertussis than is present in the pediatric vaccines. A reduced amount of diphtheria toxoid is used in the adult preparation because both the amount of toxoid and increasing age are associated with more severe reactions to vaccination. Adults who are unimmunized should be given a series of three doses (0.5 mL intramuscularly) of Tdap, with the second dose 4 to 8 weeks after the first, and the third dose 6 to 12 months after the second. A booster should be given every 10 years thereafter. All travelers should know when they were last immunized and stay current with booster doses.

From the standpoint of tetanus prevention, care of wounds is crucial. The tetanus-prone wound, contaminated with dirt or feces or caused by puncture, crush, avulsion, or frostbite, should be cleaned and debrided appropriately. Persons with tetanus-prone wounds should receive 250 units of TIG intramuscularly (for all ages) if their immunization history is unknown or their immunization series is incomplete. These persons should also receive a dose of Tdap and complete an immunization series. Persons fully immunized and given an appropriate booster before a tetanus-prone wound should not receive TIG. If they have not received a booster within 5 years, however, they should receive a dose of Tdap.

MAJOR PROTOZOAN INFECTIONS OTHER THAN MALARIA

AFRICAN TRYPANOSOMIASIS

Trypanosoma brucei rhodesiense (East Africa) and *T. brucei gambiense* (West Africa) are important infectious diseases in Africa

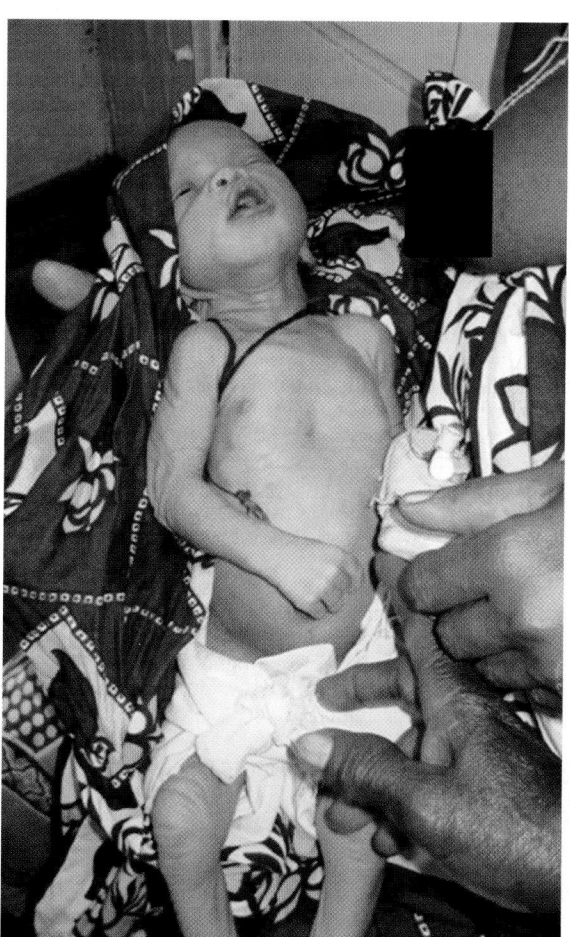

FIGURE 81-3 Neonatal tetanus in Kenya.

and have provided remarkable insights into the importance of antigenic variation as a strategy used by parasites to avoid the immune response.[69] *T. brucei gambiense* causes African sleeping sickness, and *T. brucei rhodesiense* causes an acute disease that may end in heart failure. The parasites are transmitted to humans by tsetse flies (*Glossina* spp.) in sub-Saharan Africa. Metacyclic promastigotes are injected into the bloodstream through the saliva of the biting tsetse fly and divide into long slender forms in the bloodstream. These eventually differentiate into short stumpy forms, which are taken up in the blood meal of the tsetse. Once in the fly, the parasite differentiates into procyclic forms. It takes approximately 3 weeks for the protozoa to develop into infective metacyclics within the tsetse fly. Approximately 10,000 human cases are reported each year. In East Africa, animals such as antelope, bushbuck, and hartebeest serve as reservoirs. In West and Central Africa, humans are the only reservoir.[44,99]

Clinical Manifestations

The initial sign of infection is a nodule at the site of the tsetse fly bite. This lesion becomes erythematous and painful over 1 week and usually recedes after several days. Dissemination of the trypanosome throughout the body causes clinical symptoms, notably fever, headache, and severe malaise. On physical examination, enlarged supraclavicular and posterior cervical lymph nodes are noted. This phase of illness lasts several days and is followed by an asymptomatic period of several weeks. The acute phase may then recur. In the case of *T. brucei gambiense* infection, symptoms are less severe and evolve into a syndrome characterized by behavioral changes and chronic somnolence. *T. brucei rhodesiense* infections cause severe anemia, frequent episodes of fever, and eventual heart failure and severe CNS involvement. Both forms have high fatality rates. Without treatment, infected patients die within weeks to months after *T. brucei rhodesiense* disease, and within a few years from *T. brucei gambiense* disease.[19]

Diagnosis

Definitive diagnosis depends on identification of parasites in blood, lymphatics, or CSF. Thick blood smears and buffy coat preparations should be prepared with Giemsa stain and examined for the presence of trypanosomes. CSF should be subjected to centrifugation and the sediment examined for parasites. Associated laboratory abnormalities include anemia, monocytosis, and elevated serum and CSF IgM levels.

Management

Suramin (available from the CDC) should be used for treatment of early *T. brucei rhodesiense* infection, although the drug may cause proteinuria. A test dose of 100 mg intravenously (IV) is first given to detect possible idiosyncratic reactions. If tolerated, 1 g should be given on the initial day of treatment and 3, 7, 14, and 21 days later. If CNS involvement is diagnosed or strongly suspected (CSF lymphocytosis and elevated IgM), melarsoprol (available from the CDC) should be administered. This drug should be given at 2 to 3.6 mg/kg/d IV for 3 days. After 1 week with no drug given, additional injections of 3.6 mg/kg/d IV for 3 days are given. Repeat again after 1 week with no drug given. This arsenical compound is toxic, causing encephalopathy and exfoliative dermatitis, and should be used only in a controlled hospital setting. For early *T. brucei gambiense* infection, pentamidine (4 mg/kg body weight intramuscularly, up to 300 mg/kg given over 7 days) is the treatment of choice. Eflornithine, 100 mg/kg every 6 hours for 14 days, should be used for more advanced cases of this infection.

SOUTH AMERICAN TRYPANOSOMIASIS (CHAGAS' DISEASE)

Trypanosoma cruzi is transmitted to humans by triatomids that live in the cracks of mud-built homes in Central and Latin America. These insects are common in areas of Brazil, Venezuela, and Argentina with poor socioeconomic development. The infection has been reported as far north as the southern United States.

Clinical Manifestations

Affected individuals generally do not recall initial contact with the insects, when triatomid feces containing the protozoan organisms are deposited on broken skin or mucous membranes and then multiply within local macrophages. The macrophages rupture and elicit an inflammatory reaction that appears as a nodule with slightly painful satellite nodules or draining lymph nodes. A symptomatic phase, characterized by fever and diffuse lymph node enlargement, develops. Hepatosplenomegaly may also occur. In severe cases, acute myocarditis, pericarditis, or endocarditis is seen. After several months, the acute phase resolves, and chronic disease appears, characterized by cardiomyopathy, megaesophagus, or megacolon.[74] It is rare for the traveler to develop these signs or symptoms.

Diagnosis

Diagnosis during the acute phase may be made by demonstration of parasites in leukocytes in Giemsa-stained blood smears. Amastigotes of *T. cruzi* may also be present in biopsy specimens of lymph nodes or muscle. Elevated IgM antibody titers to *T. cruzi* (performed by the CDC) also support the diagnosis. In the chronic phases of Chagas' disease, the clinical findings of cardiomyopathy, megaesophagus, or megacolon, in concert with isolation of *T. cruzi* from blood, support the diagnosis. To detect trypanosomes in blood, uninfected triatomids are permitted to feed on the patient's forearm for 30 minutes. The insects are then kept for 30 days, and the intestinal contents of the insect inspected for *T. cruzi*. If negative, the examination may be repeated 60 days later. This test is positive in about 50% of cases. Serologic tests, including complement fixation anti–*T. cruzi* antibodies, are useful but may also be positive in long-term residents of endemic areas.

Management

Acute Chagas' disease is treated with nifurtimox, 8 to 10 mg/kg body weight orally per day in four divided doses for 120 days. The drug is available from the CDC. Chronic disease manifestations are treated with supportive or palliative therapies, including heart transplantation for severe cardiomyopathies.

LEISHMANIASIS

Humans may be infected by *Leishmania* species that cause three clinical syndromes: cutaneous, mucosal, or visceral leishmaniasis. These intracellular parasites are transmitted by phlebotomine sandflies. Various forms of the infection occur throughout Latin and Central America, Africa, the Middle East, and Asia (Figure 81-4).[75] Cutaneous lesions are caused by *Leishmania tropica*, *L. major* and *L. aethiopica* (Old World species), and by *L. mexicana*, *L. amazonensis*, *L. braziliensis*, *L. panamensis*, *L. guyanensis*, and *L. peruviana* (New World species).

Cutaneous disease begins as a small ulcer with raised borders. Ulcers can persist as nodules or papules. In the chronic phase, these nonhealing ulcers frequently become secondarily infected by bacteria.[98] Mucosal leishmaniasis is typically caused

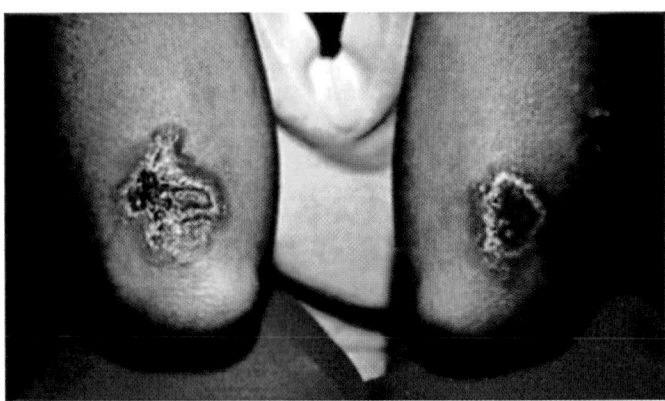

FIGURE 81-4 Old World leishmaniasis. *(Courtesy Richard Kaplan.)*

by *L. braziliensis, L panamensis,* and *L. guyanensis.* It begins as a single nodule, and months to years after the cutaneous lesion heals, progresses to the oropharyngeal or nasal mucosa, where it causes severe destruction. This disease occurs primarily in residents of the Amazon basin. Visceral leishmaniasis (kala-azar) is caused by *L. donovani, L. infantum,* and *L. chagasi.* Affected individuals generally do not recall an initial skin lesion. Several months after inoculation, fever, abdominal discomfort, and weakness develop and become progressively more severe. Nausea and vomiting are protracted, the skin becomes dry and dark, and abdominal distention with hepatosplenomegaly eventually appears.

Diagnosis is made by demonstration of the presence of the parasite in tissue biopsy or needle aspiration of affected tissue. Serologic testing is usually positive in mucosal or visceral leishmaniasis (available at the CDC). Treatment is indicated for mucosal and visceral leishmaniasis; liposomal amphotericin B is the only FDA-approved treatment. Protection from sandfly bites prevents the disease. All forms of leishmaniasis are rare in travelers and nonresidents of endemic areas.

MAJOR HELMINTHIC INFECTIONS

Worm infections are common among travelers to developing countries, especially in those who spend time in rural areas. However, unlike many viral and protozoan infections, helminths rarely cause life-threatening disease, and infested persons are often asymptomatic.

SCHISTOSOMIASIS

Three major species of schistosomes infect humans: *Schistosoma mansoni, S. haematobium,* and *S. japonicum. S. mansoni* infection occurs in South America and Africa. *S. haematobium* infection occurs primarily in Africa, especially Egypt and East Africa. *S. japonicum* infection is present exclusively in the Far East. Schistosomiasis is transmitted by freshwater snails. These snails release cercariae that penetrate the skin of humans. The cercariae rapidly transform into schistosomulae, which migrate to the lungs and eventually the portal (in the case of *S. mansoni* and *S. japonicum*) or vesical (in the case of *S. haematobium*) venous system to differentiate into adult worms. Fecund female worms release eggs, which may be passed in feces or urine. Miracidia released from this stage may then infect snails in water used for bathing, washing clothes, or other communal activities.

Clinical Manifestations

Signs and symptoms of infection vary among the three schistosome species. The initial presentation of acute *S. mansoni* infection may include fever, anorexia, weight loss, and abdominal pain. This unusual symptom complex, which occurs in individuals with heavy infection, has been referred to as "Katayama fever" and appears 18 to 60 days after exposure.[78] Travelers with light or moderate exposure, however, usually have no specific signs or only mild local dermatitis (swimmer's itch) associated with contact with cercariae, the infective stage of the parasite released by snails (Figure 81-5). In persons with established infections, the prevalence of clinical manifestations is low. Most individuals have no signs specifically attributable to *S. mansoni* infection. Hepatomegaly or splenomegaly, attributable to portal hypertension after granulomatous reactions to eggs deposited in the liver, occurs in 15% of patients. Eggs may also embolize to the lungs and induce granulomatous lesions and cor pulmonale. Those at greatest risk are persons who have the heaviest intensity of infection as judged by fecal egg counts. These complications may ultimately result in esophageal and GI varices, which cause acute blood loss.

Manifestations of *S. japonicum* infections are similar to those of *S. mansoni* infections, except that Katayama fever appears to be more frequent in the former case. In addition, there is a unique manifestation of *S. japonicum* infection attributable to embolization of eggs to the brain. Generalized or jacksonian seizures are the major signs of cerebral schistosomiasis. Because *S. haematobium* adult worms inhabit the venous system of the

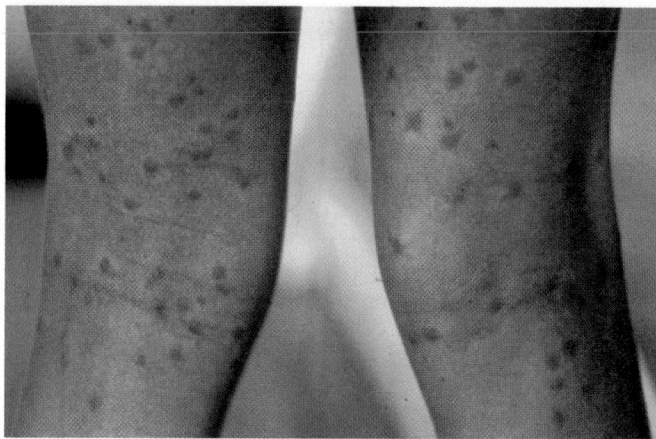

FIGURE 81-5 Mild local dermatitis associated with contact with cercariae, the infective stage of *Schistosoma* spp. released by snails. *(From Ryan ET, Wilson ME, Kain KC: Illness after international travel, N Engl J Med 347:505, 2002.)*

genitourinary tract, signs and symptoms of this helminth infection are primarily secondary to granulomatous reactions to eggs present in the ureters and bladder wall. Dysuria and hematuria have been reported in many individuals who reside in endemic areas.

Treatment and Prevention

Treatment for all *Schistosoma* species is a one-time dose of praziquantel at 40 to 60 mg/kg, depending on the species (*S. japonicum* should be treated with 60 mg/kg of praziquantel). Patients with intense reactions may benefit from a course of oral corticosteroids.

The major risk to travelers is encountered when exposure to large numbers of cercariae occurs by bathing in freshwater that contains infective snails. Cases of transverse myelitis have been reported in these circumstances. Appropriate preventive measures include counseling to avoid bathing or swimming in freshwater in endemic areas.

FILARIASES

Three major types of human filariasis exist. Infections caused by *Onchocerca volvulus* are manifest primarily as skin and eye diseases. *Brugia malayi* and *Wuchereria bancrofti* cause lymphatic filariasis. *Loa loa* infection may cause skin disease. Each of these is described separately because their ecologies and manifestations are distinct.

Onchocerciasis

Onchocerca volvulus is transmitted to humans by the bite of *Simulium* species of blackflies in Central America and West and Central Africa. Infective, or third-stage, larvae eventually develop into adult worms contained in deep subcutaneous nodules that are asymptomatic and may be palpable. Microfilariae are released from adult female worms and cause dermatitis as they migrate through the skin. The organisms have a propensity to invade the eye (especially the anterior chamber and cornea), where they cause blindness. Diagnosis is based on prolonged residence in an endemic area (e.g., Peace Corps volunteers) and parasitologic identification in skin snips or slit-lamp examination of the eye. Treatment is with ivermectin to clear microfilariae.[86] For children and adults, 150 mcg/kg of ivermectin is given as a single oral dose every 6 months.

Lymphatic Filariasis

Brugia malayi and *Wuchereria bancrofti* are transmitted by mosquitoes. Infective larvae eventually develop into lymphatic-dwelling adult worms, which release microfilariae into the bloodstream. Although chronic infection and recurrent exposure are associated with a wide variety of clinical manifestations,

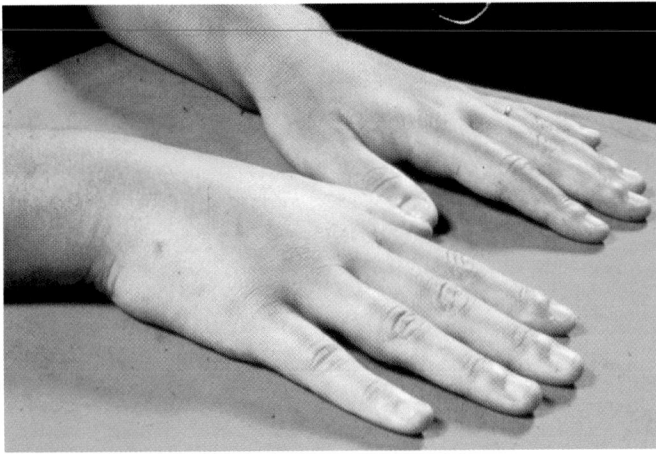

FIGURE 81-6 Calabar swellings of loiasis (loaiasis). *(From Ryan ET, Wilson ME, Kain KC: Illness after international travel, N Engl J Med 347:505, 2002.)*

including tropical pulmonary eosinophilia, acute lymphangitis, and elephantiasis, these manifestations are rare in nonresidents of endemic areas. The only definitive diagnostic test is identification of parasites in the bloodstream. Because nonresidents and many residents who are infected may not have detectable parasitemia, other laboratory studies (eosinophilia, elevated serum IgE level) must be used as aids in diagnosis. Diethylcarbamazine (6 mg/kg/day in three doses for 12 days) is the treatment.[86]

Loiasis (Loaiasis)

Loa loa is transmitted to humans by the bites of tabanid flies that live along river edges in Central and West Africa. Microfilariae migrate in the bloodstream, whereas adult worms migrate in cutaneous tissues. The major disease manifestation is Calabar swellings, which are characterized as egg-sized or smaller raised lesions, predominantly over the extremities, that are tender and surrounded by edematous skin (Figure 81-6). They may migrate and last several days. Migration of the worm across the eye is known as loiasis, loa loa, or African eye worm (Figure 81-7). The pathogenesis may be related to migration of adult worms or release of antigens that elicit immunologic hypersensitivity reactions. Treatment is with diethylcarbamazine, 6 mg/kg/day in three doses for 21 days. Diethylcarbamazine must be administered with caution, because it can cause serious side effects, such as encephalitis and retinal hemorrhages, in patients with loiasis; the risk is increased with high microfilarial loads (>8000 microfilariae/mL).[71]

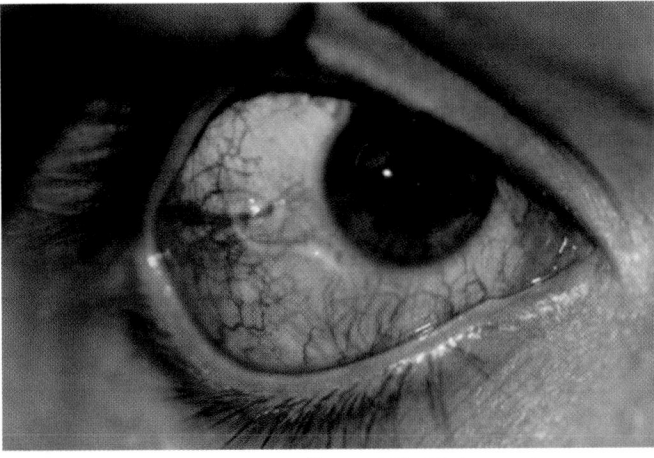

FIGURE 81-7 Loiasis. *(From Moffett S, Wills CP: Images in emergency medicine: Young man with foreign-body sensation in the right eye—loaiasis (African eye worm), Ann Emerg Med 55:578, 2010.)*

INTESTINAL HELMINTH INFECTIONS

Ascariasis

Approximately 25% of the world's population is infected with *Ascaris lumbricoides*. Although this nematode contributes significantly to morbidity in children with poor nutrition, it generally does not cause significant health problems for the traveler. The helminth is transmitted by eggs contained in ingested pieces of soil, such as may be found on vegetables grown in countries with poor hygienic conditions. It is not limited to tropical climates and occurs in North America and Europe. Ingested eggs enter the small intestine. Larvae leave the eggshell to penetrate the mucosa and eventually enter the bloodstream and lymphatics. Between 1 and 5 days after infection, they enter the liver and, at about 14 days, the lungs. The larvae then rupture through the alveoli, ascend the trachea, and return to the intestine on being swallowed. In the small intestine, adult males and females develop into macroscopic worms (12 to 25 cm long). Eggs passed via feces continue the life cycle.

Ascaris infection is often asymptomatic, but several syndromes are associated with tissue and intestinal phases of infection. Persons who are recurrently exposed may develop pulmonary ascariasis, characterized by cough, wheezing, eosinophilia, and fleeting pulmonary infiltrates on chest radiographic examination. Children may have intestinal or biliary tract obstruction caused by infestations with large numbers of worms from repeated ingestion of *Ascaris* eggs. Intestinal symptoms are seen mainly in persons with heavy infection, an uncommon situation in the traveler.

Diagnosis of ascariasis may be made by identification of one of several parasite stages. Adult ascarids occasionally migrate from the mouth or anus. Ascaris larvae may rarely be observed in sputum or gastric washings. The most common means of diagnosis is identification of eggs in feces. Eggs are ovoid, 35 to 70 mm in diameter, and consist of an outer white shell and brownish ovum internally. The eggs are not produced until approximately 9 weeks after infection. Intestinal ascariasis is treated with albendazole or mebendazole. An alternative regimen that avoids the use of benzimidazoles (e.g., for treatment of pregnant women) is pyrantel pamoate (11 mg/kg to a maximum of 1 g).[14]

Hookworm

Ancylostoma duodenale and *Necator americanus* infections occur most often in the tropics but also in temperate climates where sanitation is poor. Hookworm is second only to *Ascaris lumbricoides* in terms of the number of people infected. Humans are infected percutaneously by third-stage larvae in the soil. The larvae enter the bloodstream, pass to the lungs, and rupture the alveolar lining, eventually to ascend the trachea and descend the esophagus to differentiate into adult worms. These adult worms contain cutting plates on the anterior end and feed on host blood obtained through their attachment sites in the upper small intestine. Each *N. americanus* infection causes an estimated 0.03 mL of blood loss per day, whereas the *A. duodenale* hookworm consumes 0.26 mL per day. Iron deficiency anemia, especially in persons with low iron intake, is the major clinical manifestation of hookworm infection.

The diagnosis may be made by identification of hookworm eggs in feces. The eggs are round, 40 to 60 mm [1.6 to 2.4 inches] in diameter, and have a "smoother" shell than do *Ascaris* eggs. Although multiple drugs are effective in treatment, albendazole is most readily available. Supplemental iron should be given to persons when necessary. Infection with hookworm is rare in the traveler from a developed country. Migrating animal hookworms, such as *Ancylostoma braziliense* and *Ancylostoma caninum*, may create serpiginous lesions in superficial tissues of humans (Figure 81-8).[14]

Strongyloidiasis

Strongyloides stercoralis infection occurs in tropical and temperate regions. The infection is initiated by contact with soil containing infective third-stage larvae. The helminth follows a route within the host similar to that described for hookworms. In

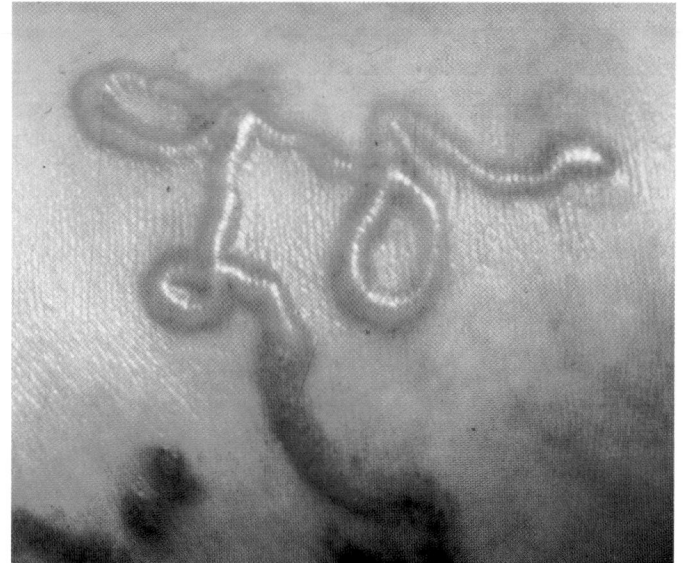

FIGURE 81-8 Migrating animal hookworms, such as *Ancylostoma braziliense* and *Ancylostoma caninum*, may create serpiginous lesions in superficial tissues of humans. *(From Ryan ET, Wilson ME, Kain KC: Illness after international travel, N Engl J Med 347:505, 2002.)*

neous or intestinal manifestations. The former are urticarial lesions around the buttocks and waist that last 1 to 2 days. These are secondary to penetration of larvae present in the feces. Other symptoms include indigestion, abdominal cramps, and diarrhea. Diagnosis is made by identification of larvae in fresh stools or GI washings. Rhabditiform larvae 250 mm long and 10 to 20 mm wide are most often observed, although filariform larvae may also be present. Treatment is with ivermectin, 200 mcg/kg as a single oral dose for 1 to 2 days.[80]

ENTEROBIASIS

Enterobiasis, or pinworm infection, exists in all parts of the world. Eggs are passed from female worms in the colon. Infection is transmitted by ingestion of *Enterobius vermicularis* eggs, which develop into gravid adult female worms in the large bowel. The infection is especially common in crowded settings where sanitation is poor. The diagnosis may be made by identification of adult worms migrating along the perianal area or by eggs deposited in the same area. Eggs are detected by applying a piece of sticky cellophane tape to the area and inspecting it microscopically. Treatment is with pyrantel pamoate (11 mg/kg [maximum 1 g] as a single oral dose), mebendazole (100 mg as a single oral dose for all ages, to be repeated 2 weeks later), or albendazole (400 mg as a single oral dose for all ages, repeated 2 weeks later). Repeated treatments as a result of reinfection in crowded settings are frequently required.[85]

REFERENCES

Complete references used in this text are available online at expertconsult.inkling.com.

addition, there is an autoinfection cycle in which larvae released in the intestine may penetrate the mucosa directly and then migrate through the liver and lungs. This occurs only in immunocompromised individuals. Many persons with *S. stercoralis* infection are asymptomatic. Some persons, however, have cuta-

---

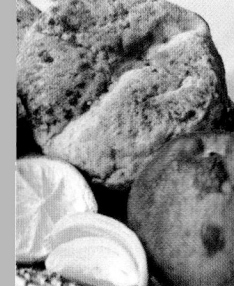

CHAPTER 82

Infectious Diarrhea from Wilderness and Foreign Travel

JAVIER A. ADACHI, HOWARD D. BACKER, AND HERBERT L. DUPONT

Acute infectious diarrhea is one of the most common and significant medical problems in any population, second only to acute upper respiratory diseases. Worldwide, diarrheal diseases caused almost 1 billion episodes of illness in 1996.[188] Rates of illness among children in developing areas of the world range from 5 to 15 episodes per child per year, with diarrhea being the most important cause of morbidity and mortality in many regions. Readily available oral rehydration solutions prevent large numbers of dehydration-associated deaths from acute diarrhea, especially in developing areas, but invasive bacterial enterocolitis (caused by *Shigella* and *Campylobacter* spp.), persistent diarrhea (defined as illness lasting 14 days or longer), malnutrition, and increased susceptibility to other infections still cause significant morbidity and mortality.[188] Specific groups of U.S. populations, including international travelers to developing regions, gay males practicing unsafe sex, non–toilet-trained toddlers in some day care centers, and mentally impaired residents of custodial institutions, can have rates of diarrhea approximating those in the developing world.

Clinical features of acute diarrheal illnesses often do not permit differentiation of a specific etiologic agent, but fortunately the majority of these infections do not require specific treatment. We formulate a clinical approach to self-therapy that is likely to minimize the complications and suffering caused by these illnesses. For this discussion, "travelers" includes business or pleasure travelers as well as wilderness and adventure travelers.

GENERAL PRINCIPLES OF ENTERIC DISEASE
EPIDEMIOLOGY

Fecal-oral contamination through ingestion of contaminated water and food (waterborne or food-borne) is the usual route of transmission of the enteric pathogens causing acute infectious diarrhea. (See Chapter 88 for further details on the relationship among enteric infections, safe drinking water, and sanitation.)

The relative importance of food and water depends mainly on location and precautions taken. The majority of pathogens that cause traveler's diarrhea (TD) or wilderness-acquired diarrhea can be either food-borne or waterborne; however, waterborne pathogens from drinking untreated surface water or from inadvertent ingestion during recreational water activity account for most infectious diarrhea acquired in the U.S. wilderness. Prevention of infection includes proper sanitation and water disinfection.

Person-to-person transmission is seen with pathogens that have small infectious doses, such as *Shigella* spp., hepatitis A virus, *Giardia*, and noroviruses. These infections are most common in populations whose habits expose them to high levels of pathogens (e.g., infants in day care centers, homosexuals, persons with minimal access to water); prevention includes adequate handwashing and personal hygiene. Other, less common routes of fecal-oral transmission are through aerosols (some viruses), contaminated hands or surfaces, and sexual activity.

In areas of Africa, Asia, and Latin America where satisfactory sanitation is lacking, diarrhea remains the leading cause of infant morbidity and mortality. Good sanitation is related to a much lower incidence of infectious diarrhea in industrialized areas. Travelers to foreign countries and wilderness areas often leave behind their customary methods of sanitation, such as flush toilets and safe tap water, and do not have proximity to advanced medical care.

Outbreaks of infectious diarrhea in day care centers among non–toilet-trained toddlers are associated with low-inoculum organisms, including *Shigella, Cryptosporidium, Giardia,* and viral pathogens. Hospitals, especially intensive care units and pediatric wards; institutions for mentally handicapped patients; and nursing homes are also locations with a high incidence of diarrheal diseases. *Clostridium difficile* is the most important definable pathogen in these settings.[165] *Salmonella* spp., rotavirus, and enteropathogenic *Escherichia coli* may on occasion cause nosocomial outbreaks.

Antimicrobial therapy is indicated for moderate to severe TD or when a specific bacterial or parasitic pathogen is identified (see later for details). Recent use of an antimicrobial agent (or cytotoxic agent) is frequently associated with *C. difficile* infection in debilitated hospitalized patients.[77]

In the developing world, children under 5 years of age have the highest morbidity from diarrhea, and infants under 1 year of age experience the highest mortality rates.[43] The enteropathogens more common in childhood infectious diarrhea are rotavirus, enterotoxigenic *Escherichia coli* (ETEC), enteropathogenic *E. coli* (EPEC), enteroaggregative *E. coli* (EAEC), *Campylobacter* spp., and *Giardia*. Residents in industrialized countries have only one to two bouts of diarrhea per person per year, with no difference between age groups. Complications, including death, are more common in elderly persons.[125]

Organisms are shed in stool during asymptomatic and symptomatic infection and for a period after illness. Long-term fecal shedding or chronic carrier states are reported to be important only for typhoid fever; however, parasites may be persistently shed in intestinal protozoal infections, such as amebiasis, giardiasis, and cryptosporidiosis. Carriers may act as reservoirs for spreading infection, even in areas with low infection risk. A few enteric pathogens have animal reservoirs and are spread to exposed persons. These include *Salmonella* spp., *Yersinia, Campylobacter, Giardia, Balantidium coli, Sarcocystis,* and *Cryptosporidium.*

Most cases of acute diarrhea are caused by infectious microorganisms, including bacteria, viruses, and protozoa. Fungal agents have rarely been reported. Table 82-1 lists the etiologic agents often associated with travel to developing tropical areas or with wilderness travel in an industrialized region. Food-borne illness may consist of food "poisoning" or food "infection." In food poisoning, an intoxication results when toxins produced by bacteria are found in food in sufficient concentrations to produce symptoms. A rare cause of food poisoning that results in paralysis is botulism, caused when the neurotoxin of *Clostridium botulinum* is ingested. Other food-borne pathogens are viruses, including rotavirus and small, round viruses (e.g., noro-

viruses, astrovirus), and intestinal protozoal agents, including *Giardia, Entamoeba histolytica,* and *Cryptosporidium.*

Food intoxication, caused by ingestion of preformed toxins from *Staphylococcus aureus* or *Bacillus cereus*, typically has a short incubation period (2 to 7 hours) and causes common source outbreaks involving multiple persons.[44] Infection and diarrhea caused by a living enteropathogen must first traverse the stomach and infect the small bowel or colon, explaining a longer incubation period of 14 or more hours, and usually more than 1 day.

Immunocompromised patients, including those with advanced infection by the human immunodeficiency virus (HIV), are prone to infection by a wide variety of enteropathogens, to develop infectious diarrhea, and to experience recurrent infections. Advanced acquired immunodeficiency syndrome (AIDS) is associated with chronic diarrhea secondary to ultrastructural changes in gut morphology and malabsorption, or because of reduced immunity and coinfection with enteropathogens. The pathogens responsible in advanced AIDS include *Mycobacterium avium-intracellulare* complex, *Cryptosporidium, Giardia, Isospora, Cyclospora, Microsporidium,* cytomegalovirus, herpes simplex virus, and HIV itself (so-called AIDS enteropathy). Treatment of HIV with highly active antiretroviral therapy (HAART) and treatment of the enteric infection(s) are associated with improved symptomatology and decreased rates of infection.

PATHOPHYSIOLOGY

Three intestinal mechanisms lead to acute diarrhea. The most common pathophysiologic mechanism in acute infectious diarrhea is alteration of fluid and electrolyte movement from the

TABLE 82-1 Enteropathogens Found in Tropical and Wilderness Travel

Agents	Travel to Developing Tropical Regions	Wilderness Travel or General Incidence in Industrialized Regions
Bacteria		
Enterotoxigenic *Escherichia coli*	Yes	Increasing with food imported from developing countries
Enteroinvasive *E. coli*	Rarely	Rare outbreaks
Enteroaggregative *E. coli*	Yes	Growing importance as a pediatric pathogen in diarrhea
Salmonella spp.	Yes	Yes
Shigella spp.	Yes	Yes
Campylobacter spp.	Yes	Yes
Vibrio cholerae	Limited	Not currently
Yersinia enterocolitica	Rare	Limited
Aeromonas spp.	Yes	Yes
Plesiomonas shigelloides	Yes	Rarely
Viruses		
Norovirus	Yes	Yes
Rotavirus	Yes	Decreasing due to routine vaccine use
Hepatitis A	Yes	Yes
Protozoa		
Giardia lamblia	Yes	Yes
Entamoeba histolytica	Yes	Rarely
Cryptosporidium spp.	Yes	Yes
Cystoisospora belli	Regional importance	Rarely
Cyclospora cayetanensis	Limited	Rarely
Microsporidia		
Balantidium coli	Limited	Rarely
Sarcocystis	Limited	Rarely
Blastocystis hominis	Limited	Rarely

TABLE 82-2 Bacterial Enteropathogens: Virulence Properties

Pathogen	Virulence Properties
Vibrio cholerae	Heat-labile enterotoxin
Vibrio parahemolyticus	Invasiveness (?), enterotoxin, hemolytic toxin
Enterotoxigenic Escherichia coli	Heat-stable and heat-labile enterotoxins, colonization factor antigens
Enteroinvasive E. coli	Shigella-like invasiveness
Enteroaggregative E. coli	Enteroadherence, virulence characteristics associated with toxin production and local inflammation
Salmonella spp.	Cholera-like toxin, invasiveness
Shigella spp.	Shiga-like toxin, invasiveness
Campylobacter jejuni	Cholera-like toxin, invasiveness
Aeromonas spp.	Hemolysin, cytotoxin, enterotoxin
Yersinia enterocolitica	Heat-stable enterotoxin, invasiveness
Clostridium difficile	Toxins A and B, binary toxin
Clostridium perfringens	Preformed toxin
Bacillus cereus	Preformed toxins: short-acting like S. aureus and long-acting like C. perfringens
Staphylococcus aureus	Preformed toxin

serosal to the mucosal surface of the gut (secretory diarrhea). This alteration may occur as a result of cyclic nucleotide stimulation (as a second messenger) or by an inflammatory process that is associated with release of proinflammatory cytokines. The second mechanism is malabsorption or presence of nonabsorbable substances in the lumen of the bowel, including lactase deficiency and AIDS-associated malabsorption. The third mechanism of diarrhea is altered intestinal motility. Secretory mechanisms best explain acute infectious diarrhea, whereas malabsorption and altered motility are more important in chronic forms of diarrhea, such as tropical and nontropical sprue, Whipple's disease, intestinal scleroderma, irritable bowel syndrome, and inflammatory bowel disease. Table 82-2 shows the virulence factors of the most important enteric pathogens related to infectious diarrhea.

In secretory diarrhea, the unformed stools are usually of large volume and small in number (characteristically less than six bowel movements per day). Stools do not contain blood, and fever is unusual. Examples of pathogens in this group are Vibrio cholerae, ETEC, preformed enterotoxins, noroviruses, rotavirus, Giardia, and Cryptosporidium. Dehydration is the major complication, especially in the extremes of age. Without adequate therapy, secretory diarrhea can be followed by renal insufficiency.

Invasive pathogens involving the distal ileum and colon damage the mucosa and elicit an inflammatory response associated with secretory diarrhea and colitis. In this form of colitis, stools are typically liquid and small-volume, and may contain blood and many leukocytes. The common microorganisms in this group are Shigella, Salmonella, EIEC, Shiga toxin–producing E. coli (STEC) including E. coli O157:H7, Yersinia enterocolitica, Campylobacter spp., Aeromonas, Vibrio parahaemolyticus, and E. histolytica. Complications include dehydration and systemic involvement, especially in children with malnutrition.[156]

TRAVELER'S DIARRHEA

Traveler's diarrhea is the most important travel-related illness in terms of frequency and economic impact. Point of origin, destination, and host factors are the main risk determinants.[194] Although the same infections can be contracted domestically, international travel is more often associated with enteric infection and diarrhea, particularly when traveling to developing tropical regions. The 2% to 4% rate of diarrhea for people who take short-term trips to low-endemic areas (e.g., United States, Canada, Northwestern

Europe, Australia, Japan) may be related to more frequent consumption of food in public restaurants, increased intake of alcohol, or stress. This rate of diarrhea increases to about 10% for travelers from these low-endemic areas to northern Mediterranean areas, China, Russia, or some Caribbean islands. The incidence increases as high as 40% to 50% for short-term travelers from low-risk countries to high-risk countries (developing tropical and subtropical regions of Latin America, Southeast Asia, and Africa). More than 100 million persons travel each year from industrialized countries to high-risk areas, resulting in more than 30 million travelers with diarrhea.[45] Multiple episodes of diarrhea may occur on the same trip. Attack rates remain high for the first 4 weeks in a country of risk,[57] then decrease, but not to the levels of local inhabitants. Immunity to ETEC infection, either asymptomatic or symptomatic, occurs after repeated or chronic exposure, which supports the feasibility of developing a vaccine.[74]

Although any food-borne or waterborne enteropathogen can cause TD, bacteria are the most common etiologic agents among persons traveling to high-risk areas. The bacterial flora of the bowel changes rapidly after arrival in a country with high rates of TD. At least 15% of travelers remain asymptomatic despite the occurrence of infection by pathogenic organisms, including ETEC and Shigella.[160]

DEFINITION

Traveler's diarrhea refers to an illness contracted while traveling, although in 15% of patients, symptoms first occur after returning home. Most clinical studies define TD as passage of three or more unformed stools in a 24-hour period in association with one or more enteric symptoms, such as abdominal cramps, fever, fecal urgency, tenesmus, bloody-mucoid stools, nausea, and vomiting.[49]

ETIOLOGY

Because the incidence of TD partly reflects the extent of environmental contamination with feces, the etiologic agents are pathogens causing illness in local children. Table 82-3 provides a list of etiologic agents important in TD. Twenty-five years ago, specific pathogens were found in only 20% of cases. Currently, etiologic agents can be identified in up to 80% of TD episodes.[106] In most studies, however, causative pathogens are not identified in 20% to 40% of cases. In most of these patients, antimicrobial therapy shortens illness, suggesting that this subset of diarrhea is caused by undetected bacterial pathogens.[56] Overall, the major etiologic agents and their frequency of isolation are remarkably similar worldwide.

Worldwide, ETEC is the most common cause of TD,[183] accounting for about one-third to one-half of cases. EAEC has been identified as the second most common bacterial cause of TD, causing up to 30% of cases in some areas of the world.[3] One study found that food is the source of both types of E. coli. Viable ETEC and EAEC were identified in hot sauces served on the table in popular restaurants in Guadalajara, Mexico.[4] Shigella and Campylobacter species cause around 20% of illness and Salmonella 4% to 5%, with other culprits being Vibrio, Aeromonas, Plesiomonas, viruses (10%), and parasites.[183] Specific pathogens may predominate at a particular time or location.

CLINICAL SYNDROMES

Table 82-4 outlines the major syndromes in patients with enteric infection. The typical clinical syndrome of TD secondary to the major infectious causes (e.g., ETEC) begins abruptly with abdominal cramping and watery diarrhea. Most cases are mild, consisting of passage of one to two unformed stools per day associated with tolerable symptoms that do not interfere with normal activities. Approximately 30% of affected persons experience moderately severe illness, with three to five unformed stools per day and distressing symptoms forcing a change in activities or itinerary. Only 1% to 3% of persons with TD occurring in Latin America or Africa experience febrile dysenteric illness,[67,134] whereas approximately 9% of travelers with diarrhea acquired in

TABLE 82-3 Major Pathogens in Traveler's Diarrhea (Travel to Developing Tropical Regions)

Agent	Frequency (%)	Distribution
Bacteria	**50-80**	
Enterotoxigenic *Escherichia coli*	5-50	Developing countries, tropical areas, infants, travelers
Enteroaggregative *E. coli*	5-30	Infants, worldwide
Salmonella spp.	1-15	Worldwide
Shigella spp.	1-15	Worldwide
Campylobacter jejuni	1-30	Worldwide, more common in Asia
Aeromonas spp.	0-10	Worldwide, especially Thailand, Australia, Canada
Plesiomonas shigelloides	0-5	Worldwide
Other	0-5	
Viruses	**0-20**	
Rotavirus	0-20	Worldwide, children 6-24 months
Norovirus	1-20	Worldwide, cruise ships
Protozoa	**1-5**	
Giardia lamblia	0-5	Worldwide, zoonosis, alpine areas
Entamoeba histolytica	0-5	Developing and tropical countries, especially Mexico, India, western and South Africa, parts of South America
Cryptosporidium parvum	0-5	Worldwide, including cooler developed countries
Unknown	10-40	

For details on published studies, see reference 183.

the Indian subcontinent of Asia develop this more serious form of illness.[195] Symptoms lasting more than 1 to 2 weeks suggest a protozoan etiology such as *Giardia*, *E. histolytica*, *Cryptosporidium*, or other parasite.[47] TD should be considered a self-limited nonfatal condition, but it may lead to chronic illness[47] and postinfectious irritable bowel syndrome (PI-IBS).[152,198]

An important part of initial assessment is to measure hydration, including determination of vital signs (orthostatic pulse, blood pressure), mental status, skin turgor, hydration of mucous

TABLE 82-4 Clinical Syndromes in Enteric Disease

Syndrome	Agent
Acute watery diarrhea	Any agent, especially with toxin-mediated diseases (e.g., enterotoxigenic *Escherichia coli*, *Vibrio cholerae*)
Febrile dysentery	*Shigella*, *Campylobacter jejuni*, *Salmonella*, enteroinvasive *E. coli*, *Aeromonas* spp., *Vibrio* spp., *Yersinia enterocolitica*, *Entamoeba histolytica*, inflammatory bowel disease
Vomiting (predominant symptom)	Viral agents, particularly noroviruses, preformed toxins of *Staphylococcus aureus* or short-acting toxin of *Bacillus cereus*
Persistent diarrhea (>14 days)	Protozoa, small bowel bacterial overgrowth, inflammatory or invasive enteropathogens (*Shigella*, enteroaggregative *E. coli*)
Chronic diarrhea (>30 days)	Small bowel injury, inflammatory bowel disease, postinfectious irritable bowel syndrome, Brainerd diarrhea

membranes, and urine output. Dehydration is most common in pediatric and elderly populations.

Fever is a reaction to an intestinal inflammatory process. High fever suggests a pathogen invasive to the intestinal mucosa, which classically includes bacterial enteropathogens such as *Shigella*, *Salmonella*, and *Campylobacter* spp. Fever can also be produced by strains of EIEC, *V. parahaemolyticus*, *Aeromonas*, *C. difficile*, and viral pathogens.

Vomiting as the predominant symptom in a traveler usually suggests norovirus infection.[6,116] Vomiting is also seen in "food poisoning" secondary to consumption of preformed enterotoxin produced by *S. aureus* or *B. cereus*.

Dysentery is defined as passage of small-volume stools with gross blood and mucus. Common causes include *Shigella*, *C. jejuni*, *Salmonella*, *Aeromonas*, *V. parahaemolyticus*, *Y. enterocolitica*, EIEC, STEC, *E. histolytica*, and preexisting inflammatory bowel disease.

Abdominal examination in persons with TD often shows mild tenderness but should not demonstrate signs of peritoneal irritation. Rectal examination may reveal tenderness in enterocolitis, and patients may have painful external hemorrhoids as a result of excessive number of bowel movements.

Some enteric pathogens produce both diarrheal and systemic diseases. These include hemolytic-uremic syndrome related to infection with shigellosis or STEC, glomerulonephritis related to *Y. enterocolitica* (Reiter's syndrome), and sepsis seen with bacteremic salmonellosis caused by *Salmonella typhi*, *Salmonella paratyphi*, and nontyphoid strains of *Salmonella*.

PERSISTENT AND CHRONIC DIARRHEA

Diarrhea and abdominal complaints frequently persist after the traveler returns home.[141] Up to 3% of persons with TD from high-risk areas develop persistent diarrhea.[47] *Persistent* diarrhea is defined as illness lasting 14 days or longer, whereas diarrhea is considered *chronic* when it lasts 30 days or longer. The etiology of persistent or chronic diarrhea differs from acute diarrhea; important causes include protozoal parasites (*Giardia*, *Cryptosporidium*, *Cyclospora*, *E. histolytica*), bacteria (*Salmonella*, *Shigella*, *Campylobacter*, *Y. enterocolitica*), lactase deficiency induced by a small bowel pathogen (*Giardia*, rotavirus, or norovirus), and small bowel bacterial overgrowth syndrome secondary to small bowel motility inhibition (from enteric infection) or to antimicrobial use. Occasionally, other parasitic enteric infections can cause more persistent illness. These include *Strongyloides stercoralis*, *Trichuris trichiura*, and severe infection by *Necator americanus* or *Ancylostoma duodenale*. In rare cases, more protracted diarrhea may be a prominent symptom in persons with schistosomiasis, *Plasmodium falciparum* malaria, leishmaniasis, or African trypanosomiasis.

When chronic diarrhea follows a bout of TD, a pathogen is not identified, and the patient fails to respond to empirical antimicrobial therapy, activation of an underlying condition such as inflammatory bowel disease, celiac disease, or PI-IBS should be considered. Even with eradication of microbial pathogens with antimicrobial therapy, bowel habits may not return to normal for several weeks. This represents slow repair of damaged intestinal mucosa. Small bowel bacterial overgrowth has been identified in patients with persistent diarrhea after an episode of TD. In the 1980s, an idiopathic form of chronic diarrhea emerged called Brainerd diarrhea, named after the city in Minnesota where the first outbreak was identified.[155] The known vehicles of transmission of Brainerd diarrhea are raw (unpasteurized) milk[155] and untreated water, such as well water.[157] There is no diagnostic test or therapy, and the diagnosis is suspected based on the epidemiologic history (exposure to unpasteurized milk or untreated water just before onset of illness). Although the average duration of Brainerd diarrhea is 2 years, the condition invariably resolves.

The approach to evaluate persistent or chronic diarrhea in travelers should begin with diagnostic tests for conventional bacterial pathogens in stools and at least three parasitologic evaluations of freshly passed stools. Dietary modification in all cases should initially include avoidance of milk and dairy products because of the possibility of lactase deficiency. Treatment

TABLE 82-5 Indications for Laboratory Test in Diarrheal Diseases and Possible Diagnoses

Laboratory Test	Indication	Diagnosis/Agent
Fecal leukocytes or fecal lactoferrin, fecal calprotectin	Moderate to severe cases	Diffuse colonic inflammation, invasive or inflammatory bacterial enteropathogen
Stool culture	Moderate to severe diarrhea, fever, persistent diarrhea, fecal leukocytes or lactoferrin (+), male homosexual	Any bacterial enteric pathogen
Blood culture	Enteric fever, sepsis	*Salmonella*, less likely *Campylobacter* spp., *Yersinia*
Parasite examination	Persistent diarrhea, travel to specific areas, day care centers, male homosexuals	Any protozoan parasite
Parasite enzyme immunoassay	Persistent diarrhea, travel to specific areas, day care centers, male homosexuals	*Giardia, Entamoeba histolytica, Cryptosporidium*
Amebic serology	Persistent diarrhea, liver abscess	*Entamoeba histolytica*
Rotavirus antigen	Hospitalized infants (<3 years old).	Rotavirus
Clostridium difficile toxin by EIA or PCR	Antibiotic-associated diarrhea, especially occurring in hospital	*C. difficile*

EIA, Enzyme immunoassay; *PCR*, polymerase chain reaction.

should be specific, following the results of microbiologic tests. Because most of these chronic forms of diarrhea are self-limited, it is unwise to employ empirical antibiotics in these patients. If all tests are negative, some experts will prescribe a single limited empirical trial with metronidazole for possible *Giardia* infection, because three tests may still miss 10% of infections. A better choice than metronidazole for empirical treatment of parasitic infection is nitazoxanide, which offers coverage for multiple parasitic pathogens.[104]

LABORATORY TESTS AND PROCEDURES

In clinical practice, laboratory testing is reserved for ongoing illness after the patient returns home, when empirical treatment is unsuccessful, for persons with moderate to severe diarrhea, and those with persistent illness. Persons with milder forms of diarrhea usually need only clinical evaluation; etiologic assessment is unnecessary.

Several laboratory tests are useful in evaluating patients with diarrheal disease (Table 82-5). Presence of fecal leukocytes is a reliable indicator of diffuse colonic inflammation. For moderate to severe illness, this is the most rapid, useful test and ideal screening procedure. A large number of neutrophils per high-power field using dilute methylene blue or trichrome stains (which also helps with identification of parasites) can be helpful in making an etiologic diagnosis of *Shigella, Salmonella*, or *Campylobacter* spp. (Figure 82-1).[88] Other organisms and conditions that may lead to presence of fecal leukocytes are *C. difficile, Aeromonas, Y. enterocolitica, V. parahaemolyticus*, EIEC, idiopathic ulcerative colitis, and allergic colitis.

Lactoferrin is found in granules of neutrophils and can be identified in fecal samples by commercial immunoassay method (Leuko-Test, TechLab). This test does not require a freshly collected stool sample or experienced technician, and is a more sensitive marker of inflammation than microscopic examination of fecal leukocytes.[22]

Bacterial infection is specifically diagnosed by stool culture, although routine stool testing identifies few pathogens. A routine laboratory should be able to recover *Shigella, Salmonella*, and *Campylobacter* and, if specifically requested, *V. cholerae, V. parahaemolyticus, Aeromonas, Y. enterocolitica*, and *C. difficile* from a stool culture. The major indication for performing a stool culture is the presence of febrile, dysenteric disease.

Blood culture(s) should be performed in all patients hospitalized with gastrointestinal (GI) illness or those with significant fever, especially when combined with a high degree of systemic toxicity. Systemic infections by *S. typhi* and non-*typhi Salmonella, Shigella, Campylobacter fetus*, and *Y. enterocolitica* may be diagnosed by blood culture.

Patients with persistent TD should be studied for presence of parasitic infection. Immunologic techniques to detect antigens of protozoan parasites are more efficient than are stool examinations for ova and parasites, and are in common use for parasites inhabiting the duodenum (e.g., *Giardia, Cryptosporidium, E. histolytica*, Microsporidia). At times, intestinal parasites are better detected using a sample from duodenal aspiration or intestinal biopsy.[86,133]

In select cases, particularly clinical colitis and diarrhea persisting for 14 days or longer, flexible sigmoidoscopy or colonoscopy should be considered to study colonic lesions and collect samples for culture and microscopy. Lower GI tract endoscopy is particularly useful when stools contain many leukocytes per high-power field. Colonic mucosal changes may not be specific, except when pseudomembranes are sought in *C. difficile* infection. In homosexual male patients with acute diarrhea, examination of the distal colon may show evidence of proctitis (mucosal inflammation in the distal 15 cm of the colon), proctocolitis (inflammation beyond 15 cm), or enteritis. If there are no leukocytes in the stool or if colonoscopy is negative, esophagogastroduodenoscopy (EGD) should be considered, looking at duodenal mucus for *Giardia lamblia*. Tests for malabsorption and biopsy of the small bowel mucosa may be useful in making a diagnosis.

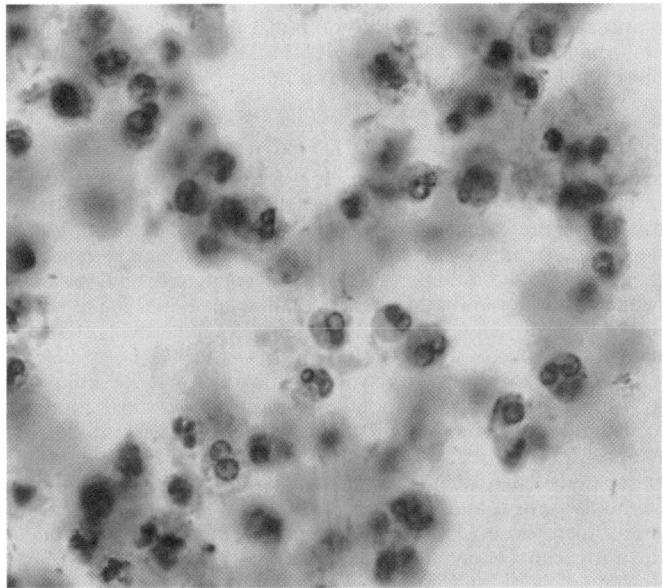

FIGURE 82-1 Methylene blue stain of a fecal smear from a patient with bacillary dysentery (×400). Numerous polymorphonuclear leukocytes are present. This indicates the presence of diffuse colonic inflammation.

Polymerase chain reaction (PCR) methods are being developed for diagnosis of various forms of diarrhea. Often, a number of pathogens are included in a multiplex approach to diagnosis.[11] PCR methods are sensitive, but in the presence of asymptomatic infection that is so common in travelers eating contaminated food, may yield a false-positive test.[46] Licensed multiplex PCR diagnostics will lead to an increased level of pathogen detection in all settings. The methodology is extremely sensitive, and we will find many false-positive results while sorting out disease etiology that will initially present clinicians with complex therapeutic decisions.

TREATMENT

Outpatient treatment with instructions for oral rehydration can be used in the vast majority of adults and children. Rehydration is particularly important in persons with cholera-like diarrhea or when diarrhea is seen in extremes of age. Significant dehydration from diarrhea in travelers is unusual.

Treatment with intravenous (IV) fluids is indicated for the following:

- Patients with hypotension
- Inability to retain oral fluids
- Systemic compromise (high fever and toxicity)
- Moderate toxicity or dehydration, and severe underlying disease
- Severe diarrhea at extremes of age

Supplemental nutrition is beneficial (essential in undernourished populations) and can be given as soon as fluid deficit losses are replaced, usually after the first 4 hours. In more severe forms of acute diarrheal disease, the intestinal tract may not be able to process complex dietary products, so patients are often told to avoid solids and eat easily digested foods. As stooling decreases and appetite improves, staple foods such as cereals, bananas, crackers, toast, lentils, potatoes, and other cooked vegetables are well tolerated and can be gradually added to the diet to facilitate enterocyte renewal, with subsequent progression to white meats, fruits, and vegetables. Dairy products and red meat are recommended only after diarrhea has resolved, usually after 2 to 3 days. Only foods and drinks that prolong diarrhea or increase intestinal motility should be avoided. Examples include foods that contain lactose, caffeine, alcohol, high fiber, and fats. Breastfeeding of infants should be continued or resumed as soon as possible. Patients with TD should avoid excessive physical activity to reduce the risk of fluid loss and dehydration.

Fluid status in the field should be assessed by physical signs related to hydration, including pulse, hydration of mucous membranes, skin turgor, and urine output. Urine color and volume are excellent measures. For travelers in the wilderness or tropics, fluid replacement must equal basic needs plus volume of diarrhea plus estimated sweat loss.

Symptomatic Therapy

Symptomatic medications are useful for treatment of milder forms of diarrhea, because they decrease symptoms and allow patients to return more quickly to normal activities. Lactobacillus preparations and yogurt are safe, but evidence is insufficient to establish their value in the therapy of TD. Adsorbent agents bind nonspecifically to water and other intraluminal material and make stools more formed. They have limited value for treatment of acute diarrhea.

The most useful drug for symptomatic therapy is the antimotility drug loperamide. In addition to slowing intestinal motility, loperamide and other antimotility drugs alter water and electrolyte transport, probably affecting both secretion and absorption. Compared with placebo, antimotility drugs reduce the number of stools passed and duration of illness by about 80%.[50,54] The usual initial dose of loperamide is 4 mg. If diarrhea continues, the drug can be given in additional doses of 2 mg after each unformed stool, not to exceed 8 mg/day. Loperamide is not given for more than 2 days. Diphenoxylate with atropine is less expensive than loperamide but has greater central opiate effects, a danger in case of accidental overdose by a child, and more side effects without antidiarrheal benefits because of the atropine,

which is added only to prevent drug overdose. Tincture of opium or paregoric opium preparations are rapidly and equally effective and offer modest relief of symptoms. A major problem with this class of drugs is postdiarrhea constipation, so only the loading dose should be employed if these medications are used.

Antimotility drugs should never be used alone in patients who have dysenteric diarrhea, because inhibition of gut motility may facilitate intestinal infection by invasive bacterial enteropathogens.[58] However, this theoretical deleterious effect does not appear to be an issue when loperamide is used concurrently with an effective antimicrobial agent.[65,66,201] Antimotility drugs should not be given to children younger than 3 years.

Probiotics have been tested for treatment and prevention of infectious diarrhea. Several meta-analyses of randomized controlled trials have noted a modest effect on frequency and duration of diarrhea. Probiotics may also be of value for antibiotic-induced diarrhea and PI-IBS. Different types of probiotic bacteria are available in capsules, powder, therapeutic yogurts, and other modalities. Effective dosage is not well delineated, and the number of live microorganisms is unreliable. Probiotic preparations have not been effective in preventing TD.[209] New intestine-specific probiotics are likely to be identified as the intestinal microbiome is better characterized.

Because increased secretion of water and electrolytes is the major physiologic derangement in acute watery diarrhea, therapy aimed at this effect is appealing. Aspirin and other nonsteroidal antiinflammatory drugs (NSAIDs) inhibit secretion,[164] but their safety is a concern because of gastric mucosal toxicity. The salicylate moiety of bismuth subsalicylate reduces the number of stools passed and duration of diarrhea by about 50%, altering secretion in the intestine. Bismuth subsalicylate also has antimicrobial and antiinflammatory properties. New compounds are being developed that have antisecretory properties without motility effects.[39,55] Table 82-6 summarizes the recommended dosages of available symptomatic treatments.

Antimicrobial Therapy

Although most enteric infections do not require antibiotics, empirical antimicrobial therapy is indicated in acute TD and febrile dysenteric illness, because of the importance of *Shigella* and *Campylobacter* as etiologic agents of this syndrome. Travelers with acute diarrhea and mild symptomatology usually do not need empirical antimicrobial therapy and can be treated with oral fluids and saltine (soda) crackers. Travelers with acute diarrhea and moderate symptoms serious enough to change an itinerary and cause great inconvenience[191] should be treated with empirical antimicrobial therapy or symptomatic therapy with loperamide or bismuth subsalicylate. Finally, travelers with more severe symptoms with any degree of incapacitation or with dysentery should be treated with empirical antimicrobial therapy immediately after passage of the first unformed stool (Table 82-7).[49] Loperamide can be given with the antibacterial drug for faster clinical response.[60] Therapy for specific infections is discussed in the corresponding sections (Table 82-8).

TABLE 82-6 Nonspecific Drugs for Therapy of Traveler's Diarrhea in Adults	
Agent	**Therapeutic Dose**
Loperamide	4 mg initially; if nonresponsive, can give 2 mg (one capsule) after each loose stool, not to exceed 8 mg (four capsules) daily; do not use in dysenteric or febrile diarrhea
Bismuth subsalicylate	30 mL or two 262-mg tablets every 30 minutes for eight doses; may repeat on day 2
Probiotics	Dose according to package, because products and formulations vary. Daily dose may make diarrhea less severe and shorten its duration; consider for prevention of antibiotic-associated diarrhea

TABLE 82-7 Empirical Treatment and Evaluation of Traveler's Diarrhea in Adults

Clinical Manifestations	Recommendations*
Watery diarrhea with mild symptoms (no change in itinerary)	Oral fluids and symptomatic therapy (can give antibiotics† or loperamide)
Watery diarrhea with moderate symptoms (change in itinerary but able to function)	Symptomatic treatment with loperamide and empirical antibiotic† treatment after passage of first unformed stool
Watery diarrhea with severe symptoms (incapacitating)	Antibiotic† after passage of first unformed stool
Dysentery or fever	Azithromycin, 1000 mg in single dose; loperamide is not recommended.
Persistent diarrhea (>14 days)	Parasite examination and stool culture; consider gastrointestinal evaluation.
Vomiting, minimal diarrhea	Oral fluids, and consider using bismuth subsalicylate.
Diarrhea in pregnant women	Fluids and electrolytes; if severely ill, treat with azithromycin, 500 mg once daily for 3 days.

*Treatment should be self-initiated during travel without evaluation.
†Antibiotic options include ciprofloxacin, 500 mg twice daily for 1-3 days; or other fluoroquinolone for 3 days; or azithromycin, 1000 mg in a single dose.

Fluoroquinolones, azithromycin, and rifaximin have adequate activity against bacterial enteric pathogens to be considered useful for empirical therapy of TD.[51] Ciprofloxacin is often the least expensive drug known to be effective. Problems with this drug[210] are ineffectiveness for fluoroquinolone-resistant *Campy-*

TABLE 82-8 Antimicrobial Therapy for Organism-Specific Diarrhea in Adults

Diagnosis	Recommendation
Enterotoxigenic and enteroaggregative *Escherichia coli* diarrhea	Rifaximin, 200 mg tid for 3 days *or* Ciprofloxacin, 500 mg bid for 1-3 days *or* Other fluoroquinolone for 3 days *or* Azithromycin, 1000-mg single dose
Cholera	Doxycycline, 300-mg single dose
Systemic salmonellosis (typhoid fever or bacteremic infection)	Ciprofloxacin, 500 mg bid for 5-7 days *or* Levofloxacin, 500 mg qd for 7-10 days
Salmonellosis (intestinal nontyphoid salmonellosis without systemic infection)	Antimicrobial therapy controversial if systemically ill (high fever and toxicity) or in a high-risk group: sickle cell anemia, age <3 mo or >64 yr, taking corticosteroids, undergoing dialysis, those with inflammatory bowel disease (if decision to treat, use regimen as for Systemic salmonellosis)
Shigellosis	Ciprofloxacin, 500 mg bid for 3 days *or* Levofloxacin, 500 mg bid for 3 days
Campylobacteriosis	Erythromycin, 500 mg qid for 5 days *or* Azithromycin, 500 mg qd for 3 days, or 1000 mg in single dose

bid, Twice daily; *qd,* daily; *qid,* four times daily; *tid,* three times daily.

lobacter strains,[204] depletion of gut flora,[108] predisposing to *C. difficile* infection,[147] and damage to articular cartilage.[136]

Azithromycin is a good alternative for treatment of acute TD. It is given in a single dose of 1 g for TD.[204] Its main use is treatment of dysenteric and febrile TD. Azithromycin has the advantage of being approved for pediatric TD (5 mg/kg/day for 3 days). Rifaximin (200 mg three times daily) was approved in 2004 by the U.S. Food and Drug Administration (FDA) for treatment of TD caused by noninvasive *E. coli* in patients 12 years and older. Rifaximin is as effective as ciprofloxacin for treatment of watery diarrhea caused by noninvasive bacterial causes of TD.[61] Modification of an orally administered, poorly absorbed rifamycin molecule that concentrates in the distal small bowel and colon may increase the drug's activity against invasive bacterial pathogens.[63]

Travelers to high-risk regions should carry an antibacterial drug for treatment of bacterial diarrhea.[51] A symptomatic drug, such as loperamide, may also be included for immediate relief of symptoms. If both drugs are employed in acute TD, persons should be instructed to take loperamide only if they do not have fever and are not passing grossly bloody stools. The duration of antimicrobials needed in TD appears to be short for the absorbed drugs, which are fluoroquinolones or azithromycin. For rifaximin therapy, a full 3 days of treatment should be undertaken. An ideal approach is to have both rifaximin and azithromycin in the travel medicine kit. Rifaximin should be used with watery diarrhea (90% of illness likely to be seen), but when bloody stools are passed and fever is present, azithromycin should be taken.

PREVENTION AND PROPHYLAXIS

Food, Beverage, and Personal Hygiene

Food and water transmit the pathogens that cause infectious diarrhea and TD.[4,203,215] When diarrhea occurs, however, the exact source cannot be determined. Being careful about what is eaten is recommended and may be helpful in reducing the occurrence of illness,[118] but dietary habits usually cannot be rigidly controlled.[185] Food in developing countries is often contaminated with fecal coliforms and enteropathogens.[215] *V. cholerae* remains viable for 1 to 3 weeks in food,[70] and *Salmonella* can survive 2 to 14 days in water or in the environment at large in a desiccated state.

Risk of illness is lowest when most meals are self-prepared and eaten in a private home, intermediate when food is consumed at public restaurants, and highest when food is obtained from street vendors.[17] The following standard dietary recommendations for prevention are based more on known potential vehicles for transmission of illness than on strong evidence.

1. Avoid tap water, ice made from untreated water, and suspect bottled water. Bottled and carbonated drinks, beer, and wine are probably safe. Boiled or otherwise disinfected water is safe. Tap water in high-risk countries is difficult to implicate in TD, but has been shown to contain enteric bacteria and pathogenic viruses and parasites.[12] Bottled carbonated beverages are considered safe because of the antibacterial effects of the low acidity. Alcohol in mixed drinks does not disinfect contaminated ice cubes unless the alcohol content is at very high and potentially unsafe concentrations.[40]

2. Avoid unpasteurized dairy products. These may be the source of infection with *Salmonella, Campylobacter, Brucella, Listeria monocytogenes, Mycobacterium* spp., and others.[163]

3. Avoid raw meat and vegetables. Raw vegetables in salads may be contaminated by fertilization with human waste or by washing in contaminated water. Anything that can be peeled or have the surface removed is safe. Fruits and leafy vegetables can also be disinfected by immersion and washing in iodinated water or by exposure to boiling water for 30 seconds. Povidone-iodine 10% has been suggested as a practical disinfectant for water in the field in a wilderness setting[90] (see Chapter 88). Raw seafood, including traditional dishes such as ceviche and sashimi, has been associated with increased risk of TD. Shellfish concentrate enteric organisms from contaminated water and can carry hepatitis A, noroviruses, *Aeromonas hydrophila, Y. enterocolitica, V. cholerae,*

and *V. parahaemolyticus*. Raw fish can carry parasites such as *Anisakis simplex*, *Clonorchis sinensis*, and *Metagonimus yokogawai*. Raw meat is a source of *Salmonella* and *Campylobacter* and is the vehicle for *Trichinella*, *Taenia saginata*, *Taenia solium*, and *Sarcocystis*. Although adequate cooking kills all microorganisms and parasites, if food is left at room temperature and recontaminated before serving, it can transmit *Salmonella*, *Shigella*, ETEC, or EAEC. Food served on an airplane, train, boat, or bus may have been catered in the country of origin. Problems of food hygiene pertaining to these forms of public transportation may be related to employee handling of food, even in the United States.

Generally safe foods are those served steaming hot, dry items such as bread, freshly cooked food, foods that have high sugar content (e.g., syrups, jellies, jam, honey), and fruits that have been peeled.

Sanitation and hygiene are among primary means of prevention for residents in developing areas and for wilderness groups. The role for prevention for most travelers is more difficult to demonstrate. Cruise passengers using regular handwashing with soap and water can see reduction in norovirus gastroenteritis, whereas alcohol-based hand sanitizers may not be effective.[126] Regular use of alcohol hand sanitizers did not appear to offer any protection against either diarrhea or respiratory tract infection in travelers in one study,[95] undoubtedly because of the enormous dose of diarrheogenic *E. coli* needed to cause illness. Handwashing and cleaning of cookware may be useful in preventing diarrhea in wilderness backpackers where low-inoculum pathogens may be seen.[23]

Chemoprophylaxis

Chemoprophylaxis with antibiotics was shown in the 1950s and 1960s to effectively prevent TD among international travelers.[114] This was the first evidence that bacterial pathogens were the most important causes of TD. Preventive antibiotics may be recommended for trips of 2 weeks or less to high-risk regions and will require a prescription from a physician (Table 82-9).

Because of safety and efficacy, rifaximin is the optimal drug when prophylaxis is employed: the dose is one 200-mg tablet twice daily with major daily meals. Another effective dosage formulation of rifaximin is a 550-mg tablet taken once during breakfast each day of the trip.

Several non-antimicrobial agents have been studied for prevention of TD, with some found to be minimally effective. Lactobacilli have been tested on the assumption that they are safe and favorably modify intestinal flora, but they did not invariably reduce the incidence of TD and provided protective efficacy only up to 47%.[91] Of the non-antibiotic drugs, only bismuth subsalicylate (BSS), the active ingredient in Pepto-Bismol, has been shown by controlled studies to offer reasonable protection and safety.[52,64] The currently recommended dose of BSS is two tablets with each meal and two tablets at bedtime, or two tablets four times a day (2.1 g/day) while in a high-risk region for trips of 2 weeks or less. Mild side effects include constipation, tinnitus, and temporarily blackened tongue or stools. BSS should not be used by someone with aspirin allergy or in young children. The precise mechanism by which BSS prevents diarrhea is still unknown. Salicylate released during dissociation in the stomach exhibits antisecretory activity after exposure to bacterial enterotoxin on intestinal mucosa, and bismuth salts have antimicrobial activity.[83]

Immunoprophylaxis

Spurred by emergence of in vitro resistance among enteropathogens to antimicrobial agents, including the fluoroquinolones, and with the knowledge that persons develop natural protection against TD as they remain in a high-risk area, vaccines are being developed to prevent TD. Several vaccines are being or have been developed for protection against rotavirus, *Shigella*, *V. cholerae*, and ETEC. The vaccine most relevant to TD is ETEC, since it is the most important cause of TD and typically occurs during the first 2 weeks in a country of risk.[2] An orally administered ETEC vaccine is marketed as Dukoral in many European countries. The vaccine uses a recombinant form of the binding subunit of cholera toxin that resembles the heat-labile toxin of ETEC (LT). The vaccine was successfully employed in a study of Finnish travelers to Morocco.[158] The vaccine fails to immunize against the nonantigenic heat-stable toxin of ETEC (ST). A study of the effectiveness of Dukoral in preventing TD provided evidence that the vaccine might be expected to prevent two of seven (28%) cases of TD if routinely employed.[127] Adding whole cells containing gut attachment fimbriae of ETEC has been one approach to increase the spectrum of activity of this oral vaccine. Making sure the correct fimbrial adhesin is included in the vaccine is a challenge of this approach.[176]

BACTERIAL ENTEROPATHOGENS

ESCHERICHIA COLI

The diarrheagenic *E. coli* represent a heterogeneous group of organisms that belong to one taxonomic species, but have different virulence properties, epidemiologic characteristics, and clinical features. At least six groups have been characterized, based on genotypic or phenotypic markers.[145] Discussed here are the pathotypes of diarrheagenic *E. coli* important in TD.[216]

Enterotoxigenic E. coli

First identified in the 1970s, ETEC strains were shown to produce one or two enterotoxins that act on the small intestine through different cyclic nucleotide pathways showing different time responses in the gut.[145] One of these toxins is a heat-labile cholera-like toxin (LT), a high-molecular-weight protein immunologically and physiologically similar to cholera toxin. Human ETEC strains also have a low-molecular-weight, poorly antigenic toxin that is heat stable (ST).[170] One common method for diagnosis of ETEC is identification of specific DNA plasmid sequences using a hybridization technique.[145] More recently, PCR has been used to improve the level of detection.[8,15,75,205,207,216] ETEC has worldwide distribution and is the major cause of TD, accounting for 30% to 40% of cases in series from Latin America, Africa, and southern Asia (Indian subcontinent).[183] It also accounts for a large percentage of enteritis in local pediatric populations of developing countries, where contaminated food and water are the primary sources of infection. Person-to-person spread is infrequent because of the large infectious dose (10^6 to 10^{10} organisms).[55]

TABLE 82-9 Prophylactic Medications for Prevention of Traveler's Diarrhea*

Agent	Protective Efficacy	Prophylactic Dose	Comment
Bismuth subsalicylate	65%	30 mL or two 262-mg tablets before meals and at bedtime	Safe, temporary darkening of stools and tongue
Fluoroquinolones	90%	Ciprofloxacin, 500 mg once daily	Side effects and toxicity unacceptable considering expected benefit; concern with development of antibiotic resistance
Rifaximin	70%-80%	Rifaximin, 200 mg twice daily with meals	Safe, nonabsorbable, no increased resistance; should be considered the standard agent for prophylaxis during high-risk travel

*Not generally recommended for healthy travelers able to carry out preventive measures; to be used in special situations (see text) and for no longer than 2 weeks.

Enteroinvasive *E. coli*

As with *Shigella*, EIEC strains possess the property of bowel mucosa invasion, resulting in microabscesses and ulcer formation. Because of the presence of the same invasive plasmid and other antigens of *Shigella*,[121,171] EIEC must be considered in the differential diagnosis of febrile dysenteric diarrhea. EIEC strains cause a small fraction of TD cases.[212]

Enteroaggregative *E. coli*

The EAEC strains are an important cause of TD in all regions of the world.[3] These strains adhere to HEp-2 cells in a typical aggregative, "stacked brick" pattern. Several bacterial markers have been studied as possible diagnostic aids, but no single marker is present in all strains.[96,98,105] Some studies suggest that EAEC should be considered a phenotypically and genotypically heterogeneous group.[24,36,98,122,144,145] Although the pathophysiology of EAEC is not completely understood, presence of multiple virulence factors and stimulation of inflammatory cytokines/chemokines have been described.[22,84,97-99,105,107,143,218] EAEC has been associated with acute and persistent diarrhea in children living in developing countries.[32,96,148,180,218]

Diffusely Adherent *E. coli*

These strains show a diffuse, nonaggregative adherence pattern to HEp-2 cells. There is limited evidence that these strains are causes of TD[138,206] and diarrhea in children in developing countries.[79]

Laboratory culture cannot differentiate the various diarrheagenic strains of *E. coli* from normal bowel flora or from one another. Specialized assays, such as DNA probing and HEp-2 adherence technique, are specifically used for research purposes.[144] New serologic and molecular diagnostic techniques under investigation may become available in the future to differentiate these organisms.[8,12,16,75,129,146,167,190,207]

Most cases of *E. coli* diarrhea are brief and self-limited (see Antimicrobial Therapy, earlier). Treatment is with rifaximin, ciprofloxacin, or azithromycin. EIEC should be treated as for shigellosis with 3 days of therapy with a fluoroquinolone or 1 g of azithromycin in a single dose.

SALMONELLA

Salmonella infections may result in four different clinical syndromes: gastroenterocolitis, enteric (typhoid) fever, bacteremia with focal extraintestinal infection, and asymptomatic carriage.[20,179] Gastroenterocolitis and typhoid fever are the two most important forms for travelers. Although the incubation period for typhoid fever is usually 1 to 2 weeks, it is only 8 to 48 hours for intestinal infections with nontyphoid *Salmonella*.[161] Nausea, vomiting, malaise, headache, and low-grade fever may precede abdominal cramps and diarrhea. Stools are usually foul and green-brown to watery, with variable amounts of mucus, blood, and leukocytes. Cholera-like fluid loss or dysentery with grossly bloody and mucoid stools occurs less often. The acute phase lasts only a few days. Asymptomatic excretion of organisms in the stool continues for 4 to 8 weeks; chronic carriers are rare. Infants younger than 3 months experience longer illnesses (average, 8 days) with more complications. Among all ages, transient bacteremia is common, accounting for significant isolation of *Salmonella* types from blood. Fever and malaise occurring more than 1 week after resolution of diarrhea suggest a complication or another diagnosis.[110,161] In healthy adults, *Salmonella* bacteremia occurs in 5% to 8% of infections and is not distinguishable from other causes of sepsis.

Diagnosis is made by isolation of *Salmonella* from stool or blood cultured onto selective media (MacConkey or *Salmonella-Shigella* agar). Supportive treatment with fluids is sufficient therapy for most cases of uncomplicated *Salmonella* enterocolitis. Antimicrobial therapy is indicated for persons who have symptomatic *Salmonella* infection with fever, systemic toxicity, or bloody stools. Fluoroquinolones are the treatment of choice for most forms of systemic salmonellosis because they shorten duration of illness. Doses are the same as those recommended to treat shigellosis, although treatment is continued for 7 days (14 days if patient is immunosuppressed). For known intestinal salmonellosis, antibiotics are used only in the more severely ill patients or when bacteremia is suspected.

Immunity to *Salmonella* is serotype specific. Vaccines have not been successful for nontyphoid *Salmonella* because of the number of serotypes. For typhoid fever, immunoprophylaxis is available with two licensed vaccines. The first is a live-attenuated strain Ty21a that is given as one oral dose every other day for four doses.[9,78] The second is an inactivated Vi polysaccharide preparation given as a single parenteral immunization.[1] Both preparations are of approximately equal cost and effectiveness.

SHIGELLA

Shigellae are nonmotile, nonsporulating, gram-negative rods in the Enterobacteriaceae family. There are four species or groups: A (*Shigella dysenteriae*), B (*Shigella flexneri*), C (*Shigella boydii*), and D (*Shigella sonnei*); the first three contain numerous serotypes. Fecal-oral contamination is the mode of spread, most often from contaminated food in the case of TD. With an infectious dose as low as 10 to 200 organisms, person-to-person spread also occurs.[62] The essential virulence factor of *Shigella* is invasiveness associated with a large (120- to 140-megadalton) plasmid. As with most enteric pathogens, infection with *Shigella* may be asymptomatic, mild, or severe. In the classic form of shigellosis, after 1 to 3 days of small bowel disease, colonic involvement causes progression to clinical dysentery. In the dysenteric form, the volume of stools decreases and the frequency increases, with passage of up to 20 to 30 movements a day, containing gross blood and associated with fecal urgency and often tenesmus. Fever is common in dysenteric cases and found in up to one-half of cases of shigellosis. Mild abdominal tenderness is also common, but without peritoneal signs.

Laboratory tests often show mild leukocytosis with increased number of immature granulocytes. If colitis is present, microscopic examination of the stool shows countless neutrophils. Diagnosis is made by stool culture on selective media (MacConkey or *Salmonella-Shigella* agar), which is positive in most infected patients.[59] Patients with fever and dysentery should be treated with absorbed antimicrobial agents, including fluoroquinolones or azithromycin. The current dosage recommendations for fluoroquinolones are norfloxacin (400 mg twice daily), ciprofloxacin (500 mg twice daily), or levofloxacin (500 mg once daily), for a total of 3 days. Single-dose therapy is probably effective in milder forms of illness. For children, azithromycin (10 mg/kg/day for 3 days) or a 3-day course of a fluoroquinolone can safely be used, even though this class of drugs is not approved for use in children.

CAMPYLOBACTER

The organism is a small, curved, gram-negative rod, formerly classified as *Vibrio*. *Campylobacter jejuni/coli* strains are widespread in the environment, most often spread from contaminated food. The most important source for human illness is poultry, but epidemics have also been associated with ingestion of raw milk.[18,19] *C. jejuni* has been isolated from surface water and can survive up to 5 weeks in cold water, ensuring its potential for wilderness waterborne spread. Person-to-person spread occurs but is uncommon. The prevalence of *C. jejuni* as a cause of TD varies with geography and time of year. TD secondary to *C. jejuni* is more prevalent in Southeast Asia and accounts for about 3% of cases in rainy summertime and in up to 15% of cases during drier wintertime.[18,135,178] All segments of the small and large intestine may be affected in intestinal campylobacteriosis. The incubation period of *C. jejuni* enteritis is 2 to 7 days. Clinical symptoms are extremely variable and nonspecific. Patients often have a 1-day prodrome of general malaise and fever, followed by abdominal cramps and pain that herald the onset of diarrhea, with up to eight bowel movements a day. Diarrhea is initially watery, followed by passage of stools that are bile stained or bloody. *C. jejuni* infection has been associated with occurrence of Guillain-Barré syndrome.[18,100,140,169] The mechanism of development of this postinfectious complication relates to molecular mimicry, with development of antiganglioside antibodies stimulated by infection by specific strains of *Campylobacter*.[80]

Definitive diagnosis is made by stool culture on a selective medium (e.g., Skirrow, Butzler, Campy-BAP), with isolation rates directly related to severity of disease. *C. fetus* may be grown from the blood in patients with systemic illness. Treatment is primarily supportive with oral fluids; dehydration is usually mild. Early antibiotic therapy appears to be effective in intestinal campylobacteriosis.[18] The antibiotic of choice is erythromycin or azithromycin.[82,119]

VIBRIOS

Cholera is a severe form of watery diarrhea often associated with dehydration. The disease is caused by *V. cholerae* O group 1 (O1), a motile, curved, gram-negative rod. These microorganisms have two major biotypes, classic and El Tor, which produce similar clinical illnesses, and each one contains two main serotypes, Ogawa and Inaba.[175] Non-O1 *V. cholerae* strains also produce diarrheal illness, but they show less potential for epidemic disease.[111,120] Most cases of gastroenteritis caused by noncholera vibrios have been associated with ingestion of raw seafood. Cases have been reported from travelers, particularly after visits to coastal areas of Southeast Asia and Latin America. *V. parahaemolyticus* causes 70% of cases of food-borne gastroenteritis in Japan (where large amounts of raw seafood are eaten), leads to sporadic outbreaks in the United States, and is a common cause of TD in Thailand.[21] After passing through the stomach, the organism multiplies and colonizes the small bowel. The local effects of enterotoxin account for the pathophysiology of cholera. No pathologic changes are noted in the intestinal wall. Some cholera infections are asymptomatic, and 60% to 80% of clinical cases present as mild diarrhea that never raises suspicion for cholera.[94]

After an incubation period of 2 days (range, 1 to 5 days), fluid accumulates in the gut, causing intestinal distention and diarrhea. Diarrhea may begin as passage of brown stools but soon assumes the translucent, gray, watery appearance known as "rice water" stools. In serious cases, stool volume may reach 1 L/hr, leading to severe dehydration, acidosis, shock, and death. Vomiting may occur as a result of gut distention or acidosis.[111,175]

The clinical syndrome caused by noncholera vibrios is not characteristic. Intestinal illness is associated with diarrhea, abdominal cramps, and fever, with nausea and vomiting in about 20% of cases. Diarrhea may be severe, with up to 20 to 30 watery stools per day. In outbreaks of *V. parahaemolyticus* infection, explosive diarrhea associated with abdominal cramps and nausea is often described, with vomiting in about 50% and fever in about 30% of cases. A dysentery-like syndrome with mucoid bloody diarrhea is often seen in disease outbreaks.[21] Infections are usually brief, lasting an average of 3 days, with spontaneous resolution.

Diagnosis for any of the *Vibrio* strains can be made by stool culture on suitable media (e.g., thiosulfate-citrate–bile salts–sucrose [TCBS], agar). Vibrios can survive for 1 week on a stool-saturated piece of filter paper sealed in a plastic bag, before placing it in the culture media.[111] *V. cholerae* infection can also be diagnosed using a darkfield microscopic examination of fresh stools, which may reveal the characteristic helical vibrio in motion.

Aggressive replacement of fluid and electrolytes is the cornerstone of therapy for cholera, especially in severe cases. Severe untreated cholera has 50% mortality, which may be reduced to 1% with appropriate treatment. Children are at higher risk for complications and death. In severe cholera, antibiotics shorten duration of diarrhea and excretion of organisms, and reduce fluid losses, but are not as important as fluid therapy. Oral antibiotics can be started within a few hours of initial rehydration. The drug of choice is doxycycline, 300 mg as a single dose in adults or 50 mg/kg/day in four divided doses for children. Treatment of patients infected with noncholera vibrios should also focus on fluid replacement. Little information exists on the benefit of antibiotic therapy for GI disease, but antimicrobials may be reasonable in dysentery-like cases or prolonged illness. The same antimicrobial agents used in cholera could be used against this infection.

The current parenteral cholera vaccine has no antitoxin activity and is only about 50% effective in reducing attack rates over a 3- to 6-month period for persons living in endemic areas. It is not recommended for travelers to endemic areas.[111] Outside the United States, two additional vaccines are available: an oral killed whole-cell–cholera toxin recombinant B subunit (WC-rBS) and an oral live-attenuated *V. cholerae* vaccine (CVD 103-HgR), both with 60% to 100% rate of protection against *V. cholerae* O1 for at least 6 months. They are not active against *V. cholerae* O139.[173] A bivalent (CVD103-HgR plus CVD 111) oral vaccine has been shown to be more effective than the monovalent vaccine.[10,13,87,202]

AEROMONAS SPECIES AND PLESIOMONAS SHIGELLOIDES

Aeromonas species and *P. shigelloides* are gram-negative, facultative anaerobic, nonsporulating rods. Their normal habitats are water and soil, and these bacteria have been implicated in a variety of human illnesses, most often gastroenteritis.[92,93,103,211] Clinical illness associated with enteric infection by *A. hydrophila* varies from acute to chronic diarrhea and from passage of watery stools to dysentery with colitis.[103,181,208] *Aeromonas* strains are susceptible to antibiotics used to treat TD. *P. shigelloides* has been associated with recent travel and ingestion of raw or inadequately cooked shellfish. *Plesiomonas* may cause dysenteric illness suggestive of an invasive organism, but its pathogenic mechanisms remain poorly defined.[93] *Plesiomonas* is susceptible to anti-TD antibiotics.

VIRAL ENTERIC PATHOGENS

Noroviruses have been shown to be important causes of approximately 10% of TD cases.[6,30,101,116] These viruses are highly infective (10 to 100 organisms per inoculum), and infection is spread by common-source vehicles with a propensity for secondary person-to-person spread (high secondary attack rate).[89] Humans are the only known carriers of noroviruses. *Norovirus* is known as the "cruise ship virus" based on its importance in that setting. Between 20% and 67% of norovirus outbreaks have been associated with food.[28,149] After a cruise ship has experienced a norovirus outbreak, this infection can continue to be a problem on future trips with the involved ship, despite extensive sanitization.[101] *Norovirus* has also been a recurrent problem among groups rafting the Colorado River. Transmission is followed by an incubation period of 24 to 48 hours, and illness begins abruptly with vomiting, abdominal cramps, and diarrhea. Stools are watery without blood or leukocytes. Other common symptoms include low-grade fever, malaise, myalgias, respiratory symptoms, and headache. Illness is almost always mild and self-limited, lasting 1 to 2 days. Complications and mortality are extremely rare and usually involve elderly and debilitated patients. Immunoassays and molecular techniques (reverse-transcriptase PCR) are available for detection of these small, round RNA viruses in stool.[6,29] Vaccine development for noroviruses is in a very early stage.[117]

INTESTINAL PROTOZOA

Protozoal infections may be pathogenic or commensal (having little or no effect) for the human host. Although acute self-limited diarrheal illness may occur, only a small proportion of cases of acute TD are caused by parasites. Symptoms are nonspecific, and diagnosis is often made on stool examination. Most protozoal infections are suspected on the basis of subacute or chronic GI symptoms, which may fluctuate over time.

Several factors have increased the prevalence of intestinal parasites in the United States and worldwide: an increase in immunocompromised patients, who frequently become infected by these organisms; improvement in diagnostic techniques; increase in group settings (day care centers and nursing homes); more frequent international travel; and in the United States, increased immigration of people from developing countries.[113,133]

All intestinal protozoa are transmitted by the fecal-oral route. Thus, infection rates are highest in areas and groups with poor sanitation, close contact, or particular customs favoring transmission. These reemerging infections have been related to large outbreaks of communicable diseases in the United States, often secondary to water contamination.[217] In addition to spread by food, water, and person-to-person contact, mechanical vectors such as flies may also spread these organisms. Transmission of intestinal protozoa is favored by a hardy cyst, which is passed in the feces of an infected host. In addition to an infective cyst, the life cycle for most intestinal protozoa includes a trophozoite, which is responsible for reproduction and pathogenicity. Only a single host is required, except for *Sarcocystis*, which requires ingestion of raw meat from an intermediate host. Zoonotic spread to humans has been documented for *Giardia, Cryptosporidium, Entamoeba polecki,* and *Balantidium coli.*

As with enteric bacteria, symptoms from infection by intestinal protozoa depend on the level of bowel colonized. Those colonizing the small intestine, such as *Giardia* and coccidia (see *Cryptosporidium*), cause a wide spectrum of GI complaints, including malabsorption (resulting in foul stools and flatulence) and weight loss in persistent infections. Although many protozoa are capable of superficial mucosal invasion, only *E. histolytica* and *B. coli*, which colonize the colon, can ulcerate the bowel wall, cause dysentery, and spread to other tissues.[86] Most infections are asymptomatic and self-limited in immunocompetent persons, but can be persistent and severe in immunocompromised hosts. Table 82-10 summarizes treatment of intestinal protozoal infections.

Prevention of infection is focused on interruption of fecal-oral transmission and is similar to other bacterial and viral causes of TD, including personal hygiene, water disinfection, basic food precautions, and care in food preparation. Currently, no vaccines are available for enteric protozoan infections, although there are efforts to develop a vaccine for *E. histolytica.*

GIARDIA LAMBLIA

Giardia lamblia (also known as *Giardia intestinalis* or *Giardia duodenalis*) is a flagellate protozoan. Classification of *Giardia* species remains controversial, but there are at least six species and other genotypes, primarily distinguished by host. *G. duodenalis* is the species of major concern for human infection.[5]

TABLE 82-10 Antiparasitic Therapy for Giardiasis	
Adult Treatment	**Pediatric Treatment and Other Drugs**
Tinidazole, 2000 mg single dose	Tinidazole, 50 mg/kg single dose
or	
Nitazoxanide, 500 mg bid for 3 days	Children age 1-4 yr: nitazoxanide, 100 mg bid for 3 days;
or	Children age 4-11 yr: nitazoxanide, 200 mg bid for 3 days
Metronidazole, 250 mg tid for 5-7 days or 2 g/day in a single dose for 3 days (high dose has more side effects),	Metronidazole, 15 mg/kg/day divided tid for 5-7 days
or	
Albendazole, 400 mg single dose or qd for 5-7 days (single dose less effective),	Albendazole, 10 to 15 mg/kg qd for 5-7 days
or	
Diloxanide (Furamide), adults and children age 12 yr and older: 500 mg tid for 5-10 days	Children up to age 12 yr: diloxanide, 20 mg/kg/day in three divided doses for 5-10 days

Data from references 25, 26, 33, 69, 72, 76, 85, 130, 142, 150, 153, 159, 162, 172, 182, 187, 189, and 213.
bid, Twice daily; *qd,* daily; *tid,* three times daily.

Giardia is the most common protozoal intestinal parasite isolated worldwide, including in the United States. Prevalence ranges from 3% to 7% in the United States to 30% or more in developing areas with poor sanitation. All age groups are affected. In the United States, a seasonal peak in cases coincides with the summer recreational water season and likely reflects increased outdoor activities and exposures, such as camping and use of communal swimming venues (e.g., lakes, rivers, swimming pools, water parks).[217]

Persons at increased risk for infection reflect the fecal-oral transmission through food, water, and person-to-person contact with a low infectious dose, including (1) travelers to disease-endemic areas; (2) children in child care settings; (3) close contacts of infected persons (family or household contacts); (4) persons who ingest contaminated drinking water, recreational water (lakes, rivers, and pools), or untreated surface water (backpacking or camping); (5) persons who have contact with infected animals; and (6) men who have sex with men.

Giardia accounts for a small percentage of TD. Because of the relatively long incubation period and persistent symptoms, *Giardia* is more likely to be found as the cause of diarrhea that occurs or persists after returning home from travel to a developing region.

Epidemiologic studies suggest acquired resistance, with lower rates of infection and illness among residents of endemically infected areas compared with visitors, and among adults compared with children; however, reinfection occurs.

Natural Reservoirs

Giardiasis usually represents a zoonosis and has been detected in almost all classes of vertebrates, including domestic animals and wildlife, including beavers, cattle, dogs, cats, rodents, and sheep. Although *G. intestinalis* infects both humans and animals with cross-infectivity, molecular epidemiology suggests that the role of zoonotic transmission to humans and importance of animal contamination of food and water may be less than previously thought.[217]

Transmission and Infectious Dose

Giardia infection is transmitted by the fecal-oral route and results from ingestion of *Giardia* cysts through consumption of fecally contaminated food or water or through person-to-person (or, to a lesser extent, animal-to-person) transmission. The cysts are infectious immediately on being excreted in feces. Infected persons have been reported to shed 10^8 to 10^9 cysts in the stool per day and to excrete cysts for months. The infective dose of *Giardia* for humans is low; 10 to 25 cysts caused infection in 8 of 25 individuals; more than 25 cysts caused infection in 100%. Infectivity apparently depends on both host and parasite factors.[153] Person-to-person spread may be the most common means of transmission for humans. Areas and populations with poor hygiene and close physical contact have higher rates of infection, and infection of other household members is common. Venereal transmission occurs through direct fecal-oral contamination.

Water is a major vehicle of infection in community outbreaks, usually in small water systems that use untreated or inadequately treated surface water, and may play a significant role in U.S. wilderness travelers who develop intestinal illness.[112,217] Cysts retain viability in cold water for as long as 2 to 3 months. Giardiasis has been called "backpacker's diarrhea" because of the common association with alpine mountain waters.

Pathophysiology and Clinical Presentation

The pathophysiologic mechanisms of diarrhea and malabsorption in giardiasis are poorly understood, and more than one mechanism, including altered gut motility and hypersecretion of fluids, is probably involved. Most small bowel biopsies in human patients demonstrate minimal or no changes. Enterotoxins have not been found.[153,162]

Most infections are asymptomatic, but carriers can excrete high numbers of cysts in stools. The attack rate for symptomatic infection in the natural setting varies from 5% to 70%. Correlation between inoculum size and infection rates has been noted, but not with numbers of cysts passed or severity of symptoms.

The incubation period averages 1 to 2 weeks, with a mean of 9 days. A few people experience abrupt onset of explosive watery diarrhea accompanied by abdominal cramps, foul flatus, vomiting, low-grade fever, and malaise. This typically lasts 3 to 4 days before transition into the more common subacute syndrome. In most patients, onset is more insidious and symptoms are persistent or recurrent. Stools become mushy, greasy, and malodorous. Watery diarrhea may alternate with soft stools and even constipation. Upper GI tract symptoms, typically exacerbated postprandially, accompany stool changes, but they may be present in the absence of soft stool. These include midabdominal and upper abdominal cramping, substernal burning, acid indigestion, sulfurous belching, nausea, distention, early satiety, and foul flatus. Constitutional symptoms of anorexia, fatigue, and weight loss are common. Unusual presentations include allergic manifestations such as urticaria, erythema multiforme, and bronchospasm. Some *Giardia* infections are associated with chronic illness. Adults may have a long-standing malabsorption syndrome and marked weight loss, and children may have failure-to-thrive syndrome.[68,86]

Immunologic responses are effective in the majority of infections, because spontaneous clinical recovery is common with or without the disappearance of organisms. Average duration of symptoms in all ages ranges from 3 to 10 weeks. Both cellular and humoral responses to *Giardia* have been demonstrated.

Diagnosis

Direct stool examination may be used when newer immunologic tests are not available. Cyst passage is extremely variable and not related to clinical symptoms, so multiple stool collections (i.e., three stool specimens collected every other day) increase test sensitivity. One stool sample will allow detection of 60% to 80% of infections, two stool samples will allow detection of 80% to 90%, and three stool samples will allow detection of more than 90%. Trophozoites may be found in fresh, watery stools (Figure 82-2) but disintegrate rapidly. Stools should be preserved in a fixative, such as polyvinyl alcohol, or a formalin preparation if not immediately examined. In the office, fresh stool can be mixed with an iodine solution (e.g., Gram's iodine) or methylene blue and examined for cysts on a wet mount. Many antibiotics, enemas, laxatives, and barium studies mask or eliminate parasites from stools, so examinations should be delayed for 5 to 10 days after these interventions. Trichrome stain is better than the formalin-ether concentration technique for identification of protozoal cysts and trophozoites. Another noninvasive office test is duodenal mucus sampling using a string test (Enterotest), which has reported sensitivity of 10% to 80%. Duodenal biopsy is a sensitive test, but rarely necessary.[133] Direct fluorescent antibody (DFA) testing is an extremely sensitive and specific detection method and is considered the gold standard by many laboratory workers. Immunologic tests on stool are replacing direct microscopy because they are much easier and require less experience to interpret. Immunoassays using enzyme-linked immunosorbent assay (ELISA) or enzyme immunoassay (EIA) on stool approach 100% sensitivity and specificity. Other molecular techniques are available but not commonly used in clinical settings.

Treatment

Because of the difficulty and expense of confirming the diagnosis in some patients, a therapeutic trial of drugs may be attempted when suspicion is high. In the field, it is reasonable to initiate presumptive treatment for *Giardia* for secretory diarrhea (non-dysentery) lasting more than 1 week that does not respond to a trial of antibiotic therapy.

Symptomatic patients should be treated for comfort and to prevent development of chronic illness. Asymptomatic carriers in nonendemic areas should be treated when identified because they may transmit the infection or develop symptomatic illness. No drug is effective in all cases. In resistant cases, a longer course of two drugs taken concurrently has been suggested. Relapses occur up to several weeks after treatment, necessitating a second course of the same medication or an alternative drug. Malabsorption usually resolves with treatment, but persistent diarrhea may result from lactose intolerance or a syndrome resembling celiac disease, rather than from treatment failure.

The three groups of drugs currently being used are nitroimidazoles (metronidazole, tinidazole, albendazole, ornidazole, nimorazole), nitrofuran derivatives (furazolidone), and acridine compounds (mepacrine, quinacrine).[26,76] Tinidazole and nitazoxanide (Alinia) have similar or better effectiveness (average, 85% to 90%) than does metronidazole and have been approved by the FDA for this use in the United States. Tinidazole is licensed for children older than 3 years, and nitazoxanide is available in suspension for children as young as 1 year. Albendazole has comparable effectiveness with metronidazole and is often used outside the United States because of its broad activity against other parasitic worms.[189] Other alternatives include furazolidone, which results in cure rates between 80% and 96% and is also available as a pediatric suspension. Paromomycin (Humatin) is a nonabsorbable drug that is recommended for pregnant women or for use in severely symptomatic individuals. Quinacrine (Atabrine) achieves high cure rates, but it is no longer available in the United States because it produces frequent and potential severe side effects, especially in children, and safer medications are available. Mebendazole and ornidazole are two other nitroimidazoles that have been used successfully, but less data are available for these drugs. Treatment of giardiasis has been extensively reviewed.[76]

ENTAMOEBA

The genus *Entamoeba* contains many species. Six that can reside in the human intestinal lumen are *E. histolytica*, *E. dispar*, *E. moshkovskii*, *E. polecki*, *E. coli*, and *E. hartmanni*. *E. histolytica* is the only species definitely associated with clinical pathology in humans. The others are considered commensal; however, *E. polecki* and *E. moshkovskii* have been suspected of causing lower intestinal symptoms in cases involving heavy infection.[71] In addition, isoenzyme analysis has recognized 22 different zymodemes of *E. histolytica*, which may explain geographic differences in rates of invasive disease.[166]

Epidemiology and Risk

Entamoeba histolytica is found worldwide. Similar to *Giardia*, transmission is fecal-oral through person-to-person contact or contaminated food or water. Cysts remain viable outside the body for weeks to months, unlike the fragile trophozoites. Unlike *Giardia*, there is no zoonosis, and the reservoir of infection is human. Approximately 12% of the world's population is infected,

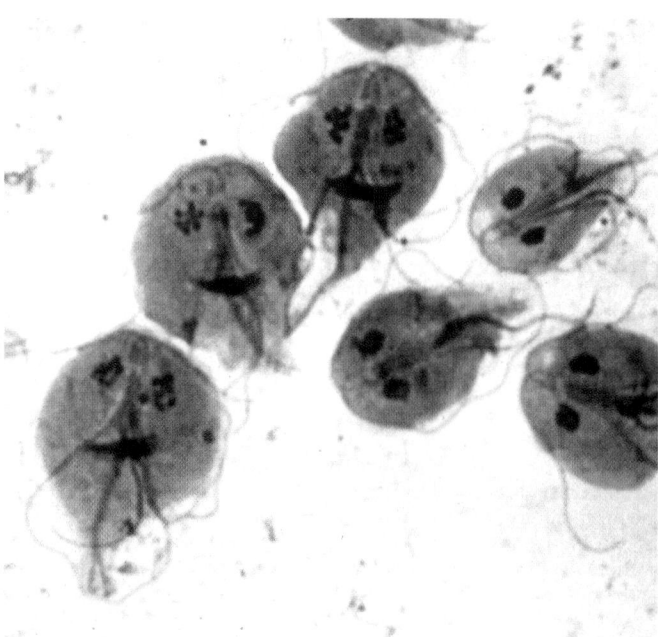

FIGURE 82-2 *Giardia* trophozoites seen in culture. The finding of cysts or trophozoites in a patient with diarrhea is sufficient to make a tentative diagnosis of giardiasis. *(Courtesy D. Lindmark.)*

although this figure may include *E. dispar*, which is not pathogenic. Higher prevalence in tropical countries is related to increased risk of fecal-oral contamination, which depends on sanitation, cultural habits, crowding, and socioeconomic status.[192] *E. histolytica* is a leading cause of death by parasitic infection worldwide. The World Health Organization (WHO) estimates that *E. histolytica* infects 500 million people per year, causes disease in 50 million, and kills 100,000 individuals annually. Importation of infections by travelers and immigrants accounts for most cases in the United States and other temperate countries. Amebiasis accounts for less than 1% of TD cases.

Pathophysiology and Clinical Course

The pathogenicity of *E. histolytica* is still not well understood. Invasion may be a function of motility, soluble toxins, cysteine protease, or lytic enzymes.[177,192] The cecum and ascending colon are most frequently involved, followed by the rectum and sigmoid colon, with lesions of increasing severity and depth of inflammation and ulceration. Extraintestinal spread is hematogenous. Abscesses containing acellular debris develop primarily in the liver but may involve the brain and lung.

The incubation period ranges from 1 to 4 months. Although 80% to 99% of infections result in asymptomatic carriers, a spectrum of GI diseases may result, with considerable variation in severity. Most often, colonic inflammation without dysentery causes lower abdominal cramping and altered stools, sometimes containing mucus and blood.[102] Weight loss, anorexia, and nausea may be present. Symptoms usually fluctuate and persist for months. The subacute infection may evolve into a chronic, nondysenteric bowel syndrome with intermittent diarrhea, abdominal pain, weight loss, and flatulence. Dysentery may develop suddenly after an incubation period of 8 to 10 days or after a period of mild symptoms. Affected persons may have frequent passage of bloody stools, tenesmus, moderate to severe abdominal pain and tenderness, and fever.[168,192]

Amebic liver abscess is the most common and serious complication from hematogenous spread. Individuals can present with liver abscess months to years after travel or residency in an endemic area. The disease should be suspected in anyone with an appropriate exposure history (residency or travel in an endemic area) presenting with fever, right upper quadrant pain, and hepatic tenderness.

The fatality rate for amebic dysentery and its complications is about 2%. Complications of intestinal involvement develop in 2% to 20% of patients and include perforation, toxic megacolon, and ameboma, which is an annular inflammatory lesion of the ascending colon containing live trophozoites. A postdysentery syndrome can occur in patients with acute amebic dysentery and can be confused with ulcerative colitis. Asymptomatic carriers of *E. histolytica* can develop invasive disease, but more often the infection resolves spontaneously.

Humoral antibodies increase with invasive disease and persist for long periods. Although they do not protect against reinfection or bowel invasion, they may prevent recurrent liver infection. Mucosal immunity may provide some protection against recurrent intestinal infection with *E. histolytica*; once the infection is cleared, recurrence is unusual. However, asymptomatic cyst shedding and active GI illness may persist for years, indicating lack of consistent immune response in the intestinal lumen. Oral vaccines and DNA-based vaccines have been successfully tested in animal models, but human testing has not been done, and no vaccine is currently available.[192,193]

Diagnosis

Routine screening of asymptomatic persons of high-risk groups is not cost-effective, except perhaps for food handlers and persons returning from an extended stay in endemic countries. The diagnosis of invasive amebiasis is most frequently attempted by a combination of microscopy of a fecal specimen, serologic testing, and where indicated, colonoscopy and biopsy of intestinal amebic lesions or drainage of a liver abscess. Where available, detection of *E. histolytica*–specific antigen and DNA in stool and other clinical samples (ELISA[42]) may replace microscopic stool examination, which is complicated by morphologically similar, nonpathogenic species. Antigen detection using ELISA is both rapid and technically simple to perform and can be used in laboratories that do not have molecular facilities, making it appropriate for use in the developing world, where amebiasis is most prevalent.[200]

Serologic tests are not useful for identifying asymptomatic carriers but are positive in 85% to 95% of patients with dysentery and 90% to 100% of patients with liver abscess. In combination with ultrasound or other abdominal imaging, serology is helpful for diagnosis where PCR is not routinely available. Because they do not distinguish between current and prior infections, serologic tests are more useful in developed countries with low incidence of infection. The combination of serologic tests with detection of the parasite (by antigen detection or PCR) offers the best approach to diagnosis.[71] New antigen detection techniques can differentiate between *E. histolytica* and *E. dispar*. PCR techniques have been developed and show greater than 95% sensitivity and specificity.

Diagnosis of intestinal amebiasis by microscopic identification of cysts or trophozoites in stool still plays a significant role where other techniques are not available. Mucus from fresh stools or sigmoidoscopic scrapings and aspirates mixed with a drop of saline may show trophozoites if examined within 1 hour. For delayed examination, stool must be preserved in polyvinyl alcohol or other fixative and may be examined later with trichrome stain. Fecal shedding of cysts is irregular, but three stools on alternate days identify most infections. Sigmoidoscopy or colonoscopy is useful for viewing the pathologic lesions and obtaining selective samples of mucus and biopsies of mucosal ulcers, which usually contain organisms. Finding cysts does not confirm the diagnosis of symptomatic intestinal amebiasis. The key to establishing the diagnosis is finding motile trophozoites with ingested red blood cells. It is rare to identify *E. histolytica* in stool samples from patients with liver abscesses.

Culture techniques are available but not generally used in clinical laboratories because they are expensive and time-consuming.

Treatment

There are multiple benefits to treatment of *E. histolytica* infection, including reducing the infectious period, length of illness, risk of transmission to others, rates of severe illness, and preventing complications of invasive disease.[37] U.S. guidelines suggest that asymptomatic carriers should be treated because a cyst passer represents a potential health hazard to others, and reinfection in the United States is uncommon. Moreover, asymptomatic colonization with *E. histolytica*, if left untreated, can lead to invasive disease. Treatment of amebiasis is based on location of infection and degree of symptoms. Medications are divided into tissue amebicides (e.g., metronidazole, tinidazole, emetine, dehydroemetine, chloroquine), which are well-absorbed drugs that combat invasive amebiasis in the bowel and liver, and poorly absorbed drugs (e.g., iodoquinol, paromomycin, diloxanide furoate) for luminal infections. In general, treatment is effective for invasive infections but disappointing for intestinal colonization. The current drug of choice for asymptomatic carriers is iodoquinol. Side effects are mild and consist of abdominal pain, diarrhea, and rash. Diloxanide furoate (Furamide) is another drug of choice, but in the United States, it is classified as an investigational drug, available only through the Centers for Disease Control and Prevention (CDC). Paromomycin is also effective. Although metronidazole has been used in asymptomatic carriers with 90% success, most reserve this drug for invasive and symptomatic infections[14,166] (Table 82-11).

Invasive disease is treated with a tissue-active drug, followed by a luminal agent (in the same dosages as for asymptomatic infection). Tinidazole or metronidazole are the drugs of choice for oral therapy of amebic dysentery or liver abscess. Tinidazole has slightly better effectiveness and fewer side effects than does metronidazole. Other nitroimidazoles that have been tested include ornidazole, nitazoxanide, and secnidazole. Emetine and dehydroemetine are used parenterally in severe cases of amebiasis, primarily extraintestinal, followed by iodoquinol for 20 days. These two drugs have frequent systemic side effects, including development of cardiac arrhythmias requiring hospitalization for

TABLE 82-11 Therapy for Infectious Diarrhea Caused by Protozoa*

Diagnosis	Recommendation	
	Adult Dose	Pediatric Dose and Other Potential Treatment Drugs
Entamoeba histolytica Treatment for asymptomatic cyst excretion	Iodoquinol, 650 mg tid for 20 days *or* Paromomycin, 500 mg tid for 7 days	Children: iodoquinol, 10-13.3 mg/kg tid for 20 days Children: paromomycin, 25 mg/kg/day in three doses for 7 days
E. histolytica Treatment of diarrhea	Metronidazole, 750 mg tid for 5 to10 days *or* Tinidazole, 1000 mg bid for 3 days *or* Secnidazole, 2000 mg single dose Followed by: Iodoquinol, 650 mg tid for 20 days *or* Paromomycin, 500 mg tid for 7 days	Children: metronidazole, 50 mg/kg/day in three doses for 10 days Children: tinidazole, 50 mg/kg/day in three doses for 3 days Children: secnidazole, 30 mg/kg/day single dose
Cryptosporidiosis	Nitazoxanide, 500 mg bid for 3 days In severe cases or patients with AIDS, consider: Nitazoxanide, 500 mg bid for 2 weeks Paromomycin, 500-750 mg tid or qid for 2 weeks	Children: nitazoxanide Age 12-47 mo: 100 mg (5 mL) bid for 3 days Age 4-11 yr: 200 mg (10 mL) bid for 3 days Adult alternatives: Azithromycin, 1200 mg qd for 4 weeks Albendazole, 400 mg bid for 7-14 days
Cyclosporiasis	TMP/SMX, 160 mg/800 mg bid-qid for 7 days In patients with AIDS, follow with: TMP-SXZ, 160 mg/800 mg 3 times per week	Children: TMP/SMX, 5 mg/25 mg/kg/day for 7 days
Cystoisosporiasis	TMP/SMX, 160 mg/800 mg qid for 10 days, followed by: 160 mg/800 mg bid for 3 weeks Pyrimethamine, 75 mg qd, with folinic acid, 10 mg (or divided dose bid), for 2 weeks	Alternatives: Pyrimethamine, 25 mg, and sulfadoxine, 500 mg (Fansidar) *or* Ciprofloxacin, 500 mg bid for 7 days
Microsporidiosis	Albendazole, 400 mg bid for 2-4 weeks In patients with AIDS: follow with chronic suppression	
Balantidium coli (symptomatic)	Tetracycline, 500 mg qid for 10 days *or* Metronidazole, 750 mg tid for 5-10 days *or* Iodoquinol, 650 mg tid for 20 days	Children: metronidazole, 35-50 mg/kg/day in three divided doses for 5 days Children: iodoquinol, 30-40 mg/kg/day (max 2 g) in three doses for 20 days
Blastocystis hominis (symptomatic)	Nitazoxanide, 500 bid for 3 days *or* Metronidazole, 750 mg tid for 5-10 days	Children: nitazoxanide Age 12 to 47 mo: 100 mg (5 mL) bid for 3 days Age 4 to 11 yr: 200 mg (10 mL) bid for 3 days
D. fragilis	Paromomycin 25-35 mg/kg/d PO in 3 daily doses/d for 7 days *or* Metronidazol 500-750 mg PO tid for 10 days *or* Iodoquinol 650 mg PO tid doses for 20 days	Paromomycin 25-35 mg/kg/d PO in 3 daily doses/d for 7 days *or* Metronidazole 30-50 mg/kg/d PO tid for 10 days *or* Iodoquinol 30-40 mg/kg/d (max 2 g) PO in 3 daily doses for 20 days

See Table 82-10 for treatment of giardiasis.
*Effectiveness of many antiparasitic agents is not well demonstrated for each protozoan infection.
bid, Twice daily; *qd*, daily; *qid*, four times daily; *tid*, three times daily; *TMP/SMX*, trimethoprim/sulfamethoxazole.

cardiac monitoring. Because this class of drugs is related to ipecac, the drugs also cause vomiting.

Successful resolution of symptoms from *E. polecki* has been reported with metronidazole followed by diloxanide furoate, in the same dosages as for amebiasis.

CRYPTOSPORIDIUM

Cryptosporidium is a coccidian parasite related to *Toxoplasma* and *Plasmodium*. Other coccidia capable of causing human intestinal infection include Microsporidia, *Cyclospora*, and *Isospora*. In the environment, *Cryptosporidium* exists as a hearty, 5-mm-diameter oocyst containing four sporozoites. As with *Giardia*, the cysts are infectious when excreted. Humans and animals are infected by ingesting oocysts, which travel through the gut lumen to the small intestine, where they release the sporozoites.[27,31,34,35,38,85,115,137,151,172,187]

Epidemiology and Risk for Wilderness and International Travelers

The epidemiology and transmission of *Giardia* and *Cryptosporidium* spp. are similar. *C. parvum* causes a ubiquitous zoonosis with worldwide distribution. *Cryptosporidium* infects a wide variety of domestic and wild animals. *C. hominis*, the human pathogen, is important and underappreciated.[174] Molecular analysis has revealed at least 14 species of *Cryptosporidium* that are distinguished primarily, but not solely, by host and cannot be distinguished by morphology. It is a reemergent enteric pathogen in humans. Prevalence of infection in human populations varies from 0.1% to 3% in cooler, developed countries (Europe, North

America) to 0.5% to 10% in warmer countries (Africa, Asia). The infection has been described in persons who have contact with animals, such as veterinarians and farmers; infants in day care centers; travelers to endemic areas; and patients who have AIDS or who are otherwise immunocompromised. It has infected large numbers of individuals in community-wide waterborne outbreaks.[217] *Cryptosporidium* poses a risk to wilderness users because oocysts are found widely in surface water and have high degree of resistance to chlorine.[123,124] The infective dose of *Cryptosporidium* for humans is low (mean, 132 cysts in a human challenge trial), similar to that seen with *Giardia* spp.[48] Fecal-oral contamination is the mode of transmission. The different routes of transmission are waterborne, especially in large community outbreaks; person-to-person, especially in day care centers, custodial institutions, and hospitals; food-borne; sexual, with no association with specific behavior; and zoonotic.

Pathophysiology and Clinical Course

The pathophysiologic mechanisms of diarrhea and malabsorption are not completely understood. The parasites may activate cellular and humoral immune and inflammatory responses, leading to cell damage and ultimately producing malabsorption and osmotic diarrhea.

Clinical manifestations depend on the patient's immune status, but asymptomatic infection occurs in both normal and immunocompromised hosts. In immunocompetent persons, the usual incubation period of *Cryptosporidium* is from 5 to 28 days. Symptoms consist of watery diarrhea associated with cramps, nausea, flatulence, and at times, vomiting and low-grade fever. The syndrome is generally mild and self-limited, lasting 5 to 6 days in some groups (range, 2 to 26 days). In contrast, immunocompromised hosts experience more frequent and prolonged infections, with profuse chronic watery diarrhea, malabsorption, and weight loss lasting months to years. Fluid losses can be overwhelming in a fulminant cholera-like illness, with high mortality. Cyst passage in stool usually ends within 1 week of resolution of symptoms but may persist for up to 2 months after recovery. Reinfection of an immunocompetent person has been documented. Rarely, *Cryptosporidium* can infect other organ systems, including the respiratory system, liver and biliary system, and stomach, particularly in immunocompromised persons.

Diagnosis

Oocysts can be routinely found in stools in intestinal infections, even though shedding may be intermittent. Concentration techniques and staining with modified acid-fast, Giemsa, or Ziehl-Neelsen techniques facilitate identification of *Cryptosporidium* oocysts. The Enterotest is also useful to diagnose cryptosporidiosis. Newer immunologic techniques (immunofluorescence, EIA) to detect antigen in stools are faster and have adequate sensitivity and excellent specificity.

Treatment

Because this disease is usually mild and self-limited in immunocompetent hosts, supportive care in some cases may be sufficient. Treatment is indicated for severe disease in otherwise healthy people and in immunocompromised patients with illness. Nitazoxanide is the most useful drug for treating cryptosporidiosis (see Table 82-11). Paromomycin and azithromycin have also shown some effectiveness against *Cryptosporidium*. Roxithromycin, ionophores, sulfonamides, and mefloquine have also been tested against cryptosporidiosis, especially in patients with AIDS and chronic diarrheal disease, with variable but generally positive effects.

The most effective prevention in HIV patients is HAART that supports the immune system.

CYSTOISOSPORA BELLI

Cystoisospora belli is a coccidian protozoal parasite. It is an uncommon cause of diarrhea in humans, but its prevalence, as with *Cryptosporidium*, has been increasing in immunocompromised patients. Ingested oocysts release sporocysts in the small intestine that develop into trophozoites.[35,81,130,133,162,213]

Epidemiology and the Risk for Wilderness and International Travelers

Humans are the only host (although there are a few reports in dogs), and infections are transmitted by fecal-oral contamination through direct contact with food and water, so rates are typically higher in settings with high density of people, close contact, or poor hygiene. *C. belli* is endemic in areas of South America, Africa, and Asia. The prevalence is not precisely known, but ranges from 0.2% to 3% in U.S. patients with AIDS and from 8% to 20% in Haitian and African patients with AIDS. Infection rates in otherwise healthy persons with diarrhea are usually low. Most cases have been identified in tropical regions among natives, travelers, and the military.

Pathophysiology and Clinical Course

The life cycle and pathogenesis of *C. belli* are similar to those of *Cryptosporidium*. The organism invades mucosal cells of the small intestine, causing an inflammatory response in the submucosa and variable destruction of the brush border.

In immunocompetent persons, *C. belli* infection may be asymptomatic or may cause mild transient diarrhea and abdominal cramps. Other symptoms include profuse watery diarrhea, flatulence, anorexia, weight loss, low-grade fever, and malabsorption. Generally, infection is self-limited, ending in 2 to 3 weeks, but some persons have symptoms lasting months to years. Infections in immunocompromised patients tend to be more severe and follow a more protracted course. Rarely, acalculous cholecystitis or reactive arthritis has been reported. Recurrences are common.

Diagnosis

Diagnosis can be made by identification of immature oocysts in fresh stool. However, excretion may occur sporadically and in small numbers, so concentration techniques are usually required. Staining with modified Ziehl-Neelsen can also be useful. When stools are negative, the organism can be recovered from the jejunum through a biopsy or string test. Unlike the other intestinal protozoa, *C. belli* may cause eosinophilia.

Treatment

Successful treatment has been reported with trimethoprim-sulfamethoxazole (TMP-SMX) (see Table 82-11). Other options are pyrimethamine with folinic acid, metronidazole, and nitazoxanide (for patients allergic to sulfonamides). In patients with HIV infection, chronic lifetime suppression therapy is indicated with either TMP-SMX or pyrimethamine plus folinic acid daily.

CYCLOSPORA CAYETANENSIS

Cyclospora species were initially thought to be blue-green algae (cyanobacteria-like organisms). The life cycle and pathogenesis of *C. cayetanensis* are not completely understood. Oocysts need about 7 to 15 days to sporulate and become infectious, so they are not immediately infectious on passage.[7,35,81,131,154,162,184,197]

Epidemiology and the Risk for Wilderness and International Travelers

Cyclospora cayetanensis has been shown to be an important cause of acute and protracted diarrhea. Fecal-oral transmission occurs through food, water, and soil. The organism is endemic in many developing countries in all continents. There are numerous reports of *Cyclospora* infection with diarrhea in travelers to Nepal, Haiti, Peru, and Guatemala. In the United States, most of the outbreaks have been food-borne, associated with ingestion of contaminated imported raspberries. Humans are the only known reservoir; there is conflicting evidence for a zoonosis.

Pathophysiology and Clinical Course

The onset of diarrhea is usually abrupt, with symptoms lasting 7 weeks or even longer. Other symptoms include anorexia, nausea, flatulence, fatigue, abdominal cramping, and weight loss. In patients with AIDS, the duration may be longer and severity greater.

Diagnosis

Small, spherical organisms can be detected in fresh or concentrated stool. They show variable staining with acid-fast methods, but stain best with carbolfuchsin. Phase-contrast microscopy and autofluorescence are also useful in the diagnosis. A PCR method is used primarily for research.

Treatment

The treatment of choice is TMP-SMX. This treatment provides rapid clinical and parasitologic cure, with few recurrences. In patients with AIDS, chronic suppression with TMP-SMX may be required. Ciprofloxacin has been used successfully in persons with sulfa allergy (see Table 82-11).

MISCELLANEOUS PARASITIC AGENTS

Microsporidia

More than 100 genera and 1000 species of microsporidia exist in the phylum Microspora. Most species infect insects, birds, and fish. Only 12 species have been reported to infect humans, and of these, only two, *Enterocytozoon bieneusi* and *Encephalitozoon intestinalis*, have been found to cause diarrhea in humans. Microsporidia are obligate intracellular protozoa.[33,35,41,73,81,128,133,139,186,213,214]

Transmission is thought to be fecal-oral or urinary-oral and the infection zoonotic. Spores are environmentally resistant, so waterborne transmission also occurs. Prevalence of microsporidiosis in patients who have AIDS and chronic diarrhea is 7% to 50%. Diarrhea from microsporidia has been reported in travelers to the tropics. Clinical manifestations of intestinal microsporidiosis are chronic diarrhea, loss of appetite, weight loss, malabsorption, and fever. Acute self-limited diarrhea has been reported in immunocompetent hosts. Other infections include keratoconjunctivitis, hepatitis, peritonitis, myositis, central nervous system infection, urinary tract infections, sinusitis, and disseminated disease.

Diagnosis involves trichrome staining of concentrated stools or intestinal biopsy sampling. Electron microscopy is considered the gold standard. Immunologic and molecular biologic techniques are still under evaluation. The most effective drug against most species is albendazole (400 mg twice daily for 2 to 4 weeks). Other drugs that show different efficacies include atovaquone, metronidazole, furazolidone, azithromycin, itraconazole, and sulfonamides.

Sarcocystis

Few human infections with *Sarcocystis* have been reported.[35,81,182,213] Infection may be asymptomatic or associated with diarrhea, abdominal pain, nausea, and bloating. Symptoms typically improve within 48 hours of onset of illness. Diagnosis is based on identification of cysts in concentrated feces. No specific treatment has been established, but TMP-SMX and furazolidone have had variable efficacy (see Table 82-11).

Balantidium

Balantidium coli is a rare pathogen in humans.[182,213] It is the largest and only ciliated protozoa that infects humans. The life cycle involves only trophozoite and cyst stages. Many aspects of the epidemiology are unclear. Pigs appear to be the primary reservoir, although other animals have been implicated. There is no intermediate host. Transmission is fecal-oral, and water is the most common vehicle. Infection is most common in tropical and subtropical regions with poor hygiene. Clinical features resemble those of amebiasis, with a spectrum including asymptomatic infection, chronic intermittent diarrhea of variable intensity, acute dysentery with mucosal invasion, and rarely, metastatic abscesses. Diagnosis is made by observing the organism in a wet mount sample of stool. Trophozoites are seen much more often than are cysts. Recommended treatment is tetracycline or metronidazole. Nitazoxanide is an alternative (see Table 82-11).

Blastocystis

The role of *Blastocystis hominis* in diarrheal disease is still controversial.[132,196,199,213] The life cycle of *B. hominis* continues to be debated. The organism is frequently identified in stool samples by its characteristic appearance, but often is not directly correlated with symptoms, which might be caused by other, undetected pathogens. However, well-defined outbreaks of *B. hominis* have been reported. Treatment is not warranted in asymptomatic infections. When found in large numbers as the sole pathogen, *B. hominis* is suspected as the potential etiologic agent of diarrheal illness. In these cases, therapy may be attempted with nitazoxanide or metronidazole (see Table 82-11).

Dientamoeba

Dientamoeba fragilis occasionally causes diarrhea, occurring characteristically in tropical regions.[109,182,213] It may be found in stools of persons without enteric symptoms. Because cyst forms have not been identified, the mode of transmission remains unknown. Illness caused by the parasite typically resembles giardiasis. Identification can be done from stool samples, a fixative, and almost any type of stain. Treatment of *D. fragilis* is effective with iodoquinol and tetracyclines. There are also reports of successful treatment with metronidazole, paromomycin, and secnidazole[182,213] (see Table 82-11).

REFERENCES

Complete references used in this text are available online at expertconsult.inkling.com.

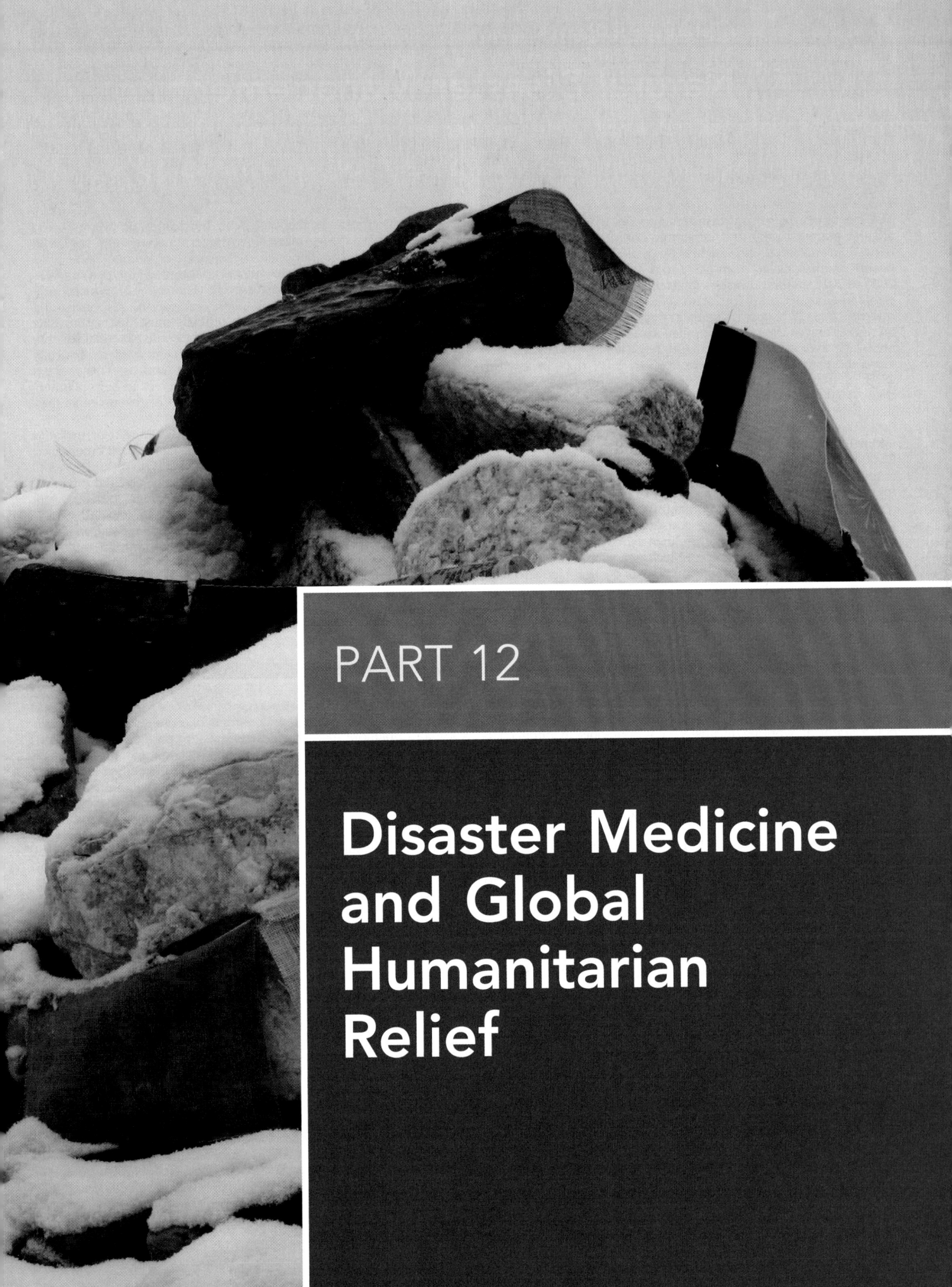

PART 12

Disaster Medicine and Global Humanitarian Relief

The frequency of natural disasters appears to be increasing, as are the human health and economic consequences that follow them.[46] From 2000 to 2015, nearly twice as many natural disasters occurred annually as from 1980 to 1995[34] (Figure 83-1). From 2006 to 2015, natural disasters affected approximately 165 million people per year worldwide, at an average annual cost of approximately U.S. $128 billion.[34] The data suggest that economic impacts are increasing as the size of populations increase in hazard-prone areas; the average costs of damages per disaster (in U.S. dollars) were more than 75% higher in 2000 to 2015 than in 1980 to 1995.[15,34] In that same time period, natural disasters claimed more than 745,000 lives.[24] The 2010 earthquake in Haiti killed more than 230,000 people, injured more than 200,000, and displaced more than one million from their homes. The Japan earthquake and tsunami of 2011 killed at least 18,000 people, injured at least 27,000, and displaced more than 400,000. Critical examination of responses to these tragic events has improved proposed tactics for future disaster responses.[21]

In addition to advances in organizational systems and medical practices used in disaster responses worldwide in the past decades, new technologies are increasingly available to the public and to responders, and are having a significant impact on disaster responses. Because the public has greater access to real-time information using networked systems, communication and response strategies are changing. Social media (e.g., Facebook and Twitter) and newer crowdsourcing platforms (e.g., Ushahidi) can augment situational awareness of both professional responders and the general public by providing real-time data regarding the event, locations of victims, and many specific health needs[57] (Video 83-1).

There is significant potential overlap in the skills of providers trained in wilderness and disaster medicine, with both groups being adept at working in austere environments in often challenging conditions, providing clinical care with limited resources, and being able to improvise when needed in order to best support health.[58]

SCOPE OF THE PROBLEM

Many different definitions of *disaster* have been proposed, but a common theme among most definitions is that disasters create needs that outstrip the resources immediately available to respond. The Centre for Research on the Epidemiology of Disasters in Brussels describes a disaster as a "situation or event which overwhelms local capacity, necessitating a request to a national or international level for external assistance."[25] Disasters can be natural or technological, and technological disasters can be accidental or intentional. Within the realm of natural disasters, the general categories are (1) biologic (transmissible pathogens, insect infestations, toxins), (2) geophysical (earthquakes/tsunamis, volcanoes, dry mass movements), (3) hydrologic (floods, wet mass movements), (4) meteorologic (storms), (5) climatologic (extreme temperatures, droughts, wildfires), and (6) extraterrestrial (meteorites/asteroids).[23] From 2000 to 2015, an average of 419 natural disasters was reported annually worldwide. These disasters occurred in more than 120 countries, but more than a third of all natural disasters occurred in just five countries (China, United States, Indonesia, the Philippines, and India). The most frequent types of disasters were hydrologic (50.9%), meteorologic (26.5%), climatologic (13.4%), and geophysical (9.4%). Disaster events may occur suddenly, with little to no warning, as is the case with earthquakes and volcanic eruptions; may occur with some warning, as is the case with hurricanes or cyclones and floods; or may evolve more slowly over time, as is the case with many transmissible pathogen outbreaks.

Taking a rational approach to preparing for all types of disasters requires using the disaster cycle (Figure 83-2), which traditionally has four phases: planning, mitigation, response, and recovery. In the planning phase, officials must first assess data available to them to examine the likelihood and potential severity of all of the hazards facing their region, as well as critically examine their current readiness for those hazards. This process is called a hazard vulnerability analysis; it serves to help planners logically prioritize planning efforts and use of resources as they prepare for potential emergencies.

Once emergency managers have completed and/or updated a hazard vulnerability analysis, they can examine their emergency response plans and systems to see how those plans and systems can best be improved for the known threats faced by the region. In the mitigation phase, emergency managers and other leaders take steps to limit the scope of damage for anticipated events they cannot fully prevent. Examples of effective mitigation activities include using improved building codes to help buildings withstand earthquakes, designing floodways to divert water away from population centers and other vital areas in the community, and building tornado safe rooms in highly vulnerable areas. Essential actions in the response and recovery phases are discussed.

HEALTH CONSEQUENCES OF DISASTERS

Disasters can produce a wide range of potential health effects on a population; many of these effects are predictable. Although categories and specific types of potential natural hazards may vary greatly, the potential public health and medical needs of at-risk populations generally do not vary.[27,44] Required public health and medical interventions following a disaster typically depend more on the severity of the disaster than on than on the specific event itself; some exceptions are related to the types of acute injuries sustained from different types of events.

In nearly all disasters, people, especially those displaced from their homes, require replacement of water, sanitation, shelter, and food. Inadequate access to water within a population can produce health consequences within days, as can inadequate access to shelter, depending on the weather conditions. Inadequate sanitation and lack of food produce more delayed, but no less profound, effects on the health of the community. Exacerbation of chronic illnesses is also a commonly observed health consequence following a disaster. This often arises from a combination of factors, including health stress from the event itself, disrupted access to usual medical care, and inadequate access to pharmaceutical supplies. Mental health concerns are also common following disasters, although the type and severity vary depending on the type and severity of the disaster, population affected, and other variables.

Outbreaks of infectious diseases following a natural disaster are often mentioned as a primary health concern; however, "the relationship between natural disasters and communicable diseases is frequently misconstrued."[79] In disasters with large numbers of fatalities, there is a common fear that dead bodies are a potential source of disease for the community. However, the evidence suggests that among those killed by the (noninfectious) natural

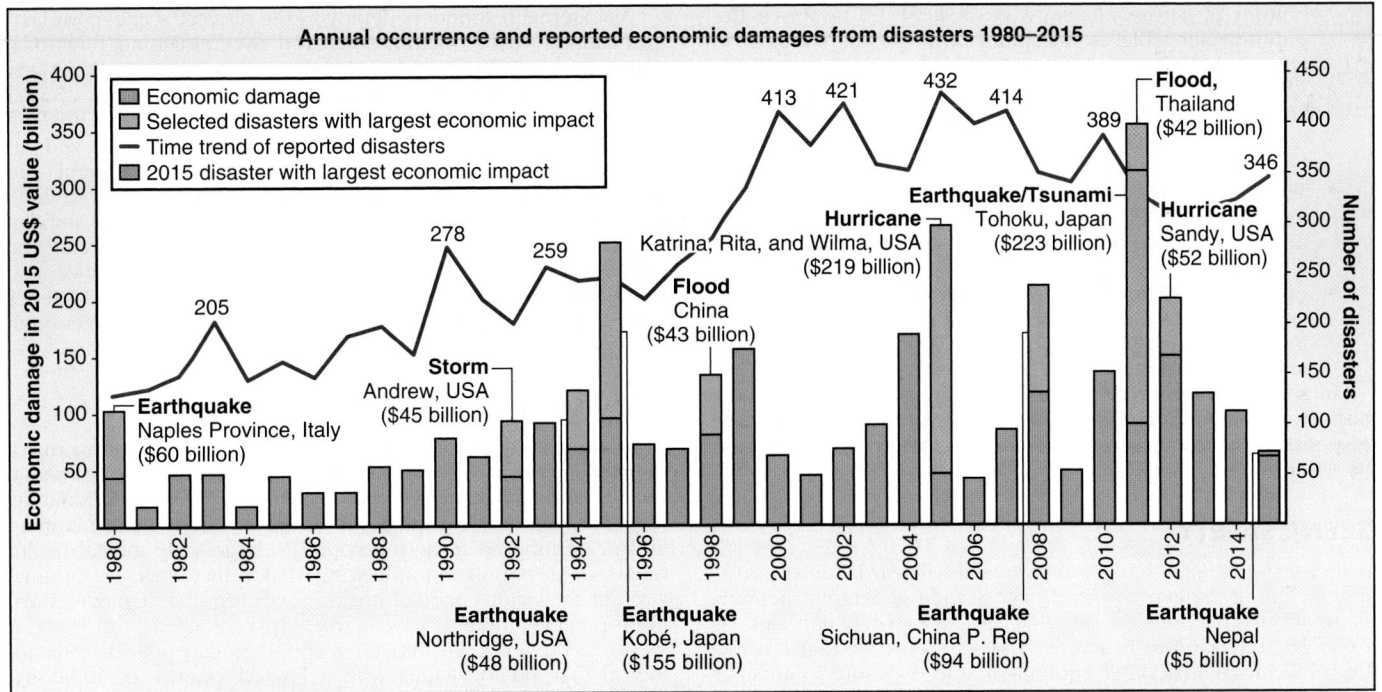

FIGURE 83-1 Annual occurrence and reported economic damages in disasters from 1980 to 2015. *(From Centre for Research on the Epidemiology of Disasters/United States Agency for International Development, CredCrunch 41 February 2016: cred.be/publications.)*

disaster itself, the risk of transmission of acute illness from the bodies of the deceased is extremely small.[52] In fact, the greatest risk factors for acute outbreaks of infectious disease depend on the characteristics of the displaced population and the care that they receive following the disaster. The key variables that influence the true likelihood of infectious disease outbreaks include the underlying immunization rates of the displaced population and their access to health care, as well as the degree of crowding in mass shelters and the distance of water supplies from shelters and latrines.[79] Diarrheal outbreak risks are highest when shelters are overcrowded, clean water is not available, and sanitation systems are inadequate and/or improperly located. Outbreaks of measles and other vaccine-preventable illness among displaced persons have been noted when vaccination rates are low. Malnutrition is also a risk factor for transmissible disease among displaced persons, although this is much more common following prolonged armed conflicts than after natural disasters.[62]

Acute injury and illness are the health consequences that most depend on the type of disaster. For example, earthquakes may produce more crush injuries, requiring greater attention to orthopedic and spinal care in the response, whereas floods may produce more near-drownings, hypothermia, and contaminated wounds among survivors.[3,60]

HEALTH AND THE MEDICAL RESPONSE TO NATURAL DISASTERS

A successful medical response to disasters requires meeting the health needs of the entire population affected by the disaster, not just the needs of those acutely injured by the event. Traditionally, much medical planning has focused on mass casualty planning and mass trauma care; however, the health consequences of disrupted access to primary care, poor sanitation, limited access to clean water and food, and crowding in shelters must also be considered.[79] The Sphere Project was established in 1997 as a voluntary initiative among humanitarian organizations to improve the quality of humanitarian assistance and response and to address the basic health concerns following disaster. The Sphere Handbook, *Humanitarian Charter and Minimum Standards in Humanitarian Response,* is one of the most internationally recognized and accepted documents delineating core principles and minimum standards in disaster health and humanitarian response.[64] Key minimum standards of note in the 2011 handbook that are relevant to health and medical disaster responders include[64]:

- Affected persons must be aware of key public health risks, and be able to adopt measures to prevent deterioration in hygienic conditions, as well as to use and maintain the provided facilities.
- All people must have safe and equitable access to sufficient water for drinking, cooking, and personal and domestic hygiene. Average water use for drinking, cooking, and personal hygiene in any household is at least 15 L per person per day; average drinking water needed for survival is 2.5 to 3 L per person per day.
- The habitat, food preparation and service areas, public centers, and areas around drinking water sources must be free from human fecal contamination. Latrines must be at least 30 m away from any groundwater source, and the

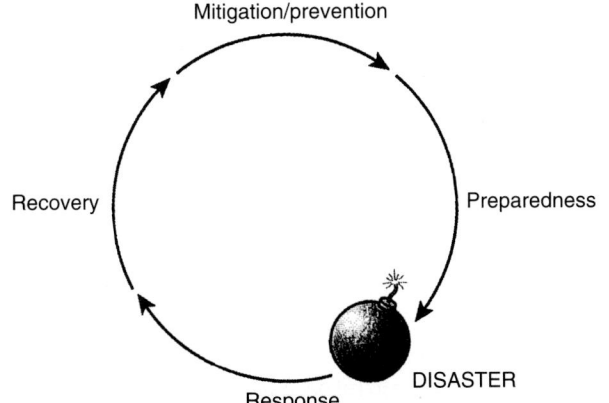

FIGURE 83-2 The disaster cycle. *(From Ciottone GR: Introduction to disaster medicine. In Ciottone GR, Biddinger PD, Darling RG, et al, editors: Ciottone's disaster medicine, 2nd ed, St Louis, 2016, Elsevier.)*

bottom of latrine pits must be at least 1.5 m above the groundwater table. A maximum of 20 people should use any single toilet.

- All disaster-affected people should have the knowledge and means to protect themselves from disease and nuisance vectors that are likely to cause significant risks to health or well-being.
- The environment should not be littered by solid waste, including medical waste. Affected persons should have the means to dispose of their domestic waste conveniently and effectively.
- People should have an environment in which health risks and other risks posed by water erosion and standing water, including storm water, flood water, domestic wastewater, and wastewater from medical facilities, are minimized.

In addition to ensuring provision of the affected population's basic health and hygiene needs, there are additional specific response considerations of which the medical professional must be aware.

SCENE SAFETY

A disaster scene may have numerous safety hazards for responders, including dangerous travel over a wide geographic region; injury from collapsed or unstable structures or falling debris; exposure to hazardous materials, smoke, or dust; excessive noise from machinery and other equipment; and exposure to adverse weather or unfamiliar and/or dangerous environments. Workers may suffer fatigue and dehydration.[31] There may be security concerns in conflict zones or if there is significant civil unrest. The phase of search and rescue of survivors is an especially dangerous phase of the response; Chapter 55 discusses this phase in detail. Medical responders must have access to appropriately trained personnel who are able to assess for the presence and significance of safety threats, so everyone is aware of risks and able to minimize them. Formal appointment of an appropriately trained safety officer at the disaster scene is a commonly recognized best practice. Responders must also have access to any necessary personal protective equipment for use in the response, provided that they are appropriately trained to wear the personal protective equipment and medically suited to use it.

PROVISION OF ACUTE CARE

It is commonly said that "all disasters are local," meaning that the initial medical care following any disaster will be provided by local emergency medical services, hospital, and community responders available in the area.[53] This can produce significant challenges for local medical and public health systems, because the majority of injuries and deaths occur at the time of the disaster event, generally before external assistance can be mobilized to deploy to the scene. Many of the acutely life-saving interventions needed after disasters must be performed quickly. For example, the demand for acute medical services is highest in the first 12 hours to 3 days following an earthquake.[3] Strategies that local systems may use to provide necessary care include a combination of working harder (e.g., calling in more staff, providing greater throughput, or working longer hours), simplifying care (using medical austerity), and/or adopting a triage ethic that potentially limits care. Depending on the degree of mismatch between resources and needs, the focus of postdisaster care may change from individual care to public health efforts, with an explicit goal of doing the greatest good for the greatest number of people. Debates continue regarding altering standards of care during disaster relief efforts. In the United States, concerns have been noted about provider credentialing, malpractice considerations and coverage, and changing standards of care in disaster or emergency situations.[4,5] A transparent, medically and ethically sound triage system is necessary to determine a victim's medical needs and to best match them with available resources. The level of austerity is determined by availability of health care personnel, supplies, and equipment at the disaster treatment site, and varies throughout the disaster as available resources and needs evolve.

As external responders deploy to the disaster scene, coordination among relief organizations and the remaining functional components of the local health infrastructure is essential. Many different types of field hospitals have been deployed to disaster situations, from improvised tents staffed with medical teams and limited equipment to highly functional modular systems with an operating room, intensive care unit, emergency department, and other dedicated facilities. Some internationally deployed field hospital facilities are owned and operated by national military services but are sometimes used in a humanitarian context. The intention is to use these facilities to assist with resuscitation and stabilization of acutely injured disaster victims, but recent studies have questioned whether they can be deployed quickly enough to effectively serve this purpose.[78]

PROVISION OF MENTAL HEALTH CARE

A growing body of evidence has shown that exposure to major disaster events is a risk factor for experiencing adverse mental health and substance abuse problems.[30,32,56] Unfortunately, however, medical planning for disasters often omits planning and/or training on how to respond to large-scale mental health needs of a population following major incidents.[35,63] Optimal support for victims' mental health needs requires deployment of appropriately trained psychiatrists, psychologists, and social workers; however, all disaster responders can provide psychological first aid to victims with a limited amount of additional training. Psychological first aid is a "humane, supportive response to a fellow human being who is suffering and who may need support,"[83] and is supported and recommended by the World Health Organization, the Sphere Project, and numerous other humanitarian organizations. Psychological first-aid action principles can be found in Figure 83-3 and involve the following themes:

- Providing practical care and support that does not intrude
- Assessing needs and concerns
- Helping people to address basic needs (e.g., food and water, information)
- Listening to people but not pressuring them to talk
- Comforting people and helping them to feel calm
- Helping people connect to information, services, and social supports
- Protecting people from further harm.

SUPPORT FOR PRIMARY CARE AND LONG-TERM CARE

Disasters can substantially limit an affected population's local medical care system through direct physical damage to medical facilities, equipment, and supplies; overload of facilities with acutely injured victims; and displacement of patients and medical

LOOK
- Check for safety
- Check for people with obvious urgent basic needs
- Check for people with serious distress reactions

LISTEN
- Approach people who may need support
- Ask about people's needs and concerns
- Listen to people and help them to feel calm

LINK
- Help people address basic needs and gain access to services
- Help people cope with problems
- Give information
- Connect people with loved ones and social support

FIGURE 83-3 Psychological first-aid action principles. (*From World Health Organization, War Trauma Foundation and World Vision International: Psychological first aid: guide for field workers, Geneva, 2011, World Health Organization.*)

personnel away from their usual sites of medical care.[61] Disasters often disrupt the population's access to usual sites of primary care, as well as to specialty care sites, such as dialysis centers or substance abuse treatment clinics. This can produce adverse health outcomes, especially if patients cannot have access to care for diabetes, high blood pressure, heart failure, and other chronic disorders.[45,50,59] There is growing awareness that medical responders need to be able to support, but not replace, the local primary health care infrastructure while it is being reconstituted following a disaster. Although this function has traditionally received less attention than the function of providing acute trauma and injury care, the provision of primary care is very important to the overall success of a disaster response and is in need of further study and planning measures.

CARE OF THE DECEASED

As previously mentioned, rumors regarding the health threats caused by dead bodies are common following a disaster among both the general population and some responder groups. Inappropriate actions, such as creating mass graves for the deceased, have been observed in disasters as a response to such poor information. These actions can disrupt proper identification of victims and cause additional emotional trauma for survivors. As much as possible, bodies should be cared for with great respect, and care for the deceased should foster trust between the community and disaster responders. Burial is generally an appropriate method of disposal; deference should be given to local cultural customs whenever safely possible. The World Health Organization lists the following important principles when dealing with fatalities in a disaster situation[82]:

- Give priority to the living over the dead.
- Dispel myths about health risks posed by corpses.
- Identify and tag corpses.
- Provide appropriate mortuary services.
- Reject unceremonious and mass disposal of unidentified corpses.
- Respond to the wishes of the family.
- Respect cultural and religious observances.
- Protect communities from transmission of medical epidemics.

CARE FOR VULNERABLE POPULATIONS

Disasters disproportionately affect the world's poor, marginalized populations and nations, which bear the brunt of the health effects.[10,11,17,55] Any group or population considered to be at higher risk for poor outcomes in the wake of a disaster is considered vulnerable. Commonly, this includes households headed by women and children, older adults, the disabled, and persons with preexisting mental illness. Unfortunately, however, because of physical and social barriers, these populations are often excluded from the planning and preparation process before disasters strike, and they often cannot get critical goods and services following a disaster. Preventing exploitation of these groups (e.g., sexual and gender-based violence, human trafficking) requires security, active surveillance programs, responsive community services, and engaged authorities.

ORGANIZATIONAL SYSTEMS FOR DISASTER RESPONSE

THE INCIDENT COMMAND SYSTEM AND THE NATIONAL INCIDENT MANAGEMENT SYSTEM

The Incident Command System (ICS) is an incident management framework designed to support efficient and effective management of disaster and other emergency events that is now widely used by governmental, nongovernmental, and private organizations across the United States. The ICS originally arose in the 1970s after the U.S. Congress noted numerous systemic failures in a response to severe wildfires in southern California, including poor communication, incompatible leadership structures among organizations, and lack of coordination of response plans by similar agencies. To address these failures, Congress funded development of what is now the ICS, which allows more effective interagency communication, integration, and coordination.[28] Principal features of the ICS include use of common terms, a unity of command, management by objective, a manageable span of control, and flexible organizational structure to respond to any size or type of incident.[72] *Unity of command* means that in order to maintain clear authority and lines of communication, each individual participating in the response has only one supervisor. *Management by objective* means that the incident response objectives are clearly and explicitly identified by the command leadership, and are agreed upon and followed by all persons operating within the ICS for a fixed period of time (the operational period). The recommended *manageable span of control* means that any supervisor within the ICS organizational chart has three to seven subordinates.

The ICS became the national standard for public safety, emergency medical services, hospitals, and many other organizations in 2004 when it was included as a fundamental tenet of the National Incident Management System, and its use became a requirement of federal preparedness funding.[54] The ICS has been adapted for specific settings, such as hospitals and schools, and has been recommended as a global incident management system by the United Nations.[13,26,70]

The ICS uses a flexible, scalable organizational structure that includes a command team and four functional areas (Figure 83-4):

- Command: Responsible for overall management and direction of the incident; sets the response strategy

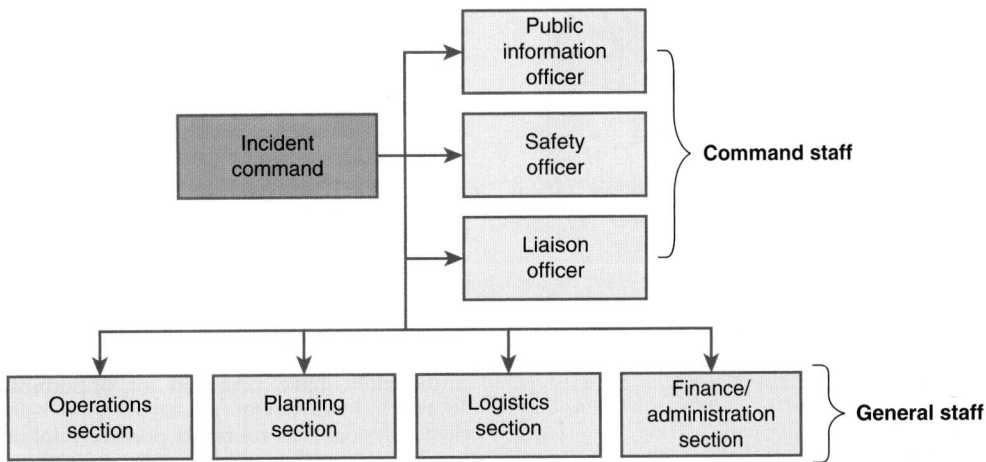

FIGURE 83-4 The incident command system. *(From Federal Emergency Management Agency: emilms.fema.gov/IS200b/ICS01summary.htm.)*

- Operations: Conducts tactical response activities, such as search and rescue, patient care, medical evacuation, or fire suppression
- Planning: Collects and evaluates response information; supports situational awareness throughout the entire ICS structure; is responsible for creating and updating an incident action plan that is followed by all personnel
- Logistics: Manages and procures supplies, facilities, transportation, and other needed resources to support the response tactics and responders
- Finance and Administration: Oversees financial management, timekeeping, and related administrative management functions; is typically activated for longer-term or complex incidents

When multiple organizations or jurisdictions have overlapping legal authority or jurisdiction for an event, a *unified command* is established. The unified command provides a mechanism for incident commanders representing multiple organizations to work within a single integrated command structure that shares a common set of incident objectives.[72] The unified command improves coordination and communication and allows organizations to work together without ceding individual "authority, responsibility, or accountability."[72] A unified command has been set up in many major domestic disasters, including the multistate responses to Hurricane Katrina and the *Deepwater Horizon* oil spill.[14,29]

As mentioned earlier, the ICS is just one part of the larger National Incident Management System in the United States, which provides a nationwide model for how all levels of government and the private sector can collaborate in all types of emergencies.[72] Such collaboration ideally starts long before any disaster event occurs. The preparedness cycle (Figure 83-5) illustrates that disaster preparedness is an iterative cycle in which response partners are continually planning, training, testing, and evaluating their systems so they can identify gaps and problems well in advance of the incident. Numerous after-action reports following successful responses to incidents have cited collaborative planning, training, and exercising as the building blocks that helped to forge relationships and build trust, improving overall management.[14,47]

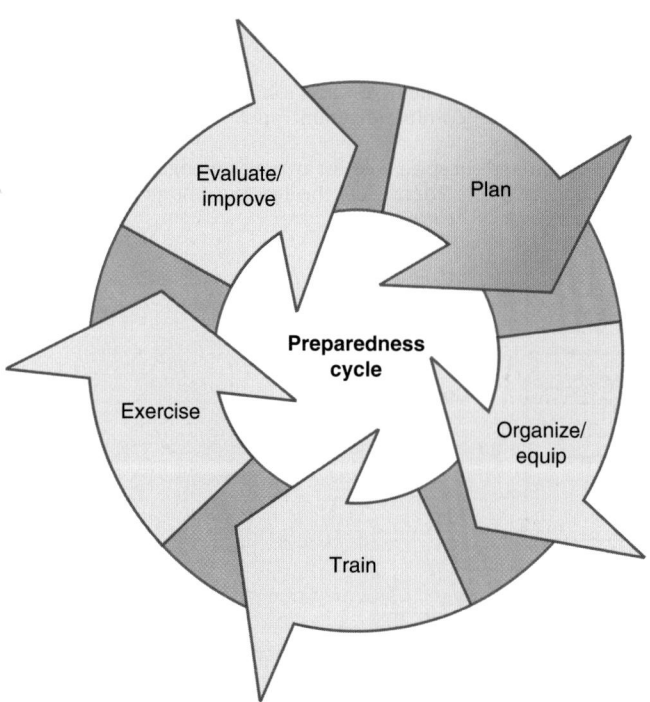

FIGURE 83-5 The preparedness cycle. *(From Federal Emergency Management Agency: fema.gov.)*

THE UNITED NATIONS CLUSTER APPROACH FOR GLOBAL HUMANITARIAN RESPONSE

The ICS is the standard incident management framework used in the United States, but different structures are often used in non-U.S. disasters, especially when responders from many countries combine in the response. Global and domestic disaster response systems share many goals, including improving multiagency coordination, forming flexible organizational structures to meet the needs of the incident, and reducing duplication of efforts. However, unlike a domestic incident management system, which can be mandated by national legislation, the multiple and diverse agencies that respond to a global disaster "cannot be forced to work within the parameters of a common plan—ultimately, [leaders] must persuade the majority of the value of a cohesive approach."[9] Global disaster response agencies and personnel must also respect the sovereignty of the nation affected by the disaster. Therefore, any global disaster response system must be respectful of the affected nation's people and government by being flexible enough to take a supporting or leading role, depending on the nation's coordination capacity and requests for assistance.[40,66]

The United Nations' cluster approach was formally adopted in 2005, and has served since then as the primary framework used in global humanitarian disaster responses, designed to promote preparedness, accountability, and predictability. Prior to its adoption, many global responses suffered from shortcomings in quality and timeliness of the response, isolation of planning and preparedness measures among key agencies, and lack of clarity about roles and responsibilities, among other challenges.[2] Essential humanitarian principles that accompany the cluster approach have also been developed. These are meant to guide all of the response systems and activities operating within the cluster system so they can be effective, regardless of the context in which they are applied.[41,68]

A *cluster* is a group of humanitarian organizations (that may or may not be associated with the United Nations) working in each major sector, such as shelter or health, of a humanitarian response. A designated agency leads the response for each cluster at the global level and at the country level (Figure 83-6). Each cluster lead agency has responsibility for coordinating activities before, during, and after a disaster to most effectively meet the needs of affected people. Clusters at the global level are involved in building preparedness and technical capacity through development of standards, tools, and protocols; providing training and technical assistance for all levels of responders; sharing best practices and lessons learned; and facilitating partnerships among the cluster's participating agencies.[37] When a disaster occurs, a cluster may be activated if the government of the affected nation is too overwhelmed or constrained to coordinate a response. Country-level clusters engage in collaborative planning, implementation, and monitoring of cluster strategies. They prepare needs assessments and suggest solutions and priorities to the humanitarian coordinator, to whom all cluster lead agencies are accountable. Using a flexible and modular approach, only those clusters that address an identified gap are activated during a disaster; they are deactivated when the need subsides and/or when the local government becomes able to address the need. Any humanitarian organization participating in a cluster shares the responsibility with the lead agency to meet the humanitarian needs of the affected nation and a responsibility to adhere to common standards. Some of these standards include commitment to humanitarian principles, capacity and willingness to contribute to the cluster's response plan, and commitment to participate in and work cooperatively with the cluster to ensure optimal use of available resources.[40]

Real-world disasters in which the cluster approach has been used since 2005, such as the Pakistan (2005) and Haiti (2010) earthquakes, have provided an opportunity to evaluate the approach. Involvement of local authorities and institutions in the cluster system was found to positively influence the short-term and long-term effects of the response, particularly when national agencies had sufficient capacity and were assigned to lead clusters. Early identification and involvement of local leaders also

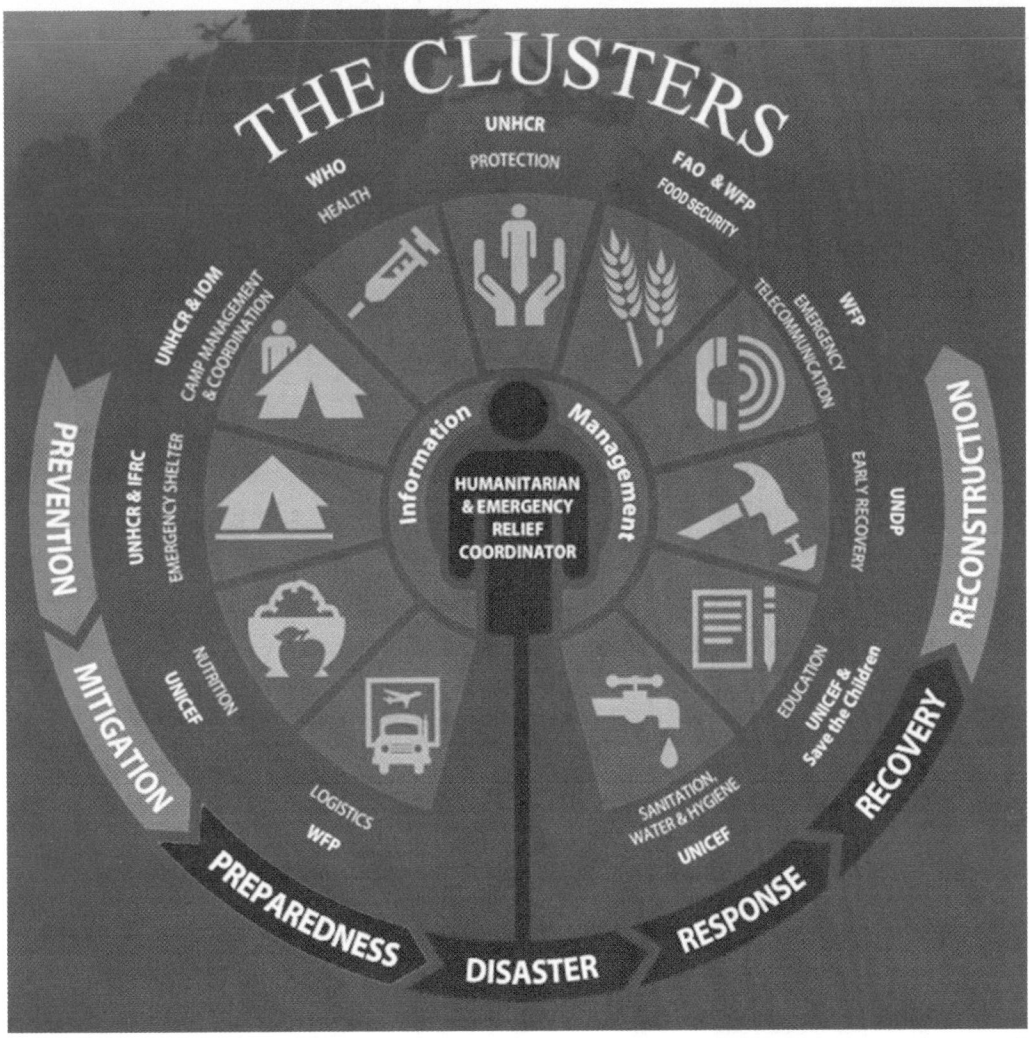

FIGURE 83-6 The United Nations cluster system. (*From United Nations Office for the Coordination of Humanitarian Affairs: unocha.org/what-we-do/coordination-tools/cluster-coordination.*)

appeared to have a positive impact on the transition to recovery and reconstruction. However, noted challenges with local integration of the cluster system included exclusion of local agencies by not conducting meetings or sharing materials in the local language, as well as negative consequences of aid actions that, in some cases, ignored and/or competed with local efforts.[1,7,33] Evaluators also noted challenges with insufficient training and lack of support for cluster leaders, as well as high rate of turnover among participating nongovernmental organizations. They also noted that cluster meetings were too long and too frequent. In 2011, a set of improvements known as the transformative agenda included measures to strengthen leadership in the cluster approach, an emphasis on augmenting rather than replacing existing capacities, and attempts to simplify cluster processes.[38]

CORE ACTIVITIES OF THE DISASTER RESPONSE AND RECOVERY PHASES

Although they are often thought of as separate, the phases of disaster response and recovery are, in fact, overlapping and range from immediate life safety activities through actions to support long-term physical and social recovery of a community (Figure 83-7). Complexity and duration of each phase can vary substantially, depending on type and scope of event, resources available to respond, and overall resiliency of the community.[71,73]

When advance notice of a severe natural event is available, as may be the case with certain floods, wildland fires, and hur-ricanes, the disaster response can begin before the hazard arrives. Activities may include issuing public information and warnings, taking emergency protective measures, such as creating sandbag barriers, prepositioning critical supplies or personnel, and evacuation of personnel from vulnerable areas. Once the hazard impact occurs, immediate life safety priorities take precedence, including search and rescue operations and provision of first aid and emergency medical services. In many disasters, local organizations and civilian bystanders are often the initial responders called on to deliver most of the immediate life-saving care before outside resources can be mobilized. This underscores the need for local and personal preparedness, as well as for community-based disaster response training.[6,8,76]

Successful disaster responses are generally able to stabilize the situation following the initial event and prevent secondary disasters, such as spread of communicable diseases,[43] death or illness from exposure,[1] and other long-term negative health consequences.[81] This phase may be referred to as the short-term recovery or emergency relief phase and involves meeting the immediate needs for food, water, shelter, sanitation and hygiene, clothing, and medicine. Family reunification and fatalities management may also occur at this time. As short-term recovery efforts continue, planning begins for longer-term recovery efforts involving local and external agencies, and formal disaster assessments occur.[48] Formal disaster assessments are rigorous processes designed to support the best use of recovery resources and allow for coordinated recovery strategies to take shape across the community.[39] As early recovery progresses, subtle but

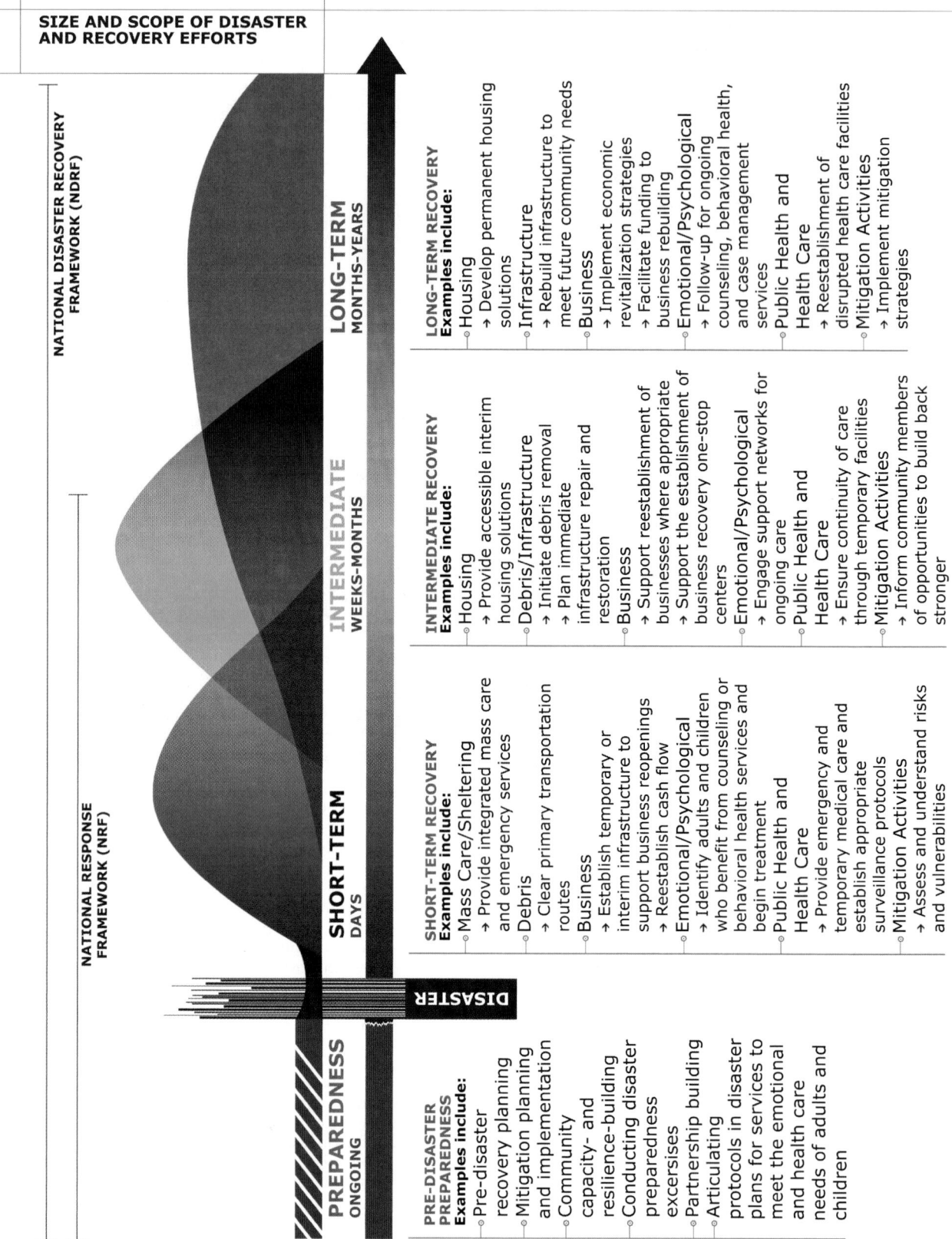

FIGURE 83-7 The disaster response and recovery continuum. *(From Federal Emergency Management Agency: fema.gov/pdf/recoveryframework/ndrf.pdf, 2011, p. 8.)*

significant changes occur. For example, moving persons from a temporary shelter to temporary housing allows individuals and communities to reestablish more normal predisaster routines.[48]

Medium-term to long-term recovery includes reconstruction of permanent physical structures. The purpose of this reconstruction is not simply to restore previous structures and systems, but to identify and implement lessons learned to mitigate against future hazards.[48] Support for local leadership and primacy, fostering inclusive partnerships, and informed decision making based on needs and vulnerability assessments are cross-cutting principles for U.S. domestic and international humanitarian recovery efforts.[18,71]

PROFESSIONALIZATION OF THE DISASTER RESPONSE

In the past several years, there has been growing recognition that disaster medical assistance personnel and the organizations sponsoring their deployment can cause harm to the affected population, even when intentions are good. Deployment of foreign personnel with improper training for the needed medical services, economic displacement of local medical providers and businesses by free international aid resources, and poor accountability of organizations to the crisis-affected state and local authorities have all been described in humanitarian medical responses to disasters. To acknowledge this, the Sphere Project has developed four protection principles for responding humanitarian agencies, the first of which is that they "should ensure that their actions do not bring further harm to affected people."[64] Additionally, the Sphere Handbook notes important trends in the professionalization of disaster response, including:

- A growing conceptual and operational focus on local and national responses with the awareness that affected populations must be consulted and the response capacities of the crisis-affected state and national agencies and institutions must be reinforced
- More proactive accountability of humanitarian action, in particular, accountability to affected populations, but also more proactive coordination, including within the humanitarian reform process (cluster approach), under the auspices of the interagency standing committee
- An increased focus on protection issues and responses
- Increasing awareness of potentially large-scale forced migration due to climate change–induced disasters and an awareness that environmental degradation increases vulnerability
- The recognition that poor urban populations are growing rapidly and that they have specific vulnerabilities, in particular, related to the money economy, social cohesion, and physical space
- New approaches to aid, such as cash and voucher transfers and local purchases, replacing in-kind shipments of humanitarian assistance
- An increased recognition of disaster risk reduction as both a sector and an approach
- An increased involvement of the military in humanitarian response, a set of actors not primarily driven by the humanitarian imperative, requiring the development of specific guidelines and coordination strategies for humanitarian civil–military dialogue
- An increased involvement of the private sector in humanitarian response requiring similar guidelines and strategies as the civil-military dialogue.[64]

SOCIAL MEDIA AND MOBILE TECHNOLOGY IN DISASTERS

Rapidly expanding global access to the Internet and social media platforms and widespread availability of mobile phones have had a remarkable effect on disaster response in the past decade. Online tools allow greater information sharing among affected populations and responders. This has significantly improved situational awareness, empowered community members, and given rise to a new type of emergency responder: the digital humanitarian. Researchers have recently categorized social media functions in disasters into 15 categories, such as providing and receiving disaster preparedness information, sending and receiving requests for help or assistance, raising awareness and donations, and implementing traditional crisis communication activities, providing a helpful framework to study and discuss this expanding topic.[36]

The 2010 Haiti earthquake was an early example of an evolving disaster response in the digital age. The Ushahidi open-source platform established a Haiti page just 2 hours after the earthquake occurred, and allowed thousands of online volunteers from around the world to monitor, categorize, and map

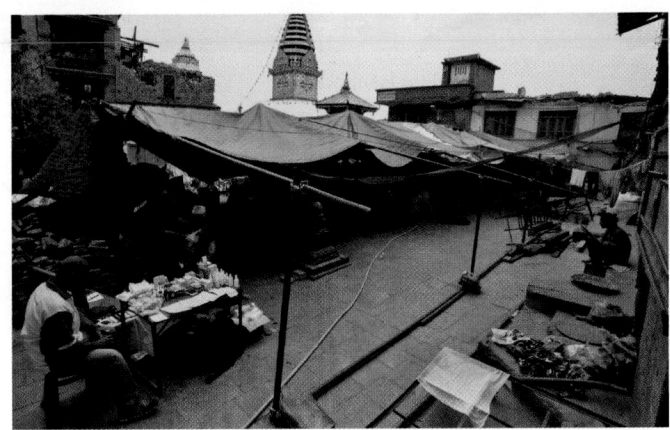

FIGURE 83-8 Disaster medical care in Kathmandu, Nepal. *(Courtesy Jon Brack.)*

information collected from survivors on the ground. This information was used by responding agencies to quickly match resources with needs.[57] Responses to subsequent natural disasters, including the earthquakes in Chile (2010) and Nepal (2015) (Figures 83-8 and 83-9) and Supertyphoon Yolanda (2013), have used digital humanitarians, and many of them are now part of formally activated networks to review, verify, and translate digital information into usable data.[20,22]

Governmental agencies have also increasingly embraced social media platforms, including Facebook, Twitter, and YouTube, and mobile devices to communicate about disasters before, during, and after they occur.[19,51] The Federal Emergency Management Agency, for example, has created a smartphone application that provides general disaster preparedness information, and real-time weather alerts, and allows individuals to find shelters, apply for aid, and submit disaster reports. Tools such as the Google Person Finder, Facebook Safety Check, and Red Cross Safe and Well allow individuals to report their status and reconnect with loved ones.

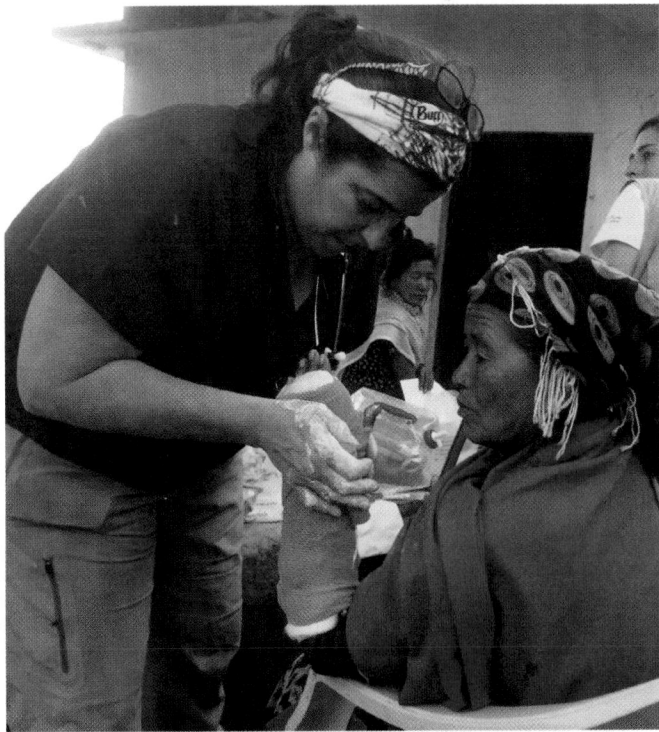

FIGURE 83-9 Nursing care in Dhading, Nepal. *(Courtesy Sheila Preece.)*

TABLE 83-1 Responder Self-Care

	Individual Actions*	Organizational Measures†
Predisaster care	Personal assessment of current physical and emotional health, training and competency for the job at hand, family preparedness and ability to cope with responder's absence and assignment, employer support and preparedness for responder's absence	Has written policy for staff stress management Conducts predeployment screening and assessments Conducts predeployment training and stress education
Care during disaster deployment	Self-monitor and maintain boundaries Maintain contact with friends, family, colleagues, as possible Work with partner or in teams Take breaks Avoid use of food and substances as a support	Monitors staff stress response Provides ongoing stress management training and support Provides crisis support for critical or unusual sources of severe stress Provides practical and emotional end-of-assignment support
Postdisaster care	Seek out and give social support Consider participating in an organized debriefing Maintain contact with colleagues from deployment Pay attention to health, nutrition, rekindling relationships Make time for sleep, exercise, and leisure activities	Has policies and capabilities to provide postassignment support to staff

*Data from National Child Traumatic Stress Network and National Center for PTSD. Psychological first aid field operations guide, 2nd ed, appendix 3: Provider care, 2006. http://www.ptsd.va.gov/professional/manuals/psych-first-aid.asp; and U.S. Department of Health and Human Services. A guide to managing stress in crisis response professions. DHHS pub no 4113. Rockville, MD, 2005, Center for Mental Health Services, Substance Abuse and Mental Health Services Administration.
†Data from Antares Foundation. Managing stress in humanitarian workers: guidelines for good practice, 3rd ed, 2012: www.antaresfoundation.org.

Nongovernmental relief organizations are using social media and mobile devices in new and effective ways to collect and manage donations to support their response efforts. The American Red Cross raised U.S. $32 million for Haiti relief efforts by inviting donors to text "Haiti" to their office and contribute $10 each, as compared with raising only $130,000 via mobile phone donations following Hurricane Katrina 5 years earlier.[84] Following Hurricane Sandy, an Amazon.com "wedding registry" was created, allowing individuals to donate specific items, such as flashlights and diapers, requested by a grassroots relief network.[42] The recovers.org platform, developed by residents of a Massachusetts community hit with an EF3 tornado, convenes government organizations, aid organizations, and individuals on a common platform to directly match needs and resources (https://www.ted.com/talks/caitria_and_morgan_o_neill_how_to_step_up_in_the_face_of_disaster).

However, with the many potential applications of social media in disasters, researchers and practitioners urge that advance planning is necessary to be most effective.[36,51] Organizations should strongly consider establishing a social media presence before a disaster, establishing training and staffing plans for social media use during a disaster, coordinating with partners for consistent messaging, and engaging with active social media discussions during the response and recovery phases, including correcting the spread of false rumors in real time.[74] The United Nations Office for the Coordination of Humanitarian Affairs has proposed hashtag standards for emergencies, in the hope of organizing information in a way that makes it easier for responders to find and act upon the information. This was inspired in part by the emergence of standardized hashtags during widespread floods in the Philippines in 2012. #RescuePH requested a rescue, #ReliefPH requested and shared relief resources and information, #FloodPH reported flooded locations, and #SAFENOW allowed users to update prior requests.[67]

RESPONDER SELF-CARE

Many health care workers responding to natural disasters will find the experience challenging and meaningful, but the reality of a disaster deployment can include exposure to trauma, violence, long hours, austere working and living conditions in an unfamiliar environment, and concern about family and work responsibilities at home. It is important that potential disaster responders understand, prepare for, and continuously manage the potential effects of stress during their response and afterward. Common stress reactions can be behavioral (e.g., irritability, hypervigilance), physical (e.g., chronic fatigue, weight loss or gain), psychological (e.g., feeling heroic, guilty, or grief-stricken), cognitive (e.g., memory problems, difficulty making decisions), and social (e.g., isolating, difficulty receiving or accepting support).[69] These are normal reactions to abnormal situations. Mild to moderate stress reactions can improve one's immediate performance, and most disaster workers recover from them in the months following deployment.[49,75] Posttraumatic growth is a long-term benefit some disaster workers experience following a deployment; this can manifest itself in an "increased sense of mastery, self-efficacy, control, [and a sense of truly making a difference]."[12,69] On the other hand, disaster responders returning from deployments can experience depression, burnout, anxiety, and posttraumatic stress disorder; the percentages of these reactions vary by event and individual background.[16,49,77] Factors such as prior mental health issues, lack of appreciation and recognition, poor team functioning, lack of social support, and being a volunteer, rather than a professional, responder are associated with negative postdisaster mental health effects.[49,65]

Ideally, responder self-care takes place before, during, and after a deployment and occurs on both the individual and organizational level. Examples of self-care activities at both levels are included in Table 83-1. Good self-care also protects the responder from becoming an additional disaster casualty and placing additional burdens on already-strained resources. Available programs and policies in place to support responder well-being are helpful references to include when a person is trying to decide whether to respond to a disaster and/or with which organization he or she may choose to deploy.[80]

REFERENCES

Complete references used in this text are available online at expertconsult.inkling.com.

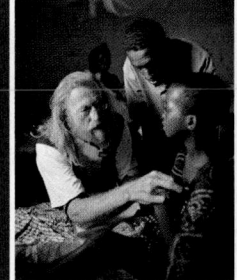

CHAPTER 84

Global Humanitarian Medicine and Disaster Relief

BRUCE LAMPARD, KEVIN COPPOCK, KIRSTEN N. JOHNSON, STEPHANIE KAYDEN, JOANNE LIU, MARILYN McHARG, LISA K. ODDY, PARVEEN K. PARMAR, MATTHEW C. SPITZER, AND RAGHU VENUGOPAL

Health care professionals engaging in wilderness medicine have many personal and professional qualities ideally suited for international humanitarian and disaster medicine. These individuals are able to cope with environmental extremes and rugged situations, and are by nature adaptable and practical (Figure 84-1). Such health care providers appreciate human diversity and thrive through altruism.

This chapter outlines many of the major medical and nonmedical issues pertaining to serving as an aid worker in humanitarian emergencies, disasters, and related crises. It is geared to medical providers from all related allied disciplines. This field is in constant evolution; readers are encouraged to consult the cited online references for up-to-date information.

The aid work community is rife with differing opinions and debate on critical issues. The concepts and opinions written in this chapter should serve to foster personal and professional reflections. The chapter is a framework for exploring humanitarian and disaster work. It is important to realize that comprehensive graduate studies are dedicated to this topic. It is our hope that this chapter will inspire readers to engage in aid work, which is a unique, important, and rewarding component of wilderness medicine.

SURVEY OF KEY EVENTS AND MEDICAL PROBLEMS

Events and disasters requiring humanitarian support have occurred throughout human history and will continue to occur. These events vary in location, impact, and responses. This section of the chapter provides an overview of some of the more notable types of events.

ARMED CONFLICT

The seeds of humanitarianism can be traced back to the social justice movements of the 19th century, such as abolitionism and missionary efforts. Many, however, place the origin of modern humanitarian action in 1859 with the Battle of Solferino in northern Italy.[4] Franco-Sardinian and Austrian forces engaged in combat, leaving 6000 persons dead and 35,000 wounded or missing. A young Swiss businessman, Henry Dunant, and the local population did their best to care for the injured in the Castiglione church. Dunant's experiences led him to create an organization called the International Committee of the Red Cross (ICRC), which would go on to protect and assist persons wounded in war. Dunant's work eventually led to the Red Cross and Red Crescent Movement, which is composed of the ICRC, the International Federation of the Red Cross and Red Crescent Societies (IFRC), and national societies from virtually every country in the world. The principles that governed these societies later became the basis of the Geneva Conventions,[18] which outline the protection and care needed for civilians and prisoners in times of armed conflict. The ICRC led the way for provision of humanitarian emergency aid in the 20th century, but did not remain the only leader for long.

In the wake of the First World War, Save the Children was created in the United Kingdom, to feed children starving throughout Europe. The International Rescue Committee had its roots in 1933, assisting Germans suffering under the Hitler regime. In 1942, the Oxford Committee for Famine Relief, later Oxfam, campaigned for food supplies to be sent through an allied naval blockade to starving women and children in enemy-occupied Greece during the Second World War. Following World War II, a number of American charities banded together to form the Cooperative for American Remittances to Europe (CARE) and sent small packages of food and relief to recipients in Europe. The United Nations (UN) was formed in 1945, and many of its humanitarian arms were set up soon after: UNICEF to assist children, the UN High Commissioner for Refugees, and the World Food Programme. In the late 1960s, a group of French physicians working for the ICRC in the Nigerian Biafra conflict became frustrated by the organization's confidential, reserved style of operations and its passivity in the face of mass starvation. In 1971 alongside some journalist colleagues, they formed Médecins Sans Frontières (MSF), or Doctors Without Borders.[27] Since Solferino, armed conflict has always played a central role in humanitarian actions, whether workers are responding to the consequences of conflict or being influenced by the logic and operations of conflict.

The Cold War had a major impact on humanitarian events because proxy wars were fought in such nations as Mozambique, Angola, Afghanistan, Ethiopia, and Somalia. These conflicts led to an explosion in the numbers of refugees crossing international borders. Refugee camps swelled in the 1980s and 1990s and still persist. Many aid organizations "cut their teeth" and matured serving these needy populations.

Numerous protracted conflicts continue to be foci for humanitarian organizations; some have been going on for years or decades. For example, South Sudan has been engulfed in a civil war since the 1980s, and the Democratic Republic of Congo is still suffering through a conflict, at one point labeled Africa's World War, that tragically began on the heels of the Rwandan genocide in 1994. Each of these conflicts takes up a major proportion of the human and financial resources of certain large international aid agencies; the inherent dangers are obvious. There are many other examples, such as conflicts in Afghanistan, Somalia, Colombia, and the Central African Republic.

At times, aid has not been easily rendered for reasons not immediately made public. In the 1984 famine in Ethiopia, during which one million people died, the Ethiopian government forcibly moved its people from drought-prone areas. Later, it was learned that this was done for political reasons, to suppress a rebel movement. In the catastrophic refugee camps of the eastern Democratic Republic of Congo, formed after genocide in Rwanda in 1994 (Figure 84-2), some humanitarian agencies came to believe that the aid provided was being manipulated by the same forces that had conducted the genocide. In these situations, aid agencies have withdrawn their services once workers are convinced that resources are being misused for political ends rather than to genuinely help those in greatest need. Strong-arm regimes persist to this day, forcing aid organizations to make difficult

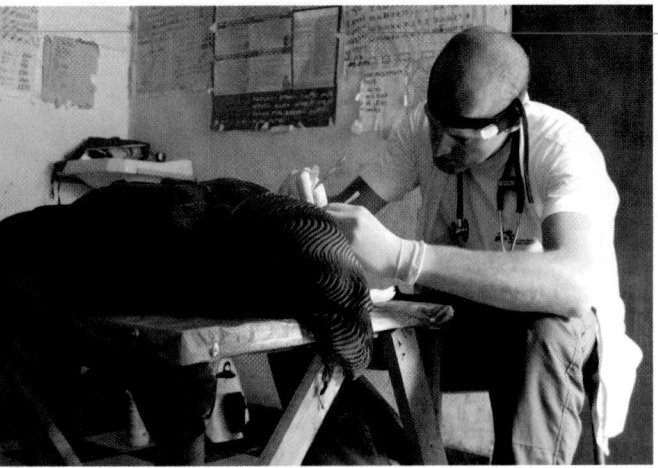

FIGURE 84-1 Médecins Sans Frontières aid worker performing a minor surgical procedure in Ethiopia, 2008. *(Courtesy Damien Follet, Médecins Sans Frontières.)*

choices between reporting what workers see on the ground and obtaining government permission to continue providing aid to suffering populations.[27]

The notion of "military humanitarianism" grew from crises in which Western military forces became increasingly involved in providing humanitarian assistance. In 1991, following ousting of the Iraqi regime from Kuwait, the Kurdish exodus to the north of Iraq led to a massive relief operation involving foreign governments. In 1992, interclan warfare in Somalia led to an ill-fated operation led by the U.S. military to secure the region and deliver aid. The 1990s were marked by rupture of the former Yugoslavia, war in Bosnia, and war in the former Serbian province of Kosovo. Events included the July 1995 execution of 7000 persons in the UN "safe haven" of Srebrenica. Later, a "humanitarian war" consisting of aerial bombing was led by Western governments and the North Atlantic Treaty Organization (NATO) to aid the former Serbian territory of Kosovo; the war arguably contributed to displacement of more than one million Albanians. NATO's use of the word *humanitarian* to justify its actions has been disputed.[27] "If an appeal to humanitarian considerations can justify both a medical aid operation and a military campaign, doesn't that suggest that aid workers and international troops represent two sides of the same coin?"[36] The consequences of military humanitarianism for aid organizations became even clearer in Afghanistan following the U.S.-led invasion after 9/11 and subsequent occupation of the country by NATO. Stark examples involved deployment of special forces in civilian dress who claimed to be on a humanitarian mission and threatened to suspend aid to populations in southern Afghanistan if the people refused to provide information about the Taliban and al-Qaeda. Such actions led to a dangerous blurring of the lines of identities

and intentions, leaving it difficult to distinguish aid efforts from political or military actions. The end results were loss of aid workers' lives and formation of a climate in which it was much more difficult to negotiate access to suspicious populations.

Beyond Afghanistan, recent conflicts in Iraq, Syria, and Somalia have been marked by extreme insecurity for aid workers. These crises also typify the polarized and growing anti-Western context in which Western coalition military forces are operating or seeking influence.[27] For MSF, the problems peaked in 2013 in Somalia, arguably the world's most failed state; after delivering humanitarian assistance there for 22 years, MSF finally had to withdraw completely from the country. Aid organizations have yet to find a way to minimize risks and provide safe access in such highly insecure places. Until they do, it is the populations left behind that suffer.

In response to armed conflicts over decades, specialized medical and surgical skills have been developed and refined. The importance of improved logistic abilities of aid organizations has had a significant impact on their effectiveness. Public health efforts, such as preemptive measles vaccinations, epidemiologic tools for detecting epidemics, and curative medical approaches, have evolved enough that significant problems of morbidity and mortality can be predicted and diseases prevented and treated. Medical care available in complex conflict settings has improved to the extent that human immunodeficiency virus/acquired immunodeficiency syndrome (HIV/AIDS) and tuberculosis have been successfully treated in areas such as the eastern Democratic Republic of Congo and south Sudan.[27]

POPULATION DISPLACEMENT

People may be forced to leave their homes due to violence or natural disasters. Once they have decided to do so and cross an international boundary, they officially become refugees and are guaranteed certain rights and protections under international law. Most, however, do not cross an international boundary, and they become internally displaced people within their home country. They remain under the protection of their own government, even though that government may have been the cause of their flight. Internally displaced people are among the world's most vulnerable people.

As of January 2014, the number of displaced persons due to conflict surpassed 50 million, with 16.7 million refugees, mostly from Palestine, Syria, Afghanistan, and Somalia, and 33.3 million internally displaced people, notably from Syria, Sudan, Iraq, Colombia, Democratic Republic of Congo, and South Sudan[15] (Figure 84-3). Another 22 million people were newly displaced

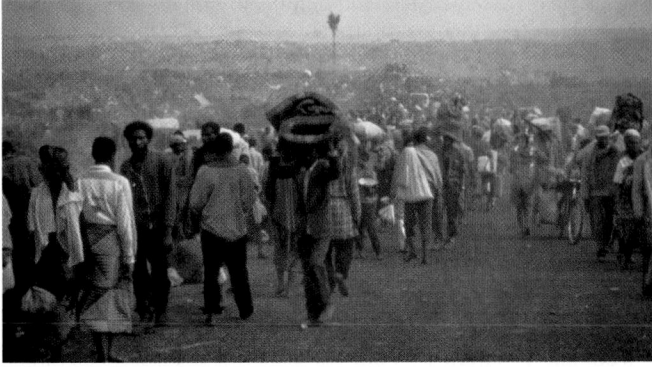

FIGURE 84-2 Massive exodus of refugees toward Goma, Zaïre, 1994. *(Courtesy B. Press, Médecins Sans Frontières.)*

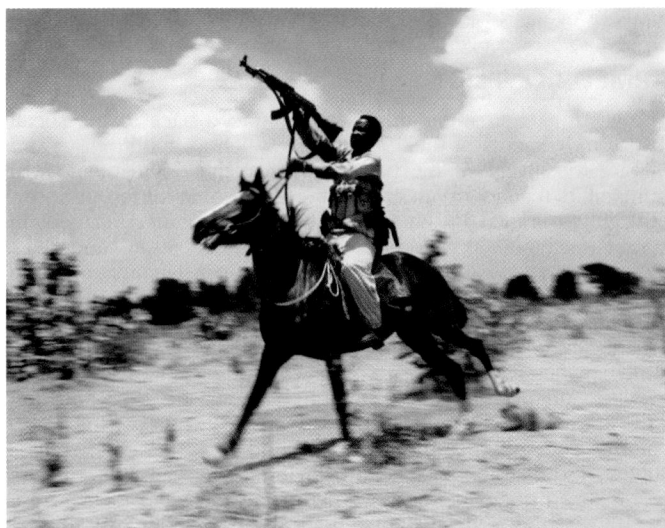

FIGURE 84-3 Violence and targeted attacks by armed elements on civilians led to the displacement of hundreds of thousands in the Darfur region of Sudan, 2004. *(Courtesy Espen Rasmussen, Médecins Sans Frontières.)*

in 2013 as a result of natural disasters, mostly in the Philippines, China, and India.

The priorities in refugee emergencies are outlined in the section on Needs in Humanitarian Crises later in this chapter.[20]

NATURAL DISASTERS

Major natural disasters (see Chapter 86) have occurred throughout human history. International nongovernmental organizations (NGOs) previously played minor roles while military forces provided most of the aid. This scenario has changed dramatically in recent years.

The history of natural disasters is one of devastating losses of life. Floods in China in 1931 killed between 1 and 4 million persons. Severe storms also take their toll. The 2008 cyclone in Myanmar killed more than 80,000 and displaced more than 2 million inhabitants.[33] In November 2013, more than 6000 persons died and another 4 million were displaced as Typhoon Haiyan struck the coasts of the Philippines.[12]

Earthquakes have wreaked particular destruction. In December 2004, a major earthquake in the Indian Ocean caused a tsunami that affected numerous Asian countries and killed 230,000 persons. Although some national governments were able to care for their own populations, the international response was massive. It was also apparent that unless an organization was already present on the ground at the time of the disaster, the possibility that an organization could become operational within 24 to 48 hours was limited to a select few that had plans in place for a surge in need and logistic stockpiles of needed food and goods. Even with such a capacity for response, it can be challenging to determine which ports or airstrips are not damaged, especially because other first-response organizations are attempting to do the same. This was the case in Nepal following the earthquakes that occurred in close succession in April and May of 2015.

In January 2010 an earthquake devastated Haiti, a nation that was already perhaps the most desperate and neglected nation in the Americas (Figure 84-4). During the disaster, 60% of the country's existing health care facilities were destroyed and 10% of medical personnel either were killed or left the country. The human death toll was 220,000, and much of the infrastructure of the nation was lost. Although the immediate focus was on major surgical and intensive medical care, basic primary care was needed for thousands with minor injuries and chronic medical problems. The psychological trauma was widespread, especially due to aftershocks. Countless lives were saved by the efforts of the overall response. Lessons about coordination and leadership

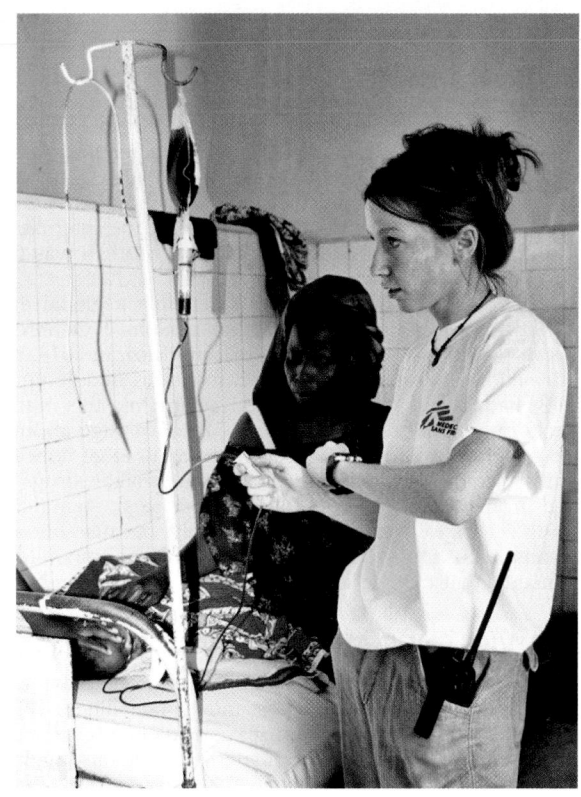

FIGURE 84-5 Malaria treatment of a child with antimalarials and blood transfusion in Ivory Coast, 2003. (*Courtesy Peter Casaer, Médecins Sans Frontières.*)

were still to be learned, however,[14] especially when hundreds of aid workers, many of whom did not have appropriate expertise or training, from many organizations were arriving. Haitians and state systems were excluded from decision making, and there was little understanding of how to provide acute care in the densely populated urban areas or, later on, care for the victims of a cholera epidemic.

On March 2011, an earthquake occurred off the coast of Japan, triggering a tsunami and subsequent nuclear reactor meltdown. It is instructive to bear in mind that wealthy countries are not immune from crisis; a humanitarian response took place in that highly developed country.

DISEASE EPIDEMICS

By definition, disease epidemics occur when new or resurgent cases of a certain disease, in a given human population and during a given period, substantially exceed what is expected based on recent experience. Medieval history recounts epochs of plague killing millions of persons. Influenza in the early 1900s killed between 50 and 100 million persons; from 1956 to 1958, flu epidemics killed another 4 million. Smallpox swept across the world for centuries before vaccination resulted in its eradication. Measles continues to kill approximately 164,000 persons annually and remains a serious concern in regions with crowded and malnourished populations. In some refugee camps, measles vaccine is provided along with vitamin A, which reduces the impact of the infection. Malaria epidemics persist worldwide, particularly in sub-Saharan African. Rapid antigen detection tests and artemisinin-based antimalarial medications have improved diagnosis and disease management (Figure 84-5).

Numerous other disease epidemics have occurred and continue to occur. Global cholera pandemics have killed millions across all continents, despite the treatment, fluid replacement, being straightforward. Meningococcal meningitis can be epidemic in the "meningitis belt" of sub-Saharan Africa, from Senegal to Ethiopia. Mass treatment and vaccination campaigns are required once the disease burden hits epidemic proportions.

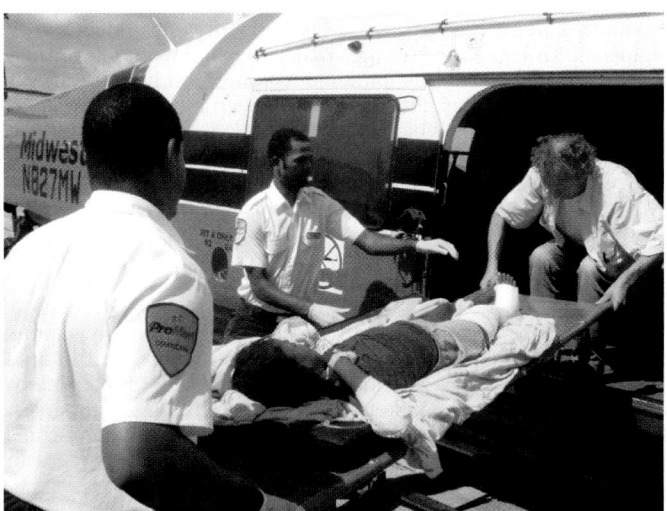

FIGURE 84-4 An 8-year-old girl is transferred by MSF for specialized surgical care to Santo Domingo following initial surgical attention in Haiti following the 2010 earthquake. (*Courtesy Stefaan Maddens, Médecins Sans Frontières.*)

Currently, efforts are under way to vaccinate residents of the entire meningitis belt region in order to eradicate the illness. In March 2014, the largest epidemic ever seen of Ebola viral hemorrhagic fever occurred. It affected primarily Guinea, Liberia, and Sierra Leone; cases were found in Nigeria, Mali, Senegal, Spain, the United States, and the United Kingdom. After the onset of the epidemic, more than 25,000 people were infected, of whom more than 40% died. Whether because of lack of expertise or fear, and aside from a few notable exceptions, the international response to support West Africa during this outbreak was tragically too little, too late.

The current HIV/AIDS pandemic is certainly a global emergency, with at least 35 million infected persons.[39] Of infected persons worldwide, 71% are in sub-Saharan Africa. In 2013, more than 11 million HIV-positive people in low- and middle-income countries had access to antiretroviral treatment; this number represents only 36% of the total need. Global outrage about the high cost of HIV/AIDS treatment inspired a surge of concerted activism. Subsequently, the price of antiretroviral drugs has dropped from about $15,000 to $150 per year, significantly improving access to treatment. Unfortunately, because one-third of persons with HIV/AIDS are coinfected with tuberculosis; resurgence of that disease has also become a global problem.

SEXUAL VIOLENCE AND MENTAL ILLNESS

Victims of disasters and humanitarian crises around the world continue to endure sexual violence and mental illness (Figure 84-6). In settings where the rate of sexual violence is high, as in conflict zones and refugee camps, dedicated teams might be created to provide assistance, with staff working in the community to raise awareness of the problem of sexual violence and to promote social and legal support. In 2013, MSF treated more than 11,000 victims of rape; these statistics are likely incomplete because patients experience shame and fear about reporting rape, are stigmatized, and have logistic problems in seeking care.[21]

Due to armed conflict, displacement, neglect, and disaster, persons in crisis are increasingly recognized to suffer mental health consequences. Providing psychosocial support to victims of trauma may help reduce the incidence of long-term psychological problems. Psychosocial care focuses on supporting a community to develop its own culturally appropriate coping

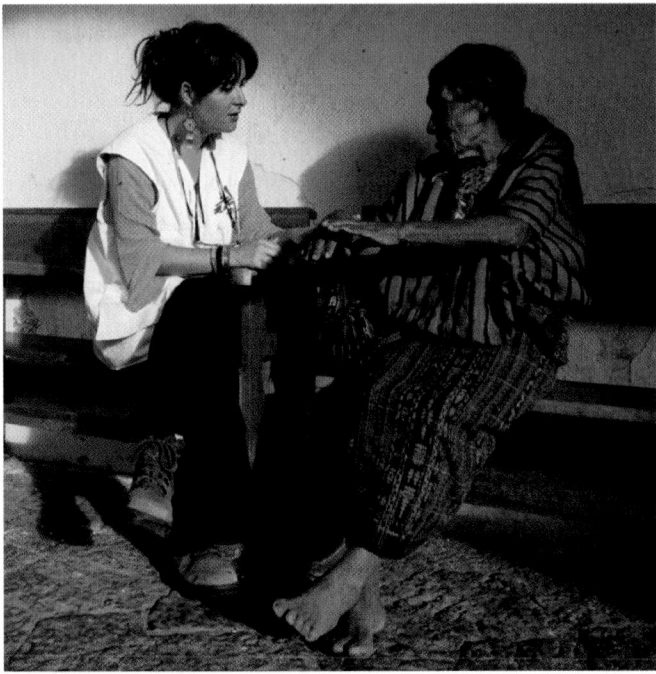

FIGURE 84-6 Mental health assistance is provided to victim of tropical storm Stan in Guatemala, 2005. *(Courtesy Marco Baroncini, Médecins Sans Frontières.)*

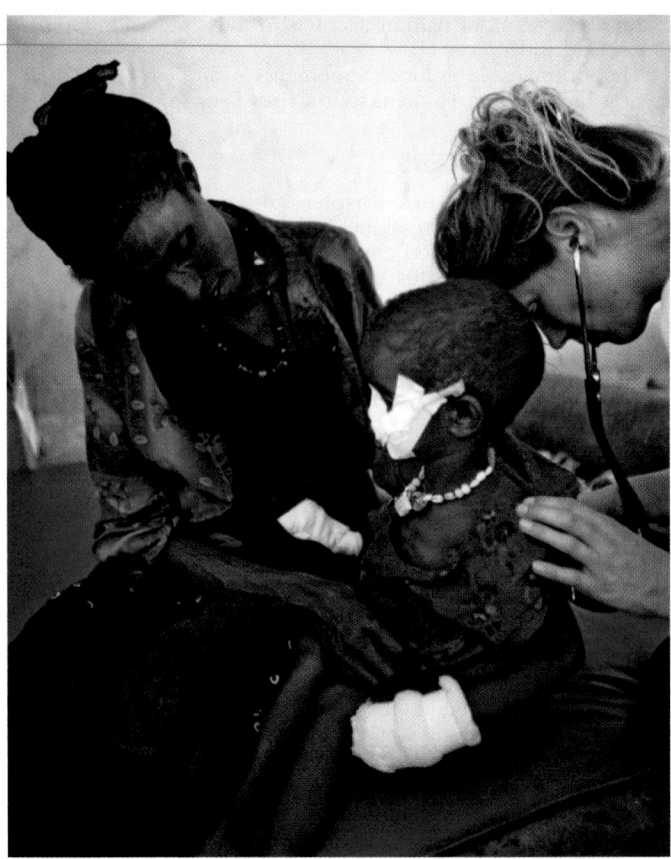

FIGURE 84-7 3-year-old girl receiving treatment for kala azar and malnutrition in Somalia, 2004. Bandages on the hands and face are in place to prevent the child from removing the nasogastric tube. *(Courtesy Espen Rasmussen, Médecins Sans Frontières.)*

strategies after trauma. In some instances, psychiatric care for select individuals may also be needed.

FAMINE AND MALNUTRITION

Famines continue to cause significant rates of morbidity and mortality (Figure 84-7). Malnutrition is involved in nearly half of all deaths of children under 5 years of age, or almost 3 million per year.[34] Although it is easy to think of famine as a result of lack of food, it is rarely that simple. Factors such as conflict, resource scarcity, climate change, and governmental policies play significant roles. One of the major developments from the 2005 famine in Niger was implementation of ready-to-use therapeutic foods such as Plumpy'Nut (a peanut-butter—like food requiring no water), which became available on an outpatient basis (Figure 84-8). This intervention became a substitute for admitting patients to traditional therapeutic feeding centers, where they would have obtained a watery milk-based refeeding treatment.

NEGLECTED DISEASES

Rare and/or neglected diseases cause serious crises in various parts of the globe. Because these diseases are not well known and receive less media attention, they often do not represent an enticing or lucrative market for commercial drug companies. Hence, there are often few options available for treating victims of such diseases, such as human African trypanosomiasis (African sleeping sickness), Chagas' disease, and leishmaniasis.

EMERGING URBAN CONTEXTS

New contexts requiring humanitarian assistance will continue to arise. Rapid urbanization has led to increased violent conflict in

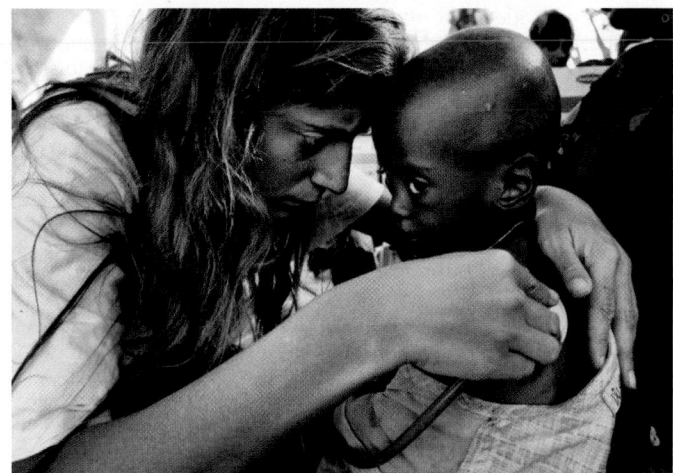

FIGURE 84-8 MSF aid worker examines a child with severe malnutrition in Ethiopia, 2008. Children without medical complications are treated on an ambulatory basis. *(Courtesy Francesco Zizola, Médecins Sans Frontières.)*

zone. These include the affected population, national government and local groups, UN, armed actors, foreign governments, Red Cross, NGOs, religious or faith-based organizations, private corporations, donor agencies, and academic institutions. Each organization has specific capabilities, limitations, and niches. The usual agencies responding to medical needs include a state ministry of health, the World Health Organization (WHO), and medical NGOs.

First and foremost, it is the ministry of health that is officially responsible for health care of the population. If humanitarian medical agencies are operating, it must be assumed that the ministry of health has been overwhelmed in one or more of its capacities. In certain cases, ministry of health staff may be unable, uninterested, or unwilling to work in the affected area because of the level of violence or the presence of hostile antigovernment forces. In other circumstances, the ministry of health may have been virtually nonfunctional before the crisis. This is most often true for provision of accessible, quality primary health care. The ministry of health may not have the level of expertise or the required human, financial, and material resources to provide medical care required to adequately respond to the crisis.

The WHO is often present in the affected country before a crisis. This organization provides technical advice and supports training. It sometimes provides administrative capacity or medical and logistic resources to the ministry of health. During a crisis, the WHO continues in this advisory role while taking on other responsibilities. Most prominently, it works with the ministry of health to coordinate the emergency response. At times, the WHO takes the lead on the coordination role, especially in the first phases of an emergency or in nations where the ministry of health lacks the capacity or interest.

Medical NGOs, such as MSF, Medical Emergency Relief International, the International Rescue Committee, the International Medical Corps, and Médecins du Monde, usually focus on patient treatment during a crisis. These organizations have well-developed logistic supply systems for drugs and medical materials managed by staff knowledgeable in logistics and pharmacists. NGOs have pools of international medical staff, including nurses, general physicians, and specialists such as epidemiologists, psychologists, and surgeons. Activities are coordinated by experienced operations staff that oversee the assignments and manage relations with other actors (Figure 84-10). When possible, the majority of NGO workers, medical or nonmedical, are nationals from the affected country, and they often work in ministry of health hospitals and clinics (Figure 84-11). NGOs frequently pay stipends to ministry of health staff in these facilities. This compensation provides extra motivation to support the increased workload and to enable quality control and greater efficiency; it also runs the risk of creating a "brain drain" from local health systems. NGOs ensure a constant supply of essential medical materials and

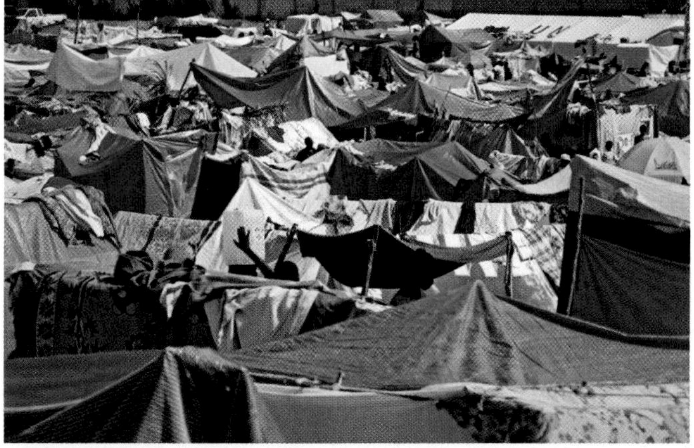

the vast slums of cities such as Port-au-Prince in Haiti, Rio de Janeiro in Brazil, and Tegucigalpa in Honduras. Street children and marginalized populations are victims of such settings. These contexts are in part driven by criminal violence. However, in some countries, such as Colombia, urbanization and slum growth are driven as much by political conflict as by criminal elements; both lead to indigenous people leaving rural areas for cities.

Responding to natural disasters and epidemics in urban settings is more difficult than in rural or lightly populated settings. Not only is there a higher impact purely because of the numbers of people involved, but gaining a solid understanding of stakeholders and power dynamics is more complicated. The 2010 Haiti earthquake and the cholera outbreak that followed were excellent examples of how much aid organizations still need to learn (Figure 84-9).

ACTORS DURING EVENTS: THEIR CAPABILITIES, LIMITATIONS, AND USUAL ROLES

The number of agencies responding to humanitarian crises has greatly increased in the last three decades. However, it is common to see a "standard" set of organizations and actors in a crisis

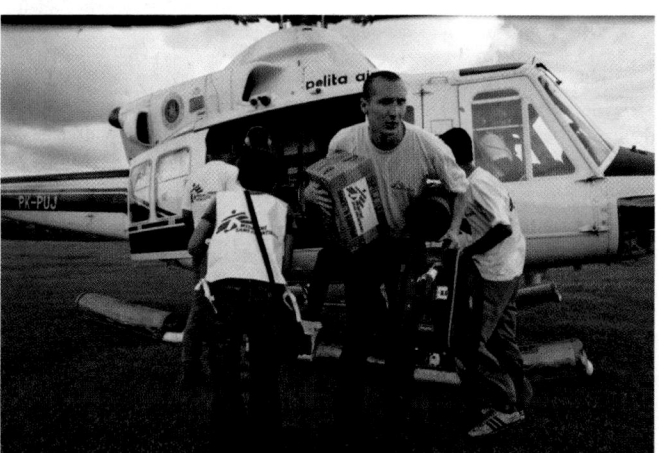

FIGURE 84-9 Many lost their homes and were displaced following the 2010 Haiti earthquake. Shelter construction was a major problem. *(Courtesy Paul Cabrera, Médecins Sans Frontières.)*

FIGURE 84-10 Aid workers brought rice, water, and essential supplies to isolated areas affected by the 2004 Indian Ocean tsunami, and then returned to the base station with patients requiring treatment (Indonesia, 2005). *(Courtesy Francesco Zizola, Médecins Sans Frontières.)*

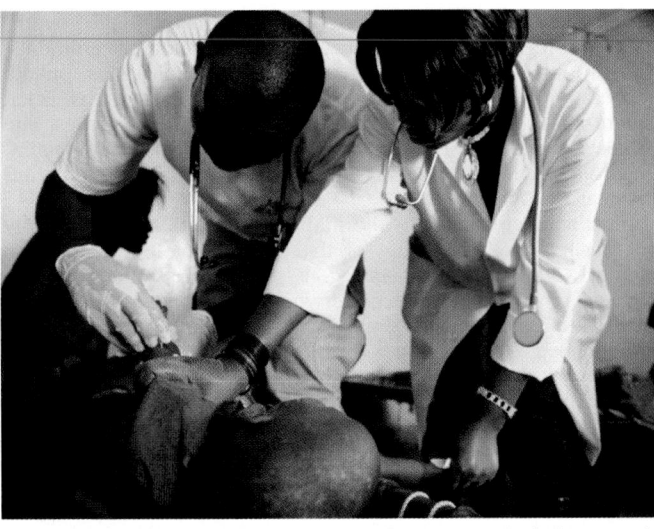

FIGURE 84-11 NGO workers caring for a patient with cholera in collaboration with the national ministry of health in Lusaka, Zambia, 2010. *(Courtesy Robin Meldrum, Médecins Sans Frontières.)*

drugs, and help to improve water and sanitation systems of health care facilities. They seek to maintain a constant power supply and work in other essential sectors necessary to ensure safe and quality health care management within the facility. In many cases, the NGO essentially takes over management of the hospital, although striving to be tactful and to respect preexisting management structures.

In cases in which a ministry of health hospital has been abandoned or destroyed, medical NGOs will usually either take over the abandoned facility until the ministry of health can return or will convert existing suitable buildings into temporary health structures. In some cases, NGOs set up full medical services in an inflatable or container-based hospital. In some settings, as during cholera outbreaks, NGOs set up separate medical structures outside the hospital to ensure proper disease containment.

In certain circumstances, medical NGOs provide primary health care through mobile clinics (Figure 84-12). This is essentially outpatient care for people spread out in smaller groups within the affected region. Mobile clinic teams can be converted into mass vaccination teams when there are outbreaks of contagious diseases, such as yellow fever, measles, or meningitis.

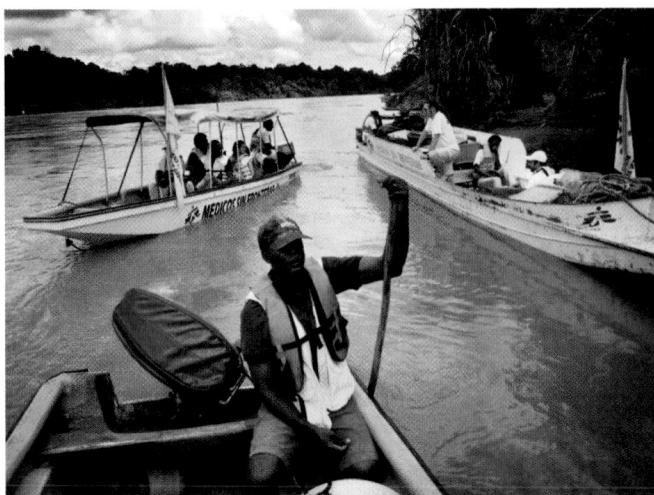

FIGURE 84-12 MSF sexual and reproductive mobile health care outreach team in Colombia, 2007. *(Courtesy Francesco Zizola, Médecins Sans Frontières.)*

NGOs provide more than curative care. Depending on their mandate, they may be equipped for preventing deterioration of the overall health condition of the population. They do this by providing shelter, water, sanitation, food and nutrition, nonfood items (e.g., soap, sanitary napkins, buckets, blankets), education, and protection. Improving palliative care is also a growing concern.

Humanitarian UN organizations specialize in specific types of essential services and populations. The UN Children's Fund, or UNICEF, supports activities such as the provision of vaccines to the ministry of health for access by NGOs. UNICEF also provides medications to health care facilities and increasingly supports therapeutic treatment of acutely undernourished children.

The UN High Commission for Refugees coordinates relief activities and provision of essential services to refugees and internally displaced populations. As much as possible, it funds NGOs to provide basic services to the refugee population. The commission also supplies shelter support, such as tents and other essential material, and often offers expert advice. It negotiates living space for refugees, protects refugee rights in the host country, and undertakes assessments when new displacements occur.

The World Food Programme provides foods, such as maize, oil, sugar, and pulse (food crops harvested for their dry seeds), to populations in crisis. Most of these foods are donated by donor countries, but increasingly, food is purchased locally or regionally. The World Food Programme normally oversees food transport from its source to the disaster zone. In line with this often massive network involving logistics, the World Food Programme can take the lead in providing air transport for UN and NGO aid workers to areas that are difficult or hazardous to reach by road.

The UN Population Fund is involved in reproductive health, gender equality, and strategies to promote healthy population growth. It specifically supports the ministry of health and other government sectors in providing safe maternal care. The International Organization for Migration assists displaced people, often through provision of shelter and the orderly and humane migration of persons in transit.

To varying degrees, all UN agencies limit the scope of their direct implementation of field operations because of high personnel costs, high levels of bureaucracy, and security restrictions. NGOs are therefore seen as essential service providers that take contacts from UN agencies to implement and provide basic services to populations in need.

Certain NGOs have developed specializations in certain sectors. Action Contre la Faim, or Action Against Hunger, specializes in food distribution and nutrition activities. CARE has developed expertise in camp management, food and nonfood item distributions, and shelter provision. Save the Children and Plan International focus on education, child protection, and primary health care services. The German government organization Gesellschaft für Technische Zusammenarbeit is often involved in logistics and mechanical support for UN and NGO vehicle fleets.

Many religious or faith-based NGOs, such as World Vision, Catholic Relief Services, Adventist Development and Relief Agency, Lutheran World Relief, and the Mennonite Committee, are active during the crisis phase of emergencies. These organizations tend to have a longer-term, developmental approach to their interventions and are well suited to carry on a project once the work is handed over by the more immediately responsive humanitarian medical agencies that focus on the emergency phase of a crisis.

During a crisis, the Red Cross can often mobilize volunteers to assist with the response. National Red Cross or Red Crescent Society members are involved in many sectors and phases of emergency response, including distribution of food, nonfood items, and water and the provision of primary health care, shelter, and sanitation. The IFRC specializes in a rapid response to natural disasters. In conflict zones, the ICRC is also involved in a variety of activities. Most notably, these include emergency surgical response for war wounded, reuniting separated families, and monitoring conditions of prisoners of war and prisons. The ICRC is not an NGO, but rather, a charter organization with a special

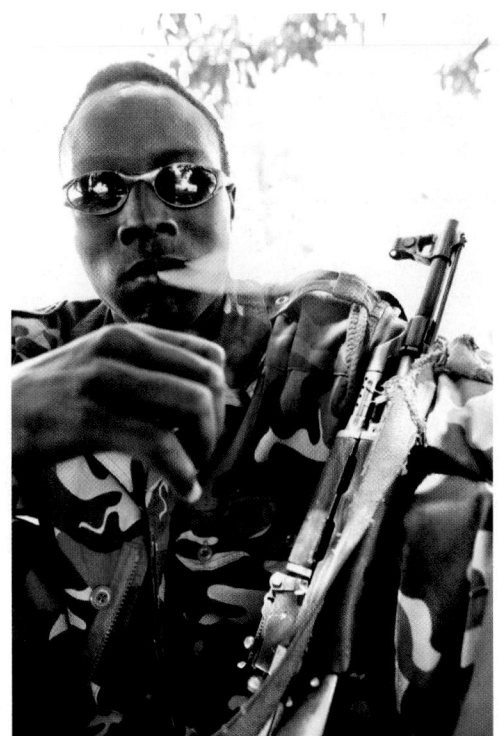

FIGURE 84-13 Sudanese Janjaweed fighter poses in a small village in Darfur, Sudan, at the border with Chad, 2004. *(Courtesy Espen Rasmussen, Médecins Sans Frontières.)*

international mandate to monitor the respect of international humanitarian law in armed conflict.

Other organizations focus on advocacy and human rights protection. Oxfam International (originally, the Oxford Committee for Famine Relief) increasingly specializes in advocacy and in-depth analysis of the vulnerability of affected populations. Organizations such as Human Rights Watch and Amnesty International collect testimony and do research on the plight of persons affected by crises, especially in cases where abuse occurs. The International Crisis Group provides detailed analysis of a given crisis situation and the factors that contribute to its deterioration or improvement.

Foreign governments provide funding for many of the activities mentioned. Most NGOs and all UN organizations rely on this funding. A few organizations, such as MSF, are (at least for the most part) financially independent and do not rely on government-sourced funds.

Armed groups can figure prominently in a crisis zone (Figure 84-13). These can include UN or other foreign forces, domestic military forces, and domestic or foreign police forces. Also present may be nonstate actors, such as antigovernment forces or forces involved in armed actions in many states. For the most part, armed groups allow relief agencies to operate unobstructed. Police and military forces, whether foreign or domestic, can play an important role in providing stability to the affected region. At the same, time, armed elements can also destabilize any context and create fear and suffering in the host population, especially if they rob, rape, steal, and kill, as has occurred in eastern Congo. Foreign troops, including UN forces, have an interest in facilitating and sometimes even undertaking, relief activities. Aid agencies often appreciate the remarkable logistic capabilities of these forces, but are also often reticent to collaborate too closely with an armed group.

Undisciplined armed groups, or armed actors hostile to the objectives of the aid agency or the aid agency donors, can hinder the provision of aid. The threat of armed robbery, extortion, or physical violence from such groups imposes security risks that restrict the movement of aid workers and the procurement and provision of essential supplies and materials.

MOTIVATING FACTORS FOR ORGANIZATIONAL INVOLVEMENT

Motivations for involvement during crises and disasters influence theoretical and practical objectives. The overall vision of an organization dictates how it will prioritize precious resources and time. It influences interactions with the affected population and other actors. It affects how and from whom organizations raise funds. For example, some aid organizations have few reservations about using full-page, "flies in the eyes" advertisements to portray starving children to aggressively raise money. Other organizations depict beneficiaries with greater dignity and strive to raise only the funds they can immediately spend. Both approaches have merits and challenges. An organization's goals influence the type of field in which it wants to operate (e.g., strictly in an emergency situation or later, in a developmental context or during the transition between the two) and with whom the organization affiliates or partners. Goals influence public positioning, as well as how and with whom organizations conduct advocacy.

A variety of motivating factors stimulate organizational involvement in crises (Figure 84-14). As with any organization, there are sometimes detailed objectives and operational priorities that may work at cross-purposes. For example, agencies involved in medical assistance or public health in a crisis share a common purpose: to save lives through provision of essential health care services. However, interpretation of this purpose is rarely straightforward because it is influenced by the traditions, culture, and motivation of the agency. For example, some NGOs strongly believe in hands-on provision of medical care to individual patients. In contrast, other NGOs would rather build their capacity or train operators, leaving the day-to-day medical care to local actors. Both approaches have legitimacy; prospective aid workers should align themselves with an approach they prefer. Another type of tension occurs between curative care and public health approaches. For example, some aid organizations believe that the best way to address the HIV pandemic is to directly treat infected persons, whereas others place more emphasis on public education and prevention efforts.

Some medical aid actors, for example, Médecins du Monde (Doctors of the World), are motivated to raise public awareness of the plight of the population. This is equal in importance to and sometimes has an even greater impact than provision of medical care, depending on the context. This tension poses a dilemma for most medical relief personnel. Should the organization undertake advocacy and public condemnation of abuses and gross neglect? Doing so could compromise the agency's neutrality in the face of armed actors that control violence, making it more

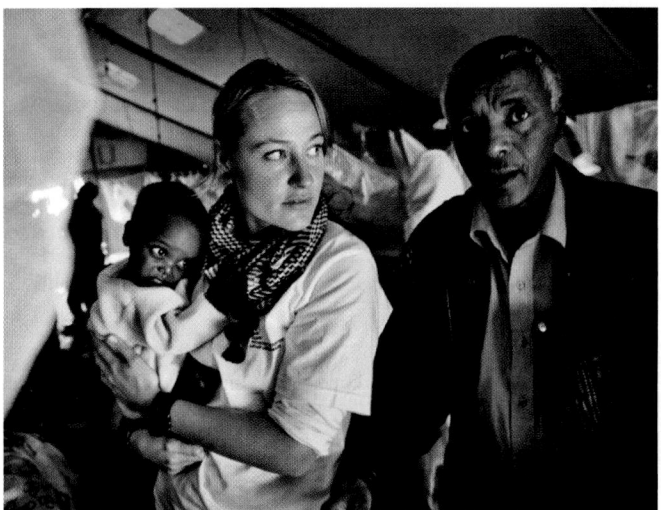

FIGURE 84-14 MSF aid worker with a child with severe malnutrition in Ethiopia, 2008. *(Courtesy Francesco Zizola, Médecins Sans Frontières.)*

difficult to safely provide medical services. Speaking out can result in the organization being expelled by a government not wanting to face criticism.

Other NGOs, such as the Save the Children Fund, are rights-based organizations, that is, they are motivated to uphold human rights. These organizations view the provision of their services as meeting the basic rights of the affected population and affording some protection against abuse to the population.

The ICRC was founded on international humanitarian law. Members are the primary defenders of the laws of war and proactively promote respect for these laws among armed groups. They favor neutrality and thus do not take sides in a conflict. Although this affords them unparalleled access, it limits their public advocacy.

Other organizations are motivated by religious beliefs and principles. Christian Aid, World Vision, Catholic Relief Services, and Islamic Relief are examples. By and large, these agencies do not have the objective to proselytize, other than by example.

Foreign governments are motivated by a combination of "enlightened self-interest," public pressure, and quasi-humanitarian motivations. In a major natural disaster, the citizens of a nation may desire to see their government doing something to help. In other cases, the foreign government may be expressing a humanitarian ideal they feel is intrinsic to their culture and society; however, if the stakes are high, self-interest will always prevail. The notion of enlightened self-interest simply means, "by helping others, we help ourselves." For example, military medical personnel may be required to provide services to a population located in a strategic region or area. In this case, the primary motivation to provide the service may be to gather intelligence and to garner the sympathy of the population (to win "hearts and minds"). In this way, foreign governments can also isolate insurgents trying to use the population as cover, as well as fulfilling other strategic purposes.

The UN can follow a similar logic, although its motivation is one of collective security, well-being, and stability. Depending on the circumstances, the UN may proactively align its agencies and (as much as possible) the NGOs, so that all efforts contribute to the desired end. This integration of efforts and conditioning of aid on strategic objectives, rather than on existing needs of the population, may be criticized by more independent NGOs.

NEEDS IN HUMANITARIAN CRISES

Humanitarian crises most often happen in the countries least able or least willing to deal with them, because of underlying poverty, lack of resources and infrastructure, or political instability. Thus the needs in a crisis situation go well beyond medical care. The following is an outline of needs commonly seen during disasters and crises, including displaced populations in camp settings.[20,26]

INITIAL ASSESSMENT

Prior to undertaking any humanitarian intervention, a thorough, rapid assessment must be conducted. This initial assessment addresses each of the sectors listed below and identifies the current situation, existing and necessary resources, interventions needed, and possibilities for specific interventions. The first phase of an initial assessment occurs within a matter of days and includes collection of both quantitative and qualitative data. Further details on how to conduct an initial assessment follows later.

Water and Sanitation

Depending on the ambient conditions, human beings without water to drink will die from dehydration in a matter of hours to days. Consumption of contaminated water leads to transmission of pathogens, often leading to fatal diarrhea and other infectious diseases. Transmission of disease most often occurs from drinking water contaminated by human feces; thus water and sanitation are intimately linked. The Sphere Project (described in more detail later) sets out the following guidelines for water and sanitation.[30]

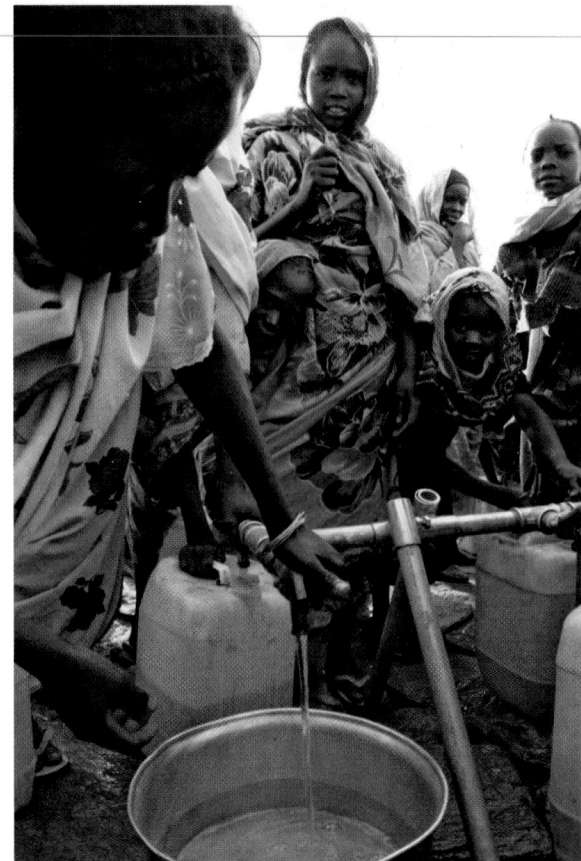

FIGURE 84-15 Internally displaced Sudanese women and girls wait a long time at a water tap stand to collect clean water in Sudan, 2004. (*Courtesy Stefan Pleger, Médecins Sans Frontières.*)

Water. Each individual should have, on average, 15 L/day of clean water for drinking, cooking, and personal hygiene (Figure 84-15). In an emergency situation, one may start by providing 5 L/day, making provisions to supply more water as soon as possible. In a stabilized setting, the goal is to supply each individual with 20 L/day. Water-gathering points must be within 500 m (1640 feet) of each household, with individuals queuing no longer than 15 minutes and able to fill their 20-L containers in 3 minutes or less. Taste and cultural acceptability of the water source must be taken into consideration.

Sanitation. A maximum of 20 people should use each toilet. Toilets, generally latrines, should ideally be provided for each household and segregated by sex (Figure 84-16). In an acute emergency, it may be necessary to build large pit latrines until more private, permanent structures can be built. Toilets should be no more than 50 m (164 feet) from homes, and they should be clean and well maintained.

Cultural acceptability is crucial when constructing latrines. If men, women, and children do not feel comfortable using the toilets provided, they will defecate elsewhere, near homes and water sources, leading to the spread of disease. Additionally, security concerns must be taken into account when latrines are constructed. In multiple-refugee settings, women have been sexually assaulted while using poorly lit, insecure public latrines.[28]

Food and Nutrition

Food shortages and acute malnutrition are common in humanitarian crises. Often, crises occur in areas with a high baseline prevalence of malnutrition prior to the emergency. Providing adequate, culturally appropriate nutrition is a key part of any humanitarian response. This includes not only providing an adequate supply of food (estimated to be approximately 2100 Kcal/day by Sphere guidelines)[30] but also identifying those

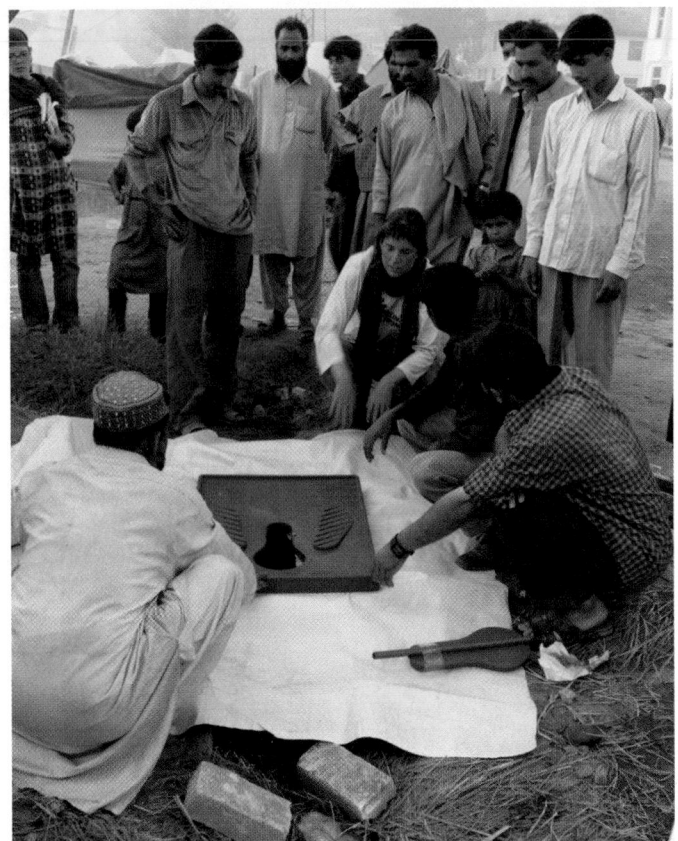

FIGURE 84-16 Logistics staff build latrines in Muzaffarabad, Pakistan, where thousands of displaced people had arrived following an earthquake in northern Pakistan, 2005. *(Courtesy Stephan Grosse Rueschkamp, Médecins Sans Frontières.)*

populations suffering from acute micronutrient or macronutrient malnutrition and designing programs to address the needs of these populations.

The initial assessment should identify the global acute malnutrition rate, in order to determine what sort of supplementation programs are needed and to identify populations at risk (e.g., children under 5 years of age, pregnant and nursing mothers, the chronically ill). Micronutrients, such as vitamin A, should be provided to populations exhibiting symptoms or at risk for deficiency. Whenever possible, local food sources should be used to provide nutrition to the population in crisis. The ICRC's *Nutrition Manual for Humanitarian Action* provides an excellent reference for provision of nutrition and treatment of malnutrition.[24]

Shelter, Security, and Site Planning

Hundreds, if not thousands, of people can be displaced by conflict or natural disaster. One of the first priorities of any humanitarian response is to provide adequate shelter, essential nonfood items, and adequate security to the displaced population. Sphere standards suggest that temporary shelters provide a minimum of 3.5 m² of covered space per person, ensure adequate access to essential needs, such as water, toilets, and health care facilities, and keep families and social networks intact whenever possible.

Provision of culturally acceptable nonfood items, including clothing, bedding, pots, plates, utensils, soap, and burial materials, is required where appropriate. Adequate lighting, gender-separated latrines, and adequate camp security are essential (Figure 84-17). Camps must be protected from invading forces and on-site crime. The site on which the camp will be built must also meet specific criteria, including a gradient of no more than 6% and proximity to a water supply and a transport route.[30]

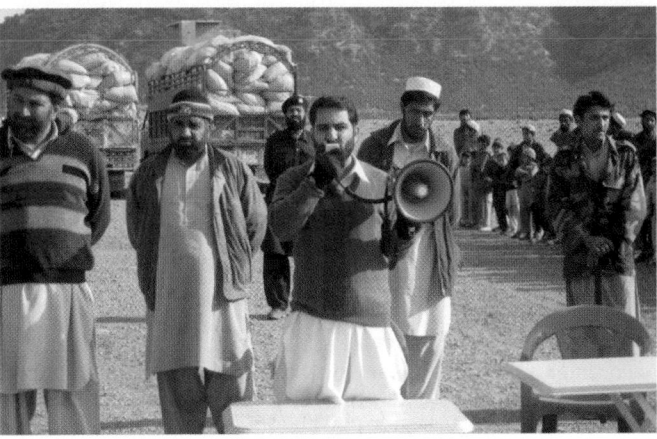

FIGURE 84-17 Nonfood items are distributed by NGOs to people fleeing violence in an isolated region in northern Pakistan, 2010. *(Courtesy Médecins Sans Frontières-France.)*

HEALTH CARE IN THE EMERGENCY PHASE

Health care needs in a crisis can result from epidemic, acute, and chronic medical illness, malnutrition, and traumatic injuries resulting from a natural disaster or conflict (Figure 84-18). MSF suggests a health care system be constructed to provide necessary curative treatment, reduce suffering from disease, and be capable of carrying out case findings. The health care system should have the ability to treat a large number of patients, provide access to various levels of care, and contribute to public health surveillance. Finally, it should provide both preventive and curative services and be flexible enough to adapt quickly to a highly dynamic situation.[20] Health care facilities should be equipped to care for various types of disease, including surgical disease, mental health disorders, obstetric conditions, and chronic diseases such as HIV and tuberculosis. Staff members should have a working knowledge of diseases commonly seen in refugee and crisis settings.

Control of Communicable Diseases and Epidemics

The MSF's *Refugee Health: An Approach to Emergency Situations* estimates that up to 95% of deaths among refugees in crisis are due to preventable diseases such as measles, diarrhea, respiratory illnesses, and malnutrition.[20] Epidemics can be caused by these diseases, as well as by malaria, meningococcal meningitis, typhus, hepatitis, encephalitis, and hemorrhagic fevers such as yellow fever and dengue. These communicable diseases may arrive in the camp with the host population, or they may be new to the

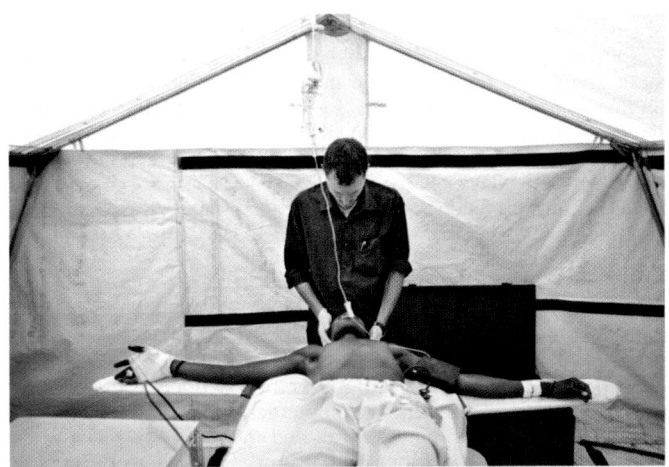

FIGURE 84-18 18-year-old Darfur refugee who has been shot in the hand is prepared for surgery in Chad, 2004. *(Courtesy Espen Rasmussen, Médecins Sans Frontières.)*

displaced persons and endemic to the area of the encampment. Overcrowding, malnutrition, and poor sanitation lead to increased transmission, which can have devastating consequences.

In order to prevent epidemics, mass vaccination campaigns, particularly for measles, must be carried out early in the crisis. Robust and sensitive surveillance systems must be implemented, and protocols for prevention, diagnosis, and treatment of potentially epidemic disease must be widely available. Laboratories to identify potentially epidemic disease must be identified early, and adequate medications and medical supplies must be readily available. Refer to *Communicable Disease Control in Emergencies: A Field Manual* by the WHO for further guidance.[8]

Public Health Surveillance

According to the U.S. Centers for Disease Control (CDC), "Public health surveillance refers to the collection, analysis, and use of data to target public health prevention. It is the foundation of public health practice."[7]

A public health surveillance system should collect demographic, mortality, morbidity, needs, and program activity data.[20] The system should be as simple as possible and allow for rapid identification of threats to public health. Additionally, this system should assist in the planning of the intervention, including what populations are most at risk, what areas to target, the size of the impending threat, and other factors. A robust public health surveillance system should allow for ongoing monitoring and evaluation of the program at the field level, and all information gleaned from the system should be easily and rapidly used at the program level. Most often, data will be collected at health centers and selected community centers. For a detailed discussion of public health surveillance systems, refer to the "Surveillance" section in *Communicable Disease Control in Emergencies: A Field Manual* by the WHO.[8]

HUMAN RESOURCES AND TRAINING

Adequate numbers of trained staff are crucial for a successful response to a humanitarian crisis. Unfortunately, in the acute phase, adequate staff is often lacking. Generally, a mixture of national and expatriate personnel will work together during a given response, with the assistance of selected staff from the refugee/displaced population. This draws from MSF's *Refugee Health: An Approach to Emergency Situations.*[20]

As with any sector, the first step is to perform an assessment to determine needs, based on planned interventions. For example, staff will likely be needed for each of the sectors mentioned in this section, including for health centers, feeding centers, security, surveillance, and community outreach. The recently displaced will often include many potentially qualified staff. However, it is important to seek proof of qualifications whenever possible and to respect local employment laws when hiring refugee/displaced staff. The recently displaced may, quite understandably, be tempted to overstate qualifications in order to obtain more resources.

Once appropriate staff members have been recruited, assessment of needed training is the next step. For example, training on mass vaccination campaigns for measles can be implemented. Training can take on the form of formal classes or apprenticeships as necessary. It is important to clearly outline the salary, hours of work, days off each week, vacation time, and so forth in a contract for each employee, in accordance with national/local laws.

Coordination and Logistic Support

Almost all modern humanitarian operations will have a field logistician to manage a refugee/displaced camp's needs. The number of staff members on the logistics team can equal or exceed that of the medical staff. Logistics is defined as the science of organization, planning, and implementation. Logisticians are responsible for keeping medical and nonmedical inventories stocked, ensuring the function of camp facilities, coordinating transportation of materials and staff, and providing security. Without adequate logistic support, a program is doomed to fail (Figure 84-19). The importance of the work of the logistics team,

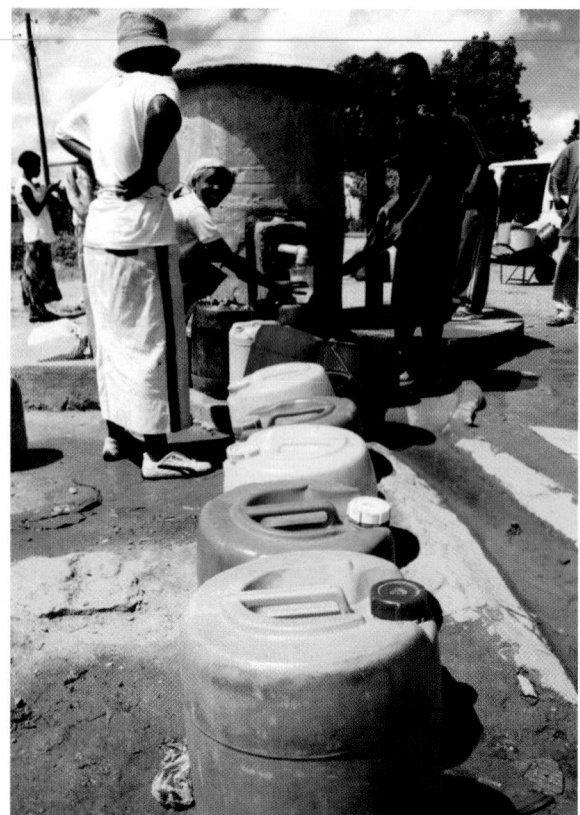

FIGURE 84-19 Following the outbreak of cholera in Zimbabwe, NGO logisticians constructed "elephant" pumps near Harare that operated 24 hours per day, providing water for up to 5000 persons, 2009. *(Courtesy Joanna Stavropoulou, Médecins Sans Frontières.)*

which often takes place behind the scenes, cannot be overstated. Courses on logistics in emergencies are provided by many organizations, including MSF, ICRC, RedR UK, Massachusetts Institute of Technology, and a number of other universities and NGOs.

IDENTIFYING HEALTH CARE NEEDS FOLLOWING A DISASTER AND SETTING UP A HUMANITARIAN INTERVENTION

BACKGROUND

Information gathering is recognized as the crucial first step in assessing the needs of a population affected by a disaster.[6] Initially, a limited amount of information obtained on site will suffice to guide relief efforts.[32] This information must be obtained quickly and must include health indicators. The art and science of this public health intelligence is the disaster application of *rapid epidemiologic assessment (REA)*, which, when related specifically to health, is termed the *rapid health assessment (RHA)*.

Over the last two decades, REA protocols have been standardized and specialized for use in natural disasters and complex humanitarian emergencies and are now incorporated into all major humanitarian organizations' field manuals (Box 84-1). In addition to collecting information on disaster impact, displaced persons, health care facilities, and entire health sectors, REAs provide estimates of population size and composition, mortality rates, nutrition and health status, and environmental risks that may affect health in the future.[6] By assessing the impact of disasters on health, REA information enables the mapping of affected communities, examining the public health impact of the emergency, and reviewing availability of local resources.[6] These data serve as the initial step in development of an ongoing health

BOX 84-1   List of Organizations with Rapid Health Assessment Protocols*

Rapid Health Assessment Protocols for Emergencies (WHO)
Handbook for Emergencies (UNHCR)
Assisting in Emergencies (UNICEF)
Handbook for Delegates (FRC)
Humanitarian Charter and Minimum Standards in Disaster Response (Sphere)
Refugee Health (MSF)
Rapid Health Assessment of Refugees or Displaced Populations (Epicentre)
Field Operations Guide (OFDA)
Famine-Affected, Refugee, and Displaced Populations: Recommendations for Public Health Issues (CDC)

Additional References Consulted

War and Public Health (ICRC)
A Framework for Survival (Center for International Health and Cooperation)

*See Internet Resources for online locations of each organization's RHA protocol.
From Bradt DA, Drummond CM: Rapid epidemiological assessment of health status in displaced populations: an evolution toward standard minimum essential data sets, *Prehosp Disast Med* 17:178, 2003.
CDC, Centers for Disease Control and Prevention; ICRC, International Committee for the Red Cross; IFRC, International Federation of the Red Cross and Red Crescent Societies; Sphere, Sphere Project; MSF, Medécins Sans Frontières; OsFDA, Office of U.S. Foreign Disasters Assistance; UNHCR, United Nations High Commissioner for Refugees; UNICEF, United Nations Children's Fund; WHO, World Health Organization.

information system and in design of targeted and appropriate health interventions. Additionally, the data collected in ongoing REA assessments permit humanitarian organizations to evaluate and monitor programs, and to advocate and build the capacity for affected populations.

PRINCIPLES FOR HEALTH ASSESSMENT IN DISASTERS AND CRISES

The objective of a health-related humanitarian intervention during the acute phase of an emergency is to reduce the numbers of deaths and to stabilize the population's health situation. In order to do this, data must be rapidly collected. Exacerbation of baseline health needs, additional health needs, and emerging health needs (Figure 84-20) must be differentiated. Health indicators, such as mortality and malnutrition rates, must be determined in the early stages of the emergency. The RHA is a key instrument in all these processes. It is a collection of subjective and objective information that measures the damage and identifies the needs and the level and type of response.[29] The RHA is based more on qualitative than quantitative data and thus can be subject to biases, as well as measurement and sampling errors.[29] However, it is the first step in a continuous process and provides the basis for comprehensive follow-up assessment missions.

The main methods employed in any RHA are:[29]

Review of existing information
Interviews
Observation
Rapid surveys

Several key questions must be answered by the RHA:[29]

Is there an emergency or not?
What are the type, impact, and possible evolution of the emergency?
What is the most severely affected geographic area and catchment population?
What is the main health problem?
What is the existing response capacity?
What are critical information gaps for follow-up assessments?
What are recommended priority actions for immediate response?
What are the resources needed to implement those priority actions?

The type of disaster and its context both affect the assessment. Because each type of disaster is associated with different consequences (e.g., floods are often associated with food shortages that can affect baseline malnutrition rates), the RHA should be tailored to the disaster. According to the UN Global Health Cluster, there are six categories of disaster and complex humanitarian emergencies that have a far-reaching negative impact:[29]

Rapid-onset natural disasters (e.g., floods, earthquakes, tropical storms, volcanic eruptions)
Slow-onset (natural) disasters (e.g., drought, famine, desertification)
Technologic disasters (e.g., pollution, spillage, explosion, fire)
Complex humanitarian emergencies (e.g., armed conflict)
Epidemics (e.g., cholera, meningitis, measles, hemorrhagic fever)
Sudden, large population movements

After the assessment is completed, results are compiled and analyzed, and a report drafted that includes recommendations for action. A summary of key activities for the assessment is:

Planning the mission
Field visits
Analysis
Report writing
Dissemination

Given the dynamic nature of the disaster or complex humanitarian emergency, the results of the RHA are only valid for a limited period, so results should be disseminated within 2 weeks after the start of the emergency.[29]

The Assessment Process

Planning.   To undertake an RHA, four main basic preconditions must be fulfilled that affect all frameworks for humanitarian action.[29] These preconditions are unimpeded access, security, relevant expertise, and availability of funding for the intervention(s).

Visas and security clearance must be obtained for both national and international staff. Local customs must be respected and local authorities contacted for permission to conduct the assessment. Teams must be briefed on security protocols and provided with evacuation plans and maps with global positioning

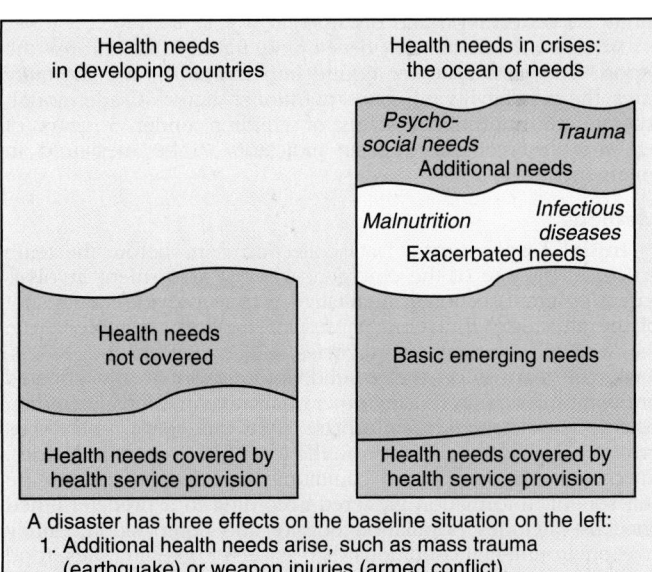

FIGURE 84-20 The "Ocean of Needs" in a humanitarian emergency. *(From Michael M: Global health cluster rapid health assessment guidelines, 2007: 2. wpro.who.int/internet/files/eha/toolkit/web/health-cluster-approach.html.)*

system coordinates if possible. Site visits may be day trips or longer, according to the number of sites and distances, and transportation, including drivers and fuel, may need to be arranged.

Team. The assessment team should be a multifunctional, multidisciplinary group whose members have various areas of expertise and organizational representation. The group should include a mix of genders, nationals/internationals, and insiders/outsiders.[23,29] The team should be deployed to perform the assessment within hours to days after the alert. Sufficient time must be reserved for in-country briefing of the whole team and familiarization with the RHA tools. This is especially important if the team includes translators. In most cases, team members should be properly identified with badges from their organization and should travel in vehicles marked with the organization's logo; however, for security reasons, this is not always the case. Gender issues may need to be considered; female team members may be required to interview female respondents. Teams must be briefed on local customs and clothing. Women may be required to cover their heads, and clothing must always be modest.

Tools. The RHA consists of data gathered from a number of sources. In this way, information can be triangulated, which helps to minimize the potential for bias and measurement error. The RHA framework includes reviewing existing information, interviewing, observation, and rapid health surveys.[29]

Existing information includes reports by the UN agency, NGO, and other groups; maps; demographic statistics from census data; and administrative data (e.g., ministry of health data, clinical records, and health indicators gathered by health services and programs).[29]

Interviews are semistructured and normally held with key informants, selected because they possess specific information or are representative of a category of the affected population.[29] Focus group interviews may also be conducted. These provide a large body of information in a relatively short period of time.

Observation is also called direct observation and entails examining the environment, infrastructure, events, relationships, and people in order to produce information on the general status of the population and to provide context.[29] A useful form of direct observation is a *transect walk,* which is a relaxed stroll with key informants through an area of interest. This provides an opportunity for observation and discussion.[29]

Surveys are crucial for developing figures that inform the report. They are used to inquire into morbidity and mortality rates, the case fatality ratio, and nutritional status.[29] Crude mortality rate and nutritional status of children under 5 years of age are the recognized basic indicators to be measured in emergencies.

Methods

Initial Assessment. Data collection starts before the team arrives at the site of the emergency. Initial assessment involves gathering cross-sectional, qualitative data to provide a snapshot of the affected population. It uses information assembled from the Internet, government agencies, UN agencies, and NGOs. Once the team is on the ground, information on the affected population is acquired using other qualitative methods, including participant observation, informant style interviews, and focus groups. Available materials from the local government ministries, international agencies, and community-based organizations are still sought. Information gathered according to a predetermined checklist includes population density and composition, family size, environmental conditions such as vector breeding sites, food availability, and types of disease.[6]

Surveys and Sampling Methods. Cross-sectional household surveys are a key component of REAs (Table 84-1). Survey questions are based on the objectives and outcomes that need to be measured, including mortality and malnutrition rates.

Sampling methods include probability and nonprobability sampling. The two most common categories of nonprobability sampling are convenience sampling and purposive sampling. Convenience sampling relies on sampling the respondents most easy to assess. Consequently, this is the type most often used in emergency situations.[29]

TABLE 84-1 Characteristics of Rapid Health Assessments, Cross-Sectional Household Surveys, and Surveillance Methods Used to Assess Populations Affected by Humanitarian Emergencies

	Assessment	Survey	Surveillance
Objective	Rapid appraisal	Medium-term appraisal	Analytic appraisal
Data type	Qualitative	Quantitative	Quantitative
Units	Community	Household	Community
Method	Observation, interviews, focus groups	Sample with survey	Periodic, standardized

Courtesy Kirsten Johnson, MD, McGill University.

Probability sampling methods are simple random sampling, systematic random sampling, stratified random sampling, and cluster sampling. The first three methods require lists of individuals, households, or the population at hand. These lists are often difficult to obtain in a complex emergency because of the high level of disorder and movement of people. The fourth method, cluster sampling, only requires a map of the area with approximate estimates of the relative sizes of the population units. This method of sampling is also valued for its simplicity, reasonable validity, and precision. For these reasons, cluster sampling is the most commonly used method of probability sampling in humanitarian emergencies.[38]

Cluster sampling methods require estimation of the population. This can be obtained from census data, maps, aerial photographs, or satellite imagery. For example, using aerial photographs to map a refugee camp provides a visual layout of the entire area. This area is then divided into smaller sections. The density is determined by counting the number of people populating one of the smaller segments. The total population is then determined by multiplying the number of sections in the total area by the number of people counted in the first segment. This method has been found to have reasonable accuracy and is commonly used in the field by MSF and other major NGOs.

Cluster sampling that has been validated for immunization and nutrition studies uses the 30×30, two-stage sampling methodology, or some derivative of this method.[38] The first stage requires grouping the population into smaller geographic units, such as villages, and then choosing these units, or clusters, proportional to the population size (the recommended number of clusters is at least 30, but this can be increased if subgroup analysis is intended). The second stage requires selection of households and then individuals, who are asked to participate in the survey within each cluster; the recommended number is at least 30. The choice of 30 clusters is based on statistical considerations for stability and distribution of means and proportion, whereas the choice of 30 individuals per cluster is based on the number of individuals necessary to have sufficient precision and who can be reasonably measured in a single day.[38]

Data Analysis. The RHA should use standards against which needs can be measured in order to define aid priorities calculated on the basis of need alone. There is widespread agreement to use crude mortality rate and the nutritional status of under-5s as common indicators, to which the under-5 mortality rate is often added.[38] Additional key basic indicators are shown in Table 84-2.

Acute malnutrition is estimated by the weight-for-height index or the mid–upper arm circumference. When using the weight-for-height index, children with an index of less than 80% of the median are considered moderately malnourished and children with index scores of less than 70% are severely malnourished.[31] A global acute malnutrition rate of more than 10% is considered critical; if it reaches 20%, immediate humanitarian intervention is needed.[29]

The estimate of population size can be used to establish mortality rates. The most specific indicator of the health status

TABLE 84-2   Common Indicators of Population Mortality in Emergencies

Indicator	Simplified Formula	Common Application
Crude MR	Deaths ÷ (population at risk × period of time)	Always presented
Age-specific MR	Deaths in age group ÷ (population in age group at risk × period of time for those within the age range)	Under-5 mortality rate (U5MR)
Group-specific MR	Deaths in subgroup ÷ (subgroup populations at risk × period of time)	MR among males/females; among unaccompanied children; among displaced persons vs. residents; in a special ethnic group
Period-specific MR	Deaths during subperiod ÷ (population at risk during subperiod × duration of subperiod)	Monthly MR; MR during epidemic period; MR before/after displacement
Cause-specific MR	Deaths due to given cause ÷ (population at risk × period of time)	MR due to violence; MR due to disease causing epidemic
Proportionate mortality	Deaths due to given cause ÷ total deaths (*not* a rate)	Proportion of deaths due to violence; proportion due to disease causing epidemic
Case-fatality ratio (CFR [or rate])	Deaths due to given cause (disease) ÷ total cases of given disease	CFR of cholera, measles, severe malaria; important during epidemic
Excess MR (total number of excess deaths)	Observed MR − expected noncrisis MR (× population at risk × period of time)	

From Checchi F, Roberts L: Interpreting and using mortality data in humanitarian emergencies: A primer for nonepidemiologists, Humanitarian Practice Network No. 52, September 2005, p 5. MR, mortality rate.

of the affected population is the crude mortality rate, which is typically expressed as deaths per day per 10,000 persons.

A rule of thumb for the emergency threshold is a doubling of the norm of the mortality rate. However, the baseline crude mortality rate varies by location and may not be readily available. In developing countries, the baseline crude mortality rate is normally between 0.4 and 0.6 per 10,000 persons per day.[30,31] The crude mortality rate is considered elevated if it is higher than 1 death per 10,000 per day; it is deemed critical when deaths exceed 2 per 10,000 per day.[31] This number is doubled for all children under 5 years of age. Therefore, the under-5 crude mortality rate is considered elevated at more than 2 deaths per 10,000 per day and severe if there are more than 4 deaths per 10,000 per day. Age-specific mortality rates should be obtained as soon as possible and disaggregated into age-groups of less than 12 months, 1 to 5 years, 6 to 14 years, 15 to 45 years, and over 45 years, thus allowing for better targeted programs.

Knowing the cause-specific mortality rates is paramount for effective planning of interventions. Standard case definitions of communicable and noncommunicable diseases common to complex emergencies should be used in order to identify the immediate health problems. Part of the purpose of the RHA is to identify risk factors for, and outbreaks of, disease, in addition to other factors that will result in high death rates. Determining the cause of death not only helps to prioritize and establish appropriate interventions, but also enhances accuracy of monitoring these programs over time. Baseline disease surveillance systems need to be established as early as possible, along with a system to promote communication of data between agencies and the local government.

Reporting

The RHA report must be clear, standardized, action oriented, timely, and widely distributed. A model outline might include the following headings:[29]

    Executive summary
    Assessment
    Background
    Affected population
    Needs and resources
    Capacities
    Current responses
    Conclusions
    Recommendations
    Budget required and international aid needed
    Forthcoming reports
    Annexes (maps, health facility description, narratives)

Program Development: the Logical Framework

RHAs are designed to be the initial phase of a continuum that informs humanitarian action. Usually, donors are prepared to allocate resources on the basis of the limited information that the RHA provides. Consequently, programs must be constructed that follow the recommendations put forward in the RHA report but also with the flexibility to change based on ongoing surveillance, monitoring, and evaluation measures.

Initial programs should focus on the most significant causes of illness and death. In complex humanitarian emergencies, these normally are diarrheal disease, acute respiratory tract infections, measles, malaria, and trauma (Figure 84-21).

Many strategies can be used to approach program design. The logical framework (log frame) is commonly employed in humanitarian emergencies because it breaks down a complex set of activities and enables a snapshot view of the goals a project or program aims to accomplish.[19] This approach requires thought about objectives and encourages identification and use of measurable indicators.[19] It provides a focus for people involved in different activities to see how their roles and actions fit into a bigger picture.[19]

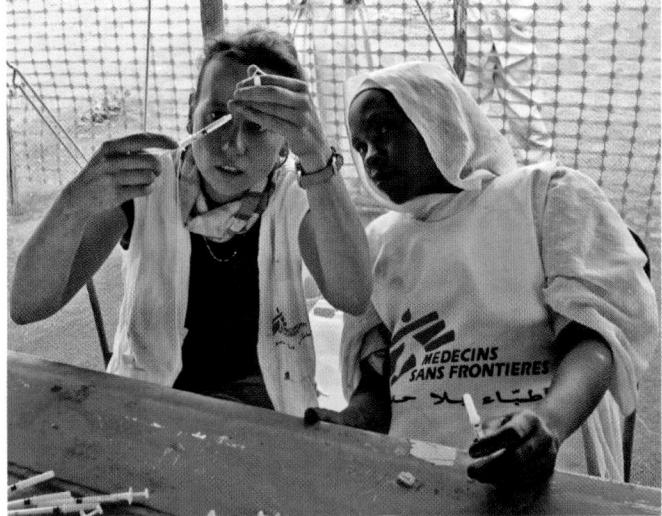

FIGURE 84-21 Relief workers prepare for a measles vaccination campaign in Darfur, Sudan, 2004. (*Courtesy Kris Torgeson, Médecins Sans Frontières.*)

TABLE 84-3 Logical Framework Matrix*

Objective (Narrative Summary)	Indicators	Sources of Verification	Assumption
Goal (overall objective)			
Purpose (outcome)			
Outputs (results)			
Activities			

*See text for an explanation of the "log frame" matrix, shown here.
From Grove N, Zwi AB: Beyond the log frame: a new tool for examining health and peace-building initiatives, *Dev Pract* 18:66, 2008.

The log frame is described as a "matrix which summarizes the main elements of a program and connects them to one another."[11] The log frame in its most basic form consists of a matrix, with the rows corresponding to a hierarchy of project objectives (goal, purpose, output, activities) and the columns used to describe the objective (narrative summary), indicators, sources of verification, and critical assumptions (Table 84-3).[19]

The matrix is intended to reflect a "vertical logic." The first column, starting from the bottom, should tell a "feasible means-to-ends narrative" about a project or program.[19] It describes how a set of activities (such as training technicians and building wells) produces an output (increased quantity of water) that is related to a defined purpose (providing access to more clean drinking water for a village) that in turn contributes to a goal (reduced morbidity and mortality from water-related diseases).[19] At the same time, the log frame provides a "horizontal logic" that

outlines how progress toward each objective can be measured and verified; it also identifies any external factors that may affect or impede the ability of the project to reach its objectives[19] (Figure 84-22).

As a program is being designed and implemented, coordination and communication between relief organizations and the local population are critical. Responding organizations too often create programmatic plans without involving the host population. Assistance programs should be assessed for suitability, both to the population and context of the emergency.

Surveillance, Monitoring, and Evaluation

Data collection employing standardized surveys should be continued periodically in order to create an effective surveillance system. Specific information in the context of a complex emergency that must be assessed on a regular basis includes, but is not limited to, population demographics, mortality rates, nutritional status, identification of vulnerable groups, and review of all the external interventions that are being implemented. Surveillance systems should be monitored for trends. Spikes in rates of disease, malnutrition, or death indicate the need for program changes or shifting of resources to meet changing needs. Increases can also be used to advocate for additional resources. Decreases in rates are measures of a program's success.

PUTTING SERVICES IN PLACE AND MOBILIZING RESOURCES

Effective coordination of humanitarian assistance is crucial for saving lives, helping victims, and encouraging local coping mechanisms. Humanitarian emergency situations are characterized by widespread and urgent needs, competing priorities, destroyed or damaged infrastructure, rapid influx of relief workers and

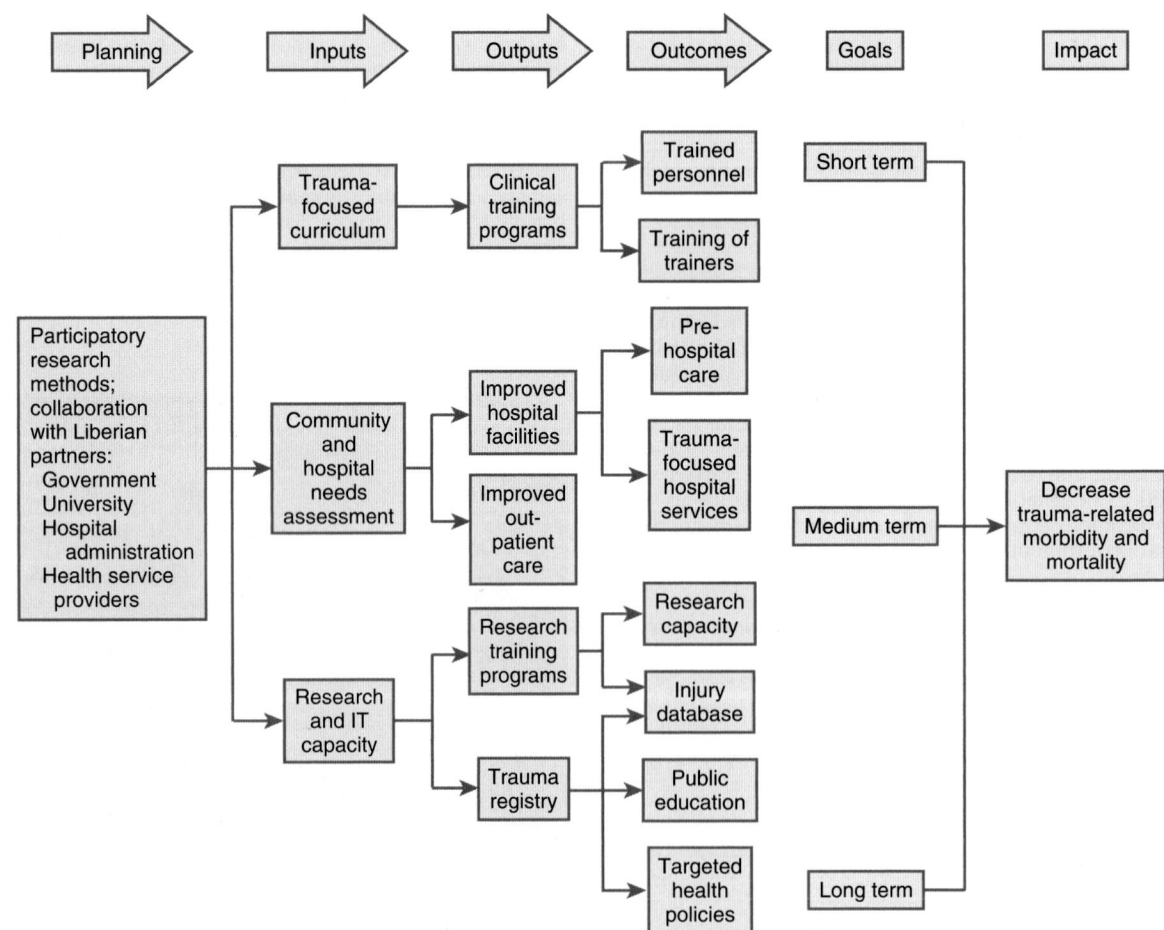

FIGURE 84-22 An example of a logic model for a proposed trauma system in Liberia. *(Courtesy Kirsten Johnson, MD, McGill University.)*

humanitarian aid, and great pressure on national authorities and civic institutions.[3] An emergency situation frequently risks slipping into chaos.

Weak or absent coordination in humanitarian crises could result in gaps in services for affected populations, duplication of efforts, inefficient use of resources, political and other impediments, and slow reactions to changing conditions. By contrast, effective coordination allows entities to harmonize their responses. When coordination works, humanitarian aid efforts become greater than the sum of their parts.

Other than coordination, mechanisms that should be in place to facilitate the humanitarian response include:

Rapid deployment of qualified personnel

Stand-by logistic support, including telecommunications equipment, specially equipped field vehicles, medical supplies and drugs, cold chain and personal support kits

Funding

THE AID WORKER IN THE HUMANITARIAN CRISIS

MOTIVATING FACTORS FOR PERSONAL INVOLVEMENT IN HUMANITARIAN EVENTS AND DISASTERS

It is worth asking why a health care professional who is capable, respected, and experienced would leave his or her home, job, and loved ones to work in a challenging, exhausting, and possibly dangerous destination. And why do it for months to years with little or no salary? Hardened aid workers would joke that they are crazy. Generally, this is only a little bit true.

There are many reasons to depart for the field; for most persons, there is a combination of factors. Though these motivations are usually intense and well-intentioned, there can be contradictory effects. For example, committing to work for the benefit of those in need overseas can develop strong field skills and experience, but can contribute, at least temporarily, to becoming out of date or less well adapted to the medical skills and knowledge required for work at home. Volunteerism is often commended and comes with considerable rewards, but lack of anticipation and preparation can result in financial and career difficulties. Personal discoveries are made and deep personal connections are forged while working in such challenging contexts, but friendships and relationships at home can be affected. Providing medical relief to persons in profound need is the primary motivation for most health care professionals (Figure 84-23). The medical act can be understood to exist in two interconnected parts: The first part is the concrete action, such as a consultation or surgical procedure, and the second part is being with patients, accompanying them physically and emotionally. Both parts are challenged in the field when resources are limited, time is short, and the number of patients and complexity of context become overwhelming. Aid workers practice "bearing witness" in their own ways; in doing this work, they recognize what James Orbinski, the former International President of MSF, wrote in *An Imperfect Offering*, "Humanitarianism is about more than medical efficiency or technical competence. In its first moment, in its sacred present, humanitarianism seeks to relieve the immediacy of suffering and most especially of suffering alone."[25]

Humanitarian principles are touchstones for many who go into the field. These include independence, neutrality, impartiality, humanism, compassion, empathy, and solidarity (Table 84-4). Individuals differ in the emphasis they place on each of these ideals, and their understanding and practice evolves over the course of many deployments. Personal and organizational experiences can and should lead to their being discussed, debated, and questioned regarding how we understand and apply the various principles, adapt them, and even sometimes contradict them.

A sense of responsibility to fellow human beings or commitment to social justice often contributes to an individual's decision to deploy, and may be based on personal philosophy, or moral, religious, or spiritual grounds (Figure 84-24). When medical

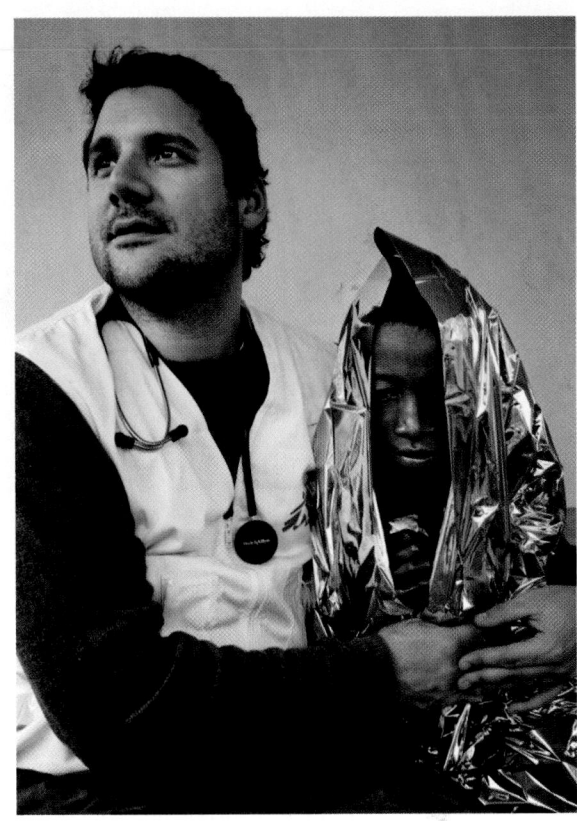

FIGURE 84-23 MSF aid worker with a child with severe malnutrition in a rewarming survival blanket in Ethiopia, 2008. (*Courtesy Francesco Zizola, Médecins Sans Frontières.*)

action and associated services alone are unable to meet needs; when patients, health care workers, and facilities are specifically targeted; or when the aid worker or NGO perceives that the conditions of a population would benefit if shared with a larger audience, then these convictions, in relation to humanitarian

TABLE 84-4	Fundamental Humanitarian Principles
Humanity	Humanitarian assistance is provided without discrimination to prevent and alleviate suffering wherever it may be found. Its purpose is to protect life and health, and to ensure respect for the human being.
Impartiality	Humanitarian assistance makes no discrimination as to nationality, race, religious beliefs, class, or political opinions. It endeavors to relieve the suffering of individuals, being guided solely by their needs, and to give priority to the most urgent cases of distress.
Neutrality	In order to continue to enjoy the confidence of all, humanitarian assistance may not take sides in hostilities or engage at any time in controversies of a political, racial, religious, or ideologic nature.
Independence	Humanitarian assistance must always maintain its autonomy by resisting any interference, whether political, ideologic, or economic, capable of diverting it from the course of action laid down by the requirements of humanity, impartiality, and neutrality.
Voluntary	Humanitarian assistance is not prompted in any manner by desire for personal, political, or financial gain.

Excerpted from International Committee of the Red Cross: The Fundamental Principles of the Red Cross and Red Crescent, ICRC publication 1996 ref. 0513: icrc.org/eng/assets/files/other/icrc_002_0513.pdf.

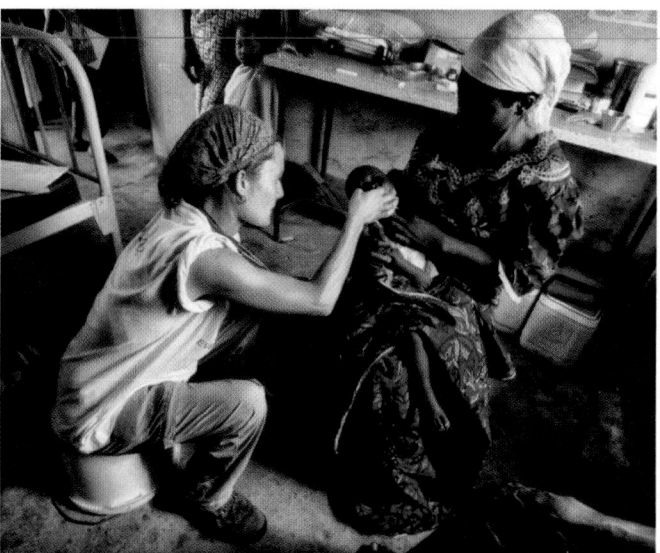

FIGURE 84-24 Aid worker examines a child in the midst of a nutritional crisis in the southeastern region of the Central African Republic, 2009. (*Courtesy Jaume Codina, Médecins Sans Frontières.*)

principles, may justify a more concerted advocacy, and sometimes speaking out publicly on behalf of patients.

Although most contexts allow considerable local, personal, or private advocacy, public speaking out must be carefully considered if carried out. There are many competing interests and ulterior motives in the field, and various actors may perceive the situation differently. The local community and local authorities, government representatives, nonstate actors, and one's own patients and staff can have strong reactions to public speech and action, with potential repercussions for the safety of patients and health care workers, and even (though rarely) for the ability to continue providing assistance at all.

It is important for persons considering aid work to realize that any conditions placed on victims can limit delivery and effectiveness of care. Aid work is compromised if made conditional on political support, military cooperation, or religious affiliation. This can subvert assistance and negate the humanitarian nature of action, leading to increased danger for patients and workers, and diminished ability to help those most in need. The personal motivations of aid workers may vary greatly, but the strategy and practice of assistance should be unconditional and based on need alone.

Despite popular media representations and some public perceptions, aid workers do not aim to be, and fortunately are not, saints, angels, or heroes. Humanitarian aid workers are of course very much human and, as such, are flawed, complicated, and have mixed or ambivalent feelings about what they do and how they do it. During their time in the field, they will undoubtedly experience joy and fulfillment, but also boredom, frustration, and even personal crises.

Certain personal motivations can be limiting or even harmful. Some aid workers view going to the field as a type of medical tourism or adventurism. Undoubtedly, medical skills can enable one to travel widely and have a "cross-cultural experience," but this attitude toward aid work tends to voyeurism, trivializing patients and their situation. Other aid workers seek the "helper's high," the positive feeling that comes from doing something "good." Others have "check-mark syndrome"; for them, working in an emergency situation is just one more box to tick off on their list for doing it all. Both of these attitudes are inherently self-serving, and treat patients as a means to a personal end.

Some persons perform aid work to "find themselves." This can be part of forming an identity, finding a cause in which to believe, or finding a raison d'être into which to channel one's time, skills, and passion. This can resonate constructively for persons who have long trained and worked in a rigid and rigorous medical environment, where they question their contribution.

For others, humanitarian work is about "testing oneself" by engaging in self-sacrifice and seeking a challenge. In aid work this is often possible because one must often depend on clinical skills over technology, and workers are required to deliver effective care with limited resources.

For some, aid work serves as a flight from a negative situation. There may be professional frustration with medical practice in a developed country with a burdensome or wasteful health system. Some may be disillusioned with the values and way of life in their home society, and seek something more meaningful personally and professionally. Persons who deploy to leave behind personal problems or conflicts should be aware that "wherever you go, there you are."

Many workers find that when they are in the field with patients, they find a better understanding of the human condition. To do this work is to enter into the possible beauty and brutality of the lives of others. Aid work allows discovery of important differences, and challenges a person's ideas about the world. Workers discover what people have in common and what may transcend distance, language, and culture.

PROFESSIONAL CHARACTERISTICS OF THE AID WORKER

Qualities that support field work include professional preparation, understanding the project context, and teamwork and management skills. These characteristics are enhanced by a clear mission purpose and the desire to provide the best medical assistance.

A key foundation for effectiveness in the field is the highest possible level of clinical skills, which is even more relevant in places with the fewest resources. There is no substitute for superb medical practice, because humanitarian assistance aims to provide the best possible care, not a "better than nothing" approach. Although work in the field is growing more technical and more specialized over time, aid workers should ideally have well-rounded medical skills and be capable of managing patients with a poor premorbid state who are decompensating. Patients often present at or near the point of death, so procedural and resuscitation skills are essential. Relevant capacities derive from the fields of pediatrics, infectious diseases, emergency medicine, obstetrics and gynecology, surgery including trauma care, family and community medicine, wilderness medicine, and mental health (Figure 84-25). Tropical medicine training is recommended. Medical knowledge is not often the major limiting factor in aid work, although it is perhaps what most providers worry about, particularly on their first mission. Colleagues from the area or region can be an invaluable resource, providing the aid worker is respectful and able to listen. There are increasingly available in-field resources, and technical assistance is commonly available from the capital city coordinating team or from headquarters via

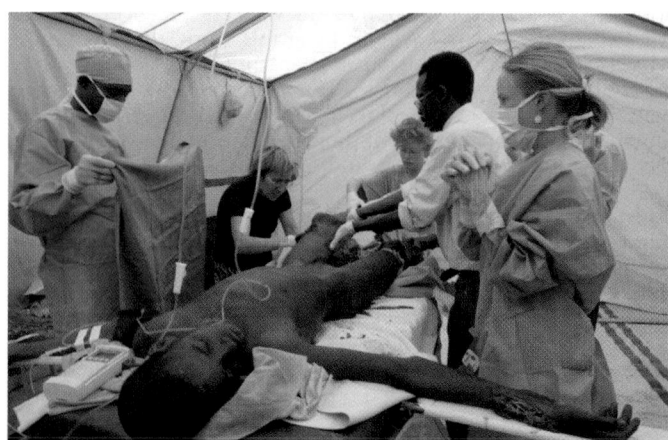

FIGURE 84-25 Victim of a land mine at the Chad-Sudan border is prepared for surgery by a multidisciplinary international team in 2004. (*Courtesy Francesco Zizola, Médecins Sans Frontières.*)

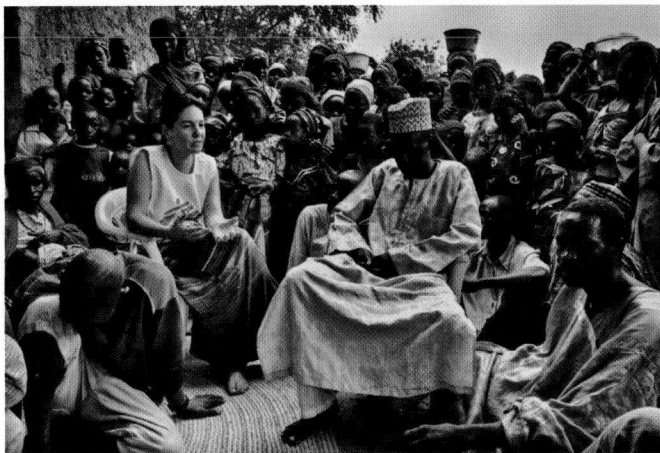

FIGURE 84-26 Aid workers meet with village elders to explain the importance of mothers bringing malnourished children to medical attention in Djibouti, 2010. *(Courtesy Claude Mahoudeau, Médecins Sans Frontières.)*

the Internet, email, mobile phone, or satellite phone. Prior professional experience in resource-poor settings is valuable, including in an underserved or isolated location in one's home country.

Communication skills are vital. French, English, Spanish, and, increasingly, Arabic are commonly used languages. Improving language skills before deploying helps aid workers function as part of a team and understand subtleties missed in translation. In many projects, communication with patients requires less common local languages and dialects. There may be multiple languages spoken in the same location, especially among displaced populations. At the very least, it is useful to learn key phrases, such as greetings, expressions of gratitude, and simple medical questions, in the local dialect. This fosters good will and creates the precious moments when one can speak directly to patients. A key skill is knowing how to best work in translation (Figure 84-26). One model, based on the Refugee Medical Clinic at the San Francisco General Hospital, includes these guidelines: forming an alliance with one's interpreter and positioning that person to allow the aid worker to remain face to face with the patient; asking the interpreter to provide the aid worker with culturally relevant information; and making best efforts to keep eye contact with the patient in order to address him or her directly. Ask the interpreter to speak in the first person, translate literally, and use short, simple sentences that minimize addition of jargon and metaphors.[9]

Having a professional approach to field placement begins with keeping one's availability up to date. Prospective aid workers should also allow a reasonable time frame for an assignment and "down time" both before and after the deployment to deal with the unexpected. The human resources officer has the primary responsibility for matching the right person to the right position, but aid workers should ask questions and carefully review background papers and the job description while remaining adaptable to the reality that is met on arrival in the field. There should be congruence between the phase of the project and how the aid worker fits into it. It is important to realize that there is no obligation to accept the mission offered if you perceive that you are not a good fit for the position or cannot accept the conditions and/or overall security situation. Aid workers should clearly communicate with human resources personnel, ask questions and raise concerns where pertinent, and remain flexible.

Clinical, leadership, and management capacities evolve over multiple field assignments, as the aid worker may take on higher levels of responsibility. All of these qualities may be required during a single mission and even on a first mission. It is not uncommon to be in a position of authority, although this is shifting somewhat as national or local staff have risen in responsibility within some organizations.

Appropriate behavior, given the local context, is important in patient care, staff interactions, and relations with the community. For example, modest dress including specific local dictates, or wearing a laboratory coat may be expected and necessary. One should strive always to be respectful and courteous. The qualities of listening before speaking and understanding before acting, although not always possible, are part of establishing good relations. It may take a long time to firmly grasp one's role in a project, and it is often worth being patient as the process unfolds.

Comprehending the local context is crucial. This includes spending time with local authorities and the community. One should become familiar with the medical and social hierarchy and the relationship between traditional leaders and government officials. There are benefits to getting to know diverse members of the community. For example, when the single ancient electric generator at the camp breaks down, it is invaluable to know the person who can fix it. Knowing the traditional midwife who delivered half the children in the town may be a path to understanding causes and solutions to poor maternal outcomes.

A respectful bedside manner is important, despite possible chaos or lack of medical facilities and equipment. Even in capable, well-intentioned hands, preserving patient dignity can be challenging when medical services are overwhelmed (Figure 84-27). Proactively seek the ideas of locally based staff and beneficiaries. They know the population best, have been there before, and will continue to manage care after you leave. Avoid any condescending or patronizing behavior because it can feed thorny political and social issues, including past experiences with colonization, military occupation, and regional tensions.

The ability to work cooperatively with others is crucial. The team will cross nationalities and languages, medical specialties, and nonmedical backgrounds. Individuals should recognize the value of different perspectives and support them. Effective teams invest in team building and collaboration, and conduct regular meetings. Informal meetings can sometimes take the form of having tea, a warm beer, or a meal together at a staff member's home or in a neutral location. This informality helps set aside personal and political differences and deepens interpersonal links. Teaching one's responsibilities to others also helps develop a beneficial redundancy within the project. This is especially useful when workers are away on a break or leave the project. It is always best that no single person become indispensable.

Management skills are required of those in leadership positions, which is commonplace even among inexperienced first-mission aid workers. However, these skills are not often well developed among medical providers. Ideally, projects should have dedicated "project coordinators," who lead the team overall

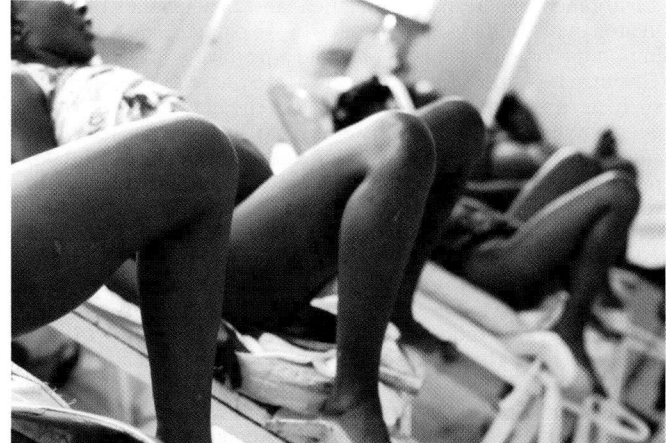

FIGURE 84-27 Jude Anne Hospital, Port-au-Prince, Haiti. In the absence of affordable maternity care elsewhere, six women safely deliver at the same time at this NGO hospital. Unfortunately, women in labor must sometimes wait on the floor for an empty bed. Those who have just delivered have no choice but to pack and leave minutes after delivering, 2007. *(Courtesy Julie Remy, Médecins Sans Frontières.)*

with more formal management skills. However, all health staffers need to work in a systematic and deliberate way, set priorities, and ensure timely follow-through on tasks. In our home societies, most clinicians rely on support staff, administrators, and managers to plan, organize, and ensure a smoothly functioning medical system. In the field, these responsibilities may likely fall on the shoulders of medical aid workers; not being prepared for this is commonly cited as a deficit among expatriates. Health care professionals should have basic management skills, including being able to anticipate human resources and material needs for the project based on the medical goals. They should be able to develop job descriptions, hire and fire staff, schedule staff, and supervise and evaluate team members. Aid workers need to enforce best practices based on evidence-based medicine when available, while individualizing care and looking for improvements to better outcomes, teaching, and learning from colleagues. They should mediate staff and patient concerns in a fair and transparent manner, acknowledging that optimal working conditions will likely never occur. Aid workers should treat all staff equally and fairly and always avoid playing favorites.

Leadership skills are relevant not only for heads of mission or project coordinators. At all levels, there is a need for self-reliance and initiative. Aid workers need to look ahead, assess risk, and anticipate changes in the context so as to best adapt interventions to what is needed. This follows from observing, drawing from past experience, asking questions and listening, collecting information widely, making time for analysis and reflection, and capturing and putting together the best ideas. In aid work, with its difficult contexts and many challenges, building strategic vision and carrying it out will require all of this and more of you and your team.

TYPICAL DAILY FIELD RESPONSIBILITIES OF HEALTH CARE WORKERS

The heavy workload of medical staff during aid missions is a reality; however, intense periods of work are sometimes punctuated by inactivity or even boredom. The field activities of medical staff are diverse, so being flexible is paramount. A useful attitude is to have one's sleeves rolled up and be ready to do whatever it takes to attend to the needs of the victims of a crisis. For example, if the logistics team is working around the clock to process a massive international shipment of aid goods, it engenders goodwill and teamwork for the medical staff to also help move boxes (Figure 84-28).

The expatriate staff can set the tone for the work environment. Nonetheless, the vast majority of medical and nonmedical work in disasters is done by national staffers who are hired from the affected population. It is critical to create a collaborative working environment where national staffers and beneficiaries of aid are treated with dignity and respect by expatriate staff. It is also important for expatriates to promote a positive work-life balance. This may be impossible during the acute phase of an emergency, such as an earthquake, tsunami, or cholera outbreak, where every moment of action can equate to lives saved. Outside of such situations, however, working at a breakneck speed, taking no breaks, and burning out prematurely are best avoided. Setting realistic goals, realizing that you cannot "save the world," and taking care of yourself are often not accomplished by overzealous but well-intentioned aid workers. Inability to follow a reasonable pace can lead to premature burnout, rapid turnover of staff, disruption of the medical program, and unnecessary stress within the team. If one aid worker cannot rest, it makes it harder for others to rest. The realistic aid worker knows that no one can do it all and derives satisfaction from small daily achievements in a chaotic work environment (Figure 84-29).

Field duties vary depending on the qualifications, job description, and local situation. Among physicians, a key factor determining one's role is the ability to perform surgery. Nonsurgical physicians typically lead the care of pediatric and adult patients with nonsurgical conditions and ambulatory services for specific conditions, such as tuberculosis, HIV, and sexual violence. Nurses serve in various settings, including hospitals, operating theaters, mobile clinics, specialized clinics for conditions such as

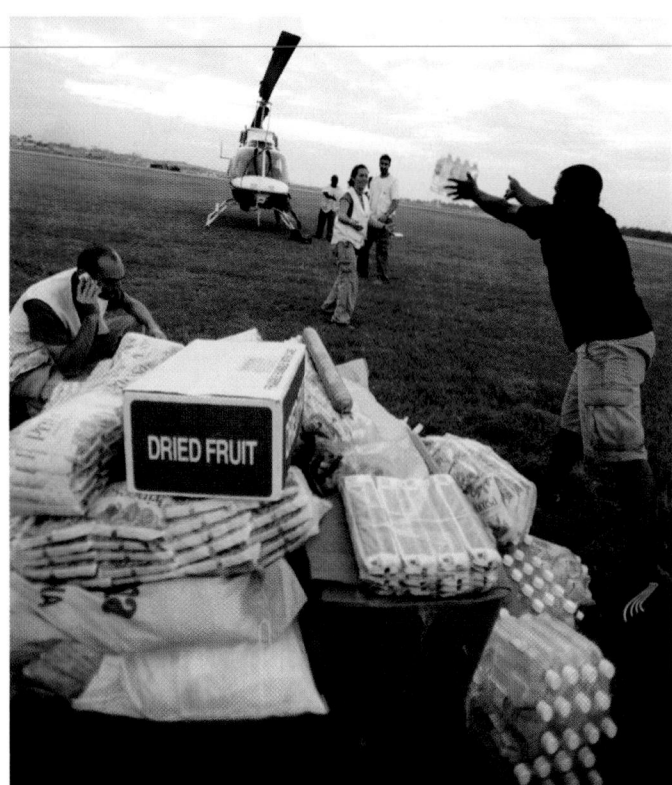

FIGURE 84-28 Aid workers unload supplies from a helicopter following the 2010 earthquake in Haiti. (*Courtesy Julie Remy, Médecins Sans Frontières.*)

tuberculosis and HIV, and primary health centers. In some aid organizations, expatriate physicians play a largely clinical role and expatriate nurses play a more managerial role.

Expatriate medical staffs have hands-on medical and paramedical duties. A key role is attending to the sickest patients requiring the most acute medical care, using what is available and realistic in the particular disaster setting. Expatriate staff should be present for patients requiring resuscitation or a high level of medical care. However, this category of patients should not necessarily be given undue attention at the expense of usually high numbers of ambulatory patients. In all cases, it is important to work alongside the local staff to make the best

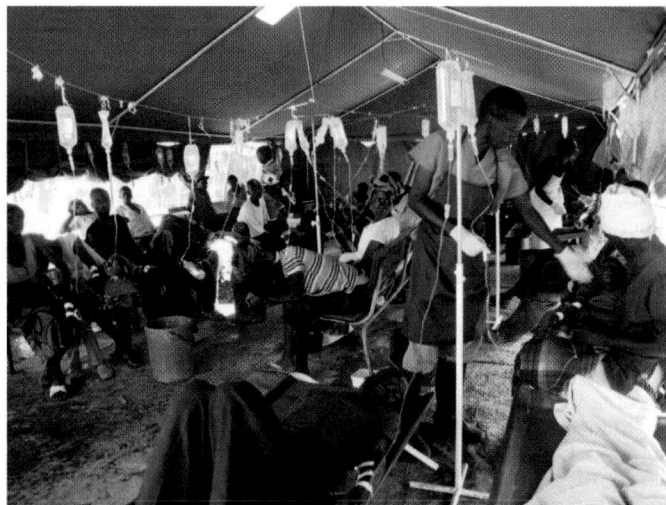

FIGURE 84-29 Patients with cholera receiving intravenous hydration in a makeshift treatment center in Kadoma, Zimbabwe, 2009. (*Courtesy Médecins Sans Frontières Germany.*)

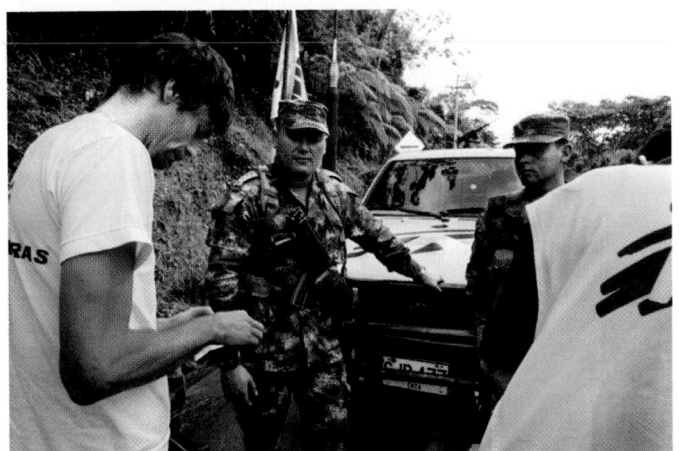

FIGURE 84-30 MSF mobile health team negotiates access with military officers in Colombia, 2007. *(Courtesy Juan Carlos Tomasi, Médecins Sans Frontières.)*

diagnosis possible and provide the highest level of care, while balancing cost, feasibility, sustainability, and other considerations, such as security. For example, urgently transferring a patient with a surgical abdomen to a higher level of care on insecure roads at night may not be possible. Should an untoward event, such as a kidnapping, carjacking, or armed attack on patients, families, or staff occur, an attempted patient transfer may jeopardize the overall humanitarian intervention. An untoward security event can shut down an entire project, depriving hundreds or thousands of patients of needed care. Security often supersedes medical considerations. Therefore security-sensitive final decisions such as patient transfers are often made with nonmedical project coordinators and coordination staff in the capital city (Figure 84-30).

Medical care begins with a decision about the goals of the medical program. In most cases, everything cannot be done, and difficult choices have to be made. Goals can include provision of basic ambulatory medical care at the expense of not aiding the sickest, or offering a secondary or tertiary level of care, leaving primary care to other actors. These decisions are not always easy and may require negotiation with the affected population, MOH, stakeholders, and other NGOs. However, in many "silent" disaster settings in remote locales, there are few other actors, in which case the medical priorities come down to undertaking a needs assessment, making difficult decisions, and doing the best one can with available resources. Compromises are common, but they should be minimized as much as possible.

Patient triage is required during an acute disaster. Medical staff must decide which patients are candidates for immediate medical aid, which can wait, which should be directed to other aid providers, and which should be palliated. The healthy, loud, and influential will often jump to the front of a queue of patients waiting to be seen in an outpatient clinic at the expense of children, older adults, women, and the marginalized. Instituting triage based on sound criteria ensures that the sickest are aided first and those that are turned away are not the most vulnerable. Such tools include the WHO integrated approach to childhood illnesses[37] and pediatric emergency triage and treatment guidelines currently being implemented. A healthy skepticism about seemingly well patients should exist. Foreign aid organizations that distribute free medications become an attractive target for malingering individuals hoping to obtain pills that can be later sold in the market.

Medical care of admitted and ambulatory patients can be conducted by both expatriate and national staff (Figure 84-31). These activities can be conducted by different types of medical providers. The exact delegation of medical duties will depend on the skills and availability of medical providers, as well as local custom and program design. Expatriate doctors often supervise ward rounds. An early morning ward round with discharges

makes room for new admissions that will flow from primary health clinics during the day. During ward rounds, there optimally should be some clinical teaching. National staff have often worked independently for a number of years and may have advanced medical and surgical skills and be more knowledgeable on certain topics than are expatriates, so knowledge sharing is important.

All aspects of the medical program require expatriate supervision and involvement in order to ensure quality, appropriateness, and impartiality of the aid provided. Ambulatory outpatient care should not be minimized in priority. The outpatient department often sees hundreds of patients per day, so small changes in protocol or policy can significantly change the quality of care and costs incurred. A priority should be standardization of medical care; a number of guidebooks exist that have been translated into multiple languages and are available for free on the Internet (refbooks.msf.org/). Medical staff hired in the affected country may have had limited formal medical or nursing education, so a priority for expatriate staff should be to ensure a consistent level of knowledge and skill among the national staff, as well as enforcement of the use of standard medical protocols and pharmacopeia that meet international standards.

Evacuating the critically ill or those requiring specialized services creates difficult decisions that should involve the expatriate medical staff. These decisions often require significant input from nonmedical staff who best understand logistic and security situations. Evacuation is often not possible, so aid workers must be prepared to improvise care with available resources (Figure 84-32). Consultation via email, satellite phone, and radio may be available to gain advice from colleagues with more experience.

Provision of medical care to expatriate and national staff themselves is often done by the expatriate "medic" (physician or nurse). Aid workers often become ill, and protecting their health is a priority. Infectious diseases, such as diarrhea, cellulitis, and malaria, are common, as are symptoms related to stress and

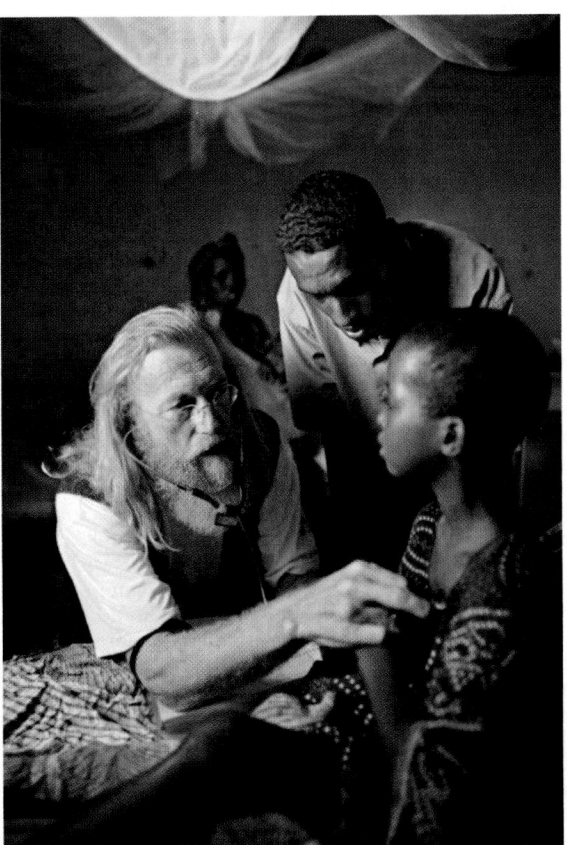

FIGURE 84-31 Expatriate medic conducts ward rounds at an MSF medical facility in southwestern Somalia, 2006. *(Courtesy Espen Rasmussen, Médecins Sans Frontières.)*

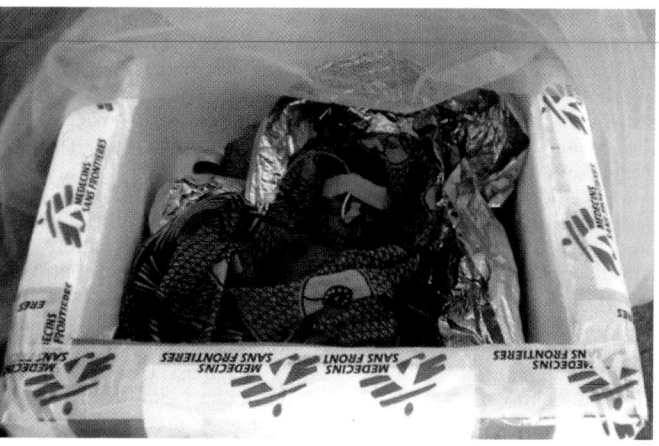

FIGURE 84-32 A premature newborn is cared for in an improvised incubator made from a styrofoam box in the Central African Republic, 2009. (*Courtesy Raghu Venugopal, Médecins Sans Frontières.*)

overwork. Certain medical duties, such as the care of victims of sexual assault, may emotionally overwhelm aid staff, so preventive counseling for aid workers may be required. Medics need to monitor the work and nonwork environments in order to safeguard team health. Although the set-up and maintenance of housing, eating, and cooking areas often falls to the logistics staff, medics should keep an eye out for problems in these areas because they can seriously affect team health and the ability to retain staff. Use of illicit drugs or excessive alcohol drinking is not uncommon in a stressful environment. These may violate national laws and result in jailing or expelling of aid staff. Persons not coping well who turn to substance abuse may require counseling and support, time off, disciplinary action, or removal from the field.

Daily activities include management of staff employed from the affected country. During design of the medical program, a list of required human resources is developed. Medical workers to be hired include physicians, nurses, nurse's aides, orderlies, pharmacists, and hygiene staff. Job descriptions and contracts need to be formulated with the aid of human resources officers. Often, prospective medical staff need to be quickly screened, interviewed, and hired. Aid workers should be cognizant of the impact their employment practices may have on the local economy and health worker market. Often, local employers and the Ministry of Health cannot "compete" with the salaries offered by international aid organizations. This can result in an exodus from local organizations. However, it may result in improved use of underutilized or undersupported medical providers.

National staff may possess extensive medical knowledge and skills. Others require education about standardized medical practices. Coaching and mentoring of staff into positions of increasing responsibility is typical. A careful balance of delegation of medical tasks to national staff followed by supervision is necessary. Staff require evaluations; in some cases, change of position, warning, or dismissal may be necessary if performance is not adequate. In a community with rebels, warlords, fighting clans, and lawlessness, such employment decisions can be a tricky situation because employees may be related to belligerents of conflict. Any termination of an employee's contract should be done with prudence and consultation with human resources to prevent retaliation.

All staff must strive to ensure that theft of resources be minimized, because this is a common and serious problem in aid work. The work of pharmacists, stock-keepers, and guards must be scrutinized fairly and carefully to guard against the reality of theft, corruption, and misdirection of aid. Local staff may face pressure from gangs and other armed elements to steal.

Nonclinical duties include generation of information systems and data evaluation. Key data points include number of daily consultations and daily rates of morbidity and mortality. Also monitored are syndromes suggestive of emergence of epidemic

disease (e.g., cases of watery diarrhea that may suggest a cholera outbreak). Most NGOs have a standard format of recording and list of data points for which they require monthly record keeping. Data packages exist for management of specific conditions, such as HIV (e.g., the Follow-up and Care of HIV Infection and AIDS in MSF). Deaths should be reviewed by the responsible medical officers and means sought to improve quality of medical care where appropriate.

Organizing daily medical care involves scheduling staff, including at night and on weekends. Where there is no preexisting medical facility, aid workers may have to physically set up wards. Other services and structures that require set up and scheduling include the operating theater, pharmacy, laboratory, and medical storeroom. Isolation space needs to be set aside for patients with communicable diseases such as gastroenteritis, cholera, dysentery, TB, or hemorrhagic fever. The logistics staff most likely will set up ancillary services, including a place for patients and their families to toilet, bathe, dispose of waste, cook food, obtain clean water, and wash clothes.

Advocacy on behalf of the affected population facing the crisis is a key role of aid workers. Medics are in close daily contact with patients and families. This places them in a unique position to learn about their struggles and needs. Aid workers should take time to speak to beneficiaries about nonmedical issues and understand their realities. Advocacy can take the form of requesting more services from one's own organization, the host government, or other aid agencies. It can include speaking out in one's home society about the crisis in order to bring attention to the situation. Speaking out can take the form of a press release, news conference, presentation to peers or government officials, or written communication in the medical or lay press. Some aid workers maintain a blog during their overseas service (msf.ca/en/staff-and-patients-blogs). Blogs can generate awareness, but should be conducted with attention to security considerations and in consultation with coordination staff within one's organization.

Aid workers should continuously reanalyze the relevance of their presence and intervention. It should be asked whether the resources spent in one's project could be better spent elsewhere. This is often not easy or comfortable, and it raises concerns among the beneficiaries of aid and national staff, who often do not want to see resources diverted elsewhere. However, just as every project opens, it also must eventually close. Aid workers should thus keep in mind possible exit strategies and opportunities to transition to appropriate partners. Finally, aid workers should always strive to find the neediest population. This may require conducting outreach and assessments of neighboring communities and maintaining good communication links with local actors, other aid agencies, the government, and the host population.

HOW TO BECOME INVOLVED AND STAY INVOLVED

Once the health care worker is interested in aid work, there are several steps that can lead to becoming involved and remaining committed to a unique and demanding endeavor. Becoming involved should first include analyzing one's own motivations for being an aid worker. Ideally, motivations should be altruistic and driven solely by a desire to aid the victims of a crisis. Financial, personal, professional, community, and academic rewards can be part of and follow aid work, but these should be secondary motivating factors. Aid work attracts all kinds of people—a common caricature is of "misfits, mercenaries, and missionaries." Try not to be one of these.

Networking with colleagues and experienced aid workers is useful. These contacts often have pearls of wisdom that can apply to an intended clinical practice setting, including how to plan time away from one's usual employment and information on aid organizations seeking particular medical skills.

Internet-based research on aid organizations is essential. Inevitably, there will be advantages and drawbacks to each aid organization. No aid organization is perfect, and few can do everything for everyone. It is key to contact human resources

BOX 84-2 Select Humanitarian Organizations Involved in Health Care Delivery

Action Contre la Faim (Action Against Hunger)
ACF, a global humanitarian organization committed to ending world hunger, works to save the lives of malnourished children while providing communities with access to safe water and sustainable solutions to hunger: actionagainsthunger.org

Alliance for International Medical Action
ALIMA operates a new model for responding to humanitarian crises. It brings together the medical expertise of international humanitarian aid workers with that of national medical organizations and global research institutions to provide quality medical care to people in need: alima_ong.org/en/

International Committee of the Red Cross
The ICRC is an impartial, neutral, and independent organization with an exclusively humanitarian mission to protect the lives and dignity of victims of armed conflict and other situations of violence and to provide them with assistance: icrc.org/en

International Federation of the Red Cross and Red Crescent Societies
The world's largest humanitarian organization, the IFRC carries out relief operations to assist victims of disasters, and combines this with development work to strengthen the capacities of its member National Societies: ifrc.org/en

International Medical Corps
The IMC works to relieve the suffering of those affected by war, natural disaster, and disease by delivering vital health care services that focus on training and helping devastated populations return to self-reliance: internationalmedicalcorps.org

International Rescue Committee
The IRC helps people whose lives and livelihoods are shattered by conflict and disaster, through provision of health care, infrastructure, learning, and economic support: rescue.org

Médecins Sans Frontières (Doctors Without Borders)
MSF is an international, independent, medical humanitarian organization that delivers emergency aid to people affected by armed conflict, epidemics, natural disasters, and exclusion from health care: msf.org

Partners in Health
PIH strives to achieve two overarching goals: to bring the benefits of modern medical science to those most in need of them and to serve as an antidote to despair: pih.org

Save the Children
Save the Children ensures that children affected by floods, famines, earthquakes, and armed conflict get life-saving medical aid, shelter, food, and water: savethechildren.org

World Vision International
WVI is a global Christian relief, development, and advocacy organization dedicated to working with children, families, and communities to overcome poverty and injustice, through transformational development, emergency relief, justice promotion, partnerships, and public awareness: wvi.org

---

obstetrics and gynecology, tropical medicine, HIV/AIDS and tuberculosis care, mental health, public health, dermatology, and dentistry. Additional assets include basic skills in biostatistics, epidemiology, and use of common spreadsheet and database programs. Enrolling in language courses and gaining language proficiency increases the likelihood of being deployed.

Exposure to austere, impoverished environments is an important preparatory consideration. Aid work is often in rural environments with limited or no access to telecommunications, modern comforts, and the company of friends and family. Spending time in such an environment can be helpful in determining whether one will be comfortable and thrive in a similar setting.

Redeploying can be challenging and is ideally driven by an ongoing humanitarian concern to serve those in need. Persons who redeploy are often those who had a satisfying initial experience and were able to meet the personal and professional challenges they encountered. In other cases, priorities such as being close to one's family, having children, financial considerations, maintaining relationships with loved ones, and occupational decisions take precedence over another deployment. Some find repetitive aid missions financially difficult or even impossible, because many charitable organizations do not provide compensation or only a limited stipend.

Continuing involvement in aid work should include reassessment of one's knowledge base, skills, and attitudes. A mission often highlights potential areas for personal and professional development. For example, strategies to cope with boredom and stress can be fine-tuned during a return home. An aid worker may wish to gain more surgical skills, or expertise in relevant fields such as vaccination and nutrition. A number of aid organizations offer courses to returned staff. Some of these courses are linked to a return of service in the future. An aid worker may wish to pursue additional training through university-based courses in areas such as tropical medicine, pediatrics, or other topics.

HOW TO PREPARE FOR A MISSION

Preparing for a humanitarian mission can be daunting. One is expected to perform in an austere, high-stress environment with limited resources. Each humanitarian worker's abilities and limits are different based on his or her training, personality, and experiences. Before signing up, it is crucial that each individual determine whether he or she will be able to function adequately in the setting of a crisis. It is best for all involved if any hesitations are dealt with *before* the mission begins.

Preparing to Deliver Medical Care in a Crisis

A medical provider in a humanitarian crisis will likely be responsible for the care of hundreds, or even thousands, of patients. Whether responding to the needs of a population affected by armed conflict or to a disaster in the days and weeks following an earthquake, one will encounter patients with acute traumatic injuries. Poor roads and lack of public safety further generate trauma. Sooner or later, an even larger burden of medical disease will surface, including infectious diseases, common pediatric illnesses, chronic disease that has worsened in the context of the emergency, and obstetric and gynecologic diseases. Ideally, the aid worker's skill set is suited to dealing with such a broad range of medical problems.

It is crucial to remember, however, that public health needs are often greatest immediately following a humanitarian crisis. Diseases not often encountered in one's normal practice can cause large epidemics that lead to a high level of death and disability (Figure 84-33). Before deployment, try to learn about prevention, diagnosis, and treatment of diseases that may cause epidemics during acute crises (Box 84-3). In addition to these diseases, common illnesses include HIV/AIDS, tuberculosis, and malaria. Clinical guidelines can be very useful. The deploying NGO will often provide clinical guidelines tailored to its own formulary and the setting. If this is not available, the MSF *Clinical Guidelines* are useful (refbooks.msf.org/). In addition, some smaller textbooks with information on tropical diseases are available (Box 84-4).

---

officers in different organizations to learn more about the nature of the group's objectives and operations, as well as how one might fit with that group. A list of international humanitarian organizations is found in Box 84-2. Some organizations offer seminars, webinars, and informal presentations about their work. A useful opportunity is to attend a presentation from a returned field worker. Experienced field workers can relate "the good, the bad, and the ugly" of the organization one aims to join, with specific examples from their missions.

Some aid organizations have local fundraisers and events to raise the level of public awareness about aid work. These events will often be staffed by ex–field volunteers and office staff and are forums to learn more about the aid organization.

Getting involved should include assessment of one's medical skills. It may be important to gain additional skills before deployment. Relevant skills include trauma and wound care, pediatrics,

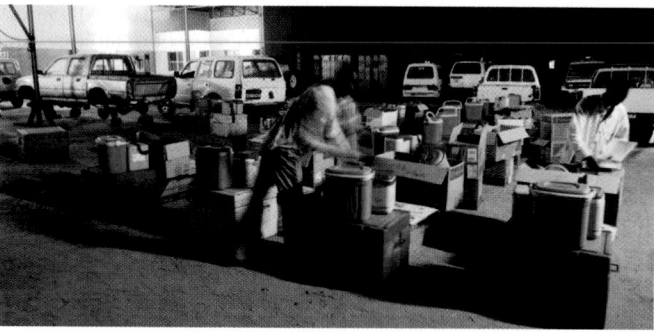

FIGURE 84-33 Logistics staff members prepare cool boxes filled with vaccines to respond to a meningitis outbreak in Dosso, Niger, 2009. (*Courtesy Olivier Asselin, Médecins Sans Frontières.*)

Medical professionals may be asked to implement basic public health interventions, such as vaccination campaigns. They may also give input on construction of latrines and water distribution points. These activities require significant support from logistics experts. International guidelines for these basic needs are outlined in the Sphere standards.[30]

BOX 84-3 Causes of Epidemic Disease in Acute Crises

Measles
Typhus
Cholera and other bacterial and nonbacterial infectious diarrheal
  diseases
Meningococcal meningitis
Relapsing fever
Typhoid fever
Respiratory illnesses, viral and bacterial
Influenza
Hepatitis A and E
Leishmaniasis
Malaria
Scabies
Hemorrhagic fevers (Ebola fever, yellow fever, dengue fever)
Plague
Japanese encephalitis
Whooping cough
Tetanus
Poliomyelitis
Conjunctivitis
Guinea worm

From Médecins Sans Frontières: *Refugee health: an approach to emergency situations*, Oxford, England, 1997, Macmillan Education, pp 145-152.

BOX 84-4 Suggested Readings in Tropical Medicine and Public Health in Crises

Brent A, Davidson R, Seale A: *Oxford Handbook of Tropical Medicine*, Oxford, England, 2014, Oxford University Press.
Beeching NJ, Gill GV: *Lecture Notes on Tropical Medicine*, Oxford, England, 2014, Blackwell Publishing Ltd.
Médecins Sans Frontières Reference Books (various): refbooks .msf.org.
Perrin P: *H.E.L.P. Public Health Course in the Management of Humanitarian Aid*, Geneva, Switzerland, 2001, International Committee of the Red Cross.
Connolly MA, editor: *Communicable Disease Control in Emergencies: A Field Manual*, Geneva, Switzerland, 2005, World Health Organization: who.int/iris/bitstream/10665/96340/1/92415 46166_eng.pdf.
WHO Technical Report Series 985: *The Selection and Use of Essential Medicines: Report of the WHO Expert Committee, 2013*, Geneva, Switzerland, 2014, World Health Organization: who.int/iris/bitstream/10665/112729/1/WHO_TRS_985_eng .pdfs/.

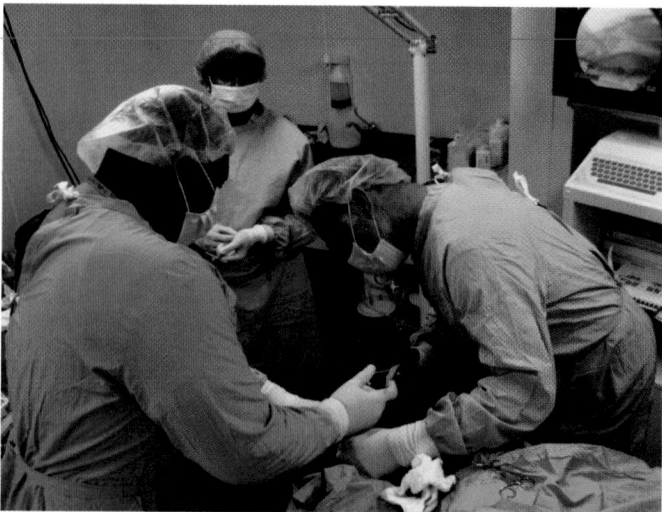

FIGURE 84-34 National and expatriate aid workers perform surgery following the 2010 Haitian earthquake. (*Courtesy Richard Accidat, Médecins Sans Frontières.*)

Because there is often a lack of ancillary and support staff, it can be helpful to know how to perform basic nursing and laboratory duties, such as starting intravenous lines, mixing an oral rehydration solution, examining blood smears for malaria, or using a hematocrit machine. It is critical to be flexible, eager to learn, and willing to assist any and all members of the team when necessary.

Working Outside One's Skill Set

In crisis settings, aid workers are sometimes asked to provide care for which they are not fully trained. For example, one may be asked to perform a dental or surgical procedure for the first time. In these situations, it is necessary to use good judgment, follow standard medical ethics, and "first, do no harm." Whenever possible, the most experienced and highly trained practitioner should provide the relevant care at all times. If possible, arrange for the patient to be transferred to a trained provider. It is not ethical for an inexperienced practitioner to perform a surgical procedure when a general surgeon is available within a reasonable distance (Figure 84-34). The crisis setting is not an excuse for an inexperienced or untrained provider to learn or perform procedures for "practice." Bad outcomes that could have been prevented or dealt with in other ways do not escape observation in the field. Local hostility, lawsuits, and expulsion of the aid worker by the NGO—or expulsion of the NGO itself from the country—are all possible consequences of reckless medical misadventures and unnecessary risk taking. For example, allowing a logistician to do a lumbar puncture is not acceptable. When faced with a surgical emergency such as a perforated viscus, it is better for someone who is not a surgeon to begin administering antibiotics and fluids, place a nasogastric tube, and arrange urgent transfer to an operating theater. Performing a laparotomy for the first time in the field when there are other options is simply not acceptable.

However, on occasion one must attempt to provide aggressive and invasive care in order to save a life or limb. For example, this might be massive debridement for necrotizing fasciitis or amputation for a severely traumatized or infected limb with bony involvement and necrosis. In these rare cases, several texts are available that may help guide these procedures (Box 84-5). As would be appropriate in any setting, be sure to have a conversation with the patient and, if present, the patient's family, clearly explaining your abilities and limitations, as well as the reasons you will be performing this procedure, although it is out of the scope of your normal practice.

Dealing With Death

In crisis settings, patients can be extremely ill, and treatment options are often limited. Unfortunately, not everyone can be saved. Despite heroic efforts, many patients die. Be prepared for this before you arrive, and take the time to debrief and check in with members of your team when there is time.

Behavior and Expectations

Having appropriate expectations before deployment can help reduce stress and improve one's ability to function. It is important to be able to live, work, and thrive in austere conditions. Food may run out, bathing may consist of no more than dousing from a bucket of cold water, and the toilet may be a hole in the ground. Resources for clinical and personal needs are often extremely limited in a crisis setting. Expect very little to be available and for systems and roles to break down.

Health professionals need to be watchful for signs that they are beginning to present with stress; then, techniques that have helped them manage stress in the past must be implemented. Before deployment, identify the healthy ways in which you can deal with stress. Exercise, walking, meditation, reading, and keeping a journal are examples. Remember that often it is unsafe to exercise outside, so consider indoor exercises, such as yoga, tai chi, stretching, or skipping. Humanitarian staff must prepare for isolation. It is often extremely difficult to communicate with family or friends. Bring along good books, a deck of cards, movies, and seasons of your favorite TV series to watch on your laptop. With the isolation comes cramped living and working conditions. Find ways to be with yourself when you need solitude. Close the door, put on headphones, use earplugs, or go for a long walk (if it is safe). It is best to avoid smoking, excessive drinking, and unsafe sex, and it is usually forbidden to use illicit drugs or engage with sex trade workers. Many organizations require humanitarian staff to sign a code of conduct before deployment.[17]

Emotions, such as frustration and anger, are normal responses to poorly functioning systems, poor resources, and an extreme level of human suffering; however, this anger is counterproductive. Try to function as professionally as possible, particularly with national staff and those from other regions, who may be accustomed to a different work ethic and pace when delivering medical care.

Adequate sleep, nutrition, hygiene, and hydration go a long way in reducing stress and improving the ability to function in a difficult setting. Whenever possible, attend to your own needs while caring for others. Most humanitarian organizations have publications on managing stress in crises.[2,16] Keep these references stowed away in your computer or bag, because you will likely find them useful.

PRACTICAL CONSIDERATIONS

Getting Oriented

Before deployment, it is important to understand the local situation, conflict, and culture as completely as possible. Humanitarian staff should contact others who have served in the region in similar roles. Seek out reports from missions carried out in the region by relevant international organizations. Several online

resources, such as the British Broadcasting Company country profiles (news.bbc.co.uk/2/hi/country_profiles/default.stm) and the CDC's travelers' health website (nc.cdc.gov/travel/), can provide political, cultural, and health information. Travel guidebooks often provide concise, readable summaries of a country's history and cultural norms, and relevant chapters can often be downloaded inexpensively online.

Deploying organizations will often provide a formal orientation and security briefing. Following the agency and team security protocols is a nonnegotiable absolute must. Not following security protocols is the surest way to be disciplined, fired, or sent home. By endangering one's own safety by not following guidelines, one jeopardizes the team, patients, and mission itself. The UN Office for Project Services provides a useful online training in UN security protocols, which are often in effect in crisis settings (training.dss.un.org/courses/login/index.php). Staff should understand security and evacuation protocols before deployment. For example, UN evacuation flights allow only one bag weighing 12 kg or less if a person is evacuated emergently.

Several books document the experiences of medical and nonmedical staff in humanitarian crises; these books help give a sense of what to expect in this unique setting (Box 84-6).

How to Pack

Pack light, but be sure to take essential items that will not be available in the destination country. The packing list in Appendix A serves as a guide. Consult with staff on the ground to complement this list. Key items include personal medications (e.g., malaria prophylaxis, daily medications, pain relievers, and sleeping pills), personal documents with additional photocopies, proof of evacuation and medical insurance, and proof of vaccination. Many countries will not allow entry without proof of updated yellow fever vaccination. Consult a travel clinic and the CDC website for necessary vaccinations several weeks before deployment. During the intervals between deployments, keep immunizations up to date.

Additional Training

Several courses offered internationally can help physicians and other health care workers to work in a humanitarian emergency (Tables 84-5 and 84-6). Consult the deploying NGO for additional recommended courses. Several universities offer courses in global public health, humanitarian aid, and tropical diseases. A master of public health degree can often be helpful in these settings. Short courses in tropical diseases are available at the Gorgas Memorial Institute of Tropical Medicine in Peru (gorgas.dom.uab.edu/), the Burnet Institute in Australia (burnet.edu.au/home), and the London School of Hygiene and Tropical Medicine (lshtm.ac.uk/). Emergency physicians may pursue a fellowship in International Emergency Medicine (see iemfellowships.com). Courses in relevant languages can also be helpful and are widely available.

Practical Tips on How to Have a Good Mission

It is important to realize that no matter what the length or intensity of the predeparture briefing, one will only really know about the conditions when on the ground at the scene. If it is a first mission, it is better to do more rather than less preparation.

Personal Matters. Embarking on a field mission is the start of a very intense journey (Figure 84-35). The personal impact is

TABLE 84-5 Select North American Master's Degree and Certificate Programs in Humanitarian Assistance

School	Location	Degrees Offered	Website
American Public	Charles Town, WV	Master of Arts (MA) in Emergency and Disaster Management	apu.apus.edu/academic/programs/degree/ 1200/master-of-arts-in-emergency-and -disaster-management-capstone-option
Andrews	Berrien Springs, MI	Master of Science in Administration (MSA) in Community and International Development with an emphasis in Disaster Preparedness Master of Social Work (MSW) with a Certificate in Emergency Preparedness	andrews.edu/grad/programs/
Benedictine	Lisle, IL	Certificate in Emergency Preparedness	online.ben.edu/online-graduate-certificates/ emergency-preparedness
Boston	Boston, MA	Master of Public Health (MPH) with an emphasis in Managing Disasters and Complex Humanitarian Emergencies Certificate in Managing Disasters and Complex Humanitarian Emergencies	bu.edu/sph/students/resources/guides/2014 -2015-concentrators-guides/global-health -concentrators-guide-2014-15/mph-degree -requirements/concentration-courses/ emphasis-areas/managing-disasters-and -complex-humanitarian-emergencies/
California State	Vallejo, CA	Master of Science (MSc) in Transportation and Engineering Management with a concentration in Humanitarian Disaster Management	csum.edu/web/industry/graduate-studies/mste
Columbia	New York, NY	Certificate in Public Health and Humanitarian Assistance	mailman.columbia.edu/academics/degree -offerings/mph/full-time-mph/certificates/ public-health-and-humanitarian-assistance
Fordham	New York, NY	MA in International Humanitarian Action International Diploma in Humanitarian Assistance International Diploma in Operational Humanitarian Assistance International Diploma in the Management of Humanitarian Action International Diploma in Humanitarian Leadership	legacy.fordham.edu/academics/programs_at _fordham_/international_humani/graduate _program/
George Brown College	Toronto, ON, Canada	Certificate in Emergency Management	coned.georgebrown.ca/owa_prod/cewskcrss. P_ProgArea?area_code=PA0046
Georgetown	Washington, DC	Certificate in Refugees and Humanitarian Emergencies	isim.georgetown.edu/academics/refugees
George Washington	Washington, DC	MA in International Development Studies with a specialization in Humanitarian Assistance	elliott.gwu.edu/international-development -studies/humanitarian-assistance
Georgia State	Atlanta, GA	Graduate Certificate in Disaster Management	pmap.gsu.edu/programs/graduate/certificates/ graduate-certificate-in-disaster-management/
Harvard	Cambridge, MA	MPH with a concentration in Humanitarian Studies, Ethics, and Human Rights Humanitarian Studies: Theory and Practice Program	humanitarianacademy.harvard.edu/about-you/ students/hsph-graduate-concentration -certificate-program hhi.harvard.edu/graduate
Johns Hopkins	Washington, DC	MPH with a concentration in Humanitarian Assistance and Health and Human Rights Certificate in Humanitarian Assistance Certificate in Health Emergencies in Large Populations	jhsph.edu/research/centers-and-institutes/ center-for-refugee-and-disaster-response/ education_training/degrees/
Justice Institute of British Columbia	New Westminster, BC, Canada	Emergency Management Certificate	jibc.ca/programs-courses/schools-departments/ school-public-safety/emergency-management -division/academic-programs/emergency -management-certificate
Massachusetts Institute of Technology	Cambridge, MA	Master of Engineering (MEng) in Logistics	scm.mit.edu/program
Royal Roads	Victoria, BC, Canada	MA in Conflict Analysis and Management MA in Disaster and Emergency Management MA in Human Security and Peace-building	royalroads.ca/prospective-students/programs/ humanitarian-studies
Ryerson	Toronto, ON, Canada	Certificate in Disaster and Emergency Management	ce-online.ryerson.ca/ce/calendar/default.aspx ?section=program&sub=cert&cert =DISMAN00&mode=program

TABLE 84-5   Select North American Master's Degree and Certificate Programs in Humanitarian Assistance—cont'd

School	Location	Degrees Offered	Website
Tufts	Medford, MA	MA in Humanitarian Assistance	fic.tufts.edu/education/maha/
		MSc in Food Policy and Applied Nutrition in the Humanitarian Assistance specialization at the Friedman School of Nutrition Science and Policy	nutrition.tufts.edu/academics/fpan
Tulane	New Orleans, LA	MPH in Disaster Management	tulane.edu/publichealth/ehs/mph.cfm
		Certificate in Disaster Management and Resilience	tulane.edu/publichealth/academics/disaster -management-and-resilience-certificate.cfm
Uniformed Services University of the Health Sciences	Bethesda, MD	Disaster Preparedness Program	cdham.org/disaster-preparedness-program -dpp
University of British Columbia	Vancouver, BC, Canada	Master of Arts in Planning (MAP) or Master of Science in Planning (MScP) with focus area on Disaster and Risk Management Planning	scarp.ubc.ca/focus-area-disaster-and-risk -management-planning
University of Connecticut	Storrs, CT	Online Master of Professional Studies in Humanitarian Services Administration	hrm.business.uconn.edu
University of Denver	Denver, CO	MA in International Studies with a graduate certificate in Humanitarian Assistance	du.edu/korbel/humanitarian-assistance/index .html
University of Hawaii	Honolulu, HI	Certificate in Disaster Management and Humanitarian Assistance	durp.hawaii.edu/Disaster%20Management.html
University of Massachusetts Boston	Boston, MA	Online certificate program in Global Post-Disaster Reconstruction and Management	umb.edu/academics/caps/corporate/disaster -reconstruction
		Online Graduate Certificate in Global Post-Disaster Studies	umb.edu/academics/caps/certificates/global -post-disaster
University of South Florida	Tampa, FL	MPH in Disaster Management and Humanitarian Relief	health.usf.edu/publichealth/onlineprograms/ omph_gdmhr.htm
		Graduate Certificate in Disaster Management	usf.edu/innovative-education/programs/ graduate-certificates/fully-online.aspx
		Graduate Certificate in Humanitarian Assistance	
University of Wisconsin	Madison, WI	Disaster Management Diploma	dmc.engr.wisc.edu/Diploma/index.lasso
York	Toronto, ON, Canada	Master of Disaster and Emergency Management	dem.gradstudies.yorku.ca

From Walker P, Russ C: Professionalising the humanitarian sector: a scoping study, Enhancing Learning and Research for Humanitarian Assistance (ELRHA), April 2010: elrha.org/uploads/Professionalising_the_humanitarian_sector.pdf.

immense, particularly if the destination is a war zone or other type of humanitarian crisis. Experiencing grinding poverty in an isolated region facing chronic neglect can be difficult as well. With that in mind, when deploying, it is important that any matters at home, including family and interpersonal relationships, are resolved so that they do not generate added stress while in the field. Organizing home-related affairs before departing will better allow the aid worker to use what little personal time exists

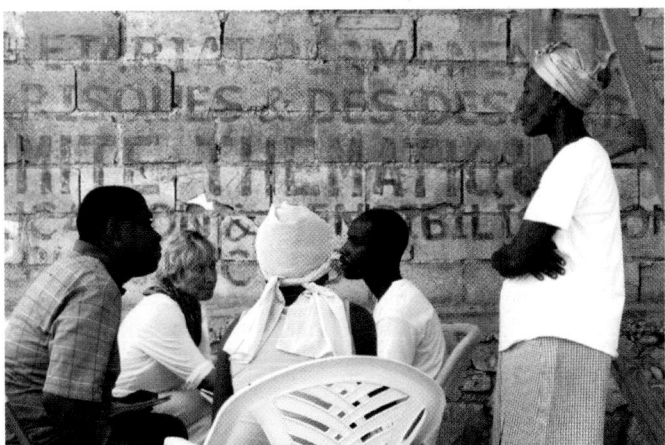

FIGURE 84-35 Aid workers provide mental health services following the 2010 earthquake in Haiti. (*Courtesy Richard Accidat, Médecins Sans Frontières.*)

in the field in a relaxing way that will feed positively into meeting the demands of the assignment. Ensure that all financial obligations (e.g., bills) are paid or otherwise resolved before departure. These matters should be settled in a way that does not require your input while on assignment.

It is wise to consider taking a vacation before deployment. This can minimize the pressures that go along with preparing for the field mission, while building energy for what lies ahead. Being well rested for the nonstop orientation and work will go a long way toward creating the possibility for a positive experience.

Before leaving, speak with others currently working in the field or with those who have worked there previously. If the organization does not mention this possibility, be sure to ask about it, because it is possible. This is an important way to find out about the living and working conditions, the people you will meet, and the work itself.

It is essential to have a positive attitude, because stress, ill will, and cynicism are common in emergencies. Try to maintain a genuine sense of optimism and healthy sense of humor. A positive attitude rubs off on teammates. Persons who are negative can drag down a team.

Be respectful of others. No matter where someone is from and no matter how you feel about their beliefs, religion, ethnicity, or nationality, do your best to keep an open mind and be supportive.

Remember that you are a guest in a foreign land. A courteous and considerate approach to local traditions, customs, and laws is central not only to showing respect but to creating the basis for open and meaningful relationships. Meeting others from different cultures is truly a privilege. Although people in distant lands may not have the same luxuries, technical gadgets, or formal education, they usually possess more in other areas of life and on other levels. The key to success is being open to this and discovering the beauty and wisdom of different cultures. Although aid workers may see the worst in humankind while working in a crisis, they will also see and experience the best (Figure 84-36). Appreciating the best is an important key to navigating through what will be a very difficult and challenging, but extremely rewarding mission.

Perhaps the most difficult challenge will be working and living as a team. Aid workers do not have the luxury of choosing their team, and organizations do not have the luxury of matching personalities. Team tensions are inevitable and the greater your emotional maturity, the better off you and your team will be.

In a war zone, external checks and balances around what is morally correct are minimal. Due process is replaced by atrocities and human rights violations. Aid workers must rely on their own internal moral compasses in these environments. Awareness of this can assist in reinforcing good decisions around one's behavior and interactions with others. Linked to this, it is important to appreciate the power balance that exists between expatriates and others. Individuals who work for aid organizations represent wealth from the perspective of most beneficiaries and community members. Although aid workers may feel that they are "roughing

TABLE 84-6 Humanitarian Training Centers, Organizations, and Resources

Sector	Name of Organization	Comments	Location	Website
Professional associations	Professionals in Humanitarian Assistance and Protection	Professional association of humanitarian workers with focus on policy and international humanitarian law	Geneva	phap.org/
	Global Humanitarian Health Association	Professional association of humanitarian health workers	Canada	Coming soon; in the meantime, go to humanitarianstudies initiative.org or humanitarianu.com
	Humanitarian Logistics Association	Professional association of logisticians	UK	humanitarianlogistics.org/
	The International Society of Physical and Rehabilitation Medicine	Global agency for physical and rehabilitation medicine	Switzerland	isprm.org
	World Association for Disaster and Emergency Medicine	Professional association for the global improvement of prehospital and emergency health care, public health, and disaster health and preparedness	USA	wadem.org
	World Public Health Nutrition Association	Professional association for public health nutritionists		wphna.org
General information on humanitarian aid and relief and training	AlertNet	News and training information		alertnet.org/theevents/ training/
	ReliefWeb	News and training information		reliefweb.int
	IRIN	Regional news		irinnews.org
	People in Aid	Resources, information, and links	UK	peopleinaid.org
	Humanitarian Practice Network (HPN)	Research and articles pertaining to the humanitarian sector	UK	odihpn.org
	OSCAR (UK information service for World Mission)	Resources, training, and links	UK	oscar.org.uk
	UN Office for the Coordination of Humanitarian Affairs(OCHA)	News and resources		unocha.org/
	Inter-Agency Standing Committee (IASC)	Standards, policy papers, news, and resources		humanitarianinfo.org/iasc/
Security and safety	RedR	Security short courses	London, UK	redr.org
	Bioforce	Security courses (French)	Vénissieux, France	bioforce.asso.fr
	Centre for Safety	Mine awareness	Nieuwegein, The Netherlands	centreforsafety.org
	Centurion Risk Assessment Services	Hostile environment and first aid (NGO and diplomats)	Hants, UK	centurionsafety.net
	OnCourse	Security, driving courses	Uganda, Kenya	oncourse4wd.com
	Essential Field Training	Security courses (French)	Switzerland	essential-field-training.org
	Merlin	Security short courses	UK	merlin.org.uk

TABLE 84-6 Humanitarian Training Centers, Organizations, and Resources—cont'd

Sector	Name of Organization	Comments	Location	Website
Medical	International Health Exchange (IHE) (often in partnership with RedR)	Link for short courses	London, UK	ihe.org.uk
	Centre for International Child Health	MSc and short courses	Melbourne, Australia	rch.org.au/cich
	Liverpool School of Tropical Medicine	Postgraduate, short courses, MSc	Liverpool, UK	lstmed.ac.uk
	Leeds Beckett University	MSc Public Health, Health Promotion	Leeds, UK	leedsbeckett.ac.uk
	Christian Medical Fellowship	Short courses, preparation for field work	London, UK	cmf.org.uk
	London School of Hygiene and Tropical Medicine	Short courses, MSc	London, UK	lshtm.ac.uk
	Institute of Tropical Medicine	Short courses, MSc	Antwerp, Belgium	itg.be
	Queen Margaret University College	Postgraduate, short courses, MSc	Edinburgh, UK	qmu.ac.uk
	Swiss Tropical and Public Health Institute	Postgraduate, short courses, MSc	Basel, Switzerland	sti.ch
	Deutsches Institut für Ärztliche Mission	Short courses, preparation for field work, German only	Tübingen, Germany	difaem.de
	Uppsala University	Short courses	Uppsala, Sweden	kbh.uu.se/imch
	Universitätsklinikum und Medizinische Fakultät Heidelberg	Short courses	Heidelberg, Germany	hyg.uni-heidelberg.de/ithoeg/teaching/short/short.htm
	InterHealth	Services	London, UK	interhealth.org.uk
	International Rescue Committee (IRC)	Short courses	New York	theirc.org/phce
	International Committee of the Red Cross (ICRC), HELP Courses	Short courses	Geneva, Switzerland	icrc.org
	Teaching-aids at Low Cost (TALC)	Teaching resources	Harpenden, Hertfordshire, UK	talcuk.org/
	Merlin	Same courses as IHE	London, UK and Washington, DC	merlin.org.uk
Nutrition	Action Against Hunger		Multinational	acf-international.org
	The Emergency Nutrition Network		Dublin, Ireland	ennonline.net
Water and sanitation	RedR Training Department	Short courses, onsite courses, resources	London, UK	redr.org
	Loughborough University	MSc	Loughborough, UK	lboro.ac.uk
	International Water and Sanitation Center (IRC)	Short courses and resources	The Netherlands	irc.nl
	NETWAS	Short courses, onsite courses	Nairobi, Kenya	netwas.org
	SKAT	Resources		skat.ch
	Department of Water and Sanitation in Developing Countries (SANDEC)	Short courses (English and German)	Switzerland	sandec.ch
	UN World Bank, WatSan Programme	Resources, short courses	Nairobi, Kenya	wsp.org
	Kenya Water for Health Organisation	Resources, short courses	Nairobi, Kenya	kwaho.org
	Water Supply and Sanitation Collaborative Council	Resources		wsscc.org
	Cranfield University		Cranfield and Shrivenham, UK	cranfield.ac.uk
Logistics	RedR Training Department	Short courses, onsite courses, resources	London, UK	redr.org
	Merlin	Short courses, onsite courses, resources		merlin.org.uk
	Bioforce	Short courses, logistics studies (French)	Vénissieux, France	bioforce.asso.fr

Continued

Sector	Name of Organization	Comments	Location	Website
Management and leadership	Centre for Health Planning and Management			keele.ac.uk
Humanitarian aid, relief, and development	University of Wolverhampton, Centre for Rural Development and Training (CRDT)	Program management and development	UK	wlv.ac.uk/crdt
	Sphere Project	Standards, resources, trainings	Geneva, Switzerland	sphereproject.org/
	Humanitarian U	Online certificate-based professional courses	Canada	humanitarianu.com
	Canadian Consortium for Humanitarian Training (CCHT)	2-week intensive competency-based entry-level certification course annually in May	Canada	humanitarianstudies initiative.org
	Leadership Academy	Training courses and resources	London, UK	humanitarianleader shipacademy.org
	Disasterready.org	Online training courses	USA	Disasterready.org
	Enhancing Learning and Research for Humanitarian Assistance (ELRHA)	Training courses and resources	UK	elrha.org
	Brunel University		Uxbridge, Middlesex, UK	brunel.ac.uk
	Centre for Development and Emergency Practice (CENDEP), Oxford Brookes University		Oxford, UK	brookes.ac.uk
	NOHA, Joint European Master's in International Humanitarian Action		Present in France, Germany, Ireland, Belgium, The Netherlands, Spain, and Sweden	nohanet.org
	University of Geneva, MS in Humanitarian Action		Programme Plurifacultaire Action Humanitaire (ppAH), Geneva, Switzerland	
	CIHC International Diploma in Humanitarian Assistance (IDHA)		Michel Veuthey, Academic Director, Geneva, Switzerland	cihc.org
	Centre for Development Studies (CDS)		Swansea, UK	swansea.ac.uk
	Centre for Health Economics		York, UK	york.ac.uk
	Christian Community Development		Korntal-München, Germany	aem.de
	International Disaster and Relief Training (IDART)	Customized trainings	Austin, TX	training2go.org/
	University of Liverpool	Diploma in Humanitarian Assistance	Liverpool, UK	liverpool.ac.uk
	Humanitarian Academy at Harvard	Short Courses	Cambridge, MA	humanitarianacademy .harvard.edu
	Global Human Rights Education and Training Centre	Online courses in human rights education		hrea.org/learn/ humanitarian-action -and-disaster-relief/
	Advanced Training Program on Humanitarian Action (ATHA)	Online and face-to-face trainings and webinars	Boston, MA	atha.se
	Imara International Humanitarian Group	Online and face-to-face trainings	Argentina	fundacion-imara.org
Monitoring and evaluation	International Institute of Rural Reconstruction		Philippines, Kenya, USA	iirr.org/
	RedR		London, UK	redr.org
	Overseas Development Group		Norwich, UK	uea.ac.uk/dev/

From Walker P, Russ C: Professionalising the humanitarian sector: a scoping study, Enhancing Learning and Research for Humanitarian Assistance (ELRHA), April 2010: elrha.org/uploads/Professionalising_the_humanitarian_sector.pdf.

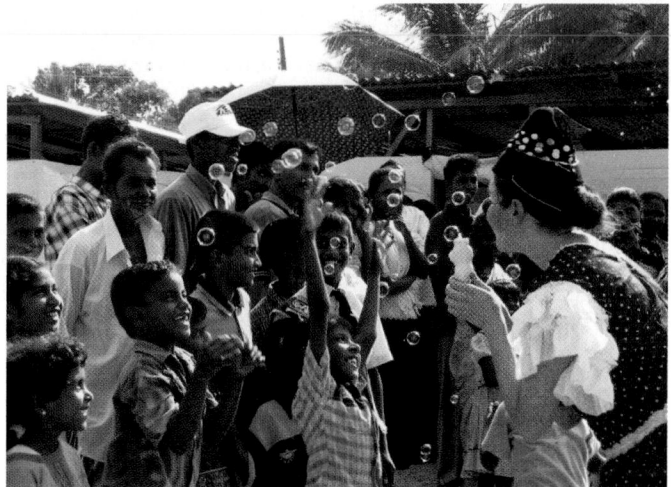

FIGURE 84-36 Payasos Sin Fronteras (Clowns Without Borders) working alongside Médecins Sans Frontières in Ampara, Sri Lanka. Performances and spectacles were organized in camps and schools to help children and youngsters overcome the trauma following the 2004 Indian Ocean tsunami, 2005. (*Courtesy Médecins Sans Frontières Spain.*)

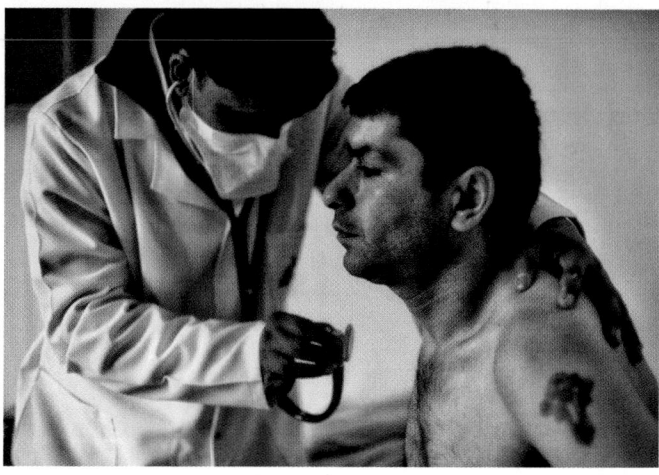

FIGURE 84-38 MSF doctor examines a patient with drug-resistant tuberculosis in Abovian, Armenia, 2010. Many patients are unable to complete the grueling therapy. (*Courtesy Bruno De Cock, Médecins Sans Frontières.*)

it" in the field, whatever they have represents more wealth than most local peoples can hope to amass in a lifetime. This affects the dynamic of the relationship and needs to be carefully examined and understood in order to avoid inadvertently abusing one's position.

Professional Matters. Much of an aid worker's success will be based on the relationships forged while on a mission (Figure 84-37). Handling this well from the start is extremely important. Persons from Western countries often have the misconception that they possess superior knowledge and that they will be imparting their wisdom to others. Although job titles may indicate something of this nature, do not be fooled. Expatriates do most of the learning, particularly on first missions.

It is important to remember that most of the local staff have been doing their work for years, and have seen expatriates come and go. It is always a good starting point in a conversation to ask local staff members how long they have worked for the organization, because this will acknowledge the desire to learn from their experience and knowledge, while also offering one's own services. It is crucial to understand what is already in place and why it has been put in place. New international staff usually

come into a project with great motivation and ambition. This can be misguided into changing work processes too quickly and without sufficient thought about what has been done before. Talking to staff and finding out the background will save much effort by zeroing in on what really needs input in a way that is effective and sustainable.

One of the most difficult aspects will be the seemingly impossible choices to face on an almost daily basis. There will be too many patients and not enough time or resources to meet all medical needs. The tragedies will be enormous and emotionally intense (Figure 84-38). It will not be possible to do everything, or to do everything well. Although aspirations will be high, expectations need to be realistic. One's well-being and capacity to sustain effort depend on this realization. Know your limits, and know that whatever you accomplish is more than if you were not there at all. Aid workers can only do their best, and whatever that is, it makes a difference for those treated. Somehow, one needs to let go of the rest without giving up hope. The aim is to be realistic, appreciate the successes, learn from the failures, and keep advancing in a way that can be sustained.

CONSIDERATIONS WHEN RETURNING HOME

The challenges involved in returning home from a mission need to be taken seriously in order to work through the experience to a positive conclusion. In the process of responding to a humanitarian crisis, aid workers often are changed, whereas persons at home have, for the most part, continued on common, everyday paths. There will be genuine and polite curiosity about one's experience, but often the experience will be too foreign for most nonparticipants to relate, in particular on a level that is sufficiently supportive (Figure 84-39).

Support that comes from family and friends will be limited in time and understanding. Do not expect too much. They remember you from before, and they will give support based on their prior experiences. Family and friends are only parts of the reentry process. Being able to tell your stories, both pleasant and unpleasant, freely and in detail will allow you to process the experience. This requires reaching out to like-minded field workers. Seeking out others who have done similar work is helpful in reflecting on experiences and working through them in a healthy way. Relying on professional psychosocial support is wise, because it is not possible to work in a war zone or humanitarian crisis and not face traumatic stress at some level. Ideally, the mental health professional with whom you consult will have experience in posttraumatic stress disorder. Some aid workers develop anxiety and depression and need assistance from a physician, psychologist, or psychiatrist. Alternative healing arts should be considered.

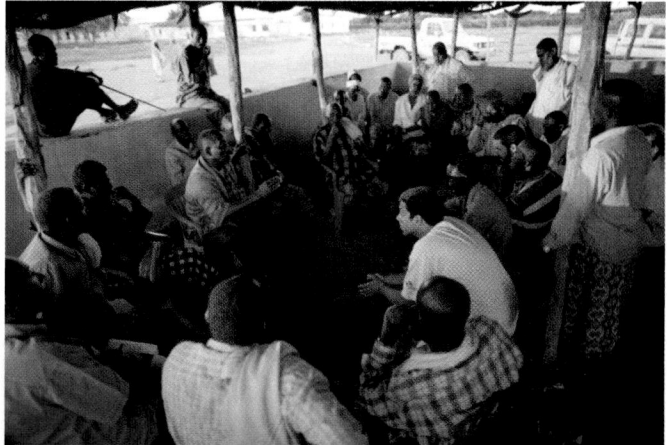

FIGURE 84-37 A field coordinator meets with members of the local community following the opening of a mother-child health care unit in the Bakool region, Somalia, 2006. (*Courtesy Espen Rasmussen, Médecins Sans Frontières.*)

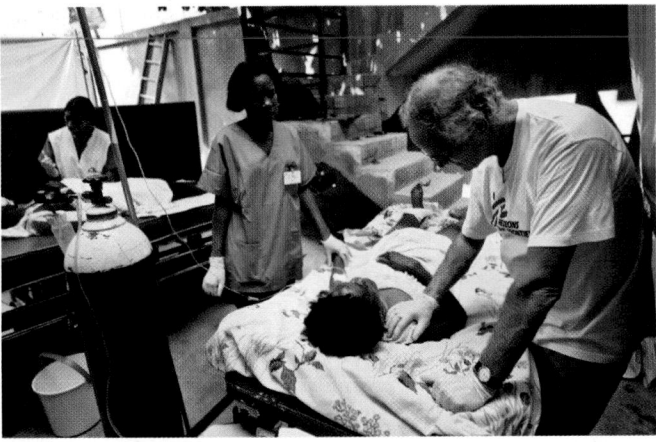

FIGURE 84-39 Haitian, German, and British physicians attend to patients in an outdoor makeshift ward following the 2010 Haitian earthquake. (*Courtesy Julie Remy, Médecins Sans Frontières.*)

After returning, reverse culture shock may occur. One may see his or her home society, culture, and relative wealth from a different perspective. One may question societal values. Over time, as one readjusts to being home, this feeling usually eases. When aid workers are engaged in relief work over a number of years, reverse culture shock will lessen because their thinking evolves around the relativity of pain and suffering and they come to accept the fact that they cannot personally take responsibility for global wrongs. Some aid workers quickly learn that although they cannot change the world, they *can* change lives, and that fact alone is settling. Some experienced aid workers simply quit comparing the perplexing and stark differences between justice and reality in the field and at home. Others use it as a basis for continued motivation to contribute to aid work.

Planning "down time" after returning home is important to recover physically, mentally, and psychologically. As tempting as it may to be to jump into another mission, it is better in the long run to take time between missions and become rooted again in one's home society. Some experienced aid workers believe it is helpful to have something or someone important "to return home to." Too many consecutive aid trips can lead to burnout and a loss of "anchors" in life. Staying involved in relief work over many years is possible, but requires pacing and keeping a strong support network at home. This can only be accomplished by taking time off between field assignments.

Whenever possible, it is important not to become financially dependent on humanitarian work. Financial dependence may mean not being able to take sufficient time off at home in between assignments.

Even if one is a medical professional, it is important to seek medical care for posttravel illnesses rather than self-diagnosing or self-treating. For example, if fever develops within the first months after returning, make sure to seek medical attention and give an accurate travel history. Tropical diseases can manifest weeks or months after returning home. It is easy to disconnect the disease from travel. Even if one only suffers what would normally be considered a viral upper respiratory tract infection, it is not worth taking the risk of ignoring it, because it could be malaria. Some aid workers routinely schedule a medical check-up with blood and stool sample analysis upon their return home.

Activities After Returning From a Mission

Aid workers find themselves with numerous choices of activities in which to engage after a mission. Some choose to present their experience to schools, universities, and government officials. Trainees in the health professions are particularly keen to learn from persons who have recently been on a mission. Colleagues at work may appreciate a presentation, and sharing one's hard work in a disaster setting can provide realistic inspiration for others wanting to go on a future mission.

Aid organizations often ask returned workers to meet with prospective donors and the general public. Workers back from the field are natural spokespersons for the organization and its work. Aid organizations often receive numerous requests for speakers from conferences and community groups. An organization may involve returnees in their recruiting efforts by having them speak with prospective future aid workers. Aid organizations also require boards of trustees or directors. Although governance may not be as exciting as is field work, it is a key part of running a charitable organization.

Some aid organizations try to promote a vibrant culture of debate and discussion within home society associations. These groups can also serve as social and professional networking opportunities to share experiences and cope with stress and isolation upon returning home. Remaining involved can strengthen a connection with an aid organization, and for some, increase the likelihood that they again work overseas.

Because returning home after a mission is not easy, some NGOs host peer support groups, which can be a rewarding way for former field workers to remain involved by helping colleagues who have had difficult field experiences. A few returned workers seek full-time or part-time employment within the organization in a head office, or seek employment with another aid organization or government bureau. Experienced workers may seek more senior voluntary positions in which they are coordinating or providing technical advice to less experienced aid workers. Many returned aid workers take courses in areas in which they would like to improve their skills.

Some returned aid workers remain engaged by writing about their work in the medical or lay press, others display photos of their mission, and a few even create art using material from their mission. The majority of aid workers enjoy coming home. Still, many have difficulty making sense of the vast disparity between the brutal reality and difficulties of their field experience and the relative prosperity, security, and comfort of life in their home society.

EVOLUTION OF THE HUMANITARIAN SYSTEM

The world is facing increased natural disasters and complex emergencies with an increase in the severity of impact on populations in terms of morbidity and mortality, forced migration, and competition for resources (Figure 84-40). This will, in turn, create increased demand for humanitarian responses; there is already unprecedented growth in this sector. In 2014, funding for international humanitarian responses totaled more than U.S. $22 billion, of which one-quarter came from private donors and the remainder from governments.[10] On average, humanitarian NGOs

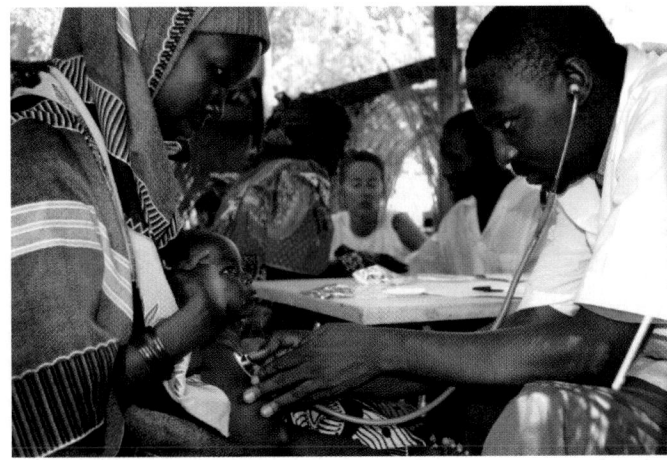

FIGURE 84-40 MSF nurse examines a child suffering severe malnutrition in the Zinder Region of Niger, 2007. (*Courtesy Karine Klein, Médecins Sans Frontières.*)

account for roughly one-third of this expenditure, and are thus major players in terms of volume of aid.[1] More than 4000 humanitarian NGOs exist worldwide, but 40% of the spending is carried out by only five (MSF, Catholic Relief Services, Oxfam, Save the Children, and World Vision International). It is estimated that in 2010, there were well over 200,000 humanitarian aid workers globally.[1] This workforce is believed to be growing at an annual rate of 6%.[35] The humanitarian sector "supply" numbers are clearly significant.

EFFORTS TOWARD IMPROVING RESPONSES TO NEEDS IN THE FIELD

Meeting the demand for humanitarian response requires careful application of lessons learned, strengthening of standards for responses, and increased attention to current training courses, certification programs, and professionalization. As the numbers of disasters and complex humanitarian emergencies increase, there needs to be a focus on enhancing quality and accountability in terms of service delivery in the field. One of the ways to do this is to ensure that humanitarians are properly trained before they provide assistance. A long-term vision is to create a professional body that accredits standardized training programs and oversees individual practice. Some efforts aimed at improving responses are already in place; a few of these are outlined in the following sections.

The Sphere Project

The Sphere Project, which has been running in various forms since 1997,[30] is an initiative to define and uphold the standards by which the global community responds to the plight of people affected by disasters. Sphere does this through a set of guidelines that are set out in the *Humanitarian Charter and Minimum Standards in Humanitarian Response* (universally known as the Sphere Handbook). Its rights-based approach outlines minimum standards that apply to each of the main sectors of response: water, sanitation, and hygiene promotion; food security and nutrition; shelter, settlement, and nonfood items; and health action. The Sphere Handbook also includes core standards and protection, the Humanitarian Charter, and references to all the contributing documents and texts.

United Nations Reform: The Cluster Approach

The response that followed the 2004 Indian Ocean tsunami was uncoordinated, duplicative, and competitive, and resulted in haphazard distribution of resources and provision of unneeded goods and services.[5] It became evident that a major problem in provision of relief and recovery was lack of coordination (Figure 84-41). As a result of this lesson, the Interagency Standing Committee of the UN Office for the Coordination of Humanitarian Affairs formed a series of clusters that encouraged operational agencies involved in international disaster responses to plan and operate together. The Department of Health Actions in Crises of the WHO was assigned as the lead of the Global Health Cluster; the Global Health Cluster brings many of the humanitarian and UN agencies that relate to health care to the table to identify how they can better coordinate their activities. A similar cluster organizational structure has been implemented in many countries. Some aid agencies have chosen to have selective involvement in the clusters approach and also continue with bilateral relationships with other actors, citing that accountability to the UN can, in selective contexts, lead to a loss of independent humanitarian action and access.

Humanitarian NGO Professionalization

The NGO community has improved its effectiveness in a number of ways, including interorganization coordination and training programs for staff. It also engages in research to inform programs (e.g., MSF's operational research center, Epicentre). Recent developments also include generation of the Code of Conduct for Health Systems Strengthening.

The NGO Code of Conduct for Health Systems Strengthening is in response to recent growth in the number of international NGOs associated with the increase in aid flows to the health sector.[13] This Code is intended as a tool for service organizations and eventually, for funders and host governments. The Code serves as a guide to encourage NGO practices that contribute to building public health systems and to discourage those that are harmful.[13] The document was drafted by a group of activist and service delivery organizations, including Health Alliance International (the convening organization), ActionAid International USA, African Medical and Research Foundation, Equinet, Health Global Access Project, Oxfam Great Britain, Partners in Health, People's Health Movement, and Physicians for Human Rights.

The articles of the Code of Conduct are as follows:[13]

NGOs will engage in hiring practices that ensure long-term health system sustainability.

NGOs will enact employee compensation practices that strengthen the public sector.

NGOs pledge to create and maintain human resources training and support systems that are good for the countries where they work.

NGOs will minimize the NGO management burden for ministries.

NGOs will support Ministries of Health as they engage with communities.

NGOs will advocate for policies that promote and support the public sector.

TRAINING AND CERTIFICATION

Several groups have attempted to define disaster medicine competencies, but few have been based on the science of disaster medicine. Currently, not even the actual domain of disaster medicine is clear, which makes it virtually impossible to reach agreement on who needs to know what in order to function during a disaster or to develop practical response plans.[5] Many organizations operate independently, which has led to inconsistency and confusion. Thus far, no international consensus has been reached about which competencies are required in order to receive credentials to work at some specific level in disaster medicine. Currently, there is no mechanism to accredit organizations to do what they say they can do.[5] There are no internationally accepted guidelines and no standards have been agreed on; hence, no competencies based on science and supposed best practices are available for dissemination and implementation.[5]

There are many NGO and academic training programs worldwide. Within the WHO Department of Health Actions in Crises, organizations and institutions that offer training programs are identifying core competencies for humanitarian workers. These must incorporate not only the minimum knowledge and skills required but also the behavior and the moral and ethical motivations that should be present for an individual to be considered

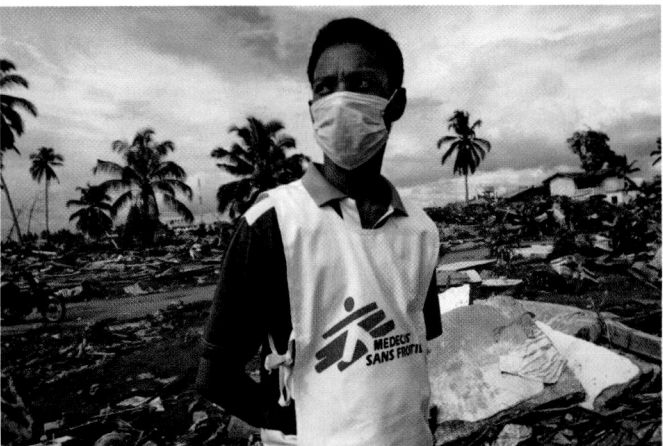

FIGURE 84-41 A relief worker assesses medical needs following the Indian Ocean tsunami, 250 km (155 miles) from Banda Aceh, an area accessible only by boat or helicopter (Indonesia, 2005). *(Courtesy Francesco Zizola, Médecins Sans Frontières.)*

competent to work in the humanitarian sector.[35] These academic and operational stakeholders plan that a certification process will be developed that will create a scale of recognized professional qualifications. Finally, in order for humanitarian aid to be truly professionalized, it is necessary to create a professional association for humanitarian workers, an academic studies association, and an association of humanitarian organizations that could institutionally support and legitimize the professional accreditation.[35]

CURRENT CHALLENGES, CONTROVERSIES AND KEY FUTURE ISSUES

By their nature, aid workers tend to respond immediately and reactively, placing themselves where need is great and working in the present moment of that need. For individuals and the organizations aiming to provide humanitarian and emergency medical assistance, and for those who support them and others who receive their assistance, waiting for the next crisis to occur is getting behind the curve. Both leaders and workers on the ground have to review and question past experience and decisions, critically analyze current situations and trends, and refuse to accept the status quo. Looking ahead, the challenges and difficulties are many, but it is in confronting them that we may improve our medical actions and have greater impact in the field.

GROWTH AND ITS EFFECTS

The number of actors in the humanitarian sector and size of aid organizations have grown tremendously, as have the financial resources used and the ambitions for goals to be achieved. Public awareness of humanitarian efforts has increased greatly as well. Through modern communication systems, media giants, and power of social networks in information sharing and advocacy, there is increasing awareness of growing needs around the globe, even during small distant crises.

Growth of the sector is frequently regarded as a good thing. The supposition is that the bigger an organization is and the more personnel it has, the more that can be done. Although this is often true, questions are asked about the effects and implications of that growth and the reality of what is actually being accomplished on the ground. In the 2010 earthquake disaster in Haiti, there was massive disorganization as hundreds of aid organizations arrived to create what has been called an aid circus (Figure 84-42). The various agencies jostled each other and "planted their flags" for a piece of the action; the result was what

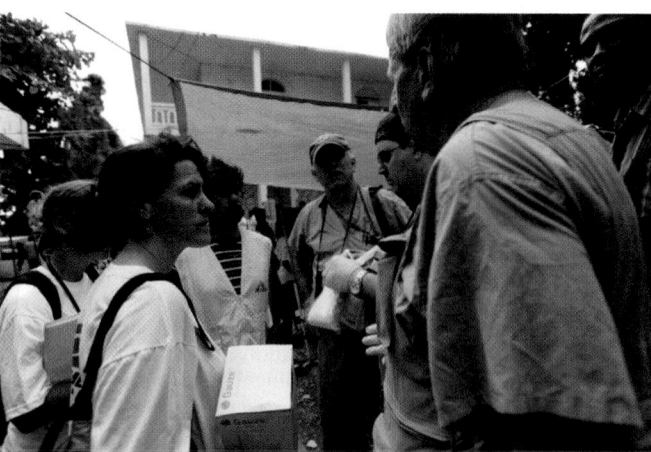

FIGURE 84-42 Aid workers in Jacmel, Haiti, following the earthquake discuss who will do what function, 2010. *(Courtesy Julie Remy, Médecins Sans Frontières.)*

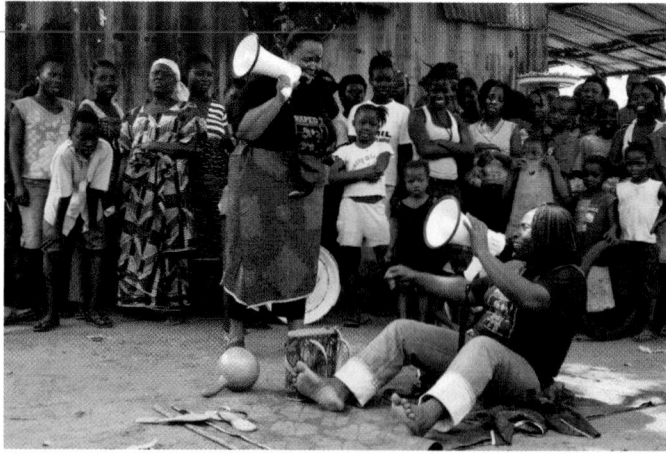

FIGURE 84-43 A health promotion and outreach team performs a street play that informs the public about what can be done following sexual assault in Liberia in 2009. *(Courtesy Alessandra Vilas Boas, Médecins Sans Frontières.)*

some have dubbed a "second disaster." Some, but not all, of the organizations were "start-ups," and their activities were not well coordinated. Many groups with good intentions lack the funding, technical expertise, and on-the-ground capacity to deliver timely and sustainable results.

Growth of an organization usually causes the headquarters to enlarge and the administration to increase, which can raise overhead costs and reduce the proportion of funds going to the field. More levels of hierarchy are introduced, and leaders are more removed from the field. Large organizations may be able to provide a robust response, but not always swiftly or with the ability to adapt quickly. The necessary professionalization of aid work has resulted in an increased organizational structure and more regulations. Although the priority of the individual medical act still exists, it must compete with many complex business issues, such as taxes, lawsuits, employment contracts, and labor disputes.

Financial, human, and intellectual resources are required to support the growth of professional agencies. More money is needed annually, more resources are needed to raise it, and more money is kept in reserve for future crises. The pool of human resources can be stretched, especially at coordinator levels that require more capability and experience. Medical leadership is hard to nurture, requiring retention over years and willingness to take on management, administrative, and planning roles.

Aid organizations can change or lose focus as they grow, shifting toward mid-term and long-term projects, public health or development-type programs, and advocacy-only work because these orientations seem to have the benefit of increased program stability and less security risk. The humanitarian sector as a whole has demonstrated more conservative decision making, and its coordination efforts are seen as sometimes slow and poorly effective. The result, as described in the 2014 MSF study "Where Is Everyone: Responding to Emergencies in the Most Difficult Places,"[22] is that in acute emergencies, and in places with challenges affecting security and logistics, there can be a near absence of both UN agencies and international NGOs. The 2014 Ebola epidemic, notwithstanding the degree of technical expertise required for a response, was a clear example of this trend of inadequate international response. The response arrived, but it was exceedingly late.

LOCAL PEOPLE AND LOCAL CAPACITY

Relief work on the ground is primarily carried out by staff from the country facing the crisis (Figure 84-43). In some instances, they are autonomous local implementing partners; at other times, local staff are hired directly by the international organization. In the latter instance, competition for the best local staff is common, with "international" salaries sometimes distorting the local economy, attracting talented staff away from the Ministry of Health or local organizations. Working relationships between international and local staff are often collegial and highly positive. However, a frequent complaint from local staff is the "revolving door" of expatriates who come and go on short missions, changing the medical program immediately upon arrival, sometimes with little experience or knowledge of how the current situation came into existence. Expatriates with little experience can be put in positions of maximal medical authority and then exercise it poorly, despite local staff having more experience and relevant skills to lead the medical team. Aid agencies have slowly evolved to elevate these local colleagues into supervisory positions, acknowledging their expertise and capacity. These "national staff workers" are increasingly being expatriated to work in other countries in need. This may benefit the organization as well as the destination country. Although it can temporarily be a drain on the home nation, the investment can return the staff member with valuable experience and increased skills and knowledge.

Local relief organizations have expanded. Some provide an excellent standard of care, and continue to work when international NGO access is limited or cut off. Others have lacked the skill and experience for implementation of programs, or do not have the impartiality and neutrality to work in a conflict or politically contested area.

The local or host community can often provide critical services to the population in danger. This adds up to a greatly increased domestic capacity to deal with the crisis. Depending on the country and context, this could be a high technical level of medical personnel, families who extend their homes and food, or community workers who help build and maintain such interventions as water and sanitation systems. Increasingly, lack of skilled medical workers in many of these contexts is met by task shifting or training lay personnel to provide health services and resources. Examples are peer groups for HIV medication adherence and initiation of treatment, community-based malaria diagnosis and treatment programs, and community management of malnutrition through locally produced supplemental food products. Even in emergency situations, it behooves the aid organization to spend sufficient time getting to know the local community, in order to capitalize on the local capacity, refine program choices based on local needs, and maximize local acceptance of the organization's presence. Avoiding paternalistic interactions with the community requires careful attention and ongoing discourse. In the end, developing a meaningful level of accountability to the beneficiaries and communities would benefit all involved.[4]

MEDICAL QUALITY AND ACCESS TO CARE

Improving the quality of medical interventions is a constant discussion in humanitarian assistance. Manuals have been refined and international standards established. These are of practical help in the field, but do not define the ultimate goals of medical care. One end of the spectrum is broad-based basic care that treats the most people at the least cost. Emphasis is placed on prevention and simple treatments of basic illnesses. Such cost-effective measures include distributing oral rehydration solution packets to treat children with diarrhea. At the other end of the spectrum is managing the most challenging clinical problems and pushing the limits of the field (Figure 84-44). Examples include using internal fixation for fractures; treating infections such as HIV in unstable conflict settings; improving therapy for multidrug-resistant TB, human African trypanosomiasis, and Chagas' disease; treating noncommunicable diseases such as hypertension and diabetes; and transporting inflatable hospitals, surgeons, and anesthetists to the field in the urgent hours after a natural disaster.

Amidst the interest in medical advances and running large programs, some basic yet vital contributors to quality can be overlooked. Examples include the quality of nursing assessments and patient surveillance, staff hand washing, sterile dressing changes, hospital hygiene, skillful triage, patient education,

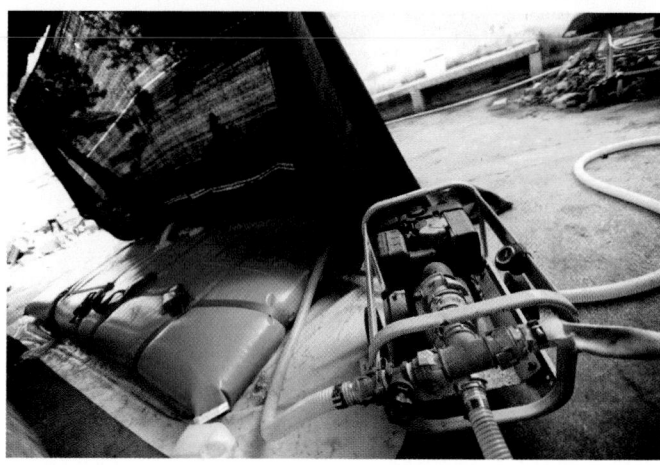

FIGURE 84-44 Water pump and water bladder equipment used for kidney dialysis at Port-au-Prince General Hospital following the 2010 earthquake in Haiti. (Courtesy Julie Remy, Médecins Sans Frontières.)

follow-up, and adherence counseling (Figure 84-45). There is little quality of care without these simple interventions. Improving adherence to evidence-based best practices in the fields of global health and disaster medicine can go some distance to reducing rates of morbidity and mortality in humanitarian projects. However, dissemination of such information to medical staff remains scattered and inconsistent.

A major barrier to medical care is access to essential medicines, biologics, and diagnostics adapted to low-income settings. Players in this arena include the pharmaceutical industry, patient rights groups, universities and other research institutions, the World Trade Organization, the WHO, and governments with variable policies that sometimes prioritize patients and the public health benefit while at other times favor protecting intellectual property and private business interests. Approaches and proposals to improve access to life-saving medications include policies allowing compulsory licenses for drug production, public campaigns to influence government and company policies, public-private partnerships for drug development, patent pools for therapeutic molecules, and a foreign currency exchange tax to be used for global health.

Problematically, medical data are often restricted from broad use by researchers or the public. Medical research in low-income

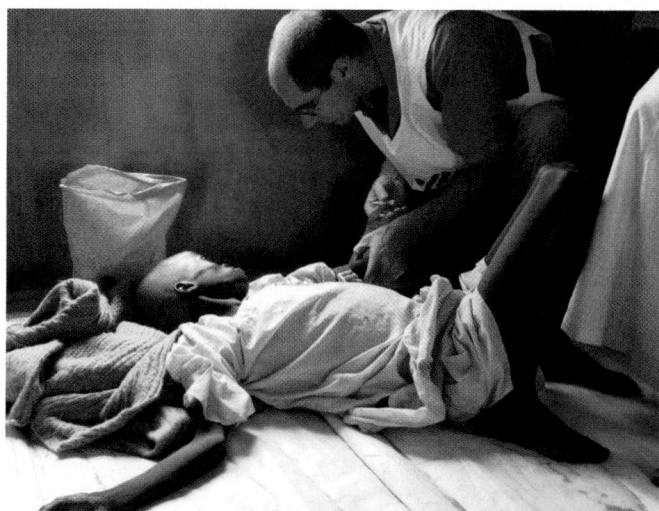

FIGURE 84-45 An aid worker inserts an intravenous line to care for a 13-year-old patient in Darfur, Sudan, 2004. (Courtesy Stephan Grosse Rueschkamp, Médecins Sans Frontières.)

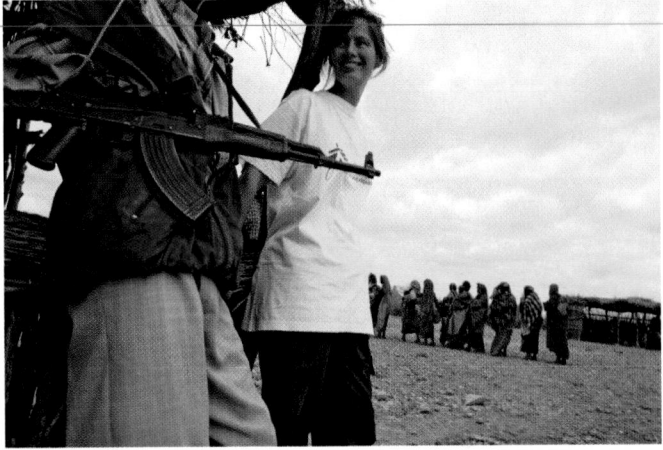

FIGURE 84-46 A doctor talks with an armed guard during a nutritional screening in Somalia in 2004. *(Courtesy Espen Rasmussen, Médecins Sans Frontières.)*

countries and from relief work is still published predominantly in proprietary journals, which own and charge for information. Nonetheless, there has been some change among private and public institutions toward collaboration and sharing of drugs and data, and proliferation of online, open-access journals is an encouraging trend.

SECURITY, INSECURITY, AND POWER IN THE FIELD

By its very nature, relief work involves an element of danger, and in some contexts that risk is considerable (Figure 84-46). The number of serious incidents continues to rise each year, with few exceptions. Causative factors include the violence inherent in conflict, societal breakdown, and criminal activity. Other reasons are political manipulation, terrorization as a tool of war, direct targeting for personal or strategic reasons, anti-Western or anti-foreigner sentiment, and an unsafe infrastructure, such as roads and buildings. Other factors at play may be underdeveloped contacts and local relations; vastly differing perceptions of the context among aid workers, belligerents, community residents, and authorities; inexperience on the part of field workers to deal with critical incidents or threats; lack of information; and the extent of personal exposure in the field.

In the past few years, there have been increasing incidents of direct targeting of patients, health care facilities, and health care personnel by militant groups. In response, the ICRC has formed the Health Care in Danger project. Some argue that the targeting represents a breakdown of respect for international humanitarian law by state and nonstate actors, specifically in regard to provisions for protection of noncombatants and civilians. Others note that throughout the long history of war, there has usually been little acceptance of neutral parties by belligerents in a conflict, and that the ability to provide relief or assistance in such settings has always been a matter of negotiation. In the field, NGOs have no choice but to believe in and endeavor to negotiate the "humanitarian space" in which to work, whether based on international law, humanitarian principles, or the measured compromise of those principles in the realpolitik that recognizes the motivations and self-interests of warring parties.

HUMANITARIANISM AND ENVIRONMENTALISM

There is near universal agreement that global climate change is an important issue, although there is variability in predictions of how soon and to what degree it might occur. If global climate change occurs, it is predicted to exacerbate flooding and drought, contribute to shortages of food and drinking water, and cause migration of populations and violent conflicts over limited resources. A more immediate concern is environmental degradation, such as poisoning of land by oil or mineral extraction companies, diversion or consumption of water and pollution of air by manufacturing industries, and destruction of natural resources by belligerents or depletion of them by populations themselves. Some argue that environmentalism encompasses humanitarianism. If a person is going to be able to deliver assistance to another person, the planet Earth must be able to house and sustain its population. Developing effective stewardship of the environment is necessary for continuing humanitarianism and responding to disasters. However, there is a natural tension between environmentalism and emergency humanitarian relief. Aid to populations in distress is necessarily focused on immediate and short-term protection of a highly vulnerable population, and its tools and actions may directly contrast with environmentalism's broader target population and longer-term goals. Environmental protection, taken to an extreme, could mean seriously limiting aid work. Aid work is messy. Airplane flights need to occur, all-terrain vehicles to run, and generators to spew out smoke. If a million people are displaced from their homes and they cut down a forest for shelter and fuel, is such an act justified so that the million can survive?

Although the priority of humanitarian relief must be saving lives, there are ways to carry out its actions that are environmentally friendly. Transportation costs are reduced if workers are deployed for longer times and plans are made for supplies needed. Hybrid car fleets and solar-powered energy reduce fossil fuel use and waste production. Lighter weight, recycled, or prefabricated building materials can spare critical local resources. The greening of humanitarianism can lead to immediate and long-term improvements, depending on how we answer the questions it raises for us. How do we minimize the impact on the environment by a displaced population and our aid efforts, thereby helping those suffering from contamination or lack of these resources? How can large relief organizations, in headquarters and in the field, reduce their own waste and production of carbon? Can we connect the principles and practice of humanitarian assistance to the preservation and regeneration of that which supports all of us?

HUMANITARIAN ETHICS AND MORALS

Although medical humanitarian workers perpetually act by definition, an ongoing debate and ever-evolving understanding of their ethics and morals must remain a critical component of these actions. What is right and wrong in a particular emergency or critical context? What can and what must we do to respond? In trying to answer these questions, we root ourselves in the person-to-person individual medical act, attempting to care for and bear witness to the other. We practice an ethic of refusal–refusal to accept the lack of humanity, refusal to accept unnatural and untimely deaths, and refusal to remain silent when speaking out may be the best way to save lives. We act, as James Orbinski said in his MSF Nobel Prize acceptance speech, "in the hope that the cycles of violence and destruction will not continue endlessly."

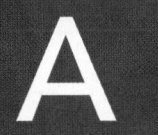

APPENDIX A

Suggested Packing List

DOCUMENTS

Passport* (plus copy)
Visa* (plus copy)
Immunization card* (plus copy)
Air ticket* (plus copy)
Letter of invitation by NGO*
Medical evacuation insurance card* (plus copy)
Health insurance card*
Trip cancellation insurance*
International calling card*
Driver's license (consider an international driver's license)*
ATM/credit cards (may not work)*
Cash (generally U.S. currency, but check with contacts)*
Copy of medical school diploma
Copy of medical license
Curriculum vitae and/or resume
Hospital identification badge
Business cards
Extra passport photos
Address/contact list* (see below)

GIFTS TO BRING YOUR TEAM

Chocolate
Cheese
Newspapers
Movies
Comfort foods (relevant to the cultures of teammates)
Coffee
Gift packages for your teammates from their families sent to you before departure

ADDRESS OR CONTACT LIST*

Field supervisor and local contacts
Arrival and airport contacts
Local embassy
Family and friends
Lost ATM or credit card reporting
Medical evacuation company
Health insurance company
Local airline office
Travel agent

GEAR

Money belt*
Day pack
Alarm clock (that runs on batteries)
Headlamps or flashlights*
Mosquito net
Sunglasses
Sleep sack
Rain protection
Duct tape
Swiss Army knife (not for carry-on)
Sewing kit

---

*These items should be packed in your carry-on bag.

Earplugs
Pocket tissues (toilet paper)*
Baby wipes
Luggage locks (for hotel, not flight)
Quick-dry travel towel
Flip-flops or shower sandals
Bandana or scarf
Travel clothesline
Laundry detergent
Sink stopper
Zip-lock bags
Water purifier or disinfection tablets
Phrasebook
Travel guide*
Stethoscope
White coat, surgical scrubs (where applicable)
Pocket medical references

ELECTRONICS

Laptop and power cord*
Electrical adapters and converter*
Surge protector
Flash drive*
Unlocked cell phone and charger*
Music player and charger*
Camera and memory cards*
Other cables and adapters
Handheld calculator
Extra batteries

FIRST-AID KIT

Sunscreen
Insect repellent
Antimalarial prophylaxis
HIV postexposure prophylaxis
Alcohol-based hand sanitizer
Traveler's diarrhea antibiotic(s)
Antidiarrheal
Laxative
Acetaminophen or ibuprofen
Decongestant
Antihistamine
Albuterol inhaler
Prednisone
Fluconazole
Bacitracin ointment
Antiemetic
Vitamins
Oral contraceptive and emergency contraceptive
Condoms
Adhesive bandages
Blister dressings
Alcohol wipes
Cloth tape
Wound closure strips
Safety pins
Tweezers
Spare eyeglasses or contact lenses
Sunglasses
Sutures and needle driver
Nitrile gloves

TOILETRIES

Toothbrush and toothpaste
Dental floss
Shampoo and soap
Comb and brush
Razor and shaving cream
Deodorant
Contact lens kit
Eyeglasses (and spare)
Sunscreen
Makeup
Mirror
Lotions and creams
Lip balm
Tampons
Facecloth
Prescription medicines*

EXTRAS

Notebook, journal, and pens
Photos from home
Gum, candy, and protein bars
Instant coffee packages and teabags
Magazines and novels
Playing cards and games
Textbooks and equipment donations

REFERENCES

> **Complete references used in this text are available online at expertconsult.inkling.com.**

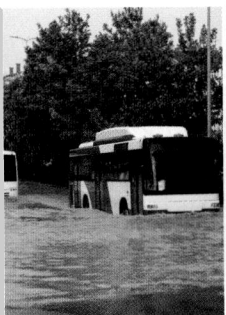

CHAPTER 85

Natural and Human-Made Hazards: Disaster Risk Management Issues

SHEILA B. REED

The term *hazard* is usually applied to a rare or extreme event in the natural or human-made environment. Hazards can include latent conditions representing future threats that can adversely affect human life or property to the extent of causing a disaster or major disruptive situation. Natural hazards are caused by biologic, geologic, seismic, hydrologic, or meteorologic processes in the natural environment and include drought, flood, earthquake, volcanic eruption, and severe storms. When natural hazards affect vulnerable human settlements, structures, and economic assets, they can be disastrous, disrupting the normal functioning of a society and necessitating extraordinary emergency interventions to save lives and the environment.

Human-made hazards are derived from human interactions with the environment, human relationships and attitudes, and the use of technology. For example, transportation accidents, petrochemical explosions, mine fires, building collapses, oil spills, hazardous waste leaks, and nuclear power plant failures are disasters in which the principal and direct causes are human actions. Many hazards have both natural and human components. Desertification results from arid conditions, erosion, and overgrazing; landslides may occur from poorly planned construction on unstable hillsides; and flooding may be caused by dam failures.

The distinction between many natural causes of hazards and the contributions of humans to disastrous situations is becoming increasingly blurred. As populations grow and expand, pressure on land resources may force settlement in vulnerable areas, where hazards such as volcanic eruptions, earthquakes, or floods can become major disasters. When disasters strike major population areas or where disaster-affected people must gather in camps or other common areas to receive relief services, incidences of disease have the potential of becoming epidemics because of overcrowding. Drought may contribute to famine in areas where food shortages result from combinations of lack of rainfall, displacement of people, and lack of access to food supplies. The widely publicized focus on the impacts of climate change emanates from studies of the effects of climatic conditions and environmental pollution. Variables in studies of global warming form such complex interactions that even computerized models have difficulty predicting the outcomes, lending possible substantiation for delays in addressing the causes. Hazards with a combination of causes result in complex disasters and often in complex emergencies. Conflicts, for example, in Syria, Iraq, and Afghanistan, create environmental disasters as well as disastrous consequences for the population in terms of death and displacement.

Whatever their causes, disasters have serious political, economic, social, and environmental implications. In less developed areas, disasters can severely set back or reverse developmental efforts. Disasters generally cause greater rates of mortality and morbidity among women and children, who are 14 times more likely than men to die during a disaster.

DISASTER RISK REDUCTION AND MANAGEMENT

This chapter covers 12 hazards, each with significant geophysical components, and discusses their causes, characteristics, predictability, adverse effects, and risk reduction measures. Hazards are viewed from a perspective of seeking means to reduce risks to vulnerable people and societies. The disaster risk reduction approach highlights causes of vulnerability and relates them closely to risk factors in society, such as poverty and economic development. The socioeconomic forces that make people vulnerable to disasters are likely to result from long-term trends. The study of disaster risk management, which formerly focused on natural hazards, now encompasses a range of slow-onset and rapid-onset disasters and their natural and human causes.

Activities associated with the conceptual framework of disaster risk reduction have gained wide usage by governments since the World Conference on Disaster Reduction in Kobe, Japan, in 2005 and have been strengthened in the follow-on World Conference on Disaster Risk Reduction in 2015 in Sendai, Japan. Disaster risk reduction aims to reduce the probability of disasters by using methods that are financially, environmentally, and culturally sensitive and by using mitigation methods that are agreed on through public consultation. The practice of disaster risk reduction encompasses all aspects of preventing, planning for, responding to, and recovering from disasters, including predisaster and postdisaster activities. A critical feature is training communities to allow them more direct responsibility for disaster reduction and creating resilience that allows societies and systems to effectively and efficiently resist, accommodate, and recover from the effects of disasters. Another key component is improving on unsustainable predisaster conditions through well-planned disaster recovery programs. The essential components of a disaster risk reduction framework are:

Risk awareness and assessment, including hazard analysis and vulnerability and capacity analysis, including analysis of possible impacts related to gender and age

Knowledge development, including education, training, research, and information

Public commitment and institutional frameworks, including organizational, policy, legislative, and community actions

Application of measures, including environmental management, land-use and urban planning, protection of critical facilities, application of science and technology, partnership and networking, and financial instruments

Early warning systems, including forecasting, dissemination of warnings, preparedness measures, and reaction capacities

Selection of management options depends on the type of hazard and its characteristics. Box 85-1 lists the elements usually found in a disaster preparedness plan for sudden-onset hazards, such as earthquakes, tsunamis, volcanic eruptions, tropical cyclones, and floods. Preparedness measures for slow-onset disasters, such as drought, include early warning systems that alert authorities to precursory conditions and allow preparations to avert food and water shortages.

SLOW-ONSET VERSUS RAPID-ONSET HAZARDS

The distinction between slow-onset and rapid-onset hazards is useful because the methods to deal with them often differ. Rapid-onset hazards often occur with violent intensity and have profound effects on the surrounding environment, resulting in measurable numbers of casualties and damage. Slow-onset climatic changes brought on by deforestation, drought, desertification, or environmental pollution change the suitability of different parts of the world for human habitation, and affect agriculture and flora and fauna. The effects of slow-onset disasters

are often insidious. Their impact can be measured only through environmental studies and in terms of reduction in quality of life and productivity for the affected population. Variables include levels of public attention to the hazards and the ability of the government to deal with them. Typically, threats become mitigated by slow movement away from hazards; for example, many of the 11,000 residents of the Pacific island nation of Tuvalu have left the country because the island is being "swallowed" by rising sea levels.

Between 1994 and 2013, 6873 natural disasters were recorded worldwide. They claimed 1.35 million lives (average 68,000 per year) and affected 218 million people. Earthquakes (and their associated tsunamis) killed more people than did all other types of disasters combined. Other primary killers were tropical cyclones and floods. Most deaths have been concentrated in a relatively small number of communities, predominantly in poorer nations of Africa, Asia, Latin America, and Oceania. In comparison, North America, Europe, Japan, and Australia have long-term average annual death tolls due to disasters that rarely exceed a few hundred persons. Although comprehensive data for economic losses from rapid-onset hazards are difficult to obtain, a few examples illustrate the scale of the problem. Annual worldwide losses from tropical cyclones are estimated at between $6 billion and $7 billion. For landslides, the comparable figure exceeds $1 billion. These figures only hint at the impact of such disasters on the affected human population. The eruption of Colombia's Nevado del Ruiz volcano in 1985 killed approximately 22,000 people and left 10,000 more homeless. An earthquake in Bam, Iran, in December of 2003 claimed at least 30,000 lives and destroyed 80% of the city. The 2005 Atlantic hurricane season caused record damages of $100 billion. Hurricane Katrina alone, in August of 2005, killed 1417 people in three U.S. states, displaced 1.5 million, and caused $75 billion in damages.

The relative human, economic, and social impacts of rapid-onset disasters are usually greatest in smaller, poorer nations. The 1985 earthquake in Mexico City caused economic losses equivalent to about 3.5% of Mexico's gross national product. Hurricane Allen in 1980 caused losses in St Lucia equivalent to 89% of the island nation's gross national product and destroyed 90% of its banana crop, which normally accounts for 80% of the country's agricultural output. One of the strongest storms in recent history, Hurricane Mitch in 1998, devastated the economies and infrastructures of Honduras and Nicaragua. From 1994 to 2013, high- and upper-income countries experienced 56% of global disasters but lost 32% of lives, whereas low- and lower-income countries experienced 44% of global disasters but suffered 68% of deaths. The disparity is further illustrated by average death rates, with more than three times the number dying in lower-income countries: 332 deaths for poor countries versus 105 for the richer countries. Economic losses from rapid-onset hazards are increasing at a fast pace. In the United States, damage to buildings from earthquakes, tropical cyclones, and floods was estimated to increase from approximately $6 billion in 1978 to more than $11 billion in 2000 without additional loss reduction measures. At this same time, it was estimated that a major earthquake in Tokyo would probably kill more than 30,000 people, cause the collapse of 60,000 houses, and set fire to more than 400,000 homes.

Slow-onset disasters take an even greater toll, but precise figures are difficult to establish. Drought currently affects more people than does any other disaster. Droughts affected more than 1 billion people, or 25% of the global total of persons affected by disasters, between 1994 and 2013, but represented only 5% of disaster events. Approximately 41% of drought disasters were in Africa, indicating that low-income countries are overwhelmed even though drought early warning systems are in place. In the United States, drought leads in economic impact, causing losses of $6 billion to $8 billion per year. Worldwide, droughts have led to famines, resulting in large numbers of deaths and displacements. Increasing desertification in arid areas may be contributing to droughts. Desertification, or decline in biologic productivity, extends to 70% of total productive arid lands (3.6 billion acres worldwide) and may adversely affect the quality of life for 10% of the world's population, including urban dwellers.

BOX 85-1 Essentials of a Preparedness Plan for Rapid-Onset Disasters

1. Identification and mapping of the hazard zones; registration of valuable and movable property
2. Identification of safe refuge zones to which the population and critical movable assets will be evacuated in case of danger
3. Identification and maintenance of evacuation routes
4. Identification of assembly points for persons awaiting transport for evacuation
5. Means of transport and traffic control
6. Shelter and accommodation in the refuge zone
7. Inventory of personnel and equipment for search and rescue
8. Hospital and medical services for treatment of injured persons
9. Security in evacuated areas
10. Formulation and communication of public warnings and procedures for communication in emergencies
11. Longer-term recovery plans (e.g., social services for trauma victims)
12. Provisions for revising and updating the plan

Climate change associated with global warming is predicted to occur over the next 100 years as a result of increased atmospheric carbon dioxide (CO_2) caused by the burning of fossil fuels, deforestation, and generation of methane. Ultimately, sea levels will rise and coastal cities worldwide will be inundated. A rise of 1 m (3.3 feet) in sea levels could flood 15% of the arable land in Egypt's Nile Delta and completely submerge the tiny islands of the Maldives, currently inhabited by 200,000. Hundreds of millions of people will also be affected if increased ultraviolet radiation is delivered to Earth's surface as a result of stratospheric ozone depletion caused by continued release of chlorofluorocarbons (CFCs).

Although global warming and ozone depletion are threats that may become more evident in the future, other forms of environmental pollution, such as water and air pollution, have immediate effects on life today. Massive oil spills, such as the 2010 leakages in the Gulf of Mexico, make headlines, and adverse health effects are seen from contamination and smog. Deforestation, particularly in the tropical rainforests, is highly significant. In addition to its contribution to possible global warming, loss of forested land increases vulnerability to droughts, landslides, and floods.

ASSESSING VULNERABILITY AND RISK

Not all hazards become disasters. Whether or not a disaster occurs depends on the magnitude, intensity, and duration of the event and vulnerability of the community. For example, a severe earthquake is not a disaster unless it significantly disrupts a community by creating large numbers of casualties and substantial destruction. Effective disaster risk management requires information about magnitude of the risk faced and how much importance society places on reduction of that risk. Risks are often quantified in aggregated ways (e.g., a probability of 1 in 23,000 per year of dying in an earthquake in Iran). The importance placed on the risk for a hazard is likely to be influenced by the nature of the risks faced on a daily basis. For instance, in Pakistan, where communities are regularly affected by floods, earthquakes, and landslides, people use their meager resources to protect against what they perceive to be the greater risks, such as disease and irrigation failure. In California, where the risk for disease is low, communities choose to initiate programs against natural disasters.

Vulnerability is defined as the conditions determined by the physical, social, economic, and environmental factors that increase the susceptibility of communities to the impact of hazards. Roles of men and women in society are also determinants of how each will be affected by different hazards, and how they will cope and recover from disasters. Many aspects of vulnerability cannot be described in monetary terms and should not be overlooked. These include personal loss of family, home, and income, along with related human suffering and psychosocial problems. Although communities in developed nations may be as prone to hazards as those living in poorer nations, wealthier communities are often less vulnerable to damage. For example, although both southern California and Managua, Nicaragua, are prone to earthquakes, California is less vulnerable to damage because of strictly enforced building codes, zoning regulations, earthquake preparedness training, and sophisticated communications systems. In 1971, the San Fernando earthquake in California measured 6.4 on the Richter scale but caused minor damage and 58 deaths, whereas an earthquake of similar magnitude that struck Managua 2 years later reduced the center of the city to rubble, killing approximately 6000 people. Similarly, in wealthy countries, drought and resulting loss of food production and groundwater are managed by use of food surpluses and treated water, but drought in poor nations often leads to deaths from famine, as well as sickness and death from contaminated water supplies.

DISASTER MITIGATION STRATEGIES

Mitigation is the effort to reduce loss of life and property from the impact of a disaster by taking action before the next disaster. Mitigation measures are most effective when all citizens understand local risks and make choices to support investments in long-term community and personal well-being. Where resources for mitigation are limited, they should be directed toward protecting the most vulnerable elements. Vulnerability also implies a lack of resources for rapid recovery.

For most risks associated with natural geophysical hazards, such as volcanic eruptions, tsunamis, and tropical cyclones, little or no opportunity is available to reduce the hazard itself. In these cases, emphasis must be placed on reducing the vulnerability of the elements at risk. However, for technologic and human-made hazards or slow-onset hazards, such as environmental pollution and desertification, reducing the hazard is likely to be the most effective mitigation strategy.

Two key aspects of mitigation are risk analysis and risk reduction. Risk analysis may include hazard mapping and multihazard mitigation planning. Risk reduction measures include floodplain management, safety programs, and hazard reduction programs. Mitigation actions by planning authorities and communities to reduce vulnerability can be active, in which desired actions are promoted through incentives, or passive, in which undesired actions are prevented by use of controls and penalties. Discussion of mitigation options follows.

ENGINEERING AND CONSTRUCTION

Engineering measures range from large-scale engineering works to strengthening individual buildings and implementing small-scale community-based projects to incorporate better protection into traditional structures, such as buildings, roads, and embankments.

PHYSICAL PLANNING MEASURES

Careful placement of new facilities, particularly community facilities such as schools, hospitals, and infrastructure elements, plays an important role in reducing the settlement vulnerability. In urban areas, deconcentration of elements especially at risk is an important principle. Specific procedures include hazard mapping and development of a master plan containing land use control guidelines. Hazard occurrence probabilities can be extrapolated from historical data and used to create hazard maps to show regional variation. Hazard mapping can be detailed by an inventory of people or things that are exposed or vulnerable to the hazard. In France, a plan called the Zones Exposed to Risks of Movements of the Soil and Subsoil produces landslide hazard maps at scales of 1 : 25,000 or larger that are used as tools for mitigation planning. The maps portray degrees of risk for various types of landslides, including activity, rate, and potential consequences.

ECONOMIC MEASURES

The linkages among different sectors of the economy may be more severely disrupted than the physical infrastructure. Diversifying and strengthening the economy are important ways to reduce risks. Within a strong economy, governments can use economic incentives to encourage individuals or institutions to take disaster mitigation actions. Increasing emphasis is being placed on securing contributions from the private sector to disaster risk reduction. Following the Indian Ocean tsunami of 2004, many beachside hotels in Thailand augmented awareness programs for clients and local communities and contributed to strengthening warning systems.

LEGISLATION, MANAGEMENT, AND INSTITUTIONAL MEASURES

The countries most affected by the 2004 Indian Ocean tsunami (Indonesia, Sri Lanka, Thailand, and the Maldives) have passed new disaster legislation that sets out general parameters for preparedness, response, and recovery. The resulting laws stipulate roles and responsibilities for members of government disaster systems, such as ministries and municipalities. These governments have also elaborated standard operating procedures and initiated drills. Myanmar (Burma) enacted a Natural Disaster Management Law in July 2013 and approved establishment of a Disaster Management Training Center in the Ayeyarwady Region, hardest hit by Cyclone Nargis in 2009. Creating disaster protection takes time and requires support from programs of education, training, and institution building to provide the required professional knowledge and competence. Improved forecasting and development of warning systems are critical protective measures.

SOCIETAL MEASURES

Mitigation planning should aim to develop a "safety culture" in which all members of society are aware of the hazards they face, know how to protect themselves, and support the protection efforts of others and the community as a whole. Specifically, these societal measures include conducting community education programs and planning and practicing evacuation procedures.

THE NATURE OF HAZARDS

Some hazards exist naturally, and others are partially rooted in natural systems. Many of these occur infrequently or affect only small populations. One example is the eruption of toxic gases from several volcanic lakes in Cameroon that killed 2000 people in 1984 and 1986. Other rare events, such as meteor impacts, may occur only once every few centuries. Additional widespread but minor phenomena that damage property but do not generally cause loss of life include land subsidence and sinkholes. Some hazards, such as snowstorms, often occur in areas that are prepared to deal with them, and thus they rarely become disasters.

This chapter discusses hazards that affect large populations and that can be categorized as follows:

Geologic hazards—earthquakes, tsunamis, volcanic eruptions, landslides

Climatic hazards—tropical cyclones, tornadoes, floods, drought, winter storms

Environmental hazards—environmental pollution, deforestation, desertification

To plan appropriate responses to implement emergency medical care and other measures to save or restore the physical and mental health of affected populations, governments and communities first need to understand the causal phenomena, characteristics, predictability of the hazards, and factors that contribute to vulnerability. Examination of the hazard's effects on humans, property, and the environment can promote measures to prevent or lessen casualties and destruction.

GEOLOGIC HAZARDS

EARTHQUAKES

Earthquakes are among the most destructive and feared of natural hazards. They may occur at any time of year, day or night, with sudden impact and little warning. They can destroy buildings in seconds, killing or injuring the inhabitants. Earthquakes not only destroy entire cities but may destabilize the government, economy, and social structure of a country.

Causal Phenomena

Earth's crust is a rock layer varying in thickness from a depth of about 5 to 10 km (3.1 to 6.2 miles) under the oceans to 70 km (43.5 miles) under the continents. The theory of plate tectonics holds that seven or eight major and many minor crustal plates, varying in size from a few hundred to many thousands of kilometers, "ride" on Earth's mobile mantle. When the plates contact each other, stresses arise in the crust. Stresses occur along the plate boundaries by pulling away from, sliding alongside, and pushing against one another. All these movements are associated with earthquakes.

Faults are areas of stress at plate boundaries that release accumulated energy by slipping or rupturing. Elastic rebound occurs when the maximum point of supportable strain is reached and a rupture occurs, allowing the rock to rebound until the strain is relieved (Figure 85-1). Usually, the rock rebounds on both sides of the fault in opposite directions. The point of rupture is called the *focus* and may be located near the surface or deep below it. The point on the surface directly above the focus is termed the *epicenter* (Figure 85-2).

The energy generated by an earthquake is not always released violently and can be small or gradual. Minor Earth tremors are recorded daily in the United States, but whether these are caused by the same processes that can level a city is not known. Most damaging earthquakes are associated with sudden ruptures of the crust.

Characteristics

The actual rupture process may last from a fraction of a second to a few minutes for a major earthquake. Seismic (from the Greek *seismos*, meaning "shock" or "earthquake") waves are generated. These last from less than one-tenth of a second to a few minutes and cause ground shaking. The seismic waves propagate in all directions, causing vibrations that damage vulnerable structures and infrastructure elements.

There are three main types of seismic waves. The body waves (P, or primary, and S, or secondary) penetrate the body of Earth, vibrating quickly (Figure 85-3). P waves travel at an average of about 6 km per second (kps) (3.7 miles per second [mps]) and provide the initial jolt that causes buildings to vibrate up and down. S waves travel about 4 kps (2.5 mps) in a movement similar to the snap of a whip, causing a sharper jolt that vibrates structures from side to side and usually results in the most destruction. Surface waves (L waves) vibrate the ground horizontally and vertically and cause swaying of tall buildings, even at great distances from the epicenter.

The earthquake focus depth is an important factor in determining the characteristics of the waves. The focus depth can be deep (from 300 to 700 km [186 to 435 miles]) or shallow (< 70 km [43 miles]). Shallow-focus earthquakes are extremely damaging because of their proximity to the surface. The earthquake may be preceded by preliminary tremors and followed by aftershocks of decreasing intensity.

Earthquake Scales

Earthquakes can be described by using two distinctly different scales of measurement demonstrating magnitude and intensity. The earthquake magnitude, or amount of energy released, is determined by using a seismograph, which records ground vibrations. The Richter scale mathematically adjusts the readings for distance of the instrument from the epicenter. The Richter scale is logarithmic; an increase of one magnitude signifies a 10-fold increase in ground motion, or about 30 times the energy. Thus, an earthquake with a Richter magnitude of 7.5 releases 30 times more energy than one with a 6.5 Richter magnitude. The smallest quake to be felt by humans was of magnitude 3.0. The largest earthquakes that have been recorded under this system are 9.5 (Chile, 1960) and 9.25 (Alaska, 1969).

The *moment magnitude scale* is a successor to the Richter scale and is most often used to estimate large earthquake magnitudes. Theoretically, all magnitude scales should yield approximately the same value for any given earthquake. However, measurement of the great Indian Ocean earthquake that occurred on December 26, 2004, generating a tsunami that killed more than 280,000 people, produced estimates by various institutions using different scales. The current official magnitude is generally considered to be 9.1 to 9.3. It was the third-largest earthquake ever recorded on a seismograph, with the longest duration of faulting between 8.3 and 10 minutes.

The earthquake intensity scale measures the effects of an earthquake where it occurs. The most widely used scale of this type is the Modified Mercalli Intensity Scale, which expresses the intensity of earthquake effects on people, structures, and Earth's surface in values from I to XII (Table 85-1). Another, more explicit, scale used in Europe is the Medvedev-Sponheuer-Karnik scale.

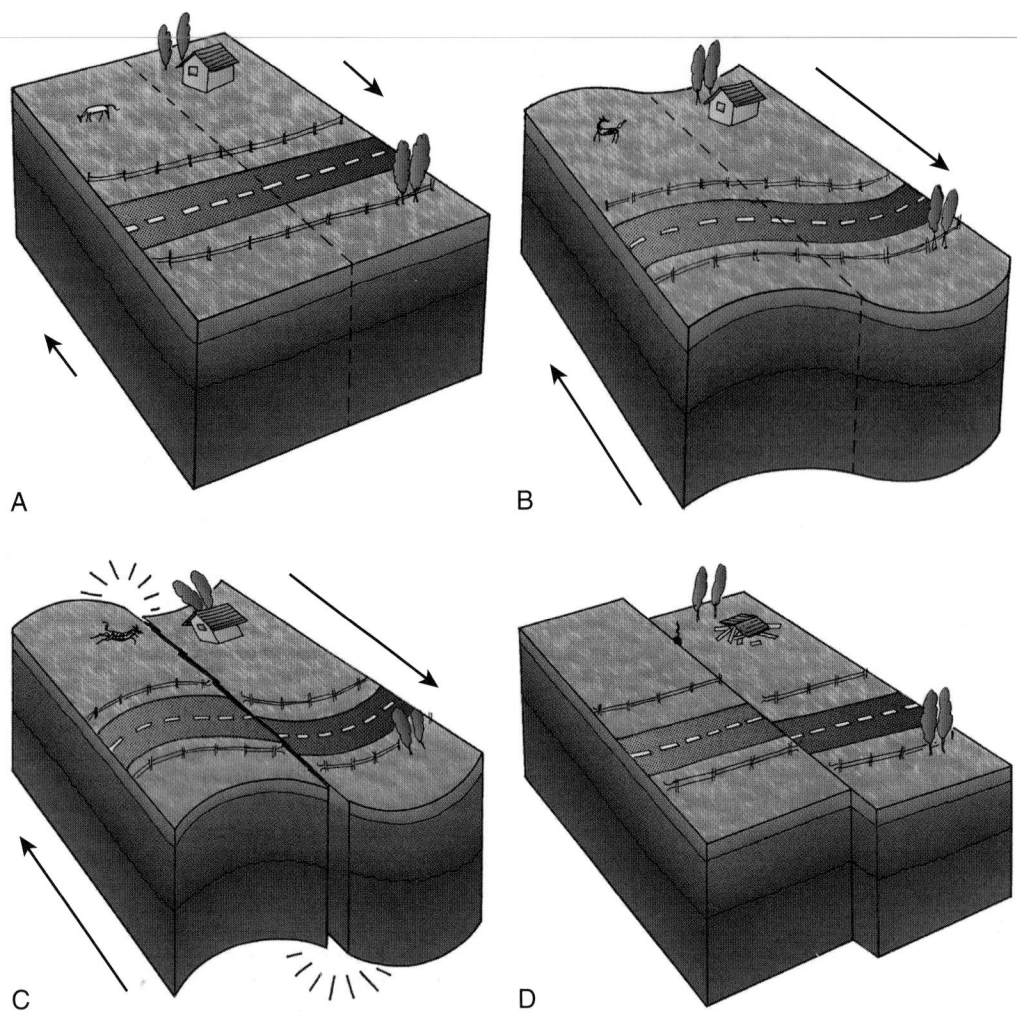

FIGURE 85-1 Elastic rebound in earthquake. **A,** Forces build up over time. **B,** Crust deforms. **C,** Crust snaps. **D,** Plates slide.

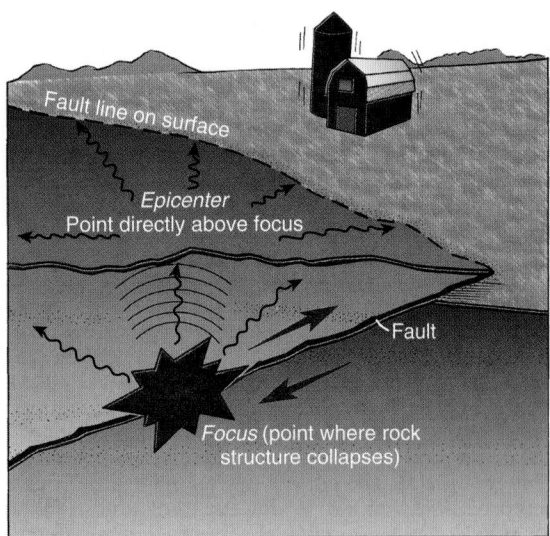

FIGURE 85-2 Motion of Earth's plates causes increased pressure at faults where the plates meet. Eventually, the rock structure collapses, and movement occurs along the fault. Energy is propagated to the surface above and radiates outward. Waves of motion in Earth's crust shake landforms and buildings, causing damage. *(Courtesy Disaster Management Center, University of Wisconsin–Madison.)*

Location and Predictability

Most earthquakes (95%) occur in well-defined zones near the boundaries of the tectonic plates. These areas bordering the Pacific Ocean are called the circum-Pacific belt. Areas traversing the East Indies, the Himalayas, Iran, Turkey, and the Balkans are called the Alpide belt. Earthquakes also occur along the ocean trenches, such as those around the Aleutian Islands, Tonga, Japan, and Chile and within the eastern Caribbean. Some earthquakes occur in the middle of the plates, possibly indicating where earlier plate boundaries might have been. These have included the New Madrid earthquake in 1811 and the Charleston earthquake in 1816 in the United States, the Agadir earthquake in 1960 in Morocco, and the Koyna earthquake in 1967 in India.

Earthquake prediction was a constant preoccupation for early astrologers and prophets. Some signs of earthquake noted by observers were buildings gently trembling, animals and birds becoming excited, and well water turning cloudy and smelling bad. Although some modern scientists claim the ability to predict earthquakes, the methods are still controversial. In fact, no earthquake has ever been precisely predicted. Rather, probabilities are calculated. For example, over the next 30 years, there is a 67% chance of an earthquake in the San Francisco Bay area. Earthquakes that have not been predicted include the 1995 earthquake in Kobe, Japan, which killed more than 5000 people, and the 2011 Tohoku earthquake. The high probability of a devastating earthquake in the Kathmandu Valley had long been discussed. The Gorkha earthquake (7.8 magnitude) in Nepal of April 2015 released some of the tectonic strain; nevertheless, considerable seismic pressure still exists in the region.

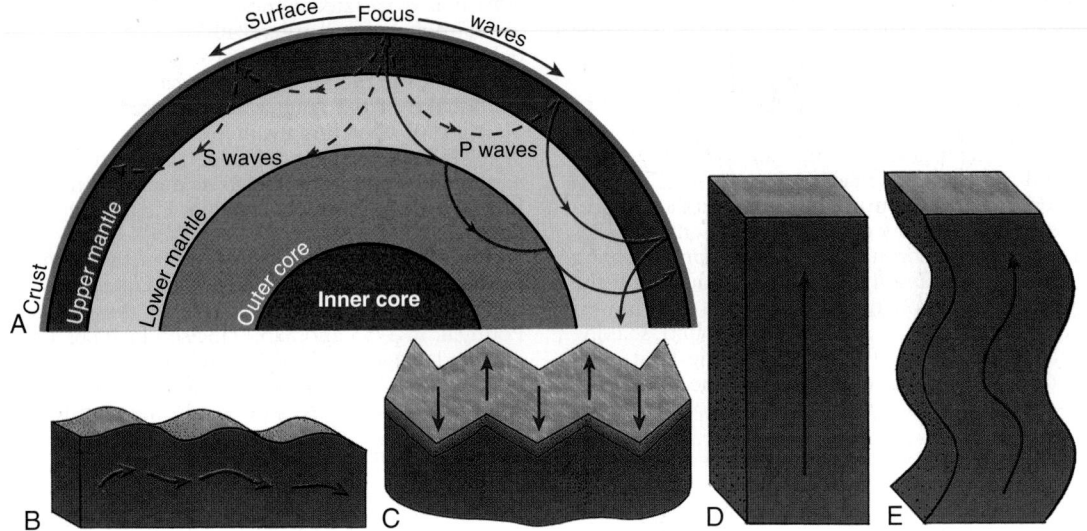

FIGURE 85-3 A, Propagation of seismic waves in an earthquake. Surface waves vibrate the ground horizontally (**B** and **C**) and vertically (**D** and **E**).

Fortunately, mechanical observation systems make it possible to issue warnings to nearby populations immediately after detection of an earthquake. Reasonable risk assessments of potential earthquake activity can be made with confidence based on the following:

Knowledge of seismic zones or areas most at risk, gained through study of historical incidence and plate tectonics

Monitoring of seismic activity by use of seismographs and other instruments (the U.S. Geological Survey monitors global seismic activity through 2150 seismic stations)

Use of community-based, scientifically sound observations, such as elevation and turbidity of water in wells and radon gas escape into well water

The island of Hispaniola, shared by Haiti and the Dominican Republic, has a history of destructive earthquakes. In January 2010, a magnitude 7.0 earthquake occurred approximately 25 km (16 miles) west-southwest from the capital city Port-au-Prince at a depth of 13 km (8.1 miles). Two years before this, scientists had detected signs of growing stresses in the fault that forms a boundary between the Gonave microplate and the Caribbean plate to the south, specifically the Enriquillo-Plantain Garden fault system, which includes much of Haiti. They warned Haitian officials that the fault was capable of causing a 7.2 magnitude earthquake, only slightly stronger than the actual 7.0 earthquake that eventually occurred. Unfortunately, 2 years is little time to prepare for such an event in a country like Haiti, which endures

TABLE 85-1	Modified Mercalli Intensity Scale of 1931
Scale	**Description**
I	Not felt except by very few persons under especially favorable circumstances.
II	Felt only by a few persons at rest, especially on upper floors of buildings. Delicately suspended objects may swing.
III	Felt quite noticeably indoors, especially on upper floors of buildings, but many people do not recognize it as an earthquake. Standing motor vehicles may rock slightly. Vibration similar to passing of truck. Duration estimated.
IV	During the day felt indoors by many but outdoors by few. At night some awakened. Dishes, windows, doors disturbed; walls make creaking sound. Sensation resembles heavy truck striking building. Standing motor vehicles rocked noticeably.
V	Felt by nearly everyone; many awakened. Some dishes, windows, etc., broken. A few instances of cracked plaster. Unstable objects overturned. Disturbances of trees, poles, and other tall objects sometimes noticed. Pendulum clocks may stop.
VI	Felt by all; many frightened and run outdoors. Some heavy furniture moved; a few instances of fallen plaster or damaged chimneys. Damage slight.
VII	Everybody runs outdoors. Damage negligible in buildings of good design and construction, slight to moderate in well-built ordinary structures, considerable in poorly built or badly designed structures. Some chimneys broken. Noticed by persons driving motor vehicles.
VIII	Damage slight in specially designed structures, considerable in ordinary substantial buildings with partial collapse, great in poorly built structures. Panel walls thrown out of frame structures. Fall of chimneys, factory stacks, columns, monuments, and walls. Heavy furniture overturned. Sand and mud ejected in small amounts. Changes in well water. Persons driving motor vehicles disturbed.
IX	Damage considerable in specially designed structures. Well-designed structures thrown out of plumb, greatly in substantial buildings with partial collapse. Buildings shifted off foundations. Ground cracked conspicuously. Underground pipes broken.
X	Some well-built wooden structures destroyed. Most masonry and frame structures with foundations destroyed; ground severely cracked. Rails bent. Landslides considerable from river banks and steep slopes. Shifted sand and mud. Water splashed (slopped) over banks.
XI	Few, if any, (masonry) structures remain standing. Bridges destroyed. Broad fissures in ground. Underground pipelines completely out of service. Earth slumps and land slips in soft ground. Rails bent greatly.
XII	Damage total. Practically all works of construction are damaged greatly or destroyed. Waves seen on ground surface. Lines of sight and level are distorted. Objects are thrown upward into the air.

widespread poverty and lacks resources for preparedness and mitigation. A legacy of poor building standards has increased vulnerability and cannot be easily remedied.

Earthquake Hazards

Earthquakes produce many direct, and sometimes indirect, effects. Landslides, flooding, and tsunamis are considered secondary hazards and are discussed later in this chapter.

Fault Displacement and Ground Shaking. Fault displacement, either rapid or gradual, may damage foundations of buildings on or near the fault area or may displace the land, creating troughs and ridges. The March 2011 Tohoku earthquake off the coast of Japan was the fifth strongest on record (9.0) and moved the entire island of Honshu 8 feet eastward. Ground shaking causes more widespread damage, particularly to the built environment. The extent of the damage is related to the size of the earthquake, closeness of the focus to the surface, buffering power of the area's rocks and soil, and type of buildings being shaken. The Northridge, California, quake in 1994 was one of the most costly, producing $44 billion in damage, due to the position of the event directly below a population center.

Aftershocks may cause further damage and may recur for weeks or even years after the initial event. The Kashmir earthquake (also known as the Northern Pakistan earthquake) occurred on October 8, 2005, and registered 7.6 on the moment magnitude scale. Affecting three countries, this earthquake killed more than 90,000 people. Between October 2005 and February 2006, there were more than 978 aftershocks of magnitude 4.0 or above.

Ground Failure and Soil Liquefaction. Seismic vibrations may cause settlement beneath buildings when soils consolidate or compact. Certain types of soil, such as alluvial and sandy soils, are more vulnerable to failure. Liquefaction is a type of ground failure that occurs when saturated soils lose strength and collapse or become liquefied. During the 1964 earthquake in Nigata, Japan, the ground beneath earthquake-resistant buildings became liquefied, causing the buildings to lean up to 45 degrees from vertical. Most of these buildings were later jacked upright and reoccupied. In the 2001 earthquake in the Bhuj area of Gudjarat, western India, many reservoir dams were damaged because of water-saturated alluvial foundations.

Lateral Spreads and Flow Failure. Lateral spreads involve the lateral movement of large blocks of soil as a result of liquefaction in a subsurface layer. During the 1964 Alaska earthquake, more than 200 bridges were damaged or destroyed by lateral spreading of flood plain deposits toward river channels. In the 1906 San Francisco earthquake, major pipelines were broken by lateral spreading, hampering efforts to fight fires. In 1989, the Marina District in San Francisco, built on soft landfill, was damaged by lateral spreading from the Loma Prieta earthquake.

Flow failure, in which either a layer of liquefied soil rides on top of another layer or blocks of intact material ride on top of liquefied soil, can be catastrophic. Some of the most damaging flow failures have occurred underwater in coastal areas, carrying away large sections of port facilities and generating large sea waves. Some flow failures on land have been as much as a mile in length and breadth, such as those induced by the 1920 earthquake in Gansu, China, which killed 200,000 people.

Landslides and Avalanches. Slope instability may cause landslides and snow avalanches during an earthquake. Steepness, weak soils, and the presence of water may contribute to vulnerability from landslides. Liquefaction of soils on slopes may lead to disastrous slides. The most abundant types of earthquake-induced landslides are rockfalls and rockslides, usually originating on steep slopes. The Kashmir earthquake of 2005 was characterized by numerous landslides that blocked access by assistance organizations to people in high mountain areas. The Nepal earthquake of April 2015 triggered avalanches on Mt Everest, killing 19 members of various climbing expeditions at the south base camp, the highest death toll in 1 day related to Everest climbing.

Tsunamis. Tsunamis may be generated by undersea or near-shore earthquakes and may break over the coastline with great destructive force. The Indian Ocean tsunami of December 2004 that devastated Banda Aceh, Indonesia, was generated by an earthquake occurring 240 km (149 miles) off the coast of Sumatra at the boundary between the Indian and Burmese tectonic plates in the Sumatra-Andaman subduction zone. A second earthquake of 8.7 magnitude occurred along the same fault in March 2005, but this event produced a much smaller tsunami (4 m [13 feet] versus 9 m [30 feet] in height). The December 2004 earthquake ruptured a longer segment of the fault and occurred in much deeper water, creating a larger movement of the sea floor.

Fires. One of the most destructive consequences of an earthquake is fire, particularly in urban centers. Great postearthquake fires played a major role in the destruction of Lisbon, Portugal, in 1755 and San Francisco in 1906, and caused considerable damage in Kobe, Japan, in 1995. The million wooden buildings in Tokyo pose a major risk of fire if an earthquake strikes, as is predicted to occur in the next few decades.

Typical Adverse Effects

Ground shaking can damage human settlements, buildings, infrastructure elements (particularly bridges), elevated roads, railways, water towers, water treatment facilities, utility lines, pipelines, electricity-generating facilities, and transformer stations. Aftershocks can do great damage to already weakened structures. Significant secondary effects include fires, dam failures, and landslides, which may block waterways and cause flooding. Flooding may also be caused by seiches (back-and-forth wave actions in bays) or by failures in dams and levees. Damage may occur to facilities that use or manufacture dangerous materials, resulting in chemical spills. Communications facilities may break down. Destruction of property may have a serious impact on shelter needs, economic production, and living standards of the affected community. Depending on their level of vulnerability, many people may be homeless in the aftermath of an earthquake.

The casualty rate is often high, especially when earthquakes occur in areas of high population density, particularly when streets between buildings are narrow, buildings are not earthquake resistant, the ground is sloping and unstable, or adobe or dry stone construction is used, with heavy upper floors and roofs.

Casualty rates may be high when quakes occur at night because the preliminary tremors are not felt during sleep and people are not tuned in to receive media warnings. In the daytime, people are particularly vulnerable in large unsafe structures such as schools and offices. Casualties generally decrease with distance from the epicenter. As a rule of thumb, quakes result in three times as many injured survivors as persons killed. The proportion of dead may be higher with major landslides and other secondary hazards. In areas where houses are of lightweight construction, especially with wood frames, casualties are generally much fewer, and earthquakes may occur regularly with no serious, direct effects on human populations.

The most widespread acute, serious medical problems are broken bones. Other health threats may occur with secondary flooding, when water supplies are disrupted (earthquakes can change levels in the water table) and contaminated water is used or water shortages exist, and when people are living in high-density relief camps, where epidemics may develop or food shortages exist.

In the aftermath of the Colombia earthquake of January 1999, which most heavily affected the city of Armenia, the death toll was 1185 and 160,000 people were left homeless, most in urban areas. In Armenia, where 60% to 70% of homes had been destroyed, movement was restricted by fallen debris and unemployment rose from 12% to 35%. People were living in unsatisfactory shelters made with plastic sheeting. Many migrated from the area to other places that could not absorb them. Although the international response to aid Colombia was strong, the overwhelming need continued to pose problems. Five weeks after the earthquake, supplies of food, clean drinking water, and shelter materials were still urgently required. Hygiene and sanitation services and essential medicines were desperately needed. Social services were required to work toward normalizing the lives of victims, especially children. In Gujarat, India, where

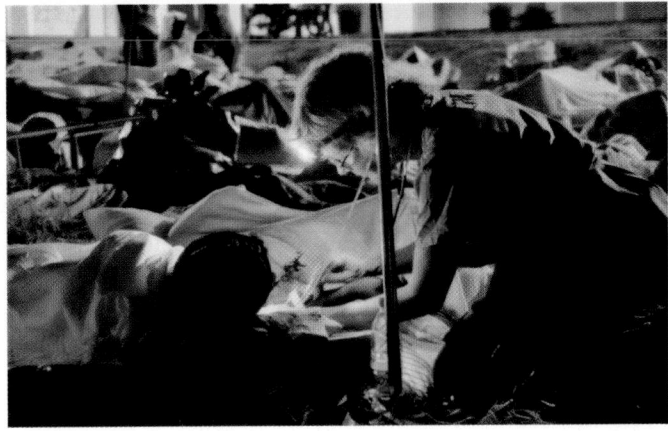

FIGURE 85-4 Nurse attending earthquake casualties in Haiti. *(Courtesy Pan America Health Organization.)*

30,000 people died in 2001, assistance agencies struggled for years to help rebuild the more than 300,000 houses that were lost. In the Kashmir earthquake of 2005, 3.3 million persons were left homeless in Pakistan, and many of them were at risk of dying from the winter cold and spread of disease.

The January 2010 Haiti earthquake affected an estimated 3 million people. It killed approximately 100,000 persons and injured approximately 300,000, although estimates of casualties widely vary. More than 1 million Haitians were left homeless. Vital elements of the infrastructure that were necessary for responding to the disaster, including air, sea, and land transport facilities and communication systems, were severely damaged or destroyed. Treatment of the injured was hampered by the lack of hospitals and morgue facilities; bodies were left to decay on the streets for many days. International assistance was offered in abundance, but the logistic capabilities in Haiti for receiving emergency aid were limited. Doubtless, more lives were lost as a result of this vulnerability (Figures 85-4 and 85-5).

Earthquake Risk Reduction Measures

Earthquake warning systems currently in use warn of an earthquake that has already occurred. Examples include those that notify the high-speed trains in Japan, which if derailed would cause hundreds of deaths. One minute before the 2011 Tohoku earthquake was felt in Tokyo, 1000 seismometers sent out warnings that saved many lives. In California, it is technically feasible to develop a system that could warn Los Angeles up to a minute before the arrival of the seismic waves, allowing certain preventive actions, such as taking cover, to occur. However, because predicting the location, time, and magnitude of earthquakes is

still likely many years away, warning systems and earthquake prevention measures are currently not reliable alternatives to preparedness. Preparedness actions include the following:

Locating critical facilities such as hospitals and communications systems in safe locations, as through microzonation.

Creating and enforcing building codes, building earthquake-resistant structures, and retrofitting older buildings: In Afghanistan, many new mud brick homes built by assistance organizations for returnees after 2003 were fitted with economical and relatively simple corner wall and ceiling braces and window lintels that reduced their vulnerability to ground shaking and collapsing roofs (Figure 85-6).

Providing public education about the earthquake risk and ways of personally adjusting to it: Education in the form of drills in schools and government buildings helps to spread the preparedness attitude. People may choose to buy insurance, although it is likely to be expensive due to the high risks. Probably the most effective measures are personal and family plans for protecting lives and property, including exactly what to do when ground shaking begins.

Risk Reduction in China. The 2008 Sichuan earthquake in China, also known as the Great Wenchuan earthquake, resulted in more than 88,000 dead and missing persons, with 4.8 million persons left homeless. The epicenter was near Chengdu city in central China; however, most casualties were in rural towns and villages. Thousands of schoolchildren died due to shoddy school construction, and the giant panda habitat was threatened. Rescue efforts were hindered by high terrains and rainstorms.

The China Earthquake Administration and the other disaster management bodies in China documented lessons with international support in joint publications. These lessons have been incorporated into intensive mitigation measures undertaken by the government nationwide in the aftermath of the earthquake. An example is the European Union–China Disaster Risk Management cooperation, which supports joint training for search and rescue and establishment of protocols and coordination mechanisms.

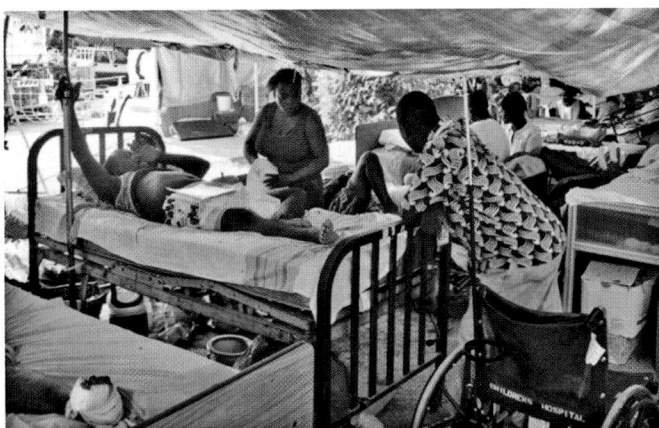

FIGURE 85-5 Makeshift hospital in Haiti. *(Courtesy Pan America Health Organization.)*

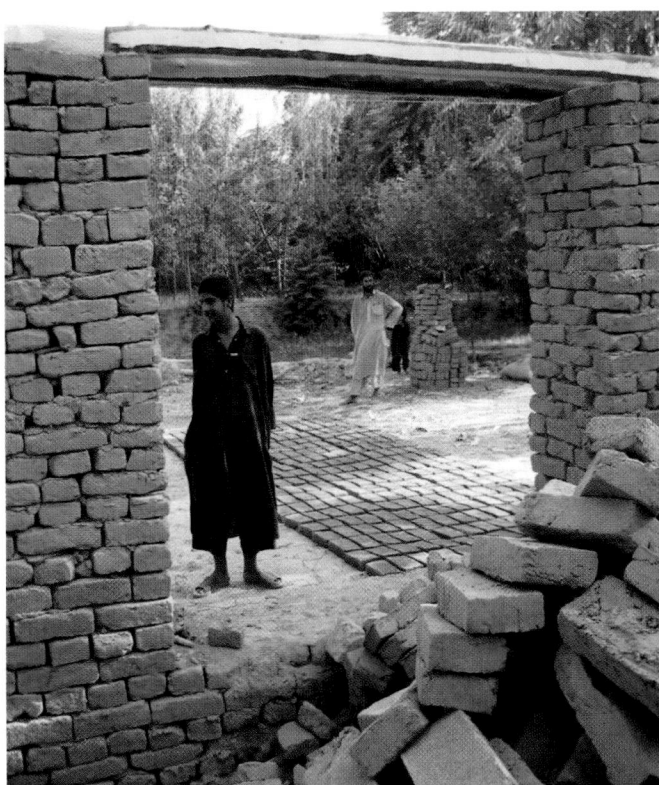

FIGURE 85-6 Earthquake-resistant lintels in Afghanistan. *(Courtesy Sheila B. Reed.)*

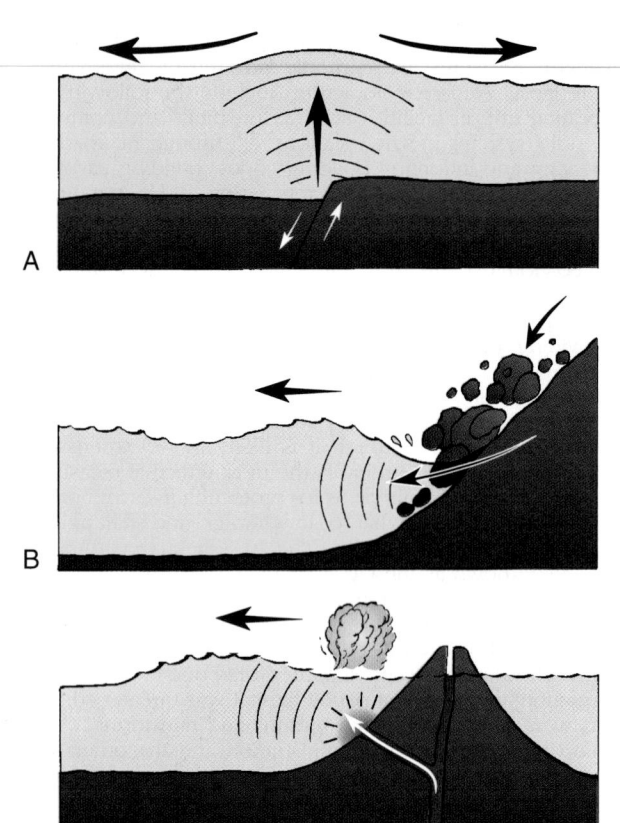

FIGURE 85-7 Tsunamis are produced in three ways. **A,** Fault movement on the sea floor. **B,** Landslide. **C,** Submarine explosion from volcanic eruption.

TSUNAMIS

Tsunami is a Japanese word meaning "harbor wave." Although tsunamis are sometimes called "tidal waves," they are unrelated to the tides. The waves originate from undersea or coastal seismic activity, landslides, and volcanic eruptions. They ultimately encroach over land with great destructive power, often affecting distant shores.

Causal Phenomena and Characteristics

The geologic movements that cause a tsunami are produced in three major ways (Figure 85-7). The foremost cause is fault movement on the sea floor, accompanied by an earthquake. The second most common cause is a landslide occurring underwater or originating above the sea and then plunging into the water. The highest tsunamis ever reported were produced by a landslide at Lituya Bay, Alaska, in 1958. A massive rockslide produced a wave that reached a high-water mark of 530 m (1740 feet) above the shoreline. A third cause of a tsunami is volcanic activity, which may uplift the flank of the volcano or cause an explosion.

Tsunamis differ from ordinary deep ocean waves, which are produced by wind blowing over water. Normal waves are rarely longer than 300 m (984 feet) from crest to crest. Tsunamis, however, may measure 150 km (90 miles) between successive wave crests. Tsunamis also travel much faster than ordinary waves. Compared with the normal wave speed of around 100 km/hr (62 mph), tsunamis in the deep water of the ocean may travel at the speed of a jet airplane—800 km/hr (497 mph). Despite their speed, tsunamis increase the water height only 30 to 45 cm (12 to 18 inches) and often pass unnoticed beneath ships at sea. In 1946, a ship's captain on a vessel lying offshore near Hilo, Hawaii, claimed he could feel no unusual waves beneath him, although he saw them crashing on the shore.

Contrary to popular belief, a tsunami is not a single giant wave. A tsunami can consist of 10 or more waves, termed a *tsunami wave train.* The waves follow each other in 5- to 90-minute intervals. As tsunamis approach the shore, they travel progressively slower. The final wave speed depends on the water depth. Waves in 18 m (59 feet) of water travel about 50 km/hr (31 mph). The shape of the near-shore sea floor influences how tsunami waves behave. Where the shore drops off quickly into deep water, the waves are smaller. Areas with long shallow shelves, such as the major Hawaiian Islands, allow formation of very high waves. In the bays and estuaries, seiches, in which the water sloshes back and forth, can amplify waves to some of the greatest heights ever observed.

On shore, the initial sign of a tsunami depends on what part of the wave first reaches land; a wave crest causes a rise in the water level, and a wave trough causes a recession. The rise may not be significant enough to be noticed by the general public. Observers are more likely to notice the withdrawal of water, which may leave fish floundering on the exposed sea floor. A tsunami does not always appear as a vertical wall of water, known as a *bore,* as is typically portrayed in drawings. More often, the effect is that of an incoming tide that floods the land. Normal waves and swells may ride on top of the tsunami wave, or the tsunami may roll across relatively calm inland waters.

The flooding produced by a tsunami may vary greatly from place to place over a short distance, depending on the submarine topography, shape of the shoreline, reflected waves, and modification of waves by seiches and tides. The Hilo, Hawaii, tsunami of 1946, originating in the Aleutian Trench, produced 18-m (59-foot) waves in one location and waves of only half that height a few miles away. The sequence of the largest wave in the tsunami wave train also varies, and the destructiveness is not always predictable. In 1960 in Hilo, many people returned to their homes after two waves had passed, only to be swallowed up in a giant bore that, in this case, was the third wave.

Predictability

Tsunamis have occurred in all oceans and in the Mediterranean Sea, but the majority of them occur in the Pacific Ocean. The zones stretching from New Zealand through East Asia, the Aleutians, and the western coasts of the Americas all the way to the South Shetland Islands are characterized by deep ocean trenches, explosive volcanic islands, and dynamic mountain ranges.

Prior to 1946, the recorded effects of tsunamis included only local casualties and significant damage. The Tsunami Warning System (TWS) was developed in Hawaii shortly after the 1946 Hilo tsunami and is headquartered in the Pacific Tsunami Warning Center in Honolulu. There are 26 member countries in the Pacific basin. The TWS works by monitoring seismic activity from a network of seismic stations. A tsunami is almost always generated by an undersea earthquake of magnitude 7.0 or greater. Therefore, special warning alarms sound when a quake measuring 6.5 or more occurs anywhere near the Pacific. A tsunami watch is declared if the epicenter is close enough to the ocean to be of concern. Government and voluntary agencies are alerted, and local media are activated to broadcast information. The five nearest tide stations monitor their gauges, and trained observers watch the waves. With positive indicators, a tsunami warning is issued.

The TWS met with general success in saving lives during the tsunamis of 1952 and 1957 in Hawaii. In 1960, however, two major earthquakes occurring a day apart rocked the coast of Chile in South America. The first registered 7.5 on the Richter scale and produced a small but noticeable wave in Hilo Bay. The second registered a stunning 8.5, more than 30 times the energy of the first, and authorities predicted generation of a large, destructive tsunami. When the waves hit Hilo, 15 hours after the earthquake, not all the public had taken the warnings seriously, and 61 people were killed. About 7 hours later, the tsunami struck Japan, killing 180. By the time that information of conditions in Chile reached the TWS, three giant waves had already destroyed villages along an 805-km (500-mile) stretch of coastal South America, arriving only 15 minutes after the earthquake.

Lack of an effective warning system has been blamed for the extensive loss of life from the tsunami generated in the Indian Ocean in December 2004. Over 290,000 people are estimated to have died in 11 countries, and thousands more remain missing. Tsunamis have been relatively rare in the Indian Ocean, and the area has no international warning system. The first tsunami-generated wave crashed into Sumatra only 30 minutes after shaking from the earthquake had subsided. The tsunami ultimately traveled nearly 5000 km (3107 miles) to Africa. In contrast to stronger preparedness levels in the Pacific countries, citizens and tourists were not fully aware of the dangers and many watched from the beach with catastrophic results. In Kobe, Japan, the World Conference on Disaster Reduction in January of 2005 laid the groundwork for the first tsunami warning system in the Indian Ocean, much of which was positioned in recent years. Indonesia has set up costly and sophisticated tsunami warning systems and carried out numerous drills. However, 400 people were killed in an October 2010 tsunami on the Mentawai Islands, indicating that those most at risk are not able to receive warnings through communications systems or cannot flee from a tsunami generated close to shore.

Vulnerability

The following major factors contribute to vulnerability to tsunamis:

A growing world population, increasing urban concentration, and larger investments in the infrastructure, particularly in coastal regions, with some settlements and economic assets in low-lying coastal areas

Lack of tsunami-resistant buildings and site planning

Lack of a warning system or lack of sufficient education for the public to create awareness of the effects of a tsunami

Unpredictable intensity of tsunamis

Typical Adverse Effects

The force of water in a bore, with pressures up to 10,000 kg/m², can raze everything in its path. The flooding from a tsunami, however, affects human settlements most, by water damage to homes, businesses, roads, and infrastructure elements. Withdrawal of the tsunami also causes significant damage. As the water is dragged back toward the sea, bottom sediments are scoured out, causing piers and port facilities to collapse and sweeping out the foundations of buildings. Entire beaches have disappeared, and houses have been carried out to sea. Water levels and currents may change unpredictably, and boats of all sizes may be swamped, sunk, or battered (Figures 85-8 to 85-10). The 2011 Tohoku earthquake generated a major tsunami that struck Sendai, Japan, traveling 10 km (6 miles) inland and precipitating nuclear accidents in the Fukushima Daiichi Nuclear Power Plant. Level-seven meltdowns occurred in three reactors. More than 100,000 persons were evacuated and not able to return

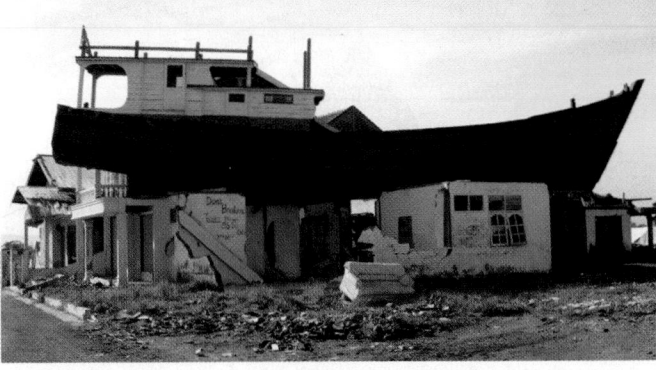

FIGURE 85-9 Boat perched on a house near Banda Aceh, Indonesia, following the December 2004 tsunami. (*Courtesy Sheila B. Reed.*)

to their homes due to continuously leaking radiation. Due to rapid evacuation and quarantine of the meltdown area, no deaths have yet been attributed to this nuclear accident, which was the second most serious on record (after Chernobyl in 1986). The earthquake and tsunami resulted in 15,900 deaths, with 2500 persons still missing. Most deaths were from drowning due to the tsunami, and very few from the earth shaking. Japan's stringent building codes and early warning system effectively stopped high-speed trains and factories; residents received cell phone warning texts.

Casualties and Public Health. Deaths occur principally from drowning as water inundates homes or neighborhoods. Many people may be washed out to sea or crushed by the giant waves. Injuries occur from battering by debris. Little evidence exists of tsunami flooding directly causing large-scale health problems. Rapid effective assistance to the Banda Aceh (Indonesia) area in early 2005 prevented widespread outbreaks of disease in displacement camps (Figure 85-11). Malaria mosquitoes may increase because of water trapped in pools. Open wells and other groundwater may be contaminated by saltwater and debris or sewage. Normal water supplies may be inaccessible for days because of broken water mains.

Crops and Food Supplies. Flooding and damage by tsunami waves may result in the following:

Harvests may be lost, depending on the time of year

Land may be rendered infertile from saltwater incursion from the sea

Food stocks not moved to high ground are damaged

Animals not moved to high ground may perish

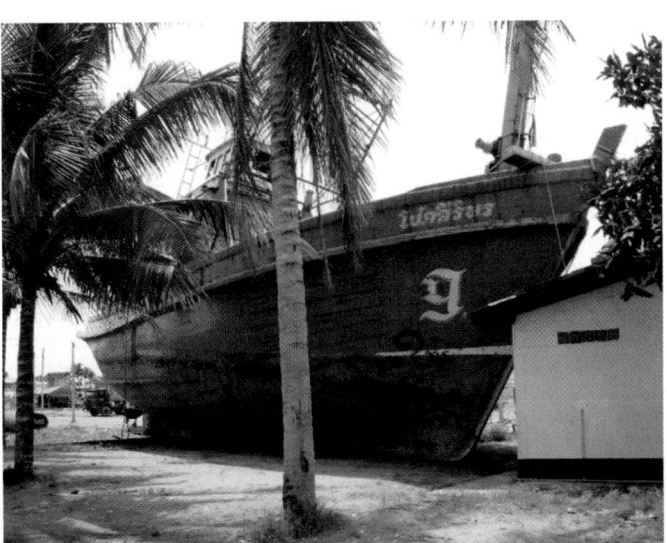

FIGURE 85-8 Ship washed ashore in tsunami, December 2004, in Ko Lanta, Thailand. (*Courtesy Sheila B. Reed.*)

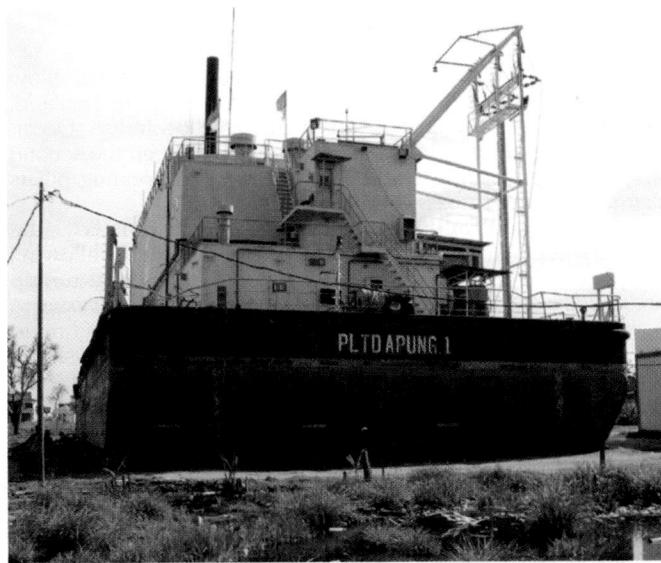

FIGURE 85-10 Generator ship washed ashore 2.3 miles inland, near Banda Aceh, Indonesia. (*Courtesy Sheila B. Reed.*)

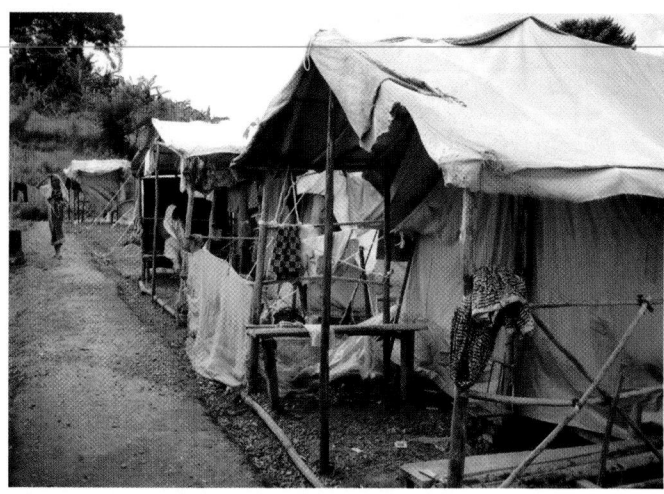

FIGURE 85-11 Displaced people in temporary settlements in Aceh Province, Indonesia. *(Courtesy Sheila B. Reed.)*

Farm implements may be lost, hindering tillage

Boats and fishing nets may be lost

In July 1998, an earthquake of magnitude 7.0 occurred close to the northwest coast of Papua New Guinea. Although the tremor was felt over a large area, no earthquake damage was reported. Only 10 minutes after the quake, however, the first of three 7- to 10-m (23- to 33-foot) waves came ashore in Sandaun Province. The tsunamis struck at high speed after dark and penetrated up to 1 km (over half a mile) inland, totally destroying villages and vegetation along 50 km (31 miles) of the coast. Of the 9000 people affected, more than 2000 died, mainly as a result of being battered by debris as they were swept away by the water.

Tsunami Risk Reduction Measures

Strategies to reduce vulnerability to tsunamis include warning systems, structural design, mapping and land use, and education.

Warning Systems. Tsunami warning systems generally include a network of seismographs to determine the depth and magnitude of submarine and coastal earthquakes, tidal gauges to measure unusual rises and falls in sea level, and a network of sensors connected to floating buoys. The Tsunami Early Warning System (TEWS) in the Indian Ocean and Southeast Asia aims for a comprehensive end-to-end warning system encompassing all aspects of disaster risk reduction.

Structural Design. Tsunamis that are only 1 m high on land can exert physical pressures that cannot be withstood by structures and buildings. Improved design is needed that will allow incursion of water with minimal impact to buildings. In Thailand, new homes for persons displaced in the 2004 Indian Ocean tsunami were designed so that living quarters are on the second floor and the ground floor consists mainly of supporting pillars that allow water to pass through.

Mapping and Land Use. Tsunami run-up maps indicate the possible levels at which a tsunami can travel inland, allowing people to take precautions when they are in a potential run-up area, such as while visiting a beach. Mapping exercises also serve to show the actual damage from a past tsunami, contributing to the understanding of what allowed protection of certain shorelines, such as coastal mangroves or plantation trees. This information contributes to land use planning. Tsunami inundation maps take into consideration potential earthquake sources, factors that will speed or reduce the tsunami, and the probability of a tsunami occurring.

Education. Public education is a major saver of lives because misconceptions regarding tsunamis are likely to place people at greater risk. Lives were saved in Thailand and Indonesia in the 2004 Indian Ocean tsunami because some people recognized that the receding seawater was a warning and urged people to flee rather than stay and watch the waves. Indonesia installed broadcast tower warning systems in Aceh province in 2005 and 2006. Residents in Banda Aceh initially panicked when the alarms sounded, causing chaos on the roadways; some towers were destroyed by angry residents in reaction to false alarms. However, after some practice, families are now more aware of how to act when a tsunami watch or warning is issued. In Japan, warnings for earthquakes and tsunamis are routine and people react appropriately because they know that even false alarms are meant to save lives. The large loss of life in the 2011 Sendai, Japan, tsunami is attributed to the unanticipated power of the earthquake and tsunami, as well as residents having no memory of such a large tsunami. The seawalls in Sendai were only approximately 3 m (9.85 feet) high, but the tsunami rose to more than 40 m (131 feet) in some areas; the presence of the seawalls may have provided a false sense of security such that residents did not see the need to move farther inland.

VOLCANIC ERUPTIONS

A volcano is a vent or chimney to Earth's surface from a reservoir of molten rock, called magma, deep in Earth's crust (see Chapter 17). Approximately 500 volcanoes are active (have erupted in recorded history), and many thousands are dormant (could become active again) or extinct (are not expected to erupt again). On average, about 50 to 60 volcanoes erupt every year; only about 150 are routinely monitored. Since 1000 AD, more than 300,000 people have been killed directly or indirectly by volcanic eruptions, and currently about 10% of the world's population lives on or near potentially dangerous volcanoes. Japan's Mt Fuji and Italy's Mt Vesuvius each pose a threat to well over a million people.

Volcanology, the study of volcanoes, has experienced a period of intensified interest after five major eruptions in the 1980s and early 1990s: Mt St Helens in Washington state in the United States (1980), El Chichón in Mexico (1982), Galunggung in Indonesia (1982), Nevado del Ruiz in Colombia (1985), and Mt Pinatubo in the Philippines (1991). Although the Mt St Helens eruptions were predicted with remarkable accuracy, predictive capability on a worldwide basis for more explosive eruptions has not been achieved. No recognized immediate precursors to the eruption of El Chichón were known. It caused the worst volcanic disaster in Mexico's history and killed approximately 2000 people. In Colombia, despite sufficient warnings, ineffective implementation and evacuation measures resulted in more than 22,000 deaths from the eruption of Nevado del Ruiz. Galunggung erupted for 9 months, disrupting the lives of 600,000 people. Despite a major evacuation effort from Mt Pinatubo, 320 people died, mainly from collapse of ash-covered roofs. A study of these eruptions underscores the importance of predisaster geoscience studies, volcanic hazard assessments, volcano monitoring, contingency planning, and enhanced communications between scientists and authorities. The world's most dangerous volcanoes are in densely populated countries where only limited resources exist to monitor them, such as Mt Nyiragongo in the Democratic Republic of the Congo.

Causal Phenomena

The basic ingredients for a volcanic eruption are magma and an accumulation of gases beneath an active volcanic vent, which may be either on land or below the sea. Magma is composed of silicates containing dissolved gases and sometimes crystallized minerals in a liquid-like suspension. Driven by buoyancy and gas pressure, magma, which is lighter than surrounding rock, forces its way upward. As it reaches the surface, the pressures decrease, enabling the dissolved gases to effervesce, pushing the magma through the volcanic vent as the gases are released.

The chemical and physical composition of magma determines the amount of force with which a volcano erupts. Magmas that are less viscous allow gas to be released more easily. More viscous magma, perhaps containing a greater concentration of solid particles, may confine these gases longer, allowing greater pressures to build up. This greater pressure may lead to more violent eruptions. The structure of the volcano is also a

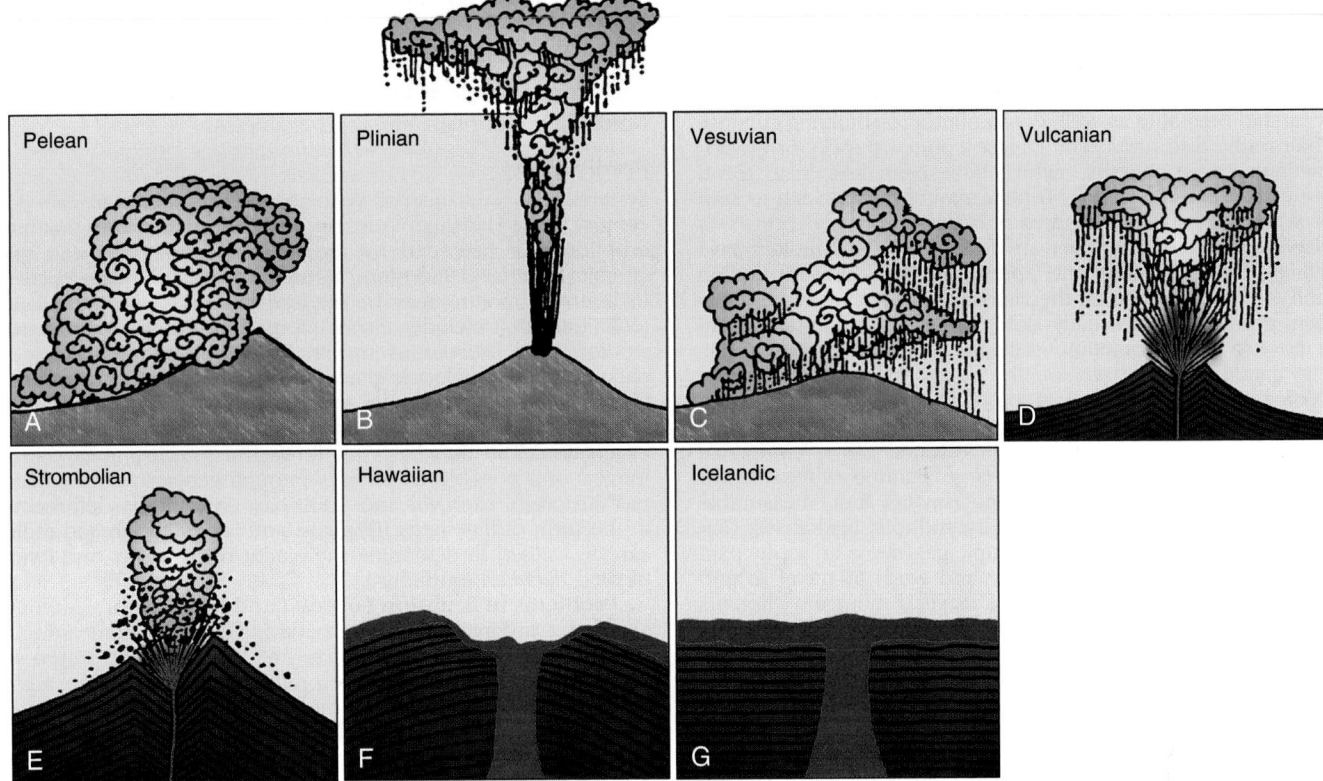

FIGURE 85-12 Eruption types. **A,** Pelean. **B,** Plinian. **C,** Vesuvian. **D,** Vulcanian. **E,** Strombolian. **F,** Hawaiian. **G,** Icelandic. *(Modified from United Nations Development Programme: Introduction to hazards, ed 3, New York, 1997, Disaster Management Training Programme, UN Office for the Coordination of Humanitarian Assistance.)*

determinant of its explosivity. Mt Calbuco in Chile is a stratovolcano that is built up of many layers of lava, and it is also an andesite rock volcano, with lavas containing 50% to 60% silicon dioxide. Calbuco erupted in April 2015 after more than 40 years of dormancy and sent a plume of volcanic ash 10 km (6.2 miles) into the sky. Volcanic eruptions may be described as follows in descending order of intensity (Figure 85-12).

Pelean Eruptions. This is the most disastrous type of eruption. The hardened plug at the volcano's throat forces the magma to blast out through a weak spot in the volcanic flank. The great force of the blast devastates most objects in its path, as occurred in the Mt St Helens eruption of 1980.

Plinian Eruptions. As the pressure on the magma is released, a violent upward expulsion of gas can extend far into the atmosphere. In 1991, Mt Pinatubo sent a plume of tephra 30 km (19 miles) above the surface.

Vesuvian Eruptions. As in the eruption of Mt Vesuvius in Italy in 79 AD, this type is very explosive and occurs infrequently. The explosion of built-up magma discharges a cloud of ash over a wide area.

Vulcanian Eruptions. Lava forms a crust over the volcanic vents between eruptions, building up the volcano. Subsequent eruptions are more violent and eject dense clouds of material. The Paricutin, Mexico, volcano originated in a cornfield in 1943 and eventually covered 260 km² (162 miles). A major eruption occurred in 1947.

Strombolian Eruptions. Gases escape through slow-moving lava in moderate explosions that may be continuous. Volcanic "bombs" of clotted lava may be ejected into the sky, as occurred in the 1965 eruption of Irazu in Costa Rica. Mt Yasur, a Strombolian volcano in Vanuatu, has erupted many times an hour for 800 years and is a major tourist attraction.

Hawaiian Eruptions. The lava is mobile and flows freely. Gases are released quietly, as in the Kilauea, Hawaii, volcano, which has continued to erupt since 1983.

Icelandic Eruptions. Similar to the Hawaiian type, lava flows from deep fissures and forms sheets spreading out in all directions, as in the Laki, Iceland, eruption of 1783.

Characteristics

No international scale exists to measure the size of volcanic eruptions. The volcanic explosivity index estimates the energy released in a volcanic eruption, based on measurements of the ejected matter, height of the eruption cloud, and other observations. The volcanic explosivity index scale ranges from 0 to 8. The largest eruption recorded was the Tambora volcano in Indonesia in 1815, which had a volcanic explosivity index of 7.

The primary volcanic hazards are associated with products of the eruption: pyroclastic flows, air-fall tephra, lava flows, and volcanic gases. The most destructive secondary hazards include lahars, landslides, and tsunamis.

Pyroclastic Flows. Pyroclastic (meaning "fire-broken" in Greek) flows are the most dangerous of all volcanic phenomena because there is virtually no defense against them. They are horizontally directed explosions or blasts of gas containing ash and larger fragments in suspension. They travel at great speed and burn everything in their path. The flows move like a snow or rock avalanche because they contain a heavy load of dust and lava fragments that are denser than the surrounding air. Gas continues to be released as they travel, creating a continuously expanding cloud.

Pyroclastic flows are responsible for the majority of deaths associated with volcanic eruptions. The pyroclastic flows from the Mt St Helens eruption in 1980 moved at rates up to 870 km/hr (541 mph), and pyroclastic deposits found 2 days after the blast at the foot of the mountain registered temperatures of more than 700° C (1292° F). The greatest distance recorded of such flows in historical times is 35 km (22 miles).

Air-Fall Tephra. Tephra smaller than 2 mm is classified as ash. Almost all volcanoes emit ash, but emissions vary widely in volume and intensity. Heavy ashfalls can cause complete darkness or drastically reduce visibility. Fine material from great eruptions may travel around the world and affect the world climate. Clouds of dust and ash can remain in the air for days or weeks and spread over large distances, causing difficulty in driving and breathing as well as contributing to building collapse and air traffic disruption. The largest tephra are rocks or blocks, sometimes called "bombs," which have been known to travel more than 4 km (2.5 miles). Tephra may be hot enough to start fires when it lands on structures or vegetation.

Lava Flows. Lava flows are formed by hot, molten lava flowing from a volcano and spreading over the surrounding countryside. Depending on the viscosity, a flow may move a few meters per hour. It is usually slow enough that living creatures can move to safety. Sometimes the edges break off, causing small, hot avalanches.

Volcanic Gases. Gas is a product of every eruption and may also be emitted by the volcano during periods of inactivity, either intermittently or continually. Volcanic gas is composed mostly of steam. Often present are large amounts of toxic sulfur dioxide and hydrogen sulfide and smaller but measurable amounts of toxic hydrochloric and hydrofluoric acid gases. CO_2 is often a major component of volcanic gas and is an asphyxiant because it is much denser than air and tends to travel to and through low-lying areas and valleys. Several mountain climbers and skiers in Japan were overcome by hydrogen sulfide fumes in a valley near the Kusatsu-Shirane volcano, and eventually an alarm system was installed. In 1986, approximately 1800 people were asphyxiated by gas bursts from crater lakes in Cameroon.

Lahars and Landslides. Enormous quantities of ash and larger fragments (tephra) accumulate after an eruption on the steep slopes of a volcano, sometimes to a depth of several meters. When mixed with water, the volcanic debris is transformed into a material resembling wet concrete that flows easily downhill. *Lahar* is an Indonesian word for debris flows or mudflows. A primary debris flow is caused by eruptive activity, such as melting of snow and ice by hot volcanic materials, and a secondary debris flow results when heavy rainfall saturates the deposits.

The rate of flow is affected by its viscosity, volume of mud and debris, and slope and character of the terrain. The velocity may reach 100 km/hr (62 mph), and distance traveled may exceed 100 km (62 miles). Mudflows and debris flows can be very destructive. They have buried entire towns, such as Armero, Colombia. They can silt up waterways, causing floods and changing river courses.

Landslides and debris avalanches are common where stress from intruding magma causes fractures along cracks in the volcano. Ground deformation from swelling and hardening of volcanic material can produce landslides.

Tsunamis. Tsunamis, described previously, are generated by movement of the ocean floor, possibly caused by a volcano. In a study of volcanic eruptions in the past 1000 years, human fatalities resulting from indirect tsunami wave hazards were as significant as those from pyroclastic flows and primary mudflows.

Location

The distribution of volcanoes, as with earthquakes, is determined by the location of geologic forces involving the tectonic or crustal plates. About 80% of the active volcanoes are located near subduction boundaries. Subduction volcanoes occur where denser crustal plates are shoved beneath less dense continental plates, which occurs in most of the Pacific Ocean, especially in the area along the rim, known as the Pacific Ring of Fire. Subduction volcanoes are found in the United States in the Cascade Range of the Pacific Northwest and further north in the Aleutian Islands off Alaska. The ring of subduction volcanoes continues along the Aleutian Trench to Japan, stretching south to the Philippines and Indonesia. Many volcanoes are located beneath the ocean, and submarine eruptions may cause tsunamis and other effects.

Rift volcanoes occur at divergent zones where two distinct plates are slowly being separated, in areas such as Iceland and East Africa; they account for about 15% of active volcanoes. Hot

spot volcanoes are located where crustal weaknesses allow molten material to penetrate, but not necessarily on the plate boundaries. These isolated regions of volcanic activity exist in about 100 places in the world. The Hawaiian Islands, in the middle of the Pacific plate, and Yellowstone Park, within the North American plate, are good examples.

Predictability

Systematic surveillance of volcanoes, begun early in the 20th century at the Hawaiian Volcano Observatory, indicates that most eruptions are preceded by measurable geophysical and geochemical changes. Short-term forecasts of future volcanic activity in hours or months may be made through volcano monitoring techniques that include seismic monitoring, ground deformation studies, and observations and recordings of hydrothermal, geochemical, and geoelectric changes. By carefully monitoring these factors, scientists were able to issue a high-confidence forecast of the 1991 Mt Pinatubo eruption, allowing a largely successful evacuation. The best basis for long-term forecasting (a year or longer) of a possible eruption is through geologic studies of the past history of each volcano. Each past eruption has left records in the form of lava beds. Deposits and layers of ash and tephra can be studied to determine the extent of the flows and length of time between eruptions.

Problems in Eruption Forecast and Prediction. Although significant progress has been made in long-term forecasting of volcanic eruptions, monitoring techniques have not progressed to the point of yielding precise predictions. For the purposes of warning the public and avoiding false alarms that create distrust and chaos, ideal predictions should provide precise information concerning the place, time, type, and magnitude of the eruption. The importance of enhanced communications between scientists and authorities is also emphasized. Despite sufficient warning, evacuation orders were not issued by local authorities, which resulted in more than 22,000 deaths from lahars produced by Nevado del Ruiz. The eruption of Mt St Helens was adequately monitored and forecasted, but the main explosion still surprised authorities because the volcano did not exhibit expected signs before eruption and because the blast was lateral rather than vertical; 57 people who remained in the danger area were killed. In the past decade, Iceland, which is home to 35 active volcanoes, has been able to successfully forecast approximately two-thirds of eruptions.

The greatest constraint to predictability is lack of baseline monitoring studies, which depict the full range of characteristics of the volcano. Accumulating baseline data may require study of the volcanic activity over thousands of years. Interpretation of baseline data enables differentiation of the precursory pattern of an actual eruption from other volcanic activity, such as intrusion of magma under the surface, which is sometimes termed an *aborted eruption*. Before the 1982 eruption of El Chichón, virtually nothing was known of its history of frequent and violent eruptions. No monitoring was conducted before or during the brief eruption.

Developing countries suffer the greatest economic losses from volcanic eruptions. More than 99% of deaths caused by an eruption since 1900 have been in developing countries. Because of shortages of funds and trained personnel, monitoring is also poorest in these countries.

Vulnerability

Rich volcanic soils and scenic terrains attract people to settle on the flanks of volcanoes. These people are more vulnerable if they live downwind from the volcano, in the path of historical channels for mudflows or lava flows, or close to waterways likely to flood because of silting. Structures with roof designs that do not resist ash accumulation are vulnerable even miles from a volcano. All combustible materials are at risk.

Typical Adverse Effects

Casualties and Health. Deaths can be expected from pyroclastic flows and mudflows and to a much lesser extent from lava flows and toxic gases. Injuries may occur from the impact of falling rock fragments and from being buried in mud. Burns to the skin, breathing passages, and lungs may result from exposure to steam and hot dust clouds. Ashfall and toxic gases may cause respiratory difficulties for people and animals. Nontoxic gases of densities greater than air, such as CO_2, can be dangerous when they collect in low-lying areas. Water supplies contaminated with ash may contain toxic chemicals and cause illness. Deaths have also occurred indirectly from starvation and from tsunamis.

Settlements, Infrastructure, and Agriculture. Complete destruction of everything in the path of pyroclastic or lava flows should be expected, including vegetation, agricultural land, human settlements, structures, and bridges, roads, and other elements of infrastructure. Structures may collapse under the weight of ash, particularly if the ash is wet. Falling ash may be hot enough to cause fires. Flooding may result from waterways filling up with volcanic deposits or from melting of large amounts of snow or glacial ice. Rivers may change course because of oversilting. Ashfall can destroy mechanical systems by clogging openings, such as those in irrigation systems and airplane and other engines. Communication systems could be disrupted by electrical storms developing in the ash clouds. Transportation by air, land, and sea may be affected. Disruption in air traffic from large ash eruptions can have serious effects on an emergency response.

Crops in the path of flows are destroyed, and ashfall may render agricultural land temporarily unusable. Heavy ash loads may break the branches of fruit or nut trees. Livestock may inhale toxic gases or ash. Ash containing toxic chemicals, such as fluorine, may contaminate grazing lands.

The Caribbean island of Montserrat has undergone volcanic activity for years. In June 1997, the famous Soufrière Hills volcano erupted, causing at least nine deaths. The resulting pyroclastic flows buried and destroyed seven villages. Only one-third of the island is now considered relatively safe. In 2002, in the Democratic Republic of the Congo, lava poured from the Nyiragongo volcano, devastating the city of Goma and forcing 300,000 to flee, some crossing the border into Rwanda. A multi-donor funded observatory was ultimately established to monitor the volcano, which emits 12,000 to 50,000 metric tons of sulfur dioxide each day.

Volcanic Eruption Risk Reduction Measures

Strengthening forecasting, initiation or expansion of volcanic monitoring, creation of emergency response plans, and establishment of effective communications and warning systems are the most effective measures to reduce the risk from volcanic hazards. As the description in the next section indicates, people may not fully accept the validity of warnings because of their own perceptions of the likelihood of hazards and adverse effects. Even those who accept the warnings may be willing to take risks to guard their livelihoods, homes, and possessions.

Despite Precautions, People Took High Risks in the Mt Merapi Eruption. The greatest population densities in Indonesia occur in the region south and east of Mt Merapi in central Java, where the soil is enriched by volcanic ash and debris. Institutionalized monitoring of volcanic activity has been ongoing since 1920. Evacuation alerts can be issued when telemetered rain gauges and radar installations at Merapi show that rainfall intensity and duration have reached a critical threshold known to trigger lahars. Preparedness measures for the Mt Merapi volcanic area have been cited as examples of good practice. These include evacuation maps, provincial and district disaster management teams (including subdistrict military units and police units), and other response organizations such as nongovernmental organizations. Evacuation routes to shelters in safe areas are clearly marked, and global positioning system coordinates are available for the evacuation area, health facilities, and warning towers. In 2006, as a response to the escalating alert levels for volcanic activity on Mt Merapi, local authorities in Yogyakarta and Central Java took steps to prepare the people at risk, warned vulnerable families to be vigilant, and asked some to move to safer areas; 20,000 people were evacuated. However, there was reluctance on the parts of some to leave their homes until the Alert 4, Code Red (signifying compulsory evacuation) was issued, because they feared losing livestock and belongings.

Beginning in mid-September of 2010, seismic activity increased, culminating in repeated outbursts of lava and ashes. In late October, eruptions became increasingly violent and continued into November. Large eruption columns formed, causing numerous pyroclastic flows down the heavily populated slopes of the volcano. Merapi's eruption was said by authorities to be the largest since the 1870s. More than 350,000 people were evacuated from the affected area. However, many persons remained behind or returned to their homes while the eruptions were continuing; 353 people were killed during the eruptions, many as a result of pyroclastic flows. The mountain continued to erupt until November 30, 2010. On December 3, 2010, the official alert status was reduced from Alert 4 to Alert 3 because the eruptive activity had subsided.

LANDSLIDES

Landslides are a major threat each year to human settlements and infrastructure elements. *Landslide* is a general term covering a wide variety of landforms and processes involving the downslope movement of soil and rock. Although landslides may occur with earthquakes, floods, and volcanoes, they are much more widespread and over time cause more property loss than any other geologic event.

Causal Phenomena

Landslides result from sudden or gradual changes in the composition, structure, hydrology, or vegetation of a slope. These changes may be natural or caused by humans, and they disturb the equilibrium of the slope's materials. A landslide occurs when the strength of the material in the slope is exceeded by the downslope stress. The resistance in a slope may be reduced by the following:

Increase in water content, caused by heavy rainfall or rising groundwater

Increase in slope angle, for new construction or by stream erosion

Breakdown or alteration of slope materials, from weathering and other natural processes, placement of underground piping for utilities, or use of landfill

Downslope stress may be caused by the following:

Vibrations from earthquakes (triggering some of the most disastrous landslides), blasting, machinery, traffic, or thunder

Removal of lateral support by previous slope failure, construction, or excavation

Removal of vegetation by fires, logging, overgrazing, or deforestation that causes loosening of soil particles and erosion

Loading with weight from rain, hail, snow, accumulation of loose rock or volcanic material, weight of buildings, or seepage from irrigation and sewage systems

Characteristics

Landslides usually occur as secondary effects of heavy storms, earthquakes, and volcanic eruptions. However, mining caused the largest nonvolcanic landslide in North American history at the Bingham Canyon Mine in Utah in 2013. The materials involved in landslides are divided into two classes: bedrock and soil (earth and organic matter debris). A landslide may be classified by its type of movement (Figure 85-13).

Falls. A fall is a mass of rock or other material that moves downward by falling or bouncing through the air. These are most common along steep road or railroad embankments, steep escarpments, or steeply undercut cliffs, especially in coastal areas. Large individual boulders can cause significant damage.

Slides. Resulting from shear failure (slippage) along one or several surfaces, the slide material may remain intact or break up. In 2010, a mudslide caused by heavy rains in Gansu, China, resulted in more than 1400 deaths.

Topples. A topple is caused by overturning forces that rotate a rock out of its original position. The rock section may have settled at a precarious angle, balancing itself on a pivotal point from which it tilts or rotates forward. A topple may not

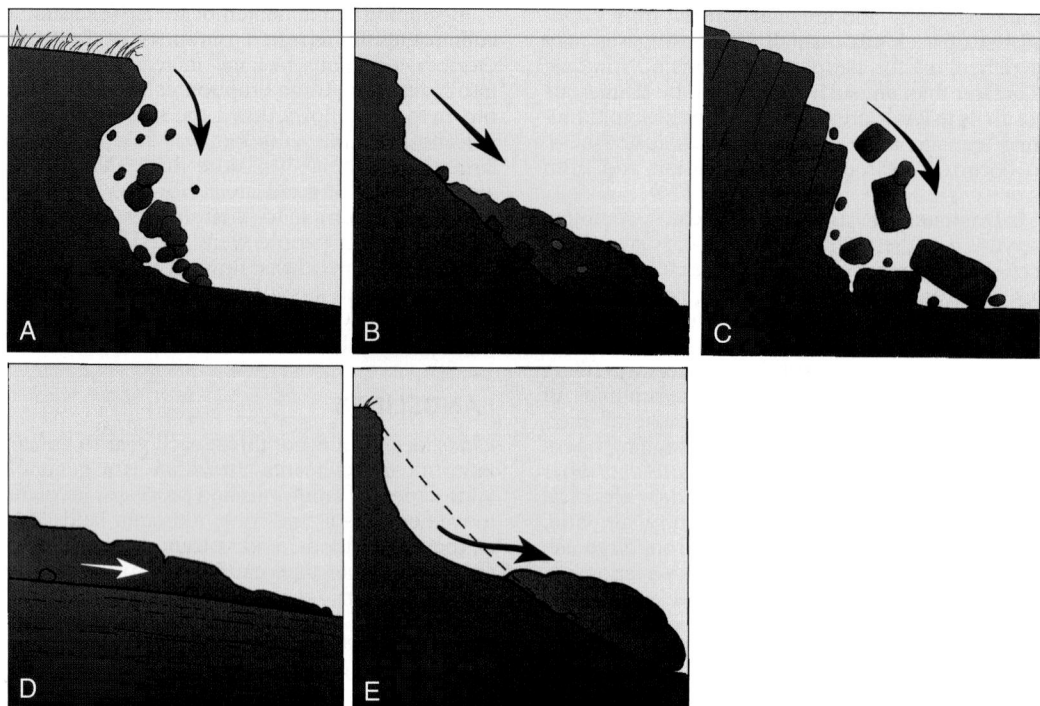

FIGURE 85-13 Landslides classified by type of movement. **A**, Fall. **B**, Slide. **C**, Topple. **D**, Lateral spread. **E**, Flow.

involve much movement, and it does not necessarily trigger a rockfall or rockslide.

Lateral Spreads. Large blocks of soil spread out horizontally by fracturing off the original base. Lateral spreads generally occur on gentle slopes, usually less than 6%, and typically spread 3 to 5 m (10 to 16 feet), but may move from 30 to 50 m (100 to 160 feet) where conditions are favorable. Lateral spreads usually break up internally and form numerous fissures and scarps. The process can be caused by liquefaction, in which saturated loose sands or silts assume a liquefied state. A lateral spread is usually triggered by ground shaking (as with an earthquake). During the 1964 Alaskan earthquake, more than 200 bridges were damaged or destroyed by lateral spreading of floodplain deposits near river channels.

Flows. Flows move as a viscous fluid, sometimes very rapidly, and can cover several miles. Water is not essential for flows to occur; however, most flows form after periods of heavy rainfall. A *mudflow* contains at least 50% sand, silt, and clay particles. A *lahar* is a mudflow that originates on the slope of a volcano and may be triggered by rainfall, sudden melting of snow or glaciers, or water flowing from crater lakes. A *debris flow* is a slurry of soils, rocks, and organic matter combined with air and water. Debris flows usually occur on steep gullies. Very slow, almost imperceptible flows of soil and bedrock are called *creeps.* Over long periods, creeps may cause telephone poles or other objects to tilt downhill.

Casualties. Catastrophic landslides have killed many thousands of persons, such as the debris slide on the slopes of Huascaran in Peru triggered by an earthquake in 1970, which killed more than 18,000 people. In January 1989, only 6 weeks after an earthquake killed 25,000 people in Armenia, another quake struck the Republic of Tajikistan, 50 km (31 miles) southwest of the capital city of Dushanbe. This quake registered 5.8 on the Richter scale. The earthquake triggered a landslide of hillside soils that had become wet with melted snow. The liquefied soil spilled downhill and eventually covered an area about 8 km (5 miles) long and 1 km (0.6 of a mile) wide. The total volume of mud was more than 10 million m³. The epicenter of the earthquake was located in the village of Sharora. This village and several others were engulfed with mud that killed 200 persons and left 30,000 homeless. Mud deposits reached a height

of 25 m (82 feet) in Sharora, causing rescue efforts to be abandoned. The area was later declared a national monument. The world's largest historic landslide occurred during the 1980 volcanic eruption of Mt St Helens. The volume of material was 2.8 km³.

Recent large-scale landslides (and their causes and characteristics) have included Leyte, Philippines, in 2006 (rockslide and debris avalanche from heavy rains; 1100 deaths); Sichuan, China, in 2008 (Wenchuan earthquake, magnitude 8.0; 15,000 landslides and 20,000 deaths from landslides); East Cairo, Egypt, al-Duwayqa rockslide in 2008 (destabilization due to human-made construction and temperature regime changes; 107 deaths and 400 persons missing); Bududa, Uganda, in 2010 (debris flows after heavy rains: more than 400 deaths and 200,000 displaced persons); and Rio de Janeiro, Brazil, in 2010 (debris flows from heavy rainfall; 350 deaths). A tragic outcome occurred when the 2013 North India floods resulted in massive debris flow landslides that killed people trapped in houses by flood waters. Entire villages disappeared and more than 5000 people perished, mainly in Uttarakhand. Heavy rains in 2014 in Hiroshima prefecture caused the deadliest landslides in 42 years in Japan . In these two cases, the public did not receive timely warnings to avert casualties.

Predictability

The velocity of landslides varies from extremely slow (< 0.06 m/year) to extremely fast (> 3 m/sec), which might imply a similar variation in predictability. In absolute terms, however, predicting the actual occurrence of a landslide is extremely difficult, although situations of high risk, such as forecasted heavy rainfall or seismic activity combined with landslide susceptibility, may lead to estimation of a time frame and possible consequences.

Estimation of landslide hazard potential includes historical information on the geology, geomorphology (study of landforms), hydrology, and vegetation of a specific area. Structural features that may affect stability include sequence and type of layering, lithologic changes, planes, joints, faults, and folds. The most important geomorphologic consideration in prediction of landslides is the history of landslides in a given area.

The source, movement, amount of water, and water pressure must be studied. Climatic patterns combined with soil type may cause different types of landslides. For example, when monsoons occur in tropical regions, large debris slides of soils, rocks, and

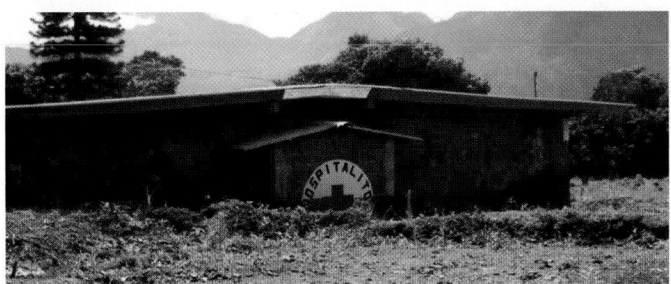

FIGURE 85-14 Former hospital in Santiago Atitlán, Guatemala, buried during mudslide. *(Courtesy Paul S. Auerbach, MD.)*

organic matter may occur. Plant cover on slopes may have either a positive or negative stabilizing effect. Roots may decrease water runoff and increase soil cohesion; conversely, they may widen fractures in rock surfaces and promote infiltration. In Nepal in 2002, a heavy monsoon season caused flooding and landslides, killing 500 people. The vulnerability to landslides was increased by the proximity of most communities to slopes and the poor quality of housing. A tragic slide in Santiago Atitlán, Guatemala, which partially buried its hospital and killed hundreds of people, on October 5, 2005 (Figure 85-14) was caused by torrential rains from Hurricane Stan combined with vulnerability of the location on the slopes of a volcano. Landslides may be expected to increase in number with other impacts of climate change. Along with more intense and extreme rainfall, the growth in population in many developing countries may increase the numbers of casualties related to landslides.

Vulnerability

Settlements built on steep slopes, in weak soils, on cliff tops, at the base of steep slopes, on alluvial outwash fans, or at the mouth of streams emerging from mountain valleys are all vulnerable. Roads and communication lines through mountainous areas are in danger. In most types of landslides, damage may occur to buildings even if foundations have been strengthened. Infrastructural elements, such as buried utility lines or brittle pipes, are vulnerable. The province of Badakhshan in Afghanistan is becoming more vulnerable to landslides and mudslides, especially during the winter snowmelts, due to increasing deforestation. Impoverished communities suffered deadly mudslides in 2014 and 2015.

Typical Adverse Effects

Anything on top of or in the path of a landslide will be severely damaged or destroyed. In addition, rubble may damage lines of communication or block roadways. Waterways may be blocked, creating a flood risk. Casualties may not be widespread, except in the case of massive movements caused by major hazards such as earthquakes and volcanoes.

In addition to direct damage from a landslide, indirect effects include loss of productivity of agricultural or forestlands (if buried), reduced real estate values in high-risk areas and lost tax revenues from these devaluations, adverse effects on water quality in streams and irrigation facilities, and secondary physical effects, such as flooding.

Fatalities have resulted from slope failure in cases where population pressure has prompted settlement in areas vulnerable to landslides. Casualties may be caused by collapse of buildings or burial by landslide debris. Worldwide, approximately 600 deaths occur per year, mainly in the circum-Pacific region. The estimate for loss of life in the United States is 25 to 50 lives per year, greater than the average loss from earthquakes.

Landslide Risk Reduction Measures

Landslide management is a well-developed science in many countries. Landslides can be mitigated where sufficient resources are available. Basic reduction measures include terrain mapping, susceptibility analysis, stability analysis, and monitoring and warning systems. Warning systems include (1) sensors placed on a possible landslide path, (2) calculation of the stability of a slope

and monitoring of the groundwater level, and (3) detection of early stages of landslide movement using sensors and inclinometers that generate detailed data sets. One major challenge is finding effective ways to manage landslides in developing countries. A further challenge centers on the fact that landslide risk mitigation may need to take into consideration changing environmental conditions, for example, looking more critically at areas underfilled with potentially degrading permafrost and the possibility of increased sediment loads and channel instability in rivers.

CLIMATIC HAZARDS
TROPICAL CYCLONES

The World Meteorological Organization (WMO) uses the generic term *tropical cyclone* to cover weather systems in which winds exceed gale force (minimum of 34 knots or 63 km/hr). Tropical cyclones are rotating, organized systems of clouds and thunderstorms with intense low-pressure circulation, originating over tropical or subtropical waters. Winds of hurricane force (63 knots or 117 km/hr) mark the most severe type. They are called hurricanes in the Caribbean region, the United States, Central America, and parts of the Pacific; typhoons in the northwestern Pacific and eastern Asia; severe cyclonic storms in the Bay of Bengal; and severe tropical cyclones in southern Indian, South Pacific, and Australian waters. For easy identification and tracking, the storms are generally given alternating masculine and feminine names or numbers that identify the year and annual sequence.

Tropical cyclones are the most devastating of seasonally recurring rapid-onset natural hazards. Between 80 and 100 tropical cyclones occur around the world each year. Devastation by violent winds, torrential rainfall, and accompanying phenomena, including storm surges and floods, can lead to massive community disruption. Official death and damage records for tropical cyclones include thousands of individual events. In Bangladesh alone, the deadliest tropical cyclone on record, Cyclone Bhola in 1970, killed between 300,000 and 500,000 people, although the exact death toll will never be known. Also in Bangladesh, deaths were recorded at 140,000 persons near Chittagong in 1991, and 3500 persons died in Cyclone Sidr in 2007. In the United States, damages approached $10 billion from Hurricane Gilbert (1988) and Hurricane Hugo (1989). Damages from Hurricane Andrew in Florida and Louisiana in 1992 totaled $16 billion. Hurricane Katrina, in August 2005, killed 1417 people in three states and caused $75 billion in damages.

In 2008, Cyclone Nargis struck Burma (Myanmar), killing more than 145,000 people, devastated the delta, which is the "rice basket" of the country, and destroyed the country's former capital and largest city, Yangon. Cyclone Nargis set several records: deadliest natural disaster in Burmese history, costliest cyclone originating in the north Indian Ocean on record, and second-deadliest northern Indian Ocean cyclone in recorded history.

Causal Phenomena

The development cycle of tropical cyclones may be divided into three stages: formation and initial development, full maturity, and modification or decay. Depending on their tracks over the warm tropical seas and proximity to land, tropical cyclones may last from less than 24 hours to more than 3 weeks (the average duration is about 6 days). Their tracks are naturally erratic but initially move generally westward and then progressively poleward into higher latitudes, where they may make landfall, or into an easterly direction as they lose their cyclonic structure.

Formation and Initial Development Stage. Four atmospheric and oceanic conditions are necessary for development of a cyclonic storm (Figure 85-15):

A warm sea temperature (> 26°C [78.8°F] to a depth of 60 m [197 feet]) provides abundant water vapor in the air by evaporation.

High relative humidity (degree to which the air is saturated by water vapor) of the atmosphere to a height of about

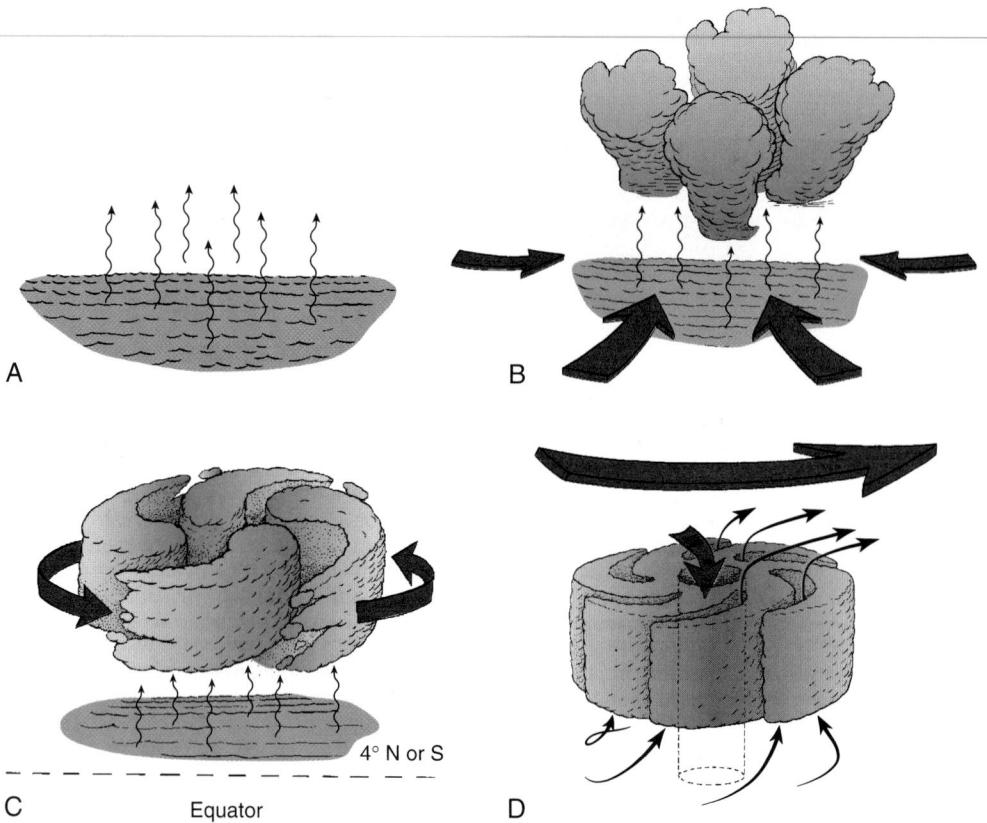

FIGURE 85-15 Cyclone formation. **A,** Warm seas (> 26°C [78.8°F]) cause rising humid air. **B,** Cooler high-altitude temperatures cause formation of cumulonimbus clouds. The surrounding air moves toward the central low-pressure area. **C,** Cumulonimbus clouds form into spiraling bands. The Coriolis effect causes winds to swirl around the central low-pressure area. **D,** High altitude dispels the top of the cyclonic air system. Dry high-altitude air flows down the "eye." Hurricane force winds circle around the eye.

7000 m (23,000 feet) facilitates condensation of water vapor into water droplets and clouds, releases heat energy, and induces a drop in barometric pressure.

Atmospheric instability (an above-average decrease of temperature with altitude) encourages considerable vertical cumulus cloud convection when condensation of rising air occurs.

A location of at least 4 to 5 latitude degrees from the equator allows the influence of Earth's rotational force to take effect (Coriolis effect) and induces cyclonic wind circulation around a low-pressure center.

The atmosphere can usually organize itself into a tropical cyclone in 2 to 4 days. This process is characterized by increasing thunderstorms and rain squalls at sea. Meteorologists can monitor these processes with weather satellites and radar from as far as 645 m (400 miles) away from the storm. The existence of favorable conditions for cyclone development determines the cyclone season for each monitoring center. In the Indian and south Asian region, the season is divided into two periods, from April to early June and from October to early December. In the Caribbean region and United States, tropical storms and hurricanes reach their peak strengths in middle to late summer. In the Southern Hemisphere, the cyclone season extends from November to April or May, but occasionally cyclones occur in other months in lower latitudes.

Maturity Stage. As viewed by weather satellites and radar imagery, the main physical feature of a mature tropical cyclone is a spiral pattern of highly turbulent, giant cumulus thundercloud bands. These bands spiral inward and form a dense, highly active central cloud core that wraps around a relatively calm and cloud-free "eye." The eye, where light winds occur, typically has a diameter of 20 to 60 km (12 to 37 miles) and appears as a black hole or dot surrounded by white clouds.

In contrast to the light wind conditions in the eye, the turbulent cloud formations extending outward from the eye accompany winds of up to 250 km/hr (155 mph), sufficient to destroy or severely damage most nonengineered structures in the affected communities. These strong winds are caused by a horizontal temperature gradient that exists between the warm core of the cyclone (up to 10°C [18°F] higher than the external environment) and the surrounding areas, resulting in a correspondingly high gradient of pressure.

Decay Stage. A tropical cyclone begins to weaken, in terms of its central low pressure, internal warm core, and extremely high winds, as soon as its sources of warm moist air begin to ebb or are abruptly cut off. This would occur during landfall, by movement into higher latitudes, or through influence of another low-pressure system. The weakening of a cyclone does not mean that danger to life and property is over. When the cyclone hits land, especially over mountainous or hilly terrain, widespread riverine and flash flooding may last for weeks. The energy from a weakening tropical cyclone may be reorganized into a less concentrated but more extensive storm system, causing widespread violent weather.

Characteristics

Tropical cyclones are characterized by their destructive winds, storm surges, and exceptional level of rainfall, which may cause flooding.

Destructive Winds. The strong winds generated by a tropical cyclone circulate clockwise in the Southern Hemisphere and counterclockwise in the Northern Hemisphere, while spiraling inward and increasing toward the cyclone center. In the Northern Hemisphere, the storms are classified as tropical depressions (maximum sustained winds of 61 km [38 miles] per hour); tropical storms (63 to 117 km [39 to 73 miles] per hour); hurricanes

(119 km [74 miles] per hour or higher); and major hurricanes (179 km [111 miles] per hour or higher).

Wind speeds progressively increase toward the core as follows:

150 to 300 km (93 to 186 miles) from the center of a typical mature cyclone, winds of 63 to 88 km/hr (39 to 54.7 mph)

100 to 150 km (62 to 93 miles) from the center, storm force winds of 89 to 117 km/hr (55 to 73 mph)

50 to 100 km (31 to 62 miles) from the center, winds in excess of hurricane force, 117 km/hr (73 mph) or greater

20 to 50 km (12 to 31 miles) from the center, the edge of the inner core containing winds 250 km/hr (155 mph) or greater

As the eye arrives, winds fall off to become almost calm, but they rise again just as quickly as the eye passes and are replaced by hurricane force winds from a direction nearly the reverse of those previously blowing.

The Beaufort scale is used to classify the intensity of the storms. It estimates the wind velocity by observations of the effects of winds on the ocean surface and familiar objects. Both the United States (Saffir-Simpson Hurricane Scale; Box 85-2) and Australia (Cyclone Severity Categories) use country-specific scales that estimate potential property damage in five categories. The Philippines has increased its typhoon warning signal numbers from three ranges of wind speeds to four in order to take into account the lower standards of building structures and regional variations. Typhoon Haiyan, known in the Philippines as Typhoon Yolanda, was one of the strongest tropical cyclones ever recorded, killing at least 6300 persons in November 2013; it was the strongest at landfall and in terms of 1-minute sustained wind speed. It was assessed as a Category 5 Super Typhoon on the Saffir-Simpson scale, making six landfalls in the Philippines before exiting into the South China Sea. It subsequently struck Vietnam as a severe tropical storm.

Storm Surges. The *storm surge,* defined as the rise in sea level above the normally predicted astronomic tide, is frequently a key or overriding factor in a tropical storm disaster. As the cyclone approaches the coast, the friction of strong onshore winds on the sea surface, in combination with the "suction effect" of reduced atmospheric pressure, can pile up seawater along a coastline near a cyclone's landfall well above the predicted tide level for that time. In cyclones of moderate intensity, the effect is generally limited to several meters, but exceptionally intense cyclones can cause storm surges up to 8 m (26 feet).

Of the countries experiencing cyclonic storms, those most vulnerable to storm surges are characterized by low-lying land along the closed and semienclosed bays facing the ocean. These countries include Bangladesh, China, India, Japan, Mexico, the United States, and Australia. Most of the casualties from the 1970 Bhola cyclone occurred from drowning in the storm surge. Prevailing onshore winds and low pressures from winter depressions in nontropical latitudes, as in countries bordering the North Sea, are also subject to storm surges that require substantial mitigation measures, such as dikes.

Rainfall Events. The world's highest rainfall totals over 1 to 2 days have occurred during tropical cyclones. The highest 12- and 24-hour totals, 135 cm (53 inches) and 188 cm (74 inches), respectively, both occurred during cyclones at La Réunion, an island in the southwestern Indian Ocean. The very high specific humidity condenses into exceptionally large raindrops and giant cumulus clouds, resulting in high precipitation rates. When a cyclone makes landfall, the rain rapidly saturates even dry catchment areas, and rapid runoff may explosively flood the usual water courses as it creates new ones.

The relationship between rainfall and wind speed is not always proportional. For instance, if the atmosphere over land is already saturated with moisture, rainfall will be strongly enhanced, and the cyclone will weaken slowly. If the atmosphere is dry, the rainfall will be greatly reduced, and the cyclone will decay faster. Thus landfall of even a relatively weak tropical cyclone may result in extensive flooding, as occurred in 2004 with Hurricane Jeanne, which had weakened to a tropical storm and dumped torrential rain on Haiti, killing 3000 people.

BOX 85-2 Saffir-Simpson Potential Hurricane Damage Scale

The Saffir-Simpson Hurricane Scale is a 1 to 5 rating based on the hurricane's present intensity. This is used to give an estimate of the potential property damage and flooding expected along the coast from a hurricane landfall. Wind speed is the determining factor in the scale, because storm surge values are highly dependent on the slope of the continental shelf and the shape of the coastline, in the landfall region. Note that all winds are using the U.S. 1-minute average.

Category 1 Hurricane
Winds 64 to 82 knots or 119 to 153 km/hr (74 to 95 mph). Storm surge generally 1.2 to 1.5 m (4 to 5 feet) above normal. No real damage to building structures. Damage primarily to unanchored mobile homes, shrubbery, and trees. Some damage to poorly constructed signs. Also, some coastal road flooding and minor pier damage.

Category 2 Hurricane
Winds 83 to 95 knots or 154 to 177 km/hr (96 to 110 mph). Storm surge generally 1.8 to 2.4 m (6 to 8 feet) above normal. Some roofing material, door, and window damage of buildings. Considerable damage to shrubbery and trees with some trees blown down. Considerable damage to mobile homes, poorly constructed signs, and piers. Coastal and low-lying escape routes flood 2 to 4 hours before arrival of the hurricane center. Small craft in unprotected anchorages break moorings.

Category 3 Hurricane
Winds 96 to 113 knots or 178 to 209 km/hr (111 to 130 mph). Storm surge generally 2.7 to 3.7 m (9 to 12 feet) above normal. Some structural damage to small residences and utility buildings with a minor amount of curtainwall failures. Damage to shrubbery and trees with foliage blown off trees and large trees blown down. Mobile homes and poorly constructed signs are destroyed. Low-lying escape routes are cut by rising water 3 to 5 hours before arrival of the center of the hurricane. Flooding near the coast destroys smaller structures, with larger structures damaged by battering from floating debris. Terrain continuously lower than 1.5 m (5 feet) above mean sea level may be flooded inland 13 km (8 miles) or more. Evacuation of low-lying residences with several blocks of the shoreline may be required.

Category 4 Hurricane
Winds 114 to 135 knots or 210 to 249 km/hr (131 to 155 mph). Storm surge generally 4 to 5.5 m (13 to 18 feet) above normal. More extensive curtainwall failures with some complete roof structure failures on small residences. Shrubs, trees, and all signs are blown down. Complete destruction of mobile homes. Extensive damage to doors and windows. Low-lying escape routes may be cut by rising water 3 to 5 hours before arrival of the center of the hurricane. Major damage to lower floors of structures near the shore. Terrain lower than 3 m (10 feet) above sea level may be flooded requiring massive evacuation of residential areas as far inland as 10 km (6 miles).

Category 5 Hurricane
Winds greater than 135 knots or 249 km/hr (155 mph). Storm surge generally greater than 5.5 m (18 feet) above normal. Complete roof failure on many residences and industrial buildings. Some complete building failures, with small utility buildings blown over or away. All shrubs, trees, and signs blown down. Complete destruction of mobile homes. Severe and extensive window and door damage. Low-lying escape routes are cut by rising water 3 to 5 hours before arrival of the center of the hurricane. Major damage to lower floors of all structures located less than 4.5 m (15 feet) above sea level and within 450 m (500 yards) of the shoreline. Massive evacuation of residential areas on low ground within 8 to 16 km (5 to 10 miles) of the shoreline may be required. Only three category 5 hurricanes have made landfall in the United States since records began: the Labor Day Hurricane of 1935, Hurricane Camille in 1969, and Hurricane Andrew in 1992.

From The National Oceanic and Atmospheric Administration—National Weather Service, National Hurricane Center, Tropical Prediction Center, Miami, Florida, 2006: nhc.noaa.gov/aboutsshs.shtml.

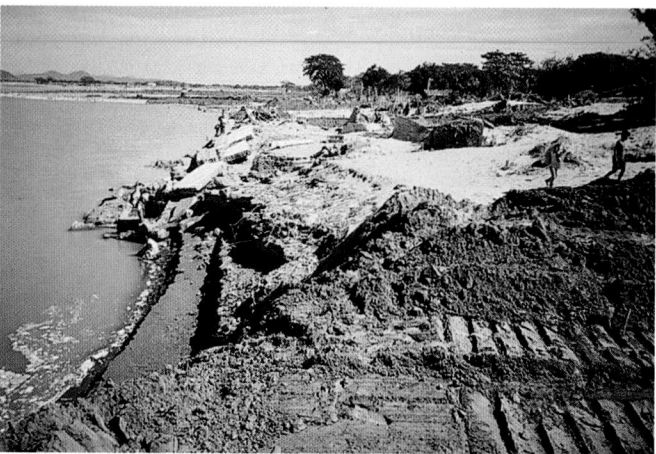

FIGURE 85-16 Aftermath of Hurricane Mitch in Honduras in 1998. *(Courtesy Paul Thompson, InterWorks.)*

Deadly Hurricanes

The 1998 Atlantic hurricane season, from June 1 to November 30, was one of the deadliest in 200 years, killing more than 10,000 people in eight countries and causing billions of dollars in damage. Fourteen named storms, four more than average, formed in the Atlantic Ocean, Caribbean Sea, and Gulf of Mexico. Of these, 10 became hurricanes. Hurricane Georges followed a path across the U.S. Virgin Islands, Puerto Rico, the Dominican Republic, Haiti, and Cuba, killing more than 500 persons and causing $5 billion in damages. Hurricane Mitch moved across Central America, killing an estimated 10,000 persons in Honduras and wiping out the country's infrastructure (Figure 85-16). Mitch regenerated as a tropical storm and then passed over south Florida.

The 2005 Atlantic hurricane season, however, was the most active season on record, lasting into January 2006. Twenty-seven tropical storms formed, of which 15 became hurricanes. Of these, seven were major hurricanes, five becoming Category 4 and three reaching Category 5. Hurricane Wilma was the most intense ever recorded in the Atlantic. It caused at least 1918 deaths and record damages of over $100 billion. Hurricanes Dennis, Emily, Katrina, Rita, and Wilma struck Mexico, Cuba, and the United States (Florida, Alabama, Louisiana, Texas, and Mississippi). The most catastrophic effects of the season were felt in New Orleans, where hurricane Katrina caused a storm surge that breached levees and flooded most of the city. Katrina started as an extremely powerful Category 5 storm off the coast but weakened to Category 4 when it hit New Orleans. Because it dropped rapidly in intensity, New Orleans experienced significantly less wind damage than might have been expected from a Category 5 storm.

Hurricane Sandy was the deadliest and most destructive hurricane of the 2012 Atlantic hurricane season. After Katrina, it was the second most costly in U.S. history and the largest in diameter. In the United States, Hurricane Sandy affected 24 states, including the entire Eastern Seaboard; its effects were felt westward to the Appalachian Mountains and even into Michigan and Wisconsin. Before its landfall in the United States, Sandy first hit Jamaica, followed by Cuba and the Bahamas; it also affected Haiti, the Dominican Republic, and Puerto Rico. Flooding in Haiti killed at least 54 persons and made 200,000 others homeless. Jamaica suffered loss of electricity for 70% of its residents and $100 million in damages.

Predictability

Tropical cyclones form in all oceans of the world except the South Atlantic and South Pacific east of 140 degrees W longitude. Nearly one-quarter form between 5 and 10 degrees latitude from the equator and two-thirds between 10 and 20 degrees latitude. It is rare for tropical cyclones to form south of 20 to 22 degrees latitude in the Southern Hemisphere; however, they occasionally form as far north as 30 to 32 degrees in the more extensive warmer waters of the Northern Hemisphere. They are mainly confined to the warmer 6 months of the year but have occurred in every month of the year in the western North Pacific. Of concern is the influence that climate change might have on the frequency and severity of tropical cyclones by virtue of raising sea surface temperatures and contributing to rising sea levels. Warm sea surface temperatures influence cyclone development, and warmer ocean waters increase hurricane intensity.

The locations, frequencies, and intensities of tropical cyclones are well known from historical observations and, more recently, from routine satellite monitoring. Tropical cyclones do not follow the same track, except coincidentally over short distances. Some follow linear paths, others recurve in a symmetric manner, and still others accelerate or slow down and seem stationary for a time. For this reason, predicting when, where, and if a storm will hit land is often difficult, especially with islands. Typhoon Parma in the Philippines in 2009 made three consecutive landfalls in the same area, which experienced winds of typhoon strength for 15 consecutive hours. In general, the difficulty in forecasting increases from lower to higher latitudes, whereas the margin of error in determining the cyclone center decreases as landfall approaches.

Special warning and preparedness strategies for evacuation from offshore facilities or closure of industrial plants must relate the costs and benefits of those strategies against the uncertainties of precision in the forecasts. For general community purposes that require a minimum 12 hours of preparedness time, the imprecision in forecasting the location of landfall within 24 hours should be generally tolerable, bearing in mind that highly adverse cyclonic weather usually commences about 6 hours before landfall of the cyclone. In the United States, a *hurricane watch* is issued when a hurricane is likely to strike within 36 hours, and a *hurricane warning* notifies of possible landfall within 24 hours. In September 2004, a Category 4 hurricane, Ivan, caused heavy damage to Jamaica, Grand Cayman, and the western tip of Cuba, and directly hit the Caribbean island of Grenada, home to 90,000 people. The island had not experienced a major hurricane in 40 years. Citizens received warnings in advance but generally did not have adequate preparedness measures in place. Remarkably few (39) died, but 90% of housing was damaged or destroyed (Figures 85-17 and 85-18).

Regrettably, progress in reducing forecasting errors has remained slow in the last two decades despite huge investments in monitoring systems. However, substantial progress has been made in the organization of warning and dissemination systems, particularly through regional cooperation. The activities of national meteorologic services are coordinated at the international level by the WMO. Forecasts and warnings are prepared within the framework of the WMO's World Weather Watch program. Under this program, meteorologic observational data

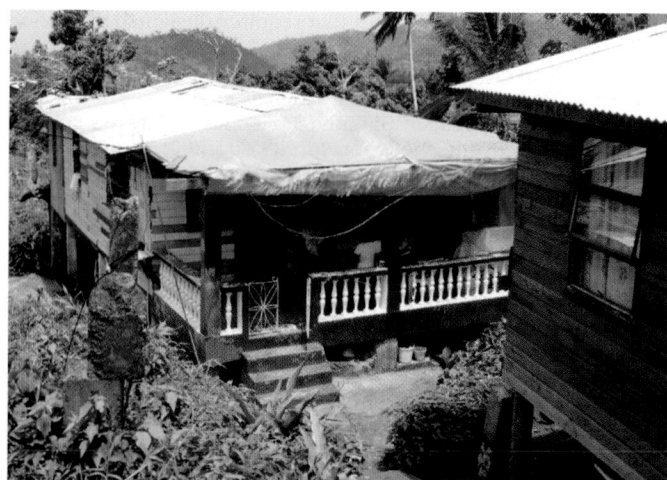

FIGURE 85-17 Damage in Grenada from Hurricane Ivan, September 2004. *(Courtesy Sheila B. Reed.)*

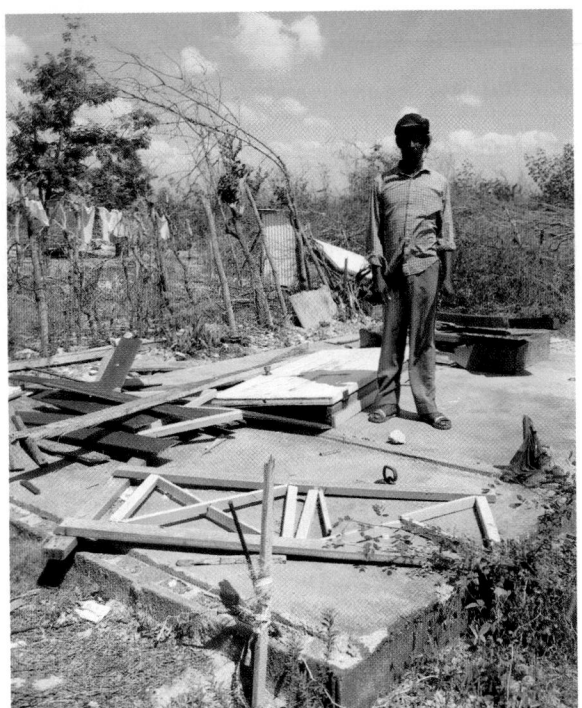

FIGURE 85-18 A man standing on the site of his house in Jamaica, destroyed by Hurricane Ivan, September 2004. *(Courtesy Sheila B. Reed.)*

are provided nationally, and data from satellites and information provided by the regional centers are exchanged around the world. The World Weather Watch system includes 8500 land stations, 5500 merchant ships, aircraft, special ocean weather ships, automatic weather stations, and meteorologic satellites. A tropical cyclone is first identified and then followed from satellite pictures. A global telecommunications system relays the observations.

Ultimately, however, national services are responsible for providing forecasts and warnings to the local population regarding tropical cyclones and the associated winds, rains, and storm surges. Unfortunately, many of the less developed countries, where most deaths from tropical cyclones occur, do not possess state-of-the-art warning systems.

Vulnerability

Human settlements located in exposed, low-lying coastal areas are vulnerable to the direct effects of a cyclone, such as wind, rain, and storm surges. Settlements in adjacent areas are vulnerable to floods, mudslides, or landslides from the resultant heavy rains. The death rate is higher where communications systems are poor and warning systems are inadequate.

The quality of structures determines resistance to the effects of the cyclone. Those most vulnerable are lightweight structures with wood frames, older buildings with weakened walls, and houses made of unreinforced concrete block (Figure 85-19). Infrastructural elements particularly at risk are telephone and telegraph poles and fishing boats and other maritime industries. Hospitals may be damaged, reducing access to health care and essential drugs.

Typical Adverse Effects

Structures are damaged and destroyed by wind force, through collapse from pressure differentials, and by flooding, storm surges, and landslides. Severe damage can occur to overhead power lines, bridges, embankments, nonweatherproofed buildings, and roofs of most structures. Falling trees, wind-driven rain, and flying debris cause considerable damage.

Casualties and Public Health. Relatively few fatalities occur because of the high winds in cyclonic storms, but many people may be injured and require hospitalization. Storm surges may cause many deaths but usually cause few injuries among survivors. Because of flooding and possible contamination of water supplies, malaria organisms and viruses may be prevalent several weeks after the flooding.

Water Supplies. Open wells and other groundwater supplies may be temporarily contaminated by flood waters and storm surges. They are considered contaminated by pathogenic organisms only if dead people or animals are lying in the sources or if sewage is present. Normal water sources may be unavailable for several days.

Crops and Food Supplies. The combination of high winds and heavy rains, even without flooding, can ruin standing crops and tree plantations. Food stocks may be lost or contaminated if the structures in which they were held have been destroyed or inundated. Salt from storm surges may also be deposited on agricultural lands and increase groundwater salinity. Fruit, nut, and lumber trees may be damaged or destroyed by winds, flooding, and storm surges. Plantation-type crops, such as bananas, are extremely vulnerable. Erosion can occur from flooding and storm surges. Food shortages may occur until the next harvest. Tree and food crops may be blown down or damaged and must be harvested prematurely.

Communications and Logistics. Communications may be severely disrupted as telephone lines, radio antennas, and satellite dishes are brought down, usually by wind. Roads and railroad lines may be blocked by fallen trees or debris, and aircraft movements may be curtailed for at least 12 to 24 hours after the storm. Modes of transportation, such as trucks, carts, and small boats, may be damaged by wind or flooding. The cumulative effect of all damage is to impede information gathering and transport networks.

Preparedness Measures Take Root After Cyclone Nargis in Burma (Myanmar)

Cyclone Nargis, a Category 4 cyclone, struck Burma in May 2008, killing 145,000 and severely affecting 2.4 million people. Wind speeds reached 200 km/hr. More than 750,000 houses, 4000

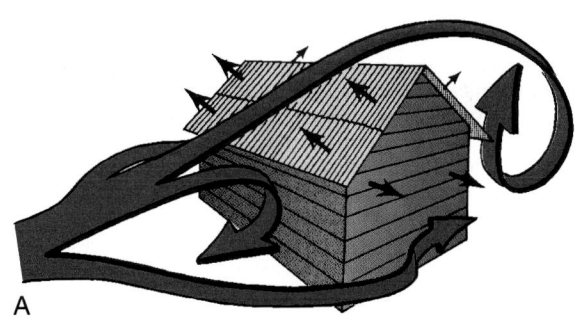

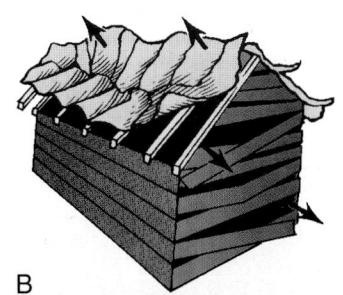

FIGURE 85-19 How high winds damage buildings. **A,** Wind blowing into a building is slowed at the windward face, creating high pressure. The airflow separates as it spills around the building, creating low pressure or suction at the end walls, roof, and leeward walls. **B,** The roof may lift off and the walls blow out if the structure is not specially reinforced. *(Courtesy Disaster Management Center, University of Wisconsin–Madison.)*

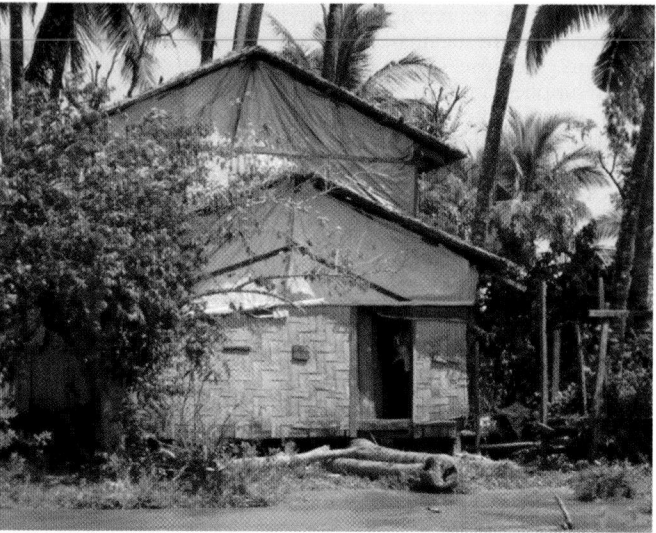

FIGURE 85-20 Plastic sheeting repair to houses after Cyclone Nargis in Burma (Myanmar). *(Courtesy Sheila B. Reed.)*

schools, and 630 health facilities were destroyed or badly damaged. More than 60% of the total rice paddy fields were submerged; millions of livestock animals were killed; and stored food, seed stocks, boats, and equipment were destroyed. The cyclone, and the flooding that followed, damaged close to 13% of ponds used for drinking and household water in Yangon and up to 43% of ponds in Ayeyarwady Division. The damage caused by Cyclone Nargis was found to be on a scale nearly equivalent to that suffered by Aceh in Indonesia, one of the most affected areas hit by the 2004 Indian Ocean tsunami.

Recovery efforts in the 2 years following Cyclone Nargis helped to restore a large percentage of agricultural productivity in Burma, although rebuilding of houses (Figure 85-20) and infrastructure elements was notably slower due to insufficient resources to implement the national recovery plan. Extensive environmental damage from the cyclone was also weakly addressed. However, disaster risk reduction measures were augmented by communities with the support of the government and assistance organizations. Many communities formed disaster management committees, promoted raising awareness, and developed evacuation plans for families and livestock (Figure 85-21). Committees and programs were established to replant mangroves and tree plantation barriers. Steps are being taken to strengthen hazard risk mapping, early warning systems, and

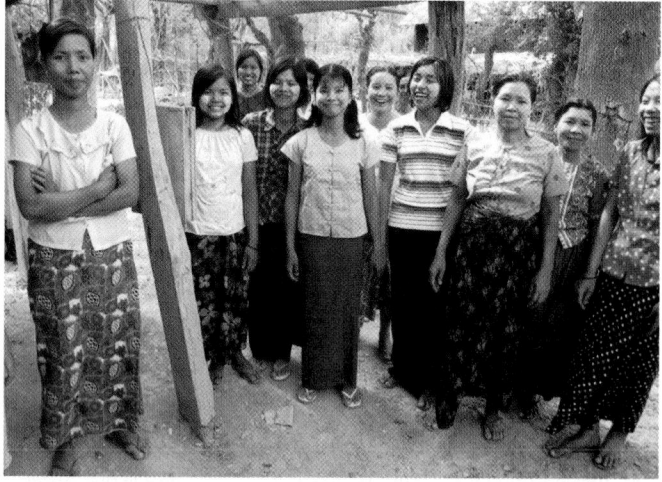

FIGURE 85-21 Women's group for disaster risk reduction in Burma. *(Courtesy Sheila B. Reed.)*

scientific research to underpin national disaster risk reduction policies.

Cyclone Risk Reduction Measures

The primary ways to reduce property damage from cyclones are accurate forecasting, sufficient warning, and establishment of evacuation procedures and building codes. As described earlier, significant challenges exist in forecasting the behavior of cyclones and other severe wind storms. Another major challenge is altering the perception of people who live in coastal areas regarding the danger from cyclonic activity. People may ignore the dangers for various reasons: lack of experience in hurricanes and cyclones, insufficient understanding of the hazard, repeated false alarms, or incorrect landfall predictions that breed complacency.

TORNADOES

A tornado is the most dramatic example of a class of storms that includes thunderstorms and hailstorms; collectively, this class is often known simply as severe local storms. Tornadoes are sometimes referred to as "twisters" in the United States. Severe local storms, which may be a few miles to a few tens of miles in diameter, are often accompanied by unusually strong, gusty winds that can cause severe damage, by heavy local rain that can cause flash floods, and by lightning, hail, and sometimes tornadoes. These intense vortices may be only a few hundred feet in diameter but can contain winds in excess of 483 km/hr (300 mph), capable of tearing roofs off houses and lifting houses, trees, and vehicles hundreds of feet through the air. Tornadoes have been known to occur in swarms, with as many as several dozen affecting an area of hundreds of thousands of square miles in a single day. A new 1-day record was set in the United States on January 21, 1999, when 38 tornadoes were hatched in Arkansas, surpassing the previous record of 20 statewide. Before early September 2015, 29 tornadoes had already occurred in the Chicago area, setting a record for the most tornadoes in 1 year in the warning area.

Causal Phenomena

Tornadoes and other severe local storms result from intense, local atmospheric instability, usually caused by solar heating of Earth's surface, which causes intense convective columns. A tornado is a vortex in which air spirals inward and upward. It is frequently, but not always, visible as a funnel cloud hanging part or all of the way from the generating storm to the ground. The upper portion of the funnel consists of water droplets, and the lower portion usually consists of dust and soil being sucked up from the ground. The funnel size may range from a few meters to a few hundred meters in diameter and from 10 m (33 feet) to several kilometers high. The funnel may undergo changes in appearance during the tornado's lifetime. There may be a single well-defined funnel, multiple funnels, or funnels that appear to consist of several ropelike strands. Tornadoes may be as loud as the roar of a freight train. For a vortex to be classified as a tornado, it must be in contact with both the ground and the cloud base. Scientists have not yet created a complete definition of the word; for example, there is disagreement about whether separate touchdowns of the same funnel constitute separate tornadoes.

Tornadoes are the most violent events associated with thunderstorms. They have been observed on every continent except Antarctica but are most frequent and fierce in the United States. As many as 1200 tornadoes may strike the United States each year, mostly in the central plains (sometimes called Tornado Alley) and southeastern states, although they have occurred in every state, mostly in the spring and summer. Of all the natural hazards in the United States, thunderstorms with associated winds, rain, hail, and lightning rank first in number of deaths, second in number of injuries, and third in property damage. The Netherlands, followed by the UK, has the highest average number of tornadoes per area of any country, but most are small and cause only minor damage.

Various types of tornadoes include the landspout, multiple vortex, and waterspout. The most common type of tornado is small and lasts only a minute or two, causing minor damage over a track often less than 90 m (300 feet) wide and 1.6 to 3.2 m (1 to 2 miles) long. Most tornado-related deaths, injuries, and property damage are caused by relatively infrequent, large, and long-lasting tornadoes with paths more than 1 mile wide and more than 100 miles long over several hours. There are several different scales for rating the strength of tornadoes. The Fujita (F) scale rates tornadoes by damage caused, but this has been replaced in some countries by the updated Enhanced Fujita (EF) scale. An F0 or EF0 tornado, the weakest category, damages trees, but not substantial structures. An F5 or EF5 tornado, the strongest category, rips buildings off their foundations and can deform large skyscrapers. The similar TORRO (T) scale ranges from a T0 for extremely weak tornadoes to T11 for the most powerful known tornadoes.

Predictability

Although conditions favorable to tornado formation can often be predicted a number of hours in advance, the areas in which these conditions are found may cover hundreds of thousands of square miles. It is impossible to predict where individual tornadoes will occur. When a warning is issued, a tornado has already formed, and the threatened population may have only a few minutes to take cover. In the United States, when tornadoes are considered likely within a well-defined region, a *tornado watch* is issued. When a tornado is actually detected, either visually or on radar, a *tornado warning* is issued. The U.S. National Weather Service has trained more than 290,000 Skywarn severe weather spotters across the United States; Canada has a similar program. When severe weather is anticipated, local weather service offices request that these spotters look out for severe weather and report any tornadoes immediately, so that the office can warn of the hazard. Storm spotters are needed because radar systems such as NEXRAD do not detect tornadoes. The radar systems merely detect "signatures" that hint at the presence of tornadoes. Radar may give a warning before there is any visual evidence of a tornado or imminent tornado, but ground truth from an observer can either verify the threat or determine that a tornado is not imminent. The spotter's ability to see what cannot be detected by radar is especially important as distance from the radar site increases, because the radar beam becomes progressively higher in altitude further away from the radar, chiefly a result of Earth's curvature, and the beam also spreads out.

Vulnerability

Most injuries from tornadoes are caused by flying or falling debris, usually from destroyed structures. The quality of structures will determine resistance to the effects of the tornado. Those most vulnerable are lightweight structures with wood frames, older buildings with weakened walls, mobile homes, and houses made of unreinforced concrete blocks. Thorough education regarding taking shelter from flying debris is essential to reduce deaths and injuries. Public education regarding the hazard is important to dispel myths. For example, opening house windows has not been shown to reduce damage even though this is a widespread belief; taking shelter under highway overpasses is not a safe way to wait out a tornado, contrary to some beliefs. On the other hand, taking shelter in a basement, under a staircase, or under a sturdy piece of furniture has been shown to increase chances of survival. Tornadoes have been known to cross major rivers, ascend mountains, affect valleys, and damage city centers. As a general rule, no area is safe from tornadoes, though some areas are less susceptible than others.

Examples of Tornado Outbreaks

The most extreme tornado in recorded history was the Tri-State Tornado, which roared through parts of Missouri, Illinois, and Indiana on March 18, 1925. It was likely an F5, although tornadoes were not ranked on any scale during that era. It holds records for longest path length (352 km [219 miles]), longest duration (about 3.5 hours), and fastest forward speed (117 km/hr [73 mph]) for a significant tornado anywhere on Earth. In addition, it is the deadliest (695 persons killed) single tornado in U.S. history. A tornado that struck Joplin, Missouri, in May 2011 killed 158 people and injured more than 1000 others, packed winds in excess of 200 mph, and stayed on the ground for more than 22 miles. The deadliest tornado in world history was the Daulatpur-Saturia tornado in Bangladesh on April 26, 1989, which killed approximately 1300 people. In Bangladesh, at least 19 tornadoes in its history have killed more than 100 people per event, almost one-half of the total deaths in the rest of the world.

The most extensive tornado outbreak on record was the Super Outbreak, on April 3 and 4, 1974, when 147 tornadoes struck Illinois, Indiana, Michigan, Ohio, West Virginia, Virginia, Kentucky, Tennessee, North Carolina, South Carolina, Georgia, and Alabama, killing 335 people, injuring more than 5500, affecting more than 27,000 households, and causing more than $600 million in damage. More than one-half the deaths were caused by fewer than 5% of the tornadoes. The worst of these struck Xenia, Ohio. It cut a swath of destruction one-half mile wide and 16 miles long, killed 34 people, injured 1150, and damaged or destroyed 2400 homes.

The year 2008 overtook the year 1998 as the deadliest tornado season in the United States, with 2192 tornadoes reported, 1691 confirmed (the most being in Kansas at 187), and 125 associated fatalities. Nine other tornado-related fatalities were reported elsewhere in the world: three in France, two each in Bangladesh and Poland, and one each in Russia and China. After a long lull in activity, a series of intense storms and associated cold fronts tracked across the Midwest, starting late on December 30, with most of the activity on December 31, New Year's Eve, 2010. Early that morning, an EF3 tornado touched down in Washington County, Arkansas, destroying houses and killing at least four people. In nearby Benton County, Arkansas, another tornado caused significant damage and injuries.

Tornado Risk Reduction Measures

The main means to prevent damage and casualties from tornadoes remains forecasting and warnings to urge the public to take protective measures. Scientists still do not know the exact mechanisms by which most tornadoes form, and occasional tornadoes still strike without a tornado warning being issued. More research is needed to refine existing knowledge. In the United States, many universities and government agencies, such as the National Severe Storms Laboratory, private-sector meteorologists, and National Center for Atmospheric Research, are actively seeking answers using various sources of funding, both private and public.

FLOODS

Throughout history, people have been attracted to the fertile lands of the floodplains, where their lives have been made easier by proximity to sources of food and water. Ironically, the same river or stream that provides sustenance to the surrounding population also renders humans vulnerable to disaster by periodic flooding. Flooding occurs when surface water covers land that is normally dry or when water overflows normal confinements. The most widespread of any hazard, floods can arise from abnormally heavy precipitation, dam failures, rapid snowmelts, river blockages, or even burst water mains. However, floods can provide benefits without creating disaster and are necessary to maintain most river ecosystems. They replenish soil fertility, provide water for crop irrigation and fisheries, and contribute seasonal water supplies to support life in arid lands.

Every year in Bangladesh, large tracts of land are submerged during the monsoon season, a normally beneficial process that deposits a rich layer of alluvial soil. The floods originate from three great river systems in the Himalayan mountains: the Ganges, Brahmaputra, and Meghna. In Bangladesh, the flood of 1974 affected 50% of the land; 27,500 persons perished from subsequent disease and starvation. Fortunately, timely arrival of food aid averted a famine crisis. In 1998, high sea levels and silting from increased deforestation upriver contributed to massive floods, killing 1500 people and causing $2 billion in damages. Farms were inundated and 26,000 cattle perished, destroying livelihoods for millions. In the aftermath of the flooding, cases of diarrheal diseases reached epidemic proportions, with 50,000 cases reported daily. The risk for other diseases, such as hepatitis, typhoid fever, and measles, was elevated because of contaminated water supplies. Destruction of almost 4 million hectares of crops and partial damage to 3 million hectares left a shortfall in annual grain requirements of 1 million tons and placed the population at risk of famine. India also suffers frequent catastrophic floods, the most recent being in October 2009, when flooding occurred across South India. It was one of the worst floods in the area in the last 100 years, killing 250 people and leaving 500,000 homeless.

In 2007, the United Nations (UN) reported the "floods of Africa" to be one of the worst flood events in recorded history, affecting 14 countries; 250 people were killed and 2.5 million others were affected by the disaster. Warnings of waterborne diseases and locust infestations were issued. The countries most affected were Ghana, Sudan, Ethiopia, Uganda, and Rwanda. In November 2009, record-breaking amounts of rain were dumped on Cumbria, England, and Cork, Ireland, causing minor floods in Cork and major floods in Cumbria. During the floods, waters reached a UK record of 2.4 m (8 feet) deep in Cockermouth, Cumbria.

Pakistan Flood Disaster of 2010

In 2010, from mid-July until mid-August, all four of Pakistan's provinces (Balochistan, Khyber Pakhtunkhwa, Punjab, and Sindh), as well as the Azad Jammu and Kashmir Region of Pakistan, flooded during the monsoon rains when dams, rivers, and lakes overflowed, killing at least 1750 people, injuring 2500, and affecting 23 million. The flood is considered the worst in Pakistan's history, and the number of individuals affected by the flooding exceeds the combined total of those affected by the 2004 Indian Ocean tsunami, the 2005 Kashmir earthquake, and the 2010 Haiti earthquake. The flooding eventually affected about one-fifth of the country (nearly 62,000 square miles, an area larger than England) and formed what was called by some the largest freshwater lake in the world. Six weeks after the floods began, as rivers continued to devour villages and farmland in the southern province of Sindh, losses of crops, seed for the next planting season, and livelihoods were predicted. The UN Relief Web reported in January 2011 that millions of flood-affected people had still not received food and medicines, primarily because of inadequate relief resources and some villages being cut off from assistance by the flood waters.

Causal Phenomena

The most important cause of floods is excessive rainfall. Rain may be seasonal and occur over wide areas or may be the result of localized storms; the latter produce the highest-intensity rainfall. Some storms are attributed to atmospheric and oceanic processes, such as the El Niño southern oscillation or strong jet streams. Melting snow is another major contributor.

Types of Floods

Flash Floods. Flash floods are usually defined as floods that occur within 6 hours of the beginning of heavy rainfall. This type of flooding requires rapid local warnings and immediate response by affected communities if damage is to be mitigated. Flash floods are normally a result of runoff from a torrential downpour, particularly if the catchment slope is unable to absorb and hold a significant part of the water. Other causes of flash floods include dam failure or sudden breakup of ice jams or other river obstructions. Flash floods are potential threats, particularly where the terrain is steep, surface runoff is high, water flows through narrow canyons, and severe rainstorms are likely.

River Floods. River floods are usually caused by precipitation over large catchment areas, by melting of the winter accumulation of snow, or by both. The floods take place in river systems with tributaries that may drain large geographic areas and encompass many independent river basins. In contrast to flash floods, river floods normally build up slowly, are often seasonal, and may continue for days or weeks. Factors governing the amount of flooding include ground conditions (amount of moisture in the soil, vegetation cover, depth of snow, cover by impervious urban surfaces such as concrete), and size of the catchment basin (Figure 85-22).

Coastal Floods. Some flooding is associated with tropical cyclones (also called hurricanes and typhoons). Catastrophic flooding from rainwater is often aggravated by wind-induced storm surges along the coast. Saltwater may flood the land by one or a combination of effects from high tides, storm surges, or tsunamis. As in river floods, intense rain falling over a large

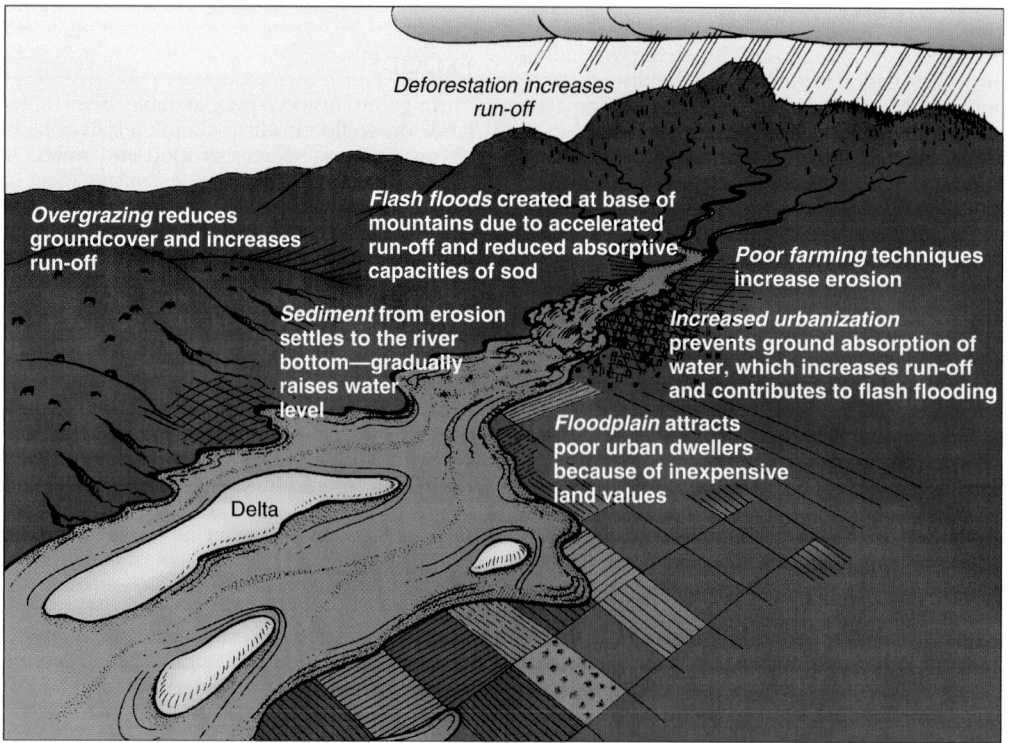

FIGURE 85-22 Flooding and its causes. *(Courtesy Disaster Management Center, University of Wisconsin.)*

geographic area will produce extreme flooding in coastal river basins.

Contribution by Humans

Floods are naturally occurring hazards but can become disasters when they affect human settlements. The magnitude and frequency of flooding often increase because of human actions. Settlement on floodplains contributes to flooding disasters by endangering humans and their assets. However, economic benefits of living on the floodplain outweigh the dangers for some societies. Population pressure is now so great that people have accepted the risk associated with floods because of the greater need for a place to live. In the United States, billions of dollars have been spent on flood protection programs since 1936. Despite this, the annual flood hazard has become greater because people have built on floodplains faster than engineers can design better flood protection. The Mississippi River, which had been protected by 5600 miles of levees, flooded in 1993, affecting nine states. Some 70% of levees failed to protect against the record rainfall.

Urbanization contributes to urban flooding. Roads and buildings prevent infiltration of water, so runoff forms artificial streams. The network of drains in urban areas may deliver water and fill natural channels more rapidly than natural drainage routes, or drains may be insufficient and overflow. Natural or artificial channels may become constricted by debris or obstructed by river facilities, impeding drainage and overflowing the catchment areas. Failure to maintain or manage drainage systems, dams, and levees in vulnerable areas also contributes to flooding. Central Europe experienced severe flooding in 2002 and incurred $18 billion in damages, with the cities of Dresden and Prague particularly affected.

Deforestation and removal of root systems increase runoff. Subsequent erosion causes sedimentation in river channels, which decreases their capacity.

Catastrophic flooding may become worse in the United States and has become more frequent in the Midwest over the last 50 years. In the summer of 2014, the Midwest was inundated with 2 months' worth of rainfall in just 1 week, submerging farms and killing crops. A Federal Emergency Management Agency assessment found that due to rising seas and more severe storms, flooding in certain areas of the United States may increase by as much as 45%.

Predictability

Riverine flood forecasting estimates the river level stage, discharge, time of occurrence, and duration of flooding, especially of peak discharge at specific points along river systems. Flooding resulting from precipitation, snowmelt in the catchment system, or upstream flooding is predictable from 12 hours to as much as several weeks ahead of events. Forecasts issued to the public result from regular monitoring of the river heights and rainfall observations. Flash flood warnings, however, depend solely on meteorologic forecasts and knowledge of local geographic conditions. The very short lead time for development of flash floods does not permit useful monitoring of actual river levels for warning purposes.

Flood hazard mapping supports flood management plans, land use planning, emergency evacuation plans, and increased public awareness. For comparison with previous flood events and conversion to warning information, assessment of the following elements should be included: flood frequency analysis, topographic mapping and height contouring around river systems with estimates of water-holding capacity of the catchment area, precipitation and snowmelt records, soil filtration capacity, and, if in a coastal area, tidal records, storm frequency, topography, coastal geography, and breakwater characteristics.

An effective means of monitoring floodplains is through remote sensing techniques. The images produced by satellites can be interpreted to map flooded and flood-prone areas. Other efforts to improve forecasting are being implemented by UN organizations, such as the WMO (using its World Weather Watch program), and the Global Data Processing System. These systems are strategic when flood conditions exist across international boundaries. The great majority of river and flash flood forecasts, however, depend on observations made by national weather services for activation of flood alert warnings.

Vulnerability

As with other hazards, perceptions by the general public of the flood hazard have improved by using flood mapping and public awareness campaigns. People in flood-prone areas in developing countries may assume high risks due to overcrowding and the need to use the land for livelihood purposes.

At notable risk in floodplain settlements are buildings made of earth or with soluble mortar, buildings with shallow foundations, or buildings that are nonresistant to water force and inundation. Infrastructural elements at particular risk include utilities, such as sewer systems, power and water supplies, and machinery and electronics belonging to industrial plants and communications groups. Of great concern are food stocks and standing crops, confined livestock, irreplaceable cultural artifacts, and fishing boats and other maritime industries.

Other factors affecting vulnerability are lack of adequate refuge sites above flood levels and accessible routes for reaching those sites. Also, lack of public information about escape routes and other appropriate response activities renders communities more vulnerable. Vietnam, which has 3444 km (2149 miles) of coastline and a complex and ancient system of sea dikes, is chronically vulnerable to floods. The government is promoting a strong institutional network to support citizens to "live with floods," reducing their vulnerability and providing social safety nets to assist with recovery.

Typical Adverse Effects

Structures are damaged by receiving the force of impact of flood waters, floating away on rising waters, becoming inundated, collapsing because of undercutting by scouring or erosion, and being struck by waterborne debris.

Damage is likely to be much greater in valleys than in open, low-lying areas. Flash floods often sweep away everything in their path. In coastal areas, storm surges are destructive both on inward travel and on outward return to the sea. Mud, oil, and other pollutants carried by water are deposited and ruin crops and building contents. Saturation of soils may cause landslides or ground failure.

Casualties and Public Health. Currents of moving or turbulent water can knock down and drown people and animals in relatively shallow depths. Major floods may result in large numbers of deaths from drowning, particularly among young and weak persons, but generally inflict few serious, nonfatal injuries requiring hospital treatment. Slow flooding causes relatively few direct deaths or injuries, but often increases the occurrence of snakebites.

Endemic disease will continue in flooded areas, but little evidence exists of floods directly causing any large-scale additional health problems besides diarrhea, malaria, and other viral outbreaks 8 to 10 weeks after the flood.

Water, Crops, and Food Supplies. Open wells and other groundwater supplies may be contaminated temporarily by debris carried by flood waters or by saltwater brought in by storm surges. They are contaminated by pathogenic organisms only if bodies of people or animals are caught in the sources or if sewage is present. Normal sources of water may not be available for several days.

Food stocks may be lost by submersion of crop storage facilities, resulting in immediate food shortages. An entire harvest may be lost, along with animal fodder, resulting in long-term food shortages. Grains quickly spoil if saturated with water, even for a short time. Most agricultural losses result from inundation of crops or stagnation of standing water, as in the 1988 Bangladesh flood.

Large numbers of animals, including draught animals, may be lost if they are not moved to safety. This may reduce availability of milk and other animal products and services, such as preparation of the land for planting. These losses, in addition to possible loss of farm implements and seed stocks, may hinder future planting efforts.

Floods bring mixed results in terms of their effects on the soil. In some cases, land may be rendered infertile for several years after a flood because of erosion of topsoil or salt permeation, as in the case of a coastal flood. Heavy silting may have adverse effects or may significantly increase fertility of the soil.

In coastal areas, where fish provide a source of protein, boats and fishing equipment may be lost or damaged.

On the positive side, floods may flush out pollutants in the waterways. Other positive effects include preserving wetlands, recharging groundwater, and maintaining river ecosystems by providing breeding, nesting, and feeding areas for fish, birds, and wildlife.

Flood Risk Reduction Measures

The major means of addressing flooding is through prevention. However, people may be lured to the floodplain with false hopes of avoiding floods. Most dams and channels are not strong enough to withstand the heaviest water pressures and if they break down, flooding can be catastrophic. Furthermore, as levees and other physical barriers age, they become more likely to fail. European countries employ a variety of means to reduce the flood risk, such as a series of reservoirs in France called Les Grands Lacs de la Seine (or Great Lakes), which help to remove pressure from the Seine during floods (especially during the regular winter flooding); protection from sea flooding by a huge mechanical barrier across the Thames River in London; underground canals that drain part of the flow of the Adige River in northern Italy; and a series of flood defenses in The Netherlands called the Delta Works, with the Oosterschelde Dam as its crowning achievement.

Because flooding may be beneficial to environmental regeneration, the challenge is to allow this while also ensuring personal and economic safety. The concept of integrated flood management, developed by the WMO in 2004, embraces floodplain land use that does not have adverse environmental impacts. Aspects include (1) integrated flood control that considers social and ecologic processes, (2) prioritization of floodplain land use, (3) integration of local stakeholder concerns, (4) a flexible approach to flood control, and (5) extensive continuous monitoring of flood control measures and flooding events. Since 2005, when Hurricane Katrina struck, flood prevention measures in New Orleans have included $14 billion spent for upgraded levees, floodwalls, and gates to form an integrated system that is designed to withstand the kind of storm that might occur every 100 years. Coastal restoration efforts are also under way to help reduce the risks to southeast Louisiana. The test came in 2012 when Hurricane Isaac struck. The system spared residents serious flooding. However, there would still be risks if an every-100-year type of storm were to occur, because the metro system is not totally protected and some communities are not covered by the federal system of flood control. Storms so intense that they occur only every 500 years are also possible; they would seriously challenge the system if rainfalls of as much as 13 inches in 24 hours were to develop.

DROUGHT

Of all natural disasters, droughts potentially have the greatest economic impact and affect the greatest number of people. They invariably have a direct and significant impact on food production and the overall economy. Because of the slow onset of droughts, their effects may accumulate over time and linger for many years. Their impact may be less obvious than that of other natural hazards but may be spread over a wider geographic area. Because of the pervasive effects of droughts, assessing their impact and planning assistance become more difficult than with other natural hazards.

No universal definition exists for drought. In general, drought is temporary reduction in water or moisture availability that is significantly below the normal or expected amount for a specified period. Because droughts occur in nearly all regions of the world and have varying characteristics, however, working definitions must be regionally specific and focus on the impacts that result from discrepancies between the supply and demand for water.

Droughts are most often associated with low rainfall and a semiarid climate. However, they also occur in areas with normally abundant rainfall. Humans tend to stabilize their activities around the expected moisture environment. Thus, after many years with above-average rainfall, people may perceive the first year of average rainfall as a drought. A rainfall level that meets the needs of a pastoralist may constitute a serious drought for a farmer growing corn. To define drought in a region, it is necessary to understand both the meteorologic characteristics and human perceptions of drought.

Types of Droughts

Meteorologic Drought. Meteorologic drought results from a shortfall in precipitation and is based on the degree of dryness relative to the normal or average amount, and on the duration of the dry period. This comparison must be specific to each region and may be measured against daily, monthly, seasonal, or annual rainfall amounts. Meteorologic drought usually precedes the other types of drought.

Hydrologic Drought. Hydrologic drought involves reduction of water resources, such as streams, groundwater, lakes, and reservoirs. It involves data on availability and off-take rates in relation to the normal operations of the system (domestic, industrial, irrigated agricultural) being supplied. One impact is competition between users for water in these storage systems.

Agricultural Drought. Agricultural drought is the impact of meteorologic and hydrologic droughts on crops and livestock production. It occurs when soil moisture is insufficient to maintain average plant growth and yields. The impact of agricultural drought is difficult to measure because of the complexity of plant growth and possible presence of other factors that may reduce yields, such as pests, weeds, low soil fertility, and low crop prices.

Famine drought can be regarded as an extreme form of agricultural drought in which food shortages are so severe that large numbers of people become unhealthy or die. Famine disasters have complex causes, such as civil war or external conflict, chronic food insecurity, or inflicted food insecurity due to political manipulation. Although scarcity of food is the main factor in a famine, death can result from other complicating influences, such as disease or lack of access to water and other services. Most deaths related to famine occur in the semiarid areas of sub-Saharan Africa. It was hoped that the lessons learned in mitigating the famine droughts in Ethiopia and Sudan in 1984 and 1985, where an estimated 900,000 people died, would prevent similar tragedies in the future. However, subsequent devastating famines occurred in Somalia in 1991 to 1992 (300,000 deaths); in North Korea in 1996 (200,000 to 3.5 million estimated deaths); again in Sudan in 1998 (70,000 deaths); again in Ethiopia in 1998 to 2000; and again in Somalia in 2011 to 2012. The Second Congo War from 1998 to 2004 caused approximately 3.8 million deaths, mainly from starvation and disease. Famine also occurred in six West African countries in 2012 due to the Sahel drought.

Socioeconomic Drought. Socioeconomic drought correlates supply and demand of goods and services with the three other types of drought and emphasizes the relationship between drought and human activities. When the supply of some goods or services, such as water, hay, or electric power, is dependent on weather, drought may cause shortages. During the drought of 2014 to 2015 that affected western U.S. states, snow shortages caused closures and severe reductions in business in ski areas; Tahoe City, California, experienced a snow deficit in the winter of 2014 to 2015 of 132.9 inches (338 cm).

Causal Phenomena

The reasons for deficiency of precipitation are not well understood. Dry seasons are typical in the tropics, when land and water reservoirs dry up and wildlife migrate to seek more fertile areas. Displacement of the normal path of the jet stream may steer rain-bearing storms elsewhere.

Recent research has focused on teleconnection, or linkages to global interactions, between the atmosphere and the oceans. Sea surface temperature anomalies influence heat and moisture, such that warm surface water may create air conditions favorable for cyclone formation. A large-scale sea surface temperature anomaly is linked to the El Niño southern oscillation events in the Pacific. These involve periodic (every 2 to 7 years) invasion of warm surface waters into the normally colder waters off the coast of South America. Droughts of 1982 to 1983 in Africa, Australia, India, Brazil, and the United States coincided with a major El Niño.

Human causes of drought, which include land use practices that give rise to desertification, such as deforestation, overcultivation, overgrazing, and mismanagement of irrigation, are thought to result in greater persistence of drought. Traditional drought-coping systems in Africa, such as pastoralists' use of seasonal grazing lands and farmers' use of fallow periods, have been reduced because of population pressures and economic policies (see Desertification, later). The global climate changes under way are expected to trigger more agricultural droughts, especially in developing countries, although global rainfall as a whole may increase.

Droughts vary in terms of intensity, duration, and coverage. Droughts tend to be more severe in drier areas of the world because of low mean annual rainfall and longer duration of dry periods. In dry areas, drought builds up slowly over several years of poor rainfall. Dry conditions in the African Sahel over a 16-year period led to widespread famine in 1984 to 1985. The quarter-century of drought conditions in the Sahel was interrupted by heavy rains in 1994. The effect of drought on food security depends, among other factors, on the size of the area affected by drought, as well as overall size of the country. Larger countries, such as India and Brazil, are rarely completely affected by drought, but smaller countries may be totally affected (Figure 85-23). In Syria in 2009 and 2010, 300,000 families moved to Damascus, Aleppo, and other cities in what constituted one of the largest internal displacements in the Middle East prior to the outbreak of conflict in Syria in 2011. This was due to rainfall averaging between 45% and 66% less than normal in three eastern provinces. Worldwide food availability may be adversely affected by drought in nations that export grain.

Severe droughts that plagued China during the spring of 2010 affected 10 regions of southwestern China, as well as parts of Southeast Asia, including Vietnam and Thailand. Resultant dust storms in March and April affected much of East Asia. This drought has been referred to as the worst in a century in southwestern China. The China Meteorological Administration recorded temperatures averaging 2°C warmer than normal over 6 months, and one-half the average precipitation for the past year across the region. The higher temperatures and drop in precipitation were unprecedented since at least the 1950s. The effects of El Niño were believed to have contributed to the drought, which may have been exacerbated by global warming and resulting climate change.

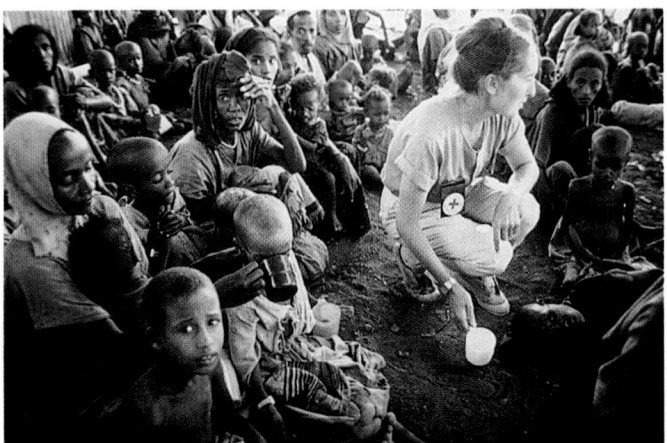

FIGURE 85-23 Victims of drought in Ethiopia. (*Courtesy United Nations.*)

Predictability

Modern meteorologic monitoring and telecommunications systems can prevent casualties from drought-induced food shortages. The slow onset of drought allows a warning time, usually several months, between the first indications and when the population will be affected. In 1987, satellite imagery and rainfall reports indicated areas within Ethiopia with below-normal moisture and allowed timely intervention to avert a major food shortage. Longer-term prediction requires analysis of a century of rainfall data, which do not exist for some parts of the world. The WMO has established a base in Niamey, Niger, to promote regional training on agricultural production and drought response. The UN International Strategy for Disaster Reduction convened panels of experts to steer development of the integrated Drought Early Warning System, which focuses on strengthening data networks and data sharing on drought indicators.

Most countries in sub-Saharan Africa have installed famine early warning systems after the 1980s drought. The UN Food and Agriculture Organization Global Information and Early Warning System and the USAID-sponsored Famine Early Warning System issue regular bulletins on rainfall, food production, and famine vulnerability. These systems rely on satellite remote sensing to detect a reduction in vegetation. In addition to the unique vantage point and condensed view, remote sensing provides a permanent historical record. The National Oceanic and Atmospheric Administration satellites provide twice-daily coverage of the planet's surface. These data are available at many receiving stations around the world. The administration has developed crop-monitoring technology for large areas of the Sahel.

Vulnerability

Although drought is more likely in dry areas with limited rainfall, physical factors, such as the moisture retention of soil and timing of rains, influence the degree of crop loss. Dependency on rainfed agriculture increases vulnerability. Farmers unable to adapt with repeated plantings may experience crop failure. Populations dependent on livestock without adequate grazing territory are also at risk. Farmers dependent on stored water resources or irrigation are more vulnerable to water shortages and may face competition for water.

Drought-related effects are more severe in countries with yearly food deficiencies and in systems that largely rely on subsistence-level farming and pastoralism. Food shortages have the greatest impact where malnutrition already exists. Most deaths related to food shortages occur in the semiarid countries of sub-Saharan Africa, whereas in more developed countries the consequences are largely economic. Adverse effects may be more serious where the drought response has not been adequately planned and where assistance measures may be poorly targeted or ineffective. There are indications that incidences of drought may increase, although this remains controversial. In any case, it is certain that societal vulnerability to drought is on the rise in many parts of the world.

Typical Adverse Effects

The effects of drought can be grouped as economic, environmental, and social. Economic effects include losses in crops, dairy and livestock, timber, fisheries, national economic growth, and income for farmers and others. Decreased tourism, loss of hydroelectric power and increased energy costs, increased food prices, unemployment, and losses of revenue to governments are other economic effects. Environmental effects include fires and dust storms; damage to animals, fish, and plant species and habitat; wind and water erosion of soils; reduced water quality or altered salinization; and reduced air quality from dust and pollutants. Social effects include food shortages (malnutrition, famine), loss of human life, conflict between water users, health problems from decreased water flow, decline in living conditions, increased poverty, social unrest, and population migration for employment.

Drought Risk Reduction Measures

A number of drought mitigation activities focus on restoring or conserving water resources. These include cloud seeding to induce rainfall, desalination of seawater for irrigation or consumption, rainwater harvesting or collection and storage of rainwater from roofs or other suitable catchments, recycling water (such as wastewater that has been treated and purified for reuse), building canals or redirecting rivers in massive attempts at irrigation within drought-prone areas, and outdoor water use restriction.

As described earlier, drought monitoring is critical for forecasting and warning and can help to prevent human-made drought. For instance, analysis of water usage in Yemen revealed that the water table (underground water level) has been put at grave risk by overuse to fertilize khat, the largest cash crop. Land use measures include carefully planned crop rotation to help minimize erosion and allow farmers to plant fewer water-dependent crops during drier years.

WINTER STORMS

Winter storms feature strong winds, extreme cold, ice storms, and heavy snowstorms. These are often deceptive killers because most deaths are indirectly related to the storm, such as those from traffic accidents and hypothermia. In the United States, of deaths related to ice and snow, about 70% occur in automobiles, and 25% are people caught out in a storm. The majority are men older than 40 years. For deaths related to cold, 50% are people over 60 years old, more than 75% are males, and about 20% occur in the home.

When temperatures are below freezing, everyone is at potential risk from winter storms. In areas of the world where roads are rarely maintained to mountainous areas, such as Nepal, Iraq, and Russia, local populations cope by storing provisions for the winter months. In more heavily populated areas, individual and societal precautions must be taken to avoid the effects of winter storms. The cost of cleaning up after winter storms and loss of business during the storm can have significant economic impact. The winter of 2010 to 2011 in Europe began with an unusually cold November caused by a cold weather cycle that started in southern Scandinavia and subsequently moved south and west over both Belgium and The Netherlands and into the west of Scotland and northeast England. Cold weather and record snowfalls resulted in airport closures and cancellations of hundreds of flights due to the snow itself, leading to backups in connecting flights throughout Europe, stranding thousands in November and again in December. The January 2015 North American blizzard, unofficially named Winter Storm Juno, affected Canada and the central and eastern United States, moving on to Greenland and Western Europe. Snow emergencies were declared in six states and travel bans enacted in four of them, as well as in New York City. Up to 88 cm (34.5 inches) of snow fell in Worchester, Massachusetts, the largest storm accumulation on the city's record.

Causal Phenomena

Cold air and below-freezing temperatures in the clouds and near the ground are necessary to make snow and ice. Moisture is needed to form clouds and precipitation. The source of moisture may be air blowing across a body of water, such as a large lake or the ocean. *Lift,* or the required force needed to raise the moist air to form the clouds and cause precipitation, can occur when warm air collides with cold air and is forced to rise over the cold dome. The boundary between the warm and cold air is called a *front.* Lift might also occur from air flowing up a mountainside.

Strong Winds. Strong winds that sometimes accompany winter storms can create blizzard conditions with blinding wind-driven snow, severe drifting, and a dangerous windchill factor. Strong winds with these intense storms and cold fronts can knock down trees, utility poles, and power lines. Storms near the coast can cause coastal flooding and beach erosion, as well as sink ships at sea. Winds descending from mountains can gust to 160 km/hr (100 mph) or more, damaging roofs and other structures.

The windchill factor is based on the rate of heat loss from exposed skin caused by combined effects of wind and cold. As the wind increases, heat is carried away from the body at an accelerated rate, driving down the body temperature. Animals are also affected by windchill.

Extreme Cold. Extreme cold often accompanies a winter storm or is left in the aftermath. What constitutes extreme cold varies in different areas. For example, in areas unaccustomed to winter weather, temperatures at the freezing mark may be considered extreme. Freezing temperatures can cause severe damage to citrus fruit crops and other vegetation.

Prolonged exposure to cold can cause frostbite (damage to body tissue caused by tissue being frozen) or hypothermia (low body temperature) (see Chapters 6 and 9). Infants and elders are most susceptible.

Ice Storms. Even a small amount of ice poses a significant hazard to motorists and pedestrians. Accumulations of ice can bring down trees, electrical wires, telephone poles and lines, and communication towers. Communication and power can be disrupted for days while utility companies work to repair extensive damage.

Snowstorms. Snow may fall as flurries, showers, squalls, blowing snow, or blizzards, the last where winds over 56 km/hr (35 mph) and blowing snow reduce visibility. The 1993 "superstorm" that reached from Canada to Central America was manifest as a blizzard in most of the affected areas. In the United States, the storm was responsible for 300 deaths and loss of electric power to more than 10 million persons. Sleet (raindrops that freeze into ice pellets before reaching the ground) can accumulate and cause problems. Heavy snow can immobilize a region and paralyze a city. Travelers can be stranded and emergency services disrupted. In rural areas, homes and farms may be cut off for days, and livestock may die if unprotected. The probability of avalanches increases in the mountains.

Predictability

Although winter storm patterns are known in most areas of the world, predicting the intensity and characteristics of winter storms is not an exact science. The effects of El Niño on the winter storm patterns of 1998 are still being debated. Typical U.S. storm patterns include the "nor'easter," which affects the mid-Atlantic coast to New England from low-pressure areas off the Carolina coast. Research is continuously under way to improve forecasting tools and techniques. For example, the Center for Analysis and Prediction of Storms at the University of Oklahoma provides feedback for the National Weather Service, National Aeronautics and Space Administration, and Department of Defense.

The capacities of most national weather services allow individuals and public services to prepare for winter storms. Winter storm watches and warnings and winter weather advisories are normally issued in most vulnerable areas. In the 2015 Winter Storm Juno, the mayor of New York City received criticism for shutting down the subway system when much less snow fell than was predicted because he had relied on models that were 50 miles off target. However, previous "nor'easters" had resulted in heavier, more disabling snowfalls for the city.

Vulnerability

Lack of a preparedness plan by individuals and communities and lack of understanding of the effects of winter storms increase vulnerability. Failure to heed warnings, lack of communication facilities to receive warnings, and insufficient preparation to cope with the cold or possible isolation from heavy snow can lead to casualties. For example, a person stranded in a vehicle or home during a winter storm without a storm survival kit or without adequate heat, food, or water may become hypothermic or dehydrated. Lack of protection for the infrastructure, utilities, and houses can result in damage, loss of service, and roof collapse from heavy snow. Downed trees may later cause forest fires. Motorists unaccustomed to driving in winter storms cause more accidents. People living in uninsulated or unheated buildings are at greater risk for hypothermia.

The 1998 Ice Storm

A storm of unprecedented impact began on January 5, 1998, and ultimately damaged about 18 million acres of rural and urban forests throughout Maine, New Hampshire, Vermont, upstate

New York, and southeastern Canada. The storm severely affected the dairy industry, maple sugar industry, small businesses, public facilities, and infrastructure elements. Power outages lasted for up to 23 days. Thousands of people required shelter for an extended period, and nine people died in the United States.

The causal factors of the storm were both natural and human-made. The population and urbanization had recently increased in the area. Cold surface temperatures were overrun by a warm moist tropical air mass, resulting in record rainfall of 5 to 15 cm (2 to 6 inches). Below-freezing temperatures caused the rain to freeze on contact, producing ice accumulations of more than 7 to 10 cm (3 to 4 inches). These factors were intensified by the long duration and significant scope of the storm, resulting in severe flooding and ice damage. Much of the damage could not be assessed until the spring thaw. As a result of the storm, the Federal Emergency Management Agency reviewed the mitigation measures in place and made new recommendations.

ENVIRONMENTAL HAZARDS

ENVIRONMENTAL POLLUTION

The world population, now around 7.3 billion, is expected to reach 9.7 billion by 2050. Despite the pressures placed on natural resources by the expanding population, many poor countries still desperately need the benefits accompanying industrialization and economic growth. In general, people in developing countries are much more vulnerable to the effects of environmental degradation because they are poorer and depend more directly on the land.

Causal Phenomena

Various parts of the environment are subjected to the effects of toxic (poisonous) chemicals produced in manufacturing, such as paint and metal production, and the burning of fossil fuels, such as gasoline, coal, and oil. Some of these chemicals are heavy metals, such as lead, which are essentially nondegradable. Other toxic compounds, such as pesticides, are purposely introduced into the environment. Toxic chemicals may accumulate and affect the quality of air and water. Other pollutants of importance are from biologic sources, such as human waste, soil sediments, and decaying organic matter.

Air Pollution. Much of the world's urban population breathes polluted air at least part of the time. China, the United States, Russia, India, Mexico, and Japan lead the world in air pollution emissions. Sulfur dioxide, a major pollutant, is a corrosive gas harmful to humans and the environment. Electricity generation using fossil fuels is the key source of sulfur dioxide in industrialized countries. In developed countries the burning of fossil fuels also contributes to its creation. Other air pollutants include nitrogen oxides, CO_2, and lead, mainly from vehicle exhaust. China surpassed the United States as the biggest producer of CO_2 in 2007.

Marine Pollution. Sewage is the major cause of ocean pollution. Raw sewage containing human excreta and domestic wastes is disposed of in large quantities directly into the ocean. In the summer of 1993, thousands of ocean beaches were closed in the United States because of high levels of pathogens from human and animal waste. Industrial effluents are also piped into the ocean.

Other pollutants include marine litter, oil spills, and dumped chemical compounds, such as those containing mercury and radioactive substances. In April 2010, the *Deepwater Horizon* offshore drilling rig exploded in the Gulf of Mexico. Oil began to leak at the wellhead more than 1400 m (5000 feet) below the surface, ultimately spilling more than 4.8 million barrels of oil, or 205.8 million barrels of crude oil, before the flow was completely stopped in September 2010. The event surpassed by 20 times the *Exxon Valdez* disaster of 1989 in Alaska's Prince William Sound as the largest oil spill in history originating in U.S. waters. Efforts were made to dilute, disperse, and contain the oil, but as much as 75% of the oil remains unaccounted for. The environmental damage affected eight U.S. national parks and more than 400 animal species that live in the Gulf islands and marshlands.

The spill had short-term and long-term impacts on fishing revenue owing to closure of shrimping waters and loss of 20% of juvenile bluefin tuna (which were already declining in numbers) in the area, and on tourism in Louisiana.

Freshwater Pollution. Human waste and other domestic wastewaters are often discharged directly into nearby bodies of water, particularly in urban areas. In developing countries, this waste may be completely untreated. Industrial effluents from paper-making, chemical, metal-working, textile, and food-processing industries reach bodies of water by direct discharge or by leaching from dumps. In August 2015, the abandoned Gold King Mine in Colorado discharged an initial 3 million gallons of contaminated water, and then continuously 500 gallons a minute into the Animas River, which posed a danger to humans and animals due to arsenic content.

Clearing the land for agriculture and using irrigation, fertilizers, and pesticides have seriously affected water quality in many countries. Unprecedented deforestation has led to soil erosion, causing accelerated runoff and sediment deposits in riverbeds. The sediment level in rivers may increase 100-fold in deforested areas during rainy seasons.

Runoff of nitrogen from fertilizers, particularly in industrialized nations, renders some water unfit to drink without treatment. Use of irrigation systems may lead to increased salinity of water sources and saltwater intrusion on coastal areas where water is withdrawn. Approximately 25% of the world's pesticide production is used in developing countries, mainly on cash crops. Accumulations of pesticide toxins are found in food, soil, and water. Although data from Africa are lacking, studies in Asia indicate that rivers and lakes in Indonesia and Malaysia have very high levels of polychlorinated biphenyls and some pesticides.

Ozone Depletion. Ozone is a form of oxygen composed of three atoms of oxygen. Most atmospheric ozone is concentrated in the upper atmosphere, or stratosphere. The ozone layer ranges from 13 to 40 km (8 to 25 miles) above Earth. Ozone screens out harmful wavelengths of ultraviolet radiation that originate from the sun, protecting life on Earth (see Chapter 16). Ultraviolet light is associated with increased nonmelanoma skin cancer, ocular cataracts, and deterioration of the retina and cornea. In addition, oceanic phytoplankton are reduced, with damage to fish larvae and young fish. Because fish provide on average approximately 14% of the animal protein consumed worldwide (60% of that in Japan), the impact could be significant. A hole in the ozone layer has been detected over Antarctica. This hole appears seasonally and is roughly the size of the United States. Thinning of the ozone layer is caused by fluorinated gases, mainly CFCs, chemicals used in refrigeration, foam products, and aerosol propellants. Although they make up a fraction of greenhouse gases, they account for 20% of the warming trend caused by radioactive trapping potential (10,000 times greater than that of CO_2).

The 1987 Montreal Protocol, an international agreement to reduce ozone depletion, was ratified by 170 countries and has successfully led to decreased ozone-depleting chemicals in the lower atmosphere. Hydrofluorocarbons were largely developed to replace CFCs as required by the Montreal Protocol. However, hydrofluorocarbons are potent greenhouse gases with a long atmospheric life and may also contribute to global warming.

Climate Change and Global Warming. For the past several decades, the climate of Earth has been changing rapidly as a result of warming of the troposphere. Scientific evidence indicates that there has been warming of the atmosphere in the last 35 years that has manifested in an increase in sea surface temperatures; widespread melting of snow, glaciers, ice sheets, and permafrost; and a significant increase in the rate of sea level rise. Over the past 50 years, the average global temperature has increased at the fastest rate in recorded history; the 10 warmest years in the 134-year record have all occurred since 2000, with the exception of 1998, and the year 2014 was the warmest on record. Put in perspective, the climate of Earth over the past 3.2 million years has fluctuated greatly, with glacial and warmer interglacial intervals and accompanying adjustment by ecosystems and living creatures. A present concern is whether the changes are occurring too rapidly to allow adjustments to take place.

One explanation for global warming is the *greenhouse effect,* which is used to describe the role of atmospheric gases (such as CO_2, methane, and water vapor) in trapping radiation that would otherwise leave the atmosphere. Without this canopy of gases and clouds, the temperature of Earth would be extremely cold. The atmospheric gases therefore behave similarly to a greenhouse.

Since the beginning of the Industrial Revolution in the late 18th century, CO_2 in the atmosphere has increased by almost 25%, mainly from combustion of coal, oil, natural gas, and gasoline. A strong scientific consensus states that buildup of greenhouse gases is warming the global atmosphere. Computer models used to examine the climatic effects of increasing CO_2 suggest that if it doubles, global surface temperatures would increase on average by 1.5° to 4.5°C (2.7° to 8.1°F).

Because burning of fossil fuels is the primary cause of global warming, developed countries are mainly at fault, and poorer countries are more likely to be the victims. However, scientists estimate that between 15% and 20% of greenhouse gases (mainly CO_2) are generated by deforestation, a trend occurring at a devastating rate in developing countries, particularly in tropical rainforests. Trees play a vital role in recycling CO_2 by taking it in, transforming it chemically, storing the carbon, and releasing oxygen into the air. When trees are cut down, left to decay, or burned, they release stored carbon into the air as CO_2. Recently in Central Africa, virgin rainforests were found to have air pollution levels comparable to those in industrial areas. A major cause of this pollution is smoke from fires that rage for months across huge stretches of land. These fires are set to clear shrubs and trees for production of crops and grasses. The effects of acid rain (pollutants that are held in the clouds and fall back to Earth in rainwater) and air pollution in Europe, Canada, and the United States also contribute to increased CO_2.

Another greenhouse gas is methane. Methane is generated by bacteria as they break down organic matter. It is emitted largely by landfills, cattle, and fermenting rice paddies. The concentration of methane gas in the atmosphere has doubled in the past 200 years, mainly because of expanded animal husbandry and rice cultivation, more landfills, and leaking natural gas pipelines.

The single biggest factor in vulnerability to climate change is poverty. Climate change will most greatly affect poor communities across Africa, Asia, and South America.

Characteristics and Typical Adverse Effects

Air Pollution. Pollution of the troposphere (lower atmosphere) is damaging to agricultural crops, forests, aquatic systems, buildings, and human health. Primary pollutants often react to form secondary pollutants (acidic compounds), a frequent cause of environmental damage. The following effects are possible:

Crop and vegetation damage by injury to plant tissue, increasing susceptibility to disease and drought

Decline in forests caused by leaf damage by acidic compounds, acidic soils, and stresses of multiple pollutants

Damage to aquatic ecosystems so that they no longer support life

Degradation of building materials, such as metal, stone, and brick

Adverse impact on human health by damage to respiratory tracts

Marine Pollution. Marine pollution has the following major effects:

Spread of pathogens from human wastes, including viruses and protozoa, that cause hepatitis, cholera, typhoid, and other infectious diseases

Release of nondegradable materials, such as plastics and netting, which may injure marine mammals

Oil pollution from oil spills

Spread of hazardous chemicals and radioactive substances into the marine ecosystem, where they may accumulate in seafood

Freshwater Pollution. Freshwater pollution results in the following adverse effects:

Untreated wastewater carrying viruses and bacteria from human feces into human drinking water, which can result in illness or even in infant deaths

Eutrophication, or decay of organic matter, which decreases oxygen levels in water, upsetting the balance of the aquatic ecosystem

Adverse health effects in persons drinking untreated water from tainted sources

Water acidification, which reduces water's capacity to support aquatic life

Runoff sediment from eroded soil deposits in drainage basins, reducing basin capacity and exacerbating flooding

Salinization from irrigation, with harmful effects on downstream agriculture

Pesticides and fertilizer chemicals, which accumulate in water and affect tissues in living organisms

Global Warming. The impacts of global warming are still uncertain. Computer models are unable to make reliable predictions of regional changes. In all likelihood, the changes will lead to an increase in disasters, including those caused by drought, floods, tropical cyclones, and tornadoes. The following changes may occur.

Rise in Sea Levels. Melting of the Arctic ice sheets and alpine glaciers could cause the seas to expand and sea levels to rise. Depending on the degree of global warming, the seas may rise 30 cm to 2 m (12 inches to 7 feet) by 2075, jeopardizing coastal settlements and marine ecosystems. A rise of 1 m (3.28 feet) in sea levels could flood 15% of arable land in Egypt's Nile Delta and would flood 12% of Bangladesh, displacing 11 million people. The tiny island of the Maldives, inhabited by 200,000, would be submerged (Figure 85-24).

Climate Change. Natural disasters, such as superhurricanes, could become common. A temperature increase of a few degrees in tropical seas can intensify hurricane production. The warmer oceans may increase the El Niño phenomenon near the coast of Peru. The El Niño southern oscillation inhibits phytoplankton growth, causes fish and shellfish to migrate or die, and forces

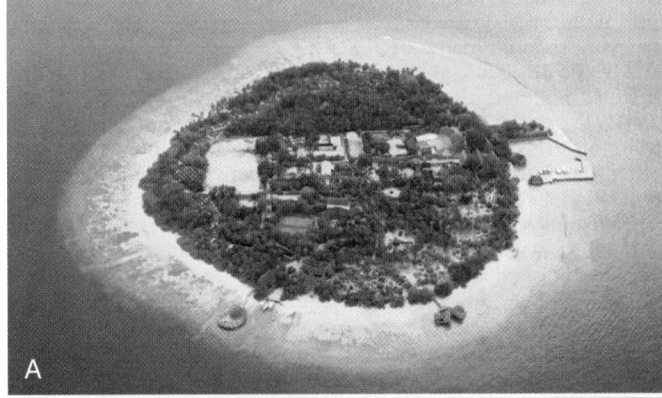

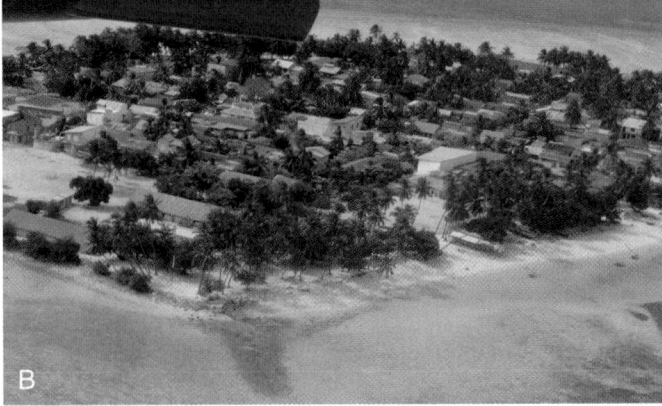

FIGURE 85-24 Islands with diminishing shorelines in the Maldives. *(Courtesy Sheila B. Reed.)*

higher forms of life (e.g., birds, humans) dependent on this sea life to migrate or die.

Other climatic changes could lead to warmer and drier conditions in middle latitudes, higher temperatures in semitropical and tropical areas, and higher rates of evaporation. Rainfall patterns may also change. The combined effects of increased CO_2 and climate changes may alter plant and animal productivity. Plants may grow faster and larger but may have reduced nutritive value.

Changes in Ecosystems. In warmer climates, grasslands, savannas, and deserts may expand, rendering them vulnerable to increased degradation through erosion and fire. Animal species that do not adapt to the temperature increases may have to relocate to survive, which would be difficult, given population pressures on land. Plant species unable to adapt would perish.

Public Health Impact. Global warming may affect mortality rates because of heat stress and may increase the incidences of respiratory diseases, allergies, and reproductive illnesses. Geographic ranges of vector-induced diseases (e.g., mosquito-borne malaria, yellow fever) and parasitic diseases might increase.

Measurement of Pollutants

Air and Water Pollutants. Pollutants are measured worldwide, but to a much lesser degree in developing countries. The most comprehensive data collection system is the Global Environment Monitoring System of the UN Environmental Programme, which provides data on sulfur dioxide and particulate matter in urban air and contaminants in water resources. Pollution production is related to per capita consumption, so that as countries develop, pollution tends to increase.

Ozone Depletion. Ozone levels are regularly monitored annually all over the world, especially in the Southern Hemisphere, where a seasonal ozone hole opens over Antarctica every year. As of 2002, there were 5791 kilotons of CFCs in existing products, such as refrigerators, air conditioners, aerosol cans, and others. However, the ban on CFCs and reduction in other fluorocarbons should result in a smaller ozone hole by 2040. By 2100, the ozone hole may completely disappear, assuming full compliance with the Montreal Protocol.

Greenhouse Effect. Greenhouse gas emissions are regularly measured throughout the world. Even if the exact levels of future greenhouse emissions were available, however, predicting the effects on global climate would be difficult. Climatic models are used to study climate change, but the models differ in their interpretation of the various interactions in Earth's systems, partly because information put into the system is incomplete; however, linkages between variables are becoming more clearly understood.

Environmental Pollution Risk Reduction Measures

Air and Water Pollution. Most nations are acting individually to control air pollution. However, since the 1986 Chernobyl Nuclear Power Plant accident in Ukraine, transboundary pollution has been recognized as an environmental hazard necessitating a multinational approach. Basic goals are to set ambient air quality standards that measure pollutants away from the source, set controls on acceptable levels, and require that every source of an air pollutant meet certain emission limits. In some cases, technologies still need to be developed to make these goals possible.

Pollution control of coastal areas in the past has proved that recovery is possible to some extent. The banned pesticide DDT, which had been found in many forms of marine life, is now decreasing in concentration. Most strategies for protecting the oceans must address broader ranges of pollutants from sewage to industrial effluents. More national and international efforts should focus on establishing the policy for protection of coastal areas. The *Deepwater Horizon* oil spill of 2010 in the Gulf of Mexico illustrated certain management issues related to offshore drilling. Government regulatory agencies were not fully aware of the cost-saving measures used by the companies involved; these measures were deemed directly responsible for causing the disaster. More strict regulations need to be imposed and monitored.

Improvement of soils can decrease the possibility of water contamination by toxic chemicals and decrease runoff, thereby lessening silting and sedimentation of waterways. Establishing

terraces and contour bounds, stabilizing sand dunes, building check dams, and planting trees and shrubs can help to stabilize soil. Watershed mapping, management, and protection are also of vital importance in ensuring a safe and plentiful drinking water supply. Proper systems to dispose of human waste should be promoted.

Regulations must be established and enforced by government agencies to protect citizens against the toxic effects of pesticides and other chemicals. Improvement of soils will also help to absorb and degrade toxins. Further studies must be made on the effects of pesticide residues. Farmers may use crop types resistant to pests or an integrated approach to pest management requiring less pesticide.

Ozone Depletion. International cooperation to limit CFC emissions should reduce production and use of CFCs in industrialized nations by 50% from 1986 levels, with developing countries allowed to increase their use slightly. Research is addressing the need for developing CFC substitutes, for minimizing loss to the atmosphere, and for recycling. Countries can regulate import and use of aerosols and disposal of refrigeration units.

Climate Change and Global Warming. All countries need to work together to minimize the effects of climate change as it directly affects our daily lives and health and the survival of species. The UN Framework Convention on Climate Change of 1994 has 194 participating states and organizations. Its ultimate objective is to achieve stabilization of greenhouse gas concentrations in the atmosphere at a level that is not dangerous. The Kyoto Protocol of 2005 is linked to the UN Framework Convention on Climate Change and sets compulsory emission targets for industrialized countries. The Bali Action Plan (2008) focused on ways to adapt to climate change and enhanced access by developing countries to predictable and sustainable financial resources for adaptation. The basic steps that need to be taken include:

Significantly reduce greenhouse gases in the next decade by enacting the needed regulatory, technologic, and behavioral changes, such as regulations to curb pollution from traffic emissions and industry

Reduce the rate of deforestation; plant trees to solve community needs for wood, such as fuel wood, or to provide profits for individual farmers with agroforestry

Increase energy production and use; promote energy efficiency in urban areas, and support renewable energy sources, such as wind, water, geothermal, and solar power; these may be of great use in areas where no electricity sources exist

Education is a vital tool for environmental awareness. By understanding relationships of ecosystems and long-term effects of degradation, people are motivated to act. Women's groups in India have established a tree protection lobby. Their motto is "trees are not wood," a concept that promotes trees as a vital part of the ecosystem, providing CO_2 exchange in the air and a root system to hold down the soil. Education regarding the environment should begin in children's early years. Education for adults may take place in farmers' cooperatives, women's cooperatives, and village settings or may accompany programs to distribute seeds and tools.

Saving the Arctic

The Arctic Ocean, a semienclosed ocean surrounded by land and composed mainly of snow and ice, is warming at a rate twice as fast as the rest of the world, partly due to black carbon pollution. Black carbon is a component of soot that peppers the snow and ice with heat-absorbing black particles. The changes are affecting the land and livelihoods of Native Alaskan coastal communities and melting the Greenland ice sheet, driving sea level rise. Over the past 7 years, snow and ice coverage has been the least ever recorded. Other pollutants affecting the Arctic include Arctic haze from long-range pollutants and bioaccumulation of polychlorinated biphenyls in Arctic wildlife and people.

The Arctic Counsel is an eight-nation body, chaired by the United States, established to take the reins about the fate of the Arctic. U.S. regulations on diesel fuel may help to reduce black carbon emissions; however, these cuts may be undermined by resumption of oil exploration in Alaska.

DEFORESTATION

Deforestation is removal or damage of vegetation in a region that is predominantly tree covered. Deforestation is a slow-onset hazard that may contribute to disasters caused by flooding, landslides, and drought. Deforestation reaches critical proportions when large areas of vegetation are removed or damaged, harming the land's protective and regenerative properties. The rapid rate of deforestation in some parts of the world is a driving force in the yearly increase of flood disasters in these areas.

Changes reported by the Food and Agriculture Organization in its Global Forest Resources Assessment 2015 indicated encouraging news, namely, that the global rate of deforestation has decreased and substantial progress has taken place in forest management. Over the past 25 years, the forest area has decreased by approximately 3.1%, but there are positive trends for reduction in forest loss. Although there was annual global deforestation of 7.6 million hectares between 2010 and 2015, there was an annual gain of 4.3 million hectares. This resulted in a net decrease of 3.3 million, compared with 9.4 million deforested hectares per annum in the 1990s. The biggest forest area loss continues to be in the tropics, particularly South America and Africa, although those rates have also decreased substantially in the past 5 years. Forests coming under management plans have increased from 27% of production forest in the 1990s to 52% of the total forested area in 2010.

The countries with the highest net loss of forest area between 2010 and 2015 are Brazil, Indonesia, Myanmar, Nigeria, Tanzania, Paraguay, Zimbabwe, Democratic Republic of the Congo, Argentina, and Venezuela. Those with the highest net gain of forest area during this period were China, Austria, Chile, the United States, the Philippines, Gabon, Laos, India, Vietnam, and France. Globally, natural forest area (also an indicator in biodiversity) is decreasing, and planted forest is increasing. Natural forest accounts for 93% of the total forest area in 2015.

The average per capita forest area has decreased from 0.8 hectare to 0.6 hectare per person during the years 1990 to 2015. Forests provide subsistence and income for nearly 1.6 billion people; the economic benefits must be considered while planning management programs. Although the amount of forestland coming under protection or conservation is growing, the future still poses problems because of rapidly increasing pressures of development and exploitation.

Causal Phenomena

The principal causes for loss and degradation of forests are conversion to other land uses (mainly agriculture and grazing) and overexploitation of forest products (industrial wood, fuel wood).

Underlying the obvious causes are fundamental problems in development, such as the use of inefficient agricultural practices (e.g., overgrazing), insecure land tenure, rising unemployment, rapid population growth, and failure to regulate and preserve forestlands. Contributing factors are air pollution, storms, pests, and diseases. A significant contributing cause in the 1990s was the number of wildfires that occurred in the western United States, Ethiopia, the western Mediterranean, and Indonesia.

Conversion of Forests to Agricultural Land. The major cause of forest loss is the spread of farming. Land may be cleared for commercial ventures such as sugar cane, coffee, or rubber plantations, which are principal causes of deforestation in Central America. In tropical rainforests, both legal colonists and squatters (i.e., illegal settlers) are trying to farm the former jungle lands, where soil conditions are fragile. Up to 90% of the nutrients are in vegetation rather than in the soil. When the forest is cut and burned, a nutrient surge occurs in the soil, lending initial fertility. After cropping and exposure to sun and rain, however, soil fertility rapidly declines, and the area becomes unproductive, perhaps prompting the farmer to slash and burn new forest areas.

Many indigenous people in the Amazon Basin, Central Africa, and Southeast Asia still practice shifting cultivation techniques, allowing fallow periods between cropping for soils to regenerate. This practice becomes unsustainable if populations increase to the extent of forcing people into smaller areas. Insecure land tenure or fixed land titles may also force overuse of the land.

Because of crowded conditions in cities and farm areas, many people migrate to areas of marginal fertility, where they must keep moving their fields to produce sufficient food. Where this occurs, the migrant farmer may damage timber, wildlife, and human resources. In Venezuela, a country that has a high rate of unemployment and rising numbers of landless peasants, 30,000 families live and farm in national parks, forest reserves, and other legally protected areas. An influx of cultivators who settled on the watershed above the Panama Canal has caused increased silting of a major reservoir that supplies Panama City.

In Central and South America, large areas of tropical forest have been cleared to create grazing lands. A major portion of this can be attributed to economic enterprises designed for meat production. The Brazilian government has granted large land concessions to domestic and foreign corporations wanting to raise cattle in the Amazon area. In Central America, virgin forest is being destroyed by ranchers who intend to export beef to the United States.

Overexploitation of Forest Products. Extensive logging in humid tropical forests, particularly in Asia and in temperate and mountainous forests, is conducted by large multinational corporations for export or to fill building needs in cities. The procedure usually involves either clear-cutting or creaming (selective logging) of the forest's small proportion of valued species. Creaming, even though it is a less radical alternative to clear-cutting, causes significant damage to vegetation and wildlife that is not apparent from statistics. A study in Indonesia revealed that logging operations damaged or destroyed about 40% of trees left behind. The roads created by logging operations may encourage settlers to enter the forest and begin slash and burn agriculture, so that eventually, even more of the forest is lost.

Firewood collection can contribute to the depletion of tree cover, particularly in lightly wooded areas. Because of a lack of alternative fuels and fuel-efficient stoves, this is especially a problem in Africa and in Asian highland countries such as Nepal. In areas of dense woods, dead material may fill local requirements for fuel. The outright destruction of trees for fuel occurs most commonly around cities and towns, where commercial markets for firewood and charcoal exist. Well-organized groups and individuals bring fuel wood by vehicle, pack animal, and cart into many cities, hastening local deforestation.

Fuel Wood Crisis. About 100 million people in developing countries cannot meet their minimum needs for energy, and almost 1.3 billion consume fuel wood resources faster than they are being replenished. In parts of West Africa, some urban families spend one-fourth of their income on wood or charcoal for cooking. In India, firewood is subsidized for the poor to prevent starvation.

Characteristics

Trees play a vital role in regulating Earth's atmosphere, ecosystems, and weather systems. They recycle CO_2, a gas now increasing in the atmosphere and thought to contribute to global warming. They release moisture to the air, thus contributing to rainfall and moderating the local and global climate. Their roots trap nutrients, improve soil fertility, and trap pollutants, keeping these from the water supply. Trees provide habitats for species, engendering diversity. They nurture traditional cultures by giving shelter, wood, food, and medicinal products. These benefits are lost as trees are destroyed.

The root systems of vegetation help retain water in the soil, anchor the soil particles, and provide aeration to keep soil from compacting. When vegetation dies, the nutrients go back to the soil. When root systems are removed, soil becomes destabilized. Water tends to flow off the top of the soil instead of percolating in, and carries valuable topsoil along with it. This soil eventually forms sediment in the drainage basins.

Deforestation poses the most immediate danger by its contribution to the following hazards:

Destabilized soils are more susceptible to landslides and may increase landslide risk in areas vulnerable to earthquakes and volcanoes.

Loss of moisture from deforestation may contribute to drought conditions, which in turn may trigger famines. Soil nutrients may also be lost through erosion of topsoil, resulting in decreased food production and possible chronic food shortages.

Erosion and dry conditions, combined with loss of vegetation and soil compaction, result in desertification and unproductive lands.

Dryness may accelerate spread of fires.

Loss of CO_2 from dying trees and fires may add to global warming.

Deforestation of watersheds, especially around smaller rivers and streams, can increase severity of flooding, reduce stream flows, evaporate springs in dry seasons, and increase the amount of sediment entering waterways.

Of all the hazards associated with deforestation, flooding may be the most serious. Usually, curative measures (e.g., dredging and dam building) rather than preventive measures are taken to solve flooding problems. As flooding worsens in developing countries, more attention is given to protection of watersheds. In India, flood damages between 1953 and 1978 averaged $250 million per year. Today, even more people live in flood-prone areas. Flood problems may not be lessened without reforestation of the increasingly denuded hills of northern India and Nepal.

Predictability

Forest resource data are being generated at a greater frequency. As of 2014, 112 countries had national forest inventories, covering 82% of the forested areas. Data are lagging in the topics and low-income countries. Measurement and monitoring of forested areas may be conducted through ground-level sampling and aerial or satellite surveys. Each method has drawbacks. Ground sampling is tedious and difficult to extrapolate, aerial surveys are expensive, and satellite imagery poses difficulty in distinguishing forests from other vegetation. Combinations of methods usually produce the best results.

Vague definitions in the study of deforestation continue to make exact determinations and forecasting difficult. According to the World Wildlife Fund's "Living Forests Report" of 2015, up to 170 million hectares of forest could be lost between 2010 and 2030 in the Amazon, Atlantic Forest and Gran Chaco (Amazon Basin), Borneo, Cerrado (Brazil), Choco-Darien (Central America), Congo Basin, East Africa, East Australia, Greater Mekong, New Guinea, and Sumatra. In addition to forest loss, productivity of forest is another sustainable indicator that needs to be measured. Forest degradation may be gauged in terms of loss of any of the goods and services that forests provide, such as fiber, food, habitat, water, carbon storage, and other protective and sociocultural values. This measurement is not an exact science, but the Food and Agricultural Organization is studying the economic benefits from forests and how to improve them with policy measures linked to the benefits.

Typical Adverse Effects

The specific impacts of deforestation include:

Loss of soil fertility in the tropics and loss of productive capacity

Soil erosion and deposition of sediment

Increased runoff

Reduction in rainfall and increase in temperature

Destruction of biodiversity and traditional cultures

Loss of "free" and extracted goods, such as fuels, food, and medicines

Exacerbation of other disasters

Economic Impact. Most developing countries are already importers of forest products, especially paper. Because the amount of wood and wood products available per person in the world is falling and thus their prices are increasing, and because of shortages of foreign currencies, import of forest products may be increasingly prohibitive for these countries. Commercially marketed firewood is becoming scarcer, and prices are climbing. Wood for construction is also scarce in many countries, which adversely affects availability of housing.

Deforestation Risk Reduction Measures

Various types of forest management, reforestation, and community participation can reduce deforestation. Over the past 25 years, countries have significantly increased knowledge of their forest resources, and most governments now recognize the vital importance of national forestry programs. Foresters help people meet their basic needs for forest products, and not always from the traditional forest or concentrated woodlot. Farmers who practice reforestation on their lands contribute effectively to the environment. Reforestation has become intrinsically interwoven with other government policies that affect the population. Forestry therefore should be considered an integral part of land use and natural resource planning sectors of government.

Forests should be viewed by governments as capital resources to be managed. Management of the system should discourage concessionaires who have been given rights to sell wood obtained from property belonging to the government or others from practices that are not sustainable. Good management encourages highly selective harvesting without undue waste of remaining trees, especially in tropical forests. Involvement of communities in forest management is now a significant feature of national forest policies throughout the world. Forest management policies must consider the need to protect forests in conflict areas and to avoid exacerbating conflict over forest resources. For any country to address its loss of forests and ensure that forests will yield economic benefits well into the future, following steps must be taken:

Forest law or basic forest policy must be written that clearly states the objective of long-term sustainable management of the forest.

Forest regulations or management guidelines must be written and followed.

Sufficient financial and human resources must be allocated.

Forest management must be considered in the broadest sense of land use planning to include solutions for people as well as for trees. Compromises between complete destruction of the forests and complete conservation might entail regulated clearing of forests for shifting cultivation, habitation, or hunting; voluntary and intentional protection of forests or individual species by designating areas for reserves or national parks; and enrichment of the forest with species from other places. The last option may be considered risky, because pests and other problems specific to certain species may accompany introduction of nonnative species.

Many unresolved scientific issues in forest management remain. How can the ever-expanding areas of secondary vegetation and degraded soils be managed to be more productive for the local people? Because most primary forests have disappeared, what type of forest can be established that would be stable and productive and that would ensure the conservation of biologic diversity? What further types of basic ecologic research are needed to manage natural forests? How can the benefits from forest utilization effectively reach communities?

DESERTIFICATION

Desertification is defined as land degradation in arid, semiarid, and dry subhumid areas, resulting mainly from human actions. Poor land use is a significant contributing factor, but desertification can also be caused by natural cycles of climate change. It affects both developed and developing regions, including Africa, the Middle East, India, Pakistan, China, Australia, Eastern Europe, Central Asia, the central and southwestern United States, and many Mediterranean countries. A slow-onset disaster, desertification worsens conditions of poverty, brings malnutrition and disease, and destabilizes the social and economic bases of affected countries.

Causal Phenomena

Climate Conditions. Vulnerability to desertification and severity of its impact are partially governed by climatic conditions of an area. The lower and more uncertain the rainfall, the greater is the potential for desertification. Other influencing factors are seasonal patterns of rainfall and high temperatures that increase evaporation, land use, and the type of vegetation cover.

The world's drylands, which are inhabited by more than 2.1 billion people, are found in two belts centered approximately on the Tropic of Cancer and the Tropic of Capricorn (23.5 degrees north and south of the equator, respectively) and cover 41% of Earth's surface. More than 80% of the total area of drylands is found on three continents: Africa (37%), Asia (33%), and Australia (14%). The drylands can be further classified into hyperarid, arid, and semiarid zones, depending on the average amount of rainfall received per year. Other factors, such as temperature and soil conditions, must be considered when determining the dryness ratio.

Both natural and human-derived climatic changes may contribute to desertification. Natural effects, such as long-term climatic cycles and the basic geometry of the earth and the sun, have resulted in drier conditions in the Sahara. Human influence is associated with the predicted global warming trend and local climatic changes, in which deforestation has reduced moisture-holding capacity of soil and decreased cloud formation. The result is less rainfall and higher temperatures.

Despite the common misperception that desertification is caused by the desert advancing itself, land degradation can occur at great distances from deserts. Desertification usually begins as a spot on the land where land abuse has been excessive; from that spot, land degradation can spread outward with continued abuse (Figure 85-25). Desertification does not cause drought but may result in greater persistence of, or susceptibility to, drought. Drought, on the other hand, contributes to desertification and increases the rate of degradation. When the rains return, however, well-managed lands recover from droughts with minimal adverse effects. Land abuse during periods of good rains and its continuation during periods of deficient rainfall contribute to desertification.

Poor Land Use Management. Desertification can be caused by five main types of poor land use, degradation, and removal of vegetation: overcultivation, cash cropping, overgrazing, deforestation, and poor irrigation practices.

Overcultivation. Overcultivation damages the structure of the soil or removes vegetation cover, leaving the soil vulnerable to erosion. Reasons for overcultivation include drought, increasing demand for food because of population growth, cropping on

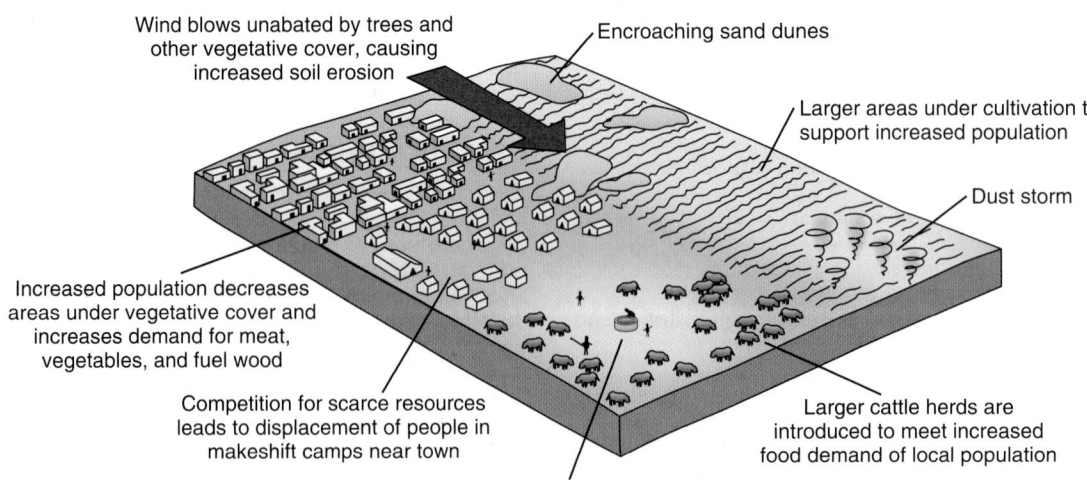

Healthy region

Winds are slowed down by vegetation, reducing wind erosion at ground level

Clouds form, causing local rains

Moisture from living vegetation evaporates, forming rain clouds

Small fields and crops supportable by regular rainfall

Trees give shade, fodder, and fuel wood for local village

Viable rangelands support small herds of grazing cattle

A

Desertified region

Wind blows unabated by trees and other vegetative cover, causing increased soil erosion

Encroaching sand dunes

Larger areas under cultivation to support increased population

Dust storm

Increased population decreases areas under vegetative cover and increases demand for meat, vegetables, and fuel wood

Competition for scarce resources leads to displacement of people in makeshift camps near town

Spot desertification starts around well due to abuse by people, livestock, and erosion

Larger cattle herds are introduced to meet increased food demand of local population

B

FIGURE 85-25 Comparison of healthy and desertified regions. (*Modified from United Nations Development Programme,* Introduction to hazards, *ed 3, New York, 1997, Disaster Management Training Programme, UN Office for the Coordination of Humanitarian Assistance.*)

marginal rangelands unsuitable for long-term production, land tenure restrictions confining sectors of the population to marginal lands, mechanized farming, and expansion of cash cropping.

Cash Cropping. Although a large part of agricultural production in developing countries fills subsistence needs, some cash crops are grown for foreign exchange. Unfortunately, a feature of most cash crops is their extreme demand for nutrients and optimum conditions. Degradation of land occurs directly through improper management of such crops and indirectly by displacing subsistence crops and pastoralism to marginal lands.

Overgrazing. Overgrazing is a major cause of desertification (rangelands account for 90% of desertified lands) and occurs when too many animals are pastured. The number of cattle in Niger, for example, increased an estimated 450% between 1938 and 1961 and an additional 29% by 1970, when the majority were killed by starvation. Livestock density increases when herd sizes grow too large in wet years and cannot be sustained in dry years. Lucrative markets for meat, such as Nigeria and the Middle East, have resulted in cattle ranches, where concentrated activity threatens land, with poor returns for the investment.

Better veterinary care has decreased mortality rates. Deep wells increase availability of water, allowing larger, less mobile herds that congregate in the well area and degrade the vegetation and soil.

Deforestation. Land is cleared for agriculture, livestock, and fuel wood production. Deforestation is the first step toward desertification, removing vegetative barriers and exposing land to sun, wind, and rain. In Africa, demands for fuel wood and charcoal exert considerable stress on wood resources.

Poor Irrigation Management. The concept of using irrigation to ward off the threat of crop failure during drought has been promoted by many development agencies. Ironically, poor management of irrigation projects has been a cause of desertification. In some cases, productivity falls and soils become salinized, alkalinized, or waterlogged. The major problem is usually inadequate drainage, and damage may be irreversible. A key example is the Greater Mussayeb irrigation project in Iraq, begun in 1953. By 1969, waterlogging was widespread, and two-thirds of the soil was saline. In 1970, a project to reclaim the salinized land was begun; because of technical and organizational limitations, the project was not successful. Egypt, Iraq, and Pakistan have lost more than 25% of their irrigated areas to salinization and waterlogging.

Role of Government Policy. Population growth and economic expansion also contribute to desertification. As populations grow, government and multilateral policies must promote increased food production through appropriate technologies that prevent soil degradation and erosion. Government policy should also address the causes of poverty, or disadvantaged peoples will place more stress on land to obtain needed resources. Some governments choose to expand cash crop cultivation to improve foreign currency holdings rather than promote food security for the poor, or they fail to resolve conflicts over scarce resources. Policies may mandate land uses that are difficult to enforce and that result in breakdown of customary land tenure or natural resource management institutions.

Characteristics

The two main characteristics of desertification, degradation of soil and degradation of vegetation, have the same result: reduction of productivity.

Degradation of Vegetation. Vegetation in arid lands adapts to the cycle of water availability by adjusting its growth. The drier the area, the farther apart plants grow. Some plants grow only during rainy seasons. Degradation of vegetation occurs initially in the early stages of desertification with deforestation, but continues after soil fertility declines.

The two main forms of vegetation degradation are overall reduction of density of the vegetation cover, or biomass, and a more subtle change in types of vegetation to less productive forms. For example, rangeland perennial grasses may be replaced by less palatable annual varieties, or more saline-tolerant crops, such as barley, may be substituted for traditional crops because of low yields from waterlogging and salinization.

Degradation of Soil. Soil degradation occurs in four major ways: water erosion, wind erosion, soil compaction, and waterlogging, which result in salinization and alkalinization.

Water Erosion. Vegetation normally protects soil from being washed away by rain and also from splash erosion by raindrops. The raindrops move the soil particles and pack them together on the surface, sealing the pores and thereby decreasing infiltration and increasing runoff. Sheet erosion is a more serious form of erosion in which fine layers of topsoil carrying soil nutrients are washed away. Unless the nutrients are replenished artificially, crop yields decline. Gullies are created by the runoff and, unless reclaimed by conservation measures, render the land unusable.

Wind Erosion. Wind erosion occurs when finer components of the soil, such as silt, clay, and organic matter that contain most of the nutrients, are blown away, leaving behind the less fertile sand and coarse particles. Sand itself may start to drift, forming dunes, but this accounts for a minor proportion of the effects of wind erosion. Strong winds may form dust storms that damage crops by shredding leaves.

Soil Compaction. Nearly complete compaction can occur when soil of poor structure is compressed by heavy machinery or by hooves of large herds of animals. A less serious form of compaction, called *surface crusting,* results when high-speed mechanical cultivation or dry season cultivation turns particles into thin powder, which then forms a crust when pelted with raindrops. Crusting and compaction make the soil less permeable for germination of new plants.

Waterlogging (Salinization and Alkalinization). These effects result from poor management of irrigation and water supplies in general. When the soil is waterlogged, the upward movement of saline in groundwater leaves salt on the surface when the water evaporates.

Predictability

Desertification is a direct socioeconomic threat to more than 200 million people and a less direct threat to 700 million, but data are still insufficient to quantify the extent of the problem and its progression. It leads to estimated losses in agricultural production of $42 billion. Databases are incomplete or do not exist for many countries. More information is needed on the characteristics and status of dryland ecosystems. Understanding climatic changes, including effects of possible global warming, is crucial to predictability. Socioeconomic indicators showing trends in human health, income, and welfare must be collected to understand related issues.

The International Soil Reference and Information Centre and UN Environmental Programme support the Global Assessment of Soil Degradation, which uses a geographic information system to access data for different areas of the world and estimate land degradation.

Rate and Scope

Although the numbers remain controversial, yearly losses to desertification are estimated at 1 to 1.3 million hectares of irrigated land, 3.5 to 4 million hectares of rain-fed cropland, and 4.5 to 5.8 million hectares of rangeland. These estimates represent an increase of 3.4% from estimates in 1994, indicating that the situation is worsening. The area of desertification is thought to be increasing at about 60,000 km^2 per year. The Global Assessment of Soil Degradation estimates for extent of desertification between 1983 and 1990 were 20% of dryland soil.

Desertification affects drylands in more than 110 countries but is concentrated in Asia and Africa, which together account for 70% of all desertified land. Scientists have tried to quantify the areas desertified on a worldwide basis. The physical damage can be measured in reduced productivity of soils and loss of vegetation. The number of casualties cannot be scientifically extrapolated, but deaths occur, directly from famine or indirectly from reduced standards of living.

Desertification Risk Reduction

The Secretariat of the UN Convention to Combat Desertification, an organization with 193 countries as parties by 2009, works with governments to highlight national focal points to communicate with scientific communities, civil society organizations, the public, and other stakeholders on matters related to desertification, land degradation, and drought. A number of innovative methods are in use to help mitigate desertification, but a great deal more effort and resources are required to stop progression. Mitigation measures should be included in national action plans to address agricultural development, drought, deforestation, and loss of biodiversity, among others. Educating children in schools and community members about the desertification hazard and dangers of deforestation is critical, as are supporting planting of seedlings and promoting other local mitigation measures. Solutions to the need for cooking fuel include solar ovens and efficient wood-burning cook stoves, which have helped to relieve pressure on the environment; however, these may be too costly for the poor to afford unless they are subsidized.

Techniques to improve and rejuvenate soil include the use of seawater that is desalinated and pumped inland. Fixating the soil is often done through use of shelterbelts, woodlots, and windbreaks. A "Green Wall of China," eventually intended to stretch more than 5700 km (3500 miles) in length (nearly as long as China's Great Wall), is being planted in northeastern China to protect deserts created by human activity. Soil enrichment and restoration of its fertility are often accomplished by planting such foods as grains, barley, and dates, as well as legumes, which extract nitrogen from the air and fix it in the soil. Sand fences can also be used to control drifting of soil and sand erosion.

ACKNOWLEDGMENTS AND RESOURCES

This chapter builds on the original teaching concept developed in Introduction to Hazards, *third edition (1997), a module prepared by this contributing author and by InterWorks of Madison, Wisconsin, for the UN Development Programme's Disaster Management Training Programme and the UN Office for the Coordination of Humanitarian Assistance. Another background document is* Natural Hazards: Causes and Effects, *a course text published in 1986 by the Disaster Management Center at the University of Wisconsin–Madison.*

SUGGESTED READINGS

Complete suggested readings used in this text are available online at expertconsult.inkling.com.

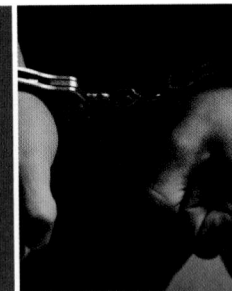

CHAPTER 86

Global Crimes, Incarceration, and Quarantine

MICHAEL VANROOYEN AND SHAWN D'ANDREA

Most physicians and medical personnel practice in relatively safe and stable environments, although some health care providers have chosen to work in conflict or other crisis settings that involve some degree of political instability and personal danger. To health care workers interested in working internationally, remote climates may seem inherently dangerous, but the opposite is often the case. For example, a rural setting in Sudan may be remote and relatively austere but is likely to be safe and secure; alternatively, working in the inner city of Nairobi, Kenya, may be much more dangerous.

Traveling and working in conflict areas or regions with significant political or social volatility requires a far more detailed understanding of the unique attributes of conflict areas. Judging whether a certain geographic region is dangerous requires significant knowledge of that area's unique political, economic, social, and cultural context. It is important to realize the relative risk of travel itself, as well as the likely causes of illness and death among travelers. The most frequent killers of travelers are cardiovascular disease and accidental injuries (most commonly motor vehicle accidents). As this chapter reviews the unique risks to workers in hostile geopolitical environments, conflict settings, war zones, and unstable social environments, it is important to keep in mind the more predictable risks of accidents and underlying health issues in travelers, in order to plan and deploy mitigation strategies.

There is very good evidence that health care workers and humanitarians working in areas of modern conflict around the world have a significantly increased risk of being killed or injured as a result of violent causes. One needs to determine the degree of risk that accompanies spending time in any particular locale. Determination of the degree of danger is a complex and dynamic process, and cannot be adequately ascertained solely from media reports or U.S. State Department travel advisories. The risk of an adverse event while traveling is closely linked to the traveler's behaviors and abilities to adapt to the shifting political and security environments in regions that may be inherently dangerous as a result of military presence, differing ethnicities, and political volatility. The contents of this chapter cover a range of considerations for travelers and aid workers traveling to settings affected by social or political instability. This information is not intended to substitute for comprehensive training programs in safety and security provided by aid organizations, the United Nations, and academic and other institutions. The authors strongly recommend that any individual considering travel to or work in such environments obtain comprehensive safety and security training.

HOSTILE GEOPOLITICAL ENVIRONMENTS AND POLITICAL INSECURITY

Certain locations frequented by civilian travelers and international workers are known to be more dangerous than others. Modern conflict over the last two decades has increasingly victimized civilians and nonwarring parties, including women and children. International workers and local and foreign staff of humanitarian agencies have been increasingly targeted for crime and other hostile activities. The conduct of war has changed considerably during the last decades in the following ways:

INCREASING NUMBERS OF VIOLENT REGIONAL ETHNIC CONFLICTS

As the Cold War era ended, the new world order quickly gave rise to a variety of ethnic tensions devoid of superpower arbitration. During the 1990s, civil conflicts erupted in the Balkans, Central Asia, and the Middle East and throughout Africa. At the time of writing, the world has more than 40 ongoing armed conflicts.[9] Many of these conflicts are intrastate struggles, with many deemed ethnic or religious wars. These conflicts are in contrast to previous international cross-border conflicts launched as proxy wars between the United States, the Soviet Union, and other neocolonialists. The net result of modern civil conflict has been massive-scale refugee emergencies and public health disasters as well as an influx of foreign workers. In addition to formally defined intrastate and international armed conflicts, there are many countries with levels of violence reflected in violent death rates that exceed those of countries at war. For example, domestic gang conflict and drug trafficking in countries in Latin America, such as Honduras, are thought to be among many factors that contribute to markedly elevated rates of homicide in the region that exceed those of many countries in the midst of internationally recognized armed conflict.[21,26]

CIVILIAN CASUALTIES

Drafting of the Geneva Convention and adoption of the tenets of international humanitarian law and codes of conduct in war have not stemmed the tide of human rights abuses and deliberate targeting of civilians during the past three decades. There is ongoing debate regarding the exact impact of war on civilian populations, but reports consistently demonstrate that the civilian population bears a very high burden of morbidity and mortality in conflict.[22] Although causes of death include violence, most deaths occur from communicable diseases and other preventable illnesses.[2] Attacking and controlling civilian populations has been a method of securing territory in conflicts, as in Darfur, the Democratic Republic of the Congo, and Syria. Civilians and foreigners can be targeted by combatants or used to advance a political or ideologic agenda.

HUMAN RIGHTS ABUSES

Violations of human rights often accompany wars. Recent conflicts have seen adoption of practices that are grave human rights abuses, including forced labor, child soldiers, sexual slavery, and the weaponization of rape. Asymmetric warfare is when one party has significant weaknesses in terms of deployable resources and therefore turns to nontraditional methods of warfare to exploit the weaknesses of the other side. Tactics used by weaker parties include insurgency, terrorism, and methods to control territory by human rights abuses, sexual violence, and child exploitation. Asymmetric warfare creates a very unstable environment for civilian workers, who can be exploited by loosely aligned militias for political and military gain.

DANGER BY GEOGRAPHY: THE WORLD'S MOST DANGEROUS PLACES

Assessment of the level of danger of a city, country, or region requires broad examination of a range of factors and cannot be determined by any single variable, such as homicide rate. A 2012 report of aid worker security noted a steady increase of attacks, including kidnapping of aid workers, since 2002. The majority of incidents are reported to have taken place in a relatively few countries, including Afghanistan, Somalia, South Sudan, Pakistan, and Sudan. Humanitarian response organizations should provide a security assessment for personnel intending to deploy to a given region.[5]

BOX 86-1 Countries With Highest Aid Worker Murder Rates From 2006 to 2010	
Somalia	Pakistan
Sri Lanka	Sudan
Central African Republic	Yemen
Chad	Occupied Palestinian Territories
Afghanistan	Democratic Republic of Congo

Adapted from *Aid Worker Security Report 2014: Unsafe passage: road attacks and their impact on humanitarian operations*, Humanitarian Outcomes, 2014, New York: aidworkersecurity.org/sites/default/files/Aid%20Worker%20Security%20Report%202014.pdf.

BOX 86-2 Countries With the Highest Murder Rates in 2012	
Honduras	Belize
Venezuela	Guatemala
Jamaica	Lesotho
Colombia	South Africa
El Salvador	Trinidad and Tobago

Data from World Health Organization: Global Health Observatory Data Repository: Homicide estimates by country (2012): apps.who.int/gho/data/node.main-amro.VIOLENCEHOMICIDE?lang=en.

In contrast to countries known to be especially dangerous to aid workers, other regions, such as the Caribbean basin, are home to cities with the highest homicide rates in the world. Travelers to such areas should be aware of the increased risk of exposure to and victimization from violence. Box 86-1 lists the aid worker murder rates from 2006 to 2011, in contrast with Box 86-2, which shows the countries with the highest homicide rates for the overall population in 2012.

REASONS FOR ENHANCED PERSONAL RISK IN POLITICALLY UNSTABLE REGIONS

Increasing Civilian Nongovernmental Organization Involvement in Unstable Regions

Escalation of ethnic and intrastate conflicts during the early 1990s after the conclusion of the Cold War led to a significant increase in civilian nongovernmental organization involvement in active conflict settings. The number and size of these organizations grew significantly during this period (Figure 86-1). They employed a large number of civilian health professionals in areas of active conflict, including the former Yugoslavia, the Great Lakes region of Africa, Somalia, and West Africa. Civilian medical and public health personnel found themselves working in settings with

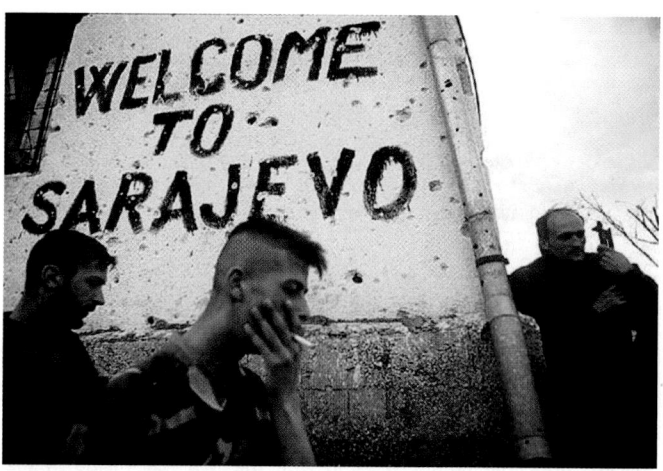

FIGURE 86-1 Bosnian soldiers watch the frontlines. Sarajevo, 1992. *(From* Welcome to Sarajevo, 1997. *Copyright Miramax Film NY, LLC.)*

active combatants, migratory populations, and international military forces, and the humanitarian needs were of a large scale.

Targeting of Civilians on the Basis of Nationality

During the post-9/11 era, following the war in Iraq, ongoing war in Afghanistan, and ongoing internal conflict in Syria, it has become increasingly difficult for Western workers to travel in several regions that are dominated by persons who are ideologically opposed to Western involvement. Although the dynamics of this change are complicated and beyond the scope of this chapter, the net result is that an American traveling in the Palestinian territories, Lebanon, Pakistan, Afghanistan, and regions of North Africa and the Middle East must consider these risks very carefully, understand local political nuances, and take the appropriate safety precautions.

Targeting Aid Workers

Intentional targeting of civilian aid workers and erosion of neutrality exemplify major changes in the recognition of the neutrality of Western aid organizations. Analysis of 382 aid worker deaths from 1985 to 1998 revealed the alarming fact that most (68%) were intentional, resulting from aggravated assault and murder. The second leading cause of death (17%) among these individuals was motor vehicle accidents.[12] Annual aid worker security reports have shown a steady rise in the number of violent attacks on workers, with 2013 noted to have the greatest number, a total of 250 incidents affecting 260 aid workers and resulting in 155 deaths. Countries with the greatest numbers of attacks on aid workers in 2013 included Afghanistan, Syria, South Sudan, Pakistan, Sudan, Somalia, Democratic Republic of the Congo, Kenya, Central African Republic, and Yemen.[6]

Restricted Access in Politically Unstable Regions

There remain several regions that are quite restrictive with regard to the numbers and types of travelers allowed into their countries. North Korea remains one of the most highly restricted countries; increasing restrictions apply to travel in countries such as Eritrea and Sudan (especially outside Khartoum). Travel restrictions remain in effect (often for obtuse reasons) in Cuba and Iran; travel to these regions may require special arrangements.

Working in settings of active conflict or social disruption caused by political instability creates high-risk situations that require a deep understanding of regional politics and local people of influence. In many of these settings, travelers encounter informal militia groups, banditry, and obstructed access. It is essential to become familiar with the range of possible threats before encountering them (Figure 86-2). Such information is frequently most reliably gathered from local sources.

Weapons

At least one aspect defining a hostile environment for travelers and health care workers is the presence of a variety of weaponry.

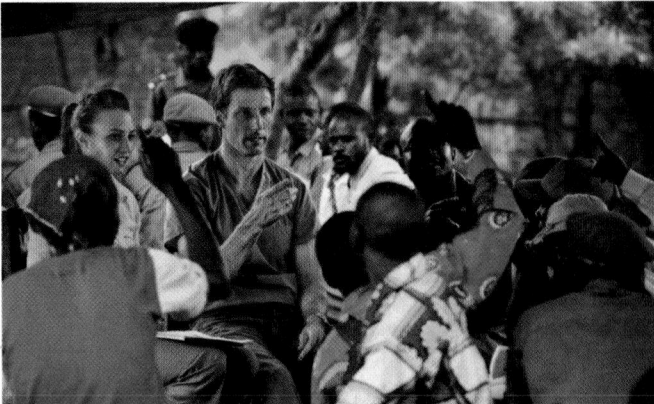

FIGURE 86-2 The author working with the Mai Mai militia in the Eastern Democratic Republic of the Congo. (*From Harvard World Media and Justin Ide.*)

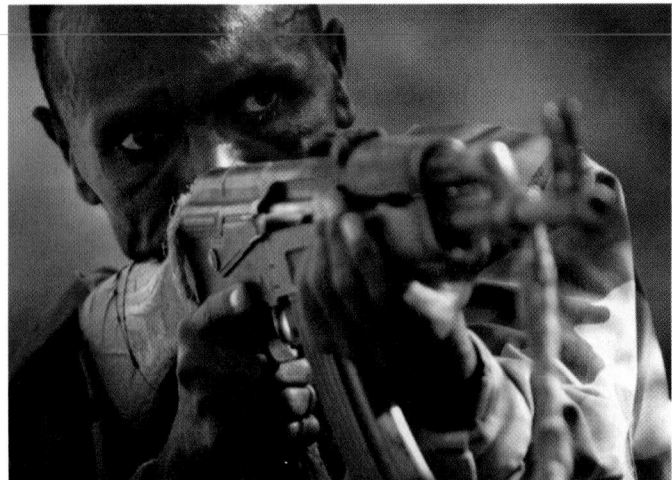

FIGURE 86-3 The AK-47. Ethiopian National Defense Force 1st Lieutenant Ayella Gissa takes aim with an AK-47 assault rifle on a simulated enemy. (*From Chief Mass Communication Specialist Eric A. Clement, U.S. Navy. March 5, 2007.*)

The most common weapon-related threat to international tourists, health care workers, and explorers is a gun in the possession of someone willing to use it for ill gain. Guns are used to protect and intimidate people and to create a threatening environment. Police, military, local militia, security personnel, and civilian gun owners create a dangerous environment for travelers. In a 2002 review of the impact of small arms assaults on aid workers, it was found that more than 220 United Nations civilian staffers have died as a result of malicious acts since 1992, and at least 265 have been taken hostage while serving in United Nations operations. This is added to the thousands of assaults on aid workers and foreign travelers in politically insecure areas, which have resulted in hundreds of deaths.[14]

The most commonly encountered weapons in most conflict areas are personal assault rifles, primarily variations of the Russian-made AK-47 (the name *AK-47* refers to "automatic Kalashnikov, 1947," for its designer, Mikhail Kalashnikov, and the first year of its production).[10] Because of their simplicity, durability, dependability, and ease of assembly, variations of the AK-47 are used more readily throughout the world than all others combined (Figure 86-3). In some regions of the world, an AK-47 can be purchased for as little as $50 to $100. Handguns are also frequently encountered weapons. They are considered close-range or self-defensive weapons, and are commonly found among military and "irregular" militias.

Encountering individuals or groups, whether they are members of a formal military group or an informal militia, with weapons is a common occurrence. As a civilian working in an unstable setting, protection is accomplished by presenting oneself and one's organization as civilian and interested in providing impartial assistance. When an individual encounters groups with weapons, it is essential to develop a clear line of communication with an unambiguous message that he or she is a civilian, is unarmed, and is not a party to the politics of the setting. It is never recommended that civilians carry a weapon. Carrying a firearm identifies a person as a possible threat and thus removes the perception of neutrality. However, it may be necessary to employ armed guards in certain situations to protect a vehicle, staff member, home, or office. The decision to employ armed guards needs to be made in a local context and by someone with deep local and regional experience.

Risk Reduction Strategies for Situations in Which There Are Armed Combatants. When traveling or working in a region that has armed combatants, there are some simple ways to avoid getting into trouble:

Do Not Carry a Gun. This may seem like simple logic, but a number of travelers who work or recreate in exotic locations feel that they will be safer when armed. This logic is almost always false. Carrying a gun, as it turns out, is by far more likely to lead to an adverse event or even death.

Avoid Places Where There Is a Danger of Being Injured. Certain locations are notorious places for explosive and gun-related violence. These include large political gatherings, checkpoints, and border crossings. The less time spent in these locations, the more likely an individual is to avoid being targeted or caught in the crossfire.

Avoid Confrontations With Local Militias or Thugs. This includes avoiding areas described above, as well as avoiding provoking military or paramilitary personnel by walking outside past curfew, taking photos of guards or military installations, or displaying an attitude that is less than polite when being questioned by militia.

Avoid Celebrations Where Guns Are Being Fired. Bullets shot off in celebration can return to Earth (or skull) at 152.4 m/sec (500 feet/sec). Celebrations in crowded areas, where those reveling in the moment are shooting bullets up in the air, are treacherous settings. Three-quarters of the injuries that occur in these situations are to the head, and many of these lead to death.

Stay Low to the Ground. For situations in which there is shooting nearby, immediately drop to the floor or get down as low as possible and crawl to a sheltered location. Do not run, and do not attempt to use a weapon unless trained and equipped to do so. If it is necessary to move, crawl along the floor and find a place to hide, preferably near a concrete wall or large solid objects.

Land Mines and Unexploded Ordnance

Travelers to areas that have historically suffered from conflict should be aware of the very real threat of land mines and unexploded ordnance. This is especially the case in regions that are currently stable but have been contested in the recent past. An estimated 60 countries worldwide remain contaminated with land mines, which cause approximately 4000 casualties annually.[7] Countries with the highest numbers of land mine injuries since the year 2000 include Afghanistan, Colombia, Cambodia, Iraq, Somalia, Ethiopia, Democratic Republic of the Congo, Sudan, Chad, South Sudan, and Sudan.[8]

Mine Types. Mines are a multibillion-dollar weapons industry. There is a wide range of antipersonnel mines produced internationally, from large antitank mines to "toe poppers" and other small devices that are intended to maim rather than kill. In general, mines are designed to injure (not kill), create terror, and disrupt military targets by injuring soldiers. They can be detonated by direct pressure, vibration, or trip wires, sending high-velocity projectiles of metal, dirt, and debris into the tissues and bones of victims (Figure 86-4). Antipersonnel land mines continue to threaten civilians and noncombatants, despite a growing number of conventions intended to ban them.

Effects of Land Mines on Populations and Health. Land mines represent both an immediate health risk and a delayed threat. More than 110 million land mines have been deployed worldwide. Between 1999 and 2009, more than 73,000 land mine casualties were reported, of which more than 70% were civilian casualties.[8] The epidemiology of land mine injuries is not known, but case fatality rates are very high. Land mine injuries pose a major problem for health care providers, who may be poorly equipped to manage the severe penetrating trauma, blast injuries, and consequent infections and gangrene. Trauma from land mine injuries requires high-level surgical services and can monopolize health care resources.

Another major problem with land mines is that they outlast any conflict, and their removal is difficult and costly. The reality of land mines is that no one truly knows how many exist or where they are located. Despite the activities of de-mining programs, land mines cause significant economic, social, and psychological disruption to communities.

Risk-Reduction Strategies When Traveling in Regions That Are Mined. It is important for international travelers, aid workers, and tourists to be aware of mine threats in many places in the world. Travel agencies will not be aware of these hazards, but there may be significant mine threats in regions frequented

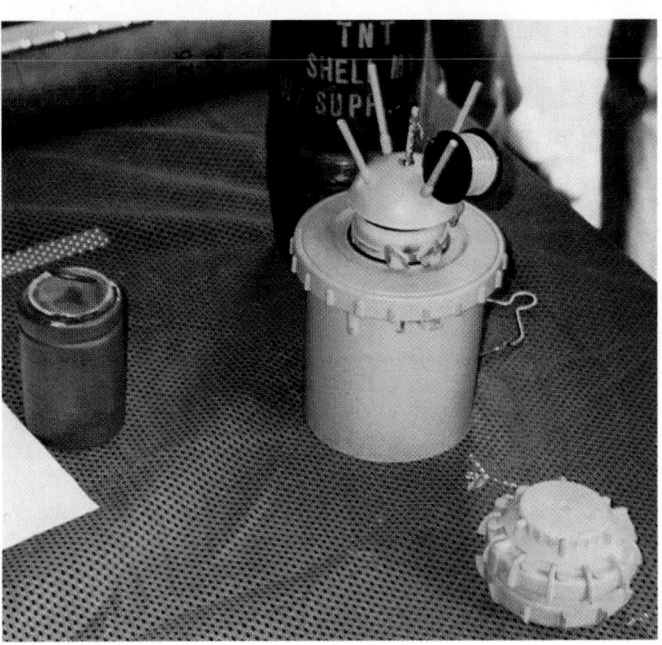

FIGURE 86-4 Land mines. From left to right, M14, Valmara 69, and VS-50. *(From Nation Defense Days, Esplanade des Invalides, Paris, France, September 24 and 25, 2005.)*

by travelers. Some of the steps travelers can take to avoid mined areas are listed in Box 86-3.

Banning Land Mines. The 1997 Ottawa Treaty, or Mine Ban Treaty (formally the Convention on the Prohibition of the Use, Stockpiling, Production and Transfer of Anti-Personnel Mines and on their Destruction), completely bans all antipersonnel land mines.[7] It has been signed by 162 countries since 1997, but only antipersonnel mines are covered. Mixed mines, antitank mines, remote-controlled M18 Claymore mines, and antihandling devices (i.e., booby traps) are not covered by the treaty.[7,8] Among the 35 nations that have yet to sign the treaty are China, Russia, India, and the United States.[7]

HIGH-RISK SITUATIONS FOR INTERNATIONAL TRAVELERS

When traveling to regions affected by political instability, it is important to be aware of particular settings that may create

---

BOX 86-3 Avoiding Mine Risks

- Obtain information about the country in which you will be traveling. There are a number of Internet sites useful for determining the regional risks of unexploded ordnance; see the-monitor.org/index.php/publications.
- Consult local officials if traveling or working in a mined region. If you are with a guided group, ask your guide about mine risks.
- Stay on well-traveled roads and paths. Do not leave the paved areas of the road—not even to walk along the side of the road to take a photograph. Avoid being the first person or vehicle in a convoy that is going into a region that may be freshly mined. Follow behind larger vehicles, and allow them to be at least 100 m (328 feet) ahead of you.
- If you have a flak jacket and are working in a mined area, sit on the jacket while driving.
- Never touch or handle suspicious items or devices, and do not pick up objects that appear to have a military function as souvenirs. Many tourists to prior conflict areas have been injured when collecting souvenirs that turned out to be unexploded ordnance.

dangerous situations for travelers. Many of these situations are avoidable by recognizing them and planning in advance what to do if they are encountered.

CHECKPOINTS

Checkpoints and military barriers are notoriously high-risk places. Checkpoints can be as simple as a local militia man with or without a uniform (but almost always carrying a weapon) standing in the middle of the road, or an official barricade with sandbags, concrete barriers, razor wire, and guard stations with an organized military presence. In general, checkpoints indicate an area of passage into areas controlled by military forces. In conflicts where child combatants are present, child soldiers may also be present at checkpoints. These areas are often points of high traffic and high tension. Avoid them if possible.

INFORMAL ROADBLOCKS

Informal roadblocks are different than official military checkpoints. Informal roadblocks are often set up by robbers or carjackers, and are most often encountered in tourist areas or on roads leading from a city to a tourist destination. These should be anticipated and avoided. Plan the travel route carefully, particularly if traveling between urban areas on narrow roads without a local driver. If an informal roadblock is encountered, either turn around or move beyond it as quickly as possible.

DEMONSTRATIONS

Crowds, demonstrations, and protests are particularly high-risk events and should be avoided whenever possible. Driving through an agitated crowd as a foreigner is potentially dangerous and can result in theft, assault, or worse. If there is a demonstration or a crowd in the street that is obstructing the route, stop the vehicle, back up or turn around, and take an alternate route (Figure 86-5).

RISK-REDUCTION STRATEGIES FOR TRAVEL BETWEEN BORDERS AND MILITARY CHECKPOINTS

Because checkpoints and guard stations are placed at frequently crossed borders, many cannot be avoided. If an individual has to cross at a manned barrier, a good strategy is to spend as little time as necessary in the vicinity of the checkpoint. Travelers should pay close attention to signs and instructions around a checkpoint and follow instructions carefully. Approach the checkpoint slowly in the vehicle, and stop when directed to do so. Keep hands visible, and remain in the vehicle unless asked to step out. Remain polite and business-like, and have appropriate documents available. If questioned, remain calm, and avoid sudden movements or erratic behavior.

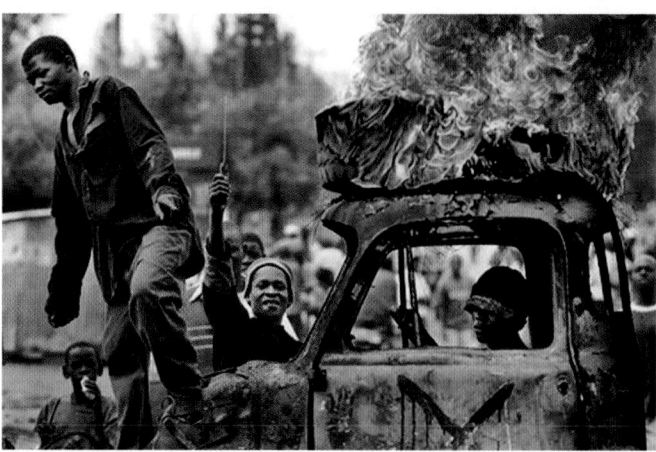

FIGURE 86-5 Roadblock during an ethnic clash in Kisumu, Kenya. *(With permission from dailymail.co.uk/news/article-510828/Kenya.)*

GLOBAL CRIMES: PATTERNS AND IMPLICATIONS FOR TRAVELERS

Changes in global patterns of crime and criminal behavior reflect both historic roots of criminal activity and the growing influence of globalization. Criminal activities during the 21st century involve high-tech tools to advance criminal networks; computer technologies are used to market and track the illegal drug trade, coordinate the laundering and smuggling of money, and create networks of communication and exchange for trafficked goods, services, and people. The high volume of global travel and shipping via air, ground, and sea has created additional challenges for addressing the movement of people and contraband. Economic disparities create greater incentives for people to participate in illegal activity and thus create entire populations that are at risk of falling prey to exploitation.

Failed states and weak governance in many nations create an environment in which the economy is largely based on crime. From the illegal mining of minerals and diamonds in the Democratic Republic of the Congo to opium cultivated in Afghanistan to the sex-slave trade in Asia, crime and trafficking have grown and prospered in a global economy. According to the United Nations Millennium Project, transnational organized crime continues to expand despite attempted multinational counterstrategies. There is an estimated volume of illicit trade of well over $1 trillion per year, generated in part by counterfeiting and intellectual property piracy at $654 billion, the global drug trade at $411 billion, and human trafficking and prostitution business totaling $240 billion.[18]

THE SCOPE AND ARRAY OF GLOBAL CRIME

Human Trafficking and Sex Slavery

The practice of profiting from the sale and exploitation of women and children has expanded into a modern-day slave trade that extends throughout Eastern Europe, Southeast Asia, and West Africa into Indonesia, Thailand, Malaysia, Europe, Japan, and the United States. Trafficking of persons, including prostitution and slavery, is more prevalent today than at any time in human history. Current worldwide estimates suggest that there are an estimated 21 million victims of human trafficking.[19] International sex tourism feeds the sex-trade industry and has expanded into a multibillion-dollar global industry. The trafficking trade ranks second in dollar income after drug smuggling. Millions of trafficked people, mostly poor women and children, are moved each year into the sex industry and become forced laborers.[16]

Advice to foreign workers and travelers regarding trafficking is simple. Do not participate in the commercial sex trade or frequent brothels, massage parlors, or similar venues. Such participation directly fuels the sex-trade industry and abduction of young women and children. The only ways to enforce a ban on such practices are to remove demand and place economic and political pressure on nations that support these industries.

Terrorism

One definition of the word *terrorism,* as used by the U.S. government, is "premeditated, politically motivated violence perpetrated against noncombatant targets by sub-national groups or clandestine agents usually intended to influence an audience."[3] The use of the word *terrorist* is often contextual, and has been expanded considerably to include many of the activities aimed at combating efforts of those doing the naming. Regardless of the application or misapplication of the term, *terrorist activity* typically refers to acts that target those persons viewed as being related to an occupying power or those nearby the target.

As terrorist networks have expanded and become more organized, the threat of attacks has increased. Terrorist groups can employ chemical and biologic weapons, bombs and explosive devices, nuclear materials, and, as was seen during the September 11, 2001, attacks on the World Trade Center and the Pentagon, use of commercial aircraft as weapons. Terrorism and use of indiscriminate violence against civilian populations continue to be major threats worldwide. During travel to selected regions of the world, terrorist threats may be aimed directly at travelers

BOX 86-4 Strategies to Reduce the Risk of Terrorist Attack When Traveling to High-Risk Areas

- Schedule direct flights, if possible, and avoid stops in high-risk airports or areas.
- Try to minimize the time spent in the public area of an airport, which is a less protected area. Move quickly from the check-in counter to the secured areas. Upon arrival, leave the airport as soon as possible.
- Refuse unexpected packages. Keep an eye out for abandoned packages, briefcases, or other suspicious items. Report them to airport authorities, and leave the area promptly. Avoid obvious terrorist targets, such as places where Westerners are known to congregate, including nightclubs, shopping malls, and tourist destinations.
- Keep a mental note of safe havens, such as police stations, hotels, and hospitals. Develop a plan of action for what you will do if a bomb explodes or if there is gunfire nearby.
- Select your own taxicabs at random. Do not take a vehicle that is not clearly identified as a taxi. Compare the face of the driver with the one on his or her posted license. Check for loose wires or other suspicious activity around your car. Drive with car windows closed in crowded streets, because bombs can be thrown through open windows.
- If you are ever in a situation where somebody starts shooting, drop to the floor or get down as low as possible. Do not move until you are sure that the danger has passed. Do not attempt to help rescuers, and do not pick up a weapon. If possible, shield yourself behind a solid object. If you must move, crawl on your stomach.

or used in places likely to be frequented by travelers, such as large hotels and resorts with high concentrations of international tourists. Most terrorist attacks are the results of site evaluation and careful planning. Just as a car thief will first be attracted to an unlocked car with the key in the ignition, terrorists are looking for the most accessible targets. Therefore, the chances are slight that a tourist traveling with an unpublished program or itinerary would be the victim of terrorism.

Terrorist activities may appear to be random and unpredictable, but there are several precautions that travelers can take to avoid such attacks. The first such protection is to avoid traveling to areas that are prone to terrorist acts, such as high-risk regions in Iraq, Afghanistan, and Pakistan. It is also advisable to avoid destinations that have a known record of terrorism, kidnapping, or politically motivated assault on civilians, such as selected cities in Mexico, Colombia, and Brazil. Other precautions include minimizing time spent in airports, shopping malls, large markets, nightclubs, and other places frequented by tourists.

Risk-Reduction Strategies for Terrorist Attacks. Reducing the risk of a terrorist attack requires a series of precautions that can provide some degree of protection. These precautions may serve as practical and psychological deterrents to would-be terrorists; see Box 86-4.

Kidnapping and Hostage Situations

Kidnapping has become a profitable industry as foreign businesses expand their reach into emerging markets. Numbers of kidnapping and abduction incidents worldwide are notoriously difficult to ascertain, partly because up to half of all kidnappings are not reported to the authorities; most of these involve businessmen, children of parents in custody disputes, or victims of politically motivated abductions. Countries with the highest numbers of kidnappings include Mexico, India, Pakistan, Iraq, and Nigeria. Regions with the highest incidence of kidnapping are Africa (34% of total reported kidnappings), followed by the Middle East (30% of total reported kidnappings). Most abducted victims are local nationals; Africa and the Middle East have the highest percentages of foreign national abduction victims, at 65% and 33%, respectively.[11]

Kidnapping is most commonly used as a means of extortion, either from the local population or from wealthy expatriates living abroad. Some of the most common ongoing kidnapping

threats are in regions in which there is a large Western industrial presence and rich foreign workers. In some settings, kidnapping for political purposes is also a major threat; this includes kidnapping of Western aid workers and journalists as a terror tactic in Iraq and Syria.

Being taken hostage, whether for political or economic reasons, is a rare but terrifying occurrence. Each hostage situation is unique and requires a tailored approach by authorities. Regardless of the variations of a hostage situation, the U.S. government's position remains that it will negotiate but not make concessions (e.g., payments) to kidnappers. U.S. government officials employ diplomatic processes and engage resources of the host country to secure the safety and release of hostages.

Risk-Reduction Strategies in Kidnapping or Hostage Situations. The U.S. Department of State provides instruction to personnel who might find themselves in a possible hostage situation. Much of this advice is predicated on the notion that the most dangerous times for any hostage are during abduction, when assailants are tense and anxious, and at any time there is a rescue attempt.

Although each hostage situation is different, there are general considerations to keep in mind. At the outset of a terrorist incident, terrorists are typically tense and high strung and may behave irrationally. They are prone to erratic and potentially violent behavior. Particularly during the early stages of a hostage situation, it is extremely important that the hostage remain calm and alert and control his or her own behavior. Some recommendations for behavior in the event of a hostage situation are outlined in Box 86-5.[4]

Piracy and Threats While Traveling at Sea

Piracy is a criminal act involving theft or violence at sea perpetrated by persons who are not affiliated with a government. Recent high-profile media reports of Somali pirates have brought attention to the phenomenon of piracy and the widespread degree of violation of national and international laws. Piracy is rampant and flourishing in East African and Southeast Asian seas, and is a significant consideration for commercial vessels, large cruise ships, and even smaller private vessels. Seaborne piracy targeting commercial and industrial ships has created a global criminal enterprise leading to worldwide losses of $13 to $16 billion per year. Many of these attacks occur in the waters between the Red Sea and Indian Ocean, off the Somali coast, and in the Strait of Malacca near Singapore.[17]

The International Maritime Bureau reports that the major type of violence during an act of piracy is hostage taking, commonly

BOX 86-5 Advice for Abductees in Hostage Situations

- Avoid resistance and sudden or threatening movements. Do not struggle or try to escape unless you are certain of being successful. Do not try to be a hero; this could endanger yourself and others.
- Consciously put yourself in a mode of passive cooperation. Talk normally. Do not complain; avoid belligerency; and comply with all orders and instructions.
- If questioned, keep your answers short. Do not volunteer information or make unnecessary overtures.
- Make a concerted effort to relax. Prepare yourself mentally, physically, and emotionally for the possibility of a long ordeal.
- Try to remain inconspicuous. Avoid direct eye contact and the appearance of observing your captors' actions.
- Avoid alcoholic beverages. Eat what they give you, even if it does not look or taste appetizing, and keep consumption of food and drink at a moderate level. A loss of appetite and weight is normal.
- If you are involved in a lengthier and drawn-out situation, try to establish rapport with your captors, and avoid political discussions or other confrontational subjects.
- Establish a daily program of mental and physical activities.
- Think positively, and avoid a sense of despair. You are a valuable commodity to your captors, and it is important to them to keep you alive and well.

for ransom. In 2006, there were 239 attacks during which 77 crew members were kidnapped and 188 taken hostage. Of these attacks, only 15 resulted in murder. In 2007, attacks by pirates rose by 10% to 263 attacks. There was a 35% increase in reported attacks involving guns. Crew members that were injured numbered 64, as compared with just 17 in 2006. Attacks continued to escalate in 2009 and 2010, and piracy is expected to be an ongoing problem for international trade and tourism.[20]

As in any major international criminal activity, the best protection is avoiding confrontation in the first place. In the case of piracy, ensure that the commercial or industrial vessel has an appropriate monitoring capacity when traveling in international waters near unstable settings, such as the coastal waters near Somalia and regions in Southeast Asia. If a civilian traveler is a victim of abduction at sea, the same principles of personal protection apply as are listed elsewhere in this chapter.

INCARCERATION AND QUARANTINE

INCARCERATION AND DETENTION: A GLOBAL PERSPECTIVE

International travelers and foreign workers rarely experience meaningful encounters with the foreign legal system. However, for those who do, the experience will likely be transformative. In 1994, Michael Fay, an 18-year-old American convicted of vandalizing cars and stealing road signs in Singapore, received international attention after being sentenced to 4 months in jail, a $2200 fine, and six strokes on the buttocks with a rattan cane. President Bill Clinton protested Fay's extreme punishment and asked the government of Singapore for clemency in his case; Fay's punishment was later reduced to four strokes in a concession to President Clinton. On May 5, 1994, Michael Fay received four strokes of the cane across his bare buttocks at Queenstown Remand Centre.[13] Although Singapore's criminal laws appear severe in contrast with American ideas of human rights, the punishment exacted on Fay served as a stark reminder that U.S. citizens residing or traveling in a foreign country are subject to the laws of that country. It is therefore the responsibility of every individual traveling abroad to understand foreign laws and regulations and to obey them.

Criminal activity in other nations can lead to severe consequences. Even relatively innocent actions such as purchasing antiques, taking photographs of a government installation, or minor traffic infractions may have serious ramifications. Thousands of Americans are arrested and detained abroad each year, with a large number of these individuals held on drug charges. Laws and regulations in foreign countries may differ significantly from those in the United States, and may not provide the protections or due process that Americans consider routine. Penalties for breaking the law in foreign nations can be more severe than in the United States for similar offenses. For example, in certain countries, drug convictions can result in life imprisonment or the death penalty.

Travelers who are arrested abroad may face confinement without being charged with a crime. Few countries provide trial by jury or even legal representation. Being accused of a crime abroad may involve months of incarceration in prisons that lack basic necessities such as reasonable nutrition, sanitation, or access to clean water. Physical punishment and abuse by guards and other prisoners are also possible.

If an individual is arrested, he or she should immediately ask to speak to a consular officer at the nearest U.S. embassy or consulate. Under international agreements, the U.S. government has the right to provide consular assistance at the request of the detainee, can provide the detainee with a list of attorneys, and can help him or her to contact family or friends. The U.S. government can also monitor the detainee's health and welfare and the conditions under which he or she is being held.[23]

DRUG OFFENSES ABROAD

Production, processing, and distribution of illicit drugs remain threats to the national security of many nations, and involve roughly half a trillion dollars in annual revenues. The illegal drug trade creates a climate of violence in many areas of the world that leads to economic and social instability. International travelers may be exposed directly to the illicit drug trade through the acquisition of illegal drugs, or be indirectly affected by theft or violence.

Every year, several hundred Americans are arrested abroad on drug charges. Persons caught with illegal drugs in a foreign country are subject to the drug laws of that country and not those of their home countries. Ignorance of the law is no excuse. In many countries, the burden of proof is on the accused to show that he or she is innocent of the charges. Every aspect of a drug arrest abroad can be different from U.S. practice. For example, few countries provide a jury trial, and many countries imprison accused offenders while they are awaiting trial, sometimes in solitary confinement, which can last for several months. It would be no surprise to find that many foreign prisons lack even minimal comforts, including beds, toilets, and adequate food. Foreign prisoners may also suffer physical abuse, confiscation of property, degrading treatment, and extortion. If convicted, one can face extremely harsh sentences ranging from fines and jail time to years of hard labor or even the death penalty.

QUARANTINE

Quarantine is the voluntary or compulsory isolation of a person or animal to contain the spread of a dangerous illness or disease. The term *quarantine* is derived from the Italian word *quarantena,* meaning "forty-day period." Quarantine has been used for decades to contain the spread of infectious diseases, and is actively used in many countries to control exposure to diseases with epidemic and pandemic potential. Quarantining people often raises questions of civil rights, especially in cases of compulsory confinement or segregation from society, such as that of Mary Mallon (i.e., Typhoid Mary), a carrier of typhoid fever who spent the last 24 years of her life under quarantine.

Quarantine Within the United States

Recent outbreaks of disease, including influenza, Middle East respiratory syndrome, and Ebola virus disease, have heightened concerns for worldwide spread of disease. In the United States, the Centers for Disease Control and Prevention (CDC) has a permanent presence of personnel in U.S. Quarantine Stations at 20 U.S. ports of entry and land border crossings in major cities where international travelers arrive. The stations are part of a comprehensive quarantine system network that serves to limit introduction of infectious diseases into the United States and to prevent their spread. The stations are staffed with quarantine medical and public health officers from the CDC, who decide whether ill persons can enter the United States and what measures should be taken to prevent the spread of infectious diseases.[1]

The CDC has the legal authority to detain any person who may have an infectious disease that is considered to be quarantinable. These diseases include cholera, diphtheria, infectious tuberculosis, plague, smallpox, yellow fever, viral hemorrhagic fevers, severe acute respiratory syndrome, and pandemic influenza. The CDC has the authority to deny ill persons with these diseases entry into the United States or to require them to be admitted to a hospital or confined to home for a certain amount of time to prevent the spread of disease[1] (Figure 86-6).

The 2013 West Africa Ebola virus disease outbreak brought the issue of isolation and quarantine of health workers into the public spotlight. Multiple expatriate health workers who may have been infected with the Ebola virus in West Africa (and some who were infected) required repatriation to the United States. During the response to the outbreak, U.S. state lawmakers mandated a wide range of self-isolation policies for returning health workers. Some of these policies were more restrictive than CDC recommendations, causing frustration and social isolation of health care workers. Depending on the insurance carrier, evacuation insurance held by many international travelers and aid workers may have exclusion policies for evacuation

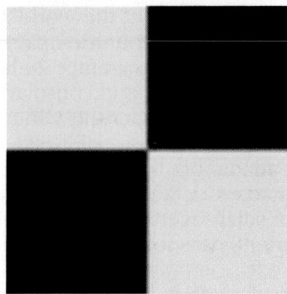

FIGURE 86-6 The "Yellow Jack" signal flag, which is flown in a harbor when a ship is under quarantine.

in the event of specific infectious diseases such as Ebola virus disease. When considering deployment with an organization in response to an emerging infectious disease, it is essential that the volunteer vet the response organization's evacuation and security plans and resources. Health care workers responding to international epidemics of emerging infectious disease should be aware that when they return to the United States, they may be subject to legally mandated restrictions on work, social activity, and travel.

Quarantine Abroad

The U.S. Department of State cannot demand immediate release of private American citizens who have been detained or quarantined abroad in accordance with local public health regulations and legal authorities. Every effort will be made to assist American citizens, but U.S. government offices overseas are unable to provide medications or administrative assistance. After the pandemic subsides and travel resumes, the U.S. Department of State can once again provide full consular services to American citizens, including routine repatriation assistance.[24]

If a traveler is overseas during the outbreak of a global pandemic, travel restrictions may limit his or her ability to return to the country of origin until travel restrictions are lifted. Given this possibility, all expatriate workers and travelers, especially those deploying to work in relief efforts in the event of an infectious disease pandemic, should anticipate the possibility of travel restrictions. Depending on the nature of the epidemic, responders may need to follow social distancing guidelines, including avoiding public gatherings and physical contact with other individuals.[15]

SAFETY AND SECURITY STRATEGIES FOR TRAVELERS

The decision to travel in an area of conflict or recently ended conflict, a region that is subject to political or military turmoil, or a country affected by an emerging infectious disease is a serious one. The more complicated the situation at the destination, the more one needs to make advance arrangements and judge the overall personal risk. International travelers and foreign workers must address the risks that they will face when crossing borders. The traveler needs to take into consideration a number of complex and dynamic features, including the risk of theft, abduction, or encounters with militia or with those who are hostile to an international presence.

International travelers, particularly expedition travelers, often have a strong motivation to press onward and continue their journey despite warning signs. The tendency of novice adventurers to blindly keep moving forward can lead one to ignore warning signs and discard pragmatism and sound judgment. The seasoned traveler, particularly one with experience in conflict settings, will be able to discern when to continue onward and when to pause and consider a new strategy. Before describing specific strategies for travelers, it is useful to consider some of the ways that people—even expert travelers—can get into trouble.

APPROACHES THAT MAY BE COUNTERPRODUCTIVE

Being Overconfident

Unrealistic optimism is a common bias in many adventure or expedition travelers, and contributes to the assumption that the ultimate outcome in any situation will be positive. This can lead to overconfidence during one's assessment of a situation. A guide with limited experience may display overconfidence because he or she has traveled to the area before without any problems. This mindset can cause one to ignore signs of danger or potentially explosive situations.

Escalating Activities

Linked to overconfidence is the notion of escalation, where one proceeds forward despite poor results. This may arise from wanting to salvage a project or an expedition or out of a desire to validate a series of poor prior decisions to get a project back on track. This commonly occurs when attempting to reach a destination despite delays, changes in weather, and the uncertainty of traveling at night in unfamiliar settings. A guide may promote risk taking to enhance his or her image, give himself or herself a sense of purpose, or create the image that he or she is in charge of the situation.

Relying on Limited Information

Making judgments about risk in a complex environment requires knowledge of the geography, political climate, and immediate threats. Those who are invested in the progress of an expedition may have limited knowledge and may be unwilling to consider things that they deem as unknowns. Risk taking also occurs as a result of pressure from headquarters, when people in leadership positions who are not in the field create pressure to "press forward" and "get the job done" without knowing the conditions on the ground. In general, decisions about field safety must be made by field personnel who are experiencing the sense of threat or uncertainty rather than by remote leadership with an unrealistic agenda.

Becoming Desensitized to Risks

For individuals or organizations in areas of relatively high risk, basic precautions and safety measures may become mundane and unimportant. Perceptions of risk can diminish, even if the true threat has not changed or is increasing. International relief personnel commonly face—and become immune to—daily threats and security issues because they become routine. In such cases, it is useful to develop and adhere to an established security protocol so that individuals or teams do not develop a sense of complacency.[15]

TRAVELING AND WORKING IN A CONFLICT ZONE: INDIVIDUAL CONSIDERATIONS

Civilians should only consider the prospect of traveling or working in an active war zone under well-defined circumstances, such as with a reputable relief organization or another organization that has significant logistic and security capabilities. In addition to the strategies discussed throughout this chapter, travelers may wish to consider the following strategies:

CONTACTS AND RESOURCES

When traveling to regions affected by conflict, it is important to have local contacts and resources. Be cautious about discussing the itinerary with strangers, and remain vague about personal matters, family members, and finances. When traveling in regions with militia or in tense political climates, make an extra effort to ensure personal security by attending to the issues noted in Box 86-6.

Many seasoned travelers working in conflict areas find it useful to register with the nearest U.S. embassy or consulate through the U.S. State Department's smart traveler enrollment

BOX 86-6 Checklist for Personal Security While Traveling

- Arrange an alternative to your hotel or lodging so if you are forced to flee, you have a safe haven.
- Establish contact with someone local who can be trusted, and keep his or her contact information handy.
- Make a special note of United Nations compounds, international organizations, and high-end hotels as possible destinations if you are in trouble.
- Remain aware of people loitering around your hotel or people who keep reappearing to assist you. Remain friendly, but avoid discussing personal matters, your itinerary, or your program.
- Do not leave personal or business papers in your hotel room, and keep copies of your documents in an alternate location.
- Avoid predictable times and routes of travel, and report any suspicious activity to local police and the nearest U.S. embassy or consulate.
- Be sure of the identity of visitors before accepting riders or opening the door of your hotel room or any vehicle.
- Do not meet strangers at unknown or remote locations.
- Make a plan in the event that there is a bomb blast, gunfire, or sudden military activity in or around your hotel. Check exits and access routes in advance.

program website at step.state.gov. Registering with U.S. authorities allows individuals to be contacted in the event of rapidly developing political situations, and can assist the government in evacuation or tracking of individuals if such persons become trapped or unable to move as a result of insecurity or military threat. Providing a detailed itinerary, copies of one's passport, and multiple contact numbers can assist the consulate with locating an individual during an emergency.

ASSISTANCE FOR VICTIMS OF CRIME OVERSEAS

If an individual is the victim of a crime overseas, the Overseas Citizens Services of the U.S. Department of State's Bureau of Consular Affairs is committed to assisting American citizens who are traveling, working, or residing abroad. Government officials known as *consuls* or *consular officers* at embassies and consul-ates in nearly 250 cities throughout the world are responsible for assisting U.S. citizens in foreign countries. Consular duty personnel are available for emergency assistance 24 hours a day, 7 days a week, at embassies, consulates, and consular agencies overseas and in Washington, DC. To contact the Office of Overseas Citizens Services in the United States, call 1-888-407-4747 from the United States or Canada or 1-202-501-4444 from outside the United States or Canada. Contact information for U.S. embassies, consulates, and consular agencies overseas can be found at travel.state.gov/content/passports/english/emergencies/victims .html.

Consuls and consular agents can help American crime victims with issues such as replacing lost or stolen passports, contacting family and relatives, obtaining medical care, and providing information about the local criminal justice system and victim assistance programs. Consular officials do not investigate crimes or provide direct legal advice, but can refer interested parties to local attorneys.[25]

SUMMARY: TRAVELING AND WORKING IN POLITICALLY INSECURE REGIONS

International travelers, expeditions, and humanitarian organizations may venture into regions that are affected by war or political instability. Traveling to a conflict area or war zone is complex and requires a detailed understanding of the political and military context and the potential for threats to personal security. It is essential to work with reputable agencies that have a significant presence on the ground and understand the risks of the region. Significant advance preparation is required. Diligent attention to the details of personal security, situational awareness, and contingency planning is essential when traveling to countries or regions in the midst or the aftermath of armed conflict.

REFERENCES

Complete references used in this text are available online at expertconsult.inkling.com.

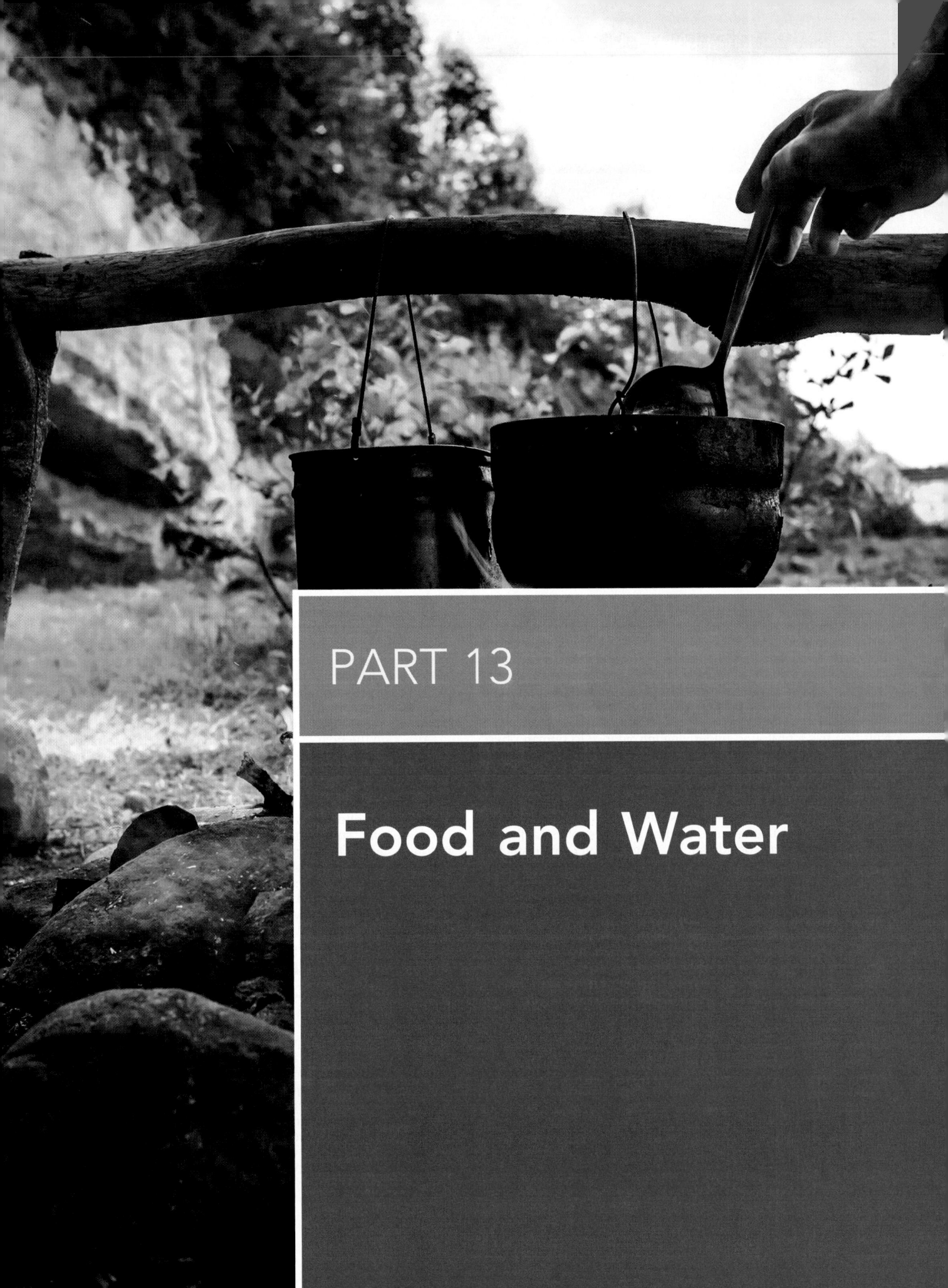

PART 13

Food and Water

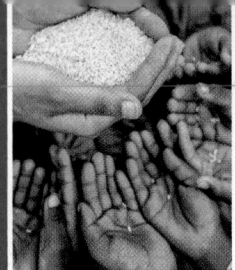

CHAPTER 87

Nutrition, Malnutrition, and Starvation

STACIE L. WING-GAIA AND E. WAYNE ASKEW

How does it feel to starve?

I am hungry. I am always hungry. ... At times I can almost forget about it but there is nothing that can hold my interest for long. ... I am cold. ... My body flame is burning as low as possible to conserve precious fuel and still maintain my life processes. ... I am weak. I can walk miles at my own pace in order to satisfy laboratory requirements, but often I trip on cracks in the sidewalk. To open a heavy door, it is necessary to brace myself and push or pull with all my might. I wouldn't think of throwing a baseball and I couldn't jump over a twelve inch railing if I tried. This lack of strength is a great frustration. It is often a greater frustration than the hunger ... and now I have edema. When I wake up in the morning my face is puffy. ... Sometimes my ankles swell and my knees are puffy. ... Social graces, interests, spontaneous activity and responsibility take second place to concerns about food. ... I lick my plate unashamedly at each meal even when guests are present. ... I can talk intellectually, my mental ability has not decreased, but my will to use my ability has.

Observations by a test participant, Minnesota Starvation Study, After 24 weeks of semistarvation (1570 kcal/day, 24% weight loss) (In *The Biology of Human Starvation*, vol. II)[75]

IMPORTANCE OF NUTRITION IN STRESSFUL ENVIRONMENTS

Nutrition has a profound underlying importance to human physiologic homeostasis and functioning in everyday life; it becomes even more important when humans work or recreate in particularly challenging or "extreme" environments.[10] The central role of nutrition is often underappreciated in wilderness expedition planning. Many wilderness enthusiasts do not consider food as critical as gear and equipment, medical supplies, physical fitness, and other logistical considerations. In temperate environments, where food and water are plentiful and resupply is feasible, the importance of nutrition may seem to diminish compared with other aspects of wilderness medicine. However, when a stressful physical environment is superimposed on the physically demanding tasks associated with wilderness activities, the role of nutrition rapidly becomes of prime importance for maintenance of performance and prevention of disease and injury, as evidenced from the description of Napoleon's disastrous 1812 winter retreat from Moscow:

The ice and deep snow with which the plains of Russia were covered, impeded ... calorification in the capillaries and pulmonary organs. The snow and cold water, which the soldiers swallowed for the purpose of allaying their hunger or satisfying their thirst ... contributed greatly to the destruction of these individuals by absorbing the small portion of heat remaining in the viscera. The agents produced the death of those particularly who had been deprived of nutriment.

Baron D. J. Larrey, inspector general, Napoleon's military medical staff (In *Hypothermia and Warfare: Napoleon's Retreat from Moscow, 1812*)[113]

Fortunately, situations encountered in wilderness activities are usually less "grim" than those faced by Napoleon's army. There is usually some food available, and few enter these environments completely unprepared. However, misfortune, combined with suboptimal or haphazard nutritional planning, can spell disaster for even the best-prepared adventurer. A wrong turn on the trail, injury, unanticipated terrain, unexpected storm, or downed airplane can deplete or isolate a victim from anticipated food sources. Food becomes an overriding consideration in a survival situation, particularly as the supply is exhausted. Although a shortage of food is certainly of concern, it does not necessarily imply impending disaster. Humans are remarkably adaptable and can subsist on poor dietary patterns for prolonged periods without disastrous effects on health and performance. As long as some baseline level of energy intake is present, at least a minimal intake of vitamins and minerals will be ensured, forestalling the eventual onset of malnutrition and clinical nutrient deficiency states. Hunger is not comfortable; optimism wanes, weight loss results, and physical and cognitive performances suffer, but a food-deprived individual can still function for an extended time. One purpose of this chapter is to review some of the physical and mental consequences of suboptimal nutrition that might be anticipated under varying degrees of food restriction. The medical planner can use this information to anticipate limitations in expedition progress or capabilities and to recognize the state of health of rescued victims of starvation or food restriction. Equally important is the proper way to re-aliment a patient after a prolonged period of unintentional starvation. This can be critically important in a rescue situation, where transport of a patient to a medical facility requires several days of refeeding en route.

Although the goal of expedition food planning is to meet daily energy and micronutrient requirements, it is not always possible to provide optimal nutrition because of logistic or situational constraints. Three nutritional states or situations may be anticipated or encountered in the wilderness: (1) ideally, optimal nutrition for effective functioning in environmental extremes; (2) frequently, suboptimal nutrition, potentially leading to malnutrition; and (3) in some instances, complete lack of nutrition or starvation. Dietary planning for wilderness expeditions and emergencies is discussed in the following sections, along with some specific food and nutrient items that may be particularly useful in wilderness environments and expeditions.

ENVIRONMENTAL STRESS AND NUTRIENT REQUIREMENTS

The physical and physiologic conditions of an individual (e.g., body weight, strength, coordination, fluid and electrolyte balance, core temperature) play a significant role in determining nutritional requirements to maintain physiologic homeostasis. These conditions also directly influence survival time, especially when humans are deprived of food or water. The most important nutrient is water.[9] If an adequate supply of water is not available, all discourse on the physiology of starvation and malnutrition is pointless, because death from dehydration will occur before depletion of energy stores. Humans can survive food deprivation for extended periods—weeks or even months—depending on their level of body fat. A nonobese adult may live as long as 60 to 70 days while fasting in a clinical setting.[66] At the end of this time, almost all body fat and one-third of lean body mass would

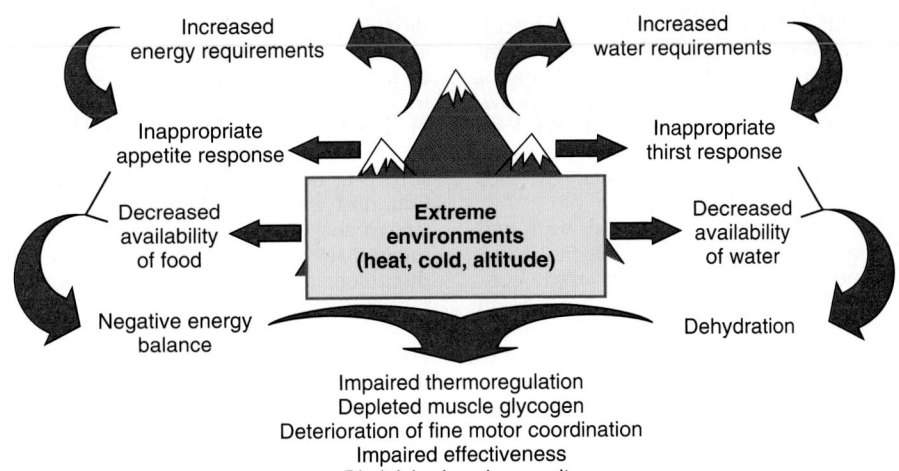

FIGURE 87-1 The influence of extreme wilderness environments on food and fluid intake and on physical and mental performance. *(Redrawn from Askew EW: In Hickson JF Jr, Wolinski I, editors: Nutrition in exercise and sport, Boca Raton, Fla, 1989, CRC Press, pp 367-384.)*

be lost.[65] James Scott, a victim of unintentional situational starvation, was marooned in a snow cave in the Himalayas with water but no food. He survived 43 days without food while losing one-third of his body weight, although he was near death at the time of rescue.[129] Death from starvation in nonobese individuals is imminent when approximately 50% of body weight has been lost. This usually corresponds to a body mass index (BMI) of 12 kg/m^2, although under some circumstances, a BMI of as low as 11 may be encountered before death.[37]

Unlike food deprivation, time to death after complete water deprivation is measured in days; estimates range from 6 to 14 days, depending on the rate of body water loss, which is influenced by environmental temperature, humidity, and activity level.[65] Water is critical because more so than any other nutrient, water is responsible for maintaining homeostasis of the internal environment.[9] It provides an aqueous medium to transport heat from cells to blood, to solvate and pass nutrients between blood and cells, to serve as a medium for intracellular reactions, and to transfer metabolic products for redistribution or excretion via urine. Both the quantity of reactants and the volume of fluid in which they are dissolved influence cellular chemical reaction rates; thus, imbalances in hydration status can alter cellular and tissue function, such as the body's ability to regulate temperature. Muscle contraction depends on transformation of chemical energy (ATP) to mechanical energy. Almost three-fourths of the energy used for muscle contraction is released as heat. Unless localized heat production from metabolism and muscle contraction is dissipated, the heat burden can be structurally damaging to enzymes or other proteins. Water absorbs heat produced at the cellular level and transfers it to the surface of the skin, where it can be dissipated to the external environment. Moreover, hypohydration can impair neuromuscular control, which is associated with increased risk of injury during demanding physical tasks in an extreme environment.[42] The importance of water is discussed in greater detail in Chapter 89. The focus of this discussion is energy restriction and assumes an adequate supply of water. For planning purposes, most wilderness expeditions require 3 to 5 L (about 3 to 5 qt) of potable water per person per day.

The environment has a primary role in determining survival under food and fluid restriction circumstances. Advances in food processing, preservation, and nutrient fortification have resulted in development of modern camping foods and the military equivalent, field rations, that can support health and performance in a variety of temperate environments, even if they are not consumed to complete caloric adequacy.[91] However, nutrition that was marginally adequate in a temperate environment may rapidly become inadequate in wilderness environments characterized by extreme temperatures, terrain, and physical demands.[90,92] Rodahl

and Issekutz[124] observed, "While short-term nutritional deficiencies in men at room temperature appear to have little or no detrimental effect on the capacity to do short-term, heavy work, there is a marked reduction in physical work capacity when a nutritional deficiency or nutritional stress is superimposed on a cold stress." Superimposed stressors, such as extreme heat, cold, altitude, sleep deprivation, physical exertion, and food restriction, influence nutrient requirements[7] and can jeopardize performance.[10,50,86,90,92,95] Figure 87-1 shows the complex interrelationship between environment and nutrition, and its effect on human physiology and performance. Stressors in the form of environmental extremes can have serious consequences on health and performance. Proper nutrition can help counter detrimental environmental influences on physical and mental performance.[2-7]

Energy and fluid deficits arising from the interaction of environment and nutrition can negatively impact physical[50] and mental[95] performance. Volitional physical activity and mood can suffer under caloric deprivation, depending on the magnitude and duration of the restriction. Motivation may be more acutely influenced by undernutrition than is actual physical performance.[95] Nutritional deficits may have a greater effect on what individuals are *willing to do* (i.e., on their perceived mood, symptoms, and self-motivation) than on what they *can do* (psychomotor performance).[134]

Nutritional Considerations in Planning for Wilderness Activities

Current American national nutritional recommendations are revised periodically and can be found in the most recent dietary reference intakes (DRIs) published by the Institute of Medicine, National Academies.[69] The DRIs are reference values for nutrient intakes that can be used to assess and plan diets for healthy people.[111] Publications that list DRIs can be obtained through the National Academies website (http://www.nap.edu/catalog.php?record_id=11767) and the National Institutes of Health website (http://ods.od.nih.gov/Health_Information/Dietary_Reference_Intakes.aspx).

The DRIs include four categories: estimated average requirement (EAR), recommended dietary allowance (RDA), adequate intake (AI), and tolerable upper limit (UL). EAR is the nutrient intake level estimated to meet the needs of 50% of healthy individuals in a particular life stage or gender group. RDA, calculated from the EAR, is the nutrient intake level sufficient to meet the needs of 97% to 98% of healthy individuals in a particular life stage or gender group. AI is an estimate of adequate intake based on observation or experimentally determined estimates when an EAR cannot be established. AI and RDA are similar but not identical. The UL is the highest daily consumption level of a nutrient; when UL is exceeded, the nutrient poses a risk of adverse health effects. In general, for nutritional planning for wilderness expeditions, the basic daily diet should meet or exceed the DRI recommendations, especially for prolonged wilderness excursions or expeditions. In the short term (<10 days), adequate energy provision is likely to be the predominant dietary concern. In the long term (>10 days), certain nutrients (vitamins and minerals) may assume more critical or primary roles in environmental extremes than they might normally fulfill in everyday life.

The effect of environmental stressors, such as cold, heat, and altitude, on vitamin and mineral requirements have been a focus of considerable military and civilian research.[8] Research conducted primarily in the post–World War II era and the Korean conflict established that vitamin and mineral requirements are not significantly increased by cold exposure, although caloric requirements for thermogenesis and work may be elevated to varying degrees, depending on the cold challenge, clothing ensemble, and level of physical exertion.[92] Work in cold environments can be adequately supported by various combinations of fat, carbohydrate, and protein, although certain combinations of macronutrients may be more beneficial than others in helping a person withstand cold exposure.[4] As an example, Mitchell and colleagues[101] demonstrated that cold tolerance (the length of time body core temperature could be defended during a controlled cold challenge) was favored by previous diets high in fat as opposed to diets higher in carbohydrate or protein. Subsequent research has indicated that the macronutrient source is less important in the cold than consuming enough total daily calories to support activity and thermogenesis.[4,57] In fact, humans demonstrate great versatility in fuel selection for physical work, including shivering thermogenesis.[31] This "metabolic flexibility" is important for sustaining both voluntary and involuntary muscular contraction. Although humans are physiologically engineered to utilize various combinations of macronutrients in the diet, in some cases a particular calorie source may possess some degree of metabolic advantage. Specific nutrient recommendations for optimal performance in specific environments are discussed under the section on tailoring diet to a specific environment.

Food and Adaptive Thermogenesis.

When environmental temperature declines, the body must compensate to maintain homeostasis by reducing heat loss and increasing heat production. Mild cold exposure, even without increased physical activity, elevates energy expenditure (i.e., heat production) in warm-blooded mammals, including humans.[76,88,155] This process, called *adaptive thermogenesis*, or regulated production of heat by the body, is influenced by environmental temperature and diet.[88] Figure 87-2 depicts the major sources of metabolic heat production in mammals. Heat can be generated from both shivering thermogenesis (ST) and nonshivering thermogenesis (NST) through synthetic, oxidative, and metabolic uncoupling processes. Mitochondria, the organelles that convert food to carbon

dioxide (CO_2), water (H_2O), and adenosine triphosphate (ATP), are fundamental in mediating these effects on energy dissipation in response to an energy-demand stimulus.[61] The greatest contributor to heat production is ST, which is supported by oxidation of carbohydrate, protein, and fat. Historically, NST, fueled primarily by brown adipose tissue (BAT), was thought to be a minor source of heat production. In recent years, however, the contribution of NST to cold-induced thermogenesis has been demonstrated and represents an area that may be susceptible to dietary manipulation, unlike ST.[26] The role of nutrients and BAT is discussed further in the following section on thermogenic nutrients.

Adaptive thermogenesis is a complex cascade of cell-signaling events primarily regulated by two major hormonal effectors: β-adrenergic agents and thyroid hormone. Thyroid hormones are major endocrine controllers of energy expenditure.[61] Thyroid hormones are critical in providing a vigorous response to cold exposure and sustaining that response by providing glucose and fatty acids to fuel energy production and thermogenesis.[136] Thyroid hormone acts synergistically with catecholamines of the sympathoadrenal system during cold adaptation and high energy output and, conversely, with low energy output when energy demands should be reduced, such as during starvation.[136] Physiologic stimuli, such as cold exposure, elicit these thermogenic hormones, which in turn interact with specific cellular tissue ligand-activated nuclear receptors called peroxisome proliferator-activated receptors (PPARs) in brown and white adipose tissue, liver, heart, and skeletal muscle. PPARs act as fatty acid sensors to control many metabolic pathways essential for energy homeostasis.[153] PPARs are mainly expressed in white and brown adipose tissue, where they control expression of several proteins involved in upregulation of lipid metabolism, subsequent energy generation, and thermogenesis. Peroxisome proliferator-activated receptor gamma coactivator-1α (PGC-1α) is a tissue-specific transcriptional coactivator protein that interacts with the nuclear receptor PPAR-γ. This permits interaction of this protein with multiple transcription factors, thus serving as a coactivator that enhances the activity of many nuclear receptors and coordinates cellular transcriptional programs important for energy metabolism and energy homeostasis. PGC-1α can interact with, and regulate the activities of, cyclic adenosine monophosphate (cAMP) response element binding protein and nuclear respiratory factors involved in energy metabolism and thermogenesis. Uncoupling protein-1 (UCP1) is found in the mitochondria of BAT and is used to generate heat by NST. Adrenergic and thyroid hormones have an impact on energy dissipation and subsequent heat production by the mitochondria in BAT and skeletal muscle through a complex signaling mechanism involving PGC-1α, PPAR-γ, and UCP1.[119] PPAR-γ is a nuclear receptor, subject to transcriptional coactivation by PGC-1α, which plays a central role in regulation of cellular energy metabolism. PGC-1α is induced

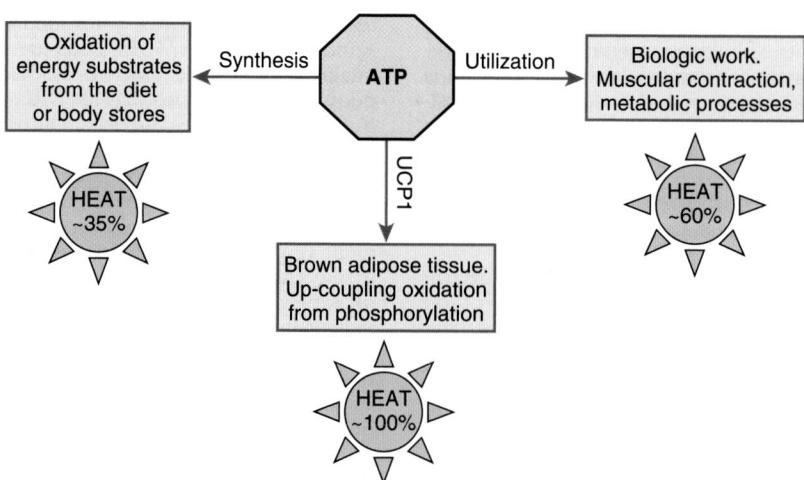

FIGURE 87-2 Energy-transforming pathways and heat production.

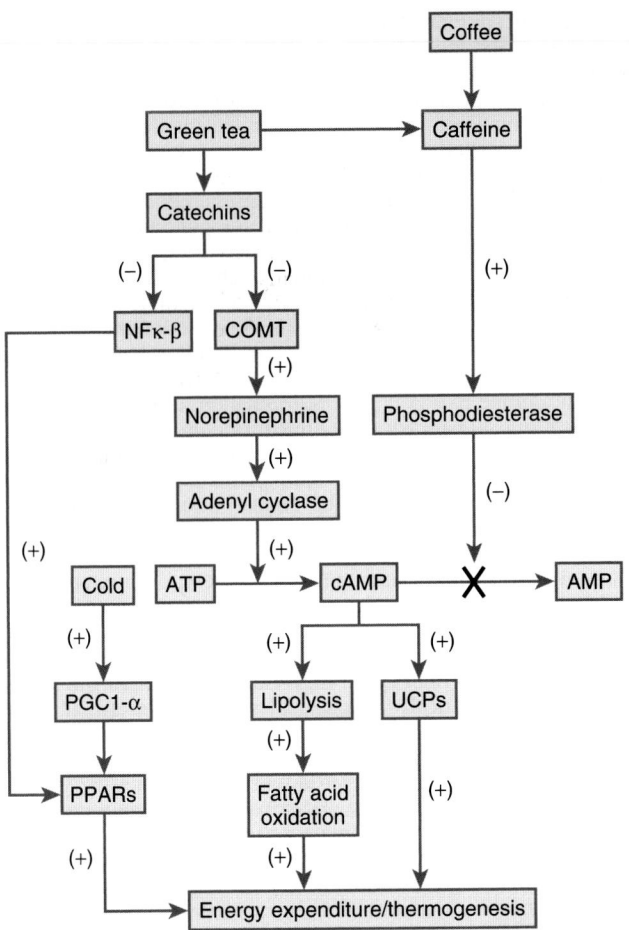

FIGURE 87-3 Cell signaling, activation of thermogenesis, and mechanism of green tea and coffee stimulation of thermogenesis. *NFκ-B,* Nuclear factor kappa B; *COMT,* catechol O-methyltransferase; *PGC1-α,* peroxisome proliferator-activated receptor gamma coactivator-1α; *PPAR,* peroxisome proliferator-activated receptors; *UCP,* uncoupling protein; *ATP,* adenosine triphosphate; *cAMP,* cyclic adenosine monophosphate; *AMP,* adenosine monophosphate. *(Modified from Hursel R, Westerterp-Plantenga MS: Thermogenic ingredients and body weight regulation,* Int J Obes 34:659, 2010.)

by cold exposure, linking this environmental stimulus to adaptive thermogenesis.[84] Induction of increased mitochondrial activity through activation of PGC-1α results in an increase in oxidative-type muscle fibers, which in turn leads to enhanced resistance to muscle fatigue and increased tolerance to cold.[81] PGC-1α is expressed at high levels in tissues where mitochondria are abundant and oxidative metabolism is active, such as BAT, heart, and skeletal muscle.[119] Figure 87-3 shows the schematic relationship of these cell-signaling and response elements and their potential interaction with cold, caffeine, and catechins.

Potential Thermogenic Nutrients. Although considerable research has been conducted on the effects of basic cell-signaling mechanisms on gene activity in response to thermogenic stimuli, less applied research has been conducted on thermogenic nutrients and whole-body cold tolerance. Older studies of food and cold tolerance have largely used core temperature responses to actual cold exposure along with dietary intervention; more recent cold tolerance research has incorporated aspects of basic cell signaling in response to specific food-derived components. Most notably, resveratrol, a plant polyphenol found in abundance in sources such as grapes and Japanese knotweed, has been shown in rat models to induce mitochondrial activity through activation of PGC-1α, which increases oxidative-type muscle fibers, thus increasing resistance to fatigue and cold tolerance.[81] Unfortunately, human resveratrol cold tolerance studies are lacking. However, if the rat model research has applicability to human

cold tolerance, resveratrol may be potentially beneficial for facilitating strenuous cold-weather activities. It is unlikely that the food products containing resveratrol could be consumed in quantities adequate to exert a similar effect to that seen in the supplemented rat model. However, numerous concentrated resveratrol supplements, and even food bars containing as much resveratrol as 50 glasses of wine, are commercially available, making a comparable dose level of resveratrol perhaps feasible for human ingestion.

More research has focused on manipulation of macronutrients—carbohydrate, protein, and fat—to enhance cold tolerance by increasing shivering thermogenesis. However, predicting significant effects of macronutrients on cold tolerance based on the thermic effect of food (specific dynamic action of carbohydrate, fat, and protein) has not proved to be a reliable indicator of ability of the body to resist cold exposure. Cold tolerance and diet studies are often complicated by interactions of energy depletion, exertional fatigue, and sleep deprivation. Although partitioning the relative contributions to thermoregulation impairment under multistressor environments is not possible, it is clear that the frequently encountered conditions of negative energy balance, fatigue, and sleep deprivation can impair thermoregulation, and that this impairment can be corrected relatively rapidly by rest and adequate feeding.[159] Dietary approaches involving adjusting the amount and frequency of meals in the cold, amount of total fat in the diet, and inclusion of caffeine/ephedra, capsaicin, and green tea seem to be the most practical approaches to augmenting thermogenesis in the cold. Blondin and associates[25] suggested that coingestion of carbohydrate sources utilizing different metabolic pathways (e.g., glucose, fructose) may be a practical dietary method to facilitate carbohydrate oxidation during cold exposure to support ST. An applied dietary application of these findings might be to put honey (high in fructose) on other high-carbohydrate foods that release glucose, such as a biscuit, bagel, or oatmeal.

Research on the NST properties of green tea seems to provide support for tea as a historically favored hot beverage for cold-weather and high-altitude expeditions. In obesity research investigating the possible thermogenic role of green tea in conjunction with caloric restriction for weight loss, green tea was found to stimulate thermogenesis in a manner that cannot be completely attributed to its caffeine content, which is relatively low.[45,46,59] The exact mechanism by which green tea stimulates NST is not clear but may involve several mechanisms, such as increased recruitment of BAT and/or enhanced BAT activity following recruitment.[26] The two primary active compounds in green tea are caffeine and catechin polyphenols, with the most active catechin being epigalocatechin gallate (EGCG). Both caffeine and catechins have separate but distinct roles in promoting thermogenesis. Caffeine inhibits the enzyme phosphodiesterase, which prevents degradation of cAMP. Cyclic AMP increases lipolysis, which provides additional fatty acids for eventual oxidation.[68] Catechins inhibit the enzyme catechol O-methyltransferase (COMT), which degrades catecholic compounds such as norepinephrine. COMT inhibition results in higher, more sustained levels of norepinephrine, which in turn produces a more sustained lipolytic response to support increased energy expenditure. Catechins also inhibit nuclear factor kappa B (NF-κB), a transcription factor that normally regulates PPARs. Upregulation of key enzymes involved in fatty acid oxidation by PPARs increases energy expenditure and enhances stimulation of fatty acid release afforded by elevated cAMP. Finally, catechins have a direct effect on expression of several uncoupling proteins that also can influence thermogenesis by uncoupling or decreasing the efficiency of oxidative phosphorylation.[78,88] Caffeine potentiates these catechin effects. The role of green tea and coffee in enhancing energy expenditure (thermogenesis) is shown schematically in Figure 87-3.

Other thermogenic "nutrients" may also have application in cold tolerance. Capsaicin is the major pungent compound found in certain pepper species and a common spice in many food products. It has been studied with mixed results for its thermogenic properties and influence on increasing fat oxidation.[138] Capsaicin is believed to increase thermogenesis by enhancing catecholamine secretion from the adrenal medulla through activation of the central nervous system (CNS), resulting in β-adrenergic stimulation.[68] It may also upregulate certain uncoupling proteins in response to catecholamine release.[94] Polymorphisms in the receptor and promoter regions of genes of individuals may explain variability in capsaicin stimulation between individuals[68] and equivocal results reported in the literature.[58,64,138]

Another thermogenic "nutrient" to consider is brown adipose tissue. BAT has been extensively studied in infants and animals under a variety of conditions. It helps maintain body temperature. It was formerly thought that this energy-rich and heat-generating tissue regresses with age.[82,83] Discovery that humans contain more BAT than previously thought,[40,151] and that cold exposure activates BAT thermogenic activity in humans,[150] has stimulated BAT research in adult humans. The unique uncoupling properties of BAT that make it such an efficient heat-producing organ may also be shared by other tissues, such as skeletal muscle. Wijers and colleagues[155] found that mitochondrial uncoupling in skeletal muscle during cold exposure may be one mechanism facilitating cold-adaptive thermogenesis in humans. Blondin and associates[26] found that daily cold exposure increases both the amount and the metabolic activity of BAT in humans, suggesting a potential nonshivering contribution to cold-induced thermogenesis. Dietary or pharmacologic approaches to stimulating BAT activity may be a promising way to turn on heat production during cold exposure. Future research on metabolic and dietary control of adaptive thermogenesis may have particular relevance to diverse metabolic outcomes, such as obesity and weight loss research, as well as human cold tolerance. Identifying ways to potentiate the NST activity of BAT through cold acclimation and pharmaceutical or dietary compounds may prove to be an important mechanism to improve cold tolerance.[26]

Tailoring Fat, Carbohydrate, and Protein to Different Environments. Although the most important nutritional concern in challenging environments, aside from water, is total energy intake, when wilderness activities shift from a cold-weather environment at sea level to cold-weather environment at moderate or high altitude, the macronutrient balance in the diet should be reconsidered. Although fat is an efficient and well-tolerated energy source during sustained, but relatively low-power-output, cold-weather activities at sea level, it is not as well tolerated at high altitude, at least in non–fat-adapted sojurners.[5] Substituting carbohydrate for fat and, to a certain degree, for protein can theoretically provide metabolic advantages to the individual's critical oxygen economy when working at altitude.[3] Carbohydrate is a more efficiently metabolized fuel at altitude than is fat because it is already partially oxidized (i.e., it contains a higher ratio of oxygen atoms to carbon atoms) and therefore requires less oxygen to combust its carbon skeleton to CO_2, H_2O, and energy. Metabolizing carbohydrate for energy requires approximately 8% to 10% less inspired oxygen than is required to obtain a similar amount of energy from fat. A high-carbohydrate diet can reduce symptoms of acute mountain sickness, enhance short-term high-intensity work and long-term submaximal efforts, and lower the effective "felt" elevation by as much as 300 to 600 m (984 to 1969 feet) by requiring less oxygen for metabolism.

Initial altitude exposure frequently results in anorexia and subsequently reduces energy and carbohydrate intake.[30] Anorexia (and thus food intake) usually improves with time and acclimatization (3 to 7 days at altitude), but, depending on the altitude, may never match that at sea level. Weight loss and performance decrements are quite common under these conditions. Carbohydrate supplementation of the diet at elevations exceeding 2200 m (7218 feet), particularly with carbohydrate-containing beverages, is usually an effective method to increase carbohydrate and total energy intakes.[3,30,48,110] Some,[39] but not all,[145] studies of carbohydrate supplementation at altitude have demonstrated a decrease in adverse symptoms resulting from acute altitude exposure. Enhancement of short-term, high-intensity performance,[31] as well as long-term, submaximal performance,[3,14,110] by carbohydrate supplementation has also been noted in some studies involving altitude exposure. The beneficial effects of carbohydrate at altitude most likely depend on the type of exercise performed

(intensity and duration) and the degree of prior muscle glycogen depletion experienced by the test participant, because of varying degrees of anorexia.

Muscle glycogen is related to the caloric adequacy of an individual's prior diet; carbohydrate intake usually parallels the overall dietary intake of the antecedent diet.[3] It is a good plan to consume a mixed diet with snacks high in carbohydrate. The most effective form of carbohydrate supplementation in environmental extremes is usually liquid beverages; people will drink when they are reluctant to eat.[3,14,30,48] Increasing fluid intake along with carbohydrate intake is also beneficial at altitude, where increased fluid losses occur as the result of diuresis and of respiration in the dry (low-relative-humidity) atmosphere.[9]

Recently, the "dogma" of high-carbohydrate diets being superior in all cases to high-fat diets, particularly in the case of sea level endurance exercise, has been challenged. Noakes and colleagues[108] questioned why the almost universal recommendation for athletes engaged in prolonged submaximal endurance exercise is a high-carbohydrate diet, particularly since work at less than 50% maximum oxygen consumption ($\dot{V}O_2max$) is well supported by fat oxidation. Furthermore, work at higher intensity can be accomplished without penalty if the athlete is already adapted to a high-fat diet.[116] Similar to the carbohydrate recommendations for athletes, the recommendation for work at high altitude is, with few exceptions,[116] for a high-carbohydrate diet.[14,39,100] Although direct comparisons of the beneficial or detrimental effects of high-fat to high-carbohydrate diets at altitude are lacking, theoretically at least, fat seems to be at a disadvantage. Recent comparisons of a high-fat versus a high-carbohydrate diet at rest and exercise at sea level suggest that pulmonary oxygen uptake kinetics associated with high-fat diets may attenuate microvascular blood flow and subsequent oxygen delivery.[121] If this is the case, one might expect the oxygen delivery problem to be even more magnified at altitude. It could be speculated that prior adaptation to a high-fat diet might lessen the microvascular blood flow attenuation, but for now, this is conjecture, and the high-carbohydrate diet remains the "most reliable" recommendation for work at altitude.

The "Right" Macronutrient Mix for Work at Altitude. There are two schools of thought regarding the most advantageous mixture of dietary macronutrients for work at altitude. Some believe that food preferences change greatly as elevation increases during the climb, and that carbohydrate becomes more palatable to the anorexic appetite. Others believe that once appetite recovers from the initial period of altitude acclimatization, the relative proportions of carbohydrate and fat in the diet are not as important as eating to energy demands to prevent loss of lean body mass. Early work published by Teasdale[147] and later advocated by Pugh[120] and Consolazio[39] favored carbohydrate for work at altitude largely because of its structural oxygen content; carbohydrate is more highly oxidized than is fat or protein and therefore theoretically should require less atmospheric oxygen (which is, in effect, reduced with the decreased barometric pressure at altitude) for its metabolism to CO_2 and ATP. This line of reasoning also agrees with what we know about the need for glycogen replenishment. Glycogen stores would be important energy providers for intense physical climbing work at altitude if one was working at a high percentage of $\dot{V}O_2max$. However, as Teasdale[147] aptly noted in "The Diet Problem for Mountaineers in the Himalayas," the actual amount of work in foot-pounds done at altitude is usually self-limited and may be relatively low compared with that at sea level; the real problem is not the amount of energy expended, but rather oxygen availability. Teasdale[147] recommended that climbers should seek a diet "demanding as little oxygen as possible," accomplishing this by ingestion of carbohydrate at frequent intervals. He also was one of the first to point out the oft-encountered "vicious" cycle of human physical deterioration at altitude: loss of appetite–partial starvation–metabolism of climbers' fat stores for energy–ketoacidosis–further anorexia and loss of appetite–loss of weight–deteriorated physical performance. This cycle of events, along with dehydration, is depicted schematically in Figure 87-1. Many of these situational/physiologic turning points leading to physical performance decrements can happen in other extreme environments, but the climber at high altitude seems to experience these adverse factors sooner and to a more significant degree than do workers in other environments. Washburn[154] emphasizes that dietary carbohydrate becomes particularly more critical as altitude increases above 3048 m (10,000 feet), and Consolazio and associates[39] identified carbohydrate as an important factor in lessening the initial severity of altitude illness. Although early observations by Pugh[120] and subsequent research by other investigators seem to indicate that carbohydrate is better "tolerated" or preferred at altitude, other studies in normobaric[125] and hypobaric hypoxic conditions[123] have failed to show a carbohydrate "preference" at altitude.[12] In a study of climbers on Mt Everest, Reynolds and co-workers[123] expected carbohydrate consumption to increase with increasing altitude but surprisingly found that retort pouch packages of high-fat sausages seemed to be preferred under cold, high-altitude conditions. This preference could be caused by a true preference for fat or simply the ease of utilization of the heat in a pouched food product. However, just because high-fat foods gain some acceptance in the cold, and perhaps even at high altitude, does not necessarily mean that carbohydrate loses its importance for glycogen repletion and maintenance of blood glucose levels needed for periods of high-power energy output. The most important consideration regarding fueling heavy physical work in the cold or in combination of cold and altitude is, as Washburn[154] stated, "Plenty of good food is of vital importance." "Good food" that is appetizing and served warm is likely to be consumed and therefore subsequently beneficial. Perhaps the real advantage of carbohydrate at altitude is more evident early in the ascent and, as climbers become more acclimated to the altitude, the exact macronutrient composition of the diet may be of lesser importance than individual climber food preferences.

ENERGY: HOW CRITICAL IS IT?

When planning for a prolonged wilderness outing, the following question should be asked: "If we run short on food, will we suffer severe consequences in our progress along our route and experience difficulty carrying our heavy packs?" For optimal performance, *total energy intake,* especially carbohydrate intake, is the key for sustaining high-level work capacity for extended periods. However, performance across a broad spectrum of backcountry tasks, including load-bearing work, is not always severely degraded by *short* periods of suboptimal energy and carbohydrate intake. A review of the effect of energy restriction on military work performance indicated that soldiers can maintain relatively normal work capacities for short periods (<10 days) of food restriction.[50] The Minnesota starvation studies conducted during World War II demonstrated that energy deficits resulting in loss of less than 10% of body weight did not greatly impair physical performance; however, underconsumption of calories for longer periods producing continued loss of body weight created significant deficits in physical performance,[146] as evidenced by observations of one participant in the 1570-kcal/day, 24-week semistarvation study, resulting in 24% body weight loss: "Then came February twelfth, the starting date of semistarvation … only two meals a day from now on. For the first two weeks the new life was fun. I was losing weight, of course, but I still had lots of energy. Then came the day when I lost my 'will to activity'—I no longer cared to do anything that required energy."

The degree of reduction of work capacity depends on the degree of caloric restriction, carbohydrate content of the food available, and power output demanded by the work. Studies of food restriction in military scenarios have revealed that restricted energy and dietary carbohydrate content over a 30-day period supported light to moderate activity level without evidence of greatly impaired physical performance capabilities.[15] On the other hand, longer periods (8 weeks) of caloric restriction coupled with higher levels of energy expenditure (U.S. Army Ranger training) have been associated with significantly reduced physical performance capacity.[107]

Because experimental conditions and performance measures differ between research studies, it is difficult to draw conclusions about the relationship between energy deficit and performance. Some indicators of performance, such as grip strength, appear to be well preserved until nutritional status is severely compromised. Other measures, such as maximal lift test, maximal jump height, isometric leg extension, and maximal oxygen uptake, appear to be more sensitive predictors of impaired performance.[71] In general, in nonobese individuals, strength seems to be rather well maintained at a hydrated body weight loss of up to 5%. This may be good news for wilderness travelers who are concurrently on a gradual weight loss program. Shedding fat actually "lightens the load" without diminishing strength. However, when dieting or restricting food results in loss of *lean* body mass, performance decrements result. Aerobic capacity and strength are reduced when loss of body weight exceeds 10% in a hydrated individual over 4 or more weeks, although this could occur sooner depending on the degree of caloric restriction, rate of weight loss, and initial body composition. Friedl[50] reviewed the influence of reduction in body weight resulting from reduced food intake on muscle strength and aerobic capacity and concluded that changes in $\dot{V}O_2$max in response to modest caloric restriction generally influence performance to a lesser degree than do reductions in muscle strength in response to weight loss. The primary concern of weight loss from inadequate energy consumption occurring during extended wilderness activities appears to be loss of muscle strength, which is influenced by an individual's initial body composition, rate of weight loss, composition of weight loss, and health status. Significant loss of muscle strength can be expected after a 5% to 10% body weight loss over 3 days (primarily from low glycogen or fluid loss) to 12 weeks (primarily from loss of lean body mass) under conditions of severe energy deficit. Significant declines in aerobic capacity can also occur after weight losses of this magnitude, but the decline in aerobic capacity appears to have relatively little effect on individual performance at moderate (<50% $\dot{V}O_2$max) sustainable workload levels.[50] In practical terms, this may mean that a gradual trek to the summit may not be precluded by a prior food restriction accompanied by significant loss of body weight, but that a short-term, all-out push for the summit to avoid impending severe weather would most likely be compromised.

Factors other than strength and aerobic capacity should also be considered when evaluating the effects of energy restriction on performance. Although weight losses of 6% or less over periods of 10 to 45 days generally do not produce significant degradations in cognitive performance,[134] mood may be adversely affected by caloric restriction.[36,97] However, long-term reduced consumption resulting in a 50% caloric deficit may significantly degrade cognitive performance.[95] Reduced food intake, when coupled with other stressors such as high rates of energy expenditure and sleep deprivation, can impair immune function.[69,80,86]

Carbohydrates: Critical for Performance of High Work Output

Both the length of time provided for dietary adaptation to carbohydrate restriction and the amount of carbohydrates in the diet can influence the level of aerobic endurance performance.[2] Aerobic endurance performance can be reduced by 40% after only 4 days on a calorically adequate but low-carbohydrate diet (i.e., with carbohydrates providing 10% of the kilocalories).[53] When a diet that was calorically adequate, but only 5% carbohydrates, was fed for 2 weeks, performance was also reduced, but only by approximately 15%, presumably because of metabolic adaptations to the shift in energy sources that occur with time.[118] Carbohydrate is important to performance, but the impact of any reduction in dietary carbohydrate intake depends on (1) period of time during which it is reduced, (2) absolute level of carbohydrate in the diet, and (3) power output ($P = F \times D / T$) needed to accomplish the task at hand. The latter point regarding power output requirements is an important consideration in provision of food for wilderness activities. Since much wilderness activity is usually recreational and not competitive, self-paced work and lowering of power requirements by increasing the time over which the work is accomplished is a feasible approach that can result in less reliance on carbohydrates and more reliance on a "slower-burning" fuel, such as fat.

Reduced carbohydrate intake, more than reduction of any other macronutrient (with the exception of water), can negatively influence muscle glycogen levels and endurance.[2] There is abundant evidence in the sports nutrition literature to permit extrapolation to similar wilderness activities and to conclude that certain types of performance, such as backpacking, cross-country skiing, and climbing, may be influenced by an acute shortage of carbohydrates in the diet, depending on the intensity of the workload (% $\dot{V}O_2$max) in which the individual is engaged. Inadequate carbohydrates in the diet, coupled with successive days of intense prolonged exercise, results in gradual reduction of glycogen stores, deterioration of performance, and increased perception of fatigue. Perceived or "felt" exertion for certain wilderness activities, such as load-bearing work, may reasonably be assumed to be a function of the dietary carbohydrate intake and its subsequent effect on muscle glycogen levels. To avoid fatigue and extend or enhance performance, carbohydrates may be ingested before, during, and after moderate- to heavy-intensity aerobic exercise.[70] This requires daily consumption of a minimum of 5 g of carbohydrate per kg body weight,[130] with ultralong (>4 hours), moderate-intensity exercise requiring as much as 8 to 12 g carbohydrate/kg/day.[28] For a 77-kg (170-lb) person, this equates to approximately 620 to 924 g of carbohydrate per day. To put this into perspective, a review of typical dietary carbohydrate intakes of male soldiers fed a variety of rations during 18 field studies in temperate, hot, and cold environments revealed intakes ranging from 244 to 467 g/day.[18] Similar data are not as well documented for nonmilitary wilderness activities, but a recent study of Mt Everest base camp trekkers revealed a carbohydrate intake of only 3 g/kg/day (325 g/day), far below the level needed for optimal glycogen stores and physical performance.[156] Most people do not selectively consume low-carbohydrate diets during wilderness activities, but total carbohydrate intake is often low because of its relationship to total energy intake and because of limited high-carbohydrate food choices. Some backpackers seek to maximize food and caloric density because of the weight of, and space available in, their packs. Calorie-dense food item choices that achieve this goal are often high in fat and relatively low in carbohydrates. Inadequate food consumption in military field exercises has been ascribed to poor ration palatability and variety, menu boredom, not enough time to eat or prepare meals, anxiety, and intentional dieting to lose weight.[91] Similar factors may be operative in wilderness expeditions. Countermeasures to reduce the effect of these factors should be taken into consideration during ration planning. To sustain short-term performance, a shortfall of energy (calories) is not as significant a concern as the lack of carbohydrate.[50] Table 87-1 lists current carbohydrate recommendations for daily fueling and recovery.

Field studies of carbohydrate intake and performance are difficult to conduct because of the many uncontrolled variables encountered outside the laboratory. Therefore, definitive field studies demonstrating a positive effect of dietary carbohydrate supplements on wilderness performance are limited.[6] However, existing field studies suggest a benefit of carbohydrate intake on performance. In one field study, participants in the Medical Expedition 2008 Hidden Valley Expedition to Nepal ingested either a 10% carbohydrate solution ad libitum (+3.5 g carbohydrate/day) or a placebo at 5152 m (16,900 feet) throughout the 22-day expedition. During the expedition, study participants completed a mountaineering time trial and multiple submaximal exercise, incremental-step tests. The carbohydrate-supplemented group was 17% faster than the placebo group during the time trial, with 18% reduction in perceived exertion.[110]

Although data from actual field studies are limited, data from studies conducted in well-controlled laboratory settings suggest that carbohydrate supplementation benefits performance. To test whether soldier performance would benefit from carbohydrate supplementation under simulated field operations, 18 physically fit U.S. Army Special Operation Forces soldiers were fed a controlled diet designed to simulate a "typical" daily dietary intake of carbohydrate and protein encountered during field operations (327 g carbohydrate/day, 201 g fat/day, and 118 g protein/day, 3657 kcal/day). The soldiers exercised daily (11 days total) under conditions designed to simulate field energy expenditure patterns (intermittent- and sustained-activity patterns of varying intensity levels). Each study participant received one of three beverage supplements during the program: placebo (0 g carbohydrate), carbohydrates (180 g carbohydrate) ingested once a day immediately after exercise, or carbohydrates divided into several doses ingested after the morning exercise session and at intervals during the afternoon exercise session. A decrease in respiratory exchange ratio in all treatments was observed, indicating that the soldiers were experiencing a carbohydrate shortage in response to the field simulation and were consequently utilizing fat to sustain energy expenditure. However, provision of supplemental carbohydrates permitted a higher level of physical performance or aerobic power to be attained. Run times to exhaustion were increased approximately 6% with the single carbohydrate feeding and 17% with the divided-dose administration. The ingestion pattern of the carbohydrate supplement as well as the carbohydrate itself appeared to influence performance, indicating that a supply of easily consumed carbohydrates (supplement or food) ingested before, during, and after field activities is an effective method to sustain or boost physical performance.[104]

Fat: A Special Place in Wilderness Exploration?

Historically, wilderness explorers and expeditions have relied heavily on foods higher in fat content than recommended by current sports nutrition and healthy dietary guidelines. One early 20th-century explorer, Vilhjalmur Stefansson, became such a strong advocate of meat-based high-fat diets that he volunteered himself for an unusual experiment in 1928.[85,141] Stefansson consumed an all-meat diet for 1 year with no detectable adverse medical consequences. Stefansson's championing of high-fat diets for work in cold regions led to a World War II–era U.S. Army and Canadian test of a high-protein and high-fat pemmican diet (low in carbohydrate) for work in the cold, but results were not encouraging.[73] Predictable fatigue occurred when the high-fat, low-carbohydrate diet was abruptly thrust on the soldiers. At the time, this study was offered as an argument against including pemmican in the cold-weather military diet. Despite the military's lack of enthusiasm for high-fat food, Arctic explorers have relied on pemmican for nutritional support during cold-weather polar expeditions.[142]

Although we now know that a period of time is required for metabolic adaptation to a high-fat diet,[115,116] the dispute continues concerning suitability of high-fat diets.[108,121] A review of numerous studies and the composition of diets and experimental conditions under which they were conducted indicates that two factors are critical to satisfactory utilization of high-fat diets: prior adaptation to fat in the diet and the power or exertion level at which individuals were required to work.[114] Humans permitted to adapt gradually to increasing levels of fat in the diet for approximately 3 weeks can function much better than if the dietary change is

TABLE 87-1 Carbohydrate Recommendations for Fueling and Recovery

Daily Fueling	Amount Of Carbohydrate
Moderate exercise (1 h·day^{-1})	5-7 g·kg^{-1}·day^{-1}
High exercise (1-3 h·day^{-1})	6-10 g·kg^{-1}·day^{-1}
Very high exercise (4-5 h·day^{-1})	8-12 g·kg^{-1}·day^{-1}
Acute Fueling Strategies	
Carbohydrate loading (events >90 minutes)	10-12 g·kg^{-1}·day^{-1} for 36-48 hours
1-4 hours before exercise	1-4 g·kg^{-1}
During sustained exercise (>1-2.5 hours)	30-60 g·h^{-1}
During ultralong exercise (>2.5-3 hours)	Up to 90 g·h^{-1}
Recovery (<8 hours between exercise bouts)	1-2 g·kg^{-1}·h^{-1} for 4 hours

From Burke LM et al: Carbohydrates for training and competition, *J Sports Sci* 29(Suppl):S17-S27, 2011.

abrupt. High-power outputs require the capacity for repeated bursts of anaerobic metabolism, which is best fueled by carbohydrates (i.e., via glucose and glycolysis). Efficient fat metabolism depends on readily available oxygen; the ability for oxygen uptake necessary for fat oxidation becomes limiting at high-power outputs. Military studies of dietary fat content confirm that a subcaloric, relatively high-fat diet (1976 kcal/day; 46% fat) can maintain moderate physical performance (including load-bearing work) for up to 30 days.[15,86] Practical physical and situational constraints, such as caloric density, weight-per-volume considerations, prior experience, work level intensity, and local availability of food, seem to affect usefulness of relatively high-fat provisions used in support of wilderness expeditions.[3,49]

Although not an ideal energy source for high-power-output competitive sporting events, fat can serve admirably as a concentrated energy source for outdoor activities requiring low-power but sustained work performance over longer periods. This is because low-power but sustained work, such a carrying a loaded backpack along a trail at a comfortable pace, can usually be accomplished aerobically at a moderate % $\dot{V}O_2$max effort that can be energetically powered largely by fat oxidation without dipping deeply into glycogen reserves. Although fat has received a somewhat tarnished health image over the past 40 years by an imperfectly understood relationship with atherosclerosis and coronary heart disease, we have gradually come to understand that there is significant interaction between the type of fat (fatty acid composition) and the individual's habitual level of physical exertion. Simply put, fat intake becomes particularly problematic when highly saturated fat (e.g., C-16:0 palmitic acid) is habitually consumed without accompanying daily high rates of energy expenditure. Anthropologic support for this concept can be found by examining cardiovascular disease in early Arctic populations that subsisted on a largely meat diet, where fat was a highly prized commodity. No one would consider classically made pemmican a "health" food, because of its high-saturated-fat content. Although pemmican is historically considered to be an ideal trail food for cold-weather expeditions because of its caloric density and resistance to spoilage, no one advocates a long-term habitual diet based on pemmican. Pemmican consumption is largely self-limited—acceptable for its purpose in the backcountry for defined periods but not acceptable as a staple in daily life. There is little scientific evidence that short periods (usually <1 month) of a high-fat diet has an irreversible effect on cardiovascular health, although a single high-fat meal can acutely influence endothelial response to the meal ingestion, causing narrowing of the arteries supplying blood to the extremities.[106] From such observations and epidemiologic studies linking long-term high dietary fat intakes to increased incidence of heart disease, we project that repeated insults of this nature may ultimately lead to increased deposition of lipid in the intima of arteries.[22,137] All indications, however, lead to the conclusion that we really do not know the time course required for high-fat diets to take a toll on our arteries, particularly if the periods of high fat consumption are intermittently imposed and further complicated by the level of caloric expenditure during these periods, as well as the type of fat consumed. Existing wilderness studies indicate that ingestion of high-fat diets do not adversely affect blood lipids and may in fact improve them.[41] The amount and type of fat in wilderness provisions remains largely a personal choice balanced against logistic constraints and the requirement for caloric density.

Washburn[154] stated that diets consisting of high levels of fat can be tolerated well by individuals doing heavy exercise in extreme, cold environments. He also wrote that diets for work in cold weather at low altitude can rely heavily on fats for energy. Because the usual diet of most humans now is generally higher in carbohydrates than fats, it is advisable that a gradual transition to a higher proportion of calories in the diet from fat be accomplished over a few weeks before embarking on an expedition. Enzyme adaptation to a higher-fat diet can help prepare the individual to optimally metabolize and utilize increased fat in the diet. Drury and associates[44] studied the metabolic effects of a diet high in fat and protein under cold-weather field conditions and found distinct adaptation to diets of this nature. Initially, blood

glucose drops sharply because of the low amount of carbohydrate in the diet, but levels out in the low-normal range after 2 to 3 days. Ketone excretion rises over the same period in response to the high levels of fat being oxidized for energy, peaking about the same time (3 days) as when glucose decrease levels out, returning to normal levels after about 9 days. Two weeks should be considered the minimum amount of time to adapt to a high-fat, low-carbohydrate diet before utilizing it as the main daily food routine during expeditions.[115]

Early explorers utilized pemmican and other high-fat, high-protein foods as staples for their expeditions, partially from observations of the dietary patterns of native people and partially from logistic considerations of weight/volume and perishability. Evidence that pemmican is not just an "antiquated dietary anachronism" has been demonstrated by current use of pemmican by Arctic adventurers Several food supply houses still manufacture and supply various versions of pemmican to outdoor enthusiasts. Persons desiring to prepare their own pemmican can do so quite easily using a kitchen food processor and readily available supermarket products. Numerous Internet guides to pemmican making can be easily accessed (e.g., http://www.traditionaltx.us/images/PEMMICAN.pdf). Pemmican is energy dense, well preserved without refrigeration, and can be a versatile energy source, especially during long days on the trail when little time or daylight is available for leisurely food preparation. It lends itself well as a cold snack on the trail. When added to a pot of hot water and mixed with a nutritious grain such as quinoa or brown rice, pemmican becomes a hot, filling meal (generically referred to by Arctic explorers as "hoosh") that can provide protein, fat, and carbohydrate at the end of a difficult day. Table 87-2 lists some nutritious carbohydrate grains that compliment a meal of pemmican "hoosh."

Protein and Maintenance of Lean Body Mass and Performance

Considerable discussion of the proper amount of protein to maintain muscle mass, prevent wasting, and sustain performance under conditions of physical stress exists in the literature. However, despite all the controversies, recommendations concerning the amount of protein in the diet have changed little since the World War I era, as evidenced by the 1919 report by Murlin and Miller[103]:

The amount of protein ... sufficient to repair all of the wastes of the body and to supply an adequate reserve is 13% of the total energy intake. It seems a matter of indifference to the muscles whether they receive their energy from carbohydrate or from fat. ... Hard muscular work therefore can be done on a diet high in carbohydrate or on a high fat diet. It is of general experience, however, that muscular work is done with less effort if there is a plentiful supply of carbohydrate.

Thirteen percent of the energy intake translates to an intake of 65 g of protein per day on a modest energy intake of 2000 kcal/day, or 130 g of protein per day on a more strenuous 4000-kcal/day energy intake. Quantities of dietary protein in the range of

	TABLE 87-2 Nutrient Contents of Some Common Grains to Add to a Pemmican "Hoosh"*				
Grain	**Energy (kcal)**	**Protein (g)**	**CHO (g)**	**Fat (g)**	**Fiber (g)**
Quinoa	374	13	69	6	6
Amaranth	374	14	66	7	15
Rice (white)	379	8	84	0	2
Rice (wild)	357	15	75	1	6
Oats (oatmeal)	375	10	78	4	7
Wheat (couscous)	376	13	77	1	5
Corn (grits)	347	9	79	1	5

Values from http://www.elook.org/nutrition/grains/.
CHO, carbohydrate.
*Note: Serving size = 100 g = 3.5 oz = approximately 1/2 cup.

TABLE 87-3 Protein Requirements Based on Activity

Activity Level	Recommended Daily Protein Intake
Sedentary adult	0.8 g/kg
Recreational athlete (low to moderate training volume and intensity)	1.0 g/kg
Endurance athletes	1.2-1.4 g/kg
Ultraendurance athletes	1.2-2.0 g/kg
Strength athletes	1.2-1.7 g/kg

From Dunford M, Doyle JA: Proteins. In *Nutrition for sport and exercise*, 3rd ed, Stamford, Conn, 2015, Cengage Learning, p 174.

65 to 135 g/day are rather easy to obtain, even for the most casual ration planner (e.g., one stick of beef jerky or one serving of peanut butter contains 6 to 8 g of protein).

Protein and Maintenance of Muscle Mass When Energy Intake Is Inadequate. The current RDA for daily protein intake for a sedentary adult is 0.8 g/kg body weight. For moderately active individuals, the recommendations are slightly higher at 1.0 g/kg and continue to increase for highly active individuals (Table 87-3). Even at the proposed maximum amount of 2.5 g/kg,[23] protein intake is relatively easy to obtain under normal conditions (i.e., adequate food availability, temperate climate). Protein considerations seem to be subordinate to the metabolic "jockeying" of fat and carbohydrate for prominence in energy provision during cold-weather and high-altitude operations. Protein is generally assumed to be of less nutritional importance from an energy standpoint. However, protein becomes of greater metabolic importance when energy demands are not being met (caloric restriction). Such situations are often encountered in wilderness settings in physically challenging environments. Recent studies of maintaining lean body mass during caloric restriction suggest that increasing protein intake may be helpful in maintaining muscle protein synthesis and muscle mass despite low-energy and relatively low-carbohydrate intakes.[19,112,117] Diets providing 80% of the energy actually expended (20% caloric shortfall) for periods up to 10 days have been shown to decrease muscle protein synthesis by 19% and, perhaps more importantly,

to reduce levels of cell-signaling proteins specific to protein synthesis.[112] Further, a caloric deficit of 40% for 21 days has been shown to upregulate the ubiquitin proteasome system, which is the primary stimulus for protein catabolism.[33] Current research indicates that if prolonged energy deficits cannot be avoided, such as during several days of inadequate food intake, nitrogen retention and maintenance of lean body mass are better preserved with accompanying protein intakes approximately twice the usually recommended RDA of 0.8 g/kg (1.6 g/kg/day). This adds retrospective credibility to the customary use of high-protein food items, such as pemmican and jerky, as ration staples by early wilderness explorers, who often found themselves in situations where it was not possible to eat a full day's ration (adequate kcal) for extended periods.

In situations where it is difficult to consume large amounts of protein, it may be more beneficial to focus on the amino acid profile of the food consumed. Branched-chain amino acids (BCAAs), in particular leucine, are important for muscle protein synthesis and may be good nutritional tools to help preserve lean body mass under energy restriction.[19] Leucine serves both as a substrate for protein synthesis and as an important signaling nutrient for regulating protein metabolism. Leucine has been shown to stimulate protein synthesis through the mammalian target of rapamycin (mTOR) and, at the same time, decrease protein degradation through inhibition of the ubiquitin proteasome pathway.[54] The unique metabolic property of leucine to prevent muscle protein loss under catabolic situations suggests that whey protein products high in leucine and other BCAAs may have application in wilderness nutrition during food preparation. The efficacy and human tolerance of leucine-rich proteins, such as whey, in support of maintaining or increasing muscle mass suggest that efficacy of leucine depends in part on the presence of other BCAAs. Indeed, leucine-rich proteins have been shown to be more efficient than leucine supplementation alone.[19] Extension of the beneficial leucine-specific effects reported in the literature involving exercise, malnutrition, weight management, and prevention of the sarcopenia of aging may apply to the situation of inadequate energy intakes in wilderness activities. Leucine may be of particular importance for activities at high altitude, where the combination of caloric restriction, low protein intake, and hypoxia work together to suppress mTOR activation and thus protein synthesis (Figure 87-4). Limited research suggests that

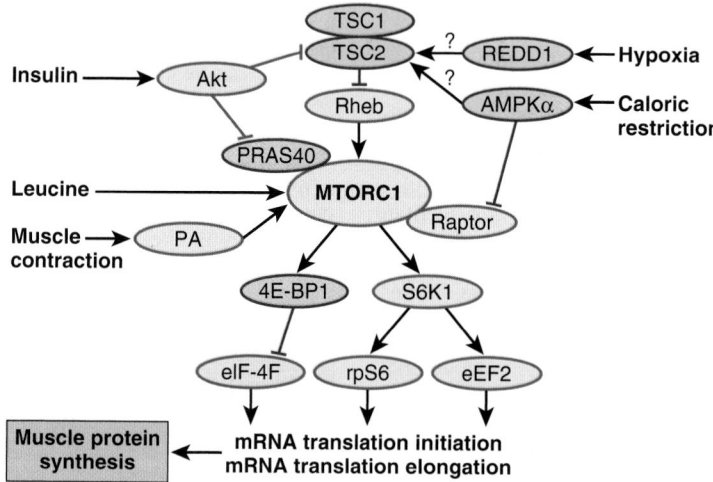

FIGURE 87-4 A simplified schematic diagram of the mammalian target of rapamycin complex 1 (mTORC1) signaling pathway and proposed cellular regulation of muscle protein synthesis in response to hypoxia, caloric restriction, insulin, muscle contraction, and leucine. Proteins in *green ovals* are positive regulators of mTORC1 and muscle protein synthesis, and proteins in *red ovals* are negative regulators of mTORC1 and/or muscle protein synthesis. *TSC1*, Tuberous sclerosis complex 1; *TSC2*, tuberous sclerosis complex 2; *Rheb*, Ras-homologue enriched in brain; *REDD1*, gene regulated in DNA damage responses and development; *AMPKα*, AMP-activated protein kinase alpha; *PRAS40*, proline-rich Akt substrate 40; *Raptor*, regulatory-associated protein of mTOR; *S6K1*, p70 ribosomal S6 kinase 1; *rpS6*, ribosomal protein S6; *eEF2*, eukaryotic elongation factor 2; *4E-BP1*, 4E binding protein 1; *eIF-4F*, eukaryotic initiation factor 4F; *PA*, phosphatidic acid; *Akt*, protein kinase B. (From Wing-Gaia SL: Nutritional strategies for the preservation of fat free mass at high altitude. Nutrients 6(2):665-681, 2014.)

TABLE 87-4 Pemmican Fortified with Unflavored Whey Hydrolysate Powder

Food Item	Grams	Energy (kcal)	CHO (g)	Saturated Fat Content (g)	Total Fat Content (g)	Protein (g)	Leucine (g)
Pemmican Standard Recipe Without Whey Protein							
Beef jerky	255	390	7	2.4	5	79	5.8
Beef tallow	60	2232	0	26.9	59.1	0	0
Cranberries, dried	115	354	95	0.1	1.6	0.1	0
Total	430	2976	102	29	65.7	79.1	5.8
Per 1000-kcal meal	144	1000	34.3	9.7	22.1	34.4	1.95
Pemmican Modified Recipe With Whey Protein							
Beef jerky	255	390	7	2.4	5	79	5.8
Beef tallow	60	2232	0	26.9	59.1	0	0
Cranberries, dried	115	354	95	0.1	1.6	0.1	0
Whey protein powder	56	220	4	2	4	42	4.6
Total	486	3196	106	31.4	69.7	121	10.4
Per 1000-kcal meal	152	1000	33.2	9.8	21.8	37.9	3.25

CHO, Carbohydrate.

BCAA and in particular leucine may be helpful for attenuating loss of body weight and lean body mass.[128,156] (See review[157] for a full discussion of muscle wasting at altitude.)

As a practical matter, a powdered whey protein supplement rich in leucine would take up little room in the pack and might be useful to incorporate into the diet on days that eating to caloric demand is not possible. Excess leucine and other BCAAs ingested beyond those required for protein synthesis and cell-signaling roles would also serve a beneficial role as an alternate supply of glucose through their conversion by gluconeogenesis to glucose. Food sources of leucine include brown rice, beans, meat, nuts, soy flour, milk, and whole wheat, although these food products might not elevate plasma leucine levels efficiently if consumed in small quantities. Whey protein supplements high in leucine are more practical and commercially available in powdered (flavored and unflavored) and food bar form. Food bars containing whey protein are particularly convenient items to increase protein and leucine intakes throughout the day. Unflavored powdered whey protein can be added to other food preparations, such as stews, soups, or pemmican, to arrive at a high-protein, high-leucine food product. Some sports gels also have leucine and BCAA, but often the dose is fairly low. Recommended supplemental doses of leucine generally range from 2 to 3 g of leucine/day. Balage and Dardevet[19] summarized human clinical trials involving as much as 7.9 g of leucine supplement/day for up to 4 months without adverse effects. Gleeson[56] observed that acute intakes of BCAA supplements of as much as 10 to 30 g of BCAA were associated with no adverse effects. Table 87-4 provides a recipe and nutrient content for whey-fortified pemmican containing approximately 3 g of leucine per 1000 kcal compared with pemmican prepared without whey powder. Consistency of the pemmican can be varied as desired by adjusting the amount of melted fat added to the pemmican. The unflavored whey protein flavor is largely masked by the customary pemmican ingredients. It should be noted that pemmican itself, by virtue of its endogenous leucine content from the dried meat (jerky), is an excellent dietary source of leucine even before whey protein supplementation. Pemmican, aside from its concentrated calorie source and adaptability to various nutritional modifications, also has the added advantage of a favorable weight/volume consideration for packing for extended backpacking trips. Figure 87-5 shows a visual comparison of the volume of 1 day's ration of 4000 kcal from pemmican versus typical commercial dehydrated backpacking food products.

VITAMINS AND THEIR RELATIONSHIP TO HEALTH AND PHYSICAL PERFORMANCE

Vitamins are complex essential organic micronutrients that function in growth, maintenance, and metabolism. Vitamins act as coenzymes in metabolic reactions, and vitamins E and C and

β-carotene (the precursor of vitamin A) act as protective antioxidants. Considerable oxidative stress may be experienced while working in environmental extremes.[7,11] High rates of energy expenditure, ultraviolet (UV) light exposure, and reduced dietary availability of foods containing antioxidants can cause excessive oxidative stress. Supplementing the diet with a vitamin and mineral mixture containing antioxidants to combat these stresses may be a more immediate concern than supplementation to prevent vitamin deficiencies (e.g., scurvy), which take a relatively long time to develop.

Prevention of vitamin deficiencies is one of the most misunderstood aspects of short- and long-range nutrition planning. Body stores of some vitamins (primarily the water-soluble vitamins) are limited, and under prolonged periods (i.e., weeks, not days) of dietary restriction, vitamin deficiencies can be manifested. This is rarely the case, however, for individuals consuming a mixed diet supplying close to the daily energy requirement. Although not routinely encountered, it is possible to develop a state of tissue depletion of thiamine, riboflavin, and pyridoxine in as short a time as 11 weeks by consuming a calorie-adequate, but vitamin-deficient, experimental diet composed of common food products.[149] Deficiencies of this nature do not develop over

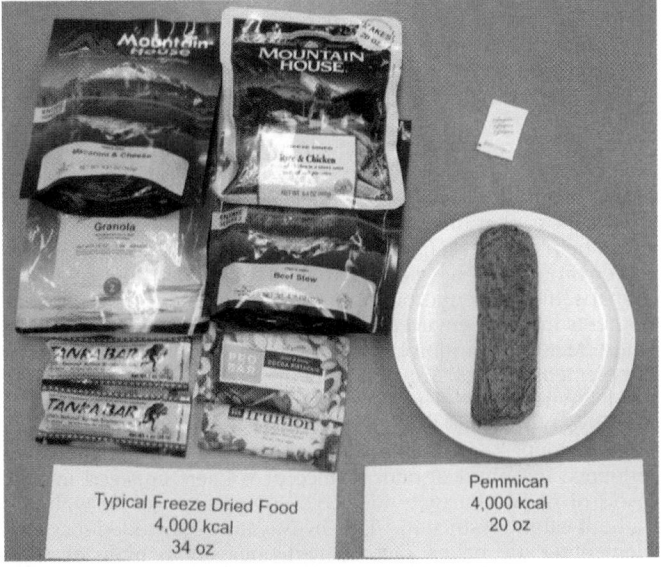

FIGURE 87-5 Comparison of volume and weight of 1 day's selection of food (~4000 kcal) in the form of typical dehydrated backpacking food items, compared with a bar of pemmican (sugar packet shown for reference).

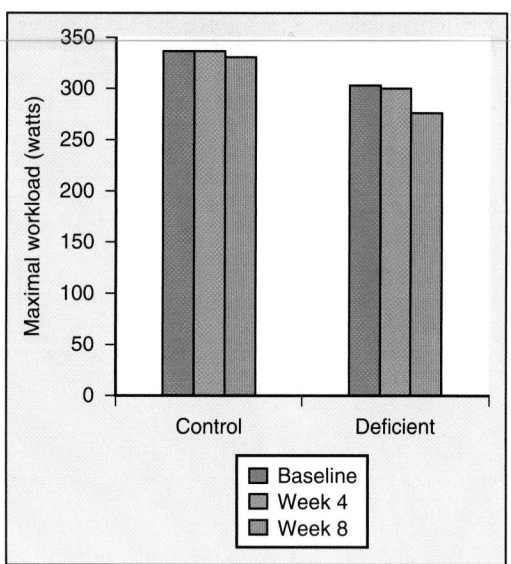

FIGURE 87-6 Impact of restricted vitamin intake on functional performance in humans. Experimental conditions: diet, 3070 kcal; thiamine, 28% RDA; riboflavin, 31% RDA; vitamin B₆, 16% RDA; vitamin C, 10% RDA. Performance test is workload achieved during incremental cycle ergometer testing. *(Data from van derBeek EJ, van Dokkum W, Schrijver J, et al: Thiamin, riboflavin, and vitamins B-6 and C: Impact of combined restricted intake on functional performance in man, Am J Clin Nutr 48:1451, 1988; and van derBeek EJ, van Dokkum W, Wedel M, et al: Thiamin, riboflavin and vitamin B-6: Impact of restricted intake on physical performance in man, J Am Coll Nutr 13:629, 1994.)*

BOX 87-1   Four Stages in the Development of a Vitamin Deficiency

1. **Preliminary Stage**
   - Inadequate amount because of poor dietary patterns or altered availability in the diet.
   - Commonly encountered after short-duration (<30 days) wilderness activities with poor nutritional planning.
   - *Consequence:* None except danger of progressing to stage 2.
2. **Biochemical Deficiency Stage**
   - The body's pool of the vitamin is decreased.
   - May be encountered after long-term (>30 days) wilderness activities accompanied by suboptimal daily nutrient intakes.
   - *Consequence:* Rates of enzyme catalyzed reactions may be slightly altered.
3. **Physiologic or Subclinical Deficiency Stage**
   - Can be detected by functional tests.
   - May be encountered after extended periods of consuming foods low in vitamins or periods of food restriction.
   - *Consequence:* Performance may be impaired slightly.
4. **Clinical Deficiency Stage**
   - Specific symptoms manifested; physical signs clinically detectable.
   - May be encountered after starvation or extended periods of food deprivation.
   - *Consequence:* Possible impairments of both health and performance.

the short term; they are not caused by a few days of suboptimal vitamin intake. Van der Beek and colleagues[148,149] studied the maintenance of human physical performance with varying degrees of vitamin restriction. Dietary vitamin deficiencies in persons consuming restricted vitamin intakes significantly less than the RDAs were manifested slowly, particularly in terms of physical performance impairments. Diets containing restricted intakes of thiamine (28% RDA), riboflavin (31% RDA), pyridoxal phosphate (16% RDA), and ascorbate (10% RDA) resulted in less than a 20% decrement in cycle ergometer performance (maximal workload) after 8 weeks at this level of restriction (Figure 87-6).

The relatively small change in performance decrements in response to vitamin restriction can be contrasted with more immediate effects of acute or long-term dietary carbohydrate restriction on physical performance. Manifestation of physical performance impairment is much more sensitive to the amount of carbohydrates in the diet in the short term (1 to 3 days) than it is to the vitamin, protein, or fat content of the diet (6 to 8 weeks).[2]

It can be generalized that development of a vitamin deficiency has four stages (Box 87-1), which involve a continuum of physiologic manifestations.

The possibility that certain nutrients (in particular, vitamins) might help people adapt to, or function more efficiently in, stressful environments has long intrigued explorers and scientists. Perhaps the most thorough study of the interaction between nutrients and the environment was conducted in the 1953 field study "Medical Nutrition Laboratory Army Winter Project: Vitamin Supplementation of Army Rations under Stress Conditions in a Cold Environment—The Pole Mountain Wyoming Study." The objective of this study was to determine if supplementation with large quantities of ascorbic acid and B-complex vitamins would influence the physical performance of soldiers engaged in high levels of physical activity in a cold environment, both with and without caloric restriction.[8] The investigators concluded that supplementing the mixed diet of men engaged in high levels of physical activity in the cold, with or without caloric restriction, did not result in significantly better physical performance.

Thus, it appears reasonable to conclude (at least from a performance standpoint) that vitamin supplementation in the wilderness environment is not nearly as critical as are total energy and carbohydrate provision. This does not mean, however, that dietary vitamin intakes should be ignored. Including a multivitamin and mineral supplement is a practical preventive measure, particularly in high-altitude environments, where considerable oxidative stress is induced. Box 87-2 summarizes conditions under which vitamin supplementation may be recommended.

Antioxidant Nutrients

Certain vitamins, such as vitamins E and C, may have important functions beyond their conventional essential roles, such as preventing degradation of the immune response, attenuating oxidative stress, and maintaining red blood cell flexibility and oxygen delivery under conditions of increased oxidative stress. In general, prolonged exposure to elevated levels of oxidative stress should be avoided because of its association with chronic disease and cellular organelle damage. In this context, it is worth noting that oxidative stress biomarkers are not only elevated while at altitude, but also can remain elevated for up to 3 days on return to sea level.[62] Although increased oxidative stress is a concern for prolonged sojourns at altitude,[11,62,99] little research can be found to support antioxidant supplementation to enhance performance or to lessen functional decrements (e.g., muscle fatigue) at altitude.[55,67] Consuming balanced meals that contain antioxidant nutrients should be adequate to control excessive free radical production because exercise itself leads to adaptations that suppress free radical production.[43] Because oxidative stressors may be encountered during wilderness activities, and because the quantity and antioxidant content of the foods are often uncertain, it seems prudent to include a multivitamin supplement with antioxidant properties among the food supplies. This nutritional

BOX 87-2   Conditions That Might Warrant Vitamin Supplementation

- Energy intake is below 1200 to 1600 kcal/day.
- Meals are routinely missed.
- Extremely poor or bizarre eating habits are practiced.
- Oxidative stressors (ultraviolet light exposure, high rates of energy expenditure, lack of fruits/vegetables in diet) are high.
- Under physiologic conditions requiring increased nutrient needs, such as pregnancy or lactation.

Supplement Facts

Serving Size 1 softgel

Amount Per Softgel	% Daily Value
Vitamin A 10,000 I.U. 100% as Beta Carotene	200%
Vitamin C 250 mg	417%
Vitamin E 200 I.U.	667%
Zinc 7.5 mg	50%
Selenium 15 mcg	21%
Copper 1 mg	50%
Manganese 1.5 mg	75%

FIGURE 87-7 Antioxidant supplements can contain a variety of nutrient components designed to act as sacrificial antioxidants (e.g., vitamin C) or as cofactors in antioxidant enzyme systems (e.g., selenium). The supplement shown is typical of many basic antioxidant formulations containing vitamin and mineral antioxidant components. (*Copyright 2007 by Mosby, Inc., an affiliate of Elsevier Inc.*)

insurance is inexpensive and takes up little space. Figure 87-7 shows the composition of a typical antioxidant vitamin and mineral supplement. A popular alternative to the typical antioxidant supplement is a food (fruit and/or vegetable)–based extract (Figure 87-8).

MINERAL SUPPLEMENTS: ELECTROLYTES, HEMATOPOIESIS, AND BONE HEALTH

The mineral content of the diet is usually not a primary concern, provided that a mixed diet that meets energy requirements is consumed daily. Supplemental calcium and iron are considerations for female travelers, as discussed in the next section. Sodium in hot environments is an exception, because it is lost during activities producing excessive sweating (see Chapter 89). Hyponatremia can occasionally be encountered in unanticipated scenarios such as a cold environment.[160] With appropriate acclimatization to heat (and resultant renal sodium conservation), the amount of sodium required in the diet for work in the heat is reduced. Laboratory studies have shown that heat acclimatization

Supplement Facts

Serving Size 1 Capsule

	Amount Per Serving	% Daily Value
Acai Berry Extract (Euterpe oleracea) (standardized to 10% phenolic acid)	125 mg	-
Noni Fruit Extract 8:1 (Morinda citrifolia)	125 mg	-
Pomegranate Fruit Extract 5:1 (Punica granatum)	125 mg	-
Wolfberry (goji) Fruit (Lycium barbarum) (freeze-dried concentrate typically containing 60% polysaccharides)	125 mg	-
Mangosteen (Garcinia mangostana) (fruit)	125 mg	-
*Daily Value not established.		

Supplement Facts

Serving Size 1 Tablet

	Amount Per Tablet	% Daily Value
Vitamin C (as ascorbic acid)	100 mg	167%
Resveratrol (from 200 mg Polygonum cuspidatum 8% total resveratrols) (Tiger cane)	16 mg	-
Grape Seed Extract (Vitis vinifera) (95% polyphenols)	50 mg	-
Grape Skin Extract (Ancellota lambrusco) (30% polyphenols)	100 mg	-
Green Tea 5:1 Extract (Carmellia sinensis) (45% polyphenolics)	200 mg	-
*Daily Value not established.		

FIGURE 87-8 Examples of phytochemical antioxidant supplements containing naturally occurring polyphenols that can be effective free radical quenchers. Many of these fruit- or vegetable-extract antioxidant formulations can have higher ORAC (oxygen radical absorption capacity) values than do conventional vitamin/mineral antioxidant supplements.

can occur when as little as 4 to 8 g of salt (NaCl) is ingested per day.[1] The amount of NaCl required for safe work in the heat depends on the degree of prior heat acclimatization and amount of sweat loss.

Altered dietary patterns or excessive sweating can influence sodium balance. Starvation can lead to plasma volume depletion when sodium in the circulation is insufficient to allow osmotic forces to retain water.[65] When nonacclimatized humans are exposed simultaneously to acute food restriction and high sweat rates, the resulting excessive loss of sodium can lead to dizziness, syncope, and collapse. These problems can be avoided by ensuring that extra salt is included in the food provisions for wilderness expeditions and that salt is available to season food during and after high sweat losses.

Another form of sodium deficit is dilutional hyponatremia caused by overhydration with fluids in conjunction with lower-than-normal sodium intake or excessive sodium loss in sweat. Hyponatremia caused by overconsumption of fluids is extremely rare when regular meals are consumed. Hyponatremia is a complication of overhydration in wilderness environments where food is neglected and water overzealously emphasized. It has been described for hot,[16,17] cold,[160] and high-altitude[140] environments. Calorie deprivation can alter sodium intake. In addition to reduced intake of sodium with food, severe caloric restriction leads to marked natriuresis.[114] Increased loss of sodium in turn leads to depletion of fluid volume, impaired cardiovascular function, and reduced work capacity, further exacerbating the effects of energy restriction. Increased aldosterone levels in response to reduced plasma volume can also lead to accelerated potassium wasting.[114]

For insurance and safety considerations, include 5 g (about two typical restaurant serving packets) of table salt for every day in the field packed with the food supplies. If necessary for fluid replacement after excessive sweating, this extra salt can be used to make a dilute electrolyte beverage by adding 0.5 tsp (2 to 3 g salt) to 1 qt of water. Excess sodium should be avoided because its excretion increases metabolic water demands.[5]

SPECIAL NUTRITIONAL REQUIREMENTS FOR FEMALE WILDERNESS TRAVELERS

Although our understanding of the differences between male and female nutritional requirements is incomplete, gender differences exist for certain nutrients, such as iron, calcium, folate, and vitamin B_6, under normal environmental living conditions.[102] Differences are particularly notable for women using oral contraceptives[93] and those who are pregnant or lactating.[34] The health implications for pregnant travelers planning a trip to altitude are beyond the scope of this chapter; they should consult a knowledgeable pediatrician or obstetrician.

Investigations of nutritional requirements at environmental extremes have been conducted on men, but comparatively little research has been directed toward women. The few studies that have been done suggest that dietary nutrient intakes of women at moderate altitude are similar to those at sea level,[77] implying that specific gender requirements that exist at sea level may be even more important at altitude, particularly if there is scarcity of nutrient-dense foods or if appetite is blunted. Some gender-specific nutrient requirements are known. For example, research in the late 1960s found that female military service members deployed to locations at moderate to high altitude required supplemental dietary iron for optimal support of the hematopoietic response to hypoxia.[60] Subsequently, research on iron requirements and the thermogenic response to cold have also identified iron as a key micronutrient for women in cold environments.[21,89] Because of their smaller body size, women usually consume fewer total food calories than men and thus are at increased risk for reduced vitamin and mineral intake. Fortunately, the need for these vitamins and minerals (with the exception of iron) is related to lean body mass, and women usually have a lower lean body mass than men.

Because the choice of available foods may be limited during expeditions into the wilderness, female travelers should include a multivitamin supplement in their provisions. It should contain

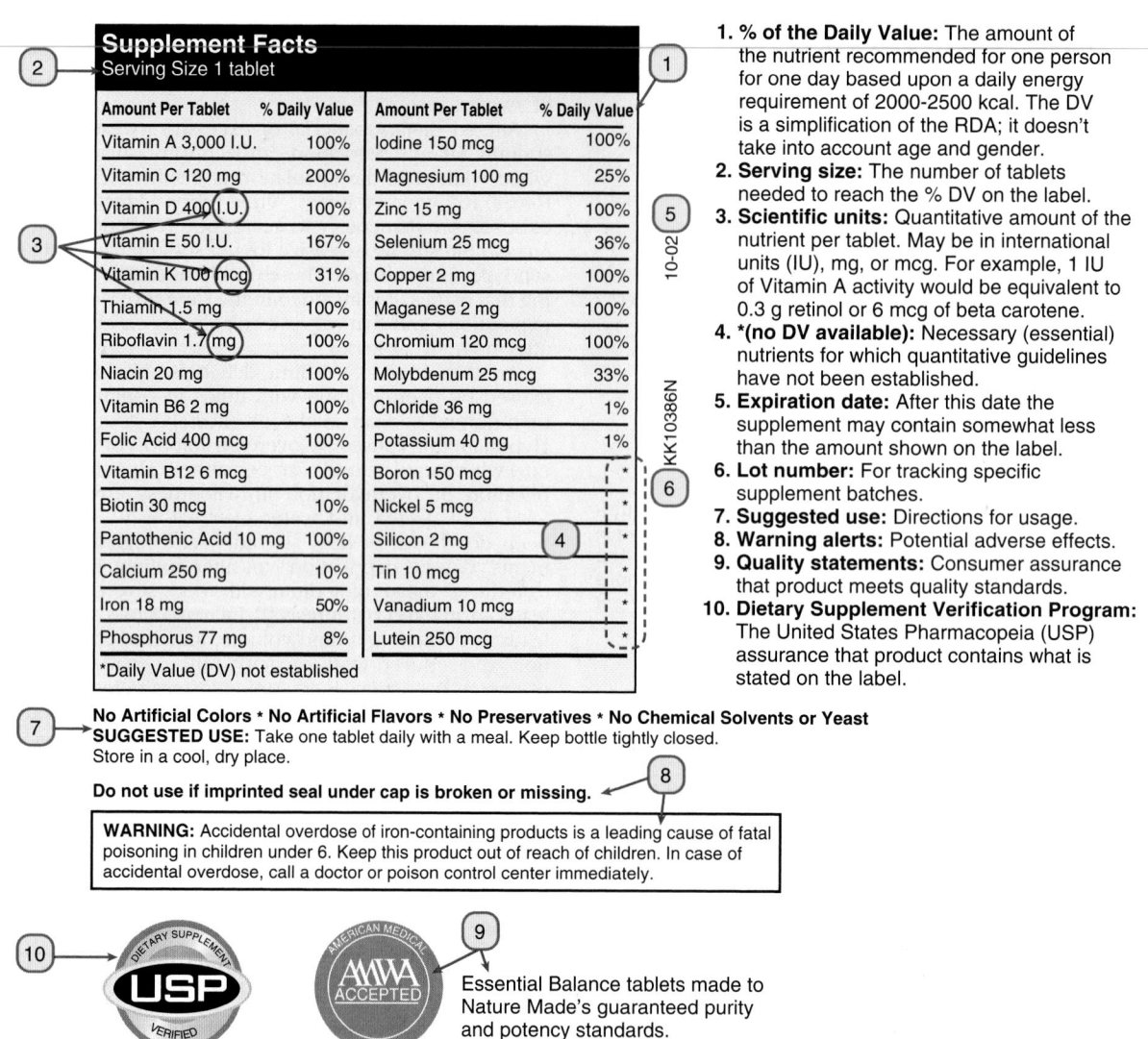

Supplement Facts
Serving Size 1 tablet

Amount Per Tablet	% Daily Value	Amount Per Tablet	% Daily Value
Vitamin A 3,000 I.U.	100%	Iodine 150 mcg	100%
Vitamin C 120 mg	200%	Magnesium 100 mg	25%
Vitamin D 400 I.U.	100%	Zinc 15 mg	100%
Vitamin E 50 I.U.	167%	Selenium 25 mcg	36%
Vitamin K 100 mcg	31%	Copper 2 mg	100%
Thiamin 1.5 mg	100%	Maganese 2 mg	100%
Riboflavin 1.7 mg	100%	Chromium 120 mcg	100%
Niacin 20 mg	100%	Molybdenum 25 mcg	33%
Vitamin B6 2 mg	100%	Chloride 36 mg	1%
Folic Acid 400 mcg	100%	Potassium 40 mg	1%
Vitamin B12 6 mcg	100%	Boron 150 mcg	*
Biotin 30 mcg	10%	Nickel 5 mcg	*
Pantothenic Acid 10 mg	100%	Silicon 2 mg	*
Calcium 250 mg	10%	Tin 10 mcg	*
Iron 18 mg	50%	Vanadium 10 mcg	*
Phosphorus 77 mg	8%	Lutein 250 mcg	*

*Daily Value (DV) not established

10-02

KK10386N

1. **% of the Daily Value:** The amount of the nutrient recommended for one person for one day based upon a daily energy requirement of 2000-2500 kcal. The DV is a simplification of the RDA; it doesn't take into account age and gender.
2. **Serving size:** The number of tablets needed to reach the % DV on the label.
3. **Scientific units:** Quantitative amount of the nutrient per tablet. May be in international units (IU), mg, or mcg. For example, 1 IU of Vitamin A activity would be equivalent to 0.3 g retinol or 6 mcg of beta carotene.
4. ***(no DV available):** Necessary (essential) nutrients for which quantitative guidelines have not been established.
5. **Expiration date:** After this date the supplement may contain somewhat less than the amount shown on the label.
6. **Lot number:** For tracking specific supplement batches.
7. **Suggested use:** Directions for usage.
8. **Warning alerts:** Potential adverse effects.
9. **Quality statements:** Consumer assurance that product meets quality standards.
10. **Dietary Supplement Verification Program:** The United States Pharmacopeia (USP) assurance that product contains what is stated on the label.

No Artificial Colors * No Artificial Flavors * No Preservatives * No Chemical Solvents or Yeast
SUGGESTED USE: Take one tablet daily with a meal. Keep bottle tightly closed. Store in a cool, dry place.

Do not use if imprinted seal under cap is broken or missing.

WARNING: Accidental overdose of iron-containing products is a leading cause of fatal poisoning in children under 6. Keep this product out of reach of children. In case of accidental overdose, call a doctor or poison control center immediately.

Essential Balance tablets made to Nature Made's guaranteed purity and potency standards.

FIGURE 87-9 Annotated multivitamin and mineral supplement label showing some key components and pertinent information. Nutrients are expressed as a percentage of the daily value (DV), which is the amount of nutrients recommended for daily consumption by most adults needing 2000 to 2500 kcal/day.

at least 50% of the female RDA for iron, zinc, folate, vitamin B6, and calcium. Antioxidant nutrients (see Vitamins and Their Relationship to Health and Physical Performance, earlier), including extra vitamins C and E and perhaps certain carotenoids, such as lutein and zeaxanthin, provide additional insurance against oxidative stress. Figure 87-9 shows the composition of a typical multivitamin and mineral supplement. The values shown reflect the daily value (DV) of the nutrients, that is, the recommended daily amount for most adults needing 2000 to 2500 kcal/day.

Multivitamins often contain relatively low amounts of calcium compared with the female RDA of 1000 to 1300 mg/day, so it may be beneficial for female travelers to include an additional bioavailable calcium supplement containing 250 to 500 mg of calcium per dose. Commercially available chocolate- or caramel-flavored calcium "chews" are convenient and contain a small amount of carbohydrate, as well as "bone-friendly" nutrients such as vitamins D and K. The U.S. RDA for calcium intake for adults younger than 50 is 1000 mg daily, and people older than 50 should ingest 1200 mg daily. Calcium supplements are best taken in small (no more than 500 mg) divided doses throughout the day. If an iron supplement is being taken in a multivitamin or by itself, it is best not to take it at the same time as the calcium supplement, because absorption of each is unpredictable and may be less than optimal in the presence of the other.[122] If an individual is traveling to high altitude, it is recommended

that serum ferritin be measured to determine iron status. If iron status is low, supplementation should be implemented before departure.

Nutrients in a vitamin-mineral supplement should be close to the DV level ($\leq$100%). This ensures adequate intake of major micronutrients with minimal risk of adverse nutrient interactions. Synthetic vitamins are structurally the same as, and cost less than, so-called natural vitamins, with the exception of vitamin E. Generic brands are also generally less expensive and equally effective. Addition of herbs, enzymes, or amino acids accomplishes little but adds cost. Some supplements containing phytonutrients extracted from plants may be appropriate when the logistics of the trip offer little or no chance to secure fresh fruits and vegetables. A source of information on vitamin and mineral supplements is ConsumerLab, which provides independent test results and information to help consumers and health care professionals evaluate health, wellness, and nutrition products. The results of its tests, including brands that have passed testing, are available at www.consumerlab.com.

Supplements can lose potency over time, so check the expiration date on the label. Figure 87-9 provides guidance for reading and interpreting supplement labels. The initials USP (for the testing organization U.S. Pharmacopeia) or words such as "release assured" or "proven release" indicate that the supplement is easily dissolved and absorbed.

NUTRITIONAL DEPRIVATION: MALNUTRITION AND STARVATION

DEFINITIONS

There is little uniformity in the terminology used to describe the physiology of human starvation. Hoffer[65] has suggested the following definitions:

Fasting: Total absence of food intake.

Starvation: Physiologic condition that develops when macronutrient content is inadequate for a prolonged period.

Semistarvation or food restriction: The more commonly encountered condition of some food intake, but of insufficient energy and protein provision.

Malnutrition: General term for the condition resulting from long-standing inadequate consumption of nutrients, abnormal absorption of nutrients, or unusual demands on certain nutrients; usually involves suboptimal food intake or consumption of food of poor nutrient density, resulting in micronutrient and macronutrient deficiencies.

Protein-energy malnutrition (PEM): Result of inadequate intake of energy, protein, or both for prolonged periods. Two related types of PEM are *marasmus* (primarily energy deficiency) and *kwashiorkor* (primarily protein deficiency). Both forms occur across a spectrum of situational and environmental conditions and exhibit many of the same symptoms. PEM is frequently a consequence of starvation, but all starvation does not necessarily lead to PEM. Development of PEM depends on body energy reserves, length of the fast, age, and presence or absence of disease. PEM is unlikely to be encountered by most wilderness travelers; a possible exception is within indigenous populations in certain Third World locations. When malnourished indigenous people are encountered in wilderness travels, caution should be exercised about sharing food. These individuals may not be accustomed to ingesting large quantities of food replete with sodium, and there may be consequences to overeating (see Feeding Victims of Starvation, later).

Cachexia: Wasting that results from metabolic stress and loss of appetite. It is sometimes called *cytokine-induced malnutrition* to distinguish it from simple food deprivation in the absence of stress. Inanition of advanced-stage cancer patients is an example of cachexia.

MALNUTRITION IN A WILDERNESS SETTING

This discussion is limited to the metabolic and physiologic consequences of starvation or energy restriction that might be encountered in wilderness settings, including unplanned emergencies that result in shortage of food, and wilderness rescue operations of victims of unintentional starvation. In these settings, duration of food restriction is usually, but not always,[129] of shorter duration than that associated with hunger encountered during famine, war, crop failure, and disease.

Solomons[139] has stated that malnutrition simply means "bad" nutrition and has listed six possible causes of nutrient deficiencies leading to malnutrition: reduced intake, decreased absorption, decreased utilization, increased destruction, increased wastage, and increased requirement. Primary malnutrition is caused by reduced intake of food. This is the most frequently encountered cause of malnutrition in wilderness settings. Reduced food intake, along with increased nutrient requirements, can contribute to development of nutrient deficiencies during expeditions under extreme environmental conditions. Secondary causes of nutrient deficiencies are less frequently encountered but can contribute significantly if disease or illness strikes the wilderness traveler.

Malnutrition develops in stages that usually require considerable time to manifest. As seen in cases of vitamin deficiency, the first changes reflect diminished dietary intake, with resultant reduced blood and tissue levels of nutrients, followed by intracellular changes in biochemical functions. Eventually, if the malnutrition is unrelieved, physical symptoms develop. These effects can include oral lesions, rashes, petechial hemorrhages, ecchymoses, pigmentation changes, and edema. People who undergo prolonged semistarvation experience hunger, weakness, lack of drive, mood changes, osteoporosis, hypoalbuminemia, edema, decreased muscle mass, alopecia, hypotension, and poor wound healing. Impaired immune function, decreased resistance to infection, and prolonged recovery from injury are all consequences of long-term food restriction.[35,51,80,132,133]

STARVATION

Starvation is the physical condition brought about by inadequate consumption, absorption, or retention of protein and dietary energy from carbohydrate and fat.[66] Starvation can be acute or chronic, as well as total or partial. Different forms of starvation are similar but not identical. Starvation can result from disease or simply from lack of food. It can ultimately manifest as a disease (PEM) or, if not prolonged, as nonpathologic weight reduction. The metabolic adaptations that occur in the progression of starvation depend on whether there is acute energy restriction or chronic undernourishment as a result of long-term low-energy intake.[131]

Acute Energy Restriction

The rapid progression of events that occur in response to acute energy inadequacy (e.g., a 50% shortfall of food during the second week of a 2-week backpacking trip) is shown in the first three steps in Figure 87-10. The body reacts quickly to energy shortage by utilizing readily available muscle and liver glycogen stores. Progression to the final steps of organ decompensation and death would be encountered only after complete starvation for several weeks. Following food restriction when the body's carbohydrate stores have been depleted, glucagon level rises, insulin level falls, and the process of gluconeogenesis accelerates, converting noncarbohydrate precursors, such as lactate, glycerol, and amino acids, to glucose in order to maintain blood glucose level and prevent hypoglycemia (Figure 87-11).

These metabolic principles are expressed in more detail in Figures 87-12 and 87-13. Data used to prepare this classic scheme of carbon flux during starvation are based largely on the work of Cahill,[31] who studied metabolic aspects of starvation in humans. Reduction in carbohydrate intake and resultant reduced glucose provision during food restriction is in large part compensated for by accelerated gluconeogenesis. The carbon skeletons of 100 g of protein from endogenous tissue sources can ultimately provide approximately 55 g of carbohydrate after metabolic transformations. The glycerol from 100 g of mobilized fat can yield 10 to 15 g of carbohydrate by gluconeogenesis.[29] As glycogen is depleted, catecholamine production rises simultaneously, facilitating fatty acid mobilization from adipose depots. Once mobilized, fatty acids are taken up by muscle in proportion to their concentration in blood and are oxidized for energy. The

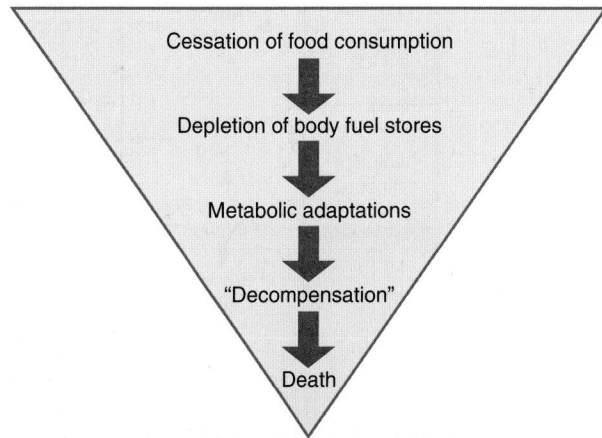

FIGURE 87-10 Sequence of events during prolonged starvation. If the fast is not terminated and energy reserves are depleted, internal organ systems ultimately used for energy will fail (decompensation), resulting in death. (*Copyright 2007 by Mosby, Inc., an affiliate of Elsevier Inc.*)

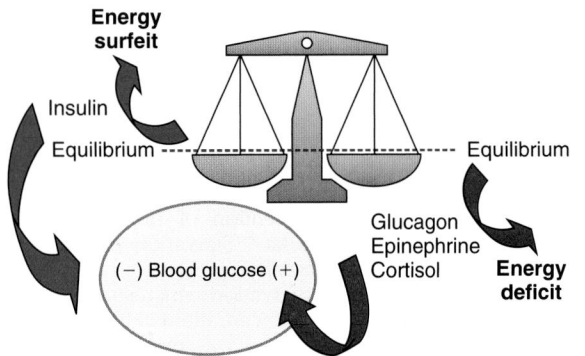

FIGURE 87-11 Influence of energy balance on hormonal control of blood glucose. When food is consumed after ingestion, insulin is released, lowering blood glucose. When no food is consumed and blood glucose drops, gluconeogenic hormones are released, and endogenous sources are used to raise blood glucose levels. *(Copyright 2007 by Mosby, Inc., an affiliate of Elsevier Inc.)*

metabolic events of a short-term fast are shown in Figure 87-12. The major difference between short- and long-term fasts is in the shift of carbon source for energy production. As the duration of the fast increases, the amount of glucose oxidized decreases and the amount of ketone bodies oxidized increases.

Long-Term Energy Restriction

Prolonged fasting is characterized initially by increased protein catabolism for gluconeogenesis, followed by increased production of ketone bodies as a consequence of fat mobilization for energy demands. A fast longer than 2 to 3 days exhausts liver glycogen and uses up about half the muscle glycogen stores.[65] Thereafter, glucose utilized by the body (in the absence of food consumption) must be synthesized from endogenous precursors through gluconeogenesis. The appearance of large amounts of ketone bodies in the blood, breath, and urine results from a low

insulin-to-glucagon ratio accompanying a prolonged fast and massive fatty acid mobilization from adipose tissue.

Ketone bodies are a metabolic consequence of vigorous fatty acid oxidation engendered by starvation in the absence of significant carbohydrate intake. Production of acetoacetate and β-hydroxybutyrate increases significantly during the first 7 to 10 days of fasting and stabilizes after 2 to 3 weeks.[24] Ketone bodies can be increasingly used for energy by muscle and brain as energy restriction becomes prolonged. Even a short-term fast elicits significant production of ketone bodies (see Figure 87-12); however, ketone body production may be virtually abolished if a minimum of 150 g of carbohydrate is ingested daily to supply the brain with glucose for energy.[29,65] Normally, in the fed state, ketone body oxidation accounts for provision of less than 3% of the total energy requirement. Longer periods (7 to 10 days) of fasting are accompanied by a greatly increased level of circulating ketone bodies, which can provide as much as 40% of the total energy expenditure and greater than 50% of the brain's energy requirement.[29,65] The switch to using ketone bodies for energy in the brain is believed to be controlled by the concentration of ketone bodies in the blood rather than being a direct hormonal effect on the brain.[24] Metabolic changes during a long-term (e.g., a 30-day) fast are depicted in Figure 87-13.

With increasing duration of the fast and depletion of muscle and liver glycogen, ketones and glucose derived from gluconeogenesis from amino acid carbon skeletons contribute to energy requirements of the brain. As starvation is prolonged and ketone bodies become the predominant fuel, less and less glucose is used, thereby reducing the amount of protein that must be catabolized to support gluconeogenesis. Blood levels of BCAAs (leucine, isoleucine, valine), which are preferred amino acid substrates for muscle energy metabolism, double by 3 to 5 days of fasting but fall during prolonged fasting. These BCAAs are believed to augment gluconeogenesis until fat metabolism has adapted to fasting.[24] The amino acid glutamine has special importance during fasting. It assumes the roles of energy source as a precursor of glucose and as a transporter of amino acid nitrogen in the form of ammonia (NH_3) from tissues to the kidneys for excretion. Urea is the major nitrogen excretory product in the urine during the fed state, but it becomes much reduced as the

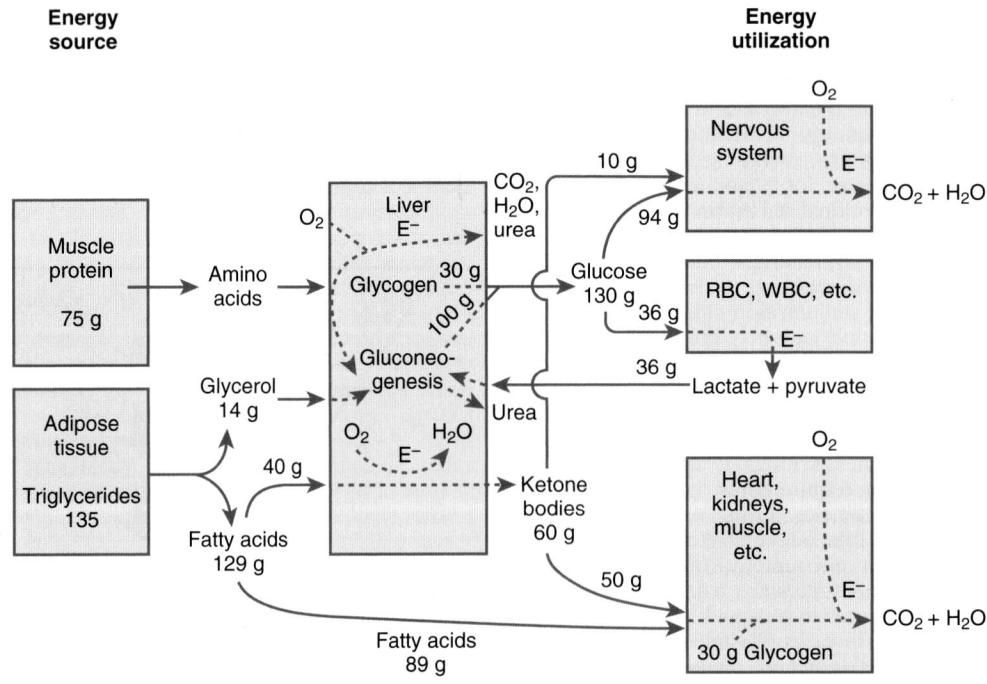

FIGURE 87-12 Fuel utilization in short-term starvation. Metabolic rates in grams per day after a 24-hour fast. Energy expenditure, 1800 kcal/day (7.53 MJ/day); respiratory quotient, 0.76. E^-, Oxidative formation of energy (ATP). *(Original data from Cahill GF Jr: Starvation in man, N Engl J Med 282:668, 1970. Algorithm redrawn from Bursztein S, Elwyn DH, Askanazi J, Kinney JM: Energy metabolism, indirect calorimetry, and nutrition, Baltimore, 1989, Lippincott Williams & Wilkins.)*

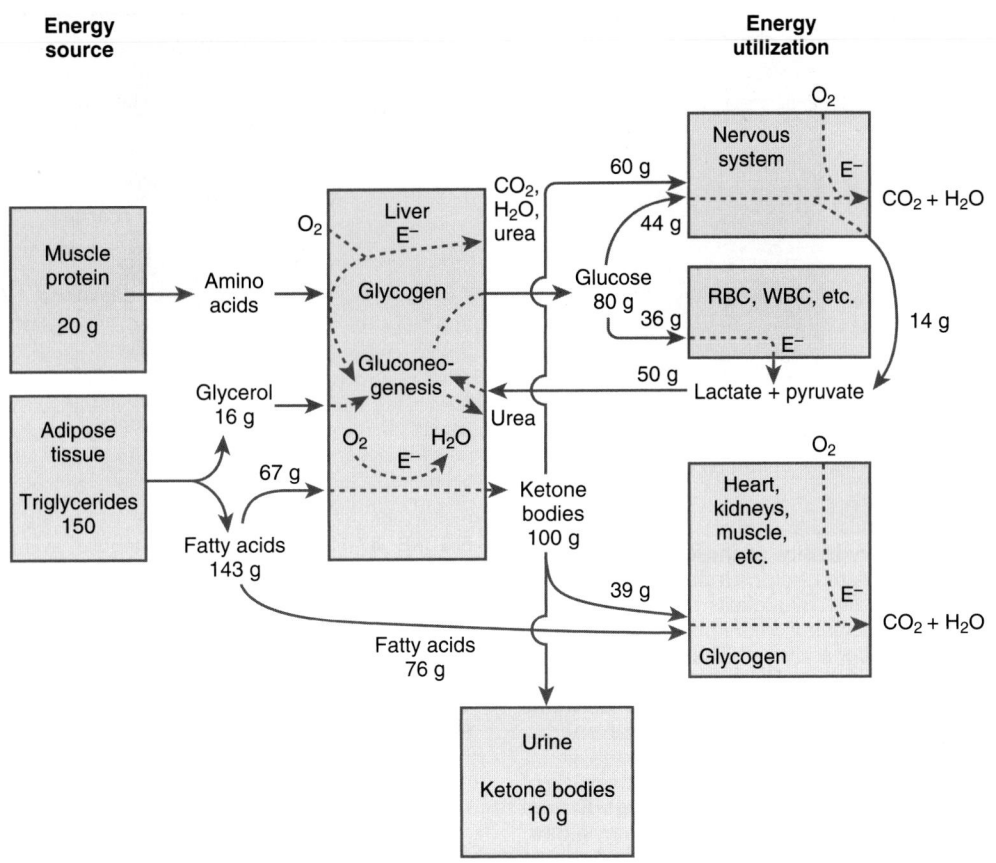

FIGURE 87-13 Fuel utilization in long-term starvation. Metabolic rates in grams per day after a prolonged fast of 5 to 6 weeks. Energy expenditure, 1450 kcal/day (6.07 MJ/day); respiratory quotient, 0.74. E^-, Oxidative formation of energy (ATP). *(Original data from Cahill GF Jr: Starvation in man, N Engl J Med 282:668, 1970. Algorithm redrawn from Bursztein S, Elwyn DH, Askanazi J, Kinney JM: Energy metabolism, indirect calorimetry, and nutrition, Baltimore, 1989, Lippincott Williams & Wilkins.)*

fast progresses and ammonia nitrogen increases. The increase in ammonia nitrogen serves to buffer ketoacids during their excretion via the urine, as well provides an excretory route for nitrogen. Glutamine is released from muscle during fasting (NH_3 formed from amino acid deamination by muscle is subsequently transaminated to glutamate to form glutamine) and serves as both a special energy source for the gut and a gluconeogenic substrate for the kidney. With increasing ketone body production, the liver reduces its rate of gluconeogenesis, and the kidney becomes the major organ of gluconeogenesis, producing more than one-half the body's glucose requirement.[24] Glutamine is the predominant substrate for kidney gluconeogenesis and provides the NH_3 required to buffer ketoacid excretion produced by ketogenesis from fat oxidation.[24]

Fortunately, muscle proteolysis does not continue at the typically high initial rate of negative nitrogen balances (10 to 12 g/day during the first 7 to 10 days of fasting). After 7 to 10 days of fasting, adaptation in the nitrogen economy of the body reduces nitrogen loss in the urine to less than one-half the initial rate.[65] Although the signal that causes muscle to reduce its catabolic rate is not well understood, it is probably related to the shift to ketone body utilization in the brain and to fatty acid oxidation in muscle during this same period. When adaptation to food restriction is not successful or food restriction is too severe, nitrogen can be lost from both central (visceral) and peripheral (skeletal muscle) sites. Development of central protein deficiency can lead to anergy and hypoalbuminemia. Reduced plasma albumin lowers plasma oncotic pressure, which permits fluid to migrate out of the vessels into the extracellular space, resulting in edema of the extremities. Edema is not present in all cases of starvation, but the presence of edema indicates severe metabolic stress and central protein deficiency and is a potentially dangerous condition.[65]

The net result of short- and long-term metabolic adaptations in energy restriction is increased efficiency of the body's metabolism. When body weight decreases 8% to 10% over a 14-day period, basal metabolic rate (BMR) can decrease about 21%. This short-term decrease in BMR is greater than would be predicted if it were caused solely by the loss of metabolically active lean tissue mass. Reduction in BMR during energy restriction occurs in two different phases.[24] Initially, there is decrease in BMR not attributable to changes in body weight or body composition. This is presumably an attempt by the body to conserve energy by increasing its metabolic efficiency despite reduced energy intake. Then, with continued energy restriction, BMR decreases further because of loss of metabolically active tissue. Several physiologic mechanisms operate to downregulate metabolic activity in the active tissue mass and to increase its metabolic efficiency. The decreased energy flux reduces activity of the sympathetic nervous system and lowers secretion and activity of three thermogenic hormones: catecholamines, T_3 (triiodothyronine), and insulin. Other energy-requiring activities, such as the sodium-potassium pump and futile metabolic cycling (e.g., phosphorylating and dephosphorylating metabolic intermediates), may also be reduced during starvation, further conserving energy.

HIERARCHY OF TISSUE UTILIZATION DURING STARVATION

There is a hierarchy of fuel source utilization during starvation. During an extended period of fasting, the mass of muscle and adipose tissue is more likely to be reduced than that of the viscera.[131] Important internal organs, such as the liver, show no evidence of dysfunction after 7 days of fasting,[126] whereas muscle cell mass decreases linearly with severity and duration of a fast.[131] Adipose mass decreases along with muscle, but not as rapidly

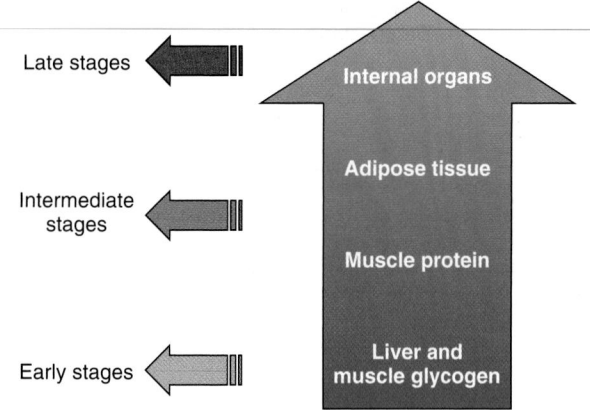

FIGURE 87-14 Energy sources during progressive stages of starvation. Note the hierarchy of the progression of utilization of energy sources.

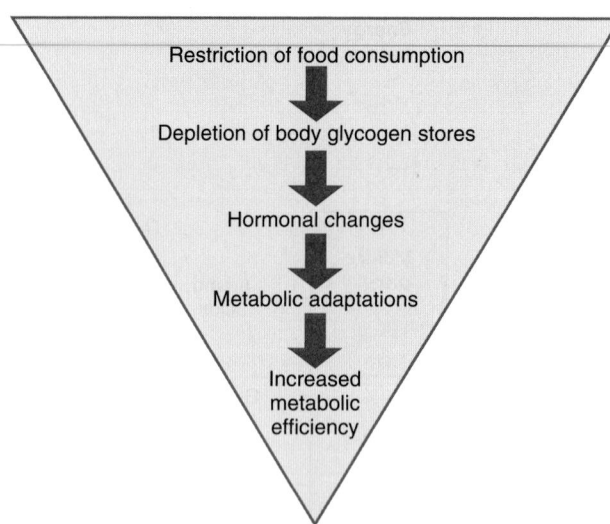

FIGURE 87-15 Sequence of metabolic events during short-term energy restriction or starvation. In the short term, metabolic efficiency increases to compensate for an energy deficit.

initially, because of the caloric density of the energy of the fat depot and low amount of associated water. Hoffer[66] has estimated that during a typical 3-week fast that elicits a weight loss of 350 g/day, the shed tissues are composed of approximately 125 g of lean tissue and 200 g of adipose tissue. The body defends a certain amount of body fat as essential for nerve sheath insulation, brain neurolipids, cell membrane integrity, and hormone synthesis. Figure 87-14 shows the general hierarchy of energy-source utilization during progressive starvation.

The largest energy reserves are found in the largest organs of the body: muscle (~28 kg) and adipose tissue (~15 kg). Critical internal organs, such as the liver, brain, heart, and kidneys, have a collective mass of less than 9 kg and are not good fuel-source candidates, because they begin to lose critical functions when they become energy sources during starvation (decompensation). Table 87-5 shows the body reserves that can be drawn on for energy during fasting for a sedentary 70-kg (154-lb) man.

SEQUENCE OF EVENTS DURING STARVATION

Sex hormone synthesis is depressed during extended periods of food restriction,[51,52] because reproduction is not a high priority during starvation. As the fast progresses, eventually even visceral organs begin to be used for energy as the body decompensates or "feeds on itself." During a prolonged fast, the body initially undergoes the series of events depicted in Figure 87-15.[24] The initial steps are similar to those of short-term energy deficiency (see Figure 87-10), but if starvation continues, metabolic adaptations ultimately fail, leading to a grim conclusion: the body has expended its reserves and enters the decomposition, or final stage, of metabolic self-destruction. Organ failure and death are the ultimate outcomes of starvation unless nutritional intervention occurs before decompensation (internal organ catabolism, loss of integration of function of bodily systems, and deterioration of homeostasis).

THE LIMITS OF HUMAN STARVATION AND FACTORS INFLUENCING SURVIVAL

There were horrific changes in my body. My buttocks were bones jutting against skin. I could no longer warm my hands by nestling them between my thighs. Now I could push a clenched fist between my legs without touching either thigh. I continually felt nauseated. The nausea became so severe I retched uncontrollably. This went on night after night. Death was closing in. My body was conceding defeat.

James Scott's observations near the end of a 43-day period of starvation while lost in the Himalayas[129]

Loss of Fat and Lean Body Mass

The body fat of humans can be considered beneficial when viewed in the context of surviving starvation.[87] A decreasing level of body fat approaching 6% loss is a harbinger of impending lean body mass deterioration in the fasting individual.[3,87] Essential fat stores (in bone marrow, heart, lungs, liver, kidneys, intestine, muscle, cell membranes, and central nervous system) are necessary for maintenance of life and prevention of decompensation. Essential fat stores constitute 3% to 4% of body weight.[109] Total body fat depletion in previously nonobese individuals occurs at approximately 50% body weight loss. In fasting uncomplicated by disease, the time until death is largely determined by the size of fat stores and the time to reach the 3% level of essential fat. Fat stores protect function.[109] Low fat stores per se are not the cause of death, but their diminution contributes to breakdown of homeostasis and impairment of physiologic function. Typical fat stores in humans vary but are typically between 10 and 15 kg (including 2.1 kg of essential fat), or approximately 27% of body weight. A well-nourished adult has sufficient fat energy stores to sustain life for 60 to 70 days. Death has been reported sooner in voluntary hunger strikers and may be related to simultaneous fluid restriction and lack of the will to live. A loss of greater than 50% of the lean body mass is also predictive of death. From a practical standpoint, the remaining body fat and protein reserves in a starving individual are difficult to measure accurately. A more practical measurement is the body mass index (BMI), calculated as body weight (kg)/height^2 (m^2). BMI is easy to obtain and a convenient method to assess risk of mortality in severely starved individuals. Before the war and famine in Somalia, the lowest BMI compatible with life was thought to be 13 in males and 11 in females.[63] Collins[37] collected data at Baidoa, Somalia in 1992 at the Concern Worldwide Adult Therapeutic Centre, where many victims of starvation were treated. He found that a BMI of 10

TABLE 87-5 Utilizable Energy Stores in a Sedentary 70-kg (154-lb) Man

Energy Source	Mass (kg)	Energy (kJ)
Fat	15	590
Protein (muscle)	6	100
Glycogen (muscle)	0.15	2.51
Glycogen (liver)	0.075	1.25
Plasma glucose	0.020	0.33
Plasma free fatty acids	0.0003	0.012
Plasma triglycerides	0.003	0.125

Data from Cahill GF Jr: Starvation in man, *N Engl J Med* 282:668, 1970.

TABLE 87-6 Demographics and Mortality Rates in the Donner Party, 1846-1847

	Frequency: N (%)	Mortality Rate: n/N (%)
Total party	90 (100)	42/90 (47)
Age (yr)		
<5	19 (21)	11/19 (58)
6-14	21 (23)	2/21 (10)
15-34	34 (38)	16/34 (47)
>35	14 (16)	11/14 (79)
Gender		
Male	55 (61)	32/55 (58)
Female	35 (39)	10/35 (29)

Data from McCurdy SA: Epidemiology of disaster: The Donner party, *West J Med* 160:338, 1994.

could be compatible with life under conditions of specialized hospital care, possibly explained by somatotype and the warm climate. However, other races in colder climates may face death before reaching the low BMI level noted in Somalia.[37]

Age and Gender Differences in Survival From Starvation

Persons possessing the most limited body reserves, such as older adults and very young children, are at increased risk for early mortality during extended periods of starvation. Children have increased nutrient requirements for growth and develop deficiency symptoms rapidly when faced with severe food restriction.

Starving women have not been studied in the same controlled manner as men. However, observational evidence of unintentional situational starvation involving both men and women seems to indicate that women may possess certain metabolic or cultural advantages over men, which may lead to a reduced incidence of mortality from severe starvation. Such evidence comes from wartime and famine, when there has been disproportionate survival of women over men.[50,109] Although situational circumstances have been suggested to account for these differences, studies of the Mormon handcart trek[20] and the Donner party[143] support the conclusion that women are at lower risk for mortality under nutritionally stressful situations. McCurdy[96] examined the mortality pattern in the Donner party, which became trapped with inadequate food supplies in the Sierra Nevada Mountains during the winter of 1846-1847. The demographic mortality data derived by McCurdy indicate that in general, very young children and males had the highest risk for mortality during starvation (Table 87-6).

The influence of gender on starvation may be attributable, at least in part, to certain metabolic advantages possessed by women, such as a higher initial level of body fat and subsequent reduced loss of protein and lean body mass during fasting. Lowell and Goodman[87] proposed that protein sparing in skeletal muscle during prolonged starvation depends on availability of lipid fuels that may provide energy and attenuate the rise in catabolic hormones during starvation. They also suggest that fatty acids may specifically modulate breakdown of myofibrillar protein, independent of their oxidation as a fuel, thus causing a direct muscle-sparing effect during prolonged starvation. Other factors may contribute. Women generally have lower body mass and less lean body mass to maintain than do men, as well as more subcutaneous fat, which may have insulation value during cold exposure. Gender-related cultural behavior, such as performance of strenuous and high-risk tasks (e.g., the men usually pulled the handcarts during the Mormon pioneer trek west from Missouri to Utah), may also play an important role.

FEEDING VICTIMS OF STARVATION

With modern sophisticated means of communication, highly trained search and rescue teams, and air evacuation resources, rescue of a lost or injured person in a wilderness environment usually is relatively rapid. One study reported that 50% of search and rescue missions were completed within 3 hours, 81% within 12 hours, and 93% within 24 hours.[79] Whereas the rescue of the starving Donner party from the Sierra Mountains in 1847 took 4 months,[96] evacuation of the nutritionally depleted Mike Stroud and Ranulph Fiennes from Antarctica in 1993 took 1 day.[144] Although Stroud and Fiennes voluntarily prolonged their period of starvation before requesting evacuation, most individuals do not have to spend more than a weekend, or at most a few days longer than anticipated, in uncomfortable circumstances. Some food likely will be available to the stranded person because most people do not enter the wilderness totally unprepared. The individual may have consumed the initial food supply and then fasted for several days before rescue or, if disciplined, may have restricted or rationed food intake for several days. Helicopter evacuation can place the rescued individual in a hospital within hours of rescue. The worst-case scenario might be the rescue of a severely injured or ill person who could not or would not eat for an extended period and could not be evacuated by helicopter.

Refeeding victims of short-term starvation is less complicated and dangerous than refeeding victims of prolonged starvation (e.g., James Scott, who was stranded in the Himalayas for 43 days without food[129]). Victims of prolonged starvation subsisting in a catabolic state have dramatically altered blood mineral and protein levels, which can be rapidly perturbed by refeeding large quantities of a normal mixed diet. The flood of nutrients with osmotic properties can lead to dangerous fluid compartment shifts. Among the numerous complications, cardiovascular and pulmonary overload caused by a rapid increase in plasma volume after fluid and nutrient ingestion can result in pulmonary edema and multisystem organ failure. The most common cause of death from refeeding is cardiac arrhythmias.[27]

The specific physiologic and metabolic effects induced by refeeding (the refeeding syndrome; Table 87-7) depend on the individual's existing metabolic state and body composition, as well as the composition of the refeeding diet.[65] Because the refeeding syndrome typically is not recognized, the National Institute for Health and Clinical Excellence (NICE) developed guidelines for identifying high-risk patients[105] (Box 87-3). Refeeding syndrome must be avoided in severely wasted individuals, particularly during the first week of nutritional repletion.[66] Hypophosphatemia, the predominant perturbation of refeeding syndrome, can occur within a few hours of reintroducing food, particularly carbohydrate, to a starved person. In addition, hyponatremia, hypocalcemia, hypomagnesemia, severe anemia, and impaired membrane and cardiovascular function are all possible complications.[27] The priority for re-alimentation of individuals lost in the wilderness for an extended time at risk of refeeding syndrome is first to correct fluid and electrolyte imbalance and to curtail ongoing protein catabolism. Ideally, electrolytes (particularly phosphorus, potassium, calcium, magnesium) would be assessed and normalized before refeeding and then monitored. However, this is an unlikely option in the wilderness setting. After assessing the risk for refeeding syndrome (see Box 87-3),

BOX 87-3 NICE Guidelines for Identification of Patients at High Risk of Refeeding Syndrome

The patient has one or more of the following:
- Body mass index (kg/m²) <16
- Unintentional weight loss >15% in the past 3-6 months
- Little or no nutritional intake for >10 days
- Low levels of potassium, phosphate, or magnesium before feeding

Or the patient has two or more of the following:
- Body mass index <16
- Unintentional weight loss >10% in the past 3-6 months
- Little or no nutritional intake for > days
- History of alcohol misuse or drugs, including insulin, chemotherapy, antacids, or diuretics

From National Institute for Health and Clinical Excellence (NICE): Nutrition support in adults: Clinical guidelines CG32, 2006. www.nice.org.uk/page .aspx?o=32.

TABLE 87-7 Suggested Refeeding Strategy for Individuals at Risk for Refeeding Syndrome

Day	Calorie Intake	Supplements
1	10 kcal/kg/day (5 kcal/kg/day for extreme cases: BMI 14 or no food for 15 days) Carbohydrate: 50%-60% Fat: 30%-40% Protein: 15%-20%	Prophylactic supplement: PO_4^{2-}: 0.5-0.8 mmol/kg/day K^+: 1-3 mmol/kg/day Mg^{2+}: 0.3-0.4 mmol/kg/day Na^+: 1 mmol/kg/day (restricted) IV fluids restricted (maintain zero balance) Oral or IV thiamine: 300 mg 30 minutes before feeding; maintenance dose: 100 mg/day during feeding
2-4	Increase by 5 kcal/kg/day. If low or no tolerance, stop or keep minimal feeding regimen.	Monitor vital signs, ECG, electrolytes, glucose, prealbumin, body weight, urine output. Administer thiamine + B complex orally or IV until day 3.
5-7	20-30 kcal/kg/day	Monitor as above. Maintain zero fluid balance. Consider iron supplement from day 7.
8-10	30 kcal/kg/day, or increase to full requirement.	Monitor as above.

Compiled from Boateng AA, Sriram K, Meguid MM, Crook M: Refeeding syndrome: Treatment considerations based on collective analysis of literature case reports, *Nutrition* 26:156-167, 2010; and Khan LUR, Ahmed J, Khan S, MacFie J: Refeeding syndrome: A literature review, *Gastroenterol Res Pract* 2011:1-7.
BMI, Body mass index; *ECG*, electrocardiogram; *IV*, intravenous(ly).

the rescuer should administer 200 to 300 mg of oral or intravenous (IV) thiamine (B_1) before feeding the victim any food. Some rescue workers carry this vitamin with them. If unavailable, a multivitamin may suffice, although the thiamine dose would most likely be lower than the recommended refeeding prophylactic dose. Food should not be introduced at a rate greater than 10 kcal/kg/day, and for the critically malnourished victim, no more than 5 kcal/kg/day. The NICE guidelines recommend that refeeding begin at no greater than 50% of the victim's energy requirements if significant weight loss has occurred and if no food has been consumed in more than 5 days.[105]

Fortunately, most rescues happen quickly, and the rescuer need not be reluctant to offer normal food to most victims of short-term (3- to 5-day) starvation without significant weight loss. The most common problem may be that the individual wants to eat too much too soon. This problem is usually self-correcting. The individual may be very hungry, weak, and dehydrated. The victim should first be reassured and then checked for injuries, illness, and dehydration. Juices, soups, instant oatmeal, granola bars, and small pieces of jerky slowly chewed along with the fruit juice are all good choices to return the digestive system to processing food while simultaneously supplying fluid, sodium, potassium, protein, and carbohydrate. Frequent small feedings are best. Sports drinks (if available) are a good choice for simultaneous rehydration, because they provide carbohydrates for energy and electrolytes that may be needed for plasma volume expansion.

It is not uncommon to encounter waterborne or food-borne illness in a backcountry rescue scenario.[16] Rescued victims may be suffering from diarrheal disease as well as starvation. Oral rehydration solutions similar to those used to treat diarrheal disease can be used in wilderness rescue for extremely dehydrated individuals.[16] IV saline and dextrose may be needed for those unable to eat because of shock, injury, or vomiting. IV normal saline should be administered to maintain a "zero" fluid balance (fluid intake and output are equal), starting with 20 to 30 ml/kg and adjusting as necessary.[27] Caution should be used with IV dextrose administration in persons at risk for refeeding syndrome because of the increased risk of hyperglycemia. If in doubt, a lower concentration (10%) of IV dextrose solution should be given.[158] Table 87-8 shows the composition of the World Health Organization's oral rehydration solution.

It is important to ensure that the kidneys are capable of normal function. Fluids should continue to be offered until the victim is able to urinate every 2 to 3 hours, and then a more aggressive re-alimentation program can be followed. If the individual does not seem to be especially dehydrated and at low risk for refeeding syndrome, dilute fruit juices or sports drinks containing 5% to 10% carbohydrate and about 20 mEq (about 1.2 g) Na^{2+} per liter are reasonable rehydration fluids. Water is appropriate. Additional sodium can be provided by liberally salting the solid food offered. A simple rehydration solution can be made by adding 1 tsp of table salt and 8 tsp of sugar to 1 L of boiled water (http://rehydrate.org/solutions/homemade.htm). Sports drinks usually contain 10 to 25 mEq of Na^{2+} and 2 to 5 mEq K^+ per liter. Bouillon cubes are a good source of sodium and convenient to carry. One bouillon cube contains about 1000 mg of Na^{2+} (44 mEq). Although providing sodium to a moderately depleted individual is beneficial and desirable for restoring plasma volume, this should be approached much more cautiously in victims of prolonged and severe malnutrition, to avoid overly rapid expansion of plasma volume that could lead to congestive heart failure.[65] Bananas are excellent sources of K^{2+} (450 mg per banana), but because they are perishable, are seldom available to a rescue party. Dried banana chips are a good alternative (152 mg K^{2+}/oz), easily included in the rescue provisions.

Depending on the severity of malnutrition and risk of refeeding syndrome, after being corrected for hydration status and electrolyte balance, the victim should be placed on a moderate-protein, high-energy diet for an ideal weight gain of 2-3 pounds per week.[98] Although there is no consensus on the "best" re-alimentation diet, some diets are likely more appropriate than others for re-alimenting starvation victims.[65] For example, a diet high in sodium and carbohydrate fed to a severely malnourished individual may cause a rapid and large increase in extracellular volume, resulting in peripheral edema as well as fluid accumulation in the heart and lungs. A low-protein, high-energy diet may make sense initially, but if continued, may cause an increase in

TABLE 87-8 Composition of World Health Organization Oral Rehydration Solution*

Solution	Glucose (g/L)	NaCl (g/L)	KCl (g/L)	Trisodium Citrate† (g/L)	Osmolality
WHO oral rehydration	20.0	3.5	1.5	2.9	310

*Preparation information available at http://rehydrate.org/ors/the_salts_of_life.htm#ORS%20Formula (commercially available from Jianas Brothers Packaging Co, 2533 SW Blvd, Kansas City, MO 64108).
†If trisodium citrate is not available, 2.5 g of common baking soda can be substituted.[16]

fat mass without the desired increase in lean tissue mass. A high-protein diet may arrest nitrogen loss, but will not lead to simultaneous replenishment of fat stores. High-protein diets are also not appropriate (at least initially) for severely starved individuals encountered during relief work in famine-stricken areas. Collins and associates[38] reported decreased mortality and increased weight gain in malnourished, edematous adults in Somalia ingesting an 8.5% protein diet compared to the higher, 16.5% protein diet. Guidelines for patients recovering from anorexia nervosa that may also apply to malnourished rescue victims suggest an energy intake of less than twice an individual's basal energy expenditure (and less than 70 to 80 kcal/kg/day) and a protein intake of less than 1.5 to 1.7 g/kg/day, with a typical range of 1.0 to 1.5 g/kg/day.[98] As stated by Mehler and colleagues,[98] the best course of action when re-alimenting a starved victim is to "start low and advance slow."

NUTRITION PLANNING FOR WILDERNESS ACTIVITIES

PRACTICAL CONSIDERATIONS

Nutrition planning is an important aspect of wilderness logistics. One difficulty is that the amount of food carried is often constrained by the space it occupies and its weight. A daily food ration of 4000 kcal for men and 3500 kcal for women will adequately encompass most moderate- to high-energy expenditure situations. If it is known that the task will be hard physical work in the cold, 4000 to 6000 kcal/day may be needed. Generally, an energy allowance of 45 to 55 kcal/kg/day will cover energy needs for most moderate to moderately heavy levels of exertion (e.g., for a 70-kg individual [154-lb] anticipating moderate work levels, 50 kcal/kg/day × 70 kg body weight = 3500 kcal/day).[10] Table 87-9 lists some typical energy targets for food planning appropriate for temperate-weather backpacking activities.

These are only approximate guidelines because it is impossible to establish energy requirements that cover all genders, body sizes, workloads, and environments. More specific nutrient guidelines for food planning can be adapted from the U.S. military target nutrient content for operational rations, which can be viewed in its entirety at www.apd.army.mil/pdffiles/r40_25.pdf. Military field ration nutrient content has been established to meet the needs of a relatively young, active population and is applicable in most circumstances to nutritional support for many wilderness outdoor activities. The standards for daily ration content shown in Table 87-10 are based on current RDAs and can be used by wilderness planners to ensure a reasonably balanced and nutrient-adequate diet to support high levels of physical activity on any particular trek.

The macronutrient composition of food is usually less important than the total energy content, except when heavy efforts are required over short (2- to 3-day) periods, during which carbohydrate content may be the most important nutritional consideration. If a high level of performance (sustained or repeated high levels of power generation, such as working at greater than 60% $\dot{V}O_2$max for prolonged periods) is anticipated, carbohydrate should be emphasized over fat (see Table 87-1 for carbohydrate recommendations). If weight of the provisions is an overriding consideration, maximal caloric density may be important, and fat

TABLE 87-9 Daily Calorie (kcal) Guidelines for Hikers*

| Body Weight (lb/kg) | Backpacking | | |
	Light Hiking	Light	Heavy
100-120/45-59	2000	2500	3500
130-150/59-68	2500	3000	4000
160-180/73-82	3000	3500	4500
190-200/86-91	3500	4000	5000

*Modify according to work level and prior experience.

TABLE 87-10 Nutritional Planning Guide for Field Rations

Nutrient	Unit of Measure*	Daily Ration
Macronutrients		
Energy	kcal	3600
Protein	g	91
Carbohydrate	g	494
Fat	g	140
Vitamins		
Vitamin A	mcg RE	1000
Vitamin D	mcg	5
Vitamin E	mg	15
Vitamin K	mcg	80
Vitamin C	mg	90
Thiamine (B$_1$)	mg	1.2
Riboflavin (B$_2$)	mg	1.3
Niacin	mg NE	16
Vitamin B$_6$	mg	1.3
Folic acid	mcg DFE	400
Vitamin B$_{12}$	mcg	2.4
Minerals		
Calcium	mg	1000
Phosphorus	mg	700
Magnesium	mg	420
Iron	mg	15
Zinc	mg	15
Sodium	mg	5000-7000
Potassium	mg	3200
Selenium	mcg	55

Based on reference dietary intakes for active military personnel (AR 40-25 Nutrition Standards and Education, Headquarters, Department of the Army, Washington, DC, 2001).
*Units: 1 mcg RE = 1 mcg retinol (3.33 IU) or 6 mcg (10 IU) β-carotene; 1 mcg cholecalciferol = 40 IU vitamin D; 1 mg vitamin E = 1 mg RRR-α-tocopherol; 1 mg NE = 1 mg niacin or 60 mg dietary tryptophan; 1 mcg DFE = 1 mcg food folate or 0.5 mcg synthetic folate.

may be emphasized over carbohydrate, particularly in cold environments. Lower levels of power generation (working at a slow and steady sustained rate at less than 50% $\dot{V}O_2$max) can usually be adequately supported by higher levels of dietary fat. Individuals who intend to subsist on diets containing greater than 50% of the energy from fat usually require a metabolic adaptation period of approximately 2 weeks to adjust to the higher level of dietary fat.[114,115] Most trail rations consisting of a typical mixed macronutrient content (50% carbohydrate, 35% fat, 15% protein) weigh approximately 1.4 to 2.7 kg (3 to 6 lb) (food for 1 day), depending on the degree of dehydration of the food. Thus, a 7-day backpacking trip may require 9.5 to 19 kg (21 to 42 lb) of food (excluding potable water). An acceptable level of protein content of the diet should provide 1.0 to 2.0 g/kg/day, depending on activity level (see Table 87-3 for protein recommendations). Protein beyond the required amount may be an inefficient source of energy, requiring more water for urea excretion as amino acids are deaminated, nitrogen is excreted as urea, and carbon skeletons are used for energy. The water burden of excess protein is not an overriding consideration if water is abundantly available, but is an important factor in arid environments.

Palatable and nutritious backpacking foods are available at most outdoor stores specializing in camping gear. Some thought (and label reading) must be put into selecting and combining these individual food items. A simple approach is to purchase packaged military food such as the meal, ready-to-eat (MRE), which contain a balanced macronutrient, vitamin, and mineral profile. A typical MRE packet supplies approximately 1250 kcal (13% protein, 36% fat, and 51% carbohydrate) and weighs about 0.6 kg (1.25 lb). MREs require no special handling or preservation and can be eaten cold or hot; their shelf life is 3 years at

80° F (27° C). Information about military rations can be found at www.dscp.dla.mil/subs/rations/rations_book.pdf. Further information regarding practical aspects of backcountry and expedition food planning can be found in the publications *NOLS Backcountry Nutrition*[126] and *Nutritional Support for Expeditions.*[13]

FOOD BARS

Some outdoor minimalists choose to ignore nutritional planning and travel with their favorite, easily consumed snack foods. This haphazard approach to nutrient requirements may work for a time but could dispose the individual to potentially important nutrient deficiencies over time or at the very least to palate fatigue. Commercial food (sports) bars are generally a better choice than candy bars and other junk food items, because they are usually nutrient fortified and less prone to melting in the pack.

Food bars might be considered the modern equivalent of the early explorer's pemmican (dried meat pulverized with fat and sometimes berries). Food bars are not as energy dense as pemmican but are certainly more palatable and nutritious. Food manufacturers have combined the camper's old standby of candy bars and trail mix into conveniently packaged and easily carried bars that usually have a good nutrient profile and may be fortified with selected vitamins, minerals, and protein. Most commercial food bars designed for sports nutrition or meal replacement are suitable for wilderness activities, although the low-carbohydrate bars may not be an appropriate choice. For unanticipated wilderness rescue operations, food bars are a good no-preparation, eat-on-the-move energy source for both rescuers and the rescued. Some companies target outdoor activities in their marketing, but the composition of their products is similar to that of others, so their claims may not be meaningful. The main considerations in food bar selection should be stability in the pack or pocket, palatability, and protein and carbohydrate content. If they are fortified with vitamins and minerals, food bars can supplement other foods. The advantages of food bars as nutrition supplements are that they consume little pack space, are a quick energy source, and are convenient when no time is available for a meal on the trail or severe weather precludes food preparation.

Most food bars contain significant amounts of carbohydrate, protein, and fat (Table 87-11). A bar containing 45 g of carbohydrate, 9 g of protein, and 4 g of fat provides approximately 240 kcal of energy. Most are rather low in fat, because they are aimed at replenishing glucose and glycogen supplies during and after sports performance. The food bar market is very competitive, so some manufacturers include "unique" nutrients or herbal compounds to appeal to the buyer. The nutritional merit of some of these additions is questionable. Additions include vitamins, minerals, and other potentially beneficial nutrients such as phytochemicals (antioxidant nutrients); medium-chain triglycerides (as an alternate energy source); branched-chain amino acids (as fuel for muscle); soy protein (an anticancer agent); ginseng (to combat stress); ginkgo biloba (to improve circulation); and choline (to improve concentration).

Selecting Food Bars

A typical energy or nutrition bar weighs about 60 g and contains 40 to 45 g of carbohydrate, 10 to 15 g of protein, and about 5 g of fat. Food bars are not dehydrated but usually have low water content, approximately 25% water by weight. Check labels for calorie and nutrient content, because these vary.

Food bars claiming to be "energy bars" tend to have more carbohydrates, whereas "low-carb" and diet bars contain fewer carbohydrates. This reduced calorie claim is usually based on net carbohydrate content, such as fiber and sugar alcohols, which may not contain caloric value. Generally, these carbohydrates do not provide as much energy as do normal food carbohydrates, and they elicit a smaller insulin response. Sugar alcohols (i.e., polyols, such as maltitol and lactitol) that impart a sweet taste are technically carbohydrates and are common in low-carbohydrate bars because, compared with sugars such as glucose, they have fewer calories and less impact on blood sugar

TABLE 87-11 Food Bar Standards for Wilderness Activities

	Amount	Comments
Nutritional Content		
Carbohydrate	40-50 g/bar	To replenish glycogen stores
Fiber	3-5 g/bar	To prevent constipation
Protein	10-25 g/bar	High-quality protein such as casein or soy may be useful in emergencies when other protein sources are not available.
Fat	Variable	Usually not critical; higher-fat bars are more calorie dense.
Vitamins	Approximately 30% RDA	Not normally needed, but can provide insurance; antioxidant vitamins E and C are most important.
Minerals	Approximately 30% RDA	Ca^{2+}, Mg^{2+}, and Zn^{2+} are the most important, although women may benefit from supplemental Fe^{2+}, especially at altitude.
Other		
Stability	—	Low melting point in heat is determined by trial and error.
Palatability	—	Provide variety to avoid taste fatigue and increase food intake.

RDA, Recommended dietary allowance.

and insulin levels. These elements of low-carb dieting do not necessarily support high-level performance on a backpacking trip. Unlike other sugars, sugar alcohols are digested primarily in the large intestine by bacterial fermentation and, consequently, may promote gas or have a laxative effect, not a desirable attribute on the trail or in the tent. If the wrapper of a bar states that net carbohydrates are only 2 g but the Nutrition Facts panel shows 20 g of carbohydrates, there are 18 g of sugar alcohols, glycerin, or fiber in the bar. High-protein bars are designed to be higher in protein. Look at the label for protein sources. High-quality casein, whey, egg, and soy protein are desirable "boosters" of the natural protein content of the basic ingredients in a food bar. Meal-replacement bars have a balance of carbohydrates, proteins, and fats similar to that of a typical mixed meal. Before hitting the trail, be sure to taste-test food bars. Some are more palatable than others.

Typically, food bars may have the vitamins and minerals or other ingredients found in a dietary supplement. Nutrition bars can provide many nutrients needed on a daily basis and may be eaten as an energy boost or a vitamin/mineral supplement, but are not recommended as a total substitute for food except in certain situations, such as a rainy day on the trail or a late camp. They are best eaten as a quick-energy snack along the trail. If fortified with the vitamins and minerals found in a multivitamin pill, food bars can also be considered a multivitamin supplement. However, it is advisable to keep track of the amounts of nutrients being ingested from the bars in addition to the amounts from other foods and supplements, to avoid exceeding recommended upper limits. Some products contain ingredients a consumer may not want in a food bar. A product that claims to be a "dietary supplement," or that provides a Supplement Facts panel instead of a Nutrition Facts panel, may contain ingredients not normally expected in food. Supplementary ingredients are not necessarily undesirable, but consumers should be aware of vitamins, minerals, herbs, or other special ingredients. For example, some products include caffeine in the form of coffee extract, guarana, or green tea. Even cocoa and chocolate contain some caffeine. Caffeine may be desirable in some circumstances, but it can enhance the action and increase the side effects of other stimulants, such as bitter orange (*Citrus aurantium*). An independent evaluation of the nutritional properties of many current commercially available food bars can be found at https://www.consumerlab.com/reviews/High_Protein_Bars_Low-Carb_Diet_Bars_Energy_Bars_and_Meal-Replacement_Bars/Nutrition Bars/ (subscription required for full report).

EMERGENCY FOOD SUPPLIES

Emergency food supplies of 250 to 350 kcal per person per day should be included in addition to the calculated caloric needs. These should be packed or carried separately from the main food items in case the main food supply is lost or destroyed. A stash of individually packaged food bars, jerky, dehydrated soup mixes, and hard candy provides an energy buffer that is reassuring even if it is not used. A bottle of multivitamins, extra salt packets, and water disinfection supplies are also advised. These small items may not seem important at the time of preparation, but that perception changes rapidly in an emergency. Finally, the most carefully planned food supply does little good unless it is eaten. Include foods that are palatable and comforting to the traveler. Do not overlook the morale-boosting aspects of a hot meal prepared on the trail.

REFERENCES

Complete references used in this text are available online at expertconsult.inkling.com.

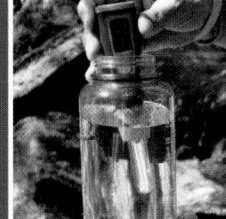

CHAPTER 88
Field Water Disinfection

HOWARD D. BACKER

Waterborne disease is a risk for international travelers who visit countries that have poor hygiene and inadequate sanitation and for wilderness users or travelers drinking surface water in any country, including the United States. Natural water may be contaminated with organic or inorganic material from land erosion, dissolution of minerals, decay of organic vegetation, biologic organisms that reside in soil and water, industrial chemical pollutants, and microorganisms from animal or human biologic waste.[71,118] The main reason for treating drinking water is to prevent gastrointestinal illness from fecal pollution with enteric pathogens.[309] Appearance, odor, and taste are not reliable to estimate water safety. Natural organic and inorganic material may not cause illness but can impart unpleasant turbidity, color, and taste to the water (Box 88-1).

Of the 1700 million square miles of water on Earth, less than 0.5% is potable.[336] Global warming is accelerating deterioration of the remaining potable supplies,[184] and emerging waterborne pathogens create the need to reevaluate detection and disinfection methods.[227,309,345] Chemical contamination of groundwater is increasing at an alarming rate in the United States and worldwide from industrial, agricultural, and individual sources. Except for certain pristine alpine or other remote water sources, virtually none of the surface water in the United States is drinkable without treatment.[184] According to the *National Water Quality Inventory Report* by the U.S. Environmental Protection Agency (EPA), as of 2004, bacterial contamination was the leading cause of river and stream impairment; mercury contamination was the leading cause of impairment in lakes, ponds, and reservoirs. Overall, about 40% of surveyed U.S. rivers, lakes, and estuaries are too polluted for basic uses such as fishing and swimming.[2] Disasters, such as floods and hurricanes, often overwhelm treatment facilities and contaminate groundwater, requiring point-of-use disinfection.[286] The World Health Organization (WHO) reports that 780 million people still lack access to an improved drinking water supply, and 2.4 billion people lack access to improved sanitation.[227,338]

BENEFITS OF WATER TREATMENT

Methods for treating water are found in Sanskrit medical lore, and pictures of apparatus used to purify water appear on Egyptian walls from the 15th century BC. Boiling and filtration through porous vessels, sand, and gravel have been known for thousands of years. The Greeks and Romans also understood the importance of pure water.[214] Sanitation, including water treatment, is considered one of the 10 great public health achievements that helped conquer infectious disease as a main cause of mortality in the United States.[48] As the percentage of the U.S. urban population served by water treatment utilities increased after 1900, the annual death rate from typhoid fever decreased.[284]

Drinking-water treatment processes provide enormous benefits with minimal risk. Without filtration and disinfection, waterborne disease would spread rapidly in most public water systems served by surface water.[79,322] The combined roles of safe water, hygiene, and adequate sanitation in reducing diarrhea and other diseases are clear and well documented. WHO estimates that 94% of diarrheal cases globally are preventable through modifications to the environment, including access to safe water.[346] Recent studies of simple water interventions in households of developing countries clearly document improved microbiologic quality of water, 30% to 60% reduced incidence of diarrheal illness, enhanced childhood survival, and reduction of parasitic diseases; much of this progress is independent of other measures to improve sanitation.* Several excellent evidence-based reviews analyze the recent large body of work in this area.[22,68,227]

From a global health perspective, water and sanitation improvements are cost-beneficial in all developing regions in the world.[132,150] Although the combination of improved water quality and sanitation has the greatest effect, improvement in water quality alone has a beneficial effect on health and can reduce incidence of diarrheal disease by more than one-third.[68,69,297,298]

In contrast to extensive evidence from developing areas of the world, there are few data to demonstrate benefits of water disinfection in the U.S. wilderness. Boulware[31] demonstrated that drinking untreated water correlated with higher rates of diarrhea among Appalachian Trail hikers.

---

*References 10, 68, 82, 105, 109, 149, 191, 192, 212, 250, 251, 259, 260, 297, 298.

BOX 88-1 Chapter Outline and Shortcuts

- For summary of each technique, see boxes in specific sections.
- For comparison of various techniques, see text and Tables 88-16 to 88-18.
- For details of products, see the appendices.

Methods of Water Disinfection That Can Be Applied in the Field	Page
Heat	1992
Physical removal	1994
Sedimentation	1994
Coagulation-flocculation	1994
Granular activated carbon	1995
Filtration	1995
Reverse osmosis	1997
Chemical disinfectants	1998
Chlorine	2002
Iodine	2003
Mixed species (electrolysis)	2007
Chlorine dioxide	2007
Hydrogen peroxide	2007
Potassium permanganate	2007
Citrus	2008
Silver	2008
Copper-zinc	2008
Nanoparticles (TiO_2)	2008
Ultraviolet light and solar	2009

RISK OF WATERBORNE DISEASE TRANSMISSION

The long list of pathogenic microorganisms capable of waterborne transmission is similar to that of potential etiologic agents of traveler's diarrhea (see Chapter 82); almost all enteric pathogens and opportunistic pathogens that are transmissible by the fecal-oral route can be transmitted through water (Box 88-2). Separating the contribution of waterborne transmission of these pathogens from food-borne and person-to-person transmission is impossible; the latter two are probably more common. In developing countries, 15% to 20% of diarrhea is estimated to be waterborne. Surprisingly, this is similar in developed countries, where as much as 15% to 30% is attributed to municipal drinking water.[113,309]

Risk for waterborne illness depends on the number of organisms consumed, which is determined by the volume of water, concentration of organisms, and treatment system efficiency.[38,77,148] Additional factors include virulence of the organism and defenses of the host (Table 88-1). Infection and illness are not synonymous; the overall likelihood of illness for all three categories of microorganisms (bacterial, viral, protozoan) is 50% to 60%. Death from enteric pathogens is unlikely in healthy, well-nourished persons, except with a few specific organisms (e.g., *Escherichia coli* O157:H7, *E. coli*: 0104:H4, or, in pregnant women, hepatitis E). In malnourished individuals, especially young children, many

TABLE 88-1 Estimated Infectious Dose of Enteric Organisms

Organism	Infectious Dose
Salmonella	10^5
Shigella	10^2
Vibrio	10^3
Enteric viruses	1-10
Giardia	10-100
Cryptosporidium	10-100

Data from Hurst C, Clark R, Regli S: Estimating the risk of acquiring infectious disease from ingestion of water. In Hurst C, editor: *Modeling disease transmission and its prevention by disinfection*, Melbourne, 1996, Cambridge University Press, pp. 99-139.

BOX 88-2 Waterborne Enteric Pathogens

Bacteria
Escherichia coli
Shigella
Campylobacter
Vibrio cholerae
Salmonella
Yersinia enterocolitica
Aeromonas

Viruses
Hepatitis A virus
Hepatitis E virus
Norovirus
Poliovirus
Miscellaneous viruses (>100 types; e.g., adenovirus, enterovirus, calicivirus, echovirus, astrovirus, coronavirus)

Protozoa
Giardia lamblia
Entamoeba histolytica
Cryptosporidium
Blastocystis hominis
Isospora belli
Balantidium coli
Acanthamoeba
Cyclospora

Parasites
Ascaris lumbricoides
Ancylostoma duodenale (hookworm)
Taenia spp. (tapeworm)
Fasciola hepatica (sheep liver fluke)
Dracunculus medinensis
Strongyloides stercoralis (pinworm)
Trichuris trichiura (whipworm)
Clonorchis sinensis (Oriental liver fluke)
Paragonimus westermani (lung fluke)
Diphyllobothrium latum (fish tapeworm)
Echinococcus granulosus (hydatid disease)

Data from references 113, 118, 262, 284, and 319.

other pathogens, including *Vibrio cholerae* and *Cryptosporidium*, can lead to infectious causes of death. Total immunity does not develop for most enteric pathogens, and reinfection may occur.[148] Several nonenteric waterborne organisms have high case fatality rates. These include *Legionella* (respiratory) and *Acanthamoeba* (neurologic).

Waterborne outbreaks do not give a complete picture of the potential for waterborne illness. Most outbreaks of waterborne diseases are not identified because not enough people become ill, providing an insensitive mechanism for detecting water contamination. When an outbreak is identified, it is very difficult to prove conclusively that the source was waterborne. The supply may have been only transiently contaminated, water samples from the time of exposure are seldom available, some organisms are difficult to detect, and almost everyone has some exposure to water.[313,349]

The data on concentration of microorganisms in surface water show widely varying values, but the testing is insufficient for risk assessment and dose-response models. Instead, infectious dose data and statistical techniques have been used to devise models for determining risk.[148] These models cannot be applied unless the microbial content of water is known. Pathogenic microorganisms clearly exist in most raw source waters, especially in surface waters.[322] Most microbiologic testing is done on community water intake sources and sewage treatment effluent. Less information is available for more remote water sources.[78,274,343]

Improved detection techniques using enzyme immunoassay (EIA) and polymerase chain reaction (PCR) may give a much more accurate picture of the specific microbes and degree of water contamination.[309] Testing may not be representative, however, because excretion and loading of microbial contaminants are dynamic and change over time.

TABLE 88-2 Water and Spread of Disease

Type	Mechanism	Examples	Prevention
Waterborne	Fecal contamination of drinking water by infectious organisms	Typhoid fever, cholera, campylobacteriosis, giardiasis, hepatitis A	Sanitation and disinfection of water
Water-washed	Person-to-person fecal-oral spread via direct contact, food, and water (all these are also waterborne)	Shigellosis, amebiasis, ascariasis, eye (trachoma) and skin infections	Handwashing and personal hygiene
Water-based	Organism or agent that lives in water	Schistosomiasis, dracunculosis, parasitic worms	Prevention of exposure from bathing
Water-related	Spread by insects that breed in water or collecting water	Malaria, sleeping sickness, yellow fever, dengue	Insect protection and piped water

Data from Bradley D: Health aspects of water supplies in tropical countries. In Feachem R, McGarry M, Mara D, editors: *Water, wastes and health in hot climates,* New York, 1977, Wiley, p 3; and Steiner T, Thielman N, Guerrant R: Protozoal agents: What are the dangers for the public water supply? *Annu Rev Med* 48:329, 1997.

Surface water is subject to frequent, dramatic changes in microbial quality as a result of activities on a watershed. Storm water causes deterioration of source water quality by increasing suspended solids, organic materials, and microorganisms. Some of these contaminants are carried by rain from the atmosphere, but most come from ground runoff. In water sources downstream from towns or villages, storms may overload sewage facilities and cause them to discharge directly into the receiving water. Some organisms (e.g., *Legionella pneumophila, Vibrio cholerae*) exist as natural organisms in water.[301]

The source of fecal contamination in water may be either human or animal. Some bacterial pathogens (*Shigella, Salmonella typhi*) occur exclusively in human feces, whereas others (*Yersinia, Campylobacter,* nontyphoid *Salmonella*) may be present in wild or domestic animals. No enteric viruses excreted by animals have been shown to be pathogenic to humans.[256] Derlet and colleagues[94,95] found that wilderness water sources in the California Sierra Nevada with significant amounts of human or animal activity are more likely to be contaminated with bacteria.

DEVELOPING COUNTRIES

In tropical areas and developing countries, water has a complex relationship with spread of disease. Bradley[32] presents a useful classification (Table 88-2), and Steiner and associates[302] proposed adding the category "water carried" for infections resulting from accidental ingestion in recreational water. Globally, 88% of the 4 billion annual cases of diarrheal disease are attributed to unsafe water and inadequate sanitation and hygiene. About 2 million people, most children under 5 years of age, die annually from illnesses associated with unsafe drinking water or inadequate sanitation.[113,135,334,346] Other estimates put the disease burden from water-related diseases, sanitation, and hygiene at 4% of all deaths and 5.7% to 7% of the total disease burden occurring globally.[36,249]

Substantial progress has been made in the past 20 years toward the goal of safe drinking water and sanitation worldwide, particularly in Asia and Latin America. Two billion people gained access to improved water from 1990 to 2010, but 780 million (11%) still lack a safe water source. Also, access to improved sanitation increased from 49% to 63% of the global population, but 2.5 billion people still lack this public health infrastructure. Africa and Oceania are the regions with the greatest need for improvement. More than 750 million persons still practice open defecation, the largest number residing in India and Africa.[227,337]

In certain tropical countries, the influence of high-density population, rampant pollution, and absence of sanitation systems means that available raw water is virtually wastewater.[60] Only 30% of waste from India's cities is treated before disposal, the rest flowing into surface or ground waters. More than 800 million Indians lack a household water connection, relying on public taps, wells, or surface sources.[66] Contamination of tap water in many urban areas should be assumed because of antiquated and inadequately monitored disposal, disinfection, and distribution systems.[80] Recent studies of household point-of-use water treatment in developing countries and refugee camps provide evidence of extensive coliform contamination in these settings.[62,82,97,127,152,259] Rai and associates[252] found coliforms in almost 90% of 506 samples in Nepal, similar for tap, well, or natural tap water. Kravitz and colleagues[171] found that water in Lesotho villages was nonpotable because of bacteriologic contamination, whether taken from unimproved or improved sources. In Sierra Leone, more than 75% of stored water in the household had high levels of coliform contamination, even when initially drawn from an improved source.[70] Gil and associates[127] found coliforms in almost 50% of water samples in the highlands of Peru and diarrheagenic *E. coli* in 33%.[127]

Water from springs and wells and even commercial bottled water may be contaminated with pathogenic microorganisms.

UNITED STATES AND DEVELOPED COUNTRIES

Developed countries such as the United States still face substantial challenges to ensure potable water in households and to maintain quality of water sources.[113,184,284,309] Improved community water supplies are still responsible for some outbreaks of gastrointestinal (GI) illness. Based on studies comparing rates of diarrheal illness in households with and without effective water filters, Colford and associates[72-74] have estimated that 4 to 11 million cases of acute GI illness annually are attributable to public drinking water systems in the United States.

The etiology of waterborne disease outbreaks from treated drinking water is different from untreated sources, with more respiratory disease caused by *Legionella* and a mix of bacterial, virus, and protozoan pathogens resulting in gastroenteritis.[349] Waterborne pathogens account for most outbreaks of infectious diarrhea acquired in U.S. wilderness and recreation areas (Box 88-3).[79] In both public and surface water supplies, there has been

BOX 88-3 Enteric Pathogens in U.S. Wilderness or Recreational Water

Commonly Reported
Giardia
Cryptosporidium

Occasionally Reported With Firm Evidence for Waterborne
Campylobacter
Hepatitis A
Hepatitis E
Enterotoxigenic *Escherichia coli*
Escherichia coli O157:H7
Shigella
Enteric viruses (especially norovirus, enteric adenovirus)

Unusual Occurrences, Waterborne Suspected
Yersinia enterocolitica
Aeromonas hydrophila
Cyanobacteria (blue-green algae)

an increase in the number of outbreaks caused by protozoan pathogens. *Giardia* is one of the most common waterborne infections, but *Cryptosporidium* epidemics have been identified with increasing frequency.[79,134,136,273] Enteric bacteria are responsible for a relatively small but consistent proportion of waterborne outbreaks in the United States,[275] but less frequently than are protozoa. Bacteria linked to water ingestion include *Salmonella, Campylobacter, Shigella sonnei, Plesiomonas shigelloides,* and *E. coli* O157:H7.[46,47,50,349]

In recreational areas, a distinct seasonal variation is seen, with the majority of cases from recreational areas occurring during summer months.[79] This is probably a result of both increased contamination and increased number of persons at risk.

Risk for GI disease to wilderness users is determined primarily by indirect evidence based on surveys.[31,349] Derlet and colleagues[90-95] have performed extensive testing for bacterial contamination of wilderness waters in the California Sierra Nevada. Human pathogenic bacteria were uncommon, but other enteric bacteria as indicators of contamination were found and associated with animal grazing, pack animals, and high levels of human activity.

RECREATIONAL CONTACT

Inadvertent ingestion during recreational activities of water not intended for drinking is a risk for swimmers and white-water boaters. The microorganisms that cause infection are those that require only a small dose. Recreational water activities have resulted in giardiasis, cryptosporidiosis,[45,49,52,350] typhoid fever, salmonellosis, shigellosis, *E. coli* O157 infection,[107] viral gastroenteritis, and hepatitis A, as well as in wound infections, septicemia, and aspiration pneumonia from *Legionella*.[79] Between 2005 and 2006, a total of 78 outbreaks associated with recreational water were reported, involving 4412 persons and resulting in 116 hospitalizations and five deaths.[350] Most outbreaks occurred in treated water venues such as pools and water parks. Of these, the majority were caused by parasites, predominantly *Cryptosporidium*, and a only few by *Giardia*, reflecting *Cryptosporidium* resistance to chlorine disinfection.[52] Bacterial contamination in treated water sources (including hospitals and hotels) most often resulted in respiratory disease caused by *Legionella* rather than in GI illness. In untreated recreational water, most often lakes and ponds, bacteria (*Shigella* and *E. coli* O157:H7) and norovirus were much more common than protozoa. These were predominantly small, inland water bodies without external sources of contamination, suggesting swimmers were the source. At least one case of usually fatal neuroinvasive disease caused by *Naegleria fowleri* is reported each year from untreated recreational water.

SPECIFIC ETIOLOGIC AGENTS

Viruses

The infectious dose of enteric viruses is only a few infectious units in the most susceptible people.[200,333,343] The risk for infections from enteric viruses is estimated to be 10 to 10,000 times higher than bacteria at the same level of exposure.[309] Hepatitis A virus (HAV), norovirus, and rotavirus are the main viruses of concern for potable water supplies. Norovirus may be the most infectious of all enteric viruses.[308] Not surprisingly, norovirus was the most commonly identified enteric virus in waterborne outbreaks in Finland.[199] All serotypes of adenovirus (besides enteric alone) are excreted in feces, so contaminated water could be a source of exposure for any type, through ingestion, inhalation, or direct contact with the eyes. Outbreaks of adenovirus have been associated with drinking water and contact with recreational water, including swimming pools.[208] In addition to HAV, waterborne transmission of hepatitis E is suspected in outbreaks among travelers from Asia.[42,162,289] Many other viruses are capable and suspected of waterborne transmission, and more than 100 different virus types are known to be excreted in human feces.[124,274] The most frequent waterborne illness (acute infectious nonbacterial gastroenteritis of unknown etiology) in the United States may be caused by undetected viruses; estimates of

viral waterborne illness are 6.5 million cases annually.[79,113,200,293] Enteroviruses have been detected, even in finished water from sewage treatment plants, with measurable levels of free residual chlorine.[125]

All surface water supplies in the United States and Canada contain naturally occurring human enteroviruses.[336] Even remote surface lakes and streams tested in California showed disturbing levels of viral contamination.[124] Widespread enteric viral contamination was found at multiple sites in a popular recreational canyon in Arizona. Viruses included poliovirus, echovirus, coxsackievirus, rotavirus, and other unidentifiable viruses and exceeded the recommended state level for recreational water use in several areas. Virus levels correlated with human activity but not with excess levels of standard coliform indicators.[274] In 2002, a series of outbreaks involving more than 130 individuals was reported on 17 different Colorado River rafting trips. Laboratory evaluation of effluent from portable toilets found norovirus, which was also isolated from river water at Lee's Ferry. No specific risk factors were identified in individuals or trips, and it was concluded that risk was likely from the river water.[139] Outbreaks have continued to occur regularly in Grand Canyon river trips, many linked conclusively to norovirus.[158,195]

No evidence exists of human immunodeficiency virus (HIV) transmitted via a waterborne route, and no epidemiologic evidence exists of casual transmission by fomites or by any environmentally mediated mode.[266] There has never been a documented case of influenza virus infection associated with water exposure, although hygiene may be a factor in transmission. Free chlorine levels of 1 to 3 mg/L are adequate to disinfect avian, H1N1, or other influenza viruses.

Protozoa

Six protozoa that cause enteric disease and may be passed by waterborne transmission are *Giardia lamblia, Cryptosporidium parvum, Entamoeba histolytica, Cyclospora cayetanensis, Isospora belli,* and the microsporidia.[113,198] The first two are the most important for wilderness travelers. *Cryptosporidium* is an emerging enteric pathogen that has overtaken *Giardia* as the most common waterborne protozoa.[43,113,350] Many aspects of *Cryptosporidium* epidemiology and transmission appear similar to *Giardia*. Ten *G. lamblia* cysts may result in infection, and the infectious dose of *Cryptosporidium* is on the order of 10^2 oocysts.[99,261] Waterborne transmission of *E. histolytica* is common in developing countries. *Cyclospora* has been epidemiologically linked to waterborne transmission in the United States and Nepal, but the reservoir and host range are not known. Unlike *Giardia* and *Cryptosporidium*, *Cyclospora* is not infectious when passed in feces and requires up to 2 weeks in the laboratory to sporulate.[291] Surface water is a common environmental source for microsporidia; however, the route of infection is unknown. *Naegleria fowleri* is a waterborne protozoan that enters the body through the nasal epithelia during swimming in contaminated surface water and causes meningoencephalitis.

***Giardia* and *Cryptosporidium*.** *Giardia* cysts have been found as frequently in pristine water and protected sources as in unprotected waters.[137,153,267,275,276,299] Repeated sampling of "negative" sources invariably produced positive results.

A zoonosis with *Giardia* is known, with at least three different species; the extent of cross-species infection is not clear.[16,341] Many of the species apparently capable of passing *Giardia* cysts to humans, including dogs, cattle, ungulates (deer), and beaver, are present in wilderness areas. Forty percent of beavers in Colorado were infected and shedding 1×10^8 cysts per animal per day. All 386 muskrats found were infected. Up to 20% of cattle examined were infected.[137] Beaver have been implicated in multiple municipal outbreaks of giardiasis. Samples from Rocky Mountain National Park[175,215] and the California Sierra Nevada[299,304] show a direct correlation between numbers of cysts and levels of human use or beaver habitation. In Yukon, Canada, 13 of 61 scat samples from various wild animals yielded *Giardia* cysts.[269]

Even with a low infectious dose, environmental cyst recovery data indicate that the risk for ingesting an infectious dose of *Giardia* cysts is small.[352,353] However, the likely model that poses a risk to campers is pulse contamination—a brief period of high cyst concentration from fecal contamination. Beaver stool and human stool may contain 1×10^6 cysts/g. Stream contamination from a beaver has been calculated to reach 245 cysts/gallon.[153] This is consistent with outbreaks in recreational water caused by human contamination.[51,52,242] In this instance, small amounts of water may cause infection, similar to an outbreak among lap swimmers from inadvertent water ingestion in a fecally contaminated pool.

Cryptosporidium oocysts are found widespread in surface water, and the cyst is durable in the environment. A large zoonosis is evident. Environmental occurrence appears ubiquitous.[182,272,273] *Cryptosporidium* is now found more frequently than *Giardia* in surface water, although in smaller numbers; it is the most common contaminant in treated recreational water and has resulted in large outbreaks in municipal water systems.[41,87,134,194,350]

Parasitic Organisms

Parasitic organisms other than protozoa are seldom considered in discussions of disinfection. Infectious eggs or larvae of many helminths are found in sewage, even in the United States.[258,287] The frequency of infection by waterborne transmission is unknown, because food and environmental contamination or skin penetration is more prevalent.[344]

The most obvious risk is from nematodes, with no intermediate hosts, that are infectious immediately or soon after eggs are passed in stool. *Ascaris lumbricoides* (roundworm) is transmitted by ingestion of the eggs in contaminated food or drink. In endemic areas, 85% of the population is infected; this leads to daily global environmental contamination by 9×10^{14} eggs.[344] *Ancylostoma duodenale* (hookworm) usually infects as larvae penetrate the skin of the foot, but it also may be acquired by mouth. Oral entry of the larvae causes pulmonary (Wakana) disease. *Necator americanus* (hookworm) does not appear to be infectious by the oral route.

Taenia solium (pork tapeworm) is infectious to humans in cyst or egg form. Eggs passed in stool are ingested in food or water and develop into tissue cysts, often in the brain, resulting in cysticercosis.

Echinococcus granulosus (dog tapeworm) can use humans as intermediate hosts. Eggs from the feces of an infected dog or other carnivore are ingested in food and water. Hydatid disease generates cysts in the liver, peritoneum, and other sites.

Fasciola hepatica (liver fluke of herbivores and humans) is normally acquired by ingestion of encysted metacercariae on water plants or free organisms in water.

Cercariae of schistosomiasis, which live in fresh water and normally enter through skin, can enter through the oral mucosa. The cercariae are killed by stomach acid.

Dracunculus medinensis (guinea tapeworm) is a tissue nematode of humans and causes the only such disease transmitted exclusively through drinking water.[354] *Dracunculus* larvae are released in water from subcutaneous worms on the legs of infected bathers or water-gatherers. Larvae are ingested by a tiny crustacean (*Cyclops* spp.), which acts as the intermediate host and releases infectious larvae when ingested by humans. Worldwide eradication of dracunculosis has nearly been accomplished.

Bacterial Spores

Bacterial spores can cause serious wound and gut infections but are not likely to be waterborne enteric pathogens. *Clostridium* is ubiquitous in soil, lake sediment, tropical water sources, and the stool of animals and humans.[135,282] *Clostridium botulinum* and *Clostridium perfringens* type A food poisoning are not waterborne because they require germination of spores in food by inadequate cooking, then production of an enterotoxin, which is ingested. *C. perfringens* type C causes enteritis necroticans, probably through in vivo production of an enterotoxin, and thus has the potential for waterborne transmission in the tropics. However, the epidemiology of these infections in the United States, as in infant botulism, is related to food-borne sources.

Algae

Cyanobacteria, formerly known as *blue-green algae,* grow rapidly in water rich in organic matter during warm weather and produce toxins that pose a health risk to humans, pets, and wildlife. Effects depend on the type of cyanobacterium and level of exposure through dermal contact or aspiration, as well as ingestion. Adverse effects include skin and eye irritation or GI upset. At higher levels, exposure can result in serious illness, including hepatotoxicity (from microcystin toxins) or neurotoxicity. The algae are readily visible and would dissuade most humans from drinking, so it poses more of a threat to animals or small children from recreational ingestion.[37]

Chemical Hazards

Chemical hazards are also an alarming source of pollution in surface water. Wilderness users must consider removal of chemical, as well as microbiologic, contaminants. The greatest risks to wilderness travelers are pesticides from agricultural runoff and heavy metals from old mine tailings. "Fracking" (hydraulic fracturing) to recover shale oil poses a new risk.[145] Industrialization proceeds worldwide without adequate environmental protection. A vast array of toxins are sold with little concept of safe use and no means of safe disposal. Inorganic chemicals in drinking water include common salts, heavy metals, asbestos, fluorides, nitrates, radionuclides, and heavy metals (arsenic, copper, iron, lead, selenium). Natural organic chemicals predominate from soil runoff, forest canopy aquatic biota, and human and animal wastes. Synthetic organic matter includes pesticides, herbicides, and chemicals from industrial or human activities.[322] Major underground aquifers are becoming contaminated. Streams and rivers in rural areas are contaminated by individual carelessness, leaching landfills, and agricultural runoff. Numerous pesticides have been found in runoff and rivers in agricultural areas of the U.S. Midwest.[211] Atmospheric spread has resulted in pesticides being found in remote wilderness lakes and in acid rain.

Persistence of Enteric Pathogens in the Environment

Once environmental contamination has occurred, a natural inactivation or die-off begins. However, enteric pathogens can retain viability for long periods[276,322] (Table 88-3). Factors promoting survival of microorganisms are pH near-neutral (between 6 and 8) and cold temperatures, which contribute to the risk for transmission in mountain regions. In temperate and warm water, survival is measured in days, with densities of infectious agents decreasing by 90% every 60 minutes. However, tropical water differs from temperate water because it contains nutrients that create a microbiologically rich environment. Coliform bacteria can survive several months in natural tropical river water and may even proliferate. Survival of other bacteria is also prolonged: about 200 hours in tropical compared with 30 hours in temperate water. *E. coli* and *V. cholerae* may occur naturally in tropical waters and are capable of surviving indefinitely.[80,135,238] As a rule, viruses persist longer than enteric bacteria in water.[331] Norovirus remained infectious in room-temperature water stored in the dark for 61 days, and virus RNA remained detectable in water for more than 3 years.[285]

Most enteric organisms, including *Shigella*, resist freezing.[96] *Salmonella typhi* can survive for up to 5 months in frozen debris and ice.[336] HAV survives 6 months at below-freezing temperatures.[312] *Cryptosporidium* may be able to survive 1 week or more in home freezers.[302] Viruses persist well on chilled, acidified, frozen foods and foods packed under modified atmosphere or in dried conditions.[12]

Natural Purification Mechanisms

It is widely believed that streams purify themselves and that certain water sources are reliably safe for drinking. These concepts have some truth but do not preclude the need for disinfection to ensure water quality (Box 88-4).

Storms usually deteriorate surface water quality by washing solids, organic materials, and microorganisms into water sources; however, rainwater can also flush streams clean by dilution and by washing microbe-laden bottom sediments downstream.[118,135] Every stream, lake, or groundwater aquifer has limited capacity to assimilate waste effluents and storm water runoff entering the drainage basin. Self-purification is a complex process that involves settling of microorganisms after clumping or adherence

TABLE 88-3 Viability of Enteric Pathogens in Water

Organism	Conditions	Survival	Reference
Vibrio cholerae	Cold	4-5 wk	Felsenfeld, 1965[108]
	Tropical	>1 yr	Perez-Rosas, 1989[238]
Campylobacter	Cold	3-5 wk	Blaser, 1980[29]
	Temperate stream	3-10 days	Singh, 1990[290]
Escherichia coli	Temperate stream	13 hr	Singh, 1990[290]
	Tropical	>1 yr	Perez-Rosas, 1989[238]
Salmonella	Temperate stream	Half-life 16 hr	Perez-Rosas, 1989[238]
Yersinia	Temperate stream	540 days	Singh, 1990[290]
Shigella	Temperate stream	Half-life 22 hr	Singh, 1990[290]
	Freeze/thaw	Yes	Dickens, 1985[96]
Enteric pathogens	Freeze/thaw	Yes	Dickens, 1985[96]
Salmonella typhi	Ice/frozen debris	5 mo	White, 1992[336]
Viruses	Cold	17-130 days	Sattar, 1978[281]
			WHO, 1979[343]
Enteric viruses	15°-25°C (59°-77°F) water	6-10 days	Rose, 1996[276]
Enteric viruses	4°C (39.2°F) water	30 days	Rose, 1996[276]
Norwalk virus	Groundwater, 25°C (77°F) kept in dark	61 days	Seitz, 2011[285]
Enteric adenovirus	Cold	Months	Mena, 2009[208]
Hepatitis A virus	Cold	1 yr	Biziagos, 1988[25]
			Thraenhart, 1991[312]
	Fresh, sea, wastewater	12 wk	Biziagos, 1988[25]
	<0°C (32°F)	6 mo	Thraenhart, 1991[312]
Giardia	Cold	2-3 mo	Bingham, 1979[23]
			DeReigner, 1989[89]
	15°C (59°F) lake, river	10-28 days	DeReigner, 1989[89]
Entamoeba histolytica	Cold	3 mo	Chang, 1953[59]
Microsporidia	4°C (39.2°F)	>1 yr	Marshall, 1997[198]
Cryptosporidium	Cold	12 mo	Current, 1985[86]
Ascaris eggs	Wet or dry	6-9 yr	WHO, 1981[344]
Hookworm larvae	Wet sand	122 days	WHO, 1981[344]

WHO, World Health Organization.

to particles, sunlight providing ultraviolet (UV) destruction, natural die-off, predators eating bacteria, and dilution. Environmental factors include water volume and temperature, hydrologic effects, acid soil contact, and solar radiation. The process is time dependent and less active during wet periods and winter conditions. Hours needed in flow time downstream to achieve a 90% bacterial kill by natural self-purification vary with pollution inflow and rate of water flow. They have been measured at approximately 50 hours in the Tennessee River, 47 hours in the Ohio River, and 32 hours in the Sacramento River, all in summer.[118]

Storage in reservoirs or lakes also improves microbiologic quality, with sedimentation as the primary process. A 100- to 1000-fold increase in fecal coliform bacteria can be found in bottom sediments compared with overlying water. This removal must be considered temporary, influenced by recirculation of organisms trapped in bottom sediments.[89,117] In optimal conditions, 10 days of reservoir storage can result in 75% to 99% removal of coliform bacteria, and 30 days can produce safe drinking water. Generally, 80% to 90% of bacteria and viruses are removed by storage, depending on inflow and outflow, temperature, and no further contamination. Cysts, with a larger size and greater weight, should settle even faster than bacteria and viruses.[5]

Groundwater is generally cleaner than surface water because of the filtration action of overlying sediments, but wells and aquifers can be polluted from surface runoff. Spring water is generally of higher quality than surface water, provided that the true source is not surface water channeling underground from a short distance above the spring.

Drawing conclusions from the preceding factors is difficult. The major factor governing the amount of microbe pollution in surface water is animal and human activity in the watershed.[95] The settling effect of lakes may make them safer than streams, but care should be taken not to disturb bottom sediments when obtaining water.

STANDARDS FOR WATER DISINFECTION

Because coliform bacteria originate primarily in the intestinal tracts of warm-blooded animals, including humans, they are used as indicators of possible fecal contamination.[135] Although compelling reasons exist for testing other organisms before determining the safety of drinking water, cost and relative difficulty in testing for viruses and protozoa are major obstacles to expanding routine water testing, so coliform remains the worldwide standard

---

BOX 88-4 Water Quality: Key Points

- In general, cloudiness indicates higher risk for contamination and lower effectiveness of chemical and UV disinfection techniques; however, in remote wilderness water, most sediment is inorganic, and clarity is not an indication of microbiologic purity.
- The major factor determining amount of microbe pollution in surface water is human and animal activity in the watershed.
- Streams do not purify themselves but may dilute a limited source of contamination.
- Settling effect of lakes may make them safer than streams, but care should be taken not to disturb bottom sediments when obtaining water.
- Groundwater sources (springs and protected wells) generally have lower microbiologic contamination because of the filtration action of overlying sediments but may have more chemical contamination.

indicator organism. In the United States, the EPA still considers coliform a useful indicator, but coliform bacteria occur in large numbers in many water distribution systems that have no problem with waterborne disease.[327] Therefore, the EPA is moving to *E. coli* as a more specific indicator of human and animal contamination. In addition, contamination with other organisms has become common, resulting in expansion of U.S. regulations to test for organisms such as *Cryptosporidium*. Molecular probes should make this process much easier but may not indicate infectivity.[214,309]

The basic federal law pertaining to drinking water is the 1974 Safe Drinking Water Act, which was expanded and strengthened by amendments in 1977, 1986, and 1996.[214,349] Additional rules were added in 1989, 1996, 1998, and 2006.[50,262] The EPA Revised Total Coliform Rule (2013) sets maximum contamination level goals of zero for waterborne pathogens but allows a more practical maximum contamination level (MCL) as an enforceable standard. It also establishes a systems approach to monitoring and testing.[321] WHO guidelines are regarded internationally as the most authoritative framework on drinking water quality.[347]

All standards acknowledge the impracticality of trying to eliminate all microorganisms from drinking water, allowing a small risk for enteric infection.[38,262,293,329] Risk models are used to predict levels of illness and desired levels of reduction, with the reality that large numbers of people in the United States have increased susceptibility to enteric infections because of decreased immunologic competency.[262] For example, EPA and Canadian guidelines suggest *Giardia* cyst removal with the goal of ensuring high probability that consumer risk is no more than one infection per 10,000 people per year.[38,256,262] The concept of risk is important for wilderness travelers as well, because it is impossible to know the risk of drinking the water in advance, and it may not be practical to eliminate all risk with treatment.

Generally, the goal of treatment is to achieve a 3- to 5-log reduction in the level of microorganisms; treatment must reduce *Giardia* or *Cryptosporidium* by 99.9% (3 log) and enteric viruses by at least 99.99% (4 log).[255]

STANDARDS FOR PORTABLE DISINFECTION PRODUCTS

The EPA and National Sanitation Foundation (NSF International) are the primary agencies that set standards for disinfection products and protocols for testing to meet these standards. NSF, the Public Health and Safety Company, is a not-for-profit, nongovernmental organization and world leader in standards development and product certification. EPA standards and NSF Protocol P231 (Microbiological Purifiers) were used to create NSF Protocol P248 (Emergency Military Operations Microbiological Water Purifiers) to test individual water purifiers for field military operations. Other pertinent NSF protocols include UV (P55), Reverse Osmosis (P58), and Point of Use (P53).

EPA Registration

Mechanical Filters. Until recently, no testing criteria were mandated for EPA registration. The EPA does not endorse, test, or approve mechanical filters; it merely assigns registration numbers. However, registration requirements distinguish between two types of filters: those that use mechanical means only and those that use a chemical, designated as a *pesticide*. Standards were developed to act as a framework for testing and evaluation of water purifiers for EPA registration, as a testing guide for manufacturers, to assist in research and development of new units, and as a guide for consumers.[327]

Filter Testing. Current registration of mechanical filters requires only that the product make reasonable claims and that the location of the manufacturer be listed; no disinfection studies are required. However, many companies now use the standards as their testing guidelines. For mechanical filters, the standards should be applied only for those microorganisms against which claims are made, such as protozoa and bacteria only for most filters. Despite criticisms of the methodology and inconsistencies and loopholes in the reporting process, EPA standards are currently the best means to compare filters.

The EPA standards include performance-based microbiologic reduction requirements, chemical health limits for substances that may be discharged, and stability requirements for chemical(s) sufficient for the shelf life of the device. The unit should signal the end of effective lifetime (e.g., by terminating discharge of treated water) or give simple instructions for servicing or replacing within measurable volume, throughput, or time frame. There are currently no national guidelines for removal of chemicals by portable filters.

The EPA standards require that "challenge water" seeded with specific amounts of microorganisms be pumped through the filters at given intervals during the claimed volume capacity of the filter. Between bacteriologic challenges, different test waters without organisms are passed through the unit. Water conditions are specified to include average and worst-case conditions; the latter are 5°C (41°F) with high levels of pollution, turbidity, and alkaline pH. Testing must be done with bacteria (*Klebsiella*), viruses (poliovirus and rotavirus), and protozoa (*Cryptosporidium* has replaced *Giardia*). A 3-log reduction (99.9%) is required for cysts, 4-log reduction (99.99%) for viruses, and 5- to 6-log reduction for bacteria. Testing is done or contracted by the manufacturer; the EPA neither tests nor specifies laboratories.

To be called a "microbiologic water purifier," the unit must remove, kill, or inactivate all types of disease-causing microorganisms from the water, including bacteria, viruses, and protozoan cysts, so as to render the processed water safe for drinking. An exception for limited claims may be allowed for units removing specific organisms to serve a definable environmental need, such as removal of protozoan cysts.

CHEMICAL METHODS

Products that are used for treating municipal or private water supplies for drinking are considered pesticides and must be registered by the EPA Office of Pesticide Programs. Registration signifies the following:

- The composition is such as to warrant the proposed claims.
- The labeling and other material required to be submitted comply with the requirements of the act.
- The method will perform its intended function without unreasonable adverse effects on the environment.
- When used in accordance with widespread and commonly recognized practice, the method will not generally cause unreasonable adverse effects on the environment.

Thus, EPA registration implies only that the "pesticide" agent is not released into the water at unsafe levels.[7,40] This is less stringent than for filters that contain halogens.

The NSF and American National Standards Institute (ANSI) perform testing of products. Their certification is based on the following: (1) reduction claims on the label are true; (2) the product does not add anything harmful; and (3) the product label, advertisements, and literature are not misleading (info .nsf.org/certified/DWTU).

DISINFECTION METHODS: DEFINITIONS

Disinfection, the desired result of field water treatment, means removal or destruction of harmful microorganisms[201] (Box 88-5). Technically, disinfection refers only to chemical means such as halogens, but the term is also applied to heat and filtration and ultraviolet irradiation. *Pasteurization* is similar to disinfection but specifically refers to the use of heat, usually at temperatures below 100°C (212°F), to kill most pathogenic organisms. Disinfection and pasteurization should not be confused with *sterilization,* which is destruction or removal of all life forms.[178] The goal of disinfection is to achieve potable water, indicating only that a water source, on average over a period of time, contains a "minimal microbial hazard," so that the statistical likelihood of illness is acceptable. Water sterilization is not necessary, because not all organisms are enteric human pathogens.[142] *Purification* is removal of organic or inorganic chemicals and particulate matter to eliminate offensive color, taste, and odor. The term

BOX 88-5   Definitions of Water Disinfection Terms

Clarification: Techniques that reduce turbidity of water.
Coagulation-flocculation: Removes smaller suspended particles and chemical complexes too small to settle by gravity (colloids).
Contact time: Length of time that the halogen is in contact with microorganisms in the water.
Disinfection: A process that kills or destroys almost all disease-producing microorganisms, with the exception of bacterial spores. As applied here, refers to pathogenic waterborne microbes and is the desired result of water treatment.
Enteric pathogen: Microorganism capable of causing intestinal infection after ingested; may be transmitted through food, water, or direct fecal-oral contamination.
Halogen: Oxidant chemical (primarily chlorine and iodine) that can be used for water disinfection.
Halogen demand: Amount of halogen reacting with impurities in the water.
Potable: Implies "drinkable" water, but technically means that a water source, on average, over a period of time, contains a "minimal microbial hazard," so that the statistical likelihood of illness is acceptable.
Purification: Removal of organic or inorganic chemicals and particulate matter to improve offensive color, taste, and odor. Sometimes used by other sources to indicate microbiologic removal.
Residual halogen concentration: Amount of active halogen remaining after halogen demand of the water is met.
Reverse osmosis: A process of filtration that uses high pressure to force water through a nanopore semipermeable membrane that filters out dissolved ions, molecules, and solids.
Sterilization: A process by which all forms of microbial life, including bacteria, viruses, protozoa, and spores, are destroyed.

is frequently used interchangeably with disinfection, but purification as used here may not remove or kill enough microorganisms to ensure microbiologic safety.[334]

HEAT

Heat is the oldest means of water disinfection. It is used worldwide by residents, travelers, and campers to provide safe drinking water. In countries with normally safe drinking water, it is often recommended as backup in emergencies or when water systems have become contaminated by floods or a lapse in water treatment plant efficacy. Fuel availability is the most important limitation to using heat. One kilogram of wood is required to boil 1 L of water.[60] For wilderness travelers without access to wood, liquid fuel is heavy (Box 88-6).

Heat inactivation of microorganisms is exponential and follows first-order kinetics. Time plotted against temperature yields a straight line when plotted on a logarithmic scale.[159] The "thermal death point" is reached in shorter time at higher temperatures, whereas lower temperatures are effective with a longer

BOX 88-6   Heat as Water Disinfection Method

Advantages	Disadvantages
Does not impart additional taste or color to water	Does not improve taste, smell, or appearance of poor-quality water
Single-step process that inactivates all enteric pathogens	Fuel sources may be scarce, expensive, or unavailable
Efficacy is *not* compromised by contaminants or particles in the water, as with chemical treatment and filtration	Does not prevent recontamination during storage
Can pasteurize water without sustained boiling	

Relative susceptibility of microorganisms to heat: protozoa > bacteria > viruses.

contact time. Pasteurization uses this principle to kill enteric food pathogens and spoiling organisms at temperatures between 60° and 74°C (140° and 165.2°F), well below boiling.[115] Pasteurization is not intended to kill all pathogenic microorganisms in the food or liquid. Typical pasteurization processes include heating to 63° to 65°C (145.4° to 149°F) for up to 30 minutes and flash pasteurization using high temperature–short time at 71° to 72°C (159.8° to 161.6°F) for 15 to 30 seconds.[201] This will kill 99.999% of viable microorganisms in milk or in fruit or vegetable juice. Therefore, the minimum critical temperature for waterborne pathogens is well below the boiling point, 100°C (212°F).[151]

Microorganisms have varying sensitivity to heat; however, all common enteric pathogens are readily inactivated by heat (Table 88-4). Bacterial spores (e.g., *Clostridium* spp.) are the most resistant; some can survive 100°C (212°F) for long periods but are not likely to be waterborne enteric pathogens. Boiling does not depend on water quality as does filtration or chemical disinfection. Heat kills or inactivates all enteric waterborne pathogens, regardless of whether they are freely suspended or present in particles.[284]

Parasitic eggs, larvae, and cercariae are all susceptible to heat. For most helminth eggs and larvae, which are more resistant than cercariae and *Cyclops* (the copepod that carries *Dracunculus*), the critical lethal temperature is 50° to 55°C (122° to 131°F).[287] Protozoal cysts, including *Giardia* and *E. histolytica*, are very susceptible to heat. *Cryptosporidium* is also inactivated at these lower pasteurization levels.

Common bacterial enteric pathogens (*E. coli*, *Salmonella*, *Shigella*) are killed by standard pasteurization temperatures of 55°C (131°F) for 30 minutes or 65°C (149°F) for less than 1 minute.[115,224] Studies have confirmed the safety of water contaminated with *V. cholerae* and *E. coli* after 10 minutes at 60° to 62°C (140° to 143.6°F) or after boiling water for 30 seconds.[130,264]

Viruses are more closely related to vegetative bacteria than to spore-bearing organisms[159] and are generally inactivated at 56° to 60°C (132.8° to 140°F) in 20 to 40 minutes or less.[3,239,307,316] Inactivation at higher temperatures is similar to that of vegetative bacteria. Death occurs in less than 1 minute above 70°C (158°F), as confirmed in milk products.[305]

Given its environmental stability and clinical virulence, HAV is a special concern. Data from food industry studies confirms susceptibility of HAV and other enteric viruses to heat at pasteurization temperatures, even in milk and other products with solids that shield the virus.[12] Widely varying data probably result from different models for virus infectivity and destruction and from the use of various test media.

BOILING TIME

The boiling time required is important when fuel is limited. The previous recommendation for treating water was to boil for 10 minutes and add 1 minute for every 305 m (1000 feet) in elevation. However, data indicate this is not necessary for disinfection. Evidence indicates that enteric pathogens are killed within seconds by boiling water and rapidly at temperatures above 60°C (140°F). In the wilderness, the time required to heat water from 55°C (131°F) to boiling temperature works toward disinfection. Therefore, any water brought to a boil should be adequately disinfected.[294] An extra margin of safety can be added by boiling for 1 minute or by keeping the water covered for several more minutes, which will maintain high pasteurization temperature without using fuel, or allowing it to cool slowly. Although the boiling point decreases with increasing altitude, this is not significant compared with the time required for thermal death at these temperatures (Table 88-5).

In recognition of the difference between pasteurizing water for drinking purposes and sterilizing to kill all microbes for surgical or laboratory purposes, many other sources, including WHO, now agree with this recommendation to simply bring water to a boil. The U.S. Centers for Disease Control and Prevention (CDC) and EPA still recommend boiling for 1 minute to add a margin of safety.[44] Other sources still suggest 3 minutes of boiling time at high altitude to give a wide margin of safety.[53,117,273,323]

TABLE 88-4 Data on Heat Inactivation of Microorganisms

Organism	Lethal Temperature/Time	Reference
Giardia	55°C (131°F) for 5 min	Jarroll, 1984[156]
	100°C (212°F) immediately	Bingham, 1979[23]
	50°C (122°F) for 10 min (95% inactivation)	Ongerth,1989[232]
	60°C (140°F) for 10 min (98% inactivation)	
	70°C (158°F) for 10 min (100% inactivation)	
	55°C (131°F)	Aukerman, 1989[8]
Entamoeba histolytica	Similar to Giardia	
Nematode cysts, helminth eggs, larvae, cercariae	50°-55°C (122°-131°F)	Shephart, 1977[287]
	65°C (149°F) for 1 min, 50°C (122°F) for 30 min	
Cryptosporidium	45°-55°C (113°-131°F) for 20 min	Anderson, 1985[6]
	55°C (131°F) warmed over 20 min	
	64.2°C (147.6°F) within 2 min	Fayer, 1994[106]
	72°C (161.6°F) heated up over 1 min	
Escherichia coli	55°C (131°F) for 30 min	Frazier, 1978[115]
	60°-62°C (140°-143.6°F) for 10 min	Neumann, 1969[224]
Salmonella, Shigella	65°C (149°F) for <1 min	
Vibrio cholerae	60°-62°C (140°-143.6°F) for 10 min	Rice, 1991[264]
	100°C (212°F) for 30 sec	
E. coli, Salmonella, Shigella, Campylobacter	60°C (140°F) for 3 min (3-log reduction)	Bandres, 1988[13]
	65°C (149°F) for 3 min (all but a few Campylobacter)	
	75°C (167°F) for 3 min (100% kill)	
E. coli	50°C (122°F) for 10 min ineffective	Groh, 1996[130]
	60°C (140°F) for 5 min	
	70°C (158°F) for 1 min	
Viruses (multiple potential food-borne)	56°C (132.8°F) for 30 min	Tuladhar, 2012[316]
	73°C (163.4°F) for 3 min (>4-log reduction)	
Viruses	55°-60°C (131°-140°F) within 20-40 min	Alder, 1992[3]
	70°C (158°F) for <1 min	
Hepatitis A	98°C (208.4°F) for 1 min	Krugman, 1970[173]
	85°C (185°F) for 1 min	Thraenhart, 1991[312]
	61°C (141.8°F) for 10 min (50% disintegrated)	
	60°C (140°F) for 19 min (in shellfish)	Peterson, 1978[240]
	60°C (140°F) for 10 min	Baert, 2009[12]
	75°C (167°F) for <0.5 min	Bidawid, 2000[20]
	80°C (176°F) for 3 min; 85°C (185°F) for ≤1 min (in various food products)	
Hepatitis E	60°C (140°F) for 30 min	Thraenhart, 1991[312]
Bacterial spores	>100°C (212°F)	Alder, 1992[3]

IMPROVISATION

Hot Tap Water

Although attaining boiling temperature is not necessary, it is the only easily recognizable end point without using a thermometer. Other markers, such as early bubble formation on the bottom of the pot, do not occur at a consistent temperature. When no other means are available, the use of hot tap water may prevent traveler's diarrhea in developing countries. Neumann[224,225] cultured samples from the hot tap water of 17 hotels in west Africa with water temperature ranging from 57° to 69°C (134.6° to 156.2°F) and found no coliform bacteria in 15 samples; one sample yielded a single colony and another sample two colonies. As a rule of thumb, water too hot to touch fell within the pasteurization range. Bandres and associates[13] measured hot tap water temperature in 14 hotels in four different countries outside the United States. Most temperatures were 55° to 60°C (131° to

140°F), but one was 44°C (111.2°F), one was 65°C (149°F), and several were 52°C (125.6°F). The authors concluded that hot water from taps would not be safe to drink. Groh and colleagues[130] showed that tolerance to touch is too variable to be reliable, because some people found 55°C (131°F) too hot to touch.

From these studies, one can conclude that if water has been sitting in a tank near 55° to 60°C (131° to 140°F) for a prolonged period, enteric pathogens will be significantly reduced, likely to potable levels. Neumann's suggestion (using water too hot to touch) is reasonable if no other method of water treatment is available.

Solar Heat

Pasteurization has been successfully achieved using solar heating. Bottom temperatures of 65°C (149°F) have been obtained for at least 1 hour in up to three 3.7-L jugs. Exposure to full sunshine in Kenya destroyed E. coli in 2-L clear plastic bottles within 7 hours if the maximum temperature reached 55°C (131°F). No thermal inactivation occurs below 40°C (104°F). Inactivation using solar heat is a combination of thermal and UV irradiation.[21,160,203] A solar cooker constructed from a foil-lined cardboard box with a glass window in the lid can be used for disinfecting large amounts of water by pasteurization. Most often, clear plastic bottles are placed on a reflective metal surface. This is a low-cost method for improving water quality, especially in refugee camps and disaster areas,[204,207,268] and is effective even with high turbidity[4] (see Ultraviolet Light, later).

TABLE 88-5 Boiling Temperatures at Various Altitudes

Altitude (ft)	Altitude (m)	Boiling Point
5000	1524	95°C (203°F)
10,000	3048	90°C (194°F)
14,000	4267	86°C (186.8°F)
19,000	5791	81°C (177.8°F)

PHYSICAL REMOVAL

TURBIDITY AND CLARIFICATION

River, lake, or pond water is often cloudy and unappealing. *Turbidity* (cloudiness) is an optical measurement of light scattering as it passes through water. Visibility in water with turbidity of 10 nephelometric turbidity units (NTU) is about 75 cm (30 inches) and with 25 NTU is 25 cm (10 inches). Turbidity is caused by suspended organic and inorganic matter, such as clay, silt, plankton, and other microscopic organisms. High turbidity is often associated with unpleasant odors and tastes, most often caused by organic compounds and metallic hydroxides with a much smaller particle size.[71,181] Clay-organic complexes may also carry pesticides or heavy metals. Bacteria, as well as viruses, may be adsorbed to particulate matter or may be embedded in it, and in highly contaminated water, microorganisms tend to aggregate and clump. In one study, 17% of turbidity particles contained attached microbes, averaging 10 to 100 bacteria per particle.[181] Organisms in the centers of these conglomerates are afforded some protection from disinfectants. Even the flocculate produced by a chlorination-flocculation tablet may harbor viable organisms.[244] Therefore, removal of turbidity and particulates may be important in preventing chemical or infectious illness.

Of 106 samples from various sources in 13 developing countries, 33% exceeded 5 NTU and 64% exceeded 1 NTU, which is the maximum turbidity level set by the EPA before water chlorination.[176] As expected, turbidity was lower in improved sources, but only 5 in 22 of these urban water sources had any detectable free chlorine residual. Household studies in developing countries indicate that most consumers find water with less than 5 NTU esthetically acceptable for drinking. The EPA has set a turbidity standard for treated drinking water at less than 0.3 NTU 95% of the time.[321]

Clarification to remove turbidity can be accomplished by simple settling, chemical processes, or filtration (Box 88-7). It is the first step in municipal water treatment, and when needed, is an important initial step in field- or household-level disinfection, before using the final treatment method of filtration or chemical disinfection; clarification greatly improves the efficacy of these techniques.[185,283] Even if turbidity is caused by benign inorganic particles, such as clay, removal is desirable for improving esthetic quality of the water. Filtration can remove larger particles, but cloudy water can rapidly clog a filter. Sedimentation and coagulation-flocculation are other clarification techniques rou-

---

BOX 88-8 Coagulation-Flocculation

Advantages	Disadvantages
Highly effective to clarify water and remove many microorganisms and some other contaminants	Unfamiliar technique to many consumers
Improves efficacy of filtration and chemical disinfection	Adds extra step unless combined flocculent-disinfectant tablet
Inexpensive and widely available	
Simple process with no toxicity	

Relative susceptibility of microorganisms to coagulation-flocculation: protozoa > bacteria = viruses.

---

tinely used in municipal disinfection plants that can be easily applied in the wilderness for pretreatment of cloudy water, which is then disinfected by microfiltration or halogenation. Coagulation-flocculation and filtration are also used to remove *Giardia* and *Cryptosporidium* cysts that are more resistant to chlorine. Early experiments with water heavily contaminated with feces containing HAV demonstrated that filtration and sedimentation alone did not prevent infection, but reduced severity of the illness. Water pretreated with coagulation, settling, and filtration and subsequently disinfected with 0.4 ppm of residual chlorine was noninfectious, whereas water chlorinated to 1 mg/L without pretreatment remained infectious.[222,223] Thus, removing particulate matter decreases the number of microorganisms and halogen demand.[161,221,248]

SEDIMENTATION

Sedimentation is the separation of suspended particles large enough to settle rapidly by gravity, such as sand and silt. Water is allowed to sit without agitation. After sediment has formed on the bottom of the container, the clear water is decanted or filtered from the top. The time required depends on the size of the particle. Generally, 1 to 3 hours are adequate for large particles such as inorganic sands and silts. Microorganisms, especially protozoan cysts, eventually settle, hastened by attachment to organic biologic particles; reductions up to 90% may be achieved within 1 to 2 days.[60,206] However, the organisms are easily disturbed during pouring or filtering. Reservoirs take advantage of sedimentation to improve microbiologic quality. In conclusion, sedimentation is often effective in reducing water turbidity and will improve microbiologic quality, but is not recommended as the sole means of disinfection.

COAGULATION-FLOCCULATION

Smaller suspended particles and chemical complexes too small to settle by gravity are called colloids. Most of these can be removed by chemical precipitation, known as coagulation-flocculation (C-F), a technique that has been used to remove unpleasant color, smell, and taste in water since 2000 BC. This technique is used routinely in large municipal disinfection plants, but is simple enough to be used at the household level and outdoors[82,259,294] (Box 88-8).

Coagulation is achieved with addition of an appropriate chemical that alters the physical state of dissolved and suspended solids, causing particles to stick together on contact because of electrostatic and ionic forces.[71,322] Aluminum salts (alum), iron, and lime (alkaline chemicals principally containing calcium or magnesium and oxygen) are frequently used, readily available coagulants. Rapid mixing is important to obtain dispersion of the coagulant. The second stage, *flocculation,* is a purely physical process obtained by prolonged gentle mixing to increase interparticle collisions and promote formation of larger particles. The flocculate particles are large enough that they can be removed by sedimentation or by filtration with relatively large pore size, including a tightly woven cloth.[180]

To clarify water by C-F in the field, add 10 to 30 mg of alum per liter of water. The exact amount is not important, so it can be done with a pinch of alum, lime (calcium oxide), or both for

---

BOX 88-7 Summary of Water Clarification Techniques

Technique	Process	Uses, Advantages
Sedimentation	Settling by gravity of large particulates	Requires only time Improves water esthetics
Coagulation-flocculation	Removes suspended particles, most microorganisms, some dissolved substances	Simple process, easily applied in field Greatly improves water quality Improves efficacy of filtration and chemical disinfection
Activated carbon (charcoal)	Removes organic and some inorganic chemicals	Removes toxins such as pesticides and many heavy metals, and removes chemical disinfectants Improves taste and esthetics of water
Filtration	Physical and chemical process	Removes microorganisms and particulates; nanofiltration may remove chemicals and monovalent ions (salt). Charcoal stage may improve taste and remove chemicals.

each gallon of water, using more if the water is very cloudy. Next, stir or shake briskly for 1 minute to mix the coagulant, then agitate gently and frequently for at least 5 minutes to assist flocculation. Settling requires at least 30 minutes, after which the water is carefully decanted or poured through a cloth or paper filter. The process can be repeated, if necessary.

During the process of C-F, protozoan cysts and bacteria act as particles and viruses react as colloidal organic particles, with removal of 1 to 2 log of these microorganisms.[180] C-F removes most coliform bacteria (60% to 98%),[81] viruses (65% to 99%),[85,253,293] *Giardia* (60% to 99%), helminth ova (95%),[287] heavy metals, dissolved phosphates, and minerals.[71,190,322,343] Organic and inorganic compounds may be removed by forming a precipitate or by adsorbing onto aluminum hydroxide or ferric hydroxide floc particles.[322] Coagulation generally removes large molecules that absorb poorly on granular activated carbon (GAC).[9]

Despite removal of most microorganisms, a subsequent disinfection step is advised. Products combining flocculants with chlorine provide a two-step process that removes turbidity and allows effective disinfection by chlorine.[259]

Toxicity

Questions have been raised concerning the association of aluminum with central nervous system (CNS) toxicity in mammals, but these effects have been observed only after exposures other than ingestion. Most of the aluminum in alum is removed with the floc. A report from the National Academy of Sciences concluded that aluminum in drinking water does not present a significant risk.[322] Alum is a common chemical used by the food industry in baking powder and for pickling. It can be found in some food stores or at chemical supply stores.

Alternative Agents

Many inorganic and organic compounds can be used as a coagulant, including lime (calcium oxide) or potash (from wood ash).[152] In an emergency, bleaching powder, baking powder, or even the fine white ash from a campfire can be used.[319] Other C-F agents used traditionally by native peoples include seed extracts from the nirmali plant in southern India, moringa plants in Sudan, crushed almonds, dried and crushed beans, and rauwaq (a form of bentonite clay).[60]

ADSORPTION

Adsorbents, such as charcoal, clay, and other types of organic matter, have been used for water treatment since ancient times.[179] These processes are often combined with filtration or coagulation, because these substances are used as the filter media and also can act as coagulants.[294] Clays can decrease turbidity and microbes in water by about 90% to 95%, but adsorption is not the main action of ceramic or clay filters. Vegetative matter, including burnt rice hulls and activated (burnt) coconut shell, also have adsorptive capacity.

Granular Activated Carbon

Granular carbon (i.e., charcoal) is widely used for water treatment and medical detoxification. Activated carbon is a natural material derived from bituminous coal, lignite, wood, coconut shell, and other materials that are activated by steam and other means. When activated, charcoal's regular array of carbon bonds is disrupted, yielding free valences that are highly reactive and that adsorb dissolved chemicals.[119,277] GAC is the best means to remove toxic organic and inorganic chemicals from water (including disinfection byproducts) and to improve odor and taste.[221,322] Thus, it is widely used in municipal disinfection plants and in home under-sink devices. GAC also removes radioactive contamination.

Many, but not all, viral particles, bacteria, and protozoan cysts are removed by GAC filters, primarily by adherence to GAC,[141,221] and some cysts are trapped in the matrix.[190] GAC does not kill microorganisms; in fact, bacteria attach to and colonize charcoal, where they are resistant to chlorination because the chlorine is adsorbed by the GAC.[179,221,322] This bacterial contamination has not been found to be harmful because the usual heterophilic

bacteria are not enteric pathogens. Enteric pathogens have been shown to survive on GAC, but if an active biofilm exists, the pathogens are rapidly displaced by heterophilic bacteria and fail to become established. Therefore, nonpathogenic bacterial colonization is encouraged in municipal plants.[257] However, these properties of carbon indicate that it will not reduce pathogenic microbes in water over an extended period, and an alternative means of disinfection should always be used.

Eventually, the binding sites on the carbon particles become saturated and no longer adsorb; some molecules are released as others preferentially bind.[221] Unfortunately, no reliable means are available to determining precisely when saturation is reached. Filters using charcoal in compressed block form as the filter element may clog before the charcoal is fully adsorbed. Presence of unpleasant taste or color in the water can be the first sign that the charcoal is spent. To test the activity of the charcoal, one may filter iodinated water or water tinted with food coloring. With regular use, the lifetime of GAC is probably measured in months; it is substantially longer with infrequent use. GAC can be "recharged," but this is not practical for small-quantity use.

Granulated activated carbon is best used after chemical disinfection to make water more palatable by completely removing the halogen[221,336] and other chemical impurities that result in bad odor and taste. For point-of-use field filters, activated carbon is used in granular or powder form, or extruded into a block that acts both as a depth filter and an adsorbent. Block carbon is more effective than granular carbon because the passages are smaller, forcing closer contact with the carbon. Ingested particles of charcoal are harmless. With increasing industrial and agricultural contamination of distant groundwater, final treatment of drinking water with GAC may be important for some wilderness users.

FILTRATION

Filters are appealing because of their simplicity and suitability for commercial production. Portable water treatment products are the third highest intended purchase of outdoor equipment, after backpacks and tents.[157] Filtration is a standard step in municipal disinfection and widely used in the food and beverage industry, as well as many other industrial processes. Many different types of media, from sand to vegetable products to fabric, have been used for water treatment throughout history in various parts of the world. Filters have the advantages of being simple and requiring no holding time (Box 88-9). They do not add any unpleasant taste and may improve taste and appearance of water. However, they require space and add weight to packs or baggage. All filters

---

BOX 88-9 Filtration

Advantages	Disadvantages
Simple to operate	Adds bulk and weight to baggage
Mechanical filters require no holding time for treatment (water is treated as it comes out of filter)	Most filters not reliable for adequate removal of viruses
Large choice of commercial products	Expensive relative to chemical treatment
Adds no unpleasant taste and usually improves taste and appearance of water	Channeling of water or high pressure can force microorganisms through the filter.
Rationally combined with halogens for removal or destruction of all pathogenic waterborne microbes	Eventually, clog from suspended particulate matter; may require some maintenance or repair in field
Different pore sizes available determine removal of microorganisms and smaller substances, including sodium (salt)	Smallest pore sizes (nanofilters, as in reverse osmosis) require higher pressure
Effectiveness not dependent on water temperature	Freezing water within filter element will compromise or destroy some filters.

Susceptibility of microorganisms to filtration: protozoa > bacteria > viruses.

eventually clog from suspended particulate matter, present even in clear streams, requiring cleaning or replacement of the filter. As a filter clogs, it requires increasing pressure to drive the water through, which can force microorganisms through the filter. A crack or eroded channel allows passage of unfiltered water. Bacteria can grow on filter media and potentially result in increased water contamination, but illness has not been demonstrated.[354] Silver is often incorporated into the filter media to prevent this growth, but it is not totally effective (see Silver, later.)

Filtration is usually a dual process: physical (separation of particles from liquid) and chemical (attachment of microorganisms to the medium). Many variables influence filter efficiency, including the characteristics of the filter media and the water, as well as flow rate. Filtration can reduce turbidity, bacteria, algae, viruses, color, oxidized iron, manganese, and radioactive particles.[85]

Many filters constructed with various designs and materials are marketed for field use. Surface, membrane, hollow-fiber, and mesh filters are very thin with a single layer of fairly precise pores, whose size should be equal to or less than the smallest dimension of the organism. These filters provide little volume for holding contaminants and thus clog rapidly, but can be cleaned easily by washing and brushing without destroying the filter. Maze or depth filters depend on a long, irregular labyrinth to trap the organism, so they may have a larger pore or passage size. Contaminants adhere to the walls of the passageway or are trapped in the numerous dead-end tunnels. Granular media, such as sand or charcoal, diatomaceous earth, or ceramic filters, function as maze filters. A depth filter has a large holding capacity for particles and lasts longer before clogging, but it may be difficult to clean effectively because many particles are trapped deep in the filter. Flow can be partially restored to a clogged filter by back flushing or surface cleaning, which removes the larger particles trapped near the surface. For ceramic filters, surface cleaning is highly effective but removes a tiny layer of the filter medium. Hollow-fiber and pleated filters rely on large surface area to avoid clogging by particles.

The size of a microorganism is the primary determinant of its susceptibility to filtration (Table 88-6 and Figure 88-1). Filters are rated by their ability to retain particles of a certain size, which is described by two terms. *Absolute rating* means that 100% of a certain size of particle is retained. *Nominal rating* indicates that

TABLE 88-6 Microorganism Susceptibility to Filtration

Organism	Average Size (μm)	Maximum Recommended Filter Rating (μm)
Viruses	0.03	N/S
Escherichia coli	0.5 × 3-8	0.2-0.4
Campylobacter	0.2-0.4 × 1.5-3.5	Same as above
Microsporidia	1-2	N/S
Cryptosporidium oocyst	2-6 (mean 5)	1
Giardia cyst	6-10 × 8-15	3-5
Entamoeba histolytica cyst	5-30 (average 10)	Same as *Giardia*
Cyclospora	8-10	Same as *Giardia*
Nematode eggs	30-40 × 50-80	20
Schistosome cercariae	50 × 100	Coffee filter or fine cloth
Dracunculus larvae	20 × 500	Coffee filter or fine cloth

N/S, Not specified.

more than 90% of a given particle size will be retained. Filter efficiency is generally determined with hard particles (beads of known diameter), but microorganisms are soft and compressible under pressure. Waterborne pathogens often adhere to larger particles or clump together, making them easier to remove by physical processes.[206] Therefore, observed reductions are often greater than expected based on their individual sizes.[294]

In general, portable filters for water treatment can be divided into *microfiltration* with pores down to 0.1 μm, *ultrafiltration* that can remove particles as small as 0.01 μm, *nanofiltration* with pore size as small as 0.001 μm or less, and *reverse osmosis* with pore size 0.0001 μm or less. Microfilters are effective for removing protozoa and bacteria, algae, most particles, and sediment, but allow dissolved material, small colloids, and some viruses to pass through. Ultrafiltration membranes are required for complete removal of viruses, colloids, and some dissolved solids. Nanofilters can remove other dissolved substances, including

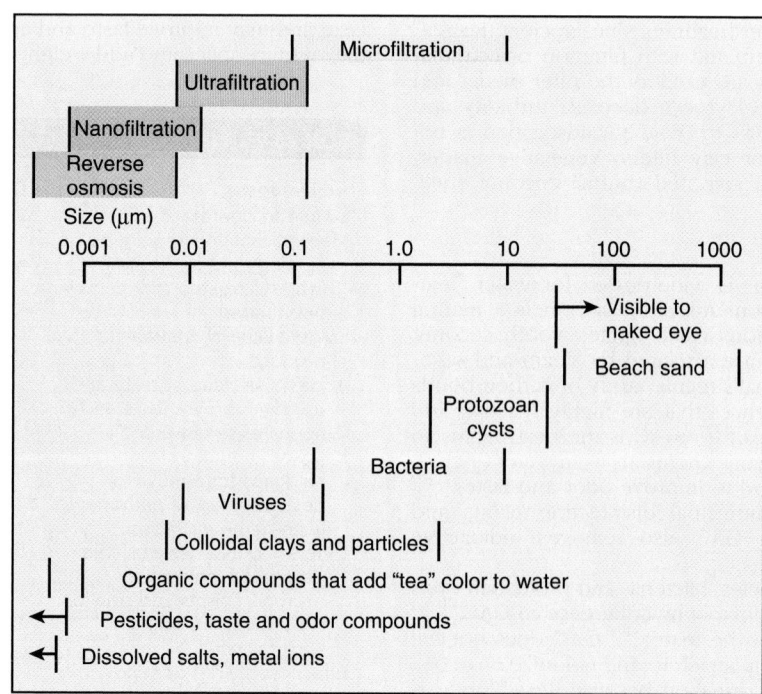

FIGURE 88-1 Relative size of microorganisms determines susceptibility to mechanical filtration. Mechanical filters span a wide range of pore sizes.

salts (sodium chloride) and endotoxins from water. Reverse osmosis removes monovalent ions (desalination) and almost all organic molecules.[180,201] All filters require pressure to drive the water through the filter element; the smaller the pore size, the more pressure required.

Simple portable filters are a reliable means to remove protozoan cysts and bacteria.[19] A microfilter membrane with a pore size of 0.2 μm can remove enteric bacteria. *Giardia* and *E. histolytica* cysts are easily filtered, requiring a maximum filter size of 5 μm. *Cryptosporidium* cysts are somewhat smaller than *Giardia* and more flexible; 57% are able to pass through a 3-μm membrane filter, so a filter with 1- to 2-μm pores is recommended.[273] Helminth eggs and larvae, which are much larger, can be removed by a 20-μm filter. *Cyclops* (the water-dwelling copepod that ingests the larva and transmits dracunculosis) can be removed by passage through a fine cloth.[287]

Adsorption and aggregation during passage through microfilters reduce viruses.[65,294] Virus particles may adhere to the walls of diatomite (ceramic) or charcoal filters by electrostatic chemical attraction, which can be enhanced by a coating on the filter or a positive charge.[104,120,123,126,257] Viruses in heavily polluted water often aggregate in large clumps and become adsorbed to particles or enmeshed in colloidal materials, making them amenable to filtration.[253,322] Thus, turbidity (cloudiness from contaminants) may help remove pathogens with filtration, whereas it inhibits chemical disinfection. In one study, however, only 10% of total virus particles detected were recovered on 3- to 5-μm pore prefilters, suggesting that most were not associated with the suspended sediment.[228] Furthermore, adsorbed viral particles can be subsequently dislodged and eluted from a filter because of competitive binding and competing electrostatic forces.[120,247,315] Good ceramic filters now remove 99% to 99.9% of viruses, but the fourth log required by water treatment units remains a challenge. First Need filter has been able to meet the EPA standards for water purifiers, including 4-log removal of viruses, apparently through use of a charged media[123,126] (see Appendix A at the end of this chapter). Ultrafilters, such as Sawyer 0.02-μm hollow-fiber filter (or nanofiltration and reverse osmosis), can mechanically filter viruses. In general, however, microfilters should not be considered adequate for complete removal of viruses, except with special equipment.[334]

Reverse Osmosis

A reverse-osmosis filter uses high pressure (100 to 800 psi) to force water through a semipermeable membrane that filters out dissolved ions, molecules, and solids.[322] This process can desalinate water, as well as remove microbiologic contamination. If pressure or degradation causes breakdown of the membrane, treatment effectiveness is lost. Even *Giardia* cyst passage has been shown to occur in a compromised reverse-osmosis unit.[83]

Small, hand-pump reverse-osmosis units have been developed. Their high price and slow output currently prohibit use by land-based wilderness travelers, but they are important survival items for ocean travelers. Battery- or power-operated units are standard equipment on large boats. The U.S. Department of Defense uses large-scale mobile reverse-osmosis units for water treatment. These are considered the most fuel-efficient mobile units, producing the highest-quality water from the greatest variety of raw water qualities, capable of producing potable water from fresh, brackish, or salt water, as well as from water contaminated by nuclear, biologic, or chemical agents. The military units use pretreatment, filtration, and desalination, then disinfection for storage.[319]

Forward Osmosis

Osmotic pressure also can be used to draw water through a membrane to create highly purified drinking water from low-quality source water, including brackish water. These products use a double-chamber bag or container with the membrane in between. A high-osmotic substance is added to the clean side, which draws water from the dirty side. Because some form of sugar and/or salt is often used to create osmotic pressure, this may result in a sweetened solution similar to a sports-electrolyte drink (see Appendix A).

Choice of Filter (See Preferred Technique and Appendix A)

Because of their use at the household level in developing countries, ceramic filters have been tested most extensively.[104] They are effective at reducing turbidity and improving microbiologic quality, second only to chlorine for reducing microbial contamination.[21,65,67,298] Many designs function by gravity, an advantage for developing countries. As with all types of filters, results depend on the characteristics of the materials (e.g., ceramic, diatomaceous earth), water quality, product engineering, and prior extent of filter use.

There are extensive data on the effectiveness of filtration in other settings, but few data are available to compare different filters for field use. Most data for portable filters are from testing contracted by the filter manufacturer, and almost all filters perform well. Schlosser and colleagues[283] tested three hand-pump filters (Katadyn Mini Ceramic, First Need Deluxe, and SweetWater WalkAbout), all of which removed 3 log (99.9%) or more of viable bacteria, leaving none in the effluent.[180] Effectiveness often varies from laboratory to actual product use in the field.[354]

The military preventive medicine group has enumerated requirements for individual filters for field use.[318] Choice should be based on anticipated water quality, number of persons to be served, mode of travel and need for portability, and availability of power source. Hollow-microfiber filters, adapted from medicine and industry, are a recent addition to point-of-use field filtration.

For domestic use and in pristine protected watersheds where pollution is minimal and the main concerns are bacteria and protozoan cysts, microfiltration can be used as the only means of disinfection. For foreign travel and for surface water with high levels of human use or sewage contamination, higher levels of filtration or supplemental methods should be used.[104] Ultrafiltration or nanofiltration, now available with hollow-fiber technology, or reverse osmosis is an alternative. Otherwise, additional treatment with heat or halogens before or after filtration guarantees effective virus removal.[257] One rational use of filtration is to clear the water of sediment and organic debris, allowing lower doses of halogens with more predictable residual levels.[221] Microfilters are also useful as a first step to remove parasites and *Cryptosporidium* organisms that have high resistance to halogens. Bacteria can grow in filters, so filter media are sometimes coated with silver to prevent bacterial growth on the surface, but this does not maintain sterility (see Silver, later).

Improvised Filters

Filtration using simple, available products is of interest for use in developing countries and in emergency situations.[294] Rice hull, ash filters, crushed charcoal, sponges, and various fabrics have all been used. Typically, bacteria and viruses can be reduced by as much as 50% to 85% and larger parasites by 99%, depending on the media. Fine woven cotton fabric is effective at removing larger parasites, such as schistosome cercariae, *Fasciola* species, and guinea worm larvae.

The effectiveness at decreasing turbidity may be used as an indicator that any filter material will reduce microbiologic contamination (see Turbidity and Clarification, earlier). A comparison of three locally available clarification techniques (cloth filtration, settling/decanting, and sand filtration) on turbidity and chlorine demand demonstrated that all three mechanisms reduced turbidity: cloth filtration, 1% to 60%; settling/decanting, 78% to 88%; and sand filtration, 57% to 99%. Sand filtration and settling/decanting, but not cloth filtration, were effective at reducing chlorine demand compared with controls.[169] Lantagne and associates[177] noted that in a small number of surface water samples tested with moderate turbidity (>2 NTU), cloth filtration reduced turbidity by 18% to 52%.

Kozlicic and associates[170] tested five commonly available household materials (newspaper, filter paper, cotton, four-layer gauze, and white cotton cloth) for filtration efficiency. Newspaper performed poorly, being too slow. Cotton cloth performed best for both physical and microbiologic parameters of water (although the latter was poorly studied). The authors incidentally noted that melted snow with the top 4 to 5 cm (1.6 to 2 inches) removed was a better-quality water source than rainwater from roof runoff.[170]

Biosand Filters

Sand filters employ a technology that has been proved over centuries of time and is still used widely in municipal plants and at the household and community level. When constructed properly, they are very reliable, but with slow flow rates. Sand filters are highly effective at removing turbidity (in one study, reduced from 6.2 to 0.9 NTU) and improving microbiologic quality (99% efficacy).[98,255] Sand filters are constructed by forming layers of aggregate increasing in size from the top to the bottom. The top layer is very fine sand, and the bottom layer consists of large gravel. The container needs an exit port on the bottom. Water on the top layer forms a biolayer where microorganisms "eat" the pathogens that pass through them. Over time, the biolayer grows to the point where it will not allow any water to pass through. At this point, the layer needs to be removed by either drying out the layer and then removing it, or stirring it up and removing dirty water from the top[21] (Figure 88-2).

The optimum depth of a community or household sand filter is 2 m (6.6 feet), with diameter determined by the volume of water needed; however, a sand filter can be improvised with stacked buckets or barrels. For example, an emergency sand filter can be made in a 20-L (5.3-gal) bucket, composed of a 10-cm (4-inch) layer of gravel beneath a 23-cm (9.1-inch) layer of sand; a layer of cotton cloth, sandwiched between two layers of wire mesh, separates the sand and gravel layers.[169]

CHEMICAL DISINFECTANTS

HALOGENS (CHLORINE AND IODINE)

Worldwide, chemical disinfection is the most widely used method for improving and maintaining microbiologic quality of drinking water. Chemical disinfectants used for water disinfection are strong oxidants. *Halogens*, chiefly chlorine and iodine, are the most common chemical disinfectants used in the field. Chlorine dioxide is now available for small-use field applications and gaining acceptance. Germicidal activity results from oxidation of essential cellular structures and enzymes.[57,178,201,221,226] Halogenated amines may be synthesized by white blood cells as part of the body's natural defenses to destroy microorganisms.[335] The disinfection process is determined by characteristics of the disinfectant, the microorganism, and environmental factors.[59,144,218]

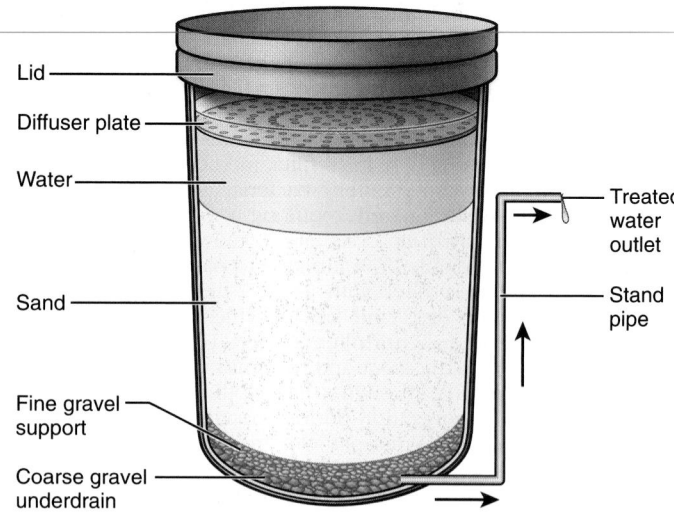

FIGURE 88-2 Biosand filter can be improvised from local materials. This may not function as well as an optimally constructed and operated biosand filter, but will significantly improve clarity and microbial content of the water.

Dilute solutions do not sterilize water. The relative potency of common disinfectants to inactivate waterborne microbes is as follows:

ozone > chlorine dioxide > electrochemically generated mixed-species oxidant > free chlorine or iodine > chloramine

Ozone and chlorine dioxide are discussed later under Miscellaneous Disinfectants.

Variables With Chemical Agents

Understanding the principal factors of chemical disinfection allows intelligent and flexible use (Table 88-7).

Concentration and Contact Time. The major variables in the disinfection reaction are amount of disinfectant (concentration) and exposure time of the microorganism to the disinfectant (contact time). Concentration of disinfectant in water is measured in parts per million (ppm) or milligrams per liter (mg/L), which

TABLE 88-7	Factors Affecting Halogen Disinfection	
	Effect	**Compensation**
Primary Factors		
Concentration	Measured in milligrams per liter (mg/L) or the equivalent, parts per million (ppm); higher concentration increases rate and proportion of microorganisms killed.	Higher concentration allows shorter contact time for equivalent results. Lower concentration requires increased contact time for equivalent levels of kill.
Contact time	Usually measured in minutes; longer contact time ensures higher proportion of organisms killed.	Contact time is inversely related to concentration; longer time allows lower concentration.
Secondary Factors		
Temperature	Cold slows reaction time.	Some treatment protocols recommend doubling the dose (concentration) of halogen in cold water, but if time allows, exposure time can be increased instead, or the temperature of the water can be increased.
Water contaminants, cloudy water (turbidity)	Halogens reacts with organic nitrogen compounds from decomposition of organisms and their wastes to form compounds with little or no disinfecting ability, effectively decreasing the concentration of available halogen. In general, turbidity increases halogen demand.	Doubling the dose of halogen for cloudy water is a crude means of compensation that often results in a strong disinfectant taste on top of the taste of the contaminants. A more rational approach is first to clarify water to reduce halogen demand.
pH	The optimal pH for disinfection is 6.5-7.5. As water becomes more alkaline, approaching pH 8.0, much higher doses of halogens are required.	Compensating for pH is not necessary for most surface water.

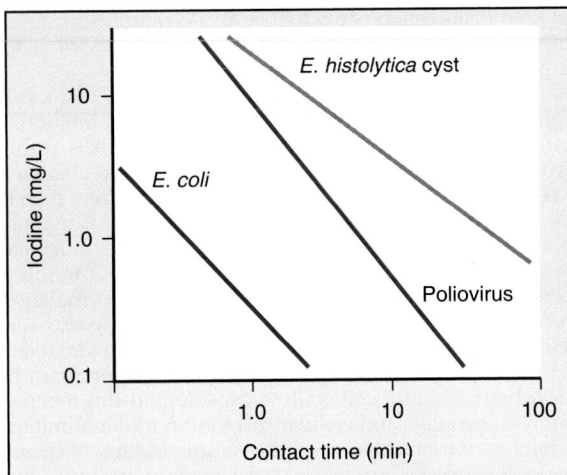

FIGURE 88-3 Relationship of halogen concentration and contact time for a given temperature and pH. The first-order chemical reaction results in a straight line over most values for each microorganism and halogen compound. *(Data from Chang SL: The use of active iodine as a water disinfectant, J Am Pharm Assoc 47:417, 1958; and Water and Sanitation for Health [WASH] Project: Report on mobile emergency water treatment and disinfection units, WASH Field Report No 217, 1980, Arlington, Va.)*

are equivalent. Contact time is usually measured in minutes but ranges from seconds to hours. In field disinfection, halogen (iodine or chlorine) concentrations of 1 to 10 mg/L for 10 to 60 minutes are generally effective.

Theoretically, the disinfection reaction follows first-order kinetics. The rate of the reaction is determined by the initial concentration of reactants, and a given proportion of the reaction occurs in any specified interval.[144,336] This means that concentration and time are inversely related, and their product results in a constant for specified disinfectant, organism, percent reduction of viable microorganisms, and given conditions of water temperature and pH: concentration × time = constant (Ct = K)[180,336] (Figure 88-3). When concentration and contact time are graphed on logarithmic coordinates, a straight line results. This means that concentration and time can be varied oppositely and still achieve the same result.[14] In field disinfection, this can be used to minimize halogen dose and improve taste or, conversely, to minimize the required contact time.

In reality, the disinfection reaction deviates slightly from first-order kinetics, and Ct values do not follow the exponential rates described by the empirical equation because microorganisms do not act as chemical reagents ($C_n t = K$). An initial lag period may be seen before inactivation begins (e.g., because of penetration of the cyst wall), and inactivation declines for more resistant organisms or those shielded by aggregation or other particles[131,137,144] (Figure 88-4).

Contaminants. Organic and inorganic nitrogen compounds from decomposition of organisms and their wastes, fecal matter, and urea complicate chemical disinfection and must be considered in field water treatment. Vegetable matter, ferrous ions, nitrites, sulfides, and humic substances also affect oxidizing disinfectants.[100,221,336] These contaminants react, especially with chlorine, to form compounds with little or no disinfecting ability, effectively decreasing the concentration of available halogen.

Halogen Demand and Residual Concentration. Halogen demand is the amount of halogen reacting with impurities. The concept applies to all chemical disinfectant agents. Residual concentration is the amount of active disinfectant remaining after demand of the water is met. To achieve microbial inactivation in aqueous solution with a chemical agent, a residual concentration must be present for a specified contact time. Failure of chlorination in municipal systems to kill cysts or other microorganisms is usually caused by difficulty maintaining adequate residual halogen concentration and contact times, rather than by extreme resistance of the organism.[303]

Halogen demand and residual concentration in surface water are the greatest uncertainties in field disinfection and may account for laboratory efficacy being better than field effectiveness because of variability in source water.[185] Nitrogen appears in most natural waters in varying amounts, which relate directly to the sanitary quality of water. Cysticidal dose of halogens is strongly affected by the level of contamination in otherwise clean water.[59,129,303] Scant data are available on halogen demand of surface water (Table 88-8). Clear water is assumed to have minimal demand and cloudy water high demand. Surface water in the wilderness contains 10 times the organic carbon content of aquifer groundwater. The green or brown color in stagnant ponds and lakes, and in tropical and lowland rivers is usually caused by organic matter with considerable halogen demand. In some cases, such as runoff after storms and snowmelt, cloudy water may be caused by inorganic sand and clay that exert little halogen demand, but in general, chlorine demand rises with increased turbidity.[181] In addition, particulate turbidity can shield microorganisms and interfere with disinfection[85,161,181] (see Turbidity and Clarification, earlier).

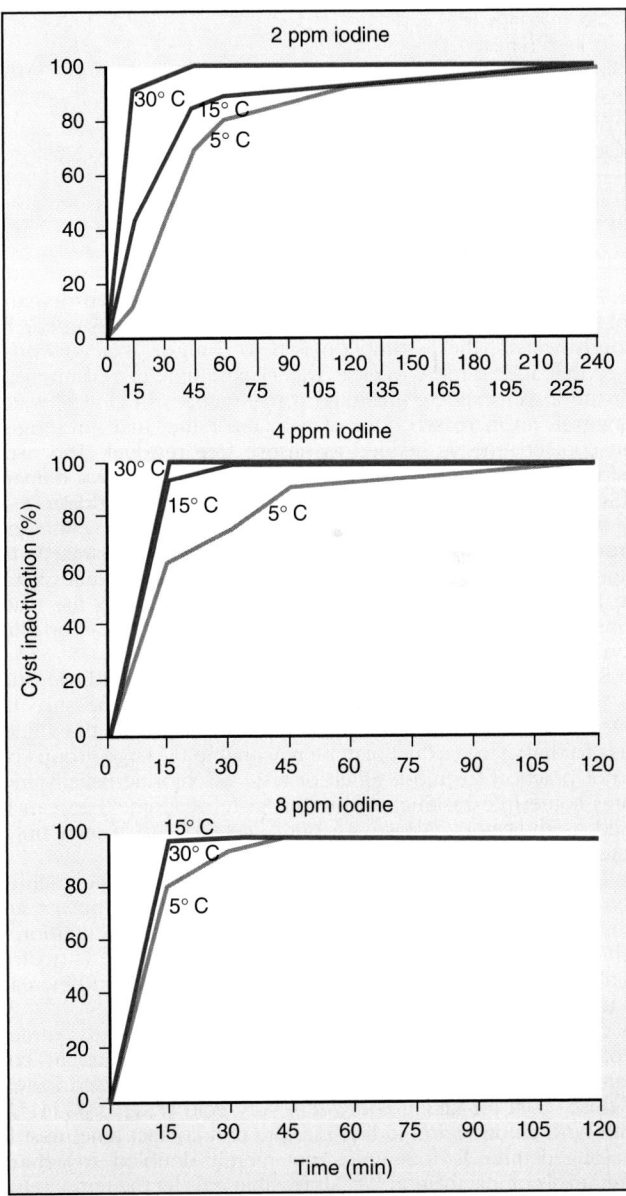

FIGURE 88-4 Effect of concentration and temperature on *Giardia* cyst inactivation by iodine. Low concentrations are effective at cold temperatures with prolonged contact time. *(From Fraker LD, Gentile D, Krivoy D, et al: Giardia cyst inactivation by iodine, J Wilderness Med 3:351, 1992.)*

TABLE 88-8	Halogen Demand of Surface Water	
Source	Halogen Demand (mg/L)	Reference
Cloudy river water, Portland, Oregon	3-4	Jarroll, 1980[154]
Cloudy water from clay particles	None	Chang, 1953[59]
Clear water with 10% sewage added	2	Chang, 1953[59]
Lily pond and turbid river water	5-6	Chang, 1953[59]
Colorado River; cloudy from inorganic sand, clay	0.3	Tunnicliff, 1984[317]
Unspecified surface waters	2-3	Culp, 1974[84]
Municipal wastewater	20-30	Culp, 1974[84]
High-elevation spring	0.3	Ongerth, 1989[231]
Western river	0.7	Ongerth, 1989[231]
Six watersheds in western Oregon	0.4-1.6	LeChevallier, 1981[181]
Small stream, Australia	1.3	Thomson, 1985[311]
Bolivian village (well and collected rain)	2	Quick, 1999[251]
Spring and well water, Haiti	≤1	Colindres, 2007[75]
Raw surface water from different sources in six different states	<1 to 17 (mean 6)	Lantagne, 2014[177]
Cloudy surface water (ponds, rivers)—household water sources in western Kenya	100-150	Crump, 2005[82]

The initial dose of halogen must consider halogen demand. For clear alpine waters, 1 mg/L demand can be assumed; for cloudy waters, the assumption is 3 to 5 mg/L. If a method is used that adds 4 mg/L to clear water, extra time can compensate for the lower expected residual concentration; in cloudy water, however, an increased dose of halogen, rather than prolonging the contact time, is needed to ensure free residual. The usual field recommendation to compensate for the unknown demand of cloudy water is a double dose of halogen (adding 8 to 16 mg/L). This crude means of compensation often results in a strong halogen taste on top of taste from contaminants. If the cause of turbidity is uncertain, the water should be allowed to sit; inorganic clay and sand will settle out, clarifying the water considerably. Other means of clarification, such as C-F or filtration, significantly reduce halogen demand.

Several simple color-strip tests are available for field use, such as those used for swimming pools and spas to measure the amount of free (residual) halogen in water. Testing in the wilderness for halogen residual may be reasonable for large groups but is not practical for most. Smell or taste of chlorine usually indicates some free residual. Color and taste of iodine also can be used as indicators. Above 0.6 ppm, a yellow to brown tint is noted.[336]

Temperature. Temperature influences rate of the disinfection reaction.[100,178,221] Cold water affects germicidal power and must be offset by longer contact time or higher concentration to achieve comparable disinfection.[128] The common rule is twofold to threefold increase in inactivation rate per 10°C (18°F) increase in temperature.

Temperature can be estimated in the field. Some treatment protocols recommend doubling the dose of halogen in cold water, but if there is no urgency, time can be increased instead of dose. Data for killing *Giardia* in very cold water (5°C [41°F]) with both chlorine and iodine indicate that contact time must be prolonged three to four times, not merely doubled, to achieve high levels of inactivation.[114,138] If feasible, raising the temperature by 10° to 20°C (18° to 36°F) allows a lower dose of halogen and more reliable disinfection at a given dose.

pH. Halogen oxidizes in water to form several compounds, each with different disinfection capabilities. The percentage of each halogen compound is determined by pH. The optimal pH

for halogen disinfection is 6.5 to 7.5.[59,217] As water becomes more alkaline, approaching pH 8.0, much higher doses of halogens are required.

Although pH can be measured in the field, the relationship is too complex to allow meaningful use of the information. Most surface water pH is neutral to mildly acidic, which is within the effective range of any chemical agent used. On the alkaline side, some surface water with pH 7.0 to 8.0 begins to affect the chemical species of chlorine, favoring less active forms.[144] Certain desert water is so alkaline that halogens would have little activity; however, these waters are usually not palatable. At this time, compensating for pH is not necessary. Tablet formulations of halogen have the advantage of some buffering capacity.

Susceptibility of Microorganisms. The final variable is the target microorganism. Sensitivity to halogen is determined by the diffusion barrier of the cell wall or capsule and the relative susceptibility of proteins and cellular respiration to denaturation and oxidation.[57,221] Organisms, in order of increasing resistance to halogen disinfection, are enteric (vegetative) bacteria, viruses, *Giardia* cysts, bacterial spores, *Cryptosporidium* oocysts, and parasitic ova[54] (Tables 88-9 and 88-10). For example, *Entamoeba histolytica* cysts are 160 times as resistant as *E. coli* and nine times as resistant as hardier enteroviruses to chlorine (HOCl). Virucidal residuals of iodine (I_2) and HOCl are 5 to 70 times higher than bactericidal residuals.[57,180,221,320] Relative resistance between organisms is similar for iodine and chlorine. The physical state of the microbes also determines their susceptibility. Microbes that are aggregated in clumps or embedded in other matter or organisms may be shielded from disinfectants.

Bacteria. All vegetative bacteria are extremely sensitive to halogens. Inactivation involves oxidation of enzymes on the cell membrane and does not require penetration.[336] Little modern work has focused on bacterial agents because they are more sensitive than viruses and cysts, and little difference is evident between the bacterial pathogens.[144] Although halogens were first used to disinfect water during cholera epidemics in 1850, recent cholera epidemics prompted review of data that reaffirmed the susceptibility of *Vibrio cholerae* to low levels of chlorine and iodine.[80] *Campylobacter* has susceptibility similar to that of other enteric pathogens.[29]

Bacterial spores, such as *Bacillus anthracis*, are relatively resistant to halogens, but with chlorine, spores are not much more resistant than are *Giardia* cysts.[14,336] Quantitative data are not available for iodine solutions, but iodine kills spores. Fortunately, sporulating bacteria do not normally cause waterborne enteric disease.[142]

Viruses. Enteroviruses are more resistant than are enteric bacteria,[221] but they constitute such a large and diverse group of organisms that generalization is especially difficult.[58,178,322] Most studies have used poliovirus, a phage virus, or coxsackievirus. The mechanism of action for halogen inactivation of viruses has not been resolved. It is not clear whether the oxidant injures protein on the shell, a process similar to bacterial inactivation,[35] or penetrates the protein capsid by chemical transformation and then attacks the nucleic acid core, as in cyst inactivation.[336] Clumping and association of viruses with cells and particulate matter are thought to be significant factors affecting viral disinfection, causing departure from first-order kinetics.[102,295,325] Cell-associated HAV was 10 times more resistant than was dispersed HAV.

Most viruses tested against chlorine have shown resistance 10 times greater than that of enteric bacteria, but inactivation is still achieved rapidly (0.3 to 4.5 minutes) with low levels (0.5 mg/L) of chlorine.[102,325] Recent work with norovirus has refuted claims that it is highly resistant to chlorine.[164,288] Current data suggest that HAV is not significantly more resistant than other enteric viruses.[129,241,296,312] In one test using iodine tablets, HAV was inactivated under difficult conditions more readily than was poliovirus or echovirus.[295,296]

Cysts and Parasites. Protozoal cysts are considerably more resistant than are enteric bacteria and enteric viruses, probably because of cysts' physiologically inactive outer shell, which the disinfectant must penetrate to be effective.[57,336] Halogens can be used in the field to inactivate *Giardia* cysts (see Figure 88-4).[320] Testing on *G. lamblia* indicates similar sensitivity to both

TABLE 88-9 Disinfection Data for Chlorine*

Halogen†	Organism	Concentration (mg/L)	Time (min)	pH	Temp	Disinfection Constant (Ct)	Reference
HOCl	*Escherichia coli*	0.1	0.16	6.0	5°C (41°F)	.016	White, 1992[336]
FAC	*Campylobacter*	0.3	0.5	6.0-8.0	25°C (77°F)	0.15	Blaser,1986[28]
FRC	20 enteric virus	0.5	60	7.8	2°C (35.6°F)	30	Briton,1980[34]
Free Cl	6 enteric viruses	0.5	4.5	6.0-8.0	5°C (41°F)	2.5	Engelbrecht, 1980[102]
Free Cl	Norovirus	1	10	6.0	5°C (41°F)	10	Shin, 2008[288]
		5	20 sec			1.66	
FRC	Hepatitis A virus	0.5	1	6.0	25°C (77°F)	0.5	Grabow, 1983[129]
Free Cl	Hepatitis A virus	0.5	5	6.0	5°C (41°F)	2.5‡	Sobsey, 1975[293]
HOCl	Amebic cysts	3.5	10		25°C (77°F)	35	Chang, 1970[57]
FRC	Amebic cysts	3.0	10	7.0	30°C (86°F)	30	Stringer, 1970[303]
Free Cl	*Giardia* cysts	2.5	60	6.0-8.0	5°C (41°F)	150	Rice, 1982[263]
Free Cl	*Giardia lamblia* cysts	0.85	90	8.0	2°-3°C (35.6°-37.4°F)	77	Wallis, 1988[332]
Free Cl	*Giardia muris* cysts	3.05	50	7.0	5°C (41°F)	153	Rubin, 1989[279]
Free Cl	*G. muris* cysts	5.87	25	7.0	5°C (41°F)	139	Rubin, 1989[279]
Free Cl	*Giardia*			6.0	0.5°C (32.9°F)	170	Hibler, 1987[138]
Free Cl	*Giardia*			6.0	5°C (41°F)	120	Hibler, 1987[138]
Free Cl	*Cryptosporidium*	80	90			7200	Korich,1990[168]
FRC	Schistosome cercariae	1.0	30	7.0	28°C (82.4°F)	30	WHO, 1981[344]
Free Cl	Nematodes	2-3	120			(Not lethal)	NAS, 1980[221]
Free Cl	Nematodes	95-100	30			(95% lethal)	NAS, 1980[221]
FRC	*Ascaris* eggs	200	20	5.0	37°C (98.6°F)	2000	Krishnaswami, 1968[172]

FAC, Free active chlorine; *FRC*, free residual chlorine; *Free Cl*, free chlorine; *HOCl*, hypochlorous acid; *NAS*, National Academy of Sciences; *WHO*, World Health Organization.
*Also see reference 54. For Ct values of chlorine for *Giardia*, also see reference 320.
†These represent nearly equivalent measurements of the residual concentration of active chlorine disinfectant compounds.
‡Four-log reduction. Most experiments use 2- to 3-log (99% to 99.9%) reduction as the end point.

iodine and chlorine.[156] Lower temperature decreases effectiveness of halogens on *Giardia*: longer contact time is required in cold and dirty water.[121,137,153,295] Review literature frequently attributes exaggerated resistance of *Giardia* to halogens.[143] Jarroll and colleagues[154,155] tested two chlorine methods and four iodine methods for effectiveness against *Giardia* cysts. All methods were effective in warm water, but only two methods destroyed all cysts in cold water in recommended doses. Higher doses or longer contact times would make all these methods effective.

Cryptosporidium oocysts differ greatly from other protozoan cysts and are highly resistant to halogens. The Ct constant for *Cryptosporidium* in warm water with chlorine has been estimated to be 9600.[45] Other data demonstrated 90% inactivation with 80 ppm of chlorine after 90 minutes, 14 times more resistant than

Giardia cysts.[168] Recent data using hypochlorous acid demonstrate a maximum inactivation rate for *Cryptosporidium* of 49% after 120 minutes.[237] The current recommendation for decontaminating chlorinated swimming pools is 20 mg for 9 hours (Ct 10,800).[39] From 65% to 80% of *Cryptosporidium* oocysts were inactivated after 4 hours by two iodine tablets in "general case" water.[121] This implies that 3-log inactivation could have been achieved after 3 to 4 more hours. Although halogens can achieve disinfection of *Cryptosporidium* in the field, this is not practical.[86,273,284,336] Resistance of *Cyclospora* and microsporidia is not well studied, but the oocysts are similar to *Cryptosporidium* and thus may resemble this protozoan more than they do *Giardia*. Both *Cryptosporidium* and *Giardia* are susceptible to chlorine dioxide.[54,168,237]

TABLE 88-10 Disinfection Data for Iodine

Halogen*	Organism	Concentration (mg/L)	Time (min)	pH	Temp	Disinfection Constant (Ct)	Reference
FRI	*Escherichia coli*	1.3	1	6.0-7.0	2°-5°C (35.6°-41°F)	1.3	National Academy of Sciences, 1980[221]
I₂	Amebic cysts	3.5	10		25°C (77°F)	35	Chang, 1970[57]
I₂	Amebic cysts	6.0	5		25°C (77°F)	30	Chang, 1970[57]
I₂	Amebic cysts	12.5	2		25°C (77°F)	25	Chang, 1970[57]
FRI	Poliovirus 1	1.25	39	6.0	25°C (77°F)	49	Berg, 1964[17]
FRI	Poliovirus 1	12.7	5	6.0	25°C (77°F)	63	Berg, 1964[17]
I₂	Poliovirus 1	1	6	7.0	18°C (64.4°F)	6	Berg, 1964[17]
I₂	Coxsackievirus	0.5	30	7.0	5°C (41°F)	15	Berg, 1964[17]
I₂	Amebic cysts	8	10	4.0-8.0	23°C (73.4°F)	80	Chang, 1953[59]
I₂	Bacteria, viruses	8	20		0°-5°C (32°-41°F)	160	Chang, 1953[59]
FRI	*Giardia* cysts	4	15	5.0	30°C (86°F)	60†	Fraker, 1992[114]
FRI	*Giardia* cysts	4	45	5.0	15°C (59°F)	170†	Fraker, 1992[114]
FRI	*Giardia* cysts	4	120	5.0	5°C (41°F)	480†	Fraker, 1992[114]

*FRI (free residual iodine) and I₂ (elemental iodine) are nearly equivalent measurements of the residual concentration of active iodine disinfectant compounds.
†100% kill; viability tested only at 15, 30, 45, 60, and 120 minutes.

Schistosome cercariae are susceptible to low concentrations of chlorine.[339] Limited data on parasitic helminth larvae and ova indicate the presence of such high levels of resistance that chemical disinfection is not useful.[172,221,287] However, these are not common waterborne pathogens and can be readily removed or destroyed by heat, filtration, or coagulation-flocculation.

Disinfection Constant. Given all the variables, the best comparison of disinfection power is the disinfection constant (Ct). Disparate results may be caused by lack of standardized experimental conditions of pH, temperature, chemical species of

TABLE 88-12 Recommendations for Contact Time With Halogens in the Field

Concentration of Halogen	Contact Time in Minutes at Various Water Temperatures		
	5°C (41°F)	15°C (59°F)	30°C (86°F)
2 ppm	240	180	60
4 ppm	180	60	45
8 ppm	60	30	15

Note: Data indicate that very cold water requires prolonged contact time with iodine or chlorine to kill *Giardia* cysts. These contact times have been extended from the usual recommendations in cold water to account for this and for the uncertainty of residual concentration.

TABLE 88-11 Water Disinfection Techniques and Halogen Doses

Iodination Techniques	Add to 1 Liter or Quart of Water	
	Amount for 4 ppm	Amount for 8 ppm
Iodine tablets	0.5 tab	1 tab
Tetraglycine hydroperiodide		
EDWGT		
Potable Aqua		
Globaline		
2% iodine solution (tincture)	0.2 mL	0.4 mL
	5 gtt*	10 gtt
10% povidone-iodine solution†	0.35 mL	0.70 mL
	8 gtt	16 gtt
Saturated solution: iodine crystals in water	13 mL	26 mL
Saturated solution: iodine crystals in alcohol	0.1 mL‡	0.2 mL

Chlorination Techniques§‖	Amount for 5 ppm§§	Amount for 10 ppm
Sodium hypochlorite (household bleach 5%)	0.1 mL	0.2 mL
	2 gtt	4 gtt
Sodium hypochlorite (household bleach 8.25%)	1 gtt	
1% bleach (CDC-WHO Safe Water System)¶	8-10 gtt	
Calcium hypochlorite** (Redi-Chlor [0.1-g tab])	0.25 tab	0.5 tab
Sodium dichloroisocyanurate (NaDCC)†† (Aquatab, Kintab)		1 tab (8.5 mg NaDCC)
Chlorine plus flocculating agent (Chlor-Floc)		1 tab‡‡

EDWGT, Emergency drinking water germicidal tablet.
*Measure of a drop varies from 16-24 gtt/mL; standard 20 gtt/mL is used here.
†Povidone-iodine solutions release free iodine in levels adequate for disinfection, but scant data are available.
‡Measure with dropper or tuberculin syringe.
§Recommended concentration of chlorine for emergency point-of-use water treatment varies across health agencies, but generally does not exceed 5 mg/L. For long-term household use in developing areas, CDC Safe Water System establishes a maximum of 2 mg/L, which is the limit of taste tolerance for many people (see reference 176).
‖For treatment of large volumes, see reference 319 for TB MED 577, or see formula to calculate in reference 176.
¶Safe Water System for long-term routine household point-of-use water disinfection recommends a hypochlorite dose of about 2 mg/L in clear water and 4 mg/L in slightly turbid water. This results in a low yet effective target residual concentration with acceptable taste, but requires testing in a particular water source to ensure sufficient residual.
**Concentrated source of hypochlorite available as granules or tablets; useful for treating larger volumes of water; often used to treat swimming pool water.
††Available in different strengths to treat different volumes of water. Check packaging to determine proper dose.
‡‡Yields 8 ppm.
§§In usual situations, EPA recommends a target residual of 4 mg/L. For household use, CDC recommends less than 2 mg/L. Many of the recommended emergency doses exceed this threshold.[177]

halogen, and species of microorganism or by different techniques for concentrating, counting, and determining viability of organisms.[144,221] The latter is especially a problem for cysts and viruses, which cannot be cultured easily.[281] The end point for disinfection effectiveness is now standardized by the EPA guidelines; most past studies used 99.9% for all organisms, with some using 99% or 99.99%. Differences between laboratory and field conditions also make extrapolation from data to practice inaccurate and suggest the need for a safety factor in the field. Despite variation, Ct remains a useful and widely used concept; values provide a basis for comparing effectiveness of different disinfectants for inactivation of specific microorganisms.[144,180,320] To use halogens for disinfection, a consensus organism (the most resistant target) determines the Ct.[144,178,336] For wilderness water, this has been protozoan cysts. Resistance of *Cryptosporidium* will not raise the threshold for halogen use; rather, it will force an alternative or a combination of methods to ensure removal and inactivation of all pathogens.

CHLORINE

Chlorine has been used as a disinfectant for 200 years. Hypochlorite was first used for water disinfection in 1854 during cholera epidemics in London and was first used continuously for water treatment in Belgium in 1902. It is currently the preferred means of municipal water disinfection worldwide and the preference of CDC and WHO for individual household disinfection of drinking water where there is no community-level treatment. It is also recommended for emergency disinfection following disasters or other disruption in community treatment.[176] Extensive data support its use (see Table 88-9).[21,54,336]

Chemistry

Chlorine reacts in water to form the following compounds[100,201,336]:

$$Cl_2 + H_2O \rightarrow H^+ + Cl^-$$

$$HOCl \rightarrow OCl^- + H^+$$

At neutral pH, negligible amounts of diatomic chlorine are present. The major disinfectant is hypochlorous acid (HOCl), which penetrates cell and cyst walls easily. Dissociation of HOCl to the much weaker disinfectant hypochlorite (OCl⁻) depends on temperature and pH. In pure water at pH 6.0, 97% of chlorine is HOCl; at pH 7.5, the HOCl/OCl⁻ ratio is 1:1; and above pH 7.5, OCl⁻ predominates.[336] The combination of these two compounds is defined as free available chlorine. Both calcium hypochlorite (Ca[OCl]₂) and sodium hypochlorite (NaOCl) readily dissociate in water, allowing the same equilibrium to form as when elemental chlorine is used.[178,336] Chloride ion (Cl⁻, NaCl, or CaCl₂) is germicidally inactive. In addition, chlorine readily reacts with ammonia to form monochloramines (NH₂Cl), dichloramines, or trichloramines, referred to as *combined chlorine*. Chloramines have weak disinfecting power and are calculated as a disinfectant

TABLE 88-13 Chlorine Dose for Large-Volume Water Disinfection

$$
\begin{aligned}
\text{Dose } (mg_{Cl}/L_{water}) = &\left(\text{Bleach concentration (\%)} \times \frac{10,000\ mg_{Cl}/L_{Cl}}{1\%} \right.\\
&\left. \times \text{Bleach added } (mL_{Cl}) \times \frac{1\ L_{Cl}}{1000\ mL_{Cl}} \right)\\
&/(\text{Volume of water } (L_{water}))
\end{aligned}
$$

From Lantagne D, Person B, Smith N, et al: Emergency water treatment with bleach in the United States: the need to revise EPA recommendations, *Environ Sci Technol* 48(9):5093-5100, 2014.

in municipal sewage plants.[144,201,217,221,336] In field disinfection, however, these compounds are not considered, and only free residual chlorine should be measured. At doses of a few milligrams per liter and contact times of about 30 minutes, free chlorine generally inactivates greater than 99.99% of enteric bacteria and viruses.[297] The CDC-WHO Safe Water System for household disinfection in developing countries provides a dosage of 1.875 or 3.75 mg/L of sodium hypochlorite with a contact time of 30 minutes, sufficient to inactivate most bacteria, viruses, and some protozoa that cause waterborne diseases (http://www.cdc.gov/safewater/).[169] Chlorine bleaches organic matter, making water sparkling blue, as in swimming pools.[336]

Toxicity

Acute toxicity to chlorine is limited; the main danger is irritation and corrosion of mucous membranes if concentrated solutions (e.g., household bleach) are ingested. Numerous cases have been reported of short-term ingestion of very high residuals (50 to 90 ppm) in drinking water; one military study used 32 ppm for several months without adverse effects.[336] Animal studies using long-term chlorination of drinking water at 100 to 200 ppm have not shown toxic effects.[221]

Sodium hypochlorite is not carcinogenic; however, reactions of chlorine with certain organic contaminants yield chlorinated hydrocarbons, chloroform, and other trihalomethanes, which are considered carcinogenic.[221,322] Public health regulations limit residual chlorine in public systems to decrease ingestion of trihalomethane. The concern is now fueled more by public fears than by scientific conclusion.[336] The risk for death from infectious diseases if disinfection is not used is much greater than any risk from chlorine disinfection byproducts.[265,322,347] These compounds are not likely to form in clean wilderness surface water, because the organic precursors are not present.

Products and Techniques for Chlorination

Free chlorine is the most widely available and affordable of chemical water disinfectants.[297] For household or field water treatment, free chlorine can be obtained in liquid, granular, and tablet forms or generated from electrolysis of salt (Appendix B; for dosage information, see Tables 88-11 to 88-13). Tablets have the advantage of easy administration and can be salvaged if the container breaks. However, they lose effectiveness with exposure to heat, air, or moisture. No significant loss of potency results from opening a glass bottle intermittently over weeks, but activity is rapidly lost after a few days of continuous exposure to air with high heat and humidity. To extend shelf life, many tablets are individually wrapped in foil.

Superchlorination-Dechlorination. The process of superchlorination-dechlorination with different reagents is used in some large-scale disinfection plants to avoid long contact times and to remove tastes and smells. High doses of chlorine remove or oxidize hydrogen sulfide and some other chemical contaminants that contribute to poor taste and odor. This method of chlorination can readily be adapted to field use. High doses of chlorine are added to the water in the form of calcium hypochlorite crystals to achieve concentrations of 30 to 200 ppm of

free chlorine. These extremely high levels are above the margin of safety for field conditions and rapidly kill all bacteria, viruses, and protozoa and could kill *Cryptosporidium* with a contact time of several hours or overnight. After at least 10 to 15 minutes, several drops of 30% hydrogen peroxide solution are added. This reduces hypochlorite to chloride, forming calcium chloride (a common food additive), which remains in solution, as follows:

$$Ca(OCl)_2 + H_2O_2 \rightarrow 2HOCl + Ca^{2+}(OH^-)_2$$

$$Ca(OCl)_2 + H_2O_2 \rightarrow CaCl_2 + 2H_2O + 2O_2$$

Excess hydrogen peroxide reacts with water to form oxygen and water. Chloride has no taste or smell. Hydrogen peroxide is also a disinfectant.[201]

The minor disadvantage of a two-step process is offset by excellent taste. Measurements to titrate peroxide to the estimated amount of chlorine do not need to be exact, but some experience is needed to balance the two and achieve optimal results. This is a good technique for highly polluted or cloudy water and for disinfecting large quantities. It is the best technique for storing water on boats or for emergency use. A high level of chlorine prevents growth of algae or bacteria during storage; water is then dechlorinated in smaller quantities when ready to use.

The two reagents must be kept tightly sealed to maintain potency of the reagents. Properly stored, calcium hypochlorite (70% available chlorine) loses only 3% to 5% of available chlorine per year. Hydrogen peroxide 30% is corrosive and burns skin, so should be used cautiously. There is currently no commercial formulation; however, the ingredients can be easily obtained and packaged in small Nalgene bottles.

IODINE

Iodine has been used as a topical and water disinfectant since the beginning of the 20th century.[178,201] Iodine is effective in low concentrations for killing bacteria, viruses, and cysts and in higher concentrations against fungi and even bacterial spores, but it is a poor algicide[59,128,221] (see Table 88-10 and Figures 88-3 and 88-4). Iodine has been used successfully in low concentrations for continuous water disinfection of small communities.[167] Despite several advantages over chlorine disinfection, iodine has not gained general acceptance because of concern for its physiologic activity. Recently, the European Union stopped the sale of iodine products used for water disinfection.

Chemistry

Iodine is the only halogen that is a solid at room temperature. Of the halogens, it has the highest atomic weight, lowest oxidation potential, and lowest water solubility. Its disinfectant activity in water is quite complex because of formation of various chemical intermediates with variable germicidal efficiency. Seven different ions or molecules are present in pure aqueous iodine solutions, but only elemental (diatomic) iodine (I_2) and hypoiodous acid (HOI) play major roles as germicides. Diatomic iodine reacts in water to form the following compounds[59,128]:

$$I_2 + H_2O \rightarrow HOI + I^- + H^+$$

I_2 is two to three times as cysticidal and six times as sporicidal as HOI, because it more easily diffuses through the cyst wall. Conversely, HOI is 40 times as virucidal and three to four times as bactericidal as I_2, because inactivation of organisms depends directly on oxidation potential, without involving cell wall diffusion.[57] Their relative concentrations are determined by pH and concentration of iodine in solution.[59] At pH 7.0 and 0.5 ppm of iodine, the concentrations of I_2 and HOI are approximately equal, resulting in a broad spectrum of germicidal action. At pH 5.0 to 6.0, most of the iodine is present as I_2, whereas at pH 8.0, 12% is present as I_2 and 88% as HOI. At higher concentrations of iodine, more HOI is present. Under field conditions, I_2 is the major disinfectant for which doses are calculated.[59]

Iodide is important because it readily forms when reducing substances are added to iodine solution. Iodide ion is without any effect for water disinfection and also has no taste or color, but is still physiologically active.

Toxicity

The main disadvantage of iodine is its physiologic activity, with effects on thyroid function, potential toxicity, and allergenicity.[236] Acute toxic responses generally result from intentional overdoses of iodine, with corrosive effects in the GI tract leading to hemorrhagic gastritis. Mean lethal dose is probably about 2 to 4 g (0.07 to 0.14 oz) of free iodine or 29.6 to 59.1 mL (1 to 2 oz) of strong tincture.[111] Iodide is absorbed into the bloodstream but has minimal toxicity (thus its use for radiographic imaging).

Sensitivity reactions, including rashes and acne, may occur with usual supplementation levels of iodine. Given the physiologic necessity of iodine, it is not clear why some people react to certain forms of the substance, such as iodized salt. As with other sensitivity reactions, these may occur with very low doses. Acute allergy to iodide is rare and manifests as individual hypersensitivity, such as angioneurotic and laryngeal edema.[236]

Chronic iodide poisoning, or iodism, occurs after prolonged ingestion of sufficiently high doses, but marked individual variation is seen. Symptoms simulate upper respiratory illness, with irritation of mucous membranes, mucus production, and cough.

Thyroid Effects of Iodine Ingestion. Iodine is an essential element for normal thyroid function and health in small amounts of 100 to 300 mcg/day. Excess amounts can result in thyroid dysfunction. Maximum safe level and duration of iodine ingestion are not clearly defined, making it difficult to provide recommendations for prolonged use in water treatment.

Most persons can tolerate high doses of iodine without development of thyroid abnormalities,[33] because the thyroid gland has an autoregulatory mechanism that effectively manages excessive iodine intake. Initially, excess iodine suppresses production of thyroid hormone, but production usually returns to normal in a few days.

Iodine-induced hyperthyroidism can result from iodine ingestion by persons with underlying thyroid disease or when iodine is given to persons with prior iodine deficiency.[33,278] During the worldwide campaign to eliminate endemic goiter and cretinism, 1% to 2% of residents developed hyperthyroidism from small amounts of dietary iodine supplementation. Groups at higher risk were older adults, Graves disease patients (especially after antithyroid therapy), and patients taking pharmacologic sources of iodine. Hyperthyroidism has been reported from iodine use as a water disinfectant in two travelers. Both were from iodine-sufficient areas and had antithyroid antibodies, suggesting underlying thyroiditis; one had a mother and sister with Hashimoto's thyroiditis.[187]

Iodine-induced hypothyroidism or goiter is much more common from excessive iodine intake. Hypothyroidism is attributed to prolonged suppression of thyroid hormone production induced by excess iodine levels, but the mechanism through which iodide goiter is produced is not well understood. The incidence of goiter varies and does not correlate well with quantity of iodine or with the level of hypothyroidism. Goiters were discovered among a group of Peace Corps volunteers in Africa and were linked epidemiologically to the use of iodine resin water filters.[114,165] Forty-four (46%) of the volunteers had enlarged thyroids, but 30 of these had normal thyroid function tests.

Iodine-induced hypothyroidism or goiter may occur with or without underlying thyroid disease but is more common in several groups[33,278,340]: (1) those with underlying thyroid problems, including prior treatment for Graves disease or subtotal thyroidectomy; (2) fetuses and infants, from placental transfer of iodide from mothers treated with iodides; (3) persons with subclinical hypothyroidism, especially older adults, in whom the incidence is 5% to 10%; and (4) patients with excessive iodide from medications (formerly potassium iodide; currently amiodarone).

Neonatal goiter is especially worrisome because it can lead to asphyxia during birth or hypothyroidism with mental impairment. Daily intakes as small as 12 mg have been reported to produce congenital iodide goiters, but generally, much higher doses are required.

Dose-Response or Threshold Level. The reported incidences of goiter, hypothyroid effects, and hyperthyroid response vary so widely that they provide no clear dose limits.[236] These

data and other controlled trials of high doses have been reviewed.[11] The use of iodine for decades as a field water disinfectant by military and civilian populations without reports of associated clinical thyroid problems suggests that the risks are minimal and would be outweighed by the risk for enteric disease. Biochemical assays show that changes in thyroid function tests are common with excess iodine intake; however, changes in thyroid function usually remain subclinical. All changes reverted to normal within weeks to months without persistent thyroid disease.

Studying longer duration of ingestion, Freund[116] found minimal changes and no clinical problems when water with 1 mg/L of iodine was used to disinfect water at a prison for up to 3 years. Referring to the same project, Thomas and colleagues[310] reported that after 15 years of ongoing iodine use at 1 mg/L, iodinated water caused no decrease in serum concentrations of thyroxine (T_4) below normal values and no allergic reactions. Patients with prior thyroid disease had no recurrence with iodinated water; four patients with active hyperthyroidism were treated in standard fashion, and their condition remained well controlled despite the extra iodine intake. Also, 177 inmates gave birth to 181 full-term infants, and no neonatal goiters were detected.

The military studied long-term toxic effects of iodine, adding sodium iodide to drinking water at a naval base for 6 months.[216] The estimated daily dose of iodine per person was 12 mg for the first 16 weeks and 19.2 mg for the next 10 weeks. No evidence of functional changes or damage in the thyroid gland, cardiovascular system, bone marrow, eyes, or kidneys was noted. No increase in skin diseases, sensitization to iodine, or impaired wound healing or resolution of infections was evident.

Recommendations. The 2001 U.S. Department of Agriculture (USDA) Recommended Dietary Intake suggested an upper limit of 1.1 mg/day for adults, weight-adjusted for children. WHO did not set a guideline value for iodine in drinking water, because of a paucity of data and because it is not recommended for long-term disinfection.

The EPA and WHO, supported by the American Water Works Association (AWWA), have recommended iodine use for water disinfection only as an emergency measure for short periods of about 3 weeks. However, this period of short use appears arbitrary. The European Union revoked approval of iodine for water purification on October 25, 2009, and it can no longer be sold for this purpose.

Available data suggest the following:
- High levels of iodine, such as those produced by recommended doses of iodine tablets, should be limited to periods of 1 month or less.
- Iodine treatment that produces a low residual (1 mg/L or less) appears safe, even for long periods, in people with normal thyroid function. This would require very low doses of iodine added to the water or an activated charcoal stage to remove residual iodine.
- Persons planning to use iodine for a prolonged period should have their thyroid gland examined and thyroid function measured to ensure that a state of euthyroidism exists.
- The following groups should not use iodine for water treatment because of their increased susceptibility to thyroid problems:
  - Pregnant women
  - Persons with known hypersensitivity to iodine
  - Persons with a history of thyroid disease, even if controlled by medication
  - Persons with a strong family history of thyroid disease (thyroiditis)
  - Persons from areas with chronic dietary iodine deficiency

Products and Techniques for Iodination

Several formulations of iodine are available for field use. (See Tables 88-10 and 88-15 for efficacy, Table 88-11 for dosing, and Table 88-14 and Appendix B for details on commercial products, including tablets and crystalline iodine.)

Resins. Iodine can be bound to an inert resin to create a disinfectant with unique properties. These are considered "demand disinfectants" because iodine transfers from the resin

TABLE 88-14 Iodine Solutions

Preparation	Iodine (%)	Iodide (%)	Type of Solution
Iodine topical solution	2.0	2.4 (sodium)	Aqueous
Lugol solution	5.0	10.0 (potassium)	Aqueous
Iodine tincture	2.0	2.4 (sodium)	Aqueous-ethanol
Strong iodine solution	7.0	9.0 (potassium)	Ethanol (85%)

to the microorganism on contact, aided by electrostatic forces, but limited amounts of iodine dissolve in the water. Iodine binds to the wall or capsule, penetrates, and kills the organism. This effectively exposes the organisms to high iodine concentrations and allows reduced contact time compared with dilute iodine solutions. Residual iodine concentration in the water depends on the properties of the resin, temperature of the water, and presence of an activated charcoal stage.

Resins have proved effective against bacteria, viruses, and cysts but not against *C. parvum* oocysts or bacterial spores.[197] When *Cryptosporidium* oocysts were passed through a triiodide resin column, most were retained in the resin column, probably by electrostatic attraction to the resin. Of those that passed through, only a small percentage were inactivated within 30 minutes by the iodine.[324]

Data suggest that both contact time and iodine residual are important for optimal results.[110,196,197] Fifty percent of *Giardia* cysts were viable 10 minutes after passage through a triiodine resin. Viable *Giardia* cysts could be recovered in 4°C (39.2°F) water 40 minutes after passage through an iodine resin.[196] A simple resin filter failed to pass the EPA protocol for "worst-case" water unless water was passed through the filter twice. The data implied that a holding (contact) time could have achieved the desired results.[122] The Canadian health department, challenging an in-line triiodine resin with highly polluted water, also found that a 15-minute contact time was necessary for warm water and 30-minute contact time for cold water.[6,103] The EPA conducted tests of triiodide resin against *E. coli* but not against other organisms, for which it relied on independent testing. It concluded that the product depends on a 0.2 ppm residual and that additional testing would be necessary below this level.

Resins are chemically and physically stable during conditions of dry storage at room temperature. Aqueous suspensions or resins retain biocidal potential for 15 years. No alteration in activity was observed after dry storage for 1 month at 50°C (122°F).[197]

Iodine Resin Filters. Iodine resins have been used for water disinfection in household or small systems and incorporated into filter designs for field use. Iodine filters are generally designed with two stages in addition to the iodine resin. A microfilter, generally 1 µm, effectively removes *Cryptosporidium*, *Giardia*, and other halogen-resistant parasitic eggs or larva. Because iodine resins kill bacteria and viruses rapidly, limited contact time is required for most water.[122] Addition of a third stage of activated charcoal removes dissolved residual, which may decrease efficacy.[196,314] In the United States, inconsistent results of product testing under variable conditions led to withdrawal of most filter models from the market. It was not clear whether failure to achieve desired results was related to inadequate contact with the resin or insufficient contact time with iodine residual. Resins are now being used in point-of-use household devices in other countries with generally good but variable microbial removal or inactivation. Significant levels of residual iodine are noted without a charcoal stage.[66]

Given some of the variability in results and uncertainty of mechanism of action, the U.S. outdoor gear companies have abandoned iodine resin–containing portable hand-pump filters, and only drink-through bottles remain on the U.S. market. Other products may still be available outside the United States or through Internet retailers.

CHLORINE VERSUS IODINE

A large body of data proves that both iodine and chlorine are effective disinfectants with adequate concentrations and contact times, except for dealing with *Cryptosporidium*.[142] Under identical water test conditions and using recommended dose and contact time, chlorine and iodine tablets are similar in their biocidal activity[243] (see Tables 88-9, 88-10, and 88-15). A few investigators have reported data suggesting ineffectiveness of common halogen preparations. Jarroll and associates[155,156] tested six methods of field disinfection and found that none achieved high levels of *Giardia* inactivation at the recommended dose and times. However, this failure simply reflected the need for longer contact times in cold water.[188] Ongerth and colleagues[232] tested seven chemical treatments for *Giardia* inactivation in clear and turbid water at 10°C (50°F). None achieved 99.9% reduction in 30

TABLE 88-15 Data on Efficacy of Chlor-Floc and Iodine Tablets

Halogen	Dose	FRC (mg/L)	Time (min)	Temperature	Organism	Log Reduction	Reference
Chlor-Floc	1 tab or 2 tabs	4-7	5	10°-20°C (50°-68°F)	Bacteria	6	Powers, 1994[244]
		4-14	20	10°-20°C (50°-68°F)	*Giardia muris*	3	
			5	10°-20°C (50°-68°F)	Rotavirus	4	
			20	10°-20°C (50°-68°F)	Poliovirus	Inadequate	
	1 tab		12	25°C (77°F)	Poliovirus	Inadequate	
Globaline	2 tabs		20	Various	Bacteria	6	
			45	5°C (41°F)	*G. muris*	3	
			20	5°C (41°F)	Rotavirus	4	
			60	5°C (41°F)	Poliovirus	60	
AquaPure	2 tabs	7-11	40	5°C (41°F)			Powers, 1992[246]
	1 tab		30-40	15°-25°C (59°-77°F)	Bacteria	6	
				15°-25°C (59°-77°F)	Rotavirus	4	
				15°-25°C (59°-77°F)	Poliovirus	2	
			20	15°-25°C (59°-77°F)	*G. muris*	2	
Globaline	2 tabs	10	60	15°C (59°F)	*Giardia*	3	Powers, 1991[245]
	1		180	5°C (41°F)	*Giardia*	3	
	2		120	5°C (41°F)	*Giardia*	3	
Iodine tablets	1 or 2	8-16	60	5°-25°C	Hepatitis A	4	Sobsey, 1991[295]
		8	60	5°C (41°F)	Poliovirus, echovirus	Insufficient	
		16	60	5°C (41°F)	Poliovirus, echovirus	4	

minutes. All iodine-based chemical methods were effective at 8 hours, but none of the chlorine preparations was effective, even after this extended time. Although these results after 30 minutes in cold water are to be expected, the 8-hour results do not conform to other experimental data on chlorine. Unfortunately, the authors did not test for residual halogen, although initial levels achieved should have been effective, and they did not test at regular time intervals to determine when the iodine methods had achieved the target reduction of organisms. Schlosser and co-workers[283] found that sodium hypochlorite tablets, sodium dichloroisocyanurate tablets, and iodine in ethanol used according to package instructions removed 2 to 3 log of bacteria in clear water, but less in turbid river water. This suggests the need for clarifying dirty water before halogen use and, if possible, providing extra contact time in any situation.

Iodine has some advantages over chlorine. Of the halogens, iodine has the lowest oxidation potential, reacts least readily with organic compounds, is least soluble, is least hydrolyzed by water, and is less affected by pH, all of which indicate that low iodine residuals should be more stable and persistent than corresponding concentrations of chlorine.[85,128,167,221] The major disadvantage is its physiologic activity.

Taste

Objectionable taste and smell are the major problems with acceptance of halogens. Most objectionable taste in treated water is derived from dissolved minerals, such as sulfur, and from chlorine compounds, chloramines, and organic nitrogen compounds, even at extremely low levels.

People are familiar with the taste of chlorine compounds; tap water usually contains 0.2 to 0.5 ppm of chlorine, swimming pools 1.5 to 3.0 ppm, and hot tubs 3.0 to 5.0 ppm. Most persons familiar with the faint taste of chlorine in water note a distinct taste at 5 ppm and a strong, unpleasant taste at 10 to 15 ppm.[271] With the promotion of chlorination for household use, focus groups on taste testing have found that the majority of CDC-WHO Safe Water System users are comfortable drinking water with a free chlorine residual of up to 2 mg/L; however, there is significant regional variation in the acceptable maximum residual, and many found the taste objectionable and unsuitable at 3 to 4 mg/L.[176] The higher sodium hypochlorite dosages necessary to ensure maintenance of chlorine residual in turbid waters exacerbate the taste and odor concerns.[169]

Elemental iodine at 1 mg/L is undetectable. Most persons can detect iodine solutions at 1.5 to 2 mg/L but do not find it objectionable.[26,85,117] Distinct taste and odor are produced by 8 ppm of iodine; however, tablets yielding these concentrations were preferred by military personnel over tincture of iodine in equivalent doses.[59,218]

Taste tolerance or preference for iodine over chlorine depends on the individual. Opposite preferences have been documented when direct comparisons are done.[229,246] Informal taste tests suggest that most persons prefer the taste of iodine to chlorine at concentrations typically used in the field. In addition, iodine forms fewer organic compounds that produce highly objectionable taste and smell.

Taste can be improved by several means (Box 88-10).

Minimizing Dose. The relationship between halogen concentration and time allows use of the minimum necessary dose, with a longer contact time (see Tables 88-9 and 88-10).

Theoretically, doubling the contact time allows a 50% reduction of halogen dose at any level. Although this relationship holds true at the higher field doses of halogens, as the levels drop, the reaction departs from mathematical models, and the straight-line graph has a "tail" (see Figure 88-4). This departure from strict first-order kinetics and the uncertainty of halogen demand in field disinfection mean that a margin of safety must be incorporated into contact times at lower doses.

Of all standard iodine doses, iodine tablets yield the highest dose (8 mg/L with an intended contact time of 10 minutes in warm water). The tablets cannot be broken in half but can be added to 2 qt instead of 1 qt of water to yield concentrations consistent with the other preparations. The recommended doses of the liquid iodine preparations yield 4 mg/L. Because even

BOX 88-10	Improving the Taste of Halogens

Decrease dose and increase contact time.
Clarify cloudy water, allowing decreased halogen.
Remove halogen.
Use granular activated charcoal to remove disinfectant.
Chemical reduction techniques
- Ascorbic acid
- Sodium thiosulfate
- Chlorination-dechlorination (uses hydrogen peroxide)

Alternative Techniques
Heat
Filtration
Chlorine dioxide
Ultraviolet irradiation
Photocatalytic (TiO_2)

clear surface water has some halogen demand, this dose of 4 mg/L should generally not be reduced for surface water, but for backing up tap water in developing countries or prefiltered water, the dose may routinely be cut in half for an added dose of 2 ppm with a few hours of contact time.[114,138,178] A similar approach can be used for chlorination methods. None of these concentrations will destroy *Cryptosporidium* oocysts.

Temperature and organic matter in the water may be manipulated. Increasing the temperature of the water, especially when initially near 5° C (41° F), decreases the Ct constant (see Tables 88-9, 88-10, and 88-15 and Figure 88-4). Filtering water before adding halogen improves the reliability of a given halogen dose by decreasing halogen demand, allowing a lower dose of halogen.[221] Sedimentation or coagulation-flocculation cleans cloudy water and lowers the required halogen dosage considerably, in addition to removing many of the contaminants that contribute to objectionable taste.

Dehalogenation. Halogen can be removed from water after the required contact time. Activated charcoal removes iodine or chlorine, allowing standard or even high doses to be used without residual taste. The relative instability of chlorine in dilute solutions can be used to decrease taste over time. Chlorine residual in an open container decreases 1 mg/L in the first hour, then 0.2 mg/L in the next 5 to 8 hours, for a total of 2.0 to 2.5 mg/L in 24 hours. UV light also depletes free chlorine.[336]

Alteration of Chemical Species (Reduction). Several chemical means are available to reduce free iodine or chlorine to iodide or chloride that have no color, smell, or taste. These forms have no disinfection action, so the techniques should be used only after the required contact time. In superchlorination-dechlorination, hydrogen peroxide "dechlorinates" water treated with calcium hypochlorite by forming calcium chloride.

Two other chemicals that may be safely used with any form of chlorine or iodine are ascorbic acid (vitamin C) and sodium thiosulfate. Ascorbic acid is widely available in crystalline or powder form. Grinding up tablets that have binders may cloud the water. Ascorbic acid is a common ingredient of flavored drink mixes, which accounts for their effectiveness in covering up the taste of halogens.[229,271] Sodium thiosulfate similarly "neutralizes" iodine and chlorine. A few granules in 1 qt of iodinated water decolorizes and removes the taste of iodine by converting it to iodide. In reaction with chlorine, it forms hydrochloric acid, which is not harmful or detectable in such dilute concentration. Thiosulfate salts are inert in vivo and poorly absorbed from the GI tract. Sodium thiosulfate is available at chemical supply stores.

Copper-zinc alloys act as catalysts to reduce free iodine and chlorine through an electrochemical reaction (see Copper and Zinc, later).

MISCELLANEOUS DISINFECTANTS
PEROXYGENS

Peroxygens are strong oxidizing agents with potent antimicrobial activity that incorporate various active forms of oxygen.[201]

Ozone

Ozone is an unstable form of oxygen, with the chemical formula O_3. In solution, it decays to O_2, producing free hydroxyl radicals. Both ozone and the hydroxyl radicals are two of the most powerful oxidants and thus are effective disinfectants, so they are widely used in municipal water treatment plants.[24,180,201,227,336] Ozone and chlorine dioxide are the only chemical disinfectants that have been demonstrated effective against *Cryptosporidium* in typical concentrations.[19,64,168,235,237]

Advantages of ozone disinfection are that it has high efficacy against all groups of microorganisms and that it produces very few disinfection byproducts.[19] Ozone is a colorless gas manufactured by passing air or oxygen through a high-voltage current discharge. The resulting ozone-rich gas is then dissolved in water, but it is not stable. Clearly this is not conducive to small, point-of-use generation, so consumers should be skeptical of techniques claiming to rely on ozone. Because it is not chemically stable after generation, no form of ozone can be used for point-of-use applications in the field.

Chlorine Dioxide

Chlorine dioxide (ClO_2), a potent biocide, has been used for many years to disinfect municipal water and in numerous other large-scale applications. Until recently, the benefits of chlorine dioxide have been limited to large-scale applications, because it is formulated as a volatile gas that must be produced on-site with sophisticated chemical-generation equipment. Newer methods enable cost-effective and portable ClO_2 generation and distribution for use in an ever-widening array of small-scale applications (Box 88-11).

For point-of-use treatment of water, chlorine dioxide is produced on site from the reaction of sodium chlorite with acid.[24,294] For example:

$$5NaClO_2 + 4HCl \rightarrow 4ClO_2 + 5NaCl + 2H_2O$$

Chlorine dioxide is not as unstable as ozone but does not produce a lasting residual. It does not form chlorinated compounds in the presence of organics and is efficacious over a wide pH range. Byproducts of chlorine dioxide are chlorite (ClO_2^-) and chlorate (ClO_3^-).

Chlorine dioxide has no taste or odor in water. It is capable of inactivating most waterborne pathogens, including *C. parvum* oocysts, at practical doses but at extended contact times of 2 to 4 hours.[64,168,219,237] It is as least as effective a bactericide as chlorine and far superior as a virucide.[201,336] There are several commercial point-of-use applications using chlorine dioxide in liquid or tablet form (see appendices at the end of this chapter).

MIXED-SPECIES DISINFECTION (ELECTROLYSIS)

Passing a current through a simple brine salt solution generates free available chlorine, as well as other "mixed-species" disinfectants that have been demonstrated effective against bacteria, viruses, and bacterial spores.[280] The process is well described and can be used on both large and small scales. It is practical and economic enough to be useful in developing areas of the world. The exact composition of the resulting solution is not well delineated because many of the compounds are evanescent and unstable. The main effect is probably caused by a combination of ClO_2, ozone, superoxides, and hypochlorous acid, giving the resulting solution greater disinfectant ability than a simple solution of sodium hypochlorite.[201] It has even been demonstrated to inactivate *Cryptosporidium*.[330] (See product appendices for more information.)

HYDROGEN PEROXIDE

Hydrogen peroxide (H_2O_2) is a strong oxidizing agent but considered a weak disinfectant for use in water treatment.[30,221,351] It is used widely as a preservative in the food industry, attractive because the byproducts are oxygen and water. In high doses (35% to 50%), H_2O_2 is a sterilant used in industry for medical and food equipment; for odor control in sewage, sludges, and landfill leachates; and for many other applications. Hydrogen peroxide is popular as a wound cleanser. It is considered nature's disinfectant because it is naturally present in milk and honey, helping to prevent spoilage.

Small doses (1 mL of 3% H_2O_2 in 1 L water) are effective for inactivating bacteria within minutes to hours, depending on the level of contamination. Tested against seven bacterial strains, hydrogen peroxide killed 1×10^6 colony-forming units per milliliter overnight, with 80% kill in 1 hour. Viruses require higher doses and longer contact times. It is a promising sporicidal agent in high (10% to 25%) concentrations.

Solutions lose potency in time, but stabilizers can be added to prevent decomposition.[30]

Although hydrogen peroxide can sterilize water, it is not widely used as a field water disinfectant, perhaps because of a lack of data for protozoan cysts and quantitative data for dilute solutions, and because the high concentrations known to be effective are very caustic. H_2O_2 may be used synergistically in combination with many other disinfectants and processes.

POTASSIUM PERMANGANATE

Potassium permanganate is a strong oxidizing agent with some disinfectant properties. It is used in municipal disinfection to control taste and odor. It has been used in a 1% to 5% solution as a drinking water disinfectant[218] and is still used for this purpose in some countries, as well as for washing fruits and vegetables.

Bacterial inactivation can be achieved with moderate concentrations and contact times (45 minutes at 2 mg/L, 15 minutes at 8 mg/L). A 1:5000 (0.5%) solution controlled *V. cholerae* and *S. typhi* contamination of fruits and vegetables. The virucidal action has been tested, but without titrations of virus that remained after various periods of contact time, so the rate of action is not known. In most instances, however, a 1:10,000 solution destroyed the infectivity of virus suspensions in 30 minutes at room temperature; 30 mg/L was effective in inactivating HAV within 15 minutes.[312]

Although potassium permanganate clearly has disinfectant action and is frequently used in some parts of the world, it cannot be recommended for point-of-use water disinfection unless it is the only means available, because quantitative data are not available for viruses, and no data are available for protozoan cysts. Packets of 1 g to be added to 1 L of water are sold in some countries. A French military guide from 1940 instructed users: "To sterilize water, use a solution of 1 gram of $KMnO_4$ for 100 grams of water. Add this solution drop by drop to the water to sterilize until the water becomes pink. The operation is considered sufficient if the water remains pink for half an hour."[61] The solutions are deep pink to purple and stain surfaces. The chemical leaves a pink to brown color in water at concentrations above 0.05 mg/L. Small deposits of brown oxides settle to the bottom of the water container. A few drops of alcohol will cause this residual color to disappear.

BOX 88-11 Chlorine Dioxide (ClO_2)	
Advantages	**Disadvantages**
Effective against all microorganisms, including *Cryptosporidium*	Solutions not stable, so do not expose tablets to air, and use generated solutions rapidly.
Low doses have no taste or color	No persistent residual, so ClO_2 does not prevent recontamination during storage.
Field products now available for individual and small-group field use and simple to use	Sensitive to sunlight, so keep bottle shaded or in pack during treatment.
More potent than equivalent doses of chlorine	
Less affected by nitrogenous wastes	

Relative susceptibility of microorganisms to chlorine dioxide: bacteria > viruses > protozoa.

CITRUS

Citrus juice contains limonene, which has biocidal properties. It is one of several essential oils and plant extracts that are used as disinfectants, cleaners, deodorizers, and antiseptics. Lemon or lime juice has been shown to destroy *Vibrio cholerae* at a concentration of 2% (equivalent of 2 tbsp/L of water) with a contact time of 30 minutes. A pH of less than 3.9 is essential, which depends on the concentration of lemon juice and the initial pH of the water.[88] Lime juice also killed 99.9% of *V. cholerae* on cabbage and lettuce and inhibited growth of *V. cholerae* in rice foods, suggesting that adding lime juice to water, beverages, and other foods can reduce disease risks.[294] More research is needed before this can be recommended as more than an ancillary or emergency measure. Commercial products using citrus cannot be recommended as primary means of water disinfection. It has been used to enhance solar UV disinfection.[112]

METALS

Metals form positive ions in water, which is the basis for their antimicrobial effects.[201] The metals most often used, silver and copper, are considered "heavy" metals and have the problems of bioaccumulation and toxicity, as with other well-known toxic metals, including mercury, arsenic, and lead.

Silver

Silver ion has bactericidal effects in low doses. Although widely used as a disinfectant, the literature on antimicrobial effects of silver is confusing and contradictory.[147,193,221,336,342] Concentrations in water less than 100 parts per billion (ppb) are effective against enteric bacteria. The reaction follows first-order kinetics and is temperature dependent.

At the recommended concentration of 50 ppb for water treatment, disinfection requires several hours. Experimental results indicate 18% survival of *E. coli* at 3 hours at 40 mcg/L. *S. typhi* was reduced more than 5 log at 50 mcg/L with a 1-hour exposure; poliovirus was not reduced at 50 mcg/L with a 1-hour exposure.[15] Data on silver for disinfection of viruses and cysts indicate limited effect, even at high doses.[57,221]

Silver is physiologically active. Acute toxicity does not occur from small doses used in disinfection, but argyria, which is permanent discoloration of the skin and mucous membranes, may result from prolonged use. For this reason, a maximum limit of 50 ppb of silver ion in potable water is recommended, with an upper limit of 10 g per lifetime (NOAEL—no observed adverse effect level). This would be reached only after drinking 3 L/day containing 0.1 mg/L over 70 years. WHO acknowledges that the daily intake of silver when used to maintain the bacteriologic quality of drinking water can constitute the major route of oral exposure but states, "It is unnecessary to recommend a health-based guideline value because [silver] is not hazardous to human health at concentrations normally found in drinking water."

Large-scale use of silver for water disinfection has been limited by cost, difficulty controlling and measuring silver content, and physiologic effects. Short-term field use is limited by its marked tendency to adsorb onto the surface of any container (resulting in unreliable concentrations) and interference by several common substances. Calcium, phosphates, and sulfides interfere significantly with silver disinfection. Organic chemicals, amines, and particulate or colloidal matter may also interfere, but no more than with chlorine.

Nevertheless, water disinfection systems using silver have been devised for spacecraft, swimming pools, and other settings.[336] The advantage is absence of taste, odor, and color. Persistence of residual silver concentration allows reliable storage of disinfected water. Silver can be supplied through a silver nitrate solution, desorption from silver-coated materials, or electrolysis. When coated on surfaces, silver acts as a constant-release disinfectant that produces aqueous silver ion concentrations of 0.006 to 0.5 ppm, which are sufficient to disinfect drinking water.[197] Because of this attractive feature, silver-based devices are being designed and tested in developing countries. In Pakistan, a nylon bag with silver-coated sand was designed to place in earthenware pitchers that store water. Silver incorporated into alum is also being tested in India.[60] Low levels of chlorine may be synergistic with silver.

Use of silver as a drinking water disinfectant has been much more popular in Europe, where silver tablets (Micropur) are sold widely for field water disinfection. They have not been approved by the EPA for this purpose in the United States, but they were approved as a water preservative to prevent bacterial growth in previously treated and stored water. Micropur Forte tablets release free chlorine for disinfection and silver for prolonged persistence of antimicrobial activity (see Appendix B at the end of this chapter).

Since bacteria grow on filter media or membranes, the filter is usually impregnated or coated with silver to inactivate pathogens that pass through the filter pores or to limit bacterial growth in the filter itself (bacteriostatic). Ceramic filters coated with silver have higher removal rates of bacteria, and filters that had been just recoated with silver initially yielded much higher disinfection efficiencies but were not able to sustain them.[15,22,119] However, filter cartridges impregnated with silver still become colonized with heterotrophic bacteria, and effluent bacterial populations are about as large as units without silver. These bacteria have not been linked to increased illness.[15,104,119,257] Colonization of filters with pathogenic coliform bacteria has not been demonstrated, but protective effect cannot be attributed to silver impregnation.[104,257]

Copper and Zinc

Copper is most frequently used as a molluscicide, algicide, and fungicide, although it is also bactericidal in very low concentrations and is virucidal.

Kinetic degradation fluxion (KDF) is a high-purity copper-zinc formulation that uses the basic chemical process of oxidation-reduction (redox) to remove chlorine, heavy metals (e.g., lead, mercury), iron, and hydrogen sulfide from water supplies. Its main actions are through its strong redox potential of 500 mV because of the propensity to exchange electrons with other substances. The redox reactions change contaminants into harmless components: chlorine into chloride (removing the taste of chlorine or iodine from treated water), soluble ferrous cations into insoluble ferric hydroxide, and hydrogen sulfide into insoluble copper sulfide. Up to 98% of lead, mercury, nickel, chromium, and other dissolved metals are removed by KDF simply by bonding to the media. KDF controls buildup of bacteria, algae, and fungi and is used for this purpose in GAC beds and carbon block filters, extending the life of carbon and improving its effectiveness.

KDF or copper alone has bacteriostatic with some bactericidal activity; microorganisms may be killed by the electrolytic field and by formation of hydroxyl radicals and peroxide water molecules.[193] Although KDF has been ruled a "pesticidal device" by the EPA, it should not be used as the sole means of water treatment and is best combined with filtration or chlorination.

KDF media can be manufactured as granules, fine steel wool–like media, or brushes with wire bristles. Currently, this technique is mostly applied in industrial settings and household in-line filters. No portable products are currently designed for the outdoor market.

NANOPARTICLES: SOLAR PHOTOCATALYTIC DISINFECTION

Nanoparticles are particles between 1 and 100 nanometers (nm) in size with unique properties as adsorbents, catalysts, and sensors that have led to their exploration in many fields of science. Several nanomaterials have been shown to have strong antimicrobial properties and are being evaluated for use in water disinfection and purification. They are not strong oxidants themselves, and are relatively stable in water and nontoxic. Nanomaterials are already being used widely in industrial purification, but they show great potential for point-of-use applications as well. There are three categories of antimicrobial nanoparticles: naturally occurring substances, including chitin obtained from arthropod shells; metals and metal oxides, including silver (nAg), titanium dioxide (TiO_2), and zinc oxide (ZnO); and synthetic engineered materials, such as fullerene (nC60) and carbon nanotubes (CNT).[174,186] The metals are of particular interest for water disinfection applications because they can be activated by UV light to produce potent oxidizers.

Titanium dioxide has the advantage of activation by UVA rays in sunlight. High-energy, short-wavelength photons from sunlight promote the photochemical reactions. In addition to being an excellent disinfectant for various microorganisms, this process is unique in its ability to break down complex organic contaminants and most heavy metals into carbon dioxide, water, and inorganic substances, which is driving considerable research for industrial processes and large-scale water treatment. TiO_2 antimicrobial properties have been studied for their effect for more than 20 years. Recent work demonstrated inactivation of *Cryptosporidium*.[306] For field water disinfection, nanoparticles coated with TiO_2 can be integrated into a plastic bag and remain active for hundreds of uses[27] (see Appendix A).

ULTRAVIOLET LIGHT

Ultraviolet lamp disinfection systems are widely used to disinfect drinking water at the community and household levels (Box 88-12).[180] In sufficient doses, all waterborne enteric pathogens are inactivated by UV radiation (UVR). UVC light in the range of 200 to 280 nm is the most effective. The germicidal effect of UV light is the result of action on the nucleic acids of bacteria and depends on light intensity and exposure time.[55] Bacteria and protozoan parasites require lower doses than do enteric viruses and bacterial spores. However, all viruses, including hepatitis A and norovirus, are susceptible, with relatively minor differences, and follow similar kinetics.[140] Bacteria (vegetative cells) are significantly more susceptible to UVR than are viruses. *Giardia* and *Cryptosporidium* are susceptible to practical doses of UVR and may be more sensitive because of their relatively large size.[19,140,189]

In sufficient doses, UV irradiation can also remove odors and dechlorinate. UV treatment does not require chemicals or affect the taste of the water. It works rapidly, and excessive dosing to the water presents no danger; in fact, it is a safety factor. UV irradiation with lamps requires a power source and is costly. UV light has no residual disinfection power; water may become recontaminated, or regrowth of bacteria may occur.[104] Particulate matter can shield microorganisms from UV rays. A portable field unit is now available and has been shown to be effective in reducing bacteria and viruses (see Appendix A in this chapter).

Solar Disinfection

There is now strong evidence that UV irradiation by sunlight in the UVA range can substantially improve microbiologic quality of water and reduce diarrheal illness in developing countries. Because of its negligible cost and simplicity, solar disinfection (SODIS) is being rapidly adopted in many developing countries. McGuigan and colleagues[204] have published an excellent review. Recent work has confirmed efficacy and optimal procedures of the SODIS technique[55,76,230,294] (Box 88-13). Transparent bottles (e.g., clear plastic beverage bottles) are exposed to sunlight for a minimum of 4 to 6 hours, but some investigations demonstrate improved benefit from several sequential days. Multiple studies

BOX 88-13 Solar Disinfection (SODIS)

Advantages	Disadvantages
Utilizes sunlight	Requires clear water
Requires no special equipment or power; relies on local resources and renewable energy	No residual effect; does not prevent recontamination during storage
Improves the microbiologic quality of drinking water; including protozoan cysts	Does not improve water esthetics
Simple in application; can be used at household level in developing countries or refugee camps	Requires multiple bottles to treat large volumes of water; use maximum 2-L bottle.
Does not change the taste of water	Requires strong, direct, abundant sunlight, with prolonged exposure; dose low and uncontrolled
Can be used in austere environments	

Relative susceptibility of microorganisms to SODIS: protozoa > bacteria > viruses.

demonstrate reduction of enteric bacteria, viruses, and protozoan cysts, and some data exist for reduction of bacterial spores.[166,203,205,298] With a water temperature of 30°C (86°F), 6 hours of middle-latitude midday summer sunshine are required to achieve a 3-log reduction of fecal coliforms.[207]

Ultraviolet irradiation and thermal inactivation were strongly synergistic for solar disinfection of drinking water in transparent plastic bottles that was heavily contaminated with *E. coli* for temperatures above 45°C (113°F). Above 55°C (131°F), thermal inactivation is of primary importance.[202,204] Whereas thermal inactivation is effective in turbid water, UV effects are inhibited.[4,151,160,268] If cloudiness is obvious, the plastic bottles need to be exposed for 2 consecutive days to produce water safe for consumption. However, if water temperatures exceed 50°C (122°F), 1 hour of exposure is sufficient to obtain safe drinking water. The treatment efficiency can be improved if the plastic bottles are exposed on sunlight-reflecting surfaces such as aluminum or corrugated iron sheets. Use of a simple reflector or solar cooker can achieve pasteurization temperatures of 65°C (149°F). Effects can also be enhanced by adding small amounts of hydrogen peroxide, lemon juice, or lime juice.[112] Oxygenation induces greater reduction of bacteria, so agitation is recommended before solar treatment in bottles.

Various types of transparent plastic materials are good transmitters of light in the UVA and visible range of the solar spectrum. Plastic bottles are made of either polyethylene terephthalate (PET) or polyvinylchloride (PVC). The use of bottles made from PET instead of PVC is recommended because PET contains fewer additives than PVC. Glass bottles are not used for SODIS because the transmission of UVR through glass is determined by its content of iron oxide; ordinary window glass of 2-mm thickness transmits almost no UVA light. Because UVR is reduced at increasing water depth, the containers used for SODIS should not exceed a water depth of 10 cm (4 inches). Aged or heavily scratched plastic bottles show reduced UV transmittance, which in turn can result in less efficient inactivation of microorganisms.[207]

In summary, where strong sunshine and clear water are available, solar disinfection of drinking water is an effective, low-cost method for improving water quality and may be of particular use in refugee camps and disaster areas.[207]

COMPARATIVE STUDIES AND PREFERRED TECHNIQUES

Presumably, standard protocols for product testing in experienced laboratories would provide comparable and reproducible results. However, studies that directly compare techniques or products often yield results that vary widely from the individual product testing. Actual efficacy in the field or household setting of developing countries vary significantly from laboratory

BOX 88-12 Ultraviolet (UV) Irradiation

Advantages	Disadvantages
Effective against all microorganisms	Requires clear water
Imparts no taste	Does not improve water esthetics
Portable device now available for individual and small-group field use and simple to use	No residual effect; does not prevent recontamination during storage
Can use UV rays from sunlight in austere conditions (see Box 88-13)	UV lamps are expensive and require power source.

Relative susceptibility of microorganisms to UV irradiation: protozoa > bacteria > viruses.

Treatment Process	Pathogen	Optimal Log Reduction*	Expected Log Reduction†	Diarrheal Disease Reduction‡
Ceramic filters	Bacteria	6	2	63% (51%-72%) for candle filters
	Viruses	4	0.5	46% (29%-59%) for bowl filters
	Protozoa	6	4	
Free chlorine	Bacteria	6	3	37% (25%-48%)
	Viruses	6	3	
	Protozoa	5	3	
Coagulation/chlorination	Bacteria	9	7	31% (18%-42%)
	Viruses	6	2-4.5	
	Protozoa	5	3	
Biosand filtration	Bacteria	3	1	47% (21%-64%)
	Viruses	3	0.5	
	Protozoa	4	2	
SODIS	Bacteria	5.5	3	31% (26%-37%)
	Viruses	4	2	
	Protozoa	3	1	

Data from multiple studies, analyzed and summarized by Sobsey, 2008.[298] Also, data from references 22, 66, 220, and 294 and Table 7.8 in WHO, 2011.[347]

SODIS, Solar disinfection.

*Skilled operators using optimal conditions and practices (efficacy); log reduction: pretreatment minus post-treatment concentration of organisms (e.g., 6 log = 99.999% removal).

†Actual field practice by unskilled persons (effectiveness); depends on water quality, quality and age of filter or materials, following proper procedure, and other factors.

‡Summary estimates from published data; vary with consistency and correct use of technique, integrity of techniques (e.g., cracked filter), and other household sanitation measures.

effectiveness because of variations in source water clarity and levels of contamination.[185] Data for the effectiveness of water disinfection techniques for wilderness travelers are essentially all done in the laboratory and not in field settings during actual use. On the other hand, many studies have recently been done on point-of-use devices in households and refugee settings in developing countries, where contamination and the risk for illness are many times higher; thus, techniques can be evaluated for both microbiologic reduction under real use and reduction of illness attributable to water treatment[22,66,220,294] (Table 88-16). These techniques for the developing world are necessarily low cost, simple to use, and include some improvised methods, which make them particularly valuable for survival, disaster, or other austere situations characterized by suboptimal conditions and supplies. Furthermore, the need for household point-of-use water treatment in developing countries is stimulating innovative approaches to disinfection that combine multiple treatment steps in series, as is done in municipal plants. For those tasked with engineering water solutions for communities or populations in austere environments, point-of-use methods were found to be more effective than were source solutions.[68,176]

Several studies comparing halogens are noted earlier in the Iodine versus Chlorine section.[142,154,156,243,283] Lee and Lee[183] compared iodine, chlorine dioxide, mixed oxidants, and UVR for disinfection of coccidian oocysts to represent *Cryptosporidium* and found that only UVR consistently inhibited sporulation. Iodine in recommended contact times was little better than controls, and chlorine dioxide left almost one-quarter of oocysts viable in moderately contaminated water and was similar to controls in highly contaminated water. One important factor may have been the large number of organisms added to the water, which greatly exceeded likely levels encountered in surface water. Betancourt and Rose[19] reviewed methods for removal of *Cryptosporidium* and found UVR and filtration effective. Sobsey and colleagues[298] reviewed data for point-of-use methods for household disinfection in developing countries. All methods had high levels of optimal effectiveness, but their actual efficacy was much less over time, likely impacted by inconsistent use. Verma and Arankalle[331] evaluated eight different higher-technology household disinfection units sold in India, each using some combination of filtration, iodine resin, chlorination, and UVR. Average removal of hepatitis E virus was 1 to 3 log, except for a hollow-fiber membrane unit that achieved 6.5-log removal. This study highlights incorporation of common disinfection techniques into household appliances for point-of-use water treatment and the discrepancy between optimal and actual efficacy for these devices, which would certainly apply to field units as well. Similarly, another study compared ceramic filters and iodine resin household devices and found high levels of bacterial removal, but that reduction of viruses and microspheres did not meet standards of EPA protocols.[67] One recently developed household device that does not require power and combines the complementary methods of filtration and disinfection did meet EPA criteria for microbiologic reduction.[67]

Although the gap between optimal and actual efficacy is disturbing, it is reassuring that in actual field conditions, all point-of-use techniques will greatly decrease the number of microorganisms and risk for illness[66,68,185,298] (see Table 88-16). As in any wilderness medical situation, some basic assessment must be done of the likely level and type of contamination, methods of disinfection available, and tolerance of risk.

PREFERRED TECHNIQUE

Field disinfection techniques and their effects on microorganisms are summarized in Table 88-17. The optimal technique for an individual or group in the wilderness or traveling in developing countries depends on the number of persons to be served, space and weight available, quality of source water (Table 88-18), personal taste preferences, and availability of fuel. The most effective technique may not always be available, but any method should greatly reduce the load of microorganisms and reduce the risk for illness. A multibarrier approach for drinking water treatment, in which a combination of various disinfectants and filtration technologies are applied for removal and inactivation of different microbial pathogens, will provide a lower risk for microbial contamination.[19] Other excellent summaries of disinfection methods are available.[180,201]

A combination of clarification using coagulation-flocculation (C-F) and filtration followed by chlorination remains the standard for municipal water treatment worldwide. The CDC and WHO also promote chlorine for household-level point-of-use disinfection in the developing world.[297,347]

In austere situations such as disasters or refugee camps, hypochlorite (household bleach) also is widely recommended.[101,176,177] However, in an attempt to simplify for a broad range of people and to provide a margin of safety, the recommendations may lead to either inadequate or excessive concentrations. For cloudy

TABLE 88-17	Summary of Field Water Disinfection Techniques				
	Bacteria	**Viruses**	**Giardia/Amebae**	**Cryptosporidium**	**Nematodes/Cercaria**
Heat	+	+	+	+	+
Filtration	+	+/–*	+	+	+
Halogens	+	+	+	–	+/–†
Chlorine dioxide	+	+	+	+	+/–†
UV	+	+	+	+	No data available
TiO₂ photocatalytic	+	+	+	+	No data available

*Most filters make no claims for viruses, but may remove up to 99%. Reverse osmosis and hollow-fiber ultrafiltration technology would be effective. General Ecology also has some data for virus removal.
†Eggs are not very susceptible to halogens but are very low risk for waterborne transmission.

water, chlorination-flocculation packets are the best and simplest method. If chlorine is not available, the SODIS technique or sand filters can be used with improvised materials.

For environments with a high-quality, low-risk source water, any of the primary techniques is adequate, with the understanding that the limitation for halogens is *Cryptosporidium* oocysts and that microfilters may not remove all viruses. Surface water, even if clear, in undeveloped countries where there is human and animal activity should be considered highly contaminated with enteric pathogens. Optimal protection requires heat, ultra-filtration, UV irradiation, or a two-stage process of filtration and halogens. Chlorine dioxide and photocatalytic TiO₂ are currently the only one-step chemical processes available. Even in the United States, water with agricultural runoff or sewage plant discharge from upstream towns or cities must be treated to remove *Cryptosporidium* and viruses. Water receiving agricultural, industrial, or mining runoff may contain chemical contamination from pesticides, other chemicals, and heavy metals. A filter containing a charcoal element is the best method for removing most chemicals.

Water from cloudy, low-elevation rivers, ponds, and lakes in developed or developing countries that does not clear with sedimentation should be pretreated with C-F and then disinfected with heat or halogens. Tablets combining C-F and chlorination are readily available and have extensive testing to demonstrate effectiveness.[82,97,243,259] Filters can be used but will clog rapidly with silted or cloudy water. A sand filtration unit can be improvised.[169] C-F will also remove some chemical contamination.

The preferred method of treatment for the military, when large-scale equipment can be brought to the site, is a reverse-osmosis water purification unit (ROWPU), because it can produce high-quality water from a low-quality source. For smaller groups, the military relies mainly on monitored chlorine. Individual means include iodine tablets, Chlor-Floc tablets, and chlorine liquid bleach.[319]

Chemical agents need to be used when water will be stored, such as on a boat, in a large camp, or for disaster relief. When only heat or filtration is used before storage, recontamination and bacterial growth can occur. Hypochlorite still has many advantages for stored water, including cost, ease of handling, and minimal volatilization in tightly covered containers.[213] A minimum residual of 3 to 5 mg/L should be maintained in the water. Superchlorination-dechlorination is especially useful in this situation because high levels of chlorination can be maintained for long periods, and when ready for use, the water can be poured into a smaller container and dechlorinated. Iodine works for short-term but not prolonged storage, because it is a poor algicide. Silver has been approved by the EPA for preservation of stored water. Chlorine dioxide does not maintain a residual concentration.

On oceangoing vessels where water must be desalinated during the voyage, only reverse-osmosis membrane filters are adequate. Water in the storage tanks should then be chlorinated.

In survival or austere situations such as disasters or refugee camps, hypochlorite (household bleach) or chlorination-flocculation packets may be available.

PREVENTION AND SANITATION

Studies in developing countries have demonstrated a clear benefit in the reduction of diarrheal illness and other infections from safe drinking water, sanitation, and hygiene (WASH).[68,149,191,210,250,251,260,297] Although a benefit can be demonstrated for the WASH interventions independently, the benefit is greater when all are applied together, especially with appropriate education.[60] Wilderness travelers essentially live in conditions similar to the developing world, without running water or sanitation. Unfortunately, many wilderness travelers confuse the continuing need for hygiene with the need to relax their standard of cleanliness.

TABLE 88-18	Choice of Method for Various Source Water		Developed or Developing Country	
	"Pristine" Wilderness Water with Little Human or Domestic Animal Activity	**Tap Water in Developing Country**	**Clear Surface Water Near Human and Animal Activity***	**Cloudy Water**
Primary concern	*Giardia*, enteric bacteria	Bacteria, *Giardia*, small numbers of viruses	All enteric pathogens, including *Cryptosporidium*	All enteric pathogens plus microorganisms
Effective methods	Any single-step method† Low-risk water; many would choose to drink untreated	Any single-step method† Risk varies depending on country; judgment required for decision to treat	1. Heat 2. Filtration plus halogen (can be done in either order) 3. Hollow-fiber ultrafiltration 4. Chlorine dioxide 5. Ultraviolet (commercial product, not sunlight)	CF followed by second step (heat, filtration, or chemical)

*Includes agricultural runoff with cattle grazing or sewage treatment effluent from upstream villages or towns.
†Includes heat, filtration, halogens, chlorine dioxide, and ultraviolet irradiation.
CF, Coagulation-flocculation.

HANDWASHING

Personal hygiene, mainly handwashing, prevents spread of infection from food contamination during preparation of meals.[209] A widely publicized study in the United States demonstrated that only 67% of Americans wash hands after using a public toilet. No one with a diarrheal illness should prepare food. A study of Appalachian Trail hikers showed that water disinfection, routine handwashing, and proper cookware cleaning were all associated with decreased diarrhea.[31] A *Shigella* outbreak among river rafters on the Colorado River was investigated and assumed to be waterborne from adjacent Native American communities, but was finally traced to infected guides who were shedding organisms in the stool and contaminating food through poor hygiene.[209] Simple handwashing with soap and water purified with hypochlorite (bleach) significantly reduced fecal contamination of market-vended beverages in Guatemala.[292] Gil and colleagues[127] tested water and objects in the kitchen in rural Peru and demonstrated widespread contamination.

Extensive research in the developing world demonstrated that treated water is often recontaminated before use, and proper storage techniques that prevent contact with hands and objects can decrease this risk for contamination.[70,297,348] Narrow-mouth jars or containers with water spigots are the best means to prevent contamination from repeated contact with hands or utensils.[259,270,292] In a refugee camp, using only a simple, improved bucket that did not allow dirty hands or a ladle to touch the water, there was 69% reduction in mean fecal coliform levels in the household water and 31% less diarrheal disease in children under 5 years of age among the group.[270]

KITCHEN AND FOOD SANITATION

Sanitation should extend to the kitchen or food preparation area.[191] In addition to handwashing, dishes and utensils should be disinfected by rinsing in chlorinated water, prepared by adding enough household bleach to achieve a distinct chlorine odor. Hargreaves[133] tested various combinations of wash and rinse water in three-bowl systems to determine what worked best for cleanliness, bacterial disinfection, and residual smell or taste of disinfectant. The optimal combination was water plus detergent in bowl 1 to remove the majority of food residue and grease; water with 10 mL of added bleach in bowl 2 to remove the remaining food residue and provide disinfection; and plain water in bowl 3 to remove residue of disinfectant. This is a variation of the most common method that adds the disinfectant to bowl 3 instead of bowl 2. If there is insufficient water or containers to provide a three-bowl system, omit bowl 3.

Washing fruits and vegetables in purified water is a common practice at all levels, from individual to the food industry. Washing has a mechanical action of removing dirt and microorganisms while the disinfectant kills microorganisms on the surface. However, neither reaches the organisms embedded in surface crevices or protected by biofilm or other particulate matter, which is why it is safer to peel most fruits and vegetables with rough skins.[163] When lettuce was seeded with oocysts, then washed and the supernatant examined for cysts, only 25% to 36% of *C. parvum* and 13% to 15% of *C. cayetanensis* oocysts were recovered in the washes. Scanning electron microscopy detected oocysts on the surface of the vegetables after washing.[233] A review of washing lettuce with various disinfectant solutions shows that high concentrations usually reduce level of viruses by 1 to 3 log.[12] Chlorine, iodine, or potassium permanganate is often used for this purpose in higher concentrations than would normally be palatable for drinking water. In the United States, chlorine wash at 20 to 200 ppm is the most common sanitizing treatment used by the fresh-produce industry and could also be used in the field by wilderness and remote area travelers.[234] Many newer technologies such as irradiation are available for the food industry but are not applicable in the field.

HUMAN WASTE DISPOSAL

The ultimate responsibility for wilderness travelers is proper sanitation to prevent contamination of water supplies from human waste. Some suggest that campers smear feces on rocks. Desiccation occurs, and UV rays in sunlight eventually inactivate most microorganisms, but rain may first wash pathogens into a water source.[63] Moreover, it will be repulsive to other campers. In the Sierras, feces left on the ground generally disappeared within 1 month, but it was not known whether disinfection occurred before decomposition or whether the feces washed away, dried, or were blown in the wind.[254] Despite more rapid decomposition in sunlight rather than underground, burying feces is still preferable in areas that receive regular use.

In the soil, microorganisms can survive for months.[326] A Sierra Club study found more prolonged microorganism survival in alpine environments.[254] The investigator marked group latrines in alpine terrain and returned 1 to 2 years later to dig test trenches. He found a thin crust of decomposition covering unaltered raw waste with high coliform bacteria counts. Microorganisms may percolate through the soil. Most bacteria are retained within 51 cm (20 inches) of the surface, but in sandy soil, this increases to 23 to 30 m (75 to 100 feet);[319] viruses can move laterally 23 to 92 m (75 to 302 feet).[281] When organisms reach groundwater, their survival is prolonged, and they often reappear in surface water or wells.[326]

The U.S. military and U.S. Forest Service recommend burial of human waste 20 to 30 cm (8 to 12 inches) deep and a minimum of 30 m (100 feet) from any water.[319,328] Decomposition is hastened by mixing in some dirt before burial. Shallow burying is not recommended because animals are more likely to find and overturn the feces. Judgment should be used to determine a location that is not likely to allow water runoff to wash organisms into nearby water sources. Groups larger than three persons should dig a common latrine to avoid numerous individual potholes and inadequate disposal. To minimize latrine odor and improve its function, it should not be used for disposal of wastewater.

In some areas, the number of individual and group latrines is so great that the entire area becomes contaminated. Therefore, sanitary facilities (outhouses) are becoming common in high-use wilderness areas. Popular river canyons require camp toilets, and all waste must be carried out in sealed containers.

REFERENCES

Complete references used in this text are available online at expertconsult.inkling.com.

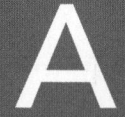

APPENDIX A

Water Disinfection Devices and Products for Field Use

Product lines are continuously evolving, and prices change frequently and vary widely. Prices quoted represent a current range from Internet advertising.

For most of these products, claims are substantiated only by company-sponsored and company-designed testing. Some results have been extrapolated to similar products. Products are tested using a standardized Environmental Protection Agency (EPA) protocol: depending on claims, filters must demonstrate removal or inactivation of 10^3 cysts (99.9%), 10^4 viruses (99.99%), and 10^6 bacteria under varying water conditions of temperature and turbidity. Few objective, comparable test results for these products are available. (See Comparative Studies and Preferred Techniques, earlier.)

Filter capacity is highly variable, depending on clarity of water. Numbers cited for capacity are usually based on clear water; testing using slightly turbid river water and following manufacturer instructions for cleaning reveals markedly different values. For all filters, it is recommended to pump dilute bleach solution through the unit after each trip and dry thoroughly before storage to decrease bacterial growth in the filter.

APPENDIX A

Product	Price	Structure/Function
Katadyn Endurance Series		http://www.katadyn.com
		Endurance filters contain a 0.2-μm ceramic candle filter, silver impregnated to decrease bacterial growth. Large units also contain silver quartz in center of filter.
Pocket Filter (Figure 88-5)	$300-370	Hand pump; 40-inch intake hose and strainer, zipper case; in-line carbon cartridge available; size: 10 × 2.4 inches; weight: 20 oz; flow: 0.75-1 L/min; capacity: 50,000 L.
Combi (Figure 88-6) Accessories: prefilter bottle adaptor, carrying bag	$175-$220	Small hand pump with ceramic filter and activated charcoal granule stage; with the optional "PLUS" package, the Combi can be connected to a water faucet for use in campers, cottages, or boats. Size: 2.4 × 12 inches; weight: 21 oz; flow: 1.0 L/min; capacity: up to 50,000 L; charcoal capacity: 200 L.
Expedition (Figure 88-7)	$1250-$1500	Large hand pump with steel stand for medium to large groups; size (packed in case): 23 × 6 × 8 inches; weight: 12 lb; flow: 4 L/min; capacity (per filter element): up to 100,000 L.
Ceradyn (Figure 88-8) and Gravidyn	$295-320	Gravity drip from one plastic bucket to another with three ceramic candle filter elements. Ceradyn uses ceramic candle filters, whereas Gravidyn filter candles combine ceramic and activated carbon elements; size: 18 inches × 11 inches diameter (26 inches high when assembled), 10-L water container; weight: 7 lb; flow: 4 L/hr; capacity: up to 150,000 L.
Siphon filter (Figure 88-9)	$65-$80	Gravity 0.2-μm ceramic siphon filter element without reservoir bag that can be used to make a gravity system out of any water container. Place one or more Siphon filter elements into a container, and let the water run through the hose into a lower-positioned vessel. Size: 6.3 × 2.6 inches; weight: 16 oz; flow: 5 L/hr; capacity: about 20,000 L.
Katadyn Backcountry Series		
Vario (Figure 88-10)	$95	Hand pump; 0.2-μm pleated glass fiber filter with 143-square-inch surface area, ceramic prefilter, and activated charcoal stage; attaches directly to water bottle; size: 7.5 × 4.0 inches; weight: 15 oz; max flow: 2 L/min (36 stokes/L); capacity: 2000 L.
Hiker and Hiker Pro (Figure 88-11)	$60-85	Hand pump; 0.2-μm pleated glass fiber with 107-square-inch surface and activated carbon core; size: 6.5 × 2.4 × 3 inches; weight: 11 oz; flow: 1 L/min (48 strokes/L); capacity: 750 L.
Gravity Camp and Base Camp (Figure 88-12)	$80-$100	Gravity filter with a 0.2-μm glass fiber filter (Hiker filter cartridge) plus granular charcoal; includes dirty water reservoir bag and tubing; Gravity Camp bag 6L, Base Camp Pro 10L; size: 10 × 6 × 2 inches; weight: 11 oz; flow: 2 L/min; capacity: 1500 L.
Katadyn Ultralight Series		
Mini (Figure 88-13)	$90-$110	Smaller, lighter hand pump; 0.2-μm ceramic filter with activated carbon; 31-inch intake hose and strainer, hard plastic enclosure and pump; size: 3.2 × 7 × 2 inches; weight: 8 oz; flow: 0.5 L/min; capacity: approx 7000 L.
Water Bottles		
MyBottle (Figure 88-14)	$40-$60	Drink-through bottle with either two stage: 0.2-μm fiberglass filter and activated carbon cartridge, or three-stage purifier cartridge with filter for protozoa, pentaiodide iodine resin (ViruStat), and activated carbon; weight: 10 oz; size: 10 inches high, 24 oz; capacity: up to 26 gal.
Microfilter	$40	Hand pump with 0.2-μm ceramic depth filter; size: 3.2 × 7 × 2 inches; weight: 8 oz; flow: 0.5 L/min; capacity: approx 2000 gal.

Continued

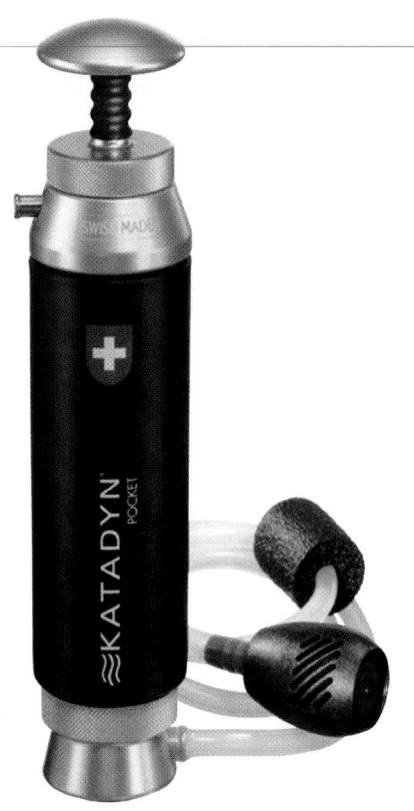

FIGURE 88-5 Pocket Filter. *(Courtesy Katadyn.)*

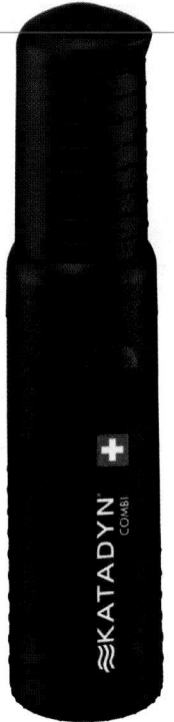

FIGURE 88-6 Combi. *(Courtesy Katadyn.)*

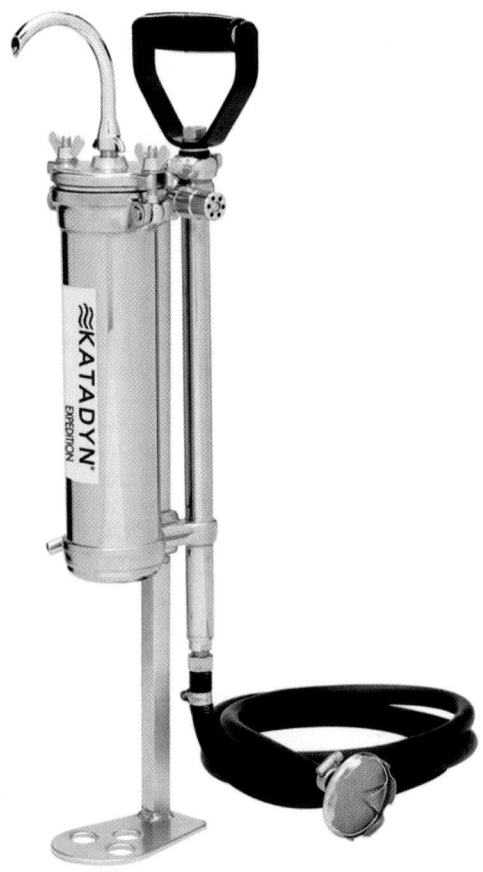

FIGURE 88-7 Expedition Filter. *(Courtesy Katadyn.)*

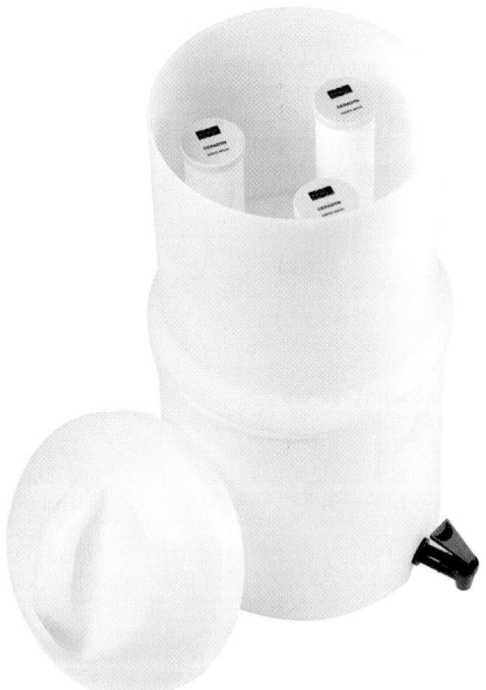

FIGURE 88-8 Drip Ceradyn. *(Courtesy Katadyn.)*

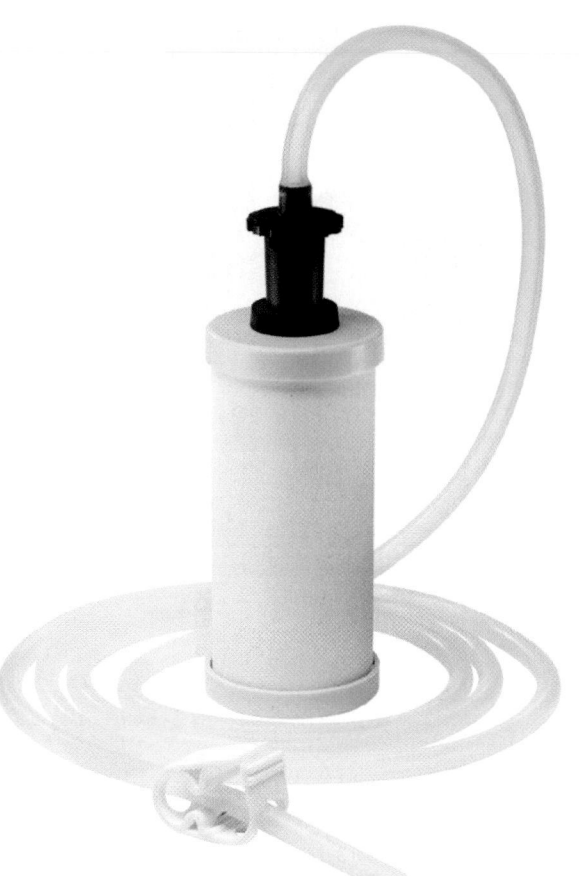

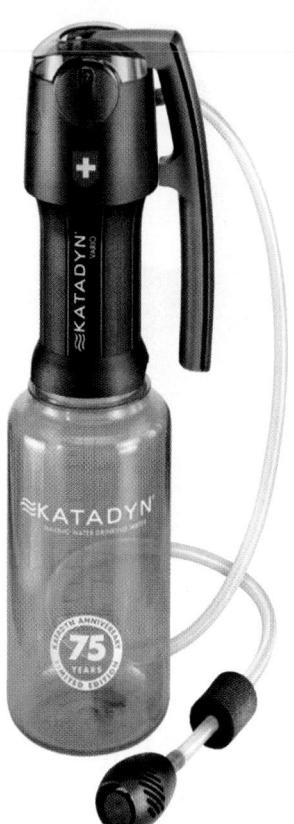

FIGURE 88-10 Vario Filter. *(Courtesy Katadyn.)*

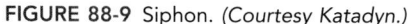

FIGURE 88-9 Siphon. *(Courtesy Katadyn.)*

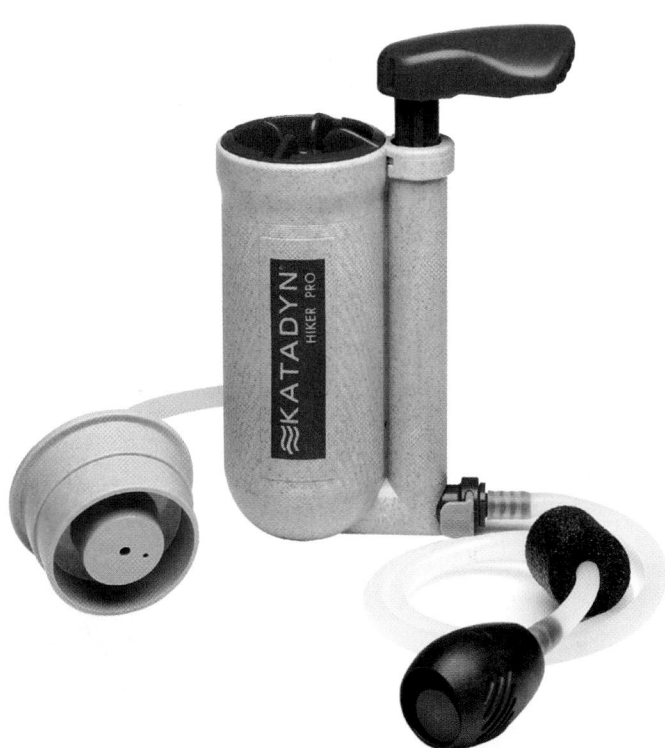

FIGURE 88-11 Hiker Pro. *(Courtesy Katadyn.)*

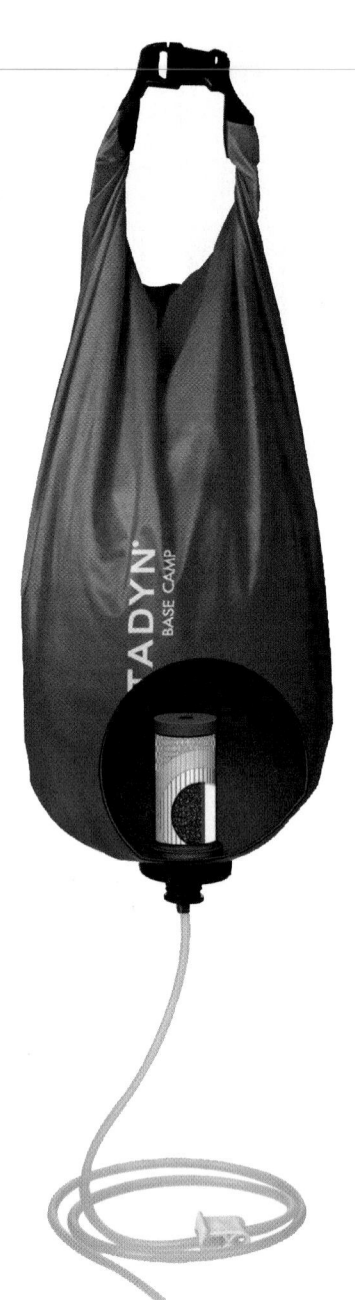

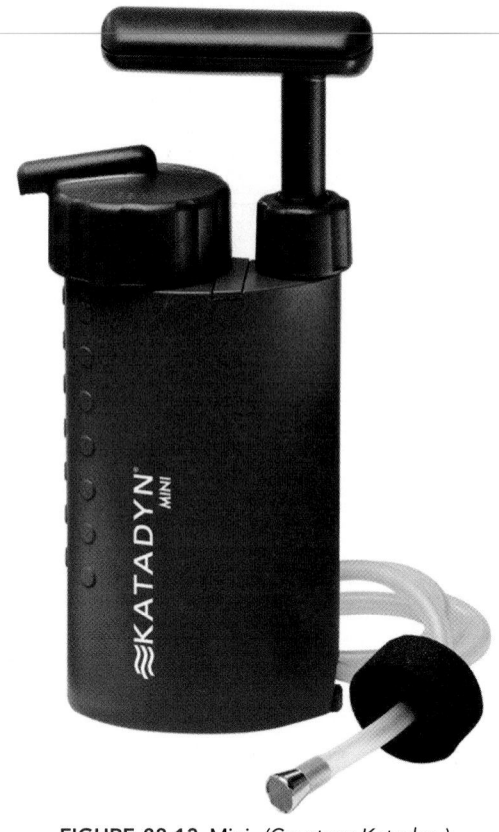

FIGURE 88-13 Mini. *(Courtesy Katadyn.)*

FIGURE 88-12 Katadyn Base Camp (cutaway view). *(Courtesy Katadyn.)*

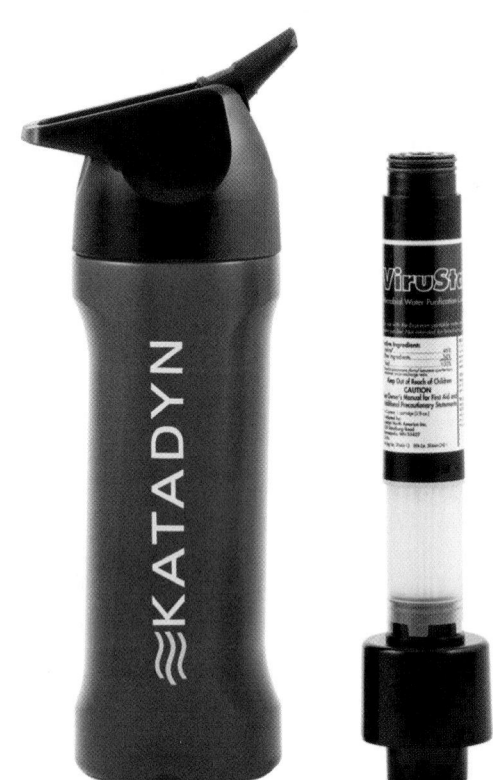

FIGURE 88-14 MyBottle Purifier. *(Courtesy Katadyn.)*

Katadyn Claims

Endurance series and Mini with ceramic and carbon filter elements remove bacterial pathogens, protozoan cysts, parasites, and nuclear debris. Clarifies cloudy water. If filter clogs, brushing the filter element (which can be done hundreds of times before needing to replace the filter element) can restore flow, or filter elements can be replaced. Claims for removal of viruses by ceramic filters not made in the United States. Pocket Filter has a lifetime warranty.

Vario and Hiker are microfilters designed for high-quality surface water. They will eliminate *Giardia, Cryptosporidium*, and most bacteria; activated carbon core "reduces chemicals and pesticides, plus improves taste of water." Filters with large surface area are "guaranteed not to clog for 1 year."

MyBottle with iodine resin filter passed EPA tests to remove 3-log cysts, 4-log viruses, and 6-log bacteria. Patented ion-release technology and carbon scrubber dramatically reduce residual iodine.

Comments

Well-designed, durable products that are effective for claims. However, high filter volume capacity is optimistic and not likely to be achieved filtering average surface water. *Backpacker* magazine field tests found the flow comparatively slow, requiring more energy to pump and frequent cleaning. Abrading the outer surface can effectively clean ceramic filters; after multiple cleanings, it is necessary to use the gauge to indicate when filter thickness becomes too thin.

Pocket Filter is the original individual or small-group filter design. Metal parts make it durable, but the heaviest for its size. Expedition filter is popular for larger groups, especially river trips, where weight is not a factor. Complete virus removal cannot be expected, although most viruses clump or adhere to larger particles or bacteria that can be filtered. Silver impregnation does not prevent bacterial growth in filters.

Ceramic candle filters have been independently tested in household use in developing countries and shown to reduce turbidity and bacteria to WHO target levels for safe drinking water.[65]

Vario and Hiker were designed for the domestic backpacking market with higher water quality, where cysts and bacteria are threats, but viruses are less of a problem. The Hiker received top ratings by *Backpacker* magazine for field tests evaluating user-friendliness. These filters may be used with a halogen disinfectant for international travel or conditions, where high levels of contamination are possible.

MyBottle filter with iodine resin is currently the only water bottle or filter product available with iodine resin (see text). Drink-through design limits to single-person day use. The filter design with charcoal removing residual iodine and ingestion directly from the filter allows no contact time and may not provide complete viral protection in all situations.

Katadyn Desalinators
Reverse Osmosis Filters

Desalinator Survivor 06 (Figure 88-15)	$1000	Hand-operated pump, reverse-osmosis membrane filter with prefilter on intake line; size: 2.5 × 5 × 8 inches; weight: 2.5 lb; flow: 40 strokes/min yields 0.9 L/hr.
Survivor 35 (Figure 88-16)	$2200	Hand-operated pump, reverse-osmosis membrane filter with prefilter on intake line; size: 3.5 × 5.5 × 22 inches; weight: 7 lb; flow: 30 strokes/min yields 4.5 L/hr.
PowerSurvivor 40E PowerSurvivor 80E	$4000 $5000	Small, power-operated models in this line of reverse-osmosis filters; uses only 4 amps, so can run for extended periods on 12-volt power source; converts to manual operation in emergencies; pump size: 6.8 × 16.5 × 15.5 inches; prefilter 12 × 6 inches; weight: 25 lb; flow: 5.7 L/hr (1.5 gal/hr); 80E size: 6 × 16 × 14 inches; weight 34 lb; flow 12.9 L/hr (4.0 gal/hr).

Claims

Reverse-osmosis units desalinate, removing 98% of salt from seawater by forcing water through a semipermeable membrane at 800 psi. In the process, microorganisms are filtered out. The manual operation of these units makes them unique and useful for survival at sea or for use in small craft without power source.

Comments

Reverse-osmosis units are nanofilters capable of removing sodium molecules, as well as all microorganisms, including viruses. They are included here for sea kayaking and small-boat journeys in open water. These units can obviate the need for relying solely on stored water or can be carried for emergency survival. Reverse-osmosis filters currently are not practical for land travel because of cost, weight, and flow rates; however, the U.S. military uses truck-mounted reverse-osmosis filters on land for their ability to handle brackish water and remove all types of microorganisms. Note that the company does not make claims for viral removal because they assume that the membrane is imperfect and some pores will be imprecise, perhaps allowing viral passage. Higher-flow power models are available from the company (Model 80E, 160E).

British Berkfeld   U.S. distributor: James Filter
http://www.jamesfilter.com/

Berkey Filters

Product	Price	Structure/Function
Models include: Travel, Big Berkey, Royal, Imperial, Berkey Light (Lexan, not stainless steel)		A line of stainless steel stacked bucket filters that operate by gravity drip and can accommodate variable numbers of candle filter elements. There are two types of filter elements: (1) ceramic with carbon core and silver impregnation, and (2) compressed carbon impregnated with silver (Black Berkey). The size of the lower reservoir varies from 1.5-6 gal. Price varies by size and number of filter elements. Flow depends on number of filter elements.
SS-4	$220	Stacked stainless steel containers with four 7-inch ceramic filters with activated carbon core; gravity flow; size: 20 × 8.5 inches (15 inches when nested); weight: 6.0 lb; flow: 24 gal/day; 2-gal capacity of lower container, capacity: 6000 gal.

Continued

FOOD AND WATER

PART 13

British Berkfeld Claims and Comments

Ceramic filter is 0.9 µm absolute, but filters >99.99% of particles larger than 0.5 µm. Removes 100% cysts and 4- to 5-log bacteria. Complete protection requires chlorine treatment as the first step. Black (compressed carbon) filters remove 4- to 5-log cysts and bacteria.

The bucket filters are excellent for stationary base camps or expatriate homes. Ceramic candle filters will perform better than the carbon ones.

AquaRain Filter Systems		http://www.aquarain.com
AquaRain 200 (Figure 88-17)	$160-200	Stainless steel containers (3 gal each) with one to four silver-impregnated ceramic filters with
AquaRain 400 (Figure 88-18)	$240-320	carbon core; gravity flow; size: 22 × 10.25 inches; weight: 10 lb; flow: 1 gal/hr with four elements, 16 gal/day with two; capacity: 30,000-60,000 gal.
		Price depends on size and number of filter elements.

AquaRain Claims and Comments

Filter has 0.2-µm absolute pore size, removes 100% cysts and 4-log reduction of bacteria. Ceramic elements can be cleaned 200 times before replacement. Similar design as Berkfeld and Katadyn bucket drip filters, although ceramic elements differ slightly. No claims for viruses.

Ceramic candle filters have demonstrated efficacy in household use in developing countries, even removing most viruses due to aggregation with other microorganisms.[65]

Product	Price	Structure/Function
General Ecology		http://www.generalecology.com
		All filters contain 0.1-µm (0.4-µm absolute) Structured Matrix filter in removable canister.
First Need XLE Portable Water Filter (Figure 88-19)	$100-$130	Hand pump with intake strainer; outflow end connects directly to common water bottle and adapters available for Platypus bottles; self-cleaning prefilter float; size: 6 × 6 inches; weight: 15 oz; flow: 2 L/min; capacity: 600 L.
Trav-L-Pure (Figure 88-20) (Carrying case included)	$230	Filter and hand pump in rectangular housing (1.5-pt capacity); pour water into housing, then pump through prefilter and microfilter; size: 4.5 × 3.5 × 6.75 inches; weight: 22 oz; flow: 1-2 pt/min; capacity: 100-400 L.
Trav-L-Pure Camper (Figure 88-21)	$85	Trav-L-Pur canister with attachment to hose bib for recreational vehicles and trailers requires water pressure of 20 psi; flow: 0.5 gal/min (1.9 L/min); capacity: 570 L.
Base Camp (see Figure 88-12)	$700	Stainless steel casing and hand pump connected by tubing; size: canister 4.1 × 8.8 inches, pump 1.5 × 10.5 inches; weight: 3 lb; flow: 2 L/min; capacity: 500 gal. Also available with electric pump and can be hooked up in series to provide higher capacity and flow.

General Ecology has an extensive product line of larger-capacity filters for use on cars, boats, aircraft, and other situations requiring high-volume output where power is available. These use the Seagull IV purifier cartridge with a pump that pushes water through the system and a prefilter that can be cleaned. They can be operated off regular current or vehicle battery.

Claims

First Need Filter is a proprietary blend of materials, including activated charcoal. "Microfiltration" with 0.1 µm retention (0.4 µm absolute) "removes bacteria and larger pathogens" (cysts, parasites). "Adsorption and molecular sieving:" carbon absorbers remove chemicals and organic pollutants that cause color and taste; cavities in surface of adsorption material draw particles in deeper. Does not remove all dissolved minerals or desalinate. Proprietary process also creates ionic surface charge that removes colloids and ultrasmall particles through "electrokinetic attraction." Has passed laboratory tests as a purifier under single-pass conditions without added chemicals or hold time, reducing rotavirus test virus by 10^4 as well as bacteria by 10^6 and *Cryptosporidium* by 10^3.[3,126]

Comments

Reasonable design, cost, and effectiveness. All units use the same basic filter media. Most testing with *Escherichia coli* and *Giardia* cysts show excellent removal. Although they have not tested with hepatitis virus, testing with rotavirus and poliovirus indicate effectiveness against viruses. Charcoal matrix will remove chemical pollutants. Despite viral claims, recommend caution in highly polluted water; prior disinfection with halogen or clarification with coagulation-flocculation would provide additional security, and coagulation-flocculation would extend filter life, whereas filter carbon would subsequently remove halogen. The filter cannot be removed to clean, although it can potentially be back-flushed; so it must be replaced when clogged. Soft intake tubing collapses under pressure of pumping.

Product	Price	Structure/Function
Cascade Designs and MSR		http://www.cascadedesigns.com/MSR
MiniWorks EX (Figure 88-22)	$90	Hand pump, cylindrical ceramic filter with block carbon core, porous foam intake filter, and 10-µm stainless steel wire mesh screen; pressure-relief valve releases at 90-95 psi; storage bag (2 or 4 L) attaches directly to outlet of pump; size: 2.75 × 7.5 inches; weight: 16 oz; flow rate: 1 L/min (85 strokes/L); capacity: 400-2000 L (400 L under average conditions).
SweetWater Microfilter (Figure 88-23)	$90	Lexan body and pump handle; 80-µm metal prefilter; in-line 4-µm secondary filter; labyrinth filter cylinder of borosilicate fibers removes pathogens to 0.2 µm; granular activated
Purifier Kit with Microfilter, purifier solution and Platypus water bag	$90	carbon; safety pressure-relief valve; end-of-life indicator; outflow tubing has universal adapter that fits all water bottles; optional input adapter that attaches to sink faucet while traveling; size: 7.75 × 2 inches; weight: 11 oz; flow: 1.25 L/min (75 strokes); capacity: 750 L.
SweetWater Purifier solution	$10	A chlorine-based purifier solution containing 3.5% sodium hypochlorite; add 5 drops to each liter of filtered water, mix for at least 10 seconds, and wait 5 minutes.
HyperFlow (Figure 88-24)	$100	Hand pump using 0.2-µm hollow-fiber filter; attaches directly to top of water bottle for pumping; maintenance kit and replacement cartridges available; size: 7 × 3.5 inches; weight: 7.4 oz; flow: 3 L/min (1 L/20 strokes); capacity: about 1000 L.

Continued

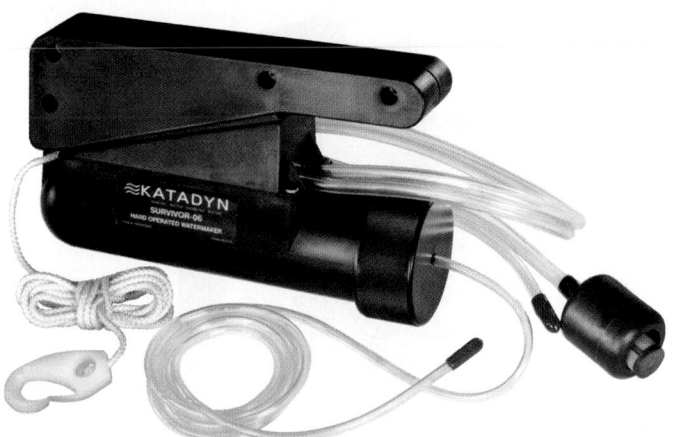

FIGURE 88-15 Survivor 06. (Courtesy Katadyn.)

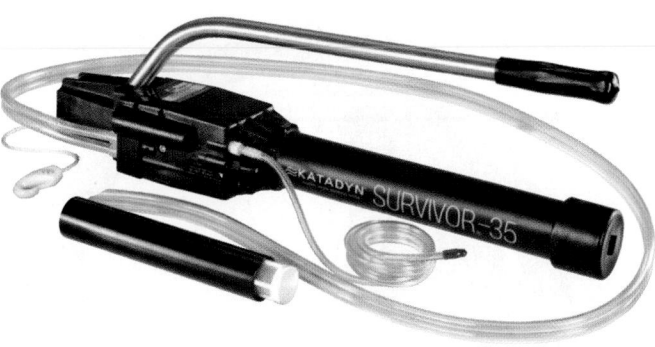

FIGURE 88-16 Survivor 35. (Courtesy Katadyn.)

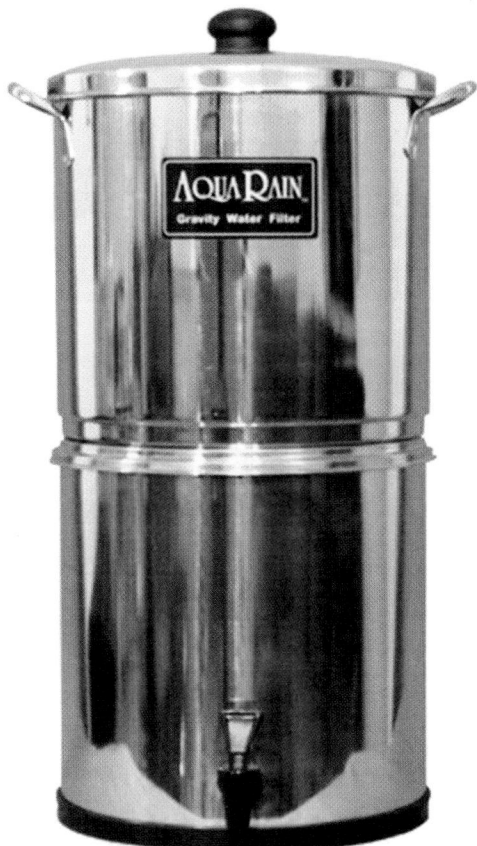

FIGURE 88-17 AquaRain 200. (Courtesy AquaRain.)

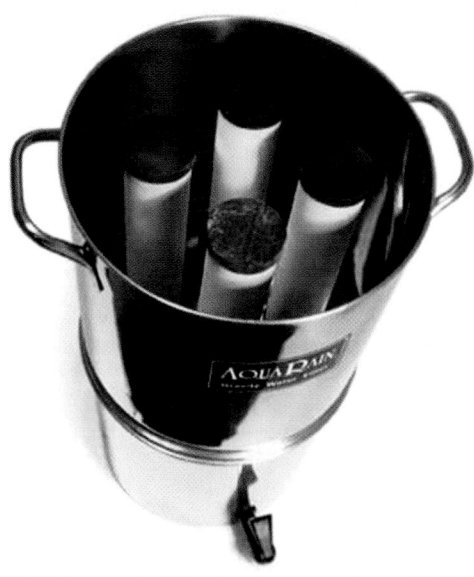

FIGURE 88-18 AquaRain 400, showing ceramic candle filters. (Courtesy AquaRain.)

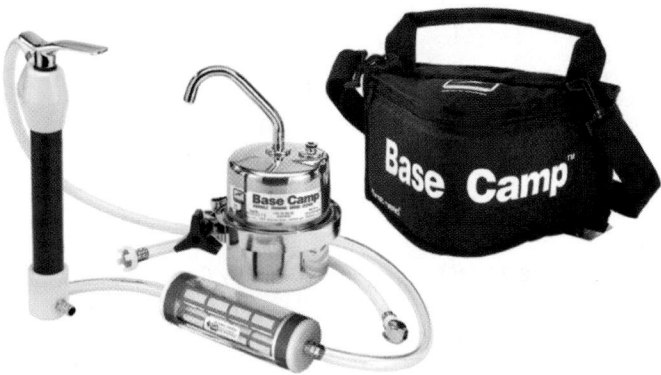

FIGURE 88-19 First Need Base Camp Filter. (Courtesy General Ecology.)

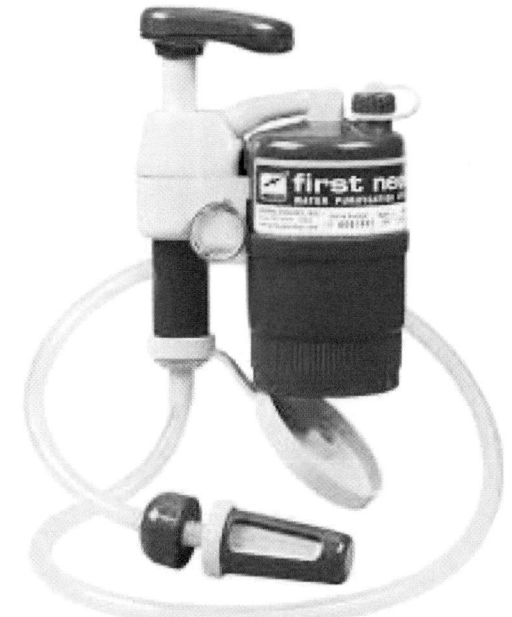

FIGURE 88-20 First Need XLE. (Courtesy General Ecology.)

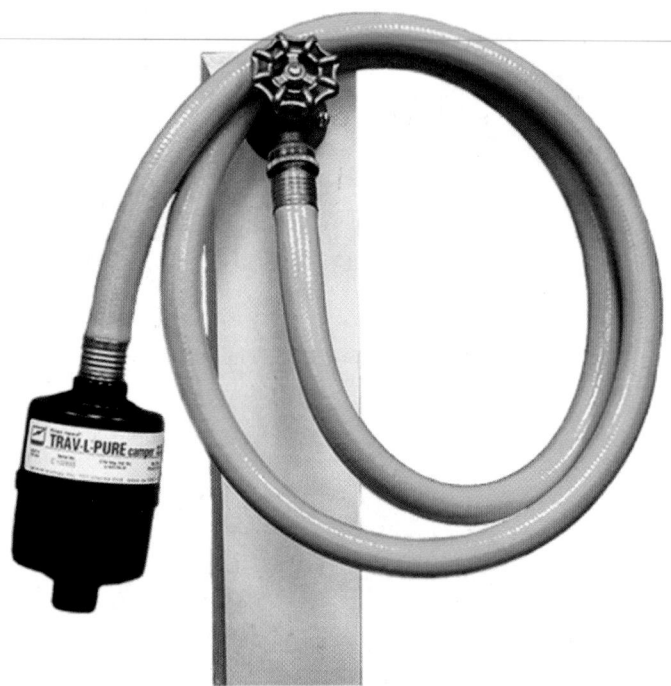

FIGURE 88-21 Trav-L-Pure Camper Canister. *(Courtesy General Ecology.)*

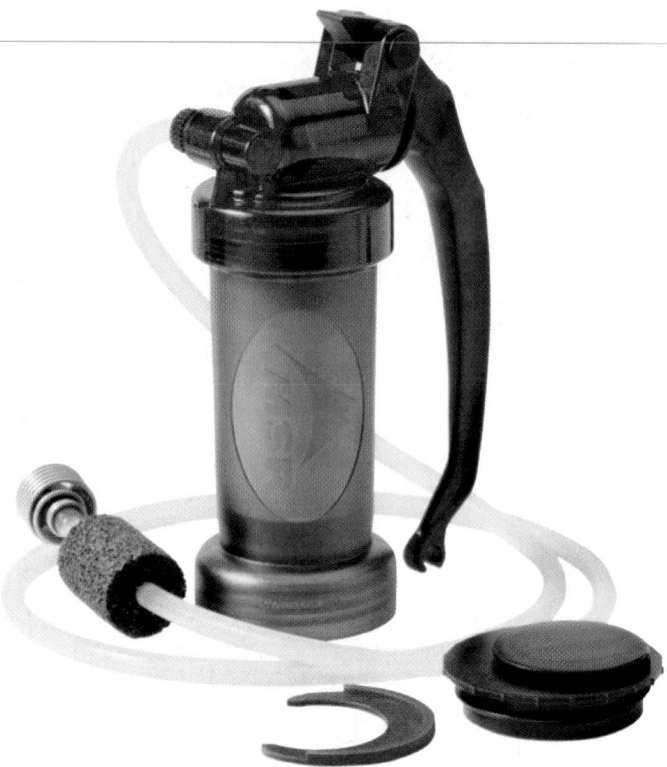

FIGURE 88-22 MSR Miniworks EX. *(Courtesy Cascade Designs.)*

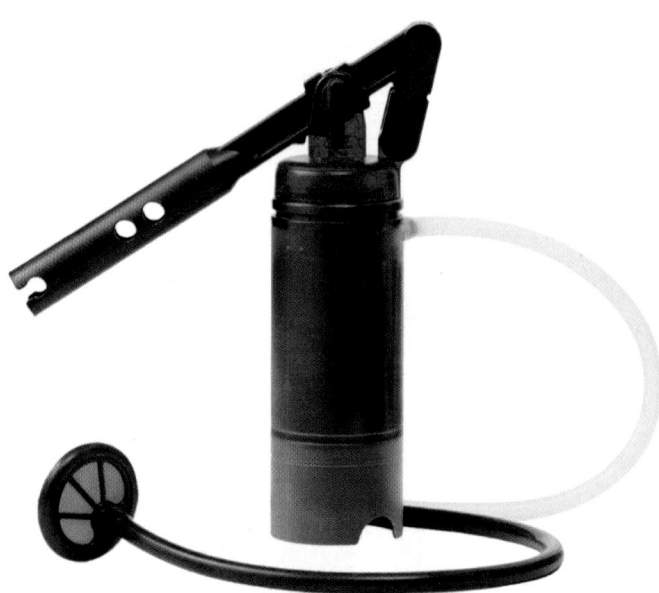

FIGURE 88-23 SweetWater Microfilter. *(Courtesy Cascade Designs.)*

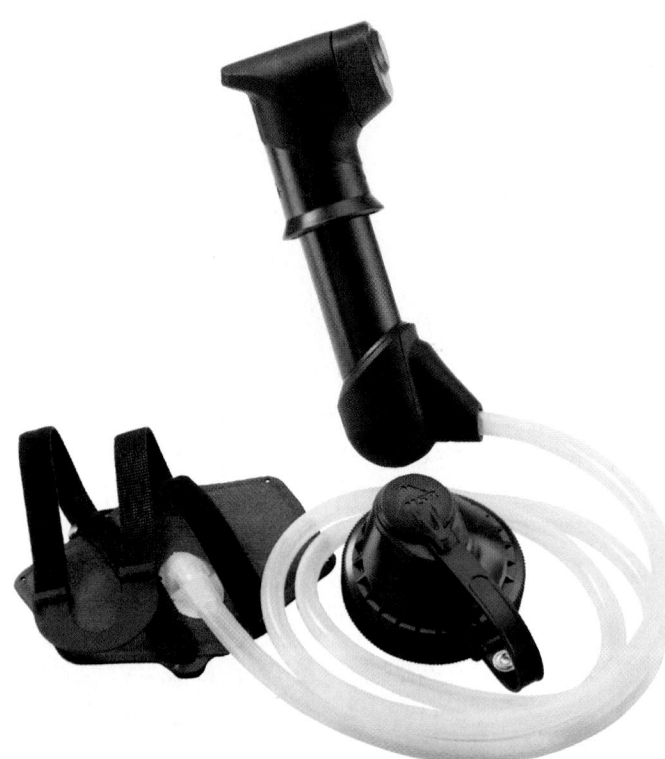

FIGURE 88-24 MSR HyperFlow. *(Courtesy Cascade Designs.)*

APPENDIX A—cont'd

AutoFlow (Figure 88-25)	$120	Gravity drip filter using hollow-fiber filter cartridge; size: 4 × 6 inches; reservoir capacity: 4 L; weight: 13.8 oz; flow: 1.75 L/min; capacity: about 1500 L/cartridge.
Platypus CleanStream Gravity Filter (Figure 88-26)		0.2-μm hollow-fiber filter cartridge gravity drip in-line system or can be used in personal hydration pack system; size: 1.8 × 5.7 inches; weight: 13.7 oz; flow: 4 L in under 2.5 min; capacity: about 1500 L.
SE200 (Figure 88-27)	$239	Recently available, Community Chlorine Maker, manufactured for developing countries. Electrochemical generation of chlorine and other disinfectant species using table salt and current from a 12-volt battery or main power source. Each 5-min run generates enough disinfectant to treat 55 gal with residual concentration of 2-ppm free hypochlorite.

Cascade Designs and MSR Claims
MiniWorks EX
Fully field-maintainable, meaning that all elements can be removed, cleaned, and replaced. Removes protozoa (including *Giardia* and *Cryptosporidium*), bacteria, pesticides, herbicides, chlorine, and discoloration. Meets EPA standards for removal of cysts and bacteria. Ceramic filters reduced turbidity from 68.8 NTU to 0.01 NTU. Carbon has been shown to reduce levels of iodine from 16 mg/L to <0.01 mg/L for at least 150 L.

SweetWater Filter
Eliminates *Giardia, Cryptosporidium,* and other critical bacterial and protozoan pathogens, pollutants, heavy metals, pesticides, and flavors. Cartridge accessory. Lighter, more compact and durable than comparable models, and easiest to clean or replace. The company recycles filter cartridges.

HyperFlow and AutoFlow
Effective against bacteria, particles, and protozoa, but not against viruses, chemicals, or toxins.

Comments
MiniWorks EX
Very good filter design and function. Prefilters protect more expensive microfilter. Effective for claims; high quality control, and extensive testing. No claims are made for viruses, although clumping and adherence remove the majority (currently 2- to 3-log removal, but not 4-log required for purifiers). Reservoir bag that attaches to outflow for filtered water storage is convenient. Filter can be easily maintained in the field; maintenance kit and all replacement parts available. Ceramic filters can be cleaned by abrading outer surface many times without compromising the filter. A simple caliper gauge indicates when filter has become too thin for reliable function.

SweetWater
Well-designed filter at a reasonable price. Pressure-release valve indicates when filter needs cleaning, but this can be a problem as the filter clogs. A brush is provided for cleaning, and cartridges are replaceable.

HyperFlow and AutoFlow
These use microtubule, hollow-fiber technology that can provide higher flow rates with less pressure, which makes them amenable to gravity systems. HyperFlow is the first hand pump with microtubules, but others are likely to follow.

SE 200
The SE200 replaces the smaller Miox unit that used the same technology, generating current from small disk batteries. The science has been known for some time and is used in large commercial processes (http://www.miox.com). Although difficult to measure various disinfectant species generated, testing has confirmed that disinfectant activity is greater than with comparable concentrations of sodium hypochlorite. Cascade Designs is being safe and conservative in their claims, basing them solely on hypochlorite generation. http://www.cascadedesigns.com/msr/global-health/se200/product

Product	Price	Structure/Function
Sawyer Products		http://www.sawyerproducts.com/
PointONE biologic filter and Point Zero Two Purifier filter cartridges		0.1-μm (absolute) hollow-fiber membrane filter, composed of a cluster of microtubules. Purifier filter has 0.02-μm fiber filter. Water is drawn through the walls of the tubules by suction, gravity, or pressure applied by squeezing a bottle; both filter cartridges can be adapted as in-line cartridge for backpack water systems, gravity drip, faucet in-line systems, or polycarbonate drinking bottle with filter. Activated charcoal prefilter cartridge included for optional use; flow: depends on method used, about 1.5 L/min, 5 gal/30 min via gravity feed system; 30 mL/sec from drink-through; capacity: 1 million gal, but depends on clarity of source water. The two types of filters are available in a variety of products and combination packages, including drink-through bottles and in-line hydration systems; gravity drip, faucet attachments, and bucket filter adapter. As yet, there are no hand pump units. Products below may not be complete representation.
All in One	$70	0.1-μm filter can be used with 32-oz squeeze bag, drinking sports bottle, bucket adapter kit, faucet adapter.
Complete Purifier system (Figure 88-28)	$95-$220	Gravity drip system using either 0.1- or 0.02-μm filter with 2 bags (dirty and clean), available in 2-L, 4-L capacity.
Filter Bucket Adapter 0.1 or 0.02 (Figure 88-29)	$60-$130	Kit to attach filter cartridge to a plastic bucket or barrel for gravity drip; comes with hole cutter, adapter, and tubing to construct system. Either 0.1- or 0.02-μm cartridge can be used; flow: estimated up to 170 gal/day.
Squeeze Water Filter (includes 12-, 16-, and 32-oz pouches, water filter, and pop-up drinking spout)	$40	0.1-μm hollow fiber filter cartridge attaches to bags that can be squeezed to maximize flow. Squeeze water into water bottle or drink directly from the filter; weight: 3 oz; capacity: 1 million gal.

Continued

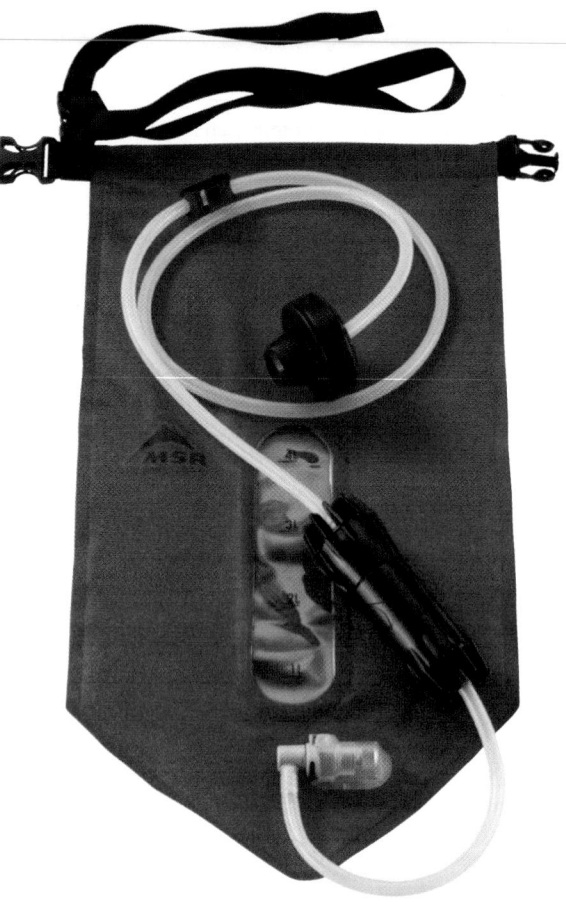

FIGURE 88-25 MSR AutoFlow. *(Courtesy Cascade Designs.)*

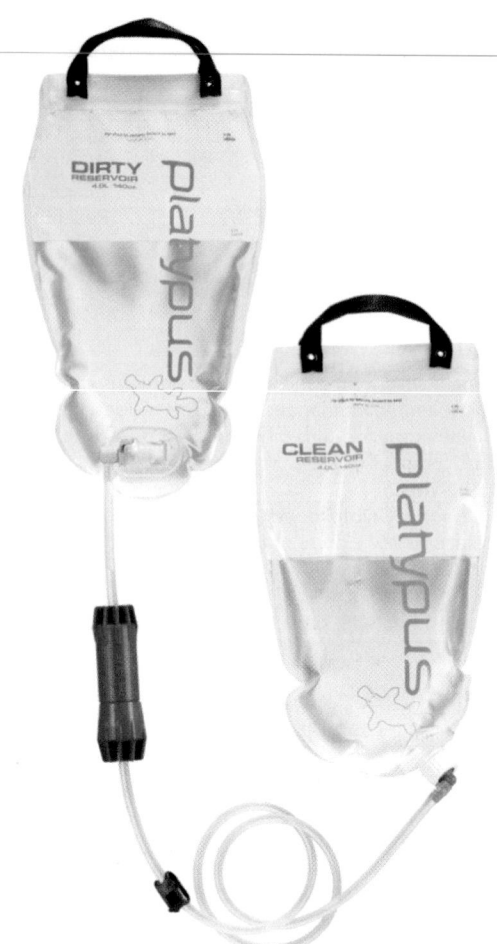

FIGURE 88-26 MSR Platypus CleanStream Gravity Filter. *(Courtesy Cascade Designs.)*

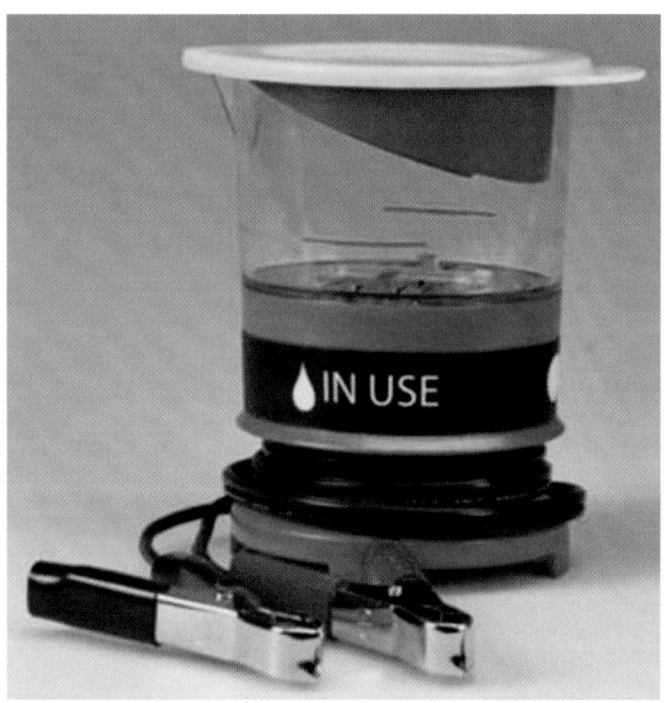

FIGURE 88-27 Cascade Designs and PATH SE200. (Developed with multiple global health NGO partners for developing-world communities.) *(Courtesy Cascade Designs.)*

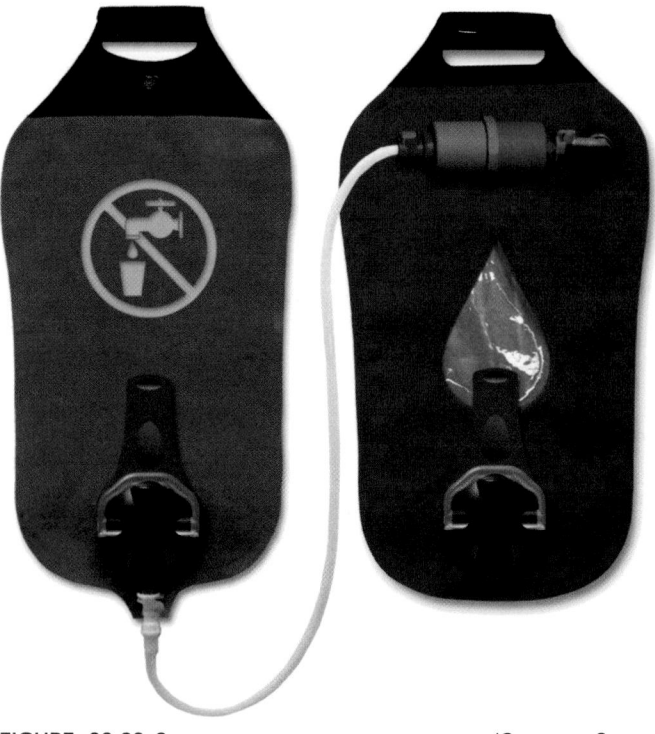

FIGURE 88-28 Sawyer water treatment system. *(Courtesy Sawyer Products.)*

PointONE 10" Filter Unit	$700	Filter cartridge and regulator with 0.1-μm absolute hollow-fiber membrane that attaches in-line to water line or plumbing; for school, hospital, and other settings with high-volume needs; regulator allows safe cleaning of the filter by back washing at an exact pressure; size: 10 inches long; flow: 5000 gal/day.

Claims

Microtubule technology (Figure 88-30) allows unprecedented flow rates and 0.1- or 0.02-μm absolute filtration. Highest level of biological filtration available on the market today; exceeds EPA standards. GAV prefilter removes lead, chlorine, odors, and taste sediment, whereas the microfilter removes bacteria, protozoa, and cysts. Biologic filters; 0.1-μm filter removes 7-log (99.9999%) bacteria and 6-log protozoa, but makes no claims for viruses; add chlorine to kill viruses. The Point Zero Two absolute purifier removes 99.99999% of bacteria, 99.9999% of protozoa and cysts, and 99.9997% of viruses from the water. It is impossible for any bacteria, protozoa, cysts, and viruses to pass through the filter.

Filters can be back-washed and are able to handle 40 psi, so they can be attached to faucets.

Comments

This technology has been used in industrial and medical processes, but only recently adapted to field water treatment. The Microfilter and Ultrafilter were carefully designed and tested. They are highly versatile, because designed as a cartridge that can be used in various systems from drinking bottles, to gravity drip systems, to in-line household systems. They offer a potential advantage over other water bottle filters because the hollow-fiber technology provides faster filtration with less pressure. The charcoal cartridge compromises some of this low-pressure flow, so is supplied separately for use only when needed. This is the first low-pressure ultrafilter to claim viral removal through mechanical filtration alone. The million-gallon guarantee is based on the large surface area of the tubules.

Bucket filter is a particularly creative application to these filters, with many applications in rural or developing countries.

Product	Price	Structure/Function
Hydro-Photon Inc		http://www.steripen.com/
SteriPEN Classic Traveler (Figure 88-31) (Comes with a thermoformed nylon carrying case)	$50-70	Portable, battery-operated (4 AA-lithium) ultraviolet (UV) water disinfection system. Disinfects up to 16 oz of clear water in less than 1 minute and 32 oz in 90 sec by stirring UV element in water; weight: 5.5 oz, with batteries; size: 7.6 × 1.5 × 1.5 inches; capacity: lamp lasts 8000 treatments; lithium batteries, 200 treatments.
AdventurerOpti	$90	Uses 2 CR123 batteries and is significantly smaller and lighter than Classic; weight: 3.8 oz; size 6.1 × 1.5 × 1 inches.
Ultra (LCD display) (Figure 88-32)	$100	Uses internal rechargeable lithium ion battery; weight: 5 oz; size: 7.3 × 1.6 × 1.3 inches; lamp life is 8000 cycles and can expect up to 100 uses from batteries.
Freedom	$100	Smallest and lightest unit, rechargeable battery through computer USB, AC outlet, or solar charger; weight: 2.6 oz; size: 5.1 × 1.4 × 0.8 inches; capacity: 40 treatments/charge; battery and UV lamp life: 8000 16-oz (0.5-L) treatments (1-L volumes disinfected by treating twice).
Sidewinder	$100	1-L bottle fits into unit with hand crank that generates UV light without batteries; weight: 16.6 oz; size: 8.6 × 5.5 × 3.8 inches; capacity: 8000 1-L treatments.

SteriPEN Claims

Highly effective against bacteria, viruses, and protozoa, including *Cryptosporidium* oocysts. UV light delivered destroys viruses, bacteria, and protozoa in 0.5 L (16 oz) of water in 48 sec or 1 L (32 oz) in 90 sec. Unit automatically turns off lamp after UV dose is delivered. Dose counter indicates when lamp replacement is necessary. In units that run on AA batteries, the recommendation is to use lithium, not alkaline batteries.

Testing demonstrates that Steri-PEN meets the EPA standards as a microbiologic water purifier.

Steri-Pen Comments

In general, UV light for water disinfection is well established from extensive scientific research and widely used for water treatment in large and medium-size applications, most of which require a fixed power and light source. The use of this portable technology is currently limited to small volumes of clear water; however, the potential is great for further advances that will increase its uses in the field. The price of some units has already decreased. Currently, one could do slightly larger volumes with multiple cycles. The testing for this device can be found on the website. Since particulates block the UV rays and shield microorganisms, testing was only successful in clear water, not in EPA "worst-case scenario" water unless prefiltered with microfiltration.[1] Therefore, users must prefilter or clarify cloudy water. The simplicity and rapidity of this technique are appealing.

Product	Price	Structure/Function
Puralytics Photocatalytic Titanium Dioxide Nanoparticles		http://www.puralytics.com
SolarBag	$90	3-L food-grade clear plastic bag with clear top and black backing and a coating of TiO_2 nanoparticles inside. Bag is filled with water and placed in sunlight, which activates the TiO_2 to catalyze a reaction to form active disinfectants (see text). The bag has backpack and handle straps to carry to and from water source; inlet debris filter; can be hung for water storage and water dispensed by a valve into canteen or pot as required. For disinfection, bag is placed flat or hanging in direct sunlight; disinfection requires 1-2 hr on sunny day and 2-4 hr on cloudy day; for unknown water sources, a food-safe dye can be used as a tracer and timer—when the color has cleared, the water has been purified. Dry weight: 100 g; size: 3 L; capacity: 250 L; shelf life: >2 yr.

Continued

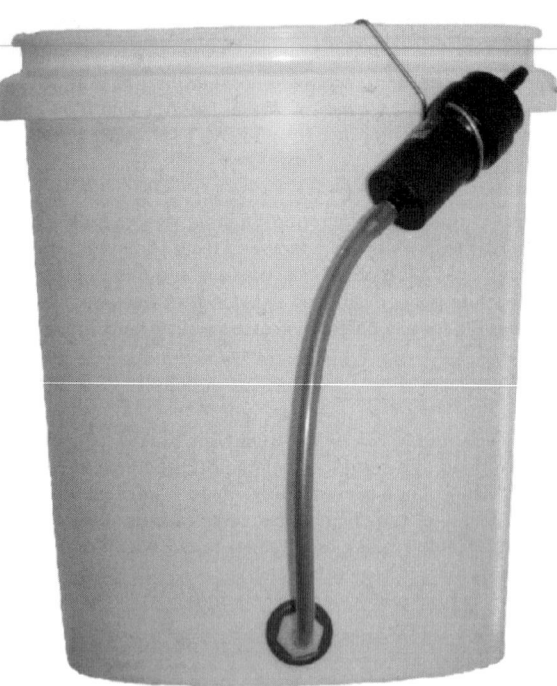

FIGURE 88-29 Sawyer bucket filter. *(Courtesy Sawyer Products.)*

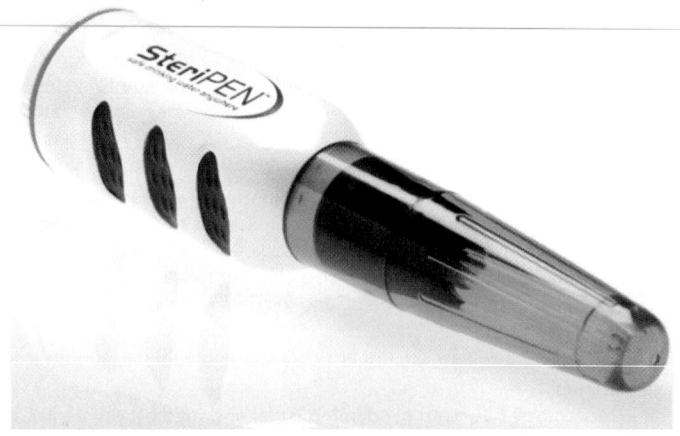

FIGURE 88-31 SteriPEN Classic. *(Courtesy Hydro-Photon.)*

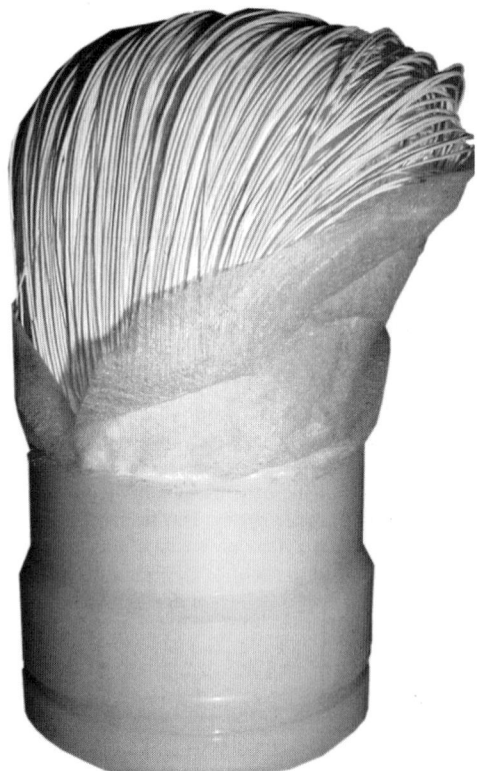

FIGURE 88-30 Microtubules in Sawyer filter cartridge. *(Courtesy Sawyer Products.)*

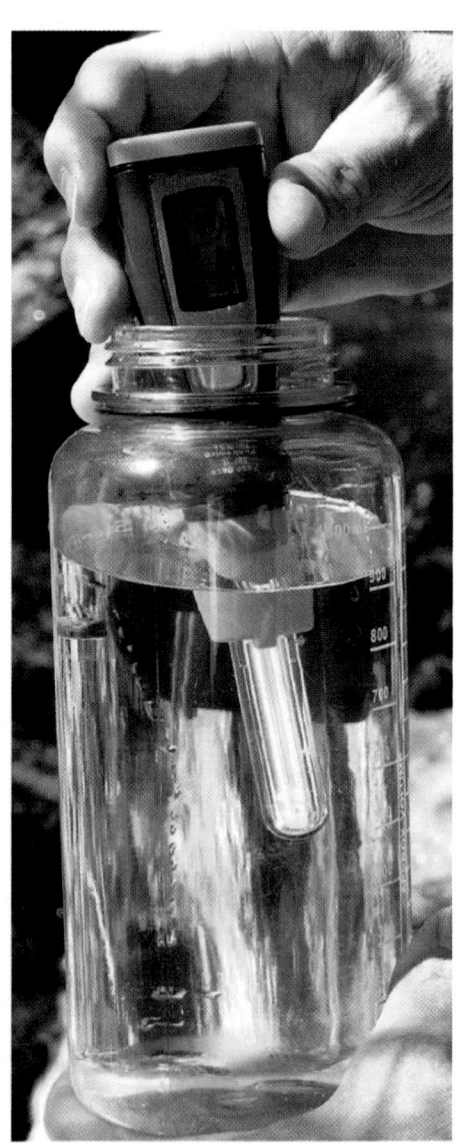

FIGURE 88-32 SteriPEN Journey. *(Courtesy Hydro-Photon.)*

Shield 500 and 1000	$9500	High-volume unit that uses UV LEDs to activate nanotechnology mesh; size: 28 × 8 × 19 inches; weight: 89 lb; flow: 200-500 gal/day; power: 640 watts; pressure 15-60 psi; life span: 10 yr. Model 1000: 500-1000 gal/day.

Claims

Works through multiple photochemical processes. Selected wavelengths of UV light generate hydroxyl radicals (OH^-) without chemical additives. Disassociates and eliminates organic compounds from the water. Reduces heavy metal to less toxic, more elemental state and irreversibly adsorbs heavy metals, including mercury, lead, chromium, and arsenic. Disinfects pathogens more effectively than standard UV irradiation. After 2 hours in the sun on an 80° F sunny day, process will reduce 7-log bacteria, 5-log viruses, 90% heavy metals, and 90% organic compounds.

Comments

This is a new and promising technology for field water disinfection and purification (see section on nanoparticles). Significant testing and literature is available because it has multiple applications in industrial and community-level water treatment. Independent testing demonstrated effectiveness against *Cryptosporidium*.[306] Blue food dye is supplied to ensure continued function of bag.

Product	Price	Structure/Function
Hydration Technology Innovations (HTI)		
http://www.htiwater.com/hti.html		
X-Pack	$64	A plastic pouch with two compartments separated by a semipermeable membrane that provides ultrafiltration to 0.0005 μm (5 Å); fill one side with dirty or contaminated suspect water; add to the other side a specially formulated syrup supplied with the kit that contains salts and sugars.
Ten 2-oz sports drink syrup charges and dye tabs	$16.50	
		Volume: 1.8 L; weight: 3 lb, includes syrup charges; flow: 1 L/4 hr, can produce a total of over 5 L of hydration drink per day; capacity: 32 L; good for a total of 10 days of use after first use.
LifePack	$35	Single filter, six 2-oz syrup charges; 5-day filter life; 1.8-L bag capacity; 3 L/day.
SeaPack	$85	Dual-chamber pouch, 1.8-L capacity each, separated by semipermeable membrane with nominal pore size of 3-5 Å; flow: 0.5 L/5 hr at 20° C (68° F); capacity: 4 L from seawater, or up to 24 L from freshwater; filter life: 10 days.
Includes eight 4-oz syrup charges		
Expedition	$299	Dual-reservoir water bladder for use with clean or contaminated water; uses osmotic filter cartridge that works by forward osmosis from osmotic syrup; one 4-oz (0.12-L) syrup pouch will filter about 2.5 L of water; capable of filtering fresh to brackish water; clean reservoir volume: 3.0 L, dirty reservoir volume: 2.5 L; flow: about 0.8 L/hr; filter life: 30-90 days (clean weekly).
Includes ten 4-oz syrup pouches, cleaning kit		
HydroWell	$389	Dual 20-L cans with osmotic filter built into a standard water can cap; forward osmosis driven by one sports syrup pouch that fits into the cap; one syrup pouch will filter one 20-L can of fresh to brackish water; flow: about 1.2 L/hr; filter life: 30-90 days (clean weekly).
Includes twenty 14-oz syrup pouches, cleaning kit		

Claims

Forward osmosis—water is driven across the membrane, not by hydraulic pressure, but by osmotic pressure created by a standard sport drink powder on the clean side of the membrane. This syrup is formulated much like the concentrate for a typical sports drink containing about 4% sugar (this compares with some other sports drinks at 6% and soda at 12%). Capable of filtering highly turbid water (tested to 800 NTU). Minimum 3-yr shelf life when stored below 32.2° C (90° F).

Comments

Forward osmosis is based on sound technology, and these products provide a good solution for disaster supplies or survival cache with long shelf life. Less optimal when on the move, although the bags could be primed and carried throughout the day while filtering. For those who prefer fresh water, the resulting sweetened solution is a major disadvantage. Simple filters or chemical solutions are lighter and faster for fresh water but cannot handle brackish water as can some of the HTI products.

Large-Scale Field Products

The following are included as examples of multistage products that are available for large-volume field water treatment. This is not a comprehensive list of products, and many others are available, including trailer-mounted reverse-osmosis systems. These products require a power source and may require truck or trailer for transportation. Most chemical systems can be scaled up through using large containers or water bladders and multistation distribution systems.

Global Hydration Water Treatment Systems

http://www.globalhydration.com/canpure-water-purification-system.htm

Can Pure Water Purification System	Dual-process purification system incorporating six-stage microfiltration system and UV disinfection; optional residual chlorination using NaDCC tablets. Model 4: size: 23 × 23 × 24 inches; weight: 82 lb; output: 8500 L/day (2245 gal/day); power requirements: small generator (130 watts), can also be run on 12-volt DC or 120-volt AC. Model 5: size 23 × 23 × 29 inches; weight 83 lb; output: 5000 gal/day. Water Miracle: size: 40 × 40 × 86.6 inches; weight: 660 lb; output: 12,720 gal/day.
Various models available	

Complete stand-alone water treatment system designed to produce potable water in remote field conditions and in emergency and disaster situations. Compact; portable; capable of running off gas or diesel generator without electricity or gravity.

Continued

First Water Systems	http://firstwaterinc.com
Responder, Outpost, Villager	All M-line (mobile) units use high-strength UV bulb for disinfection with in-line prefilter for large particulates, a 0.2-μm sediment filter to reduce turbidity, and carbon block for improving taste and smell; all units can be supplemented with residual chlorination system; run off a variety of power sources, including solar, battery, or generator.
	Water bladder and distribution system available; filling station enables either four or six lines of people to obtain water at any given time. Aqua Bags for transport of clean water are 3-gal heavy-gauge food-grade plastic bags that weigh about 20 lb when full.
Responder	Portable model with canister configuration that runs on solar, on-board 12-volt battery, AC or DC power; size: briefcase size, 20 × 17 × 9 inches; 45 lb, including wheeled case; flow: 4 gal (16 L)/min, or about 600 gal (2500 L)/day per battery.
Outpost-4	Semiportable model water purification system runs exclusively off integrated solar system and an on-board battery; size: fits in the back of a pickup truck, SUV, minivan, mounted on wheeled frame; weight: 160 lb; flow: 4 gal (16 L)/min, or about 600 gal (2500 L)/day per battery (enough water for 1000 persons per day with multiple batteries).

Comments

The UV system forces the water to circulate around the UV bulb twice, providing significantly greater "contact time" and greater ability to neutralize biologic contamination. Cigarette lighter plug adapters for additional battery power and AC power. Using multiple batteries extends the usable time and the amount of water produced. All filters easily detach for rapid cleaning or replacement.

APPENDIX B

Chemical Disinfection Products

See text for further discussion of chemical disinfectants.

IODINATION

IODINE SOLUTIONS

Iodine solutions commercially sold as topical disinfectants contain iodine, potassium or sodium iodide in water, and ethyl alcohol or glycerol (see Table 88-14). Iodide improves stability and solubility but has no germicidal activity and adds to the total amount of iodine ingested and absorbed into the body. "Decolorized" iodine solution contains iodide and should not be used for water disinfection.

IODOPHORS (POVIDONE-IODINE)

These solutions bind diatomic iodine to a neutral polymer of high molecular weight, giving the iodine greater solubility and stability with less toxicity and corrosive effect.[56,128] Povidone-iodine is a 1-vinyl-2-pyrrolidinone polymer with 9% to 12% available iodine. The iodophors are routinely used for topical disinfection, because they have less tissue toxicity than iodine solutions. Povidone is nontoxic.

In aqueous solution, povidone-iodine provides a sustained-release reservoir of halogen; free iodine is released in water solution depending on the concentration (normally, 2 to 10 ppm is present in solution). Data indicate persistence of about 2 ppm of free iodine at a 1:10,000 dilution,[128] equivalent to 0.1 mL (2 drops) added to 1 L of water. One report found these compounds similar in germicidal efficiency to other iodine-iodide solutions.[56] Conflicting values for available iodine and free iodine in dilute solutions result from the complex chemistry of povidone-iodine.[18,146]

CRYSTALS (SATURATED SOLUTION)

Because of limited solubility in water, iodine crystals may be used to generate an iodine solution for disinfection. A small amount of elemental iodine goes into solution (no significant iodide is present); the saturated solution is used to disinfect drinking water. Water can be added to the crystals hundreds of times before they are completely dissolved. Because iodine crystals evaporate in air, always keep covered with water.

To formulate this solution at home, put 4 to 8 g (exact amount does not matter) of crystalline iodine in a 1- or 2-oz bottle, and fill with water. An alternative technique is to add 8 g of iodine crystals to 100 mL of 95% ethanol. Increased solubility of iodine in alcohol makes the solution less temperature dependent and allows much smaller volumes to be used (8 mg/0.1 mL), which can be measured with a 1-mL syringe or dropper (2 drops). Residual iodine can be removed with granular activated carbon.

Product

Polar Pure

http://www.polarequipment.com/

Price: $15.00

Widely available through suppliers of outdoor products

Formulation: Eight grams of iodine crystals in a 3-oz glass bottle filled with water; 30- to 50-μm fabric prefilter provided; "trap" in bottle to catch crystals when pouring off water; capacity: 2000 qt; weight: 5 oz.

Instructions: The bottle cap is used to measure iodine solution: one capful is approximately 6.5 mL. Directions and color-dot thermometer are printed on the bottle. Recommended dose: 2 capfuls if iodine solution is 20°C (68°F) yields 4 ppm of iodine when added to 1 qt of clean water. To shorten contact time, warm water to 20°C (68°F) before adding iodine.

Comments

Saturated aqueous solution of crystalline iodine is an excellent and stable source of iodine. Recommendations are adequate for clear, warm water; however, because it is not feasible to warm all water, extend contact time to 1 to 2 hours for very cold water. Temperature of the iodine bottle also affects the concentration of iodine in the saturated solution (200 ppm at 10°C [50°F], 300 ppm at 20°C [68°F], 400 ppm at 30°C [86°F]),[59,128] which is the reason for the color-dot thermometer on the bottle. In the field, it may be easier to warm the bottle in an inner pocket than to estimate temperature and adjust the dose. The supernatant should be carefully decanted or filtered to avoid ingestion of the crystals;[353] this is aided by the weight of the crystals, which causes them to sink. Many people prefer crystalline iodine because of its large disinfectant capacity, small size, and light weight. The absence of iodide decreases total amount of iodine ingested. The glass bottle can break, and there are anecdotal reports of freezing in very cold temperatures.

Iodine in alcohol is a viable option that allows for much smaller doses because of higher solubility of iodine in alcohol. Currently, there is no commercial product, but it can easily be formulated at home.

IODINE TABLETS

The tablets contain tetraglycine hydroperiodide, which is 40% I_2 and 20% iodide.[56,218] They were originally developed by the military for individual field use because of their broad-spectrum disinfection effect, ease of handling, rapid dissolution, stability, and acceptable taste.[229,245,271]

One tablet contains 20 mg of tetraglycine hydroperiodide that releases 8 mg/L of elemental iodine into water; both diatomic iodine (I_2) and hypoiodous acid (HIO) are released. An acidic buffer provides a pH of 5.5 to 6.5, which supports better cysticidal than virucidal capacity but should be adequate for both. Tablets have the advantages of easy handling and no danger of staining or corroding if spilled. They are stable for 4 to 5 years under sealed storage conditions and for 2 weeks with frequent opening under field conditions, but they lose 30% of the active iodine if bottles are left open for 4 days in high heat or humidity.

Products

Potable Aqua (Wisconsin Pharmacal Co, Jackson, Wisconsin)
  http://potableaqua.com/
  Price: 50 tablets, $6.00; with PA Plus Neutralizing tablets, $9.00
  Widely available through suppliers of outdoor products
  Also sold as Globaline and EDWGT (emergency drinking water germicidal tablets)
  Instructions: One tablet is added to 1 qt of water. In cloudy or cold water, add two tablets. Contact time is only 10 to 15 minutes in clear, warm water; much more in cold, cloudy water (see Tables 88-10 to 88-12).
  To remove taste and color of iodine, add one tablet of Potable Aqua PA Plus, mix, and wait 3 minutes. PA Plus should be used *after* the 30-minute waiting period for Potable Aqua.
  If the tablets are gray or dark brown in color, they are still likely to be effective. If they are light green or yellow, it means they are probably no longer effective. An opened bottle should not be kept for more than 1 year.

Comments

This method was developed by the military for troops in the field. Advantages are unit dose and short contact time, but these concentrations create strong taste that is not acceptable to many wilderness users. The military requirements dictated a short contact time (10 minutes in clear, warm water), thus the relatively high concentration of iodine (8 to 16 ppm). With adequate contact time and moderate temperatures, one tablet can be added to 2 qt of water to yield 4 ppm of free iodine (see Table 88-15). Rather than use two tablets in cloudy water, clarify the water first.

PA + Plus "neutralizing" tablet contains approximately 45 mg of ascorbic acid (vitamin C), which converts iodine to iodide and removes the taste and color of iodine but has no disinfecting action. However, iodide is physiologically active, so concerns about toxicity or physiologic activity remain. For short-term use, iodine is safe and removing the taste is a major benefit. Ascorbic acid powder can be purchased at many health food stores and used to neutralize any iodine disinfecting solution.

CHLORINATION

Free chlorine is available from several compounds and widely available in liquid and tablet formulations. (See text discussion and Tables 88-11 and 88-12.)

Chlorine test strips or meters are widely available for large groups or disaster/community situations when testing for adequate chlorine residual is desired. Simple, inexpensive field test kits or swimming pool test kits with color strips are widely available from many different manufacturers to ensure adequate residual chlorine.

SODIUM HYPOCHLORITE

Household Bleach

Liquid household bleach is a sodium hypochlorite solution, most often 5.25%, but more recently 8.25%. It has the convenience of wide availability, low cost, and good stability. Sodium hypochlorite solutions are vulnerable to significant loss of available chlorine over time. Stability is greatly affected by heat and light. The 5% solution loses about 10% available chlorine over 6 months at 21.1°C (70°F) and freezes at 4.4°C (40°F). The liquid is corrosive and stains clothing if the bleach container breaks or leaks in a pack. Sodium hypochlorite solution in a squeeze dropper bottle is paired with several portable microfilter products to ensure viral disinfection (e.g., SweetWater Viral Stop).

The U.S. Centers for Disease Control and Prevention (CDC)–World Health Organization (WHO) Safe Water System promotes products worldwide with 1% sodium hypochlorite for water disinfection.[176] Recent evaluation indicates that the CDC Safe Water dose may be inadequate in organic-laden water,[101] whereas the U.S. Environmental Protection Agency (EPA) recommendations for emergency use of household bleach are too high, especially with household bleach concentration increasing to 8.25%.[177]

CALCIUM HYPOCHLORITE (DRY CHLORINE)

Calcium hypochlorite is a stable, concentrated, dry source of hypochlorite frequently used for chlorination of swimming pools. The usual formulation contains 70% concentration of chlorine. Calcium hypochlorite is inexpensive and available in tablets or granules through chemical supply or swimming pool supply stores; one common brand is HTH, but there are many commercial products.

Redi-Chlor (Gripo Laboratories, New Delhi, India)
  http://www.gripolabs.com
  50 tablets in blister packs
  Price: $9.95
  Multiple strengths, including: 0.5 g, 1.0 g, 2.0 g, 2.5 g, for treating 20, 80, 200, 240 L, respectively
  Available from multiple suppliers
  Formulation: Redi-Chlor tablets come in different sizes and can be broken in half or fourths to treat different quantities of water. Recommended dose results in 2 to 5 mg/L residual chlorine. Add more for very cold water or if faint chlorine smell is not detected after contact time. Available in blister packs of 50 0.1-g tablets that treat 1 gal per tablet or 0.25-g tablets that treat 5 gal per tablet.
  Instructions: For situations where many water containers are to be disinfected, it is easier to use a concentrated disinfecting solution. EPA instructions: Add and dissolve one heaping teaspoon of high-test granular calcium hypochlorite (approximately 0.25 oz) for each 2 gal of water. The mixture will produce a stock chlorine solution of

approximately 500 mg/L (100 to 200 times desired strength for drinking). To disinfect water, add the chlorine solution in the ratio of one part of chlorine solution to each 100 parts of water to be treated. This is roughly equal to adding 1 pt (16 oz or approximately 0.5 L) of the stock chlorine solution to each 12.5 gal (50 L) of water to be disinfected.

See U.S. military instructions[319] and Table 88-13 for more details for dosing calcium hypochlorite for various strengths of chlorine and volume of water.

Comments

This is a convenient source of concentrated hypochlorite, which can also be used for superchlorination (see text).

HALAZONE TABLETS

Aquazone (Gripo Laboratories, New Delhi, India)
www.gripolabs.com
100/250/500/1000 tablets in plastic container or 50/60 tablets in blister packs
Tablets contain a mixture of monochloraminobenzoic and dichloraminobenzoic acids.[100] Each tablet releases 2.3 to 2.5 ppm of titratable chlorine.[229]

Comments

These tablets have been criticized because the alkaline buffer necessary to improve Halazone dissolution decreases disinfectant efficiency, requiring unacceptably high concentrations and contact times (6 tablets yield 15 mg/L with recommended contact time of 60 minutes) for reliable disinfection under all conditions.[271] The shelf life is 6 months; potency decreases 50% when stored at 40° to 50°C (104° to 122°F). A new bottle should be taken on each major trip or changed every 3 to 6 months. Halazone has mainly been replaced by newer tablet formulations of chlorine.

SODIUM DICHLOROISOCYANURATE

Sodium dichloroisocyanurate (NaDCC) is a stable, nontoxic chlorine compound that releases free active chlorine and forms a mildly acidic solution, which is optimal for hypochlorous acid, the most active disinfectant of the free chlorine compounds. Free chlorine is in equilibrium with available chlorine that remains in compound, providing greater biocidal capacity. NaDCC is more stable and provides more free active chlorine than other available chlorine products for water disinfection.

Manufacturers and Product Formulations

Gripo Laboratories (New Delhi, India)
http://www.gripolabs.com/nadcc_tablets.html
Tablets available in sizes to treat 1 to 100,000 L
Kintab (Bioman Products) (Mottram, Hyde, Cheshire, UK)
http://www.bioman.co.uk
Aquatabs (Medentech, Wexford, Ireland)
Six tablet strengths: 3.5, 8.5, 17, 33, 67, and 167 mg, depending on the volume to be treated, in individual foil-wrapped packets or strips. Larger quantities are available in tubs.
Also available through Global Hydration Water Treatment Systems (Kakabeka Falls, Ontario, Canada)
http://www.globalhydration.com/aquatabs-water-purification-tablets.htm
Packs of 24 or 50 tablets to treat 1 L/tab or 30 tablets to treat 20 L (5 gal)/tab
Pristine (Advanced Chemicals Ltd, Port Coquitlam, BC, Canada)
http://www.pristine.ca/

Formulation and Instructions

When dissolved in 1 L of water, each effervescent tablet releases 10 mg of free chlorine; 50% of the available chlorine remains in compound and is released as free chlorine as solution is used up by halogen demand. Aquatab also makes slow-dissolving tablets for larger quantities of water that contain trichloroisocynuric acid (TCCA), which acts similar to NaDCC.

Disinfection of clear surface water is accomplished at 10 mg/L in 10 minutes, 1 mg/L for tap water and 2 to 5 mg/L for well water. NaDCC is also used to wash fruits and vegetables in concentrations of 20 mg/L or higher.

The tablets have a 3- to 5-year shelf life.

Comments

This is a good source of chlorine available in multiple doses and formulations, including individually wrapped tablet form; higher-concentration tablets allow for disinfection of large volumes of water or for shock chlorination of tanks and other storage systems. Tablets have been shown to be effective for household use in developing countries.[65]

CHLORINATION-FLOCCULATION

Tablets contain alum and 1.4% available chlorine in the form of sodium dichloro-s-triazinetrione with proprietary flocculating agents. Bicarbonate in the tablets promotes rapid dissolution and acts as a buffer. One 600-mg tablet yields 8 mg/L of free chlorine.

Testing by the U.S. military demonstrated biocidal effectiveness similar to iodine tablets under most conditions.[243,244,246] Extended contact time was necessary for complete viral removal in some of the tests. Because of the ability to flocculate turbid water, the action was superior to iodine in some poor-quality water. The method is optimal for humanitarian disasters, where available surface water is often highly turbid.[97] Testing in households in developing countries demonstrates reduction of diarrhea episodes with proper use.[62,82,259]

Chlor-Floc (Deatrick & Associates, Alexandria, Va)
30 tablets individually sealed in foil packets; weight: 1.6 oz.; capacity: 30 L (8 gal)
Price: $9.00
Widely available through camping, military surplus, and survival websites
Formulation/instructions: One tablet for the clarification and disinfection of 1 L of water from polluted sources at temperatures of 25°C (77°F). At 5°C (41°F), use two 600-mg tablets to provide 2.8% available chlorine. To strain the sediment, pour the water through the cloth provided. The tablets are stable for 3 years if stored out of the heat in their packaging.
At 25°C (77°F), add 1 tablet; wait 7 minutes. At 15°C (59°F), add 1 tablet; wait 15 minutes. At 10°C (50°F), add 1 tablet; wait 15 minutes. At 5°C (41°F), add 2 tablets; wait 15 minutes.
1. Add 1 or 2 tablets (600 mg) to 1 L (1.1 qt) of water.
2. Shake for 1 minute to make sure that the tablets dissolve completely.
3. Wait for 7 to 10 minutes (or the necessary time), then strain through a piece of broadly woven cloth (e.g., T-shirt material) into clean container.
4. The clarified water is now ready for drinking.
5. If water is still murky, add an additional 0.5 tablet, and repeat steps 2 and 3.
After decanting, the water looks much clearer and is left with a free chlorine residual that produces microbiologically safer water without pronounced chlorine taste or odor.[62]
PUR Purifier of Water (Proctor & Gamble)
www.pghsi.com
Instructions: Sachet of powder containing ferric sulfate as a coagulant and calcium hypochlorite as a disinfectant. Add one sachet to 10 L of water, and agitate vigorously. After the flocculants have settled to the bottom, filter through a clean cotton cloth, and wait 20 minutes to drink.
This product is available to large relief organizations for use outside the United States in disaster and conflict situations. They will also begin distribution for individual users in the developing countries.

Comments

This is one of the individual field methods for U.S. military troops and suggested for potential use in developing countries by WHO.

PUR has been used at the household level in many developing world communities and disasters.[62,75,81,82,259] It is an excellent one-step technique for cloudy and highly polluted water (see Table 88-15). Souter and colleagues[300] demonstrated that this technique reduced bacteria (14 types) by 8 log, *Giardia* and *Cryptosporidium* by 3 log, and arsenic by 99.8%.

Alum and ferric sulfate are widely used flocculants that cause suspended sediment, colloids, and many microorganisms to clump, settle to the bottom, and readily be filtered or strained. Most *Cryptosporidium* oocysts would be removed by the flocculation. Some chlorine reacts with contaminants and is inactivated. It is important to confirm some chlorine taste and smell at the end of the contact time. For added safety, prolong the contact time up to 1 hour in cold, polluted, and dirty water.

In clear water without enough impurities to flocculate, the alum causes some cloudiness and leaves a strong chlorine residual. After treatment, water should be poured through a special cloth to remove flocculants and decrease turbidity.

Both products have undergone extensive testing in field situations.

CHLORINE DIOXIDE

Chlorine dioxide (ClO_2) is routinely used in large-scale water treatment applications, as a volatile gas that is generated on site. Chemical methods for generating ClO_2 using either tablet or liquid formulations are also available for point of use in the field. Advantages of ClO_2 are greater effectiveness than chlorine at equivalent doses and the ability to inactivate *Cryptosporidium* oocysts with reasonable doses and contact times.[219]

TABLETS

Katadyn Micropur MP-1
http://www.katadyn.com/usen/katadyn-products/
Price: 20 tablets, $8.00; 30 tablets, $12.95
Available through many suppliers of outdoor products

Potable Aqua Chlorine Dioxide Water Purification Tablets
Wisconsin Pharmacal Co, Jackson, Wis
Price: 20 tablets, $10.00; 30 tablets, $14.00
Available from many outdoor suppliers

Aquamira (McNett Corp)
http://www.aquamira.com/

Pristine
Advanced Chemicals Ltd, Port Coquitlam, BC, Canada
http://www.pristine.ca/
Tablets in blister packs
Price: 12 tablets, $8.00; 24 tablets, $14.00; 50 tablets, $24.00

Formulation and Instructions

The primary chemical reaction that produces ClO_2 in Katadyn MP-1 tablets is the acid-chlorite reaction using sodium acid sulfate as the acid, a well-known reaction for ClO_2:

$$5NaClO_2 + 4NaHSO_4 \rightarrow 4ClO_2 + NaCl + 2H_2O + 4Na_2SO_4$$

A small amount of chlorine in the tablet also catalyzes the otherwise sluggish reaction.

These tablets generate ClO_2 only when coming into contact with water. Shortly after a tablet is immersed into water, a saturated solution of the soluble solid constituents forms within the matrix of the tablet. ClO_2 is rapidly formed within the pores and then carried into the bulk solution by CO_2 effervescence, which ensures that the resultant solution is well mixed without the user having to agitate the container. After the ClO_2 gas is released, the material reduces into common salts.

Katadyn company product testing shows killing of bacteria and viruses within 15 minutes in any water conditions and inactivation of *Giardia* and *Cryptosporidium* within 30 minutes in clear warm water and 4 hours in cold and dirty water. One tablet is used for treating 1 qt or 1 L of water. Instructions are to insert rapidly into water after removing from the package and avoid exposure to sunlight during disinfection contact time.

Comments

This is an important addition to chemical methods for field disinfection. Several products have met the criteria for EPA registration as an antimicrobial water purifier. The extended contact time in cold, dirty water ensures that sufficient ClO_2 is generated and adequate residual remains for sufficient time to treat water in all conditions. Where possible, clarify the water to improve taste and esthetics, and warm the water to reduce contact time. Available tests appear well designed with multiple controls. There is also documentation that residual ClO_2 concentrations were well maintained during the recommended contact times. ClO_2 does not have extended persistence in water, so it should not be used to maintain microbiologic purity of stored water. Sunlight breaks down ClO_2, so for optimal effect, keep the water bottle in a dark location, such as inside a pack or bag, during disinfection time. For some reason, having these companies release testing data for their ClO_2 products is difficult, so efficacy of particular products cannot be assured.

LIQUID CHLORINE DIOXIDE PRODUCTS

Aquamira (McNett Corp)
http://www.aquamira.com/
Pristine (Advanced Chemicals Ltd, Port Coquitlam, BC, Canada)
http://www.pristine.ca/
Personal size: two 1-oz plastic bottles; capacity: up to 120 L (30 gal) of water; $15.00
Pristine also makes 2-oz bottles ($17.00) and larger packages for relief agencies to disinfect large quantities.
Aquarius Bulk Water Treatment
http://www.advancechemicals.ca/Aquarius-Bulk-Water-Treatment-System
Includes 10 kits of Pristine solution to treat 50,000 L
Available as a system with Terra Tank water bladders (5000- to 10,000-L capacity), Honda pump to fill the bladders, mixing and injection units, and six- to eight-spigot water-dispensing system.
The system is packed in metal chests and weighs 200 lb.

Formulation and Instructions

A stabilized solution of ClO_2 is mixed with phosphoric acid, which activates the chemical and is then mixed with water for disinfection. Contact times for inactivation of *Cryptosporidium* by Pristine range from 15 minutes in warm water using a triple dose to 7 hours using a single dose in very cold water. The two solutions are mixed together in a mixing cap and added to the water for treatment.

Comments and Claims

The chemistry of generating ClO_2 through a similar method is well described. Aquamira solution was not able to meet EPA purifier standards in cold, dirty water. Currently, claims for the solution include "kills odor causing bacteria and enhances taste of stored water." The Canadian liquid product, which appears to be the same, makes full claims, including *Cryptosporidium*. Given the volatility of ClO_2 and slow reaction times, concentrations may be variable because of the mixing process and time delay. Cold and dirty "worst-case" test water may be an issue in disaster situations but is not often encountered by wilderness users.

Aquamira tablets are registered as an EPA purifier, suggesting that tablets are the more stable and reliable form of chlorine dioxide.

MIXED-SPECIES DISINFECTION

SE200 Community Chlorine Maker (Cascade Designs/MSR, Seattle, Wash)
http://www.solutionsforwater.org/wp-content/uploads/2012/03/SE200-Entrepreneur-Fact-Sheet.pdf

Comments

The SE200 was developed by PATH (international nongovernmental organization/NGO) and Cascade Designs as a low-cost, portable, battery-powered, easy-to-use electrochlorination device that creates a concentrated chlorine solution to treat water effectively. The device uses salt, water, and a 12-volt DC battery to create 60 mL of a 0.75% chlorine solution, enough to treat up to 200 L of water over a 7-minute operation cycle (see Appendix A for more information).

Electrolysis of salt to produce chlorine has been used for more than a century. Passing a current through a simple brine salt solution generates free available chlorine, as well as other "mixed-species" disinfectants that have been demonstrated effective against bacteria, viruses, and bacterial spores.[280] The process is well described and can be used on both large and small scale (http://www.miox.com/). Mixed oxidants behave similar to chlorine dioxide and ozone, although these disinfectants are difficult to detect in finished water using usual methods. Cascade Designs bases the effect of the SE200 solution solely on the hypochlorite generated, which is the main residual, measurable species; however, the resulting solution has greater disinfectant ability than a simple solution of sodium hypochlorite, including inactivation of *Cryptosporidium*.[330]

SILVER

Micropur Forte Tablets (Katadyn)

http://www.katadyn.com/chen/katadyn-products/

Available as tablets, liquid, or powder and in various quantities for individual or large-scale use.

One tablet treats 1 L of clear water.

Claims: Eliminates bacteria and viruses in 30 minutes and *Giardia* in 120 minutes; conserves drinking water for up to 6 months; can be used in plastic or glass but not all metal containers. Shelf life: 5 years in original packaging and if stored under 25°C (77°F). Cloudy water can weaken the effect of chlorine and silver ions. Use filter for cloudy water.

Comments

Widely available in Europe, but not marketed in the United States, these tablets contain silver chloride 0.1% and NaDCC 2.5%. The chlorine kills viruses, bacteria, and *Giardia*. The silver adds to the disinfection capacity, as well as preventing recontamination if water is stored for up to 6 months. Contact time is 20 to 120 minutes, depending on the temperature of the water. Shelf life is 5 years, stored in cool, dry conditions.

Micropur Classic (Katadyn)

This product releases only silver ions.

Available in two sizes of tablets (for 1 qt or 5 qt), liquid (10 drops/gal), or crystals for treating larger quantities of water.

Claims: Conserves clear water for up to 6 months; deactivates bacteria after 2 hours of contact. The silver ions cling to the cell walls of microorganisms, thus hindering their growth; affected by some metal containers. Shelf life: tablets/powder, 10 years from manufacture date; liquid, 5 years.

Comments

Although having proven antibacterial effects, silver tablets are not licensed as a water purifier in the United States; however, they are widely used in Europe for this purpose. In addition to poorly documented effects on many different types of microorganisms, there is some difficulty controlling the residual concentration and concern over chronic effects (see section on metals and silver). The product that contains only silver without chlorine makes no claims for viruses and protozoa, because concentrations may not be adequate to kill these organisms. It has EPA approval to be marketed in the United States as a "water preservative" to maintain bacteria-free water for up to 6 months. Silver has the advantage of having no taste, color, or odor. Because of these and additional attractive qualities, other applications with silver are being developed and tested, including nanoparticle materials.

MISCELLANEOUS PRODUCTS

The following products *cannot* be recommended because of insufficient effectiveness data.

Traveler's Friend (NutriBiotic)

Description: Extract from citrus (grapefruit) seeds in 10-mL or 30 mL plastic dropper bottle. Recommended dose (drops/qt): 5 to 10 for filtered water, 10 to 15 for ice water, 10 to 20 for tap water, and 15 to 25 for untreated water. Allow 30 minutes for contact time.

Claims: "All natural treatment for drinking water." Nontoxic, noncorrosive; proved effective as disinfectant for bacteria, viruses, and protozoa. Claims also made for a multitude of health uses, from skin and nails to scalp.

Comments

Citrus extract is known to have some bacteriostatic effect (see text). This product was introduced into the health market and is now looking for a broader uses. Company data from independent laboratories support bactericidal and virucidal effects. However, protozoal tests were done with trophozoites, not cysts. The data have gaps, and too much of the marketing is testimonial to allow a recommendation at this time.

Aerobic Oxygen and Aquagen

http://www.oxygenforlife.net/index.html

Comments and Claims

According to company claims, these products contain other forms of oxygen electrolytes that kill harmful bacteria in stored water and have multiple health benefits when ingested in water or used topically. The company asserts that the product does not contain chlorine dioxide or hydrogen peroxide, but rather uses some unspecified, proprietary, stabilized electrolytes of oxygen. The implication is that it uses free oxygen radicals, but these are not chemically stable. Company-sponsored testing claims effective against *Salmonella*, cholera, *E. coli*, *Streptococcus*, *Pseudomonas*, *Staphylococus* A, and *Giardia*. No dose-time response has been developed to compare the product with other disinfectants.

Aerobic Oxygen was initially introduced into the health food market but is now being offered to the general travel market. It is advertised not only as a water disinfectant, but also for qualities from strengthening the immune system and energizing to curing headaches and tropical fish diseases.

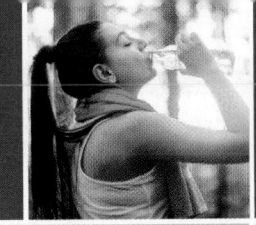

CHAPTER 89

Dehydration and Rehydration

ROBERT W. KENEFICK, SAMUEL N. CHEUVRONT, LISA R. LEON, AND KAREN K. O'BRIEN

Body fluid balance is controlled by physiologic and behavioral actions.[51,100] However, when there is lack of fluid availability, exposure to extreme environments, or illness, inability to maintain fluid balance can seriously jeopardize health and ability to perform.[100] This chapter presents an overview of topics surrounding hydration, dehydration, and rehydration. The terms euhydration, hypohydration, and hyperhydration are used. *Euhydration* defines a "normal," narrow fluctuation in body water content; *hypohydration* and *hyperhydration* define, respectively, a general deficit and a general surfeit in body water content beyond normal. The term *dehydration* specifically defines the condition of hypertonic hypovolemia brought about by net loss of hypotonic body fluids. Isotonic or hypotonic hypovolemia, manifest by large losses of solute and water, is defined simply as *hypovolemia*.[92,127] Table 89-1 lists the two principal forms of body water deficit and the physiology and particular circumstances associated with each.

BODY WATER, FLUID TURNOVER, AND FLUID REQUIREMENTS

Total body water (TBW) is the principal chemical component of the human body and represents 50% to 70% of body mass[8] for the average young adult male. It is regulated within ±0.2% to 0.5% of daily body mass.[3,40] Body water is required to sustain the cardiovascular and thermoregulatory systems and to support cellular homeostasis. Although "normal" hydration is achieved with a wide range of water intakes by sedentary and active people across the life span, homeostasis of body water can be difficult to maintain when challenged by strenuous physical work, heat stress, or illness. Despite population variability in age, body composition, and physical fitness, it is important to note that variability in TBW is accounted for almost entirely by body composition, since lean body mass contains about 73% water and fat body mass consists of about 10% water.[223] Trained athletes have relatively high TBW values by virtue of having high muscle mass and low body fat. In contrast, obese individuals with the same body mass as their lean counterparts have markedly smaller TBW volumes. Any absolute fluid deficit has more severe consequences for individuals with smaller TBW volume.

Daily water balance depends on the net difference between water gain and water loss.[100] Approximately 5% to 10% of TBW is turned over daily[171] through obligatory (nonexercise) fluid loss. Water gain occurs from consumption (liquids and food) and production (metabolic water), whereas water losses occur from respiratory, gastrointestinal (GI), renal, and sweat losses. Water lost by respiration is influenced by inspired air and pulmonary ventilation. Importantly, the volume of metabolic water produced during cellular metabolism (~0.13 g/kcal) is approximately equal to respiratory water losses (~0.12 g/kcal),[52,140] which results in water turnover with no net change in TBW. GI tract losses tend to be negligible (~100 to 200 mL/day); however, certain illnesses, such as diarrhea, can lead to loss of large amounts of fluid and electrolytes. The ability to vary urine output represents the primary means to regulate net body water balance across a broad range of fluid intake volumes and losses from other avenues. Water losses in urine approximate 1 to 2 L/day. However, urine output volumes may be larger or smaller depending on daily fluid consumption and activity.[100] Minimum outputs of approximately 20 mL/hr and maximal volumes of approximately 1000 mL/hr are possible.

Net body water balance (loss = gain) is regulated remarkably well day to day as a result of thirst and hunger, coupled with ad libitum access to food and beverages, which offset water losses.[100] Although acute mismatches between fluid gain and loss may result from illness, environmental exposure, exercise, or physical work, it is a reproducible phenomenon that intakes are generally adequate to offset net loss from day to day.[54] It is recognized, however, that after significant body water deficits, such as those associated with physical work or heat stress, many hours of rehydration and electrolyte consumption may be needed to reestablish body water balance.[208] For example, if hypohydrated by more than about 4% of total body mass, it may take more than 24 hours to fully rehydrate through water and electrolyte replacement.[5,147] Although daily strenuous activity in a hot environment can result in mild water balance deficits even with unlimited access to food and fluids,[12,208] adherence to recognized water intake guidance[12,35,189] minimizes water deficits, as determined by daily body mass stability.[40]

An adequate intake (AI) for daily total water is 3.7 L and 2.7 L for adult males and females, respectively.[100] Of these prescribed volumes, 20% of the AI for water is found in food eaten during meals and snacks and the remaining 80% (~3 L for males and 2.2 L for females) can come from beverages of all types. Daily water intake, however, varies greatly for individuals and between groups. For example, daily water needs of sedentary men are approximately 1.2 to 2.5 L[2,155] and increase to approximately 3.2 L if performing modest physical activity.[93,95] Compared to sedentary adults, active adults who live in a warm environment are reported to have daily water needs of approximately 6 L,[229] and highly active populations have been reported to have much higher values.[184] Data are limited regarding fluid needs for women, but typically they exhibit lower daily water turnover rates than their male counterparts. In general, fluid requirements vary based on an individual's body size, activity level, and the environment in which the person works, lives, or performs.

HYDRATION ASSESSMENT

Human hydration assessment is a key component for prevention and proper treatment of fluid and electrolyte imbalances.[47,127,164] When fluids are limited, illness strikes, or if there is exposure to extreme environments, cumulative fluid deficits can threaten homeostasis, health, and performance.[127,189] Health is also threatened by fluid deficits that can increase the risk of serious heat illness and by fluid surfeits that increase the risk of hyponatremia.[33,141] In many clinical and most sports and wilderness medicine situations, hypertonic hypovolemia occurs when there is net loss of hypotonic body fluids. However, substantial solute (electrolyte) can also be lost in situations involving heavy work where heat stress induces profuse sweating, during cold or high altitude exposure, and in numerous illnesses and disorders (e.g., gastroenteritis, hyperemesis, diuretic treatment, dialysis) producing isotonic or hypotonic hypovolemia.[47,127,189] Appreciation for the different types of body fluid losses that occur in response to illness, fluid restriction, or exposure to extreme environments is fundamental to proper hydration assessment[47,127] (see Table 89-1).

Most circumstances involving strenuous work in austere environments require formation and vaporization of sweat as a principal means of heat removal. Thus, when sweat losses result in body water deficit, there is a predictable rise in extracellular tonicity, which modulates renal function and urine composition in accordance with the body water deficit.[177] The basic principles

TABLE 89-1 Two Principal Forms of Body Water Deficit

Form	Physiology	Circumstances
Hypertonic hypovolemia	Body water loss > solute loss Movement of water from ICF to ECF space Partial restoration of ECF space	Sweat loss (exercise, environmental heat stress, or fever) Inadequate fluid intake Osmotic diuresis caused by glucosuria
Isotonic hypovolemia	Isotonic loss of body water and solute No net movement of water among body fluid compartments Larger contraction of ECF space than equivalent hypertonic body water deficit	Cold or high-altitude exposure Gastrointestinal losses (diarrhea, vomiting) Diuretic therapy

ECF, Extracellular fluid; *ICF,* intracellular fluid.

of body fluid regulation provide the framework for using blood (osmolality, sodium, fluid regulatory hormones) and urine (osmolality, specific gravity, color) as principal body fluid hydration assessment measures. Similarly, because humans maintain a relatively stable TBW pool despite diverse factors (e.g., climate, activity, dietary solute load) that affect water requirements,[100] acute changes in body mass may be used to accurately measure dehydration across medical disciplines.[17,40,222] Physical signs and symptoms (dizziness, headache, tachycardia, capillary refill time, sunken eyes, skin turgor) only manifest when fluid losses are severe and become debilitating.[74,217] These findings are too nonspecific to be useful in athletic settings[134] because they share symptoms indicative of other ailments (e.g., acute mountain sickness), and their use in assessment could lead to an incorrect diagnosis.

All hydration assessment methods vary greatly in applicability because of limitations such as the necessary circumstances for reliable measurement, principles of operation, cost, and complexity.[100,164] Table 89-2 lists advantages and disadvantages of numerous approaches and should be consulted when deciding on the choice of hydration marker. Definitive hydration assessment requires monitoring changes in hydration state. Although change can provide good diagnostic accuracy, it requires a valid baseline, control over confounding variables, and serial measurements.[43,135] Large population heterogeneity in part explains why there are presently few hydration status markers that display potential for high nosologic sensitivity from a single, more practical measure.[43,120] Although Table 89-3 provides euhydration thresholds for the most useful hydration assessment measurements, these measures require considerable methodologic control, expense,

TABLE 89-2 Hydration Assessment Techniques Summary

Technique	Advantages	Disadvantages
Complex Markers		
Total body water (dilution)	Accurate, reliable (gold standard)	Analytically complex, expensive, requires baseline
Plasma osmolality	Accurate, reliable (gold standard)	Analytically complex, expensive, invasive
Simple Markers		
Urine concentration	Easy, rapid, screening tool	Easily confounded, timing critical, frequency and color subjective
Body mass	Easy, rapid, screening tool	Confounded by changes in body composition
Other Markers		
Blood		
Plasma volume	No advantage over osmolality (except	Analytically complex, expensive, invasive, multiple
Plasma sodium	hyponatremia detection for plasma sodium)	confounders
Fluid balance hormones		
Bioimpedance	Easy, rapid	Requires baseline, multiple confounders
Saliva	Easy, rapid	Highly variable, immature marker, multiple confounders
Physical signs	Easy, rapid	Too generalized, subjective
Tilt test (orthostatic challenge)	Rapid	Highly variable, insensitive, requires tilt table or ability to stand
Thirst	Positive symptomatology	Develops too late and is quenched too soon

From Cheuvront SN, Sawka MN: Hydration assessment of athltetes, *Sport Sci Exchange* 18:1, 2005.

TABLE 89-3 Biomarkers of Hydration Status

Measure	Practicality	Validity (Acute vs. Chronic Changes)	Euhydration Cutoff
Total body weight	Low	Acute and chronic	<2%
Plasma osmolality	Medium	Acute and chronic	<290 mOsmol
Urine specific gravity	High	Chronic	<1.020 g/mL
Urine osmolality	High	Chronic	<700 mOsmol
Urine color	High	Acute and chronic	<4
*Body weight	High	Acute and chronic	<1% change

From Cheuvront SN, Sawka MN: Hydration assessment of athletes, *Sports Sci Exchange* 18:1, 2005.
*Potentially confounded by changes in body composition during very prolonged assessment periods. Fluid balance should be considered adequate when the combination of any two assessment outcomes is consistent with euhydration.

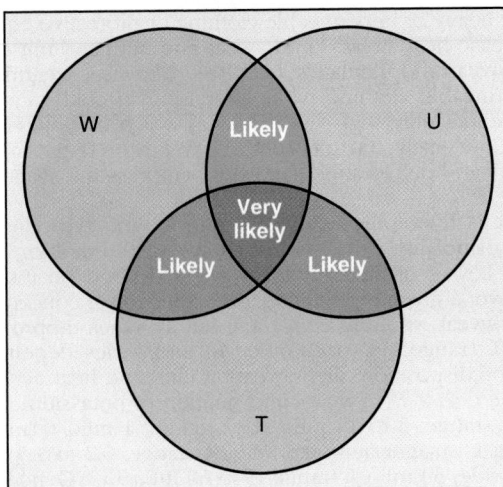

FIGURE 89-1 When two or more simple markers of dehydration are present, it is likely that a person is dehydrated. If all three markers are present, dehydration is very likely. *T*, Thirst; *U*, urine; *W*, weight. *(From Cheuvront SN, Sawka MN: Hydration assessment of athletes, Sport Sci Exchange 18(1):1-5, 2005.)*

and analytical expertise and may not be practical, day-to-day hydration monitoring of athletic sojourners.

There is no scientific consensus on how best to assess hydration status in a field setting. In most field settings, however, additive use of first morning body mass measurements in combination with some measure of first morning urine concentration and gross thirst perception provides a simple and inexpensive way to dichotomize euhydration from gross dehydration resulting from sweat loss and poor fluid intake. This approach is represented using a Venn diagram decision tool[47] (Figure 89-1). It combines three of the simplest markers of hydration: body mass (weight), urine, and thirst (WUT). No marker by itself provides enough evidence of dehydration, but the combination of any two simple self-assessment markers can indicate when dehydration is likely. The presence of all three makes dehydration very likely. The balance between science and simplicity in the choice of these measures for field hydration assessment is outlined next.

Urine Concentration

Urinalysis is a frequently used clinical measure to distinguish between normal and pathologic conditions. Urinary markers for dehydration include urine volume, urine specific gravity (USG), urine osmolality (U_{Osm}), and urine color (U_{Col}). Urine is a solution of water and various other substances. Thus, its concentration varies inversely with volume, which is reduced with dehydration. Urine output generally approximates 1 to 2 L/day but can be increased by an order of magnitude when consuming large volumes of fluid.[100] This large capacity to vary urine output represents the primary avenue to regulate net body water balance across a broad range of fluid intake volumes and losses from other avenues. Whereas quantification of urine volume is impractical on a daily basis, quantitative (USG, U_{Osm}) or qualitative (U_{Col}) assessment of its concentration is much simpler. As a screening tool to dichotomize euhydration from dehydration, urine concentration (USG, U_{Osm}, U_{Col}) is a reliable assessment technique[12,20,207] with reasonably definable thresholds.

In contrast, urine measures often correlate poorly with "gold standards" such as plasma osmolality and fail to reliably track documented changes in body mass corresponding to acute dehydration and rehydration.[114,170] When acute fluxes in body water occur, changes in plasma osmolality that stimulate endocrine regulation of renal water and electrolyte reabsorption are delayed at the site of the kidney.[170] It is also likely that drink composition influences this response. Drinking large volumes of hypotonic fluids results in copious urine production long before euhydration is achieved.[211] Urine concentration measurements can be confounded by diet, which may explain large cross-cultural

differences in urine osmolality.[128] Using the first morning void following an overnight fast minimizes confounding influences and maximizes measurement reliability.[12,207] Urinalysis of specific gravity, osmolality, and color can therefore be used to assess and distinguish euhydration from dehydration as long as the first morning void is used.

Inexpensive and easy-to-use commercial instruments are available for assessing USG and conductivity (osmolality equivalent);[20,207] a urine color chart is also available.[12] The simplest of these, color, is included in the Venn diagram. Under ideal circumstances, the urine (first morning) should be in a clean, clear vial or cup and the color assessed against a white background. Urine color can be compared against a urine color chart or assessed relative to the degree of darkness. Paler color urine (similar to lemonade) indicates adequate hydration; the darker yellow/brown the urine color (similar to apple juice), the greater the degree of dehydration. Assessing urine that has been diluted in toilet water or while in midflow may alter urine color. When in less-than-ideal conditions, urine in a urinal is less dilute. In the field, snow can provide a suitable background. Figure 89-2 presents example photos of urine color with corresponding numeric color,[12] USG, and urine osmolality values.

Body Mass

Body mass is a measurement often used in both laboratory and field environments for rapid assessment of an athlete's hydration changes. Changes in acute hydration are calculated as the difference between preexercise and postexercise body mass. The level of dehydration is best expressed as a percentage of starting body mass rather than as a percentage of TBW, since the latter ranges widely.[100] Using this technique implies that 1 g of lost mass is equivalent to 1 mL of lost water. As long as TBW loss is of interest, failure to account for carbon exchange represents the only small error (~10%) in this assumption.[44] Indeed, acute body mass changes (water) are frequently the standard against which resolution of other hydration assessment parameters are compared in the laboratory. In fact, if proper controls are made, body mass changes can provide a more sensitive estimate of acute TBW changes than do repeat measurements by dilution methods.[94]

There is also evidence that body mass is a sufficiently stable physiologic parameter for potential daily fluid balance monitoring, even over longer periods (1 to 2 weeks) that include strenuous exercise and acute fluid flux.[40,119] Young, healthy men undergoing daily exercise-heat stress maintain a stable first morning body mass as long as they make a conscious effort to replace exercise sweat losses.[40] Similarly, ad libitum intake of food and fluid will balance sweat losses incurred with regular exercise, resulting in a stable daily body mass.[119] Over longer time frames, changes in body composition (fat and lean mass) that occur with chronic energy imbalance are also reflected grossly as changes in body mass, thus limiting this technique. Clearly, if first morning body mass stability is used to monitor changes in hydration, it should be used in combination with another hydration assessment technique (e.g., urine concentration) to dissociate gross tissue losses from water losses if long-term hydration status is of interest.

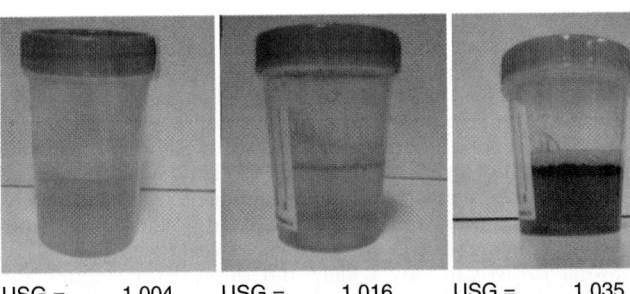

USG = 1.004	USG = 1.016	USG = 1.035
Osmolality = 105	Osmolality = 522	Osmolality = 1252
Color = 2	Color = 4	Color = 7

FIGURE 89-2 Samples of first morning urine with urine specific gravity (USG), associated osmolality (mmol/kg), and color values.

Although genuine thirst develops only after dehydration is present and is alleviated before euhydration is achieved,[92,100] thirst is one of the few reliable subjective feelings reported by humans in response to fluid restriction.[209] Plasma osmolality near 295 mmol/kg will produce an arginine vasopressin (AVP) level of approximately 5 pg/mL, which results in maximal urine concentrating capacity. The average plasma osmolality at which thirst is stimulated above baseline is also approximately 295 mmol/kg.[177] If we assume that a normal resting plasma osmolality of 285 mmol/kg becomes concentrated to 295 mmol/kg, the ratio 285/295 multiplied by a normal 42 L TBW gives an estimated 40.5 L, or 1.5 L TBW deficit, which is 2.1% dehydration for a 70-kg (154-lb) person. This is consistent with general observations of thirst insensitivity below a "threshold" fluid deficit (that thirst develops late). However, it is important to recognize that there is substantial individual variability in the plasma osmolality "set point" and the osmotic thresholds for AVP release and thirst perception. For example, Robertson and colleagues[178] report as much as a 10-fold difference between individuals in the slope of the line relating AVP to plasma osmolality. Clearly, thirst is a qualitative tool for hydration assessment, but positive thirst symptoms coupled with at least one additional Venn diagram marker suggests an increasing likelihood of dehydration.

Although plasma osmolality and TBW measurements are the hydration assessment measures for large-scale fluid needs,[100] no consensus exists for using one approach over another in a field or athletic setting. In most circumstances, using first morning body mass combined with some measure of first morning urine concentration (USG, urine osmolality and/or color) offers simple assessment and allows ample sensitivity (low false-negative) for detecting meaningful deviations in fluid balance (>2% body mass). This approach is represented using a Venn diagram decision tool[47] (see Figure 89-2). Again, it combines three of the simplest markers of hydration (WUT); no single marker provides enough evidence of dehydration, but two markers mean dehydration is likely, and all three make dehydration very likely. In a field setting, where a scale may not be available for body weight measures, the combination of first morning urine color and thirst may provide reasonable indication of the presence of dehydration.

SWEAT AND SWEAT PREDICTION

Muscular contractions involved with activity/exercise produce metabolic heat that is transferred from the active muscles to blood and then the body core. Subsequent body temperature elevations elicit heat loss responses of increased skin blood flow and increased sweat secretion so that heat can be dissipated to the environment.[198,200] Heat exchange between skin and environment is governed by biophysical properties dictated by surrounding temperature, humidity and air motion, sky and ground radiation, and clothing.[77] When ambient temperature is greater than or equal to skin temperature, evaporative heat loss accounts for all body cooling. Eccrine sweat glands secrete fluid onto the skin surface, permitting evaporative cooling when liquid is converted to water vapor. Sweat glands respond to thermal stress primarily through sympathetic cholinergic stimulation, with catecholamines having a smaller role in the sweat response.[200]

The rate of sweat evaporation depends on air movement and the water vapor pressure gradient between the skin and environment, so in still or moist air, sweat does not evaporate readily and collects on skin. Sweat that drips from the body or clothing provides no cooling benefit. If secreted sweat drips from the body and is not evaporated, higher sweating will be needed to achieve evaporative cooling requirements.[41,198] Conversely, increased air motion (wind, movement velocity) facilitates evaporation and minimizes wasted (dripping) sweat.[41]

Sweat losses can vary widely and depend on amount and intensity of physical activity and environmental conditions.[85,205] In addition, a number of factors can alter sweat rates and ultimately fluid needs. Heat acclimatization results in higher and more sustained sweating rates. Similarly, aerobic exercise training has a modest effect on enhancing sweating rate responses.[198,200]

Wearing heavy or impermeable clothing or protective equipment can increase heat stress[133] and sweat rate but can limit evaporation of sweat and ultimately heat loss. Likewise, wearing heavy or impermeable clothing while exercising in cold weather can elicit unexpectedly high sweat rates,[73] which can increase fluid needs. Conversely, factors such as wet skin (e.g., from high humidity) and dehydration can act to suppress the sweating rate response.[198]

Sweat is hypotonic relative to plasma and typically half of plasma osmolality (~145 mmol/kg vs. 290 mmol/kg, respectively).[53] Losses of electrolytes in sweat depend on total sweat losses (over a given period) and sweat electrolyte concentrations. Typical sweat sodium concentration averages approximately 35 mEq/L (range, 10 to 70 mEq /L) and varies depending on genetic predisposition, diet, sweating rate, and heat acclimatization state.[6,26,54,75,210,224] Sweat concentration of potassium averages 5 mEq/L (range, 3 to 15 mEq /L); calcium, 1 mEq/L (range, 0.3 to 2 mEq/L); magnesium, 0.8 mEq /L (range, 0.2 to 1.5 mEq/L); and chloride, 30 mEq/L (range, 5 to 60 mEq/L).[26] Gender, maturation, and aging appear to have no discernible effect on sweat electrolyte concentrations,[138,148] although dehydration can increase sweat concentrations of sodium and chloride.[146] Sweat glands reabsorb sodium and chloride by active transport, but ability to reabsorb these electrolytes does not increase proportionally with the sweating rate. As a result, sodium and chloride concentrations of sweat increase as a function of sweating rate.[6,54] Heat acclimatization improves ability to reabsorb sodium and chloride; thus, heat-acclimatized individuals usually have lower sweat sodium concentrations (e.g., >50% reduction) for any given sweating rate.[6]

Sweat rates differ among various work activities and individuals.[198] Specifics on determining individual sweat rate and fluid requirements are covered later in the fluid replacement recommendations section. Figure 89-3 depicts generalized modeling approximations for daily sweating rates as a function of daily metabolic rate (activity level) and air temperature.[100] Metabolic rate and air temperature have marked effects on water needs. In addition to air temperature, environmental factors (e.g., relative humidity, air motion, solar load, protective clothing) influence heat strain and water needs.

Central to water consumption planning is the ability to predict water needs accurately in a variety of environmental conditions, with varying activity levels, loads, clothing ensembles, and personal protective equipment. Therefore, accurate water planning tools are helpful to minimize the logistical burden of water

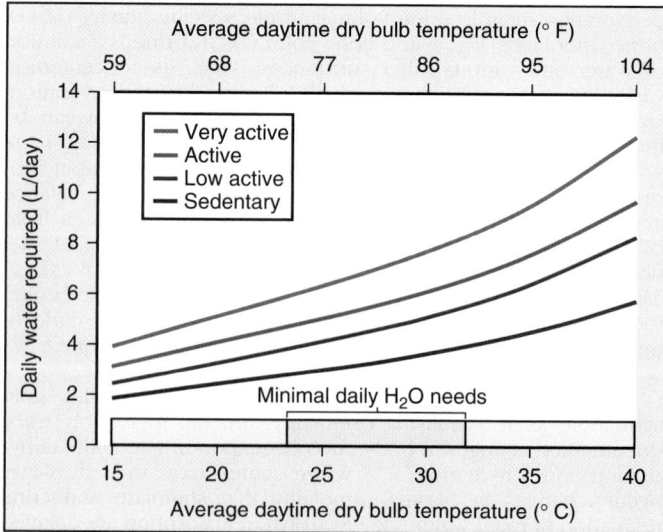

FIGURE 89-3 Generalized modeling approximations for daily sweating rates as a function of daily metabolic rate (activity level) and air temperature. *(From Institute of Medicine: Dietary reference intakes for water, potassium, sodium, chloride, and sulfate, Washington, DC, 2005, The National Academies Press.)*

transport while sustaining hydration. To calculate water needs, knowledge of sweat losses is critical, particularly for active populations and when exposed to heat stress.

The Shapiro equation has been used extensively to estimate sweating rates and calculate daily water needs.[205] This model calculates sweat rate (M_{sw}, expressed as g • m^{-2} • h^{-1}) and thus fluid needs as:

$$M_{sw} = 27.9 \times E_{req} \times (E_{max})^{-0.455}$$

where E_{req} is required evaporative cooling (in W/m^2), and E_{max} is maximal evaporative cooling capacity. E_{req} is calculated from metabolic heat production, clothing heat transfer characteristics, and the environment. E_{max} is derived from vapor transfer properties of the clothing worn and the environment. However, this equation has been shown to have limitations,[46] in that it often overpredicts fluids needs when exercise is longer than 2 hours, when improved uniforms and body armor are worn, and when high-intensity activity takes place in lower air temperatures. To address the need for improved prediction accuracy, Gonzalez and colleagues[84,87] developed and validated an updated algorithm (piece-wise [PW] model) that better predicts observed sweat losses (i.e., drinking water needs) in cool, temperate, warm-hot, high-altitude, and transient solar load environments. This new algorithm is based on metabolic demands, clothing, biophysical parameters, and environmental conditions, as with the legacy equation,[205] but expands the range of relevant environments, metabolic rates, and mission duration and includes modern clothing ensembles (e.g., body armor) potentially to provide estimates of water needs in both training and operational scenarios. Figure 89-4, from Jay and Webb,[101] depicts the adjustment to the sweat loss values yielded by the corrected Shapiro equation derived by Gonzalez and co-workers.[85] However, use of this updated algorithm is limited to individuals with extensive training in thermal biophysics and ultimately requires numerous measurement inputs.

The U.S. Army Research Institute of Environmental Medicine (ARIEM) recently developed and validated the equation just discussed that accurately predicts sweat losses (i.e., drinking water needs).[84,87] However, use of this newly developed equation was limited to experts trained in the art to produce tabled doctrine.[188]

The military user community requested greater simplicity and flexibility for predicting water needs in real time. Thus, the goal of the project was to incorporate the newly developed water prediction equation into a "smart phone" application that has been termed the Soldier Water Estimation Tool (SWET) (Figure 89-5). This smart phone application has reduced the number of inputs by the user from about 25 to five, which pertain to activity level, clothing worn, temperature, relative humidity, and cloud cover. The application provides the user with the amount of water required for the specified conditions in liters per hour. Additionally, a "Mission Planner" tab adds the option to include the total number of people and total time of the mission. The Mission Planner then calculates and reports total water needs in liters, 1-qt canteens, 2-qt canteens, and gallons.

Future work in this area may be required to increase the applicability of sweat rate prediction equations, in particular under conditions with variable solar loads, in lower air temperatures of approximately 15°C (59°F), with clothing having low water vapor permeability, or with specialized equipment (e.g., American football), and with individuals possessing greater body mass and surface areas.[101]

PHYSIOLOGIC CONSEQUENCES OF DEHYDRATION

By virtue of tonicity and volume changes, dehydration has negative consequences on thermoregulation and performance. Dehydration is caused by voluntary fluid restriction, insufficient rehydration after daily activity, or physical activity/exercise in the form of thermoregulatory sweating. The most common form of dehydration during exercise in the heat is a water deficit without proportionate sodium chloride loss.[191] Individuals often start an exercise task with normal TBW and dehydrate over an extended duration. In some situations, however, an individual might initiate activity/exercise with a body water deficit because the interval between exercise sessions is inadequate or chronic fluid intake is insufficient to replace losses. During multiple-day treks or expeditions where individuals take part in prolonged daily sessions of activity/exercise, possibly in hot conditions, a fluid

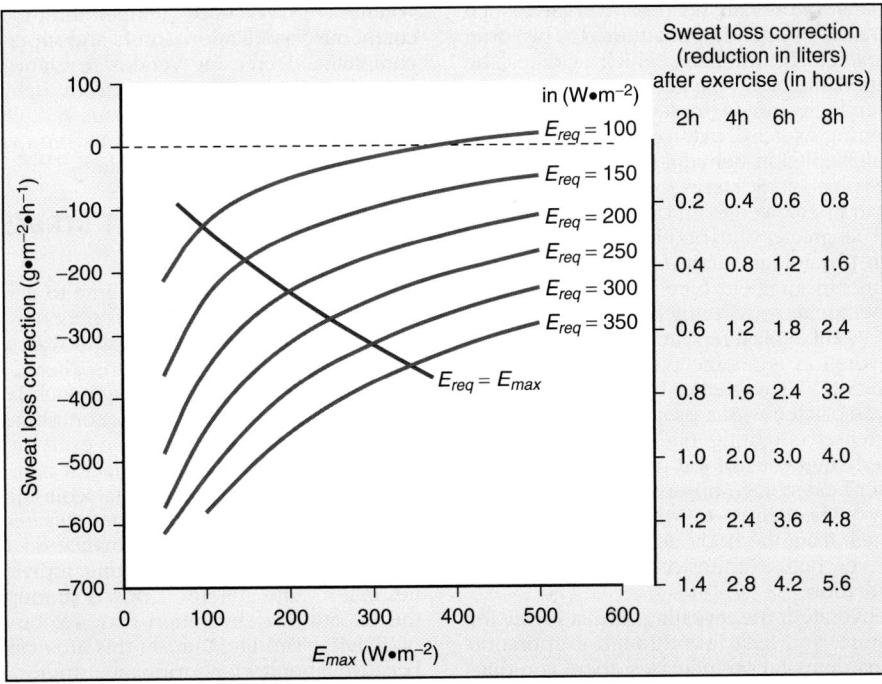

FIGURE 89-4 Sweat loss correction, where E_{req} is the amount of evaporation required to achieve heat balance, and E_{max} is the maximum rate of evaporation possible. The range of validity: E_{req} >50 W/m^2 and <360 W/m^2; E_{max} >20 W/m^2 and <525 W/m^2. Calculations for reference male with body surface area of 1.8 m^2. (From Jay O, Webb P. Improving the prediction of sweat losses during exercise, J Appl Physiol 107:375, 2009.)

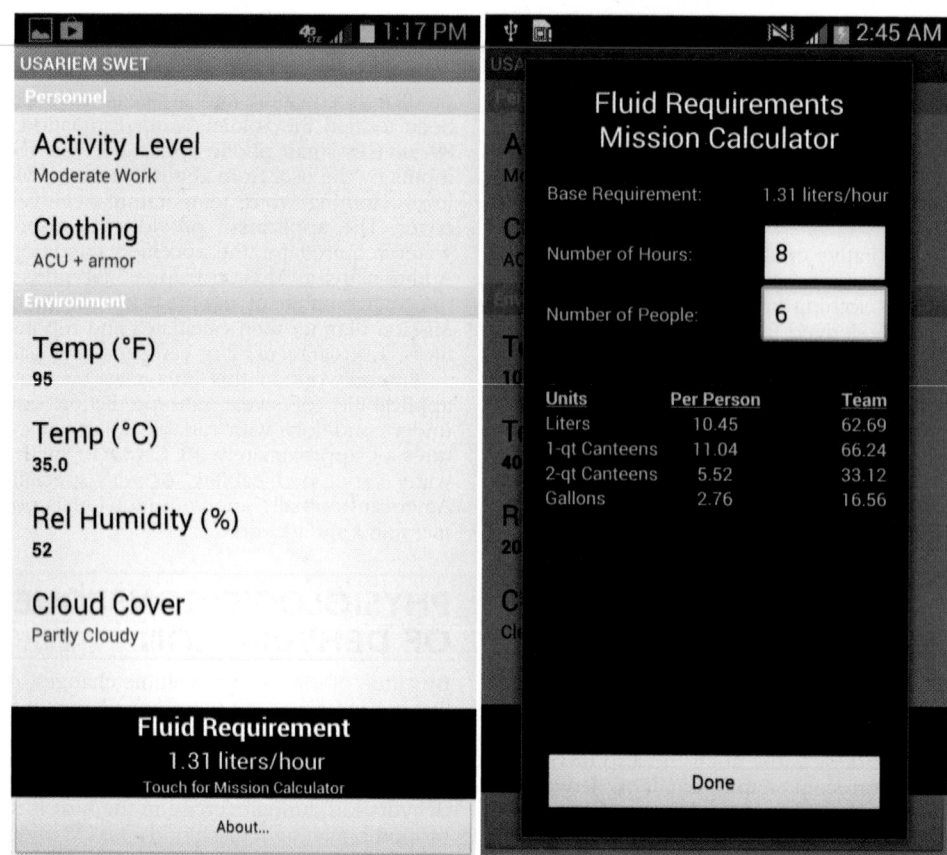

FIGURE 89-5 Soldier Water Estimation Tool (SWET). Main screen and Mission Planner screen.

deficit may be carried from one activity/exercise session to the next or from one day to the next.[83] In addition, individuals medicated with diuretics may be dehydrated before initiating exercise. Use of medications, such as acetazolamide taken prophylactically or while at altitude for acute mountain sickness, can have such an effect (and may increase risk for hyponatremia). This drug causes the kidneys to excrete bicarbonate, which acidifies the blood, increasing ventilation and blood oxygen content; however, it also increases fluid and electrolyte losses. If large sodium chloride deficits occur during exercise, extracellular fluid volume contracts and causes "salt depletion dehydration."

Dehydration increases physiologic strain, as measured by core temperature, heart rate, and perceived exertion responses during exercise-heat stress.[191] The greater the body water deficit, the greater is the increase in physiologic strain for a given exercise task.[4,142,143,201] Dehydration can augment core temperature elevations during exercise in temperate environments[30,154,195] as well as in hot environments.[50,193,203] The typical reported core temperature augmentation with dehydration is an increase of 0.1 to 0.2°C with each 1% of dehydration.[192] The greater heat storage associated with dehydration is associated with a proportionate decrease in heat loss. Thus, decreased sweating rate (evaporative heat loss) as well as decreased cutaneous blood flow (dry heat loss) are responsible for greater heat storage observed during exercise when hypohydrated.[69,70,151] The degree to which each of these mechanisms dissipates heat from the body depends on environmental conditions. However, both avenues of heat loss are unfavorably altered by dehydration.

When a person is dehydrated, the sweating rate is lower for any given core temperature, and heat loss through evaporation is reduced. In addition, as dehydration increases, there is reduction in total body sweating rate at a given core temperature during exercise-heat stress.[201] During submaximal exercise with little or no thermal strain, dehydration results in increased heart rate and decreased stroke volume, typically with no change in cardiac output relative to euhydration levels.[186,214] The addition

of heat stress in combination with dehydration during exercise results in decreased blood volume, reducing central venous pressure (CVP) and cardiac output,[111,147] and creates competition between the central and peripheral circulation for limited blood volume.[150,183] As body temperature increases during exercise, cutaneous vasodilation occurs and superficial veins become more compliant, decreasing venous resistance and pressure.[183] Effects of reduced blood volume (from dehydration) and increased blood displacement to cutaneous vascular beds (from heat stress) are decreased CVP and venous return and, ultimately, cardiac output below euhydration values.[152,194]

ENVIRONMENTAL HEAT STRESS, DEHYDRATION, AND PERFORMANCE

Physiologic factors that contribute to dehydration-mediated aerobic exercise performance decrements include increased body core temperature, increased cardiovascular strain, increased glycogen utilization, and perhaps altered central nervous system (CNS) function.[159,191,200] Although each factor is unique, evidence suggests that they interact to contribute in concert, rather than in isolation, to degrade aerobic exercise performance.[40,191,200] The relative contribution of each factor may differ depending on the specific activity, environmental conditions, heat acclimatization status, and athletic prowess, but elevated hyperthermia probably acts to accentuate the performance decrement.

In a field or wilderness setting, individuals may perform activities that require anaerobic power or muscular strength. However, the impact of dehydration may not be consistent for each type of activity. The literature in this area can be difficult to interpret because laboratory performance studies are often conducted with small numbers of participants (≤10 per study) and may be statistically underpowered to detect small but important effects. A recent comprehensive review of the dehydration/performance literature used a novel approach to assess endurance and strength or power exercise dehydration studies.[45] This less conservative

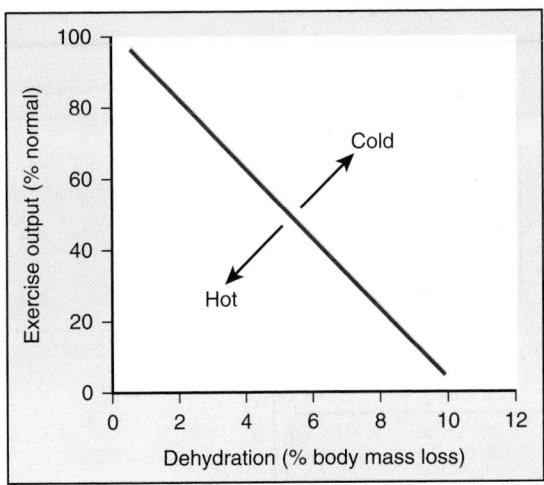

FIGURE 89-6 Percent decrement in exercise performance relative to percent dehydration (body mass loss). *(Redrawn from Adolph EF: Physiology of man in the desert, New York, 1947, Interscience.)*

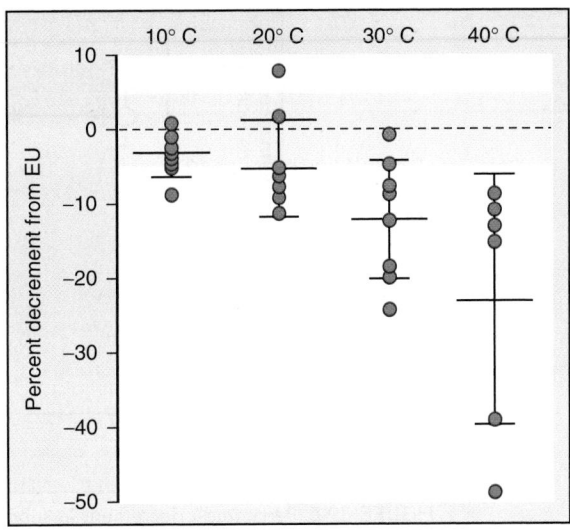

FIGURE 89-7 Percent decrement in total work performance relative to euhydration (*EU*) trial for all participants (*n* = 32) in 10°, 20°, 30°, and 40°C (50°, 68°, 86°, and 104°F) environments. Data are means; bars are 95% confidence interval. Shaded area represents coefficient of variation (±5%) based on performance variability measured during 2-week familiarization sessions.

approach counted the number of studies reporting a reduction in performance independent of *p* value with the assumption that the results should be 50% if caused solely by chance. The results were 53/60 negative performance observations (88%) for endurance exercise of 2% or greater body mass loss. For strength and power, 177/276 negative observations (67%) were observed, which coincides with findings that strength and power are negatively affected by dehydration, although to a small degree.[104]

Dehydration greater than 2% of body mass has been shown to degrade aerobic exercise performance in temperate-warm-hot environments.[36,42] As the level of dehydration increases, aerobic exercise performance is degraded proportionately.[100] The critical water deficit (>2% body mass for most individuals) and magnitude of performance decrement are likely related to environmental temperature, exercise task, and the individual's unique biologic characteristics (e.g., tolerance to dehydration). Therefore, some individuals are more or less tolerant to dehydration. Adolph and Dill[4] were among the first to document that during long-duration exercise in temperate or slightly warm environments, thermoregulatory sweating leads to progressive dehydration and results in lower exercise output (Figure 89-6). They derived this figure from limited exercise capability data and heart rate responses from a variety of exercise, heat stress, and dehydration conditions.

Exercise tasks that primarily require aerobic metabolism and that are prolonged are more adversely influenced by dehydration than are exercise tasks that require anaerobic metabolism or muscular strength and power.[196] The greater the level of dehydration, the greater is the magnitude of cardiovascular and thermoregulatory strain.[88] It has previously been demonstrated that high levels of aerobic fitness and acclimatization status provide thermoregulatory advantage. However, dehydration seems to cancel this protective effect during exercise-heat stress.[29,137,197] A comprehensive review of a number of studies that investigated the impact of dehydration on physical exercise capacity and maximal aerobic power found that in the majority of studies, exercise capacity decreased with levels of dehydration of as little as 1% to 2% body mass, although maximal aerobic power was not altered.[187] In addition, reduction in exercise capacity when dehydrated was further accentuated by heat stress.[58,158,169] In temperate environments, body water deficits of less than 2% body mass did not have a significant impact on maximal aerobic power. In a hot environment, however, a small to moderate water deficit (≥2% body mass) resulted in a large decline in maximal aerobic power.[58,158] A review of studies that observed the effects of progressive dehydration (>2% body mass) specifically on aerobic exercise performance found that in environments above 30°C (86°F), aerobic exercise performance was decreased by 7% to 60%.[42] It also appears that the magnitude of the effect increases as exercise extends beyond 90 minutes. Overall, this review

found that the impact of dehydration on prolonged work efforts is magnified by hot environments and probably worsens as the level of dehydration increases.

Few investigations have studied the impact of dehydration on aerobic performance across a range of environmental temperatures. Cheuvront and co-workers[39] observed 8% reduction in total work during a cycling time trial when dehydrated by 2% or more of body mass in a 20°C (68°F) environment. However, in a 2°C (35.6°F) environment, no effect of dehydration was observed. Kenefick and associates[108] reported decrements in aerobic performance (15-minute cycling time trial) of −3%, −5%, −12%, and −23% in 10°C (50°F), 20°C (68°F), 30°C (86°F), and 40°C (104°F) environments, respectively, when volunteers were dehydrated by 2% or more of body mass. Figure 89-7 depicts the change in performance relative to euhydrated trials and relative to the coefficient of variation (test variability; shaded area) of the cycling test itself. Mean values that lie inside the shaded area are considered to be within the "noise" of the test and those that lie outside are considered to be meaningful. Based on the findings, it would appear that the temperature cusp where dehydration of 4% of body mass altered aerobic exercise performance occurred at 20°C (68°F). It is important to note that these reported results are the minimal decrements in performance that could be expected. Greater decrements could be expected during more prolonged work or with greater levels of dehydration (Figure 89-7).

Table 89-4 depicts the decrement in aerobic time trial (<60 minutes) performance across a continuum of environmental

TABLE 89-4 Percent Decrement in Aerobic Exercise Performance (Compared to Temperate) Across a Continuum of Environmental Temperatures and at ~3000 m With and Without Dehydration (≥2% Body Mass)

Environment	Euhydrated	Dehydrated
Cold (2°-10°C; 36-50°F)	—	~3%[39,108]
Temperate (~20°C; 68°F)	—	~5% to 7%[39,108]
Warm (~30°C; 86°F)	~8%[221]	~12%[108]
Hot (~40°C; 104°F)	~17%[65]	~23%[108]
Altitude (~3000 m; 9843 ft)	~11% to 15%[37,76]	~33%[37]

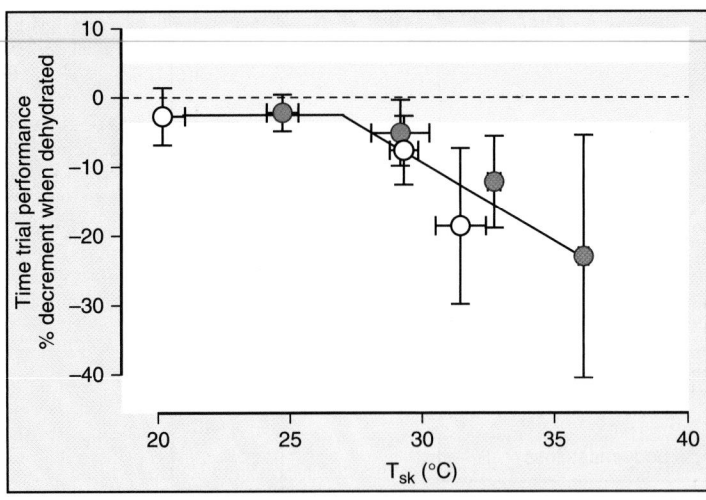

FIGURE 89-8 Percentage decrement in submaximal aerobic performance from euhydration as a function of skin temperature (T_{sk}) when dehydrated by 3% to 4% of body mass. Data are means (error bars are 95% confidence intervals) compiled from three studies,[39] employing similar experimental procedures and time trial (TI) performance tests. Filled circles represent 15-minute tests; open circles represent 30-minute tests. At a T_{sk} intercept of about 27°C (80.6°F), the percentage decrement in aerobic exercise performance declines linearly by about 1.3% for each 1°C rise in T_{sk}, similar to the single study of Kenefick et al. *(Data from Castellani JW et al: Effect of hypohydration and altitude exposure on aerobic exercise performance and acute mountain sickness, J Appl Physiol 109(6):1792-1800, 2010; Cheuvront SN et al: Hypohydration impairs endurance exercise performance in temperate but not cold air, J Appl Physiol 99:1972-1976, 2005; and Kenefick RW et al: Skin temperature modifies the impact of hypohydration on aerobic performance, J Appl Physiol 109(1):79-86, 2010.)*

temperatures and at an altitude of about 3000 m (9843 feet) with and without hypohydration (>2% body mass loss). Without any degree of dehydration, certain environments (warm-hot, altitude) have a negative impact on aerobic exercise performance. It is important to note that in combination with these environments, dehydration further degrades aerobic exercise performance, and that with longer-duration exercise (>60 minutes), greater degradations in performance can be expected. However, by maintaining a well-hydrated state, the contribution of dehydration to degradation in exercise performance can be alleviated.

One explanation for the impact of dehydration on exercise performance is that during exercise in the heat, sweat output often can exceed water intake and lead to overall loss of body water and reductions in plasma and blood volume. The amount of body fluid lost through thermoregulatory sweating can vary widely but usually is in the range of 0.5 to 1.5 L/hr. The upper limits for fluid replacement during exercise-heat stress are set by the maximal gastric emptying rates, which have been reported to be 1.0 to 1.5 L/hr for the average adult,[139,149] but are reduced by exercise-heat stress and dehydration.[33] Although gastric emptying may or may not be sufficient to maintain hydration (depending on sweating rate), people tend to drink only after thirst develops. As presented earlier, the sensation of thirst appears at about 295 mmol/kg,[177] or about 2% of body mass loss. Thus, a significant amount of fluid loss occurs before the sensation of thirst drives fluid intake. During activity, if fluid intake occurs after signaled by thirst sensation and is less than fluid loss through thermoregulatory sweating, the outcome is progressive dehydration.

Thus, during exercise in the heat with high sweat rates, there is the simultaneous problem of reduced plasma volume from dehydration while skin blood flow requirements are elevated. This dual perturbation of reduced plasma volume and elevated skin blood flow secondary to sweating is likely an important physiologic mechanism (via the cardiovascular system) contributing to impaired aerobic performance. As a result of blood pooling in the skin and reduction in plasma volume, cardiac filling is reduced, and larger fractional utilization of oxygen is required at any given workload.[14] Ultimately, these responses have a negative impact on exercise/work performance, particularly in warm-hot environments.

Figure 89-8 plots the impact of dehydration on submaximal aerobic performance from several hypohydration studies,[39] complied by Sawka and associates.[190] These studies employed similar procedures over a broad range of skin temperatures (T_{sk}) from 20° to 36°C (68° to 96.8°F). Segmented regression was used to approximate the statistical T_{sk} threshold for performance impairment using individual study data points ($n = 53$ paired observations). The threshold that best minimized the residual sums of squares was shown as 27.3°C. Warmer skin accentuated performance impairment by about 1.5% for each additional 1°C rise in T_{sk}. Therefore, as ambient conditions become warmer and elevate cutaneous vasodilation, the adverse impact of dehydration is clearly demonstrated.[190]

The negative impact of dehydration on work performance can increase risk in a field or wilderness setting. Dehydration, in combination with heat stress, reduces maximal oxygen uptake, increases relative effort, and reduces work output. When dehydrated, an individual will not be able to trek as far or as fast compared to when the person is euhydrated. For example, when on a hike, dehydration can increase the duration of time required to complete the hike beyond what is to be expected for a given distance and terrain, especially in warm-hot environments. In the scenario of a day hike or a hike to a destination, this increases the time to complete the hike and could result in a hiker being caught outdoors in adverse weather or overnight unprepared.

DEHYDRATION AND WORK PRODUCTIVITY

As previously discussed, during physical work in the heat, sweat output often exceeds water intake, which leads to body water losses. Bishop and colleagues[23] observed that, in simulated industrial work conditions, encapsulated protective clothing produced sweating rates up to 2.25 L/hr. Likewise, wearing protective equipment such as full or half face masks can make fluid consumption more difficult and further contribute to dehydration in the workplace. Firefighters wear heavy protective clothing and are exposed to intense heat. Rossi[182] reported that firefighters wearing protective clothing and equipment while performing simulated work tasks in the heat can have sweat rates up to 2.1 L/hr. Also, workers often not only become dehydrated on the job, but may start the workday with a fluid deficit. Brake and co-workers[25] observed fluid losses and hydration status of miners under thermal stress while working extended shifts (12 hours). By measuring urine specific gravity at the start of a work shift, they observed that 60% of the miners reported to work dehydrated, and that their hydration status did not improve during the shift.

While many studies have observed the effect of dehydration on physical work capacity, few studies have observed dehydration's impact on manual labor productivity. Wasterlund and colleagues[227] studied forest workers in a 15°C (59°F) environment in two scenarios: (1) participants consumed fluid sufficient to maintain a normal hydration state and (2) participants consumed limited fluid, which resulted in 0.7-kg body mass loss (>1% dehydration). The measure of productivity was the amount of time to stack and debark 2.4 cubic meters of pulpwood. When workers were dehydrated, productivity of stacking and debarking pulpwood was reduced by 12%.

DEHYDRATION AND COGNITIVE PERFORMANCE

Cognitive (mental) performance, which is important when concentration, skilled tasks, and tactical issues are involved, has been shown to be degraded by dehydration and hyperthermia in some studies.[96,179] The evidence is stronger for a negative effect of hyperthermia than for mild dehydration on degrading cognitive/mental performance,[49] but the two are closely linked when performing exercise in warm-hot weather. The relative hyperthermia associated with dehydration could diminish psychological drive[28] or perhaps alter CNS function independent of temperature. Adolph and Dill[5] reported that dehydrated subjects fainted more quickly when faced with a change in body posture (orthostatic challenge test). Likewise, Carter and colleagues reported that individuals going from a seated to a standing posture who were dehydrated by more than 2% of body mass from heat exposure exhibited significant reduction in cerebral blood flow velocity and possibly cerebral oxygen availability. Intracranial volume is altered in response to dehydration,[63] although the exact functional consequence of this is unknown. However, despite these orthostatic and cerebrovascular changes, the plausibility of dehydration altering cognition on physiologic grounds (osmolality, volume) appears small.

Some studies reported that as little as 2% dehydration has been associated with impaired visual motor tracking, short-term memory, attention, and arithmetic efficiency,[90] as well as greater tiredness, reduced alertness, and higher levels of perceived effort and concentration. In contrast, other studies have reported no effect on cognitive function with 4% dehydration, even when combined with heat exposure.[66] Equivocal findings in this area could be caused by study differences, such as dehydration methods, or the residual effects of dehydration, which include fatigue or hyperthermia. In fact, reviews of the dehydration and cognition literature suggest that future research in this area should focus on the possible confounding effects of methods used to achieve dehydration (e.g., exercise heat exposure).[91,121] Differences in the choice of cognitive test(s) or lack of test familiarity may also be blamed.[22] It should be noted that studies reporting significant alterations in cognition with dehydration as low as 1% to 2% of body mass[10,48,79,90] did not establish a well-hydrated baseline.

Another important point not often considered is absence of a genuine physiologic mechanism by which dehydration might impair cognitive function. In general, dehydration by less than 2% body mass would shrink the intravascular space by less than 200 mL and raise plasma osmolality by less than 5 mmol/kg. Much larger changes in plasma osmolality are required to increase blood-brain barrier permeability,[172] which would not be possible with the levels of dehydration achieved in most of the dehydration and cognition literature. Neural activity is closely related to cerebral blood flow (CBF),[81] but CBF is maintained at rest after intracellular[31] and extracellular[181] dehydration of 2% to 3% of body mass. Dehydration can reduce CBF transiently when an orthostatic challenge is imposed,[31,181] but this effect relates only to the risk for syncopal episodes in low-tolerance individuals.[175] As previously discussed, the measured effects of mild dehydration on brain volume are also inconsistent.

It is generally acknowledged that dehydration has a negative effect on mood state and can produce unpleasant symptoms such as dry mouth, thirst, and headache. Many studies investigating the impact of dehydration on cognition consistently report alterations in mood state, such as perceived tiredness,[218] alertness,[153] fatigue, confusion, anger, and depression.[1,10,48,78,79,90,166] Kempton and colleagues[107] demonstrated that very mild dehydration (<2% body mass) did not impair cognitive performance or cerebral perfusion but did increase measures of mental sedation. Dehydration also produced a stronger increase in the frontoparietal blood oxygen level–dependent response during an executive function task, suggesting that higher levels of neuronal activity were required (and called on) to achieve the same performance. Physiologic effects of dehydration (change in plasma osmolality by >5 mmol/kg) are associated with strong sensations of thirst that have been associated with increases in activity in certain regions of the brain (on fMRI),[61,62,185] which supports the concept that these sensations can be distracters and necessitate greater brain activity to perform the same task.[107] This ability to overcome the negative effects of stressors and maintain an effective level of performance is termed *cognitive resiliency*. This resiliency in cognitive performance has been reported even with dehydration to 4% of body mass and when exposed to cool, warm, and hot environments. Negative mood states have been reported to enlist greater effort,[212] and thus individuals may elicit greater effort and detailed attention when in negative mood states such that decisions are unaffected by dehydration. Therefore, symptomatologic distracters associated with dehydration may be a more probable explanation for impairment in cognitive function reported with dehydration. Equivocal findings related to dehydration and cognition thus may be more likely caused by the variation in cognitive resiliency. This may help to explain why some people are able to maintain cognitive function,[66] whereas others are more easily disturbed.[11,228]

Whether caused by symptomatologic distraction, some as-yet unknown mechanism related to dehydration, or the combined effect of heat and dehydration, a greater number of accidents have been reported in the summer months.[225] When these accidents occur in wilderness situations, medical help may not be readily available, with dire consequences. Accidents such as trips or falls (possibly related to orthostatic intolerance as a result of dehydration) can result in broken bones, lacerations, or death (fall from a height). Accidents occurring during expeditions or when mountaineering can be traced to a poorly made initial decision (symptomatologic distraction resulting in mental fatigue, reduced alertness, and concentration) that led to subsequent poor decisions, further compounding the severity of the situation.

DEHYDRATION AND HEAT-RELATED ILLNESS

Dehydration increases the risk for heat exhaustion[4,136,202] and is a risk factor for heatstroke.[33,68,89,174] Other factors, such as lack of heat acclimatization, certain medications, genetic predisposition, and illness, often play a large role.[33,64] Historically, unexpected cases of heat-related illness were attributed solely to dehydration, because dehydration has been shown to impair thermoregulation and increase cardiovascular strain. However, it is now suspected that previous sickness or injury might increase susceptibility to serious heat illness.[105] Dehydration was present in about 17% of all heatstroke hospitalizations in the U.S. Army over a 22-year period.[33] In a series of 82 cases of heatstroke in Israeli soldiers, dehydration was present in 16% of cases.[68] Team physicians for American football clubs have observed during summer practice that dehydration, occasionally caused or exacerbated by emesis, contributes to heatstroke.[64,176] Dehydration has been associated with reduced autonomic cardiac stability,[34] altered intracranial volume,[63] and reduced CBF velocity responses to orthostatic challenge.

HYPONATREMIA

Hyponatremia describes a state of lower-than-normal blood sodium concentration, typically less than 135 mEq/L. It is also used to describe a clinical syndrome that can occur when there is rapid lowering of blood sodium, usually to a level below 130 mEq/L and accompanied by altered cognitive status. This is a serious medical condition that can result in death. Exercise-associated hyponatremia results from prolonged work (typically >5 hours), where sweating is the primary means of heat dissipation. Because sweat contains not only water but also small quantities of electrolytes, there is a progressive loss of water, sodium, chloride, and potassium. Hyponatremia most often occurs when individuals consume low-sodium drinks or sodium-free water in excess of sweat losses (typified by body mass gains), either during or shortly after completing exercise. However, drinking sodium-free water at rates near to or slightly less than the sweat rate can theoretically produce biochemical hyponatremia when coupled with progressive loss of electrolytes. Reductions in solute concentration of extracellular fluid promote water movement from the extracellular space into cells. If this fluid shift is of sufficient magnitude and occurs rapidly, it can congest the lungs, and result in brain swelling and altered CNS function. Signs and symptoms of hyponatremia often mimic those of heat injury and include confusion, disorientation, loss of faculties, headache, nausea, vomiting, aphasia, loss of coordination, and muscle weakness. In general, hyponatremia can be distinguished from heat injury by the presence of repetitive vomiting, abdominal distention, and production of copious clear urine. Complications of severe and rapidly evolving hyponatremia include seizures, coma, pulmonary edema, and cardiorespiratory arrest.

Hyponatremia tends to be more common with long-duration activities and is precipitated by consumption of hypotonic fluid (water). Figure 89-9 illustrates the interaction between drinking rate (water only) and plasma sodium concentration for a 70-kg (154-lb) individual in a 28°C (82°F) hiking environment at a moderate pace (6 km/hr), drinking at three different rates (200, 400, and 600 mL/hr); graph A predicts the percent change in body mass over time for the three drinking rates, and B predicts expected plasma sodium concentration. The slowest drinking rate (200 mL/hr) over the duration of the hike (12 hours) predicts an elevated plasma sodium level well above that of asymptomatic hyponatremia (135 mEq/L). However, this drinking rate also results in a greater than 4% level of dehydration, a level of fluid loss that would substantially degrade performance (yellow zone, Figure 89-9A). Because the drinking rate is well in excess of sweating rate, the fastest drinking rate (600 mL/hr) actually results in a body mass gain and is predicted to result in asymptomatic hyponatremia within 5 to 6 hours of activity and symptomatic hyponatremia (sodium <130 mEq/L; yellow zone, Figure 89-9B) by 10 hours. It is important to note that predicted changes in plasma sodium concentrations are different for individuals of greater or lesser body mass and with varying sweat rates and sweat sodium concentrations. For example, in individuals who lose large amounts of sodium in their sweat ("salty sweaters"), matching fluid intake to sweat loss may still result in hyponatremia from progressive sodium loss over long-duration activity.[141] Overdrinking hypotonic fluid is the mechanism that leads to exercise-associated hyponatremia. In general, consumption of water without electrolytes should never exceed 11 L (12 qt) during a single episode of rehydration. Consumption of electrolyte-supplemented beverages should substantially delay or prevent this outcome.

Exercise-associated hyponatremia has been observed during marathon and ultramarathon competition,[59,97,213] military training,[80,163] and recreational activities.[16] In athletic events, the condition is more likely to occur in females and slower competitors, both of whom gain weight (from drinking) during the event. Severity of symptoms is related to the magnitude by which serum sodium concentration falls and the rapidity with which it develops. If hyponatremia develops over many hours, it might cause less brain swelling and less adverse symptoms.[112] Unreplaced sodium losses contribute to the rate and magnitude of sodium dilution and in certain situations (e.g., salty sweaters) may be the primary reason for development of exercise-associated hyponatremia.[141,145] Nausea, which increases arginine vasopressin (AVP; antidiuretic hormone) secretion, along with exercise-heat stress, which reduces renal blood flow and urine output, can negatively

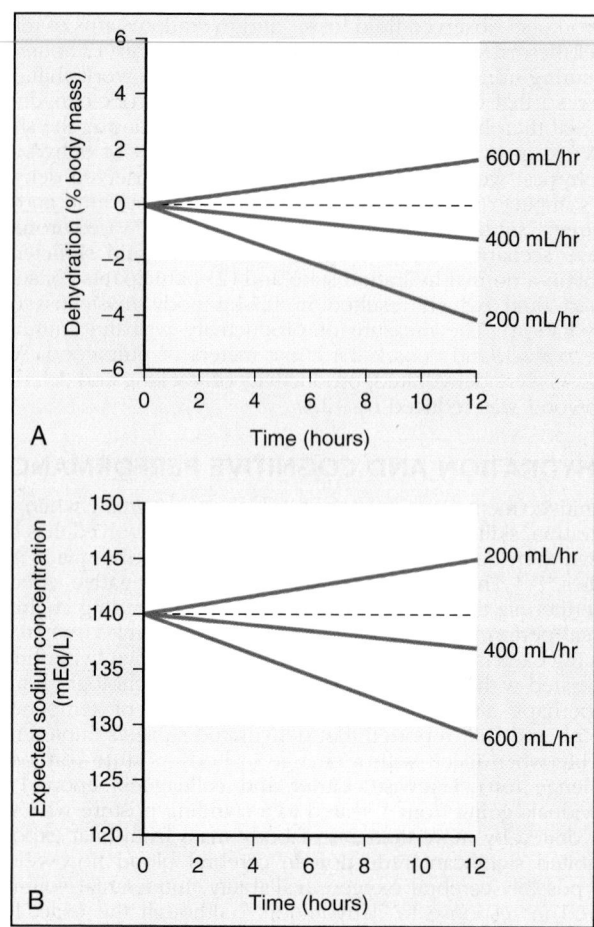

FIGURE 89-9 Prediction of the percentage change in body mass (**A**) and plasma sodium concentration (**B**) over 12 hours for three drinking rates, 200, 400, and 600 mL/hr for a 70-kg (154-lb) individual, in 28°C (82°F) hiking at 6 km/hr. The yellow zone in graph **A** represents the area where a substantial degradation in performance can be expected. The yellow zone in **B** represents the plasma sodium concentration where symptomatic hyponatremia will occur. (*Calculations from Montain SJ, Cheuvront SN, Sawka MN: Exercise associated hyponatraemia: Quantitative analysis to understand the aetiology, Br J Sports Med 40(2):98-105, 2006.*)

affect the ability of kidneys to rapidly correct the fluid-electrolyte imbalance.[233] The syndrome can be prevented by not drinking in excess of sweat rate and by consuming salt-containing fluids or foods when participating in exercise events that result in many hours of continuous or nearly continuous sweating.

DEHYDRATION AND LIMITS OF SURVIVAL

Severe elevations in blood osmotic pressures are incompatible with life. Just as hyponatremia (blood hypoosmolality) can produce fatal brain swelling, severe hypernatremia (hyperosmolality) can produce fatal brain shrinkage. The physical forces of each can produce tearing of intracerebral veins, leading to cerebral hemorrhage.[9] Although other pathologic outcomes of severe dehydration may also have fatal consequences, the effects of hyperosmolality on CNS function have long been suspected as primary.[24]

Acute elevations in plasma osmolality to greater than 350 mmol/kg produce neurologic symptoms such as seizures and coma in animals; death in humans has been consistently observed in patients with plasma osmolality greater than 370 mmol/kg.[9] Postmortem analysis of human vitreous humor samples in cases of death from dehydration show marked sodium elevation (>170 mmol/L).[126] By using the formula $2.1 \times Na^+$ to estimate osmolality,[98] a value of 357 mmol/kg is obtained. It therefore appears that a plasma osmolality value of 350 mmol/kg can be considered as an approximate limit for human survival.

The level of lethal dehydration (plasma osmolality >350 mmol/kg) and the time required to reach it can be estimated. If we assume that a 70-kg (154-lb) person possesses 42 L of body water and has a resting plasma osmolality of 285 mmol/kg, the degree of pure water loss required to concentrate plasma osmolality to the lethal limit is $(285/350) \times 42 = 34.2$ L, or 7.8 L. However, since electrolytes are also lost in urine and sweat, a reasonable correction can be applied (7.8/0.94), which yields 8.3 L. This gives a level of dehydration of almost 12% body mass and 20% of TBW. Although higher estimates have been made (~20% body mass), it is cautioned that as much as half of fasting weight losses derive from nonwater sources.[27] Under fasting conditions, Brown and colleagues[27] estimate that urine losses will stabilize at 0.5 L/day after the first day. The remaining losses from sweat depend on environmental temperature and body heat production.

Under hospitable indoor conditions, obligatory urine[27,100] and insensible sweat losses[100,115] add up to approximately 1.2 L/day, which makes survival without water possible for almost 7 days. This is longer than the 100-hour rule of thumb (~4 days)[168] but highly dependent on environmental and behavioral factors. For example, in a worst-case desert scenario where there are 10 hours of daytime high-temperature (>40° C [104° F]) environmental exposure and 14 hours of nighttime temperature(<20° C [68° F]) exposure, approximately 3.0 L/day of sweat loss can be added to the 0.5 L/day losses of urine when at rest.[27] This would limit survival to about 2.5 days. If the lost desert sojourner were to travel by night (14 hours) on foot through sand[82] at 4.8 km/hr (3 miles/hr) and rest unshaded during the day, 8.6 L/day of fluid losses[27,85] would limit survival to less than 1 day (23 hours). If traveling by day and night, sweat losses of approximately 0.60 L/hr (daytime) and 0.40 L/hr (nighttime)[85] would limit survival to about 16 hours. In each case, the distance covered would be about the same (42 to 48 miles).

DEHYDRATION AND SUSCEPTIBILITY TO COLD INJURY

A common response to cold exposure is cold-induced diuresis (CID), an increase in urine production associated with shift in fluid centrally induced by vasoconstriction.[199] In addition, when in a cold environment, attention to replacement of fluid losses is often neglected. If skin temperatures fall significantly, thirst is less noticeable in cold compared to hot weather.[110] In addition, individuals may voluntarily not drink fluid in an effort to decrease the need to urinate brought on by CID. Given the fluid loss brought on by CID, attenuation of thirst when exposed to cold,

and voluntarily not ingesting fluid, dehydration can result. Dehydration in the cold may be more important during heavy exercise when core temperature is elevated and blood flow to skin increases to dissipate heat. If individuals in the cold are heavily clothed and traversing in snow (resulting in high metabolic rates),[165] they may overheat more readily and increase fluid losses because of thermoregulatory sweating. During cold-weather outdoor activities, individuals can still become dehydrated by 3% to 8% of their body mass.[72] For these reasons, maintaining hydration is important when performing work in cold environments.

Dehydration in a cold environment does not appear to have the same impact on exercise performance as in temperate or warm-hot environments. Recent data show that if skin temperatures are low, 4% dehydration has no effect on cycling performance in the cold.[39] However, if cold strain is minimized by clothing, thereby maintaining skin and core temperatures near those observed in temperate or even hot environments, dehydration will likely degrade performance.[72] Dehydration does not alter heat conservation, heat production, or CID responses[161,162] and thus does not appear to increase likelihood of peripheral cold-associated injuries. However, lack of significant impact on exercise performance and injury does not negate the importance of maintaining hydration while in a cold environment. Little is known regarding the impact of long-term, chronic dehydration similar to that experienced on long-duration expeditions/missions in cold environments, where water availability is limited and sense of thirst is diminished. Individuals should drink adequately during endurance activity to replace fluid losses and prevent dehydration, even when in a cold environment. When returning to a warm environment, individuals who have free access to food and fluid will rehydrate on their own. When in the field, ice and snow can be melted. However, the source of ice or snow should be known, because only clean snow or ice should be melted for drinking water. If unsure, water melted from snow or ice should be properly disinfected.

FLUID REPLACEMENT (BEFORE, DURING, AFTER)

The U.S. Army has developed fluid replacement and work-pacing guidelines that incorporate work intensity, environment, work-to-rest cycles, and fluid intake, as shown in Table 89-5.[144] These guidelines use wet bulb globe temperature (WBGT) index to mark levels of environmental heat stress and emphasize the need for sufficient fluid replacement during heat stress and concern for the dangers of overhydration. WBGT uses

TABLE 89-5 Fluid Replacement Guidelines for Warm-Weather Training (Applies to Average Heat-Acclimated Soldier Wearing BDU)

Heat Category	WBGT Index (°F)	Easy Work Work/Rest (min)	Easy Work Water Intake (qt/hr)	Moderate Work Work/Rest (min)	Moderate Work Water Intake (qt/hr)	Hard Work Work/Rest (min)	Hard Work Water Intake (qt/hr)
1	78°-81.9°	NL	½	NL	¾	40/20 min	¾
2 (green)	82°-84.9°	NL	½	50/10 min	¾	30/30 min	1
3 (yellow)	85°-87.9°	NL	¾	40/20 min	¾	30/30 min	1
4 (red)	88°-89.9°	NL	¾	30/30 min	¾	20/40 min	1
5 (black)	>90°	50/10 min	1	20/40 min	1	10/50	1

Fluid intake should not exceed 1.5 qt/hr or 12 qt/day.
BDU, Battle dress uniform; NL, no limit to work time per hour; WBGT, wet bulb globe temperature.
The work/rest times and fluid replacement volumes will sustain performance and hydration for at least 4 hours of work in the specified heat category.
Individual water needs will vary ±0.25 qt/hr. Rest defined as minimal physical activity (sitting or standing), accomplished in shade if possible.
Wearing body armor: add 5° F to WBGT index.
Wearing mission-oriented protective posture (MOPP, chemical protection) overgarment, add 10° F to WBGT index.
Easy work: Weapon maintenance; walking hard surface at 2.5 miles/hr, ≤30-lb load; manual handling of arms; marksmanship training; drill and ceremony.
Moderate work: Walking loose sand at 2.5 miles/hr, no load; walking hard surface at 3.5 miles/hr, ≤40-lb load; calisthenics; patrolling; individual movement techniques (e.g., low crawl, high crawl); defensive position construction; field assaults.
Hard work: Walking hard surface at 3.5 miles/hr, ≥40-lb load; walking loose sand at 2.5 miles/hr with load.

environmental variables, such as solar radiation, humidity, and ambient temperature, in its calculation; automated systems for WBGT measurement are commercially available. The fluid replacement guidelines in Table 89-5 were designed to be simple and practical for use with large cohorts in situations where determining individual sweat rates would be impractical. These recommendations specify an upper limit for hourly and daily water intake, which safeguards against overdrinking and water intoxication. However, it is recommended that individuals performing endurance activities validate their sweat rates, because the guidelines do not account for individual variability.

AMERICAN COLLEGE OF SPORTS MEDICINE FLUID REPLACEMENT RECOMMENDATIONS

Current knowledge regarding exercise with respect to fluid replacement is presented in the 2007 American College of Sports Medicine (ACSM) Position Statement on Exercise and Fluid Replacement.[189] The position statement summarizes current knowledge regarding exercise with respect to fluid and electrolyte needs and the impact of imbalances on exercise performance and health. The statement stresses that individuals have varying sweat rates, and as such, fluid needs for individuals performing similar tasks under identical conditions can be very different. The ACSM Position Statement provides recommendations for hydration before, during, and after exercise/activity.

Before Exercise

The objective is to begin the physical activity euhydrated and with normal plasma electrolyte levels. If sufficient beverages are consumed with meals and a protracted recovery period (8 to 12 hours) has elapsed since the last exercise session, the person should already be close to being euhydrated.[100] However, if the person has sustained substantial fluid deficits and has not had adequate time or fluids/electrolytes in quantities sufficient to reestablish euhydration, an aggressive prehydration program may be merited. When hydrating before exercise, the individual should slowly drink beverage (e.g., ~5 to 7 mL/kg body mass, 350 to 490 mL for a 70-kg individual) at least 4 hours before the exercise task. If the individual does not produce urine, or the urine is dark (highly concentrated), the individual should slowly drink more beverage (e.g., another ~3 to 5 mL/kg body mass, 210 to 350 mL for a 70-kg individual) about 2 hours before activity. By hydrating several hours before exercise, there is sufficient time for urine output to return toward normal before activity. Consuming beverages with sodium (20 to 50 mEq/L) or small amounts of salted snacks or sodium-containing foods at meals will help to stimulate thirst and retain the consumed fluids.[131,173,208]

Hyperhydration can be achieved either by overdrinking or ingesting fluids (e.g., water) that expand the extracellular and intracellular spaces. Simple overdrinking usually stimulates urine production,[100] and body water rapidly returns to euhydration within several hours.[71,160,208] This means of hyperhydrating greatly increases the risk of having to void during activity/exercise[71,160] and provides no clear physiologic or performance advantage over euhydration.[106,116,117] In addition, hyperhydration can substantially dilute and lower plasma sodium[71,160] before starting exercise and therefore increase the risk of dilutional hyponatremia if fluids are aggressively replaced during exercise.[141] Enhancing palatability of ingested fluids is one way to help promote fluid consumption before, during, or after exercise. Fluid palatability is influenced by several factors, including temperature (preferred at 15° to 20°C [59° to 68°F]), sodium content, and flavoring.

During Exercise

The objective is to drink enough fluid to prevent excessive dehydration (>2% body mass loss from water deficit) during exercise by replacing sweat losses to help sustain performance. The amount and rate of fluid replacement depend on individual sweating rate, exercise duration, and opportunities to drink. Individuals should periodically drink (as opportunities allow) during activity if it is expected they will become excessively dehydrated from not drinking. Care should be taken in determining fluid replacement rates, particularly for prolonged exercise lasting longer than 3 hours. The longer the exercise duration, the greater are the cumulative effects of slight mismatches between fluid needs and replacement, which can exacerbate dehydration or dilutional hyponatremia.[141] Weight gain due to excessive fluid intake should be avoided. It is recommended that individuals monitor body mass changes during training/activity to estimate sweat loss during a particular exercise task. This allows customized fluid replacement programs to be developed for each person's particular needs.

The Institute of Medicine also provides general guidance for composition of "sports beverages" for persons performing prolonged physical activity in hot weather.[99] It recommends that fluid replacement beverages should contain about 20 to 30 mEq/L of sodium (chloride as the anion), 2 to 5 mEq/L of potassium, and 5% to 10% of carbohydrate.[99] The need for these different components (carbohydrate and electrolytes) depends on the specific exercise task (e.g., intensity and duration) and weather conditions. The sodium and potassium help replace sweat electrolyte losses, sodium also helps stimulate thirst, and carbohydrate provides energy. These components also can be consumed using nonfluid sources such as gels, energy bars, and other foods.

Carbohydrate consumption can be beneficial to sustain exercise intensity during high-intensity exercise events of 1 hour or longer, as well as less intense exercise/activity sustained for longer periods.[21,56,57,103,230] Carbohydrate-based sports beverages are sometimes used to meet carbohydrate needs while attempting to replace sweat water and electrolyte losses. Carbohydrate consumption at a rate of 1 g/min maintains blood glucose levels and exercise performance.[56,57] Most typical sport beverages contain carbohydrate sufficient to achieve this goal if drinking 1 L per hour or less. It should be noted that this rate of carbohydrate consumption was observed in highly fit, elite athletes. Most individuals would not work or perform exercise at a high enough intensity or for long enough duration to utilize 1 g/min. The greatest rates of carbohydrate delivery are achieved with a mixture of simple sugars (e.g., glucose, sucrose, fructose, maltodextrin). If fluid replacement and carbohydrate delivery are to be met with a single beverage, the carbohydrate concentration should not exceed 8%, or may even be slightly less, because highly concentrated carbohydrate beverages reduce gastric emptying.[102,226] Finally, caffeine consumption might help to sustain exercise performance[55] and likely will not alter hydration status during exercise.[57,231]

After Exercise

If recovery time and opportunities permit, consumption of normal meals and snacks with a sufficient volume of plain water will restore euhydration, provided the food contains sufficient sodium to replace sweat losses.[100] If dehydration is substantial (>2% body mass) with a relatively short recovery period (<12 hours), an aggressive rehydration program may be merited.[130,131,208]

Failure to sufficiently replace sodium losses prevents return to a euhydrated state and stimulates excessive urine production.[130,157,207] Consuming sodium helps retain ingested fluids and stimulates thirst. Sodium losses are more difficult to assess than water losses, and it is well known that individuals lose sweat electrolytes at vastly different rates. Drinks containing sodium, such as sports beverages, may be helpful, but many foods can supply the needed electrolytes. A little extra salt may be added to meals and recovery fluids when sweat sodium losses are high. Table 89-6 presents the electrolyte content of common sport drinks, tablets, and powdered additives.

Individuals looking to achieve rapid and complete recovery from dehydration should drink about 1.5 L of fluid for each kilogram of body mass lost. The additional volume is needed to compensate for increased urine production accompanying rapid consumption of large volumes of fluid.[207] Therefore, to maximize fluid retention, fluids should be consumed over time (and with sufficient electrolytes) rather than be ingested in large boluses.[113,232] Using intravenous fluid replacement after exercise may be warranted in individuals with severe dehydration, nausea, vomiting, or diarrhea, or who for some reason cannot ingest oral fluids.

TABLE 89-6 Electrolyte Content of Common Sport Drinks, Tablets, and Powdered Additives That can be Used to Help Replace Electrolytes Lost During Activity/Exercise

Product	Serv Size	CHO (g)	Na^+ (mg)	K^+ (mg)	Ca^{2+} (mg)	Mg^{2+} (mg)
CeraSport	8 fl oz	5	200	100	0	0
Ensure	8 fl oz	42	200	460	375	62.5
Elete Electrolyte Add-in	½ tsp	0	125	130	0	45
EleteTablytes	1 tablet	0	150	95	40	30
Gatorade (G2 Series)	8 fl oz	14	110	30	0	0
Gatorade (Pro Series)	8 fl oz	14	200	90	0	0
Lucozade Sport Lite	8 fl oz	5	0	0	92.5	0
Nutrilite	8 fl oz	14	110	30	0	0
Pedialyte	8 fl oz	6	253	192	25	2.5
Powerade	8 fl oz	14	100	25	0	0
Powerade Zero	8 fl oz	0	55	35	0	0
Vitaminwater Essential	8 fl oz	13	0	70	50	0
Vitalyte	8 fl oz	10	68	92	2.1	1.6

CHO, Carbohydrate.

Education

Alleviating dehydration should involve a combination of strategies that include assessment, education, and inclusion of practices that encourage fluid intake. Education is a vital component to help individuals maintain hydration before, during, and after activity. Informing individuals, especially those who perform work/activity in a hot environment, about hydration assessment, signs and dangers of dehydration, and strategies in maintaining hydration can help to reduce incidences of dehydration. Brake and associates[25] reported that individuals working in a thermally stressful environment were better able to maintain hydration when they were educated about dehydration, assessed their hydration state, and used a fluid replacement program while performing work.

MODIFYING FACTORS

Diet

One important aspect of an education and hydration program should stress the importance of consuming meals. Meal consumption is critical to ensure full hydration on a day-to-day basis.[3,4,211] Eating food promotes fluid intake and retention.[100] Sweat electrolyte losses can be replaced during meals in most individuals.[124,157,208] De Castro[60] observed food and fluid intake of 36 adults over 7 consecutive days and concluded that the amount of fluid ingested was primarily related to the amount of food ingested, and that fluid intake independent of eating was relatively rare. In addition, Maughan and colleagues, among others, reported that meals play an important role in helping to stimulate the thirst response, causing intake of additional fluids and restoration of fluid balance. Using established meal breaks may help replenish fluids and can be important in replacing sodium and other electrolytes.

Caffeine and Alcohol

Caffeine is contained in many beverages and foods. Recent evidence suggests that caffeine consumed in relatively small amounts (<180 mg/day) will likely not increase daily urine output or cause dehydration.[13] Maughan and Griffin[129] reviewed the literature on the effect of caffeine ingestion on fluid balance and concluded that doses of caffeine equivalent to the amount normally found in standard servings of tea, coffee, and carbonated soft drinks appear to have no diuretic action, and that their consumption will not result in fluid losses in excess of the volume ingested. Therefore, there would appear to be no clear basis for refraining from caffeine-containing drinks in situations where fluid balance might be compromised.

Alcohol can act as a diuretic, particularly at high doses, and can increase urine output. Therefore, alcohol should be consumed in moderation, particularly during the postexercise period, when rehydration is a goal.[206]

Facilities and Clothing

Anecdotal statements and interviews reveal that individuals will purposefully not drink fluid (voluntary dehydration) in certain situations, such as when bathroom facilities are not available, when in cold environments where exposure to the environment may be an issue, or when clothing systems are difficult to remove. Although logistical factors and conditions in the field may complicate access to facilities, a number of alternatives (e.g., toilet tents) can help to address this issue and reduce the practice of voluntary dehydration.

Gender

Women typically have lower sweating rates and electrolyte losses than men.[15,197,204] Women appear to be at greater risk than men to develop symptomatic hyponatremia when competing in longer-duration events such as marathon or ultramarathon races.[7,97] This risk can be alleviated by not overdrinking fluid.

Age

Older (>65 years) persons are generally adequately hydrated.[100] However, there is an age-related blunting of thirst response to water deprivation,[118,125,180] making older persons more susceptible to becoming dehydrated.[118] Older adults have age-related increases in resting plasma osmolality and are slower to restore body fluid homeostasis in response to water deprivation[167] and exercise[125] than are younger adults. If given sufficient time and access to water and sodium, older adults adequately restore body fluids.[123,125] Older persons are also slower to excrete water following fluid loads.[122,125,215,216,220] This slower water and sodium excretion increases sodium retention, which may lead to increased blood pressure.[123]

While thirst sensitivity to a given extracellular fluid loss is reduced in older adults, osmoreceptor signaling remains intact.[125,215,216] The osmotic and volume stimuli that result from dehydration impart important drives for thirst and drinking in older adults, just as in younger people.[18] Older adults should be encouraged to rehydrate during or after exercise.

Prepubescent children have lower sweating rates than adults, with values rarely exceeding 400 mL/hr.[19,138] However, sweat electrolyte content is similar (or slightly lower) in children compared with adults.[19] Lower sweating rates in children are probably the result of smaller body mass and metabolic rate, depending on age. Thermoregulatory sweating is not fully developed until adolescence.

Older adults and young children represent the extremes within the population, but regardless of age, if attention is paid to hydration guidelines, overdrinking will not occur, and hydration can be maintained.

ACKNOWLEDGMENT AND DISCLAIMER

The authors wish to thank Katherine M. Mitchell for her editorial assistance.

The views, opinions, and findings in this report are those of the authors and should not be construed as official U.S. Department of the Army position, policy, or decision unless so indicated by other official designation.

REFERENCES

Complete references used in this text are available online at expertconsult.inkling.com.

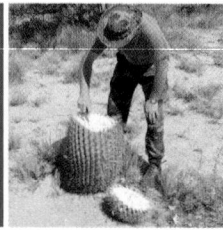

CHAPTER 90
Living Off the Land

PETER KUMMERFELDT AND DENISE M. MARTINEZ

A survivor's ability to "live off the land" is in large part determined by the person's capacity to procure, prepare, and store food and water, as well as have a basic understanding of human nutritional needs. Meeting a person's nutritional needs is significant in the context of wilderness survival and living off the land. Human survival has always been held hostage to its own nutritional needs, and the success of the human species is directly related to a continued emphasis on achieving a balanced diet.[1,21]

ACHIEVING A BALANCED DIET

The Dietary Reference Intake for energy for moderately active men age 19 to 50 years is 2900 kilocalories per day, and for moderately active women of the same age group, 2200 kcal/day[8] (Table 90-1). Energy needs increase with greater physical activity and decrease in ambient temperature. Current dietary recommendations set forth by the U.S. Food and Drug Administration (FDA) call for daily intake of energy-yielding macronutrients to be composed of 60% carbohydrates, 30% fat, and 10% protein.[12] The U.S. Department of Agriculture (USDA) also suggests that food choices be based on variety and balance, with emphasis on plant foods, primarily grains.[23] However, these recommendations may not have realistic application to wilderness survival and living off the land. To better understand the probable composition of daily energy-yielding nutrients under these conditions, we can look at the macronutrient intakes of hunter-gatherers.

Anthropologic analyses of hunter-gatherer diets show that 45% to 65% of their macronutrients were derived from animal food, both hunted and fished. The remaining 35% to 55% was made up of wild plants. It is also estimated that the average macronutrient composition of hunter-gatherers was 38% to 49% fat, 20% to 31% protein, and 31% carbohydrate.[3] For hunter-gatherer societies living at more than 40 degrees latitude north or south, there was increasing latitudinal dependence on fished animal foods and decreased dependence on plant foods. Although hunter-gatherer diets were composed primarily of animal foods with a high intake of fat, field studies of 20th-century hunter-gatherers showed them to be generally free of the signs and symptoms of cardiovascular disease.[2]

Whatever the dietary intake comes to be in wilderness survival and living off the land, there are commonsense considerations to achieving a balanced diet. Of these, *variety* is probably the most important. Variety can help ensure that the requirements for energy-yielding macronutrients (fat, protein, and carbohydrates) and micronutrients (vitamins and minerals) are met. Variety essentially translates to a balance between the intake of animal and plant foods. This balance depends on factors of climate, competition, and food-type availability, and is worth every effort to attain.

ESSENCE OF SURVIVAL

Historically, people who foraged for food from the environment were victims of aircraft accidents isolated in far-off regions of the world. They needed to supplement meager rations—the food in their pockets and possibly the food contained in a survival kit (if they had one). Castaways who washed up onshore after their boats sank were forced to collect food from the coastal environment. Others who have scavenged for food included people who became lost, although most of these were seldom lost long enough for lack of food to become a real life-or-death issue. For those who were not found within the typical 72-hour window, the ability to recognize and gather locally available wild food may have enhanced their ability to fend off assaults of the environment and prolonged their lives. Anecdotal reports of these survivors describe how many of them scavenged for berries, roots, and various forms of animal life to satisfy their hunger. Gathering food from the environment becomes important when people find themselves unable to obtain food from conventional sources, and a long-term survival situation is anticipated.

There are other circumstances in which being able to gather wild foods could prove very valuable. For example, during periods of civil unrest, particularly when traveling overseas, it is possible to find oneself in a situation in which grocery stores, supermarkets, and other sources of food are not accessible. Being able to forage for food could provide a viable alternative to jeopardizing safety by coming into contact with unfriendly locals. Knowing how to procure food could be a valuable skill in areas where natural disasters have caused extensive damage to the affected community's infrastructure and food supply. Being able to live off the land and consume unusual foods could also become important if one is taken hostage by a terrorist or criminal group. Self-sufficiency in the gathering of food and water could be particularly important to an escaped hostage attempting to return to friendly hands, as opposed to depending on hostile locals or terrorist sympathizers. In each of these situations, one may need to live off the land to augment provisions, or, in a worst-case scenario, to replace food that is no longer available.

Although being able to gather food can be important, a person should not believe that he or she would be able to live off the land indefinitely. Believing that foraging for one's own food is possible in all situations is not realistic. The time of year, environment, inadequate knowledge, lack of skill, and injury may

TABLE 90-1 Recommended Dietary Allowances for Energy

Gender	Age (yr)	Kilocalories per Day*
Male	11-14	2500
	15-18	3000
	19-24	2900
	25-50	2900
	50+	2300
Female	11-14	2200
	15-18	2200
	19-24	2200
	25-50	2200
	50+	1900

*Based on light to moderate activity levels.

severely limit a person's capability to forage for food. In fact, it may be more beneficial to limit activity by not aggressively searching for food than to expend the limited amount of energy stored in the body trying to procure food that may provide only meager energy.

Most survival manuals contain many pages devoted to identification of edible and toxic plants, techniques used to trap animals for food, and primitive fishing methods used to procure aquatic animal life. The techniques usually described are usually those used by indigenous people who still live off the land for their sustenance. The techniques depicted are presented as though they are methods that the average person could use when in an emergency and needing food. The fallacy lies in the belief that, based on a diagram or two accompanied by a paragraph of narrative, the techniques can be learned, remembered, and then used by the reader at some later date. More often than not, the techniques described *cannot* be learned by reading a book. A lifetime of training (or certainly months of practice) is needed for the techniques to become truly effective for the individual. Few people are willing to devote the time needed to develop expertise in the use of primitive food-gathering methods to a level of proficiency necessary in a survival situation.

During certain periods of the year in many parts of the world, very little, if any, natural food is available. The local people in these areas stockpile sufficient food to last through the lean times until natural sources of food are once again available. Even a well-trained and equipped survivor who arrives during these "lean times" is hard pressed to live off the land and can only hope that rescuers arrive promptly.

Living off the land is usually thought of as a task required to maintain life during a long-term survival experience in a remote corner of the world while awaiting rescue. Although this scenario occasionally happens, most of the survival experiences in North America are short term, during which the need to gather food from within the environment is not a survivor's primary focus. However, even in a short-term experience, knowing how to live off the land could prove beneficial to the survivor's physiologic need for food and psychological peace of mind. In some instances, being able to live off the land could mean the difference between surviving and dying.

The methods presented in this chapter are simple, practical, require a minimum of equipment, and most importantly, relatively easy to use in the field. Some practice will be required, but these procedures and techniques do not require a huge investment of time to develop basic skills.

WATER PROCUREMENT AND PREPARATION

Beside the need for energy-yielding macronutrients and micronutrients, the requirement for water must not be overlooked, because water is the most essential substance. Current recommendations on water intake recently released by the Institute of Medicine suggest daily intake of about 11 cups of total water for women and 16 cups for men.[7] These recommendations are based on the assumption that about 80% of a person's daily water intake comes from drinking beverages and the other 20% comes from water contained in food. Prolonged physical activity, heat exposure, extreme cold, and higher altitude increase water losses and therefore may raise daily fluid needs.

Many survivors begin their emergency already dehydrated (hypohydrated) and continue to dehydrate further when water supplies are limited and the quality of available water is suspect. There have been cases in which individuals needed water but, because of their fear that the water source was contaminated with *Giardia*, *Cryptosporidium*, or other harmful pathogens, delayed drinking or chose not to use the water at all. As a general rule, particularly in North America, because dehydration can very quickly reduce a survivor's ability to function efficiently and safely, it is usually better to drink the impure water. If the water was contaminated, the onset of symptoms will be days away. Hopefully, by then the individual will have access to medical care for treatment. Remember, doctors can cure giardiasis or cryptosporidiosis, but they can't cure "dead"! It should also be noted that gastrointestinal problems usually attributed to drinking contaminated water are in fact more often a result of poor personal hygiene habits.

The need to maintain body water levels and the physiologic impact of dehydration have been well documented in the medical literature (see Chapters 12, 13, and 89). In priority order after shelter and defending body temperature, the need to locate, procure, treat, and store water is the survivor's next most important need. Although water is important in every environment, lack of water becomes critical very quickly in hot, dry environments. Dehydration is also a critical problem at high altitude and at high latitudes where ice and snow must be melted to produce water. People who travel in these areas frequently have great difficulty obtaining water because of the hassles involved in collecting snow and ice, often under extreme weather conditions, and then having to produce the heat needed to melt it. In hot arid regions, where no surface water exists and only infrequent precipitation occurs, depending on tanks, springs, or other natural sources for water is a very questionable practice. Experienced desert travelers abide by the adage, "If you don't have it with you, you won't have it!" Lack of water in extreme conditions can lead to incapacitation within hours and death within days. Locating sources of water should be an important priority for the survivor.

FINDING AND COLLECTING WATER

Throughout much of North America, water is usually available from open sources of water, such as lakes, ponds, rivers, and streams, and can usually be obtained fairly easily. Despite this abundance of water, there have been cases in which survivors were unable to reach a water source because of their injuries.

Fundamental to finding water is recognition that it will always seek the lowest level possible and that, if present, some form of vegetation most likely indicates its presence. A good strategy to locate water is first to find a vantage point from which it is possible to scan the surrounding countryside. A person should slowly and methodically search for any indicators of water, such as green vegetation, birds flocking to specific areas, trails left by domestic or wild animals, and even large rock formations from which springs may originate or where water can become trapped. Human-made sources of water, such as windmills, tanks, dams, and irrigation canals, might also be observed. Look for water in low-lying areas, such as depressions, sinks, or tanks, where rainfall or melting snow is likely to collect. Water can often be found in these areas long after the last precipitation, especially if the areas are shaded. In arid areas where there is little vegetation to obstruct a person's view, a pair of binoculars can save a lot of walking.

Green Vegetation

Although the presence of any living vegetation is an indicator of subsurface water, the amounts of water are usually minuscule, and it is not available in sufficient quantity to justify any expenditure of energy in an attempt to dig for it. Most arid-area plants survive because their deep roots extend well below the earth's surface to gather small quantities of water available in the soil. Although it may not be appropriate to dig for this water, the process of plant transpiration can be capitalized on to collect a significant amount of water in a relatively short time. This process is described later.

Animal Trails

Most animals require water at regular intervals, usually once a day. By observing the movement of animals, it may be possible to determine the specific location of nearby water sources. Distinct trails are developed over time by both wild and domestic animals that travel to and from water sources on a regular schedule. Pay attention to forks in animal trails, because they often indicate the direction of a water source. If an animal trail forks into two trails, it is possibly leading a person away from a source of water. Conversely, if trails come together, an individual may be walking toward a source of water or food. Even though the direction to a water source can be determined, the distance to that source may be too far for the survivor to realistically reach on foot. Birds and animals have far greater capability to travel long distances without water than does a human. Consequently, it is usually better to stay in one place, as opposed to wandering around the desert looking for uncertain water sources.

Bird Movement

Most birds require water at least once per day. By watching their movement, especially in morning and evening hours of the day, a general direction of a water source may be determined. Once again, the urge to travel must be weighed against unknown distances and the questionable quality of water sources.

Open Water Sources

Collecting water from open sources is usually the easiest method available to the survivor. However, caution should be exercised. Lakeshores and the edges of rivers can be hazardous. Crashing waves, swift-moving water, undercut riverbanks, and unstable footing can all create problems. Swampy shorelines; heavy vegetation; lakes, streams, or ponds surrounded by cliffs; other difficult terrain; or unsafe ice conditions may preclude a person from getting close enough to a water source. Don't risk life and limb trying to climb or reach the water's edge when safer strategies can be used. Tie a line to a water bottle or container of some type and throw it or lower it into a water source from a safe location or vantage point. Because most water containers do not come with a reliable attachment point when the container is uncapped, make one by duct-taping a loop of parachute cord or nylon line to the side of the water container (Figure 90-1). Do not use the retaining strap that connects the cap to the water bottle for this purpose. In many cases, this strap will break or pull free from the full bottle as it is being retrieved from the water source, resulting in loss of the bottle.

In some instances, water sources may be very muddy or silty and need filtering or settling before they can be used (Figure 90-2). Rivers originating from glaciers carry large amounts of "glacial flour" that should be removed before consumption (Figure 90-3). This is best accomplished by allowing the water to settle overnight and then filtering it through fabric before drinking.

The water in some lakes, particularly those in the western United States, contains high concentrations of calcium carbonate and calcium bicarbonate in solution, which make the water nonpotable. Lakes of this nature are usually easy to identify because the calcium salts that are leached from the ground are deposited in the form of white powder around the perimeter of the lake as the water evaporates (Figure 90-4). Water containing high concentrations of calcium carbonate and bicarbonate tastes terrible and should not be consumed.

Water collected from rivers and streams should not be considered "pure" (Figure 90-5). *Giardia*, *Cryptosporidium*, and other harmful pathogens found in water sources are not deactivated by aeration or exposure to ultraviolet rays. All water

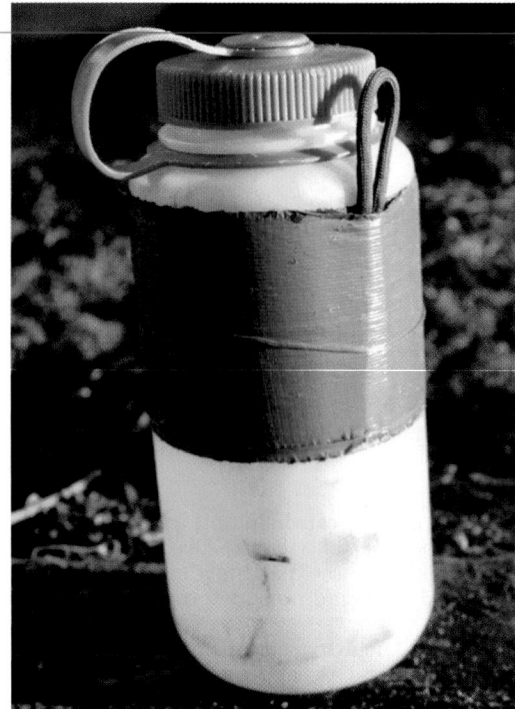

FIGURE 90-1 Attach a lanyard loop to your water bottle. *(Courtesy Peter Kummerfeldt.)*

should be disinfected and purified using methods described in Chapter 88.

Seeps and Springs

The quantity of water produced by seeps and springs varies tremendously. In some cases, the amount will be only a few teaspoons per hour (Figure 90-6). In other cases, gallons of water can flow from the ground in minutes (Figure 90-7). Where the quantities are small, the flat edge of the opening of a plastic bag can be used to scoop the water from a shallow source, or if it is flowing, to collect the water as it runs into the bag. A short piece of vinyl aquarium hose also works well for sucking water from shallow collections or to recover water from narrow cracks in the rocks.

Tanks

After a rain, water collects in low-lying areas and may be found long after the last storms have passed through the area (Figure 90-8). Check out any depressions, sinks, or other low places

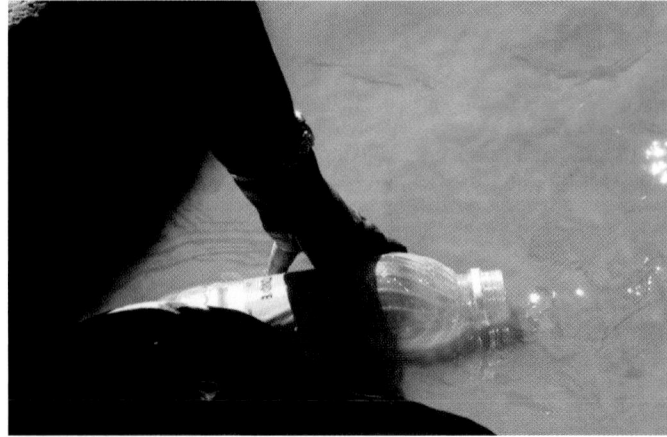

FIGURE 90-2 Muddy water should be allowed to settle and then be filtered. *(Courtesy Peter Kummerfeldt.)*

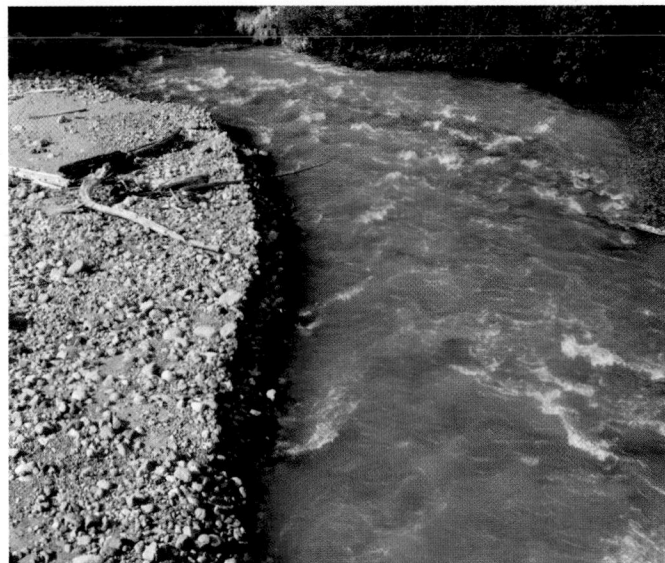

FIGURE 90-3 Rivers originating from glaciers are discolored by the glacial "flour" they are carrying. This water should be allowed to settle before filtering. (Courtesy Peter Kummerfeldt.)

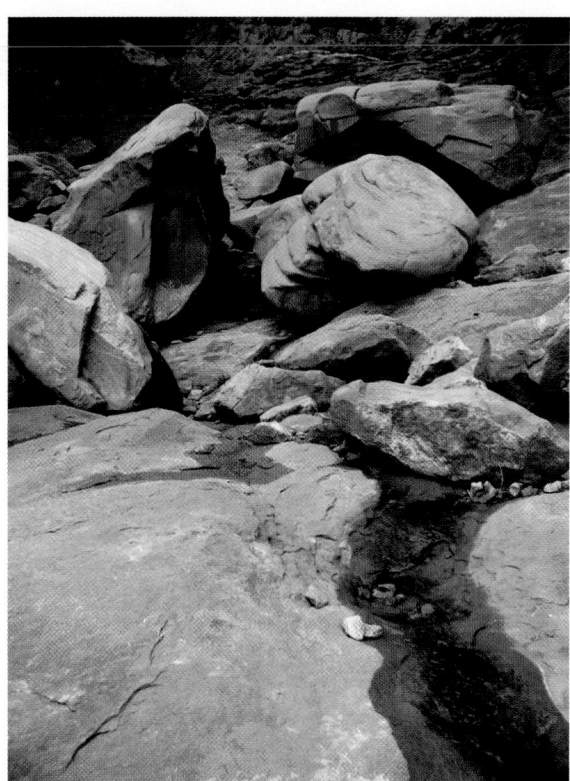

FIGURE 90-6 Desert seep. (Courtesy Peter Kummerfeldt.)

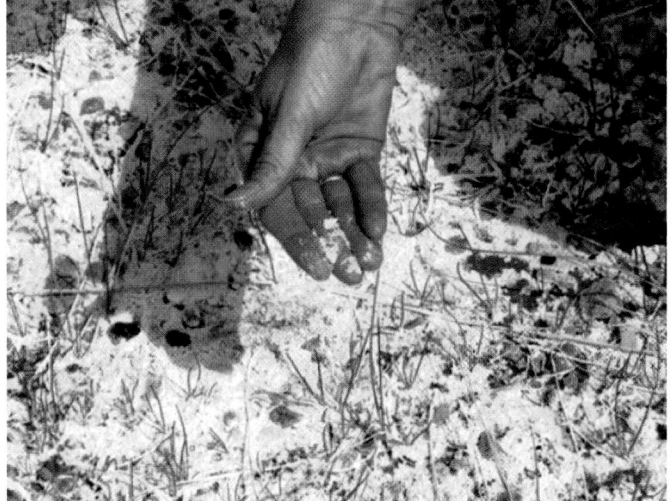

FIGURE 90-4 Calcium salts leached from the soil are a common sight around many western U.S. lakes. (Courtesy Peter Kummerfeldt.)

where water could gather. Remember, the presence of vegetation and animals could provide a clue to the presence of a water source. Water sources like these should be checked carefully because they are frequently contaminated with debris that has been washed into the drainage. Finding the remains of animals that have died nearby or in the water, animal droppings, or other similar contaminants necessitates boiling, using halogens, or a filtration system designed to disinfect water (see Chapter 88).

Wells

It may be possible to locate abandoned open wells from which water may be obtained. Usually, the rope and bucket used to lift water from these wells will be missing, and a person will have

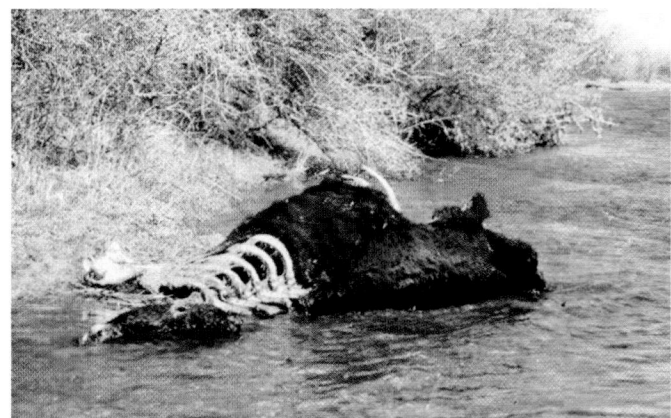

FIGURE 90-5 All water should be disinfected if possible before it is consumed. (Courtesy Peter Kummerfeldt.)

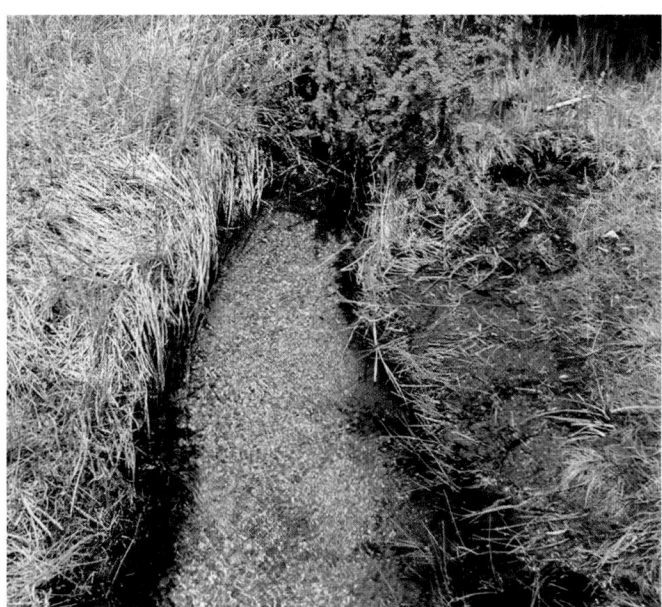

FIGURE 90-7 Desert spring. (Courtesy Peter Kummerfeldt.)

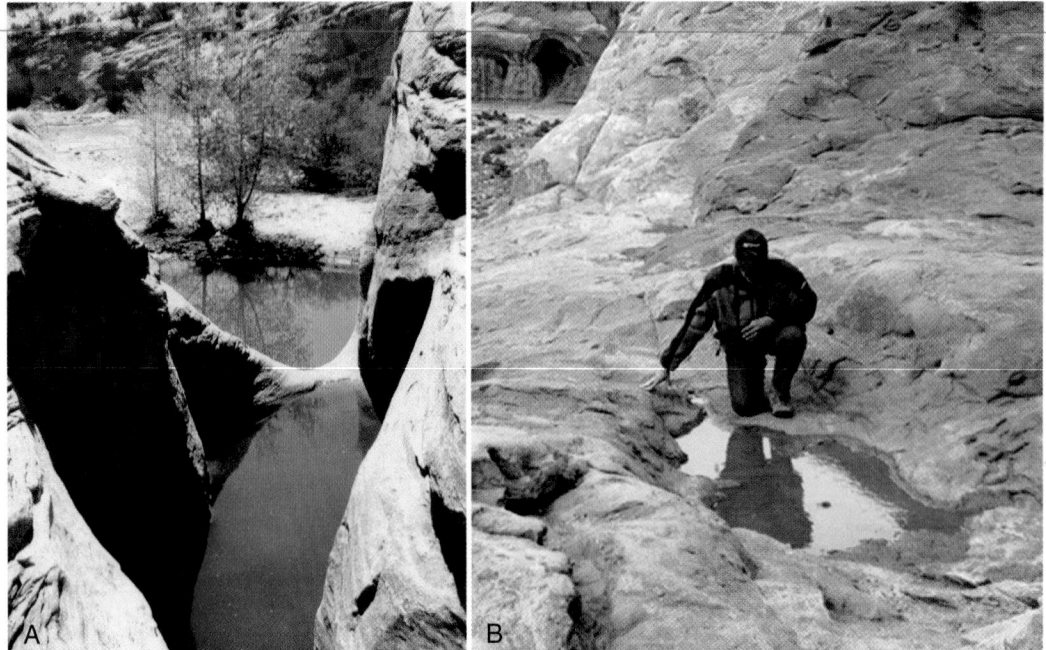

FIGURE 90-8 After rainfall, water can be found in desert tanks **(A)** and other depressions **(B)**. *(Courtesy Peter Kummerfeldt.)*

to improvise a means to lowering a container down into the well to retrieve the water. With a closed well, where the pump handle is present but secured, or where the water is piped to another location, it may be necessary to dismantle or damage the plumbing to access the water. This may not be possible without tools.

Windmills

Windmills that could provide a ready source of water are a common sight across North America, especially where little surface water exists (Figure 90-9). Typically, the water pumped to the surface is collected in a nearby tank or pumped directly into a trough from which livestock can drink (Figure 90-10). If this is not the case, it may be necessary to dismantle or damage the pipes associated with the windmill to gain access to the water. Without tools, this may not be possible.

Guzzlers

In arid areas, particularly in the western and southwestern United States, state wildlife agencies and conservation organizations have installed rainwater collectors called *guzzlers*. These water tanks can hold hundreds of gallons of water long after seasonal rains have passed (Figure 90-11). A guzzler consists of a concrete, metal, or fiberglass apron designed to gather precipitation and feed it into a holding tank, where it remains until it is consumed by thirsty animals or evaporates.

Dew

Dew forms on clear nights when the air temperature decreases and the water held in vapor or air suspension condenses on cool metal surfaces or on vegetation. Dew can be collected as it drains

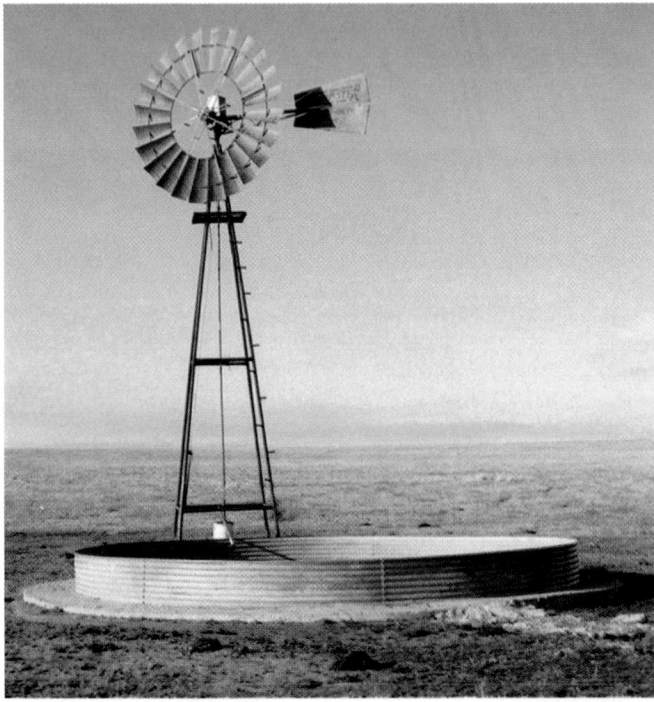

FIGURE 90-9 Windmills are a common sight across the arid regions of the western United States and may provide a survivor with a source of water. *(Courtesy Peter Kummerfeldt.)*

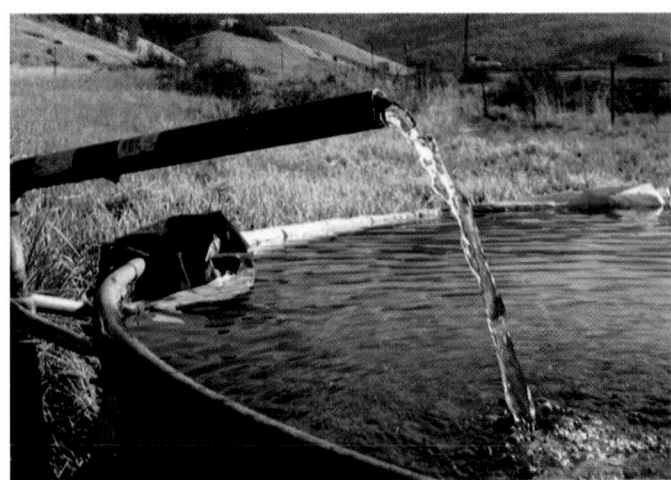

FIGURE 90-10 Water pumped from the ground by windmills may be readily available to a survivor. *(Courtesy Peter Kummerfeldt.)*

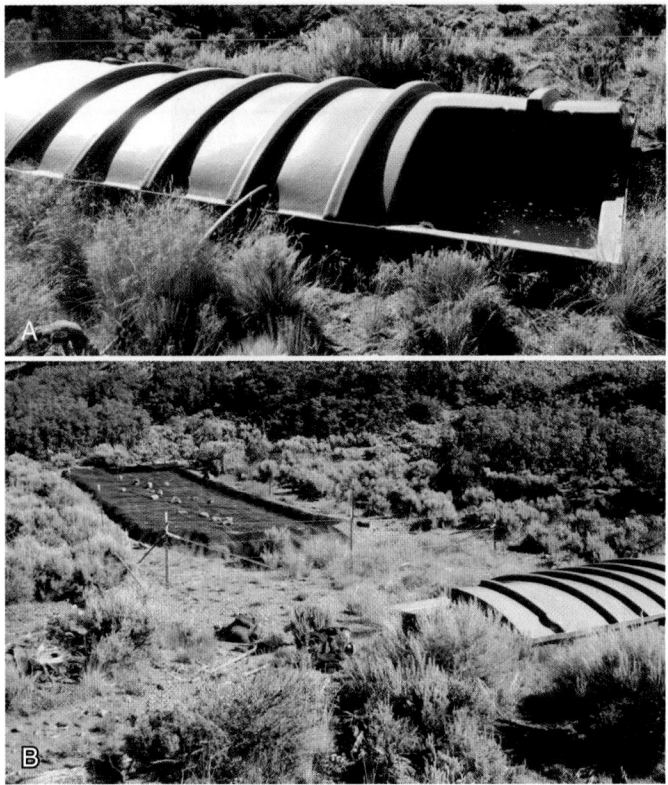

FIGURE 90-11 **A** and **B**, Guzzlers collect and store rainwater for wild-life and others in need of water. *(Courtesy Peter Kummerfeldt.)*

from inclined surfaces on which it has formed, or it can be sponged up using an absorbent material. Campers' towels are one of the best materials for collecting dew (Figure 90-12). These highly absorbent towels quickly absorb moisture and can then be wrung out into a container or squeezed directly into a person's mouth. A sponge is also very useful for collecting dew. Dew must be collected early in the morning before it is evaporated by the sun's heat.

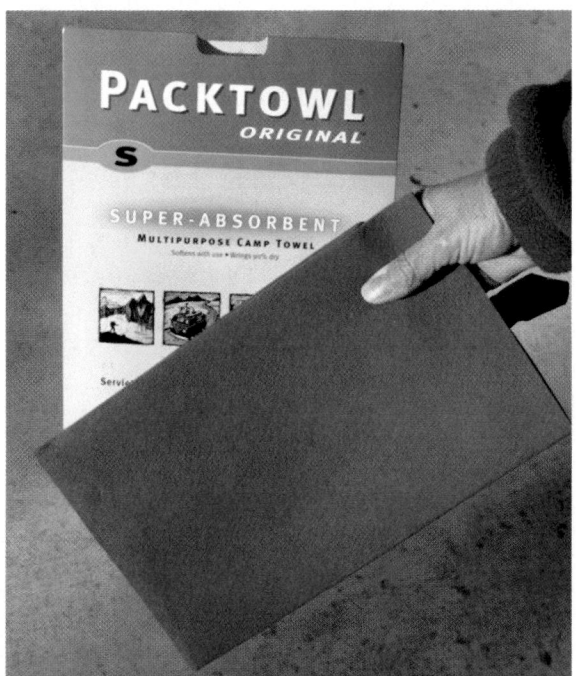

FIGURE 90-12 Campers' towels are very useful for soaking up dew or water from shallow sources. *(Courtesy Peter Kummerfeldt.)*

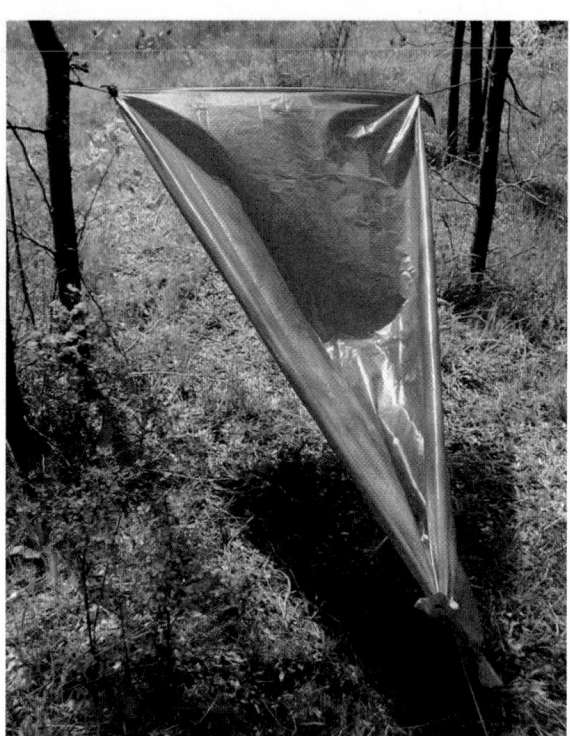

FIGURE 90-13 A plastic bag, sheet of plastic, or other material erected as shown is a very efficient method to collect large amounts of rain-water quickly. *(Courtesy Peter Kummerfeldt.)*

Rain

Rainwater can be easily collected by erecting a flat surface (Figure 90-13). Water collects on the upper surfaces of any material (it need not be waterproof) and drains to the lowest point, where it is collected.

Snow

For a normothermic person, there is no reason not to "eat" snow as an auxiliary source of water. However, for a person close to being hypothermic or who is already hypothermic, eating snow may increase loss of body heat and exacerbate the medical condition. Survival case studies reflect that individuals who chose to eat snow frequently experienced cuts and abrasions to the mouth mucosa as a result. If snow is the only source of water on hand, and no alternative methods are available to melt it, the snow should be collected, compacted by hand, and consumed in small enough quantities for heat within the mouth to melt the snow.

When snow falls and settles on the ground, it undergoes constant metamorphosis. During very cold periods, there may be very little moisture in the dry, fine, or wind-blown snow that accumulates on the ground. Over time, as snow accumulates, the weight of the upper layers of snow and the earth's latent heat cause the snow closer to the ground to change. It becomes more granular in nature and more like ice than snow. When comparing equal volumes of snow, snow collected from lower levels near the ground produces more water than does snow collected near the surface (Figure 90-14). Also, less heat will be needed to convert this snow to water.

Water Machine. The most efficient technique to convert snow into water is with what military survival schools call "a water machine" (Figure 90-15). A bag made from any available porous fabric (a T-shirt with the neck and armholes sewn shut has been used) is filled with snow and ice and hung near, but not directly over, a fire. The fire's radiant heat melts the snow in the bag and the water runs down to the lowest point of the bag, where it drains into a container. Continually refilling the bag with snow prevents it from burning. Gallons of water can be produced quickly and safely using this method. The following are the major advantages of using the water machine method:

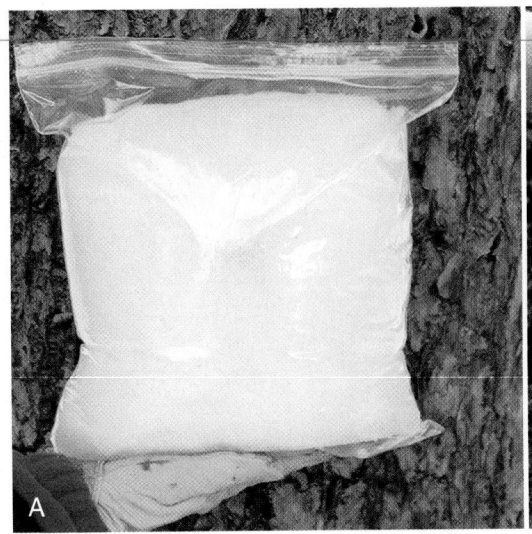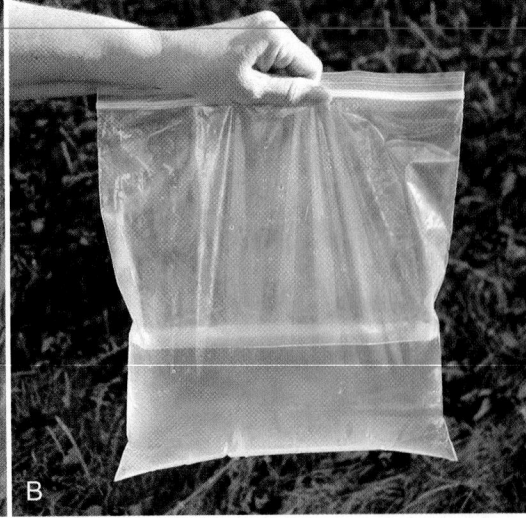

FIGURE 90-14 Melting granular snow contained in a 1-gallon zipper-lock bag **(A)** produced the water shown on the right **(B)**. *(Courtesy Peter Kummerfeldt.)*

- Once the water machine is loaded with snow and positioned, no further action is needed until the bag needs to be filled with additional snow.
- A water machine works while a person is busy with other tasks. This saves energy.
- All the debris (e.g., leaves, grass, twigs, insects) commonly found in snow is filtered out by the cloth as the water drains into a container.

- A metal container, normally needed to melt snow over a fire, is not required when using this method.

Traditionally, snow is melted by placing it in a metal container and then applying heat (Figure 90-16). Several problems soon become apparent when using this method:

- The size of container is usually quite small, which limits the amount of snow that can be melted at one time.
- When heat is applied to the container, the snow directly in contact with the heat at the bottom of the container melts and is converted to steam. This steam is absorbed by the remaining snow, leaving a space in the bottom of the container. If the snow is not constantly stirred and pressed into the container, it is possible to scorch the bottom of the container and even to melt the solder used to seal the seams.

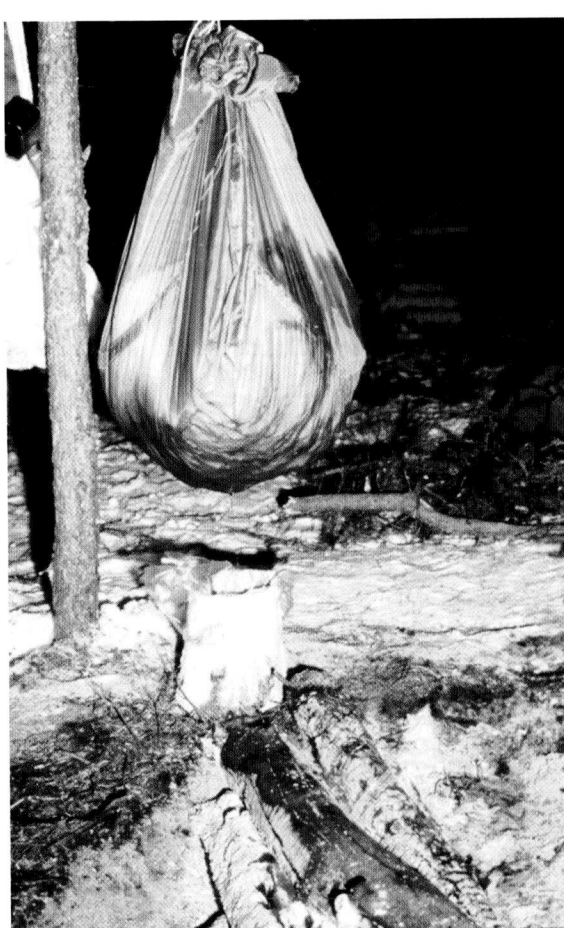

FIGURE 90-15 Water machines are the best method to use to quickly convert snow into water. *(Courtesy Peter Kummerfeldt.)*

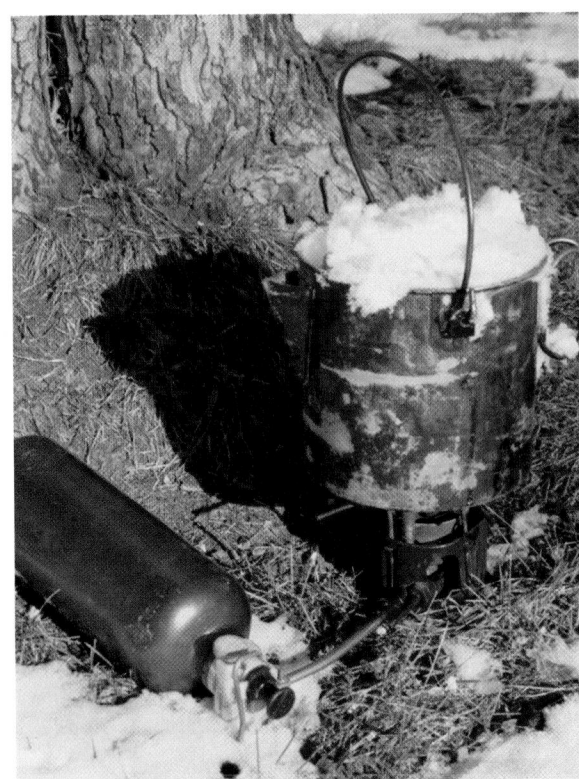

FIGURE 90-16 Melting snow in a pot is a very inefficient, time-consuming method of obtaining water from snow. *(Courtesy Peter Kummerfeldt.)*

- Using this method requires constant attention.
- The water produced using this process tastes unpleasant (smoky) and often contains ash and other debris from the fire.
- The system is inefficient, increases the likelihood of being burned, and often results in damaged clothing.

Using Body Heat to Melt Snow.   This is a very slow, inefficient method of procuring water. If this process is the only one available, a small quantity of snow (several cups) is placed in any available waterproof container. Preferably, this should be a soft plastic water bag, zipper-type bag, or other similar container that is then placed between layers of clothing. Because the amount of heat needed to convert snow to water is large and the amount of body heat available is finite, only small quantities can be melted at a time. Large quantities of snow will not melt fast enough to provide the survivor any benefit. Large quantities of snow may also cool the body too much.

Using the Sun to Melt Snow.   Another method, frequently used in winter recreation, involves using a sheet of black plastic. A thin layer of snow placed on a piece of black plastic (or other dark-colored waterproof fabric) positioned in the sun will melt. The waterproof material should be positioned on an incline so that the melt water runs to the lower edge of the fabric and drains into a container (Figure 90-17).

Digging Holes to Collect Subsurface Water

Even though water is not visible on the surface of the ground, it may still be present in the soil in sufficient quantity to be collected. Locate low-lying areas where water is most likely to have accumulated, and dig down until damp layers of soil are located (Figure 90-18). Over time, water may seep into the hole, where it can be collected. If no indicators of the presence of subsurface water are present, dig a hole in the outside bend of a dry river bed. Look for a location where the centrifugal force of water flowing down river has eroded the outer bend of a curve and created a depression, where the last remnants of water flowing down the river will have accumulated.

Beach Wells

In a coastal, saltwater environment, it is possible to locate water sources near a beach that are fresh and potable. A hole dug behind the first line of sand dunes adjacent to the high-water mark will often fill with fresh water. Fresh water, which is less dense than sea water, will collect in the hole. Holes dug in sandy soils are very tenuous and tend to cave in constantly, which may make it necessary to shore up with driftwood the sides of any hole dug in sandy areas (Figure 90-19).

Solar Stills

Solar stills use a sheet of plastic and the sun's heat to capture evaporation from soil or plants or to distill nonpotable water. The water evaporates from its source (e.g., soil, plants, urine), condenses on the plastic sheet, and runs down the sheet into a collector, from where it is retrieved (Figure 90-20).

Solar stills are *not* a reliable method of obtaining water in arid areas. The quantity of water produced by a solar still depends on the amount of water contained in the ground. Because desert soils tend to hold little or no water, the amount that a survivor

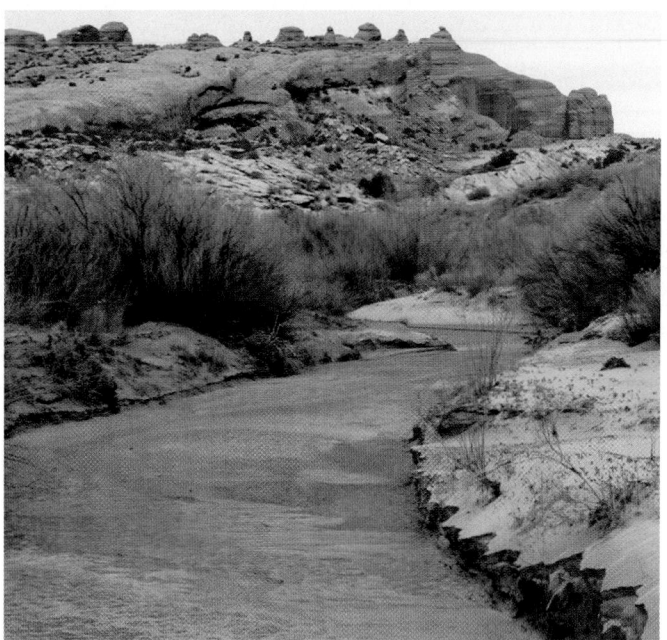

FIGURE 90-18 Damp, low-lying areas are ideal sites to dig for water. *(Courtesy Peter Kummerfeldt.)*

is likely to obtain must be balanced against the amount lost in the sweating process while constructing the device. In most cases, a person will likely lose more water than can be recovered from the still. Even if a solar still is constructed in ground that is saturated with water, its productivity in relation to the amount of effort expended is still questionable. If the ground is saturated, the other methods of water procurement described here will most likely work.

Water from Vegetation

A person's ability to collect water trapped by plants or contained within them can be a valuable aid to combating dehydration. Once again, a line must be drawn between methods that are practical and those based more on myth. Extracting water from a barrel cactus is a classic example of a survival "myth." Barrel cacti have been long featured in survival literature as a reliable source of water in arid regions (Figure 90-21). Several issues make this practice very questionable. First and most important, the quantity of fluid that can be extracted from a barrel cactus is very limited. Second, the fluid that is removed is not beneficial and may in fact be detrimental to an individual's health. Third, accessing the interior of a barrel cactus requires a substantial knife or other cutting tool. The outer skin of the cactus is very tough and covered with long spines. Barrel cactus should *not* be considered a source of water.

Water Vines

Throughout tropical and subtropical regions of the world, vines can be found that can provide a reliable supply of pure water when other sources are not available. Water-producing vines varying in size from pencil thickness up to the thickness of a male adult's forearm can even be found throughout much of the southeastern United States. Select vines with a large diameter. The greater the thickness of the vine, the more water it is capable of producing. Because water vines are woody and tough, they can be difficult to cut. A sharp knife or, better yet, a machete, will be needed to sever the vine.

To determine whether a vine is a suitable water source, the outer layers of the vine should be deeply scored with a knife. Vines that exude a white latex sap or a colored or foul-smelling sap should be avoided. If no sap is observed, or if the sap observed is clear and without aroma, a section of the vine can be cut as a water source. A 24-inch-long piece of vine should be cut by severing the higher end first and then cutting the lower end. If the lower end is cut first, the water contained within the

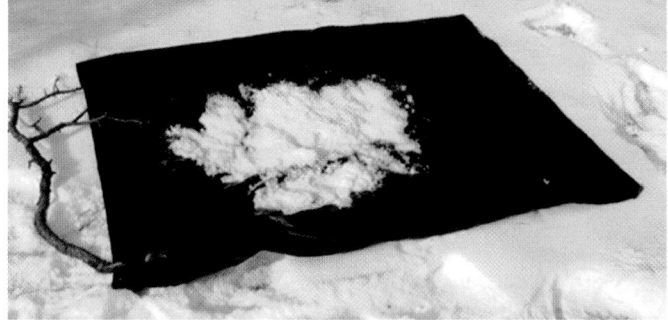

FIGURE 90-17 Solar heat and a sheet of black plastic can be used to melt snow. *(Courtesy Peter Kummerfeldt.)*

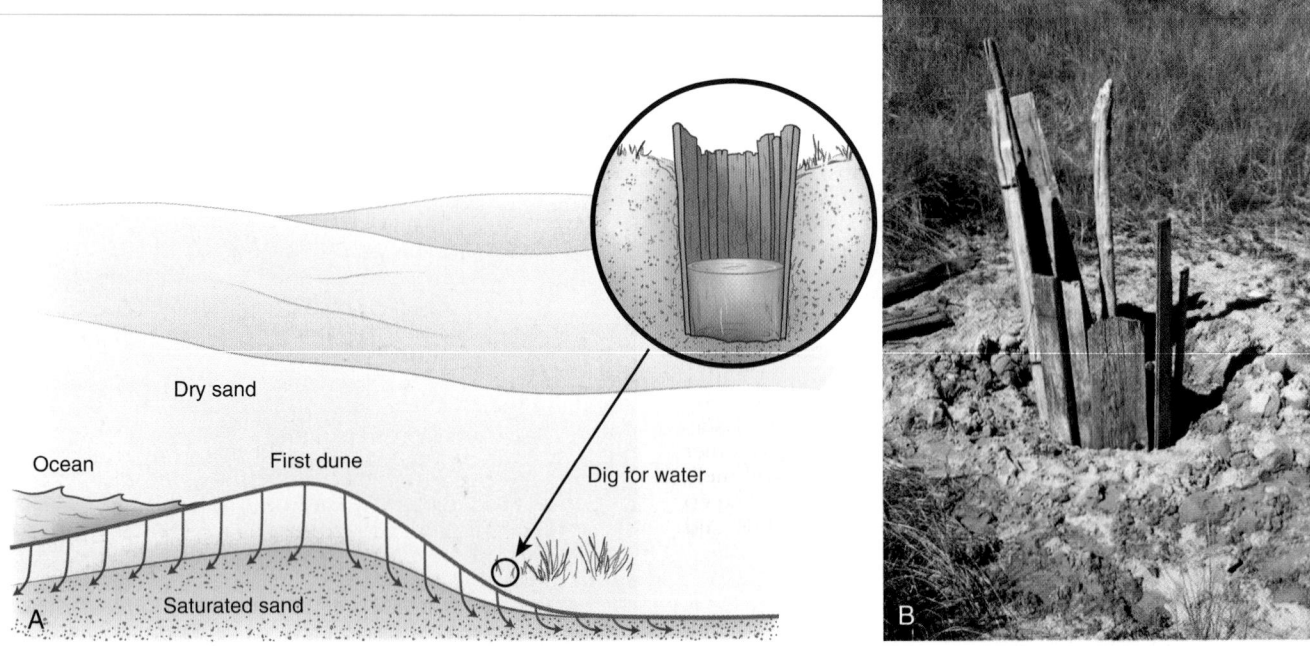

FIGURE 90-19 Beach wells dug behind the first sand dunes adjacent to the shore can produce potable water. *(Right courtesy Peter Kummerfeldt.)*

vine is drawn up by capillary action, and much less water will drain out by the time that the upper end is severed. This becomes apparent when the available knife is not large enough to cut through the tough vine quickly. In a test conducted in Florida by one of the authors (PK), a 24-inch by 4-inch section of water vine produced more than 1 cup of water.

Once detached, the section of vine is held vertically, and the water contained within the vine is allowed to drain into a container (perhaps a cupped hand), where it should be further evaluated. Liquid that is colored should not be consumed. Liquid that has an unpleasant aroma, other than a faint "woody" smell, also should be discarded. A small amount of the water should be tasted. Water that has a disagreeable flavor, other than a slightly "earthy" or "woody" taste, should not be used for drinking. This source could be used to satisfy external hygiene needs. If the water is still being considered for consumption, a small amount should then be held in the mouth for a few moments to determine if there is any burning or other disagreeable sensation.

If any irritating sensation occurs, the water should be discarded. Ultimately, plant liquid that looks like water, smells like water, and tastes like water can be safely consumed in large quantities without further purification (Figure 90-22).

Transpiration Bags

The use of clear plastic bags to enclose living vegetation and capture the moisture transpired by the leaves can be an effective method of collecting water (Figure 90-23). A plant's survival depends on its ability to gather water from the soil. This water is passed up through the plant's roots, stems, and branches and is finally released as water vapor back to the atmosphere through pores in the leaves. This process is called *transpiration*. Water vapor is captured by enclosing as much living vegetation as possible within a clear plastic bag and sealing the opening shut with a cord or duct tape. The vegetation should be given a vigorous shake before placing it in the plastic bag to remove any insects, bird droppings, or other materials that might contaminate the

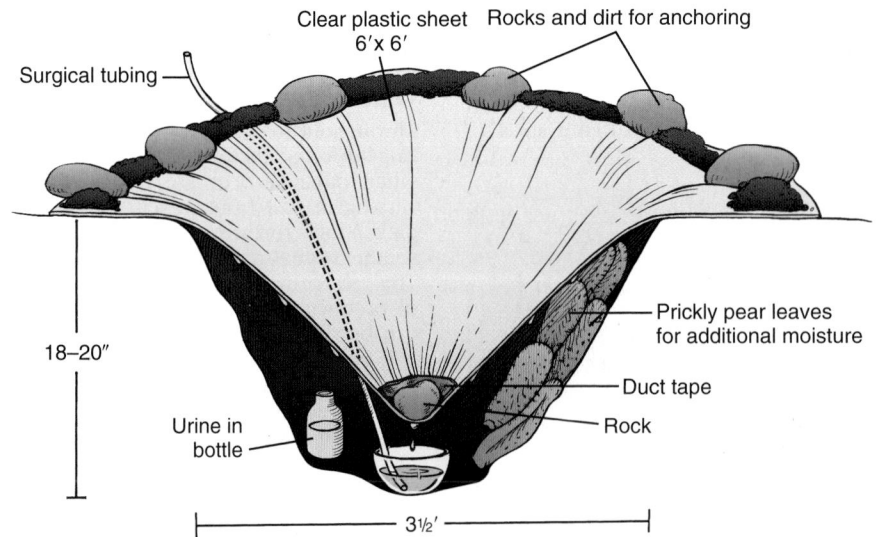

FIGURE 90-20 Solar stills are not a reliable procedure for obtaining water from the ground.

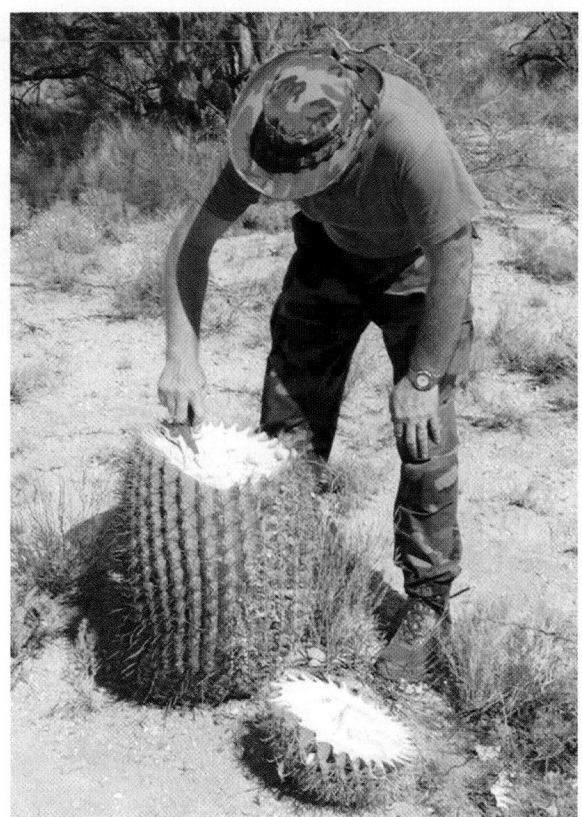

FIGURE 90-21 Barrel cacti do not contain water or water substitutes. *(Courtesy Peter Kummerfeldt.)*

water. Within a short period, water will begin to condense on the inner surface of the bag and collect into water droplets. Over hours, the droplets accumulate and drain to the lowest point.

The quantity of water obtained in this manner depends on the amount of water in the ground and the type of vegetation used. Other factors that determine water production include the amount of sunlight available, clarity of the plastic bag, and length of time the process is allowed to work. It is not uncommon to find that 2 or 3 cups of water, and sometimes much more, have accumulated over a 6- to 8-hour daylight period (Figure 90-24). This water is contamination free and does not require further purification.

Transpiration bags do not work at night, and they do not work well when opaque or colored bags are used. The process of transpiration slows down when it becomes dark. Depending on the temperature, the plastic bag can be left in place for 2 to 3 days, at which point the leaves become damaged by the heat that develops inside the bag, causing the process to stop. The water that collects can be removed from the bag by disassembling the apparatus and pouring out the water, or by punching a small hole at the lowest point in the bag and allowing the water to drain out. Neither of these procedures is optimal because one requires that the bag be reassembled and the other necessitates repairing the hole in the plastic bag. The best way to remove the water without disturbing the bag is to insert a length of vinyl aquarium hose through the neck of the bag down to the lowest point where water will collect. The water can then be sucked out or possibly siphoned into a container. When enclosing vegetation in the plastic bag, it is advisable to place a chicken egg–sized stone in the lower corner where the water will collect. The weight of the stone creates a separation between the enclosed plant life and the water and precludes the plant saps from leaching into the water.

Using the transpiration process is a practical method of collecting water in desert areas, but it is also useful in other areas where surface water is not available. Unlike deserts in other parts of the world, a considerable amount of vegetation is found

in North American deserts. This is vegetation that may be used in the transpiration bag process. Most vegetation in desert areas is thorny, so considerable care should be taken to keep these thorns from tearing the plastic bag. Desert willow, a nonthorny shrub commonly found throughout the American southwest, is an excellent source of water. The poplar family of trees, including aspen and cottonwood, found in more temperate areas, is another good source when using this method of water procurement. Because the trees and shrubs that produce the most water are deciduous (lose their leaves in winter), the transpiration bag process is limited to the time of year when vegetation is in leaf.

HOW LONG A PERSON CAN LIVE WITHOUT FOOD

Other than external factors, such as wind, precipitation, and temperature extremes, individual physiology and tenacity to live remain the primary determinants for survival without food or with limited caloric intake. An obese person carrying a large amount of body fat who arrives in a survival situation will have more fuel to burn than will a thin person. Other factors notwithstanding, this individual should live longer. Skinny but determined survivors might live longer than expected because of their tenacity.

A distinction must be made between having no food available and having limited supplies. If consumption of food is lower than the rate at which energy is expended, the body uses its reserves of fat, carbohydrates, and proteins at a pace directly related to the rate at which the energy is depleted. Without any food, most people die within 40 to 60 days. Self-imposed food fasts, such as those endured in Irish prisons by IRA militants, ranged from 50 to 60 days with no caloric intake before death. When sleep deprivation and danger are combined with little or no food, a person's awareness, judgment, and ability to concentrate decrease rapidly. Individuals attempting to survive with little or no food become apathetic, lethargic, confused, and indifferent. Consequently, they are unlikely to stay alive for long in a physiologically challenging environment.

How long a person can live without any food varies tremendously. In adult volunteers who fasted for 30 to 40 days, weight loss was marked (25% of initial body weight). During more prolonged starvation, weight loss may reach 50% in adults and possibly more in children. Loss of organ weight is greatest in the liver and intestine, moderate in the heart and kidneys, and least in the nervous system. Emaciation is most obvious in areas where prominent fat deposits normally exist. Muscle mass shrinks, and bones protrude. The skin becomes thin, dry, inelastic, pale, and cold. The hair is dry and sparse and falls out easily.

Most body systems are affected. Achlorhydria and diarrhea are common. Heart size and cardiac output are reduced, the pulse slows, and blood pressure falls. Respiratory rate and vital capacity decrease. The main endocrine disturbances are gonadal atrophy, loss of libido in men and women, and amenorrhea in women. Intellect remains clear, but apathy and irritability are common. The victim feels weak. Work capacity is diminished because of muscle destruction and eventually is worsened by cardiorespiratory failure. Anemia is usually mild, normochromic, and normocytic. Reduction in body temperature frequently contributes to death. In famine edema, serum proteins are usually normal, but loss of fat and muscle results in increased extracellular water, low tissue tensile strength, and inelastic skin. Cell-mediated immunity is compromised, and wound healing is impaired. Total starvation is fatal in 8 to 12 weeks. For more information on starvation, see Chapter 87.

The season and weather establish additional constraints on a survivor's longevity. In a benign setting, with warm temperatures both day and night, no precipitation, plenty of water available, and wood for a fire, the physiologic need for food is not as great. On the other hand, a survivor in a cold, wet, and windy environment, with inadequate clothing and no shelter, fire, or food to generate heat, will quickly succumb to hypothermia. With food, survival outcome for an individual is still not guaranteed. However, provided that other priorities are met, life may continue long enough for a survivor to be found alive.

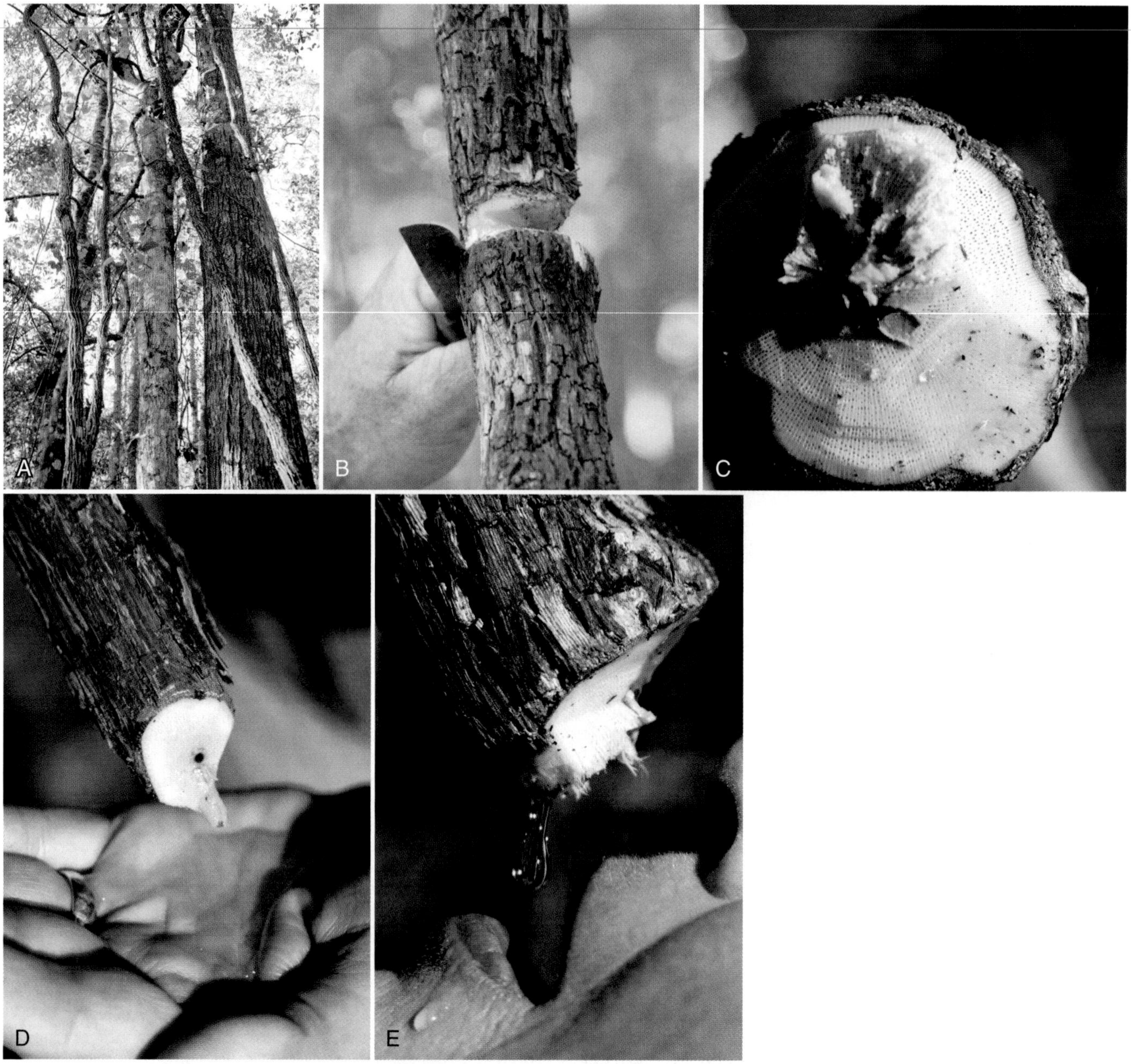

FIGURE 90-22 A to E, Water vines contain large quantities of water that can be recovered by cutting out a 60-cm (24-inch) section and draining the water into a container. *(Courtesy Peter Kummerfeldt.)*

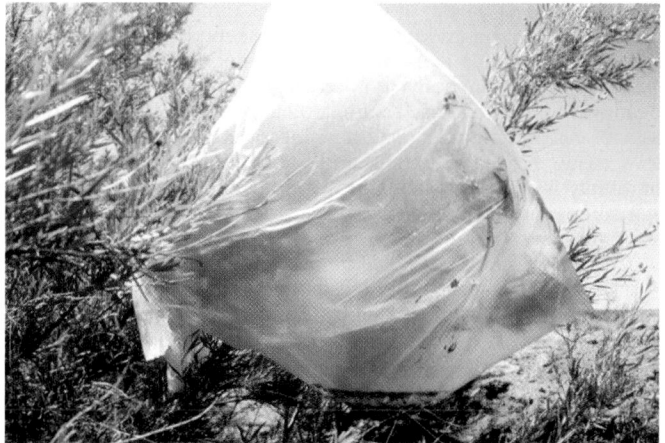

FIGURE 90-23 Transpiration bag collecting the water transpired by desert willow. *(Courtesy Peter Kummerfeldt.)*

In a cold environment, generating heat to preserve body core temperature can be very difficult without adequate food intake. Shivering, which is a primary mechanism by which the body generates heat, rapidly depletes glycogen stored in the liver and muscles unless adequate food is available. Lacking sufficient clothing and food to protect against environmental insult, survivors must rely on their ability to build a shelter and start a fire to maintain core temperature.

Survival situations demonstrate the law of diminishing returns. During the initial hours of an emergency situation, survivors are in the best condition they will enjoy during their survival experience. The impact of the environment and the lack of food, water, and sleep result in continuous degradation of the body's ability to function normally and eventually take a toll on the survivor's ability to accomplish the tasks needed to survive. Any "heavy work" should be accomplished early. Strength, mobility, balance, and dexterity diminish as each day passes. The survivor's objective is to delay this degradation for as long as possible through intelligent use of practical food- and water-gathering techniques, and in so doing, increase the chances of being rescued alive.

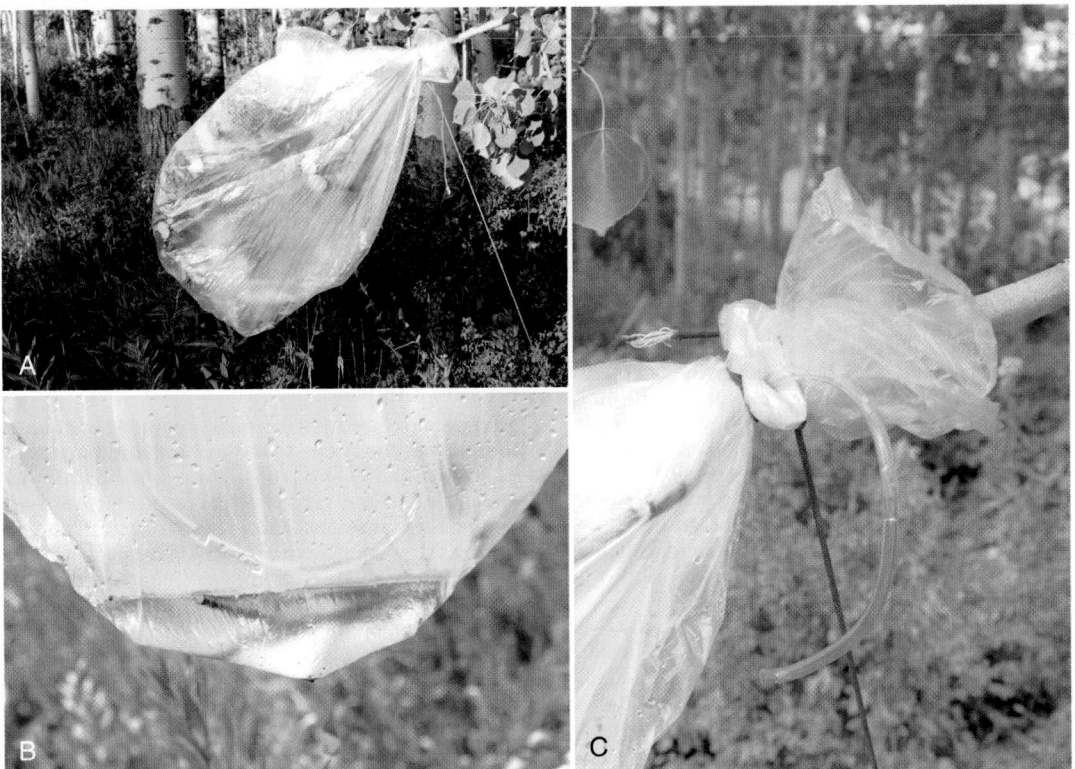

Figure 90-24 Enclose a large amount of leafy vegetation in a clear plastic bag and seal the neck **(A)**. Water transpired by the plant condenses on the inner surfaces of the bag and drains to the lowest point **(B)**, where it can be sucked out using a piece of vinyl hose **(C)**. *(Courtesy Peter Kummerfeldt.)*

The ability to select, gather, and prepare natural foods, even in short-term experiences, is valuable physiologically, but perhaps even more so psychologically. When gathering food, survivors are actively involved in surviving, contributing to their own well-being. Although the amount of food gathered may be small, the satisfaction derived from catching a fish, snaring a squirrel, or gathering a hatful of edible berries can be a great morale builder.

People who are used to having all their food come from packages, cans, or other containers may need to overcome their reluctance to eat nontraditional foods that now come packaged in skin, hair, scales, or feathers. These aversions cause people to avoid consuming available wild foods that would enhance their chances of survival. Reluctance to eat insects, for example, is based in large part on the Western cultural belief that insects are "dirty" and that eating insects is done only by those who cannot afford better food. Additionally, the vast quantities of processed food available in developed countries have produced feeding habits in which people only consume the very best of the available foods and discard the rest. Survivors will not be so fortunate that they can pick and choose what they eat. They may have to capitalize on *any* potential food that comes their way.

Procuring wild foods involves procedures and techniques that some might view as cruel, unethical, or even illegal. For example, with the exception of trapping fur-bearing animals during legal seasons and the use of traps by licensed animal control personnel to remove "problem" animals, the use of snares to obtain food is against the law. Trapping and snaring techniques have been determined to be illegal because they are so effective and because they are virtually impossible for wildlife managers to monitor. Their effectiveness is the very reason they are highly recommended for survival. Under normal circumstances, federal, state, and local laws and regulations govern procuring food from the environment. Killing animals for food outside of prescribed hunting seasons is forbidden. Gathering plant foods and killing animals is specifically prohibited in national parks and other similar sanctuaries. Accepted hunting conventions also disfavor killing females with babies and younger animals. When faced with starvation and the choice between killing an animal and digging up enough plant bulbs to make a meal, it becomes a question of common sense. The survivor should gather necessary food and leave legal issues to be sorted out after the fact. It is extremely unlikely that a survivor who could clearly demonstrate a legitimate need would be charged with an infraction of the law. This does not mean that, in a short-term survival experience, it is appropriate to disobey the law, particularly if there are reasonable alternatives.

Feeding oneself in a long-term survival experience may necessitate harvesting and butchering wild game animals. These skills were once common in Western culture but now are uncommon. To some people, the act of taking any life is reprehensible, so even in a survival situation, when faced with killing an animal for food, they will have great difficulty or even may be unable to accomplish the task. Most often, however, hunger drives survivors to carry out what they need to do to stay alive.

When considering what should be eaten in a survival situation, some people focus all their efforts on plant foods. This misguided approach may be the result of advice given in out-of-date survival manuals and from well-intentioned, but ill-informed, writers of contemporary "how-to-survive" articles. Many of these articles devote numerous pages to identification and use of plants to sustain life. Except for the short term, it is almost impossible to survive indefinitely on gathered plant life alone, even if it is available. Fats and proteins provided by eating meat are far more sustaining than are the carbohydrates provided by eating vegetable matter. If plant and animal foods are both available, survivors should attempt to balance their diets by consuming fat, proteins, and carbohydrates in order to maintain health for as long as possible.

SUCCESS STORIES

Despite the difficulties of living off the land, survival for long periods is still possible when little or no food is available. Helen Klaben[11] and Ralph Flores survived 49 days in the Yukon in a wrecked aircraft on four 105-g (3.75-oz) cans of sardines, two 198-g (7-oz) cans of tuna fish, two 0.5-kg (1-lb) cans of mixed fruit salad, one 0.5-kg (1-lb) box of saltines, five small pieces of chocolate, and 30 g (2 tablespoons) of Tang. Bob Gotchen survived for 58 days during the winter following a forced landing in Northwest Territory, eating only a few mouthfuls of frozen fish and losing 74 lb (33 kg) in the process. James Scott survived under a rocky ledge in the Himalayas for 43 days during the winter without food before being rescued. In 1972, a Uruguayan soccer team stranded in the Andes by a crash landing survived for the next 72 days with little food. In 1979, Brent Dyer and Donna Johnson walked out of the Idaho wilderness 19 days after their plane crashed.

In the last two instances, the survivors, lacking other foods, consumed the flesh of humans who had died in the accidents. Despite their psychological disinclination to eat the flesh of another person's body, it was something that they did in order to survive. Based on the accounts of these incidents, published in *Alive: The Story of the Andes Survivors* by Piers Paul Read[18] and *The Sacrament: A True Story of Survival* by Peter Gzowski,[6] it could be argued that the small amounts of human flesh they ate were of minimal physiologic benefit but of significant psychological value. Although there is no physiologic reason why human flesh should not be consumed in an emergency, we are unwilling to do so as a result of our cultural beliefs and the long-standing prohibition against cannibalism. Eating the flesh of another human to survive after that person has died accidentally is not necessarily the wicked act of a demented person. Rather, it is a last choice, a means to an end, for a starving survivor.

WILD ANIMAL FOODS

Food available to a survivor may come from many sources, including snacks or other incidental food that survivors may have placed in their pockets, emergency food contained in survival kits, and last but not least, food that might be obtained from the surrounding environment. The ability to procure natural foods from the land depends on the following:

- Knowledge of natural foods available for each season in the relevant geographic region
- Some degree of proficiency in food-gathering methods and techniques
- Physical ability to gather food
- Availability of equipment needed to gather food or ability to improvise the equipment
- Skills needed to prepare food for consumption

Knowing the environment and the techniques to procure and prepare animal life for food could prove crucial to the successful conclusion of any survival situation. This section discusses the techniques a survivor might use to harvest and prepare commonly available animal life found throughout much of North America.

MAMMALS

All mammals are edible, but because of larger mammals' size, their ability to injure or kill the survivor, and the survivor's lack of a means to kill them, it is unrealistic to count on them all as a food source. Historically, survivors have targeted the rodent family (squirrels, muskrats, porcupines, marmots, nutria, rats, and mice) and other smaller mammals, such as rabbits and hares, for food. These animals may be captured or killed with the simple equipment and basic food-gathering skills possessed by any prepared survivor.

Rabbits and Hares

Members of this animal family are found in almost every environment, from the Arctic to the tropics, and have served as the main course for many survivors' dinners. Rabbit and hare populations are cyclic; at the peak of their reproductive cycle, they can be extremely numerous and easy to catch. This is especially true during the winter months, when they pack defined trails through the snow. This is a well-known characteristic of snowshoe hares, which are found throughout the northern portions of the United States, Canada, and Alaska.

Some people are reluctant to eat rabbit. This preference is sometimes based on cultural traditions. In the West especially, rabbits are thought of as "Easter Bunnies" or as "pets" and not as a food source. Additionally, because rabbit meat is not a common product for sale in the supermarket, people conclude that it is not a "good" food item. In other parts of the world, rabbits and hares are accepted meat sources. They certainly should be welcomed as a food item by a survivor. As with most wild animals, they contain very lean, high-protein, low-fat meat.

Simple loop snares described later in this chapter are an effective means to procure rabbits and hares. Properly set out in large numbers (at least 15 snares for every animal you expect to catch), loop snares work constantly for the survivor while other tasks are being accomplished. Rabbits and other small animals usually die quickly when caught in a snare. However, if the animal is found to still be alive when the snare is checked, it can be killed quickly by striking its cranium with a stout stick or by dislocating the neck vertebrae. Dislocating the vertebrae can be quickly accomplished by lifting the animal by its hind legs and then forcefully striking its neck directly behind the ears with the stick. Unconsciousness and death result instantaneously.

Once dead, the animal is suspended head-down by tying a line to one of its rear legs and then tying this line to an anchor (Figure 90-25). To remove the hide, begin tearing the skin away from legs and tail and then proceed to separate it from the body

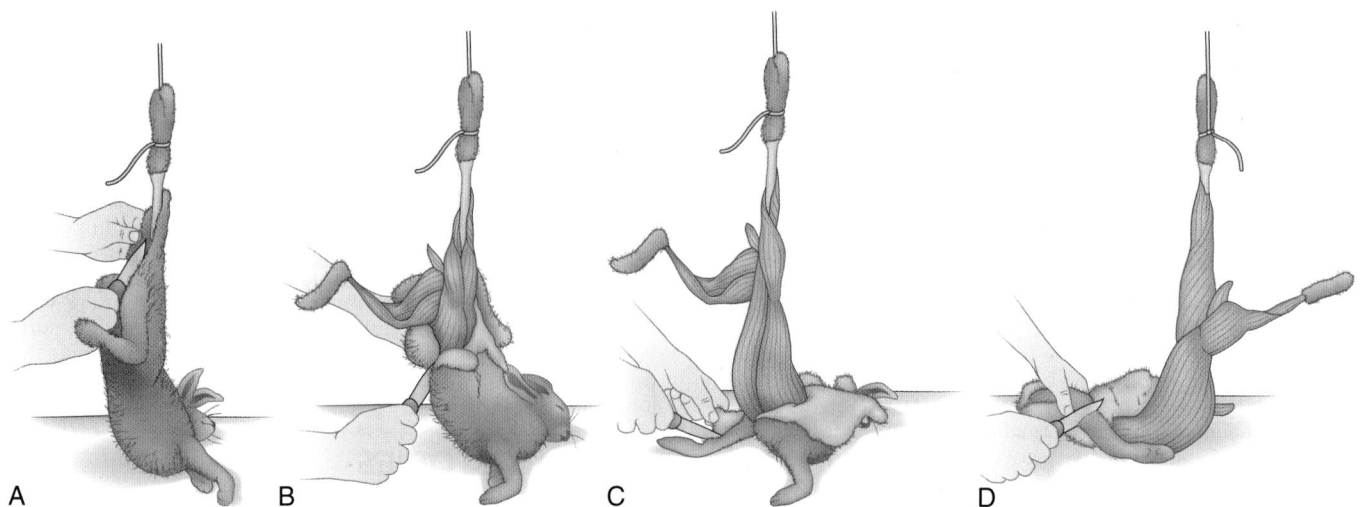

FIGURE 90-25 A to D, Anchoring one leg of the animal being skinned facilitates quick removal of its skin (see text).

by working the pelt over the forelegs and tearing it free from the front feet. Peel the hide free from the body until the only remaining attachment point is around the animal's neck. Use a knife to sever any remaining neck tissue and cut between the vertebrae if necessary. The hide can also be quickly removed from the body by cutting or tearing the skin at the midbody point and then grasping each side and pulling in opposite directions. Discard the head, hide, and feet. Lacking a knife, one can separate the head from the remainder of the carcass by grasping the head in one hand and the carcass in the other and pulling in opposite directions.

Once the skin is removed, the rabbit's entrails need to be removed. Open the abdomen by cutting through the belly muscles along a midline incision extending from pelvis to sternum. Without a knife, the skin and belly muscle tissue can be opened by tearing it with your fingers. Once this is done, locate and carefully remove the bladder intact, especially if it contains urine. The remainder of the internal organs, including the lungs and heart, can then be lifted out of the abdominal cavity and from within the chest walls. A minimum of cutting is necessary with a knife, but if one is not available, these organs can also be torn out. The carcass should then be washed with water (if available) and wiped free of any residual blood or other body fluids using a cloth or available vegetation.

Rabbits, hares, and other small animals are usually cut into pieces before cooking. However, in a survival situation, the animal can be left intact and cooked whole using the cooking methods described later in this chapter. Cooking the meat preserves it and provides the survivor with the option that portions not immediately consumed can be saved for later meals. Generally, the heart, liver, and kidneys are not eaten. However, there is no reason not to consume these organs, especially when food is limited. These organs and the head should be retained and added to any other available ingredients for a "survival stew."

Rabbits and hares are susceptible to tularemia and parasites, so if any snared animal appears to be in poor health, sluggish, or behaving unnaturally, the animal should not be handled or consumed. Rabbits and hares are also well known for serving as hosts to fleas and ticks, both of which will leave the host's body soon after it dies. It may be a good idea not to handle a freshly killed animal extensively for several hours. If you allow the animal to cool, pests will vacate the body.

Rodents

Despite the common aversion to eating rodents such as rats and mice, they can be an easily attainable and a valuable food source in a survival situation. They are widespread in distribution, usually found in large numbers, and can often be procured without the need for complex trapping procedures. Rodents commonly available to survivors in North America include squirrels (both ground and tree squirrels), porcupines, beavers, nutria, muskrats, groundhogs, prairie dogs, marmots, and a wide variety of rats and mice (Figure 90-26). Of this list, the only rodents that North Americans generally accept as food items are members of the tree squirrel family, which are frequently hunted and eaten, particularly in eastern parts of the United States. Groundhogs in the southeastern United States and prairie dogs and marmots in the West are still considered appropriate food. In other parts of the world, particularly developing nations, other types of rodents, including rats and mice, are used as a good source of protein. Other than our prejudices against eating rats and mice, there are no differences between types of rodents as to their edibility. They can all be used as a food source.

Rodents are prepared using the same procedures as those used to prepare rabbits and hares. With larger rodents, especially beavers and porcupines, the skin is tough and firmly attached, so removing it requires a sharp knife. When skinning a porcupine, considerable care should be taken to ensure that the sharp quills do not cause injuries. Puncture wounds caused by porcupine quills are painful and tend to become infected.

Larger Mammals

Large mammals may be available to a survivor, but lack of a rifle or shotgun usually limits sources to the smaller animals. It might

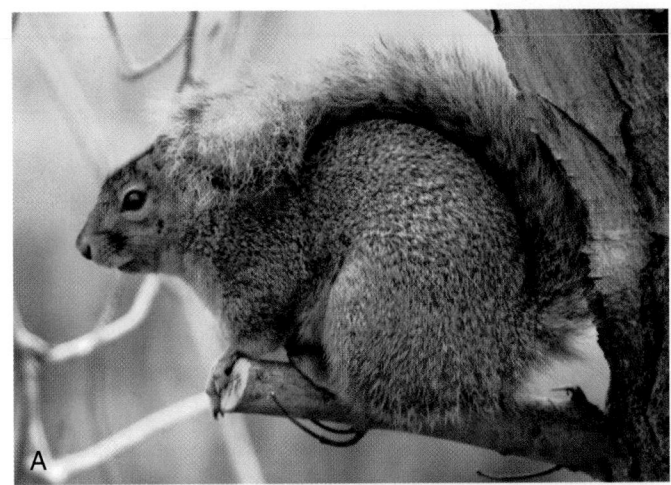
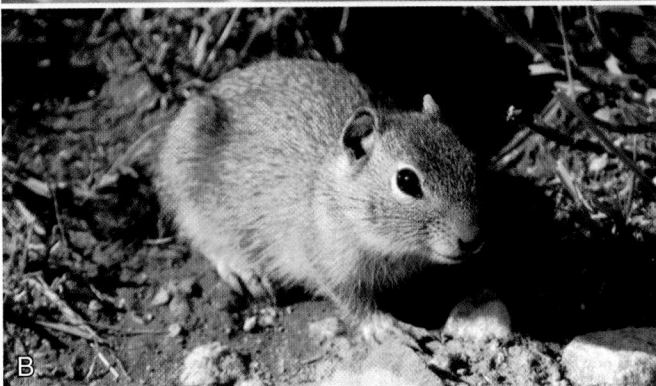

FIGURE 90-26 Rodents. **A,** Red squirrel. **B,** Uinta ground squirrel. *(Courtesy Peter Kummerfeldt.)*

be possible to salvage meat from the remains of larger animals that have been killed by predators or that died from natural causes. However, great care should be taken to ensure that predators are not in the vicinity when approaching a carcass. Most predators, particularly bears and mountain lions, will attempt to cover the remains of their kills or claimed animal carcasses with vegetation and soil. Covering the remains hides it from other predators and scavengers. A disturbed area surrounding a mound of earth and vegetation should serve as clear warning to the human survivor that a predator is nearby, and the area should be avoided.

BIRDS

Birds are found in every environment and vary in weight from ounces to many pounds. Although all birds are edible, a number of species are not particularly appetizing. Birds that feed on fish and other aquatic animal life, as well as those that feed on carrion, are generally not considered desirable to eat. They can be eaten if no other food is available and if the survivor can tolerate the unpleasant odor and disagreeable taste of the meat. Skinning, rather than plucking the feathers, on these birds can reduce some of the unpleasant taste.

Because domesticated versions of wild birds make up a considerable portion of the meat eaten in a typical American diet, survivors are less likely to experience food aversion if they use birds as a food source. Wild game birds (turkeys, grouse, ducks, and geese) are similar to the domestic versions. Species of birds belonging to the gallinaceous (chicken-like) family (e.g., grouse, pheasant, chukar, turkey, and partridge [Figure 90-27]) are often included in the diets of survivors. In remote areas where there is little contact with humans, ruffed grouse, spruce grouse, and ptarmigan in particular are very trusting in their behavior and may allow a person to approach close enough to catch them by hand. In less remote regions where they are more wary, these

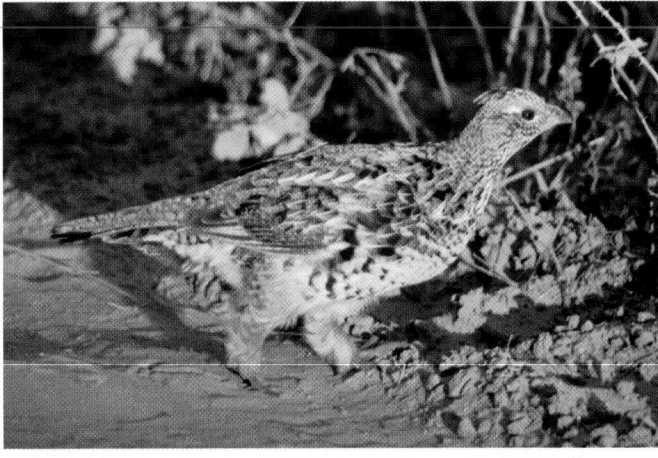

FIGURE 90-27 Grouse, ptarmigan, pheasant, and other gallinaceous birds often allow a person to approach closely. *(Courtesy Melissa Anderson.)*

birds can still be killed or captured relatively easily using techniques described later. Waterfowl, such as ducks, geese, and swans, are another group of birds that have helped to sustain survivors. Waterfowl are much more cautious and generally will not allow a person to approach. However, in the spring, when waterfowl molt and are unable to fly, they can be chased down and caught by hand or driven into nets erected close to the ground. They also can be killed or captured using the equipment and survival methods of gathering food described later. The families of birds collectively referred to as "game birds" provide much more meat by weight than do the nongame species. This is primarily because they have developed large breast muscles, or pectorals, which account for about 15% to 20% of the bird's weight. Smaller birds of the songbird varieties are edible, but when the feathers and internal organs are removed, not much meat remains.

All birds' eggs are edible (Figure 90-28), and if collected early in the incubation process, can be consumed in the same manner as a chicken egg. If incubation has progressed to the point where a "chick" has formed, the egg may still be eaten. However, to avoid aversion to this food source, the contents of the egg may have to be added to a "survival stew." Determining the state of maturation of the eggs in a nest is a difficult process. If a nest is located, leave the existing eggs in place, marking each egg if possible with a pencil mark or mud smear. On returning the following day, it is easy to determine which eggs are the newly

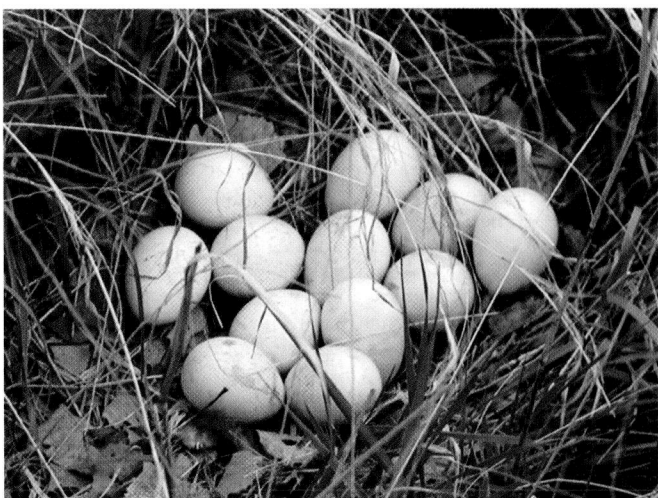

FIGURE 90-28 Wild turkey nest. All birds' eggs are edible and are best eaten before the embryos have developed. *(Courtesy Peter Kummerfeldt.)*

laid ones. Any unmarked eggs should be "fresh" and can be cooked in the same manner as any domestic chicken egg. Always leave a few eggs in the nest to encourage the parent birds to return.

Preparation of birds for consumption is straightforward. Most methods used to catch a bird also result in its death. However, in the event that a bird is captured alive, the simplest method to kill it is to cut off the head after stunning it with a solid stick. Birds can be either skinned or plucked. Grouse, turkeys, pheasants, and other "chicken-like" birds are easy to skin, whereas ducks and geese should be plucked. Once waterfowl are plucked, the remaining pinfeathers can be singed off by holding the carcass over the flames of a fire.

Having skinned or plucked the bird, cut off the head, neck, feet, and wings. To remove the internal organs, create an opening from the vent to the middle of the breast cartilage. All the viscera can be extracted through this opening by inserting a hand or fingers, depending on the size of the bird, into the cavity. Tear loose the organs from their attachment points in the abdomen and thorax. Some birds use a crop to store food until it is transferred to the gizzard, where it is ground into pieces small enough to be digested. The crop is located in a V-shaped cleft in front of the breast and is easily removed by separating this food-filled pouch from the carcass by either pulling it or cutting it free with a knife. Once the feathers and the internal organs are removed, the outer body and interior should be thoroughly washed to remove any remaining blood or other body fluids that contribute to putrefaction.

An alternative method to quickly separate the "meatier" portions of the bird from the carcass without a knife is demonstrated in Figure 90-29. The bird's breast is first exposed by tearing through the skin. The bird is then placed on its back on the ground. Place a foot on each wing and pull the breast free from the rest of the carcass by grasping it with both hands and pulling firmly straight away from the back.

Birds can be cooked whole or in pieces using any one of the cooking methods described later.

INSECTS

The practice of entomophagy, the eating of insects, is well established in many parts of world, especially developing countries in Africa, Asia, and Central and South America. In these regions, insects have long been considered either a staple part of the diet or a delicacy. Although insects are not a component of a typical American diet, they can provide a valuable food source for the survivor. More than 1400 varieties of insects found around the world are edible.[17] Among those more commonly eaten by humans are grasshoppers, crickets, ants, beetles, butterflies, moths, dragonflies, and termites (Figure 90-30).

Not all insects are edible. Some contain powerful pharmacologic toxins that would cause significant illness if consumed; some insects (and other arthropods) can cause physical harm to the survivor. Spiders, scorpions, centipedes, millipedes, bees, hornets, and hairy caterpillars should be avoided. Because some insects harbor internal parasites, it is best to cook all of them before eating.

Advantages of eating insects include the following:
- Insects are usually easy to find.
- No sophisticated equipment or special skills are required to gather insects.
- Insects are often found in large quantities.
- Insects are nutritious and provide fats and proteins.
- Insects do not require extensive preparation before consumption.

Grasshoppers, crickets, and locusts are found throughout the world in a wide variety of environments (Figure 90-31). More than 1000 species of grasshoppers are found in North America. Grasshoppers contain 40% to 50% protein[19] and are best collected in the early morning when cold temperatures make them lethargic and easy to catch. Once captured, they should be left in a container overnight to purge. Then the head and any attached viscera, the smaller forelegs, the distal section of the hind legs, and the wings are removed before cooking. The insects can be

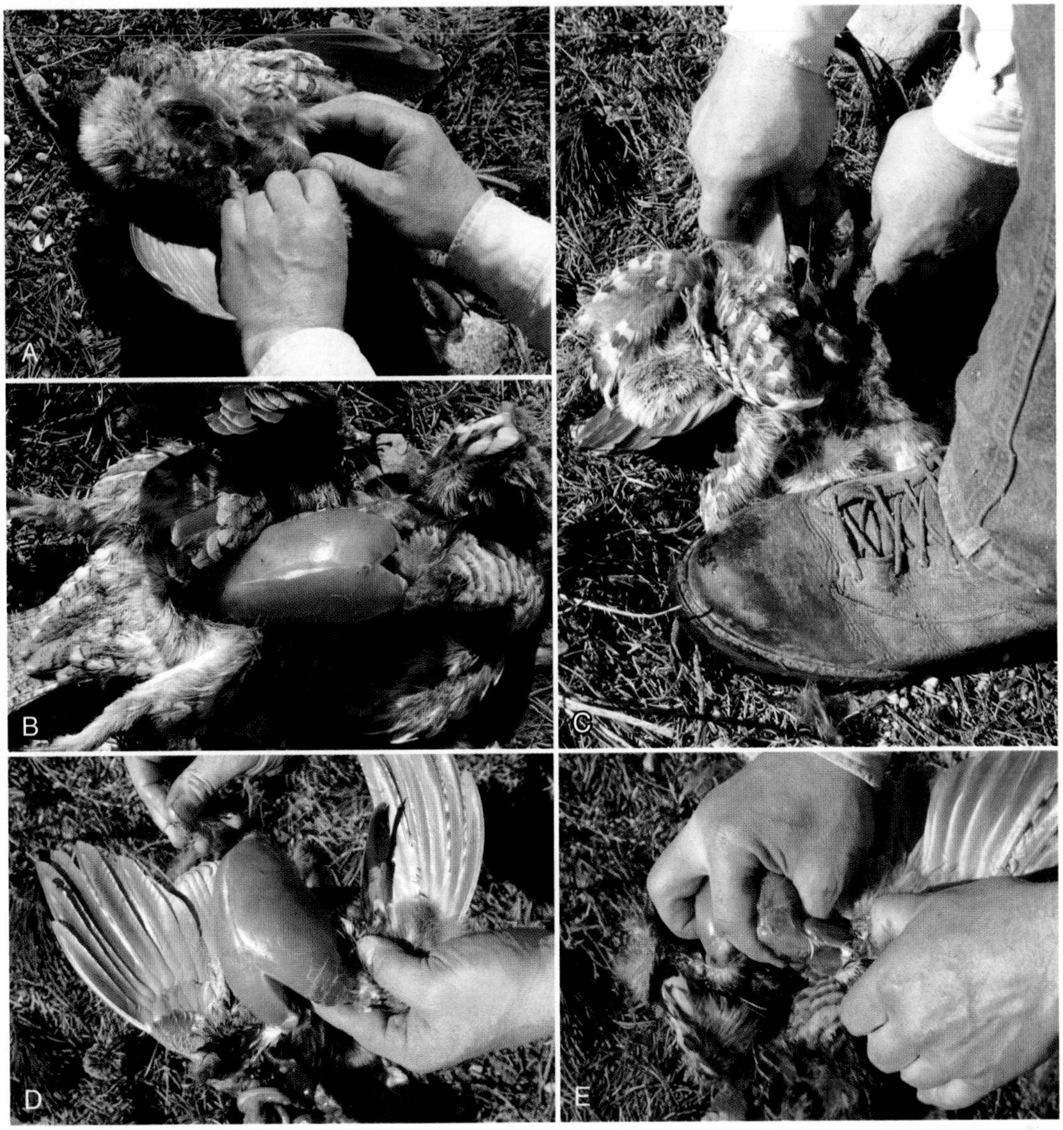

FIGURE 90-29 **A** to **E,** Removing the breast and leg meat from a grouse without using a knife. *(Courtesy Melissa Anderson.)*

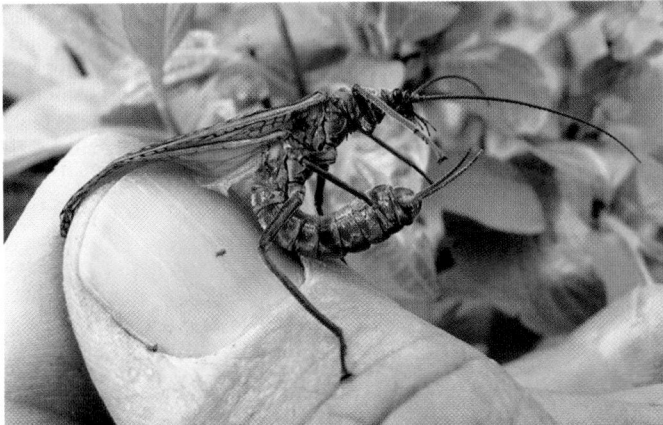

FIGURE 90-30 Salmon fly. More than 1400 species of insects found around the world are edible. *(Courtesy Peter Kummerfeldt.)*

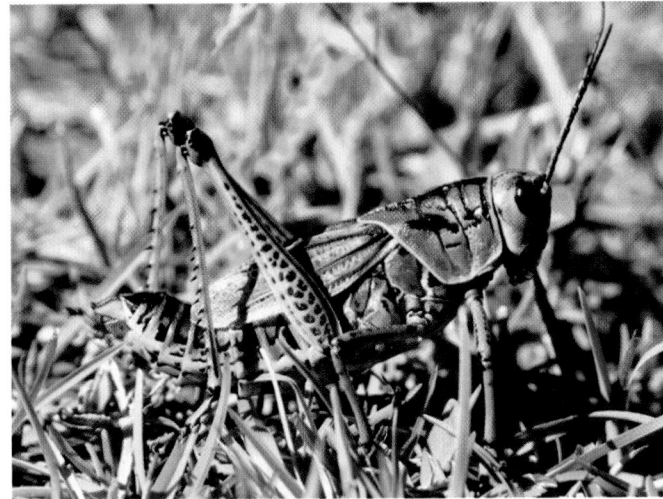

FIGURE 90-31 Grasshoppers are among the most commonly eaten insects. *(Courtesy Peter Kummerfeldt.)*

placed in the coals of a fire and roasted until crisp or baked in hot sand beside or below a fire. Grasshoppers can also be roasted by skewering several on a stick and holding them over the flames of a fire. A stew can be produced by adding grasshoppers and edible vegetation to a pot of boiling water and cooking them until the vegetation is tender. Crickets are prepared and cooked in the same way.

Termites can often be collected in large quantities, drowned in water, sun-dried, and then roasted over low heat. Prepared in this manner, they will keep for many months.

Butterfly and moth larvae are rich in protein (37%) and fat (13.7%) and are edible. The larvae can be roasted over a fire or boiled and then roasted.

Earthworms should be placed in water and allowed to purge before they are consumed. Once purged, they should be dried in the sun or over low heat and then added to other ingredients of a survival stew.

Beetles and beetle larvae are edible and are eaten around the world nearly as often as are grasshoppers and locusts. The insects should be roasted in the coals of a fire and then consumed. The indigestible head, legs, wings, and wing cases are best removed before the insect is cooked.

Snails are edible, easy to collect, and simple to prepare. Dropping snails into boiling water and allowing them to blanch for about 5 minutes facilitates removal of the meat from the shell. Snails can be eaten "as is" or added to a survival stew.

Ants require no preparation other than removing the mandibles before they are eaten.

REPTILES

Reptiles include turtles, terrapins, snakes, alligators, crocodiles, and lizards. Because they are cold blooded, some of these animals hibernate and consequently are not available year-round.

Turtles have long been used as a food source. With the exception of a few species, all forms of sea turtles, freshwater turtles, terrapins, and land tortoises are edible. Musk and yellow mud turtles both have glands that produce a strong-smelling scent and because of this are unsuitable for food. Turtles found in North America, including the alligator snapping turtle and common snapping turtle, are all considered good to eat. The alligator snapping turtle can weigh up to 200 lb (90.7 kg), and the common snapping turtle can weigh as much as 50 lb (22.7 kg).

The only practical way to kill a turtle is to cut off its head. The next step is to cut off the feet. This involves three steps: (1) with a sharp knife, cut the skin free from the shell around each leg, the neck, and the tail; (2) peel the skin free from each leg and the neck; and (3) sever each leg and the neck free from the body. The remainder of the edible portions of the turtle contained within the shell can then be withdrawn through one of the openings. With soft-shell turtles, the ventral shell can be separated from the dorsal shell by cutting through the tough cartilage that holds the two shells together. This exposes the internal organs, which can then be removed. Using a knife, separate the meat from the bones and trim off any fat as you do so.

Lizards, which vary in size from minute geckos to crocodiles more than 6 m (20 feet) long, are all edible. From a practical point of view, the smaller varieties provide little nourishment, so survivors are well advised to focus their attention on larger, more common species. Some lizards, such as the Gila monster found in a few southwestern U.S. states and the Mexican beaded lizard found in Mexico, have a venomous bite and should not be pursued as a food source (Figure 90-32). When catching other species of lizard, no special care is required. However, although they may not be venomous, they still can bite, and some have claws. Preparing lizards for a meal requires a sharp, strong knife. If it is not already dead, kill the lizard by cutting off its head. Open the abdomen and thorax to remove the internal organs. The feet should be removed and carcass rinsed with water. A lizard's skin is very firmly attached to its body and can be difficult to remove unless pieces of the body are boiled for at least an hour. Once cooked in this manner, the skin separates from the

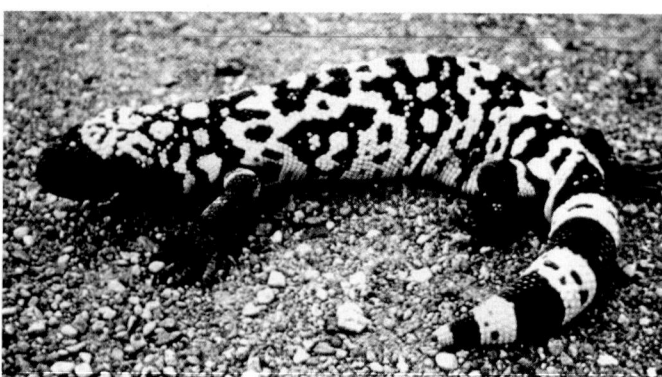

FIGURE 90-32 Because Gila monsters are venomous, they should not be considered a food source. Other, nonvenomous species can be eaten. *(Courtesy Peter Kummerfeldt.)*

body without difficulty. The lizard can be consumed after this or, to improve the flavor, can be roasted over the coals of a fire.

Alligators, crocodiles, and caimans, the largest members of the reptile family, are dangerous to humans and should not be considered as food unless they are small and can be handled safely. Small alligators and crocodiles can be caught by hand (Figure 90-33). They should be prepared in the same manner as other lizards. Most of the edible meat available from alligators and crocodiles is located in the tail and along either side of the spine. Because female crocodiles guard their nests and are very protective, caution should be exercised when attempting to catch small crocodiles or when attempting to gather crocodile eggs from the nest.

Snakes, both venomous and nonvenomous, are edible. One should proceed very cautiously when attempting to capture and kill a snake for food. A snake is best killed by pinning it to the ground with a long stick and then cutting off its head with a sharp knife. Take care not to be bitten and envenomed by a severed head. To remove the animal's skin, make an incision beginning at the vent and extending the full length of the body. By tying a piece of string to the snake's body at the head end and pulling against this anchor, the skin can be easily and quickly removed. A second slit is then made to access the snake's internal organs. These should be removed. Cook 2.5- to 5-cm (1- to 2-inch) sections of the snake using any of the techniques described later.

AMPHIBIANS

Frogs found around water throughout the United States are all edible. However, as a general rule, only the larger species provide sufficient meat to justify the effort expended in pursuing them. Brightly colored frogs found in Central and South America are highly toxic and should be avoided. The most efficient method of catching frogs is to "gig" or spear them using a two- or three-pronged spear point attached to the end of a 1.8-m (6-foot) or longer pole. Frogs can also be caught using fishing

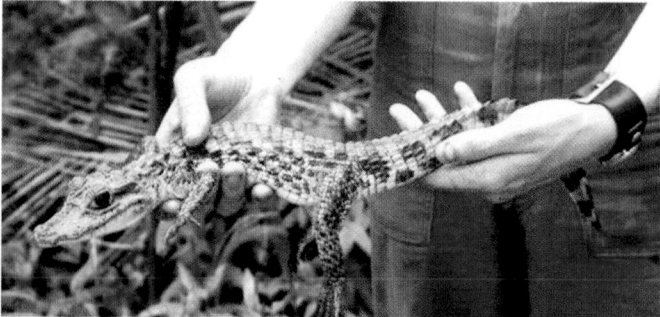

FIGURE 90-33 Small crocodiles may be easy to catch and can be eaten. *(Courtesy Peter Kummerfeldt.)*

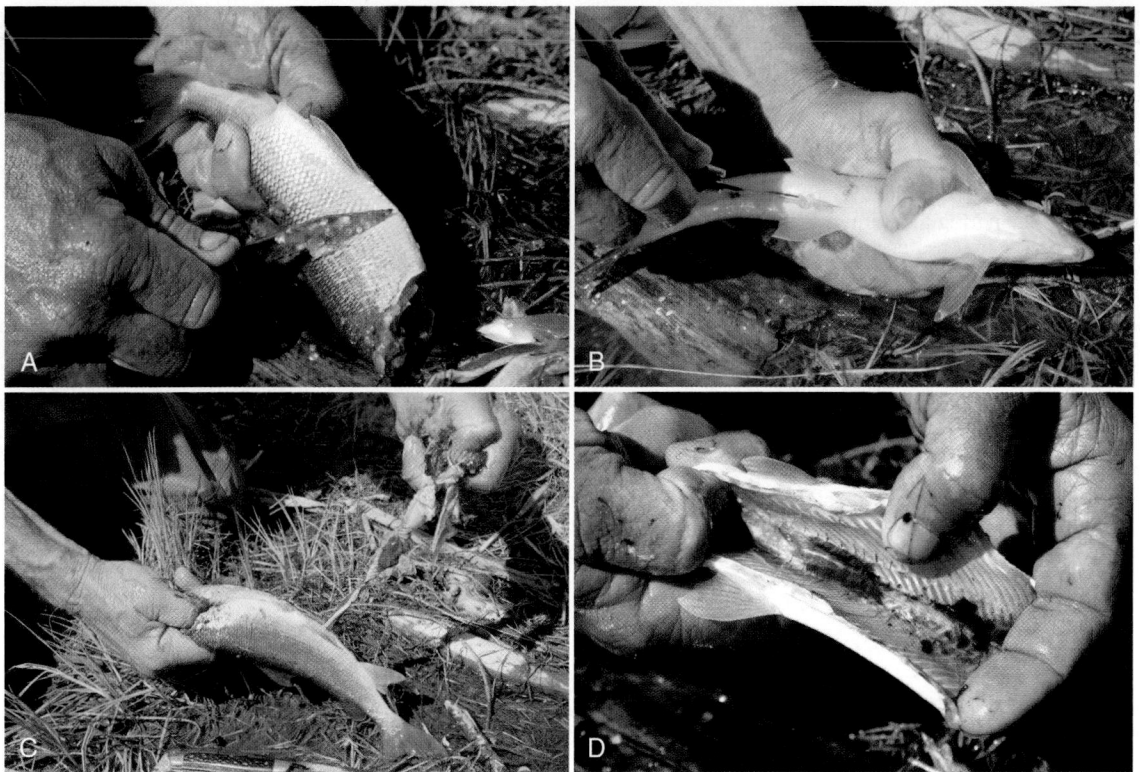

FIGURE 90-34 **A** to **D,** Scaling and cleaning a fish. *(Courtesy Peter Kummerfeldt.)*

line and a hook baited with an insect. Catching frogs by hand should be avoided because this method expends far more energy than is returned by the relatively small amount of flesh provided. To kill a frog, sever the spinal cord behind the head with a sharp knife and then remove the skin. Cut off the feet and discard them. The frog's meaty hind legs are the parts usually eaten, but the entire carcass, once skinned, has good food value. Frogs are best soaked in cold water for several hours and then cooked.

Toads secrete a toxin through their skin and are considered inedible. Unlike frogs that are most frequently found around riparian areas and waterways, toads are dry-land animals. Use this habitat preference as a differentiator when collecting frog-like animals for food.

FISH

Of all the animals available to a person trying to live off the land, fish are likely to be the most abundant and easiest to catch. They are also one of the few relatively available sources of fat—a food component not present in large quantities in any of the other smaller land animals that a survivor is likely to procure. Fish are often available year-round and can be caught using less sophisticated equipment than that needed to procure landforms of animal life. Fish of many species can be found in almost every water system throughout the world. Few bodies of water are completely barren.

All freshwater fish are edible, even varieties that are not usually used for food in North America, such as carp, suckers, and gar. Because fish tend to decompose quickly, they are best eaten soon after removing them from the water. All fish should be cooked before eating because some species are known to carry parasites, such as the *Anisakis* worm. This includes both freshwater and saltwater varieties. Depending on the species, scaling a fish is usually the first step in preparing it for a meal. Scaling is best done using a knife and scraping the skin from the tail toward the head of the fish. In some species, including trout, the scales are very small and do not need to be removed before cooking. Other species of fish, such as catfish, are better skinned. A cut is made through the skin behind the gills completely around the body of the fish. The skin is then pulled from the

body until only the white flesh remains. A Leatherman multitool or a similar tool with pliers jaws is particularly helpful in accomplishing this task.

With all the scales or skin removed, the viscera are removed by opening the abdominal cavity and removing all the internal organs. Once they are removed, a dark band of material is visible lying along the spine just below the vertebrae. This material, the posterior kidney, must be removed, which is usually accomplished by slitting the membrane that covers the kidney and scraping it out using a thumbnail or a sharpened end of a stick (Figure 90-34). Rinse the cleaned fish with water to remove all remaining blood, slime, and other materials to enhance flavor and delay putrefaction. Be especially careful when cleaning all spiny-rayed fish (e.g., bass, perch, catfish) because the spines in their fins can cause puncture injuries that may be painful or easily become infected. Do not eat the head, spinal cord, or liver of tropical fishes, and become familiar with unusual forms of seafood poisoning, such as occurs from eating puffer fish (see Chapter 78).

CRUSTACEANS

Crayfish inhabit most water systems, both still and moving, throughout much of North America. They can be gathered by turning over rocks in a river or by dangling bait, such as a piece of meat, into the lower levels of a waterway. Crayfish are attracted to the scent given off by the meat and will grab it with a powerful claw and hang on until lifted from the water. Other than pulling off the head after it has cooked, no additional preparation is needed for this food source. They can be dropped into boiling water and left until they turn red. When no container is available, crayfish can be cooked in the coals of a fire. Most edible meat will be found in the tail, with small portions also found in the large claw.

MOLLUSKS

Freshwater mollusks, commonly called mussels or "freshwater clams," live in many freshwater systems and are easily collected by hand. All varieties are edible. Although mollusks are very "chewy," they are nutritious, filling, and easy to gather. They must be thoroughly boiled to destroy harmful organic life absorbed by the animal. Certain shellfish should be avoided during toxic seasons and conditions (see Chapter 78).

METHODS OF PROCURING ANIMALS FOR FOOD

Snaring is one of the most productive methods available for procuring animal food. Snaring techniques for animals, birds, and fish are fairly easy to learn, require a minimum of equipment, and most importantly, once set up, continue to work while the survivor is busy performing other tasks. Although there are traps that will kill or hold large animals, such devices usually require considerable energy and expertise to assemble. Survivors should concentrate their efforts on catching small mammals, birds, and fish, which usually are more abundant, less wary, and require less complicated techniques for capture.

Simple Noose Snares

The simplest form of snare is a noose made from wire, fishing line, cable, parachute line, or other similar material placed over the entrance to an animal's burrow, along its trail, or near a watering or feeding area. The snare must be securely anchored so that when the animal is snared around the neck, foot, or body, it either dies from strangulation or is held in place until the device is checked. In many parts of the world, a simple loop snare is a wildlife poacher's method of choice for illegally procuring animals. This effectiveness makes use of a simple loop snare the food procurement method of choice for survivors trying to live off the land. Successful snaring depends on a person's knowledge of the animals' habits, ability to read signs left by the animals, ability to construct snares from available resources, and knowledge about where one is most likely to catch an animal. Snaring efforts should be focused on larger members of the rodent family, such as tree squirrels, ground squirrels, marmots, muskrats, woodchucks, porcupines, and prairie dogs. A word of caution: this family of animals, deer mice in particular, is a known host for fleas that transmit a variety of infectious agents (see Chapter 45).

For the inexperienced survivor, setting out many simple noose snares provides the best opportunity to procure food. First, construct an "eye" in the end of a length of wire by twisting the wire back around itself several times. Twist the loop that is created into a figure-8 and then bend the upper loop into the lower loop as shown in Figure 90-35. The opposite end of the wire is then passed back through the eye, forming a loop that is adjusted according to the size of the animal being sought. Although simple loop snares can be made from many materials, soft brass wire, aircraft safety wire (0.51 mm [0.02 inch]), or braided picture-hanging wire are best (Figure 90-36). Picture-hanging wire, floral stem wire, and bead wire are available from many hobby shops and are sold either by the pound or by the spool in a variety of gauges; 13.5 m (15 yards) of 24-gauge wire

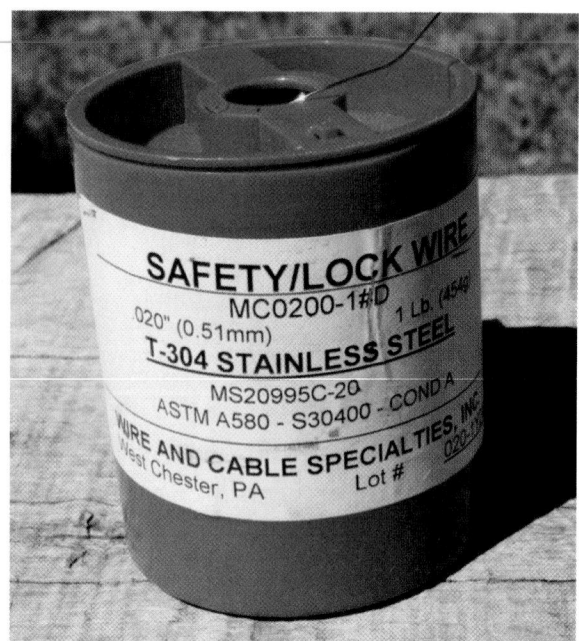

FIGURE 90-36 Suitable wire for snares can be found in hobby shops, automobile parts stores, and picture-frame galleries. *(Courtesy Peter Kummerfeldt.)*

should be included in a survival kit. This wire is strong, flexible, and difficult for an animal to gnaw through when trapped. The wire should be supple enough to shape into a loop, yet stiff enough to retain the loop shape when it is positioned. Simple loop snares made from string, parachute line, shoelaces, and other similar materials may work, but more often than not, the animal is able to free itself and escape before the snares are checked. When materials other than wire are used, noose snares must be checked at least three times a day (morning, noon, and evening) to kill any snared animals that are still alive before they are able to chew through the noose and escape. When wire is used, the trap should be checked in the morning and in the evening. Commercial snares, which could be included in a survival kit, are available. Because they use a locking mechanism that only slides one way (tighter), they are even more effective than those that might be improvised (Figure 90-37).

It is important to study animals in the area. Look for their signs, such as dung, footprints, food remnants, den sites, hair, or other indicators of their movement or presence. Try to determine

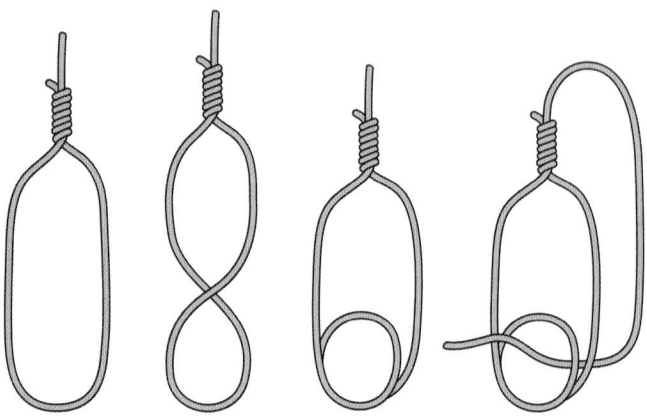

FIGURE 90-35 Snare wire "eye." Twist the loop into a figure-8, and then bend the upper loop into the lower loop as shown.

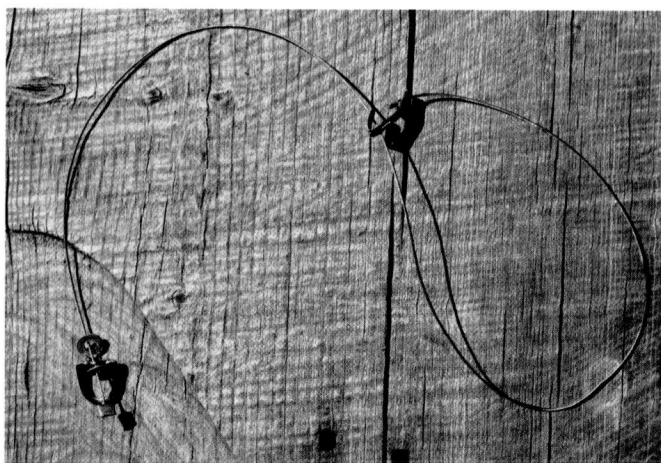

FIGURE 90-37 Unlike an improvised wire snare, Thompson Self-Locking Snares have a locking device that prevents an animal from escaping once it is held. *(Courtesy Peter Kummerfeldt.)*

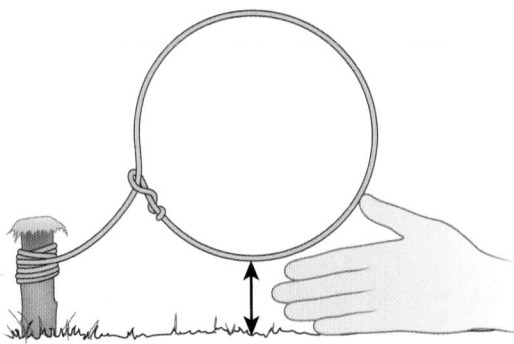

FIGURE 90-38 A rabbit snare loop should be about 10 cm (4 inches) in diameter and positioned 3 to 4 fingers-width above the ground.

their size, time of day they move, height above the ground they carry their head, size of their head, and other useful information that might assist in their capture. When constructing the snare, the size of the loop should be large enough to pass over the animal's head, but not so large that the animal can pass right through the loop. For a rabbit or hare, the noose should be fist-sized, and the lower edge of the loop should be placed 3 to 4 fingers-width above the ground (Figure 90-38). The wire should be secured to a nearby branch or stick, which prevents the animal from leaving the area once held by the snare. As the animal moves down the trail or emerges from or enters a den, its head passes through the noose, which tightens around its neck (Figure 90-39). The animal usually will lunge forward in an effort to free itself, and thus be strangled. During the summer months, it may be difficult to clearly identify where animals are moving. Because of this, it may be more appropriate to identify burrows or feeding areas in which to place snares (Figure 90-40). Using vegetation to hide the snare and funnel animals into it increases the catch rate. During the winter months, squirrels, rabbits, and hares often use the same trail through the snow as they move from one location to another. These are ideal sites to position loop snares (Figure 90-41). The packed trail guides a rabbit or squirrel directly into the loop. Once held, depending on the temperature, animals usually cool quickly and die. It may be necessary to thaw out a carcass before it can be skinned.

It is wise to situate snares in a pattern, known as a *trap line*, so that they can be easily found when checking for snared

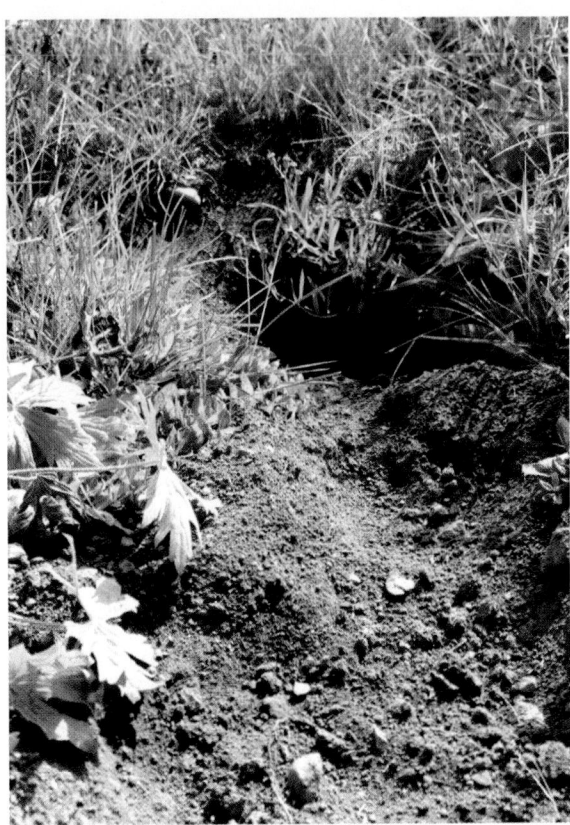

FIGURE 90-40 In the summer, it may be difficult to tell where animals are moving. Locate their burrows or dens and place snares in the entryway. *(Courtesy Peter Kummerfeldt.)*

animals. Tying a flag to a nearby branch also expedites locating a snare, especially after snow has fallen. Knowing where each snare is located saves energy otherwise wasted in hunting for difficult-to-find snares, and also reduces the likelihood of contaminating the area with human scent, which may discourage animals from moving through the locale.

It is possible that a captured animal will be found still alive and only restrained by the noose. In this situation, it must be dispatched as quickly and humanely as possible. The expedient way to accomplish this is to use a stout club and strike the animal's head forward of the ears on the upper surface of the skull. Once is usually sufficient, but check for signs of life before

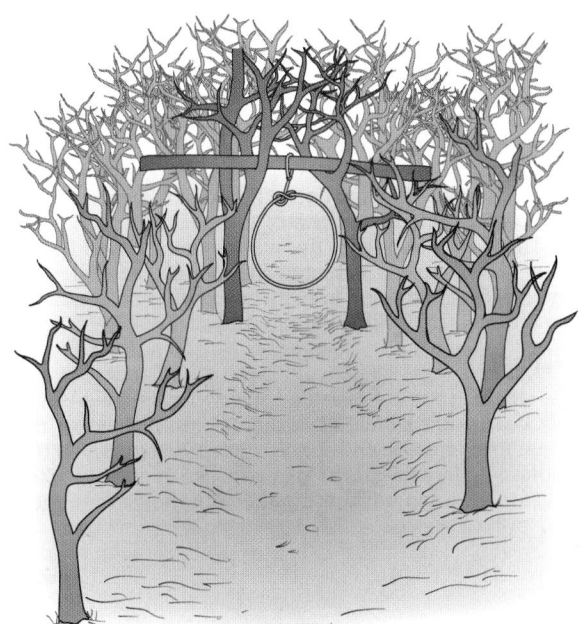

FIGURE 90-39 A snare should be situated on a game trail, preferably in a location that is naturally confined.

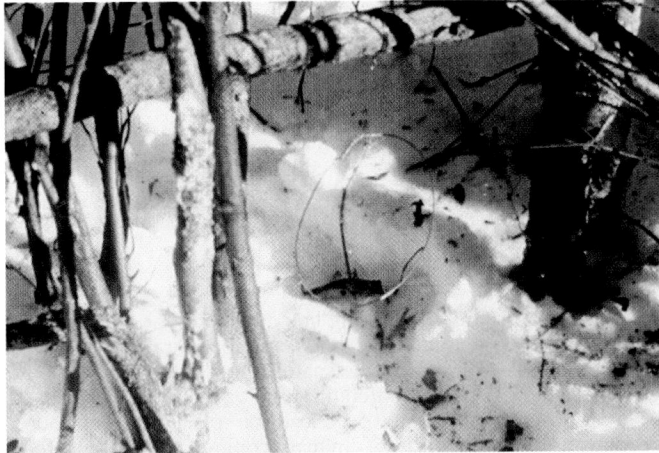

FIGURE 90-41 During the winter, snowshoe hares pack very distinct trails in the snow. These are ideal places to locate one or more snares. *(Courtesy Peter Kummerfeldt.)*

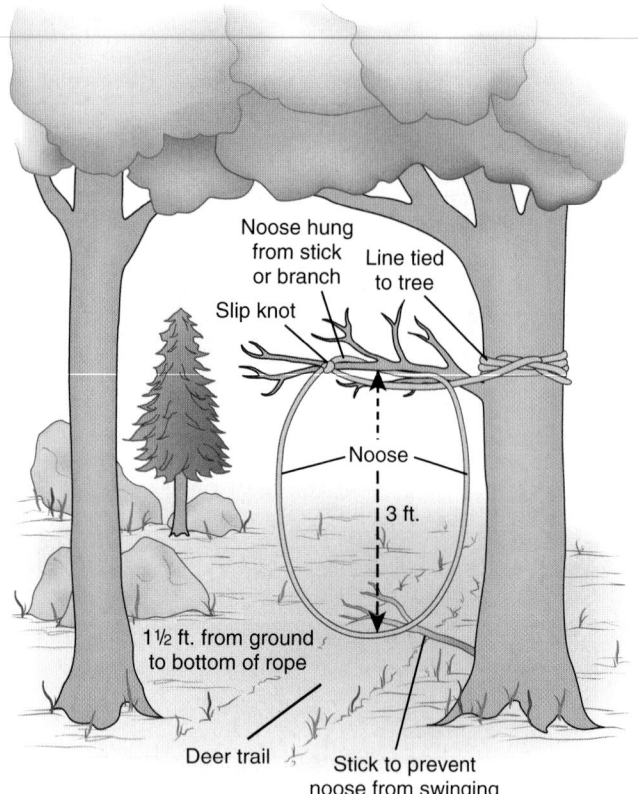

Deer snare

FIGURE 90-42 Parachute cord or similar material can be braided to make a snare that is strong enough to hold larger game.

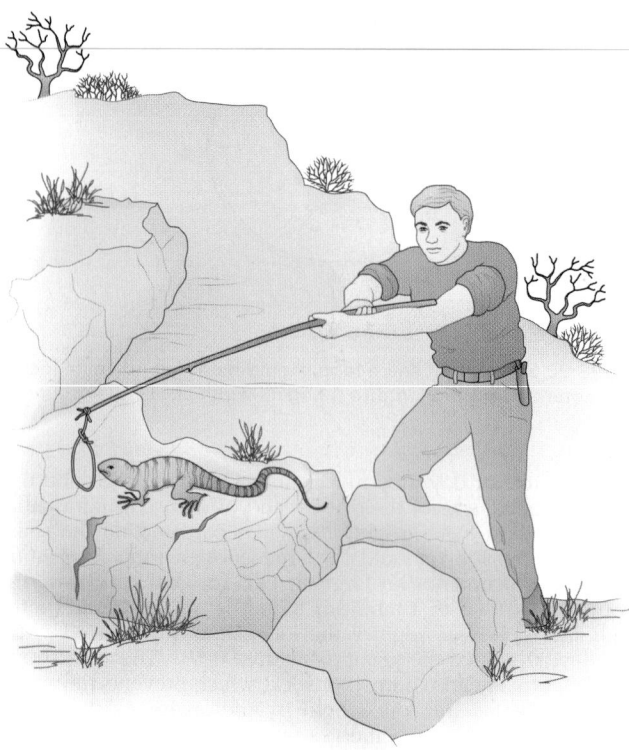

FIGURE 90-43 A wire noose attached to the end of a long stick is an effective device for catching birds, lizards, fish, and snakes.

handling the carcass. A second blow may be necessary. Be careful, because any animal, regardless of size, can inflict a serious bite if handled.

For larger animals, a stronger noose is necessary. This can be made by twisting two strands of wire together and then forming a loop from the doubled wire, or by using nooses made from braided parachute line or similar materials. Tie a secure fixed loop in the end of the line using either an overhand loop knot or a bowline and then position the loop over a game trail (Figure 90-42). Tie the opposite end to the trunk of a nearby tree or stout overhead branch. It may be necessary to use vegetation to hold the noose open when using very supple materials. A good rule of thumb is that it will take at least 15 snares to successfully catch one animal.

An animal may escape after being snared. It may be caught by one or both hind feet and may manage to escape by twisting the wire until it breaks. Predators, both four-legged and winged, will quickly find and eat a snared animal, leaving little for the human survivor. This is another reason why it pays to check traps frequently. Also, the loop may be disturbed or moved out of place without catching an animal. This usually happens because the snare has been set too close to the ground or the loop is too small. As with virtually all skill development, practice builds proficiency.

Baited Snare

A simple loop snare with a long line attached to the end can be positioned where animals or birds are feeding. Bait is placed within the circumference of the snare. When the animal (or bird) steps into the noose, the watching survivor pulls the loop closed. Many nooses attached to pegs can be placed throughout a feeding area where birds or animals congregate. As they feed, their legs become entangled in the snares. A snare could also be placed where an animal would have to reach through a noose to retrieve bait and become snared as it did so.

Noose Stick

A noose made from wire or nylon monofilament can be attached to the end of a pole, then passed over a bird's head and pulled tight to capture it. This method of snaring birds is most useful when trying to catch any of the grouse family (ruffed grouse, sage grouse, dusky grouse, spruce grouse, and ptarmigan). These birds can often be approached very closely and will allow a noose to be passed over their head. The noose stick can also be used to catch lizards and other reptiles (Figure 90-43).

The noose stick can be made in two ways. Construct a noose about 15 cm (6 inches) in diameter, and attach the opposite end of the wire or monofilament directly to the end of a pole by wrapping the wire around one end of the pole several times and then around the main body of the snare to secure it (Figure 90-44). The distance between the pole and the noose should be about 25 cm (10 inches). To catch a bird, the noose is passed over its head, and when the pole is lifted, the bird strangles. The second method requires a longer piece of wire, or a combination of a wire noose and other line. The end of a piece of wire or line is wrapped around the end of the pole and secured (Figure 90-45). The opposite end of the wire is then passed back under the wraps, and a noose is created. To use this method, the noose is passed over a bird's or lizard's head, or even around a fish, and then closed by pulling on the end of the wire.

Squirrel Pole

Using a single strand of brass or steel wire, make a small loop about 6.35 cm (2.5 inches) in diameter in one end of the wire and attach the opposite end to the lower side of a 1.8-m (6-foot)–long pole (Figure 90-46). Snares are situated every 20 cm (8 inches) along the length of the pole, with the lower edge of the

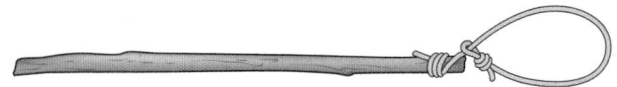

FIGURE 90-44 Noose stick with slip loop.

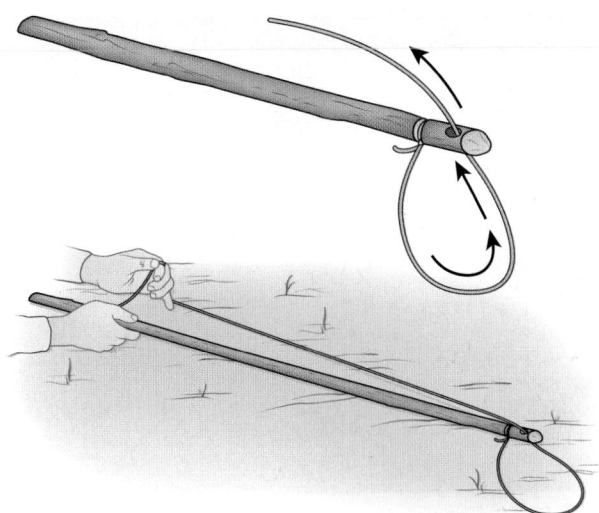

FIGURE 90-45 An alternative method of assembling a slip loop.

loop positioned about 5 cm (2 inches) above the limb. The pole with the attached loops is then leaned against a tree or used to bridge a space between two trees where squirrel activity has been observed. Squirrels are inclined to take the line of least resistance and will run up, down, or across the pole. Once they become snared in a loop, they usually fall off and are strangled. To condition the squirrels to use the pole, it can be prepositioned

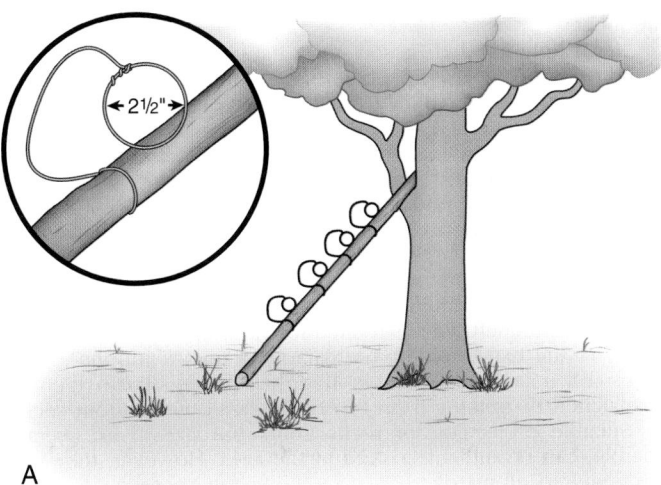

A

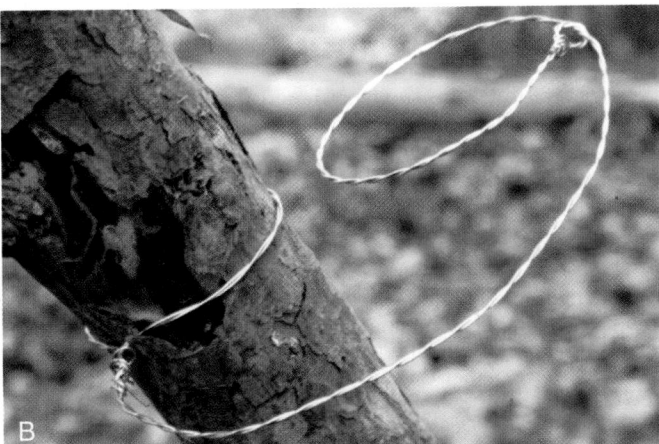

B

FIGURE 90-46 Squirrel pole. *(Bottom courtesy Peter Kummerfeldt.)*

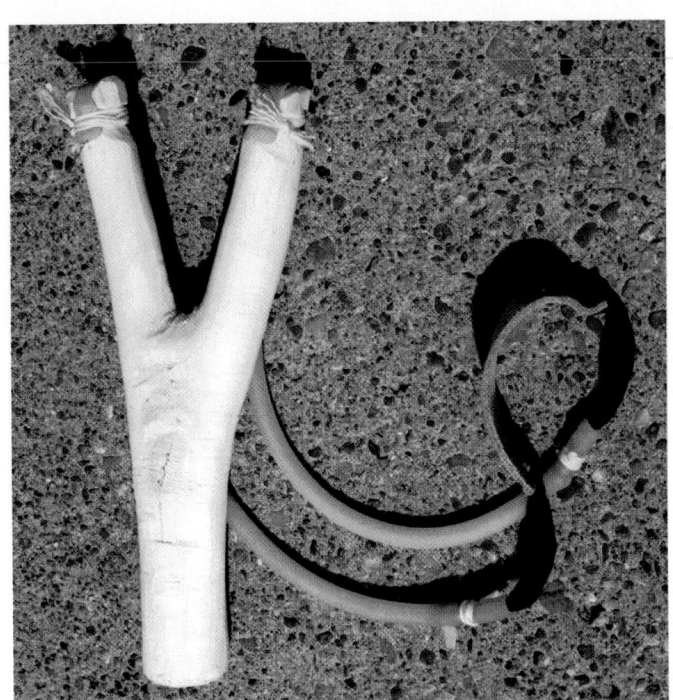

FIGURE 90-47 Sim Lovejoy "flip" or catapult. *(Courtesy Mr. Sim Lovejoy.)*

before attaching the snares for several days. Once the animals become accustomed to taking the shortcut, the snares can be attached. The wire snares should be long enough so that when snared, the squirrel hangs well below the pole and is unable to reach up and grasp the underside of the pole or to touch the ground with its hind legs when hanging. It is quite common to snare several squirrels at a time by using this method. They are inquisitive animals and will investigate another squirrel that has become snared and become trapped themselves in one of the remaining snares. A series of loop snares placed along a tree limb will work in the same fashion as the squirrel pole.

Catapult (Slingshot or Flip) Hunting

In its simplest form, a catapult, or "flip" as it is known in the southeastern United States, consists of a Y frame made from wood or metal with two pieces of surgical tubing tied to each end of the fork and a soft leather pouch attached to the other end of the surgical tubing pieces (Figure 90-47). Although catapults are often called by the misnomer "slingshot" in some regions of the United States, a catapult should not be confused with a sling, which consists of two long thongs attached to a leather pouch. Placing a golf-ball-sized stone in the pouch, the pouch and thongs are twirled overhead, and when one of the thongs is released, the stone is launched toward a target. With a catapult, which is much easier to use and much more accurate than a sling, the projectile is launched by stretching surgical tubing and then releasing the pouch propelling the projectile toward the target.

A properly constructed catapult is one of the best weapons available with which to gather animal food. Catapults are relatively small devices; are powerful, accurate, and inexpensive to make or buy; and use projectiles that can be picked up from the ground. With practice, a person with a catapult is quite capable of killing any of the smaller animals and birds that the individual is likely to encounter.

Commercially available catapults come in many varieties, including the simple forked-stick type and "hi-tech" versions that are even equipped with laser sights (Figure 90-48). Catapults that come with a folding handle are especially suitable for inclusion in a survival kit. Perhaps the best option available is to preassemble the surgical tubing and leather pouch or to buy commercially available catapult replacement parts and include those

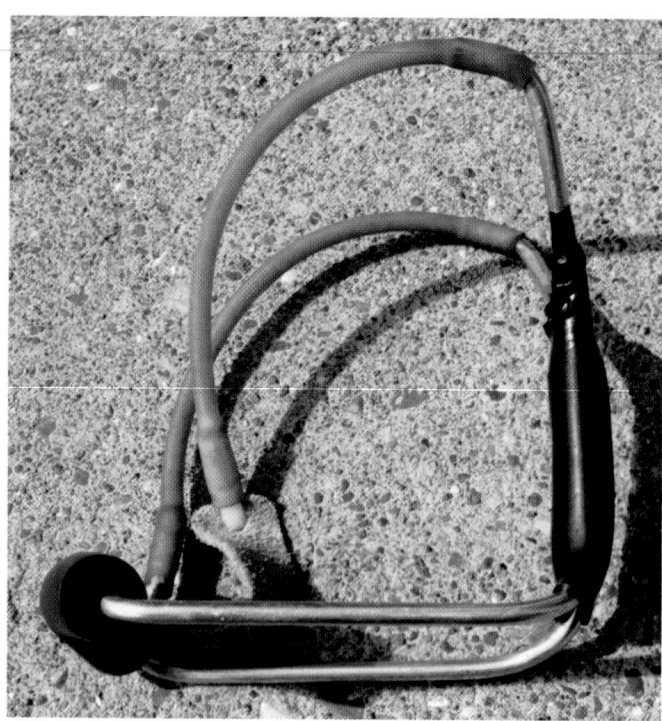

FIGURE 90-48 Commercial "wrist rocket" style of catapult. *(Courtesy Peter Kummerfeldt.)*

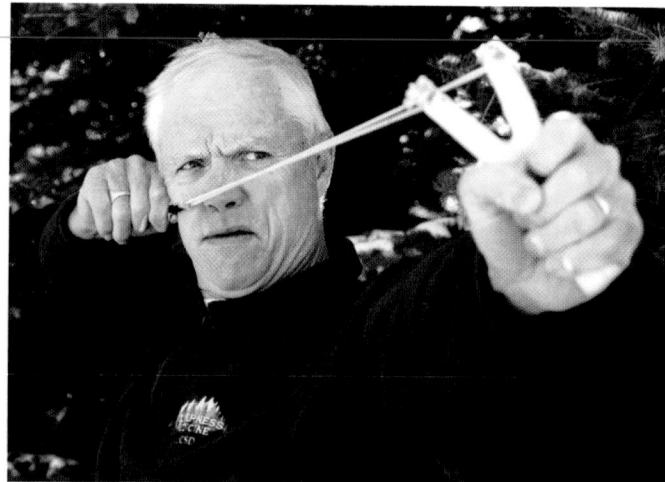

FIGURE 90-50 Firing a catapult. Eye protection is advised. *(Courtesy Peter Kummerfeldt.)*

in an emergency kit. A forked stick is then cut on-site to assemble the catapult (Figure 90-49).

The catapult user will quickly realize that should the surgical tubing snap when under tension, facial or eye injuries may result. The use of protective eye equipment is highly recommended. Inspect the condition of the tubing frequently when using the catapult, and replace it immediately if any sign of deterioration is present.

Although it is possible to kill larger animals with a catapult, more suitable-sized targets include rabbits, hares, squirrels, and most birds. With animals of this size, clean, humane kills can be made out to ranges of about 25 m (~27 yards). For the inexperienced catapult hunter, closer is always better. Many animals, especially those not traditionally hunted, will allow a person to get close if the approach is quiet and slow. Rabbits, grouse, and pheasants in particular are inclined to stay put, giving the hunter an excellent opportunity to get within range before taking a shot. This is especially true in remote parts of the country where animals that are not commonly pursued allow much closer approaches than they might in an area where hunting is frequent.

For a right-handed person, the catapult is grasped in the left hand. A projectile is slipped into the pouch and held in place using the thumb and index finger of the right hand. When the target is within range, the pouch is held at the anchor point, which is usually the base of the ear, the bend of the jaw, or the corner of the mouth. The left arm is extended, stretching the rubber between the pouch and the frame (Figure 90-50). Stretching the rubber produces the energy needed to launch the projectile toward the target and kill the animal on impact. The target's head is centered in the V of the catapult's frame, and when it is properly aligned, the pouch is released. As the pouch is released, the left wrist is rotated forward, or "flipped," to avoid injury to the hand holding the catapult frame. If hit, the animal is usually killed outright, but if only stunned, it can then be dispatched by striking it on top of the head with a stout stick.

Suitable projectiles, or rocks about the size of an average marble, can be difficult to find in the field. However, they may be acquired along riverbanks or along the shoreline of lakes, where the erosive action of water produces smooth, round stones.

Freshwater Fishing

As a general rule, the survivor should focus efforts on catching smaller fish rather than the larger ones. Smaller fish are not as wary or conditioned and are more likely to be caught using improvised fishing equipment. They are also less likely to break improvised fishing equipment.

When the rules that limit how fish can be caught in a recreational setting are preempted by the priority of surviving, a person can take advantage of otherwise-illegal techniques such as gill netting, spearing, and snaring. These are methods that require uncomplicated, simple equipment. They are techniques that can be used with little practice and that offer the best chance of procuring food. In a survival situation, the simplest fishing techniques are usually best.

Although it is possible to improvise fishhooks from many materials, the results are often crude and too large for most freshwater fishing and are not strong enough to withstand the

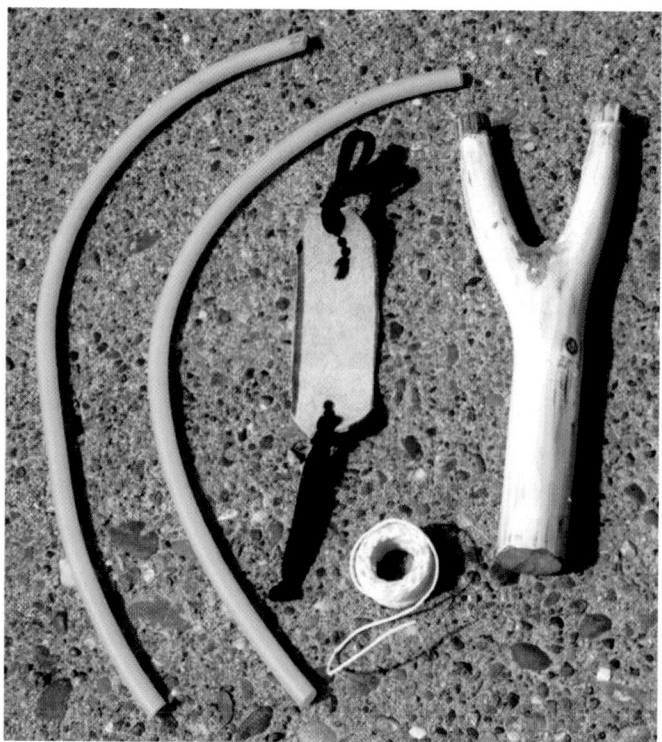

FIGURE 90-49 Catapult parts can be placed in a survival kit and then assembled on-site. *(Courtesy Mr. Sim Lovejoy.)*

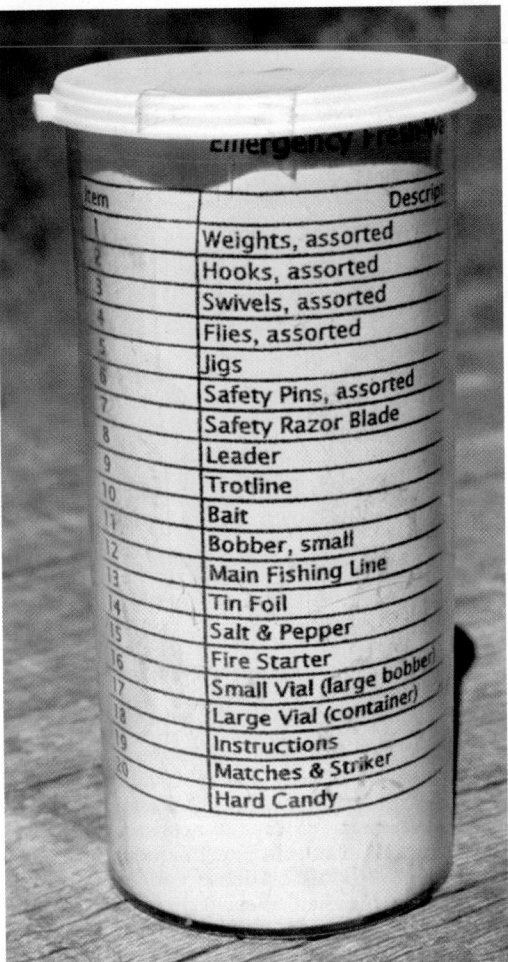

FIGURE 90-51 Commercial survival fishing kit. *(Courtesy Peter Kummerfeldt.)*

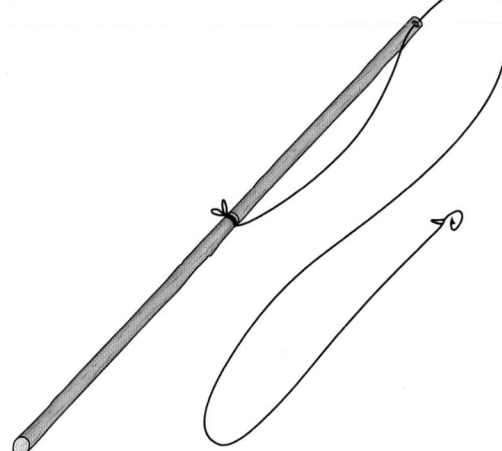

FIGURE 90-52 Improvised fishing pole.

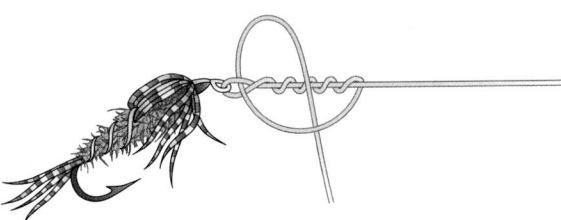

FIGURE 90-53 Improved clinch knot.

are large enough to be gathered and then impaled on a small hook. Aquatic insect life can also be gathered by seining the water with an improvised net, such as one made from a shirt (Figure 90-54). Stand on the upstream side of the net, and disturb the streambed with your feet. Insects washed free from the gravel will be flushed into the waiting net. This method usually produces larger aquatic life that can be used for bait. Other insect life suitable for bait, such as grasshoppers, crickets, and worms, can usually be found along the lakeshore or riverbank.

struggles of a fish trying to escape. Fishing line can be improvised by unraveling clothing, twisting fibers from various plants together, or using other available line. However, the effectiveness of improvised fishing line is far inferior to the quality and strength of monofilament line. For these reasons, commercial fishing equipment, including line, hooks, split shot, flies, lures, and a commercial fish spear point or a trident frog gig, should be parts of every survival kit. Prepackaged, commercially assembled emergency fishing kits are available (Figure 90-51). These come in varieties suited for saltwater fishing or use in lakes and rivers.

Pole fishing allows the user to reach out from the bank and place a baited hook exactly where it is most likely to attract a fish. For trout and similar-sized fish, cut a pole 1.8 m (6 feet) long with a 2.5-cm (1-inch)–thick butt from willow, alder, or other similar shrub. The size of the targeted fish determines the thickness of the pole needed, whereas the springiness of the material selected reduces the chance of the line breaking as the fish struggles to free itself. The line, which should be one and a half times the rod length or slightly longer, is attached at two points. The first attachment point should be the midpoint of the pole and the second at the tip. In this way, if the tip of the pole should break as a fish is being landed, the line is still attached at the lower point, and the fish, along with the hook and line, is not lost (Figure 90-52). When tying on a hook or lure, use a clinch knot (Figure 90-53).

Bait can usually be found either in the water or in the surrounding area. Try to determine the types of natural foods that the fish are eating by examining the stomach contents of the first fish caught, and if possible, use these same foods for bait. Examine the underside of rocks lifted from the river for any insect life. Most of the insects observed will be very small, but some

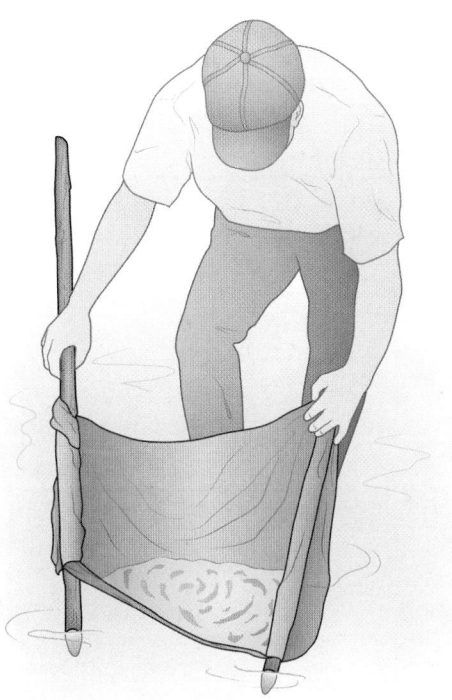

FIGURE 90-54 Seine net improvised from a shirt.

In moving water, it is usually best if the bait is cast upstream and allowed to drift with the current along the streambed. This simulates a free-floating insect or one that has fallen into the water and drowned. At the end of the drift, the bait is removed from the water and recast to a new drift line. This cast-and-retrieve process is repeated until a fish is caught. In still or slow-moving water, a bobber made from a piece of wood or other buoyant material should be used with the bait suspended below it. The distance between the bobber and the bait is adjusted until a bite is detected. Because 98% of fish feeding is below the surface, position the bait close to or right on the bottom of the river. A fish taking the baited hook will disturb the bobber, which is the primary indicator that there is a bite or hooked fish. The line is lifted quickly and the hooked fish removed from the water. To ensure that the fish is not lost, place an improvised net below it or use an improvised gaff to assist in recovery of the fish. Sliding the fish up onto the bank rather than lifting it from the water will reduce the chances of the line breaking and the fish escaping with the fishhook. In most situations, flies or bait fished below the surface will catch more fish than those presented on or closer to the water surface.

An improvised **dip net** is a very useful food-gathering tool. The net can be used to scoop up speared fish, to land those caught on a hook and line, or even to catch fish at a constricting point in a waterway. Small fish can often be caught using a dip net improvised from a shirt. Two poles attached to the sides of a shirt can be used to scoop out minnows and other small fish (see Figure 90-54).

Hand fishing works well in smaller, shallower rivers where fish take shelter beneath undercut stream banks, under sunken logs, and around other river debris. When hand fishing, the person enters the water some distance above the spot where undercut banks are likely to shelter fish. Moving downriver, the person muddies the water and drives the fish downstream. Concentrating the fish in this way increases the odds of catching one. The individual then lies on the bank above a likely hideout and, moving slowly so as not to scare the fish, reaches into the water and carefully feels for any fish that may be present (Figure 90-55). Most fish, trout in particular, will tolerate being lightly handled. When the person touches the smooth skin of the fish, it is quickly pinned to the underside of the bank or to the bottom of the river, and then, when the body is firmly grasped, the fish is flipped out onto the bank. Trying to grip the fish by the gills or some other part of its anatomy underwater is usually not successful.

Other hand fishing methods include "noodling," whereby the person reaches into underwater holes in the riverbank or under sunken logs for catfish. Once a fish is detected, the person grasps its lower lip or gills and hauls it from the water. This process is not without risk because the resting areas favored by catfish are

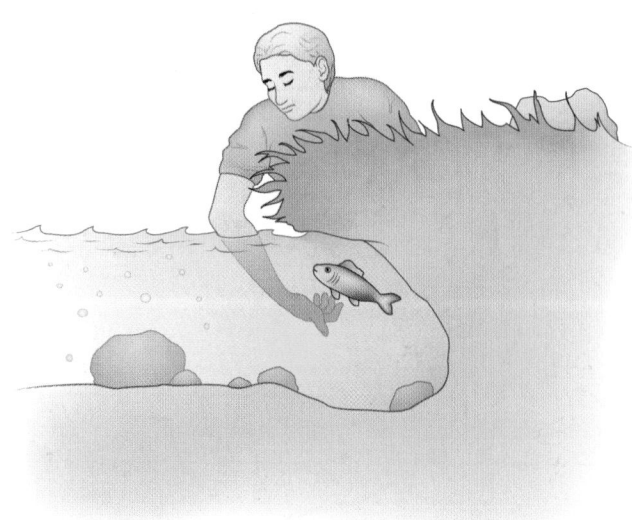

FIGURE 90-55 Hand fishing.

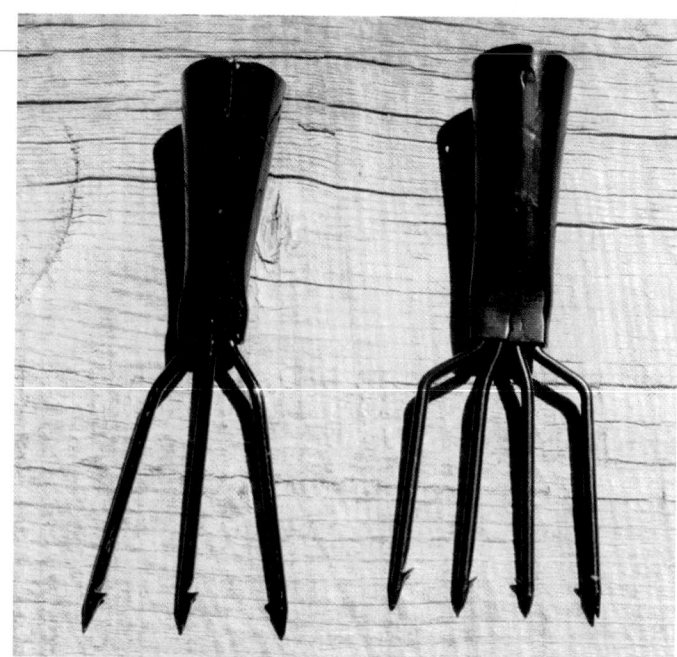

FIGURE 90-56 Fish or frog trident points, also called "gigs." *(Courtesy Peter Kummerfeldt.)*

also those favored by turtles. This can result in a nasty bite. In the United States, catfish habitat is also water moccasin (cotton-mouth snake) habitat.

Spear fishing is an effective technique available when fish are found in large schools or dense concentrations that make hitting a target much easier. Spear fishing is also a useful technique where fish can be seen, but the water is too deep for hand fishing, or where fish are too wary to be approached closely. In addition to fish, spears can also be used to procure a variety of other animals, such as frogs, lizards, and snakes. Although spear points can be improvised, the success of spear fishing largely depends on the availability of a commercial spear point. A trident point is one of the most versatile food-gathering devices available to the survivor and should be included in a survival kit (Figure 90-56). The spear point is easily attached to one end of a 2.4-m (8-foot)–long pole using a small nut and bolt (which usually come with the trident when purchased) inserted through the holes in the spear point and through the shaft of the spear.

Even though a commercial spear point may not be available, it may be possible to improvise one from available pieces of hardwood. Sharpen the end of the shaft with a knife and then harden it by turning the now-pointed end in the flames of a fire. An improvised spear should be used to impale a fish, pinning it to the river bottom, and then lifting it out by hand. Although many fish will escape this method, some will die from their injuries and may float to the surface, where they can be recovered.

To use a fish spear effectively, hold the spear point just below the surface of the water rather than standing poised with the spear held over the shoulder while waiting for a fish to come by. Placing the spear point just below the water surface reduces the aiming problems caused by water refraction and greatly increases the odds of striking the fish.

The fisherman moves slowly from a downstream position toward a resting fish or waits patiently for a fish to come within range. When within reach, the fish is impaled with a quick strike and pinned to the river bottom. Rather than lifting the fish directly from the water using the spear point, thereby risking not only the loss of the fish but also the spear point, reach down and grasp the fish with your free hand and lift it while it is attached to the spear point.

Hand line fishing greatly extends the reach of the fisherman. Many yards of line can be wrapped around a line holder, which is then unwrapped before the fisherman casts a baited hook into

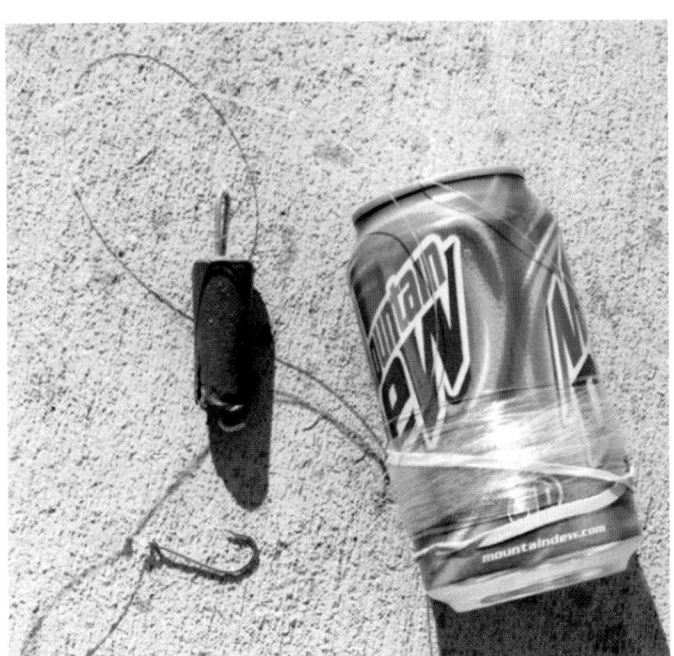

FIGURE 90-57 Beverage can hand line. (*Courtesy Peter Kummerfeldt.*)

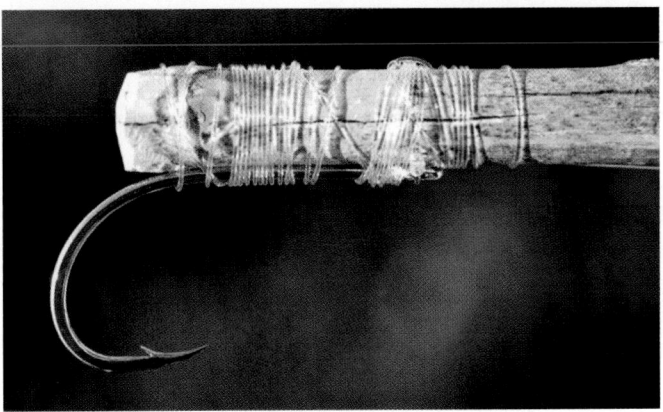

FIGURE 90-58 Improvised gaff made from a large fishhook. (*Courtesy Peter Kummerfeldt.*)

the water. Hand lining requires a substantial weight attached to the line to pull the baited hook out into deeper water, where it is allowed to remain until located and taken by a fish. When hand line fishing, the line is held in the fingertips awaiting the feel of a fish taking the bait, when the line is withdrawn quickly and the fish hooked. With a fish on, the line is quickly retrieved hand-over-hand until the fish is landed. When casting, as the bait is thrown, line control can become a problem, so tangles are common. This problem can be resolved by winding the line around the base of a beverage can or similarly shaped smooth object. The base of the can is then pointed toward the open water, and the line is cast. The weight pulls the line off of the can, and the baited hook flies out free of tangles (Figure 90-57). As the line is retrieved, it is once again wound onto the can until the next cast is made.

With **snaring,** as with snaring land animals, a wire loop attached to the end of a stout pole can be used to catch fish. Select wire that is strong enough to overcome the struggles of the snared fish (or, if limited in choice of wire, select smaller fish). The wire must also be supple enough to close quickly but stiff enough to retain the loop as it is passes through the water and over the fish's body. Attach one end of the wire to a 1.8-m (6-foot)–long pole, and create a loop in the other end large enough to pass over the head of the fish. The distance between the end of the pole and the loop should be about 30 cm (12 inches). The fisherman then approaches a resting fish from directly behind (downstream) and slowly passes the noose over its head, moving the noose toward the fish's midsection. With some fish, it may work better to pass the noose from behind and over the fish's tail. When positioned properly, the pole is then lifted, tightening the noose, and the fish is removed from the water.

Gaffing involves a large fishhook lashed securely to a long pole, which can be used to snag a resting fish and lift it from the water. To prevent the loss of the hook, should the pole break when landing larger fish, attach a length of line to the hook eye and tie it off to the stronger midpoint of the pole (Figure 90-58). Gaffing is particularly effective when fish are confined and can be approached carefully from the bank or by wading. Approach the fish slowly from downstream, and when within reach of the gaff, place the hook close to a "thick" part of the fish and strike upward quickly. Expect the fish to struggle vigorously and attempt to free itself from the hook. As quickly as possible, remove the fish from the water and strike its head above the eyes with a stout limb to kill it.

The methods discussed to this point require the active participation of a person. Sometimes, considerable amounts of energy can be expended using these techniques. These methods also expose a survivor to existing weather conditions, contact with cold water, and depending on the fishing methods used, risk for becoming hypothermic. From a survival perspective, better fishing techniques would reduce the amount of energy expended by the survivor, reduce exposure to inclement weather conditions, and limit contact with cold water while increasing the chances of catching a fish. The following are examples of passive fishing techniques that, once constructed, work for the survivor with little further expenditure of energy.

Given the time, materials, and ability, it is possible to improvise a **gill net.** However, it is much wiser to include a small (1.21 m × 3.66 m × 6.35 cm [4 feet × 12 feet × 2.5 inches]) commercially available gill net in a survival kit (Figure 90-59). The net can be used to trap fish and can also be erected on land to trap small animals and birds. Floats, made from pieces of wood or other buoyant material, need to be attached along the length of the upper edge of the net, and weights, made from stones, attached to the lower edge. Some experimentation will be necessary to find a balance where the floats remain on the surface while the stone weights fully extend the net into the depths of the water. It is better to use many smaller stones as weights than to use a few larger ones. The net is then placed in still or slow-moving water, anchored, and left to trap passing fish (Figure 90-60). The net can also be placed in a naturally constricted location or in a narrow point in the waterway created by the survivor from logs and rocks. To expedite catching fish, a person

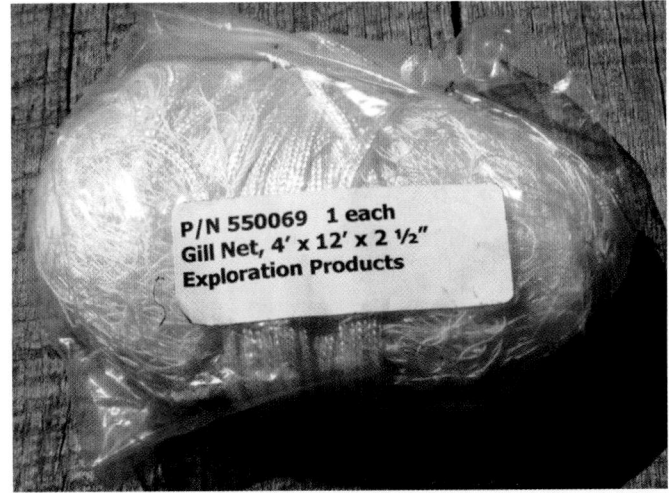

FIGURE 90-59 Commercial survival gill net. (*Courtesy Peter Kummerfeldt.*)

Floats
Weights

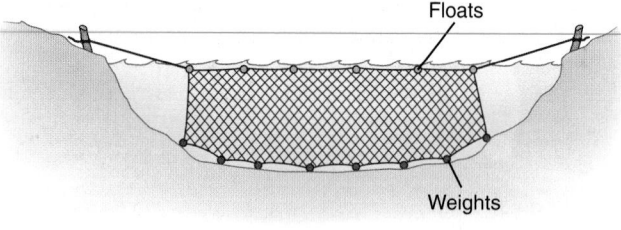

Block the whole of a smaller stream with a net.

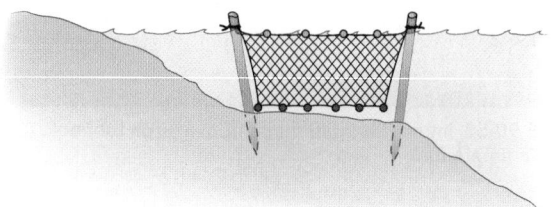

Gill net set between the beach and the main drop-off in a lake.

Fishing with nets

FIGURE 90-60 Setting a gill net to catch fish in slow-moving or still water.

would enter the water upstream of the net and move noisily downstream, scaring fish into the trap. Gill nets used in moving water must not be left in the river unattended. Debris floating downstream will collect in the net and soon destroy it. The net should be checked at least once a day and more often if the floats are seen bobbing or being drawn underwater, indicating trapped fish or river debris entangled in the net.

Set lines are usually a single hook attached to a length of line. One end is tied to an anchor onshore, and a baited hook is tied to the other end, which is cast into the water (Figure 90-61). The line can also be tied to a branch or other similar anchor point overhanging the water. The branch serves as a "fishing rod" and plays the fish until the fisherman retrieves it. Multiple set lines placed along a riverbank or along a shoreline provide the best opportunity to catch fish with the least amount of energy expended. Lines with multiple hooks attached along the length of the fishing line can also be assembled and used to catch fish. Commercial "trigger" devices, such as Speedhooks (Figure 90-62), greatly improve the fisherman's chances of hooking a fish. These devices are spring-loaded and automatically set the hook when a fish nibbles the bait. Set lines should be checked several times a day to rebait any empty hooks and to remove fish that have been hooked before other predators eat them.

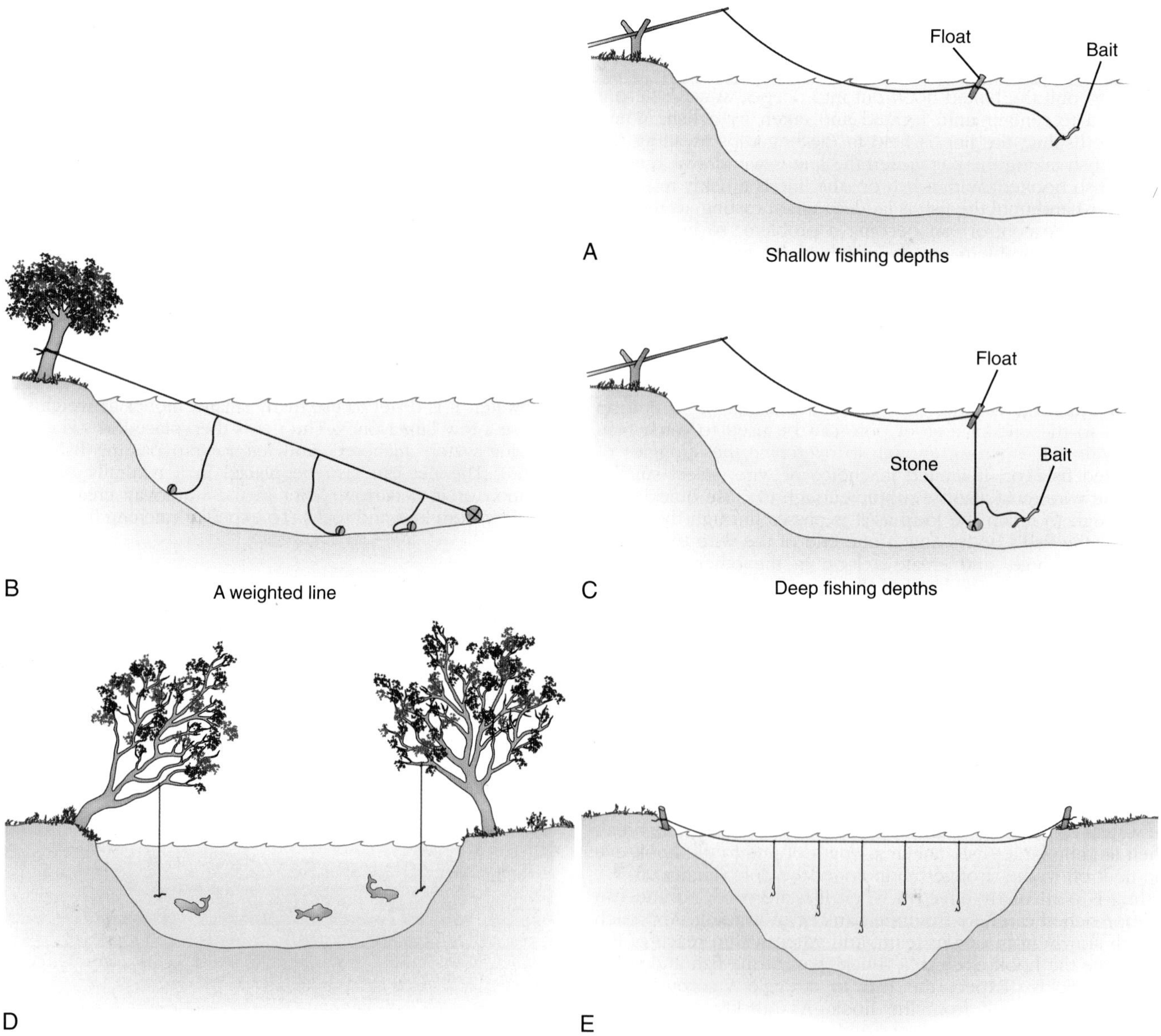

Float
Bait
A
Shallow fishing depths
B
A weighted line
Float
Stone
Bait
C
Deep fishing depths
D
E

FIGURE 90-61 **A** to **E,** Set lines.

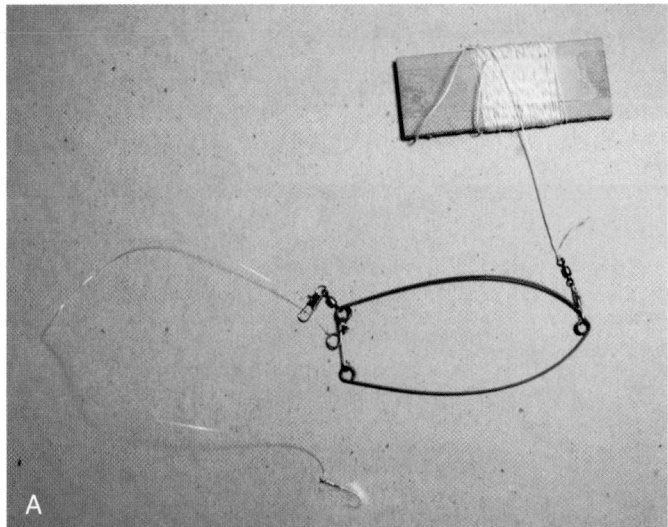

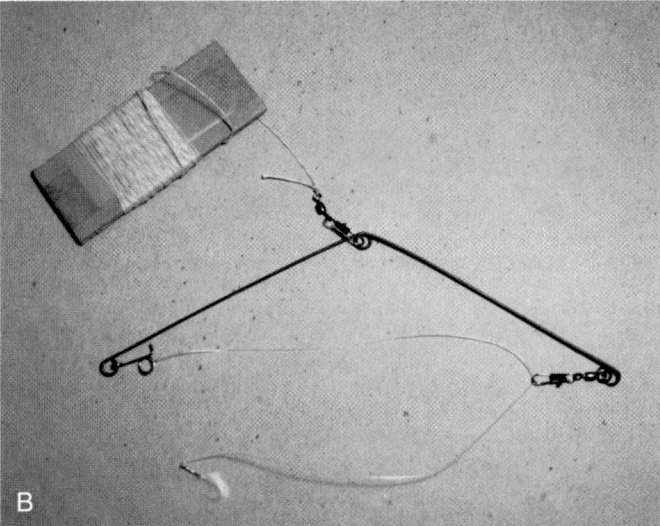

FIGURE 90-62 Commercial Speedhooks. Set position **(A)** and sprung position **(B)**. *(Courtesy Peter Kummerfeldt.)*

Survival Firearms

Having a firearm—rifle, shotgun, or handgun—with you in a survival event greatly increases your chances of becoming a more effective "hunter-gatherer." There is a big difference between trying to kill a rabbit 20 yards away with a slingshot and killing it with a .22-caliber rifle or a shotgun. Firearms eliminate the need to approach close to a potential food source. With a rifle, if one has decent stalking skills, it is possible to approach within the firearm's effective range without the targeted animal being becoming aware of human presence. A person will need to be more active when hunting with a firearm, so it is important to weigh energy expenditure against the caloric return from any animal procured.

With the decision to carry a firearm comes the responsibility to develop the proficiency necessary to be safe and to acquire adequate marksmanship and hunting skills. With good coaching, the degree of skill needed to become an accurate shot with a rifle can be achieved relatively quickly. The degree of accuracy required with a shotgun is not as critical, so proficiency may be achieved more quickly than with a rifle. The same cannot be said for handguns. To be used effectively as a food-gathering tool, or for personal defense, a handgun requires considerable time at the target range before any reasonable degree of skill can be achieved.

Knowing how to use a firearm safely and effectively is the proper first step. To further increase the possibility of putting food in the pot, it is necessary to study the activities of the animals in the area. Being able to anticipate the behavior of animals increases the chances of being in the right place at the right time. There is no shortcut to achieving this skill. Time spent in the field observing the activities of small game animals that one day might become a meal is time well spent.

A survival firearm intended for food gathering should be lightweight and compact, easy to use, easy to maintain, small caliber, and accurate to about 100 yards (91 m). Using these criteria, the best choices are shotguns and .22-caliber rifles. Because handguns are much more difficult to shoot accurately, they are not recommended as "food-gathering devices."

One of the most useful survival firearms is a combination .22-caliber rifle/20-gauge shotgun (Figure 90-63), such as those made by Savage Arms Company. A .22-caliber barrel is stacked on top of the 20-gauge shotgun barrel. The user can easily choose which barrel to use before pulling the trigger, either a single projectile or a mass of shot to dispatch the animal.

Hunting Guidelines

1. Be careful with any weapon. Despite its small caliber, a .22 bullet can travel over a mile and still cause injury.
2. Keep the weapon in good working order. Pay particular attention to ensuring that the barrel does not become clogged with dirt, snow, or other debris. A blocked barrel may explode, causing serious damage to the weapon and injuries to the user.
3. Limit targets to smaller animals and birds. The .22 rifle or shotgun is quite capable of killing larger animals when bullet placement is perfect, but it likely that the inexperienced hunter will be much more successful procuring rabbits, squirrels, grouse, etc.
4. Do not aim the weapon at any animal unless you are planning to kill it.
5. Get as close as possible to the animal you are trying to kill, increasing the likelihood of a fatal shot.
6. Squeeze the trigger only when the animal is motionless. Do not shoot at moving targets.
7. Fire from the steadiest position available. Always use an available resting object for a prop to steady your aim and maximize accuracy in order to make an effective and humane kill.
8. Hunt within established regulations and hunting seasons; however, if you are in a life-or-death survival situation and need food, it is unlikely that you would be cited for killing an animal out of season.
9. Always make sure to positively identify your target.

Because of the possibility of encountering predatory animals in Canada, Alaska, and some parts of the lower 48 states, the need for a having a survival weapon takes on the aspect of self-defense. In this instance, a handgun of .44 caliber or higher, rifle of .375 caliber or higher, or 12-gauge shotgun with slug ammunition makes more sense. Because calibers such as these tend to destroy too much meat, they are not as good for killing smaller game for food, but they better serve the need of self-defense.

When transporting firearms across state and international borders, comply with all international, federal, and state regulations. The book *Traveler's Guide to the Firearms Laws of the Fifty States* provides a wealth of information regarding travel with firearms within the United States.

WILD PLANT FOODS

Plants have always been valuable sources of food and nutrients. They are readily available throughout most of the world and are often easily procured. Foraging of wild plants, usually considered weeds, has seen people through many wars, famines, and droughts.[10,13] Studies demonstrate that wild plants are a good source of food in survival situations, allowing survivors to perform hard and prolonged physical work during periods of restricted food intake.[13] They can increase daily food mass by fivefold.[15] Wild plants are a critical component for wilderness survival and living off the land.

Wild plants are packed with a plethora of nutrients, particularly B vitamins, ascorbic acid (vitamin C), and antioxidants. Studies show that wild plants have significantly higher nutrient

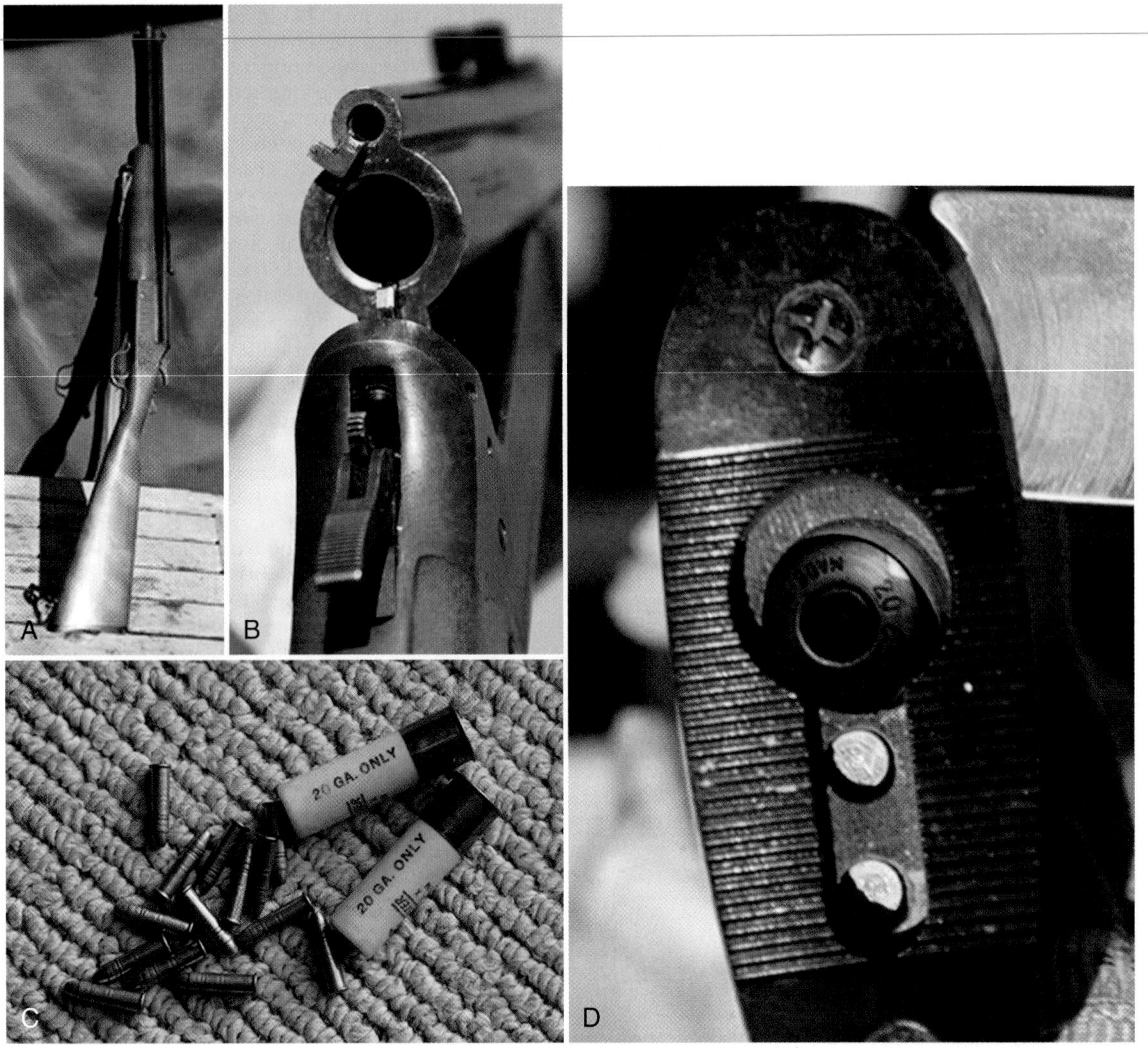

FIGURE 90-63 **A,** Savage .22/20 gauge "over and under" survival firearm. **B,** Breech showing .22-caliber barrel stacked on top of 20-gauge shotgun barrel. **C,** .22-caliber and 20-gauge ammunition. **D,** Butt plate showing ammunition stored in the stock.

ratios than do cultivated varieties.[5,14,16] It is believed that the longevity factor in the Mediterranean diet may indeed be the consistent and continued dietary integration of wild plants.[22] Of the 80,000 known edible plant species, only about 200 are cultivated regularly, and only three (corn, wheat, and rice) function as staples in modern Western societies.[20]

PROCUREMENT OF WILD PLANT FOODS

When one is harvesting wild plants, careful consideration must be given to identification, procurement, preparation, toxicity, and plant abundance (Figure 90-64). When considering plant abundance, it may once again be best to look at the practices of hunter-gatherers. Scientific analysis has shown that hunter-gatherers likely prioritized the collection of wild plants to provide the greatest ratio of energy capture to energy expenditure, in what has been called "optimal foraging."[3] Optimal foraging would clearly be advantageous to any wilderness survival situation and living off the land.

Before heading into the wilderness, it is wise to familiarize yourself with the types and abundance of edible wild plants that grow in the particular region in which you will be traveling. Because it would be impossible to list the tens of thousands of known edible plants throughout the world, this chapter concentrates only on the most common. Tables 90-2 to 90-6 list some

Text continued on p. 2085

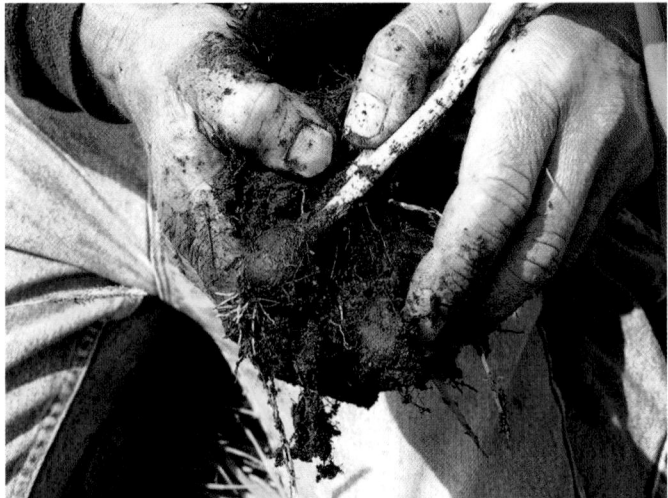

FIGURE 90-64 Gathering blue camas bulbs for a meal. *(Courtesy Peter Kummerfeldt.)*

TABLE 90-2 Temperate Region Wild Plants

Scientific Name	Common Name	Photo	Edible Part(s)	Special Preparation
Acer saccharinum *Acer saccharum*	Maple	Courtesy Denise Martinez.	Sap, young leaves, inner bark	Boil sap to concentrate sugars. Young leaves can be eaten raw or cooked. Inner bark should be boiled. Can also be dried, ground, and added to flour to make bread.
Allium spp.	Wild onion, wild garlic, wild chive	Courtesy Denise Martinez.	Young leaves, bulbs	All can be eaten raw or cooked.
Amaranthus spp.	Amaranth, pigweed	Copyright iStockphoto.com/y-studio.	Seeds, young shoots, leaves	Seeds can be eaten raw, cooked, or roasted. Can also be ground into flour. Shoots and leaves can be eaten raw or cooked. Will concentrate toxic levels of nitrates if grown in contaminated soils under drought conditions.

Continued

TABLE 90-2   Temperate Region Wild Plants—cont'd

Scientific Name	Common Name	Photo	Edible Part(s)	Special Preparation
Chenopodium spp.	Lamb's-quarter, goosefoot, quinoa	Copyright iStockphoto.com/DaisyLiang.	Leaves, seeds	Leaves can be eaten raw or cooked. Seeds must be boiled to remove saponins.
Cichorium intybus	Chicory	Copyright iStockphoto.com/BasieB.	Roots, young leaves, flowers, flower buds	Leaves, flowers, and flower buds can be eaten raw or cooked. Roots taste best when cooked in several changes of water.
Cirsium vulgare	Thistle	From Peterson LA: *A field guide to edible wild plants of eastern and central North America*, Peterson Field Guide Series No 23, Boston, 1977, Houghton Mifflin, color plate 10. Copyright 1977 by Lee Peterson. Reprinted by permission of Houghton Mifflin Company. All rights reserved.	Young shoots, stems, leaves, receptacle	All can be eaten raw or cooked.

TABLE 90-2 Temperate Region Wild Plants—cont'd

Scientific Name	Common Name	Photo	Edible Part(s)	Special Preparation
Hemerocallis spp.	Day lily	Courtesy Denise Martinez.	Roots, young shoots, flower buds, flowers	Young roots can be eaten raw. Older roots must be cooked. Young shoots, flower buds, and flowers can be eaten raw or cooked.
Malva neglecta	Mallow, cheeseweed	Courtesy Denise Martinez.	Young shoots leaves, flower buds, flowers, unripe fruit	All can be eaten raw or cooked.
Medicago sativa	Alfalfa	Courtesy Denise Martinez.	Leaves, flowering tops	All can be eaten raw or cooked.

Continued

TABLE 90-2   Temperate Region Wild Plants—cont'd

Scientific Name	Common Name	Photo	Edible Part(s)	Special Preparation
Pinus spp.	Pine	Courtesy Denise Martinez.	Young shoots, inner bark, male inflorescences, pine nuts, sap	All can be eaten raw or cooked. Inner bark best when gathered early in the year. Pine nuts best when roasted. Sizes differ depending on species. Sap can be used as cough drops.
Polygonum bistorta	Bistort		Roots, young shoots, leaves	Roots are best when cooked. Young shoots and leaves can be eaten raw or cooked.
Portulaca oleracea	Purslane	Courtesy Denise Martinez.	Roots, leaves, stems	All can be eaten raw or cooked. Best when cooked.
Pteridium aquilinum	Bracken fern		Very young fronds	Cook in several changes of water. Fronds contain ptaquiloside, the high consumption of which has been linked to esophageal cancer.[9] Fronds also contain thiaminase, which destroys thiamine (vitamin B_1) in the body.
Quercus spp.	Oak	Courtesy Denise Martinez.	Acorns	Some species have sweet acorns, which can be roasted or eaten raw. Most other species have bitter acorns, which are best when chopped and boiled in several changes of water.

TABLE 90-2   Temperate Region Wild Plants—cont'd

Scientific Name	Common Name	Photo	Edible Part(s)	Special Preparation
Rosa spp.	Wild rose	 Courtesy Denise Martinez.	Petals, rosehips	All can be eaten raw or cooked.
Rubus spp.	Blackberry, raspberry, dewberry	 From Letcher Lyle K: *The wild berry book: Romance, recipes, and remedies*, Minocqua, Wis, 1994, NorthWord Press, p 43. Copyright Larry West.	Berries, leaves	Berries can be eaten raw or cooked. Leaves can be used for tea, although excessive consumption can induce labor.
Rumex crispus	Sorrel, curly dock	 Courtesy Denise Martinez.	Leaves, seeds	Boil leaves in several changes of water. Seeds must be removed from their astringent hulls.

Continued

TABLE 90-2 Temperate Region Wild Plants—cont'd

Scientific Name	Common Name	Photo	Edible Part(s)	Special Preparation
Sagittaria latifolia	Arrowhead, Wapato	Courtesy Denise Martinez.	Tubers at end of rhizomes	All can be eaten raw or cooked.
Taraxacum officinale	Dandelion	Courtesy Denise Martinez.	Roots, leaves, flower buds, flowers	All can be eaten raw or cooked.
Trifolium repens	Clover	Courtesy Denise Martinez.	Leaves, roots, inflorescences, seeds	All can be eaten raw or cooked. Seeds can also be used for sprouting.
Typha latifolia	Cattail	Courtesy Denise Martinez.	Roots, base of leaves, young shoots, unripe inflorescences, pollen, seeds	All can be eaten raw or cooked. Remove green outer leaves to find white, tender base. Unripe inflorescences can be roasted like corn on the cob. Seeds can be obtained by removing down.

TABLE 90-2   Temperate Region Wild Plants—cont'd

Scientific Name	Common Name	Photo	Edible Part(s)	Special Preparation
Urtica dioica	Nettle	 Courtesy Denise Martinez.	Young shoots and leaves	All can be eaten raw or cooked. Protect hands and arms while harvesting to avoid contact dermatitis. Stinging is reduced when nettle is wet. Avoid eating excessive amounts of old leaves because they can lead to kidney lesions.
Vaccinium spp.	Blueberry, huckleberry, bilberry, cranberry	 From Letcher Lyle K: *The wild berry book: Romance, recipes, and remedies*, Minocqua, Wis, 1994, NorthWord Press, p 58. Copyright Brett Baunton.	Fruit	Can be eaten raw or cooked.

TABLE 90-3   Desert Region Wild Plants

Scientific Name	Common Name	Photo	Edible Part(s)	Special Preparation
Agave parryi	Agave	 Courtesy Denise Martinez.	Trunk	Dig up trunk before flower stalk appears. Chop off leaves at base and cook for several days. Flower stalk, flower buds, and flowers are also edible. They taste best when cooked.

Continued

TABLE 90-3   Desert Region Wild Plants—cont'd

Scientific Name	Common Name	Photo	Edible Part(s)	Special Preparation
Cereus giganteus	Saguaro		Fruit	Can be eaten raw or cooked. Fruit falls to ground when ripe. Use stick to dislodge fruit if still attached.
Echinocactus horizonthalonius	Barrel cactus, visnaga	 From Huey GHH, Houk R: *Wild cactus*, New York, 1996, Artisan, p 23.	Pulp (hydration and food), fruit	All can be eaten raw or cooked. To obtain fluid: chop off top, mash pulp inside stem, and then strain fluid through cloth.
Opuntia ficus-indica	Prickly pear, cholla	 Courtesy Denise Martinez.	Fruit, young joints	All can be eaten raw or cooked. Plant is best gathered with a three-pronged stick. Glochids (bristles) are best removed by rubbing in sand or scrubbing in running water.

TABLE 90-3 Desert Region Wild Plants—cont'd

Scientific Name	Common Name	Photo	Edible Part(s)	Special Preparation
Yucca baccata	Yucca	 Courtesy Denise Martinez.	Flower stalk, flower buds, flowers, fruit	Flower stalk tastes best when cooked. The remainder can be eaten raw or cooked.

TABLE 90-4 Arctic Region Wild Plants

Scientific Name	Common Name	Photo	Edible Part(s)	Special Preparation
Arctostaphylos uvaursi	Bearberry, kinnikinnick	 Courtesy Denise Martinez.	Fruit, leaves	Fruit can be eaten raw or cooked. Leaves can be used to make tea.
Cetraria islandica	Iceland moss	 From Department of the Army: *The illustrated guide to edible wild plants*, Guilford, Conn, 2003, Lyons Press, p 53.	All parts	Boil in several changes of water.
Empetrum nigrum *Papaver nudicaule*	Crowberry Arctic poppy	 From Letcher Lyle K: *The wild berry book: Romance, recipes, and remedies*, Minocqua, Wis, 1994, NorthWord Press, p 141. Copyright Joy Spurr.	Fruit Leaves, petals, flower buds, seeds	Can be eaten raw or cooked. Can be eaten raw or cooked.

Continued

TABLE 90-4   Arctic Region Wild Plants—cont'd

Scientific Name	Common Name	Photo	Edible Part(s)	Special Preparation
Salix arctica	Arctic willow	Copyright iStockphoto.com/RONSAN4D.	Young shoots	Can be eaten raw or cooked.

TABLE 90-5   Tropical Region Plants

Scientific Name	Common Name	Photo	Edible Part(s)	Special Preparation
Bambusa spp.	Bamboo		Young shoots	Can be eaten raw or cooked.
Colocasia esculenta	Taro	Courtesy Denise Martinez.	Root	Must be thoroughly cooked.
Maranta arundinacea	Arrowroot	Copyright iStockphoto.com/SUSANSAM.	Root	Remove outer skin and cook thoroughly.

TABLE 90-5 Tropical Region Plants—cont'd

Scientific Name	Common Name	Photo	Edible Part(s)	Special Preparation
Psophocarpus tetragonolobus	Goa bean	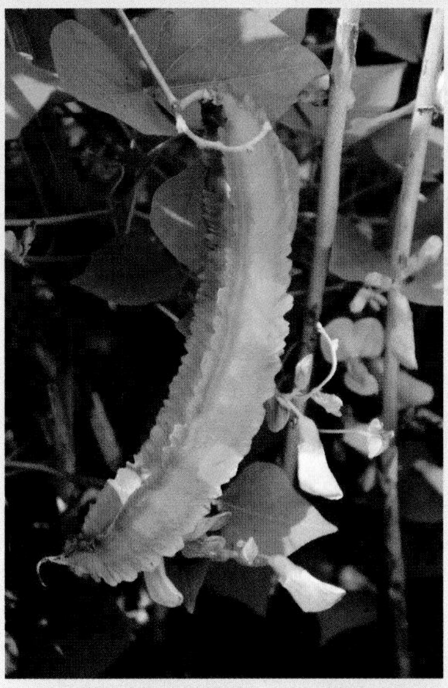 Copyright iStockphoto.com/karimitsu.	Young pods, mature seeds, root	Seeds should be parched and roasted. Other parts can be eaten raw or cooked.
Ziziphus jujuba	Jujube, Chinese date	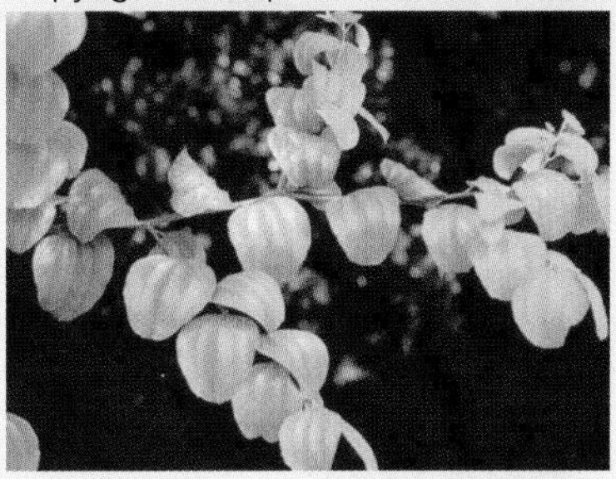 From Department of the Army: *The illustrated guide to edible wild plants*, Guilford, Conn, 2003, Lyons Press, p 37.	Fruit	Can be eaten raw or cooked. Tastes best when dried.

TABLE 90-6 Sea Plants

Scientific Name	Common Name	Photo	Edible Part(s)	Special Preparation
Alaria esculenta	Dabberlocks	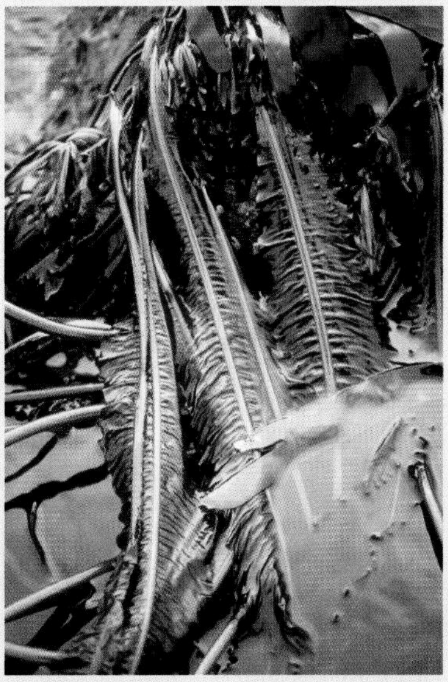 From http://www.surialink.com.	Leaves	Dry in sun or over fire. Crush and make into soup.

Continued

TABLE 90-6   Sea Plants—cont'd

Scientific Name	Common Name	Photo	Edible Part(s)	Special Preparation
Chondrus crispus	Irish moss, carrageen moss	From http://www.sb-roscoff.fr.	Leaves	Dry in sun or roast over fire. Crush and make into soup.
Palmaria palmata	Dulse	From http://omp.gso.uri.edu.	Leaves	Dry in sun or roast over fire. Crush and make into soup.
Porphyra spp.	Nori, laver	From http://www.solpugid.com.	Leaves	Dry in sun or roast over fire.

of the most common edible wild plants that can be found in specific regions of the world and how these plants are prepared. Many of these plants are easy to identify; others will take practice. Take every opportunity to practice identifying edible plants in the wilderness and in the city. Because of the challenges associated with properly identifying mushrooms and other fungi, they have been intentionally left off of the plant list. It is highly recommended that one avoid consuming fungi in a wilderness survival situation.

Understanding plant identification and toxicity is required for consumption of any wild plant. Many plants are poisonous (see Chapter 65). Tasting or swallowing even a small portion can result in severe cramping, diarrhea, rash, intestinal and metabolic disorders, and even death. When in doubt of the potential edibility of a wild plant, look for the common indicators of toxicity listed in Box 90-1.

If you have come across an unknown plant that does not exhibit any of the potentially poisonous characteristics, you can then apply the Universal Edibility Test (Box 90-2). Before testing a wild plant for edibility, make sure there is enough of the plant available to make the testing worthwhile. Test all parts of the plant separately for edibility, because some plants have both edible and inedible parts. Do not assume that a part of a plant that proved edible when cooked is edible when raw. Also, the

---

BOX 90-1   Seven Common Indicators of Plant Toxicity

1. Milky or discolored sap
2. Beans, bulbs, or seeds inside pods
3. Spines, fine hairs, or thorns
4. Dill-, carrot-, parsnip-, or parsley-like foliage
5. Almond scent in woody parts and leaves (likely contains cyanide)
6. Grain heads with pink, purple, or black spurs
7. Three-leaved growth pattern

BOX 90-2 Universal Edibility Test

1. Test only one part of a potential food plant at a time.
2. Separate the plant into its basic components—leaves, stems, roots, buds, and flowers.
3. Smell the food for strong or acrid odors. Remember that smell alone does not indicate whether or not a plant is edible or inedible.
4. Do not eat for 8 hours before starting the test.
5. During the 8 hours you abstain from eating, test for contact poisoning by placing a piece of the plant part you are testing on the inside of your elbow or wrist. Usually 15 minutes is enough time to allow for a reaction. If there is a reaction, eliminate the plant part as a food option.
6. During the test period, take nothing by mouth but the plant part you are testing and purified water.
7. Select a small portion of a single part and prepare it the way you plan to eat it.
8. Before placing the prepared plant part in your mouth, touch a small portion to the outer surface of your lip to test for burning or itching.
9. If after 3 minutes there is no reaction on your lip, place the plant part on your tongue, holding it there for 15 minutes.
10. If there is no reaction, thoroughly chew a pinch and hold it in your mouth for 15 minutes. *Do not swallow.*
11. If no burning, itching, numbing, stinging, or other irritation occurs during the 15 minutes, swallow the food.
12. Wait 8 hours. If any ill effects occur during this period, induce vomiting and drink copious amounts of water.
13. If no ill effects occur, eat 0.25 cup of the same plant part prepared the same way. Wait another 8 hours. If no ill effects occur, the plant part as prepared can be assumed to be safe to eat.

same plant may produce different reactions in different people. Bees that feed primarily on the nectar of plants (e.g., rhododendron) that are toxic to humans can produce poisonous honey (e.g., "mad honey"). Although this is extremely rare, it is worth noting if you come across a beehive in the wild.

PREPARATION OF WILD PLANT FOODS

Some wild plant foods can be eaten raw or with minimal preparation, but most need to be boiled in several changes of water to render them safe and palatable. Unfortunately, boiling often results in reduction of soluble vitamins and a plant's nutritive value. If you are unable to boil a wild plant, crush the edible plant part, put it in a sock, and securely place it in a running river for 1 or 2 days. This will help leach the astringent and bitter phytochemicals from the plant. You can do this in conjunction with boiling to help reduce preparation time.

COOKING METHODS

When possible, all wild animal foods should be thoroughly cooked before they are eaten to kill any parasites and to make the meat more palatable.

Roasting is probably the easiest way to cook a piece of meat, but is the least desirable of methods because much of the meat's nutritional value is destroyed or drips away when it is cooked in this manner. Despite this, it may be the only method that can be used when no container is available. Skewering the meat on a hardwood stick and then holding it over the flames is an expedient method to quickly cook animals, fish, or insects (Figure 90-65). Choose the stick carefully. Wood that is nonresinous is best because coniferous wood (pines, spruces and firs) may impart an unpleasant taste to the meat while it is being cooked. When using green wood, such as willow or alder, remove the bark before inserting it into the meat. By using wooden pegs, meat can also be pegged onto a slab of wood and placed near a fire, where the radiant heat will slowly cook the meat. In a rare circumstance, the wood may impart a toxin, so be familiar with toxic plants.

If a metal container is available, **boiling** is an excellent method to prepare food for consumption, especially if the broth that is created is also consumed. Alternatively, a bowl can be hollowed out of a piece of wood, which is then filled with water and the food to be cooked. Stones heated in a fire are then placed into the bowl with the food. The hot stones heat the water, and the food is cooked. As the stones cool, they are replaced with more hot ones taken from the fire. Do not use stones taken from a stream bank or other wet areas because they may explode when heated. Water contained in the rocks is converted to steam; the steam expands and explosively fractures the rock.

Baking is another effective way of cooking wild foods because the process is slow and much of the nutritive value is retained.

In *clay baking*, birds (with the feathers on) and fish (with the skin and scales) can be packed in mud or clay and then placed in the coals of a fire to bake. When using this method to cook a bird, the clay must be massaged into the feathers and the entire animal covered with a layer of clay several inches thick. Cooking time depends on the thickness of the clay and the size of the animal being cooked. Sixty minutes is usually sufficient. After this time, the hard clay shell can be broken away, exposing the cooked flesh. The skin, scales, or feathers will come away with the clay, leaving only the cooked flesh beneath.

For an *earth oven*, a hole about 2 feet deep and 2 feet square (or larger, depending on the quantity of food to be cooked) is dug, and a large hot fire is built in the hole. The fire is allowed to burn down until only coals remain and is then covered with a layer of soil. The food to be cooked is wrapped in a layer of cloth or packed in vegetation and placed in the hole. The hole is then filled in with the remaining soil and the oven left for 2 to 3 hours. After the prescribed period has elapsed, the soil is removed, and the package containing the food is carefully lifted out. Be careful when opening the oven because hot soil and steam can cause serious burns. The cooked bundles of meat and vegetation can be very fragile. Be watchful that the food is not contaminated with soil as it is taken out of the oven. Placing the wrapped food in the earth under a burning fire is a variation of this method.

Where the quantity of food is large, or an animal's carcass is to be cooked intact, a larger hole and more heat are required. For a *rock oven*, the hole is lined with rocks, and a fire is built within it. When the fire subsides, a layer of soil is placed over the hot rocks, the wrapped food is inserted, and the hole is covered with soil. Allow at least 2 hours to elapse before opening the oven to determine whether the food is cooked.

The process described above can also be used in a seashore environment. For a *sand oven*, a hole is dug in the sand, lined with rocks, and heated. The food, fish, crustaceans, shellfish, and so forth are wrapped in seaweed, placed in the hole, and left for 2 to 3 hours before removal.

Broiling foods can be achieved by placing a thin layer of flat stones over hot coals and then laying the food to be broiled on top of the stones. Meat can also be broiled by placing it on a flat rock and propping it close to a fire. Radiant heat will cook the meat. It may be necessary to turn the meat over at least once to ensure that both sides are cooked.

BASIC FOOD PRESERVATION

Most foods cannot be stored for any length of time in the wilderness without deterioration in freshness, palatability, and nutritive value. The main causes of this deterioration are microbial growth, enzyme action, and insect damage.[4] Techniques such as drying and freezing can help reduce the causes of deterioration and prolong the time that a food can be saved and eaten.

Of these techniques, drying is probably the most feasible method used in wilderness survival and living off the land. To dry meats, thinly slice them and place them across a stick or on a plank. Place them in a warm area with low humidity. You can also place them in direct sunlight. Turn meats regularly to ensure that the pieces dry throughout. Herbs (leafy plants) can be gathered and bound by their stems and hung upside down. Herbs

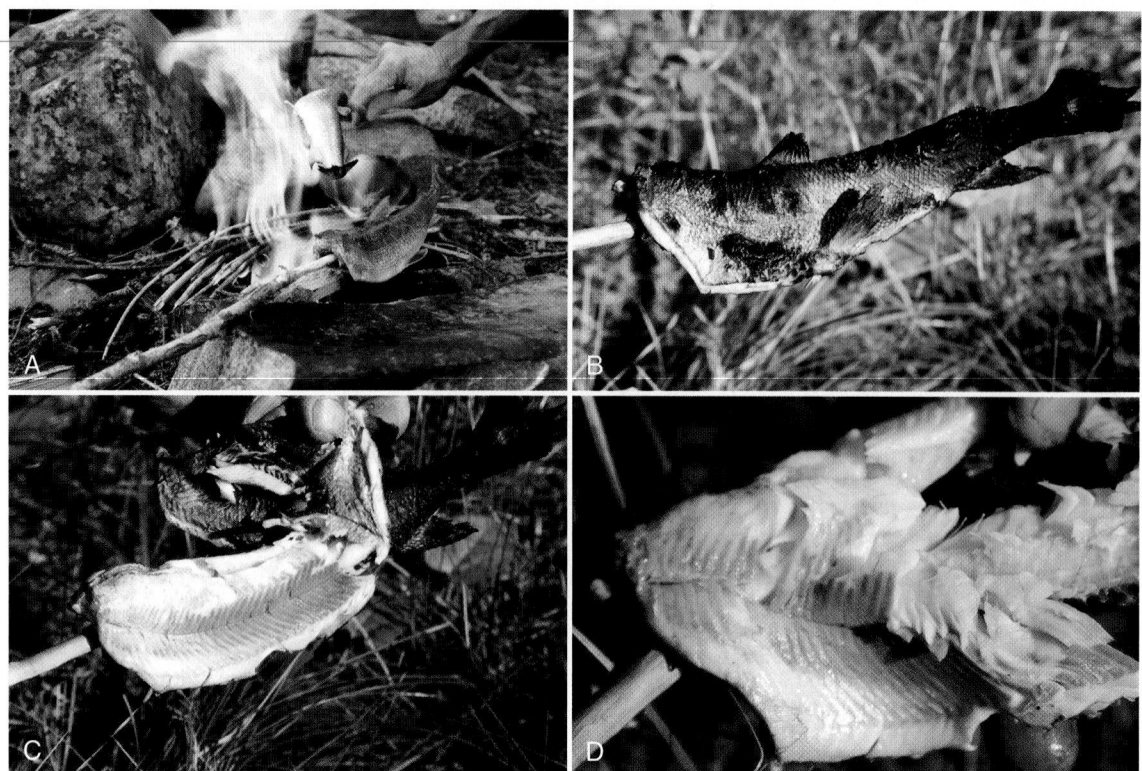

FIGURE 90-65 **A** to **D,** Roasting a fish on a stick. *(Courtesy Peter Kummerfeldt.)*

are best dried away from direct sunlight. Fruits and vegetables can be cut into small pieces and dried like meats. A screen can be made of any thin fabric, such as a light-colored T-shirt, to reduce the possibility of pest infestation. The screen should be placed so that it thoroughly protects, but does not touch, the drying food. All food should be dried in low-traffic areas free of dust.

If freezing food is a possibility, it is important to wrap the food well before freezing to avoid dehydration and cellular damage.[4] Ideally, the wrapping material should neither crack and become brittle at low temperatures nor absorb water, blood, or oil. Wrap the food with the inside of an animal hide. Foods to be frozen should be buried deeply to avoid the effects of light, changes in ambient temperature, and animal predation.

REFERENCES

Complete references used in this text are available online at www.expertconsult.inkling.com.

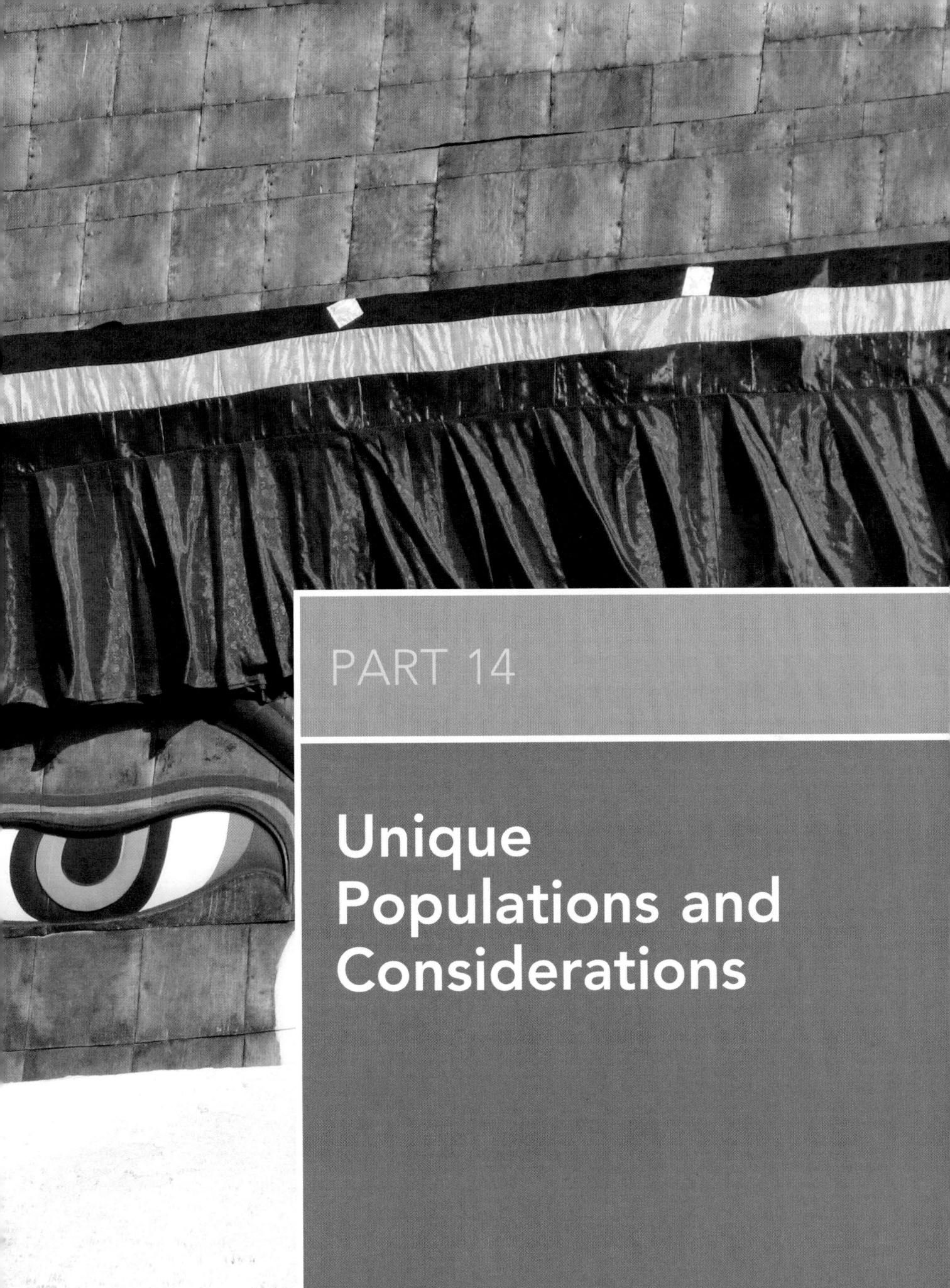

PART 14

Unique Populations and Considerations

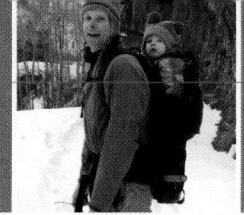

CHAPTER 91
Children in the Wilderness

JUDITH R. KLEIN

Once the realm of a few adventurous individuals, the wilderness today attracts an ever-broader range of explorers. This includes many in the pediatric age group, as parents seek to share the joys and lessons of wilderness travel with their children. In 2014, of the more than 45 million people participating in backpacking and camping, nearly 27% were younger than 18 years old.[75] Millions of children annually visit national parks and recreation areas.

Wilderness travel with children requires special preparation and places extra demands on parents. However, it also affords unique opportunities. Parents and children interact in a setting distant from the stresses of work and school. Isolated from the distractions of television and modern life, children experience new environments, interact with individuals of different cultural heritages, and participate in activities that enrich their lives. They learn to appreciate the beauty and delicate nature of the wilderness. These activities also bring families together as they learn to rely on one another for support and entertainment.

Physicians and other health care professionals can encourage and facilitate such undertakings by providing preventive health and treatment guidelines for families planning wilderness travel with children. This chapter focuses on how children differ from adults and how to prevent, recognize, and treat the medical problems children are likely to encounter in wilderness settings.

Wilderness travel may also involve travel to foreign countries. The number of families traveling outside the United States, particularly to developing countries, is on the rise, as is the number of families relocating abroad for prolonged periods. This chapter reviews risk avoidance techniques during travel, pediatric travel immunizations and prophylaxis, common pediatric medical problems seen during travel to and within developing countries, and specific issues that arise in children with chronic medical conditions.

WHAT MAKES CHILDREN DIFFERENT?

SIZE AND SHAPE

Children are distinct from adults in physical, physiologic, and psychological ways. The most obvious difference is size. During development, children may grow from the average 3-kg baby to a 60-kg adolescent, a 20-fold difference. Accordingly, medications and fluids must be calculated on an individual basis, based on the weight of the child. Table 91-1 lists average weights for age.

This variation in size also influences a child's risk of developing serious complications from envenomations. Many snakes, spiders, scorpions, and poisonous marine animals deliver the same dose of venom regardless of the victim size. Children often experience greater toxicity because of an increased dose of venom per kilogram of body weight.

Children have a larger surface area–to–body mass ratio than do adults. For example, a 3-kg infant has 2.5 times more body surface area per unit of weight than a 60-kg adult. The head, which is the part of the body most often left exposed, also takes up a larger proportion of the child's body (Figure 91-1). As a result, children experience greater exposure to environmental factors, such as cold, heat, and solar radiation. They are also more likely to suffer toxic effects from topical agents, such as medications.

MUSCULOSKELETAL SYSTEM

The musculoskeletal system in children differs from that in adults in several important ways. A child nearly doubles in height between birth and 2 years, and again between 2 and 18 years. In some respects, this rapid growth makes a child's bones much more flexible and forgiving. Because of the active osteogenic potential of the periosteum, nonunion or permanent angulation deformities at the metaphysis are unusual in children. For the same reason, fractures in the pediatric population heal quite rapidly. For example, a fractured femur typically heals in 3 weeks in a newborn, compared with 20 weeks in a 20-year-old. The strong, pliable periosteum also allows for greenstick and buckle fractures, which are not seen in the adult population. These fractures with their intact periosteum are quite stable, with little swelling or crepitus. If nondisplaced, they are often incorrectly dismissed as sprains.

Another key difference between the musculoskeletal systems of children and adults is that children have an open growth plate, or physis, at the ends of long bones. The physis connects the metaphysis to the epiphysis and consists of soft cartilaginous cells that have the consistency of rubber and act as shock absorbers (Figure 91-2). They protect the joint surfaces from suffering the grossly comminuted fractures seen in adults. However, because the growth plate is more vulnerable to injury than are the strong ligaments or capsular tissues that attach to the epiphysis, a true sprain in a child is rare. Any significant juxtaarticular tenderness in a child should be assumed to be a growth plate injury and immobilized accordingly. Such an injury is most common at the ankle (lateral malleolus), knee (distal femur), and wrist (distal radius). Physeal fractures have been classified into five Salter-Harris groups (see Figure 91-2). Salter-Harris I and II fractures generally heal without complications. Salter-Harris III and IV fractures often require open reduction of displacement to realign the joint and growth plates and to permit normal growth. A Salter-Harris V fracture has a poor prognosis; impaction and crushing of some or all of the growth plate may result in a bony bridge that inhibits further growth or causes unequal, angulated growth. Consequently, any significant injury, especially if it involves the growth plate, requires full evaluation in a medical facility.

CARDIOVASCULAR AND RESPIRATORY SYSTEMS

Basic physiologic parameters change greatly during the transitions from infancy to childhood to adulthood. Recognizing these differences is important to avoid unnecessary and potentially harmful interventions in healthy children, and to intervene aggressively when abnormal vital signs are truly present. For example, a blood pressure of 70/35 mm Hg, pulse rate of 160 beats/min, and respiratory rate of 50 breaths/min are considered ominous vital signs for an adult. However, these vital signs are normal in a 2-month-old infant. Although blood pressure readings may not be available in a wilderness setting, it is possible to assess the general appearance, work of breathing, respiratory rate, pulse, peripheral circulation, and mental status of an ill child. These observations can accurately predict how sick a child is. In general, infants and children have higher respiratory and heart rates and lower blood pressures than do adults. The normal values for various age groups are presented in Table 91-2. It is important to note that children can often maintain a normal blood pressure in the face of significant fluid or blood losses (30% to

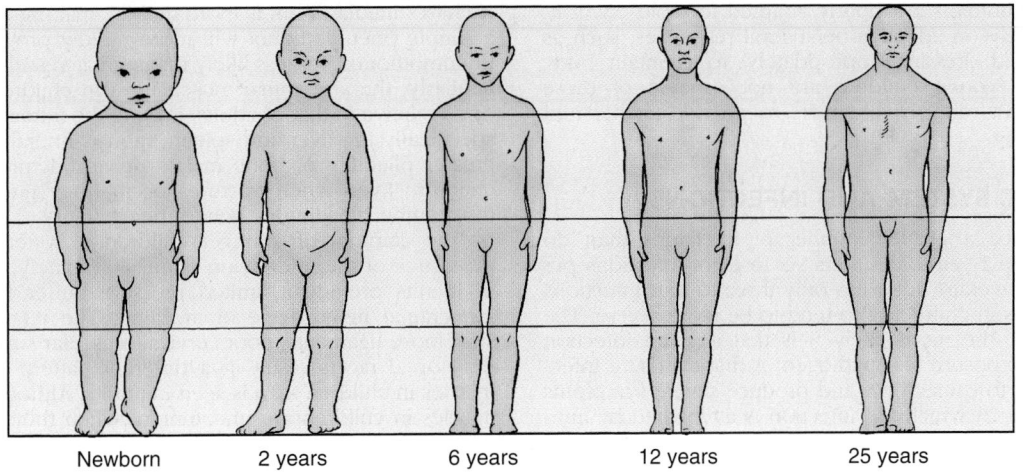

FIGURE 91-1 Body proportions.

Newborn   2 years   6 years   12 years   25 years

TABLE 91-1	Average Weight for Age	
Age	**Weight**	
yr	**kg**	**lb**
1	10	22
3	15	33
6	20	44
8	25	55
9	30	66
11	35	77
13	45	100

From U.S. Centers for Disease Control and Prevention National Center for Health Statistics: cdc.gov/nchs.

40% of total blood volume). Once the blood pressure drops, children can deteriorate very rapidly. Therefore, prompt and aggressive fluid resuscitation is essential when other signs of dehydration or volume loss (e.g., tachycardia, increased capillary refill time, cool extremities, poor urine output, decreased mental status) are present.

THERMOREGULATION

Because environmental extremes are often encountered when traveling in wilderness areas, it is important to recognize that thermoregulation is less efficient in children than in adults. A number of physiologic and morphologic differences make children more susceptible than adults to heat illness. During exercise, children generate more metabolic heat per unit of mass than do

adults. Children also have a lower cardiac output at a given metabolic rate, resulting in a lower capacity to convey heat from the body core to the periphery. Because they have a larger surface area–to–body mass ratio, children also gain heat more rapidly from the environment than do adults when ambient temperature exceeds skin temperature. In hot environments, cooling from conduction, convection, and radiation ceases to be effective, leaving evaporation (sweating) as the only effective means of heat dissipation. Unfortunately, children have a lower capacity for evaporative cooling, likely because of decreased sweat volume, regional differences in sweat patterns, and a higher sweat point (the rectal temperature when sweating starts).[55] Finally, children acclimatize to hot environments at a slower rate than do adults.

Children are also at greater risk for hypothermia. Their larger surface area–to–body mass ratio causes them to cool more rapidly than adults in cold environments. Children also have less subcutaneous fat and, therefore, less body insulation. Infants, in particular, have an inefficient shivering mechanism. This makes them particularly vulnerable to cold environments because shivering is the primary means of generating extra heat when humans are

TABLE 91-2	Age-Specific Resting Heart Rate and Respiratory Rate*	
Age	**Heart Rate (beats/min)**	**Respiratory Rate (breaths/min)**
0-5 mo	140 ± 40	40 ± 12
6-11 mo	135 ± 30	30 ± 10
1-2 yr	120 ± 30	25 ± 8
3-4 yr	110 ± 30	20 ± 6
5-7 yr	100 ± 20	16 ± 5
8-11 yr	90 ± 30	16 ± 4
12-15 yr	80 ± 20	16 ± 3

*Mean rate, ± 2 SD.

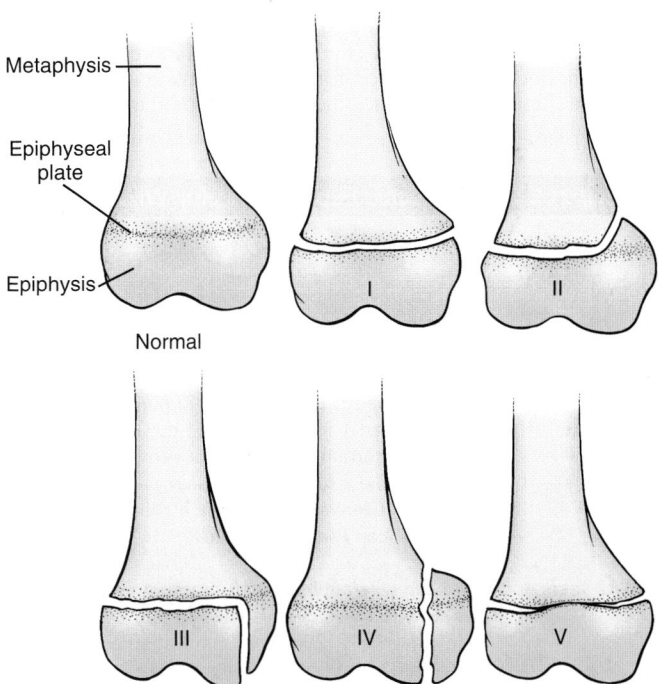

Metaphysis

Epiphyseal plate

Epiphysis

Normal   I   II

III   IV   V

FIGURE 91-2 Salter-Harris classification of physeal fractures (I to V).

cold.[7] In general, humans are poorly adapted for cold environments and must rely on adaptive behavioral responses, such as seeking shelter and dressing appropriately, to maintain body heat. Infants and young children are not capable of these responses and must rely on caregivers to provide shelter and appropriate clothing.

IMMUNOLOGIC SYSTEM AND INFECTIONS

Children experience a greater number of infections than do adults. The average 1-year-old suffers six to eight infections per year, whereas the average adult has only three to four infections per year. Infections in children also tend to be more severe. The younger the child, the more likely it is that a given infection represents a first exposure to a pathogen. A first-exposure infection is more likely to cause fever and produce severe symptoms than is reexposure, in which the infection is attenuated by antibodies produced from the first exposure. Young children are also less likely to have cross-reacting antibodies from previous infections with antigenically related organisms. When present, cross-reacting antibodies serve to attenuate the immunologic response to an infection, thereby mitigating symptom severity.

Many common respiratory bacterial or viral infections tend to produce more severe symptoms in children because of anatomic differences. The pediatric bronchioles, eustachian tubes, and larynx are narrower, and are, therefore, more easily obstructed by edema and mucus. This obstruction worsens symptoms, prolongs clearance of infection, and increases the risk for secondary infection. Pertussis (whooping cough) is a classic example of the difference in severity of infection between children and adults. Nearly 20% of infants with pertussis have severe complications, such as apnea, pneumonia, seizures, or encephalopathy. In contrast, adult pertussis, although a common cause of chronic cough, is generally indistinguishable from a common cold.

TYPES OF TRAUMATIC INJURIES

Blunt trauma is the leading cause of disorders and death in children ages 1 to 18 years. Closed head injuries are responsible for 80% of pediatric trauma deaths.[58] Although pedestrian and motor vehicle accidents are the source of many of these injuries, falls and accidents leading to drowning are close behind. Children differ from adults in their susceptibility to injuries from blunt trauma, and the nature of their injuries differs as well. As a consequence of its smaller size and conical shape, the airway of a child is more prone to obstruction. Obstruction can also occur because of the child's relatively large tongue and floppy epiglottis or the presence of mucus. A child's rib cage is more pliable and hence provides less protection for the lungs; this makes rib fractures uncommon but increases the risk for pulmonary contusion.

A child's mediastinum is more mobile, making it more likely that a simple pneumothorax will more rapidly progress to a tension pneumothorax, but less likely that a great vessel injury will occur. Similarly, the abdominal musculature in children is underdeveloped relative to that of adults, leaving the intraabdominal organs, specifically the liver and spleen, more vulnerable to injury. This greater pliability of bone makes pelvic fractures uncommon in children. Even when fractures occur, they rarely result in life-threatening bleeding or genitourinary injury.

The cranium of younger children is softer and hence less protective of the underlying brain. Fortunately, open fontanelles in infants provide a limited pressure buffer for children with intracranial hemorrhage or swelling. The relatively large head size, loose ligaments, poor cervical muscular support, and underdeveloped facets result in a different pattern of cervical spine injuries in children than is seen in adults. Although cervical spine injuries in children are uncommon, when they occur, they tend to be higher in the cervical spine and may involve injuries not visible with conventional radiography or computed tomographic (CT) scanning—thus the acronym SCIWORA, for spinal cord injury without radiographic abnormality. The term SCIWORA is somewhat of a misnomer, however, because although these injuries are not visible on radiograph or CT scan, the vast majority can be visualized with magnetic resonance imaging.

GENERAL CONSIDERATIONS AND EXPECTATIONS FOR CHILDREN IN WILDERNESS TRAVEL

Children of different ages have different needs and abilities. Expectations regarding distances of travel, pace, and safety issues vary depending on age (Table 91-3). This section explores key issues regarding wilderness travel with children of various ages and provides general expectations for each age group.

CHILDREN IN THE FIRST 2 YEARS OF LIFE

Travel Expectations

Because they are typically carried, children in their first 2 years can travel long distances, depending on the adult's hiking abilities. They do, however, place extra demands on their caregivers and require attention and care nearly all of their waking hours. Most children in this age group are content in front carriers (infants of < 6 months) or back carriers (older infants and toddlers weighing < 15 to 20 kg) and can easily travel for hours at a time. However, because of the increased risk of illness and limited communication skills, infants must be watched closely for signs of infection, hypothermia, hyperthermia, and altitude illness. Parents must be prepared to give prompt treatment

TABLE 91-3	Age-Specific Expectations for Wilderness Travel	
Age	**Expectation**	**Safety Issues**
0-2 years	Distance traveled depends on how far an adult may go with child in carrier	Provide safe play area (e.g., tent floor, extra tarp laid out) for child; put bells on child's shoes; be aware that child may put things found outside in mouth
2-4 years	Child is at a difficult age; child can hike 1-2 miles on own and needs to stop every 15 minutes	Dress child in bright colors; give child a whistle to carry and teach child how to use it (three blows for "I'm lost")
5-7 years	Child can hike 1-3 hours/day and cover 3-4 miles over easy terrain; needs to rest every 30-45 minutes	Child carries a whistle; child can carry own pack with mini–first-aid kid, flashlight, garbage bag, and water
8-9 years	Child can hike a full day at an easy pace and cover 6-7 miles over variable terrain; if child is 1.2 m (> 4 feet) tall, can use framed pack	Same as for age 5-7 years, plus adult can teach child to use a map and find a route; preconditioning can be done by increasing maximal distances by < 10%/week; watch for overuse injuries; keep weight of pack at < 20% of child's body weight
10-12 years	Child can hike a full day at a moderate pace and cover 8-10 miles over variable terrain	Same as for age 8-9 years, plus child can expand role for route planning and can learn to use a compass
Teens	Teen can hike 8-12 miles or more at an adult pace; while growth spurt is occurring, there may be a decrease in teen's pace or distance hiked	Same as for age 10-12 years, plus teen can expand survival and wilderness first-aid knowledge

or evacuate to seek medical attention should signs of serious illness develop. Evacuation plans should be formulated before departure.

Entertainment in this age group is simple. A few small toys (attached to the carrier on a short string), the natural surroundings, and a little parental attention provide ample amusement. A toddler can spend hours examining rocks, leaves, and sticks and rarely tires of a parent's undivided attention. If a child is comforted by a pacifier, it can be attached to the child's shirt or carrier, with extras packed if replacements are needed.

Safety

As babies become more active with rolling, crawling, and then walking, they require constant attention. Bells attached to their shoes may function as an alerting device, ringing when they are on the move. These children often "graze," putting everything they come across into their mouths. When they are not being carried or directly observed, it is best to have a child-proofed area for them to play in, such as a tent floor or an extra tarp. Toxic ingestions are common in this age group, and parents should be vigilant to avoid unwanted objects or plants landing in the child's mouth. Toddlers are often attracted to and fearless of water. Children of this age should never be left unattended near even the smallest streams or ponds because they can drown in even a few inches of water.

Food and Drink

Nourishment in the first 2 years is fairly simple. Infants in their first 4 to 6 months require only breast milk or formula. As long as the mother remains healthy, breastfeeding is the safest and most convenient way to feed an infant. However, if the mother is not nursing or not available, formula may be used. Formula is most conveniently carried in a powdered form and mixed as needed. The water for formula may be boiled or otherwise disinfected once a day and stored in individual bottles with airtight lids. The powder for the formula is added just before feeding. Any unused, reconstituted formula should be discarded after 2 to 3 hours at room temperature.

Baby cereals can be carried conveniently in a dry form to be mixed with formula or breast milk. Dry cereals mixed with breast milk or formula have a higher nutritional value than ready-to-feed cereals in jars. Jars of commercial pureed foods may be carried, but the empty jars must be packed out. Squeeze tubes of infant food are more convenient for all but the shortest ventures. Once a jar or tube of baby food has been opened, it should be used for only that meal. Without refrigeration, opened containers of baby food spoil quickly. Some families prefer to bring a hand grinder and make their own pureed foods.

By age 9 to 12 months, many babies are eating finger foods. Parents should be cautioned to avoid any firm round foods on which a baby may choke, such as peanuts, candies, whole grapes, or hot dogs. Up to 1 year of age, honey should be avoided because of an increased risk of botulism. Parents may also want to avoid citrus fruits, which may cause rashes around the mouth and in the diaper area. Any new food should be tested at home prior to travel to be certain the baby will accept it when away from home.

All water for drinking must be disinfected by boiling, halogenation, ultraviolet light, and/or the use of small-pore/chemical filters, depending on the water source. Chronic iodine poisoning and neonatal goiter have been associated with prolonged ingestion of large amounts of iodine, although small amounts ingested for short-duration water disinfection appear safe. It is worth noting that infants and small children often reject the taste of iodinated water. Iodine must be kept out of reach of small children; severe acute toxicity can occur with an ingestion of just 2 to 4 g. Because of toxicity issues and iodine's limited efficacy against *Cryptosporidium,* boiling, filtering, or ultraviolet (UV) light is the preferred form of water disinfection for infants and small children.

Diapers

Most children under the age of 2 years are in diapers, either disposable or cloth. Soiled diapers in a wilderness environment require special care. Thin paper diaper liners may be purchased to help collect the stool. The stool and liner should be buried in a trench at least 15 cm (6 inches) deep and 60 m (197 feet) from any water source. If disposable diapers are used, they should be packed out after the stool has been removed and buried. The used disposable diaper should be placed in a double bag for packing out. To reduce weight, urine-soaked diapers may be set out in the sun to dry. Avoid superabsorbent diapers, because they often are left on babies much longer than they should be and can lead to serious diaper rash. Also, these diapers cannot be dried out as easily and, consequently, add significant weight for the rest of the trip.

On longer trips, some families prefer to use cloth diapers, which may be washed out and reused. Cloth diapers must be changed more frequently, because they are not as absorbent. Washing cloth diapers is labor intensive, time consuming, and requires an abundant supply of water. A washbasin is needed, and the diapers must be washed in hot soapy water. The diapers should be rinsed at least twice to remove irritating soap residue, and the wastewater dumped where it will not pollute, at least 60 m (197 feet) from any water source.

Equipment

Because infants and young children are not capable of extended hikes, they are typically transported in carriers. Most front carriers work well from infancy until an age when babies can sit fairly well, typically 6 to 9 months (Figure 91-3). It is important that a front carrier extend up high enough in the back to completely support a young baby's head. Once a child is sitting well, back carriers are more comfortable (Figure 91-4). Back carriers function on the same principle as framed backpacks, redistributing the weight off the shoulders and onto the hips. Many back carriers are able to stand alone and can double as a highchair. Children must be strapped into back carriers, because it is easy for a child to be catapulted out of a carrier if the adult bends over or falls.

Sleeping bags are available for infants and toddlers, but should not be used for babies under the age of 1 year to avoid entanglement and possible suffocation. In a warm climate, a sleep sack is a safer alternative for nighttime; in a colder environment, an insulated snowsuit with hood or hat should suffice (Figure 91-5). Avoid placing diaper-clad infants into a sleeping bag with an adult; apart from safety concerns, accidents or a leaky diaper can create very unpleasant sleeping conditions. Children, including young infants, also need their own sleeping pads. Such pads protect them from hard, rough ground under the tent and insulate them from the cold ground.

Shoes for young children should protect their feet and allow for full range of movement. The best shoes for toddlers are lightweight and flexible. They need shoes that stay on well, because children can flip their shoes off while in a carrier. Velcro-strapped shoes stay on well and are easy to put on and take off. Because children often lose shoes, an extra pair should be included.

CHILDREN 2 TO 4 YEARS OF AGE

Travel Expectations

Children 2 to 4 years old are the most challenging to take into the wilderness. Two-year-olds become easily frustrated and throw temper tantrums, often as a result of the collision between adult restrictions and their desires for independence and control. By 2 years of age, children are becoming too heavy to carry for prolonged periods, but they are still incapable of hiking long distances on their own. They are just gaining bladder and bowel control, and accidents are frequent. Despite these difficulties, wilderness trips with this age group can be successful with appropriate planning, preparation, and adjustment of expectations.

A key ingredient to successful wilderness trips with small children is to keep things slow, simple, and flexible. This is the age of independence and assertion. The children need to be given some control and allowed to set a pace. Adults should encourage young children to express their natural curiosity and

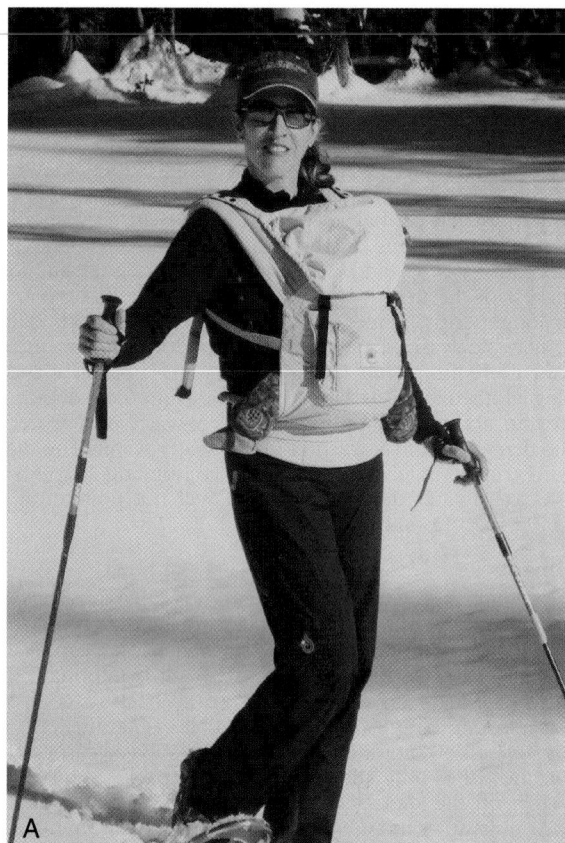

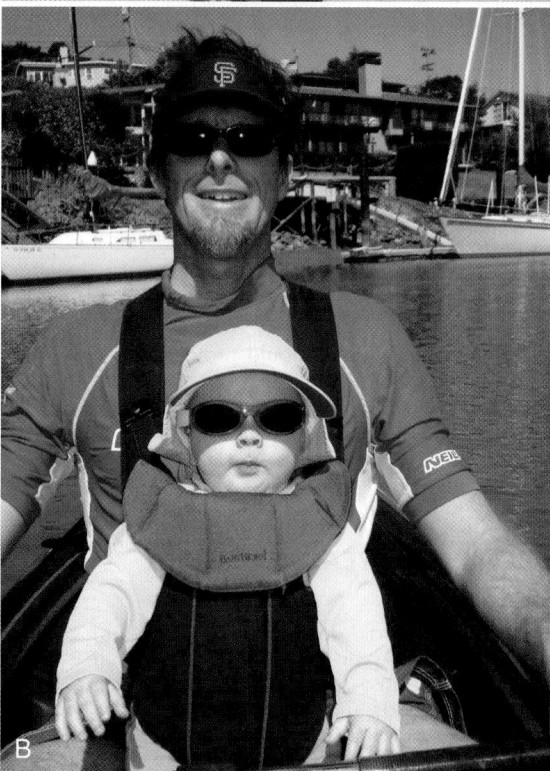

FIGURE 91-3 Infants in front carriers. *(Courtesy Judith R. Klein, MD.)*

enthusiasm for the outdoors by letting them stop to explore their surroundings. Parents can enjoy rediscovering nature through the eyes of their children by exploring rocks and tide pools and observing a caterpillar's crawl. Parents should expect to stop at least every 10 to 15 minutes while hiking. If a diversion or a stimulus is needed to get the children hiking again, parents can

begin a story or favorite song and continue it while hiking. An alternative for those willing to carry a small electronic device and headphones is an audiobook. Recorded stories are an extremely effective distraction for children in this age group, particularly if the terrain is less interesting or the day longer than expected (Figure 91-6). Overall, with patience and plenty of time, parents can expect children in this age group to travel 1 to 2 miles (1.6 to 3.2 km) under their own power over easy terrain.

Safety

Unfortunately, 2- to 4-year-olds are notorious for exploring the environment either by wandering off or by trying to become a backcountry gourmet. Young children must be watched closely and cautioned to keep wild mushrooms, plants, berries, and other inedible or toxic items out of their mouths. Children should be kept within sight at all times because their desire to explore often defies good judgment and exceeds their physical abilities. Although attacks are rare, mountain lions may view small children as easy prey and can strike quickly. Parents should, therefore, discourage their children from wandering ahead unaccompanied. Toddlers should also be encouraged to step only where they can see (i.e., on top of logs rather than over them) to avoid any unsuspecting reptile or large insect.

When selecting a campsite, dangerous features such as steep drop-offs and fast, deep water should be avoided. Children should be dressed in brightly colored clothing, so they are more easily located if they become lost. As children get older, they may carry a whistle to call for help when they are lost. The standard distress signal is three blows to indicate "I'm lost" or "I need help"; the response is two blows to indicate "help is coming." Parents should teach children to stay put once they discover they are lost and wait to let help come to them. If children panic and start running when they realize they are lost, they increase the chance not only of getting injured but also of traveling farther from the family. The concept of "hug a tree" will be described later in the chapter.

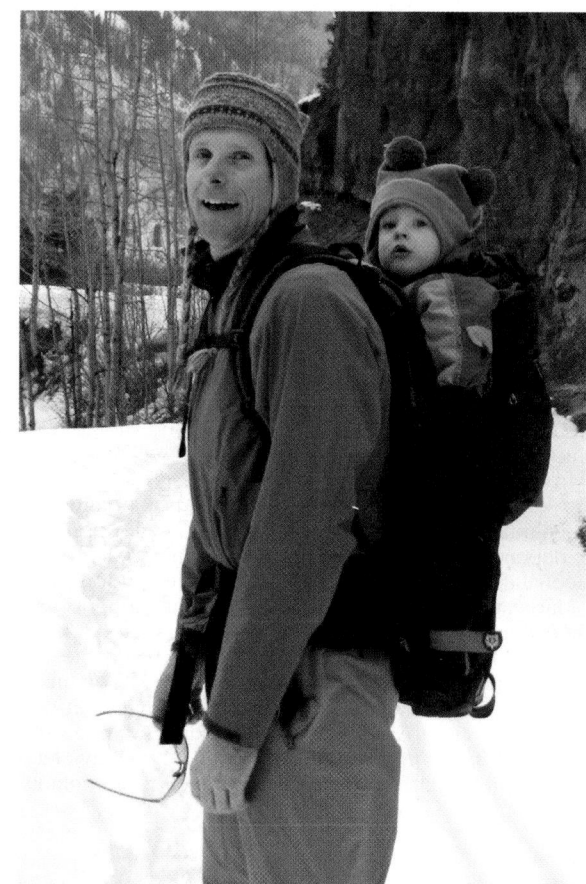

FIGURE 91-4 Toddler in back carrier. *(Courtesy Judith R. Klein, MD.)*

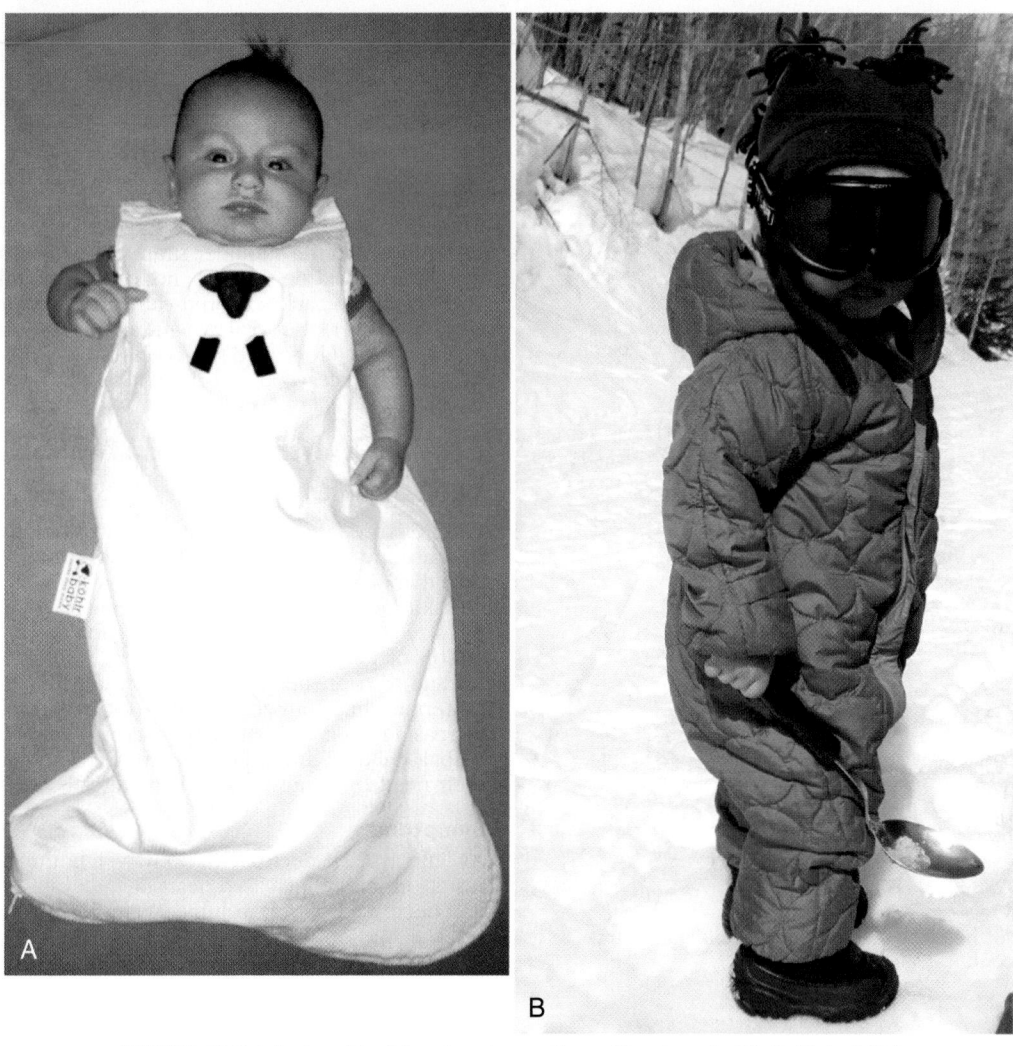

FIGURE 91-5 Infant and toddler sleeping options. *(Courtesy Judith R. Klein, MD.)*

Food

The diet of 2- to 4-year-olds is usually quite simple but very individual. They tend to have strong preferences and dislikes. Unfortunately, many children at this age do not care for the convenient "all-in-one-pot" cooking common around campfires. Foods should be tested at home first to be sure they are acceptable to the child. Nutritious snacks, such as raisins, granola bars, bagels, nut butters, string cheese, and fruit bars, can be packed. These snacks may become a child's meal. Small children should not be given items on which they may choke, such as peanuts, grapes, hard candies, or hot dogs. At least one adult member should be trained in basic cardiopulmonary resuscitation (CPR) and know how to assist a choking child.

Toileting

Most children become toilet trained by the end of their third year. However, accidents are common and parents need to be prepared with extra dry clothing that is readily accessible. Children should be taught correct toileting procedure for the wilderness environment. Stools should be deposited at least 60 m (197 feet) from a water source, buried in a hole approximately 15 cm (6 inches) deep, and completely covered. Many families carry a special trowel for this purpose. Some groups staying in one location for more than a day dig a specific toileting trench, 30 to 45 cm deep, to be used multiple times. They then add enough dirt after each use to cover all waste. Children need help learning to squat over the trench and to bury their stools.

It may be years before children gain reliable nighttime bladder control. Cotton and down sleeping bags should be avoided because they lose their insulating abilities and take a long time to dry. Fortunately, many synthetic bags are available, with fills such as Primaloft and Climashield, which maintain warmth and loft when wet. Once again, children at this age should sleep in their own sleeping bags to avoid sharing nighttime accidents with parents or caregivers.

CHILDREN OF SCHOOL AGE (5 YEARS AND UP)

Travel Expectations

Once children enter kindergarten, their abilities and attention span increase dramatically. This enables them to participate more actively in many outdoor activities. Children are hungry for knowledge and readily absorb information about nature and outdoor activities. They enjoy being included in initial planning, as well as in field activities, such as setting up camp, cooking, purifying water, and cleaning up. School-age children can understand maps and often enjoy following their progress from one point to another. This is an ideal age to explain to them the rules of survival in, living in, and traveling through wilderness areas. The examples and rules parents set for appropriate behavior in the wilderness at this age become lessons engraved for a lifetime.

When parents are planning hiking trips, it is important that they have appropriate expectations for children's evolving abilities (see Table 91-3). Children enrolled in organized sports activities are likely to have greater endurance in the wilderness. A child's hiking ability can be estimated by walks around the neighborhood or in a local park. If this practice becomes a

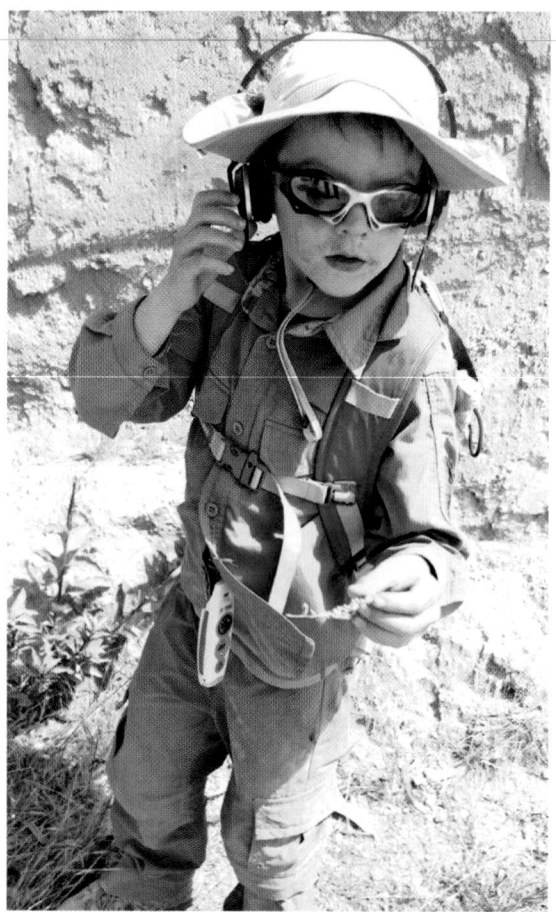

FIGURE 91-6 Use of headphones and audiobooks during treks and travel. *(Courtesy Judith R. Klein, MD.)*

first-aid kit (adhesive bandages, wipes, personal medication), insect repellent, and other survival items (e.g., pocket knife, flint and steel) as they learn to use them. The maximal weight of these packs should be 20% of the child's body weight until he or she has had significant backcountry experience and can comfortably carry more. Once children reach 4 feet (1.2 m) in height, they can be fitted for a framed backpack. Internal-frame backpacks tend to be more comfortable than external-frame packs. When a backpack is properly fitted, the waistband should rest at the hips and the shoulder strap should be adjusted so that the weight is carried on the hips, not on the shoulders (Figure 91-7). With a framed pack, children can carry even more of their own gear. However, the total weight should be gradually increased to allow the child to become comfortable with heavier loads and should not exceed 30% of the child's body weight.

ENVIRONMENTAL ILLNESSES

DEHYDRATION

Children are at greater risk of dehydration than are adults. Because the surface area–to–body mass ratio of a child is greater than that of an adolescent or adult, insensible fluid losses through the skin account for a larger percentage of total fluid losses as the size of the child decreases. In addition, the sodium concentration of children's sweat is generally less than that of adults, leading to a greater relative free water loss. Infants are unable to report thirst, an important marker of fluid deficit, thereby increasing their risk of dehydration. Even once they become verbal, children are often preoccupied and fail to report or meet their need for fluids, even when water is freely available.

Symptoms

As little as a 2% decrease in body weight through free water loss results in mildly increased heart rate, elevated body temperature, and decreased plasma volume. Water losses of 4% to 5% of body

routine, children become preconditioned, increase their endurance, and learn to pace themselves. More importantly, parents can learn what to expect and can test methods for motivating their children. It is better to underestimate than to overestimate a child's ability. Parents should also remember that children, like adults, have good and bad days, so allowances should be made.

Safety

School-age children can learn to become more self-sufficient and in tune with their surroundings. They can be taught to recognize landmarks in their environment, so they are less likely to become lost. Such landmarks can be pointed out, and children should be encouraged to view their surroundings from different angles so that they can find their way back if they stray off. Children should periodically turn around so they can see where they came from, as well as where they are going. As children advance in school years, they can learn survival skills, such as how to maintain warmth, build shelters, secure food and water, and use a signal mirror, map, and compass. As with the previous age group, they should carry a whistle and know how to use it appropriately.

Equipment

Children like to feel important, capable, and independent. These feelings are enhanced if they are allowed to carry some of their own gear. Even 5-year-olds like to carry their own soft backpacks. Items they can carry in the packs include snacks, a favorite small toy, extra clothing, sunscreen, a flashlight or headlamp, a small trash bag (excellent to wear for warmth or rain protection), and a whistle. As a child grows, the contents of his or her backpack should reflect his or her increasing independence, with more self-care and survival items. In addition to the preceding items, children may wish to carry their own water bottle, mini–

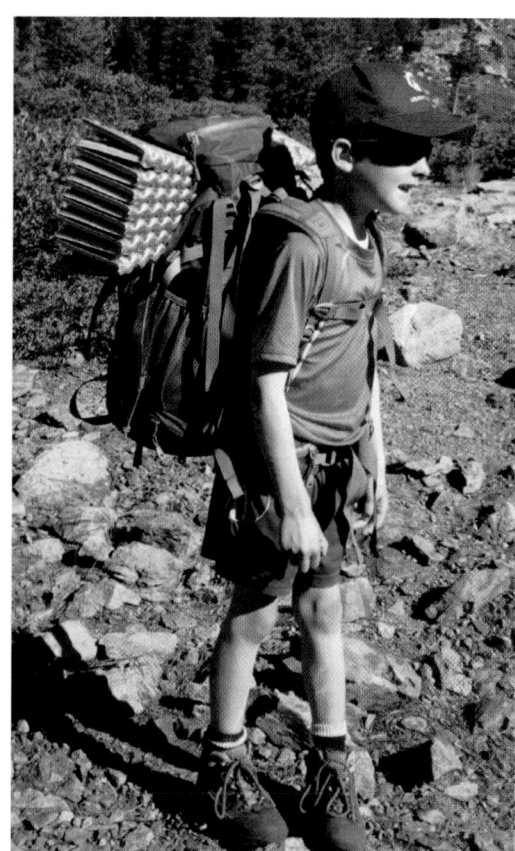

FIGURE 91-7 Backpack fit for a child. *(Courtesy Judith R. Klein, MD.)*

weight reduce muscular work capacity by 20% to 30%.[55] Symptoms of dehydration include weakness, fatigue, nausea, vomiting, and, ultimately, lethargy. In a young child, the first sign may be irritability and loss of appetite. Dehydration also predisposes a child to other environmental hazards, such as hypothermia, hyperthermia, and acute mountain sickness (AMS).

Treatment

It is the caregiver's responsibility to provide fluids and coax the child to drink frequently. For short (<2-hour) periods of activity, water is as efficacious a rehydration solution as are carbohydrate-electrolyte drinks.[55] That being said, a small amount of juice or other sweetener diluted in a larger volume of water may enhance the fluid intake of a child. Avoid undiluted juices or heavily sweetened drinks because they can worsen dehydration; the high carbohydrate load in these drinks promotes osmotic diuresis. A child eating a normal diet does not require electrolyte replacement unless sweating is prolonged or excessive. By closely monitoring a child's urine output, fluid deficits can be recognized and promptly managed. A child with decreased urine output or dark, concentrated urine needs extra fluids.

HYPOTHERMIA

Children cool more rapidly than do adults because they have a relatively large surface area and often lack the knowledge and judgment to initiate behaviors that maintain warmth in a cold environment (see Chapter 7). In addition, they have a more difficult time maintaining body temperature in cold climates, predominantly because they do not shiver as effectively.[7] As a result, parents participating in cold weather recreation with children should be able to recognize, treat, and, preferably, prevent hypothermia and frostbite.

Hypothermia is defined as core body temperature below 35°C (95°F). At this temperature, the body no longer generates enough heat to maintain body functions. The condition is considered mild when core temperature is 33° to 35°C (91° to 95°F); moderate at temperatures between 28° and 32°C (82° and 90°F); and severe when it is less than 28°C (82°F). The signs and symptoms of hypothermia are listed in Table 91-4, although these may be quite variable. The most important clue to significant hypothermia is altered mental status. An infant may become lethargic and difficult to arouse. An older child may be shivering, stumbling, or appear confused. These signs merit prompt treatment for hypothermia. Of note, the presence or absence of shivering is not a reliable marker of the severity of hypothermia. Physicians should also caution parents that hypothermia can develop at moderate ambient temperatures if adverse climatic conditions are compounded by illness, fatigue, dehydration, inadequate nutrition, or wet clothing.

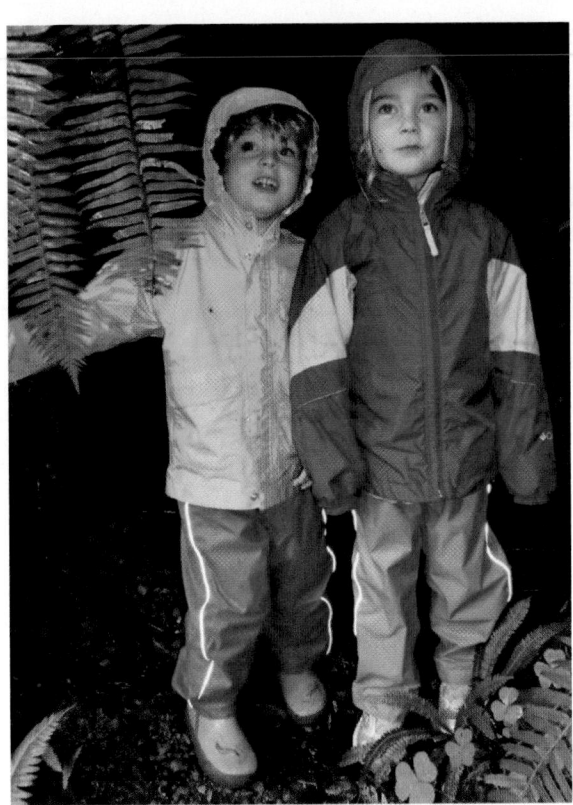

FIGURE 91-8 Layering of clothing for cold environments. *(Courtesy Judith R. Klein, MD.)*

Prevention

When preparing for cold weather activities, children should dress in layers to allow clothing to be added or subtracted as necessary (Figure 91-8). This avoids excessive perspiration while maintaining warmth. An inner, wicking layer should be followed by a middle, insulating layer and, finally, by an outer, protective layer.

Because children generally avail themselves of any opportunity to get wet, clothing that maintains low thermal conductance when moist is particularly important. Conductive heat loss may increase 5-fold in wet clothing and up to 25-fold if the child is completely immersed in water. Traditional wool retains warmth when wet because of its unique ability to suspend water vapor within the fibers; however, it is heavier than synthetics and takes much longer to dry. Cotton has a high thermal conductance that increases greatly when wet and is, therefore, a poor choice for wilderness activities in cold weather. Synthetic materials (polypropylene, Capilene, Thermax, CoolMax) wick moisture away from the skin and dry quickly, making them ideal for an inner layer. Finely woven merino wool also provides these same advantages as a wicking layer. The middle, insulating layer may incorporate wool, polyester pile or fleece, down, or similar materials. Finally, windproof and water-resistant outer garments (e.g., Gore-Tex) decrease heat loss from convection and keep children dry. Hats and mittens are also essential; the uncovered head of a child dissipates up to 70% of total body heat production at an ambient temperature of 5°C (41°F).[7]

Treatment

For the hypothermic child, field rewarming begins with limiting further exposure to the cold environment. Find immediate shelter for the child. Wet clothing should be removed, and the child's head and neck should be protected from further heat loss. Place the child together with a normothermic person in a sleeping bag insulated from the ground to provide external warmth. Hot water bottles, insulated to prevent burns, may also be placed at the axillae, neck, and groin. If the child is alert, oral hydration with warm fluids containing glucose repletes glycogen and corrects

TABLE 91-4 Signs and Symptoms of Hypothermia*		
Rectal Temperature		**Signs and Symptoms**
Mild	33°-35°C (91°-95°F)	Sensation of cold, shivering, increased heart rate, progressive incoordination in hand movements, development of poor judgment
Moderate	28°-32°C (82°-90°F)	Loss of shivering, difficulty walking or following commands, inappropriate (for the outside temperature) undressing, increasing confusion, decreased arrhythmia threshold
Severe	<28°C (<82°F)	Rigid muscles, progressive loss of reflexes and voluntary motion, hypotension, bradycardia, hypoventilation, dilated pupils, increasing risk of fatal arrhythmias, looks as if death is imminent

*Data from adult subjects.

dehydration, which frequently accompanies hypothermia. Signs of severe hypothermia (e.g., severe lethargy or confusion, diminished pulses) dictate immediate evacuation as conditions permit. Rescuers should handle the victim gently to prevent precipitating arrhythmias.

FROSTBITE

Localized cold injury can result in frostbite (see Chapter 9). Predisposing factors include wet skin, constricting garments that hinder blood circulation, fatigue, dehydration, contact with cold surfaces, and wind. If the skin temperature drops below 10°C (50°F), cutaneous sensation is generally abolished and injury may go unnoticed. Skin cooled to −4°C (24°F) freezes.

Frostbite has traditionally been divided into degrees of injury, much like burns. Determination of the depth of injury should occur 24 to 48 hours after rewarming; prior to this, frostbitten skin generally appears hard and feels numb. Skin with superficial frostbite is typically swollen, pink or erythematous, painful, somewhat warm, and often blistered. Sites with deep frostbite are cooler, not edematous, pale, anesthetic, and do not have blisters or bullae. In children, frostbite that extends into bone may affect the growth plate and result in skeletal deformities.[7] Verbal children will frequently report cold hands and feet, but adults should be vigilant about checking extremities and noses and ears of nonverbal children, particularly those poorly visible in back carriers. A mirror, frequently used, can assist in this regard. Reports of small children developing frostbite and hypothermia while being carried on the backs of adults engaged in outdoor winter pursuits are not infrequent.

Treatment

All wet and constricting clothing should be removed and hypothermia treated aggressively. Rapid rewarming, the primary treatment for frostbite, should be initiated as soon as possible. This is best accomplished by immersion of the frostbitten area in water warmed to 40°C (104°F). This temperature maximizes the rewarming speed while preventing thermal burn injuries. Thawing usually takes 30 to 45 minutes and is complete when the skin is soft and pliable. Field rewarming is indicated unless evacuation is imminent and rapid; however, great care should be taken to avoid refreezing. Refreezing causes far more damage than delayed thawing, because of formation of ice crystals in connective tissue. Vigorous rubbing should be avoided because it is ineffective and potentially harmful to skin. After thawing, proper wound care is essential. Frostbitten sites should be kept clean, ruptured bullae debrided, and the area dressed in a bulky dressing. Oral ibuprofen and topical *Aloe vera* facilitate healing. Evacuation to a medical facility skilled in the management of frostbite is essential.

HYPERTHERMIA

Families participating in wilderness activities in hot climates must take special precautions to avoid heat illnesses (see Chapters 12 and 13). Children do not tolerate the demands of exercise in the heat as well as do adults. They generate more heat per kilogram and are less able to disperse heat from the core to the periphery. Parents planning wilderness ventures with children in hot climates can follow some simple guidelines for avoiding heat illness. The most obvious guideline entails reducing the duration and intensity of activities under conditions of high climatic heat stress. Likelihood of heat illness depends on relative humidity, wind velocity, and radiant heat, as well as standard dry-bulb thermometer temperature. Figure 91-9 gives a rough guide for activity levels based on temperature and relative humidity.

Prevention

Children should be fully hydrated before prolonged exercise and actively encouraged to drink fluids at regular intervals.[55] Infants and neonates are most vulnerable to heat illness. Under high climatic heat stress, infants fed undiluted cow's milk or formula may develop marked salt retention and dehydration. They should

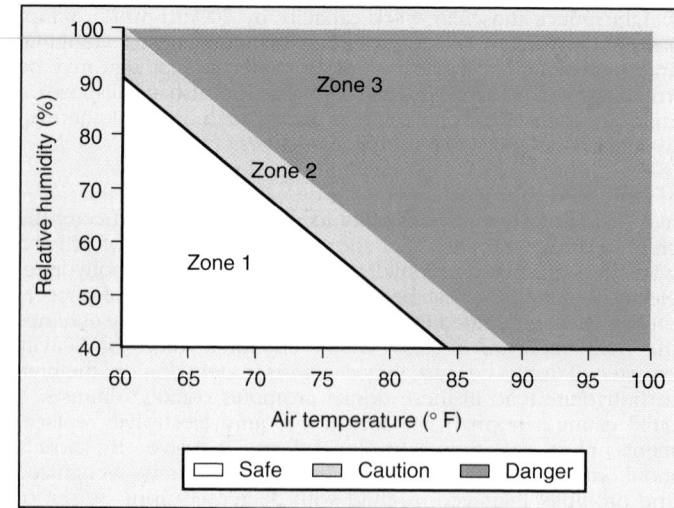

FIGURE 91-9 Activity levels based on temperature and relative humidity.

be given extra water or dilute feedings. The lower osmolar load of breast milk appears to protect against heat illness and hypernatremia.

Because their mechanism of evaporative heat loss (sweating) is immature relative to that of an adult, children should be encouraged to engage in activities in the shade to maximize other means of dissipating heat, such as radiation (skin-to-air gradient). Also, because sweat evaporated from clothing contributes less to cooling than does sweat evaporated from skin, children should be changed out of sweat-soaked clothing and wear dry, lightweight, loose-fitting clothing. As exemplified by cultures that inhabit the desert (e.g., Bedouins of Saudi Arabia), full-coverage, lightweight, and light-colored clothing items provide the most protection from heat. Finally, children acclimatize to heat more slowly than do adults, often taking 10 to 14 days to fully adapt. Intensity and duration of exercise should gradually be increased over this period.

Symptoms and Treatment

Early signs and symptoms of heat illness include flushing, tachycardia, weakness and lethargy, mild confusion, headache, and nausea. Vomiting often occurs in children. Sweating may be present or absent and should not be relied upon as a clinical indicator of the severity of hyperthermia. If heat illness develops, children should be removed from obvious sources of heat, including direct sunlight, and have their clothing removed. Convective cooling can be increased in the field by vigorous fanning after spraying or sprinkling the victim with water. Ice packs or cold compresses placed on the groin, axillae, and scalp will aid cooling. Cool-water immersion is probably the most effective means of rapid field cooling if the child's head position can be controlled. If the child is alert, dehydration should be corrected with oral fluids. Progression of symptoms or failure to respond to treatment mandates immediate evacuation.

SUN DAMAGE

Hazards of overexposure to sunlight include sunburn, photoaging, skin cancer, and phototoxic and photoallergic reactions (see Chapter 16). Climatic changes, such as global warming and ozone degradation, have increased these hazards.[10] Preventing ultraviolet damage to skin should begin in childhood, because 50% to 80% of a person's lifetime sun exposure occurs before 18 years of age.[9,30] Adolescence is the period when children are most at risk. In one study, 83% of children 12 to 18 years old reported at least one sunburn per summer; 36% reported three or more sunburns per summer.[30] Recent evidence suggests that the risk of developing malignant melanoma increases significantly with the number of sunburns in childhood.[23] This risk is even higher if a child is light-skinned with a propensity to burn rather than tan. Tolerance to sun exposure is determined by the amount of melanin in skin and ability of skin to produce melanin in response to sunlight. In general, children have lower melanin levels and thinner skin than do adults and are at greater risk for sun damage.

The ultraviolet (UV) wavelengths UVA and UVB are principally responsible for the harmful effects of solar radiation. UVB is primarily responsible for suntan and sunburn and also promotes development of skin cancer and skin aging. UVB increases 4% for every 300-m gain in elevation above sea level. Therefore, a backpacker at 3000 m will have a 40% increase in UVB exposure. UVA, which is 10 to 100 times more abundant than UVB, is only 0.001 as potent at inducing sunburn. It is also less affected than is UVB by changes in season or solar zenith angle. UVA is primarily responsible for photosensitivity reactions and solar urticaria. It also contributes to skin cancer and skin aging. A number of drugs often used in adolescence, such as tetracycline, vitamin A derivatives (Retin-A, Accutane), and nonsteroidal anti-inflammatory drugs, increase the risk of photosensitivity reactions and the need for UVA protection. Consequently, it is important to use sunscreens that protect against both UVA and UVB.

The harmful effects of UV radiation from the sun can be reduced if parents are educated regarding the dangers of sun exposure and encouraged to use sun-protective clothing and sunscreens early in their children's lives. One study demonstrated a 60% reduction in childhood sunburns with good parental role-modeling and sunscreen vigilance.[61] Regular use of sunscreen with a sun protection factor (SPF) of at least 15 for the first 18 years of life reduces a person's lifetime risk of developing non-melanoma skin cancer by 78%.[54]

Prevention

The most effective means of preventing sun damage is using protective clothing and avoiding excessive sun exposure. Midday hours (10 AM to 4 PM), particularly around highly reflective surfaces (e.g., water, sand, snow), at high altitude and at the equator are the most dangerous in terms of quantity of UV exposure. Shady areas should be used for activities during these times. Hats with wide brims and neck drapes help to protect the face and neck from sun exposure (Figure 91-10). Clothing made from tightly woven fabrics is more protective than clothing made from loosely woven fabric. For example, loosely woven fabrics, such as those used in most T-shirts, have an SPF of only 5. Most clothing loses more of its sun protective effect when wet. Several manufacturers are marketing high-SPF (25 to 50) protective clothing (coolibar.com; sunprotectiveclothing.com). This specialized clothing is cool and lightweight, dries quickly, and can maintain its full SPF capabilities when wet (see Figure 91-10). Caution is advised on overcast days, because 80% of the sun's rays still reach the earth even when the sun is not visible.[54] In addition,

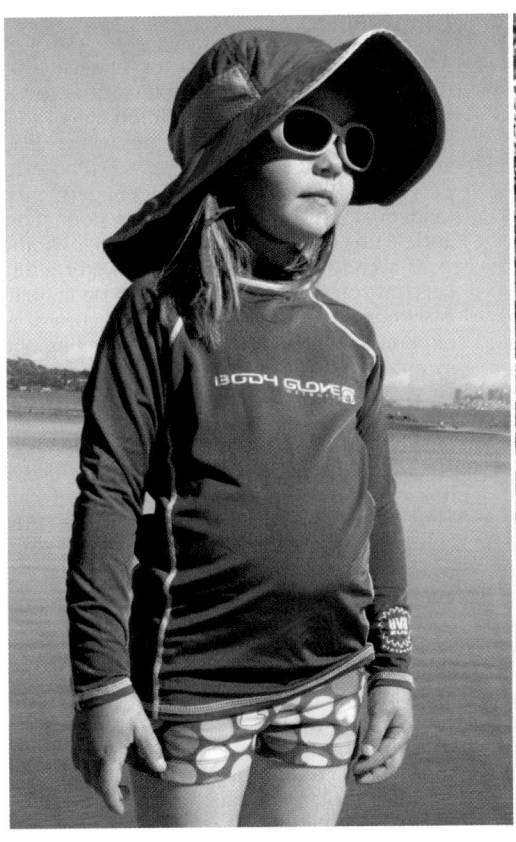
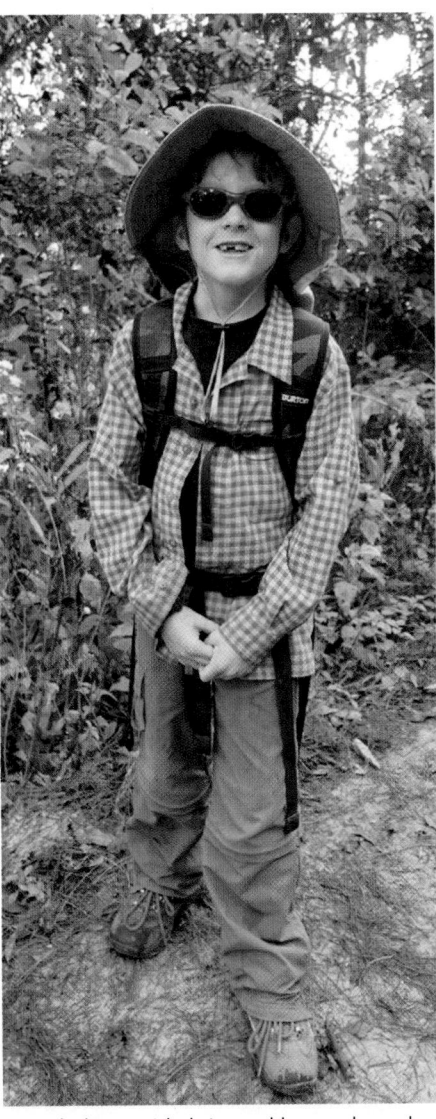

FIGURE 91-10 Options for appropriate sun wear: protective clothing, wide-brimmed hat, and sunglasses. *(Courtesy Judith R. Klein, MD.)*

because clouds filter out heat from infrared rays, children feel more comfortable and tend to stay out longer, thereby increasing their overall UV exposure.

Proper eye protection is often overlooked in infants and young children. Excessive UV light, particularly during snow and water activities, can result in UV keratitis (see Chapter 48) with even brief exposures. Properly fitting sunglasses that transmit less than 10% of UV rays should be part of a child's outdoor activity armamentarium (see Figure 91-10). Side shields and polarizing lenses are particularly important in snow conditions.

Sunscreens

Sunscreens formulated with a variety of different agents to prevent UV damage to the skin include physical blocks, chemical blocks, and antioxidants. Physical blocks, such as zinc oxide and titanium dioxide, reflect UV light and do not penetrate the skin. Chemical blocks prevent UV light from entering the skin, and are themselves absorbed into the epithelium. Chemical blocks have ingredients that block UVB or UVA, or both. Agents that block UVB include PABA, cinnamates, salicylates, and anthranilates; those that block less potent UVA rays include avobenzone and the anthranilates. Benzophenones, oxybenzone, and the physical blocking agents protect against both UVA and UVB.[54] Antioxidants present in sunscreens include vitamins C and E, resveratrol, and pomegranate. These agents help to repair skin damage. Sunscreens that combine protective ingredients with antioxidants are the most effective. The sun protection factor (SPF) is a measure of a sunscreen's effectiveness. It is measured in terms of the minimal dose (in length of time) of UV radiation required to cause skin erythema. Sunscreens with SPF 30 or higher provide a superior degree of photoprotection and almost completely prevent cellular changes seen with sunburn.[54]

Overall, there is little difference between child and adult sunscreens except for price. Parents should select sunscreens based on ingredients. Physical blocks are preferred for children because they are difficult to wash or rub off and do not degrade in the sun. Therefore, they do not need to be reapplied as frequently as do chemical sunscreens. In addition, they are much less likely than chemical sunscreens to be absorbed through skin because of their larger particle size. Several studies have suggested that certain chemical sun filters (notably benzophenones, cinnamates, camphor and parabens) may act as endocrine disrupters when absorbed through the skin of developing children, in particular affecting reproductive hormones.[43] This emerging body of evidence provides yet another reason to choose physical sunblocks for children during sensitive periods of development.

Apply a thick coat of sunscreen at least half an hour before outdoor activity. Sunscreens must be applied in adequate quantity to provide the SPF indicated on the bottle.[69] Select a sunscreen with a SPF of at least 15, but preferably greater than 30. Waterproof sunscreens are preferred if children are anywhere near water, because these products maintain efficacy for up to 80 minutes of water immersion. Sunscreens should be reapplied at least every 2 hours (or more frequently) during prolonged water immersion or excessive sweating. Cream and lotion sunscreens provide coverage superior to spray-on formulations because they can be applied evenly and in the quantities required to provide effective sun protection. Attention should be focused on applying ample sunscreen to vulnerable areas, such as the nose, shoulders, and dorsum of the feet. Infants younger than age 6 months should be outfitted with hats and protective clothing and should be placed in the shade (Figure 91-11). Sunscreens in this age group should be limited to small areas of skin only, because infant skin is thin and chemically sensitive.

Treatment

When sunburn occurs, the mainstays of treatment are cool compresses, topical antipruritics, and nonsteroidal antiinflammatory drugs. Topical *Aloe vera* cream or gel often provides a soothing effect for an uncomfortable child. Further sun exposure should be avoided while the skin is healing. As always, prevention is superior to any treatment.

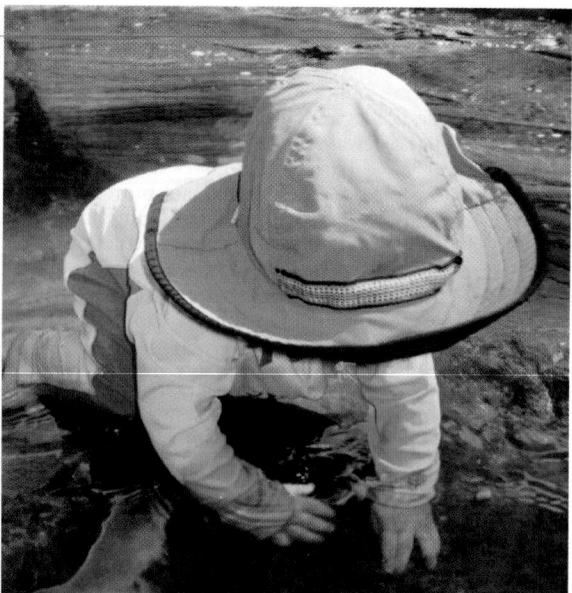

FIGURE 91-11 Infant wearing clothing with full sun protection. (*Courtesy Judith R. Klein, MD.*)

DROWNING

According to the Centers for Disease Control and Prevention (CDC), drowning (see Chapter 69) is the second leading cause of injury-related death in children ages 1 to 14 years in the United States.[85] Worldwide, drowning is the leading cause of death among boys ages 5 to 14 years.[85] Those most at risk are unsupervised toddlers and male teenagers, in particular, those with inadequate swimming skills and poor judgment. Complications and deaths result from asphyxiation, hypothermia, and/or trauma.

If a child is pulled from the water after a submersion event, cervical spine precautions should be maintained unless the event is witnessed and no trauma has occurred. All children who have experienced a period of near drowning should be observed for symptoms, have vital signs taken, and have their lungs auscultated. Respiratory distress, vital sign abnormalities, and rales on physical examination are indications for transport to a medical facility.[77] If the child is apneic or pulseless, CPR should be initiated immediately, with emphasis on effective ventilation, because this condition is the primary cause of cardiopulmonary arrest. Five rescue breaths should be given prior to initiating chest compressions because initial ventilation may be difficult due to water in the alveoli. The child should be transported to an emergency care facility as quickly as possible. All wet clothing should be removed and rewarming initiated.

Prognostic assessments based on the initial appearance of the child should not be made in the field, particularly in the setting of cold water immersion. Reduction of brain temperatures by 10° C (50° F) during drowning decreases adenosine triphosphate consumption by 50%, doubling the time that the brain can survive intact during a period of apnea.[77] Survival with good neurologic outcome has been documented in children with prolonged (> 40 minutes) submersion in cold water. The exception to this would be a drowning event in a remote wilderness area, where transport and evacuation times may be extremely long. That being said, emphasis in the field should be on rapid rescue and immediate CPR.

Prevention

Preventive measures are critical to reduce the number of drowning and near-drowning incidents. Most importantly, children should be taught to swim at an early age and learn to "read" the water and make appropriate judgments regarding water safety. They should be taught to swim with a buddy, particularly in moving and deep water. Young children should always be supervised by an adult skilled in CPR and water rescue. Use of a personal flotation device (PFD) is highly encouraged until the child is a strong swimmer capable of treading water for prolonged periods. Air- or foam-filled toys, such as rings or noodles, or floats placed on the arms should not be used in place of PFDs. Cold water, rapidly moving current, water hazards, and large waves should be approached with extreme caution and only by strong swimmers.

HIGH-ALTITUDE ILLNESS

High-altitude illness (see Chapter 1) can be viewed as a continuum from acute mountain sickness (AMS) to life-threatening conditions such as high-altitude pulmonary edema (HAPE) and high-altitude cerebral edema (HACE). AMS usually develops within 24 hours of ascent. The incidence and severity of AMS depend on individual susceptibility, as well as rate of ascent and altitude attained. In one study, 37% of children who ascended rapidly to 3500 m developed AMS.[11] Studies have shown mixed results in terms of the relative incidence of AMS in children versus adults, but children may more susceptible to hypobaric hypoxia than are adults.[56]

Symptoms

Children need to be queried frequently for the onset of symptoms because they are less likely to speak up and report symptoms than are adults. The cardinal symptoms of AMS are throbbing headache, anorexia, and malaise. Children are particularly prone to nausea and vomiting. Other symptoms include dizziness and fragmented sleep. Infants may display nonspecific findings, such as irritability, poor feeding, and sleep disturbance. As AMS worsens, headaches become more severe, and nausea and anorexia progress to vomiting. Dyspnea at rest and confusion and ataxia mark development of the life-threatening conditions HAPE and HACE, respectively.

Prevention

The safest and most effective method of preventing high-altitude illness is to allow for acclimatization via graded ascent. No precise, scientifically proved guidelines exist, given the markedly variable individual susceptibility to altitude illness. However, general recommendations for children (and adults) without altitude experience are listed in Box 91-1. After day trips to higher altitude, children should return to lower altitude to sleep in order to aid acclimatization. The sleeping altitude is particularly important with regard to development of symptoms. A high-carbohydrate diet and plenty of fluids can also help reduce the risk of high-altitude illness.

Acetazolamide has been convincingly shown to reduce the incidence of AMS in adults.[24] Pretreatment with this agent mimics the acclimatized state by inducing hyperchloremic metabolic acidosis, allowing for inducing published studies of its efficacy in children, but clinical experience suggests that it is beneficial. The primary indication for acetazolamide prophylaxis in children is a history of recurrent AMS despite graded ascent.[56] Acetazolamide is given at 5 mg/kg/day, in two divided doses, up to a maximum daily dosage of 250 mg. It should be started 24 hours before ascent and continued for 3 to 5 days while at maximal altitude. It can be discontinued once descent has begun. Side effects include nausea, mild somnolence, and paresthesias that can be particularly bothersome in children. Ibuprofen as a prophylactic agent for AMS has also been examined in several studies in adults only. The presumed mechanism of action of ibuprofen is modulation of the inflammatory cascade that leads to AMS. Taken on the day of initial ascent until peak altitude is reached, ibuprofen at 600 mg three times a day (10 mg/kg/dose in children) has been shown to reduce the incidence of AMS relative to both placebo and acetazolamide.[48,62] Dexamethasone prevents or reduces symptoms of AMS in adults, but its use is discouraged in prevention of AMS in children, because it masks early symptoms of AMS and thereby encourages continued ascent. Ginkgo biloba has also been studied as an herbal alternative to acetazolamide for prevention of AMS; its efficacy is uncertain because of variability in commercially available formulations.[45] Salmeterol, an inhaled long-acting β-agonist, has been studied as a prophylactic agent against HAPE in adults, but has not been evaluated in children.

Treatment

Treatment of mild AMS requires prompt recognition of symptoms, cessation of ascent, and allowing time for acclimatization. Proceeding to higher altitude in the presence of symptoms is strongly contraindicated and may lead to the life-threatening conditions HAPE and HACE. Symptomatic therapy includes rest, acetaminophen for headache, and adequate hydration. Ondansetron (Zofran) may be used to relieve nausea and vomiting. Dystonia in response to phenothiazines, such as promethazine, occurs disproportionately in young children, so these agents should be avoided. Ondansetron is given orally at 0.1 to 0.15 mg/kg up to 4 mg every 4 hours. If symptoms resolve, the child may continue to ascend slowly. However, if symptoms progress or fail to improve, descent is mandatory. Although descent should proceed as far as necessary for improvement, 500 to 1000 m is often sufficient. If immediate descent is not possible, oxygen should be administered. Studies examining dexamethasone and acetazolamide for treatment of AMS suggest that both are effective.[24] Dexamethasone should be reserved for patients with moderate to severe AMS or HACE. Symptoms of HACE or HAPE demand immediate descent and possible evacuation to a medical facility.

BITES AND STINGS

Bites and stings occur commonly in the pediatric age group. In 2012, the American Association of Poison Control Centers reported that more than 20,000, or roughly one-third, of reported bites and stings occurred in individuals under the age of 20 years.[57] Remarkably, no fatalities were reported in this age group. This emphasizes the need for appropriate triage to determine which children require aggressive therapy so that potentially harmful field interventions can be avoided.

Dangerous interactions between children and surrounding fauna can be limited by judicious use of protective clothing, sturdy footwear, appropriate chemical barriers, and education. These principles apply to snakes, bees, wasps, yellow jackets, mosquitoes, and ticks.

Snakebites

Of the 8000 venomous snakebites that are estimated to occur in the United States each year, about 20% occur in people under the age of 20 years.[57] Deaths from domestic snakebites are uncommon, with none reported in children in the 2012 Annual Report of the American Association of Poison Control Centers. More than two-thirds of bites in children are on the lower extremities; these are predominantly in younger children walking or running over rocks and in brush. Most snakebites can be prevented. Children should be instructed not to handle snakes, not to reach blindly into crevices, and to avoid turning over rocks and fallen limbs. A useful adage is that hands and feet should never go where the eyes cannot see. When walking through endemic areas, hikers should stay on trails and wear long, loose pants and boots that extend above the ankle (see Figure 91-10). Campsites should be on open ground, away from wood piles or rock piles.

If a bite occurs, the child should back well away from the snake and be calmed. Agitation and movement of the bitten

---

BOX 91-1 Preventing High-Altitude Illness

Avoid abrupt increases of more than 500 m in sleeping altitude per night above 2500 m.
Spend 2 or 3 nights at 2500 to 3000 m before ascending further.
Climb high; sleep low.
Drink sufficient fluids.
Eat high-carbohydrate foods.
Avoid artificial sleep aids (e.g., diphenhydramine).
Consider using prophylactic acetazolamide.

extremity might promote venom circulation. The wound should be cleansed rapidly and any constricting items of clothing or jewelry removed. The bitten extremity should be immobilized and positioned at the level of the heart. No incision over the bite should be made. Mechanical suction (e.g., Sawyer extractor) is ineffective at removing snakebite venom and can worsen tissue ischemia in the 99% of endemic snakebites that are inflicted by members of the crotalid family (rattlesnakes, cottonmouths, copperheads).[2] Advanced techniques for potentially limiting venom spread, particularly with exotic snake envenomations, are discussed in detail in Chapters 35 and 36. All victims of potentially poisonous snakebites should be transported to a medical facility for prompt evaluation, local wound care, and possible antivenom administration. Crotalidae Polyvalent Immune Fab antivenom (CroFab, BTG International) has been shown to be safe and effective in children, particularly if administered early.[31]

HYMENOPTERA STINGS

Hymenoptera (bees, wasps, hornets, and ants) stings are the most common cause of envenomations in children (see Chapter 41). Although Hymenoptera venom possesses intrinsic toxicity, the amount delivered is small and multiple stings are necessary for significant human morbidity. However, the venom components are potent antigens capable of producing anaphylaxis mediated by immunoglobulin E in sensitized individuals. Although children appear less susceptible to systemic reactions than are adults, physicians should educate parents in the management of Hymenoptera stings, particularly if a child has previously had a severe reaction.

Hymenoptera stings usually produce local pain, swelling, and erythema. If a stinger is embedded, it should be removed as quickly as possibly by whatever means available, because the speed of removal of the stinger is far more important than the method of extraction.[84] Within 20 seconds, 90% of the contents of the venom sac are discharged into the victim, and 100% within 1 minute.[12] Applying ice or cool compresses reduces pain and swelling. Elevation and immobilization are indicated for large local reactions on extremities. In older children, oral antihistamines may provide additional symptomatic relief.

Early signs of a systemic reaction include generalized pruritus, urticaria, angioedema, bronchospasm, and laryngeal edema. Presence of these signs or symptoms mandates immediate medical evaluation. Aqueous epinephrine (1:1000) is the drug of choice for systemic sting reactions and should be administered in the field if available (0.01 mg/kg intramuscularly up to 0.3 mg). Epinephrine is easily delivered in the field with an EpiPen or EpiPen Jr. These contain a spring-loaded automatic injector that delivers 0.3 mg (EpiPen) or 0.15 mg (EpiPen Jr) of epinephrine IM when triggered by pressing the device against the thigh. The EpiPen Jr. is appropriate for children up to 15 kg, and the regular EpiPen is appropriate for larger children and adults. Carrying two EpiPens is recommended because transport times to definitive medical care are often longer than the effective half-life of a single dose. In addition, in a dire situation, an extra dose of epinephrine can be accessed from an EpiPen by cutting away the autoinjector mechanism and using the syringe and needle directly. Because up to one-half of all patients with anaphylactic reactions have no forewarning, epinephrine belongs in all wilderness medical kits.

Mosquito Bites

Mosquitoes not only present a high nuisance potential but also serve as vectors of disease (see Chapter 39). A number of steps can be taken to avoid mosquito bites (Box 91-2). A proper wardrobe that provides an excellent physical barrier is the first defense. This should include ankle-high footwear, pants cinched at the ankles or tucked into socks, a long-sleeved shirt, and a full-brimmed hat. Mosquito head netting draped over a child's hat will protect the face and neck. Mosquito netting, especially in the sleeping area, has been found to reduce the mosquito attack rate by 97%.[15]

Repellents containing DEET (N,N-diethyl-m-toluamide) are effective against mosquitoes, ticks, black flies, and many other

---

BOX 91-2   Mosquito Avoidance

Wear hat, long-sleeved shirt, and pants. Tuck pants into socks.
Minimize outdoor activities at dusk.
Use mosquito netting to cover the heads of children and the sleeping area.
Soak or spray clothing, netting, and screens with permethrin (Permanone or Duranon).
Use insect repellents with picaridin or < 35% DEET on exposed skin only, avoiding children's hands.
Apply repellents over any other creams such as sunscreen to minimize absorption and maximize the repellent effect.
Keep repellents out of reach of small children.

DEET, N,N-diethyl-m-toluamide.

---

arthropods. DEET works by providing a vapor barrier that presents the insect with an offensive odor and a bad taste. DEET has an extensive safety record; over 50 years, there have been only 43 case reports of toxicity.[42] These rare toxic effects are more common with high concentrations and include dermatitis with erythema, bullae, and skin necrosis, and, even more rarely, meningoencephalitis. A large study based on data from the American Association of Poison Control Centers refuted the commonly held belief that children are more susceptible to DEET toxicity. The study demonstrated that children actually have less severe outcomes after DEET exposures than do adults.[8,42] Although products containing 100% DEET are commercially available, long-acting formulations of less than 30% to 35% DEET appear equally effective in protecting against mosquitoes, with much less potential for toxicity.[60,80] Although available data do not permit precise safety guidelines, infants younger than 6 months should avoid DEET, but those older than 6 months can use products with up to 30% to 35% DEET. The repellent effect can last up to 8 hours, but heavy perspiration or swimming should prompt reapplication every 6 to 8 hours. Dawn and dusk are particularly risky times; outdoor activities should be limited at these times if possible. Parents should not allow children under 8 years old to apply DEET to themselves, because of the risk of DEET exposure to the eyes or mouth in this age group. Repellent should not be applied over lacerations, wounds, or irritated skin because of increased risk of absorption. DEET products can be applied over other creams to maximize the repellent effect. Combination sunscreen and repellent products should be avoided, because the instructions for use of the two ingredients are different (e.g., sunscreen requires more frequent application) and because sunscreens may increase skin absorption of DEET. In addition, some studies have shown that DEET can degrade sun-filtering chemicals, thereby decreasing the SPF of the sunscreen.[42] Parents should also be cautioned to keep DEET out of reach of small children, because ingestion may be fatal.

Picaridin (e.g., Natrapel) is an alternative to DEET. Commonly used in Europe and Australia, it is odorless, minimally toxic, and considered by the World Health Organization (WHO) and the U.S. Environmental Protection Agency to be an effective insect repellent. Although picaridin does not have the lengthy record of efficacy and safety of DEET, concentrations of up to 20% are considered effective against a broad array of biting insects for up to 8 to 10 hours. Picaridin is not recommended for children under 2 years of age. Botanical products have increasingly been marketed as safer, more "natural" alternatives to chemical repellents. These include oil of lemon eucalyptus, lavender oil, soybean oil, and geraniol oil. In various studies, oil of lemon eucalyptus has been shown to be as effective against mosquitoes, biting flies, and gnats as low-concentration (7% to 15%) DEET products.[42] It is not particularly effective against ticks. Where data are available, the other oils appear to be even less effective.[80] Although natural products may be acceptable in areas where mosquitoes do not carry disease, in U.S. areas with persistently active West Nile virus disease and tick-borne diseases, and certainly in much of the tropical developing world where malaria and dengue fever are endemic, these products are inadequate. Also, the above oils have been associated with aspiration pneumonitis when accidentally ingested by young children. They are not recommended for children under 3 years of age.

The pesticide permethrin, available as a 0.5% spray or soaking liquid (Permanone, Duranon Tick Repellent), is safe and effective against arthropods, especially ticks. Unlike DEET, permethrin requires direct contact with insects in order to repel, so should not be applied to skin. Permethrin should be applied to clothing, bed sheets, and netting for maximum efficacy. Permethrins as a class have low toxicity in mammals. The combination of DEET applied to exposed skin and permethrin treatment of clothing is particularly effective in protecting against mosquito and tick bites. This combination can reduce mosquito bites by up to 99% for up to 8 hours.[52] The protective effect of mosquito netting is also greatly enhanced when it is impregnated with permethrin. These effects are longer lasting with permethrin soaks (up to 20 washings) than with permethrin spraying (5 washes) of clothing and netting. Alternatively, clothing, bed nets, and bed sheets are available that are made of fabric already treated with permethrin and effective for 25 washings (buzzoffoutdoorwear.com).

West Nile virus (WNV) disease continues to be a concern across the United States, with over 30,000 cases and 1500 deaths reported from 48 states by 2010.[87] During 2012, another major outbreak occurred with nearly 6000 new cases. Infection is uncommon in children; they represent only 5% of known WNV cases. WNV disease is a zoonotic disease transmitted from animal hosts to humans via infected *Culex* mosquitoes. Most infected individuals are asymptomatic, but 20% develop a mild nonspecific febrile illness and 20% to 25% develop a maculopapular rash lasting less than a week. Overall, 9% of reported cases had neurologic involvement, mostly in adults. Protection against bites during the active daytime hours of the *Culex* mosquito is the only means of prevention of WNV-related disease in humans.

Tick Bites

Like mosquitoes, ticks serve as vectors for disease, most notably Lyme disease (see Chapter 42). Lyme disease is rare on the Pacific coast but endemic in the northeastern United States, where up to 30% to 50% of *Ixodid* ticks are carriers.[27] As global temperatures rise, the northern range of the *Ixodid* tick is expanding, so we are likely to see more cases extending into Canada. The number of cases in the United States each year has leveled off at nearly 35,000 cases reported to the CDC in 2013.[66] Children between the ages of 5 and 9 years have the highest incidence of Lyme disease, likely because of extended outdoor play.[89] Transmission of the Lyme spirochete, *Borrelia burgdorferi,* typically requires 48 to 72 hours or more of tick contact. Therefore, tick checks should be conducted regularly while traveling through wilderness areas. If a tick is found embedded in skin, it should be grasped with forceps close to the skin surface and gentle traction applied. Using alcohol or an open flame for removal is strongly discouraged, because these techniques do not tend to work and can induce tick salivation or regurgitation into the wound.

After tick removal, parents should observe the child for appearance of a large erythematous or targetoid annular lesion at the bite site within 7 to 10 days, but occasionally as long as 30 days. This rash, erythema migrans, either painful or pruritic, is characteristic of early localized Lyme disease. If neglected, the rash spreads and fever, neurologic symptoms, and arthritis may develop. Treatment for early-stage Lyme disease in children 8 years of age or younger is amoxicillin 40 mg/kg/day (for a maximum dose of 1500 mg) divided into three doses for 14 to 21 days; for children older than 8 years of age, doxycycline is given at 2 mg/kg (for a maximum dose of 100 mg) twice a day for 14 to 21 days. A vaccine against Lyme disease is no longer commercially available. Some infectious disease experts have advocated antibiotic prophylaxis for individuals over 8 years of age if tick exposure exceeds 36 hours and if the prevalence of the spirochete in ticks in the area is more than 20%.[89] Prophylaxis, if given, is doxycycline 4 mg/kg in a single dose, up to a maximum of 200 mg. As with mosquitoes, clothing and chemical barriers, such as DEET and permethrin, are the first lines of defense against ticks and the diseases they carry. Children should be dressed in light-colored clothing for outdoor play so ticks are more visible during tick checks.

LOST CHILDREN AND SURVIVAL

It is common, but preventable, for children to become lost in the wilderness. Children should be taught to recognize landmarks and to turn around and look backward periodically to familiarize themselves with the terrain. Those who are capable of reading a compass and topographic map should carry these items at all times. Young children should wear brightly colored clothing to facilitate a search should they become lost. They should carry a whistle around their necks and be taught the universal signal for help: three blasts in a row. It should be emphasized to the child that the whistle is intended for emergency use only. Portable two-way radios can also be used for emergency communication if a child is lost. Depending on the model, the range can extend 2 to 5 miles, but mountains and ridges can cause interference. As soon as they are able to carry a backpack, children should be equipped with survival items. A flashlight, bottle of water, extra food, and a few brightly colored garbage bags can make all the difference for a child forced to spend several hours or a night out in the wilderness. Also, every child should carry a piece of paper with his or her parents' names, address, and phone number on it. Older children who venture out without their parents should always tell an adult where they are going, with whom, and when they expect to return.

A few programs, such as Hug-a-Tree (gpsar.org/hugatree. html), instruct children in the basics of survival when lost. The title of the program is intended to remind children of three important tenets of survival when lost: stay in one place to facilitate any search, take advantage of the natural shelter provided by a tree, and feel the security and calming effects of a large natural protector. By hugging a tree and not wandering around, children can work on making signals out of rocks or branches, thereby indicating their location. Children should be taught to make themselves look big and noisy (coats or arms in the air, blow a whistle) or to lay down with arms out if they hear a helicopter. Children should learn to avoid getting wet (e.g., wear a garbage bag if it is raining and avoid rivers or lakes), to wear a hat, and to stuff pine needles or dry grass into their clothes to insulate themselves if they become chilled. Children can practice making temporary shelters out of logs, branches, and leaves and thereby experience the warmth and protection provided by these natural features. They should avoid lying directly on the ground and should use leaves and branches to insulate themselves from the cold earth or snow. Children should be advised not to eat anything with which they are not familiar. The program also reminds children that there are no animals "out there" in the United States that will hurt them (e.g., "lions, tigers, bears") and that they should yell at any noises that they hear. Finally, children should be reminded that they will not be punished for getting lost and that lots of people will be looking for them, so they should just stay put. Parents should be encouraged to mobilize search and rescue resources early, before time and foul weather obscure a child's tracks.

Older children and adolescents who plan on spending time in the wilderness should be encouraged to participate in a program that teaches basic survival and first-aid skills. Several organizations, such as Lifeschool's Go Adventures in Bodega, California (goadventure.org/), and the National Outdoor Leadership School (NOLS: nols.edu) provide instruction for children. Lifeschool is intended as an introduction to the backcountry for children ages 12 to 18 years, whereas NOLS provides more technical instruction in various forms of wilderness travel, in addition to first-aid and survival training.

HOMESICKNESS

Most children experience some degree of distress when faced with separation from home, particularly when they are not accompanied by a parent. Predisposing factors to the depression and anxiety referred to as homesickness include young age, little prior separation experience, high parental separation anxiety, great perceived distance from home, few initial positive experiences after separation, preexisting anxiety or depression, and little perceived control over the situation.[78] Parents should be encouraged to introduce short periods of separation from home and family, leading up to longer periods. They should discuss the exciting aspects of any future adventure and encourage active decision making regarding activities and the destination. Parents should also try to alleviate their own separation anxiety and ensure positive early postseparation experiences for their child.[78] The presence of familiar faces, such as friends or favorite playmates, can significantly reduce a child's feeling of homesickness. Activities that include a child's favorite games and meals will be remembered by the child as fun experiences in which he or she would like to reengage. Through careful planning and coordination, parents can do much to allay the fear and anxiety of children as they travel away from home.

FOREIGN TRAVEL WITH CHILDREN

Visits to foreign countries provide superb educational, social, and cultural experiences for children. According to the CDC, an estimated 2.2 million U.S. children traveled abroad in 2010, a number that has steadily increased.[80] Traveling to wilderness or rural areas within developing nations entails not only the risks of wilderness travel but also those of poor sanitation conditions with exposure to bacteria, viruses, protozoa, and helminths not usually seen in the developed world. Although there is little consensus among experts, parents should be made aware of the greater risks of traveling to a developing country with a child under 2 years of age. This increased risk is the result of incomplete immunizations, an underdeveloped or naive immune system, poor hygiene practices (e.g., hands to mouth), and age- and weight-based contraindications for vaccinations and various medications.

It is the role of some physicians to provide guidance and information to parents planning foreign travel. Emergence and widespread availability of the Internet has provided physicians and travelers with easily accessible and up-to-the-minute guides to disease outbreaks, immunizations, and symptoms and treatments for various tropical diseases. Reliable sources for this type of information are listed in Table 91-5.

Preparation for foreign travel with children includes identification and avoidance of risky endeavors, administration of appropriate immunizations and prophylactic medications, knowledge of common childhood diseases and the means of treating them, understanding prevalent tropical diseases in the area of travel, and, finally, comprehensive follow-up after the trip with an informed physician. Physicians should be aware of the impact of foreign travel on children with chronic medical conditions.

GENERAL RECOMMENDATIONS FOR TRAVEL WITH CHILDREN

Physicians should emphasize to families that risk avoidance is the most important aspect of safe travel. The basic tenets of safe foreign travel with children are listed in Box 91-3. Parents should select modes of transportation, activities, and overnight settings carefully to avoid unnecessary hazards. Because traumatic injury

---

BOX 91-3   Risk Avoidance During Travel

Select appropriate settings: supervised swimming, safe campsites, protective devices.
Protect skin: sunscreen, repellents, protective clothing, closed shoes.
Eat and drink cleanly: water disinfection, careful food selection, "boil it, peel it, cook it, or forget it."
Avoid bugs and wild animals: clothing, netting, repellents, vigilance, safe practices.

---

is the leading cause of disorders and deaths among children, prevention is key. Protective devices, such as car seats, helmets, PFDs, and protective clothing and pads, should be used as often as possible (Figure 91-12). Do not assume that any of these items is available in the destination country. Freshwater swimming should be avoided in developing countries to prevent parasitic infections, such as schistosomiasis. Where swimming is appropriate, parents should provide close supervision. Drowning is the second leading cause of death among pediatric travelers.[80] Skin protection is also vital in the outdoors, particularly in tropical environments. Wearing closed shoes and avoiding play directly on the ground can prevent infections with various hookworms, *Strongyloides,* and other parasites that enter through the skin. Closed shoes also protect feet from injuries that can result in wounds infected with *Staphylococcus aureus* and other organisms that grow vigorously in the tropics. Clothing should be selected carefully based on ambient temperature and expected conditions. Even in hot, sunny climates, light, high-SPF clothing should cover as much body surface as possible to provide protection from parasites, insects, and UV light. Sunscreen should be used liberally and reapplied every few hours, particularly after swimming.

Parents should be advised to take great care in selecting foods and safe drinking water for themselves and their children, who are particularly vulnerable to disease (Box 91-4). All foods should

BOX 91-4   Prevention of Food-Borne and Waterborne Diseases

Wash hands thoroughly before eating or preparing food.
Eat only well-cooked vegetables, meat, and seafood.
Eat only fruit that can be peeled.
Drink only disinfected or boiled water, carbonated drinks, hot teas, or coffee.
Drink or eat only pasteurized dairy products.
Avoid ice cubes or use only those made from disinfected water.
Breastfeed infants.
Prepare formula with disinfected or boiled water.
Brush teeth with disinfected water.
Choose well-cooked foods prepared freshly in front of you.

TABLE 91-5   Resources for Current Safe Travel, Immunizations, and Malaria Prophylaxis Recommendations

Resource Name	URL	Comments
U.S. Centers for Disease Control and Prevention (CDC)	cdc.gov	General website
	cdc.gov/travel/	Index of travel information, vaccines, disease outbreaks by destination country
	cdc.gov/mmwr	*Morbidity and Mortality Weekly Report* online (international bulletin on disease outbreaks)
	cdc.gov/travel/yellowbook/2014/chapter-7 -international-travel-infants-children/vaccine -recommendations-for-infants-children	Vaccine recommendations for traveling children
World Health Organization	who.int/en/	Latest information on disease outbreaks
Travel Medicine Providers	tripprep.com	Vaccinations, epidemics, travel medicine providers
Travel Internationally with Your Kids	travelwithyourkids.com/	Parent-friendly website with much practical information

and especially around mealtimes, successfully interrupts the fecal-oral passage of disease. Hand sanitizer with an alcohol content of more than 60% is an alternative when hand washing is not convenient.

Parents should focus efforts on avoiding contact between children and insects or wild animals. Mosquitoes and ticks can be avoided by limiting outdoor activities between dusk and dawn and by wearing protective clothing and repellent (see Box 91-2 and Figure 91-10). As mentioned previously, DEET is an effective repellent but should not be used at concentrations greater than 35% in children because of the risk of toxicity.[42,80] Children's hands should be free of DEET to prevent accidental eye and mouth contact. Picaridin is an alternative repellent with efficacy against mosquitoes, ticks, and biting flies but has a shorter track record of success. As mentioned earlier, botanical oil repellents should not be used where there is a heavy concentration of biting insects and where these insects carry disease. Outer clothing and bed netting should be treated with permethrin. Check for ticks daily when in tick-infested areas. Children should be warned to watch where they place their hands and feet (e.g., not in crevices, unattended shoes, unchecked sleeping bags) to avoid the unexpected arthropod or snake.

IMMUNIZATIONS

Foreign travel with children requires advance planning because vaccines recommended for travel to certain countries may take up to 6 weeks to complete. The CDC website (cdc.gov/travel) provides up-to-date information on immunizations and prophylaxis based on the following:

Countries of travel
Length of time in each country
Location of destinations (rural versus urban)
Time of year
Types of lodging and eating facilities
Previous immunizations
Age and weight of the child

Vaccines may be categorized as routine (hepatitis B, polio, diphtheria-tetanus-pertussis, *Haemophilus influenzae* B, pneumococcus, rotavirus, measles-mumps-rubella, varicella, hepatitis A, meningococcus), seasonally or geographically indicated or required (influenza, yellow fever, typhoid, immunoglobulin), and indicated for extended stay (Japanese encephalitis, rabies)[82] (Table 91-6). Indications, dosages, and schedules for administration of these immunizations are listed in Table 91-7. The risk of acquiring diseases covered by many routine childhood immunizations is greater when traveling to developing countries because of inconsistencies in local immunization practices and subsequent loss of herd immunity. Children who have not completed their primary series of immunizations may require acceleration of the vaccination schedule or extra doses to maximize protection before travel. The minimum age at which some vaccinations can be given is listed in Table 91-7. In addition, seasonal influenza A vaccine should be given to all children older than 6 months

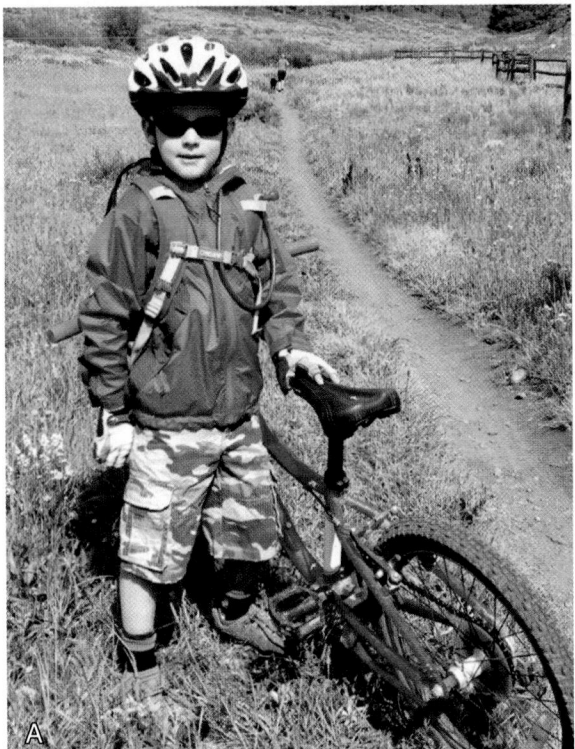

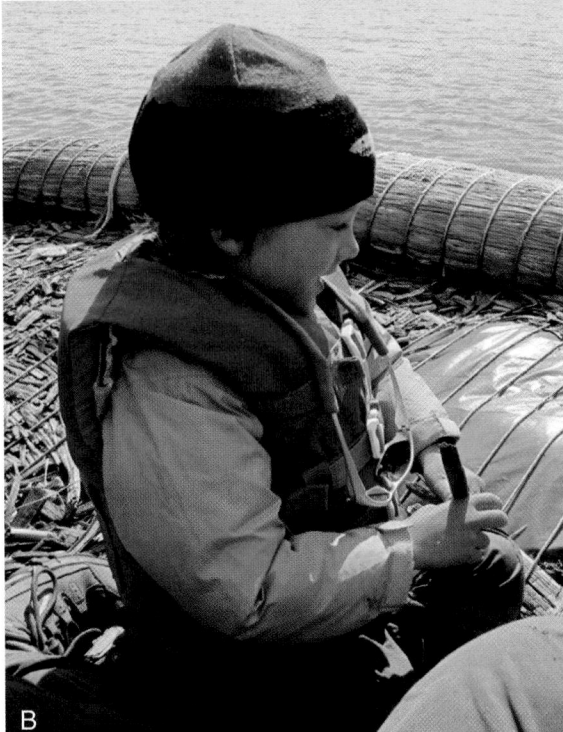

FIGURE 91-12 Proper use of helmet (**A**) and personal flotation device (**B**). *(Courtesy Judith R. Klein, MD.)*

be well-cooked, canned, or peeled. All milk products should be either pasteurized or boiled to avoid diarrheal illness and tick-borne encephalitis. Water should never be consumed from the tap; only water that is bottled, has been boiled for 1 minute, or has been treated with UV light (SteriPEN) or a chemical (iodine) and microfiltered (0.2-μm pore size) should be ingested. In certain areas, even bottled water is suspect. Breastfeeding is safest for young infants. If formula is used, only properly disinfected water should be used for its preparation. Finally, proper and frequent hand washing, particularly with infants and toddlers

TABLE 91-6	Categories of Vaccines for Children
Type of Vaccine	**Examples**
Routine	Hepatitis B, polio, diphtheria-tetanus-pertussis (DTaP), *Haemophilus influenzae* B (Hib), pneumococcal (PCV-13), rotavirus (RotaTeq), measles-mumps-rubella (MMR), varicella virus (VZV), hepatitis A, meningococcal
Required or seasonally or geographically indicated for travel	Yellow fever, typhoid, meningococcal, influenza (seasonal), immunoglobulin
Extended stay	Rabies, Japanese encephalitis

From U.S. Centers for Disease Control and Prevention: cdc.gov/travel/yellowbook/2014/chapter-7-international-travel-infants-children/vaccine-recommendations-for-infants-children.

traveling during influenza season, which is December to April in the Northern Hemisphere and April to October in the Southern Hemisphere. Rotavirus vaccine is also strongly recommended for young infants traveling abroad. Rotavirus is the most common cause of acute gastroenteritis in young children, with 80% of children infected by the age of 5 years prior to vaccine introduc-

tion.[17] In the developing world, it is responsible for the deaths of more than half a million children per year under 5 years of age. As with many other diseases, children are more likely to develop acute gastroenteritis while traveling, so vaccination is an important preventive tool. Finally, the vaccine against meningo-coccus, now routine in adolescents, should be administered to

TABLE 91-7 Recommended Vaccines for Pediatric Travelers

Vaccine	Recommended Age at Vaccination (Earliest Possible Age)	Dosing Schedule	Comments and Contraindications
Routine Vaccinations			
Polio (IPV) (intramuscular)	2 mo (6 wk)	2, 4, 6-12 mo and 4-6 yr	Oral polio vaccine is no longer recommended because of risk of inactivated virus–associated paralytic polio in undiagnosed immunocompromised infants
Diphtheria-tetanus–acellular pertussis (DTaP)	2 mo (6 wk)	2, 4, 6, 15-18 mo and 4-6 yr	Large retrospective study indicated no increased risk of autism with DTaP
Tetanus-diphtheria-pertussis (Tdap)	10 years	Booster every 10 yr	Replaces dT to improve waning pertussis immunity
Haemophilus influenzae type B (Hib) polysaccharide conjugate	2 mo (6 wk)	2, 4, 6, 12-15 mo	Typically given as combination with DTaP; three or four doses depending on vaccine used
Pneumococcus (PCV-13): 13-valent conjugate	2 mo (6 wk)	2, 4, 6, 12-15 mo	Use protein polysaccharide vaccine (PPSV) for certain high-risk groups more than 5 yr old
Rotavirus (RotaTeq or Rotarix) live oral	2 mo (6 wk)	2, 4, 6 mo	Must give first dose before age 15 weeks (risk of intussception increases if first dose is given after 15 wk of age); two or three doses depending on type of vaccine used
Hepatitis B inactivated viral antigen	Birth	3 doses: 0, 1, 6 mo	Some protection after just one or two doses
Measles-mumps-rubella (MMR)	12-15 mo (6 mo)	12-15 mo booster at 4-6 yr	Give at least 2-3 weeks before any immunoglobulin; give one dose before international travel if 6-11 mo of age; give two doses 4 weeks apart if > 12 mo of age
Varicella live attenuated virus	12 mo	12 mo-12 yr: 12-15 mo booster at 4-6 yr > 12 yr: two doses, 4-12 wk apart	Give at least 2-3 wk before any immunoglobulin; may be given with MMR at different sites; avoid if child is immunocompromised
Hepatitis A inactivated virus	12 mo	Two doses, 6-12 mo apart	Preferred for hepatitis A protection if child is ≥ 2 yr (WHO recommendation is child ≥ 1 yr); effective in 4 wk; one dose enough for travel; two doses needed for long-term protection
Meningococcus (Menactra, Menveo, Menomune; MenHibrix for meningococcal groups C and Y and *H. influenzae* type B)	2 yr (9 mo)	9-23 mo: two doses Menactra, 3 mo apart > 2 yr: one dose any vaccine type	Recommended for all adolescents 11-20 yr Use for central Africa, Nepal, and epidemic areas Some efficacy of MenHibrix for children > 3 mo
Seasonally or Geographically Indicated or Required Vaccines			
Seasonal influenza A inactivated virus (intramuscular)	6 mo	If first vaccination, give two doses, 1 mo apart; otherwise, give single dose	Influenza season is December to April in Northern Hemisphere and April to October in Southern Hemisphere
Seasonal influenza A live attenuated virus (intranasal)	5 yr (2 yr)	Single dose	Live attenuated vaccine is given only to healthy, nonasthmatic, nonimmunocompromised children
Hepatitis A: immunoglobulin	Birth	0.02 mL/kg	Hepatitis A protection for those < 1 yr or > 1 yr and travel commencing in < 2 wk; beware of timing with live virus vaccines; effective for 3 mo
Yellow fever live virus	9 mo (6 mo)	Single dose given at least 10 days before departure; booster is given every 10 yr	Required for parts of sub-Saharan Africa and tropical South America; may give at 6-9 mo if infant is traveling to epidemic area, but there is a risk of vaccine-related encephalitis
Typhoid (ViCPS) intramuscular polysaccharide	2 yr	Single dose; booster every 2 yr	Important for Latin America, Asia, and Africa; vaccine is not a substitute for eating and drinking cleanly; only 50% to 80% effective
Typhoid (Ty21a) oral live attenuated	> 6 years	One capsule every 2 days for 4 days; booster every 5 years	Only 50% to 80% effective

TABLE 91-7 Recommended Vaccines for Pediatric Travelers—cont'd

Vaccine	Recommended Age at Vaccination (Earliest Possible Age)	Dosing Schedule	Comments and Contraindications
Vaccines for Extended Stay			
Japanese encephalitis inactivated virus	1 yr (2 mo)	At 0, 28 days; last dose > 10 days before travel; unclear booster interval	Indicated for parts of India and rural Asia if stay > 1 mo; no safety data for children < 1 yr of age; high rate of hypersensitivity
Rabies HDCV (Imovax) or PCEC (RabAvert)	Birth	Days 0, 7, 21-28 if child will be in endemic area for > 1 month	If child has been exposed and previously immunized, repeat either vaccine 1 mL IM days 0, 3 If child has been exposed but not previously immunized, • Give rabies immunoglobulin (RIG) 20 IU/kg as much as possible at site of exposure and the rest IM • Give either vaccine 1 mL IM on days 0, 3, 7, 14

Data from Centers for Disease Control and Prevention: Vaccine recommendations for infants and children: cdc.gov/travel/yellowbook/2014/chapter-7-international-travel-infants-children/vaccine-recommendations-for-infants-children.

all children older than 9 months of age traveling to endemic areas or locales with regional epidemics. If travel to such an area is essential for a younger child, the vaccine MenHibrix has some, albeit modest, efficacy in infants as young as 3 months.[82] Generally, children younger than 9 months should avoid travel to such areas. For families planning more prolonged stays, particularly in rural areas, the primary rabies vaccination series should be considered. Rabies is more common in children than adults, likely due to greater animal contact. Children are also more likely to be bitten on the face, increasing the likelihood of transmission due to a greater vascular supply in this area. If a bite occurs, it should be washed immediately with soap, water, and dilute iodine and the child should be taken to medical attention for primary vaccination and rabies immunoglobulin (if they have not previously been vaccinated).

In the United States, hepatitis A vaccine is recommended for children older than 1 year of age. For children younger than age 1 year or for those unable to receive this vaccine more than 2 weeks before travel, immunoglobulin can provide passive hepatitis A prophylaxis. Administration of immunoglobulin interferes with the humoral response to some of the live attenuated virus vaccines, such as the measles-mumps-rubella and varicella vaccines. If immunoglobulin is given first, these vaccinations should be delayed by at least 6 weeks, and preferably by 3 months, to obtain an adequate immunogenic response.[82] When both are needed for travel, it is best to give the measles-mumps-rubella or varicella vaccine first; the immunoglobulin can be given closer to the time of travel, at least 2 weeks and preferably 4 weeks later. Immunoglobulin does not interfere with antibody production after oral polio or yellow fever vaccines and may be given at the same visit. Yellow fever vaccination is often a requirement for travel to certain countries in Africa and South America. Infants older than age 9 months can receive this live virus vaccination, but younger infants are at risk for vaccine-related encephalitis and should not travel to areas where yellow fever is endemic.[82]

Ideally, a medical visit to discuss travel plans and start immunizations should be made 6 weeks before travel. As mentioned previously, not all immunologic agents recommended for travel are compatible and some require multiple doses. Therefore, selection of immunizations to be given at any one time and the interval between immunizations are important. Table 91-8 presents recommendations for the timing and sequence of specific travel immunizations. In general, all toxoid, recombinant, inactivated, and live attenuated vaccines may be given simultaneously. Live attenuated vaccines should be given either simultaneously or at least 30 days apart to avoid reduced immunoreactivity to each vaccine.

PROPHYLAXIS: MALARIA

In 2013, there were 198 million cases of malaria worldwide, with 584,000 deaths, the majority in sub-Saharan Africa.[88] Children younger than 5 years are particularly vulnerable and represent more than 80% of the fatalities from this disease. In Africa, malaria is responsible for 20% of all childhood deaths. The risk of acquiring malaria (see Chapter 40) during visits to developing countries in the tropics is significant. Even areas where the overall risk is relatively low may have foci of intense transmission. The number of cases of malaria diagnosed in the United States is steadily rising, with nearly 2000 cases reported in 2011.[53] Of these patients, nearly 70% came from sub-Saharan Africa, 22% from Asia, and 8% from Caribbean nations. Fifteen percent of these cases involved children under the age of 18 years. Of note, children with malaria can rapidly develop high levels of parasitemia and are, therefore, at greater risk of severe complications, including shock, seizures, coma, and death.

Protective measures to prevent mosquito bites help interrupt transmission of malaria but are not foolproof (see Box 91-2). Therefore, chemoprophylaxis is highly recommended for travelers to countries where malaria is endemic. *Plasmodium falciparum* (64%) and *Plasmodium vivax* (28%) are the two species

TABLE 91-8 Recommended Timing and Sequence of Nonroutine Immunizations for Foreign Travel*

4-6 Weeks Before Departure	1 Week After Initial Visit	7-10 Days Before Departure
Hepatitis A (need second dose 6-12 months later)	—	Immunoglobulin for hepatitis A prevention if vaccine not given
Yellow fever	—	
Typhoid ViCPS or Ty21a	—	
Meningococcal	—	
Japanese encephalitis		Japanese encephalitis
Rabies	Rabies	Rabies

*Give only immunizations indicated for area of travel, length of stay, and age of child.
Simultaneous administration of routine and travel-related vaccines is acceptable with the exception of measles-mumps-rubella vaccine or varicella vaccine with immunoglobulin. Administer immunoglobulin at least 3 weeks after these live virus vaccines.

TABLE 91-9 Malaria Chemoprophylaxis

Medication	Indications and Contraindications	Dosage
Chloroquine (Aralen) (liquid form Nivaquine not available in United States)	Travel to chloroquine-sensitive areas (Caribbean, Central America north of Panama, Middle East)	5 mg base/kg every wk up to 300 mg starting 1 wk before exposure until 4 wk after exposure; 10 mg/mL form available outside United States
Mefloquine (Lariam) (250 mg tab)	Travel to chloroquine-resistant/mefloquine-sensitive area; do not use in setting of epilepsy, psychiatric illness, cardiac arrhythmias	Give every week starting 1 wk before exposure until 4 wk after exposure Dosage: < 9 kg: 5 mg/kg/week 10-20 kg: 1/4 tab every wk 20-30 kg: 1/2 tab every wk 30-45 kg: 3/4 tab every wk > 45 kg: 1 tab every wk
Atovaquone (A) plus Proguanil (P) (Malarone) Pedi tab: 62.5 mg A/25 mg P Adult tab: 250 mg A/ 100 mg P	Travel to chloroquine- or mefloquine-resistant areas; contraindicated if creatinine clearance < 30 mL/min; give 2 days prior to exposure through 7 days after exposure	5-8 kg: 1/2 pedi tab every day 8-10 kg: 3/4 pedi tab every day 10-20 kg: 1 pedi tab every day 20-30 kg: 2 pedi tab every day 30-40 kg: 3 pedi tab every day > 40 kg: 1 adult tab every day For emergency treatment: take four times usual prophylaxis dose listed above every day for 3 days if NOT used for prophylaxis
Doxycycline	Travel to chloroquine- or mefloquine-resistant areas; > 8 yr of age only; beware of photosensitivity	2 mg/kg/day up to 100 mg/day for 1-2 days before exposure and for 4 wk after exposure
Artemether-lumefantrine (Coartem 20/120)	Emergency treatment if medical assistance > 24 hours away and malaria suspected; NOT for prophylaxis	5-15 kg: 1 tab every day for 3 days 15-25 kg: 2 tabs every day for 3 days 25-35 kg: 3 tabs every day for 3 days > 35 kg: 4 tabs every day for 3 days
Primaquine	Prevention of relapse with *P. vivax* or *P. ovale*; use after prolonged stay in malaria-endemic area; avoid if glucose-6-phosphate dehydrogenase deficient	0.5 mg/kg/day for 14 days

Data from Centers for Disease Control and Prevention: Information for health care providers: Malaria: cdc.gov/travel/yellowbook/2014/chapter-3-infectious-diseases-related-to-travel/malaria.

most often responsible for malaria. The most lethal plasmodium, *P. falciparum,* has developed widespread resistance to chloroquine and in some areas (extreme northern and southern Thailand, Cambodia, Myanmar), resistance to mefloquine.[52] Therefore, the choice of prophylactic agent is based primarily on the presence of resistant malaria in the area of travel. The age, weight, and medical history of the child are additional determinants of the appropriate prophylactic agent. Table 91-9 lists the available options for malaria chemoprophylaxis.

If a child is traveling to a chloroquine-sensitive area, such as the Caribbean, parts of Central America, or the Middle East, chloroquine is the drug of choice. Chloroquine prophylaxis should be given weekly, starting 1 week before travel, and continued for 4 weeks thereafter. Chloroquine passes through breast milk, but not in sufficient quantities to protect an infant. Therefore, a breastfed infant should receive chloroquine prophylaxis in standard recommended doses (see Table 91-9). Chloroquine is not readily available in a liquid form in the United States. The powder, which is extremely bitter, may be suspended in a syrup or mixed with food. Instant pudding effectively masks the bitter taste and makes the medicine more palatable. An acceptable-tasting chloroquine liquid (Nivaquine) is available outside the United States. Chloroquine should be kept out of the reach of children. As little as 300 mg may be fatal in small children.[72] If a toxic chloroquine ingestion occurs, the child should be transported promptly to a medical facility.

For children traveling to chloroquine-resistant areas, the next question is whether they are traveling to an area that is also mefloquine resistant. This includes parts of Myanmar (Burma), Cambodia, and Thailand. If the area is mefloquine sensitive, then mefloquine (Lariam) is a good option. The advantage of mefloquine is that the dose is given weekly, from 1 to 2 weeks before travel until 4 weeks after return. It should be avoided in children who weigh less than 5 kg and in those with psychiatric illnesses,

epilepsy, or underlying cardiac arrhythmias. If the area is mefloquine resistant (or is mefloquine sensitive but contraindications to mefloquine exist or parents prefer not to use mefloquine), the two options are atovaquone plus proguanil (Malarone) or doxycycline. Malarone is approved in the United States for children weighing more than 5 kg, but requires daily administration. It must be taken 2 days before entry into a malarial area and continued for 7 days after leaving. It is contraindicated in the setting of severe renal impairment (creatinine clearance < 30 mL/min). Atovaquone-proguanil and mefloquine are available only in tablet form, but tablets may be administered crushed. Alternatively, a compounding pharmacist may prepare the child's dose in a gelatin capsule and the contents of the capsule can be placed in food just prior to administration. Doxycycline is indicated for children older than age 8 years traveling to mefloquine-resistant areas or with contraindications to mefloquine or atovaquone-proguanil use. It must be given daily. It is started 1 to 2 days before and continued for 4 weeks after travel to a malarial area. Side effects include diarrhea and photosensitivity. With all antimalarials, particularly those given daily, timing of medication ingestion is critical. Medications should be taken at the same time each day or week, to avoid a drop in blood levels below the level of efficacy. Given the difficulties in administering medications to children, weekly dosing (mefloquine) may be preferable when this is an option. The importance of proper prophylaxis against malaria cannot be overemphasized. In a review of pediatric malaria cases, 75% to 100% of patients had received no or inadequate chemoprophylaxis.[22,76]

Families traveling to remote areas where malaria is endemic but where medical care may not be immediately available should consider carrying a treatment regimen for the disease, to be administered if their child develops an acute febrile illness. This medication is not intended to be a replacement for definitive medical care; it is simply a temporizing measure. This treatment may be either atovaquone-proguanil if it is not being used for prophylaxis or artemether-lumefantrine (Coartem). Full guidelines for medication choice and dosing regimens are found on the CDC website.[36] Of note, artemisinin-derived agents are not generally used for prophylaxis, because the short half-lives of these drugs would require multiple daily doses.

Primaquine is an antimalarial drug used to prevent emergence of *P. vivax* and *Plasmodium ovale* after heavy or prolonged (many months) exposure to mosquitoes. Routine chemoprophylaxis does not kill the exoerythrocytic stages of these *Plasmodium* species. Primaquine is taken daily for 2 weeks after leaving a malarial area. Primaquine should not be given to anyone with glucose-6-phosphate dehydrogenase deficiency.

TRAVEL-RELATED PROBLEMS

Next to boredom and restlessness, motion sickness and eustachian tube dysfunction are the most common problems encountered by children during travel. Parents can minimize the first two problems by preparing small activity packs or bags with paper, pencils, crayons, stickers, cards, travel puzzles, or small toys. Once at their destination, children most frequently suffer from diarrhea, fevers, rashes, and respiratory tract infections.[37] Parents should be aware of the basic elements of diagnosis and treatment and the indications for immediate medical attention.

MOTION SICKNESS

Motion sickness can occur with air, land, or sea travel (see Chapter 70), particularly in children ages 2 through 12 years. Emotional upset, noxious odors, and ear infections can make symptoms worse. Children experiencing motion sickness are often pale and diaphoretic, and feel nauseated and weak. They may vomit, but this does not provide prolonged relief. Children known to be susceptible to motion sickness should be seated in the middle or near the front of the boat, plane, or car, where motion is minimized. They should be encouraged to look at objects far away and avoid focusing on close objects, such as books. Some children get significant relief from using headphones to listen to music or stories.

Dimenhydrinate (Dramamine, 1 to 1.5 mg/kg) administered 1 hour before departure and repeated every 6 hours can help patients known to be prone to motion sickness. If dimenhydrinate is not available, diphenhydramine (Benadryl, 1.25 mg/kg every 6 hours up to 50 mg/dose) is also effective. Both medications may cause drowsiness, and diphenhydramine occasionally causes paradoxic excitability in children. Scopolamine patches, commonly used in adults, should not be used in children, because they are particularly susceptible to the side effects of belladonna alkaloids. It has been postulated that this particular administration system might release too much scopolamine and, consequently, produce serious side effects in children.

EUSTACHIAN TUBE DYSFUNCTION

Eustachian tube dysfunction is the result of disequilibrium between pressure in the eustachian tube and the surrounding atmospheric pressure. If atmospheric pressure rises (e.g., with descent in an airplane) and the pressure within the tube does not rise as quickly as the ambient pressure, the eustachian tube becomes compressed. If compressed enough, the eustachian tube cannot equalize pressure in the middle ear with that of the environment, resulting in a sense of compression on the outer aspect of the tympanic membrane. Far more children than adults (nearly 15% of the pediatric population) suffer from this problem, because of the relatively smaller, and hence more compressible, pediatric eustachian tube. Swallowing often helps relieve the pressure disequilibrium and may be facilitated by drinking, sucking on a pacifier, or, for the breastfed infant, nursing. Older children may wish to chew gum or yawn to equalize middle ear and atmospheric pressure. Contrary to popular belief, decongestants are not useful with eustachian tube dysfunction in children and should generally be avoided in young children.

TRAVELER'S DIARRHEA

Traveling to wilderness areas or developing countries requires leaving behind modern sanitation facilities and reliably disinfected tap water. Unfortunately, this places travelers at increased risk for diarrheal illness (see Chapter 82). Up to 60% of children younger than age 3 years develop prolonged diarrhea (> 10 days) during travel in tropical or subtropical areas.[3,14] This risk is highest in young visitors to Africa and India, followed by travelers to Asia and Latin America. Young children are at greater risk for traveler's diarrhea (TD) and its complications because of their relatively poor hygiene, oral exploration, immature immune systems, higher gastric pH, more rapid gastric emptying, and difficulties with adequate hydration.

TD is defined by the National Institutes of Health as a twofold or greater increase in the frequency of unformed stools, or any number of such stools when accompanied by symptoms of fever, abdominal cramping, vomiting, or blood or mucus in the stools. In small children, the course tends to be more severe and prolonged, lasting from 3 days to 3 weeks.[3,79] Most cases of TD (>80%) are caused by bacteria, followed by parasites (10%) and viruses (5% to 8%) (Table 91-10). Enterotoxigenic *Escherichia coli* alone is responsible for 50% of TD cases.[79] *Campylobacter* and *Shigella* are also prominent causes of TD, along with rotavirus and norovirus. *Giardia* is by far the most common parasitic cause of TD and more indolent in onset.

Prevention

Standard recommendations for prevention of TD are based primarily on known potential sources for transmission of illness (see Box 91-4). Transmission is through fecal-oral contamination, with water, food, and fingers the most common vehicles. Careful selection and preparation of food and beverages can decrease the risk of acquiring TD. As mentioned previously, washing hands thoroughly before eating decreases bacterial carriage and serves as a reminder to children of the need for precautions. If soap is unavailable, gross particles can be rinsed off with water and the hands then cleansed with a hand sanitizer that is more than 60% alcohol based. The "boil it, cook it, peel it, or forget it" rule implies that all raw vegetables and salads should be avoided, meats and seafood be well cooked, and fruits properly peeled. See Chapter 88 for a complete discussion of water disinfection.

Using antibiotics to prevent TD in children is not recommended by the CDC due to concerns about adverse drug effects and the development of drug resistance. Bismuth subsalicylate (Pepto-Bismol) has been shown in adults to be an effective form

TABLE 91-10 Causes of Traveler's Diarrhea in Children

Agent	Examples
Preformed toxin	Enterotoxigenic *Escherichia coli**
	Staphylococcus aureus
	Bacillus cereus
Viral	Rotavirus*
	Norovirus*
	Adenovirus
	Enterovirus
	Influenza virus
	Hepatitis virus
Bacterial	*Shigella**
	*Campylobacter**
	Salmonella
	Enteroinvasive *E. coli*
	Yersinia enterocolitica
	Vibrio cholerae
Parasitic	*Giardia lamblia*
	Entamoeba histolytica
	Cryptosporidium

*Most common.

BOX 91-5   Signs of Dehydration

Mild to Moderate (5% to 10%)
Irritability/restlessness
Sunken eyes/fontanelle
Dry mucous membranes
Very thirsty
Decreased urine output

Severe (>10%)
Lethargy
Very sunken eyes
Very dry mucous membranes
Unable to take liquids orally
Cool, mottled extremities
Rapid, thready pulse
Tachypnea
No urine output for several hours

BOX 91-6   Homemade Oral Rehydration Solutions

Glucose-Based Solutions*
1 teaspoon (5 mL) salt
8 teaspoons (40 mL) sugar
1 L disinfected/boiled water

Rice Cereal–Based Solutions*
1 teaspoon (5 mL) salt
1 cup (50 g) rice cereal
1 L disinfected/boiled water

Data from rehydrate.org.
*Can be used directly or diluted in half to reduce osmolarity. Add mashed banana to rice cereal–based solution to add K$^+$. Solutions left without refrigeration for more than 12 hours should be discarded.

of chemoprophylaxis against TD. The few small studies in children have demonstrated modest, if any, efficacy.[3,90] Therefore, and because of the risk of administering salicylates to children, using bismuth subsalicylate for TD prevention in children, particularly those younger than age 3 years, is not recommended. Probiotic agents, such as *Lactobacillus acidophilus,* have been shown to be effective for prevention and treatment of TD in children.[4,13,70] The mechanism of action of these nonpathogenic live microorganisms is not entirely clear, but most likely involves competition with pathogens for intestinal receptors and nutrients, improving immune function in the gut, increasing intestinal acidity, reducing intestinal permeability, and/or production of chemicals by the probiotic agent with efficacy against pathogens.[4] *Lactobacillus* is available over the counter; the dosage is one tablet or capsule a day for children younger than age 2 years, and two a day for children older than 2 years. Capsules can be opened and the contents placed in food or drink for children unable or unwilling to take pills.

Treatment

The major cause of illness and death in infants and small children with diarrhea is dehydration.[3,79] Signs of dehydration in children are listed in Box 91-5. According to the WHO, dehydration is best categorized as mild to moderate, or severe. This distinction is based on changes in behavior and mental state, quality of the mucous membranes, presence of oliguria or anuria, changes in vital signs, and evidence of decreasing peripheral perfusion. Parental assessment of dehydration using urine output, tearing, and fontanelle contour has been shown to be accurate.[3,20] Children young enough to be wearing diapers should have some urine output at least every 8 hours. If they do not, they are very likely dehydrated.

The cornerstone of treatment for TD is oral rehydration therapy (ORT), which if instituted early, can be used alone in 90% to 95% of cases.[5] It is as effective as intravenous hydration in mild to moderate dehydration caused by gastroenteritis. ORT is often tolerated by children who are vomiting if it is administered frequently in small quantities. The truly dehydrated child will typically drink an oral rehydration solution (ORS) eagerly. Parents traveling to developing countries or wilderness areas with children should carry powdered ORS or a recipe for a homemade solution (Box 91-6). Powdered ORS is readily available in most developing countries in pharmacies and drugstores. Most available ORS is glucose-based. In the past, the standard WHO ORS was not particularly effective in reducing stool frequency and volume. By reducing the osmolarity of an ORS, stool frequency in children with noncholera diarrhea is reduced and ORS requirements may be reduced by as much as 20%.[5] Many studies have looked at the efficacy of rice-based ORS relative to the WHO standard and reduced-osmolarity ORS. Rice-based ORS is less expensive and often better tolerated by children, particularly those in nations where people consume a great deal of rice. The rice-based ORS (e.g., CeraLyte: ceraproductsinc.com) has a slightly lower osmolarity and higher concentration of organic solutes, two aspects that promote enhanced absorption of Na$^+$ and water.[33] Although rice-based ORS appears superior to standard WHO ORS in several studies, there have not been studies with sufficient power to demonstrate any difference in efficacy relative to the reduced-osmolarity ORS. Therefore, either rice-based ORS or reduced-osmolarity WHO ORS can be used. All ORSs should be discarded 12 hours after reconstitution when left at room temperature, and after 24 hours if they have been refrigerated.

For rapid treatment of mild to moderate dehydration, 50 to 100 mL/kg of ORS should be administered over the first 4-hour period to rehydrate the child. An additional 10 mL/kg can be given for each diarrheal stool and 5 mL/kg for each episode of emesis. If vomiting develops, most children will tolerate ORS if a small volume (5 to 10 mL) is given every 5 minutes. Reduced-osmolarity ORS contains 75 mEq/L of sodium, 1.5% glucose, and 20 mEq/L of potassium (Table 91-11). If a solution with more glucose is used, the osmotic pressure exerted by the carbohydrate in the intestinal lumen produces fluid losses greater than the amounts of fluid absorbed, thereby exacerbating diarrhea. Most colas, sports drinks, and juices contain 6% to 15% carbohydrate and are not appropriate rehydration solutions. Once a child has been rehydrated, ORS may be rejected, and

TABLE 91-11   Field Treatment of Dehydration

	Low-Osmolarity Glucose-Based Oral Rehydration Solution*	Ceralyte, Rice Cereal–Based Oral Rehydration Solution*	Apple Juice
Volume	50-100 mL/kg/4 hours	Same	Not recommended
Electrolytes			
Na$^+$ (mEq/L)	75	50-90	0.4
Glucose (%)	1.5-2.5	4	12
K$^+$ (mEq/L)	20	20	44
HCO$_3^-$ (mEq/L)	30	30	None
Osmolarity (mOsm/L)	245	220	730

Data from Atia AN, Buchman AL: ORS in non-cholera diarrhea, Am J Gastroenterol 104:2596, 2009.
*Add 10 mL/kg or about 4 oz for each diarrheal stool and 5 mL/kg or about 2 oz for each bout of emesis.

regular liquids can be resumed. There is no scientific basis for any highly restrictive diet during and following diarrhea, including the popular BRAT diet (bananas, rice, apples, toast). Feeding of solid food, particularly complex carbohydrates and yogurt, should be resumed as soon as vomiting resolves. Solid food promotes enterocyte regeneration and reduces duration of diarrhea.[2,4] Foods (e.g., juice) with high concentrations of simple sugars can exacerbate diarrhea because of their high osmotic load, as can lactose-containing foods due to transient lactase deficiency.[51] Both should be avoided in the recovery phase.

Although oral hydration is the cornerstone of therapy for TD, medications may occasionally be helpful. Children with large volumes of diarrhea can develop zinc deficiency. Zinc is important not only for cellular immunity but also for maintenance of gut mucosal cells. Zinc deficiency can lead to a vicious cycle of increasing duration and severity of diarrhea. Zinc supplementation in acute diarrhea has been shown to reduce the duration of diarrhea and the ORS requirement.[47,90] Presently, the WHO recommends zinc supplementation (20 mg/day for 10 to 14 days for children ≥ 6 months of age and 10 mg/day for children < 6 months of age) with ORS in children in the developing world with acute diarrheal illness.[47] Given current evidence, this recommendation should be followed by young travelers with acute diarrhea.

The American Academy of Pediatrics does not support the use of antimotility agents in children because of concern for ileus and decreased mental status. However, a recent Cochrane Database review demonstrated a modest benefit of loperamide in children, reducing the duration of diarrhea and the stool frequency.[20] High-volume, frequent, and prolonged diarrhea can not only lead to significant dehydration but also significant perianal skin breakdown and superinfection in children still in diapers. Based on this and other data, antimotility agents, specifically loperamide (Imodium) should be considered in children over the age of 3 years. The dosage is 1 to 2 mg for the first dose followed by 1 to 2 mg after each loose stool with a maximum of 3 mg daily in 3- to 5-year-olds, 4 mg daily in 5- to 8-year-olds, and 6 mg daily in 8- to 12-year-olds. Diphenoxylate (Lomotil) is not recommended, because its use has been associated with toxic megacolon in individuals with bacterial invasive diarrhea. Other antidiarrheal agents, such as bismuth subsalicylate or attapulgite, have not been convincingly shown to be effective in children and should be avoided, given the dangers of aspirin products in children under the age of 12 years.[3,20,79]

Empirical treatment with antibiotics for TD is safe and effective in reducing TD severity and duration in adults and children, but concern about adverse effects and development of bacterial resistance has made recommendations for pediatric use inconsistent. Currently, the CDC recommends using antibiotics in children to reduce duration of diarrhea acquired in areas with high rates of TD, particularly cases with fever, bloody stool, and/or abdominal distention.[79] Caution is advised if shiga-toxin producing *E. coli* is suspected, because antibiotics can increase the risk of hemolytic-uremic syndrome. With increasing bacterial resistance to trimethoprim-sulfamethoxazole, azithromycin is now the drug of choice for treatment of bacterial diarrhea.[3,79,90] The dosage is 10 mg/kg/day up to 500 mg a day for 3 days. In children over 12 years of age, ciprofloxacin at a dose of 15 to 20 mg/kg (maximum 500 mg) every 12 hours for 3 days may be used. Bacterial resistance to quinolones is increasing, particularly in Southeast Asia, making azithromycin the best choice.[79,90] Severe dehydration, high fever, failure of ORT, failure of antibiotic therapy for bloody diarrhea, or altered mental status require prompt medical attention and administration of intravenous fluids for rehydration (Box 91-7). Typhoid fever caused by *Salmonella typhi* should be managed initially in a hospital setting with a quinolone, azithromycin, or a third-generation cephalosporin, such as ceftriaxone, depending on regional resistance patterns and the appearance of the child.[50,81]

CONSTIPATION

Although not as serious a problem as diarrhea, constipation can be a significant and uncomfortable issue for children

---

BOX 91-7 Indications for Seeking Immediate Medical Attention for Children With Diarrhea

Severe dehydration
High fever
Failure of oral rehydration therapy
Failure of antibiotic treatment for bloody diarrhea
Altered mental status
Suspicion of typhoid fever

---

during travel. Several factors can contribute to development of constipation:

Change in diet
Decline in fruit, vegetable, and water consumption because of sanitary concerns in developing countries
Viral illnesses
Dehydration

Constipation is defined as decrease in stool frequency and increased firmness of the stool. Firm stool is more difficult to pass and can result in painful anal fissures and hemorrhoids. Children who experience anal pain during defecation may choose to retain stool, exacerbating the constipation problem.

The best approaches to constipation are prevention and, if that fails, early management. To prevent constipation, parents should provide safe fruits and vegetables or dried prunes for their children and should actively encourage clean water consumption. Anal fissures and hemorrhoids should be managed with sitz baths, vitamin A and D ointment, and antiinflammatory hemorrhoidal creams such as Anusol. If these approaches fail, bulk stool softeners (e.g., Metamucil) and, in extreme cases, hypertonic phosphate enemas (e.g., Fleets) or polyethylene glycol (Miralax) can be used in children older than 1 year. Laxatives are not generally recommended, because chronic use can actually result in paradoxic constipation. If constipation is accompanied by severe abdominal pain, distention, vomiting, or fever, children should be brought to medical attention for further evaluation.

ABDOMINAL PAIN

Abdominal pain is a common complaint in children. The causes range widely, from extremely benign viral infections or constipation to serious or life-threatening conditions such as appendicitis or ectopic pregnancy. Caregivers accompanying children into the backcountry or to developing countries should be taught the basic indications for seeking medical treatment for this complaint. Abdominal discomfort accompanied by vomiting or diarrhea may be observed for 12 hours with appropriate hydration. If the pain worsens or fails to resolve, or the child develops high fever, vomiting for more than 24 hours, focal abdominal tenderness, or abdominal distention, the child should be brought to medical attention. If a child complains of suprapubic pain and dysuria, a 7-day course of antibiotics (e.g., cephalexin or ciprofloxacin in older children) may be administered for presumed bladder infection. If the symptoms do not improve in 2 to 3 days, or if high fever or back pain develops, the child should be brought to medical attention because these symptoms suggest pyelonephritis. In adolescent girls, the presence of lower abdominal pain, amenorrhea, or vaginal bleeding suggests the possibility of ectopic pregnancy. If this is suspected, immediate medical evaluation is indicated.

RESPIRATORY INFECTIONS AND OTITIS MEDIA

Respiratory tract and otolaryngologic infections are very common in the pediatric population. The majority of infections, including acute otitis media, sinusitis, pharyngitis, croup, bronchiolitis, and bronchitis, involve the upper respiratory tract. The vast majority of these are viral in etiology; a minority are the result of infections with *Streptococcus pneumoniae*, *Haemophilus influenzae*, or *Moraxella catarrhalis*.[71,91] Because definitive diagnoses based on otoscopy and auscultation of the lungs often cannot be made in the course of wilderness travel, parents must rely on symptoms and the presence of fever to determine whether treatment is necessary. Presence of high fever plus otalgia for more than 2 days, or sore throat without cough or rhinorrhea, probably merits both antimicrobial and symptomatic treatment. Mucopurulent nasal discharge lasting longer than 10 days may indicate a bacterial cause of sinusitis and also merits antibiotic therapy. It should be noted, however, that acute otitis media and streptococcal pharyngitis cases typically resolve without intervention.[71,91] Furthermore, antibiotic treatment of upper respiratory tract infections, such as bronchitis, bronchiolitis, croup, and most cases of pharyngitis, does not shorten the course, minimize symptoms, or decrease complications. If streptococcal pharyngitis is suspected on the basis of absence of cough or coryza and the presence of fever, cervical lymphadenopathy, and tonsillar exudate, then antibiotic therapy may be warranted. Antibiotics for streptococcal pharyngitis mildly reduce duration of disease, incidence of suppurative complications, such as peritonsillar abscess, and incidence of rheumatic fever.

With increasing use of antibiotics, bacterial resistance to these agents has risen dramatically. Forty to fifty percent of *S. pneumoniae* isolates now produce beta lactamase. Introduction of the 13-valent pneumococcal vaccine has changed the microbial representation in acute otitis media, with *H. influenzae* and *M. catarrhalis* now more common.[41] Nonetheless, minimal inhibitory concentration testing has demonstrated sensitivity of these bacterial agents to high-dose amoxicillin, even among resistant strains. First-line therapy for suspected bacterial acute otitis media or sinusitis is, therefore, high-dose amoxicillin at 80 mg/kg/day divided into two doses per day. Second-line therapy is high-dose amoxicillin-clavulanate (80 mg/kg/day divided into two doses per day) or cefuroxime (15 mg/kg twice a day). Uncomplicated acute otitis media in children older than 2 years may be treated for 5 to 7 days; otherwise, the standard treatment for acute otitis media is 10 days, and for sinusitis 14 days.[16] Suspected streptococcal pharyngitis can be treated for 10 days with amoxicillin, or for 5 days with azithromycin (10 mg/kg on day 1; then 5 mg/kg/day on days 2 to 5).

Often more important for patients than antibiotics are medications for symptomatic relief. Judicious use of acetaminophen (15 mg/kg every 4 hours) and/or ibuprofen (10 mg/kg every 6 to 8 hours) along with a topical analgesic (e.g., antipyrine-benzocaine otic drops) is strongly recommended.

If influenza is suspected based on the season of the year, regional epidemics, and symptoms (e.g., high fever, respiratory symptoms, myalgias), parents should consider administering oseltamivir (3 mg/kg/dose twice daily) to high-risk children. High-risk children are those younger than age 5 years (particularly < 2 years), with chronic lung or other organ dysfunction, who are immunocompromised (e.g., infection with human immunodeficiency virus, diabetes), or are taking long-term aspirin therapy.[40] Treatment is most effective in reducing length and severity of disease if it is given within the first 48 hours of illness. Any child with suspected influenza who appears ill or has signs of lower respiratory tract infection should immediately be given oseltamivir and taken to the nearest medical facility.

Coughing is a common symptom associated with viral upper respiratory infections in children. A cough may persist for weeks after resolution of other viral symptoms. Its persistence is not an indication for antibiotics unless pertussis is strongly suspected based on exposure, severity of cough (plus persistence), and vaccination history. Generally, antitussives such as dextromethorphan are not recommended for children due to concerns regarding the effects of narcotic products on young children. Humidifiers and steam from a running shower have anecdotally provided significant relief for coughing children, particularly at night when the cough tends to worsen. Several studies have also looked at the salutary effects of honey on a pediatric cough and found it to be equivalent in efficacy to traditional antitussives.[74] Honey should not be used in children under the age of 1 year because of the risk of botulism. If there is concern for foreign body aspiration or if the child has a significant voice change or signs of

respiratory distress, caregivers should bring the child to immediate medical attention.

FEVER OF UNCLEAR ETIOLOGY

High fever that develops in a child during the course of foreign travel may be the result of a common infection (e.g., viral syndrome, pharyngitis) or a manifestation of a tropical disease. Box 91-8 lists the indications for prompt medical attention in a child with fever. The leading tropical cause of fever in travelers to Africa is malaria. If malaria is suspected, the child should immediately be taken to the closest medical facility because most cases of illness and most deaths related to malaria occur in children. If a medical facility cannot be reached within 24 hours, any child weighing more than 5 kg (11 lb) should be given atovaquone-proguanil or artemether-lumefantrine as standby treatment, as previously described and indicated in Table 91-9.[36]

In adult and child travelers to most other parts of the world, dengue is the most common cause of tropical fever.[37] Unfortunately, 95% of dengue cases worldwide are among children under the age of 15 years.[83] The result of a mosquito-borne arbovirus, dengue is characterized by fever, headaches, a maculopapular rash, and myalgias. Symptoms range from mild fever to hemorrhagic shock, with infants younger than 1 year and children between the ages of 4 and 9 years at greatest risk of severe disease.[83] With the exception of hemorrhagic dengue, treatment of dengue fever is purely symptomatic. The southeastern United States and Hawaii have substantial populations of dengue-carrying *Aedes aegypti* mosquitoes that cause sporadic cases. Mosquito avoidance is the best approach to preventing disease. Unlike the malarial vector, the mosquitoes bearing dengue are most active during the daytime, so protective clothing and repellents should be used during all of the child's waking hours. There is no prophylaxis or vaccine available to prevent dengue.

Typhoid fever, caused by the bacteria *Salmonella enterica* serotype *Typhi*, is another common cause of tropical fever in children. The risk is highest among travelers to southern and Southeast Asia (6 to 30 times as high).[81] Onset of the disease is insidious with gradually increasing fever, headache, and anorexia; diarrhea develops later in the course of the disease. Children who appear ill may have invasive typhoidal disease and should be treated in a medical facility. Resistance to antibiotics is rising in developing countries, but strains are typically susceptible to azithromycin and third-generation cephalosporins (e.g., ceftriaxone). Quinolones, once the mainstay of therapy, are becoming less effective and are generally not indicated in children under 12 years of age.[1] Transmission of typhoid is strictly fecal-oral between human hosts, so thorough hand washing is essential. Food and water precautions mentioned previously should be observed. Two vaccinations are available to prevent typhoid fever and are 50% to 80% effective in preventing disease. The Vi capsular polysaccharide vaccine (ViCPS) is recommended for children over 2 years of age and consists of a single dose of vaccine administered 2 weeks prior to travel. A booster is required every 2 years. An alternative is an oral, live attenuated vaccine (Vivotif) that consists of a series of four capsules, with one taken every other day. Repeat dosing is required every 5 years. This vaccine is not recommended in children under 6 years of age.

HEADACHE

Headache is a common travel-related problem in the adolescent population. The most common causes of headaches in children are viral illnesses, migraines, dental infections, sinusitis, tension, or fatigue. Life-threatening causes of headache, such as meningitis, spontaneous or posttraumatic intracranial bleeding, or mass lesions, should be considered in any child with this complaint. Parasitic diseases, such as dengue fever and malaria, can also cause severe headache.

A child with a tender tooth or tenderness to palpation of the sinuses should be managed with analgesics (e.g., acetaminophen or ibuprofen) and antibiotics. Dental infections respond well to amoxicillin and a visit to the dentist for definitive management. (See Respiratory Infections and Otitis Media, earlier, for information on antibiotic treatment of sinus infections.) If a child has had a previous migraine headache or has a history that is classic for migraine (e.g., unilateral headache, aura, visual scotoma, photophobia, nausea, family history of migraine), analgesics and rest in a quiet, dark room are appropriate first-line therapies. Caffeine in the form of a strong cup of coffee is also a helpful improvisational treatment for migraine headaches. If a child's headache is accompanied by high fever, neck stiffness, vomiting, confusion, neurologic abnormalities, or a recent history of trauma, the child should be brought to medical attention immediately.

CONJUNCTIVITIS

Conjunctivitis, or "pinkeye," is a common pediatric problem. Most conjunctivitis in children is either allergic or infectious (e.g., adenovirus, *Staphylococcus, Streptococcus,* or *Haemophilus*). Itching and clear discharge suggest an allergic cause best treated with a topical or systemic antihistamine (e.g., diphenhydramine). Absence of itching, along with a slightly thicker or colored discharge from one or both eyes, is more consistent with an infectious cause of conjunctivitis. Distinguishing between viral and bacterial causes can be very difficult, so all patients with suspected infectious conjunctivitis should be treated with a topical antibiotic, such as erythromycin ointment (four times a day for 7 days), or polymyxin B sulfate plus trimethoprim (Polytrim) ophthalmic solution (1 drop every 3 hours for 7 days). Drops are preferred when the child is willing to accept them because they do not obscure vision. Eye discharge should be wiped from the eye with a warm moist cloth, and contact precautions should be exercised to prevent spread of what is a very infectious condition until the discharge resolves.

If the presence of a foreign body in the eye is suspected or there is chemical exposure to the eye, a drop of topical ocular anesthetic, such as proparacaine, should be applied and the eye flushed vigorously with water. Caregivers should then administer oral analgesics to the child and apply topical antibiotic ointment or solution for 24 to 48 hours. If the foreign body sensation persists after 1 to 2 days, there is likely to be a retained foreign body and the child should be brought to medical attention. In addition, the presence of eye pain, periorbital swelling, fever, photophobia, or visual blurring with or without a history of antecedent eye trauma or contact lens use suggests a more serious diagnosis and should prompt immediate medical attention.

RASHES

Identification of rashes in children is an art. Although parents cannot be expected to become familiar with all types of rashes, they may be able to distinguish common rashes from potentially dangerous exanthems. Petechial, purpuric, or mucosal lesions are markers for potentially serious diseases and should prompt parents to seek medical attention immediately. Standard dermatology textbooks with photographs can be used to instruct parents to recognize common viral exanthems and rashes caused by varicella, scabies, and contact dermatitis (e.g., poison oak or poison ivy). Scabies can most safely be abolished with permethrin. Contact dermatitis often can be simply treated with 1% hydrocortisone cream and diphenhydramine (see Chapter 64). When dermatitis covers the face, genitals, or large portions of the child's skin, systemic corticosteroids may be indicated.

LACERATIONS

Soft tissue injuries are extremely common among children, particularly as they become more ambulatory. All wounds should be thoroughly irrigated with clean water and explored to ensure that no foreign bodies remain. Children with lacerations that require suturing should be brought to medical attention. In general, lacerations should not be sutured in the backcountry or in a remote area, outside a medical facility, because of the risk of infection. Such lacerations should be covered with a water-resistant dressing, splinted if located over a joint, and observed. If no evidence of infection develops over 4 to 5 days, the laceration may be repaired by delayed primary closure. One exception is a laceration to the face. The face has an excellent blood supply and infections are rare. After thorough irrigation via a 14-gauge intravenous catheter attached to a syringe, relatively superficial facial wounds can be approximated with adhesive wound closure strips and then repaired with tissue glue. Scalp lacerations that are relatively superficial and uncontaminated can also be repaired after thorough irrigation. The most straightforward technique that can be used in children with hair longer than 3 cm is that of hair apposition. Strands of hair are taken from each side of the wound, twisted to achieve wound closure, and "locked" in place with cyanoacrylate glue (Figure 91-13).

If a wound becomes infected, it should be kept elevated and warm compresses applied. Given the rising incidence of methicillin–resistant *Staphylococcus aureus* (MRSA), antibiotics effective against this bacteria should be initiated promptly. Trimethoprim-sulfamethoxazole is an excellent agent. The dose is 8 to 10 mg/kg/day of the trimethoprim component divided twice daily. This is often paired with cephalexin 25 to 50 mg/kg/day (maximum 4 g/day) divided into two doses per day to cover *Streptococcal* infection. Doxycycline (2 mg/kg/day divided into two doses per day) is an option for children over 8 years of age and offers good coverage for *Staphylococcus* and some coverage for *Streptococcus* species.

ANIMAL BITES

Bites from stray dogs and other animals are more frequent during travel to the developing world. Prevention techniques primarily involve keeping children away from stray dogs and other wild

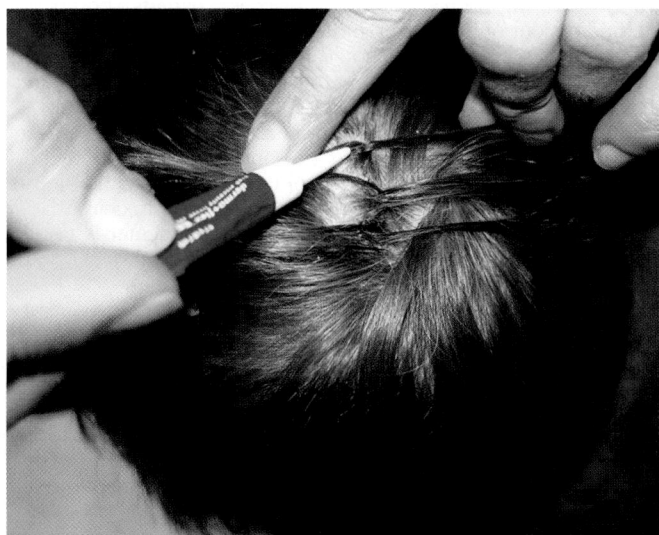

FIGURE 91-13 Hair apposition technique for scalp wound closure. *(Courtesy Judith R. Klein, MD.)*

animals and a strict "no feeding of animals" rule. Sleeping areas should be protected from bats, which are frequent carriers of disease. If a bite occurs, it should be irrigated copiously. In general, lacerations from animal bites should not be repaired primarily, with the exception of certain facial wounds. All victims of animal bites should receive antibiotic prophylaxis, ideally with amoxicillin-clavulanate (80 mg/kg/day divided into two doses) or azithromycin (10 mg/kg on day 1; then 5 mg/kg/day for 5 days) in individuals who are allergic to penicillin.[26]

Rabies is endemic in many parts of the world, including much of South and Central America, India, Southeast Asia, and the Phillipines.[65] Unlike in the United States, where bats and raccoons are the most common carriers, in the developing world, domesticated animals, such as dogs and cats, are most frequently implicated in rabies transmission. Current CDC guidelines recommend that children traveling to endemic areas for more than a month or those who will be spending a great deal of time outdoors should receive rabies prophylaxis prior to travel.[65] All animal bites that occur in areas endemic for rabies, no matter how superficial, require postexposure rabies prophylaxis (see Table 91-7 for the schedule of vaccination). Any contact between a child and a raccoon, bat, fox, or skunk in an endemic area should be considered a high-risk event and treated with rabies postexposure prophylaxis. If a bite occurs in a child who has been previously vaccinated, two more doses of the vaccine should be given. If a bite occurs in a child with no preexposure vaccination, the child should begin the four-dose rabies vaccination series *and* receive rabies immunoglobulin (HRIG: 20 IU/kg with as much as possible in and around the wound and the remainder intramuscularly in a large muscle).

POISONING

In their first few years of life, children explore the environment with their hands and mouths. Plants, flowers, mushrooms, and medications, including those in the pediatric first-aid kit, are all potentially tasty treats to a toddler. Travel into the wilderness expands the repertoire of available objects for a child to orally explore. In an urban environment or during travel in the United States, a call to a poison center (1-800-222-1222) can provide immediate information regarding the dangers of a particular ingestion and the possible need for emergency evaluation and treatment. In the wilderness and when traveling abroad, particularly in developing countries, this is rarely an option. Because it is unrealistic to expect a parent to know whether a certain medication, cosmetic, plant, or mushroom is toxic, the best advice is prevention.

All medications and cosmetics should be kept out of reach and stored in child-resistant containers. One should never try to encourage a child to take a medication by referring to it as "candy." During forays into the wilderness, parents should not let toddlers out of their sight and should explain to their children why plants or mushrooms should not be put in their mouths. If a child's skin or eyes are exposed to a toxic substance, the area should be flushed vigorously with clean water for 15 to 20 minutes. Ipecac syrup, a powerful emetic and once a mainstay of home treatment for ingested poisons, is no longer recommended by the American Academy of Pediatrics. If a child ingests a plant, mushroom, or medication with a level of toxicity that is unknown to the caregiver, and calling a poison center is not an option, the child should be taken to a medical facility for evaluation.

FOREIGN BODIES

In addition to exploring the world around them with their mouths, toddlers and even young school-age children enjoy placing objects into their noses and ears. Such objects, particularly if they are organic in nature, can result in infection of the sinuses and external ear, respectively, and should be removed promptly.

Objects that are easily visible in the nose near the nares can be removed by two caregivers. While one person holds the child's head motionless, the other carefully removes the object with forceps or tweezers. If the object is not near the nares or cannot be easily visualized, a "mouth-to-mouth" technique can be used to try to remove the object. While occluding the uninvolved nare with one finger, the parent should place her mouth over the child's mouth and blow hard several times. Ideally, this creates enough pressure to expel the object from the nasal passage. If an object is lodged in the child's ear, it is best removed with forceful irrigation with clean, warm (37°C [99°F]) water using a bulb syringe. If the object is an insect and the tympanic membrane is not perforated, the ear should first be filled with isopropyl alcohol for several minutes to kill the insect prior to irrigation. If these techniques fail to remove the foreign body from the child's ear or nose, the child should be brought to medical attention so that the object can be removed by direct visualization under proper procedural sedation.

SPECIAL CONSIDERATIONS FOR CHILDREN WITH CHRONIC MEDICAL PROBLEMS

ASTHMA

Parents of children with asthma face unique challenges when traveling into the wilderness or to the developing world. In both situations, access to medical care may be limited and parents may need to treat exacerbations that would normally require advanced medical attention. In addition, exposure to known asthma triggers, such as tobacco and specific allergens, may not be as controllable while traveling. A study of adult adventure travelers demonstrated that the major risk factors for asthma exacerbations while traveling include poorly controlled asthma prior to departure and intensive physical exertion.[21]

To prepare for travel, parents should work with their pediatrician to stabilize their child's asthma to the extent possible. Any physical exertion planned should be graded so that the child's response can be gauged and activities scaled back as necessary. In locales with heavy particulate pollution or in settings with significant tobacco exposure, the child's activities should be limited. In addition to packing extra canisters of the child's inhalers and an extra spacer or aerochamber, parents should carry a course of high-dose steroids for administration during an acute exacerbation not responding immediately to an inhaled bronchodilator (e.g., albuterol). Options for steroids include prednisone or prednisolone (2 mg/kg on day 1, then 1 mg/kg on days 2 to 5, up to a maximum of 60 mg/day) or dexamethasone (0.6 mg/kg/day for 2 days, up to a maximum of 10 mg/day). For children 5 years and older, a peak flow meter is a useful item to assist in gauging the severity of an asthma exacerbation. For families with children with life-threatening asthma (i.e., prior intubation), an EpiPen is an essential first-aid kit item.

DIABETES

Traveling with a child with diabetes requires thorough advance preparation and vigilance throughout the trip. Families traveling to the developing world or remote areas should assume that no supplies or medications will be available at their destination and should travel with sufficient insulin, syringes, alcohol wipes, lancets and test strips, and a spare glucometer. Urine test strips can be extremely useful for parents trying to decide whether their child needs to be evacuated to medical care if traveling in a remote location. The presence of ketones in the urine in a diabetic child who appears ill mandates immediate medical evaluation. Parents should also prepare a list of medical providers and/or hospitals capable of providing medical assistance to their child should the need arise.

Diabetic children should be encouraged to drink fluids frequently, particularly at high altitude and in warm climates. Parents of diabetics should always carry glucose tablets and small snacks that they know their child will eat. Older children should carry these items for themselves. Daily trip planning should guarantee that meals and snacks are not skipped by a diabetic child. Parents should also be aware that with the increased activity that occurs during travel, insulin dosing may need to be reduced to prevent hypoglycemia. Finally, diabetic children are at greater risk for infections, particularly those of the skin. All wounds should be thoroughly cleaned with soap and clean water. Any redness, warmth, or edema should be treated with antibiotics, preferably trimethoprim-sulfamethoxazole to cover MRSA. Marine wounds require quinolones and animal bites require amoxicillin-clavulanate to cover specific organisms. Diabetic children with wounds that progress despite oral antibiotics should receive prompt medical evaluation.

SICKLE CELL DISEASE

For children with sickle cell disease, the focus during travel should be on prevention. Parents should be aware of the triggers for pain crisis, and emphasize hydration and hygiene to prevent diarrheal illness. Travel to high altitude should in general be avoided, because of the possibility of altitude-related hypoxia resulting in a pain crisis. If a crisis develops, the child should be treated with rest, oral hydration, and appropriate pain medications (ibuprofen or narcotics). If this therapy is ineffective or if the crisis involves chest or abdominal pain, parents should seek immediate medical attention for their child.

Fever is a common and significant problem for children with sickle cell disease. By the age of 1 year, children with this disease are effectively asplenic as a result of sickling-related infarction. As a consequence, infections with encapsulated organisms normally cleared by the spleen can rapidly lead to sepsis. Vaccinations against *H. influenzae, Streptococcus pneumoniae,* and *Neisseria meningitidis* are the first line of defense. In addition, the American Academy of Pediatrics recommends penicillin prophylaxis (125 mg twice a day) for sickle cell patients under the age of 5 years to effect a significant (85%) reduction in pneumococcal bacteremia.[39] Children with sickle cell disease who develop fever should receive prompt medical attention. If this is not immediately available, initiate treatment with an antibiotic, such as amoxicillin-clavulanate (80 mg/kg/day divided into two doses). Children under the age of 5 years are at particularly high risk for sepsis.

CONGENITAL HEART DISEASE AND PULMONARY HYPERTENSION

Traveling with children with cardiac or pulmonary problems can be a challenge. During flight, most airline cabins are pressurized to allow a fraction of inspired oxygen (FiO_2) of 0.17 to 0.18 as opposed to the typical FiO_2 of 0.21 at sea level. Depending on the nature and severity of the child's disease, this may require arranging for an oxygen tank and delivery apparatus during flight. Travel to high altitude should be cleared by the child's primary or specialty physician for the same reasons. Respiratory infections are more common during travel. Because of the potentially significant impact of seemingly minor respiratory infections (e.g., influenza) on children with cardiopulmonary disease, hand hygiene is particularly important to prevent inoculation with infected secretions via hand-to-nose and hand-to-eye contact. An emergency plan should be available for every country on the child's itinerary, including a specialist contact and full description of the child's condition and health care needs.

EPILEPSY

Traveling with children with epilepsy involves early pretrip planning. Every effort should be made to get the child's seizures under control with medications, ideally with a 3- to 6-month seizure-free period prior to departure. In addition to a child's typical triggers for seizures (e.g., missed medication doses, fever, dehydration), travel to distant lands may involve jet lag and sleep deprivation, both of which can precipitate an event. Parents of an epileptic child should allow extra time on arrival at a destination for acclimatization to a new time zone and for adequate sleep. The child's activities during travel should be selected carefully, because rescue after a seizure event may be challenging in remote locations in the developing world. Parents should also

be encouraged to carry a generous supply of the patient's antiepileptic medications, assuming that these might not be available at the destination. In addition, a rescue medication, such as rectal diazepam (0.3 to 0.5 mg/kg), should be included in the medical kit in case the child has a lengthy (> 5 minutes) seizure or multiple seizures. Children with seizures in the setting of trauma or high fever, who do not return to the baseline mental status within an hour or two following the seizure, or who have atypical or multiple seizures within a short period of time, should be brought to medical attention.

TRAVELING WITH INFANTS AND NEONATES

A family traveling with an infant should be particularly vigilant about monitoring their child's state of health. Infants become hypothermic, hyperthermic, septic, and dehydrated more rapidly than do adults or older children. A thermometer and appropriate lubricant should be included in the medical kit for monitoring rectal temperature. Digital thermometers are recommended, because they are less likely to break, are easy to read, and acquire a temperature reading three to four times faster than does a glass thermometer. Rectal temperature above 38°C (100.4°F) in a child younger than age 3 months requires immediate medical evaluation.

Infants are less tolerant of problems that generate excess mucus. Until the age of 6 months, infants are obligate nose breathers, so obstruction of the nasal passages with mucus can cause significant respiratory distress. A bulb syringe is handy for suctioning mucus from the oropharynx and nasal passages. A few drops of saline solution (1/4 tsp of salt in 1 cup of water) instilled into the nares a few minutes before aspiration helps to loosen mucus. Nasal aspiration should be reserved for times of most need, such as before feeding and sleep, because the procedure is irritating to a child. Other uses for a clean bulb syringe include flushing foreign bodies from ears and administering enemas.

Away from the conveniences of home, diapers tend to be changed less frequently. Diaper rash can become a problem. A barrier cream containing zinc oxide may be helpful, and should be used at the first sign of irritation. If the rash progresses to intense erythema with satellite lesions despite appropriate cleaning and barrier cream use, an antifungal cream, such as miconazole or clotrimazole, should be applied two to three times a day until the rash resolves. The child should also be left for a few hours each day without a diaper to make the perineal area less hospitable to fungus. Children with severe diarrhea can develop diaper-area dermatitis from irritant stool. These children should be treated with a topical antiinflammatory, such as 1% hydrocortisone topped by a barrier cream.

In very young infants, 3 to 12 weeks of age, colic can be a challenging and vexing problem. A few hours of inconsolable crying a day is not uncommon in this age group, but should still prompt investigation. If the infant is feeding well, urinating and stooling regularly, and has neither fever nor rash, the most likely cause for this recurrent, seemingly inconsolable crying is colic. Colic is defined as a pattern of daily paroxysms of irritability and crying without a significant identifiable cause. The pathophysiology of colic is not clear but has been postulated as immaturity in the gastrointestinal or nervous system, response to maternally ingested foods in breastfed babies, or a product of over- or understimulation of an infant. Colicky infants can often be soothed with rocking motions and close parental contact. Gentle abdominal massage can also be helpful. Breastfeeding mothers should consider eliminating caffeine, spicy foods, citrus, and/or dairy from their diets. Colic typically resolves by 3 to 4 months of age.

Box 91-9 outlines indications for immediate medical evaluation of young infants. As mentioned previously, parents are strongly advised against traveling to the developing world with children under the age of 2 years. Immature immune systems, an incomplete vaccination status, contraindications to prophylactic medications and travel vaccines, and frequent hand-to-mouth

Appearance of being ill
Fever in a child < 3 mo of age
Respiratory distress or apnea
  Capillary refill time > 2 sec and/or no urine output in 8 hr
Lethargy/persistent irritability
  Vomiting > 24 hr
Bloody stools
Rash: vesicles, petechiae, or purpura

BOX 91-10 Pediatric Wilderness Medical Kit: Basic Supplies

- Identification and basic health information for child: past medical history, medications, allergies, blood type, weight
- First-aid supplies: adhesive bandages, gauze pads, gauze roll, tape, nonadherent dressings, moleskin/Spenco 2nd Skin/New-Skin, benzoin, steri-strips, cyanoacrylate glue, alcohol wipes, povidone-iodine solution for dilution and disinfection, safety pins, tweezers, lightweight malleable splint (SAM splint), syringe (20-35 mL), and 14-gauge plastic catheter for wound irrigation
- Powdered oral rehydration solution (homemade or commercially available formula that meets the World Health Organization recommendations)
- Sunscreen: SPF 15 or greater
- Insect repellent: DEET < 35% or picaridin
- Whistle for child
- For infant < 3 months: rectal thermometer, bulb syringe

DEET, N,N-diethyl-m-toluamide; SPF, sun protection factor.

contact make infants and very young children extremely susceptible to disease. Only essential travel should be undertaken.

PEDIATRIC WILDERNESS MEDICAL KITS

When a family travels in remote areas, the medical kit must be adapted to meet the special needs of children. Items carried vary depending on the ages of the children, preexisting medical conditions, length of travel, specific environmental conditions likely to be encountered, and medical sophistication of the adults. Although there is considerable room for individual preference in assembling a medical kit, certain items are essential for management of problems commonly encountered during wilderness travel with children (Box 91-10).

To reduce weight and bulk, medications selected for a wilderness medical kit should have multiple uses (Table 91-12). For example, diphenhydramine is effective for allergic symptoms, pruritus, motion sickness, nausea, and insomnia. Desitin, best known for its use in preventing diaper rash, is an excellent sunblock, because it contains 40% zinc oxide. A broad-spectrum antifungal cream, such as miconazole or clotrimazole, covers not only tineal infections (ringworm, jock itch, and athlete's foot) but also *Candida* infections (diaper rash and vaginitis). Medications in liquid form should generally be avoided because they add excess weight to the medical kit and can leak. If an infant under the age of 6 months is traveling, liquid medications can be carried in light- and leak-proof powder form. Most children are able to chew tablets once their first molars are present (by about 15 months). Before that time, chewable medications or tablets can be crushed between two spoons and mixed with food. If a child dislikes the taste of a medication, it may be camouflaged

in food such as instant pudding, which is easily carried in powdered form.

Painful musculoskeletal injuries are a potential complication of wilderness activities, so pain medication for children should be included in every medical kit. Acetaminophen not only relieves minor aches and pains but also is effective for fever control. It is well tolerated by most children and available in many pleasant-tasting forms for children unable to swallow pills: chewable 80- or 160-mg tablets, elixir (160 mg/5 mL), and concentrated drops (80 mg/0.8 mL). Ibuprofen is effective for pain and fever control. Its duration of action is 6 to 8 hours, compared with 4 to 6 hours for acetaminophen. Ibuprofen is available in many forms: infant drops (40 mg/mL), children's elixir (100 mg/5 mL), 50- or 100-mg chewable tablets, and 100- or 200-mg caplets. Analgesics that contain narcotics are generally not recommended for children, particularly for the first few years of life, due to respiratory depression. Many recent studies suggest that such analgesics are no more effective for severe pain in children than ibuprofen given in the proper dosage.[64]

Two or three antibiotics will treat most bacterial infections encountered in children. The ages of children traveling, their allergies or chronic medical conditions, their intolerance of medications, and past experience, as well as knowledge of the disease prevalence or epidemics at the travel destination, must be taken

TABLE 91-12 Pediatric Medications in the Wilderness Medical Kit

Medication	Indication	Dose
Topical Medications		
Antiseptic ointment (e.g., bacitracin or polymyxin)	Superficial skin infections	Apply as directed qd to tid
Topical corticosteroid (e.g., 1% hydrocortisone)	Contact or atopic dermatitis, insect bites, sunburn	Apply to affected areas bid to tid (use sunscreen aggressively; avoid > 1% corticosteroid on face)
Antifungal cream (e.g., clotrimazole or miconazole)	Yeast at diaper area, groin, scalp, feet; ringworm	Apply bid for 7-10 days and for several days after rash has resolved
Desitin cream	Sunblock, diaper-area erythema	Apply thick coat as sunscreen or thin coat for diaper area
Permethrin (Elimite)	Scabies, lice, treatment for clothing and mosquito netting	Apply 5% cream from chin to soles of feet and wash after 8-14 hr; do not use in children < 2 mo of age or on eyes, nose, mouth
Anesthetic eye drops (e.g., proparacaine)*†	Removal of superficial ocular foreign body	1 drop in affected eye for removal of foreign body; must patch eye for protection for at least 1 hr
Antibiotic eye ointment (e.g., erythromycin)† or drops (e.g., polymyxin B sulfate plus trimethoprim [Polytrim])†	Purulent conjunctivitis, suspected corneal abrasion	Ointment: thin line upper lid margin tid to qid; Drops: 1 drop every 3 hr for 7 days

TABLE 91-12   Pediatric Medications in the Wilderness Medical Kit—cont'd

Medication	Indication	Dose
Antipyrine-benzocaine otic drops†	Ear pain (otitis externa or media); avoid if < 3 mo or tympanic membrane rupture suspected	3-4 drops in affected ear every 2-3 hr as needed to relieve pain
Oral Medications		
Diphenhydramine 12.5 mg/5 mL elixir 25- or 50-mg capsules	Allergy symptoms, pruritus, insomnia, nausea, motion sickness	1.25 mg/kg/dose every 6 hr (up to 25-50 mg/dose); may cause paradoxic restlessness in children
Acetaminophen 80 mg/0.8 mL drops 160 mg/5 mL elixir 80- and 160-mg chewable tabs	Fever control, pain	15-20 mg/kg every 4-6 hr up to 650 mg/dose
Ibuprofen 40 mg/1 mL drops 100 mg/5 mL elixir 50- or 100-mg chewable tabs 100- or 200-mg caplets	Fever control, pain, antiinflammatory	10 mg/kg/dose every 8 hr up to 600 mg/dose
Dimenhydrinate (Dramamine) 12.5 mg/5 mL elixir 50-mg chewable tabs	Motion sickness	1-1.5 mg/kg/dose 1 hr before departure and every 6 hr after; may cause drowsiness
Oral Antibiotics (as Appropriate for Age of Child)		
Amoxicillin†	Acute otitis media, sinusitis, pharyngitis, pneumonia	80 mg/kg/day in divided dose bid for 10 days if < 5 yr or for 5 days if > 5 yr 125- or 250-mg chewable tabs 250-mg capsule
Amoxicillin-clavulanate (Augmentin)†	Penicillin-resistant organisms, acute otitis media, sinusitis, animal bites	80 mg/kg/day in divided dose bid 200- and 400-mg chewable tabs 200 and 400 mg/5 mL elixir
Azithromycin (Zithromax)†	Acute otitis media, sinusitis, pharyngitis, pneumonia, traveler's diarrhea, skin infections, animal bites	10 mg/kg on day 1, then 5 mg/kg/day for 4 days 125 and 250 mg/5 mL elixir 250-mg tabs (best)
Ciprofloxacin (Cipro)†	Not first line < 18 yr due to adverse effects: urinary tract infection, traveler's diarrhea, wounds acquired in an aquatic environment	20-30 mg/kg/day in divided dose bid up to 500 mg bid 100-, 200-, 500-mg tabs
Trimethoprim-sulfamethoxazole (Septra)†	Suspected methicillin-resistant *Staphylococcus aureus* skin infection 80/400 SS tab; 160/800 DS tab	8-10 mg trimethoprim/kg/day in divided dose bid > 2 months old
Oseltamivir (Tamiflu)†	Influenza treatment (12 mg/mL susp 30-, 45-, 75-mg caps)	Not recommended < 3 mo old; treat for 5 days 3-12 mo: 3 mg/kg/dose twice daily > 12 mo or < 15 kg: 30 mg bid 15-23 kg: 45 mg bid 24-40 kg: 60 mg bid > 40 kg: 75 mg bid
Other Preparations		
Epinephrine (premeasured)† 0.15 mg EpiPen Jr 0.3 mg EpiPen	Anaphylaxis, severe asthma	0.15 mg intramuscularly up to 15 kg (33 lb); 0.3 mg intramuscularly if > 15 kg (> 33 lb)
Oral rehydration packet	Dehydration	See Table 91-11 for administration guidelines
Foreign Travel		
Loperamide 1 mg/5 mL 1 mg caps	Nonbloody diarrhea, minimally febrile, significant diarrhea older than age 2 years	13-20 kg (29-44 lb): 1 mg tid; 20-30 kg (44-66 lb): 2 mg bid; > 30 kg (> 66 lb): 2 mg tid;
Appropriate malaria prophylaxis†	—	See Table 91-9 if indicated†
Zofran ODT† 4 mg tab	Nausea/vomiting, dehydration	6 mo-1yr: 1 mg 1-4 yr: 2 mg > 4 yr: 4 mg
Travel to High Altitude		
Acetazolamide (Diamox)† 30 or 50 mg/mL suspension 125-mg tab	Recurrent acute mountain sickness despite graded ascent	5 mg/kg/day divided bid up to 250 mg/day

*Administration of this medication by other than trained medical personnel is strongly discouraged, given the risk of overuse and subsequent worsening of eye injury; if significant eye irritation persists, medical attention must be sought to evaluate for corneal injury.
†Available by prescription only.

into account when antibiotics are selected. Given increasing bacterial resistance to common antibiotics, choices should be reevaluated periodically to ensure that infections likely to be encountered can be successfully treated with these agents. All oral antibiotics require a prescription. Amoxicillin is available in pleasant-tasting chewable tablets (125 and 250 mg) and in powdered form for suspension (125 and 250 mg/5 mL). Because of current resistance patterns, high-dose therapy with 80 mg/kg in divided doses, twice daily, is indicated. Amoxicillin is familiar to and well tolerated by most children. Amoxicillin-clavulanate provides excellent coverage when a penicillin-resistant organism is suspected for recurrent pharyngitis, soft tissue infections, animal bites, and other infections. The most common side effect is diarrhea, but this is reduced with newer formulations. Both are available in 200- and 400-mg (amoxicillin component) chewable tablets and as 200 and 400 mg/5 mL liquid. Azithromycin (Zithromax) is a long-acting macrolide without the gastrointestinal side effects of erythromycin. It is effective for treating otitis media, sinusitis, pharyngitis, lower respiratory tract infections, TD, skin infections, typhoid fever, and common animal bites. It is particularly useful in children with penicillin allergies. Because of its broad utility, azithromycin is an excellent antibiotic choice for a pediatric medical kit. Dosing is extremely convenient because of azithromycin's long half-life; a dose of 10 mg/kg on day 1 is followed by 5 mg/kg/day for a total of 5 days. Ciprofloxacin has broad-spectrum coverage and is useful for treatment of bacterial diarrhea, complex urinary tract infections, typhoid fever, and wounds acquired in an aquatic environment. Its use has not been approved for children younger than age 18 years in the United States because of a potential problem with arthropathic effects on weight-bearing joints. However, a study involving more than 600 children found only a 1.3% rate of reversible arthralgia and no evidence of arthropathy.[1] Nonetheless, ciprofloxacin should not routinely be recommended for children unless a special situation arises in which the benefits of its use outweigh the risks (e.g., complex pyelonephritis, typhoid fever). Trimethoprim-sulfamethoxazole (Septra) is a sulfa antibiotic useful against skin infections where MRSA is a concern. In many areas, the presence of MRSA in infected wounds and cellulitis is so high that the recommendation is to always use an agent with bactericidal activity against MRSA. The dose is 8 to 10 mg/kg/day of the trimethoprim component in divided doses twice daily. Finally, for children younger than age 5 years, those with chronic medical conditions, or those receiving long-term aspirin therapy who will be traveling in areas with influenza activity, parents should consider including oseltamivir (Tamiflu) in their medical kit.[40] It is available in suspension or capsule form. The dose is 3 mg/kg/day in two divided doses.

Parents of children with special medical conditions should carry a pertinent medical summary and have resources to gain access to specialty physicians in the destination countries. A generous supply of necessary medications with instructions for caregivers and consulting physicians on treatment plans for various complications should be included in the medical kit. An extra supply of all essential medications should be kept with either the parents or the patient in case the medical kit gets lost or separated from the patient when the medication is needed. Some travelers in areas endemic for hepatitis B or C and acquired immunodeficiency syndrome carry their own needles and syringes for emergency use. The International Association for Medical Assistance to Travelers (iamat.org) maintains a directory of qualified physicians worldwide who speak English.

ENVIRONMENTAL CONCERNS AND CHILD HEALTH

Because of their physical, physiologic, and cognitive immaturity, children are particularly vulnerable to adverse health effects from environmental hazards. Children breathe more air, drink more water, and eat more food per unit of body weight than adults. They play more outdoors and have more life-years during which to suffer any long-term ill effects of environmental degradation and climate extremes. It is estimated that by 2100, there will be an additional 60,000 to 250,000 pediatric deaths each year due to health conditions related to climate change.[6,10]

Specifically, children are more susceptible to thermal stresses that can lead to dehydration and hyperthermia, particularly during exercise. Higher average temperatures may further increase this risk. The rates of sunburn in children and of subsequent melanoma are likely to rise. Warmer temperatures typically result in higher levels of ozone and other air pollutants. Because children tend to spend more time outdoors and have higher minute ventilation, increased air pollution can significantly affect children with asthma and other respiratory diseases. Warmer winters and rising carbon dioxide levels may result in earlier and more abundant release of pollens derived from grasses and other plants, which could increase incidence and severity of atopic syndromes in children.[10] Higher temperatures, along with changes in humidity and flood frequency, are likely to result in significant increases in vector- and rodent-borne disease transmission. Recent modeling experiments suggest that global distribution of malaria, a disproportionate killer of children, is likely to expand over the coming decades.[18,63] The rate of dengue virus replication in *A. aegypti* mosquitoes increases directly with temperature. Higher global temperatures may result in a higher infection rate, particularly in children who are less able to protect themselves from mosquitoes. Tick-borne diseases may become more prevalent as flooding expands the rodent population that is an integral part of the tick life cycle. Extremes of precipitation, specifically flooding, increase the likelihood of drinking contaminated water and contracting waterborne gastrointestinal illnesses. As discussed previously, children suffer disproportionate rates of morbidity and mortality from acute gastroenteritis.

If for no other reason than preserving our children's health, it is incumbent upon us to mitigate these effects of fossil fuel consumption. Physicians and other health care professionals can educate communities about the impacts of climate change on child health and emphasize the need for policies supportive of a clean, healthy environment.

REFERENCES

Complete references used in this text are available online at expertconsult.inkling.com.

CHAPTER 92

Women in the Wilderness

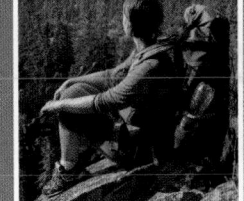

RENEE N. SALAS AND SUSAN ANDERSON

> Travel not only stirs the blood … it also gives birth to the spirit.
> Alexandra David-Neel, French explorer and writer (1868-1969), who walked 2000 miles (3220 km) across the Himalayas to enter Lhasa at the age of 55 in 1924

Women travel to remote areas of the world at all stages of life. Wilderness travel health issues vary according to a woman's life stage and style. Travel may include adolescent women kayaking in Amazonian jungles, pregnant women climbing 5000-m (16,000-foot) peaks, and senior researcher scientists working for a year in Antarctica.

Wilderness experiences may increase a woman's self-esteem. Physical activity has numerous health benefits for women, including stress reduction and prevention of osteoporosis, heart disease, diabetes, breast cancer, cognitive decline, osteoporotic fractures, and depression.[41,54,149] Women defy daily prior boundaries in outdoor achievement. Companies have taken notice. Active clothing and recreational equipment designed specifically for women represent a multibillion-dollar industry.

Problems unique to women can diminish the wilderness experience or place travelers at risk. Wilderness travel health recommendations for a particular woman should consider her age and life stage, background and health history, level of fitness, itinerary, and planned activity. Physicians and other health care providers can assist women embarking on wilderness experiences by providing individualized prevention and treatment guidelines. Because wilderness journeys may include travel to remote locations, special considerations for wilderness travel to developing countries are discussed.

GENDER-BASED RESEARCH

In 2001, the Institute of Medicine of the National Academy of Sciences released the report "Exploring the Biological Contributions to Human Health: Does Sex Matter?"[112] The institute's report was the first significant review of biomedical research to date related to sex and gender differences. The report confirmed the importance of gender and recommended more funding for multidisciplinary research to address issues of gender and health in all areas of medicine.

Since then, women's health- and gender-based research initiatives have been developed at academic institutions and organizations around the world. New training programs and fellowships have grown exponentially, and more journals, textbooks, and other related publications have focused on women's health and gender medicine.[30,31,131-133,150,183,210,211]

Wilderness medicine research exploring gender issues is increasing (e.g., study of effects of extremes of environment on fertility and pregnancy outcome). Pregnant women who live at altitude experience a high rate of fetal intrauterine growth restriction (IUGR). Ramifications of this for pregnant short-term travelers to altitude are being studied. Certain infectious diseases (e.g., malaria, typhoid, and amebiasis) carry special risks for women (e.g., an accelerated or more severe course), especially during pregnancy.[180] Women exposed to schistosomiasis by swimming, canoeing, or rafting may become infected. Female genital schistosomiasis can lead to subtle genital tract inflammatory changes that increase the risk of future infertility.[65,72,74,86,106,183,210] For a woman, exposure to certain environmental extremes or pathogens at a particular stage of life may lead to severe long-term consequences.

Many practical questions need to be answered. What is the safety of recommended immunizations and medications for a specific itinerary in pregnancy? What is the risk for deep thrombosis in a breast cancer survivor taking tamoxifen who wants to trek over a 5500-m (18,000-foot) mountain pass? Do antimicrobials prescribed for malaria chemoprophylaxis or for self-treatment of traveler's diarrhea interfere with efficacy of oral contraceptive pills? Gender and life-stage issues are important when considering a woman's risks for wilderness and environmental exposure, preventive measures, treatment options, and possible long-term complications.

PRE–WILDERNESS TRAVEL WOMEN'S HEALTH ASSESSMENT

Key areas to address for any female wilderness traveler are outlined in the pre–wilderness travel checklist for women (Box 92-1). Priorities are to identify each patient's life-stage and medical issues that could be exacerbated by physical demands and the wilderness setting. Environmental and infectious disease risks should be assessed. Consider the duration of the excursion, need for additional conditioning and acclimatization, and any difficulty in gaining access to sophisticated medical care.

Prior to undertaking physically challenging activities or prolonged remote travel, women should undergo a thorough medical assessment (Box 92-2). The physician collects historical information and performs a comprehensive physical examination, with special attention to the genitourinary tract, breasts, and cardiovascular, respiratory, and musculoskeletal systems. Laboratory screening should be guided by the patient's age, medical status, and risk factors. Consider assays for hemoglobin and hematocrit, thyroid panel, urinalysis, urine culture, pregnancy test, Pap smear, and screening for sexually transmitted infections (STIs) and hepatitis. In women more than 40 years of age, consider an electrocardiogram with stress testing and pulmonary function tests. In women with a strong family history of breast cancer, consider a mammogram. Bone densitometry should be considered in perimenopausal and postmenopausal women and in young women with a history of fractures or abnormal menses consistent with a hypoestrogenic state.

Recommendations for a medical kit should be adapted to life-stage and health needs. Provide maintenance medications for optimal control of medical conditions for the planned duration of travel, emergency needs, and expected dose adjustments. Review contraceptive needs and options. Include basic supplies for hygienic and anticipated therapeutic needs related to menses, the urinary tract, and vaginitis. Suggestions are given in Table 92-1 and Box 92-3.

After the medical evaluation, a final risk assessment should be discussed with guidelines for prevention and treatment versus adaptation of the itinerary to decrease any particular risk.

WHAT MAKES WOMEN DIFFERENT?
GENDER-RELATED PERFORMANCE

Gender-specific differences in anatomy and physiology are mainly due to hormonal differences that vary across the life span. Typically, women are smaller than men, have less lean muscle

BOX 92-1   Pre–Wilderness Travel Checklist for Women

Current age or life stage
Personal level of risk taking
Itinerary
Gender-specific recommendations related to:
   Environmental risks
     Altitude, heat, cold, water, etc.
     Preventive measures
   Infectious disease risk
     Vaccine-preventable diseases
     Chemoprophylaxis
     Personal protective measures
   Sports and exercise
     Level of fitness
     Equipment
Practical issues
   Genitourinary issues
     Menstruation or dysfunctional uterine bleeding
     Contraception and emergency contraception
     Breast health
     Vaginal health
     Urinary tract issues
     Sexually transmitted infection risk
   Pregnancy
     Planned or unplanned
     Lactation
   Perimenopausal and menopausal issues
Medical issues
   Past medical history
   Long-term travel
     Pap smear and mammogram
     Copy of electrocardiogram if older than 50 years or cardiac history
Psychological issues
Cultural issues
Personal safety issues
   Self-defense training
   Personal protection devices
Wilderness medicine kit
Emergency plans
   Medical and evacuation insurance
   Copy of medical data

BOX 92-3   Supplies for the Medical Kit for Women

Menstrual supplies
   Calendar to keep track of menses
   Supplies and devices
     Pads, tampons, menstrual cups
     Towelettes, plastic disposal bags, matches
     Premenstrual symptom medications
     Dysfunctional uterine bleeding medications
Urinary voiding
   Medications for urinary tract infections and burning
   Toilet tissue, towelettes
   Funnels, paper or plastic
   Pads for incontinence
   Urinary dipstick to screen for infection
Vaginitis
   Self-treatment medications (yeast, bacterial vaginosis)
   pH paper
   Vaginal speculum and gloves if trained medical professional on expedition
Contraception
   Contraception options
   Emergency contraception
   Chart to keep track of pills, patches, or ring use
   Timer, special wristwatch or cell phone "alarm"
Pregnancy tests
Perimenopausal and menopausal issues
   Stress incontinence, pads
   Atrophic vaginitis, vaginal moisturizers and lubricants
Pregnancy supplies
   Prenatal vitamins
   Blood pressure cuff
   Urine protein and glucose strips to screen for diabetes and preeclampsia
   Urine leukocyte esterase strips to check for urinary tract infection
Supplies for lactation
   Breast pump
   Nipple cream
   Self-treatment, mastitis
Personal safety
   Alarms
   Pepper spray
   Other self-defense measures

BOX 92-2   Assessment of a Woman's Health: Screening Highlights

Menstrual History
Age at menarche, regularity, characteristics, timing, extent of blood flow (length, amount), intermenstrual bleeding, perimenstrual symptoms (e.g., dysmenorrhea, headache, premenstrual syndrome), plans for managing periods (hygienic, therapeutic)

Sexual History
Age at coitarche, number of partners, sexual orientation, sexually transmitted infections, contraceptive history, plans for sexual activity in the wilderness, dyspareunia

Gynecologic History
Ovarian cysts, uterine fibroids, endometriosis, cervical dysplasia, surgical history, pelvic pain, vaginal discharge, vaginal infections and treatment, pregnancy and complications

Breast
Galactorrhea, discharge, masses, surgery

Gastrointestinal System and Urinary Tract
Ulcers, irritable bowel syndrome, gallbladder disease, constipation, urinary tract infections, nephrolithiasis, stress incontinence, urgency incontinence

Musculoskeletal System and Skin
Injuries (exercise related and accidents), limitations, muscle cramps, joint pain and swelling, arthritis, rashes, acne, sun sensitivity, hirsutism, hair loss

Exposure to Abuse
Battering, sexual harassment, sexual assault

Habits
Smoking, alcohol, illicit drug use

Current Problems
Condition, medications, status of control, complications

Immunizations
Measles, mumps, rubella, polio, diphtheria, tetanus, hepatitis, others

Family History
Thyroid disease, hypertension, autoimmune disorders, diabetes, breast and gynecologic malignancies, osteoporosis

Allergies
General, drug related, bite and sting sensitivities

Nutritional
Eating disorders, weight changes, food sensitivities, dietary preferences (e.g., vegetarianism), caloric intake, assessment of mineral and vitamin intake in diet, supplements (e.g., iron, vitamins, calcium), including homeopathic compounds

TABLE 92-1 Medications for the Medical Kit for Women*†

Indication	Medication	Dosage
Dysmenorrhea	Ibuprofen	200 mg PO 3 tabs q 6-8 hr
Headache/pain/fever	Acetaminophen	325-650 mg PO q 6 hr; max 3 g/24 hr
Nausea and vomiting	Promethazine (tablet or suppository)	12.5-25 mg PO or per rectum q 4-6 hr prn for nausea
	Ondansetron ODT (orally dissolving tablet)	4-8 mg SL (under the tongue) q 6-12 hr prn for nausea
Urinary tract infection	Nitrofurantoin	100 mg PO BID for 5 days
	Ciprofloxacin	250-500 mg PO BID for 3 days (for pyelonephritis, 500 mg BID for 7-14 days)
	Trimethoprim-sulfamethoxazole	160 mg/800 mg PO BID for 3-5 days
Pyelonephritis: Nitrofurantoin does not have appropriate renal penetration and thus should not be used. Other antibiotics listed can be used for an extended length of treatment (7-14 days) when pyelonephritis is clinically suspected.		
Urinary analgesic	Pyridium	200 mg PO TID for 2 days prn for burning
Yeast vaginitis	Miconazole cream or suppository	One applicator qhs for 1-7 days
	Fluconazole	150 mg PO single dose
Bacterial vaginosis	Metronidazole tablets	500 mg PO BID for 7 days
	Tinidazole	1 g PO qd for 5 days
		2 g PO qd for 2 days
	Metronidazole vaginal gel/clindamycin vaginal cream	One applicator qhs for 3-7 days
Menstrual regulation or breakthrough bleeding	Oral contraceptive pills	1 qd
	Conjugated estrogen	2.5 mg PO qd
	Medroxyprogesterone acetate	5-10 mg PO qd (For abnormal uterine bleeding, duration is 5-10 days starting day 16 or 21 of menstrual cycle.)
Nutritional supplements	Ferrous sulfate	325 mg PO qd-TID
	Calcium carbonate	1000-1250 mg PO qd
	Multivitamin	1 PO qd

BID, Twice daily; PO, by mouth; prn, as needed; q, every; qd, daily; qhs, at bedtime; TID, three times daily.
*These recommendations are in addition to the ones recommended for a general medical kit in Chapter 102.
†Suggested medications or equivalent depending on tolerance, allergy history, and patient preferences.

mass, and have 8% to 10% more fat mass for a given body size. These differences are attributed to increased estrogens in females and increased androgens in males. Females reach physiologic and skeletal maturity and achieve peak height at an earlier age than do males. Women have a larger surface area–to–body mass ratio. The blood volume and hemoglobin, stroke volume, and cardiac output are all lower in women. These and other factors contribute to lower maximal aerobic power (even for similar training status) in women. $\dot{V}O_2$max is the gold standard as an index of cardiorespiratory fitness. Women of comparable training status usually have $\dot{V}O_2$max values that are 5% to 15% lower than those of men. Correction of $\dot{V}O_2$max values for lean body mass does not correct the discrepancy between genders completely, which may relate to lower hemoglobin concentrations in women, leading to less oxygen-carrying capacity.[66]

Estrogen and progesterone influence ventilation and thermoregulation during exercise. Women have a smaller lung capacity than men, which may limit women's extreme exercise performance. Control of ventilation is influenced by progesterone that increases the central ventilatory drive and affects breathing responsiveness during exercise and at altitude.[66]

Thermoregulatory control is affected by the menstrual cycle. In the menstrual cycle's luteal phase, when progesterone and estrogen are elevated, thresholds at which cutaneous vasodilation and sweating are initiated increase approximately +0.5° C (+1.8° F) as compared with the early follicular phase, when these hormones are low. These subtle thermoregulatory differences across the menstrual cycle have not been found to affect exercise performance. Physiologic mechanisms that affect adaptation and performance in women are subtle. There is substantial biologic variability among individuals.[2,123]

GENDER-RELATED ISSUES CONCERNING ENVIRONMENTAL EXPOSURE

Women and Altitude

Differences in how men and women respond to altitude are thought to be hormonally mediated. Adaptation to high altitude involves a series of physiologic responses triggered by hypoxemia. The sigmoidal shape of the oxyhemoglobin dissociation curve prevents a drop in the oxygen saturation below 90% in healthy persons until an altitude of approximately 2400 m (8000 feet) is reached. At higher altitudes, hypoxia stimulates respiratory, cardiovascular, and hematologic changes influenced by degree and duration of hypoxia.

Increased minute ventilation (i.e., increased tidal volume and respiratory rate) is the central initial response to high altitude. This hypoxic ventilatory response (HVR) is mediated by carotid body chemoreceptors that respond to a decrease in arterial oxygen pressure (PaO_2) and signal the medullary respiratory center to increase ventilation. The HVR has been closely related to adequacy of acclimatization and risk for developing acute mountain sickness (AMS).[185] The degree of HVR to a given PaO_2 varies among individuals and is genetically influenced. The HVR is inhibited by respiratory depressants (e.g., alcohol and sedatives) and stimulated by respiratory stimulants (e.g., caffeine and cocoa). Progesterone is a potent respiratory stimulant and acts primarily through activation of peripheral arterial chemoreceptors. Progesterone is produced by all steroid-forming glands (e.g., ovaries, testes, adrenal cortex, corpus luteum, and placenta).

The effect of hormones on ventilatory control is debated.[43,179] Some studies have shown no gender variation between hypoxic sensitivity differences; others have shown a difference.[45,143,159,175] Evidence suggests that the HVR is less pronounced in women. This has been attributed to testosterone's ability to increase the chemoreflex.[60,156,170,208,213] There does not appear to be any difference between the sexes in the hypercapnic ventilatory response.[117,175] Women appear to be less susceptible to periodic breathing during sleep at altitude, possibly because of a decreased chemoreflex sensitivity to hypoxia.[60,140] Acetazolamide reduces periodic breathing during sleep in both sexes.[60] Extended altitude exposure in women causes a decreased $\dot{V}O_2$max but no change in the maximal heart rate and work capacity.[84] In one study, women had a 13% decrease in $\dot{V}O_2$max versus 17% in men.[44]

No gender difference exists in the incidence of AMS. The AMS incidence is not affected significantly by the menstrual phase.[93]

Even in the menstrual cycle's luteal phase, when progesterone levels increase as much as 10-fold, no difference has been observed between males and nonpregnant females in AMS incidence.[98] Early studies reported an increased incidence of pulmonary edema in men. These studies were skewed by a vast predominance of male subjects and may not reflect a true gender predilection.[91,99,141] Women have a higher incidence of peripheral edema at high altitude.[98] Extended high-altitude exposure is known to cause decreases in body weight, from 0% to 5% of fat free mass. Women were found to have a smaller fat loss than males and to adapt more slowly.[84,223]

Women incur a risk of physical trauma and delayed medical care during remote travel. Evidence, recommendations, and guidelines for pregnant women traveling to altitude are discussed in the pregnancy section.

Women and Hot and Cold Environments

Because of a lower basal sweat rate, women rely more heavily on circulatory mechanisms for heat dissipation in hot environments.[186] In hot, humid environments (e.g., jungle), a lower sweat rate allows females to adapt more easily and decreases the risk for dehydration.[32] In hot, arid environments (e.g., desert), if adequate fluid replacement is available, a higher sweat rate is advantageous because perspiration decreases the hyperthermia risk. Following acclimation to dry heat, women's sudorific response begins to equal that of men. With similar acclimatization and physical training, women tolerate physical activity in hot environments as well as do men. Women planning wilderness expeditions to hot, dry destinations are advised to plan a 1- to 2-week acclimation period in a hot environment. In general, heat tolerance depends more on cardiovascular fitness than on gender.

In moderately cold environments, women typically adapt better than men, partly because they have a thicker layer of subcutaneous fat. At extremely cold temperatures, women may be at a disadvantage because of decreased muscle mass. Although adaptation to cold environments depends more on body size, physical fitness, and degree of acclimation than on gender, exercise performed during cold exposure may be more effective in maintaining body heat in women than in men.[146] Primary Raynaud's syndrome precipitated by a cold environment is more common in women and may result in numb or painful extremities, typically of the digits. Rewarming an affected area is therapeutic. Preventive measures (e.g., wearing gloves and using hand and boot warmers before exposure) are helpful. Treatment with a calcium channel blocker (e.g., nifedipine) remains a widely used therapy, although evidence of its efficacy is not conclusive.[82] Suggested treatment doses are nifedipine IR (immediate release) tablets 10 to 30 mg orally three times a day or nifedipine SR (sustained release) tablets 30 to 90 mg orally once a day, titrated to symptom relief. Other treatment options include topical 1% nitroglycerin or L-arginine, sildenafil, L-arginine, and botulinum toxin A.[113,129]

GENDER-RELATED ISSUES CONCERNING INFECTIOUS DISEASES

Wilderness travel may increase exposure to infectious diseases. Gender-related anatomic or physiologic differences (e.g., pregnancy) can influence the risk.[135,193] Women should update routine and travel-related immunizations prior to becoming pregnant. Maternal vaccination decreases the risk to the unborn child. Preconception immunizations are preferred to vaccination during pregnancy. Because as many as 50% of pregnancies are unplanned, women of reproductive age should be encouraged to update their regular and travel-related immunizations at all routine visits. Travel-related infections (e.g., malaria and hepatitis E) for which there are no preventive immunizations can create increased risks during pregnancy.

To advise women on infectious risk issues, especially for long-term or adventure travel to endemic and remote areas, consider the geographic location; mode of transmission, clinical manifestations, and diagnosis of possible infections; how infections might affect a pregnancy or lead to changes in the female genital tract; and other gender-related issues.

Schistosomiasis is caused by the *Schistosoma* trematode and is believed to infect nearly 200 million individuals in 76 countries.[94A,148] Female genital schistosomiasis has been associated with a wide range of pathologies (e.g., infertility, miscarriage, preterm delivery, and increased susceptibility to superinfections and human immunodeficiency virus [HIV]).[125,172] Women may have lesions of the vulva, vagina, cervix, uterus, and fallopian tubes. The risk for schistosomiasis in female adventure travelers and expatriates living in endemic areas is considerable.[67,134,198,215] Nearly all cases occur in individuals who travel to Africa, with an additional risk factor being a month or more of travel.[148] Centers for Disease Control and Prevention (CDC) investigators found a high incidence of schistosomiasis among expatriates in Malawi. Of 917 persons serologically tested, 302 (33%) had the schistosomal antibody. Of these, 292 (93%) had the antibody to *Schistosoma haematobium*.[65] After recreational exposure (e.g., swimming, wading, kayaking) in the Nile River in Uganda, 17% had evidence of schistosome infection. Physicians may be confronted with parasitic infections causing gynecologic pathologic conditions. This occurs not only in women who have lived in endemic countries but also in women who travel to subtropical countries for work or wilderness expeditions.[74] Women should be educated about the risk of female genital schistosomiasis and the need to avoid exposure to it.[72] The diagnosis is made by microscopic identification of parasite eggs in stool or by serologic tests in lesser infections, where egg shedding may be inconsistent. Antibody tests do not distinguish between prior and current infections. The CDC has an excellent test for *Schistosoma mansoni* (i.e., FAST-ELISA). The World Health Organization recommends preventive chemotherapy with praziquantel on a yearly basis for high-risk populations living in endemic areas, but not for women who travel to endemic regions.[219] Although this recommendation does not prevent infection or development of the disease, it seems to decrease the incidence and severity of complications, and reduces egg production. Praziquantel acts against mature schistosome parasites. It is most effective if taken after the parasite has developed to the adult stage, which is at least 4 to 6 weeks after exposure. Recommended dosing for praziquantel is 40 mg/kg/day orally divided into one or two doses for 1 day for *S. haematobium*, *Schistosoma intercalatum*, and *S. mansoni*. Praziquantel 60 mg/kg/day divided into two or three doses for 1 day is recommended for *Schistosoma japonicum* and *Schistosoma mekongi*. An alternative treatment choice for *S. mansoni* is oxamniquine 15 mg/kg orally one time.[81] Using praziquantel as a postexposure prophylaxis (PEP) pill to prevent schistosomiasis immediately after a high-risk freshwater exposure is not effective and not recommended for travelers. More information on testing and diagnosis can be found through the CDC Parasitic Diseases Branch at 1-404-718-4745 or at cdc.gov/parasites/schistosomiasis.

PRACTICAL ISSUES FOR WOMEN DURING WILDERNESS TRAVEL

Women between the ages of 10 and 50 years menstruate on average once a month, with a high degree of individual variability. Women should be prepared to experience changes in their cycle and premenstrual symptoms during wilderness travel. Changes in exercise, diet, sleep patterns, and time zones can affect the hypothalamic-pituitary axis and cause menses to become irregular or cease. It is helpful for women on long-term expeditions to chart their cycles. Follow guidelines in cases of amenorrhea or dysfunctional uterine bleeding.[4,25,62,] Reproductive-age women sexually active with men should carry pregnancy tests to rule out pregnancy if they miss a menstrual period. Consider the best options for feminine hygiene products (e.g., product weight, bulk, and disposal options) for a particular trip. A number of alternative menstrual products are available, including soft reusable intravaginal rubber cups (Keeper, DivaCup) (Figure 92-1). Another option is a menstrual cup (Instead Softcup). Although sold for a single use, it can easily be washed and reused. Feminine hygiene products can also be used for wilderness first aid or survival. Tampons may be used as a medical bandage, nasal packing for epistaxis, crude water filter, fire fuel, cord, or ear plugs. Menstrual pads have many of the same applications, as well as potential to act as a compression dressing for wound management (Figure 92-2).

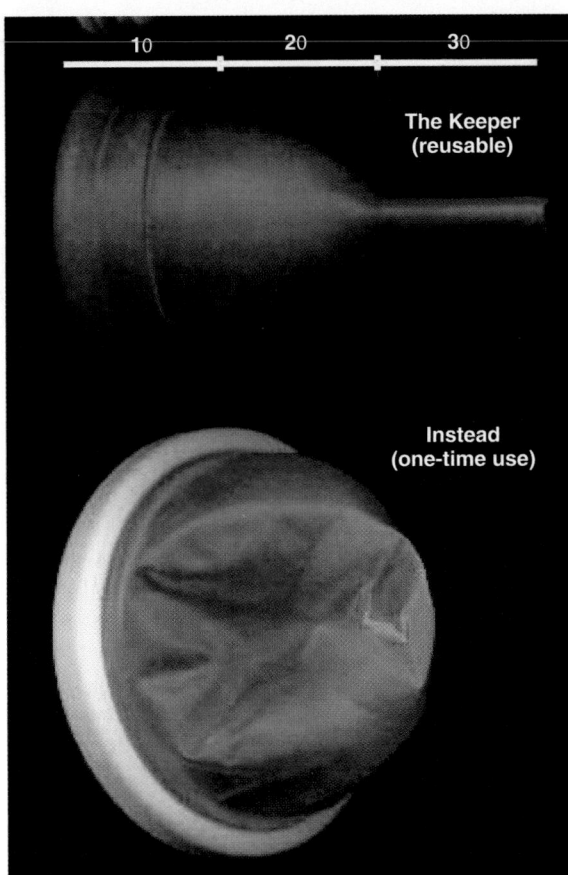

FIGURE 92-1 Options for feminine hygiene. *(Courtesy Harry Finley: mum.org/MenCups.htm.)*

DYSMENORRHEA

Women may experience premenstrual symptoms while traveling, even if they have never experienced symptoms before. Include medications for self-treatment of these symptoms (e.g., ibuprofen) in the medical kit.

CONTROLLING THE MENSTRUAL CYCLE

Some women prefer not to have a menstrual period during long-distance trekking, bicycling, or other endeavors. Options to control the menstrual cycle include oral contraceptives (OCs) or using a contraceptive patch or ring without a hormone-free interval. "Tri-cycling" involves taking three to four cycles continuously by not observing the pill-free days. This decreases the need for menstrual supplies and reduces premenstrual symptoms. Women should be warned that a small amount of breakthrough bleeding may occur, because the endometrium may not remain stable without the physiologic curettage of the pill-free interval.[62]

Another option to decrease menstrual bleeding is to try a method of contraception that leads to endometrial thinning over time and amenorrhea. Examples of such methods include progestin-only pills, Depo-Provera, or the progesterone intrauterine device (IUD) (Table 92-2). In some women, progestin-only contraception may be less predictable for cycle control and lead instead to irregular bleeding or spotting between menses. If a progestin-only method is chosen, start at least 3 to 6 months in advance of departure in order to evaluate menstrual cycle effects.

MENSTRUAL CYCLE DISTURBANCE

Menstrual cycle disturbance is one of the most frequent reasons a woman seeks medical care.[108] Among highly trained athletes and in environments that impose extreme physical and psychological demands, disturbances can be found in more than 50% of women not taking OCs. Menstrual problems during long-distance hiking were found to be the most common complaint of women

backpackers. A study of backpackers on the Appalachian Trail found that 87% of women with regular menstrual cycles prior to travel had menstrual abnormalities while backpacking.[50] High altitude, in combination with other stressors (e.g., time change, cold, and weight loss) is likely to modify the menstrual cycle.

Understanding menstrual cycle abnormalities requires a basic understanding of the normal menstrual cycle (Figure 92-3). In premenopausal women, progesterone and estrogen fluctuate. Normal cycles occur at regular intervals, require ovulation, and typically average 28 days (range 21 to 35 days). By convention, the menstrual cycle's first day corresponds to the first day of menstrual bleeding. This typically lasts approximately 4 days (range 3 to 7 days). Menstrual bleeding represents desquamation of functional endometrium, results from progesterone withdrawal in the absence of conception during the previous cycle, and coincides with recruitment of a new group of primordial follicles for maturation. The first menstrual cycle stage (i.e., up to the time of ovulation) is referred to as the *follicular phase* or *endometrial proliferative phase*. In the early follicular phase, estrogen and progesterone levels are low. In the *late follicular phase* (also called the *preovulatory phase*), typically days 8 to 11, there is a brief surge in estrogen levels, which promotes ovulation. The second menstrual stage is the *luteal phase* or *endometrial secretory phase*. After ovulation, estrogen and progesterone levels peak (typically days 19 to 21) and then decrease until the following menstrual phase. Throughout the menstrual cycle, pulsatile release of gonadotropin-releasing hormone (GnRH) by the hypothalamus occurs hourly during the follicular phase and every 1.5 hours during the luteal phase. Factors that disrupt normal pulsatile release of GnRH or reduce the pituitary ability to respond are the major contributors to menstrual cycle abnormalities in premenopausal women.[51] In women who use OCs, or contraceptive patches or rings, hormone levels are elevated during use of active hormone pills (or patch or ring) for 3 weeks and decreased during the week of placebo (no pill, patch, or ring) use. After menopause, levels of circulating estrogen and progesterone decrease substantially. Estrogen replacement (or combined estrogen and progestin) increases levels of these hormones.

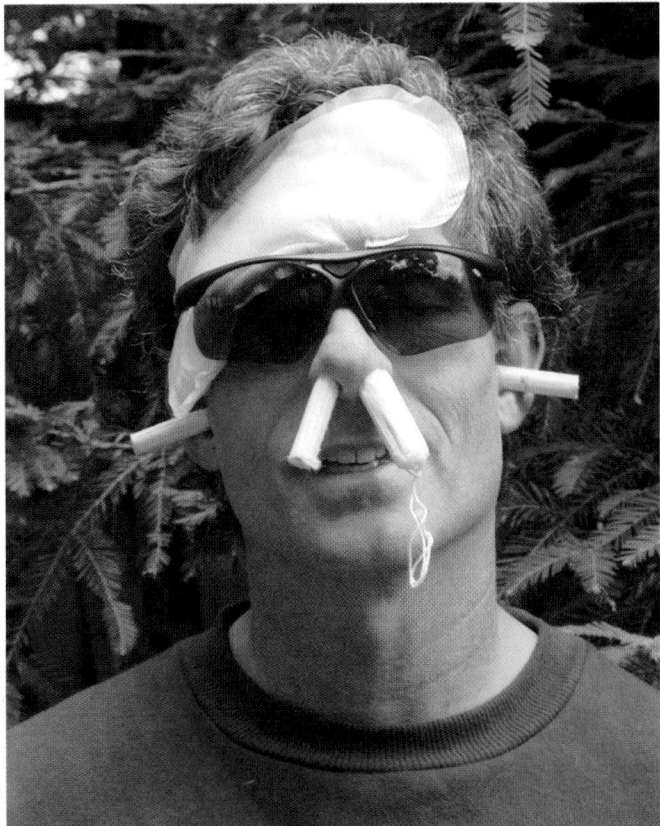

FIGURE 92-2 Multiple uses of feminine hygiene supplies in the wilderness. *(Courtesy Susan Anderson.)*

TABLE 92-2 Common Contraceptive Choices

Methods	Mechanism	Advantages/Disadvantages	Wilderness Travel Issues
Barrier Methods			
Spermicides, creams, jellies, foams, melting suppositories, sponges, foaming tablets, films	Surface-active agents that damage the cell membranes of sperm, bacteria, and viruses.	Chronic exposure may cause mucosal injury that increases risk for HIV transmission.	Available over the counter. Store in cool dark place.
Sponge	Polyurethane sponge containing nonoxynol-9. Sponge traps and absorbs semen before sperm reach cervix. Leave in place for 6 hr after intercourse.	One size. Over the counter. Moisten with water before insertion. Loop for removal. Do not wear longer than 30 hr owing to rare risk for toxic shock syndrome.	Available over the counter. Use disinfected water for moistening in countries with questionable water supply. Protects for 24 hr no matter how many times intercourse occurs.
Cervical cap	Mechanical barrier. Requires spermicide.	Requires clinician fitting. Can use for up to 48 hr. Small risk for toxic shock syndrome. Small risk for cervical dysplasia.	Easy to carry. Rubber may deteriorate in heat and humidity.
Diaphragm	Dome-shaped rubber cup. Use with spermicide. Protection for 6 hr.	Requires clinician fitting. Insert extra spermicide with repeated intercourse. After use, leave in for 6 hr.	Carry in climate-resistant case. Spermicide may not be available in developing countries.
FemCap	Silicone rubber sailor hat–shaped cap intended for use with a spermicide.	Latex free. Two sizes; clinician fitting required. Can be worn up to 48 hr.	Easy to carry. In the future, may be used with spermicide and microbicide for protection against STIs.
Condom			
Female condom (Reality)	Polyurethane pouch. Spermicide not required. One use only.	Can be inserted 8 hr prior to intercourse.	Female controlled. Does not deteriorate in heat and humidity. Bring own supply.
Male condom	Latex Polyurethane Lambskin/natural	Possible allergy. Do not use oil-based lubricants. Thinner and stronger. More resistant to deterioration. Can use oil-based lubricants. Small pores permit passages of viruses (hepatitis B virus, herpes simplex virus, HIV). Use ONLY for contraception. Brands and materials differ in quality.	Quality varies from country to country. Bring supply from reliable source of latex and polyurethane types. May break down in heat and humidity. Estimated to last 1 mo in wallet; check expiration date. Use emergency contraceptive if condom breaks, no backup method in place (i.e., OC pill, diaphragm, sponge). Store in cool, dry place.
Hormonal Methods			
Combined pill: estrogen + progesterone Many different types: Monophasic Triphasic Continuous use	Inhibition of ovulation by blocking LH surge. Thickens cervical mucus to prevent sperm penetration to upper genital tract. Inhibits capacitation of sperm, limits ability of sperm to fertilize egg. Slows tubal motility, delaying sperm transport.	Increased menstrual cycle regularity. Less blood loss. Less cramping. Reduces ectopic pregnancy. Less pelvic inflammatory disease. Fewer cysts or fibroids. Less endometriosis. If nausea and vomiting, need to take backup method or consider placing pill in vagina for absorption (still use backup method). May use as emergency contraception; check instructions. Slight increase in risk for DVT and stroke, especially in smokers.	Convenient, effective, easy to carry. Need to take every 24 hr. May use to delay menses by starting next package of active pills after 3 wk of previous package, or use "continuous use" package. Risk breakthrough bleeding with continuous use. Consider drug interactions. Rare risk of DVT. Bring own supply. Research availability of OC pills and/or other method of contraception to use if OC pills lost or stolen.*
Transdermal patch (Ortho Evra)	Matchbook-size device placed on skin. One patch/wk for 3 wk, followed by 1 wk patch free. Each 20-cm² patch contains 6 mg norelgestromin and 0.75 mg ethinyl estradiol.	Side effects and contraindications similar to those of combined OC pills. Better compliance than with OC pills. Place on nonexposed area of skin.	Better compliance due to weekly dosing. Absorption not affected by gastrointestinal illness.

TABLE 92-2 Common Contraceptive Choices—cont'd

Methods	Mechanism	Advantages/Disadvantages	Wilderness Travel Issues
Vaginal ring (NuvaRing)	Flexible and colorless vaginal ring used for 3 wk followed by 1 wk ring free. Releases combination of progestin with estrogen for absorption across vaginal wall.	Side effects and contraindications similar to those of combined OC pills. Leave ring in place for 3 wk. Do not remove for intercourse. Ring can be removed for up to 3 hr without losing efficacy. If > 3 hr, need backup method for 7 days.	Better compliance due to dosing. Less breakthrough bleeding. Absorption not affected by gastrointestinal illness.
Nestorone/ethinyl estradiol contraceptive vaginal ring (awaiting FDA approval)	2¼-inch-diameter ring similar in design and mechanism to NuvaRing. 103 mg Nestorone/17.4 mg ethinyl estradiol. Use for 3 wk, followed by 1 wk ring free. Designed for 13 cycles (1 year) of use.	Leave ring in for 3 wk. One ring is effective for up to 1 year. Does not require health care visit for placement.	Ideal for extended international travel, especially in settings with few resources. Keep in safe place during week off so as not to lose method of contraception. Bring backup ring for extended travel in case lost or misplaced.
Progestin-Only Methods			
Progestin-only pills	Inhibition of ovulation (may occasionally ovulate). Thickened and suppressed cervical mucus. Suppression of midcycle LH and FSH.	Use if cannot take estrogen. Take same type of pill every day (no pill-free week). Decreased menstrual cramps, less bleeding. Can use if breastfeeding. Decreased risk of thrombotic complications. Older women, smokers can use.	Need to be prepared for irregular bleeding. MUST take pill at same time every day (set alarm to help with time zone changes).
Depo-Provera	150 mg by intramuscular injection or 104 mg administered subcutaneously every 3 mo. Blocks midcycle LH hormone surge and inhibits ovulation.	Good choice for women who cannot take estrogen. Good compliance. Side effects: weight gain, menstrual irregularities, acne, mood changes, decreased libido, decreased bone density. Not possible to discontinue immediately.	Use if compliance issues (e.g., unable to remember OC pills). Contraceptive coverage for 3 mo. If travel > 3 mo, need to get injection or switch method. Need to be prepared for irregular bleeding.
Implanon or Nexplanon (second generation)	4-cm long implant that releases progestin etonorgestrel at a rate of 60 mcg daily. Suppresses ovulation, thickens cervical mucus, leads to atrophic endometrium.	3 years of contraception. Can be reversed any time by removing this one implant. Menstrual cycle disturbances.	Great option for travel. Lasts 3 years.
Progering	Progestin-only vaginal ring. Each ring releases 10 mg progesterone daily.	Replace every 3 mo or once a year, depending on formulation. Safe for lactating women.	Easy for travel.
Intrauterine Device			

Three approved for use in the United States (others available worldwide)	Inhibition of sperm migration, fertilization, and ovum transport.
	Creates environment that is spermicidal by provoking a sterile inflammatory reaction that is toxic to sperm and implantation.
		Option for nullgravid and multiparous women at low risk for STIs who desire short-term contraception.
		Small risk of IUD-induced infection:
		  At insertion
		  More than one partner
		Option for women with
		  History of diabetes
		  History of DVT
		  who are breastfeeding
			Long-term contraception for 5-10 years
			Need fewer supplies for contraception.
			Need to know how to check for string.
			Need backup method if falls out.
			Need to protect against STIs.
			Need medical evaluation for missing string
			Excessive vaginal bleeding
			Abdominal pain
			Vaginal discharge
			Pregnancy

ParaGard T 380A Copper	T-shaped polyurethane frame holding 380 mg of exposed surface of copper.	Increased menstrual bleeding and cramping may occur in first few months following insertion; relieved with NSAIDs.	Effective for 10 years. Need fewer supplies.

Continued

TABLE 92-2 Common Contraceptive Choices—cont'd

Methods	Mechanism	Advantages/Disadvantages	Wilderness Travel Issues
Mirena—levonorgestrel-releasing intrauterine system (LNG-IUS)	T-shaped with a polydimethylsiloxane sleeve delivering 20 mcg levonorgestrel. Size: 32 mm horizontally by 32 mm vertically by 4.75 mm insertion tube	Less bleeding and cramping due to effect of levonorgestrel.	Effective for 5 years. Need fewer supplies.
Skyla—levonorgestrel-releasing intrauterine system (LNG-IUS)	Similar to Mirena system in design and mechanism. 14 mcg of levonorgestrel per day. Size: 28 cm horizontally by 30 mm vertically by 3.8 mm insertion tube.	Smallest IUD marketed to adolescent and nulliparous women.	Effective for 3 years.
Methods of Contraception Undergoing Clinical Trials			
Microbiocide/spermicidal creams (e.g., ACIDFORM)†	Combination spermicidal and microbiocide to be used alone or with barrier methods above.	Dual protection against pregnancy and STIs.	
Transdermal spray contraception	Daily progestin-only "spray-on" contraceptive. Progestin Nestorone inhibits ovulation.	Metered-dose aerosol delivers preset amount. Absorbed immediately. Safe for breastfeeding women.	
Transdermal gel	Two versions: Nestorone (19-norprogesterone derivative) only. Combination estradiol and norprogesterone.	Application in periumbilical region.	Cutaneous contamination could limit absorption when showering limited.
Disposable diaphragms (Duet with BufferGel)	Diaphragms that release spermicide/microbicide. They may be used up to 24 hr with multiple acts of intercourse.	Easy to use.	No extra spermicide/microbicide required.

DVT, Deep vein thrombosis; FDA, Food and Drug Administration; FSH, follicle-stimulating hormone; HIV, human immunodeficiency virus; LH, luteinizing hormone; OC, oral contraceptive; STI, sexually transmitted infection.
*See ec.princeton.edu/worldwide/default.asp#country.
†See Bayer LL, Jensen JT: ACIDFORM: a review of the evidence, Contraception 90(1):11-18, 2014.

CAUSES OF ABNORMAL UTERINE BLEEDING

Understanding the physiology of the normal menstrual cycle and differential diagnosis of dysfunctional uterine bleeding at each phase of a woman's reproductive life will help to diagnose and manage these conditions.

Abnormal uterine bleeding (AUB) is any aberration in the normal menstrual bleeding pattern in premenopausal women or any bleeding episode in postmenopausal women. The most common causes of AUB are problems related to pregnancy and hormonal contraceptive therapy. Initial evaluation of AUB in any premenopausal woman includes a pregnancy test (i.e., urine or serum screen for human chorionic gonadotropin [hCG]), regardless of contraceptive history. Non–pregnancy-related causes of AUB include uterine and extrauterine causes.

The history helps identify a presumptive cause and empirical therapeutic approach for AUB, particularly in the absence of laboratory resources. The pertinent history includes age at onset of menses, regularity of menses, usual length of menses and blood flow, perimenstrual symptoms, medical problems, a basic review of endocrine symptoms, and a history of any prior pregnancies, STIs, and surgeries.[108] Characterize the current complaint, including changes in the frequency of bleeding, amount of flow, new symptoms, relationship to activities, recent sexual history, systemic symptoms, weight change, change in medications or use of other health-related products, and change in exercise patterns.

OVULATORY WOMEN

When a premenopausal woman with consistent, regular cyclic menses presents with a progressively increasing amount and duration of menstrual flow, the most common causes are uterine fibroids, particularly submucosal (i.e., just beneath the endometrium) fibroids, endometriosis, and adenomyosis (i.e., endometriosis of the uterine muscle wall). These conditions are frequently associated with progressive dysmenorrhea and are more likely to occur with advancing age. Consider medications (e.g., estrogen, tamoxifen, warfarin, nonsteroidal antiinflammatory drugs) or homeopathic compounds as possible causes of AUB. An abrupt change in duration or amount of blood flow suggests either a corpus luteal cyst (often associated with unilateral lower abdominal discomfort) or acute pelvic inflammatory disease (PID) that is often accompanied by more diffuse abdominal pain and systemic symptoms. In ovulating women, endometrial hyperplasia is unusual and uterine or ovarian (estrogen-secreting) malignancies are rare. Perimenopausal women who are still ovulatory may have progressively more frequent menses accompanied by changes in flow and duration, with or without the underlying causes noted above.

Evaluate women with intermenstrual or postcoital bleeding for cervicovaginal infections (e.g., bacterial vaginosis (BV), yeast, trichomoniasis, and condylomas). Endocervical polyps, cervical dysplasia, and invasive cervical carcinoma can lead to profuse coital bleeding and dyspareunia. Acute pain with coitus not accompanied by bleeding is more likely due to PID, ovarian cyst rupture, or adnexal torsion.

ANOVULATORY WOMEN

Anovulatory uterine bleeding is more common than are ovulatory abnormalities among women who partake in wilderness experiences. Divide anovulatory bleeding problems into those occurring with adequate estrogen and those accompanied by low estrogen production. Women with adequate estrogen stores are often characterized by hypersecretion of gonadotropins and frequent heavy bleeding (e.g., polycystic ovary syndrome). OCs help stabilize the endometrium and decrease the menstrual flow.

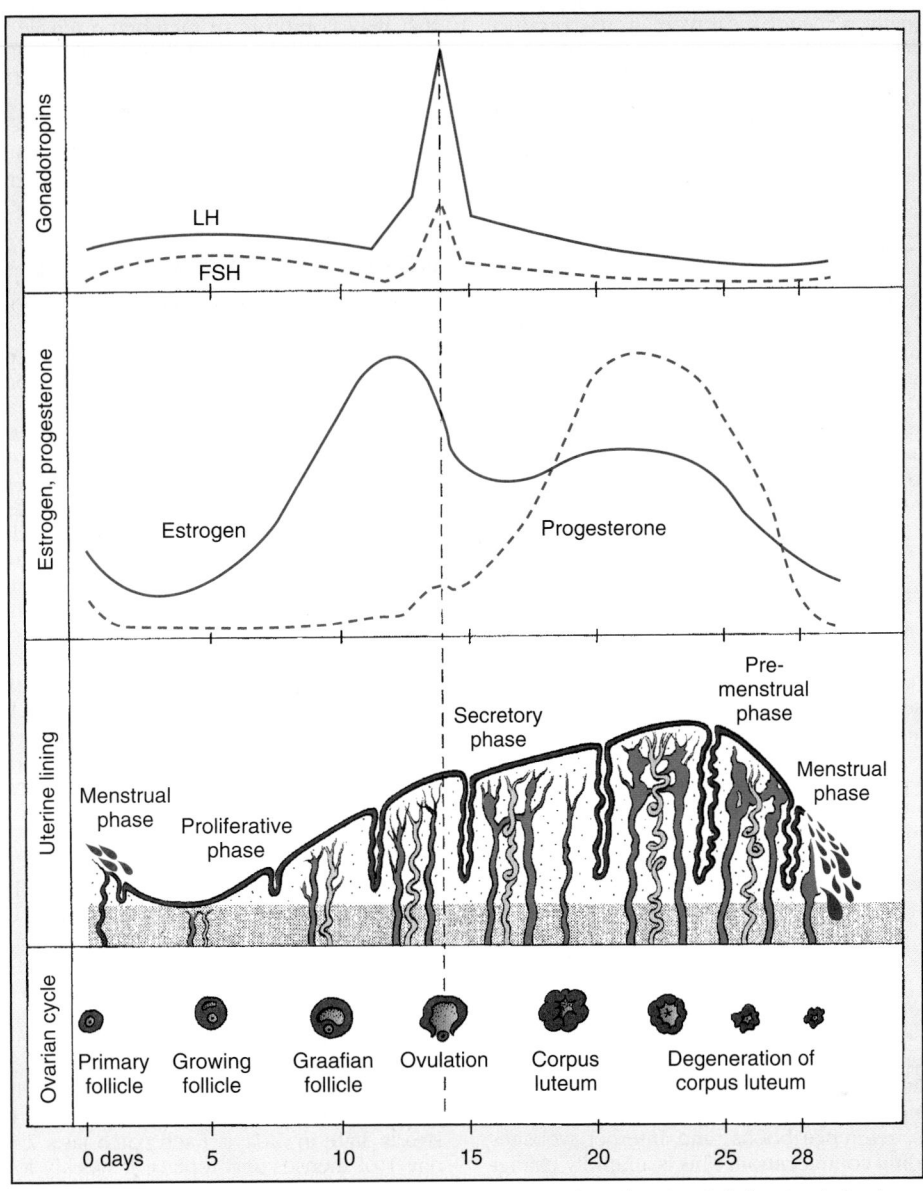

FIGURE 92-3 Normal human ovarian and endometrial (menstrual) cycle. FSH, follicle-stimulating hormone; LH, luteinizing hormone. *(Modified from Shaw ST Jr, Roche PC: Menstruation. In Finn CA, editor: Oxford reviews of reproduction and endocrinology, vol 2, Oxford, United Kingdom, 1980, Oxford University Press.)*

Anovulation can be caused by inadequate release of pituitary gonadotropins that leads to decreased estrogen production and presents as amenorrhea. Amenorrhea can be a symptom of the female athletic triad historically defined by disordered eating, amenorrhea, and osteoporosis.[114] More recent consensus statements use a more encompassing diagnostic term, relative energy deficiency in sport (RED-S), because there are more impaired physiologic states with this condition than those listed in the triad. RED-S has also been exhibited in males.[157] More commonly, anovulatory cycles and amenorrhea result from changes in a woman's usual routine of sleep, diet, and exercise patterns, all of which are extremely common to a wilderness experience.

The American College of Obstetrics and Gynecology guidelines for workup of acute abnormal uterine bleeding can be found at acog.org/Resources-And-Publications/Committee-Opinions/Committee-on-Gynecologic-Practice/Management-of-Acute-Abnormal-Uterine-Bleeding-in-Nonpregnant-Reproductive-Aged-Women.[25]

To evaluate vaginal bleeding in the wilderness, it is critical to differentiate a true emergency (e.g., ectopic pregnancy or miscarriage) from a more benign cause that can be stabilized and evaluated later. If the pregnancy test is positive, immediate medical evacuation should be arranged. If the pregnancy test is negative and there is no other evidence of an anatomic abnormality or systemic illness, vaginal bleeding is likely a form of dysfunctional uterine bleeding. Use the following measures to attempt to stop bleeding until further evaluation can be obtained.

For women without contraindications to estrogen or progestin, hormonal therapy with either estrogen or progestin or a combined hormonal preparation may be used to stabilize the endometrial lining. One option is to take an OC pill containing 30 to 35 mcg of ethinyl estradiol every 4 to 6 hours until bleeding is under control, and then continue taking one tablet a day until the 21 active pills are finished. A few days later, synchronized withdrawal bleeding will occur. A woman may opt to continue taking one OC pill a day to prevent withdrawal bleeding until evaluation can be obtained. Although the mechanism of action of a bolus of estrogen and progesterone is not well understood, its effect is thought to be mediated by accelerated proliferation of the endometrial basal layer that seals the bleeding vessels.

In perimenopausal women with irregular bleeding, a low-dose OC containing 20 mcg ethinyl estradiol may be tried. Advantages include predictable cycle control, reliable contraception, decrease in perimenopausal symptoms (e.g., mood swings, irritability, decreased libido, and hot flashes), and possibly prevention of accelerated bone and mineral loss during perimenopausal years.

Menopause is associated with amenorrhea as a result of cessation of ovarian estrogen production and inactive atrophic endometrium. Occasionally, a menopausal woman may produce sufficient estrogen from peripheral conversion of ovarian and adrenal androgens to stimulate the endometrial lining and cause resumption of bleeding. Postmenopausal bleeding can also be due to atrophy. Although postmenopausal bleeding is usually mild and does not need emergent treatment, a medical evaluation is important to rule out more serious causes (e.g., underlying malignancy).[4]

PREGNANCY TESTS

Pregnancy tests are helpful to evaluate amenorrhea, vaginal bleeding, pelvic pain, and other symptoms that may be related to a pregnancy. Pregnancy tests should be carried in the medical kit. Urine pregnancy kits are not always available in remote areas, and outside developed countries, test reliability can vary. Pregnancy test kits have limited shelf lives. Check expiration dates. Environmental extremes can also affect test accuracy. Observe manufacturer's recommendations regarding storage. As with most self-diagnostic tests, review test procedures with the woman before travel.[69]

CONTRACEPTIVE OPTIONS DURING WILDERNESS TRAVEL

Address contraceptive options for all women wilderness travelers of reproductive age (see Table 92-2). Contraceptive options include lower-dose OC pills, several new oral progestins, progestin-only implants, and a progestin-bearing IUD. Certain delivery methods (e.g., contraceptive patch and vaginal ring) are excellent options for wilderness travelers. They do not require daily compliance with taking a pill at the same time every day or rely on drug absorption that could be affected by a gastrointestinal (GI) illness (e.g., nausea, vomiting, or diarrhea). Contraceptive efficacy is improved with use of the contraceptive patch or ring, and there is less risk for irregular bleeding due to fluctuating hormone levels.[47,103]

The best contraceptive method for a particular woman depends on the planned activities and itinerary. Consider accessibility and ease of use, weight and bulk, effects of extremely hot or cold environments, effects of immersion into water, and method reliability under perfect and imperfect use.

Wilderness medicine providers should take advantage of current journal articles, reference books, and Internet websites with information regarding contraception. This is a rapidly changing field.[3,47,68, 85,103,128] Relevant websites include the

American College of Obstetrics and Gynecology at acog.org,
Hormonal Birth Control at acog.org/publications/patient _education/bp159.cfm,
International Planned Parenthood Federation at ippf.org, and the Princeton Emergency Contraception site at ec.princeton.edu.

In women already using a contraceptive method, evaluate the method's ease of use and reliability as well as any special recommendations concerning use during travel. Begin any new method several months before travel, especially if planning overseas or remote travel or a long-term assignment. Backup methods should be discussed. The International Planned Parenthood Federation maintains a worldwide guide to contraceptives and a list of family planning clinics. The Princeton Emergency Contraception website also lists emergency contraception (EC) options available worldwide.

BARRIER CONTRACEPTIVES

The most common barrier contraceptives used during travel include the diaphragm, cervical cap, sponge, vaginal spermicide, and male condom.[103] Barrier contraceptive methods have a reassuring safety profile (limited to latex allergy and method failure resulting in pregnancy), but all have disadvantages for regular use in a wilderness setting. Even under ideal use, failure rates with a spermicidal foam or gel are relatively high (estimated at 20% to 30% with "typical use" and 6% to 20% with "perfect use.") Barrier devices may be susceptible to extremes of heat or cold

that may compromise membrane tensile strength and effectiveness. Some couples find these methods inconvenient and messy enough to discourage compliance in environments not conducive to cleanup. Bulk and weight complicate transport of sufficient spermicidal compound. Barrier methods decrease the risk for STIs, including gonorrhea, chlamydial infection, and HIV transmission, but offer variable protection against human papillomavirus or genital herpes simplex virus, even if used correctly.

HORMONAL CONTRACEPTIVES

Combination (estrogen and progestin) OCs, either monophasic or multiphasic, offer the most reliable, convenient, and cost-effective risk-to-benefit ratio for healthy reproductive-age women. Consider previous experience of use, complications of therapy, menstrual history, and skin type. Failure rates with optimal use are extremely low (1%) but may be worsened by difficulty with compliance or GI illness during travel. Common side effects include nausea, vomiting, weight gain, and breakthrough bleeding. In most patients, breakthrough bleeding decreases with consistent use, and there is no need to change the brand of OC as a result. Potential benefits of OCs include normalization of cycles, fewer midcycle ovulatory (e.g., mittelschmerz) and perimenstrual (e.g., dysmenorrhea, headaches) symptoms, lighter menstrual flow, suppression of ovarian cyst formation, reduced risk for endometrial cancer, prevention of osteoporosis, and increased bone mass. Condoms must still be used to prevent STIs. Major contraindications include a history of thromboembolic disease, certain autoimmune disorders with thromboembolic risk factors, uncontrolled hypertension, hepatic dysfunction, diabetes with complications, and cigarette smoking.

TRANSDERMAL HORMONAL CONTRACEPTION

The U.S. Food and Drug Administration (FDA) approved the first transdermal contraceptive patch in 2001. The contraceptive patch is a matchbook-sized device that is placed on the skin (abdomen, upper outer arm, buttocks, or upper torso but not the breasts). It consists of a three-layer matrix with an outer polyester protective layer and a medicated adhesive layer that contains the contraceptive steroids. A clear, polyester release liner, which protects the adhesive layer, is removed before application. The patch releases 22 mcg of ethinyl estradiol and 150 mcg of norelgestromin daily. Hormones are absorbed into the blood and reach a steady state in 2 days. Each patch lasts 7 days. Apply a patch on day 1 of menses and replace it weekly for 3 weeks. No patch is used during the fourth week. Place each patch at a different site. The efficacy is similar with various application sites. Contraceptive efficacy is not thought to be affected by humid climates, vigorous exercise, exposure to saunas, or water baths. The patch has similar side effects to OCs. In addition, users may experience occasional mild to moderate application-site reactions and an increased incidence of breast tenderness during the first few months of use. Most women have found the patch to be more convenient than a daily pill when traveling, and it is easy to check to make sure it is in place. To discard a used patch, fold it in half and discard it in solid waste garbage. Do not flush it down a toilet. There are no hormonal peaks and troughs. Oral antibiotic use is not believed to interfere with efficacy. The FDA has issued a warning about Internet sales of counterfeit contraceptive patches.[73]

VAGINAL RING

The NuvaRing is a soft, flexible, and transparent ring made of an ethylene vinyl acetate copolymer. It has an outer diameter of 54 mm and cross section of 44 mm. Two steroid reservoir cores in the ring provide daily hormone release of 15 mcg of ethinyl estradiol and 120 mcg of etonorgestrel (an active metabolite of desogestrel). The NuvaRing provides hormone bioavailability comparable with an OC (e.g., desogestrel ethinyl estradiol [Ortho-Cept]). The device is inserted in the vagina and removed after 3 weeks. Following one "ring-free" week, a new ring is inserted. If the ring is expelled accidentally, it can be washed and reinserted.

If the ring is out for more than 3 hours, a backup contraceptive method is recommended. Advantages include good contraceptive efficacy with continuous release, leading to better compliance. The ring does not depend on GI absorption, so will continue its effectiveness despite GI illness.[92] Side effects are rare, and include prolonged menstrual bleeding, vaginal discomfort, and foreign-body sensation. Use of common antibiotics (e.g., amoxicillin and doxycycline) does not appear to affect the efficacy.[78]

INTRAUTERINE DEVICES

An IUD is a highly effective and convenient form of contraception, especially for parous women in a monogamous relationship. Women who cannot take estrogens (i.e., history of breast cancer, thromboembolism, diabetes, or breastfeeding) are candidates for an IUD.[15] The IUD should be inserted at least 3 months before departure, because complications occur most often within the first month after insertion. IUDs are occasionally associated with increased menstrual flow, dysmenorrhea, intermenstrual spotting, and expulsion. However, the Copper T 380A IUD (ParaGard) and the levonorgestrel systems, or LNG-IUS (Mirena/Skyla), carry minimal risks for these side effects. Mirena releases approximately 20 mcg of levonorgestrel per day, approximately 10% of that provided by a levonorgestrel-containing OC. The Mirena requires replacement every 5 years, and the Skyla is replaced every 3 years. The Copper T 380A IUD is effective for 10 years or longer. For certain women, an IUD is a great option for wilderness travel.[10]

The IUD's most serious risk, affecting less than 1% of users, is an acute or indolent pelvic infection that might become clinically significant in the wilderness. The risk is greatest within the first month after IUD insertion or replacement and among women at increased risk for STIs. Women with multiple partners, previous pelvic infections, unrecognized chlamydial infection or gonorrhea, recurrent episodes of bacterial vaginosis, or tobacco use are at highest risk. When acute PID occurs with lower abdominopelvic pain, peritonitis, purulent vaginal discharge, and fever, remove the IUD immediately by simple traction on the string protruding from the external cervical os. Start a broad-spectrum antibiotic. Evacuation is mandatory when the device cannot be removed. Pelvic infection should be suspected, even without fever and peritoneal signs, if irregular bleeding occurs, particularly when accompanied by pelvic discomfort and discharge. When the IUD is removed at this stage, infections may respond to therapy with oral or parenteral antibiotics.[10]

Another potentially serious risk for IUD users is pregnancy, occurring in approximately 1 in 1000 users per year with the levonorgestrel systems. Both intrauterine and extrauterine pregnancies can occur with an IUD in place. The latter is more common, but the risk is still only half that of women who use no contraception. Confirmed or suspected pregnancy in a woman with an IUD is an indication for immediate evacuation.

EMERGENCY CONTRACEPTION

Emergency contraception (EC) is defined as a method of contraception that women can use after unprotected intercourse or contraceptive failure to prevent pregnancy (Table 92-3). EC should be used when desired in cases of unprotected intercourse, contraceptive failure, or sexual assault. EC should be included in every woman's wilderness medical kit. It decreases a woman's risk for pregnancy from approximately 8% to 1% or 2%. The Princeton Emergency Contraceptive website (ec.princeton.edu) has an excellent review of EC options, commonly asked questions, and a chart of dosing options for specific OC brands being used as EC, as well as OC options available in different countries.[23,103,130]

Three major categories of EC are available worldwide: progestin-only pills, estrogen-progestin combined OC pills, and nonhormonal options.[68,128] Nonhormonal options include a selective progesterone receptor modulator (ulipristal acetate, or Ella), copper IUD insertion, and mifepristone (only available in select countries). Ulipristal acetate is more effective than levonorgestrel and combined pill regimens, and maintains its efficacy for up to 5 days.[27] EC options available in most countries include a progestin-only option (i.e., levonorgestrel) or estrogen-progestin combination OC pills. Studies have shown that Plan B (i.e., levonorgestrel) is equally effective when both doses of pills (1.5 mg total) are taken at the same time, rather than when the 0.75-mg tablets are taken 12 hours apart.[103] The "one-dose" option may improve compliance and effectiveness. Plan B is better tolerated than are other ECs that contain estrogen. In the United States

---

TABLE 92-3 Emergency Contraceptive Methods*

	No. of Pills per Dose	Ethinyl Estradiol (µg)	Levonorgestrel (µg)	Instructions
Progestin Only				
Levonorgestrel (Plan B)	1 tab	0	750	Take 2 tabs (150 µg Levonorgesterl) as soon as possible within 120 hr of risk.
Ovrette	20 tab	0	750	Take 20 tabs (150 µg Levonorgesterl); then take 20 pills 12 hr later. May take both doses at once.
Combined Over-the-Counter (take first dose within 72 hr of risk)				
Alesse	5 pink	100	500	Take first dose as soon as possible.
Lo/Ovral	4 white	120	600	Take second dose 12 hr later.
Nordette	4 orange	120	600	May need antiemetic medication.
Levlen	4 orange	120	600	
Levora	4 white	120	600	
Seasonale	4 pink	120	600	
Tril-Levlen	4 yellow	120	500	
Triphasil	4 yellow	120	500	
Trivora	4 pink	120	500	
Nonhormonal Options				
Ulipristal Acetate (Ella)	30 mg	Progestin receptor modulator with antiprogestin activity.		No change in efficacy with time if taken within 120 hr.
Copper IUD	Insertion of single IUD	Sterile inflammatory reaction creating spermicidal environment not conducive to implantation.		Insertion within 120 hr.
Mifepristone	10-50 mg	Synthetic steroidal antiprogesterone/ antiglucocorticoid.		Available only in Armenia, China, Russia, and Vietnam.

*See emergency contraceptive website for current recommendations and for options available worldwide: ec.princeton.edu/worldwide/.

and Canada, progestin-only ECs are available over the counter and uliprital acetate (Ella) is available by prescription. Complete EC as soon as possible, preferably within 72 hours after unprotected intercourse. Ulipristal acetate is effective up to 120 hours after unprotected intercourse. New data indicate that all EC options may be effective for up to 120 hours.[94,130] Although inserting a copper IUD has the best efficacy, this is not feasible in a wilderness environment. Administer an antiemetic when using OCs containing estrogen and progesterone. If there are persistent nausea and vomiting, EC pills may be administered vaginally.[23]

Following EC use, initiate a combined hormonal method (e.g., OC pill, patch, ring). Two to three weeks later, perform a urine pregnancy test to rule out pregnancy. In pregnancies following EC, combined hormonal contraception use has not been found to increase teratogenic risk.[47]

SPECIAL ISSUES RELATED TO HORMONAL CONTRACEPTIVES AND WILDERNESS TRAVEL

Changes in Time Zone

Many low-dose OC formulations are time sensitive. Failure to take a pill in a timely manner because of time zone changes or a change in schedule could result in ovulation. Use a wristwatch or mobile phone alarm dedicated to OC dosing control for precise determination of 24-hour intervals.

Absorption of Oral Contraceptives

Nausea, vomiting, or diarrhea during travel may decrease pill absorption. If vomiting occurs within 3 hours of taking a pill, take another. If a replacement pill cannot be retained, use a backup contraceptive method for the rest of the month (equivalent to missing a pill). If the missed pill was less than 7 days from the end of the monthly package, consider eliminating the pill-free interval and starting the next package right away. For continued nausea and vomiting, some clinicians recommend inserting the OC pill into the vagina for absorption, although efficacy has not been evaluated in clinical trials. Estrogens are absorbed better through the vaginal mucosa than through the GI tract.[6,38] For women at risk for GI illness during travel, a contraceptive patch or a ring is ideal.

Drug Interactions That May Affect Oral Contraceptive Efficacy

A common question is whether antibiotics affect OC efficacy. OC metabolism is increased by any drug that increases liver microsomal enzyme activity. Despite numerous case reports of penicillins, tetracyclines, metronidazole, and nitrofurantoin causing contraceptive failure in humans, the general consensus of large-scale studies is that antibiotics other than rifampin do not lower steroid blood concentrations[34,103,107,126,203] However, individual women have been shown to have decreased ethinyl estradiol levels while taking antibiotics. Because these women cannot be identified in advance, most clinicians and the OC package insert take a conservative approach and advise women to use a backup method of contraception when taking antibiotics.[77] Recent data suggest that contraceptive patch and ring efficacy are not affected by concurrent antibiotics.[78]

GENDER AND RISK FOR VENOUS THROMBOEMBOLISM: CONTRACEPTION, PREGNANCY, AND BEYOND

The incidence of venous thromboembolism (VTE) in young women is estimated to be 1 to 3 per 10,000 per year.[19] Pregnancy increases this risk three- to five-fold. Low-dose contraceptives increase the risk three- to four-fold.[137] The association between pregnancy and VTE is well established. Pulmonary embolism is one of the leading causes of peripartum mortality.[202] Increased VTE risk is also associated with hormone replacement therapy and estrogen-antagonist therapies. These exposures are unique (i.e., pregnancy and OCs) or nearly unique (i.e., estrogen agonist and antagonist therapies) to the female gender.[155] The VTE risk may be important to consider in some wilderness settings (e.g., high-altitude expeditions) that may include risk factors (e.g., immobility due to bad weather).

OCs are believed to effect thrombosis by altering endogenous coagulation and fibrinolytic systems. OC use is associated with increases in prothrombin, fibrinogen levels, and factors VII, VIII, and X, and with decreases in factor V levels. Use of OCs is associated with a twofold to threefold increase in the risk for VTE. Use of third-generation OC drugs containing gestodene, desogestrel, drospirenone, or cyproterone acetate as the progestin component likely confers up to a six-fold greater risk than use of second-generation preparations.[138] This may be due to a greater estrogen effect. Expert consensus statements deem this risk to be acceptable.[26,192] Inform patients of possible risks and make joint decisions that are best for each individual case. Obese patients and smokers are also at increased risk.[207]

The term *hormone replacement therapy* refers to use of a variety of estrogen or combined estrogen and progestin formulations prescribed to relieve menopausal symptoms and prevent osteoporosis. Effects of hormone replacement therapy on the coagulation system appear to be similar to those of OCs, with evidence for increased markers of coagulation, factor VII levels, and activated protein C resistance, and a decrease in antithrombin levels.[178]

Two selective estrogen receptor modulators are used. Tamoxifen is used primarily for adjuvant treatment of breast cancer, and raloxifene has been approved for prevention of osteoporosis. Both are approved for breast cancer prevention.[209] Although these agents have antiestrogenic properties, they also have partial agonist effects at selected receptors and might be expected to have some of the same side effects and associated risks as do other estrogens. The Breast Cancer Prevention Trial[88] reported a threefold increased risk for pulmonary embolism and no significant increased risk for deep vein thrombosis among women with breast cancer receiving tamoxifen. Aromatase inhibitors, also used for treatment and prevention of breast cancer, are associated with a lower incidence of venous thrombosis than is tamoxifen.[29,209]

Pregnancy is a well-recognized risk factor for thromboembolic disease. Physiologic changes that occur during pregnancy pose several risks for VTE. Hypercoagulability results from increased levels of fibrinogen and several clotting factors (II, VII, VIII, IX, X, XII), as well as decreased levels of inhibitors of coagulation (e.g., protein S). Altered coagulation persists throughout pregnancy and for up to 6 weeks postpartum. Venous stasis occurs from hormonally induced increases in venous distensibility and capacity, as well as vena cava compression by the gravid uterus.[202] Vascular injury resulting from childbirth, especially cesarean birth, further escalates the risk for peripartum VTE. Cesarean birth is associated with an increased incidence of VTE compared with vaginal delivery. Other risk factors for VTE during pregnancy include obesity, advanced maternal age, parity, whether a woman has had prolonged bed rest, the presence of infection or thrombophilia, and a history of VTE.

Exposure to high altitude has been reported as a potential risk factor for thromboembolic events, because of hypoxia, polycythemia, dehydration, cold, and periods of venous stasis, but data are limited.[97] VTE risk from the use of OCs or other types of hormonal therapy has not been systematically studied at high altitude. As a precaution, women planning high-altitude excursions who desire hormonal contraception should consider a combination pill containing the lowest dose of ethinyl estradiol (20 mcg) or its equivalent or a contraceptive patch or ring.[118,144] Contraceptive options for women at high risk of thrombolic events include an IUD or a progestin-only method.[15]

If a thrombotic or thromboembolic event is suspected, aspirin therapy may be started empirically while awaiting medical evacuation. Aspirin prophylaxis has been shown to reduce the incidence of VTE and pulmonary embolism in high-risk medical and surgical patients, but no studies have evaluated aspirin in reducing deep vein thrombosis/pulmonary embolism related to altitude or air travel.[177]

BREAST HEALTH

Women should examine their breasts for masses before travel. Women older than 40 years of age and women with a strong family history of breast cancer should have a breast examination and mammography screening. Although there are reports of self-diagnosis and treatment in the field,[105] a breast mass would ideally be evaluated before travel to a remote location. A woman who has had a prior mastectomy and lymph node dissection with resulting lymphedema may want to use an arm sleeve to decrease swelling during air travel and extended backpacking or trekking expeditions.[102] These women should be taught how to recognize cellulitis and how to treat it with appropriate antibiotics.[195]

There have been no large studies on breast implant safety at altitude or during scuba diving. In one small study evaluating breast implants in simulated dives, there were no ruptures, but morphologic distortions occurred in some implants. Repetitive stress associated with the total number and depth of dives may decrease the implant life span.[80,96] Test any clothing and sports equipment ahead of time for breast comfort. Sports bras are helpful for many women. Issues pertinent to breastfeeding are discussed in the section on pregnancy.

URINARY TRACT ISSUES

Women are prone to urinary tract infections (UTIs) during wilderness travel. Contributing factors include dehydration, less frequent urination owing to lack of convenient toilets, fewer available facilities for hygiene, and increased sexual activity. Sexual intercourse increases the risk for UTI at all ages because of urethral massage, which introduces bacteria into the urethra and bladder. Voiding after intercourse lessens this risk. The UTI risk is increased during pregnancy because of urinary stasis and ureteral compression by the uterus. UTIs in older women may be due to changes in the urogenital epithelium. Women of all ages should be taught to recognize symptoms of UTI and how to self-treat with oral antibiotics and a urinary analgesic agent. Urinary dipsticks to check for leukocytes and nitrites may be carried in a medical kit.

Measures to prevent UTIs include adequate hydration and urination when needed, even if there is no facility or object behind which to seek privacy. Some women find squatting positions to be awkward. It may be helpful to practice deep knee bends before the trip. Women should consider attire (e.g., a free-flowing skirt) that would both facilitate squatting and add privacy. A number of plastic and paper funnels have been designed to assist women to urinate while standing (Figure 92-4). These methods require practice. To use, place one's back to the wind and point the funnel downward while leaning slightly forward.

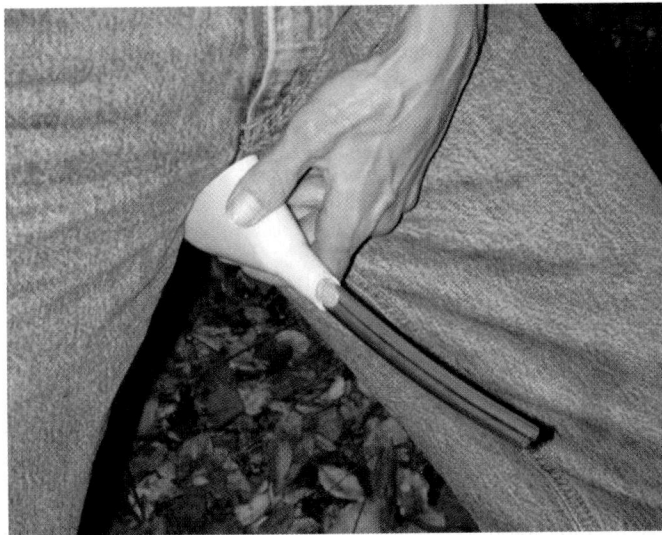

FIGURE 92-4 Urine director. *(Courtesy Susan Anderson.)*

If wearing pants, make certain that zippers or other openings are long enough to accommodate the device. Funnels are especially useful in extremes of cold weather and high altitude when wearing a skirt or pulling down pants is undesirable. Funnels may be connected to a longer tube that is attached to a container for urine storage (traveljohn.com) if it is too cold to urinate outside the tent or during a long road trip. One product (e.g., the Whiz) mixes an antibacterial agent into the plastic and coats the device so that it repels fluid and is easily cleaned. The device may be hand washed or cleaned in a washing machine.

Options for reusable and/or disposable female urine devices include:

Freshette: freshette.com
GoGirl: go-girl.com
Lady Elegance P Ez
Sheewee: shewee.com
Traveljohn: traveljohn.com
Urinelle
Urifemme: urifemme.com
WHIZ all-terrain director: whizproducts.co.uk

Patients with stress incontinence or bladder control should consult a physician specializing in female urinary tract problems before the trip. For minor symptoms, pelvic floor exercises and a supply of panty liners may prove helpful. Older women may experience vaginal dryness and urinary frequency or urgency without dysuria. Data suggest that estrogen vaginal cream, vaginal rings, or a low-dose pill inserted intravaginally may decrease urogenital dryness and frequency symptoms.[33,39,40]

VAGINAL DISCHARGE OR ITCHING

Environmental conditions and constraints on hygiene during wilderness travel promote changes in a woman's vaginal ecosystem that may result in increased vaginal discharge and vulvar itching and irritation. Because diagnostic capabilities in the wilderness are limited, clinical features (Table 92-4) can help guide diagnosis and treatment. Women should be taught self-diagnostic skills and carry appropriate treatment. Even if a woman has never had a vaginal infection, she should be prepared for this possibility, especially during extended itineraries. Advise women to seek medical evaluation if the symptoms do not improve with self-treatment. The normal vaginal pH is less than 4.5 (a range of 3.8 to 4.2 is common). The most common causes of vaginitis during wilderness travel are yeast infection, BV, and chemical irritation.

VULVOVAGINAL CANDIDIASIS

Symptomatic yeast infections are often referred to as vulvovaginal candidiasis. About 80% to 90% of these result from overgrowth by *Candida albicans*. Risk factors for yeast infections include pregnancy, hormonal therapy, recent antibiotic use, corticosteroid therapy, postovulatory phase of menstrual cycle, frequent coitus, condom use, and intravaginal use of spermicidal compounds.[11]

The most common complaint of women with vulvovaginal candidiasis is vulvar pruritus or burning, not vaginal discharge. In more severe cases, redness, irritation, burning, soreness, swelling, and external dysuria are variably present. Characteristic white, flocculent, and adherent discharge ("cottage cheese") is often diagnostic but is not consistently present or visible externally. Yeast discharge is thicker than that seen with BV or trichomoniasis, is usually not frothy or malodorous, and often has a pH of 4.5 or less unless a mixed infection is present. In the emergency department, approximately 50% of yeast infections are confirmed by direct microscopic examination of discharge diluted in saline. Diagnosis is most reliably accomplished by detection of budding yeast hyphae or spores using a slide preparation with 10% potassium hydroxide added to lyse background epithelial cells and bacteria.

Treatment consists of azole derivatives, many of which (e.g., butoconazole, clotrimazole, miconazole, tioconazole) are available over the counter as topical creams, vaginal tablets, and suppositories. Therapy periods range from 1 to 14 days depending on the formulation and infection severity. Treatment regimens

TABLE 92-4 Differential Diagnosis of Vulvovaginitis

Factors	Normal	Bacterial Vaginosis	Vulvovaginal Candidiasis	Trichomoniasis	Atrophic Vaginitis	Other
Discharge	White, clear, finely granular	Gray-white, thin, homogeneous, adherent, frothy	White, thick, curd-like, adherent	Gray to yellow-green, occasionally frothy, adherent	Thin, clear to serosanguineous	Normal
pH	3.8-4.2	>4.5	≤4.5	>4.5	>4.5	3.8-4.2
Amine odor	Absent	Present	Absent	Variably present	Usually absent	Absent
Primary complaints	None	Malodorous discharge	Pruritus, irritation	Severe pruritis, discharge, dyspareunia, dysuria	Burning, soreness, dyspareunia	Burning, irritation, swelling, soreness
Microscopic appearance	Normal epithelial cells, lactobacilli	"Clue cells," no WBCs	Budding yeast, hyphae, spores	Trichomonads, many WBCs (PMNs)	Small, round (parabasal) epithelial cells, many PMNs	Normal
Other findings and diagnostic features	None	Minimal vulvar involvement	Vulvar and vaginal erythema, predisposing medical conditions	Intense vulvovaginal erythema, "strawberry cervix," other STIs	Atrophy of vulva and vaginal epithelium	Highly variable

PMNs, Polymorphonuclear neutrophil leukocytes; STIs, sexually transmitted infections; WBCs, white blood cells.

of at least 3 days' duration result in a greater initial response rate and a decreased chance of immediate recurrence. Symptoms related to inflammatory vulvar involvement respond most rapidly to topical creams, although application may be accompanied by burning pain. Oral fluconazole (150 mg, single dose) is a convenient therapeutic agent to include in the basic pharmacopoeia of a wilderness expedition. Women with frequent recurrences or predictable outbreaks at specific times in their cycle (most often premenstrually) should consider prophylactic weekly suppressive therapy with fluconazole (150 mg orally) or clotrimazole (1% intravaginal applicator).[191] To treat local symptoms, a low-potency steroid cream can be used in conjunction with a topical antifungal.

BACTERIAL VAGINOSIS

Bacterial vaginosis (BV) is the most common cause of vaginitis in women of childbearing age.[11] The most common complaints of women with BV are discharge and odor, itching, and irritation of the vulva and vagina. More than half of women with BV do not complain of symptoms or are unaware that symptoms result from a treatable condition. BV is believed to result from a disturbance in the normal vaginal flora, whereby the normal level of hydrogen peroxide–producing lactobacilli is replaced by less dominant organisms.[189] Discharge accompanying BV is typically thin, watery, grayish white, frothy, and homogeneous (not flocculent), uniformly coating the vaginal walls and introitus. More than 50% of women with BV complain of a fishy odor, particularly during menstruation and immediately after unprotected sexual intercourse. Blood and semen can alkalinize the vagina and volatilize a variety of amines (e.g., cadaverine) produced by anaerobic organisms.

BV diagnosis is confirmed by the presence of three of the following: discharge, pH greater than 4.5, release of amines (fishy odor) when discharge is exposed to 10% KOH ("whiff test"), and microscopic detection of "clue cells" (epithelial cells coated with bacteria) in saline solution. The microscopic appearance of pure BV is characterized by few, if any, leukocytes and a few motile and curved rods (lactobacilli). BV is treated with metronidazole, which can be administered orally (500 mg twice daily for 7 days) or as a 0.75% vaginal gel (once daily for 5 days). These regimens have initial response rates in excess of 90%. Tinidazole is a second-generation nitroimidazole with a longer half-life than metronidazole. The recommended oral dosage schedules are 1 g/day for 5 days or 2 g/day for 2 days. Clindamycin (300 mg orally twice daily for 5 to 7 days or 2% vaginal gel daily for 7 days) has comparable efficacy, but is expensive, has deleterious effects on normal vaginal lactobacilli, and increases the risk for

pseudomembranous enterocolitis (a rare side effect that could be life-threatening in the wilderness). There may be treatment failures with any of the options above.[11]

TRICHOMONAS VAGINITIS

Trichomonas vaginalis is a single-celled parasite that causes vaginitis in 2 to 3 million women annually in the United States.[217] It is predominantly sexually transmitted and is found most often in individuals with multiple sex partners and those with a history of or current STIs. Diagnosis and treatment of a woman and her sex partner are best accomplished at a screening visit before departure on a wilderness excursion. Unlike BV and yeast vaginitis, detection of *T. vaginalis*, even in asymptomatic women, is an indication for treatment and more complete STI screening.

The most common complaints include severe vulvovaginal pruritus, dyspareunia, and dysuria. Physical examination often reveals intense vaginal erythema and petechial cervical lesions (i.e., "strawberry cervix"). Vaginal discharge is typically gray or yellow-green, somewhat cloudy, and variably frothy and malodorous. The presence of frothy and malodorous discharge frequently indicates a mixed infection with the amine-producing organisms seen in BV. The vaginal fluid pH is elevated, typically above a numeric value of 5.0, and frequently exceeds a value of 6.0.

Because of diagnostic difficulties in the wilderness, empirical therapy is justified. Options include metronidazole administered as a single 2-g oral dose; in severe cases or cases that are not resolved by a single dose, it is given for a week (500 mg orally twice daily) or longer. Tinidazole given as a single dose of 2 g orally is also an option. For optimal results, sexual partners should be treated simultaneously and sexual activity stopped during therapy. To minimize GI side effects, metronidazole or tinidazole should be taken with plenty of water. This may not reduce the unpleasant metallic taste, but may reduce the risk for nausea, vomiting, and gastric irritation. Because a disulfiram-like effect is possible, alcohol should be avoided while taking metronidazole or tinidazole. Metronidazole 0.75% vaginal gel is not appropriate for treatment of trichomoniasis.[190]

ATROPHIC VAGINITIS

A decrease in estrogen levels during perimenopause and menopause can cause vaginal atrophy. This effect can also occur in hypoestrogenized premenopausal women (e.g., some amenorrheic athletes and women taking ovarian suppressive therapy with GnRH agonists). Thinning of vaginal epithelium due to a lost estrogen effect is the presumed cause. Reduced epithelial cell glycogen, an important substrate for lactobacilli, leads to increased vaginal pH and alterations in flora with subsequent overgrowth of nonacidophilic organisms. Symptoms include burning or soreness, dyspareunia, and watery or even serosanguineous vaginal discharge. Typically, the vaginal mucosa is uniformly erythematous and may have areas of petechiae. The vaginal pH usually exceeds a numeric value of 5.0 (often 6.0 to 7.0), and microscopic evaluation of discharge reveals small, round, immature epithelial cells (parabasal cells), increased neutrophils, and a paucity of lactobacilli. Treatment includes the use of topical or oral estrogen replacement therapy.[167] Treatment with low-dose topical estrogen (cream, ring, or tablet) usually provides complete relief of symptoms within weeks. In the interim, women may obtain relief with use of vaginal moisturizers and lubricants (e.g., Astroglide, Replens).

NONINFECTIOUS VULVOVAGINITIS

Vulvovaginitis due to environmental exposures can cause local irritation. It may be of greater significance when the ability to attend to personal hygiene is limited.[100] Common causative agents include latex condoms, spermicidal compounds, soaps, detergents, fabric softeners, deodorant products, menstrual pads and tampons, and topical medications such as antimycotics and povidone-iodine. Exclude an infectious cause and identify the source of the reaction to make the diagnosis. Once a potentially offending cause is identified (e.g., recent change in laundry detergent), exposure is avoided and symptoms can be treated (i.e., pain relief, antihistamines, sitz baths). Topical corticosteroid creams may be tried, but in rare instances, they may exacerbate symptoms.

SEXUALLY TRANSMITTED INFECTIONS

If a woman has a new discharge or pelvic pain following a sexual encounter, she may have a sexually transmitted infection (STI) and should be evaluated as soon as possible. Discussion of safe-sex practices and risks associated with STIs pertinent to the destination should be included in the pre–wilderness travel visit.[104]

Women are at a higher risk for acquiring an STI from infected men than men would be from infected women. Long-term complications related to STIs include PID, chronic pelvic pain, and infertility. To prevent acquisition of STIs, women should avoid casual sex and always practice safe sex by using condoms, no matter what other means of contraception are used simultaneously. High-quality latex condoms are an essential part of a sexually active traveler's medical kit, regardless of gender. A male or female condom made of polyurethane is an effective alternative for persons allergic to latex. Patients with a history of genital herpes simplex virus infection should bring a supply of antiviral medication (e.g., acyclovir, valacyclovir) to treat an outbreak during travel.

NONOCCUPATIONAL POSTEXPOSURE HIV PROPHYLAXIS

Women should be educated about the availability of postexposure HIV prophylaxis for high-risk sexual exposures or sexual assault.[63,169,176,204] If a woman is traveling to a remote area, include the initial week of treatment in the traveler's medical kit. Travelers should check with the CDC (cdc.gov) or World Health Organization (int/hiv/topics/prophylaxis/en/) for the latest information on nonoccupational postexposure HIV prophylaxis recommendations. The National HIV/AIDS Clinician Consultation Center at the University of California, San Francisco, operates the National Clinicians' Postexposure Prophylaxis Hotline. The hotline is available 24 hours a day, 7 days a week (1-888-448-4911) or one can use the website at nccc.ucsf.edu/clinician-consultation/pep-post-exposure-prophylaxis/. Ideally, one should do research and obtain an option for a personal HIV postexposure prophylaxis starter kit prior to travel so testing can be started immediately following a high-risk exposure while waiting for a consultation. Home testing kits for HIV are available in many countries.

Sensitivity and specificity of these tests vary. HIV testing should be repeated with a reliable laboratory analysis.[8,196]

PERSONAL SAFETY

Women of all ages should take a self-defense course. There are many personal self-defense devices available, such as pepper spray (made from cayenne pepper), Mace (tear gas), capsules that let out a pungent odor, and sound devices or alarms. One should also consider carrying a portable smoke alarm because they are not provided in many international accommodations.

SEXUAL ASSAULT

Sexual assault of women in the wilderness is assumed to be rare but is probably underreported. One in every three women will be physically, sexually, or otherwise abused in her lifetime.[220] Wilderness morbidity and mortality statistics are limited, but one study of eight National Park Service areas in California over 3 years reported only one incident of sexual assault.[152] Many wilderness incidents are likely not reported. Overall, only 7% of all rapes are estimated to be reported.[46] All women should be prepared and practice measures to prevent assault.

The best defense against sexual assault is not going into the wilderness with unfamiliar people. The chance of meeting an assailant is quite low. A woman traveling into the wilderness alone or with someone she does not know well is advised to tell friends or family exactly where and with whom she is traveling and when she anticipates returning.

If sexually assaulted, women are advised to seek medical attention as soon as possible. Most emergency departments can evaluate and treat sexual assault victims. It may be impossible to reach a medical facility for many hours or even days, but an attempt should be made to preserve potential evidence. Women are advised to avoid douching, gargling, brushing teeth, or changing clothes. If clothes are removed, they should be placed in a paper bag and brought to a medical facility. The CDC recommends STI prophylaxis, postexposure prophylaxis for HIV, and EC for women at risk.[63,204] Posttraumatic stress counseling should also be offered.

WILDERNESS TRAVEL DURING PREGNANCY

Many women involved in wilderness activities expect to continue their adventures at all stages of pregnancy. These women understand the benefits of exercise and the positive effects that participating in a wilderness experience have on their general health and well-being.[18] However, pregnancy is considered a relative contraindication to wilderness activities unless access to medical care is available or provisions are made for rapid evacuation. Review the pregnant traveler's itinerary and assess for risks relating to the destination or specific activity that may be a risk to the mother or fetus. Counsel pregnant travelers to take preventive measures or consider an alternative plan. Although a successful prior pregnancy is a relatively good predictor of outcome after the first trimester, pregnancy is unpredictable. A pregnant woman should consider potential risks of unexpected complications and how she would feel if the outcome resulted in preventable maternal or fetal morbidity and mortality.

Information on the pregnant traveler is based on small studies, anecdotal information, and extrapolation from nonpregnant travelers. Evidence-based recommendations are lacking for pregnant women.

PRE–WILDERNESS TRAVEL EVALUATION DURING PREGNANCY

Box 92-4 is a checklist for pregnant travelers. Basic questions to ask when counseling pregnant women prior to travel to remote places include[31]:

What are the medical and obstetric risks associated with wilderness travel?

BOX 92-4   Checklist for Pregnant Travelers

Pretravel Risk Assessment
Stage of gestation
Obstetric risk factors
Medical risk factors
Destination risk considerations
  Access to care
  Medical services available during transit and at destination
  Emergency evacuation insurance
  Review emergency signs and symptoms: vaginal bleeding, abdominal pain, contractions, proteinuria, headache with visual change, severe edema and/or accelerated weight gain, decreased fetal activity, and rupture of membranes
  Due to infectious disease
  Chloroquine-resistant *Plasmodium falciparum* malaria
  Outbreak of disease requiring a live virus vaccine
  Outbreak of disease for which no vaccine is available and that has a high risk for maternal and fetal complications and death
  Due to food and water exposure
  Due to insect exposure
  Due to environment
  Exercise risk
  Altitude
  Heat
  Cold
  Open-water bodies
  Dehydration

Recommendations
Medical insurance and evacuation coverage
Immunizations to reflect actual risk for disease and probable benefit
Medications: review safety during pregnancy
Preventive measures
  Medical kit adaptations for pregnancy and infant care
  Plans for emergency delivery and infant resuscitation
  Emergency delivery kit
  Infant resuscitation kit
Postpone wilderness travel if risks outweigh benefits, or adapt itinerary to decrease risks

---

What medical services are available during transit and at the intended destinations?

What does health insurance cover for a woman who is out of the area for delivery or pregnancy-related complications?

What are the signs of serious pregnancy-related illness for which emergency medical help should be sought?

What are some general guidelines to follow for medical management of illness that will safeguard a pregnant woman and her fetus?

Are required and recommended immunizations for the proposed itinerary safe in pregnancy?

What medications are safe in pregnancy?

Are there special concerns related to environmental conditions or activities?

Is the woman prepared for a "wilderness delivery"?

Is there need for an infant resuscitation kit?

Pre–wilderness travel preparation starts with a review of the woman's obstetric and medical history. Health practitioners who advise pregnant women should work closely with a woman's obstetrician to assess potential benefits and risks involved in a particular wilderness trip. Any history of pregnancy problems (e.g., vaginal bleeding, preterm labor, or chronic illness) increases the risk. Categories of potential high-risk pregnancies for which travel should be delayed or the itinerary adjusted are summarized in Box 92-5. The obstetric history should be reviewed for complications for which there may be a high risk of recurrence (e.g., preterm labor, premature rupture of membranes, pre-eclampsia, gestational diabetes, fetal growth restriction, group B hemolytic streptococcal infection, UTI, chorioamnionitis, blood group isoimmunization, thromboembolic event, surgical delivery, and postdelivery complications). Perform a complete physical examination.

Laboratory evaluation before departure includes standard blood tests recommended by the ACOG: complete blood count, blood type, antibody screen (and screen of partner if the woman is Rh negative or isoimmunized), and basic serologic measurements (rapid plasma reagin, rubella, hepatitis B, HIV). Serologic screening for varicella and herpes simplex virus 2 should also be considered in the woman with no history of varicella or genital herpes because of the potential for first-time outbreaks during pregnancy in women with unrecognized infection. Individuals at risk and those not previously evaluated should also be offered hemoglobin electrophoresis to assess for hemoglobinopathies. Urinalysis and urine culture are performed because of the high frequency of asymptomatic infections during pregnancy that can complicate outcomes. Vaginal fluid should be assessed for BV because treatment early in pregnancy may prevent premature rupture of membranes and preterm labor. Perform a Pap smear. A woman beyond 10 weeks' gestation should undergo routine genetic and biochemical screening (e.g., maternal serum α-fetoprotein, estriol, hCG) to assess for certain congenital and chromosomal abnormalities. Abnormal biochemical markers may indicate complications (e.g., fetal growth restriction and pre-eclampsia) due to early abnormalities in placentation that can become clinically significant later in gestation. These conditions also increase the risk for premature delivery, as well as for maternal and fetal complications and death.[16,17,22]

Screen for diabetes. Gestational diabetes with a previous pregnancy is associated with increased risk during subsequent gestations. Proper dietary counseling and regular blood sugar monitoring with a portable plasma glucose monitor should be conducted throughout the pregnancy. Insulin, sufficient syringes, and alcohol wipes should be included with basic medical supplies in the event that glycemic control deteriorates. The goal is to maintain fasting plasma glucose levels at 90 mg/dL or less and lower than 120 mg/dL 2 hours after meals. Physical conditioning reduces the risk for developing diabetes during pregnancy. Women with pregestational diabetes of any duration should have a baseline electrocardiogram and possibly an echocardiogram before participation in any wilderness-related activities.

All pregnant wilderness travelers should have an obstetric sonogram before departure.[22] Early in the pregnancy, ultrasonography can accurately confirm gestational age, viability, intrauterine location, and number of fetuses. It may also rule out the

BOX 92-5   Potential Contraindications for Wilderness Travel During Pregnancy

Obstetric Risk Factors
Extremes of maternal age
Vaginal bleeding this pregnancy
Multiple gestation this pregnancy
Fetal abnormalities or growth issues (IUGR)
History of gestational diabetes or hypertension
History of miscarriage, preterm labor, abnormal implantation of placenta, or premature rupture of membranes

Medical Risk Factors
History of thromboembolism
Cardiac disease
Severe anemia
Medical disease requiring ongoing assessment and medication such as diabetes, pulmonary disease, or renal disease

Risk Factors at Wilderness Destination
Lack of access to medical care
High altitude
Disease requiring a live virus vaccine (e.g., yellow fever, measles)
Mefloquine-resistant *Plasmodium falciparum* malaria
Epidemic of infectious disease leading to high-risk maternal and fetal illness
Natural disasters

Risk Factors Due to Sports Activity
Scuba diving
High risk for trauma

presence of an ectopic pregnancy, adnexal mass, abnormal placental implantation, or molar pregnancy. Second-trimester ultrasonography can estimate gestational age and assess major fetal abnormalities, location of the placenta in relationship to the cervix, cervical length, and integrity of the internal cervical os. Beyond 20 weeks' gestation, normal fetal growth and blood flow patterns in umbilical and middle cerebral arteries can be assessed by Doppler velocimetry. Normal results indicate a lower risk for complications (e.g., IUGR, preeclampsia, and preterm labor). Findings that significantly increase maternal or fetal risk are contraindications to travel.

Counseling on the timing of wilderness activity should be done, although no interval during pregnancy is considered absolutely safe. Guidelines of the American Association of Obstetricians and Gynecologists state that the safest time to travel is during the second trimester because the pregnancy is established and extra weight is not usually a functional limitation for the mother.[21] Risk for miscarriage is highest during the first trimester. The first trimester is also when effects on a fetus from medications or vaccines needed by the mother would be greatest. The primary risks in the third trimester are complications (e.g., bleeding, preeclampsia, and preterm labor and delivery).

One of the most important considerations for a pregnant woman planning wilderness travel is assessment of available options in case of an emergency. The complete itinerary should be evaluated with attention to both availability and quality of medical care during transit and at the final destination. Access to high-quality care during travel is essential in case of preterm labor or an unexpected complication of pregnancy.

Pregnant women traveling to a more remote area or to a less developed country should review their health insurance policy coverage guidelines. An additional travel health and evacuation insurance policy that provides a worldwide 24-hour medical assistance hotline number may need to be purchased. This service would provide telephone contact with medical personnel to help arrange emergency medical consultation and treatment, monitor care, and provide emergency evacuation to a more advanced medical facility if necessary. Patients must be aware that medical evacuation can take hours to days from remote locations. Each policy must be reviewed carefully to make sure that it covers expenses associated with a normal pregnancy (e.g., delivery), as well as with the possible complications of pregnancy (e.g., miscarriage early in pregnancy or third-trimester preeclampsia). Policies should also cover expenses associated with emergency care of the fetus and newborn.

Teach pregnant patients warning signs of potentially serious problems (e.g., bleeding, passing tissue or clots, abdominal pain or cramps, rupture of membranes, decreased fetal movement, headache, or visual changes) and develop a plan for what they should do if these occur. Each woman should carry a copy of her medical record (including blood type and Rh) and her physician's phone number, fax number, and email address. This information may be helpful for routine questions or if there is an emergency.

PHYSIOLOGIC CHANGES ACCOMPANYING PREGNANCY

Normal physiologic changes of pregnancy (e.g., reduced exercise and heat tolerance, elevated heart rate related to physiologic anemia, and increased plasma volume) may have an impact on wilderness travel. Within weeks of conception, hormonal changes accompanying pregnancy result in physiologic adaptations affecting every organ system. Increased progesterone has smooth muscle relaxation effects to maintain uterine quiescence, but also contributes to vasomotor instability, hypotension, gastric reflux, and constipation. Estrogens stimulate hepatic production of many hormone-binding globulins and of coagulation factors II, V, VII, VIII, IX, X, and XII, and fibrinogen that contributes to the hypercoagulable state of pregnancy and increased risk for VTE.[19]

Cardiovascular Adaptation

Pregnancy affects maternal hemodynamics by inducing increases in blood volume, heart rate, and stroke volume, and decrease in systemic vascular resistance. Cardiac output increases 30% to 50% by the end of the first trimester owing to an increase in stroke volume secondary to an increase in preload. Gradual increases in the maternal heart rate usually peak between 24 and 28 weeks' gestation. Uterine blood flow increases from 50 mL/min to more than 500 mL/min, corresponding to an increase from approximately 1% to 20% of total cardiac output. Systemic vascular resistance decreases primarily from the low-resistance placental vascular bed, which is the equivalent of a large arteriovenous shunt. Peripheral vasodilatory effects of progesterone, estrogen, and other factors also contribute. These hemodynamic changes help to provide the circulatory reserve necessary to provide nutrients and oxygen to the mother and fetus at rest and during moderate exercise.[7,75]

Changes in Blood Volume

The total blood volume increases 40% to 50% during normal pregnancy because of rapid expansion of the plasma volume. A disproportionate increase in plasma volume over red cell mass results in so-called physiologic anemia of pregnancy. Physiologic effects of hypervolemia and anemia during pregnancy have several benefits. Decreased blood viscosity (from greater increases in plasma than red cell volume) results in reduced resistance to flow, facilitating placental perfusion and lowering cardiac work. The increase in blood volume ($\approx$ 50% higher than in nonpregnant women) provides some reserve against normal blood loss occurring during parturition. Most of the increased cardiac output is distributed to the placenta to provide nutrients to the fetus, to the kidneys for excretion of maternal and fetal waste products, and to the skin to assist in maternal temperature control.[7]

Respiratory Status

Respiratory system changes during pregnancy help to compensate for physiologic anemia to maintain fetal and maternal homeostasis. Progesterone directly stimulates the respiratory center and increases carbon dioxide sensitivity, resulting in a 30% to 40% increase in tidal volume (TV). The respiratory rate (RR) does not change significantly, but as a result of TV changes, the minute ventilation (i.e., TV $\times$ RR) increases 25% to 30%, despite a slight decrease in total lung capacity. A 20% reduction of functional residual capacity due to decreased expiratory reserve volume and residual volume characterizes the relative hyperventilation with compensated respiratory alkalosis. Many of these changes are completed by the end of the first trimester. Their sum is a dramatic 50% increase in alveolar ventilation, increased PaO_2, 30% increase in 1-minute oxygen uptake, and significant decrease in the partial pressure of carbon dioxide. The overall effect is to increase the oxygen-carrying capacity of maternal blood to accommodate fetal and maternal metabolic needs, while facilitating diffusion of carbon dioxide from the fetus. For the wilderness traveler, these changes lead to higher oxygen saturation under hypoxic conditions (e.g., high altitude).

Urinary System

Significant changes in the urinary system account for many complaints and complications of pregnancy (e.g., urinary frequency, incontinence, and increased risk for UTIs). In the first trimester, ureters become dilated, elongated, and more tortuous, presumably under the influence of progesterone. Further dilation of proximal ureters occurs when the uterus reaches the level of the pelvic brim at about 20 weeks' gestation and compresses the ureters, resulting in the first presentations of pyelonephritis. This more often occurs on the right than the left owing to dextrorotation of the uterus by the descending colon. Vesicoureteral reflux occurs secondary to decreased ureterovesical junction competency and contributes to an increased risk for an upper tract infection. This is exacerbated by a progressive decrease in bladder capacity and doubling of intravesicular pressures (from 10 to 20 cm H_2O) during gestation. These factors also contribute to frequent complaints of urinary incontinence in pregnant women.

Integumentary and Musculoskeletal Status

Integumentary and musculoskeletal changes can have significant effects on a pregnant wilderness traveler's well-being. Increased estrogen leads to proliferation and dilation of small arterioles in the skin to help compensate for the increased need to remove heat generated by the maternal and fetal metabolism. Because of these inherent changes, pregnant women have a limited capacity to respond further to heat stress and are at an increased risk for hyperthermia in hot and humid environments. Estrogen and other pregnancy-associated hormones also increase skin sensitivity to damage by sun exposure, particularly in fair-skinned individuals. Some pregnant women have a predisposition to skin hyperpigmentation in a nonuniform distribution because of excessive melanin deposition in the dermis and epidermis. This is enhanced by sun exposure and often affects the face (melasma), midline abdomen (linea nigra), nipples, axillae, and perineum. It may require a prolonged period for resolution after delivery or may never resolve completely.[75]

Weight gain, weight redistribution, and ligamentous relaxation may pose risks even to well-conditioned pregnant women.[24] Weight gain during pregnancy is approximately 9 to 16 kg (20 to 35 lb). Some weight gain is important during pregnancy to avoid a catabolic state and may be more important to highly conditioned athletes that enter pregnancy with limited fat stores. Increased weight stresses the skeleton and ligaments and may accumulate more rapidly than conditioning can handle. Much of the weight gain is contributed by uterine and fetal growth, resulting in forward displacement of the center of gravity. This is usually accompanied by progressive lower spine lordosis and increased strain on spinal ligaments, disks, and paravertebral muscles. When lumbar lordosis is exaggerated, traction and compression on the sciatic nerves can cause significant pain and weakness in the buttocks and lower extremities. Lower spine changes are frequently followed by compensatory flexion of the cervical spine. This can place traction on the median and ulnar nerves, resulting in upper extremity pain, paresthesias, and weakness.[49]

Challenges of weight gain are accompanied by dramatic changes in ligamentous support throughout the body. Under the influence of relaxin and other hormones, ligaments become more compliant and hydrophilic. Benefits of this include relaxation in the sacroiliac joints and symphysis pubis to facilitate delivery, but hormonal effects on other ligaments can lead to complications. For example, fluid retention by the wrist's flexor retinaculum can cause median nerve compression. This results in carpal tunnel syndrome, a common complaint of pregnancy. This may be more than just a nuisance to the wilderness traveler because pain and hand weakness can compromise activities that require hand strength and endurance (e.g., rock climbing, canoeing). Pelvic girdle instability, accompanied by weight gain, can cause a shift in the center of gravity and spinal lordosis leading to gait and balance disturbances interfering with enjoyment of many wilderness activities such as hiking or skiing. These changes also lead to an increase in the severity of trauma accompanying falls. Maternal trauma remains one of the leading causes of fetal death, typically due to placental abruption or preterm labor.[52,71] The anterior cruciate ligament is especially prone to severe trauma; injury is three to four times more likely in women, and the ligament is especially susceptible to trauma in the active pregnant woman.[214] Difficult terrain poses a risk to pregnant wilderness travelers.

Changes in Immune Status: Response to Infection and Vaccines

Pregnancy results in a number of changes in the maternal immune system. Evidence suggests that there is a reduction in cell-mediated immunity during pregnancy. Pregnancy results in increased susceptibility (or predisposition to more severe disease) to a number of infections in which the cell-mediated immune response is important (e.g., malaria, typhoid, amebiasis, coccidioidomycosis, leishmaniasis, filariasis, leptospirosis, leprosy, trypanosomiasis, listeriosis, and tuberculosis).[127,135,147,171] Determine the risk for these infections when the itinerary is being reviewed. In contrast, infections in which the humoral system is the most important response show no increase in susceptibility to infection. B-cell numbers and function do not appear to be reduced during pregnancy.

Immunizations During Pregnancy and Lactation.

Women should be vaccinated before pregnancy. Risks and benefits of immunizations during pregnancy must be weighed against the maternal risk for illness, likelihood of adverse fetal outcomes if the mother becomes ill, and risks associated with vaccines. Risks for immunizations during pregnancy are largely theoretical.[124] When the risk for disease exposure is high, benefits of vaccinating pregnant women usually outweigh potential risks.[1,79,87,90,158,173,197,206,221]

Breastfeeding is not a contraindication to most vaccinations, with the possible exception of yellow fever (YF) vaccine. Three cases of YF vaccine–associated neurologic disease have been documented in breastfed infants whose mothers received the vaccine.[58] It is not clear if transmission occurred via breast milk. Breastfeeding mothers should be advised not to travel to a zone endemic for YF if such travel will require administration of YF vaccine. For a woman trying to conceive, it is recommended that she wait for 1 month after receiving a live virus vaccine (e.g., measles-mumps-rubella, varicella, YF) to become pregnant. If a woman receives a vaccine and later finds out that she is pregnant, there is no indication for termination of the pregnancy.[1]

Ideally, avoid vaccinations during the first trimester because of uncertain effects on the developing fetus. Serologic studies for hepatitis A and B, varicella, measles, and rubella may be checked to assess the potential risk for infection. In general during pregnancy, inactivated vaccines are safe but live vaccines are contraindicated. Tetanus and diphtheria toxoids and influenza vaccine are routinely given during pregnancy. Hepatitis A and B, Japanese encephalitis, meningococcal, rabies, and typhoid fever (inactivated) vaccines may also be administered during pregnancy if there is risk for exposure to these infections.

YF vaccine safety during pregnancy is unknown, but the vaccine has been administered to hundreds of pregnant women without increased risk versus the general population.[124,218] There is concern for decreased seroconversion rates if vaccination is given later in pregnancy. If the risk for YF infection is low but proof of immunization is required, a medical waiver can be given. If the risk for YF is high and travel unavoidable, administer the vaccine. A small study of pregnant women inadvertently given YF vaccine did not find adverse fetal or maternal outcomes.[197] As of June 2016, YF vaccine recommendations will change to advising that one dose of YF vaccine will provide lifetime immunity.[58] Prudence recommends that YF vaccine be given to all women of reproductive age prior to pregnancy who might travel to a zone endemic for YF during their lifetime. This would avoid the theoretical concerns associated with YF vaccine administration during pregnancy. All vaccines are listed as category C under the FDA pregnancy categories (Table 92-5).[1]

MEDICATIONS DURING PREGNANCY

Food and Drug Administration Guidelines

The FDA has developed a set of guidelines to categorize drugs, vaccines, and toxoids with regard to developmental toxicity and adverse fetal outcome. Assessments are based on the degree to which available information has ruled out a risk to the fetus balanced against potential benefits to pregnant woman (Box 92-6). Most medications fall under FDA category C. Few double-blind studies have been done in pregnant women to categorize drugs.

Other Resources for Information on Medications During Pregnancy

Physicians advising pregnant women should have ready access to references related to medication use during pregnancy. The text *Drugs in Pregnancy and Lactation*[53] includes reproductive literature reviews relevant to drugs and immunizations. Each medication is categorized by FDA risk classifications. There are Internet resources with information on the teratogenic risk of particular medications or vaccines. Table 92-6 lists some of the medications commonly used by pregnant women during travel.

TABLE 92-5 CDC Recommendations for Vaccination During Pregnancy*

Vaccination of Pregnant Women Is Recommended

Hepatitis B	Recombinant or plasma-derived	Recommended for women at risk of infection.
Influenza	Inactivated whole virus or subunit	All women who are pregnant in the second and third trimesters during the flu season (*Northern Hemisphere*: October to May; *Southern Hemisphere*: April to September; *tropics*: year round) and women at high risk for pulmonary complications regardless of trimester.
Diphtheria-tetanus	Toxoid	If indicated, such as lack of primary series, or no booster within past 10 years.
Diphtheria-tetanus-pertussis (TDaP)	Toxoid-acellular	TDaP should be given during each pregnancy, preferably during the third trimester at 27 to 36 weeks to maximize maternal antibody response and passive antibody transfer to infant. However, it may be given at any time.
Hepatitis A	Inactivated virus	Data on safety in pregnancy are not available. Because hepatitis A vaccine is produced from inactivated hepatitis A virus, theoretical risk of vaccination should be weighed against risk of disease. Consider immune globulin rather than vaccine.

Pregnancy Is a Precaution, and Under Normal Circumstances Vaccination Should Be Deferred; Vaccine Should Only Be Given When Benefits Outweigh Risks

Japanese encephalitis	Inactivated virus	Data on safety in pregnancy are not available. Pregnant women who must travel to an area where risk is high should be vaccinated when theoretical risks are outweighed by risk of disease.
Meningococcal meningitis	Polysaccharide	Meningococcal conjugate vaccine (MCV4) is preferred for adults. However, there are no data on safety and immunogenicity in pregnant women. Polyvalent meningococcal meningitis vaccine (MPSV4) can be administered during pregnancy if the woman is entering an epidemic area. Indications for prophylaxis are not altered by pregnancy; vaccine recommended in unusual outbreak situations.
Pneumococcal	Polysaccharide	Safety of pneumococcal (PPV23) vaccine during the first trimester has not been evaluated, although no adverse events have been reported after inadvertent vaccination during pregnancy. Women with chronic diseases, smokers, and immunosuppressed women should consider vaccination.
Polio, inactivated	Inactivated virus	Indicated for susceptible pregnant women traveling in endemic areas or in other high-risk situations.
Rabies	Inactivated virus	Indications for postexposure prophylaxis not altered by pregnancy. If risk of exposure to rabies is substantial, preexposure prophylaxis may also be indicated.
Typhoid (ViCPS)	Polysaccharide	If indicated for travel to endemic areas.
Typhoid (Ty21a)	Live bacterial	Data on safety in pregnancy are not available; theoretical risk because live-attenuated.
Yellow fever	Live attenuated virus	Use caution. Safety of yellow fever vaccination in pregnancy has not been studied in a large prospective trial. Pregnant women who must travel to areas where risk of yellow fever infection is high should be vaccinated and their infants should be monitored after birth for evidence of congenital infection and other possible adverse effects resulting from yellow fever vaccination. Pregnancy may interfere with the immune response to yellow fever vaccine. Consider serologic testing to document a protective immune response to the vaccine. Avoid in breastfeeding mothers unless travel to high endemic region is unavoidable.†

Pregnancy Is a Contraindication to Vaccination; Vaccine Should Not Be Administered to Pregnant Women

Tuberculosis (BCG)	Attenuated mycobacterial	Contraindicated because of theoretical risk of disseminated disease. Skin testing for tuberculosis exposure before and after travel is preferable when risk of possible exposure is high.
Measles-mumps-rubella	Live attenuated virus	Contraindicated. Vaccination of susceptible women should be part of postpartum care. Unvaccinated women should delay travel to countries where measles is endemic until after delivery. Unvaccinated pregnant women with a documented exposure to measles should receive immunoglobulin within 6 days to prevent illness.
Human papillomavirus	Recombinant quadrivalent	Contraindicated. Vaccine has not been causally associated with adverse outcomes of pregnancy. However, additional information is needed for further recommendations.
Varicella	Live attenuated virus	Contraindicated. Vaccination of susceptible women should be considered postpartum. Unvaccinated pregnant women should consider postponing travel until after delivery, when the vaccine can be given safely.

Vaccine/Immunobiologic		Use
Immune globulins, pooled or hyperimmune	Immune globulin or specific globulin preparations	If indicated for preexposure or postexposure use. No known risk to fetus.

*Adapted from Vaccines and immunizations: Guidelines for vaccinating pregnant women; and Travel and other vaccines, CDC health information for international travel: cdc.gov/vaccines/pubs/preg-guide.htm.
†See Brunette GW, editor: CDC health information for international travel 2016, New York, 2016, Oxford University Press.

BOX 92-6   U.S. Food and Drug Administration Use-in-Pregnancy Classifications

Category A: Adequate and well-controlled studies in women show no risk to the fetus.

Category B: No evidence of risk in humans. Either studies in animals show risk, but human findings do not, or, in the absence of human studies, animal findings are negative.

Category C: Risk cannot be ruled out. No adequate and well-controlled studies in humans, or animal studies are either positive for fetal risk or lacking as well. Drugs should be given only if the potential benefit justifies the potential risk to the fetus.

Category D: There is positive evidence of human fetal risk. Nevertheless, potential benefits may outweigh the potential risks.

Category X: Contraindicated in pregnancy. Studies in animals or humans, investigations, or postmarketing reports have shown that fetal risk far outweighs any potential benefit to the patient.

INFECTIOUS DISEASE RISK

Pregnancy causes immune system adaptations. Pregnant women have been found to have increased severity of infections when they suffer influenza, hepatitis E viral infection, or herpes simplex virus infection.[127] Pregnancy leads to both increased susceptibility to and severity of malaria from *Plasmodium falciparum*, and increased susceptibility to listeriosis.

Food-Borne and Waterborne Disease

The main concern with traveler's diarrhea during pregnancy is dehydration that can compromise placental blood flow and adversely affect the fetus. Reduced gastric acidity during pregnancy may predispose to GI illness. Boiling water is the most effective and safest method of disinfection. Iodination of water is not recommended, because of risk of fetal goiter. Other options are chlorination, a filter containing three elements (i.e., microfiltration, activated charcoal, and iodine resin), or ultraviolet light exposure (e.g., SteriPEN). Iodine resins transfer iodine to microorganisms that come into contact with the resin but leave little

TABLE 92-6   Medication Use During Pregnancy and Lactation

Medication	Category	Issues During Pregnancy	Issues During Lactation
Analgesics/Antipyretics		*Try nonpharmaceutical methods first to treat pain such as rest, ice, heat, massage.*	
Acetaminophen	B	Safe in low doses short term.	Compatible
Aspirin	C/D	Avoid first and last trimester. Has been associated with premature closure of ductus and excessive bleeding. Low-dose aspirin (60-80 mg) may be used for preeclampsia.	Use caution
Nonsteroidal antiinflammatory (Ibuprofen, Naproxen)	B/D	Should not be used in first and last trimesters owing to effects on premature closure of ductus and effects on clotting. Not teratogenic.	Compatible
Codeine	C/D	Use cautiously as may cause respiratory depression and withdrawal symptoms in fetus if used near term.	Compatible
Hydrocodone	C/D	Use cautiously as may cause respiratory depression in infant if used near term.	Use caution
Antibiotics for URI, UTI, GI, Skin, Other		*Use antibiotics only if strong evidence of bacterial infection.*	
Amoxicillin, amoxicillin + clavulanic acid (Augmentin), amoxicillin + sulbactam (Unasyn)	B	Safe. Use for treatment of otitis media, sinusitis, streptococcal pharyngitis.	Safe
Azithromycin	B	Safe. Use for bronchitis, pneumonia, gastroenteritis (*Campylobacter, Shigella, Salmonella, Escherichia coli*).	Use caution
Cephalosporins	B	Safe. Use for otitis, streptococcal infections, sinusitis, pharyngitis.	Use caution. Can be used to treat mastitis.
Clindamycin PO or Clindamycin vaginal cream	B	Safe. Use for bacterial vaginosis (BV) orally or locally in second or third trimester; avoid in first trimester.	Compatible
Ciprofloxacin, other quinolones	C	Controversial. Sometimes used short term in severe infections and/or long term in life-threatening infections (e.g., anthrax). May be used if potential benefit justifies risk to fetus.	Compatible
Dicloxacillin	B	Safe. Use for skin infections.	Safe. Used to treat mastitis.
Doxycycline, tetracycline	D	May cause permanent discoloration of the teeth during tooth development, including the last half of pregnancy, infancy, and childhood until 8 years of age.	Avoid
Erythromycin (base or state)	B	Safe. Use for bacterial causes of URI.	Compatible
Nitrofurantoin	B	Drug of choice for UTI in pregnancy.	Use caution
Penicillin	B	Safe.	Safe
Sulfonamides	B/D	Safe. However, not recommended in third trimester owing to risk for hyperbilirubinemia and kernicterus.	Avoid
Trimethoprim	C	Avoid	Use caution
Gastrointestinal			
Antidiarrheal		*Replacing fluid lost is key.*	
Atropine sulfate diphenoxylate hydrochloride (Lomotil)	C	Use only if severe symptoms.	Avoid
Loperamide (Imodium)	C	Use only if severe symptoms.	Compatible

Medication	Category	Issues During Pregnancy	Issues During Lactation
Nausea/vomiting, esophageal reflux		*Encourage supportive measures first rather than medications: crackers upon arising, frequent small meals, protein meal at bedtime.*	
Antacids	B	May use sparingly for symptoms as needed.	Safe
Bismuth subsalicylate (Pepto Bismol)	C/D	Avoid as contains bismuth and salicylate.	Use caution
Cimetidine, ranitidine, omeprazole	B/C	Safe. Study during the first trimester found it is not associated with an increase in congenital malformations.	Use caution
Ondansetron (Zofran)	B	Use for hyperemesis gravidarum.	Use caution
Metoclopramide (Reglan)	B	Safe in small doses.	Use caution
Dimenhydrinate (Dramamine)	B	Safe for severe nausea.	Use caution
Phenothiazines (Compazine)	C	Often clinically used for nausea and vomiting of pregnancy despite class rating.	Avoid
Promethazine (Phenergan)	C	Often clinically used for nausea and vomiting of pregnancy despite class rating.	Avoid
Acupressure (Sea-Bands)		Safe.	Safe
Emetrol (fluid replacement)	B	Safe. Oral solution.	Safe
Ginger	C	Safe.	Use caution
Meclizine	B	Safe for treatment of severe nausea and vomiting.	Compatible
Pyridoxine (B$_6$)	A	Safe. Used for nausea.	Compatible
Constipation		*Increase fiber and fluid in diet first.*	
Bisacodyl	C	Safe to use occasionally.	Use caution
Milk of magnesia	B	Safe in small amounts.	Safe
Psyllium hydrophilic mucilloid	C	Safe.	Compatible
Hemorrhoids		Increase fiber and fluid in diet.	
Anusol HC suppositories	C	Safe.	Use caution
Antihistamines and Related Respiratory			
URI, congestion, cough		*Symptomatic treatment: steam, rest, fluids.*	
Chlorpheniramine	B	Use cautiously for severe symptoms.	Use caution
Cetirizine (Zyrtec)	B	Safe. Nonsedating but use cautiously.	Use caution
Diphenhydramine (Benadryl)	B	Safe. Use cautiously.	Use caution
Loratadine (Claritin)	B	Safe. Nonsedating but use cautiously.	Compatible
Dextromethorphan	C	Probably safe. Use in small amounts.	Compatible
Guaifenesin	C	Probably safe. Use only if needed.	Use caution
Pseudoephedrine (Sudafed)	C	Avoid in first trimester. Use cautiously.	Compatible
Saline nasal spray	A	Safe.	Safe
Topical nasal decongestants			
Oxymetazoline (Afrin)		Safe. Do not use for more than 3 days.	Safe
Asthma, allergy			
Inhaled bronchodilators (Albuterol)	C	Safe for use of wheezing during pregnancy.	Unknown
Inhaled steroids (Fluticasone)	C	Use if indicated.	Safe
Nasal steroids (Fluticasone)	C	Use if indicated.	Safe
Antimalarials			
Artemether-lumefantrine (Coartem)	C	Used in second and third trimesters for treatment of severe malaria.	Use caution. Excreted in breast milk. Infant still needs own chemoprophylaxis.
Mefloquine (Lariam)	C	Avoid during first trimester unless unavoidable travel to high-risk area. Safe in second and third trimesters for high-risk travel.	Use caution. Excreted in breast milk. Infant still needs chemoprophylaxis.
Chloroquine	C	Avoid in first trimester unless traveling to high-risk area.	Use caution. Excreted in milk in small amounts. Infant still needs chemoprophylaxis.
Atovaquone, proguanil (Malarone)	C	Avoid in first trimester.	Use caution. Safe if infant is > 11 kg (24 lb) or if benefit for mother outweighs possible risk.
Doxycycline	D	Contraindicated for malaria prophylaxis. May be considered for treatment of severe infections.	Avoid
Primaquine	C	Do not administer during pregnancy because of the possibility the fetus may be G6PD deficient. If a causal cure with primaquine is indicated, continue to suppress with chloroquine (or other chemoprophylaxis) until delivery.	Use caution
Proguanil	C	Not associated with teratogenicity. Not effective as a single agent.	Use caution

Continued

TABLE 92-6 Medication Use During Pregnancy and Lactation—cont'd

Medication	Category	Issues During Pregnancy	Issues During Lactation
Insect Repellent			
DEET		Safe. Use sparingly as directed.	Compatible
Antiparasitics			
Albendazole	C	Teratogenic in animal studies. Avoid during first trimester. Treat after delivery if possible. May be indicated for serious infections.	Use caution
Metronidazole	B	Contraindicated during first trimester. Use in second and third trimesters only if clearly indicated.	Use caution. Single dose: hold breastfeeding 12-24 hr.
Antivirals			
Acyclovir	B	Use when indicated.	Compatible
Altitude Sickness			
Acetazolamide (Diamox)	C	Do not use during first trimester. Use only if benefit outweighs risk.	Use caution
Dexamethasone (Decadron)	C	May use if needed for treatment for altitude illness.	Avoid
Calcium Channel Blockers (Nifedipine)	C	Use only to treat severe symptoms of pulmonary edema.	Use caution
Water Disinfection		*Use chemical (halogenation), mechanical (filtration), or energy (boiling, UV).*	
Iodine	D	Avoid. May lead to goiter and fetal hypothyroidism.	Avoid

Data from Briggs G, Freeman R, Yaffe S: *Drugs in pregnancy and lactation*, Baltimore, 2010, Lippincott Williams & Wilkins; Micromedex Online; American Academy of Pediatrics, 2010; and Lexi-Comp Online UptoDate.
GI, gastrointestinal; G6PD, glucose-6-phosphate dehydrogenase; URI, upper respiratory infection; UTI, urinary tract infection.

iodine dissolved in the water. Meat should be well cooked and all dairy products (including cheeses) pasteurized to decrease the risk for toxoplasmosis, listeriosis, and other food-borne pathogens.

Treatment of GI illness during pregnancy should emphasize oral rehydration. Pharmacologic measures are limited. First-line treatment should include vitamin B_6 or vitamin B_6 plus doxylamine. Treatment with ginger may be considered as a nonpharmacologic option.[27] Ondansetron (category B) is an antiemetic commonly used to treat nausea and vomiting of pregnancy, and is a very effective drug to treat emesis associated with gastroenteritis. Products containing bismuth and salicylate (e.g., Pepto-Bismol) are associated with the risks of congenital malformations (bismuth) and fetal bleeding (salicylate). To control frequency of bowel movements with severe diarrhea, consider use of the antimotility drugs loperamide or diphenoxylate (category B). Antimicrobial choices are limited. Fluoroquinolones (category C) are not recommended, although data from inadvertent exposure during pregnancy do not show an association with adverse outcomes. Adverse effects have been shown in animals but not in humans. Azithromycin (FDA category B) is safe in pregnancy. Cefixime and other cephalosporins are safe during pregnancy, but their effectiveness is unclear.[53]

Vector-Borne Disease: Malaria

Most studies on malaria during pregnancy have been performed in endemic areas. These studies have demonstrated that pregnant women have increased susceptibility to *P. falciparum* infection during pregnancy compared with nonpregnant women. Pregnancy also increases the clinical severity of P. falciparum malaria in women, both with and without preexisting immunity.[160] Preferential sequestration of parasitized red blood cells in the placenta and suppression of selected components of the immune system during pregnancy can result in IUGR, premature delivery, anemia, fetal loss, maternal death, or congenital malaria.[76] Maternal and perinatal mortality rates markedly increase with infection.

Pregnant wilderness travelers need to scrutinize their itinerary for risk to themselves and their fetus. If a woman is pregnant or plans to become pregnant and cannot defer travel to a high-risk area, appropriate chemoprophylaxis and maximal personal protective measures are essential.[57,61,89,184] Mefloquine-resistant strains of *P. falciparum* are increasing worldwide. In these geographic areas, there is no ideal safe option for prophylaxis, and travel should be strongly discouraged.

Personal Protective Measures. Pregnant women should use a combination of physical and chemical barriers (Figure 92-5). Permethrin (or deltamethrin) may be used to treat clothing, and *N,N*-diethyl-*meta*-toluamide (DEET) in a concentration of 30% to 35% may be used on exposed skin. DEET crosses the placenta in small amounts but has not been associated with adverse fetal effects when used as directed. Picaridin 20% and lemon eucalyptus 20% (p-menthane-3,8-diol) are effective insect repellents when applied to skin. Clothing pretreated with permethrin is available.[57]

Pregnancy may lead to "increased attractiveness" to mosquitoes. This may relate to physiologic changes during pregnancy (e.g., greater body heat and surface area) that provide a greater host signal for the mosquito. Human behavioral factors (e.g., more frequent trips outside the tent to urinate) may give mosquitoes a prolonged opportunity to attack.[139]

Chemoprophylaxis. Options for chemoprophylaxis and their uses and contraindications during pregnancy and lactation are listed in Table 92-6. For travel to chloroquine-sensitive malaria areas, chloroquine can be prescribed. Chloroquine has been used for decades for prophylaxis and treatment of chloroquine-sensitive malaria without adverse fetal or maternal effects. For travel to chloroquine-resistant *P. falciparum* areas, travel should be deferred during pregnancy if possible. If travel is unavoidable, mefloquine is the only available antimalarial currently recommended. Limited studies in the second and third trimesters have not found increased rates of stillbirth or congenital malformations. Postmarketing surveillance suggests that first-trimester use is also safe.[165] Doxycycline and primaquine are contraindicated in pregnancy. Atovaquone-proguanil is not currently recommended for prophylaxis during pregnancy due to insufficient data. If a pregnant traveler is unable to take mefloquine chemoprophylaxis, the CDC Malaria Hotline (1-855-856-4713), answered during Eastern Standard Time business hours, should be consulted for guidance. Each pregnant woman should carefully consider the impact of acquiring a severe case of malaria that may result in a poor fetal outcome.[166,184] If a pregnant woman

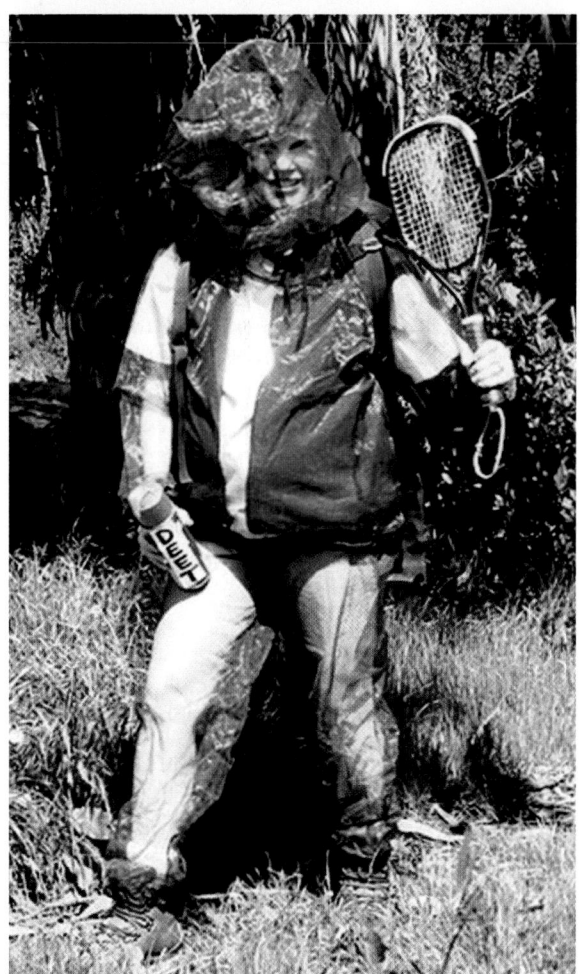

FIGURE 92-5 Personal protective measures during pregnancy. *(Courtesy Susan Anderson.)*

symptoms of acute infection are fever, conjunctivitis, arthralgias, and maculopapular rash.[64b] Only 20% of infected patients develop these self-limited and nonspecific symptoms, which typically last a week. Death is extremely rare. Consumer testing for infection is not commercially available. Reverse transcriptase polymerase chain reaction (RT-PCR) and IgM antibody assays can be performed at the Centers for Disease Control and Prevention (CDC) if infection is suspected.[64c] Diagnosed or suspected Zika virus infection should be reported to the appropriate state health officials. Treatment is supportive. Given that dengue and chikungunya viruses can be present as co-infections, nonsteroidal antiinflammatory drugs should be avoided to prevent hemorrhagic complications.[64b]

Maternal-to-fetal intrauterine transmission has been implicated, as Zika virus RNA has been detected in amniotic fluid of fetuses with microcephaly.[165a] Mouse models support this hypothesis. Given the risk for neonatal microcephaly, all pregnant women who have traveled to an endemic region within 2 weeks of development of two or more of the following symptoms—fever, maculopapular rash, arthralgia, conjunctivitis—should be tested.[64b,64c] Testing persons possibly exposed should also be offered within 2 to 12 weeks, even if they are asymptomatic, and in particular whenever an ultrasound examination shows fetal microcephaly or intracranial calcifications. Serial ultrasound examinations should be completed if a pregnant woman tests positive for Zika virus infection. As of the writing of this chapter, there is no vaccine. Therefore, prevention is essential. Because the virus can be sexually transmitted, pregnant women should abstain from sexual intercourse or use proper protection against sexually transmitted disease with any partner who might have been exposed or infected.[64a]

SPORTS AND WILDERNESS ADVENTURE RISKS DURING PREGNANCY

Exercise During Pregnancy

Exercise during pregnancy is recommended for most women. Potential benefits and possible risks of particular exercises have been reviewed.[7,54,149] Unless there are other medical or pregnancy-related contraindications (e.g., risk for premature labor, incompetent cervix, multiple gestation, bleeding), exercise and recreational training should be encouraged throughout pregnancy. Precautions should be taken to avoid prolonged exposure to extremes of temperature, dehydration, hypoglycemia, prolonged anaerobic conditions, and excessive skeletal stress.

Even well-conditioned athletes experience limits on strenuous activity because of hemodynamic changes of pregnancy. Exceeding this limit could have deleterious effects on the fetal status because of decreased uterine perfusion, increased uterine contractions, maternal acidosis, and hypoglycemia. Mild to moderate exercise is not associated with increased pregnancy loss. Running and other endurance sports may divert uterine blood flow and should be done with care as pregnancy progresses.

The ACOG provides the following recommendations for exercise during pregnancy:[7,24]

Maintain the maternal heart rate at less than 140 beats/min during exercise

Limit strenuous activity to less than 15 minutes

Avoid a core temperature higher than 38°C (100.4°F)

Do not exercise in the supine position after the fourth month

Altitude and Pregnancy

The current literature regarding pregnancy and altitude has been obtained from research involving permanent residents of high altitude.[83,115,120] Studies of high-altitude residents indicate that pregnancy and altitude act together to increase ventilation. Arterial oxygen saturation in the pregnant woman is higher due to increases in ventilation.[154] In general, hypoxic conditions compromise uteroplacental circulation and cause placental hypoxia and IUGR. Women of ethnic groups with multiple generations living at extreme altitude (≈ 4300 m [14,000 feet]) display relatively increased uterine artery blood flow and higher birth weights than those found in recent immigrants (e.g., ethnic

develops malaria and it is after hours, the CDC Emergency Operations Center (1-770-488-7100) can be used to speak with a CDC malaria branch expert. Initial treatment guidelines are available on the CDC website cdc.gov/malaria/diagnosis_treatment/clinicians3.html.

Hepatitis E

Hepatitis E is a major cause of hepatitis outbreaks in India, Nepal, China, Pakistan, Africa, and countries of the former Soviet Union, and cases are also reported from Central America and Southeast Asia. Viral transmission occurs through fecal-oral exposure. Most outbreaks result from fecal contamination of drinking water. In nonpregnant women, severe disease occurs in less than 1% of individuals. Hepatitis E infection acquired during pregnancy, however, has a mortality rate of 15% to 25%.[64,161] Third-trimester hepatitis E infection is associated with fetal complications and death. Causes of increased severity during pregnancy are not known. A vaccine is being tested in clinical trials.[205] Passive immunization with immune globulin is not effective in preventing hepatitis E infection.[109] Ideally, pregnant women should not travel to an area with a high risk of hepatitis E until after delivery.

Zika Virus

Zika virus infection has rapidly emerged as a significant public health issue. Because of its association with neonatal microcephaly, infection with this virus has important ramifications for pregnant women.[105a,151a] The virus is believed to be transmitted primarily by *Aedes* species of mosquitoes, particularly *Aedes africanus*, *A. aegypti*, and *A. albopictus*.[64d] The four key

Tibetan versus immigrant Han Chinese women on the Tibetan plateau.[56,121,122,194,216,225] A study in women residing in Colorado found that uterine artery blood flow was lower at high altitude (3100 m [10,000 feet]) than at low altitude (1600 m [5200 feet]), which could decrease fetal oxygen delivery.[224] Placental changes due to altitude exposure have not been conclusively studied in short-term travelers.[5]

Pregnancy-induced hypertension and preeclampsia are more common in women living at high altitude.[120] Infant birth weights are lower at high altitude compared with weights of infants born at sea level. Low oxygen tension and pressure changes result in IUGR and an increased risk for premature labor in women who spend most of their pregnancy above 2500 m (8200 feet).[5] Studies done on pregnancy at high altitude have demonstrated that chronic hypoxia plays a key role in causing IUGR and pre-eclampsia. Genetic factors have been identified that may relate to an underlying susceptibility to complications of pregnancy and fetal life.[154] Although exercise during pregnancy has been shown to be safe and is recommended for all healthy women, little is known about the combined effects of high altitude and exercise during pregnancy. Maternal hyperventilation and an elevated blood hemoglobin concentration maintain the resting arterial oxygen content at or above sea level values. During exercise, arterial hemoglobin saturation falls, which decreases the oxygen content. Uterine blood flow is likely to decrease further during exercise in proportion to the intensity and duration of exercise. A combined reduction in arterial oxygen content and uterine artery flow suggests that fetal oxygen delivery is compromised during exercise at altitude.[83] If the maternal skeletal muscles and the uteroplacental circulation are competing for the blood supply, exercise has the potential to cause fetal hypoxia or preterm labor at high altitude.[114] More studies are needed to evaluate the combined effects of altitude and exercise on pregnancy in short-term sojourners. Due to a paucity of experimental data, recommendations regarding exercise during pregnancy at elevations higher than 1600 m (5200 feet) are based on the synthesis of available information regarding the independent effects of high altitude and exercise on utero-placental oxygen delivery.[83] For a nonsmoking woman with an otherwise normal pregnancy who is traveling to altitudes up to 2500 m (8200 feet) in the second half of pregnancy, there is little risk for fetal complications.[110] There are no data on safety at higher elevations. One study of pregnant sojourners at a moderate altitude of less than 2500 m (8200 feet) found that the incidence of AMS during pregnancy did not differ from that in nonpregnant women.[164] As for high-altitude residents, increased incidence of preeclampsia, gestational hypertension, and placental abruption in women who stay at higher altitudes for periods of weeks to months has been reported. Infants of women found to have preeclampsia were at increased risk for IUGR.[153]

Altitude alone does not determine fetal oxygen stress. Diseases that decrease the maternal (and fetal) PaO_2 and arterial oxygen saturation (e.g., HAPE, lung disease, smoking, and other disorders of oxygen transport) can place the fetus at greater risk.

A medical commission from the International Climbing and Mountaineering Federation reviewed the research to date on women and altitude and published a consensus paper[115] and official recommendations at their website (theuiaa.org).[116]

Recommendations for Pregnant Women Traveling to a High Altitude

First trimester: Short stays (hours to days) at altitudes up to 2500 m (8200 feet) without heavy exercise.
  Healthy pregnant women in the first trimester with good access to care may go to altitudes of 1600 m (5200 feet) to 2500 m (8200 feet). Plan to allow 2 to 3 days to acclimatize.
  Women at an increased risk for spontaneous abortion should avoid altitude exposure during the first trimester.
  Women with risk factors for preeclampsia or placental abruption, or who are carrying fetuses at risk for IUGR, should not go to a high altitude, even for short stays.
Later trimesters: Short stays (hours to days) at altitudes up to 2500 m (8200 feet) without heavy exercise pose little risk to the pregnancy or of fetal complications during the second half of pregnancy.

Contraindications for going to altitude after 20 weeks of pregnancy include:
  Chronic hypertension or other factors that increase the risk for preeclampsia
  Preeclampsia
  Impaired placental function (e.g., ultrasound diagnosis of partial abruption, clots)
  IUGR
  Maternal cardiac or pulmonary disease
  Anemia
  Smoking
Any trimester: Exercise
  Mild to moderate exercise: Plan at least 2 to 3 days for acclimatization before exercising at an altitude higher than 2500 m (8200 feet).
  Strenuous exercise: Plan at least 2 weeks for full acclimatization before strenuous exercise and avoid heavy exertion at higher altitudes.
  Most would advise against travel to altitude after 36 weeks because of lack of access to optimal care.
Any trimester: Longer stays at high altitude (2500 m [8200 feet])
  There is increased risk for preeclampsia, placental abruption, and IUGR.[130,154,175,177]
  All women should be monitored for signs and symptoms of preeclampsia, placental pathology, and fetal IUGR.
  Prenatal visits should include blood pressure monitoring, urine protein check, and Doppler ultrasound monitoring of the uterine artery for waveform and volumetric flow.
  For "prenatal self-checks," women should be taught how to take their own blood pressure, screen for urine protein and glucose, and assess for other early symptoms of preeclampsia.
  Women at risk should be identified and referred for advanced health care services immediately.
  Ideally, maternal artery and fetal umbilical arterial waveforms and growth after 20 weeks should be followed in high-risk women.

Acute Mountain Sickness

Considerations about acute mountain sickness (AMS) in pregnancy include:
  AMS incidence does not differ between pregnant and nonpregnant women.[164]
  There are few data on treatment of AMS during pregnancy.
  Strict guidelines for acclimatization should be followed as outlined above.
  Acetazolamide and other sulfonamides are contraindicated during the first trimester due to studies demonstrating teratogenicity in animals and are not recommended after 36 weeks due to increased risk for neonatal jaundice.[59]
  If a pregnant woman has symptoms of AMS, theoretical risks of medication must be weighed against symptoms.
  Descent and oxygen therapy are the preferred treatment.
  Use of acetazolamide or dexamethasone may be considered on an individual basis.

There are no studies on skiing while pregnant, although for a normal healthy pregnancy, there is likely little risk during the first trimester. Access to care is the most important issue in case of an emergency. Women skiing later in pregnancy are at higher risk due to increased weight, change in their center of gravity, and increased joint laxity that may predispose to falls, with subsequent placental disruption, ligament ruptures, or other devastating consequences. Short-term travel to a favorite mountain escape with adequate resources is probably safe for a pregnant adventurer with a normal pregnancy. More research is needed to evaluate risks of intense exercise at altitude during pregnancy.[35,36,83,115]

Water Sports During Pregnancy

Swimming and snorkeling are safe during pregnancy and considered to be an excellent form of exercise for pregnant women.[119] Scuba diving is potentially hazardous. The fetus is at risk from nitrogen bubbles in the fetal-placental circulation during decompression on ascent. Most authorities consider pregnancy a contraindication to diving.[48,59,70,200]

Diving is compromised by increased abdominal girth, difficulty breathing due to engorgement of mucous membranes of the nose and oropharynx, and increased buoyancy secondary to fat deposition. Higher levels of body fat also increase the risk for decompression sickness because nitrogen tends to be retained in these tissues. Dyspnea may be exaggerated and lead to panic even in experienced divers.

As with exertion at high altitude, pregnant women may have limited ability to maintain anaerobic metabolism for prolonged periods because of fetal needs. Pregnant women should also limit prolonged nondiving immersion in cold water that might lead to hypoventilation and hypothermia. Effects of scuba diving on pregnancy have been reviewed in detail.[59] Advice for a woman who finds out she was pregnant during the time she was diving is to not terminate the pregnancy. There are case reports of normal pregnancies despite continued diving. If a pregnant woman insists on diving, it is recommended that she not dive below a depth of 18 m (60 feet) and only remain underwater for half the recommended Navy dive table times.[70] CDC recommendations advise against diving in pregnancy owing to increased risk of air embolism.[58]

Waterskiing, jet skiing, and other water sports that might force water into the vagina and cervix and increase the risk for miscarriage or peritonitis are not recommended activities during pregnancy.[142]

Heat and Pregnancy

Safe limits for exposure to heat during pregnancy have not been established. Acclimation to environments characterized by high temperatures, particularly with high humidity, may be especially difficult for pregnant women and may pose a fetal risk. Hyperthermia has been shown to be teratogenic in various animal models. A higher incidence of birth defects, particularly neural tube defects, has been found among offspring of women who experienced first-trimester hyperthermia by environmental exposure or febrile illness.[151] Later in pregnancy, the fetus depends on maternal abilities to eliminate excess heat. Elevated ambient temperature decreases ability of the pregnant woman to dissipate heat. Elevated humidity decreases the contribution of perspiration to heat loss. Together, these factors increase the risk for an elevated maternal core temperature that further raises the fetal metabolic activity and heat generation. Hyperthermia, particularly with dehydration and loss of electrolytes, increases the risk for premature labor.[37,182,212] Fetal stress, due to decreased uterine perfusion secondary to compensatory peripheral vasodilation and depletion of intravascular volume, further increases the likelihood of preterm labor. Pregnant women exposed to hot climates should pay particular attention to remaining well hydrated.

Data regarding effects of exercise on core temperature are limited. To date, hyperthermia associated with exercise has not been found to be teratogenic in humans. It is recommended that pregnant women avoid hot tubs and saunas.[199,201]

Exposure to Venomous Animal Bites and Stings

Venomous animal bites and stings during pregnancy may have serious effects on the fetus and mother. Snakebite in pregnant women has caused reported fetal death rates ranging from 20% to 40% since 1966.[55] There have been no formal epidemiologic studies on the effect of antivenom on fetal development. Although a large percentage of fetal deaths occurred in mothers who received antivenom, deaths may have been related to the severity of the bite rather than to the therapy. Risks of untreated significant maternal venom poisoning outweigh any theoretical concerns about antivenom risks to the unborn child. "What is good for the mother is good for the fetus."[55]

Envenomation during pregnancy should be reported to a poison control center and to the pharmaceutical company that produces the antivenom so that information on medical management and fetal outcomes can be evaluated and lead to evidence-based recommendations. More research is needed to evaluate the risk-to-benefit profiles of snake, spider, and scorpion antivenoms on pregnant women, embryos, and fetuses.

Remote Wilderness Travel During Pregnancy

Prolonged wilderness excursions during pregnancy, particularly those extending into the late second and third trimesters, should include preparations for ongoing assessment and emergency delivery. Routine antepartum care usually includes visits to a health care provider at least monthly until 26 to 28 weeks, every 2 weeks thereafter until 36 weeks, and then weekly until delivery. Beyond the due date, more frequent visits and fetal monitoring are often recommended. Routine visits focus on uterine activity, vaginal discharge, abdominopelvic pain, headaches, symptoms of UTI, current medications, and fetal activity.[75]

A basic antepartum examination includes measurements of blood pressure, weight, and uterine size (height of the uterine fundus above symphysis) and subjective assessments of peripheral edema and reflexes. Urine is tested at each visit with a multitest strip that provides estimates of glycosuria, proteinuria, pH, and presence of nitrites. For wilderness travelers, elevated pH and presence of nitrites may be associated with a UTI. In Rh-negative women with Rh-positive partners, Rh antibody screening is often repeated at 26 to 28 weeks, before administration of Rh immune globulin for prophylaxis against third-trimester sensitization. If an Rh antibody screen cannot be performed, Rh immune globulin should be administered empirically. Maternal hemoglobin and hematocrit are frequently measured in each trimester to assess the need for iron supplementation. If hemoglobin testing cannot be performed, consider empirical supplemental iron during pregnancy unless the woman has a contraindication (e.g., hemochromatosis). All pregnant women should take prenatal vitamins.[75]

PRENATAL CARE IN THE WILDERNESS

Basic supplies for pregnant wilderness travelers include a diary to record progress; reminders of scheduled testing and complications; a tape measure, stethoscope, and sphygmomanometer; urine test strips; and supplies of prenatal vitamins and iron. Other supplies may include a glucometer with test strips, calcium supplements, and basic medications for the most common pregnancy complaints. These include an oral antiemetic (e.g., orally dissolving ondansetron tablets [Zofran ODT]) or suppository (e.g. promethazine or prochlorperazine) for nausea and vomiting, acetaminophen for headaches and pain, stool softener for constipation, and antibiotics for UTIs and vaginitis. In addition to basic medical supplies, pregnant women should have changes in clothing size and possibly shoe size.

Ideally, delivery in the wilderness should not be planned. If delivery in the wilderness is a possibility, special preparations need to be made (Box 92-7), including plans for emergency evacuation and infant resuscitation if needed.

COMPLICATIONS DURING PREGNANCY

Miscarriage

Women who are pregnant or become pregnant for the first time while in the wilderness are at high risk for complications. About 15% to 25% of all pregnancies abort spontaneously during the first trimester, and this number may exceed 60% to 70% in the true primigravida.[181] Reasons may be related to immunologic naiveté to paternal antigens expressed by the fetal tissues. In contrast, isolated miscarriages in women who have successfully carried pregnancies often result from chromosomal abnormalities. Impending first-trimester miscarriages are usually preceded by embryonic demise and accompanied by reduction or loss of early pregnancy-related symptoms (e.g., breast tenderness and nausea). Bleeding and uterine contractions eventually occur and accompany expulsion of products of conception. Under most circumstances, hemorrhage during miscarriage is self-limited and not life-threatening, but at times can be heavy. Risk factors for significant hemorrhage include fetal death not preceding the event, miscarriage late in the first trimester or during the second trimester, or prolonged or incomplete expulsion.[162] Half of women with first-trimester vaginal bleeding will continue to have viable pregnancies. However, this is difficult to assess in the wilderness.[188] Spontaneous abortion after the first trimester is much riskier but less common. It also can result from chromosomal abnormalities or fetal anomalies but is more likely to be caused by chorioamnionitis, UTI, severe abnormalities of placentation, poorly controlled maternal medical conditions, or cervical incompetence.

BOX 92-7 Supplies for Management of Wilderness Delivery

Standard Supplies
Clean towels
Surgical sponges
Surgical gloves
Speculum
Umbilical cord clamps
Suction bulb
Suture kit
Scalpel
Scissors
Syringes and needles
Local anesthetic
Injectable oxytocin
Injectable and oral methylergonovine
Oral analgesics (e.g., ibuprofen, acetaminophen with codeine)
Oral broad-spectrum antibiotic
Sanitary napkins
Neonatal mask and suction
Self-inflating bag/valve/mask resuscitator (Ambu bag)
Reusable uterine balloon tamponade device to control postpartum hemorrhage

Optional Supplies
Injectable magnesium sulfate
Intravenous fluids and administration supplies
Injectable narcotic
Naloxone
Misoprostol
Prostaglandin $F_{2\alpha}$
Injectable antibiotic

Acute and significant blood loss in a physiologically hostile environment can compromise the endurance of the most highly trained individual. Under wilderness conditions, control of significant maternal hemorrhage accompanying miscarriage may be difficult unless provisions, facilities, and medical supplies are available. Uterine curettage is most often used to complete evacuation of the uterus when medical facilities are available. Once empty, uterine involution, spontaneous or aided by uterine massage, is usually sufficient to impede bleeding from the implantation site. In the absence of the ability to perform curettage, treatment with methylergonovine (0.2 mg orally or intramuscularly) can enhance uterine contractions, accelerate expulsion of products of conception, and promote uterine involution to maintain hemostasis while plans for evacuation are being made. Methylergonovine should not be used in patients with hypertensive disorders, underlying vascular disease, and certain cardiac abnormalities unless the benefits clearly outweigh the risks of acute generalized vasoconstriction. As an alternative, the prostaglandin F_{2a} drug carboprost tromethamine (250 mcg intramuscularly) or misoprostol (400 to 600 mcg orally or sublingually) can be administered to stop uterine bleeding with less risk for cardiovascular compromise. Dosing depends on the indication and whether it is given orally, sublingually, or vaginally (misoprostol .org/File/dosage_guidelines.pdf).[95]

Ectopic Pregnancy

Far more dangerous than miscarriage, ectopic pregnancy must always be considered a life-threatening emergency that requires immediate medical attention.[20] Ectopic pregnancy refers to implantation at any location outside the uterine cavity, most often (>95%) within the fallopian tube. Hemorrhage resulting from ectopic pregnancy is still the leading cause of first-trimester maternal death. Ectopic pregnancy incidence has tripled over the past 30 years and now exceeds 1 in every 100 pregnancies. This increase is directly proportional to the increased incidence of acute and chronic PID. The most common predisposing risk factors include a history of infections, multiple sex partners, early age at onset of sexual activity, delayed childbearing, and previous IUD use. Independent risk factors are a history of abdominal and tubal surgery, including previous tubal sterilization procedures,

endometriosis, diethylstilbestrol exposure, and pregnancy by assisted reproductive interventions. Regardless of the cause, prior ectopic pregnancy increases the risk for another ectopic pregnancy approximately 10-fold. A woman with a history of ectopic pregnancy should not intentionally plan to conceive again in the wilderness and should have intrauterine pregnancy confirmed ultrasonographically before departure.

Most women with a tubal ectopic pregnancy become symptomatic before 12 weeks' gestation and present with complaints of abdominal pain and altered menses. Early pregnancy symptoms may be minimal or absent. Pain often begins unilaterally with sudden onset and is usually severe and distinguishable by its persistence and intensity from intermittent cramping pain accompanying miscarriage. Clinical findings include tender adnexal mass, nontender cervix, small to slightly enlarged nontender uterus, and absence of high-grade fever. Low-grade temperature elevation to 38° C (100.4° F) may occur in as many as 20% of women with ectopic pregnancy. When intraperitoneal hemorrhage accompanies tube rupture, pain becomes diffuse, with peritoneal signs of tenderness, guarding, and rebound. Shoulder pain from diaphragmatic irritation may be present. Pelvic examination at this point usually elicits discomfort with movement of the cervix and uterus. Fullness of the cul-de-sac posterior to the uterus and abdominal distention suggest significant intraperitoneal blood loss. See Chapter 109 for details on ultrasonographic assessment of pregnant patients under austere conditions. In the pregnant patient with acute abdominal pain, ultrasonographic evidence of abdominal free fluid indicates the presence of an ectopic pregnancy until proven otherwise.

Vaginal bleeding accompanying an ectopic pregnancy usually follows a variable period of amenorrhea. It often begins with minimal flow of blood darker than that seen during miscarriage and results from inadequate progestational support of the decidualized endometrium. Uterine cramping may ensue, with passage of organized clot and tissue in the form of a decidual cast resembling products of conception, leading to a mistaken diagnosis of spontaneous abortion. Cessation of pain is typical with completion of a miscarriage. In an ectopic pregnancy, pain typically continues despite passage of a decidual cast. With rupture of an ectopic pregnancy, heavier, bright-red bleeding may occur vaginally. If accompanied by significant intraperitoneal hemorrhage, this may rapidly result in hemodynamic decompensation that can only be controlled surgically. Differential diagnosis of ectopic pregnancy includes normal intrauterine pregnancy with a corpus luteal cyst or hemorrhagic corpus luteum, threatened or incomplete abortion, PID, adnexal torsion (usually associated with adnexal enlargement from a benign or neoplastic process), endometriosis, UTI or ureteral stone, degenerating fibroid, and appendicitis. Although simultaneous intrauterine and ectopic pregnancies were once considered extremely rare, the incidence is now estimated at 1 in 6000 in the general population and higher than 1 in 100 among recipients of assisted reproductive techniques. Diagnosis of ectopic pregnancy is considered presumptively in any woman with a positive pregnancy test, abnormal bleeding, and abdominal pain. In a full-service medical care facility, the first step in management is to assess serum hCG levels and ascertain location of the pregnancy. Intrauterine pregnancy can usually be confirmed by transvaginal ultrasonography once the serum hCG level exceeds 1000 mIU/mL, corresponding to 3 to 4 weeks after conception or 5 to 7 weeks from the last normal menstrual period. Absence of a visualized intrauterine pregnancy at hCG levels of 1000 to 1500 mIU/mL or greater suggests ectopic pregnancy. However, some normal intrauterine pregnancies may appear later on ultrasound. In an urban setting, if the fetus is not visualized and the patient is asymptomatic, it may be reasonable to monitor with serial hCG levels and ultrasonograms. However, in a wilderness setting that precludes the ability to perform ultrasonography and quantitative determinations of hCG, plans for evacuation must be made at the first suspicion of the diagnosis of ectopic pregnancy.[20,75]

Later Pregnancy Complications

Complications that cause bleeding at 20 weeks' gestation or later cannot be optimally managed in most wilderness settings

Placenta previa
Placental abruption
Preterm labor
Premature rupture of membranes
Chorioamnionitis
Preeclampsia, eclampsia, HELLP syndrome (hemolysis, elevated liver function enzymes, and low platelets)

(Box 92-8). Plans should be made for immediate evacuation. Second- and third-trimester bleeding could simply be the result of cervical effacement, labor, cervical polyps, coital trauma, or vaginitis, but it could also be much more serious (e.g., placenta previa or placental abruption).[75,168] Historical information and physical findings may suggest a cause, but definitive care is required to rule out potentially life-threatening diagnoses.

Placenta Previa. Placenta previa results from placental implantation in the lower uterine segment over or near the internal cervical os. It occurs in approximately 1 of 200 births. The risk increases with age and parity, cigarette smoking, multiple gestations, submucosal fibroids, history of multiple dilation and curettage procedures, and prior cesarean delivery. The classic presentation of placenta previa is painless, sudden, heavy, and bright-red vaginal bleeding.[187] It may occur with exertional activity, straining on the toilet, or intercourse but also occurs at rest with no obvious precipitating factor. No internal vaginal examination should be done, because this may worsen the bleeding.[168]

Placental Abruption. Placental abruption is defined as separation of the placenta from the maternal interface before delivery. One of the most common causes is trauma. Risk factors include hypertensive disorders (e.g., preeclampsia, chronic hypertension), other chronic diseases with vascular compromise (e.g., diabetes, renal disease, certain autoimmune disorders), coagulation disorders (presence of lupus anticoagulants or anticardiolipin antibodies, proteins S and C deficiencies, factor V Leiden, antithrombin III deficiency), trauma, chorioamnionitis, advanced maternal age, and multiparity. Placental abruption is highly variable in presentation, depending on the location and extent of separation and hemorrhage. About 80% of placental abruptions result in visible bleeding accompanying the onset of other symptoms. Unlike placenta previa, abruption is usually accompanied by a sudden onset of sharp pain. The pain may be focal and continuous, intermittently intensifying with frequent uterine contractions and irritability that usually accompany and can extend placental separation.[75]

Premature Labor. Despite advances in obstetric and neonatal care in the past 50 years, rates of preterm delivery, defined as delivery before 37 completed weeks' gestation, have not changed. Rates range from 8% to 10% of all pregnancies in the United States. Premature labor is still the leading cause of perinatal complications and death. Only half of women who experience preterm labor, defined as regular uterine contractions resulting in progressive cervical change (as assessed by effacement, dilation, and softening) actually progress to preterm delivery. Symptoms of preterm labor include mild and menstrual-like painful uterine contractions, intermittent low back pain or pressure, pelvic pressure, increase in vaginal discharge resulting from effacement with compression of endocervical glands or leaking of amniotic fluid, and bloody "show." Common risk factors for preterm labor and delivery include premature rupture of membranes, subclinical or overt chorioamnionitis, UTI, preeclampsia, multiple gestation, hydramnios, dehydration, constipation, chronic stress, and incompetent cervix.[18,75] The pregnant wilderness traveler is at risk for several of these factors (e.g. UTI, dehydration) and should strive to reduce their occurrence.

Thorough evaluation and management of preterm labor cannot be done in most wilderness settings. Empirical measures can be taken, however, based on symptoms and palpation of uterine contractions while awaiting evacuation or preparation for delivery (if evacuation is delayed or impossible). If vaginal bleeding is present, pelvic examination should be avoided unless placenta previa has been previously excluded and sterile supplies are available. If done by an experienced person, cervical examination should determine dilation, effacement, and consistency, as well as station and presentation of the baby. Once it has been concluded that the woman is in preterm labor and evacuation is required, do not repeat examinations unless delivery appears imminent. If she clearly has ruptured membranes, note the characteristics (clear, bloody, meconium stained) of the fluid but do not perform an internal vaginal examination, to minimize the risk for introducing infection. Plans should be made for evacuation at any initial signs of premature labor. If premature labor cannot be stopped before evacuation, guidelines for management of delivery are described below.

Preeclampsia. The diagnosis of preeclampsia is based on the triad of hypertension, proteinuria, and edema.[13] Hypertension is defined as systolic blood pressure of 140 mm Hg or higher or diastolic blood pressure of 90 mm Hg or higher measured on two separate occasions 6 or more hours apart or persistent elevations above baseline. Proteinuria is defined as 0.3 g or more of protein in a 24-hour urine collection, which usually corresponds with "1+" (30 mg/dL) or greater on a urine dipstick test. Edema is considered significant for a diagnosis of preeclampsia only if it is generalized or if the woman has had a sudden weight gain of 2.27 kg (5 lb) or more in a week. Diagnosis of preeclampsia requires the presence of hypertension with proteinuria or the presence of edema, or both. Women meeting these criteria have at least mild preeclampsia. If preeclampsia is suspected, plans should be made for immediate evacuation from the wilderness setting.

Diagnostic criteria for severe preeclampsia require only one of the following: systolic blood pressure of 160 mm Hg or higher or diastolic blood pressure of 110 mm Hg or higher on two occasions at least 6 hours apart; proteinuria (5 mg/24 hours or higher); oliguria (400 mL/24 hours or less); persistent epigastric pain; pulmonary edema or cyanosis; impaired liver function of unclear cause; thrombocytopenia (100,000 platelets/mL of blood or less[21]); and eclampsia (grand mal seizures). Most cases of severe preeclampsia are associated with IUGR or abnormalities of fetal umbilical (increased resistance) arterial flow consistent with relative placental insufficiency and decreased resistance in maternal middle cerebral arterial flow. Eclampsia is a major cause of maternal and fetal complications and death worldwide, occurring in 1 in 2000 pregnancies in the United States. Although difficult to anticipate, presence of visual disturbances, severe headache, irritability, epigastric or right upper quadrant pain, nausea and vomiting, and cerebral dysfunction must be considered predictors of eclampsia. If a woman has early signs of preeclampsia, she should be evacuated because she may progress to severe eclampsia with high rates of morbidity and possible death.[13] Field management should include bed rest until evacuation can be arranged.

EMERGENCY DELIVERY

Although a delivery should never be planned for a wilderness expedition, unexpected delivery may occur. A pregnant woman traveling after 20 weeks' gestation should consider emergency provisions and plans. The travel location, duration of stay, and distance dictate the extent of these plans. Consider the distance to medical care facilities, convenience of evacuation routes, ease of communication, and availability of evacuation support. Any woman planning a wilderness excursion should review detailed emergency plans with her physician and expedition partners. Some considerations are reviewed briefly below.

If a woman goes into labor unexpectedly on a trip, the health care provider or person with the most childbirth experience that is willing to assist in the delivery should be identified as the team leader and "midwife." Participatory roles for other members of the party should be defined in cooperation with the pregnant woman. Requests for privacy and intimacy should be respected to the extent possible.

By necessity and practicality, delivery in the wilderness dictates a laissez-faire approach. Excessive intervention (e.g., repeated cervical examinations, artificial rupture of membranes, augmentation of uterine contractions by oxytocin or nipple

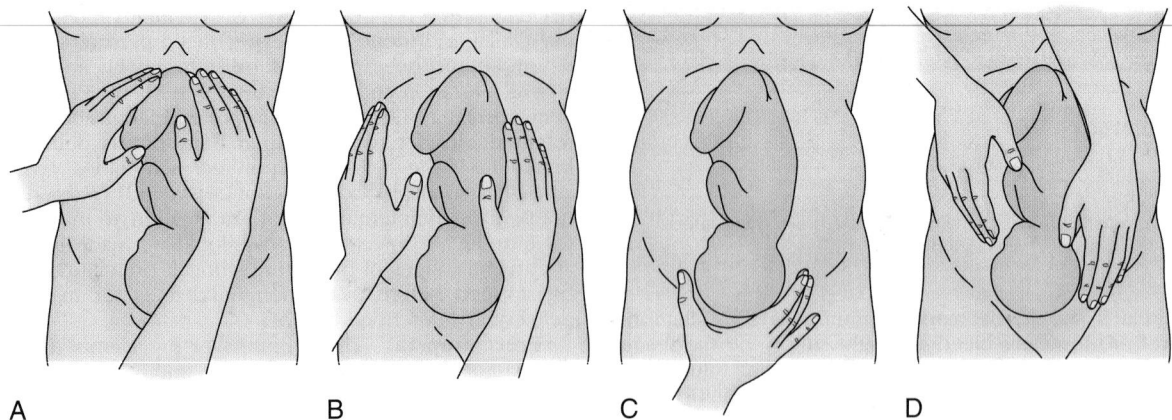

FIGURE 92-6 Ascertaining fetal position by Leopold's maneuvers. **A,** Assess part of fetus in upper uterus. **B,** Ascertain location of fetal back. **C,** Identify presenting part. **D,** Determine descent of presenting part.

stimulation, manual cervical dilation) is neither warranted nor appropriate because delivery cannot be expedited for concerns of fetal distress, and such intervention may increase maternal and fetal risks. Prepare a clean, comfortable, and quiet site for the delivery. If clean and sterile supplies and medications are available, these should be brought to this location and inventoried by the team leader (see Box 92-7). Make clean towels, clothing, bedding, soap, and clean water readily accessible.

The fetal position should be determined. In late third-trimester pregnancies, this can be accomplished by external abdominal palpation using Leopold's maneuvers (Figure 92-6).[13] In preterm pregnancies, this may first require internal digital examination, but determining the fetal position is extremely important because the risk for malpresentation (i.e., breech, transverse, or compound lie) is inversely proportional to the gestational age, as is the disparity between the fetal head and abdominal circumferences. Digital examination should not be done in a wilderness setting unless sterility can be ensured because of the risk of introducing infection. At term, the incidence of breech presentation is about 3%, whereas it may exceed 25% before 30 weeks' gestation. If the woman reports fetal activity, or if this is visible or palpable on abdominal examination, evaluation of the fetal heart rate can be assessed. Fetal activity frequently diminishes with the onset of labor. If the woman or examiner cannot detect fetal activity, assess viability by auscultation. A stethoscope or the ear can be positioned over the location of the baby's back and shoulder. Auscultation with a stethoscope bell placed on the abdomen with minimal pressure is usually more sensitive than using the stethoscope's diaphragm. The normal fetal heart rate at term falls between 120 and 160 beats/min. In most wilderness situations, once viability is confirmed, further auscultation is probably unnecessary and may even provoke anxiety because of inherent difficulties of fetal heart rate detection with unamplified methods, subtle changes in fetal position, descent of the presenting part, and increasing discomfort of labor as it progresses.

In early stages of labor or with spontaneous rupture of membranes in the absence of regular uterine contractions, rest, fluid intake, and frequent light meals should be encouraged. Activity should be restricted until the fetal head is engaged, because too much activity prior to this point might result in umbilical cord prolapse and fetal distress. Prophylactic antibiotics should be started, especially when there has been preterm premature rupture of membranes, or rupture of membranes prior to 37 weeks' gestation. Antibiotic regimen recommendations are as follows:

- Rupture ≥12 hours without signs of infection or labor: Amoxicillin 3 g/day in three divided doses for 5 to 7 days (Note: Do not use amoxicillin/clavulanate because of the increased incidence of necrotizing enterocolitis in neonates).
- Rupture ≥12 hours in labor without signs of infection: Ampicillin 2 g IV for one dose, and then 1 g every 4 hours until delivery. No further antibiotics.
- Rupture of membranes (no time requirement) with signs of infection with/without labor: Ampicillin 2 g IV every 6 hours and metronidazole 500 mg IV every 8 hours and gentamycin

3-5 mg/kg daily. Continue IV antibiotics for 48 hours after fever resolves, and then continue amoxicillin 3 g/day PO in three divided doses and metronidazole 500 mg PO every 12 hours for a total of 10 days of treatment.[73a]

Digital cervical examination is not necessary and is contraindicated with amniotic membrane rupture because of the risk of infection. As labor becomes more active, as gauged by increased frequency, regularity, strength of uterine contractions, pelvic pressure, and discomfort level, the safest approach is to limit oral intake to clear liquids only. The GI tract becomes quiescent with active labor. Because vomiting is not unusual, especially during the "transition" phase of labor, clear liquids minimize discomfort and decrease the risk for aspiration. Intermittent ambulation may also decrease discomfort associated with contractions and can be continued, if the woman desires, until she feels the need to push. During this time, she should also be reminded to empty her bladder because she may not be able to differentiate the sensation of needing to void from that of pressure from the presenting fetal part. A full bladder not only adds to the discomfort of labor but also can impede descent of the baby into the pelvis and prolong parturition.

Although some women become irritable as labor intensifies before complete dilation and do not want to be touched, others appreciate low-back or extremity massage between contractions. Breathing and relaxation techniques to distract, maintain composure, and preserve energy that will be required during the second stage of labor are also beneficial. During labor, no oral pain medication should be given. Parenteral intravenous narcotics, although acceptable, should be administered sparingly unless naloxone is available to manage fetal depression that may result.

When the woman begins to feel involuntary efforts to push with contractions, cervical examination should be performed with a clean or sterile glove or freshly washed hands. At the same time that cervical dilation and effacement are assessed, the presenting fetal body part should be identified and its station determined in relation to the ischial spine. If the cervix is completely dilated and effaced so that no cervical tissue is palpable between the presenting part and the vaginal wall, the first stage of labor is complete and the woman can begin pushing with contractions. If the cervix is not completely dilated, encourage the woman not to push with contractions so that she does not become exhausted or risk entrapping the cervix between the presenting part and pelvis. Cervical entrapment can lead to cervical edema and thickening. It is more commonly due to cephalopelvic disproportion. If membranes have ruptured, note the presence or absence of meconium. If membranes have not ruptured, they should not be ruptured intentionally, particularly if the baby is premature or in a breech presentation.

Once the cervix is completely dilated, the desire to push may become involuntary, and pain is less of an issue until the moment of delivery. Pushing is done only with uterine contractions. At the onset of a contraction, the woman takes in a deep breath and then exhales. Then she takes in and holds another deep breath, bearing down without releasing air as if straining to have a bowel movement. Most contractions are long enough to permit two or three attempts at this maneuver. Proper pushing is evident by expansion of the introitus and rectum during the effort and should not be accompanied by tensing of the extremities. Once the contraction is over, she should expel any held air and begin restful breathing, trying to relax completely to conserve energy and recover for the next contraction. The woman may push in any position in which she feels comfortable. However, she should avoid lying flat on her back because uterine compression of the inferior vena cava can lead to maternal hypotension and decreased uterine perfusion. Common positions include semirecumbent, with the back and head elevated and legs drawn up or supported at the knees during contractions; lateral recumbent, with the superior leg flexed and supported during contractions; squatting; sitting; kneeling on all fours; and standing while being supported from behind around the torso. These positions can also be used for the actual delivery, as long as the attendant has adequate access. Once the presenting part reaches, distends, and remains at the vaginal introitus between contractions, final preparations are made for delivery. A delivery position should be selected that allows control of the presenting part, protection of the perineum, and room to accomplish completion of the birth with as little trauma to the baby as possible. Delivery should be performed during a contraction.[75]

COMPLICATED DELIVERIES

Vertex Delivery

The most common fetal presentation is the cephalic (or vertex) presentation, with the fetal head facing the perineum (occiput anterior) (Figure 92-7). When the perineum begins to distend with a contraction, instruct the woman to bear down. Intentional cutting of an episiotomy in a wilderness setting is not recommended. Spontaneous lacerations are more likely to occur along less vascular tissue planes and less likely to extend into the rectum. Support the perineum between the rectum and the introitus using the index finger and thumb of the nondominant hand. Maintain the fetal head in flexion until the crown has just begun to clear the symphysis. Instruct the woman to stop pushing while the attendant exerts steady inward and upward pressure at the perineum against the fetal chin, thereby extending the head and completing its delivery while protecting the perineum. Once delivered, the fetal head will usually rotate laterally to align itself with the shoulders. Clean the infant's mouth and nose by bulb aspiration or simple swabbing with a clean gauze or cloth. This step is especially important when meconium is present to prevent aspiration of this fluid when the baby is free to take its first breaths. Once the oropharynx is cleaned, palpate the fetal neck to rule out the presence of a nuchal cord. If present, one or more loops of umbilical cord are often loose enough to be slipped

over the baby's head before completion of the delivery. If they cannot be slipped over the head but are not tight, the baby can frequently be delivered through the loops. If the cord is tightly applied around the neck, the attendant should doubly clamp or tie a section of one loop, cut between the clamps, and then deliver the baby. Fashioning clamps may require creativity, depending on your resources. One could use fishing line, rope, a shoestring, or organic matter if absolutely necessary.

In the final stages of delivery, the woman resumes pushing while steady downward (toward the maternal sacrum) traction is applied with hands cupping both sides of the fetal head. When the anterior shoulder has cleared the symphysis, the perineum should again be supported while the head is elevated and the posterior shoulder delivered. The rest of the baby's body usually follows without effort. The baby is held below the perineum (to prevent loss of blood to the placenta from the baby) while the oropharynx is again cleaned and the baby dried. Usually, rubbing the baby dry is sufficient to stimulate breathing and crying. The umbilical cord should be doubly clamped or tied and then severed. The baby should be thoroughly dried and wrapped in clean, dry, and warm fabric with its head covered and given to the mother if she desires. If the baby does not cry within 10 to 15 seconds after delivery, has obvious airway obstruction, or is premature, the umbilical cord should be cut immediately and resuscitative efforts begun.

Shoulder Dystocia

If there is difficulty delivering the anterior shoulder (shoulder dystocia) by the method outlined, immediate steps should be taken to accomplish this. True shoulder dystocia occurs in less than 1% of deliveries and is rare in uncomplicated labors, but is a substantial cause of fetal and maternal distress or complications. Shoulder dystocia is often anticipated when the fetal head snaps back tightly and fails to rotate after its delivery. If available, other individuals can assist. Throughout the steps necessary to accomplish delivery, excessive traction on the fetal head is avoided because it may stretch the brachial plexus, resulting in Erb's or Klumpke's palsy. First, position the woman so that the buttocks are elevated to allow at least 12 inches of free space beneath the perineum to maneuver. Flex both legs upward to the chest (McRobert's maneuver) while the woman is supported in a semirecumbent position. Attempt delivery again by downward traction on the fetal head.[75]

If the shoulder is still impacted against the symphysis, apply pressure with the fist or heel of the hand just above the symphysis in the midline. This may reduce dystocia sufficiently to accomplish the delivery. Assistants should not push on the uterine fundus, because this can further impact the shoulder. If these maneuvers fail, an episiotomy should be cut to admit several fingers or the hand beneath the posterior shoulder. Once

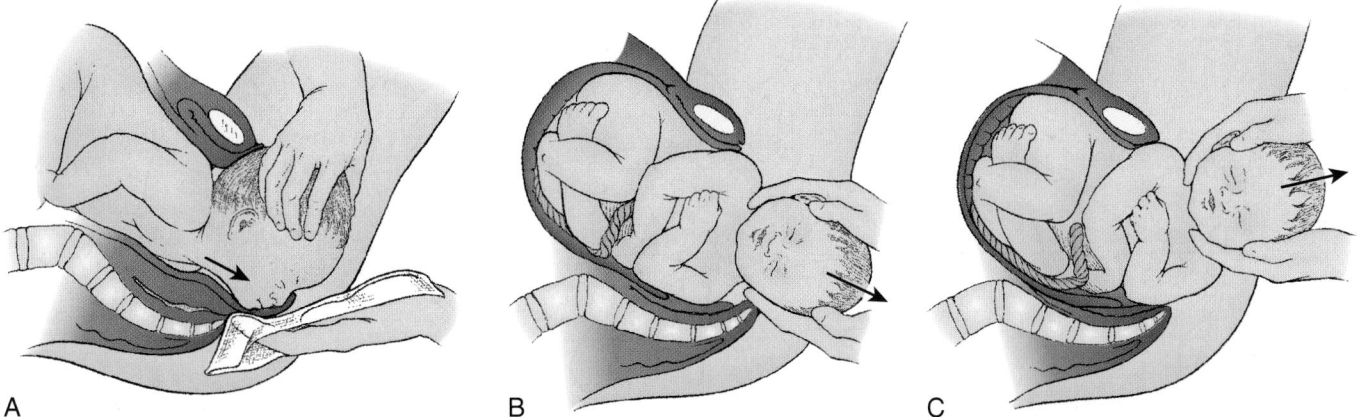

FIGURE 92-7 Management of vaginal vertex delivery. **A,** Control delivery of fetal head by upward pressure on the chin with countertraction on the occiput until the symphysis is cleared. **B,** Delivery of anterior shoulder by downward traction on the fetal head. **C,** Delivery of posterior shoulder by upward traction on the fetal head. *(Modified from Pritchard JA, MacDonald PC: Williams obstetrics, ed 16, New York,1980, Appleton Century Crofts.)*

the hand has been inserted, rotate the baby by applying pressure to the shoulder and scapula (Wood's maneuver). The corkscrew rotation will deliver the posterior shoulder as it turns anteriorly, the anterior shoulder will dislodge, and the baby can be delivered without further difficulty. If this rotational maneuver fails, the posterior arm is delivered by grasping it along the forearm and sweeping it across the chest and out the vagina. This technique may fracture the humerus or clavicle but may prevent infant death because of inability to complete a delivery. Once the posterior arm is out, the anterior shoulder can usually be displaced downward, or the baby can then be rotated, allowing completion of the delivery. This approach is preferable to intentionally fracturing the clavicle, which can be technically difficult and does not provide as much room for the delivery.

If the baby is in a vertex presentation but facing the symphysis (occiput posterior), the labor is often more prolonged and uncomfortable, particularly in the woman's lower back. The delivery is basically accomplished as described, except the final maneuvers to deliver the fetal head are extension first, then flexion. Perineal and introital trauma is a greater risk with an occiput posterior delivery. Management of this fetal presentation by the wilderness birth attendant should be a minor challenge compared with delivery of a breech baby.

Breech Delivery

Because most wilderness deliveries are "unexpected" and more likely to be premature, the baby will also more likely be in a breech lie (Figure 92-8). Other than chance and prematurity, the greatest risk factors for a baby to be in a breech presentation are unsuspected congenital fetal anomalies, chromosomal abnormalities, and maternal uterine abnormalities. Each of these adds a new level of challenge to the birth attendant. Under the best of

circumstances, delivery of a breech versus a vertex presentation carries a threefold to fourfold greater risk for morbidity resulting from prematurity, congenital abnormalities, and trauma at delivery. Delivery trauma often results from the relatively larger fetal head and smaller body circumference of a premature infant. This disproportion can lead to head entrapment and is especially difficult when the fetal body has negotiated an incompletely dilated cervix.

Breech babies come in many forms: frank breech (hips flexed, knees extended, buttocks presenting), complete breech (both hips and both knees flexed, buttocks and feet presenting), incomplete breech (one hip flexed, one hip partially extended, knees flexed, buttocks and feet presenting), and footling breech (hips and knees extended, feet presenting). Regardless of the form, the approach in a wilderness setting demands patience. No effort should be made to deliver a breech baby until the presenting part is visible at the introitus and the cervix is completely dilated. Membranes should not be artificially ruptured in breech presentations. As the amniotic sac balloons into the birth canal, it helps to dilate the cervix completely. This facilitates descent of the baby through a lubricated smooth surface against which the body can freely move and cushions the umbilical cord against compression in the birth canal.

When the cervix is completely dilated, instruct the woman to push. Regardless of the type of breech presentation, the safest course is to allow the body to be extruded to at least the level of the umbilicus by maternal efforts alone. This increases the chance that the fetal head has begun to pass through the pelvic inlet. For a baby in a frank or complete breech lie, deliver the posterior leg by gently grasping the thigh and flexing the leg at the knee as it is rotated medially and toward the introitus. Rotate the baby to face the ground with the baby's back toward the

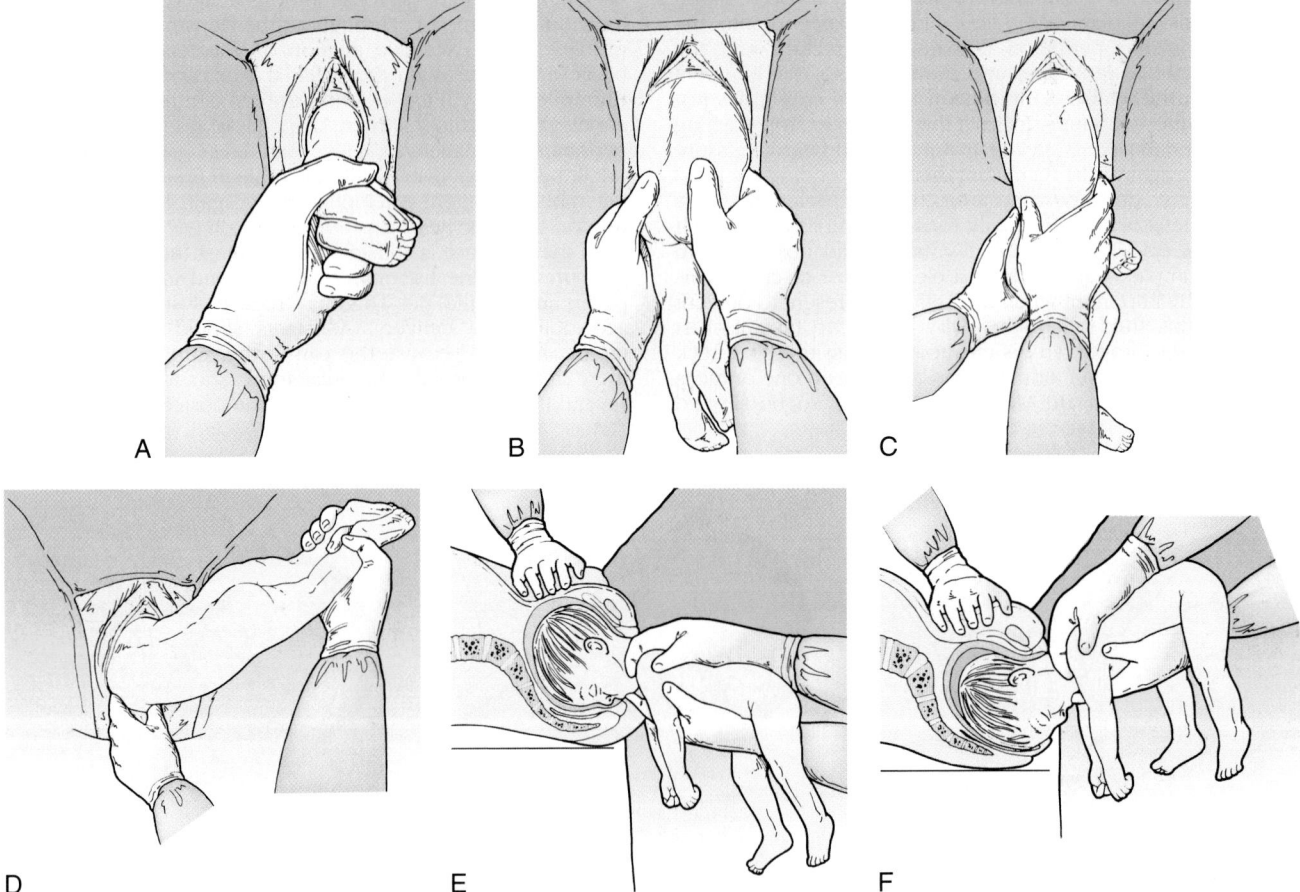

FIGURE 92-8 Management of vaginal breech delivery. **A,** Downward traction at ankles until buttocks clear the introitus. **B,** Traction on pelvic girdle until an axilla becomes visible. **C,** Delivery of posterior shoulder and arm. **D,** Delivery of anterior shoulder and arm with downward traction. **E,** Cradling baby on a forearm, a finger is inserted into mouth or against chin. **F,** Delivery completed by outward traction while maintaining fetal head in a flexed position. *(Modified from Pritchard JA, MacDonald PC: Williams obstetrics, ed 16, New York, 1980, Appleton Century Crofts.)*

sky. Rotate the baby another 45 degrees in the same direction to facilitate delivery of the other leg using the technique described for the first leg. Legs and buttocks can be wrapped in a clean towel to provide a firmer grip and decrease infant trauma. Subsequent delivery is the same as for a footling breech presentation. Grasp the upper legs on each side, with the index fingers crossing the infant's pelvic girdle and both thumbs positioned just above the crease of the buttocks. Use gentle side-to-side rotational motion over an arc of 90 degrees outward and downward, and apply traction while the mother pushes, until the upper portion of a scapula is visible at the introitus. With the baby's body rotated 45 degrees toward the opposite side, use flexion and medial rotation across the chest to deliver the arm. Rotate the baby to the opposite side in the same position, and deliver the other arm. If assistants are present, they should help the woman into the McRobert's position with hyperflexion at the hips to maximize space between the symphysis and sacrum.[75]

Maintaining the baby in the same plane as the vagina, the birth attendant reaches palm up between the baby's legs and into the vagina, supporting the baby's entire body on the forearm while placing the second and fourth fingers over the infant's maxillae and placing the middle finger into the mouth or on the chin. The other hand is positioned over the infant's upper back so that those fingers are overlying each shoulder. If there is sufficient room, the middle fingers can be applied to the fetal occiput. Then with the woman pushing, flex the baby's head downward and complete the delivery. Firm suprapubic pressure can help to maintain the head in flexion. During this final stage, do not elevate the baby's body more than 45 degrees above the plane of the vagina to avoid hyperextension of the head. If the fetal head cannot be delivered because the cervix is incompletely dilated, cut the cervix at the 2- and 10-o'clock positions (Dührssen's incisions) to provide sufficient room to complete the delivery. Once delivered, if the baby breathes and cries spontaneously or with minimal stimulation, delay cutting the umbilical cord while the baby is dried. This allows some of the blood retained in the placenta from umbilical vein compression (common with breech deliveries) to return to the baby. If infant response is limited, immediately clamp and cut the umbilical cord and start neonatal resuscitation.

NEONATAL RESUSCITATION

The first steps in neonatal resuscitation are to dry the baby thoroughly, keep the baby warm, and clear the nose and mouth of excess fluid. Assess the respiratory effort and heart rate (by auscultation or palpation at the base of the umbilical cord). If the baby is breathing spontaneously with a pulse greater than 100 beats/min, keep the baby warm and observe. If the pulse falls below 100 beats/min and the respiratory effort is poor, the next step is to improve ventilation. If further stimulation of the baby by rubbing with a towel or flicking the heels fails to elicit improvement in respiratory effort and pulse, the next step is to provide ventilatory support. This ideally is via application of positive-pressure ventilation with a neonatal mask and Ambu bag (preferably with oxygen). If available, perform gentle (15 to 30 cm H_2O) and rapid (40 to 60 breaths/min) ventilation for 30 seconds and then reassess heart rate. If no equipment is available, place the resuscitator's mouth over the infant's nose and mouth, and deliver rapid shallow breaths at a rate of 30 to 40 breaths/min. If this restores the heart rate and respiratory effort, observe the baby for deterioration in status and repeat the maneuvers as necessary until support is available.[28]

If the baby's heart rate falls below 60 beats/min, full infant cardiopulmonary resuscitation (CPR) should be started. Cardiac compression is performed by (1) placing both thumbs on the sternum just above the xiphoid and facing the fetal head, (2) gently stabilizing this position with the other fingers around the chest, and (3) supplying compressions to a depth of 0.5 to 0.75 inches (1.2 to 1.9 cm) at a rate of about 90 per minute. Care should be taken not to deliver compression to the baby's ribs. Continue ventilation simultaneously as described. If the heart rate after 30 seconds of chest compressions is 80 to 100 beats/min, continue the resuscitation with ventilatory support only. If the heart rate is more than 100 beats/min, discontinue CPR and observe. If the heart rate is still less than 80 beats/min, continue CPR. See the latest neonatal and pediatric resuscitation guidelines from the American Heart Association and American Academy of Pediatrics (aap.org/nrp/) or the World Health Organization.

DELIVERY OF PLACENTA

After the baby is delivered and stabilized, redirect attention to the mother. The first step is to assess the status of placental separation. The heel of the nondominant hand is placed just above the symphysis to hold the uterus in position, and then the fingers are cupped to apply pressure to the uterine fundus while providing gentle, steady downward traction on the umbilical cord. If this maneuver does not promote placental separation, as indicated by a gush of bleeding, lengthening of the cord, and descent of the placenta into the vagina, interrupt these efforts until these signs ensue. When the placenta does descend, instruct the mother to once again push to complete the third stage of labor. By rotating the placenta several times once it has passed through the introitus, complete extrusion of the attached chorioamnionic membranes usually results. If there are signs of placental separation but resistance to extraction, place a hand in the vagina and into the cervix. If the placenta is filling the cervix, it should be grasped and gently extracted. If the placenta does not separate spontaneously or is adherent to the uterine wall (placenta accreta), no effort should be made to separate it manually in a wilderness setting because this could precipitate uncontrollable hemorrhage.[111] Excessive traction on the umbilical cord also could result in uterine inversion, causing vasomotor collapse and hemodynamic decompensation.[12,18]

Once placental expulsion has occurred, gently massage the uterus through the abdominal wall to promote contraction and involution. Usually this is sufficient to control hemorrhage from the placental bed. If this is ineffective, it may be necessary to explore the uterus manually for a retained placenta while compressing the fundus externally until it contracts. Additional measures to aid uterine involution and control bleeding include nipple massage to promote endogenous release of oxytocin and one of the following: administration of oxytocin (10 units/mL intramuscularly); methylergonovine, an ergot derivative (0.2 mg intramuscularly or orally every 2 to 4 hours); prostaglandin F_2 carboprost tromethamine (250 mcg intramuscularly); or misoprostol. The optimal dose and route of administration of misoprostol are unclear. Doses of 200 to 1000 mcg have been administered via oral, sublingual, and rectal routes, or using a combination of routes. If none of these measures is successful, and if bleeding from a laceration has been eliminated as a source, the uterus can be packed with clean sponges or towels until additional medical assistance arrives.[12] Use of a reusable intrauterine balloon tamponade device consisting of a condom-covered Foley catheter attached to a syringe has been associated with marked decreases in maternal death from postpartum bleeding in austere environments.[163] Once the placenta is removed and uterine bleeding controlled, assess and repair maternal injury. The most common sites of lacerations are the perineum, periurethral tissues surrounding the external meatus, lower vagina, and cervix. Significant cervical lacerations in unhurried deliveries are rare unless uncontrollable pushing has occurred before complete dilation. Other lacerations from a spontaneous delivery usually occur along tissue planes that do not disrupt vital areas. They will heal naturally or can be repaired later. Significant bleeding at any of these sites can usually be easily controlled by direct pressure. If available, application of ice packs to the perineum for the first 12 to 24 hours after delivery provides relief.

RESOURCES FOR OBSTETRICS IN REMOTE SETTINGS

Médecins Sans Frontières has published a downloadable manual on "Obstetrics in Remote Settings." This manual is intended for nonobstetricians working in remote settings where medical resources are lacking and reviews much of the information described above related to pregnancy, delivery in remote situations, possible complications, infant resuscitation, and postpartum care. It has excellent diagrams for persons interested in more details (http://refbooks.msf.org/msf_docs/en/obstetrics/obstetrics_en.pdf).

Goals are to protect the mother's life, limit the functional sequelae of pregnancy, and deliver the child in the best possible condition. The manual is not meant to teach advanced diagnosis and management, but to present basic concepts most likely to assist those practicing in difficult conditions. For the wilderness provider, the manual is a good review of warning signs to consider during pregnancy, delivery, and postpartum periods.

BREASTFEEDING

Unless the baby is too premature or too unstable to nurse, breastfeeding should be encouraged as soon as possible after birth. Benefits include promotion of uterine contractions that control hemorrhage at the placental insertion site; encouragement of maternal-newborn bonding; provision of safe, easily digestible, and balanced nutritional support for the baby; and transmission of antibodies (immunoglobulin A) that protect the enteric mucosa against invasion by colonizing bacteria.[9]

During the first 24 hours after delivery, frequent brief feedings (every 2 to 3 hours; 5 minutes on each breast, alternating first breast) are recommended. Although only a small amount of breast fluid (colostrum) is present initially, it contains electrolytes, minerals, and a high concentration of protein and protective immunoglobulin A antibodies. Increase the length of time spent breastfeeding and the intervals between feedings as milk production is established over the next 2 to 3 days. Feeding schedules are typically 10- to 15-minute periods on each breast 8 to 12 times per day. It should be made clear to the mother that babies are not restricted to this regimen.

Instruct breastfeeding women to drink plenty of fluids (2 L/day); increase their caloric intake by 500 to 600 kcal/day, including a total protein intake of 60 to 70 g/day; and consume foods rich in calcium (1200 mg/day).

Breastfeeding Practicalities

Several conditions can interfere with breastfeeding or cause maternal frustration. Breast engorgement 48 to 72 hours after delivery, signifying the onset of milk production accompanied by lymphatic obstruction, can cause pain and low-grade fever, interfere with the baby latching on, and inhibit milk letdown. Frequent feedings and warm compresses just before nursing help to stimulate milk letdown. Cool compresses after nursing, a supportive nursing bra, and acetaminophen usually provide symptomatic relief until milk production and newborn consumption are in equilibrium and lymphatic obstruction is resolving. Engorgement usually resolves within 24 to 48 hours.

Sore and cracked nipples are a frequent complaint of women nursing for the first time. Short, frequent feedings with several rotations between breasts at each sitting can be beneficial. After each feeding, gently cleanse with water and apply a small amount of milk expressed from the breast and spread around the areola to dry to help protect the nipples. Lanolin formulations designed for breastfeeding women can be used as well. Place dry absorbent nursing pads over the nipples between feedings. If contact with clothing or even the nursing pads creates discomfort, breast shells can be used to prevent surface contact. Occasionally, nipple shields can be beneficial for the mother, as well as for the infant who has difficulty latching onto the breast.

Mastitis occurs in 2% to 3% of lactating women and should not be confused with breast engorgement. Mastitis rarely occurs until at least 3 to 4 weeks postpartum.[145] Unlike breast engorgement, mastitis is usually unilateral and accompanied by localized pain, erythema, brawny edema, fever, and malaise. It is more common among women who report painful and cracked nipples and who participate in vigorous exercise- and work-related upper body activities. Encourage these women to empty their breasts by nursing or pumping before these activities and to wear a properly fitting and supportive bra as preventive measures. Women who develop mastitis should continue to nurse from the affected breast and may benefit from warm compresses and pumping between nursing. They should be placed on a course of antibiotics (e.g., dicloxacillin 500 mg or cephalexin 500 mg

four times daily) for 10 to 14 days, with coverage for *Staphylococcus* and *Streptococcus* species and *Escherichia coli*, the most common bacterial isolates from affected breasts. Failure to improve or worsening while on this regimen, as determined by consolidation, widening of erythema and induration, and abscess formation, occurs in 10% to 15% of women. Incision and drainage may be required.[145] Consider treatment for antibiotic-resistant organisms (e.g., methicillin-resistant *Staphylococcus aureus*).

For the breastfeeding mother who is traveling without her infant, a breast pump can be used to maintain milk production and prevent engorgement and mastitis. Manual, battery-powered, and electric breast pumps are available.[67]

Medications During Breastfeeding

Physicians treating breastfeeding mothers should have access to relevant and accurate sources providing data on medication safety during pregnancy and breastfeeding.[53,67,93]

Useful References on Medication During Breastfeeding

The Committee on Drugs of the American Academy of Pediatrics publishes a list of drugs and chemicals transferred into human milk. The list is updated on a regular basis. The statement may be found online at aap.org. *Medications and Mother's Milk*, by Thomas Hale, is an excellent reference that provides an alphabetical list of medications with references at the end of each review.[101] This source calculates a theoretical infant dose of medication that a breastfed infant might receive. An article entitled "Breastfeeding Travelers: Precautions and Recommendations" is also an excellent review on this topic.[67]

Because no randomized controlled trials exist on the safety of medications during lactation, any medication given to a lactating woman should be carefully considered. Most routinely prescribed drugs are safe to use during lactation. Short-acting drugs administered after a feeding have the least opportunity to be excreted into milk. Few drugs are absolutely contraindicated while breastfeeding. With important exceptions, most categories of medications are safe for mothers to take without discontinuing breastfeeding. Most medications have no effect on the milk supply or on infant health (see Table 92-6). Lactating mothers may safely receive nearly all vaccinations because most strains of live viral vaccines are not known to be transmitted in breast milk. The exceptions are attenuated rubella virus and YF vaccines. Infants are usually not infected by the vaccine strain of rubella. There are reports that women who are vaccinated for YF and then breastfeed an infant may increase the risk of neurologic disease in the infant, as discussed earlier.[58]

WILDERNESS HEALTH ISSUES FOR WOMEN OVER 50 YEARS OF AGE

Women are traveling to remote areas of the world at all stages of life. One of the fastest-growing subgroups in adventure travel is made up of older adventuresses, or women over 50 years of age. Older women may begin to have more personal freedom as their children leave home, as relationships change through death or divorce, and/or as there may be more flexibility in their professional lives as they acquire seniority and more financial stability. The oldest traveler to contact the CDC traveler's health team was 99 years old. There are many reasons to push physical and emotional boundaries, including planning a trip as escape from an intense professional or personal life, recovering from an illness, learning a new sport (e.g., mountain climbing or kayaking), volunteering their skills, or further exploring of the world. For a woman recovering from breast cancer or a personal loss, the ability to summit a mountain or to participate in another new arena of exploration can build confidence and self-esteem. The opportunity to travel with partners or friends, with their adult children, or "solo" for the first time, is empowering. A wealth of data support the benefits of physical and intellectual activity and exploration to prevent and ameliorate disease as a person ages.[136,174] Chapter 93 addresses the topic of elder wilderness travelers. Box 92-9 is a useful checklist for older female explorers to consider.

BOX 92-9 Checklist for the Older Adventurers

Review itinerary
Review past medical history and medications carefully
Address concerns related to medical history and plan preventive
   measures as indicated
Immunizations
   Risk versus benefit
   Issues related to immunogenicity of vaccines in the older adult
Chemoprophylaxis
Environmental
   Heat, cold, performance data in the older individuals
Menopausal issues
   Estrogen replacement therapy
   Osteoporosis prevention
   Incontinence, urinary tract infection, constipation, other
Sexually transmitted infection prevention
Medical kit
Safety and security issues
Pre–wilderness travel evaluation: electrocardiogram, mammogram,
   Pap smear
Medical and evacuation insurance

Twenty years from now you will be more disappointed by the things that you didn't do than by the ones you did do. So throw off the bowlines. Sail away from the safe harbor. Catch the trade winds in your sails. Explore. Dream. Discover.
Mark Twain

ACKNOWLEDGMENTS

Thanks to Bertha Chen, MD, Associate Professor, Department of Obstetrics and Gynecology, Stanford University School of Medicine, and to Stanford librarian Christopher Stave.

REFERENCES

Complete references used in this text are available online at expertconsult.inkling.com.

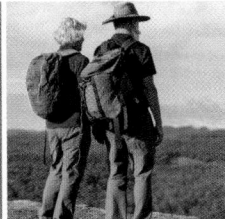

CHAPTER 93
Older Adults in the Wilderness

CHRISTOPHER R. CARPENTER AND NOUSHAFARIN TALEGHANI

DEFINITION OF OLDER ADULT

Despite rapid advances in understanding the molecular and physiologic attributes of aging, no consensus exists on when a person becomes "old." Every person ages chronologically, but the phenotypic expression of biologic aging is highly variable between persons. Individuals routinely defy preconceptions of aging by appearing younger or older than their chronologic age. Aging is associated with a measurable physiologic decline in most organ systems, however (Table 93-1). The key concept is that exacerbations of chronic illnesses, which increase with aging, are the main risk for the elderly wilderness adventurer, not age alone.[31] One recommendation is to classify people according to chronologic age: (1) *athletic old* (younger than 55 years), (2) *young old* (55 to 75 years of age), and (3) *old old* (older than 75 years of age).[131] By focusing only on chronologic age, however, one fails to recognize the nonuniform functional changes that take place during the passage of years or the residual effects of remote illnesses and injuries. A more accurate and comprehensive classification system consisting of three separate components is preferred: (1) *chronologic,* describing a simple time-based classification of years; (2) *pathologic,* describing morphologic and anatomic changes associated with disease or degenerative processes; and (3) *functional,* describing changes in function resulting from impairment.

The functional classification of individuals is based on an idealized bell-shaped distribution curve that places participants in one of five categories labeled alphabetically: (A) high-performance persons, (B) healthy vigorous persons, (C) healthy deconditioned persons, (D) persons with risk factors, and (E) persons who are manifestly ill. Specific aerobic capacity, defined as the maximal physical work capacity, can be derived from graded exercise testing. Other specific functional characteristics can be determined from testing physical modalities in a human performance laboratory, cardiac rehabilitation center, or physical or occupational therapy unit. This classification is useful for matching an individual with various wilderness activities according to physical and environmental demands.

Individuals who plan to participate in wilderness ventures probably have already been through a form of natural selection. For example, a person who aspires to participate in an expedition to Mt Everest will probably have already participated in a similar activity and will have proved his or her capacity to function at an extreme level of performance. This person would most likely be in participant group A or B. An individual who is healthy but has not recently been involved in vigorous activities and become "deconditioned" may be in group C. The motivation may be a desire to reaffirm youth or vigor in some form of exciting or hazardous activity. These individuals deserve the scrutiny of alert organizers, with perhaps an assessment before the venture in order to consider risk factors or occult health problems.

Particular attention should be directed toward any individual at risk of illness or injury (group D), even though manifested evidence of disease may not be apparent. For example, cardiovascular risk factors identified upon interview and examination, such as smoking, a fat-laden diet, and high blood pressure, may warrant a detailed medical examination to determine the level of functional capacity considered safe for that individual. An examination may disclose the presence of diseases, asymptomatic or symptomatic. Group E includes persons with definite manifestations of illness. Supervised outdoor activities can still be of value for such persons and have on occasion been used as a form of physical therapy and rehabilitation for persons with various illnesses, including cardiovascular disease. Persons in this category should be treated as individuals for their assessment and require a high degree of medical evaluation and supervision.

TABLE 93-1 Age-Related Biologic Changes and Their Functional Consequences

Organ System	Age-Related Anatomic Changes	Age-Related Physiologic Changes	Age-Related Functional Consequences
General	Decreased organ and muscle mass	Decreased organ function; decreased oxygen consumption	Decreased flexibility, endurance, and maximal performance
Cardiovascular	Fibrosis of arterial media; thickening of arterial intima; sclerosis of arterial valves (especially aortic and mitral); elongation and tortuosity of aorta	Decreased maximal heart rate of 6-10 beats/min per decade; decreased β-adrenergic responses; increased left ventricular ejection fraction; decreased arterial compliance	Decreased cardiac output of 20% to 30% by age 70 years; decreased maximal physical work capacity; orthostatic hypotension; decreased endurance; syncope; shortness of breath
Lungs	Decreased lung elasticity; decreased activity of cilia; reduced cough reflex	Decreased vital capacity of approximately 30 mL/yr after age 30 years; microaspiration	Shortness of breath; cough; aspiration pneumonia
Kidneys	Increased number of abnormal glomeruli	Decreased glomerular filtration rate; decreased renal blood flow; decreased urine concentration; compensatory reduction in muscle mass, neutralizing creatinine elevation; proteinuria	Delayed response to salt or fluid restriction; nocturia
Genitourinary	Prostatic enlargement; vaginal/urethral mucosal atrophy	Urinary retention (increased residual volume); bacteriuria; atrophic vaginitis	Nocturia; tenesmus; incontinence; urinary tract infection
Gastrointestinal	Atrophic mucosa; atrophic taste buds; anorectal incompetence	Decreased salivary flow; decreased gastric hydrochloric acid; decreased hepatic function; decreased motility	Regurgitation with aspiration; food intolerances; constipation; incontinence; modified appetite, food intake, and motility
Hematologic/immune	Bone marrow fibrosis; metaplasia	Decreased bone marrow reserve; decreased T-cell function; antibody dysfunction	False-negative immunologic skin tests; false-positive laboratory immune tests (e.g., rheumatoid factor and antinuclear antibody)
Musculoskeletal	Decreased height, weight, lean body mass, muscle, and bone density; sarcopenia	Loss of skeletal calcium; reduced elasticity in connective tissue; decreased viscosity of synovial fluid	Loss of cartilaginous surfaces; hypertrophic changes in joints; increased ratio of fat to muscle mass; osteoporosis; failure to thrive; loss of muscle mass and strength of 20% by age 65 years
Endocrine	Osteoporosis; vertebral collapse; changes in fluid volumes	Altered glucose homeostasis; decreased thyroid and testosterone hormone, renin, aldosterone production, and vitamin D absorption; increased antidiuretic hormone	Hyperglycemic response to stress; diabetes mellitus; hyponatremia; hyperkalemia; osteopenia; osteoporosis; impotence
Nervous	Reduced brain mass; decreased cortical cell count	Decreased brain catechol and dopamine synthesis; impaired thermal regulation	Decreased nerve conduction; impaired cerebral and cognitive functions; dementia; depression; forgetfulness; sleep changes; loss of agility; impaired balance; falls; hypothermia, hyperthermia; sensory impairment, including taste, smell, vision, hearing, and touch
Eyes	Decreased translucency of lens; decreased size of pupil; increased intraocular pressure; macular degeneration; arcus senilis	Decreased accommodation; need for increased illumination; susceptibility to glare	Decreased vision, including color and night vision; impaired accommodation; presbyopia
Ears	Loss of auditory neurons; atrophy of cochlear hair cells	Decreased hearing, especially tones higher than 2000 Hz; decreased directional discrimination; vestibular dysfunction	Loss of hearing; loss of click pitch hearing and constant discrimination; balance impairment with falls
Skin	Flattening, atrophy, and attenuation in dermal collagen, rete pegs, and cytoplasm of basal keratinocytes	Decreased skin thickness; risk for dermoepidermal separation; loss of elasticity	Decreased resistance to tearing

WHY AND HOW SOME OLDER ADULTS VENTURE INTO THE WILDERNESS

In addition to an unprecedented post–World War II population explosion, 20th century advances in medical science and hygiene dramatically altered the age composition of the persons who make up Western civilization. In 1900 the median age in the United States was 23 years, increasing to 30 years in 1950, 33 years in 1990, and 36 years in 2000. Senior citizens over age 65 years in the United States increased from 35 million (12.4% of the general population) in the year 2000 to 71 million (19.6%) in 2030. The "old-old" represent the fastest-growing segment of society; octogenarians numbered 9.3 million (3.3%) in 2000 and will reach 19.5 million (5.4%) by 2030.[24]

Many aging adults adopt active and adventurous lifestyles and activities, using time and disposable income that were not available when they were younger. For example, the number of adults over age 50 who reported mountaineering accidents increased five-fold between 1980 and 2010, during a period when the overall population of that age group increased from 26% to 32%.[113] Wilderness fatalities in older adults have been reported in diverse outdoor activities ranging from caving[134] to hiking.[45] Personal reasons given by elders for venturing into the wilderness are enjoyment of nature, physical fitness, tension reduction, tranquility and solitude away from noise and crowds, experiences with friends, enhancement of skill and competency, and excitement or even the thrill of risk-taking.[107]

For elders, the physical and environmental demands of certain activities may be excessive. The physical workload of a wilderness venture depends on its nature and characteristics of its component parts. For example, is the venture a walk or a climb? What is the nature of the terrain? What is the altitude? What is the ambient temperature? It is prudent for elders to examine plans for prospective wilderness ventures and to select activities consistent with their personal capacity, skill, and tolerance. Wilderness activities can be classified according to their physical, technical, and environmental characteristics. The skill, judgment, and capacity of all participants, elders included, can be matched with the characteristics of the venture to determine whether individual capacity is adequate for the demands.

CLASSIFYING "FITNESS FOR ADVENTURE" BY AGE, HEALTH, AND FUNCTIONAL STATUS

Active older adults seeking wilderness adventures generally are more fit, vigorous, and health conscious than the general population. Not surprisingly, wilderness medicine research implies that older adults exposed to environmental challenges are often at less risk (or at least not at increased risk) in high-altitude situations[68,98,119,124] and tropical regions.[127] However, some older adults are at medical risk when exposed to new environmental challenges. Classifying wilderness ventures according to demands required by the activity is helpful. A useful classification includes (1) extreme-performance ventures, (2) high-performance ventures, (3) recreational activities, and (4) therapeutic activities (Table 93-2). The physiologic attributes of the elderly adventurer can be qualitatively categorized (Table 93-3). In conjunction with the activity classification and objective assessment of underlying disease and physiologic capacity learned via the history and physical examination (Box 93-1), experts can categorize the individual adventurer risk prior to wilderness exposure (Table 93-4).

As an example of this classification scheme, a 58-year-old who has coronary artery disease and angina with a stent in place is symptomatic during a graded exercise test. This individual would be functionally classified as

Chronologic: 58 years of age
Pathologic: stented coronary artery disease
Functional: symptomatic (angina) 6 metabolic equivalent of task (6-MET) maximal physical work capacity

This person is manifestly ill and is considered class E. Such pre–wilderness exposure classifications by clinicians provide a basis for recommendations about the risk of extreme environment exposure and optimal management of underlying medical conditions. Clinicians experienced in wilderness medicine and travel medicine can use this classification scheme in conjunction with an individual patient's preferences, goals of care, and anticipated destinations to provide efficient preexposure preventive planning, advice, and prescribing (Box 93-2).

ENVIRONMENTAL STRESSES AND OLDER ADULTS

Environmental variables encountered in the great diversity of outdoor wilderness activities may produce significant physiologic stresses. These variables include extremes of heat and cold, high altitude, water immersion, tropical humidity, desert aridity, and ultraviolet exposure. The common denominator in nearly all wilderness ventures is physical activity, often at extreme levels. To compound the complexity of physical activity influenced by environmental stress, the physician may care for a senior afflicted with subclinical or manifesting disease. When the physiologic demands from environmental stresses are added to the increased and prevalent degenerative conditions and diseases associated

TABLE 93-2 Classification of Wilderness Ventures

Class	General Description	Examples
1	Extreme-performance ventures	High-altitude mountaineering, such as a Mt Everest climb or other Himalayan trekking
2	High-performance ventures	Remote hunting activities, particularly at high altitude or under stresses of heat, dust, or cold
		Jungle trekking
3	Recreational activities	Trail walking is generally considered recreational, but because of endurance demands and environmental risks, it may present physiologic hazards
		Other activities that may fit this classification:
		Alpine hiking
		National park trail walking
		Forest-based orienteering
4	Therapeutic activities	For more than a century, physical activity has been recommended for certain individuals with cardiovascular disease and other physical limitations to improve their functional capacity

TABLE 93-3 Classification of Participants in Wilderness Ventures

Group	General Description	Examples
A	Individuals with demonstrated ability to engage in high-performance activities	Athletes in training; Mountaineers continually active and in training; Workers involved with heavy physical tasks
B	Healthy, vigorous individuals	Athletes; Active hunting guides
C	Healthy, deconditioned individuals	Young to middle-aged, healthy business and professional people who are moderately active
D	Individuals with risk factors	Individuals at risk because of age, lifestyle, smoking, excessive alcohol consumption, or factors not under their control; most elders are in this group
E	Individuals who are manifestly ill	People at any age with chronic illness or physical limitations, such as heart disease, diabetes, or neuromuscular or orthopedic problems

BOX 93-1 Components of the Medical Examination

1. **Personal characteristics,** which provide a profile of the subject regarding age; gender; education; occupation; status as volunteer or recruit; history of a recent or remote similar venture; use of tobacco, alcohol, drugs, or steroids; history of psychological or interpersonal problems, especially during wilderness ventures; and history of participation in athletics.
2. **Historical features,** such as illness, with particular emphasis on cardiovascular, pulmonary, musculoskeletal, and neurologic problems; problems associated with a previous venture; intolerance to altitude, heat, or cold; psychological problems; accidents; and pertinent family history.
3. **Medical examination,** including examination of heart rate, blood pressure, precise cardiac examination (including auscultation); examination of peripheral pulses and carotid arteries; auscultation of the chest; abdominal palpation with rectal examination; musculoskeletal system with range of motion of joints and back; and height and weight.
4. **Physiologic examination,** which is only rarely required, depends largely on the nature of the venture and may range from simple simulation of the planned activity to functional aerobic testing for $\dot{V}O_{2max}$ using a treadmill, cycle, or step ergometry. Functional testing with electrocardiographic monitoring is frequently used for diagnostic testing and for predicting cardiovascular response to exercise. Testing by running for speed or endurance and evaluation of dynamic strength and agility are rarely used but are interesting during skill assessment. Testing for hypoxic ventilatory response may be primarily of research interest but nonetheless should be considered if precision is needed for elders going to high altitude.
5. **Psychological interviews** largely depend on the skill and technique of the examiner and should attempt to uncover a history of previous difficulties with group interaction and team activities, or fears related to physical and environmental stress.

BOX 93-2 Older Adult Checklist Prior to and During Wilderness Exposure

Seek medical advice before trip and avoid travel if unstable medical condition exists

Obtain requisite age-appropriate immunizations for regions traveled

Exercise months before major trips to ensure physical fitness for potentially harsh environmental exposures

For remote locales, purchase travel insurance

Do research on airline travel restrictions on medications and medical devices; request necessary documentation from physician

Consult physician or pharmacist regarding regular medications and:

    Potential interactions with medications used to treat travel-related infectious illnesses or high-altitude sickness

    Respiratory depressant effects

    Medication effects on cognition, acclimatization, thermoregulation, and exercise tolerance.

    Appropriate storage of medications

    Review time zone changes and medication schedule

Bring extra doses of medications and carry emergency supply separate from main travel equipment; travel with companions who you inform of existing medical conditions and the location of key medications and medical equipment

Permit time for acclimatization to temperature and altitude

Schedule time for nutrition and hydration

Wear MedicAlert bracelet at all times

with aging, the risk for illness and injury is increased. The complete package of age, conditioning, environment, nature of the activity, and experience must be considered when an elder is advised or treated in the wilderness.

ALTITUDE

Increasing personal wealth and renewed interest in outdoor activities have led increasing numbers of adventurers of all ages to explore mountain climbing, trekking, and skiing. In 1999 an estimated 100 million tourists worldwide visited high altitudes,

15% of whom were over age 60 years.[16] Increasing altitudes decrease atmospheric pressure and the partial pressure of oxygen such that at 5500 m (18,000 feet) of altitude, atmospheric pressure is half that of sea level. Although the elderly demonstrate reduced ventilatory and heart rate responses compared with younger individuals,[81] the respiratory system adapts within 2 days, and the heart rate and metabolic responses adapt within 1 week.[16] The hypoxic ventilatory response is an essential defense mechanism against high-altitude hypoxia; dopamine is the neurotransmitter responsible for the carotid body chemoreceptor response to hypoxia. Older adults demonstrate decreased dopamine receptor sensitivity during short-term adaptation to altitude.[126]

Exposures to the relative hypoxia of high altitude are a risk in all age groups for high-altitude pulmonary edema (HAPE) and high-altitude cerebral edema (HACE), discussed more fully in Chapters 1, 2, and 3.[60,108] Aging reduces physiologic components of the gas exchange process that maintain oxygenation, such as

TABLE 93-4 Construction of the Medical Examination of Prospective Participants in Wilderness Ventures

Classification of Characteristics of Participants	Classification of Venture			
	1. Extreme Performance	2. High Performance	3. Recreational	4. Therapeutic
A. Demonstrated high performance	2, 3, **5***	2, 3, **5**	2	†
B. Healthy, vigorous	2, 3, 4, **5**	2, 3, **5**	**2**	**2**
C. Healthy, "deconditioned"	1, 2, 3, **4, 5**	2, 3, **4, 5**	2, **4**	2, **3, 4**
D. Risk factors	1, 2, **3, 4, 5**	1, 2, **3, 4, 5**	2, **3, 4**, 5	2, **3, 4, 5**
E. Illness	†	†	1, 2, **3, 4, 5**	1, 2, **3, 4**, 5

Category of components (from Box 93-1):
1. Personal data
2. Historical data
3. Medical findings
4. Physiologic assessment
5. Psychological evaluation

*A reason for classifying wilderness ventures and participants is to help design an examination that assesses the most important data, depending on the physical status of the individual and the nature of the venture. All categories listed in Box 93-1 should be considered in the examination, but those shown here in **bold** numbers are of prime importance and should be emphasized.

†Individualized assessment indicated.

Data from Decentennial state population changes by age, Stat Bull Metrop Insur Co 73:30, 1992; and Erb BD: Determining medical suitability for wilderness ventures. In Domej W, Schobersberger W, Waanders R, Berghold F, editors: Jahrbuch 2005, Innsbruck, Austria, 2005, Austrian Society for Alpine and High Altitude Medicine.

vital capacity and hypoxic ventilatory drive.[60] Older persons are known to have a lower arterial partial pressure of oxygen (PO_2) because of thickening of the pulmonary alveolar-capillary membrane.[81] The risk for altitude sickness among elders is increased by a poor physical condition, alcohol intake, preexisting pulmonary disease, medication, and excessive activity within the first 12 hours after arriving at altitude. Alcohol tolerance is variable, so total abstinence during a wilderness venture is recommended. It is prudent to avoid sedatives and hypnotics at high altitude.

The physical manifestations and optimal management of HAPE and HACE in older adults are not clearly understood. This is in part because older adults are often excluded from altitude studies that include younger, more vigorous subjects. For example, studies evaluating the sharpened Romberg test as a screen for acute mountain sickness extended only to age 65 years,[76] and randomized trials of ibuprofen[53,91] and acetazolamide[12] excluded older adults. However, as summarized below, most high-altitude illness studies suggest that older adults are not at increased risk for HAPE or HACE.[68,98,119,124]

Honigman studied the general population at moderate altitude (2000 to 3000 m [6500 to 9750 feet]) at ski resorts in Colorado. Predictors of mountain sickness included chronic residence at an altitude greater than 1000 m (3250 feet) before a high-altitude venture, underlying lung problems, previous history of acute mountain sickness ($p < 0.05$), and, surprisingly, age younger than 60 years.[68] One hypothesis for identification of older age as a protective factor against mountain sickness is self-selection among the small group of elderly individuals who are exposed to altitude and activity; wilderness medicine enthusiasts likely represent a healthier subset of all older adults. Another possibility is that elders require more time to ascend and thus are more diligent with regard to acclimatization.

Roach and colleagues studied 97 older men and women (ages 59 to 83 years) over a 5-day period in Vail, Colorado at a moderate elevation of 2500 m (8200 feet). They concluded that it was generally safe for older men and women with underlying, asymptomatic cardiovascular and lung disease to make short sojourns to moderate altitudes. In particular, they suggested that hypertension was not a contraindication for travel to moderate altitudes, although blood pressure should be closely monitored and antihypertensive medication continued as prescribed. Of note, their subjects had a short stopover at a lower altitude, and the authors acknowledge that selection bias may have played a role in this particular study.[119]

Although older adults do not appear to be at increased risk for illness related to high altitude, they are more likely to require emergency evacuation when it occurs.[83] Therefore, prior to embarking on wilderness adventures with high-altitude exposures, prudent and specific considerations for individuals with preexisting pulmonary,[94,4] cardiovascular,[4] neurologic,[7] ocular,[96] endocrine,[15] and other conditions[102] are required. For example, safety of high-altitude trekking in high-functioning, physically fit individuals after coronary artery bypass surgery has been the subject of debate, without any clear consensus.[8,50,70,118] In fact, in the 1930s, hypobarism was used as a stress test to diagnose occult coronary artery disease.[86] The question for the physician screening an asymptomatic individual prior to high-altitude exposure must therefore be to accurately label the patient's cardiovascular status (and coronary circulation) as "normal." An electrocardiogram alone has a positive predictive value of 0.0001% for such individuals and should not be the sole marker of a "normal heart"; instead, preventive prealtitude cardiac screening should include a careful history of the usual activity level, symptoms with this activity, and education about appropriate ascent rates and acclimatization.[84,118]

The cerebral effects of high altitude include headache, acute mountain sickness, cerebral edema, and cerebral vasospasm. This last effect may manifest as transient ischemic attacks or transient global amnesia.[139] High-altitude exposure may impair memory, perception, cognitive flexibility, and psychomotor responsiveness, which can lead to poor decision making and preventable tragedies in patients.[120] These effects are magnified by fragmented sleep.[137] Disorientation and confusion related to HACE are not uncommon in younger populations initially exposed to high altitude[6]; 33% of acutely ill community-dwelling older adults (albeit not those who trek mountains) frequently demonstrate cognitive impairment if formally tested.[20] Therefore, as noted later in this chapter, it is important to have a sea-level objective cognitive baseline test for comparison when symptoms arise at high altitude.[65] Altered mental status in older adults can also occur on descent, as reported in the case of an experienced 85-year-old mountaineer with thiazide-related hyponatremia and hyperactive delirium.[29]

Acetazolamide is the drug of choice for prophylaxis against periodic breathing[61] and acute mountain sickness. When prescribing for the elderly, drug-drug and drug-disease interactions are important to consider (Table 93-5).[95,108] Elders may experience side effects, such as weakness, nausea, and paresthesias, with large doses of acetazolamide; therefore, caution is encouraged. In addition, acetazolamide compromises exercise capacity during early acclimatization in older persons.[12] Characteristics of elders who are vulnerable to altitude illness are listed in Box 93-3. Age-appropriate preventive measures for high-altitude illness are suggested in Box 93-4.

COLD

Cold exposure (discussed more fully in Chapters 7 to 11) is poorly tolerated in older adults. Unfortunately, the Wilderness Medical Society practice guidelines for hypothermia and frostbite do not evaluate age-related risk factors for cold injuries.[100,143] The complex mechanisms that control body temperatures in elders are not as responsive as in younger people due to age-related changes in multiple organ systems, as well as the effects of certain medications (Box 93-5).[30] Research suggests that age may not influence thermosensitivity upon immersion into cold water.[54] With aging, the metabolic rate is diminished. When associated with age-related reduction in muscle mass, the shivering response is blunted and there is reduced capacity for heat generation. In addition, the peripheral vasoconstrictive response to cold is diminished. Systolic hypertension through stimulation of the sympathetic nervous system is exaggerated in a cold environment.

BOX 93-3 Characteristics of Elders Vulnerable to Altitude Illness

1. Abrupt ascent in altitude from near sea level to 3000 m (9750 feet) or higher, without an extra night for acclimatization for every additional 600 to 900 m (1950 to 2900 feet) of continuing ascent
2. History of previous episode of altitude sickness
3. Preexisting lung disease characterized by decreased capacity and decreased hypoxic ventilatory response
4. Preexisting cardiovascular disease
5. Metabolic abnormalities associated with diabetes and renal disease
6. Medication that influences respiratory drive
7. Low physical functional capacity
8. Obesity

BOX 93-4 Prevention of Altitude Sickness in Elders

1. Avoid strenuous physical activity at altitude if there is a history of acute mountain sickness.
2. Limit the intensity of physical activity in the presence of cardiovascular disease.
3. Limit physical activity in the presence of pulmonary disease, especially if there is decreased vital capacity.
4. Avoid significant physical activity for at least 12 hours after arrival at an altitude of 2500 m (8100 feet) or more above sea level, and delay physical activity for an additional 24 hours for every gain of 600 to 900 m (1950 to 2900 feet) in altitude.
5. Be aware of all medications and their effects on hypoxic ventilatory drive.
6. Use carbonic anhydrase inhibitors (acetazolamide) according to recommendations of the venture leaders, considering the altitude, medical history, and other medications.

TABLE 93-5 Issues Related to Dosages of Medications Used for Prevention and Treatment of Altitude-Related Illness in Aging Adults

Medications	Renal Insufficiency	Hepatic Insufficiency	Other Major Dosage Issues
Acetazolamide	Avoid with GFR < 10 mL/min, metabolic acidosis, hypokalemia, hypercalcemia, or recurrent nephrolithiasis	Acetazolamide contraindicated	Avoid in patients receiving long-term aspirin or with FEV$_1$ < 25% predicted; caution with sulfa allergy; avoid concurrent use of topiramate, potassium-wasting diuretics, and ophthalmic carbonic anhydrase inhibitors
Dexamethasone	No contraindications	No contraindications	Expect ↑blood glucose in diabetics; avoid in patients at risk of peptic ulcer or upper GI bleeding; caution in patients at risk for amebiasis or strongyloidiasis
Nifedipine	No contraindications	Best to avoid; if necessary, administer at reduced dose (10 mg twice daily) of sustained-release version	Caution in patients at increased risk of GI bleeding or with gastroesophageal reflux; caution in patients taking medications metabolized by CytP450 3A4 and 1A2 pathways; caution using concurrently with other antihypertensive medications
Tadalafil	If GFR 30-50 mL/min give 5 mg/day; if GFR < 30 mL/min, give no more than 5 mg	Child's class A and B maximum 10 mg/day; Child's class C, do not use tadalafil	Increase risk of gastroesophageal reflux; avoid concurrent use of nitrates or α-blockers; caution in patients taking medications metabolized by CytP450 3A4 pathway
Sildenafil	Dose adjustment if GFR > 30 mL/min	Dose reduction recommended starting at 25 mg 3 times a day; avoid use in patients with known esophageal or gastric varices	Avoid in patients with known varices; avoid concurrent use of nitrates or α-blockers; caution in patients taking medications metabolized by CytP450 3A4 pathway
Salmeterol	No contraindications	Best to avoid	Potential for adverse effects in patients with arrhythmia-prone coronary artery disease; avoid concurrent use of β-blockers, monoamine oxidase inhibitors, or tricyclic antidepressants

FEV$_1$, forced expiratory ventilation; GFR, glomerular filtration rate; GI, gastrointestinal.
Adapted from Luks AM, Swenson ER: Medication and dosage considerations in the prophylaxis and treatment of high-altitude illness, Chest 133:744-755, 2008.

The cardiac workload is increased; consequently, in the presence of coronary artery disease, angina is frequently precipitated by exertion and cold. Four avoidance factors for persons with coronary artery disease, the "four Es of angina," are *exertion, emotion, eating* excessively, and *exposure* to cold.

Exhaustion added to hypoglycemia and dehydration compounds the problem of impaired metabolic function, making the elder individual more vulnerable to the effects of cold. Adequate food intake is essential for maintaining body heat and may become critical. Other physical environmental influences, such as wind, humidity, ultraviolet and infrared radiation, and altitude, should be factored into the exposure equation.[115] The wind chill index provides a useful teaching device for reminding explorers about the hazards of combined cold and wind. The classic combination of cold, dampness, wind, and exhaustion may prove fatal, especially in an elder with decreased physical reserves.

Medical conditions such as cardiovascular disease, metabolic diseases such as hypothyroidism and diabetes, compromised nutritional status, and modified thermoregulatory responses resulting from central nervous system disease or medication may influence heat conservation and contribute to hypothermia. Heat loss may also be increased by damp, wet clothing. All persons should be cautioned to carry ample clothing for changes after saturation with moisture.

Peripheral vasoconstriction, the fundamental mechanism for heat conservation, may be enhanced to some small degree by long-term exposure to cold. When an older adult recognizes personal intolerance to cold, he or she may begin a program of gradual increase in exposure to cold. Prevention of cold injury, however, is best achieved through a learning process derived from experience.[123] Elders should never venture unaccompanied into the cold wilderness. Judgment, orientation, and independent responsibility may be impaired in elders who find themselves lost in the cold or in a rescue situation. Some useful preventive measures are suggested in Box 93-6.

HEAT

Heat-related illnesses range from heat edema to life-threatening heat stroke (see Chapters 12 and 13).[87,90] Acute management of heat-related illness is identical to that for younger populations.[39,142] Tolerance to heat depends on characteristics of the

---

BOX 93-5 Causes of Older Adult Vulnerability to Cold Exposure

1. Peripheral vascular disease (impaired vasoconstriction)
2. Hypertension (perhaps cold induced)
3. Heart disease, including coronary artery disease, decreased cardiac output, congestive heart failure
4. Metabolic diseases (diabetes, obesity, hypothyroidism)
5. Hematologic disorders (anemia, dysproteinemias)
6. Pulmonary disease (cold-induced asthma, chronic obstructive pulmonary disease)
7. Drugs and alcohol
8. Medications, particularly β-blockers and tranquilizers

BOX 93-6 Prevention of Cold Injury in Older Adult Adventurers

1. Avoid exhaustion during wilderness ventures.
2. Limit exposure.
3. Carry and wear adequate clothing, including rain gear.
4. Stay dry and avoid damp undergarments from excessive sweating.
5. Maintain adequate nutrition with high carbohydrate intake and fat. Carry adequate food for the trip.
6. Maintain adequate fluid intake. Do not consume snow or ice.
7. Participate in a physical training program before the expedition.
8. Pay attention to medication effects.
9. Avoid alcohol and illicit drugs.
10. Always maintain access to an adequate shelter.

BOX 93-7   Attributes of Older Adult Vulnerability to Heat Exposure

1. Obesity
2. Decreased physical functional capacity
3. Infrequent heat exposure
4. Altered thermoregulatory center in the hypothalamus or insensitive skin sensors
5. Metabolic and serum electrolyte abnormalities
6. Heart disease, coronary artery disease, pulmonary disease, diabetes, and renal disease
7. Peripheral vascular disease
8. Multiple medications, often in combination: anticholinergics, antipsychotics, tranquilizers, and β-blockers
9. Alcohol

host, including health status, medications taken, frequency and duration of exposure, history of recent acclimatization, and prevalent environmental factors. Elders in a hot wilderness setting may have personal host characteristics, in addition to the environment, that further limit tolerance and safety (Box 93-7). The person's weight; a fractionated body mass; cardiovascular, renal, or pulmonary problems; and the presence of various medications may influence the individual response to heat.

Regulation of body heat may be affected by altered function of the thermoregulatory center located in the anterior preoptic hypothalamic nuclei, by deranged skin sensors, or by medications used to treat various diseases. These include anticholinergics, beta-adrenergic blockers, antipsychotic medications, and major tranquilizers. Side effects influence adaptation of sweat mechanisms to thermal stress. Diuretics may produce hypovolemia with loss of adequate subcutaneous circulation for heat dissipation. Because older adults in general consume more medications than do younger persons, it is very important to approach heat injury from a position of prevention.

The cardiovascular system plays a major role in heat regulation through heat dissipation. Circulatory abnormalities, peripheral vascular disease, hypertension, and reduced cardiac output may modify heat dissipation, resulting in vulnerability to heat injury. The physical work capacity, as measured by maximal oxygen consumption ($\dot{V}O_{2max}$), decreases 5% to 15% per decade after age 25 years. β-adrenergic blockers and calcium channel blockers may also influence cardiac output by modifying the heart rate and myocardial contractility.

To prevent heat-related illness associated with wilderness activities in older adults (Box 93-8), it is sometimes helpful to suggest a regular exercise program in the heat for the purpose of adaptation. A regular program consisting of 60 to 100 minutes of low-intensity exercise per day for 7 to 14 days at tolerable heat levels before the planned exposure should result in significant adaptation in normal individuals. The exercise level should require oxygen consumption of less than 50% of the individual's $\dot{V}O_{2max}$. Experience teaches that a degree of adaptation results from frequent and extended periods of exposure. Acclimatization to heat yields a generally improved response to exercise. Physiologic responses to adaptation include lower heart rate, enhanced tolerance to physical activity, predictable core temperature in response to heat stress, increased sweat rate, and decreased sodium loss through sweating.

Additional environmental factors, such as high humidity, high winds, and infrared and ultraviolet radiation exposure, may

BOX 93-8   Prevention of Heat Injuries in Older Adults

1. Assess health status, with particular emphasis on history, cardiovascular status, obesity, and previous history of problems associated with heat exposure.
2. Maintain adequate hydration.
3. Maintain adequate nutritional status: food, fluid, and electrolyte intake.
4. Participate in a proper acclimatization program.

modify levels of an individual's tolerance to heat, partly through skin changes. It is valuable to teach individuals to be aware of the environment and associated responses such as warmth, coldness, or dampness in the skin.

TRAVEL MEDICINE AND OLDER ADULTS

As the population increases, older people have the opportunity to travel for longer periods and to destinations that are quite different from those to which they have become accustomed. Compared with younger populations, elders tend to have more ongoing medical issues and also have certain limitations related to the aging process. However, most of the time, ongoing medical issues do not contraindicate or impede travel. Older adults traveling to exotic locales or more adventurous destinations often choose to use a managed tour so that a tour manager (and often a tour doctor or nurse) conducts much of the logistical planning. Even on managed tours, older adults frequently seek medical advice for gastrointestinal, respiratory, dermatologic, and cardiovascular symptoms.[127,128] Anticipating and preventing medical complications is prudent for older adults exploring far-away locales, especially patients with preexisting medical conditions.[111] Travelers should seek the advice of medical specialists related to their specific medical condition(s), as well as a travel medical physician, prior to embarking on a wilderness or exotic trip. Travelers should also ensure that their medical insurance covers them in a foreign country.

Many elderly travelers require vaccinations and seek guidance from a primary care provider. Physicians routinely confront clinical decisions about which patient to vaccinate, assessing vaccination safety for particular patients, and estimating the level of protective efficacy likely to be offered by a vaccine(s).[3] Aging is associated with alterations in immune responses (Figure 93-1), which may lead to clinically significant changes in safety, immunogenicity, and protective efficacy of certain vaccines.[78] Immune senescence and diminished vaccine efficacy are associated with loss of B-cell activity, although changes in T-cell function are the dominant age-associated cellular dysfunctions in the immune system.[78] In the future, new approaches to augment efficacy of traditional vaccinations, such as viral vectors for antigen delivery, DNA-based vaccines, and toll-like receptor agonists, may improve immunoprotection following vaccination.[138]

Leder and colleagues evaluated existing data regarding the effects of age on responses after immunization to vaccines generally administered before travel. The specific vaccines included hepatitis A, typhoid, yellow fever, encephalitis, and rabies vaccines. Additional vaccines discussed were many routine vaccines frequently administered before travel, including tetanus-diphtheria-toxoid, hepatitis B, pneumococcal, and influenza vaccines. The authors noted diminished serologic responses to hepatitis A and rabies vaccines in older individuals, as well as increased toxic effects following yellow fever vaccination.[82] However, many of the vaccines currently in use—in particular, many of the vaccines given prior to travel—have never been specifically studied in elderly subjects, and many questions remain unanswered. Existing evidence suggests that immune responses are at least in part age dependent. This could translate into a requirement for altered vaccine schedules for elderly persons, such as those used for many vaccines administered to infants. Additional studies need to be conducted to ascertain the schedules. These issues are becoming increasingly important as the number of elderly persons in the population increases and they travel to exotic destinations.

MEDICAL EXAMINATION FOR OLDER ADULTS PLANNING WILDERNESS TRAVEL

There are two important occasions when wilderness medical leaders should consider a health and medical evaluation for older adult adventurers: (1) during the planning phase before the

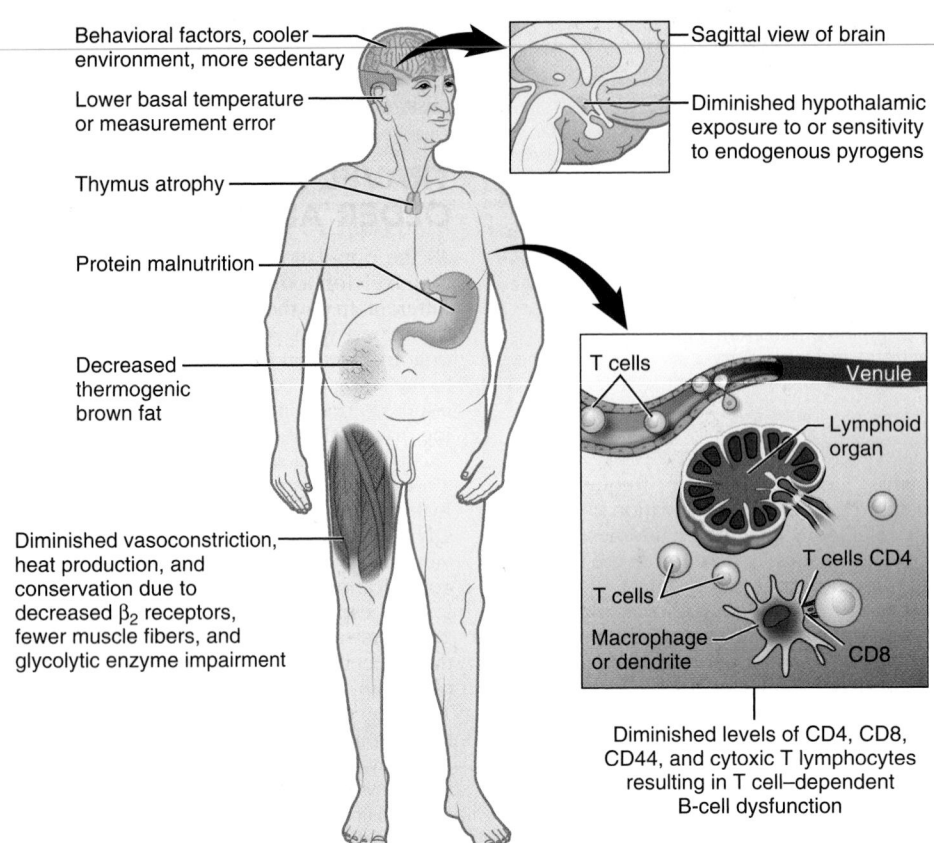

FIGURE 93-1 Factors associated with a diminished older adult response to thermoregulation and immune response. *(From Katz ED, Carpenter CR: Fever and immune function in the elderly: In Meldon SW, Ma OJ, Woolard R, editors: Geriatric emergency medicine, New York, 2004, McGraw-Hill, Figure 9-1, p 59.)*

venture and (2) in response to symptoms that occur during or after the venture. Components of the pretrip evaluation are based on the characteristics of the individual and on the nature of the proposed venture. By the time an individual qualifies for designation as an older adult, that person has usually made some arrangements for medical care, examination, and advice. However, as older adults consider venturing into the wilderness, there is often confusion or insecurity about the prospect of what medical issues might become important. A formal prewilderness clinical examination may be helpful to prevent or anticipate medical problems. The content of a medical examination, consisting of any or all of the five categories listed in Box 93-1, matches characteristics of the individual with characteristics of the venture and identifies components of the medical examination that may be needed (see Table 93-4). Wilderness leaders indicate that the most important part of the medical examination before a wilderness adventure is an in-depth interview by an examiner experienced in medical care *and* the nature of the venture, so the most appropriate screening physician may not be the patient's primary care physician. However, if the primary care physician is the only available screening physician, then it is advisable to seek input from persons who have experienced the anticipated environmental hazards and understand the physiology of the older adult's underlying comorbidities. After the interview, appropriate medical, laboratory, radiographic, and physiologic studies may be performed. The remainder of this chapter reviews age-related changes in specific organ systems pertinent to the medical evaluation prior to wilderness adventures.

CARDIOVASCULAR DISEASE

Age-related changes in the cardiovascular system affect the heart rhythm, myocardial pump function, and afterload. With aging, there is a progressive reduction in the number of pacemaker cells in the sinoatrial node, increase in myocyte cell volume per nucleus in both ventricles, increase in peripheral vascular resistance, and increase in aortic impedance from loss of elasticity. Increased levels of circulating catecholamines are associated with aging, especially with stress, but β-adrenergic–induced vasodilation decreases with age. This is important for exercise tolerance in elders.

The presence of pump failure, either systolic or diastolic, may be indicated by recent weight gain, shortness of breath, orthopnea, or ankle edema. The patient with symptomatic heart failure should limit remote wilderness ventures to activities that do not cause excessive shortness of breath, breathing through an open mouth, or excessive fatigue. Peripheral vascular disease, claudication, symptomatic carotid disease, and aortic aneurysm warrant caution with regard to the difficulty of return or evacuation in the event of incapacity.

Cardiac rhythm disturbances range from the nuisance effect of premature systoles to significant rhythm disturbances, such as atrial fibrillation, to potentially life-threatening ventricular arrhythmias. An older adult who is aware of symptoms related to an arrhythmia should seek evaluation by a physician before a wilderness adventure. The evaluation should include history of the onset of symptoms and initiating factors, medications taken, physical examination with emphasis on auscultation of the mitral and aortic valves, electrocardiogram, ambulatory monitoring if there is a history of heart disease or light-headedness, and possibly echocardiogram. For persons with atrial fibrillation, structural heart disease, and an appropriate rate response to exercise, activities consistent with the limitations of the structural heart disease are allowed. Persons with atrial fibrillation requiring anticoagulation should not participate in activities risking physical contact and injury, in particular head trauma.

Valvular pathology, especially aortic and mitral valve issues, may be recognized by auscultation and confirmed by echocardiography. The patient with a prosthetic cardiac valve may be at risk during prolonged adventures with exposure to inclement weather, infectious diseases among fellow travelers, or diseases among the local populace.

CORONARY ARTERY DISEASE

A heart attack is the ultimate medical emergency and frequently mimics other environmental catastrophes, such as high-altitude illness.[5] In the United States, millions of individuals suffer myocardial infarctions annually, 30% of whom do not survive. Of these, 50% die within the first hour of the onset of chest pain. Because the myocardium depends almost entirely on aerobic metabolism, the workload is reflected in the myocardial oxygen consumption. Delivery of oxygen to the myocardium depends on the coronary blood flow. Hence, integrity of the coronary arteries is essential for a viable response to wilderness stresses. Remoteness and delay in instituting treatment in wilderness settings render myocardial infarction to be of high risk for poor outcome in many cases. If a victim survives the first hour, which may be the time required to initiate a search and rescue, there may be a maximum 85% chance of survival, using urban statistics.[38]

Only one-half of people with myocardial infarction have symptoms beforehand, and acute myocardial infarction can be difficult to recognize,[110] but asking about the history and risk factors during a medical history might help clinicians risk-stratify an older adult's chances of a myocardial infarction before the wilderness adventure. However, exercise testing in asymptomatic patients without risk factors for coronary artery disease is not usually indicated.[71] Subgroups of cardiac patients with pre-existing pulmonary hypertension, uncompensated congestive heart failure, unstable angina, recent myocardial infarction, severe anemia, or decreased arterial oxygen saturation are at higher risk than are other cardiac patients.[133] The history should include detailed assessment of risk factors for coronary artery disease. Knowledge of the existence and extent of coronary artery disease will influence recommendations for the nature and level of activity, expected tolerance to environmental stresses, and recommendations as to the degree of remoteness, level of exertion, and environmental factors that the individual should endure in the proposed wilderness adventure. Activity prescriptions target heart rate rather than workload.[105] A series of philosophical discussions dealing with the limitations of wilderness activities in people who have undergone cardiac surgery appeared in a series of letter exchanges and editorials in the *Journal of the American Medical Association*.[8,50,70,118] The conclusion places the decision-making process squarely on the clinical judgment of the cardiologist on a case-by-case basis.[118]

Because there is no absolutely risk-free activity for a person with significant cardiovascular disease, prevention is the fundamental principle for reducing risk. Before vigorous outdoor activity by an older adult, the physician should:

- Understand the individual's wilderness activity plans
- Based upon contemporary geopolitical conditions, weather patterns, and the epidemiologic status of infectious diseases, anticipate exertional and environmental stressors
- Recognize a history of coronary artery disease and other illnesses, and the use of medications
- Be prepared to make specific recommendations regarding physical activity and exposure

There are currently no published guidelines to aid in advising older individuals intending to venture into the wilderness, but the American College of Sports Medicine provides exercise and physical activity recommendations.[26] High-level recommendations suggest that older adults are able to engage in acute aerobic or resistance exercise and experience positive adaptations to exercise training. In addition, individuals vary widely in how they adapt to exercise; the variability is likely related to the individual lifestyle and genetic factors.

HYPERTENSION

Hypertension is an important marker for potential cardiovascular problems.[73] Complications include angina, myocardial infarction, left ventricular hypertrophy, heart failure, stroke (both ischemic and hemorrhagic), and renal failure. The most widely accepted values of blood pressure considered to represent hypertension are systolic pressure above 140 mm Hg or diastolic pressure over 90 mm Hg. Treatment of hypertension prior to a wilderness adventure is recommended. However, common antihypertensive medications are associated with significant side effects that can alter the physiologic adjustment to environmental stressors and interact with common pharmacologic therapies for high-altitude illness and infectious diseases. Diuretics deplete volume and are associated with hypokalemia and hyponatremia. β-adrenergic blockers reduce the adaptive capacities of the heart rate and thermoregulation. Calcium channel blockers are frequently associated with headache, flushing, and edema.

DERMATOLOGIC DISORDERS

Thin Skin

Normal aging of skin leads to atrophy, decreased elasticity, and impaired metabolic and reparative responses. These changes are different from photoaging, which is due to sun exposure. As the epidermis becomes thinner and the dermoepidermal junction flattens, the skin becomes fragile and subject to shear stress.[103] This is why removing an adhesive from an older person's skin can dislodge the epidermis and why bleeding into the space between the dermis and epidermis occurs more frequently, as evidenced by bruising from seemingly mundane contact.

Additional changes that occur in an older individual's skin include delayed wound healing due to thinning of the dermis with decreased vascularity.[55] The ability to deliver heat to the skin for excretion is impaired. Combined with the loss of subdermal fat that decreases insulation, this leads to inability of older persons to conserve heat as well as can younger persons. Sensory perception of the skin decreases, leading to increased risk for injury.

Vitamin D synthesis declines with aging; outdoor activity benefits older adults by reducing the likelihood of inadequate levels of this vitamin.[44] Unfortunately, sun exposure is also associated with risks. Photoaging that is not due to physiologic skin aging produces cosmetically undesirable changes in skin, making it look wrinkled, yellow, and rough. These changes can sometimes be reversed by topical treatments with retinoic acid and refraining from sun exposure. Sunscreen with a high sun protection factor (SPF) should be applied liberally. The Skin Cancer Foundation considers SPF of 15 or higher acceptable ultraviolet B protection for normal everyday activity, and SPF of 30 or higher acceptable for extended or intense outdoor activity. Such sunscreens also provide some protection against ultraviolet A wavelengths, although the SPF rating refers only to ultraviolet B protection.[88]

Onychomycosis

Onychomycosis is nail infection caused by any fungus, including yeast and nondermatophyte molds. In one study, most patients were noted to have toenail involvement, mostly due to a dermatophyte.[58] Although onychomycosis is usually a cosmetic concern to patients, it can also cause physical discomfort. Toenails are most likely to give hikers problems in the wilderness. Risk factors that have been associated with onychomycosis include older age, tinea pedis, diabetes, and genetic predisposition.[49]

Potassium hydroxide examination of a scraping from under the nail is followed by culture as the general diagnostic approach. Traditional topical therapies are usually ineffective for clearing the primary infection; even oral therapy is associated with a high rate of treatment failure or reoccurrence.[34,56,57] Nevertheless, treatment is often dictated because morbidity associated with the infection, especially with comorbidities such as diabetes, is high. Oral terbinafine is considered first-line therapy because data suggest greater efficacy and fewer side effects.[59] Oral itraconazole is also effective. Onychomycosis should be treated in patients with a history of cellulitis or diabetes or those who are experiencing discomfort. During oral therapy, monitoring liver function is important because these drugs can be hepatotoxic. Newer therapies include laser application, broad-spectrum antifungals such as albaconazole, nail lacquers, or ionophoretic drug delivery, which is a low-level electrical current used to enhance absorption of topical medications.[13,104]

DENTAL ISSUES

Dentures are removable false teeth made of acrylic or metal. They fit snugly over the gums to replace missing teeth. Complete dentures are used when all the teeth are missing; partial dentures are used when some natural teeth remain. A dental bridge spans the gap created by one or more missing teeth. Bridges are contructed of two or more crowns for the teeth on either side of the gap. These false teeth are called pontics, and can be made from gold, alloys, porcelain, or a combination of these materials. The bridges are supported by natural teeth or implants.

Caring for dentures and dental bridges in the wilderness can be challenging. Common denture or bridge problems often stem from poor oral hygiene. To avoid problems such as gum and mouth irritation, stomatitis, or cheilitis, brush and floss often and use proper technique to keep dentures clean. Bridges rely on the health of surrounding teeth, so daily brushing is essential. Mouth infections can occur. Stomatitis is caused by *Candida* and often goes unnoticed until red lesions appear in the mouth. Cheilitis (also called cheilosis) is a painful infection that causes inflammation and cracking at the corners of the mouth, caused by overgrowth of yeast. Yeast can accumulate in moist areas of the mouth if dentures do not fit properly or are not properly cleaned and stored.

In addition to proper oral hygiene and making sure that dentures fit well, it is also important to maintain dentures. This includes not sleeping with dentures, handling them with care, and cleaning them daily. Tips for cleaning dentures in the wilderness include:

- Soak dentures overnight in a denture cleaner (warm water can be used as a substitute if no denture cleaner is available, but hot water that will alter the shape of the denture should not be used)
- Use a soft-bristled brush or special denture-cleaning brush to thoroughly clean dentures every morning before inserting them into the mouth
- Never use powdered household cleaners or bleach on dentures
- Never use toothpaste on dentures because it is too abrasive
- Lacking any proper cleaning solution in the wilderness, use a very small amount of soap and copious water

When dentures are not in the mouth, they should be stored in denture-cleaning solution or warm water. Carrying a small container for dentures when in the wilderness is the best way to keep them clean and safe when not in the mouth. In the event of serious facial injury, the first responder should examine the mouth carefully for fractures of dentures or displaced dental appliances, which could cause respiratory obstruction.

GASTROINTESTINAL DISORDERS

Among the most common gastrointestinal problems affecting older adults are constipation and diverticulitis.[85] Physical activity and a high-fiber diet reduce symptomatic diverticular disease.[1] Constipation is a frequent complaint among 33% of adults over age 60 years in the Western hemisphere.[32] A difference exists between the medical definition and an older adult's perception of constipation and their need for laxatives.[33] Normal frequency of bowel movements ranges from three defecations per day to three per week. Laxatives are used by 15% to 30% of elders on a regular basis. When such individuals find themselves in the wilderness, away from the convenience of their bathrooms, alteration in bowel habits may occur, sometimes to the point of fecal impaction. Diverticulitis may flare at such times, requiring dietary change, stool softeners, and antibiotics.[136] It is prudent to obtain a detailed history of bowel habits and medications before embarking on a wilderness venture. Dietary fruit, fiber, and grain combined with stool softeners for older adults during a wilderness adventure may help prevent fecal impaction, rectal fissures, hemorrhoid bleeding, fecal incontinence, and chafing.

Gastrointestinal disorders noted among older adults may include malignant disease of the colon and pancreas, gastric ulceration that may bleed, especially after nonsteroidal antiinflammatory drug (NSAID) ingestion, and *Helicobacter pylori* infection.[85] A surgical emergency may arise from an incarcerated or strangulated inguinal or ventral hernia.

In elders, diarrhea contracted in Third World countries may be severe, leading to dehydration, gastrointestinal bleeding, or perforation of a hollow organ.[129] Some evidence indicates that older travelers adhere more closely to sanitary water sources and are less likely to report diarrhea.[2] Exacerbations of diverticulitis or acute cholecystitis (with or without pancreatitis), persistent or unusual abdominal pain, vomiting, bleeding, or worsening dehydration are reasons for ending the adventure and initiating evacuation to medical care. When traveling to remote locales, it is prudent for certain expeditions to carry intravenous fluids and consider appropriate antimicrobial prophylaxis or medications for presumptive treatment of infectious diarrhea.

GENITOURINARY DISORDERS

Elders are particularly vulnerable to urinary tract disorders, including infection, obstruction, and ureteral, renal, or bladder stones. Bladder infection in women is common in remote settings because of dehydration and difficulty with hygiene.[66] Incontinence after hysterectomy is frequent, and discomfort from chafing and bladder infection may be present. It is prudent for women to carry medicated skin pads and cotton diapers. Men may incur bladder infection from benign prostatic hypertrophy with obstruction. Anticholinergic medications may induce bladder relaxation with subsequent retention. Terazosin hydrochloride, an α_1-selective adrenoreceptor blocking agent, may improve urine flow in instances of obstruction resulting from benign prostatic hypertrophy by reducing bladder outlet obstruction without affecting bladder contractility. On extended trips in remote areas, it may be prudent to carry a catheter for emergency relief of acute urinary retention.

Dehydration from fluid loss or inadequate oral replacement may precipitate infection. Adequate fluid intake is the key to genitourinary health in the wilderness, so it is particularly important to caution the participant about water quality.

MENOPAUSE

Menopause is a normal phenomenon associated with aging. Rather than occurring as a discrete, definable event, the menopause transition may take place over a period of several years, beginning around 40 years of age or as late as 55 years of age. Also known as the climacteric, this is a time in life when the opportunity for leisure activities may be greatest. Women who participate in wilderness activities must deal with the symptoms and somatic changes of menopause in addition to the physical and environmental stresses of the wilderness.

Symptoms that foretell the onset of menopause include vasomotor flushing, night sweats, insomnia, vaginal dryness, and variations in menstrual cycle and flow. Convention accepts that 12 months of cessation of menses is a confirmation of menopause.

As ovarian production of estrogen declines, the androgen : estrogen ratio changes dramatically. Gonadotropin feedback results in increased follicle-stimulating hormone in a range of up to 30 MIU/mL. Progesterone secretion is variable and may either increase or decrease.[132] Resulting anatomic changes from these hormonal alterations may affect lipid ratios, the coronary arteries, cortical and trabecular bone, and changes in body fat distribution with a shift in fat toward the center of the body. Changes in cognitive functions have also been reported.

In the past, hormonal replacement therapy was often used for menopausal or postmenopausal women or those who underwent surgical hysterectomy, based upon three classic indications: (1) for symptoms related to estrogen deficiency (vasomotor symptoms or genitourinary tissue atrophy); (2) to prevent or treat osteoporosis; and (3) for prevention of cardiovascular morbidity and mortality, all of which may occur in the wilderness setting. Hormone replacement therapy is much more controversial today because compelling research indicates that it significantly increases the risks of coronary artery disease and breast cancer.[25,114]

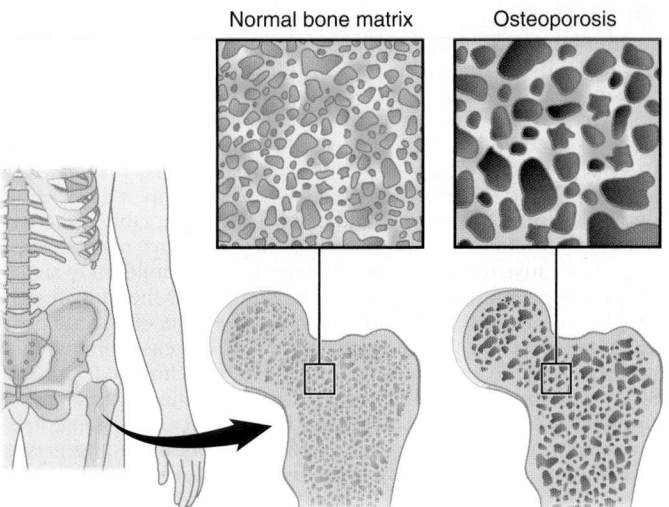

| Normal bone matrix | Osteoporosis |

FIGURE 93-2 This artistic rendition of normal and osteoporotic bone demonstrates the striking difference in bone density and histologic microstructure. *(Redrawn from Nucleus Medical Media, Kennesaw, Georgia; with permission from MedlinePlus Medical Encyclopedia: nlm.nih.gov/medlineplus/ency/imagepages/17156.htm.)*

MUSCULOSKELETAL DISORDERS

Musculoskeletal disorders are common among elders. Age-related musculoskeletal system changes include decreases in lean body mass and increases in total body fat, with loss of muscle mass due to decreasing numbers of muscle fibers; this also reduces muscle strength.[23] Another important physiologic change is loss of skeletal bone mass and density (osteoporosis; Figure 93-2). Osteoporosis occurs earlier in women, during the postmenopausal period, but by age 60 years, men and women have equal rates of bone loss. Bone integrity declines with aging. The combination of decreased bone integrity with diminishing bone mass reduces bone strength, increasing skeletal fragility and susceptibility to fractures caused by less kinetic injury than that needed to fracture bones of younger patients.[23] The lifetime risk of fractures in women after age 50 years is 17.5% for hip fractures, 16% for vertebral fractures, and 16% for wrist (Colles) fractures. Men over age 50 years carry a lifetime fracture risk of 6% for hip fractures, 5% for vertebral fractures, and 2.5% for wrist (Colles) fractures.[92]

The aging joint undergoes degenerative changes in its components. Cartilage has very little ability to heal. Injuries to cartilage tend to accumulate with age, leading to irreversible damage and osteophyte formation, developing into hypertrophic osteoarthritic changes in joints of the extremities and spine. Skeletal muscle undergoes age-related changes with loss of muscle mass. Changes in hormones, growth hormone/insulin-like growth factor-1, androgen:estrogen ratio, cytokines and growth factor, interleukin-6, and free radical production may be related to atrophic changes.[52]

Osteoarthritis, the most common form of arthritis, affects millions of U.S. older adults.[48] The prevalence of arthritis and osteoarthritis both increase with age.[52] In the wilderness, joint stress associated with extended hiking, injuries from repetitive motion, falls, and other trauma, when superimposed on the aging body, can induce functional impairments. Limitations in mobility from pain lead to loss of success or even to significant hazards during wilderness ventures.

A detailed musculoskeletal history and physical examination, with emphasis on prior and present symptoms, are of value for any older adult contemplating physical activity, and essential for any older adult planning remote wilderness activities. Treatment of arthritis in a layered stepwise manner begins with rest, acetaminophen, NSAIDs, and topical capsaicin.[52] Older adults must be cautioned about gastric irritation from NSAIDs and their danger in the presence of comorbid conditions and anticoagulant therapy. Intraarticular corticosteroids may help reduce inflammation.

Before and after the onset of symptoms, weight reduction and physical therapy, including progressive resistance training, aerobic conditioning, and spa therapy, may be effective in treatment or when preparing for a wilderness adventure. Corsets, braces, and canes prescribed by the treating specialist should be used, but the layperson is cautioned against self-prescription. A conditioning program before the wilderness adventure may help prevent musculoskeletal problems or may precipitate symptoms that alert the individual to a problem not previously recognized. It is better for symptoms to occur at home and serve as a warning for potential untoward events than for them to occur in a location far from medical care. Because degenerative changes in the lumbar and cervical spine may become symptomatic, it is appropriate to carry a backpack during a conditioning program before a hiking adventure. At least one, and preferably two, hiking sticks are recommended for hiking activities.

Arthroplasty

Age-related musculoskeletal changes lead many individuals to consider arthroplasty, a trend that is increasing around the world with an aging society.[36,69,117] Hip and knee replacement surgery are the most frequent joint replacement surgeries and are cost-effective.[116] However, patients vary in their willingness to undergo joint replacement when weighing anticipated benefits and pain alleviation against postoperative functional recovery and hospitalization.[72] Individuals engaged in high-impact activities such as mountaineering and skiing are generally motivated to resume outdoor activities as soon as possible following arthroplasty. Prosthetic joints have a reduced loading capacity without biologic adaptability. High-impact sports may increase wear, but regular and moderate activity increases the longevity of total hip arthroplasties.

Several considerations merit discussion with patients contemplating wilderness adventures prior to or following hip arthroplasty: First, experts generally agree that low-impact sports, such as level surface walking or bicycling, stair climbing, swimming, and golf, can be resumed within 7 months following surgery without restrictions. Higher-impact activities, such as mountaineering, are less liberally recommended.[135] Second, minimally invasive hip arthroplasty represents one surgical approach to reduce recovery times and safely permit resumption of high-impact activities, although orthopedic studies do not report long-term outcomes.[112,121] Third, patients and surgeons should inform the rehabilitation team of the objective to return to high-impact activities, such as mountain sports, during the postoperative recovery phase. Patients should not anticipate becoming involved in a high-impact activity after joint replacement unless they were engaged in that same activity prior to arthroplasty. Fourth, in planning wilderness adventures following hip or knee replacement, patients should avoid routes with foreseeable hazards, such as ice or slippery slopes that lead to hard falls. Although each postarthroplasty patient's capacity to engage in high-activity sports should be assessed individually, general contraindications to participation in these activities include revision surgery, prior prosthesis dislocation, deep wound infection, prosthesis instability, osteoporosis, significant pain with sports practice, or gluteal muscle insufficiency.[112]

Spinal Stenosis

Spinal stenosis is the clinical syndrome of neurogenic claudication secondary to narrowing of the lumbar spinal cord canal, and manifests as lower back pain with radiation to the legs; this impairs walking.[79] Narrowing can occur in the central spinal canal or in the neural foramina. Pain is exacerbated by lumbar extension and improved with lumbar flexion. Patients are comfortable sitting and less comfortable with prolonged walking. Weakness that limits function is uncommon. The sensitivity of computed tomography scanning or magnetic resonance imaging for lumbar spine stenosis exceeds 70%.[41] Twenty percent of persons over age 60 years have imaging evidence of spinal stenosis with no symptoms.[10,75] Most symptomatic patients managed nonoperatively report no progression over 1 year. Studies evaluating surgical decompression versus nonoperative management do not demonstrate a significant benefit with either approach.[74] Active postoperative rehabilitation improves functional recovery.[99] No studies have identified the ability to return to wilderness adventure pursuits with operative or nonoperative management of spinal stenosis.

Foot Problems

Bunions, or hallux valgus, are bony joint deformities at the distal base of the first metatarsal. The main sign of a bunion is the big toe pointing toward the other toes on the same foot, which may force the first metatarsal to protrude outward. Symptoms may include pain and swelling over the big toe exacerbated by pressure from wearing shoes; hard, callused, and red skin caused by overlap of the big toe and second toe; sore skin over the top of the bunion; and changes to the shape of the foot, making it difficult to find properly fitting shoes.

Treatment of bunions is generally first with properly fitted shoes, followed by orthotics, followed by surgery as needed.

FALLS AND RESULTING INJURIES

One of the most important sequelae of aging is an increased risk of falls and injuries related to falls. A fall is an unintentional, sudden descent to a lower level. Most geriatric falls occur from standing or when arising from a sitting position. Approximately 27% of independent community-dwelling adults over age 65 fall each year, and the rates of injurious falls are increasing faster than the overall rates of falls in older adults.[51] Falls occur due to a complex interplay of intrinsic factors (balance and gait stability, motor strength, reaction time, visual impairment) and extrinsic factors (environmental hazards, medication side effects). Most falls in community-dwelling adults occur in or around the home, and 20% cause serious injury.[97] Unfortunately, many elderly fall victims do not receive guideline-directed clinical care,[122] likely because of a combination of an inadequate capacity to predict future falls,[18,51] insufficient fall prevention interventions, and incomplete incorporation of implementation science principles into fall injury prevention efforts.[21] Multiple fall risk stratification instruments exist,[18,51] yet most remain without convincing validation. For example, in older adults presenting to an emergency department for evaluation after a fall, two instruments have been derived to risk-stratify individuals for future falls, but neither has been validated. Furthermore, neither instrument identifies individuals at increased risk for future falls; instead, both instruments only identify those at lower risk for future falls.[18] Nonetheless, one of these instruments is depicted in Box 93-9 because it may represent a simple method in the field to assess a future risk of falls in wilderness settings following an accidental standing-level fall.[22]

SENSORY SENESCENCE

Senses serve as a warning system for hazards in the wilderness. The five classic sensory "instruments" of vision, smell, taste, touch, and hearing (including its vestibular function) send signals to the central nervous system during interpretation of the physical environment. With age, sensory organs undergo functional degeneration. Up to 75% of elders have visual and auditory impairments not reported to their physicians. Changes may be subtle. The aging rule is that after age 30 years, there is a 1% loss per year of physiologic function in most organ systems.

BOX 93-9 Carpenter Instrument for Stratification of Six-Month Fall Risk Among Older Adults in the Emergency Department

Presence of nonhealing foot sore?
Any fall in last 12 months?
Inability to cut own toenails?
Self-reported depression?

More than one "yes" response in a community-dwelling older adult indicates an increased risk for falls.

Vision Issues

Acute, subacute, and chronic ophthalmologic issues should be evaluated by an ophthalmologist prior to embarking on a wilderness adventure.[96] Complete healing after eye surgery should be confirmed before the adventurer heads into the wilderness, especially with altitude changes. Visual acuity decreases because of morphologic changes in the lens, choroid, retina, macula, rods and cones, and other neural elements and by an increase in intraocular pressure. Night vision and color vision are notably decreased after age 50 years. Hypoxia, to which the elder's eye may be sensitive, may cause tunnel vision. This can be a valuable body signal, indicating an altitude that may be hazardous for the individual.

The most troublesome ophthalmologic effects of age are glaucoma and changes in refractive power. Increased intraocular pressure may be associated with halos and declining vision. This is a serious medical condition warranting continuing care by an ophthalmologist. Manifestations and treatment of far-sightedness range from purchasing a pair of nonprescription reading glasses to elaborate multipower prescription lenses and surgical correction of lens abnormalities. Negotiating rough terrain may be difficult while wearing bifocals. An older person walking on a wooded trail may be unable to see roots or rocks in his or her path. Trifocals and various lens designs have been tried, but experience suggests that trail glasses should be configured for distance, with separate reading glasses for close-up work such as map reading. Paradoxically, corrective lens use has been associated with an increased fall risk in multiple studies.[37,40,64]

Taste Issues

Some lingual papillae are lost because of age, diminishing the ability to taste. Salivary secretion is reduced. Dentures may cover secondary taste sites. Because olfactory bulbs also undergo atrophy with age, combined taste and olfactory sensory deprivation may account for decreased "pleasure" of trail food taste.

Touch Issues

In addition to assisting in the fine movement needed for technical work, sensitivity of touch against a hostile environment may be lifesaving. For example, conventional wisdom holds that the threshold for feeling a gentle breeze against the cheek is about 5 miles per hour. Impairment of cold awareness, which originates from stimuli at the end bulbs of Krause in the skin, along with age-attenuated metabolic adaptation to cold, can interfere with signals that alert an individual to assume cover from the weather.

Hearing Issues

According to the National Institute on Deafness and other Communication Disease, one-third of the population age 65 to 74 years reports difficulty hearing, a percentage of individuals that increases to 50% by age 75 years. Hearing loss can be debilitating, leading to increased risk of falls and less awareness of danger while driving because one is less aware of surroundings. Hearing loss can also lead to social isolation. Most cases of hearing loss in adults are from damage to the inner ear, with the two most common causes of that damage being aging and chronic exposure to loud noises. Middle and outer ear causes of hearing loss are often reversible and include such causes as impacted cerumen, fluid buildup from infection, or use of certain ototoxic medications. Older adults often have a mix of both types of hearing loss. Acoustic trauma may cause permanent reduction in sensitivity to high-frequency sounds. Failure to hear the "click pitch" of consonants may obscure communications because consonants often are found at the beginning and end of words. Speech in that circumstance may be heard as a continuous drone of vowels.

Problems with sound localization may result in loss of directional hearing. An aging brain cannot process confused sound signals as accurately. Add tinnitus and a hostile environment, and the hearing sense loses its value as an important survival tool. The vestibular apparatus is especially valuable for balance and stability; combined with proprioception, it may provide a "biologic gyroscope" of crucial importance. Increasing age seems to be associated with more frequent episodes of vestibular dysfunction, including vertigo.

Hearing aids dramatically reduce auditory deficits, improving the ability to hear, speak, and resume normal activities. Devices that amplify sound are integral to management of hearing impairment and include hearing aids, portable devices that can be used to amplify the sound coming from speakers at public events, and devices such as cochlear implants. Unfortunately, less than half of the elderly population with hearing impairment uses a hearing aid.[89,130] The first step in providing hearing amplification is to determine if the individual will benefit from hearing aids, based on audiogram results, lifestyle, motivation for use, and the individual's expectations.

A common misconception is that hearing aids restore normal hearing (much as corrective lenses restore sight). Hearing aids improve hearing by 30% to 60% at best. The goal of these devices is not to restore hearing but to significantly improve the ability to communicate and the quality of life. Digital hearing aids and the older analog hearing aids are the most popular hearing devices prescribed by audiologists. Hearing aids are useful for enhancing volume, sound direction, and pitch discrimination. Traditional analog hearing aids have limitations, especially in high-frequency ranges, obscuring click pitch discrimination. Digital devices, some with a range of 500 to 6000 Hz, provide increased clarity and sound quality and can enhance volume, as well as directionality, a valuable warning signal in the wilderness setting. Programmable units can be changed according to needs, such as listening to music and background noise reduction. Unilateral hearing loss can be improved by "cross-over" hearing aids. Less expensive versions available without a prescription include personal sound amplifiers, which are over-the-counter products with fewer features and less functionality than offered by more sophisticated fitted devices. However, personal sound amplifiers are significantly less expensive ($35 to $50 U.S. versus several thousand dollars) and a reasonable solution for individuals with a mild hearing deficit who are not ready for the high cost of a prescription fitted device, and may represent an alternative for wilderness travelers who do not want to risk losing expensive appliances. Travelers with significant hearing loss should consult an audiologist about anticipated outdoor activities to determine the best approach.

In the wilderness setting, a hearing aid user must be cautious to prevent sweat, rain, and other moisture from entering the components. A drying kit containing desiccating crystals is available and should be carried by anyone wearing a hearing aid while in the wilderness.

TREMORS

Tremors are rhythmic, involuntary body movements. Once considered a benign accompaniment of aging, tremors are now recognized as an abnormal and sometimes controllable component of growing older.[47] Essential tremor is the most common movement disorder; it affects up to 20 million individuals in the United States, with worldwide population prevalence estimates ranging from 0.4% to 6.3%.[93] Other forms of tremor include physiologic (low amplitude, high frequency), Parkinson disease, medication-induced, lesional (multiple sclerosis, stroke, cerebellar), dystonic, and psychogenic. Tremors can occur at rest or with activity. Physiologic tremors become more pronounced with stimulants (methylphenidate, dextroamphetamine, caffeine, nicotine, β-agonist inhalers), sleep deprivation, and stress. Ethanol withdrawal can also cause or exacerbate tremors. Action tremors include postural (noted while holding a position against gravity), kinetic (noted with volitional movement), intention (amplitude increases with targeted movement), task-specific, or isometric (noted with muscle contraction against resistance without movement). Tremor should be distinguished from other involuntary movement disorders, including dystonia, chorea, dyskinesia, myoclonus, and asterixis.[47]

Identifying the cause of tremor can be important before or during a wilderness adventure. Before traveling, understanding the cause, likely precipitants, and effective treatments for tremor empowers the screening physician and patient to plan proactively for fine motor tasks that might require companion assistance, medications, and situations to avoid. During the wilderness experience, recognizing the cause and preexisting nature of tremors permits medical personnel to avoid unnecessary evaluations for other causes while understanding available treatments, if necessary. The neurologic examination is essential to distinguish essential tremor from that of Parkinson disease, as well as other forms of movement disorder. Imaging and laboratory tests are generally not required to diagnose the origin of tremor. Bradykinesia, rigidity, masked face, muffled speech, or asymmetric arm swing or stride length while walking suggest Parkinson tremor. Over one million individuals live with Parkinson disease in the United States. The annual incidence for ages 64 to 74 years is 1%, compared with 3.1% for ages 74 to 85 years and 4.3% for persons over age 85 years.[43] Worldwide, there is a tendency for Parkinson disease to develop in individuals over age 60 years, males, and nonsmokers.[42] Differentiating Parkinson disease from essential tremor is quite important because Parkinson disease is an independent risk factor for falls.[51] In addition, Parkinson disease medication management using dopaminergic agents is quite different from that for other forms of tremor.[27] First-line medical management for essential tremor is propranolol or primidone.[47]

NEUROPSYCHIATRIC AND SUBSTANCE ABUSE DISORDERS

Situational stresses are often superimposed on environmental stresses during wilderness ventures. Difficulties with group interaction, changes in rational thought in individuals with organic brain disease, or behavioral upheaval from bipolar states can jeopardize health and safety not only of an individual but of an entire group.

Drug abuse[46] and alcohol use disorders[77] occur in aging adults. Subtle alcoholism may evolve into full-blown withdrawal psychosis during a hypoxic event or during extreme physical exertion. Drug use in elders may not necessarily be "recreational," but withdrawal from ethical drugs may still be quite severe.[35] Leaders of wilderness ventures must recognize the danger of disruptive psychiatric problems and attempt to prevent them by careful screening before the venture.

As people age, a variety of cognitive disorders becomes apparent, including progressive dementia, acute confusional states such as delirium, and cognitive disorders resulting from psychiatric syndromes. Table 93-6 distinguishes delirium from dementia.[62] The cause of dementia is not uniform and includes Alzheimer disease, cerebrovascular disease, Lewy body dementia, and frontotemporal dementia, as well as multiple forms of reversible "pseudodementia" such as vitamin B_{12} deficiency, depression, and hypothyroidism.[9,28] The most common cause of dementia is Alzheimer disease, afflicting 26.6 million individuals worldwide in 2006 and projected to affect 1 in 85 persons by 2050.[14] In the United States, the cost of dementia care was $604 billion in 2010; if these expenses represented the gross domestic

TABLE 93-6 Features Distinguishing Delirium From Dementia

Characteristic	Delirium	Dementia
Onset	Hours to days	Months to years
Course	Waxing and waning	Stable
Inattention	Present	Usually absent
Altered level of consciousness	Usually present	Typically absent
Disorganized thinking	May be present	Typically absent
Sleep-wake cycle	Present	Typically absent
Perceptual disturbances and hallucinations	May be present	Typically absent
Reversible cognitive decline	Usually reversible	Rarely reversible

Han JH, Wilber ST: Altered mental status in older patients in the emergency department, Clin Geriatr Med 29:101-136, 2013.

TABLE 93-7 Distinguishing Features of Different Forms of Dementia and Conditions That Mimic Dementia

Characteristic	Delirium
Alzheimer disease	Early: gradual memory loss with preserved level of consciousness, subtle language errors, worsened visual-spatial perception Midstage: apraxia, disorientation, impaired judgment Late stage: aphasia, apraxia, agnosia, inattention
Vascular dementia	Loss of cognitive function correlated with cerebrovascular events, stepwise deterioration; may present in individuals with "silent" strokes
Lewy body dementia	Mild parkinsonism with unexplained falls, hallucinations and delusions, fluctuating cognition, extreme sensitivity to extrapyramidal side effects of antipsychotic medications
Frontotemporal dementia	Onset often before age 60, language difficulties common, prominent personality changes often with behavior disturbances such as impulsivity or aggression
Depression, major	Anhedonia, hopelessness; diminished self-worth, appetite, and libido
Medications	Benzodiazepines, barbiturates, anticholinergics, other sedative-hypnotics
Traumatic brain injury	Features vary by site of injury; personality and mood changes common
Normal-pressure hydrocephalus	Gait instability, urinary incontinence, psychomotor slowing and apathy

Adapted from Blass DM, Rabins PV: In the clinic: dementia, Ann Intern Med 148:ITC4-1-ITC4-16, 2008, Table 1, p ITC4-5.

product of a nation, the nation would have the world's 18th largest economy.[140]

Table 93-7 differentiates the features of various forms of dementia.[9] Although the impact of various forms has not been formally evaluated in wilderness settings, theoretically, different issues can be anticipated in planning such adventures. Early Alzheimer dementia is characterized by gradual memory loss, language errors, and declining visual-spatial perception, so these individuals could manifest short-term memory deficits by failing to inform the wilderness medicine clinician about pertinent health issues or forgetting key recommendations before or during a wilderness adventure. Vascular dementia manifests as stepwise deterioration correlated with cerebral ischemic events; the specific cognitive deficit varies with the anatomic distribution of the ischemic injury. Lewy body dementia is characterized by Parkinsonism, frequent falls, hallucinations, and fluctuating cognition, all of which could present extreme hazards to a patient and travel companions during a wilderness adventure. Frontotemporal dementia often presents before age 60 years; memory is preserved early in the course of disease but personality changes, such as impulsivity and apathy, become apparent that may be hazardous during a wilderness adventure. By understanding the specific dementia diagnosis, wilderness medicine clinicians, patients, and their travel companions can plan adventures more appropriately, including activities to avoid, anticipated supervision requirements, medications to avoid, and communication requirements for outside clinicians who may need to care for acute illnesses or injury.

Early dementia is often undetected by primary care physicians without focused case finding.[17] In fact, the U.S. Preventive Services Task Force finds insufficient evidence to support routine cognitive screening in primary care settings.[106] However, focused cognitive screening may be important for older individuals planning a wilderness adventure. Cognitive symptoms may be precipitated in vulnerable individuals by physical or environmental stresses of the wilderness.[29] The two usual sources of information concerning the status of a patient are the patient's family and the patient herself or himself. It is rare for a family member to approach the physician with concerns about the cognitive function of a relative; thus, an interview and brief mental status testing using validated instruments should be included in the medical examination.[19] Multiple dementia screening instruments exist, none of which are diagnostic when used alone.[67] Several examples of validated and appropriately brief screening instruments and scoring instructions are provided in Box 93-10, including the informant-based AD8,[19] Short Blessed Test,[19,80] Brief Alzheimer Screen,[19,101] and Clock-Drawing Test.[109] An abnormal dementia screen should prompt referral to a neurocognitive psychologist or neurologist for definitive imaging and evaluation. Delirium screening tests differ from dementia screening tests.[141] Brief delirium screening tests appropriate for office or wilderness use include the Brief Confusion Assessment Method (Figure 93-3).[63] Acute delirium is a neurologic emergency and should prompt immediate evacuation to an appropriate medical facility. A cognitive interview should provide the examiner with insight into prior cognitive skills and personality traits to serve as a baseline. Included should be the nature of the patient's memory at that time, interval since onset of symptoms, nature of onset (slow or sudden), and current state of cognitive function. Initial laboratory testing for persons with abnormal cognitive screening should include a comprehensive metabolic profile, complete blood count, thyroid-stimulating hormone level, and vitamin B_{12} level; additional tests might include the rapid plasma reagin assay, HIV testing, toxicology and heavy metal screens, and erythrocyte sedimentation rate.[9]

PHARMACOLOGY, PHARMACOKINETICS, AND POLYPHARMACY

Older people are major consumers of all categories of medications. The health status and pharmacokinetics of elders influence drug choices, dosages, prospects for adverse reactions, and

---

BOX 93-10 Brief Dementia Screening Tests

AD8 Dementia Screening Interview
  If the patient has an accompanying reliable informant, the informant is asked the following questions:
  Has this patient displayed any of the following issues? Remember that a "yes" response indicates that you think there has been a change in the last several years caused by thinking and memory (cognitive) problems.
  Problems with judgment (e.g., falls for scams, makes bad financial decisions, buys gifts inappropriate for recipients)?
1. Reduced interest in hobbies or activities?
2. Repeats questions, stories, or statements?

3. Trouble learning how to use a tool, appliance, or gadget (e.g., computer, microwave, remote control)?
4. Forgets correct month or year?
5. Difficulty handling complicated financial affairs (e.g., balancing checkbook, figuring income taxes, paying bills)?
6. Difficulty remembering appointments?
7. Consistent problems with thinking and/or memory?
  Each affirmative response is 1 point. If the score is 2 or higher, the risk for cognitive impairment is considered high.

BOX 93-10 Brief Dementia Screening Tests—cont'd

Short Blessed Test

Instructions to the patient: Now, I would like to ask you some questions to check your memory and concentration. Some of them may be easy and some of them may be hard.

	Correct	Incorrect
1. What year is it now?	0	1
2. What month is this?	0	1

3. Please repeat this name and address after me:
   John Brown, 42 Market Street, Chicago
   John Brown, 42 Market Street, Chicago
   John Brown, 42 Market Street, Chicago
   (underline words repeated correctly in each trial)
   Trials to learn _____ (if unable to do in 3 trials = C)

	Correct	Incorrect
4. Without looking at your watch or clock, tell me what time it is. (If response is vague, prompt for specific response within 1 hour.)	0	1

5. Count aloud backward from 20 to 1. (Mark correctly sequenced numerals; if patient starts counting forward or forgets the task, repeat instructions and score 1 error.)   **0 1 2 Errors**
   20 19 18 17 16 15 14 13 12 11 10 9 8 7 6
   5 4 3 2 1

6. Say the months of the year in reverse order. (If the tester needs to prompt with the last name of the month of the year, 1 error should be scored; mark correctly sequenced months.)
   D N O S A JL JN MY AP MR F J   **0 1 2 Errors**

7. Repeat the name and address you were asked to remember.
   (John Brown, 42 Market Street, Chicago)   **0 1 2 3 4 5 Errors**
   _____, _____, _____, _____

			Final Item Score
Item	Errors	Weighting Factor	
1		× 4	
2		× 3	
3		× 3	
4		× 2	
5		× 2	
6		× 2	

Sum Total (range 0 to 28) =
0-4 = normal cognition
5-9 = questionable impairment
≥10 = impairment consistent with dementia

Brief Alzheimer Screen

Instructions to the patient: I would like to ask you some questions that ask you to use your memory. I am going to name three objects. Please wait until I say all three words; then repeat them. Remember what they are because I am going to ask you to name them again in a few minutes. Please repeat these words for me: APPLE TABLE PENNY
(May repeat names 3 times if necessary, repetition not scored.)

Did the patient correctly repeat all three words?	YES	NO
1. What is the date? (D)	Correct	Incorrect

2. Name as many animals as you can in 30 seconds. (A) _____ (number)
3. Spell "world" backward. (S)
   Number correct
   0 1 2 3 4 5
4. Three-item recall. (R)
   Number correct
   0 1 2 3

Brief Alzheimer Screen = (3.03 × R) + (0.67 × A) = (4.75 × D) + (2.01 × S)
A score of 26 or lower is consistent with dementia.
Clock-Drawing Test
Scores above 2 suggest dementia.

1. Perfect

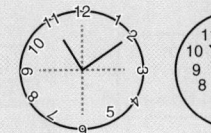

2. Minor visuospatial errors
   Examples
   • Mildly impaired spacing of times
   • Draws times outside circle
   • Turns page while writing numbers so that some numbers appear upside down
   • Draws in lines (spokes) to orient spacing

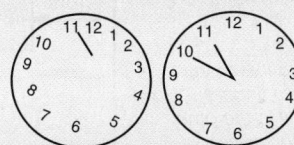

3. Inaccurate representation of 10 after 11 when visuospatial organization is perfect or shows only minor deviations.
   Examples
   • Minute hand points to 10
   • Writes '10 after 11'
   • Unable to make any denotation of time

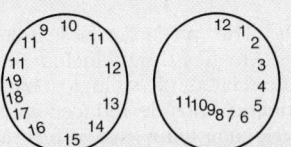

4. Moderate visuospatial disorganization of times such that accurate denotation of 10 after 11 is impossible.
   Examples
   • Moderately poor spacing
   • Omits numbers
   • Perseveration – repeats circle or continues on past 12 to 13, 14, 15 etc.
   • Right-left reversal – numbers drawn counter clockwise
   • Dysgraphia – unable to write numbers accurately

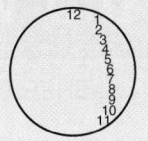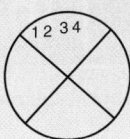

5. Severe level of disorganization as described in 4.

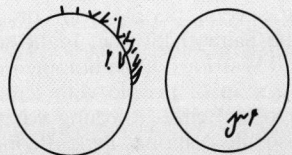

6. No reasonable representation of a clock Exclude severe depression or other psychotic states.
   Examples
   • No attempt at all
   • No semblance of a clock at all
   • Writes a word or name

Adapted from Carpenter CR, Bassett ER, Fischer GM, et al: Four sensitive screening tools to detect cognitive impairment in geriatric emergency department patients: Brief Alzheimer Screen, Short Blessed Test, Ottawa3DY, and the caregiver-completed AD8, Acad Emerg Med 18(4):374-384, 2011; and from http://tinyurl.com/ClockDrawingTest2015.

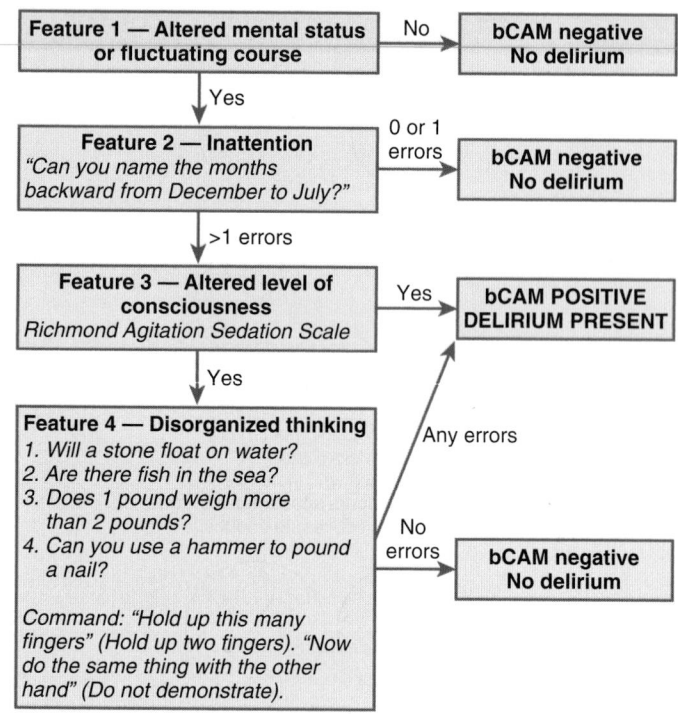

Feature 1 — Altered mental status or fluctuating course → No → **bCAM negative** No delirium

↓ Yes

Feature 2 — Inattention "Can you name the months backward from December to July?" → 0 or 1 errors → **bCAM negative** No delirium

↓ >1 errors

Feature 3 — Altered level of consciousness *Richmond Agitation Sedation Scale* → Yes → **bCAM POSITIVE DELIRIUM PRESENT**

↓ Yes

Feature 4 — Disorganized thinking
1. Will a stone float on water?
2. Are there fish in the sea?
3. Does 1 pound weigh more than 2 pounds?
4. Can you use a hammer to pound a nail?

Command: "Hold up this many fingers" (Hold up two fingers). "Now do the same thing with the other hand" (Do not demonstrate).

Any errors → **bCAM POSITIVE DELIRIUM PRESENT**

No errors → **bCAM negative** No delirium

FIGURE 93-3 Brief Confusion Assessment Method and Delirium Triage Screen. *(From Han JH, Wilson A, Vaselevskis EE, et al: Diagnosing delirium in older emergency department patients: validity and reliability of the delirium triage screen and the brief confusion assessment method, Ann Emerg Med 62:457-465, 2013.)*

therapeutic goals. The physician assessment of older adults before wilderness activities should include a careful review of all medications.[11] Age-related physiologic changes that may influence pharmacokinetics include reduced gastric acid production and altered gastric emptying that affect absorption; reduced splanchnic blood flow that affects first-pass (or presystemic) clearance; reduced body water, serum albumin, body fat, and body mass that affect protein binding; changes in hepatic size and blood flow that affect hepatic clearance; and reduced glomerular filtration rate and renal tubular function that affect renal clearance.[125] As a result, physicians recognize that it is usually prudent to begin with a lower starting dose and lower maintenance dose of certain prescribed medications in older patients.

CONCLUSION

Older adults are exploring wilderness environments with increasing frequency because they enjoy the fellowship, camaraderie, and adventure of these activities. Unfortunately, health risks associated with high-performance activities increase with age because of altered physiologic function, unrecognized impairments, or the cumulative effects of illnesses and their treatment. To reduce risks, appropriately screened older adults should be advised to temper their enthusiasm with the caution derived from the wisdom of experience. Importantly, a healthy respect for risk should not become a fear that precludes beneficial and desirable wilderness experiences. "Old" is not synonymous with "unable." The golden years hold many opportunities for adventure. We concur that the optimist sees sunset as sunrise in reverse.

ACKNOWLEDGMENTS

The authors are indebted to Kenneth Brummel-Smith, MD, and Alan Lazaroff, MD, from the American Geriatrics Society for sharing their experiences, advice, and wisdom in reviewing this chapter.

REFERENCES

Complete references used in this text are available online at expertconsult.inkling.com.

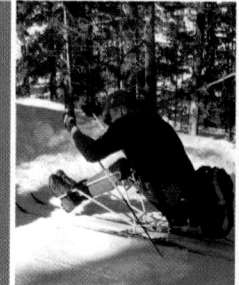

CHAPTER 94
Persons With Disabilities in the Wilderness

SUSAN B. SHEEHY

A blind climber reached the summit of Mt Everest. A group of people, including several people with disabilities, rafted the Middle Fork of the Salmon River in Idaho and camped on its banks. A Wounded Warrior double amputee completed a triathlon in Hawaii. A group of people with tetraplegic spinal cord injuries scuba-dived in Belize. A young paraplegic male scaled El Capitan in Yosemite National Park. People with disabilities who participate in outdoor activities express feelings of significant accomplishment and increased self-confidence. Those who accompany them express deeper understanding of the abilities of people with disabilities, feelings of personal growth, and gratefulness for being able to witness such significant and life-changing accomplishments.

Why would people with disabilities want to participate in wilderness activities? Their reasons are the same as those of able-bodied people. They want to experience the beauty of the wilderness and challenge themselves. They possess the same competitive spirit as do able-bodied people and often work diligently to build endurance, strength, speed, and the skills to transfer to wilderness activities. People with disabilities do not want the wilderness environment altered to meet their accessibility needs. Rather, they want it preserved in its natural state.[47] It is essential to provide information about opportunities for wilderness adventures, including organizations that have programs for people with disabilities and the types of programs they offer, places where disabled persons can obtain appropriate equipment and guides/helpers, preparations needed before a trip, and things to consider during a trip.

The benefits of wilderness adventures for people with disabilities are increased self-efficacy, deeper understanding of personal abilities and capabilities, improved functional independence, satisfaction in succeeding at challenges, new opportunities, greater social adjustments, improved physical and psychological health, building like-minded relationships, deeper appreciation for nature, the positive reactions of family members, and spiritual benefits.[63] People with disabilities who participate in wilderness activities experience outcomes that result in positive outlooks on their personal lives, work, and family relationships. *"Study results on integrated wilderness adventure programs indicate that these programs are successful therapies for persons with disabilities with low morale, showing an increase in self-awareness, personal goals, interpersonal relationships, and nature appreciation."[88]*

PEOPLE WITH DISABILITIES IN THE WILDERNESS

Wilderness is defined as a remote geographic location more than 1 hour from definitive medical care.[27] There are numerous wilderness opportunities available to people with disabilities. Many organizations offer equipment, guides, and activities for all ages and most levels of disability regardless of ability to pay. Many people with disabilities take part in activities that were previously thought impossible. Wheelchair users can rock climb and people with tetraplegia are able to swim with sharks. People with amputations can hike and run trails. People with hearing loss can raft rivers, and people with vision loss can climb mountains. These activities require significant knowledge about the disability and possible complications and detailed pretrip planning.

One cannot hike a trail if one cannot reach the trail. However, with adaptive devices, the trail may become accessible. As long as safety is a priority, people with disabilities can take part in many outdoor activities with the help of friends, guides, and adaptive equipment. Wilderness activities for people with disabilities can help to dispel the myths of limitations and reveal realities about abilities of people with disabilities (Figure 94-1).

PREPARATION FOR A WILDERNESS ADVENTURE

Many wilderness activities require no special adaptation for people with disabilities, and others can be adapted to meet special needs. Adaptive equipment should be viewed as assistive devices that help a person supersede physical limitations and/or provide extra safety measures.

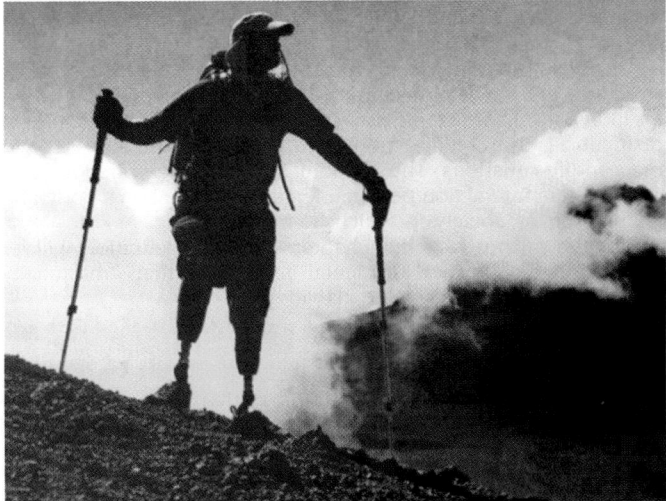

FIGURE 94-1 Double amputee hiking a mountain trail. (*Courtesy the Borden Institute, Ft Detrick, Maryland.*)

TABLE 94-1	General Considerations in Planning for a Trip by a Disabled Person
Topic	**Considerations**
Risk assessment and precautions	Diagnosis-specific potential complications during the trip
Limitations of the condition	Functional; cardiac; respiratory; elimination; psychological
Medical clearance	Physician authorization to participate
Personal care needs	Self-care; requires some assistance; requires complete assistance
Environmental hazards	Hazards specific to the condition
Available resources during the trip (including evacuation plan)	Location of resources; how to gain access to resources; time and distance to resources
Regulations specific to area	Special requirements or permits for use of assistive devices
Weather conditions	Short-term and long-range weather forecast; especially important for climbers, those using motorized vehicles, and those wearing prosthetic devices

As needed for an able-bodied person, it is important to train appropriately and specifically for any physical activity. It is essential to match adaptive devices to the participants' needs, body types, and skill levels. Inappropriate adaptive equipment (fit or type) may result in physical injury or adversely affect physical ability and inhibit performance. People with disabilities and chronic illnesses are at risk for any of the hazards usually associated with an activity, to which are added unique potential complications associated with a disability or illness. Health care providers accompanying people with disabilities in the wilderness must be equipped with the knowledge, ability, and equipment to manage all aspects of complications. In preparation for a safe and successful wilderness experience, plans must include anticipation of potential medical complications, knowledge of treatment protocols, and appropriate supplies, equipment, and medications.

Careful planning for the entire experience is essential and must include assurance that others on the trip are in agreement with and involved in pretrip planning. Anticipate any challenges that are expected or may occur and be prepared to address them, including emergency medications and treatment modalities related to the disability and an evacuation plan. Ensure that the person with the disability participates in planning for the trip to the extent possible, including taking part in a physical conditioning program and having a full understanding of physiologic limitations and risk factors (Table 94-1).

WORLDWIDE WILDERNESS PROGRAMS FOR PERSONS WITH DISABILITIES

Education and adventure groups have expanded their programs to be inclusive of people with functional limitations. There are customized programs that incorporate outdoor activities such as hiking, running, camping, rafting, canoeing, kayaking, caving, scuba diving, hunting, fishing, skiing, bicycling, and rock climbing. The national organization specific to a given disability or sport can be used as a reference point to explore wilderness opportunities, regardless of one's ability level.

In Canada, a nationwide campaign was launched by 250 communities with the goal of promoting public awareness of the fact that people with disabilities can function independently within society.[26] By 1992, more than 600 additional communities joined the effort. The British Mountaineering Council of the United Kingdom lists all the adventure clubs in the UK for climbers, hill

TABLE 94-2 Prevalence of Disability for Selected Age Groups: 2005 and 2010

Category	2005		2010	
	Number	%	Number	%
All ages	**291,099,000**	**100%**	**303,858,000**	**100**
Disabled	54,425,000	18.7	56,672,000	187
Severely disabled	34,947,000	12.0	38,284,000	12.6
Age ≥ 6 years	**266,752,000**	**100**	**278,222,000**	**100**
Needed personal assistance with an ADL or IADL	10,996,000	4.1	12,349,000	4.4
Age ≥ 15 years	**230,391,000**	**100**	**241,682,000**	**100**
Disabled	49,069,000	21.3	51,454,000	21.3
Severely disabled	32,771,000	14.2	35,683,000	14.8
Vision impairment	7,793,000	3.4	8,077,000	3.3
Severe vision impairment	1,783,000	0.8	2,010,000	0,8
Hearing impairment	7,809,000	3.4	7,572,000	3.1
Severe hearing impairment	993,000	0.4	1,092,000	0.5
Age 21-64 years	**170,349,000**	**100**	**177,295,000**	**100**
Disabled	21,141,000	16.5	29,479,000	16.6
Severely disabled	18,705,000	11.0	20,286,000	11.4
Age ≥ 65 years	**35,028,000**	**100**	**38,599,000**	**100**
Disabled	18,132,000	51.8	19,234,000	49
Severely disabled	12,942,000	36.9	14,138,000	36.6

Adapted from 2010 U.S. Census Report: census.gov.
ADL, Activity of daily living; *IADL,* instrumental activity of daily living

walkers, and mountaineers and indicates which ones are accessible to people with disabilities. There are many other organizations across the United States and in other countries that offer similar services. Outward Bound in the United States (outwardbound.org) offers an 8-day course, "Activate," where persons with disabilities can experience the full range of activities typical of an Outward Bound course for able-bodied people.

PREVALENCE OF DISABILITY IN THE UNITED STATES

Approximately 19% of the U.S. population (56.7 million people) lives with some level of disability. Of these, approximately 38.3 million have severe disabilities.[72] In addition, of the estimated 2 million young men and women who were deployed to Iraq and Afghanistan between 2001 and 2014, there have been more than 60,000 wounded in action (fractures, shrapnel wounds, burns, traumatic brain injuries, spinal cord injuries, loss of vision and/or hearing, amputations, and other injuries resulting in nerve damage and paralysis, leading to permanent disabilities).[18] These young men and women are returning home to heal and reintegrate. Wilderness activities can help to rebuild confidence, inspire undertaking new adventures, and regain a sense of self-worth (Tables 94-2 and 94-3).

TABLE 94-3 Number of People in the United States With Specific Disabilities (U.S. Census, 2012)

Specific Disability	Number of People
Vision loss	8.1 million
Hearing loss	7.6 million
Mobility challenges	30.6 million
Lifting/grasping challenges	19.9 million
Severe depression/anxiety	7.0 million

A BRIEF HISTORY OF DISABILITIES, DISABILITY TERMINOLOGY, AND DISABILITY ETIQUETTE

The definition and descriptions of disabilities have evolved over millennia. The ancient Greeks thought that sick people were inferior.[7] Plato determined that "deformed offspring" should be put away in some mysterious unknown place.[33] Early Christian doctrine spoke to a person being diseased as a means of purification on the road to grace and not to be disgraced or punished.[7] In the 16th century, however, Luther and Calvin preached that people who were mentally retarded or who had other disabilities were possessed by demons.[49] Hobbes wrote that 19th century Darwinism supporters believed that protecting the "unfit" would be a barrier in the process of natural selection of the fittest.[37]

The first mention of disabilities in the United States was in the Military Laws of the United States Army, where the policy for pensions and compensation for disabilities and deaths were defined. *Disabled* was defined as "any degree of personal disability which renders the individual less able to provide for his subsistence ... a disability may properly be said to be permanent when it appears to be chronic or of indefinite future duration."[46]

The word *disability* is defined as "an inability to pursue an occupation because of a physical or mental impairment; lack of legal qualifications to do something; disqualification, restriction, or disadvantage; incapacitated by illness or injury; physically or mentally impaired in a way that substantially limits activity, especially in relation to employment or education" (*Merriam-Webster,* 2015). Disabilities were previously defined as physical impairments that occurred as results of accidents, illnesses, and congenital conditions. Currently they are described as multidimensional, to include physical, mental, and emotional conditions that restrict both physical and social activities.

For purposes of this chapter, the Americans with Disabilities Act (ADA) of 2008 (a federal law) definition will be used. The ADA states that a person with a disability is "any person who has a physical or mental impairment that substantially limits one or more major life activities, has a record of such impairment, or is regarded as having such an impairment."[4] Several federal agencies have defined disabilities within the parameters of their targeted programs. The ADA Amendment Act of 2008 defined major life activities as "... caring for one's self, performing manual tasks, seeing, hearing, eating, sleeping, walking, standing, lifting, bending, speaking, reading, learning, concentrating, thinking, communicating, and working" ... and further defines a major life activity to include ... "the operation of a major bodily function, including but not limited to, functions of the immune system, normal cell growth, digestive, bowel, bladder, neurologic, brain, respiratory, circulatory, endocrine, and reproductive functions."[4]

The World Health Organization summarized its definition of disability with the following, "Disabilities is an umbrella term covering impairments, activity limitations, and participation restrictions. An impairment is a problem in body function or structure; an activity limitation is the difficulty encountered by an individual in executing a task or action; while a participation restriction is a problem experienced by an individual in involvement in life situations. Thus disability is a complex phenomenon reflecting an interaction between features of a person's body and features of the society in which he or she lives."[78]

For the purposes of this chapter, the ADA definition will be foundational: a physical or mental impairment that substantially limits one or more major life activities.[4]

DISABILITY ETIQUETTE

Most people with disabilities are sensitive to terms used to describe their disabilities. Terminology can cause one to place unintentional restrictions on persons with disabilities. Do not use terms such as "disabled person" or "the amputee." S/he is "a person with a disability" and/or "a person with an amputation." People in wheelchairs should not be referred to as "wheelchair bound." Rather, they are "people who use wheelchairs."

If you see someone with a disability struggling to complete a task, ask if you may be of help or how you can be of help; do not assume the person wants your help.

BARRIERS THAT RESTRICT PEOPLE WITH DISABILITIES

Barriers that restrict people with disabilities from wilderness activity participation may be personal, attitudinal, physical, or psychological. The person with a disability may lack self-confidence, have low self-esteem, be isolated, have difficulty finding acceptance, and lack the finances and transportation to avail themselves of wilderness programs and equipment (Box 94-1).

WILDERNESS LEGAL AND LEGISLATIVE ISSUES

In 1990, the Americans with Disability Act (ADA) was signed into law.[73] It is considered by many to be the civil rights legislation for people with disabilities that prohibits discrimination based on someone's ability and the person's need for accommodations and accessibility. The bill's primary sponsor was Senator Tom Harkin (D-IA), whose deaf brother was present in the Senate gallery when his brother's speech was simultaneously delivered vocally and in American Sign Language. The Act was further amended in 2008[4] to clarify definitions of disabilities and broaden the scope of the law.

Until the ADA was enacted, the Wilderness Act of 1964,[76] in particular Section 4C, had provisions that essentially prohibited people with disabilities who required motorized assistive devices from gaining access to wilderness environments. "… [T]here should be no temporary road, motor vehicles, motorized equipment or motor boats, no landing of aircraft, no other form of mechanical transport, and no structure or installation within any such area."

The ADA defines people with disabilities[73] as:
1. People with physical or mental impairments that substantially limit one of more of their major life activities
2. Those with a record of such impairments
3. Those being regarded as having such impairment

Disability is recognized by the ADA as a multidimensional and complex entity involving physical, emotional, and mental elements of functioning and includes restrictions in participation in social activities and being able to participate in the environment where one lives, works, and plays. This expanded definition of disability has led to federal funding to increase opportunities for people with disabilities so that they are able to be productive in the workplace and participate in physical activities. It provides for persons with disabilities being able to use necessary assistive devices, such as wheelchairs, respiratory assist devices, and service dogs, in the wilderness.

The National Council on Disabilities prepared a report for the President and the Congress on accessibility for people with disabilities as determined in Section 507(a) of the ADA and the Wilderness Act. "In general—Congress reaffirms that nothing in the Wilderness Act is to be construed as prohibiting the use of a wheelchair in a wilderness area by an individual whose disability requires use of a wheelchair, and consistent with the Wilderness Act, no agency is required to provide any form of special treatment or accommodation, or to construct any facility or modify any conditions of lands within a wilderness area to facilitate such use." It went on to say that the National Park System is not mandated to alter trails, campsites, footbridges, or make other accommodations within the National Parks and that motorized wheelchairs that are designed for indoor use and for use in pedestrian areas may be used in wilderness areas, but that other motorized vehicles, such as all-terrain vehicles, may not be used on lands within the National Wilderness Preservation System.[52]

Prior to the Wilderness Preservation Act and the ADA, the Architectural Barriers Act of 1968 and Section 504 of the Rehabilitation Act of 1973 (amended in 1978) mandated that the National Park Service policy would ensure the highest feasible level of accessibility in all visitor and management buildings and facilities, provided that the nature of both the area and the facility remained intact.

PREPARING PEOPLE WITH DISABILITIES FOR WILDERNESS ADVENTURES

In the spirit of the 1948 London Olympic Games, Sir Ludwig Gutmann from the Stokes Mandeville Hospital arranged for a wheelchair competition. It was met with such enthusiasm that the Stokes Mandeville Games became a regular occurrence and precursor to the current Paralympic Games,[17] which demonstrate the athleticism of people with disabilities.

Over the last several decades, people with disabilities have been encouraged to participate in more activities. There has been a great deal of focus on assisting people to achieve personal goals despite their disabilities, with much emphasis on exercise. The keys to safe wilderness adventures are maximizing functional independence and minimizing health risks. Prior to participating in a wilderness experience, a functional assessment should be completed to plan for the trip and to understand the limitations of the person with a disability. Of particular importance is assessment of the level of independence, ability to transfer or ambulate, level of mobility with and without adaptive equipment, and proficiency in using adaptive equipment.

Fitness programs for people with disabilities typically focus on improving cardiovascular endurance and increasing muscle strength and range of motion. The American College of Sports Medicine has proposed that problem-oriented exercise management be used to develop custom exercise programs for people with a variety of physical challenges and disabilities.[3] Problem-oriented exercise management uses exercise testing to identify physiologic dysfunction in such areas as mobility, strength, and endurance. It provides information to guide training and integrates exercise into medical management plans with attainable goals. A cognitive assessment may also be helpful to estimate the ability for skills acquisition and awareness of safety issues. A number of cognitive assessment tools, such as the Mini-Mental State Examination, are available for practitioner use.

The goals of preparticipation examinations are to assess, educate, and prevent. Appropriate physical screening must take place to rule out contraindications for a given activity and to develop a list of precautions. One should assess the physical capacity to understand and perform physical requirements for a specific activity; educate the participant about exercise preparation and potential medical risks; provide information to both participant and team members about the participant and potential safety risks; take into consideration the effects of medications; weigh the risks, costs, and benefits of a specific activity; and determine the costs associated with training requirements.

There are no standard guidelines that define how many people are required to safely support a person with a disability

Food
Water disinfection equipment
Diet-specific food
Electrolyte replacements

Gear
Durable medical equipment
Adaptive equipment for specific sports

Activities of Daily Living
Adaptive devices
Toileting supplies: catheters, suppositories, plastic bags with zip
   closure, wipes, toilet paper, nonlatex gloves

Sleeping
Appropriate padding; warmth, pillows, foam

Head
Hat, cap with visor, sunglasses, goggles, bandana

Upper Body Clothing
Long-sleeve shirts, warm jacket, hoods, scarfs, waterproof jacket,
rain poncho

Lower Body Clothing
Extra dresser , long underwear, waterproof pants, bathing suit, wet
suit

Hands
Mittens, gloves, hand warmers*

Feet
Socks (liners and heavy weight), foot warmers*

Accessories
Appropriate backpack, first-aid kit, insect repellent, sunscreen, lip
gloss, trash bags (heavy-weight black trash bags for insulation),
instruction books, emergency phone numbers, cell phone,
evacuation plan

Medications and Lotions
Prescription medications (bring extra), antibiotics, eye drops,
normal saline (for irrigation), anti-diarrheals, laxatives, analgesics,
antacids, topical steroids, sunscreen, antihistamine, epinephrine,
calamine lotion

*Do not use hand or foot warmers if there is loss of sensation and heat of the
pack cannot be sensed by the user

What are the potential complications of the disability or condition?
Which complications associated with this disability or condition
   commonly affect this individual?
How is the complication managed at home?
Will the wilderness environment be the cause of possible
   complications?
How can the complication be prevented?
What specialty equipment is necessary to prevent complications?

With solid planning, team support, and proper equipment, a wilderness experience for a person with a disability can be safe and enjoyable (Box 94-4).

CHECKLIST FOR PREPARATION FOR A TRIP

Participant education: Brief all participants about specifics of the trip. Provide details to the person with a disability.

Pretrip planning: Discuss every aspect of the trip and determine what needs to be accomplished prior to the trip, including physical preparation; obtaining permits, necessary equipment, supplies, assistive devices, and special equipment; and incorporating dietary requirements.

Prevention: Discuss possible complications specific to the participant's condition and plan preventive measures.

Fitness and conditioning prior to departure: Discuss the amount of time required and specific ways to prepare for the physical requirements of the trip.

Hygiene during the trip: Determine methods for toileting and bathing during the trip, to include any special equipment.

Guidance required during the trip: Determine who will be the designated guide for the disabled person and which members of the trip can provide extra assistance as needed.

Expectations: Review trip activities and minimum to maximum expectations of all members of the trip.

Medical clearance: Obtain medical clearance if necessary.

Immunizations: Ensure that routine immunizations are current and obtain those that are specific to the region in which the trip will take place.

Medications: Bring prescription medications, including broad-spectrum antibiotics, eye drops, antidiarrheal and anticonstipation medications, analgesics, antacids, and topical steroids.

Address fears: Address and acknowledge fears, such as concerns about snakes or other animals that might be encountered, heights, claustrophobia.

Protection: Bring supplies to prevent sunburn and protect the traveler from rain, snow, heat, cold, and insect bites. Plan for frequent rest stops within the time and mileage goals to allow for position changes and stretching. Apply sunscreen of the appropriate sun protection factor (SPF) to any exposed body areas. Cover large areas with clothing. Take extra precautions if the person is taking medications that increase sun sensitivity (see Box 94-2).

Check frequently for hypothermia
Maintain adequate hydration by drinking plenty of liquids
Maintain the same eating schedule as that of home
Bring enough medication to last at least 3 days beyond the length
   of the trip
Bring a family member or personal care attendant if needed
Let other key people who are not coming on the trip know the
   planned itinerary and overnight locations

National Center on Physical Activity and Disability, Department of Disability and
Human Development: General guidelines for an outdoor experience, 2011,
Chicago, 2011, College of Applied Health Sciences, University of Illinois:
nchpad.org.

in the wilderness. It may take as few as one or a team of five or more people, depending upon the person's disability, ability, and strength of each team member. Every situation is unique and therefore requires careful planning and determination of resources. Common sense thorough preplanning is essential.

The first step is to define the nature of the activity, where it will take place, and for how long it will last. One then factors in the season and weather conditions. Determine the accessibility to and within the site and any special equipment that may be necessary. Inquire about the condition of pathways and trails, especially for use by mobility assist devices.

There may be disruption of normal activities of daily living. This may result in frustration and discomfort. Ask the participant if he or she has had prior difficulties with heat or cold. Someone on the trip team must receive and understand all pertinent medical information, including medications, signs and symptoms, possible complications, and treatments. The caregiver should be prepared to make medical decisions and initiate interventions, and determine when medical evacuation is necessary. This necessitates knowledge about the rescue and evacuation process supported by possession of communication devices such as satellite phones or emergency personal radio beacons (Box 94-2).

Answers to these questions will assist trip planners in acting to prevent complications rather than needing to react when a complication occurs. Should a complication occur, they will be fully prepared to intervene (Box 94-3).

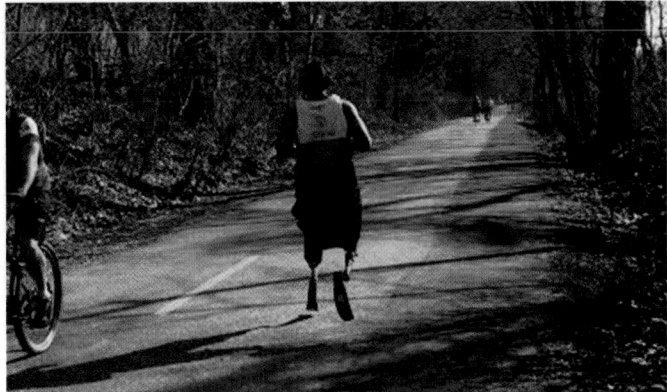

FIGURE 94-2 Master Sargent Cedric King, double amputee, training for a long-distance cross-country run. (*Courtesy MSGT Cedric King.*)

SELECTED DISABILITIES WITH WILDERNESS CONSIDERATIONS

PERSONS WITH CHALLENGES TO MOBILITY

There are more than 9.9 million people over the age of 15 years who have upper body mobility limitations, including difficulties with physical tasks. In addition, there are more than 30.6 million people over the age of 15 years who have lower body mobility limitations while walking, transferring, and climbing stairs. There are more than 3.6 million permanent wheelchair users, and 1.6 million permanent crutch, cane, or walker users.[72]

In addition to the source of the immobility, there are common secondary complications of immobility that include shoulder, back, and wrist pain, poor sleep patterns, spasticity, muscle atrophy, low self-esteem, depression, and weight issues. All of these should be considered when preparing for a wilderness adventure. Common wilderness challenges for people with mobility issues are steep grades, uneven terrain, adverse weather conditions, and inability to use assistive devices in certain situations.

PERSONS WITH AMPUTATIONS

There are more than 1.7 million people in the United States living with amputations (Figure 94-2).[79] Eighty-two percent of new amputations occur as a result of vascular system issues in the elderly population. Of these, 97% are lower extremity amputations, with 25% above the knee and 27.6% below the knee.[5] Other amputations occur as the result of trauma or malignant diseases. Amputations are one of the signature injuries of the recent Middle East wars due to mounted (in vehicles) and dismounted (foot patrol) encounters with improvised explosive devices. Approximately 1558 (6%) of the U.S. casualties in the post-9/11 wars resulted in amputations of one or more limbs.[15]

People who undergo amputations are fitted with prosthetic devices early in their recovery periods and discouraged from using wheelchairs except in cases of extreme fatigue or stump wounds. Because of the high volume of young military personnel with amputations, significant research has been focused on better design and function of upper and lower limb prosthetics. Due to rapid advances in technology, people with amputations are able to increasingly become more active and independent and are able to participate in a wide range of activities. Evolution of advanced prosthetics and bionics has enabled people with amputations to grasp, ambulate, run short and long distances, dance, hike, climb, cycle, swim, and do most anything able-bodied people can do (Figures 94-3 and 94-4).

The functional level of a person with an amputation depends upon several factors, including the initial injury, how the remaining part of the limb heals and how much is viable, the potential for rehabilitation, type of prosthetic that is appropriate for the patient, and joint function as it relates to the wound.[16,35] Age, rather than level of amputation, appears to be what influences

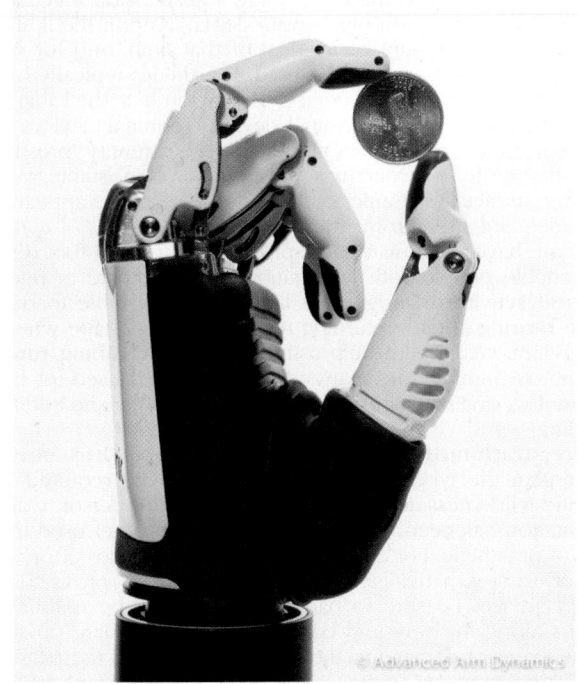

FIGURE 94-3 The bebionic hand. (*Courtesy Advanced Arm Dynamics.*)

participation in wilderness activities. The functional level also depends upon the psychological response of the person to the injury, because losing a limb is a very personal loss and adjustment to the loss often takes time. Early engagement in activities often affects the outlook and willingness to continue to participate in such activities.

Prosthetics

Most limb prosthetics have a socket that connects to the residual limb and transmits forces associated with movement. The limb

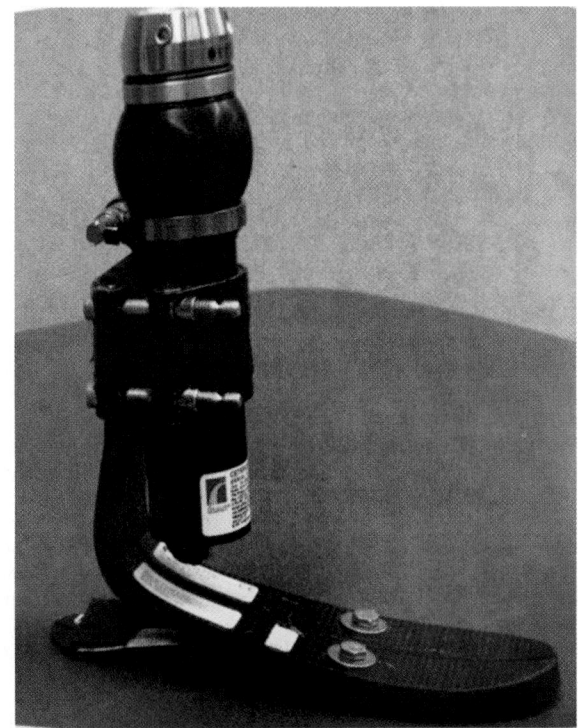

FIGURE 94-4 Dynamic-response prosthetic foot. (*Courtesy Diest and Associates Prosthetic Centre, Pretoria, South Africa, and Össur, Inc.*)

prosthetic attaches to the body using a suspension mechanism. The type of suspension mechanism depends upon the limb that is affected, the amount of residual of that limb, and for which activities the prosthetic will be used. Prosthetics typically have a pylon, joint, and terminal device. The pylon is a shell that connects the socket to the terminal device. Terminal devices have different functions. For example, lower extremity prosthetics have five basic foot functions: shock absorption; stable weight-bearing surface; anatomic joint function; cosmetic appearance; and adequate strength for the activity.

There have been many new prosthetic knee and foot designs that enable people with amputations to participate in rigorous physical activities. Designs are lightweight and able to deform when bearing a load, returning to their original shape when the load is lightened. There are prosthetics for rock climbing, running, cycling, swimming, and many other activities. If used for hiking or running, one may consider using larger sockets and additional padding.

Preparation of Prosthetics Before a Trip. It is important to preplan the types of prosthetics that will be required for a specific wilderness adventure, ensuring that the person with the amputation has been fitted and has had time to get used to that type of prosthetic. For questions about specific types of prosthetics for various activities, one should consult a prosthetist for expert advice. Be sure to pack tools that may be required for repairs along the way and consider bringing a spare prosthetic in the event of damage to the original one. Keep the prosthetic dry if it is not meant for water sports. Elastomeric skins are available to cover and protect prosthetics.

A good way for someone with an amputation to condition aerobically without high impact to the residual limb is cycling or swimming. There are several different types of swimming prosthetics, making it easier to maintain parallel trunk and shoulders, to propel, and to enter and exit the water. Most below-the-knee swim prosthetics are hollow and fill with water when submerged to decrease buoyancy. A hole drilled in the ankle area allows water to drain upon exit from the water. Upper extremity prosthetics have similar use principles as lower extremity prosthetics. Above-knee swim prosthetics have quick-release lock mechanisms that allow the user to walk on land. Many persons with amputations prefer to swim without a prosthetic device. It is possible to use swim fins with certain water prosthetics.

Check all prosthetic components frequently. Consider a change of training routine prior to the wilderness adventure in order to adapt to a new prosthetic. Ensure that the fit and suspension are good and that the prosthetic has the proper amount of shock-absorbing capacity. If more-rigorous-than-normal activities are required, the person with the amputation should train accordingly. If a new prosthetic device is required, be sure it is used prior to the trip to ensure proper fit and comfort.

Adaptive devices are available for various sports, such as skiing, using a three-track ski or single ski (sit-ski, monoski, or regular ski with two outriggers) that can be used both by amputees and by people with paraplegia. With appropriate training, proper assistance, and adaptive equipment, healthy people with amputations may develop the ability to perform almost any wilderness activity (Figure 94-5).[21]

Discomfort Caused by Prosthetics. Swelling of the distal segment of the residual limb is usually due to a socket that is too tight, causing venous outflow obstruction. If the socket is too loose, swelling will occur to fill the empty space. Protection of the skin under the prosthetic depends upon the specific construction of the prosthetic. Some prosthetics employ a traditional stockinette, some use silicone "socks," and others use a vacuum technique that suspends the stump without the distal part of the stump touching prosthetic material. If blisters or abrasions occur on the stump during the trip, remove the prosthetic and treat the injured area immediately. The prosthetic should not be worn until the blisters and/or abrasions are treated and deemed safe to bear pressure and friction. An alternate form of mobility, such as a wheelchair, must be provided.

Causes of prosthetic discomfort can be poor fit, inadequate suspension, and shock-absorbing qualities less than what are

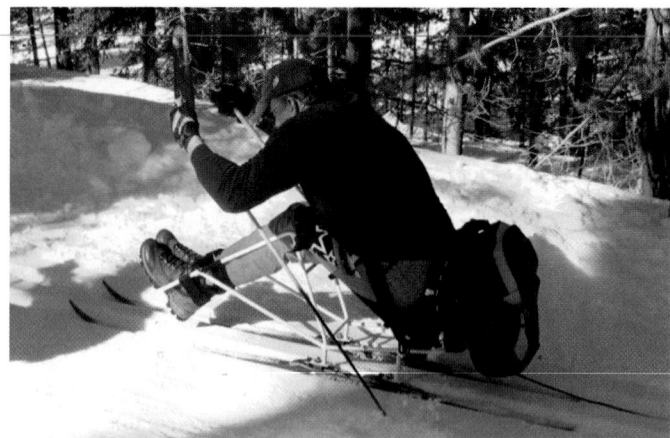

FIGURE 94-5 Single-track cross-country skier at Ski for Light, 2005. (*Courtesy Craig Gray.*)

required for a particular sport, any of which can result in blisters, abrasions, pressure sores, edema, and back pain.

As with any other athlete, be cognizant of hypothermia or hyperthermia and various forms of dehydration. Because of an absent limb, especially a lower limb, temperature control may be challenging, because excessive perspiration may occur on other parts of the body, resulting in hypothermia and dehydration. Replace wet clothing and stump socks with dry apparel, and pay particular attention to fluid intake and systemic hydration.

PERSONS WITH CEREBRAL PALSY

Most people with cerebral palsy have muscle imbalances, difficulty with balance and posture, and vision, speech, and swallowing issues. They are readily prone to dehydration and exhaustion. Many have cognitive disabilities; others have excellent cognition but lack the ability to communicate via speech. If speech recognition or simulation devices are available and accompany the participant on an adventure, ensure that a battery source is available for the duration of the trip.

Trip Preparation

Persons with cerebral palsy require varying levels of assistance depending upon the severity of their condition. It is essential for persons who wish to participate in wilderness activities to prepare for the trip by exercising to strengthen muscles, increase range of motion, and increase endurance levels. Seventy-five percent of people with cerebral palsy are independent with activities of daily living, mobility, and communication.[74] The Cerebral Palsy International Sports and Recreation Association developed a classification system based on functional abilities.[13] The classification system also includes other conditions characterized by nonprogressive brain lesions, such as stroke, brain injuries, and tumors.

Challenges During the Trip

Low-intensity exercises, such as walking, may prove to be much more intense for people with cerebral palsy. They are more likely to injure the shoulders, hands, knees, and ankles.[67] They are also more prone to dehydration and exhaustion due to the excess energy required for simple physical activities and needed to overcome increased tone. Dehydration commonly leads to constipation, electrolyte imbalance, muscle inefficiency, and renal insufficiency. Be particularly cognizant of the need for frequent hydration, and ensure that there are ample fluids available. Pace activities to avoid exhaustion, which may lead to decreased muscle coordination. Select activities that can be adjusted in intensity and pace, such as walking, hiking, backpacking, swimming, and cycling, and take frequent rest stops.

PERSONS WITH MULTIPLE SCLEROSIS

There are approximately 400,000 people in the United States living with multiple sclerosis and approximately 10,000 newly diagnosed cases each year. It most commonly affects people between the ages of 18 and 50 years. Symptoms may be blurred vision, balance issues, weakness in extremities, numbness, tingling, vertigo, spasticity, cognitive impairment, emotional changes and depression, altered gait, and problems with balance, coordination, bladder control, and sexual function The course of the disease is variable, ranging from death within 5 years (5% of people diagnosed) to one "episode" in a lifetime.[55]

Preparation for and Challenges During the Trip

Prior to a wilderness trip, physical conditioning to improve endurance is essential. During the trip, avoid elevated body temperatures and excess humidity, because both have been associated with worsened symptoms of multiple sclerosis. Cold temperatures may cause an increase in spasticity and other symptoms. Mobility and cognition problems may be exacerbated during a trip, so be prepared to provide an alternate mobility modality, such as a wheelchair.

Bladder issues typically involve urinary frequency, retention, and/or incontinence. Be prepared to manage these situations, especially when restrooms are not readily available. Consider urinary devices specifically designed for use during travel, such as the Lady J and Freshette. Additional disposable bowel and bladder management devices can be found at www.traveljohn.com.

PERSONS WITH SPINAL CORD INJURIES

There are approximately 276,000 people in the United States living with spinal cord injuries (SCIs) (Figure 94-6), and 12,500 new cases each year. Seventy-nine percent are males. The average age at injury is 42 years, due to the high number of elder persons who sustain SCIs as a result of a fall. However, the largest percentage is typically young adolescents to young adults.[56]

Injuries range from cervical to thoracic to lumbosacral injuries. People with injuries in the cervical area typically have tetraplegia, affecting the upper extremities, lower extremities, chest, and abdomen (including bowel and bladder). Injuries at level C4 or higher may affect a person's ability to breathe without assistance due to loss of diaphragmatic innervation. Spinal cord injuries in the thoracic and lumbar regions usually result in paraplegia, affecting the abdomen (including bowel and bladder) and lower

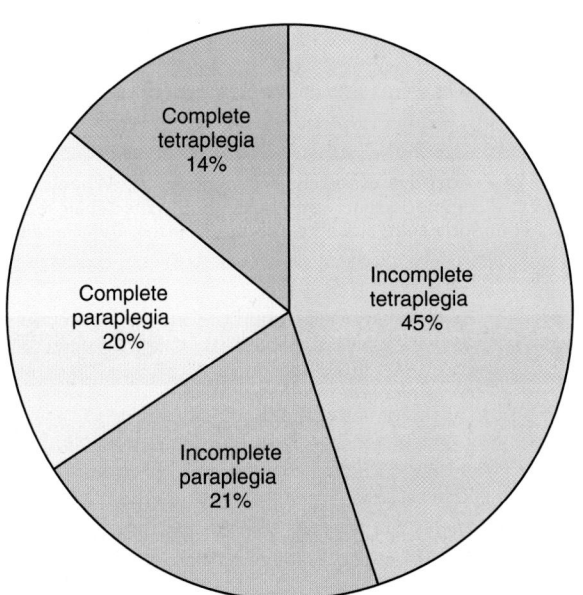

FIGURE 94-6 Types of spinal cord injuries.

extremities. If the SCI is complete, there will be no distal motor or sensory function. If the injury is incomplete, there may be some motor and/or sensory function at or below the level of the injury. The extent of recovery depends upon the extent of damage to the spinal cord.

Trip Preparation

Because of advances in adaptive equipment and rehabilitation programs, with preplanning, people with spinal cord injuries can now be safely and actively involved in many types of wilderness activities.

If a mobility device will be used, consider how the device will be broken down or compactly packed to allow for transport. If flying, contact the airline to obtain information about size specifications and limitations, and to obtain a "medically necessary" tag so the equipment does not count against the allowed baggage amount. Check with wilderness areas to ensure that mobility devices are permitted. Special permission may be required for use of power wheelchairs or other mobility assist devices. Bring inflatable mattresses, material for extra soft sleep surfaces and padding, and medications that are prescribed, intended for a bowel regimen, and needed for emergency purposes.

Training before the trip should focus on cardiovascular conditioning using such equipment as hand cycles, VitaGlide, or NuStep, strength and endurance training, and familiarity with equipment that will be used during the trip. New equipment should be broken in before the trip. Each member of the team should plan to spend time with the person with the disability prior to the trip so that familiarity and comfort are not issues during the trip. Identify roles and responsibilities and learn about the specific needs of the individual. Pretrip planning includes discussions with the participant about the current skin condition, how the person handles urination and a daily bowel program, and if the person will require a care provider during the trip.

Challenges During the Trip

Secure the paralyzed areas of the person, such as a limb or the upper body, to the equipment to avoid inadvertent injuries, and recheck them frequently. Pad equipment straps, such as climbing harnesses, parachute harnesses, scuba buoyancy-control devices, and other unpadded straps, to avoid pressure injuries. Protect sleep pressure areas and remember to clear stones, twigs, and other debris from sleep areas.

Protect the skin from dryness by applying moisturizer each night, paying particular attention to the hands and fingers. Ensure that gloves are durable and intact, fit well but are not constricting, are soft and smooth on the inside, and are warm and water repellent. Mittens are warmer than gloves but are not as flexible for various purposes. Carry several pairs of gloves, and change them if they become wet. If hands become cold, small hand warmers or heat packs can be used (never directly against the skin) to provide warmth. Pay special attention to the hands; check for dryness, hangnails, cuts, open scrapes, and bruises.

Persons with SCIs may have lost the sensation to cold and may therefore need protection from frostbite. Ensure that clothing and other protective equipment provide warmth and functional usability. It may be necessary for someone with an SCI to wear clothing and shoes or boots of a larger size than usual so that layers of clothing or socks can be worn underneath to provide insulation. Frequent checking of hands, fingers, feet, and toes for warmth and adequate circulation is essential. Remove any wet clothing, socks, and foot gear immediately. Take extra caution around the campfire to prevent burns to areas that lack sensation. Do a complete visual skin inspection at least once a day. Maintain medication routines and remember to pack special dietary foods. Dietary intake should be kept as close to normal as possible to avoid changes in bowel function. Changes in activity, fluid intake, and food intake may cause diarrhea or constipation. If new foods are necessary for the trip, they should be introduced into the diet well in advance of the trip.

Despite one's best efforts, the wilderness activity may disrupt a regular SCI bowel program. Factors that may influence the desire to maintain a regular bowel routine are wearing multiple layers of clothing and not wanting to undress, necessity to pack out all human waste, lack of private space, and being otherwise occupied. Fecal elimination in the wilderness can be well managed with preplanning and practice. Most manual wheelchairs can be adapted to become commodes. The chair seat fabric can be cut to accommodate the size of a toilet seat–sized hole. The edge of the fabric should be stitched or enforced with duct tape to avoid fraying. Velcro is sewn around the edges of the seat where the "cover" will be attached. The hole can be covered by using fabric of the same type and size as the original seat to cover the entire seat base, attached with Velcro tape to cover the hole. A padded cushion is placed on top of the cover. When needed as a commode, the user is transferred off the chair, the padded cushion and "cover" are removed, and the user is returned to the chair prepared to urinate or defecate (Figure 94-7).

Several options can be employed to collect the feces, urine, and wipes. If it is not in an area where waste must be carried out, the commode seat can be placed over a pit or cat hole. If a pit is not permitted, urine and feces can be collected in a large plastic bag under the chair. The bag can be draped over a bucket for stability. Light-weight absorbent kitty litter can be placed in bags prior to the trip to absorb odor and liquids. Carry biodegradable toilet paper, wipes, and sanitary products. Anything not biodegradable must be packed out. If the participant uses a power wheelchair, converting it to a commode chair will not possible due to the chair components located directly under the seat. Consideration should be given to bringing a manual chair that has been converted to a commode chair, or a portable commode to which the participant can be transferred, for toileting.

Special consideration must be given to maintenance of normothermia, protection of skin, bowel and bladder programs, and prevention and treatment of autonomic dysreflexia. Attention should be given to body areas that lack sensation, especially at pressure points. Do not use chemical heat packs on areas that lack sensation. Frequent (every 30 minutes) weight shifts are essential to prevent pressure sores.

Autonomic dysreflexia, also known as *hyperreflexia,* is a life-threatening medical condition that requires immediate intervention. Autonomic dysreflexia is an exaggerated and unopposed sympathetic response to a noxious stimulus below the level of the injury that results in extreme hypertension, sudden-onset severe headache, and diaphoresis above the level of the injury. It may occur at any time in people with SCIs at or above the level of T6. Untreated or delayed treatment of autonomic dyslexia may result in cerebral or subarachnoid hemorrhage.

Recognize the signs and symptoms and be prepared to intervene immediately (Boxes 94-5 and 94-6).

Other potential complications of SCIs that may occur in wilderness environments are pneumonia, atelectasis, pressure sores, lower extremity edema, deep vein thrombosis (DVT),

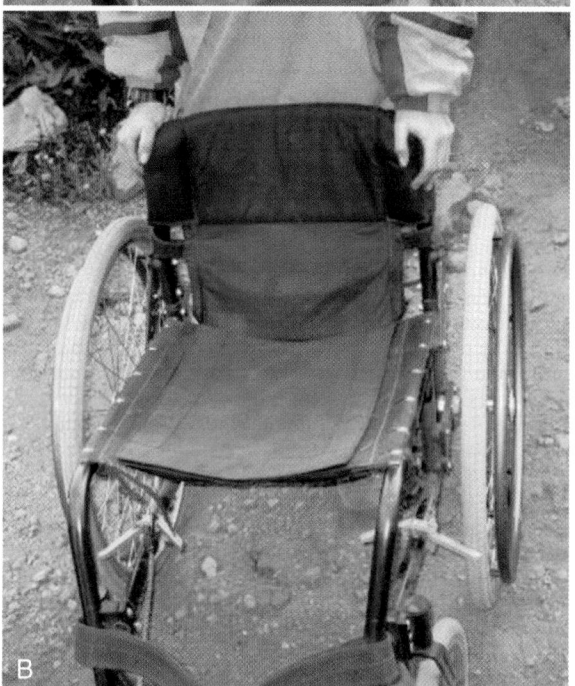

FIGURE 94-7 Adaptive wheelchair commode. **A,** Wheelchair seat modified to a commode seat; open position. **B,** Wheelchair seat modified to a commode seat; closed position. *(Courtesy Jeff Pagels.)*

BOX 94-5   Common Causes of Autonomic Dysreflexia

Bladder distention
Fecal impaction or constipation
Tight shoes or belt
Ingrown toenail
Insect bite
Exposure to extreme temperatures
Menstrual cramps
Intercourse
Pregnancy, labor, ectopic pregnancy, ovarian cyst
Vaginal inflammation
Appendicitis
Renal calculi
Gallstones

BOX 94-6   Emergency Interventions for Autonomic Dysreflexia

Sit the person as upright as possible
Eliminate the cause of the dysreflexia as soon as possible
Always check for a distended bladder and empty as soon as possible
Loosen belt or any tight clothing and remove shoes
Give nifedipine (Procardia) 10 mg initially (swallow capsule whole) or nitroglycerin 0.4-mg spray (metered dose) or sublingual tablet
Consider clonidine (Catapres), captopril (Capoten), prazosin (Minipress), or labetalol (Normodyne) as directed

urinary tract infection (UTI), hypothermia, and heat-related illness. Pay particular attention to respiratory effort, because most people with complete cervical injuries have compromised breathing resulting from loss of function of thoracic and abdominal muscles. Coughing and clearing the airway may be extremely difficult. DVT prevention includes adequate hydration and range-of-motion exercises, or repositioning legs to a nondependent position. Sitting in a position where the legs are dependent for long periods of time results in stasis and increased potential for DVT.[67]

Bowel and bladder management of SCI patients in the wilderness requires strict adherence to a schedule. Options for bladder management are intermittent catheterization using hydrophilic-coated catheters, indwelling catheters, or external "Texas" catheters. Catheterization techniques such as the Credé maneuver are not ideal in wilderness settings. In order for intermittent catheterization to be successful, the urethral sphincter must remain constricted to retain urine while the bladder remains relaxed to be able to collect urine. Participants may be taking oxybutynin chloride (Ditropan) or tolterodine tartrate (Detrol) to relax the bladder.

If intermittent catheterization is selected as the bladder regimen of choice, pay strict attention to urinary output at each catheterization to determine the appropriate amount of fluid intake to avoid dehydration or overdistention of the bladder. Catheterization frequency may require adjustment based on increased fluid intake or excess fluid loss as a result of exercise or perspiration and/or diuresis due to exercise or altitude. The urinary volume per catheterization should be below 500 mL. If urinary leakage occurs between catheterizations, the cause may be UTI, bladder or sphincter problems, or a change in fluid intake amount. Handwashing using soap and water, antiseptic wipes, or waterless hand sanitizer is key to prevention of UTIs. Catheters should be hand washed with soap and water, air dried, and stored in paper (not plastic) bags if reuse is the plan.

Consider using touchless catheters. A touchless catheter is contained within a collection device. It becomes lubricated as it passes through the prelubricated outlet on the collection bag prior to insertion through the urethra. After draining the bladder, the catheter is withdrawn and slipped back into the collection bag. The bag is recapped and the entire bag and contents can be discarded in accordance with wilderness protocols.

Reflex voiding can be accomplished in males if there is an intact sacral micturition reflex. Bladder filling triggers sacral efferent nerves to cause involuntary bladder contractions. Voiding occurs because of intermittent sphincter relaxation during bladder contractions. A condom catheter (Texas catheter) is worn at all times and is the collection device of choice. The collection device should be cleaned or changed once a day and the penis washed and allowed to dry for 20 to 30 minutes before reapplication of the catheter. Secure the drainage tube carefully and change the connection site each day if taped to the skin. Complications may include a leaking condom, skin breakdown, UTI, urethral fistula, inadequate bladder emptying, high intravesical voiding pressures, and autonomic dysreflexia.[43]

If there is detrusor sphincter dyssynergy, suprapubic bladder tapping, using an alpha-adrenergic blocker (e.g., tamsulosin HCl [Flomax], doxazosin [Cardura], or terazosin HCl [Hytrin]), botulinum toxin injections, urethral stents, or sphincterotomy may be necessary to effectively empty the bladder.

PERSONS WITH SENSORY CHALLENGES

Persons With Vision Loss

Low-vision blindness is one of the most common disabilities; in the United States, it occurs in 3.3 million people 40 years of age or older.[72] Low-vision blindness is defined as a best corrected vision of less than 20/40 in the best eye. Blindness is defined as a best corrected vision of less than 20/200.

Leading causes of vision loss are refractive errors, corneal opacities, age-related disease such as macular degeneration, cataract, and optic nerve atrophy. Refractive errors may be due to nutritional deficiencies or metabolic abnormalities. Corneal opacities occur due to infectious diseases and trauma.

Decreased visual acuity usually results in less physical activity, fewer social interactions, emotional distress, and a lesser quality of life.

Trip Preparation. People with vision loss may be able to perform at high physical levels with the help of adapted equipment guides, support groups, and social training opportunities provided by people who understand the disability. Prior to the trip, spend time with the participant to learn about his ability to navigate independently, or with assistance or guidance, and the types of assistive devices required. Determine how instructions are to be given and what special equipment will be required.

Exercise may increase visual loss due to glaucoma; it will improve when exercise ceases. Be particularly aware that altitude blindness may occur, especially above 10,000 feet, if ascent occurs in the early postoperative period following LASIK surgery.

Challenges During the Trip. Allow the participant as much independence as is safe. Be the person's eyes and vividly describe surroundings, including obstacles and hazards. Offer assistance, support, and encouragement.

Users of long white canes often experience neck and back pain due to the need to maintain an extreme upright "stiff" posture, shoulder pain while keeping the elbow in toward the chest, and wrist and forearm pain due to repetitive "sweeping" of the cane using only a forearm and wrist movement (Figure 94-8). These anatomic position requirements make it difficult to hike steep or winding trails without assistance.

Persons With Hearing Loss

Thirty-six million people in the United States (17% of the population) have some degree of hearing loss. High-frequency hearing loss has occurred in 26 million Americans between the ages of 20 to 69 years because of frequent sustained exposure to loud sounds or noises produced by leisure or work activities.[72] This is especially prevalent in military members and veterans who have been exposed to blasts and loud explosions.

People who are hard of hearing (at 35 to 69 decibels) have difficulty understanding speech without use of an assistive device.

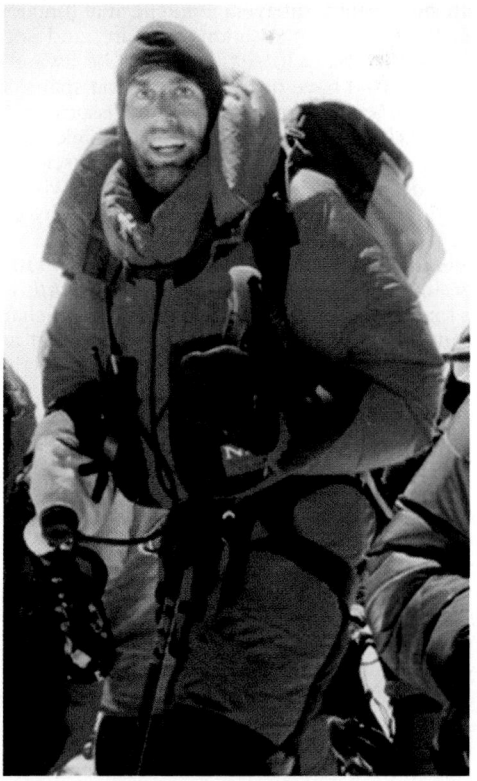

FIGURE 94-8 Eric Weihenmayer, the first blind climber to reach the summit of Mt Everest. *(Courtesy Luis Benitez.)*

The National Institute on Deafness and Other Communication Disorders reports that only 1 in 5 people who would benefit from a hearing aid wears one.[54] People who have hearing loss above 70 decibels are unable to understand speech, so hearing aids are not helpful for them.[8]

Trip Preparation. People with hearing losses may use lip reading, sign language, hearing aids, or other amplification systems. In preparation for a wilderness trip, consider the type of communication assistance needed. Someone with hearing loss may also have difficulty with speech, reading, and writing. Visibility of lips for lip reading or hands for signing may not be possible much of the time in the wilderness, so it is essential that alternative forms of communication, such as touch, large hand signals, or writing, be determined prior to the trip.

Challenges During the Trip. During the trip, communicate face-to-face whenever possible. Gain the person's attention using a light touch on their shoulder or via a visual sign. Maintain eye contact whenever possible and speak directly to the listener. Remember to bring along writing utensils and a white board or paper. If you do not understand what the person is saying, do not pretend that you do. Let the person know you do not understand. Make sure that assistive devices and/or amplifiers are available if appropriate. Carry extra batteries for hearing aids. If possible, try to have an interpreter available. Learn to take your time communicating and allow time for questions.

American Sign Language (ASL) is the most common form of sign language. It is important to know that ASL is not English; it is a visual and spatial language that has its own grammatical structure and syntax. Learn some common signs and/or bring along a poster with pictures of common hand signals that can be selected and a finger alphabet that can be copied (Figure 94-9; https://www.start-american-sign-language.com/).

PERSONS WITH COGNITIVE CHALLENGES

Approximately 15.2 million adults (6.3% of the U.S. population) experience cognitive, mental or emotional disabilities; 1.2 million adults and 2.7 million children have learning disabilities.[72]

Persons With Intellectual Disabilities

People with significantly subaverage intellectual functioning may have difficulty with communication, self-care, and social skills. They may lack the ability to self-direct and be aware of health and safety issues, and have decreased attention spans. They may require assistance with adaptive skills, safety issues, and environmental concerns. They may not be able to think concretely or determine risks. In addition, they may have muscle imbalances and balance and posture issues. They often have visual, speech, and swallowing challenges and are prone to dehydration and exhaustion.

The International Classification of Diseases, 11th edition, working group proposes replacing the term *mental retardation* with terms for a group of developmental conditions characterized by significant impairment of cognitive functions that are associated with limitations of learning, adaptive behaviors, and skill.[36] Four levels of severity reflect the extent of intellectual impairment: mild, moderate, severe, and profound.

People with intellectual development delays may exhibit delays in language development, poor memory skills, difficulty in understanding and practicing social skills, difficulty in problem solving, and delays in self-care and self-help skills. They may also lack social inhibitions.

Wilderness experiences for people with intellectual development disorders may enhance learning opportunities and produce enjoyable interactions with the environment. Levels of support vary across four dimensions: intellectual ability and ability to adapt, psychological and emotional concerns, physical and health concerns, and environmental issues.

Persons With Autism

Autism spectrum disorder and *autism* are terms used for a range of complex disorders involving brain development. Adults and children with autism spectrum disorder may exhibit the following characteristic verbal and nonverbal communication difficulties:
- Difficulty with social interactions
- Repetitive behaviors
- Intellectual disabilities
- Lack of motor coordination
- Physical health issues (e.g., sleep and gastrointestinal disturbances, ranging from constipation and diarrhea to inflammatory bowel disease) and seizure disorders

They may excel in such areas as art, math, music, and visual skills; 40% of persons on the autism spectrum have exceptional visual, musical, and academic skills. Approximately 25% are nonverbal, but can learn to communicate via other means, such as pictures, sign language, and electronic word processors.[6]

One in 68 U.S. children has been identified as being on the autism spectrum. It is more common in male children than females, with data showing 1 in 42 boys and 1 in 189 girls diagnosed. The apparent recent increase is partially explained by the increased awareness of the presence of autism leading to recognition and diagnosis, and possibly by environmental factors. A very small number (15% to 20% of cases) appear to be associated with genetic conditions, such as fragile X syndrome, tuberous sclerosis, Angelman syndrome, and chromosome 15 duplication.[12]

Many people with autism have difficulty understanding that others have a different perspective from theirs. They have difficulty understanding emotions or gestures, such as hugging or smiling, and are hypersensitive or hyposensitive and underresponsive to touch or sound. Many who speak do so in single words or repeat the same phrases, or repeat what they hear (echolalia). Mildly affected children may develop a significantly large vocabulary but have great difficulty forming sentences and maintaining significant communication. Movements, gestures, and expression may not match what they are thinking or saying. Repetitive behaviors may include body rocking, hand flapping, jumping, running, rearranging objects, and repeating words or phrases.

Trip Preparation. Children and adults on the autism spectrum range from mildly to severely affected. Consideration of inclusion in a wilderness activity must be carefully discussed and meticulously planned by the person's family in collaboration with any counselor and healthcare team. A wilderness adventure may not be appropriate for everyone. That being said, an outdoor adventure or wilderness experience may be of great value in providing learning and socialization opportunities in a natural environment. The focus of an outdoor adventure program for a person with mild autism might include maximizing social skills and experiencing new physical challenges. Personal motivation may be one of the primary obstacles to ongoing participation and cooperation in a given activity.

The wilderness may provide a positive environment for occupational and physical progress and for opportunities that promote growth and development in social and emotional aspects of life. Levels of support with wilderness activities must be considered based on the level of intellectual functioning and adaptive skills, psychological and emotional status, physical and health status, and appropriate environmental opportunities for the person in question. Support may be required intermittently, on a limited basis, or continuously.

Persons With Traumatic Brain Injuries

Traumatic brain injuries (TBIs), ranging from mild to severe, are among the most common causes of disability in the United States. They occur in more than 2.5 million people annually, resulting in 2,213,000 emergency department visits, 283,630 hospitalizations, and 52,844 deaths.[12,64] TBIs may have accompanying emotional and behavioral issues, mobility disorders, and cognitive impairment, including memory deficits, impulsive behaviors, emotional instability, and sleep disorders. In addition, 30% to 60% of persons with TBIs have traumatic vestibular pathology and may experience vertigo, disequilibrium, ataxia, and reduction of perceptual function.

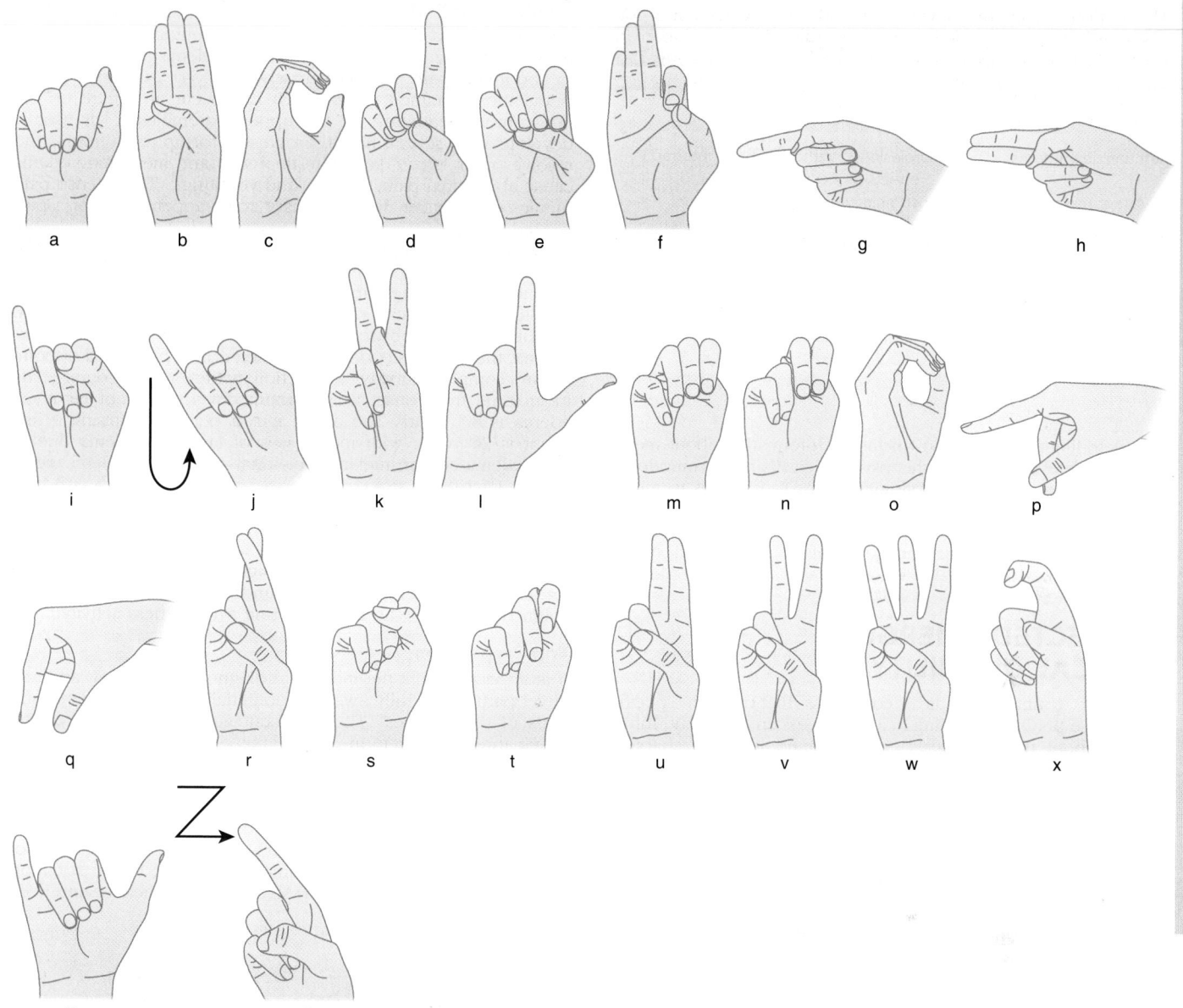

FIGURE 94-9 American Sign Language Finger Alphabet. *(Courtesy National Institutes of Health.)*

Trip Preparation.   It is essential to have complete information about the person and the injury. Medical clearance must be obtained prior to a wilderness adventure. Ensure that all instructions are written as well as spoken. Bring a full supply of all routine and other necessary medications. Be familiar with effects and side effects of medications, especially psychopharmacologic medications.

People with mild TBIs may become fatigued more easily in the wilderness. Pretrip aerobic and neuromuscular training may improve locomotor efficiency. Offering outdoor opportunities may lead to better physical and emotional well-being and reduce concurrent depression.

Ataxia may interfere with a person's ability to independently perform activities of daily living, such as eating, hygiene and toileting, and ambulation. Adaptive equipment, such as weights or cuffs, may help with stabilization. Medications, such as propranolol, used to treat tremor, may limit the cardiovascular response to exercise and therefore may be somewhat counterproductive when rigorous exercise is expected.

PERSONS WITH PSYCHOLOGICAL OR MENTAL HEALTH CHALLENGES

The DSM-5 development website (dsm5.org) proposes the following new definition of mental disorder: "A behavioral or psychological syndrome or pattern that occurs in an individual that reflects an underlying psychobiological dysfunction, the consequences of which are clinically significant distress (e.g., a painful symptom) or disability impairment in one or more important areas of functioning. It must not be merely an expectable response to common stressors and losses (for example, loss of a loved one) or a culturally sanctioned response to a particular event (for example, trance states in religious rituals) that is not primarily a result of social deviance or conflicts with society."[21]

Trip Preparation

The success of a wilderness adventure for someone with a psychological or mental health condition will more likely be ensured if there is thorough pretrip preparation that includes gathering

TABLE 94-4 Psychopharmacologic Medications and Possible Side Effects

Psychopharmacologic Medication	Side Effects
Antianxiety agents	Drowsiness; withdrawal; heightened effects of alcohol
Antidepressants	Insomnia; weight gain; dizziness
Antipsychotics	Gait disturbances secondary to tardive dyskinesia; dehydration
Beta-adrenergic blockers	Slow heart rate
Fluphenazine (Prolixin)	Increases blood pressure
Haloperidol (Haldol)	Increases heart rate; possibly lowers blood pressure; prolongs QT interval

complete illness information (including information about medications), determination of the psychological and/or emotional status, assessment of the physiologic status as it relates to medications and medication side effects, and the person's understanding of what such a trip entails. Psychopharmacologic agents may affect cardiovascular function, gait, balance, and mood (Table 94-4).

A SELECTED EMERGENT MEDICAL DISABILITY

There are countless medical conditions that require specific knowledge pertinent to being in a wilderness environment. Information about these diseases can be found in other chapters throughout this book. No matter what the disease, common sense should prevail. Pretrip planning and conditioning are always essential. Select activities that are safe and within the abilities of the participant. Consider complications that might occur while in the wilderness and be prepared to intervene. Always think about hypothermia and hyperthermia, dehydration, sunburn, and heat-related illnesses. Carry routine and other medications that may be required. Plan for adaptive equipment and dietary and elimination needs. Obtain medical clearance when required. Be realistic and honest with the participant and be certain to keep expectations within abilities and limitations.

HEREDITARY ANGIOEDEMA OCCURRING IN THE WILDERNESS

Hereditary angioedema (HAE), somewhat similar to idiopathic anaphylaxis, manifests gradually, painfully, and without the typical anaphylactic dermatologic manifetations.[28] It is caused by deficiency of the plasma protein C1 esterase inhibitor (C1-INH).[10,28,79] The term *angioedema* describes localized, transient, and episodic edema of deeper layers of the skin and intestinal mucosa characterized by abdominal pain, skin swelling, and life-threatening upper airway obstruction.[10] Abdominal pain is caused by plasma extravasation and subsequent edema in affected areas.[32] Episodes may be provoked by emotional stress, infection,[24] localized trauma (particularly injection of a local anesthetic, surgery, or trauma),[42] dental procedure,[39] or exercise.[22] Laryngeal edema can cause immediate life-threatening airway obstruction and is the major source of death related to HAE. Historically, the mortality rate for attacks involving the upper airway exceeds 25% in untreated patients.[39] Angioedema manifests as swelling of the extremities in 75% of patients and swelling of the face and throat in 30%. Abdominal pain is a major symptom, occurring in 93% of patients.[39]

HAE has been estimated to affect 1 in 10,000 to 50,000 persons.[22,28,38] Although urticaria and angioedema are common problems that affect nearly 20% of the general population, true HAE occurs in approximately 2% of the U.S. population.[22] Of all angioedema cases, HAE accounts for only 0.4%.[39]

Clinical Presentation

The skin and gastrointestinal tract are more commonly involved than the airway. The ratio of laryngeal edema to skin swelling to abdominal pain is approximately 1 : 70 : 54. Cutaneous edema is the most common symptom. It can occur anywhere on the body, most frequently on the upper extremities.[22,24] It usually develops over several hours, progresses for up to 36 hours, and resolves over 1 to 3 days. Intestinal wall and mesenteric edema cause abdominal pain, nausea, and vomiting.[65] The intense pain mimics peptic ulcer disease, biliary colic, appendicitis, or a perforated viscus.[22,39]

Edema of the upper airway is a medical emergency. The individual with airway involvement may first experience a full or tight sensation in the throat, dysphagia, and/or voice alteration.[21] Soft tissue edema can rapidly result in stridor and progress to complete airway obstruction.[22] Following the onset of angioedema, the patient's condition can deteriorate from mild discomfort to complete airway obstruction within a few hours.[29] The mean time from onset to maximum development of laryngeal edema is 8.3 hours. The mean age of persons suffering a first event is 26 years, with most cases of laryngeal edema due to angioedema occurring in individuals ages 11 to 45 years (Figure 94-10).[29]

The relatively short time frame from onset to full development of symptoms is significant for wilderness adventurers because the first episode of HAE-associated laryngeal edema may occur as a result of increased exercise. Significant advanced planning for airway management must be undertaken for anyone with a diagnosis of HAE who is considering a wilderness activity.

Trip Preparation

It is imperative that the individual diagnosed with HAE and any travel partners be fully aware of potential triggers and manifestations of the disease.[10] The treatment goal is prevention of the attack through long-term prophylaxis. Therapeutic intervention after an episode begins is aimed at reducing the severity and/or duration of the attack. Because vigorous activities can precipitate HAE attacks, Elnicki[22] suggests that a short course of anabolic steroids before the planned event may lessen frequency and severity of attacks.

A person with HAE must immediately bring to the attention of travel partners the onset of HAE symptoms. The face and neck

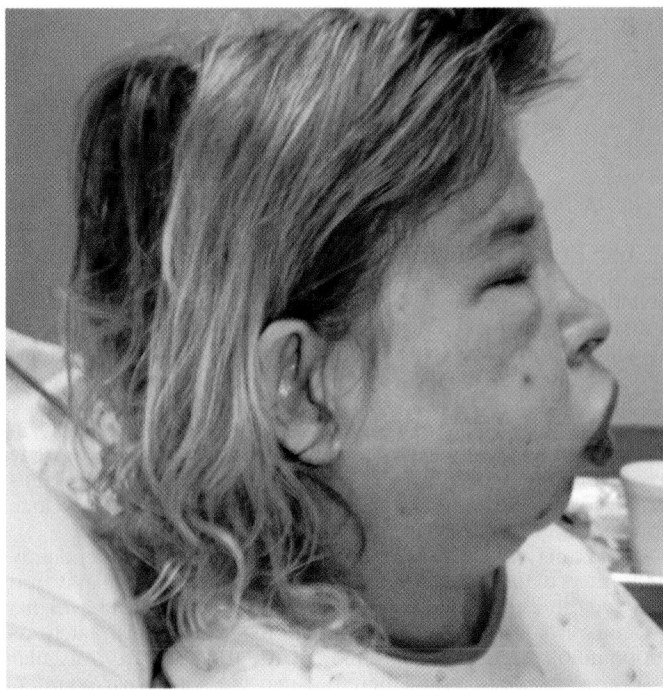

FIGURE 94-10 Hereditary angioedema, lateral view. (*Courtesy Sheryl Olson.*)

should be closely monitored for edema and signs of airway involvement. The possibility of the need for airway management should be anticipated. Nebulized racemic epinephrine is the emergency drug of choice to decrease upper airway edema during an attack. For anaphylaxis-induced hereditary angioedema, inject epinephrine intramuscularly into the anterolateral mid-aspect of the quadriceps muscle. Initial dose for adults is 0.2 to 0.5 mL (0.2 to 0.5 mg) of 1:1000 dilution (1 mg/mL) epinephrine. The dose may be repeated every 5 to 15 minutes. Pediatric dose is 0.01 mg/kg (to a maximum total dosage of 0.3 mg) of 1:1000 dilution epinephrine.

If airway obstruction becomes severe and ventilation is compromised, advanced airway management, such as endotracheal intubation or cricothyrotomy, becomes essential. Even though an individual with known HAE may have had no prior episodes of airway obstruction, it is advisable to have equipment, medications for rapid sequence intubation, and a person skilled in their use, available for advanced airway management. Rapid sequence intubation allows for an opportunity for early intubation if the person is in severe respiratory distress while still conscious and alert.

The trachea should be intubated before laryngeal edema becomes so severe that intubation would be very difficult to achieve. If endotracheal intubation cannot be achieved, cricothyrotomy is the emergency surgical procedure of choice. This must be accompanied by airway maintenance equipment once the procedure has been completed. Without life-saving airway maintenance, the first episode of HAE may be fatal.[10]

Acute management goals include decreasing duration and severity of signs and symptoms after onset. An episode of abdominal colic may require narcotics to relieve symptomatic pain. Extreme edema of the extremities or abdomen may indicate vascular fluid loss. Intravenous fluid replacement should be considered. The awake and alert patient who does not have airway compromise or dysphagia should be encouraged to increase oral fluid intake until symptoms resolve.

An algorithm for treatment of HAE was developed in 2003 through consensus of European and North American investigators, patient care providers, patient group representatives, and individual patients.[11] Fresh frozen plasma would be the first-line intervention in a hospital setting. Anticoagulant therapy may prevent recurrent or ongoing thromboembolic occlusion of the circulation.[22] Heparin 30,000 units can be administered in aerosolized form via a nebulizer during an acute attack.[24]

At the first recognition of airway involvement, C1-INH concentrate, if available, should be given as soon as possible. In one study, use of Cinryze, a nanofiltered C1 inhibitor concentrate, when used in treatment of acute angioedema related to HAE, significantly shortened the median time to unequivocal relief of symptoms when compared with placebo. When used for prophylaxis, Cinryze significantly decreases the number of attacks.[80]

Long-term management of HAE consists of therapeutic prophylaxis to minimize frequency and severity of attacks. Individuals who experience frequent symptoms may require daily suppressive therapy with an androgen steroid, such as danazol (Danocrine), stanozolol (Winstrol), oxymetholone (Anadrol-50), or oxandrolone (Oxandrin). Persons with frequent severe attacks of HAE should be discouraged from participating in wilderness activities until the frequency of attacks is controlled.[45]

Challenges During the Trip

Known causative stimuli should be prevented or eliminated whenever possible. In the wilderness, it is especially important to pad pressure points that may trigger an acute attack. Every sport involves certain unique pieces of equipment that can result in pressure on parts of the body. When hiking or skiing, special attention should be paid to the feet. Trail shoes, hiking boots, and ski boots should fit well and be broken in prior to the wilderness adventure. Shoes and boots have tongue flaps and seams that may cause a pressure point. One-piece liners that are heat-molded to the foot and ankle eliminate pressure points. Check to ensure that socks are form fitting and wrinkle free.

Backpacks should be appropriately fitted. Waist belts should be wide and well-padded to distribute weight evenly, preventing pressure points on the iliac crests. Shoulder straps should be padded and fit the shoulders so as not to exert pressure on the axillae. A chest strap at the level of the sternum can aid in decreasing pressure of the lateral aspects of the shoulder strap. The backpack should be worn and gradually weighted during training, to increase weight and endurance tolerance.

River sports require use of helmets and paddles. Attention must be given to pressure points on the head, chin, and mandible. Gloves should be worn to protect hands from blistering during paddling.

ADAPTIVE SPORTS

Most outdoor activities have methods and adaptive equipment to make them available to persons with a disability. The website abilities.com has information on sports and sports organizations and clubs that have programs for people with disabilities, ability expositions around the country, and information about participating in sports activities, regardless of ability or experience level. The website nolimitstahoe.com lists several videos ("No Barriers," "Beyond Barriers," "Wheels of Fire," and "Courageous Climber") that demonstrate how people with disabilities participate in climbing, skiing, kayaking, surfing, sailing, diving, and hang gliding. Several selected outdoor sports are now discussed.

RIVER SPORTS: CANOEING, KAYAKING, AND RAFTING

Watercraft, such as canoes, kayaks, and rafts, offer opportunities for persons with disabilities to access wilderness environments and enjoy activities on lakes, streams, rivers, and oceans. If arm mobility is good, solo navigation in a craft may be possible. If arm mobility is not good, partnering with someone is an option. Before the wilderness experience, time should be spent at a swimming pool or small water space practicing entering and exiting the craft, navigating it, and learning and practicing what to do in the event of a capsize or ejection event. Ski or hiking poles may provide assistance with entering and exiting watercraft and the water.

Determination of the degree of difficulty of rapids or projection of wave size to be encountered should be made in advance. Regardless of size or degree, a personal flotation device and helmet should be worn at all times. Both of these items are mandatory on commercial whitewater activities. In a typical ejection situation in rapids, the person ejected is instructed to float on his or her back with legs together and feet forward.

If the person does not have leg movement, the common practice is to strap the legs together at the knees so that they stay together in the event of ejection, avoiding the possibility of legs getting trapped below the water's surface. A pull buoy can be attached to the strap. Do not tighten the strap to the point where circulation is compromised. Also, be sure to tuck in any loose ends of the strap.

Check frequently for cold water surrounding the legs and lower trunk and protect the participant from hypothermia. Standard seats in kayaks and canoes commercially offered typically provide a place to sit and something to lean against. If a craft has only a bench seat, consider securing a well-padded seat to the bench that has a back rest and side supports to provide pelvic stability and back support unless the participant has sufficient balance and trunk and leg strength to maintain a sitting position without using a seat and backrest. Trunk and pelvis stability are essential to be able to effectively paddle. The group Disabled Adventurers (disabledadventurers.com) has created a number of adaptive devices to enable people with disabilities to use kayaks (Figure 94-11). Instructions are located on the group's website so that some of their ideas can be built by users.

CLIMBING

Adaptive climbing (rock and ice) has become increasingly popular over the past two decades. It was pioneered in the late

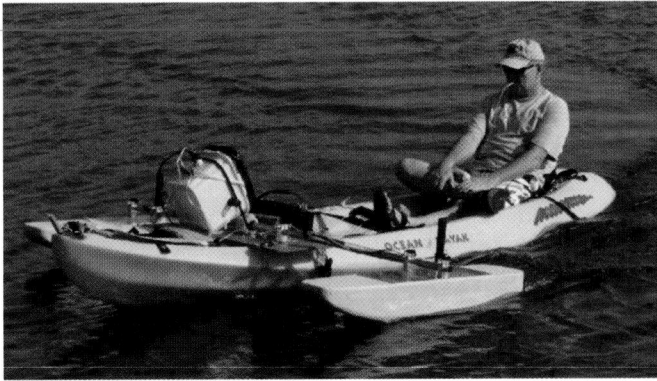

FIGURE 94-11 Motorized kayak with sip-and-puff steering device. *(Courtesy Mark Theobald, Disabled Adventurers:* disabledadventurers. com.)

1980s by extreme athlete Mark Wellman, who was the first paraplegic to summit the 3000-foot granite face of El Capitan in Yosemite National Park. He had to perform 7000 pull-ups to reach the summit.[75] The first U.S. Paraclimbing Competition took place in 2013, and the International Federation of Sports Climbing Paraclimbing World Cup competition occurred in September 2014.[40]

Climbing can increase confidence, help to develop problem-solving and adaptation skills, increase independence, and improve self-awareness and willingness to trust. Many persons who suffer from posttraumatic stress disorder (PTSD) and/or TBIs have benefited greatly from climbing, as have persons with motor, sensory, and cognitive deficits. Physiologically, when climbing, a person with a disability can learn to use muscle groups in different ways and enhance fine and gross motor skills.

Persons with motor, vision, and hearing disabilities have been able to participate in climbing activities. Blind climbers rely on their sense of touch to identify the next handholds. Climbing can be accomplished using appropriate adaptive equipment, such as harness or pulley systems, prosthetic climbing feet, prosthetic knees, and specialized protective equipment, such as padded chaps to protect legs.[37] Many climbing clubs and organizations have programs using climbing walls specifically for training people with disabilities, such as the Adaptive Climbing Group of Brooklyn[1] and Paradox Sports in Boulder, Colorado.[57] They also arrange for climbing adventures.

HAND CYCLING AND TANDEM RECLINING CYCLES

Hand cycling has become a popular outdoor sport for people with lower motor impairments. Special cycles are available that are designed for use by persons with various disabilities. Racing, off-road, and mountain bike models are available that have adjustable seats and seat heights, hand-operated brakes, and tires appropriate for the terrain. Pedaling is accomplished by arm cranking (Figure 94-12).

Hand cycles come in a variety of styles. They are land vehicles that typically have one steerable front wheel powered by hand cranking and two coasting or stabilizing rear wheels. The brakes are located on the hand grips. Hand cycles used for rough terrain typically have two front wheels and one rear wheel.

Tandem reclining cycles can be used by a nondisabled cyclist pedaling and steering in the front seat and a disabled cyclist who is able to pedal, such as a blind cyclist, in the rear seat. If this type of cycle is used, be sure to attach safety flags on the rear of the cycle so that motorists can clearly see the cycle when it is on a road or trail (Figure 94-13).

The motivational documentary/video "Crank It Up!" is the story of three paraplegic men who hand crank specially designed hand cycle mountain bikes on the very dangerous and challenging White Rim Trail in Canyonlands, Utah (nolimitstahoe.com).

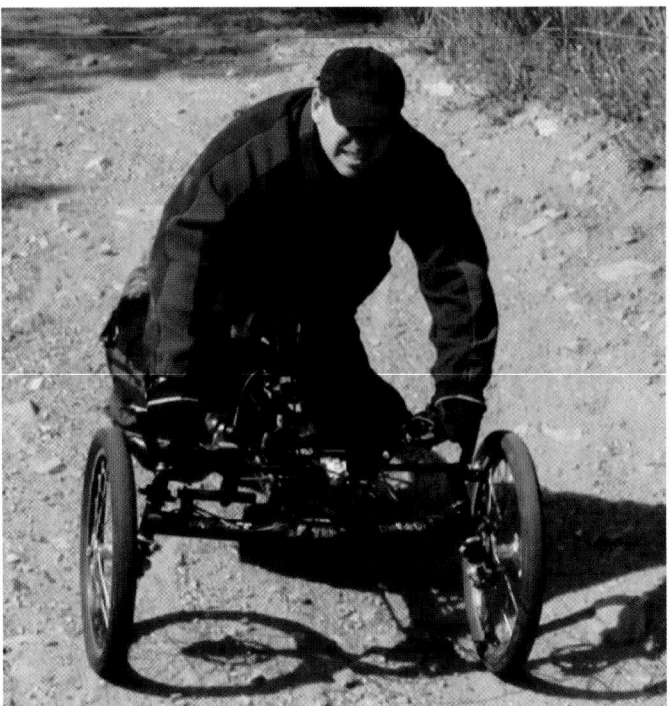

FIGURE 94-12 Jeff Pagels pedaling the one-off wheelchair on a rough road where vehicles require four-wheel drive. *(Courtesy Sheryl Olson.)*

HIKING

Hiking is something that can be done by many people with disabilities. Hiking may assist with balance, stability, and depth perception, and provide leverage for an extra push. The key to successful hiking is conditioning prior to the hike. New hikers who are disabled should check with their primary care providers to obtain medical clearance to participate in the activity. Persons with lower limb amputations should check with their prosthetists to be certain that they have the proper prosthetic and fit for hiking.

Begin by walking on flat surfaces, and progress to gentle hills, then more difficult hills and increasingly steep and long sets of stairs. Cardiac exercises should be added to the regime, along

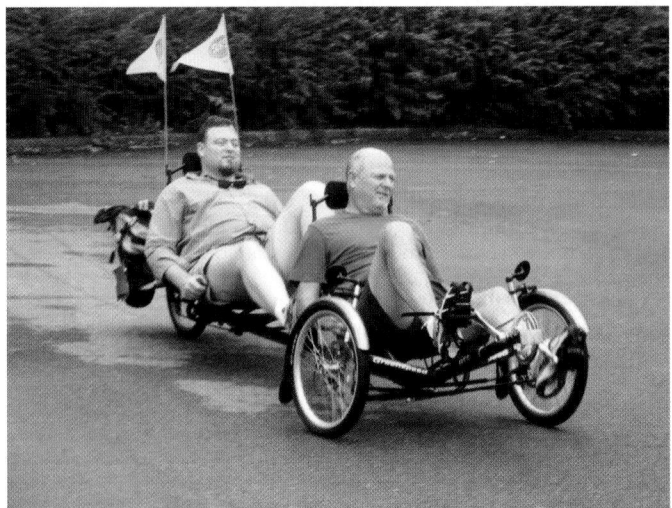

FIGURE 94-13 Blind rear seat cyclist on a tandem cycle. *(Courtesy the Borden Institute [US Army] from the "Warrior Transition Leader: Medical Rehabilitation Handbook.")*

with leg strengthening using power lifting and weight training to strengthen the core and abdominal muscles.

Proper footwear is essential. Wear shoes or boots that provide stability and cushion the feet to absorb shock. Warm socks of good quality that will wick away moisture and prevent blisters are essential. Bring extra pairs in the event of excess moisture. Amputees should wear prosthetic socks to prevent blisters and pressure sores and allow for stump expansion.

Dressing in layers is important to adjust for temperature changes. The first layer should be a lightweight synthetic garment that wicks moisture away from the body. The second layer should be an insulation layer, such as fleece, wool, down, or a synthetic fabric. The third layer should be water and wind resistant. Be sure to pack sunscreen, sunglasses, and a protective hat.

HORSEBACK RIDING

Horseback riding (also known as *hippotherapy* when used as a physical therapy modality) is an activity that provides physical exercise as well as the psychological benefits of a person with a disability experiencing an outdoor environment. It improves self-confidence and self-esteem. One can expect to see improved muscle strength in the chest and back and improved core strength. One study demonstrated that as few as 8 minutes of hippotherapy in children with cerebral palsy resulted in significant improvement of symmetry of muscle activity.[5] Riding assists range of motion, joint flexibility, and balance when the rider is coached to focus on posture and body alignment.

People with multiple sclerosis have mixed results when horseback riding. Some benefit because it improves retaining functional ability while on the horse and afterwards. For unknown reasons, others with the same diagnosis experience worsened symptoms of the disease. Be sure to assess riders before, during, and after riding at each session.

HUNTING

In some states, it is permissible for a person with a disability to hunt from a vehicle. There are mobility devices and hunting equipment that can be adapted to the special needs of the person with a disability, including camping equipment and hunting blinds. Wheelchairs must be appropriate for the type of terrain that will be traversed. The Action Trackchair (actiontrackchair.com) is an off-road wheelchair that can maneuver over sand, mud, snow, grassy fields, and wooded trails. It has tank-like tracks that rotate in a continuous loop, to provide continuous extraction (Figure 94-14).

Several other types of wheelchairs are suitable for use by hunters who are disabled. The Extreme 4 × 4 (Mobility USA [mobility-usa.com]) is a power chair equipped with either large off-road tires or tracks. It has a camouflage option and can be fitted with gun mounts. The Go-Getter wheelchair can be attached to a four-wheeler. The Landed All-Terrain Wheelchair has large tires and can navigate over mud, sand, gravel, and snow. There are several companies that can customize all-terrain vehicles and motorcycle sidecars to accommodate physically disabled people and can install motorized ramps on larger vehicles to transport motorized assist devices.

Power-assist wheelchairs help propel wheelchairs where the user prefers a manual chair but is not strong enough to propel it themselves. There are wheelchairs that can be converted from a seated position to a standing position (thestandingcompany.com).

Guns, rifles, and bows and arrows should be securely attached in a position where a person with tetraplegia can easily use them. If there is gross arm movement but no hand and finger movement, a device can be rigged to a firearm between the trigger and the person's arm so that the trigger can be pulled. Bow-and-arrow equipment can be adapted to the special needs of the disabled hunter. Physically Challenged Bowhunters of America provides and/or recommends adaptive products (pcba-inc.org).

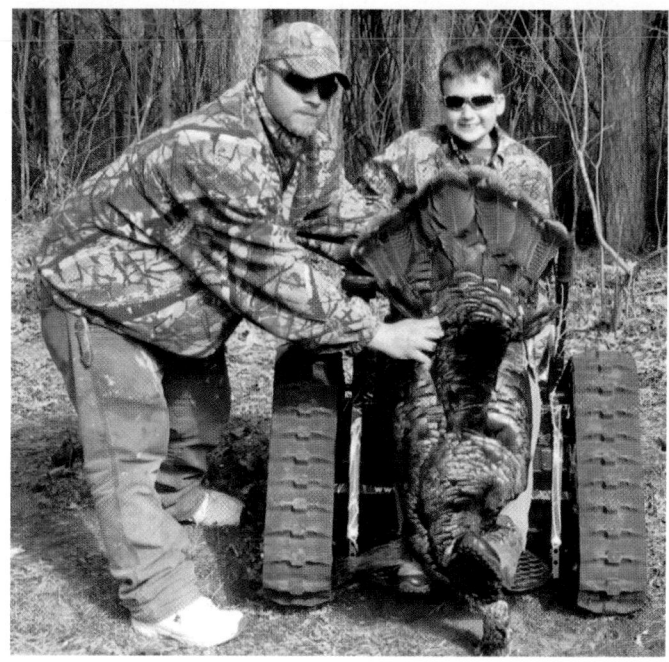

FIGURE 94-14 Teddy Perron and father Troy Perron after a successful wheelchair hunt. *(Courtesy Stephanie Perron.)*

The following are examples of adaptive equipment:
Activity trays and hand controls (beadaptive.com)
Binocular and flashlight holds (bigskyimagination.com)
Duck and game calls (hands free) (woodswise.com)
Rifles (custom) (randyscustomrifles.com)
Rifle scope (wheelchair mounted) (riflevision.com)
Rifle rests (hands free) (sr77.com)
Toilet systems (cleanwaste.com)
Wheelchair-accessible game blinds (ameristep.com)

SCUBA DIVING

Persons with many different disabilities can enjoy scuba diving.

Scuba Diving for Persons With Spinal Cord Injuries and Amputations

People with SCIs or amputations may enjoy the freedom of constraints from gravity when scuba diving. Most can meet the criteria for scuba certification with the assistance of a dedicated dive assistant who can help with flooding, clearing, and removal of the face mask if needed. Neoprene wetsuits should be custom fitted to the person with a disability, accounting for amputated limbs.

Balance Challenges. Because balance may be a challenge for the person with an SCI because of inability to use arms and legs to make trunk adjustments, counterweights may be added to achieve symmetric balance. The weights should be carefully positioned to maintain gravity along the center axis of the body.[58] They should constantly be monitored for readjustment to maintain desired body position.

Neoprene wetsuits and boots may increase the tendency for legs to rise toward the surface. Strap the legs together, and weight them near the ankles to prevent uncontrolled floating. Adjust weights to accommodate surface floating, ascent, and descent. Keep a record of use of weights and locations in a dive log for future reference.

Thermal Issues. Due to loss of thermoregulation, people with SCIs may be at risk for hypothermia while in the water. Plan for preventive and/or intervention measures in the dive preparation plan. Exposure to cold water may increase sympathetic nervous system activity, predisposing individuals with SCIs at and above level T6 to autonomic dysreflexia.[70]

A full-length wetsuit with a hood and dive booties should be worn to prevent hypothermia and unexpected direct contact with ocean life. Foot fins are not necessary for paraplegics and tetraplegics. However, hand fins can be quite advantageous for navigation for paraplegics. Consider use of a thin nylon or polyester body suit prior to donning the wetsuit to make donning the wetsuit easier. Wearing gloves should also be considered.

Anxiety. A person with limited physical capabilities may have anxiety about diving because of the fear of not being able to move in event of an emergency. It is very important that the person with the disability practice in a pool with complete scuba equipment and a dive buddy to develop familiarity with the equipment, experience flotation without gravity, and develop complete trust in his or her dive assistant.

The first pool session should focus on balance and weight distribution to adjust body position and develop a comfort level. Practice entering and exiting the water from a dive platform or boat. Practice with someone lifting the diver who is disabled onto the platform or boat. It may be necessary to remove weights and the air tank before attempting to lift the person onto the platform or into the boat. Leave the buoyancy compensation device in place to be able to use the handholds during the lift. Entry into the water can be made from the beach by carrying, or using a large, wheeled water device, boogie board, or surfboard.

Other Equipment and Considerations. A second-stage scuba regulator should be easy to purge and breathing resistance be adjustable. Ensure that the regulator is easily accessible and attached to the front of the buoyancy compensation device in the event of dislodgment.

A diver with a lower leg amputation should consider wearing a weight-integrated buoyancy compensation device rather than a weight belt. A weight-integrated buoyancy compensation device is less confining and allows better mobility in the water. It requires great finesse to control body movements when only one fin can be worn. The diver should be able to choose the fin that works best, perhaps a split fin or stiff fin.

The diver should empty his or her bladder prior to entering the water, because descent increases body pressure and diuresis. A person with an SCI may not sense a full bladder; there is a risk for autonomic dysreflexia.

Be aware of the strength of the current and possibility of having to swim against the current during the dive. The disabled diver may be capable of swimming into a strong current.

Scuba Diving for a Visually Impaired Person

Blind divers, with greater acoustic adaptation, often express joy at being able to hear the sounds of the underwater world not typically heard by sighted divers. They feel the currents, water pressures, and slight changes in water temperatures, and appreciate those unique opportunities.

The buoyancy compensation device, tank, and regulator require no special adaptation for the visually impaired diver. Diving can be safely accomplished with a dive buddy to monitor the dive time and tank pressures. Discuss the direction of the dive in relation to underwater currents prior to the dive. The blind diver may lead with the sighted diver tracking, or the sighted diver can lead with the blind diver following the sound of air bubbles. Both divers should have a tank-banger for communication. Establish a simple code prior to the dive. For example, two bangs could mean, "go to your right"; three bangs could mean, "go to your left." Be sure to establish a code to call for immediate help.

The dive buddy should never lose sight of the blind diver. If separation occurs, the tank-banger can be used to establish communication if the divers are within an audible distance from one another. Without proprioception input in an environment without gravity, a blind diver may become disoriented in relation to upright and upside-down positions. Reorientation can occur by placing a hand over the air bubbles as they leave the regulator to feel the direction in which they are rising in order correct the body position.

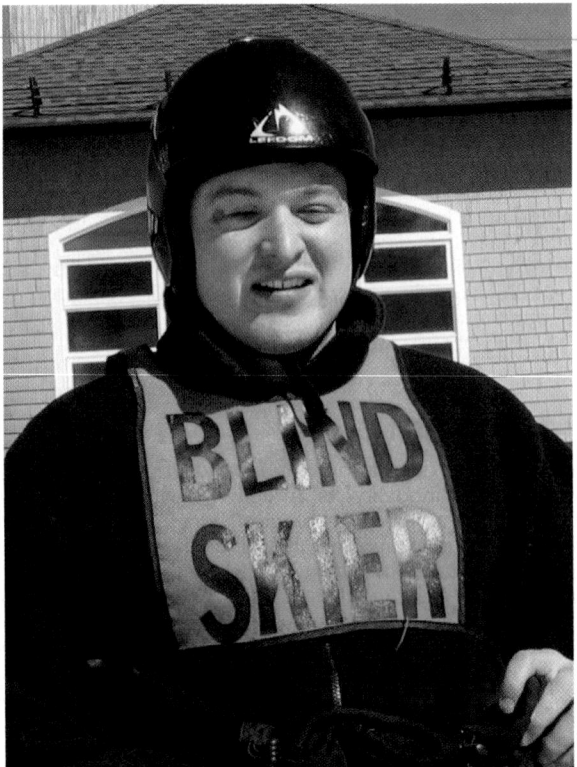

FIGURE 94-15 Blind skier preparing for a ski run. *(Courtesy the Borden Institute [US Army] from the "Warrior Transition Leader: Medical Rehabilitation Handbook.")*

Scuba Diving for a Person With Hearing Impairment

There is no contraindication to scuba diving for the hearing-impaired individual. In fact, if there is more than one hearing-impaired diver in the group and they both sign (ASL), they will have a better way of communicating when underwater than non–hearing-impaired individuals.

SKIING

A wide variety of skis are available for disabled skiers. Monoskis, sit-skis, toboggan skis, and cross-country skis allow for a variety of terrain, both alpine and cross-country, to be available to disabled skiers. Monoskis may have hydraulically controlled up-and-down positions. Sit-skis are usually constructed from fiberglass and use short poles with picks for the skier to be able to start, turn, and stop. Persons with bilateral amputations can use four-track skis, which have two skis and two outriggers. Skiers with SCIs or amputations, those who are blind or have hearing loss, and those with other disabilities have been able to enjoy the thrill of skiing. The national organization Ski for Light[66] offers ski lessons and assistants for vision-impaired skiers and persons with other disabilities (Figure 94-15).

In the spring of 1993, Matt Wellman was the first paraplegic to traverse the Sierra Nevada mountain range on a sit-ski. His 4-day journey took him across Ellery Lake on the east side of the Sierra, where he ascended over Tioga Pass to finish at Crane Flat on the west side of the Sierra.

ASSISTANCE DOGS

Several types of dogs are trained to assist people with various disabilities. Typically, breeds of assistance dogs are German shepherds, golden retrievers, and Labrador retrievers, selected because of their intelligence, loyalty, attentiveness, empowerment, and size. That being said, the type and size of dog selected should depend upon the expected work to be accomplished by the animal.

There are therapy dogs, service dogs,[23] leader dogs (also known as guide dogs for the blind and seeing-eye dogs), hearing dogs,[34] seizure dogs,[19] diabetes alert dogs,[26] and companion dogs for persons with PTSD. Assistance dogs bring many benefits and companionship to their owners.[62] For many people, the assistance dog gives them a reason to continue with their struggles, to get out of bed and out of the house each day. People with disabilities who have assistance dogs are able to make new friends easily because dogs are generally loved by most people.[41,46]

Therapy dogs are specially trained primarily to visit patients in hospitals and nursing homes. They are sociable, gentle, and calming and bring smiles to the faces of persons they visit.

Service dogs are trained to assist people with mobility, sensory, and other types of disabilities. They are professionally trained to accomplish tasks (sometimes up to 28 individual tasks[23]) for one individual, such as to open doors, assist with dressing, retrieve items, and navigate outdoors and inside the home.

Leader dogs or *guide dogs* for the blind are trained to assist people with limited or no vision. The first known assistance dogs were trained after World War I to assist soldiers returning from the war with vision loss.[62]

Hearing assist dogs, which are typically smaller size than other assistance dogs, are trained to alert people who are deaf to important sounds, such as a baby's cry, ringing telephone or doorbell, or smoke detector alarm. They are trained to respond to their human partner's voice and hand signals.

Seizure alert dogs are astute at recognizing an impending seizure and trained to protect their human partner when he or she seizes. The size, breed, and gender of this assistance dog is irrelevant, as long as there is a bond between the dog and its partner.

Diabetic alert dogs are trained to sense impending hypoglycemia and to notify their human partners. Diabetic alert dogs are relatively new to the class of assistance dogs; the first diabetic alert dog was trained in 2003.[26]

PTSD assistance dogs are the newest members of the assistance dog group. They are usually large dogs and are matched with military members or veterans who have been diagnosed with PTSD. The dogs provide companionship and a calming influence on their partners and alert and respond when there is a PTSD crisis event. The use of these specially trained dogs has become more prevalent for people with PTSD and depression in civilian communities.

People with disabilities who are partnered with assistance dogs may take their dogs along with them on wilderness trips. Be sure to check the Transportation Security Administration (TSA) website for rules and regulations pertaining to travel with an assistance dog (tsa.gov/travel/special-procedures) and for guidelines and rules for passing through security clearance. Carry paperwork that identifies and verifies that the animal is an assistance animal. Labeling on the dog's harness is also expected. TSA officers have been trained not to communicate, distract, interact, play, feed, or pet service animals and to ask permission before touching the service animal or its belongings. The TSA recommends advising the security officer on how to best achieve screening (i.e., side-by-side, dog in front, dog behind) when passing through the metal detector as a human-dog team. If the alarm goes off, secondary screening will occur. The officer will obtain permission from the handler before touching the dog or its belongings.

Three other U.S. federal agencies that may be encountered when traveling with a service animal are the U.S. Department of Agriculture, Animal and Plant Health Inspection Service (APHIS), and Veterinary Services. Cooperate fully and advise the inspectors about how to interact with the animal and how to accomplish the desired tasks. An APHIS-accredited veterinarian can complete an international health certificate and certify that the animal is in good health, conduct tests, and record test results. A completed international health certificate must be endorsed by a Veterinary Services area office for export of the animal from the United States. Information about the Veterinary Services office for individual states can be found at aphis.usda.gov/import_export/index.shtml.

Become familiar with the import rules for animals when traveling outside the United States. Contact the country's embassy to determine rules specific for service animals for the country where travel is planned. A list of consulates can be found at the U.S. Department of State website state.gov. The APHIS website on animal welfare offers excellent references to find state regulations, foreign country requirements, disease restrictions, and U.S. Customs and Border Patrol publications on pets (aphis.usda.gov/aphis/home/).

Contact the destination wilderness location regarding regulations about assistance dogs. Check with a veterinarian for rules and regulations for travel and wilderness, such as immunization requirements and preventive measures. Since passage of the ADA, assistance animals are defined as "any guide dog, signal dog, or other animal individually trained to do work or perform tasks for the benefit of an individual with a disability, including, but not limited to, guiding individuals with impaired vision, alerting individuals with impaired hearing to intruders or sounds, providing minimal protection or rescue work, pulling a wheelchair, or fetching dropped items."[2] Service animals are in a class of their own and not considered to be pets. Therefore, they are permitted to go where other pets are not allowed.

On occasion, park superintendents may close a specific area of a park to service animals if it is deemed that the service animal may pose a direct threat to the health and safety of people or wildlife.

Remember to pack animal-specific supplies, such as food, special harnesses, water, bowls, play toys, and sleep surfaces.

OPPORTUNITIES FOR WILDERNESS ADVENTURES

There are hundreds of websites that offer information about adaptive equipment, organizations, teachers, coaches, and guides, and activities for people with disabilities. Here is a list of organizations that offer opportunities in specific outdoor sports:

RESOURCES FOR WILDERNESS SPORTS

Archery
United Foundation for Disabled Archers
320-634-3660
uffdaclub.com

USA Archery
719-866-4576
teamusa.org/USA-Archery

Canoeing
American Canoe Association—Disabled Paddlers
703-451-0141
americancanoe.org/?page=Courses_Adaptive

Cycling and Racing
Hand Crank Racing Association
530-244-3577
shasta.com/geneva/CrankRace/

Hand Cycle Racing
757-422-1912
handcycleracing.com

Wheelchair Motorcycle Association
508-583-8614
iandr.mwcil.org

Horseback Riding
American Hippotherapy Association
970-818-1322
americanhippotherapyassociation.org

National Center for Equine Facilitated Therapy
650-851-2271
nceft.org

Professional Association of Therapeutic Horsemanship International (PATH Intl.),
800-369-7433
pathintl.org/

Hunting, Shooting, and Fishing

Amateur Trapshooting Association
618-449-2224
shootata.com

Buckmasters American Deer Foundation
334-215-3337
buckmasters.com/

Disabled Hunters Resources
huntingpa.com/disabledhunters.html

Fishing Has No Boundaries
800-243-3462
fhnbinc.org

Mountain States Chapter, Paralyzed Veterans of America
800-833-9400
mscpva.org/shooting.html

National Skeet Shooting Association
800-877-5338
nssa-nsca.org

National Wheelchair Shooting Federation
877-865-4893
livingwellwithadisability.org

NRA Disabled Shooting Services
703-267-1495
nchpad.org

Outdoor Buddies Hunting Program
719-783-9044
outdoorbuddies.org

Physically Challenged Bowhunters of America
855-247-7222
pcba-inc.org

Wheelin' Sportsmen (National Wild Turkey Federation)
800-THE-NWTF
nwtf.org/wheelin

Rock Climbing

Lover's Leap Guides
530-318-2939
loversleap.net

Montana Mountaineering
208-420-6842
montanamountaineering.org

Rowing and Sailing

U.S. Rowing Association
800-314-4ROW
usrowing.org

Sailing
footeprint.com/sailingweb

Running

Achilles Track Club
212-354-0300
achillesinternational.org/

Scuba Diving

Handicapped Scuba Association International
949-498-4540
hsascuba.com

International Association for Handicapped Divers
iahd.org

Snowboarding and Skiing

National Ability Center
435-649-3991
discovernac.org/

Sitski Extreme Adaptive Sports
908-313-5590
sitski.com

Snowmass Village
800-SNOW-MASS
gosnowmass.com/

U.S. Ski and Snowboarding Association—Disabled
435-649-9090
usskiteam.com/

Swimming

USA Swimming
719-866-4578
usaswimming.org

Water Skiing

Water Skiers with Disabilities Association
usawaterski.org

REFERENCES

Complete references used in this text are available online at expertconsult.inkling.com.

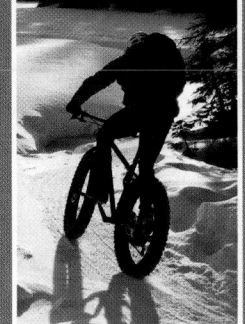

CHAPTER 95

Physiology of Exercise, Conditioning, and Performance Training for Wilderness Adventure

ROBERT B. SCHOENE

For millions of years, humans have survived in wilderness environments. It is only in the last few millennia that socialization has led to what we call "civilization." Modern life has formed a construct for human existence that has largely overcome the need for competence in survival. However, there are still populations that rely on physical capabilities and resourcefulness to survive on planet Earth, most of which is still wilderness (Figure 95-1).

Many people now seek their ancestral origins with an ineffable call to return to oceans, mountains, deserts, and rivers in all corners of the globe. It is this yearning to seek both solitude and fellowship with other kindred spirits that takes us from what we call civilization to wilderness. Some persons are prepared with skills to thrive in the wild but others wander unprepared to endure the unavoidable physical stresses that one may encounter.

This chapter addresses the physical and psychological challenges faced in the wilderness and attempts to offer insights into the best ways to prepare for survival, enjoyment, and the ability to thrive.

MENTAL AWARENESS

Especially during the past three decades, there has been growing interest in seeking adventure to experience wilderness via guided trips, group ventures, and solo forays. The press and popular literature have recounted these experiences for the general public, many of whom would otherwise have little concept of adventure and the attendant risks. The romantic notion of rafting a remote river, trekking in the Himalayas, or riding a camel in the Sahara Desert does not often anticipate the possibility of 2 weeks in torrential rain on a cold river, biting snow and altitude illness, contaminated food and diarrhea, or even a camel bite. The western traveler is often a person who comes from a comfortable home and who assumes that he or she will be cared for—or even rescued, if necessary—and then transported home with a minimum amount of inconvenience to be able to recount his or her adventures with persons who are similarly ignorant of the actual risks.

To enjoy the wilderness, one must accept that occasional hardships are frequent aspects of adventures. Therefore, self-reliance or group reliance is critical, and a modicum of medical and survival skills must be obtained. Reading the great tales of survival and studying survival theories can be helpful, but mental preparation cannot be taught solely in the classroom and library; it must be learned and then practiced until one becomes experienced. Thus, one should strive to learn, know oneself, accept the risks of the adventure, and become a strong member of the team; being unprepared may put many participants at risk.

PHYSICAL CONDITIONING

Wilderness adventures require a wide range of physical capabilities. Rather than being a specialized endeavor where one particular form of conditioning will ensure success, wilderness travel is varied and at many times unpredictable, and requires strength, flexibility, endurance, speed, and mental resourcefulness. Each of us begins our training with a different dose of each of these

characteristics and must do our best to optimize them. Having the strength to pull a colleague out of a crevasse or drag oneself with a broken ankle up a steep trail may be essential for survival. Having the reflexes and speed to avoid rockfall or grab a teammate before he or she falls into a river may mean the difference between life and death. Having the endurance to hike for days out of the mountains to initiate a rescue for an injured friend will minimize that friend's exposure to cold or heat.

This chapter deals primarily with aerobic fitness and exercise physiology with an emphasis on high-altitude fitness, because adaptation and exercise performance in that environment carry with them concepts universally applicable to all wilderness endeavors.

AEROBIC FITNESS

The best way to prepare for any form of wilderness venture is to be in the wilderness on a regular basis. However, for most persons who are not professional river or mountain guides, it is not possible to be active in these terrains every day. Thus, we need to improvise and incorporate physical training into our busy schedules so that when we enter the wilderness, we are prepared.

The concepts of aerobic fitness are similar for champion and recreational athletes. The parts of the "engine" are the same; it is the quality and fine-tuning that are different. Three essential characteristics are the maximum oxygen consumption ($\dot{V}O_2max$), lactate or anaerobic threshold (which defines sustainable work), and efficiency. These factors are interrelated in a way that results in effective performance, and each is trainable. The interrelationships result in improved endurance, the most important overall factor for enjoyment and survival in the wilderness.[42]

MAXIMUM OXYGEN CONSUMPTION

Oxygen consumption ($\dot{V}O_2$) is defined by the Fick equation:

$$\dot{V}O_2 = \text{Cardiac output} \times \text{Extraction of oxygen}$$

Cardiac output is equal to the heart rate multiplied by the stroke volume. Oxygen extraction is the difference between the content of oxygen of the arterial and mixed venous blood (i.e., the amount of oxygen that is used as blood traverses tissue beds). The metabolic response of exertion is limited by cardiac output and the limits of oxygen extraction, both of which can be modulated with training. The role of $\dot{V}O_2max$ and its various considerations are discussed by Levine.[48]

$\dot{V}O_2max$ is the fingerprint of an individual's physiology. It is a reproducible marker of fitness in an individual that varies depending on training, altitude, and illness. The many genetic factors (i.e., polygenic) that contribute to a person's $\dot{V}O_2max$ make it highly unlikely that any one individual could be endowed with all of the necessary genes.[76] One's $\dot{V}O_2max$ is influenced by both inherited and environmental factors.[8] What remains to be explained is the observation that, among sedentary subjects in family groups who were maintained on a supervised aerobic exercise program for 20 weeks, there was great variability in how much $\dot{V}O_2max$ could be improved[7] (Figure 95-2). The

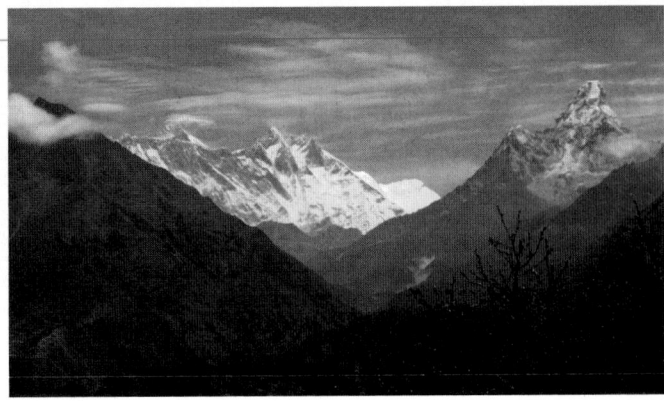

FIGURE 95-1 View in the Khumbu region of Nepal, with Mt Everest, Mt Lhotse, and Mt Ama Dablam appearing most prominent. (*Courtesy Robert B. Schoene.*)

improvement in $\dot{V}O_2$max ranged from negative values to 30% improvement, and these various levels of improvement were grouped in family clusters. Further data from this series of studies looked at age, race, gender, and initial fitness and found that all subjects experienced gains in $\dot{V}O_2$max, but with a great deal of variability and little correlation among the aforementioned factors that contributed to those gains. It is clear that there are limits in training to improve $\dot{V}O_2$max. In other words, a "normal" individual with a $\dot{V}O_2$max of 42 mL/kg/min may be able to improve his or her $\dot{V}O_2$max to the high 40s mL/kg/min but will never be able to approach the 75 to 85 mL/kg/min range of high-performance middle- to long-distance athletes, who chose their parents well.

What parts of one's aerobic capacity can be trained? Considering the Fick equation, it becomes apparent that an increase in cardiac output or improved extraction of oxygen, or both, will improve $\dot{V}O_2$max. In fact, both things happen, but it is clearly the heart that can be trained more by increasing its stroke volume and improving its muscular strength.[22,31] Thus, the heart rate necessary to achieve an appropriate cardiac output for any given metabolic rate is lower in the trained state as compared with the untrained state. Although the maximum heart rate does not

change with training, resting and submaximal heart rates are lower and can be used as simple markers to monitor training. Although the elements of oxygen extraction somewhat improve, the heart's stroke volume conveys increased ability to perfuse large volumes of muscle mass such that, with training, there are increased capillary and mitochondrial densities and optimization of the components of oxidative metabolism.[3,30,36,37]

It is fascinating to put human physiology in perspective with the rest of the animal kingdom. Normal humans in the age range of 20 to 40 years have a $\dot{V}O_2$max somewhere around 40 mL/kg/min, and accomplished endurance athletes have one in the range of 70 to 85 mL/kg/min; alternatively, some large mammals have extraordinarily high aerobic capacities. For instance, horses have $\dot{V}O_2$max values that range from 134 mL/kg/min in standardbred horses[2] to 160 mL/kg/min in thoroughbreds.[46,52] The North American pronghorn antelope is said to have values as high as 300 mL/kg/min. Although thoroughbred horses were bred several hundred years ago to be great aerobic athletes, the antelope's evolutionary strategy is to have exercise capabilities that optimize its chance of preserving the small family groups that live on an open plain full of predators (i.e., the pronghorn can run sustainably at 80.5 km/hr [50 mi/hr]).

Does $\dot{V}O_2$max correlate with being able to go faster, last longer, jump higher, climb faster, or survive better in the wilderness? The answer is "yes and no." Certainly, the high-performance endurance athlete needs to have a large aerobic capacity, but even in this group, there is heterogeneity in $\dot{V}O_2$max and performance. This indicates that there are other components of physical characteristics that translate into endurance and performance and that are also influenced by training. Most athletic events attract athletes that share certain phenotypic characteristics that, as with animals in nature, result in some homogeneity; in addition, among people who venture into the wilderness—including even among elite high-altitude climbers—there is a great deal of phenotypic heterogeneity. Regardless of the lack of a strong correlation between $\dot{V}O_2$max and performance in the wilderness, there is one precept that is sacrosanct: The body must translate energy expenditure into sustainable and efficient mechanical output.

THRESHOLD OF SUSTAINABILITY

Exercising at the highest possible sustainable workload results in the best individual performance. The point in progressive exercise above which the level of intensity cannot be sustained has been given many names. *Anaerobic, ventilatory,* and *lactate thresholds* are the most commonly used terms, although none clearly defines the phenomenon well. At any given point of training or health, the threshold is fairly reproducible. The term *lactate threshold* (LT) will be used for sake of this discussion. It is important to understand that the LT—more than $\dot{V}O_2$max—can be trained to move to a higher level of intensity; this translates into a functional increase in endurance and performance, whether in athletic endeavor or wilderness adventure.

The onset of unsustainable work intensity essentially involves a shift of fuel supply within the cell. At workloads below the LT, free fatty acids are the primary oxidative fuel. Above the LT, when the oxidative turnover of free fatty acids cannot keep up with the demand for adenosine triphosphate, glycolysis occurs. Muscle glycogen is broken down as fuel, with lactic acid being produced at a rate beyond the body's ability to use it.[41,61] Blood lactate levels correlate with the intensity of work and thus are inversely correlated with the duration of a competitive event (Figure 95-3).

For example, a 10,000-m runner may have only a slightly elevated blood lactate level as compared with the resting level as he or she slowly depletes muscle glycogen; alternatively, an 800-m runner will have a markedly elevated blood lactate concentration at the end of the race, because glycolytic signaling is invoked early at high levels of exertion. With sustained aerobic training, use of free fatty acids, which is abundant, is shifted to higher intensities and functionally spares muscle glycogen. The point at which lactate starts to rise in the blood is quite variable, but usually occurs at about 60% of $\dot{V}O_2$max in untrained

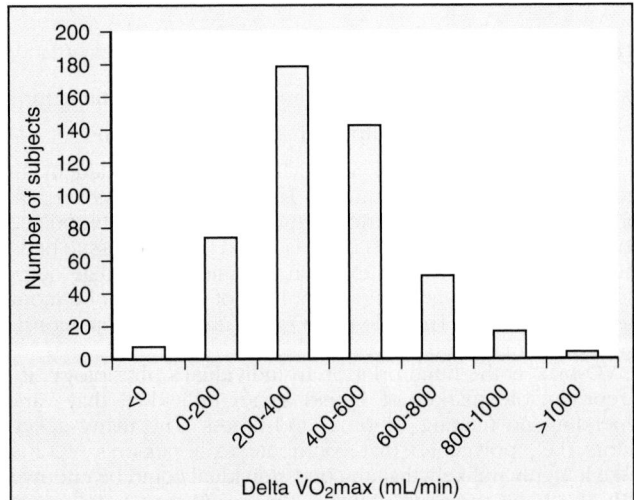

FIGURE 95-2 Distribution of 481 subjects by classes of increase (δ) in maximum oxygen consumption ($\dot{V}O_2$max) as compared with baseline levels. (*From Bouchard C, An P, Rice T, et al: Familial aggregation of VO(2max) response to exercise training: results from the HERITAGE Family Study, J Appl Physiol 87:1003, 1999.*)

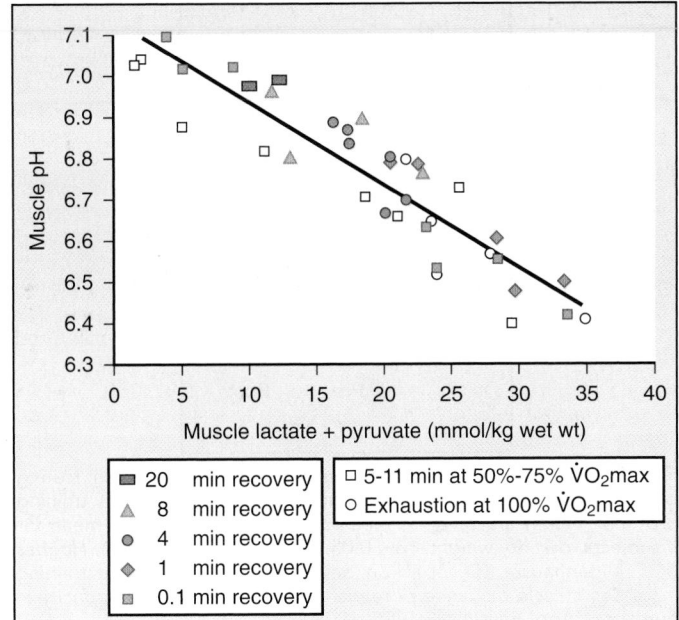

FIGURE 95-3 Linear relationship between the amount of muscle lactate and pyruvate as compared with muscle pH. Data are combined from different exercise intensities and different durations of recovery after exercise to exhaustion. *(From Robergs RA, Ghiasvand F, Parker D: Biochemistry of exercise-induced metabolic acidosis, Am J Physiol Regul Integr Comp Physiol 287:R502, 2004; and Sahlin K, Horris RC, Nylind B, et al: Lactate content and pH in muscle samples obtained after dynamic exercise, Pflugers Arch 367:143, 1976.)*

individuals; in highly trained individuals, this point may come at 75% to 85% of $\dot{V}O_2$max. In the trained individual, this difference is due both to improved convection of oxygen with a high cardiac output and increased capillary density, as well as to distribution of muscle fiber types with improved oxidative efficiency.

Lactate has often been portrayed as the culprit that leads to fatigue. However, two misconceptions about this need to be corrected. First, as long as there is blood flow, the LT is actually not associated with mitochondrial hypoxia or anoxia. "Anaerobic" metabolism is not occurring. Convection of oxygen to the cell, and diffusion gradients from the blood across the cell membrane into the cytosol and from the cytosol into the mitochondria, are adequate to supply oxygen for oxidative phosphorylation. Second, it is not accumulation of lactic acid that causes muscle fatigue or pain during exhaustive exercise. More likely, muscle fatigue is accumulation of the associated hydrogen ion when progressively increasing amounts of pyruvate being delivered to the mitochondria cannot undergo oxidation, thus leading to the generation of lactic acid and the associated hydrogen ion.

IMPROVING HUMAN PERFORMANCE

MALLEABILITY OF THE LACTATE THRESHOLD

Understanding the top end of the body's physiology is only the beginning of understanding the translation of energy potential into endurance, efficiency, and performance. This next section stresses the importance of sustainable work, which is the key to engaging in any wilderness endeavor. Sustainable work is defined as the level of exertion that can be sustained for many minutes, hours, or days. It is an intensity of exertion that is below one's LT. Levels of intensity above the LT are reserved for more explosive events in sport or flight of less than a few minutes' duration, such as the 100-m to 800-m events in track and field. In the wild, the short spurt of energy exerted by a cheetah to capture prey is above the animal's LT and not sustainable, which is why the gazelle sometimes wins.

The ability of a muscle to sustain work is related to its oxidative capacity. This capacity is quite malleable, and depends on the level of the muscle's activity while it is engaged.[20,35] Among high-level athletes, oxidative capacity can be several-fold greater than among untrained individuals. Functionally, then, competitive endurance athletes have inherently high $\dot{V}O_2$max levels, and can perform sustainable work at a much higher percentage of their maximum capacity. For example, an international cyclist may have a maximum work capacity of 550 watts and be able to sustain 450 watts of work during an hour-long hill climb. This is an extraordinary level of work output. A more usual and quasi-sedentary individual may have a maximum workload of 200 watts and be able to sustain 50% to 60% of that work intensity, which is considered to be "normal."

In highly specialized athletes, such as cyclists, the muscle mass involved in the effort has been shown to be progressively recruited in a way such that the oxidative stress is balanced and shared.[14,16] As much as 25% of the cyclist's muscle mass can be spared on a rotating basis, which reduces the oxidative stress of muscle fibers, thus prolonging the onset of the LT. This phenomenon may perhaps be a way to acquire more endurance, delay fatigue, and promote efficiency. Furthermore, with a finite fuel supply, this strategy would preserve glycogen stores and delay the onset of glycolysis (and thus production of lactate).

Functioning "at the edge" of performance requires delicate juggling of aerobic and anaerobic metabolism. This success translates into activities like running an efficient marathon, where 10% of the activity may be above the LT, or being able to hike as quickly as possible out of the high mountains to effect a rescue for a fallen colleague without collapsing from fatigue.

The crux of cellular oxidative metabolism is convection of oxygen to the cell by the circulation, diffusion of oxygen across the cell membrane into the cytosol, and then diffusion of oxygen into the mitochondria. The actual diffusion gradient necessary to get oxygen to the mitochondria is on the order of 2 to 3 mm Hg at each of these steps.[66] Thus, perfusion rather than hypoxemia per se is a limiting factor. Therefore, one of the most important adaptive steps is augmenting blood flow through angiogenesis of the microcirculation. In this regard, in two studies, highly trained cyclists and triathletes with comparable values of $\dot{V}O_2$max were exercised at 88% of their maximum aerobic capacity until fatigue.[14,15] There were two patterns that showed a shorter and longer time to fatigue. The athletes with more endurance had a substantially greater capillary density than did the athletes who fatigued earlier, despite comparable maximum aerobic capacities. Because both groups were highly trained, it is not clear whether, in certain athletes, there is some inherent propensity for greater signaling of angiogenesis that comes from training. The authors speculated that this augmented perfusion may be important not only for the convective phase of oxygen but also for providing a greater volume of the effluent portion of metabolic by-products.

Another study looked at subtle factors that contribute to fatigue at very high levels of exercise and found that very small changes in energy expenditure when a person is at exercise intensities of greater than 80% of $\dot{V}O_2$max can lead to rapid onset of fatigue.[53] Therefore, it is critical for an athlete—whether on the field or in the wilderness—to know the location of his or her "edge" so there is some reserve for optimally finishing an activity.

TRAINING EFFECT ON THE LACTATE THRESHOLD

Much has been written since the late 1970s about plasticity of the LT. It behooves any athlete to be able to perform at the highest percentage of his or her maximum aerobic capacity. One of the first studies to look at the effect of aerobic training on the LT involved nine sedentary men who performed 9 weeks of supervised endurance training for 45 minutes per day for 4.1 days per week.[17] There was a comparable untrained control group. The exercise group increased its LT by 44% expressed as absolute $\dot{V}O_2$, and 15% expressed as $\dot{V}O_2$max. $\dot{V}O_2$max also increased 25%. The maximum work rate increased 28%, with decreases in the ventilatory equivalent seen at submaximal levels of work. The volume of work was similar in the test group, so the study

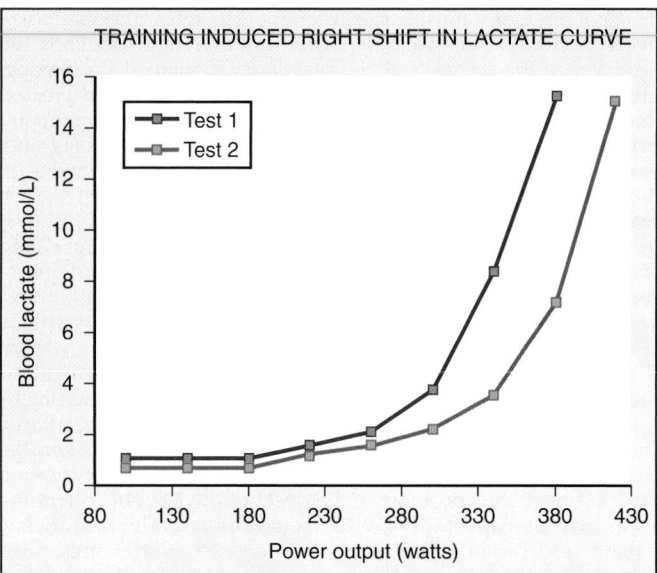

FIGURE 95-4 Training moves the lactate threshold to a higher level of sustainable work.

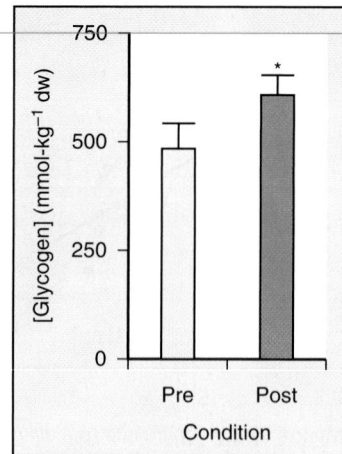

FIGURE 95-5 Muscle glycogen concentration measured in resting biopsy samples obtained before and after a 2-week sprint training protocol. Values are given as mean ± standard error of the mean for 8 subjects. dw, dry weight. *$p < 0.05$. (*From Burgomaster KA, Hughes SC, Heigenhauser GJ, et al: Six sessions of sprint interval training increases muscle oxidative potential and cycle endurance capacity in humans, J Appl Physiol 98:1985, 2005.*)

did not answer the following questions (Figure 95-4): How much volume is necessary to induce these changes? If some work is good, is more or less better?

The focus of studies then became the effect of volume versus intensity of work on the aforementioned variables, all of which had important implications for performance and health.[27] As understanding of endurance training expanded, there was emerging and ongoing interest in the effects of other types of training, such as interval training (IT), which for many years had been a standard training technique for athletes. IT can take many forms, but is usually described as a series of intense training bouts above the LT, interspersed with recovery periods. Middle distance and endurance athletes perform some level of endurance (i.e., below LT) training every day and then add IT sessions 2 to 3 days per week. Historically, with IT, the time and volume of training have been thought to be able to be markedly reduced. The thinking has been that very intense exercise levels signal greater changes in muscle oxidative capacity, which otherwise would not be stimulated by endurance-oriented aerobic training. Most studies have been done in athletes who were already engaged in active training, so one of the questions that arose was whether IT could add further benefits to performance for athletes who were already performing at a highly trained level.

Several studies have looked at a number of variations on the IT theme and its effect on performance, LT, serum lactate, time to exhaustion, muscle physiology, and so forth. One study enrolled seven trained male distance runners and added 3 days of intense levels of training (i.e., > 95% heart rate maximum) per week for 8 weeks.[1] The results showed no change in $\dot{V}O_2$max, but there was improvement in 10,000-m times, increased time to exhaustion on a set treadmill pace and incline, decreased serum lactate concentrations at 85% and 90% maximum heart rate, and correlations of the decrease in lactate with improvements in performance times. In another study among recreationally active young males, a mere six bouts of four to seven "all-out" Wingate tests spread out over 2 weeks (with recovery days in between) resulted in a 100% increase in cycle endurance time, with muscle biopsies showing a 26% increase in muscle glycogen and a 38% increase in citrate synthase, both markers of muscle oxidative capacity[11] (Figures 95-5 and 95-6).

These two studies provide an interesting contrast in that intense training improved the already trained athletes somewhat and the modestly trained recreational athletes a great deal.

Another study divided 16 active young males into intense IT and endurance training groups that were followed for 2 weeks. The time commitment for the two groups was 2.5 hours and 10.5

hours, respectively. Training results for both groups were similar in that they showed improved time trial times and similar changes in markers of oxidative capacity and buffering capacity in muscle biopsy samples after the training intervention[26] (Figure 95-7).

In a study of a somewhat similar design and intent with more outcome variables, this same investigative group showed comparable improvements in performance, endurance time, and oxidative markers in muscle biopsies[10] (Figure 95-8). After 4 weeks of speed IT in a group of healthy recreationally active subjects, similar findings resulted when compared with those of an endurance group, and the ratio of muscle to capillary to fiber was similar in both groups.[39]

Thus, training intensity was heralded as an important part of overall training.[14] From a practical standpoint, for busy lives, efficiency of training may be an important consideration; thus, this is a significant finding.

These studies are only a few of the better examples of a large body of literature looking at endurance versus intense or interval styles of training. For wilderness activities, the lessons are crucial. Endurance training in the classic sense is the core of training philosophy, but the adventurer also wants to be able to perform at the highest sustainable level that can be created by following

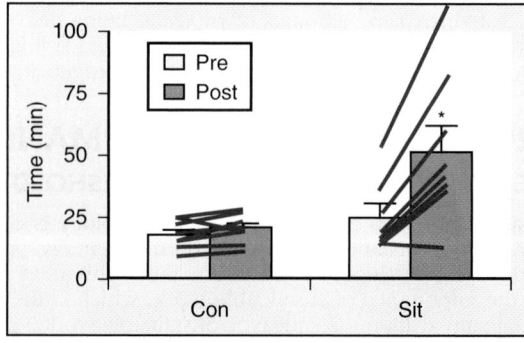

FIGURE 95-6 Cycle endurance time to fatigue before and after a 2-week sprint training protocol (training group; *Sit*) or equivalent period without training (control; *Con*). Values are given as mean ± standard error of the mean for 8 subjects. Individual data are also plotted for all subjects in each group. *$p < 0.05$. (*From Burgomaster KA, Hughes SC, Heigenhauser GJ, et al: Six sessions of sprint interval training increases muscle oxidative potential and cycle endurance capacity in humans, J Appl Physiol 98:1985, 2005.*)

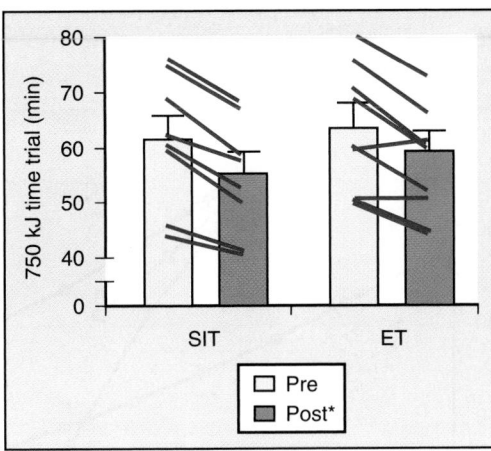

FIGURE 95-7 750-kJ cycling time trial performance before (Pre) and after (Post) six sessions of sprint interval training (SIT) or endurance training (ET) over 2 weeks. $*p \leq 0.05$ as compared with pretraining values (main effect for time). The lines denote individual data for eight subjects in each group. (From Gibala MJ, Little JP, van Essen M, et al: Short-term sprint interval versus traditional endurance training: similar initial adaptations in human skeletal muscle and exercise performance, J Physiol 575:901, 2006.)

a training routine that is reasonable and realistic (i.e., compatible with one's other life responsibilities). If it can be accommodated, inclusion of 2 to 3 days of IT per week can be an important addition to endurance training.

From a practical standpoint, how does one perform IT? First, if one has never done that type of training, it is important to realize that it is an intensity of exercise that is not particularly comfortable. Thus, when exercising for minutes at a time above LT, at about 40 seconds into the exercise interval, it will feel like it is time to stop. One should design an IT session and stick to

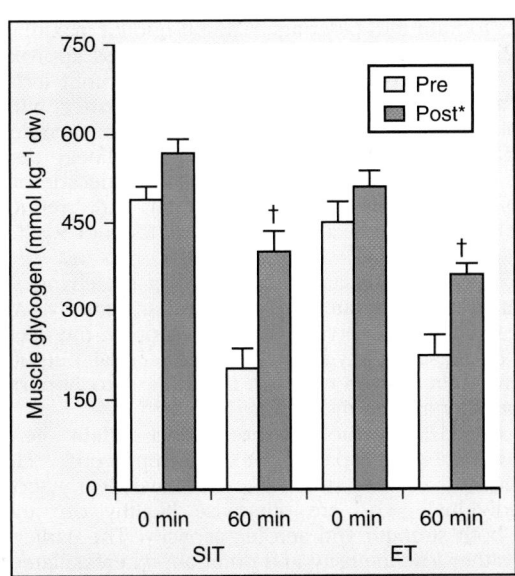

FIGURE 95-8 Muscle glycogen concentration measured at rest and during cycling exercise that consisted of 60 minutes at 65% peak oxygen consumption before (Pre) and after (Post) 6 weeks of sprint interval training (SIT) or 6 weeks of endurance training (ET). Values are given as mean ± standard error of the mean (n = 10 per group). dw, dry weight. *Main effect for condition ($p < 0.05$) such that posttraining (Post) > pretraining (Pre). †Condition (Pre and Post) × Time (0 and 60 minutes) interaction ($p < 0.05$) such that Post 60 minutes > Pre 60 minutes in both groups. (From Burgomaster KA, Howarth KR, Phillips SM, et al: Similar metabolic adaptations during exercise after low volume sprint interval and traditional endurance training in humans, J Physiol 586:151, 2008.)

it, especially through the last few seconds. Intervals can easily be incorporated into one's usual routine. Always include an aerobic warm-up and cool-down period. Whether on a bike or on foot, on a trail or road, find a modest hill that takes 1 to 2 minutes to "sprint" up; then slowly jog down and repeat. Start out with a single interval, and then, over the course of a few weeks, build up to 10 intervals. Improvement and familiarity with the new territory of anaerobic training will come rapidly. Start out with one interval day per week, and then increase to two interval days per week over a couple of months. It is felt important not to train above LT every day, because adequate recovery time is essential.

There are a couple of ways to achieve recovery between intervals. One can arbitrarily state that there will be a certain number of intervals of 1 to 2 minutes' duration, with 2 to 3 minutes between intervals assigned for recovery. For instance, one can run 400-m intervals and walk 200 m between each of them. Whatever one does, my best advice is to stick to it compulsively. A more physiologic way to recover is to use a heart rate monitor. Make sure that, at the end of each interval, a near-maximum heart rate is attained. The maximum heart rate is a person's actual maximum heart rate rather than the "220 beats/min minus age" number that is often used but is only vaguely accurate. Determining the maximum heart rate is actually not as easy as it sounds, because most people do not reach it in a reproducible manner. The heart rate at a true anaerobic interval could be considered the maximum heart rate, or one can do a formal cardiopulmonary exercise test during which a trained observer can look for the heart rate at a plateau of $\dot{V}O_2$max. At the end of each interval, one should walk or cycle slowly until a certain desired postrecovery heart rate is achieved, at which point the next interval may begin. Determining the recovery heart rate will likely take some trial and error. It should be defined as the heart rate after recovery from which the next interval can be done at very close to the previous pace. For example, one may run 400-m intervals and reach a maximum heart rate of 180 beats/min and then undergo a recovery walk. Then, for example, when a heart rate of 110 beats/min is reached, the next interval is started. There are obviously much less rigorous ways to perform interval work, but engaging in the creative design process will make one's workouts more fun and varied.

A more tolerable regimen has been proposed by Gliemann and colleagues.[29] The routine they studied involves intervals of a minute in duration, beginning with the first 30 seconds at a sustainable but hard intensity, followed by 20 seconds above the LT, and then 10 seconds of all-out effort. The number of intervals can be increased over time. Their studies showed similar improvement in fitness and performance, and production of vascular endothelial growth factor (VEGF), a marker of microvascular angiogenesis. They propose that this ramped format of IT is more tolerable than and just as beneficial as an intense minute at maximum effort.

EFFICIENCY OF MOVEMENT

In the final step to understanding movement over ground or water, energy must be turned into work with some degree of efficiency (i.e., using the biomechanics of the body to optimize the energy generated by oxidative metabolism). Most of that biomechanical efficiency is inborn. There are many athletes who are so efficient that their excellent performance may be achieved with a less-than-elite aerobic capacity. By the same token, there are many individuals with prodigious $\dot{V}O_2$max levels and high LTs with suboptimal biomechanics such that their transformation of energy to movement prohibits them from performing at an elite level. This is contrasted with high-altitude mountaineers who have high (but not extraordinary) levels of $\dot{V}O_2$, whose efficiency of movement and high LTs allow them to move quickly and efficiently for hours.

A fascinating example of efficient energy expenditure comes from a study at 4700 m in Tibet, where the authors did maximal exercise testing for 17 Tibetans native to the area and 14 recently migrated Han Chinese. Although the Han had higher $\dot{V}O_2$max values than did the Tibetans (i.e., 36 versus 30 mL/kg/min), the

Tibetans generated significantly higher work output (i.e., 176 versus 150 watts) at those maximum $\dot{V}O_2$ levels, LTs at higher percentage of $\dot{V}O_2$max (i.e., 84% versus 62%), and lower blood lactate concentrations.[25] There is ongoing speculation as to whether these characteristics are genetic or adaptive; however, regardless of the mechanism of these differences, the Tibetans appear to be ideal work machines at high altitude, and they are able to perform more efficient work with less energy expenditure. Thus, the question arises: Can we train ourselves not only to be more fit but also more efficient (i.e., the perfect adaptation for the wilderness adventurer)?

There are a number of studies demonstrating that—with aerobic, anaerobic, and resistive training—modest improvements in work efficiency can be attained. In a previously cited study,[39] speed endurance training in competitive runners resulted in 5.7% to 6.6% lower oxygen consumptions at three set levels of speed on a treadmill compared with endurance-trained runners. In another training study in runners comparing endurance and IT for 4 weeks,[6] many of the measured variables, including $\dot{V}O_2$max, were unchanged. The most notable finding was that, at maximum energy expenditure (which was unchanged between the two groups), velocity was significantly higher in the runners who had used IT, suggesting greater running economy. Although the topic of exposure to intermittent hypoxia will be discussed more later in this chapter, it is worthy of brief mention to note that, in one study, college track athletes were randomly assigned to 29 days of low-altitude normoxia, constant simulated high altitude (3000 m), or nocturnal hypoxia. Although there were no changes in $\dot{V}O_2$max, hemoglobin, endurance, or LT, the athletes exposed to intermittent nocturnal hypoxia showed about 5% improvement in running economy at a high race speed.

The mechanisms for these improvements are only speculative, but some insight may be gained from a study looking at work efficiency in highly trained cyclists. The investigators looked at work related to caloric expenditure and found a positive correlation with type I (aerobic) muscle fiber types taken from thigh muscle biopsies.[16] Of note was the large range (i.e., 32% to 76%) of type I fibers in these athletes. One of the potential mechanisms of energy cost saving with intense training of any type may be a decrease in ventilatory demand and thus the work of breathing, which, although modest, may be critical to performance.[24] The addition of explosive strength to normal endurance training in competitive runners as compared with ongoing endurance training resulted in improved 5000-m times, which correlated with the improvement in running efficiency. It has even been suggested that ongoing training and competition by a repeat Tour de France winner have resulted in improved efficiency.[14] Although the improvements in efficiency are modest in most of these studies, such improvements may be critical not only to competitive athletes but also to survival in a wilderness environment.

AGING AND TRAINING

As one ages, wisdom—more than speed—in the wilderness may be one's saving grace, but it does not preclude ongoing commitment to conditioning. There is a wealth of literature about the effects of aging on muscle and aerobic performance; a brief summary is important to include here, because so many of us will continue to venture into the wilderness. It is difficult to define old age, but one could say that it begins with the later part of the sixth decade, when there seems to be an inexorable decrease in aerobic capacity and strength. There is another phase of aging, called *senescence,* when there is a profound and irretrievable decline in mitochondrial function, muscle mass, and cardiac compliance. The topic of master athletes and the underlying physiologic mechanisms accounting for the decline in aerobic capacity with age despite rigorous training are also important areas for aging wilderness adventurers to consider.[71]

Almost all organs involved in exercise show declining elasticity and flexibility with age. For example, in the lungs, there are decreased compliance and elastic recoil, decreased respiratory muscle strength, greater gas exchange heterogeneity, and decreased chemosensor sensitivity. These changes result in a greater

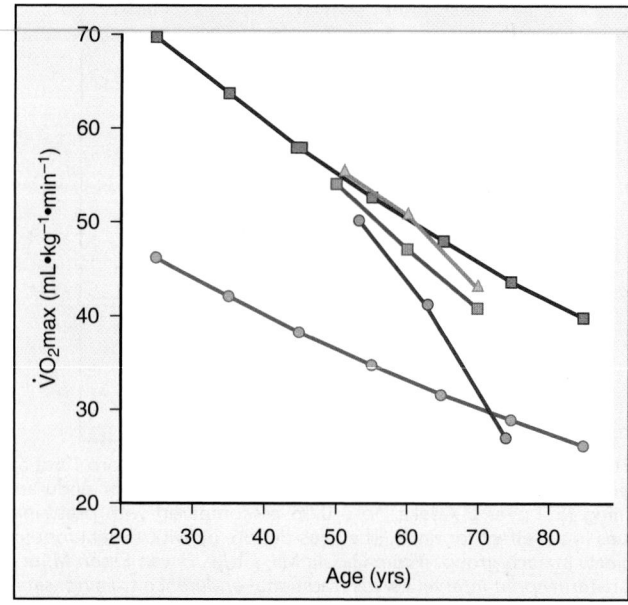

FIGURE 95-9 Maximum oxygen consumption ($\dot{V}O_2$max) of older endurance athletes who continued to train at a high (■), moderate (■), or low intensity (●) after 10-year and 20-year follow-ups (present study). Curves for athletes (▲) and untrained healthy persons (●) are cross-sectional norms. *(From Heath GW, Hagberg JM, Ehsani AA, et al: A physiologic comparison of younger and older endurance athletes, J Appl Physiol 51:634, 1981.)*

work of breathing with exercise, impingement on expiratory flow limitation, enhanced tachypnea with smaller tidal volume, higher-frequency breathing pattern, and potential hypoxemia.

The heart also loses elasticity as the ventricles stiffen and impair end-diastolic filling. In addition, there is a reduction of maximum heart rate. This reduction can be minimized if one continues to train into older age. The oft-quoted maximum heart rate of 220 beats/min minus age is but a gross approximation taken from the cross-sectional data of mostly unfit individuals. There is a decline in peripheral vascular compliance, which may play a role in further hindering blood flow and oxygen delivery.[58] Some of the earlier data also suggested a linear decline in $\dot{V}O_2$max beginning sometime during the third decade of life,[18,40] but subsequent studies have shown that little reduction in $\dot{V}O_2$max occurs from the age of 20 years to the mid-50s if athletes continue active training[57,72] (Figure 95-9).

The cross-sectional data certainly reflect the changes in lifestyle that come with families, jobs, and geography. Although $\dot{V}O_2$max declines in everyone at a certain point, the decline is a result of decreases in oxygen delivery and cardiac output as well as a decrease in oxygen use with declining mitochondrial function, especially among the truly elderly.[5,47,68]

It also used to be thought that, after a certain age, neither strength nor aerobic capacity could be improved.[4,19] However, many studies over the last two decades have clearly shown that older individuals who are otherwise healthy can train and improve both strength and aerobic capacity. The earlier studies were of rather low intensity and duration; whereas, later studies showed that substantial gains could be made with higher intensity and longer duration of training. These gains can translate into practical function in any wilderness environment.

Comparing the decline in $\dot{V}O_2$max between masters and sedentary subjects more than 60 years old, Rogers and colleagues[64] showed that, with ongoing aerobic training, older individuals could decrease the decline per decade in $\dot{V}O_2$max from 10% to 5%. Kohrt and colleagues[45] took 110 untrained men and women between the ages of 60 and 71 years, measured their prestudy $\dot{V}O_2$max, and then had them perform 9 to 12 months of walking or running 4 days per week for 40 minutes per session at 80% of their predicted maximum heart rates. Men and women improved their maximum values by 26% and 23%, respectively. When they were divided into three equal age groups, there also was similar improvement. In terms of improvements, these values are comparable with those seen among younger subjects.

Conley and colleagues[13] engaged sedentary healthy men and women between the ages of 65 and 92 years in 4 months of both aerobic and strength training and used $\dot{V}O_2$max testing, Cybex strength measurements, muscle biopsies, and nuclear magnetic resonance spectroscopy to measure creatine phosphate dynamics before and after training. They compared the results of these subjects with those of healthy controls, and found substantial improvements in all of the outcome variables, which were equal in percentage of improvement to those obtained with younger subjects.

These studies are a few of many that have confirmed two important facts: (1) older healthy individuals can be trained in both endurance and strength to a degree comparable with those of younger subjects; and (2) individuals who continue to train throughout life can slow the inevitable rate of decline in aerobic capacity. As is true for younger individuals, it is the total amount of work done that is the important factor for the making of aerobic gains. The American Academy of Sports Medicine recommends approximately 250 to 300 kcal per session. The energy expended is a combination of duration and intensity that must add up to the recommended total. In other words, 40 to 50 minutes of moderate walking would be comparable with 20 to 30 minutes of jogging or slow running for these elder groups.

HIGH ALTITUDE AND EXERCISE

During the summer of 1968 in Mexico City, three world records were set in track and field, and one favored American miler was soundly defeated. Tommie Smith (200 m), Lee Evans (400 m), and Bob Beamon (long jump) set records that stood for decades. Jim Ryun, the favorite in the 1500 m, was beaten by Kip Keino from Kenya. Aside from the fact that the first three were serendipitously some of the greatest sprinters and jumpers of all time, part of their advantage may have been the slightly thinner air at the altitude of 2200 m (Figure 95-10).

Alternatively, Jim Ryun and the American middle-distance hopes were dashed. The burning questions then became the following: Was Ryun not acclimatized to the higher altitude? Was there something special about Keino's being born and raised at that altitude in Kenya? These questions set off an intense interest in high-altitude training, which was thought to be the answer for improved aerobic performance. Initially, no one thought of any potential deleterious effects of training at higher altitudes. As has been discussed previously, in spite of certain acknowledged benefits, training at such altitudes does not allow one to reach the intensity of training that is necessary for improved aerobic fitness and higher sustainable workloads. Prudent investigators started a series of studies to answer these questions more precisely. In fact, before the 1988 Seoul Olympics, the American road cycling coach wanted to take the team to an altitude of more than 3700 m for 2 weeks right before the games, which were to be held at sea level. Fortunately, he was prevailed upon to not do so. By that time, it was clear that there was a decrease in intensity of work that athletes were able to do at those altitudes. High intensity of work, as has been noted previously, is needed for greater gains in aerobic capacity and beneficial alteration of the LT.

EFFECT OF HIGH ALTITUDE ON EXERCISE

The next two sections of this chapter cover the effects of altitude on exercise as well as the positive and negative aspects of training at high altitude (Figure 95-11). Both topics have important implications for wilderness travel, much of which occurs in the cold, thin air. Chapter 1 covers the broad topics of high-altitude acclimatization and illness.

All levels of climbers dream of scaling the world's highest peaks. Those who are successful at high-altitude climbing are athletes whose characteristics are not uniform. However, as is true of other elite athletes, certain traits are necessary.[33,56,60,74]

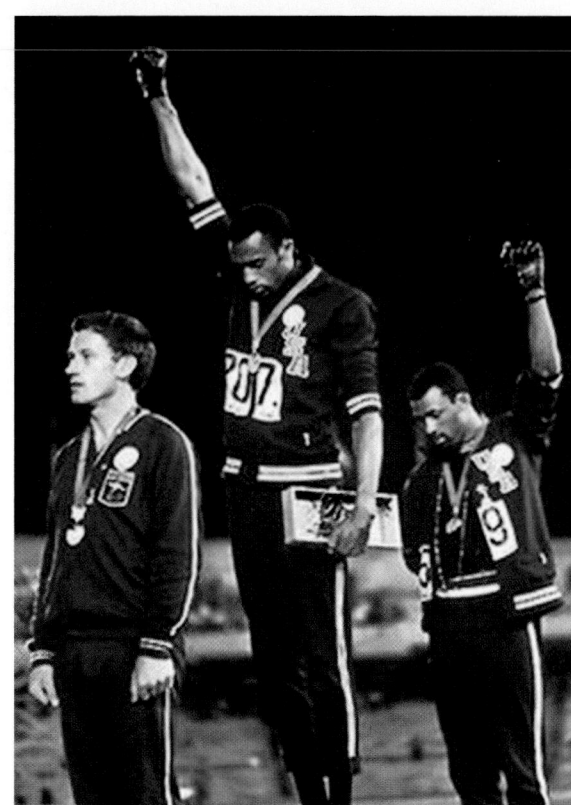

FIGURE 95-10 Peter Norman, Tommie Smith, and John Carlos at the award ceremony for the 200 m race at the 1968 Summer Olympics in Mexico City, an altitude of 2200 m (7218 feet).

Many of the same physiologic limitations are encountered to a lesser degree at more moderate altitudes frequented by trekkers and adventure travelers, but for both groups, an understanding of the common hindrances is quite important.

Anyone who has sojourned quickly to 3000 m or higher cannot exert themselves without dyspnea and exercise limitation. With acclimatization over time, the limitations discovered at 3000 m can be substantially diminished.[34] At altitudes of 3500 to 8000 m, sea-level performance cannot be attained despite prolonged adaptation. Although the fraction of oxygen in the earth's atmosphere is constant at 0.2093, the barometric pressure and thus the content of oxygen decreases as one ascends. For example, with some variation depending on the weather, the

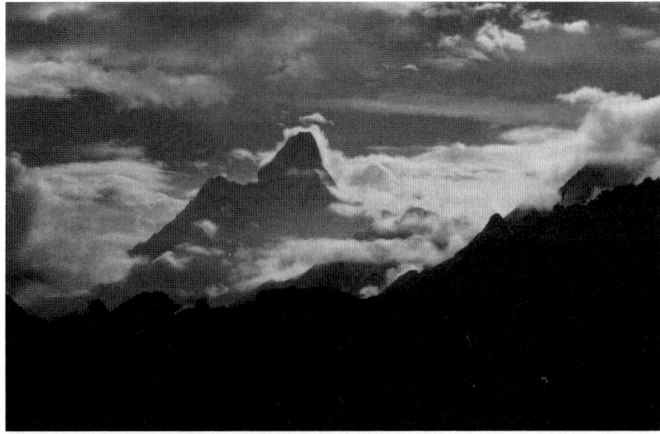

FIGURE 95-11 Mt Ama Dablam in the Khumbu region of Nepal. (Courtesy Robert B. Schoene.)

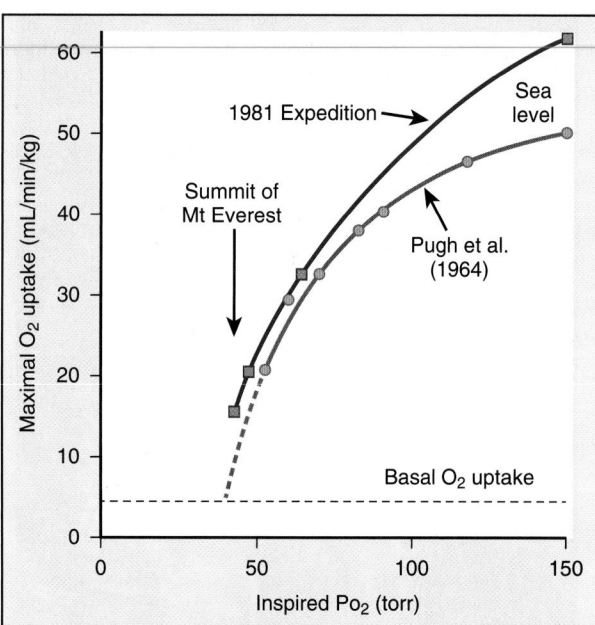

FIGURE 95-12 Maximum oxygen (O_2) consumption plotted against inspired partial pressure of oxygen (PO_2). The present data (■) are contrasted with measurements (●) made previously by Pugh. Note that, although the curve derived from the data in the present study is only slightly shifted to the left, because of the steepness of slope, gain in maximum oxygen uptake at extreme altitudes is substantial. *(From West JB, Boyer SJ, Graber DJ, et al: Maximal exercise at extreme altitudes on Mount Everest, J Appl Physiol 55:688, 1983; and Pugh LG: Cardiac output in muscular exercise at 5800 m (19,000 feet), J Appl Physiol 19:441, 1964.)*

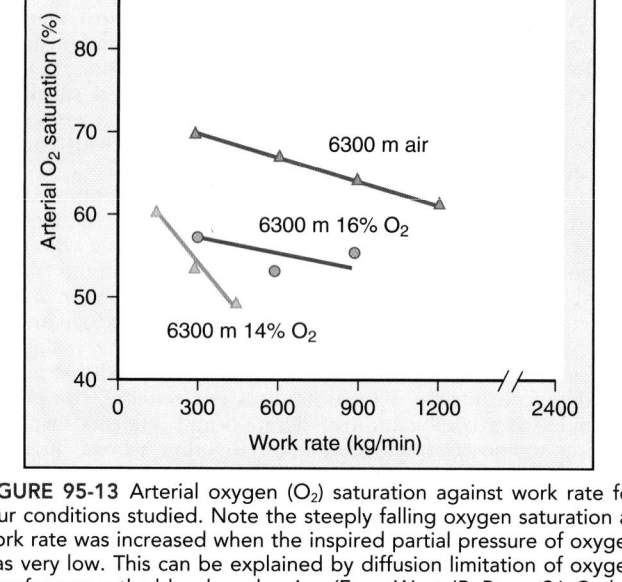

FIGURE 95-13 Arterial oxygen (O_2) saturation against work rate for four conditions studied. Note the steeply falling oxygen saturation as work rate was increased when the inspired partial pressure of oxygen was very low. This can be explained by diffusion limitation of oxygen transfer across the blood-gas barrier. *(From West JB, Boyer SJ, Graber DJ, et al: Maximal exercise at extreme altitudes on Mount Everest, J Appl Physiol 55:688, 1983; and Sutton JR, Reeves JT, Wagner PD, et al: Operation Everest II: oxygen transport during exercise at extreme simulated altitude, J Appl Physiol 64:1309, 1988.)*

barometric pressure at sea level is approximately 760 mm Hg, whereas, at the summit of Mt Everest (as measured by Chris Pizzo on October 23, 1981), the barometric pressure was 253 mm Hg. Thus, at the summit, there is approximately one-third of the amount of oxygen available for aerobic activity as compared with sea level.[75] With less oxygen available in the air, there is a decrease in oxygen availability at each step of the delivery of oxygen from air to the lungs to the blood to the tissues and mitochondria. As a climber ascends, his or her $\dot{V}O_2$max decreases[70,73] (Figure 95-12), and the speed of ascent and sustainable work rate decrease.

One of the limiting factors is the increased work of breathing that occurs for any given level of energy expenditure. For example, the ventilatory equivalent is almost four times greater at 6300 m than it is at sea level.[12,67] Thus, blood flow necessary to perfuse the muscles of respiration is stolen from the muscles of locomotion. Furthermore, because of a diffusion limitation of oxygen from air to the blood at high altitude, the higher one ascends, the greater the amount of oxygen desaturation with exercise (Figure 95-13).

The body at high altitude goes through a complex series of adaptations that do their best to optimize delivery and use of oxygen, despite less availability. The breadth of acclimatization involves a progressive increase in ventilation that is immediate and goes on for weeks; an improvement in ventilation and perfusion match in the lungs and thus gas exchange, which occurs over the course of several hours; an increase in oxygen-carrying capacity as a result of an increase in red blood cell production through erythropoiesis that occurs within 10 to 14 days; and an improvement in tissue oxidative capacities over a number of weeks to months.

For persons going to high altitudes, the most important thing to remember is that everyone's rate of adaptation at each of these steps is different, which results in a range of time for adaptation. Thus, when on a trek, everyone with enough time to do so should adapt well and be equal in terms of acclimatization and

fitness; however, it is difficult to predict who will be a slow versus fast adapter. Sometimes the individual who feels less well at the beginning may be the best acclimatized at the end.

In terms of training for high-altitude ventures, other than being generally fit, there is not much a lowlander can do to prepare. Chapter 1 suggests rates of ascent to minimize the chances of getting altitude illnesses. These rates are similar to those needed for people to gain acclimatization and fitness. The most common mistake is to take too little time for a trip to the Himalayas or the Andes—or even a week-long ski trip to Colorado. A rigid schedule that does not allow sufficient time for acclimatization is dissatisfying at best and dangerous at worst. Having been preexposed to high altitude before going on a challenging trek is always beneficial, but usually neither feasible nor practical.[55] Such issues have become important considerations for military personnel, who may need to ascend rapidly for certain operations.[54]

HYPOXIC TRAINING

Interest in training at high altitude for low-altitude athletic events has not abated over the last four decades. What started as a positive assumption turned into an area of intense research to try to answer whether living or training at high altitude is beneficial for low-altitude competition. Some of these principles apply not only to competitive events but also to travel and adventure to high altitudes. The purpose of altitude training and intermittent hypoxic training is to induce some physiologic adaptation from hypoxia that is presumably beneficial to endurance performance.[51]

When it finally dawned on trainers and coaches that full-time hypoxic exposure might not be beneficial, a number of methods were tried to get "enough" hypoxic exposure without having too much. Levine and Stray-Gundersen[50] set out on a prolonged series of experiments in accomplished runners. The study design included four groups: (1) athletes who lived and trained at low altitude (LLTL); (2) those who lived high and trained high (LHTH); (3) those who lived low and trained high (LLTH); and (4) those who lived high and trained low (LHTL). Part of the rationale for such a design was to test the hypothesis that training at high altitude does not allow an athlete to achieve as intense a training effect as he or she could achieve at lower altitude. The altitude exposure of the LHTL group was 4 weeks of 20 hours per day at 2500 m. The upshot from these series of studies was that the athletes who improved their $\dot{V}O_2max$ and 5000-m times were in the LHTL group, and this improvement correlated with those who had an erythropoietic response. The increase in $\dot{V}O_2max$ corresponded precisely with the increase in oxygen-carrying capacity. However, even in the LHTL group, there were responders and nonresponders, which were differentiated by improvements in 5000-m race time. The responders' improvements corresponded with whether they had an erythropoietic response. Levine contends that there is a threshold (i.e., specific hypoxic dose) that is necessary to inducing these responses and that, in a number of previous studies, the dose may not have been long or high enough.[49] In his discussion, he reminds the reader that the mechanism of response to hypoxia is signaled by hypoxia-inducible factor-1α and that this protein is one of the most evanescent proteins of gene transcription described in the body: when the hypoxic stimulus is removed, hypoxia-inducible factor-1α immediately disappears. Thus, all subsequent gene transcription ceases, and no further growth factors (e.g., erythropoietin) are stimulated. The hypoxic exposure must be intense and sufficiently prolonged to keep the cycle going. Not everyone responds, and the gains are minimal among those who do. So is it all worth it?

Many athletes think it is worth it. The urge to excel has led to "hypoxic sleeping tents" that can be purchased. With such a tent, the athlete can sleep in his or her bed and dial in progressive altitudes for weeks of "natural acclimatization and blood doping." This trend has led to a number of studies of intermittent hypoxia (i.e., normobaric or hypobaric) to see if effects similar to those obtained at true altitude could be found. Julian and colleagues[43] exposed athletes to progressive normobaric hypoxia (i.e., a fraction of inspired oxygen of 0.11%) for 2 weeks for 70 minutes each day and found no changes in performance or erythropoietic markers. Using normobaric hypoxia (i.e., a fraction of inspired oxygen of 14.5%) for 6 weeks, Zoll and colleagues[77] divided runners into two groups: LLTL and LLTH. They looked at performance (i.e., $\dot{V}O_2max$ and time to exhaustion) and muscle biopsies to evaluate markers of hypoxic transcription and oxidative phosphorylation. With the LLTH design, the researchers found a modest improvement in $\dot{V}O_2max$ (5%), a remarkable improvement in time to exhaustion (26%), and substantial increases in the transcription factors and markers of oxidative phosphorylation. Gore and colleagues[32] exposed athletes to a simulated altitude of 4000 to 5500 m for 3 hours per day on 5 days per week for 4 weeks and found an increase in erythropoietin but no increase in markers of red cell production. With a similar design, this same research group studied swimmers and found no improvement in swimming times with the intermittent hypoxia.[63] They concluded that the "hypoxic dose" was not adequate enough.

Other studies have shown similar modest or negative results with various paradigms of altitude training. Siebermann et al.[69] used normobaric hypoxia simulated to 3000 m for 16 hours per day for 4 weeks. They found no difference in physiologic markers and performance between the low-altitude and simulated high-altitude exposure. On the other hand, Saugy and colleagues[65] used hypobaric hypoxia and compared findings with exposure at comparable altitude and duration to subjects in normobaric hypoxia, and found a modest improvement in the normobaric hypoxia group. The mechanism of the difference is not clear.

Not all intermittent hypoxic studies have been negative. Katayama and colleagues[44] exposed a small group of runners to a simulated altitude of 4500 m for 90 minutes per day three times per week for 3 weeks. In the hypoxic group, they found improvements in running time and time to exhaustion as well as lower $\dot{V}O_2$ levels at submaximal exercise levels, with no other changes

in hemodynamic or hematologic variables. Thus, the authors contended that this type of exposure led to an improvement in running efficiency. However, they did not offer any insight into the mechanism of presumed efficiency. Humberstone-Gough and colleagues[38] compared a group living high and training low (LHTL) with intermittent hypoxic training, and found a greater increase in hemoglobin as well as improved running efficiency and speed in the LHTL group. Another construct was utilized by Faiss and colleagues[23] in athletes from team sports. They used intermittent hypoxic exposure to repeat sprint training during hypoxia, and found decreased fatigue in the interval-trained athletes. Presumed improvement in efficiency was invoked as the mechanism of improvement.

So, are all of these manipulations much ado about nothing? There seems to be a benefit in performance for some athletes who are "responders," but clearly the "dose" and duration of the hypoxic exposure have to be adequate. That dose is a tedious one to determine, and such efforts may only be worthwhile for highly competitive athletes. As for those who venture into the mountains, remember to go slowly and enjoy the scenery.

ARTIFICIAL TRAINING METHODS: BLOOD TRANSFUSION

With the advent of competitive wilderness events (e.g., endurance high-altitude races, "X-games," speed climbs), the use of dangerous and arguably unethical methods to improve one's performance has inevitably emerged. This is not surprising given the presence of such methods in other sports for decades or perhaps even centuries. Although there is no role for such interventions in wilderness activities or competitions, a short comment on one of the most egregious approaches is warranted.

There is a surfeit of information on blood transfusions ("doping") and erythropoietic medications.[21,28,62] The interest in enhancement of performance by increasing oxygen-carrying capacity with extra red blood cells was brought to attention via the 1968 Mexico City Olympics and then into the 1970s, when certain middle-distance Scandinavian track athletes were suspected of blood doping. Subsequent data supported the benefit of increased red blood cell mass and improved aerobic performance.[9] Such augmentation was achieved by either autologous or allogeneic transfusions, and later when recombinant erythropoietin (EPO) was developed. Administration of this drug was rampant in a number of sports venues, most notoriously European cycling. Although the benefit of increased red cell mass was acknowledged, the philosophy that, "If some is good, more is better" led to fatal complications in a number of young athletes, because the downside sequelae of increased red blood cell mass were increased blood viscosity, strokes, and death.

Both the scientific community and international sports governing bodies have rallied to try to prevent such abuse and minimize the physical risk to young, vulnerable athletes. Detection of both blood doping and EPO has reached a scientific level of sophistication such that most athletes, when properly screened, can be discovered.

It is the opinion of this author that to summit Mt Everest, win a high-altitude endurance race, or be publically acclaimed as a champion in an extreme sport, one should compete and perform within the boundaries of "fair means." To do otherwise clearly sometimes incurs unacceptable risks of injury and death, because the wilderness environment in and of itself can accentuate dehydration, hemoconcentration, and subsequent medical consequences, including death. As emphasized earlier, one should go to the wilderness for enjoyment, fellowship, and self-fulfillment.

REFERENCES

Complete references used in this text are available online at expertconsult.inkling.com.

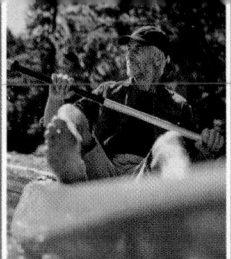

CHAPTER 96
Exercise, Conditioning, and Performance Training

JOLIE BOOKSPAN

A surprising number of exercise and conditioning activities do not build function for daily life, the trail, or survival in the wilderness. Sets and repetitions of stretches and exercises do not change poor movement ergonomics or repair injuries. Some reinforce movement habits leading to increased injury, which may be mistaken for overtraining and pain syndromes. Stretches and exercises are most beneficial when they directly train and practice real-life function and healthful biomechanics. This chapter covers healthy, functional training for lifetime health, pain prevention, and healthier wilderness travel.

FITNESS AS A LIFESTYLE

To many people, fitness means stopping "real" life to do repetitions of motions in a gym with poor similarity to movement patterns in daily life or sport, and then returning to moving with poor ergonomics, bending in unhealthful ways dozens of times daily, and slouching when standing, sitting, and moving. Fitness as a lifestyle does not necessarily mean working out or going hiking. It is how one moves in all regular daily activities everywhere, sometimes called functional movement. Where conventional exercises are sometimes not healthy and will not prevent poor movement that injures, functional fitness adds strength, mobility, injury prevention, awareness, stretch, and other benefits that would otherwise not be achieved. Gymnasium training can be helpful or harmful, depending on the nature and quality of the exercises, stretching routines, and workouts taught and performed.

Changing exercises into healthy functional movement is a large and inspiring area of rethinking and retraining. Instead of sitting and moving slouched and then stopping to stretch to relieve the resulting pain, one should sit, stand, and lift properly to enact exercise and muscle length as a lifestyle, and prevent pain in the first place. Instead of isolated abdominal exercises, one should employ a neutral spine posture that uses abdominal muscles to prevent an unhealthful spine angle during running and movements of daily living; this deploys substantial functional abdominal exercise in daily standing and moving. It is important to be active, but not as a different, inconvenient part of the day. Ordinary daily actions to bend, move, lift, reach, and balance, when changed to healthful patterns, provides healthy, built-in exercise as a lifestyle.

SPECIFICITY

Strength, power, muscular endurance, balance, and cardiovascular fitness engage different body systems. Each develops through different practices. Working one part, such as arms or legs, or one system, such as strength or flexibility, does little to develop other parts or systems.[9] Running, for example, creates cardiovascular, metabolic, and structural changes specific to running but not necessarily to hanging from rock ledges. Trained runners may exhaust themselves during long swims, and paddlers during climbs, even though all may have high aerobic capacity. Another example is a common weight-lifting practice of lifting at slow speed. This does not train the more rapid joint angle movement needed in common wilderness, daily life, and rescue situations.[13] Slow lifting can build strength, just as can any weight lifting, but not power that depends on speed, or injury-prevention capability that comes from training

for rapid stabilization. To get off a ridge before bad weather hits, and be fast and safe when these attributes are most needed, one needs to train different body parts and systems to work together.

It is best to train as needed for function, and to train abilities together. Wilderness skills and activities of daily living are multisystem, multijoint, multispeed, and multifunctional entities. The wilderness often demands endurance, strength, power, and balance simultaneously (e.g., holding healthy joint positioning under the weight of a pack while crossing a rope bridge, descending carrying a stretcher on skis or in foul weather, rock hopping, escaping a flash flood, or hiking with small children).

STRENGTH, MUSCULAR ENDURANCE, AND POWER

Strength is generally defined as how much a person can move or carry in a single or a few efforts. Muscular endurance is how long one can continue being strong. Power in a fitness setting is how quickly one can be strong; power is work per unit of time.

The ability to perform strength, endurance, and power tasks depends on the individual level of fitness, workload, type of work, exercise efficiency, and leverage, and on whether the work is external, such as carrying weights,[54] or internal, such as carrying oneself,[176] which varies with body weight. On ascents, a heavy person may work harder and closer to his or her maximum than does a lighter person of similar fitness or even of lesser fitness, depending on the workload. Internal work such as hiking and climbing may favor the smaller, lighter person. For external work such as that involved in a portage, rescue, and hauling gear, a larger person of high muscular fitness may have an advantage. Several factors influence advantage more than do strength and size.

Different activities require different ratios of strength to muscle contraction speed. A higher strength component compared with speed of contraction (e.g., used during portage and rock climbing scrambling) is strength-dominated power.[9] Kicking with fins, swimming, running, jumping, and deploying safety equipment primarily employ speed-dominated power.[125] Many situations, such as navigating rapids, require both strength and speed in constantly changing proportions.

Abdominal Muscles and the Core

It is a common assumption that strong abdominal or other muscles support the back, spine, or body, for certain activities. However, abdominal strength or endurance does not automatically support any structures or reduce the incidence of back pain. The word *support* is often used without understanding what the muscles actually do. Merely being strong or tight does not effect any change or support. Actual support entails a voluntary and specific change in vertebral and pelvic angles to reduce loading and pain-producing positioning.[20] For the abdominal muscles to support the back, it means they need to move the spine away from an injurious into a healthful angle that can be maintained during movement and standing. Merely strengthening muscles by conventional exercises does not accomplish that.

Abdominal muscles do not lend a special "support" function different from other muscles. Like any other skeletal muscles, abdominal muscles pull on the bones to which they are attached. Specifically, abdominal muscles pull the ribs and pelvis to bend (flex) the spine forward. The times during which one needs abdominal muscles to pull to flex the spine forward is not when lying on the back, but when standing, walking, running, carrying loads, and during all other movement (even some instances of sitting), not to bend forward but enough to prevent the spine from hyperextending into compressive hyperlordosis (swayback). Hyperlordosis increases the lower spinal curve, compressing posterior vertebrae and associated facet joints. Hyperlordosis is a major cause of "mystery" lower back pain felt after prolonged periods of upright position because of the compressive loading from the acutely pinched lumbar angle. Sitting and bending far forward temporarily stretches the compressed painful area, giving rise to mistaken practices of forward bending to cure back pain, rather than stop the damaging cause of allowing the painful hyperextended posture. It should be noted that in certain circumstances of anatomic abnormality, such as spinal stenosis, slightly bending forward for a moment can provide pain relief and is diagnostic. Using a neutral spine can also provide this in many cases.

Hyperlordosis means too much inward curve to the lower (lumbar) spine. It is not a structural problem but an unhealthful and easily changed bad posture. Tightening or strengthening abdominal muscles does not change a hyperlordotic spine angle or prevent return of the resulting pain. Preventing the overly large arch of hyperlordosis by moving the pelvis and lumbar spine to a neutral angle discontinues unhealthful loading and the cause of that specific pain.

Maintaining a neutral spine posture employs voluntary use of abdominal muscles. Strengthening abdominal muscles through exercises does not cause or promote a neutral spine. Through practice, abdominal muscles are in constant use to flex the spine sufficiently to habitually maintain a neutral spine posture.

It does not take great core strength to transform a hyperlordotic to a neutral lumbar spine. Therefore, even smaller people can tolerate a heavy pack with less strain, whereas someone with a strong core who stands with an increased lordotic arch (hyperlordosis) imposes a high load on vertebral facets[107] and disks[23] from the weight of the upper body and the pack on the unfavorable vertebral angle. The person who uses core muscles to prevent an injurious spinal angle will acutely reduce back pain, and prevent its return without exercise or medical treatments.[21] To feel the change from hyperlordosis to a neutral spine posture, try the following and refer to Figures 96-1 to 96-3 for change of hyperlordosis to neutral:

- Stand with your back against a wall. Touch the heels, buttocks, and upper back to the wall. Notice if you have a large space between your lower back and the wall, and/or if you need to lift ribs to enable your upper body to touch the wall. If this causes back pain, you may have a hyperlordosis component. Reducing this to neutral spine will immediately reduce lower back compression and therefore pain.
- Change the large lumbar space to neutral spine posture by gently pressing the lower back closer toward the wall, reducing the large arch. Tuck hips as if starting a crunch, without curling the upper body forward. Do not tighten hip or abdominal muscles or curl your upper body away from the wall. Learn to stand comfortably upright, not bent forward. If previous pain existed from too high an angle, low back pressure should be gone by reducing the angle to neutral. Do not tighten abdominal muscles or flatten your lower back completely against the wall. Reduce a large inward curve to make the curve smaller and feel how the spine and pelvis moves without tightening to achieve the movement.
- Now try again to stand with your back against a wall, this time also touching (or approximating) the back of your head to the wall. Notice if you need to increase the lower back arch or lift ribs to allow your head to touch or come closer to the wall. If this causes lower back pain, you may have a hyperlordosis component, and reducing it to neutral as described above would help.

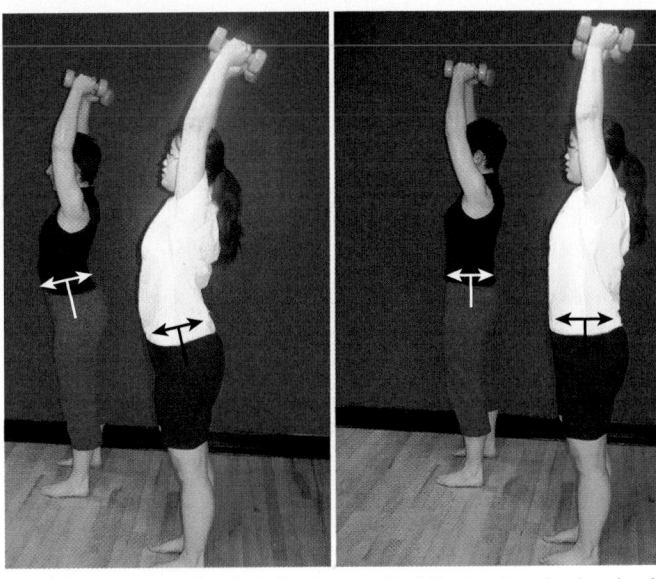

FIGURE 96-1 Hyperlordotic lumbar angle shifts load to the low back (left). Hyperlordosis components include tilting the pelvis anteriorly and/or leaning the upper torso rearward (thoracic leanback). To reduce hyperlordosis to neutral spine posture, tuck the pelvis until it is vertical and bring the upper body forward until it is upright (right). Moving the spine to neutral and maintaining neutral spine posture (not strengthening or tightening) is how abdominal muscles prevent back pain.

- If you cannot reduce hyperlordosis and still maintain the back of your head touching the wall or close enough to it to stand comfortably upright and vertical, your anterior chest and/or anterior hip may be too tight to allow healthful upright standing. Use the functional stretching section that follows for stretches to address these issues. Until then, learn the movement to reduce a significant lumbar hyperlordosis to a smaller healthier neutral spine angle without

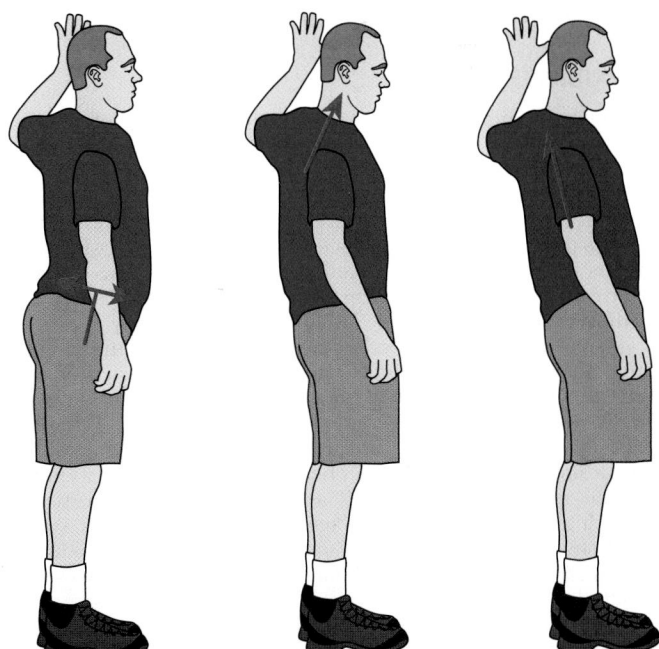

FIGURE 96-2 Restore muscle length to the anterior chest to prevent tightness that favors unhealthful and painful neck and upper back positioning. Maintain a vertical pelvis position (center). Avoid hyperlordosis caused by a flexed, anteriorly tilted hip (left), forward head (center), and hyperlordosis by deploying thoracic leanback and/or pushing the pelvis forward (right).

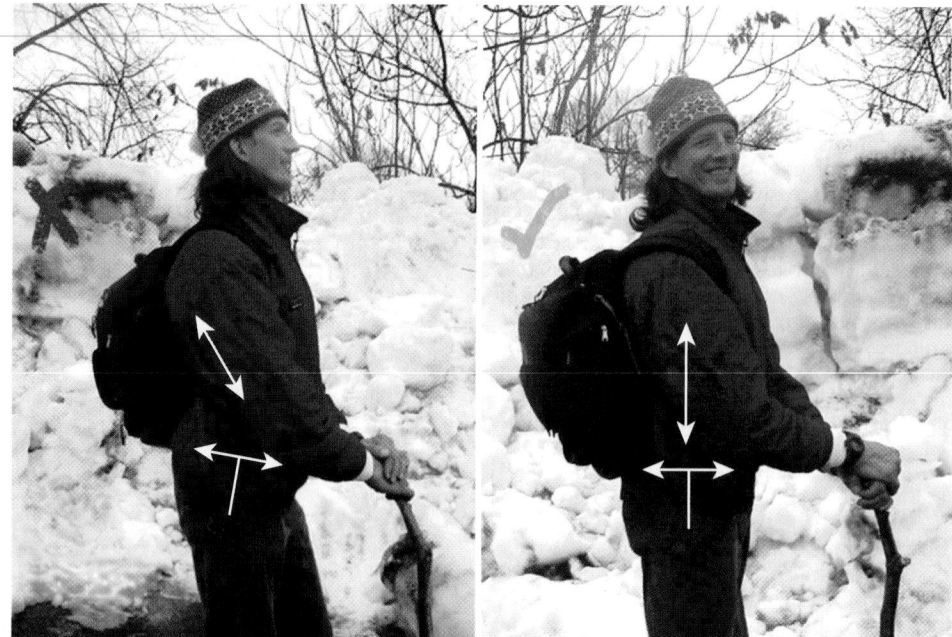

FIGURE 96-3 Hyperlordosis *(left)* shifts the load to the low back joints *(facets)* and is not necessary to balance the pack. Instead, pull upper body to an upright position and tuck the hip to achieve a neutral spine posture and vertical pelvis position, which shift body and pack weight off the lumbar facets and into core musculature *(right)*.

the back of your head against the wall, so that you can put a healthier spine angle and more ergonomic position to immediate use on the trail.

Use abdominal muscles functionally in this way to reduce a hyperlordotic spine during all activity, particularly when lifting overhead and carrying loads, whether in the gym or wilderness (see Figure 96-1). When performed correctly, this reduces loading and pain from functional poor posture, [21] as well as increased vertebral sheer attributed to spondylolisthesis.[24] See Conditioning, later, for functional retraining of core muscles.

FLEXIBILITY

Flexibility training is said to reduce the incidence of activity-based injury.[131] One proposed mechanism is increased muscle length before reaching a tearing point,[137] probably from change in the viscoelastic properties of muscle-tendon units.[178] Another is reduced tendon organ activation.[120] However, the number of injuries that continue to occur seems to dispel the idea of stretching, as it is commonly practiced, as preventive.[150] The disparity seems to lie in how stretching is commonly accomplished, and in movement patterns used during exercise and daily life.

Most conventional stretch practices exacerbate the original problem of pain and dysfunction from excess thoracic kyphosis and stretch weakness of the back and hips. After rounding forward all day over the computer, desk, steering wheel, handle-bars, or backpack, more forward rounding is neither healthful nor desired. The widespread phenomenon of forward bending for the majority of stretching and exercise creates a widely occurring lack of extension range of motion needed to simply stand straight, often resulting in chronic low-grade aches, injury, and wear and tear from habitual unhealthy ergonomics and positioning.

To understand functional flexibility for healthy muscle length for all activities, try the following test to see if you can comfortably stand up straight:

- Stand against a wall with the back of your head, shoulders, hips, and heels touching the wall. A small space remains between your lower back and the wall. Check the following to see if you are too tight to stand comfortably upright:

Do you have to increase the lumbar arch or lift your ribs to touch your head against the wall? Does your chin jut forward or lift up? Is it too uncomfortable to stand upright against the wall? That means you cannot stand comfortably upright with healthy muscle length in real life.

- When lying supine, can you rest comfortably flat with both legs straight without a pillow under the head or knees?

Anterior muscle tightness of the chest and hip are often the limiting factors in being able to stand comfortably upright in a healthy position. A tight, rounded anterior chest and shoulders contribute to neck, upper back, and shoulder pain.[71] Tight anterior hip muscles, common in people who use flexion-dominated exercises, change the normal angle of the hips and low back, inhibiting normal standing, walking, and running, and add a large share of low back pain.[46] Tight hip muscles, calf muscles, and Achilles tendons contribute to walking duck-footed, or toe-out.[151] The resulting change in gait and stance may wear on ankles, knees,[80] hips, and big toe,[151] and contribute to bunion formation.[142] Tight feet add to some, but not all, causes of plantar fasciitis.[162] Tight hamstrings may be prone to strains. It has been reliably established that tight hamstrings are not related to back pain. It is also found that high hamstring flexibility is not statistically correlated with a reduced incidence of back pain.[26] Constant hamstring stretches by bending forward from a standing or sitting position is associated with an increased incidence of disk injury. See the Conditioning section for functional stretches to remedy these issues.

CONDITIONING

This section covers specific functional exercises for health during wilderness travel.

FUNCTIONAL CONDITIONING

Training in the manner used for actual activity is called functional exercise. Strength increase through lifting weights by isolating specific muscles with discrete exercises does not train the multifunctional movement needed to prevent injury, for example, when opening a window or carrying a heavy pack. Many people accustomed to running on a treadmill or elliptical trainer later turn an ankle on uneven terrain because they have not trained balance, proprioception, stabilization muscles, changing direction, push-off phase, and so on.

An effective approach to training for wilderness skills is to change the practice of exercise for each body part to integrated, functional motion for real-life health and physical ability. Instead of using a treadmill, walk and move over uneven ground for movement and balance training to reduce the risk of sprain on uneven footing and unstable slopes. Use muscles to hold the neck, back, and legs in healthy positions all the time, rather than slumping under heavy packs, for built-in, functional exercise and injury prevention. Climb stairs and hills, not a stair-climber machine, to train for the hills. Use good bending technique, covered below, for the innumerable activities of daily living, to strengthen and accustom the body to needed movement. Lift, move, lunge, walk, and squat to prepare for portaging, hauling, climbing, hoisting, and squatting.

STRENGTH, ENDURANCE, AND POWER FOR WILDERNESS PREPAREDNESS

To increase strength, lift a weight heavy enough to produce muscle failure after 8 to 10 lifts in each manner needed for each task. Continuously lifting a weight light enough to be moved or lifted more than 10 times increases muscular endurance. Lifting the same weight faster trains power.

For external work of dragging sleds, building shelters, rescuing, and carrying gear and packs, train by carrying and moving real-life loads in functional movement patterns at varying speeds, while maintaining healthy positioning of the back, neck, and knees.

To develop muscular ability to move your body for hiking, climbing, skiing, and hauling up inclines, practice lifting your body at varying speeds for various repetitions with pull-ups, push-ups, lunges, and squats. Lifting external weight improves strength, but the joint and muscle mechanics of lifting weights are different from moving one's body against the ground or overhead support. To progress, lift yourself while wearing a backpack or other weight. Loading in addition to body weight also trains the important skill of safely moving under the weight of external loads.

Climbing with packs and other skills requiring both internal and external strength to lift and haul is best trained with intelligent cross-training to optimize several fitness components. Vary lifting and training workouts to avoid injury and stagnation.

Upper Body

Push-Ups. Push-ups are functional for strengthening, for endurance if done as many repetitions, for skill in maneuvering body weight, and when done properly, for training the neutral spine posture. Push-ups are effective, convenient, and easy to improve. A supplemental benefit is to strengthen forearms and wrist bones. One of three main sites of osteoporosis is the wrist. Although principal movers for push-ups are the arm and chest muscles, the back, hip, and core are needed to produce and hold a neutral spine posture and prevent hyperlordosis. Push-ups without preventing hyperlordosis do not train stabilization or exercise core muscles, and transfer body weight to the lumbar spine. Use a mirror when possible to determine positioning. To do push-ups with healthful ergonomics, follow these guidelines:

- During the entire range of push-up movement, tuck the pelvis to reduce the low back arch, as if beginning a crunch. When abdominal muscles are used enough to straighten the back, you will feel them working. The more tuck, the more abdominal involvement. Do not bend at the hip to the extent that the posterior hip lifts upward. Hold a straight position with a minimal lumbar curve throughout the push-up.
- Hold the head and neck straight in line with the back, without drooping.
- Keep the upper back straight, not hunched or rounded.

- Keep the elbows slightly bent at the top of the push-up, not locked straight. Do this as well when holding the top push-up position, called a "plank." If the arms are too weak to support the body weight, strengthen them, but do not add to elbow injury by holding them locked in extension.
- Keep weight distributed over the entire hand to strengthen the wrist without compressing the joint.
- When proficient in holding a neutral pelvis during slow push-ups, increase power with increasingly rapid executions of single push-ups, and then multiples. Try to push off quickly and powerfully so that you can clap your hands. Try pushing off enough to lift the feet as well while safely executing jumping push-ups that maintain back posture. Land with shock absorption, without increasing the lumbar arch on landing. Keep hips tucked to neutral without lifting them.
- Push-ups can be done in inventive ways that simulate extreme wilderness situations; for example, one can do push-ups with one foot lifted, both feet propped on a bench, both hands on a medicine ball or exercise ball that rolls, or even hands and feet on two separate medicine balls or other rolling object. Use abdominal muscles to prevent low back arch, not by tightening, but by moving the spine into neutral spine posture without pelvic rotation.
- Prop feet on increasingly high supports until the position is vertical like a handstand. Do small elbow bends, like upside-down push-ups. Work up to holding a handstand without a wall, doing full dips.

Holding a tucked push-up position even for a few seconds without increased lumbar arch and hyperlordosis may be difficult; such a finding makes it clear why the posture sags under body weight throughout the day, pressuring the lower spine joints and soft tissue. Properly done push-ups train spine positioning in the manner needed for real-life neutral posture, and for wilderness situations of carrying loads with healthy ergonomics. If full push-ups cannot yet be done, start with a high plank to train the neutral spine posture. Make increasing efforts to dip down and push back up. Done correctly, you will feel much abdominal, back, and arm activity.

Pull-Ups. Pull-ups are functional training for hauling yourself up, an often-needed outdoor skill. Hang from a bar, door jam, or tree limb for pull-ups.

- Tuck hips under, as described for push-ups. This lordosis-reducing maneuver specifically trains core muscles in a functional manner with the bonus of training a neutral standing posture.
- If full pull-ups cannot yet be done, start with hanging from a bar to train grip, arms, and neutral spine posture. Make increasing efforts to pull. Use a step to boost the initial lift; then pull up the lower body weight unassisted.
- Avoid exclusive use of machines that allow pull-ups using less than body weight. These machines prevent needed training of hanging against full body weight.
- To practice for special climbing situations, hang feet on another overhead support while doing pull-ups. Reducing weight on arms assists pull-ups while adding tilt and stabilization components.

Lower Body

An average day entails hundreds of bending actions for household and work activities. Instead of doing sets and reps of artificial lunges and squats, use the same advised bending actions for the hundreds of bends that can occur daily.

Squats. The squat is a functional strengthener, enhancing the ability to lift, carry, jump, and rise from the ground quickly and easily, and while carrying loads. Functional movement trains a wide range in the amount of squat and whole-body movement. This combines balance, posture, strength, flexibility, and specific movement skills to prevent pain and injury to the knees and back that arise from bad bending.

One can transform all the different daily actions of retrieving objects from the floor and surfaces of various heights into many dozens of functional squats. Done with unhealthy positioning, squats may accumulate damage to the back and knees. Done properly, squats strengthen legs while training for a good bending position.

Practice at first with a mirror to observe positioning:

- Stand facing the mirror with feet apart, and observe your knees.
- Bend both knees, keeping both heels firmly touching the floor.
- As you squat, notice if you allow knees to sway inward of the feet. Use lateral thigh muscles to pull knees over feet.
- Stand sideways to the mirror and watch your knees in side view while squatting. Notice if your knees slide forward. Look down and pull knees back until you can see your toes. Hips should move back without arching the back. Keep hips tucked to neutral spine posture, not increased in arch. Increasing the arch was a fitness fad for many years, but as with all hyperlordosis, it added back pain and reduced use of core muscles.
- Keep kneecaps in line with the direction of the feet.
- Keep weight distributed around the entire soles of the feet, not tilting inward onto the arches.

Each time you bend daily, use the squat, always keeping both heels fully touching the floor for functional built-in Achilles tendon stretch. If you keep both feet and knees facing forward, you will achieve this stretch. If you are not able to maintain fully the advised feet and knees position, at least keep the knees facing in the same direction as the feet.

- To progress, perform squats while lifting a judicious amount of weight with each squat. Try lifting weights to develop other muscle groups by performing curls, bench and military presses, overhead lifts, shrugs, and lifts to the side and to the front, among others. Maintain healthful knee, back, and neck posture. Notice if you arch the low back to lift overhead. Prevent that sort of arching by tucking hips to neutral and bringing your upper body more upright.
- Standing (neutral spine posture) places less load on the back than if the weight is carried while sitting. Therefore, instead of sitting to perform biceps curls or other lift, stand or combine repetitions of curling the weight with repetitions of squatting.
- If you use a barbell, hold the weight across the chest. Avoid weight behind the neck unless practicing the fireman's carry or other required task. Observe the neck and spine position.
- Try upside-down squats (leg presses) lying on your back, lifting your pack or a friend with your legs. Do not curl your back, because this stresses intervertebral disks. Keep your hips firmly on the ground.

Apply healthy knee and foot posture for all daily bending and walking. Do not be daunted if it takes time to solidify these habits, but stick with it, because using muscles is important. Get built-in daily bending as a lifestyle, instead of as isolated sets and reps and then returning to bad bending the rest of the day.

Avoid squatting on the balls of the feet with heels raised. An acute knee angle under the body weight pries the knee joints, depending on the size of one's thighs. Certain meniscal injuries of professional baseball catchers are caused by repetitive squatting on toes.[8] To sit in a full squat to rest, or for toileting, keep heels on the floor, a customary sitting posture in much of the world. Squatting with heels down is a functional Achilles tendon stretch.

Lunges. The lunge functionally strengthens the ability to lift oneself to a stand while carrying an overloaded pack or rescued friend, to duck in order to dodge falling rocks, and to climb difficult terrain. Use the lunge for a healthy way to bend and pick up things. Done properly, lunges are beneficial to knee strength and health. The lunge is often done with unnecessary strain on the knee and back, and/or with ineffective use of muscles.

To perform healthy and effective lunges, do the following:

- The key to healthy lunges is torso and knee position. Reduce lower back overarch by tucking the hip, as if starting a crunch, to neutral spine posture. Done correctly, you will immediately feel stretch increase in your rear anterior hip and lower spine.
- Keep your body weight centered between both legs, not leaning toward the front leg.
- Lift the rear heel with the foot straight, not turned out, and bend both knees to lower directly down.
- Keep the front knee over the front heel as you lower. Do not let the front knee slide forward.
- Lower further as you progress, anywhere from an inch to almost to the floor. Keep the rear knee off the floor. Keep the body upright as you lower and rise.
- Use lateral thigh muscles to keep the front knee over the front heel, not sagging or tilting inward (knock-knee, or valgus knee).
- Keep feet in position and do lunges one after the next without moving the feet.
- Practice landing from jumps in proper lunge or squat form. Do not let the body weight fall inward on your knees or arches. Land with soft shock absorption using the torso, thigh, lower leg, and gluteal muscles. Learn to hold proper posture during jumps to train power, strength, and speed, while reducing injury potential. Add sequential jumps and landings for plyometric training (see Power and Plyometrics, later).
- To progress, lift hand weights with each lunge: curls, presses overhead, shrugs, and lifts to the side and the front. Keep good knee, back, and neck posture. Do not arch your back to overhead lift. This multisegmental activity simulates actual daily needs, such as lifting baskets and children, and trains lifting skills for the trail.
- Practice lunges first slowly, and then more quickly (and carefully), to train functional speed and power.

Abdominal and Core Muscle Conditioning

Strengthening core muscles is commonly thought to solve back pain by correcting muscle weakness. On scrutiny, core strengthening has not been found to reduce pain[70] or effect any greater relief than does aerobic exercise or nonstrength programs.[1,57,101] Exercising abdominal and torso muscles does not alter the poor mechanics that are the source of pain.[116] Tightening and clenching muscles is not functional and in fact inhibits optimal muscle use. Using abdominal and core muscles to reposition the spine to reduce hyperlordosis to a neutral angle is how the abdominal muscles unload the facets and support the back.[20] Using abdominal muscles to flex the spine sufficiently to prevent hyperlordosis when standing, running, and lifting overhead gives functional abdominal exercise during most daily activities.

Crunches, and other common flexion-based exercises, may increase strength, but not functional strength for standing and lifting in the upright position of real activity.[20] Holding neutral spine posture against a stationary or moving load is the key to learning how to use abdominal and core muscles for back pain and posture control. For effective abdominal muscle strengthening specific to daily life and trail ergonomics, try the following:

Isometric Abdominal Muscles Retraining Drill

- Lie face up on the floor holding a pair of light dumbbells. Hold legs straight, not bent at the knee, to simulate standing.
- Extend your arms with biceps next to your ears, holding dumbbells approximately an inch off the floor. Notice if your ribs lift and your lower spine arch increases. Press the lumbar spine to the floor. You will feel the load shift to the abdominal muscles.
- The key to using abdominal muscles is to prevent the ribs from lifting, or the low back from arching from the floor. Press ribs downward.
- Raise and lower the dumbbells to about an inch from the floor as many times as you can (at least 8 to 10 times), continuously using abdominal muscles to keep the lower

back from rising from the floor at any point during the exercise. Keep breathing.

- When you have mastered controlling torso positioning during slow arm movement, increase the speed of raising and lowering the weights. Raise the weights no more than a few inches from the floor. If you can see them, they are too high. As the weight lowers, the momentum and weight will encourage lifting the ribs and arching to shift the work of the exercise from the abdominal muscles to the vertebral joints. Use abdominal muscles to prevent this. This abdominal exercise also works the arms and back. The benefit is to learn to use abdominal muscles to hold safe, effective, and functional neutral spine posture when using the rest of your body.
- It is commonly repeated that knees must be bent to protect the back. However, normal standing and function during real activity are not done with knees bent. Bent knees do not protect the back. Using core muscles to maintain a neutral vertebral angle is what prevents a painful angle and load.[20]
- You may feel the thighs lift if your anterior hip is tight. A tight anterior hip is another problematic result of flexion-based exercise systems. If your anterior hip muscles are too shortened to allow flat supine lying down (or prone without increasing the lumbar arch), you are too tight for standing upright with straight legs, as needed for ordinary life.
- Use this straight-leg exercise (isometric abdominal muscles) to retrain use of these muscles to hold the spine and pelvis in position when standing, and to lengthen the anterior hip muscles to normal extension needed for upright activity and comfortable supine positioning.

Using Neutral Spine Posture and Preventing Hyperlordosis for Push-Ups, Planks, and Pull-Ups. This was described earlier. Tuck hips to neutral. Without the tuck to remove low back overarch, core muscles are not in use, and body weight shifts to the vertebral joints (facets). To add resistance to training functional neutral spine posture, do the following:

- Hold a neutral spine push-up position with one arm raised to or above ear level. Keep the body level, not turned. Raise the opposite leg, keeping a straight neutral spine posture.
- Do neutral spine push-ups on a medicine or exercise ball. Practice holding a neutral torso posture, using abdominal and core muscles to train healthy postural habits. Do not take a good exercise adjunct, like a ball, and lose benefits by doing crunches on it.
- Do push-ups with neutral spine posture and one leg out to the side 90 degrees and parallel to the floor. To progress, lift the opposite arm to the side.
- Remember neutral spine posture during pull-ups. It is common to sway the lumbar spine to make the pull easier. Tuck hips and spine while hanging, and while pulling up.

Using Bands and Cables While Standing With Neutral Spine Posture. Pulling cables connected to weights is a common exercise. Without maintaining the spine and pelvis in neutral position as described above, you will miss the majority of the exercise, and practice injurious faulty posture during exercises. Neutral spine posture during various arm directions against resistance of cables provides large core muscle training, when used to maintain spine position.

Using abdominal muscles does not mean "sucking them in," "tightening," or "pressing your navel to your spine." Breathing and healthy movement are restricted or impossible with tightened abdominal muscles, and tightening does not change the poor posture that loads the low back. To understand this, try the following: tighten abdominal muscles as commonly taught. Press your navel to your spine. Tighten the entire area. Note that such tightening would not be possible or useful for daily activity. Next, stand with arched posture. Tighten the abs and surrounding musculature. Note that posture does not change. Stop tightening the area so that movement is unrestricted. Tuck the spine and hips to remove the lordotic arch, straightening

posture. Train the abdominal musculature for wilderness activity by using muscles to hold healthy spine and pelvic positioning under load, during standing, lifting, and movement. Neutral spine posture (preventing hyperlordosis) provides efficient exercise at the same time as retraining posture and back pain prevention habits.

Hands and Wrists

Hands and wrists require strengthening and training for daily use and wilderness needs of grabbing, holding, lifting, hanging, pulling, belaying, carrying, and rescuing.

- Open jars. Wring wet clothes. Work with clay. Squeeze things. Give massages. Use pliers and screwdrivers. Saw wood.
- Hang from a bar or tree limb to strengthen grip. Increase the time held. Hang from fingers, then fewer fingers, and different groupings of fingers. Perhaps, eventually, hang from one finger.
- Carry groceries with hands, not a cart. Do not lean back when carrying. Stand straight, torso tucked using core muscles (see Abdominal and Core Muscle Conditioning, earlier).
- Carry suitcases and other items with handles, arms by your sides, holding with finger grip (farmer's carry). Carry heavy dumbbells across the room (lifting and setting down properly, using legs, not bending forward). Use a farmer's carry on unwieldy items like plate weights and heavy books like encyclopedias, as if they were suitcases.
- Train the pinch grip and holding grip strength of fingers and palm by carrying partially inflated medicine balls of different weights or rubber balls filled with water.
- Do push-ups to strengthen wrists and arms, and become accustomed to holding and pushing weight with your hands. Keep weight on the whole hand and fingers, not concentrated on the wrists.
- Do push-ups, or hold the push-up position on fingertips, then fewer fingers, and groupings of fingers.
- Use fingers to push and pull things.
- Instead of hanging directly from a pull-up bar, loop a towel over the bar. Grip the towel at each end and hang to train grip for climbing and rescue.
- Hang from door jams and oddly shaped overhead structures for finger grip training.
- Instead of first gripping and then lowering body weight, jump up to hang from fingers, to practice unexpected situations requiring quick, sure grasp.
- Get rest and stretch fingers back (extension) between intense periods of finger grip and handgrip training to prevent tendon irritation.
- Regularly stretch fingers back softly, and open fingers as widely as possible.

Feet and Ankles

Feet and ankles need exercise but are often overlooked in fitness routines. Tight, weak feet and ankles are more likely to cramp, hurt, strain, and develop plantar fasciitis[103,183] and deformed toes. When the big toe joint does not extend normally when walking (hallux rigidus, or stiffness in the first metatarsophalangeal joint), it alters gait and posture, reduces needed plantar stretch, and promotes hallux valgus (big toe bent away from midline) and bunion. Altered gait may affect the hip and low back dynamics. Weak, unused toes easily deform and curl. Toes must be straight and strong for balance and healthy gait. Weak, overly stretched ankles without a good proprioceptive sense of neutral position are prone to recurrent sprains.

Feet are easy to condition because they routinely bear body weight, giving built-in opportunities to retrain positioning using foot and ankle musculature and proprioceptive skills. Healthful foot and ankle training uses accustomed activities with attention to using foot, ankle, and leg muscles to hold foot and ankle positioning, instead of letting muscles atrophy in tight or supportive shoes. Here is how:

- Keep feet facing straight ahead for gait. Parallel gait builds needed, functional stretch to the fascia and Achilles tendon with each step. Gait with feet and legs turned outward contributes to hip and knee pain, bunion and valgus toe formation, and is often mistaken for "flat feet" because it weights the medial edge of the feet, thereby pronating, everting, and flattening arches. Toe-in strains the foot, knee, and hip, and affects normal gait.

- Maintain neutral ankle position and prevent eversion and pronation (arch flattening) by deliberately using lateral ankle and thigh muscles to reposition the feet and ankles to neutral level position. Many cases of flat feet are acquired pronation sequelae (bad posture and weak, untrained muscles), not a structural problem.
- Learn to preserve arch and ankle stability without supportive shoes or devices. When standing on the ball of the foot (tiptoe), do not allow ankle inversion, which would tilt toward the small toes. Keep body weight over the big toe and second toe. Practicing neutral ankle on "tiptoe" position deliberately prevents inversion.
- Stretch feet daily using the lunge and bending of the squat, described earlier. Keep the back foot facing straight forward, not turned even slightly outward, or stretch that benefits the foot and calf will be lost. Lift the heel to stretch the bottom of the foot. When stretching the sole of the foot with your hands, stretch the entire sole, not just the toes.
- When you lift weights, stand with feet, ankles, and knees in healthful position, as described above.
- To add function, balance, and strength, lift weights standing on one leg in a healthful position. One-legged standing presents a greater challenge to prevent knee torsion (usually adversely rotating medially) and hold a healthful position.
- Put the toes and forefoot under something weighty such as a door, your other foot, or a friend, and lift the toes and foot.
- Play hopscotch. Hopscotch was possibly developed for Roman soldiers to exercise their feet and ankles. Do other fun combination balancing and hopping games.
- Have fun with balance exercises while training healthy foot and ankle positioning (see Balance Skills for the Trail, later). They strengthen and train ankles and feet in ways needed for normal life and to keep balance on narrow, rocky, uneven, and slippery trails.
- Stand on one foot for increasingly long periods while preventing slouching in other segments. Move the other leg in inventive directions at varying speeds.
- If toes do not move freely, or shoes make toes touch closely to each other, the shoes are too tight for daily wear. Practice moving toes in all directions often. Stretch toes with your hands and by using your foot muscles. When standing, do not clench toes, or lift toes from the ground. Avoid heeled shoes; they are prone to deform feet and are detrimental to posture and gait, affecting the kinetic chain from feet to back and neck.
- Hold foot and ankle posture comfortably level against pronation and supination by using your own muscles. Do not wear a tight boot to do what your own muscles and kinesthetic sense can and should practice doing. Do not let foot muscles atrophy from the disuse caused by a tight, supportive shoe.
- Keep feet facing straight ahead, not turning in or out, except where terrain requires pivoting. Allow the foot to bend at the toe knuckles and push off the ball of the foot, not the sides of the toes. For slopes, heel-first walking often works best. When descending stairs, come down toe-first, and then bring the heel down. Do not crash down on heels. Bend knees for shock absorption with each step.

POWER AND PLYOMETRICS

Plyometrics are exercises designed to train muscles for quick powerful moves.[18] The muscle is first quickly stretched under load (contracted eccentrically) and then immediately forcefully contracted concentrically. Examples are push-ups with a clap

between each pair, and rapidly jumping over a line of boxes with quick deceleration crouches between each pair. Plyometric exercises stress muscles and associated attachments more than do other exercises.[55] Learning and maintaining healthy joint positioning and good shock absorption are the keys to safety during plyometric training. Here are some training examples:

- Throw and catch a heavy ball against a (sturdy) wall or in the air in a quick succession of forceful throws and quick deceleration catches, fully bending the arms. Many small children love being thrown in the air and safely caught. Remember safety for all in this exercise. Do not arch the low back when throwing or catching. Keep hips tucked, using torso muscles to handle the load, not the low back. Do not lean back when standing and throwing overhead (see Abdominal and Core Muscle Conditioning, earlier).
- Jumping is a natural plyometric exercise. Use healthful foot, ankle, and knee positioning and neutral spine posture.
- Lie on your back, feet in the air. A partner leans heavily on your feet. Bend your knees to do leg presses. When the partner and you are secure in healthful positioning, press strongly enough to fling the partner off the surface of the feet (a few inches to start); then catch him or her again on the feet, bending knees before straightening knees to press him or her away from you into the air.

STRETCHING FOR WILDERNESS PREPAREDNESS

Heavy packs and difficult terrain may tempt one to adopt poor body positioning. Sagging usually occurs in directions already favored by tightness. Strain and injury often result, confused with overtraining. Fitness classes are filled with people stretching, often in unhealthy ways that emphasize the injurious positioning that first caused their tightness, pain, and injuries. Flexibility training, whether in a gym or during actual daily life movement, needs to retrain muscle length so that you no longer stand, sit, and move with strained unhealthful positioning, rather than holding arbitrary poses for set lengths of time. The main areas to stretch for functional wilderness health and ergonomics are the anterior shoulder and chest, hamstrings, hips, and feet. Stretches should be functional, which means they will support how you move in real life.

Anterior Shoulder and Chest

- Stand upright near a wall with arms relaxed at your sides. Notice if your thumbs point toward each other. This internal arm rotation usually indicates pectoral shortening. Note that trying to hold arms with thumbs facing forward instead of inward may feel tight or unnatural, because tightness prevents it. Next, stand with your back against a wall, touching heels, buttocks, upper back, and the back of the head. Notice if this aligned standing is uncomfortable or if you increase lower spine lordosis instead of having sufficient muscle length to stand reasonably upright.

To restore healthy resting length to the anterior chest, try these stretches:

- Anterior (pectoral) stretch: Face the wall and pull one bent elbow out to the side, with the inside of the arm against the wall. Turn your body and feet away from the wall and use the wall to gently brace the inside of the elbow. Feel the stretch in the anterior chest muscles. Do not hunch or tighten the shoulder. Hold for a few seconds on each side. Drop the arms and observe thumb positioning, which this stretch should correct by lengthening the previously tight anterior chest. Restored functional anterior muscle length should now allow comfortable straight standing against the wall, with heels, hips, back, and the back of the head touching (see Fitness as a Lifestyle, earlier). Do this stretch in the morning, before exercise, and throughout the day to restore healthy shoulder and head positioning (see Figure 96-2).

- Top of the shoulder (trapezius) stretch: Remain with your back against the wall, and the back of your head touching the wall. Place one hand behind the opposite hip, as if in an opposite pants pocket. Slide your free arm down toward the knee, keeping the back of your head touching the wall and allowing your neck to stretch comfortably. Do each side for a few seconds each. Do not lean forward. Try the preceding wall-stand posture check again. It should become even more comfortable and possible.
- A stretch that is both diagnostic and therapeutic for tightness is to lie flat on your back without a pillow under either the head or knees. Do not lift your chin or arch your back. Practice a relaxed straight posture. Can you put your arms straight out to the side on the floor without arching your back? Can you bend your elbows keeping your hands against the floor? Can you relax your upper arms against your ears, still touching the floor without arching your back? Many people are so round shouldered that this is uncomfortable or impossible. Use the two preceding stretches.
- Lie supine with a small rolled towel or pillow between your shoulders. Retract your shoulders to the floor over this roll without arching the low back.
- Lie face down, hands at sides and off the floor. Slowly lift your upper body a few inches, and then lower it. Feel the lift from your upper chest, not by lifting your chin. Notice if you bend from the neck. Your intent is to keep your neck in neutral position and feel the range of motion from your chest. This upper back extension is an effective postural strengthener that combines the range of motion. As you progress, move hands to the side and then overhead.

Hip and Thigh

- The squat and lunge described in the strengthening section are important functional stretches. Done as described, the lunge stretches the anterior hip and thigh, Achilles tendon, and foot. For both, tuck your pelvis to vertical position and spine to neutral posture. For the lunge, you should immediately feel the crucial hip flexor stretch when you tuck to neutral position. When used for daily bending and reaching, you gain hundreds of built-in stretches daily.
- For deep lateral rotators, lie supine with knees bent, both feet on the floor. Cross one ankle over the opposite knee. Move the foot on the floor away from the midline until a deep stretch is felt. Gently press the crossed knee away. Hold briefly, and then gently drop both legs to each side. Repeat with the other ankle crossed. For this stretch in a chair, sit up with one ankle crossed over the other knee. Press the crossed knee down. Sit upright and lift the head up, chin held in.
- An effective low back and hip strengthener that includes a functional stretch is good bending using the squat. For all daily bending where you use a partial squat, keep both heels down and the upper body upright. You will get hundreds of built-in functional stretches daily.
- To stretch the quadriceps while standing, hold one foot behind you. Tuck the pelvis to vertical and spine to neutral position. Arching the back will lose the stretch.
- For better quadriceps stretch, stand on one leg, and bend the knee of the other leg in such a way that you hold the foot behind the body. As soon as you change the pelvis angle to vertical and simultaneously attain a neutral spine posture, you will feel a better quadriceps stretch.

Hamstrings

Hamstring flexibility or tightness is not correlated with back pain when one is standing or running, sitting (usually), or exercising.[26] It is also not true that tight hamstrings pull the pelvis posteriorly. Many people with tight hamstrings tilt the pelvis anteriorly and stand with hyperlordosis, which would not be possible with a tight posterior pull.

Lack of hamstring flexibility reduces the capacity to sit on the floor with the feet together and outstretched without rounding the back, which in turn, unequally loads the lumbar intervertebral disks. The result is that many people sit (and stretch) rounded because tightness makes slouching more comfortable and customary than does a healthy position.

Stretching the hamstrings can restore the resting length sufficient for healthy sitting with legs outstretched and for functional use of hamstring length needed for kicks, leaps, dancing, climbing moves, and other real-life ranges of motion.

Bending forward from a standing position is not healthy for low back structures.[146,170] To stretch hamstrings without forward bending, try the following:

- The most functional hamstring stretch, meaning the way you need hamstring length for real activity, is to stand upright on one leg and lift the other straight out in front of you. Make sure your standing foot is facing straight forward, not turned out, even a small amount. If it is turned, then either hop to straighten it or put your other foot down, adjust, and figure how to lift one leg without twisting the other foot. This will be healthy training for walking, running, and other movement. Lift to any height that creates stretch in the hamstring.
- A hamstring stretch lying on the floor is to lie flat and lift one leg, pointing the foot to the sky. Keep the other leg straight and flat on the floor. Notice if your anterior hip is so tight that the leg on the floor lifts also. Include anterior hip stretches by lunges, described earlier, until remedied. Keep the shoulders and neck relaxed on the floor. Do not round the back and call it a leg stretch. Another hamstring stretch is the "downward dog," described next.

Achilles Tendon and Foot

- A common Achilles tendon stretch is to lunge toward a wall. It is ineffective when done with the hip flexed and protruding posteriorly instead of vertically. Bring the hip forward, as if trying to touch it to the wall. Keep the back foot straight, not turned out, or the stretch is lost and the medial knee bears the pressure.
- A more effective Achilles tendon stretch is standing with one heel pressing toward the wall at about shin height. Stand no more than fingertip distance from the wall and stand upright (see Hamstrings, earlier). Keep the hip tucked and back foot straight, not turned outward.
- An effective built-in Achilles tendon stretch is to use squats with heels firmly on the floor and feet facing forward aligned with the knees for routine bending.
- The downward dog is an effective multijoint stretch with body weight supported on the hands, protecting the back. Put the hands and feet on the floor, hands far forward of the feet as if starting a push-up and weight mostly on the hands. Keeping the feet where they are, lift the hips up in the air, pushing the hips backward until the heels relax to the floor. Arch the back, rather than letting it round or hunch. Relax the head downward. Keep the feet straight, not turned, with weight on the rims, not the arches. Push the fingers forward with straight, not locked, elbows.
- During daily walking and movement, do not let the body weight fall inward to the arches; keep weight on the sole of the foot. Point toes straight ahead. This prevents uneven and unhealthy stretch forces that gradually deform the feet, ankles, and knees. Make sure the straight leg posture continues through the knee and hip, to prevent straightening the foot from overstraining another part higher up the kinetic chain.

FLEXIBILITY-ENHANCING TECHNIQUES

Several methods augment stretching gains. Stretch regularly. Be warm before stretching.[58,175] *Warming up* means raising the body temperature, because elasticity increases with temperature.

Active warming is accomplished more quickly and effectively with a few push-ups and lunges than with light jogging. Do not be afraid of exercise without air conditioning. Within limits, warmer environments help. Passive warming in a hot tub or shower, or locally applied heat, can help prepare for movement, although direct activity should also be part of a warm-up.

A quick technique to improve immediate flexibility is called push-pull, contract-relax, or proprioceptive neuromuscular facilitation.[50] While holding a given stretch at a maximal comfortable stretch, push (contract) against resistance in the direction opposite the stretch for 4 or 5 seconds without moving or reducing the stretch, to fatigue the muscle. Then pull (relax) into the stretch. Use this technique slowly and safely for any desired stretch.

BALANCE SKILLS FOR THE TRAIL

Balance is easily and highly trainable, but often overlooked. Good balance is crucial for ease of movement, independence, variety of activity, and preventing falls, ankle sprains, and slips on the trail. Injury and disuse diminish balance, which is a use-it-or-lose-it skill. Vicious cycles grow of poor balance, injury, and decreasing activity because of inability and reduced activity. Recurrent ankle sprains are often a matter of lack of retraining foot and ankle proprioceptors that give information about positioning. Weak untrained ankles turn without warning muscles to regain balance and footing. Many balance exercises are isolated, but balance for real life is multifactorial; training needs to address function.

Examples of basic, low-level functional balance needed for health include the ability to put on hosiery and shoes while standing, to step over a pile of clothes on the floor without falling or spilling a cup of water, descending narrow basement stairs holding a laundry basket in both hands without holding the railing, and standing from a chair or the floor without using your hands. Average balance skills include the ability to leap over a puddle or hole in the street and land lightly on the other foot, or safely climb a stepladder without hands and change an overhead light bulb without holding on. High functional balance skill examples are the ability to walk through a rushing rocky stream and rescue a child on a rock.

Try the following in a safe environment with good limb mechanics:

- Stand to exercise. It is functional and healthier for the back than sitting to lift weights or stretch.
- When you lift weights, stand on one foot (at a time) in a healthful position practicing balance and stabilization.
- Be able to balance while lifting or climbing without needing supportive shoes or devices.
- Lift free weights. Instead of standard linear lifts, make figure-8 and other irregular patterns for stabilization and balance. Repeat standing on one foot and then the other. Do not let your weight fall inward on your arches. Maintain good foot posture by using muscles and balance.
- Throw and catch things standing on one foot. Then, throw and catch standing on the ball of one foot.
- Practice balancing on one foot, one knee, or one knee and hand while on the floor simulating climbing or camping activities.
- Practice rising up from the floor and then back down in a smooth manner. Repeat without using hands. Repeat while holding a package.
- For balance and flexibility, stand to put on and take off pants, socks, and shoes.
- Stand on tiptoe. Keep ankles straight and your weight on the entire ball of the foot, not teetering on the outside of the foot or inverting the ankle. Raise and lower 10 times.
- Raise and lower on the ball of only one foot. Maintain a healthy foot and ankle position with weight centered over the big and second toes, not tilting toward the small toes. When proficient, try balancing with eyes closed.
- Walk over uneven ground. Then walk a line on uneven ground. Walk backward on uneven ground.

- Walk a line sideways. Cross the feet, first one in front and then the other behind (grapevine walking). Practice on uneven ground.
- Hop on a line and then hop the line backward, advancing to hopping on uneven ground.
- Slalom hop a line, and then slalom hop the line backward.
- Try going without trekking poles before the first climb.
- Hop from one line, space, marking, or crack in the sidewalk or ground to the next such indicator. When landing from any hop or jump, use shock absorption by bending the knees and using muscles to slow and pad the landing.
- Kneel on a large exercise ball. Stand on rolling surfaces. Walk on fence rails. Use a skateboard and balance board. Skate.

DEVELOPING SPEED FOR WILDERNESS SITUATIONS

Wilderness conditions often require the ability to react, move, grasp, or run quickly. Speed training aids outdoor activities, from catching falling equipment or companions, to paddling around unexpected logs, to running from bees. Each person has different muscle fiber distributions that favor speed, strength, or endurance. Some have a greater distribution of slow, oxidative (type I) fibers, which are highly fatigue resistant and benefit from long steady efforts. Others may have a greater percentage of fast-twitch fibers (type IIb), favoring bursts of strength and speed. Both types respond to training. Individuals with a predominance of slow-oxidative fibers may need to train speed as a corrective countermeasure.

The way to be fast is to train fast. The practice of slow weight-lifting, sometimes called super slow, is a limited way to train with weights. Slow training increases the total time spent lifting, so it increases strength, but does not develop speed for moving heavy objects. Similar strength and endurance gains can be made from lifting weights more quickly and using more lifts, so that the total muscle work remains the same. As the amount of weight lifted quickly increases, the power component increases. When speed training, maintain posture and a safe lifting technique. Injury potential rises with speed of movement, which is another reason to properly train speed. Following are a few examples of speed games to increase speed of movement. With each, imagine application to wilderness performance situations.

- Run a short distance (e.g., 15, 25, or 50 yards) at maximal speed. Rest 10 seconds. Repeat 10 times. Work to increase speed.
- Run quickly enough to keep a hat or piece of paper placed on your chest from falling, requiring a minimum speed for the duration of this drill. Vary distances using this technique.
- Have a friend point a flashlight beam at the ground, moving it quickly from point to point. Jump quickly to each new point. Try jumping with both feet and hopping with one foot.
- Kneel or squat and try the above game using your hand, grabbing or tapping at the flashlight beam on the floor. Do a few dozen points, and then change hands.
- Have a friend hold a piece of paper near your hand and drop it without warning. Practice catching it.
- Practice moving a heavy weight quickly, both body weight and external weight. Do one push-up at high speed, rest, and repeat, until reaching 10 push-ups. Practice lifting your pack, or throwing and catching a weighted ball (medicine ball). Notice and preserve a healthful spine position.
- Do 8 to 10 push-ups quickly without stopping and without letting your low back arch or hitch upward.
- Try lunges quickly, first singly, then in groups.
- Punch (or grab to simulate catching something) as fast as possible. Then repeat twice in rapid succession. Then repeat three times, then four, and so on, until you can punch or grab like a machine gun. Bring the elbow all the

way back to your side each time, like a piston, or like sawing wood.
- Quickly sit or kneel on the floor, and rise to a stand. Try this (safely) wearing your pack.
- Have a friend poke at your feet quickly with a (nonsharp) stick or squirt you with a water pistol. Jump and duck to avoid hits.
- Practice throwing a heavy ball or rescue device. Carefully practice throwing and catching heavy thrown objects.
- Devise other speed games that simulate real-life needs and varying proportions of speed and strength (e.g., assemble gear, break camp, don rescue clothing, dodge hurtling objects).

CONDITIONING FOR SPECIAL ENVIRONMENTS

To handle predicted thermal environments, train in the cold or heat. For a 30-mile hike, practice covering the entire distance. For a journey at night, train to some extent during those hours. For extended caving, accustom yourself to lengthened wake cycles and lack of external circadian cues. Teach your system what to expect. Cross-train, taking into consideration all anticipated interacting environmental conditions of wilderness travel.

Heat

Because exercise in the heat (see Chapters 12 and 13) can be an enormous cardiovascular load, aerobic fitness is a major factor in heat tolerance.[37] Exercise in high heat may be expected during desert treks, ultramarathons, and jungle expeditions, when working in tropical medical clinics, and during other vigorous activities (or even sedentary situations) in deserts and tropics. Exercising in heat accomplishes heat acclimatization more effectively than does heat exposure without exercise.[118]

Fitness training in heat produces several adaptations. One is expansion of blood plasma volume.[147] Increased blood is pumped with each beat, supplying blood simultaneously to muscles for exercise and skin for cooling. Increased plasma volume increases the sweat reservoir and functions as a heat sink, absorbing heat without an increase in body temperature. Sweating begins earlier, at a higher rate, and with greater electrolyte conservation.[153] With increased fluid available for cooling and muscular activity, a fit, heat-acclimated person's core temperature will not rise as high at rest[30] or at the same exercise intensity as that of a nonacclimated person.[110] The well-conditioned body produces more of several protective heat-shock proteins, further increasing tolerance to heat exposure.[114] Physical training can negate the decrease of heat tolerance with age.[6]

Heat adaptation occurs quickly, with dramatic changes in the first 4 to 5 days. Acclimatization is nearly complete in 1 to 2 weeks of continuous exposure to exercise in the heat.[123] Acclimatization does not occur if time is spent in air-conditioned environments. A protective environment prevents discomfort and heat illness, but such a microclimate reduces acclimatization and heat conditioning. With reduced physical conditioning, adaptations are lost over several weeks.[6]

Physical training in a cool environment improves tolerance to exercise in the heat and the rate of heat acclimatization, but not as much as does training in the heat.[122] To condition for high exertion in extreme heat, spend time in environments matching expected temperatures. Ease into activity, gradually increasing exercise intensity and duration. Stay well hydrated and consume appropriate amounts of electrolytes. For a single exertion in the heat, precooling with air-conditioning or cold baths attenuates a rise in core temperature[19] and provides a margin for increased heat accumulation before overheating occurs.[75] Because precooling provides no acclimatization to exercise in the heat and will not prevent heat illness, it is best used when one is already acclimatized. Some people training for ultramarathons in heat use a sauna while wearing heat-trapping clothing. When they travel by automobile, they close windows and turn on the heater to increase acclimatization time. They avoid air-conditioning for sleep or rest, and wearing cooling garments when training. Such training should be approached slowly and extremely carefully, with full understanding and education about health-preserving methods to avoid dangerous dehydration or potentially catastrophic increases in body temperature. This is exemplified by episodes of fatal heatstroke in athletes and soldiers. To condition for milder heat, spend increasing periods in the target environmental temperature, avoiding air-conditioning. Gradually increase physical activity, closely matching expected conditions. At all times be aware of the signs and symptoms of heat-related illnesses, and make every attempt to be under constant observation and/or supervision.

Cold

To increase cold tolerance and prepare for cold conditions (see Chapter 6), spend increasingly long times exposed to the temperatures and humidity expected, while training to levels of physical activity at or greater than expected levels. Stay well fed, hydrated, and rested to be able to train hard, because cold tolerance is reduced by calorie deficit[56,73] and exertional fatigue.[182] With that knowledge, also train for situations when you will be cold, hungry, and tired.

Cold acclimatization involves at least three adaptations, with the extent of each varying between individuals and with exposure. Shivering begins at lower body temperatures after heat is generated without shivering.[105] There may be simultaneously increased[138] and decreased skin temperature,[47] depending on circumstances and anatomic location.[89] In some cases, skin blood flow increases to keep extremities warm and resist cold injury.[139] In other cases, it decreases to reduce heat loss.[140] For example, skin temperatures of Australian Aborigines[31] and Arctic dwellers[94] were found to be lower while they slept than those of the unacclimatized European investigators. It is also the case that different people regulate body temperature to different set points.[96] A third hallmark of cold-acclimatized people is improved ability to sleep in the cold.[29] Cold acclimatization is noted in indigenous people at their cold residential climates (e.g., in the African Kalahari, Australian desert, and Tierra del Fuego in southern Chile). Many sleep outdoors nearly naked in freezing temperatures. When long-term exposure ends, cold adaptation lessens. Cold tolerance decreases with dehydration, lack of sleep, and food deprivation.

The relationship between fitness and cold is not as marked as that between fitness and heat tolerance. However, structural and metabolic changes that occur with exercise training benefit cold tolerance. A fit person tolerates a lower body temperature than does an unfit person before the onset of shivering, and can generate more heat through shivering.[16] Increased muscle mass in trained athletes increases metabolic heat production ability[17] and insulation, better maintaining body temperature without shivering.[181] Physical fitness allows exercise at a higher intensity to generate heat. Cold tolerance is improved to a greater extent by exercise in cold conditions than from exercise alone. For example, seasonal acclimatization[74] occurs in people working outdoors in the cold and fishermen who immerse their hands in cold water to tend their winter nets.

Altitude

Please see Chapter 1.

Scuba Diving

Being in good physical condition is beneficial for divers, even though sport diving is not generally rigorous (see Chapter 71). Fitness reduces the risk of several diseases affecting general health, increases the tolerance to heat and cold, increases the ability to lift and carry gear, and reduces the chance of sudden death from unaccustomed exertion. Physical fitness can improve diving safety and the ability to dive more comfortably, possibly making the difference between a safe diving trip and a diving accident. Divers with preexisting small lung cysts or end-expiratory flow limitation may be at risk of pulmonary barotrauma, but physical fitness or training does not appear to be a factor in susceptibility.[160] Whether one's physical condition (or how much) may relate to the risk of decompression sickness is not firmly established. Anecdotally, the risk is higher in poorly conditioned divers, which may relate to lack of strength or swimming ability for handling situations that incur decompression problems. A 2014 case-control study of the relative importance of risk factors found the highest major item was "shortness of breath after heavy exercise during the dive."[157] Higher body fat may predispose to a risk for decompression sickness, but there is not a firm correlation. It may be that fatter subjects in studies of risk were in poorer physical condition, had a higher incidence of fatty blood vessels that compromise circulation, or were older. It also is not known if the risk involves total body fat or percentage of body fat. For example, a 54.4-kg (120-lb) woman with 20% body fat has 10.9 kg (24 lb) of fat, whereas an 81.6-kg (180-lb) man with 15% body fat carries 12.25 kg (27 lb) of fat.

To condition for diving, swim with fins regularly. Wear tanks or simulate tanks by increasing the resistance to forward movement by tilting a kickboard to increase the presented surface area, and by using devices such as drag suits, webbed gloves, tethers, and other commercial and home-made resistance tools. Maintain speed and finning mechanics. On land, lift, carry, and walk around wearing tanks, a weight belt, and other gear. Avoid bending over to pick up gear while wearing tanks. Bend and lift properly using the legs. Practice climbing ladders wearing gear to simulate boat diving.

PERFORMANCE AND INJURY

The most common wilderness injuries are not due to avalanches, stings, bites, or heat or sun; they are the same aches, pulls, strains, and pains that often occur from poor body mechanics and injurious exercise practice.

AVOIDING EXERCISE INJURIES

Many common exercises do not train the body to move in functional ways, or are in themselves not healthful movements and may reinforce unhealthful movement patterns and injuries. Resultant avoidable pain is misidentified as overuse, or attributed to a structural but unrelated finding on radiograph. Some otherwise useful exercises are rendered ineffective or injurious if carried out with commonly accepted but poor ergonomics. One common practice is to make an exercise easier by transferring the body weight to the joints through slouching, rather than doing the muscular work of holding the body in a healthy position. Examples include lifting weight overhead by increasing the lumbar arch and tilting the pelvis forward, instead of preventing a hyperlordotic lower spine, and maintaining a neutral spine posture (see Abdominal and Core Muscle Conditioning, earlier); allowing the knee and ankle to tilt medially under a load, rather than countering with leg muscle repositioning; craning the neck while exercising or lifting; and lack of muscle use for intrinsic shock absorption when stepping down from terrain, stairs, or a step bench. Allowing body weight to sag into joints instead of using supporting muscles negates the benefit of the exercise, and wears joints. Poor positioning (bad ergonomics) during lifting may be associated with a higher rate of exertion.[43] The following paragraphs describe maintaining healthy positioning to avoid injury from exercise.

Healthier Spine Positioning

Flexion (forward bending) and hyperlordosis are two common injurious spine positions encountered in daily life and exercise. Flexion imposes injurious unequal loading of the lower spine.[146,170] Much of an ordinary day is spent slouching and rounded over desks, computers, handlebars, and steering wheels, and bent under packs for hiking. The ubiquitous practice of forward bending during certain fitness exercises and stretches contributes to cumulative disc degeneration and soft tissue injury. Hip hinging (hip flexion while keeping the back straight) is not a healthy bending practice. Forward bending for conventional stretching may stretch back muscles, but at the price of pressure

on intervertebral disks and soft tissue, whether done with a straight or rounded back.[146]

Standing, Walking, and Running. Hyperlordosis during standing, walking, and running is a common contributor to low back pain from upright ambulation.[20] Low back arch may increase from tilting the pelvis forward or leaning the thoracic cage backward, or both.[22] Learn to identify components of hyperlordosis. The pelvis should be vertical, and not tilted or pushed forward. The upper body should be vertical, and not leaning back from the lumbar spine. Maintain neutral spine posture. Consciously use abdominal muscles without tightening them, to pull the pelvis to vertical position and the upper body to an upright and vertical position (see Figures 96-1 and 96-3).

Lifting Loads. Instead of sitting to lift weights for exercise, stand for functional strength, practice stabilizing a weight, and practice using neutral spine posture while resisting loads.

Lift weights up from the floor with knees bent over the feet, with the upper body as upright as the weight allows, without inducing hyperlordosis. Lift weights overhead with an upright, vertical upper body, without inducing hyperlordosis.

Carrying Loads. Unhealthful positioning includes forward rounding and hyperlordotic arching.[88] Injury potential is not as much from the weight of the pack or asymmetric distribution of the load[135] as from not maintaining healthful positioning or properly using muscles to counter the pull of the load.[20] Maintain neutral spine posture against the weight of carried objects by consciously using abdominal muscles to pull the pelvis into vertical alignment and a more upright upper body (see Figure 96-3).

When lifting and carrying weights, do not allow the low back to increase the arch under the load. A hyperlordotic arch transfers body weight plus the weight of the load to the low back.[107] Reduce the arch to neutral spine posture by tucking the hips and ribcage, as if starting a crunch until upright. The abdominal muscles gain functional exercise to achieve and maintain neutral spine posture. For anterior loads such as a heavy basket, a child in arms, armful of firewood, or any significant weight, notice if you lean the upper body backward at the lumbar curve. Instead, bring the upper body to upright and tuck the pelvis to vertical and neutral position. Neutral spine posture gives built-in functional abdominal exercise without tightening or flexing. For posterior loads such as packs, notice if you hunch forward, lean back, or hitch to the side to offset the load. Use the above technique to straighten the posture and prevent hyperlordosis. When pushing or pulling heavy loads, or reaching or lifting overhead, use neutral spine posture to prevent poor spine dynamics. Convert gear to a built-in core-muscle trainer.

Stretch and Exercise

Stretch hamstrings in functional way without forward bending (see Flexibility-Enhancing Techniques, earlier). Instead of forward bending to exercise abdominal and core muscles, such as those used in conventional abdominal training classes or Pilates classes that emphasize flexion, use functional training exercises (see Abdominal and Core Muscle Conditioning, earlier).

Healthier Knee Positioning

Letting knees sway medially (valgus knee [genu valgum]) or rotate medially (torsion) strains the medial knee,[106] wears upon cartilage,[40] and interferes with normal muscle use and kneecap tracking.[159] Poor limb positioning, biomechanics, and ergonomics, known to be related to lower limb pain, are not prevented or remediated by conventional strengthening and knee rehabilitation programs. Simple voluntary repositioning, from unhealthful to healthful joint angles, prevents injury from misuse.[25,26] Stand and step with feet parallel, not turning toe-in or toe-out, where terrain allows. Stand and step with feet and knees facing the same direction. Watch for and correct kneecaps that face medially (knee torsion) rather than forward in the same direction of the feet. When walking, running, and stepping up stairs and rocky terrain, prevent medial knee sway (valgus knee). Use thigh muscles to align knees comfortably over the feet, without slouching inward. Keep the knee over the foot, not tilting forward of the foot. Step onto the whole foot where possible, pushing through the heel, not only the front of the foot. Allowing the knee to shift far forward and stepping up onto the ball of the foot increases the transfer of body weight through the knee joint rather than within the thigh musculature. When stepping down, step lightly. Use conscious muscle control to decelerate. Bend knees with descent for shock absorption.

Healthier Neck Positioning

In daily standing, sitting, and ambulating, a common unhealthful habit is to slouch so that the head and neck tilt or round forward of the body line. The resulting "forward head" is a widespread cause of neck and upper body pain, mistakenly called "stress" and "upper crossed syndrome." Lifting the chin while tilting the neck forward compounds hyperextension of the cervical spine. These are simply bad postures. Looking high overhead is a common position during exercise and stretching, and for wilderness activities of stargazing, belaying, rock climbing, scouting, and drinking from a canteen. The same two poor positioning habits are common. One is to tilt the neck and head forward when looking upward, and to lift the chin, thereby hyperextending one cervical segment, rather than distributing extension throughout the upper vertebral column. Another is to increase the low back arch (hyperlordosis) instead of extending the spine at the upper back. Chronic hyperextension in both the lower spine and neck is a factor in disk degeneration,[33] shears intervertebral disks between the vertebrae,[121] causes facet pain, and promotes a cycle of a forward head position, overly stretched and weak structures, and neck and shoulder pain. Lengthen and unround from the upper back to look upward, keeping the chin in. Lift from the shoulders and chest without arching the low back or tilting the chin forward. Prevent the neck from jutting forward at an angle. Forward head posture commonly results in neck, shoulder, and upper back pain,[69] often mistaken for "stress." The forward head also rotates the shoulder forward, interfering with raising the arm and thereby contributing to impingement.[67] Get the needed range of motion more through straightening the upper spine, not by leaning the torso rearward or lifting the chin. Be aware of the difference between bringing rounded shoulders to neutral position while maintaining the upper body vertical, and leaning the entire upper body rearward. Test the head and neck posture by standing against a wall. The heels, hips, upper back, and back of the head should all comfortably touch without increasing the lumbar or cervical arch, or bringing the chin upward or forward. See the stretching section, Anterior Shoulder and Chest, earlier, to remedy tightness that prevents upright standing posture.

For driving or sitting, move the seat forward rather than rounding the body forward. Instead of perching toward the front of the chair, sit at the chair back. Rather than rounding the lower back against the seat back, use a roll to maintain a neutral lower spine, only if needed, depending on the chair design, and lean the upper body back against the seat back (see Long Sitting in an Automobile, later). "Ergonomic" chairs do not make you sit well; you do that yourself. You can sit well on a bucket, or in injurious way in an expensive ergonomic seat.

AVOIDING INJURIES FROM STRETCHING

Just as not all foods are healthy, neither are all stretches. Many persons practice the same poor positioning as already used all day, imposing unhealthful twist or load on joints and soft tissue, deforming or injuring them over time. Shoulder stands and the yoga plow position (lying on the upper back, legs overhead, with the cervical and thoracic spine in weighted flexion) promotes stretch deformation of the posterior longitudinal ligament,[180] bone spurs, and the common injurious posture of forward head and round shoulders. Overstretched ligaments are plastic, not elastic. They do not return to normal length and cannot hold vertebrae in position or function as a firewall to intervertebral disks. The posterior force of the forced flexion under the body's weight may eventually degenerate and herniate cervical disks and promote bone spurs.[146,170]

Skip the common shoulder stretch typified by bending forward with arms lifted behind with clasped hands. The resultant unsupported, weighted lumbar flexion promotes disk degeneration and herniation. Forced shoulder hyperextension overloads the constitutionally susceptible anterior shoulder capsule. Several yoga stretches involve twisting at the knee, or lying back on folded, twisted knees, forcibly lengthening the collateral ligaments, and twisting menisci and other supporting structures. Avoid assisted stretches where anyone presses your back into a rounded position or flexion. Avoid vigorously oscillating knees (butterfly knees) when sitting with bent knees and soles of feet touching. Do not let anyone stand on or push your knees to facilitate stretching.

Add extension stretches to learn to "unround" the upper spine and prevent chronic thoracic kyphosis. When leaning back to stretch, whether standing, sitting, or lying, lift from the upper body rather than jutting the chin forward and bending at the neck. Keep a neutral neck. When sitting cross-legged, notice the ankle. Externally rotate from the hip rather than inverting the lateral ankle (turning the sole medially or upward). Overstretching lateral ligaments leaves the ankle prone to inversion sprain.

Stretch muscles, not joints. Do not force joints into such ligament laxity that they no longer seat properly. Not all joint laxity is instability. There is a difference between a healthful flexible joint and an unstable joint. Unstable joints wear and tear. In a suddenly forceful situation, weak, unstable joints may be predisposed to pulls or dislocations.

Hard stretching just before an athletic event may reduce the tendinous stiffness that assists elastic recoil in high-exertion situations,[90] reducing maximal force development.[136] Rather than stretching to maximize length before competitive events, use stretches described under Conditioning, earlier, to regain functional muscle length for healthy ergonomics. Similarly, chronically holding a muscle in a stretched position weakens it. Chronic slouching and lengthy sitting weaken the lengthened muscles of the back and posterior hip. Slouching is a stretch, but not a beneficial one. Avoid compounding the problem by avoiding forward rounding and bending.

BACK PAIN PREVENTION DURING LONG TRAVEL TO THE WILDERNESS

Neck and back pain from sitting poorly in airline seats far exceeds the incidence of deep vein thrombosis. Vehicle seats often have concave backs. Long sitting in lumbar, thoracic, and cervical flexion pressures intervertebral disks and soft tissue. A pillow behind the head exacerbates flexion. Sitting stresses disks to a higher extent than does standing, and poor sitting posture amplifies strain. Travel to the wilderness can involve sitting long hours while driving or flying. Try the following for better sitting mechanics to easily prevent strain:

Use of Lumbar Roll

A lumbar roll fills the space between a too-concave chair back and the lumbar spine so that you can sit relaxed and comfortably in neutral spine posture. However, not all seats and chairs need a lumbar roll. A lumbar roll that is too large or inflexible, or positioned incorrectly, can be uncomfortable or unhealthful. To test lumbar roll function and appropriate size, sit in a chair with your entire back against the back of the chair. Place your forearm behind you at the lumbar level between your low back and the chair. Lean your upper back against the chair back so that the low back does not press your arm, but rests lightly. Correct placement and size of the roll should feel comfortable. Your forearm is usually about the right size for a lumbar roll, depending on how hollow is the chair back. A small towel, article of clothing, or inflatable pillow makes an inexpensive lumbar roll that packs flat and is lightweight. Do not use a roll to force yourself into an unnaturally straight or arched posture.

Long Sitting in an Automobile

Use a lumbar roll, as described. Car seats that are positioned too far back from the steering wheel encourage hunching and leaning forward to hold the wheel. If needed, slide the seat position forward. Tilt the seat to a slight backward slant if needed. With hips all the way against the rear of the seat, see if you can lean back comfortably against the seat, instead of rounding forward. If you feel neck strain, then recheck and correct if you are tilting the neck forward or straining in any direction to be "straight." During rest breaks, do not add to the long flexion of sitting with more flexion stretches. Use comfortable extension stretches instead, described earlier in the flexibility section.

Buses and Flights

Commercial transport seats are often concave, encouraging prolonged, forced flexion.

Where needed, use two pillows for forming a lumbar roll (described above), one in the inward space of the low back, and the second in the overly curved thoracic space left by the extreme concavity of the seat. Lean back to an upright position, rather than rounded forward. Sometimes, one long pillow or folded article of clothing turned vertically can suffice. Make sure it is comfortable. For in-flight sleeping, lean back while preventing as much rounding of the neck and low back as feasible. Flights sometimes have a video message encouraging in-seat stretching. Often the advice is to forward bend. Instead, extension is indicated to counter long periods of flexion. Stretch the shoulders back, not forward. Pull the chin in while leaning back. Press hands to the thighs, and lift the chest to extend the upper spine with the chin held neutral, not forward. Extend the legs as much as space allows, lift the hips, and extend the back, pushing on feet and armrests. Breathe deeply every so often. Pump feet. Squeeze the knees together and apart, upward and downward against the hands. Open and shut the hands. Squeeze the shoulder blades back. Get out of the seat. Try anterior chest stretches (see Flexibility-Enhancing Techniques, earlier) and various lunges with a neutral pelvis (see Hip and Thigh, earlier). Walk around as often and long as feasible.

SORENESS AFTER EXERTION

Anyone, even highly trained competitive athletes, can be sore after hard activity. Soreness develops in the days following activity, rather than during activity, so is called delayed-onset muscle soreness. Mechanical stress initiates a chain of events. At the time of effort, cell membrane damage in muscle fibers disrupts calcium homeostasis.[5] Abnormal influx of the ion inhibits cellular respiration in the mitochondria. Lack of adenosine triphosphate starves structures, activating lysosomal proteases[41] that degrade and release proinflammatory cytokines[152] and other serum proteins[32] that induce inflammation. Free radicals promote release of arachidonic acid from cell membranes.[145] Arachidonic acid (an omega-6 fatty acid) is converted by cyclooxygenase-2 (COX-2) into proinflammatory prostaglandins,[111] which, along with histamines and kinins, accumulate in the interstitium, stimulate nociceptors, and cause pain.[5]

An inflammatory response begins the healing process by attracting polymorphonuclear neutrophils.[41,100] Activation of the complement system may also contribute to mobilization of neutrophils.[34] The inflammatory process is self-regulated by a balance of proinflammatory and antiinflammatory mediators.[44] The extent and magnitude of the response are determined by the presence or absence of both types of mediators.[111] The result of this balance is that a person is stiff, sore, and weak for 1 to 5 days.

Numerous products and protocols are claimed to prevent or reduce exertional soreness. None are completely successful. Although soreness is often more pronounced with eccentric contraction (lengthening under tension), soreness results with sufficient stimulation after all types of muscular contraction.[72]

Concentric muscular contraction is contraction that shortens muscles, for example, contracting the biceps to lift a load. Concentric contractions against a high load, such as ascending while carrying a heavy pack, create conditions for soreness, particularly in the most exercised muscles, such as the hamstring, gluteal, and calf muscles. After hard swims, soreness may occur in the latissimus dorsi and leg extensors, depending on the stroke. Isometric contraction maintains the muscle at one length while under tension, for example, gripping a rock ledge. Soreness after technical climbing is common in wrist and forearm flexor muscles. Eccentric muscular contraction is contraction while the muscle lengthens. When lowering a pack to the ground, the biceps lengthens while in a high contractile state, to guide the load at the chosen speed and direction. The high load of eccentric muscle contraction of descending slopes is often felt primarily in the decelerating muscles of the thigh, shins, and ankles, particularly when stepping down hard and not using muscles to decelerate and absorb shock during gait.

Sometimes pain is not soreness, but injury from strained muscle fibers due to poor posture, efforts above tolerance, or joints twisted into harmful positions. During exertion, if pain, tearing, or pinching is felt in a joint, or a feeling like electricity radiates down a limb, that is probably an injury process. Similarly, if joints feel hot, swollen, or sore after effort, that may signify an injury. Soreness from carrying packs with poor body ergonomics, such as forward head, round shoulders, and torso hunched against the load of packs or the cold, is often felt later in the neck, upper back, and shoulders. Pain from a hyperlordotic lower spine under the load of a pack is often felt focally in the low back and posterior hip.

Specific warm-up or stretching before activity does not prevent delayed soreness,[72] but deployed properly after activity may help alleviate soreness. Stretch affected areas gently (see Conditioning, earlier), and keep sore areas moving. Eat food with antiinflammatory components to perhaps soothe the inflammatory component of delayed soreness. Such foods include leafy green vegetables, cherries, and blueberries, which contain quercetin (a plant pigment belonging to the flavonoids); curcumin (turmeric); ginger; and plant foods containing resveratrol (especially grape skins). Several foods with essential fatty acids, including omega-3, are known for antiinflammatory properties: flaxseeds, pumpkin seeds, olive oil, and fermented soy products. These are light and easily carried as fresh food or supplements for wilderness travel.

The science supporting these recommendations is evolving. The yellow spice curcumin inhibits two proinflammatory mediators, tumor necrosis factor alpha and interleukin-1 (IL-1).[35] Antiinflammatory properties of resveratrol in grape skins[156] and ginger[95] act via suppression of the proinflammatory catalyst COX-2. Green tea contains the polyphenolic compound GTP, found to inhibit the proinflammatory cytokine IL-1.[115] Salicylic acid is a chemical produced by plants to protect themselves from pathogens, and is responsible for the antiinflammatory action of aspirin. Organic vegetables were found to have higher concentrations of salicylic acid (117 ng/g) than did nonorganic vegetables (20 ng/g), possibly because they were less likely to be protected from infection.[12]

Arachidonic acid, a component of human nutrition, is also a precursor of prostaglandins involved in the inflammatory response. Avoid proinflammatory foods that promote arachidonic acid in excess, such as foods containing omega-6 fatty acids, which are converted by COX-2 into prostaglandins[111] and leukotriene B_4.[145] Sources of proinflammatory mediators include peanuts, beef, chicken, and eggs.[145] Another food popularly implicated as proinflammatory is sugar. Diets heavy in inflammatory components may produce what is described as the "diet-induced proinflammatory state."[145]

FITNESS MYTHS

Myth: Walk and run toe-out, because that is the natural direction of the foot and leg muscles.

Fact: Toe-out (duck foot) position may signal tightness in the plantar fascia, metatarsal phalangeal joints, Achilles tendon, calf, and/or external rotators of the thigh in a cycle of tightness and loss of the stretch that is normally obtained from a straight position during gait. Slight anatomic differences in femoral position usually do not factor in the many degrees of turnout commonly seen, except for major hip pathologies. Toe-out walking imposes a high degree of strain on the feet, ankles, knees, and hips. It contributes to pronation, bunion formation, and the cycle of tightness. It decreases the push-off phase by pressing medially off the big toe rather than the ball of the foot and all toes, reducing speed and jumping ability. Without addressing the cause of deviation in gait, simply forcing parallel gait may lead to other complications. Stretch and retrain gait to keep legs parallel and body weight on the sole, not arches, for standing, walking, jumping, and movement.

Myth: High-top shoes and elastic bracing prevent ankle sprain.

Fact: The main predisposing factors in repeat sprains are disuse atrophy and lack of proprioception and balance sense caused by "supportive" shoes that do not promote stabilizing body weight with ankle and foot postural muscles. Hard stabilizing shoes also contribute to knee and leg pain,[149] and prevent normal foot and fascia stretch. Prevent ankle sprain with balance and kinesthetic retraining for foot and ankle positioning (see Feet and Ankles, earlier).

Myth: Women are more prone to lower body injuries than are men.

Fact: Several studies have identified training, biomechanics, and fitness, not gender, as primary injury risk factors. Data from army recruits showed that those of lower physical fitness had a consistently higher injury rate. When comparing men and women of equal aerobic fitness, rates of injury were similar.[78] In a study of 861 Army recruits, the higher rate of injuries among women "appears to be explained by physical fitness" rather than sex differences.[14] More confirming data came from a 13-year study of 60,000 high school athletes in 18 sports. "What we have here is not a gender issue, but instead a classic combination of training error and [lack of] physical fitness."[133]

Myth: Devices and pills that increase heart rate or blood flow without exercise can improve aerobic fitness.

Fact: Claims are made that head-standing, massage, or lying head-down improves circulation to the head, or that heating the body or holding a yoga stretch increases the heart rate, conferring aerobic benefit. Increased heart rate and local blood flow alone do not benefit cardiovascular status. Situational fright and moving the legs of a person lying in bed raise the heart rate, but are neurogenic rather than cardiogenic increases. Raising the body temperature through a hot shower or tub or sweating in a sauna suit increases the heart rate through skin vasodilation to shed heat. Blood pressure decreases, with consequent increase in the heart rate to maintain pressure. There is no aerobic benefit to overheating or sweating, and caloric expenditure is not raised. Improve aerobic ability through regular moderate-to-high–energy exercise, such as biking, swimming, rowing, skating, dancing, sprinting, and skiing, repeated regularly over time.

Myth: Older people need less exercise.

Fact: Exercise becomes more important and protective with aging. Deconditioning over years is often confused with aging. Regular exercise, functional stretching, and balance practice slow physical decline and can confer gains equivalent to stopping or reversing years of aging. Older people who exercise, move, balance, and stretch have many of the functional characteristics of a chronologically younger person. They can reach, bend, and move easily, negotiate uneven sidewalks and other terrain, and carry their own gear. The antiaging effect of exercise is effective in all age groups. Geriatric populations on exercise programs show improved strength and mobility. Physical gains often eliminate the need for walkers, wheelchairs, and canes, and

self-sufficiency returns. Many people do not crouch or sit on the floor because they are too weak to get up. That is not aging, but the need to regain strength to do it. Even critically ill people receiving assisted movement have a shortened recovery time, fewer bedrest-related illnesses, and a reduced need for sedatives. Exercise and skills practice are the keys to independence and retention of physical ability.

PERFORMANCE ENHANCEMENT

PERFORMANCE-ENHANCING DRUGS AND NUTRIENTS FOR EXERCISE AND EXPEDITIONS

Foods to increase physical ability have been sought throughout history. Indigenous and mountain people have long used stimulant plants such as coffee, kola, khat, betel nut, and coca to withstand cold, hypoxia, hunger, and fatigue. Aztec warriors hoped to increase bravery by eating the hearts of brave enemies. Berserkers were Norse warriors legendary for savagery and reckless frenzy in battle; they ate *Amanita muscaria* mushrooms. Dervishes whirled longer by drinking coffee. Before the first Olympic games in 776 BC, athletes used wine to enhance performance by dulling pain; concoctions of wine and substances from strychnine to cocaine were used in later Olympic games. Amphetamines were long given to soldiers to delay fatigue, and were widely used in medical practice until recently. Today, ergogenic aids include stimulants, muscle growth promoters, energy substrates, and oxygen utilization enhancers. They range from healthy to dangerous and illegal.

Methylxanthines

Methylxanthines are a class of stimulant alkaloids found in plants, including coffee, tea, cocoa, guarana, yerba mate, and kola (cola). They may be humankind's most commonly consumed drugs. Animals also seek them out. In South America, animals chew coca leaves, and goats in the Middle East are credited with originally showing the effects of eating coffee seeds to humans. (Although popularly called coffee beans, coffee seeds look like, but are not, true beans.) Methylxanthines are purinergic, acting on purine neurotransmitters such as adenosine.[143] They elevate cyclic adenosine monophosphate in several tissues, including the brain, with stimulant, diuretic, and vasodilator properties.[77] All xanthines have a similar stereochemistry, but each has unique properties. In various products promoted for health and energy, they are often combined (stacked), yielding compound effects.

Caffeine

Caffeine is the primary methylxanthine in coffee and kola nut, from which many cola sodas are made, and is present in smaller amounts in chocolate and tea. It was probably discovered in the Stone Age, and has been widely used ever since for its effects. Caffeine increases endurance and is particularly used for long endurance events.[63] How caffeine helps athletic performance is still studied and debated. Caffeine is thought to help endurance by directly stimulating the central nervous system, increasing plasma epinephrine,[134] which enhances excitation-contraction coupling mechanisms.[158] Some work shows epinephrine-induced enhanced free fatty acid oxidation for fuel,[129] which in turn spares muscle glycogen,[154] whereas others dispute lipid mobilization by caffeine[62,166] and show ergogenic effects of caffeine without an increase in plasma epinephrine.[64,166] Caffeine decreases the perception of effort, perhaps through adrenocortical axis stimulation,[93] which promotes cortisol and β-endorphin release.[42,92] The caffeine molecule is similar to the depressant molecule adenosine. As a competitive antagonist of adenosine receptors, caffeine replaces adenosine.[155] Reported effects on short-duration intense anaerobic activity are inconclusive about whether power or endurance is aided. Positive effects are attributed to increased motor unit recruitment[98] and resistance to fatigue through mobilization of intracellular calcium from the sarcoplasmic reticulum.[158] Although caffeine in isolation increases endurance, some work suggests that the effects do not extrapolate fully to coffee, perhaps because of components present in coffee that moderate the effect.[63] Caffeine with phenylpropanolamine interacts adversely, increasing the risk of hemorrhagic stroke.[28] Phenylpropanolamine is used as a decongestant and weight-control drug. The U.S. Food and Drug Administration banned this drug combination in 1983. Habitual caffeine users do not derive ergogenic effects from usual amounts of caffeine. Dependence and withdrawal symptoms, often severe, are common.

Theophylline

Theophylline is the methylxanthine in tea leaves, along with a small amount of caffeine and theobromine.[61] Theophylline is a smooth muscle relaxant, diuretic, cardiac stimulant, and vasodilator; it is used to treat asthma and other obstructive pulmonary disease. Theophylline delays skeletal muscle fatigue[102] and is thought to increase aerobic endurance through increased blood glycerol levels without increase in plasma epinephrine.[66] A study of Mt Everest base-camp expeditioners found no evidence that tea acts as a diuretic in regular tea drinkers, even at high altitude where fluid balance is stressed, or that it exerts a positive effect on mood.[144]

Theobromine

Theobromine is the primary methylxanthine in chocolate. Other compounds in cocoa include caffeine, serotonin, histamine, tryptophan, tryptamine, tyramine, phenylethylamine, octopamine, and anandamide.[127] Theobromine is found in smaller quantities in the kola nut. It is a weak diuretic, bronchodilator, and stimulant, and may increase mood and motivation to work.[117] Dark chocolate contains higher levels of theobromine than does lighter chocolate, along with substantial amounts of flavonoids and phenolics, possibly good for the heart. The healthiest way to use theobromine on the trail is in unsweetened cocoa, rather than in sweetened candy.

Guarana

Guarana is made from the crushed seeds of *Paullinia cupana*, a South American vine. It is considered to be as potent as caffeine (often called herbal caffeine), with similar effects.[3] However, guarana may not contain caffeine, but rather, the isomer guaranine.[15] Coffee contains between 1% and 4% caffeine. Guaranine is reported to either contain or be the equivalent of 5% caffeine. It contains lower amounts of the methylxanthines theophylline and theobromine.[132] Guarana is frequently found in herbal and nutritional supplements and has been used for energy and headache relief. Use is linked to unpleasant overstimulation, and withdrawal to weakness and depression.

Yerba Mate

Yerba mate is a South American tea-like beverage made from mate *(Flex paraguariensis)*, an evergreen holly. Among other plant substances and vitamins, mate contains a small amount of xanthines, primarily mateine, and smaller amounts of theophylline and theobromine. Mateine is a simple stereoisomer of caffeine, but has distinct effects. Like other xanthines, it relaxes smooth muscle airways and peripheral blood vessels, and is a mild diuretic. Central nervous system effects are disputed.[53] Although the xanthines in mate occur in minute amounts, they attract much speculation regarding possible benefit. Anecdotal claims are that persons with caffeine sensitivities seem able to drink mate for stimulation without insomnia and irritability. The cytotoxic and antioxidant activities of components in mate are speculated to confer a possible anticancer benefit,[128] but at least three studies link mate consumption with oropharyngeal or esophageal cancer.[59,60,148]

CHOLINERGIC STIMULANTS (TOBACCO, ARECA, AND LOBELIA)

Cholinergic agents stimulate nerve cells or fibers that employ acetylcholine as a neurotransmitter. They cause cardiac inhibition, vasodilation, gastrointestinal peristalsis, and other parasympathetic effects.

Nicotine

Nicotine is an alkaloid found in various plants, especially tobacco. It is poisonous, but in small doses is used for its stimulant effects. These effects have long been used to combat hunger and fatigue in various difficult environments, although nicotine has not been specifically found to enhance physical ability. It has mixed effects because it stimulates both the sympathetic and parasympathetic systems.[184] It is used in various forms, usually as chewing or smoking tobacco. Nicotine patches and gum have been used to try to boost alertness.

Betel Nut

Betel nut *(Areca catechu)* is a mild stimulant habitually chewed by many millions of people, primarily in Asia. It contains the alkaloids arecoline and guvacoline. Chewers, known by their reddish black teeth, primarily chew the areca nut wrapped in betel leaf, with mineral lime often added as a catalyst. The lime hydrolyzes the arecoline and guvacoline into arecaidine and guvacine, which are strong inhibitors of γ-aminobutyric acid (GABA) uptake. Aromatic phenolic compounds stimulate release of catecholamines. As a result of complex interactions, betel chewing affects parasympathetic, GABAergic, and sympathetic functions.[39] The dilute plant alkaloids are chewed over hours and slowly absorbed through the mucous membranes of the mouth to furnish a subtle stimulation and not-so-subtle parasympathetic salivation.

Lobelia

This plant, also called asthma weed, wild tobacco, pukeweed, and vomit wort, is another parasympathetic agent used in folk medicine to aid breathing, and more recently as a source of chromium.[99] It is found in several "health" tonics, with side effects reported to be difficulty breathing, rapid heartbeat, low blood pressure, diarrhea, vomiting, dizziness, and tremors.

SYMPATHOMIMETIC STIMULANTS: MONOAMINERGIC SUBSTANCES (AMPHETAMINES, COCA, KHAT, AND EPHEDRA)

Sympathomimetics mimic the sympathetic nervous system and stimulate release of noradrenaline and adrenaline. They enhance alertness and reduce hunger and mental and physical fatigue. Examples are amphetamines, coca, khat leaves, and ma huang (ephedra). Overstimulation is common, with addiction to some resulting in various unhealthy effects.

Amphetamines

Methamphetamine (Methedrine), levoamphetamine (Benzedrine), and dextroamphetamine (Dexedrine) are collectively known as amphetamines. Intense stimulation is followed by withdrawal depression, fatigue, and rebound appetite as neuronal dopamine stores, peaked by use,[38] are depleted in the mesolimbic pleasure center of the brain.[10] Development of amphetamines in the United States was first supported as a substitute for Chinese ephedra. Amphetamines were at one time prescribed to soldiers and widely used in clinical medicine to combat weight loss, asthma, depression, Parkinson's disease, hyperactivity in children, and travel sickness. They have been used for their alerting, enjoyable effects, and to reduce hunger and fatigue. Users may experience abnormally high or irregular heart rates, elevated blood pressure, and, sometimes, mental states resembling paranoid schizophrenia. Abdominal cramps, incoordination, dizziness, dry mouth, nausea, and vomiting may also accompany initial use. Chronic users are found to have structural deficits in several brain areas.[161] Acutely, amphetamines increase the risk of hyperthermia by two mechanisms: increased endogenous heat production and decreased heat dissipation due to peripheral vasoconstriction.[85] Deaths in the heat have resulted in endurance athletes and soldiers,[65,171] and in a 12-year-old taking appetite suppressants.[85] Amphetamines usually physically and psychologically addict the user after about 12 weeks, with abusers increasing doses from 10 to 1000 times to retain effects. Although amphetamines extend endurance, they are counterproductive to healthful wilderness travel. Over-the-counter (OTC) supplements marketed for weight loss and energy continue to be manufactured with amphetamine-like substances, with periodic reports of injury and death. However, the dependence created is an underreported health and economic concern.

Coca

Leaves of the South American shrub *Erythroxylum coca* contain from 0.1% to 0.9% of the alkaloid cocaine. Cocaine is a powerful cardiovascular stimulant that blocks catecholamine reuptake and prolongs effects of released neurotransmitters.[104] Release of norepinephrine increases blood pressure[163] and arrhythmias.[68] Resulting catecholamine depletion leads to intense depression (cocaine crash).[86] Sudden heart attack may occur in an otherwise healthy person.[91,126,167] Until the early 1900s, cocaine was widely sold OTC in tonics, toothache cures, and patent medicines. Combined with alcohol, cocaine alkaloid yields cocaethylene, a potent reinforcing compound, becoming a popular ingredient in wines such as Vin Mariani. As an export drug, cocaine is extracted in a paste from soaked, mashed coca leaves, often in the form of cocaine hydrochloride salt, with high percentages of cocaine. Addictive and socially and medically unhealthy, cocaine is unsuitable and profoundly unwise for athletic efforts.

Khat

Khat grows in eastern Africa and southern Arabia. It is frequently chewed for amphetamine-like stimulatory effects and to reduce fatigue and appetite. Khat releases catecholamines from presynaptic storage.[83] Leaves of the khat bush contain the alkaloid cathinone, which functions like amphetamine, and a milder form of cathinone, cathine,[173] one of the alkaloids found in ephedra. Cathinone increases blood pressure, heart rate, and psychostimulation.[27] Both cathinone and cathine are controlled substances (cathinone is schedule I and cathine is schedule IV).

Ephedra (Ma Huang)

Ephedra is a plant native to Pakistan, China, and northwestern India. The three ephedra species, *Ephedra sinica, E. equisetina,* and *E. intermedia,* are collectively known by their Chinese name, ma huang. The ephedra plant has two main active compounds: ephedrine (2-methylamino-1-phenyl-1-propanol) and pseudoephedrine.[172] Ephedrine and pseudoephedrine are both sympathomimetic, with effects similar to amphetamine but to a lesser degree. Unlike pseudoephedrine, ephedrine mediates effects through circulating epinephrine[48] and is a bronchial dilator used in treating asthma. Many now-banned "energy" and weight loss products contained one or more of the several forms of ephedra. Ephedrine can have several nervous system effects, such as insomnia, tremors, anxiety, and seizures.[124] Effects do not always depend on the dosage. Ephedra is associated with a small number of cases of cardiovascular toxicities attributed to sympathomimetic adrenergic effects, including myocarditis, arrhythmias, myocardial infarction, cardiac arrest, and sudden death.[119] The hypertensive effect is postulated as a factor in the increased risk of stroke.[112] Ergogenic effects are debated and risks do not seem to show that ephedra is advantageous for wilderness travel. The FDA banned ephedra in December 2003.

OTHER STIMULANTS

Ginseng

Ginseng collectively refers to several different plant species from various countries, each with possibly unique effects. The main active agents are ginsenosides, which are triterpene saponins. It is usually the root that is used, with active agents varying with species of plant, age, location, and method and timing of harvest and processing. Because of ginseng's adaptogen and stimulant qualities, it is used in many candies, pills, and drinks, with numerous claims. Investigations have found that many ginseng preparations contain other stimulating compounds, usually caffeine, and that ginsenoside content varies greatly, with some preparations containing none at all, making interpretation of claims difficult. Although some animal studies show effect, in many human studies there does not seem to be ergogenic effect on oxygen consumption, respiratory exchange ratio, minute ventilation, blood lactic acid concentration, heart rate, perceived exertion,[49,113] exercise time, workload, plasma lactate, or hematocrit.[4] A study reviewing clinical trials showed no beneficial effect on physical performance, psychomotor performance, cognitive function, immunomodulation, diabetes mellitus, or herpes simplex type II infections.[168] Excess may result in diarrhea, nervousness, blood glucose changes, and insomnia. Ginseng may potentiate or interact adversely with caffeine, phenelzine (Nardil),[79] warfarin (Coumadin),[164] and monoamine oxidase inhibitors.[109]

Anabolic Steroids

Anabolic steroids are controlled drugs with growth-promoting and androgenic effects. They improve athletic performance when strength is a primary component, and when used with intense training programs and adequate nutrition. For ergogenic effect, anabolic steroids are taken at 10 to 100 times the therapeutic dose for medical conditions. A large black market exists for controlled medical and veterinary anabolic steroids, such as Trenbolone, which is used to increase the weight of cattle. A related steroid is tetrahydrogestrinone, a designer anabolic steroid derived from gestrinone, a European drug for endometriosis. Several popular steroids have progestogenic activity. Others are aromatizing (synthesize estrogens), including methandrostenolone (Dianabol), boldenone (Equipoise), and to a lesser extent fluoxymesterone (Halotestin). Users seeking to avoid estrogenic side effects or recover depressed testosterone production after a cycle of steroid use may "stack" (combine) antiestrogens (aromatase inhibitors or receptor blockers) such as aminoglutethimide (Cytadren) and clomiphene (Clomid). The pattern of increasing a dose through a cycle is referred to as pyramiding. The risk for injury increases, because tendons and ligaments do not strengthen at the same rate as muscle. Side effects can be common and injurious. One study indicates that reports of hepatotoxicity may be overstated[45]; however, other adverse effects of anabolic steroids seem to be documented, including apoptosis of skeletal muscle,[2] cardiovascular damage,[108] decreased endogenous androgen production and testicular atrophy,[87] thrombotic phenomena such as strokes, myocardial infarctions, and limb loss,[51,52] uncontrolled behaviors,[7] and dependency behavior and withdrawal depression.[84]

ANABOLIC (GROWTH-PROMOTING) NONSTEROIDS

DHEA

Dehydro-3-epiandrosterone (DHEA) is a weak intermediate steroid, the most abundant naturally made in the body. DHEA is manufactured from cholesterol, mostly in the adrenal glands, and to a lesser extent in the ovaries and testes. DHEA converts to dozens of hormones, including estrogen and testosterone in both men and women. DHEA levels wane with age and certain illnesses, leading to the question of whether restoring those levels can mitigate effects of age and disease, even though it is unknown if lowered DHEA causes such problems. Although DHEA is commonly purchased in hopes of enhancing strength, gains are not confirmed in controlled investigation.[81] The estrogenic potential seems to produce results in the laboratory for women to restore lost bone and absent menstrual periods. Before taking DHEA, one should have blood levels checked for deficiency.

Androstenedione

Androstenedione (andro) is made in the body from DHEA. Androstenedione is a precursor molecule (prohormone) of both testosterone and estrogen. Which hormone pathway it takes depends on several factors, including the percentage of body fat; a high percentage of body fat increases estrogenic potential. Androstenedione is accepted as an aromatizer, being readily converted to estrone. Popularity seems to stem from its status as a precursor to testosterone. For perspective, cholesterol is also a precursor molecule to testosterone, but eating it does not increase testosterone. Reports from gyms and androstenedione manufacturers state that athletic ability is always greatly helped. Studies do not find ergogenic potential.[81] Some studies show increased strength, but no more than in control groups with matched exercise without androstenedione. Another study found no increase in plasma testosterone and no anabolic effect on muscle protein in young men.[130] Supplementation may suppress endogenous production. OTC androstenedione supplements have sometimes been found to contain elements not on the label that can cause a positive drug test for other banned substances.

Creatine

As quickly as ATP is used for fuel in cells, it is rebuilt for more activity using phosphocreatine, stored mostly in skeletal muscle, and a smaller amount of free creatine. Use of supplemental creatine to fuel intense, short efforts is behind sales of creatine monohydrate, the synthetic form of endogenous creatine phosphate. Creatine seems to assist repetitive, high-intensity, short-term efforts with brief recovery.[165] Whether creatine is an important adjunct for extended exercise is debated. Individual variation is wide.[82] Advice to eat steak, fish, and pork, which contain creatine, is misguided because creatine denatures during the cooking process. Creatine (methylguanidine-acetic acid) is an amino acid made in the liver, pancreas, and kidneys from arginine and glycine, which are obtained from balanced meals, including vegetarian meals. The ergogenic effect of creatine supplementation seems to be counteracted by caffeine.[165] Long-term effects of supplementation are not known.

FOODS

Carbohydrates

Ingested and stored carbohydrate is ergogenic, providing fuel and delaying fatigue during intense, long-duration exercise, and aiding recovery after exercise.[174] The larger the body's carbohydrate stores, the longer exercise can be extended before fatigue, depending on the fitness level. Depletion of blood glucose and stored carbohydrate is related to fatigue and reduced athletic ability.[169] Storing muscle glycogen is accomplished by hard physical training and restocking muscles by eating healthy carbohydrate, preferably within the first 30 minutes after a bout of exertion.

Vitamins and Minerals

No evidence supports vitamin or mineral supplementation as ergogenic. Supplementation is useful when nutritional deficiency exists,[177] for athletes in weight-restricted events, or for extended and extreme wilderness travel with inadequate nutrition. However, increasing intake will not improve physical ability with adequate nutrition. Oversupplementation may alter utilization of other micronutrients. Supplementation to offset poor eating habits is not a healthy solution.

Bee Pollen

Bee pollen claims include various effects, from vague vitality to specific athletic improvements. Bee pollen has nutritional components, but it has not been experimentally shown to enhance any aspect of athletic performance[179] or to have any effect on the level of physical stimulation.[76] It may provoke allergic reactions in susceptible people.

WATER

Water is an overlooked athletic ability aid. Although possessing no ergogenic chemical or property, water is a necessary, inexpensive, and easy fluid replacer for healthy functioning, heat balance, and recovery from exercise. Drinking too much will not enhance health, and in extremes, can result in dilutional hyponatremia (see Chapter 89).

Fitness Water, Fitness Carbo, and/or Protein Drinks With "Buzz"

Many packaged "health" and sports drinks contain stimulants of many kinds—ginseng, guarana, and caffeine among them. These are advertised as energy drinks and vitality enhancers. Check the label. Remember that they are stimulants with associated health risks. Also note if they contain refined sugar, hydrogenated fat, dyes, flavors, and fillers.

Alerting and Wakefulness Adjuncts

Products (e.g., nicotine) may increase alertness or stimulation without augmenting the physical ability to do work and thus may be represented as ergogenic without being work-enhancing. Some, such as amphetamines, provide global stimulation but then require recovery sleep, becoming counterproductive in settings requiring good health. Products such as modafinil (Provigil [U.S.] or Alertec [Canada]) and adrafinil aim to focus on wakefulness and vigilance by targeting specific sleep-promoting areas of the suprachiasmatic nuclei,[141] without binding to dopaminergic or adrenergic receptors.[36,97] These drugs are labeled for narcolepsy, with the intended use being wakefulness during an ordinary day, followed by a normal night's sleep. Off-label use as a lifestyle drug, to extend wakefulness for stretches of 40 hours and more without the need for recovery sleep, seems to be increasing among those seeking advantage in an ultramarathon, the military, or a competitive workplace. Prolonged sleep deprivation is known to depress immune function. Animals in experiments and humans deprived of sleep by torture have psychotic effects and die from infections. The effects and safety of these drugs over extended periods are not yet known.[11]

REFERENCES

Complete references used in this text are available online at expertconsult.inkling.com.

CHAPTER 97

Wilderness and Endurance Events

DAVID A. TOWNES AND BRANDEE L. WAITE

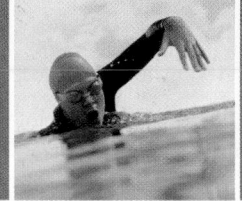

Perhaps the earliest record of an endurance event may be traced back to ancient Greece in the 5th century BC. The Persians invaded Greece in 490 BC, landing in Marathon, a small town about 26 miles from Athens. Seriously outnumbered by the Persians, the Athenians sent messengers to cities throughout Greece requesting assistance. Legend has it that after the battle, a man named Pheidippides was sent from Marathon to Athens to bring word of the Greek victory. He covered the 26-plus miles on foot, only to drop dead after proclaiming *"Niki!"* ("victory"). Debate continues among historians about what really occurred. For instance, there is evidence that Pheidippides was actually sent from Marathon to request help and that news of the victory was delivered by a man named Eukles.[35] Although the exact details remain unclear, when the modern-day Olympic games were inaugurated in Greece in 1896, the legend of Pheidippides served as inspiration for the marathon. That first marathon covered a distance of 40 km (24.85 miles), the distance from Marathon Bridge to Olympic Stadium.[36]

During the next 28 years, the marathon continued to evolve. In the United States, the Boston Athletic Association held its first marathon on April 19, 1897, to commemorate the famous ride of Paul Revere on that date in 1775. For the Olympic Games in London in 1908, the marathon distance was changed to 26 miles, the distance from Windsor Castle to White City Stadium, with an additional 385 yards added so that the race would finish in front of the royal family's viewing box. Finally, in the 1924 Olympic Games in Paris, the distance was set at 26.2 miles, establishing the modern-day marathon distance.[36] Today, hundreds of marathons are held throughout the world each year.

The past quarter-century has seen tremendous growth in the popularity not only of marathons but other endurance events, including cycling events, triathlons, ultratriathlons, and ultramarathons. In addition, advances and improvements in outdoor equipment, along with relatively efficient and affordable travel, have allowed increased participation in such activities as adventure travel, backcountry skiing, mountain biking, mountaineering, orienteering, rock climbing, sea kayaking, scuba diving, snowboarding, trekking, and white-water rafting and kayaking.

The growth of these activities, along with continued popularity of endurance events, has led to development of activities that combine aspects of both. Wilderness multisport endurance events, also referred to as *adventure races* or *multisporting,* have soared in popularity throughout the world, with increasing numbers of events and participants each year.

This chapter emphasizes development of a medical support plan for wilderness and endurance events, including adventure races, cycling events, marathons, and triathlons. This information should prove useful for persons charged with provision of medical care for these activities, as well as for those participating in the events.

TYPES OF EVENTS

ADVENTURE RACES

In adventure races or wilderness multisport endurance events, athletes compete over a course that requires performance of multiple disciplines that may include caving, fixed-line mountaineering, flat- and white-water boating, hiking, in-line skating, mountain biking, navigation and orienteering, technical climbing and ropes skills, trail running, and trekking. Races are categorized by duration into sprint (< 6 hours), intermediate (6 to 12 hours), long (12 to 36 hours), and expedition (> 36 hours) length.

Adventure racing began in the early 1980s with the first large, well-organized events, including the Coast-to-Coast, started in New Zealand in 1980, and the Alaska Wilderness Classic, started in 1983. These were followed by other well-known events, including New Zealand's Raid Gauloises and the Southern Traverse, begun in 1989 and 1991, respectively. The Eco-Challenge introduced adventure racing to the United States in 1995. The Primal Quest, started in 2002 in Telluride, Colorado, brought adventure racing more into the mainstream of American sports through network television coverage. In addition to these expedition-length races, there are countless shorter races throughout the world, for example, the Tough Mudder, a 1-day 10- to 12-mile obstacle course held in over 50 locations worldwide in 2015. In the United States, the U.S. Adventure Race Association (USARA), established in 1998, serves as the governing body for adventure racing (see usara.com). The inaugural USARA Adventure Race National Championship was held in 2000 in California. The first Adventure Race World Championship was held in 2001 in Switzerland.

Expedition-length adventure races are competitive team events that require at least one member of the four- or five-person team to be the opposite gender of the other teammates. Teams race together, with each team member completing each discipline along the course. The course may cover hundreds of miles and take up to 10 days or more to complete.

In many expedition-length adventure races, teams are provided maps and the Universal Transverse Mercator coordinates for each checkpoint and transition area (where teams change disciplines) through which they must pass, but there is no set course between checkpoints and transition areas. Unique to these events, it is left to the team to decide the best route between checkpoints, depending on their strengths and weakness. Whereas one team may opt to go around a ridge, another may go over it. In addition, there are no built-in rest periods, and once the race begins, teams may race around the clock. An individual team must strategize if and when to rest.

When teams in expedition-length events are racing on the course, they are governed by a set of instructions called the "rules of travel." These rules dictate multiple aspects of the race, such as where and when a team may travel on paved roads, existing trails, or water. For example, white-water travel is often prohibited at night in the interest of safety. In addition, the rules of travel specify safety equipment that must be used for each discipline, including mandatory use of personal flotation devices while on the water and helmets while riding bicycles.

The rules of travel also dictate several aspects of the event pertaining to medical care that should be included in the medical support plan. They govern use of medications, including performance-enhancing substances, specify penalties for use of medical resources during the race, and outline criteria for medical withdrawal from the event.

A breach of the rules of travel results in a penalty for the offending team. Minor infractions, such as travel on an unapproved section of paved road, might result in additional hours being added to the team's total time at the end of the race. Major infractions, such as not wearing a helmet during a mountain bike section or use of a banned substance, may result in disqualification.

The team to complete the course with the fastest time after all penalties have been allocated is declared the winner. In many events, prize money is awarded to the top teams.

CYCLING EVENTS

Organized endurance cycling events are often noncompetitive group rides or events designed to raise money for charity. These are normally staged, multiday events with participants riding during the day and resting at night. Several investigations have demonstrated that those in charge of medical provision for these rides must be prepared to treat a wide variety of injuries and illnesses. Because many of these events are designed to raise money for charity, the general health and experience of the participants may be more varied than in other endurance events.

USA Cycling, the governing body for mountain biking in the United States, sanctioned more than 3000 cycling events in 2013 (see usacycling.org); however, this represents only a fraction of the events held annually.

In cycling, perhaps more than in other endurance sports, the use of performance-enhancing substances (actual and alleged use) has been a major issue at both the professional and amateur levels. A medical support plan for all events should include a description of the banned substance policy, testing procedures, if any, and rules for disciplinary action for any violation.

MARATHONS AND ULTRAMARATHONS

Marathons are perhaps the most popular endurance events. Standard marathons cover 26.2 miles (42 km), whereas ultramarathons may be 100 miles (160 km) or more. In 2013 there were more than 1100 marathons held in the United States, with approximately 541,000 finishers, compared with approximately only 300 marathons in 2000 (see runningusa.org/marathon-report-2014). In 2012, an estimated 60,000 people finished ultramarathons in the United States, compared with 10,000 finishers in 1990.

USA Track and Field (USATF; see usatf.org) is the national governing body of long-distance running and is a member of the International Association of Athletics Federations (IAAF; see iaaf.org), which sets the rules of competition for all officially sanctioned long-distance running events in the United States and throughout the world. However, the majority of marathons in the United States are non-USATF events.

USATF rules of competition allow for sanctioned medical assistance for participants by authorized official event personnel. Current rules do not stipulate specific penalties or disqualification for acceptance of medical assistance, so long as it does not alter the scheduled time of competition for any athlete, interfere with other athletes in the competition, or incorporate use of illegal or banned substances, technology, or devices that may give the athlete an unfair competitive advantage. A medical official may choose to remove an athlete from competition if the official feels it is medically necessary for safety of the athlete or for safety of other athletes in the competition. Use of intravenous (IV) fluids or other medications during competition (as long as they are not banned substances) are not specifically listed as grounds for disqualification, but they may be subject to review. Additional rules about clothing, shoes, and athlete interactions with race officials, if breached, may result in disqualification (iaaf.org/about-iaaf/documents/rules-regulations).

Although many uncertified events incorporate the same rules, it is imperative that medical providers and athletes familiarize themselves with the rules of a particular event. In general, ultramarathons are not under the governance of the USATF, and rules for these events may be vastly different from those for standard marathons. Some marathons and ultramarathons allow for pacing, in which a noncompeting individual may run alongside a competitor to help the runner keep a certain pace. In other races this is strictly prohibited. Most standard marathons do not enforce time penalties. However, ultramarathons often have rules similar to those for adventure races, where rule infractions may carry time penalties, which are added to the runner's finishing time.

TRIATHLONS

Triathlons, which consist of swimming, cycling, and running, are held in various lengths:

sprint length: a 400- to 800-m [0.25- to 0.5-mile] swim, a 16- to 24-km [10- to 15-mile] bike, and a 5-km [3.1-mile] run);

international or Olympic length: 1500- m [0.9-mile] swim, 38- to 43-km [24- to 27-mile] bike, and 10-km [6-mile] run); and

Ironman, or ultratriathlon: 4-km [2.4-mile] swim, 180-km [112-mile] bike, and 34-km [26.2-mile] run that may last many hours, or days in the case of staged races.

USA Triathlon (USAT) is the governing body for triathlons in the United States (see usatriathlon.org).

The first recorded competitive triathlon was the Mission Bay Triathlon held in San Diego, California, in 1974. It was intended as no more than a break in the normal grind of training for marathons and 10-K races. In 1978, several participants in that first event combined three of Oahu's endurance events (the Waikiki Rough Water Swim, the Around-Oahu Bike Ride, and the Honolulu Marathon) into one race that we now know as the Ironman Triathlon, the most famous event in the sport.

Most triathlons require participants to wear a swim cap and allow goggles, but forbid use of fins, snorkels, paddles, or other devices during the swim. In addition, many allow swimmers to wear wetsuits. To maximize safety during the swim, rescue personnel in boats patrol the water to offer assistance to any swimmer in need. During the bike section, all participants are required to wear a helmet. Regulations about drafting during the bike section vary by event. Most events also have rules about what is allowable and required during the "transition zones," when competitors switch from swimming to cycling, and again from cycling to running.

Most races allow for medical assistance by official event personnel, although rules among events vary and often intentionally leave room for individual interpretation. For example, the rules for the 2014 Ironman Triathlon state that while there is no penalty for receiving a medical evaluation, IV fluid administration results in disqualification (see ironman.com). Although many unsanctioned events use USAT rules as guidelines, medical providers and participants must understand the rules of the specific race in which they are involved. It is often helpful to have medical providers participate in development of these rules.

MEDICAL SUPPORT FOR WILDERNESS AND ENDURANCE EVENTS

With growing popularity of wilderness endurance events has come increasing demand for medical support for these activities. Provision of medical care for wilderness and endurance events represents a unique area of wilderness and event medicine. This chapter reviews the basics of medical support for wilderness and endurance events and suggests strategies for developing a medical support plan for these activities. Although many general aspects of provision of medical support apply to all events, the complexity of certain events (especially adventure races) often warrants additional resources. Adjustments need to be made in anticipation of the type, amount, and severity of anticipated injuries and illnesses. In addition, logistics, communication, emergency medical services, and search and rescue protocols should be tailored to the specific event.

MASS GATHERINGS

Information from the study of mass gatherings serves as a background for the provision of medical support for wilderness and endurance events. A significant amount of variation exists in the literature concerning the definition of a mass gathering. In some cases, it has been defined as an event with more than 1000 participants; in others, an event is not considered a mass gathering unless there are more than 25,000 participants.[8,31]

Provision of medical support for any event begins with development of a medical support plan. Several authors have described this process for mass gatherings.[9,23,27] The basic goals are to provide rapid access and triage, stabilization and transport of seriously injured or ill patients, and on-site care for minor injuries and illnesses.[8] Nine important elements of planning are attendance or crowd size, personnel, medical triage and facilities, communication, transportation, medical records, public information and education, mutual aid, and data collection.[23]

General recommendations have been made about the location and staffing of on-site medical facilities at mass gatherings. One group of investigators recommends that advanced life support (ALS) units be in place so that the response time from collapse to ALS care is 5 minutes or less for all participants under all conditions.[44] Others have suggested the goals of basic first aid in 4 minutes, ALS care in 8 minutes, and evacuation to a medical facility within 30 minutes.[41] For staffing, it has been suggested that minimum staffing for every 10,000 participants be a two-person team consisting of registered nurses, emergency medical technicians, or paramedics, or a combination of all three.

In terms of on-site medical care provision, events may be divided into four categories, classes, or types. Category I events are those in which spectators remain seated for a set period of time or for the duration of the event. Common examples include stadium sporting events and concerts. In category II events, such as golf tournaments, Mardi Gras or Carnival celebrations, and state fairs, spectators are mobile and may become participants in the events. A large geographic area and participants often outnumbering spectators characterize category III events, which include charity walks, bicycle rides, marathons, and triathlons.[34] In addition, because of the extreme nature and unique challenges in providing medical support for adventure races and similar endurance events, several authors have labeled these events category IV events.[6,51,52,54] In general, categories III and IV events do not meet the participant number criterion of mass gatherings.

Most existing investigations of medical support involve categories I and II events, with a smaller number of investigations of categories III and IV events. Most investigations of categories I and II events include the frequency and type of injuries and illnesses treated, rate of utilization of on-site medical services, and rate of transfer to local care facilities. Their goal has been to determine what factors influence the type and frequency of injuries and illnesses in order to better anticipate needs and establish appropriate guidelines and standards of care. Much information in these investigations is anecdotal and descriptive; several studies have concluded that there is no standard of care for emergency medical services at mass gatherings.[2,8,41,44]

The incidence of true medical emergencies at mass gatherings appears to be relatively small. In one large study, 75% of medical encounters involved respiratory illnesses, heat-related injuries, and minor problems such as sunburn, blisters, and headache. Asthma was the most common reason for required acute medical intervention.[3]

The relationship between attendance (crowd size) and utilization of on-site medical services is unclear. Several studies have found that overall utilization grew with attendance but that the utilization rate did not increase and, in some cases, actually decreased, with larger attendance.[2,9,58] Rate of utilization of on-site medical services varies widely among events, ranging from 0.14 to 90 patients per 1000 participants, with most events reporting 0.5 to 2 patients per 1000 participants.[2,8,44]

Crowd (participant) demographics, event type, and availability of alcohol and drugs may also be used to help estimate utilization of medical resources. Studies demonstrate that when alcohol is readily available, there is an increase in medical problems related to intoxication.[2,31] In contrast, during a Papal visit, one would expect less intoxication but more cardiac-related problems.[27]

Overall, a number of factors may influence the utilization rate and type of medical care required. These include type and duration of the event, weather, availability of alcohol and drugs, and crowd demographics, including average age, density, and mood.[2,3,31]

WILDERNESS AND ENDURANCE EVENTS

Although the basic influence of attendance, temperature, and relative humidity on utilization of medical resources is likely to be similar across all events, caution should be used when applying utilization rates from categories I and II events to categories

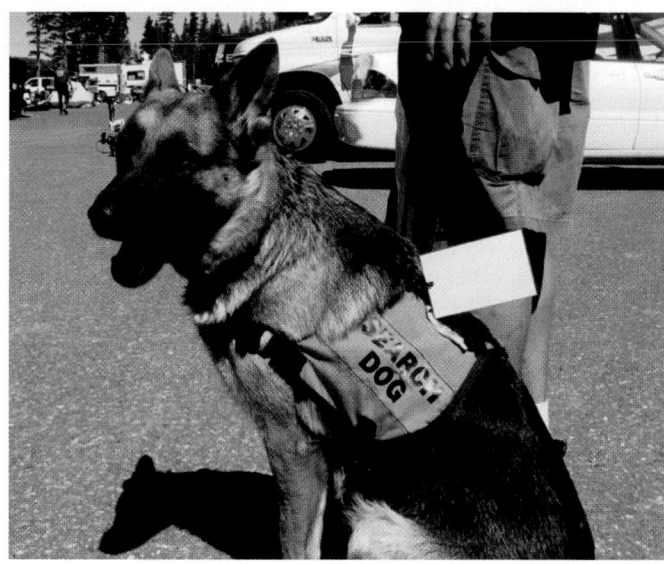

FIGURE 97-1 Adventure races represent a unique area of wilderness and event medicine because they have no set course and technical search and rescue may be required. *(Courtesy David Townes, MD.)*

III and IV events. Compared with categories I and II events, utilization rates of on-site medical resources are likely to be higher for category III events and significantly higher for category IV events.

Appropriate on-site medical support for wilderness and endurance events is important to help ensure health and safety of participants. As popularity of wilderness and endurance events grows, courses are longer and more demanding, events are held in more remote and exotic locations around the world, and the potential increases for illness and injury.

Wilderness and endurance events often occur in rough and remote terrain where communication may be difficult, transport time to definitive care prolonged, and technical search and rescue required. In some wilderness events, the entire course is set, whereas in others there is no set course between checkpoints and transition areas. In events with no set course, the exact location of each team may be unknown. In addition, many of these events are not staged, resulting in hundreds of miles separating lead teams from the back of the pack (Figure 97-1). Categories III and IV events present additional challenges for provision of medical care and represent a new and important area of event and wilderness medicine.

DEVELOPMENT OF A MEDICAL SUPPORT PLAN

Provision of medical support for any event begins with development of a medical support plan. The importance of early planning, organization, and good communication cannot be overemphasized.[55] For any event, the medical support plan should be based on anticipation of needs. This begins with estimation of number of patients and type of injuries and illnesses that will require treatment in both best-case and worst-case scenarios. It is often helpful to review utilization of medical resources for similar events that have been held.[27]

Development of a medical support plan should be done under direction of the event's medical director. The primary responsibilities of the medical director are the health and safety of participants. The medical director may be a physician, paramedic, emergency medical technician, nurse, or other medical professional. Ideally, this individual should have prior experience as a medical director for similar events and will serve as care provider, planner, advisor, educator, and liaison with the community.[19] It is essential that the director be familiar with the location of the event, including the capability of local emergency medical services (EMS), local health care facilities, and in the case of category IV events such as adventure races, local search and rescue (SAR) system. Medical support plan development should begin several months to a few years before the event, depending on event complexity.

Development of a medical support plan begins with careful review of the course, including its location, disciplines required, time of year, and climate conditions, including precipitation, temperature, and humidity. In this way, occurrence and type of injuries, illnesses, endemic diseases, and environmental emergencies, such as dehydration, heat and cold illness, and altitude illness, can be roughly anticipated. High temperature and relative humidity can have a major effect on utilization of on-site medical resources. Both of these factors are associated with increases in demand for on-site medical services; however, humidity has a greater effect than does temperature. During mass gatherings, availability of water influenced the incidences of dehydration and heat illness.[2,8,27]

In general, the medical support plan should be comprehensive and outline all aspects of medical support, including a complete list of medical supplies, equipment, and personnel (Box 97-1). Treatment and transfer protocols should be clearly outlined, assigning any penalties for receiving medical care and establishing indications for medical disqualification or withdrawal from the event. It is important that the medical support plan be based on estimates of the type and frequency of injuries and illnesses expected in both best and worst case scenarios.

In some of the locations where these events occur, especially category IV events, there are inherent difficulties in communication, travel, and general logistics. It may be unrealistic to assume that local EMS, health care facilities, and SAR will be able to handle the potential increased burden and demand for services imposed by the event.

The basic goal of the medical support plan should be to provide definitive treatment for minor illnesses and injuries, establish initial stabilization, and facilitate transfer for more severe illnesses and injuries[52] (Figure 97-2). It is fundamental that the medical support plan be based on anticipation of need. For the event medical director, adventure races and other category IV

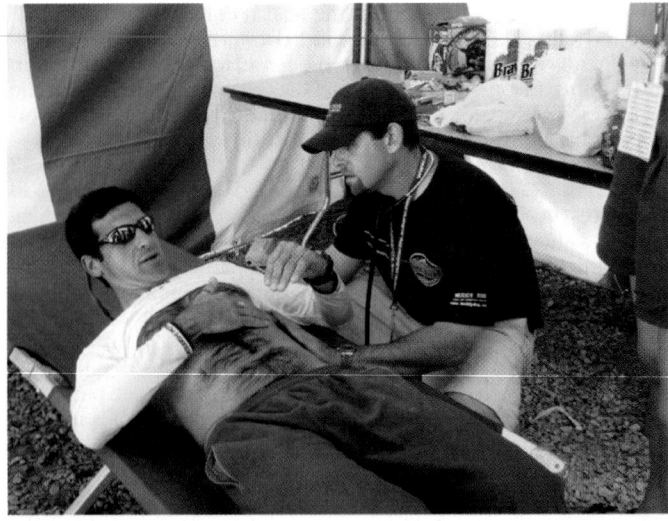

FIGURE 97-2 In wilderness and endurance events, the basic goal of the medical support plan should be to provide definitive treatment for minor illnesses and injuries and to provide initial stabilization and facilitate transfer for more severe situations. (*Courtesy David Townes, MD.*)

events present the greatest challenge in medical support plan development, often occurring in sparsely populated rural or very remote, rugged wilderness terrain. Although there are resources and even consensus guidelines for some events to assist the medical director in developing the medical support plan, the body of knowledge is still incomplete and anticipating medical needs thus remains a challenge.[24] Available information demonstrates that medical providers should be prepared to treat a wide variety of injuries and illnesses.[15,54]

BOX 97-1   Suggested Medical Equipment and Supplies for Wilderness and Endurance Events

Foot Care
Coban self-adherent wrap
Elastikon tape
Hypafix tape
Leukotape
Moleskin
New-Skin

General
Alcohol pads
Blankets
Cotton swabs
Examination gloves (S/M/L)
Flashlight and battery
Hand cleaner, sterilizer, and sanitizer
Instant cold packs
Portable bed or cots
Sharps and needle boxes
Sphygmomanometer
Stethoscope
Syringes and needles (3 mL/22 gauge/
    1 inch)
Tape (varying sizes)
Thermometer (oral and rectal)
Tongue depressors
Utility towels

Intravenous Fluids
Angiocatheters (18- and 22-gauge)
Fluids: Normal saline (1 L bags)
IV starter kits
IV tubing kits

Medications
Injection
Diphenhydramine (Benadryl)
D50 (dextrose in water)
Epinephrine
Ketorolac
Lidocaine (1% or 2%)
Promethazine

Inhaled
Albuterol

Oral
Acetaminophen
Antihistamine
Hurricane gel
Nonsteroidal antiinflammatory drugs
Antidiarrheal drugs
Prednisone
Pseudoephedrine (Sudafed)

Topical
Antibiotic or antiseptic ointment
2% lidocaine (Xylocaine) jelly
Hydrocortisone cream
Ophthalmic antibiotic

Miscellaneous
Duct tape
Fans and water sprayers
Foley catheters
Nasal packing
Pregnancy test kits

Orthopedic
Elastic bandages
Cardboard splints
Finger splints
SAM splints

Respiratory
Ambu bags
Laryngoscope and blades
Endotracheal tubes (varying sizes)
Nebulization pipes
Oxygen masks
Oxygen tanks
Oxygen tank regulators
Oxygen tubing

Trauma and Transport
14-gauge angiocatheters
Backboard
Cervical collars
Head immobilizers
Strap kits

Wound
Bandages (varying sizes)
Dressing (4 × 4, rolled gauze)
Masks with eye shields
Needles for irrigation
Normal saline for irrigation (500-mL bags)
Sterile gloves
Steri-strips
Suture kits
Suture (3.0, 4.0, 5.0, 6.0)
Forceps
Wound (tissue) glue

Modified from Townes DA: Wilderness medicine: strategies for provision of medical support for adventure racing, *Sports Med* 35:557, 2005.

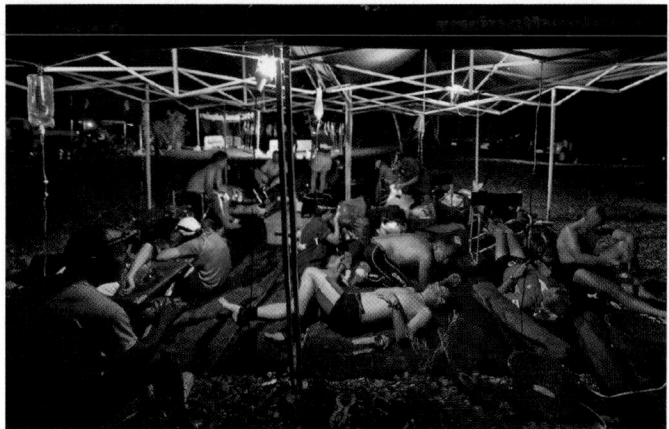

FIGURE 97-3 Overnight medical care administered at ultramarathon in the Australian outback, a hot and humid environment. *(Courtesy of Chris Lusher for RacingThePlanet.)*

PERSONNEL, EQUIPMENT, SUPPLIES, AND LOGISTICS

The type, amount, and placement of personnel, equipment, and supplies varies among events. The medical support plan should include clear and comprehensive descriptions of these components for each individual event.

For most endurance events, medical care is administered along the course at medical stations or within medical tents (Figure 97-3). In triathlons and adventure races, medical care is often administered at "transition areas," where racers change from one discipline to another. In adventure races, medical care may also be administered at designated checkpoints along the course where it is anticipated that medical care may be required.

Standard marathons and triathlons often have medical tents positioned every 1 to 3 miles. Ultramarathons normally have medical tents spread further apart, positioned every 5 to 10 miles along the course. During endurance cycling events, medical tents are positioned every 10 to 20 miles. Positioning of medical tents during adventure races is more variable, reflecting terrain variability in the courses. In a typical 400-mile-long adventure race, there may be up to 10 medical stations.

Personnel

On-site medical personnel should be able to recognize and initiate treatment for routine injuries and illnesses, major and minor trauma, environmental conditions, and endemic diseases. Ideally, they should have experience in wilderness and event medicine. Essential skills include patient assessment, establishing IV access, administration of fluids and medications, and packaging of patients for transfer or evacuation. Personnel might include physicians, paramedics, emergency medical technicians, physician assistants, nurse practitioners, and/or wilderness first responders. At a minimum, staffing each medical station should include one or more individuals with excellent patient assessment skills and the ability to establish IV access and administer medications. Because of the high incidence of foot problems among race participants, the authors have found it extremely useful to include personnel with expertise in foot care whenever possible.

Equipment and Supplies

The medical support plan should include a comprehensive list of medical supplies. The list should be available at each medical tent or station so that inventory can be maintained and personnel will not waste time looking for items that are not available. A sample supply list is shown in Box 97-1. Substitutions, adjustments, additions, and subtractions should be made based on the particular event. It is useful to have all supplies packaged in durable carts, with the location of supplies standardized so that each cart is as similar as possible (Figure 97-4). This allows personnel to move from one medical station to another and easily locate supplies. Supplies should be packaged in clear plastic bags

and labeled (with an index card inside the bag) to aid in organization, especially when supply carts are moved over rough terrain from one point to another. Equipment and supply needs should be anticipated and adjustments made in the number of supplies at each medical station. Examples include anticipating that foot care supplies will be in high demand after a long trek, but less so after a kayaking section of the course; or predicting that skin lubricant or antifungal creams will be in higher demand during the latter part of the endurance event. Cycling events and mountain biking sections of adventure races events may require more bandaging and wound care supplies due to the higher potential for large abrasions sustained from falls while cycling. Each aid station should prepare a portable "go bag," to be carried in the event that a medical team needs to leave the tent in order to treat a patient in the field.

Thorough and careful review of the course allows a medical director to estimate of the type and number of environmental injuries and illnesses that will require treatment during the event. For example, if the course requires travel at high altitude, the medical support plan should include a protocol for treatment of altitude illness. This might include indications for oxygen, medications such as dexamethasone, and the use and location of a Gamow-type hyperbaric bag.

Even with the best planning, the wide variety and variability of these events—especially adventure races—makes it impossible to precisely predict the injury and illness pattern for any one event. In the authors' experience, there may be significant year-to-year differences in the same event. During the 2002 Primal Quest, a large number of participants developed shortness of breath and wheezing during the event, requiring treatment with β-adrenergic agonists, even though only a few athletes reported a history of exercise-induced asthma. In contrast, during the 2003 Primal Quest, very few athletes required use of these drugs; however, poison ivy on a section of the course rendered prednisone in short supply.

Logistics

One of the biggest challenges in providing medical support, especially for adventure races, is the logistics of equipment, supplies, and scheduling of personnel. Because medical stations will

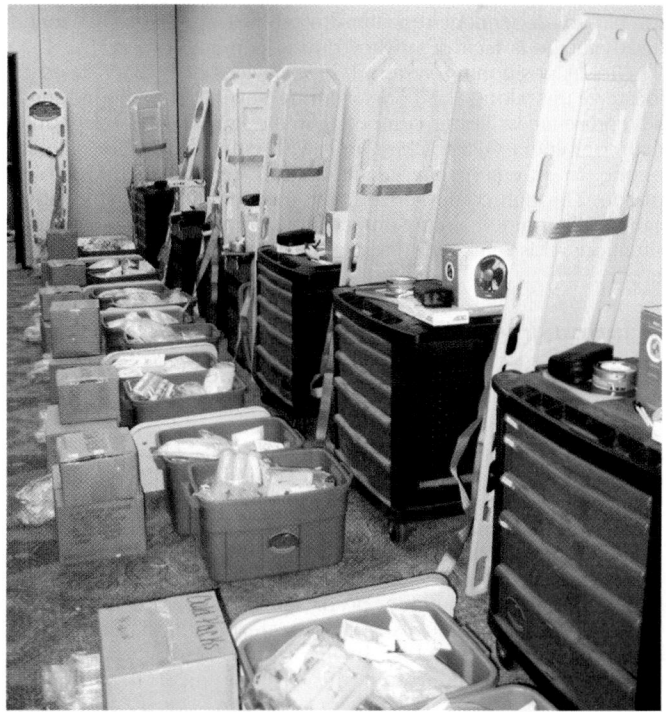

FIGURE 97-4 Medical supplies should be packed in durable carts that can be easily moved from one location to another. *(Courtesy David Townes, MD.)*

need to be open as the fastest teams reach them and remain in duty until the slowest teams have passed, this is a dynamic process. It is impossible to predict the exact timing before the event and thus important to build sufficient flexibility into the schedule to allow for uncertainty. This should be clearly outlined in the medical support plan with a time schedule and location for all personnel, medical supplies, and equipment. It is important to include packaging, transportation, and set-up time for equipment and supplies. In addition, during adventure races lasting several days or more, personnel should be given mandatory time off.

Ideally, personnel and equipment should include full-time, on-site, ALS-staffed ambulance and helicopter support. Every effort should be made to have an ALS ambulance on site, especially in remote locations where the local EMS response may be prolonged. If a medically equipped helicopter is not available, one option is to ensure that the helicopter used for general transportation and media is also prepared to evacuate and transport ill and injured participants if necessary.

COMMUNICATION

An important challenge in providing medical support for wilderness and endurance events is communication among athletes, race staff, medical staff, and EMS and SAR personnel. Communication is especially important between race participants and medical personnel in the event of an emergency. Given the rugged terrain and remote locations in which some categories III and IV events take place, communication can be difficult and unreliable.

Communication options include cellular phones, satellite phones, and radios. Each system has advantages and disadvantages, and the best modality depends on the individual situation. The advantages of cellular phones include widespread availability and direct, private, person-to-person communication. However, cellular phones are limited by network availability, making them useless in many situations. Satellite phones offer better coverage, but are expensive, relatively large and heavy, and unreliable under certain conditions. In addition, they generally require the caller to remain in one place with an unobstructed view of the sky to minimize the chance of dropping the call. Radios are usually readily available and offer reliable coverage in a variety of conditions. One disadvantage of radios is the need for battery-dependent repeaters to cover large areas. A second disadvantage is lack of privacy during communication.

Global positioning system (GPS) devices have been used to locate teams along the course during several expedition-length adventure races. Teams competing in the Primal Quest carry units that combine a GPS tracking unit with either a radio or satellite phone. In an emergency, teams notify race officials by radio or phone. Through computerized GPS tracking, their exact location can be determined almost immediately. In addition to emergency situations, this tracking system is used to follow progress of the event.

EMERGENCY RESPONSE

The medical support plan should include a protocol for notification of medical personnel of any medical emergency on the course. During standard and ultradistance triathlons, marathons, and cycling events, this is often a relatively straightforward process. A participant with a minor or moderate illness or injury is encouraged to continue or return to the nearest aid station or medical tent for medical assistance. Participants in these types of events generally do not carry phones or radios while they are competing. If the injury or illness is more severe and limits the athlete's ability to continue, he or she must rely on other competitors to notify officials at the nearest medical tent, or be assisted by roving mobile medical personnel or ambulances driving along the course, if this type of medical support is available.

Adventure races present a more complex set of challenges in identification and location of ill and injured participants. In the interest of simplicity, it may be useful to develop and employ a

TABLE 97-1 Emergency Classification for Adventure Races		
Emergency Classification	**Description**	**Examples**
I	Requires no evacuation; patient will proceed to next medical tent for evaluation	Laceration
II	Requires evacuation; not life threatening	Ankle injury or likely fracture
III	Requires immediate evaluation; life threatening	Head injury

three-part classification system for injury and illness (Table 97-1). Athletes often carry phones or radios during these events and use this system when notifying race and medical personnel of an emergency. The medical support plan should include a protocol for notification of medical personnel of any medical emergency on the course. In one commonly used example, a class I emergency, such as a laceration, requires no evacuation, and the athlete will proceed to the closest medical station for evaluation and treatment. A class II emergency, such as an injured ankle, requires evacuation, but is not life threatening. A class III emergency requires immediate evacuation, as in the case of a head injury.

In the event of a medical emergency, athletes are instructed to first notify race personnel of their team number and the emergency classification number. The purpose of this system is to allow athletes to quickly identify themselves and communicate the severity of the situation to medical personnel. It is important to relay information quickly and accurately because communication systems may be unreliable or inconsistent and could potentially break down at any given time. Thus it is crucial to ensure that the most important facts are sent and received immediately; additional details can be provided if communication remains intact.

ACCEPTANCE OF MEDICAL CARE

One area of controversy among medical personnel, event organizers, and athletes involves penalties for acceptance of medical support during an endurance event. Administration of IV fluid is a commonly cited example. If acceptance of IV fluid results in disqualification, athletes may push themselves too hard in an attempt to remain in the event. If IV fluid is administered without penalty, racers may request it at every opportunity to gain a theoretical competitive advantage. The authors and several race directors of both categories III and IV events use an "IV fluid rule" intended to allow fair and safe competition. This should be tailored for each individual event. For example, the IV fluid rule used during the Primal Quest expedition-length adventure race is shown in Box 97-2. As more events are held and investigations about the advisability of IV hydration are undertaken, such rules may be refined.

BOX 97-2 Intravenous Fluid Rule Used During the Primal Quest, 2002 to 2008
Athletes who receive intravenous (IV) fluid are automatically penalized 4 hours. The penalty period begins with the completion of the last liter of fluid.
Athletes requiring more than 2 L of IV fluid at one time (one medical station) or any amount of IV fluid at more than one time (multiple medical stations) will be automatically disqualified from the event.
All athletes who require IV fluid must be evaluated and medically cleared by the race medical director or his or her designee before returning to the race. Return to the race will occur only after the 4-hour penalty has been served.

From Townes DA: Medical support plan: Primal Quest 2002, unpublished.

MEDICAL DISQUALIFICATION

A potential conflict arises when the medical team and an athlete disagree about the athlete's ability to continue to race safely. In adventure races and other team endurance events, one strategy the authors have found helpful in this situation is to explain the concerns to the other seven members of the team (the four crew members and three remaining racers, in the case of adventure races). They will often help convince their ill or injured teammate to withdraw from the race. Sometimes these individuals agree that their teammate should not continue, but are unable or unwilling to convince the athlete to stop. In these cases, the team may look to the medical director for help. The medical director for the event should have the final say about whether an athlete is able to continue the race. This should be clearly explained to all race participants prior to the competition, and they should sign a release form indicating their acceptance of this policy.

EMERGENCY MEDICAL SERVICES AND SEARCH AND RESCUE TEAMS

It is essential to identify local ground and air ambulance services, SAR services, care facilities, and hospitals and trauma centers (and their capabilities) for each location along the course (Figure 97-5). Expedition-length adventure races may cover multiple hospital, trauma center, and EMS and SAR jurisdictions. At each medical station, there should be a folder containing the location and contact information for the resources specific to that medical station. It should also include the location and description of the medical station that will be readily understood by local providers. For example, when requesting a local ambulance, it will be more efficient to describe "Spring Valley Camp Ground, off of County Road 14" rather than "medical tent 5." In this way, any medical personnel, even without local knowledge, are able to quickly request services and communicate accurately. It is also important to determine whether a national emergency network such as 9-1-1 is available and whether it can reached by an out-of-area cellular phone. The importance of working with local providers cannot be overemphasized. It is strongly recommended that a member of the local EMS community act as a liaison between the race and local medical community. This individual is often helpful in determining what EMS, SAR service, or care facility should be utilized.

LEGAL CONSIDERATIONS

Important considerations in development of a medical support plan for any event include licensing, liability, and insurance coverage for medical personnel. The necessary requirements vary depending on location. Because events are held throughout the world, no single set of standards is applicable to every situation. It is essential to understand and adhere to the requirements of the specific location, and it may be beneficial for the medial director and race organization to solicit expert legal advice.

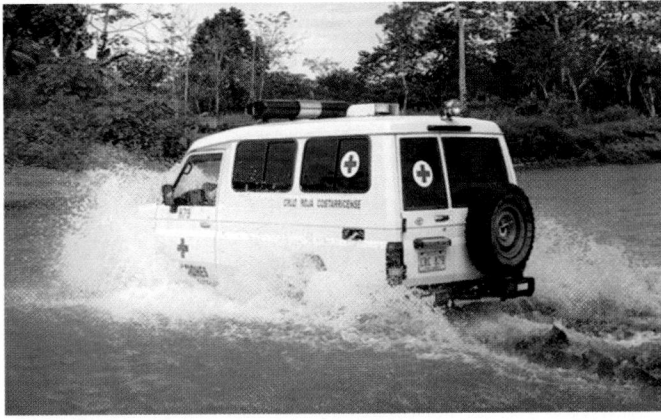

FIGURE 97-5 Medical transport for a wilderness event needs to be predetermined for the entire course. *(Courtesy David Townes, MD.)*

In addition to basic issues of licensing and liability, several questions should be considered. Is the liability different for a volunteer compared with someone who is paid? If medical personnel are covered under the general liability policy of the event, do they require additional insurance? What is the validity of liability waivers signed by race participants? What constitutes the practice of medicine? For instance, does a volunteer who applies a dressing to a blister need to be licensed to do so? Do all medical personnel need to be licensed, or just the medical director? If controlled substances are included in the medical kits, what additional measures are required? The answers to these questions depend on the laws that govern the location of the event.

INJURIES AND ILLNESSES BY EVENT TYPE

CYCLING EVENTS

The most common reasons to need medical care during cycling events include dehydration, heat illness, and soft tissue injuries. During the 1996 California AIDS Ride,[17] heat-related illness accounted for 31% of encounters, followed by pulmonary complaints (12%) and orthopedic problems (9%). During the 2001 Midwest AIDS Ride,[53] dehydration accounted for 35% of encounters, followed by orthopedic problems (27%), skin and soft tissue problems (10%), ophthalmologic problems (6%), gastrointestinal problems (6%), respiratory problems (4%), head and neck problems (3%), allergic reactions (3%), cardiac problems (2%), psychiatric problems (<1%), and other problems (4%). The most common orthopedic problem was overuse injury of the knee, primarily due to iliotibial band syndrome.[17,53] Fortunately, major trauma is rare. This is likely in part because of mandatory helmet use and protection from traffic provided by these events.

Because a large percentage of injuries sustained during endurance cycling events are overuse injuries resulting from inadequate training or conditioning, it may prove useful to send educational material directed at proper training techniques to the participants well in advance of the event.

TRIATHLONS

The overall injury rate for triathlons has been calculated at 13% to 25% of participants.[26] Each of the three disciplines is associated with a fairly unique set of injuries.

The swimming section of triathlon events has the greatest potential for death. It is essential to have sufficient rescue boats with qualified personnel in the water. Fortunately, the swimming section is associated with the fewest overall problems, accounting for only 3% of medical visits in one study.[26] Besides drowning, hypothermia is the greatest risk during the swimming section. Mandatory use of wetsuits may reduce this incidence. Blunt trauma from being kicked in the water and corneal irritation or abrasion from trauma, goggles, and defogging solutions are not uncommon. In addition, jellyfish stings, sea urchin punctures, coral lacerations, and aspiration have all been reported.[48] Leptospirosis has also been described in triathlon participants.[11]

The biking section is associated with trauma, including fractures, sprains, and abrasions, or "road rash." Biking accounts for 7% to 10% of triathlon injuries.[26] Occurrence of significant injury is reduced by rules that require helmet use and do not allow drafting.

The running section at the end of the triathlon is associated with the largest demand for medical assistance. In fact, 75% of medical care is delivered in the last 8 hours of the event, with 75% of this amount delivered at the finish. Many of these injuries and illnesses are due to dehydration and electrolyte abnormalities.[26]

MARATHONS AND ULTRAMARATHONS

In a 12-year study of the Twin Cities Marathon in Minneapolis and St Paul, Minnesota, 90% of medical encounters occurred at the finish line. The most common reason was exercise-associated

TABLE 97-2 Injury and Illness Rates in Multiday Ultramarathon Runners (% of Medical Tent Visits by Diagnosis)

Diagnosis	Marathon	Multistage Ultramarathon Major[a]	Multistage Ultramarathon Minor
Medical Illnesses			
Exercise-associated collapse[b]	59%	56.5%	3.9%
Altitude sickness	—	0	1%
Serious medical diagnosis[c]	0.14%	1.6%	0.1%
Other medical diagnosis[d]	0.48%	0	2.4%
Musculoskeletal Injuries			
Bursitis	—	1.6%	1%
Sprain	1.3%	3.2%	2.3%
Strain	14.3%	1.6%	2.4%
Tendinitis	—	11.3%	10.3%
Other[e]	0.28%	4.8%	2.6%
Skin Disorders			
Abrasion	1.9%	0	3.9%
Blister	19.9%	16.2%	57.8%
Cellulitis	—	1.6%	0.7%
Subungual hematoma	—	1.6%	9.5%
Other[f]	—	0	2.1%

[a]Major = unable to complete race; Minor = able to continue in race
[b]Hyperthermia, normothermia, hypothermia
[c]Hyponatremia, hematuria, renal stone
[d]Blurred vision, conjunctivits, diarrhea, dyspepsia, epistaxis, hematochezia, insect bite, neuropathy, pharyngitis, upper respiratory infection
[e]Fracture, metatarsalgia, contusion, costochondritis, laceration, splinter
[f]Callus, nail avulsion, rash, paronychia, wart

collapse (59%), followed by skin problems (21%), musculoskeletal problems (17%), and other medical problems (3%).[38] The mechanism of collapse at the end of a marathon may be due to postural hypotension from inadequate venous return secondary to decreased skeletal muscle massage when the competitor abruptly stops running.[33] Sudden cardiac deaths have been reported during marathons, but they are exceedingly rare.[30] About half of these cases occurred in individuals with preexisting cardiac disease.[14] Heat illnesses, including heat exhaustion and heat stroke, occur more commonly in participants who are not properly acclimatized, especially during events in warmer climates. Injury and illness rates during multiday ultramarathon races are shown in Table 97-2.

ADVENTURE RACES

Injuries and illness are common during adventure races. Many are minor, and relatively few result in withdrawal from an event.[5,50,54] Most injuries involve skin and soft tissues.[5,15,54] In a survey of 223 adventure race athletes, 73% reported at least one injury (acute or chronic) during the 18 months before the survey.[15] This is comparable with overall (acute and chronic) injuries reported during orienteering and standard triathlons, although lower than in ultraendurance triathlons, in which injury rates as high as 90% have been reported. In the survey, 44% of advanced, 35% of intermediate, and 19% of beginner racers reported acute injuries. Chronic injuries were more common, reported in 59%, 54%, and 56% of athletes, respectively.[15] Acute injuries are considerably more common during adventure races as compared with triathlons. Some of the difference has been attributed to lower extremity injuries sustained during maneuvering over unstable terrain and the inherent risks of mountain biking. In the survey, the most common site of acute injury was the ankle, followed by the arm and shoulder, knee, and lower back.[15]

In a prospective cohort study of injuries and illness treated during the Primal Quest expedition-length adventure race held in 2002 in Telluride, Colorado, 243 medical encounters and 302 distinct injuries and illnesses were reported among the 248 athletes who participated. Of the 179 (59%) injuries and 123 (41%) illnesses reported, skin and soft tissue injuries were the most common (48%), with blisters on the feet representing the single most frequent reason to utilize on-site medical resources (32.8%).[54] A complete list of injuries and illness by type, number, and frequency is given in Table 97-3.

Although injury was more common overall, illness resulted in more medical withdrawals from the event. Of the 28 athletes who withdrew for medical reasons, 60% withdrew because of illness. Respiratory illness, including upper respiratory infection, bronchitis, and reactive airway disease–asthma, were the most common (32.1%) medical reasons to withdraw, followed by dehydration (25.0%), altitude illness (14.3%), skin and soft tissue problems (14.3%), orthopedic problems (10.7%), and genitourinary problems (3.6%).[5] In a similar study, the only medical withdrawal from a 2-day wilderness multisport event was due to reactive airway disease in the setting of a viral respiratory infection.[5]

Reactive airway disease–asthma appears to be a common cause of illness during adventure races. The relatively high incidence observed may be partially explained by changes in respiratory function in participants. This has been demonstrated by several investigations. In a study of two consecutive years of a wilderness multisport endurance event, measurements of oxygen saturation (SaO_2), forced expiratory volume in 1 second (FEV_1), and forced vital capacity (FVC) were taken before and after the event and at 45-minute intervals during the event. During the event, there was a progressive decline in both FEV_1 and FVC from the starting line to the finish. At the finish, the FEV_1 had declined by 22% to 25% and FVC had declined by 14% to 22% over the 2 years of the study. Changes in SaO_2 were less dramatic.[40] A similar study of 25 adventure race athletes found a mean decrease in FEV_1 of 15.1% and FVC of 13% between the start and finish of the event. Fourteen (56%) of these athletes had a decrease in FEV_1 and FVC of more than 10%, and seven (28%) had a decrease of more than 20%.[39] A decline in respiratory function has been described in other endurance athletes but to a lesser degree.[21,28,29] Possible explanations for these findings include bronchospasm, airway inflammation, muscle fatigue, and pulmonary edema.

Complicating the understanding of reactive airway disease–asthma observed during adventure races is the fact that many events have sections that occur at high altitude. In an investigation of the 2002 Primal Quest, the incidence of altitude illness requiring medical treatment was 14.1%. Most cases were acute mountain sickness (13.3%). Only 0.81% of cases were high-altitude pulmonary edema. The potential role of altitude illness in exacerbating or alleviating other respiratory problems remains a concern.[50]

Previous studies have demonstrated improvement in asthma at high altitude. Explanations offered for this observation include reduction in pollen and pollution, and increase in cortisol levels

TABLE 97-3 Injuries and Illnesses During the Primal Quest, 2002

Type of Injury or Illness	Number of Cases (n = 302)	Percentage of Cases
Skin or soft tissue	145	48.0
Respiratory	55	18.2
Altitude (acute mountain sickness, high-altitude pulmonary edema)	36	11.9
Orthopedic	29	9.6
Dehydration	21	7.0
Gastrointestinal	6	2.0
Head, ears, eyes, nose, throat	5	1.7
Genitourinary	3	1.0
Other	2	<1.0

From Townes DA, Talbot TS, Wedmore IS, et al: Event medicine: injury and illness during an expedition-length adventure race, *J Emerg Med* 27:161, 2004.

at high altitude.[1,7] Other studies have found that exercise at altitude may exacerbate acute mountain sickness.[37] Further studies are necessary to fully understand the interaction between reactive airway disease–asthma, respiratory tract infections, and altitude illness during adventure races.

In addition, injuries and illnesses due to environmental exposure are common during adventure races. A study of Australia's Winter Classic, a 2-day event, found that 21% of participants developed symptoms consistent with exposure.[5] During the Primal Quest in 2003, 25% of medical withdrawals were attributed to dehydration or heat illness.[54]

SPECIFIC INJURIES AND ILLNESSES: ENDEMIC DISEASE

Another potential source of illness during wilderness and endurance events is endemic disease. The literature includes descriptions of everything from isolated cases to widespread infections affecting large numbers of participants.

In the 1997 Raid Gauloises held in Lesotho and Natal, South Africa, 13 French athletes were diagnosed with African tick-bite fever. This rickettsial disease is caused by *Rickettsia africae* and transmitted by *Amblyomma* ticks. Signs and symptoms included fever, headache, multiple inoculation scars, regional lymphadenopathy, and rash.[16]

Another potential infection during endurance events is leptospirosis. Leptospirosis is a bacterial zoonotic infection associated with exposure to water or soil that has been contaminated by wild and domestic animals, which serve as reservoirs and transmit the infection by shedding the causative organism, *Leptospira interrogans,* in urine. The illness is characterized by symptoms that include fever, chills, myalgias, headache, conjunctival suffusion, abdominal pain, vomiting, diarrhea, and rash. This may progress to aseptic meningitis, jaundice, renal failure, hepatic failure, and hemorrhage. The syndrome of fever, meningismus, and renal and hepatic failure is referred to as *Weil's disease.* The incubation period is most commonly 5 to 14 days, but ranges from 2 to 30 days. Mild infections can be treated with tetracycline and severe cases with IV penicillin (see Chapter 34).

The most widely publicized outbreak of leptospirosis occurred during the Eco-Challenge-Sabah 2000 adventure race held in Malaysian Borneo.[12,13,42,48] Of 304 athletes competing, 189 were contacted, of which 80 met the case definition for leptospirosis. No deaths were reported. Risk factors identified were kayaking or swimming in the Segama River, swallowing water from the Segama River, and spelunking (caving). Swimming in the Segama River was the only risk factor independently associated with illness. Of the 20 athletes who reported taking doxycycline for prophylaxis of malaria or leptospirosis, four (20%) developed symptoms of leptospirosis. When this rate was compared with those not taking doxycycline and adjusted for exposure, doxycycline use was determined to be protective; however, the difference was not significant.[42] Leptospirosis infections have also been attributed to participation in an adventure race in Guam, triathlons in Illinois and Wisconsin, white-water rafting in Costa Rica, and an endurance-length "swamp" adventure race in Florida.[10,11,20,47]

Myiasis, infestation of humans by fly larvae, has been reported during an adventure race. In a 2001 race in the Para State jungle region of Brazil, an athlete fell and sustained a wound that was infested with a third-stage larva of the New World screwworm fly *Cochliomyia hominivorax.* Although most cases of myiasis are benign, infestation by invasive species like the screwworm may result in extensive tissue damage, pain, and even death, because the larvae have powerful oral hooks that can invade cartilage and bone.[43]

In 2012, there were 22 cases of *Campylobacter coli* infection (4 confirmed and 18 probable) among participants in a 2-day adventure race in Nevada. A case control study identified inadvertent swallowing of muddy surface water as a significant risk factor.[57]

Wilderness and endurance events are held in a wide variety of locations and conditions. Given the potential for participants to become ill during or after the event, it is essential that the medical director be familiar with endemic diseases for a particular event related to its location, time of year, and current environmental conditions.

MAJOR TRAUMA

Major trauma has occurred during wilderness and endurance events, resulting in significant injuries and death.[25] Fortunately, the incidence is low, but because of potential complications and death, the medical support plan should include equipment, supplies, and personnel to provide initial stabilization and treatment of major trauma. It should also include a protocol for evacuation and transport developed in close conjunction with local EMS and, in the case of adventure races, local SAR personnel. Obtaining appropriate personnel and equipment may require a significant financial commitment by the race organization. The medical director must emphasize the importance of these resources and insist on having them, even though they may go unused. Examples include full-time paramedic-staffed ALS ambulances, helicopters, and other rescue vehicles. Litters and Gamow-type hyperbaric bags can represent a significant expense for some events. The medical support plan should specify the location of these limited resources and their movement during the event. For example, it may be necessary to "leapfrog" ambulances from one location to another during the event to deploy resources most effectively. This planning should be done prior to beginning the event.

FOOT CARE

Foot-related problems (see Chapter 25), particularly blisters, are perhaps the most common reason to seek medical care during wilderness and endurance events (Figure 97-6). In one investigation during an adventure race, foot blisters were the most common reason to seek care, accounting for 53% of medical encounters.[54]

Staffing and supplies should reflect the high incidence of foot-related problems. Ideally, the medical team should include providers with expertise in foot care. At a minimum, all providers should have a basic understanding of foot and blister care (see Chapter 25).

There seem to be as many different techniques for prevention and treatment of blisters as there are feet. Athletes use duct tape, antiperspirants, petroleum jelly, and multiple newer products designed specifically for blister prevention. In a text dedicated to the subject, the authors list 159 ways to prevent blisters.[56] Despite the variety of preventive methods, susceptibility to blisters varies. Although some athletes remain blister-free with little effort, others suffer from blisters no matter what measures are taken.

Treatment of blisters begins before they form. All blisters begin as "hot spots" that should be treated with tape or one of many blister products on the market. If the athlete is no longer

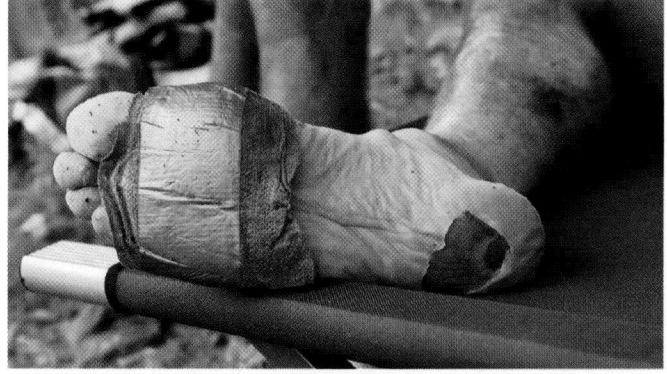

FIGURE 97-6 Self-administered forefoot blister treatment with medical team debridement of deep heel blister in an ultramarathon runner. *(Courtesy of Chris Lusher for RacingThePlanet.)*

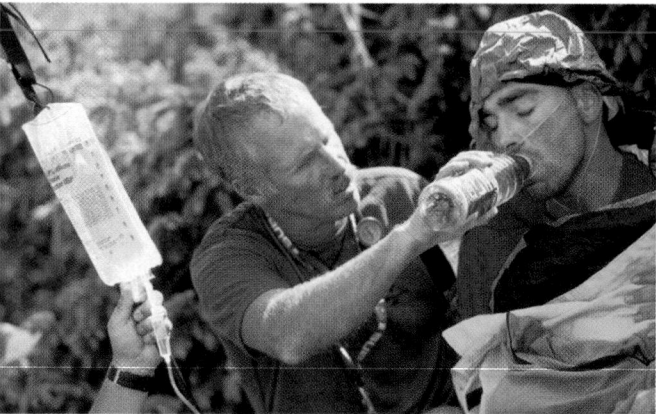

FIGURE 97-7 Dehydration and hyponatremia are common in wilderness and endurance events. *(Courtesy Tim Holstrom.)*

continuing in the event, blisters need not be drained unless they are infected. If the athlete plans to continue, however, it may be necessary to drain the blister to allow application of a dressing that will stay in place. The blister can be drained with any sterile sharp object, such as a needle, blade, scissors, or nail clipper. Ideally, a small hole is made in the blister to drain the fluid and the overlying dead skin is left in place. After the area has been cleaned, it should be dressed with tape or a blister care product. Blisters should be monitored closely for infection.

DEHYDRATION AND HYPONATREMIA

Dehydration and hyponatremia are common during wilderness and endurance events, especially marathons and triathlons. Medical team members should be familiar with the recognition, diagnosis, and treatment of these disorders (Figure 97-7). During the Hawaii Ironman Triathlon, dehydration was the most common reason to receive on-site medical care, and hyponatremia the most common electrolyte disturbance. Dehydration with hyponatremia is rare in races lasting less than 4 hours, and becomes more common in races lasting longer than 8 hours.[22]

Hyponatremia is defined as a serum sodium level of less than 135 mEq/L associated with malaise, disorientation, hyperreflexia, nausea, and fatigue. More severe cases may result in seizures, stupor, coma, and death. Seizures have been reported in a tri-athlete with a serum sodium level of 116 mEq/L, and rapid neurologic deterioration and encephalopathy in ultramarathon runners.[18,46,49]

Hyponatremia occurs when free water intake exceeds free water loss. In the endurance athlete, this is thought to occur in two distinct ways, although there is some debate about the exact cause of exercise-associated hyponatremia. Several authors have suggested that hyponatremia is a result of net water gain during exercise secondarily associated with sodium loss through sweat.[22] Others have attributed it to salt depletion due to massive sweat losses associated with net dehydration.[22] Additional studies have demonstrated that hyponatremia may occur in the setting of dehydration or overhydration.[45]

In a study of 605 participants in the New Zealand triathlon, 58 (18%) were found to be hyponatremic. Of these, 18 were symptomatic, and 11 were severely hyponatremic, defined as having serum sodium of less than 130 mmol/L. The serum sodium concentration following the race was inversely related to weight change during the event. That is, athletes with hypernatremia were dehydrated, but athletes with severe hyponatremia were generally overhydrated. The relationship between mild hyponatremia and hydration status was less clear. Some athletes with mild hyponatremia were dehydrated, but others were overhydrated. It would appear that the mechanisms for mild hyponatremia in the endurance athlete include fluid overload or large salt losses through sweat, or a combination of the two.[45]

Whatever the mechanism, it is important to be aware of both dehydration and hyponatremia in triathlon participants. There are various recommendations to help reduce the incidence of dehydration and hyponatremia. These include (1) athletes should have 0.5 L of fluid intake for each pound (0.45 kg) lost during an event, (2) during races lasting more than 4 hours, athletes should use some form of sodium replacement (1 g/hr), (3) athletes from cooler climates should give themselves a week to acclimatize and should increase salt intake by 10 to 25 g/day, and (4) IV fluid therapy for races longer than 4 hours should be 5% dextrose in normal saline, and for races less than 4 hours, it should be either 5% dextrose in normal saline or 5% dextrose in 0.5 normal saline.[22] Studies of marathon runners have suggested that replacement of sodium at a rate of 20 mEq/hr and potassium at 8 mEq/hr will maintain normal blood levels.[32]

More recently, the Wilderness Medical Society published guidelines for treatment of exercise-associated hyponatremia. These recommendations encourage competitors to drink according to thirst rather than a predetermined schedule in order to avoid overhydration.[4] Additionally, in evaluating a symptomatic competitor, if a blood electrolyte measurement is available on-site and the sodium level is less than 135 mmol/L, the recommendation is to administer an IV bolus of 100 mL of 3% saline, repeated every 10 minutes up to three doses or until neurologic symptoms subside, while preparing for transport to a hospital setting.[4] These guidelines also suggest that if no point-of-care testing is available, one should place an IV line only and give oral hypertonic solution; avoid giving hypotonic solution because of the risk of further lowering the sodium level.[4] Difficulty arises in the absence of point-of-care testing because the symptoms of hyponatremia and dehydration may be similar but different interventions are needed for the two disorders. When in a very remote location (> 4 hours to definitive medical care) without point-of-care testing, one must rely on clinical assessment and judgment to make a diagnosis and treat accordingly. Providers should use caution because there are risks associated with administration of either hypertonic or hypotonic solution in a given context.

REFERENCES

Complete references used in this text are available online at expertconsult.inkling.com.

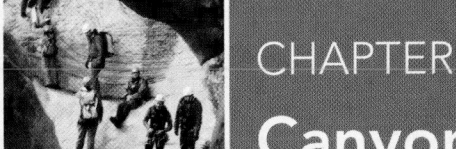

CHAPTER 98
Canyoneering and Canyon Medicine

GIACOMO STRAPAZZON AND GORDON L. LARSEN

Canyoneering (referred to as *canyoning* in Europe) is the term used for a recreational activity involving travel through canyons using a variety of techniques and technical skills. Canyoneering is physically challenging and may require any combination of down-climbing, rappelling down waterfalls, swimming through cold pools and swiftwater, escaping keeper potholes, and using advanced ropework. Navigational skills are essential. This chapter provides an overview of pertinent aspects of canyoneering, namely, canyon environment and potential hazards, progression techniques and necessary equipment, common injuries and illnesses, medical interventions and equipment, and companion rescue and SAR operational considerations. For more information about details of technical rescue, see Chapter 56.

CANYONEERING
HISTORICAL PERSPECTIVE

Canyoneering is at least several hundred years old. Native American cultures (e.g., peoples from Ancestral Puebloan and Fremont) that settled inside natural caves at the base of canyons were likely the true pioneers of canyoneering. Early American explorers and settlers were also reported to have been faced with a maze of canyons in the southwestern regions of the United States.[58] Canyoneering first emerged for recreational exploration in Europe in the late 19th century after the father of modern caving, Édouard-Alfred Martel, explored the Bramabiau cave in France.[14] In 1893, Armand Janet and Lucien Briet became famous due to their explorations in the Verdon region in France and the Sierra de Guara region in Spain.[14] Recreational exploration of canyons was not common during the World Wars, but gained importance again in the 1960s. In 1977, Pierre Minvielle published the first canyoneering guide *Grottes et canyons, les 100 plus belles courses et randonnées*,[32] which marked the beginning of recreational canyoneering in France. Soon the first commission for canyoneering was established within the French Federation of Speleology.[14]

Zion National Park in southern Utah is the most popular region for canyoneering in the United States. Recreational canyoneering in this region began in the 1960s. The term *canyoneering*, as employed to refer to the modern form of recreational exploration in canyons, was not used until the 1990s, when it appeared in the book *Canyoneering: The San Rafael Swell* by Steve Allen.[1] In 1993, two scout leaders were tragically killed on a group excursion in Zion National Park as a result of being caught in hydraulics at the base of a waterfall. The survival story and eventual evacuation of the lone scout group after four cold nights on a ledge in Kolob Canyon in Zion National Park raised public awareness about canyoneering.[3] Over the past decades, canyoneering has become one of the fastest-growing wilderness recreation activities. Development of specialized equipment and techniques has facilitated commercial operations and exploration of increasingly more difficult canyons. The associated increase in rescues led to establishment of specially trained and equipped SAR teams.

Demographics

In the United States, canyoneering is most common in the sandstone slot canyons of the Colorado Plateau, but canyons also exist in the Cascade, Rocky Mountain, San Gabriel, and Sierra Nevada ranges. Canyons are also present offshore on the Hawaiian islands. Over the past 15 years requests for access permits in Zion National Park increased so rapidly that the park services had to develop new usage plans. Remarkably, a 5-year increase in usage of 500% to 1200% in the most popular areas was reported by park officials.[48] Canyoneering seems to attract younger people and more females than other types of wilderness recreation, for example, mountaineering. However, in a web-based survey of 38 members of American and Australian canyoneering associations, almost 90% of respondents were male. Equally, the average level of experience was 6.5 years with 25 canyoneering days per year.[48] These results were based on a small sample of individuals and may not be reflective of a larger population or other regions. In a larger investigation, over a 5-year period in Sierra de Guara, Spain, 8019 canyoneers in 1648 groups were surveyed; 62% of canyoneers were male, with a median age of 32 years (standard deviation 12 years).[5] The majority of canyoneers were in groups of 6 to 10 members, and typically each group had planned the descent before the excursion using canyoneering guides and maps. However, a staggering 73% of those canyoneers sampled were not registered members of a recognized mountain or sport association; nonmembers were reported as less likely to adhere to recommendations regarding individual safety equipment.[5]

Despite any safety concerns, canyoneering has also become popular outside the United States and Europe; for example, in Australia, New Zealand, Japan, and Brazil; as well as on tropical islands (La Reunion Island, French West Indies, and Madeira, Portugal) and in high-altitude mountain ranges (Andes, Himalayas).[4]

CANYON ENVIRONMENT

Of all SAR operations in U.S. National Parks in 2005, the second most frequent rescue location was canyons; only rescues in mountainous terrain above 1500 m (5000 feet) were more common.[22] A *canyon* can be defined as a deep, narrow valley or gorge with steep sides or cliff walls and vertical drops. Canyons can be found as features in mutiple rock types, for example, limestone, granite, sandstone, and basalt (Figure 98-1). They exist on every continent, at any altitude, and in any environment (deserts, rain forests, mountains). The form of a canyon is largely determined by past and present water flow. Over time, action of water and gravel, through erosion, can carve deep channels and other formations in the rock. Water flow over these formations determines the dynamic elements of a canyon. The exact water regime in a canyon depends largely on seasonal trends in climate and geography of the region and tributary catchments. Changes in water flow typically occur during periods of snow melt, glacial melt, and rainfall.

Recognizable features within the canyon environment are important for correctly assessing the mode of safe progression. A *pool* is a deep spot in a streambed. A *pothole* is a bowl-shaped depression in the rock surface that has been carved by swirling actions of stones. A pothole can be dry or filled with water (Figure 98-2). Deep pools, or potholes, are common where the water swirls against canyon walls. A *waterfall* is a place where water flows over a vertical drop, and it is probably the most characteristic feature of wet canyons. A drop over a smooth sloping surface forms a natural *water slide* (or *toboggan*) when wet. An *eddy* is a horizontal reversal of water flow caused by a protrusion from the bank, a turn, or an obstacle (see Chapter 62, Whitewater Medicine and Rescue).[38] An *eddy fence* is the boundary between the downstream water flow and the stalled or reversing water of an eddy. A *hydraulic* is a low-pressure area that draws water from a higher-pressure area downstream.

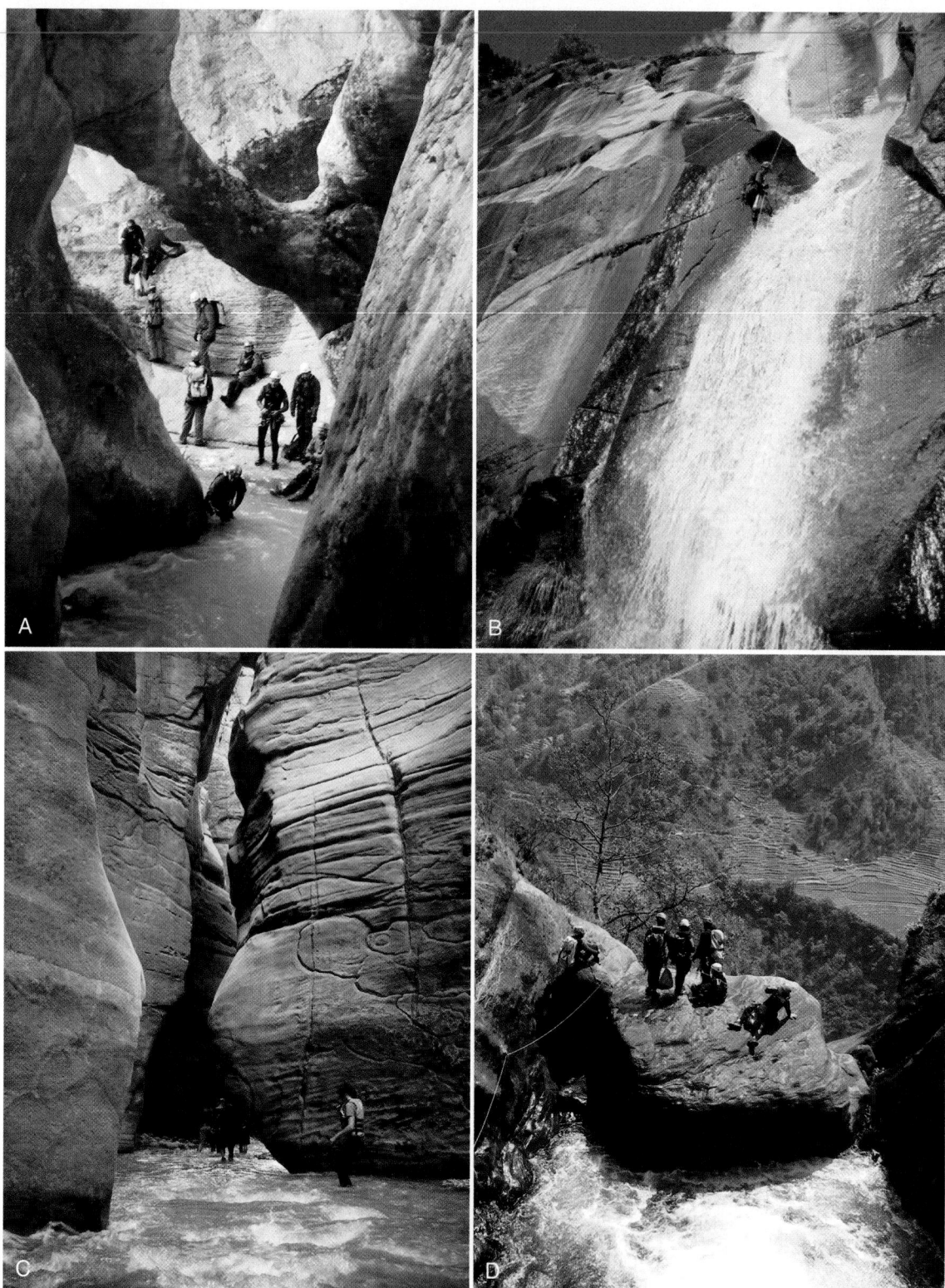

FIGURE 98-1 A, Limestone wet canyon. **B,** Granite wet canyon. **C,** Sandstone slot canyon. **D,** Himalayan canyon. *(Courtesy Erwin Kob.)*

Hydraulics are more commonly associated with rivers, but dangerous hydraulics also exist in wet canyons, typically at the base of a waterfall or water slide (Figure 98-3).

CANYONEERING HAZARDS

The main hazard during descent in a dry canyon is falling, either due to incorrect rope techniques or falling debris. The main hazards in a wet canyon are water and wet surfaces.[44] As water level rises (e.g., in a more narrow section), speed and power of the current increase exponentially. When speed is doubled, the force of the water against an object in the current is quadrupled. Canyoneers are subject to these forces while walking, swiftwater swimming, sliding, and descending under a waterfall. Hydraulics can cause trapping and drowning (Figure 98-4).[44] Canyoneers fixed on a rope can get trapped in a hydraulic. Jammed debris

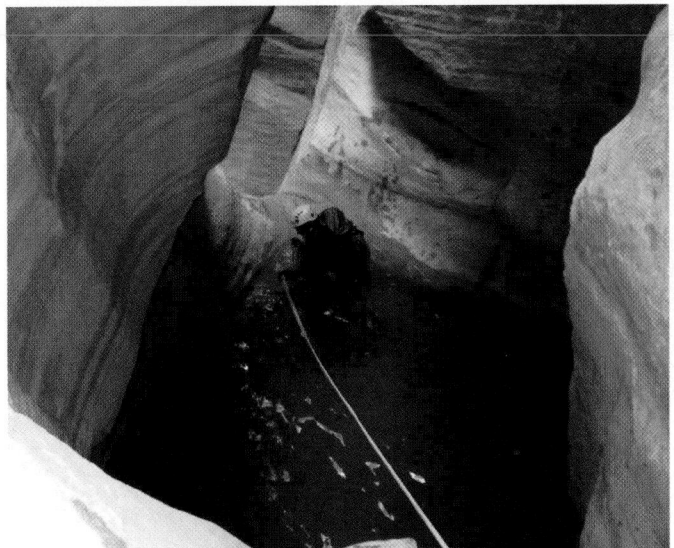

FIGURE 98-2 A pothole filled with water. (*Courtesy Gordon Larsen.*)

can create a *strainer* (sieve) and may not be visible in dirty water or in a pool or pothole. Pools and potholes can hide water traps, but are avoidable with good navigation techniques. A water trap can be recognized in advance, when the outflow is not equal to the inflow in a pool (see Figure 98-4).[44]

A *flash flood* is the sudden rise of water in a canyon, which may occur within minutes or even seconds. Heavy rainfall in the catchment of the canyon (that could be many kilometers distant) is the most common reason (Figure 98-5). Flash floods can also result if a hydroelectric dam is opened, or a natural dam collapses. Floods can occur in both dry and wet canyons.[44] In one widely publicized incident in 1999, 21 tourists on a commercial canyoneering trip drowned in Saxetenbach Gorge, Switzerland.[46] In another incident, seven adults were killed in a flash flood in Zion National Park on September 14, 2015. The party was in Keyhole Canyon, a popular and short slot canyon, when a fierce afternoon thunderstorm dumped more than an inch of rain over the upper drainage of the canyon in less than an hour. There were no survivors and some of the bodies were found miles downstream. Such incidents can be prevented with knowledge of the forecast and weather conditions. Changes in weather conditions (approaching thunderstorms) and/or water (color, clarity, level, presence of floating debris) may be indicators of a potential flash flood. If any of these signs appear, canyoneers

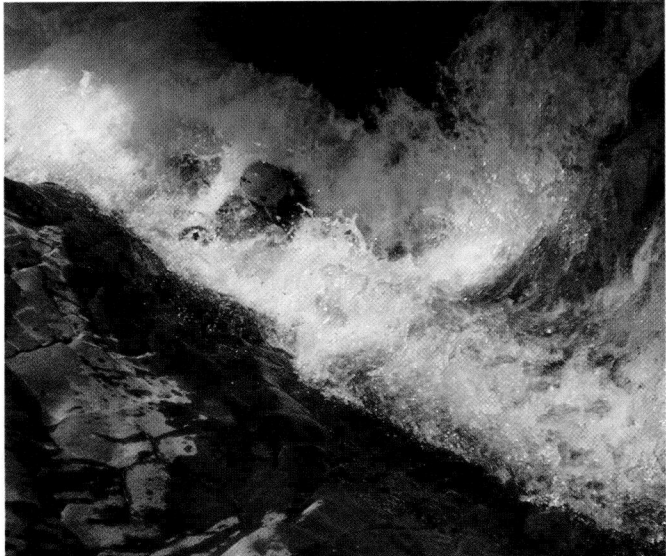

FIGURE 98-3 Hydraulic at the base of a low drop. (*Courtesy Erwin Kob.*)

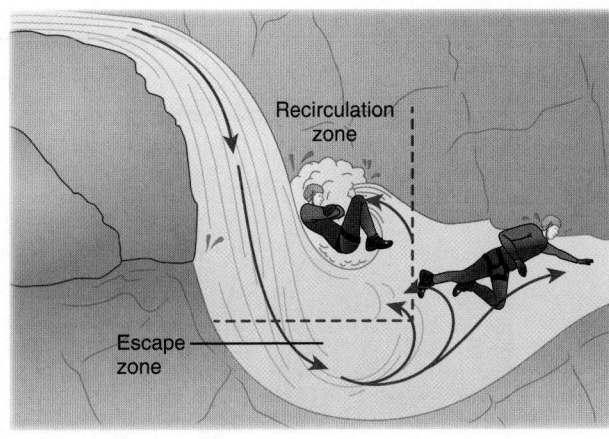

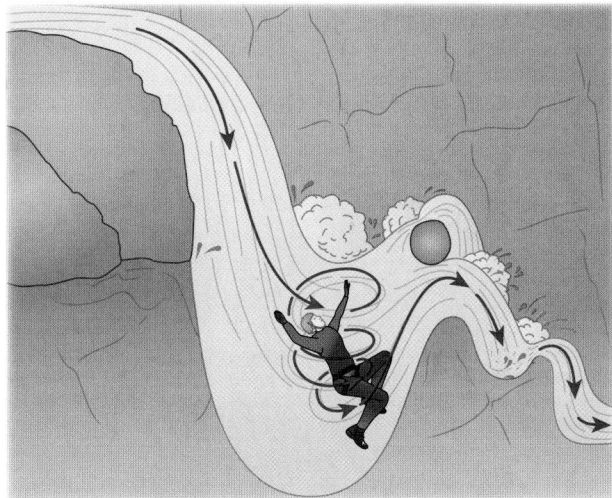

FIGURE 98-4 **A,** Hydraulic with a canyoneer escaping from the pool. **B,** Pothole with a water trap (water outflow is not equal to inflow in the pool).

should move to higher ground immediately and stay there until conditions improve. Canyons do not provide sufficient protection from lightning during thunderstorms.

Environmental risks while canyoneering include accidental hypothermia and heat-related illnesses, potentially even during the same trip. Extreme temperature differentials are possible, depending on sun, water, and wind exposure of different canyon sections. For example, outside temperature can exceed 38°C (100°F), while shaded pools in a narrow slot canyon can be as cold as 6°C (43°F). Hypothermia is a risk regardless of season and is not necessarily recognized by the victim. Immersion in water causes rapid heat loss by conduction/convection that is increased with wind, immobilization, and exhaustion.[11] Risk of immersion hypothermia is present in water colder than 25°C (77°F)[30] and is more severe in water colder than 15°C (59°F). Some technical canyons require extremely strenuous efforts, which can lead to dehydration followed by heat exhaustion, especially if there are alternating wet and dry sections. Heat stroke is an advanced stage of heat exhaustion and can be exacerbated by long exposure and exertion time.[9]

Traveling to and from remote drop-in and exit points can be challenging and risky and requires careful planning. Canyoneers may be exposed to extreme temperatures, thunderstorms, and wild flora (e.g., cacti) and fauna. Venomous snakes, scorpions, spiders, and fire ants can be encountered.[48] Tick-borne diseases may be a risk, especially if skin is exposed while a person is traveling to and from a canyon. Water can be infected by various agents of zoonosis due to deposition by wild animals. Dead animal carcasses are encountered frequently in canyons and can be a source of water contamination. Water can also become contaminated during flooding from upstream human settlements.

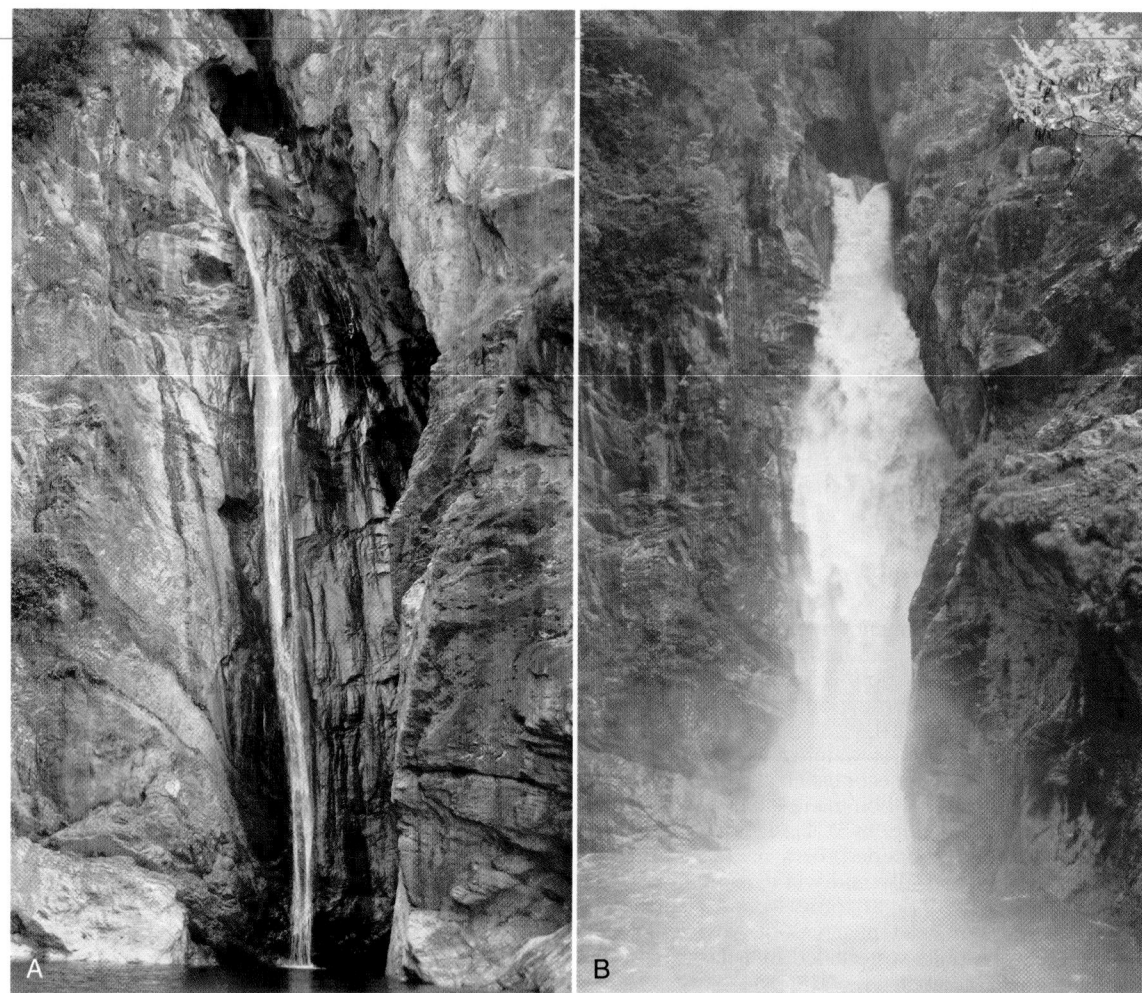

FIGURE 98-5 A, Normal canyon water flow. A canyoneer can rappel well away from the water flow. **B,** Flash flood. *(Courtesy Erwin Kob.)*

EQUIPMENT

Canyoneering is considerably more damaging to the body, clothing, and hardware than are most wilderness activities (with perhaps the exception of caving). A balance between personal safety and protection and freedom of movement is the most important consideration when choosing clothing for canyoneering. Having the right equipment[7,39,44] and knowing how to use it in progression techniques are essential for personal safety and accident prevention. Existing data show that many groups are not equipped even with minimum personal or safety equipment.[5]

Complete canyoneering equipment includes helmet, shoes specifically designed for canyoneering, wetsuit or drysuit (and personal flotation device [PFD] if necessary), harness, specialized descender, ascender, lanyard, webbing, carabiners, pulleys, slings, whistle, knife for cutting ropes, dive googles and snorkel, headlamp, survival kit (Box 98-1), packs and rope bags, drybags and kegs, canyoneering ropes, and other hardware (Figure

98-6).[7,44] A full description of canyoneering hardware can be found in technical canyoneering manuals[7,26,44] and in Chapter 56, Technical Rescue, and Chapter 108, Ropes and Knot Tying.

Climbing or mountaineering helmets with Conformité Européenne (CE) certification (preferably Union Internationale des Associations d'Alpinisme [UIAA]) should be used. Helmets for canoeing and kayaking without Comité Européen de Normalisation (CE EN) 12492 certification are not considered appropriate equipment for canyoneering.[44] Helmets should be lightweight and adjustable, with a durable shell and expanded polystyrene foam liner for flotation. A helmet adapted to allow attachment of a headlamp is considered preferable.

Shoes specifically designed for canyoneering (e.g., Bestard 0880 Canyon Guide; Five Ten Canyoneer 3) are essential and may reduce the risk of accidents and injuries (primarily falls and lower extremity injuries). In a recent French study, 80% (inexperienced) injured canyoneers were not wearing canyoneering shoes.[13] Appropriate footwear comprises a sole that provides traction on both wet and dry surfaces, good fit with proper ankle and foot support, rapid draining, and narrow profile to permit jamming and close-in edging.

Wetsuits offer whole body insulation via application of a layer of foamed neoprene directly next to the skin, thus allowing reduction in heat conduction away from the body.[38] Full-body wetsuits guarantee better freedom of movement; however, proper fit and adequate stretch are important considerations. Wetsuits that comprise two parts, when worn in conjunction with a set of waterproof overalls and a jacket, are particularly useful in canyons with both dry and wet sections. The disadvantages of wearing a wetsuit while canyoneering are manifold, namely, the additional weight (particularly when wet), volume, and limited protection against

BOX 98-1	Minimum Survival Kit for Canyoneering*
First-aid kit	Replacement batteries
Rescue foil	Hat
Garbage bag	Socks
Duct tape	Gloves
Waterproof matches or lighter	Metal cup
Candle	Food
"Cyalume"	Water disinfectant
Small headlamp	

*Materials are kept in a keg (3.6 L [7.6 pt]).

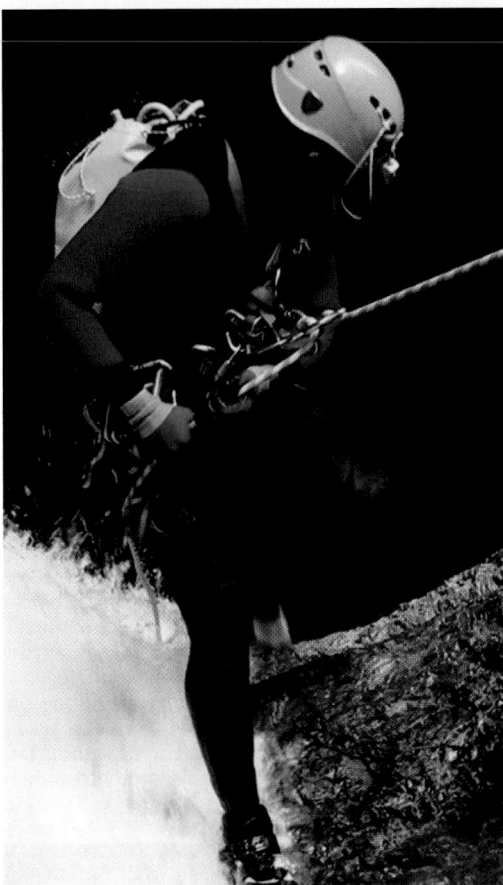

FIGURE 98-6 Standard personal equipment of a canyoneer in a wet canyon. From top to bottom: helmet with whistle, wetsuit with shears in a chest pocket, descender with multiple braking options, harness with mechanical devices and carabiner slings (also for backup), gloves for hand protection, and canyoneering shoes. (Courtesy Erwin Kob.)

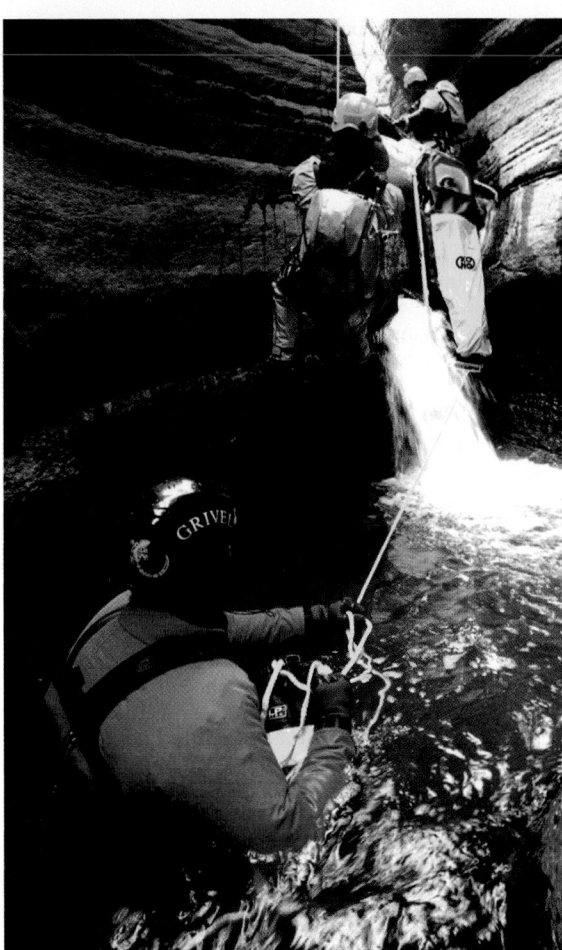

FIGURE 98-7 SAR team members wearing drysuits and PFDs during a rescue operation with prolonged water exposure. (Copyright KONG Italy. Courtesy Michael Kammerer: kong.it/.)

cold air when wet. Neoprene gloves, socks, and hoods are useful additions for thermal insulation and protection.

Alternatively, drysuits insulate by preventing water from entering via tight seals around the hands, feet, and neck.[38] These are full-body suits comprised of waterproof material and usually worn with thermal undergarments. Drysuits are effective in extreme conditions and commonly used during long operations, or specifically night SAR activities (Figure 98-7). The disadvantage of wearing a drysuit is the additional expense and the fact that they do not function if punctured, protect from impacts, or provide flotation.[38,44]

A canyoneering harness (e.g., Edelrid Iguazu; Petzl Canyon) also requires additional consideration and slight adaptation compared to most climbing harnesses. There should be a reinforced attachment point, positioned high and horizontally, for enhanced canyoneering specific functionality. The vertical configuration of the belay loop on a climbing harnesses tends to twist the rappel device 90 degrees to the intended angle of use, making rope handling more awkward.[44] A removable and replaceable seat cover can protect the wetsuit and harness from abrasion.

Descenders have multiple braking options and can be placed on the rope without removing it from the harness. The Petzl Pirana is formed as a figure-eight but tends to prevent a lark's head hitch around the body. The Petzl Pirana also reduces rope twisting without decreasing the braking friction. The Sterling ATS and Kong OKA are rappel devices similar to the Petzl Pirana, but provide additional friction and can be used for rescue maneuvers. The Black Diamond ATC-XP is popular in the United States; it should be avoided in wet canyons with hydraulics and waterfalls. At least one member of a canyoneering group should bring mechanical ascenders, and every canyoneer should carry a few

slings (usually made of Kevlar), to make soft cams such as Prusik, Klemheist, or Bachmann knots. Slings (and other mechanical devices for ascent and descent) are necessary when there is a knot in the rope or in emergency situations.[44] Whistles are used for communication during progression and ropeworks (Table 98-1). Whistles should be attached to the helmet or PFD. Only whistles that function if wet are suitable; avoid whistles with a cork ball. Carry knives or shears attached to the harness or in a

TABLE 98-1 SUDOT Whistle Signals for Canyoneering Communication During Ropework

Command	Whistle Signal	Meaning or Action
Stop!	One blast	Stop all movement until further instruction is provided
Up	Two blasts*	Often used to signal that the rope is too long
Down	Three blasts*	Often used to signal that the rope is too short or that a person is stuck on the rope
Off rope/ rope free	Four blasts*	Canyoneer is clear of the rope and it is available
Trouble/help!	Continuous blast	General emergency signal

Modified from ASTM F1768-97(2014): Standard guide for using whistle signals during rope rescue operations, ASTM International, 2014, West Conshohocken, Pennsylvania: astm.org.
*In Italy, commands are codified in a different way.

chest pocket. A throw bag should be carried in canyons with swiftwater (see Chapter 62, Whitewater Medicine and Rescue).[38] PFDs that provide mobility and comfort (e.g., type III PFD worn by paddlers) are suitable.[38]

PROGRESSION TECHNIQUES

Canyoneering has been referred to as the decathlon of wilderness activities. A typical progression scenario includes squeezing by or scrambling over lodged boulders, navigating deep potholes or swiftly moving streams, and rappelling down waterfalls up to 30 m (98.5 feet). Special techniques have been developed from climbing, caving and swiftwater swimming, and are important for personal safety and accident prevention. The correct use of standardized equipment and techniques ensures a balance between rapid descent and controlled progression and risk management.

Progression Without a Rope

Progression without a rope includes many techniques, namely, scrambling, climbing, sliding, jumping, swimming (also in swiftwater), and deep wading (Figure 98-8). Scrambling is common in sections with debris or rough terrain. Standard climbing techniques (often adapted or improvised) are often used to enter and exit a pothole, down-climb a chimney, or reach an emergency evacuation point. Jumps and slides are part of the attraction of canyoneering, but a pool or pothole should always be assessed first for hazards. Jumps are done in a vertical position with the arms close to the body and knees slightly bent.[44] This position prevents typical canyoneering injuries, such as shoulder dislocation, vertebral compression fracture, lower extremity injury, and

head trauma. Jumps can be useful to avoid hydraulics and other dangerous situations. To pass a hydraulic when the eddy fence is too far in advance to jump over it, jump into the turbulence (whitewater) and move downstream of the hydraulic (see Figure 98-4). If passing a hydraulic, a group member should be positioned with a throw bag or be prepared to use other swiftwater techniques for companion rescue. Sliding is done in a crouched position with the back elevated from the rock, legs straight, toes up, and arms close to the body or crossed on the chest. Packs are usually thrown in advance to reduce the impact in shallow pools or potholes. Floating and wading techniques are used to move with or across the main flow of water and during rescue.[38] The position for floating is with feet downstream if there are undercut rocks, or upstream if there are strainers.

Progression With a Rope

Standard rope techniques for progression use releasable rappels. Rappel and rope techniques used by climbers and canyoneers have many similarities and differences (Figure 98-9). Rappelling in a dry canyon can be comparable to rappelling in traditional climbing. The rope is threaded through the anchor and rappelling is done on both strands with a descender and a secondary conditional self-belay (e.g., autoblock knot, Petzl Shunt) as a backup. This method should be avoided in wet canyons because there is an increased risk that the canyoneers will encounter hazards, such as drowning, hypothermia, and suspension syndrome, if they become stuck on the rope in a waterfall feature (Figure 98-10). In wet canyons, rappelling is commonly done on a single strand, without a secondary conditional self-belay as a backup. A knot block (or a blocked figure-eight descender) is placed against the rappel metal ring and secured with a carabiner.[44] The

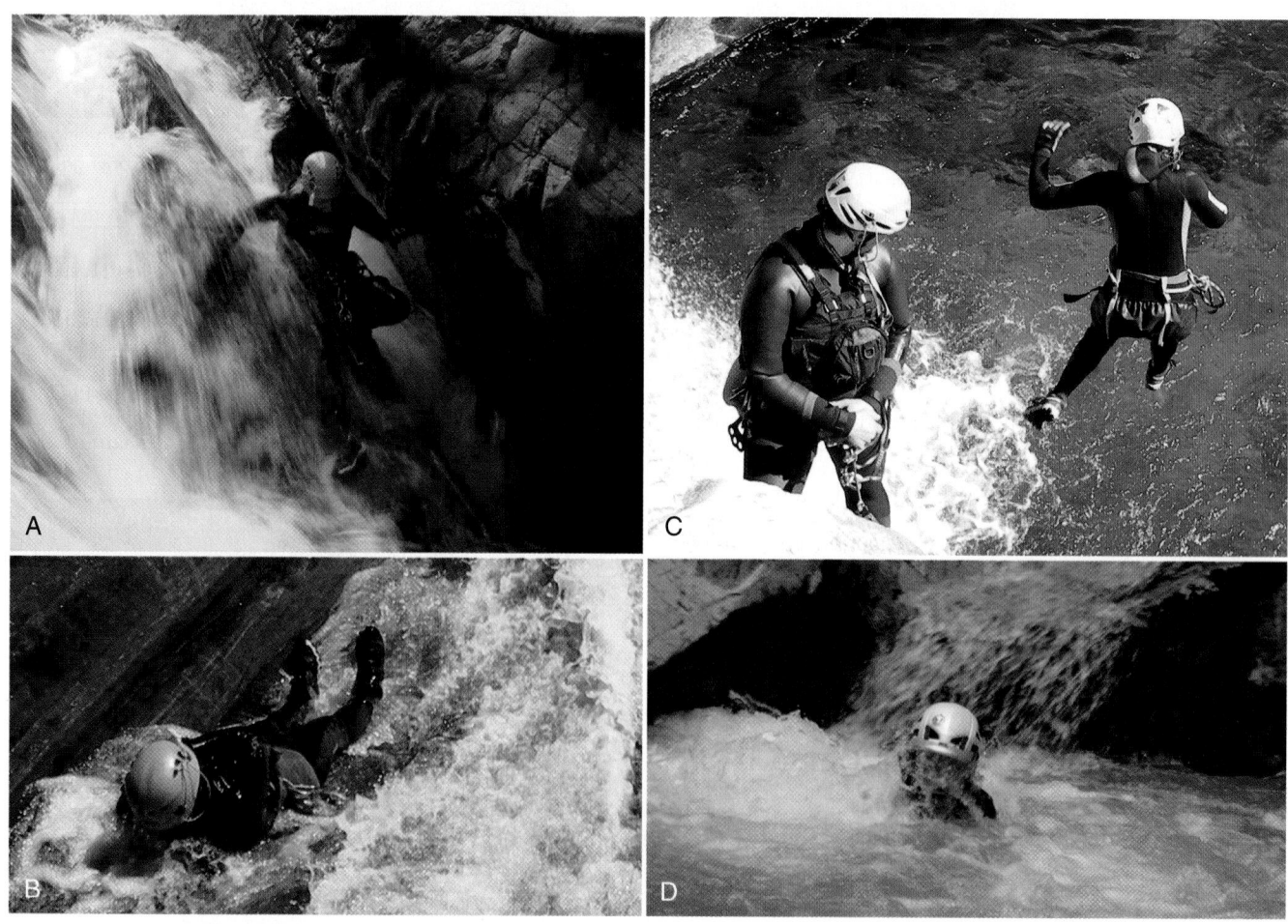

FIGURE 98-8 Progression without a rope. **A,** Scrambling in a wet area with debris (tree). **B,** Sliding on a water toboggan with arms crossed on the chest. **C,** Jumping in a clear pool feet first (correct) with one arm too far from the body (incorrect). **D,** Swiftwater swimming in a hydraulic. (**A-C** *Courtesy Erwin Kob;* **D** *courtesy Oskar Piazza.*)

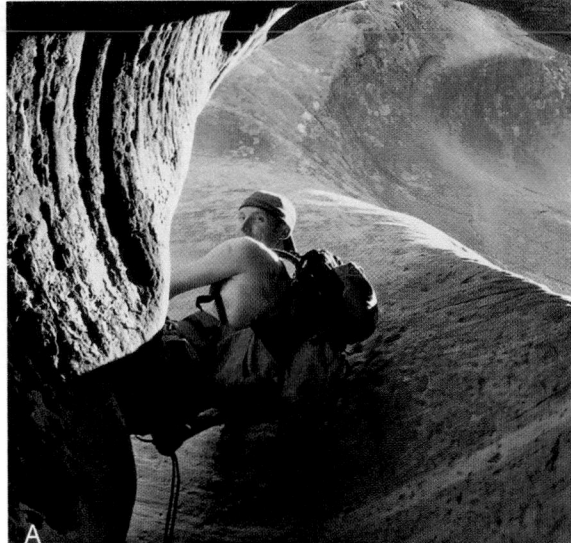

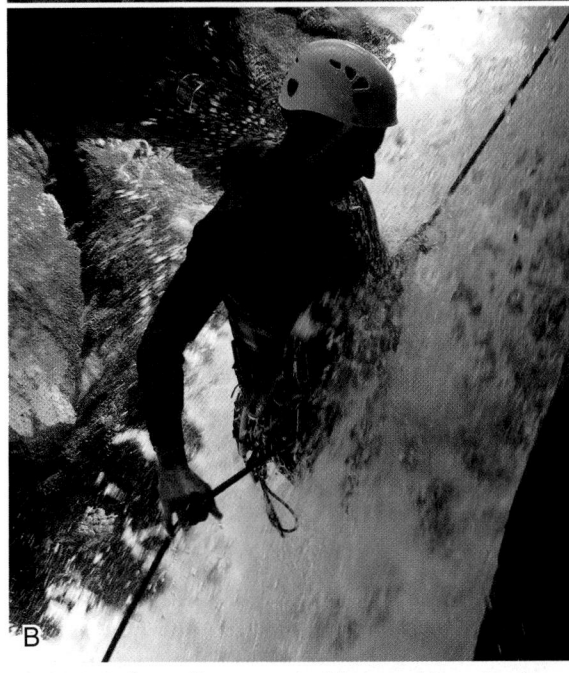

FIGURE 98-9 A, Rappelling on a double strand in a dry slot canyon (with high risk of falling debris and skin abrasion). **B,** Rappelling on a single strand in a waterfall (with the risk of being stuck and of hypothermia). *(Courtesy Gordon Larsen [A] and Erwin Kob [B].)*

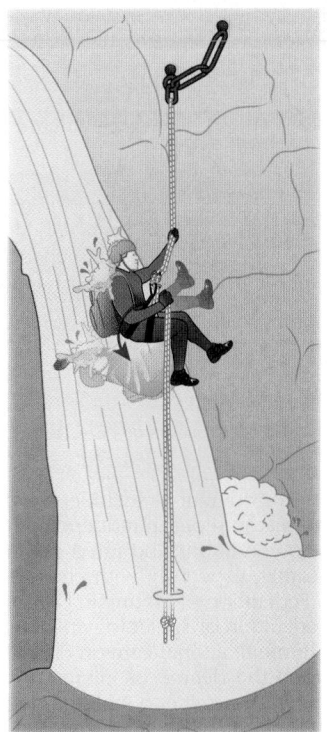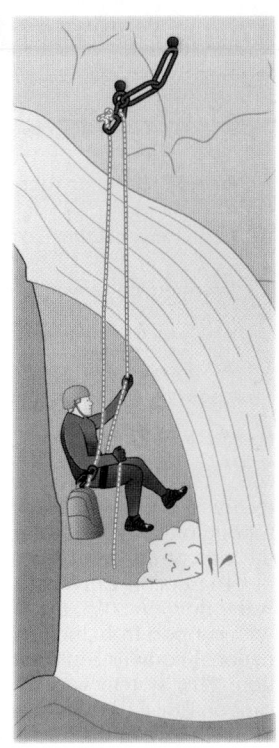

FIGURE 98-10 A, Incorrect rappelling on a double strand with an autoblock knot in a wet canyon with a pack on the shoulder. **B,** Correct rappelling on a single strand blocked on the anchor and with a pack attached to an equipment loop with a carabiner-on-carabiner technique.

Ascending techniques are similar to those used in caving but are not that common in canyoneering. They are used when backtracking to exit the canyon, when releasing a stuck rope, or for self-rescue maneuvers.

CANYON CLASSIFICATION AND MAPPING

Canyons have varying levels of difficulty. However, to date, classification of canyoneering routes has been widely discussed but with little consensus. There is general acceptance that a classification system must contain several key considerations of equal importance, such as location, access routes, and required

first strand is used for descent and the second strand is usually brought down by the last person. This allows rope retrieval and is important in case of self-rescue or companion rescue. Ropes should be positioned in a way to reduce friction and rope damage. Ideally, the rope should be kept above the water where possible. Equally, it is important to avoid use of a final knot, as this could become trapped in hydraulics at the base of a waterfall or a slide.[44] There are several other special considerations for rappelling, such as guided rappels to avoid obstacles during the descent, or a single strand blocked on a figure-eight descender controlled by a companion to reduce rope damage (Figure 98-11). Complete details about progression techniques can be found in technical canyoneering manuals.[14,44]

Large potholes are common in many canyons and especially in sandstone slot canyons. *Keeper potholes* are large, circular potholes too deep to scramble out of and with water too deep to stand in. There are several improvised systems designed to allow escape from keeper potholes, including hooks attached to long poles to aid climbing and weighted bags that are thrown over an edge.[7]

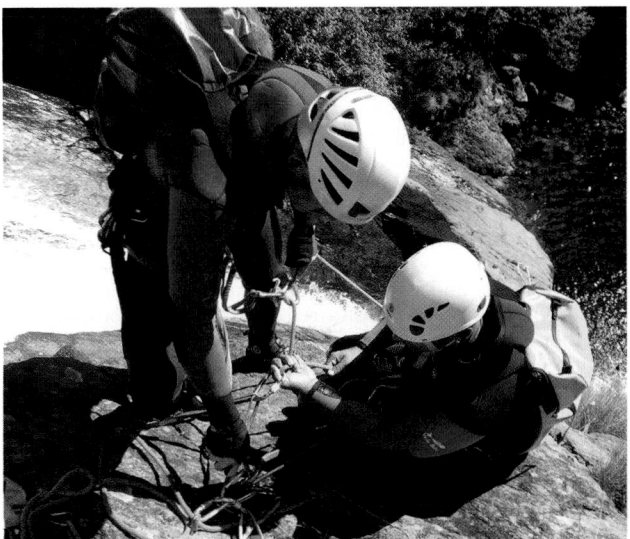

FIGURE 98-11 Rappelling on a single strand controlled by a companion with a Petzl Pirana descender to reduce rope damage on rocks. *(Courtesy Oskar Piazza.)*

TABLE 98-2 American Canyoneering Association Classification of Canyons

Terrain and Technical Ropework	Water Volume and Current	Time and Commitment (Optional)	Risk and Seriousness (Optional)
1, Canyon hiking, no rope	A, Dry or wading up to waist, no swimming	I-II, Half day	G-PG, General audiences or parental guide suggested
2, Basic canyoneering, scrambling	B, Swimming in still water; wet disconnects; no current	III-IV, Full day	R, Risky (not recommended for beginners; solid technical skill required)
3, Intermediate canyoneering, rappelling	C, Currents and waterfalls	V-VI, Multiple days	X-XX, Extreme or double extreme (serious injuries or death if error in techniques or judgment)
4, Advanced-expert canyoneering, advanced ropework, and problem solving	—	—	—

Modified from Haro JL, Samsó L: Les cotations: Les cahiers de l'EFC [serial online] 1:20-26, 2010: fedme.es/salaprensa/upfiles/675_F_es.pdf.

technical knowledge. Additional considerations include seasonal topographical water volume and meteorological influence within the canyon environment. Canyon conditions and rated difficulty of progression can vary significantly, especially with changes in water flow. In 2005, the French Federation of Mountain Climbing, with support from the French Federation of Speleology plus other national commissions, adopted a multifactorial canyon classification. This system was based upon the degree of interest in the canyon (local [*] to international [****]), combined with the degree of technical difficulty, overall exposure risk, and progression length.[15] The degree of exposure or length of canyon route is classified on six levels (I to VI). This classification is dependent on length of time required to traverse the chosen section or sections and ease of exit strategy throughout the canyon route. Classification of the degree of difficulty of canyon progression is determined under optimal canyon conditions, i.e., during the season where the least extreme environmental factors are reported and the canyon is considered most accessible. Level of difficulty describes both technical (vertical) difficulty and water (aquatic) difficulty. Vertical ("v") and aquatic ("a") difficulty are described in seven classes. This class system ranges from very easy (1) to extremely difficult (7). Since its inception in 2005 by the French, this classification in its entirety has subsequently been adopted by most canyoneering associations in Europe.[19] A similar classification proposed by the American Canyoneering Association is currently used in both Zion National Park and the Colorado Plateau region. This classification places emphasis on two main considerations, plus two optional factors for enhanced interrogation of the canyon route. Primary considerations are related to canyon terrain and the corresponding level of technical ropework proficiency needed. Secondary considerations are focused on canyon water volume and current presence. Finally, the optional factors for consideration include progression time, commitment, and risk assessment (Table 98-2).[7,19] For example, Mystery Canyon in Zion National Park is classified as *** III v3 a1 or as 3B III, and Imlay Canyon in Zion National Park as **** IV v5 a3 or as 4B IV R (according to French and American classifications, respectively).

Reaching a canyon may require navigational skills in remote or extreme environments; it is critical to know GPS coordinates of drop-in and exit points. It is also important to record time of access, descent, and exit; number of rappels; maximum length of a rappel (and presence of a re-belay); suggested rope length; and other information specific for the route (e.g., special technical and personal equipment, possible escape points). Canyoneering maps show a longitudinal section of the canyon with waterfalls, slides, pools, and other important progression elements (Figure 98-12).

CANYON MEDICINE

EPIDEMIOLOGY OF INJURIES AND ILLNESSES

Injuries to the lower extremities are common, mainly because progression without ropes involves jumps or slides and walking or scrambling on wet surfaces. Data show that fractures (lower extremities and spine or thorax) followed by sprains (mostly to the lower extremities) and dislocations (mostly to the upper extremities) account for the majority of injuries requiring a SAR operation. In a 10-year (1999 to 2009) retrospective analysis of canyon rescues in Aragon, Spain, traumatic injuries were reported in 419 (81%) patients.[45] Isolated injuries of extremities were more common than spine or multiple injuries. The most common injury location was the lower extremity (74%) (Table 98-3).[45] Similar data were obtained from 362 patients rescued in canyons in France between 1998 and 2001; the most common injury location was the lower extremity (50%, of which 72% were fractures and 24% were sprains). Injuries to the spine, thorax, and abdomen accounted for 16%, whereas upper extremity injuries accounted for only 10% (57% dislocations, 38% fractures).[42] Similarly, in Zion National Park between 1999 and 2002, the most common injury location was the lower extremity.[48] Between 1997 and 2002 in La Reunion Island, France, a popular tropical canyoneering region, the most common injury location was also reported to be the lower extremity.[10] Regional discrepancies in injury patterns may be due to differences in environmental factors, type of rescue included in the sample (companion rescue and/or SAR operations), and changes in equipment and progression techniques over time.

Medical and environmental illnesses were reported in 49 (9%) patients in Spain (see Table 98-3)[45] and 25 (12%) patients in

TABLE 98-3 Type of Injury and Illness in Canyoneers (n=520) Rescued in Search and Rescue Operations in Aragon, Spain, from 1999 to 2009

Injury or Illness	n	Type	n (%)*
Traumatic injury	419		
		Head/face	5 (1.1)
		Spine/back	39 (9.2)
		Upper extremity	51 (12.6)
		Lower extremity	310 (74.0)
		Thorax	2 (0.4)
		Abdomen	1 (0.2)
		Pelvis	2 (0.4)
		Multiple	9 (2.1)
Medical or environmental illness	49		
		Drowning	16 (32.7)
		Heat-related illness	25 (51.0)
		Hypothermia	1 (2.0)
		Medical illness†	7 (14.3)
Uninjured	50		
Total	518‡		

Modified from Soteras I, Subirats E, Strapazzon G: Epidemiological and medical aspects of canyoning rescue operations, Injury 46(4):585-589, 2015.
*% refers to each category of injury or illness.
†Anaphylaxis (n=1), anxiety (n=1), coronary syndrome (n=2), dizziness (n=1), exhaustion (n=1), seizures (n=1).
‡Data were missing for two cases.

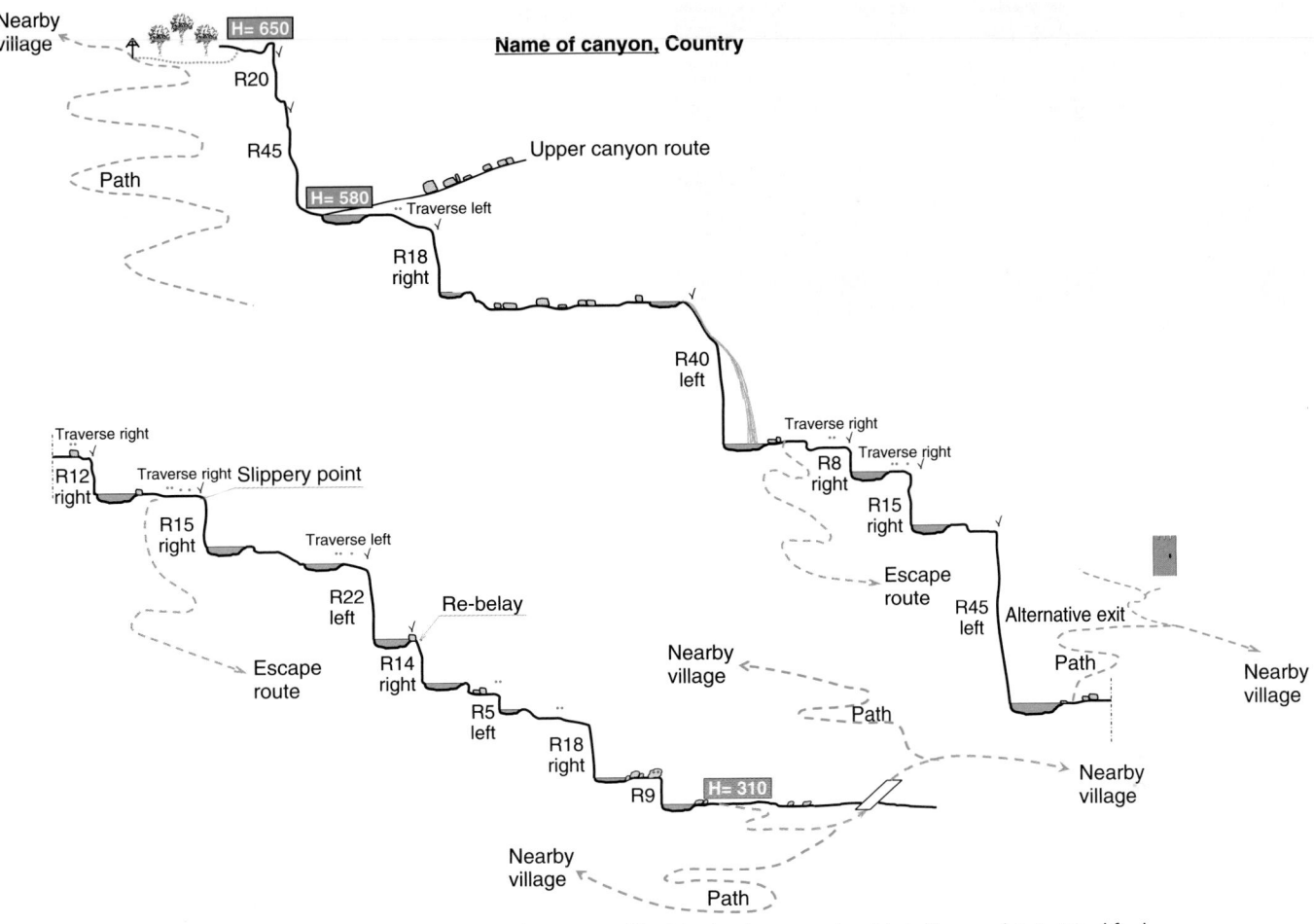

FIGURE 98-12 Longitudinal section of a canyon. H, altitude above sea level (m); R, rappel (m). *(Modified courtesy Erwin Kob.)*

France.[42] In Spain, heat-related illnesses were the most common illness (51%), followed in descending order by drowning (33%), medical illnesses (14%), and accidental hypothermia (2%).[45] Similarly, in La Reunion Island, heat-related illnesses were the most common, followed by accidental hypothermia, drowning, and medical illnesses.[10] In general, most patients rescued from canyons probably have mild to moderate accidental hypothermia or heat injury, but the incidence remains unknown because most cases are unreported. A web-based survey of American and Australian canyoneers[48] compared with European canyoneers[42,45] showed a higher frequency of environmental illnesses resulting from both warm and cold exposure. In European data, accidental hypothermia was reported in only a minority of cases, though it is probably present but not documented in many patients with traumatic injuries. The prevalence of accidental hypothermia in canyoneering patients with traumatic injuries is likely similar to that in other trauma situations (e.g., car accidents). In Germany, secondary hypothermia (defined in this study as core body temperature < 36°C [96.8°F]), occurred in nearly 50% of trauma patients and in 98% of entrapped patients rescued by a helicopter emergency medical service.[23] Other reported medical illnesses included cardiac arrest and thermal shock, anaphylaxis, panic attack, seizures, syncope, and infectious diseases.[10,18,25,31,42,45,51]

Medical and environmental illnesses are reportedly less frequent than are traumatic injuries, but are often more severe. The same web-based survey of American and Australian canyoneers found a higher frequency of severe environmental illnesses compared with traumatic injuries, reported as the average incidence of the injury or illness seen or suffered in a canyoneering career (6.5 years, with 25 days per year of canyoneering).[48] Equally, in Spain, the percentage of patients in SAR operations with a potential or actual life-threatening injury or illness (i.e., predefined as a National Advisory Committee for Aeronautics [NACA] score ≥ 4)[8] was reportedly higher for medical and environmental illnesses than for traumatic injuries

(96% vs. 47%).[45] Within those patients, approximately 95% were classified as having a Glasgow Coma Scale score of 15.[45] Nevertheless, the patient's clinical status may worsen with prolonged exposure and a long alert or delayed evacuation. Potential or actual life-threatening injuries (NACA: 4 to 6), were found in 28 (5%) patients.[45] Correspondingly in France, a similar survey revealed that head trauma and multiple injuries were more severe in the majority of the reported cases.[42]

Fatalities occurred in 3% to 5% of canyon rescue operations.[10,42,45] Drowning and traumatic injuries were considered the primary causes of fatalities in France, Spain, and tropical regions.[10,42,45] In Spain, 19 (4%) patients were pronounced dead at the scene (NACA: 7): 9 patients from traumatic injuries, 8 from drowning, and 2 with cardiac arrest due to coronary syndrome. The causes of death were similar in France and tropical regions.[10,42] In comparison, the cause of death is not commonly reported in the United States, but unpublished data from Zion National Park demonstrate similar trends in reported fatalities.

MECHANISM OF INJURIES AND ILLNESSES

Errors in progression techniques or negligence cause most injuries and illnesses in canyoneering (Figure 98-13). In France, for example, 70% of SAR operations reportedly involved an incident directly caused by errors in progression techniques, whereas the remaining 30% where considered a result of negligence alone.[42] In correspondence, research related to the incidence of accidents in canyon environment in Italy indicated that the majority of requests for SAR assistance are due to inexperience.[17] Data from a 5-year survey in Sierra de Guara, Spain, showed that only 69% of canyoneering groups had at least one technically proficient canyoneer.[5] The most common mechanisms that cause canyoneering incidents are jumps, falls and slips, and rappelling. In France, jumps reportedly caused 35% of incidents, followed by falls and slips (32%) and rappelling (13%).[42] Incident reports

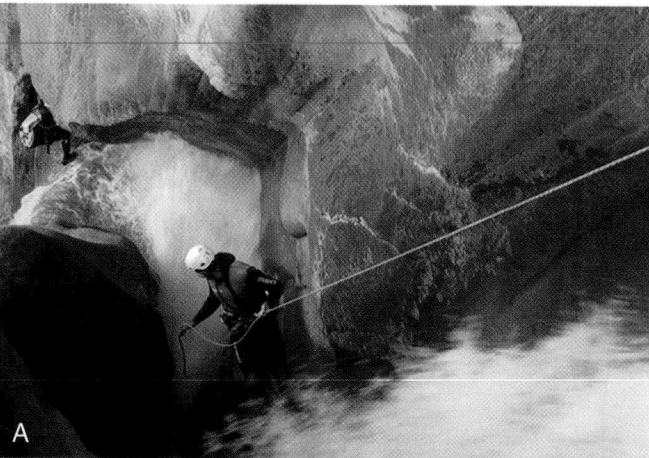

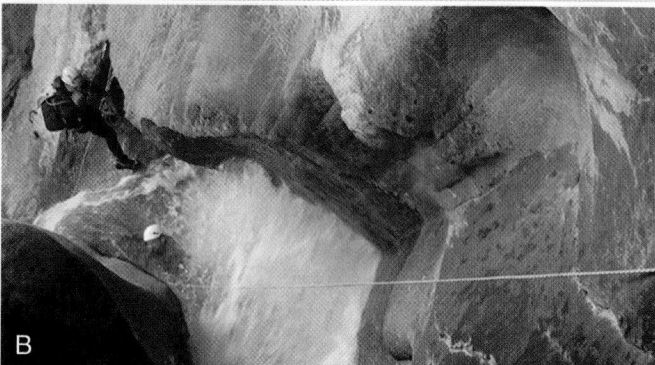

FIGURE 98-13 **A,** Navigation and technical skills are essential. **B,** Canyoneer can avoid getting stuck or losing control of the rope when crossing the water flow while rappelling. *(Courtesy Erwin Kob.)*

from La Reunion Island demonstrate similar determinant mechanisms of injury.[10]

Falls, Jumps, and Other Traumatic Mechanisms

Jumps, and falls or slips caused moderate to severe traumatic injuries in 13% and 25% of cases, respectively.[42] Table 98-4 shows some of the most common errors in progression technique, and the associated mechanism of injury and possible injury. For example, calcaneal, tibial plateau, acetabular, and vertebral compression fractures are possible after incorrectly estimating the depth of a pool prior to a jump. Knowledge of the mechanism of injury is helpful for on-site diagnosis and decision making during a rescue.

Abrasions, blisters, and lacerations are common minor injuries caused by impacts during sliding and jumping and not wearing appropriate clothing, such as gloves, long-sleeved clothing, shoes, and neoprene socks. Abrasions due to flora and cacti have also been reported in approximately one in three canyoneers per year of activity.[48] Other common traumatic injuries include damage to the outer ear due to helmet-related mechanical strain incurred while jumping; bruised testicles from water impact after high jumps (especially with poor jumping technique); and several minor orthopedic problems from errors in ropework. Burns on the fingers and palms may occur in canyoneers who grab ropes after losing control on rappels without a secondary conditional self-belay (e.g., autoblock knot) as a backup.

Barotrauma in canyoneering is a consequence of quick pressure changes during jumps. Without equalization of pressure, it can occur at depths of approximately 1 m (3.3 feet), which is possible with a jump from approximately 6 m (19.7 feet). Damage is caused by pressure differences between air- or gas-filled spaces in the body and incompressible structures. Barotrauma is covered in detail in Chapter 71, Diving Medicine. Pain can develop in the ear during ascent because of pressure from expanding gas that is not released through the eustachian tube. It can result in clinical symptoms, including vertigo and tinnitus. The sinuses are the second most common site of barotrauma.

Environmental Exposure

Heat loss in water is 25 times greater than in air, and heat loss by conduction increases as thermal gradients increase in cold water. Several experimental studies have found significantly faster cooling rates for healthy human volunteers wearing wetsuits or drysuits in rough or turbulent water compared with calm water (see Chapter 8, Immersion into Cold Water).[47] Decreased heat production due to exhaustion or immobilization increases cooling, even in healthy canyoneers. Decreased heat production from immobilization and/or impaired thermoregulation from injuries (e.g., central nervous system trauma) should be suspected in all injured canyoneers. The hazards of cold water are independent of the season or ambient air temperature.

Drowning primarily occurs when a person is trapped underwater, but can also occur after a person jumps into a cold pool. Mistakes while swimming or rappelling are common causes. Prolonged exposure to cold water affects neuromuscular activity.

TABLE 98-4	Canyoneering-Specific Mechanisms Associated with Particular Traumatic Injuries	
Errors in Progression Technique	**Mechanism of Injury**	**Possible Injury**
Jump in a pool or pothole without checking the depth or for debris	Landing flat on the feet from a height	Calcaneus, tibial plateau, acetabulum, vertebral compression fractures
Jump in a pool or pothole	Fall on the outstretched arm	Posterior dislocation of the shoulder
Fall on a wet surface	Fall, landing on the outstretched arm or with the elbow beneath the body	Fracture of the radial head
Fall on a wet surface	Fall on the outstretched arm	Posterior dislocation of the shoulder
Fall on a wet surface	Forced dorsiflexion of the wrist	Fracture of the scaphoid, lunate dislocation, perilunar dislocation, Colles fracture
Slip on a wet surface	Ankle inversion force	Fracture of any of the three malleoli, fracture of the base of the fifth metatarsal
Slip on a wet surface	Rotatory ankle force	Fracture of any of the three malleoli, disruption of the anterior tibiofibular ligament with proximal fibular fracture (Maisonneuve injury)
Slip on a wet surface	Inversion or medial or lateral stress to the forefoot; axial load on the metatarsal heads with the ankle plantarflexed	Midfoot dislocation (Lisfranc injury)

Modified from Menkes JS: Initial evaluation and management of orthopedic injuries. In Tintinalli JE, editor: Tintinalli's emergency medicine, 7th ed, New York, 2011, McGraw Hill, pp 1783-1796.

There is initially decreased sensation in the hands and fingers and decreased coordination of gross and fine motor control, followed by loss of muscular power. In France, 25% of reported fatalities were due to incorrect execution of rappelling technique, which left canyoneers trapped in the flow of a waterfall (e.g., incorrect positioning of the pack can cause rotation backward under the water) (see Figure 98-10).[42] When an unconscious patient is found in a waterfall, drowning should be differentiated from severe hypothermia and/or suspension syndrome.

Staying longer than planned in a canyon can increase the risk of being caught in a flash flood. Flash floods on the Colorado Plateau have been concomitant with several drowning fatalities and associated trauma incidents.[3] Similarly, flash floods were responsible for 50% of fatal accidents in France between 2004 and 2008.[35]

Immersion in pools and potholes, especially with low or no water flow and in summer months, poses a risk of zoonosis. Outbreaks of leptospirosis have been reported after canyoneering in tropical and subtropical regions.[25] Giardiasis and other zoonoses can occur. Water exposure can worsen an infection or cause infections of the eyes and other mucous membranes. A case of anterior uveitis was reported in a patient after canyoneering in the French West Indies.[31] Heavy rainfall and flooding may increase human exposure to contaminants and waterborne pathogens.

A recreational hand dermatitis called *canyoning hand* may result from repeated water immersion with subsequent periods of drying and contact with abrasive rock.[12] Prolonged skin wetting causes destruction of the stratum corneum and cutaneous erosions. Skin lesions are found only on the fingertips and palms, and include erythema, punctate erosions, and edema on the fingertips and thenar and hypothenar eminences (Figure 98-14). This condition can be prevented by wearing gloves. Otitis externa (swimmer's ear) is a common but poorly documented skin injury related to water exposure. This can usually be resolved by limiting further exposure to water and/or treatment with topical antibiotic solutions (see Chapter 76, Aquatic Skin Disorders).

There are no reported cases in canyoneering of severe non-freezing cold-induced injuries, such as trench (immersion) foot.[33]

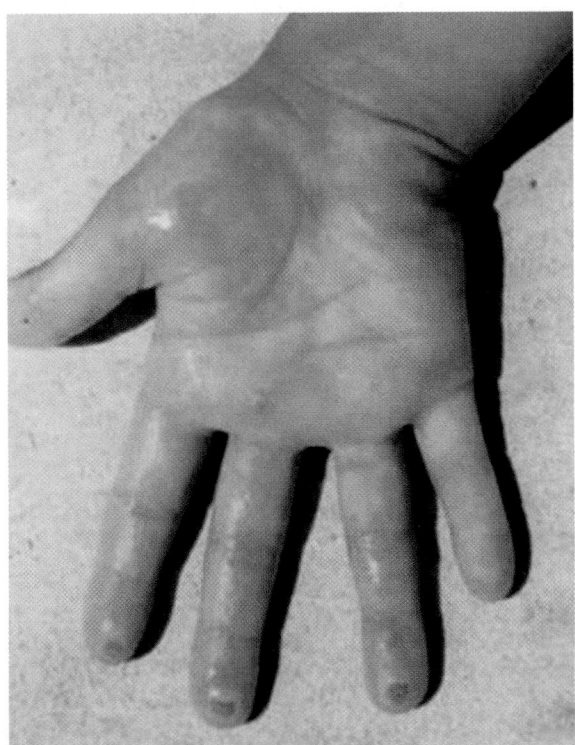

FIGURE 98-14 Canyoning hand, showing erythema and erosions on the fingertips and thenar and hypothenar eminences. *(From Descamps V, Puechal X: "Canyoning hand": a new recreational hand dermatitis. Contact Dermatitis 47:363-364, 2002.)*

However, severe nerve damage associated with nonfreezing cold-induced damage in other settings has been seen after prolonged exposure.[54] The combination of cold and wet over prolonged periods could lead to similar skin damage in canyoneering; the lower the water temperature, the faster a nonfreezing cold-induced injury could occur. This can be prevented by wearing specific canyoneering shoes, waiting in a dry place if stranded, and staying active to promote blood flow to the feet.

Heat-related illnesses due to heat injuries, dehydration, and strenuous physical effort are possible and may be exacerbated by drysuits and wetsuits. A case of exertional rhabdomyolysis complicated by mild acute renal failure has been reported from a canyoneering environment. Associated clinical signs and symptoms included progressive weakness in the extremities, myalgia, cramps, and gross pigmenturia.[49] Neoprene allergic dermatitis due to chemical additives used in rubber processing has been described in divers and therefore may be anticipated in canyoneers.

MEDICAL MANAGEMENT

Recommendations and protocols for patient assessment and emergency care in canyons are based on standard principles of wilderness trauma care. Safety evaluation and risk assessment are equally important to companion rescuers and SAR teams, both to prevent accidents and carry out rescue operations. Basic management steps are to (1) control the situation and assess the possible risk for SAR team members and/or companions; (2) obtain an overview of the patient situation; (3) move the patient to a safe and stable place; (4) perform a primary survey; (5) resuscitate the patient if necessary; (6) perform a secondary survey; (7) make a definite plan; and (8) package the patient for evacuation.[2,6,41] These steps may have to be adapted or improvised depending on the environment and situation. Care should be appropriate and sustainable throughout a rescue. Medical monitoring is critical. The U.S. Department of the Interior, National Park Service, underlines that "Medical personnel should be educated [...] to the realities of patient care limitations in the technical environment."[39] Table 98-5 shows proposed medical interventions according to rescue technique and environment.[39] The most common on-site medical interventions in all Spanish SAR operations over a 10-year period are shown in Table 98-6.[45] Splinting or immobilization and analgesia were the most common on-site medical interventions (71% and 34% of rescued canyoneers, respectively). Reduction of dislocations was done in 7% of patients. Vascular access was obtained in 6% of patients and followed by fluid administration in most cases. Chest tube insertion was never performed. Oxygen was administered in 4% of patients, but no advanced airway control was executed despite the presence of a physician in all cases. Cardiopulmonary resuscitation was performed on four patients, but vasoactive drugs and defibrillators were not used. Medical interventions were reportedly similar in La Reunion Island.[10] Specifications for canyon rescue are described in detail within the following paragraphs to promote a comprehensive understanding of treatment limitations within this difficult environment.

Risk Assessment and Safety

During canyon rescue, risk assessment primarily refers to risks imposed by water (Figure 98-15).[57] If a canyoneer becomes stuck and falls unconscious while rappelling down a waterfall, there is immediately a high risk of drowning and the priority is a pickoff (not resuscitation). In this scenario, if the risk is unacceptable for rescuers, the patient should be lowered using a second rope with a "cut and lower" procedure. Similarly, if an unconscious canyoneer becomes trapped in a hydraulic, the personal safety of the rescuer entering the water is the priority, followed by quick recovery of the patient and subsequent effective treatment. If the patient did not fall from a height, the reported incidence of spine injury in drowning is low (0.009%).[56] However, when removing the patient from the water, immobilization of the patient remains critical, where rescue is not impeded. On removal from the water, and if possible, the patient should be transferred to a safe and stable place and insulated fully from cold and water

TABLE 98-5 Medical Interventions According to Rescue Technique and Environment That Can Be Found in Search and Rescue Operations in Canyons

Intervention	Low-Angle Maneuvers*	High-Angle Maneuvers†	Helicopter Short-Haul or Hoist‡	Water or Swiftwater Rescue
BLS airway	R	T	R	T
BLS vital signs	R	N	N	N
Splinting or bandaging	R	T	R	T
Tourniquet	R	R	R	R
Spinal immobilization	R	N	R	R
Medication IN, IM, or PO	T	T	T	T
Medication IV or IO	T	N	N	N
Chest decompression	T	T	T	T
ALS airway	T	T	T	T

Modified from Thompson J: Medical considerations. In Phillips K, editor: Technical rescue handbook, 11th ed, U.S. Department of the Interior, National Park Service, 2014, pp 230-243.
ALS, advanced life support; BLS, basic life support; IM, intramuscular; IN, intranasal; IO, intraosseous; IV, intravenous; N, not practical in this setting; PO, oral; R, recommended skill; T, training strongly recommended.
*Rough terrain or debris with an angle less than 20 degrees.
†Terrain with an angle greater than 20 degrees to vertical.
‡Technical maneuvers with no complex ground rescue.

(Figure 98-16). Under these conditions, hypothermia can result within a short period, even within a neoprene suit.[57]

Drowning Management

Drowning incidents in canyons can be different than in other bodies of water (see Chapter 69, Drowning and Submersion Injuries). Victims are usually found floating or entrapped in hydraulics or in a waterfall, and high-impact injuries are more common. Once the patient is out of the water, immediate ventilatory support and early chest compressions result in a better prognosis and outcome in patients in cardiac or ventilatory arrest.[55] It is advisable to be in a dry place when defibrillating and to first dry the chest.[55] Advanced treatment by the SAR team can be further complicated if oxygen and/or continuous positive airway pressure are not available. Vomiting is a common complication for rescue breathing or chest compressions[29] and therefore continuous clinical monitoring is required. Rapid cooling due to immersion in cold water may offer a protective benefit and prolong the time after which resuscitation can still be successful. This is particularly qualifiable in cases where the patient cooled before becoming hypoxic (caused by closure of the glottis or after inhalation of water into the lungs).[55]

Patient Assessment

Debris and steep or rough terrain can make physical examination difficult. In this scenario, the patient should be placed in a horizontal position by being positioned perpendicular to the slope. The patient should be insulated from the ground. It is possible to layer ropes, canyoneering packs, aluminum foil, and garbage bags to make a comfortable and insulated surface (and improvised spinal immobilization). The medical examination may be more difficult if the patient is wearing a wetsuit, but the first assessment should be as complete as possible. A vertical incision in the wetsuit provides access for examination (or intervention)

TABLE 98-6 On-Site Medical Interventions in Canyoneers (n=520) Rescued in Search and Rescue Operations in Aragon, Spain, from 1999 to 2009

Intervention	n	%
Oxygen administration	19	3.7
Airway management	0	0.0
Intravenous lines	31	6.0
Analgesics*	175	33.7
Intravenous fluid administration	27	5.2
Vasoactive drugs†	0	0.0
Basic life support	4	1.5
Reduction of dislocations	35	6.7
Splinting or immobilization	370	71.2
Hypothermia prevention	10	1.9
Antibiotics	0	0.0

Modified from Soteras I, Subirats E, Strapazzon G: Epidemiological and medical aspects of canyoning rescue operations, Injury 46(4):585-589, 2015.
*Morphine or analogs (n=81), nonsteroidal antiinflammatory drugs (n = 74), pyrazole derivatives (n = 41), tramadol (n = 19), ketamine (n=4).
†Epinephrine, ephedrine, atropine.

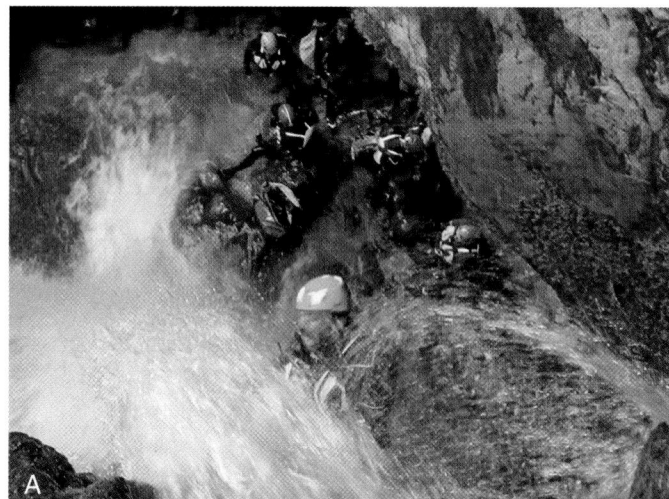

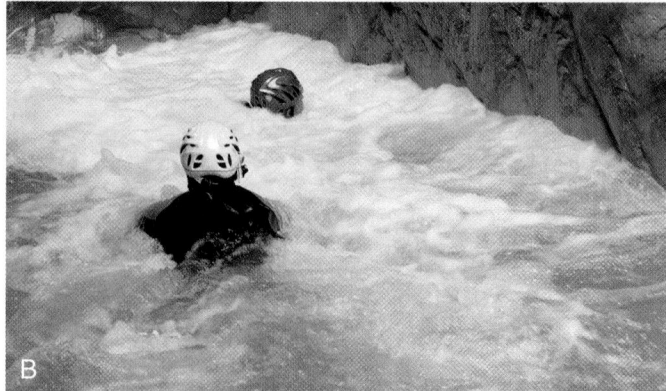

FIGURE 98-15 Risk assessment and safety in rescue operations includes knowing where you are going, how to get there, and what understanding safety is. **A,** Safety in rappelling. **B,** Safety in swiftwater. *(Courtesy Oskar Piazza.)*

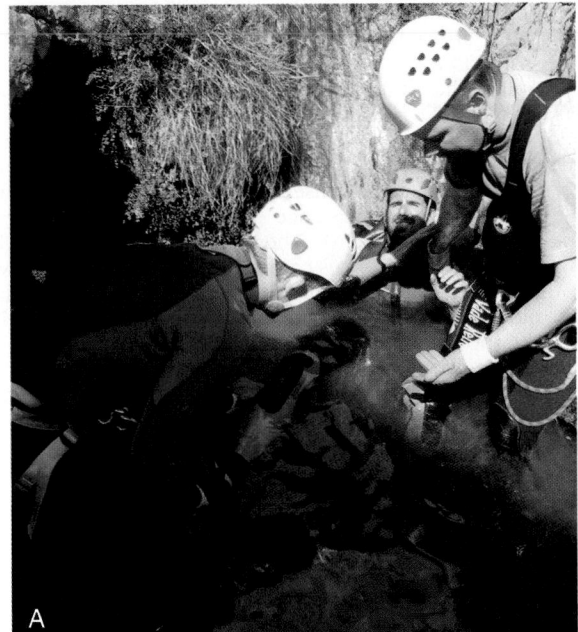

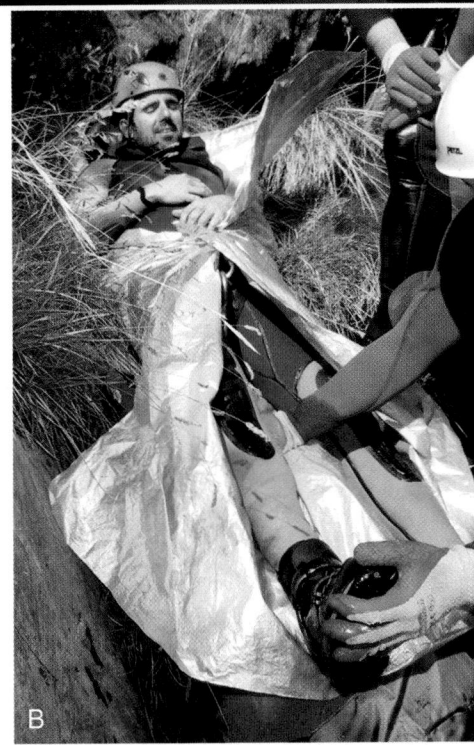

FIGURE 98-16 Principles of patient assessment. **A,** Removal from the water (and immobilization in trauma) is the first priority. **B,** Find a safe and stable place. Keep the patient insulated from the ground. *(Courtesy Inigo Soteras.)*

and can be closed afterward with bandages or duct tape. This limits the degree of exposure of the patient. Pulses and other vital signs should be sought for at least 60 seconds when hypothermia is suspected.[11] On-site differentiation of drowning, severe hypothermia,[11] and/or cardiac arrest related to suspension syndrome (if the patient was rescued from a rappel)[34] can be difficult.

Hypothermia Prevention

All patients should be assessed for accidental hypothermia, because measures to prevent development or exacerbation of hypothermia are critical to patient prognosis and should be taken immediately. Removing the patient from the water is the first priority. Subsequently, wind chill can cause further cooling of

the patient by evaporation of moisture. Early application of adequate insulation on-site is crucial to limit heat loss. Removal of wet clothing is generally suggested, but can be difficult in the canyon environment. A study demonstrated that mean skin temperature in healthy persons wearing wet clothing increased with addition of a vapor barrier under an ordinary ambulance blanket at an ambient temperature of 5°C (41°F; wind speed of 3 m/s [7 mph]),[52] conditions that are similar to those in the bottom of a canyon. A vapor barrier can be easily fashioned from a garbage bag (Figure 98-17), which when combined with a dry insulating layer is more effective than bubble wrap or other rescue foils (see Figure 98-17). This method is effective even when the patient is still wearing wet clothing.[24,52] Cold exposure can be reduced by moving the patient into a tent and insulating him from the ground. In the interim, a neoprene hood or cap can be used to minimize heat loss from the head. However, if the patient is in cardiac arrest, a hood or heating the head is not appropriate. High-calorie food and warm, sweet fluids should be given to a conscious patient. A 10-point scale has recently been developed to evaluate thermal discomfort in conscious patients.[28]

Pain Management

Analgesia administration should be a priority when moving the victim to a safe and stable environment after a water rescue or pickoff from a waterfall. A nasal Mucosal Atomizer Device (MAD) may be useful to administer analgesia (e.g., ketamine) and other

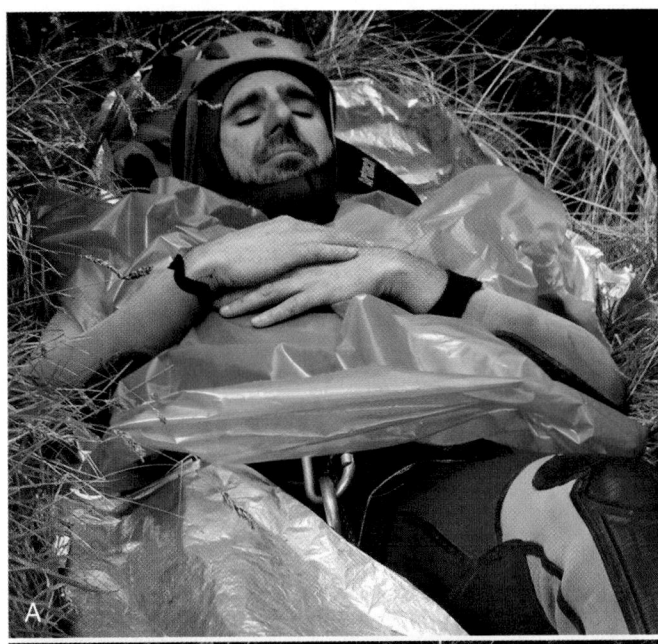

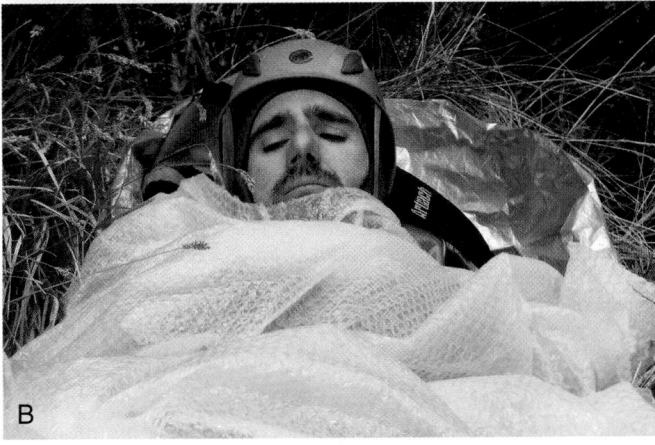

FIGURE 98-17 Hypothermia prevention is a priority. **A,** Insulation with a garbage bag. **B,** Insulation with bubble wrap. *(Courtesy Inigo Soteras.)*

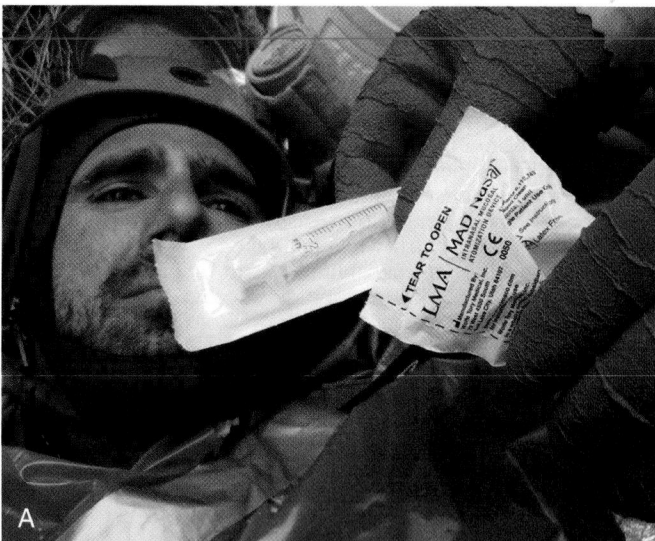

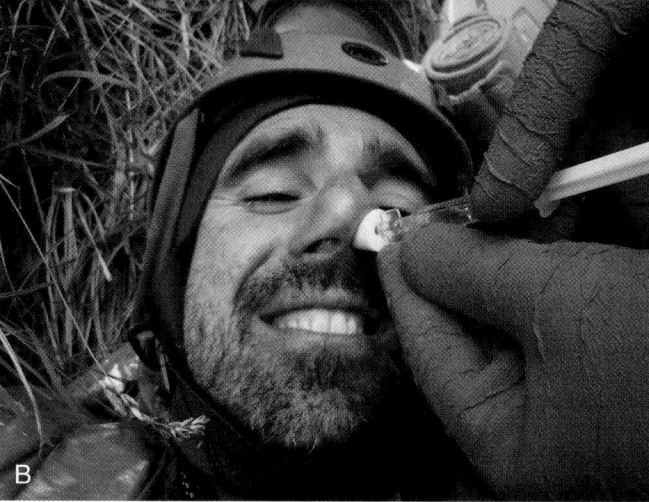

FIGURE 98-18 Administration of analgesia with a MAD device. **A,** Materials required. **B,** Administration. *(Courtesy Inigo Soteras.)*

above the knee; or (3) the humerus slightly anterior to the lateral midline of the arm at the greater tubercle (with the patient supine and the arm adducted, elbow bent, and hand on the umbilicus). After cleaning the skin, the needle is angled respective to the site as follows: (1) perpendicular to the humerus; (2) slightly superior on the anterior femur; or (3) slightly inferior on the tibia. For manual insertion, the needle (stabilized in the palm with the index finger on the skin) is inserted with a twisting motion until there is a decrease in resistance and a crunching sound (the distance is usually > 1 cm). Thereafter, the stylet should be removed. Proper placement is confirmed by one of the following: the catheter stands at a 90-degree angle to the skin and is firmly seated; blood is seen at the hub of the catheter; or fluid flows freely with no evidence of extravasation.[43] Once placed, the needle needs to be secured and checked. Flushing with lidocaine 2% (0.5 mg/kg) over 1 minute should be considered prior to fluid infusion and medication administration. Systemic analgesia, such as fentanyl, is a good drug for intraosseous infusion. In the field, a practical method is to give fluids and drugs as boluses using the 60-mL syringe before moving the patient. During patient transport, the intraosseous site should be checked for fluid extravasation every 30 minutes, as well as before and after every drug administration. An intraosseous needle should be replaced with an intravenous line as soon as possible. Intraosseous infusions prolonged beyond 24 hours are associated with increased risk of osteomyelitis.

Hemorrhage and Wound Care

Management of severe bleeding does not differ from that undertaken in other wilderness settings (see Chapter 21, Wound Management). There is always increased risk of infection in an aquatic environment. Preventing infection is fundamental, even with minor scratches and abrasions. Wound irrigation is crucial for optimizing wound healing, as long as there is sufficient pressure and volume. Use irrigation volumes of approximately 100 mL/cm of wound length, using sterile or potable water, except if the bleeding is profuse. Antibiotic prophylaxis should be administered for severe wounds if the expected time from injury to definitive care is greater than 2 hours.[43] Interestingly, despite this recommendation, this practice seems to be uncommon in established practice; for example, antibiotic prophylaxis was never administered in a 10-year period of SAR operations in Spain.[45] Before evacuating the patient, if there is risk of water contact, where possible all dressings and bandages should be covered with plastic wrap (Figure 98-19). The patient should be reassessed for comfort, distal circulation, sensation, and motor function in affected extremities.

Splinting and Reduction

Reduction and splinting maneuvers on-site may be appropriate when evacuation is difficult (Figure 98-20). Reduction is indicated for any suspected fracture or dislocation with a decreased distal pulse, or a deformity affecting the ability to adequately splint and/or transport (in particular for a long transport).[43] The dynamics of the accident should be evaluated in each case to assess the risk of associated fractures. However, on-site reduction, especially of shoulder dislocation, is usually safe and should be done immediately. Medical personnel should use the technique with which they are most familiar, but should also be up to date and proficient in alternative procedures used in difficult situations or terrain. As with wound care, the splinted area can be covered in plastic wrap to create a waterproof seal (Figure 98-21). Duct tape can also be used on the dressings for additional protection, taking care not to place it circumferentially. Once the splint is applied the patient should be reassessed regularly for comfort, distal circulation, sensation, and motor function in affected extremities.

Patient Packaging

It is important to package the patient before evacuation. This includes stabilization, immobilization, and preparation for transport (Figure 98-22). To guarantee correct packaging: (1) place the stretcher horizontally and close to the patient; (2) open the waterproof bag and straps; (3) place the patient in the stretcher; (4) close all straps gently (starting from the thorax and moving

drugs rapidly. The technique can be used in a patient in any position, but may be less effective if the nasal passage is obstructed. To use this device, a syringe (3 mL) is filled and the MAD is attached to the tip of the syringe; the syringe is pretested before insertion into one nostril and depressed with sufficient force to atomize the medication (Figure 98-18).[43] Up to 1 mL per nostril per dose is suggested (the dose should be repeated in the other nostril if giving more than a single dose). One possible side effect is choking. It is important to first check for nasal obstruction and adjust dosage if the patient is hypothermic. Moreover, it is important to be informed about specific drug doses when using an "alternative" pain management route. Regional nerve blocks are a valuable option for analgesia, but require special expertise due to environmental and logistical factors (e.g., limited monitoring options and long evacuation times).[16]

Alternative Routes for Fluid Administration

It can be difficult to obtain vascular access on-site in a hypothermic and/or hypovolemic patient. Intraosseous access may be used as an alternative route for drug and fluid administration. Intraosseous access can be placed manually or via a driver and needle set (EZ-IO). Common sites include the proximal tibia, distal anterior femur, and proximal humerus; fractured bones or contaminated sites should not be used.[43] The manual equipment includes a 16- or 18-gauge intraosseous needle, 5-mL syringe, 60-mL syringe, and intravascular fluid. Appropriate insertion sites include (1) the proximal tibia 2 cm below and medial to the tibial tuberosity (with a rope or a pack under the knee); (2) the distal anterior femur 3 cm above the patella on the anterior midline

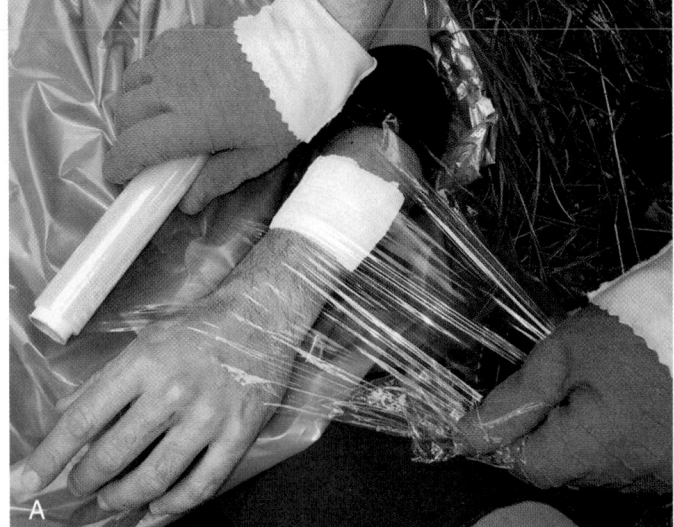

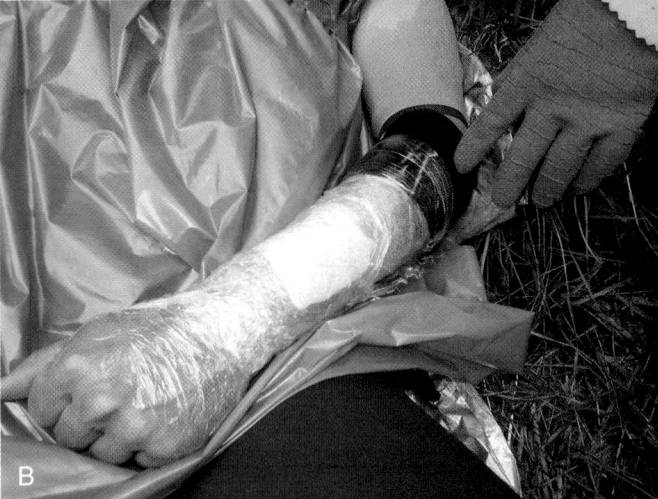

FIGURE 98-19 Improvised wound care dressings. **A,** Plastic wrap can be used as an outer layer. **B,** Waterproof wrapping is essential during water transport. *(Courtesy Inigo Soteras.)*

toward the feet) and adapting to injuries; (5) rotate the stretcher vertically and recheck that the straps are secure; (6) close the waterproof bag and external straps; and (7) confirm that the float valve is working.[44] Packaging is considered correct if it prevents further injuries and ensures patient comfort during evacuation.

MEDICAL EQUIPMENT

First-Aid Materials for Canyoneers

Every canyoneering group should have at least one first-aid kit and be prepared and trained to use it. A web-based survey of

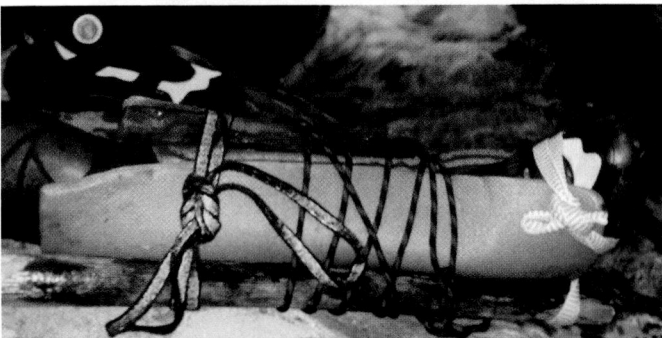

FIGURE 98-20 Improvised splint of an ankle injury with slings, sleeping mat and wood. *(Courtesy Erwin Kob.)*

American and Australian canyoneers found that nearly 90% of respondents carried a first-aid kit, mostly containing wound care materials and analgesics.[48] Space is limited in canyoneering packs, but it is advisable to also include SAM Splints, duct tape, aluminum foil, and garbage bags; these simple additional materials are adequate for most minor injuries and hypothermia prevention. A first-aid kit should be kept in a keg with the survival kit (Figure 98-23).

Medical Equipment for Search and Rescue Teams

There are some general recommendations for technical medical kits for canyon rescue, although the exact contents may differ based on personal or institutional preferences. The International Commission for Mountain Emergency Medicine (ICAR Medcom) suggests that equipment be stored and transported in floatable canyoneering packs. Specialized containers (drybags or kegs) can be used to ensure that all materials are kept dry; in addition, sterile equipment should be stored in sealed individual plastic bags that are checked and changed regularly.[27] Water damage is the main risk for medical equipment and materials. Backup packaging with sealed individual plastic bags is important to minimize this risk. Medical-kit bags are generally divided by application: airway management and ventilation, circulation with hemorrhage control, analgesia and medication, and splinting and immobilization (ikar-cisa.org/ikar-cisa/documents/2011/ikar2011 1027000798.pdf).[27] The airway management and ventilation bag should specifically contain a handheld suction device to clear airways, extension tubing with an interposed bacterial filter for ventilation maneuvers, nasogastric tube to empty the stomach in case of drowning, and other standard materials and backup devices. A cost-effective solution to extend oxygen use and minimize weight is the Oxymizer oxygen conserver with a B(M6) aluminum oxygen cylinder, or the Trek S portable aerosol system.[39] Intraosseous infusion systems should be included in the bag. The medication bag should contain antibiotics in case of wound contamination by water or long rescue times. Benzodiazepines and antiemetics should also be routinely carried, because they are the second most commonly used drug in canyon rescue (after analgesics).[45] SAM Splints are a valuable addition to the bag for splinting and immobilization; they are lightweight, reusable, and versatile, and can be formed into an improvised cervical spine collar. Neoprene splint kits usually contain 5 aluminum-bar–coated neoprene splints, which are malleable and allow quick immobilization; however, weight and volume can limit their use in ground rescue operations. Elastic bandages are preferred to adhesive tape because they work when wet. The Kendrick Extrication Device is a valuable immobilization device that can be used for spine immobilization during pickoff from a waterfall, or moving the victim to a safe and stable environment. A special harness that encloses both the patient and the Kendrick Extrication Device is used for hoist evacuations.[37]

Electronic devices should be avoided, although a portable pulse oximeter and heart rate monitor may be useful. Materials to prevent hypothermia are important. A thermometer for core temperature measurement is essential to accurately assess severity of hypothermia.[50] A drybag containing a monitor and automated external defibrillator should be available when managing critically injured patients.

Organization of Equipment Packs

SAR team members involved in the first response should have one pack for medical assessment and treatment and two packs for rope and swiftwater progression (Figure 98-24).[44] The medical pack should be organized according to the modality of assessment and treatment. Equipment for trauma care, hypothermia prevention, nutrition, and splinting and immobilization should be carried.[40]

The technical rescue medical kit should also be modular, and is carried by medical personnel of the SAR team. The National Park Service adopted a similar organization of medical equipment in which bags with basic and advanced materials are brought to the site depending on the level of care needed. The usefulness of routinely carrying advanced airway management equipment

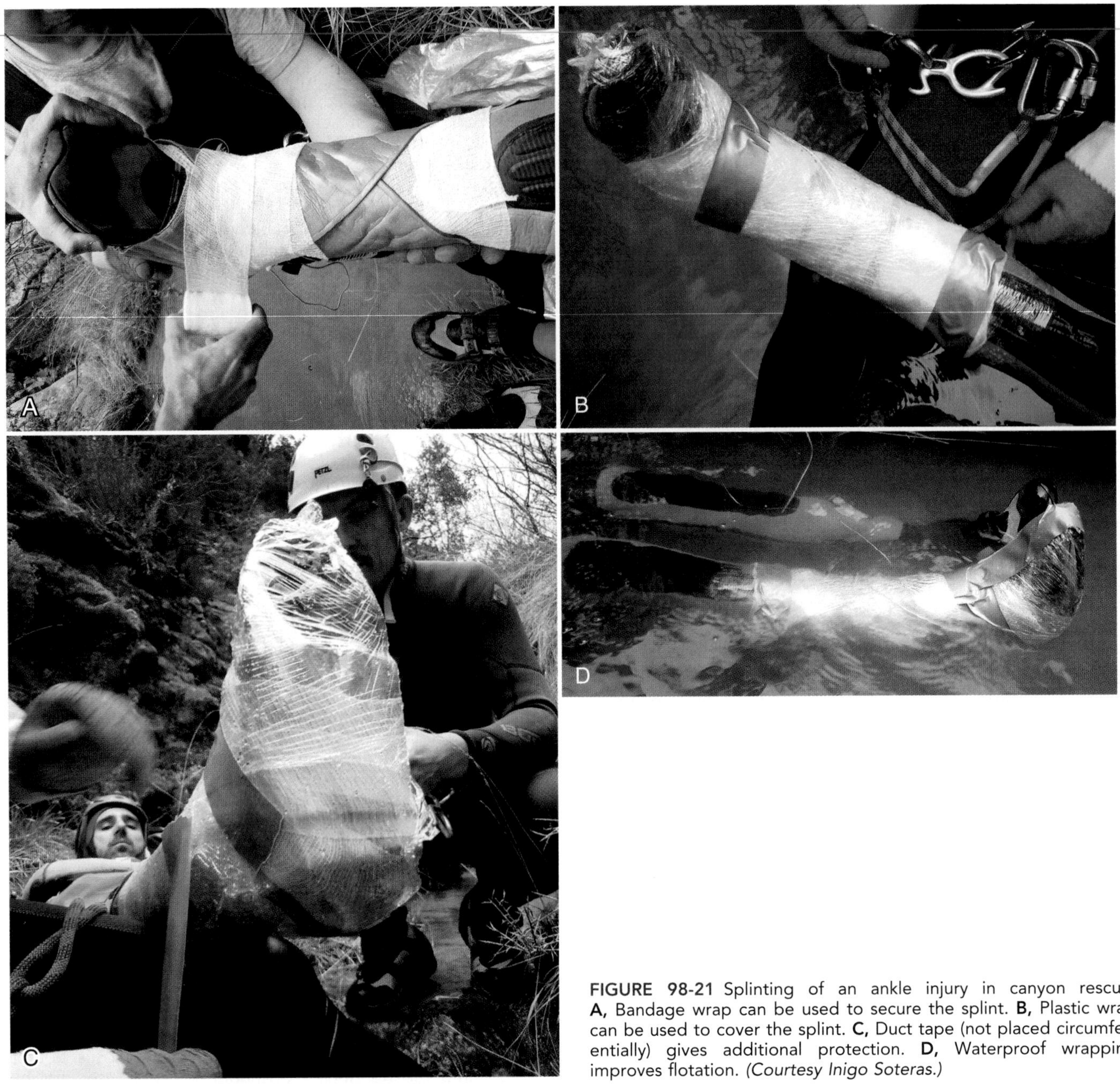

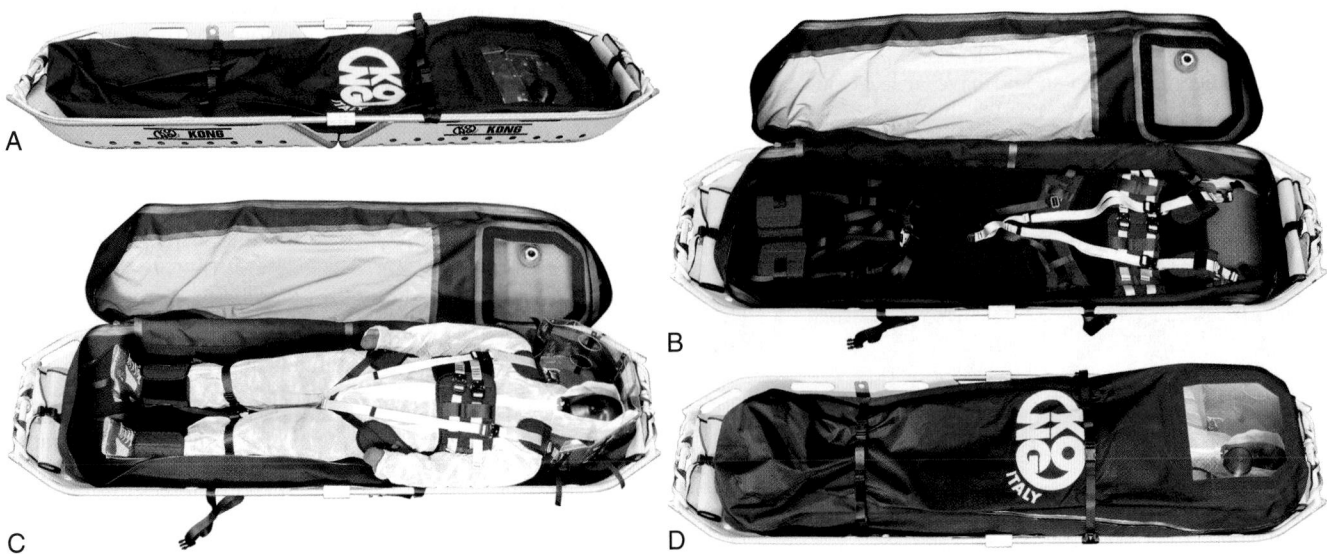

FIGURE 98-21 Splinting of an ankle injury in canyon rescue. **A,** Bandage wrap can be used to secure the splint. **B,** Plastic wrap can be used to cover the splint. **C,** Duct tape (not placed circumferentially) gives additional protection. **D,** Waterproof wrapping improves flotation. *(Courtesy Inigo Soteras.)*

FIGURE 98-22 Patient packaging. **A,** Kong 911 Canyon stretcher placed horizontally. **B,** Open waterproof bag with straps inside. **C,** Dummy placed inside and fixed with straps. **D,** Waterproof bag and external straps closed. *(Copyright KONG Italy. Courtesy Michael Kammerer: kong.it/.)*

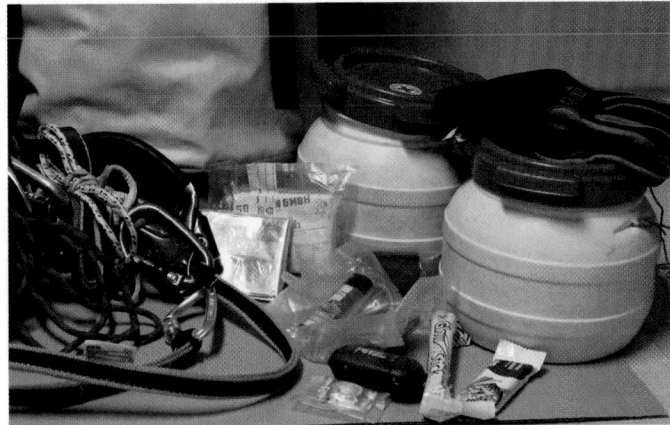

FIGURE 98-23 Canyoneering survival kit items should be kept in kegs, and equipment should be stored in sealed plastic bags. *(Courtesy Giacomo Strapazzon.)*

has been debated. It may be reasonable to have it available when there is an advanced life support provider.

Canyon Stretcher

Canyon stretchers should have the following features: (1) buoyancy; (2) ability to keep the patient dry; (3) ability to protect the victim from impact or collision; (4) suitability for sliding transport; and (5) suitability for rope transport. Some models use a removable float on a standard mountain-rescue stretcher to make a floatable stretcher that maintains the head of the supine patient above the water.[44] These models are not ideal in swiftwater or waterfalls because they do not guarantee sufficient protection for the patient. Other models are based on inflatable systems; the advantage being that they can be used in larger rivers with big pools, with the disadvantage being the risk of puncture and lack of rigid head protection.[38] A model developed with the Italian National Technical School for Canyoneering Rescue (CNSAS-SNaFor) can be positioned at an angle to adapt to the terrain, is buoyant, and has a built-in waterproof bag to keep the victim dry. The Kong 911 Canyon stretcher is designed to fully enclose the patient and has a float valve for water-based transportation (see Figure 98-22). This model has an aluminum-and-fiberglass shell to protect the victim from impact or collision, and has a transparent shield made of polycarbonate to protect the head.[44] Although the watertight seal is designed to allow relatively easy access to the patient, it can induce claustrophobia and prevent continuous communication. Medical personnel and stretcher attendants should continuously monitor the patient through the transparent shield and maintain radio communication. When using this model it is particularly important to open the bag and reevaluate the patient periodically, ideally every 10 minutes or less.[44] Internal webbing on stretchers helps secure the patient quickly and enables low- and high-angle operations. There are special accessories for stretchers for hoist evacuations. Similar to cave stretchers, many models can be disassembled into two pieces for easier transportation.[44]

EVACUATION

Evacuation Planning

Reaching the exit point of a canyon with an injured or ill patient can be a challenge. In Spain, 63% of SAR operations required technical proficiency over terrain with some grade of difficulty, mainly for incidents in a site with moderate to extremely difficult access. Six percent of SAR operations were done by ground rescue without air-based rescue, either due to adverse weather conditions (e.g., low clouds, rain, strong wind) or during night operations.[45] Data from France and La Reunion Island are similar.[10,42] Risk assessment is important in planning an evacuation strategy. The weather forecast should be continuously monitored during the rescue. It is preferable to transport without a stretcher if possible and plan a dry evacuation with alternative

transport, unless the rescue time is largely reduced with water transport (Figure 98-25). Artificial high directionals or hoists are techniques to evacuate an injured patient from a cliff wall. Technical details on canyon evacuations are covered in Chapter 56, Technical Rescue. If an advanced life support intervention is necessary for the patient's survival, risks versus benefits of the intervention are evaluated by the medical and technical leaders of the operation. It is usually preferable to avoid a night rescue (when the patient is not critically injured), if the operation can be suspended and resumed in the morning. When the canyon is located in a remote area, an external health post can provide valuable logistical and emergency support to emergency medical services teams.

Medical Considerations in Evacuation

The patient must be placed correctly in the stretcher before evacuation and transport (Figure 98-26). It is important to take measures (e.g., pillows and medications for prevention of decubitus lesions) to prevent complications associated with prolonged transport. Fluid and medications are given as boluses before transport. During evacuation, monitoring for possible complications or deterioration of clinical status is critical and should be done using all available means. Do not rely only on electronic devices. Medical personnel are not always within monitoring distance (e.g., when transporting the patient over a highline or

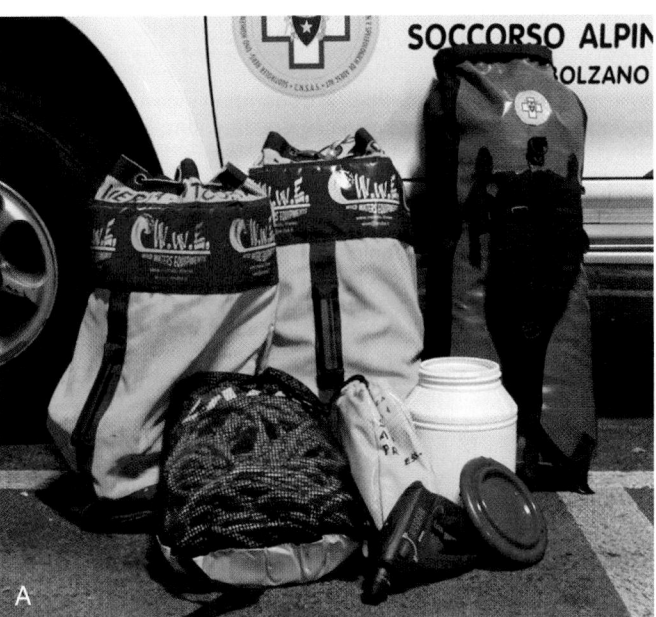

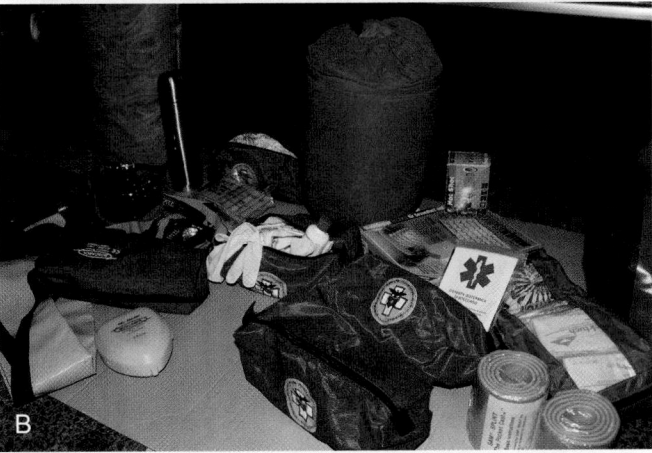

FIGURE 98-24 Organization of the first-response equipment according to standards of the Italian CNSAS canyon rescue team. **A,** *Left to right:* two packs for rope and swiftwater progression and one pack for medical assessment and treatment. **B,** Contents of a medical pack. *(Courtesy Giacomo Strapazzon.)*

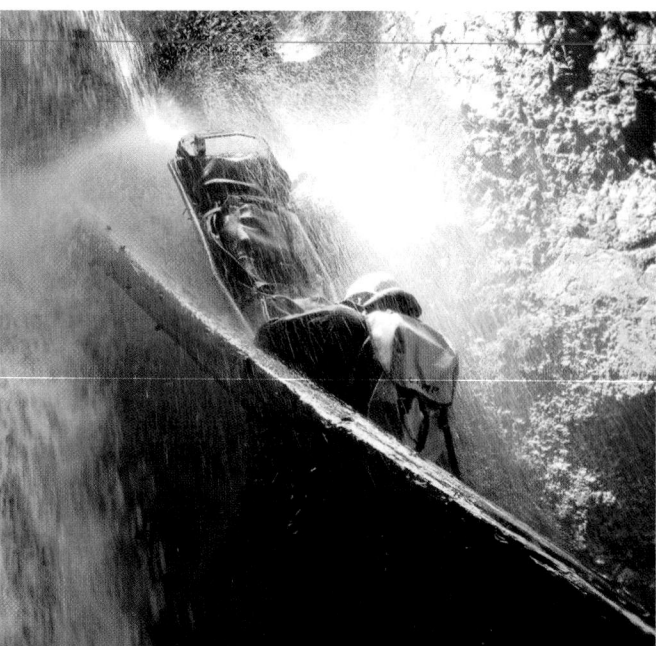

FIGURE 98-25 Transportation of a canyon stretcher in a waterfall by a SAR team member. *(Courtesy Erwin Kob.)*

in a waterfall) (see Figure 98-25). Continuing measures to prevent hypothermia are important, as is documenting information on the rescue and medical interventions.

Technical Materials for Evacuation by Search and Rescue Teams

Complete rescue equipment in Italy includes specific packs for rescue rigging (one pack for highline installation, one pack for drilling, and two packs for rope and swiftwater progression) and for evacuation with a stretcher (one pack for stretcher management, two packs with ropes for stretcher progression, and two packs for rope progression of the rescue team).[44]

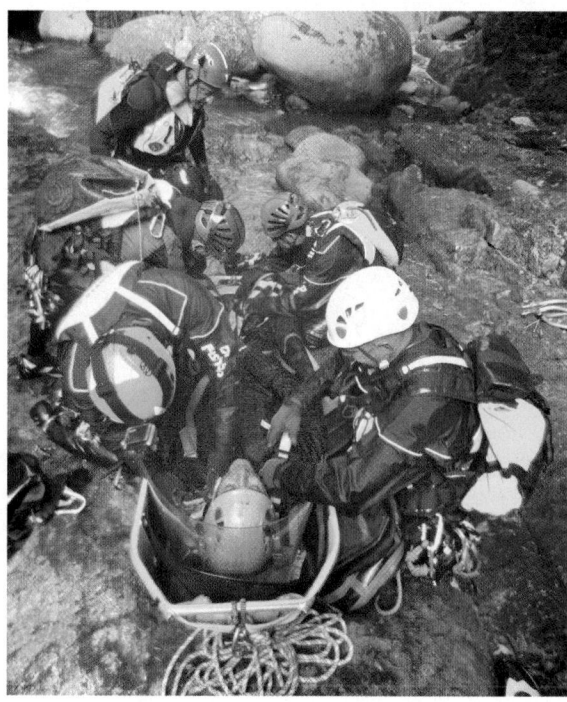

FIGURE 98-26 Assessment for correct placement of a patient in the stretcher before transport. Stretcher attendants should take care that the patient is not hit by carabiners and slings during the operations. *(Courtesy Oskar Piazza.)*

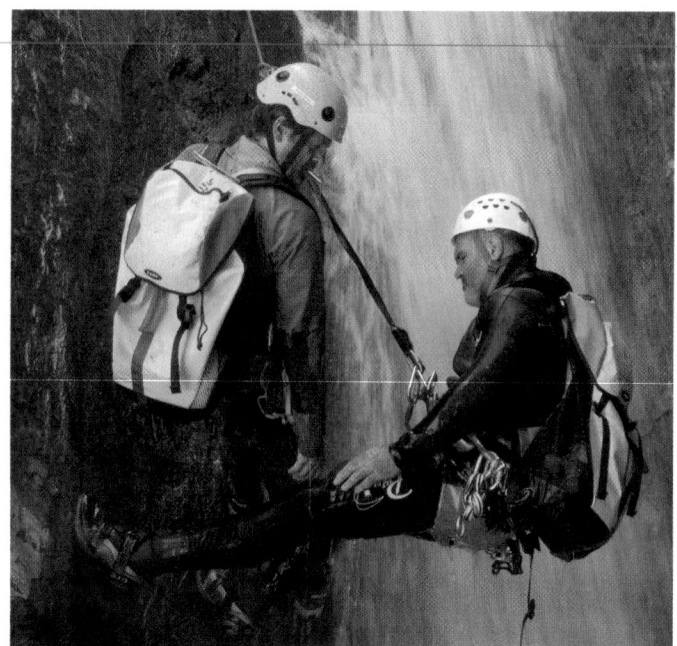

FIGURE 98-27 Communication of rescue orders during a SAR operation using a whistle. *(Courtesy Oskar Piazza.)*

Communication Equipment During Evacuation

Communication equipment is essential in canyoneering rescue. Standard whistle signals (Figure 98-27; see Table 98-1) and swiftwater hand signals are also used in canyoneering.[38] A SAR team member will commonly be posted in the canyon as a "radio relay" with one or more handheld radios. Waterproof field radios allow communication between different SAR team members in the canyon and between air and ground support teams. Radios should have at least an international protection level against liquid ingress (retain function after immersion for 30 minutes at a depth of 1 m).[44]

RESCUE

Companion Rescue

Companion rescue refers to management of an incident by fellow group members. Companion rescue can be lifesaving; wilderness basic life support and first-aid training should be included in canyoneering courses. Companion rescue is quite common, occurring in up to 50% of cases in a web-based survey of American and Australian canyoneers.[48] Incident management by companions is not well documented, although management of minor injuries, such as minor cutaneous and orthopedic injuries, seems to be common (Figure 98-28).

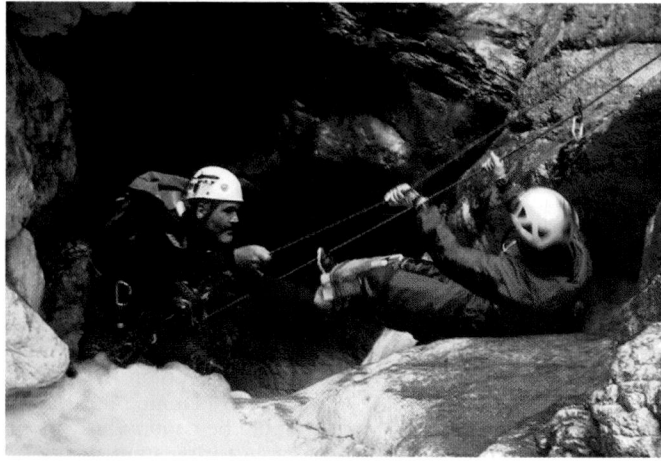

FIGURE 98-28 Companion rescue of a team member with an improvised splint. *(Courtesy Erwin Kob.)*

ICAR Medcom published recommendations on minimal requirements for medical training for professional guides (ikarcisa.org/ikar-cisa/documents/2011/ikar20111027000798.pdf).[57] These recommendations should be considered basic principles for any group leader, even those without professional certification. Canyoneering guides must be technically competent and have specific knowledge of water and helicopter rescue in canyons. Guides must also be familiar with the local SAR organization and proficient in delivering expected standards of patient care in the wilderness. In brief, emergency extrication of a person stuck on a rope is possible with a few additional carabiners and slings, and emergency rescue from swiftwater is possible with a throw bag if canyoneers have proper technical knowledge.

Companion rescue has particular importance in drowning incidents. The chance of successful resuscitation decreases with time; thus, prompt care by companions is crucial. Immediate ventilatory support and early chest compressions result in better prognosis and outcome in patients in cardiac or ventilatory arrest, but should be started when the patient is out of the water.

Search and Rescue Operations

Demographics of Search and Rescue Operations. Canyoneering incidents accounted for 2% of SAR operations in U.S. National Parks in 2005 (mountaineering also accounted for 2%). However, this proportionately small percentage of rescues belies the fact that the number of responses to canyoneering incidents doubled between 2003 to 2004 and 2005 to 2006.[20] Canyoneering incidents account for an even higher percentage of SAR operations in popular canyoneering regions (Figure 98-29). For example, it is one of the most common reasons for SAR operations in Utah's National Parks (up to 50% in Zion National Park and 27% in Glen Canyon National Recreation Area between 2001 and 2005).[21] In Italy and Spain, there was a concurrent reported increase in canyon rescue operations and higher percentage of SAR operations in popular canyoneering regions.[17,45]

SAR operations show seasonal peaks that reflect trends in recreation. In Zion National Park and surrounding regions, most incidents occur between May and November, with the highest peaks at the end of summer and beginning of autumn. At higher latitudes, most operations occur in July and August (canyoneering incidents accounting for 50% of cases in Spain; approximately 67% of cases in France).[42,45] In La Reunion Island, rescues are most common when canyoneering conditions are best and during the most popular vacation period.[10] Tourists and locals are equally involved in these incidents; for example, on La Reunion Island, one-third of all SAR operations involved tourists, one-third involved locals, and one-third were unknown.[10] In Spain, the demographics of rescued canyoneers reflect the entire population of canyoneers in that region; there is not a particular demographic category that has a higher frequency of incidents.[5,45] However, 23 (5%) patients were under the age of 16 years. Data from France were similar.[42]

Comparatively, most emergency calls involve nonguided groups as opposed to guided groups (nonguided groups accounted for ~ 80% of calls in France and on La Reunion Island).[10,42] Alerts made by nonguided groups involved both a higher percentage of major injuries and illnesses and a person or group trapped in difficult terrain with limited evacuation options.[42]

Duration of Search and Rescue Operations. A typical scenario in Zion National Park is an incident occurring in the early afternoon. Cellular phone service is limited, and the narrow slot canyons also limit reception for satellite phones. A group member or another group often has to complete the canyon route and hike out to inform the park rangers. A first SAR team of rangers is sent to the incident site to assess the situation. At this time, darkness is usually approaching, and unless the patient is critically injured, rangers spend the night with the patient in location awaiting daylight and a full rescue team to complete evacuation. If the victim is critically ill or injured, the rescue and evacuation operation continues through the night, despite the potential risk to the SAR team.

Data from European SAR groups demonstrate similar rescue procedures and concurrent rescue durations. In France, mean rescue duration from the incident to admission to an acute care facility (or evacuation of uninjured patients) was 170 minutes

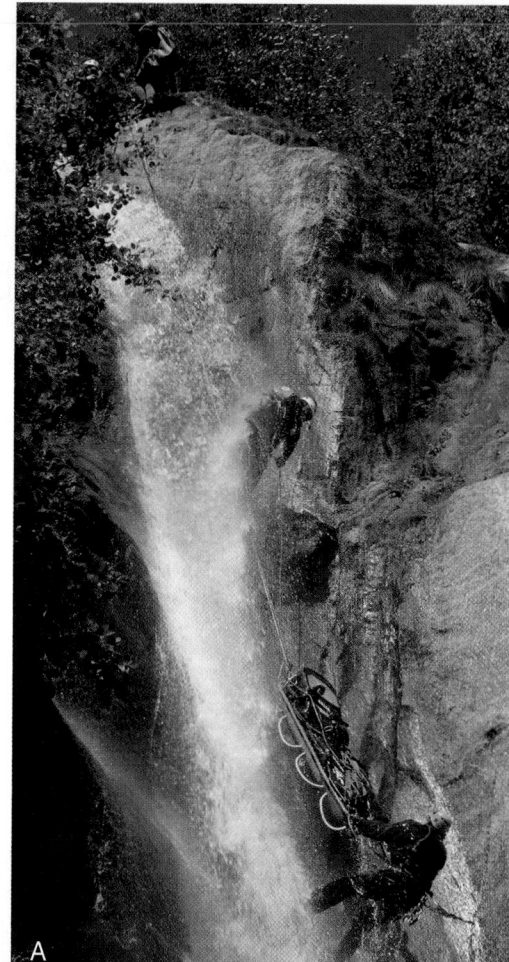

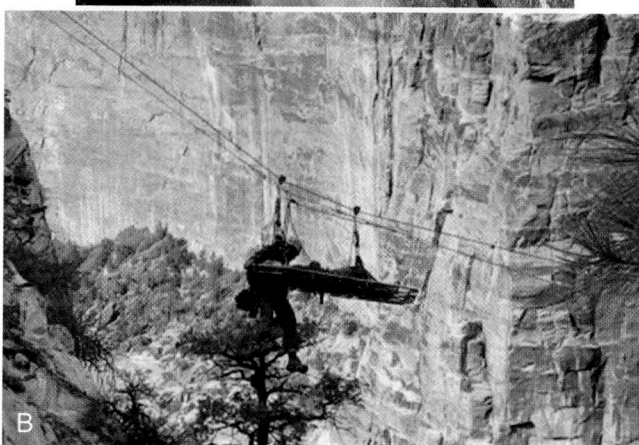

FIGURE 98-29 Transport of a stretcher by a SAR team. A, High-angle terrain in a wet canyon. B, Highline in a dry canyon. (*Courtesy Oskar Piazza [A] and Gordon Larsen [B].*)

(range, 35 to 1140 minutes).[42] Long SAR operations were either due to delay in response time or prolonged rescue effort at the scene of the incident. The mean time to the emergency call was 83 minutes (range, 1 to 980 minutes). Similar to the scenario described in Zion National Park, in many cases delays incurred during response to an incident and subsequent rescue efforts were due to problems with electronic communication, lack of group proficiency, and long exit routes. Understanding the challenges of the canyon environment, alternative escape routes, and contact strategies with the local SAR organization can speed up rescue operations. The time from the incident to the emergency call for nonguided canyoneers was nearly double that for professionally guided groups.[42] The mean scene time was 104 minutes (range, 10 to 725 minutes) and approximately 86 minutes with the exclusion of extreme values. In Spain, the median time from emergency call to admission to an acute care facility (or evacuation for uninjured patients) was 90 minutes (range, 10 to 860 minutes).[45] Almost 50% of SAR operations in Spain involved ground rescue with or without air rescue support.[45] Helicopter-supported rescue can reduce this time. Successful hoist operations during canyon rescues have been reported.[36] Helicopters that are equipped with a hoist or a short-haul can transport the SAR team with all necessary rescue and medical equipment directly to the site or to the nearest possible access site.[53] In France and on La Reunion Island, air rescue was also common (alone or in combination with ground rescue), but up to 20% of SAR operations involved only ground rescue.[10,42] Despite the observation that most of the injuries in canyoneering are of mild to moderate severity, duration of the potential rescue scenario probably justifies on-site presence of an emergency medical technician, paramedic, or physician.

Financial Costs of Canyon Rescue. Financial costs of canyon rescue are high. The Zion National Park Service was among the U.S. National Park Service units with the highest total and average SAR operation costs in 2005.[20] Many U.S. National Parks have introduced permits for technical canyoneering trips to reduce the number of incidents. Although Zion National Park does not charge for SAR operations, ambulance transfer and hospital care are expensive. Personal health insurance is strongly recommended for canyoneers.

Education of Search and Rescue Teams for Canyon Rescue. In the United States, SAR operations in slot canyons usually involve the National Park Service. Occasionally local agency rescue teams, usually county-based teams, are called to support a rescue. There are no specific canyoneering courses or guidelines used in the United States or by the National Park Service, but rescue teams working in regions with canyons have become familiar with canyon rescue. In France in the 1990s, the mountain rescue organization implemented specific training and rescue protocols for SAR teams involved in canyon rescue operations. In 2005, the Italian mountain rescue founded the CNSAS SNaFor with certified national instructors and specific training for rescuers as standard.

SAR team members (and companions) should be able to perform patient assessment and treatment at the basic level of an emergency medical technician. The ICAR Medcom developed specific recommendations for use of medical equipment.[27] The National Park Service developed emergency medical protocols for SAR teams in the United States.[39,43] Rescue personnel are trained in basic emergency medical technician care, and many National Park rangers complete a rigorous emergency medical services course similar to that completed by paramedics.

ACKNOWLEDGMENTS

The authors acknowledge Emily Procter, Craig Thexton, Erwin Kob, Oskar Piazza, Gigliola Mancinelli, Inigo Soteras, and Hermann Brugger for their invaluable input.

REFERENCES

Complete references used in this text are available online at expertconsult.inkling.com.

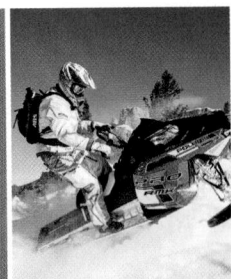

CHAPTER 99
Cycles, Snowmobiles, and Other Wilderness Conveyances

TODD W. THOMSEN

MOUNTAIN BIKES

The sport of mountain bicycling began in the 1970s when cyclists looking for new challenges began riding 1950s-era bikes (complete with balloon tires and coaster brakes) down the rocky trails of Mt Tamalpais in Marin County, California. Recognizing the need for better equipment, Joe Breeze is credited with building the first mountain bike with 26-inch knobby tires in 1977.[31] The popularity of mountain biking has grown quickly.[15] Mountain bikes accounted for 25% of all bicycle sales over the past decade. Today, sanctioned races are held in a variety of disciplines, ages, and skill levels.[38,75,97,131] Mountain biking became an Olympic sport in 1996 and achieved full Olympic status in 2000.[99,121] Approximately 40 million Americans participate in the sport annually.[74,119]

Most enthusiasts ride recreationally for fun and exercise. Mountain biking has distinct categories. *Cross-country cycling* involves traversing varied terrain, including uphill sections, and requires a great deal of aerobic fitness (Figure 99-1). Cross-country races may last several hours.[76] Participants often perform at 90% of maximum heart rate during the entire race.[75] *Downhill riding* involves high-speed descents on trails with varied terrain (Figure 99-2). Jumps and other acrobatic stunts are common and increase risk of injury.[21,35] Downhill races may last only minutes, but speeds of up to 70 miles per hour (mph) can be achieved by experts.[38] *Freeriding* focuses on tricks and jumps of downhill riding (Figure 99-3).[38] Mountain biking parks use ski lifts to carry riders up mountains. They have numerous terrain features used for jumps.[141] *Four-cross* and *dual-slalom races* are head-to-head racing events on downhill courses (Figure 99-4).[38,121] *Endurance races* last more than 6 hours. *Stage races* are long-distance events over the course of several days.[15,110]

EQUIPMENT

Mountain bike frames can range from heavy, inexpensive steel models to lightweight and expensive carbon fiber frames. Frames made of aluminum and titanium can be crafted to suit particular types of riding (e.g., cross-country and downhill).

Many mountain bikes have a front suspension fork that reduces trail vibrations and improves steering and control. Some bikes also feature rear suspensions. This increases riding efficiency and decreases trail vibrations to the rider (Figure 99-5).[58,122,149] Riders of full-suspension bicycles may experience fewer injuries.[14,121] Fat bikes have large (> 4 inches in width) low-pressure tires that allow riding in "soft" conditions (e.g., on sand or snow) (Figure 99-6).

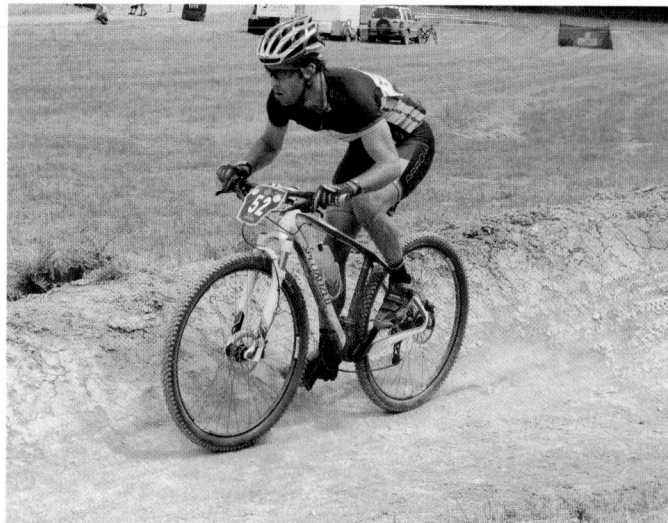

FIGURE 99-1 Cross-country mountain bike racer. Cross-country riding involves cycling over varied terrain, and often includes extended uphill sections.

Mountain bikes often are equipped with powerful disk brakes that allow braking in wet conditions and may reduce the incidence of rider injury.[121] Clipless pedal systems allow the foot to lock onto a pedal until a twisting motion of the foot releases the cleat. Clipless pedal systems increase pedaling efficiency. Failure to disengage the foot during a fall may lead to rider injury.[128]

PROTECTIVE GEAR

The majority of mountain bikers wear helmets.[14,35,38] Bicycling helmets made of expanded polystyrene foam are most commonly used.[25] Downhill and freeride cyclists frequently use full-face helmets to provide additional protection.[14] Other protective gear includes neck braces, padded thoracic jackets, padded cycling shorts, and pads for shoulders, elbows, knees, and shins (Figure 99-7).[21] Cycling gloves decrease injuries.[14] Mouth guards are rarely used, but may provide protection against dental trauma.[15] Use of protective gear should be guided by the type of riding pursued. At a minimum, a helmet, gloves, and protective eyewear should be worn.

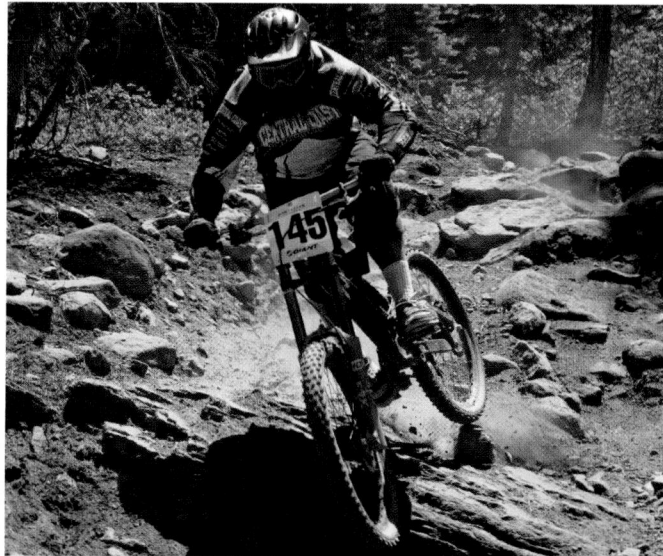

FIGURE 99-2 Downhill mountain bike racer. Downhill riding consists of cycling down steep hills at high speeds. Natural and man-made trail features and obstacles are commonly encountered. *(Courtesy Dr. Steven J. Wolf.)*

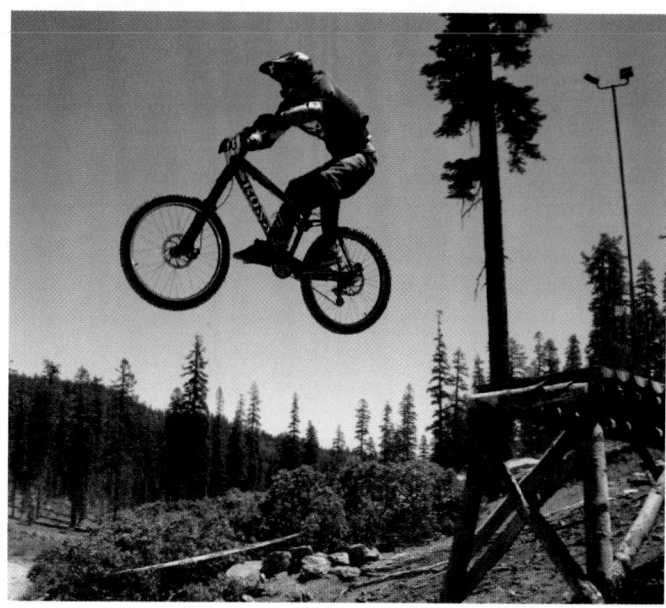

FIGURE 99-3 Freeriding is similar to downhill biking. Jumps and acrobatic stunts performed at high speeds are the focus of this discipline. *(Courtesy Dr. Steven J. Wolf.)*

MECHANISM OF INJURY

Falling Over the Handlebars

Falling over the handlebars (colloquially referred to as an *endo*) is the most common mechanism of injury in mountain biking (Figure 99-8).[35,94] This occurs when the front tire makes impact with an immobile object or when the front brake locks the front wheel and the rider continues to rotate around the pivot point of the front axle. Over-the-handlebar incidents are typically more severe than sideways falls and associated with distinct injuries that include head, neck, facial, and dental trauma.[15,38,45,95,121] If the abdomen strikes the handlebars, injury to the liver, spleen, and diaphragm may occur.[15] Fractures and dislocations of the shoulder, elbow, forearm, and wrist are common.[21,35,84,121]

Falling Sideways

The other common mountain bike injury is falling to the side (Figure 99-9). Bicycles are inherently less stable at lower speeds, which can lead to sideways falls when riding uphill over technical terrain. High-speed cornering or jumping over obstacles during descent can also lead to sideways falls. These falls tend to injure the lower extremities, although upper extremity injuries may occur if the fall is on an outstretched hand.[21,38,45]

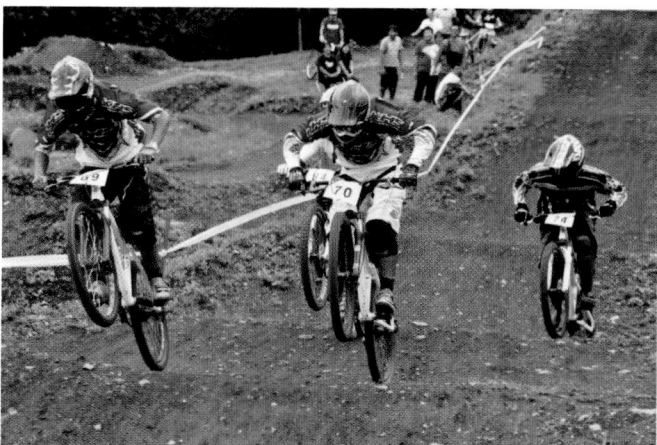

FIGURE 99-4 Four-cross racing involves head-to-head racing on downhill courses. High-speed crashes and collisions with other riders are ever-present possibilities.

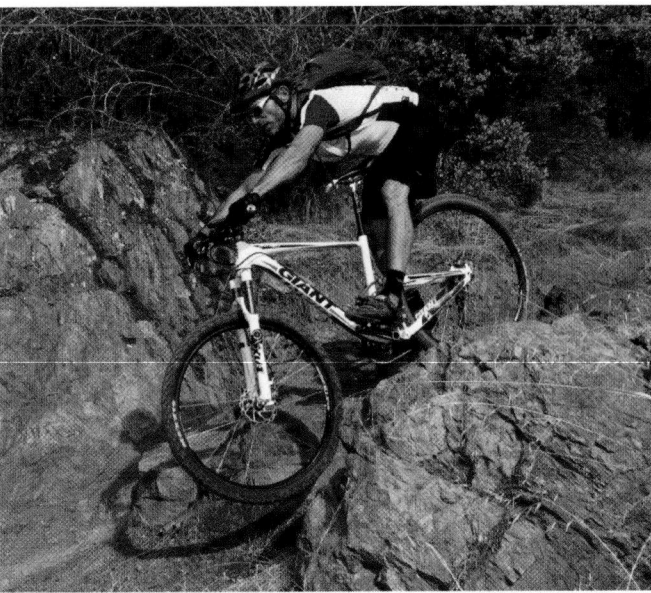

FIGURE 99-5 Modern mountain bicycles are highly specialized pieces of equipment. This bike has front and rear suspensions, disk brakes, and clipless pedals. Such features are common on today's bikes. *(Courtesy Dr. Steven J. Wolf.)*

Pedal-Related Injuries

On bikes with clipless pedal systems, if the rider fails to disengage the foot from the pedal during a fall, lower extremity injuries (e.g., soft tissue injury, femur and acetabular fractures) may result.[128] Riders using traditional flat pedals (i.e., platform pedals) are also at risk for pedal-related injury. If the foot slips, the pedal may forcefully hit the shin, causing a laceration or avulsion injury.

EPIDEMIOLOGY OF MOUNTAIN BIKING INJURIES

Injury Rates

Reliable estimates of injury rates experienced by mountain bicyclists are limited. Such injuries are likely to be underreported.[15]

In the United States, approximately 15,000 patients are treated annually for injuries related to mountain biking.[121] Common injuries are fractures, soft tissue injuries, and lacerations. Five percent of patients are hospitalized. Overall, accidents declined by 56% between 1995 and 2007. No fatalities were reported. In

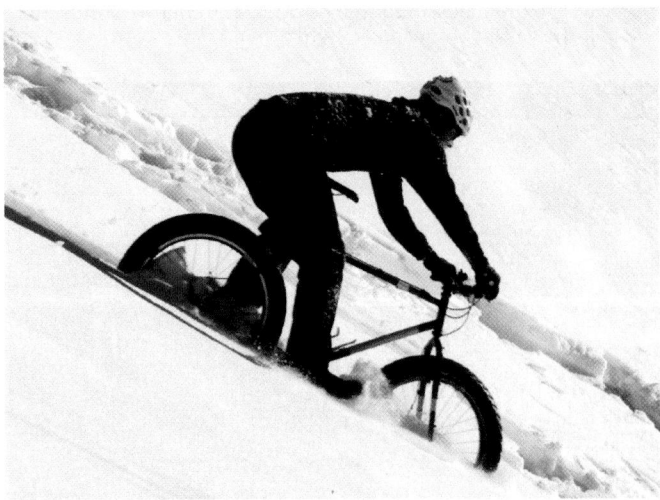

FIGURE 99-6 Fat bikes are increasingly popular versions of mountain bikes. Fat bikes have massive low-pressure tires that allow for riding in unconventional cycling environments, such as through snow and sand. *(Courtesy Anthony DeLorenzo.)*

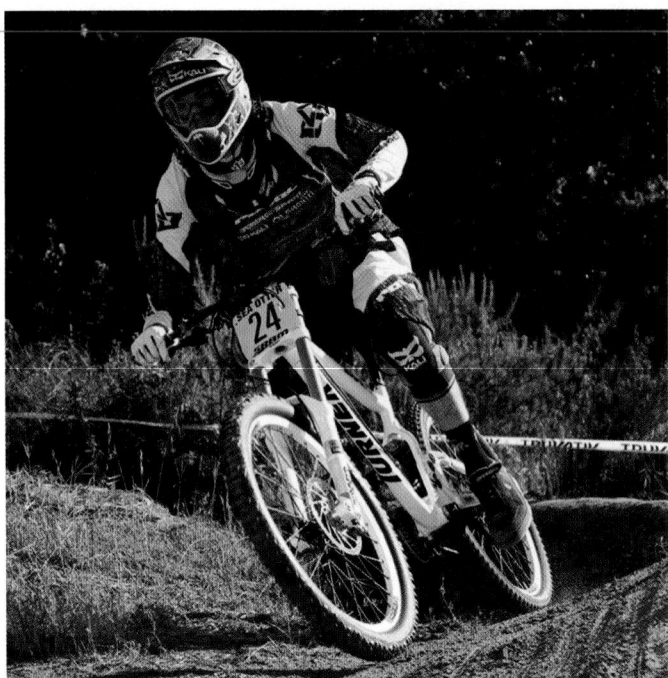

FIGURE 99-7 Protective gear. This downhill racer is wearing a full complement of protective gear. Note the full-face helmet, goggles, neck brace, arm and leg pads, and gloves. Using such equipment decreases risk of injury. *(Courtesy Dr. Steven J. Wolf.)*

one study, trauma center admissions for mountain biking injuries increased threefold from 1992 to 2002.[89]

Some studies define the rate of injuries from mountain biking in terms of injuries-per-hour-of-biking or injuries-per-biking-exposure. Recreational riders experience 1.54 injuries per 1000 biker-exposures (one biker-exposure equals one person riding a mountain bike on 1 day).[14] If one injury occurs per 1000 hours of mountain biking, that equals a risk of injury of 0.6% per year.[65] Similar results are described in a pediatric population.[15]

Mountain biking may present a higher risk of injury than other common outdoor activities. In a review of a college outdoor program, mountain biking resulted in 7.5 injuries per 1000 participant days, a higher rate than for mountain climbing, backpacking, kayaking, hiking, cross-country skiing, and snowshoeing.[64]

Age and Gender

Most mountain bikers are young men, 20 to 39 years old), and they suffer most of the injuries.[18,35,38,45,84,89,121]. Female riders may be injured at higher rates than men.[121] In a study of a large off-road race, 0.77% of women sustained injuries, versus 0.44% of men.[96] Women were 1.94 times more likely to be injured, and 4.17 times more likely to sustain a fracture.

Older patients may be at higher risk for more severe injuries than their younger counterparts. Patients more than 40 years old are more likely to suffer dislocations or to be hospitalized.[121] Patients between the ages of 14 and 19 years sustained more traumatic brain injuries (TBIs) than did all other age groups combined; this may be secondary to decreased helmet use by these riders.

Types of Injuries

Most mountain biking injuries are minor. The appendicular skeleton is more likely to be injured than is the axial spine. Hospitalization rates of injured mountain bikers are poorly documented; in one series, the rate was 16%.[14]

Minor injuries (e.g., abrasions, contusions, and lacerations) are the most commonly reported conditions and account for more than 50% of injuries. They are usually of little clinical consequence.[21,94] Fractures of the upper extremities occur in 10% to

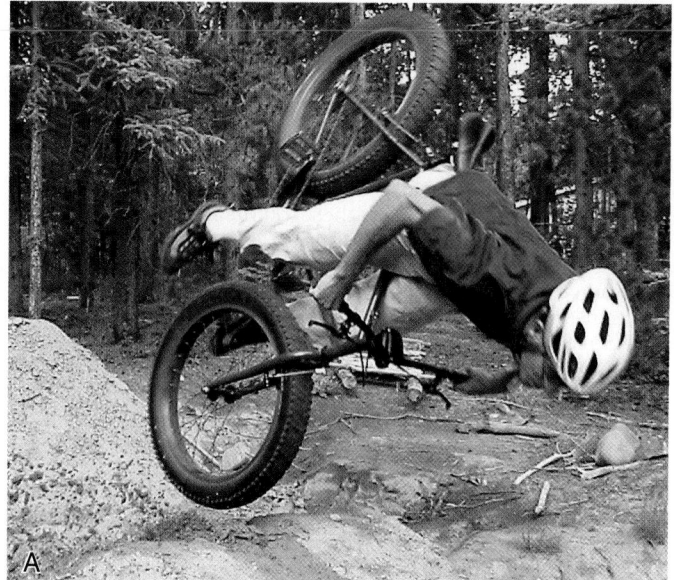

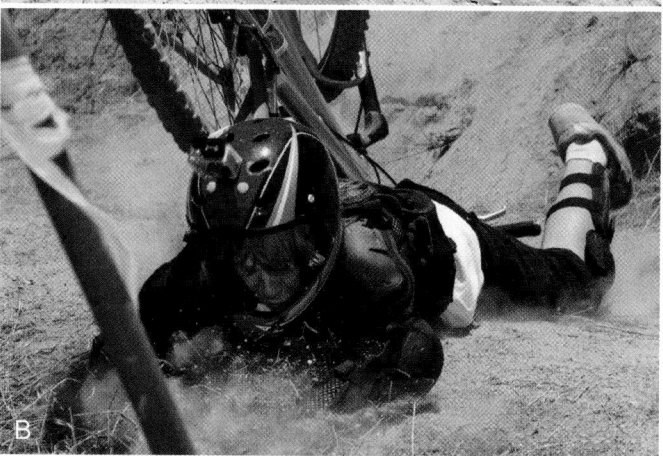

FIGURE 99-8 Over-the-handlebars mechanism of injury. **A,** Over-the-handlebar crashes occur when the front tire comes to an abrupt stop, usually after striking an immobile object or locking up the front brake. The momentum of the bike continues forward and rotates around the front axle. There is potential for substantial head, cervical spine, thoracoabdominal, and upper extremity injury. **B,** This cyclist also crashed over the handlebars. Note how the use of protective gear (full-face helmet, torso protector, and arm and leg pads) shields the biker from injury. (**A** *courtesy Anthony Lorenzo;* **B** *courtesy Dr. Steven J. Wolf.*)

20% of U.S. emergency department cases.[45,84] Lower extremity fractures occur less frequently.[21]

In a review of mountain biking injuries requiring trauma center admission in Vancouver, orthopedic injuries (46%) accounted for the majority of cases, followed by head and spine (12% each), chest (10%), abdominal (5%), and genitourinary injuries (2%).[89] Sixty-six percent of these admitted patients required operative intervention. Only one fatality was reported during this 10-year period.

Injury Rates for Different Types of Riding

Although studies of mountain biking injury rates have focused mainly on racing environments, the vast majority of injuries occur in recreational riders.[84]

Downhill mountain biking is more dangerous than cross-country riding. In two studies, downhill rates of injury were 16.8 and 43.4 injuries per 1000 hours of exposure, a rate significantly higher than the rate for cross-country riding, at 3.7 and 12 injuries per 1000 hours of exposure.[38,21] Downhill riding rates of injury decrease as rider experience increases; more injuries are sustained during competition than during practice.[21]

Cross-country racing may be more dangerous than endurance or stage racing. Lareau found that 7.2% of cross-country riders were injured during a race versus 4.7% of endurance race riders.[97] Cross-country races last about 2 hours; endurance races last longer than 6 hours. These differences may be due to the greater intensity of cross-country racing or the greater experience of endurance riders. Most injuries in the endurance and stage racers were minor (e.g., abrasions, contusions, strains, and blisters).[110]

Mountain biking has been reported to be more dangerous than road cycling. Palmer reported that mountain bikers suffered 14.4 accidents per 100,000 km cycled; city cyclists suffered 1.7 accidents per 100,000 km. Touring cyclists suffered 11.5 injuries per 100,000 km.[127] Mountain bikers are more likely to sustain fractures, dislocations, and concussions than are their road-riding counterparts.[131] Although the mechanism of injury often differed between road and mountain cyclists (e.g., being struck by another vehicle versus falling during a jump), similar types of injuries were encountered (e.g., head injury, facial trauma, and extremity injury).[140]

Causes of Mountain Biking Injuries

Rider error (e.g., poor judgment, excessive speed, and overestimation of ability) is the most common cause of injury.[21,65,94] Factors external to the rider (e.g., irregular terrain surfaces, bad trail conditions, unforeseen obstacles, and equipment failure) also are frequently blamed for crashes leading to injury.[21,94]

ACUTE MOUNTAIN BIKING INJURIES

Craniofacial, Brain, and Cervical Spine Injuries

Craniofacial injuries often occur in over-the-handlebar crashes (see Figure 99-8A). Mountain bikers are more likely to sustain facial injuries (e.g., facial bone fractures, dentoalveolar injuries, and facial soft tissue injuries) than are road cyclists.[38] One survey found that 30% of riders had suffered or knew a rider who had sustained either a dental fracture or an avulsion.[117] Most of the respondents were not aware that avulsed teeth could be reimplanted. Education about self-reimplantation in the field and routine use of mouth guards was suggested.

Rare facial injuries include a degloving injury of the oral mucosa in a cyclist who crashed during performance of an aerial stunt.[138] In one report, a foreign body perforated the tympanic membrane during a fall, resulting in trans-tympanic facial nerve injury and facial palsy.[116] Wearing a full-face helmet would likely prevent many of these injuries, especially when descending at high speed (Figure 99-10).

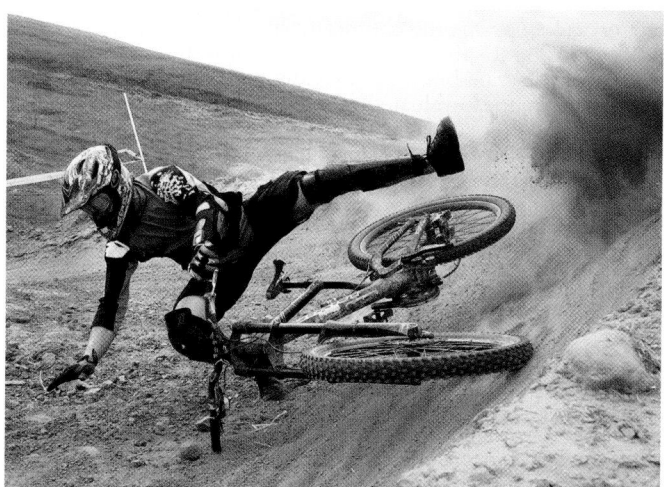

FIGURE 99-9 Fall-off-the-side mechanism of injury. Riders falling off the side of the bike are at risk for lower extremity injuries. Falls on outstretched hands, as depicted above, can lead to scaphoid fracture, distal radius fracture, and posterior elbow dislocation. (*Courtesy Dr. Steven J. Wolf.*)

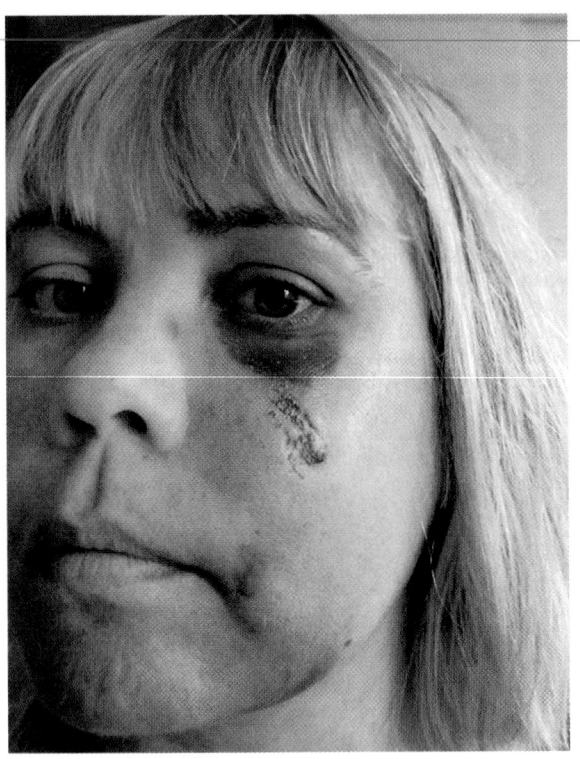

FIGURE 99-10 This mountain biker sustained facial contusions, a mild concussion, and a shoulder contusion after falling over the handlebars of her bike. The accident was caused by overzealous application of the front brake during descent. She was wearing a helmet and escaped serious injury. (*Courtesy Cynthia Froning.*)

Brain injuries (e.g., concussions and other TBIs) occur at a much lower frequency than does extremity trauma.[15,45,84,121] Intracranial hemorrhage is even more rare.[15,121] Use of full-face helmets (as compared with traditional cycling helmets) is not associated with decreased incidence of TBI.[14]

One series describes patients with symptoms consistent with benign positional paroxysmal vertigo occurring several hours after a mountain bike race.[168] Frequent vibratory impacts, repeated acceleration and deceleration, and increased gravitational forces experienced during jumping and landing were theorized to cause displacement of otoconia, leading to benign paroxysmal positional vertigo–like symptoms. All riders recovered without sequelae.

Cervical spine injuries are relatively rare. Vertebral fractures, dislocations, and spinal cord trauma (with resulting paraplegia) have been described.[15,38,84] In a review of mountain bike–related axial spine injuries evaluated at a regional spine referral center, 95% percent of patients were male. The mean age was 32.7 years.[56] Forty percent sustained spinal cord injuries; two patients remained dependent on a ventilator at the time of discharge.

Thoracoabdominal Injuries

Rib fractures are the most commonly reported thoracic injury in mountain bikers.[14] More severe chest trauma is rare; however, reports exist of these injuries, such as hemopneumothorax requiring tube thoracostomy.[84] Ortega reported a series of 11/11 cyclists with elevated cardiac troponin (cTnI) levels after a 95-km race.[125] None experienced cardiovascular symptoms. The clinical significance of this finding is unclear. Piniewska-Juraszek reported the case of a 41-year-old male cyclist who suffered ventricular fibrillation cardiac arrest during a 32-km mountain bike race.[134] The patient was successfully defibrillated in the field and ultimately diagnosed with acute anterior wall myocardial infarction due to left anterior coronary artery occlusion.

Abdominal injury is much more common than thoracic injury in mountain bikers. A common mechanism of injury is blunt force trauma from the handlebars.[15,38] The abdominal wall should be examined for a *handlebar bruise* as a sign of intraabdominal injury[57] (Figure 99-11). Solid-organ injuries (e.g., liver and spleen laceration or hematoma) are the most commonly encountered intraabdominal injuries.[15,38,120] Hollow viscus injuries (e.g., small bowel hematoma and jejunal rupture) occur less frequently.[38,148] Rare intraabdominal injuries include diaphragmatic rupture, pancreatic transection, and small bowel evisceration.[38,102,105]

Infectious gastroenteritis outbreaks after mountain bike races have been reported.[69,86,160] In these outbreaks, the race course passed through muddy fields and *Campylobacter jejuni* was identified as the source. Mud contaminated with animal feces (the source of *C. jejuni*) likely splashed onto the riders' faces or was transmitted from dirty water bottles. Rider education, provision of clean water, and attention to food hygiene at aid stations are recommended.

Genitourinary Injuries

Blunt abdominal trauma may cause renal contusion and fracture.[14,84] Traumatic arterial priapism has been reported, usually from a direct blow to the perineum by the bicycle's top tube.[53,66,77] Selective arterial embolization was required to achieve detumescence. A case of spontaneous intracavernosal hematoma in a long-distance mountain cyclist has been reported.[177] Chronic genitourinary maladies in cyclists are more common and are discussed later in this chapter.

Appendicular Skeleton Injuries

Upper Extremity Injuries. Extremity fractures are much more common than are axial injuries.[14] Upper extremity fractures occur when one falls onto an outstretched hand or uses the arm to protect the face during a fall.[15,38] Clavicle fractures are extremely common, and often incurred with a fall over the handlebars.[84] Distal radius fractures, scaphoid fractures, and elbow dislocations result from falling onto an outstretched hand[38,84] (Figure 99-12). Radial head fractures, metacarpal and phalangeal fractures, and dislocations are common.[35,136] Soft tissue injuries are also extremely common[15,35] (Figure 99-13).

Lower Extremity Injuries. Lower extremity fractures occur less frequently than do upper extremity fractures. Femur and acetabular fractures have occurred in riders falling sideways with feet still engaged in clipless pedals.[154] Tibia and femur fractures have been documented.[15,38,84] Callaghan reported a rider who sustained a Lisfranc fracture-dislocation after failing to disengage from a clipless pedal. This is reminiscent of the original 19th century description of Lisfranc injury in a soldier who fell from his horse with his boot still caught in the stirrup.[36] Soft tissue injuries of the leg are extremely common. The shin is particularly susceptible to soft tissue injury secondary to blunt trauma by rocks, undergrowth, and bicycle pedals.[15,38] Shin and knee protectors decrease incidence and magnitude of these injuries.

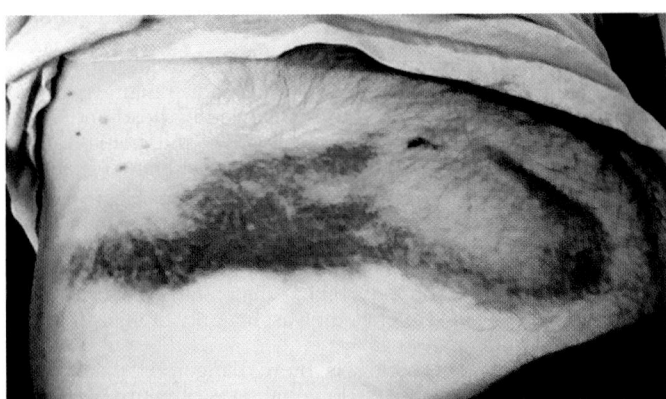

FIGURE 99-11 Handlebar bruise. Patients who go over the handlebars should be examined for a handlebar bruise. This finding indicates substantial impact between the anterior abdominal wall and the handlebars, and raises suspicion for liver or splenic injury. Hollow viscus injuries are less common.

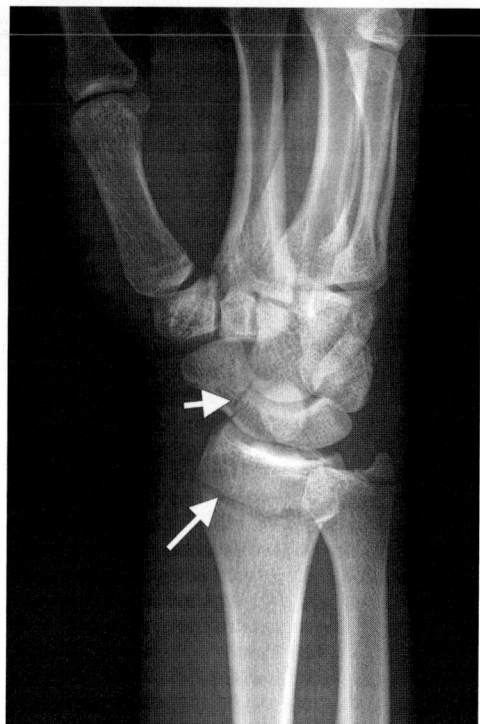

FIGURE 99-12 Distal radius and scaphoid fractures. This patient fell off his bike onto an outstretched hand. Distal radius fracture (*long arrow*) and scaphoid fracture (*short arrow*) are common injuries in this type of accident.

Electrolyte Disorders

Exercise-associated hyponatremia (EAH) is commonly seen in endurance athletes; up to 22% of marathon runners may be afflicted. Mountain bikers competing in long-distance events may be similarly at risk.[88] EAH (i.e., water intoxication) results from fluid consumption in excess of losses during prolonged exercise, and can occur up to 24 hours after the event.[44] EAH risk factors include slow pace, duration of exercise greater than 4 hours, low-body mass, preexercise hydration, use of nonsteroidal antiinflammatory drugs (NSAIDs), and extremely hot or cold environments.[44] Symptoms are nonspecific (e.g., nausea, vomiting, confusion, and headache); more severe cases present with seizures, pulmonary and cerebral edema, and death.[44] Mountain

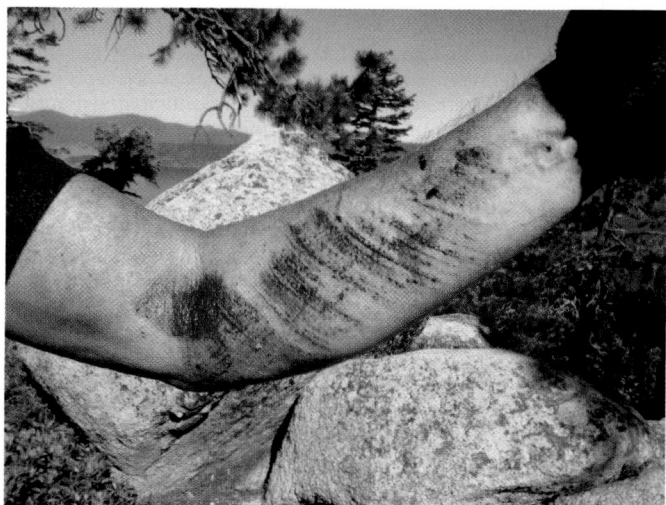

FIGURE 99-13 Soft tissue injuries, such as this abrasion, are among the most common maladies encountered in mountain biking.

cyclists competing in endurance events often carry one or two 24-oz water bottles, and may also use a backpack hydration system that can carry up to 100 oz. Aid stations offer water or other fluids. Remaining hydrated during exercise is a great concern, but avoiding overhydration is equally important.[91] Because EAH is not chronic hyponatremia, rapid correction with hypertonic saline is considered to be safe and does not risk central pontine demyelination.[88]

Despite the apparent risk of endurance mountain cyclists developing EAH, multiple reviews in the literature have failed to document its occurrence.[44,90,91,142] The reason for the low incidence in endurance cyclists versus other endurance athletes is unclear.

EAH is prevented by avoiding overconsumption of hypotonic fluids. A recommended starting point for hydration is consumption of 0.4 to 0.8 L of fluid per hour; electrolyte-containing sports drinks are likely preferable to water.[147] In the studies above, drinking to the dictates of thirst was a successful strategy.

Severe and Fatal Injuries

Severe and fatal mountain biking injuries are rare. Intracranial hemorrhage, cervical spine injuries, hemopneumothorax, blunt abdominal trauma, and fatalities have been reported in small numbers.[15,84] In a 12-year review of U.S. emergency department visits for mountain biking injuries, no fatal injuries were identified.[121] Aitken reported no fatal injuries in a review of Scottish mountain biking injuries.[14] Media reports exist of individual fatal mountain biking accidents.[37,164,173]

CHRONIC MOUNTAIN BIKING INJURIES (OVERUSE SYNDROMES)

Mountain cyclists are at risk for chronic injuries (i.e., overuse syndromes) caused by body positions sustained over extended periods while riding over rough terrain surfaces (e.g., roots, rocks, and ledges). Overuse syndromes may afflict up to 90% of competitive racers and 46% of recreational riders who cycle on a regular basis. The cervical and lumbar spine, buttocks, knees, and hands are commonly involved.[99]

Mountain bicycles for cross-country or endurance riding often have the saddle at a high position (to allow extension of the leg during pedaling) and the handlebars at the level of the saddle. Riders flex at the waist over the front of the bicycle and extend the neck (see Figure 99-1). Cervical strain and spasm frequently result.[15] Lower back strain is also common because prolonged lumbar spine flexion leads to spinal extensor muscle spasm and lumbar disk stress.[99]

Patellofemoral pain syndrome (PFP) is a common cycling-related overuse injury. Symptoms include anterior knee aching pain behind the patella, exacerbated by knee flexion and extension.[47] Risk factors for PFP syndrome include patellar misalignment (e.g., patella alta or valgus deformity of the knee).[15] PFP is theorized to be caused by microtrauma and inflammation, as well as cartilage stress.[47] Poor cycling biomechanics (e.g., inexperienced or fatigued riders) impart additional stress to the patellofemoral joint, as does riding in a gear that is too high (i.e., requires increased muscular effort). PFP syndrome may be prevented by appropriate conditioning exercises to prevent fatigue during riding and adjusting the bicycle to properly fit the rider. Consultation with a professional bike fitter may be beneficial for riders suffering from PFP.

Iliotibial band (ITB) syndrome is another common overuse injury.[15] Symptoms include lateral knee pain exacerbated by repetitive motions (e.g., cycling). ITB syndrome may be due to friction of the ITB against the lateral femoral condyle, compression of soft tissues under the ITB, and chronic inflammation of the ITB bursa.[159] Causes may include inadequate stretching, poorly fitted bicycles, and riding in too high a gear. As with PFP, prevention strategies include conditioning exercises and proper bike fitting.[15]

Hands are frequently afflicted by overuse syndromes. Both medial and ulnar nerve palsies are more common in mountain bikers than in road cyclists.[129] Ulnar neuropathy results from ulnar nerve compression within the canal of Guyon. Median neuropathy results from median nerve compression within the carpal tunnel. Both motor and sensory symptoms can result, with pain and numbness in the fingers being most common.[15] The risk can be decreased with proper bike fitting, frequent changes of hand positions during riding, use of cycling gloves, and not gripping the handlebars too tightly.[129] For more severe cases, rest, splinting, and NSAIDs may be helpful.[85] *Hypothenar hammer syndrome* (i.e., ulnar artery occlusion) results from repetitive compression of the superficial branch of the ulnar artery as it crosses the hypothenar muscles.[10,15,38] Symptoms include hand and finger numbness, tingling, cold insensitivity, discoloration of fingertips, and hypothenar pain.[10] Prevention is similar to that discussed to avoid ulnar nerve compression.

Common maladies due to bicycle seats include chafing, perineal folliculitis and furuncles, and urethritis.[15] Erectile dysfunction was described in 4.2% of mountain cyclists after a 320-km race.[54] Perineal numbness and paresthesias are common, and likely due to compressive neuropathy.[38,53] Genital ultrasonography of mountain bikers has revealed numerous abnormalities, many of uncertain clinical significance. Findings of scertoliths, spermatoceles, epididymal calcifications, hydroceles, varicoceles, and torsion of the appendix testis have been described.[15,62,113] Battaglia reported five cases of clitoral microcalcifications; none experienced sexual dysfunction.[19] In a review of professional cyclists, hemorrhoids, anal fissures, perianal abscesses, and higher sphincter pressures and sphincter hypertrophy (which could lead to defecation disorders) were documented.[146] Prevention of chronic perineal conditions may prove difficult. If a rider is experiencing perineal complaints, alternative saddles should be tried. Regular use of padded bicycle shorts is recommended. Products to reduce chafing (e.g., Body Glide antichafe balm, chamois cream, or diaper rash products such as Desitin) can help prevent and treat local irritation and saddle sores.

INJURY PREVENTION

Risk-taking activity (e.g., riding beyond ability) often leads to injury.[15,84] Mountain biking injuries might be decreased by educational programs, especially at high-risk locations (e.g., downhill mountain bike parks).[15,21] Instruction on bike handling, braking, basic bike maintenance, proper protective gear, and trail selection should be included. Riders who self-report fast riding are at higher risk for severe injury. Efforts to encourage riding at controlled speeds might reduce injuries.[141] Attention to trail design and maintenance, including removal of unsafe obstacles and modification of trails to limit the opportunity to achieve full speed, may provide additional benefit. In commonly used public lands, separation of hiking and bicycling trails can lessen the chance of injury to both hikers and bikers.[21]

Individuals can reduce risks by maintaining equipment; improperly adjusted equipment or fatigued components can lead to injury.[15] Improper bike adjustment may lead to overuse syndromes. Proper protective gear is required during mountain biking. Helmets, gloves, and protective eyewear should be worn. For downhill riders and freeriders, full-face helmets, arm and leg protection, and neck and thorax protectors should be considered. Riders experiencing symptoms of overuse syndromes should be evaluated by a professional bike fitter.

Rider fatigue is a common contributing factor to mountain bike crashes. Fatigue compromises performance, leads to loss of control, and increases susceptibility to injury.[15] Structured aerobic and anaerobic fitness training is beneficial to help the rider sustain a high workload.[158] Increased core muscle strength (i.e., trunk and abdomen) can reduce lower back overuse syndromes. Hip extensor and abductor strengthening programs can help prevent chronic knee injuries.[99] Adequate hydration and nutrition can reduce rider fatigue.[147] Adequate caloric and carbohydrate intake (1 to 1.2 g/min) optimizes performance.[83] Carbohydrate loading in the days prior to an endurance event increases muscle glycogen stores, reduces fatigue, and improves performance.[106] Protein intake while cycling is thought to prevent body mass loss, enhance thermoregulatory capacity, and improve competitive exercise performance.[23,40] Sports drinks, energy bars, and energy tablets are helpful to maintain proper fluid and caloric

BOX 99-1 Key Steps in Planning Medical Coverage for a Mountain Biking Event

Select a medical director. The medical director will be in charge of all planning activities, as well as medical activities during the race.

Review the course. Identify areas where injuries are more likely to occur.

Map out shelters, evacuation routes, landing zones for helicopters, and trailhead access for ambulances and other rescue vehicles.

Plan for anticipated weather conditions at the time of the race (such as extreme heat or cold).

Consider pre-event medical screening for participants.

Plan for the number of caregivers required at the event. Consider not only the total number of participants and anticipated injury rates but also the geographic aspects of the course.

Formulate protocols for evacuation.

Plan for and acquire necessary medical equipment.

Obtain communications equipment, and formulate communication protocols with local agencies and rescue personnel.

Provide medical staff with easily identifiable uniforms (e.g., T-shirts, jackets).

Establish a plan to keep accurate records of all medical encounters during the event.

Data from Burdick TE: Wilderness event medicine: planning for mass gatherings in remote areas, *Travel Med Infect Dis* 3(4):249-258, 2005.

intake during riding. Adequate hydration and nutrition regimens are important because decreased fatigue during riding can prevent accidents.[137]

MEDICAL COVERAGE AT MOUNTAIN BIKING EVENTS

Medical support at organized wilderness endurance events is covered in Chapter 114; the key point is an organized plan, formulated well in advance of the event. Box 99-1 reviews steps in formulating this plan. The race event plan itself deserves great attention. Mountain bike injuries are 10 times more likely to occur on downhill sections. Aid stations should be strategically located near these areas.[34] Stage races, which cover long distances over remote areas, often leave rescuers with limited access to injured athletes.[110] Ensuring that sufficient medical personnel are available to reach injured parties in a reasonable amount of time, as well as *a priori* coordination with local rescue agencies, is of paramount importance. Protocols should be developed detailing who can be treated on site and who requires evacuation to a hospital.[110] Large events in remote locations can potentially strain local emergency medical services, rescue, and hospital resources; prior coordination with these agencies is necessary.[39] The number of health care workers required for an event is a function of the number of participants, anticipated injury rates, and layout of the course.[34] Events covering large distances require more caregivers. Equipment at aid stations should reflect the anticipated injuries and illnesses (Box 99-2).[97] Soft tissue injuries and fractures are likely to occur. Common illnesses include gastrointestinal disorders, flu-like malaise, and environmental conditions. Aid stations should be stocked accordingly. Supplies that include intravenous fluids, antiemetics, antidiarrheals, and over-the-counter analgesics should be in adequate supply. Although more catastrophic injuries or illnesses are unlikely to be encountered, being prepared for them with advanced equipment is required, especially if operating in remote environments with limited access to emergency medical services or local hospitals.

SNOWMOBILES

The first snowmobile was introduced in 1923 by Joseph Armand Bombardier. It was intended as winter transportation for hunting and fishing. Snowmobiles have been used as school buses, ambulances, and war-time vehicles.[135] Snowmobiling is a popular recreational activity in North America and northern Europe. Two million snowmobiles are registered in the United States and Canada; 100,000 machines are sold annually in these regions.[78,133,162] The average snowmobiler is 44 years old and rides more than 1600 miles per season.[78] More than 3000 snowmobile clubs in North America provide safety and training programs, represent the snowmobile community in political issues (e.g., land access), and groom and maintain local trails.[12,42]

North America has 225,000 miles of groomed snowmobile trails. Riders also explore the backcountry on both private and public lands.[78] Snowmobile racing is popular. There are many types of racing, such as cross-country racing, drag racing, hill climbing, and snocross).[79] Extreme snowmobiling is the newest sector of the sport. As in motocross, riders jump and perform tricks with their vehicles over obstacles, sometimes at great speeds.[104] The risk of injury is high.

EQUIPMENT

Snowmobiles range from basic entry-level machines to high-performance vehicles (Figure 99-14). The engine size ranges from 250 to 1000 cc, and speeds up to 100 mph can be reached.[43] Snowmobiles can weigh in excess of 600 lb, which puts riders at risk for serious injury from rollover accidents.[51,133] Several categories of snowmobiles are manufactured:[7,8]

- Trail snowmobiles (i.e., entry-level snowmobiles) are ideal for riders new to the sport. They are lightweight, easy to maneuver, and moderately powered (60 to 70 horsepower [hp]).

- Performance snowmobiles have larger engines (usually over 85 hp), are heavier, and have more aggressive handling characteristics. They are less forgiving when maneuvered improperly. Use should be reserved for experienced riders.

- Touring snowmobiles are designed for two riders. Comfort takes precedence over performance. They tend to be larger and heavier than trail or performance machines.

- Mountain snowmobiles are designed for backcountry and mountain riding. They are high-horsepower machines designed to perform well in deep powder, on steep terrain, and at high altitude.

- Utility (or working) snowmobiles are designed for commercial applications (such as ski resorts, or search and rescue efforts). These machines are wider and heavier than are recreational vehicles, and perform well on trails and in heavy snow.

- Youth-specific models are designed for riders 8 years of age and older. They are lightweight, low-horsepower machines and are easy to handle. The top speed is often limited by a governor.

PROTECTIVE GEAR

With any high-speed wintertime sport, proper protection against the elements is mandatory. A traditional layering approach is ideal. Next-to-the-skin layers should be made of wool or synthetic material that can wick away moisture. Cotton should not be used. Midlayers of woolen or synthetic fabrics can be chosen according to local weather conditions.

Outer layers provide warmth and protection against wind and precipitation. They must allow for unrestricted freedom of movement and not interfere with vehicle operation. Snowmobile-specific suits, or jacket and bib pants work well. Skiing outerwear or similar items may also be worn. Outer shells made from Gore-Tex or other similar synthetic fabrics that are waterproof and windproof provide the best protection. Outerwear with built-in buoyant foam insulation (e.g., Ice Rider Jacket from Mustang Survival, Bellingham, Washington) is available, and can be life-saving in a fall through the ice.[3] Avalanche airbag systems (e.g., ABS Backpack, ABS Avalanche Rescue Devices, Inc., Langley, British Columbia) can be helpful safety items in avalanche-prone terrain (see Figure 99-14).

Helmets should always be worn, and in many states are required by law.[13] Full-face helmets designed specifically for snowmobilers are ideal. They not only protect the head and face but also provide warmth and have antifog visors to protect eyes

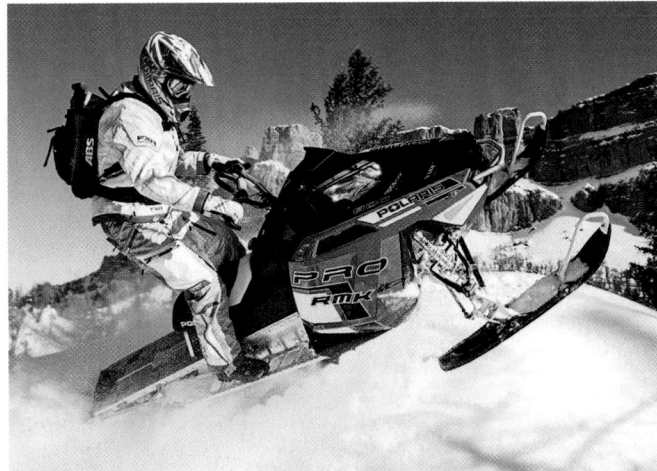

FIGURE 99-14 The modern snowmobile. Today's snowmobiles are high-performance machines, can weigh more than 600 lb, and can reach speeds above 100 mph. They are thrilling to ride but can cause injury or death. Note the full complement of protective gear worn by the rider: helmet, goggles, snowmobile suit, boots, and avalanche airbag system. (*Courtesy Polaris, Medina, Minnesota.*)

and increase visibility. Motorcycle-style helmets may be worn but often require use of goggles.[157] A review of snowmobile injuries at three trauma centers in Minnesota found that only 35% of victims were helmeted.[22] A review of traumatic injuries in Alaskan children found a similar 33% rate of helmet usage.[155] Helmets are effective at preventing central nervous system injury (odds ratio [OR] 0.28, 0.18 to 0.44), and are associated with a lower likelihood of death or permanent disability (OR .026, 0.01 to 0.67). Other studies report similar findings.[92] Potential barriers to helmet usage include discomfort, inconvenience, and lack of perceived risk.[155]

Water- and wind-resistant gloves and waterproof winter boots are required. Gloves should not be so bulky as to interfere with operation of the snowmobile. Silk, wool, or synthetic glove liners can be worn to provide additional warmth. Boots should be warm and comfortable and have rubber-lugged soles to provide traction.[157] Riders should pack a gear bag that includes personal items, safety equipment, tools, and an emergency first-aid kit[157] (Box 99-3).

MECHANISM OF INJURY

On snowmobiles, drivers are injured more frequently than are passengers.[161] Driver inexperience and poor judgment are the leading causes of accidents.[43,133] Drivers' unfamiliarity with local terrain may contribute to crashes; visitors have injury rates approximately four times higher than do local riders.[176] Excessive speed was found to be a factor in 64% of fatalities in New England in the early 2000s.[22,43] Inattentive operation (e.g., driving

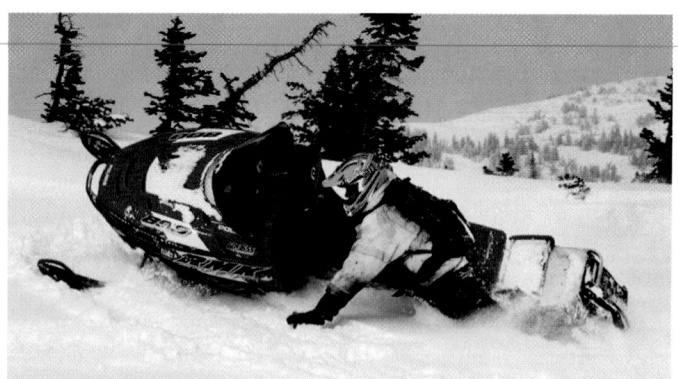

FIGURE 99-15 The most common mechanism of injury during snowmobiling is colliding with a fixed object. Rollover accidents, such as depicted here, are also frequently encountered and can lead to substantial injury, given the weight of the vehicle.

on the wrong side of a trail, jumping over barrier embankments, and negotiating curves improperly) also contributes to snowmobiling injuries.[43]

Collisions with fixed objects (e.g., trees, rocks, snowdrifts, and ice) constitute the most common mechanism of injury in snowmobile accidents.[22,26,51,82,139,162,167] These collisions occur more frequently after sunset.[43] Rollover accidents are common, and given these machines' weight, can cause significant trauma[51,82,139,162,167] (Figure 99-15). Less common mechanisms include collisions with other snowmobiles or other vehicles, driver or passenger ejection, passenger injuries while being pulled behind snowmobiles (on inner tubes or sleds), and "clothesline" accidents.[139,162,167] Clothesline injuries tend to occur in open fields, when an unexpected fence is encountered at high speed.[67] This can result in devastating facial and neck lacerations, airway trauma, and cervical and thoracic spine injuries.[51] Fall-through-the-ice accidents occur when a person is snowmobiling over insufficiently frozen bodies of water. These accidents may lead to hypothermia or drowning, and are discussed later in the chapter.[51,82,139,162,167]

Snowmobilers are at risk for environmental injury (e.g., frostbite and hypothermia). Cold ambient temperatures and high-speed wind exposures contribute. Frostbite on exposed skin is not uncommon.[123] Skin and body temperatures decrease by several degrees Centigrade after 2 hours of snowmobiling.[169] Review of specific snowmobile-related cold injuries follows later in this chapter.

EPIDEMIOLOGY OF SNOWMOBILING INJURIES

Studies of snowmobiling injuries are flawed by methodologic variability. Underreporting is likely. Approximately 10,000 to 14,000 patients are treated each year in U.S. emergency departments for snowmobiling injuries.[133,153,162] The Consumer Products Safety Commission (CPSC) estimates 110 deaths per year in the United States; other sources estimate approximately 200.[133,162] Rates of all injuries are between 2.8 and 5 injuries per 1000 registered snowmobiles per year.[133,161] Fatality rates in northern New England states have been estimated at between 1 and 1.7 deaths per 10,000 registered snowmobiles.[43]

Young men (15 to 35 years of age) account for the vast majority of snowmobiling accidents and fatalities.[24,26,60,82,135,144,153,161] In a 20-year review of accidents in Canada, males accounted for 89% of snowmobile fatalities and 81% of seriously injured persons.[167] In a similar review in Minnesota, 85% of snowmobile accident patients were male.[22] Male predominance is likely due to young men's higher participation rate and risk-taking behavior.

Most snowmobiling injuries or deaths occur during recreational activity, often on weekends. Many accidents occur after sunset, when visibility is reduced.[82,162] Injuries in the workplace (e.g., livestock herding and military exercises) are less common.[82] A review of injuries during organized snowmobile competitions

---

BOX 99-3   Recommended Snowmobiling Gear

Personal Items
Driver's license
Snowmobile safety certification card (if required by state law)
Money
Medications
Cell phone
Water
High-energy food

Safety Equipment
Compass and map
Waterproof matches, candle, fire starter
Flashlight and spare batteries
Extra ignition key
GPS unit
Small shovel
Probe and avalanche beacon (if traveling in avalanche-prone regions)
Strobe light or flares
Ice picks, kept readily available in outer pockets (if traveling over a frozen body of water; used to aid in self-extraction in case of falling through the ice)

Tools
Spare sparkplug and sparkplug wrench
Other wrenches for general repair
Screwdrivers
Pliers
Knife
Electrical or duct tape
Bungee cords
Tow rope

First-Aid Kit
Bandages
Gauze pads
Adhesive tape
Elastic wraps
Thermal or "space" blanket
Scissors
Antiseptic solution

Data from *Safe Riders: Snowmobile Safety Awareness Program*, 2014: saferidersafetyawareness.org.

(e.g., speed racing or snocross) has not been published, but accidents are common. A professional competitor died from injuries sustained in a crash during an aerial stunt in the 2013 X-Games.[30] This "best trick contest" has been dropped from X-Games motorcycle and snowmobile events.[28] Although snowmobiling activity is typically off road, one study found that 11% of snowmobile crashes occurred on roadways.[167]

Alcohol and Snowmobiling Injuries

Alcohol use is strongly associated with snowmobiling injuries and deaths. A Canadian study found that 67% of fatally injured snowmobilers tested positive for alcohol, and 80% of those had a blood alcohol level greater than 0.08% (80 mg/dL).[167] U.S. studies reveal similar findings; 44% to 64% of injured snowmobilers had consumed alcohol.[22,162] Rowe compared snowmobile-related fatalities with age- and sex-matched automobile and motorcycle fatalities; snowmobilers had a fourfold greater use of alcohol.[144] Males were more likely to have consumed alcohol.[167] Programs aimed at decreasing alcohol use when snowmobiling would likely decrease morbidity and mortality rates.

TYPES OF SNOWMOBILING INJURIES

Snowmobile accidents can be thought of as cold-weather, off-road analogs of motorcycle accidents. Riders may suffer substantial multisystem injuries, which may not be apparent on initial evaluation. Clinical management is the same as that of any multisystem trauma patient.

Head injuries are among the most commonly reported injuries; in one series, 35% of patients were reported to have sustained head injuries.[22,41,51,82,135,139,162] Head injuries may include concussion, traumatic subarachnoid hemorrhage, subdural hematoma, parenchymal contusion, and skull fracture.[153] Helmets had been worn in less than 30% of cases. They should be routinely worn.[92,155]

Extremity fractures occur in two-thirds of snowmobile crash victims.[22,167] Lower extremities are the most frequent sites of injury.[26,41,51,87,133,135,161] No fracture patterns have emerged as specific to snowmobiling. Soft tissue injuries (e.g., anterior cruciate ligament tear and acromioclavicular separation) have been reported.[87] Extremities should be splinted in the field if potential for fracture exists. A high index of suspicion for significant occult injury must be maintained.

Axial skeleton injuries are less common than are extremity fractures. Eighteen percent of injured Minnesota snowmobilers had spinal injuries.[22] In a similar review from New York, 6% sustained hip or pelvis fractures.[135] A 14-year-old boy fractured all his cervical vertebrae in a high-energy snowmobile accident.[100] He suffered no neurologic injury and was successfully treated using a halo device.

Snowmobile accidents can cause substantial thoracoabdominal trauma. In one series, thoracic injuries included pneumothorax and hemothorax (19%), pulmonary contusion (16%), rib fractures (29%), clavicle fractures (11%), and scapula fractures (3%).[135] Intraabdominal injury was less common, and included spleen (12%), liver (4%), and renal injuries (2%). A Minnesota cohort had similar injury patterns: 29% of patients sustained thoracic injury and 15% abdominal trauma.[22]

Chronic and overuse injuries related to snowmobile use are not described in the medical literature, save for a single report by Anttonen regarding *white finger syndrome*. This condition is a form of Raynaud's syndrome caused by continuous vibration to the hands.[17]

FATAL SNOWMOBILING INJURIES

The most frequent risk factors for fatal injury are male gender, alcohol use, and excessive speed.[126,139,162] Other risks include inattentive or careless vehicle operation and inexperience.[43] In northern New England, 82% of fatalities were a result of blunt trauma to the head, chest, and/or abdomen; 7% from drownings, 4% from medical causes, and 7% from unknown causes. Blunt traumatic injuries leading to death are most frequently caused by

striking a fixed object.[51,139,162] Deaths are more likely to occur on weekends and after sunset.[43,126]

PEDIATRIC SNOWMOBILING INJURIES

Many snowmobile enthusiasts consider snowmobiling to be a family sport. The majority of snowmobile owners are married with children.[139] Children may be injured while operating the vehicle or riding as a passenger.[51,118] Size, weight, and speed of modern snowmobiles predispose young riders to injury. Passengers towed behind a snowmobile (more likely to be children than adults) are at high risk for injury.[139,162]

As with adults, male children and adolescents are much more likely to be injured in a snowmobile accident than are females.[51,118,139] In a study of Norwegian youth snowmobilers, boys were more likely to adopt peer-group conformity than were girls, and were less likely to identify potential risks in snowmobiling activities.[111] Whereas girls were more likely to focus on risks and how to avoid them, boys were more focused on testing their limits while driving. Such differences likely contribute to the increased injury rates in boys.

Injury patterns are similar in pediatric victims of snowmobile injuries, compared with adults. Orthopedic injuries are most commonly reported, but blunt head, thoracic, and abdominal trauma are common.[51,118,139] Helmet use among pediatric patients ranges from 53% to 68%.[51,118] In response to concerns regarding pediatric injuries and deaths from snowmobiling, the American Academy of Pediatrics has published recommendations regarding safe use of snowmobiles[9] (Box 99-4).

FALLS THROUGH THE ICE WHEN SNOWMOBILING

Driving snowmobiles across a frozen body of water (e.g., river, lake, or ocean) is inherently risky. Falls through the ice and drowning account for between 4% and 38% of snowmobiling deaths[139,162] and are frequently reported by local media.[1,5] "Skimming" (i.e., attempting to ride a snowmobile over a section of open water) is an activity pursued by some. This activity is extremely dangerous.[43,150]

Of 307 falling-through-the-ice events in Alaska, more than 50% involved a snowmobile.[60] Sixty-eight percent of the incidents led to search and rescue operations; 35% were fatal. Most victims were men, with a mean age of 33 years. Falls through the ice occurred most frequently on rivers. Overflow conditions (i.e., water from a high tide, rain, or snowmelt that collects above surface ice and subsequently partially refreezes) was a factor in 11% of cases. The author posited that these events may become

---

BOX 99-4 American Academy of Pediatrics: Snowmobiling Recommendations

Children younger than 16 years old should not operate a snowmobile.

Children younger than 6 years old should not ride as a passenger on a snowmobile (they lack the stamina and strength to stay on).

Snowmobile manufacturers should avoid advertisements directed toward children.

Graduated licensing programs should be put in place for operators 16 years and older.

Travel at safe speed should be encouraged.

Speed governors should be used for inexperienced riders.

There is absolutely no alcohol or drug use.

Proper gear, including helmets, is mandatory at all times.

Always travel in groups of two persons or more.

Avoid ice unless its condition and thickness are known.

No more than one passenger rides on a snowmobile.

Never tow a passenger recreationally behind a snowmobile on any conveyance.

Ensure that the snowmobile is properly maintained.

Data from American Academy of Pediatrics: Snowmobiling hazards, *Pediatrics* 106(5):1142-1144, 2000.

more common in Alaska due to global warming with a shortened ice travel season. In a Minnesota review, an average of 6.3 deaths occur annually as a result of falling through the ice; half of victims were on snowmobiles.[115] In a review of 246 snowmobile-related deaths, the Canadian Red Cross concluded the majority of immersion deaths were preventable.[49]

The best way to avoid falling through the ice is to avoid crossing frozen lakes or rivers. Ice thickness can vary widely.[156] Ice thickness and quality must be evaluated before driving onto ice. Riders should not assume that tracks from prior snowmobiles ensure safe passage. The burden of establishing safe passage rests with the individual.

Evaluation of ice conditions begins before starting out. Check with local authorities, who may have knowledge of local ice conditions and routes to avoid. Ice should be qualitatively assessed before embarking. Only clear, hard ice is recommended for travel.[156] Ice that is slushy, on or near moving water, has thawed or refrozen, or is layered due to sudden temperature changes, must be avoided.[2] Ice covered by snow may be weakened because snow acts to insulate the water and may retard ice formation and growth.[2] If no apparent qualitative deficiencies are noted, the next step is to measure ice thickness.

The Minnesota Department of Natural Resources has developed ice thickness guidelines (Figure 99-16).[114] These guidelines are intended for new, clear ice only. White ice or "snow" ice is less than half as strong; thickness guidelines should be doubled for travel on white ice. These are general guidelines only. Other environmental factors may cause ice to be unsafe.

To measure ice thickness, an ice chisel, auger, or cordless drill can be used to make a hole.[114] Insert a tape measure into the hole, hook it on the bottom edge of the ice, and measure the thickness. The Minnesota guidelines recommend checking ice thickness every 150 feet. Although this may be feasible for ice fishermen, it is unreasonable to assume that persons on snowmobiles will start and stop at these intervals. Regardless, ice conditions can change rapidly over short distances. The rider choosing to travel over ice must use common sense, recheck the ice thickness as local conditions warrant, be willing to acknowledge an inherent risk of falling through, and be prepared for such an accident.

The first step in responding to falling through the ice is to remain calm. Outer clothing layers should remain on; their insulating layers trap air and can provide buoyancy. The victim should then turn and face the direction from which he or she came; ice in that direction is known to be solid enough to support a snowmobile. Ice in any other direction is of unknown thickness and quality. Place hands and arms on the surface of the ice. Screwdrivers, ice picks, or other similar objects, if kept in easily accessible outer pockets, can be used to dig into the

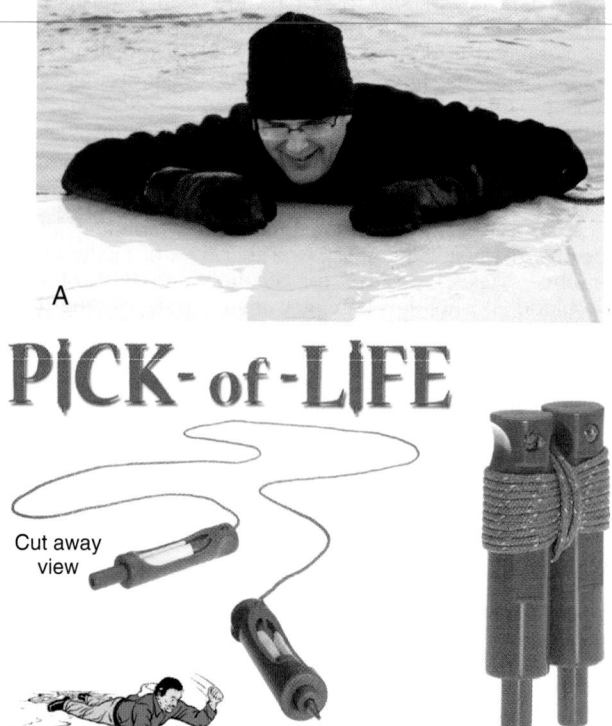

A

B

FIGURE 99-17 Falling through the ice. **A,** Self-extraction from the water up onto the surface may be difficult, if not impossible, given the slippery nature of the ice. **B,** Ice picks, long industrial nails, or screwdrivers may be used to dig into the ice to pull oneself up and out of the water. Commercially available ice picks designed specifically for this emergency are ideal and should be kept in a readily accessible outer pocket. (**A** courtesy Angel-Guard Products, Worcester, Massachusetts.)

ice and help the victim pull himself or herself out of the water (Figure 99-17). Without such devices, self-extraction may prove almost impossible because of the lack of traction. Kicking with legs while using the ice picks can aid propulsion out of the water and onto the ice surface. Once the person has been extracted, the person lies flat on the surface and rolls away from the hole. Standing up may concentrate too much weight on a minimal surface area and result in ice breakage. Once the person is safely away from the water, efforts to seek shelter, remove wet clothing, and rewarm need to be urgently pursued.[6]

Witnesses to fall-through-the-ice accidents also need to remain calm and carefully formulate a rescue plan. A call for emergency assistance should be made as soon as possible. "Preach, reach, throw, row, go," an adage familiar to lifeguards, is also sage advice in this situation:[4]

- Preach: Let the victim know you are there to help; encourage the person to fight for survival.
- Reach: If the victim is reachable from shore, extend an object such as a ladder or long pole.
- Throw: Try to toss a rope or buoyant object (such as a personal flotation device) to the victim. Encourage the victim to tie the rope around himself or herself before the victim is too weak to grasp it.
- Row: Push a light boat across the ice to the edge of the hole, get into the boat, and pull the victim in over the bow.
- Go: As an absolute last resort, and if no other possibilities for rescue exist, consider approaching the victim while lying down on the ice. Nonprofessionals without extensive preparation and specialized equipment who attempt this type of rescue are at substantial risk of themselves becoming victims.

Please see Chapters 7 to 10 for details on hypothermia, frostbite, and immersion into cold water.

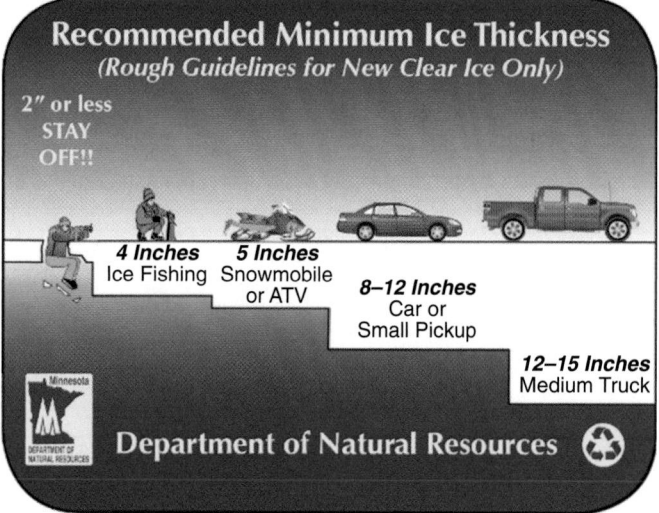

FIGURE 99-16 Ice thickness guidelines. (Courtesy Minnesota Department of Natural Resources.)

SAFETY AND RISK REDUCTION IN SNOWMOBILING

Safety rules and regulations vary greatly by jurisdiction. In Maine, there are no speed limits for snowmobiles; riders are simply mandated to "operate at a reasonable and prudent speed for conditions." In New Hampshire, the speed limit is 45 mph unless otherwise posted, and in Vermont, it is 35 mph on public lands and "reasonable speeds" on private lands.[43] Not all states have helmet laws; some require helmets only for riders less than 18 years of age.[139] Given that excessive speed and lack of helmet use are associated with snowmobiling injuries and deaths, legal and educational efforts to limit speed and mandate helmet usage appear reasonable.

Safety courses vary by jurisdiction. Many states offer free safety training courses; many do not require them. Maine does not require a safety course; New Hampshire does for persons under the age of 18 without a driver's license, and Vermonters are required to take a class if they were born after July 1, 1983.[43] Training would likely increase safety. Topics might include proper operating procedures, risks of high speed, safety gear (including the use of flotation devices), and ice safety and rescue procedures. Given the extremely high percentages of accident victims who are impaired by alcohol at the time of a crash, alcohol-related education should be investigated.[144] Targeted programs for young men (15 to 35 years old), focused on risk-taking behavior and appropriate risk-reduction strategies, may yield positive results.[135]

Safety improvement for children should include adherence to recommendations of the American Academy of Pediatrics regarding snowmobiling (see Box 99-4). Local interventions (e.g., trail maintenance programs and removal of fixed objects that may be struck) and restrictions against towing passengers might also be considered.

ALL-TERRAIN VEHICLES

All-terrain vehicles (ATVs) are popular off-road vehicles. Approximately 10.2 million ATVs are in use in the United States, with almost 700,000 new units sold each year.[61] Of ATV users, 81% are male, and 40% are less than 30 years old. ATVs specifically designed for youths are popular and make up 40% of total U.S. ATV sales.[61] In a 2001 study, approximately 7.2 million children less than 15 years of age had ridden an ATV at least once. Young ATV riders are particularly prone to injury.

ATVs are used in a wide variety of settings. In the United States, approximately 80% are used solely for recreational purposes; the remainder are used in commercial environments or in tasks as varied as farming, police and government functions, patrolling of park lands and beaches, and search and rescue operations, and as a primary mode of transportation in remote regions.[61,98] ATVs are well suited for farming and property maintenance because they are able to maneuver in rough terrain, can be fitted with accessories (such as racks, plows, and winches), and can carry larger loads and travel much faster than can a person on foot. Recreational ATV enthusiasts enjoy their vehicles on public and private lands, including designated ATV parks and trail systems (e.g., the Hatfield-McCoy Trails in West Virginia).[52,61]

EQUIPMENT

ATVs are powerful machines propelled by gas engines and capable of achieving speeds of up to 100 mph. They have high-volume, low-pressure tires, narrow wheelbases, short turning radius, and high center of gravity. These characteristics make ATVs ideal for off-road travel, but render them unstable and prone to rollover.[27] Instability is pronounced when an ATV is operated at high speeds on paved roads because it is not designed to be used in such a manner.[52] Most ATVs are intended for a single operator. Elongated straddle seats enable the user to "actively" operate the vehicle (i.e., enable the driver to shift the body weight in order to steer, climb, descend, and maintain control), a requirement for safe operation. If a passenger joins the driver on an ATV designed for one person, active control of

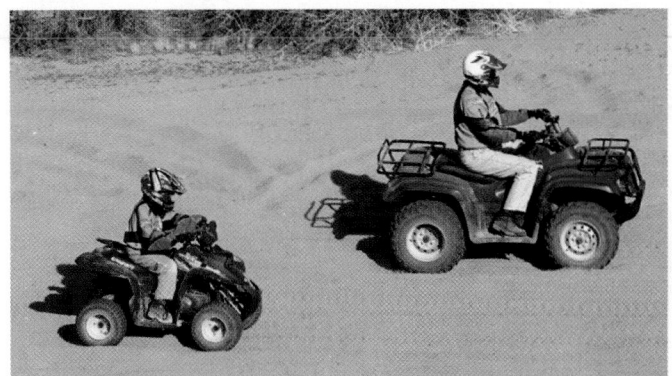

FIGURE 99-18 All-terrain vehicles (ATVs). A wide variety of ATVs are available, including sport, utility, and youth models. Children should never be allowed to operate adult-sized vehicles. They lack the strength, coordination, and judgment required to operate these vehicles safely. Many authorities believe children under the age of 16 years should not be allowed to operate any ATV, regardless of the child's size. These riders are properly equipped with helmets, protective eyewear, riding jacket, long pants, gloves, and sturdy boots.

the vehicle is compromised.[52] Original ATVs had three wheels. These were discontinued in the 1980s for safety reasons. Nearly all ATVs in use today are four-wheeled models.[48]

Multiple types of ATVs are available[61] (Figure 99-18). Sport models intended for recreational trail riding have engines that range from 90 to 1000 cc, and weigh 300 to 700 lb. Utility models are similar to sport models, but are equipped with a variety of accessories (e.g., cargo and/or gun racks) that improve utility (e.g., for farming, patrol and policing operations, camping, and hunting). Youth models are designed to make the vehicles safer for young riders; engines are less than 90 cc, and vehicle weight is less than 300 lb. Youth ATVs are equipped with governors that limit top speed to 10 to 15 mph. Transition models are available for adolescents and teenagers. Although they are larger and more powerful than youth models, these ATVs are lighter and less powerful than full-size ATVs.

PROTECTIVE GEAR AND HELMETS

Proper protective gear is mandatory when operating an ATV (see Figure 99-18). Full-length pants, long-sleeve tops, and gloves help prevent soft tissue injuries. Sturdy boots with rugged nonslip soles are required. Protective eyewear (e.g., goggles or safety glasses) should always be worn. A review of ocular injuries (e.g., eyelid lacerations, traumatic cataracts, and corneal abrasions) sustained by ATV riders found that 100% of victims were not wearing protective eyewear.[107] Protective gear and pads designed for ATV use are readily available; they include riding boots, chest and back protectors, elbow and wrist guards, goggles, kidney belts, knee and ankle guards, neck braces and supports, shoulder pads, and protective undergarments. The protective benefit of such equipment seems obvious, but studies have not been performed to evaluate efficacy.

Helmet use is supported by robust research. A properly fitting helmet approved by the Department of Transportation should be worn whenever a person is operating an ATV. Despite numerous safety campaigns, helmet usage remains low. Eighty-three percent of ATV-related fatalities in the United States involved victims who were not wearing helmets, according to recent government statistics.[61] Numerous other studies of injuries and deaths related to ATV use document similar noncompliance with helmet use.* Rates of helmet usage range from 0% to 46%; no report documents a usage rate of more than 50%.[151,152,174] Studies from New Zealand and Canada show similar results.[20,50,174]

---

*References 20, 27, 50, 55, 107, 112, 130, 143, 151, 152, 155, 163, 165, 174.

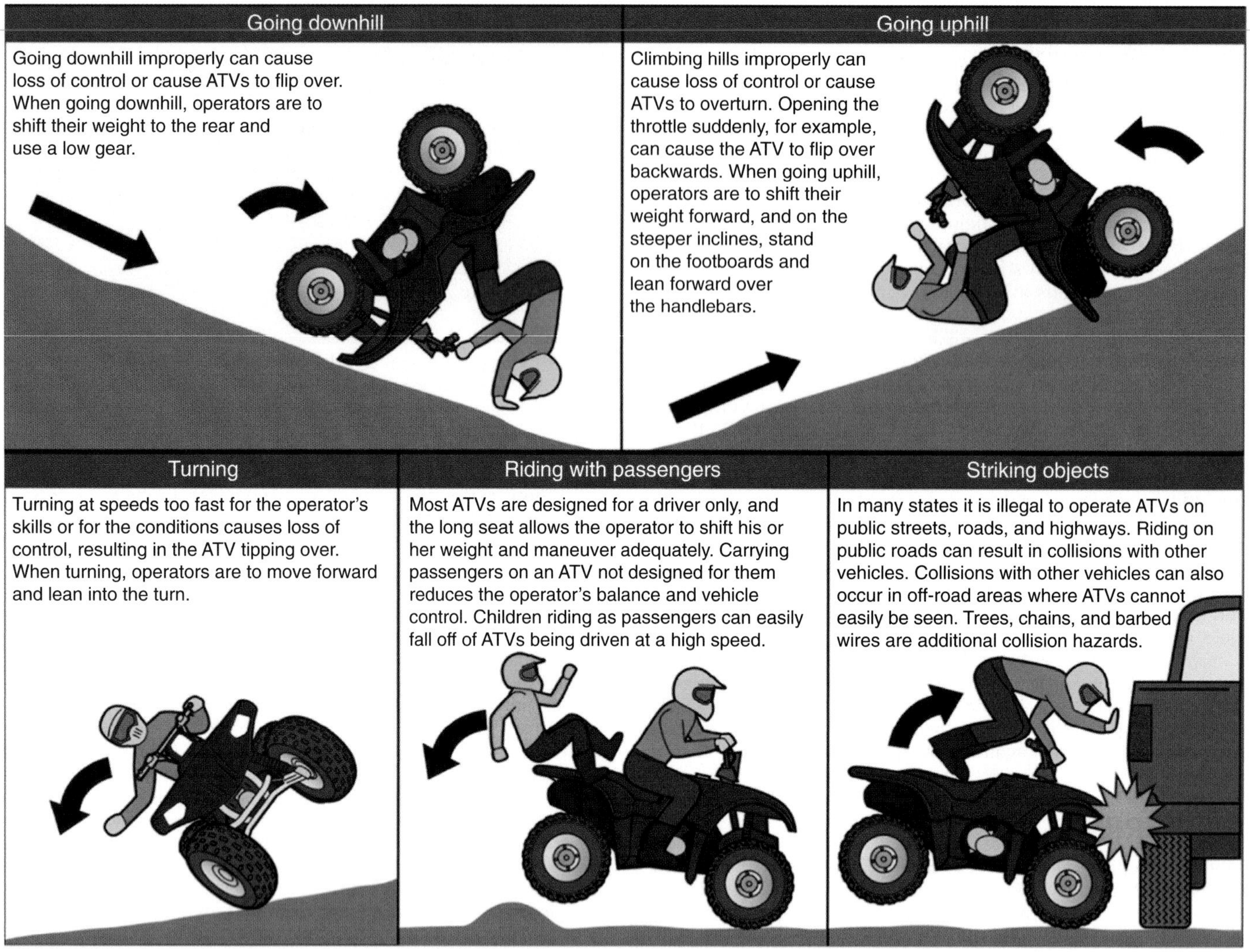

Going downhill

Going downhill improperly can cause loss of control or cause ATVs to flip over. When going downhill, operators are to shift their weight to the rear and use a low gear.

Going uphill

Climbing hills improperly can cause loss of control or cause ATVs to overturn. Opening the throttle suddenly, for example, can cause the ATV to flip over backwards. When going uphill, operators are to shift their weight forward, and on the steeper inclines, stand on the footboards and lean forward over the handlebars.

Turning

Turning at speeds too fast for the operator's skills or for the conditions causes loss of control, resulting in the ATV tipping over. When turning, operators are to move forward and lean into the turn.

Riding with passengers

Most ATVs are designed for a driver only, and the long seat allows the operator to shift his or her weight and maneuver adequately. Carrying passengers on an ATV not designed for them reduces the operator's balance and vehicle control. Children riding as passengers can easily fall off of ATVs being driven at a high speed.

Striking objects

In many states it is illegal to operate ATVs on public streets, roads, and highways. Riding on public roads can result in collisions with other vehicles. Collisions with other vehicles can also occur in off-road areas where ATVs cannot easily be seen. Trees, chains, and barbed wires are additional collision hazards.

FIGURE 99-19 Mechanism of injury in ATV accidents. *(Courtesy U.S. Government Accountability Office.)*

Data on helmet-use risk reduction are compelling. Helmets save lives and prevent injuries to the head, face, and neck.* Data on ATV crash victims in West Virginia illustrate the point.[112] Unhelmeted riders were significantly more likely to suffer head and neck soft tissue injuries (81% versus 56%), concussions (60% versus 38%), intracranial hemorrhages (22% versus 6%), facial fractures (21% versus 12%), and skull fractures (19% versus 9%). Unhelmeted riders were less likely to be discharged home from the emergency department (33% versus 45%). A review of CPSC fatality data indicates that helmets reduced likelihood of head injury among fatal crash victims by 58%.[52] A study of Alaskan children involved in ATV accidents found that helmets significantly reduced risk for central nervous system injury (OR 0.28, 95% confidence interval [CI] 0.18 to 0.44), as well as risk for death or permanent disability (OR 0.26, 95% CI 0.10 to 0.44).[155]

MECHANISM OF INJURY

Several distinct mechanisms of ATV injury cause the majority of injuries and fatalities (Figure 99-19). Collisions with fixed objects (e.g., trees, rocks, or embankments) are the leading causes of death and injury. U.S. and Canadian government statistics reveal these collisions cause 48% to 52% of fatalities.[61,167] A rollover crash is the second most common cause.[27,61,108] (Figure 99-20). An innovative review of YouTube videos and real-world ATV

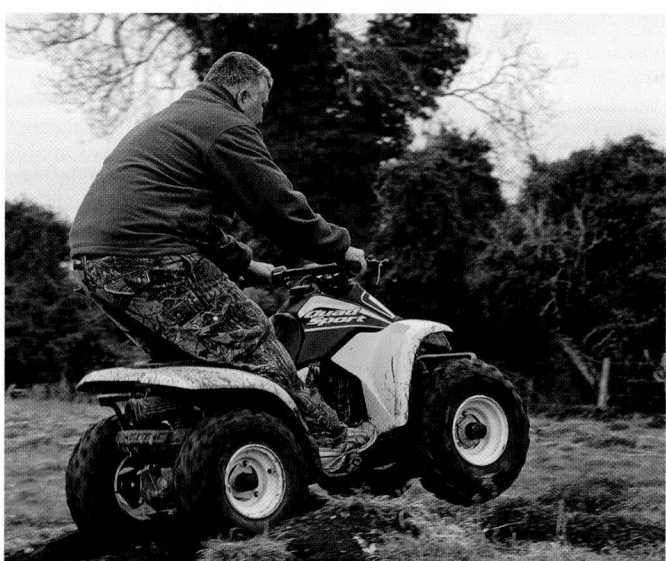

FIGURE 99-20 ATVs are prone to rollover crashes, given their high center of gravity. The vehicles may roll over even at low speeds. The rider here is particularly susceptible to head injury because he is not wearing a helmet.

*References 52, 59, 63, 72, 93, 109, 112, 130, 143, 145, 155, 165, 174.

rollover events found that ATVs rolled sideways in 47% of events, rearward in 44%, and forward in 9%.[166] Most rollovers occurred at low speeds: 86% at 10 mph or less and 53% at less than 3 mph. Seventy-nine percent of riders were uninjured, 16% sustained injuries secondary to contact with the vehicle, and 5% sustained injuries unrelated to the ATV (e.g., striking the ground). Attempts to actively dismount at the time of rollover occurred in 63% of cases; 72% of these attempts were successful. Fifteen percent of dismounters sustained injury, while 32% of riders who remained on the ATV were injured. The author concluded that active rider movements, including separating from the vehicle in the event of a rollover, were important in determining outcomes of an ATV crash. Less common mechanisms include ejection from the vehicle, unexpected terrain changes, and *clothesline injuries,* which occur when a rider runs into a wire fence at high speed (as they do with snowmobiles).[27,59,61,98]

ATVs are designed for off-road use. Their high center of gravity and low-pressure tires perform poorly on hard surfaces at high speeds. Operating these vehicles on paved roadways is a dangerous endeavor. CPSC data reveal that 60% of all ATV fatalities between 1985 and 2009 were a result of roadway crashes and accidents.[52] ATV crashes on the road are more likely to involve ATV passengers, and so have multiple fatalities. On-road ATV victims are more likely to be intoxicated and less likely to wear helmets than their off-road counterparts. Fatality Analysis Report System data regarding on-road ATV deaths provide additional insight.[172] Of 1701 reported fatalities, 1482 were drivers and 210 were passengers (the rider status was unknown in several cases). Half were teenagers or younger; 90% were male. Helmets were worn by only 13% of drivers and 6% of passengers. Forty-three percent had a blood alcohol content of more than 0.08%. Speeding was implicated in 42% of single-vehicle crashes. The most common mechanism was striking a fixed object; rollover events were common. ATVs should not be operated on roadways. Other risk-laden activities (e.g., not wearing a helmet, carrying a passenger, speeding, and consuming alcohol) further increase the risk for death.

EPIDEMIOLOGY OF ATV INJURIES

Nonfatal Injuries

In 2011, 107,500 patients were treated in U.S. emergency departments for ATV-related injuries.[48] Eighty-seven percent were treated and released. Twenty-seven percent were less than 16 years old. In 2009, the rate of injury in the United States was 37.9/100,000 riders, and was highest in the 13- to 15-year-old age group. The mean age of ATV crash victims is 27 to 30 years old. Males are involved in 70% to 80% of crashes.[29,32,55,93,145,167] Rural inhabitants are much more likely to be injured on an ATV than are their urban counterparts (227/100,000 versus 7.3/100,000); ATVs are used primarily in remote environments.[32]

Fatal Injuries

The CPSC reports 11,688 persons died from ATV accidents between 1982 and 2011.[48] Twenty-five percent were less than 16 years old, and 10% less than 12 years old. Deaths per year have increased over time; the Government Accountability Office (GAO) reported 816 fatalities in 2007, a 53% increase in 8 years.[61] ATV use tripled in the same time period. Males account for 80% to 90% of fatal accidents, and the average age is approximately 30 years old.[46,61,73,101,167] In the United States, the rate of death from ATV accidents is 0.32/100,000.[73] The death rate for males is sixfold higher than for females (0.55 versus 0.09/100,000). In Canada, the overall death rate is similar to that in the United States, at 0.3/100,000.[167] The CPSC database for 1982 to 2007 includes deaths from all 50 states in the United States, with California (504), Texas (478), Pennsylvania (459), West Virginia (444), and Kentucky (419) leading the list.

Pediatric Injuries and Fatalities

Pediatric injuries and deaths related to ATV use merit special attention. Children make up 14% to 18% of riders but 20% of ATV deaths and 33% of injuries.[61,98] Between 1996 and 2005, 320,700 children sustained an ATV-related injury; 1154 were

killed.[48] The annualized injury rate is approximately 56/100,000.[152] Injured youths are 75% to 80% male; their injury rate is twice as high as that of females.[98,152,170] An ATV operator less than 16 years old has a 33% chance of sustaining an ATV-related injury during the vehicle's lifespan.[27] Child passengers are at greater risk of death or serious injury (particularly head and neck injuries) than are child drivers.[152]

Pediatric riders figure prominently in injury and death statistics for many reasons. Most children (≈ 90% in the GAO and CPSC databases) are killed or injured while riding adult ATVs.[48,61,108] Children do not have the judgment, skill, strength, or endurance to maneuver an adult-sized ATV weighing over 700 lb. Children may not weigh enough to counter the rotational momentum of the vehicle by changing their center of gravity (i.e., they are unable to "actively" ride the ATV).[98] Many stakeholders (e.g., GAO, CPSC, public health officials, and industry representatives) agree that children should never ride adult ATVs.[48,61,152] The CPSC estimates that the risk of injury to young riders could be cut in half if they rode models designed specifically for young people.[152] Although manufacturers and distributors have agreed to prevent dealers from selling adult-sized ATVs to children, undercover checks by the GAO revealed that 70% of dealers were willing to make such a transaction.[61]

A child's risk of injury and death persists even when riding an age-appropriate ATV. Youth-sized vehicles are quite heavy and are still prone to rollover, even at low speeds. In the event of a rollover, children may not be able to extricate themselves from beneath a heavy vehicle. Children have less impulse control and are prone to taking more dangerous risks.[61] Children are likely to disregard basic ATV safety principles while riding. In a review of pediatric trauma center admissions over a 5-year period, Mazotas found that 70% of patients were not wearing a helmet, 56% had no adult supervision, 50% were double riding (i.e., carrying a passenger), 23% were riding on paved roads, and 16% were riding at night.[108]

ALCOHOL AND ATVS

Alcohol intoxication plays a central role in ATV-related injuries and deaths. Alcohol contributes to up to 50% of ATV crashes.[52,72,107,163,167] Alcohol was present in 50% of riders killed in West Virginia between 2004 and 2006, and in 88% the blood alcohol concentration was greater than 0.08%. Marijuana was detected in 11% of the victims, and opioids (7%), benzodiazepines (6%), cocaine (2%), and methamphetamine (1%) were also found.[72] A survey of Canadian youths found that 10% reported operating a vehicle after consuming alcohol or other illicit substances.[132] Respondents were more likely to engage in such behaviors if they were male, from rural communities, or from lower socioeconomic strata. A review of the Alberta Trauma Registry found alcohol to an independent predictor of mortality in ATV crashes (relative risk [RR] 2.33; interquartile range [IQR] 1.52 to 3.56).[93] The American College of Emergency Physicians has a policy statement supporting adoption and enforcement of legislation prohibiting use of alcohol or drugs while operating motorized off-road vehicles.[11] Such action is sound and should be vigorously pursued.

TYPES OF ATV INJURIES

ATV crashes lead to multisystem trauma. Soft tissue injuries and fractures are the most commonly reported injuries. Of ATV patients treated in U.S. emergency departments, 27% sustained contusions and abrasions, 23% sustained fractures, 17% had sprains and strains, and 11% had lacerations.[48] These injuries were in an upper extremity (29%), head or neck (28%), torso (22%), and leg (20%). Other reports indicate similar findings.[152,174] Fractures are present in up to 50% of ATV patients.[55,167] Sport-specific constellations of injuries have not been reported.

Head injuries are common following ATV accidents. Injury and death rates are compounded by lack of helmet use. Blunt head trauma with loss of consciousness is common.[170] Skull fractures (e.g., temporal bone, skull base, and face) are also frequently seen.[16,107] Intracranial injury (e.g., epidural hematoma, subdural hematoma, subarachnoid hemorrhage, and intraparenchymal hemorrhage) should be ruled out.[61,107] As mentioned previously, riders are at risk for ocular injury. Primary ocular trauma (e.g., subconjunctival hemorrhage, open-globe injury, or retinal detachment) has been reported.[107]

Of ATV crash patients, 5% to 20% suffer blunt abdominal injuries and 13% to 22% suffer thoracic injuries.[48,108,174] Blunt renal injuries are described.[71] Specific ATV-related thoracoabdominal injury patterns have not been well described.

Intracranial trauma and other head injuries are the leading causes of death from ATV accidents. Exsanguination (e.g., from great vessel injury or internal organ injury) also contribute substantially to death rates.[46,98,101,112] Traumatic asphyxiation (as might occur in a rollover accident when the victim is unable to self-extricate) was reported as the cause of death in 15% of Australian victims.[46]

SAFETY AND RISK REDUCTION

Risk factors for ATV-related injuries include:
- Male gender
- Age younger than 16 years
- Youth riders operating an adult-sized ATV
- Failure to wear a helmet
- Carrying a passenger
- Alcohol use or intoxication
- Driving at excessive speed
- Driving on paved roads
- Lack of training and experience[52,61,98]

ATV safety stakeholders have advocated for proper ATV training and routine use of proper safety equipment (e.g., helmets). This training is especially important because ATV operation appears deceptively easy. In communities where ATVs are widely used, local populations should be educated about a helmet's ability to decrease the risk of TBI.[29,61]

The CPSC filed a lawsuit against the five main ATV manufacturers in 1988 to encourage safety standards.[61] The resulting settlement mandated that manufacturers must:
- Stop selling three-wheeled vehicles.
- Promote and sell four-wheeled vehicles with an engine size of more than 90 cc only to riders age 16 years and older.
- Promote youth-sized models with engine sizes of 70 to 90 cc for children.
- Provide free training to all purchasers and their family members.
- Conduct nationwide safety public awareness campaigns.
- Adhere to advertising guidelines.
- Affix warning labels to vehicles.
- Develop voluntary ATV industry safety standards.

The CPSC-mandated dealer training programs must include content on safe riding practices, how to operate an ATV on hills, how to use proper protective gear, how to avoid hazards of improper operation, and other topics.[61] Although such programs are sound, real-world application may fall short. As few as 10% of purchasers may actually participate in free training.[98] ATVs are often bought second-hand or through nonauthorized dealers, so purchasers do not receive training. Even dealer compliance with the CPSC's recommendations falls short. A telephone survey of ATV dealers in Illinois found that only 75% recommended child-sized ATVs for youth participants, and only 50% offered safety training.[70] To provide further outreach to consumers, the CPSC has developed a website, ATVsafety.org, which hosts safety guidelines, injury statistics, and other useful information. The CPSC also produces television and radio public service announcements.[48]

Regional safety regulations vary greatly between jurisdictions. Thirty-two states have minimum operating ages, 28 have helmet and eye protection rules, 21 require a safety certificate, and 12 require a motor vehicle license.[61] Most states prohibit use of ATVs on roadways; others allow on-road passage but require riders to wear helmets when riding on roads.[172] The efficacy of safety legislation is uncertain. Data from the Centers for Disease Control and Prevention WONDER database show that states with no

BOX 99-5 Summary of Position Statements From Medical Societies Regarding ATV Safety

Children under the age of 16 years* should not operate ATVs, regardless of the size of the vehicle.
Use of helmets, eye protection, and protective clothing and footwear is mandatory.
Passengers should never be allowed on an ATV.
Alcohol or other intoxicants should never be consumed prior to riding an ATV.
All operators should complete a training course, including both classroom and practical sessions.
ATVs should never be ridden on paved roadways.
Riders should avoid excessive speeds, jumps and stunts, and riding after dark.

*The American Academy of Orthopedic Surgeons recommends that no one under the age of 18 years should operate an ATV.
Data from Larson A, McIntosh A: The epidemiology of injury in ATV and motocross sports, *Med Sport Sci* 58:158-172, 2012; Burd R: American Pediatric Surgical Association Trauma Committee position statement on the use of all-terrain vehicles by children and youth, *J Pediatr Surg* 44(8):1638-1639, 2009; Yanchar N: Preventing injuries from all-terrain vehicles, *Paediatr Child Health* 17(9):513, 2012.

helmet requirements had 23% more ATV-related deaths than did states with such requirements.[73] However, studies from Quebec and North Carolina found rates of helmet usage and numbers and types of injuries were unchanged after the enactment of helmet laws.[20,109] Safety programs have been implemented in populations of interest (e.g., hunters taking safety classes and high school students). Participants' awareness of safety issues appears to be heightened (as evidenced by preintervention and postintervention tests), but the impact of such programs has yet to be demonstrated.[81,124,171]

Professional medical societies (e.g., American Academy of Orthopedic Surgeons, American Pediatric Surgical Association, and Canadian Paediatric Society) have recognized the need for improved safety measures regarding ATV use.[33,98,175] A summary of their position statements is presented in Box 99-5.

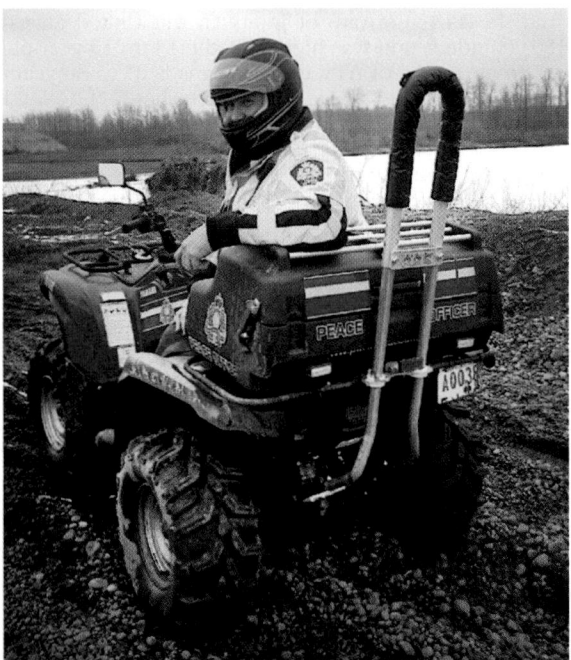

FIGURE 99-21 Crush guard. This safety device is designed to prevent the driver from being crushed by the heavy vehicle in the event of a rollover accident. Its use is not widespread, and its efficacy has yet to be determined. (*Courtesy Quadbar Safety:* quadbarsafety.com.)

Improved ATV design and engineering are other possible avenues for risk reduction. Some have advocated for redesign of seats on adult ATVs, moving them far enough from the handlebars that children cannot reach them. The backs of seats could be shortened to stop at the rear axle to decrease the possibility of carrying passengers.[80] A "safety star" system for ATVs could help guide consumers to a proper vehicle.[68] Aftermarket safety products, such as crush guards, are available (see atvlifeguards.com/ and quadbarsafety.com/); these may prevent crush injuries by allowing riders to climb out from underneath a vehicle that has rolled over[103] (Figure 99-21). The efficacy of these devices is uncertain.

REFERENCES

Complete references used in this text are available online at expertconsult.inkling.com.

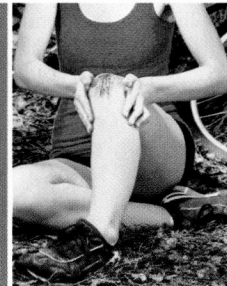

CHAPTER 100
Medical Liability and Wilderness Emergencies

CAROLYN S. LANGER AND BRIAN S.S. AUERBACH

This chapter presents a review of the legal issues that arise in the context of wilderness emergencies, with particular attention to those related to medical liability. With support from case studies, federal and state statutes, and various secondary sources, the chapter introduces basic legal concepts, including negligence, waiver of liability, and Good Samaritan laws. It also covers legal doctrines that are of critical importance to trip operators and wilderness medicine physicians alike, including the duty to warn, medical screening of trip participants, duty to rescue, standing orders, and medical record keeping.

Christopher Mance was a senior at Ohio University when he enrolled in a wilderness course as part of his outdoor studies. In fulfillment of a class requirement, Mance embarked on an overnight solo camping excursion in a secluded area. During this wilderness trip, he suffered an epileptic seizure and fell face first into a campfire. Mance sustained severe burns to his face, arms, and hands, which rendered him extensively disfigured. Ohio University knew that Christopher Mance had a history of seizure disorder, but Mance had signed a waiver of liability before the trip. He maintained that his seizure disorder was well controlled on a regimen of divalproex (Depakote), a medication he had been taking for years.[31]

What was Ohio University's obligation to warn Mance of wilderness hazards, such as a change in sleep patterns that can lower the seizure threshold? Did the waiver that Mance signed effectively release Ohio University from liability? Did a physician clear Mance to embark on this solo camping excursion? What are the legal guidelines for prohibiting participation in such a trip? If a physician had screened Mance's medical records and concluded that he could not participate, to what Americans with Disabilities Act (ADA) laws would that physician have been subjected? Should Mance or Ohio University bear the economic costs of his injuries?

In recent years, personal wealth, general interest, increased leisure time, globalization of the economy, and sophisticated marketing have led to expanded participation by the general public (with an aging population) in expeditions and cruises to remote environments, including wilderness areas. Such travel poses a higher risk for injury and illness than does travel in urban areas and often involves exposure to extreme weather conditions, limited access to medical personnel and supplies, and extended patient management because of limited medical evacuation capabilities. What are the medicolegal ramifications for tour operators and trip physicians? Historically, the probability of a lawsuit was low because participants were younger, more physically fit, and more experienced adventurers who tended to be greater risk takers with awareness of and willingness to assume these risks. However, increased involvement of a less prepared and marginally aware general population in wilderness pursuits has undoubtedly generated a concomitant increase in exposure to liability. To minimize liability, tour operators and trip physicians must implement sound risk management strategies for medical clearance, education, and provision of medical services to trip participants.

The issues described earlier highlight some of the common medicolegal concerns that arise when people are injured in the wilderness. This chapter addresses these and other legal issues that may be encountered by physicians and trip operators.

TORT LAW AND THE DOCTRINE OF NEGLIGENCE

CASE STUDY: SNAKEBITE AND MEDICAL MALPRACTICE

On August 11, a victim sustained a rattlesnake bite to the index and middle fingers of his left hand. Suction cups and a tourniquet were immediately applied, and the victim was transported to the hospital within 15 minutes. Another 15 minutes passed before Dr. A arrived. Dr. A proceeded to treat the patient by injecting antivenom into the base of the fingers bitten by the snake and into the left deltoid, despite an instruction sheet accompanying the antivenom that cautioned, "Do not inject serum into a finger or toe." Dr. A packed the patient's hand in ice and admitted him to the hospital. Two days later, the patient was sent home with instructions to keep ice on the hand.

Eight days later the victim's two fingers, hand, and arm were edematous, discolored, and odorous from gangrene. Dr. B assumed care of the patient. He applied a heating pad and injected antibiotics. On September 9, the two fingers required amputation. Is Dr. A liable for medical malpractice?

In tort law, members of society owe a duty to others to act reasonably and in a way that will not hurt another person or his or her property. In the context of wilderness medicine, redress for a private civil wrong is typically sought under a medical negligence doctrine. To bring a cause of action under a negligence theory, the plaintiff (the party filing the claim) must establish the following four elements:

1. *Duty:* The defendant has a duty by virtue of the physician-patient relationship to use due care as would a reasonably prudent physician under similar circumstances. For example, a plaintiff could argue that a trip physician owes the participants a duty to "possess and bring to bear on the patient's behalf that degree of knowledge, skill, and care that would be exercised by a reasonable and prudent physician under similar circumstances" given the prevailing state of medical knowledge and available resources.[46] To meet this duty, physicians must typically adhere to the standard of care established by the medical profession.

2. *Breach of duty:* Defendants breach their duty when they fail to conform to the duty of care or to act in accordance with norms or standards of practice. This breach may occur either through commission or omission of certain acts. For example, a physician may breach the duty of care by failing to diagnose or treat a condition (omission) or by improperly treating a patient (commission).

3. *Causation:* The plaintiff must further prove that the defendant's conduct was the direct, foreseeable, and proximate cause of the resulting injury. In other words, absent the defendant's conduct, the harm would not have occurred. Establishing causation is often the most problematic step for plaintiffs. For example, an injured traveler might allege that a trip leader or medical practitioner breached the duty of care by delaying medical evacuation, but the defendant could argue that the injury had already occurred and that any delay in evacuation neither caused nor aggravated the injury.

4. *Damages:* Finally, the plaintiff must demonstrate damages, that is, harm to the individual's person, property, or interests, for which the redress is customarily a monetary award. Awards may encompass special damages (e.g., out-of-pocket losses, medical expenses, lost earnings), general damages (pain and suffering, mental anguish, and other emotional injury), and punitive damages. Punitive damages are rare in the medical context because the plaintiff must prove that the defendant's conduct exceeded simple negligence and was intentional, grossly negligent, reckless, malicious, or fraudulent. Nonetheless, physicians should be aware that their insurance policies generally do not provide malpractice coverage for punitive damages.

Medical malpractice is a specific form of negligence occurring during execution of a physician's professional or fiduciary duties. Medical malpractice can be defined as medical care that falls below the standard of care expected of a reasonably prudent physician under similar circumstances, resulting in foreseeable harm to the patient.[44] In all negligence suits, the plaintiff bears the burden of proof in establishing the requisite four elements under a "more probable than not" standard. In other words, the plaintiff must establish that there was a greater than 50% probability that the defendant's breach of duty caused the harm.

In the snakebite case presented earlier, the first element is clearly demonstrated. Dr. A's actions established a physician-patient relationship and acceptance of the duty to render care. Establishing the second and third elements is more problematic. The court held that Dr. A did not breach his duty. The court elaborated, "There are wide variations in accepted methods of treatment of rattlesnake bites. The method of treatment chosen and used by the defendant was an acceptable method of treatment." In other words, even though physicians must act with the level of skill and learning possessed by minimally qualified members of the profession, they are judged by reference to the beliefs of the school that they follow. That is, their practice need not be followed by a majority consensus, provided that it is supported by a recognized school of practice in the medical community.

The court further held that the plaintiff failed to establish causation. Expert testimony showed that "rattlesnake bites in extremities always present some chance of tissue destruction" and that the most probable cause of tissue death in the two distal phalanges was the rattlesnake venom. Thus Dr. A was found not liable. Whether Dr. A's intervention met the standard of care and caused the ultimate amputation are debatable. Typically, though, both parties to the litigation use expert witness testimony to establish their respective positions vis-à-vis standard of care and causation issues.

Each state has its own body of statutory, regulatory, and case law in addition to federal law. Thus, although this chapter presents general legal and risk management principles, physicians should always familiarize themselves with the laws and precedents in their own states before implementing policies and procedures related to wilderness or travel medicine. Unless the trip application has a jurisdiction clause explicitly limiting the venue for litigation (often the state in which the tour outfit has its headquarters or principal place of business), a plaintiff could theoretically bring a claim in his or her own state of residence, in the state where the physician is licensed, in any state where the tour outfit conducts business or has some nexus, or in the jurisdiction where the injury occurred.

LIABILITY CONCERNS IN WILDERNESS MEDICINE

The remainder of this chapter examines how the legal doctrines apply in the unique circumstances of wilderness medicine. Not surprisingly, increased participation of the general population in adventure travel has led to higher—and in many cases unrealistic—expectations on the part of the public. Some unseasoned travelers to remote destinations anticipate the same level of medical resources (including personnel, equipment, medications, and evacuation capabilities) as those to which they have access via large, urban tertiary-care medical centers. It is therefore vital for tour operators and trip physicians to understand the duty and standard of care to which they must adhere and to educate trip participants regarding the medical risks of travel.

DUTY TO WARN AND EDUCATE TRIP PARTICIPANTS

CASE STUDY: DUTY TO WARN

A middle-aged male traveler booked a tour to Bolivia through a travel agent. In the trip brochure, the tour operator represented itself as an experienced and reputable company and stated that it researched all locations to which it arranged tours and "would care for participants from 'portal to portal.'"[42] In addition, the travel agent asked both the tour operator and local health agencies about health requirements and necessary precautions. During the trip, the traveler developed high-altitude cerebral edema after flying from Chile (at sea level) to La Paz, Bolivia (elevation 3962 m [13,000 feet]), in less than 1 hour. He subsequently sued the travel agent and tour organizer for failure to warn him of the health risks associated with his travel.

In general, there is no duty to warn of dangers that are as obvious to the participant as to the organizer. Obvious dangers might include possible seasickness or airsickness, substandard sanitation, and poor environmental conditions. Moreover, travel agents and tour operators have no duty to investigate potential vacation sites (not even those where conditions and terrain are dangerous) or lower standards of medical care in foreign countries. However, they do have a duty to warn travelers of known unreasonable risks or dangers, such as political turmoil and criminal attacks, which are foreseeable or likely to occur. Typically, to incur this duty to warn, the travel agent or tour operator must have actual or constructive notice of the hazardous condition arising from their knowledge of special circumstances (e.g., prior occurrences). In addition, travel agents and tour operators may contractually expand their duty to warn through representations made in brochures or other advertisements. In the case mentioned earlier, for example, the court recognized that tour organizers are not insurers of the safety of tourists with whom they contract and need not warn of obvious hazards. Nonetheless, in this case the travel organizer contractually expanded its obligation through its representations and brochures and created a reasonable expectation on the part of the tourist that it would research the risks of high-altitude travel and warn him of accompanying dangers.

Even in the absence of liability, trip organizers and medical practitioners have incentive to prevent travel-associated injury or illness, because they suffer financially and ethically when a tourist experiences physical or financial loss, fellow travelers are inconvenienced, or the reputation of the company or medical practice is potentially damaged. Sound risk management principles dictate that travel companies provide as much useful information as feasible to prevent adverse consequences. Companies lacking the wherewithal to research health hazards may benefit from the assistance of a medical adviser. Depending on the nature of the trip, some or all of the following information may be useful to participants:

- Environmental conditions (e.g., climate, altitude, terrain)
- Activity level (type, intensity, duration, and frequency of activity or exertion required)
- Specific health hazards (e.g., tropical diseases, marine envenomation, frostbite, heat injuries)
- General health information (e.g., safety of local food and water, local medical resources)
- Known risks (e.g., political unrest, high crime areas)
- Recommended immunizations

Whether an outfitter has an obligation to provide helmets and safety equipment depends on many factors, including anticipated hazards, experience of participants, industry practice, and so forth. However, even when the outfitter requires participants to furnish their own safety equipment, it is advisable for the outfitter to identify potential hazards and required gear. Perhaps a more pressing concern is the noncompliant participant who refuses to wear or use furnished safety gear or who otherwise acts in a reckless manner. In these instances, signed waivers may be of some value, but juries are not always sympathetic to waivers because the trip operator is sometimes perceived as being in a better position to ensure participant safety. The more prudent risk mitigation step might be to include a statement in the trip brochure or application indicating that the trip operator may, in its discretion, dismiss any participant at any time during the trip for cause, including failure to wear appropriate safety gear or to comply with safety rules, at no liability or cost to the trip operator.

MEDICAL CLEARANCE OF TRIP PARTICIPANTS

Tour operators have no duty to medically screen trip participants. Travelers have a responsibility to exercise due caution for their own safety. Nonetheless, do tour operators have the right or an incentive to screen participants? Medical clearance of travelers may serve several beneficial purposes. It can function to educate participants about potential health hazards, thereby reducing their risk for harm. Medical screening affords the participant's private physician the opportunity to more effectively manage the patient's care. It also may enable a tour operator to arrange accommodations in advance for participants with special needs. Moreover, medical clearance may reduce the tour operator's liability, costs, and inconvenience.

On the other hand, medical screening has certain disadvantages. Some authorities consider medical screening useless because a high-risk patient with a strong desire to go on a trip may ignore the inherent dangers and conceal a significant medical history (or shop around for a physician willing to grant the medical clearance). In addition, since enactment of the ADA in 1990, many tour operators fear discrimination lawsuits for medically screening out disabled persons. However, with a proper understanding of the legal issues underlying medical clearance and the ADA, tour operators and physicians can safeguard the interests of all parties involved.

THE AMERICANS WITH DISABILITIES ACT

Molly, who is a double amputee as a result of a car accident, applies to Whitewater Ventures to participate in a rafting trip. The outfitter rejects her application, claiming that she would not be able to meet their safety standards and swim independently. Frank is hearing impaired and requests that National Park Adventures (NPA) provide a sign language interpreter on a biking and hiking trip out west. NPA refuses, citing the unduly burdensome expense involved in hiring a signer. Tommy is a 10-year-old boy with autism who requires a behavior plan and one-to-one aide to support him in a parks and recreation program run by a major metropolitan park agency. The city indicates that it cannot accommodate this request because its staff lacks the required expertise to provide these services. Meghan uses a wheelchair for mobility, and is interested in participating in a mountain trek in Nepal. The adventure outfitter declines her request to provide bus transportation throughout the entire trek. Do all of these individuals have a legal right to access these recreational activities, and must the providers of these recreational opportunities offer an accommodation if needed?

For persons with and without disabilities alike, recreational, travel, and wilderness pursuits provide enjoyment and diversion and lead to enhanced fitness, self-esteem, leisure skills, social opportunities, mental well-being, and quality of life.[33] The ADA opened doors to leisure and recreational activities for persons with disabilities (see Chapter 94). Under Title II of the ADA, state and local governments may not refuse participation by a person with a disability in a service, program, or activity simply because that person has a disability.[9] Title III of the ADA prohibits all places of public accommodation and services operated by private entities from discriminating against the disabled.[10] These private entities include both for-profit businesses (such as adventure outfitters and tour operators) and nonprofit groups (such as community sporting leagues, YMCAs, and Boys and Girls Clubs).

Furthermore, an entity may not apply eligibility criteria that screen out an individual or any class of individuals with disabilities "unless such criteria can be shown to be necessary for the provision of the goods, services, facilities, advantages, or accommodations."[11] For example, "a cruise line could not apply eligibility criteria to potential passengers in a manner that would screen out individuals with disabilities unless the criteria are 'necessary.'"[12]

An entity is not, however, required to permit an individual to participate in services when the individual poses a direct threat to the health or safety of themselves or others. This determination that the participant poses a significant risk must be an individualized assessment using reasonable judgment based on current medical knowledge or the best available objective evidence. In addition, the "safety exception" may justify excluding individuals when they pose a threat to themselves. The safety exception holds that an entity may impose legitimate safety requirements that are necessary for safe operations. As an example, the regulations cite as a valid screening criterion the requirement for all participants in a recreational rafting expedition to meet a necessary level of swimming proficiency.

For screening criteria to be valid, they must be uniformly applied to all prospective participants, not merely to those with disabilities. Moreover, they must be based on actual risks, not on mere speculation, stereotypes, or generalizations about a person or class of persons with a particular disability. A tour organizer could not, for example, categorically exclude all persons with a history of angina from a high-altitude trip, but rather must afford individuals with documented, well-controlled angina an opportunity to establish their fitness and eligibility for the trip. In the case described earlier, Whitewater Ventures may require that Molly be able to swim independently, but the provider must apply this criterion to all applicants and must afford Molly the opportunity to demonstrate her ability to meet this eligibility criterion. Moreover, as a reasonable accommodation (see later), Molly could likely wear a personal flotation device, if needed, to demonstrate swimming proficiency.

Even when screening criteria are valid and the prospective participant cannot meet those requirements, a public accommodation must make reasonable modifications in policies and practices or must accommodate the disabled individual unless such modifications would cause an economic or administrative burden or would fundamentally alter the nature of the goods, services, or facilities offered. For example, in the case of Tommy described earlier, if the metropolitan park agency has a budget in the millions of dollars, the cost of hiring an outside aide to provide one-to-one support for Tommy and to develop and implement a behavior plan may not be an undue burden. On the other hand, if National Park Adventures is a small entity with annual revenues of $300,000 and only two full-time staff members, a court might find a signer to be an economic burden for such a small outfit, although the court might cite other less costly accommodations that NPA could provide to Frank, such as a written tour book. These decisions must be made on a case-by-case basis depending on the facts of the case. Similarly, a court would consider the specific facts of a case in determining if an accommodation would fundamentally alter the nature of the goods, services, or facilities. A cruise line could be required (as a reasonable modification) to provide an individual who relies on a wheelchair for mobility with a stateroom on the same level as the restaurant. However, a mountain trek would not be required to transform to a bus tour to accommodate this same individual.

MEDICAL SCREENING

To minimize the potential for discrimination claims, tour operators should provide physicians granting medical clearance as much information as possible regarding the physical demands of the trip. Tour organizers must provide detailed information concerning environmental conditions, specific health hazards, health and living conditions at the destination site, and availability of local medical resources. Companies should be as specific as possible in describing environmental conditions (e.g., altitude in feet, temperature in degrees). Trip organizers also must delineate the type, intensity, duration, and frequency of activity (e.g., bus tour, mild walking [1.6 to 3.2 km or 1 to 2 miles per day], vigorous hiking [specify distance and terrain], backpacking [specify weight of gear], trekking to remote areas [e.g., 24 hours from definitive medical care], climbing, swimming, canoeing).

The health care professional in turn must tailor the medical history and examination to the physical demands of the trip. The physician should become familiar with the patient's medical history, including any medications that could interact with the environment to which the patient is traveling. If applicable, the clinician should advise the patient to bring extra medications or medical equipment (e.g., a spare pair of eyeglasses, extra hearing aid batteries, anaphylaxis kit) in case complications or exacerbations occur. The physician also should inform the patient of applicable first-aid procedures and may also need to inform the trip organizer of special needs or accommodations.

Because patients and their physicians are sometimes hesitant to disclose confidential medical information to a travel company, medical clearance forms should emphasize functional abilities and limitations rather than diagnoses. If medical clearance forms request sufficiently detailed information about the prospective participant's medical fitness to meet the physical demands of the trip, travel companies frequently do not need to know about specific medical diagnoses. Companies that request confidential medical information should disclose this information only to employees who have a need to know and should ensure that the company medical adviser or trip physician safeguards this information in a locked file, typically at the company's offices, unless arrangements have been made for the physician adviser to store medical records at his or her private office. The company also may want to encourage high-risk patients to share medical information with trip leaders or bring along key medical records. It may be desirable for the trip physician or individual trip participants to bring along key medical documents or summaries that can easily be stored in their backpacks, particularly when traveling under Spartan conditions or to remote sites. Even though a medical adviser employed by the company or a private family physician makes determinations about medical fitness and medical clearance, the travel company bears legal responsibility for excluding disabled participants or for failing to accommodate their needs.

PROFESSIONAL LIABILITY, MEDICAL MALPRACTICE, AND GOOD SAMARITAN LAWS

In addition to complaints arising from lack of proper health warnings, injured trip participants commonly base claims on the company's failure to provide adequate medical services and facilities and negligent delivery of medical care. Historically, tour operators and cruise ships have had no obligation to ensure the health or safety of participants or to provide health care, particularly physicians' services, on trips. Trip organizers should nonetheless ascertain the appropriate standard of care for their particular circumstances by determining medical resources that other companies have provided on similar expeditions to similar destinations. Companies generally have the duty to staff trips to remote locations with personnel who have "significant training to provide adequate first aid and medical care until evacuation can be arranged."[25] Typically these staff members are emergency medical technicians (EMTs) or laypersons with basic first-aid training. Organizers of trips to locales with readily available medical care may have a lesser obligation to furnish staff trained in first aid. In the event of an adverse medical outcome, travel company employees are judged by a "reasonably prudent person" standard; that is, they have the duty to use reasonable care to furnish such aid and assistance as an ordinarily prudent person or trip leader would under similar circumstances.

Several professional medical organizations, such as the American College of Emergency Physicians and the Wilderness Medical Society, have sought to define and establish standards of care for the provision of medical services on cruise ships and expeditions. Many companies voluntarily staff physicians on their trips (and publicize that they have done so) for the comfort and convenience of the participants or to provide a competitive marketing advantage. Travel companies that advertise the presence of trip physicians and medical facilities in brochures, contracts, and other correspondence to participants or prospective participants contractually expand their obligation by creating an implied or express contract for the availability of certain medical services. At a minimum, it is expected that trip physicians will have the resources and capability to evaluate and manage emergencies and, when necessary, will arrange for more definitive care for the types of injuries and illnesses that might be reasonably anticipated on these types of trips.[6]

Who, if anyone, is liable when the physician commits medical malpractice? Is the physician protected by Good Samaritan laws? A nurse was accompanying an elementary school group on a trip to a farm in order to provide first aid and administer medication if needed. A boy who did not attend that school, but happened to be on the premises at the same time, poked himself in the eye with a wire. The nurse volunteered to look at the eye, administered ice, and reportedly instructed the boy's father to seek medical care if any problems developed. Two days later the eye was found to be infected, and after several surgeries, the boy eventually lost the eye. The boy's family sued the nurse for gross negligence. Under the Good Samaritan statute in that jurisdiction, a nurse is liable only for acts or omissions constituting gross negligence when the nurse "voluntarily and without the expectation of monetary compensation renders first aid or emergency treatment at the scene of an accident or other emergency, outside a hospital, doctor's office or any other place having proper and necessary medical equipment, to a person who is unconscious, ill or injured."[32] The court found in favor of the nurse, ruling that she was under no duty to render assistance to the child. She was on the premises to provide nursing services exclusively to the elementary school students on the class trip, which did not include the injured boy. She volunteered to help him and had no expectation of monetary compensation for such assistance.

Although Good Samaritan laws vary from state to state, most of these laws generally hold physicians and other personnel free from liability when assisting in an emergency, provided their conduct was not grossly negligent (a higher threshold than simple negligence), wanton, or willful. Other provisions common to many Good Samaritan laws include requirements to render care in an emergency or at the scene of an emergency, to act in good faith, to provide services gratuitously, and to have no pre-existing duty to the victim to respond or provide aid. For example, if a physician happens upon a stranger in need of emergent care while hiking up a mountain and provides medical care, his or her services would most likely fall within the purview of Good Samaritan laws.

On the other hand, does the physician acting as the "trip physician" lose his or her Good Samaritan protection? A typical custom in the adventure travel industry is to offer physicians generous discounts on trips in exchange for the provision of medical support for fellow participants. Many of these physicians are under the mistaken impression that they are covered by Good Samaritan laws in the event of a malpractice claim. The discounted fee, however, is the equivalent of compensation, and these physicians, along with those on straight salaries, would in all likelihood be considered independent contractors with a pre-existing duty to render medical care to fellow participants.

This potential exposure to malpractice claims has two important risk management implications for expedition physicians. First, physicians must familiarize themselves with the medical issues that they are likely to encounter on their trips and must possess the knowledge and skills to diagnose and treat relevant medical disorders. There is currently no prescriptive training, certification, or specialty requisite to serving as a trip physician. However, in determining the standard of care, a jury would expect the physician to anticipate foreseeable medical problems, assess the patient, and administer first-aid measures as would a reasonably prudent physician under similar circumstances, taking into account the remote location, extremes of environment, and limited capability to transport medical equipment on the trip. A physician employed on a cruise to known endemic areas must be familiar with diagnosis and treatment of tropical diseases. A physician with a mountain trekking group should be able to recognize signs and symptoms of high-altitude sickness and be proficient in management of this condition.

The trip physician's specialty is generally not a shield from liability. For example, a psychiatrist who holds himself or herself out as a trek physician would not be exculpated in a malpractice claim merely because he or she lacked training and experience in infectious diseases, primary care, emergency medicine, and other relevant areas. Therefore, physicians who lack the necessary skills to diagnose, treat, or stabilize basic first-aid, primary care, or emergency conditions may want to consider declining participation as a compensated trip physician because they would likely be held to the same standard of care as, for example, a primary care or emergency physician. On the other hand, specialty alone does not disqualify a physician from participating as a trip physician if he or she has acquired appropriate skills through prior participation in similar activities, conferences, previous duty in the public health service or military, and so forth. The determinative issue is how the "reasonably prudent physician" would have prepared for the trip and diagnosed and treated the patient under similar circumstances. Certifications, such as Advanced Cardiac Life Support, Advanced Trauma Life Support, and various wilderness medicine programs, are useful in demonstrating that the trip physician had training and acquired a certain level of proficiency in understanding and applying the standard of care. However, these certifications will not, in and of themselves, absolve the physician of liability, because the physician must still demonstrate that he or she adhered to the appropriate standard of care in any particular malpractice claim.

Physicians should not assume that their medical malpractice insurance policies cover claims arising out of medical services rendered on trips. Many insurance policies carry limitations on coverage for care delivered outside the scope of a physician's normal practice or beyond a certain geographic area. In these cases, trip physicians should seek extended coverage through their own insurance policies or through the tour organizer.

Both the plaintiff and defendant typically rely on expert witness testimony to identify the standard of care and offer an opinion regarding the defendant physician's adherence to that standard of care. Various state licensing boards are beginning to grapple with what their roles should be, if any, in sanctioning expert witnesses who give false or misleading testimony or who otherwise carry out their functions in a negligent manner. State licensing board policies on disciplining expert witnesses are not uniform across the country, but the American Medical Association (AMA) and many component state medical societies are advocating greater state government oversight of expert witness conduct and formal sanctioning when indicated, including possible loss of licensure. Regardless, any physicians wishing to serve as expert witnesses should closely scrutinize their qualifications and suitability to testify about wilderness medicine issues. The AMA House of Delegates has proposed the following minimum requirements for qualification as an expert witness (Policy H-265.994[3a]):

The AMA believes that the minimum statutory requirements for qualification as an expert witness in medical liability issues should reflect the following: (i) that the witness be required to have comparable education, training, and occupational experience in the same field as the defendant or specialty expertise in the disease process or procedure performed in the case; (ii) that the occupational experience include active medical practice or teaching experience in the same field as the defendant; (iii) that the active medical practice or teaching experience must have been within five years of the date of the occurrence giving rise to the claim; and (iv) that the witness be certified by a board recognized by the American Board of Medical Specialties or the American Osteopathic Association or by a board with equivalent standards.[21]

The negligence of a physician generally will not be imputed under a theory of respondeat superior (master-servant relationship) to the tour organizer or carrier. Many courts have noted that the relationship between a trip member and physician is not a traditional activity over which a cruise ship or tour organizer has control. Moreover, a shipping or travel company is not in the business of providing medical services to participants and does not possess the requisite expertise to supervise a physician brought along for the convenience of the participants. Nonetheless, once the carrier or tour organizer undertakes to hire a physician, it owes a duty to participants to exercise reasonable care in the selection of a competent and qualified physician. To the extent that the company fails to discharge this duty, it may be subject to a cause of action for the negligent hiring of an incompetent physician. Therefore, cruise lines and tour operators should ensure that trip physicians are proficient in general medical care, emergency treatment, and medical management of diseases endemic to the destination site.

Furthermore, travel companies and cruise ships should brief trip physicians on available resources, host country medical facilities, and evacuation procedures. Finally, companies should conduct formal credentialing of prospective trip physicians by verifying medical school graduation, board certification, and state licensure, and researching any history of disciplinary actions.

WAIVER OF LIABILITY

Under certain circumstances, a defendant in a lawsuit may avoid liability *even though* the plaintiff proves every element of the cause of action alleged. Such circumstances are known as "affirmative defenses," and they play a critical role in all manner of disputes; for example, well-known defenses in a criminal context include *duress, insanity,* and *self-defense.*

When negligence is alleged against an operator, physician, or other party in a wilderness setting, the defendant frequently raises the defense of *waiver of liability.* Waiver is typically achieved with a contractual release from liability, which is a signed agreement on the part of the injured party that the defendant will not be liable for injuries caused by the defendant's negligence. The naive wilderness operator might attempt to protect itself and its staff, medical and other, from liability by simply requiring its participants to sign such a contract. It turns out, however, that contractual release is not simple. Even though the legal system generally allows two willing parties to bind themselves by contract to any terms they agree on, there are many cases in which courts refuse to enforce waiver provisions.

NO WAIVER FOR GROSS NEGLIGENCE

Gross negligence is a form of negligence in which the party's failure to exercise reasonable care constitutes an *extreme* departure from the ordinary standard of conduct. It is, in some sense, a "worst" case of negligence, although still unintentional. Many jurisdictions that would allow a party to contractually release another party for ordinary negligence refuse to enforce releases for gross negligence, on the basis that such releases run contrary to public policy.

In its 2007 holding in the case of *Santa Barbara v Janeway*, the Supreme Court of California handed down a ruling that brought California law in line with the majority of states, where an agreement in the context of sports or recreational programs to release liability for gross negligence is unenforceable as a matter of policy.[8] In *Janeway*, the parents of a 14-year-old developmentally disabled child sued the City of Santa Barbara for the wrongful death of their child, Katie Janeway. Katie, who suffered from cerebral palsy, epilepsy, and other developmental disabilities, participated in a summer camp conducted by the City in 1999, 2000, 2001, and 2002. She had a history of seizures brought on by exposure to water, of which the camp administrators were aware.

On the second day of the 2002 camp, Katie suffered a seizure waiting to enter the locker room of the camp's pool. A camp counselor who had been assigned to monitor Katie while she was at the pool observed the seizure, but Katie appeared to recover quickly and was subsequently allowed to swim. The same counselor, who was supposed to be watching Katie, turned her back for a very short time and lost track of the child. The counselor had the lifeguards clear the pool, and Katie was found drowned at the bottom of the pool, approximately 5 minutes from when she had last been seen.

In the litigation that followed, the camp raised the defense of contractual waiver, based on a form signed by Katie's mother that released the camp and its employees for liability arising out of "any negligent act." The issue of whether that waiver was effective as to gross negligence came before the California Supreme Court, which found that although the wording "any negligent act" certainly included gross negligence, "an agreement purporting to release liability for future gross negligence … violates public policy and is unenforceable." In so holding, California came into line with the majority of states where the law is the same: it would go against public policy to enforce waivers for gross negligence.

OTHER BARS TO WAIVER

In addition to the common bar against waivers for gross negligence, many states prohibit releases for *ordinary* negligence under all manner of circumstances. For example, the *Janeway* court noted vast variation in the laws of different states. A majority of states bar a parent from releasing a minor's claims for negligence.[24] Vermont has voided releases for ordinary negligence in the context of recreational skiing on the basis that the ski resort is able to prevent dangerous conditions over which the skier has no control.[50] Connecticut has similarly invalidated waivers for activities that include snow tubing and horseback riding.[43] Washington State has voided agreements releasing public school districts from liability from future ordinary negligence related to interscholastic athletics.[54] New York has voided waivers in the context of auto racing, resort skiing, horseback riding, parachuting, tennis, and other recreational activities.[40] Virginia has voided *all* preinjury releases for liability.[26] Many states also bar enforcement of waivers for future negligence when such waivers are against the public interest. For example, in California, as in most states, a hospital cannot obtain releases for ordinary negligence.[53]

The above enumeration of bars to waiver is by no means exhaustive. It does give some indication, however, as to how difficult it can be to state any general rule as to what circumstances are sufficient to guarantee enforceability of a waiver. Instead, the ability of a party to obtain an effective release depends greatly on the type of activity and the state whose law is applied.

EFFECTIVE WAIVER

In light of the subtleties of waiver law, an operator cannot guarantee enforcement of its waiver; there are many steps necessary for an effective waiver that can increase likelihood of enforcement. Most important is to obtain advice of competent legal counsel regarding the following key issues:

- *Jurisdiction:* Enforceability of a waiver depends heavily on the state whose law is enforced and the activity to be covered. This is not a simple question. Consider a tour operator, such as Overland Inc. of Williamstown, Massachusetts, which operates hiking trips throughout states such as California and Vermont for high school students from all 50 states and internationally. In such complicated circumstances, only competent legal counsel can draft a waiver that is most likely to be enforced.
- *Assumption of risk:* Waivers are more likely to be enforced when they are accompanied by an acknowledgment and assumption of risk. This makes sense; whereas it may be fair to allow a party to give up claims when that party understands the risks inherent to the activity, courts are much more reluctant to enforce releases where the injured party did not acknowledge such danger.
- *Consideration:* Contracts that are not supported by a legal construct known as "consideration" are not enforceable. Consideration is best understood as meaning "value in return." For example, a woman rents skis from a shop, pays for them, leaves the building, and begins to drive away. An employee runs out and has the woman sign a release form in the parking lot. This release is likely unenforceable for lack of consideration: the woman already had gotten everything she wanted out of the deal—skis. With no value in return, the waiver is likely unenforceable. A short difference in timing would make all the difference; if the ski shop refused to hand over skis until its renters signed releases (which is standard practice in the industry), it would at least ensure that the waiver is supported by consideration.

Only legal counsel can provide proper advice on effective waiver. Depending on the nature and scope of the activity, and location of the operation, waiver may simply be impossible. In such cases, the operator may seek protection of indemnity or may take further measures to ensure that their operation and employees undertake reasonable care of the well-being of their participants. In theory, after all, waiver only comes into play when the defendant has actually been negligent.

DUTY TO RESCUE AND ABANDONMENT DOCTRINE

A physician who is on an expedition to Alaska and approaching the summit of Denali happens upon a trekker with multiple fractures and hypothermia. Does the physician have an obligation to treat the victim or attempt a rescue?

To answer that question, consider the example of David Sharp, a climber who died of severe altitude sickness and hypothermia while on Mt Everest in May 2006. Sharp lay by the side of the trail exhausted, his situation worsening, as numerous climbers trekked past him and made their summit attempts. Although a few climbers provided Sharp with supplemental oxygen, essentially he was left to die, and he perished on the mountain. David Sharp's plight and death generated international outrage over the procession of climbers who passed him by, apparently ignoring his dire condition.[34] Although moral debate ensued from this tragic story, from a legal standpoint, the climbers who walked past Sharp without offering assistance were completely within their legal rights. Sharp's case illustrates the general rule that some special relationship must exist to create a duty; conversely, without any special relationship, no duty exists.

In particular, it is well-settled law in the United States that there is no duty of a physician (or any other individual) to rescue an individual merely happened upon in need of medical care or assistance, except in certain exceptional circumstances.[57] Most notably, when an individual has created a hazardous situation that directly causes another individual harm, there *does* exist a duty for the perpetrator to rescue the victim.[47] In the case of a biking accident on a remote trail, the individual who caused the accident, through negligence or purely bad luck, has a duty to assist the injured. Louisiana has a law on the books requiring a hunter who accidentally shoots another hunter to aid in the injured party's rescue. This duty is most simply fulfilled by alerting authorities or the emergency medical system. Duty to rescue also exists with certain relationships beyond physician and patient, such as parent and minor child or in *loco parentis* baby-sitters or schoolteachers.[36]

Internationally, however, there are numerous countries that *do* obligate a duty to rescue. Generally, countries whose legal system is rooted in civil law (such as those of continental Europe, Asia, and South America) have a duty to rescue, whereas common law countries (such as the United States and other former British colonies) do not recognize a general legal duty to rescue.

HARM TO THE RESCUER

In cases where the circumstances of the rescue are caused by a party, through negligence or otherwise, the party who caused the original harm also bears legal liability for harm caused to the rescuer during the rescue. In the landmark case *Wagner v International Railway* of 1926, Justice Cardozo states that "danger invites peril ... The wrongdoer may not have foreseen the coming of a deliverer. He is accountable as if he had." Consequently, an injured rescuer may recover damages for harm sustained during a rescue attempt from the party who caused the original harm.[55]

In a wilderness context, a physician has a duty to the patients he or she agrees to treat or treats, but not necessarily to everyone he or she happens upon in his or her travels. As in an ordinary medical malpractice case, only when the physician-patient relationship is established can a plaintiff prevail in proving medical malpractice in a wilderness setting.

ABANDONMENT DOCTRINE

Once established, a physician-patient relationship is subject to abandonment principles should the relationship end. Abandonment is the unilateral termination of the physician-patient relationship by the physician without adequate notice to the patient, despite the need for ongoing medical care. In general, a physician has no legal duty to provide care for or to rescue endangered strangers. "The law imposes no liability upon those who stand idly by and fail to rescue a stranger who is in danger."[35] Moreover, abandonment occurs only in the presence of an established physician-patient relationship. Thus, the physician who refuses to enter into a physician-patient relationship and initiate treatment will not be held liable for abandonment.

Traditionally, once an individual initiated a rescue attempt, he or she could abandon rescue efforts at any time. "[The] motives in discontinuing the services are immaterial... [The rescuer] may without liability discontinue the services through mere caprice or because of personal dislike or enmity toward the [victim]."[32] However, if by giving aid the rescuer has put the victim in a worse position than before the attempt to aid, the rescuer may be liable. For example, the victim may have relied on the rescuer's efforts to his or her detriment, foregoing other opportunities to obtain assistance during the rescuer's intervention.

The best risk management tool is to assume that physicians who either implicitly or explicitly agree to treat patients create a duty to provide continuity of care. Given these circumstances, physicians can generally avoid liability for abandonment under the following conditions:

- The physician and patient mutually consent to terminate the relationship.
- The patient dismisses the physician.
- The victim no longer requires care, recovers, or dies.
- The physician dies or is disabled.
- Further rescue efforts would place the rescuer's life in danger.
- The physician gives the patient reasonable notice of his or her intent to withdraw from the care of the patient and, particularly in an emergency, continues to treat the patient until another qualified health care provider takes over the case.

Improper termination of the physician-patient relationship may lead to a cause of action for breach of contract or professional negligence, as well as for abandonment.

STANDING ORDERS AND MEDICAL KITS

There is tremendous variability in the medical expertise of trip leaders and participants and in the resources, including medical equipment and supplies, that accompany treks and trips into the wilderness. Delivery of medical care by nonphysicians represents one of the most problematic and controversial issues for trip organizers. Absent any representations to the contrary in travel brochures or other documents sent to participants, there is no implied or express contract to provide medical care to trip participants. Nonetheless, because of the nature of the business proprietor-customer relationship, trip leaders have some preexisting duties, namely, to exercise due care in the performance of their duties and in facilitating evacuations, when feasible, as would be considered reasonable under the circumstances. In other words, if they have made no claims to the contrary, trip leaders and staff have no duty to render care beyond basic first-aid services that an ordinary layperson could provide.

May a nonmedical trip leader or an EMT, paramedic, or other allied health care provider render medical services beyond the scope of his or her training or certification? One state board of registration in medicine defines the practice of medicine as:

Conduct, the purpose or reasonably foreseeable effect of which is to encourage the reliance of another person upon an individual's knowledge or skill in the maintenance of human health by the prevention, alleviation, or cure of disease and involving or reasonably thought to involve an assumption of responsibility for the other person's physical or mental well-being: diagnosis, treatment, use of instruments or other devices, or the prescription or administration of drugs for the relief of diseases or adverse physical or mental conditions. A person who holds himself out to the public as a physician or surgeon, or with the initials M.D. or D.O. in connection with his name, and who also assumes responsibility for another person's physical or mental well-being, is engaged in the practice of medicine. The practice of medicine does not mean conduct ... engaged in by persons licensed by other boards of registration with authority to regulate such conduct; nor does it mean assistance rendered in emergency situations by persons other than licensees.[13]

Consider the hypothetical example of a trekker who suffers a painful shoulder dislocation with diminished distal pulses. A nonphysician attempts a joint reduction. Successful reduction allows for a safe evacuation in the following 12 to 24 hours by hiking out with the comfort of a sling. Without reduction, a painful shoulder dislocation, especially in the setting of neurovascular compromise, would have necessitated a more urgent rescue, possibly including helicopter transport, and much higher risk to the injured person and rescuers. Such practice of medicine in the wilderness context is routinely implemented by outdoor programs without issue. Legally, most states require that an EMT or paramedic act under the supervision of a physician. Supervision usually entails direct observation, radio or telephone communication, or written guidelines, protocols, or standing orders (usually with reasonable access to a physician who can respond to questions and provide requested guidance). These statutes were enacted under the assumption that physician consultation would be fairly accessible. Even with the advent of cellular telephones and telemedicine, many trekkers and travelers to remote regions cannot easily obtain physician consultation. In general, trip leaders and staff who practice beyond the scope of their education, training, and certification could be engaging in the unlawful practice of medicine.

Even in an emergency situation, it is unclear whether Good Samaritan statutes protect trip leaders and staff. As previously discussed, travel companies and their trip leaders are to a certain extent compensated for safeguarding the safety and welfare of participants. Therefore it seems most likely that courts would use a reasonable care standard in determining the negligence of trip leaders. In other words, the court would determine how a reasonable trip leader with similar education, training, and certification would respond in similar circumstances, taking into account the emergent nature of the victim's illness or injury, remoteness of location, scarcity of medical equipment, limited means of evacuation, and inaccessibility of definitive medical care.

Many wilderness expeditions carry medical kits stocked with prescription drugs, including controlled substances. Epinephrine is one such medication, particularly germane to wilderness medicine, that has legislation supporting its use by nonmedical persons. Activist groups have worked with state legislators and EMS agencies to promote legal use of the EpiPen by trained EMTs. Although some states still lack coverage, most support EpiPen use by EMTs. In 2009, the New York State Assembly passed a bill that requires all ambulances in the state to carry EpiPens.[38] More recently, this trend has extended to public workers. For example, Arkansas passed legislation in 2009 that authorizes public sector employees, including tour operators, forest rangers, and teachers, to use EpiPens.[3] The New York Assembly took a stronger stance, enacting legislation in February of 2010 that requires these devices at all children's overnight, summer day and traveling camps.[39] Other states have followed suit. Internationally, Ottawa enacted "Sabrina's law," named after a young girl who died of anaphylactic shock at a school where the nursing office was not equipped with this lifesaving medication.[45] Generally, this legislation has been widely supported and is likely to expand further to states and countries that have not already enacted it.

Despite progressive legislation liberalizing the use of EpiPens, other medications frequently contained in wilderness medical kits do not have such coverage. Outdoor outfitters routinely carry prescription pain medications and antibiotics into the backcountry. This practice is high risk from a medicolegal perspective and generally not supported legally or covered by standard malpractice coverage. Failure of nonmedical trip leaders to provide these medications would not be considered negligence because doing so is in violation of the law, particularly when the trip organizer did not create the peril and provided adequate advance warnings to trip participants. If a nonphysician dispenses drugs, it could very likely constitute the unlawful practice of medicine. Moreover, physicians who do not accompany the travelers but who nonetheless write the initial prescriptions to stock the medical kits expose themselves to lawsuits arising out of any malpractice on the part of the trip leader with regard to use of those medications. For example, a nonmedical trip leader might improperly diagnose and dispense medications or might overlook certain drug interactions. In addition, physicians who write prescriptions to stock medical kits face the risk of being disciplined by their respective state boards of medicine for inappropriate prescribing practices, particularly if medications are dispensed to an unintended recipient or if there is an adverse event.

This legal dogma is of little comfort to trip leaders who find themselves in emergency situations. In some instances, trip leaders on overseas travel have been known to purchase or to recommend that participants purchase medications abroad that would require prescriptions in the United States. These drugs are sometimes available over the counter in foreign countries. Although the purchase and use of these medications are legal on foreign soil, travelers should be cautioned about the potential lack of guarantees regarding safety, quality, and efficacy of locally procured drugs. If the nonphysician trip leader chooses to dispense medications, whether originally stocked in the medical kit before departure from the United States or obtained abroad, a court would in all likelihood judge any adverse consequences in accordance with a "due care" standard. That is, a trip leader who dispensed medications with resultant harm to the patient would be expected to demonstrate the due care of a reasonably prudent person under similar circumstances, taking into account the emergent nature of the medical condition, remoteness of the trip, availability of definitive medical care, and so forth. To avoid potential liability, trip organizers should adhere to the following basic risk management principles:

- Do not advertise medical capabilities and resources beyond the scope of expertise of trip staff members or resources readily accessible in the country.
- Emphasize the need for trip participants to bring along an adequate supply of their own prescription drugs, and even verify that they have done so.
- Caution trip participants about the lack of safeguards concerning the safety, quality, and efficacy of medications obtained overseas.

If trip organizers choose to equip staff members with medical kits, one expert in wilderness medicine recommends that the contents of the kit be based on the following factors[19]:

- Environmental extremes encountered during the trip
- Endemic diseases
- Medical expertise of the medical officer
- Medical expertise of the expedition members
- Number of people on the trip
- Responsibility for local health care
- Length of the trip
- Distance from definitive medical care
- Availability of rescue (i.e., helicopter)

MEDICAL RECORD KEEPING IN WILDERNESS MEDICINE

Good record keeping is of paramount importance in the practice of wilderness medicine. The medical record is both a health care document and a legal document. Although storage space and the portability of written or electronic medical records on trips to remote locations are often limited, trip physicians should nonetheless strive to be as thorough as possible in documenting medical care. The medical record functions as a complete, written, and chronologic record of a patient's medical history, condition, and treatment. In medical malpractice claims, which are frequently litigated years after the alleged occurrence, these records may be the only written source from which the sequence of events and subsequent treatment can be reconstructed. Moreover, memories fade and witnesses become less available over time. Therefore courts tend to give tremendous weight to the written record and will often assume that documented events occurred and undocumented events did not occur, particularly when the oral testimonies of the litigants conflict.

Although the length and content of entries vary with the specific circumstances, notes should at a minimum include the patient's chief complaint, the results of the physical examination (including normal findings), an assessment, and treatment plan. The key point to remember in creation of medical records is that they may be used to prove or disprove that the medical practitioner adhered to the appropriate standard of care. Therefore physicians should record sufficient details to reflect their thought processes and to justify care provided under the circumstances. Moreover, physicians should document events chronologically and as soon as feasible after delivery of medical care. Once notes have been entered into the written or electronic medical record, the medical practitioner should never alter (or write or type over) the original notes. Entries should not be removed or inserted. If corrections are necessary, for written records, the physician may place a single line through the error, enter the correction, and initial and date the correction. For written or electronic medical records, the clinician may draft an addendum. Addenda should be placed after the last entry in the chart. Of course, notes should always be legible, signed, and dated by the health care provider making the entry. Upon completion of the trip, the company should treat these medical records as confidential information and place them in locked medical files, granting access to designated personnel (company medical advisers or others with a need to know) only. Some states have explicit laws or regulations that dictate the minimum period for retention of medical records. In the absence of such laws, travel companies and cruise lines should store medical records for the period of time corresponding to the statute of limitations for tort claims in their states, which, although varying from state to state, is typically about 2 to 3 years.

MEDICAL LIABILITY IN FOREIGN COUNTRIES

International travel continues to be popular. In addition to leisure travel, many medical professionals have the opportunity to provide on-call medical services for a variety of foreign excursions, including cruises, treks, and climbing expeditions. Although many of the theories of liability discussed in this chapter around the world are similar to those in the United States, there may be notable differences from domestic law.

This section should be read as a primer for any medical professional contemplating foreign travel, but is no replacement for finding a foreign attorney should the need arise. In addition to a basic overview of foreign medical liability, a physician traveling abroad should also know the basic steps for retaining a foreign attorney.

GOOD SAMARITAN LAWS ABROAD

Just as Good Samaritan laws vary from state to state, so too do they vary from country to country. Any medical professional contemplating foreign travel, whether as a physician or as a layperson, should become familiar with the laws of their destination regarding the liability assumed by coming to the aid of a person in need. Below is a short list of commonly visited countries and their respective Good Samaritan laws:

- Europe[52]
  - Great Britain: No duty to act unless there is a preexisting relationship that gives rise to the duty, but can be held liable if negligent rescue causes harm.
  - France: No duty to act, but liability can arise from any harm suffered during a rescue, unless that harm was necessary for the rescue.
  - Germany: Duty to act, but no liability for harm that occurred during the rescue.
  - Belgium: Duty to act unless there is serious danger to rescuer.
  - Finland: Duty to act, liability for harm suffered during negligent rescue.
  - Portugal: Duty to act unless serious danger to rescuer.
  - Spain: Duty to act for medical professionals; liability for harm suffered during negligent rescue.
  - Italy: Duty to act, but no liability for harm that occurred during rescue, unless due to negligence.
- Asia
  - China[29]: No duty to act, but liability can arise from harm suffered during a rescue. Good Samaritan laws are beginning to be enacted in certain provinces.[49]
  - Singapore[7]: No duty to act, but no official Good Samaritan law.
  - India[23]: No official Good Samaritan law.
  - Korea[30]: No duty to act; no liability for harm during rescue unless negligent.
  - Russia[51] Duty to act.
- Africa
  - Uganda[16]: No official Good Samaritan law.
- Australia[4]: Most territories limit liability to harm that occurs during a negligent rescue.

This nonexclusive list demonstrates the wide range of duties each country expects its citizens and visitors to uphold while within its boundaries. Countries that may share borders do not necessary share laws or legal systems; therefore, consulting a legal expert before extended travel is recommended for any medical professional.

TRANSPORTING MEDICAL SUPPLIES OVERSEAS

Many physicians, whether traveling for leisure or through contract, wish to carry their own medical supplies when traveling overseas. In general, transport of most supplies is not problematic. However, when transporting medications, in particular pain medications, care should be taken to determine the laws concerning narcotics in a particular country. Penalties for carrying restricted medications can be severe, potentially resulting in extended jail sentences or corporal or capital punishments.[28] The International Narcotics Control Board has issued several whitepapers concerning transport and regulation of narcotic medications abroad, including Model Guidelines for the International Provision of Controlled Medicines for Emergency Medical Care.[18,56]

RETAINING A FOREIGN ATTORNEY

Unless a U.S. attorney is also licensed in a particular foreign jurisdiction, the attorney cannot represent any party outside of the United States; a medical professional in need of foreign legal services must search for local counsel. Finding foreign counsel can be a daunting task, especially after a medical emergency has occurred. The U.S. Department of State[17] lists several points of consideration that should be undertaken in the search for a foreign attorney:

- Understand your attorney: Know the basic facts of your situation, but do not expect the attorney to be able to provide quick answers to a complicated question.
- Fees: Know the local currency and a general operating rate for your attorney. Many lawyers may expect payment in advance, while others may be willing to work for deferred fees. If you are planning to leave the country imminently, ensure that your attorney knows you will be leaving the country before any retainer agreement is signed.
- Method of payment: Ensure that your prospective lawyer can accept a form of payment that you can provide, whether it is the local currency, travelers' check, check, or credit card. Be aware that many banks and credit companies charge additional fees for foreign transactions.
- Progress reports: Foreign court activities and proceedings can be faster or slower than those of courts in the United States. Ensure that your lawyer will periodically update you on the progress of your case, and, if you have left the country, inform you if you need to return to the jurisdiction.
- Language: Is the foreign attorney fluent in English or your native language? Many court systems will allow for translation services, but beware of the "telephone" effect if too many parties are involved.
- Time: Find out from your prospective attorney how much time is estimated for the case to resolve.
- Travel restrictions: If you were planning to be in the foreign country for only a short period of time, ensure that the attorney explains your obligation about whether or not you must remain in the country for the duration of the case.

The Department of State cannot directly recommend a particular attorney,[18] so a physician in need of an attorney should find the nearest embassy, which should have a list of possible foreign counsel. In addition to the Department of State, both the American Bar Association (ABA)[1] and the American Society of International Law (ASIL)[2] maintain databases of information about foreign counsel that a physician can use in finding legal aid abroad.

MEDICAL CARE PROVIDED IN-FLIGHT

Not all injuries occur on the ground; a recent study estimated that a medical emergency will occur in the air once every 604 flights.[41] U.S. air carriers are obligated under federal law to provide medical kits and automatic external defibrillators on all aircraft and train crew members in their use,[5,14] but medical situations can often arise in-flight that require immediate intervention by trained medical personnel. However, positioning of the aircraft, which might be located outside the borders of the contiguous United States, can lead to legal complications not present in traditional ground location settings.

In the case of in-flight medical care rendered onboard a flight operated by a U.S. air carrier traveling over U.S. territory, responding medical professionals are granted liability protections against a potential lawsuit by the Aviation Medical Assistance Act of 1998 (AMAA), which states:

An individual shall not be liable for damages in any action brought in a Federal or State court arising out of the acts or omissions of the individual in providing or attempting to provide assistance in the case of an in-flight medical emergency unless the individual, while rendering such assistance, is guilty of gross negligence or willful misconduct.[5]

While the language of the Act does not clearly define gross negligence, flagrant disregard for a patient's health and safety is the generally accepted standard, as when an intoxicated physician treats a patient.[37] Consistent with the other U.S. medical liability principles discussed above, there is no legal duty for a physician to respond to a medical emergency that occurs during a domestic flight.

The AMAA additionally applies to international flights operated by domestic air carriers. However, the legal calculus becomes less clear on flights traveling internationally operated by international carriers. At least one U.S. court has held that the AMAA does not apply to foreign air carriers.[27] Although air carrier liability on international flights is standardized internationally by the Montreal Convention,[15,20] no such standardization exists concerning liability for the medical professional who responds to an in-flight emergency that occurs during an international flight. Generally, the country of aircraft registration determines the liability law to be applied, but the citizenship of physician or patient, along with the actual location of the aircraft at the time of the emergency, can also potentially dictate the choice of law,[22] In contrast to the United States and the United Kingdom,[48] many countries, as discussed above, impose a legal obligation for a medical professional to assist during an emergency.

Although a responding medical professional may be asked to advise the flight crew as to the status of the patient and severity of the emergency, the final decision on whether the flight should be diverted is made by the pilot commanding the aircraft. Responding professionals should always take advantage of all available ground-based medical support. Ultimately, whether legally obligated to assist or not, a medical professional providing assistance to a person in need during a flight should practice with the same level of ethics and attention to care as they would on the ground.

CONCLUSION

The services of medical professionals on cruises and expeditions can be invaluable to the safety and welfare of participants. Expanded participation of higher-risk individuals on trips to more remote regions of the world increases the liability exposure of health care providers. Legal issues, particularly causation, become more complex when medicine is practiced in these unconventional settings. By following the risk management principles outlined in this chapter, physicians can continue to provide effective care while minimizing their liability.

REFERENCES

Complete references used in this text are available online at expertconsult.inkling.com.

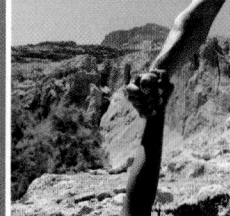

CHAPTER 101
Ethics of Wilderness Medicine

KENNETH V. ISERSON AND CARLTON E. HEINE

Ethics is the application of moral values and principles to guide human action. Providing care for others often involves intense human interactions. Thus, health care providers must frequently examine ethical issues in their work. Although the moral issues in wilderness medicine are an extension of traditional medical ethics, they are not directly comparable with the moral issues that arise either in medicine delivered in health care facilities or care delivered by urban emergency medical services. Wilderness medicine is unique, and its special attributes create unique ethical problems (Table 101-1). The working environment, concepts that involve standards of care, safety of rescuers and patients, and even the relationship between the provider and patient are different in a remote environment than in a traditional medical setting. For example, a hospital's working environment is rarely a factor considered by the hospital-based practitioner in the determination of what medical care to deliver, but the working environment is of major concern in the wilderness. Similarly, whereas patients usually have a clear legal relationship with the hospital practitioner and arrive at a hospital requesting care, neither condition is necessarily true in the wilderness setting. Even more striking are the differences between the hospital and the wilderness settings with regard to equipment availability, personnel training, need for evacuation or rescue, and provision for the safety of those involved. All of these differences can lead to unique ethical dilemmas in wilderness medicine.

This chapter provides an overview of ethical values as they apply to wilderness medicine. It describes a model for bioethical decision making in wilderness medicine, and provides examples of unique dilemmas that may be encountered in wilderness settings.

APPLICATION OF VALUES AND PRINCIPLES TO GUIDE HUMAN ACTIVITIES

Moral values are acquired throughout life from many sources, and develop into ethical action guides. In everyday situations, individuals may be unaware that these values are guiding their actions. However, when faced with situations that are rarely encountered, people may question how they should apply their

TABLE 101-1 Differences Between Hospital Practice, Emergency Medical Services, and Wilderness Medicine

Aspect of Medicine	Hospital Practice	Emergency Medical Services	Wilderness Medicine*
Environment	Controlled, known, static	Partly controlled, partly known, changeable	Uncontrolled, partly known, changeable
Patient	Known, requests care	Unknown, sometimes requests care	Unknown, sometimes requests care
Equipment	Sophisticated	Adequate	Rudimentary
Security	Safe	Usually safe	Questionable
Personnel	Highly educated, definitive care	Highly educated, basic care	Variable education, basic care
Evacuation	Rare	Built into system	Major concern
Rescue	No	Rare	Common

*Includes search and rescue.

values to solve practical problems. Such situations develop in wilderness medicine because the settings can challenge practitioners to demonstrate expertise outside the usual scope of their medical specialties.

Both patients' and clinicians' values control patient-clinician encounters. When patients express their values, clinicians can get an impression of patients' views about the necessary treatment, desired quality of life, and other complex attitudes that control willingness to seek and accept medical care. The clinician's values, both personal and professional, are also part of the relationship and sometimes conflict with the patient's values.

Ethical discussions often revolve around applying ethical principles in a consistent manner or in a way that could be applied by all practitioners in the same situation. Ethical principles or rules should be applied consistently across all scenarios. If an accepted principle is that a patient with decision-making capacity may make his or her own decisions about health care, then this principle should be applied to all situations, not just when it is convenient for the health care provider. Likewise, if the principle is universal to medical practice, then all health care providers (not just a privileged or unique group) should be able to apply it to their practices.

SOURCES OF VALUES

Moral values are the guideposts used to structure an individual's actions in life. They signify a person's duties and responsibilities, what is important to them, and how they interact with others. Thomas Aquinas said that there are three vital things for each person: "to know what he ought to believe; to know what he ought to desire; and to know what he ought to do."[1]

Moral values derive from many sources: family, society, school, religion, professional training, and related interactions. Family and religion generally guide development of values during the formative years. For nearly all people, these values form the bedrock upon which their lives are structured. Additional significant influences are the media, schooling, and society. Education broadens a child's experiences and values beyond the home. Finally, societal pressures continue to influence most individuals' value systems throughout life. Taken as a whole, different individuals' values derived from these multiple sources may conflict, leading to disagreements when ethical dilemmas arise over which action to take.

Professional schooling and interactions further refine how a person's values are applied. For example, one reason that medical students take anatomy courses is to destroy an ingrained cultural value against mutilating the dead. This allows them to accept and acquire the values of beneficial mutilation (i.e., surgery), handling the dead (e.g., resuscitation, pathology, transplantation), and invading another's body (i.e., invasive medical procedures).[9] In addition, when exposed to clinical practice, medical students, nurses, medics, and other health care providers learn to adopt the values of their preceptors. In any residency program, trainees learn intrinsic professional values, and the majority of trainees behave remarkably like the faculty.

VALUES IN MODERN BIOMEDICAL ETHICS

Another category of professional values, which is sometimes referred to as the *Georgetown bioethics catechism,* has emerged as an ideal for modern medicine, especially in the United States. These values include autonomy, beneficence, nonmaleficence, and distributive justice.

For the past four decades in the United States, the overriding professional and societal bioethical value has been a patient's autonomy. *Autonomy* recognizes an adult's right to accept or reject recommendations for his or her personal medical care (even to the extent of refusing all care) in the presence of appropriate decision-making capacity. Current bioethical opinion demands that clinicians respect patient autonomy. This is the counterweight to the long-practiced paternalism of the medical profession, wherein the physician alone determined what was good for the patient. Coupled with paternalism is coercion, which is the threat or use of violence to influence behavior or choice. The august figure in white (or in a medic's or search-and-rescue team's uniform) who implies that there will be dire consequences if medical recommendations are not followed remains a potent challenge to patient autonomy.

At the patient's bedside, *beneficence,* which is the act of doing good, and confidentiality, which is the nondisclosure of personal health information (and which was not part of the original Georgetown list), have been long-held and nearly universal tenets of the medical profession. Likewise, personal integrity—adherence to one's own moral and professional standards—is basic to ethical thought and action. One basic tenet taught to all medical students is *nonmaleficence:* "First, do no harm." This credo, often stated in its Latin form as *Primum non nocere,* derives from the historic knowledge that patients' encounters with physicians can be harmful as well as helpful. It recognizes every physician's fallibility.

The concept of comparative or *distributive justice* suggests that all individuals and groups in society should share equitably in the benefits and burdens of that society. Many society-wide decisions about the allocation of limited health care resources are based on this principle. However, it is a fallacy to extrapolate from this valid principle the idea that individual clinicians can arbitrarily limit or terminate care on a case-by-case basis simply because there exists a need to limit resource expenditures.[15]

VALUES APPLICABLE TO WILDERNESS MEDICINE

Safety or Security

Safety is wilderness medicine's primary controlling value in most circumstances. Safety begins with a measure of responsibility toward oneself, then one's companions, and finally the patient. In the unique setting of wilderness medicine, this responsibility extends to the wilderness team's safety from the environment, victims, and their own poor judgment; this is a concept more familiar to emergency medical services personnel than to health care providers in normal medical practice. However, this value is of paramount importance in wilderness medicine. Safety is the responsibility of any wilderness medical provider, even if he or she is not officially designated a provider but must take over during a medical crisis as a result of possessing special knowledge or skills. Decisions about rescue, evacuation, terminating group travel, or even attempts to perform certain medical interventions must include safety considerations.

As noted above, concerns about safety are applied in the following order: oneself, other team members, and then the patient. Ethical theory supports this hierarchy. Beneficence by medical personnel does not imply the need to endanger oneself. Indeed, if medical skills are to be useful, medical personnel must be able to render care. In addition, inherent in any leadership position is the responsibility to protect one's team. Therefore, the team members' safety is the second responsibility. Finally, the patient's safety should be ensured, but never at the expense of the medical team's safety. This is to say that, in unknown or unknowable circumstances, the medical leader may have to weigh potential risks against benefits. All risks must be considered in these "calculations," as in the case of a badly injured trekker who might survive if evacuated by aeromedical transport. If the helicopter team is willing to attempt a pickup, then the wilderness medical care provider must determine whether local conditions are sufficiently safe to justify the request, balancing the chance of benefit to the patient with potential safety risks.

One example illustrating safety issues occurred in the Pacific Northwest near Mt Baker. A group of adults and adolescents were on a hike above some snowfields when two parents and their daughter decided to glissade down one of the fields, something they had done before. As the mother and daughter sped over a crest, they dropped into a crevasse and were injured. The father pieced together what had happened and sought help. Eventually, a group of climbers was enlisted. No one was eager to descend into the trench, but one man from the climbing group agreed to be lowered on a rope, telling the group, "Just make sure you get me out."

The ethical question here is how much risk and responsibility untrained volunteers have in this type of wilderness crisis. A second issue that has to be considered is the capability of the group to attempt a rescue without endangering themselves and possibly creating the need for a second rescue. As a member of the hiking group, the father in this situation had a responsibility to help; however, because he was technically incapable of the rescue, his only responsible avenue of action was to seek help. Alternatively, bystanders have no fundamental responsibility to help or to assume any risk beyond what they are willing to assume. The man who agreed to be lowered into the crevasse would have been acting ethically if at any point in the rescue attempt he had signaled to the group to pull him up without helping the victims or if he had walked away and not allowed himself to be lowered into the trench in the first place. Despite entreaties from others, bystanders need not justify their participation or nonparticipation to anyone but themselves.[20]

In contrast, Ernest Shackelton, the appointed leader of a 19th-century attempt to be the first to reach the South Pole, had the responsibility to do his utmost to see his men safely home. During the voyage, their ship broke up in the ice, and the men had to pull lifeboats over ice to reach open sea while struggling against all odds to reach safety. Shackelton's steady and undaunted leadership is credited with helping all of his men to reach safety.[16]

A unique ethical problem that arises in wilderness settings, and that has often led to disasters, is when the team (especially the nonmedical team leader) ignores or overrides the medical person's decision. Individual team members have been harmed and multiple team members lost because factors other than the team members' safety and well-being were given priority.[14,22] Heeding the demands of safety is especially important, because the majority of people who are in the wilderness have risk-taking personalities, leading them to downplay security in favor of adventure.

Utility

In the language of ethics, utilitarian thinking plays a dominant role in wilderness ethics. Utilitarianism is the philosophy that promotes the greatest good or happiness for the greatest number of individuals. When applied to wilderness medicine, it promotes the well-being of the many over the well-being of the individual.

This can be defended by simply recognizing the unique aspects of wilderness medical practice, such as the uncontrolled environment, unfamiliarity with the patient, rudimentary equipment, and changeable situations, all of which contribute to safety concerns.

The ultimate application of utility in remote settings was described in the great survivor story of the men of the *Essex*, the doomed whaling ship that was the basis for Herman Melville's *Moby Dick*.[21] As was common after shipwrecks, the men drew lots to decide who would be sacrificed and die so that the others in the small boat could live a little longer without starvation.[24] One can argue that if all of the men consented to this process, then it was ethical, but the very nature of the situation put each man under such extreme duress that it would be questionable if any man's consent could be considered voluntary. In these types of extreme circumstances, the ethics of draconian decisions, such as survivor cannibalism, are always fraught with paradoxic ethical dilemmas.[9]

Decision-Making Capacity and Consent

Many ethical dilemmas in emergency medical care revolve around ascertaining a patient's decision-making capacity, often linked with consent to, or more often, refusal of, a medical procedure. Because a basic canon of both ethics and law, as stated by Justice Cardozo, is that "[e]very human being of adult years and sound mind has a right to determine what shall be done with his own body,"[23] these decisions about what action to take can often be made more clear by understanding what is meant by the term *decision-making capacity* and how it relates to consent. (Note that the term *competent* is often used when *capacity* is really what is meant. *Competent*, meaning "possessing the requisite natural or legal qualifications," is a legal term; competency can be determined only by the court.[19])

Capacity is always decision-specific rather than global. To have adequate decision-making capacity in any particular circumstance, a person must understand the available options and the consequences of acting on the various options, and he or she must be able to compare any chosen option against the costs and benefits related to a relatively stable framework of personal values and priorities[3,4] (Box 101-1). This last requirement is the most difficult to understand and requires a subjective interpretation. The easiest way to assess it is to ask why the individual made such a decision. Disagreement with the physician's recommendation is not in and of itself grounds for determining whether a person is incapable of making his or her own decisions. In fact, even refusal of lifesaving medical care may not prove that the person is incapable of making valid decisions if that refusal is made on the basis of firmly held religious beliefs (e.g., a Jehovah's Witness refusing a blood transfusion).

A person must be permitted to consent to or to refuse any medical intervention if he or she has decision-making capacity for that decision and if the clinician respects the patient's autonomy. Three general types of consent exist: presumed, implied, and informed. *Presumed consent*, sometimes called *emergency consent*, covers the necessary lifesaving procedures that any reasonable person would wish to have if he or she was lacking decision-making capacity; controlling hemorrhage and securing an airway in an unconscious victim of a fall are common examples. *Implied consent* is when a person with decision-making capacity cooperates with a procedure, such as holding out an arm to donate blood or to allow initiation of an intravenous line. *Informed consent* is when a person who retains decision-making

---

BOX 101-1 Components of Decision-Making Capacity

Knowledge of options
Awareness of the consequences of each option
Appreciation of personal costs and benefits of options in relation to relatively stable values and preferences

From Buchanan AE: The question of competence. In Iserson KV, Sanders AB, Mathieu D, editors: *Ethics in emergency medicine*, ed 2, Tucson, Arizona, 1995, Galen Press.

capacity is given all of the pertinent facts regarding the risks and benefits of a particular procedure, understands them, and voluntarily agrees to undergo the procedure.[11]

Questions applying to consent in the wilderness setting can be difficult. Does the victim have the capacity to understand the situation? Will decision-making capacity be questioned only if a person refuses "good" medical care? In addition (and this is unresolved even in standard medical practice), one must consider which procedures require informed rather than implied consent. The requirement to obtain informed consent varies in practice and the law from area to area. This variation stems from differing local practice standards and state laws, and disparities in physician training. Determining decision-making capacity and providing an opportunity for a patient to consent to a procedure when appropriate are crucial to respecting that patient's autonomy.

BIOETHICAL DECISION-MAKING PROCESS*

Both standard bioethics and wilderness medical ethics often involve difficult situations with no "correct" answer. Usually more than two possible actions exist. When faced with such a dilemma, how should the health care practitioner respond? Health care professionals often apply their values without much conscious deliberation: they act instinctively based on their prior behavior and training. Values are constantly (although not necessarily consistently) applied to everyday decisions. Of course, most decisions are not ethical decisions. Ethical dilemmas arise from a conflict between two seemingly equivalent values that are represented by different and mutually exclusive possible actions.

An example of a bioethical dilemma in wilderness medicine may help illustrate ethical decision making. For example, a distress call is received from anxious relatives or by radio from a plane flying over a wilderness area. The victim is in a hazardous area or, more commonly, caught in terrible weather. The clinician directing the search and rescue team must decide how to respond to the call in a setting that may put the team in danger. The standard bioethical value of beneficence directly competes with the bioethical value of safety in wilderness medicine. Each has a strong pull on the decision maker, with each value providing good arguments for sending or not sending the rescue team. Although the value of safety may often be considered paramount in the wilderness setting, the emotional and altruistic pulls of beneficence make this a difficult choice. Considering this case, a word should first be said about rights and duties in relation to health care. Although the word *rights* is glibly used in many situations, a personal right is present only if another person or society as a whole has an identifiable duty to the individual. One person has a right to receive a service from another person only when the second person has a duty and therefore an obligation to provide that service. Correspondingly, no health care practitioner has a duty to provide all of the health care that people desire or need. However, practitioners do have a duty to provide safety, when possible, for those whom they direct in wilderness settings.

Because an ethical dilemma arises when two or more seemingly correct actions appear to have equal benefits, the choice of actions should be examined first. How are these proposed "correct" actions determined in the first place? After that, which of these actions is the more ethically acceptable?

CHOOSING AN ACTION IN THE STANDARD SETTING

Jonsen and colleagues[12] suggested four groups of factors to consider when determining a course of action in the face of a bioethical dilemma in the standard clinical paradigm. These include medical indications for the action, the patient's preferences, consideration of the quality of life, and other contextual factors. These can be seen as an "ethical square," with the top two boxes (i.e., the first two factors) having more weight (Figure 101-1).

Medical indications are often more straightforward in the wilderness setting than they are in standard health care. In the wilderness, treatment is basic, injuries and illnesses are generally acute, and intervention is normally life preserving rather than death prolonging. The clinicians use standard clinical algorithms that are appropriate for their level of training and expertise. In

---

MEDICAL INDICATION

1. What is the patient's medical problem? Prognosis?
2. Is the problem acute? Chronic? Critical? Emergent? Reversible?
3. What are the goals of treatment?
4. What are the probabilities of treatment success?
5. What are the plans in case of therapeutic failure?
6. In sum, how can this patient be benefited by medical interventions, and how can harm be avoided?

PATIENT WISHES

1. What has the patient expressed about treatment preferences?
2. Has the patient been informed of benefits and risks, understood, and given consent?
3. Does the patient have decision-making capacity? What is the evidence of incapacity?
4. Has the patient expressed prior preferences, e.g., advance directives?
5. If the patient is incapacitated, who is the appropriate surrogate? Is the surrogate using appropriate standards?
6. Is the patient unwilling or unable to cooperate with medical treatment? If so, why?
7. In sum, is the patient's right to choose being respected to the best extent possible?

QUALITY OF LIFE

1. What are the prospects, with or without treatment, for a return to patient's normal life?
2. Are there biases that might prejudice the provider's evaluation of the patient's quality of life?
3. What physical, mental, or social deficit is the patient likely to experience if treatment succeeds?
4. Is the patient's present or future condition such that he or she might judge continued life undesirable?

CONTEXTUAL FEATURES

1. SAFETY ISSUES. In wilderness medicine, these are often the most important considerations.
2. Are there family issues that might influence treatment decisions?
3. Are there provider (SAR or trip member) issues that might influence treatment decisions?
4. Are there financial and economic factors (evacuation/rescue costs)?
5. Are there problems of allocations of resources?
6. What are the legal implications of treatment decisions?
7. Any provider, organization-related, or institutional conflicts of interest?

FIGURE 101-1 The ethical square. SAR, search and rescue.

remote areas, questions may arise about whether an ophthalmologist should attempt to reduce a hip dislocation or whether a nurse should attempt to establish a surgical airway. These dilemmas should, when feasible, be decided with input from the patient or a surrogate. As a matter of proper planning, behavior in critical scenarios must be decided in advance. In general, however, medical indications are clear.

Bioethicists normally feel most comfortable helping to resolve cases using only the medical indications and patients' wishes, which are all above the double line in Figure 101-1. When these factors are ambiguous, however, two other sets of factors must be considered: contextual factors and quality of life. In the wilderness setting, the primary contextual factor is safety. This may overshadow all other considerations involved in a victim's treatment. Other contextual factors include the financial implications of various treatments and the effect of various options on other trip members. In the standard medical situation, this is, admittedly, a fuzzy area. Related to these, and even more nebulous, are quality-of-life factors. These relate to the nature of a person's current and presumed future existence as viewed by others. For those who retain decision-making capacity, their autonomous decisions reflect their view of life. In the wilderness setting, time and circumstances usually do not allow clinicians to make quality-of-life judgments.

CHOOSING AN ACTION IN THE WILDERNESS

The importance of safety factors in the wilderness setting leads to the altered diagram of decision making for ethical problems in wilderness medicine (Figure 101-2). This includes three groups of factors to consider when choosing a course of action: safety, medical indications, and patient autonomy. Within this decision-making model, safety factors must be given the most weight.

Safety factors include security of the medical and rescue personnel and the victim, as well as the risks of both proposed procedures and evacuation method. As mentioned previously, medical team safety is a valid consideration because of the inherent risk-taking nature of people in the wilderness. In recent legal actions pertaining to wilderness injuries, the law has recognized a "doctrine of reasonable implied assumption of risk." This implied risk is also part of an acceptable concept of wilderness triage. Wilderness triage takes place when the same injuries or illnesses that would cause minimal morbidity in a medically sophisticated environment inevitably cause death when they occur in the wilderness. A fractured femur in the lone wilderness traveler or an abdominal gunshot wound in a remote area is often a virtual death sentence. This is a risk that wilderness adventurers take, although not always with a clear understanding of the enormity of the risk.

USING AN ALGORITHM AS A GUIDE FOR A DECISION

In bioethics, although disagreements may arise regarding the optimal course of action chosen using a specific set of values,

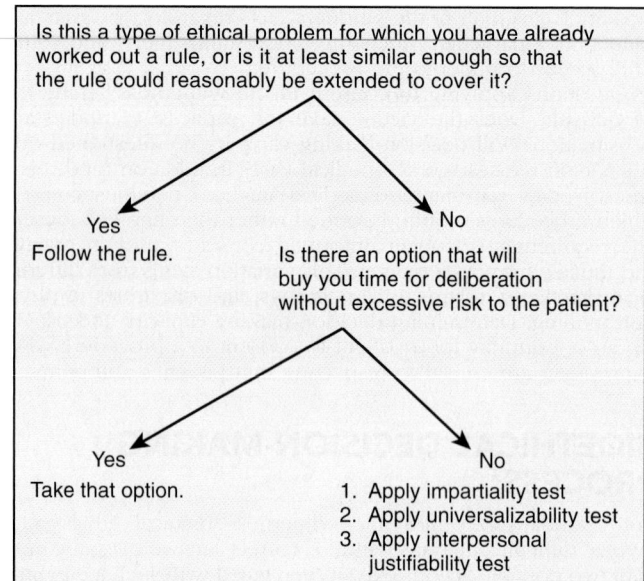

FIGURE 101-3 A rapid approach to emergency ethical problems. (*Modified from Iserson KV: An approach to ethical problems in emergency medicine. In Iserson KV, Sanders AB, Mathieu D, editors:* Ethics in emergency medicine, *ed 2, Tucson, Ariz, 1995, Galen Press.*)

general agreement often exists as to what constitutes ethically wrong actions. The method of ethical case analysis described in Figure 101-3 is designed to provide the emergency practitioner with prompt assistance for selecting an ethically correct, although not necessarily a theoretically "best," course of action.[7] This method applies equally well both in the wilderness setting and in the normal hospital setting.

The first step in using the algorithm in Figure 101-3 is to use a known precedent. This is the simplest solution to an ethical dilemma, but requires planning in advance, including reading and thinking about ethical problems. Many physicians and other health care professionals are not prepared to do this. Just as with any emergency procedure, wilderness medicine physicians and health care professionals should be prepared with a course of action for the most common ethical dilemmas likely to occur in the wilderness setting.

With no precedent, the second step is to "buy time." What action will not be harmful to the patient and will provide time for the consultation or information gathering needed to refine the action plan? In a wilderness medical setting, this might mean placing a person's arm in a sling for comfort while deciding whether an inexperienced provider should attempt to reduce a dislocation or fracture.

With no precedent on which to rely and no way to buy time, the health care professional must select a possible course of action and test it for ethical viability. The impartiality test, the universalizability test, and the interpersonal justifiability test are drawn from three different philosophical theories. First, the *impartiality test* is applied. The practitioner asks whether he or she would ask to have this action performed if he or she was in the patient's place. In essence, this is a form of the Golden Rule: "Do unto others as you would have done unto you." According to John Stuart Mill, this espouses "the complete spirit of the ethics of utility."[18] Second, the *universalizability test* asks if the health care professional would feel comfortable having all practitioners perform this action in all relevantly similar circumstances. This generalizes the action and asks whether developing a universal rule for the contemplated behavior is reasonable. This is merely a restatement of Kant's categorical imperative: "Act as if the maxim of thy act were to become by thy will a universal law of nature."[13] Finally, the *interpersonal justifiability test* asks if the practitioner can supply good reasons to others for his or her action. Will peers, superiors, or the public be satisfied with the action taken and reasons for it? This test uses David Gauthier's basic theory of consensus values as a final screen for a proposed

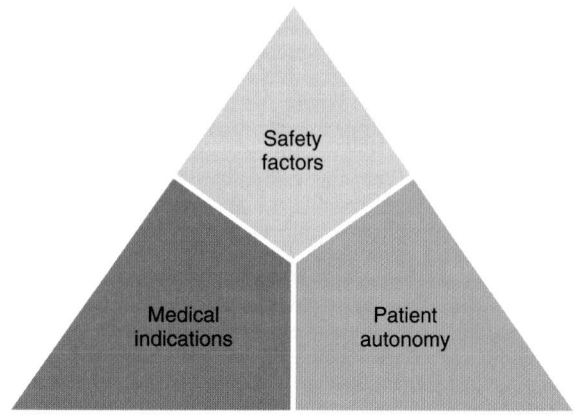

FIGURE 101-2 Wilderness medicine's ethical triangle.

action.[6] If all three tests can be answered in the affirmative, the health care professional can be reasonably assured that the proposed action falls within the scope of morally acceptable actions. However, if the proposed action fails any of these tests, the algorithm must be applied to another proposed action.

ETHICAL DILEMMAS IN WILDERNESS MEDICINE

With its unique setting and mode of practice, wilderness medicine provides practitioners with situations that are rarely seen by most other providers. These dilemmas can be grouped into three categories: standards of care, priority in care, and the decision-making process (Box 101-2). As might be expected, some of the issues in each group deal with provider-patient dilemmas, whereas others have more to do with group or governmental policies. These dilemmas have few parallels in other areas of medical practice (except perhaps battlefield medical practice or medical care during major disasters), resulting in ethical decisions that differ from those in standard medical settings. Such dilemmas include providing euthanasia for potentially nonfatal medical conditions, abandoning patients, and prioritizing medical care for original patients and rescue team members. However, the ethical decision-making process used to sort through these dilemmas is similar to that used in other settings; this is a basic truism sometimes obscured by the unique setting and issues of wilderness medical care. A limited discussion of these ethical dilemmas and the values involved follows.

STANDARD-OF-CARE DILEMMAS

Limited Resources

In the wilderness setting, resources are limited. Medical equipment is usually confined to supplies that can be carried into the field on foot, or, in some cases, by a pack animal or helicopter. Moreover, wilderness rescue personnel may have limited medical skills. The combination of limited skills and limited availability of supplies and equipment gives rise to ethical dilemmas. What should be included in wilderness medical kits? Their composition is resource allocation at its most basic. In addition, who makes these decisions?

Rarely do people consider pretrip decision making to be a part of medical care. However, it is very much a part of wilderness medicine. For example, decisions regarding the contents of

---

BOX 101-2   Ethical Dilemmas in Wilderness Care

Standard-of-Care Dilemmas
Limited resources: The standard of care differs. What should be brought into the field? How are resources distributed?
Cultural: Are Western standards of care and attitudes appropriate when treating locals in a foreign country?
Untrained personnel: How much authority is delegated to untrained personnel?

Priority-in-Care Dilemmas
Triage choices: Who should be rescued first? (Those most injured or ill? Injured or ill rescuers? Those with the best chance of survival? Women and children? Those with important information, such as scientists who have collected data? Those who do not volunteer to stay behind?)
Issues of survival
Issues of direct life-threatening situations for health care providers
Motorized vehicle restrictions and environmental protection in the wilderness areas

Decision-Making Dilemmas
Lack of availability of a surrogate decision maker or a family member
Euthanasia
Lack of an ethics consultation
Advance directives
No-rescue areas

---

medical kits made well in advance of, rather than during, triage will affect the patient's care. Although the individual wilderness traveler usually determines what is carried into the field, he or she generally fails to realize that this decision may set a limit on treatment. Any traveler planning a trip into a wilderness area must assume that the contents of the medical kit will be the only resources available for medical treatment. Although the group, a medical committee, or the medical director or advisor selects equipment for organized wilderness excursions or search and rescue teams, the selection still limits the medical care that can be given.

Although commercially available, standardized medical kits are usually designed on the basis of medical criteria, it is vital to recognize that some types of treatment will be implicitly unavailable because of what is excluded from these kits. No one is expected to carry a fully stocked emergency department into the field, but clearly identifying the ethical dilemmas that are entailed in compiling these kits helps team members with their decisions. For example, if a decision to not carry antiarrhythmic medications or a defibrillator is made and if a team member suffers a cardiac rhythm abnormality, then there will be little that can be done for him or her. Some people may omit medical kit items that could be useful, such as intravenous solutions. As the medical person on one doomed expedition to the Himalayan peak Nanda Devi recalled, "[My] irritation grew as [I] remembered [being] pressured into leaving intravenous fluids behind."[22] Such preexpedition resource decisions may jeopardize a team member.

Cultural Differences

Many wilderness emergencies occur in places outside of the United States or other Western countries. Are Western standards of care and attitudes appropriate when treating locals in a foreign country? Whose values control medical treatment and other actions?

Three circumstances may present ethical dilemmas in the delivery of medical care during expeditions to remote areas. The first is lack of cultural sensitivity. Aggressive offers to address disease or injury may frustrate or anger local patients or providers, whose methods of treatment fit within the region's cultural milieu and may be as good as or better than "modern" medicine. Temporarily replacing or upstaging traditional healers and their methods may degrade them in the eyes of the local population.

The second situation is when medical problems occur that are beyond the capabilities of an expedition's practitioners. After offering the care for which they are competent, practitioners may feel obligated to attempt treatments beyond their knowledge or abilities. An internist may face treating a gunshot wound to the chest, a psychiatrist may encounter a complicated obstetric emergency, or a paramedic may confront an epidemic. Often without any direction except a moral compass, these caregivers may be tempted to stretch their abilities beyond the limits of patient safety. Cultural ethical concerns should be considered when deciding which course of action to pursue.

The third situation relates to the larger question of the fairness of chance encounters: a woman's life is saved when a passing trekker is able to treat her pyelonephritis; after a surgeon relocates his hip, a man will continue to be able to provide for his family; and a paramedic happens to be on hand to intubate a child with epiglottitis. These situations by themselves rarely encompass ethical issues. The larger question, which may be more philosophical than practical, is how such interventions interfere with the balance of life in the area. Are chance encounters an aberration or simply a part of life? One of the most common situations in this category is a wilderness team from a developed country leaving medications behind with individuals who would not normally have access to them. Beyond the questions of the medications' efficacy, continued availability, and safety in inexperienced hands, there are the ethical concerns about altering the life balance of other cultures. Trekkers who traverse areas that others commonly visit do not face this dilemma, because medications are routinely distributed by a succession of groups. However, this question arises during expeditions that enter rarely visited areas, such as remote areas in Papua New Guinea or the Amazon Basin.

Giving Authority to Untrained Personnel

Wilderness travelers face ethical dilemmas when they encounter medical situations for which they are not trained; this is certainly not restricted to laypersons. Medics, physician assistants, nurses, and physicians may quickly find themselves out of their depth in a wilderness setting. This occurs when they treat patients with conditions comfortably treated only in an urban environment or when an illness or injury is beyond the scope of personal experience and knowledge. When deciding whether to intervene in such a situation, the person planning to help must weigh the chance of benefiting the patient (i.e., the value of beneficence) against the chance of harming the patient (i.e., the value of nonmaleficence).

The following hypothetical case illustrates both the questions raised in this type of dilemma and application of the Rapid Approach to Emergency Ethical Problems (see Figure 101-3). A backcountry excursion sets out with a medical provider who is unprepared for orthopedic emergencies. When a group member dislocates her shoulder, the provider is unwilling to go beyond his level of training by attempting shoulder relocation, although the victim (as well as the rest of the party) encourages the attempt. Another member of the party with even less training volunteers to attempt the maneuver, so the clinician is now in a double bind, seemingly forced either to overextend his skills or to acquiesce to even less knowledgeable medical care for the victim.

How could this dilemma be resolved using the Rapid Approach to Emergency Ethical Problems? The first step would be to anticipate such a situation in advance and plan a course of action. Because orthopedic trauma is common in the wilderness, any medical provider should expect to face such a situation. Note that planning may obviate this ethical dilemma, as it does in many other situations, because the provider may then acquire the requisite orthopedic knowledge and skills in advance or may abandon plans to assume this wilderness medical role. Whether or not the skill level is unchanged, the provider may also make a decision about an ethical course of action after discussing the potential problem in advance with knowledgeable peers or after acquiring information from other sources. Perhaps the provider has previously decided to act in such situations (i.e., his or her paradigm as part of the Rapid Approach to Emergency Ethical Problems). It is reasonable to base intervention on (1) determining whether the patient has appropriate decision-making capacity; (2) informing the patient fully and honestly about the apparent situation and options; and (3) acquiescing to the patient's desires, whether attempting relocation or simply securing the arm in place. Honest acceptance of the patient's autonomy to control his or her medical care often resolves a seemingly difficult ethical dilemma.

If the provider believes that the "experienced" layman offering to help has insufficient knowledge, then the provider must decide whether the paradigm case for which he or she prepared a response is similar enough to use for the current circumstances. If it is, then the dilemma is resolved, and that rule should be followed. However, if the provider believes that the current situation differs significantly from the paradigm case or if he or she has simply failed to decide in advance about an ethical course of action, then the provider should move on to trying to buy time. In the scenario presented, buying time may consist of making the patient comfortable before contacting help or thinking through the problem. Help may be available to organized wilderness excursions through radio or mobile telephone communication. The assistance may involve experienced advice about other actions that can be taken to resolve the dilemma or orthopedic advice about ways to reduce the shoulder. Sometimes, however, no help is available or not enough time can be bought to secure help. In that case, the health care provider must make a decision to act.

Using step 3, the provider attempts to choose an action that is ethically acceptable (by applying the ideas found in Figure 101-2), even if it is not the optimal action that he or she might select if more time were available to consider the problem. Possible actions in this case might include attempting reduction, allowing the layperson to attempt reduction, simply immobilizing

the victim's shoulder, leaving the victim and going for help, or ignoring the situation and leaving the decision to someone else. The provider must first choose a course of action (remembering that not deciding is also a course of action) and then decide whether the choice falls within the scope of ethically acceptable behavior. For example, if the proposed action is shoulder immobilization, the three tests of impartiality (i.e., the Golden Rule), universalizability (i.e., "Should every practitioner do as I plan to do?"), and interpersonal justifiability (i.e., "Would I be ashamed to have my actions publicized?") should be applied to this action. If the action passes all three tests, it is probably ethically acceptable and may be used. Remember that ethically acceptable actions may differ with the circumstances or the wilderness group involved.

Health care policy is another aspect of this type of ethical dilemma. Restricting medical practitioners from fully using their skills and knowledge may limit wilderness medical care. For example, paramedics are told that in some jurisdictions, on penalty of losing their licenses, they may not reduce fractures, perform cricothyrotomies, or, in a few locations, perform endotracheal intubations. Emergency medical technicians, first-aid providers, first responders, and the like are more severely restricted. Nurses may not know what procedures their licenses allow, and physicians are constantly concerned about liability. In general, many practitioners in wilderness settings feel that the laws and administrative policies under which they work restrict their actions. This attitude and their subsequent behavior may lead to substandard care for victims of wilderness injury or illness. The Wilderness Medical Society and other groups have begun working to overcome these limitations. Currently, however, an ethical dilemma may exist when practitioners face medical situations in the field that they know how to treat but that exceed their licenses or official certifications. A clear conflict may exist between the law and an individual's ethical responsibilities. Practitioners have to decide the best course of action, preferably in advance of the problem.

PRIORITY-IN-CARE DILEMMAS

Triage takes on new dimensions in wilderness settings. Ethical dilemmas easily arise when health care providers face not only triage among victims but also critical decisions about whether to help victims at all. These settings also produce situations in which rescuers or other members of the party may be placed in danger by helping an injured person.

Triage Choices: Whom to Rescue First and How to Distribute Resources

Medical practitioners, especially those in the fields of surgery and emergency care, are familiar with medical triage in which multiple patients need care and in which patients must be sorted by severity of injury, availability of resources, and possibility of successful treatment. These triage decisions have their own unique set of ethical dilemmas. Wilderness triage is unusual for several reasons and may present ethical dilemmas that are markedly different from those encountered in nonwilderness environments.

Three ethical dilemmas result from wilderness triage questions that are unlikely to occur elsewhere (with the exception of battlefield settings).[5] The first dilemma arises when the wilderness practitioner knows all the victims and may have personal ties to at least one. This is unlike normal triage scenarios and complicates any decision about who receives treatment, especially if resources are limited. For example, during an outbreak of giardiasis in a party of 12, the provider may have only enough metronidazole (Flagyl) to treat 5 people. Another more serious example would be a lightning strike in the midst of six people, with only one other individual capable of providing assistance. In each case, the medical practitioner applying triage criteria may be torn between medical and personal concerns.

A second ethical triage dilemma arises in what may be thought of as the "us-versus-them" situation. Members of both the wilderness party and the local population may be in the victim pool to be triaged. To whom does the provider owe primary responsibility? Some may argue that the implicit or explicit contract between the provider and group members warrants treating group members first. However, in the battlefield setting, which may often be analogous to the wilderness setting with regard to medical ethics, the Geneva Convention specifies that patients are always to be triaged for medical care *on the basis of medical need and the ability to treat*. Whether military caregivers follow this dictum in practice is moot. The wilderness caregiver must carefully consider this issue before venturing into the field.

Finally, ethical dilemmas arise because not all team members are equal. If triage among team members is necessary, treatment on the basis of pure medical necessity is not always realistic. In the giardiasis example, will the sickest patients be treated, or will treatment be given to the less-sick guide and translator, who are needed to lead the party safely out of the wilderness? The greatest good for the greatest number, or the concept of group safety, must prevail. This may be neither a comfortable nor an intuitively obvious decision.

An ethical dilemma also arises when a rescue team member is injured while in the field. Should rescue teams treat their injured team member before, or instead of, other victims? Wilderness rescue is an inherently dangerous operation. Although the safety record of some organized and experienced rescue groups has been excellent, this is not universal, particularly with ad hoc rescue attempts.[10] Where should the team's priorities lie? Again, an analogy can be drawn with triage parameters in emergency care. The principle of triage is that, as long as resources are available, the most seriously injured are treated first. Those who cannot be saved with available resources or be evacuated in time to be saved are given only comfort measures. This situation logically and morally prevails in wilderness medical care. However, emotion rather than reason often influences actions, so the wilderness health care provider must ensure that ethical decision making prevails.

Issues of Survival

In some situations, the lives of expedition members may be put at immediate risk if an injured person receives optimal assistance. One well-known example is high-altitude climber Simon Yates, who, while trying to lower his injured climbing partner, Joe Simpson, down to base camp in the Peruvian Andes, found himself in a situation in which he had to either cut the lowering rope tethering his partner, almost assuredly killing him, or risk also dying himself.[25] (He chose to cut the rope and, amazingly, Simpson survived.)

I couldn't help him, and it occurred to me that in all likelihood he would fall to his death. I wasn't disturbed by the thought. In a way I hoped he would fall. I knew I couldn't leave him while he was still fighting for it, but I had no idea how I might help him. I could get down. If I tried to get him down I might die with him. It didn't frighten me. It just seemed a waste. It would be pointless. ... The knife! The thought came out of nowhere. Of course, the knife. Be quick, come on, get it. ... I reached down again, and this time I touched the blade to the rope. It needed no pressure. The taut rope exploded at the touch of the blade, and I flew backwards into the seat as the pulling strain vanished. ... I was alive, and for the moment that was all I could think about. ... There was no guilt, not even sorrow. ... I was actually pleased that I had been strong enough to cut the rope. There had been nothing else left to me, and so I had gone ahead with it. I had done it. ... I was alive because I had held everything together right up to the last moment. It had been executed calmly. ... I should feel guilty. I don't. I did right.

In another example, a diver may surface too quickly and suffer an air embolism. Reviewing the ethical considerations in wilderness medicine's ethical triangle (see Figure 101-2), both medical indications and possibly patient autonomy influence the decision to rapidly transport the victim to a recompression chamber. However, even with the medical urgency of the situation, the other divers' safety mandates that the boat remain in the area until the other divers are on board. This example demonstrates again that, in the wilderness setting, security factors are primary when making ethical decisions.

Issues of Direct Life-Threatening Situations for the Health Care Provider

Health care providers in a wilderness setting often have the opportunity to rescue others, which directly supports their underlying motivation to be of help. However, situations arise in which providing help puts the caregiver or the entire team at significant risk; this has already been discussed in Safety or Security, previously. Wilderness medical leaders commonly decline entering a dangerous situation to attempt to rescue a patient. However, a more direct and powerful ethical issue arises when the caregiver must directly and explicitly sacrifice the patient for personal or team safety; this is somewhat analogous to the difference between passive and active euthanasia. For example, this occurs when a helicopter hoisting a patient encounters difficulties that endanger the craft. Standard procedure is to cut the hoist line, sacrificing the patient. In the abstract, the safety of the helicopter crew (and possibly rescuers on the ground) outweighs that of the patient. Yet in reality, the conflict between safety and beneficence may not be intrinsically clear to the health care provider; an answer in favor of safety contradicts all professional education and experiences. This conflict must be resolved in advance or within a few seconds during the event if anyone is to survive. In the analogous scenario on the battlefield, the question is raised, "How many medics do you sacrifice to save one infantryman?" The same dilemma applies to rescuers.

DECISION-MAKING DILEMMAS

Health care decisions are generally the responsibility of the adult with decision-making capacity. If a patient lacks the ability to make these decisions, health care providers normally seek a surrogate decision maker, advance directive, or counsel of a bioethics committee or colleague. These resources are rarely available in the wilderness setting, so health care decisions can therefore become more problematic. When family or close friends are present, they may act as surrogates to make decisions for the patient, but this is much less frequent in the wilderness setting than in the urban environment. The wilderness medical provider must therefore be prepared to make difficult decisions without this guidance.

Advance Directives

To allay the problems of the absence of surrogate decision makers or knowledge about a patient's wishes, health care providers for organized expeditions, especially those in which significant risk of danger exists, may want to request that each team member complete an advance directive. The normal forms for advance directives (i.e., durable power of attorney for health care, living will) may not suffice in the wilderness setting. Rather, a more specific directive should be used. It should detail how aggressive each individual would want the team to be when trying to extract him or her from a dangerous situation if the victim (1) had a reasonable chance of survival given available resources; (2) had a reasonable chance of survival but with serious physical disability; (3) had a reasonable chance of survival but with serious brain injury; or (4) had a poor chance of surviving. It should also address what to do with the body if the individual dies. Any directive given by a team member would be tempered by the need to ensure the safety of other team members, but such a directive might give the medical provider a better idea of each team member's desires. Indeed, just discussing these scenarios with the team before the trip takes place may be beneficial for elucidating attitudes and health care desires in the wilderness.

Euthanasia

Controversy continues to rage in society and medicine over the concept of active euthanasia (i.e., mercy killing). In wilderness medicine, however, euthanasia may be less ethically problematic, although it is a very sensitive issue to discuss and devastating event for those involved. Active euthanasia may be an ethically acceptable alternative for the rare situation in which a patient will die either because he or she cannot be rescued from the wilderness environment or because survival of group members would be jeopardized by attempting to evacuate or remain with him or her until help arrives. The seriously injured person on a high-altitude climb with inclement weather quickly approaching and the injured caver in a flooding cave are two examples. In these cases, euthanasia is based on the beneficence of relieving suffering in a doomed individual (although many in the medical profession believe that euthanasia violates professional principles), security for other members of the party (not creating more victims), and perhaps patient autonomy.[2]

Further complicating the preceding scenarios is the question of whether such patients should be simply left to die (i.e., passive euthanasia) or more humanely killed (i.e., active euthanasia). This question should be given serious consideration, because many incidents of passive euthanasia in wilderness settings occur, especially in high-risk or remote areas. For example, passive euthanasia has occurred several times on expeditions to Mt Everest when unconscious hypothermic climbers were left to die when conditions made it difficult or impossible to get them down.[22] The ethical question of what is best for the injured individual almost always comes into direct conflict with other team members' lack of confidence in their (or their medical person's) prognosis and their unwillingness to implement active euthanasia. Lack of certainty about a prognosis may sometimes be justified. For example, during a disastrous expedition to Mt Everest, a physician climber who was left for dead (active euthanasia was not discussed among team members) survived by eventually making it to camp on his own.

DILEMMAS IN WILDERNESS POLICIES

Ethical decision making plays a part in policies governing wilderness medicine. The values of beneficence and nonmaleficence make proposed and actual rules for wilderness medical practice untenable. These policies include when to stop searches, prohibition of motorized vehicles in wilderness areas, no-rescue areas, prohibition of environmental destruction, and restriction of medical providers' roles (see Giving Authority to Untrained Personnel, earlier).

When to Stop Searches

Without a body or corpse, it is difficult for managers of wilderness searches to know when to stop searching for someone who is presumed lost. Resource allocation decisions (i.e., distributive justice) create the contours of the solution to this kind of ethical dilemma. The parameters include available resources, probability of finding the lost person, danger to searchers, and likelihood of survivability under existing conditions. An example of such a dilemma occurred near Mt Rainier when a hunter briefly lost consciousness and became separated from his group. Fortunately, he was a strong, heavy man who could draw on fat stores for energy and warmth for several days. His hunting companions immediately began a search, followed by a formal search and rescue by a trained team the next morning. The dilemma was when to stop or pause the search because of bad weather, risks to the searchers, or the probability that the hunter was dead as a result of a preexisting heart condition. Severe weather caused the search to be halted after 4 days because of danger to the searchers, but it was to resume the next day after the weather had cleared. Before the search could be resumed, however, the victim found his way to a road, where he encountered a ranger. As this case illustrates, searches will often persist beyond the point at which the victim is believed to be dead in hopes of finding the victim alive or at least finding the corpse. It is the search leader's responsibility to continue the search process as long as it is reasonable to do so.[20]

Motorized Vehicle Restrictions and Environmental Protection in Wilderness Areas

A policy occasionally imposed on wilderness medical practice is that of no motorized vehicles in designated wilderness areas. This rule has logical roots but is enforced only intermittently. However, when it is used to hinder rescue efforts or delay needed medical care, it defeats a basic purpose of society: the assurance of citizens' welfare.

A related issue is the basic tenet of wilderness travel, which is that the environment should be left at least as pristine as it was found. However, situations arise when preservation of a wilderness area must be weighed against pain and suffering or life and death. Sometimes it may be necessary to chop down trees to make space for a helicopter pad or blast a new entry into a cave. Preservation of wilderness areas is an important goal, but so are preservation of human life and values, and the latter should not be overridden to reach a symbolic goal. Human life is a priority.

No-Rescue Areas

Perhaps the most pernicious concept proposed to govern wilderness medical care is that of the no-rescue area, into which adventurers would go with the foreknowledge that no rescue would be available.[17] This is akin to playing Russian roulette; people entering these wilderness areas put life and limb at risk while society condones and presumably enforces a requirement to not assist those in need. All explorers pushing the envelope of what is possible have entered these areas. The first men in space, and certainly Neil Armstrong and Buzz Aldrin, knew that rescue from the surface of the moon was not an option. The early mountaineers did not venture above 8000 m (26,247 feet) and expect a rescue if things went poorly. Today, the space shuttle has a backup plan, and climbers have been rescued from the highest altitudes. Is it reasonable to designate areas and to pursue adventures where no rescue would be attempted or even contemplated?

SUMMARY

Enjoying the wilderness and being capable and willing to provide care in remote settings fulfill many human desires. The challenges and decisions that sometimes need to be made can call an individual's values into question and haunt the individual for a long time. Preparing for these situations by thoughtfully selecting medical equipment, seeking out additional skills, and having difficult conversations with participants before a trip occurs can be as important as physical training. Sometimes, despite thorough preparation, unforeseeable events happen, and the decision tools presented in the algorithm in Figure 101-3 can be helpful to the provider and patient.

REFERENCES

Complete references used in this text are available online at expertconsult.inkling.com.

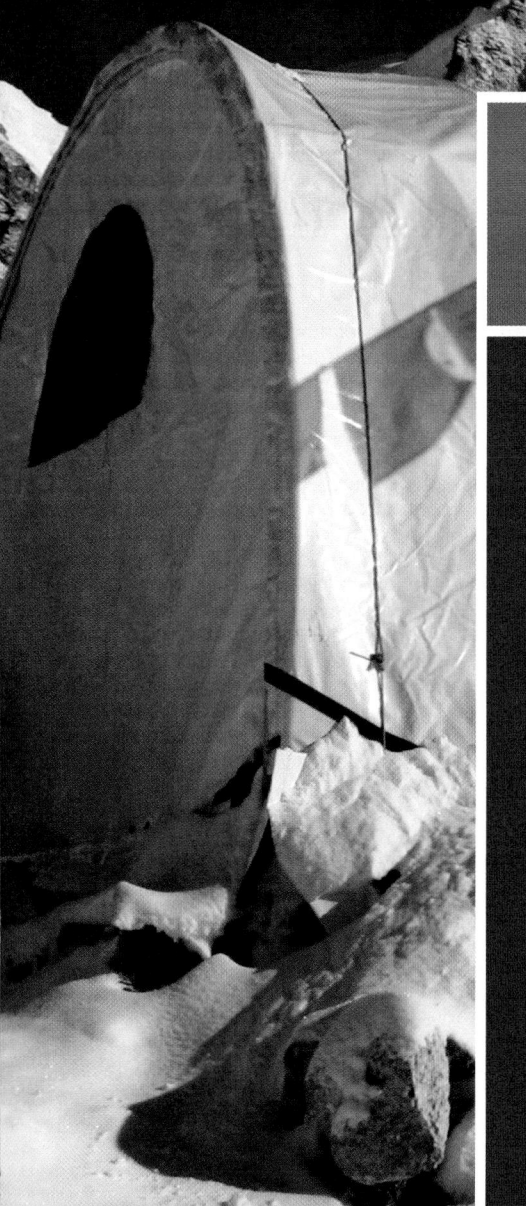

Wilderness Equipment and Special Knowledge

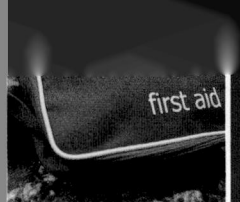

first aid

Wilderness Preparation, Equipment, and Medical Supplies

MICHAEL S. LIPNICK AND MATTHEW R. LEWIN

Wilderness travel and recreation expose individuals to illness and injury far from medical care. Travelers must be prepared to diagnose and treat frequently encountered conditions and promptly recognize when illness or injury requires evacuation. Although easily recognized, certain common problems such as blisters and diarrhea may become serious obstacles to a journey. Less frequent, more serious conditions, such as occult infection or internal traumatic injury, may be unnoticed and may threaten life or limb. In the hands of experienced personnel, appropriate trip planning and the correct supplies can greatly reduce morbidity associated with medical problems in remote settings.

This chapter primarily focuses on terrestrial travel and begins with epidemiologic considerations in trip planning. An overview of pretrip preparation includes trip personnel training, strategies for injury and illness prevention, a framework for participant medical screening, and considerations for environmental and activity-specific risks. Potential components of medical kits, strategies for kit assembly, and additional specialized equipment are then discussed. Various medications useful in wilderness settings are reviewed, followed by discussion of common medical problems encountered in the wilderness. The final section provides a sample journey to illustrate key concepts in pretrip planning, illness management, and decision making.

EPIDEMIOLOGY REVIEW

Reviewing available data on injury and illness prevalence during wilderness excursions is an important component of thorough pretrip planning. Given the relatively limited amount of existing data and large regional and temporal variations in these statistics, consultation with prior expedition leaders, local guides, and other first-hand sources specific to the planned trip location and activity are particularly important. The most extensive research to help quantify the statistical risk of injury or illness during different types of wilderness activities has occurred in the fields of high-altitude and dive medicine, with limited studies in other fields,[46] including desert,[48] tropical, and aquatic environments.

Existing data suggest that in remote environments, incidence of traumatic injury (generally of a minor nature) exceeds that of medical illness, and among backcountry fatalities, traumatic etiologies are by far the most common.[13,18,22,25,26,34,47] Data from the U.S. National Park Service (NPS), which include both front-country and backcountry data, are consistent with this observation but also suggest that among higher-acuity wilderness medical events, such as those requiring advanced interventions (e.g., IV placement, medication administration, advanced airway management), medical illnesses are responsible for a significant proportion. Between 2007 and 2011, NPS data indicate emergency medical services (EMS) events occurred 64,045 times (45.9 times per 1 million visitors) and were categorized as medical (29%), traumatic (28%), and first aid (43%). The majority (61.4%) of the 1480 fatalities during this period were traumatic; among medical events, 1.8% were cardiac arrests.[11]

Falls, drowning, and blunt trauma constitute the most common causes of wilderness fatalities.[16,22,34] For life-threatening injuries, causes of preventable prehospital deaths include unrecognized trauma, exsanguination, asphyxia (often caused by inadequate airway management) and pneumothoraces. For nontraumatic deaths, cardiovascular disease is responsible for a significant proportion. Recreational activities, such as cycling or use of all-

terrain vehicles, has been associated with significantly increased risk of injury.[8] Ice and rock climbing generate a unique array of injuries, including death from severe head trauma.

Common types of nonfatal injury include soft tissue damage (e.g., abrasions, lacerations, sprains), whereas more serious soft tissue injuries (e.g., dislocations, fractures) account for less than 5% of all trauma. The lower extremities are by far the most likely parts to be involved in minor orthopedic injuries,[30] emphasizing the importance of appropriate foot care and footwear selection.

In addition to trauma, wilderness travelers often report medical illnesses attributable to nonspecific syndromes, such as gastroenteritis or upper respiratory infections. These illnesses likely result in part from exposure to new pathogens and from travel conditions that preclude adequate preemptive hygiene measures. Other frequently reported medical problems include headache (exacerbated by high altitude), dyspepsia (from local food intolerance), dehydration, heat-related illness, dermatitis, sunburn, allergic reactions, blisters, and other integument-related problems.[6,16,30]

Environmental causes of illness predominantly relate to high altitudes and extremes of temperature and can generally be avoided with adequate planning and early recognition.[6,16,30,32]

It cannot be overemphasized that prior expedition leaders, local guides, and other first-hand sources can provide the best guidance when preparing for potential backcountry medical challenges, including availability of medications and emergency resources. This is especially true for foreign travel.

GENERAL PREPARATION

Careful evaluations of weather patterns, participant health, planned activities, rescue options, and journey duration are critical to pretrip preparation and can help guide prevention and treatment plans for anticipated injuries and illnesses (Box 102-1).

Prevention is of paramount importance when discussing management of injury and illness during wilderness recreation. Medical care may be greatly delayed, and in certain circumstances, timely, formal medical attention may not be an option.

Mode of travel, destination, duration, environment, planned activities, and the number of persons on any trip can vary to such a degree that, in reality, there is no universal planning strategy. Physicians in the office face the challenge of advising travelers about medicines and medical equipment, knowing that their patients could face decisions they are not qualified or prepared to make. Travelers and their physicians must recognize these limitations and seek appropriate consultation from experienced colleagues as well as from books, wilderness medicine courses, and myriad high-quality Internet resources (see Appendix A in this chapter).

It must be emphasized that regardless of a physician's prior wilderness medicine experience, it is essential to have detailed discussions with expedition leaders and past members regarding occurrence of various medical problems, trauma, and utility and local availability of various medical supplies on previous, similar expeditions. Local rangers and EMS personnel can provide valuable information about weather patterns and risks specific to local terrain (e.g., propensity for mudslides, flashfloods, and electrical storms). Climbers and mountaineers will benefit from reading *Accidents in North American Mountaineering,* an annual publication that describes and analyzes climbing injuries and fatalities

BOX 102-1   Pretrip Checklist for General Preparedness

- ☐ Identify and outline trip itinerary.
- ☐ Conduct pretrip medical briefing to advise participants of risks.
- ☐ Ensure physical conditioning of participants is adequate.
- ☐ Ensure medical and dental checkups up-to-date (pretrip health questionnaires).
- ☐ Review immunizations status (specific to region of travel).
- ☐ Review potential injuries and medical conditions relevant to planned itinerary, activities, and participant medical conditions.
- ☐ Review potential rescue and evacuation routes throughout itinerary.
- ☐ Review of historic and current weather conditions (National Climatic Data Center, http://www.ncdc.noaa.gov; the National Weather Service, http://www.nws.noaa.gov; The Weather Channel, http://www.weather.com).
- ☐ Obtain medical insurance with evacuation coverage (where possible).
- ☐ Share itinerary with emergency contacts and necessary authorities.
- ☐ Establish knowledge of available communication and navigation tools.
- ☐ Establish plan for clean water supply (chemical or device disinfection vs. storage).
- ☐ Obtain medical alert medallions or cards as well as emergency contact information as needed.
- ☐ Compile and review equipment and medical supplies (quantity and expiration).

occurring each year in North America (http://publications .americanaplineclub.org).

Familiarity with evacuation resources (e.g., availability of search and rescue teams), communications devices (e.g., satellite phones, cell phone coverage), and navigation devices (e.g., maps, GPS) is an important component of trip preparation. A brief discussion of various communication and navigation devices is provided later in the section on specialized equipment, with a more in-depth discussion in Chapter 106. Using satellite or cell phones to activate a rescue can expedite patient care, but neither device should be regarded as a substitute for proper preparation and sound judgment during wilderness travel.

Rescue services in most mountainous regions outside the United States require accident insurance or a substantial cash payment before helicopter transport. If traveling in these areas, expedition members should work with group leaders to ensure that appropriate rescue and accident insurance coverage is obtained for all travelers. Many insurance companies (e.g., International SOS)[24] exist for this purpose and provide medical evacuation coverage to a hospital for stabilization and then evacuation to the home country. There are also environment-specific medical evacuation options. For example, members of the American Alpine Club receive $5000 of global rescue coverage without altitude limitations.[2] Travelers should also review life insurance, credit card benefits, and personal health insurance policies for both benefits and limitations related to travel and high-risk activities.

Travelers and their physicians should take a proactive and informed approach to the places they will visit. Attention should be given to regional hazards and locally available health resources. For example, drinking water quality and treatment options, endemic infectious diseases, environmental exposures, and venomous animals should all be considered and studied. Foreigners often underappreciate the diversity and burden of endemic infectious diseases. Although infections such as malaria, yellow fever, dengue fever, and schistosomiasis are commonly known, many region-specific endemic viral diseases (e.g., Japanese encephalitis, chikungunya), parasitic infections (e.g., leishmaniasis, balamuthiasis), and devastating bacterial infections (e.g., cancrum oris [necrotizing stomatitis]) are less familiar to many clinicians. For each geographic region of travel, the trip medical officer should take appropriate steps to understand indigenous venomous animals, endemic diseases, including their prevention and treatment, and local environmental hazards, including man-made dangers, such as unexploded ordnance.

Malaria prophylaxis, when required, should be used based on the U.S. Centers for Disease Control and Prevention (CDC) or World Health Organization (WHO) recommendations (Box 102-2). In areas with mosquitoes, persons should carry mosquito nets and insect repellent containing a sufficiently high concentration of N,N-diethyl-m-toluamide (DEET; this substance can be purchased at up to 100% concentrations at most wilderness stores). Details on malaria prevention, diagnosis, and management should be reviewed before departure to endemic regions (see Chapter 40).

Travelers should receive destination-appropriate immunizations as far in advance of travel as possible. One vaccine requiring significant discussion before administration is rabies vaccine. Within the United States, rabies vaccination is only considered for those routinely exposed in close quarters to specific wild animals (e.g., veterinarians, field scientists handling bats), because (1) the disease burden of rabies is relatively low, (2) the primary animal reservoir is not in urban or domesticated animals, and (3) there is widespread availability of safe, postexposure prophylaxis. When traveling outside the United States to certain resource-constrained regions, especially India and Central and South America, a large reservoir of disease is found in urban dogs, and postexposure prophylaxis may be less readily available. Given rabies' devastating prognosis, an informed decision regarding immunization must be made based on risk of exposure and access to prompt, postexposure treatment. The CDC provides specific information about exposure criteria, postexposure prophylaxis, and recommendations for vaccination[39] (see Chapter 31).

Before the trip, consideration should be given to caffeine, alcohol, and drug dependencies. Management of such dependencies is a sensitive and complex issue unlikely to be satisfactorily resolved in a wilderness setting. Eliminating access to substances to which individuals have chronic dependencies will often cause

BOX 102-2   Guidelines for Travel in Developing Countries

Before Travel

Consult local sources of medical help; the International Society of Travel Medicine Clinic Directory is available by phone request (770-736-7060) or online (http://www.istm.org).

Obtain up-to-date travel warnings from the Travelers' Health section of the Centers for Disease Control and Prevention (CDC) website at http://wwwnc.cdc.gov/travel/.

Consider purchasing the CDC's *Yellow Book*, a reference published every 2 years primarily for health care providers who advise on international travel. This resource can also be obtained in electronic format for Android or iOS devices.

Obtain necessary vaccinations and prophylactic medications (i.e., antimalarials). Recommendations are available from the CDC (http://www.cdc.gov) and the World Health Organization (http://www.who.int). Update vaccinations for tetanus, measles, mumps, pertussis, diphtheria, and rubella as needed.

During Travel

Contact the U.S. embassy on arrival if not registered prior to trip departure. Have extra copies of essential documents, such as passports, passport photo, yellow fever vaccination documentation (where applicable), and itineraries. Carry phrase books and dictionaries with phonetic and native script translations.

Use an insect repellent containing high concentrations of N,N-diethyl-m-toluamide (i.e., DEET). Formulations approaching 100% (if such are recommended) can be readily purchased. Citronella and other homeopathic remedies for this purpose are not as effective and therefore falsely reassuring.

Avoid ice, unboiled or nonbottled water, and uncooked food.

Take caution when wading or swimming in lakes and canals.

Avoid nocturnal travel and travel during inclement weather.

Do not use unsafe means of transportation (overloaded motor vehicles, vehicles without safety restraints, unregistered or unlicensed vehicles, motorcycles [with or] without helmets).

From http://www.cdc.gov/features/travelershealth.html.

hardship. For example, caffeine withdrawal is a significant cause of headaches among recreational trekkers at high altitude and is often mistaken for a symptom of acute mountain sickness.[17] Strategies for addressing dependencies should be discussed with both the individual member and the group leader. Caffeine and alcohol intake can each result in diuresis and dehydration. Excess alcohol should be avoided because it also causes peripheral vasodilation, which can result in excessive heat gain in hot environments and heat loss in cold or wet environments. Alcohol can also interfere with acclimatization and exacerbate symptoms of acute mountain sickness and should be avoided entirely at altitudes of more than 2438 m (8000 feet). In addition, alcohol's effects on judgment and sensory perception may result in failure to acknowledge early symptoms of environmental illness and may increase risk of injury.

PRETRIP EVALUATION FOR HEALTHY PARTICIPANTS

Regardless of a traveler's overall state of health, all participants in wilderness activities have the responsibility to investigate potential health risks associated with an upcoming excursion and to seek appropriate pretrip medical counseling, preferably from their personal physician.

This discussion provides a potential framework to assist medical personnel and trip leaders in evaluating healthy participants for wilderness travel. It is important for both the travelers being screened and personnel performing the screening to recognize the purpose and limitations of the process. Pretrip evaluation of travelers should not be used to "clear" participants; even the most thorough evaluation cannot absolutely ensure health and safety in the wilderness (e.g., occult coronary artery disease, traumatic injuries). Rather, the pretrip medical evaluation should aim to identify potential harms or risks, ensure all steps have been taken to minimize these risks, and determine if the potential risks are acceptable to the traveler and trip leader.

Medical optimization or harm reduction may occur through fitness training, medication changes, further diagnostic tests, or even by recommending the traveler not participate in the planned activity. These principles apply to evaluation of both healthy participants and those with existing medical conditions.

For our purposes here, "healthy participants" are members of a trip without any known, significant past medical history and who can demonstrate tolerance of activity levels at least comparable to those planned during the proposed trip. It is often a significant challenge to identify correctly participants who are "healthy," and the excellent health of individual participants should not dissuade the expedition medical leader, trip leader, or the participants themselves from completing comprehensive trip preparation.

Each participant must provide a complete medical history, including vaccinations relevant to the area of travel, chronic diseases, history of hospitalizations, surgical history, allergies, medications, and any specific medical concerns (see Appendix B). The designated trip medical personnel or trip leader should gather and review this information and inform prospective participants of potential risks involved with the planned excursion (see Chapter 100). Trip leaders should confidentially, but frankly, discuss medical problems with each participant. This might require a formal pretrip medical evaluation by another physician if any uncertainty exists about the candidate's suitability for the trip. Safety of the individual and group are the coordinator's first priorities.

There are limited data to help guide pretrip screening recommendations for otherwise healthy individuals. Appendix B of this chapter is an example of a pretrip medical screening form that can be used to assist with such evaluation. Although pretrip medical evaluations should involve the participant, participant's primary physician, expedition leader, and designated trip medical staff, ultimately it is the participants' responsibility to pursue adequate pretrip medical preparation and evaluation.

Even the most active and healthy individuals should begin a graduated exercise program at least 2 months before departure to minimize deleterious effects of muscular, metabolic, and mental fatigue inherent to long-distance and remote travel (see Chapter 95). This is especially important for people traveling to high altitudes; aerobic capacity in a sedentary person drops approximately 4% for each 300 m (1000 feet) above the 1200-m (4000-foot) level, but the loss is only one-half as great in an aerobically fit individual.[10,21] Similarly, instruction on careful stretching of muscle groups may increase efficiency and lessen the likelihood of soft tissue injury during exertion and minor accidents, and balance and agility training can be lifesaving in slippery, mountainous environments, such as found in rain forests and mountaineering.

If excessive environmental heat is anticipated, preparatory exercise in a hot and humid environment (this can be simulated with sweat clothing) for 1 hour daily for at least 7 days before departure helps preserve plasma volume (aldosterone effect) and sweat rate while lowering myocardial oxygen demand and sweat sodium content.[14] This acclimatization will be lost within 1 week if not maintained. Such conditioning should be practiced with caution because of the risk for dehydration.

For groups without trained medical leadership, participants should address these issues with their personal physicians before departure, either in person or by questionnaires (see Appendix B).

EVALUATION OF PARTICIPANTS WITH PREEXISTING MEDICAL CONDITIONS

Travelers with complex medical conditions participate in wilderness expeditions, although few data exist to help guide pretrip screening and preparation for these participants.[19] As a general rule, all existing medical conditions should be stable (well controlled), self-managed, and discussed with the participant's personal physician in the context of the planned trip.

Wilderness expedition participants must be encouraged to disclose medical conditions to expedition medical personnel, because existing medical problems can jeopardize not only the health of the affected participant but also that of other party members. Adequate pretrip planning can help mitigate this risk.

Much of the approach to evaluating participants with preexisting medical conditions is similar to that discussed for healthy participants. Once again, these participants should provide a thorough medical history (Appendix B), and the designated trip medical personnel should review this information, perform a thorough evaluation (likely including a physical examination), and inform prospective participants of potential risks involved with the planned excursion (see Chapter 100). Additionally, careful evaluation of the participant's functional status should include a review of daily activity level and ensure the participant is able to demonstrate an activity level consistent with, or in excess of, that required by the proposed trip without worrisome symptoms such as angina, lightheadedness, or severe dyspnea. Any concerning findings during this crucial component of the evaluation may prompt further workup.

Travelers with preexisting medical conditions carry the responsibility to discuss travel plans and request recommendations from their personal physicians (see Chapter 53). The physician should speak directly to the trip coordinator, and vice versa, if there are any doubts about medical suitability for the proposed itinerary. At-risk travelers should wear medical identification bracelets and be required to obtain and manage their own medications. The trip medical provider should know about these illnesses and carry replacement medications provided by these individuals for safekeeping.

Several common medical conditions, such as chronic obstructive pulmonary disease (COPD), asthma, cardiac disease, diabetes, allergies, and seizures, warrant special consideration during pretrip planning. Pulmonary hypertension, recent pulmonary embolism, history of recurrent spontaneous pneumothorax, sickle cell disease, and sleep apnea are considered contraindications to high-altitude travel.

Generally speaking, participants with chronic medical conditions should be encouraged to bring adequate supplies for at least two to three times the planned itinerary length, erring on the side of additional reserve supplies for more severe illnesses.

These participants should also bring necessary supplies for potential exacerbations when applicable (e.g., epilepsy, COPD).

Patients with a history of seizures should continue routine medications and also carry an injectable form of benzodiazepine, such as lorazepam (Ativan). Suppositories (rectal diazepam) are appropriate if the party is traveling in a cool or cold environment or with children (see Chapter 51).

Caution should be taken when travelers with a history of COPD or asthma are attempting high-altitude travel. A plan for rapid descent is essential, because people with asthma and COPD will predictably experience greater-than-normal difficulty as a result of hypoxia and air trapping from high altitudes. Similarly, dry air, exercise, or noxious stimuli (e.g., smoke, red tide) may exacerbate COPD processes.[28] Thus, a plan for rapid treatment should be in place before departure. Exercise in cold, dry air may trigger wheezing. Poor air quality, a byproduct of fossil fuel burning or even remote volcanic activity, along with winds that can "stir up" larger particulate matter such as dust or sand, can also cause irritation. In addition to carrying a β-adrenergic agonist metered-dose inhaler, travelers with COPD or asthma should carry a 2-week course of an oral corticosteroid (e.g., prednisone) plus an appropriate oral antibiotic (e.g., fluoroquinolone, advanced macrolide, or doxycycline). Studies of aircraft pressurized to 2438-m (8000-foot) altitude reveal that people with moderately severe COPD may have significant dyspnea at this attitude. This may serve as a surrogate marker for the altitude to which such individuals can safely travel.[1,7] People with mild to moderate COPD should not sleep above 3048 m (10,000 feet) because of the potential for nocturnal desaturation. The decision to travel to altitude with existing pulmonary disease is multifactorial.[31] Great caution must be advised for patients who chronically retain carbon dioxide, because small changes in the partial pressure of inspired oxygen can cause significant changes in their ability to oxygenate adequately.

Patients with a known history of significant cardiac disease warrant special consideration before participation in wilderness activities (see Chapter 50). All such travelers should undergo evaluations by their primary care and specialist physicians before travel. During travel, these patients should continue routine medications and provide copies of their most recent electrocardiograms to trip personnel (for comparison if evacuated to a facility with ECG capability). These participants also must be instructed when to withhold medications (e.g., not to take diuretics and other blood pressure–lowering medications when lightheaded or feeling weak).

Outdoor adventure travel can provoke angina among people with underlying heart disease. There is continued debate about the evaluation and advice a physician should provide patients with cardiovascular disease. Participants must be aware that no amount of pretrip evaluation, including stress testing or even coronary artery revascularization, can guarantee prevention of cardiac events in the backcountry. For prospective travelers with unstable angina, pulmonary hypertension, congestive heart failure, or obstructive or severe valvular disease (e.g., aortic stenosis), vigorous adventure travel is contraindicated. A traveler with a history of cerebral transient ischemic attacks may be able to participate in outdoor travel if attention is given to proper hydration and use of antiplatelet agents, such as aspirin or clopidogrel (Plavix), or other anticoagulants as indicated and prescribed by the treating physician. As the number of new antiplatelet and anticoagulant medications continues to increase, trip medical personnel must carefully review each participant's medication lists to identify travelers who may be at high risk of occult hemorrhage after trauma.

Diabetic travelers should be instructed to bring an ample supply of their routine medications, a functioning and spare glucose meter, and emergency glucose supply for patients on a regimen other than biguanide-only therapy (see Chapter 53, Table 53-4). Specific recommendations vary depending on the traveler's diabetes type (1 or 2) and medication regimen (e.g., if type 2 with insulin dependence). All diabetic travelers must consult with their personal physician before wilderness travel.

Outdoor travel often disrupts the normal meal schedules of diabetic travelers. Although some individuals need less insulin when participating in high levels of exercise, such as backpacking, this phenomenon is not true for all. Diabetic persons should monitor their blood glucose at least twice a day, regardless of how good they feel, modifying their insulin and eating regimens accordingly. Other group members in close contact with insulin-dependent diabetic travelers should know that the first two interventions for an ill-appearing diabetic person are a small amount of sugar in any form (e.g., juice, granulated table sugar, candy, syrup or honey), orally or under the tongue, and measurement of blood glucose level. For persons taking oral hypoglycemic agents with hypoglycemia refractory to sublingual sugar, injectable glucagon can be a useful adjunct, provided there is the medical expertise to administer it and manage its common adverse effects. During air travel, insulin-dependent diabetic persons should take their daily dose of insulin and eat according to the local time at departure. For a diabetic person traveling eastbound across multiple time zones, the day is effectively shortened. At arrival, the person should eat and administer insulin in accordance with local time but reduce the dose by one-third. For travel westbound, the day will lengthen, and a second dose of insulin after 18 hours of travel may be administered after glucose monitoring, if indicated (see Chapter 53).

Human immunodeficiency virus (HIV) infection does not preclude safe wilderness travel if the HIV-positive person is aware of his or her degree of immunosuppression and pays meticulous attention to water disinfection and pretrip immunizations. The decision for travel must be made with involvement of the patient's personal physician.

During pretrip evaluation, participants should be informed that many prescription drugs can predispose travelers to heat-, cold-, and altitude-related illnesses and to increased risk of dehydration-related emergencies, such as kidney stones or pancreatitis related to some HIV medications. Diuretic use may lead to intravascular volume contraction, impaired heat transfer to the skin, dehydration, and potentially life-threatening electrolyte abnormalities such as hypokalemia. Travelers taking diuretics should carry a packaged electrolyte replacement (i.e., oral rehydration solution) and a source of potassium (e.g., dried bananas, potato chips). The anticholinergic action of antihistamines, phenothiazines, and tricyclic antidepressants may result in hypothalamic dysfunction and diminished sweating with subsequent hyperthermia.

Patients with serious medical allergies or active illnesses should have an appropriate medical identification bracelet, anklet, medallion, or wallet card and should store personal medications in a protected but accessible location in their pack. Patients with a history of significant allergic reactions should carry at least two epinephrine autoinjectors or injectable epinephrine with a needle and syringe (see Bites and Stings, later). At a minimum, for each patient with a severe allergy, a second member of the expedition should be aware of the allergy and its appropriate treatment in case the patient becomes incapacitated during a severe acute allergic episode. Every traveler should carry a complete personal medication list during travel, with both generic and brand names listed.

Travelers who report dental problems during pretrip evaluation should be promptly evaluated by a dentist because untreated dental pathology can become a major obstacle to a successful trip. Travelers should also be advised to see their physicians about known sleep disorders, concerns for jet lag, and existing chronic pain issues before departure.

For a complete discussion of considerations for chronic diseases and wilderness travel, see Chapter 53.

TRAINING IN FIRST AID AND WILDERNESS SAFETY

No medical specialty or training pathway provides all the skills necessary to care for the many potential and real challenges faced during wilderness travel. Many courses and certifications in wilderness first aid and safety exist, with little evidence to suggest superiority of any one training strategy for wilderness first responders.[51] Appropriate pretrip training must be tailored according to personnel background (e.g., physician vs. lay provider), trip duration, and planned activities (e.g., training in mountain rescue).

Large expeditions frequently enlist experienced medical personnel for logistics planning or even to accompany the trip, whereas most small groups trekking into the wilderness do not have access to this expertise. Even when a physician is a party member, he or she may not be specifically trained in wilderness medicine or certified in a field of medicine with skills relevant to manage commonly encountered wilderness medicine scenarios.

For physicians joining expeditions, training and current proficiency in emergency medicine likely provide the greatest breadth of applicable knowledge and skills. Physicians trained in internal medicine or family medicine might provide suitable expedition physicians with adjunctive training or experience. Anesthesiologists (skilled in resuscitation and airway management) might also be able to function in this role and often provide expertise in altitude and diving physiology. In general, current certification (or equivalency) in basic life support (BLS), advanced cardiac life support (ACLS), advanced trauma life support (ATLS), and pediatric advanced life support (PALS) is desirable. Several organizations that support wilderness recreational activities recommend personnel obtain a minimum of Red Cross standard first aid or equivalent as well as certification in cardiopulmonary resuscitation (CPR) appropriate for the age of trip participants (see Chapter 80 for additional discussion of expedition medical officer qualifications).

Before departure, the trip coordinator should review emergency supplies with the group. The person should demonstrate proper use of mechanical devices and discuss medication indications. Groups planning an extended or high-risk outing may want to conduct a mock injury evaluation and management exercise.

Participants should be encouraged to take general courses in first aid and wilderness safety, with attention to the most fundamental skills. Some agencies that offer general and specialized training in skiing, mountaineering, river rafting, and other types of wilderness medicine are listed in Appendix A.

Additional information on training programs for physicians, residents, and medical students as well as nonphysician providers can be found in Box 113-9 in Chapter 113. Locally organized programs may be found through the American Red Cross, sporting goods stores, and continuing education departments of local colleges. Larger organizations, such as the Wilderness Medical Society (WMS), offer regular conferences and workshops nationally as well as referral to a large member community of experienced clinicians, researchers, lecturers, and experts worldwide.

TRIP DURATION AND ACCESS TO MEDICAL SUPPORT

When serious illness or injury occurs, the longer the delay in obtaining advanced medical assistance, the more likely may be the irreversible loss of physiologic function, life, or limb. One must anticipate delays in care when in rural or remote areas, because the nearest physician or hospital might not be equipped to handle a major injury or illness. Furthermore, expeditions with prolonged or limited evacuation options warrant additional consideration for equipment discussed later in this chapter.

Trip leaders and medical staff should be aware of potential evacuation options, including times to the nearest health facilities, throughout the itinerary. Party members should agree in advance about simple emergency distress signals, such as whistle or flashlight signals, to facilitate rescue during the expedition if needed.

Access to timely medical care can significantly impact the immediate treatment plan. For example, when a traveler sustains a deep extremity laceration, the likelihood of infection increases with each passing hour. Clear-cut guidelines used in hospitals to determine if suturing or stapling are appropriate become unclear, including the use of prophylactic antibiotics. If the patient can reach trained and equipped medical help within a few hours, it will suffice to control bleeding, irrigate with any source of potable water, and apply a sterile dressing held in place by improvised cravats or tape. Although not sterile, water reservoirs found in many packs, such as those made by Camelbak, can be used for irrigation when no other options exist (tubing from water reservoirs has also been used to attempt endotracheal intubation). If definitive care is more than several hours away, irrigation with water containing a topical disinfectant may be desirable. If care will be delayed 6 hours or more, a decision must be made whether to close the wound before evacuating the patient (see Chapter 21). Estimated time delay depends on the type of rescue services, method of contact, terrain, weather, and number of able-bodied (i.e., carrying) people.

Manually evacuating a patient is an option but requires a relatively mobile person or generally a minimum of 6 carriers if the person is immobilized. In this regard, it is important to know if other groups might be trekking in the same vicinity. If access is controlled by permit, the administering agency should be asked about neighboring parties' itinerary, which might influence the types of equipment carried if communication is established with other groups before departure. The likelihood of mishap increases as trip duration lengthens; this is partly attributable to unpredictable weather and cumulative effects of fatigue and repetitive strain injuries. In the case of a recognized need for evacuation, medical interventions, such as improvised splints, braces, and crutches, enabling self-rescue (i.e., walking under one's own power, with or without assistance) can make the difference between minor delays and costly, multiday evacuations involving search and rescue teams.

Long trips usually involve extensive planning, significant financial investment, and time away from work and family. Nevertheless, party members may be reluctant to shorten the trip and generally favor continuing in the face of mild medical disability and equipment failure. Groups planning to be away from civilization for more than 1 week should have a maximally diversified list of medical and contingency items.

ENVIRONMENTAL RISKS: WEATHER AND TERRAIN

Weather, terrain, and activity interact to increase the risk for illness or injury. It is essential for expedition medical staff to be familiar with historic and current weather and terrain conditions for planned itineraries before departure.

Particularly hazardous situations include winter climbing, mountaineering, skiing, and travel from low- to high-humidity environments, as in the equatorial tropics. Potential obstacles must be figured into estimates of maximum delay to medical assistance. National and global historic summary data indicating temperature ranges, winds, and duration, type, and amount of precipitation can be obtained from the National Climatic Data Center (see Box 102-2). State and national park services and state climatology offices can also provide detailed information about regional conditions. Local rangers and EMS personnel may provide valuable information about weather patterns and risks specific to local terrain and should always be considered during trip planning. The National Weather Service office nearest the travel site can provide short-term forecasts and in many regions broadcasts weather information between 162.40 and 162.55 MHz VHF (see Appendix A).

Knowledge of terrain and environmental conditions is also essential when selecting everything from socks to sleeping bags. A single manufacturer can easily have dozens of similar-appearing sleeping bags with ratings from extreme cold to warm weather with varying degrees of water resistance. The proper sleeping bag can be very expensive, but choosing the wrong gear for the trip can be even more costly. Chapter 110 provides a dedicated discussion of fabric and clothing selection strategies for wilderness travel.

SUPPLIES, KIT ASSEMBLY STRATEGIES, AND SPECIALIZED EQUIPMENT

There is no universal wilderness medical kit. The only perfect kit is the one that has what you need at the moment you need it. Most commercially available kits charge a premium for packaging and branding. Although packaging and kit organization are critically important, the components of retail kits can usually be purchased piecemeal and assembled for a fraction of the cost. Kits and equipment must be modified for each trip based on factors such as duration, number of participants, planned activities, endemic diseases, environmental conditions, and distance to definitive care. When building a medical kit, it is important to include supplies that do not require expertise beyond the scope of training for available personnel.

This section provides guidance on kit assembly strategies, including what and how much to bring, how to pack and organize, and what specialized equipment is available to address specific environmental hazards. Medications for trip medical kits are discussed later.

STRATEGIES FOR PACKAGING MEDICAL KITS

Medical supplies for an expedition may be divided into five components: (1) personal medical supplies; (2) comprehensive community medical supplies; (3) devices for the medically trained traveler; (4) specialized equipment for particular environmental and recreational hazards; and (5) supplies stored in a vehicle. Strategies for compiling each of these components are discussed later.

A medical kit can be assembled by customizing kits that are already available or by starting from scratch. Budget and time constraints, as well as skill and differing levels of training, influence this process. As skill and experience level lead to increased improvisational ability, travelers will find that the amount of equipment needed and size of first-aid kits may decrease. When assembling a medical kit, it is generally advisable that travelers not bring equipment (including medications) that requires skill, knowledge, or licensure beyond that which is immediately available. Inappropriate management of injury and illness can be more harmful than sticking to basic interventions or doing nothing at all.

As with any area of wilderness medicine, resourcefulness and opportunism may be helpful for packing medical kits. Each year, catalog and Internet-based outfitters have clearance sales that include many of the items discussed here and in other chapters. In addition, high-quality and normally expensive items (e.g., laryngoscopes, watertight boxes, sunglasses) are available in new and used condition on popular public auction websites. The reader is cautioned to purchase only from reputable sellers and to inspect all purchases for integrity and functionality.

How a kit is organized is almost as important as the contents of the kit. If items cannot be quickly and easily found, especially for emergency supplies, they are of little use. Size and organization of medical kits depend on the same trip-specific factors mentioned previously, including trip duration, number of participants, planned activities, and distance to definitive care.

For expeditions with the capacity to travel with larger kits, a brightly painted, clearly marked, watertight aluminum or plastic box can serve as a container for the comprehensive community medical kit. The underside of the lid can be an ideal place to secure equipment for treating immediately life-threatening emergencies, such as respiratory distress, anaphylaxis, hemorrhage, cardiovascular disease, and tension pneumothorax (see Figure 102-2 on p. 2289). For other kit designs, it may be preferable to create an emergency response module that includes supplies for responding to immediately life-threatening emergencies (e.g., airway equipment, epinephrine, tactical tourniquet, aspirin, 14-gauge vascular access catheter, gloves, trauma shears). Small to medium-sized duffel bags can be used to group equipment by category (e.g., medications, diagnostics, wound care, emergency response) within the kit. Medications can be further compartmentalized within the duffle by creating separate, zipper-locked, heavy-duty plastic bags labeled by category (e.g., antibiotics, analgesics) and system (e.g., respiratory/allergy, cardiovascular, gastrointestinal, ear/nose/throat, genitourinary/gynecologic, dermatologic).

Miscellaneous items that are not likely to be needed urgently or frequently can be stored under the duffel bags. Other useful items, such as repair supplies (Table 102-1), should also be considered but are usually better if packed separately.

For smaller kits, a variety of vessels can be used, including small backpacks, toiletry organizers, dry bags, and military surplus bags (Figure 102-1). Regardless of the size or style chosen for a medical kit, it is highly recommended to compartmentalize supplies as much as possible. This can be done using built-in compartments or packaging related items by category or system into heavy-duty, labeled plastic bags.

Liquids, ointments, and creams can leak easily, so take special care when packing these items, or consider repackaging in well-labeled, durable plastic bottles (e.g., small Nalgene bottles).

HOW MUCH TO BRING

Duration of the outing or expedition, party size, probability of specific illnesses, and maximum interval to medical care are primary factors when considering what and how much to bring into the wilderness. No single formula can be used to calculate quantities of trip supplies. A simple but often effective approach to determining how much to bring is to calculate the dosing schedule of each medication under consideration and then multiply it by the maximum interval to medical care and the number of people who are likely to require the specified therapy at any one time.

TABLE 102-1	Repair Supplies to Consider for Wilderness Travel	
Item	**Description**	**Uses and Comments**
Multitool	Pocket tool that includes collapsible screwdrivers, pliers, awl, and saw	
Needle or sewing awl	With heavy thread: 30 g (1 oz)	Clothing and pack repair
Screwdrivers	Flat and Phillips No. 2: 88-177 g (3-6 oz)	For skis, No. 3 posidrive or filed-down No. 2 Phillips
Duct tape or reinforced strapping	2.5-10 cm (1-4 inches) wide and 1.5 m (5 yards) long; 59 g (2 oz) per person per trip	
Wire and nylon cord	Braided steel and braided nylon: 0.9-1.8 m (3-6 feet), 59 g (2 oz)	Repair of binding, boot, snowshoe, and pack
Needle-nose pliers	With wire cutters	
Vise-grip pliers	13 cm (5 inches); 148-237 g (5-8 oz)	
Awl	One multifunction knife per person per trip: 59 g (2 oz)	Repair of clothing, pack, and shelter
Glue	Two-component epoxy or meltable nylon glue stick: 30 g (1 oz)	
Spare bale and screws	Two per person per trip	Repair of ski binding
P-tex ski base stick	Meltable No. 1: 30 g (1 oz)	Repair of plastic ski base
Spare ski tip	Plastic or aluminum: 88-148 g (3-5 oz)	
Spare crampon wrench	No. 1; one per person per trip	
Knife sharpener	Diamond bar, ceramic, or stone: 59-89 g (2-3 oz)	

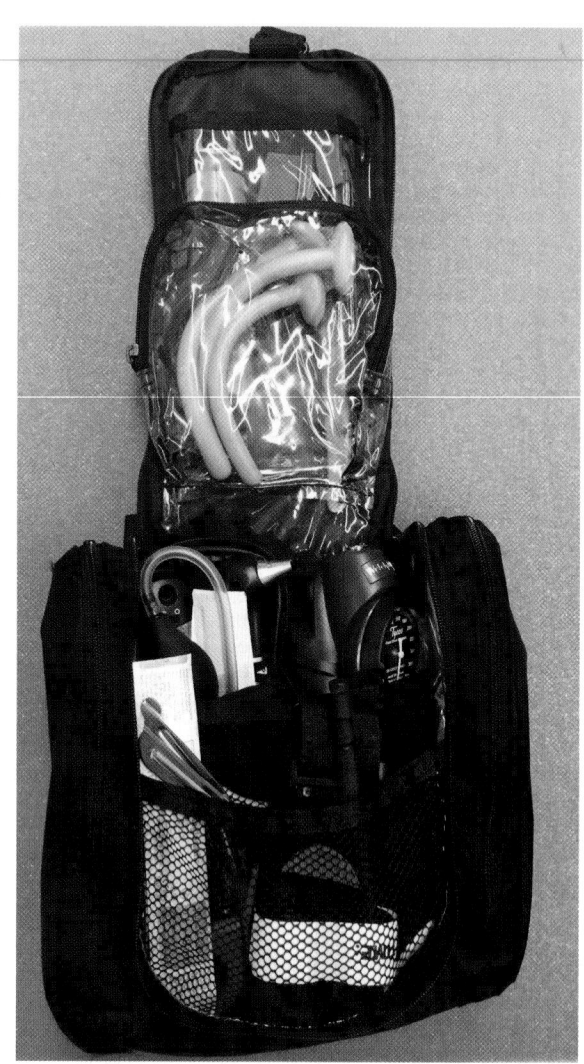

FIGURE 102-1 Example of a compact emergency response and diagnostics module made from a toiletry bag. This small kit contains emergency supplies (oral/nasopharyngeal airways, laryngoscopes, endotracheal tube, 14-gauge vascular access catheter, tactical tourniquet, epinephrine, gloves, eye protection, trauma shears, safety pins) and diagnostic equipment (pulse oximeter, sphygmomanometer, thermometer, precordial stethoscope, otoscope/ophthalmoscope, fluorescein).

For example, on a 2-week rafting trip that is 3 days away from the nearest pharmacy with 10 people, one can estimate how much metronidazole should be available for treatment of giardiasis. Assume all members become infected and require a treatment course of 5 days × 500 mg orally (PO) every 8 hours (q8h) = 15 tablets per person; 10 members × 15 tabs = 150 tabs. It is highly unlikely that all members would become infected, however, or that all would become infected at the beginning of the trip, so some participants should be able to complete medication courses with drugs obtained on returning home. Furthermore, evacuation time is only 3 days and could be done if supplies were dwindling. Thus, taking fewer than 150 tabs would be reasonable. To recalculate, if you assume only two-thirds of the trip members become infected and you bring enough only for the 3-day evacuation (7 persons × 500 mg PO q8h × 3 days = 56 tabs), you arrive at a more reasonable quantity to pack for such a trip.

The rationale for choosing which medications to bring on an excursion is based on the likelihood of injury or illness (increases with longer trip duration) and expected time frame for support and rescue. In a low-risk outing (e.g., 1-day hike), the interval to medical care is short (<4 hours), and trip duration (e.g., 1 day) places one at low risk of acquiring a medical illness that can only

be managed in the field. Because traumatic injury or a life-threatening allergic reaction is always of prime concern, even during a low-risk outing, analgesics and medications for anaphylaxis can be extremely important. A moderate-risk trek (e.g., 1-day "ski-in" with 2 nights of winter camping) will have a longer interval to medical care (e.g., 4 to 12 hours) and a trip duration that increase the chance of injury and illness. With a "ski-out" time of 4 to 12 hours plus added time to return with organized help, expectations are that an ill group member will not receive sophisticated rescue efforts until the following day. In such situations, opioids to control pain, antibiotics to prevent infection from soft tissue injuries, and antiemetic or antidiarrheal medications to control gastrointestinal (GI) upset and preserve fluid and electrolyte balances become paramount. A high-risk outing (e.g., weeklong expedition with mountain climbing) precludes seeking formal help within a 12-hour period. With such an expedition, nonemergent problems (e.g., athlete's foot, infected blisters, dermatitis, asthma, bronchitis, sinusitis) are likely to occur, limiting the performance and enjoyment of some participants. In addition to carrying the medicines and supplies noted previously for low- and moderate-risk treks, one should have treatments to manage more persistent medical illness, including a full course of oral antibiotics for respiratory, abdominal, and soft tissue infections; oral and potent topical corticosteroids for dermatologic problems; and assorted ophthalmic and otic medications to deal with bothersome infections or allergic reactions affecting vital sensory organs.

PERSONAL MEDICAL KIT

For the purposes of this discussion, "personal medical kits" are small, on-person kits of essential supplies for each trip participant. Although containing only basic supplies, these are key components of an expedition's medical armamentarium. Carrying a minimum amount of items on one's person serves two purposes: (1) redundancy of essential supplies in the event of theft, damage, or loss during travel and (2) personal supply in the event of separation from travel partners. A sudden fall, avalanche, or swamping can quickly separate a person from the group and his or her gear.

The supplies for a personal medical kit should provide protection from the elements, permit self-treatment of minor traumatic injuries, allow signaling for purposes of search and rescue, and include an adequate supply of home medications. These items typically include assorted adhesive compress strips, a knife or razor blade, butane lighter or matches (preferably the waterproof, strike-anywhere type), plastic whistle, small reflective mirror, length of thin nylon cord, bandanna (which can double as a cravat or sling), and safety pins (Box 102-3). A nonperishable source of quick, high-energy food (e.g., candy, nutrition bar) is valuable during isolation to maintain strength and morale. These items can be compactly stored inside a plastic bag or small stuff sack and may be carried in either a pocket or a small pack. Zippered, passport-size waist belts are comfortable and inexpensive options.

As noted previously, all travelers should carry some form of identification, and those with serious medical allergies or active illnesses should have an appropriate medical alert bracelet, anklet, medallion, or wallet card. A copy of one's passport can be invaluable.

Participants with any medical condition prone to acute exacerbations (e.g. asthma, diabetes, severe allergies) must carry adequate supply of necessary medications in their personal medical kit. For example, travelers with a history of bee, wasp, or other anaphylactic or anaphylactoid reactions should carry at least two preloaded syringes of 1:1000 aqueous epinephrine solution (e.g., epinephrine autoinjector). Keep such devices in a cool, dark compartment, and inform others in the party about the medicine's location and proper use. Advanced practitioners might carry a vial of epinephrine and syringes with needles to increase versatility and lower cost. Asthmatic persons should carry extra inhalers for maintenance and treatment of exacerbations.

Certain contingency "essentials" should be carried on every venture. In addition to one's personal first-aid, hygiene, and

BOX 102-3 Contents of a Personal Medical Kit

On-Person Items

- Personal prescription medications, labeled, in plastic or waterproof lightweight box
- High-priority over-the-counter medications (see Table 102-2)
- Copy of identification
- Pencil and notepad (waterproof, depending on environment)
- Hat and sunglasses
- High–sun protection factor (SPF) sunscreen and lip balm
- Topographic map and compass and basic knowledge of their use
- Multitool knife (e.g., Swiss Army, Leatherman) or razor blade
- Nylon cord
- Whistle and small reflective mirror
- Plastic cable ties
- Lighter or waterproof matches
- Poncho or large, black or orange, plastic yard waste bag
- Adhesive compress
- Alcohol-based gel (e.g., Purell) for hands
- Alcohol swabs
- Adherent bandages
- Duct tape (exterior grade, weatherproof)
- Fluorescent surveyor's tape
- Bandanna, safety pins (see Chapter 46)
- Nonperishable high-energy bar or gummy bears
- Personal hygiene material
- Survival guide or first-aid booklet
- Personal mosquito netting for sleep (when appropriate)
- Ear plugs (sleep hygiene)

clothing items, a flashlight, extra pair of sunglasses, coins, and credit card for telephone calls (although the former is becoming obsolete) should be considered. Extra clothing, food, and water should be carried in proportion to the risk associated with the trip. These nonmedical items are discussed in greater detail in Chapter 111.

A host of over-the-counter (OTC) medications may be useful for wilderness travel and considered for a personal medical kit. Some commonly required, nonprescription items of value are listed in Table 102-2 (highlighted in green and marked with †). Analgesics for trauma are high-priority medications. For mild to moderate pain, acetaminophen or a non-steroidal anti-inflammatory drug can be effective alone or in combination. Decongestants are helpful for treating symptoms associated with upper respiratory tract infections. GI complaints may necessitate antacids, antidiarrheal agents, or promotility agents.

Antiseptic cream or ointment is useful when treating superficial skin infections, and a corticosteroid ointment is valuable for treating certain rashes or contact dermatitis. Aloe vera gel is useful for treating frostbite and burns.

In general, sunburn is best avoided by complete coverage with clothing, hats, and scarves along with fastidious application of a high–sun protection factor (SPF) (i.e., SPF > 30) sunscreen and lip balm. Ultrahigh-SPF sunscreens (i.e., 70 to 100 or more) are available in the United States but not in many low- and middle-income countries and should be purchased before departure. Anticipate sharing a significant percentage of your sunscreen supply.

Text continued on p. 2287

TABLE 102-2 Select Medications for Wilderness Travel*

Drug	Formulation	Select Indications	Comments
Analgesics**			
Acetaminophen† (Tylenol, paracetamol, APAP [acetyl-para-aminophenol])	500-1000 mg PO tabs	Analgesia, fever reduction	Although OTC, this drug can have significant analgesic effects, especially when used in combination with NSAIDs, or with opiates for moderate to severe pain. Caution in patients with history of liver disease or alcoholism. Overdose can be life threatening. Many flu remedies contain acetaminophen and should be accounted for in total daily dose calculations. Paracetamol is metabolized to acetaminophen.
Ibuprofen† (Advil, Motrin)	200 mg PO tabs	Analgesia, antiinflammatory	When no contraindications, NSAIDS should be considered in combination with acetaminophen for mild to moderate pain and with opiates if necessary for moderate to severe pain. This is not to be used if GI bleeding, pregnancy, chronic kidney disease, or severe dehydration is present. NSAIDs may help prevent acute mountain sickness. Caution with total daily dose and prolonged use.
Acetylsalicylic acid† (Aspirin, Bayer, Ecotrin)	325-500 mg PO tabs	Analgesia	This is not to be used if significant bleeding is present. Can be used for antiplatelet effect in suspected ACS (preferably chewed, non-enteric-coated tabs). May be administered PR.
Hydrocodone and acetaminophen** (Vicodin, Lortab, Norco)	5 to 10 mg/325 mg PO tabs, dose limited by total daily acetaminophen dose	Analgesia	As with all opiates, may cause severe constipation. Given concern for inadvertent acetaminophen toxicity, would recommend hydrocodone or oxycodone preparations without acetaminophen. Given hydrocodone's reclassification as Schedule II and variable metabolism, oxycodone may be considered as a more reliable analgesic.
Oxycodone**	5 mg PO tabs	Analgesia	As with many opioids, significant nausea, especially when taken without food. Monitor for constipation. May cause impaired reaction time, balance, and wakefulness.

Continued

TABLE 102-2 Select Medications for Wilderness Travel*—cont'd

Drug	Formulation	Select Indications	Comments
Tramadol** (Ultram)	50 mg PO tabs	Analgesia	Use caution, because may cause CNS depression and impair reaction time, balance, and wakefulness. May increase risk of seizures, especially in patients taking several drugs, including SSRIs, TCAs, and MAOIs. Multiple interactions.
Bupivacaine (Marcaine, Sensorcaine)	0.25% solution, maximum SC dose of 2.5 mg/kg	Advanced-tier local or regional anesthesia	Use with caution on the feet, because such use may allow further skin damage to go unnoticed. Hypotension and dysrhythmias can occur at toxic doses. IV injection can be fatal. Perineural injections may be effective for tooth pain and extremity fractures, and effects may last up to 10 hours. Soak gauze with this drug for topical and dental applications.
Lidocaine (Xylocaine)	1%-2% solution for injection with or without epinephrine; maximum SC dose of 4.5 mg/kg without epinephrine, up to 7 mg/kg with epinephrine	Local anesthesia	Conventional teaching is that lidocaine with epinephrine should not be used when injecting distal extremities (i.e., fingers, nose, penis, toes, ears) because of potential for vascular compromise. Consider bringing multiple small vials; repeat use of single vials is not recommended. Local anesthetic of choice for minor procedures because of fast onset and relatively wide therapeutic window. This short-acting agent (relative to bupivacaine) may be used as an antiarrhythmic in ACLS. Toxic doses may result in seizure or cardiac arrest.
Lidocaine jelly 2%	Apply to skin as needed or 30 min before procedure; 5 mL packages	Analgesia, prophylaxis for catheter insertion	Use with caution; it may allow further skin damage to go unnoticed.
Tetracaine	0.5% solution for eye drops	Analgesia for procedures	Should not be used if etiology of injury and expert consultation unavailable, because it can worsen injury.
Morphine sulfate**	20 mg IV/IM vial	Advanced-tier analgesia	Morphine may cause nausea, vomiting, rash (histamine release), hypotension, sedation, and apnea. Administer it with an antiemetic as a precaution.
Ketamine**	50 mg/mL, 5-10 mL vial IV (alternate dosing for IM and PO available)	Advanced-tier analgesia	Anticipate increased oral secretions and potential for hallucinations. May consider premedication with antisialagogue (glycopyrrolate, scopolamine) and sedative (midazolam). Can be used only by qualified and experienced providers to achieve sedation for surgical procedures or control of severe pain with relatively less respiratory depression than opiates.
Naloxone (Narcan)	0.4-2 mg SC, IM, IV, or by endotracheal tube	Opioid overdose	Naloxone may precipitate opioid withdrawal among chronic opioid users. Rare adverse effects include pulmonary edema and seizure.
Pentazocine** (Talwin)	50 mg PO tabs	Opioid agonist-antagonist	Pentazocine still has abuse potential. IV/IM formulations also available.
Capsaicin ointment†	2 g tube	Topical analgesic for osteoarthritis	Prolonged use may result in burns. Adjunct or alternative when NSAIDs or PO medications contraindicated.
Antimicrobials			
Albendazole (Albenza)	200 mg PO tabs	Anthelmintic with broad range of activity against neurocysticercosis, echinococcosis, ascariasis, hookworm, and trichuriasis	Not to be used by pregnant patients or by children <2 years old. Consider expert consultation before administration because significant contraindications exist.
Amoxicillin/clavulanic acid (Augmentin)	875 mg/125 mg PO tabs	Animal bites, oral infections, skin and soft tissue infections, severe acute otitis media, and tonsillopharyngitis	Contraindicated in patients with penicillin allergy. Can be used in conjunction with clindamycin for suspected polymicrobial anaerobic pulmonary infections (aspiration pneumonia).

TABLE 102-2 Select Medications for Wilderness Travel*—cont'd

Drug	Formulation	Select Indications	Comments
Artemether/lumefantrine (Coartem, Riamet)	20 mg artemether, 120 mg lumefantrine PO tabs	Malaria (*Plasmodium falciparum*) treatment in chloroquine-resistant areas (check CDC.gov for guidelines)	Can be used for malaria treatment, although significant side effects and contraindications exist. Use caution when purchasing in certain regions because significant quality differences may exist between manufacturers.
Artesunate	60 mg ampule for IV or IM	Severe malaria (*P. falciparum*) treatment in chloroquine-resistant areas (check CDC.gov for guidelines)	Can be used for malaria treatment, although significant side effects and contraindications exist. May not be able to purchase in certain regions.
Atovaquone/proguanil (Malarone)	250 mg/100 mg PO tabs	Severe malaria prophylaxis and treatment in chloroquine-resistant areas (check CDC.gov for guidelines)	Use with caution in a patient with severe GI upset. This is not to be used for complicated or cerebral malaria.
Azithromycin (Zithromax)	250 mg PO tabs	Pneumonia, otitis media, tonsillopharyngitis, gonococcal infection, bacterial sinusitis, traveler's diarrhea	May cause nausea, vomiting, and QT prolongation. Single 1000 mg dose may be more effective for traveler's diarrhea than divided dosing.
Bacitracin† (ointment)	28 g, 120 g, or 454 g tube	Topical infection prevention	Can cause allergic reactions. Clear affected area before application. Many potential alternatives.
Cefazolin (Ancef, Kefzol)	1 g vials IM/IV‡	Soft tissue infection, uncomplicated cystitis, crush injuries, open fractures	Penicillin allergy is a risk factor for cephalosporin allergy.
Ceftriaxone (Rocephin)	1 g vials, powder for reconstitution IM/IV‡	Pneumonia, meningitis, gonorrhea, intraabdominal infection, pyelonephritis, sepsis	Third-generation cephalosporin. Penicillin allergy is a risk factor for cephalosporin allergy.
Cephalexin (Keflex)	500 mg PO tabs	Superficial, soft tissue infection, streptococcal pharyngitis, uncomplicated cystitis	First-generation cephalosporin. Penicillin allergy is a risk factor for cephalosporin allergy.
Chloroquine (Aralen)	500 mg PO tabs	For severe malaria prophylaxis or treatment in chloroquine-sensitive areas (check CDC.gov for guidelines)	May cause nausea and diarrhea. Significant contraindications, including caution in patients with preexisting auditory problems, G6PD deficiency, psoriasis, or seizure disorder.
Ciprofloxacin (Cipro)	250-750 mg PO tabs	Traveler's diarrhea, cystitis, pneumonia, intraabdominal infection, prostatitis, sinusitis, typhoid fever, meningitis prophylaxis (off-label use)	Fluoroquinolones are not recommended for patients <16 years old because of the risk for cartilage injury and tendinopathies. Do not give with calcium containing foods or antacids (chelates quinolones). Avoid in patients receiving concurrent corticosteroids.
Ciprofloxacin otic solution (Cetraxal)	0.2% solution, formulations with dexamethasone available	Acute otitis externa; formulation for ophthalmic applications is 0.3%	May need ear wick for administration. Warm bottle in hand before administration to avoid adverse response. Pseudomonal resistance can occur.
Clindamycin (Cleocin)	150-450 mg PO tabs	Anaerobic infections; severe soft tissue infection (off-label use), toxic shock syndrome, pelvic inflammatory disease	May be useful for suspected MRSA soft tissue infections.
Doxycycline (Vibramycin)	100 mg PO tabs	Severe malaria prophylaxis, Lyme disease, *Vibrio cholerae*, *Chlamydia*, pneumonia, bronchitis, tick-borne rickettsial disease; may be useful for unidentified infections from marine environment	Not recommended for patients <8 years old because of teeth staining. Inactivated by calcium-containing products (food and antacids). Causes significant photosensitivity and pill esophagitis (remain upright at least 30 min after ingesting with full glass of water). Expired doxycycline is considered dangerously nephrotoxic.
Erythromycin	3.5 g tube, 0.5% ointment	Bacterial conjunctivitis, uncomplicated corneal abrasion	Consider antipseudomonal coverage (quinolone drops) if contact lens wearer.

Continued

TABLE 102-2 Select Medications for Wilderness Travel*—cont'd

Drug	Formulation	Select Indications	Comments
Fluconazole (Diflucan)	150 mg PO tabs	Vaginal and oropharyngeal candidiasis; coccidioidomycosis, dermatophyte (tinea) infections	Liver toxicity may occur. May be required for female patients taking concurrent antibiotics. Topical antifungals may be sufficient for tinea infections when available.
Ivermectin (Stromectol)	3 mg tabs PO (dosing in mcg/kg, usual dose 150-200 mcg/kg)	Scabies and lice (off-label use); onchocerciasis and strongyloidiasis; cutaneous larval migrans (*Ancylostoma braziliense* or *Ancylostoma caninum*); activity against *Wuchereria bancrofti, Brugia malayi, Mansonella ozzardi,* and *Loa loa,* although not first-line therapy.	Multiple doses are not well evaluated in patients with severe liver disease. Ivermectin is often more practical and effective than topical treatment for scabies (95% effective if given in two doses).[49] May not be necessary to bring, depending on travel conditions and geography.
Levofloxacin (Levaquin)	500 mg or 750 mg PO tabs	Intraabdominal infections, pneumonia, cystitis, traveler's diarrhea (off-label use)	In the absence of ileus, same bioavailability when given PO as IV. Tendon inflammation and rupture (e.g., Achilles tendon, rotator cuff, biceps) are significant concerns. Avoid concurrent calcium-containing foods and medications. Ciprofloxacin can often be considered an alternative. Avoid in patients taking corticosteroids.
Mefloquine (Lariam)	250 mg PO tabs	Chloroquine-resistant malaria prophylaxis and treatment (check CDC.gov for guidelines)	Dosed weekly for prophylaxis. Do not prescribe to patients with prior adverse reactions to mefloquine, which may include hallucinations and night terrors. Caution in patients with significant psychiatric history.
Metronidazole (Flagyl)	500 mg PO tabs	Suspected giardiasis; severe diarrhea or diarrhea with fever, blood, or leukocytes	Alcohol consumption may cause a disulfiram-like reaction. The use of metronidazole may increase the toxicity of lithium, phenytoin, and anticoagulants.
Moxifloxacin (Moxeza)	0.5% optic solution, 3 mL bottle	Bacterial conjunctivitis, corneal ulceration	Not first-line therapy for bacterial conjunctivitis (due to emerging resistance) unless contact lens wearer, because of high incidence of *Pseudomonas* infection
Penicillin V (Pen-Vee)	500 mg PO tabs	Dental infections, streptococcal pharyngitis	Multiple broad-spectrum alternatives may be more appropriate for wilderness travel.
Permethrin (Elimite)	60 g tube, 5% cream	Scabies and head lice	See Ivermectin above and discussion of permethrin-impregnated apparel in text.
Praziquantel (Biltricide)	600 mg (scored) PO tabs	Schistosomiasis, intestinal tapeworms, cysticercosis	Limited or no activity in acute exposure (larval stage). Consider inclusion in medical kit only if prolonged (>21 day) travel to endemic regions.
Quinine (Qualaquin)	650 mg PO tabs	Malaria treatment (P. *falciparum*) in chloroquine-resistant areas (check CDC.gov for guidelines)	Quinine may prolong the QT interval. An IV form is available if patient unable to tolerate PO route. Additional concurrent therapy may be required (e.g., doxycycline).
Rabies vaccine (RVA, RabAvert)	1 mL IM (vials)‡	Postexposure and pre-exposure rabies treatment	Dosing varies based on prior vaccination history. Wound cleansing and possibly immunoglobulin (at separate IM site) also required for postexposure prophylaxis.
Rabies immune globulin (Imogam, BayRab)	20 units/kg	Postexposure rabies treatment	Local wound infiltration with immune globulin, and remainder of dose given IM at a site remote to vaccine site. Consider inclusion in medical kit based on risk.
Trimethoprim-sulfamethoxazole (Bactrim, Septra)	160 mg/800 mg tab PO tabs	Cystitis, traveler's diarrhea, soft tissue infections	Caution in patients with chronic kidney disease or sulfa allergy.
Vancomycin	1 g vial IV‡	Meningitis, sepsis, suspected MRSA infection	Can cause profound hemodynamic instability with rapid administration. Only to be used by experienced personnel. For consideration by well-equipped trips staffed by qualified personnel.

TABLE 102-2 Select Medications for Wilderness Travel*—cont'd

Drug	Formulation	Select Indications	Comments
Cardiovascular			
Amiodarone	450 mg/9 mL vial	Antiarrhythmic in ACLS	Multiple contraindications and adverse reactions, including hemodynamic collapse and fatal arrhythmia with administration. Only to be considered by expeditions with advanced medical support.
Acetylsalicylic acid† (Aspirin, Bayer, Ecotrin)	325 mg PO tabs	ACS, analgesia, antiinflammatory	Increased risk for GI bleeding and other bleeding diatheses. Preferably chewed when used for ACS. Can be given PR.
Atropine	1 mg/mL vial	Symptomatic bradycardia, ACLS	This drug causes tachycardia and stool and urinary retention.
Clonidine (Catapres)	0.1 mg PO tabs	Hypertension	Clonidine may cause drowsiness and dizziness. Can lead to rebound hypertension.
Enoxaparin (Lovenox)	80 mg/0.8 mL prefilled syringes; subcutaneous administration only; weight-based dosing differs by indication	ACS, pulmonary embolism, deep vein thrombosis	Significant risk of bleeding.
Lidocaine	10 mL 2% vial, IV	Antiarrhythmic in ACLS	Potential for significant cardiac and neurotoxicity.
Metoprolol tartrate (Lopressor)	25 mg PO tabs	SVT and ACS	May impair exercise tolerance; may cause bronchospasm and unstable bradycardia.
Epinephrine	1 mL, 0.3 mg IM q 10-15 min for anaphylaxis; 10-300 mcg IV for anaphylaxis; 1 mg q 3-5 min for cardiac arrest	Anaphylactic reaction, hypotension, cardiac arrest, severe asthma, ACLS	Special consideration must be given to appropriate dosing, dilution, and route of administration, which vary considerably between indications. Advanced training and licensure required.
Epinephrine autoinjector (EpiPen)	0.3 mg single-dose autoinjector	Anaphylactic reaction	Inject into an extremity large muscle group (usually anterolateral thigh). Requires pretrip training. Requirement for all travelers with history of anaphylaxis. EpiPen Jr. (lower dose) may be required based on weight of travelers.
Nitroglycerin (Nitrostat, Nitrolingual)	0.4 mg sublingual tabs, or inhaler, 400 mcg/spray	Angina, select exacerbations of congestive heart failure	Relief of chest pain with nitroglycerin does not identify the pain as being cardiac in origin. Nitroglycerin is heat and light sensitive with a short shelf life. May cause hypotension and potentially life-threatening interactions with phosphodiesterase inhibitors, such as those used for erectile dysfunction (e.g., Viagra, Cialis, Levitra, Silagra).
Oxygen	Titrate to effect	Respiratory distress, ACS, decompression sickness, traumatic head injury, inhalational injury	Oxygen tanks are explosive, heavy, and bulky. Oxygen storage requires special attention and regular maintenance. Can be problematic if traveling by air.
Neurologic			
Alprazolam** (Xanax)	0.25-0.5 mg PO tabs	Insomnia, anxiety	Causes sedation and can lead to respiratory compromise. Potential for abuse and withdrawal.
Clonazepam** (Klonopin)	0.25-0.5 mg PO tabs	Insomnia, anxiety	Causes sedation and can lead to respiratory compromise. Potential for abuse and withdrawal.
Dextroamphetamine (Dexedrine, Dextrostat)	5 mg PO tabs	Fatigue, difficulty concentrating	May cause nervousness, diarrhea, or loss of appetite.
Diazepam** (Valium)	5 mg PO scored tabs	Anxiety, agitation, seizures	Causes sedation and can lead to respiratory compromise. Potential for abuse and withdrawal.
Dimenhydrinate† (Dramamine)	50 mg PO tabs	Antihistamine, motion sickness	Causes CNS depression.
Etomidate (Amidate)	20 or 40 mg vial, IV injection	Rapid-sequence intubation	To be used only by trained providers planning to intubate during emergencies. Can cause hemodynamic compromise by depressing sympathetic tone.
Haloperidol (Haldol)	5 mg/mL vial; IM, IV, PO formulations available	Agitation, mania, psychosis	Dystonic reactions may occur; treat these with diphenhydramine or benztropine (Cogentin). Can cause QT prolongation.

Continued

TABLE 102-2 Select Medications for Wilderness Travel*—cont'd

Drug	Formulation	Select Indications	Comments
Lorazepam** (Ativan)	2 mg/mL IM/IV	Anxiety, agitation, seizures, alcohol withdrawal	Causes sedation and can lead to respiratory compromise. Potential for abuse and withdrawal.
Meclizine† (Antivert, Bonine)	25 mg PO tabs	Vertigo, motion sickness prophylaxis	Adverse reactions include CNS depression and blurred vision (which can impair reading and ability to perform procedures requiring fine dexterity).
Midazolam** (Versed)	10 mg/mL vial; oral syrup also available	Anxiety, procedural sedation	Must be secured as significant abuse potential and side effects.
Modafinil (Provigil)	100 mg PO tabs	Circadian rhythm disturbances, shift work (e.g., night watch), fatigue	Use with caution in patients with cardiovascular disease or a history of psychiatric disorders.
Olanzapine (Zyprexa)	10 mg PO tabs; SL/IM administration available	Agitation, mania, psychotic disorders	Can cause tardive dyskinesia, neuroleptic malignant syndrome, orthostatic hypotension, and hyperglycemia.
Scopolamine (Transderm Scop)	1.5 mg TD patch	Motion sickness prevention, antiemetic	Significant anticholinergic symptoms, including blurred vision, CNS depression, and dyshydrosis (which can impair sweating and thermoregulation).
Succinylcholine	200 mg vial	Rapid-sequence intubation	Consider inclusion in medical kit only if personnel present with advanced airway equipment, training, and licensure. Review potentially life-threatening contraindications before use.
Dermatologic			
Clotrimazole† (Lotrimin, Mycelex)	1% cream	Topical fungal infections	Multiple alternatives exist.
Hydrocortisone† (Cortaid, Hytone)	1% cream	Contact dermatitis	Hydrocortisone is not to be used to treat infections. Repeated use can cause skin atrophy, especially on face, genital area, and dorsum of hand.
Triamcinolone (Aristocort, Kenalog)	0.1% ointment	Contact dermatitis, severe itching	Triamcinolone is significantly more potent than hydrocortisone OTC, although requires prescription. It should not to be used to treat infectious rashes. Repeated use can cause skin atrophy, especially on face, genital area, and dorsum of hand. Numerous alternatives exist.
Mupirocin (Bactroban)	2% cream, 15 g or 30 g tube	Impetigo	MRSA coverage for superficial infections. Components of OTC triple-antibiotic ointments (bacitracin-neomycin-polymyxin B) may be inferior to mupirocin for impetigo.
Diphenhydramine† (Benadryl)	25-50 mg PO tabs	Seasonal allergies, allergic reactions, dystonic reactions	Causes significant impairment of psychomotor performance and cognitive function.
Metronidazole (Metrogel)	Vaginal 0.75% cream	Bacterial vaginosis	The formulation tends to separate at high temperatures; consider an oral formulation for more compact and stable transport.
Nystatin (Nyamyc)	Vaginal suppositories and creams	Vulvovaginal candidiasis, balanitis, localized skin infections	Creams and suppositories tend to melt in warm or hot environments. Fluconazole is more stable and can be taken as a single oral dose, but it belongs to Pregnancy Category C and requires prescription. Nystatin is very inexpensive.
Permethrin (Elimite, Nix)	5% cream	Scabies; head lice may be treated with a 1% permethrin rinse	This cream causes temporary stinging. Treatment may be repeated after 7 days for increased efficacy. Read notes on ivermectin adjunctive therapy.
Polymyxin B, bacitracin, and neomycin ointments† (Neosporin)	15 g packs	Lacerations, superficial skin infections	This is not a substitute for systemic antibiotics for soft tissue infections.
Silver sulfadiazine (Silvadene)	1% cream, 50 g tube	Burns, large soft tissue injuries, open fractures	Remove cream from a previous application before reapplying. This drug contains sulfa.
Tolnaftate† (Tinactin)	1% cream, gel, spray, or powder	Localized skin infections that are suspected of being fungal in origin	The safety profile is unknown for pregnancy.

TABLE 102-2 Select Medications for Wilderness Travel*—cont'd

Drug	Formulation	Select Indications	Comments
Eye, Ear, Nose, and Throat Topical Medications§			
Artificial Tears†	10 mL container	Xerophthalmia (dry eyes)	Rule out foreign body, corneal abrasion, or other pathologies before use.
Cyclopentolate (AK-Pentolate, Cyclogyl)	1% drops, 5 mL container	Snowblindness (off-label use)	Decreases pain (photophobia) by decreasing ciliary muscle spasm. Not to be used for patients who need to walk or drive. It may cause acute angle-closure glaucoma. Scopolamine 0.25% and homatropine 2%-5% may be alternatives.
Diclofenac	0.1% drops	Snowblindness	Consider using adjunct PO analgesic.
Dexamethasone, neomycin, and polymyxin ointment (Maxitrol)	Drops or ointment	Snowblindness, disabling allergic conjunctivitis	Cortisporin (neomycin, polymyxin, and hydrocortisone) may be interchangeable with Maxitrol for otic and ophthalmic irritation.
Erythromycin ophthalmic ointment (Ilotycin)	0.5% ointment, 3.5 g tube	Corneal abrasions or ulcerations	The ointment stays on the eye but blurs vision; it should be used at night or while resting. Multiple alternatives exist.
Gentamicin (Garamycin) or Tobramycin (Tobrex) drops	0.3% drops	Corneal abrasions or ulcerations in contact lens wearers	May cause chemical keratitis. Interchangeable with ofloxacin or ciprofloxacin drops in select indications.
Moxifloxacin (Vigamox)	0.5% drops	Bacterial keratitis	Fourth-generation fluoroquinolone with possibly less resistance than earlier generation meds. Increased cost.
Neomycin and polymyxin B sulfate and hydrocortisone otic suspension (Cortisporin Otic Suspension)	Neomycin 0.35%, polymyxin B 10,000 units/mL, hydrocortisone 0.5%	Otitis externa	Must avoid the use of topical aminoglycosides if tympanic membrane ruptured.
Ofloxacin (Floxin Otic)	0.3% otic solution	Otitis externa	Second-generation fluoroquinolone. Multiple alternatives exist. A wisp of cotton wool placed in the ear as a wick will draw medication into the ear canal.
Oxymetazoline (Afrin)	0.05% nasal spray	Congestion, epistaxis	This drug may be sprayed on a laceration to temporarily decrease bleeding. It causes rebound congestion with prolonged use.
Pilocarpine (Isopto Carpine)	2% drops	Acute angle-closure glaucoma	Only to be used by experienced and appropriately trained personnel.
Phenylephrine (Neo-Synephrine)	0.5%-2.5% drops	To induce mydriasis	Only to be used by experienced and appropriately trained personnel.
Polymyxin B and trimethoprim eye drops (Polytrim)	10000 units/mL solution	Corneal abrasions or ulcerations, snowblindness	Ointments can be used instead of drops, but these impair vision and should only be used when patients are resting or sleeping. Worsening eye irritation suggests chemical keratitis caused by medication.
Prednisolone	1% drops	Allergic keratitis, acute angle-closure glaucoma	Because steroids may worsen eye infections, they are typically prescribed only on advice from ophthalmologist.
Tetracaine	0.5% drops	See Analgesia section	
Timolol (Istalol)	0.5% drops	Acute angle-closure glaucoma	Significant side effects can occur; should be used only under expert consultation.
Gastrointestinal			
Bismuth subsalicylate† (Pepto-Bismol, Kaopectate)	262 mg PO tabs	Abdominal pain, vomiting, diarrhea	With this drug, the stool and tongue may turn black; excessive intake can cause salicylate poisoning. May provide good GI prophylaxis from coliform infection if taken before meals.
Docusate sodium† (Colace)	100 mg PO tabs	Constipation	Docusate may cause diarrhea and abdominal cramping. Liquid form may also be useful for cerumen disimpaction.[43]

Continued

TABLE 102-2   Select Medications for Wilderness Travel*—cont'd

Drug	Formulation	Select Indications	Comments
Famotidine† (Pepcid)	20 mg PO tabs	Peptic ulcer disease, dyspepsia	Decreased stomach pH may predispose patient to GI infections. Consider including one H_2 blocker, because this will have faster onset than PPI (even faster if combined with calcium carbonate and/or magnesium hydroxide).
Lactase† (Lactaid)	250 mg PO tabs	Lactose intolerance	Travelers with known lactose intolerance are advised to bring lactase. Transient lactose intolerance often develops after traveler's diarrhea.
Loperamide† (Imodium)	2mg PO tabs	Diarrhea	Decreases symptoms in most cases of traveler's diarrhea, but has not been adequately studied for safety in patients with bloody diarrhea. Use contraindicated with certain diarrheal illnesses.
Meclizine† (Antivert)	25 mg PO tabs	Motion sickness, nausea	See Neurologic section.
Omeprazole† (Prilosec)	20 PO tabs	Peptic ulcer disease, dyspepsia	Decreased stomach pH may predispose patient to GI infections.
Ondansetron (Zofran)	8 mg PO tabs; 4 mg/2 mL vials	Nausea, vomiting	May cause QT prolongation; limited efficacy for motion sickness–induced nausea.
Promethazine (Phenergan)	25 mg PO tabs	Nausea, vomiting, motion-sickness	Especially effective for motion sickness. Acute dystonic reactions related to promethazine can be treated with diphenhydramine or benztropine. Do not use in pediatric patients. Black Box warnings exist.
Prochlorperazine (Compazine)	5 mg PO tabs; also available PR and as solution for injection, 5 mg/mL	Nausea, vomiting	Causes sedation and dystonia; is not for use in patients <2 years old. Acute dystonic reactions related to prochlorperazine can be treated with diphenhydramine or benztropine.
Senna† (Senokot)	8.6 mg PO tabs	Constipation	Constipation can be a significant challenge for many travelers, and care must be taken before severe constipation is mistaken for more serious illness.
Witch hazel pads† (Preparation H)	Package, 10 each	Hemorrhoids	Multiple alternative antihemorrhoidal medications exist.
High Altitude			
Acetazolamide (Diamox)	250 mg PO tabs	Acute mountain sickness treatment and prevention, acute angle closure glaucoma	Acetazolamide is contraindicated for patients with sulfa allergy; it may cause vertigo, diuresis-induced hypovolemia, paresthesias, and taste changes.
Dexamethasone (Decadron)	10 mg/mL vial for IV administration	High-altitude cerebral edema, antiinflammatory for allergic reactions	Dexamethasone may cause agitation, mood disturbances, hypertension, and hyperglycemia. Takes hours to achieve maximal effect. One IV corticosteroid may be sufficient for the purposes of a medical kit; many alternatives exist.
Nifedipine (Procardia, Adalat)	30 mg PO tabs	High-altitude pulmonary edema	Do not give to patients who are hypotensive. Nifedipine can also be used to treat hypertension.
Sildenafil (Viagra)	50 mg PO tabs	May enhance cardiovascular performance at high altitude, but still experimental	May cause hypotension, headache, lightheadedness, and blue scotomata. Sildenafil is not for patients who are taking nitrates or who have a history of retinal disease.
Respiratory			
Albuterol inhaler (Ventolin, Proventil, Salbutamol)	90 mcg/puff metered-dose inhaler	Asthma exacerbation, COPD	Albuterol may cause tachycardia or provoke anxiety.
Beclomethasone (QVAR, Vanceril)	40 mcg/dose aerosol inhaler	Chronic asthma	This is one of the inhaled corticosteroids given for chronic asthma; it may have fewer systemic side effects than oral corticosteroids.
Diphenhydramine† (Benadryl)	25-50 mg PO tabs	Seasonal allergies, allergic reactions, dystonic reactions	Causes significant impairment of psychomotor performance and cognitive function.
Epinephrine (Primatene Mist)	0.22 mg/puff aerosolized	Asthma exacerbation, allergic reactions (airway edema), anecdotal use for symptomatic bradycardia	Use with caution in older adults and those with known coronary disease.
Fexofenadine† (Allegra)	60 mg PO tabs	Seasonal allergies, urticaria	Nonsedating antihistamine is useful for the treatment of nasal congestion and allergy-induced itching; it costs more than diphenhydramine, but CNS effects are less pronounced.

TABLE 102-2 Select Medications for Wilderness Travel*—cont'd

Drug	Formulation	Select Indications	Comments
Promethazine/codeine**	6.25/10/5 mL syrup PO	Persistent cough	This may be a good medication for acute gastroenteritis in adults, due to the combined antiemetic (promethazine) and antimotility actions (codeine). Black Box warnings exist.
Ipratropium (Atrovent)	18 mcg/puff inhaler	Asthma exacerbation, intranasal administration for treatment of URI symptoms	Ipratropium is not for patients with life-threatening soy or peanut allergies. Also available in combination with albuterol (e.g., Combivent).
Loratidine† (Claritin)	10 mg PO tabs	Seasonal allergies, urticaria	Potentially less impairment in psychomotor performance and cognitive function than diphenhydramine, but may be less effective[5,40]
Phenylephrine†	10 mg PO tabs	Nasal congestion	Contraindicated in patients taking MAOI. Caution in patients with hypertension. Pseudoephedrine may be used as an alternative.
Prednisone (Deltasone, Pred-Pak)	5 mg PO tabs	Asthma exacerbation, allergic reactions, severe allergic contact dermatitis (poison ivy/oak)	Short-term side effects include insomnia and anxiety. Taper may be therapeutically beneficial, although rarely required when used in doses <50 mg daily for <5 days. Monitor for vaginal and oropharyngeal candidiasis.
Pseudoephedrine† (Sudafed)	30 mg PO tabs	Nasal congestion	May have significant cardiovascular and CNS effects.
Cetylpyridinium and benzocaine† (Cepacol)	20 PO lozenges	Sore throat	Acetaminophen and ibuprofen can be helpful adjunct to treating pharyngitis. Many alternative lozenges exist.
Miscellaneous Medications			
Oral glucose† (Glutose)	20 g PO tabs	Hypoglycemia	Hard candy or naturally sweetened fruit juice may be as effective.
Dextrose solution	50%, 25g/50 mL vial	Hypoglycemia	For advanced providers where IV access is possible.
Methylprednisone (Solu-Medrol)	1000 mg/vial‡	Anaphylaxis or severe asthma/COPD exacerbation	Can be used as alternative to dexamethasone, hydrocortisone, or prednisone in select indications.
Hydrocortisone powder	100 mg/2 mL	Anaphylaxis or severe asthma/COPD exacerbation	Can be used as alternative to dexamethasone, methylprednisone, or prednisone in select indications.

ACS, Acute coronary syndrome; *ACLS*, advanced cardiac life support; *CNS*, central nervous system; *COPD*, chronic obstructive pulmonary disease; *GI*, gastrointestinal; *IM*, intramuscular; *IV*, intravenous; *MAOIs*, monoamine oxidase inhibitors; *MRSA*, methicillin-resistant *Staphylococcus aureus*; *NSAIDs*, nonsteroidal antiinflammatory drugs; *OTC*, over the counter; *PO*, by mouth; *PPI*, proton pump inhibitor; *PR*, by rectum; *q*, every; *SC*, subcutaneous; *SL*, sublingual; *SSRIs*, selective serotonin reuptake inhibitors; *SVT*, supraventricular tachycardia; *TCAs*, tricyclic antidepressants; *TD*, transdermal; *URI*, upper respiratory tract infection.

*This table is intended to serve as a list of potentially useful medications for management of commonly encountered medical scenarios in the wilderness. The table should not be used as a treatment guide or as a substitute for manufacturer labels or information contained in the *Physicians' Desk Reference*. All medications listed here must be administered by personnel with appropriate training and licensure. Selection of medications to include in a first-aid kit must be tailored to the specifics of a trip including but not limited to the itinerary, number of travelers, preexisting medical conditions, potentially encountered conditions, and region of travel.

**Providers who bring opioids and other controlled/scheduled medications should do so only if appropriate licensure and training has been obtained. Nonphysician travelers must have a prescription from their personal physician and bring appropriate documentation while traveling. Laws for controlled substances are not universal, and traveling with certain medications may even be illegal in certain destination countries.

†Does not require a prescription in the United States.

‡Requires resuspension. Read package inserts to ensure adequate supply of solution. Usually a supply of any sterile IV fluid solution can work, although some medications may require sterile water to avoid precipitation.

§Caution with multiuse ophthalmic drop applicators because contamination can be source of bacterial keratitis.

Medications highlighted in green are considered high priority with high likelihood of use during wilderness travel.

Medications highlighted in red are considered a potential priority medication with less frequent use, but with potential for preventing significant morbidity or mortality.

Medications highlighted in blue may be considered high priority depending on region of travel or preexisting medical conditions.

If a travel party will not include a community medical kit, individual travelers should consider inclusion of additional high-priority medications (e.g., broad spectrum antibiotic) for their personal medical kit.

COMPREHENSIVE COMMUNITY MEDICAL KIT

A comprehensive, community medical kit is compiled and maintained by the trip's designated medical leader. This kit includes supplies needed to manage a broad range of anticipated injuries and illnesses, with emphasis on injury management and high-priority medications (Box 102-4 and Figure 102-2; see also Table 102-2). Bulky and heavy items, including most stock first-aid and contingency supplies, should be labeled and can be distributed among group members for storage and transport if there is no designated box or bag. A medical cross symbol should be placed on compartments containing the first-aid items. Repair materials are best kept in clearly labeled stuff sacks or watertight boxes independent of the first-aid and medical supplies. In hot environments, aluminum boxes (e.g., Zarges) tend to oxidize over time and leave unpleasant residues on their contents. Thus, materials should not be stored long term in these sturdy, lightweight boxes. Durable plastic boxes, such as those manufactured by Otter and Pelican, should be considered. Although they are durable, large cases are not practical for certain expeditions because of size and weight. A variety of more portable vessels (e.g., backpacks,

BOX 102-4   Contents of a Comprehensive Community Medical Kit*

Wound and Trauma Management

Liquid soap
Alcohol-based gel (e.g., Purell) for hands
Sterile, nitrile gloves
Nonsterile gloves
Splash shield and face protection
Syringes (2, 5, 10, 20 or 30, and 60 cc [mL])
Large- and small-gauge hypodermic needles (e.g., 18 and 25 gauge)
Sterile irrigation saline
Morgan eye lenses
Alcohol pads
Antiseptic towelettes
Povidone-iodine 10% solution (Betadine) or chlorhexidine (Hibiclens)
Wound closure strips (Steri-Strips)
Tincture of benzoin (or Mastisol)
Tissue glue for wound closure (2-octyl cyanoacrylate [Dermabond])
Suture materials (2-0, 4-0 nylon or silk with cutting needle; 3-0 Vicryl with tapered needle)
Disposable skin stapler and remover
Silver nitrate sticks
Esmarch bandage, 3 × 36 inches
Disposable scalpels with No. 11 or 15 blade
Hot and cold packs
Tactical tourniquet
10 × 10-cm (4 × 4-inch) sterile dressing pads
15 × 27-cm (5 × 9-inch) sterile dressing pads
9-cm (3-inch) sterile gauze bandage
Cotton-tipped applicators
Nonadherent sterile dressing
Xeroform and petroleum jelly (Vaseline) gauze burn dressings
Elastic bandage wraps with Velcro closures
Adhesive cloth tape
Adhesive, porous paper tape (1.3 cm [0.5 inch])
Gauze roll (11.4 cm × 3.7 m [4.5 inches × 4 yards])
Adhesive bandages (Band-Aids)
Tegaderm
Eye pad and eye shield
Moleskin, Blist-O-Ban, and silver duct tape
SAM Splints (15 × 110 cm [4.4 × 36 inch])
Aluminum finger splints
Kendrick (or improvised) femur traction device
Slishman Traction Splint
Slishman Rescue Harness
Triangular (cravat) bandage and safety pins
Headlamp
Hemostats and or needle drivers (Spencer Wells)
Trauma shears
Surgical scissors
Toothed and nontoothed forceps
Chlorhexidine surgical scrub brushes
Surgicel Nu-Knit, QuickClot
Plastic finger

Cotton pledgets
Nasal balloon device
Absorbable nasal packing
Urinary catheter, 14 French (catheter bag and tubing)
Absorbable nasal packing

Medications

Select medication listed in Table 102-2 (tailored to anticipated conditions and trip duration, party size, and available space)

Miscellaneous Items

Waterproof flashlight and matches
Signal mirror/dental mirror and whistle
Plastic resealable bags (e.g., whirlpacks)
Permanent markers (e.g., Sharpie)
Notebook and record-keeping supplies (waterproof, depending on environment)
Adhesive labels
Pill bottles and cotton balls
Nail clippers
Steel sewing needles, paper clips, and safety pins
Forceps for removal of splinters and ticks
Pocketknife or multitool knife
Trauma shears
Eyelet scissors
Silver duct tape
Tongue depressors
Chemical ice packs and heating packs
Sun hats and high-SPF sunscreen and lip balm
Emergency blanket (e.g., Space blanket, Pro Tech)
N,N-diethyl-m-toluamide–containing insect repellent (e.g., REI Jungle Juice 100)
Contact lens solution and case
Digital thermometers
Commercially made oral rehydration powder packs†

Equipment

Diagnostic instruments: see Table 102-3
Specialized equipment: see Box 102-7

Dental and Ear-Nose-Throat Supplies

Oil of cloves (eugenol), 3.5 mL; combine with calcium hydroxide powder to make temporary fillings
Calcium hydroxide powder or putty
Cavit (7 g)
Intermediate restorative material
Express Putty
Wooden spatulas for mixing and applying
Paraffin (dental wax) stick
Dental floss
Dental mirror
Cotton rolls and pellets
Ear curettes (consider for trips with aquatic activity)
Ear wicks (consider for trips with aquatic activity)

*This is intended to serve as a list of potential equipment that ultimately must be tailored to the specific details of the proposed trip itinerary.
†Recommend purchase of commercially-made ORS in line with current World Health Organization (WHO) guidelines (equimolar glucose:sodium and 200-310 mOsm/L). *Oral Rehydration Salts: Production of the new ORS*, Geneva, 2006, WHO Press. http://apps.who.int/iris/bitstream/10665/69227/1/WHO_FCH_CAH_06.1.pdf?ua=1&ua=1.

military surplus bags) can be substituted and should be organized using a strategy similar to that previously discussed.

MEDICAL SUPPLIES FOR THE MEDICALLY TRAINED TRAVELER

Expeditions traveling with physicians, remote medical support (via two-way communications), or other providers with advanced training may be able to incorporate a wide variety of additional supplies that are not recommended for untrained wilderness medicine providers (Boxes 102-5 and 102-6 and Tables 102-2 and 102-3). These supplies may vary widely based on trip factors and the training background of expedition medical personnel.

Delivery of medical care by nonphysician providers, including use of certain supplies, techniques, prescription and even OTC medications, represents a controversial wilderness medicine topic from medicolegal and ethical aspects (see Chapter 100).

Designated trip medical leaders, whether physicians or nonphysicians, should generally avoid bringing supplies (including medications) they are not familiar with and not licensed to use. If access to remote, formal medical support is available (e.g., via satellite phone to dedicated medical support staff), inclusion of advanced supplies may be appropriate. Alternatively, should the risks of a trip or a participant's preexisting condition warrant inclusion of advanced equipment, the trip medical leader should seek appropriate training and certification before disembarkation.

Certain necessary skills may be acquired in advanced first-aid, paramedic, or nursing classes. Intramuscular (IM) and intravenous (IV) medications should only be administered by personnel with formal licensure and training. Inclusion of IV access supplies

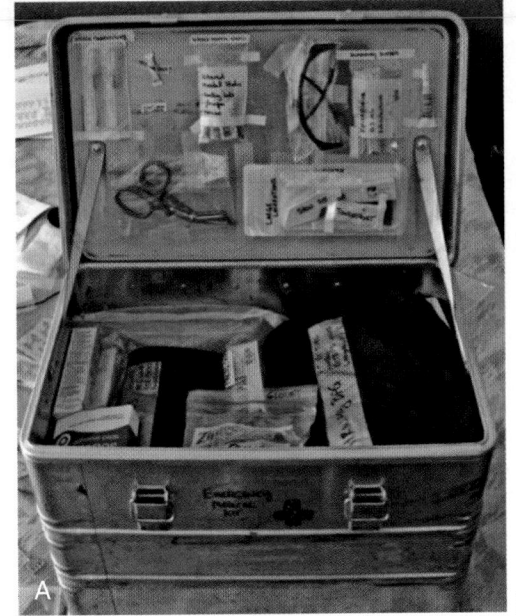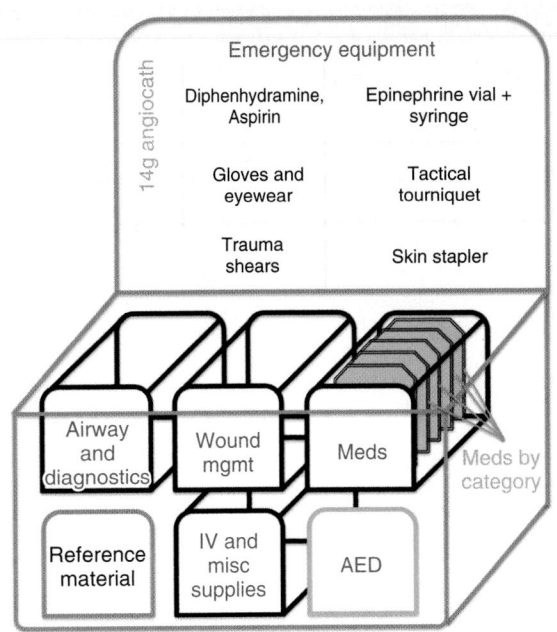

FIGURE 102-2 A, Medical kit from the Mongolian American Expedition to the Gobi Desert set up in watertight Zarges aluminum freight box. **B,** Schematic diagram suggesting arrangement for a comprehensive expedition medical kit.

and isotonic crystalloid solution may be reasonable to carry for certain expeditions. For conscious travelers with mild to moderate dehydration and no ileus, adequate rehydration can generally be accomplished using commercially available oral rehydration supplements (ORS).

Items such as surgical tools, advanced airway equipment, chest tubes, and mechanical suction devices may be appropriate for certain high-risk expeditions with adequately trained personnel. Material for splinting may be available in the surrounding environment. However, if the nature of the expedition is such that extremity injuries are possible, equipment for splinting and stabilization (e.g., Exos brace, SAM Splint, Fast Set-3 Moldable Splint Kit, Redi Universal Splint) should be considered.

The decision to bring oxygen on any trip requires special consideration. Oxygen supplies occupy significant space and weight and may have limited utility for certain expeditions (high-altitude and dive excursions being two notable exceptions). Careful review of protocols for safe transport, storage, and maintenance of oxygen must be undertaken regularly. Trip staff must be familiar with the quantity of oxygen available in the first-aid kit, use of regulators, and indications for appropriate use (e.g., routine use of oxygen in patients with suspected acute coronary syndrome and normal oxygen saturation is controversial[51]). For example, applying oxygen by face mask at 6 L/min for a

BOX 102-5 Contents of a Medical Kit for Expeditions and the Medically Trained Traveler

Medical reference materials (books, tablet, or smartphone*)
Comprehensive community first-aid kit (see Box 102-4)
Appropriate medications for select priority illnesses (see Tables 102-2)
Portable diagnostic instruments for wilderness travel (Table 102-3)
Advanced devices for the medically trained traveler (see Box 102-6)
Specialized equipment based on recreational and environmental hazards (see Box 102-7)

*When planning to use electronic medical reference material, significant limitations in battery life and Internet must be taken into consideration.

BOX 102-6 Advanced Devices for the Medically Trained Traveler*

Oral and nasopharyngeal airways
Bulb suction device
Self-inflating bag-mask ventilation device with pediatric/adult mask sizes
Oxygen supply (see text)
Laryngoscope (MacIntosh blade sizes 2, 3, 4, Miller 3)
Oral and nasogastric tubes, 14 French
Nasal cannula and nonrebreather facemask (if oxygen supply available)
Cricothyrotomy cannula or catheter (e.g., Abelson cannula) or prepackaged cricothyrotomy kit (e.g., Portex Cricothyroidotomy Kit, Nu-Trake cricothyrotomy device, Tactical CricKit)
Endotracheal tube (size 7.0 internal diameter and pediatric sizes when appropriate) and stylets
Laryngeal mask airway (LMA; sizes 3, 4, and 5)
King airway or Combitube
Gum elastic bougie
Chest tube set, 32 French (practical only on major expeditions) with capability for formal or improvised water seal
Heimlich valve
Intravenous tubing with high-flow drip chamber and spike (see Figure 19-25 for use as emergency cricothyrotomy device)†
Needles and syringes (for intravenous hydration and emergency injectables)
Intravenous catheters (assorted sizes 14, 16, 18, 20, and 22 gauge)
Sharps disposal device (biohazard disposal container)
Intravenous tourniquet
Intravenous fluid (normal saline, lactated Ringer's, or Plasma-Lyte)
Adjustable cervical collar
Automated external defibrillator (AED)
Surgical tools
Surgical or fine-dust masks, N95 mask when concern for tuberculosis (TB)

*Selection of the equipment listed here must be made at the discretion of the trip medical officer based on several factors, including level of training and space allotted for medical supplies.
†From Platts-Mills TF, Lewin MR, Wells J, et al: Improvised cricothyrotomy provides reliable airway access in an un-embalmed human cadaver model, *Wilderness Environ Med* 17:81, 2006.

TABLE 102-3 Portable Diagnostic Instruments for Wilderness Travel*

Device	Indication
Thermometer (e.g., ADTEMP 419 digital or other low-reading device)	Essential for evaluation of hypothermic and hyperthermic patients (e.g., infection, exposure).
Sphygmomanometer (blood pressure cuff)	Useful for accurate measurement of blood pressure, particularly in trauma patients and patients with tachycardia or altered mental status; may be used as an adjustable tourniquet. Ensure appropriate cuff sizes and stethoscope are also packed.
Stethoscope	Useful for auscultation of Korotkoff sounds for manual blood pressure measurement and for chest auscultation, particularly to evaluate for the presence of wheezing, pulmonary edema, or pneumothorax.
Precordial stethoscope	A precordial stethoscope with earpiece can be a useful and inexpensive tool for continuously monitoring heart rate and respiratory rate.
Urinalysis test strips (e.g., Clinitek)	Useful for evaluation of abdominal pain, urinary symptoms, ketosis, and hyperglycemia.
Chronometer (waterproof with second hand)	Useful for accurate measurement of heart rate and respiratory rate; also important when planning evacuations.
Urine pregnancy test (e.g., Baby Check, Midstream, SureStep, or one of many other generic and name brands)	Essential for evaluation of abdominal pain in women of childbearing age; a positive pregnancy test may raise the possibility of ectopic pregnancy, and immediate evacuation might be considered. These tests vary in sensitivity and may also produce false-positive results.
Pulse oximeter (e.g., Nonin)	Considerable variation exists in the quality of over-the-counter probes (https://www.ncbi.nlm.nih.gov/pubmed/27089002). Choosing a manufacturer who also makes FDA-approved (medical-grade) probes, ideally with plethysmography, is recommended (extra batteries likely needed). Keep in mind that most of these units do not feature alarms or capability to provide continuous monitoring.
Glucometer (e.g., Therasense)	Useful for routine diabetes management and for evaluation of ill-appearing diabetic individuals who may have too-low or too-high serum glucose levels.
Fluorescein dye strips	Necessary for diagnosis of corneal abrasions. The cobalt light source on an ophthalmoscope or a fluorescent light stick can be used to illuminate the fluorescein.
Magnifying glass	For foreign body identification and removal.
Otoscope	For foreign body or otalgia evaluation (infectious, inflammatory, and traumatic etiologies); consider a device with capability for pneumatic otoscopy. Do not forget specula (preferably reusable soft tips of varying sizes).
Ophthalmoscope	Devices with cobalt light filters when used in conjunction with fluorescein are especially useful for the diagnosis of corneal abrasions.
End-tidal carbon dioxide detector (e.g., Nellcor)	Colorimetric devices are available to help with confirmation of endotracheal tube placement, while quantitative digital devices remain expensive and not practical for many expeditions.
Rapid diagnostic tests	When traveling to endemic regions, purchase of rapid diagnostic kits can be useful when evaluating febrile illnesses. Several kits are available for malaria, dengue, and typhoid as well as other illnesses. These kits require a drop of blood on a test strip. Travelers must investigate sensitivity and specificity for specific manufacturers and types of organisms (e.g., *Plasmodium vivax* vs. *P. falciparum*) because this is an evolving technology, may not be FDA approved, and usually is available for purchase at pharmacies in country of travel.

FDA, U.S. Food and Drug Administration.
*Appropriate training is required for use of these devices.

nonhypoxemic patient with lower abdominal pain is not only unnecessary but also will quickly exhaust supplies. In this case, if a D-size oxygen cylinder were packed and appropriately filled before departure, at 6 L/min this tank would last only about 1 hour (425 L ÷ 6 L/min = 71 minutes). Of note, portable oxygen tanks found in many first-aid kits are significantly smaller than a D-size cylinder and expected to last for much shorter durations. Any excursion that brings oxygen should also carry a pulse oximeter, not only to appropriately identify patients in need of oxygen therapy but also to titrate therapy in order to conserve supply. All wilderness medicine providers, even with proficiency using a variety of common airway and oxygen delivery devices, should familiarize themselves with the specific equipment packed for the trip. For example, some expensive oxygen kits lack self-inflating bag-mask devices and contain (oxygen-powered) manually triggered ventilation devices (MTV) that may be unfamiliar to many providers.

Table 102-4 provides a list of proposed medical kits for specific purposes as detailed in other chapters.

SPECIALIZED EQUIPMENT FOR ENVIRONMENTAL AND RECREATIONAL HAZARDS

A host of activities, including mountain climbing, water activities, and winter expedition travel, have inherent risks that may warrant specialized equipment. This section discusses specialized items

Table 102-4 Proposed Medical Kits for Specific Purposes With Chapter References

Medical Kit Type	Reference Location	Chapter
Sample contents of a wilderness airway management kit	Box 19-5	19
Facial trauma medical kit	Box 20-1	20
Wound care first-aid kit	Table 21-8	21
Tactical personal supply module	Table 27-8	27
Tactical basic medical module	Table 27-9	27
Tactical intermediate medical module	Table 27-10	27
Tactical major trauma module	Table 27-11	27
Pain management first-aid kit	Box 47-3	47
Wilderness eye emergency kit	Box 48-1	48
Technical rescue medical kit	Appendix	56
Minimal equipment for survival first-aid kit	Appendix D	59
Medical kit for jungle travel	Box 60-1	60
Desert survival kit	Box 61-1	61
Whitewater first-aid kits	Appendix A	62
Expedition medical kit	Appendix	80
Basic emergency kit	Box 111-1	111

BOX 102-7 Specialized Equipment for Environmental and Recreational Hazards

High Altitude
Gamow bag and accessories
Pulse oximeter
Oxygen canisters, nasal cannulae, face masks, oxygen tubing, and
  connections

Cold and Avalanche Exposure
External thermal stabilizer bag
Res-Q-Air
Hot Sac
Intravenous fluid warmer
Chemical warmers (e.g., Grabber)
Electric foot warmers (e.g., Hotronic)
Low-reading thermometer
Space Thermal Reflective Survival Bag
Adhesive climbing skins
Ice axe
Adjustable ski or probe pole
AvaLung avalanche vest
Tracker DTS
Avalanche Beacon

Water Sports (Low Impact)
CPR Microshield
Water disinfection equipment (i.e., filter, iodine or chlorine,
  SteriPEN)

Water Sports (High Impact)
Cervical spine immobilizer
Pelvic immobilizer (e.g., SAM Pelvic Sling)

Bicycling
All-terrain cyclist kit
Occlusive dressings

Tropical and Third-World Travel
Pressure immobilization equipment (for snakebite)
Permethrin-containing insect repellent
Mosquito nets
Oral rehydration electrolyte powder packs
Water disinfection equipment (i.e., filter, iodine or chlorine,
  SteriPEN)

Mountain Climbing and Hiking
Prefabricated splints and pelvic immobilizer (sling)
Slishman Traction Splint (not available in United States)
Slishman Rescue Harness
Ankle brace (e.g., Aircast)

that may be needed for certain high-risk recreational activities (Box 102-7 and Appendix C).

Two pieces of potentially lifesaving equipment with applicability in almost all environments include communication and navigation devices. In the past, satellite phones and global positional system (GPS) devices were prohibitively expensive; now one can purchase or rent a GPS device or satellite phone for a reasonable cost. Many smartphones are GPS enabled and with the necessary applications are able to function for this purpose, with the caveat that battery life can be significantly limiting. There are several GPS-equipped emergency alert communication devices that can be activated solely for the purpose of emergency rescue and medical aid. When activated, these devices, as with in-home medical alert systems, globally locate the device using GPS technology and then connect the user (qualitatively or via bidirectional audio) with a 24/7 support network to direct an appropriate response.[45] These devices can be purchased at a reasonable cost, and network support can be maintained for less than one would pay for satellite telephone services. In most countries, including low- and middle-income countries, cellular telephones have good reception, sometimes even in remote areas. Many of these devices require open space to send and receive, so forested areas can severely impair their function. Once again, using satellite or cell phones to activate a rescue

can expedite patient care, but neither device should be regarded as a substitute for proper preparation and sound judgment during wilderness travel. Chapter 106 provides additional discussion of specialized navigation and communication equipment.

High-Altitude Exposure

Mountain climbing not only poses a risk for traumatic injury but also subjects the climber to altitude-related illnesses, possibly requiring portable oxygen or a pressure bag (e.g., Gamow bag).[4,15] The Gamow bag is a portable hyperbaric chamber resembling a large sleeping bag with a window (Figure 102-3). It has been shown to be effective for treatment of high-altitude pulmonary and cerebral edema. Constructed of nylon, the bag can be folded, and has a packing weight of 6.6 kg (14.5 lb). Inflated, it is 2.1 m (7 feet) long and has a diameter of 64 cm (21 inches). The bag is pressurized with a foot pump at a rate of 10 to 20 strokes per minute and has relief valves pressurized to approximately 1 kg (2 lb) per square inch, allowing venting of expired air. With pressurization, the Gamow bag simulates a descent of approximately 1000 to 2800 m (3281 to 9186 feet). In a situation such as a remote clinic with electricity, a mechanical compressor can be used to avoid the fatiguing task of foot pumping. In addition, a breathing bladder has been introduced. One end of this large nylon bag connects to a face mask, and the other end connects to one of the pressure-relief valves of the Gamow bag. The patient inhales uncontaminated air from the Gamow bag, and the exhaled air flows down a plastic tube into the bladder. This obviates the need for manual foot pumping of the bag for 15 to 30 minutes until the bladder becomes full; it is then necessary to operate the foot pump again to repressurize the bag. The bladder is an excellent adjunct for expeditions at very high altitude that are far from medical evacuation and when a prolonged period of resuscitation is anticipated. The recently developed Gamow tent operates on the same principle as the Gamow bag; it is almost 50% larger and has added height that allows a patient to sit upright.

These devices are expensive and intended for expeditions that are going to extreme altitudes (i.e., >4267 m [14,000 feet]) or dangerous situations (e.g., ice climbing on a steep glacial crevasse) that prevent rapid descent. Before using any therapy for hypoxia, physicians should be familiar with expected oxygen saturations for humans at various altitudes.

Cold Exposure

Extreme cold exposure may necessitate provision of warmed IV fluids and humidified oxygen in addition to usual supportive care. Travelers engaging in low-risk trips can use a sleeping bag wrapped with a space emergency blanket to provide a capsule that preserves heat and allows thermal recovery. The space blanket is made of a lightweight material capable of reflecting and retaining more than 80% of radiated body heat. Another helpful product is the Grabber Warmer. Useful for prevention of frostbite, this small pad undergoes a chemical reaction on exposure to air, producing heat. Grabber brand warmers can maintain a temperature of 66° C (150° F) for 7 hours or more. They can

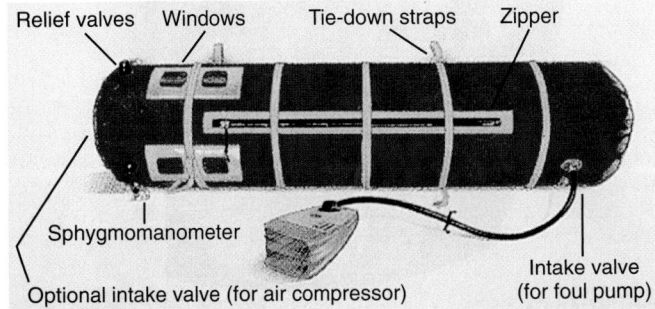

FIGURE 102-3 Gamow bag. Attached is the foot pump required to pressurize the compartment to 2 lb/in². Four windows are strategically located to permit observation, and entry is through a lengthwise zipper.

be placed in gloves, shoes, and pockets for prevention of frostbite, but should be used as directed to avoid burns because of the high temperatures that can be generated. They have also anecdotally been used (off-label) to warm IV fluids by coiling IV tubing around the warmer. In forested areas, a large plastic bag filled with leaves can provide insulation.

People involved in cold-water search, rescue, or other high-risk cold-water endeavors should consider purchase of a Hypothermic Stabilizer Bag. This product consists of an internal, high-pile fabric that wicks water to allow quick drying of hypothermic patients. The thermal properties far exceed those of an equivalent-thickness conventional down sleeping bag, and the product requires no additional insulation underneath it for support and comfort. A key feature allows the ability to perform CPR through an access window over the chest. The stabilizer's outer cover is made of water-resistant material and has carrying handles to facilitate safe patient transport.

For more remote or risky expeditions distant from medical rescue or assistance, several sophisticated products could be useful. Of value in circumstances of high avalanche danger is a lightweight vest with a breathing tube (e.g., AvaLung),[35] which permits extraction of oxygen and redirected release of carbon dioxide when an individual is trapped under snow (Figure 102-4). Such a device may prolong survival chances until the victim is found by another person appropriately outfitted with a snow shovel and an avalanche beacon or probe. For victims of severe exposure hypothermia, elevation of core temperature and prevention of further body heat loss may be critical. Inhalation of warm humidified air is now possible with portable field units, such as the battery-operated Res-Q-Air. The unit is simple to operate, has a temperature-control valve, and runs for 1 hour on battery power. It is small ($27 \times 9 \times 3$ cm [$9 \times 3 \times 2$ inches]), and weighs approximately 2 kg (4.5 lb). In the event that emergency IV fluids may be required, the Soft Sack IV Fluid Warmer can be used. This product comes in a soft, rugged, portable case and has its own battery power source. Temperature within the bag is maintained at 37° C (98° F) to keep IV fluids warm, and the bag has a protective sleeve to place over IV tubing to preserve warmth.

A Note on "Space Blankets"

"Space blankets" are plastic sheets, coated with a highly reflective material, that provide effective reflection of radiated body heat.

Radiant heat loss is a minor component of heat loss as compared with conductive, convective, and evaporative losses. A space blanket provides virtually no insulation against conductive heat loss. Without concomitant bulky insulation, it is nearly useless when placed against any cold surface. As listed in Box 102-3, the personal medical kit should include a poncho or large plastic yard waste bag (these are available in bright orange from a variety of sources, such as OutdoorSafe). Although they are equally ineffective against conductive heat loss, these large yard waste bags are more durable over time when folded and better suited as a full body vapor barrier and enclosure. Space blankets often deteriorate along crease lines, even when stored properly. In emergency situations, the waste bags are easily worn as ponchos and stuffed on the inside with leaves, moss, grass, or other naturally obtainable bulky insulation, which makes them highly effective thermal conductive barriers.

Water Disinfection

The key design features of a water disinfection system for backcountry travel include (1) adequate pore size of the filter to remove bacteria and protozoan cysts (i.e., ≤0.2 mm); (2) filter element that either has activated charcoal or is impregnated with silver or iodine for local antibacterial action; (3) pump-feed mechanism that forces water through the filter housing; (4) device that can be easily disassembled and cleaned for proper maintenance; and (5) product that is light, durable, simple to use, and can provide enough volume of clean water needed for the traveling party. Noteworthy filters that have most of these desirable features include those from Katadyn, PUR, and MSR WaterWorks. Disinfection with or without filtration may be achieved chemically with the use of iodine, chlorine, or ultraviolet (UV) radiation. Each method has benefits and shortcomings (see Chapter 88). Before the expedition, trip or medical leaders must investigate the potential likely pathogens to be eliminated, initial level of debris in the anticipated water sources, and volume of water (needed by the travel party) to be disinfected, as these are key factors for method selection. It is always advisable to have capacity for a backup method of water disinfection, such as boiling.

Bicycling

Cycling poses significantly increased risk for soft tissue injuries that may require occlusive water-based gel dressings for optimal wound care. Several prepackaged medical kits for cyclists are available. Individuals who want to modify a basic first-aid kit for treating cycling injuries should consider supplies needed to treat abrasions and minor burns. Proper wound management requires a protective pad that is nonadherent, cools the skin, and absorbs exuded fluids. Breathable water-based gels (e.g., Spenco 2nd Skin) are good for this purpose.

Mountain Climbing and Hiking

In wilderness travel above the tree line, inclusion of more advanced splinting products should be considered, but many common materials (e.g., cardboard and water bottles) provide excellent immobilization. A structural aluminum malleable SAM Splint weighs approximately 113.4 g (4 oz). The foam-coated aluminum strip unfolds to provide rigid longitudinal support. It can also be configured as a cervical collar, although an injured neck may require additional immobilization. At least two SAM Splints are required to stabilize an entire extremity. The SAM Sling is a force-controlled circumferential pelvic sling belt that is used for reduction and stabilization of pelvic fractures. The Slishman Traction Splint is a lightweight splint made from a pulley system and collapsible ski pole used as a lower-extremity traction device for femur and hip fractures. The Kendrick Traction Device is similar but uses a dedicated pole and nylon straps; it can also be used for dislocated shoulder reductions. Ankle injuries are common, and air-inflatable or gel-filled splints (e.g., Aircast) provide stability and fit comfortably in a wide range of footwear.

Protection Against Mosquito-Borne Illness

Personal mosquito netting is a requirement when traveling in tropical areas with mosquitoes, even when appropriate pretravel

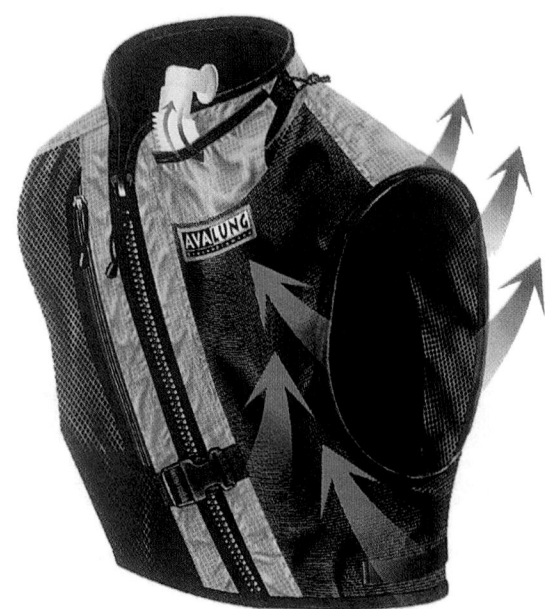

FIGURE 102-4 The AvaLung is a lightweight vest designed to improve avalanche survival. Victims are able to draw air from even a dense snowpack through the front using an air-exchange mouthpiece. A one-way valve permits exhalation of carbon dioxide, which is expelled through the back of the vest. *(Courtesy Black Diamond, Ltd.)*

BOX 102-8 In-Vehicle Emergency Supplies

First Aid, Rescue, and Survival
Comprehensive medical kit (see Box 102-4)
Large burn dressings
Boards for splint construction
Backboard, short or folding long (e.g., Junkin; see Appendix C)
Bags, large plastic
Collapsible shovel
Blankets—wool and space blankets or plastic yard waste bags (see text, Cold Exposure)
Climbing rope and hardware*
Candles, long burning
Flares
Flashlights and batteries in watertight storage
Headlamps
Food and water
Matches (waterproof) or butane-type lighter
Radio, citizens' band
Satellite phone
Global positioning system (GPS) device (e.g., Garmin eTrex, smartphone app or watch)
Rope
Saw with metal-cutting blade
Small stove, pot or coffee can, and utensils
Tarp, plastic
Toilet paper
Whistle

Automotive
Aluminum foil to cover windows
Cables to jump-start battery
Chains with tighteners, with repair links and special pliers†
Fire extinguisher
10-minute flares (at least six; can also serve as fire starters)
Industrial or welding gloves
Engine oil and extra can
Shovel, metal or Lexan, with short or collapsible handle
Tool kit
Small axe
Tow chain or cable
Wheel chock or wedge blocks
Siphon hose or hand-crank gas pump
5- and 10-gallon water cans
Propane tank with regulator and hoses
Solar panels or rolls
Car cigarette lighter adapters and cables
Country-appropriate electrical plug adapters
Spare automotive battery
Gasoline-powered generator
Propane or butane cigarette lighters
Tire pump
Flat-tire repair kit
Spare tire (2)
Tie-down straps
Extra gas (20 L)
High-lift jack and plate for jack

*Mountain terrain supplies (special training needed).
†Winter weather supplies.

vaccinations and antimalarial prophylaxis have been given. Mosquitoes are vectors for many serious illnesses, and mosquito netting is a simple and effective barrier. Netting impregnated with permethrin mosquito repellent is widely available in outdoor shops, as are long-lasting spray preparations for persons who want to treat existing clothes and equipment. Many compact and sturdy hammocks are manufactured with built-in mosquito netting. A second hammock suspended under the shadow of the rainfly allows dry storage of field gear and clothes off the ground in areas with frequent rain.

ITEMS STORED IN THE VEHICLE

When feasible, a complete emergency kit should be stored in a vehicle or at base camp (Box 102-8). This kit should also provide material necessary to manage accidents encountered along the highway and to cope with the environment if the occupants are stranded by automotive trouble or natural disaster. Several large burn dressings and a board with strapping to restrain the head and neck will fit in a standard vehicle trunk or other recess. Although only large vehicles can accommodate the usual full-length backboard, a folding backboard is available from Junkin Safety Appliance (see Appendix C in this chapter). The remaining contents of an emergency kit will fit in a medium (18 cm wide × 37 cm long × 27 cm high [6 × 12 × 9 inches]) or large (24 cm wide × 55 cm long × 43 cm high [8 × 18 × 14 inches]) military surplus ammunition box, watertight plastic box (e.g., OtterBox), or soft medic bag (e.g., CamelBak) of similar size (Figure 102-5).

MEDICAL REFERENCE MATERIAL

Ensuring access to familiar, readily understood, and comprehensive medical reference material is an important component of

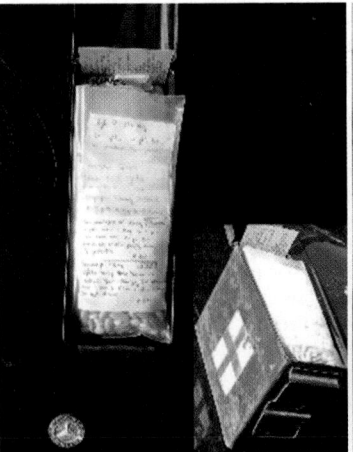
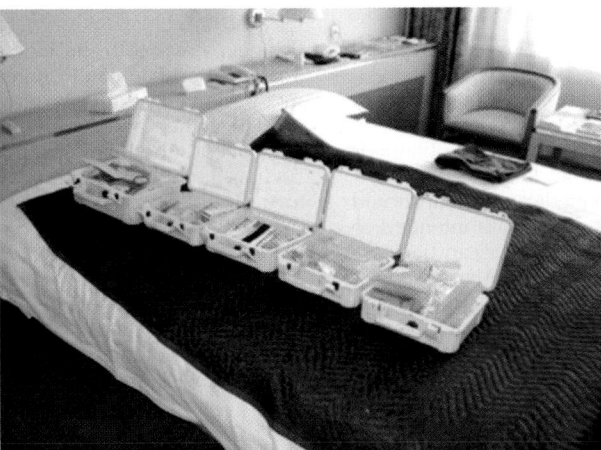
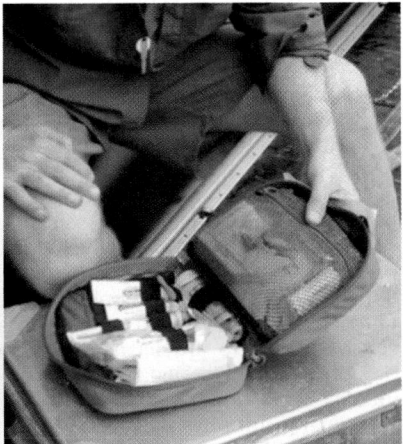

FIGURE 102-5 First-aid kits for vehicles. Medications are stored in zipper-lock bags with dosing instructions. Each kit has an inventory card. Small kits such as these are appropriate for short excursions and while driving in a caravan.

pretrip planning but does not replace appropriate training and preparation. Traditional medical reference materials have limited utility in remote settings due to weight and size constrictions but may be extremely useful when not in the field. Numerous pocket guides exist, but often lack comprehensiveness. Books such as this one can be obtained as a field guide (*Field Guide to Wilderness Medicine*) or downloaded in electronic format as an application for mobile phone or tablet devices (https://itunes.apple.com/us/app/field-guide-to-wilderness/id713382694?mt=8). In addition, a variety of other electronic resources and mobile applications are readily available and sometimes free, including applications ("apps") for drug reference (e.g., *Physicians' Desk Reference,* http://www.pdr.net/), ePocrates (http://www.epocrates.com/products), and infectious disease guides (e.g., Sanford Guide, http://www.sanfordguide.com/); Johns Hopkins Guides (http://www.hopkinsguides.com/hopkins/ub); and downloadable clinical practice manuals for resource-constrained settings (e.g., *Integrated Management of Adolescent and Adult Illness* manual[23]). Careful attention must be given to battery life and charging capability of mobile devices if electronic resources are the primary format for reference material in the field. In certain circumstances, it may be prudent also to carry printed copies of drug and other information specific to the medications in the trip first-aid kit as well as to known existing medical conditions in the travel party.

Mobile Health (mHealth) and Emerging Technologies

The number of portable, consumer electronic medical devices has skyrocketed in recent years. Many of these products are designed for and require a mobile smartphone for use, thus the term *mHealth.* These products range from portable diagnostic devices such as Bluetooth ECGs capable of email transmission, to videoconference-telemedicine consult apps, to mobile phone–based pulse oximeters and thermometers. Despite potential promise of improved diagnostics and treatment of patients, as yet the applicability of these devices in remote settings is uncertain. Careful consideration before purchasing must be given to battery requirements and device accuracy (many are not validated or formally approved for patient care), among other concerns. It is also important to keep in mind that most consumer medical devices are not certified to be used for continuous patient monitoring. As a result, these devices often turn off automatically after set periods and do not have alarms to signal abnormal values.

MEDICATIONS USEFUL IN THE WILDERNESS SETTING

PRIORITY PRESCRIPTION AND OVER-THE-COUNTER MEDICATIONS

Expedition medical officers must confront several key questions before selecting medications to incorporate into a first-aid kit:

1. What medications am I (or other members of the party) trained to administer and distribute?
2. What medications are likely to be lifesaving?
3. What medications are most likely to be needed based on the trip itinerary and personal medical histories obtained?
4. How much space exists in the first-aid kit?

Table 102-2 lists OTC and prescription medications that should be considered for wilderness excursions. This list is intended to serve as a framework from which a medical officer can begin to prioritize both OTC and prescription medications. Many medications (e.g., atropine, epinephrine, dexamethasone, nifedipine, nitroglycerin) have significant systemic effects and should generally be limited to physicians, nurses acting under the direction of a physician, or designated medical providers with appropriate training.

Primary care physicians taking care of travelers will often be asked to prescribe medicines that will be used or withheld on the basis of the judgment of someone who is not a physician (i.e., the traveler or trip leader) (Figure 102-6). Patients should be educated about appropriate and inappropriate use of

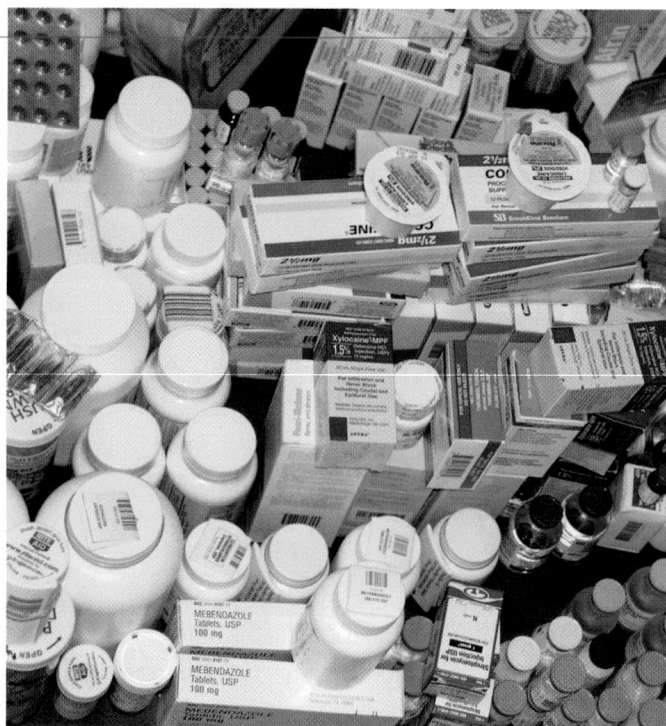

FIGURE 102-6 Medications. See Table 102-2 for a list of over-the-counter and prescription medications often considered for various types of wilderness expeditions. *(Courtesy Matthew R. Lewin.)*

medicines and encouraged to consult a local physician or communicate with a physician from their country of origin before taking any prescription medications or even certain OTC medications.

When assembling medical kits, always include copies of the manufacturer's package insert with each medicine or ensure offline electronic access using a smartphone or other device. Expedition members should visit their personal health care providers to obtain prescriptions before departure. Although sharing of medications within a group of travelers is common, it is not an activity that the prescribing physician should endorse or be responsible for unless the doctor is acting as an adviser to the entire group. All physicians should be aware of their potential liability when traveling with, prescribing medications for, or advising a travel group from a remote location.

An additional challenge facing the expedition medical officer is allocation of opioid-containing analgesics, sleep aids, and other controlled medications. Expedition members naturally hope to be as comfortable as possible and to sleep well, although these may be unreasonable expectations at times. Likewise, medical designees want to provide adequate treatment for pain and anxiety. Because of the potential for inappropriate use of these medications, it is advisable to limit access and consistently apply predetermined policies for the use of opioids and anxiolytics. All controlled substances should be kept in a secure compartment such as a zippered locking bank bag if space permits, and inventory should be regularly monitored.

Injectable drugs are rarely needed for management of wilderness-associated trauma and illness, because most emergencies can be managed by either oral or transdermal application of medicines. Intravenous medications are temperature sensitive, fragile, expire quickly, and require monitoring of vital signs because of potency and immediate onset of action. In certain circumstances, such as lengthy, remote expeditions with high-level medical support, inclusion of several injectable medications may be justified. Numerous analgesics can also be given intramuscularly.

Opioid analgesics can be used to treat pain if combining first-line analgesics (e.g., NSAIDs and acetaminophen) is inadequate. At least one oral opioid should be included in an expedition first-aid kit if a licensed provider is available.[41] Caution must be used in all travelers who are to receive opiates, but especially those with altered mental status or significant coexisting respiratory disease. Respiratory depression with limited ability to manage the airway or provide supplemental oxygen can be fatal. Oral opioids may be appropriate for moderate to severe pain. Opioids and dehydration can predispose an individual to constipation, which is an uncomfortable and potentially dangerous problem. Any patient initiating opioid therapy should be advised to also start a bowel regimen. Docusate sodium (Colace) and senna (Senokot) are acceptable first-line agents, although caution must be used with gel capsule formulations in hot environments, because melting is a common issue. Any expedition carrying opioids should also carry a reversal agent (e.g., naloxone). Travelers with chronic pain syndromes should seek appropriate analgesics and adequate supplies from their personal physician before departure.

Whenever possible, medicines should be purchased as tablets rather than capsules because of the tendency of capsules to break apart or dissolve (Figure 102-7). Under extremes of temperature, creams may become unusable, and in such environments, oral medications are preferred. For example, creams for genital yeast infections have a tendency to separate, whereas oral antifungals (e.g., fluconazole), although more expensive, are compact, stable, and may be discretely and hygienically administered.

Purchasing medications on arrival may be necessary and may save money, but must be done with caution. A study of the quality of antibiotics in a developing country found that, in approximately 30% of the products studied, the drug was either not present or present in lower dosages than stated.[38] If treatment failure poses a significant health threat, the traveler should make every effort to obtain medications from a reliable source. Although many medications that require prescriptions for purchase in high-income countries, including opioids, are available over the counter in low- and middle-income countries, the advice of a local physician may still be helpful.

Whether expired medications should be used depends on stability and safety. It is a dubious practice, but one that is widespread. The term *stability* refers to the tendency of a drug to become less potent over time. Manufacturers provide an expiration date up to which point the drug will lose more than 10% of its potency, if kept in its original closed container. After the container has been opened, the expiration date no longer applies. Retail pharmacies typically label repackaged drugs with a "beyond-use" date that is generally 1 year from the date the prescription was filled. Many drugs maintain potency of more than 90% for long after the expiration date. For example, ciprofloxacin can remain stable for several years after the expiration date, even under conditions such as high temperature and humidity. Passing an expiration date does not necessarily indicate that the drug becomes harmful for human use. Nevertheless, a known exception is tetracycline antibiotics, which degrade into toxic metabolites that can damage the kidneys.[9] For medications that are dosed to effect (e.g., those used to treat pain, gastric, respiratory, and psychiatric symptoms), decreases in potency usually present minimal risk to the patient. For medications with specific recommended doses (e.g., antibiotics, therapies for high-altitude illnesses), decreased potency could result in ineffective treatment of a serious condition. (See the text Appendix, Drug Stability in the Wilderness.)

PASSING THROUGH CUSTOMS WITH MEDICATIONS

Each medication should be labeled with the patient's name, prescribing physician's name, dosing schedule, indications, and warnings. In most parts of the world, individuals carrying properly labeled medications receive little attention at customs. For persons leading a group and carrying the community medication supply, appropriate documentation is important. To facilitate passage through customs, all medication bottles should be labeled appropriately, including "For use by the _____ Expedition only." Medical designees should carry multiple copies of their credentials and letters of purpose from their sponsoring institutions. A letter from the sponsoring institution or company that designates the carrier of the medications as the group's medical officer or physician will usually suffice.

Special caution must be used when traveling with scheduled or controlled substances because these may require special documentation or even may be illegal in the destination country. Impeccable documentation and group discussions with participating travelers before departure are critically important because certain countries have strict laws that may include harsh legal action, including long-term imprisonment or even capital punishment.

Inevitably something will be overlooked, confiscated, or needed unexpectedly. A visit to a local hospital or clinic may require creative pantomime and drawing. These visits provide helpful local medical contacts and identify appropriate sites for donation of medications and equipment, when appropriate, on return.[54] Sterile items such as disposable needles, IV tubing, and catheters may be much less expensive. It should not be taken for granted that these will be available or fit correctly on items purchased in preparation for international travel.

A dictionary of the local language is essential. Many developing countries have hospitals and training modeled after countries

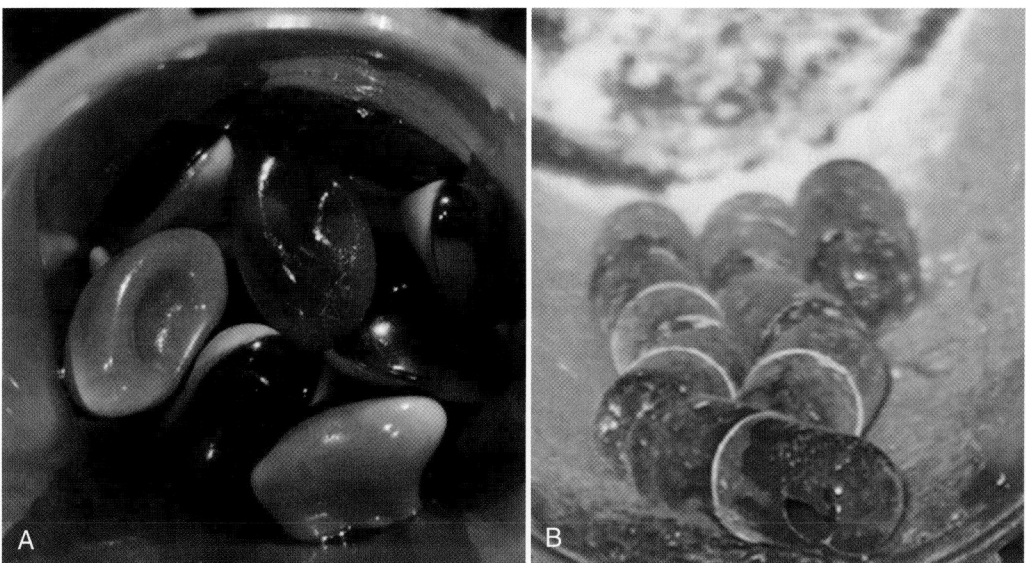

FIGURE 102-7 Gel tabs (**A**) and gelatin capsules (**B**) are susceptible to damage from heat and vibration. Consideration should be given not just to the medication, but also the dosage form.

that once occupied them. Thus, when traveling in Central Asia (e.g., Kazakhstan, Mongolia), a Russian dictionary is helpful, because a high percentage of pharmacists and physicians in this area speak Russian and read Cyrillic. Similarly, local medical providers in many parts of Africa and Southeast Asia are familiar with or fluent in French.

PREPARING FOR COMMON MEDICAL PROBLEMS IN THE WILDERNESS

Thresholds for administering medications—including analgesics, sleep agents, and antibiotics—during travel depend on practice style, supplies, and evacuation options. Treatment thresholds tend to be lower (i.e., more aggressive) in the wilderness than at home. To ensure timely care, all trip members should feel comfortable seeking consultation or clarification from the expedition's medical designee. A secure log of all patient encounters is important for both patient and physician. Preparation for common medical problems in the wilderness setting is discussed next, followed by consideration of certain challenges encountered in some low-income countries.

GASTROINTESTINAL, GENITOURINARY, AND REPRODUCTIVE CARE

Travelers should anticipate significant changes to normal hygiene practices that can potentially have negative impacts on health and morale. With adequate planning, participants can generally mitigate the potentially negative consequences of these changes. Groups camping in a delicate ecology or near freshwater should use a lightweight and portable commode with sturdy disposable plastic bags. This practice has become law when working or traveling in certain areas, such as federal land in the United States. Urine containers may be appropriate if prolonged adverse weather is a possibility. Funnel-like devices that connect to urine containers (e.g., Lady J; see Appendix C) may be helpful for women. People embarking on long journeys should be aware that their normal bowel habits are likely to change. Lack of public sanitation may compel the more fastidious to bring their own supplies of toilet paper, baby wipes, and items for treatment of perianal itching and hemorrhoids, such as pads saturated in witch hazel (e.g., Tucks) and other familiar brand-name formulations (e.g., Anusol, Preparation H). Women should predict their needs for absorbent pads and tampons based on their menstrual cycles. Knowing how and being able to squat is of vital importance and can be more difficult for men. Concepts of privacy might have to be discarded in lieu of necessity.

Some women who use oral contraceptive pills may change their cycles to avoid menstruating on long journeys. Women should discuss this possibility with their personal physicians several weeks before departure. In addition, a urine pregnancy test should be included in most medical kits.

Diarrhea and Abdominal Pain

Although most cases of diarrhea and abdominal pain are relatively benign and manageable even in a remote setting, the differential diagnosis is broad. Consideration must be given to infectious (e.g., enteric gram-negative rods, typhoid, giardiasis) and noninfectious (e.g., constipation, peptic ulcer disease, appendicitis) causes, because benign conditions, such as constipation, if not addressed early and appropriately, can cause significant impediments for travelers.

Gastrointestinal distress and traveler's diarrhea can occur during any significant geographic change (e.g., in Mexico, bismuth subsalicylate is sometimes advertised for Mexicans traveling to the United States to avoid "Uncle Sam's revenge"), but more likely when traveling in low- and middle-income countries that lack adequate water sanitation infrastructure. Whatever the etiology, careful selection of foods and drinks can decrease the risk for infection. Bottled or boiled drinks and cooked or peeled foods are less likely to contain pathogens. Conversely, cold drinks, ice cubes, and raw or undercooked foods are more likely to contain pathogens. Fomites can be highly contaminated

with feces even if people are fastidious; flies land on feces and transport pathogens from plate to plate. Treatment of traveler's diarrhea should focus on fluid replacement, consideration of antibiotics, and symptomatic treatment. Each participant should be encouraged to report the first loose stool. For select pathologies, treatment at the onset of symptoms can cut duration of symptoms from 3 days to 1 day and minimize spread of infection to others within the group. Bacterial pathogens cause about 80% of acute traveler's diarrhea, which explains why antibiotic treatment is so effective. Patients with diarrhea should increase fluid intake and avoid sharing or preparing drinks or food for others.

Patients with diarrhea who are very young or very old, have significant underlying disease, or are unable to tolerate oral fluids should seek local medical attention and evaluation; parenteral fluids may be necessary to treat these individuals. As previously mentioned, for conscious travelers with mild to moderate dehydration and no ileus, adequate rehydration can generally be accomplished using commercially available oral rehydration supplements (ORS). Oral glucose-electrolyte solutions[20,37] with equimolar glucose and sodium and osmolality of 200 to 310 mOsom/L have been shown to be as effective as IV fluid therapy in treating moderate hypovolemia associated with certain diarrheal diseases. Commercially available ORS that are in line with WHO recommendations can be obtained as powder packs for easy resuspension calculations using 1-L travel bottles.[36]

Chapter 82 provides a more extensive discussion of the principles of treatment for infectious diarrhea.

All women with abdominal pain without an obvious explanation should receive a pregnancy test. If the test is positive, the patient should seek immediate medical attention, given the risk for ectopic pregnancy. Women who know they are pregnant must notify trip medical staff and should consider ultrasound studies before travel to identify the location and number of pregnancies.

Medical attention should be considered for anyone with atypical abdominal pain. Proton pump inhibitors (PPIs; e.g., omeprazole, pantoprazole) and histamine-2 (H$_2$) receptor antagonists (e.g., famotidine, ranitidine) are typically prescribed for acid reflux and dyspepsia, but both medications cause hypochlorhydria (i.e., decreased levels of stomach acid and elevated stomach pH), which compromises defense mechanisms of the upper GI tract. Use of these medications may predispose travelers to bacterial and parasitic intestinal infections.[42] Patients taking H$_2$ receptor antagonists and PPIs should be aware of their potential to increase incidence and perhaps severity of GI infections. Temporarily stopping these medications during travel should be considered on a case-by-case basis.

All travelers should receive hepatitis A immunization prior to travel to endemic regions.

Sexually Transmitted Infections

Sexually transmitted infections are common among travelers; trip medical personnel should be able to recognize and treat common conditions. Trip medical personnel should also be prepared to decrease transmission by including ample supply of lubricated and nonlubricated synthetic condoms in the medical kit and making this supply accessible.

Expedition participants considering sexual activity with a new partner should be encouraged to carry condoms. Condoms without lubrication can also serve as waterproof pill carriers, small tourniquets, and makeshift canteens (these have sometimes been used by the British military). Chancroid is particularly prevalent in the developing world and can act as a vehicle for more serious and less treatable infections, such as HIV and herpes simplex. All travelers of reproductive age should receive vaccinations for hepatitis B and consider human papillomavirus (HPV) vaccination.

ORAL HYGIENE AND HEALTH

Mild sore throat and a foul taste are common when traveling in the mountains and in cool weather, probably because of mouth breathing, enhanced loss of moisture from the upper respiratory tract, and medication effects. Both problems can be addressed by using either hard candies or medicated lozenges (e.g., Cepacol, Chloraseptic). Saline spray can keep nasal passages hydrated. Because treatment of early caries and loose fillings (which may trap expanding air) can prevent dental demise, each party member should have a dental examination before the trip. During the trip, frequent brushing may seem impractical, but having multiple brushes available and a few small tubes of toothpaste make this less so. Flossing after meals, rinsing well with water, and chewing sugar-free gum also help to maintain oral hygiene.

Toothache is common at high altitudes and during ascent from deep dives. For painful cavities or decay, temporary filling materials (e.g., Cavit) can be obtained in small squeeze tubes and applied to a tooth with a wet cotton applicator to prevent sticking. A dental emergency in any environment, hot or cold, should not occur because of lack of preparation.

FRACTURES AND DISLOCATIONS

Splints can be improvised from cardboard, plaster, cloth, duct tape, water cans, and a phenomenal array of other materials. A number of lightweight splinting products, including moldable splints, ankle braces, and pelvic immobilizers, are available (see Box 102-7 and Mountain Climbing and Hiking, earlier). There are several types of cold packs, including chemical, flexible, and rigid. Chemical cold packs are available at most wilderness and outdoor outfitters and should be used with caution when there is a break in the skin. In general, these packs are intended for single use only. Some cold packs have the potential to cause frostbite; improper application can cause or worsen injury. Gel packs are stored in the freezer and might be seen only in large expeditions with solar- or fuel-powered generators. For areas in which a cold mountain stream is accessible, submerging the injured extremity (or legs tired from a day of hiking) is helpful.

SLEEPING AND STAYING AWAKE

Difficulty sleeping during travel is common and often caused by stress associated with a new environment or jet lag. Decreased sleep negatively impacts not only trip enjoyment but also physical performance and judgment, thereby significantly increasing a traveler's risk of injury. Medications that aid induction and maintenance of sleep can be useful, as can nonpharmacologic sleep aids, such as ear plugs, eye masks, and relaxing music. Nonpharmacologic methods should always be first line. Oral diphenhydramine is generally a safe and effective soporific. A 25- to 50-mg dose can result in sedation for approximately 6 hours. Diphenhydramine also causes mild mental impairment lasting about 2 hours, and because of its anticholinergic effect, can cause urinary retention in predisposed individuals. The medical kit may carry benzodiazepines to treat seizures. They are also effective sedatives and may be used with discretion as a sleeping medication if nonpharmacologic methods and diphenhydramine are ineffective. Patients should be warned about potential adverse effects and the possibility for abuse with benzodiazepines and other sleep remedies. Benzodiazepines should not be used with alcohol and are contraindicated in pregnancy (Pregnancy Category D), except for emergencies such as seizures. Physicians prescribing benzodiazepines to women should document the last menstrual period or require a pregnancy test in addition to a detailed discussion of the risks and benefits of these medications when sexual activity and pregnancy are possibilities.

Additional problems with sleep are experienced at high altitudes, where hypoxia, frequent awakenings, and periodic breathing are almost universal. Zolpidem (Ambien), temazepam (Restoril), acetazolamide, and a variety of other medications have each been examined for treatment of sleep problems at altitude. Drugs such as zolpidem and temazepam have been shown to subjectively improve sleep quality and decrease nocturnal variations in oxygen saturation in participants at 5300 m (17,388 feet). In addition, acetazolamide and theophylline have been shown to decrease periodic breathing. Acetazolamide can significantly reduce nocturnal hypoxia from periodic breathing.[12,52] Climbers and trekkers who have difficulty sleeping at altitude should consider a trial course of acetazolamide. If acetazolamide is ineffective, zolpidem or temazepam may be useful. Patients should be aware that the effect of benzodiazepines on daytime performance at high altitudes is unknown. In addition, patients should be cautioned against the use of temazepam, alprazolam (Xanax), or other benzodiazepines during technical ascents because of the risk for impaired judgment and performance. Nevertheless, a supply of these medications should be available for emergency use.

Some travelers will encounter situations that require staying awake for an extended period; long drives, rescues, and night watch are a few possible scenarios. For these situations, caffeine-containing drinks or OTC stimulant medications may be invaluable. Caffeine is also useful for temporary relief of caffeine withdrawal headaches and is available in 200-mg tablets, roughly equivalent to 2 cups of strong coffee. Caffeine use should be discouraged among patients with a history of seizures, high blood pressure, or heart disease. Because of the diuretic effect, patients using caffeine will need to consume additional fluids to stay well hydrated. Newer (but expensive) drugs, such as modafinil (Provigil), are becoming popular but have not been formally evaluated in the wilderness setting. In emergency situations, stimulants such as prescription amphetamine derivatives (e.g., dextroamphetamine and amphetamine [Adderall] and methylphenidate [Ritalin]), have been used successfully but carry significant risk of physical and psychiatric adverse effects, as do all stimulants. Consumption of energy drinks with alcohol is considered a risk factor for problematic drinking and impulsivity.[44]

BLISTERS AND FOOT CARE

Participants should bring footwear they have already worn and found comfortable. Socks should be kept clean and dry. At a minimum, a second pair is usually necessary, but in most cases, multiple pairs should be brought.

Identifying and addressing painful areas on the feet early can prevent blisters. There are many ways to prevent blisters by minimizing friction and pressure at "hot spots" using basic elements of the medical kit. Petroleum jelly on a gauze pad, covered by duct tape, is a reliable method of preventing or treating blisters. In addition, duct tape placed on the inner lining of shoes decreases friction between the sock and shoe; it can also be placed directly on the surface of the skin. A long-acting local anesthetic such as bupivacaine can provide exceptional relief if there is no alternative to walking, and a blister injury must be overcome. Local anesthesia may allow further tissue trauma to go unrecognized, and thus is not a solution for blisters encountered at the beginning of a multiday trip. Finally, a small square of silk, paper currency, or candy wrapper can be glued to the heel or to another pressure point. This durable method of blister care is another example of a simple, inexpensive alternative to commercial preparations, which may not be available or sufficiently durable in suboptimal conditions. Similarly, methylacrylate–based glue can be used to repair skin fissures (Figure 102-8), and abrasives can be used to reduce the size of thick, cracked callouses. People who anticipate problems with blisters should consider reading John Vonhof's book, *Fixing Your Feet,* which provides detailed information about ways to protect the feet during extended travel. (See Appendix A in this chapter and Chapter 25.)

Nail clippers are an important addition to the medical kit for people on extended journeys. For shorter trips, trimming toenails before departure reduces likelihood of injury to the toenail and surrounding soft tissue. However, caution must be taken to evert the distal nail edges among people who are prone to ingrown toenails. Hikers whose feet sweat excessively may benefit from talc or medicated powder (e.g., tolnaftate [Tinactin]; see Table 102-2). Travelers in cold and aquatic environments are especially prone to dry skin. Petroleum jelly and skin creams and lotions (e.g., Eucerin, Lubriderm, Keri) may help forestall microtrauma and epidermal cracking.

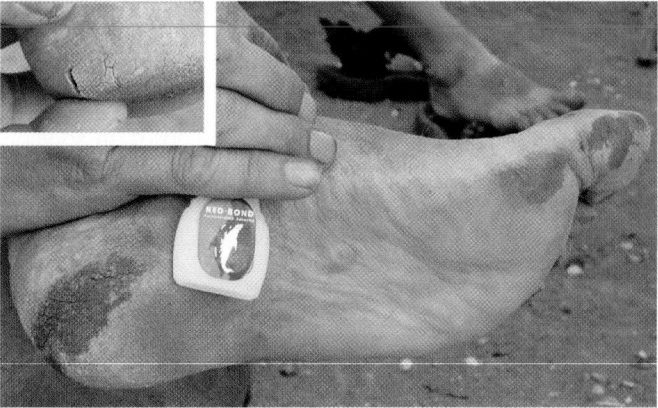

FIGURE 102-8 Methyl acrylate glues may be useful for closing skin fissures and small lacerations. Skin glues should not be used to close lacerations in cosmetically significant areas (e.g., eyebrows, eyelids).

WOUNDS

Cleanliness and hemostasis are the cornerstones of good wound care, whether in an emergency department or a remote setting. Although this chapter discusses numerous potential wound care supplies, in practice, inclusion of a few simple supplies and good improvisational skills can help ensure adequate wound management under most wilderness conditions.

The medical kit should include tactical tourniquets or a blood pressure cuff to help stop bleeding. Traditional medical teaching during the last half-century has focused on avoiding tourniquets in favor of direct pressure, arterial pressure points, and elevation. It was taught that arterial occlusive tourniquets could lead to limb ischemia and loss in an "uncontrolled" out-of-hospital setting. Although inadequately applied tourniquets can increase bleeding (if only venous but not arterial flow is occluded) and cause neurovascular injury (especially with prolonged use), military data from recent conflicts have demonstrated the safety and efficacy of appropriately applied, arterial occlusive tourniquets.[3,27,29] Direct pressure is still the preferred method for hemor-

rhage control, but when not feasible, such as limb amputation or during technical evacuation with limited manpower, tourniquets can be lifesaving. With smaller hemorrhages, nasal sprays containing vasoconstrictors can help provide hemostasis. For some injuries, particularly those that involve the scalp, closure of the wound with staples will rapidly provide hemostasis; a small "ten shot" skin stapler (e.g., ConMed Reflex, 3M Precise) is a useful addition to the medical kit.

Water for irrigation should be clean and ideally sterile, but copious irrigation with nonsterile water is preferable to no irrigation if an adequate supply of sterile water is not on hand. IV fluids may need to be conserved if rescue is not imminent. Forcefully ejecting irrigation solution from a 20-mL syringe through an 18-gauge needle generates pressures adequate to dislodge bacteria and microscopic particles from contaminated wound surfaces (Figure 102-9). A squeezable bottle with holes punched in the top or a plastic bag with small holes suffices for lower-pressure irrigation. When appropriate, surgical excision of crushed, devitalized, or severely contaminated tissue can be achieved with sharp eyelet or suture-cutting scissors from the medical kit's surgical or bandage-cutting tools.

Surgical tools may be crudely disinfected by rubbing vigorously with a prepackaged towelette containing alcohol, chlorhexidine (Hibiclens), povidone-iodine (Betadine), or benzalkonium chloride. After cleaning the instruments with alcohol or chlorhexidine towelettes, igniting the residual alcohol will provide additional disinfection. Flame sterilization until red hot or boiling may also be acceptable. Although less efficient, immersion in boiling water (for about the same duration as one boils drinking water for disinfection) can also help disinfect materials. Use of these techniques may be considered when more reliable techniques are unavailable but should not be confused with sterility.[36a] Data on the safety and efficacy of these methods are lacking.

Wound care adjuncts, including Tegaderm adhesive dressings and Spenco 2nd Skin, can be extremely useful in wilderness settings. Tegaderm is a transparent adhesive covering for clean wounds that provides a barrier to water, dust, and dirt while allowing oxygen to penetrate. It is available in a variety of sizes and can remain in place for several days provided no wound complications arise. Spenco 2nd Skin is a polyethylene oxide gel laminate that reduces friction damage to the skin underlying blisters and burns; the product may offer additional protection

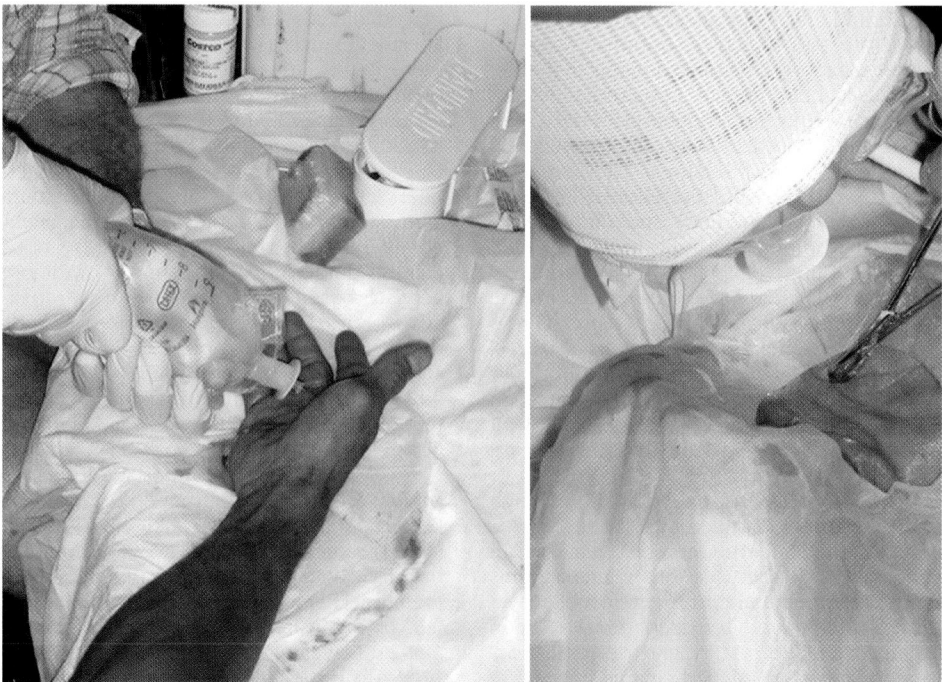

FIGURE 102-9 Water for irrigation should be clean and ideally sterile. Copious irrigation with nonsterile water is preferable to no irrigation.

by redistributing pressure and absorbing exudates. These are just two examples of many potential wound care dressings that can be helpful in remote settings.

Necessary quantities of dressings, gauze, and suture material can be calculated in a similar manner used for calculation of medication quantities (see sample calculations in Strategies for Packaging Medical Kits, earlier). However, prevalence of traumatic injury during travel should be considered. Thus, it is not necessary to bring enough packing for 10 lacerations if there are 10 people on the trip.

BITES AND STINGS

Travelers should know the signs and treatments of allergic reactions and be prepared to intervene. Epinephrine preparations, an antihistamine such as diphenhydramine (Benadryl), and oral corticosteroids are essential components of the medicine supply. As discussed earlier, individuals with a history of allergy to insect stings should carry their own epinephrine. For trained medical professionals, an inexpensive alternative to preloaded syringes is to carry a 1-cc syringe with needle and a 1-mg ampule of 1:1000 epinephrine (0.1% or 1 mg/mL) (Figure 102-10). The benefit of this approach is that a 1-mL vial provides at least three doses of epinephrine in the event of a severe reaction or reactions in multiple patients. Glass epinephrine ampules require careful handling and storage out of light.

Topical corticosteroids are especially useful for insect bites and contact dermatitis and may alleviate suffering and obviate the need for systemic drugs. Maximally potent fluorinated corticosteroid cream preparations (e.g., betamethasone, fluocinolone, fluocinonide, halcinonide) are recommended for use under the harsh circumstances of wilderness travel (see Table 102-2). Short-term use rarely causes complications, although, for the face, moderate-potency preparations, such as triamcinolone, are preferred over maximally potent formulations.

Snakebite treatment is discussed in Chapters 35 and 36.

Travelers expecting frequent exposure to snakes or dangerous marine animals, such as stonefish, might consider obtaining antivenom specific for the area of travel or knowing the location of the closest facility with the antivenom. All antivenoms, including the new formulation for rattlesnakes (CroFab), carry a significant risk for both severe allergic reaction and delayed serum sickness and thus should be administered only by people who are prop-

erly trained and equipped to handle these situations. Using an injectable cholinesterase inhibitor (e.g., neostigmine in combination with anticholinergic drug, such as atropine or glycopyrrolate) may delay or reverse the effects of a neurotoxic envenomation, such as that of a cobra or krait.

SUNBURN, SNOWBLINDNESS, AND SUNGLASSES

All travelers should use both barrier protection (e.g., hat, long sleeves) and sunscreen with an SPF of at least 30 with full ultraviolet A (UVA) and UVB light protection. Efficacy of sunscreen is diminished by sweat, water, wind, dirt, and friction. A hat and long-sleeved clothing plus sunscreen will prevent severe sunburn in most environments. Zinc oxide and titanium dioxide sunblocks or "face masks" provide additional protection in snow, high altitudes, and deserts. Modern and readily available formulations can provide remarkable sun protection without the traditional opacified coating of the skin usually seen with zinc and titanium creams. Sunscreens with compounds such as avobenzone and octocrylene should be sought, because these can protect over a broader range of the UVA and UVB spectrum.[50]

In 1997, the incidence of snowblindness (photokeratitis) among trekkers and porters in central Nepal was about 3%.[6] Snowblindness, a burn injury to the cornea, results from cumulative exposure to sunlight (see Chapter 48). If there is significant risk of eye pathology, an expedition is strongly encouraged to bring fluorescein and an appropriate light source for thorough ophthalmologic examination (see Table 102-3). Topical ophthalmic anesthesia provides pain relief and facilitates examination, but should not be given repeatedly because of increased risk for ulcer formation (see Table 102-2). Several therapies may have a role in snowblindness, including topical nonsteroidal antiinflammatory drug (NSAID) drops, antibiotic drops, and asking the traveler to rest with eyes closed in a dark location. Snowblindness is very painful, but full recovery usually occurs within 24 to 72 hours. Optimal eye protection can be achieved by wearing sunglasses with 100% UV light protection. The major variables to consider when buying sunglasses are durability, light transmission, photochromicity (i.e., darkening with increasing sun intensity), and polarization.

Although plastic lenses are lightweight, they scratch easily and are generally not recommended for extensive wilderness trekking. Glass lenses with the best photochromic properties can be coated for greater than 99% UV absorption, but are heavy, susceptible to breakage, and moderately susceptible to scratching. The most durable lenses are made of polycarbonate; these are lightweight and shatterproof. For this reason, polycarbonate is usually the preferred material for serious wilderness sports. Polycarbonate models that absorb at least 99% of UV light are manufactured by such brand names as Orvis, All Weather, Bolle, Coyote (polarized), Gargoyles, Gentex, Learjet, Oakley, Ski-Optics, Suncloud, Transitions (photochromic), and Wings. Although polarization does not protect from UV light, it reduces glare and increases contrast, making it highly desirable for winter mountaineering, skiing, and aquatic wilderness sports. External clip-on plastic polarizers are also available, and some soft contact lenses absorb UV radiation.

Because light reflects off snow and sand, sunglasses with side protection are recommended in these environments. Side shields, nose guards, and eye patches can be fashioned from almost any material. Because sunglasses are often forgotten, misplaced, or broken, for long trips, every member of the expedition should carry two pairs of sunglasses. Expedition physicians should carry extra pairs. Retention (i.e., neck) straps are recommended for virtually all outdoor activities. For water sports, a lanyard may be attached from the glasses' frame and over the back to a belt loop. In addition, the physician should know how to improvise sunglasses from available materials (e.g., by making two horizontal slits or multiple dots in an ocular barrier, such as duct tape), because loss of vision in even one member can quickly endanger the entire party.

Eye protection should be worn at all times when working with or in the vicinity of others using hand tools, machinery, or flammable substances. A loupe or other handheld lens can be

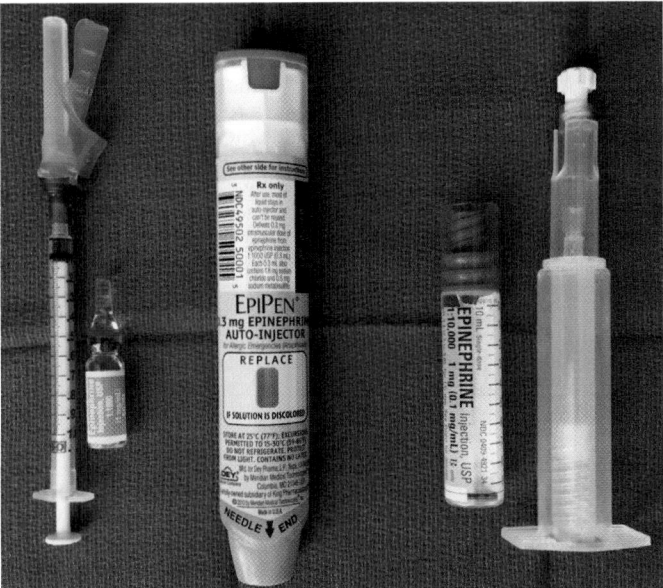

FIGURE 102-10 Three different preparations of epinephrine. *Left*, 1-mg vial of epinephrine 1:1000 and insulin syringe *Middle*, Single-use (0.3 mg, 0.3 mL, 1:1000) autoinjector device, the EpiPen. *Right*, Single-use injectable delivery device, 1:10000, 1-mg dose.

very helpful for identifying ulcerations and removing corneal foreign bodies. Sandstorms are also a common source of foreign body eye irritation. Ski and swim goggles offer good eye protection for areas where particles from tools or storms are flying at high velocity. Goggles are more effective than sunglasses with side shields for repelling dust and sand particles swirling and ricocheting in high winds.

PAIN

Pain control in remote settings should follow a multimodal approach. Medication side effects (e.g., constipation with opiates, risk of acute kidney injury with NSAIDs in a dehydrated, injured patient) and limitations in supplies (e.g., not having potent opiates or large quantities) can best be overcome with this strategy. Most individuals and groups should consider carrying at least one NSAID (e.g., ibuprofen), acetaminophen (paracetamol), and an oral opioid (e.g., oxycodone).[41] The combination of acetaminophen with an NSAID is more effective than either medication alone and may achieve analgesia comparable to some opioids. Furthermore, the combination of NSAIDs and acetaminophen can significantly reduce opioid requirement for cases of severe pain. Many drug formulations contain acetaminophen, and thus careful attention is required to avoid toxic doses of this drug (see Analgesics in Table 102-2).

When discussing analgesia in remote environments, one must include mention of ketamine. This medication can be used in oral (PO), IM, or IV forms and is unique among potent analgesic medications in that it has relatively limited respiratory or cardiovascular depression even when used at higher doses.[33] Ketamine's mechanism of action is distinct from the analgesic medications previously listed and is primarily mediated through the N-methyl-D-aspartate (NMDA) receptor. Additionally, it provides a state of hypnosis in addition to analgesia, which can be particularly useful for more painful procedures, such as minor surgeries, suturing, and fracture reductions, or extrications. Despite its favorable safety profile and long history of use in remote medical settings, ketamine should be used only by those with necessary licensure and experience. Increased secretions, hallucinations, and increased intracranial pressure are among many adverse effects that impact its safe use.

Transmucosal, transdermal, and intranasal narcotics can also be used for analgesia in the wilderness setting, although provider familiarity with dosing and availability of alternative therapies has limited popularity of these methods[41] (see Table 102-2).

SPECIAL CONSIDERATIONS

In low- and middle-income countries, donations of leftover, nonexpired medications, even in modest quantities, to a local hospital or clinic are usually greatly appreciated. Meeting with a local pharmacist or clinic before departure can be helpful for arranging a donation and engendering good will. However, donation of expired medications to even the most impoverished regions is generally considered unacceptable.[47]

Related to donation of medications is the issue of providing medical care to local people encountered during an expedition. Often, the medical designee, recognizing a significant illness in a local person, will want to provide care. Such interventions are generally beneficial and without significant cost to an expedition. The medical designee should keep in mind that this care is temporary in almost all cases and may diminish the perceived value of local healers or the existing medical system. In addition, lacking medical translation experience, the group's translator may not be able to communicate instructions effectively to patients, which may lead to dangerous misunderstandings. For example, nitroglycerin sublingual tablets might be given to a nomad with stable angina for "chest pain." The recipient might perceive this as a general pain medication and give it to a child with headache or another adult with aortic stenosis.

The medical designee will be expected to provide care for both native and foreign members of the expedition and must plan accordingly, unless the hosting team is accompanied by a local health care provider. Because these issues will directly affect

the assembly of the medical kit, they should be discussed with the group leader in detail before departure.

A SAMPLE JOURNEY

The month is March, and the goal is a 4-day climb to the summit of Mt Shasta (elevation, 4317 m [14,162 feet]) in the Cascade Mountain range. There are 17 established routes. However, during the winter, these are limited, and the team has decided to climb Avalanche Gulch, a popular route. The team consists of 10 cross-country skiers, some with significant climbing experience and others with very little. The base camp will be at 2134 m (7000 feet).

Two weeks prior to the trip, the trip leader asks all participants to complete a pretrip medical evaluation form (Appendix B). After review of the collected forms, all participants appear to have acceptable levels of baseline fitness, and no major health contraindications are discovered. The trip leader asks two participants with preexisting medical conditions to ensure adequate supply of their prescription medications and asks all participants to review recommendations for packing, including clothes, personal first-aid kit, and other appropriate gear as previously discussed. Additionally, all participants are encouraged to complete pretrip, daily aerobic and strength-training routines to ensure optimal fitness at the time of travel. Several members of the group have completed an American Red Cross advanced first-aid course, and all group members are encouraged to attend an avalanche seminar offered to the public by the National Ski Patrol System.

Before disembarkation, a briefing with all participants is held to discuss plans, contingencies, and potential risks involved. Historical weather patterns, current forecasts, and current terrain conditions are obtained from Internet sources and local park rangers and discussed at the briefing. Were a skier to become disabled en route, one of the others would remain with the victim while another two would ski out to the nearest telephone or source of help (it is no longer than an 8-hour downhill ski from the farthest point along the route in good weather). Helicopter evacuation to the nearest hospital would usually be accomplished within the next 2 to 4 hours, making the maximum interval to medical care 12 hours, weather permitting. Based on a review of historical incidents in the region, weather can delay evacuation up to several days. All team members are made aware of a satellite phone contained in the trip leader's pack. The trip poses increased risks related to trauma, cold injury, avalanche danger, snowblindness, and high-altitude illness. With the possibility of an overnight stay until rescue arrives, medicine selection focuses on pain control for traumatic injury and acute mountain sickness. Appropriate topical medicines include sunscreens and those for managing corneal injury from snowblindness. Systemic medicines of value include a limited supply of high-priority broad-spectrum antibiotics to treat infection of soft tissue injuries, plus specialized medicines for prevention and treatment of acute mountain sickness.

The trip leader must decide how much acetazolamide (Diamox) should be carried. If the acetazolamide supply is intended for both prophylaxis and treatment, if there are 10 members, and if the maximum anticipated time to rescue is 24 hours, a conservative calculation (i.e., assuming all members require treatment and that evacuation can be accomplished within 24 hours) can be estimated as follows:

Prophylaxis: 1 pill (125 mg) twice a day during 4 days of ascent for 10 people = 80 pills

Treatment: 2 pills (250 mg) twice a day for 1 day awaiting rescue for 10 people = 40 pills

Total: Prophylaxis + Treatment = 80 + 40 = 120 pills

Finally, emphasis must be placed on the recreational and environmental hazards likely to be encountered during travel. In this example, the dangers relate mainly to high altitude and cold exposure. Box 102-7 lists specialized equipment that may be of value under the conditions described. Because the peak altitude is only 4317 m (14,162 feet) and the nearby medical center has prompt helicopter evacuation abilities, a Gamow bag would not likely be useful for treating high-altitude illness. However, because of unpredictable weather and visibility, addition of the

Gamow bag to the medical kit could be considered, weight and bulk permitting. In addition, the need to carry technical equipment to provide warmed IV solutions or humidified oxygen is offset by a prompt helicopter rescue. Frostbite can occur rapidly, and each individual may want to carry a personal supply of chemical hand warmers (e.g., Grabber Warmers) because of their low weight and ease of packing. In addition, certain repair equipment should be carried (see Table 102-1). Overall, thoughtful advanced consideration of proximity to care, duration, and probability of various illnesses and injuries will guide decisions about medication selection and quantities when preparing for a wilderness outing.

APPENDIX A

Information Sources on Wilderness Emergencies and Suggested Reading

American River Touring Association, 24000 Casa Loma Road, Groveland, CA 95321; 800-323-2782; http://www.arta.org. This is a nonprofit organization that sponsors basic and leadership courses for river rafting and kayaking.

Emergency Response Institute, 4537 Foxhall Drive NE, Olympia, WA 98516; 360-491-7785; http://www.eri-intl.com. The Institute publishes books and sponsors symposia about search and rescue, emergency preparedness, survival, and outdoor leadership.

National Association for Search and Rescue (NASAR), PO Box 232020, Centreville, VA 20120-2020; 703-222-6277; http://www.nasar.org. This educational association provides conferences, symposia, and training that address search and rescue and emergency response, including communications. It also sponsors *Rescue* magazine, which is published by JEMS Communications, 1947 Camino-Vida Roble, Suite 200, Carlsbad, CA 92008; 619-431-9797.

National Climatic Data Center, 151 Patton Avenue #120, Asheville, NC 28801-5001; 828-271-4800; http://www.ncdc.noaa.gov. The Center provides historic weather summaries for U.S. and many foreign cities; there is a small fee for materials. Telephone first to determine the availability of relevant data.

National Ski Patrol System (NSP), 133 South Van Gordon, Suite 100, Lakewood, CO 80228; 303-988-1111; http://www.nsp.org. This organization sponsors training programs that address winter emergency care, avalanches, and ski mountaineering, some of which are open to the public. It also sells equipment and first-aid supplies through a catalog to its members.

National Weather Service, 1325 East West Highway, Silver Spring, MD 20910; http://www.weather.gov/. The National Weather Service site nearest the travel site can provide forecasts and in many regions provides broadcasts over National Oceanic and Atmospheric Administration Weather Radio on frequencies between 162.40 and 162.55 MHz, including 3- to 5-day forecasts and avalanche warnings.

Outward Bound Training Institute; 800-779-7935; http://www.outwardbound.com. This nonprofit educational organization uses mountain, river, and ocean wilderness settings to provide stimuli for personal development; separate leadership training courses are also available.

The Travel Doctor, 7515 Greenville Avenue, #600 Dallas, TX 75231; http://www.thetraveldoctor.com. An excellent website for travel alerts and for learning about the pitfalls of travel to different international locales. The Travel Doctor also lists prescription medications that are useful for various travel-related illnesses.

Undersea and Hyperbaric Medical Society, 10531 Metropolitan Avenue, Kensington, MD 20895; 301-942-2980; http://www.uhms.org. This is a nonprofit organization that sponsors workshops and meetings about the prevention and treatment of diving injuries and illnesses that are treatable with hyperbaric oxygen. It also publishes a bimonthly newsletter, *Pressure,* and two research publications, *Undersea Biomedical Research* and *Journal of Hyperbaric Medicine.*

Wilderness Education Association, 900 East 7th Street, Bloomington, IN 47405; 812-855-4095; http://www.weainfo.org. The Wilderness Education Association is a nonprofit educational organization that specializes in training and certifying outdoor leaders.

Wilderness Medical Society, 2150 S 1300 E, Suite 500, Salt Lake City, UT 84106; 801-990-2988; http://www.wms.org. This nonprofit organization of medical and related professionals is devoted to prevention and treatment of wilderness injuries and illnesses. The Society publishes the quarterly newsletter *Wilderness Medicine Letter,* which covers wilderness medicine meetings, literature review, field management, and position statements. It also publishes *Wilderness and Environmental Medicine* (formerly *Journal of Wilderness Medicine*), which is the official academic publication of the Society. Teaching simulations and educational lecture series are also available through the website.

Wilderness Medical Society (WMS) Practice Guidelines. Since 1987, the WMS has published Practice Guidelines for Wilderness Emergency Care on a variety of topics; published in *Wilderness and Environmental Medicine* and available online through pubmed.org.

Emergency Medicine Residents' Association (EMRA), Wilderness Medicine Division; http://www.emra.org/committees-divisions/wilderness-division/. Provides a select number of simulation scenarios and other resources.

Pretrip Medical Evaluation Form for Wilderness Travel

PARTICIPANT INFORMATION		
Name:	Email:	
Age:	Sex: ☐ M ☐ F	Weight:
Height:	Phone #:	
Home address:		
TRIP INFORMATION		
Trip Dates:	Location:	
Planned activities (climbing, cycling, etc.):		
EMERGENCY CONTACT		
Name:	Relationship:	
Address:	Phone:	
City/State/Zip:	Email:	
PRIMARY CARE PHYSICIAN CONTACT		
Name:		
Address:	Phone:	
City/State/Zip:	Email:	
MEDICAL HISTORY		
1. Allergies to food or medications (include reactions such as rash, shortness of breath):		
2. Allergies to insects and other:		
3. Current Medications (List prescription and over-the-counter medications; include dosing and scheduling; attach sheet if needed):		

4. Have you ever had any of the conditions listed below? Please check the appropriate boxes.

Diabetes?	☐ Yes	☐ No
Mental illness (anxiety, depression, other)?	☐ Yes	☐ No
Epilepsy, seizures, convulsions?	☐ Yes	☐ No
Neurologic problems (stroke/TIA)?	☐ Yes	☐ No
Heart or lung problems?	☐ Yes	☐ No
Acute mountain sickness?	☐ Yes	☐ No
Kidney or genitourinary problems?	☐ Yes	☐ No
Deep vein thrombosis (blood clot)?	☐ Yes	☐ No
Injuries or joint problems?	☐ Yes	☐ No
Fainting episodes?	☐ Yes	☐ No
Bleeding or clotting disorders?	☐ Yes	☐ No
Visual or hearing impairments?	☐ Yes	☐ No
Asthma or COPD?	☐ Yes	☐ No
Ulcers?	☐ Yes	☐ No
Metal implants?	☐ Yes	☐ No
Gastrointestinal problems?	☐ Yes	☐ No

If you answered "yes" to any of the questions above, please provide details of your condition in the space provided on the next section of this form, Medical History.

5. Medical History (List prior and current medical problems and injuries including surgeries and hospitalizations):

6. Do you have any family history of death or disability in a first-degree relative (parent or sibling) under the age of 50 from a known heart condition or any sudden death in a first-degree relative under the age of 50 for unknown reasons? ☐ Yes ☐ No

7. How often do you drink alcohol? ☐ Never ☐ Few times per month
☐ Few times per week ☐ Daily

8. Do you currently smoke cigarettes, or have you previously smoked regularly? ☐ Yes ☐ No

9. Please list any recreational drugs that you currently or recently have used:

☐ None

10. List any phobias that may affect your ability to participate in trip activities:

11. Are you able to jog 1 mile in less than 12 minutes *and* perform the level of activity planned for the trip without chest pain, feeling faint, or struggling? ☐ Yes ☐ No

12. Are you currently or possibly pregnant? ☐ Yes ☐ No | Last menstrual period: ____/____/____

VACCINATION HISTORY
(Please Attach Copy of Original Vaccination History)

Hepatitis A: ☐ Yes
(Date:(____/____/____) ☐ No
☐ Unsure

Typhoid: ☐ Yes (Date:(____/____/____)
☐ No
☐ Unsure

Hepatitis B: ☐ Yes
(Date:(____/____/____) ☐ No
☐ Unsure

Meningitis: ☐ Yes (Date:(____/____/____)
☐ No
☐ Unsure

Yellow fever: ☐ Yes
(Date:(____/____/____) ☐ No
☐ Unsure

Rabies: ☐ Yes (Date:(____/____/____)
☐ No
☐ Unsure

MMR: ☐ Yes
(Date:(____/____/____) ☐ No
☐ Unsure

Tetanus: ☐ Yes (Date:(____/____/____)
☐ No
☐ Unsure

APPLICANT SIGNATURE

I certify to the best of my knowledge that all information I have provided on this form is accurate and will notify the trip coordinator should any information change prior to my planned excursion. I recognize that it is my personal responsibility to discuss my health and fitness level with my primary care physician and to decide appropriateness and risks as pertains to the planned trip. I have been given the opportunity to ask all questions as pertains to the risks and benefits of the proposed activity.

Signature of participant: | Date:

CERTIFYING PHYSICIAN SIGNATURE *(IF APPLICABLE)*

I certify that I have reviewed the medical information provided to me by the participant listed above and (check one):

☐ I have *not* <u>found</u> any medical conditions that preclude this participant from the proposed trip.

☐ I have found medical conditions that preclude this participant from the proposed trip.

Signature of Certifying Physician *(if applicable):* | Date:

Office Phone:

Many of the products cited in this chapter can be found in outdoor equipment retail stores or pharmacies. The sources listed below are for specialized products that are referred to in the text.

Black Diamond Equipment, Ltd, 2084 East 3900 South, Salt Lake City, UT 84124; 801-278-5552; http://www.bdel.com. Black Diamond Equipment is the manufacturer of the AvaLung, which is the first and only active avalanche safety device that may enable the avalanche victim to breathe while waiting to be excavated.

Besse Medical, 9075 Centre Pointe Drive, Suite 140, West Chester, OH 45069; http://www.besse.com. Besse is a distributor of vaccines, pharmaceuticals, and medical supplies.

CamelBak Products, LLC, 2000 S. McDowell, Suite 200, Petaluma, CA 94954; http://www.camelbak.com: Tactical and medic backpacks are superb and can be customized.

Campmor, PO Box 700, Saddle River, NJ 07458; 888-CAMPMOR (888-226-7667); http://www.campmor.com. Campmor provides the Lady-J urinal guide and other camping equipment.

Chinook Medical Gear, Inc, 3455 Main Avenue, Durango, CO 81301; 800-766-1365; http://www.chinookmed.com. Chinook is one of the most complete catalog retailers for wilderness medical supplies and the carrier of the Gamow bag. It is a good beginning resource for the person who is in need of a wide variety of medical supplies.

ConMed Corporation, 525 French Road, Utica, NY 13502; 315-797-8375; http://www.conmed.com. ConMed is the maker of skin staplers and other surgical instruments.

Garmin International Inc, 1200 East 151st Street, Olathe, KS 66062; 913-397-8200; http://www.garmin.com. Garmin is the maker of a wide variety of easy-to-use global positioning system devices and instructional videos for GPS education.

Gilbert Surgical Instruments, PO Box 458, Bellmawr, NJ 08031; 856-933-2770. Gilbert is the manufacturer of the Abelson emergency cricothyrotomy cannula and other respiratory care instruments.

Grabber Performance Group, 4600 Danvers Drive SE, Grand Rapids, MI 49512; 800-518-0938; http://www.grabberwarmers .com. Grabber is the manufacturer of a variety of packaged miniature heaters with accessories that are useful for preventing cold-related injuries of the hands, feet, and face.

International SOS, Inc, 11601 Wilshire Boulevard, 5th Floor, Suite 525, Los Angeles, CA 90025; 310-828-2081; http://www .internationalsos.com. International SOS specializes in international medical and evacuation insurance.

Junkin Safety Appliance Co, 3121 Millers Lane, Louisville, KY 40216; 888-458-6546; http://www.junkinsafety.com. Junkin manufactures several folding aluminum full-length backboards, splints, and stretchers that weigh as little as 6.8 kg (15 lb). Other safety equipment produced by this company includes fire blankets and cervical spine immobilizers.

King Systems, 15011 Herriman Boulevard, Noblesville, IN, 46060; 800-642-5464; http://www.kingsystems.com.

Marmot Mountain LLC, 2321 Circadian Way, Santa Rosa, CA 95407. Marmot Mountain is a manufacturer of outdoor clothing and equipment.

MARSARS/Great Eastern Marine, Inc, 205 Myrtle Street, Shelton, CT 06484-4015; 203-924-7315 or 866-426-2423; http://www .marsars.com. MARSARS is the manufacturer of water and ice rescue equipment; a hypothermic stabilizer bag and additional accessory heat packs are available.

Mountain Safety Research, 4000 1st Avenue South, Seattle, WA 98134; 800-531-9531; http://www.msrcorp.com. This company is the manufacturer of high-performance and lightweight stoves as well as the WaterWorks filtration system.

National Ski Patrol System, Inc (NSP), 133 South Van Gordon, Suite 100, Lakewood, CO 80228; 303-988-1111; http://www .nsp.org. NSP provides various first-aid supplies and equipment for winter skiing and mountaineering that are sold by catalog to its members.

Oakley, Inc, 1 Icon, Foothill Ranch, CA 92610; 800-431-1439; http://www.oakley.com; customercare@oakley.com. Oakley specializes in outdoor-wear sunglasses for a variety of activities.

Otter Products, Bldg 1, Old-Town Square, Suite 303, Fort Collins, CO 80524; 888-695-8820; http://www.otterbox.com and http:// www.watertightcase.com. Otter manufactures a variety of watertight cases that are useful for everything from personal digital assistants to large medical kits.

Outdoor Research, 1000 1st Avenue South, Seattle, WA 98134; 800-421-2421; http://www.orgear.com. Outdoor Research sells a diverse array of tote bags, medical travel kits, and stuff sacks that are useful for international travel.

OutdoorSafe, PO Box 62039, Colorado Springs, CO 80962-2039, 719-593-5852; info@outdoorsafe.com.

Patagonia, Inc, PO Box 150, Ventura, CA 93002; 805-643-8616; http://www.patagonia.com. Patagonia is the manufacturer of Capilene underclothing as well as a variety of outdoor clothing.

Pelican Products, Inc, 23215 Early Avenue, Torrance, CA 90505; 310-326-4700 within California, 800-473-5422 outside of California; fax, 310-326-3311; http://www.pelican.com; sales@ pelican.com. Pelican is the manufacturer of watertight freight boxes as well as bright and durable headlamps.

Recreational Equipment (REI); 800-426-4840; http://www.rei.com. REI is a provider of Thermax underclothing as well as a variety of sunglasses, outdoor gear, and clothing.

Res-Q Products, Inc, PO Box 661, Quathiaski Cove, BC, Canada VOP 1N0; http://www.hypothermia.org (educational site) or http://www.hypothermia-ca.com. Res-Q Products is the maker of Res-Q-Air and IV Hot-Sack plus its accessories; the company is a provider of sophisticated equipment for the serious expedition traveler to areas of extreme cold.

SAM Splints, 4909 South Coast Highway #245, Newport, OR 97365; 541-867-4726; http://www.sammedical.com/ (accessed 2/8/16). This company is the maker of the SAM Folding Splint (4 oz) and many other splinting and first-aid products that are made for outdoor travel and first aid.

Slishman Traction Splint; http://www.rescue-essentials.com/ slishman-traction-splint-sts/ (accessed 2/8/16). This splint is available from Bound Tree Medical in the United Kingdom; it is not currently available for sale in the United States.

Travel Medicine Inc, 351 Pleasant Street, Suite 312, Northampton, MA 01060; 800-872-8633; http://www.travmed.com. Travel Medicine specializes in educational books and handy supplies for international travel; it is the source of insect repellents, clothing, and nets for mosquito protection.

Zarges Aluminum Boxes, Soanar Inc, Mayer Krieg Components, 9 Civic Square, Croydon, Victoria 3136 Australia; 61 2 9741 0192; http://www.soanar.com. This company manufactures extremely durable, lightweight, watertight aluminum freight boxes that are ideal for the storage of medical and communications equipment.

REFERENCES

Complete references used in this text are available online at expertconsult.inkling.com.

Effective emergency medical care often requires skillful administration of oxygen (O_2). Medical personnel must be familiar with oxygen's therapeutic value, indications, hazards, and techniques for maximizing delivery.

Oxygen is required for cellular metabolism, and thus for life. O_2 is a colorless, odorless, and tasteless gas that makes up 21% of Earth's atmosphere and is obtained commercially by fractional distillation of air.[4,5] Convenient delivery mechanisms allow administration of supplemental O_2 in prehospital settings. Oxygen use and storage pose some risk. Oxygen is not flammable, but rapidly accelerates fuel combustion.

INDICATIONS

Indications to use supplemental O_2 include the following[3,6]:

- Shock
- Tissue hypoxia
- Hypoxemia
- Pulmonary gas exchange impairment caused by trauma, edema, asthma, infection, or embolism
- Acute myocardial infarction (MI), cerebrovascular accident (CVA, stroke)
- Decompression illness (DCI), including both decompression sickness (DCS) and arterial gas embolism (AGE)
- Moderate to severe acute mountain sickness (AMS)
- High-altitude pulmonary edema (HAPE)
- High-altitude cerebral edema (HACE)
- Carbon monoxide (CO) poisoning
- Respiratory or cardiopulmonary arrest
- General anesthesia

Oxygen should be considered for any condition that reduces oxygenation or tissue perfusion. By reversing hypoxia and hypoxemia, O_2 may reduce edema around injury sites. In a diving-related emergency, high concentrations of inspired O_2 create a large pressure gradient between the inhaled gas and excess nitrogen in the body, helping to remove built-up nitrogen and possibly relieve symptoms of DCS.

Oxygen should be administered by providers trained in its use. The U.S. Food and Drug Administration (FDA) "regards oxygen to be a prescription drug. Nevertheless, FDA recognizes that there are many circumstances under which it would be impractical to insist that oxygen be administered only under the supervision of a physician."[20]

The FDA acknowledges the importance of oxygen in medical emergencies, stating, "The label for medical oxygen should bear the statement, 'For emergency use only when administered by properly trained personnel for oxygen deficiency and resuscitation. For all other medical applications, Caution: Federal law prohibits dispensing without prescription.'"[18]

CONTRAINDICATIONS

In an acutely hypoxic patient, there is no absolute contraindication to administration of supplemental O_2. In patients with severe chronic obstructive disease (COPD), prolonged administration of O_2 may cause hypercapnia, so close monitoring of ventilation is important.[15]

PULMONARY OXYGEN TOXICITY

If a high concentration of supplemental O_2 is administered for many hours, pulmonary O_2 toxicity is possible, particularly if a

diver with DCI subsequently requires hyperbaric oxygen therapy (HBOT). First symptoms of pulmonary O_2 toxicity are caused by tracheobronchitis, which is characterized by substernal burning, chest tightness, and cough. Continued exposure may result in dyspnea and adult respiratory distress syndrome (ARDS). Pulmonary O_2 toxicity is usually reversible with cessation of O_2 therapy or reduction in inspired concentration.[12]

Inspired O_2 partial pressure and the individual's susceptibility are key factors influencing rapidity of O_2 toxicity development. In some individuals, continuously breathing 100% O_2 at normal atmospheric pressure (1 atmosphere [atm]) may cause symptoms to appear as soon 6 hours; however, most people can safely breathe O_2 at a fractional inspired concentration (FIO_2) of 1.0 for 12 hours. Rate of onset of symptoms can be reduced by using periodic "air breaks," during which the patient breathes air for 5 to 10 minutes.

CENTRAL NERVOUS SYSTEM OXYGEN TOXICITY

Central nervous system (CNS) O_2 toxicity can only occur when a person is exposed to O_2 at ambient pressures greater than 1 atm (e.g., while diving underwater or during HBOT in a hyperbaric chamber). In hyperbaric settings, the term *absolute pressure* (ATA) can be useful. ATA is the total ambient pressure (standard atmospheric plus any additional pressure) on the system being calculated or measured. Inspired partial pressure of O_2 (PIO_2) is calculated by multiplying FIO_2 by ambient pressure in ATA ($PIO_2 = FIO_2 \times ATA$). Signs and symptoms of CNS O_2 toxicity are most likely to appear at PIO_2 greater than 1.6 and may include sweating, bradycardia, mood changes, nausea, visual field constriction, twitching, syncope, and seizures. During HBOT, implementation of periodic 5-minute air breaks reduces the likelihood of CNS O_2 toxicity. Oxygen seizures occur at 1.3 per 10,000 treatments for HBOT at 2.4 ATA (0.7 per 10,000 when hypoglycemic seizures are excluded).[7] With air breaks and a resting patient, treatment with 100% O_2 at almost 3 ATA is possible. If the individual were performing physically exerting exercise (e.g., swimming), such high concentrations would not be safe because it would raise the incidence of oxygen seizures to an unacceptable level.

EQUIPMENT

CYLINDERS

Medical O_2 cylinders are made of aluminum or steel and come in a variety of sizes (Table 103-1 and Figure 103-1). The working pressure of steel medical O_2 cylinders is 2015 pounds per square inch (psi). The working pressure of aluminum O_2 cylinders is either 2015 psi or 2216 psi, depending on the size, construction, and design.

Oxygen cylinders in the United States are usually painted green or have distinctive green shoulders (i.e., the top of the cylinder nearest the pillar valve). European Union (EU) standard requires all oxygen cylinders to have white shoulders. The cylinder's body can be green or black.

Cylinders come in two practical field sizes: D (50 cm [20 inches] in length; carries 360 L of oxygen) and E (75 cm [30 inches] in length; carries 625 L of oxygen). Time during which oxygen can be delivered is calculated by dividing tank capacity by flow rate.

In the United States, any pressure vessel transported on public roads is subject to U.S. Department of Transportation (DOT)

TABLE 103-1 Common Portable Medical Oxygen Cylinder Specifications

Cylinder Size	Alloy	Working Pressure (psi)	Volume (L, ft³)	Length (cm, in)	Diameter (cm, in)	Weight (kg, lb)
M9	Aluminum	2015	8.7, 246.3	27.7, 10.9	11.1, 4.4	1.8, 3.9
D	Aluminum	2015	15, 424.7	41.9, 16.5	11.1, 4.4	2.5, 5.5
D*	Steel	2015	14.5, 410.4	42.5, 16.75	11.1, 4.4	3.4, 7.5
Jumbo D	Aluminum	2216	22.9, 648.3	43.2, 17	13.3, 5.3	4.1, 9.0
E	Aluminum	2015	24, 679.4	65.0, 25.6	11.1, 4.4	3.6, 8.0
E*	Steel	2015	24.1, 682.0	65.4, 25.75	11.1, 4.4	4.8, 10.5

Note: Aluminum cylinder specifications provided by Luxfer Inc.
*Steel cylinder specifications provided by Pressed Steel Tank Co.

regulations. The DOT requires that cylinders undergo visual and hydrostatic testing every 5 years. Cylinders that do not pass are destroyed, and those that pass are appropriately stamped and labeled.[17] Gas suppliers will not fill cylinders that have not been appropriately tested and stamped.

VALVES

Valves for medical O_2 cylinders sold in the United States are designed to accept only medical O_2 regulators to avoid the possibility of using a medical O_2 regulator with an incompatible gas (e.g., acetylene). Two types of valves are available in the United States: CGA-870 and CGA-540. CGA-870 is also known as the "pin-index" valve and used on smaller, portable cylinders (e.g., D, E). CGA-540 is used primarily on larger, nonportable cylinders (e.g., H, M), such as those mounted in ambulances.

Outside the United States, a number of other medical O_2 valve types are manufactured and used. Adapters are available to make a U.S. pin-index regulator fit on an Australian bull-nose valve. Using adapters is discouraged by the U.S. Compressed Gas Association (CGA).

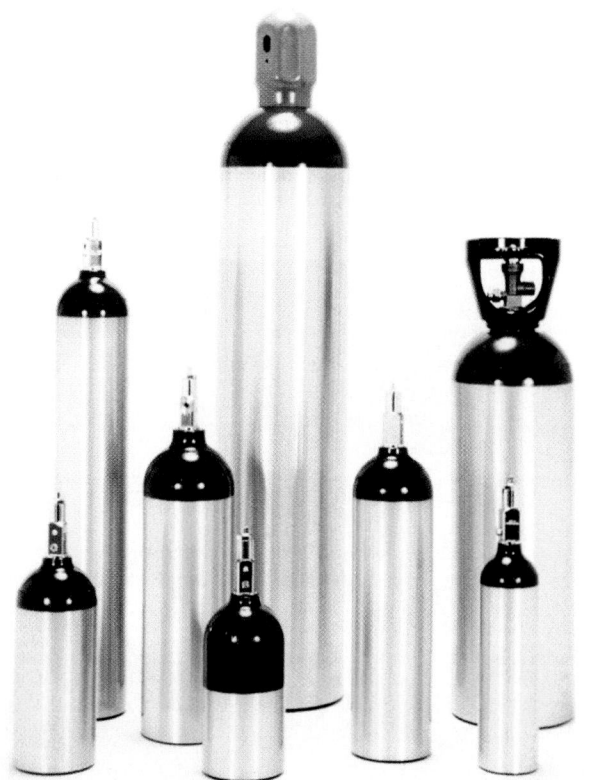

FIGURE 103-1 Oxygen cylinders come in a variety of sizes and capacities. Cylinder decisions should be based on the amount of time a person will likely need to provide care until the injured person can be brought to emergency care. *(Courtesy Divers Alert Network.)*

Some O_2 cylinders come with built-in O_2 regulators. These cylinders offer simplicity but may limit flow options.

REGULATORS

A regulator functions to reduce peak pressures within the tank to a usable O_2 flow rate. It is typically mounted directly to the cylinder with a compatible valve. A regulator consists of a pressure gauge, pressure-reducing valve, and flowmeter. It reduces the high pressure of the oxygen inside the tank (>2000 psi) to approximately 50 psi and allows delivery at flow rates between 1 and 15 liters per minute (L/min). Regulators are primarily of three types: constant flow only, demand/flow-restricted oxygen-powered ventilator (FROPV) only, or multifunction, which has both constant flow and demand/FROPV capability (Figure 103-2A).

A pressure gauge allows the user to monitor the amount of O_2 in the cylinder. In a tank with a maximum operating pressure of 2000 psi, a reading of 500 psi indicates that there remains one-quarter of the tank's O_2.

Other features may include a *diameter index safety system* (DISS) fitting for an FROPV (to prevent accidental connection of an inappropriate delivery device), constant flow controller device (either knob or gauge), or both, as with the multifunction regulator (Figure 103-2B).

DEVICES FOR ASSISTED VENTILATION

If a patient is not adequately oxygenating or ventilating, assisted ventilation devices can be used. When used on a nonintubated patient, these devices all depend on adequate mask seal to ensure optimal O_2 delivery and ventilatory support. Use of a device minimizes direct patient contact and reduces risk for disease transmission. Personal protective equipment (e.g., gloves, goggles) and standard precaution practices should always be employed.

Bag-Valve-Mask Device

A bag-valve-mask (BVM) device consists of a mask, bag, and valves that direct flow of air and O_2. As with the FROPV, different mask sizes can be used to accommodate different faces or be attached directly to an endotracheal tube (ETT). The volume of the bag is 1600 mL in most commercially available models (Figure 103-3).

Adult BVM devices should have the following features: (1) non-jam inlet valve system that allows a maximum O_2 inlet flow of 30 L/min; (2) either no pressure-relief valve or, if present, a pressure-relief valve capable of being closed; (3) standard 15-mm/22-mm fittings; (4) an O_2 reservoir to allow delivery of high O_2 concentrations; (5) nonrebreathing outlet valve that cannot be obstructed by foreign material; and (6) ability to function satisfactorily under common environmental conditions and temperature extremes.[14]

The BVM works best with supplemental O_2 but will function on room air if O_2 supply is depleted. In intubated patients, experienced health care providers may be able to "feel" decreased lung compliance.

The BVM requires training and practice to use effectively. Even with proper training, it is difficult to maintain adequate

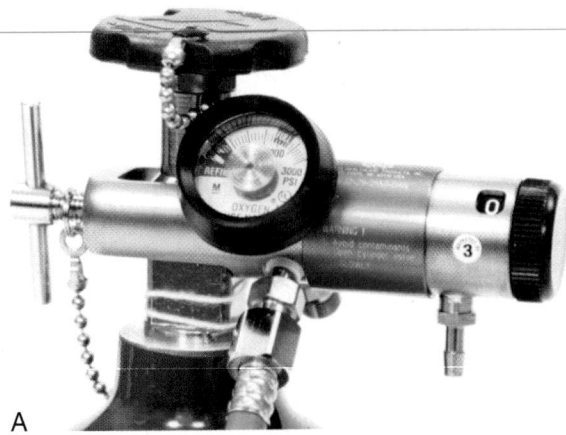

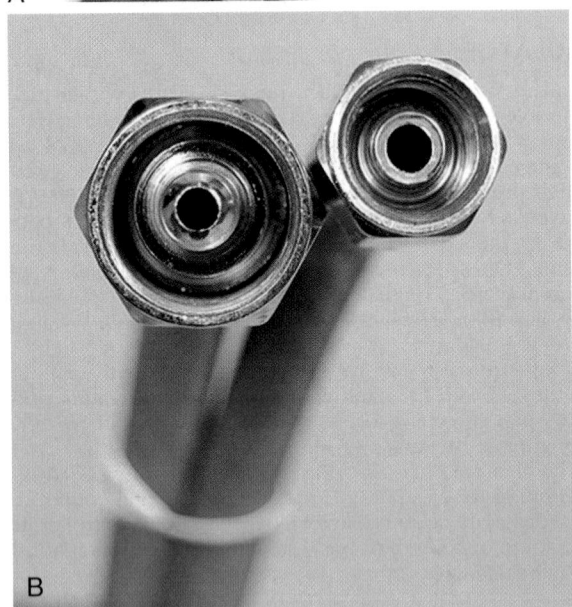

FIGURE 103-2 A, Multifunction regulators allow one to provide oxygen using a constant flow device, by demand-type device, or both at the same time. **B,** Diameter index safety system (DISS) prevents accidental connection of an inappropriate delivery device. (**A** *courtesy Divers Alert Network; **B** from Darby M, Walsh M:* Dental hygiene, *3rd ed, St Louis, 2010, Saunders. Courtesy Dr. Mark Dellinges and Cory Price.*)

a. The second rescuer should ventilate the patient by squeezing the bag with both hands. Gentle, steady force on the bag should result in chest rise.

b. If excessive force on the bag is required, or chest does not rise, have the first rescuer reassess airway patency. Reposition mask and airway. Attempt to ventilate again.

c. If ventilation still remains inadequate, check for airway obstruction; consider using an airway adjunct (e.g., nasal trumpet, oral airway) and initiating an airway obstruction protocol.

5. Ventilations should last 1 second as part of cardiopulmonary resuscitation (CPR).
6. Alternate 30 chest compressions with two ventilations.
7. Ventilate with sufficient speed and force to make the patient's lower chest and upper abdomen rise.
8. It is not necessary to empty the bag with each ventilation.
9. When providing care for an intubated patient, it is not necessary to pause and alternate ventilations with compressions. One rescuer should deliver compressions at a rate of 100 per minute, and the other rescuer (or rescuers) should deliver 8 to 10 breaths a minute (one breath about every 6 to 8 seconds).

Resuscitation Mask

A pocket-type resuscitation mask is a clear, flexible plastic mask designed to fit over the patient's mouth and nose while the health care provider ventilates by exhaling forcefully through the "chimney" (Figure 103-4). Typically, a one-way valve directs the rescuer's breath into the patient while directing the patient's exhaled breath away from the rescuer. This simple device requires minimal training and is lightweight, easily packed, and available both with and without an outlet for supplemental O_2. Presence of an O_2 inlet is preferred.[14] For the purpose of delivering adequate tidal volumes, trials have found mouth-to-mask ventilation superior to BVM devices.[17]

An adequate seal is best achieved with a mouth-to-mask device when the rescuer is positioned at the top of the patient's head. Rescuers seal lips around the coupling adapter of the mask and ventilate using both hands to hold the mask securely in position and maintain airway patency with head tilt.[19] This technique is the preferred position when two rescuers are present. When only one rescuer is present, the rescuer must be positioned at the patient's side.

When using the pocket-style resuscitation mask to deliver O_2:
1. Remove the O_2 tubing from a nonrebreather mask.
2. Stretch out the hose to be certain there are no kinks.

mask seal, maintain airway patency, and ventilate sufficient volumes (600 to 1000 mL) when only one rescuer is available. DOT National Standard Curricula (NSC) for first responders, emergency medical technicians (EMTs), and paramedics recommend the BVM be used first with two rescuers (one maintaining mask seal and patency of the airway, the other squeezing the bag). NSC recommends that use of a BVM with one rescuer should be the last choice (after all other devices and techniques) in ventilating a patient.[17]

A BVM has no overpressurization relief valve. Although rarely a concern in nonintubated patients (because of difficulty establishing a tight seal), this can be a problem in intubated patients.

To use a BVM:
1. Attach the O_2 tubing from the BVM to the constant flow barbed outlet on the O_2 regulator. Expand the bag (which is often stored collapsed).
2. Set the constant flow controller to 10 to 15 L/min.
3. Establish airway patency by direct visualization. Suction or manually clear as able.
4. Position one rescuer at the patient's head to maintain the airway and ensure mask seal.

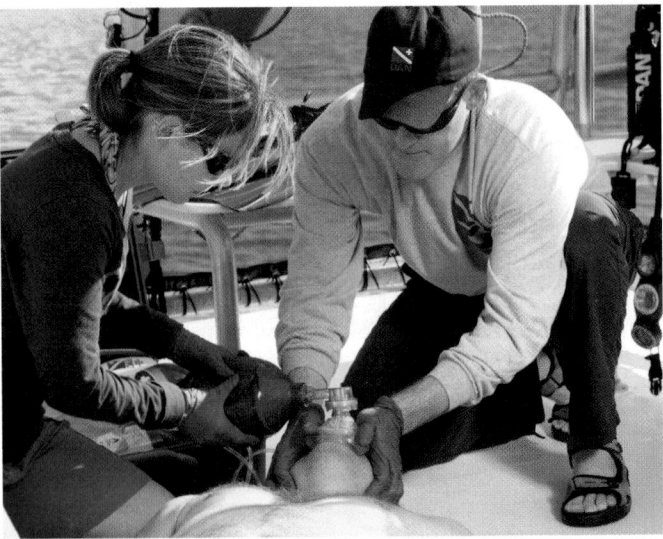

FIGURE 103-3 Bag-valve-mask (BVM) devices are often used to resuscitate an injured person using 100% O_2. BVM devices are relatively inexpensive and very effective, although they can be tiring for the user and require specific training. (*Courtesy Divers Alert Network.*)

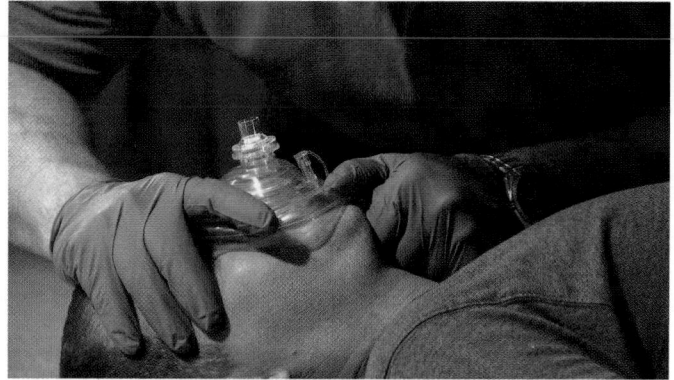

FIGURE 103-4 Resuscitation mask allows rescuers to resuscitate an injured person either with their exhaled breath or with supplemental oxygen. (*Courtesy Divers Alert Network.*)

3. Attach the O₂ tubing to the constant flow barbed outlet on the O₂ regulator.
4. Connect the other end of the tubing to the O₂ inlet on the resuscitation mask.
5. Set the constant flow controller to 10 to 15 L/min.
6. The rescuer should ensure a proper mask seal by positioning the mask over the patient's mouth and nose, lifting the jaw up into the mask.
7. The rescuer should inhale away from the mask and then breathe into the one-way valve on the mask to make the patient's lower chest and upper abdomen rise.
8. Ventilations should last 1 second as part of CPR.
9. Alternate 30 chest compressions with two ventilations.
   a. If the ventilations do not go in, reposition the patient's airway.
   b. If the ventilations still do not go in, check for airway obstruction, and initiate an airway obstruction protocol.

FROPV/Positive-Pressure Demand Valve

Older-style positive-pressure demand valves (PPDVs), such as the LSP 063-05 or Elder CPR Demand valve, function both in positive-pressure mode (pushing the button to ventilate a non-breathing patient) and demand mode.

It is a misconception that a PPDV will easily cause pulmonary overpressurization injury; this valve has fallen out of favor with some health care providers. In positive-pressure mode, all PPDVs manufactured in the United States have an overpressure relief valve that stops the flow of gas at 55 to 65 cm H₂O (a pressure at which lung overpressurization is unlikely). MTV-100 FROPV (LSP/Allied) has two overpressure-relief valves, the first set at 60 cm H₂O and the second at 65 to 80 cm H₂O.*

Earlier PPDVs were designed to meet the American Heart Association (AHA) Emergency Cardiac Care Committee (ECC) CPR guidelines before 1986, which called for "four quick initial breaths and then two quick breaths after every 15 compressions."[9] This faster rate of ventilation was equivalent to 160 L/min.

In 1986, CPR standards were changed to "two slow breaths, each 1.5 seconds in duration."[9] The standard changed again in 1992 to "two slow, full breaths, with a duration of 1.5 to 2 seconds each" (equivalent to 40 L/min).[9]

In 1993, the FROPV was introduced. Its specifications include a flow rate of 40 L/min while being used in positive-pressure mode and 115 L/min in demand mode, eliminating difficulties associated with earlier models (Figure 103-5).

A mask adapter is a standard 15-mm fitting that fits a variety of masks and can also be used directly with an ETT. A FROPV requires a supply of pressurized O₂. In intubated patients, the

health care provider will not be able to "feel" decreased lung compliance.

When using an FROPV:
1. Connect the FROPV to the DISS threaded port on the O₂ regulator.
2. It is not necessary to adjust the O₂ flow rate on the regulator.
3. Position one rescuer at the patient's head to maintain the airway and ensure a mask seal.
4. The second rescuer should ventilate the patient by depressing the button on the FROPV.
5. The second rescuer should also place a second hand on the patient's upper abdomen and lower chest to monitor chest rise.
6. Ventilations should last 1 second as part of CPR.
7. Alternate 30 chest compressions with two ventilations.
   a. If the ventilations do not go in, have the first rescuer reposition the patient's airway.
   b. If the ventilations still do not go in, check for airway obstruction, and initiate an airway obstruction protocol.

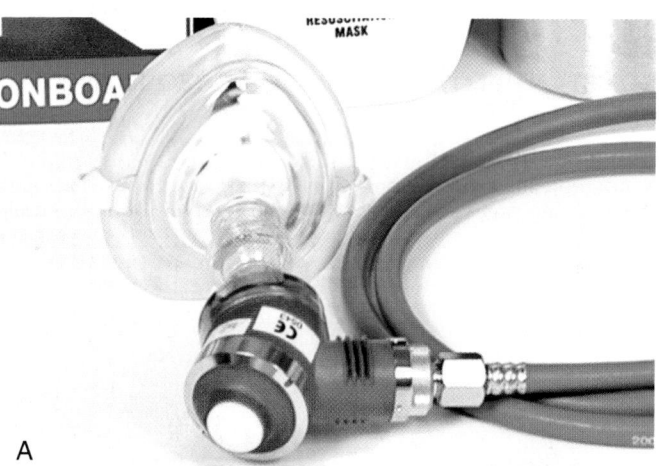

A

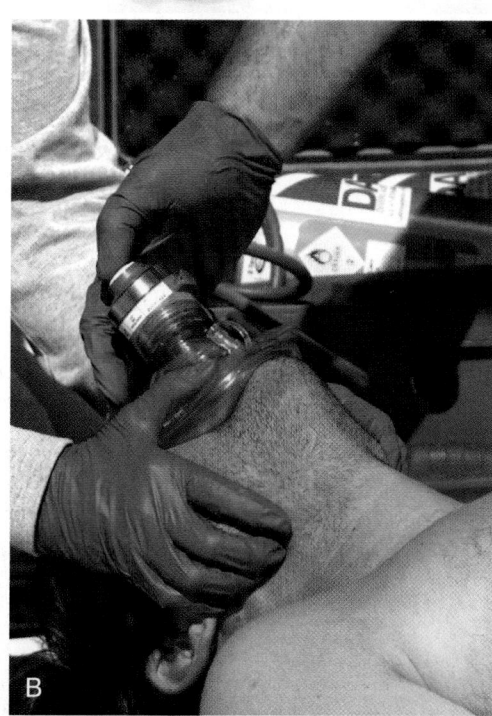

B

FIGURE 103-5 A, Flow-restricted oxygen-powered ventilator (FROPV) allows the rescuer to resuscitate an injured person using 100% O₂. FROPV devices have pressure restrictions to reduce the likelihood of harm to the patient. The ventilators are more expensive and require additional training, although they are less tiring for rescuers than a BVM device (**B**). (*Courtesy Divers Alert Network.*)

---

*Specifications from Allied Healthcare, Inc./Life Support Products.

Demand-Only, or FROPVs in Demand Mode

Use of demand mode requires spontaneous respirations. To use in demand mode, hold the mask to the patient's face. Negative pressure of inhalation opens the valve and then gas flows (Figure 103-6). Flow stops when the person stops inhaling, similar to other demand systems, such as scuba and aviation regulators. This is the first choice for O_2 delivery when there is critical need for a high concentration of inspired O_2 or gas supplies are limited.

When using a demand-only valve:

1. Connect the demand valve to the DISS threaded port on the O_2 regulator.
2. It is not necessary to adjust the O_2 flow rate on the regulator.
3. Ask the patient to breathe normally from the mask.
4. Monitor the patient to ensure breathing.
5. Watch the clear mask to make sure it fogs with each exhalation.
6. If the patient is not conscious or is breathing adequately to activate the demand-only valve, it is necessary to switch to a constant flow delivery device, such as the nonrebreather mask.

CONSTANT FLOW DEVICES FOR ADEQUATELY BREATHING PATIENTS

Nonrebreather Mask

A nonrebreather mask consists of a mask, reservoir bag, and series of one-way valves, one separating reservoir from the mask

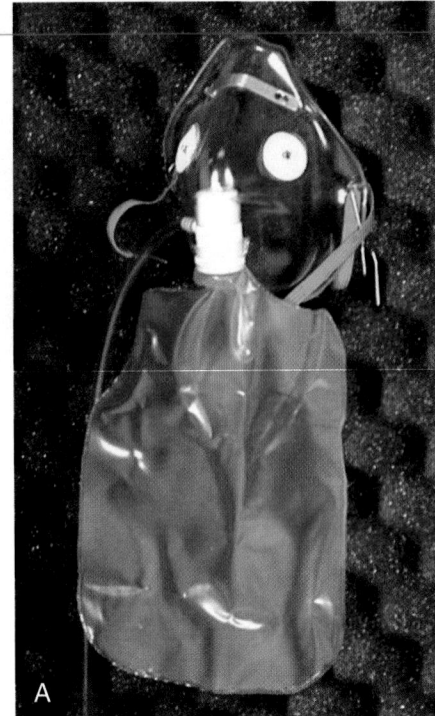

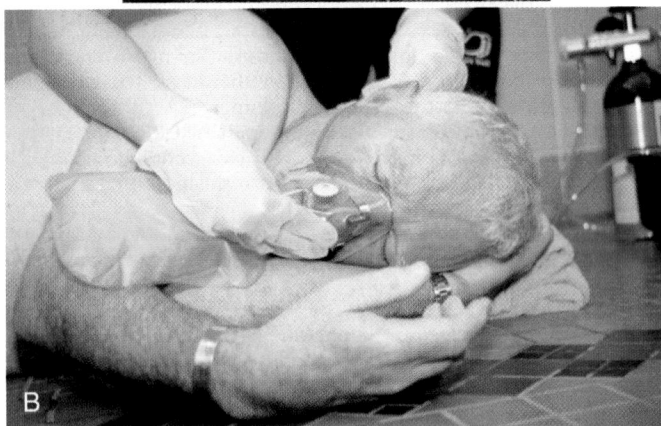

FIGURE 103-7 A nonrebreather mask (A) is the simplest O_2 delivery device. It can deliver high O_2 concentrations; however, rescuers must be careful to ensure a good mask seal, or the concentration of inspired O_2 will drop (B). It also wastes gas because O_2 flows even when the injured person is exhaling or not breathing. (Courtesy Divers Alert Network.)

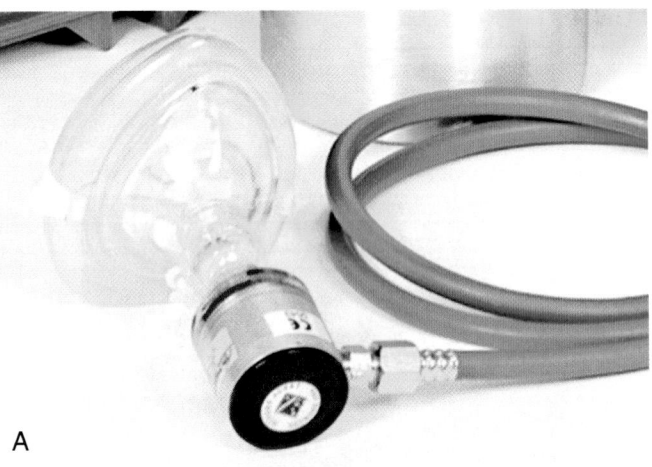

A

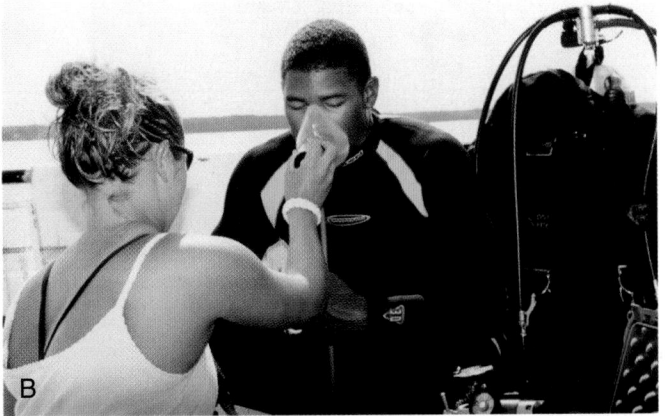

B

FIGURE 103-6 A, Demand valves deliver 100% O_2 to an injured person when he or she inhales, much like a scuba diving regulator. B, This device can be used only by conscious, breathing persons. It has the advantage of delivering high concentrations of gas and limiting waste compared with a constant flow device. (Courtesy Divers Alert Network.)

and others on the sides of the mask. O_2 constantly flows into the reservoir bag, then is inhaled. One-way valves on the sides of the mask keep ambient air from coming into the mask and diluting the O_2. Expired air goes out of the mask through valves and is prevented from entering the reservoir (Figure 103-7).

Efficiency of this system depends on mask fit, face seal, and proper functioning of valves. Under ideal conditions, this mask (when fitted with all three valves) may deliver an FIO_2 of up to 0.95. Field studies show it may deliver FIO_2 as low as 0.60, but it is still the most effective constant flow device available (except for demand regulators and O_2 rebreathers).

To use the mask, it is attached to the O_2 supply at a flow rate of 10 to 15 L/min. The reservoir bag must be inflated or "primed" before placing it on the patient; some new models are designed to be self-priming and will fill automatically when connected to the O_2 flow. Priming is done by placing a finger on the valve between the reservoir and mask while the reservoir inflates.

Masks are available with either one or two one-way valves. If the mask has only one valve (labeled as "with safety outlet"), it is a *partial rebreather* and will deliver reduced FIO_2.

Nonrebreather masks provide the highest FIO_2 of constant flow devices, but tend to waste O_2 and may not deliver a high FIO_2 under less-than-ideal conditions. Patients wearing a nonrebreather mask must never be left alone and should be carefully monitored. O_2 supply must be maintained. If not, suffocation can result.

When using a nonrebreather mask:

1. Open the nonrebreather mask packaging; stretch out the tubing to make sure there are no kinks.
2. Connect the tubing on the nonrebreather mask to the constant flow, barbed outlet on the O_2 regulator.
3. Set the constant flow controller to 10 to 15 L/min.
4. Place a thumb over the one-way valve between the mask and the reservoir bag.
5. Allow the bag to fill completely before placing the mask on the patient.
6. Position the mask over the patient's mouth and nose.
7. Pinch the nose clip over the patient's nose.
8. Pull on the elastic straps to tighten the mask to the patient's face, and pull the skin into the mask.
9. Ask the patient to breathe normally from the mask.
10. Monitor the patient to ensure breathing.
11. Watch the clear mask to make sure it fogs with each exhalation.

Nasal Cannula

A nasal cannula may be used when a patient will not tolerate a mask or when high inspired O_2 concentrations are not required.[17] A nasal cannula delivers FIO_2 of only 0.24 to 0.29.[16]

Flow rates for a nasal cannula are limited to 1 to 6 L/min. Flow rates exceeding 6 L/min are uncomfortable and may result in drying of the nasal mucosa. To use the nasal cannula, place prongs in the patient's nares and loop the tubing over the top of the ears to hold it in place. Adjust the tightness at the neck to a comfortable level.

Other constant flow masks, including partial rebreather, simple face, and Venturi masks, deliver only low levels of FIO_2 and are not recommended for prehospital use.[17] Automatic transport ventilators are not practical for remote emergency medicine.

When using a nasal cannula:

1. Open the cannula packaging; stretch out the tubing to make sure there are no kinks.
2. Connect the tubing to the constant flow, barbed outlet on the O_2 regulator.
3. Set the constant flow controller to 4 to 6 L/min.
4. Position the prongs in the patient's nostrils.
5. Position the hose behind the patient's head and tighten the straps.
6. Ask the patient to breathe normally through the nose.
7. Monitor the patient.
8. If oxygen supplies are limited, titrate O_2 flow to improved symptoms. At high altitude, maintain O_2 saturation above 90% to 92%.

OXYGEN REBREATHERS

Insufficient oxygen supplies are a common problem. All the O_2 delivery devices discussed make inefficient use of limited O_2 supplies and will require multiple portable cylinders if the transport time exceeds 1 hour (Figure 103-8). Breathing room air, a person inhales 21% O_2 and exhales 16% O_2. Under perfect conditions, using supplemental O_2, a patient would inhale 100% O_2 and exhale 95% O_2 and 5% carbon dioxide (CO_2). Rebreather devices are designed to reuse that exhaled O_2-rich air, and remove CO_2 and exchange it for additional oxygen.

Rebreather devices all have the same basic components: mask, breathing circuit (similar to anesthesia equipment), and canister with an absorbent chemical, usually soda lime.

Soda lime chemically removes CO_2 from the exhaled gas, allowing O_2 to be rebreathed.* Supplemental O_2 is added at

---

*$2NaOH + CO_2 = Na_2CO_3 + H_2O + Heat$ (from WR Grace, Inc.)

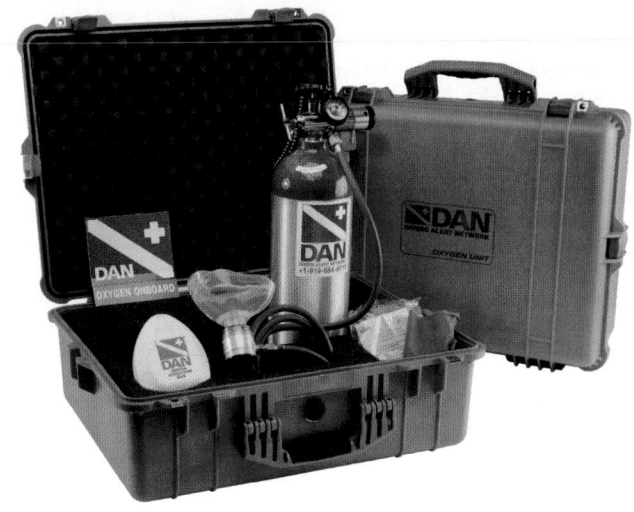

FIGURE 103-8 A typical oxygen kit created for the marine/aquatic environment includes a multifunction regulator to care for more than one injured person, along with delivery masks and a watertight case to protect the equipment. *(Courtesy Divers Alert Network.)*

approximately 1 L/min to replace metabolized O_2. Using this system, an O_2 tank that would supply a nonrebreather mask for 45 minutes, or an on demand device for approximately 1 hour, can provide a patient an FIO_2 of 0.85 to 0.99 for more than 8 hours. If oxygen supplies are limited, this device may prove invaluable.

Manufacturers recommend first oxygenating the patient before setting up the unit, then flushing the system of air, and applying the unit to the patient. Air breaks may minimize the risk for pulmonary oxygen toxicity.

Chemical reaction between CO_2 and soda lime produces heat and water, providing warmed and humidified O_2. In cold climates, this is an advantage. In hot climates, consider passing the breathing circuit hoses through cold or ice water to cool the gas.

Rebreather devices require significant training and contain parts (typically the breathing circuit and absorbent canister) that are often single-patient use. Adequate mask seal is required to function effectively; otherwise, dilution of inhaled gas with air results in a lower FIO_2. Compared with a constant flow mask, increased breathing resistance may be experienced.

Common resuscitators are systems by Wenoll, Circulox, and OXI-Saver Resuscitator.[13]

EMERGENCY OXYGEN ADMINISTRATION AT HIGH ALTITUDE

Atmospheric pressure and partial pressure of oxygen (PO_2) decrease with altitude (see Chapter 1, Table 1-2). Oxygen can be used to treat high-altitude pulmonary or cerebral edema. Definitive treatment is descent to a lower altitude. Supplemental O_2 is indicated if it will not delay descent, or if immediate descent is not possible. Increased partial pressure of available O_2 is achieved by increasing the O_2 concentration or increasing the barometric pressure.

Many climbers use O_2 when climbing above 8000 m (26,247 feet). O_2 sets for climbing, typically continuous flow open circuits with rebreather reservoirs, are suitable for emergency O_2 delivery. Pulse demand and rebreathing circuits have achieved only limited popularity because of concerns about reliability in extreme environments. A mask producing expiratory resistance or continuous positive airway pressure (CPAP) could hypothetically improve gas exchange in climbers with severe high-altitude pulmonary edema.[1]

Portable hyperbaric chambers that increase barometric pressure and therefore available O_2 are used to treat various high-altitude syndromes.[11] A patient is placed within the bag, which is inflated and pressurized, simulating a descent of 500 to 2000 m (1640 to 6562 feet). Continuous air is introduced by a high-volume foot pump and exhausted through pressure-relief valves[21] (see Chapter 2 for further details).

General anesthesia is occasionally needed for emergencies at very high altitudes. Although a trained anesthetist can safely administer general anesthesia to an acclimatized patient,[10] it is generally prudent to descend to lower areas.

OXYGEN GENERATOR SYSTEMS

Oxygen generators produced O_2 using a chemical process. O_2 concentrators typically use electrical power and are not readily portable for field use. These devices often produce 3 to 4 L/min over a 15-minute cycle, with a peak flow of up to 6 L. Although insufficient for some emergency needs, these rates can be employed to fill an O_2 cylinder to operational pressure. In established remote clinics with electrical supply, O_2 generators provide abundant O_2 stores without need for distant and costly resupply.

HOW TO ADMINISTER OXYGEN FROM A TANK (CYLINDER)

1. Place the cylinder upright. Open and close the tank valve slowly ("crack the tank") with a wrench to remove debris from the outlet.
2. Close the tank valve and attach a regulator to the tank. Tighten the regulator to the tank securely by hand. Never use a regulator without the proper oxygen washer. *Never use tape to hold a loose regulator in place.*
   a. Ideally, the depressurized regulator should remain attached to the tank at all times. This ensures that the equipment is ready to use and free of debris.
3. Open tank valve slowly, one full turn.
4. Attach an O_2 delivery device to the regulator, either to the DISS threaded port or to the constant flow nipple on the end of the regulator. Attach a breathing mask or nasal cannula to the other end of hose or tubing, if it is not already attached.
5. Adjust the constant flow controller to the desired flow rate in liters per minute when using a constant flow mask.
   a. When using a demand-style mask connected to the DISS threaded port, it is not necessary to adjust the flow rate.
   b. A regulator marking of "low" indicates 2 to 4 L/min, "medium" is 4 to 8 L/min, and "high" is 10 to 15 L/min. Flow rate for a nonrebreather mask should be no less than 6 L/min; flow rate for a nasal cannula should be no more than 6 L/min.
   c. To ensure proper oxygenation, the recipient should receive high-flow O_2 (10 to 15 L/min) whenever feasible.
6. Position the mask or cannula on the patient's face. Adjust for comfort. Observe the patient to be certain that the device is tolerated, and that the reservoir bag fills properly.

For more detailed information on airway management, see Chapter 19.

Precautions

- Never allow an open flame near an O_2 delivery system.
- Do not expose an O_2 tank to excessive heat (52° C [125° F]) or freezing cold. This prohibition may be difficult to apply when O_2 tanks are carried on mountain-climbing expeditions.
- Never direct the top of a tank valve toward anyone; a loose regulator can be blown off the top of the cylinder with tremendous force.
- Do not drop or roll a cylinder.
- Close all valves when the cylinder is not in use.

SPECIAL CONSIDERATIONS IN NONBREATHING OR INADEQUATELY BREATHING PATIENTS

Caregivers ventilating nonbreathing patients need to consider ventilatory rate, volume, flow rate or speed, pressure, and

oxygenation. Ventilations should be provided at 12 per minute for an adult (>8 years old) and 20 per minute for children and infants.[9] Health care providers may administer rescue breaths with or without supplemental O_2. If a lay provider finds a patient not breathing, full CPR should be initiated.

Volume for adult ventilations is 700 to 1000 mL. If a ventilation device do not have an overpressure-relief valve or greater volumes are administered, pulmonary barotrauma (overpressurization injury) could result. Ventilatory volumes less than 800 mL may be insufficient to inflate the alveoli, and thus gas exchange may be inadequate. Each ventilation should last 1 second (equivalent to 40 L/min). Faster ventilation rates force open the esophagus and push air into the stomach. Gastric insufflation greatly increases the risk for regurgitation and aspiration of gastric contents.[9]

A differential pressure as low as 90 to 110 cm H_2O has been demonstrated sufficient to rupture alveolar septa and to allow gas to escape into interstitial spaces.[2,3] Care must be taken not to exceed these pressures when ventilating a patient. Humans can easily generate pressures exceeding 120 cm H_2O by exhaling forcefully, and thus, according to ECC CPR guidelines, one should "blow until the chest rises" to accommodate various sizes of patients. Of devices for ventilating adult patients, only PPDV/FROPV devices have an overpressure-relief valve.

The goal of assisted ventilation is to provide O_2 to patients. With direct mouth-to-mouth or mouth-to-mask breathing, FIO_2 will be 0.16, or 16% O_2. Adding O_2 at a flow rate of 15 L/min may increase FIO_2 with a pocket mask to up to 50%. A BVM on room air is 0.21, and with O_2 at 15 L/min, up to 0.9, depending on equipment and skill of the ventilator. An FROPV delivers close to 1.0, or 100% O_2.[3,9]

Both volume and O_2 delivered by ventilation depends on airway patency and quality of mask seal. In a nonintubated patient, poor mask seal is the single most common cause of inadequate ventilation. With each ventilation, take great care to ensure airway patency and good mask seal. Use of an oropharyngeal, nasopharyngeal, or combination airway can greatly improve upper airway patency.

Current AHA guidelines recommend that if supplemental O_2 (minimum flow rate of 8 to 12 L/min with O_2 concentration of 40%) is available, rescuers skilled in BVM ventilation should attempt to deliver a tidal volume (V_T) of 6 to 7 mL/kg, or approximately 400 to 600 mL over 1 second. Because actual V_T delivered is impossible to determine, V_T can be titrated to provide sufficient ventilation to maintain O_2 saturation and produce visible chest expansion. V_T should be sufficient to cause the chest to rise. This smaller V_T may be associated with development of hypercarbia. If oxygen is *not* available, rescuers should attempt to deliver the same V_T recommended for mouth-to-mouth ventilation (10 mL/kg, 700 to 1000 mL). This V_T should result in obvious chest rise.[14]

An FROPV delivers the greatest FIO_2, making it the only device that is limited to 40 L/min flow rate (1 second in duration). Because it has an overpressure-relief valve, it may be the best choice for ventilating a person in respiratory arrest, whether or not the person is intubated. A BVM unit used by two rescuers (one to maintain the mask seal, the other to squeeze the bag) is the best alternative and preferred choice for ventilating a person in respiratory arrest.[8,17] Preferences for ventilating a person in respiratory arrest are as follows:

1. BVM unit with two rescuers and supplemental O_2
2. Resuscitation mask with supplemental O_2
3. FROPV
4. BVM unit with one rescuer and supplemental O_2
5. Mouth-to-mouth ventilation is the last choice and not an option for professional rescuers because of the risk for disease transmission.

HAZARDS

Oxygen does not burn, but it greatly accelerates combustion. Concentrated O_2 facilitates conversion of sparks or embers (e.g., lit cigarettes) into vigorous fires. O_2 should only be used in open, well-ventilated areas and never in the presence of burning materials. Use care when handling O_2 equipment to avoid allowing contaminants (e.g., petroleum products) to come in or around the orifices on the cylinder or regulator through which O_2 flows. Cylinders should not be exposed to temperatures above 52°C (125°F).

LEGAL ISSUES

The FDA regulations regarding O_2 administration equipment state that to qualify as "emergency medical oxygen administration equipment," a device must "be capable of administering a flow rate of at least 6 L/min for a period of at least 15 minutes."[19] Equipment not meeting this minimum standard may not be sold in the United States as emergency medical O_2 administration equipment.

According to FDA regulations, a medical O_2 cylinder can be filled "for emergency use only when administered by properly trained personnel for O_2 deficiency and resuscitation." For all other medical applications, "Caution: Federal law prohibits dispensing without prescription."[18]

REFERENCES

Complete references used in this text are available online at expertconsult.inkling.com.

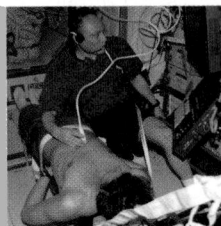

CHAPTER 104
Telemedicine in the Wilderness

JUSTIN T. PITMAN, ASHLEY KOCHANEK WEISMAN, AND N. STUART HARRIS

Telemedicine is broadly defined as the practice of medical care through any medium that separates a patient and care provider. The prefix *tele* derives from ancient Greek, "at a distance," and *medicine* from the Latin *mederi*, "to heal." Although technologic purists might balk at histories of missive-related medical consults (noted as distantly as ancient Greek and Egyptian texts) as "telemedicine," the essence of caregivers engaging in clinical assessment at a distance from their patients gives even this ancient epistolary practice reasonable claim to the first practice of telemedicine. Although the essentials of that exchange have not changed in the last 4000 years, what have changed are speed, quantity, quality, and accessibility of data that may be transmitted between patient and caregiver. In the last 20 years, the means of data acquisition and ease of transmitting vast volumes of data inexpensively from any point on the globe have expanded tremendously. Real-time data are now routinely transmitted between hospitals and distant caregivers, including video interviews, complete electronic medical records, detailed physiologic monitoring, electrocardiograms, electroencephalograms, and state-of-the-art images (e.g., ultrasound, radiography, computed tomography, magnetic resonance). Once digitized and using current communication networks, data may be readily transferred from the International Space Station (ISS) to Houston's Mission Control Center (MCC) or from Mt Everest Base Camp to any academic center (Figure 104-1).

Telemedicine techniques can provide critical services in the most remote and austere wilderness conditions, emphasizing its importance for wilderness medicine and care rendered in other austere settings. In developed urban areas, telemedicine is often used for reasons of convenience. In rural areas, telemedicine networks "take the doctor to the patient," regardless of the distance between them. Through a range of rural telemedicine projects, diagnostic and treatment expertise can be applied to a vast, sparsely settled geographic range (e.g., Alaska health networks for remote villages). Telemedicine allows greater equity of access to health care, especially for persons for "whom time and distance constitute formidable obstacles to the receipt of care."[5] Telemedicine proves a means of overcoming limitations in medical care posed by geography, financial constraints, and weather. As Bashshur and Lovett[5] predicted in 1977, telemedicine's major promise for the future is to bring health services to people "wherever it now is not possible or feasible to bring people to health services." For many in wilderness locations, this is exactly what would be intended. As recently as 15 years ago, computing technology for such devices was prohibitively expensive and only accessible by groups or individuals with large budgets. However, over the past decade, technologic evolution has produced smaller, more powerful, yet energy-efficient devices that are now within an attainable price range. With such profound and widespread accessibility, telecommunication from mobile and remote locations is now frequently practiced.

EVOLUTION OF TELEMEDICINE

Although we think of modern telemedicine as a product of recent technology, the underlying concept of communicating medical information from a distance can be traced back several centuries. Perhaps the earliest documented evidence of health information transmission originates from the African continent. Villagers used smoke signals as a way to convey the presence of serious disease or illness and serve as a warning to others to keep their distance. It has been noted from ancient Greek and Egyptian texts that practitioners used to convey information to patients through the use of a runner. Bonfires were used throughout Europe in the 1600s to transmit information regarding the bubonic plague.[10]

Until the mid-1800s, information transfer between two distant parties relied on nonelectrical means of conveyance, including smoke signals, bonfires, drum code, runners, riders, and letters. The first electronic transmission, sent via telegraph by Samuel Morse in 1844 between Baltimore and Washington, DC, signaled the birth of modern electronic telemedicine. During the American Civil War, telegraph was used to transmit information regarding casualty lists and to order medical supplies.[48] In 1875, Alexander G. Bell's first communication via telephone was to his assistant, Mr. Watson.[13] As recorded in Bell's journal, "I then shouted into the M [mouthpiece] the following sentence: 'Mr. Watson—come here, I want to see you.'" Bell had accidentally spilled battery acid on his leg and, by telephone, was able to call Mr. Watson to provide medical aid. The telephone was rapidly and widely adopted for ease of use and immediately embraced by physicians as the mainstay for both physician-physician and physician-patient communication. In 1906, Dr. Willem Leister Einthoven successfully transmitted an electrocardiogram (ECG) over telephone lines, likely the first example of telecardiology.[14]

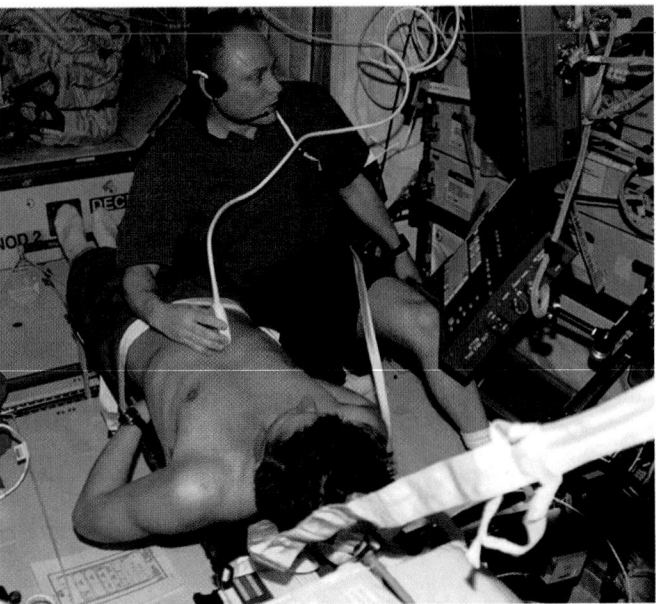

FIGURE 104-1 Ultrasound on International Space Station. Astronauts and cosmonauts practice zero-gravity abdominal ultrasound from Earth orbit. *(Courtesy National Aeronautics and Space Administration, Washington, DC. From Dulchavsky SA, Kirkpatrick AW: The surgeon's use of ultrasound in thoracoabdominal trauma. In Cameron JL, Cameron AM, editors: Current surgical therapy, 10th ed, Philadelphia, 2011, Elsevier, pp 900-905.)*

The advent of two-way radio communication soon followed. For the first time, users could communicate between distances without a hard-line connection. In 1924, *Radio News* magazine ran a futuristic cover story, "The Radio Doctor—*Maybe!*" In this story, Hugo Gernsback, an American inventor, writer, and magazine publisher, postulated development of a machine, the "teledactyl," or "distant fingers"[18] (Figure 104-2). Using the teledactyl, he hypothesized that a physician would not only be able to view his patient remotely via a two-way view screen, but using robotic arms and fingers, physically examine the patient and generate a diagnosis as if the two were present within the same room. In 1935, an Italian group led by Professor G. Guida in Rome established the International Radio Medical Center, which offered radio medical assistance to crews at sea. With government funding, it later expanded services to provide 24-hour physician support to sailors, aviators, and rural populations in Italy.[2] By the late 1930s, radio-based medical communication was extensively used in remote and wilderness areas. To serve rural populations, Australia developed the Royal Flying Doctor service, which fielded teleconsultations from remote individuals using two-way radios powered by bicycle pedal–driven dynamos.[42]

New technology soon allowed for miniaturization, mass production, and affordability of telephone and radio devices, a huge advance for future wilderness applications. In 1947, Norman Holter transmitted the first portable radio-electrocardiogram.[22] Although the machine weighed almost 38 kg (85 lb), it could be strapped to a person's back and monitor heart rate and rhythm during activities and in locations never before studied, whether the patient was cycling at full speed, skiing at altitude, or hiking in heat[36] (Figure 104-3). By 1950, radiologists in Pennsylvania and Canada had used telephone lines to transmit radiographic images. Soldiers and national parks services used portable radios to call for medical assistance and helicopter dispatch from distant field locations. Sailors were using radio to transmit ECGs and x-ray images from distant ocean sites.[33]

In the 1960s, television and video technology were first used to perform telemedicine. Physicians and medical staff at the Nebraska Psychiatric Institute used two-way closed-circuit television (CCT) to connect the institute in Omaha and the state mental hospital in Norfolk, 112 miles away, enabling consultations between specialists and general practitioners.[10,30,48] By 1967, Bird and colleagues established a two-way audiovisual microwave link between Massachusetts General Hospital and Logan International Airport.[10,48] This service was set up for remote physicians to augment medical care of an on-site 24/7 nurse-staffed clinic.

President John F. Kennedy's decision to fund the National Aeronautics and Space Administration (NASA) in 1961 proved pivotal for development of radio, satellite, and television telemedicine technologies that would eventually be applied to astronauts, adventurers, and average citizens. As a critical step in landing a man on the Moon, NASA had to answer a fundamental question: Could a human body function in space? This sparked development of new satellite-based telemedicine systems. NASA built monitoring systems capable of constantly recording real-time physiologic parameters (heart rate, respiratory rate, blood pressure, temperature) and transmitting these data to physicians regardless of the astronauts' position in Earth orbit. As flight time shifted from hours (Earth orbit) to days (lunar orbit), NASA recognized the need for the ability to diagnose and treat in-flight emergencies and began to develop more advanced medical support systems.

This realization also highlighted the need to achieve remote health monitoring for non-space-related situations. NASA, the U.S. Indian Health Service, and the Lockheed Corporation jointly sponsored the Space Technology Applied to Rural Papago Advanced Health Care (STARPAHC).[48] The project began with two Native American paramedics driving a van to deliver care to rural communities with the assistance of physicians connected by two-way microwave transmission from the regional Public Health Service Hospital.[17] This program provided the combined benefits of the "telemedicine trifecta": (1) triage decisions, (2)

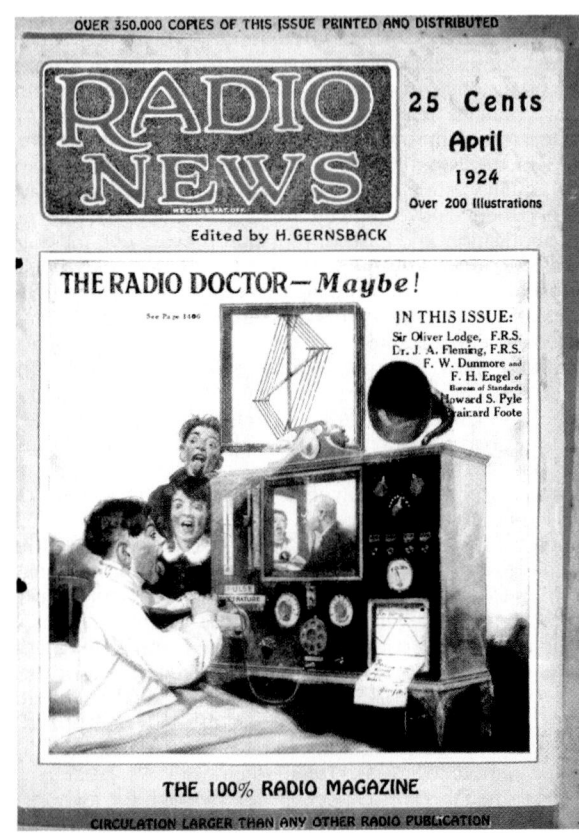

FIGURE 104-2 "Teledactyl." Diagnosis by radio: cover of *Radio News,* April 1924; "The Radio Doctor—*Maybe!*" (by Hugo Gernsback). The illustration portrays a family physician using two-way radio communication to speak with, visualize, and examine the patient.

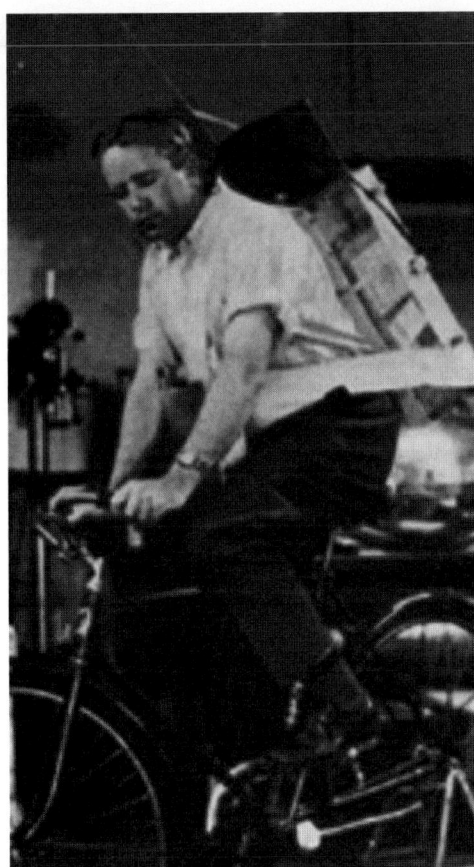

FIGURE 104-3 Tele-electrocardiography. Norman Holter demonstrating his radio-electrocardiograph while riding a bicycle in 1947, the first documented use of portable ECG monitoring. The device weighed 38 kg (84 lb). *(From Ioannou K, Ignaszewski M, MacDonald I: Ambulatory electrocardiography: The contribution of Norman Jefferis Holter, BC Med J 56(2):86-89, 2014.)*

guidance through obtaining a medical history and simple procedures, and (3) specialist consultation. NASA established standards for television telemedicine applications. NASA also led a collaboration to determine the minimal television system requirements for effective care. Their goal was to achieve the same diagnostic accuracy in a patient who was interviewed and examined by a nurse with the guidance of a remote physician (i.e., telemedicine) as in an in-person patient-physician encounter.[8,19] This project recognized that telemedicine requires the same rigorous scientific proof and quality control standards as does bedside medicine. NASA also spearheaded the first international telemedicine cooperation. In 1989, using the "Space Bridge to Armenia and Ufa," Russia provided audio, visual, and facsimile-based medical consultation to clinicians caring for earthquake victims in Armenia hospitals and later to burn victims in a railway fire in Ufa, Russia.[21] These collaborations set the precedent for international telemedicine efforts that would serve hundreds of wilderness expeditions and robust, permanent base stations in austere environments of Mt Everest and Antarctica.

Radio, television, and satellite systems created faster two-way networks that enabled telemedicine to reach remote settings. However, the links were limited; NASA scientists, Royal Flying Doctor service, and psychiatrists in Nebraska could not engage in real-time consultation outside of established channels. Several groups of American computer scientists noted this problem of limited connectivity and created a new network of computer-based interface message processors, precursors to modern routers. Their goal was to allow simultaneous communication among dozens of academic centers over a single network. In 1969, their project, initially called ARPANET, was deployed and quickly evolved from a system using a few dozen scientists with room-size computers communicating over telephone lines at a bandwidth of 56 kilobits per second (kbps), to become the current Internet, where more than 2.8 billion users communicate with handheld devices linked via cable modem at 160 megabits per second (Mbps).[38]

Faster, higher-resolution data transfer allows telemedicine to be available to an exponentially greater number of patients, adventurers, and physicians around the globe. Although data transmission time is directly proportional to distance (unidirectional transmission from Earth to Mars takes on average 14 minutes), technology exists for communication throughout the Solar System, allowing for future theoretical human exploration with medical support of Mars and other planetary bodies. On the ground, these capabilities have also rapidly changed. In 1987, a telephone line connection enabled x-ray and detailed ultrasound echocardiographic images to be transmitted from rural Nova Scotia to pediatric cardiology consultants for diagnosis and treatment advice.[15] Less than 15 years later, dial-up connection made two-way video consultation with specialists available to ailing scientists in Antarctica 24 hours a day.[7] As the World Wide Web and cellular data access have become globally available through handheld devices, it is now the case that digitized photos, radiographic images, ECGs, and audio files are universally available for education and medical advice. A trekker may download a range of advanced health care applications to a smartphone via the airport wireless Internet connection before departure and then carry the telemedicine-empowered smartphone to a remote location (Table 104-1).

TELEMEDICINE SYSTEMS ENGINEERING

The increase in telemedicine's scope is fueled by improvements in computer technology and communication networks. Telemedicine can be divided into three broad categories: store-and-forward, remote monitoring, and live streaming audio or video interaction (Table 104-2). In store-and-forward systems, patient data or consultant advice are saved and stored in an electronic medium. When timing is appropriate, these data are then uploaded via telephone, hard disk, or wirelessly, then transferred for later review. This allows for the two parties to be physically separated in both space and time and still communicate relevant data. This separation has several drawbacks. In particular, it limits caregiver ability to obtain real-time clinical history or physical examination and to provide immediate assistance with diagnosis and treatment. Currently, typical applications of store-and-forward include the use of a Holter monitor or loop recorder for arrhythmia detection, where cardiac electrical activity is stored over a period of time and as needed, uploaded from home for

TABLE 104-1 Wilderness First-Aid Smartphone Apps*

Application (App)	Device	Cost
Army First Aid by Double Dog Studios	iPhone	$1.99
First Aid by Red Cross	iPhone, Android	Free
GotoAID by Jaargon, Ltd	iPhone, Android	Free, $4.99
Pocket First Aid & CPR by American Heart Association	iPhone, Android	$1.99
SAS Survival by trellisys.net	iPhone, Android	Free, $5.99
Wilderness First Aid by Wildside Medical Education LLC	iPhone, Android	$0.99
Wilderness Survival by Jason Vance	iPhone	$1.99

*Price and app availability are subject to change.

TABLE 104-2 Types of Communication in Telemedicine Systems

Type	Mechanism	Examples	Limitations
Store-and-forward	Data stored on patient machine and uploaded to specialist. Specialist recommendations sent back.	Holter/loop monitor Radiographic images Dermatologic images	Clinical history Physical examination Time-sensitive information Inexpensive
Remote monitoring	Physician monitors patient data remotely using technologic devices.	Heart disease Diabetes Asthma	Clinical history Physical examination Moderately expensive
Live-stream communication	Live two-way communication between patient and clinician replacing in-person evaluation.	Live diagnostic consultations Procedural guidance Triage decision making Live physiologic monitoring	Reliable data infrastructure Expensive

clinical review in the office at a later date. Other uses include tele-radiology and tele-dermatology. Tele-radiology uses patient images captured in one location and then uploaded to a central server for radiologist review either from home, another state, or another country. With tele-dermatology, experts provide downloadable visual diagnosis aids for generalists to use when they encounter an unknown lesion or rash, as well as provide ability to upload digital photo documentation that can then be forwarded over the network for remote dermatology consultation.

Remote monitoring provides a means for a physician or medical provider to monitor and subsequently manage a patient from afar and is particularly helpful managing chronic diseases such as asthma, diabetes, dyslipidemia, or heart disease. Based on patient-gathered metrics (e.g., blood pressure, blood sugar, or lipid levels), remote clinicians can quickly and accurately adjust patient medications.

Lastly, telemedicine can be used to employ real-time connections, including telephone, video conferencing, and live physiologic monitoring. Real-time telemedicine is used to connect patients and physicians in rural settings with distant specialists. In acute settings, real-time telemedicine helps save lives by allowing diagnosis, triage, and treatment from highly qualified practitioners. A volunteer emergency physician staffing a remote Himalayan medical clinic may be concerned regarding a pediatric patient with fever, atypical soft tissue swelling, and rash, and via the telephone may contact a remote pediatrician to discuss physical exam findings, differential diagnoses, and whether the patient requires more urgent evaluation. In another example, to evaluate a patient with traumatic injuries, a distant clinician using a live audiovisual link could guide a field care provider inexperienced in ultrasound through the components of a focused assessment with sonography in trauma (FAST) examination and determine whether the patient may require immediate evacuation and operative intervention. Video conferencing with specialists can be used for routine consultations or follow-up appointments.[11,17] It can save patients and families time and money, improve patient satisfaction, and reduce the environmental impact of medical practice.[20]

Telemedicine systems all contain three basic data functions: acquisition, transmission, and reconstruction and interpretation (Table 104-3). Within each of these areas, any device capable of the qualities of that grouping can be used as part of a system. With current digital systems, increasing frequency of "plug and play" simplicity can be expected (Figure 104-4). For example, for data acquisition, digital medical devices and methods include voice and streaming video over the Internet, ultrasound, ECG, and text documents with past medical history, which are transmitted through any of a range of media (typically, satellite phone connection for remote, austere environments) and then reconstituted at a secondary site (usually accomplished on a standard personal computer). Although options for addition of two-way voice, real-time audio, and other methods can be made, these three essential elements exist as the backbone of every telemedicine system. Certain devices require a means of reconfiguring data (e.g., ultrasound device might need to be plugged into video-streaming device to digitize and compress the signal for transmission), but these typically can be easily and inexpensively accomplished (Figure 104-5). By mixing and matching the different components of the telemedicine system, it can be reconfigured easily to perform a myriad of tasks, whether gathering remote field data, providing local care givers with expert consultation to aid the management of chronic illness, or assisting in the decision-making process and acute management of injury or illness in an austere location.

Current devices allow certain physiologic systems to be easily monitored and data to be stored and transmitted. The devices can record physiologic signals necessary for research purposes, including electroencephalograph (EEG), ECG, respirations, spirometry, oximetry, electromyogram (EMG), and more with compact hardware that can fit in the palm of one's hand.[6] Novices, guided by experts thousands of miles away, have successfully used ultrasound systems, linked by satellite phone to a video-streaming device and laptop computer, to stream video through the Internet to assay for pulmonary edema in high-altitude climbers on Mt Everest.[37] In this example, the authors report on a telemedicine system constructed using a standard,

TABLE 104-3 The Three Required Components of a Telemedicine System

Data Acquisition	Data Transmission	Data Reconstruction and Interpretation
Physical examination by local provider Real-time history by patient Text documents Electrocardiogram Anatomic imaging (CT, MRI, ultrasound, radiography) Physiologic monitoring Electroencephalogram	Satellite phone Cellular/smartphone Internet Visual (semaphor) Radio-wave	Receiver compatible with transmitting system, most typically a computer with a display

CT, Computed tomography; *MRI,* magnetic resonance imaging.

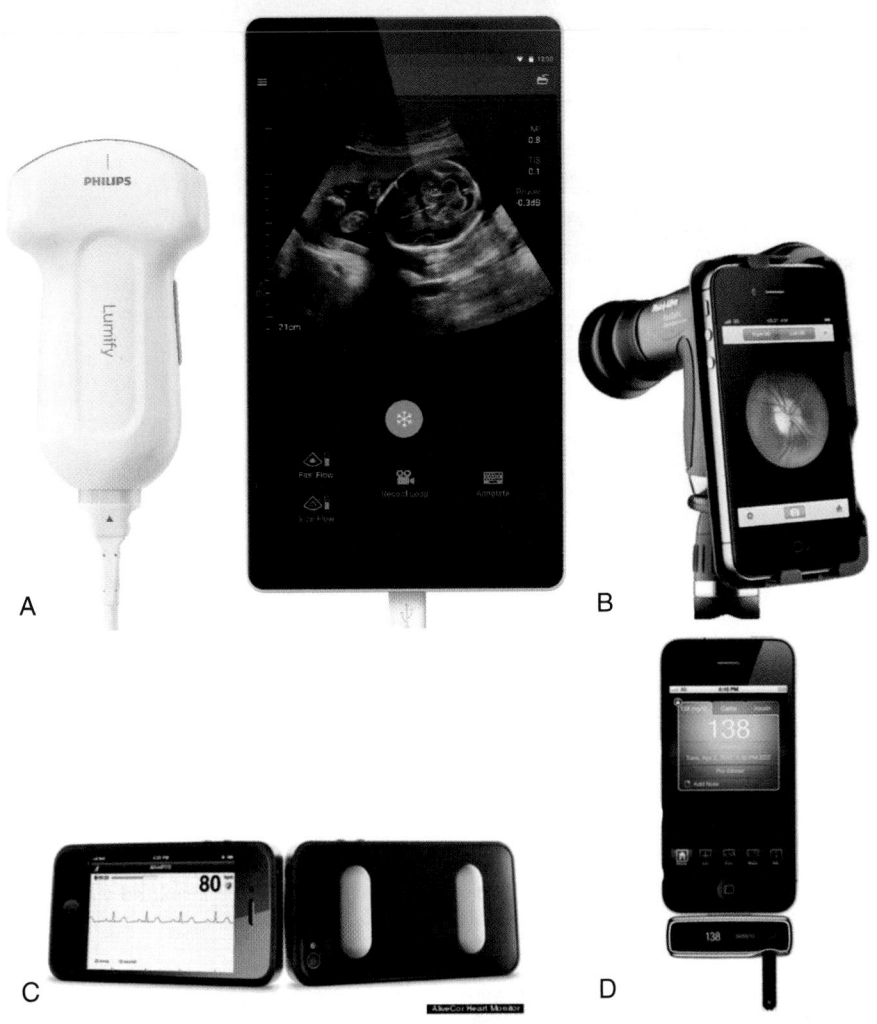

FIGURE 104-4 Smartphone telemedicine. Miniaturization of biologic sensors and medical devices allows remote monitoring or diagnostics for use in the field. **A,** The Philips Lumify, a portable ultrasound designed for a mobile smart device. **B,** WelchAllyn iExamine, an iPhone-compatible funduscope. **C,** AliveCor Heart Monitor, a smartphone-based ECG machine. **D,** Sanofi iBGStar, an iPhone-based glucometer. (*A courtesy Philips Ultrasound Inc, Andover, MA; B courtesy WelchAllyn, Skaneateles Falls, NY; C courtesy AliveCor, San Francisco; D courtesy Sanofi, Bridgewater, NJ.*)

commercially available, portable ultrasound system coupled with a two-way communications system. They describe a system remarkable in its capability and ease of use. In this study, the ultrasound operators were nonphysician climbers without ultrasound experience. A 2-minute orientation to the ultrasound machine, probe orientation, remote commands, and examination conduct was given over a satellite phone by a remote ultrasound expert just before the examination. The remote expert communicated with the climbers using bidirectional audio, reviewed streaming video output from the ultrasound, and guided the examination with the aid of a cue card to which the climbers referred (Figure 104-6). In this and other investigations, compelling evidence shows that "coupling portable ultrasound with remote expert guidance telemedicine provides robust diagnostic capability in austere locations."[37]

Each of these components of the telemedicine system can further be defined by their speed and resolution. A major defining parameter in any telecommunication network is bandwidth. *Bandwidth* is the amount of data transmitted per unit time and often the rate-determining step in a telemedicine system.[11] Speed of data transfer is usually measured in bits per second (bps). A bit is a single value in a line of computer code, and either represents 0 or 1. A byte is 8 bits in size and represents the smallest addressable memory unit; it takes 8 bits or 1 byte to form a single character of the alphabet (Table 104-4). A network connection that allows for a 1 megabit per second (Mbps) or 1000 kilobits per second (Kbps) can transfer data at the rate of 125 kilobytes per second (KBps) (Table 104-5). Transferring a 5-megabyte (MB) photograph over a 14-Kbps connection (14.4-Kbps dial-up modem) takes approximately 45 minutes. Sending the same file over a 10-Mbps connection (broadband cable modem) takes 3.8 seconds (Table 104-6). Tele–diabetic retinopathy screening requires about 5 MB per compressed diagnostic video, ultrasound requires approximately 120 KB to transmit 5 key frames per second, or about 100 MB of compressed data for a full echocardiogram, and live video conferencing with diagnostic-quality resolution requires speeds of 1 to 2 Mbps or more.[40] Meeting these bandwidth benchmarks requires capable underlying technologic infrastructure or that caregivers carry significant telecommunication equipment. For example, expeditions on Mt Everest and along the Amazon River have carried their own equipment to link with orbiting satellites.[4,27] As recently as 2014, attempts to use "3G" wireless for telehealth in rural South Africa proved unsuccessful because there was not a functional 3G cellular network, but instead a very slow general packet radio service.[9] Before deployment,

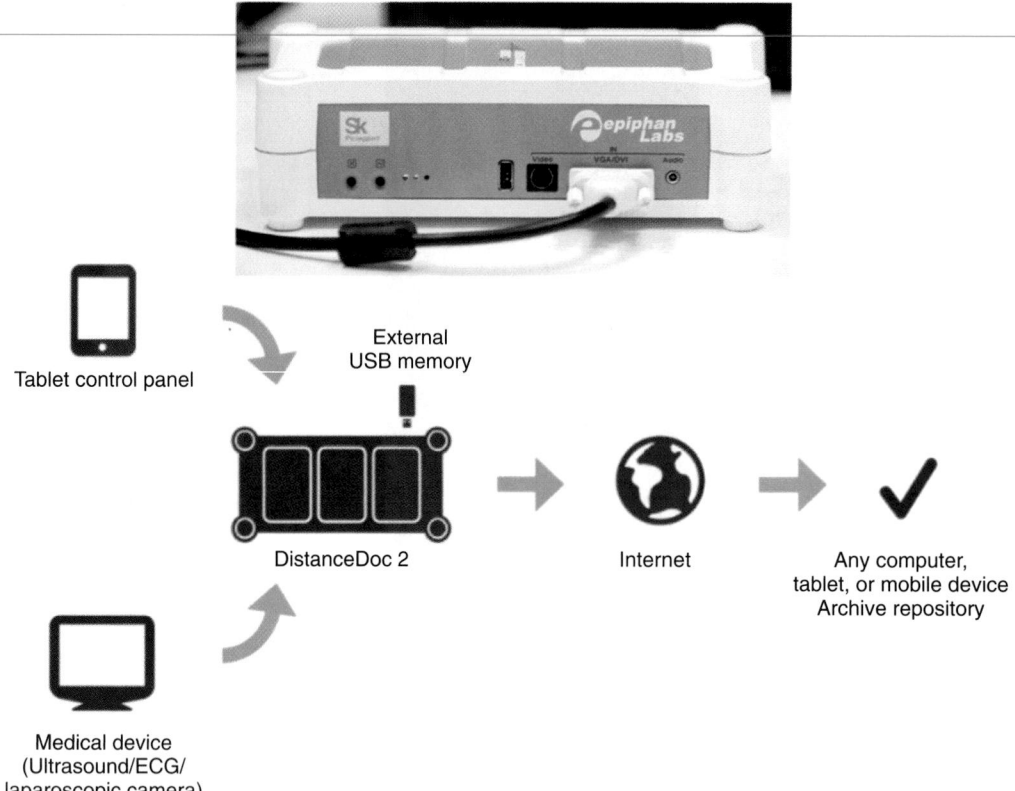

Tablet control panel

External
USB memory

DistanceDoc 2

Internet

Any computer,
tablet, or mobile device
Archive repository

Medical device
(Ultrasound/ECG/
laparoscopic camera)

FIGURE 104-5 Telemedicine made easy. Shown is the DistanceDoc, a device that allows for real-time capture of images and video from any medical device or tablet with a compatible video output. The medical device or tablet video output is connected to DistanceDoc video input. Captured images and video can then either be saved to a USB stick/internal storage or compressed and transmitted via the Internet for real-time diagnostic evaluation. *(Courtesy Epiphan Labs, Skolkovo, Russia.)*

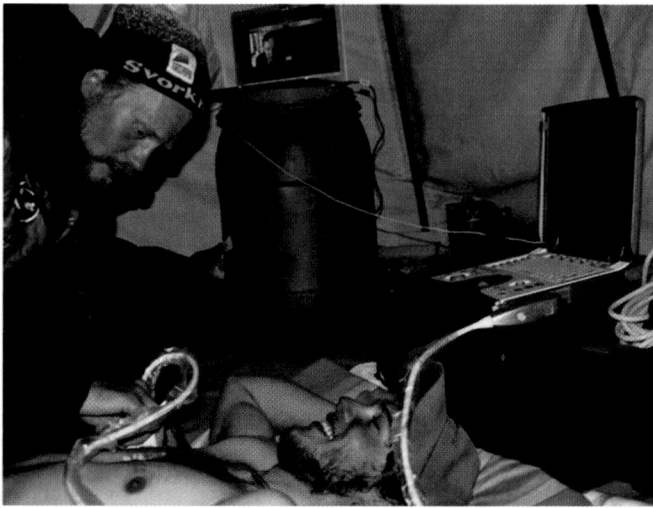

FIGURE 104-6 Telemedicine on Mt Everest. This climber is performing a thoracic ultrasound examination on a fellow climber in a tent at Advanced Base Camp using telemedical guidance. They are being led in this examination through a real-time audiovisual connection with a remote expert, visible on the computer screen on the top of the barrel in the background. *(From Otto CM, Hamilton DR, Levin BD, et al: Into thin air: Extreme ultrasound on Mt. Everest, Wilderness Environ Med 20(3):283:289, 2009.)*

TABLE 104-4	Memory Conversion		
Memory	**Abbreviation**	**Value**	**Size**
bit	b	1	0 or 1
byte	B	1	8 bits
kilobit	kb, Kb	10³	1000 bits
kilobyte	KB	10³	1024 bytes
megabit	Mb	10⁶	1000 kilobits
megabyte	MB	10⁶	1024 kilobytes
gigabit	Gb	10⁹	1000 megabits
gigabyte	GB	10⁹	1024 megabytes
terabit	Tb	10¹²	1000 gigabits
terabyte	TB	10¹²	1024 gigabytes

TABLE 104-5	Network Bandwidth	
Network	**Minimum**	**Maximum**
Dial up	2.4 Kbps	56 Kbps
ISDN	64 Kbps	128 Kbps
DSL	128 Kbps	9 Mbps
ADSL	1.5 Mbps	9 Mbps
Cable	512 Kbps	20 Mbps
Wireless	Variable depending on source	
T-1	1.544 Mbps	1.544 Mbps
T-3	43 Mbps	45 Mbps
OC3	155.52 Mbps	155.52 Mbps
Satellite	492 Kbps	512 Kbps

Data from Beal V: Types of internet connections. Webopedia, 2014. www.webopedia.com/quick_ref/internet_connection_types.asp. *Kbps,* Kilobits per second; *Mbps,* megabits per second.

TABLE 104-6 Network Transfer Rate and Theoretical Maximum Download Speed Chart*

Network Speed	Transfer Rate (MB/s)	1 MB	5 MB	10 MB	50 MB	100 MB	500 MB	1 GB	10 GB
14.4 Kbps	0.0018	9:15	46:17:00	1:32:35	7:42:57	15:25:55	77:09:37	154:19:105	1543:12:35
28.8 Kbps	0.0036	4:37	23:08	46:17:00	3:51:28	7:42:57	38:34:48	77:09:37	771:36:17
56 Kbps	0.007	2:22	11:54	23:48	1:59:02	3:58:05	19:50:28	39:40:57	396:49:31
128 Kbps	0.016	1:02	5:12	10:25	52:05:00	1:44:10	8:40:50	17:21:40	173:36:40
256 Kbps	0.032	0:32	2:36	5:12	26:02:00	52:05:00	4:20:25	8:40:50	86:48:20
512 Kbps	0.064	0:15	1:18	2:36	13:01	26:02:00	2:10:12	4:20:25	43:24:10
1 Mbps	0.125	0:07	0:39	1:18	6:30	13:01	1:05:06	2:10:12	21:42:05
2 Mbps	0.25	0:03	0:19	0:39	3:15	6:30	32:33:00	1:05:06	10:51:02
5 Mbps	0.625	0:015	0:08	0:16	1:20	2:40	13:20	26:40:00	5:26:01
10 Mbps	1.25	<0:01	0:04	0:08	0:40	1:20	6:40	13:20	2:13:20
20 Mbps	2.5	<0:01	0:02	0:04	0:20	0:40	3:20	6:50	1:06:40
50 Mbps	6.25	<0:01	<0:01	0:01	0:07	0:15	1:18	2:36	26:08:00
100 Mbps	12.5	<0:01	<0:01	<0:01	0:04	0:08	0:40	1:20	13:20

*Time listed as hh:mm:ss.
Kbps, Kilobits per second; *Mbps*, megabits per second; *GB*, gigabytes.

thorough assessment of field location infrastructure should be performed to evaluate availability and reliability of telecommunication networks; this is essential for successful implementation of telemedicine.

Telemedicine involves several logistical and ethical considerations on the part of the network and physicians providing consultation. The logistics particularly pertinent to wilderness locations are discussed later. Both parties should be aware of and should agree to certain responsibilities and availability, and should discuss a backup plan for unscheduled blackout times. Although disruptions in connectivity in remote settings can occur without warning, it is ethically unsound to begin providing a level of care that requires telemedicine and be unable to complete that care plan because of a predictable disruption in telemedicine service. This issue is further complicated in cases of medical expeditions that use telemedicine to provide medical services to isolated communities for a short time. Similar to the medical mission model, temporary telemedicine services can provide great benefit, but caution should be exercised to defer evaluations and treatments that will require follow up beyond the duration of the expedition.

On-scene medical providers and the tele-physician should be aware of the capabilities of the facility they are speaking with and give advice accordingly. Legal responsibility for patient care is shared between the on-site and telemedicine teams. Each should provide a standard of care to the best of their abilities and acknowledge the limitations of tele-practice as these arise. If at all feasible, informed consent should be obtained in the setting of procedures or decision making, explaining the use of telemedicine to assist an on-site provider. The need for lifesaving procedures may make this impossible, but every effort should be made to discuss care options with the patient in their native language before undertaking a procedure in the field or an evacuation that carries explainable risk. The ideal network for telemedicine is a secure one that preserves privacy of the patient-physician interaction, or the blindedness of observers performing clinical research. (See core guidelines for telemedicine operations at www.americantelemed.org.)

Before deployment of a telemedicine system for rural, international, or expedition use, careful thought regarding specific needs and medical goals is critical. Depending on the location of use, multiple factors must be considered, including budget, local infrastructure, unique environmental threats (cold, altitude, salt, water exposure), size, and weight restrictions (Box 104-1). Specific environmental factors to consider include sunlight availability to power solar grids, waterproofing in areas with exposure to rainfall, equipment tolerance of the cold/hypobaric conditions of high altitude, and general ruggedness of equipment to survive exposure to harsh environmental exposures to dust, wind, and other elements. Equipment specifications must be scrutinized to determine whether modifications are necessary before deployment. Caregivers must be cognizant of their destination's network communication and power grid infrastructure capabilities. If a reliable electrical infrastructure will not allow safe and reliable equipment use, alternative power supplies (batteries, solar/wind power, portable generator) will be required to operate the telemedicine system. Caregivers must be knowledgeable about the type and speed of the network connection, because speed will likely be a significant bottleneck for data transmission. If only a telephone or local area network (LAN) line connection is present, data transmission may be limited to audio, document, or e-mail, whereas cable or 3G cellular capability may allow real-time audiovisual communication and live data streaming (Figures 104-7 and 104-8).

Before investing in telemedicine technology, consideration should be given to the specific injuries and illnesses likely to occur during the deployment and what the use of telemedicine will be expected to achieve.[47] It should be determined if data requirements are most easily satisfied using a store-and-forward method, remote monitoring, or live streaming mechanism. Setting up an advanced tele-stroke neurologic consultation service for remote areas requires real-time audiovisual connectivity with two-way communication ability to allow rapid diagnostic and treatment conversations. The data and power requirements for such a service can be time and money intensive. Conversely, a wilderness expedition leader who intends to rely on infrequent use of a satellite telephone to make a triage decisions regarding management and evacuation of injured mountaineers has much less technologic demand.

For telemedicine to be successful, each participant's level of medical training should be determined and integrated appropriately. Although some procedures and treatments can be conveyed using verbal communication to a layperson (e.g., how to use a needle to perform decompression needle thoracostomy in a patient with a tension pneumothorax), others may require significant medical expertise (e.g., surgeon remotely guiding a general practitioner through an appendectomy). Certain skill sets are unable to be transferred via audio or video conferencing. It is important to recognize that if medical equipment is being brought along, there should be an individual(s) capable of using it.

Developing effective telemedicine systems in the wilderness requires one to be methodical and to take each of these features into consideration. First is a complete needs assessment. What are the expedition's most critical or common medical needs? Would they benefit from store-forward, physiologic monitoring, or live streaming telemedicine? What is the region's

BOX 104-1 Telemedicine Needs Assessment

How to Choose a Telemedicine System

1. Where will the telemedicine system be deployed?
   Environmental factors:
   - Availability of sunshine (e.g., solar power production influenced by cloud cover, natural terrain: north side of mountain in northern hemisphere)
   - Rainfall/exposure (waterproofing needs)
   - Wind/dust/vibration (ruggedness of equipment)
   - High altitude (hypobaria and cold can disable some devices)

   Is equipment suitable for deployment in particular environmental conditions?

   Does equipment require special attention or modification to maintain functionality?

2. What is the level of network and power grid infrastructure and its reliability?
   Is there reliable power, and is an alternative source needed (generator, batteries, solar array, wind power)?
   Is there access to a communications network?
   - Telephone/LAN line
   - Cellular/3G/4G LTE
   - Wireless
   - Satellite

   Network reliability and speed will dictate data transmission bottlenecks and limit efficacy of telemedicine networks requiring fast data transfer.

3. What are the objectives of telemedicine network?
   - Research
   - Rural/international medical care

- Adventure/expedition medical care
  What is the simplest and most reliable system to accomplish predetermined goals?

4. What are the size, weight, and cost limitations of system components?
   Telemedicine system must fit within size, weight, and budgetary constraints, which may represent significant restrictions on type of system.

5. What injuries/medical illnesses are expected?
   Injury/illness pattern expected:
   - In particular destination (e.g., alpine vs. desert environment)
   - In particular activity (e.g., mountaineering vs. scuba diving)
   - Chronic illness within community or expedition/crew

   Knowing expected needs of telemedicine system can allow for appropriate selection.
   Triage decision (Evacuation: Yes/No)
   Advanced medical care/procedures
   Chronic illness management

6. What is the medical training of expedition or crew members?
   What level of medical expertise is immediately available?
   Certain knowledge/skill sets cannot be transferred via communication.
   Medical equipment brought should match skill level of individuals.

---

infrastructure and the team's ability to care for and maintain equipment? What is the greatest bandwidth that can be achieved with reasonable consistency? Will the system be used for emergencies only, or routine medical care? What will be the availability and responsibility of on-site providers and telemedicine consultants? Once the expedition is capable of carrying out telemedicine, the most successful systems stress thorough understanding of the content, time, cost, and quality of proposed remote medical interactions and information exchanges, as well as in-person alternatives.[12,16,34]

MODERN TELEMEDICINE

Modern telemedicine fills three major information gaps in wilderness and rural medicine: remote specialist consultation, remote monitoring of patients, and patient and physician education. Common telemedicine specialties include radiology, cardiology, dermatology, and psychiatry, with pediatric branches of these specialties especially well represented. Among emergency specialty consultations, tele-neurology is well established and provides real-time diagnostic examinations and expert advice

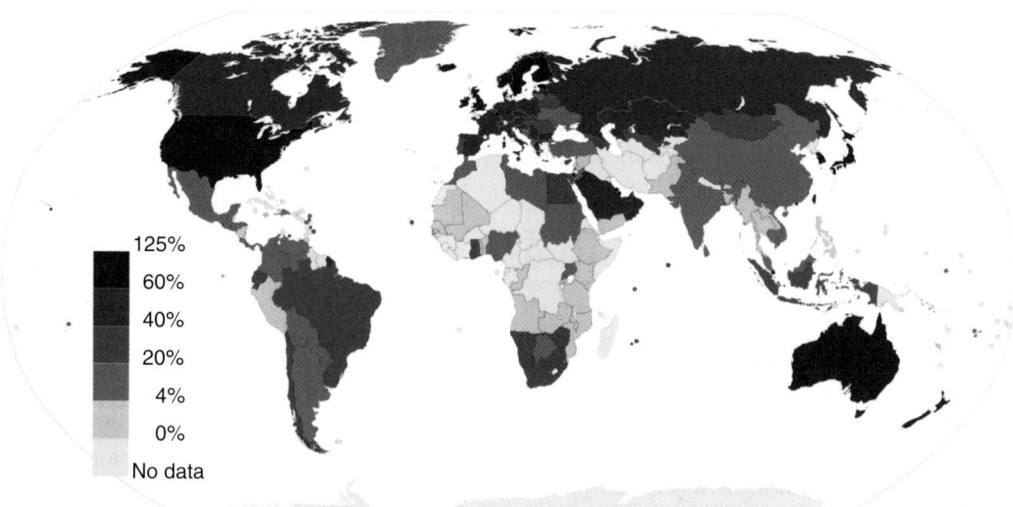

FIGURE 104-7 Global cellular 3G/LTE broadband global accessibility as of 2012. Despite the increasing size of cellular broadband networks, many areas of the world still do not have access to cellular broadband Internet connectivity. *Darker shades of blue* represent areas with high accessibility; *lighter shades* demonstrate limited access. *(Courtesy Jeff Ogden: Mobile broadband internet penetration world map, Wikimedia Commons, 2013.)*

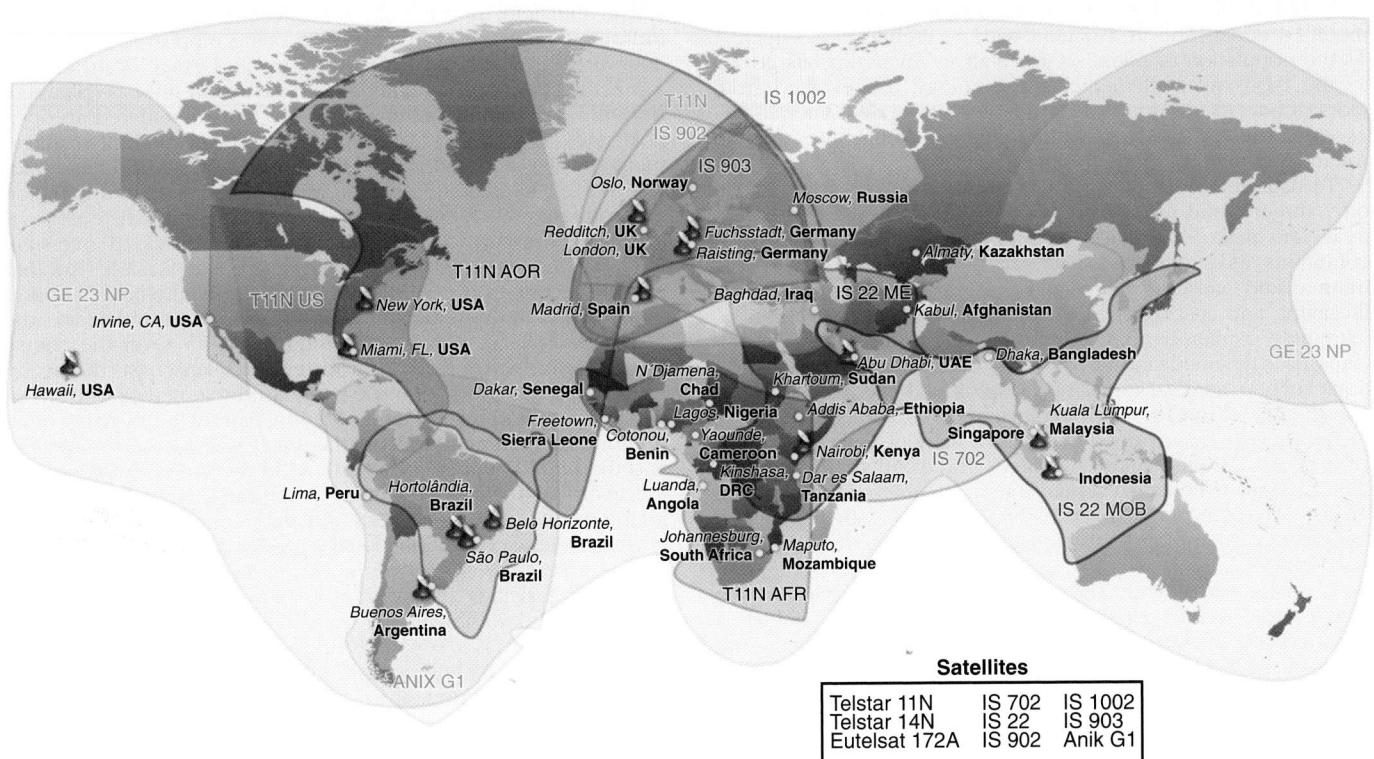

FIGURE 104-8 Satellite broadband global accessibility. With orbiting geosynchronous communications satellites, broadband Internet is now accessible from nearly every inch of the globe. *(Courtesy TEC Offshore: VSAT. TEC Offshore Marine Services Communications, 2015.* www.tecoffshore.com/communications/vsat/.)

regarding use of thrombolytic drugs for acute ischemic strokes. Other specialists who have joined the field of telemedicine include burn surgeons, orthopedists, pediatric traumatologists, and neurosurgeons.[41,43] Technology can be as complex as a dedicated video conferencing network utilizing international satellite systems, or as simple and publicly available as smartphone cameras and multimedia messaging service.[44] True telesurgery remains in developmental phases, but in 2002, surgeons in New York City put forth a compelling proof of concept by successfully completing laparoscopic cholecystectomy on a patient in Strasbourg, France via signals sent over asynchronous transfer mode (ATM) telecommunications technology to a surgical robot.[28]

Telemedicine has been rapidly adopted in intensive care units (ICUs), rehabilitation centers, and nursing facilities for remote monitoring of physiologic parameters and specialist consultations.[24] Its role in monitoring patients at home (with a goal of keeping them healthy and at home) is being fine-tuned. Modern physicians can currently monitor patient physiology to a degree and detail at a distance that Norman Holter could hardly have imagined. From home, heart failure patients can transmit daily heart rate, weight, blood pressure, and even pulmonary artery pressure to clinicians and can receive clinical advice according to algorithms that help predict exacerbations.[1,3]

Finally, telemedicine currently plays a growing role in patient and clinician education. Procedural teleconferences, such as the Boston International Live Endoscopy Course, use high-definition video and two-way audio to provide live broadcasts of thousands of procedures with real-time, interactive teaching to gastroenterologists worldwide. Similar conferences exist for surgeons and interventional cardiologists. Clinician education has improved medical student learning from live surgery teleconferences. Internet-based programs, podcasts, and simulations allied with free, open access medical education enable clinicians to access new information and question colleagues and experts.[46,35]

TELEMEDICINE IN THE WILD

Wilderness medicine draws from the telemedicine applications of specialty consultation and procedural guidance, remote physiologic monitoring, and education. It matches the needs of austere environments and expeditions with the capabilities of telemedicine technology to keep mountaineers safe, handle emergencies, and contribute to our understanding of human physiology in extreme wilderness environments. Antarctica and Mt Everest Base Camp are two notably extreme environments with highly sophisticated medical care and telemedicine support that have utilized telemedicine in several capacities and served as examples for others. Antarctic expeditions in the early 1900s recognized the need for remote medical care and brought medical supplies and expedition medical doctors with their crews. An Australian expedition in 1911-1914 pioneered the use of wireless communications to provide telemedicine support between the doctor at a sub-Antarctic base location and far-forward explorers on the ice.[25] Over time, duration of human stays on Antarctica has grown from a few challenging weeks to year-round scientific investigation. Correspondingly, the role of telemedicine has grown to help study and improve health in humans under the physical and psychological stress of continual darkness and freezing cold. Detailed research by the Australian National Antarctic Research Expeditions (ANARE), facilitated by robust medicine and telemedicine communications, has linked vitamin D deficiency to hormonal changes related to bone and behavioral health.[23] On subsequent expeditions by Australian and American teams, issues ranging from severe accidents to complications of chronic medical disease arose, for which remote expert physicians helped save lives. In the 1950s, Americans and Australians constructed permanent research facilities that included a medical ward staffed by an on-site physician with radio-based medical support. In 1961, Australian team physician Russel Pardoe under the guidance of a surgeon in Melbourne made lifesaving use of the Morse code–based telemedicine system to perform a burr hole with a modified dental drill in a patient with a cerebral hemorrhage.[25] As the population of scientists and staff in Antarctica has grown to the thousands, telemedicine technology has evolved from Morse code to continuously available high-speed Internet via geosynchronous satellites, without the blackouts that plagued Antarctic communications through the 1990s.[7]

To date, remote applications of neurology, cardiology, oncology, surgery, and anesthesiology have been used to diagnose, treat, and make evacuation or supply-drop decisions for such conditions as stroke, heart attack, breast cancer, orthopedic trauma, and gallstone pancreatitis. Telemedicine is particularly lifesaving and cost-effective in winter, when evacuation can be extremely dangerous, if not impossible. On-site general physicians used telemedicine guidance to diagnose and treat conditions such as surgical repair of ligamentous knee injuries under anesthesia, self-biopsy, and administration of chemotherapy for breast cancer. This avoided evacuation without delaying clinical care.[7,45] The United States manages three Antarctic hospitals that have been linked to tertiary medical centers (University of Texas Galveston and University of Colorado) with high-speed two-way video and audio to facilitate ongoing medical care and research.

Formal medical care and telemedicine began later in the Himalayas. Twenty years after Sir Edmund Hillary's 1953 first ascent of Mt Everest, a coalition of medical professionals and guides founded the Himalayan Rescue Association and began providing care at a high-altitude hospital with radio connection for evacuation assistance. True telemedicine on Mt Everest arrived in 1998 with a Yale University/NASA collaboration. The Everest Extreme Expedition (E3) achieved the following three goals:

1. Establishing a daily medical clinic and connecting Mt Everest Base Camp with Yale New Haven medical center in real time with two satellite telephones with sufficient bandwidth to support audio and video.
2. Physiologic monitoring of climbers at high altitudes using wearable devices.
3. Performing numerous experiments related to high-altitude physiology.

The E3 team's temporary clinic saw approximately 150 patients during their stay and used telemedicine to perform medical "rounds" each day on clinic patients and remotely monitored climbers, bringing the standard of high-altitude health care impressively close to that of lowland tertiary medical care. Numerous tests included ultrasound, digital funduscopy, cardiac and pulmonary auscultation, and even a Gram stain. These were transmitted to Yale for live, detailed evaluation, enabling numerous diagnoses (e.g., high-altitude retinopathy, pneumonia, high-altitude pulmonary edema, rotator cuff impingement) and guiding treatment.[4] Although the E3 expedition was temporary, its success stimulated additional telemedicine projects and connections between Mt Everest Base Camp and academic medical institutions for research and patient care. A subsequent series of studies by the Xtreme Everest Research Group employed telemedical physiologic monitoring and real-time data transmission to conduct high-altitude physiology research to expand understanding of hypoxia among climbers in austere environments.[29]

Another major wilderness application of telemedicine is expedition medicine. It is becoming more common for commercial and scientific expeditions to include a wilderness medicine physician in the team and to connect the team to telemedicine resources for further safety. As one of the world's premier wilderness education institutions, the National Outdoor Leadership School (NOLS) decisions involving need for acute communication and access to medical expertise in the backcountry are illustrative. As policy, NOLS now requires one electronic communication device (typically a satellite phone) as standard issue to be carried by instructors on every course. Satellite phones allow instructors with varying degrees of medical training (typically wilderness first responder or wilderness emergency medical technician) to discuss cases with expert medical control while still in the field. In addition, some form of electronic position-indicating radio beacon (EPIRB) is being employed on certain courses. EPIRBs allow rapid notification and exact localization of a potential patient if an emergency evacuation must be planned. In the Indian Himalayas, when a NOLS student suffered an open tibia fracture during a fall on glacial moraine, medical management and decision making provided from NOLS world headquarters in the United States allowed rapid stabilization and initiation of treatment. When poor weather prevented immediate evacuation, ongoing medical expertise from afar provided oversight until evacuation to definitive medical care was feasible. Another notable recent example of extensive, live telemedicine support in an area with unpredictable infrastructure and weather was the Martin Strel Amazon swim expedition in 2007. Over the course of the 66-day swim from Peru to the Brazilian coast, the group used intermittent Skype and e-mail-based telemedicine to maintain frequent and helpful contact at low bandwidth by using light, durable equipment suited for the small size of their watercraft and the humid, wet environment. As in the Yale-Everest project, the team used these modalities to conduct daily tele-rounds to keep on-site and remote medical team members abreast of daily events, weather conditions, vital signs, and physical exam findings to assess the overall health of the swimmer, a strategy that the lead physicians and swimmer believed was essential to safe and successful completion of the journey.[27]

Telemedicine is a key aid to triage and evacuations decisions on expeditions. Technologies such as continuous or intermittent physiologic monitoring, live streaming video examinations, or e-mail conversations with on-site clinicians can help remote physicians assess indications for evacuation. As ultrasound machines and smartphones with video cameras become smaller and more portable, tele-ultrasound is increasingly available and helpful in wilderness settings. Lung ultrasound in particular, with its ability to diagnose and quantify lung pathology (e.g., pneumothorax, pneumonia, pleural effusion, pulmonary edema), is simple enough to teach to nonphysicians; even a school-aged child can perform an acceptable examination when being guided by smartphone teleconference with a remote physician.[31] Cardiac and abdominal ultrasound with remote interpretation and guidance are under investigation and will likely provide helpful data regarding altitude-related pulmonary edema, pneumonia, pneumothorax, pericardial effusion, reduced cardiac function, intra-abdominal bleeding, and fracture.[32] Further study must be done to determine reliability of remote guidance for nonphysicians to perform these studies.

Additional roles for telemedicine in expeditions and military operations are found in store-and-forward smartphone applications (apps) that help on-site clinicians manage unfamiliar clinical conditions. Several apps are available to assist in triage during combat and disaster situations. One such application includes digital representation of a human body that solicits input of injuries and treatments and subsequently reviews these situations (real and simulated) to improve decision making.[39] Another smartphone app can be used by military field medics in the assessment of neurocognitive function after a blast injury or performance degradation from environmental factors to determine whether a soldier remains cognitively fit for duty.[26] The World Health Organization (WHO) and U.S. Centers for Disease Control and Prevention (CDC) offer numerous digital references for triage, disaster relief, first aid, vaccination, and infectious disease maps. Additionally, this textbook and several other wilderness medicine and first-aid references are available in digital form and can be carried to any location hospitable to smartphone, tablet, or e-reader.

REFERENCES

Complete references used in this text are available online at expertconsult.inkling.com.

STEVEN C. CARLETON

Communications to facilitate safe wilderness travel can be as simple as two-way voice transmission over handheld walkie-talkies or as complex as real-time telemedicine using a laptop computer and satellite Internet connection. Highly capable communications equipment can be reliably operated independent of the electrical grid, but this convenience extracts a cost. Gear can be expensive, fragile, bulky, and complex to operate. Portable gear may be limited in broadcast power and thus in range of transmission. Preplanning is essential. Commercial subscriptions and licensure are required to use many of the technologies of greatest utility, and national regulations must be addressed if the equipment is to be imported and used legally in countries other than the country of origin. With rare exceptions, land-based cellular phone technology is not useful in the wilderness setting; the infrastructure required for call routing is simply too limited (90% of Earth is beyond the reach of cellular phone signals).

TWO-WAY LOCAL COMMUNICATION

Local communication in wilderness relies primarily on frequency-modulated (FM) voice radio in the very-high-frequency (VHF, 30 to 300 megahertz [MHz]) and ultra-high-frequency (UHF, 300 MHz to 3 gigahertz [GHz]) portions of the radio spectrum. Unlike commercial amplitude-modulated (AM) and shortwave radio (i.e., 300 kilohertz [KHz] to 30 MHz), these frequencies do not usually benefit from ionospheric effects to increase range and are not reliable for long-range transmissions.

The most common misperception about portable radio transmission involves range. From a practical standpoint, communication with handheld radio devices should be considered to be "line of sight." The radio horizon to which these devices can effectively communicate is influenced by wattage of the transmitter, heights of the transmitting and receiving antennas, orientation of the antennas, and presence of obstructions to propagation (e.g., foliage, terrain features).[2,18] A simple equation defines the maximum theoretical range between a transmitter and receiver, where D is the distance to the radio horizon in miles; Hr is the height of the receiver in feet; and Ht is the height of the transmitter in feet[21]:

$$D = 1.33 \left[\sqrt{(2 \ Hr)} + \sqrt{(2 \ Ht)} \right]$$

For a transmitter and receiver being held with the antennas 1.8 m (6 feet) off the ground, the maximum theoretic range would be approximately 14.5 km (9 miles). The actual maximum range would reliably be only a fraction of this. By comparison, the theoretical range for communication between a ground-based transmitter and a satellite in low Earth orbit (LEO) would be several thousand miles, and the practical range would be a substantial fraction of this, as long as obvious overhead obstructions (e.g., cliff walls, forest canopies) were avoided.

As a general rule, when free of visual obstructions, the radio horizon can be considered as the distance to the visual horizon plus 10% to 15%. Propagation is maximized when antennas are elevated above ground as much as possible and visual obstructions between the transmitter and receiver are avoided. Propagation with handheld radios is also optimized when antennas are held vertically. Transmissions from the depths of a river valley might only be receivable at a distance just beyond the ridgelines of the valley's horizons, with even greater limitations if the valley is forested. In addition, there are levels of output power insuf-ficient to reach the theoretical radio horizon because of degradation of the signal (by the inverse-square law that governs all electromagnetic radiation [*path loss*]) and from ground absorption of radio waves.

When traveling in a group, the ability of members to communicate over distances of several kilometers can greatly facilitate safety. Simple radio gear can be used to locate and rescue lost or injured members or to communicate information that allows the lost or injured person to self-rescue. The Federal Communications Commission (FCC) has allocated many frequency bands for both nonlicensed and licensed use by individuals for short-distance communication within the United States. Relatively inexpensive, lightweight, highly portable, and reliable radio transceivers are available for handheld use. For optimal communication within an expedition, the channels or frequencies to be used for various purposes must be defined in advance. Establishing regular check-in times and communication schedules helps to maintain group situational awareness, rapidly recognize problems (e.g., by failure to communicate on schedule), and maximize battery life.

FAMILY RADIO SERVICE

Family Radio Service (FRS) represents a group of 14 discrete frequencies in the UHF spectrum at 2.5-KHz intervals from 462.5625 MHz to 462.7125 MHz and from 467.5626 MHz to 467.7125 MHz. The FCC has designated FRS for use by individuals and businesses for short-range, two-way communication within the United States and its territorial islands.[19] Licensure is not required, and there are no age restrictions on usage. Transmission output power is limited to 0.5 watts, transmission mode is limited to FM voice, and transmitters cannot be legally modified after purchase. Two-way communication using FRS radios is *simplex* in type, meaning that the transmitting and receiving frequencies are identical. It is estimated that there are 50 to 80 million FRS radio transceivers in circulation,[3,4] ranging in price from $20 to $400, depending on their features. Radios from different manufacturers are interoperable.

The most commonly cited limitation of FRS radio is congestion of the channels as a result of number of units in use. This is less likely to be factor in a wilderness setting. Misperceptions exist about FRS's range of reliable communications. Manufacturers often claim communication ranges of 16 to 48 km (10 to 30 miles). Although true in idealized circumstances, these conditions are unlikely to be encountered in wilderness applications. From a practical standpoint, FRS communication is reliable over distances up to several kilometers. FRS radios are generally small enough to fit in a pocket and operate with disposable batteries or rechargeable battery packs. The operating life is greatest with fresh disposable batteries. Figure 105-1 shows a pair of typical FRS/GMRS hybrid radios (*A* and *B*).

GENERAL MOBILE RADIO SERVICE

General Mobile Radio Service (GMRS) is a service designated by the FCC for two-way FM voice communication by individuals and their immediate family members within the United States and its territorial islands.[22] Most GMRS transceivers are hybrids, sharing seven of the 467-MHz frequencies (i.e., channels 8 [467.5625 MHz] through 14 [467.7125 MHz]) with FRS and having

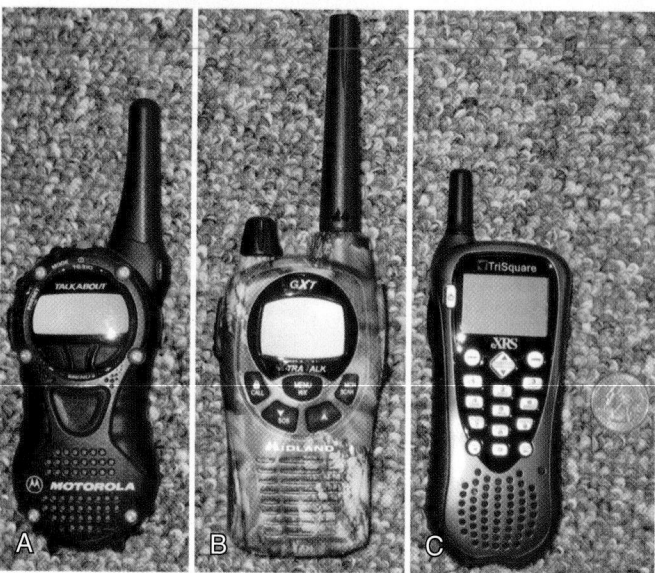

FIGURE 105-1 Several inexpensive handheld radios for short-distance communication. **A** and **B,** Hybrid Family Radio Service (FRS)/General Mobile Radio Service (GMRS) transceivers. **C,** 900-MHz (33-cm band) frequency-hopping spread spectrum (FHSS) radio. A common coin is pictured to provide scale. All three radios can be powered by rechargeable battery packs or disposable AA batteries. The FRS/GMRS radios require a license from the U.S. Federal Communications Commission (FCC) to transmit on the higher-wattage channels unique to the General Mobile Radio Service.

an additional 16 channels from 462.5500 MHz to 462.7250 MHz that are unavailable to FRS users. Unlike FRS, GMRS is licensed through the FCC. Licensure requires the applicant to be a U.S. citizen, over 18 years old, and not acting as an agent of a foreign government. An application must be approved, and a $65 application fee and $25 regulatory fee paid; online submission is available at http://wireless2fcc.gov.[7] Approval of an online application generally takes only a few days. The license is valid for 5 years. The GMRS license permits members of the holder's immediate family to communicate with the licensee without the need for separate licenses. Communication outside this restriction would require that each have a separate license.

GMRS transmitters are permitted to use up to 5 watts of output power on channels not shared with FRS. This allows clear communication with handheld units over a considerably greater range than with FRS, but still only a few miles. On the shared channels, transmitter power is intended to be restricted to the same 0.5 watts as for FRS. However, many hybrid transceivers require the user to switch manually to the lower power setting on the shared channels. Failure to do so violates FCC rules but does not disable the GMRS radio from transmitting on these frequencies at the higher wattage. In this circumstance, inequality in transmission power could result in the operator of an FRS radio being able to receive from a GMRS transmitter, but being unable to reply to the GMRS operator given the distance involved. GMRS radios built by different manufactures are interoperable (Figure 105-1A and B). In my tests using commonly available, inexpensive GMRS transceivers, clear communication in lightly forested terrain with low intervening hills was possible to a range of 4 to 5 km (2.4 to 3 miles). GMRS radios cannot be modified to extend range.

Handheld communication in GMRS is generally simplex in nature, but these radios can also be used in conjunction with mobile and fixed relay stations (i.e., repeaters) to greatly increase their range. In this circumstance, the radios operate in *duplex* mode, meaning that the transmission frequencies of the handheld unit and the repeater differ. By convention, these two frequencies are separated by 5 MHz to avoid the two signals talking over one another. As such, channels with 462-MHz frequencies are paired with channels having 467-MHz frequencies when repeaters are used. The frequency on which a receiver listens for a relayed message must correspond with that of the repeater station and not that of the original transmission. This salutary feature of GMRS can be exploited in the wilderness setting only where fixed or mobile repeaters are available. A single unit combining a mapping global positioning system (GPS) receiver with an FRS/GMRS hybrid radio exists that transmits FM voice as well as GPS coordinates of the user. This feature allows remote GPS tracking.[8] This function can be easily emulated manually if the person transmitting has a separate GPS receiver and simply reads the GPS coordinates during transmission. This practice should be part of the preplanned radio routine when check-in calls are made among expedition members during wilderness travel.

900-MHz BAND

In 2000, the FCC approved low-power, unlicensed, publicly available voice communications in the UHF band between 902 MHz and 928 MHz. Simultaneously, they issued a requirement that technical measures be taken to avoid the chaos of overuse found on other channels.[3,4,25] The solution to avoid channel overcrowding is a method called *frequency-hopping spread spectrum* (FHSS), which created an almost unlimited number of virtual channels within the 900-MHz band.[4] Radios using this digital technology continually shift among frequencies, spending less than 1 second at any given frequency. This largely eliminates multiple concurrent conversations being overheard on a given channel in areas with heavy radio traffic. Handheld FHSS radios are available at a cost of $30 to $250 (Figure 105-1C). These can use both disposable and rechargeable batteries, are highly portable, and have a practical range of about 1 to 2 km (0.6 to 1.2 miles). Repeaters for FHSS radio do not exist, and the range of the handheld units cannot be extended. The software algorithms that control the frequency hopping are proprietary, and these radios are not interoperable among manufacturers. Some models are capable of sending brief text messages to compatible receivers as an alternative to voice communication.

2-METER AND 70-CENTIMETER AMATEUR RADIO SERVICE

There are numerous highly capable, highly portable, handheld amateur radio service (i.e., ham) radios—called *handheld transceivers* or *handy talkies* (HTs)—that transmit in the VHF spectrum at 144 MHz to 148 MHz (i.e., the 2-m band), in the UHF spectrum at 420 MHz to 450 MHz (i.e., the 70-cm band), or in both (i.e., dual band) (Figure 105-2).[5] HTs typically cost from $120 to $500, depending on features. Most have removable antennae allowing the stock "rubber ducky" antenna to be easily replaced with more capable 0.625-wave, telescoping, base-loaded antenna. These greatly improve receiver performance but are slightly less portable. Most HTs use rechargeable metal hydride or lithium ion battery packs; however, optional battery trays that accept AA batteries are available for many models. The transmitter output is typically 1.5 to 5 watts. Many units can optionally transmit at lower power to extend battery life when the necessary range is short. Most dual-band units support both simplex and duplex modes, including VHF to UHF and UHF to VHF duplex. Radio communication with HTs primarily involves FM voice transmission, but these units are capable of receiving Morse code via carrier wave and voice by single side-band transmission.

The principle advantage of HTs over the handheld radios discussed earlier is range. Although the propagation characteristics of the radio waves transmitted from these devices are similar to those of the other frequencies, the receiver sensitivity and antenna efficiency tend to be better in HTs than in FRS, GMRS, and FHSS radios. Typical 2-m HT-to-HT range on flat terrain is 5 to 10 km (3 to 6 miles). When used with a repeater that has been strategically placed on elevated terrain, HT-to-repeater ranges of dozens of kilometers may be achieved, and subsequent relay from repeater to repeater can then extend the range for long-distance communication. However, as with GMRS radios, repeaters are unlikely to be available in the vast majority of wilderness settings. HTs tend to be ruggedly built, and some

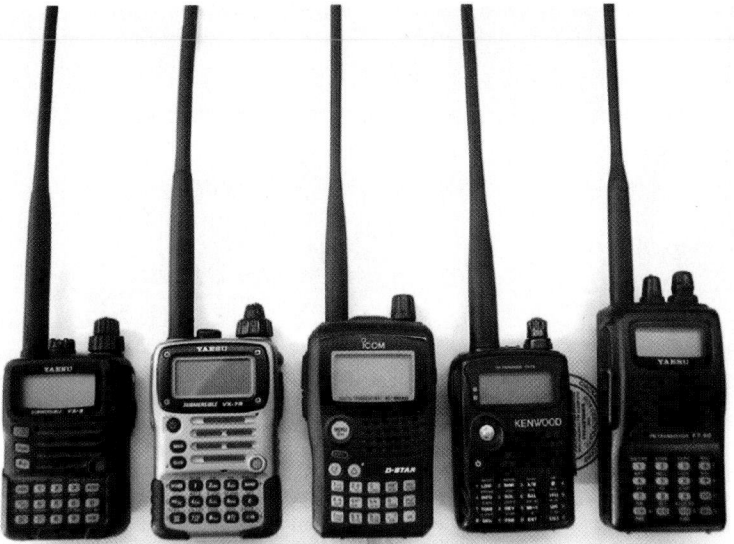

FIGURE 105-2 A selection of small, handheld handy talkies (HTs). These radios communicate on the 2-m (144-MHz) and 70-cm (420-MHz) amateur radio service bands. HTs are more capable and rugged than FRS, GMRS, and FHSS radios, but their use requires FCC licensure through a process that includes testing on radio theory, equipment, procedures, and regulations. The radios pictured here use rechargeable lithium ion batteries.

models are even submersible. Most can receive a broad range of the radio spectrum in addition to the transmitter frequencies, allowing weather broadcasts, commercial AM broadcasts, marine VHF, air band, and commercial FM radio to be monitored.

Radio communication in the United States using frequencies allocated to the amateur radio service requires FCC licensure. The most basic class of license that is sufficient for operation in the 2-m and 70-cm bands is the Technician Class license. There is no age limit or fee for licensure. Being granted a Technician Class license requires correctly answering 26 of 35 multiple-choice questions on a test covering radio theory and equipment and the regulations governing radio communication.[7] The test is administered by an FCC-approved examiner from the applicant's local area. Considerable course work or reading is required to pass the examination, but knowledge of Morse code is not required. A two-page form (FCC Form 605) must be completed and can be submitted online at http://wireless2fcc.gov. The applicant must assert he or she is not acting as an agent for a foreign government. If 2-m or 70-cm HTs are used for expedition communication, each individual using a transceiver requires a separate license.

Choice of radio equipment for wilderness communication will be guided by cost, range, battery life and type, regulations governing radio communication in the country of intended use, and licensure considerations. From the standpoint of pure utility, 2-m/70-cm dual-band HTs offer an excellent blend of range, cost, durability, and size. However, relatively few U.S. citizens hold amateur radio licenses, and the majority of individuals participating in a wilderness trip will have neither the time nor the background to acquire a Technician Class license before traveling. FRS and 900-MHz FHSS radios are inexpensive and do not require a license but have range limitations unsuitable for expeditions if members may be separated by more than a few kilometers. GMRS offers a workable compromise; the transmission power enables communication over a practical range, and licensure is simple and not prohibitively expensive.

All the forms of two-way radio communication discussed can be as simple as tuning to a prearranged channel, pushing the transmit button, and speaking into the radio microphone. The equipment for each type of service may have other functions to increase convenience and flexibility of operation, but these are not necessary for basic transmission and receipt of messages.

Other radio services available for portable use include citizens band, marine-VHF, and business-band radio. These are less practical than the alternatives previously discussed and offer no compelling advantages for terrestrial wilderness use.

A novel approach to short-range radio transmission recently became available that utilizes the user's smartphone as a communication interface. The device, goTenna, is a 2-watt VHF radio transceiver that operates at 151 MHz to 154 MHz. It pairs via Bluetooth LE with the operator's Android or iOS phone and allows transmission of text messages up to 160 characters in length, and sharing of GPS locations with any other individual within range who also has a device. Neither cellular service nor satellite communication is required for text communication. A free app allows users' locations to be displayed on previously downloaded offline maps, and text communication to be private between two individuals, shared between up to 10 members of a group, or "shouted" to any nearby person who has a unit. The range of communication varies with location; it is advertised to be approximately 4 miles in most backcountry terrain. goTenna units are sold in pairs for approximately $200 US, recharge using a USB cable, and weigh less than 2 ounces.

TWO-WAY LONG-DISTANCE VOICE COMMUNICATION

The ideal device for wilderness communication would offer the portability and convenience of a cellular telephone with worldwide coverage. As mentioned previously, land-based cellular telephony is inadequate for this task; however, satellite-based telephone services are well established and approach this ideal. It is now fairly routine to be able to call any telephone number (e.g., fixed phones, cellular phones, other satellite phones) from almost any location on Earth that has unobstructed access to the sky. Licensure is not required for use, but satellite telephones are expensive, the cost of on-air minutes is high, and their use requires preplanned subscription. Satellite phones are also expressly forbidden in some countries. These devices are unsurpassed for utility and flexibility, allowing access to any resource that is available by regular telephone, including Internet connectivity.

Numerous commercial services are available for satellite telephony. Several have near-global reach, whereas others are restricted to particular geographic areas determined by the location of their geostationary Earth orbit (GEO) satellites. All involve the use of handsets with folding antennas that are size-compatible

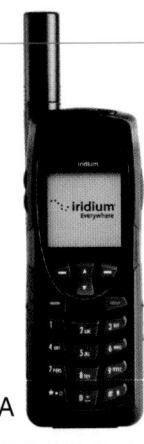
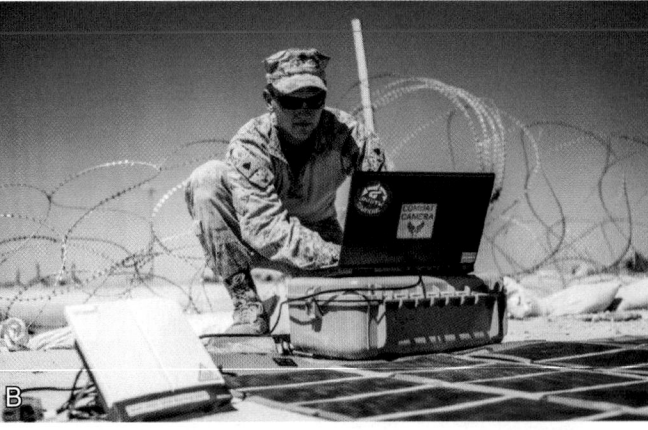

FIGURE 105-3 A, Typical satellite telephone. The antenna on most satellite phones folds for travel and must be extended and held vertically to optimize performance. Satellite phones are becoming smaller as technology evolves. **B,** Representative Broadband Global Area Network (BGAN) terminal. This device is plugged into the USB port of a laptop and oriented so that the integral antenna faces the GEO satellite for the region in question to provide satellite Internet service. A BGAN terminal allows standard voice communication and data transfer for text or e-mail and has the capacity to stream larger volumes of data at transfer rates that allow smooth, real-time video to be transmitted and received. Applications for telemedicine are promising. (**A** *Iridium 9555 Satellite Phone courtesy Chroma Communications, Inc; https:// satellitecommunications.ca/product/iridium-9555-satellite-phone.*)

with wilderness use (Figure 105-3A). Commercially available phones do not meet military standards for ruggedness, and the manufacturers make no particular claims regarding resistance to weather, water, dust, vibration, or being dropped. The latest-generation handsets cost from $500 to $1500, depending on available features; these can also be rented for temporary use at daily, weekly, or monthly rates. As for cell phone service, there is a bewildering array of rental and purchase plans and rate plans that may involve prepaid minutes or pay-as-you-go airtime. In general, calls to landline phones and cell phones are less expensive than calls to other in-plan satellite phones, whereas calls to satellite phones supported by other vendors are the most expensive. The principal service providers are described in the following sections.

IRIDIUM

The Iridium system has a constellation of 66 operational satellites in near-polar low Earth orbit (LEO). Iridium provides true global coverage. The number of satellites allows calls to be readily linked from an overhead satellite to three others and subsequently to ground stations or "gateways" in Hawaii and Arizona, reducing the potential for dropped calls. Each individual satellite has a maximum view time of about 10 minutes to a user on the ground, and passes the call to another linked satellite as the signal weakens. Because of the relatively low orbital altitude (476 miles), delay from transmission to reception (latency) is small and tends not to interrupt a normal mode of conversation.[16] Used, older-generation Iridium phones can be purchased for about $750, whereas the newest handsets cost $1400. Phones can be rented for rates that range from $3 to $10 per day. Most rate plans require a monthly fee in addition to a per-minute charge; a basic plan may cost $40 per month, with airtime costing an additional $1 to $1.75 per minute. The first generation of Iridium satellites are scheduled to be replaced beginning in 2015 by a new constellation of 66 operational satellites with six orbiting and nine ground-based spares (Iridium NEXT).

GLOBALSTAR

The Globalstar satellite system provides broad coverage but excludes the majority of the Arctic and Antarctic, sub-Saharan Africa, and parts of Asia. Globalstar uses a constellation of 60 satellites (48 operational) in LEO with an orbital inclination of 52

degrees. The system offers the same low call latency and satellite linkage as Iridium.[9] The Globalstar system is censored in China.

Globalstar-compatible handsets generally cost from $500 to $1000 and can be rented at rates comparable to those for other service providers. Recently, Globalstar began offering, through their SPOT subsidiary, handsets that are available from brick-and-mortar outdoor equipment stores. Globalstar per-minute rates vary by the region from which the call is made. There may be roaming charges in some regions.

INMARSAT

Inmarsat, based in Britain, makes use of three GEO satellites spaced more or less evenly about the planet for its current satellite telephony and Internet services. Coverage is broader than that of Globalstar but less than that of Iridium and excludes the majority of the Arctic and Antarctic as well as much of Alaska, Greenland, and Siberia. The high altitude of the GEO satellites introduces some delay into voice communication, resulting in latencies between transmission and reception of up to 0.5 second. However, the incidence of dropped calls is lower with GEO than with LEO satellites. Inmarsat appears to be concentrating its service efforts on satellite Internet connectivity.[13]

THURAYA

The Thuraya system is based in the United Arab Emirates and operates three GEO satellites that provide service to virtually all of Europe, much of Asia, Australia, and all but the southernmost portions of Africa.[27] Thuraya satellite phones are available for purchase for approximately $600 to $900 and can be rented for about $80 to $100 per week or $180 to $300 per month, exclusive of airtime. Outgoing calls cost between $2 and $12 per minute, depending on the type of phone being called; incoming calls do not incur charges. Thuraya offers an accessory for a popular brand of smartphone (SatSleeve) that converts the handset into a satellite phone with voice, e-mail, social media, and short-message service (SMS) functionality. Service is limited to the same service area as for their dedicated satellite phone handsets.[28]

Handsets for satellite telephone services discussed here generally provide 2 to 6 hours of talk time and 20 to 40 hours of continuous standby time on a battery charge. If a satellite service is selected with attention to geography and legal restrictions, and if the phone is safeguarded against damage, battery power is available, and the user can afford the charges, a satellite telephone offers the wilderness traveler the utility of a cellular phone.

SATELLITE MESSAGING DEVICES

A novel approach to satellite communication for wilderness travel is the introduction of *satellite messengers/communicators*.[6,26] These are portable, battery-powered devices that contain two elements: (1) a radio that receives continuous positional information from the Navstar GPS satellite constellation and (2) a transmitter, or transceiver, that communicates with LEO communication satellites (Figure 105-4A and B). Use requires purchase of monthly or yearly subscription plans from the companies that manufacture the devices and operate the associated communication satellites (SPOT, Inc., through their parent company, Globalstar; DeLorme, Inc., in cooperation with Iridium). These plans provide various levels of emergency response and communication. Basic satellite messengers allow travelers to be tracked online (Figure 105-4C); to "check in" with position, date, and time; to send preprogrammed one-way messages; and to initiate a rescue response by pressing an "SOS" button in case of emergency. Messages, tracking information, and requests for search and rescue (SAR) are transmitted to a monitoring center operated by the service vendor, then to the e-mail addresses or cellular phones of contacts designated by the user. Requests for emergency response also prompt notification of the user's emergency

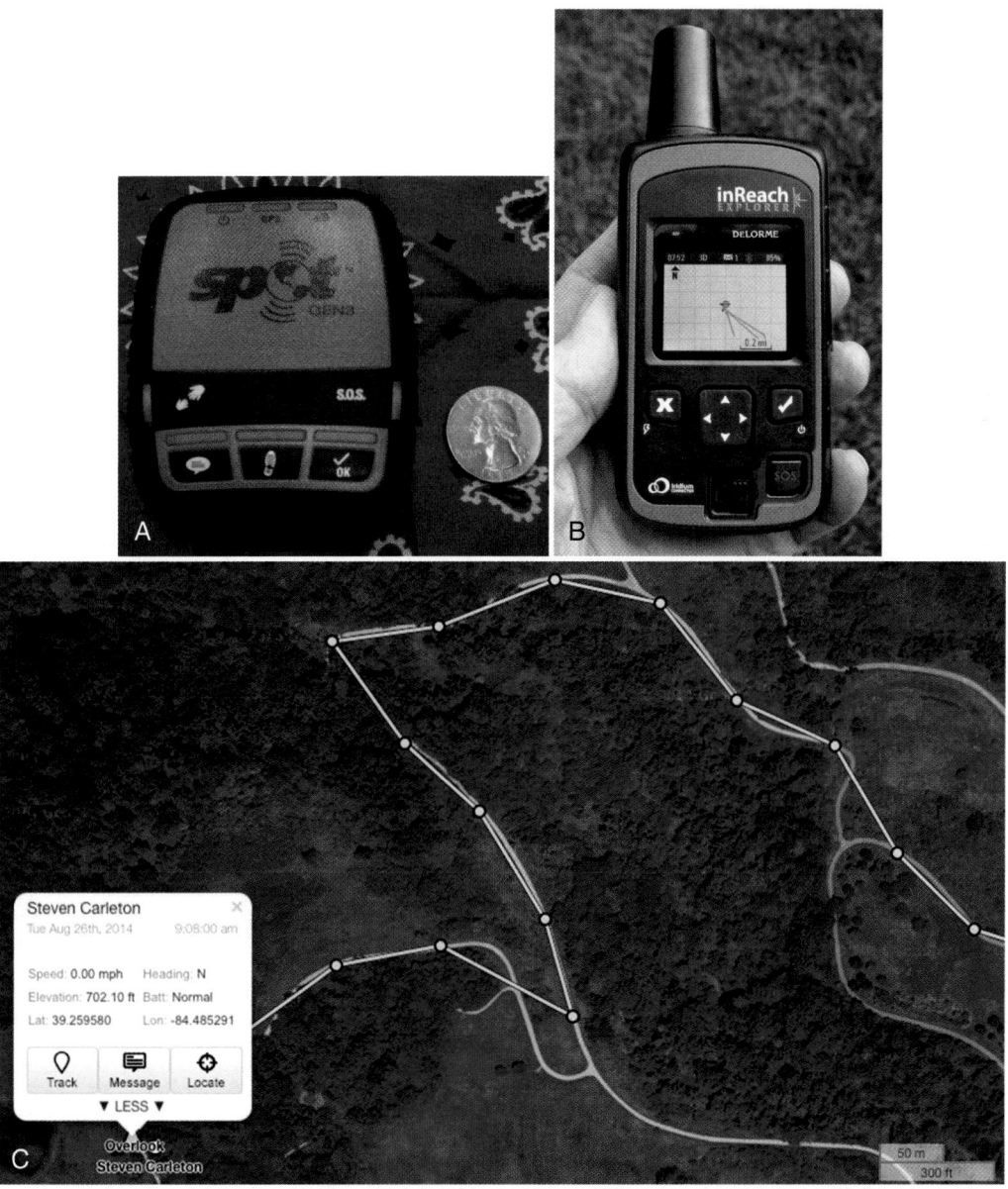

FIGURE 105-4 **A,** Satellite messenger with a common coin provided for scale. Note that the user interface consists of only four buttons and four indicator light-emitting diodes. The "HELP" and "9-1-1" buttons are recessed to prevent accidental activation. During routine use, the unit is turned on and given several minutes to establish a GPS fix, and the "OK" button in pressed to send the current coordinates and a preplanned check-in message to the cell phones or e-mail addresses of individuals designated by the user. Battery power is sufficient for hundreds of such check-in messages. **B,** Satellite communicator that permits simple GPS navigation as well as the functions described in **A.** This device also allows two-way satellite text communication using a virtual keyboard. **C,** Demonstration of the GPS tracking function supported by the device shown in **B.** GPS coordinates are sent via satellite at intervals determined by the user to a Web page that plots the user's location on a map or satellite image for each check-in time. Messages from the user can be appended to each plotted point to allow emergency contacts, family members, expedition support personnel, or media to follow the progress of a wilderness excursion.

contacts and are routed to the GEOS International Emergency Response Coordination Center, which contacts governmental emergency providers in the locale from which the transmission originated.[26] The button that initiates an emergency response is designed to minimize the possibility of accidental activation. If this occurs and is recognized, the user can rescind the request for emergency assistance by various methods. Nonetheless, numerous accidental emergency activations have occurred and represent a wasteful, potentially dangerous unintended consequence inherent to a one-button, automatic request for help.

Later-generation devices allow two-way text communication via SMS, transmission of brief e-mails, and posting of tracking information and messages to social media. Two-way communication allows transmitted tracking data to be augmented with timely status updates from the user and has the potential to reduce accidental SAR activations by allowing follow-up communication after the request for help is received. Most units capable of two-way communication pair via Bluetooth with a smartphone or tablet, which then serves as the communication interface. The advantages of convenience and familiarity offered by these external interfaces may be hampered by their fragility and limited battery life. Several models have the ability to function as standalone communicators using an on-screen, virtual keyboard as the communication interface (Figure 105-4B). These units also have full GPS functionality, allowing continuous determination of position, waypoint navigation, and some limited mapping features.

SATELLITE INTERNET

Few wilderness expeditions require access to the Internet to transmit e-mail, text, or two-way real-time voice and images. However, these functionalities exist and can be exploited for expedition media updates, technical assistance, telemedicine, and reassurance of the traveler's family and friends (see Chapter 104).

Data-enabled satellite telephones can be connected by cable to a computer to allow the phone to act as a wireless modem and permit Internet connectivity. This method of connection in effect is standard dial-up service, with data transfer rates of 2.4 kilobytes per second (KBps).[17,23] Some vendors have optional external data modules that compress the data and transmit through dedicated data servers, allowing effective transfer rates of up to 9.6 KBps over the 2.4-KBps connection. Such speeds are sufficient for transmitting and receiving e-mail or text but are impractical for transmission of large image files or real-time video. Inmarsat markets a dedicated satellite Internet service called the *Broadband Global Area Network* (BGAN) that was designed for such high-volume data streaming.[12]

A variety of manufacturers make dedicated satellite Internet terminals for use with the Inmarsat BGAN service (see Figure 105-3B). These terminals cost several thousand dollars, are comparable in size to a laptop computer, work exclusive of a satellite telephone, and have batteries that can be recharged by optional solar cells or other power sources. Battery life is 2 to 3.5 hours for voice calls or data streaming, with a continuous standby time of 36 hours. BGAN terminals can be rented. Several levels of service are offered by Inmarsat, including a standard data connection for browsing and e-mail, and multiple levels of dedicated streaming connectivity that provide data transfer rates from 32 KBps to 512 KBps.[11] These services are billed at monthly rates. For standard service, this rate may include an allocation of a specified amount of data (in megabytes [MB]) that can be transmitted without additional charge, or may be a base rate onto which any data transmissions are added as an additional fee. Typical fees are approximately $5 to $7 per MB. Data streaming with the dedicated services is generally billed by time. Transmission of 1 MB of data over a 200-KBps connection takes approximately 40 seconds.

BGAN terminals connect to a computer by a cable. The antenna, which is integral to the terminal case, is aimed in the direction of the GEO satellite serving the region. The terminal is configured using included software, and the Internet connection is established through the satellite. Once connected, browsing and data handling are the same as with any other networked computer.[11] Cautions about use of this technology are identical to those for satellite telephones: these devices are heavy, bulky,

power hungry, expensive, and illegal in some locales. BGAN is best suited to expeditions that operate from a base camp or vehicle and have a source of external power. Recently developed technology has overcome these obstacles, allowing true global access to the Internet, as well as voice-over Internet protocol (VoIP) communication via cellular phone.

SATELLITE WI-FI

In 2014, Iridium, Globalstar, and Addvalue (allied with Inmarsat) each introduced devices that establish a Wi-Fi "hot spot" (802.11 d/g/n standard) and communicate with their proprietary satellite networks. The Globalstar device (Sat-Fi) is intended primarily for vehicular and industrial applications. It requires a 12-V direct current (DC) external power supply and external antenna and measures $6.3 \times 6.3 \times 2.4$ inches. This device allows simultaneous data connections for up to eight compatible devices (Windows, MacIntosh, Android, or iOS) over a 30.5-m (100-foot) radius. Connectivity requires a proprietary application (app) to be installed on the mobile devices to be used. Data transfer rates of 9.6 KBps can be achieved under optimal conditions. This rate is sufficient for text communication via SMS, e-mail, and social media, but is very slow for image transmission or web browsing. Only a single voice call can be placed at a time. 9-1-1 calling is supported in North America. The device does not automatically upload GPS positional data to permit tracking, although this functionality is planned for the near future. The device costs approximately $1000, is available from numerous online retailers, and requires one of a menu of data and voice plans. Data rates are approximately $1.00 (US dollar/USD) per minute, but burst transmission greatly reduces the time required for messages to be sent and received. Voice rates are similar to Globalstar satellite phone rates and may include roaming charges. Although the device is more portable than a BGAN unit, it suffers from many of the same limitations for individual use.[10]

The Iridium satellite wireless hot spot (Iridium GO!) is designed specifically for wilderness operation; it measures $4.5 \times 3.25 \times 1.25$ inches, has an integral folding antenna, and is powered by internal, replaceable, rechargeable lithium ion batteries or a 5-V DC USB power supply. A full battery charge provides 7 hours of talk time and 16 hours of standby time. The unit meets military standards for ruggedness and is water and dust resistant. It establishes a data connection between a line-of-sight satellite and up to five Wi-Fi-enabled Android or iOS mobile devices that are running a downloadable, proprietary app. Connectivity is possible over a radius of 30.5 m (100 feet). The data transfer rate is 2.5 KBps under optimal conditions, a speed sufficient for text transmissions via SMS, e-mail, or social media. Download of a 100-KB image might require more than 5 minutes, and transfer of 1 MB of data might require almost 1 hour. The device is available from online retailers for $800 to $850. Service plans charge approximately $1.00 USD/min for data. Voice rates begin at $1.49 USD/min to any phone, and $0.66 USD/min to other Iridium phones. Voice rates fall as larger plans are purchased. Outgoing SMS messages are billed per message at a base cost of $0.50 USD each. Incoming messages are free. The device has a one-button emergency response activation feature. Online GPS tracking is supported similar to the satellite messengers/communicators discussed earlier.[15]

The Inmarsat-compatible device (Wideye iSavi) offers near-global coverage, except for high polar latitudes. It is intermediate in size between the Iridium GO! and Globalstar SatFi units, weighing 1.9 lb and measuring $7.1 \times 6.7 \times 1.2$ inches. It permits data transmission rates of up to 384-KBps download speed and 240-KBps upload speed and supports voice, SMS, and social media functions. The standard, rechargeable, internal, 3 amp-hour lithium ion battery allows 2 hours of continuous transmission time and 24 hours of standby time. The device costs $1350 USD. Data plans charge $2.79 USD to $5.00 USD per MB.[1]

From the standpoint of portability, support for GPS tracking, facilitation of both voice and data communication, and emergency response initiation, satellite wireless hot-spot technology approaches a practical ideal for multifunctional wilderness communication. Initial cost may be prohibitive for the individual traveler, and service costs can be daunting if discipline is not exercised in their use. The capabilities of these devices can only be realized through a paired smartphone or tablet computer, which tend to be fragile and have relatively brief battery lives. Satellite Wi-Fi and all other forms of satellite-based communication require unobstructed access to the sky. If a traveler encounters an emergency in a slot canyon, cave, or even under a particularly heavy forest canopy, these aids may be inoperable.

EMERGENCY BEACONS

Emergency beacons are a form of one-way, satellite-based communication that initiates a SAR response from governmental agencies. They have been in use for decades and are mandated by law for oceangoing ships (i.e., emergency position-indicating radio beacons [EPIRBs]) and for aircraft (i.e., emergency locator transmitters [ELTs]). More recently, this concept has been extended to land-going individuals in the form of personal locator beacons (PLBs). Before development of practical digital radio technology, EPIRBs, ELTs, and PLBs transmitted only an analog distress tone and homing signal at 121.5 MHz that was monitored by Cosmicheskaya Sistema Poiska Avariynyh Sudov–Search and Rescue Satellite Tracking (COSPAS-SARSAT) satellites. In addition to initiating SAR operations, this signal assisted with coarse radiolocation of the transmitter. Historically, the vast majority of emergency calls triggered on 121.5 MHz were false alarms or spurious activations caused by nonemergency transmissions with overlapping frequencies. This resulted in enormous resource expenditures without demonstrable benefit because of inability to identify the source of the communication to check its veracity and thus to abort an unnecessary response.[14,24]

As technology improved, a digital beacon was added at 406 MHz that transmits a distress call that includes identifying information about the transmitter. On enabled models, the signal may also include GPS coordinates of the transmitter. PLBs require registration with national authorities in the country of origin and intended use. In the United States, the registering agency is the National Oceanic and Atmospheric Administration (NOAA).[20] International registration is available through the COSPAS-SARSAT center. Registration is free, can be made online at http://www

.beaconregistration.noaa.gov or http://www.406registration.com/ibrd, allows the PLB to be linked to the identity of the user, and includes emergency contact information that can be accessed by SAR authorities on receipt of a distress call. Although false alarms from 406-MHz devices occur, the ability to identify and contact the device operator allows false alarms to be recognized and the rescue response to be aborted in approximately 70% of cases. The 406-MHz beacons' homing function is superior to that of the 121.5-MHz signals, allowing the receiving satellite to locate the source of transmission within about a 5-km (3-mile) circle.[14]

Satellite monitoring of the 121.5-MHz service was discontinued in February 2009, but PLBs that transmit on both this and the 406-MHz frequencies are still common. Commercial airliners continue to monitor 121.5 MHz, and the analog signal may be used by local SAR assets for ground-based radiolocation. Older devices that use only this frequency should be avoided.

Pocket-sized PLBs can be purchased for $300 to $600 or rented for $50 to $60 per week. PLBs typically have battery power for 20 to 48 hours of continuous operation once activated, depending on temperature. Because they communicate with satellites, PLBs avoid the range limitations encountered with ground-based, line-of-sight radio communications. They offer tremendous utility for initiating SAR operations in an emergency. However, they are inflexible. PLBs only transmit the trigger for an emergency response and the user's identification and general positional information. Media reports document frequent incidents of inappropriate SAR activations and poorly conceived expeditions by unprepared individuals who were emboldened in their travel planning by the notion that rescue was available at the touch of a button. Such an attitude ignores the cost of the emergency response and risk to rescuers and should be discouraged. As with all forms of satellite communication, use of PLBs requires unobstructed access to the sky.

REFERENCES

Complete references used in this text are available online at expertconsult.inkling.com.

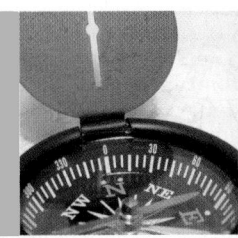

CHAPTER 106
Wilderness Navigation Techniques

STEVEN C. CARLETON

Many environmental illnesses occur as a consequence of becoming lost. Even well-prepared individuals may suffer hypothermia, heatstroke, frostbite, immersion foot, sunburn, dehydration, starvation, and a variety of other conditions if they become separated from the resources of their expedition or have an unanticipated extension of their time outdoors. The individual can minimize the possibility of becoming lost by maintaining awareness of position and direction and familiarity with local landmarks at all times during travel. This chapter discusses satellite navigation, terrestrial coordinate systems, route finding with the magnetic compass, map reading, application of celestial navigation in wilderness travel, and employment of alternative methods for recovering when lost.

All of navigation boils down to two processes: (1) determination of direction and (2) establishment of position. Awareness of position and direction permit practice of a fundamental process

in navigation, the process of "dead" (deduced) reckoning. Dead reckoning is the estimation of current location based on knowledge of the direction, rate, and time of travel from a known starting point. Whenever traveling in the wilderness, dead reckoning should be practiced so that a general awareness of position is never lost. Estimates of time of travel, rate of travel, and direction of travel should be recorded whenever possible so that the last known position and subsequent movement from that position are preserved. In the wilderness setting, determination of direction and fixing of position may be simple but can be challenging. Generally, routes and landmarks are provided by a map, but local knowledge from memory may have to suffice. Direction is often derived from a magnetic compass, but other methods of direction finding can be exploited when the compass is forgotten, lost, damaged, or unreliable. Lines of position (LOPs) are established by trails or bearings to identifiable landmarks; however, shorelines, watercourses, firebreaks, and bearings to celestial bodies or radio sources can substitute. Position can be estimated with the careful practice of dead reckoning, determined from scratch by triangulation of bearings from landmarks, or fixed with astonishing ease and accuracy with the use of a satellite navigation receiver. None of these navigational techniques is prohibitively expensive or so equipment intensive as to be incompatible with a hiker's kit. Each method requires understanding of its practice and limitations. Nothing substitutes for preparation, but effective wilderness navigation can be practiced using nothing more than the clues offered by the environment and the wits of the navigator. For travelers in the continental United States, it is significant that no site is more than 48 km (30 miles) from a road, and thus from a potential source of help.

NAVIGATION WITH THE GLOBAL NAVIGATION SATELLITE SYSTEMS

Satellite navigation systems have been in widespread civilian use for decades after implementation of the Navstar Global Positioning System (GPS) by the United States and the Global Orbiting Navigation Satellite System (GLONASS) by Russia. The European Union has partially implemented a similar system (Galileo), as have the Chinese (BeiDou). Licensing requirements and trade agreements have pressured the manufacturers of satellite receivers to make chipsets that are interoperable among these systems. Combined GPS/GLONASS receivers are currently on the market, and receivers that will be able to access all four systems are on the horizon. Although GPS has been an appropriate generic term for satellite navigation, it is now more appropriate to refer to these collective technologies as the Global Navigation Satellite System (GNSS).[3] This term will be used for general reference to satellite navigation in this chapter unless the specific features of an individual service or device are being discussed.

Space-based navigation systems use satellites as predictable extraterrestrial references for determination of terrestrial position. Calculation of position is based on circles of equal distance from the satellites. GPS consists of a constellation of 24 active satellites arrayed in six orbital planes, with four satellites per orbital plane. The orbital planes are inclined to Earth's equator by 55 degrees. The orbital paths of the satellites are nearly circular and have an altitude of approximately 20,000 km (12,425 miles; medium Earth orbit [MEO]) with an orbital period of 11 hours and 58 minutes. At any given time, five to eight satellites are available in line of sight to a GPS receiver anywhere on the surface of the earth.[13,23]

The method of position determination using GPS depends on calculation of the range between the satellite and receiver. GPS signals are transmitted on two frequencies by each satellite: L1 (1575.4 MHz) and L2 (1227.6 MHz).[11] Transmitted information includes the precise time as kept onboard the satellite by multiple atomic clocks, a satellite *ephemeris* (i.e., a catalog of predicted positions), and data concerning corrections for atmospheric propagation of radio signals and satellite clock errors. The GPS receiver decodes the positional data for each satellite and compares the timing information transmitted by the satellite with time as kept by the receiver's onboard clock. Because distance = speed × time, the transit time of the signal allows calculation of the distance between receiver and satellite.[20] At any given instant, a GPS receiver in contact with a Navstar satellite will lie on the surface of a sphere of equal distance from the satellite. The intersection of this sphere of equal distance with the earth's surface forms a circle of equal distance. The intersection of two such circles occurs at only two points, and the intersection of three such circles occurs at a single point on the earth's surface[13,23,24,34] (Figure 106-1); this is the position of the receiver. If the intersection of the sphere of equal distance of a fourth satellite is added, the approximate altitude of the receiver can be determined. Software allows the GPS receiver to choose the optimal group of four satellites for position determination among the subset of satellites within the line of sight of the receiver.

As originally configured, two levels of service were provided by GPS; the Standard Positioning Service (SPS) and the Precise

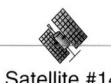

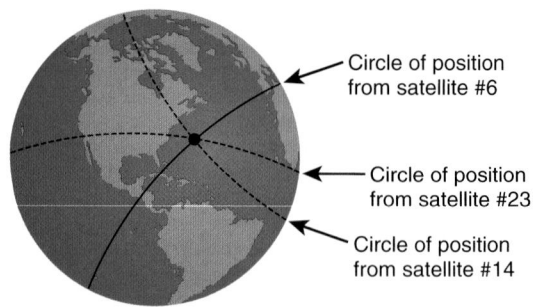
Satellite #14

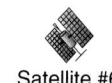
Satellite #6

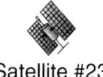
Satellite #23

FIGURE 106-1 A Global Positioning System fix from the intersection of three circles of equal distance from three separate satellites. (*From Monahan K, Douglass D:* GPS instant navigation, *Bishop, Calif, 1998, Fine Edge Productions.*)

Positioning Service (PPS). SPS provided civilian users with positional accuracy to 100 m (328 feet) 95% to 98% of the time, to 50 m (164 feet) 65% of the time, and to 40 m (131 feet) 50% of the time. The intentional inaccuracy of SPS resulted from the introduction of timing errors into the broadcast signal from the satellites on frequency L1; this degradation of precise data from the satellites is called *selective availability* and is controllable from the ground. Selective availability was formally implemented 1 year after public availability of GPS was granted in 1994 and was discontinued in 1999. There are no plans for reimplementation, and PPS is the level of service available to all military and civilian users at the time of this writing. PPS provides positional accuracy of 15 m (49 feet), velocity accuracy of 0.1 m/sec, and time accuracy of 100 nanoseconds. To comply with the requirements of safety-of-life aviation applications, the Wide Area Augmentation System (WAAS) was developed in cooperation with the U.S. Federal Aviation Administration (FAA) and Department of Transportation. WAAS consists of 25 North American ground stations that monitor and correct errors in the GPS satellite signals caused by ionospheric interference, orbital drift, and clock errors. Corrections are transmitted on the L1 frequency by geostationary satellites and can be received by enabled receivers. WAAS was implemented for general application in 2000 and for aviation safety-of-life applications in 2003. WAAS-enabled civilian GPS receivers allow less than 3-m (10-foot) horizontal and 6-m (20-foot) vertical positional accuracy 95% of the time, with 7-m (23-foot) accuracy the remainder of the time.[15] Currently, WAAS is available only in the continental United States, including Alaska, border areas of Canada and Mexico, and the surrounding coastal waters.

GLONASS has marginally better satellite coverage than GPS in high northern and southern latitudes because of its high orbital inclination to the equator (64.8 degrees). Its positional accuracy is 30 m (98 feet). GLONASS-capable receivers are less widely available than GPS receivers, but receivers capable of operating with both systems will soon become standard. The GLONASS constellation has 30 satellites (24 active, 6 spare) in three orbital planes at 120-degree intervals in longitude.

Galileo, a cooperative venture of the European Union and European Space Agency, had its initial satellite launch in 2011. Eight satellites were in place as of March 2015, with a total of 18 to be in orbit by the end of 2015. The completed constellation will consist of 30 satellites in MEO, occupying three orbital planes with an orbital inclination of 56 degrees. Galileo is intended to become operational for general use by 2016 and will be publically available and interoperable with GLONASS and GPS. Galileo will offer 1-m (3.3-foot) accuracy in position and altitude for latitudes of 75 degrees north to 75 degrees south.[14] Coverage will extend into extreme polar latitudes, although with lesser accuracy.

BeiDou, the Chinese system, became operational in greater China in 2003, offering 100-m (328-foot) accuracy. The second phase of deployment, BeiDou-2, offered regional coverage in the Asia-Pacific area with 25-m (83-foot) accuracy in late 2012. Global coverage with a constellation of five GEO and 27 MEO satellites is anticipated by 2020.[1,8]

The raw output of a GNSS receiver is in latitude and longitude to the nearest second of arc or in Universal Transverse Mercator (UTM) grid coordinates to the nearest meter. This information is somewhat abstract in isolation, but software included with the receiver permits the user to understand absolute and relative position and perform sophisticated navigational feats in the absence of other navigational aids. Even without a map or compass, GNSS allows users to determine their current position, direction, course traveled, deviation from an intended course of travel, bearing and linear distance to predetermined targets, and velocity. Hikers with GNSS devices can literally have no idea about where they are, but if they have the coordinates of where they want to go, they can find their way to safety with remarkable fidelity. Even the simplest commercially available GNSS receivers render it almost impossible to become lost over distances likely to be encountered on a hike. These receivers dispense with complex displays and have only two buttons. At the start of a hike, the user turns the unit on, allows it a brief period to acquire a fix, then pushes a button to record the coordinates of the initial position as a *waypoint*. As the hike progresses, the receiver continually determines and displays the distance and direction to the waypoint and provides an arrow that points to the waypoint (Figure 106-2). As long as the user follows the displayed arrow on the return hike, he or she will move toward

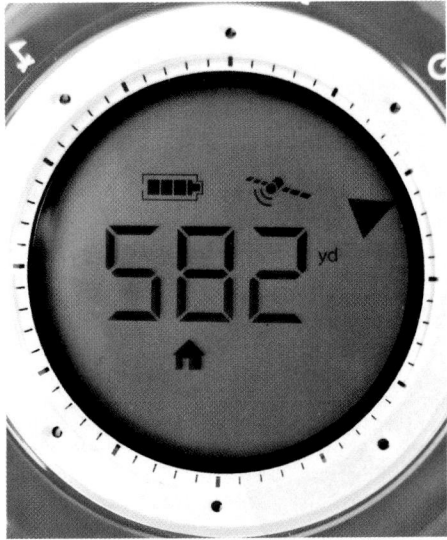

FIGURE 106-2 A simple, single-function, Global Positioning System (GPS) receiver. The screen displays the distance to a known waypoint (designated by the "house" symbol) and has an arrow on the rim that points in the direction of the waypoint. As the user hikes in the direction indicated by the arrow, the distance counts down and, in the absence of obstructions to travel, the waypoint is gained.

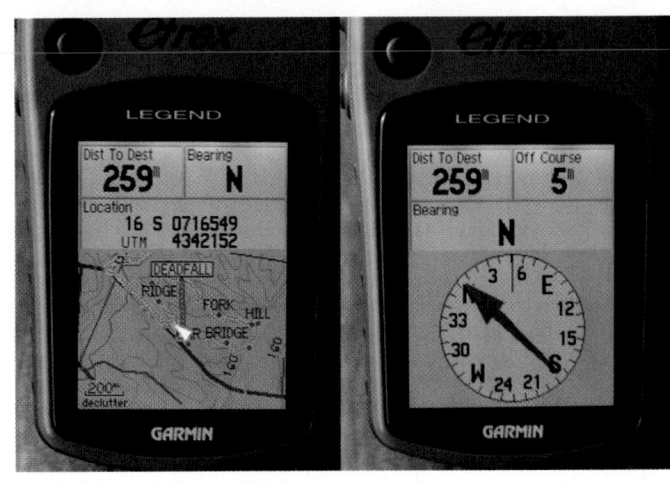

FIGURE 106-3 A typical GPS receiver showing two navigation screens. The screen on the left displays the terrestrial coordinates of the user's position in the Universal Transverse Mercator format, with a moving map that shows the current position (indicated by the ▲ symbol) and several labeled waypoints. The tracks made by the user when walking the route are shown as a continuous line of small dots. A pink line shows the bearing line from the user's starting location to a selected waypoint (i.e., "DEADFALL"). The data fields display the distance to the waypoint in meters and the true bearing to the waypoint. North is at the top of the screen. The screen on the right shows the bearing and distance to the selected waypoint and a graphic representation of the direction of travel to the waypoint. The data field in the upper right corner displays the distance in meters that the hiker is off of the line between the original position and the waypoint. If the user walks a course that minimizes the deviation from this line, the waypoint will be gained. If the user is forced to detour by terrain features, he or she can return to the line to get back on course. Note the scale indicators (i.e., meter bar at the bottom left of the screen and meter ring around the current position of the hiker).

the starting location. This type of receiver will not allow the traveler to predict or avoid impassable obstacles that may lie on the straight-line course between the current position and the goal. However, most general-purpose GNSS receivers have a "moving map" feature that solves this issue, as described later. All receivers can calculate the heading of travel and thus provide the user with a method of determining cardinal directions by walking a brief straight course.

Waypoint navigation is a feature of particular utility for wilderness travel. Waypoints can be preloaded into the GNSS receiver via the keypad or downloaded from a personal computer, or they can be added on the hike with a few keystrokes as locations of interest are encountered. Most receivers have memory capacity sufficient for storage of several hundred waypoints. A group of sequential waypoints can be stored as a route, and the actual path followed between waypoints on the outbound leg of a route can be stored as tracks. *Tracks* are the virtual equivalent of the user's footprints and are displayed on the GPS screen as a string of points or a continuous, meandering line. On the return leg of a route, the receiver can display the path defined by the tracks of the user, the bearing and distance to any selected waypoint, and the current course (Figure 106-3). Many receivers inform the user that a waypoint is near by sounding a proximity alarm and then automatically switch to the next waypoint in the route. Theoretically, these capabilities allow a hiker to follow a route in conditions of near-zero visibility when using no references other than the display of the GNSS receiver. Identification of a large number of waypoints connected by tracks on a complex route essentially allows the user to follow a "breadcrumb trail" to return to the objective[34] (Figure 106-3).

GNSS reaches its greatest usefulness when used in conjunction with a map. Many inexpensive GNSS units include low-resolution base maps with a resolution of a few hundred meters. More capable receivers often include or permit downloading of high-resolution topographic maps. Receivers with mapping capabilities display the user's current position, with any stored waypoints, routes, or tracks superimposed on the map image (Figure 106-3). When a topographic map is available—whether virtual or on paper—GNSS allows users to plot their position and route at will, determine bearings to landmarks even when the landmarks are not visible, enter the location of terrain features for use as predetermined waypoints, and precalculate the distances to be traveled during a trek. The fullest use of GNSS with a map requires understanding two frequently used terrestrial coordinate systems: the geodetic coordinate system and UTM coordinate system.

The explosion in cellular telephone technology was followed a decade later by widespread civilian access to satellite navigation. This had an unintended consequence, with a negative societal impact in countries that offered 9-1-1 or equivalent emergency call services. Replacement of landlines by mobile phones hampered the ability of emergency services automatically to determine the location of mobile callers. In recognition of this problem, the U.S. Federal Communication Commission (FCC) established a 1994 standard requiring mobile phone carriers to provide 9-1-1 service that allows location of the user to be established. The inclusion of GPS-capable chipsets in cellular phones followed. Of the 228 million cell phones sold in the United States in 2011, 90% were GPS capable. Worldwide, 40% of the 1.6 billion cell phones purchased were GPS capable. The vast majority of currently manufactured GNSS chipsets are incorporated into cell phones rather than into dedicated GNSS receivers.[5] In terms of wilderness navigation, this trend is a dual-edged sword; although satellite navigation capability is extremely widespread, the majority of the devices that offer this capability are not designed for wilderness use. They are fragile, have a relatively short battery life, and have less capable antennas than dedicated navigation receivers. Reliance on cell phones as an aid to navigation has the potential to save lives, but also to embolden otherwise unprepared travelers to venture into the wild without more appropriate gear.

GEODETIC COORDINATE SYSTEM

The geodetic terrestrial coordinates of latitude and longitude evolved in response to the requirements of navigation at sea, where identifiable landmarks may be absent for thousands of miles, and unobstructed visibility in good weather may permit identification of a landfall from a considerable distance. With this coordinate system, the earth has a North Pole and South Pole that define its axis of rotation. This axis passes through the earth's center. Any plane that passes through the center of the earth describes a circle on the surface called a *great circle*. The equator is the great circle described by the plane that passes perpendicular to the earth's axis. The great circle of a plane that contains the earth's axis is called a *meridian*. Meridians always run due north and south and converge at the poles. The Prime Meridian is the great circle that passes through Greenwich, England. Greenwich was assigned the Prime Meridian by treaty in 1884 in recognition of the work on astronomy and navigation performed at the Greenwich Royal Observatory.

The angular measurement or arc between the Prime Meridian and the local meridian passing through any other point on the planet's surface is called the *longitude* (λ) of that point. Longitude is measured in degrees, minutes, and seconds of arc east or west of the Prime Meridian, from 0 degrees through 180 degrees. Longitude bears a special relationship to time. Within reasonable standards of accuracy, Earth rotates once about its axis every 24 hours. As such, Earth moves through 360 degrees of longitude in 24 hours, that is, 15 degrees each hour and 1 degree every 4 minutes. It is this fact that establishes the conventions by which sundials work, clocks run, and time and distance are defined. It also forever links the modern practice of celestial position finding to the accurate keeping of time.

The angular measurement between the plane of the equator, as measured north or south from the center of the earth to a point on the surface, is the *latitude* (L) of that point (Figure 106-4). All points at the same latitude form a *parallel* of latitude. Latitude is measured in degrees, minutes, and seconds of arc from 0 degrees through 90 degrees north or south. As such, the latitude of the equator is 0 degrees, whereas that of each pole is 90 degrees north or south. Every point on the surface of the earth is defined by a specific longitude and latitude.

A nautical mile (i.e., 1852 m, 6076 feet, 1.15 statute miles) is the distance on a great circle that covers an angle of 1 minute of arc as measured from the center of the earth. A degree of arc

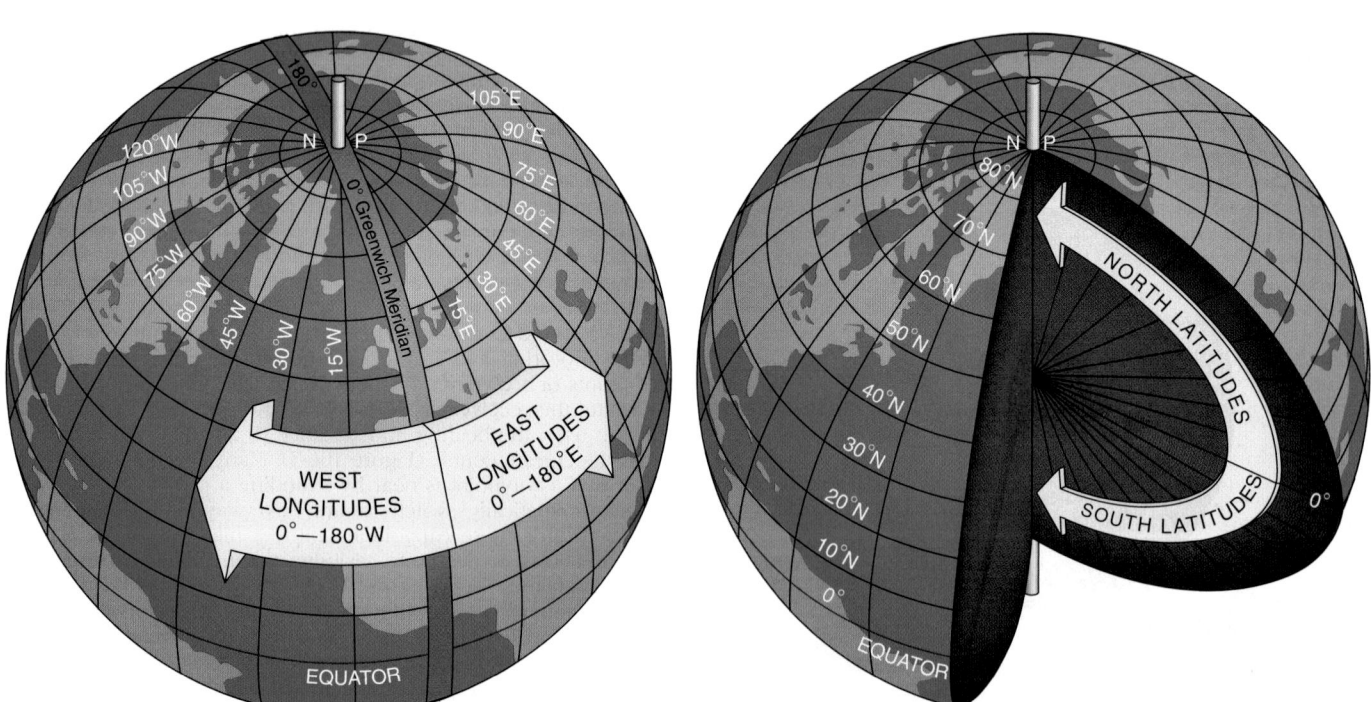

FIGURE 106-4 Meridians of longitude (including the Prime Meridian) and parallels of latitude as measured north and south of the equator in degrees of arc from the center of the earth. *(With permission from the Department of the Air Force: Survival Training Edition AF Manual 64-3, Randolph Air Force Base, Texas, 1969, Air Training Command.)*

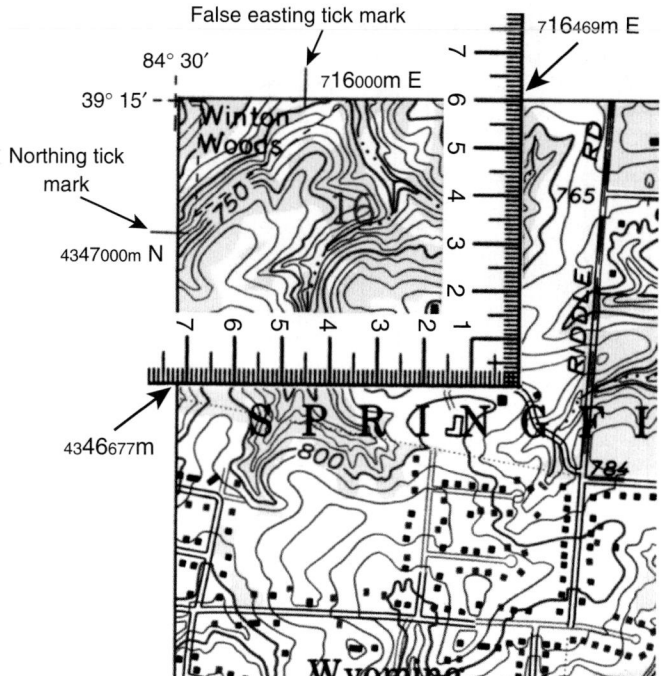

FIGURE 106-5 Portion of a United States Geological Survey 1:24,000 map showing the blue Universal Transverse Mercator tick marks on the map margin that give values for false easting ($^716^{000}$ m E) and northing ($^{43}47^{000}$ m N). A 1:24000 Universal Transverse Mercator roamer scale is superimposed on the map. The points of intersection between the arms of the roamer scale and the map margin allow the grid reference for the point at the outside corner of the roamer scale to be read.

(60 minutes of arc) is thus 60 nautical miles, and 1 second of arc is equal to about 100 feet. It must be recognized that 1 minute of latitude will always equal 1 nautical mile, whereas 1 minute of longitude will only equal 1 nautical mile at the equator. At all points north or south of the equator, 1 minute of longitude will cover less than 1 nautical mile, as a result of the convergence of the meridians toward the poles. At either of Earth's poles, one could walk through 360 degrees of longitude in only a few strides.

Latitude and longitude appear along the margins of topographic maps distributed by the United States Geological Survey (USGS) and by other national governmental organizations responsible for cartography. At each map corner, the latitude and longitude of the point defined by the intersection of the horizontal and vertical map margins is recorded in degrees, minutes, and seconds (Figure 106-5). On standard USGS 7.5- and 15-minute maps, latitude and longitude notations appear on the margins at intervals of 2.5 minutes of arc and are marked with black tick marks on the inside edges of each margin.

Although it is conceptually useful, the nautically based latitude and longitude system is less well suited to land navigation, where precision on the order of tens of meters is often required and visibility may be limited by terrain features and vegetation. In addition, calculation of a new position based on the direction and distance traveled from a known starting point requires intimidating mathematics in the geodetic system, and the interconversion of minutes or seconds of arc to meters or feet is cumbersome and confusing. For these reasons, the UTM grid or the Military Grid Reference System was adopted by the United States Defense Mapping Agency in 1947 to cope with the specific exigencies of maneuvering and delivering ordnance on land.

UNIVERSAL TRANSVERSE MERCATOR COORDINATE SYSTEM

The UTM and Military Grid Reference System grids are metric, make use of the transverse Mercator map projection in common with maps distributed by the USGS, and require no conversion

between distances expressed as angles and linear measures of distance expressed in meters (m) or kilometers (km). UTM divides the earth's surface from 80 degrees south latitude to 84 degrees north latitude into 60 south-to-north–running zones arrayed around the surface of the planet like narrow slices of an orange. Each zone is 6 degrees wide in longitude. The zones are consecutively numbered from 1 through 60 beginning at an index line, the International Date Line, and progressing eastward. Each zone is subdivided from south to north in 8-degree increments of latitude (except the northernmost zone, which encompasses 12 degrees of latitude [i.e., 72 degrees north to 84 degrees north]). The south-to-north divisions of each zone are labeled consecutively and alphabetically from C through X, excluding the letters I and O to avoid confusion with the numbers 1 and 0 (Figure 106-6). In UTM, terrestrial coordinates are expressed in meters east of a false origin and north of a latitude index line. The *false origin* for any zone is an arbitrarily assigned south-north line 500,000 m (1,640,420 feet) to the west of the central meridian of the UTM zone of interest. Progress to the east of the false origin is termed *false easting* or simply *easting*. In the northern hemisphere, the latitude index is the equator. In the southern hemisphere, the latitude index is the southern limit of strip C (i.e., 80 degrees south latitude). Progress to the north of the latitude index is termed *northing*.[7,23,40]

UTM coordinates are printed on all USGS maps produced during the past several decades. These appear as numbered blue tick marks occurring at 1-km intervals along the horizontal and vertical map margins. The numbers express UTM eastings and northings and thus increase from left to right and from bottom to top (i.e., to the right and up). By convention, the central meridian of each of the 60 UTM zones is assigned an easting value of 500,000 m E (500,000 m east of the false origin of the zone). Easting values less than 500,000 thus lie west of the central meridian for the applicable UTM zone, and easting values of more than 500,000 lie east of the central meridian for the UTM zone in question. Slight overlap (i.e., 80 km) between adjacent zones prevents negative easting values from occurring. Similarly, easting values of more than 1,000,000 are never encountered; they would lie beyond the overlap into the next zone to the east. For the northern hemisphere, northing values are expressed as meters north of the equator and range from zero to 10,000,000 m N (10,000,000 m north of the equator) (Figure 106-7). Negative values for northing are avoided for the southern hemisphere by labeling the equator as 10,000,000 m N and counting upward toward this number as one moves northward from the southern latitude index (i.e., 80 degrees south latitude).

On the horizontal margins of the map in the left upper and right lower corners, one of the last blue tick marks is labeled with a six-digit number in mixed large and small numerals (i.e., $^716^{000}$ m E in Figure 106-5). This refers to a line that is 716,000 m east of the false origin or 216,000 m east of the central meridian of the applicable UTM zone, because the false easting value is more than 500,000 (the central meridian in this example is in UTM Zone 16 at 87 degrees west longitude). Similarly, one of the blue tick marks at the right lower or left upper vertical margins of the map image is labeled with a multidigit number (i.e., $^{43}74^{000}$ m N for the left upper border), indicating a line 4,374,000 m north of the equator in UTM row S. Note that, within the six-digit false easting value and seven-digit northing value, the numerals in larger type represent thousands of meters or kilometers. UTM tick marks on a map margin between corners are labeled with three- or four-digit numbers. The last two digits, which are in large numerals, represent whole kilometers in relation to the UTM reference value given near the corner of the map. Thus, for practical purposes, when navigating within an area of several dozens to several hundreds of square kilometers, the UTM margin tick marks on any large-scale USGS map can be thought of as a simple kilometer scale. The long and intimidating numeric labels on the tick marks can be ignored (except to recognize that they indicate 1-km increments on the map margin).

Every point on the earth's surface can be described by a unique false easting and northing value; this is described as a *grid reference*. Use of the UTM grid system for plotting position

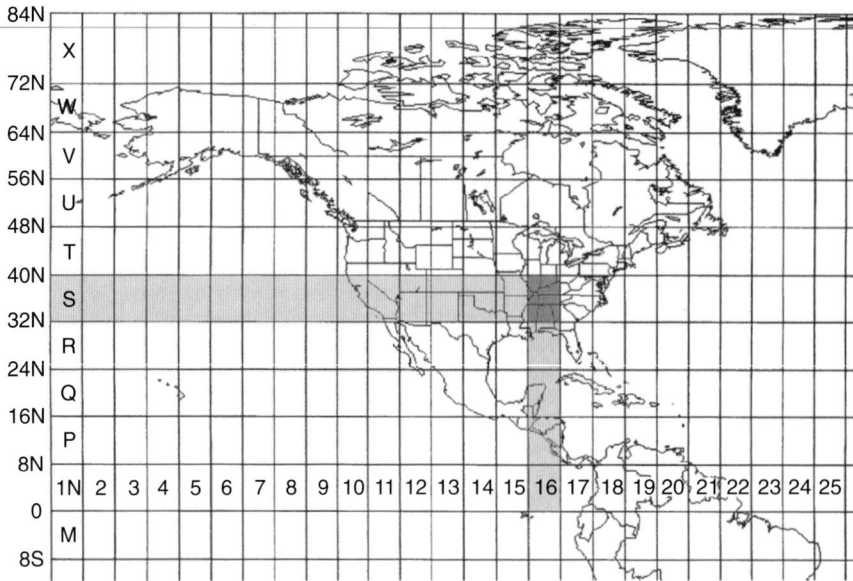

FIGURE 106-6 Map with the Universal Transverse Mercator (UTM) grid overlaid on a portion of the western hemisphere. Zone 16 and Row S are highlighted in *light gray*. The area of their intersection, designated as *16S*, is highlighted in *dark gray*. The central meridian for this zone lies at 87 degrees west longitude. The uppermost right-hand corner of the map represents the area used in the examples involving UTM coordinates discussed in the text.

based on a map is actually much simpler than its conceptual framework would suggest. Position plotting is greatly assisted by using a specialized ruler called a *roamer scale* that is compatible with common USGS map scales (see Figure 106-5). Roamer scales are included on many baseplate compasses, can be easily made from a scrap of paper, or can be printed or purchased from Internet sources. The large graduations on a roamer scale

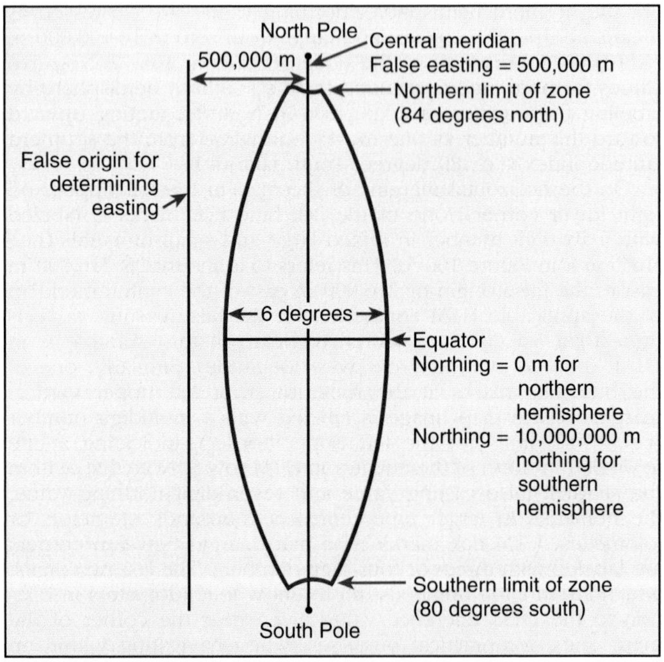

FIGURE 106-7 Diagram of a representative UTM zone showing the false origin 500,000 m to the west of the central meridian of the zone. The zone extends from 80 degrees south latitude to 84 degrees north latitude and spans 6 degrees of longitude. Note that the equator forms the index line for reckoning northing for the northern hemisphere, whereas the southern limit of the zone forms the northing index for the southern hemisphere. *(Redrawn from Cole WP: Using the UTM grid system to record historic sites.* http://www.cr.nps.gov/nr/publications/bulletins/nrb28/.)

generally denote 100-m increments, whereas the smaller divisions may represent a 10- or 20-m span. The steps for determining UTM coordinates for any point on a compatible map follow:

1. Mark the position of interest on the map with an "X."
2. Examine the margins of the map to become familiar with the three- or four-digit labels for the UTM ticks. For most hiking trips covered by a single map, or small number of maps, the UTM zone and row can be ignored.
3. Draw lines connecting tick marks of equal value on the top and bottom margins of the map. This need only be done for the area of the map surrounding the position of interest. Connect tick marks on the vertical margins of the map in the same manner. This will form a grid of 1-km squares on the desired portion of the map.
4. Position the corner of the roamer scale or ruler at the "X." Measure from the X to the nearest false easting line to the left, and record the easting value of the X. Measure to the nearest northing line below the X, and record the northing value of the X.
5. The unique position of point "X" is now known, and can serve as a reference point for subsequent navigation. This might include use as a GPS waypoint, as the position of a prominent landmark to be used for the triangulation of bearings, or to label a known starting point for the next leg of the hike.

When a degree of comfort with UTM coordinates is attained, navigation from point to point becomes much more intuitive than with latitude and longitude. Using the method just described, it is a simple matter to determine bearing and distance in meters between any two points on the map, to plot GPS waypoints on the map, or to identify a probable position based on dead reckoning from a known starting point. Note that it is standard for GPS receivers to be able to express the user's position in any of several formats, including as UTM coordinates. A location near my home has geodetic coordinates of 39 degrees and 15 minutes north latitude and 84 degrees and 30 minutes west longitude, as determined by a commonly available, inexpensive GPS receiver. With several simple key presses, the grid reference is expressed in UTM format as:

$$16S\ ^{07}16^{469}_{\ \ \ \ \ }{}^{43}_{}46^{677}$$

This indicates that the location is in UTM Grid Zone 16S (Zone 16, Row S). The meridians bounding Zone 16 are 90 degrees west longitude on the west and 84 degrees west longitude on the east. Row S is bounded by 32 degrees north latitude to the south and 40 degrees north latitude to the north. The latitude and longitude boundaries of the identified zone and row include southwestern Ohio. The numbers specifying the unique location within the zone and row must be read, per UTM convention, to the right (easting) and then up (northing). The first seven-digit number indicates that the site of interest has a false easting value of 716^{469} m E (i.e., 716,469 m east of the central meridian for the zone) or 469 m east of the 16-km tick mark on the horizontal margin of the relevant USGS map (see Figure 106-5). The second number indicates that the location has a northing value of 4346^{677} m N (i.e., 4,346,677 m north of the equator) or 677 m north of the 46-km tick mark on the vertical map margin.

For navigation in the majority of wilderness activities, the area of interest fits within a single USGS 7.5-minute square, and accuracy to within 100 m is adequate. As such, the UTM coordinates used to describe a location can be abbreviated for simplicity, including only the whole kilometers (i.e., the larger two-digit numerals) and the small digit to their immediate right (representing hundreds of meters). Do not round the last digit upward. In the prior example, the location of interest would be described in abbreviated UTM notation as easting 16^4, northing 46^6 (i.e., about 400 m east of the 16 tick mark and about 600 m north of the 46 tick mark).[7] Map usage involving the UTM coordinate system is greatly facilitated by drawing a 1-km by 1-km grid on the map using the UTM tick marks to define the whole-kilometer spacing of the grid lines.

In practice, GPS should be applied to a wilderness trek in the following manner. Before embarking on a trip, the user should choose a terrestrial coordinate system (i.e., UTM vs. latitude and longitude) and then enter into the receiver the precise coordinates of various important landmarks on the intended route of travel. The coordinates of locations of interest can be obtained from a trail guide or from a topographic map. For reasons articulated earlier, UTM coordinates offer a substantive benefit for land navigation as compared with the geodetic coordinate system. The waypoints obtained in this manner are entered, labeled, and stored within the receiver's memory. If a topographic map of the area of travel is available, a UTM grid should be drawn on the map using the method outlined previously. At the beginning of the trip, the location of the nearest town or source of assistance and the location of the trailhead where the trip is begun are entered as waypoints. The trip then progresses using the map, established trails, or the GPS receiver to follow the intended route. Tracks are recorded as the trip progresses. When pausing to camp, the position of the camp would be named and entered as yet another waypoint. At any time, the bearing and distance to any waypoint of interest are available to the user. If, in a spasm of self-reliance, the user decides to lay aside the GPS receiver and pursue traditional methods of navigation and the person becomes lost, reactivation of the receiver will allow the direction and distance to safety to be immediately determined; the tracks to the last waypoint could be retraced, or the receiver could be used to guide the person by bearing and distance to the next waypoint on the route.

Highly capable GPS receivers, including WAAS-enabled receivers, are commonly available at a price of about $100. They will fit into a shirt pocket and have sufficient battery power for 10 to 30 hours of continuous use. This is sufficient for weeks of navigation if power is used judiciously, and most models use common AA or AAA batteries. Models that incorporate onscreen topographic maps can be purchased for $200 to $700. However, GPS still suffers from important limitations. Dead batteries yield a useless receiver, so spare batteries should always be included when traveling. The receivers are relatively fragile, and many are not waterproof or even particularly water resistant. Obstruction of the sky by terrain features or heavy foliage may interfere with reception of satellite signals, which may render the receiver unable to acquire a sufficient number of satellites to provide a fix. In an era of national security risk, selective availability could be reimplemented or WAAS could be restricted, with resultant degradation of the accuracy of recreational GPS. Still, GPS is unsurpassed with regard to ease of use, accuracy, and usefulness for wilderness navigation. When applied with common sense and

routine awareness of approximate location, even the simplest GPS receiver renders it virtually impossible to become lost and effectively eliminates many of the pathfinding challenges that are inherent to wilderness travel. However, reliance on GPS as the sole navigational resource for any wilderness expedition is a grave error. As with all high-technology methodology, GPS can be easily disabled. The more self-contained methods of navigation discussed in later sections should be used whenever possible to maintain positional awareness and navigational skill in anticipation of the possibility that GPS may fail.

COMPASS NAVIGATION

The directional properties of lodestone (magnetite) were recognized by a variety of civilizations during ancient times. References to the use of a directional magnetized needle at sea appear in Chinese literature dating from the 12th century CE. Descriptions of the magnetic compass in European writings followed during the 13th century, by which time it was noted that a needle stroked on lodestone pointed to the vicinity of the North Star.[4,6,12] Discovery of the magnetic compass was a seminal event in exploration of the planet; the compass allowed reasonably accurate steering in all weather and provided the directional reference that permitted development of the process of dead reckoning.

MAGNETIC DIP, DEVIATION, AND DECLINATION

The directional properties of the compass result from interactions between magnetized iron in the compass needle and magnetic lines of force generated by metals in the earth's core. These lines of force have both a vertical and horizontal component. The vertical component is termed *magnetic inclination* or *dip*. Dip causes a compass needle to incline downward from horizontal, potentially to a degree that interferes with ability of the needle or card to pivot freely. Dip is 90 degrees at the magnetic poles and 0 degrees at the magnetic equator. Most modern compasses are manufactured to compensate for the average dip that is likely to be encountered in the region of intended use. Others allow a small weight to be moved along the indicator needle to compensate for dip in any region of use.[38]

The horizontal component of the magnetic lines of force causes the compass needle to point to the earth's north magnetic pole. It is an unfortunate fact that the earth's magnetic and geographic poles do not correspond in location. The earth's magnetic lines of force are not straight lines; rather, they meander in an irregular fashion dictated by irregularities in the density of the core. The irregular directionality of the earth's magnetic field is called *magnetic declination*. The compass needle is also influenced by local magnetic forces. These forces may result from natural sources such as ore deposits or from artificial sources such as ferromagnetic metals in vehicles, equipment, and clothing fasteners. Displacement of the compass needle resulting from local magnetic influences is termed *deviation*. As a result of magnetic declination and deviation, compasses point to geographic north only when used with care in selected locations. In general, compasses point northward but not exactly due north.

Direction in compass navigation is expressed in three ways: (1) true direction, or direction measured in reference to the earth's meridians and geographic poles; (2) magnetic direction, or direction measured in reference to the earth's magnetic poles; and (3) compass direction, or direction measured by the magnetic compass. Magnetic direction varies from true direction by the sum of declination and deviation. Compass direction varies from magnetic direction by the quantity of deviation.[10,32] The definitions of magnetic and compass direction point out the necessity of minimizing preventable sources of compass deviation when taking bearings. For practical purposes, when preventable sources of deviation are minimized and the compass is used with caution, magnetic and compass direction can be considered to be equivalent.

Wandering lines of points with equal magnetic declination can be graphed on maps and charts; these are called *isogonic lines*. Lines representing points on the surface of the earth where the magnetic declination is zero, and where magnetic north and

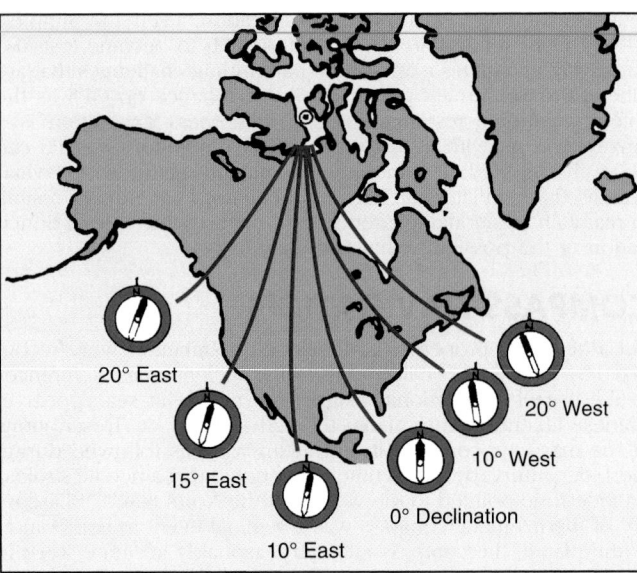

FIGURE 106-8 Schematic representation of North America showing declination at various locations as the difference between true north (i.e., "N" on the compass rim) and magnetic north (i.e., tip of the compass needle). *(From Seidman D: The essential wilderness navigator, Camden, Me, 1995, Ragged Mountain Press.)*

true north are aligned, are termed *agonic lines*. In the Americas, an agonic line follows a relatively straight and slanting course extending from the east coast of Victoria Island in north-central Canada through western Lake Superior, along the west coast of Florida, and traversing South America from the Gulf of Venezuela to the southeastern coast of Brazil. At locations east of the agonic line, the compass needle declines to the west (counterclockwise) of true north; at points west of the agonic line, the compass needle declines to the east (clockwise) of true north. By convention, magnetic declination is given a positive sign when east and a negative sign when west (Figure 106-8). Declination is quantified as the angle between true and magnetic north.

By way of example, in southwestern Ohio the current magnetic declination is negative 5.71 degrees, or approximately 6 degrees west. This means that a compass needle actually points 6 degrees to the west of true north and that the true bearing given by the needle is 354 degrees when the needle points to 360 degrees on the compass rim. Any magnetic bearing taken with a compass will thus be 6 degrees greater than the true bearing. To correct from magnetic to true, 6 degrees must be subtracted from any indicated magnetic bearing.

The mnemonic "Declination east, compass bearing least; declination west, compass bearing greatest" may be helpful for converting magnetic direction to true direction when taking a bearing. In other words, to convert from magnetic to true while taking a bearing from the compass, add east declination to the compass bearing, or subtract west declination from the compass bearing. When taking a true bearing from a map and converting it to a compass bearing to follow in the environment, subtract east declination from the true bearing, or add west declination to the true bearing. Interconversion between magnetic and true bearings is an essential skill for compass navigation. Failure to recognize this relationship will result in significant errors when following a map route by compass, because directional references on the map are based on true direction. At a location where the magnetic declination is 10 degrees, travel over a straight course derived from a map and guided by a compass will result in a 0.18-mile error for each 1 mile traveled if declination is not considered.[22]

Magnetic declination for any location can be determined by referencing the *Isogonic Chart for Magnetic Declination* produced every 5 years by the USGS, or by accessing the National Oceanic and Atmospheric Administration (NOAA) website at www.ngd.noaa.gov. In the United States, magnetic declination varies from 23 degrees East in Washington State to 22 degrees West in Maine (see Figure 106-8).[10] On standard USGS 7.5-minute and 15-minute squares, magnetic declination is indicated by a pointer next to the indicator for true north at the bottom of the map. If one does not have access to an isogonic chart, declination for any location in the northern hemisphere can be empirically determined with reasonable accuracy by comparing the magnetic bearing of north with the true bearing, as indicated by the direction to the star Polaris. Polaris lies up to 45 minutes of arc (i.e., 0.75 degrees) away from true north at some times of day, but this offset is negligible for wilderness navigation situations. Declination at any location can also be determined by comparing the magnetic bearing of a prominent landmark with the true bearing between the observer's known location and location of the landmark as read from a map.[7]

COMPASS TYPES

The three compass types used in land navigation are the fixed-dial compass, magnetic card compass, and baseplate compass (Figure 106-9). The simplest compass is the fixed-dial, which uses a magnetized needle that is balanced on a pivot and enclosed in a case and that is graduated around its periphery into 360 degrees. The magnetic card compass uses a magnetized needle or wire fixed to a circular card that is graduated around its periphery from 0 degrees to 360 degrees. The housing of the compass is marked with a line called the *lubber line* that allows magnetic bearings to be determined when the line is pointed at an object of interest. The lensatic compass used by the military, which has a lens for magnification of the compass card and sights for alignment to distant objects, is a typical magnetic card compass. The most useful compass for land navigation is the baseplate compass,[22,25,35,39] which consists of a fixed-dial compass (or capsule) mounted to a baseplate in a manner that allows the capsule to rotate in relation to the baseplate. The baseplate is marked with a line used to indicate the direction of travel. This line functions in a manner identical to the lubber line of the magnetic card compass. The capsule of the compass has an orienting arrow inscribed on its lower surface that points to the graduation denoting north on the capsule rim. On different models, this graduation may be labeled "0°", "360°", or "N". Rotation of the capsule such that the compass needle is superimposed on the orienting arrow and points to "N" on the capsule rim allows the user to easily read the magnetic bearing indicated by the direction-of-travel line. As long as the direction-of-travel line is followed and the needle remains superimposed on the orienting arrow, the user is assured of maintaining the desired magnetic bearing during travel.

Many baseplate compasses allow the orienting arrow to be adjusted relative to the rim of the capsule to compensate for

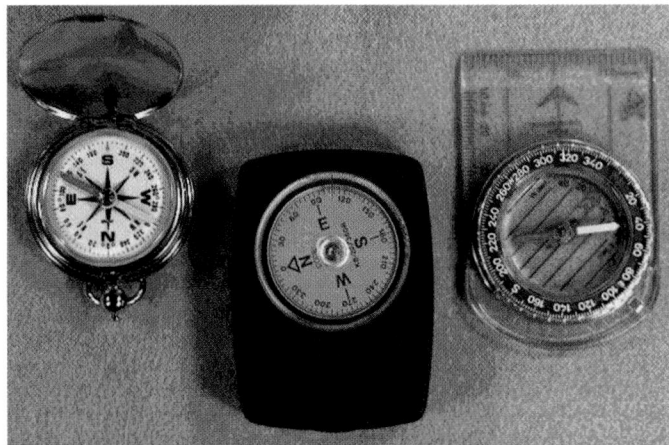

FIGURE 106-9 The three basic compass types. *From left to right:* Fixed-dial compass, magnetic card compass, and baseplate compass. Note the deviation in indicated north resulting from local magnetic influences.

magnetic declination. When the orienting arrow of such a compass is adjusted to point to the bearing of magnetic north, the "N" graduation on the capsule rim will indicate true north when the compass needle aligns with the orienting arrow. All bearings as read on the capsule rim will now represent true—rather than magnetic—direction. Baseplate compasses have other features particularly suited for use with a map, including plotting scales, a straightedge, and often a protractor and magnifier.[39]

Correction for declination when using a fixed-dial or magnetic card compass requires addition or subtraction of the declination, as appropriate, from the magnetic bearing indicated by the compass rim or lubber line.

COMPASS USE

A magnetic compass is used to establish cardinal directions, bearings for use in route finding, and back bearings for use in returning to a known starting location. The term *back bearing* refers to the reciprocal of the bearing followed on the outbound leg of a journey (i.e., outbound bearing minus 180 degrees) or the reciprocal of a measured bearing to a prominent terrain feature. Any route can be subdivided into legs that can be defined by magnetic bearing lines. Ideally, each leg should pass between prominent and identifiable landmarks that will remain recognizable even in the dark or in poor weather. However, even when weather or lighting conditions prevent visual acquisition of the landmark from a distance, careful compass work should permit the user to reach an objective. Early during the course of travel over each leg, the observer should visually check the back bearing of the direction of travel to become familiar with the view of the starting point as it will appear on the return journey. If possible, the bearing and back bearing of each leg of a route, and the landmarks defining each leg, should be recorded on paper rather than trusted to memory.

Use of a compass in this manner permits the user to return easily to the desired direction of travel if an obstacle to the intended route is encountered. The course around the obstacle is recorded as a series of legs of known direction and estimated (by stride) length. When permitted by the terrain, right-angle detours are the simplest to follow. The user returns to the intended route by traveling the reciprocal of the course of the detour for the same distance as that required for bypass of the obstacle[9] (Figure 106-10). Return to the intended course is greatly augmented by using natural ranges. A natural range is formed by two landmarks that lie along the same bearing line, with one end indicated by a landmark of intermediate distance from the viewer and one at a greater distance (e.g., a large tree or rock formation several kilometers from the viewer and the silhouette of a hill or mountain on the horizon). As the traveler deviates from the intended course, the near and far landmarks will fall out of line. When the traveler returns to the intended route, the objects forming the natural range will return to alignment.

Use of a compass with a map allows the user to orient the map to the environment and relate bearings taken from the map to bearings measured with the compass. Correction for declination is essential when the compass is used for this task if true bearings are to be used when plotting a route. However, there is no absolute need for the use of true bearings in navigation; it is important only that the map and compass agree. Agreement can be accomplished either by correcting the compass to the map or by correcting the map to the compass. If a baseplate compass with declination adjustment is used, it is relatively simple to correct the compass to the map and use true bearings for all subsequent travel. With all types of compasses, however, it is easiest to use magnetic bearings exclusively. If the declination is known or can be determined observationally, magnetic meridians can be drawn on the map to be used in place of the true meridians represented by the map margins (Figure 106-11). These magnetic meridians will form an angle with the true meridians equal to the declination angle. A map modified in this manner permits magnetic bearings (rather than true) to be taken from the map for use when following a course. The internal consistency of this method is always much less confusing than the method requiring conversion between true bearings and compass bearings. Because of the ease with which bearings may be taken from the map when it is marked with magnetic meridians, maps for use in navigational sports (e.g., orienteering) are prepared exclusively with magnetic meridians. Choice between the use of true versus magnetic bearings should be made in advance of travel to permit modification of the map. Plotting magnetic meridians on a map requires a pencil, straightedge, flat surface, and protractor; these items are unlikely to be available during a field emergency.[38,39]

To orient a map with a baseplate compass corrected for declination, the compass capsule is rotated such that "N" on the capsule rim is aligned with the direction-of-travel arrow. An edge of the baseplate parallel to the direction-of-travel arrow is then placed on one of the vertical borders of the map. The map, with the compass in place, is then rotated until the compass needle is superimposed on the orienting arrow on the base of the capsule. True north on the map is now aligned with true north on the planet.

To orient a map that has been modified with magnetic meridians using an uncompensated baseplate compass, the compass capsule is rotated until "N" on the capsule rim aligns with the direction-of-travel arrow. An edge of the compass parallel to the

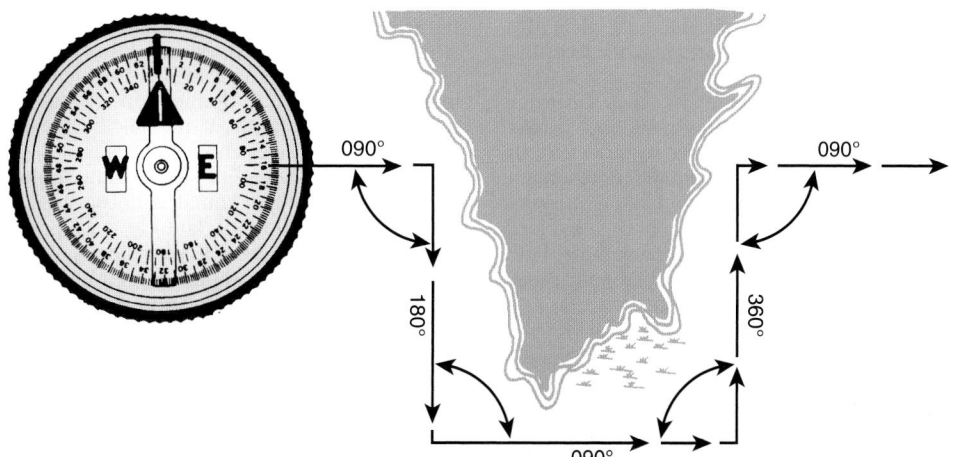

FIGURE 106-10 Use of a compass to return to an intended route when faced with an obstacle. A course 90 degrees to the intended course is walked for a known number of steps, the obstacle is bypassed, and the original course is regained by walking the reciprocal course of the initial detour for the same distance. *(From the Department of the Army: Map reading and land navigation, Field Manual 21-26, Washington, DC, 1987, Headquarters, Department of the Army.)*

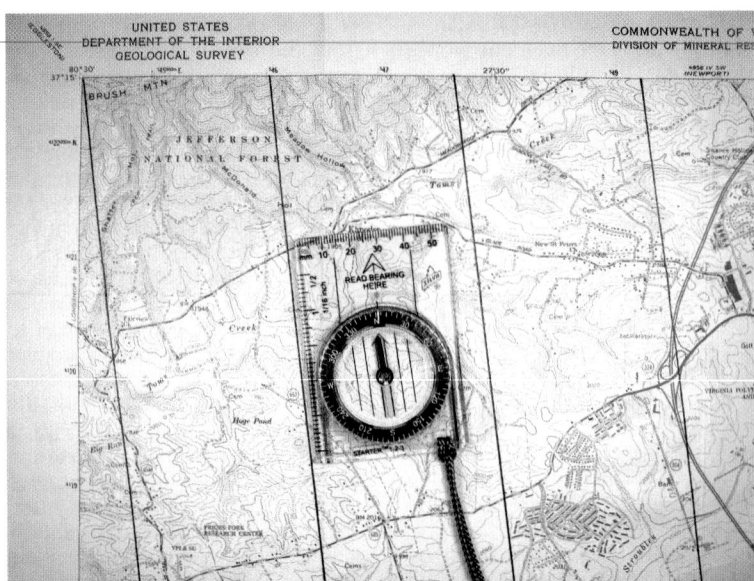

FIGURE 106-11 United States Geological Survey 1:24,000 (7.5-minute) map modified with magnetic meridians (*dark lines*). The magnetic meridians reflect the 8 degrees west declination of the area represented on the map. The compass has been placed with its edge parallel to a magnetic meridian, and the compass capsule rotated such that the orienting arrow on the bottom of the capsule points to north on the map. The map and compass were then rotated in concert to align the compass needle and the orienting arrow. The map is now oriented to the terrain, and directions as indicated on the capsule rim represent magnetic bearings to objects in the environment.

direction-of-travel arrow is placed on one of the magnetic meridians plotted on the map. The map, with the compass in place, is rotated until the compass needle is superimposed on the orienting arrow. True north on the map now corresponds with true north in the surrounding landscape.[22,35,38,39] If an uncompensated compass of another type is used, the north-south line of the compass face or lubber line is superimposed on a magnetic meridian, and the map and compass are rotated in concert until the indicator needle points to "N".

To plot and follow a bearing using a baseplate compass and map, the map is held horizontally, and a straightedge of the baseplate parallel to the direction-of-travel arrow is placed on a line connecting the starting and ending points of the leg. The compass capsule is then rotated until the orienting arrow points to north as indicated on the map. The map and compass are held together and rotated until the compass needle is superimposed on the orienting arrow. The intersection of the direction-of-travel arrow and the capsule rim now indicates the bearing of the leg, and the direction-of-travel arrow points to the objective (Figure 106-12). To follow the bearing, the user walks in the direction indicated by the direction-of-travel arrow while keeping the compass needle and orienting arrow in alignment.

When a map is oriented to the environment, back bearings from landmarks that are visible both on the map and in the landscape can be used to obtain a positional fix by resection or triangulation.[35] Each back bearing from a landmark represents a line of position (LOP) that can be plotted on the map. The point of crossing of two or more LOPs fixes the position of the observer (Figure 106-13). Alternatively, the intersection between the LOP represented by a bearing line and a shoreline, riverbank, road, firebreak, or ridgeline can be used to fix position on a map.

MAKESHIFT COMPASSES

A field-expedient compass can be fabricated with relative ease. Items containing iron, nickel, or cobalt are suitable for use as an indicator needle. Iron in the form of a steel needle, pin, wire, staple, or paper clip is most commonly available. Most of these items are magnetized as purchased. If not, they can be magnetized by stroking them on a magnet salvaged from an electric motor or radio speaker, on a magnetized screwdriver or similar item, or on a piece of silk. A dry cell also can be used to mag-

netize a needle by wrapping an insulated wire tightly around the needle and connecting the ends of the wire to the battery terminals for several minutes. There is a fire risk associated with shorting the battery terminals in this manner, and sparks and heat should be expected. Trial and error will often yield a suitable magnetizer. The indicator needle is floated in water by placing it on a wood chip, leaf, slip of paper, or small piece of cork or closed-cell foam. The container, which may be the cupped palm of the hand or a puddle, should be protected from the wind (Figure 106-14). A compass that has been so constructed will reliably indicate a magnetic north-south line. The absolute determination of direction may require external cues, such as the general direction of sunrise, sunset, or position of the sun at midday.

CELESTIAL NAVIGATION

Celestial navigation exploits the predictable relationship between the apparent positions of selected celestial bodies and surface of the earth. The influence of celestial navigation on world history is immense. Millennia before European cultures conceived of celestial navigation as a means for facilitating exploration, commerce, and military domination of the seas, the people that populated the islands of the Pacific Basin were making open-ocean voyages over thousands of miles guided by memorized "star paths."[17] The use of simple altitude-measuring devices (e.g., Greek gnomon, Arab kamal, Chinese stretch board) for the qualitative determination of latitude was practiced by mariners in antiquity. As the Age of Exploration dawned, competing governments of Western Europe devoted enormous energy to systematization of celestial navigation, funding legions of astronomers for development of coordinate systems and accurate tables of stellar, solar, lunar, and planetary positions. Instruments such as the mariner's astrolabe, quadrant, octant, and sextant permitted accurate and reproducible quantitative measurement of the altitude of celestial bodies, and accurate clocks became available to permit ready determination of longitude.[4,44]

Celestial navigation has its greatest usefulness and easiest application at sea. Standard celestial practice depends on availability of a sea horizon as a reference point for measurement of altitude. The horizon reference for land navigation is necessarily artificial (i.e., a plumb bob, bubble level, or level reflective

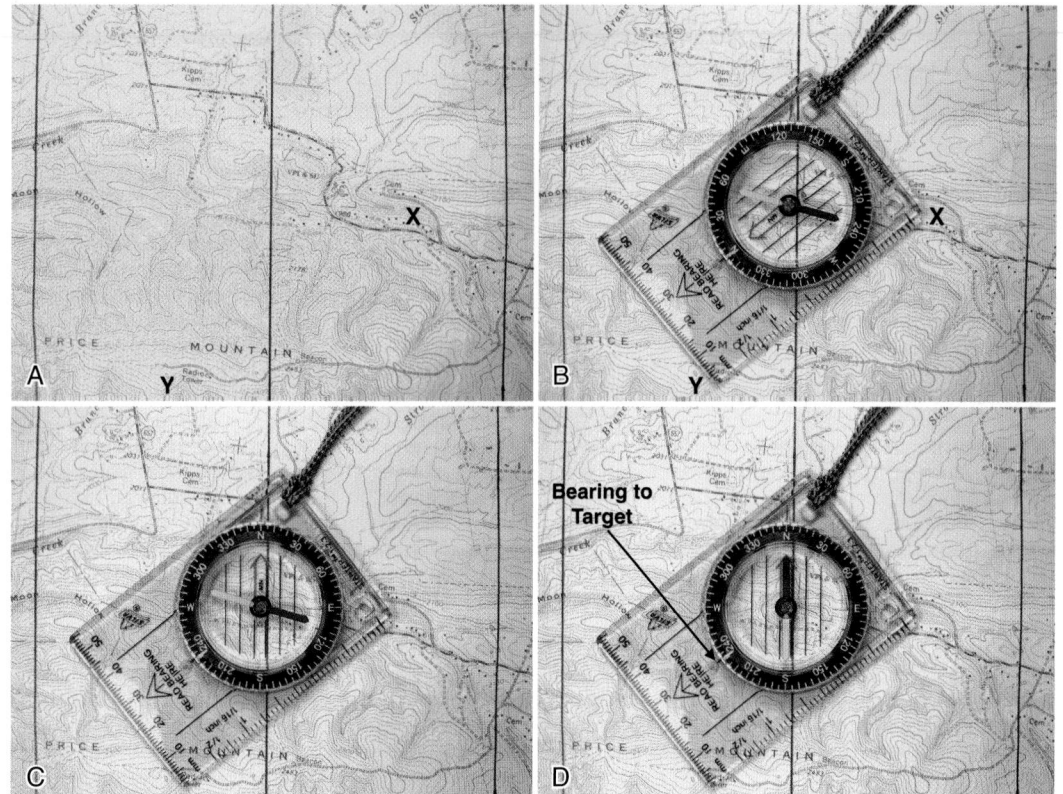

FIGURE 106-12 The steps for plotting and following a bearing using a map and compass. **A,** The current position (road junction at *X*) and destination (watch tower at *Y*) are identified. **B,** The compass is then placed on the map with an edge along the line connecting *X* and *Y*. **C,** The compass capsule is rotated so that the orienting arrow points north as indicated by the magnetic meridians drawn on the map. The compass is now oriented to the map. **D,** The compass and map are now held horizontally and rotated until the magnetic needle is superimposed on the orienting arrow. The map is now aligned to the environment, and the bearing to *Y* is indicated at the intersection of the compass capsule and the direction-of-travel arrow (232 degrees in this example). As long as the needle is kept superimposed on the orienting arrow, the direction-of-travel arrow will point toward the destination.

surface). Positions resulting from celestial fixes, even with scrupulous technique, are only approximations of the navigator's actual position. Errors of several miles are common. This is of little consequence in the open ocean, even as landfall approaches; the target destination is generally large enough to be seen from many miles away. This degree of imprecision may prove troublesome on land, but accuracy of celestial navigation should still suffice for many wilderness situations.

Although developed for use on trackless seas, celestial navigation has a long and rich tradition of use on land. With this type of navigation, Lewis and Clark established the positions of landmarks during their exploration of the American West. Various expeditions that explored the North and South Poles depended entirely on celestial observations to determine direction and position. Celestial navigation techniques can be applied in a wilderness setting at a variety of levels. Traditional celestial navigation, in which sextant observations lead to the fixing of terrestrial

FIGURE 106-13 Establishing a magnetic fix by crossing the back bearings from two prominent landmarks. This process is known as *resection*.

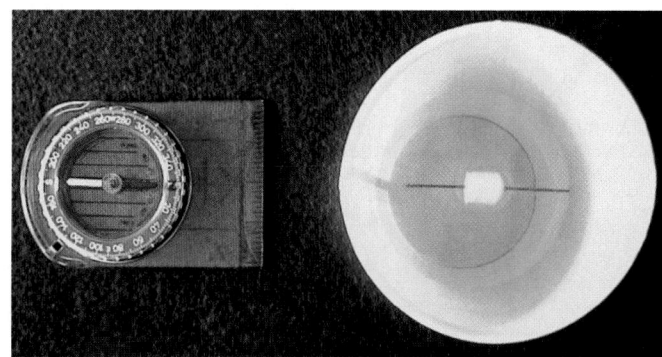

FIGURE 106-14 A makeshift compass constructed from a plastic cup, straight pin, and foam packing peanut. Note the correspondence between north as indicated by the makeshift device and the commercial compass.

position, can be accomplished with relatively little equipment but requires considerable preplanning. This methodology is unlikely to be adopted for use by the vast majority of wilderness travelers. However, simplified celestial techniques requiring little or no equipment are well suited to field-expedient navigation and can provide accurate directional information in the absence of a compass. In particular, understanding movement of the sun and several prominent stars can allow accurate route finding without recourse to technology. To understand the relationship between the position of a celestial body and the position of an observer on Earth, it is necessary to relate the coordinate systems that are used to describe celestial position and the appearance of the sky from the earth's surface (i.e., the horizon coordinate system) to the geodetic system previously discussed.

CELESTIAL COORDINATES

To a terrestrial observer, the sky appears to be an immense hollow sphere with the earth at its center, and the stars painted on its inner surface. The sphere rotates about the earth once daily. The sun, moon, and planets wander across the background of stars on concentric spheres of their own. This is exactly how the universe was described by Ptolemy during the second century CE and is called the *geocentric model*. This theory was highly popular with the Catholic Church; challenging it led to persecution of many intellectuals during the era of the Spanish Inquisition. It held sway until the 16th century, when it was replaced, gingerly, with an equally incorrect heliocentric (i.e., sun-centered) model. The geocentric model, although false, is a useful construct for ordering the heavens and is the model used for definition of celestial coordinates.

The celestial coordinate system plays off the geodetic terrestrial coordinate system. The terrestrial poles are projected outward to the surface of the imaginary celestial sphere to form the north and south celestial poles. The terrestrial equator is similarly projected outward to form the celestial equator, which is also known as the *equinoctial*. The celestial correlate to latitude is declination; this is unrelated to magnetic declination in compass use (Figure 106-15). The declination of a celestial body is the angle measured from the center of the earth (and geocentric universe)

north or south of the celestial equator from 0 degrees through 90 degrees of arc. Declinations north of the celestial equator are positive (+), whereas those south of the celestial equator are negative (−). The declinations of the celestial poles are thus +90 degrees and −90 degrees, respectively, whereas that of the celestial equator is 0 degrees. The declinations of the sun, moon, four navigational planets (Venus, Mars, Jupiter, and Saturn), and 57 navigational stars are listed in the daily pages of the *Nautical Almanac*.[12,21]

The celestial correlate to longitude is less intuitive and requires explanation. Projections of terrestrial meridians onto the celestial sphere form celestial meridians. Projection of the Greenwich meridian onto the celestial sphere forms the Greenwich celestial meridian. Projection of an observer's meridian onto the celestial sphere forms the local celestial meridian (Figure 106-15). A meridian on the surface of the celestial sphere that contains a celestial body and the celestial poles and is perpendicular to the celestial equator is called the *hour circle* of that body. Hour circles converge toward the celestial poles in a manner identical to meridians on Earth. As the celestial sphere rotates about its polar axis, the hour circles of all celestial bodies appear to rotate above a terrestrial observer, rising in the east, sweeping overhead, and setting in the west. A reference hour circle on the celestial sphere called the *first point of Aries* or the *hour circle of Aries* substitutes for the terrestrial Prime Meridian. The first point of Aries is represented by an hour circle that intersects the celestial equator at the point where the sun crosses it at the moment of the spring equinox. The angular measurement between the hour circle of a celestial body and the Greenwich celestial meridian is called the *Greenwich hour angle* (GHA) of the body. GHA is the celestial equivalent of longitude and is measured westward from the Greenwich celestial meridian from 0 degrees through 360 degrees. The Greenwich hour angle of Aries (GHA^{Aries}) is the angle between the Greenwich celestial meridian and the hour circle of Aries at any given second in time. The GHAs for Aries and for the sun and moon, Venus, Mars, Jupiter, and Saturn are listed for each hour of each day of a year in daily pages of the *Nautical Almanac*. Interpolation tables permit determination of hour angles for each second of the year.[21,32]

The GHAs of the 57 navigational stars are defined by their predictable and nearly constant relationship to the hour angle of Aries. The angular measurement between the hour circle of Aries and the hour circle of any of the navigational stars is called the *sidereal hour angle* (SHA) of that star. The GHA of each of the navigational stars is thus equal to the sum of the hour angle of Aries and the SHA of the star in question (GHA^{star} = GHA^{Aries} + SHA^{star}).

For the practice of celestial navigation, the hour angle of a celestial body is ultimately defined in reference to the observer's local celestial meridian. The angular measurement between the local celestial meridian and the hour circle of a body is the *local hour angle* (LHA) of that body. The LHA, as with the GHA, is measured westward from the local celestial meridian from 0 degrees through 360 degrees. The LHA of a celestial body equals the GHA of the body plus the observer's longitude if east, or minus the observer's longitude if west (LHA = GHA + East λ; LHA = GHA − West λ). When a celestial body is on an observer's meridian, its GHA equals the longitude of the observer's position.[4]

HORIZON COORDINATE SYSTEM

The horizon coordinate system defines celestial position from the point of view of the earthbound observer. The point on the celestial sphere directly over the observer's head is called the *zenith*; the point on the celestial sphere directly beneath the feet of the observer is called the *nadir*. The zenith and nadir lie on a line that includes the observer's terrestrial position and the earth's center. The plane that passes though the center of the earth perpendicular to this line is called the observer's *celestial horizon*. The celestial horizon lies parallel to the observer's visible horizon. Any great circle on the celestial sphere formed by a plane passing perpendicular to the celestial horizon is called a *vertical circle* (Figure 106-16). Vertical circles converge at the

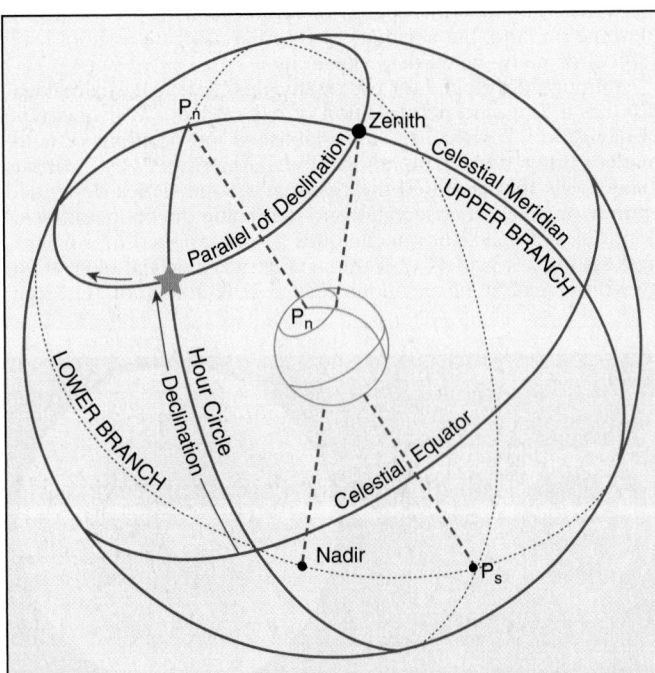

FIGURE 106-15 Diagram showing the celestial meridian of an observer on the earth's surface and the celestial meridian corresponding to the hour circle of an observed star. (*From Bowditch N: The American practical navigator: An epitome of navigation, Washington, DC, 1984, Defense Mapping Agency Hydrographic/Topographic Center.*)

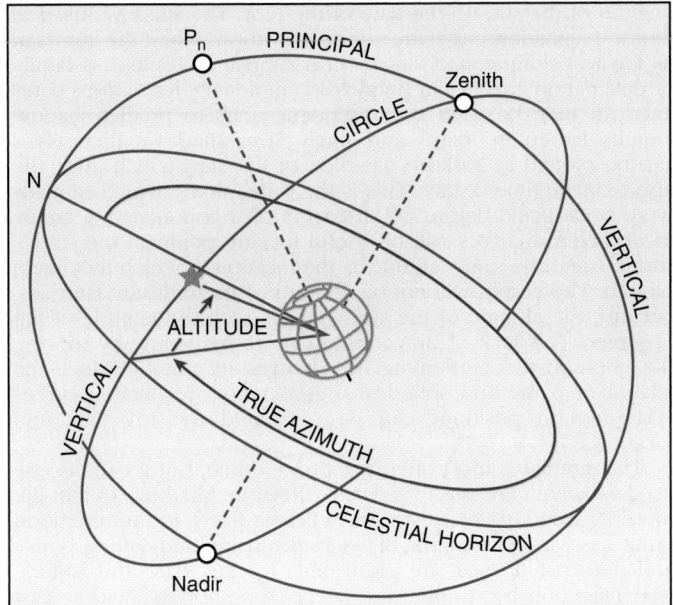

FIGURE 106-16 Schematic representation of the horizon coordinate system showing the observer's zenith and nadir, the celestial horizon, the prime and principal vertical circles, the elevated pole *(Pn)*, and the altitude and azimuth of the body being observed. *(From Hobbs RR: Marine navigation: Piloting and celestial and electronic navigation, ed 4, Annapolis, Md, 1998, Naval Institute Press.)*

the *local apparent noon* (LAN), is that moment when the sun achieves its greatest altitude. The sun is observed with the sextant for a brief period of time preceding LAN until the altitude ceases to increase and begins to fall. The maximum sextant altitude so determined is corrected using *Nautical Almanac* data to yield Ho, which is then converted to zenith distance (ZD). Zenith distance is the angular distance between observer's zenith and the body; thus, ZD = 90 degrees – Ho. The algebraic sum of ZD and the declination of the sun (d; from the *Nautical Almanac*) at the approximate time of observation gives the observer's latitude with the use of the following formulae[12,26]:

1. L = ZD + d, when L and d have the same sign and L>d.
2. L = d – ZD, when L and d have the same sign and d>L.
3. L = ZD – d, when L and d have different signs.

Because declination of the sun changes very slowly on an hourly basis, accuracy is acceptable if the sun's declination is known for merely the approximate time of observation. The noon sight requires only the sun's declination and precise altitude. Determination of latitude by meridian passage can be accomplished by observation of any celestial body of known declination, although observation is easiest with the sun.

Another extremely simple observation to determine latitude involves measuring the altitude of Polaris (also known as α *Ursae Minoris,* the *Pole Star,* or the *North Star*). Because Polaris rotates about the true north celestial pole on a very short radius (i.e., <1 degree of arc), at two times each day, the altitude of Polaris will be equal to the altitude of the true pole, and that altitude will equal the latitude of the observer. The altitude of Polaris most closely approximates the altitude of the pole—and thus latitude—when the constellations Ursa Major (the Big Dipper) and Cassiopeia are positioned as indicated by Figure 106-17. For the remainder of the day, there will be a predictable discrepancy

observer's zenith and nadir in a manner analogous to convergence of the terrestrial and celestial meridians at their poles. Three of the infinite number of potential vertical circles for any surface position are of particular importance: (1) the *principal vertical,* which is the vertical circle lying on the observer's celestial meridian; (2) the *prime vertical,* which is the vertical circle passing through points due east and west of the observer; and (3) the *vertical circle* containing a celestial body of interest (Figure 106-16).[21]

The angular measurement between an observer's celestial horizon and a celestial body is the *altitude* of that body. Altitudes are expressed in degrees, minutes, and seconds of arc from 0 degrees (the horizon) through 90 degrees (the zenith). In the traditional practice of celestial navigation, altitudes are measured using a sextant, octant, or quadrant. Altitude, as measured by an instrument in reference to the horizon, is termed *sextant altitude* (Hs), regardless of the type of instrument used. Hs, once corrected for various atmospheric and geometric factors, is then called *observed altitude* (Ho). The corrections to be applied are tabulated in the *Nautical Almanac*. The true altitude of a body can be calculated for any given terrestrial position at any instant of time using application of spherical trigonometry. This altitude is called *calculated altitude* (Hc).[4]

The other determinant of the observed position of a celestial body is angular measurement along the celestial horizon between true north and the vertical circle including the body. This angle is called the *azimuth* (Zn) of the body and is measured clockwise from 0 degrees through 360 degrees (see Figure 106-16).

CELESTIAL LINES OF POSITION

Methods for Latitude

The simplest celestial LOP is derived from the noon sight or meridian altitude of the sun. This method dominated celestial navigation from the 17th century until the late 1800s. The noon sight is simple but inflexible. It is very adaptable to wilderness navigation, requiring minimal mathematics and little equipment. The noon sight allows direct determination of latitude by measuring altitude of the sun at the moment that it passes the observer's meridian. The instant of solar meridian passage, which is called

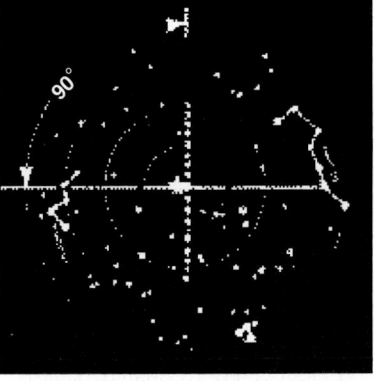

No correction

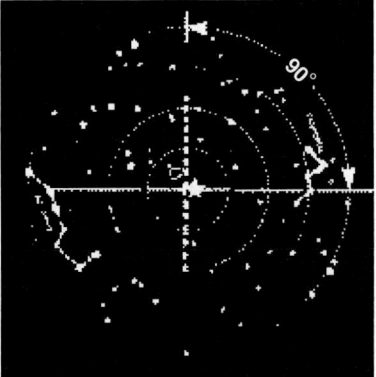

No correction

FIGURE 106-17 Diagram indicating appearance of the north circumpolar sky at the two times of day when the observed altitude of Polaris is equivalent to the latitude of the observer. *(From the Department of the Air Force: Survival Training Edition AF Manual 64-3, Randolph Air Force Base, Texas, 1969, Air Training Command.)*

between the measured altitude of the star and the latitude of the observer. The *Nautical Almanac* has a brief table that corrects for this discrepancy, allowing an observer to determine accurate latitude by the altitude of Polaris at any time when the star is visible and a suitable horizon is available. The Polaris sight requires Greenwich Mean Time (GMT) to within several minutes, a precise measurement of altitude, and data from the *Nautical Almanac*.[4,12]

The latitude obtained by the noon sight or Polaris sight represents the simplest available celestial LOP. This line can be used to determine a fix if coupled with a sight that yields longitude, or with another LOP obtained by any other method. For land navigation, this second LOP might represent a linear surface feature, compass bearing, or radio bearing that crosses the determined latitude line at a single point.

Methods for Longitude

Determination of longitude is considerably more involved than determination of latitude, requiring precise timekeeping, meticulous observation, extensive preplanning, and detailed tables of celestial data. The seminal advance in the search for a method of determining longitude was invention of the chronometer by John Harrison in 1735. With an accurate timepiece, longitude could be directly determined by measuring the altitude of any celestial body of known coordinates at a precisely known instant of time. This method, which is called *time sight,* revolutionized exploration but involves formidable mathematics. A simpler alternative exists that is adaptable to the wilderness setting. This traditional technique for establishing longitude is called *equal altitude method*. Equal altitude method requires accurate timekeeping, the ability to measure altitude with precision, and data from the *Nautical Almanac*. At a convenient interval before the meridian passage of the body (i.e., 1 to 2 hours), the altitude of the body is taken, and GMT is noted. The sextant is left at the altitude setting of the first observation. After the body passes the meridian, it is observed until it falls to the exact altitude of the first reading, and the time is again noted. Meridian passage will have occurred at the midpoint between these two times, and the GMT of meridian passage is then known. At the moment of meridian passage, LHA of the body equals zero, and GHA of the body (from the *Nautical Almanac*) equals the observer's longitude.

In theory, the instant of meridian passage could be found by noting the moment the body reached maximum altitude, achieving the same result. This is highly inaccurate in practice because of the extremely slow rate of change of altitude in the minutes immediately surrounding the LAN.[26] Other elegant and highly accurate methods exist for determining longitude and position. These use Sumner lines, a particularly flexible form of celestial LOP discovered by Thomas H. Sumner in 1837, and the altitude-intercept method discovered by Marcq Saint-Hillaire in 1875. These methods have a rich and colorful history and serve as the principal methods for celestial position finding at sea. However, these techniques are unlikely to be practiced by the land navigator and are not discussed further here. Interested readers are referred to several references for further study.[4,12,21,26,43]

CELESTIAL METHODS FOR DIRECTION FINDING

SHADOW METHODS

The axis of rotation of the earth is inclined at about 23.5 degrees from the orbital plane of the solar system. It is this phenomenon that results in the seasons; in the variable path of the sun through the sky with each season; and in the terrestrial definitions of the tropics, the temperate zones, and Arctic and Antarctic zones. The apparent path of the sun is lower in the sky, and shadows cast by the sun are longer at any given time of day in winter than in summer. A plot of the tips of the shadows cast in daylight by a vertical object (i.e., a gnomon) on any given date results in a curved line called a *declination curve*. The declination curve is so named because shadow lengths are proportional to the dec-

lination of the sun on the date of the plot. The shadows used to plot a declination curve are shortest at noon, when the sun is at its greatest altitude, and longest near sunrise and sunset. A family of declination curves can be plotted empirically for various dates and can then be used in subsequent years to predict shadow lengths for future dates and times. The shadows themselves can be plotted to indicate direction of the sun, which gives the approximate time of day. This is the principle by which sundials were constructed before the discovery of trigonometry. A family of declination curves will be useful for any point on the earth's surface near the same latitude as the location at which they were plotted. The curves will not be accurate at more distant latitudes, because the altitude of the sun changes with the latitude of the observer. This lack of universality can be overcome by moving the gnomon to compensate for changes in latitude. Since the advent of plane and spherical trigonometry, declination curves and gnomon positions can be calculated for any date and location.[36]

The sundial is most often used to tell time, but it can also be used as a sun compass to indicate direction. Shadows cast in the morning hours point westward, whereas those in the afternoon point eastward. Variations between the rising and setting points and due east or west are predictable for any date and latitude (see Direction by Amplitudes, later). The shortest shadow cast by the sun occurs at LAN and always lies on a due north-south line. Alternatively, a north-south line can be found by bisecting the angle between two points on a declination curve that are at equal distances from the gnomon. Knowing this, a sun compass can be constructed that indicates true direction with a high degree of accuracy whenever the shadow tip of the appropriately positioned gnomon lies on the declination curve for the approximate date of observation. Figure 106-18 shows such a sun compass, called a *Universal Pocket Navigator,* with a scale to compensate for the latitude of the user.[36] A copy of this sun compass, a pin or a toothpick that is more than 2.5 cm (1 inch) in length, and sunshine are all that is necessary to determine the cardinal directions with an accuracy greater than that typically achievable with a magnetic compass (Figure 106-19).

In the absence of a copy of Figure 106-18, the same principle can be applied to construct a sun compass on the fly. Any flat surface (e.g., a chip of wood, piece of bark, scrap of paper) is placed horizontally in the sun, and a gnomon of convenient length is stuck in the surface in a vertical position. The tip of the shadow cast by the gnomon is marked at various times beginning shortly after sunrise, and a curve is traced between the marks. At some point, the sun will pass the meridian, and the shadow will begin to lengthen again. A line between the base of the gnomon and the point of closest approach of the curve represents solar noon and runs due north to due south. Whether the shadow at noon points north or south depends on whether the observer is in the northern hemisphere, southern hemisphere, or the equatorial tropics. The actual direction indicated by the shadow is easily determined by noting the general direction of sunrise, which is on the eastward side of the sun compass. The remaining afternoon portion of the curve can either be completed freehand as a mirror image of the morning curve or by continued observation and marking of shadow tips (Figure 106-20). On subsequent days, the sun compass is reoriented to true north by rotating the horizontal surface until the tip of the gnomon's shadow touches the curve. A sun compass prepared in this manner is highly portable and remains accurate for many days, until there is significant change in the latitude of the traveler or in declination of the sun. New curves can be prepared on the same compass as needed.

Other methods of direction finding with the use of shadows exist but are significantly less accurate. The direction of travel of a shadow tip over 1 hour or so will point generally eastward throughout the day.[9] The accuracy of this method is degraded in direct proportion to the length of time before or after noon that the observations take place and in inverse proportion to the declination of the sun. Errors of more than 30 degrees are possible when conditions are unfavorable, such as at higher latitudes and during winter, when the path of the sun is low in the sky. However, errors incurred during morning hours will tend to be

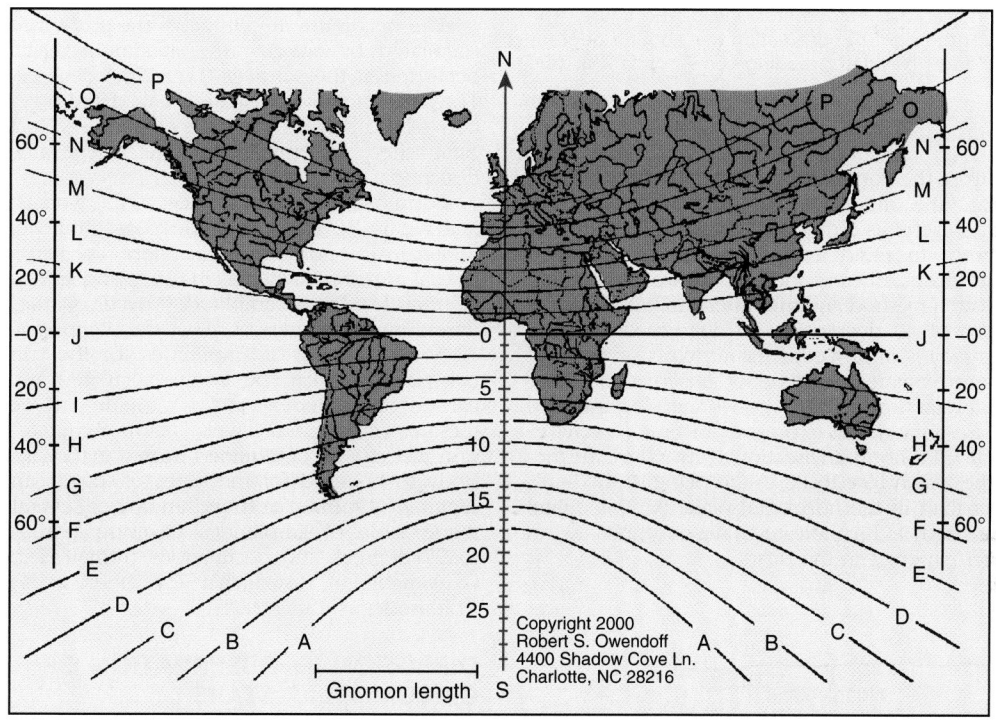

SELECTOR CHART						
NORTHERN HEMISPHERE						
Dec 22	Jan 22 Nov 22	Feb 22 Oct 22	Mar 22 Sep 22	Apr 22 Aug 22	May 22 Jul 22	Jun 22
0–N	0–M	1–K	0–J	0–I	1–G	2–F
2–N	3–M	4–K	3–J	2–I	3–G	4–F
6–N	6–M	7–K	5–J	4–I	6–G	7–F
10–P	10–N	11–K	9–J	9–H	11–F	12–E
20–P	18–N	14–L	12–J	12–H	13–F	14–E
30–Q	29–Q	23–L	18–J	18–G	21–D	21–C
Wait for rescue party			25–J	25–F	28–B	29–A
Jun 22	Jul 22 May 22	Aug 22 Apr 22	Sep 22 Mar 22	Oct 22 Feb 22	Nov 22 Jan 22	Dec 22
SOUTHERN HEMISPHERE						

Latitude rows (left and right): 0°, 10°, 20°, 30°, 40°, 50°, 60°

In the southern hemisphere, the arrow points to the south, and west (a.m.) is interchanged with east (p.m.)

FIGURE 106-18 The Universal Pocket Navigator. Enter the Selector Chart with arguments for approximate date and approximate latitude as determined from the background map. Stick a pin or toothpick vertically in the center line at the cross-mark indicated by the Selector Chart to serve as a gnomon. The tip of the gnomon should stand above the figure by the length indicated by the gnomon scale. Hold the figure horizontally, and rotate your body until the shadow of the tip of the gnomon lies on the appropriate lettered curve (as listed in the Selector Chart). The arrow now points north. *(From Owendoff RS: Better ways of pathfinding, Harrisburg, Pa, 1964, Stackpole.)*

canceled by reciprocal errors incurred during afternoon hours, as long as the rate of change in latitude while traveling is relatively slow during the period of observation.[36] The shortest shadow cast by a vertical gnomon throughout the course of the day lies on a north-south line at all latitudes. The point of closest approach of a declination curve to the gnomon may be difficult to determine accurately when the rate of change of the sun's altitude around LAN is slow. As an alternative method, a line bisecting the angle between any two shadows of equal length cast by a vertical gnomon will lie on a north-south line at all latitudes.

An ordinary analog wristwatch or pocket watch can be used to provide a rough north-south direction using the shadow technique. Because a conventional watch has a 12-hour cycle of rotation, the hour hand rotates at 30 degrees per hour, which is twice the rate of the apparent angular movement of the sun. Thus, if the hour hand of the watch is aligned with the shadow of a vertical object (i.e., the hand is pointing directly at the sun), the bisected angle between the hour hand and 12 o'clock on the dial yields a line that runs generally north to south. At times before 0600 or after 1800, the larger of the two possible angles between the hour hand and 12 o'clock should be used. This method is fraught with errors that increase in magnitude when the sun's altitude is high (i.e., in tropical or subtropical latitudes or during late-spring, summer, and early-fall months). It is also subject to errors that result from differences between zone time

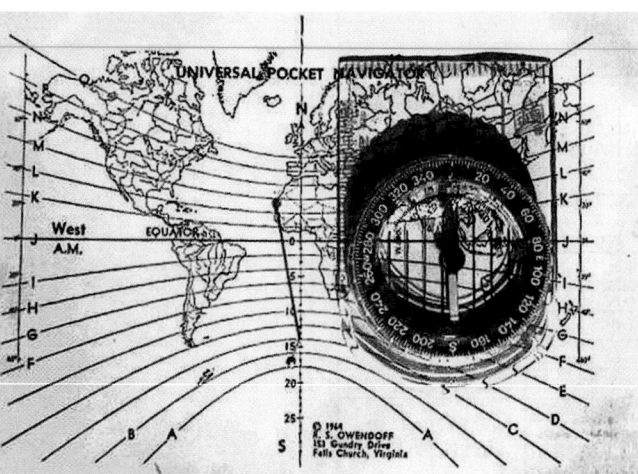

FIGURE 106-19 Use of the Universal Pocket Navigator to find north. The Selector Chart was entered with the date of October 25 and the assumed latitude of 40 degrees, yielding declination curve L and gnomon position 14. Note the correspondence between magnetic north and north as indicated by the center line of the figure. The magnetic declination at the sight of observation was about 5 degrees west. The Universal Pocket Navigator reading corresponds with true north.

and local time and from the equation of time (i.e., the difference between mean solar time and true solar time). However, the watch method can be useful as a direction finder if the potential for inaccuracy is kept in mind and if techniques are used to reduce avoidable errors. Correspondence between direction determined by the watch method and true direction will be greatest between latitudes of 40 degrees to 60 degrees during the winter months. Accuracy is improved if the watch is set to local solar time at the approximate longitude of observation rather than zone time (Local solar time = GMT + east longitude expressed in time *or* GMT − west longitude expressed in time [where 15 degrees of longitude = 1 hour]). Directional errors are further reduced by tilting the watch face to lie in the plane of the sun's apparent path rather than in the horizontal plane.[16,36,38] A digital watch may also be used if the indicated time is drawn as an analog clock face on paper or in the dust.

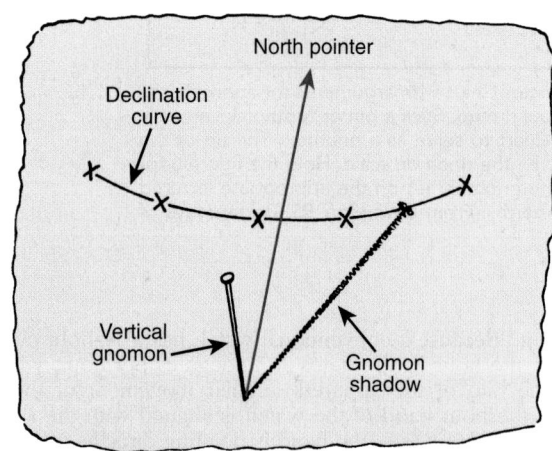

FIGURE 106-20 A makeshift sun compass inscribed on a scrap of paper. The declination curve has been empirically determined by tracing a line through points representing the tip of the gnomon shadow at various times throughout the day. On subsequent days, rotation of the figure such that the shadow tip touches the curve will orient the line connecting the base of the gnomon to the point of closest approach of the curve to point north. *(From Owendoff RS: Better ways of pathfinding, Harrisburg, Pa, 1964, Stackpole.)*

DIRECTION BY AMPLITUDES

Amplitude of a heavenly body is the angular measurement between the body when it is on the horizon and the observer's prime vertical circle. When the body is rising, amplitude is reckoned from due east; when the body is setting, amplitude is reckoned from due west. Amplitude is designated as north or south, depending on the relative position of the body on the horizon and the prime vertical circle. Amplitude will always be north when the declination of the body is positive, and vice versa. For objects of constant declination (i.e., the "fixed stars"), amplitude is constant. For the sun, moon, and planets, amplitude varies with the seasonal variations in the declination of these bodies. Knowledge of the amplitude of the sun for various dates is useful as a means of determining direction at sunrise and sunset. Amplitude of the sun is zero on the dates of the spring and fall equinoxes, and the sun rises due east and sets due west of an observer at any latitude between the Arctic Circle and Antarctic Circle on those dates.[4,12]

The formula for calculating the amplitude of any body at rising or setting (i.e., when altitude = 0) is known as Napier's rule[4,30,31]:

$$A = \sin^{-1}(\sin d / \cos L)$$

The maximum amplitude of the sun for any given latitude is calculated by entering the maximum declinations of the sun occurring at the solstices (i.e., ±23.5 degrees) into the formula.[4] The amplitude for any date is calculated by entering the declination of the sun on the date of interest. Note that directions as established by amplitudes are true (rather than magnetic) directions.

For most of the year in most of the world, the sun's amplitude lies within 30 degrees of due east and west. During fall and winter in the northern hemisphere, the sun rises and sets south of east and west, whereas in the spring and summer the opposite is true. Maximum amplitudes occur at the solstices, whereas minimum amplitudes occur at the equinoxes.

A useful table of amplitudes for the sun or other selected celestial body can be easily calculated by Napier's rule and carried on an index card to provide a directional reference in the area of intended travel. The approximate latitude of the area of travel can be determined from a map. The declinations of the body to be used for the dates of travel can be located in the *Nautical Almanac* or found on any of several websites. A ready-made table of amplitudes covering latitudes from 0 degrees to 77 degrees and declinations from 0 degrees to 24 degrees is available in Bowditch's *The American Practical Navigator,*[4] Volume II, as Table 27.

DIRECTION BY OBSERVATION OF CIRCUMPOLAR STARS

Polaris provides the most reliable directional indicator in the night sky and can be used to indicate direction within a degree of true north at any location above 10 degrees north latitude. Use of the star becomes progressively more difficult as its altitude increases above 60 degrees north because of the difficulty relating the star's azimuth to the horizon. A stick with a string tied to the end and weighted with a bolt or washer can be used to find the point on the horizon representing north in this setting. The stick is held such that the string hangs in a line from Polaris to the horizon. The point of intersection of the string with the horizon indicates north.[6]

The Big Dipper (Ursa Major) can be used to identify Polaris or true north by extending a line from the "Pointers" (i.e., α Ursae Majoris or Dubhe and β Ursae Majoris or Merak) toward the north celestial pole. These stars form the leading edge of the Dipper. The distance between them multiplied by five indicates the approximate position of Polaris. When the Dipper is low in the sky or below the horizon, a similar process can be followed in identifying north from the constellation Cassiopeia. Cassiopeia has the appearance of a flattened letter "M" when above the pole, and "W" when below. If a line drawn between the stars forming the feet of the "M" (i.e., β Cassiopeiae or Caph and ε Cassiopeiae) is assigned length *y,* a perpendicular line of length

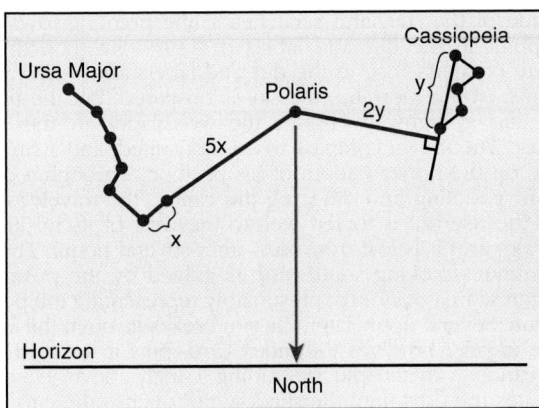

FIGURE 106-21 The azimuth of Polaris is always within 45 arc minutes of true north. Lines as indicated from the "pointers" of the constellation Ursa Major, or from the trailing star of the constellation Cassiopeia, can also be used to find north when Polaris is obscured by clouds or below the horizon. (*From Burch D:* Emergency navigation, *Camden, Me, 1986, International Marine Publishing.*)

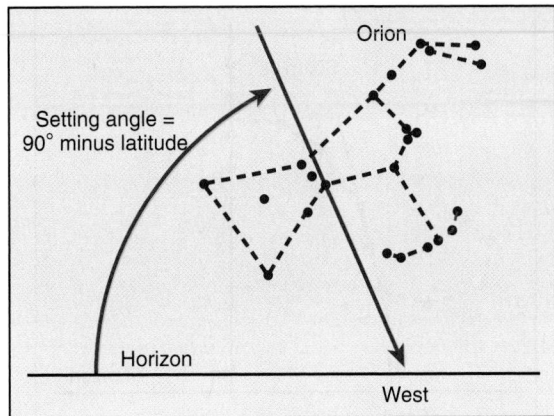

FIGURE 106-23 Determination of true west by observation of the setting point of the star Mintaka (with declination 0) in the belt of the constellation Orion. The rising point of the same star indicates true east. (*From Burch D:* Emergency navigation, *Camden, Me, 1986, International Marine Publishing.*)

2*y* extending from the trailing star indicates approximate north (Figure 106-21).

In the southern hemisphere, there is no conspicuous star that marks the south celestial pole. However, the distinctive asterism of the Southern Cross can be used to point to the approximate location of the pole and thus to indicate south. The Southern Cross consists of four stars, and the declination of the crossbar is approximately −60 degrees. The long axis of the cross lies on a line that passes within 3 degrees of the south celestial pole. The distance to the approximate pole from the star forming the base of the cross (i.e., α Crucis or Acrux) is approximately five times the length of the long axis of the cross (Figure 106-22). At latitudes where the cross is visible but the south celestial pole is below the horizon, the long axis of the Southern Cross indicates south when the constellation is vertically oriented.[6,9,39]

When the Southern Cross is below the horizon or too low in the sky for reliable observation, the bright stars Canopus (α Carinae) and Achernar (α Eridani) can be used to find south. If a line between these stars is considered to represent the base of an equilateral triangle, the apex of the triangle points to the approximate location of the south celestial pole[6,9] (Figure 106-22).

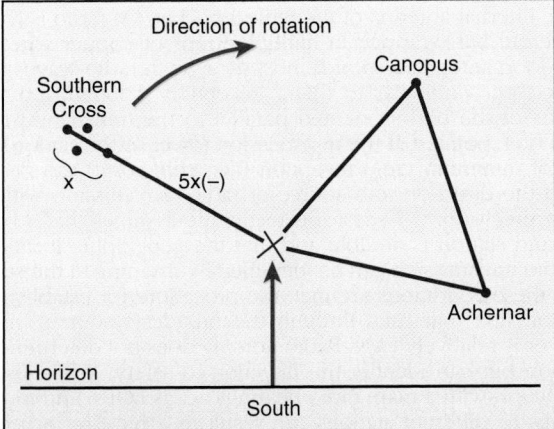

FIGURE 106-22 Determination of south by circumpolar stars. The long axis of the Southern Cross lies along an approximate radius extending from the south celestial pole at the distance indicated in the figure. The apex of an equilateral triangle with the stars Achernar and Canopus forming the vertices of the base also approximates the position of the south celestial pole. (*From Burch D:* Emergency navigation, *Camden, Me, 1986, International Marine Publishing.*)

DIRECTION BY OBSERVATION OF OTHER STARS

It should be clear from the amplitude formula that any object with a known declination of less than ±5 degrees could be used to give a reasonably accurate indication of east at the time of rising or west at the time of setting. By virtue of its brightness and of the familiarity of the constellation in which it is located, the star δ Orionis (i.e., Mintaka; declination, −0 degrees and 18 minutes) is particularly useful in this regard. Mintaka is the leading star in the belt of the constellation Orion; it rises due east and sets due west at any latitude from which it is observed (Figure 106-23). Unfortunately, the visibility of Mintaka at rising or setting is limited to the months of October through April. When the star is obscured by haze or by clouds at rising, or the time of rising is missed, location of the rising can be extrapolated. Within 1 to 2 hours of the rising time, hold a straightedge connecting the star to the horizon at the rising angle of the star, where rising angle is equal to 90 degrees minus the latitude. The point at which the straightedge touches the horizon indicates the position the star occupied when on the horizon. Because the rising and setting angles of any body are the same, the same technique can be used to determine the point on the horizon where the star will set.[6]

The constellation Scorpius is prominent in the southern sky at mid–northern latitudes during the summer. This constellation contains a distinctive reddish star, Antares (i.e., α Scorpii), at the position of the neck of the scorpion. To the east of Antares, the tail of the scorpion hangs toward the horizon. Three stars (i.e., ε, μ, and ζ Scorpii) just before the sharp bend in the tail of the figure form a nearly straight line. The stars that are the head and claws of the figure (i.e., β, δ [Dschubba], and π Scorpii) lie in a fairly straight line located immediately to the west of Antares. Configuration of the constellation is such that the stars forming the linear array of the tail point due south when the line of the head and claws has passed the meridian and is perpendicular to the horizon (Figure 106-24).[6]

In the Caroline Islands of the South Pacific, the bearings at rising and setting times of 32 prominent stars are memorized by navigators to permit determination of direction at sea. The fidelity of this "star compass" for direction finding is demonstrated by the ability of these navigators to make successful landfall on minute atolls after open-ocean voyages of hundreds of miles.[18] Memorization or recording of the rising or setting azimuths of a few prominent stars at the latitude of a planned trip will afford the same directional reference to the land navigator in case the compass or other navigational aid is lost or damaged. These azimuths could be precalculated in minutes using Napier's rule.

Finally, observation of the movement of any overhead celestial body relative to a fixed reference (e.g., a branch, guy

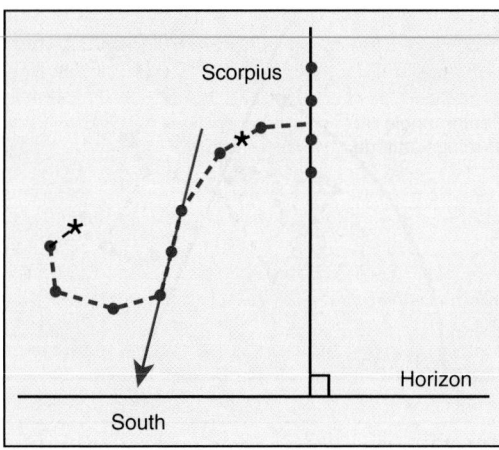

FIGURE 106-24 Determination of south by observation of the constellation Scorpius. When the best-fit line connecting the stars forming the head and claws of the figure is perpendicular to the horizon, the linear array of stars in the tail of the asterism points south. *(From Burch D:* Emergency navigation, *Camden, Me, 1986, International Marine Publishing.)*

line) over a span of 15 to 20 minutes (i.e., 4 to 5 degrees of movement) will give a reasonably accurate indication of east and west.

PRACTICAL FIELD-EXPEDIENT CELESTIAL NAVIGATION

The following discussion demonstrates the practical use of the methods just described on a hypothetical trip to one of the most remote areas in the 48 continental United States. Before leaving on a trip to the Florida Everglades in mid-May, a traveler consults a map of the intended area of travel, noting the approximate latitude (25 degrees north) of the area in question. The traveler also consults the *Nautical Almanac,* Bowditch's *The American Practical Navigator,*[4] or a website to obtain the approximate declination of the sun (18.5 degrees north) during the week of intended travel. By applying Napier's rule and using a calculator, or by consulting Bowditch,[4] the traveler notes that the sun will rise approximately 20 degrees north of due east and set 20 degrees north of due west during the trip. This information is recorded on an index card. The traveler then checks the same sources to see which easily recognized stars will be visible after sunset, near midnight, or before sunrise during the planned dates of the excursion. In this case, the traveler notes that Polaris will be visible all night and that the constellation Scorpius (see Figure 106-24) will be prominent, and almost due south, just before 1 AM. Antares, a prominent red star in Scorpius, rises shortly after twilight and has a declination of 26 degrees south. By using the formula or table, the traveler determines that the amplitude of Antares at rising will be approximately 29 degrees, and the star will rise at a bearing of about 119 degrees and set at a bearing of about 251 degrees; this information is also recorded on the index card. On the morning of arrival at the destination latitude, the traveler places the index card on a flat surface in sunlight and sticks a pin into the card so that it protrudes 1 inch above the face of the card. A sun compass is constructed by the method described earlier (see Figure 106-20), and the card and pin are then placed in a pocket.

The traveler paddles to a remote location in the park on a cloudy day and travels farther than anticipated because of an unusually high tide. He has a spill from the canoe en route, and while in the middle of the Everglades, becomes stranded when the tide recedes. He discovers that his compass and map are missing and that his watch is broken, but the index card is still in his pocket. The weather worsens, and the traveler loses all directional reference and is forced to camp. That evening, the eastern horizon clears, and Antares is observed rising at low altitude. The traveler retrieves the index card, recalls the rising

amplitude of the star, and scratches a line pointing toward the rising point in the dirt and labels it "119°". He then draws a complete compass rose in the dirt and labels all of the cardinal directions. In the morning, the sky is obscured, but the traveler recalls that a highway crosses the Everglades to the south-southeast. The drawn compass rose is consulted, and a small rise is noted on the horizon south of his position. Through a combination of paddling and dragging the canoe, the traveler moves toward the rise but is forced well to the west of its position by the terrain, and it is lost from view after several hours. The traveler continues moving southward as judged by the position of the brightest area of clouds, presumably representing the position of the sun. Several hours later, the sun breaks through the clouds, and the traveler retrieves the index card, pins it flat to the seat of the canoe with the pin protruding 1 inch above its surface, and rotates the card until the shadow tip touches the curve. The cardinal directions are now reestablished, and the traveler proceeds southeast as indicated by the sun compass. As the weather worsens, the traveler again identifies a landmark on the southern horizon and moves toward it after the shadow is lost. As night falls, the clouds thin on the western horizon, the setting sun is observed, and the cardinal directions are again established by the amplitude method. Travel progresses to the southeast. That night, the northern sky transiently clears enough for Polaris to be identified. The traveler continues southward away from the direction of the star, but becomes disoriented. During a rest period, the traveler lies on the ground and observes the movement of overhead stars for 15 minutes through a break in the overcast, reacquiring the cardinal directions. He continues southward and notices lights in the direction of travel; he then reaches the highway and is rescued by motorists.

The successful outcome in this example resulted from preparation in advance of travel and familiarity with the navigational clues offered by the environment. Being lost in the middle of a desert or in mountainous terrain during winter may represent a more desperate situation than that just described, but the methods used for recovery would be identical if sophisticated navigational aids were unavailable.

NAVIGATION WITH A POCKET RADIO

Radio transmission and reception are inherently directional. This is particularly evident with reception in the broadcast band (i.e., 500 to 1600 KHz) and is a principle that is more apparent in inexpensive portable radios than in larger, more expensive models. Exploitation of this characteristic was used extensively in aviation navigation from the 1930s through the 1950s. There are anecdotal reports of successful sailings from the west coast of the United States to Hawaii using only an amplitude-modulated (AM) radio and jet contrails as navigational aids.

The internal antenna of the typical pocket AM radio is formed by a ferrite bar wrapped in multiple loops of copper wire. This ferrite-loop antenna responds most strongly to radio-waves when oriented perpendicular to them. Reception is minimized when the axis of the bar is oriented parallel to the transmitted radio-waves (i.e., pointed at the transmission tower of the station). The point of minimum radio reception (i.e., *null point*) can be used to find the direction to a source of radio transmission with surprising precision.[6,38] Use of this technique assumes that a broadcast band station is audible and that the geographic location of the radio transmission can be identified by listening to the station. When these conditions are met, the procedure for establishing a direction line that runs through the broadcast source and the observer is relatively easy. Radio homing does not determine true direction but can identify the direction to safety. When used in conjunction with a map, radio bearings act as LOPs, and multiple bearings to different stations can result in a fix. The procedure for navigation by radio bearings follows:

1. If not known, determine orientation of the radio's internal antenna. This can be done by opening the case and looking for the antenna (i.e., a dark-gray or black bar wrapped in fine copper wire) or by rotating the radio while listening to a station and determining the plane of rotation that results in a null point (rotation about the long axis of the antenna will

not change the reception, whereas rotation perpendicular to the long axis will result in nulling).

2. Select an audible AM station and listen until the location of the station is identified. Hold the radio in a manner that allows the long axis of the internal antenna to act as a pointer. Rotate the radio parallel to the ground until the radio signal becomes faintest or disappears. Nulling of the signal can be augmented by tuning to the fringes of the station frequency if the reception is strong.

3. The actual direction to the source of radio transmission will be one of the reciprocal bearings of the LOP connecting the observer and the station location. The bearing that actually points to the radio source can be determined if the observer has even a crude understanding of his or her position relative to the station (e.g., generally north of vs. generally south of). The bearing to the broadcast source can also be determined by serially checking the null point of the station while traveling. The angle over which nulling occurs becomes greater as the signal weakens with increasing distance from the source. Thus, if the angle over which the signal nulls is widening as travel progresses, the observer is moving away from the radio source. If the angle over which the station nulls narrows as travel progresses, the observer is moving toward the source.

4. If a compass is available, determine the azimuth of the null point. Keep the compass far enough from the radio to avoid influencing the needle with the radio's metal parts. A compass allows the magnetic bearing to the station to be determined. This bearing can then be followed to safety without further use of the radio.

5. If a map and compass are available, orient the map using the compass and draw a line though the broadcast source on the map at the azimuth of the null point. Extend this line to the edges of the map. Your location is somewhere on or near this line. If you have a map but no compass and can properly orient the map by natural cues, place the radio on top of the broadcast location on the map, and rotate it until the signal nulls. Draw a line parallel to the internal antenna through the broadcast location, and extend it to the map margins. Again, your position lies somewhere on this line. When two or more stations can be tuned and identified, the LOPs connecting the observer to each radio source will cross, and a fix can be obtained at the point of crossing. The uncertainty of this fix will be least when the angle between two position lines is close to 90 degrees or when the angles among three position lines are close to 120 degrees.

ORIENTEERING AND GEOCACHING

Orienteering is a competitive sport in which an unfamiliar course is navigated using map and compass. Usually, participants are required to find a number of controls (i.e., identified sites) in a set sequence; this is called *point-to-point orienteering*. In a variant, participants have a fixed amount of time to visit as many controls as possible in any sequence; this is called *score orienteering*.[2] Orienteering is usually practiced as a cross-country footrace over a distance of kilometers or miles, but shorter courses can be set up in paved or inhabited areas for participants of differing abilities. Appropriately constructed courses can be negotiated on foot, on skis, or by bicycle or wheelchair.

Orienteering had its genesis in military land navigation exercises. The term *orienteering* was coined in Sweden in 1900 to describe a ski relay race over a distance of more than 160 km (100 miles). By the close of World War I, orienteering clubs conducting competitive meets were well established in Scandinavia. The sport rapidly gained popularity in Europe and was introduced in North America during the late 1940s. By the 1970s, the International Orienteering Federation was established to codify standards and rules.[2] Orienteering is now practiced by many thousands of people on all continents.

Orienteering has spawned several offshoot sports. *Rogaining* is a team form of score orienteering practiced over a 24- to 48-hour period, requiring overnight camping as a component. Participants set out from a central base to find as many controls as possible during the allotted time span. Return to the base for meals, rest, refreshment, or socializing is permitted. *Adventure racing* is a form of team orienteering practiced over long distances and time spans of days to weeks; it may involve running, hiking, biking, and canoeing as components.[27]

THE ORIENTEERING MEET

Orienteering meets are usually sponsored by local clubs operating under guidelines established by the International Orienteering Federation, United States Orienteering Federation (USOF), or other national federations. Events may be advertised in local newspapers or on websites maintained by the sponsoring clubs. Most events offer multiple courses to accommodate participants of varying skill and fitness levels. An internationally standardized color-coding system identifies the technical difficulty of each course (Table 106-1).[37]

The only required equipment for competitive orienteering is an orienteering compass, pencil or pen, and appropriate athletic clothing. Participants register for a course, pay a fee, and receive a start time, course map, printed description of the controls along the course (e.g., "at bend in creek"), and control card that will be marked with a coded hole punch attached to each control point. The map displays magnetic meridians, eliminating the need to correct for declination. The map may also have the controls and lines connecting them printed on it (Figure 106-25), or participants may be required to copy these features onto their map from a master map.

Several minutes before the appointed start time, the participant reports to the starting line. The starter tears a stub from the control card to allow a tally of participants on the course. The participant orients the map to the environment using the compass and visual landmarks and starts the course when told by the starter. The starter records the starting time with the participant's name or number for comparison with the finish time and

TABLE 106-1 Color-Coded Events: Standards for Competitors

Color	Length (km)	Control Sites	Type of Leg	Technical Level	Time (min)	Age (yr)
String	0.5-1.0	On the line	Along the string	Easy	10-15	3
White	1.0-1.5	On major line features and at junctions	Along line features, no route choice	Easy	15-40	6-12
Yellow	1.0-2.5	On line features and at easy adjacent features	Along line features, minimal route choice, no compass legs	Easy	20-45	8
Orange	2.0-3.5	On minor line and easy point features	Route choice with compass legs and collecting features near controls	Medium	35-55	10
Red	4.5-6.0	Same as Orange	Same as Orange	Medium	50-80	10
Green	3.5-4.5	At small point and contour features	Fine compass and contour legs, more physical	Hard	25-55	10
Blue	4.5-6.5	Same as Green	Same as Green	Hard	50-75	10
Brown	6.5	Same as Green	Same as Green	Hard	60-85	10

Modified and with permission from Renfrew T: *Orienteering*, Champaign, Ill, 1997, Human Kinetics.

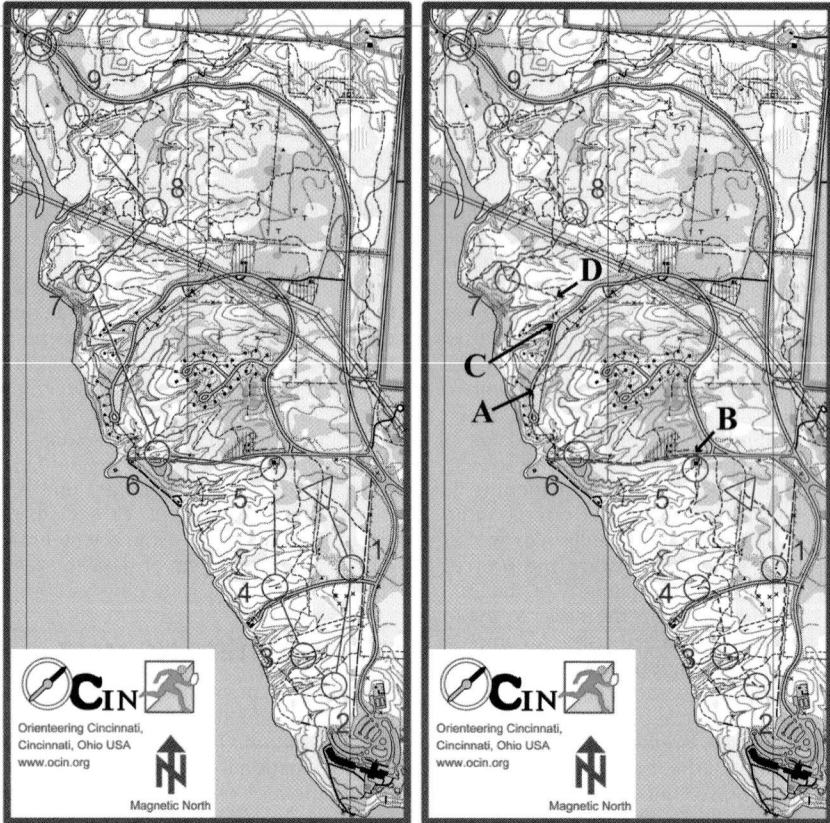

FIGURE 106-25 Paired orienteering maps for a typical yellow-level course showing the starting point as a *triangle*, the control points as *numbered circles*, and the finish point as a *double circle*. Note the magnetic meridians printed on the map as a directional reference. In the map on the left, bearing lines connect the controls but may not represent the fastest, least strenuous, or safest routes of travel. The actual route followed is shown in the map on the right. Note the use of the road segment *(A)* between Controls 6 and 7 as a handrail. The road immediately to the north of Control 5 *(B)* represents a collecting feature should the participant overrun the control. The branch in the road between Controls 6 and 7 *(C)* forms an attack point for reaching the path that leads to Control 7. On this leg, the participant deliberately aimed off to meet the path at a point known to be east of the target *(D)* so that the path could be followed in the proper direction toward the objective. *(From Michael Minium, Orienteering Cincinnati, Inc., and the United States Orienteering Federation, 2005.)*

determination of elapsed time to run the course. When running the course, the participant continually reorients the map to the environment using the compass, and the environment to the map by comparing visual cues with map features. The participant chooses a route between control points by considering terrain features and the presence or absence of readily identifiable landmarks that may assist with navigation. As the participant approaches the area of a control, the area is scanned for descriptive features and the orange and white flag that identifies the site; the control point is then located, and the participant punches his or her control card with the punch attached to the control as proof of having been there. The participant then reorients the map and progresses to the next control in sequence. This process is repeated until the course is completed. As the participant crosses the finish line, the time is recorded, and the number on the control card is checked against the stub that was collected by the starter. The card is then inspected to establish that all the control points were visited, and the course time is calculated and recorded. At the completion of the meet, the winners of each course are determined and announced, and prizes may be awarded.[2,37]

Several concepts that receive particular emphasis in orienteering are extremely useful for general map and compass navigation.[28,37] A *handrail* is a linear feature on the map that can be easily recognized in the terrain and used as a guide toward an objective. Typical handrails include paths, roads, streams, fences, shorelines, firebreaks, ridgelines, and abrupt contour changes.

When a handrail is encountered, the navigator can move along it with speed until the chosen route deviates from it or the objective is encountered. An *attack point* is a prominent and obvious feature in the terrain from which an objective can be easily located; this may be a knoll, bend in a path, narrowing in a stream, or another point feature. An attack point can be chosen in advance of travel, allowing the bearing and distance from the point to the objective to be calculated in advance. When the attack point is reached, discovery of the ultimate objective is greatly simplified. A *collecting feature* is an easily recognized terrain feature that lies beyond a desired objective. If the collecting feature is encountered, the navigator knows that the target has been passed and can retrace his or her steps to the last known position for a second attempt at the objective. *Aiming off* is a technique for reducing confusion when navigating toward a particular point that lies on a handrail feature. A common problem with land navigation involves encountering such a linear feature and then not knowing which way to turn to follow the handrail to the objective. Aiming off involves introducing a deliberate error into the bearing to the handrail so that it will be encountered at a point that is absolutely known to be to the left or right of the intended target. The navigator then follows the handrail in the direction that corrects the error and is certain to lead to the objective (see Figure 106-25).

Handrails, collecting features, attack points, and opportunities for aiming off should be determined in advance of travel by studying the map and the visible terrain. This permits selection of a route that facilitates speed, safety, and ease of travel. These features should be recorded rather than trusted to memory. Critical evaluation of the map for such features greatly increases the navigator's awareness of terrain as well as his or her competence in map reading.

ORIENTEERING FOR CHILDREN

Successful orienteering depends on an ability to apply basic land navigation skills with speed and accuracy. The skills required for completion of even simple orienteering courses are completely translatable to following a wilderness route. Note in Table 106-1 that string courses—in which participants literally follow a string, ribbon, or length of yarn strung from one control to the next—are available as an introduction for the very young. Courses classified as white, yellow, and orange are also of a length and technical level that are appropriate for children. As such, orienteering offers perhaps the most reliable and accessible avenue for teaching map and compass skills to children. Map reading, orientation of a map with a compass, orientation of a map to the environment, route selection, terrain recognition, and outdoor safety are all concepts that are compatible with training in a classroom or backyard setting. These skills can then be applied in any large indoor space or at a local park.[28]

Most orienteering clubs offer programs for teaching children. The USOF sponsors a four-step program to foster progressive mastery of necessary skills in a logical sequence.[41,42] The program begins at the Little Troll level and involves string courses. Participants complete five USOF-sponsored courses with adult assistance. At the conclusion of each course, the child receives a sticker that he or she affixes to a special card. The completed card is redeemed with the USOF for a Little Troll patch, and the child then progresses to the Chipmunk level. As Chipmunks, participants learn to be more comfortable in an outdoor setting and are introduced to map symbols, the concept of control sites, and the procedures of running a course. After completion of five USOF-sponsored white courses with adult assistance, the child receives a Chipmunk patch and advances to become a Rabbit. At the Rabbit level, knowledge of map symbols and colors is expanded, safety awareness is increased, and the child learns to orient the map to the terrain, mark his or her current location, select routes to follow, and follow a path between controls. Some adult assistance continues at this level. After completion of seven sponsored white courses, the child receives a Rabbit patch and advances to training as a Roadrunner. Training at this level occurs without direct adult assistance, although an adult follows the child on each course. Roadrunners are required to know safety rules and learn to adjust the orientation of the map as they cover the course, make independent route selections, and orienteer in sequence from control to control. After completion of another seven white courses, the child receives a Roadrunner patch and progresses to solo orienteering.[41] The International Orienteering Federation supports a similar progressive training program for children called the *Swedish Step System*.[37]

In orienteering, correction for declination is not required because the maps are prepared with reference to magnetic meridians, creating internal consistency between the map and compass. Separate training in the conversion of magnetic and true bearings is required to allow the practice of safe and comprehensive map and compass navigation.

GEOCACHING

The sports of orienteering and rogaining prohibit the use of GPS technology. The recently developed sport of *geocaching* offers an excellent opportunity for training in the use of terrestrial coordinates and GPS receivers. Geocaching is essentially a treasure hunt in a challenging environment. The sponsors of a cache leave a container or object in a concealed location identified only by latitude and longitude, or UTM coordinates. Locations of caches, relevant maps, and location descriptions are published on websites maintained by cache sponsors. Persons seeking the cache use the provided information and a GPS receiver to locate the site. When the cache is located, the participant may record the date of discovery in an enclosed logbook, if provided, and the cache is replaced. Note that the cache may be located in an easily discovered spot or in an extremely challenging position such as on a cliff face, in a tree, buried, or underwater. Many variations on the basic theme exist, including caches that contain coordinates for locating the next cache in a sequence and caches that contain hints for locating a final cache after accumulation of clues from several other caches.[19] Geocaching is greatly facilitated by the use of a WAAS-enabled GPS receiver because of increased accuracy available with this technology.

CONCLUSION

The body of literature covering the topic of navigation is immense. Many techniques for determining direction and position exist in addition to those described in this chapter, and several references catalog these methods.[4,6,16,26,30,43,44] It is sufficient to the task of navigation if the aforementioned methods are understood in terms of their practical application, even if why they work remains obscure. Practice is essential, and the reader is encouraged to increase his or her familiarity with the motion of celestial bodies, inconstancy of Earth's magnetic field, and use of a variety of common navigational aids (e.g., compass, topographic map). Inexperienced persons anticipating a backcountry trip are strongly encouraged to increase their navigational skill by participating in the sports of orienteering and geocaching. A review of land-navigation techniques, advance study of the area of intended travel, and familiarity with the appearance of the day and night skies during the planned time of travel should be routine components of preparation for any wilderness expedition.

REFERENCES

Complete references used in this text are available online at www.expertconsult.inkling.com.

GENERAL CIRCULATION AND ATMOSPHERIC PROFILE

CLIMATE CONTROLS AND RADIATION BALANCE

Equatorial regions receive a net surplus and polar regions receive a net deficit of solar radiation because of differences in solar angle and beam dissipation at the poles and the equator. This heat imbalance drives the ocean-atmosphere circulation. Heat is transported in the atmosphere primarily through convection, conduction, and advection. Convection and conduction are important in vertical atmospheric heat transport. Latent and sensible heating are the key mechanisms by which convective and conductive transport are enacted. Horizontal heat transport is achieved primarily through migration of air masses and eddy circulation.

Average global circulation on a simplified basis consists of three circulation cells. This structure is found in both hemispheres. The cell that straddles the tropics (0 degrees to ~30 degrees), known as the *Hadley cell,* is characterized by rising motion on its ascending limb along the equator and sinking motion on its descending limb at the subtropics (~30 degrees). A second cell, known as the *Ferrel cell,* has an ascending limb at the midlatitudes and descending limb at the subtropics. The third cell, known as the *polar cell,* is characterized by rising motion at the midlatitudes and subsidence at the poles.

This circulation structure results in a climate with intense convective precipitation in the regions along the rising limb of the Hadley cell. This region is identified as the *intertropical convergence zone* (ITCZ) because it is a zone where intense heating leads to convective motion and low pressure. Low-level or surface convergence and upper-level divergence result in convective precipitation in this zone. Regions along the descending limb of the Hadley cell—approximately 30 degrees north and 30 degrees south—tend to be warm and dry as subsiding air warms and dries out the air column. It is no coincidence that most deserts are found at this latitude. The midlatitudes (40 degrees to 50 degrees)—the rising limb of the Ferrel cell—have cells of low pressure and receive precipitation from storms and frontal systems. Polar regions along the subsiding limb of the polar cell are characterized by cold and relatively dry climates.

The three-division structure results in surface winds blowing from the east (easterly) out of the subtropical high-pressure zone to the low-pressure zone at the equator; winds from the west (westerly) out of the subtropical highs to the midlatitude low-pressure zone; and polar easterlies flowing from the polar high-pressure zone to the midlatitude low (Figure 107-1). Such an east-west wind direction, as opposed to north-south, prevails because of the Coriolis effect, which acts on the pressure gradient force and deflects winds to the right in the northern hemisphere and to the left in the southern hemisphere.

The tricell structure is only a simplified representation of the general atmospheric circulation. In reality, the Ferrel cell does not persist throughout the year, as does the Hadley cell. The pressure gradient at the polar front is so intense that it results in eddies that are instrumental in poleward heat transport, particularly during winter, when the equator-pole pressure gradient is at a maximum. The midlatitudes are the regions most influenced by air masses. Eddy circulation is predominant at the boundary, the *polar front,* between the Ferrel cell and the polar cell.

ATMOSPHERIC PROFILE

Lapse Rate

Temperature generally decreases with altitude in the troposphere, as evidenced by decreasing temperature as one ascends a mountain. The rate at which air cools as it rises depends on the amount of moisture in the air, as well as dynamics of the atmosphere. This rate can be estimated to be 6.5°C for every 1000-m gain in elevation, or 3.5°F for every 1000 feet.

Moisture

Humidity reflects the amount of moisture in the air, usually measured by relative humidity and dew point temperature. Relative humidity is a ratio of the amount of moisture in the air to the amount the air can hold at that temperature. Atmospheric moisture is often given as relative humidity, which must be accompanied by a temperature to be a valuable indication of the air's moisture content.

Dew point temperature is the temperature at which the air becomes completely saturated. If air is cooled to this temperature at the surface, fog will form. If air is forced to rise and cools to this temperature, clouds will form.

Heat capacity is the amount of energy required to increase the temperature of a substance. This is important because of the great difference in heat capacity of land and water. Water heats and cools much more slowly than does land, which has important implications for weather in the interior of continents, especially compared with coastal areas.

CLIMATIC REGIONS CONTROLLED BY LATITUDE: TROPICS, MIDLATITUDES, AND POLES

MIDLATITUDE AND POLAR CLIMATES

Most weather systems, such as midlatitude cyclones and thunderstorms, form at the frontal boundaries between air masses of different densities and are steered by upper-level winds, typically to the east in the midlatitudes and west above 60 degrees. This is in contrast to tropical cyclones, which are not influenced by air masses and only form over the ocean. Midlatitude cyclones are a powerful means by which air can be transported across latitudes. These differing air masses meet at boundaries called *fronts.*

Cold and warm fronts are typically oriented around a cyclone, as shown in Figure 107-2. The colder, polar air mass advances equatorward behind the cyclone at the cold front, while the warmer air mass advances poleward ahead of it behind the warm front. Typically, the faster-moving cold front catches up to the warm front as the cyclone matures and "occludes," and the cyclone begins to lose its strength as the temperature differences from which it derives its energy dissipate. Occasionally, neither air mass will be able to dislodge the other, and the front will become stationary. Stationary fronts are conducive to prolonged periods of precipitation and can serve as a focus for moisture transport and subsequent precipitation as new areas of low pressure move along the front.

These areas of low pressure have favored storm tracks that shift during the year and as larger-scale atmospheric conditions

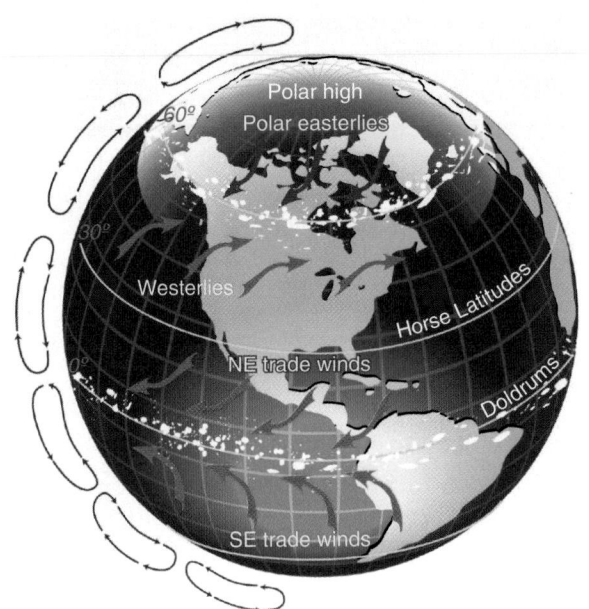

FIGURE 107-1 General circulation of the atmosphere. *(Courtesy Deborah Mioduszewski.)*

change. Often, atmospheric patterns emerge where cyclones take the same track, moving through the same areas for up to several weeks. Conversely, locations removed from these storm tracks may experience persistent fair weather associated with an accompanying anticyclone. Cyclones often form and move along the polar front, where there is a sharp contrast in temperature and moisture. During winter, the precise track of a cyclone will determine whether rain, snow, or a mixture will fall in a given location, with snow more likely on the poleward side of the cyclone and rain on the equatorward side.

These cyclones bring the most noticeable changes to sensible weather in the mid- and high latitudes. In addition to precipitation ranging from drizzle and fog to severe thunderstorms, temperature and humidity levels vary greatly in different parts of the storm. Warm and moist air is advected in behind the warm front with a shift in the wind, causing extremely uncomfortable weather in the summer and thaws in the winter. Colder, dryer, and usually breezy or blustery weather accompanies passage of a cold front as air from higher latitudes is advected in behind a departing cyclone.

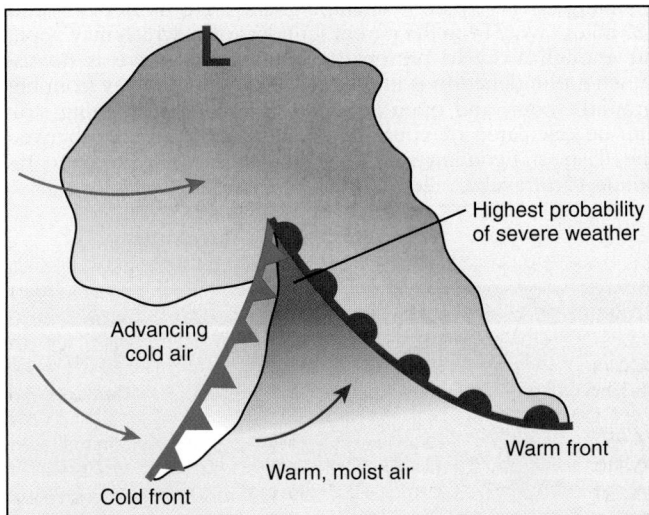

FIGURE 107-2 Midlatitude cyclone model. *L*, Low pressure. *(Courtesy Deborah Mioduszewski.)*

Midlatitude cyclones can bring ice and snow with cold temperatures. Snow occurs when the entire atmosphere is below freezing, whereas sleet (ice pellets) and freezing rain occur when there are intrusions of warmer air in the lower atmosphere. These cyclones are considered to be a blizzard when strong winds accompany the snow. These strong winds result from the gradient in surface pressure across the area and are primarily caused by the strength of the low-pressure system, with rapidly strengthening storms often generating the strongest winds. When winds are strong enough, blowing snow can generate whiteout conditions that reduce visibility to near zero and can be disorienting to anyone caught outdoors.

Ice storms often occur as snow is transitioning to rain behind a warm front and as the lighter warm air slides in above the colder air mass. This changes the precipitation to sleet, freezing rain, and finally rain when the surface temperature rises above freezing. If the surface temperature cannot rise above freezing, an extended period of freezing rain occurs and is particularly hazardous. Even the thinnest glaze of ice can be treacherous, but prolonged freezing rain accumulates as a heavy layer of ice that weighs down everything above the ground. This occurs during cold-air *damming* events when low-level cooler air is dammed against mountains and cannot be displaced, most often in the leeward side of mountain ranges (e.g., Appalachian Mountains). Ice storms are most disruptive when the temperature remains below freezing as the storm ends and remains there for days afterward.

When and where the transition between precipitation types occurs is very difficult to forecast precisely, even for meteorologists, but trends in temperature, pressure, and wind direction can provide clues. Rising temperature and dew point during snow or a mix, particularly with a south or southwest wind in the northern hemisphere, indicate that the warm front is likely approaching and precipitation will soon transition to rain. Rain with temperatures near freezing and a falling barometer may indicate an approaching cold front, in which case a change to snow is likely as the front passes when the pressure begins rising again, the wind shifts, and temperature drops.

SUBTROPICAL AND TROPICAL CLIMATES

The subtropics lie poleward of the Hadley cell, at about 35 degrees north and 35 degrees south. The subtropics are characterized by warm and dry climates. Weather in the subtropics is primarily influenced by frontal systems during the winter and spring seasons. Tropical weather systems can affect weather in the fall, particularly in the coastal lower latitudes of the subtropics. The summers tend to be hot and dry, and summer heat waves are common. These heat waves can persist for days, aided by the positive feedback among dry soils, temperature, and atmospheric subsidence (sinking air). If the antecedent winter and spring seasons were dry, it is more likely that the oncoming summer will be dry, given that land-surface processes play a significant role in driving convective processes in the subtropics.

Tropical climates are found along the rising limb of the Hadley cell. Temperature is high throughout the year, with the average coldest temperature not below 18° C (64.4° F). Convective processes and convective precipitation, typically experienced as brief periods of intense rainfall from showers and thunderstorms, dominate the climate of the tropics but are not the sole climatic phenomena found there. Monsoons and tropical cyclones can also account for a significant amount of precipitation that falls in parts of the tropics.

MONSOONS

The term *monsoon* refers to the seasonal reversal in atmospheric circulation and associated precipitation in tropical and subtropical regions. Reversal of wind direction takes place with seasonal migration of the ITCZ, which induces a temperature difference between the land surface and ocean. The land-ocean temperature difference induces a land-ocean pressure gradient that drives the monsoonal winds. Regional components of the monsoon include the tropical and subtropical regions of Asia, Australia, Africa,

South America, and southwestern North America. The onset of monsoonal rains varies among and within these regions.

TROPICAL CYCLONES

Intense convective heating, particularly in the tropics, creates regions of low atmospheric pressure characterized by clouds, showers, and locally windy conditions. If low-pressure systems form over warm oceans of the tropics and subtropics at least 5 degrees from the equator, they have the potential to develop into cyclones, which are intense, rotating low-pressure systems. Winds flow counterclockwise in the northern hemisphere and clockwise in the southern hemisphere around cyclones. Cyclones, hurricanes, and typhoons all refer to the same phenomenon. The convention is to use *typhoons* to identify severe cyclones in East Asia, *hurricanes* for severe cyclones in North America, and *cyclones* for severe cyclones over the Indian Ocean region. Cyclones form in all the major ocean basins, except the South Atlantic and Southeast Pacific. Minimum factors needed for cyclones to develop are sea surface temperatures exceeding 28°C (82.4°F) and a minimal amount of vertical wind shear. Extratropical cyclones form at frontal boundaries. After formation, tropical cyclones tend to move westward and poleward. Some cyclones, particularly in the midlatitudes, recurve and enter the westerlies. Tropical cyclones tend to dissipate on making landfall. Cyclones are classified by their intensity as follows:

- Tropical depression: winds up to 64 km/hr (39.8 miles/hr)
- Tropical storm: winds of 64 to 118 km/hr (39.8 to 73.3 miles/hr)
- Severe tropical cyclone, hurricane, or typhoon: winds greater than 118 km/hr (74 miles/hr)

These are further categorized using the Saffir-Simpson scale, ranging from category 1 to category 5 (most severe) (Table 107-1).

Tropical cyclones have spiraling bands, often termed "rain bands," of convective clouds (Figure 107-3). Intense upward motion and thus the heaviest rainfall occur within these rain bands and in the eyewall, which encircles the calm eye at the center of the storm. Wind speeds increase with each rain band toward the center of the cyclone as the pressure decreases. The wind is typically strongest in the quadrant of the cyclone where the wind direction is the same as the cyclone's motion, and weakest on the opposite side (Figure 107-3). The destructive winds of a cyclone are strongest at the coast and well above the surface, where frictional effects are minimized.

In addition to destructive winds, the greatest hazards from tropical cyclones on land include heavy rainfall and storm-surge flooding. Heavy rain and consequent flooding are always threats with cyclones, regardless of strength. This is exacerbated in mountainous regions, where mudslides and flash floods frequently result. Rainfall potential depends primarily on the cyclone's speed and access to atmospheric energy and moisture, which are typically well predicted by meteorologists but impossible to predict without these tools. The storm surge occurs primarily as the storm's persistent wind pushes water ahead of it and is experienced on the coast as a relatively gradual rise in water as the storm's center approaches. Storm surge is historically the deadliest of a cyclone's hazards but can be avoided by seeking higher ground, if possible.

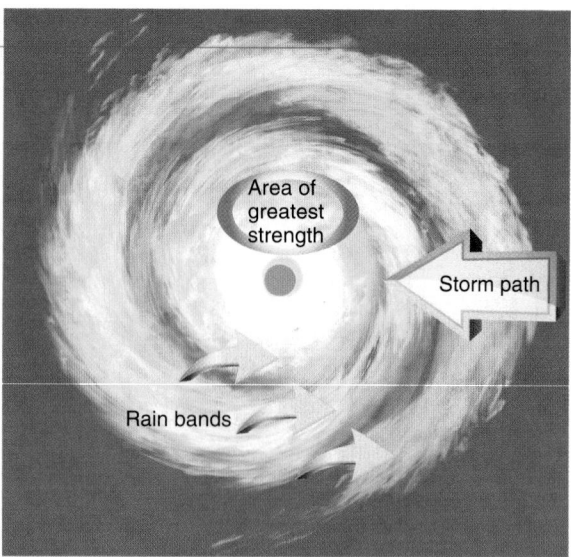

FIGURE 107-3 Tropical cyclone, motion and structure (northern hemisphere). *(Courtesy Deborah Mioduszewski.)*

THUNDERSTORMS

Thunderstorms result from atmospheric instability caused by intense convective heating processes in the tropics, and with convergence of air masses of different temperatures in midlatitudes, particularly in continental climates. Cumulonimbus clouds are characteristic features of thunderstorms, as are lightning and thunder, wind gusts, and heavy rain.

Flash flooding, the rapid flooding of low-lying areas, can occur in any location given a long enough period of heavy rain. The probability of such an event depends on the strength of the wind in the midlevels of the atmosphere as well as the moisture available to precipitate, which cannot be predicted on the ground. Intense, slow-moving, and persistent thunderstorms in upstream regions of river catchments with sharp elevation gradients may induce flash flooding in downstream regions where little or no rain falls, such as the Big Thompson Canyon Flood that killed 143 people in Colorado in 1976. Therefore, hikers should pay particular attention to the topography of the local area and the possibility of rapid, unexpected rises in nearby streams. In these regions, it is critical to have access to real-time weather alerts and ideally weather radar to monitor such storms.

One of the major dangers associated with thunderstorms is lightning (see Chapter 5). Lightning can strike more than 32 km (20 miles) away from the parent thunderstorm, which may appear far enough away to present the illusion that there is no risk. When a thunderstorm is in the area, seek shelter away from high ground, water, and open spaces. Distance to a lightning strike can be calculated by counting the number of seconds between the flash of lightning and the thunder, keeping in mind that sound can travel a mile in 4.5 seconds.

TABLE 107-1 Saffir-Simpson Scale of Tropical Cyclone Intensity

| Category | Pressure (mb) | Wind Speed | | Storm Surge | | Damage |
		km/hr	miles/hr	m	ft	
1	≥980	119-154	74-95	1-2	4-5	Minimal
2	965-979	155-178	96-110	2-3	6-8	Moderate
3	945-964	179-210	111-130	3-4	9-12	Extensive
4	920-944	211-250	131-155	4-6	13-18	Extreme
5	<920	>250	>155	>6	>18	Catastrophic

Hail may be encountered in some thunderstorms, though rarely reaching a size that is dangerous to people. Hail is formed in strong thunderstorm updrafts that can support ice chunks as the hail nuclei are accreted with more ice before becoming heavy enough to fall to the ground. Ideal conditions for hail formation are often best in continental climates and near mountain ranges, where a larger depth of the cumulonimbus cloud is below freezing and conditions promoting strong updrafts are enhanced. As such, hail occurs globally, but most frequently in central Europe, the foothills around the Himalayas and European Alps, and particularly across North America's Great Plains and Rockies. The hazards of large hailstones and long-lasting storms are much more serious for agriculture, livestock, infrastructure, and personal property, where risks are primarily economic, rather than for safety and logistics in wilderness operations.

Tornadoes are extremely dangerous weather phenomena characterized by rapidly rotating air that reaches the ground beneath cumulonimbus clouds. They are preceded by a lowering of part of the cloud base, with rotation of this base (funnel cloud) often visible. All funnel clouds do not produce tornadoes, but all tornadoes are preceded by funnel clouds. Once a tornado forms, it is not dissipated or deterred by topography, land surfaces, or human construction. Tornadoes cross over rivers and mountains and strike cities as easily as they move across the prairie. Although most tornadoes are relatively weak and short-lived (<175 km/hr [108 miles/hr] and <10 minutes), violent tornadoes are typically much wider, longer lasting, and cause the most damage. Because the greatest hazard from tornadoes is wind-blown debris, the best refuge is in the interior of a sturdy shelter away from windows. A storm shelter designed and tested specifically to withstand tornadoes offers the best protection. Both underground storm cellars and interior "safe rooms" are usually available in tornado-prone regions and are designed to withstand the strongest tornadoes. If no shelter of any kind is available, the individual is advised to lie flat in a ditch or natural culvert. Climatologically, tornadoes most often occur in the interior of continents, particularly the United States and Canada, where tornadoes tend to be more frequent and stronger than elsewhere.

Waterspouts, as with tornadoes, are columns of rapidly rotating air that are visible due to condensation of water vapor in the funnel (not water being sucked up). Some are associated with supercells and therefore can be considered tornadoes over water. However, many are called "fair-weather waterspouts" because they generally are not associated with thunderstorms. Instead, they form under large cumulus clouds in light wind conditions. Their life span is typically less than 20 minutes, winds rarely exceed 113 km/hr (70 miles/hr), and they are usually found in coastal regions. However, waterspouts can still cause considerable damage and injury, and it is advisable to avoid them or seek shelter if they come ashore.

Types of Thunderstorms

Severe thunderstorms are storms with wind speeds above 93 km/hr (58 miles/hr). Updrafts and downdrafts associated with severe thunderstorms often reinforce each other and intensify the storm.

Mesoscale convective complexes (MCCs) are roughly circular, organized storm systems composed of several thunderstorms. MCCs are common occurrences over the Great Plains region of the United States and Canada, where mesoscale (10 to 1000 km [6 to 620 miles] in diameter) atmospheric processes provide conditions suitable for reinforcement of thunderstorm complexes.

Frontal/squall-line thunderstorms tend to form parallel to and ahead of cold fronts in the presence of wind shear. They form a linear band of storm cells with a life span of about $\frac{1}{2}$ to 4 days and are often a clear visual indication on radar of an approaching cold front.

Supercell thunderstorms are violent storms that occur as isolated thunderstorms, each with a diameter of 20 to 50 km (12 to 31 miles). Supercells are the most common type of thunderstorms to generate tornadoes.

ARID CLIMATES

Arid climates are characterized by lack of moisture. These are found along subtropical high-pressure zones or in the interiors of large continents, where the influence of moisture-laden oceanic frontal systems is limited. Deserts are characteristic ecosystems of arid climates. Extreme heat, high diurnal temperature ranges, wind, and fire danger are important elements of desert climates.

Virga refers to precipitation that falls from clouds but evaporates or sublimates before reaching the ground. This can sometimes be seen as a rain shaft in the distance, with a veil of rain under the clouds becoming streaky and disappearing before reaching the ground. Virga is much more common in arid regions, since lower humidity of the air induces evaporation more readily, although hazards, such as lightning and strong downdrafts of wind, still exist.

MOUNTAIN CLIMATES

Lifting of air caused by the presence of mountains is known as *orographic lift,* which results in cooling of the air. If sufficient moisture is present, condensation takes place. Such convection can induce thunderstorm development on the windward side of a mountain (Figure 107-4). In the winter, orographic lift can both enhance and generate heavy snowfall in mountainous regions, particularly on the windward side of a mountain range. Average winter snowfall in the mountains is typically substantially greater than elsewhere for this reason, and the greatest potential for heavy snowfall occurs in regions with a moisture source upstream (e.g., lakes, oceans), such as northern Japan, the northwest coast of North America, and elevated locations in the lee of the Great Lakes.

In the presence of steep topography, convective processes may be limited to the windward side because the mountain ridge can form a wet-dry divide. Air flowing over a mountain ridge and downward along the leeward side warms and dries through the process of adiabatic compression. Thus, leeward winds are characteristically dry and warm. Such winds are known internationally as foehn winds and are given regional names in the United States, such as the Chinook winds in the lee of the Rockies and the Santa Ana winds that blow into Los Angeles.

Wind direction typically reverses twice a day in mountain climates. During the day, wind flows upslope from the valley toward the mountain. At night, winds blow downslope from the mountain toward the valley. Horizontal temperature differences that develop in complex terrain produce diurnal mountain winds. Overnight and into the early morning, cold air accumulates in valleys and causes a temperature inversion. By morning, valley bottoms are colder than mountain slopes, and a pressure gradient develops that drives upslope winds. Convective heating during the day dissipates the temperature inversion in the valleys.

Varied topography in mountain ranges results in a myriad of microclimates. Factors, such as exposure to sunshine, slope direction, elevation, and windward or leeward side of major weather systems, determine the varied characteristics of microclimates found in mountainous regions. Therefore, weather is generally more difficult to predict in the mountains and changes more frequently, especially in more exposed locations.

MARINE/COASTAL CLIMATES

The difference in heat capacity between land and ocean initiates a diurnal sea-land breeze circulation. During the day, land heats up faster than the ocean, establishing a land-ocean temperature difference that causes a pressure gradient. Wind blows toward the lower pressure over land to equalize the pressure difference. At night, land surfaces cool rapidly compared with adjacent oceans. The cycle is reversed at night, with winds blowing from the land toward the ocean to dispel the ocean-land temperature (and thus pressure) gradient (Figure 107-5).

Ocean upwelling (cold) currents, particularly along the west coasts of continents, modify climate in adjacent land areas. Summers and winters in such locations are mild because of the

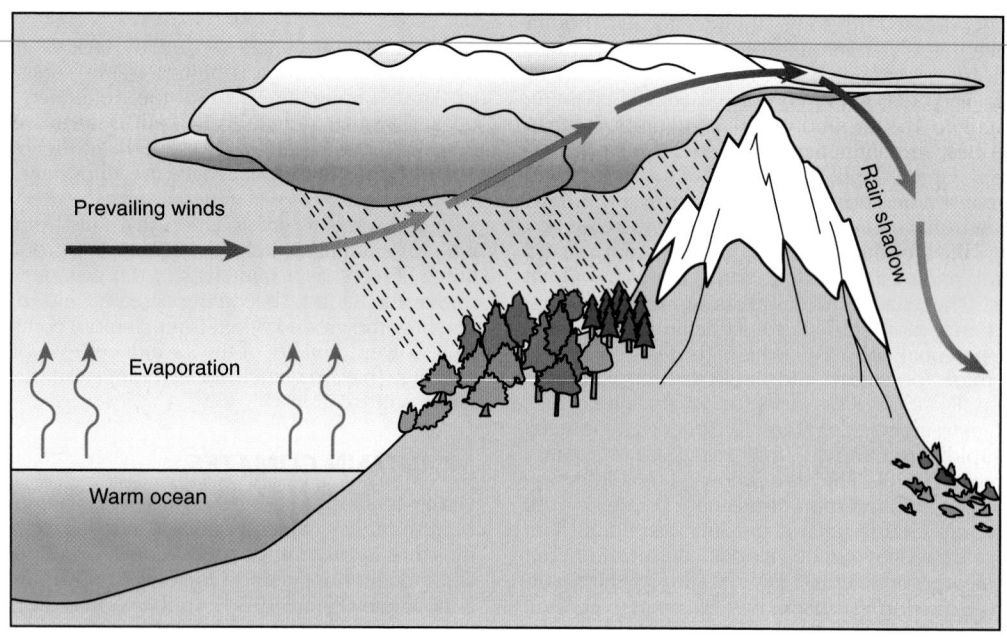

FIGURE 107-4 Orographic precipitation. *(Courtesy Deborah Mioduszewski.)*

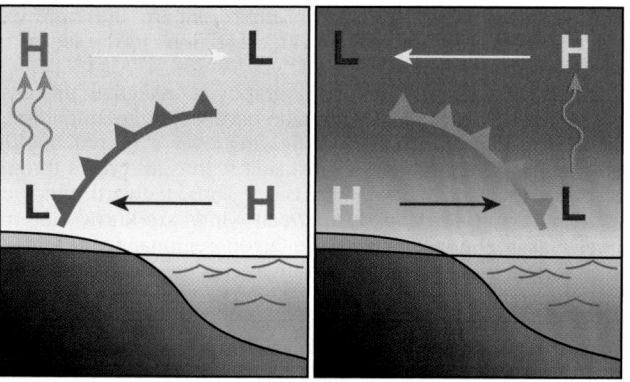

FIGURE 107-5 Land-sea breeze circulation. *H*, High pressure; *L*, low pressure. *(Courtesy Deborah Mioduszewski.)*

moderating effect of the cool water. However, these locations are also prone to low clouds, advection fog, and light rain throughout the year.

Fog is formed when the temperature drops to near its dew point or when moisture is added to the air to saturate it. *Radiation fog* is a shallow layer of fog near the surface caused by rapid cooling of the land. The air just above the land cools to its dew point and condenses, although this type of fog typically dissipates quickly in the morning as the sun rises. *Advection fog* forms when moist air is transported horizontally (advected) over a cool

surface. The surface cools the moist air to its dew point, causing condensation and fog. It is most common on land when warm air advects over a snow pack and the snow cools the air to saturation. Advection fog is most common over water and adjacent coastal locations when tropical air moves over a cool ocean current. *Upslope fog* occurs when air is forced to rise. It cools to its dew point, and a cloud forms at the surface.

HUMAN COMFORT

Wind chill refers to accelerated cooling of the human body that occurs because of atmospheric motion, particularly when temperatures are low, typically below 7°C (44.6°F). Weather forecasts often report both absolute and relative (i.e., wind chill) temperatures when wind chill is a factor.

Heat index is a metric that describes "how hot it feels" when humidity is combined with actual air temperature. During summer months, particularly in more humid regions of the world, it is important to heed forecasted heat index values when planning outdoor activities. Table 107-2 provides an indication of the danger levels associated with various values of the heat index.

Haze is reduced visibility caused by suspension of particulates in the air. Such particulates may either be aerosols (e.g., carbon particles, salt) or air pollutants (e.g., nitrogen oxides, ozone, hydrocarbons). Haze generated by atmospheric pollutants is referred to as "photochemical smog" and is often exacerbated by nearby human activity, such as coal-burning power plants and automobile traffic. Additionally, a region's topography can compound this effect. An example is the Los Angeles basin, where

TABLE 107-2	Categories of Heat Index	
Category	**Heat Index**	**Possible Heat Disorders for People in High-Risk Groups**
Extreme danger	54°C or higher (130°F or higher)	Heatstroke or sunstroke likely
Danger	41° to 54°C (105° to 129°F)	Sunstroke, muscle cramps, and/or heat exhaustion likely. Heatstroke possible with prolonged exposure and/or physical activity.
Extreme caution	32° to 41°C (90° to 105°F)	Sunstroke, muscle cramps, and/or heat exhaustion possible with prolonged exposure and/or physical activity.
Caution	27° to 32°C (80° to 90°F)	Fatigue possible with prolonged exposure and/or physical activity.

Modified from http://www.srh.noaa.gov/ssd/html/heatwv.htm.

TABLE 107-3 Air Quality Index (AQI)

AQI Levels of Health Concern	Numeric Value	Meaning
Good	0 to 50	Air quality is considered satisfactory, and air pollution poses little or no risk.
Moderate	51 to 100	Air quality is acceptable. for some pollutants, however, there may be a moderate health concern for a very small number of people who are unusually sensitive to air pollution.
Unhealthy for Sensitive Groups	101 to 150	Members of sensitive groups may experience health effects. The general public is not likely to be affected.
Unhealthy	151 to 200	Everyone may begin to experience health effects. members of sensitive groups may experience more serious health effects.
Very Unhealthy	201 to 300	Health alert: everyone may experience more serious health effects.
Hazardous	301 to 500	Health warnings of emergency conditions. The entire population is more likely to be affected.

Modified from http://www.airnow.gov/index.cfm?action=aqibasics.aqi.

surrounding mountains help keep polluted air in place and close to the surface.

Air Quality Index (AQI) is a measure of daily air quality in the context of human health. In the United States, the Environmental Protection Agency (EPA) calculates the AQI for five major air pollutants: ground-level ozone, particulate matter, carbon monoxide, sulfur dioxide, and nitrous oxide. The AQI has a range from 0 to 500, with lower values (up to 50) associated with good air quality and higher values (300 and above) associated with levels of air pollution hazardous to health. The EPA uses color-coded categorizations of the AQI to indicate possible health effects associated with different values (Table 107-3).

Vector-borne diseases, such as malaria, dengue, and hantavirus, have been linked to climatic events. In the tropics, dengue outbreaks occur at the onset of rainy seasons, such as the monsoons. Malaria and hantavirus outbreaks in certain regions of the tropics have been associated with the warm phase of the El Niño Southern Oscillation (ENSO), when increased temperature is conducive to vector breeding.

Stratospheric ozone prevents much of the sun's ultraviolet (UV) radiation from reaching the earth's surface. UV radiation that passes through the atmosphere is a health concern, primarily to eyes and skin. The two primary factors affecting risk for receiving unhealthy levels of UV radiation are angle of the sun and elevation. Higher levels of UV radiation are more likely at high elevations, where radiation has to pass through less of the atmosphere. The *sun angle* refers to both its varying angle throughout the day and its differing angles at different latitudes. At low latitudes, the sun angle remains high throughout the year, and therefore sunburn risk remains relatively high. At higher latitudes, the risk is especially high in late spring and early summer, when solar angle is highest. In either case, this risk is enhanced during the hours around solar noon. In addition, clouds only scatter solar radiation; they do not block it. This allows UV radiation to reach the surface diffusely, where it is still harmful. *Diffuse radiation* is radiation that has been scattered, usually by clouds, but that still reaches the ground. As a result, sun protection should be used even when the sun is blocked by clouds.

Stratospheric ozone is not evenly distributed around the world and tends to be thinner at higher latitudes, particularly during the spring. Therefore, care should be taken to wear sunscreen, protective clothing, and eyewear when engaged in outdoor activity, particularly in springtime in the mid- to high latitudes and year-round in the tropics.

WEATHER FORECASTING

OBTAINING DATA AND FORECASTS AND PREDICTING WEATHER IN THE NEAR TERM

Weather forecasting in the wilderness requires data collection, whether from online sources (ideal) or with what is readily available and observable. Crude forecasts can be made by monitoring clouds and basic weather variables, such as temperature, humidity, and wind direction, if this is all that is available. If online resources are available, reliable short-term forecasts can be obtained for most locations on Earth, typically provided by either private or public weather services. The primary use of online sources lies in the ability to monitor real-time weather information, such as radar, satellite, and observations, in addition to obtaining forecasts. The primary purpose of data collection outdoors should be to make a rough forecast of ensuing weather conditions in the near term through 48 hours.

Proliferation of smartphones in recent years has allowed more accessible Internet connectivity in the wilderness. This allows for current weather forecasts and real-time radar and satellite images. In addition, there are many weather applications (apps) for use on smartphones. For a complete listing of weather apps for iOS, see https://itunes.apple.com/us/genre/ios-weather/id6001?mt=8. For a list of recommended weather apps for Android phones, see www.androidauthority.com/the-9-best-weather-apps-for-android-256942/.

PORTABLE WEATHER INSTRUMENTS OF USE IN THE WILDERNESS

Barometer

Barometers are useful for assessing evolution of weather systems, especially in the midlatitudes. Changes in atmospheric pressure at one location are small in comparison with changes as one moves up or down in elevation; thus, barometers must be calibrated with changes in elevation if this is not already done automatically. In general, the value of the atmospheric pressure is much less significant than its trend over time. A steady drop in pressure indicates the possibility of stormy conditions in the near future, whereas rising pressure generally portends fair weather.

Thermometer

Portable thermometers provide indication of imminent changes in weather conditions, such as those arising from passage of a frontal system. They could also be consulted to ascertain the probability of freezing conditions and risk for hypothermia. Because these applications do not require a high degree of precision, there is no need for a costly, high-precision instrument.

Lightning Detector

Portable lightning detectors are useful for detecting lightning within a 64- to 120-km (40- to 75-mile) radius, depending on the instrument. Lightning detectors operate with varying degrees of accuracy and can be limited in their ability to describe storm position and movement. Because they operate by detecting the electromagnetic pulses of lightning, interference can occur when operating near many types of electronic devices, including car engines, appliances, fluorescent lights, and even cell phones. However, most lightning detectors now have incorporated systems to warn the user of interference and automatically mitigate it. In addition, the interference can often be minimized by moving a few meters from the source, so outdoor operation is recommended.

TYPES OF FORECASTS

Forecasts vary by timescale, ranging from weather forecasts to seasonal climate forecasts.

Weather forecasts assess the future state of the atmosphere and its constituent elements in reference to components such as temperature, wind, and precipitation. Weather forecasts are generated using numeric integrations of the equations of motion in the atmosphere. Such forecasts require accurate observations of the initial atmospheric state that are fed into numeric computer models. There are four types of weather forecasts:

- *Nowcasts:* up to 0 to 3 hours, or 6 hours in some locations
- *Short-range forecasts:* up to 48 hours
- *Medium-range forecasts:* 3 to 7 days in advance
- *Long-range forecasts:* more than 7 days in advance

Skill

Accuracy of weather forecasts quickly declines with time because of the inherent chaos of the atmosphere. The details of midlatitude cyclones and smaller-scale events are impossible to forecast accurately beyond a few days, even if the pattern that produced them is relatively easy to identify. In the tropics, forecast skill is higher during years when either phase of the ENSO phenomenon—La Niña or El Niño—is underway, because ENSO is the single most dominant mode of climate variability at the seasonal and interannual timescales.[2] ENSO-led seasonal forecast skill tends to be higher in winter and spring seasons. This is particularly so for tropical and subtropical regions. However, in the higher latitudes of the subtropics and in the midlatitudes, seasonal forecast skill can be confounded by atmospheric circulation patterns driven by phenomena (e.g., North Atlantic Oscillation) that operate at shorter timescales.

HOW TO INTERPRET FORECASTS

ACCESSING FORECASTS

There are many online resources for weather forecasts for a particular location. In any country, the authoritative source for weather forecasts is the National Meteorological and Hydrological Services (NMHS) of that country. Links to the weather forecasts for cities issued by most NMHS centers are available through http://www.worldweather.wmo.int/ on the World Meteorological Organization (WMO) website.

North America

In the United States, the National Weather Service (NWS) is responsible for all outlooks, forecasts, and advisories. Some of these responsibilities are handled by specialized centers within the organization. The National Hurricane Center (www.nhc.noaa.gov/) issues all updates on tropical weather in the Atlantic and eastern Pacific Oceans, regardless of the impact on the United States. The Storm Prediction Center (www.spc.noaa.gov/) handles all severe weather, including tornado and severe thunderstorm watches. Local NWS offices are responsible for issuing warnings on such events. Medium- to long-range discussions, outlooks, and forecasts are available from the Climate Prediction Center (www.cpc.noaa.gov/), and broader national forecasts and discussions for different regions of the country are available from the Hydrometeorological Prediction Center (www.hpc.ncep.noaa.gov/), which also provides guidance on quantitative precipitation forecasts and winter weather.

In Canada, Environment Canada (www.weatheroffice.gc.ca) is responsible for all outlooks, forecasting, and advisories. These include data and forecasts regarding hurricanes, sea ice, aviation, and air quality. Environment Canada issues watches, warnings, and special weather statements for all of Canada, including its waters.

International Forecasts

The WMO has a dedicated website for severe weather warnings for various parts of the world. Such forecasts are categorized by region (e.g., European Union: www.meteoalarm.eu/) or by weather phenomena (e.g., tropical cyclones or thunderstorms:

severe.worldweather.org/). Forecasts of severe weather in maritime regions are available through the Global Maritime Distress and Safety System (weather.gmdss.org/).

FORECAST VARIABLES

Seasonal Precipitation Forecasts

Seasonal precipitation forecasts are presented as tercile probability forecasts in the United States. Tercile forecasts are based on the assumption that precipitation in a coming season has a 33% probability of falling within one of three possible categories: below, near, or above normal. The forecast is expressed as the probability of seasonal rainfall being below normal, near normal, or above normal, or in terms of expected rainfall anomalies.

Temperature Forecasts

Temperature forecasts are issued as expected daily minimum and maximum temperatures. In countries outside the United States, the convention is to express the two values in degrees Celsius.

Humidity

Humidity forecasts are usually issued as expected relative humidity, ranging from 0% to 100%.

Wind Direction and Speed

Wind forecasts indicate direction (eight possible directions: N, NE, E, SE, S, SW, W, and NW) and speed (expressed as kilometers per hour or miles per hour). In maritime environments, the convention is to use knots (1 knot equals 1.852 km/hr [1.151 miles/hr]).

Precipitation

Precipitation is forecast as probability of precipitation (POP) and, if applicable, quantitative precipitation forecast (QPF). POP should be interpreted as the probability that precipitation will fall at any specific point. QPF is the total amount of rain (or melted frozen precipitation) expected to fall in a specified period.

FORECAST PRODUCTS

UNITED STATES

According to the NWS, a warning is issued when a hazardous weather or hydrologic event is occurring, imminent, or likely. A warning means that conditions pose a threat to life or property. An advisory is also issued when such events are occurring, imminent, or likely, but the event is not expected to be as severe. The criteria for advisories and warnings vary among different NWS offices. Events such as heat index and winter weather, including snow, ice, and wind chill, may be perceived differently in different parts of the country. A watch is issued when the risk for a hazardous or hydrologic event is increasing, but its occurrence, location, or timing is still uncertain. As time advances, a watch could be replaced by an advisory or a warning. A watch is issued when warning-level conditions are anticipated. When a watch is issued, people should proceed with a plan of action for the predicted event and continue to be alert for further information and possible warnings.

INTERNATIONAL

Regional Specialized Meteorological Centers (RSMCs) and Tropical Cyclone Warning Centers (TCWCs), established through the WMO, provide warnings on severe weather, particularly cyclones. Figure 107-6 shows locations of the RSCMs and TCWCs.

Tropical storm warnings use the Saffir-Simpson scale. Such warnings are often accompanied by a brief description of the damage likely to occur with the passage of each storm. Box 107-1 provides examples of the narrative used by the Indian Meteorological Department, responsible for RSMC-New Delhi, to describe potential damage associated with a "deep depression" (28 to 33 knots) and a "severe cyclonic storm" (equivalent to a category 4 on the Saffir-Simpson scale).

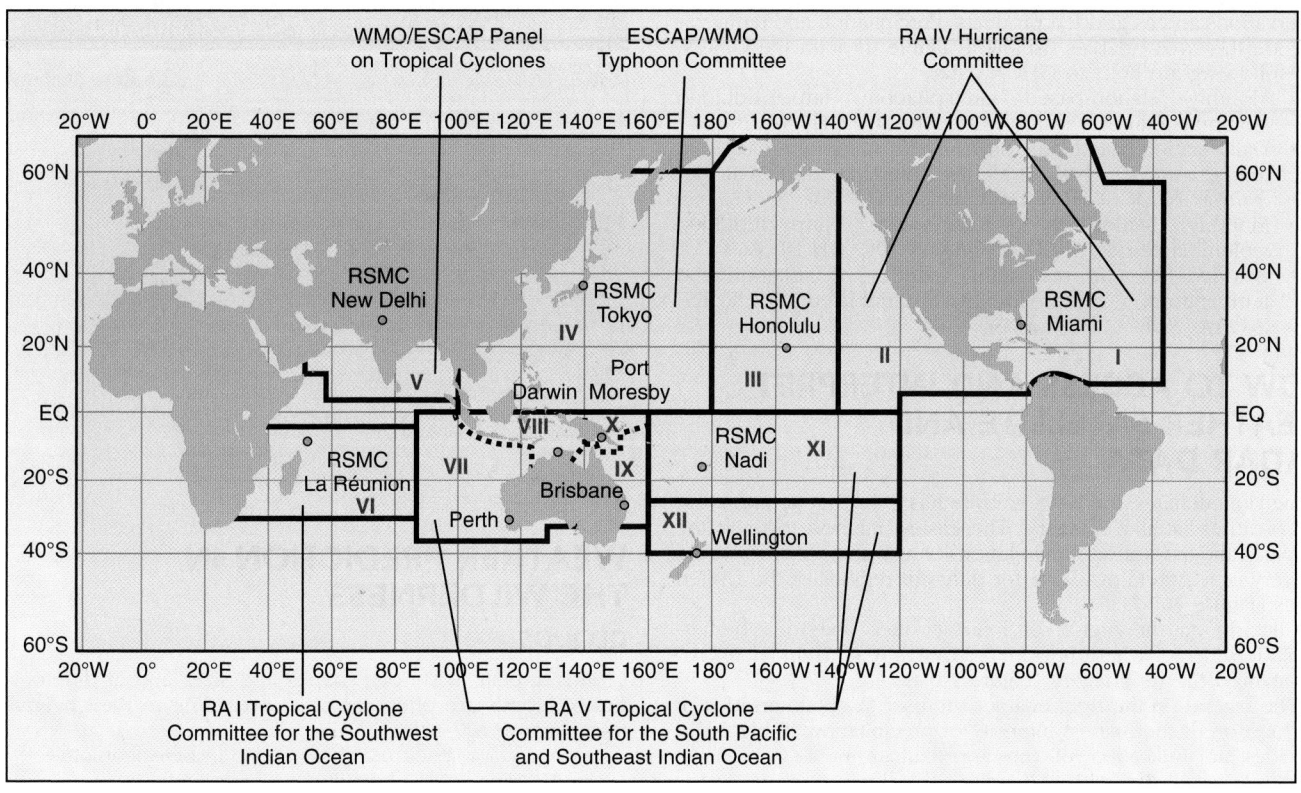

FIGURE 107-6 Location of the Regional Specialized Meteorological Centers and Tropical Warning Centers. (*From* http://www.nhc.noaa.gov/gifs/wmo-tcp2.jpg.)

HOW TO OBTAIN SURFACE OBSERVATIONS

UNITED STATES

Historic surface observations for the United States are available online through the National Climatic Data Center (www.ncdc.noaa.gov/oa/climate/climatedata.html). Station-based data are available from hourly to monthly time resolution. The data are available free of charge to e-mail users with domains ending in .edu, .k12, .gov, and .mil; otherwise, fees apply to cover processing expenses. Data are also available from automated stations and volunteer observations through the NWS. Another source of data is the volunteer network of precipitation observers known as Community Collaborative Rain, Hail and Snow; data are available at www.cocorahs.org/.

GLOBAL DATA

Surface observations from various part of the globe can be accessed through the Global Historical Climatology Network (GHCN). Such observations are available as station-based

---

BOX 107-1 Examples of Indian Meteorological Department Narratives

What is the damage potential of a deep depression (28 to 33 knots)?
What are the suggested actions?
Structures: Minor damage to loose/unsecured structures.
Road/Rail: Some breaches in Kutcha road due to flooding.
Agriculture: Minor damage to banana trees and near coastal agriculture due to salt spray. Damage to rice paddy crops.
Marine Interests: Very rough seas. Sea waves about 4 to 6 m high.
Coastal Zone: Minor damage to Kutcha embankments.
Overall Damage Category: Minor.
Suggested Actions: Fishermen advised not to venture into sea.

What is the damage potential of a super cyclonic storm (120 knots [222 km/hr]) and above?
What are the suggested actions?
Structures: Extensive damage to nonconcrete residential and industrial buildings. Structural damage to concrete structures. Air full of large projectiles.
Communication and Power: Uprooting of power and communication poles. Total disruption of communication and power supply.

Road/Rail: Extensive damage to Kutcha roads and some damage to poorly repaired pucca roads. Large-scale submerging of coastal roads due to flooding and seawater inundation. Total disruption of railway and road traffic due to major damages to bridges, signals, and railway tracks. Washing away of rail/road links at several places.
Agriculture: Total destruction of standing crops/orchards, uprooting of large trees and blowing away of palm and coconut crowns, stripping of tree barks.
Marine Interests: Phenomenal seas with wave heights more than 14 m. All shipping activity unsafe.
Coastal Zone: Extensive damage to port installations. Storm surge more than 5 m. Inundation up to 40 km in specific areas and extensive beach erosion. All ships torn from their moorings. Flooding of escape routes.
Overall Damage Category: Catastrophic.
Suggested Actions: Fishermen not to venture into sea. Large-scale evacuations needed. Total stoppage of rail and road traffic needed in vulnerable areas.

Modified from www.imd.gov.in/section/nhac/dynamic/faq/FAQP.htm#q51.

observations and as gridded products. Precipitation and temperature are the two variables usually available through the GHCN. The following are links to GHCN data:

- Monthly station-based precipitation: http://iridl.ldeo.columbia.edu/SOURCES/.NOAA/.NCDC/.GHCN/.v2beta/
- Daily station-based precipitation and minimum-maximum temperature: http://iridl.ldeo.columbia.edu/SOURCES/.NOAA/.NCDC/.GHCN_Daily/.version1/
- Monthly station-based temperature: http://iridl.ldeo.columbia.edu/SOURCES/.NOAA/.NCDC/.GHCN/.v2/
- Gridded (2° × 2° resolution) monthly precipitation and temperature: http://iridl.ldeo.columbia.edu/SOURCES/.NOAA/.NCEP/.CPC/.CAMS/

HOW TO ACCESS AND INTERPRET WEATHER SATELLITE AND RADAR DATA

In the United States, the NWS website has links to real-time radar and weather satellite imagery. The easiest method to track the passage (and associated precipitation) of a storm is to study radar imagery of a system available for different regions of the United States (Figure 107-7).

Clicking on the region of interest takes one to a higher-resolution image, where relevant warnings (e.g., thunderstorms) are marked on the imagery (Figure 107-8).

The legend on the right enables the user to obtain an idea of the location of the highest intensity of precipitation. Table 107-4 provides an indication of the approximate rainfall intensity, which is associated with the units dBZ (known as "reflected intensities" or "decibels of Z").

Satellite images enable a user to obtain a quick, large-scale estimation of where overcast/stormy conditions are located and where clear weather prevails, with a satellite loop allowing for a general extrapolation of these conditions to locations downstream (Figure 107-9).

TABLE 107-4 Doppler Radar Scale of Intensity

dBZ	Rain Rate (inches/hr)
65	16+
60	8.00
55	4.00
52	2.50
47	1.25
41	0.50
36	0.25
30	0.10
20	Trace
<20	No rain

From http://www.srh.noaa.gov/jetstream/doppler/baserefl.htm#rainrate.
dBZ, Decibels of reflectivity (Z).

WEATHER PREDICTION IN THE WILDERNESS

CLOUDS

Clouds appear in various shapes and sizes and at different altitudes. Clouds are often classified according to their height and form (Figure 107-10):

- *High clouds:* cirrus, cirrostratus, and cirrocumulus
- *Middle clouds:* altostratus and altocumulus
- *Low clouds:* stratus, stratocumulus, and nimbostratus
- *Clouds with extensive vertical development:* cumulus and cumulonimbus

Frequency of occurrence of the different cloud types differs in the tropics and higher latitudes. Cumulus is the predominant cloud form in the tropics.[1]

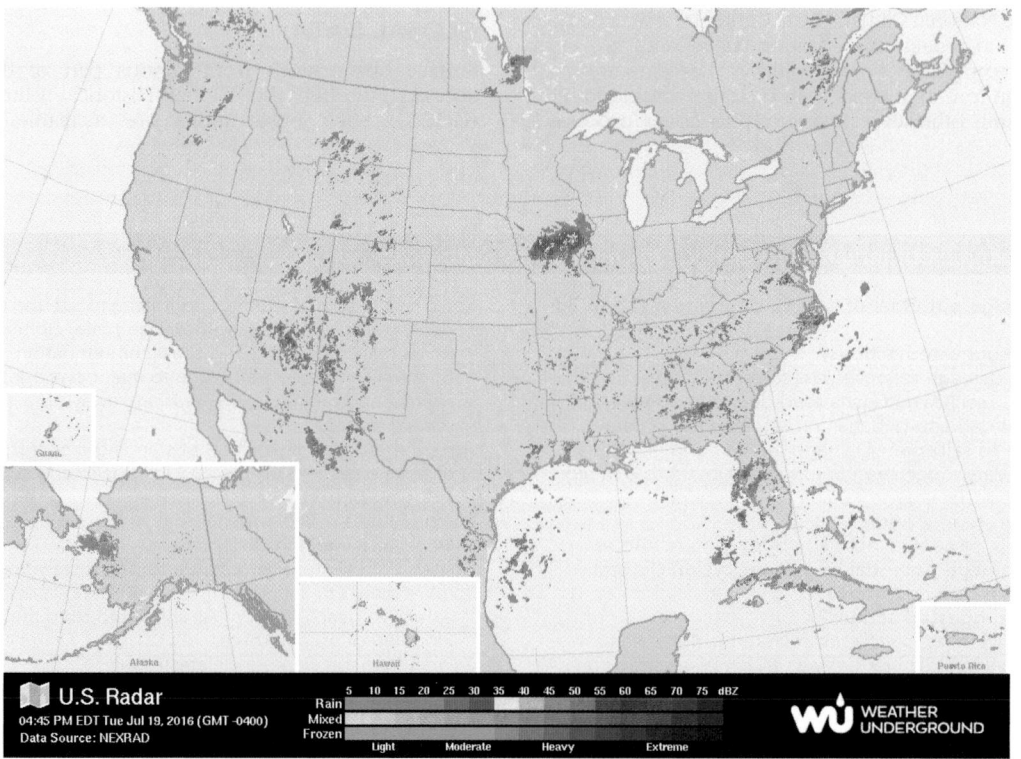

FIGURE 107-7 Example of radar imagery over the United States.

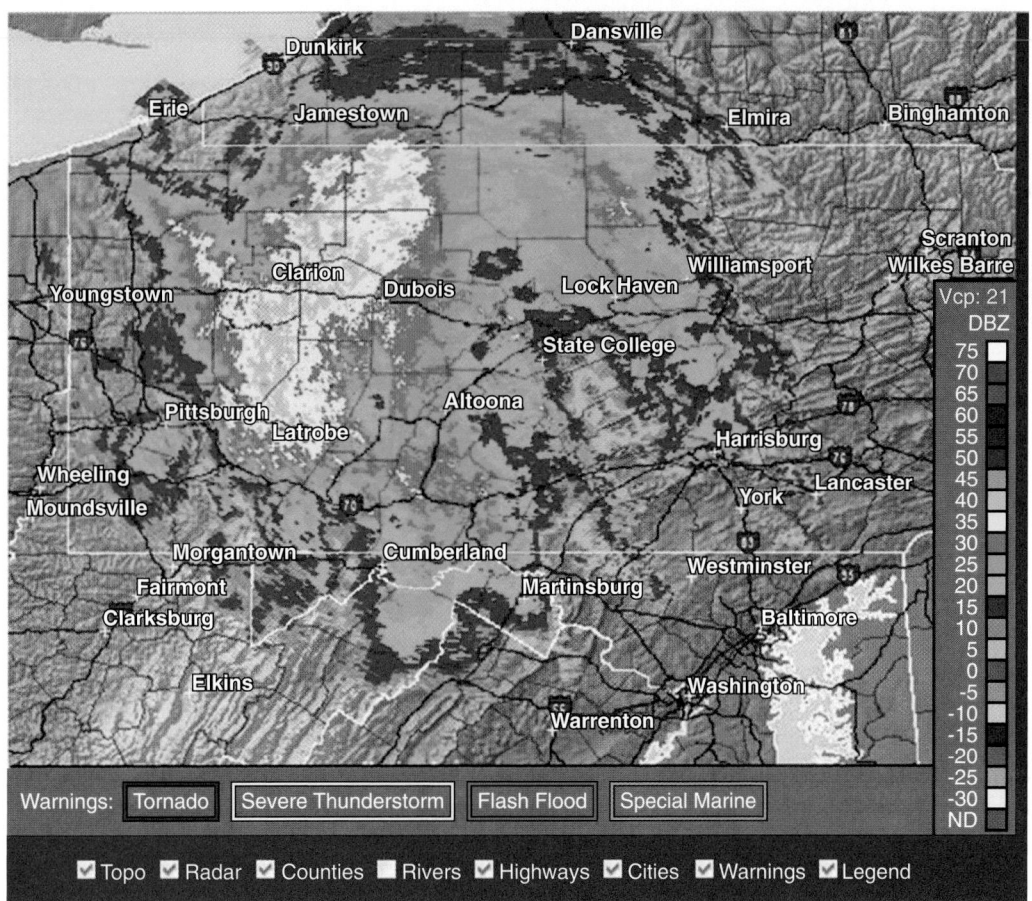

FIGURE 107-8 Example of a Doppler radar image.

GOES WESTERN U.S. SECTOR IR IMAGE

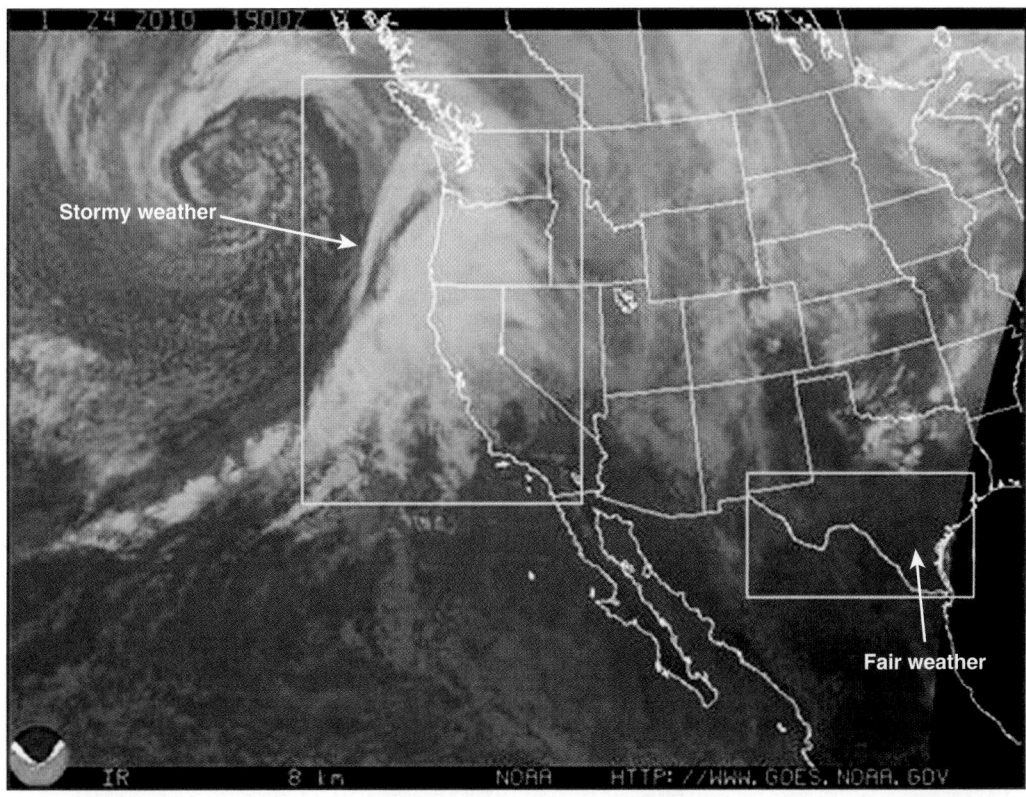

Western Conus Sector (IR Ch4)

FIGURE 107-9 Example of the usefulness of satellite imagery in capturing stormy and clear conditions.

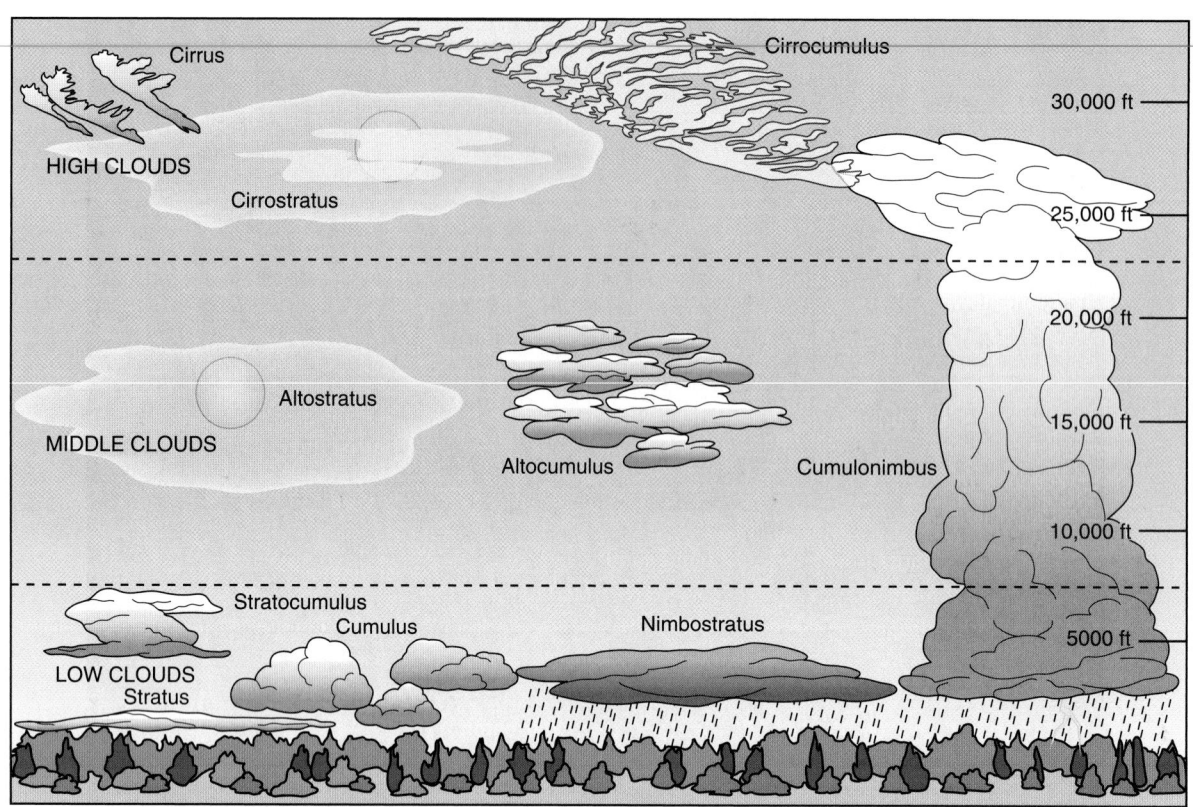

FIGURE 107-10 Guide to different cloud types.

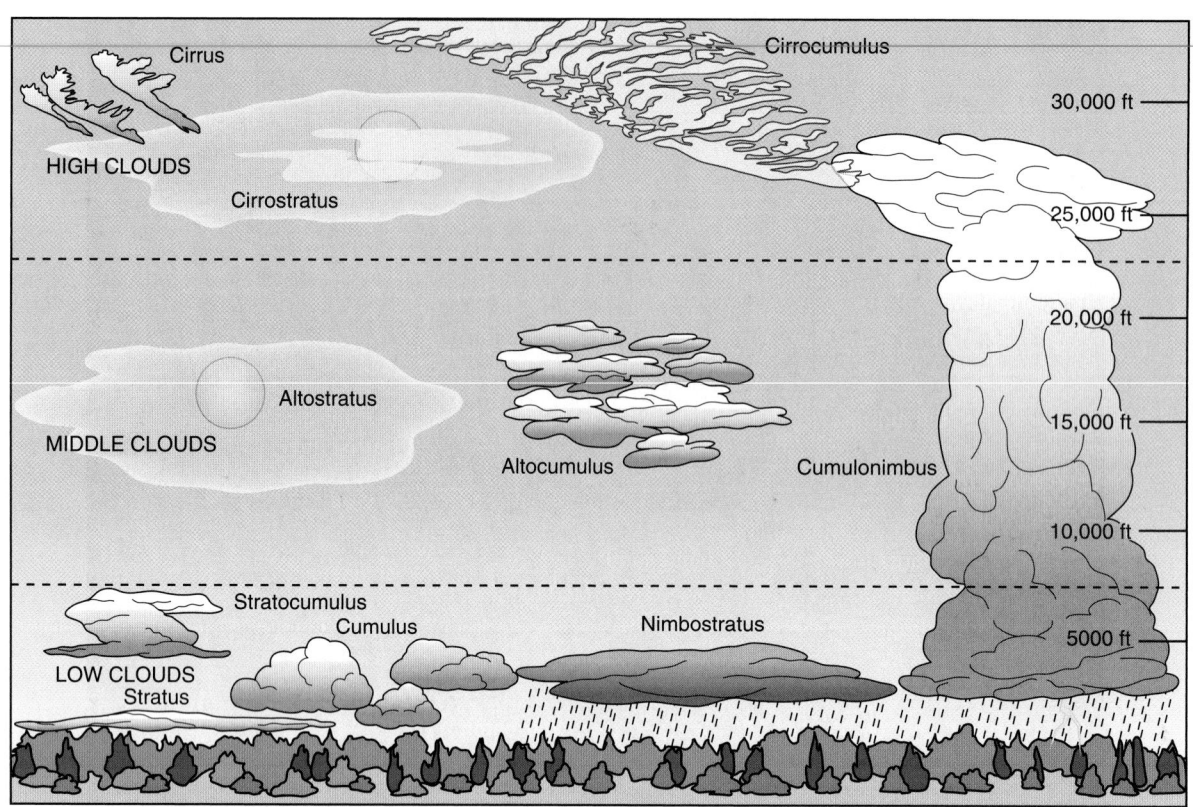

(Labels within figure 107-10: Cirrus, Cirrocumulus, 30,000 ft, HIGH CLOUDS, Cirrostratus, 25,000 ft, 20,000 ft, Altostratus, MIDDLE CLOUDS, Altocumulus, 15,000 ft, Cumulonimbus, 10,000 ft, Stratocumulus, Cumulus, Nimbostratus, LOW CLOUDS, Stratus, 5000 ft)

CLOUDS AND WEATHER

Clouds are among the best indicators of changing weather in the wilderness. Figure 107-11 shows the typical progression of clouds as a midlatitude cyclone moves through to the left of the observer, whereas a simplified version would apply when it moves to the right. Cirrus clouds are often present 1 to 2 days before a storm and serve as the earliest indication that a cyclone is approaching. They should be noted as a sign that a storm might be on its way, bearing in mind that cirrus can be associated with storms that have no appreciable impact on a location, as well as with other innocuous disturbances.

When cirrus begins to transition into a deck of altostratus, it can reasonably be assumed that the clouds are associated with a storm or front that is nearing. Stratus clouds are most frequently associated with warm fronts because they are a good indication that air is being forced to rise gradually over a wedge of cooler air, as is found in a warm front. In general, stratus clouds occur as a warmer air mass is being lifted over a cooler one; the longer this occurs, the more likely the stratus clouds are to lower and begin precipitating. Therefore, as altostratus clouds lower into a low, gray deck of nimbostratus clouds, it is a good assumption that a light, steady rain or snow will follow. Nimbostratus clouds occur in the vicinity of the warm front and near the center of low pressure, where air is being lifted.

The location of low pressure can often be assessed using a simple rule called Buys Ballot's law. When the observer stands with his or her back to the wind in the northern hemisphere, the low pressure will be to the left. This rule is reversed in the southern hemisphere and works best at higher latitudes.

The weather conditions ahead of a warm front typically include winds from the east or southeast with cool conditions and a slowly dropping barometric pressure. After the front passes, the pressure continues to drop, and the wind shifts clockwise to the south or southwest, in most regions bringing in warmer and

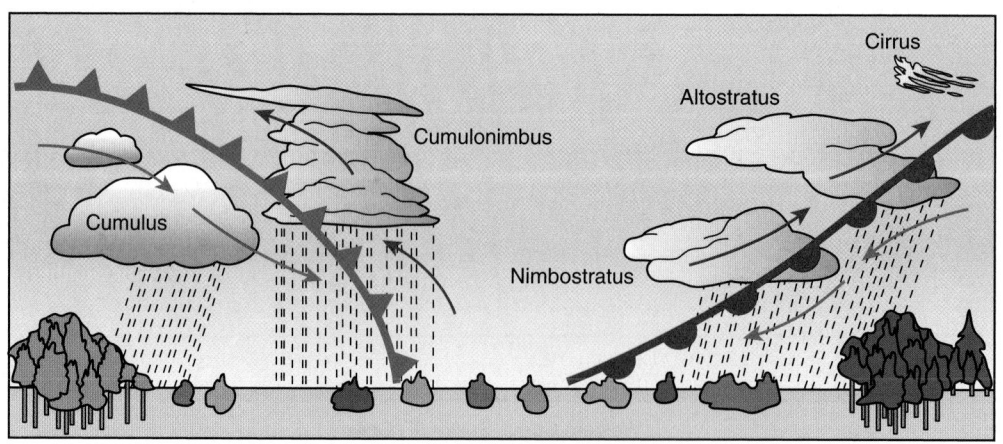

FIGURE 107-11 Progression of a midlatitude cyclone as seen from the ground.

(Labels within figure 107-11: Cirrus, Altostratus, Cumulonimbus, Cumulus, Nimbostratus)

moister air. This region of the cyclone between the cold and warm fronts is associated with the most instability, which increases the chance for showers and thunderstorms and the highest probability of severe weather (see Figure 107-2). Because there is more instability, cumulus clouds dominate this sector. In the winter, warm air can rapidly be transported into this part of the storm, changing snow and ice to rain.

Passage of the cold front is easy to observe because there are several sharp changes in weather conditions. Before its passage, wind typically blows from the south or southwest, the dew point and temperature are relatively high, and air pressure is dropping. The strongest atmospheric lift is found near a cold front, so cumulonimbus clouds with associated heavy rain and severe weather can be found at the frontal boundary. Typically, precipitation in the vicinity of a cold front does not fall for as long as it does ahead of a warm front, because the slope, and therefore area of uplift, is much steeper and narrower with a cold front. After the front passes, wind typically shifts clockwise to the west or northwest, temperature and dew point slowly drop, and air pressure rises. Strong cold frontal passages can be observed as a deck of low or midlevel clouds sharply giving way to blue sky. Clearing skies are typically observed relatively quickly after the front has passed, often with gusty winds remaining for 1 day or longer.

Dense cumulonimbus clouds in the tropics portend thunderstorms and lightning. Altocumulus and altostratus clouds are associated with disturbed weather, such as tropical cyclones, or in locations of large-scale orographic lifting.[1] Cirrus clouds often form as leftover anvils from cumulonimbus clouds. However, they can also form independently and are usually associated with upper-atmospheric cyclones. High cirrus clouds are often observed before formation of a tropical cyclone, followed by midlevel and low-level stratus clouds (see Figure 107-3). Eventually, showery precipitation from cumulus and cumulonimbus clouds arrives and increases in intensity as pressure steadily falls.

BOUNDARY LAYER STABILITY

Fronts and cyclones are not always needed for precipitation or severe weather. Strong daytime heating is all that is necessary to induce deep convection, which can occur frequently in the moister parts of the tropics and subtropics, as well as during the summer in midlatitudes. Stability of the lower atmosphere can be difficult to assess from observation, but can be useful to determine how much potential there is for thunderstorms. To achieve deep convection, air must be readily able to rise and overcome any resistance. Rising plumes of smoke or steam can give an indication of the stability of the lower atmosphere. If it rises to a certain level before spreading out horizontally, it is safe to assume that the lower atmosphere is at least somewhat stable. If nothing stops it from rising, the lower atmosphere may be quite unstable. A large amount of haze or pollution in the air is an indication of a stagnant environment where air moves very little, either horizontally and vertically. In arid regions, "dust devils" are also indication of an unstable, but dry, atmosphere. Clouds in their vertical development can be good indicators of atmospheric stability. Clouds with minimal vertical development, such as stratus and "fair-weather" cumulus, indicate a stable atmosphere. Rapidly building cumulus clouds are a good indication that the atmosphere is unstable, and showers or thunderstorms should be forecast.

BACKING AND VEERING

To aid in assessing current weather conditions, cold and warm air advection can be diagnosed by observing movement of clouds at different levels. Advection is horizontal transport of air from one location to another, bringing with it the temperature and humidity characteristics of its source region. Cold-air advection, an indication of stability and improving (but colder) weather, often follows passage of low pressure. Wind direction at different levels of the atmosphere differ in this situation; at the surface, the wind may blow from the west or northwest, but much higher in the atmosphere, the wind may be out of the southwest or west, respectively. The wind is said to *back with height*, and this is an indication of cold-air advection. Similarly, warm air advected ahead of warm fronts creates an unstable situation, because it is forced to rise over the existing air mass. At the surface, wind out of the southeast is often accompanied by a southwesterly wind at the midlevels of the atmosphere, so the wind is said to *veer with height*. Two levels of clouds with movement that veers with height is a good indication that a steady rain or snow will follow.

REFERENCES

Complete references used in this text are available online at expertconsult.inkling.com.

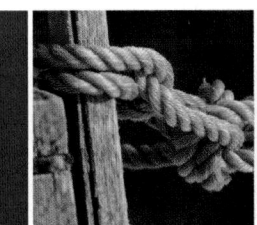

CHAPTER 108
Ropes and Knot Tying

LOUI H. McCURLEY AND THOMAS EVANS

Every wilderness traveler should be familiar with use of ropes and other tension materials (members) such as webbing and cordage. In the hands of someone who has a reasonable amount of knowledge and skill, these tools may be used to perform many functions. The ability to use software (ropes, webbing, cordage) effectively and to create the knots that make them functional is a hallmark of an avid and experienced outdoors person. These tools are often used for lashing, shelter construction, food storage (protection from wildlife), and specialized wilderness adventure activities such as climbing, canyoneering, and caving. More importantly, during an emergency, ropes, webbing, and cordage can be lifesaving resources for the person who knows how to use them properly. This chapter provides an introduction to rope, webbing, and cordage use. The interested reader should consult training manuals for further information and study.

ROPES, WEBBING, AND CORDAGE TERMINOLOGY

In terms of equipment nomenclature, rope, cordage, and webbing are classified as *software*. This term refers to the concept of soft, pliable, and "knotable" material. Any software used to support a human load should be specifically designed, tested, and approved for that purpose, whether for recreation or rescue.

Cordage is a general term used to refer to various types of cords, lines, ropes, and strings intended for use as tension members. Typically, cordage is composed of flexible intertwined fibers that are woven, twisted, braided, or otherwise formed into a round structure. In practice, particularly when referring to life safety products, cordage is used in a narrower sense. Instead, the word *rope* is used to describe a thicker tension member, such as might be appropriate for use as a primary support line, whereas cordage is reserved to describe smaller-diameter ancillary items.

Webbing is flat, unlike rope and cordage, and used to tie knots in and around locations in which rope and cordage would be damaged. The flatter shape of webbing makes it more conducive for certain functions than rope or cordage.

ROPE SELECTION CONSIDERATIONS

Selecting the right rope for the job means first and foremost understanding how a rope is affected by, and performs with, the way you use it. The following discussion provides some background for balancing these needs against available alternatives.

FALL FACTORS

Fall factors can be calculated by dividing the fall distance by the length of the rope between the load and the anchor or belay. Thus, a 0.9-m (3-foot) fall on a 2.7-m (9-foot) rope would be a fall factor of 0.3; an 0.9-m (3-foot) fall on an 0.9-m (3-foot) rope would be a fall factor of 1.0; and a 0.9-m (3-foot) fall on a 30.5 m (100-foot) rope would be a fall factor of 0.03. This calculation assumes the fall takes place in free air without rope drag across the rock face or through intermediate equipment (Figure 108-1).

The danger of a high fall factor on a low-stretch or static rope is not necessarily that the rope will break, but that the high-

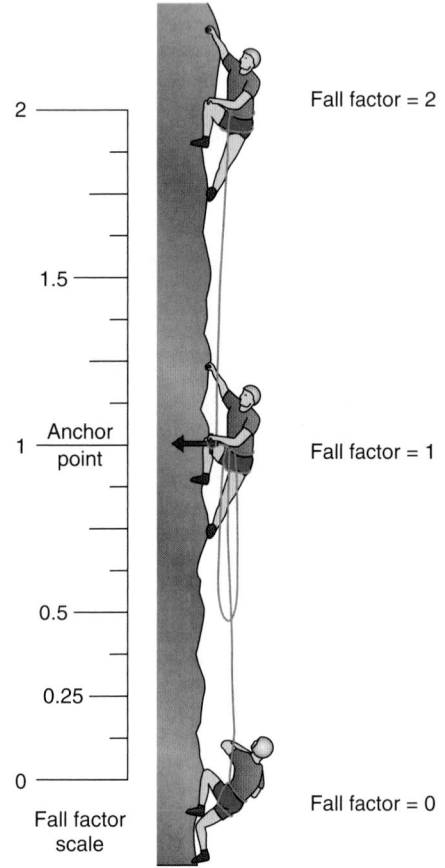

FIGURE 108-1 Fall factors.

impact forces may subject the person to great discomfort and possible injury or death. A static rope transfers more of a shock load to the anchors than does a dynamic rope, increasing damage potential. Another concern in any impact load situation is the effect such forces have on equipment, such as belay devices, rope grabs, or ascenders. Some of these devices can damage a rope when subjected to relatively low-impact forces.

At one time, the general recommendation was that a dynamic rope should be used where high fall factors were likely, whereas static rope is more suited to circumstances involving lower fall factors. However, subsequent research has shown that the concept of fall factors does not apply to static rope in the same manner as to dynamic rope, and it is better understood that force absorption is more a matter of system performance than simply a matter of rope. The study of impact forces and ways that different pieces of equipment relate to different constructions of rope when subjected to such forces is fairly complicated, but two general rules of thumb are (1) design and operate rope systems to minimize the potential for high-impact forces, and (2) exercise great caution when selecting belay methods.

ROPE DIAMETER

Just as no single type of rope is appropriate for all activities, no single size fits all conditions. Purchasing the largest rope in the hope that it will fit all situations because it is strong could lead to problems when working with the rope and auxiliary equipment. Rope strength and elongation are more critical, and size considerations should follow. However, ensure that hardware (e.g., ascenders, rappel devices) is designed for the chosen rope diameter.

ROPE STRENGTH

Rope strength is a misunderstood topic. Life safety rope strength is usually referred to as *minimum breaking strength*. Unfortunately, reported numbers do not necessarily reflect numbers adequate for comparison. Variations in test methods, as well as in analysis of results, provide little more than marketing fodder that can create great confusion.

One way to report strength is as the rope's "ultimate" or "maximum" breaking strength, which is the highest score of a given rope in a series of tests. An alternative is to list the average breaking strength of several tests. A more conservative method is to define breaking strength at a value that is two or three standard deviations (2 or 3 SD) below the average test result. Another method is to define the minimum as not greater than 10% below the average. Often, figures for tensile or breaking strength are reported with no explanation about whether they are average or minimum, or whether some other measure was used. Simply stated, the term *breaking strength* may refer to any one of these reporting methods or to another method altogether.

To add to the confusion, a number of factors affect test results. The rate at which the pull is applied to the rope, temperature, humidity, diameter of the object to which the rope is attached, and other factors all affect test results. Unless ropes are tested in exactly the same way, results cannot be directly compared. Consequently, only general comparisons are justifiable.

One common test method that has been adopted by several standards organizations is CI-1801 from the Cordage Institute. CI-1801 for life safety rope is specific and gives a common baseline from which to attain results. This standard also calls for a very conservative reporting method, wherein minimum breaking strength is defined as 3 SD below the mean of several break tests; this helps normalize results. In addition to type of construction, the strength of a rope comes from the amount of nylon used and the type of construction; similar rope constructions of the same diameter should have similar strengths if they have the same amount and quality of nylon.

Results from laboratory tests may differ greatly from rope performance in real-world applications, which cannot be consistently and accurately quantified. For example, a knotted rope loaded over a building edge may not have anything close to the rope strength measured in a laboratory.

SAFETY FACTORS

It is clear that a rope should be stronger than the force of the intended load, but how much stronger? The ratio of a rope's strength to the weight of the intended load is often called a *design factor*. If the strength of a rope is 1134 kg (2500 lb) and the intended load is 227 kg (500 lb), the design factor is 5:1. The design factor takes into consideration only the new condition of an item as it is designed to perform. When translating a design factor into a system safety factor, factors such as age, wear and tear, dry or wet conditions, and system rigging should be considered.

Because a rope system is only as strong as its weakest link, selecting a sufficiently strong rope is only the beginning. Generally, component design factors tend to be very high, often as high as 15:1. However, when all these components are joined into a larger system in the real world, the remaining system safety factor may be less than half that value.

The *system safety factor* is the ratio between the weak link in a system and the load to be applied. System safety factors also take into account the ways that loads are applied to a system. For example, redirectional pulleys, rigging angles, and mechanical advantage systems can all increase forces within a system.

As a rule, the higher the probability and consequences of failure, the higher should be the system safety factor.

SERVICE LIFE

The service life of a rope cannot be determined in advance. How long a rope lasts depends on many variables, including individual care, frequency of use, type of hardware used, speed of descent on rappels, exposure to abrasion, local climate, and type of loading. DuPont claims at least a 10-year shelf life for nylon, and rope tests have confirmed that an unused rope can last up to 10 years without significant strength loss. However, used ropes degrade more quickly.

Any rope can fail after poor care or under extreme conditions, such as shock loading and sharp edges. A shock load involving a 0.25 fall factor for a static rope or 1.5 fall factor for a dynamic rope will likely cause internal invisible damage to the rope, although damage may also be caused with lower fall factors. Regardless of how long a rope has been in service, it should be immediately discarded when it becomes cut, when abrasion has caused significant wear to the sheath, after a hard shock load, when chemical contamination is suspected, or any time there is doubt about it for any reason.

WEBBING

No discussion of ropes and tension members would be complete without mentioning webbing. As with rope, only webbing designed for outdoor use and fabricated to hold a human load should be used in applications supporting body weight. Webbing is engineered to meet one of two standards: climbing specification (climb spec) or military specification (mil spec) (Table 108-1). Climb spec webbing is stronger than mil spec webbing; however, both webbing types are strong.

TABLE 108-1 Webbing Minimum Breaking Strength by Size (Width) Noted in Pounds-Force (lbf) and Kilonewtons (kN)

Width	Minimum Breaking Strength
9.5 mm (0.375 inch)	950 lbf (4.2 kN)
12.7 mm (0.5 inch)	1000 lbf (4.4 kN)
14 mm (0.563 inch)	1500 lbf (6.7 kN)
16 mm (0.625 inch)	2250 lbf (10.0 kN)
19 mm (0.75 inch)	2300 lbf (10.2 kN)
22 mm (0.875 inch)	3100 lbf (13.8 kN)
25 mm (1.0 inch)	4000 lbf (17.8 kN)

TABLE 108-2 Cord Minimum Breaking Strength by Size (Diameter) Noted in Pounds-Force (lbf) and Kilonewtons (kN)

Diameter	Minimum Breaking Strength
4 mm (0.16 inch)	720 lbf (3.2 kN)
5 mm (0.20 inch)	1125 lbf (5.0 kN)
6 mm (0.24 inch)	1620 lbf (7.2 kN)
7 mm (0.28 inch)	2200 lbf (9.8 kN)
8 mm (0.31 inch)	2875 lbf (12.8 kN)

Webbing comes in two forms, flat and tubular. Generally, flat webbing is stronger but less abrasion resistant, whereas tubular webbing is weaker (but strong enough) and significantly more abrasion resistant. Consequently, most sport participants use tubular webbing. Flat webbing is one sheet of woven fibers; tubular webbing is a continuous tube of webbing that lays flat. To determine if webbing is tubular, cut an end open and see if it is possible to open the webbing. If there is a space inside, it is tubular.

Webbing can be made out of the same fibers as ropes; however, most webbing on the market is made of nylon or Dyneema. The most common size is 1-inch (2.5-cm) tubular webbing.

In general, webbing is used in locations where minimal stretch is desired, where tying a rope would or could cause damage, or in locations where a larger interface would help the software stay put. Webbing is inexpensive, so using webbing to sling trees or rocks is a good way to preserve rope by preventing abrasion and rubbing. Because webbing is flat, when wrapped around an object, considerable friction is created, thus preventing the webbing from becoming loose. As a result, webbing is a favorite for building anchors on and around objects, as well as for building etriers (webbing ladders) and other short tethers.

Because webbing is flat, it behaves differently when knotted, so knots such as the overhand bend or overhand on a bight are better choices for tying webbing. Except for climbing hitches, almost all knots in webbing derive from the overhand knot, usually the overhand bend (water knot) or overhand on a bight.

ACCESSORY CORD

Accessory cord, or just cord, superficially resembles rope but behaves much differently. Accessory cord may be found in a kernmantle construction, appearing almost identical to kernmantle rope, or in a braided construction. Experienced users know that kernmantle cordage can be used to support human loads when used appropriately, but braided cordage should not be used to support a human life. Kernmantle accessory cord used for life safety should meet an appropriate standard (e.g., UIAA, CEN, CI-1803) (Table 108-2). General utility cord may be strong but is not held to the same quality standards as kernmantle cordage.

Around camp, utility cordage has many uses (e.g., guy lines for tents, securing food in trees, tying equipment to backpacks). During a medical emergency, these cords can be used effectively to splint and otherwise stabilize patient injuries. However, cords should not be used for life support functions. Kernmantle cord is frequently used to build anchors (cordelette), tie climbing hitches (Prusik hitch; see Hitches, later), or other short, personal tethers. As with webbing, kernmantle cord is used in places where using rope could produce unwanted rope abrasion. Some prefer cordage because it is easier to tie knots using cord, and strands slide more easily over anchor hardware, thus making multipoint anchors easier to fabricate. As with rope, a wide variety of fibers may be used to make cordage, although nylon and Dyneema may be most common. For best results, use sewn rather than tied Dyneema cordage, because this fiber has a low coefficient of friction, allowing knots to slide out more easily (see Knot Safety, later).

ROPE FOR LIFE SAFETY

Not every rope is appropriate for every purpose; ropes used for life safety should be different from those used to make camp. Rope users should understand the characteristics of different ropes and should choose ropes with the desired characteristics for their intended function.

Ropes used in non–life safety applications are known as *commodity ropes* and can be found in hardware stores, discount stores, and one's garage. These ropes are suitable for use in noncritical applications, where rope failure is unlikely or would have relatively minor consequences.

No rope should ever be used to support a human life unless it has been engineered and built for that purpose. Stories abound of towropes being (fatally) used as climbing ropes, utility ropes coming apart when used as hand lines, and natural-fiber ropes rotting away to nothing. A good way to know a rope is designed for life safety purposes is to check whether it is certified to any life safety standards, such as those promulgated by the International Climbing and Mountaineering Federation (UIAA), Cordage Institute (CI), American National Standards Institute (ANSI), American Society for Testing and Materials (ASTM), Committee for European Normalization (CEN), or National Fire Protection Association (NFPA).

Various life safety ropes are manufactured for different applications because the desired rope priorities are different for rock climbers, mountaineers, cavers, rope access technicians, and rescue personnel. Although priorities vary, users consider similar variables but want different combinations of properties. Important performance considerations for life safety rope include the following:

- Strength
- Impact force transmitted during a fall
- Number of falls held
- Elongation
- Diameter
- Abrasion resistance
- Compatibility with other equipment
- Hand (knotability)
- Weight
- Flotation

Life safety rope users generally select rope based on whether they want a rope that stretches a little, a lot, or somewhere in between. As such, life safety rope is classified into three types: dynamic, low stretch, and static. Each of these three rope types is tested to different standards and criteria.

Although there are no cookie-cutter solutions to rope selection, some generalizations can be made. A climber who could potentially take a significant fall on a rope will opt for a higher-stretch rope for its ability to absorb the forces of a fall—a dynamic rope. A rescuer who wants to lower or raise a load without excess elongation may choose a rope with as little stretch as possible—a static rope. The user who wants a limited amount of stretch but would like at least some force-absorption capability may opt for a low-stretch rope. Therefore, to select the appropriate rope, it is important to understand the desired rope functions and performance characteristics.

STRENGTH

Strength requirements for life safety rope are most important to people who are using the rope for raising, lowering, ascending, or rappelling. Although most rope users never come close to pushing the strength limits of their equipment, a necessary margin of safety should be engineered into any system. In extreme environments or with heavy loads and complex systems, combined with safety margin requirements, creating systems with the desired safety margin can be a challenge.

Every system should be built to withstand greater than the actual force expected on the system. The difference between these two numbers is known as a "safety factor" and is expressed as a ratio. For example, a system capable of withstanding up to 5000 lb at its weakest point, but is expected to only see 1000 lb in actual use, is said to have a 5:1 safety factor. That is, the

TABLE 108-3 Rope Minimum Breaking Strength by Size (Diameter) Noted in Pounds-Force (lbf) and Kilonewtons (kN)

Diameter	Minimum Breaking Strength
7 mm (0.28 inch)	2200 lbf (9.8 kN)
8 mm (0.31 inch)	2875 lbf (12.8 kN)
10 mm (0.38 inch)	4500 lbf (20.0 kN)
11 mm (0.44 inch)	6000 lbf (26.7 kN)
12.5 mm (0.5 inch)	9000 lbf (40.0 kN)
16 mm (0.63 inch)	12,500 lbf (55.6 kN)

actual strength of the system is five times greater than the intended load.

Safety factors are most appropriately applied to the completed system, not just the rope or other individual components. What constitutes an appropriate safety factor is at the discretion of the user. When there is a low likelihood of failure with minimal consequence, a safety factor as low as 2:1 may be appropriate. Situations that involve a high probability or consequence of failure may call for a higher safety factor.

Establishing and calculating an appropriate safety factor requires significant user sophistication and high component strengths to compensate for strength reductions that occur as the equipment is integrated into a system. According to CI specifications, static and low-stretch life safety rope must meet the minimum strength requirement outlined in Table 108-3.

IMPACT FORCE

Impact force is an important consideration, especially for sport climbers who are climbing above their protection, thereby exposing themselves to a fall with significant impact potential. Dynamic ropes are typically used for such applications. They are designed to absorb energy during a fall so that the force is not transmitted to the climber or to anchorages. Dynamic ropes are tested to verify their performance using an 80-kg (176-lb) mass and are certified to either UIAA or European Committee for Standardization (CEN) standards. During these tests, the 80-kg (176-lb) mass is attached to a 2.5-m (8.2-foot) rope, anchored over an edge, then raised 2.3 m (7.5 feet) above the anchor. It is then dropped 4.8 m (15.7 feet), with the requirement that the resulting impact force be less than 12 kilonewtons (kN), or 2698 pounds-force (lbf). Despite a rope passing this laboratory test to qualify as dynamic, it should be noted that taking a 12-kN impact is not a pleasant experience and may cause injury during a real-life fall. Typical industrial fall protection standards require fall protection equipment to limit impact forces to 8 kN or less, which is also based on an 80-kg (176-lb) mass. Climbers who weigh considerably more will generate greater forces and may require larger-diameter dynamic ropes to provide proper safety and a reasonably low impact force.

When it comes to static and low-stretch ropes, impact force is an important consideration, but impact force testing is not performed in the same way as on dynamic rope, because static and low-stretch ropes are not intended for use when significant impact may occur.

NUMBER OF FALLS HELD

Number of falls held applies only to dynamic climbing rope, on which falls are anticipated. To test for this, the impact force test described previously is repeated until the rope breaks. To qualify for UIAA or CEN certification, a rope is required to sustain a minimum of five falls. The maximum number of falls achieved without breaking the rope is known as the *fall rating*. It is important to note that for this test, the impact force requirement of 12 kN or less is measured only on the first fall. After the first fall, impact force is not measured and can be any force, as long as the rope does not break. This fall rating is basically used for comparison of one rope with another when purchasing a dynamic rope; it has little to do with the actual number of falls a given rope can take in the real world of climbing. A good-quality dynamic rope can provide service for hundreds of low-impact falls. Alternatively, just because a rope is rated at 12 or 15 falls does not mean that it should be used over and over after an extremely high-impact fall has occurred (see Fall Factors, later, for estimating the impact of high-force falls on a rope).

ELONGATION

An important attribute of nylon and polyester ropes is inherent ability to absorb force. Virtually any loading of a rope results in at least some impact force, which could damage equipment and systems if the rope does not have some stretch. Using high-quality nylon and polyester life safety rope helps protect against the effects of such loading. Although absorption of impact force generally translates into a high-stretch rope, elongation poses a practical concern when heavy loads are being raised, lowered, and positioned on a vertical plane. Ropes with too much elongation require more effort to raise, may "bounce" the load, and may cause a stopped load to creep dangerously. For this reason, ropes with lower elongation are preferred for raising, lowering, and positioning heavy loads. Aramid materials, such as Kevlar, Technora, and Twaron, are most desirable because of their resistance to heat, but a secondary characteristic of these fibers is minimal elongation. Such ropes, frequently used for emergency escape from fire, should be used with great caution. There are also accessory cords and cordelettes made with ultra-high-modulus polyethylene (UHMPE) yarns, such as Spectra and Dyneema. These materials do not offer heat resistance, but feature a high strength-to-weight ratio. However, they offer almost no elongation or energy-absorbing abilities. Caution should be used during application of such superstatic ropes, because even the slightest slip could pass high-impact forces to the rope, anchors, and user, much as would a steel cable.

DIAMETER

Most life safety ropes range in diameter from 7.5 to 13 mm (0.23 to 0.57 inch). Accurate assessment and reporting of diameter are critical for these ropes. Most of the auxiliary equipment designed for use with life safety ropes is designed to function with specific rope sizes. Rope friction, ability to be gripped, and weight are also important considerations. Balancing these factors is a matter of personal preference. Some brands and constructions of rope seem fatter than others despite being advertised as the same size. How tight or loose a rope is made will change the hand (i.e., the feel) of a rope as well as the actual diameter at any given load. In addition, there are different methods of determining rope diameter from one standard to the next. Typically, for life safety ropes, some reference load is placed on the rope, the diameter is measured in several places, and an average is provided to the purchaser.

ABRASION RESISTANCE

Life safety ropes should be built for abrasion resistance on rock, ice, and industrial surfaces. This translates to better protection against cutting and damage as well as greater security. Because ropes with the best abrasion resistance generally do not also boast the softest hand, experienced rope users are often identifiable by their preference for ropes with a tighter sheath weave and stiffer characteristics.

COMPATIBILITY WITH OTHER EQUIPMENT

Auxiliary equipment selected for use with life safety rope should be selected according to purpose and with consideration of the specific rope to be used. Rope construction is important with some devices, as is sheath material, flexibility (too much or too little), rope diameter, and even sheath slippage.

HAND

The term *hand,* when applied to a rope, refers to its flexibility and handling characteristics. A rope must be manageable and easy to work with, but these terms are very subjective. An experienced user will have different priorities than will an inexperienced user. Although a soft hand and flexibility are often preferred by inexperienced rope users, ropes with the best abrasion resistance, least sheath slippage, and greatest efficiency in systems are usually those with a stiffer hand.

QUALITY

In addition to the technical considerations involved with the manufacture of life safety rope, quality is a key factor. Some user groups of life safety rope now mandate that qualifying manufacturers meet specific quality assurance criteria, such as third-party certification to a quality standard, such as the International Organization for Standardization's ISO 9001:2008 Quality Management Systems Requirements.

WEIGHT

In some use environments, such as deep caves or wet and cold canyons, the rope weight significantly alters how ropes are carried and used. Users working in environments where heavy or bulky ropes provide a hindrance often chose smaller-diameter ropes (lighter in weight) to facilitate their use. Those working in open environments, where strength is a priority, often use heavier ropes.

WATER RESISTANCE/FLOTATION

Users who work in or around water may prefer ropes that have water-resistant coatings to prevent absorption of water. Such coatings reduce water weight absorbed by rope and prevent water running off ropes and making users wet and cold. Water resistance is of most concern when flotation is a priority and weight of a soaked rope would be problematic. This is only an issue in certain environments, so is not a concern to users unless integral to their particular environment.

LIFE SAFETY ROPE CONSTRUCTION

Most life safety ropes in the 21st century are of kernmantle construction. The German word *kernmantle* means "core" (kern) and "sheath" (mantle). Kernmantle rope sheaths are braided around the core, and their design is crucial to the hand, knotability, and abrasion resistance of the rope. A tightly woven sheath is more durable than a loose weave, but this feature must be finely balanced to maintain knotability. Other variables include fiber denier (diameter), number of strands in the braid, and angle of weave.

MATERIALS

Before development of synthetic fiber ropes, the standard was rope made of natural fibers (e.g., manila). Natural-fiber rope degrades in strength even when carefully stored; it lacks the ability to absorb shock loads, lacks continuous fibers along the length of the rope, and has low strength compared with certain artificial fibers. For these reasons, natural-fiber ropes are no longer considered appropriate for life safety applications. Synthetic fibers, including nylon, polyester, UHMPE, aramides, and polyolefin, are more often used in modern rope making.

Nylon

Nylon is the most common and suitable fiber for general life safety use. Nylon is approximately 10% stronger than polyester, but nylon fiber may lose as much as 10% to 15% of its strength when wet. This strength loss is not permanent; the nylon regains its strength when it dries. In addition, nylon can handle about twice as much shock loading per pound as can polyester when both are wet.

Nylon strongly resists most chemicals, but certain acids and bleaches can cause degradation, especially in high concentrations. For the high-angle technician, the source of most damaging acids is batteries, including lead acid and "sealed" or "dry-cell" batteries. Users must scrupulously protect ropes from direct contact with batteries and exposure to acid fumes or residues that might be found in vehicle storage compartments, trunks, and garage floors. Industrial users should take special precautions for storage and handling because of chemicals used in their rescue environments.

Polyester

Polyester fibers are used in many ropes. Dacron has a melting point of approximately 249° C (480° F), which is in the range of nylon 6,6 with a melting point of approximately 269° C (516° F); the melting point of polyester is 265° C (509° F). Polyester fiber has a high tensile strength even when wet, has low elongation at break, and can be as effectively stabilized to ultraviolet (UV) light as can nylon. These factors make polyester rope well suited for marine applications (e.g., for boat-rigging lines), and make it an interesting choice for life safety applications. Whereas nylon is susceptible to degradation from exposure to acids, polyester is more susceptible to damage from alkali. Polyester fiber also has lower dynamic energy absorption, which means that it cannot handle shock loads or repeated loading as well as can nylon fiber.

Ultra-High-Molecular-Weight Polyethylene

Also known as high-modulus polyethylene (HMPE) and more commonly by trade names Spectra and Dyneema, ultra-high-molecular-weight polyethylene (UHMPE) fiber floats and has better abrasion resistance than do aramids, but still has too little stretch to absorb dynamic energy. UHMPE fibers have too low a melting point to be used safely with most rappelling equipment. In addition, they tend to be very slippery and do not hold knots well under high tension. These properties make them excellent marine ropes, as well as short runners and tethers for sport climbing applications.

Aramids

Aramids, commonly known by the trade names Kevlar, Technora, and Twaron, are extremely strong fibers, resist high temperatures, and have become popular for escape ropes when one requires smaller-diameter, higher-strength ropes with ability to withstand higher working temperatures than can nylon and polyester ropes. Aramids are very susceptible to internal and external abrasion. Because these fibers cannot absorb dynamic energy and are easier to break if bent too tightly (i.e., in a knot or rappel device), they are dangerous to use in most life safety rope applications.

Polyolefin

Polyolefin (polypropylene or polyethylene) fiber ropes are used when their flotation property is required, as for water rescue. They have good resistance to most acids; however, polyolefin fibers rapidly degrade, especially under UV light exposure. Because this fiber has low abrasion resistance, strength, life expectancy, and melting point, it is a poor choice for most life safety applications.

ROPE TYPE

The core of a kernmantle rope primarily determines its elongation, force absorption, and strength properties. The terms *dynamic, low stretch,* and *static* are technically misnomers in that all ropes are dynamic to some degree. However, these are industry-standard terms useful for relating the degree of elongation inherent in each rope type.

Dynamic Kernmantle Rope

A well-designed dynamic rope intended to absorb the shock load of a fall will also be very stretchy, with as much as 30% elongation at 10% of minimum breaking strength. Thus, a dynamic kernmantle rope would be very difficult to use effectively for positioning heavy loads (e.g., rescue load), contending with changing loads (e.g., loading patient midface on rock wall), or

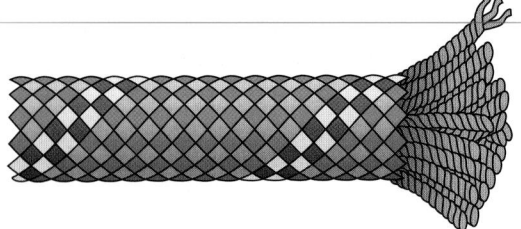

FIGURE 108-2 Dynamic kernmantle rope.

rigging into a haul system (i.e., where energy would be wasted with each pull because of the inherent elongation). This type of rope would also be very difficult to use effectively under high tension (e.g., as a highline).

Dynamic ropes also tend to have a lower tensile strength than do static or low-stretch kernmantle ropes because of the same design characteristics that allow it to stretch. Furthermore, dynamic kernmantle designs are often softer and have a lower percentage of sheath than do static kernmantle ropes, making them more susceptible to abrasion and wear (Figure 108-2).

Static Kernmantle Rope

A static kernmantle rope is designed to be very strong and to have minimal stretch (i.e., as little as 3% to 6% at 10% minimum breaking strength). For consistent strength, inner bundles run continuously and unbroken throughout the length of the rope, usually in a near-parallel manner, to reduce stretch and spin (Figure 108-3). This load-carrying core is protected from dirt, abrasion, and cutting by a tightly braided outer sheath. Static kernmantle ropes are ideal for lowering and raising heavy loads (e.g., during rescue), work positioning, fall protection, and ascending. Static ropes should not be subjected to a fall factor of more than 0.25 unless additional force-absorption provisions are made in the system.

Low-Stretch Kernmantle Rope

Low-stretch kernmantle ropes elongate 6% to 10% at 10% breaking strength, fulfilling the needs not met by highly dynamic climbing ropes or very stable, static kernmantle designs. This is achieved using a different core construction and a better sheath-core relationship, which typically gives such ropes a softer profile than that of static lines. However, these same characteristics decrease abrasion resistance and make this type of rope less desirable for positioning. Low-stretch ropes are often used for belaying heavy loads, especially where fall factor potential is low.

KNOTS IN SOFTWARE

Medical professionals encounter many knots during the course of their careers. From the square knot in a stitched laceration to neckties at administrative functions, practical and symbolic representations of knots abound.

In modern society, knots are used as a form of expression, in art, as mathematical structures, and for security purposes. Determination of "good" versus "bad" in analysis of a knot lies solely in the knot's ability to achieve the purpose for which it was created. Therefore, you may find that several of the good and clever knots you have learned are useless when it comes to functioning in the wilderness.

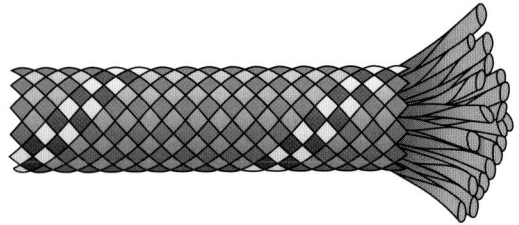

FIGURE 108-3 Static kernmantle rope.

USES

Knots are applied in the wilderness to stake out tents or shelters, tie flies to fishing lines, create suspended "bear-proof" gear caches, and occasionally tie things together.

When performing wilderness medical evacuation, knots take on great significance. Many medical professionals find themselves working alongside rescue technicians in steep terrain, where knots are used for safety of rescue personnel and patient evacuation. Improvisational medical techniques often involve knots. Knotted rope or fabric can be used to secure a splint, create a hasty patient transport device, or provide secure shelter for people in precarious environmental situations.

HOW KNOTS WORK

A knot or hitch is held together by internal friction. The friction is attained by the rope twisting and turning around itself or another object, such as a carabiner, capstan, or another rope. The geometry of the twists and turns give knots and hitches their shape, function, strength, and ultimately behavior under load. In a wilderness rescue situation, lives may depend on this skill, so experienced outdoor users should be able to select the correct knot without hesitation, tie knots correctly the first time, and tie knots with gloved hands, on muddy or icy rope, in the dark, and under stress. One should be able to determine by looking at a knot whether it is tied correctly.

Unfortunately, it has been said, "If you can't tie a knot, tie a lot," which is the genesis of the "lotta knot." In a lotta knot, the greater the mass of rope and the more twists and turns it takes in relation to itself, the higher the probability that the knot will hold. Although the theory is somewhat humorous, it is seldom effective. The lotta knot sometimes holds because the larger rope mass increases the odds of getting a bend to hold. However, there are many disadvantages to this type of knot. It uses lots of rope, is difficult to tension, and is frequently difficult to untie. It is unpredictable and may fail to perform altogether. Consequently, outdoor users should strive to learn tried-and-true knots because they are faster, more efficient, and safer to use. One hallmark of a seasoned outdoor user is basic knotcraft.

When working with software, it is critical to be aware of the material type into which the knot is tied. Some fibers have a low coefficient of friction (e.g., Spectra, Dyneema) and require special considerations when tying knots. Similarly, knots that are effective on rope do not always perform well in webbing.

KNOT TERMINOLOGY

To communicate more effectively, knot users employ discipline-specific terminology. Learning these terms will allow you to communicate more efficiently and effectively in the backcountry. For examples of these terms, see Figure 108-4.

The *working end* is the section of software used to tie the knot.

The *standing part* (or *end*) is the section not actively used to form the knot or rigging.

The *running end* (or simply the *end*) is the free end of the software.

A *line* is some software in use. For example, a rope used to rappel is called a *rappel line*.

A *bight* of rope is formed when the rope takes a U-turn on itself so that the running end and standing end run parallel to each another. The U portion, where the rope bends, is referred to as the *bight*.

A *loop* of rope is made by crossing a portion of the standing end over or under the running end. Note that a loop closes, as compared with a bight. Thus, many knots that form a loop from a bight in the standing part of the rope are named *something on a bight,* (e.g., figure-8 on a bight).

The *tail* of a rope is the typically short, unused length of rope that remains when a knot is tied.

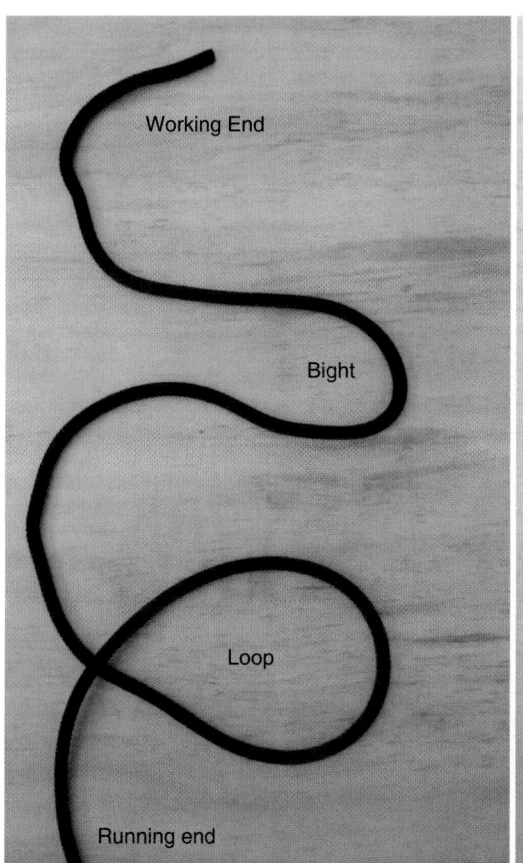
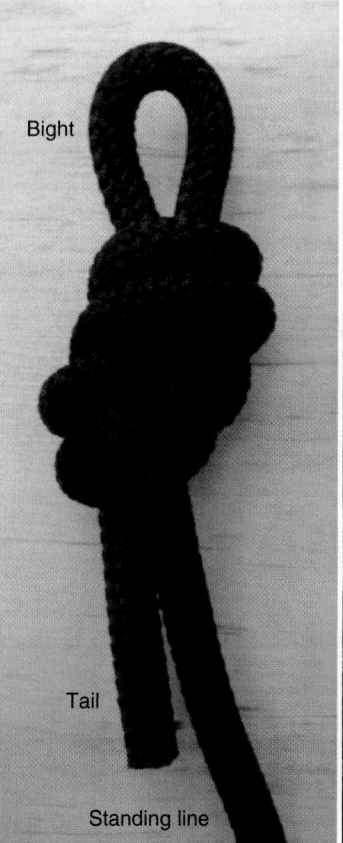
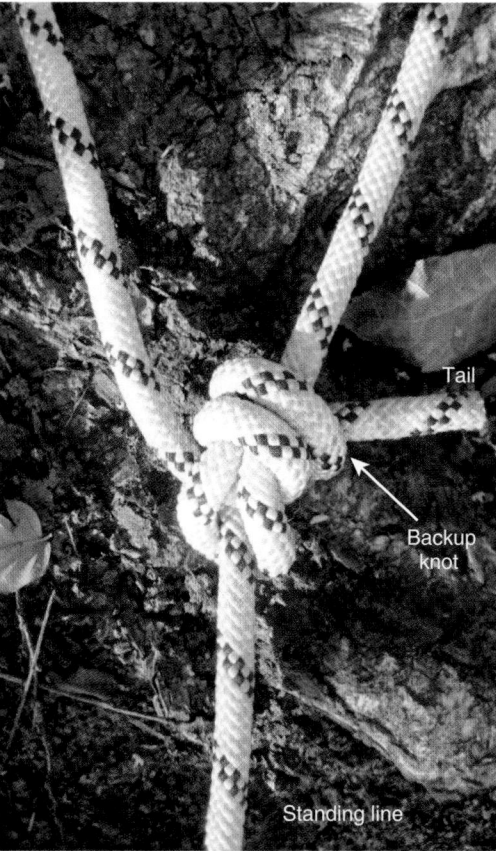

FIGURE 108-4 Knot terminology.

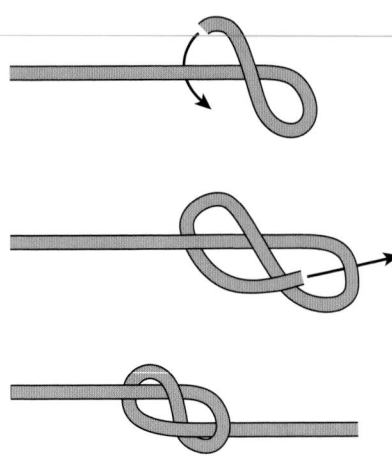

FIGURE 108-5 Figure-8 knot.

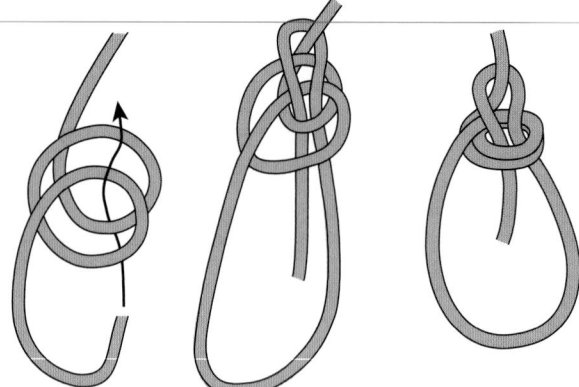

FIGURE 108-7 High-strength bowline or double bowline.

CATEGORIES OF KNOTS

The most practical way to select a knot is to evaluate what function the knot will perform. For our purposes, knots have five basic functions: (1) stopper knots; (2) end-of-line knots; (3) midline knots; (4) knots that join two ropes; and (5) safety knots.

There are knot subsets for the terminology purist. A knot tied around something (e.g., a tree, a standing rope, the rail of a litter) that conforms to the shape of the object around which it is tied, and does not hold its shape when the object around which it is tied is removed, is called a *hitch*. A knot that connects two ends of software is called a *bend*. A *loop* is a section of rope that crosses itself, and a *tied loop* is a knot that forms a fixed eye or loop in the end of a rope. Regardless of the name, basic rules apply to any of these ties.

Stopper Knots

A stopper knot is often used in rappelling. Before a rope end is lowered or thrown down for a rappel, a stopper knot is tied into the end to prevent the rappeller from rappelling off the end should the rope not reach the ground. Rappelling off the end of a rope is one of the most frequent causes of climbing injuries and is entirely preventable with stopper knots. Stopper knots perform a similar function as part of other applications.

The most common stopper knots are the *figure-8 knot* (Figure 108-5) or the *barrel knot*. When two ropes are used in tandem, the stopper knot should be tied into both lines together. A simple overhand knot (Figure 108-6) may also be used for this purpose, but its relatively low bulk makes it less desirable than a figure-8 knot.

Stopper knots, such as the figure-8 and overhand knots, are the foundations of many other knots for wilderness use. It is important to learn these before progressing further.

END-OF-LINE KNOTS

Perhaps the most common knot use is to make a loop in the end of a rope to anchor, tie in, or attach the rope to something. Bowline knots, borrowed from mariners, have been used by mountaineers for years. However, this knot can "capsize" into a slipknot quite easily when the tail is pulled; therefore, the *high-strength bowline knot* (Figure 108-7) is often preferred for life safety applications. Other variations on the bowline knot that include added safety for live loads are the simple *bowline with safety* (Figure 108-8) and the *bowline with Yosemite safety* (Figure 108-9).

A handy way to tie a mainline and backup line together for attachment to a live load, such as a litter with patient and attendant, is the *interlocking long-tail bowlines* (Figure 108-10), which consist of two simple bowlines with small loops tied to interlock, while leaving long tails for additional attachment to the litter and attendant.

Another bowline variation is the *bowline on a coil* (Figure 108-11). With its several large loops, the bowline on a coil can be used creatively, to attach a person to a belay line if a harness is not available, or create a load-distributing anchor.

Many people prefer to use variations of the figure-8 knot for multiple applications, perhaps because they prefer to learn only one knot. The figure-8 knot may be tied directly onto a bight (Figure 108-12) or may be tied as a retrace (Figure 108-13).

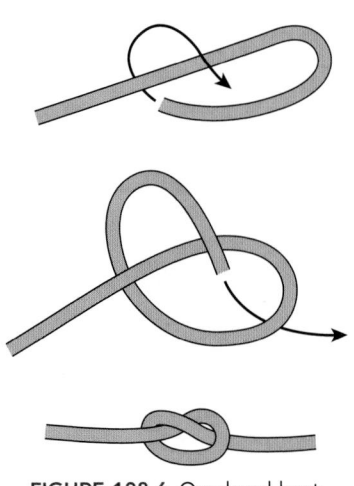

FIGURE 108-6 Overhand knot.

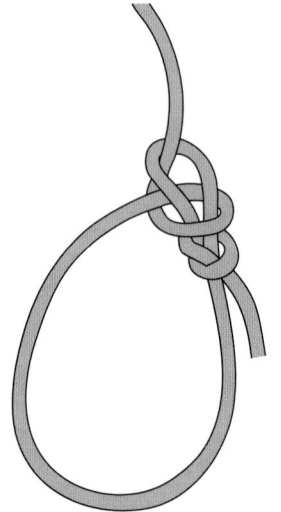

FIGURE 108-8 Bowline with safety.

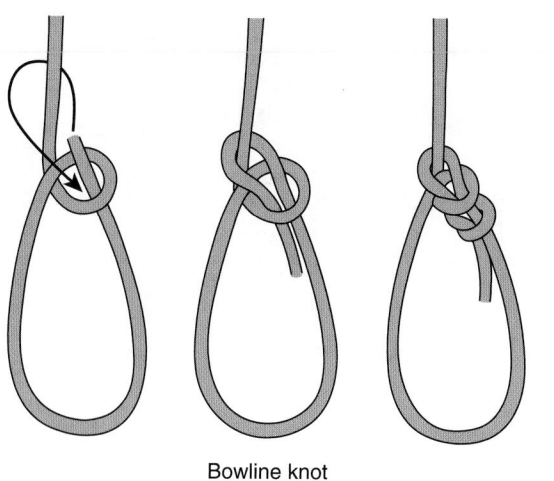

Bowline knot

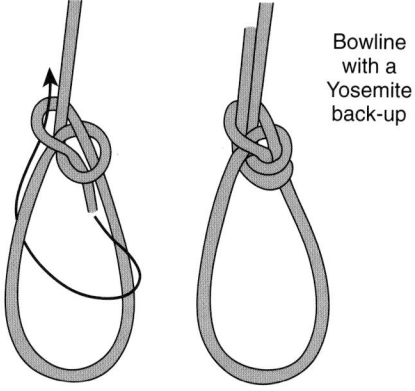

Bowline
with a
Yosemite
back-up

FIGURE 108-9 Bowline with Yosemite safety.

Although the versatile nature of the figure-8 knot is attractive, it should be noted that learning only one knot is limiting. Some people think that the figure-8 knot is easier to tie and check than other knots. In truth, the redundant nature of the figure-8 retrace can make it deceptive on visual inspection, and this factor has resulted in accidents.

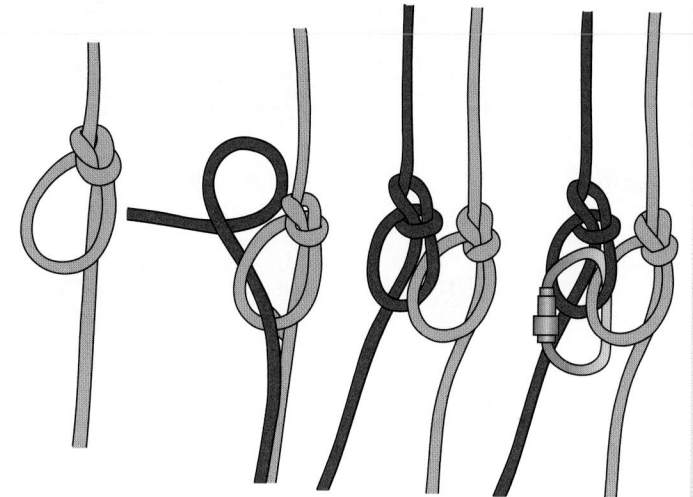

FIGURE 108-10 Interlocking long-tail bowlines.

Midline Knots

Knots are often used to form loops in the middle of a rope or for clipping into, grasping, or bypassing a piece of damaged rope. Perhaps the easiest and most common method of making such a loop is with a simple *overhand on a bight* (Figure 108-14). Alternatively, a *figure-8 on a bight* (see Figure 108-12) may be used for this purpose. Either of these options works well as long as the load is attached to the bight. However, both these loops are susceptible to deformation when not loaded. More importantly, if the rope below the knot is loaded, the knots deform, weaken, and can roll down the rope. If nothing is in the loop, it is possible for the knots to roll out of the rope entirely.

More preferable is the *butterfly knot* (Figure 108-15), particularly if the loop and the line beneath it will be placed under significant load. The butterfly can be pulled effectively either from the loop (in any direction) or from below the knot without negative effect. Caution must be exercised with this knot, because if the loop is not big enough and not loaded, it can pull out under tension.

For a quick and versatile solution to creating twin loops in the middle of a rope, a bowline can be tied on a bight of rope. The *bowline on a bight* (Figure 108-16) results in two relatively

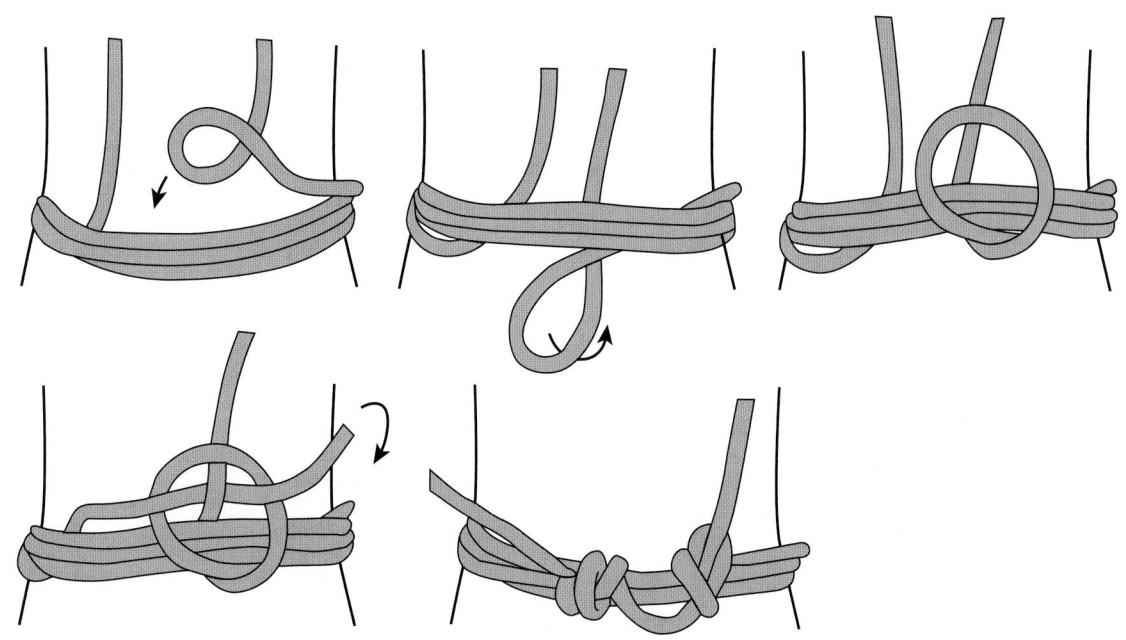

FIGURE 108-11 Bowline on a coil.

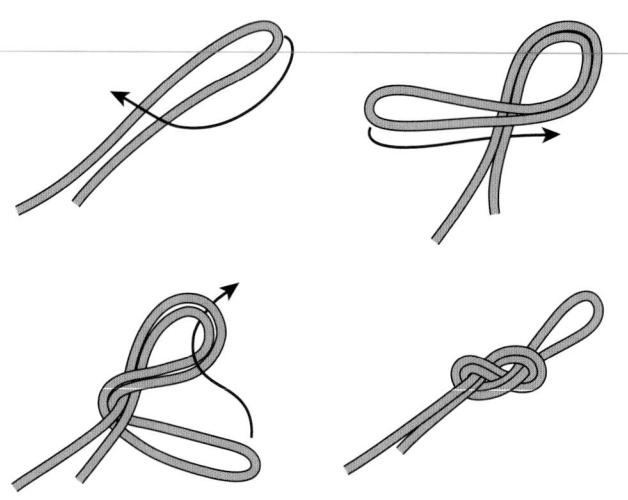

FIGURE 108-12 Figure-8 on a bight.

symmetric loops that can be used to make an emergency boat-swains chair, hand loops, or towing bridle.

Another midline knot is the *inline figure-8 knot* (Figure 108-17). It is tied with its loop in line with the direction of pull on the rope. It is possible to make a foot-and-hand loop ladder out of a single piece of rope using this knot, but it should not be used if multidirectional loading of the loop and the rope's ends is anticipated, because it can roll and capsize if pulled in

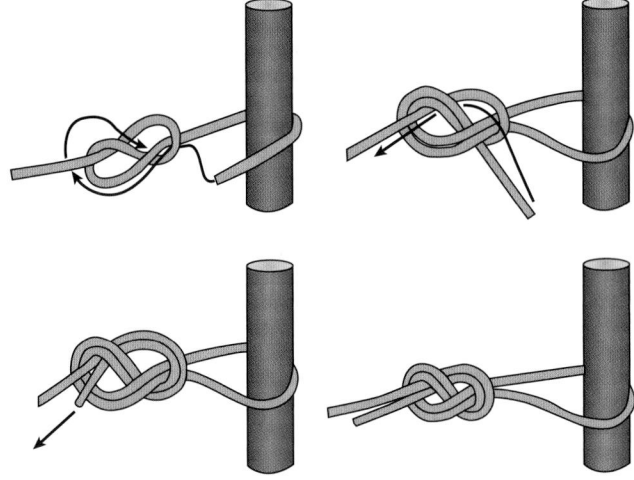

FIGURE 108-13 Retrace figure-8 on a bight.

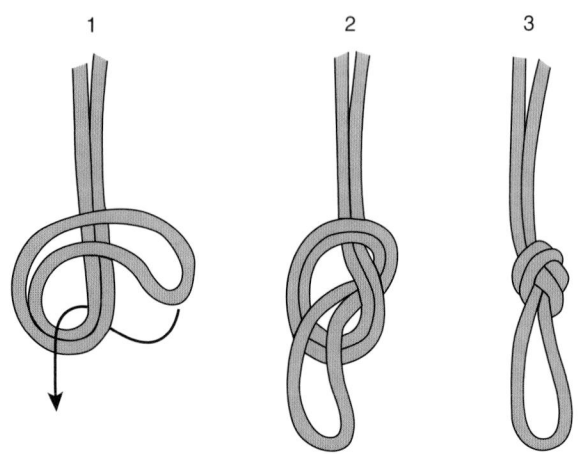

FIGURE 108-14 Overhand on a bight.

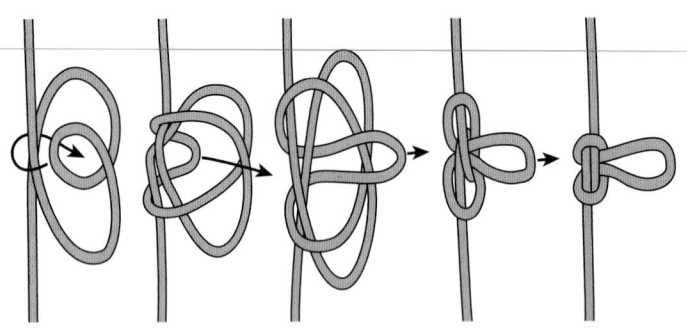

FIGURE 108-15 Butterfly knot.

the wrong direction. The butterfly knot is much better suited for multidirectional loading applications.

To create two loops quickly for equalized multiple anchor points to share a load, the *double figure-8* ("bunny ears") *knot* (Figure 108-18) can be tied midline or as an end-of-line knot. The loops or "ears" can be elongated or shortened to equalize the load between two anchor points.

Knots That Join Two Ropes (Bends)

Tying a knot that will not untie is important when joining two ropes, particularly when the ends are in places difficult to monitor.

Most people have learned to tie a *square knot* (Figure 108-19) for the purpose of joining rope ends. Although well known and easy to tie, this knot is far from secure or reliable. It can easily untie itself, either by pulling through when tightened or by shaking apart when loose. In short, the square knot should be avoided for all but decorative purposes, and when used, should be secured with safety knots on both ends.

The *overhand bend* (Figure 108-20) is a preferred choice for joining two ropes in sport climbing and canyoneering, when

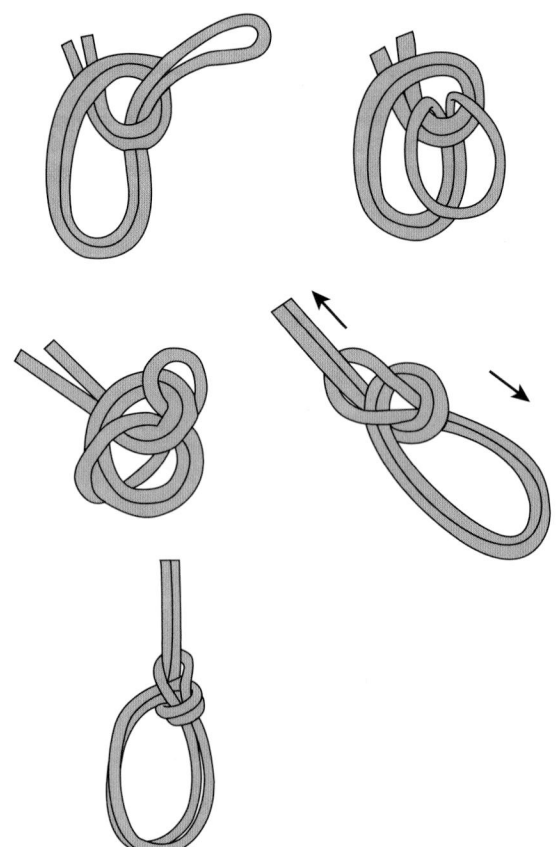

FIGURE 108-16 Bowline on a bight.

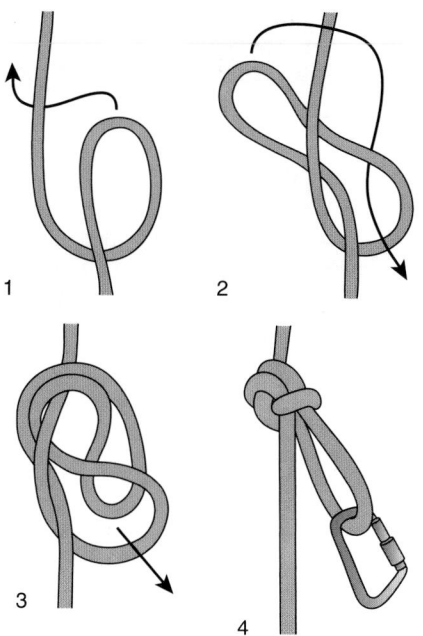

FIGURE 108-17 Inline figure-8 knot.

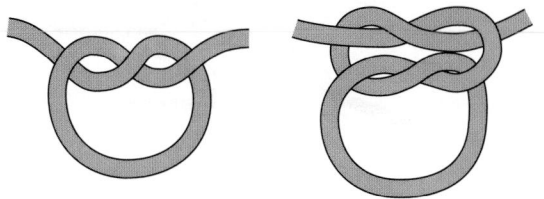

FIGURE 108-19 Square knot.

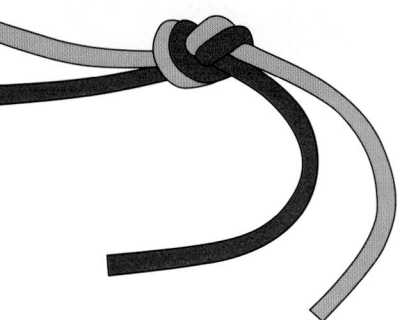

FIGURE 108-20 Overhand bend.

ropes are to be retrieved and pulled over edges. When used, this knot should be tied with extra-long tails in case the knot rolls when loaded. Because this knot may untie while in use, it is not secure enough for rescue purposes. Instead, the more secure *double fisherman's bend* (Figure 108-21) should be used. This bend is very effective for joining ropes of relatively equal diam-

eter. Care should be taken to ensure that the two halves of the bend nestle against each other, and that there is enough tail protruding from the knot to keep the knot from unraveling. This knot is also used to join two ends of a short length of cordage for use as a Prusik hitch (see Hitches, later).

When ropes of unequal diameter are joined, the *double-sheet bend* (Figure 108-22) is a more effective tie. This is a bulkier alternative that is perhaps not quite as strong, but can be easier to untie. For added security, safety knots can be tied on both sides of the bend.

The versatile figure-8 knot deserves honorable mention here. Retracing a figure-8 knot in the opposing direction, with a second

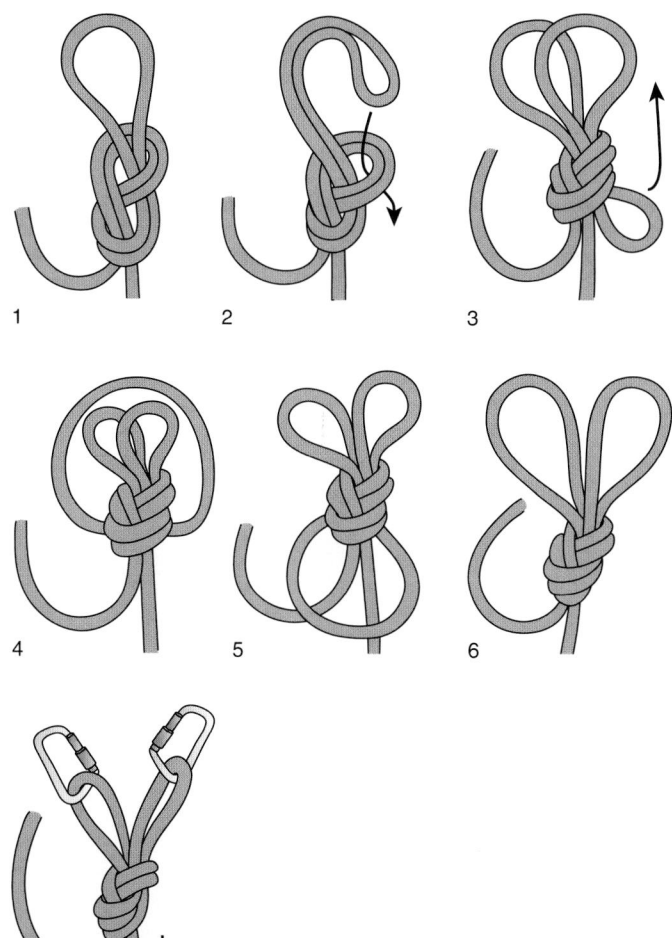

FIGURE 108-18 Double figure-8 loop, or "bunny ears."

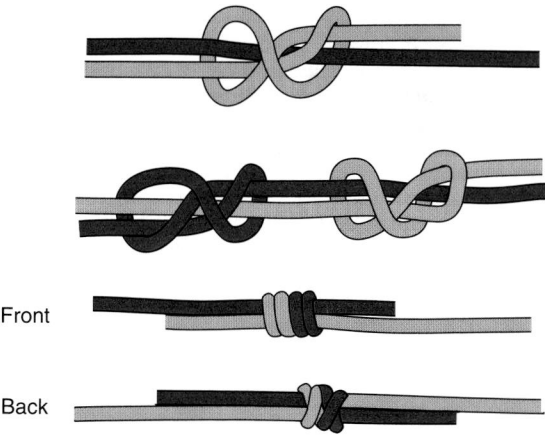

FIGURE 108-21 Double fisherman's bend, grapevine bend, or double-overhand bend.

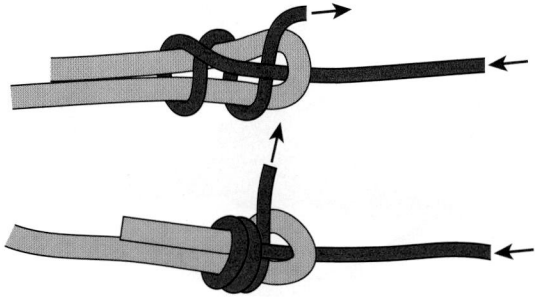

FIGURE 108-22 Double-sheet bend.

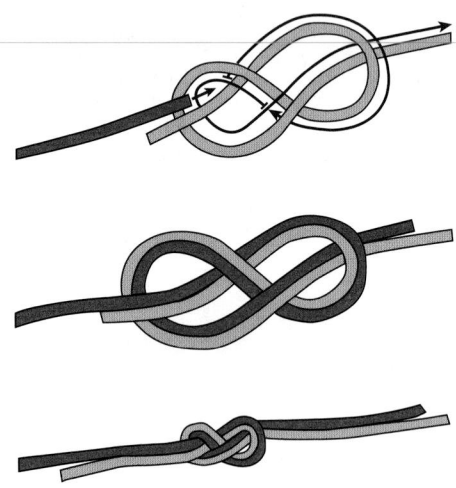

FIGURE 108-23 Figure-8 bend.

rope, results in the *figure-8 bend*, an effective means of joining rope ends (Figure 108-23). Care must be taken with this method to ensure that the rope ends exit from opposite ends of the bend. If tied simply as a figure-8 knot, this bend has a tendency to deform and pull itself apart (Figure 108-24).

Most knots work best in cordage or rope that has a rounded surface. Flat webbing and similar materials perform differently under tension. The preferred bend for joining webbing ends is known as the *ring bend*, sometimes also called the *tape knot* or *water knot* (Figure 108-25). This is most useful for forming webbing slings into a loop, but it can also be used for lashing.

Hitches

Hitching is a method of tying a rope around itself or an object in such a way that the object is integral to the support of the hitch. Consequently, hitches fall apart when the object around which they are tied is removed. There may be severe consequences when a hitch unties. Specifically, disintegration of a hitch results in immediate release of whatever load it is holding.

One of the most common hitches is the *Prusik hitch* (Figure 108-26). A Prusik hitch is a sliding hitch by which a cord can be attached to a rope and slid up and down the rope for positioning, climbing, or progress capture. However, under tension, the hitch will not slide. A Prusik hitch is created by tying a length of cordage into a loop by means of a double fisherman's bend. Wrapping the loop around the main rope and through its own loop two or three times and then pulling it tight forms the hitch.

Another common hitch used in climbing and rescue applications is the *clove hitch* (Figure 108-27). This hitch is useful when trying to shorten the distance between two objects, such as the

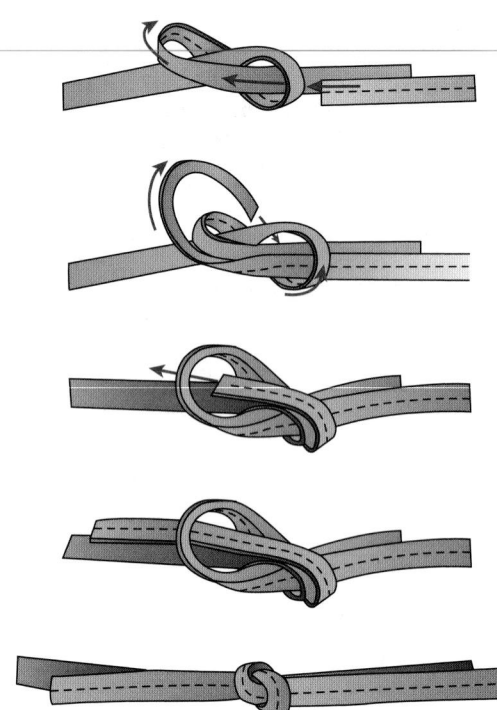

FIGURE 108-25 Ring bend or tape knot.

climber's belay and the climber or the litter rail and the rescuer. It is also useful in some lashing techniques, but can have a tendency to roll loose, which can be solved by using a stopper knot.

The *Münter hitch* (Figure 108-28), or Italian hitch, can be tied around a carabiner or pole and is used to add friction to a system, or as a belay. This hitch is particularly useful because it effectively adds friction regardless of the direction in which the rope is moving. However, care should be taken when using the hitch around a carabiner, because the moving rope tends to slip through the gate of the carabiner, rendering the hitch useless.

The *trucker's hitch* is handy for pulling cord or webbing tight across something (e.g., a load in the bed of a pickup truck, thus the name) or securing a patient snugly into a litter (Figure 108-29).

The *girth hitch* (Figure 108-30) is useful for quick attachment of a sling or rope to almost anything, although it is not very secure. Girth hitches reduce software strength by about half, so they are more appropriate when strength is not an important feature of the software connection.

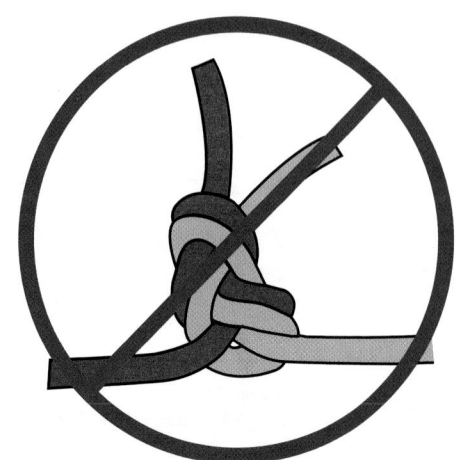

FIGURE 108-24 Incorrectly tied and loaded figure-8 bend.

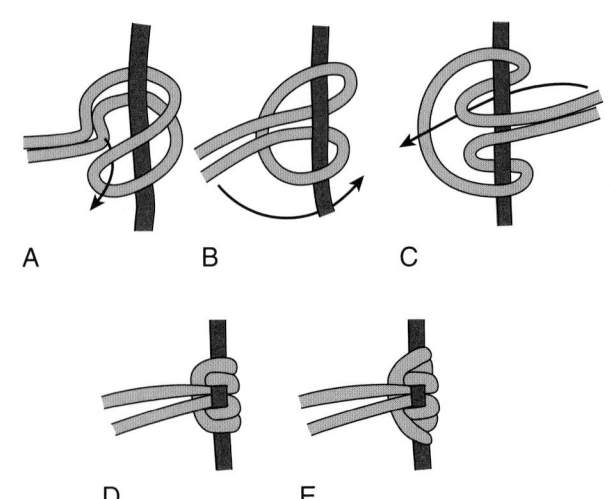

FIGURE 108-26 Prusik hitch. **A** to **C**, Tying sequence for the Prusik hitch. **D**, Two-wrap Prusik hitch. **E**, Three-wrap Prusik hitch.

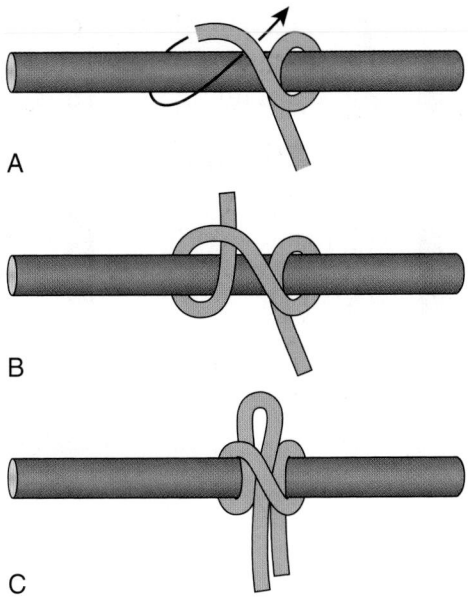

Lashing

Lashing refers to the process of binding items together, such as poles for a shelter or drag. One basic technique used when starting or finishing a lashing involves the *round turn with two half hitches* (Figure 108-31). This is a more secure but bulkier solution for lashing than is the clove hitch. There are several variations on the concept of lashing, including *square lashing* (Figure 108-32) for arranging poles to create a corner, *diagonal lashing* (Figure 108-33) for joining poles to create a triangular shape, and *sheer lashing* (Figure 108-34) for joining poles side by side. Lashings can be extremely useful tools for creating conveniences at camp as well as for emergency use in creating tripods and other mechanical aids.

Emergency Harnesses

The ability to make an emergency harness quickly out of rope or webbing is a key skill for anyone traveling into the wilderness, whether for climbing a damaged mast or belaying someone up or down a cliff. One of the simplest and easiest harnesses to tie is the *hasty diaper harness* (Figure 108-35). A simple loop of webbing is made by tying a ring bend (see Figure 108-25) in the ends of a length of webbing; alternatively, a loop of rope is made by tying a double fisherman's bend in the ends of a length of rope. The loop goes on like a diaper and closes in the front with a carabiner or screw link. There are other ways to use webbing to tie a harness, but this is the easiest way.

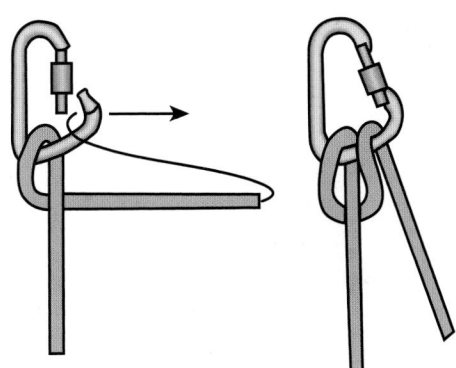

FIGURE 108-28 Münter hitch.

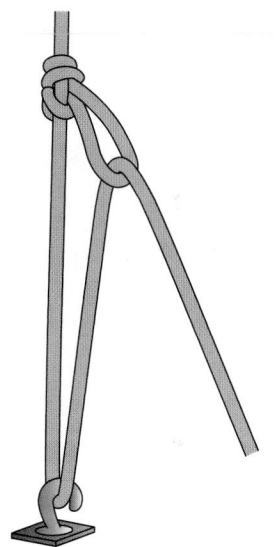

FIGURE 108-29 Trucker's hitch.

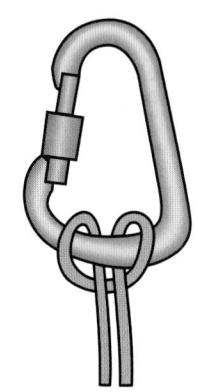

FIGURE 108-30 Girth hitch.

KNOT SAFETY

Knots should be tied, dressed, and tensioned before use. Dressing a knot involves aligning the rope strands parallel to each other so they minimally overlap in the knot. Generally, this results in a "prettier" knot that looks more orderly and can be more effectively tightened. Tensioning a knot keeps it in place and ensures that it does not slip or untie when not under tension. To ensure correct dressing and tension, every knot should be inspected visually and by touch before use, preferably by someone other than the person who tied it. Thereafter, knots should be monitored at intervals. Many knots have a tendency to loosen, and some can even change forms (e.g., into a slipknot).

A safety knot can help prevent mishaps. A safety knot is an overhand knot (see Figure 108-6) or *barrel knot* (Figure 108-36) tied into the tail of the rope after a knot is tied. The safety knot is placed to keep the original knot from deforming or unraveling.

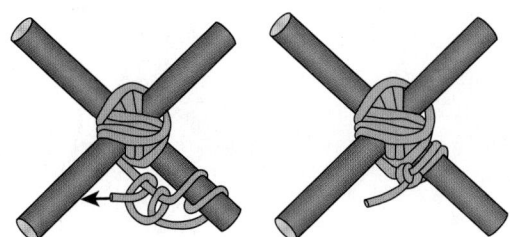

FIGURE 108-31 Round turn and two half hitches.

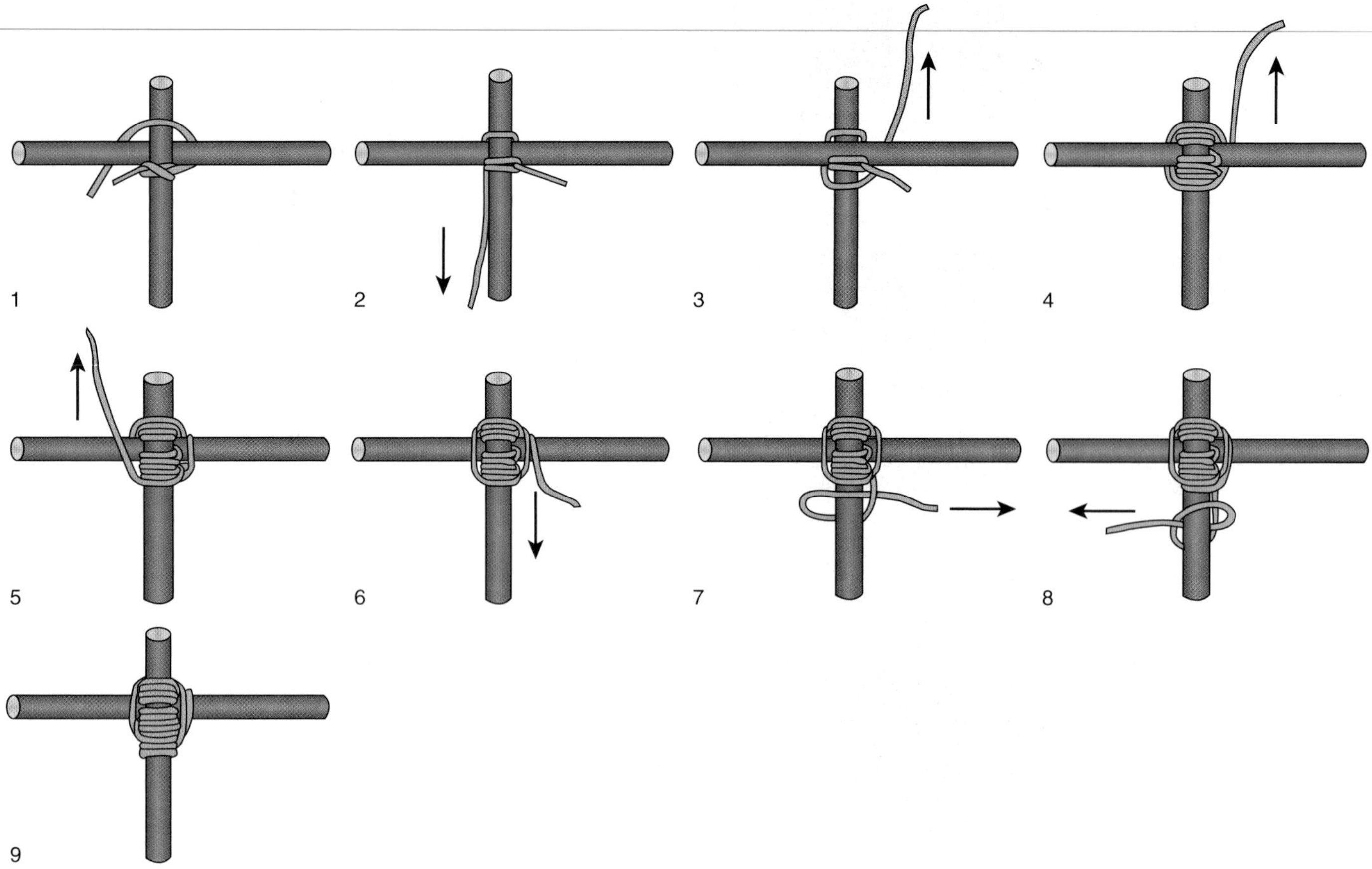

FIGURE 108-32 Square lash.

KNOTS AND SOFTWARE STRENGTH

All knots reduce software strength. The amount of strength loss is affected by tightness of the bends and the "pinching" effect of the knot on itself. The strength of a knot is directly proportional to strength of the material into which it is tied. Knot strengths are usually expressed in terms of *efficiency ratio*. A knot rated at 85% efficiency is said to maintain about 85% of the reported breaking strength of the material in which it is tied.

Some individuals and agencies have reported that any knot reduces the strength of a rope by at least 50%. This information is erroneous, because efficiency of any knot depends on which knot is used, which rope it is tied into, whether it is tied correctly, and how it is maintained. Most knots recommended for use in wilderness rescue reduce the strength of a typical rescue rope to no less than 65% of that rope's minimum breaking strength. Most commonly used knots are even more efficient and have strength in the range of 80%.

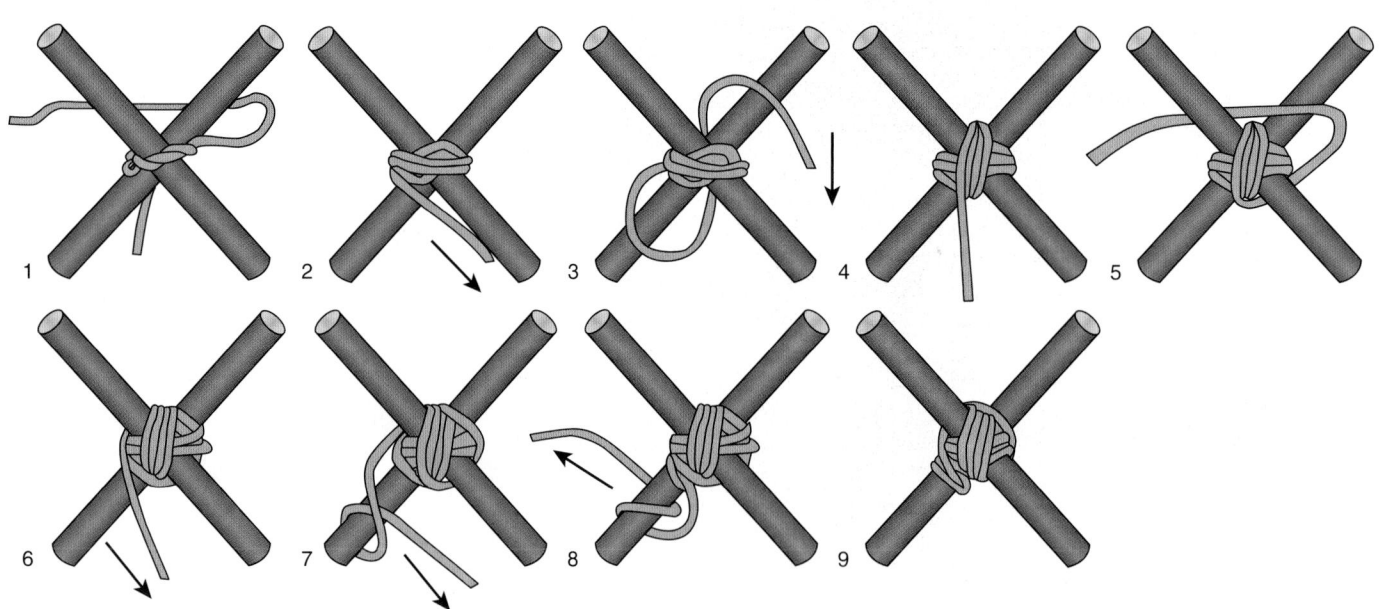

FIGURE 108-33 Diagonal lash.

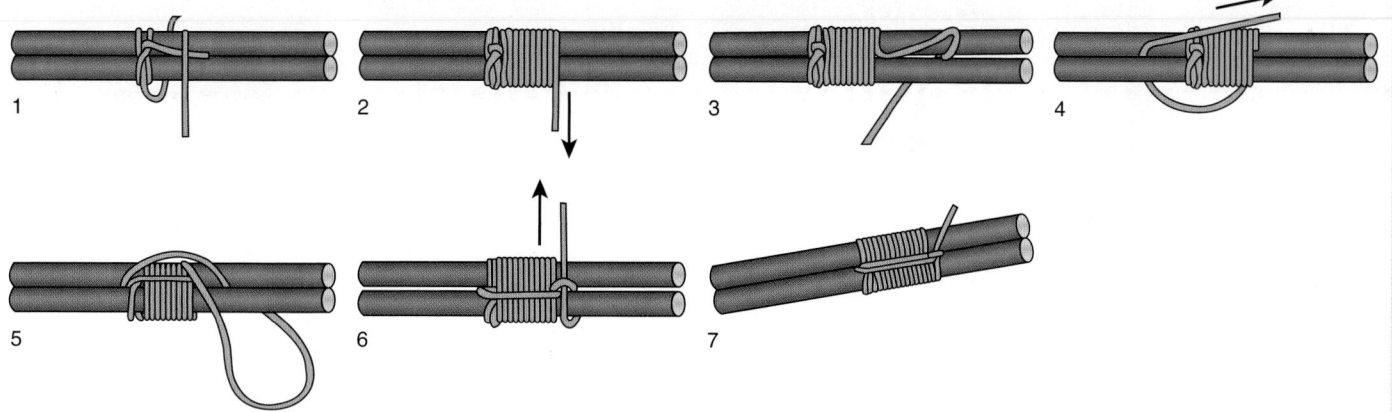

FIGURE 108-34 Sheer lash.

Unfortunately, accurate data about knot efficiencies are difficult to find. Comprehensive testing that includes statistically significant sample sizes, differences among rope fibers, rope construction, rope diameters, rope type (static vs. dynamic), loading rate (dynamic vs. slow), and other variables is nonexistent. However, enough data have been produced to provide a general idea about different knot strengths. The following data, taken from different sources and reflecting limited testing, should be referenced for trend information only.

The relative breaking strength of kernmantle design ropes is listed with the following knots:

- Double fisherman's bend: 65% to 70%
- Bowline: 70% to 75%
- Figure-8 on a bight: 75% to 80%
- Overhand knot: 60% to 65%

The best way to know the strength of a knot on a given rope is to test the knot that is to be used on the rope that is to be used. One should test enough samples to demonstrate the range of variation, which requires using enough samples to provide a reasonable margin of error.

LEARNING MORE ABOUT SOFTWARE AND KNOTS

Learning how to use software for rescue purposes requires training and personal study. A basic vertical class about rappelling and ascending a rope requires a minimum of 2 to 3 days; a rope access certification class generally requires a full week. After a basic rope skills class is completed, regular practice is required to maintain proficiency. Many excellent advanced classes in patient movement by rope or vertical rescue are offered. Anticipate at least 1 week of training for a beginning class about rope rescue. In addition to personal training, there are numerous educational materials to advance this personal study.

For more information about using ropes, webbing, and cordage in rescue-specific situations, see the fourth edition of *High-Angle Rescue Techniques* by Hudson and Vines, which can be supplemented with an education course.

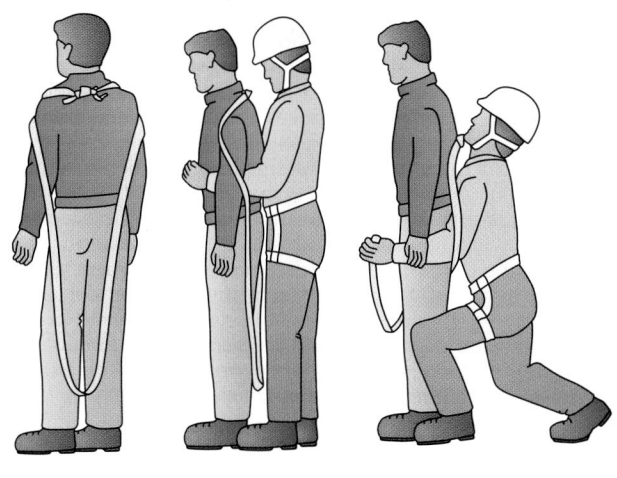

FIGURE 108-35 Hasty diaper harness.

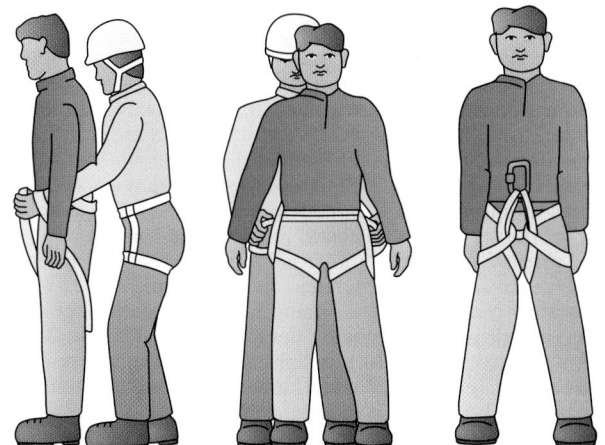

FIGURE 108-35 Hasty diaper harness.

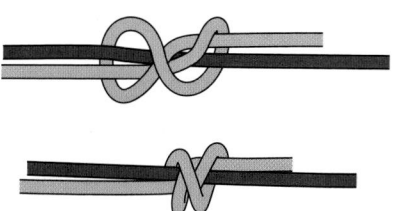

FIGURE 108-36 Barrel knot.

VICKI E. NOBLE, ALICE F. MURRAY, AND N. STUART HARRIS

Modern wilderness travelers have ready access to portable medical equipment with advanced imaging and diagnostic abilities.

In this chapter, we explain how current portable ultrasound devices offer an array of powerful diagnostic techniques for medical care in the field. We discuss ultrasound as the one form of human anatomic imaging with obvious, direct application in wilderness clinical care and research. For detailed descriptions of all ultrasound techniques, excellent texts are available dedicated to clinical ultrasound.[45,50] Our goal is to provide sufficient detail so that a provider, even with minimal training in ultrasound, can acquire and begin to apply potentially lifesaving imaging techniques while in the field. Experimental studies and routine clinical practice have established that these skills can rapidly, safely, and effectively be learned for use in austere environments, both by medical experts and nonphysicians.[22] Ultrasound images of diagnostic quality can be acquired by untrained persons under the real-time guidance of ultrasound experts thousands of miles away.[53] We provide simple instructions and representative images for various clinical ultrasound techniques that are likely to prove critical in austere environments. Because of inherent limitations of electrical power sources in austere environments, we discuss systems that can reliably power electrical devices. We discuss multiple promising research techniques using ultrasonographic imaging that are well suited for use in the field.

INTRODUCTION TO ULTRASOUND

Wilderness travelers now have access to machines that are lightweight, compact, and sufficiently robust to be carried in a daypack. Machines provide diagnostic anatomic imaging that can be interpreted in the field at costs within reach of expeditions and individuals (Table 109-1). To best utilize their capabilities, it is necessary to understand the physics of how ultrasound machines acquire and generate images. Many of the "artifacts" generated by these principles are quite useful in wilderness settings.

Sonographic imaging is based on the principle of the piezoelectric effect, defined by Pierre and Jacques Curie in 1880 as a property of quartz crystals that creates an electric potential when stimulated by a mechanical force. These same crystals produce a mechanical potential when an electric force is applied.[19] Using these properties, a modern ultrasound machine functions by applying an electrical charge to a piezoelectric crystal (in the transducer or probe) that then converts the electrical signal to a sound wave. Anatomic structures reflect these sound waves back toward the piezoelectric crystal. The crystal turns this mechanical force into an electric current, which is quantified and interpreted to produce an image.

Sound waves (as a mechanical force) require a medium. Fluid-filled structures provide an excellent medium and conduct sound easily, while air scatters the returning sound so that very little of the mechanical force is returned to the probe. Different tissues (reflecting different densities in the body) have varying abilities to conduct sound waves, known as their intrinsic propagation speeds. These propagation speeds are related to density, and therefore each tissue also has an intrinsic attenuation coefficient that modulates the speed of sound through the tissue (Table 109-2). Differences in wave propagation, refraction, and reflection are the factors that allow internal structures to be imaged. Dense structures tend to reflect sound and thus look bright on ultrasound, whereas less dense structures tend to conduct sound and look darker on ultrasound.

PROBE CONSTRUCTION AND FREQUENCY

Ultrasound machines typically have multiple probes with different frequencies and shapes, optimized for different indications (Table 109-3). High-frequency probes generate a higher number of short-wavelength sound waves per second. This generates more frequent reflections over a shorter distance, yielding a high-resolution image but shallow depth of view. Low-frequency probes generate fewer waves per second of longer wavelength. These waves travel greater distances with fewer reflections and offer more penetration but less resolution. More superficial musculoskeletal structures (e.g., bones, fractures, ligaments, tendons) are best seen with high-frequency imaging. Deeper intra-abdominal organs (e.g., spleen, heart, kidneys) are best seen with low-frequency imaging. In addition, each probe has an inherent limitation to the depth it can image. For a high-frequency probe, a maximal depth of 8 cm (3.2 inches) is typical; for a low-frequency probe, 30 cm (12 inches). In an ideal world, portable ultrasound machines available to wilderness explorers would have both low- and high-frequency options to optimize the ability to image different anatomic structures.

OVERVIEW OF CLINICAL IMAGING

Three buttons on a portable ultrasound machine are important to understand in order to optimize image quality. The first button is depth control. All machines allow adjustment of how long the machine "listens" for reflections. This influences their ability to generate an image from shallow (less time) or deeper (more time) structures. The second important button is gain control. Clinicians may think of gain as analogous to volume on a radio. By turning up gain, the "brightness" of signals displayed on the screen is increased. This can be useful to view an image on a screen under sunny conditions or if the reflected image is very dark. Third, some portable machines allow for different "modes" of ultrasound display. B-mode stands for "brightness" and is the typical gray-scale mode that generates an anatomic image. M-mode stands for "motion" and displays a representation of motion within a single anatomic plane over a linear axis of time. M-mode can be effectively used to highlight and quantify the movement of structures (e.g., physiologic lung sliding, fetal heart rate). Doppler can be used on some machines to show velocity and direction of flow. Doppler ultrasound relies on the principle of Doppler/frequency shift to sense movement of reflected ultrasound waves toward and away from the probe. This is represented either by color changes (color Doppler) or by audible or graphic peaks (spectral Doppler). Power Doppler is a form of color Doppler that uses a slightly different component of returned signal and is more sensitive in low-flow states. Power Doppler sacrifices the ability to demonstrate direction of flow to gain sensitivity in detecting lower levels of flow.

TABLE 109-1 Advantages and Limitations of Ultrasound in the Wilderness

Advantages	Limitations
Portable, lightweight, field-ready	Electronic equipment— sensitive to cold, dust, and breakage
Safe, nonionizing (allows multiple assays)	
Relatively inexpensive	Power system (or numerous batteries) required for extended backcountry use
Provides immediate data	
Easy-to-learn techniques, or to be guided from a distance using telemedicine	Requires operator to learn techniques
Allows multiple organ systems to be investigated	
Excellent flexibility for both research and clinical care	
Allows novel research investigations	

TABLE 109-2 Attenuation Coefficients in Ultrasound Images

Tissue	Attenuation Coefficient	Appearance
Air	4500	Scattered
Bone	870	Bright; reflected
Muscle	350	Moderately bright
Liver/kidney	90	—
Fat	60	Dark
Blood	9	Very dark
Fluid	0	Anechoic; none reflected

COMMON CLINICAL IMAGING APPLICATIONS

FOCUSED ASSESSMENT WITH SONOGRAPHY FOR TRAUMA

The Focused Assessment with Sonography for Trauma (FAST) examination is a standard component of initial assessment of the trauma patient. It consists of a rapid, focused ultrasound examination of the abdomen, thorax, and heart using a curvilinear 2.5- or 3.5-MHz probe. FAST examination allows prompt assessment for the presence of free fluid in the right upper quadrant (Morison's pouch), left upper quadrant (perisplenic space), suprapubic pelvis (rectovesical pouch in males, pouch of Douglas in females), pericardium, and thoracic cavity.

TABLE 109-3 Types and Ideal Uses of Different Ultrasound Probes

Type (Depth/Resolution)	Ideal Uses
Low-frequency (2-5 MHz) curved array (Excellent depth of imaging)	FAST examination
	Thoracic evaluation (for pulmonary edema)
	Cardiac views
High-frequency (8-10 MHz) linear array (Excellent resolution, limited depth)	Foreign body location
	Thoracic assessment (for pneumothorax)
	Eye evaluation, optic nerve sheath assays
	Fractures

FAST, Focused Assessment with Sonography for Trauma.

The FAST examination is indicated for patients who have sustained abdominal trauma. It has the benefit of being easily repeated as a patient's clinical condition changes. The main objective of the FAST exam is to answer whether a patient's hemodynamic instability can be attributed to fluid in the thorax, peritoneum, or around the heart. A negative FAST exam suggests that clinicians should evaluate for other sources of hemodynamic instability (e.g., spinal shock, myocardial infarctions, infection). A positive FAST exam in the hemodynamically stable patient is a warning to anticipate clinical deterioration. Especially for the novice user, FAST examination is an insensitive indicator of solid-organ injury, bowel injury, or retroperitoneal bleeding.

The FAST examination consists of four standard views: right and left upper quadrants, pelvis, and cardiac.

Right Upper Quadrant

Morison's pouch is the most dependent portion of the upper peritoneal cavity and thus is where early evidence of intraperitoneal free fluid may be discovered. To obtain this view, place the probe in the right posterior axillary line at the level of the 11th and 12th ribs (Figure 109-1). Move the probe anteriorly with sweeping, angular adjustments until a clear view of the anterior fascia of the kidney and posterior portion of the liver capsule is obtained. When looking at the right upper quadrant, it is essential that the inferior pole of the right kidney is included in this sweep, because this is the most sensitive location of the right upper quadrant evaluation in which to detect free fluid. Moreover, it is important to image the hyperechoic diaphragm in the right upper quadrant, because seeing anechoic fluid above the diaphragm— or continuation of the spine shadow above the diaphragm— demonstrates fluid in the thorax (Figure 109-2). In a normal study, intrathoracic air prevents transmission of sound waves, so the thoracic spine cannot be seen on this view. Instead, the spine and the diaphragm can be seen coming together at a point (Figure 109-3). Figures 109-4 and 109-5 show negative and positive images, respectively, of the right upper quadrant view.

Left Upper Quadrant

The left upper quadrant examination visualizes the spleen, left kidney, and perisplenic space. To obtain this view, place the probe in the left posterior axillary line between the 10th and 11th ribs (Figure 109-6). In this view, it is more important to see the perisplenic area because blood will collect around the spleen before spilling over the spleno-colic ligament into the splenorenal space. Figures 109-7 and 109-8 show negative and positive views, respectively. Again, ruling out a positive "spine sign" by seeing the spine and diaphragm meet at a point is essential to rule out anechoic fluid in the left thorax.

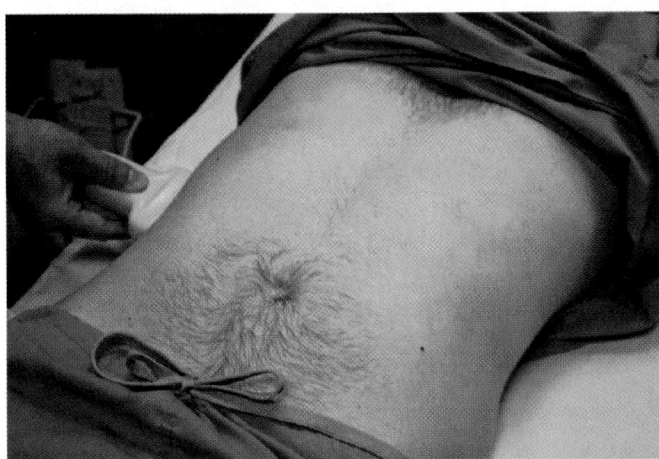

FIGURE 109-1 Right upper quadrant of FAST examination. Place the probe in the right posterior axillary line at the level of the 11th and 12th ribs. This allows the liver, right kidney (with its inferior pole), and Morison's pouch to be imaged. *(Courtesy Division of Emergency Ultrasound, Massachusetts General Hospital, Boston.)*

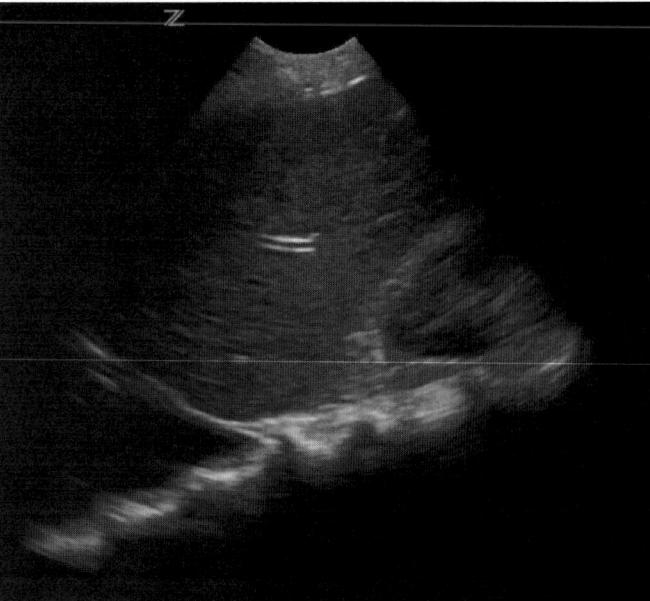

FIGURE 109-2 Presence of a "spine sign" indicates fluid in the thorax. The thoracic spine is visualized extending above the bright, white diaphragm, indicating that sonolucent fluid above the diaphragm is transmitting the sound waves through to the thoracic spine. *(Courtesy Division of Emergency Ultrasound, Massachusetts General Hospital, Boston.)*

Pelvis

The suprapubic view visualizes the most dependent section of the lower abdomen and pelvis. In males, the rectovesical pouch is visualized; in females, the pouch of Douglas is seen. These spaces are in the most dependent portion of the lower abdomen and pelvis; hence, they are where fluid is likely to collect. To obtain this view, place the probe in the midline just superior to

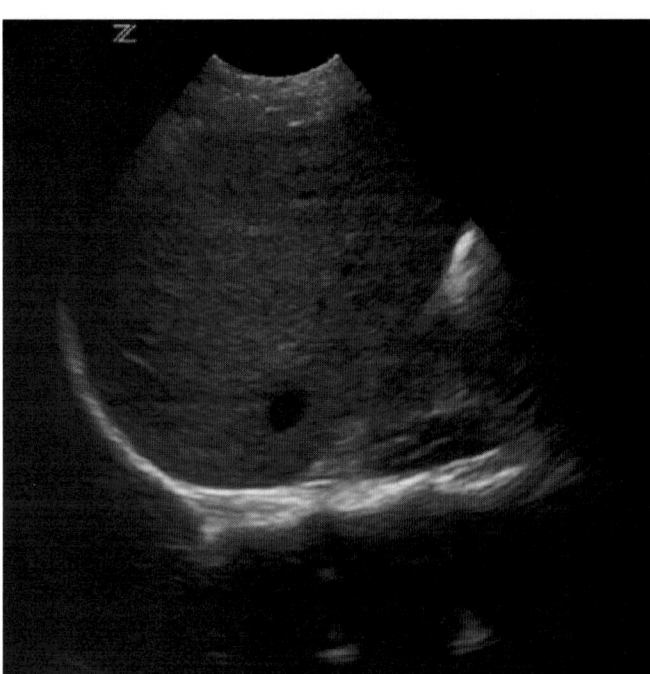

FIGURE 109-3 Lack of a "spine sign" indicates a normal thorax. The abdominal spine stops and meets the diaphragm at a point, indicating that air in the thoracic cavity is blocking the sound waves from reaching the thoracic spine. *(Courtesy Division of Emergency Ultrasound, Massachusetts General Hospital, Boston.)*

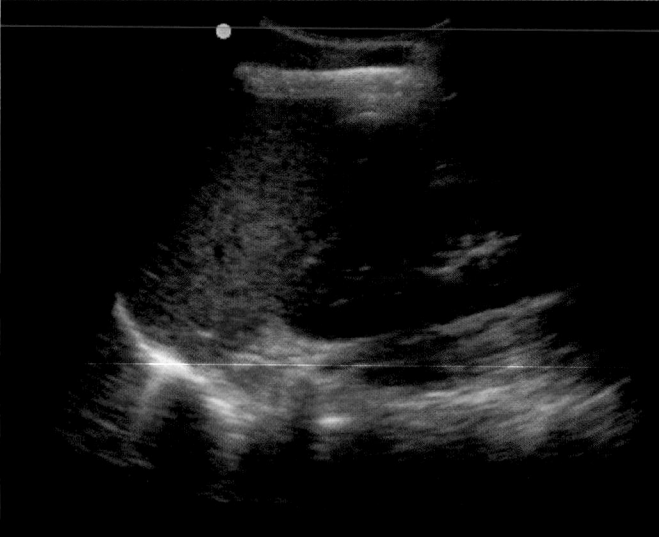

FIGURE 109-4 Right upper quadrant of FAST examination. Normal anatomy reveals the anterior fascia of the kidney *(right midscreen)* and the posterior portion of the liver capsule *(left midscreen)*. A "negative" image shows these two structures clearly and directly apposed. The brightly reflective, curvilinear line of the diaphragm is seen at the far left, lower portion of the screen. *(Courtesy Division of Emergency Ultrasound, Massachusetts General Hospital, Boston.)*

the symphysis pubis (Figure 109-9). Angle the probe toward the rectum. With the probe held in place, fan up and down and side to side until the pouch of Douglas or rectovesical space is visualized. A negative image shows each gender-specific space without evidence of hypoechoic free fluid (Figure 109-10). A positive image reveals perivesicular free fluid (Figure 109-11).

Cardiac View

Cardiac examination allows rapid assessment for pericardial fluid. It screens for fluid between the pericardium and myocardium, and in the case of traumatic injury can yield lifesaving

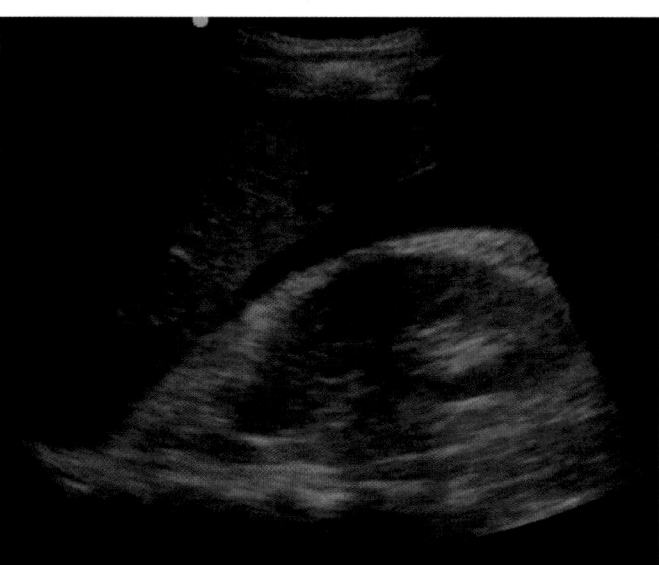

FIGURE 109-5 Right upper quadrant of FAST examination. A "positive" image for abdominal free fluid reveals a lenticular, hypoechoic, dark stripe between the liver *(midscreen)* and kidney *(top right)*. This image demonstrates why it is important to see the inferior pole of the right kidney for a complete interrogation of this space. *(Courtesy Division of Emergency Ultrasound, Massachusetts General Hospital, Boston.)*

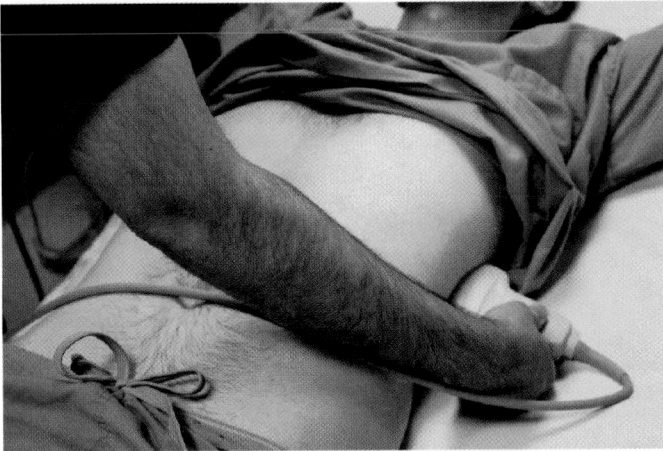

FIGURE 109-6 Left upper quadrant of FAST examination. To obtain this view, place the probe in the left posterior axillary line between the 10th and 11th ribs. This allows the spleen, left kidney, and perisplenic space to be imaged. (*Courtesy Division of Emergency Ultrasound, Massachusetts General Hospital, Boston.*)

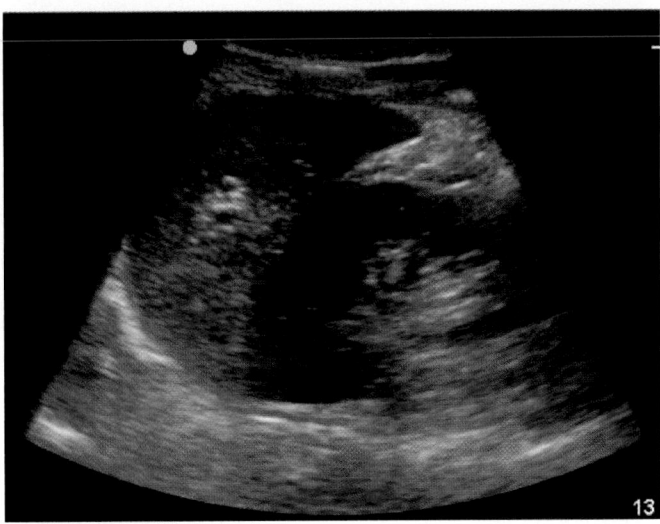

FIGURE 109-7 Left upper quadrant of FAST examination. A "negative" image reveals the spleen (*left side of screen*) and kidney (*right midscreen*) in close apposition. (*Courtesy Division of Emergency Ultrasound, Massachusetts General Hospital, Boston.*)

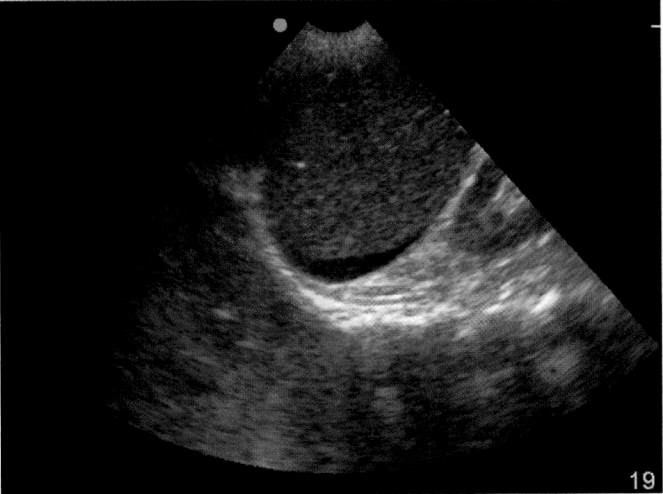

FIGURE 109-8 Left upper quadrant of FAST examination. A "positive" image for abdominal free fluid reveals a hypoechoic, dark stripe, here most notable at the inferior tip of the spleen (*center of screen*). The kidney is seen on the far right. (*Courtesy Division of Emergency Ultrasound, Massachusetts General Hospital, Boston.*)

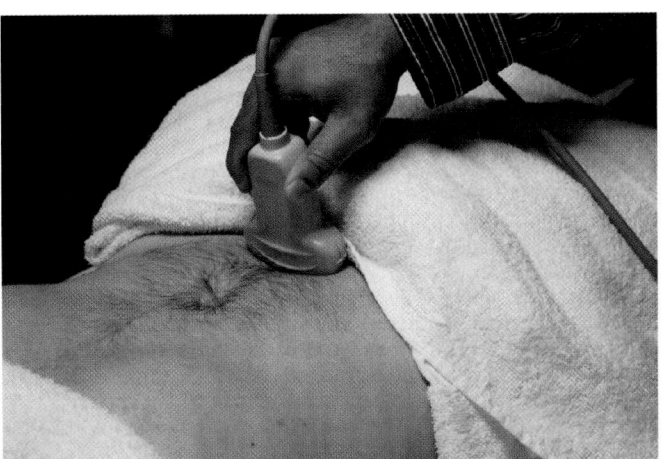

FIGURE 109-9 Suprapubic view of FAST examination. To obtain this view, place the probe in the midline just superior to the symphysis pubis. Angle the probe toward the rectum, then with probe held in place, rotate up the spine until the pouch of Douglas or rectovesical space is visualized. (*Courtesy Division of Emergency Ultrasound, Massachusetts General Hospital, Boston.*)

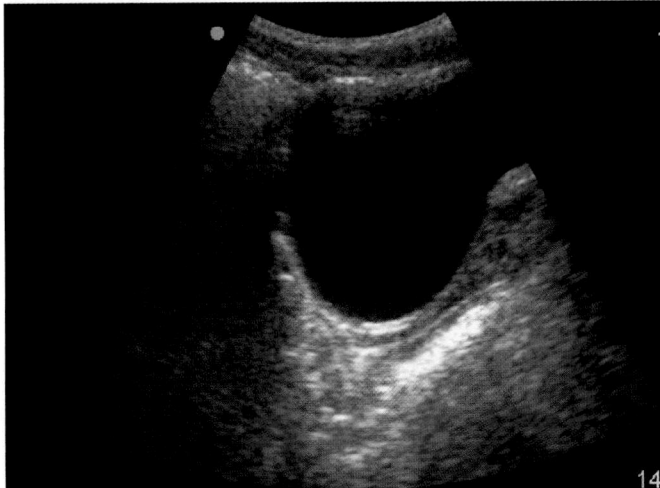

FIGURE 109-10 Suprapubic view of FAST examination. A "negative" image shows each gender-specific space without evidence of hypoechoic free fluid outside of the bladder. Here, the full bladder (globular, dark structure in *midscreen*) is visualized. There is no free fluid outside the bladder. (*Courtesy Division of Emergency Ultrasound, Massachusetts General Hospital, Boston.*)

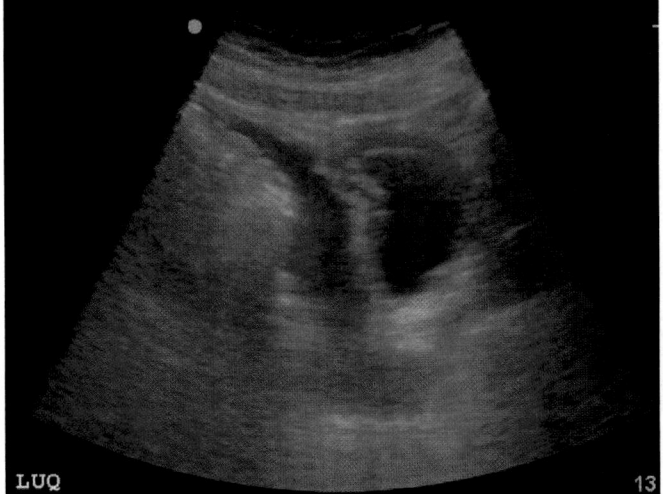

FIGURE 109-11 Suprapubic view of FAST examination. A "positive" image reveals perivesicular abdominal free fluid (irregularly shaped, hypoechoic, dark stripe) in the center of screen. The circle to the right is the partially decompressed bladder. (*Courtesy Division of Emergency Ultrasound, Massachusetts General Hospital, Boston.*)

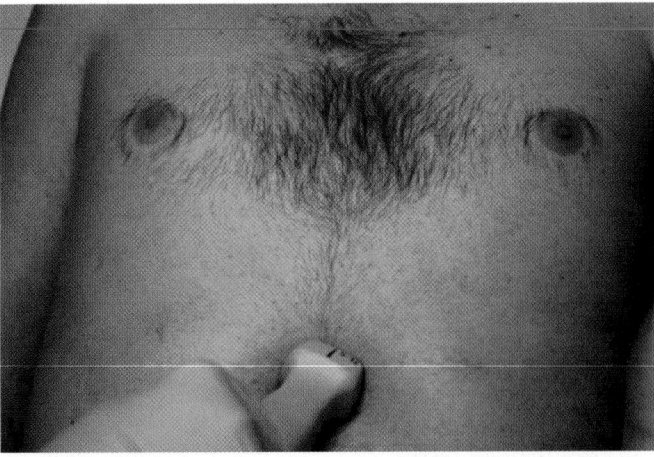

FIGURE 109-12 Subxiphoid view of FAST examination. To obtain this view, place the probe just inferior to the xiphoid process, with the angle upward under the costal margin toward the left shoulder. (*Courtesy Division of Emergency Ultrasound, Massachusetts General Hospital, Boston.*)

information. To obtain this view, place the probe just inferior to the xiphoid process, with the angle upward under the costal margin toward the left shoulder (Figure 109-12). A "negative" image for free fluid displays the echogenic, bright pericardial sac immediately adjacent to the active cardiac surface (Figure 109-13). A "positive" image for free fluid reveals a hypoechoic, dark stripe between the pericardial sac and the cardiac surface (Figure 109-14). An additional view of the heart may be obtained using the "parasternal long" cardiac view. This view can be helpful in patients who are uncooperative, obese, or in whom the clinician is trying to distinguish between pericardial and left-sided pleural fluid. To achieve this view, position the probe to the left of the sternum in the 4th to 5th intercostal space with the probe indicator pointing toward 4 o'clock (Figure 109-15). Representative negative and positive images are provided in Figures 109-16 and 109-17, respectively.

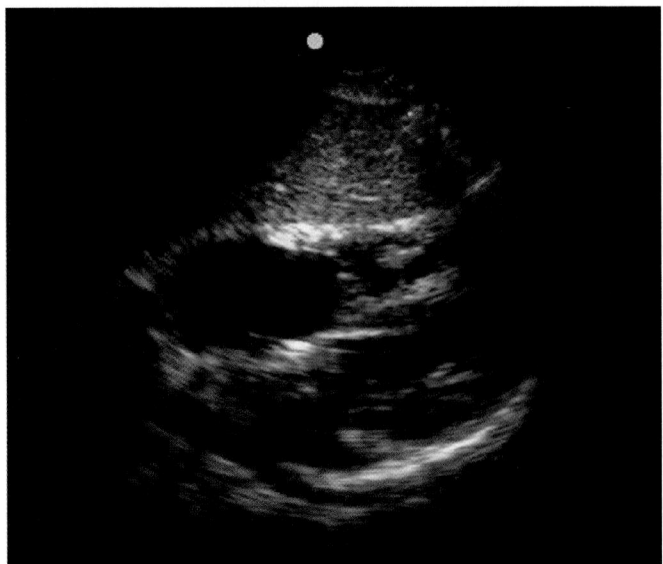

FIGURE 109-13 Subxiphoid view of FAST examination. The pericardial examination screens for fluid between the fibrous pericardium and the heart. In this "normal" study, there is no pericardial effusion. The atria are seen on the left side of the screen, the ventricles to the right. The right atrium and ventricle are at the top of the screen, and the left atrium and ventricle at the bottom. (*Courtesy Division of Emergency Ultrasound, Massachusetts General Hospital, Boston.*)

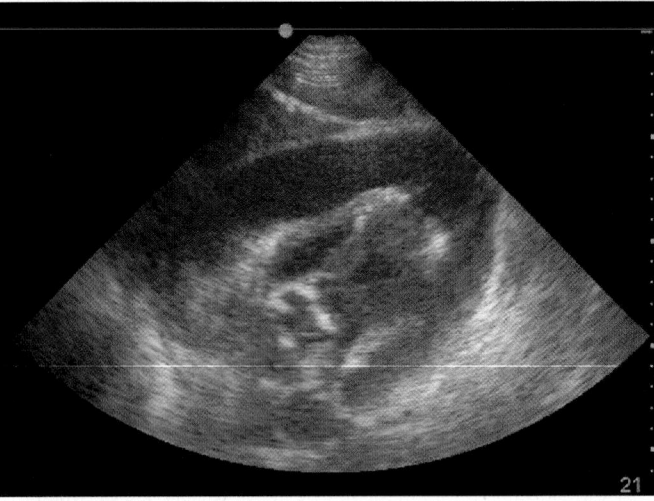

FIGURE 109-14 Subxiphoid view of FAST examination. A large pericardial effusion (dark, anechoic layer) envelops the anterior and posterior heart. (*Courtesy Division of Emergency Ultrasound, Massachusetts General Hospital, Boston.*)

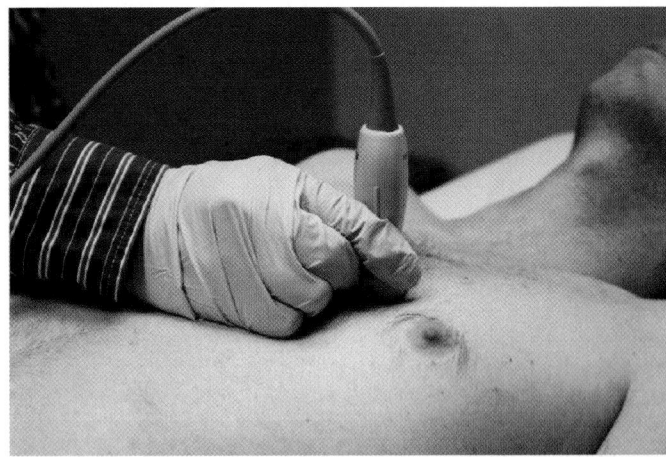

FIGURE 109-15 Parasternal long view of FAST examination. To achieve this view, position the probe to the left of the sternum in the 4th to 5th intercostal space with the probe indicator pointing toward 4 o'clock. (*Courtesy Division of Emergency Ultrasound, Massachusetts General Hospital, Boston.*)

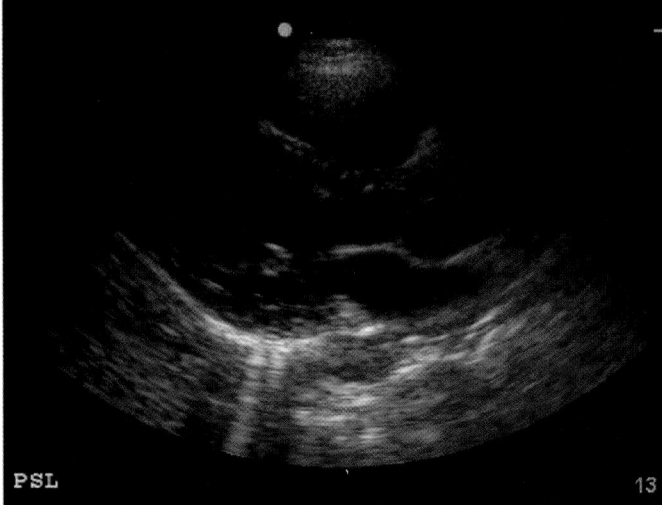

FIGURE 109-16 Parasternal long view of FAST examination. This normal anatomy reveals the left ventricle and outflow track lying horizontally in the middle of the screen. The aortic valve is seen in the right midfield of this image. The bright pericardium is directly adjacent to the myocardium, as there is no pericardial effusion. (*Courtesy Division of Emergency Ultrasound, Massachusetts General Hospital, Boston.*)

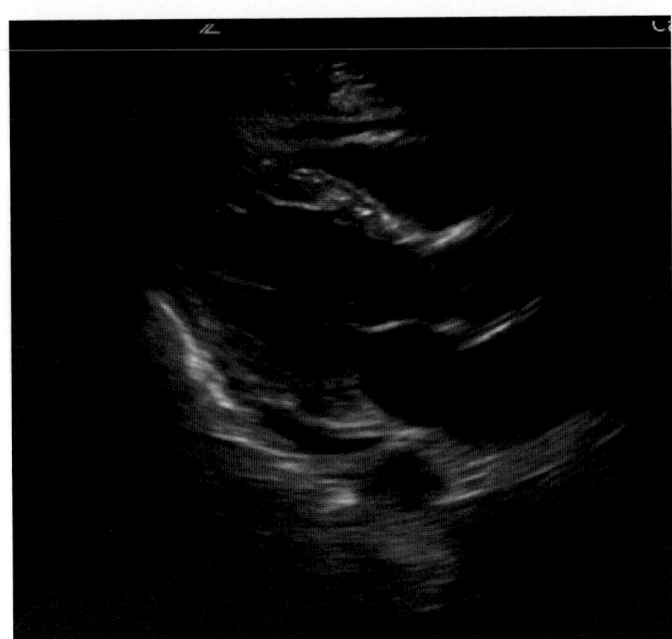

FIGURE 109-17 Parasternal long view of the heart. A large pericardial effusion (darker, hypoechoic layer) envelops the anterior and posterior heart traveling anterior to the descending thoracic aorta, thus distinguishing it from a pleural effusion, which would travel behind the descending thoracic aorta. *(Courtesy Division of Emergency Ultrasound, Massachusetts General Hospital, Boston.)*

THORACIC ULTRASOUND FOR PNEUMOTHORAX AND PULMONARY EDEMA

Ultrasound of the thorax can be used to screen effectively for pneumothorax, pulmonary edema, pleural effusion, and interstitial disease.

Pneumothorax

Ultrasound for pneumothorax can be done with either the high-frequency or the low-frequency probe. The clinician turns down the gain and decreases the depth when performing this examination so that the bright, echogenic pleural line is centered in the middle of the screen and stands out from the less echoic surrounding structures just below the rib shadow.

The scanning protocol depends on how thorough the clinician wants to be and how small a pneumothorax is suspected. For an initial screen for a hemodynamically significant pneumothorax, the probe is placed on the chest in a sagittal position in the 2nd to 3rd intercostal space in the midclavicular line and slowly moved toward the lateral chest. In real time, normal lung anatomy is revealed through two characteristic findings: presence of "lung sliding" (the sliding motion of the visceral pleura against parietal pleura with inspiration and expiration) and visualization of "comet tails." Comet tails are artifacts that appear as a bright, white line caused by the reverberation of the sound waves between the dense visceral and parietal pleurae (Figure 109-18). If air separated the visceral and parietal pleurae, it would scatter the returning sound waves, and the visceral pleura deep to the pneumothorax would be invisible. In a patient with a pneumothorax, neither lung sliding nor comet tails will be visualized. All that will be seen is the static parietal pleura. It is important to note that only the area of the lung seen under the footprint of the probe can be called "negative." When evaluating for pneumothorax, sensitivity of the ultrasound exam is increased by imaging more of the surface area of the thorax.

An additional technique to screen for the presence of pneumothorax can be accomplished using M-mode scanning. M-mode imaging produces a linear representation of movement in a single plane over a period of time. By aligning that plane through the structure of interest (in this case the pleural line), changes within that plane (e.g., lung sliding) can be readily appreciated.

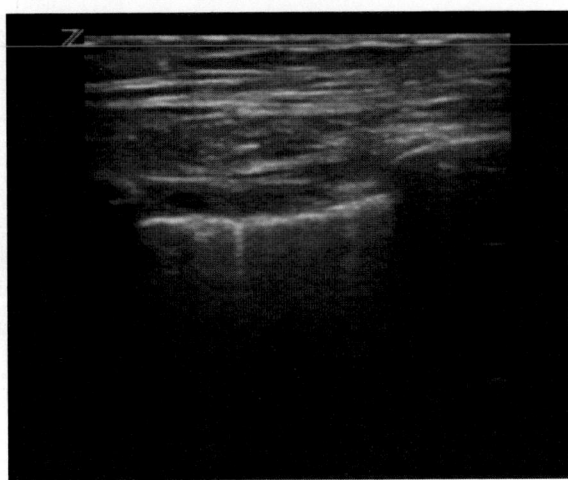

FIGURE 109-18 Normal lung anatomy. The rib shadows and comet-tail reflection are seen well here. *(Courtesy Division of Emergency Ultrasound, Massachusetts General Hospital, Boston.)*

Normal sliding movement between parietal and visceral pleurae will produce the "seashore" sign (Figure 109-19). Normal skin and intercostal muscles have minimal movement during breathing and appear as flat, stacked lines using M-mode. Below the bright, white line of the pleural surface, normal lung tissue moves, which results in this structure having a granular appearance. This image has been described as reminiscent of waves (the superficial/superior, stacked, linear portion of the image) against a beach (the deeper/lower granular portion of the image). In patients with a pneumothorax, lung tissue appears stationary and thus appears in M-mode as a series of stacked lines, just like the superficial muscle above it. This results in the "bar code" sign (Figure 109-20).

Pulmonary Edema

Ultrasound is very accurate at assessing the water content of lung tissue. However, instead of imaging the tissue directly, this

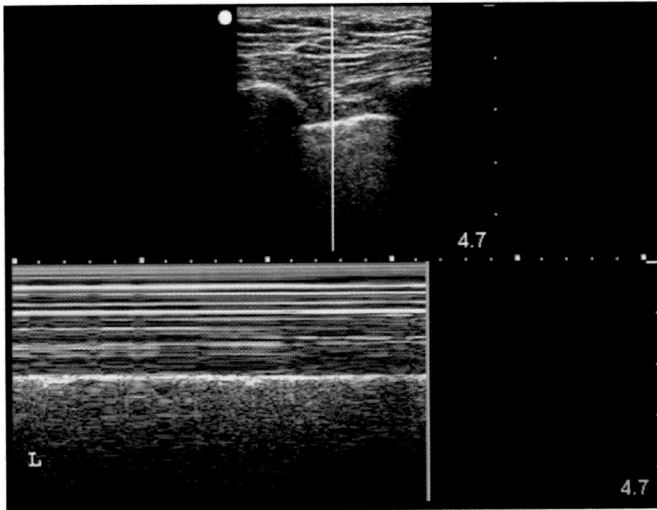

FIGURE 109-19 "Seashore" sign indicates normal anatomy with no pneumothorax. Images obtained of thorax employing B-mode imaging *(top)* and M-mode imaging *(below).* Normal skin/intracostal muscles *(top of lower image)* have minimal movement during breathing and thus appear as flat, stacked lines using M-mode. Below the bright, white line of the pleural surface, normal lung tissue does move, and this results in this structure having a granular appearance *(bottom of image).* This image has been described as reminiscent of waves *(superficial/superior, stacked, linear portion of image)* against a beach *(deeper/lower granular portion of image). (Courtesy Division of Emergency Ultrasound, Massachusetts General Hospital, Boston.)*

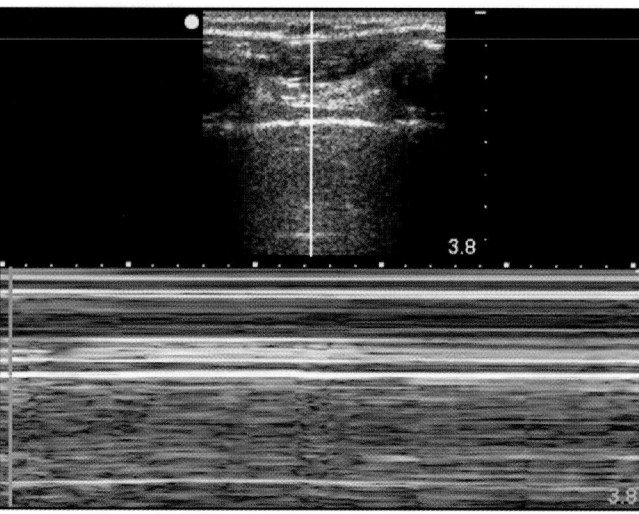

FIGURE 109-20 "Bar code" sign indicates the presence of a pneumothorax. Images obtained of thorax employing B-mode imaging *(top)* and M-mode imaging *(below)*. In a patient with a pneumothorax, the lung tissue appears stationary and thus appears in M-mode as a series of stacked lines no different than the superficial muscle above it. *(Courtesy Division of Emergency Ultrasound, Massachusetts General Hospital, Boston.)*

assessment is done by evaluating artifacts caused by the impedance difference between air-filled alveoli and fluid-filled interstitium. When the lung is well aerated and without excessive lung water, sound waves generated by a low-frequency probe bounce between the pleural line and skin, causing a horizontal artifact known as *A-lines* (Figure 109-21). If the interstitium and then the alveoli start to fill with fluid, the tissue begins to conduct sound. The reflections generated by this impedance difference (fluid and air) are called *B-lines* (Figure 109-22). B-lines are vertical reflections that originate at the pleura and must travel to at least a depth of 18 cm (7.2 inches; this is why the low-frequency probe is used). B-lines move with the pleural line during respiration.

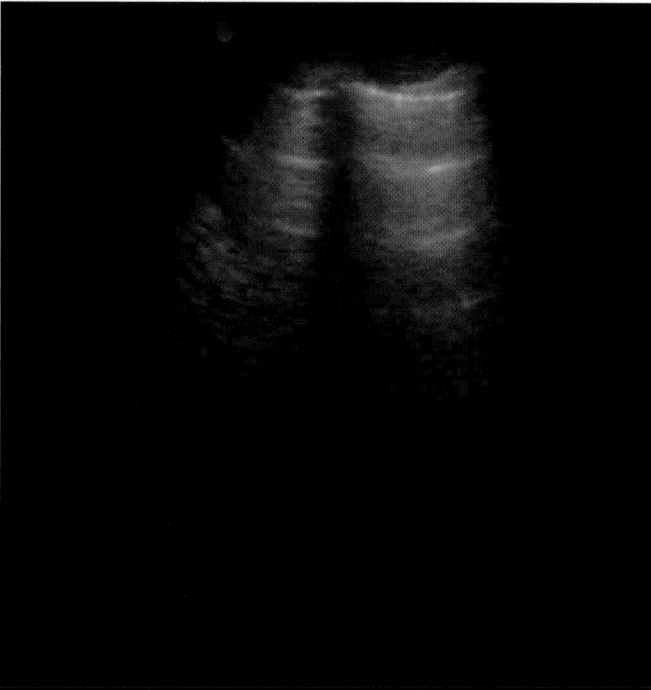

FIGURE 109-21 A-lines are a reverberation artifact between the skin and the pleura indicating an air-filled lung. *(Courtesy Division of Emergency Ultrasound, Massachusetts General Hospital, Boston.)*

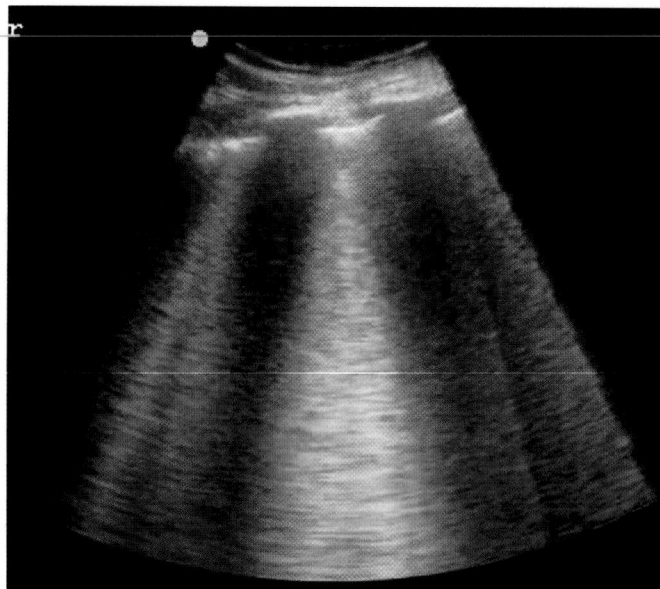

FIGURE 109-22 B-lines are vertical artifacts indicating sound is now being reflected through a fluid-filled lung. *(Courtesy Division of Emergency Ultrasound, Massachusetts General Hospital, Boston.)*

Numerous papers demonstrate that more B-lines correlate directly with increasing amounts of lung water in the lung tissue.[3,35,70] The scanning protocol usually consists of four zones for each thoracic cavity—superior and inferior midclavicular zones and superior and inferior axillary zones of the right and left thorax—to map out lung tissue and identify whether the B-line artifacts are diffuse or focal. Global assessment of mild, moderate, or severe B-lines and the pattern of interstitial fluid can reveal different clinical scenarios (i.e., diffuse findings are consistent with pulmonary edema, and focal findings with pneumonia).[71]

Presence of B-lines correlates well with natriuretic peptide levels, wedge pressures as determined by pulmonary artery catheterization, and interstitial disease on chest computed tomography (CT).[3,70] B-lines appear and resolve in minutes to hours, so ultrasound for pulmonary edema evolution is particularly useful.[49] Thoracic ultrasound scanning allows diagnosis and monitoring of pulmonary edema in both subclinical and overt high-altitude pulmonary edema (HAPE) that may affect oxygenation at high altitude (Figure 109-23). Multiple papers have described use of ultrasound for diagnosis and monitoring HAPE.[25,56] Conventional radiography is less sensitive to detect subclinical pulmonary edema and early HAPE and does not allow easy tracking of progression or resolution of fluid accumulation.[13,69] Techniques that overcome these shortcomings, such as CT or magnetic resonance imaging (MRI), are not available in the field. Ultrasound is the ideal diagnostic imaging modality for HAPE because it diagnoses subclinical disease and can be used to monitor disease progression or resolution.

MUSCULOSKELETAL ASSESSMENT

Fractures

Ultrasound to diagnose bony fractures in adults and children is well established.[18] Bones of the upper extremities, lower extremities, face and skull, sternum, and ribs have all been studied and are well suited for ultrasound imaging.[14,18,48,64,73] Ultrasound guidance for diagnosis and closed reduction of fractures is useful.[17] Persons employing large animals on backcountry travel now can access a growing body of literature on assessment of veterinary bone and joint integrity using ultrasound techniques.[13]

Technique for ultrasound assessment of bony fracture is simple. A high-frequency (7.5- to 10-MHz) linear-array probe is ideal. The depth of scan should be reduced to that needed to visualize the bony surfaces. Starting with the probe's long surface parallel to the bone, the examiner moves down the bone looking

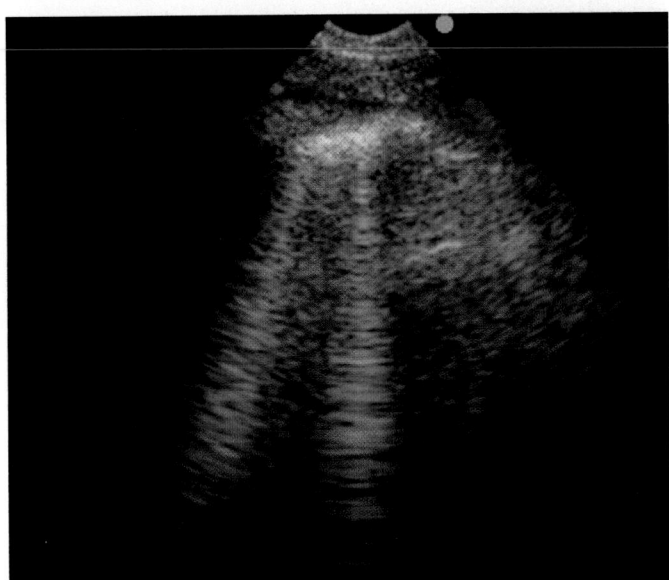

FIGURE 109-23 B-lines can be seen in this patient with high-altitude pulmonary edema diagnosed below Mt Everest Base Camp in Pheriche, Nepal. Views obtained using low-frequency curved probe and B-mode imaging. *(Courtesy Peter J. Fagenholz.)*

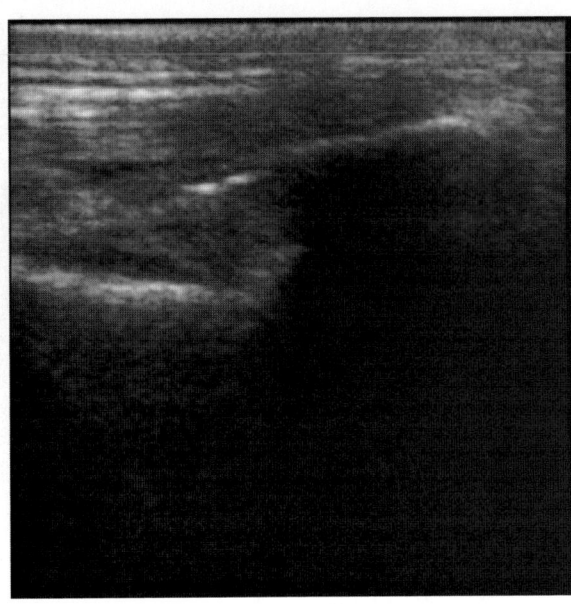

FIGURE 109-25 Ultrasound of fractured distal radius. In this "positive" study, the highly reflective bony cortex is notably irregular and approximately 1 cm (0.4 inch) displaced. In bone studies with a fracture, the site of sonographic step-off is likely to possess tactile maximal tenderness to palpation. *(Courtesy Division of Emergency Ultrasound, Massachusetts General Hospital, Boston.)*

at the linear, highly reflective (bright on the screen) bony cortex. A normal study reveals a contiguous, smooth, linear or curvilinear surface along the length of the bone (Figure 109-24). A fracture appears as a sharp, pointed step-off or break in the cortex (Figure 109-25). Clinical correlation is helpful. The site of sonographic step-off is likely to display both sonographic and tactile maximal tenderness to palpation. Skull fracture can be more difficult to discover using ultrasound because of the broad, curved surface to be studied, but excellent diagnostic images may be obtained (Figures 109-26 and 109-27).

Dislocation

Ultrasound has been demonstrated to be quite accurate for diagnosis of shoulder dislocation.[1] There is less literature supporting its use in other joint dislocations, but the principle of use would be the same.

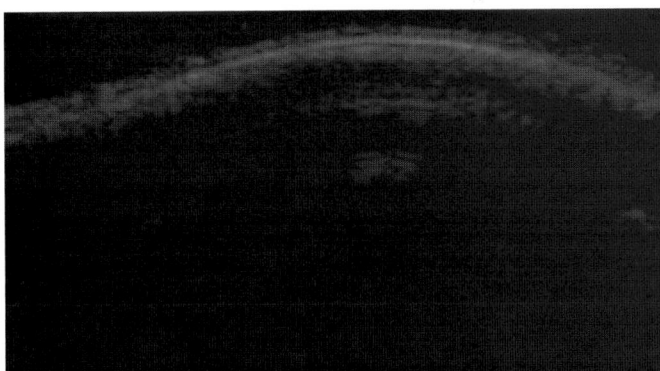

FIGURE 109-26 Ultrasound of normal pediatric skull. In this "negative" study, the contiguous, smooth, curvilinear bony cortex is seen running horizontally across the screen at approximately 0.5 cm (0.2 inch) depth. Bone views were obtained using a high-frequency (7.5 to 10 MHz) linear-array probe. *(Courtesy N. Stuart Harris.)*

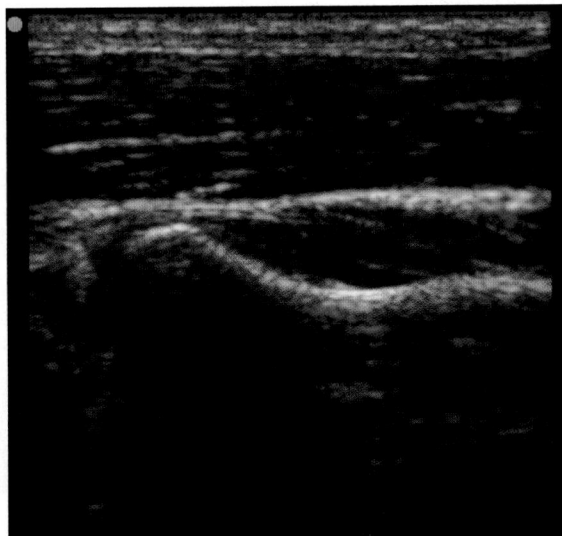

FIGURE 109-24 Ultrasound of normal distal radius. In this "negative" study, the contiguous, smooth, linear, and highly reflective bony cortex is seen running horizontally across the screen at approximately 1 cm (0.4 inch) depth. Normal (darker) muscle tissue is seen superficial to the bone. *(Courtesy Division of Emergency Ultrasound, Massachusetts General Hospital, Boston.)*

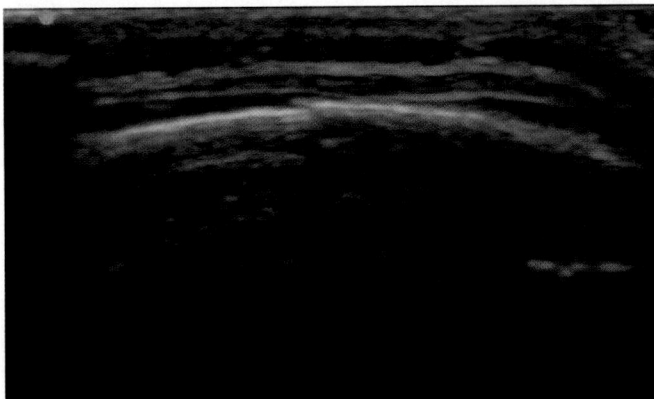

FIGURE 109-27 Ultrasound of a fractured pediatric skull. In this "positive" study, a clear break in the otherwise smooth, curvilinear bony cortex can be appreciated in the middle of the screen. *(Courtesy Division of Emergency Ultrasound, Massachusetts General Hospital, Boston.)*

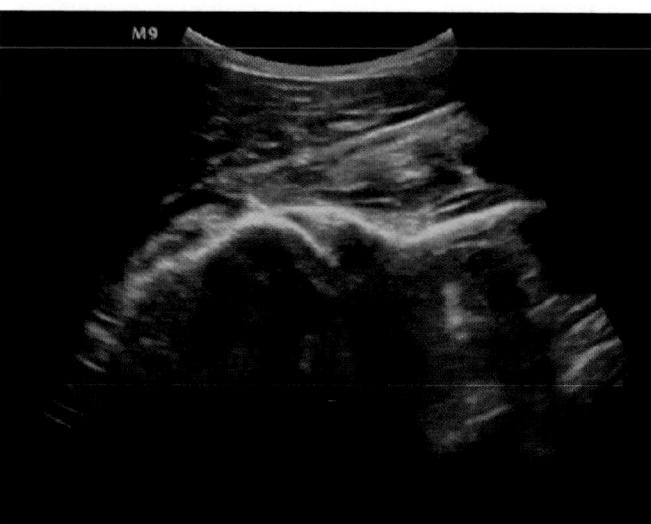

FIGURE 109-28 Normal articulation of the humeral head with the glenoid fossa. *(Courtesy Division of Emergency Ultrasound, Massachusetts General Hospital, Boston.)*

To assess for shoulder dislocation, use the curved low-frequency probe (2 to 5 MHz) and place it parallel to the top of the scapula, looking at the shoulder joint from posterior to anterior. A normally located humeral head will be seen at the level of the glenoid fossa (Figure 109-28), whereas an anteriorly dislocated shoulder will be seen at a greater depth on the screen, no longer contiguous with the glenoid fossa (Figure 109-29). Ultrasound can be used to demonstrate alignment after relocation of the affected bone.

OPTIC NERVE SHEATH ULTRASONOGRAPHY

Increased intracranial pressure (ICP) plays a role in severe high-altitude cerebral edema (HACE) and thus has long been a parameter of interest in high-altitude research. It is hypothesized that increased ICP is also associated with acute mountain sickness (AMS), but this relationship has not yet been convincingly established.[62] Lack of consistent data on ICP at high altitude largely results from a lack of sensitive, noninvasive techniques for assessing ICP. Where invasive measures have been used, the number of patients has been too small to draw meaningful conclusions.[33] However, published data have correlated symptoms of AMS with ultrasonographic assessment of optic nerve sheath diameter (ONSD). Ultrasound is a promising research tool to explore the pathophysiology of this AMS, especially because other diagnostic imaging modalities are not available in this setting.[26,11]

As measured by ultrasound, ONSD correlates with radiologic measures of increased ICP[30,38] and direct measurement of ICP in intrathecal infusion tests.[32] The physiologic basis of this technique is that increases in ICP are transmitted by cerebrospinal fluid down the perineural subarachnoid space of the optic nerve, causing expansion of the nerve sheath. Ultrasound can be used to follow this change by imaging through the eye and measuring the diameter of the shadow of the optic nerve sheath. This technique has been shown to have some interobserver variability; optimal methods for acquiring and measuring images are still being developed.[6] Nevertheless, a sufficient number of independent studies have documented correlation with radiographic and invasive measures of ICP.[11,66] At present, optic nerve sonography is an important research tool. Its clinical application, which has focused recently on identifying sensitivity and specificity of certain cutoff values for pathologically increased ICP, is still being refined. Given significant individual variability in optic nerve sheath size, using serial examinations to assess for changes within the same person or the same cohort over time may be more important than isolated ONSD values. For research purposes, small numbers of observers can be trained to minimize problems of interobserver variation.[6]

Optic nerve sheath ultrasound is usually performed with the patient supine with eyes closed. There are two acceptable imaging techniques. The first is to place an adhesive plastic dressing over the closed eyelid to keep ultrasound gel off the face and to hold the lid closed. The ultrasound gel is applied on top of the plastic. The second is to put ultrasound gel inside a thin plastic bag, into which the ultrasound probe is placed, after which the external surface of the bag is applied to the closed eyelid (Figure 109-30). A high-frequency (7- to 10-MHz) transducer is used to acquire a longitudinal, cross-sectional image of the optic nerve posterior to the orbit (Figure 109-31). The ONSD is measured 3 mm (0.12 inch) behind the retina; enlarged ONSD measurement is typically considered to be greater than 5 mm (0.2 inch). More important than absolute size are changes noted before and after intervention on the same individual (Figure 109-32).

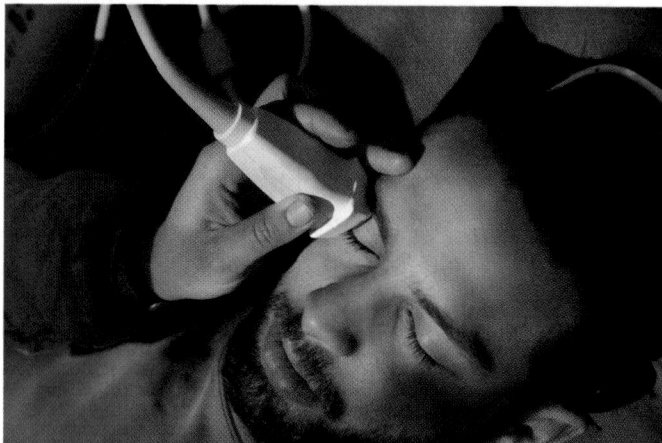

FIGURE 109-30 Optic nerve sheath diameter assay. This study is typically performed with the subject supine and with eyes closed. The probe is placed on the closed lid, typically just lateral to the center of the pupil, and adjusted until a longitudinal, cross-sectional image of the optic nerve (posterior to the orbit) is obtained. To maximize visual clarity, this figure does not show the occlusive dressing (to protect the eye), ultrasound gel, or a high frequency (7- to 10-MHz), linear probe that are typically employed. *(Courtesy N. Stuart Harris.)*

FIGURE 109-29 Anterior dislocation showing inferior displacement of the humeral head. *(Courtesy Division of Emergency Ultrasound, Massachusetts General Hospital, Boston.)*

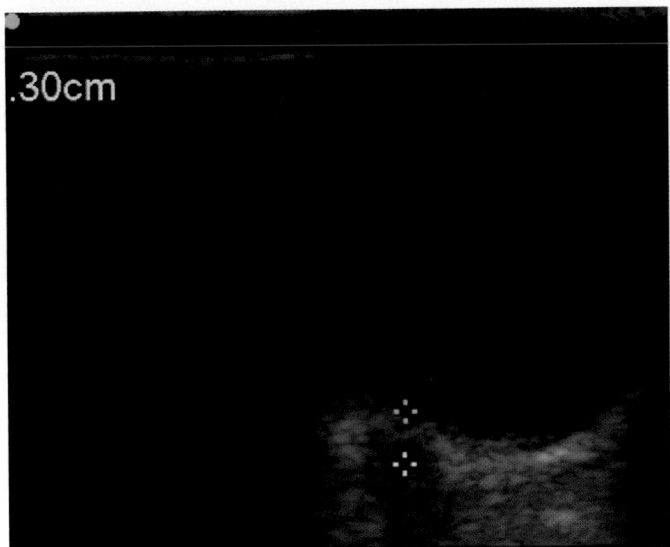

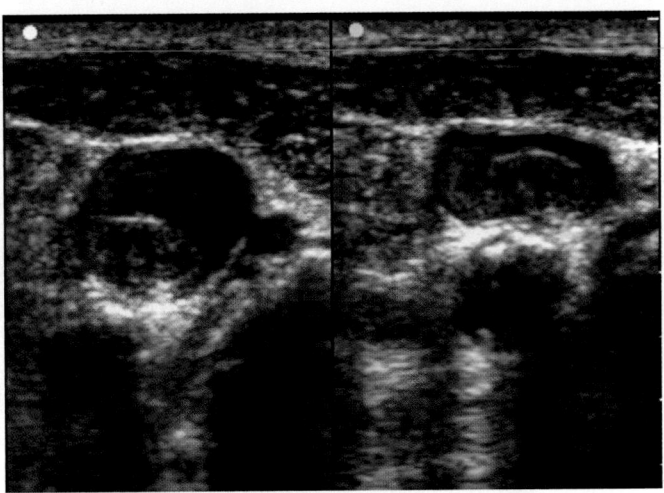

FIGURE 109-33 Vein seen with echogenic, noncompressible clot. *(Courtesy Division of Emergency Ultrasound, Massachusetts General Hospital, Boston.)*

FIGURE 109-31 Normal optic nerve sheath diameter. This "negative" study of a research participant was obtained at low elevation before climbing Mt Kilimanjaro. The patient's optic nerve sheath diameter measures a normal 4.1 mm (0.16 inch). Crosshairs mark the surface of the retina *(upper crosshairs)* and 3 mm (0.1 inch) deep to the retina *(lower crosshairs);* 3 mm (0.1 inch) is the conventional depth at which the optic nerve sheath diameter is measured in cross section. Anechoic, dark, vitreous makes up the majority of this image. *(Courtesy N. Stuart Harris.)*

DOPPLER AND BLOOD FLOW STUDIES

Doppler ultrasound allows determination of blood flow data and associated information (e.g., resistive and pulsatility indices) in any sonographically accessible blood vessel.[66] At high altitude, the effect of hypoxia on coagulation continues to generate interest.[59,67] Doppler and other techniques can be used to identify venous and arterial thromboses. The two-zone scanning protocol for evaluating the lower-extremity venous system has been well studied. A high-frequency probe is used to image the two high-turbulence zones: (1) the common femoral vein from the junction with the greater saphenous vein through the bifurcation of the

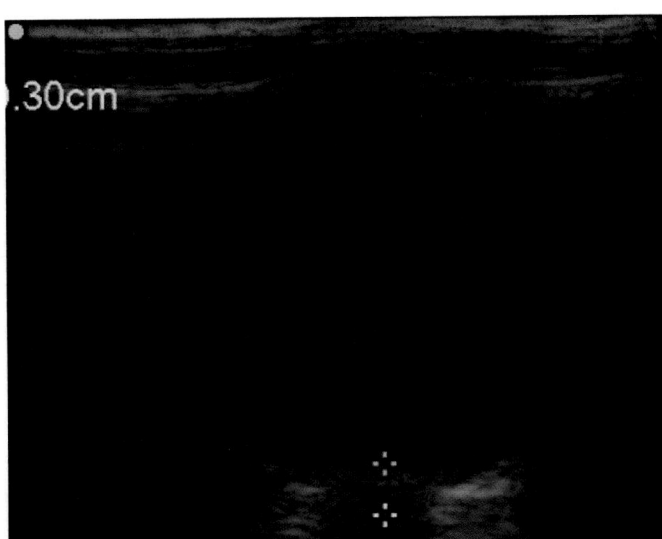

FIGURE 109-32 Enlarged optic nerve sheath diameter. This is the individual seen in Figure 109-31, but now at 5730 m (18,800 feet) in the summit crater of Mt Kilimanjaro and with severe acute mountain sickness. In this "positive" study, this patient's optic nerve sheath diameter now measures a greatly enlarged 6.5 mm (0.26 inch). In many indications, 5.0 mm (0.2 inch) may be considered as potential evidence of increased intracranial pressure. *(Courtesy N. Stuart Harris.)*

deep and superficial femoral veins, and (2) the popliteal vein through the trifurcation. Both zones should be compressed in their entirety. Inability to fully compress the vessel indicates the presence of clot[7,36] (Figure 109-33). This technique has greater than 90% sensitivity for proximal deep vein thrombosis (DVT) and approximately 50% sensitivity for distal DVT. Color flow Doppler allows assessment of clot in noncompressible vessels, such as the portal circulation vessels, which are also at risk at high altitude. This scanning protocol is technically more challenging and requires dedicated training.[5] Arterial imaging can be used when arterial thrombosis is suspected clinically. Pulse-wave Doppler is applied to measure velocity amplitude of the affected vessel and can be compared to the maximal velocities on the unaffected side (Figure 109-34).

INFERIOR VENA CAVA AND VOLUME ASSESSMENT

Techniques exist for estimating volume status by imaging the inferior vena cava (IVC), but this scanning application is most helpful in looking for volume depletion and monitoring the response to oral rehydration. This technique has been used to assess central volume status in the field at high altitude.[58a] The scanning protocol begins by placing the probe in a transverse orientation in the subxiphoid position and then rotating to the long axis, angling the probe under the costal margin, and following the IVC behind the liver into the right atrium (Figure 109-35). A flat, small-diameter IVC indicates low venous pressure (Figure 109-36).[41] A flat, volume-depleted IVC responds in real time to volume challenges by becoming more distended. This imaging technique may be used as a method to monitor a patient's response to rehydration. A distended, noncollapsible IVC indicates elevated venous pressure. This can either be the result of non–fluid-responsive pathology (e.g., heart failure) or fluid-responsive conditions (e.g., cardiac tamponade, pulmonary embolus) (Figure 109-37). Decisions regarding fluid resuscitation of patients with a distended IVC should be made after a careful cardiac evaluation.

ECHOCARDIOGRAPHY FOR PATENT FORAMEN OVALE

Echocardiographic techniques can be of great use to the high-altitude researcher when evaluating physiologic responses to altitude and hypoxia. There is good evidence that basic cardiac ultrasound imaging techniques looking for pericardial effusion, global systolic function, and dilation of the right ventricle can be mastered with focused training.[41] Techniques for detecting a patent foramen ovale (PFO), a condition associated with

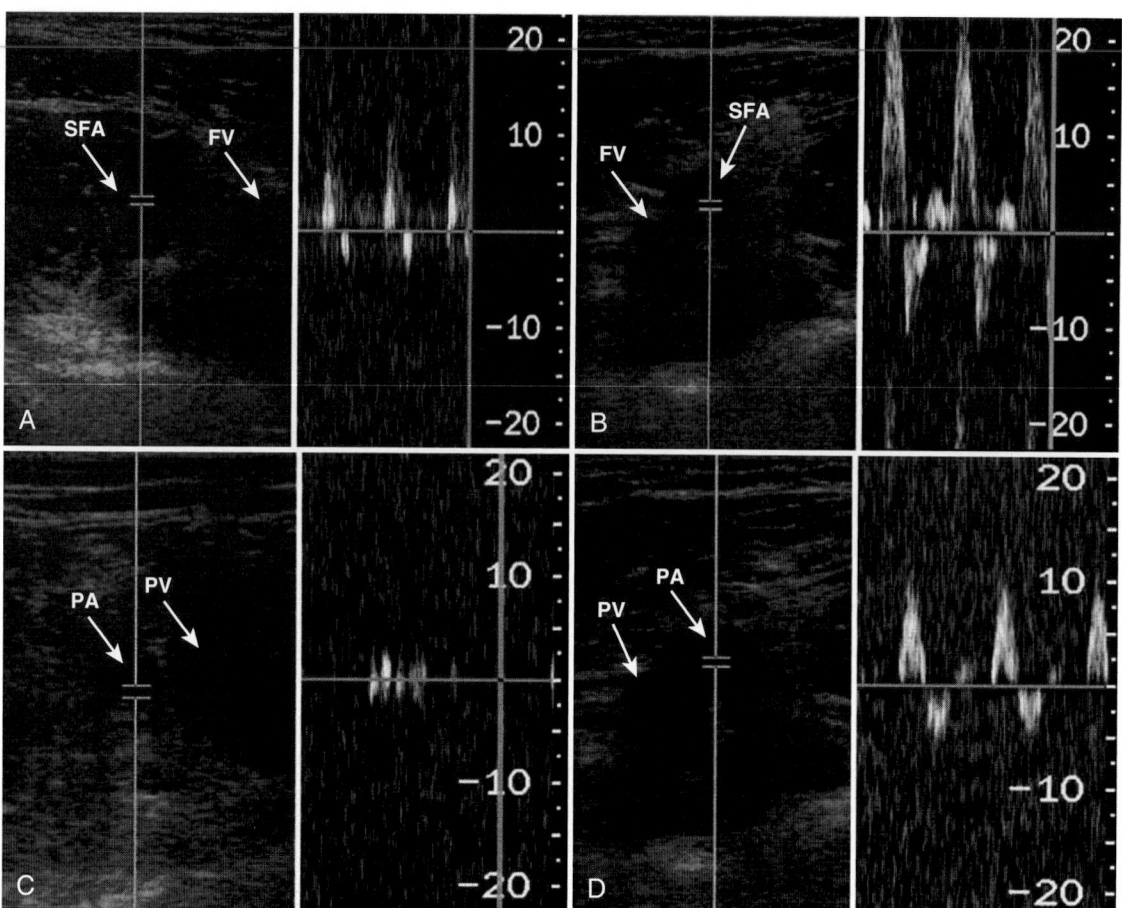

FIGURE 109-34 Two-dimensional and Doppler ultrasound images of the right and left superficial femoral and popliteal arteries. These images are from a trekker stricken with a limb-threatening arterial thrombus a day's walk below Mt Everest Base Camp. **A,** Right SFA and associated Doppler signal showing decreased flow compared with the left SFA. **B,** Left SFA and associated Doppler signal showing normal flow velocity. **C,** Right popliteal artery and associated Doppler signal showing a lack of flow. **D,** Left popliteal artery and associated Doppler signal showing normal flow. The crosshairs indicate the point at which the Doppler signal was measured. Units on the right axis are centimeters per second. *FV,* Femoral vein; *PA,* popliteal artery; *PV,* popliteal vein; *SFA,* superficial femoral artery. *(Courtesy Peter J. Fagenholz, as published in Fagenholz PJ, Gutman JA, Murray AF, et al: Arterial thrombosis at high altitude resulting in loss of limb, High Alt Med Biol 8:340, 2007.)*

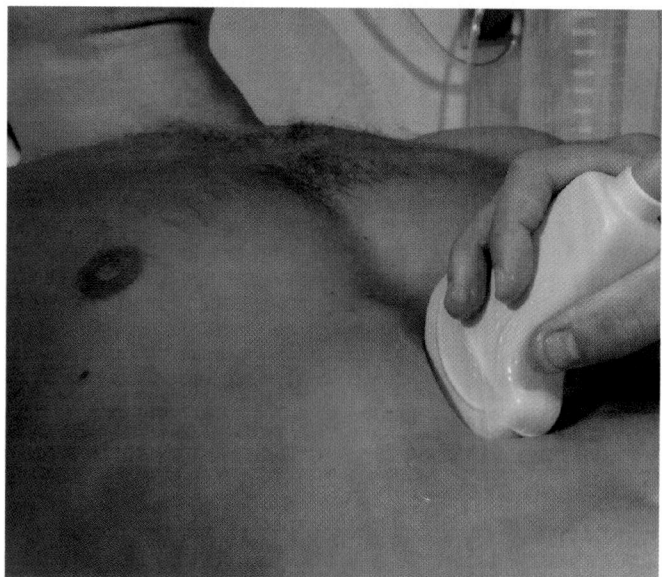

FIGURE 109-35 Probe position for inferior vena cava (IVC) exam. The IVC is usually visualized by initially placing the probe in the transverse orientation in the subxiphoid position. When the central vessels (IVC and aorta) are identified, the probe is rotated in the long axis to follow the IVC behind the liver and into the right atrium. *(Courtesy Division of Emergency Ultrasound, Massachusetts General Hospital, Boston.)*

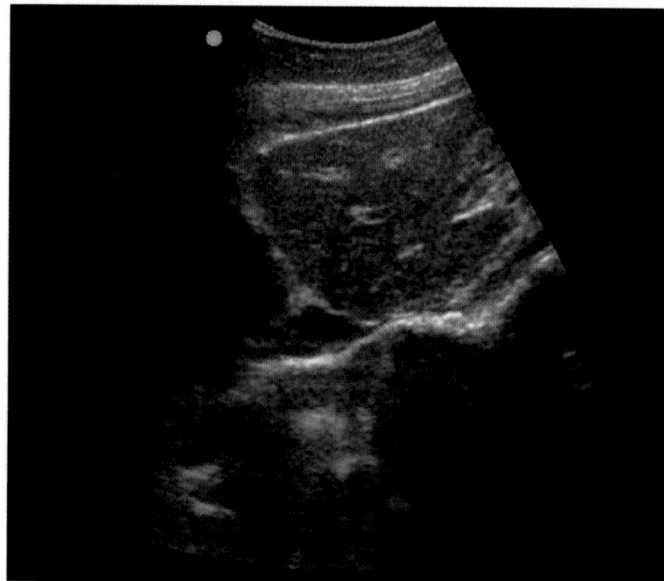

FIGURE 109-36 This inferior vena cava (IVC) is completely collapsed with inspiration, consistent with hypovolemia. *(Courtesy Division of Emergency Ultrasound, Massachusetts General Hospital, Boston.)*

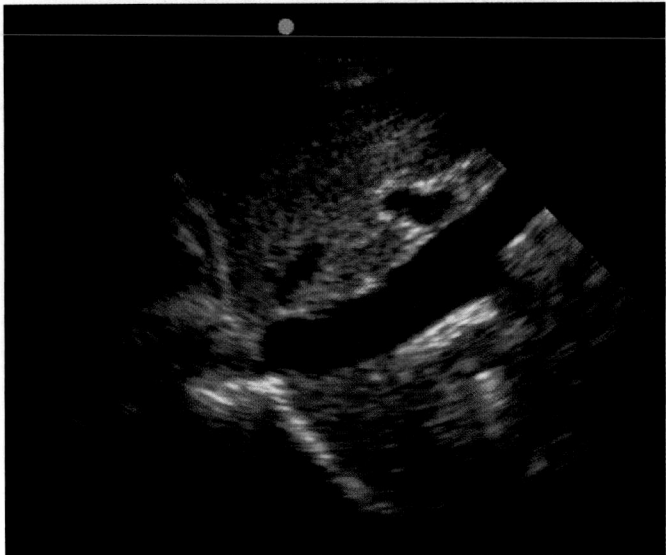

FIGURE 109-37 Inferior vena cava (IVC) image showing a distended, noncollapsible IVC. Before a decision is made about resuscitation strategies, this patient should have a cardiac ultrasound examination. *(Courtesy Division of Emergency Ultrasound, Massachusetts General Hospital, Boston.)*

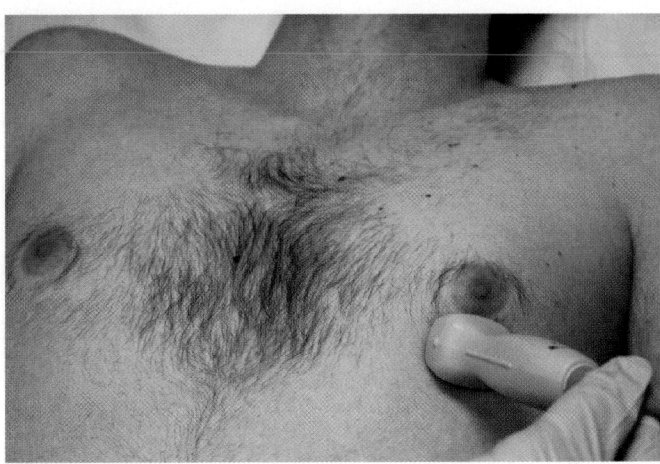

FIGURE 109-38 Probe position to obtain four-chamber apical ("apical-four") cardiac view on transthoracic echocardiography. *(Courtesy Division of Emergency Ultrasound, Massachusetts General Hospital, Boston.)*

HAPE susceptibility, can be taught with focused methods.[4] More advanced hemodynamic assessments and echocardiology evaluations require more extensive training. The technical demands of the techniques for measuring pulmonary artery pressure, cardiac output, and other aspects of cardiac function are beyond the scope of this chapter.[20,63] Readers are referred to other resources.[15,52]

Because the presence of a PFO has been associated with HAPE susceptibility, researchers will want to monitor for this condition in future HAPE studies. PFO may bear further investigation as a cause of shunting and hypoxemia at high altitude outside the setting of HAPE. Transthoracic echocardiography (TTE) and transesophageal echocardiography (TEE) techniques can be used to evaluate for PFO. TTE is less invasive and does not require sedation. Machines with harmonic imaging have made TTE as sensitive (~80%) as TEE for detection of PFO. We discuss TTE technique here.[21] Assessment for PFO is performed with a 2.5- to 5-MHz transducer. An "apical-four" image is obtained with the patient positioned in the left lateral decubitus position and the transducer placed at the point of maximal impulse of the heart apex and pointed toward the right shoulder (Figure 109-38). The atrial (and ventricular) septum should be vertically aligned in a four-chamber apical view (Figure 109-39). After intravenous (IV) injection of 10 mL of agitated saline contrast, the right side of the heart is monitored for opacification with contrast. A first injection is usually performed at rest, with three subsequent injections performed during maneuvers (e.g., cough or Valsalva maneuver) designed to increase right atrial pressure. The presence of a PFO is determined by presence of bubbles in the left side of the heart within five cardiac cycles. PFO size can be characterized as small (0 to 10 bubbles), moderate (10 to 50), or large (>50). The occurrence of bubbles after five cardiac cycles indicates intrapulmonary shunt.

PREGNANCY

Clinical obstetrics has long relied on perinatal ultrasound and a wide array of techniques for assessing the fetus. Many of these have been employed at high altitude, and there is much interest in how the fetus, placental blood flow, and maternal physiology respond to hypoxia and high altitude.[39,40] These ultrasound techniques require more advanced sonographic training and are not described here. We discuss early obstetric ultrasound imaging to assess for the presence of an intrauterine pregnancy. Second-

and third-trimester ultrasound techniques are used to assess for number of gestations, fetal lie, placental positioning, and quantity of amniotic fluid. This is only an introduction, and one should seek further guidance elsewhere for more extensive description of these techniques.

First-Trimester Ultrasound

First-trimester ultrasound should be considered in female patients presenting with a positive pregnancy test (or presumed early pregnancy, if testing is unavailable) together with concerns for ectopic pregnancy, such as vaginal bleeding, lower abdominal pain, syncope, and hypotension. The aim of the ultrasound is to demonstrate the presence of an intrauterine pregnancy (IUP) and thus decrease the post-test probability of ectopic pregnancy to near zero. Unless the patient has undergone fertility treatment, the possibility of heterotopic pregnancy is rare if an IUP is identified.

Intrauterine pregnancy is defined as presence of a gestational sac together with a yolk sac and fetal pole (with or without fetal heartbeat). If only a presumed gestational sac is visualized, a number of possibilities exist: the pregnancy is too early for the other pregnancy-related structures to be identified (in which

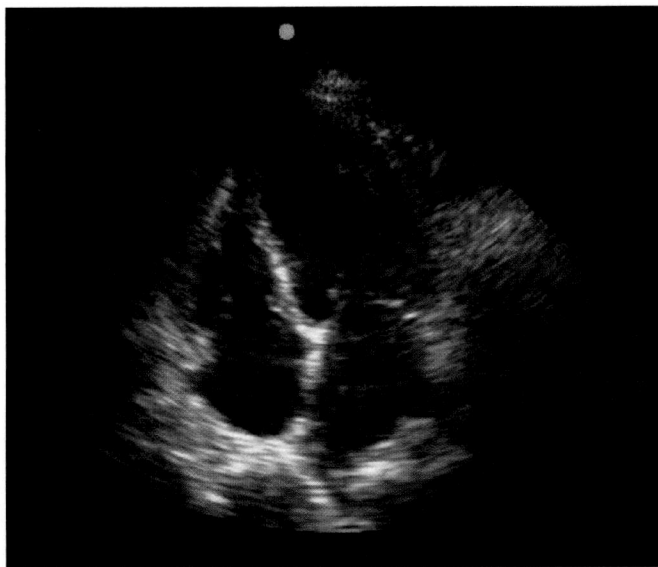

FIGURE 109-39 Image of normal "apical four." Note the vertical alignment of the septum. *(Courtesy Division of Emergency Ultrasound, Massachusetts General Hospital, Boston.)*

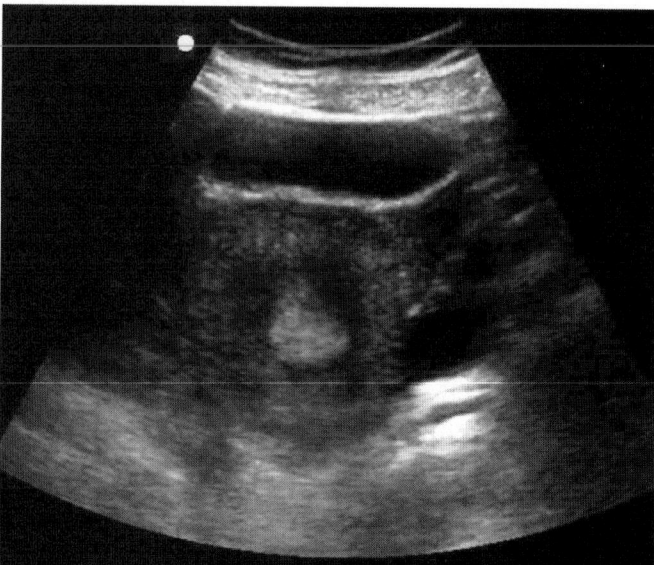

FIGURE 109-40 Transverse view of the uterus using the transabdominal probe. *(Courtesy Division of Emergency Ultrasound, Massachusetts General Hospital, Boston.)*

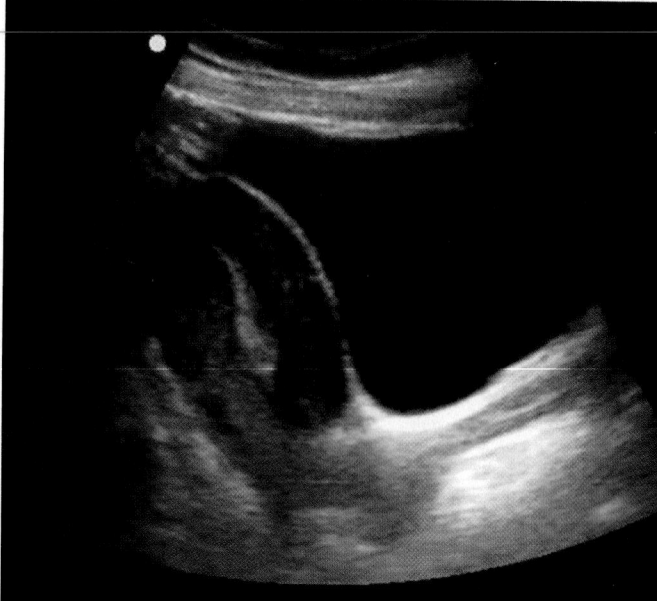

FIGURE 109-41 Longitudinal view of the uterus using the transabdominal probe. *(Courtesy Division of Emergency Ultrasound, Massachusetts General Hospital, Boston.)*

case either a transvaginal ultrasound should be performed or a repeat transabdominal ultrasound in 1 week), there has been fetal demise, or the patient has an ectopic pregnancy. In austere settings, if a patient has a positive pregnancy test and no identifiable IUP on ultrasound, an ectopic pregnancy is assumed until proved otherwise and appropriate measures taken.

Early-pregnancy ultrasound imaging in the hospital setting often employs both transabdominal and transvaginal scanning. In the wilderness setting, one will likely only have a curvilinear or phased-array probe, and therefore only the transabdominal approach will be possible. Using the curvilinear 2.5-MHz probe, the pelvis should be imaged in both transverse and sagittal planes. The probe is placed in the midline just superior to the symphysis pubis. For the transverse orientation, the probe marker is pointed toward the right side of the patient. The probe should be angled down into the pelvis in order to visualize the uterus in cross section (Figure 109-40). Fan the probe up and down to ensure that the entire uterus is visualized, looking for the presence of an IUP. Note the area posterior to the uterus—the pouch of Douglas/retrovesicular space—where fluid can be seen in the event of a ruptured ectopic pregnancy.

For the sagittal or longitudinal orientation, rotate the probe 90 degrees to have the marker pointing toward the patient's head. Angle the probe into the pelvis. Fan the probe left and right to visualize the entire uterus and cervix (Figure 109-41), looking for evidence of an IUP. Look closely at the pouch of Douglas for the presence of free fluid.

In first-trimester scanning, the gestational sac appears as a black, anechoic circular structure within the body of the uterus (Figure 109-42). The yolk sac is a small, hyperechoic circle located within the gestational sac (Figure 109-43). A fetal pole is an echogenic longitudinal structure that sits between the yolk sac and edge of the gestational sac (Figure 109-44).

If movement or flutterings are seen within the fetal pole, fetal heart rate can be measured. Press the M-mode button on the machine, then place the line over the beating heart. Press the M-mode button a second time to record movement over time across that line. The majority of machines will calculate the fetal heart rate by placing calipers from one beat to the next (Figure 109-45). Normal fetal heart rate ranges from approximately 100 to 180 beats per minute.

A FAST examination should be performed in the hemodynamically unstable patient, looking for free intraperitoneal fluid. In a supine patient, because Morison's pouch is the most dependent area, it may be the first place to visualize free fluid in the setting of a ruptured ectopic pregnancy. If fluid is seen in

Morison's pouch in a pregnant, nontrauma patient with hemodynamic instability in the wilderness setting, initiate immediate evacuation.[47]

Second- and Third-Trimester Ultrasound

In resource-limited settings, the point-of-care applications for second- and third-trimester evaluations are usually to (1) look at fetal positioning (transverse, breech, or head first), (2) identify the number of pregnancies, (3) quantify the volume of amniotic fluid, (4) identify placental positioning, and (5) estimate gestational age. In these settings, prenatal evaluation may not occur until late in the second trimester or even at the start of labor.

Fetal Positioning and Number of Pregnancies. The first two applications are to identify patients at greater risk for complications with vaginal delivery and to encourage childbirth in a

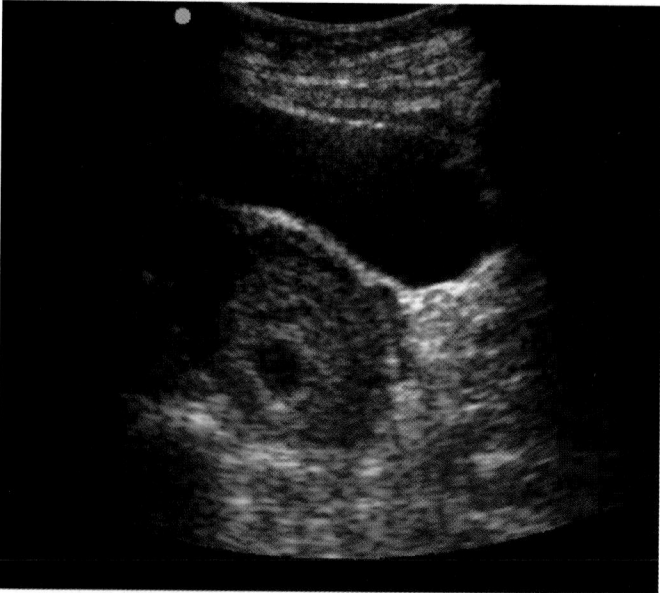

FIGURE 109-42 Image of a gestational sac. *(Courtesy Division of Emergency Ultrasound, Massachusetts General Hospital, Boston.)*

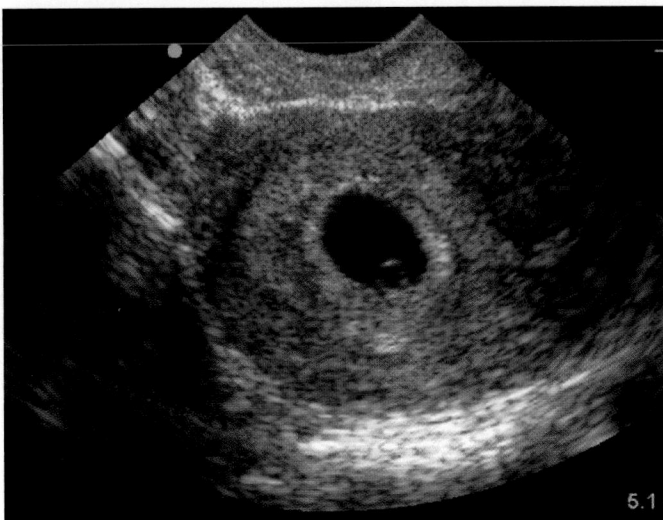

FIGURE 109-43 Image of a yolk sac, the small "sac within the sac." Occasionally, the zoom function on the ultrasound machine will need to be used to see this finding with the transabdominal probe. (*Courtesy Division of Emergency Ultrasound, Massachusetts General Hospital, Boston.*)

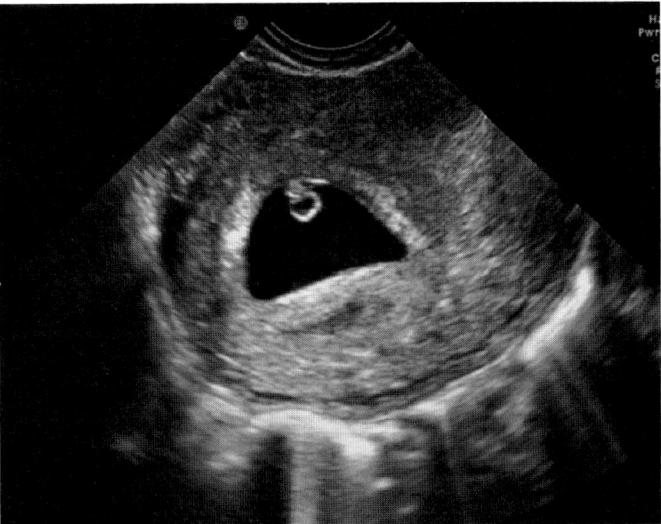

FIGURE 109-44 Image of a fetal pole. (*Courtesy Division of Emergency Ultrasound, Massachusetts General Hospital, Boston.*)

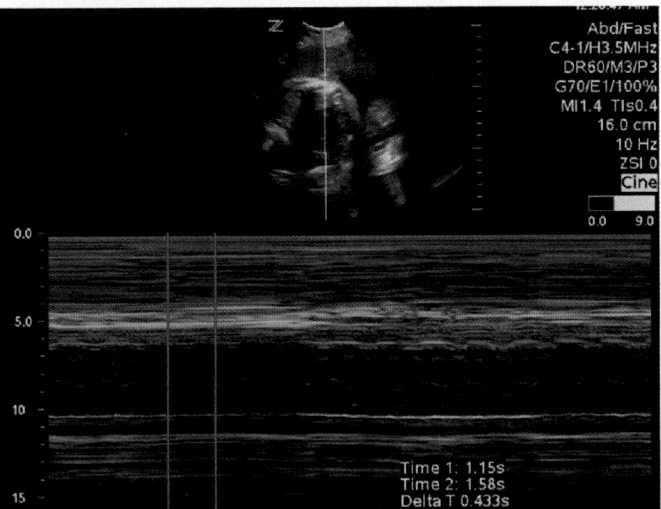

FIGURE 109-45 When calculating the fetal heart rate, M-mode imaging should always be used. (*Courtesy Division of Emergency Ultrasound, Massachusetts General Hospital, Boston.*)

center that can handle difficult deliveries. The low-frequency probe is used to examine the entire uterus to identify fetal position and number. The head is readily identifiable by the circular bright echotexture of the skull; its location relative to the external probe position identifies the position of the fetus. A common mistake with second- and third-trimester scanning is not increasing the depth of field appropriately. Inadequate depth of field prevents visualization of the entire uterus.

Amniotic Fluid Volume Assessment. Multiple techniques are described to estimate the amount of amniotic fluid. The simplest is the single deepest pocket or maximum vertical pocket technique. Using the transabdominal probe, the entire uterus is interrogated, and the largest anechoic pocket of amniotic fluid is identified. Less than 1 cm (0.2 inch) is a good predictor for oligohydramnios and thus of fetal growth restriction. More than 8 cm (3.2 inches) has been used as a marker for polyhydramnios.[42] This examination is not an emergent procedure, but rather, helps predict a complicated labor and poor fetal outcome because of ongoing issues with the pregnancy. If either of these conditions is seen, the woman should be referred to obstetric care where she can deliver in a supervised environment with surgical capacity. Oligohydramnios can be a marker of severe maternal dehydration, and thus IV hydration is recommended.[51]

Placental Positioning. To identify placental position, use the curvilinear 2.5-MHz probe to perform full interrogation of the uterus. The placenta appears as thickening of the uterine wall with a solid echotexture and should be in the anterior or superior (fundal) positioning. If the placenta is seen in the lower uterine segments, the cervix should be identified to see if the placenta fully or partially covers the cervical opening. Occasionally, this scanning technique can be augmented by performing translabial scan with the curvilinear probe. The probe is placed just external to the labia; in this position, the cervix is more readily identified. It should be stressed, however, that any woman in the second or third trimester with painless, bright-red vaginal bleeding should be assumed to have placenta previa and appropriate care measures (evacuation to a facility with surgical capacity) taken.

Gestational Age/Dating. The most useful function of second- and third-trimester ultrasound is to assist in more accurate dating of the pregnancy to facilitate better labor planning. There are several methods. First-trimester techniques usually involve measuring crown-rump length and using the ultrasound machine's software to translate this distance into gestational age (Figure 109-46). Second-trimester techniques that have shown reliable accuracy are biparietal diameter and femur

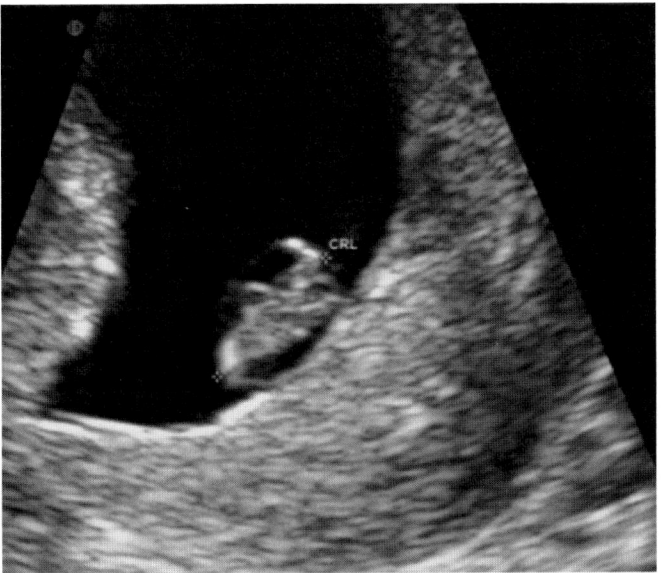

FIGURE 109-46 In this image the crown-rump length (*CRL*) is being measured, and the machine is estimating fetal age based on this measurement. (*Courtesy Division of Emergency Ultrasound, Massachusetts General Hospital, Boston.*)

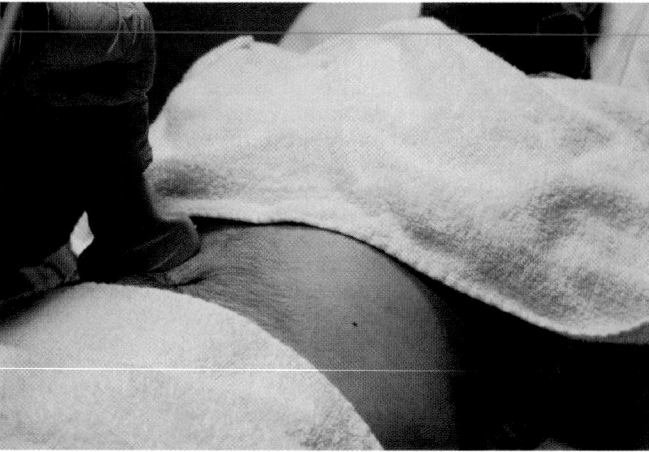

FIGURE 109-47 Probe position for right upper quadrant assessment of the gallbladder. To visualize the gallbladder, place a 2- to 5-MHz abdominal probe on the abdomen inferior to the medial edge of the right costal margin. Angle the probe toward the right shoulder, then sweep toward the patient's right flank. (*Courtesy Division of Emergency Ultrasound, Massachusetts General Hospital, Boston.*)

length measurements.[57] To ensure that correct maximal diameter for both these techniques is obtained, careful fanning through the entire structure is recommended. Machine software translates these dimensions into gestational age.

RIGHT UPPER QUADRANT ULTRASONOGRAPHY

Ultrasonography is the initial imaging test of choice to investigate for acute cholecystitis and gallbladder stones. For these conditions, in trained hands, ultrasonography has sensitivity of 90% to 95% and specificity of approximately 80%.[61]

Place a 2- to 5-MHz probe on the abdomen along the medial edge of the right costal margin (Figure 109-47). Angle the probe toward the right shoulder. Depending on the patient's degree of abdominal obesity, a moderate amount of downward pressure may be required to image under the costal margin. When the large, homogeneous mass of the liver can readily be appreciated, sweep the probe laterally toward the right flank. By using this sweeping motion, the examiner can visualize the gallbladder as an oblong, hypoechoic, cystic structure. In young patients, more anterior positioning of the gallbladder may require the probe to be pressed flat against the abdominal wall while angled toward the right shoulder. In obese patients, an abdominal approach may be difficult and an intracostal approach may be helpful. In these cases, the probe can be positioned perpendicularly to the anterior, inferior left chest wall 5 to 7 cm (2 to 2.8 inches) lateral to the sternum. The probe is pointed between the most inferior ribs and toward the back.

In each of these techniques, the gallbladder should appear in a long-axis view as a pear-shaped organ (Figure 109-48). Small, sweeping motions with the probe should ensure that the entirety of the organ is imaged. Attention should be paid to gallbladder wall thickness, presence of gallbladder stones or sludging, pericholecystic fluid, air within the gallbladder wall, and sonographic Murphy's sign (maximal tenderness when direct pressure is applied to the gallbladder as it is visualized). After completing study of the long axis, rotate the probe 90 degrees to visualize the short axis of the gallbladder. In the short axis, the gallbladder appears as a nearly spherical object. Typically, measurements of gallbladder wall thickness are achieved in the short axis.

A "negative" study for acute cholecystitis reveals an anechoic, cystic structure without stones or sludging. The wall should be crisp and clean without surrounding fluid and should be less than 3 mm (1.2 inches) thick. The gallbladder should not be tender to focal pressure directly applied through the probe (negative sonographic Murphy's sign).

In addition to identification of shadowing gallstones, sonographic findings that suggest a "positive" study for acute chole-

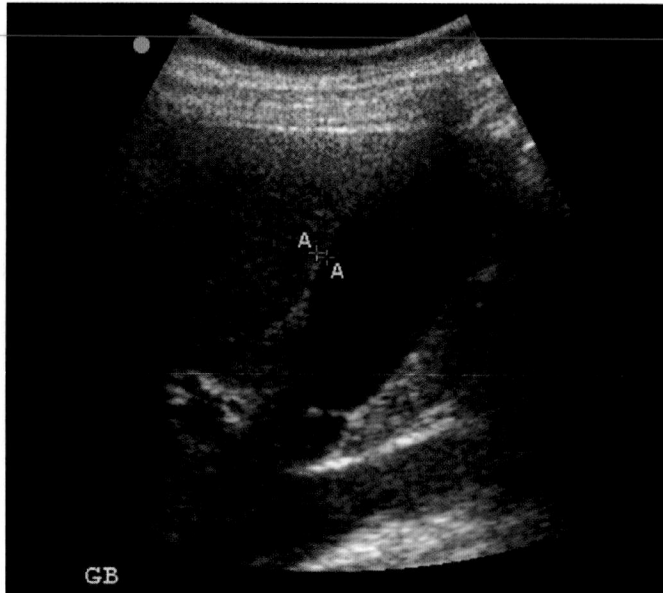

FIGURE 109-48 Normal gallbladder. A "negative" study for acute cholecystitis reveals an anechoic, cystic structure without stones or sludging. It has a nonthickened wall (<3 mm [0.12 inch]), is not surrounded by pericholecystic fluid, has no intramural gas, and is not tender to focal pressure directly applied through the probe (negative sonographic Murphy's sign). (*Courtesy Division of Emergency Ultrasound, Massachusetts General Hospital, Boston.*)

cystitis include findings of a thickened gallbladder wall (>3 mm), anechoic pericholecystic fluid, intramural gas or bright, white echogenic shadows, and a gallbladder tender to focal pressure directly applied through the probe (positive sonographic Murphy's sign) (Figure 109-49).

In cases of isolated cholecystic stones (without acute infection), the typically rounded intracystic stones are appreciated as bright, white (hyperechoic) structures with resulting dark streaks

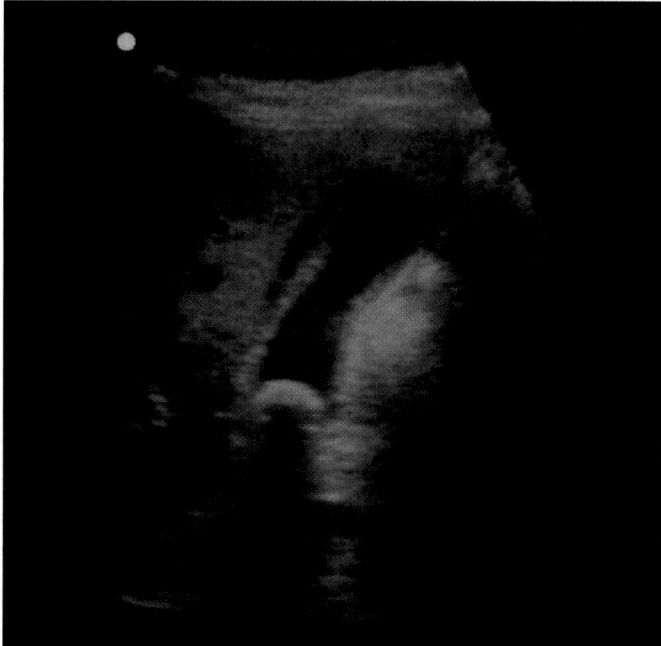

FIGURE 109-49 Acute cholecystitis. Sonographic findings that suggest a "positive" study for acute cholecystitis include findings of a gallbladder that has a thickened wall (>3 mm [0.12 inch]), is surrounded by anechoic pericholecystic fluid, has intramural gas, and is tender to focal pressure directly applied through the probe (positive sonographic Murphy's sign). (*Courtesy Division of Emergency Ultrasound, Massachusetts General Hospital, Boston.*)

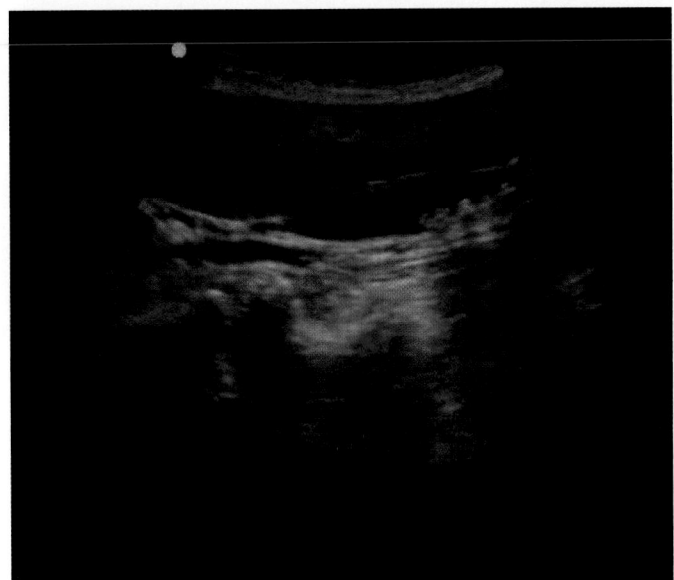

FIGURE 109-50 Isolated cholecystic stones (without acute infection). The typically rounded intracystic stones can be appreciated as bright, white (hyperechoic) structures with resulting dark streaks (anechoic shadowing) behind. *(Courtesy Division of Emergency Ultrasound, Massachusetts General Hospital, Boston.)*

(anechoic shadowing) behind (Figure 109-50). Isolated stones may be asymptomatic or may cause pain (biliary colic). Asymptomatic biliary stones and acute biliary colic are not surgical emergencies. Presence of stones with secondary signs of infection or inflammation is consistent with cholecystitis and indication for emergent intervention.

RIGHT LOWER QUADRANT ULTRASONOGRAPHY

Ultrasound is an imperfect but potentially valuable tool for imaging of the right lower quadrant. Although abdominal CT scan remains the gold standard to evaluate for acute appendicitis in much of the developed world, this is changing.[58] Benefits of ultrasound include lower cost and lack of radiation exposure. Increased training in right lower quadrant ultrasonography means that the appendix can often be visualized for acute appendicitis.[65] Sensitivity and specificity for ultrasonographic assessment of acute appendicitis are influenced by patient size, abdominal obesity, and appendiceal positioning. Unlike a right upper quadrant study, which can use the liver as a large acoustic window to view the gallbladder, anatomy surrounding the appendix is often air filled and thus may allow only limited image quality. Furthermore, unlike the gallbladder, which has consistent landmarks (immediately inferior to the liver), the position of the appendix can vary significantly within the right lower quadrant, making the study more technically difficult. If located retrocecally, the appendix is even less amenable to ultrasound imaging. For these reasons, most would consider ultrasound for appendicitis a "rule-in" test and not a "rule-out" test.[68] Good evidence suggests using an "ultrasound first" pathway for patients can limit the number of CT scans and expedite treatment.[24] Increasing evidence that uncomplicated appendicitis can often be managed nonsurgically[23,44,46] would be of additional benefit in remote locations. This experience has been described on French nuclear submarines, where ultrasound remains the imaging modality of choice for right lower quadrant assessment.[34]

Technique

Technique for right lower quadrant assessment begins by placing a 2- to 5-MHz probe on McBurney's point (situated about one-third the distance between the right anterior superior iliac spine and umbilicus; this point marks the normal position of the base of the appendix) (Figure 109-51). Sweep the probe along the line between the right anterior superior iliac spine and umbilicus. If

the appendix is still not visualized, the operator should sweep superior and then inferior to this line. Puylaert[60] described a graded compression technique for evaluating the appendix. The technique employs gradual application of significant pressure with the probe against the right lower quadrant abdominal wall. This helps to displace gas-filled bowel and to decrease the distance between the transducer and the appendix, thereby enhancing image quality. Findings suggestive of acute appendicitis include an engorged, tubular structure with an outer diameter of greater than 6 mm (0.2 inch), noncompressible lumen, periappendiceal fluid collection, shadowing appendicolith, and lack of peristalsis[60] (Figure 109-52). In patients with high clinical suspicion for disease, a nondiagnostic ultrasound should be followed by further testing.

PERIPHERAL VEINS

Sonographic guidance for placement of peripheral IV lines can prove useful in patients who have difficult vascular access. This imaging is best achieved using a high-frequency (10-MHz) linear probe.

Typical sites for placement of peripheral IV lines are the antecubital and external jugular veins, but any venous structure can be used. It should be remembered that unlike arteries, veins have thin walls, are nonpulsatile, and are readily compressible. Peripheral veins typically travel alone, whereas central veins are accompanied by arterial vessels.

To establish peripheral IV access, standard sterile technique is employed. The probe is sheathed in a sterile cover, and sterile jelly is applied to the antiseptically prepared skin. In a right-hand-dominant operator, the probe is held in the left hand. Place the probe over the vessel, 1 to 2 cm (0.4 to 0.8 inch) proximal to where the needle enters the skin, so that the site where the needle tip will enter the vessel is directly under the probe. As soon as the tip of the needle is seen entering the vessel's lumen, a "flash" of blood should be appreciated within the IV catheter. At this point, if there is only a single operator, put down the probe so that the catheter may be more easily threaded off the needle. The catheter can be appreciated in a cross-sectional view as a bright, punctuate, circular structure within the darker, circular vessel (Figure 109-53).

SPECIAL CONSIDERATIONS FOR ULTRASOUND IN REMOTE LOCATIONS

TELE-ULTRASOUND

Tele-ultrasound, one subset of telemedicine, is the practice of ultrasound whereby the patient, ultrasound machine, and

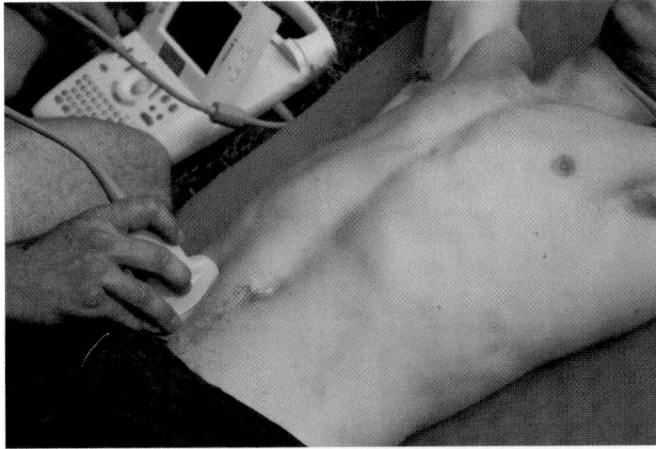

FIGURE 109-51 Probe position for right lower quadrant assessment for appendicitis. Place a 2- to 5-MHz probe on the abdomen, about one-third the distance between the right anterior superior iliac spine and the umbilicus—McBurney's point—which marks the normal position of the base of the appendix. *(Courtesy N. Stuart Harris.)*

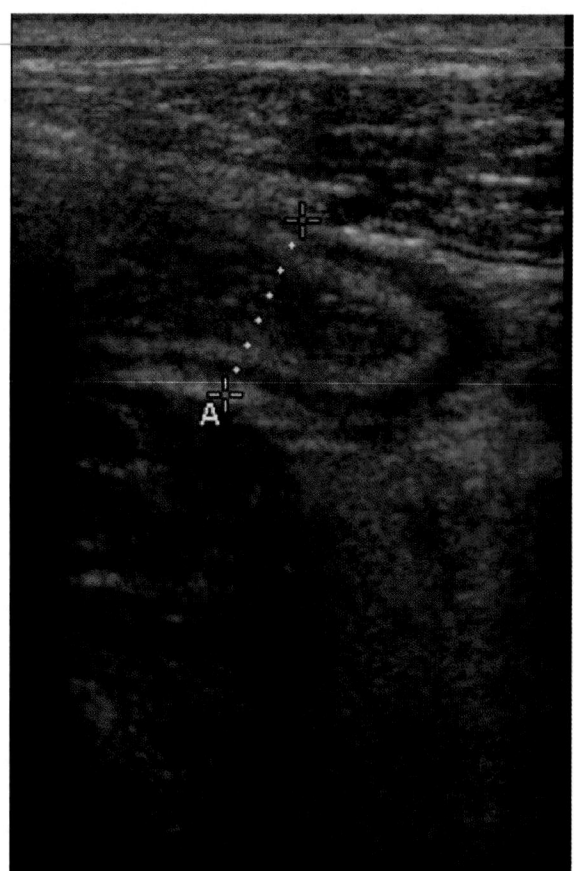

FIGURE 109-52 Acute appendicitis. Findings suggestive of acute appendicitis include an engorged, tubular structure with an outer diameter of greater than 6 mm (0.24 inch) (here seen to be 13 mm [0.51 inch]), noncompressible lumen, periappendiceal fluid collection, and lack of peristalsis. (*Courtesy Division of Emergency Ultrasound, Massachusetts General Hospital, Boston.*)

nonexpert sonographer are in a location distant from the expert sonographer. Tele-ultrasound has evolved because of decreasing costs of machines and increased expertise in the field, together with exponential increase in the speed, quantity, and quality of data that may be transmitted between the patient and caregiver. Telemedicine is discussed in Chapter 104.

Tele-ultrasound can effectively bring the expert to the bedside. Real-time relay of images allows immediate instruction as well

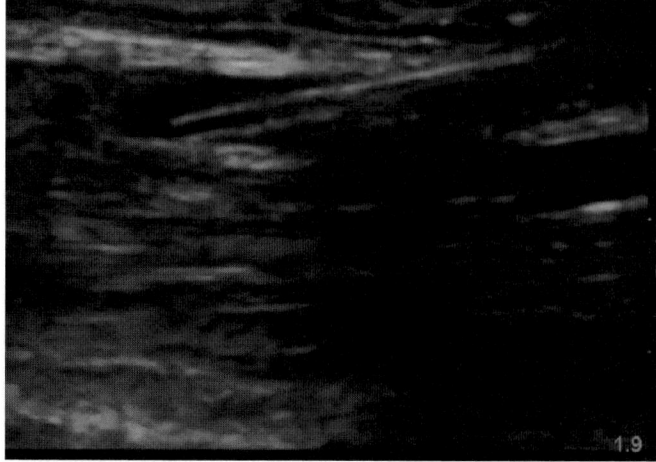

FIGURE 109-53 Peripheral vein. In this longitudinal view, the catheter can be appreciated as a bright, tubular structure within the darker vessel. (*Courtesy Division of Emergency Ultrasound, Massachusetts General Hospital, Boston.*)

as interpretation by the remote expert. In some cases, environmental or communication conditions require a brief delay, after which the expert can provide feedback and diagnoses. Studies have shown that remote experts can direct nonphysicians to perform examinations and obtain adequate images for the expert to make clinical diagnoses, thereby bringing the physician to the bedside. This is invaluable for patients living in remote rural settings or wilderness locations.

Tele-ultrasound requires a machine, means of transmitting acquired images, and a remote site capable of reconstituting images to be interpreted. To create imaging data capable of being transmitted, an ultrasound machine may be connected to a video-streaming device to allow digitization of the images and compression in order for the study to be transmitted to the remote setting. Data can then be transmitted to a distant site. Voice-over Internet protocol (VOIP) systems such as Skype (Skype Technologies S.A., Luxembourg), FaceTime (Apple Inc., United States), and Google Chat (Google Inc., United States) allow voice, together with other multimedia such as video, to be transmitted via the Internet. These programs should be downloaded onto personal computers at both settings before expeditions. By adding video, the remote expert may visualize the nonexpert's probe positioning and give instantaneous feedback and instruction, to allow acquisition of the best images possible. Research supports feasibility of these techniques by novice providers under distant expert guidance in a variety of ultrasound applications.[8,12,43]

Some of the earliest examples of successful utilization of tele-ultrasound came from aboard the International Space Station (ISS). Novice ultrasonographers (crew medical officers) with less than 3 hours of ultrasound training before departure for the ISS have been guided by experts at the Mission Control Center in Texas to successfully perform diagnostic-quality FAST, genitourinary, musculoskeletal, and ocular ultrasound examinations. In a number of these studies, a 2-second time delay was reported in video and audio transmission; however, this did not impair the expert's ability to instruct the novice, and images were always adequate for clinical decision making. Addition of ultrasound aboard the ISS has proved invaluable in management of patients at this location, enabling improved diagnosis to help guide management options, where medical evacuation has very significant consequences.[16,27,28,37]

Otto and colleagues[53] described successful use of ultrasound by nonphysician climbers guided by remote ultrasound experts at Advanced Base Camp (6400 m [20,997 feet]) on Mt Everest. This aided diagnoses of HAPE by visualizing B-lines on thoracic ultrasound. Analog ultrasound images were digitized, compressed, and transmitted via Internet to the computer of the remote expert, who then, by bidirectional radio, guided the examination.

McMurdo Research Station, one of three research stations operated by the United States Antarctic Program (USAP), has proved an ideal setting for tele-ultrasound. In this harsh environment, New Zealand, approximately 3800 km (2361 miles) distant, has the nearest tertiary care center. An ultrasound machine was acquired by USAP in 2000. Tele-ultrasound allowed problems posed by varying degrees of staff training to be overcome. A case report from McMurdo describes cardiac ultrasound performed by a physician with basic ultrasound skills on a 26-year-old patient with pleuritic chest pain suspected as pericarditis. The echocardiogram was transmitted via a DICOM-compatible software program to the radiology department at St Luke's Hospital in Denver. A report was generated and e-mailed back to the Antarctic, confirming a small pericardial effusion. A repeat ultrasound examination 4 days later under expert guidance from cardiologists based at the University of Texas, with the ultrasound machine connected via an S-video input to a PolyCom View Station, enabled live transmission of the images. In addition, a camera recorded the physician scanning the patient. Imaging confirmed a small, resolving effusion with no evidence of cardiac tamponade, enabling the patient to be managed at the research station and avoiding evacuation.[54]

In a retrospective review of all ultrasound examinations performed at two of the USAP research stations over 1 year, 66 ultrasounds were performed on 49 patients.[55] The majority (94%)

were reviewed at a later date by experts, and 6% were interpreted in real time. The majority of studies were abdominal, genitourinary, and gynecologic examinations. Ultrasound prevented intercontinental aeromedical evacuation in 25.8% of cases and had a significant effect on diagnosis and management of illness in patients at the South Pole and McMurdo research stations. The authors concluded that "ultrasound is a valuable addition to remote medical care for isolated populations with limited access to tertiary-healthcare facilities."[55]

A group in Togo designed a low-cost tele-imaging system to enable novice ultrasonographers (including midwives, nurses, and technicians) based in remote hospitals to have access to real-time tele-ultrasound expertise from hospital centers in Lome, Togo, and Tours, France.[2] Ten radiologists, nine of whom worked in Lome, covered approximately 6 million inhabitants. When high-bandwidth Internet connections were available, they used real-time transmission of ultrasound video sequences via the Internet between providers. If only low-bandwidth connectivity was available, they used a software program called LogMeIn, which enables transmission of video together with audio via the Internet. The group successfully performed real-time tele-ultrasound on 50 patients, with 1.5- to 2-second transmission delays. Image quality was reported as adequate.[2]

Power Supply Considerations

A critical concern for any ultrasound or telemedical device in the field is ensuring an adequate power supply. Limited information is readily available on how best to provide portable, reliable power in the field. To help bridge this critical gap, we briefly discuss different power supply systems that have proved effective in wilderness settings.

A practitioner seeking to use electronic equipment in a wilderness setting faces unique but surmountable problems. When used at field sites with standard current systems (e.g., well-equipped mountain huts or research hypobaric chamber facilities), whether on or off the grid, electronic equipment can be seamlessly incorporated. In foreign countries, appropriate plug and power adapters may be required. For more austere field sites, portable machines are most appropriate. These can usually run on rechargeable batteries for 1 to 5 hours.

Options for portable power supply can be divided into classifications of batteries, solar supply, and other. Light, portable solar arrays that can generate adequate power for charging an ultrasound machine and laptop computer (e.g., Brunton Solaris 26 or CT Solar Expedition Solar Package) are probably the most frequently used power sources for remote field studies. We have successfully conducted sonographic research from the base to the summit of Mt Kilimanjaro (5895 m [19,341 feet]) and Mt Denali (6168 m [20,320 feet]) while depending solely on electric current gathered from solar arrays (Figures 109-54 and 109-55). Our series of solar arrays produced a nominal output of 54 W, controlled by an electronic voltage regulator using a lead-acid battery storage system. This proved adequate for frequent assays using a SonoSite 180 and Mindray M7 ultrasound devices with routine laptop data storage backup.

The total current generated by solar arrays is influenced by many variables, including size of the arrays ("rated" current capacity) and factors that influence intensity and length of exposure to solar radiation, including season of the year; prevalence and density of cloud cover; orientation, latitude, and altitude of arrays; time of day; and ability to position arrays for adequate length of time during each day. A highly mobile expedition, which may not be able to spread out its arrays during peak daylight hours, will be at a disadvantage compared with a fixed team, because the fixed team has the entirety of a day's available solar radiation to convert to electric current. An obvious limitation of solar power generation is the presence of available solar radiation. An expedition during the dry season under equatorial sun on Mt Kilimanjaro has power-generating advantages over a similarly sized system used at high latitudes and with greater likelihood of cloud cover. Small portable windmills, human-powered crank generators, and small turbines that can take advantage of running water to provide hydroelectric power are options. The power demands of portable ultrasound

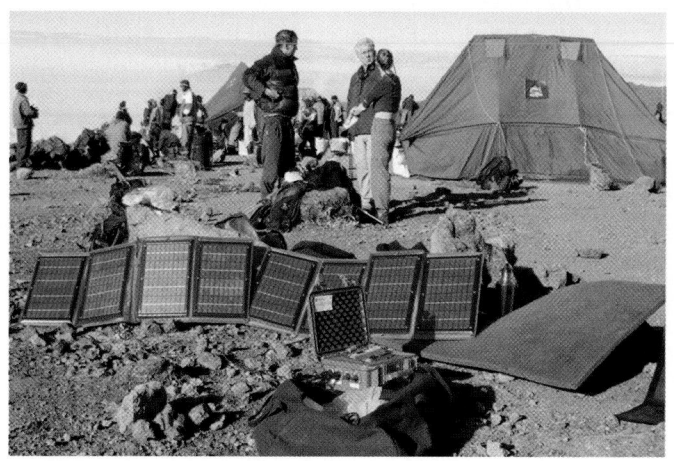

FIGURE 109-54 These rigid solar arrays provide more than 50 W of power under equatorial sun on Mt Kilimanjaro. They weigh less than 4.5 kg (10 lb). This power is controlled by an electronic voltage regulator using a lead-acid battery storage system, housed in the orange, waterproof case in the foreground (6.3 kg [14 lb]). *(Courtesy N. Stuart Harris.)*

machines and laptops are small enough that these options may be feasible.

Under any but ideal circumstances (e.g., under equatorial sun in a desert climate), solar power may be unreliable, so it is worth bringing multiple sets of batteries to be charged when solar power is plentiful and used to run the machines during less plentiful periods. Choice of batteries for these systems is critical. Variables to consider include decisions about appropriate battery size (measured in ampere-hours) and battery type (lead acid vs. lithium ion). Typical alkaline cells used by consumer electronics are insufficient. By establishing the power draw of all equipment (ultrasound and laptop power requirements are located in the manuals accompanying each machine) and then multiplying current factor (in amperes) by length of time each machine will

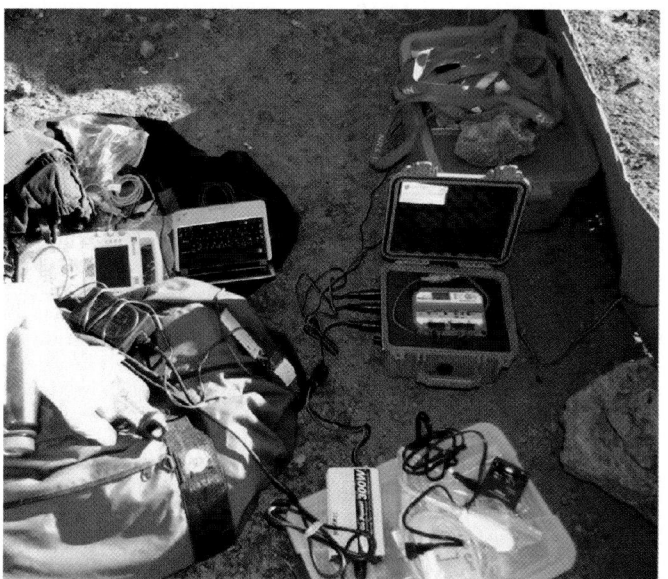

FIGURE 109-55 Electronic devices employed in the field on a solar-powered, high-altitude ultrasound research expedition on Mt Kilimanjaro in association with the U.S. Army and Explorers' Club. *Left to right,* The ultrasound unit (SonoSite 180), laptop data storage (Dell Inspiron 910), DC-to-AC converter (bright-yellow box in foreground, Go Power! 300-W converter), electronic voltage regulator with lead-acid battery storage (orange box, CT Solar.com) with 54-W solar arrays (*at far right,* CT Solar.com). Total weight of all electronic and power storage equipment was less than 18 kg (40 lb). *(Courtesy N. Stuart Harris.)*

TABLE 109-4 Advantages and Limitations of Battery Types to Power Wilderness Electronic Equipment

Battery Type	Advantages	Limitations
Lead acid	Inexpensive Internationally readily available Ease of transport on commercial airlines	Low power density (heavy/current stored) Decreased efficiency in cold temperatures
Lithium ion	High power density (relatively lightweight) Maintains effectiveness even when cold	Expensive Difficult to transport on commercial flights

be employed (in hours), reasonable estimation of battery size (in ampere-hours) can be established. Allowances for any current converters (converters are often less than 50% efficient) must be made.

Standard choices for nonsolar power supplies include "standard" sealed, lead-acid or lithium-ion batteries. Advantages of lead-acid batteries include low price, relative ease of replacement (even in the developing world), and ease of transport on commercial airlines (they can travel as checked baggage without difficulty) (Table 109-4). Disadvantages include relatively low power density (high weight of battery per unit of current compared with lithium-ion battery systems) and marked performance decreases on exposure to colder temperatures. Advantages of lithium-ion batteries include high power density (relatively lighter weight per unit of current stored than with lead-acid batteries) and higher levels of performance at the lower temperatures typically experienced at high altitude. Disadvantages include prohibition on their transport by commercial airlines (without special and expensive packaging and labeling requirements) and relatively greater expense.

Voltage and current regulators may be required to prevent overcharging and potentially destroying batteries or ultrasound machines if using solar panels that provide more that 10 W of power. Commercially available units, some of which come packaged in robust, waterproof cases specifically designed for wilderness expedition use, can contain both battery and current control systems within the armored cases and have proved reliable for high-altitude expeditions.

When a portable power supply is employed, one must account for loss of power from transformer use. Many ultrasound units in North America assume ready availability of 110- to 120-V alternating current (AC). This current is fed through a transformer to produce 10- to 20-V direct current (DC) that powers the unit. Each step of current conversion incurs a (potentially significant) loss of electrical energy, because useful energy is converted to (wasted) heat energy by the transformer. This became especially notable during our Mt Kilimanjaro research, when a series of transformers (with attendant losses in power) were required. For example, our SonoSite 180 employed a 14.4-V DC system, whereas our solar-produced, battery-stored current existed in a standard 12-V DC system (12 V is the standard current employed internationally in automobiles). Ideally, a simple DC-to-DC converter would exist to allow "direct" use of this similar DC current without conversion by DC to AC transformer. Unfortunately, unlike many common consumer electronics (from cell phones to laptops), most currently available ultrasound units do not allow direct use of standard 12-V DC systems. This requires that a wasteful series of step-up (from 12-V DC to 120-V AC) and then step-down (from 120-V AC to 14- to 20-V DC) current transformers be employed. It is hoped that ultrasound and telemedical equipment manufacturers will overcome these inefficiencies in future designs.

Careful troubleshooting before departure for the field will help ensure adequacy of the power supply and compatibility of the power system with the ultrasound machine. All critical components (some as simple as a 10¢ main fuse in some systems, without which the entire power system is unusable) must be backed up with spares.

ADVANTAGES OF ULTRASOUND IN THE WILDERNESS

Portability

Extraordinarily powerful ultrasound equipment can be carried by hand. Compared with other diagnostic imaging devices that might be considered for wilderness use (e.g., conventional radiography, CT, MRI), ultrasound machines are much more compact, lighter, and more portable (see Table 109-3). The revolution in digital and ultrasound technology and manufacturing has allowed small, laptop-sized machines to overtake the capabilities of older, larger machines for virtually every application. Because portable machines have become small, often weighing less than 4 to 6 kg (8.8 to 13.2 lb), their utility has increased for wilderness settings. In austere locations with no power source (e.g., remote alpine environment or disaster area), ultrasound devices can be powered using batteries, including portable photovoltaic arrays. A SonoSite MicroMaxx ultrasound machine used successfully on the 2007 Caudwell Xtreme Everest expedition at Camp Four on the South Col (8016 m [26,299 feet]) of Mt Everest was powered by standard MicroMaxx batteries charged at base camp and Camp Two using a combination of generators or solar power.[9] We conducted research using a SonoSite 180 machine carried to the summit of Mt Kilimanjaro (5895 m [19,341 feet]) and a Mindray M7 to the summit of Denali powered by hand-carried solar arrays. A portable ultrasound setup with batteries, power source, laptop computer for image storage and backup, and enough ultrasound gel for clinical use or research can reasonably be expected to weigh approximately 13.6 kg (30 lb) and to be carried to remote locations by a single physician or investigator. Some machines are essentially modular attachments to laptop computers or even cellphones, further reducing the need for separate pieces of equipment.

Safety and Noninvasiveness

Diagnostic ultrasound has few known risks.[29] To highlight this fact, ultrasound is the clinical imaging modality of choice for many high-risk patient populations, including pregnant women and their fetuses. Ultrasound is routinely used at the bedside for rapid assessment of critically ill trauma and medical patients. A physician with a bedside ultrasound machine can quickly and in real time assay for a range of common, acute life threats, including intraperitoneal free fluid or pericardial effusion, obviating the risks associated with delays caused by patient transport or image processing. No other clinical imaging system allows this combination of speed, safety, portability, and immediacy of result.

In many research applications, such as replacement of invasive pulmonary arterial catheterization by transthoracic echocardiography, ultrasound provides an essentially risk-free, noninvasive option to take the place of a potentially risky, invasive technique.[4] The safe, noninvasive, and painless nature of ultrasound compared with other diagnostic and research techniques encourages patient compliance and aids recruitment for research protocols by making participation more attractive to potential volunteers. For research purposes, the U.S. Department of Health and Human Services Office for Human Research Protections specifically identifies ultrasound, Doppler measurements, and echocardiography as research methodologies eligible for expedited investigational review board review, significantly easing administrative burdens and potentially shortening the time between conception and execution of studies. For research purposes, because ultrasound itself does not significantly impact participants or other experimental manipulations, sonographic monitoring can easily be added to other experimental protocols for purposes of collecting additional relevant data (e.g., monitoring additional parameters of potential interest during a drug trial) or conducting a separate parallel study. For example, we joined research conducted by U.S. Army Research Institute of Environmental Medicine collaborators and were able to assay sonographically measurable parameters (e.g., ONSD, pulmonary artery pressure) during a study originally designed to examine the effects of moderate-altitude prepositioning on combat readiness of military recruits during exposure to high altitude. Ultrasound does not employ ionizing radiation, so there is no known additive risk of repeated ultrasound exposures.

Versatility

Ultrasound machines enable immediate access to advanced diagnostic imaging. Ultrasound provides imaging of soft tissue, abdominal and thoracic organs, bone, muscle, and skin processes that can immediately and directly inform medical decision making.

For both routine clinical and specialized research purposes, a single ultrasound machine and ultrasonographer (with appropriate training) can monitor a wide range of organ systems and potential research parameters. For example, in a research project using ultrasound, multiple parameters (e.g., eyes, chest, heart) can be studied at no more cost to the clinician/researcher or risk to the patient/participant than if a single measurement were taken. Researchers studying ICP and ONSD in trekkers with severe AMS could incorporate chest ultrasound to investigate a separate hypothesis in the same cohort, while all the time having the ultrasound available to help diagnose common clinical conditions.

Cost

Ultrasound machine cost varies widely and is influenced by size, weight, image quality, and special imaging capabilities (e.g., Doppler or color flow imaging). Selecting a machine appropriate for an austere setting requires advance thinking. To ensure reliability, especially under the stresses of harsh conditions, a preference for solid-state, nondynamic systems (e.g., fixed- vs. phased-array probes) is prudent. These systems often offer the additional benefit of being more reasonably priced. It is critical for wilderness practitioners to define exactly what capabilities they will require from the device in their unique work environment so that the correct ultrasound unit can be chosen.

LIMITATIONS OF WILDERNESS ULTRASOUND

There are general drawbacks of ultrasound for wilderness use.[74] Although portable and relatively durable for in-hospital clinical use, ultrasound machines can be fragile and require careful packing and handling during transport and field use. Austere conditions place strains on ultrasound machines far in excess of what the machines ordinarily encounter in routine clinical practice. Mechanical failure has jeopardized or terminated wilderness clinical and research expeditions.[10,72]

Ultrasound machines are not easily serviced in the field. By picking a machine with the fewest movable mechanical parts (i.e., choosing fixed-array rather than phased-array probes and solid-state units rather than spinning hard discs for memory), the risk for mechanical failure can be somewhat mitigated.

Hypobaric cold (high altitude), blowing dust (alpine or desert environments), water damage (riparian or rain forest environments), salt exposure (marine environments), rough handling during transport, and other factors can quickly disable a machine (sometimes permanently), but most difficulties can be anticipated and mitigated. For example, machines should be protected in strong, well-padded rigid cases and ideally carried by a responsible person at all times. Such cases can be readily and inexpensively fashioned from rigid tool cases retrofitted with hand-cut foam padding. Pelican and other strong, waterproof cases can be customized for ultrasound devices and probes. Using such a case, one author has witnessed an ultrasound device survive a 100 foot fall from a helicopter onto a glacial surface—and remain fully functional.

To enhance effectiveness and protect the ultrasound device, it may be necessary to sleep with batteries next to the body, prepare warm water in which to soak a probe to achieve reliable functioning in the cold, or to operate the machine within a plastic bag to protect against dust. Risk of theft is real, particularly in chaotic, urban, or disaster settings. Traditional (spinning) hard drives have been implicated in machine failure at high altitude, probably caused by cold and the influence of decreased barometric pressure on internal air-filled cushioning components. Solid-state memory devices (i.e., flash cards) without moving parts are readily available for primary data storage on laptop computers and USB drives. These solid-state units should prove to be significantly more reliable than their mechanical counterparts. A plan to rapidly service or exchange malfunctioning machines should be made in advance. Bringing a backup machine is an effective hedge against malfunction. Thorough testing before field use, careful machine handling, device security, and thoughtful attention to potential site-specific problems enable a clinician or researcher to increase the likelihood of maintaining the ultrasound unit during a wilderness experience.

Before departure, sufficient ultrasound training must be completed to ensure that diagnostic-quality images and accurate measurements can be reliably obtained. Although some imaging techniques, such as quantitative echocardiography, require more extensive training, other applications, such as thoracic or long-bone applications, are straightforward and have been taught successfully in brief sessions, or even through remote expert guidance at the time of image acquisition. A growing body of evidence, both on Earth and in space, confirms that these techniques can be effectively taught to nonphysicians with minimal prior training, when guided by audiovisual linkage to expert ultrasonographers.[53]

A means to save and review images obtained in the field is typical and prudent practice. When ultrasound images are being used primarily for research purposes, great attention should be paid to the quantity and robustness of data storage options. Data storage needs are influenced by types of images that are saved (e.g., still images vs. video clips), definition of the individual images (e.g., low-definition black-and-white images from an older machine vs. color and velocity data–embedded images from a state-of-the-art echocardiography device), and total number of individual images. It is good practice to routinely back up all data, even if the ultrasound machine is capable of storing all necessary images in its memory. Most machines are accompanied by software packages that allow image downloading and handling on a personal computer. In planning data storage, it is important to be aware of the capabilities of the software. If saved images will be analyzed at a later time by a blinded observer, it is important to be sure that the imaging software is capable of allowing the necessary analysis, and that image labeling at the time of acquisition does not compromise blinding.

REFERENCES

Complete references used in this text are available online at expertconsult.inkling.com.

▋ There's no bad weather, just bad clothing.   —*SCANDINAVIAN SAYING*

Clothing as an adaptive strategy has evolved a long way from the rough animal hides of prehistoric days. Regardless of its structure, clothing serves two primary purposes: protection from the environment and optimization of thermoregulation. The metabolism of mammals produces heat. The environment demands that heat be retained or released to maintain optimum body temperature. Clothing is one of humanity's behavioral adaptations to changing temperatures that occur as a result of geographic location or environmental shift. Humans adapt modifying clothing systems or changing activity levels to conserve or reduce heat production. To this end, clothing manufacturers take advantage of fiber qualities in the design of fabrics that perform well in all conditions.

The well-designed outdoor clothing available to contemporary wilderness professionals retains or releases heat in response to the environment and individual comfort. When choosing clothing, one must consider personal comfort, weather (both immediate and near future), geographic location, and specifics of the activity. Activity is as much a driver of clothing choice as is the weather. There are vastly different requirements for aerobic or high-exertion activities than for sedentary tasks. Also, when deciding "what to wear," one must consider the duration of the outing. For example, an activity lasting weeks in a remote locale will require different clothing than a short outing close to an urban environment. For the wilderness professional, clothing is not just for personal adornment or comfort—it may also be a lifesaving tool (Box 110-1).

This chapter introduces the wilderness medical provider to the properties of fabrics and fibers used in the manufacture of clothing. The reader should be able to design a personal strategy for choosing the appropriate garment and layering system for the activity and environment to which he or she will be exposed (Figure 110-1).

FIBER AND FABRIC

With the exception of leather and hide construction, clothing is made from fabric woven from fibers. Type of fiber, density of weave, and presence of any treatments or finishes determines the properties of the fabric. The four properties of concern are thickness, reaction to moisture, thermal conductance, and tightness of weave (Table 110-1).

Fibers may be natural, synthetic, or a blend of both. In general, natural fibers are more durable and softer to the touch than are synthetics. Synthetic fibers are typically lighter and quick to dry. Blending is the act of combining different fiber types together to achieve a particular characteristic. For example, blending cotton and polyester produces a fiber with the absorbency of cotton and strength of polyester. Blends influence coloring, strength, absorbency, ease of washing, resistance to wrinkling, and ease of spinning and weaving into fabric.

NATURAL FIBERS

The most common natural fiber is cotton, frequently used in T-shirts and nontechnical clothing. It is highly hydrophilic and has poor moisture regain. Although it wicks moisture away from the skin, the fiber does not redistribute moisture to external surfaces for evaporation. Cotton absorbs and holds moisture, rapidly losing any insulative value. Cotton that is saturated retains only 10% of its original insulative value. These properties make cotton undesirable for use as an insulation layer when heat conservation is the goal. Conversely, in a warm or hot environment, cotton helps to keep a person cool. The moisture absorbed by the fabric aids in cooling by convection and conduction.

Wool and Merino Wool

Cloth woven from traditional wool or merino wool is an excellent insulating fabric. The core of wool fiber absorbs moisture and redistributes it to the fabric surface, from where moisture can evaporate. Wool's moderate affinity for absorbing moisture is balanced by excellent regain, meaning that the fabric retains warmth and does not feel cool or wet when damp. However, when it is saturated with moisture, wool feels wet.

Many people find that wool feels scratchy. Traditional sheep wool has barbs in the outer layer, or epicuticle, of the fiber. In contrast, merino wool is a much finer fiber with far fewer barbs. These ultrafine (17.5 μm in diameter) fibers make for very soft and lightweight fabric with a tight weave. These properties contribute to durability and shape retention. The fabric remains highly elastic and shrinks minimally. The fibers are antibacterial; thus, fewer odor-producing metabolites are present.

Wool, including merino wool, is spun from the fleece of sheep. Other fibers, technically not wool, including alpaca, llama, and cashmere, share many of the properties of merino wool. Alpaca and llama are *camelids*, originally from South America, and cashmere goats produce the fleece from which cashmere is spun (Figure 110-2). These wool-like fibers are frequently blended with true wool to create a soft, durable weave used for direct skin contact.

When considering its purpose for technical clothing, silk is most often used to manufacture base layers. Untreated silk retains moisture, although not to the degree of cotton. The majority of silk used for outdoor clothing is chemically treated and wicks moisture well. Silk can be blended with other fibers to smooth its texture or enhance elasticity.

Down

Down is composed of the very soft, fine feathers that insulate birds. Most birds have some down, but waterfowl have extensive layers of down as an adaptation to their environment. These insulating feathers trap air and the bird's body heat. These same properties are exploited when down is used as insulation in clothing. Natural down forms clusters resembling the head of a dandelion (Figure 110-3). The propensity toward clustering gives down its loft. As an insulating fiber, down traps heat in the air pockets of the cluster. Down's insulative value is quantified as "fill." Fill power is the number of cubic inches displaced by 1 ounce of down. Higher-fill down is composed of larger, more mature clusters. These clusters trap more air, hold more heat, and retain their shape better after compression. In general, the higher the fill value, the warmer is the garment. However, a 600-fill parka may be as warm as an 800-fill parka; it simply requires more down to achieve the insulative value.

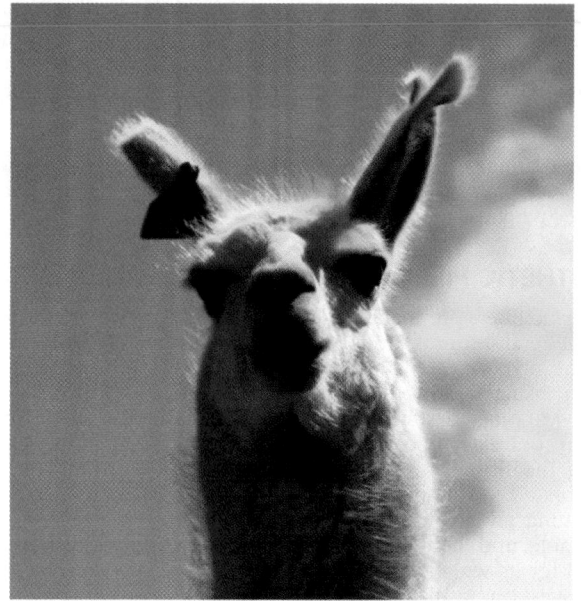

FIGURE 110-2 Argentinian llama. *(Copyright 2010, J. Dow.)*

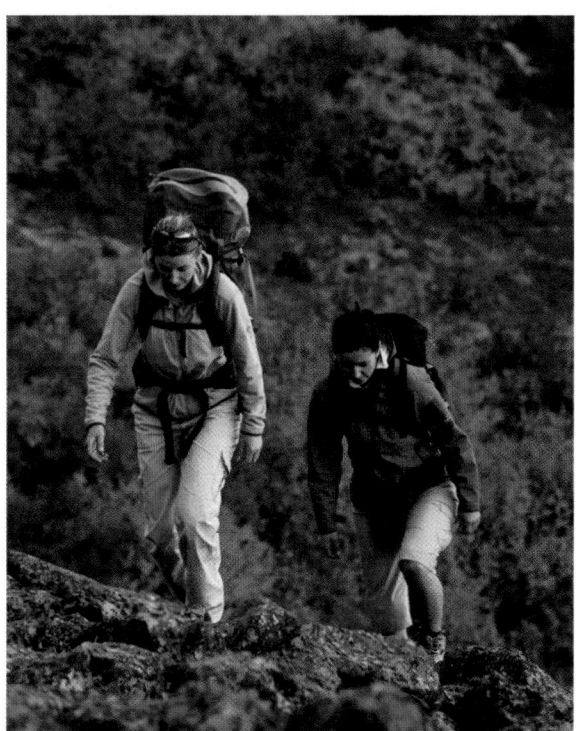

FIGURE 110-1 Alaska hiking in Arc'teryx clothing and packs. *(Copyright 2008, Arc'teryx. Courtesy Brian Goldstone.)*

Down is an ideal insulator. It is warm, lightweight, and compressible. Its greatest drawback is its hydrophilic nature, making it almost useless when wet. Manufactures have addressed this by treating down clusters with a durable water-repellant coating, preventing down from absorbing moisture. Hydrophobic down is able to retain its loft after being shaken for a minimum of 40 minutes (untreated down can withstand 22 minutes). New brands of hydrophobic down include DriDown, DownTek, and Nikwax Hydrophobic Down.

Fur, Leather, and Hides

Historically, protective clothing was made from animal products. Hides, feathers, and intestines have been used to make garments. Northern indigenous peoples continue to use fur and pelts for outerwear. Pelts and hides are water resistant, warm, and physically protective. They are also heavy and can restrict movement, demonstrating little flexibility or stretch. Traditional fur trim, which traps air around the face and wrists, has largely been replaced with synthetic and wool fleece.

Leather is the finished product of tanned animal hide, with cow, goat, and sheep being the most common. Depending on the refining process, leather can be very soft and supple, or

TABLE 110-1   Properties of Fabric

Property	Considerations
Thickness	Positive correlation to insulative value (when dry).
	Rarely more than 2.5 cm (1 inch).
Moisture	Wicking action: *hydrophilic* fabric moves moisture from the body surface to the material; *hydrophobic* fabric transfers moisture from the body across the fabric to other clothing or the air.
	Evaporative ability (rate of drying).
	Moisture *regain*: amount of moisture a fabric can absorb before it feels cold; the higher the regain, the more functional for aerobic activity in wet or cold environments.
	Amount of insulative value when wet.
Thermal conductance	The less thermal conductance, the better the heat retention and insulation.
Weave	Tighter weaves permit less wind to penetrate and decreases convective cooling; allows perspiration to accumulate between layers (may lead to conductive heat loss).

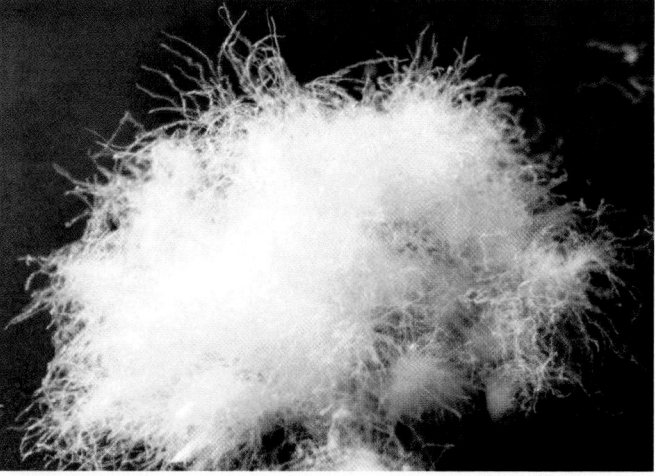

FIGURE 110-3 Down puff. *(Copyright 2010, Gary Peterson, Western Mountaineering.)*

tough, thick, and abrasion resistant. Leather is frequently used in the manufacture of footwear and gloves, capitalizing on its durability. Leather is not water resistant and saturates rapidly. It must be treated with an oil-based product, such as mink oil or Sno-Seal, in order to have any water resistance. Synthetics have replaced leather in most outdoor clothing, requiring less care while retaining durability. Abrasion-resistant nylon is used to reinforce cuffs, shoulders and elbows, replacing traditional leather patches.

SYNTHETIC FIBERS

Synthetic fibers are manufactured, not found in nature. *Polyester* is a general term for any petroleum-based fiber. Polyester fibers can be manufactured in almost any thickness or configuration. As an insulator, polyester fibers can be molded with a hollow core, trapping air that is then warmed by body heat. Unlike cotton, polyester fibers do not absorb moisture. Moisture wicks along the fiber to the surface of the fabric, from where it is evaporated. Garment manufacturers exploit this combination of insulating and hydrophobic properties. Polyester fleece is soft, washable, and durable. Bulky fleece traps air and is exceptionally warm for its weight. If woven tightly, wind and water resistance improves, but insulative value is lost. This property is showcased by W. L. Gore's Windstopper fabrics.

Polyester is formed into sheets of insulation and sewn into the layers of garments. Polyester insulation has high moisture *regain* and good evaporative qualities; however, it is not as compressible as down. The fibers eventually deteriorate and break down after repeated use and washing. As with down, synthetic insulation should not be stored compressed. Prolonged compression damages both down and synthetic fibers, causing them to lose loft and insulative value (Table 110-2).

Polypropylene was one of the first synthetic fabrics used for base layers. It wicks moisture well, has low thermal conductance, and is durable. Unfortunately, it has high odor retention and stains readily. Other synthetic fabrics, such as Capilene, Polartec, Coolmax, and REI-MTS, have largely replaced polypropylene.

Nylon, like polyester, is another manufactured polymer filament. Nylon absorbs minimal water and is highly abrasion resistant, but melts easily. Nylon can be formed into large-diameter fibers and woven into very durable fabrics, such as Cordura. This tough fabric is used to reinforce wear points, replacing the traditional leather patch. Nylon can be very tightly woven, creating a wind- and water-resistant fabric. Unfortunately, this is at the expense of breathability, so moisture condenses on the inside of the garment (Table 110-3).

TABLE 110-2 Down vs. Synthetic: Comparison of Properties

Property	Down	Synthetic
Compressibility	Excellent	Good
Insulative quality when wet	Traditional down: poor DriDown: good	Good
Weight	Lighter per volume	Heavier than down
Durability	Longer lasting with proper care	Will break down over time even with proper care
Care	Careful laundering	No special products needed
Warmth	Greater warmth-to-weight ratio	
Allergenic properties	Possible	None
Expense	High	Moderate
Drying time	Slow (traditional down) Moderate (DriDown)	Fast

Blends

Fabric manufacturers blend fibers to capitalize on the properties of each type, using natural and synthetic blends. For example, spandex is blended with wool or cotton to improve stretch and retention of shape. Wool is frequently blended with polyester to improve durability and fit.

Waterproof/Breathable Fabrics

Waterproof/breathable fabrics are designed to repel moisture and allow perspiration to escape in the form of water vapor. The combined properties help regulate body heat by keeping clothing dry, preventing perspiration accumulating within clothing and saturation from external moisture. Fabrics are made waterproof/breathable through application of laminates, coatings, and durable water-repellent finishes.

Laminates. Laminate fabrics are designed by bonding a waterproof/breathable membrane to the underside of the garment's exterior. This exterior layer is usually made of nylon fabric. If there are two layers, the fabric is designated "two-ply." The laminate may be sandwiched between two layers, creating three-ply material. This combination is more durable than two-ply

TABLE 110-3 Comparison of Fabric Properties: Synthetic, Wool, and Silk

	Synthetic	Wool	Silk
Moisture management	Excellent Nonabsorptive; transports moisture away from the skin, spreading the moisture over a large surface area to evaporate	Excellent Absorbs up to 36% of weight in moisture before releasing to the surface	Good Treated silk transports moisture; conventional silk absorbs moisture.
Drying time	Excellent Fastest	Good Slower to dry: hydrophobic properties resist moisture, and the fabric feels dry on the skin.	Fair
Temperature regulation	Fair to good	Very good More warmth than synthetics of the same thickness	Very good Performs better in cold than in hot temperatures
Odors	Poor Bacteria flourish	Excellent Naturally bacteriostatic	Fair
Stretch	Very good Retains its shape after stress	Very good	Good
Price	Good: $$$	Expensive: $$$$	Fairly good: $$
Use	For all activities: excels for rain and high heat and humidity. Wear snugly for cold weather, loosely for hot weather.	Most activities: if humidity is too high, the fabric will not dry.	Most cool-weather activities

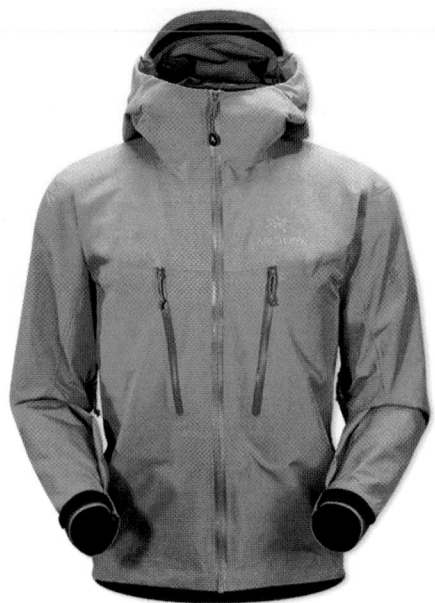

FIGURE 110-4 Arc'teryx Alpha LT hard-shell jacket. Lightweight and waterproof three-ply shell is ideal for use with a climbing harness.

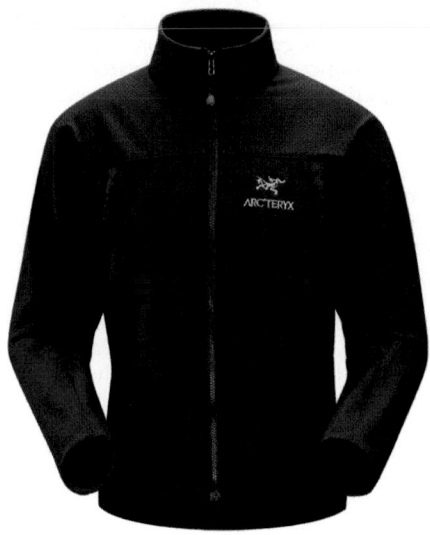

FIGURE 110-5 Arc'teryx Gamma AR. Highly breathable, insulated soft-shell jacket with shaping for enhanced mobility.

but is also heavier. W. L. Gore and Associates produced the first waterproof/breathable membrane, called Gore-Tex. This trade name is commonly, and incorrectly, used to refer to the entire category of laminate clothing (Figure 110-4). There are now many manufacturers of laminate products, but the basis of the technology is the membrane. The membrane is formed of stretched (expanded) polytetrafluoroethylene (ePTFE). The stretching process expands the ePTFE and introduces microtears (perforations) in the laminate. These openings are small enough to allow water vapor from perspiration to escape (breathability), while not allowing water droplets to enter from the outside environment (water resistance). The pores of ePTFE are 20,000 times smaller than the smallest raindrop, yet large enough to allow water vapor to pass through. Water can only penetrate ePTFE if it is applied with significant force or if the surface of the ePTFE is contaminated or soiled, leading to leakage. Gore and eVent, two of the predominant manufacturers, use different methods to address soilage. Gore applies a microthin layer of polyurethane to the laminate, designed to be porous and not affect breathability. eVent uses a proprietary method to integrate a substance into the laminate itself. By preventing soilage, the waterproof and breathable properties of the fabric are maintained.

Coated Fabrics. Coatings are liquid solutions, predominantly polyurethane, that are applied to the interior of a garment. *Microporous* coatings are formed of microscopic channels that are too small for water droplets to penetrate but porous enough to allow water vapor to escape. Channels are formed as the coating adheres to the fabric, secondary to a foaming agent or to introduced solids that cause microscopic cracks in the coating. *Monolithic* coating agents form a hydrophilic layer, transporting moisture to the surface of the garment. Microporous and monolithic coating methods are virtually indistinguishable, with some manufacturers using both methods. Coated fabrics are not as breathable as those employing laminates and are generally not as durable. They are, however, more compressible and significantly less expensive than are laminates.

Polyurethane is also used for rubberized nylon garments. These garments are not breathable because of the robust layer of polyurethane. This fabric is ideal for marine environments and sedentary activities, where sweat accumulation is not an issue for maintaining warmth.

Soft-Shell Fabrics. Soft-shell fabric is among the most widely used outerwear fabrics. This fabric excels in breathability and flexibility while demonstrating moderate water resistance. Its tightly woven outer layer and inner lining of varying insulative quality may also employ a windproof or highly water-resistant laminate. Garments of soft-shell fabric combine the properties of an insulating middle layer with a protective outer layer, making them effective tools for both temperature and moisture management. Moderately water resistant because of the tightly woven exterior and DWR finish, soft-shell garments excel when worn for highly aerobic activities when rain is not a concern (Figure 110-5).

Durable Water-Repellent Finish. A durable water-repellent (DWR) finish is applied to all waterproof/breathable fabrics after the garment is completed, enhancing water resistance without compromising breathability. The finish bonds to the fibers, not the pores, causing water to bead up and roll off the exterior. Ideally, the DWR finish forms a dense, chemical buffer, with the molecular structure forming an upright, brush-like texture. Water has a high contact angle with the finish, forming a spherical droplet. A low contact angle causes droplets to flatten into a dome-like shape, increasing the area of contact and allowing water eventually to seep into the pores of the fabric (Figure 110-6).

LAYERING

Dressing in layers enhances the wearer's ability to adapt to a changing environment, with each layer maximizing the properties of the garment's construction. Layering permits addition and subtraction of clothing, adjusting to changes in body temperature

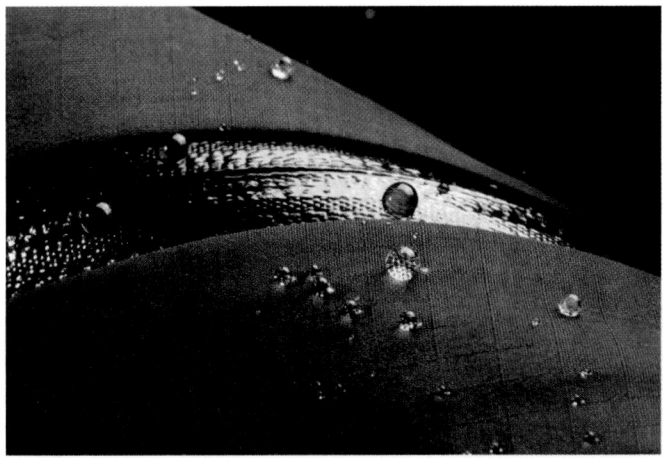

FIGURE 110-6 Watertight zipper and fabric with durable water-repellent finish demonstrates how water beads on the surface. (*Copyright 2010, Arc'teryx.*)

and metabolic output. This optimizes retention (or release) of metabolic heat and energy conservation. By adjusting layers in response to changing conditions, the wearer can either prevent sweating and overheating or prevent undesired heat loss and cooling. In anticipation of increased body heat and sweating when traveling uphill, layers can be preemptively removed and zippers lowered to promote ventilation. This prevents clothing from becoming saturated by sweat, which avoids not only an uncomfortable scenario, but also having saturated fibers lose their insulative properties. This is most important in cold environments, where insulation loss and long drying times lead to hypothermia. Removing layers in response to increased work conserves energy and moisture. In contrast to removing layers to prevent sweating, when workload decreases or the environment cools, adding layers traps metabolic heat in the insulative layers. Simple management of a personal layering system conserves energy. Layering systems permit rapid response to a changing environment, because it is easier to replace a single ruined garment than an entire suit of clothing. By layering, it is possible to pack fewer garments and still be comfortable across a range of environmental conditions and activity levels. When preparing for any excursion, participants must anticipate environmental variations such as unexpected precipitation and temperature change. A versatile layering system accommodates this eventuality.

The fit and physical properties of each layer are important. The base layer should be snug but not confining, with the middle layer fitting comfortably over it. The outer layer need only be large enough to fit over both the base and the middle layer without compressing them. Compressing the middle layer reduces its insulative properties. Seams are ideally flat-sewn. Harness and pack straps should not rub or chafe on seams or folds of fabric. Testing the fit, comfort, and effectiveness of the layering system before the adventure prevents the discomfort of poorly fitting layers and ensures that the purpose of the layering system—warmth and energy conservation—is fulfilled (Figure 110-7).

BASE LAYER

The base layer is next to the skin. It may be as sparse as briefs and a sports bra, or as extensive as full-coverage long underwear. The base layer's primary function is to regulate body temperature by retaining heat and transferring moisture away from the skin. Moisture management is established by the fiber's wicking properties. Moisture is drawn away from the skin surface by the fiber's hydrophobic properties. Moisture, through capillary action, travels the length of the fiber to the outer surface to be evaporated. Base layers must fit without imposing irritating seams or wrinkles. They should allow unrestricted movement. Well-designed insulative base layers are made from polyester, merino wool, silk, or a blend of fibers. Cotton is a poor base layer fabric because it loses its insulative value when wet.

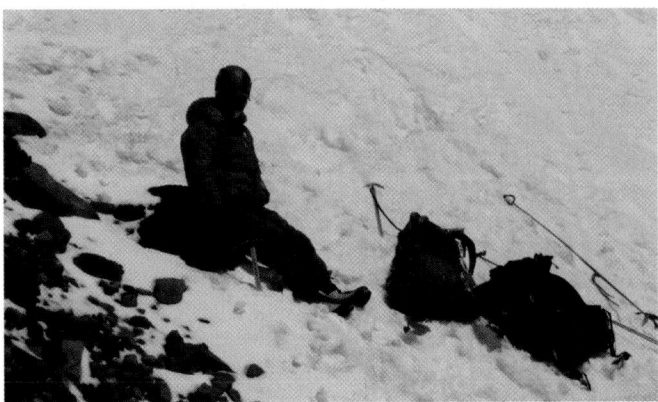

FIGURE 110-7 Although it is sunny, the cold temperatures necessitate layering well with insulating garments. Andy Rich at Camp Muir, Mt Rainier. *(Copyright 2014, J. Dow.)*

	Approximate clo Range	Garment Example
Base	0.15-0.3	Silk weight, cotton t-shirt
Lightweight	0.3-0.5	Polartec 100, Patagonia R1
Midweight	0.75-0.85	Polartec 200, MontBell Thermawrap parka, Icebreaker 150
Heavyweight	0.90-0.11	Polartec 300, Patagonia R3, Icebreaker 260-300
Expedition	≥1.4	Patagonia down pullover and most high-loft insulation

TABLE 110-4 Insulating Value of Clothing*

*The insulating value of clothing is measure in *clo*. *Clo* was first defined in 1941 as a descriptive measure of thermal protection. One *clo* is the amount of clothing necessary for a sedentary person to be comfortable at 21°C (69.8°F), relative humidity less than 50%, and with normal ventilation. A lightweight business suit is approximately 1 *clo*. The lowest *clo* value is 0.0 (a naked individual), whereas the highest practical value is 4.0 (Arctic fur clothing). Contemporary manufactures do not use *clo* as a comparative unit. Polartec grades its fleeces as 50, 100, 200, or 300 weight, and other manufacturers grade garments as light-, mid- and heavyweight. This table shows some generalities about different layer types.

Base layers are available in ultralightweight, lightweight, midweight, and expedition weight. The designation of weight varies among manufacturers and is a relative measure (Table 110-4). The choice of layer type depends on the activity and environmental conditions. In mild to moderate conditions, a lightweight or midweight layer is appropriate. In conditions of extreme cold, a heavier base layer, maximizing heat retention, is preferred. Base layers may have zippers for ventilation. If vigorous, heat-producing activity is anticipated, consider a top with a zipped neck. Lowering the zipper allows increased ventilation around the neck to release heat, and it can be quickly closed to restore protection. Bottom layers are available with overlapping flaps or zippers. With a properly fitting system, significantly less skin is exposed to cold, and harnesses do not need to be removed. One-piece base layers cover both top and bottom with a single garment. Most are designed with a long zipper to be used for ventilation and elimination. In general, these garments are suited for extreme cold, where even the chance of exposure through a waistline gap would be dangerous.

The base layer remains a key tool for temperature regulation in hot environments. The choice of a predominantly hydrophilic fabric, such as cotton, enhances evaporative cooling. Cotton's moisture retention and slow drying time are negative qualities in a cool or cold environment but are useful in a hot environment. Base layers employed in hot weather should be loose fitting so as not to retain excess body heat.

MIDDLE LAYER

The purpose of the middle layer is insulation. As with the base layer, it is chosen with consideration of the environment, activities planned, and personal metabolic needs. The middle layer may consist of multiple garments. This is most common when highly variable conditions are expected. A heavy shirt and vest or two midweight garments are significantly more versatile than a single fleece jacket. Wool is a soft and warm material, providing reliable warmth and retaining most of its insulative value when wet. Fleece and other synthetics dry relatively quickly and have a higher warmth-to-weight ratio than wool, but are bulkier. The middle layer retains heat by trapping air next to the body. Fleece garments, down, and synthetic fill jackets operate on this principle. Air is trapped in the space between fibers or feathers and is warmed by body heat. Down performs superbly in a cool, dry environment. Synthetic fiber insulation retains much of its insulative properties when wet and dries quickly. Traditional down is useless when wet, but newer, hydrophobic down garments are performing well in wet environments.

The middle layer must fit appropriately to be functional and comfortable. The design and special features of the garment should be considered. Zippers add weight and may provide entry for cold air or moisture if not protected, but they enhance ventilation and make adding or subtracting a layer easier. For example, full-zip pants can be removed without removing boots or crampons. Pockets are useful for small items but must fasten to prevent loss of items and to keep out snow and water. Zipper placement is important when considering harnesses, packs, and access to inner layers.

OUTER LAYER

The outermost layer provides protection from dirt, dust, wind, rain, and snow. Protection from wind and water does not depend on fabric thickness, but rather on tightness of weave. Unfortunately, the tighter the weave, the less breathable the garment. Therefore, moisture does not wick away from the skin or middle layers. Protective outer-shell fabrics, commonly called "hardshell," are tightly woven and abrasion resistant. Most technical outerwear is designed with laminate fabrics. Laminates allow water vapor to pass out through the micropores while not allowing droplets to penetrate. Breathability of any fabric can be overcome by vigorous exercise, because sweat condenses on the inner surface. Similarly, if exposed to very heavy rain or high-pressure water sources, water repellency may be compromised. To combat excess sweat condensation, outer layers are designed to ventilate excess moisture through vents and armpit zippers. A coated nylon rain shell or rubberized nylon shell can be considered if the wearer is sedentary or there is little activity. These garments are essentially waterproof but do not breathe or ventilate through the fabric.

Jacket and parka choices range from light wind-shells to heavy down parkas. The garment needs to fit loosely enough not to compress the middle, insulating layer, but without excess bulk that may bind packs or become caught in gear. Pockets should zip-close, be accessible, and be roomy. Zippers should be sealed or have storm flaps, and the wearer should be able to operate them wearing gloves. Drawstrings and cuffs prevent wind and snow from entering the garment. Hoods should be adjustable, fitting over the head or helmet without restricting vision or movement.

Pants should be loose enough to permit movement and should have no excess fabric to become caught in crampons, foliage, or gear. Full-length zippers, while adding weight, allow pants to be removed without removing footwear. Pockets, as with all garments, should fasten and not be bulky. The waistband should not interfere with hip belts or harnesses. Bibs can be substituted, keeping the core warmer and eliminating the chance of the waistline becoming exposed or the waistband being an encumbrance. As with base and middle layers, pants may have a full fly that zips around to the back of the garment (Figure 110-8).

MULTILAYERED GARMENTS

Multilayered garments serve as both a middle and an outer layer, with soft-shell garments being the most common. These garments are ideal for vigorous exercise when rain is not expected. Soft-shell design is water resistant because of a dense weave and DWR finish, but prolonged precipitation will overwhelm the water resistance. Once the wearer is no longer exercising, these garments may not provide adequate insulation. Manufacturers have designed insulated waterproof garments that combine a down or synthetic loft layer with a waterproof outer layer. These garments are excellent for inclement weather and nonvigorous exercise.

ACCESSORIES
HEADGEAR

Appropriate headgear is necessary in all climates, whether to protect from the environment or prevent heat loss through the scalp. Hats and caps with brims are necessary in sunny

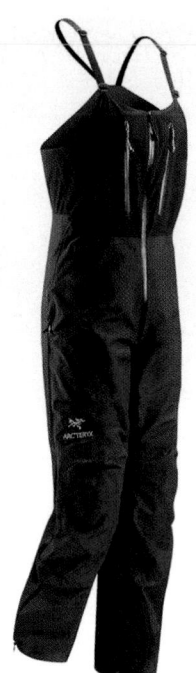

FIGURE 110-8 Arc'teryx Alpha SV Bib demonstrates protection from the weather and uses a combination of Gore-Tex Pro Shell fabric from the waist down and Schoeller Dynamic GNS stretch-woven fabric for the bib.

environments and when there are reflective sources, such as water or snow. Hats providing sun protection must have a sufficiently broad brim to shade the face, ears, and neck. Insulating headgear is made of most fabrics. As with all other layers, the anticipated environment, activities, and excursion length should be considered when choosing a hat. Knit hats are made from wool or synthetic yarns, including blends. They vary in thickness from ultralightweight to heavyweight. Hats may be lined with a wind-resistant or insulating layer. The hat should fit snugly enough to keep from shifting or blowing off, but not so tight as to constrict or be uncomfortable. Earflaps, tassels, and ties must not interfere with helmet fit, and the hat should fit comfortably under a helmet or hood of the outer layer (Figure 110-9).

NECKWEAR

Scarves, neck gaiters, and balaclavas are common types of neckwear. Scarves may range from a bandana to a long wrap. Long

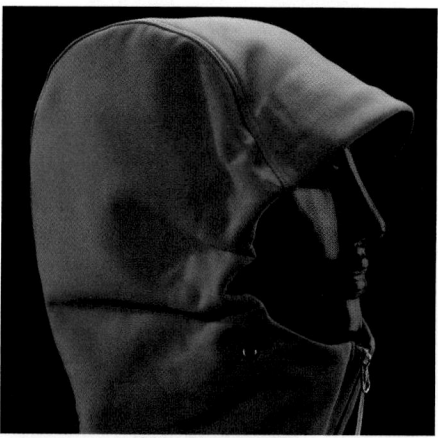

FIGURE 110-9 Arc'teryx Firee Hoody demonstrates how a well-fitting hood is adjusted to be snug around the head, protecting the face and neck while not blocking peripheral vision.

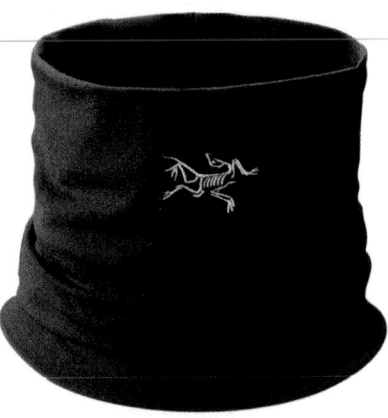

FIGURE 110-10 Arc'teryx Rho LTW neck gaiter retains warmth and will not catch in gear.

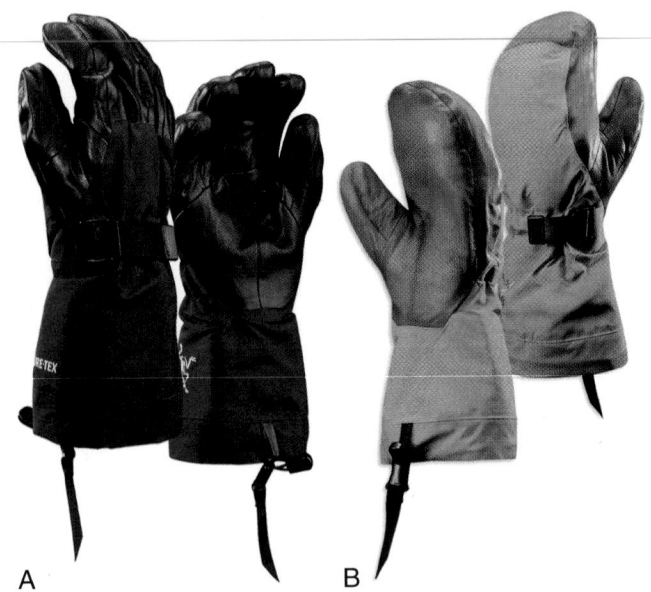

A   B

FIGURE 110-12 **A,** Arc'teryx Alpha SV glove has an outer waterproof/ breathable layer with fingers designed to articulate with maximal dexterity. This is combined with a removable Polartec WindPro liner for insulation and protection. **B,** Arc'teryx Alpha SV mitt is also a layered system with a waterproof/breathable outer shell and insulated liner. Both glove and mitten are reinforced with leather at high-wear zones.

scarves are useful for full head, neck, and face protection, especially in a hot, sunny environment. They can be cumbersome and can become entangled in hardware. Neck gaiters are tubes of fleece, wool, or other knit fabric designed to pull over the head and encircle the neck (Figure 110-10). They retain heat and protect the neck from sun, wind, and cold. Like hats, neck gaiters need to fit well, should not be too snug, and should allow helmets and other protective gear to be worn comfortably. Balaclavas can be described as long hats with an opening for the face (Figure 110-11). These are quite versatile and can be worn as a hat or can be pulled down around the neck to minimize escape of warmth or entry of cold air. Hats may have integrated skirting or tails to cover the neck while ensuring adequate airflow; these are typically seen in desert environments.

EYEWEAR

See Chapter 48.

HANDWEAR

Gloves and mittens provide protection from environmental heat, cold, ultraviolet radiation, and physical harm (e.g., thorns, abrasions, lacerations, fire, toxic substances). Handwear ranges from thin cotton, wool, or synthetic liner gloves to abrasion-resistant, waterproof, and insulated gloves and mittens for environmental

extremes. Gloves separate the fingers, allowing for increased dexterity, but are not as warm as mittens. Mittens separate only the thumb, providing maximal warmth (Figure 110-12).

Thin liner gloves permit maximal dexterity and afford some environmental protection. In extreme cold, this thin layer may protect against frostbite during brief exposures. If the liner snags or tears, it should be repaired or replaced. Following the same principles of layering, liners are frequently worn under heavier gloves or mittens. They also provide a measure of protection if the outer glove must be removed for tasks demanding more dexterity (Figure 110-13).

Gloves vary tremendously, with many hybrids of natural and synthetic materials. A glove may have a soft-shell body and leather palm, or it may be all leather or all fleece. Fleece gloves insulate well, and many are made with Windstopper laminate. Hard-shell, laminate gloves are available as shells to be worn over other glove layers or with integral insulation. Neoprene is used for gloves employed in marine and extremely wet conditions. It is common to have multiple pairs of gloves on any trip; an efficient combination of layers minimizes the number of pairs required.

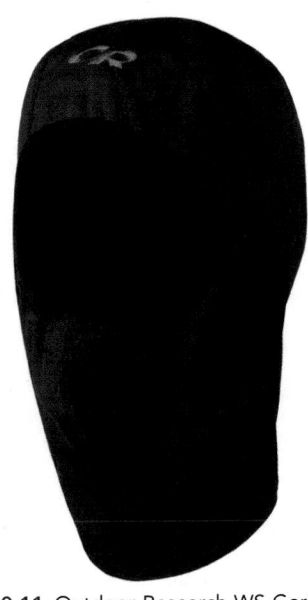

FIGURE 110-11 Outdoor Research WS Gorilla Balaclava.

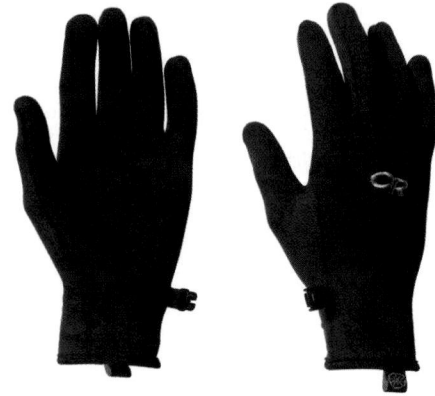

FIGURE 110-13 Outdoor Research PL Glove is designed to be soft and form fitting without restrictions. It is an ideal base layer or liner glove.

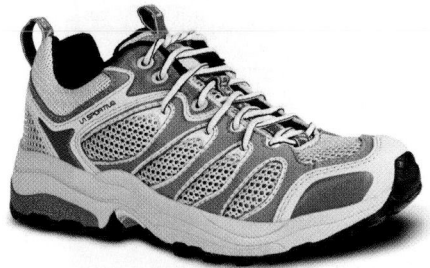

FIGURE 110-14 La Sportiva Imogene. Trail-running shoes are designed to support the foot with strategic cushioning while maintaining flexibility for uneven surfaces.

FOOTWEAR

Proper-fitting and appropriate footwear is essential for any excursion. All footwear must fit snugly enough to prevent slippage and loosely enough to allow adequate circulation. Socks are manufactured from most fibers, including wool, synthetics, and blends. Socks are also usually layered, with a thin wool or polyester sock as a liner or base layer. This provides an initial layer to wick moisture away from the skin, and if fit properly, minimizes friction that can cause blisters. The thicker, insulating sock must also fit well, with no bunching or wrinkles. Improper socks can lead to hot spots or blisters and in extreme cold may sufficiently inhibit circulation to promote frostbite. The chosen sock combination should be tried with each pair of boots and shoes to determine if the fit is correct.

Boots and shoes have become very specialized. Hiking boots are no longer heavy leather "clod-stompers" where fit was accomplished by adding pairs of socks. Professional fitting is ideal when acquiring footwear. A well-fit boot or shoe has no heel rise and adequate room at the toes to move or wiggle them. The foot does not slide forward when walking down an incline, and there are no pressure points. Some people require custom orthotic designs or molded boot liners to achieve proper fit. The sole is constructed of a rubberized polymer with a tread pattern. The tread maximizes traction on uneven surfaces. Trail shoes are designed with a flexible sole (Figure 110-14). Hiking and mountaineering boots may have a metal shank in the sole to increase stability on uneven surfaces. Full-shank boots have no flex and are the most stable (Figure 110-15).

Footwear is constructed from a wide range of materials. Most models are available with a waterproof/breathable membrane. Fabric or mesh construction is the norm for trail shoes and light hiking boots. Leather, or a similar abrasion-resistant synthetic, is frequently sewn over points of stress or common areas of wear. More substantial boots are designed with more leather or synthetic materials (less fabric and mesh), increasing stability and

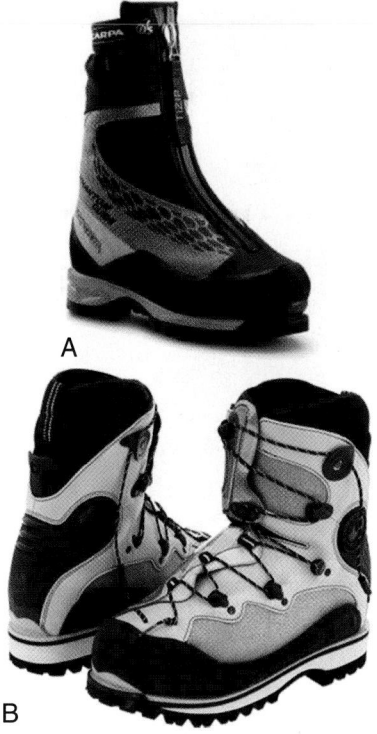

FIGURE 110-16 **A,** Scarpa Phantom Guide. Single boot with an integrated gaiter, ideal for ice climbing and high-altitude climbing, up to 5000-m (16,404-foot) peaks. Many companies are now producing "all-in-one" boots with integrated gaiter and insulation. **B,** La Sportiva Spantik. Lightweight, extremely warm double boot, ideal for 6000- to 7000-m (19,685- to 22,966-foot) peaks or high, cold mountaineering endeavors.

durability. Mountaineering boots are typically constructed of plastic or a semirigid synthetic. Boots designed for extreme cold and high-altitude conditions have removable and often custom moldable boot liners. These so-called double boots are designed to be maximally insulating while providing for a degree of dexterity while walking and climbing (Figures 110-16 and 110-17).

Gaiters and overboots are designed to protect and insulate footwear. Gaiters, tube-like constructions that cover the lower leg, are constructed of abrasion-resistant nylon with or without a waterproof/breathable laminate (Figure 110-18). Gaiters keep dirt, stones, mud, and snow out of shoes and boots. Supergaiters cover the entire boot, with a rubber rand that covers the boot rand. In addition to the protective qualities of gaiters, many supergaiters have an insulative lining that provides additional

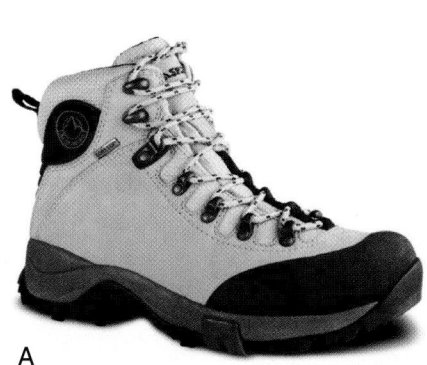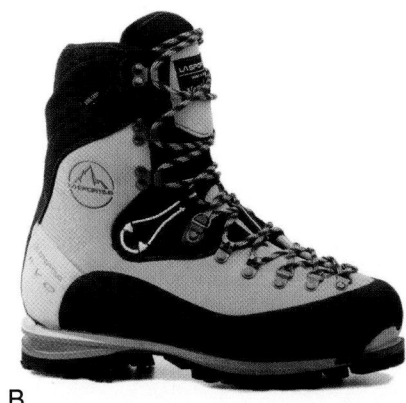

FIGURE 110-15 Two examples of boots: **A,** La Sportiva Thunder II GTX. This midweight boot is designed with Cordura and leather upper, with a Gore-Tex lining for water resistance. **B,** La Sportiva Nepal EVO GTX. This full-shank mountaineering boot is designed with silicone-impregnated leather for water resistance. The leather itself is durable and abrasion resistant.

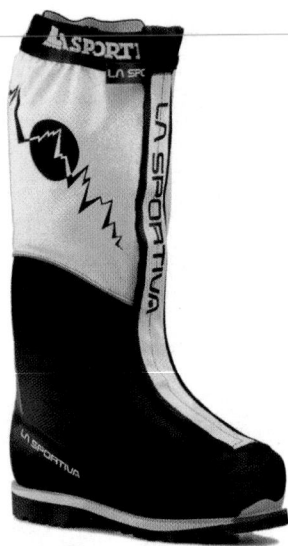

FIGURE 110-17 La Sportiva Olympus Mon EVO. This boot is designed for the most extreme conditions, with a thermal insulating inner boot and thermoreflective outer boot. The integrated gaiter protects the boot from abrasion and wear, in addition to preventing debris from entering.

thermal protection for the feet. Supergaiters leave the boot sole free, so traction is maintained and crampons do not need to be refit. Overboots cover the entire boot, providing further insulation from the cold ground. Typically, overboots have a fabric sole with no traction. Crampons need to be refit to accommodate overboots (Table 110-5).

CARE AND STORAGE OF CLOTHING

Proper care and storage of outdoor clothing prolongs garment life and maintains properties of insulation, water resistance, and breathability. Technical fabrics do not have universal care guidelines, so manufacturers' care instructions should be followed (Figure 110-19).

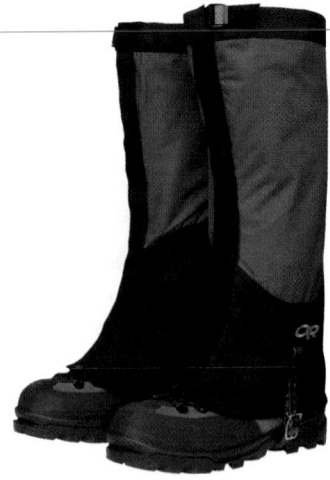

FIGURE 110-18 Outdoor Research Verglas Gaiters. Typically used over hiking or mountaineering boots to keep debris from entering the boot. Constructed of a waterproof/breathable Ventia fabric leg section and a Cordura boot section.

Any contaminant on fabric reduces its effectiveness. Soot, grease, sunscreen, dirt, and body oils contribute to garment failure. *N,N*-diethyl-3-methylbenzamide (DEET) may physically damage rayon or spandex fibers. It does not damage wool or cotton. The insect repellent picaridin does not damage synthetic or natural fibers. Soiled fabric is more susceptible to *pilling*, which is fraying of fibers in areas of friction. These abraded fibers attract more soil and enlarge. Contaminants affect the intrinsic fibers of fabric, inhibiting the wicking process and negatively affecting its water resistance and breathability.

LAUNDERING

Before laundering, the garment should be prepared by closing all zippers and sealing all hook-and-loop closures. All pockets should be inspected—a retained stick of lip balm can ruin a garment. All stains should be spot-treated by gently massaging in the proper cleaning solution. Turning the garment inside-out

Shoe Type	Common Use	Advantages and Disadvantages
Sandals	Water sports	Well ventilated and quick drying Provides protection to sole of foot Does not protect toes or top of foot
Running shoes	Trail running	Good underfoot support and traction Lightweight and ventilated Poor ankle support
Rock shoes	Rock climbing	"Sticky rubber" soles for traction on vertical surfaces Sport-specific shoe and not practical for other uses
Water shoes	Kayaking, boating	Neoprene shoes for insulation in water Rubber soles for traction Little use outside water sports
Approach shoes	Walking, easy hiking, approach to climbing areas	Lightweight with adequate traction Not designed for strenuous hikes or unstable ground
Hiking boots	Hiking, backpacking	Extensive range of design and materials Lightweight synthetic to heavy leather Full and partial shank soles for stability Excellent traction
Mountaineering boots	Mountaineering and ice climbing	Double or single boots Crampon compatible Well insulating Heavy and not ideal for hiking
Pac boots, Sorels	Insulated, water-resistant winter boots	Well insulated and water resistant Good for activities that do not require traction or maximal support

TABLE 110-5 Shoe Types and Their Uses

Fabric Care Symbols

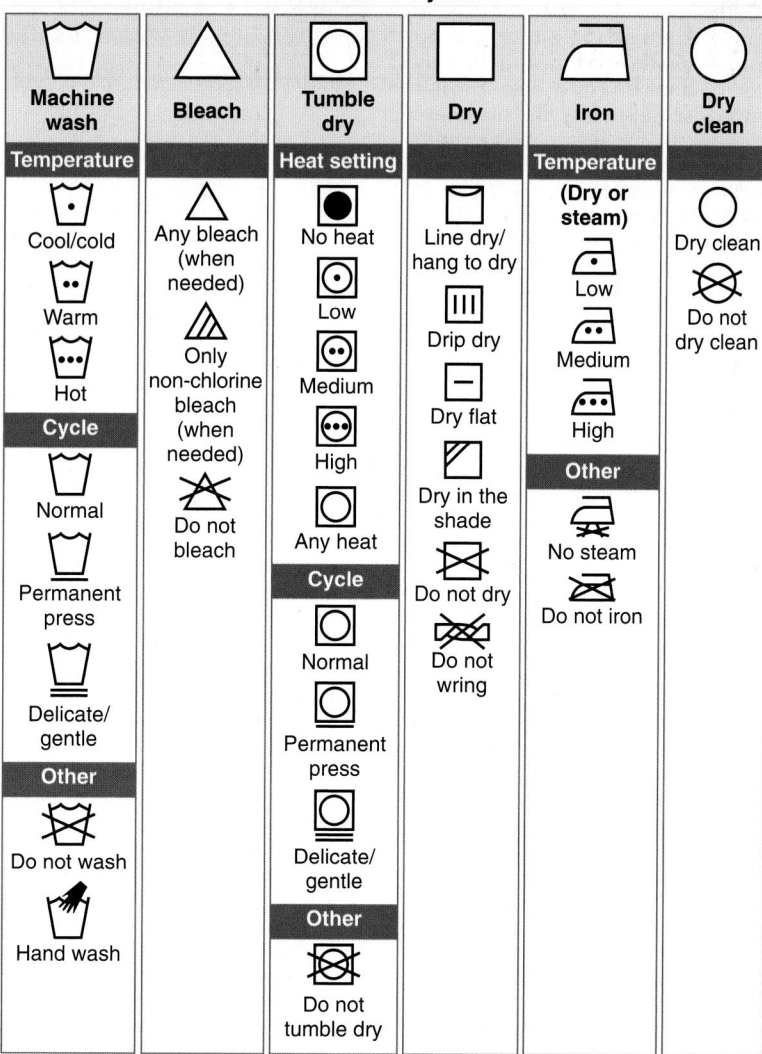

FIGURE 110-19 Laundering symbols. (*From* http://www.cleaninginstitute.org/clean_living/your_guide_to _fabric_care_symbols.asp.)

decreases abrasive damage to the outer surface. If available, a front-loading washer is preferred; the central agitator of a top-loading unit may damage clothing. Choose the correct laundry solution. Most mass-market products contain surfactants, designed to bind and lift away grease. This is helpful if the garment is not treated with a DWR finish. The surfactant does not completely rinse away and can leave a residue. This contaminant will decrease effectiveness of the DWR finish and reduce waterproof/ breathable properties of the fabric. Specialty detergents formulated for technical fabrics are designed to rinse completely and leave no product bound to the fibers. If specialty detergents are not available, use products labeled "clear," "earth-friendly," or "free," because these tend to leave behind less residue but still require an extra rinse cycle. *Do not* use fabric softener. Fabric softeners are designed to leave behind oils and fragrances, which act as contaminants on fabric. This applies to both liquid softeners and dryer sheets.

DRYING

Adhere to the manufacturer's instructions. If garments are not line-dried, use a low heat setting, and do not allow the garment to sit in the dryer when the cycle is complete. Dryer fins can become extremely hot and may melt synthetic fibers. Be cognizant of the possibility of shrinkage with wool and wool-blend garments. Cotton garments that are not preshrunk will shrink if washed in hot water or placed in a hot dryer. Preshrunk garments may still experience 2% to 3% shrinkage. To mitigate shrinkage, launder in cold water and line-dry.

DURABLE WATER-REPELLENT FINISH

All waterproof/breathable fabrics are treated with a DWR finish. For the finish to continue to be effective, manufacturers recommend washing at least yearly, and more frequently when there is obvious buildup of dirt, oils, or other contaminants. Sunscreens, lotions, and body oil that rub off onto the fabric surface decrease effectiveness of the DWR finish. Smoke specifically decreases water repellency. DWR finishes require maintenance when water no longer beads up on the surface of the garment. If the garment is clean, 10 to 15 minutes in a dryer on the low heat setting will restore the finish. DWR finish, on a microscopic level, resembles upright columns. With soilage, use, and abrasion, the columns no longer stand upright. Heat restores the upright structure of the finish. Reapplication of the DWR finish is possible with after-market products, such as Revive XTM, Sport-Wash, or NikWax. If the garment has a laminate membrane, a spray-on product is more effective. If there is no membrane, use a wash-in product.

FOOTWEAR

Boots and shoes should by well cleaned before storing. It is easy just to kick them into the closet, but dirt and organic material mechanically break down both leather and synthetic materials, decreasing longevity. Never store footwear damp or wet. Newspaper stuffed into a damp boot helps absorb moisture, but be sure to remove it. Do not put footwear in a clothes dryer; air-drying or low heat with commercial boot dryers is best. Do not apply after-market treatments unless suggested by the manufacturer because some may affect the sealants. Boots may require seam sealing and renewal of waterproofing after extended use. Leather boots require conditioners on a periodic basis. Mink oil, Sno-Seal, or similar products can restore water resistance to both leather and seams.

STORAGE

Outdoor clothing and technical fabrics should be stored uncompressed and in a dry environment. A damp basement or garage is not a good location; moisture may lead to formation of mold and mildew, damaging fabrics. Down and synthetic insulating layers lose loft, and thus insulative value, when stored compressed. Insects can damage clothing if an infestation occurs. Moths are especially damaging to wool. Cedar is a natural repellent and is available as blocks or rounds to place with the garments. Cedar-lined chests of drawers are another option. Cedar does not guarantee safety of the garment, because moths may still attack the clothing. In this case, mothballs formed from pesticides may be necessary. Mothballs are made from naphthalene (1,4-dichlorobenzene) or camphor. Camphor may be both naturally occurring, found in the wood of the camphor laurel, or synthesized from oil of turpentine. When placed in an airtight container, mothballs sublimate to vapor, killing both larvae and adult moths. Both are toxic and may be carcinogenic, necessitating that the garment be aired out for at least 1 day before use. If wool is stored in an airtight bag, be certain it is completely dry, or it will mildew.

REPAIR

Even with conscientious care and careful use, clothing becomes damaged. Patch kits available from manufacturers can be applied to maintain fabric integrity. These are far superior to the improvised fix of duct tape. Ideally, repairs are completed professionally, protecting laminates, sealed seams, and specialty zippers. Most manufacturers will repair a garment sent to them. In the field, stopgap measures include tape, fabric glue, and safety pins. Seams and rents in fabric can be temporarily repaired using a needle and polyester thread.

SPECIAL-USE CLOTHING

SUN PROTECTION CLOTHING

Protection from the sun is important both to reduce skin damage from ultraviolet radiation (UVR) and to decrease radiant heat gain in hot environments. With rare exception, clothing protects the skin from UVR by simply covering the surface. Special sun protection or "UV-blocking" garments employ a tight weave to prevent any radiation from penetrating the fabric. Any property that blocks sun, such as a tight weave or thicker fiber, improves sun protection. Stretchy garments create spaces through which UVR can penetrate. Wet garments are not as effective as dry garments at blocking UVR. Sun-protective clothing is characteristically white or pastel colored to maximize reflective qualities.

Clothing manufacturers report an ultraviolet protection factor (UPF), determined by using one of several rating systems. For comparative value, a plain white T-shirt has a UPF value between 5 and 9, whereas sun protection clothing will have UPF of 30 or greater (Table 110-6).

INSECT-REPELLENT CLOTHING

Mechanical protection offered by clothing is the first barrier to insects. Clothing that is loosely fitted prevents insects from biting or stinging through fabric, and elasticized cuffs and wrists prevent insects from migrating under clothes onto the skin. Insect-

TABLE 110-6 Ultraviolet Protection Factor (UPF) Ratings

General Rating	UPF Rating	UV Light Blocked (%)
Good	15-20	93.3-95.8
Very good	25-35	95.9-97.4
Excellent	40+	>97.5

repellent chemicals, usually permethrin, are impregnated into garment fibers. Permethrin is an odorless insecticidal compound synthesized to mimic a chemical found in chrysanthemums. It eventually washes out of the garment but is expected to maintain effectiveness for 20 to 25 washings. Products are available that can be sprayed on or used as garment soaks. Any product used should last about five washings. Follow product instructions to maximize effectiveness.

FIRE-RESISTANT CLOTHING

Nomex is the proprietary fabric used to manufacture the majority of fire-resistant clothing. It is a structural variant of Kevlar. Flight suits and some rescue gear are made from this fabric. The fire resistance may be intrinsic to the fabric, as with Nomex, or secondary to an externally applied retardant agent. The base fiber of fire-resistant clothing must not melt, which eliminates nylon as a substrate. Wool is naturally fire resistant; it is still flammable but extinguishes quickly.

VAPOR-BARRIER CLOTHING

The applications for vapor-barrier clothing are limited to extremely cold environments. Most clothing is designed to wick perspiration into the middle layers and away from the skin. In extreme cold, the middle layer may not dry, causing loss of insulative value. The premise of a vapor barrier is to keep the insulating layer dry. Perspiration is wicked into the base layer and remains there, unable to pass the vapor barrier. This leads to damp clothing next to the skin, but the insulative value of the middle layers is preserved because they remain dry. Maintaining effectiveness of the insulating layer outweighs the relative discomfort of a damp layer next to the skin.

SPORT-SPECIFIC CLOTHING

Sport-specific clothing is not necessarily better than general outdoor clothing. The basic principles of construction and fabric utilization are the same, but the clothing has design properties specific to the sport. For example, outer layers for mountaineering and ice climbing have less fabric around the waist or a much shorter torso rise to accommodate a harness. Gloves must both insulate and allow dexterity. Pockets are situated on the chest, and hand-warmer pockets are frequently eliminated. Kayaking jackets have tight-fitting or neoprene cuffs and waistbands to reduce water entry into the garment. Rock-climbing clothing is snug fitting to prevent fabric from catching in gear. Specialty rock-climbing shoes are required (Figure 110-20). Desert environments require increased sun and heat protection. Jungle and snake-infested areas demand protective boots and snug-fitting ankle and wrist cuffs.

CLIMATE-SPECIFIC CLOTHING

When preparing for any excursion, the expected environment is one of the principal factors determining clothing choice. Different clothing systems are needed for each environment, but the basic principles of thermoregulation and moisture management utilizing layering always apply. In addition to anticipating climate and weather extremes, physical features of the environment and activity to be pursued are important considerations. A hike or backpacking trip through an open forest, tundra, or grassland

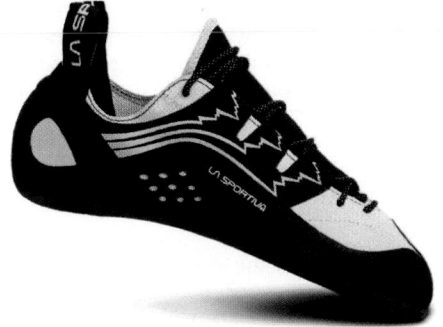

FIGURE 110-20 La Sportiva Katana Lace. Climbing shoes are the most specialized piece of rock-climbing clothing. The shoe's rubber rand permits the climber to stand on exceptionally thin edges. Climbing shoes must balance fit, comfort, dexterity, and stability.

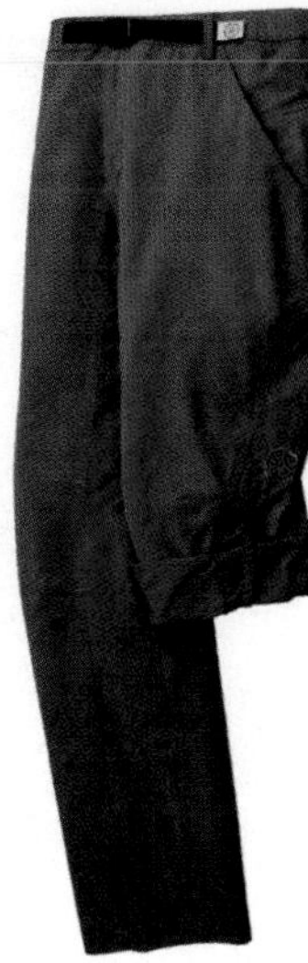

FIGURE 110-21 Outdoor Research Venture Pants. These pants offer 30+ ultraviolet protection factor protection and employ a durable water-repellent finish to shed moisture. They are designed for maximum mobility with a gusseted crotch and articulated knees. By rolling up the pant legs, these types of pants are ideal for warmer weather and expected stream crossings.

will not subject clothing to the type of damage made likely by bushwhacking and scrambling over rocks. For all climates, nylon and cotton-polyester blends offer the most abrasion-resistant fabrics. Fleece and any fabric with a loose weave will snag and tear. The need for a garment to tolerate abrasion must be balanced with the considerations for insulation (Table 110-7).

HEAT

Hot and extremely hot environments require clothing that protects from the sun and enhances cooling. Hot climates are those with sustained temperatures above 38° C (100.4° F). Extremely hot climates have temperatures above 46° C (114.8° F); the latter is typically a desert environment.

Fabrics and design of hot-weather clothing must be able to protect from the sun and keep the wearer cool. Air needs to circulate freely across the skin while the clothing shields from UVR. A fabric's ability to protect from the sun is rated as either the ultraviolet protection factor (Australia) or the clothing protection factor (United Kingdom). The fabrics are tested with a spectrometer to measure the ability to block UVR. Not all fabrics receive UV-protective ratings, but they still provide a degree of sun protection. Tightly woven fabrics are more protective than materials with a loose weave. Wet fabrics lose protective value, as do worn or abraided fabrics. Air circulation optimizes both convective and evaporative cooling. Strategically placed vents and mesh panels combined with a loose fit maximize ventilation. Many garments are designed to be "convertible," with zip-off pant legs and easily rolled-up sleeves, offering the wearer maximum versatility for changing conditions (Figure 110-21).

Thermoregulation cannot be managed by clothing alone. Behavior modification is the best strategy for cooling in conditions of extreme heat and humidity. If the environment is dry and hot, moistening the fabric enhances evaporative cooling. Exposing arms and legs promotes more rapid evaporation and convection, but sunscreen must be applied. In extreme heat, seeking shade and avoiding heavy physical activities during the hottest parts of the day are necessary precautions.

TEMPERATE

Mild temperatures, ranging between freezing and body temperature, characterize temperate climates. This broad range of environmental conditions requires clothing that accommodates the perspiration of activity during the day and provides warmth during cool nights. Unless it is exceptionally humid or rainy, most clothing dries quickly (Figure 110-22).

Lightweight, quick-drying nylon clothing provides protection from the sun and from abrasion caused by brambles and brush. Polyester-cotton blends are also highly abrasion resistant and dry relatively quickly. Long sleeves and pants may be necessary for cooler evenings or rainy conditions. A lightweight middle layer, such as fleece or a heavy shirt, coupled with gloves and hat, will stave off evening chill. Wind and water protection are accomplished with a lightweight outer layer. A jacket constructed of a waterproof/breathable laminate is most versatile. If extremely wet conditions are expected and the chance of perspiration is low, consider a coated nylon garment.

COLD

Daytime low temperatures that drop below freezing characterize cold climates. Layering systems must accommodate both the relative midday warmth and the potential for precipitation in the form of rain and snow (Figure 110-23). Clothing does not dry readily in these conditions. Efficient moisture management is imperative to maintain warmth as temperature drops. The base layer should accommodate daytime warmth and not contribute

TABLE 110-7	Climates		
	Temperature (Daytime)	**Moist or Humid Environment**	**Dry Environment**
Extremely hot	High greater than 46° C (114.8° F)	Rare	Desert in summer
Hot	High greater than 37° C (98.6° F)	Rainforest	Desert in summer
Temperate	Between 0° C and 37° C (32° and 98.6° F)	Deciduous forest, coastal forest, maritime mountain	Inland mountain, forest, desert in winter
Cold	Low below 0° C (32° F)	Coastal mountains, high-latitude mountains	Inland mountain, tundra
Extremely cold	Low below −29° C (−20.2° F)	Rare: interior northern climates with inversions (Fairbanks, Alaska)	Alpine winter, high latitude and high altitude

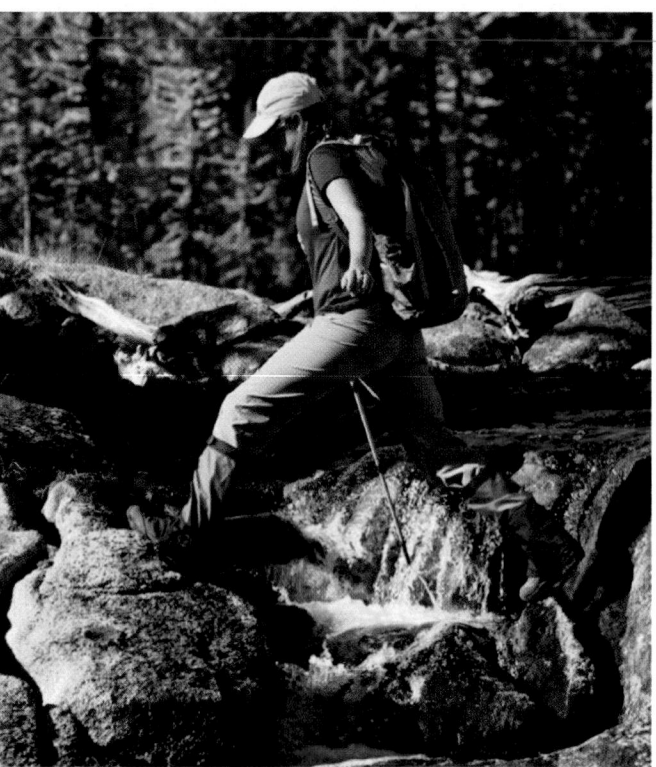

FIGURE 110-22 Stream crossing in Outdoor Research gear. *(Copyright 2010, Outdoor Research.)*

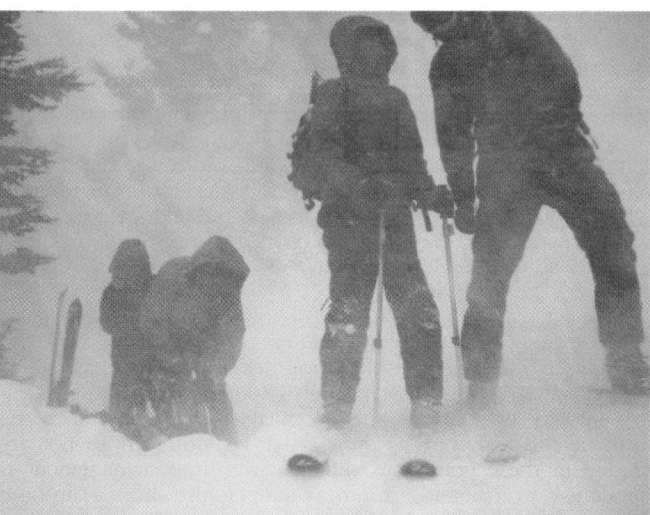

FIGURE 110-23 Anchorage Nordic Ski Patrol members were prepared for the rapid change in weather on this stormy day. Backcountry ski tour/patrol, Chugach Mountains. *(Copyright 2008, J. Dow.)*

to overheating. A lightweight or midweight pair of long underwear is preferable over heavyweight garments. Insulating middle layers that can be easily shed or added are key to maintaining comfort. Careful consideration of the garment's properties, such as the ability to vent through neck and leg zippers and ease of donning the garment over boots, harnesses, or helmets, enhances efficiency of the layering system. The outer, protective layer must be resistant to both wind and water.

Extreme Cold

Extreme cold characterizes the conditions encountered at high altitude, in glaciated terrain, or at extreme latitudes. With few exceptions, these climates are dry with precipitation in the form of snow. High-latitude coastlines and conditions that produce ice fog are the rare times that penetrating moisture is present. Wind is a major factor contributing to heat loss. Garment properties, such as draw cords and waist skirts, keep the wind from entering. All skin must be covered. Gloves, hats, and balaclavas and/or neck gaiters are necessary. Clothing must be easily layered and not constrictive so as not to lose loft. In these conditions, removing an outer layer to add insulation may not be possible. An insulating parka that fits over the outer shell solves this dilemma. This situation is frequently encountered when mountaineering. Heat generated by climbing is rapidly lost, necessitating the added insulation.

Accessories, such as gloves, hats, overboots, and gaiters, maintain warmth. Fit and insulative properties are important considerations. Gloves should have a gauntlet cuff, completely covering the wrist cuff of the outer layer. Overboots must overlap with the cuffs of pants and have no gaps. Headwear should not expose the neck or ears. This may be accomplished by using a balaclava or a combination of neck gaiter and hat. Any exposed areas should be addressed immediately. A pause in activity to maintain clothing may be annoying, but frostbite is a much greater burden.

WATER (OCEAN AND RIVER)

For activities in and around water, hypothermia is the greatest environmental danger. Neoprene garments provide excellent insulation and a degree of wind resistance. Neoprene is a synthetic material impregnated with nitrogen bubbles. This foam-like structure contributes to the insulative quality. Proper-fitting garments are snug but allow a necessary amount of water to be trapped between the wet suit and skin. The water is warmed by the body and acts as an additional insulator. The activity, expected climate, and water temperature determine the necessary body coverage and thickness of the suit. Neoprene accessories extend protection to hands, neck, head, and feet. Dry suits are especially suitable for extremely cold water. Unlike wet suits, dry suits do not let water in and are made of a thicker material, with seals at the neck, wrists, and ankles to prevent water entry. Some suits have integrated booties. Additional insulating layers can be worn under the dry suit.

SELECTED RESOURCES

Selected resources used in this text are available online at www.expertconsult.inkling.com.

JOHN R. HOVEY*

This chapter examines concepts for choosing specialized outdoor equipment. Appropriate gear can enhance speed, safety, comfort, and durability.

GENERAL CONCEPTS FOR CHOOSING EQUIPMENT

Consider these factors when choosing outdoor equipment:
- Activity
- Location of activity
- Transport to and during activity
- Duration of activity
- Budget

Individual and expedition needs guide gear choice. An extended Himalayan high-altitude expedition requires very different gear than a summertime white-water kayak day trip on the Colorado River. In the wilderness, your life might depend on your nonmedical equipment (Figure 111-1).

CHOOSING GEAR

An extensive variety of outdoor gear is available in terms of cost, materials, and quality. More expensive can mean higher-quality equipment, but not invariably. Many activities require sport-specific gear, but basic items (e.g., tents, stoves, sleeping bags) often can be used for many situations.

Weight and bulk are major factors. For car camping, a large two-burner gas stove and bulky sleeping bag are appropriate. Similarly, on trips with support vehicles, boats, or porters (e.g., research or scientific expeditions), having the latest lightweight gear may be less critical. In contrast, travelers carrying their own gear (e.g., backpackers, ski-tourers, cyclists) often want lightweight and compact versions. Alpine mountaineering-style gear perfected by long-distance hikers is lightweight, rugged, and compact. Equipment that is smaller and lighter saves energy and can lead to a safer, more enjoyable experience.

Carbon fiber, titanium, magnesium, aluminum, and plastics can be crafted into lightweight, durable, and high-performing equipment. There are trade-offs to be considered; for example, a standard aluminum avalanche probe is more durable and only minimally heavier than a new carbon-fiber probe. Lightweight gear is often less durable (e.g., a Lexan avalanche shovel is not nearly as durable as a slightly heavier aluminum shovel). Multi-function gear can be an excellent way to shed weight and space, but performance of each function may be compromised (e.g., a dedicated avalanche probe is superior to ski poles that convert to a probe) (Figure 111-2).

Practice using equipment properly is critical, especially with highly technical or complicated equipment. Simple tools are often more reliable and durable. Procure gear that is easy to adjust and repair in the field. Avoid complex gear that requires special tools for setup, repair, or maintenance. For example, choose "tool-free" crampons that adjust without a wrench or screwdriver, and use a compass with an easily adjustable declination correction. When traveling in teams, members should divide

equipment to avoid needless redundancy. Teams can split up the weight and bulk of such items as stoves, tents, medical gear, and research equipment. Plan well, but learn to improvise. Never cut corners on emergency kits or survival gear.

ESSENTIAL EMERGENCY EQUIPMENT

When planning wilderness activity, travelers should prepare a basic emergency kit. In 1906, The Mountaineers began creating a series of climbing courses and collaborations that ultimately produced the book *Mountaineering: The Freedom of the Hills*. It included a list of "10 Essentials" that was the gold standard for emergency preparedness in the outdoors.

10 Essentials: Classic list
1. Map
2. Compass
3. Sunglasses and sunscreen
4. Headlamp/flashlight
5. Knife
6. First-aid supplies
7. Fire starter
8. Matches
9. Extra clothing
10. Extra food

The advent of new technologies necessitated revision of the original list; however, the fundamental concept of preparation remains unchanged.

10 Essentials: Updated list
1. Navigation
2. Sun protection
3. Illumination
4. Repair kit and tools/power
5. First-aid supplies
6. Fire starter
7. Nutrition (extra food)
8. Hydration (safe water)
9. Insulation (clothing/sleeping bag)
10. Emergency shelter

Essential equipment may vary according to context. A basic emergency kit should include first-aid, survival, and repair materials. To determine the size and contents of an emergency kit, ask: who, what, where, when, how far, and how long?

WHO?

The number of people and level of expertise are crucial to deciding how much equipment to bring. For example, a sole medical provider on an extended trip with both young and old participants needs a large, comprehensive emergency kit. For a trip with a group of doctors and two guides (carrying kits), one might carry only a small personal kit. Number of people, medical background, medical conditions, and age of participants are factors in the determination of what to carry.

WHAT AND WHERE?

Design the kit based on activity. Although hiking, camping, backpacking, and trekking may yield similar kits, special situations deserve additional consideration. A dive expedition in Hawaii requires much different gear than an international medical

---

*This chapter is based on work by John Gookin, Christopher Van Tilburg, Marion C. McDevitt, and Nathan K. Friedline in previous editions.

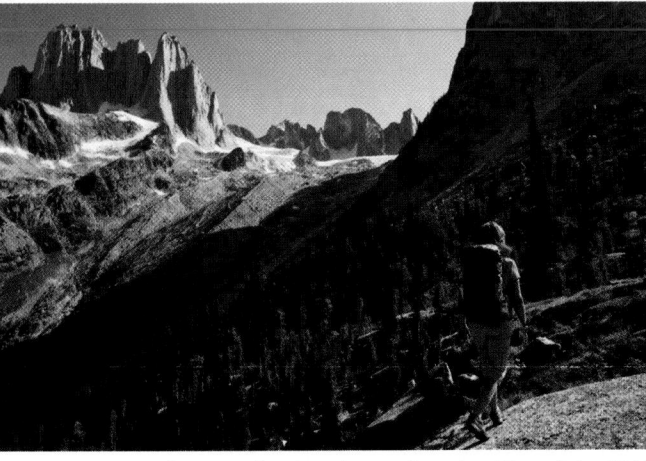

FIGURE 111-1 Hiking in the Bugaboos, Canada. *(Copyright 2010 Arc'teryx, by Brian Goldstone/Angela Percival.)*

relief program to sub-Saharan Africa. Kayakers and rafters need different equipment than cross-country mountain bikers. Persons traveling to developing countries, to high altitude, or on the ocean require specialty equipment related to climate and terrain.

WHEN?

Time of year may be a factor in determining how much gear is carried. During the winter, one may carry more survival gear and equipment for avalanche safety, snow camping, and cold-injury prevention. A summer trip in the desert may focus on sun protection, water storage, and heat mitigation.

HOW FAR? HOW LONG?

Longer trips to remote destinations mandate more advanced equipment for safety and survival. Commercially available emergency kits usually include first-aid, survival, and repair supplies. Alternatively, a wilderness enthusiast can prepare his or her own custom kit. Three basic sizes for emergency kits are generally in use.

- A basic emergency kit may be used for day outings (see Box 111-1 for an example of a basic compact kit). This includes equipment to cover one unexpected night out in mild weather. A small kit provides only the bare minimum of survival gear for food, shelter, water procurement, navigation, fire building, first aid, and equipment repair. Everyone should carry a personal emergency kit, even if there is a large group emergency kit.
- A large, multiday kit is intended for overnight climbing, backpacking, kayaking, or rafting trips that may last from 1 day to

---

BOX 111-1 Basic Emergency Kit

A basic emergency kit should include first-aid, survival, and repair materials.

First-Aid Kit

Waterproof-cloth first-aid tape is an essential first-aid item. It has a wide range of uses and is difficult to improvise in the field. A basic kit should include wound care supplies and personal protective equipment (CPR mask, gloves, face mask) at a minimum. Wilderness medicine professionals may carry more advanced supplies, tools, and medicines (see Chapter 102). This kit should also include sunscreen.

Fire-Starting Materials

Carry windproof and waterproof matches in a watertight jar with a striking swatch, lighter, or metal match (flint with steel striking blade). One may also carry fire starter, such as petroleum jelly–impregnated cotton balls or commercial fire-starting tablets.

Navigation

The bare minimum is a compass with declination correction and a topographic map. An altimeter is useful, especially in the mountains or canyons. One may choose to carry a GPS unit but should always have a compass for backup (see Chapter 106). Surveyor's tape can be used to mark dense woods. Wands (1-m [3-foot] bamboo poles with surveyor's tape on the top) are useful for marking crevasses and snow routes on glaciers.

Power

Carry extra batteries for headlamp, camera, avalanche beacon, medical equipment, GPS units, and other electronics.

Sun Protection

Carry sunscreen and sun-protective eyewear, either goggles or glasses. A sun hat and sun protection clothing are important.

Heat

Chemical hand or foot warmers are useful.

Light

Headlamp—include a spare bulb and spare batteries.

Repair Materials

The basic repair supplies can include a multitool. This should include pliers, wire cutters, screwdrivers, small knife blade, and scissors (see Box 111-4). Duct tape, 5 cm × 1.5 m (2 inches × 5 feet), rolled then squeezed flat, is extremely useful and difficult to improvise in the field. Repair materials should include thread and awl, wire or paper clips, plastic cable ties, polyurethane plastic straps, and nylon cord (3 m × 4 mm [9.8 feet × 0.2 inch]).

Clothing

Carry at least one layer more than you expect to use on the trip. Consider carrying enough clothing to survive the unexpected night out. See Chapter 110 for detailed information on clothing.

Emergency Shelter

Have the ability to improvise an emergency shelter using materials in the wilderness, or carry an emergency bivouac sack. This can be a simple, compact plastic tube shelter or even a large plastic garbage bag.

Communication

For basic communication in varied terrain or storms, a plastic whistle can be much louder than the human voice. A signal mirror is useful for communicating with rescue aircraft. Cell phones, satellite phones, VHF radios, and FRS radios can aid in emergencies.

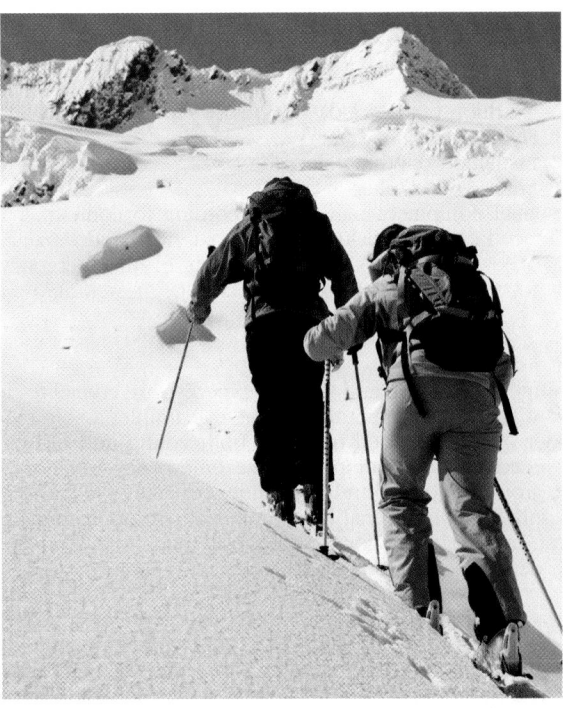

FIGURE 111-2 Ski touring in British Columbia, Canada. *(Copyright 2009, Arc'teryx. Courtesy Brian Goldstone.)*

CPR, Cardiopulmonary resuscitation; *FRS,* family radio station; *GPS,* global positioning system; *VHF,* very high frequency.

2 weeks. It anticipates advanced needs for water procurement, shelter building, and navigation. Guides, trip leaders, and outdoor professionals often carry these kits.

- Expeditions of 1 week or longer may require specialized equipment and a broad range of supplies for situations that involve large numbers of people encountering problems in extreme environments.

Information about retail emergency kits is found at www.adventuremedicalkits.com. Complete medical supplies are listed in Chapter 102. Equipment for vehicles is listed in Box 111-2.

NAVIGATION

The bare minimum navigation system is a compass with declination correction and a topographic map. Global Positioning System (GPS) technology offers many admirable features; however, it may prove unreliable. A common failure of GPS navigation is when a sufficient number of satellites cannot be acquired in dense foliage or obstructing terrain, such as in a slot canyon. In addition, batteries often do not perform adequately in temperature extremes. One should always carry a compass and appropriate map for backup (see Chapter 106).

An altimeter is useful, especially in the mountains or canyons. Wrist altimeters may use GPS or changes in barometric pressure. GPS devices are more accurate. A sudden change in barometric pressure can indicate an impending storm and allow persons additional time to find shelter. Many wristwatches now feature storm alarms.

GPS devices allow easy and accurate positioning by triangulation with satellites (Figure 111-3). GPS is most useful when used in concert with a topographic map and compass. GPS devices provide information such as velocity, bearing, and distance or deviation to next waypoint. They are available in handheld and wrist-top configurations. Handheld units have a larger screen but are more bulky than the wrist-top devices. Some display topographic maps, although at varying resolutions. Wrist-top devices may offer features such as a heart rate monitor and serve to combine a traditional training wristwatch with a GPS device. Devices are often compatible with software mapping programs (e.g., Google Earth), so users may upload information to a personal computer to track route/performance (Figure 111-3B). Wrist-top GPS units are usually synchronized to a computer, where preplanned checkpoints are established.

BOX 111-2 Suggested Emergency Equipment for Vehicles

Two spare tires
Tire jack and iron
High-lift jack
Sand and snow plate for jack
Jumper cables
Tow strap
Tow rope
Extra gas, at least 20 L (5 gal)
Extra oil, 2 L (2 qt)
Extra food and water for emergency rations
Tire pump
Snow shovel
Sand or dirt shovel
Fire extinguisher
Headlamp/spotlight
Road flares
Tie-down straps
Flat-tire repair kit: awl, rubber cement, patch, or plug material
Flat-tire repair canister: pressurized glue that inflates tire and plugs flat tire
Spare valve stems for tires
Tool kit: screwdrivers, wrench or socket set, pliers, and tongue-and-groove pliers
Repair kit: electrical tape, wire, duct tape
Tarp and spare blanket or sleeping bag
Comprehensive first-aid kit

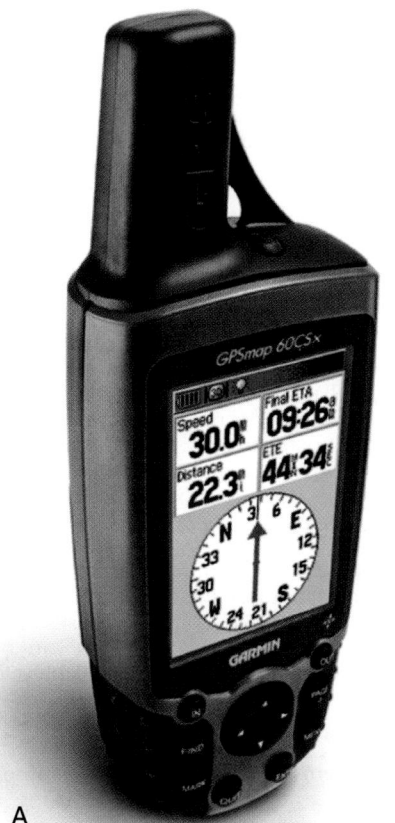

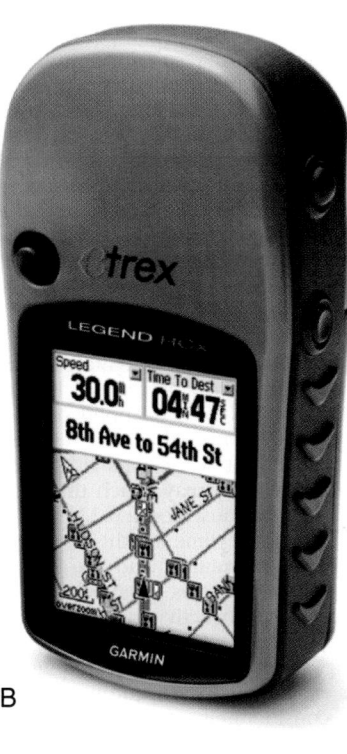

FIGURE 111-3 Garmin, a leader in GPS navigation, has many models. **A,** Garmin GPSMAP 60CSx. **B,** Garmin eTrex Legend HCx.

SUN PROTECTION

Carry sunscreen and sun-protective eyewear, either goggles or glasses. A sun hat and sun protection clothing are also important (see Chapter 16).

SUNGLASSES AND GOGGLES

Sunglasses and goggles provide visual comfort and clarity while protecting one's vision from the elements and damaging ultraviolet (UV) radiation. Glasses should fit close to the face. Broad temple arms or leather blinders can also be employed to protect against reflected light, which is important in mountain climbing or glacier travel because of higher levels of UV light.

Polarized and mirror lenses can reduce eye fatigue and improve vision. Lens color can provide functional benefit. Red, gray, green, and brown lenses decrease color distortion. Brown, orange, and yellow increase contrast. Orange and yellow increase depth perception but also increase color distortion. No one lens is ideal for any given environment, so interchangeable lenses provide an advantage. An important consideration is the percentage of light transmitted. Most sunglasses fall within a range of 10% to 30%. Dark lenses that allow a low percentage of light transmission can result in loss of vision when moving from a bright environment to one that is dark, such as when driving into a tunnel or shaded turn. Lenses with less than 10% transmission accompanied by tightly fitted side guards are needed in the extreme lighting conditions of glacier travel.

Lenses are constructed of glass or plastic. Glass and plastic are almost transparent to the visible spectrum while opaque to the UV spectrum. Glass lenses maintain superior clarity and scratch resistance but are heavier and more fragile than plastic lenses. Several varieties of plastic lenses (e.g., acrylic, polyurethane, CR-39, polycarbonate) are available. Polycarbonate is the lightest option and offers the greatest impact resistance (50 times greater than that of glass). Polycarbonate is used in aircraft windshields and is preferred for contact sports and outdoor activities.

The UV spectrum is divided into UVA (320 to 400 nm), UVB (280 to 320 nm), and UVC. UVC is entirely blocked by the atmosphere. UVA and UVB are damaging and result in significant morbidity. UV light contributes to a number of ocular disorders (e.g., cataract, pterygium, solar keratitis [snowblindness], macular degeneration). Glasses should absorb 99% to 100% of the UV spectrum at 400 nm. Glasses meeting this requirement are often labeled "UV 400." The U.S. standard is established by the American National Standards Institute (ANSI). According to ANSI Z80.3-2101, lens should have UVB transmittance of no more than 1% and UVA transmittance of no more than 0.3 times the visual light transmittance.

Several ballistic standards exist for military applications (e.g., ballistic International Standards Organization/ISO testing, ANSI test standards, MIL-STD 622 ballistic test). The United States uses ANSI criteria for basic-impact and high-impact protection. In the basic-impact test, a 2.5-cm (1-inch) steel ball is dropped on the lens from a height of 127 cm (50 inches). In the high-velocity test, a 0.6-cm (0.25-inch) steel ball is shot at the lens at 150 ft/sec. To pass both tests, no part of the lens may touch the eye. In the MIL-STD 622 ballistic test, the lens must stop a 0.22-caliber bullet fired from 6.1 m (20 feet). At the time of this writing, Oakley, Revision, Wiley X, Uvex, ESS, Pyramex, and Gargoyles manufacture sunglasses in compliance with this standard.

Consider buoyancy for any water sports activity, and ventilation and antifog coating for cold environments, where perspiration can steam up lenses. Prescription lenses help vision-impaired persons. For contact sports or other activities requiring agility and retention (e.g., kayaking), consider impact-resistant lenses and a strap to secure the frame in place.

Goggles should be judged by the same standards as glasses. Interchangeable lenses may be a convenient option. Goggles should conform to the face using hypoallergenic foam without pressure points. Fogging can impede vision. Proprietary antifog coating and adjustable ventilation can help, as can a double-layered lens. Some goggles incorporate small electric fans to evacuate moisture. Establish compatibility with the intended helmet before buying.

LIGHTS

HEADLAMPS

Headlamps permit hands-free use. Light-emitting diode (LED) technology allows lights to be compact, rugged, and lightweight with long battery life. For these reasons, LEDs have largely replaced traditional lightbulbs.

Lamps have three key properties: brightness (distance), duration (time of usable light), and shape of beam. These depend on type of bulb, shape of housing, and battery type and size. LEDs are small, have a smooth light, and use batteries efficiently. Because they are not nearly as bright as other bulbs, headlamps using LEDs usually have three or more diodes in operation simultaneously. Incandescent bulbs are becoming obsolete in headlamps. They consume moderate amounts of battery power. Halogen and xenon bulbs emit whiter and brighter light but usually consume power at much higher rates. They will also decline in use as LED units predominate in the marketplace.

With two equal AA batteries, most headlamp bulbs perform as follows:

- Xenon halogen: 3 to 4 hours on maximum power; 10 hours on less power
- Standard tungsten: 7 to 10 hours on maximum power
- LED: 30 to 40 hours on maximum power, up to 120 hours on limited power

Some headlamps have two types of bulbs: a bright xenon or halogen for important tasks that require bright light and three or more LEDs for functioning around camp or reading. These lamps can be an excellent choice for professionals. The bright light can be used for night search and rescue or identifying animals. The LED can be used for documenting research or repairing gear. New designs incorporate such features as the ability to change the main LED to a flashing mode, dim or brighten the beam electronically, switch to a red light, and lock the headlamp in a power-off mode to prevent accidental battery drainage when not in use.

A good headlamp is durable, weather resistant, and has smooth light distribution with an adjustable beam. A narrow beam with a longer range, up to 30 m (100 feet), is good for night searches or route finding. Headlamps with a wide but short beam are idea for close work (e.g., within a tent or vehicle). Waterproof lamps have gaskets to resist rain and sweat. Dive headlamps are completely sealed and submersible. Cavers often use long-lasting carbide (also called acetylene) lamps. These lamps produce and burn acetylene (C_2H_2) created by the reaction of calcium carbide (CaC_2) with water (Figure 111-4).

Batteries are disposable or rechargeable. Disposable (alkaline or lithium) batteries have a shelf life of 7 to 10 years and are less expensive. Rechargeable (nickel-cadmium or lithium-ion) batteries have a higher energy density than disposable batteries. They are expensive but cost efficient if used frequently. Large battery packs provide much longer life and may be stored on the back of the helmet or on a waist belt. Remote battery packs can also be stored under clothing and kept warm for more effective operation (e.g., during high-altitude mountaineering). Battery longevity is improved if stored cold.

FLASHLIGHTS

In the wilderness, handheld flashlights are not as useful as headlamps, because the hand occupied by the flashlight is unavailable for other tasks. For special uses (e.g., vehicle-based search and rescue), handheld spotlights can be invaluable. Rechargeable handheld flashlights are available with hand cranks.

LANTERNS

Lanterns are valuable for base camp operations or on trips with large groups when light for cooking, reading, writing, or performing activities is needed. Liquid-fuel lanterns burn white gas, a purified form of gasoline, yielding more light per pound of fuel than do battery-powered lamps. With a gas lantern, one should carry spare mantles and transport the lamp in a protective case. Mantles and glass globes are fragile, and gas must be stored

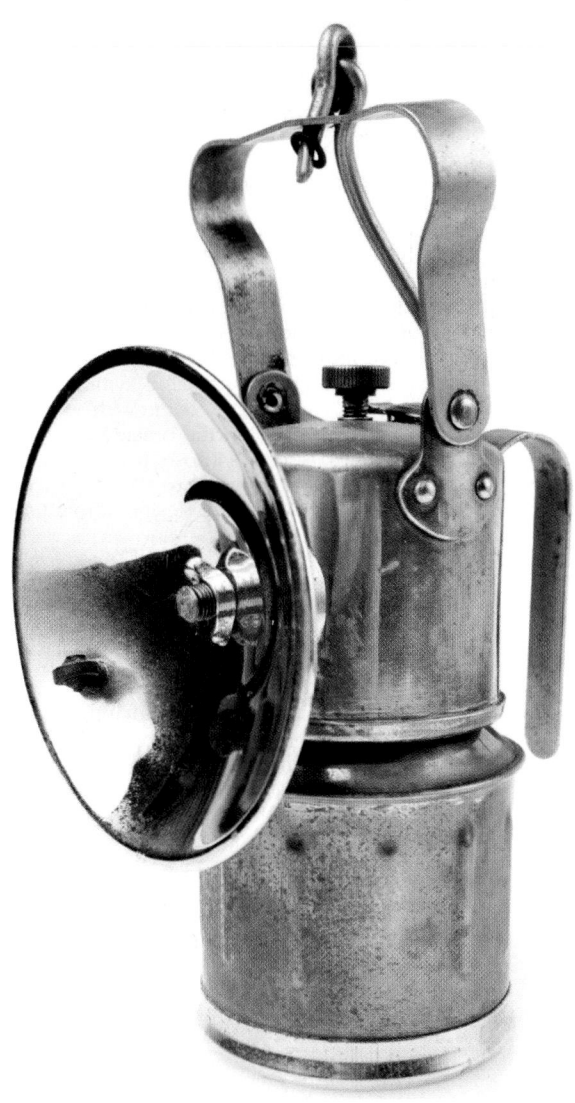

FIGURE 111-4 Old mining lamp of the carbide type. Carbide lamps are still often used in caving. *(Copyright iStockphoto.com/ fergregory.)*

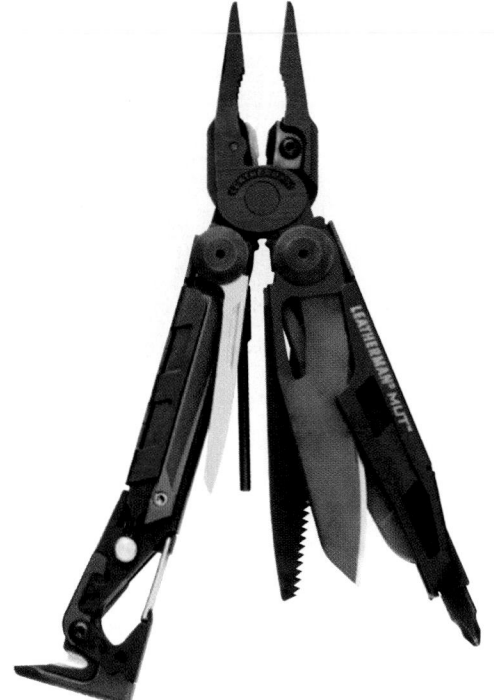

FIGURE 111-5 Leatherman MUT multitool.

Battery-operated fluorescent-bulb lanterns provide efficient, smooth, and useful light without the risks associated with fuel or the fragility of mantles or glass globes. These lanterns are replacing liquid and compressed-gas lanterns where safety (e.g., on commercial trips with campers inexperienced with the hazards of gas) and ruggedness (e.g., for international travel) are key.

Oil and kerosene lanterns are impractical for wilderness travel and rarely used.

Candle lanterns are used occasionally by campers. These are simple, reliable, and emit only enough light for limited needs (e.g., reading, eating).

Lantern Safety

Liquid-fuel and compressed-gas lanterns emit carbon monoxide (CO) and should never be used in a tent, vehicle, cave, or other enclosed space. Even in extreme-weather and survival situations, adequate ventilation must be ensured, or illness and even death by CO poisoning can occur. Any open flame (even enclosed in a glass globe) can ignite clothing, sleeping bags, or tents and should be used with extreme caution. For these reasons, many professional guides prefer battery-operated lanterns.

TOOLS

MULTIFUNCTION TOOLS

A compact multifunction tool (multitool) or a pocketknife with bottle and can openers may suffice for recreational trips. Professional guides may need a compact folding knife blade and a separate multipurpose tool with many tool components (Figure 111-5 and Box 111-4).

safely. These lanterns become very hot. Hazards associated with liquid fuel are listed in Box 111-3.

Compressed-gas lanterns run on liquefied gas (e.g., butane, propane, or a mixture of both) and are fuel efficient and light-weight. The compressed gas is contained in a cylinder and tends to be less messy than liquid gas. Per ounce, these lanterns are brighter than liquid-gas lamps but have similarly fragile globes and mantles.

BOX 111-3   Stove and Liquid and Gas Lantern Safety

Backpacking stoves often tip over. Burns are common from spilled pots of scalding water, using bare hands near a flame or frying pan, or directly from ignited stove fuel. Lantern globes become very hot. To minimize problems:
• Supervise the stove area so that no one tips a pot over.
• Do not allow people to sit in the impact area around a burning stove.
• Use a ladle instead of pouring from the pot.
• Use a handle when picking up a pot or lid.
• Do not carry a pot of boiling water.
• Do not pour boiling water into a cup that is in someone's hand.
• Place a lantern on secure location.
• Avoid cooking in an enclosed tent or snow cave. Avoid using a fuel lantern in a tent. Carbon monoxide poisoning can result in death.

BOX 111-4   Suggested Multitool Options

Awl	Saw
Bottle opener	Scissors
Can opener	Screwdriver, flat head
Corkscrew	Screwdriver, Phillips
File	Tweezers
Knife	Wire cutters
Pliers	

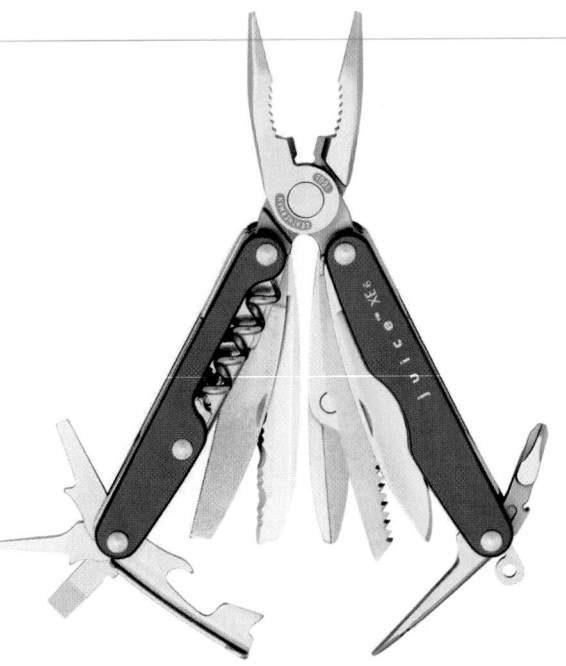

FIGURE 111-6 Leatherman Juice Xe6 multitool.

A pocketknife or a pocket multitool with pliers is sufficient for emergency use or basic camp chores. Although versatile, multifunction tools may not replace specific tools; for example, a real screwdriver may be needed to apply sufficient torque to repair a ski binding. Similarly, to repair a broken bike chain, tongue-and-groove pliers are much easier to use than small, multitool pliers. To cut a rope on the river, a boater's knife is more reliable than the small blade of a multitool.

At a minimum, a multitool should have pliers, wire cutters, knife blade, can opener, and flat and Phillips head screwdrivers. It is useful in many situations to have a saw, awl, tweezers, and scissors (Figure 111-6).

Multitools are available in two configurations. Those incorporating a pair of pliers are preferred. These tend to be heavier, but pliers are useful to repair equipment. The second style is based on a folding pocketknife (e.g., Swiss Army brand). These contain many features but rarely have effective pliers. If one carries a folding-knife style of multitool, a separate pair of pliers should be carried on longer trips.

Choose the multitool that fits your specific needs by comparing different models, as follows:
- Open all accessories. Blades that lock open generally provide more control than nonlocking blades. Blades that are difficult to open when new may be impossible to open after a few trips.
- Discern which tools will really be used.
- Test the pliers on a piece of wood or tent pole by gripping tightly. Some tools have sharper handle corners than do others; the smoother edges may provide more control, better fit, and comfort on gripping. Larger tools or with compound leverage tend to provide more gripping force.

For specific applications, one may need specific tools. Mountain bikers need bike chain repair tools, a tire pump, patch kit, extra tube, and hex wrenches. Skiers and snowboarders need a No. 3 Phillips screwdriver for binding screws. Rafters need tools, as well as a pump and patch kit, to repair a boat or an oar.

KNIVES

Generally, knives exist in two basic forms: fixed blades and folding blades. Many survival experts believe that a nonfolding, fixed-blade knife is best. Folding knives are often more practical because they can be stowed in the handle, making them more compact. Persons who prefer a folding knife usually select one with a locking blade so that more force can be applied without risk for the knife folding accidentally (Figure 111-7). A fixed-blade knife provides greater structural strength for making kindling and other maneuvers requiring force.

Blade Shapes

Knife blades have many shapes, depending on their intended use. For example:
- Hunting knives range from all-purpose utility knives to special skinning or gut hook knives for field dressing game. Large animal knives generally have longer and wider blades compared with those for upland birds and waterfowl.
- Fishing knives, such as fillet knives for field gutting and dressing fish, usually have long, narrow blades.
- Dive knives are usually straight and have symmetric blades and waterproof handles. They usually come with a specialized holster to attach to a diver's leg on the outside of a wet suit.
- Rescue and river knives, such as those used by kayakers, rafters, and canoers, are often serrated to easily cut rope and cord in emergencies. The holsters are designed to attach to a life vest.

Construction

Most blades are made from durable, high-carbon steel. High carbon content (typically 0.5% to 1.5%) makes steel strong, easy to sharpen, and hold an edge during regular use. However, it oxidizes easily and rusts with weather exposure. Many steel alloys use more or less carbon and other alloying elements to optimize performance.

Stainless steel, similar to high-carbon steel, contains enough chromium to resist stains and rust, so it is excellent for use on long trips. Surgical stainless steel is less frequently used. It has more chromium, so it is stain and rust resistant and cleans easily. However, the blade does not hold an edge as well as does high-carbon steel.

Titanium is light, durable, and resists stains well. The main drawback is that titanium is more expensive than steel.

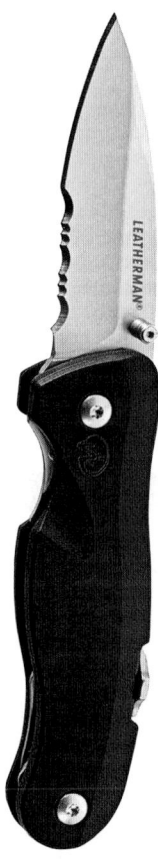

FIGURE 111-7 Leatherman Crater knife.

Ceramic, or zirconium oxide, is extremely hard and thus needs to be sharpened infrequently. However, ceramic knives are brittle and need to be sharpened with a special diamond sharpener.

Handles

The handle should be strong, easy to clean, and fit comfortably in the hand. Wood handles look nice, but plastic handles are more durable and easier to clean and sterilize. Some knives have rubberized grips; if present, these should be well bonded to the blade.

Care

Knife maintenance starts with cleaning. Even the finest stainless steel corrodes if moisture, food, or dirt remain in contact. Dirty knives should be cleaned and dried immediately. Keep knives clean in the field by wiping with a clean cloth, with the sharp side of the blade pointed away from the wiping hand. If used for food or edible game, knives should be disinfected using hot soapy water or alcohol-based cleanser. Locking knives should be lubricated with light oil as recommended by the manufacturer.

If a tool is immersed in saltwater, it should be rinsed in freshwater, dried, and then lubricated. Lubrication not only greases the joints but also displaces water. Joints may be more prone to corrosion because of electrolysis between different metals in the tool.

Keep knives sharp by using a whetstone or ceramic stick. If a knife is used excessively, it may need to be professionally sharpened. Use caution when sharpening with a whetstone to avoid thinning and reshaping the blade.

SHOVELS AND TROWELS

A small, military folding steel shovel is often adequate for emergency use on expeditions using pack animals. For vehicle expeditions or trips, a full garden spade (to shovel dirt or mud) and a large grain scoop (to move snow) may be necessary to extricate a vehicle or clear a road.

For backpacking, a small and lightweight trowel works well to dig cat holes for improvised latrines. A 10- to 15-cm (4- to 6-inch) blade is sufficient. Stainless steel trowels usually have a folding handle. Plastic trowels are not as durable, especially in rocky or hard dirt.

For backcountry snow travel, a compact snow shovel with a removable handle for storage in a backpack is necessary for avalanches, digging snow shelters, and similar uses. Shovel blades for avalanche rescue should be metal and as large as is practical.

SAWS AND AXES

Saws are necessary for vehicle trips to remove downed logs from the road or for large expeditions that need to cut downed timber for fuel. The saw attached to a multitool is sufficient only for dire emergencies. These are too small to cut firewood but may be used to cut tiny limbs for emergency shelters.

Cord saws (e.g., cable or chain saws) are suited for emergencies only. These long strands of cord, cable, or chain are gripped at both ends and pulled back and forth to cut wood.

Folding saws are approximately 20 to 30 cm (8 to 12 inches) long when collapsed. They are small enough to carry in a backpack and can effectively cut tree limbs and small trunks. The blade is stowed in a collapsed, encased position, protecting people and gear from accidental injury.

For vehicle- or pack-animal–supported expeditions, larger folding saws are available that have blades of 30 to 61 cm (12 to 24 inches) in length. A compact ax can be useful for chopping firewood.

GEAR REPAIR

Carry basic materials to repair gear. Anything that can serve as a fastener, patch, or adhesive can potentially return a broken piece of equipment to service. Box 111-5 lists typical contents for a basic backcountry gear repair kit.

BOX 111-5 Basic Backcountry Gear Repair Kit

Adhesive nylon patches for clothing, backpacks, and tents
Cable ties
Duct tape
Flat 2.5-cm (1-inch) nylon webbing
Nylon cord, 2 mm × 30 m (0.08 inch × 98.4 feet)
Safety pins
Seam adhesive for repairing clothing, backpacks, and tents
Sewing kit
Paper clips or similar wire
Tent pole splint, aluminum tube with hose clamps

FIRST-AID KIT

Medical kits should be designed based on length of trip, number of travelers, and nature of the trip. The kit should be inspected, restocked, and repacked before departure. Commercial kits are often less expensive than individually prepared kits. A custom kit may be more efficient. In the wilderness, the ability to improvise medical supplies is important. Certain components of the medical kit, such as waterproof cloth tape, are difficult to improvise. See Chapter 102 for more information.

FIRE-STARTING MATERIALS

Carry one or more fire starters, including windproof/waterproof matches in a watertight container with a striking swatch, a cigarette lighter, magnesium shaving edge and sparking insert, or a metal match (flint with steel striking blade). Consider carrying fire-starter materials such as dry tinder, candles, priming paste, heat nuggets, dryer lint, cotton balls soaked in petroleum jelly, and commercial fire-starting tablets. A fixed-blade knife without a joint between blade and handle is useful for making kindling. Anticipate how your travel plan will influence the availability of fuel sources. When climbing above tree line, wood may not be available. When traveling in a rain forest, all vegetation may be saturated from heavy rains.

FOOD

Carry extra food or energy sources. Carry extra meals and appropriate snacks (e.g., fruit, energy bars, gels, trail mix) for energy-intensive adventures. See Chapter 87 for more information.

WATER

Safe drinking water and adequate hydration are essential. Water disinfection is discussed in Chapter 88. Use a plastic or metal container for personal water storage. Many bottles (e.g., polycarbonate bottles, epoxy linings in some aluminum bottles) expose people to bisphenol A (BPA), an unhealthy additive. Use bottles that are BPA free. Additives that have not been fully tested may still be present. Because of this concern, metal bottles (e.g., aluminum, stainless steel) have become popular. Aluminum bottles require a thin layer of plastic or resin to prevent the metal from interacting with liquids in the bottle. This lining may constitute a safety issue. Stainless steel bottles do not require a liner but can impart a metallic taste to water. One should seek "food-grade" stainless steel (Figure 111-8). Consider how the bottle will be used (e.g., in a bike cage or side pocket of a backpack), and purchase one that fits. A wide mouth allows for easier filling and cleaning, but it is usually easier to drink from a narrow-mouthed bottle. Sport tops allow one-handed drinking and are popular with cyclists and hikers, but these often leak if inverted or compressed in a pack. The Platy bottle (a bag with a drinking spout) is collapsible and compact when empty.

Vinyl hydration bladders (e.g., Camelbak, Platypus) have an attached drinking tube to allow sipping without having to open a backpack or unscrew a lid. The tube has a mouthpiece that consists of a slit valve, which remains closed when not in use. The user bites the valve, opens the slit, and sucks out water. The

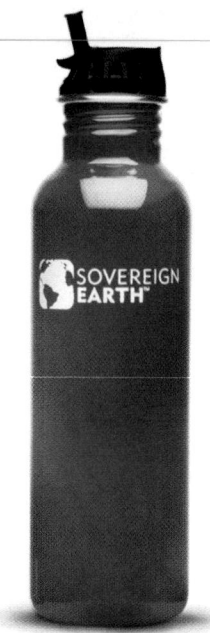

FIGURE 111-8 Drink safely with the all-steel water bottle and filter from Sovereign Earth.

TABLE 111-1 Water Bottle Comparison

Bottle Type	Advantages	Disadvantages
Single-use plastic	Convenient	Most not recycled May leach BPA Made of petroleum Not safe to reuse
Polycarbonate	Reduces waste Saves money	Nonrecyclable May leach BPA Made of petroleum May not be dishwasher safe
Aluminum	Reduces waste Saves money 100% recyclable Durable Lightweight	Liner may leach BPA Not dishwasher safe
Stainless steel	Reduces waste Saves money 100% recyclable Most durable BPA-free Dishwasher safe	Most expensive

BPA, Bisphenol A.

vinyl bags come in 1-, 2-, and 3-L sizes. Many backpacks have an internal sleeve specifically to hold a hydration bag. Drinking tubes freeze in cold conditions but are helpful in hot or moderate conditions. Neoprene sleeves help minimize frozen drinking tubes. In a cold climate, use a neoprene sleeve, and blow all the water from the tube back into the reservoir after each mouth draw (Figure 111-9A). Although not foolproof, this decreases risk of tube freezing. A backup bottle should be carried. In cold weather, put bottles in insulated sleeves (e.g., fashioned from closed-cell foam pad and duct tape). During travel, pack water bottles within a parka to prevent freezing (Figure 111-9B). At night, fill the water bottle with hot water (if approved by the manufacturer), and place the bottle inside the sleeping bag (after ensuring the bottle is securely closed and dry). This contributes heat to the sleeping bag and preserves water to drink. Thawing frozen water bottles is difficult and consumes precious fuel. Frozen water often cracks bottles and renders them useless.

Bottles should not be used for hot liquids unless specifically intended for that purpose, because chemical leaching (e.g., of BPA) may occur. Heat may damage the liners of aluminum bottles. Noninsulated bottles may become hot and cause burns. Most bottles can safely contain juices, sodas, iced tea or coffee, and energy and sports drinks. Some manufacturers claim their

bottles are "dishwasher safe," whereas others recommend hand-washing with hot water and gentle detergent. A soft brush should be used on aluminum bottles to avoid damage to the liner. Cleaning brushes and cleansing tablets are available (Table 111-1).

Larger containers (e.g., 20-L [5.3-gal] size) are usually carried in vehicles. Collapsible vinyl bottles and bags can be carried empty in a backpack and filled in camp to allow ample water for cooking, bathing, cleaning dishes, and refilling personal water bottles. Accordion-style collapsible bottles tend to crack after repeated use. Nylon-lined water bags are light and collapse when not in use. These are common gear on large expeditions when extra water storage is needed in base camp and when carrying bottles is cumbersome. Water bags are compact when empty (see Figure 111-9A).

Between trips, plastic water containers should be carefully cleaned. Soft-plastic containers and hydration bags need to be scrubbed by hand with hot soapy water and rinsed thoroughly. To disinfect and minimize mold and bacterial growth, rinse with chlorinated water (5 mL [1 tsp] of bleach in 1 L of water) and dry thoroughly. After prolonged storage, eliminate odors by washing with baking soda solution (5 mL [1 tsp] of baking soda in 1 L of water), then rinsing with water. Clean tubes and valves on drinking hoses after each use. Replace worn or excessively soiled parts.

HEAT PACKS AND HEATERS

Heat packs can prevent hypothermia and frostbite. These are available for feet, hands, and backs. Most disposable heat packs use a chemical reaction to generate heat. When the polypropylene pouch is opened and agitated, iron is exposed to oxygen, oxidizes, and produces iron oxide and heat. This reaction lasts for 4 to 8 hours. Sodium chloride acts as a catalyst, carbon disperses heat, cellulose acts as filler, and vermiculite acts as a heat retainer.

Heat packs can prevent frostbite when used in gloves and boots and can contribute to core warming if placed under the axillae, in the groin, or on the torso. Of note, the heat generated is not independently sufficient to rewarm a moderately hypothermic person. Some heat packs are configured in a belt to be worn on the low back, and some feature adhesive so they can be attached to gloves or socks. Most manufacturers recommend against using them directly on skin, to avoid risk for burns.

Electric boot heaters (e.g., for skiing, biking, hiking, or climbing boots) have small, rechargeable battery packs that fit on the back of the upper boot near the cuff. Cords run into the boot. The heating element is placed just under the ball of the foot on

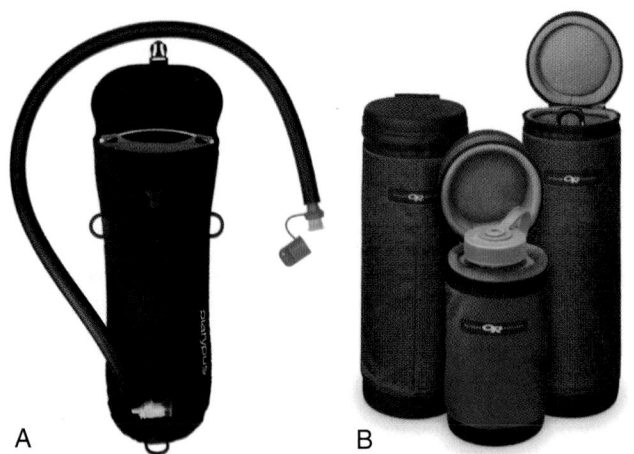

FIGURE 111-9 In cold or hot conditions, use a Platypus Insulator for your water bag **(A)** or an Outdoor Research water bottle parka for your water bottle **(B)**.

a foot bed. These heaters can provide up to 18 hours of heat production at low power. They are most useful for persons prone to frostbite and for short (e.g., 1- or 2-day) cold-weather outings, because they need to be recharged.

OPTICS

For backpacking, compact binoculars and telescopes are useful because space and weight are priorities. Larger binoculars and telescopes have a wider objective lens, better magnification, and a wider field of view but add bulk and weight, so are best suited for base camps, research stations, and vehicles.

Two numbers identify an optical device's chief properties: the first denotes magnification, the second the objective lens' diameter. The objective lens is that farthest from the eye and is measured in millimeters. A monocular described as "6 × 25" has a magnification of 6 (i.e., the object appears six times closer than with the unaided eye) and a 25-mm (1-inch) objective lens. A larger objective lens allows more light into the binocular or telescope, which is preferred for low-light situations (e.g., dawn or dusk).

Other factors are used to compare optics. *Exit pupil* describes the diameter of light (in millimeters) exiting the near lens when looking through the device at a bright light. It is calculated by dividing object lens diameter by magnification (e.g., $25 \div 6 \approx 4$). The larger the exit pupil, the more light reaches the wearer's eye, and the view is perceived as brighter, especially in low-light conditions. *Field of view* describes the width of view (in feet) at 1000 yards. It is determined by magnification and the focal lengths of the objective and eyepiece lenses. Field of view correlates with magnification. Lower magnification allows a broader field of view; higher magnification (e.g., a telescope) yields a smaller field of view. *Eye relief* is the distance from the eyepiece (in millimeters) at which the full viewing angle is visible. People who wear glasses may require eye relief of 11 mm (0.4 inch) or more to use their glasses while looking through the device.

Other factors to consider when choosing optics include:

- Lens coatings cut glare.
- Waterproof housings protect from rain or snow.
- Plastic housings, sometimes called *armor,* protect the device when stowed during travel, when dropped, and in rugged environments.
- Focus types should include one or two adjustments. One is a central focus found on binoculars and monoculars. Binoculars should have a separate focus on one eyepiece to accommodate different foci for each eye. The user first focuses the eyepiece to equalize eyes, then uses the central focus to bring the object into view.
- Zoom alters magnification and field of view. This adds weight because of additional lenses but can be useful for multipurpose binoculars and telescopes.

PACKS

One ideally should have a professional (e.g., at an outdoor store) assist in fitting any pack for correct size, type, body shape, and specific application.

LUMBAR PACKS

Lumbar packs are small and work well for brief hikes in clear weather or for carrying emergency supplies when skiing within a developed winter resort. They have the capacity to hold food, water, emergency kit, extra windbreaker, hat, and gloves.

DAY PACKS

Day packs, or rucksacks, are small packs that carry gear for a 1-day outing, usually a spare jacket, food, water, and emergency supplies. A day pack's capacity is approximately 16 L (1000 inches³). Shoulder straps and belt typically have minimum padding. They are light, compact, and often have no frame.

BACKPACKS

There are two types of backpacks: internal- and external-frame packs (Figure 111-10A). Internal-frame packs are an excellent choice for many situations. Aluminum or plastic stays are sewn into pockets inside the pack to add support. Internal-frame packs have more capacity than day packs and have thicker padding on the waist belt and shoulder straps. Compared with external-frame models, internal-frame packs are more flexible and narrower and thus easier to maneuver when hiking in tight spaces (e.g., caves, canyons, thick forests) (Figure 111-10B). Because they stay close against the body, internal-frame packs are warmer and allow better balance and maneuverability when hiking over rough terrain, skiing, or climbing. Compression straps allow the load to be cinched. This keeps the pack tighter and more stable, especially when partially full.

Top-loading packs have one large compartment that opens at the top. These generally have a drawstring closure and a lid covering the top. These packs have great capacity, sit well on the torso, and are easy to unload with the pack upright. Panel-loading packs have a large zipper on the front of the pack. These allow easy access to the entire contents of the pack.

Zippers can be convenient, but overpacking and external forces (e.g., dropping the pack) can cause the zipper to fail. Ensure your pack will still be functional if the zipper fails.

External-frame packs have a stiff aluminum tube frame on the outside of the pack. The frame holds the straps and waist belt. The nylon pack is attached to the frame. External-frame packs are more comfortable when carrying heavy loads, in that they

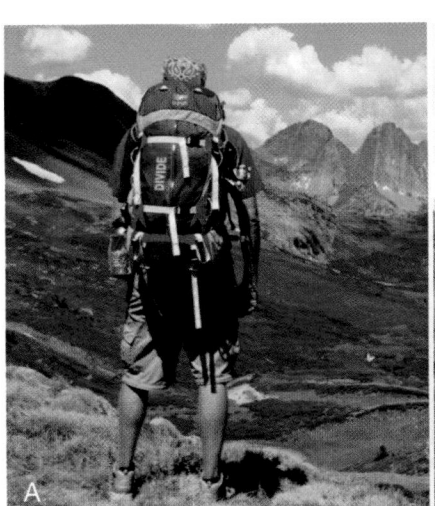
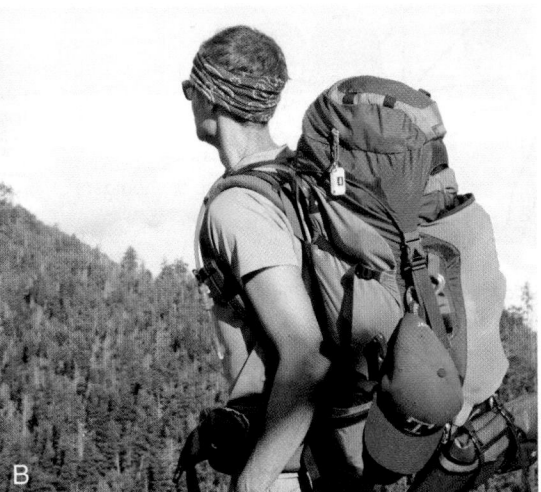

FIGURE 111-10 A, Backpacking with the Mile High Mountaineering Divide pack in the San Juan Mountains. **B,** Backpacking with Mile High Mountaineering Fifty-Two 80 pack. *(Copyright Mile High Mountaineering.)*

distribute weight efficiently between the shoulder straps and waist belt. Some people can carry more than 50% of their body weight using an external-frame pack. External-frame packs can be cooler than internal-frame packs, because the pack sits away from the wearer's back. They can be easier to pack, because they usually have multiple compartments. External-frame packs are bulkier, so are not a good choice for tight spaces, aerobic activity, climbing, airline travel, or off-trail hiking.

Choosing the right size is important. Consider what will be carried (e.g., rescue, research, or work equipment in addition to personal gear). For extended travel, 50 to 100 L, (3000 to 6000 inches³) may be needed.

Packs are designed to be used substantially full. If a pack is routinely used half full, the pack itself will weigh more than necessary and fit will be suboptimal. If the pack is not large enough, or if one needs to have easier access to certain equipment, pockets can be added. However, pockets can be unstable and are a less efficient way to carry heavy items. Gear (e.g., sleeping pads, tent poles) can be strapped to the outside the pack.

Suspension systems vary from simple webbing belt and shoulder straps to well-padded systems that wrap around the torso, customized for body shape and height. Women should use packs designed for a woman's anatomy. For full loads, choose a system that comfortably rests weight on the hips but snugly pulls the load toward the back. For larger packs, choose thick hip and shoulder padding and a fit that easily adjusts while walking to take pressure off hot spots. A padded hip belt and lumbar pad should fit snugly with ample room to tighten the belt when in the field (Figure 111-11A to C). For small day packs, choose a lightweight and comfortable suspension system that does not have more padding than needed for the relatively light load.

Ultralight materials are now being used for some packs but rarely are as durable as heavier materials.

Load-adjusting straps are helpful for packs of 50 L (3000 inches³) or more. A sternum strap brings the shoulder straps into position over the collarbones. Load-lifting straps on top of the shoulder strap bring the top of the pack closer to the shoulders. Belt-stabilizer straps at the waist bring the bottom of the pack closer to the hips. These straps should be adjusted in the field to best stabilize the pack depending on how it is loaded.

Try on a pack before purchase. Load the pack with as much weight as intended for the average trip, hoist the pack up and over obstacles, and climb up and down stairs. A professional fitter can assist with size and selection and adjust the straps and harness system (Figure 111-11D). Certain adjustments, such as shoulder strap height, can be fitted once and then not changed, but other features, such as side-load adjustment straps, should be adjusted at the trailhead and while walking. Make necessary adjustments each time a pack is put on: lean forward, and center the waist belt over the bony iliac crest. Cinch the buckle snugly. While still leaning forward, cinch the shoulder straps snugly under your arms. Stand up. If the pack has more waist belt adjustments toward the back, snug them to pull the weight into the body. Adjust the shoulder top straps to pull the load into the body and take pressure off the shoulders. These tension straps should be approximately 30 to 45 degrees off the horizontal axis and should arise from the top of the shoulder. Backpack accessories may add essential space but also add weight, needless complexity, and bulk. Packs can be made with integral map pockets, hydration bag holders, water bottle pockets, shovel pocket, crampon patch, ice ax straps, removable lids that convert to lumbar packs, and an extension cuff to extend the volume on a top-loading pack. Many packs have lash patches that allow one to strap on additional items (e.g., sleeping pads, tents, climbing gear).

Packs for special use include those in the following situations:

- Climbers and mountaineers require ice ax loops, crampon patches, and wand pockets.
- Backpackers need water bottle pockets or hydration bladder pouch and lash patches for lashing on tents or sleeping bags.
- Mountain bike backpacks are usually compact, about 4 L (250 inches³), to fit between the shoulders and not impede the rider. They are designed to carry a hydration bladder, food, emergency kit, and bike repair tools.
- Mountain rescuers and ski patrollers may need internal pockets to organize gear such as snow shovels, avalanche probes, and first-aid supplies.
- Backcountry skiers and snowboarders need straps to hold their skis or snowboard on the outside of the pack when hiking.
- Photographers need compartments lined with foam to protect equipment.
- International travelers can use compartments that stow the suspension system when intended as checked airline luggage and can use wheels for easy transport.

Packing a backpack efficiently is an art form. Nylon stuff sacks can be used to compartmentalize gear. Mesh bags or plastic ziplock freezer bags work well for small items. Pack heavy objects low and forward (i.e., close to one's back) to improve balance. Balance the pack so that left and right are equal. Store sleeping bags and bulky clothing in compression stuff sacks to reduce volume (Figure 111-12A). Minimize the amount of gear lashed on the outside, and if tied outside the pack, make sure everything is secured tightly. In wet climates, consider waterproofing the pack by lining it with a tough garbage or trash compactor bag, using a pack rain cover, or packing gear in dry bags (as used by kayakers and rafters).

DUFFELS, STUFF SACKS, AND DRY BAGS

Duffels should be large enough to hold needed equipment but not so large they are cumbersome to transport. Duffels should

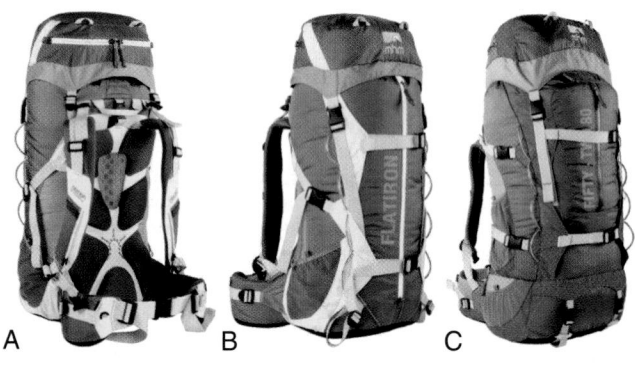

A   B   C

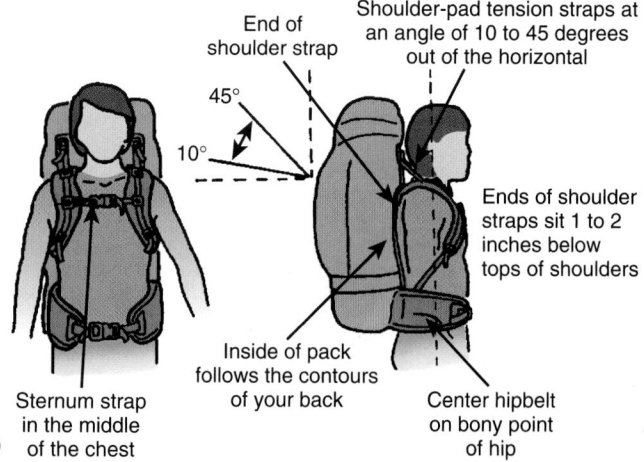

End of shoulder strap

Shoulder-pad tension straps at an angle of 10 to 45 degrees out of the horizontal

45°

10°

Ends of shoulder straps sit 1 to 2 inches below tops of shoulders

Inside of pack follows the contours of your back

Sternum strap in the middle of the chest

Center hipbelt on bony point of hip

D

FIGURE 111-11 A, Mile High Mountaineering Flatiron 38 internal-frame pack (back). B, Mile High Mountaineering Flatiron 38 internal-frame pack (front). C, Mile High Mountaineering Fifty-Two 80 Pack. D, Backpack suspension system. (D redrawn from Harvey M: The National Outdoor Leadership School's Wilderness Guide: The Classic Handbook, revised and updated, New York, 1999, Touchstone.)

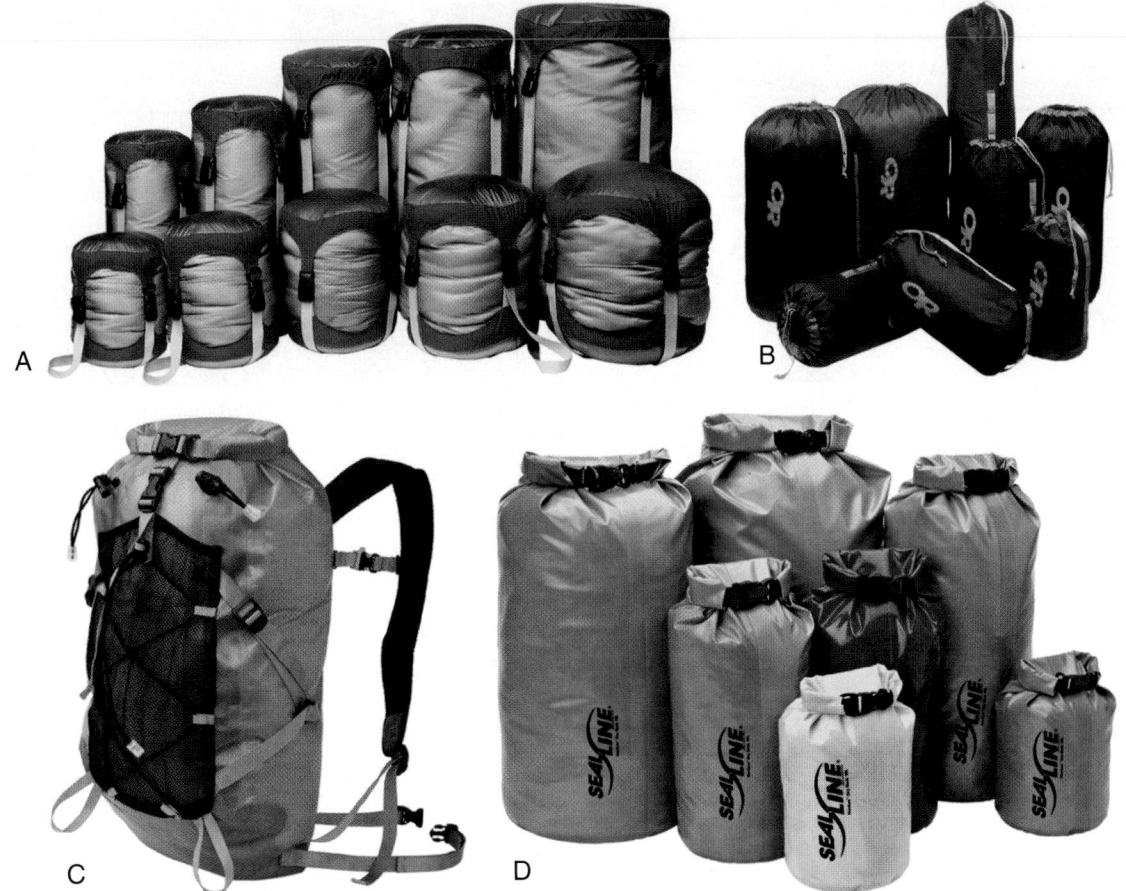

FIGURE 111-12 Organize and protect your gear using stuff sacks, compression bags, or dry bags. **A,** Outdoor Research (OR) Ultralight Compression Sack. **B,** OR Durable Stuff Sack. **C,** OR Drycomp Ridge Sack (side). **D,** SealLine Nimbus Sack group.

be constructed with heavy-duty zippers and stitching. Heavy-duty shoulder straps or straps that convert to a backpack can be helpful. Wheels add weight and can fail but are a great benefit for transporting bags in airports. Choose a size that can be reasonably carried and used. This may be as small as 25 L (1500 inches³) or as large as 170 L (10,000 inches³). Duffels larger than 115 L (7000 inches³) are usually too heavy to be carried for more than a short distance. It is often better to use two smaller packs when packing such items as ski, camping, and climbing gear.

For baggage carried in commercial airline cabins (carry-on), duffels must comply with airline restrictions. Most airlines restrict checked bags to 23 kg (50 lb), but restrictions down to 18 kg (40 lb) are not unusual on some flights. Bags should be locked with Transportation Security Administration–approved luggage padlocks.

Stuff sacks are an excellent way to organize gear packed in larger bags or packs. Some have compression straps or are packing cubes with cloth on one side and net on the other with a zipper (Figure 111-12B). Small dry bags can be useful for personal items and electronics and can be clear or opaque; clear bags allow viewing of the contents. Larger dry bags can have straps that convert the bags to backpacks (Figure 111-12C). Dry bags for river or ocean travel help ensure gear remains dry (Figure 111-12D).

ELECTRONICS

Electronics may be ubiquitous in the backcountry. Before purchasing, consider the following:
- Do they enhance the outdoor experience, improve the margin of safety, or increase emergency response capabilities?

- Are they easy to use? Some manuals are difficult to read and are complicated. Does one need the manual to remember how to operate or calibrate the device?
- Does the device still work after a week in the field? Devices can be rendered useless because of exposure to cold weather or water, or from being dropped.
- Are the batteries fresh and fully charged? (See Box 111-6.)

If an electronic device will be used, have contingency plans for emergencies. For example, when using a GPS or wrist-top electronic compass, carry a standard compass and altimeter. Consider the following:
- GPS units and GPS-equipped smartphones are small, lightweight, and easy to use. A map and compass should be carried for backup. GPS may be unreliable, especially when in a deep canyon where it is not possible to receive adequate satellite signal.
- Wrist-top computers are valuable and versatile. They often contain a compass, altimeter, stopwatch, timer, multiple alarms, barometer, and even a heart rate monitor. They can be accurate but more complicated to use than a standard nonelectronic compass.
- Family radio station (FRS) radios are inexpensive and valuable, especially for outdoor families. These small, ultrahigh-frequency (UHF) walkie-talkies are easy to use and excellent for communication within the effective range. Some ski patrols and park rangers monitor FRS channels. However, most FRS radios transmit at 0.5 to 1 W of power and have a range of only 1.6 to 3.2 km (1 to 2 miles) in clear, line-of-sight terrain. (See Chapter 105.)
- Very-high-frequency (VHF) radios are typically used by marine travelers and are also available for backcountry land travelers. In the United States, VHF radios need to be registered with

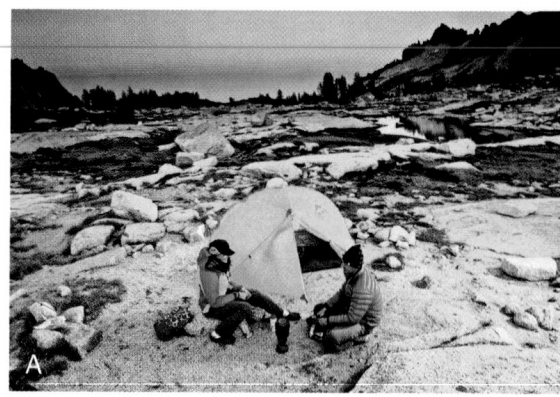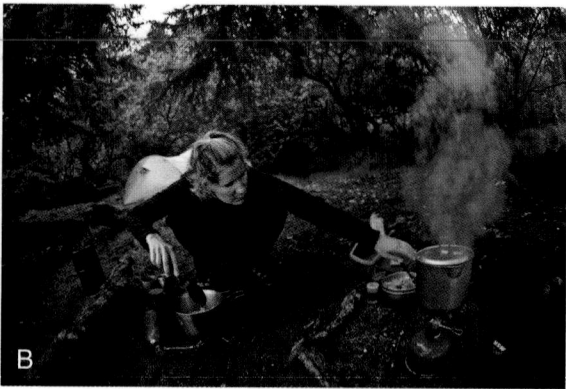

FIGURE 111-13 A, Camp is set. **B,** Cooking dinner with MSR WhisperLite stove and MSR Reactor canister stove. (**A** *copyright 2010, Outdoor Research Marketing;* **B** *copyright 2008, Arc'teryx, by Brian Goldstone.*)

the Federal Communications Commission. These usually transmit at 5 W and thus have much longer range than FRS radios. Certain channels may be monitored by local law enforcement, park service, or forest service personnel.

- Personal locator beacons (PLBs) are used by mariners and aviators. Now widely available for all backcountry travelers, the unique number is registered with an international satellite locator system. If activated, the PLB broadcasts a signal through a satellite to a ground station rescue center.
- Cell and satellite phones are common in the wilderness. Cell phones have made rescues much easier by allowing quicker and more accurate responses. However, these phones cannot always connect with a cell tower or satellite, and they exhaust batteries quickly.
- Weather radio is broadcast in the United States by the National Weather Service. The continuous broadcast operates on 162.40-, 162.475-, or 162.55-MHz VHF frequency, depending on the area, and gives detailed weather information on a continuous, round-the-clock basis that is updated daily or, in some cases, hourly.

POWER

Carry extra batteries for headlamp, camera, avalanche beacon, medical equipment, GPS units, and other electronics. Power converters may be useful when car camping and can help recharge batteries. See Chapter 109 for a more detailed discussion of how to power electronic devices using solar systems.

OVERNIGHT GEAR

For overnight wilderness travel, cooking, sleeping, and shelter equipment are necessary (Figure 111-13A). Some backpackers and climbers prefer minimal equipment to enable a faster rate of travel (e.g., by shortening and drilling holes in the handles of their toothbrushes or utensils to reduce weight). Be certain to plan for adverse weather (Figure 111-13B).

STOVES

Camp stoves are valuable to disinfect water, improve nutrition and hydration, and improve morale in foul weather by allowing for hot food and drink. In alpine environments, camp stoves may be needed to melt drinking water from snow. Stoves have varied efficiency (i.e., how much water can be boiled per unit of fuel) and heat output (i.e., how quickly they boil water). There are a variety of stove types from which to choose (Tables 111-2 to 111-4).

TABLE 111-2	Recommended Stove Type per Activity
Activity	**Stove Type**
Backpacking	Canister stove system
Winter or high-elevation use	Liquid-fuel stove
Large groups	Liquid-fuel stove
To boil water only	Canister stove system
Ultralight backpacking	Canister, alcohol, or solid-fuel stove
International travel	Multifuel stove

TABLE 111-3	Canister Stove: Advantages and Disadvantages	
Advantages	**Disadvantages**	
Easy to use	Fuel is expensive.	
Compact and lightweight	Poor cold-weather performance	
Good flame control	Reduced heat output over time	
No spilled fuel	Difficult to judge quantity of fuel remaining	
Instant maximum heat output	Canister fuel difficult to find internationally	
Burns clean	Can be unstable—small base, high center of gravity	
No priming	Not widely recyclable	

BOX 111-6 Important Tips on Battery Selection and Use

- Alkaline batteries are standard and relatively inexpensive. Name brands may provide more useful hours than budget brands. Alkaline batteries are shorter lasting and perform worse in cold environments than lithium batteries. Lithium batteries provide a constant voltage output until they fail. Alkaline batteries slowly decrease voltage output as they are drained.
- Rechargeable batteries are an option for short outings. Disposable alkaline cells yield about double the power/weight of rechargeable batteries. Lithium-ion rechargeable batteries are preferred. They do not have "memory" and thus do not need to be deep-charged; they can be "topped off" without a full discharge. Older nickel–metal hydride rechargeable batteries need to be frequently fully discharged, then recharged.
- Try to choose electronics that all use a single type of battery so that you only need to carry one type for replacement (e.g., carry a headlamp, laryngoscope, otoscope, avalanche beacon, radio, and GPS unit that all take size AA batteries). Newer, lighter electronics may use AAA, rechargeable, or camera-size batteries.
- Make sure to have a backup plan if batteries fail. For example, be prepared to navigate with a compass if a Global Positioning System (GPS) unit stops working. Remove batteries from stored electronics when trip is completed to prevent corrosive damage.

TABLE 111-4 Fuel Comparison

Fuel	Advantages	Disadvantages
White gas	Cleanest, most efficient fuel Spilled fuel evaporates quickly. Readily available in United States Best for cold weather use	Priming usually required Spilled fuel very flammable
Kerosene	Spilled fuel will not ignite easily. Fuel sold throughout world High heat output	Priming required Spilled fuel evaporates slowly. Noticeable odor
Unleaded auto gas	Most readily available in United States	Priming usually required Spilled fuel very flammable Gas additives can lead to clogging.

The simplest stove is a solid-fuel stove. These stoves burn wood, natural charcoal, or other burnable materials. They are light and compact because fuel is not carried but usually gathered at the site. They are good for emergency or limited use, especially when abundant wood is available. Variations in heat and flame may make cooking unpredictable. They are best for short trips when one is not relying on the stove for survival.

Alcohol-fuel stoves are usually aluminum with brass burners. Liquid alcohol is poured into the burner and lit. Denatured alcohol (sometimes called methylated spirits or solvent alcohol) is a mixture of ethyl and methyl alcohols and is often available in hardware stores. Isopropyl alcohol and grain alcohol (pure ethanol) can also be used. Alcohol stoves are lightweight, compact, quiet, and have no moving parts or complicated valves. They can be difficult to control and can have limited heat output (e.g., the Trangia takes 7 to 10 minutes to boil 0.65 L of water). Given their simplicity, these stoves are sometimes preferred by "ultralight" campers.

Canister stoves burn fuel from a sealed, pressurized canister containing either butane or a butane-propane blend (Figure 111-14). These stoves are easy to ignite and burn hot. They are powerful and typically boil 1 L of water in 3 to 4 minutes. They are clean burning, do not leave soot, and rarely clog. The canisters are not refillable but can be recycled. For single use, Jetboil has an efficient, lightweight, and compact system. The pot also serves as an insulated mug, eliminating the need for additional cook set or bowl/cup (Figure 111-14C). Most canisters feature a Lindal valve with standardized threading so that fuel canisters are interchangeable between brands. Canister stoves have drawbacks. In cold temperatures (<0° C [32° F]), canisters depressurize, leading to a weak or no flame. As the canister warms, it repressurizes, and function returns. Canisters may be kept warm in sleeping bags or inside coats. A windscreen should not be used with a canister stove because it can cause heat to build up around the canister and cause it to explode. Canister stoves are starting to replace white-gas stoves as the standard for backcountry travel. A 226.8-g (8-oz) canister of fuel will boil water for two people for 4 days in summer temperatures. Wind, low temperatures, and longer cooking times increase fuel consumption.

White-gas stoves burn a purified form of gasoline. Fuel-filled bottles are pressurized with a tiny pump before use (Figure 111-14D). In cold temperatures and high altitudes, they may require priming with isopropyl or ethyl alcohol before lighting. They are powerful and reliable but can be messy and smell of gasoline. They may require frequent cleaning using specialized

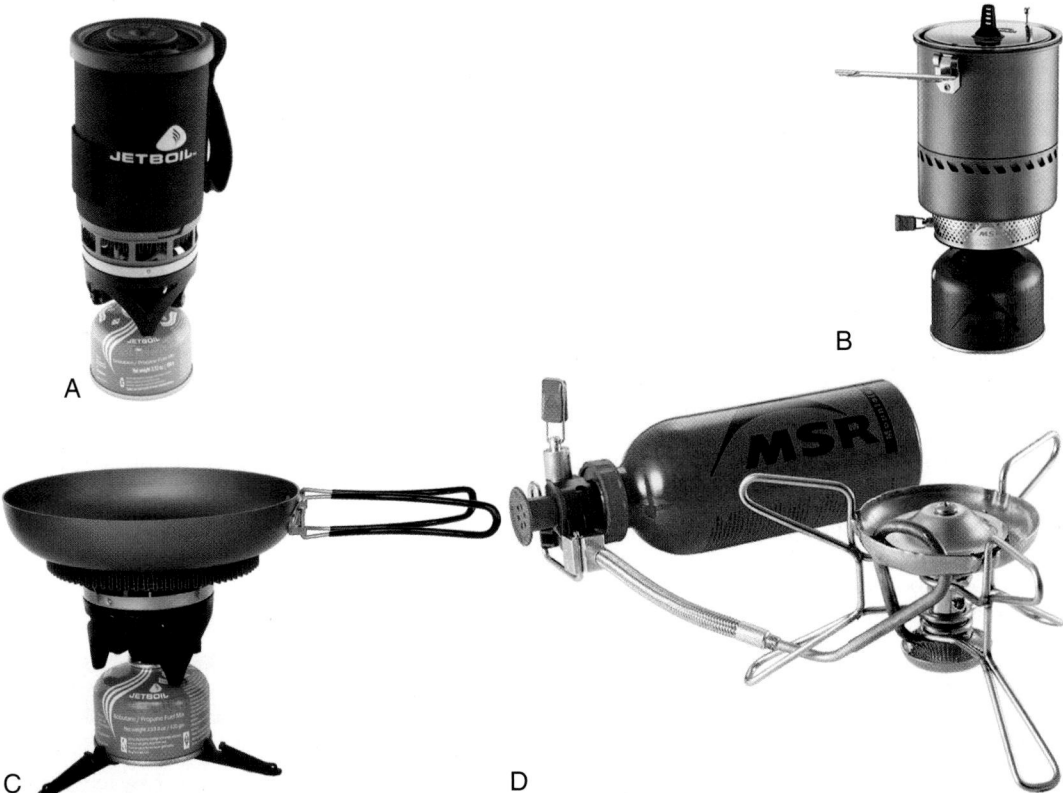

FIGURE 111-14 A, Jetboil Personal Cooking System (PCS) is an ultracompact 1-L (1.1-qt) unit, ideal for dehydrated meals, coffee or tea on the go, remote worksites, and emergency kits. Travel light. The PCS is a complete food and beverage multitool and weighs about a pound. **B,** MSR Reactor canister stove. **C,** Jetboil Ring and Fry Pan used with the Jetboil Group Cooking System (GCS). **D,** MSR WhisperLite International.

tools because of carbon deposits. Some versions have built-in cleaning tools to simplify this task. Gas is found in most camping stores, often sold as Coleman Fuel. These stoves should be used with a windscreen and heat reflector to improve heat transfer. The fuel is stored in refillable aluminum bottles of 0.3-, 0.6-, or 1-L sizes. These stoves may be slightly less powerful than canister stoves and boil 1 L of water in 4 to 5 minutes.

Gas requirements suggested by MSR are 114 mL (3.9 oz) of liquid fuel per person per day for cooking, and double that for melting snow and cooking. For an extremely cold trip, one may require as much as four times the amount of liquid fuel per person per day. Multifuel stoves are variations of the white-gas stove, with a more versatile jet that accepts a variety of petroleum-based fuels, many of which are less pure than white gas. In addition to white gas, these stoves may burn kerosene, unleaded or leaded auto fuel, or jet fuel. They are useful for international travelers who might not have access to white gas or pressurized canisters. Improved versatility may be accompanied by jets frequently clogging with carbon soot, especially with poor-quality fuel. They do not burn as hot when using fuel with impurities. Multifuel stoves should be used primarily with white gas; alternative fuels should be used in emergencies or when standard white gas is unavailable. See http://fuel.papo-art.com/ for a detailed list of international fuel names.

Dual-fitting stoves (e.g., OmniFuel stove by Primus) have fittings for both liquid fuel (similar to multifuel stoves) and pressurized canisters with a butane-propane mix. Although expensive and heavier, this stove burns any available fuel. This may be the best choice for expeditions outside the United States.

Two-burner portable camp stoves usually burn propane or white gas. They work well when camping with vehicle support, pack animals, or boats. A two-burner stove is superb for cooking large meals for groups. Propane canisters are heavier and bulkier than white-gas bottles, but propane burns cleanly and efficiently.

Once stove type has been decided, compare different brands using burn time, boil time, and liters of water boiled per 100 g (3.5 oz) of fuel. *Burn time* describes how long a stove burns using a given amount of fuel. *Boil time* is the period required to bring 1 L of 21.1° C (70° F) water to a boil. "Liters of water boiled (per 100 g of fuel)" measures fuel efficiency at full stove power. Fuel degrades when it contacts air. Fuel should be stored in an airtight container.

Accessories

The following accessories may be available for certain stoves:
- *Flame adjuster.* Many canister and liquid-fuel stoves allow flames to be adjusted from full power to simmer.
- *Auto lighter.* A small, hand-operated piezoelectric sparker ignites the flame. This can be unreliable in wind or rain. Always carry matches or a lighter for backup.
- *Cleaning tool.* Some stoves are maintenance free. However, many liquid-fuel stoves can be clogged with soot. Many models have built-in cleaning devices. Others use a cleaning tool to unclog the valve. In emergencies, a safety pin can suffice if the tool is lost, but the jet may be permanently altered and may impair function.
- *Heat reflector.* Many white-gas stoves include a heat reflector to channel heat from the flame directly to the pot. For most pressurized canister models, this is not recommended because the stove may become too hot, damaging valves and seals and posing a risk of canister rupture. Always follow the manufacturer's recommendations.
- *Windscreens* on white-gas stoves can improve transfer of heat to the pot and minimize wind-related heat loss. Windscreens for pressurized canister stoves are not recommended by the manufacturer in some cases.
- A *stove case* can help protect the stove and reduce soot transfer during transport.

It is important to be able to disconnect fuel from the stove for careful storage. Folding or collapsing the stove makes storage easier, but the stove should be simple to reassemble. Airline regulations prohibit travel with fuel. Box 111-3 includes information on stove safety.

COOK SETS

For most 1- or 2-night trips with one or two campers, a single 1-L pot is usually adequate for boiling water for morning drinks and melting snow for water. For more people, consider carrying two pots or a larger, 2- or 3-L pot. Nesting pots that fit inside each other pack well and offer more versatile sizes (e.g., 0.5, 1, and 2 L). Lids shorten cooking time and protect food from debris. A pot handle or pliers is essential to lift hot pots from burners. Cookware is constructed from aluminum, stainless steel, or titanium. Aluminum is light, inexpensive, and conducts heat well, but it is not as durable as other materials and can dent easily. Titanium is extremely light and strong, but it is expensive and does not conduct heat as well as other materials. Stainless steel is the heaviest and most durable and is scratch resistant.

Nonstick coatings are cleaned easily when adequate water and soap are available. However, sand, dirt, and utensils wear down these coatings quickly.

Specialized pots with a built-in heat exchanger (e.g., Jetboil system previously mentioned) may increase the stove's efficiency.

Cooking utensils include pot grips, serving spoon, ladle, and spatula. For personal utensils, ultralight campers carry only a spoon or spork (a spoon/fork utensil with a spoon on one end and fork on the other; the edge of the fork is serrated for cutting food). Plastic utensils are the norm because they are durable, light, and easy to clean. A small bowl and covered mug usually are adequate for personal dishes.

Dish soap and a small sponge are used to clean cook sets and utensils. Biodegradable camp soap is sold in most outdoor and camp supply stores. Camp soap, hand soap, and shampoo are available in dissolvable sheets that create suds when contacted by water.

PERSONAL TOILETRIES

Personal hygiene is extremely important in wilderness travel for group and individual health. A typical list of toiletries includes:
- Toothbrush, collapsible
- Toothpaste
- Dental floss
- All-purpose camp soap (can be used for dishes, hair, and skin)
- Alcohol-based antiseptic hand gel
- Lotion/sunscreen
- Wet wipes
- Toilet paper
- Feminine hygiene products
- Razor and shaving cream
- Compact hairbrush or comb
- Travel towel (Figure 111-15)

SLEEPING BAGS

Sleep quality is important. A warm sleeping bag can be lifesaving. New products feature higher-fill down, softer synthetics, and lighter constructions. Box 111-7 lists points of comparison for insulation. Determine the purpose of the bag, and then consider comfort, weight, and size.

When choosing a sleeping bag, consider shell material (water resistant vs. untreated nylon), fill materials (down or synthetic

---

BOX 111-7   Down vs. Synthetic-Filled Sleeping Bags, Comparing Equal-Weight Bags

Down	Synthetic
Warmer	Easy to clean and store
More compressible	Retains significant warmth when wet
Softer	Dries quicker
Longer lasting	Less expensive
	Less likely to be allergenic

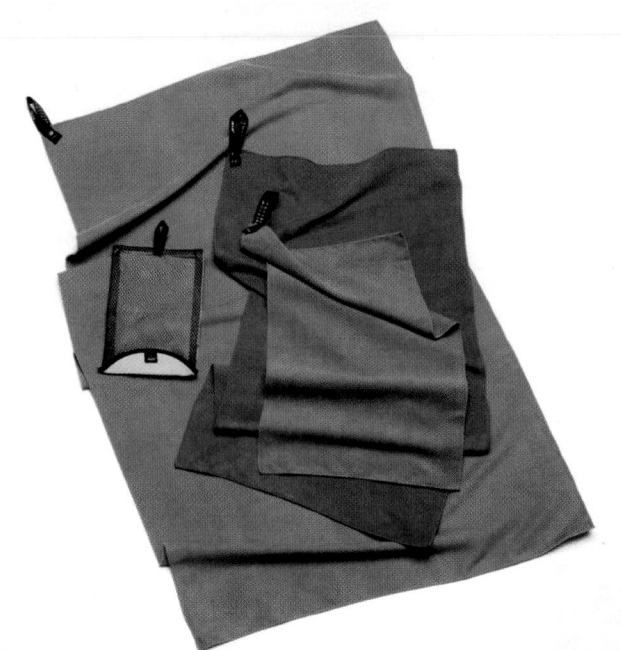

FIGURE 111-15 MSR PackTowl UltraLite. Quick-to-dry, lightweight, microfiber travel towels.

[influences weight and warmth]), shape (rectangular or mummy), and zipper options (which side, full length, coupling).

Insulation

Down. Down has no equal for warmth-to-weight ratio and compressibility. Compared with synthetic fill, down is more durable, retaining the ability to rebound to full volume over years of compression cycles. Down settles closely around the body and feels warmer and cozier than do synthetic fillers. Down is best for alpine trips where cold temperatures are encountered and is also a good choice for trips requiring light and compact gear. Down is less well suited for wet environments. Down should not be stored compressed.

Down is expensive and must be used with care. If down becomes wet, it loses its ability to insulate. Wet down takes an enormous amount of time and energy to dry out. Sleeping bag shells can be constructed from water-resistant laminates (e.g., Gore-Tex). Although these may improve weather resistance, they may not breathe well, allowing the down to become wet from perspiration. Uncoated nylon, the typical shell material for sleeping bags, breathes much better but is not waterproof. A tent or bivouac sack can be used to protect the bag from becoming wet.

Fill power provides a valuable measure to quantify the overall insulatory value of down. The volume of a 28-g (1-oz) sample of down being compressed by weighted piston is measured in a Plexiglas cylinder. The test requires controlled temperature, humidity, and preparation of the sample. If other factors are equal, a sleeping bag made with high-fill power will be lighter and more compressible than an equally warm bag filled with lower-quality down. Fill power is expressed as cubic inches per ounce. A lofting power of 400 to 450 is considered medium quality, 500 to 550 good, 550 to 750 very good, and 750+ excellent. Currently, 800+ fill is top quality; for example, 800-fill-power is warmer than 600-fill-power. For the same warmth rating, an 800-fill-power bag is the lightest.

Synthetics. Synthetic insulation does not absorb as much water as does down and continues to provide effective insulation when damp. Synthetic bags are preferred for outings where the bag may become wet (e.g., boating, rafting) or in climates where rain may be anticipated. They work well for people who frequently encounter dirty conditions and for children, because these are easy to launder. Synthetics should not be stored compressed in a stuff sack.

Synthetic insulators include polyester, polypropylene, blends, and proprietary fabrics (e.g., Polarguard, Hollofil, PrimaLoft). Synthetics are extruded petroleum-based polymers formed into *batts* or sheets of fibers to maximize the air-trapping qualities of the fiber. They provide a consistent thickness and durability to allow for use into a sleeping bag. Fiber designs include:

- *Short fiber.* Original polyester fiber fills were made of short fibers loosely arranged in a batt. This offered compressibility, but the fibers tended to shift and settle, allowing thin spots to form in the sleeping bag. Modern versions of short-fiber insulations are now bonded together.
- *Continuous filament.* Designed to prevent the thin spots seen with short-fiber fills, these batts consist of continuous filaments of polyester arranged into uniformly thick layers. They retain their shape and fiber position over time but have decreased compressibility, so tend to be bulky.
- *Microfiber.* In the last decade, development of superfine polyester (and other synthetic) fibers has improved warmth-to-weight ratios. Advanced bonding and fiber stabilization processes create compressible, lightweight synthetic fills with excellent loft, air-trapping ability, and water resistance.

From a pure warmth-to-weight basis, synthetics neither compete with top-quality down, nor are they as durable (tending to lose loft over time). When absolute warmth-to-weight is critical and environmental conditions allow, down is still the preferred choice.

Temperature

Temperature ratings vary between manufacturers, quality of down or synthetic filler, construction, design, and shell material. Choose a lightweight bag rated 30° to 45° F (−1.1° to 7.2° C) for summer fair weather, travel to the tropics, or an emergency bag for search and rescue. For three-season use below timberline, select a sleeping bag rated 20° to 15° F (−6.7° to −9.4° C). Choose a warmer bag, rated 0° F (−17.8° C), if carrying fewer clothes or if you prefer more warmth. For four-season use above timberline, consider a bag rated 5° to −20° F (−15° to −28.9° C). High-altitude expedition bags are usually rated −20° F (−28.9° C) or −40° F/C.

A sleeping bag's temperature rating is only an approximate guide to the lowest temperature at which an average person will remain warm. Although a useful adjunct to consider, in the United States the rating is assigned by the manufacturer, and variability exists across the industry. Factors that influence a rating and one's comfort at low temperatures in a sleeping bag include metabolic rate, type of sleeping pad, type of tent or shelter, amount and type of clothing worn, design and construction of sleeping bag, nutrition, and hydration status. In Europe, a standardized rating system (EN 13537) controls these variables. The European rating assumes use of one synthetic base layer worn (top and bottom), a hat, and a closed-cell foam sleeping pad of standard thickness. The results of this rating system are reported in three numbers: the upper and lower temperature limits at which a man is comfortable, and the lower temperature limit at which a woman is comfortable.

A bag's insulation value is related to the loft material and thickness. Winter and mountain expedition bags usually have 15 to 23 cm (6 to 9 inches) of loft; midweight bags may have 10 to 15 cm (4 to 6 inches) of loft; and those for summer may have 5 cm (2 inches) of loft.

The bag should be fitted to the individual's body size. A bag that is too long or wide results in dead space to be heated. Bags specific to women have greater insulation in the hip and feet areas. Mummy bags provide the most efficient shape (Figure 111-16).

Rectangular bags are bulky, allowing excess material around the legs and feet. Because they allow more space, they can be more comfortable for someone who changes positions frequently during sleep. These bags may be reasonable for car camping or if a mummy bag feels too restrictive (Figure 111-17A and Box 111-8). Consider using a sweater or coat as a "collar" at the top of a rectangular bag to prevent heat loss. Sleeping bags are sized for women (short, 5½ feet [167.6 cm]), men (regular, 6 feet [182.9 cm]), and tall (6½ feet [200.7 cm]). Bags have right- or left-sided zippers. Individual bags may be chosen with compatible

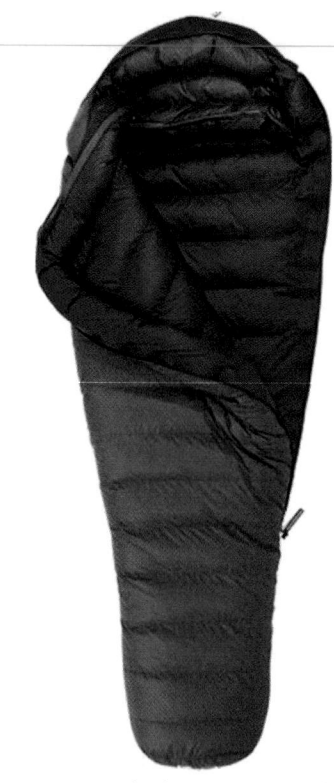

FIGURE 111-16 Standard mummy down sleeping bag.

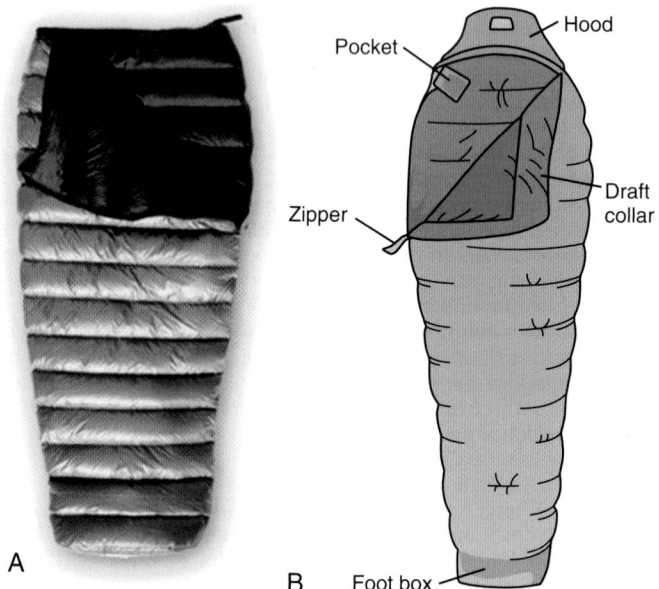

A   B

FIGURE 111-17 A, Semirectangular down sleeping bag for those who find a mummy bag too restricting. **B,** Anatomy of a sleeping bag.

BOX 111-8	Sleeping Bag Shape Comparison
Mummy	**Rectangular**
Efficient	High volume
Light	Heavy
Warm	Less warm
Expensive	Less expensive
Restrictive	Comfortable

BOX 111-9	Tips to Stay Warmer at Night

- Wear a hat to bed.
- Wear clothes to bed, especially wool or synthetic long underwear.
- Use a liner of silk or fleece.
- Use a thicker pad or two pads.
- Use a bivouac sack or outer bag.
- Consider buying a warmer tent or bag.
- Eat a high-fat snack or drink a high-calorie beverage before going to bed to provide additional calories for generating heat at night.
- Fill your water bottle with hot water—close securely, and place in sleeping bag.

zippers so that they may be connected. A full-length zipper allows better temperature regulation but adds weight.

Warmth is added to sleeping bags in other ways (Box 111-9). A draft tube is an insulated tube covering the zipper, preventing wind from entering and heat from escaping the bag. A shoulder collar seals in warmth. A hood can insulate the head and most of the face. Both should have drawstrings and should be able to cinch loosely to fully cover the user, except for the nose, mouth, and eyes (Figure 111-17B). A convertible sleeping bag provides an accessory blanket that may be zipped on in winter and off in summer.

SLEEPING PADS

A sleeping pad is critical for warmth and comfort. A thicker pad offers more insulation from the ground and may offer more comfort. A summer camper may be able to stay warm and comfortable with a pad ranging from 1.9 cm (0.75 inch) to 3.8 cm (1.5 inches). A snow camper should use a 5-cm-thick (2-inch-thick) pad for adequate insulation. Thicker pads are likely to be bulkier and heavier.

Closed-cell foam pads are the least expensive and most durable. Dense foam is filled with sealed air cells. If strapped outside a backpack, it can be exposed to the elements and still function well. Closed-cell foam does not soak up water. It provides superior insulation against the cold ground but may provide less cushioning than other pads. Alpinists, climbers, and adventure sports participants favor these pads (Figure 111-18).

Open-cell foam is similar to a sponge with tiny, open air cells. These are comfortable, lightweight, and compressible but not as durable, and they do not insulate as well as closed-cell pads. Open-cell pads can absorb large quantities of water.

A 5-cm-thick (2-inch-thick) dual-density pad provides a blend of warmth, durability, and comfort. These pads usually have thick, abrasion-resistant closed-cell foam on one side and lighter, more compressible open-cell foam for comfort on the other. They are best used in dry or sheltered conditions.

"Self-inflating" pads are preferred by many backpackers for their comfort and compatibility. These are nylon-encased open-cell foam with an air valve. The nylon shell protects the foam from absorbing water and holds air to improve insulation and comfort (Figure 111-19). Although nominally "self-inflating," they usually require a person to blow them up. These pads are often heavier than closed-cell foam pads but can be just as comfortable as open-cell pads. The amount of air in the pad can be adjusted for comfort. A small puncture can render them unusable. Always carry a patch kit, which includes a strip of adhesive-backed shell material or some nonadhesive material and rubber cement. A bike repair patch kit usually works, as may duct tape. In most environments, a ground cloth should be used to prevent punctures.

The newest generation of inflatable pads have no foam inside and use ultralight materials. They are lightweight and comfortable but not as warm as "self-inflating" pads and even more susceptible to punctures.

Pad accessories may improve comfort but add weight. Pads may have built-in pillows, separate air chambers that can be

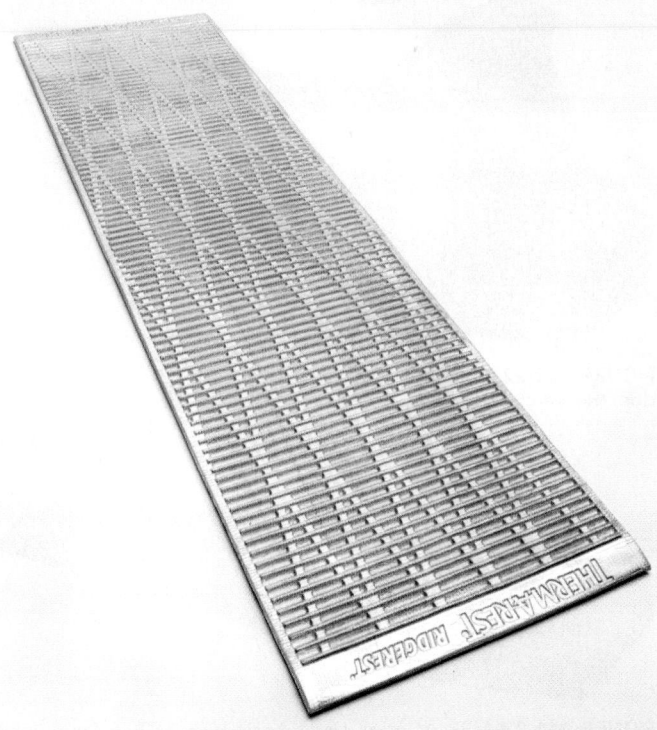

FIGURE 111-18 Therm-a-Rest-RidgeRest SOLite. The unique ridged pattern traps heat and provides more comfort than any flat-foam mattress and is practically indestructible, providing comfort you can take anywhere.

FIGURE 111-19 Therm-a-Rest sleeping pad. "Self-inflating" air mattresses come in variable thicknesses and lengths.

adjusted for comfort, and nonslip surfaces so that the sleeping bag does not slide off the pad during the night. To save weight, consider a mummy-shaped pad that matches the footprint of the sleeping bag. For use in nonwinter conditions, use a three-quarter-length pad in which the feet and forelegs hang off the pad. There are female-specific pads that have more insulation and support in the midsection and foot section.

SHELTERS

Shelters protect travelers from rain, snow, cold, heat, sun, insects, small animals, and dirt. They provide privacy in crowded areas and a place to store and operate equipment (Figure 111-20).

Construction and Design

Most tents used by wilderness professionals are freestanding; they will stand up without guy lines or stakes. The exceptions are tents or tarps used by ultralight backpackers or cyclists, where space and weight are at a premium. Nonfreestanding tents are lighter because they do not require as many poles in the design, but they require stakes and guy lines. They take longer to set up and are typically not as sturdy in wind and rain.

Almost all shelters are constructed of nylon. *Nylon* is a generic term for petroleum-based polyamide fabrics made in numerous weaves and thicknesses. It is light and strong, resists abrasion, is easy to wash, has low absorbency, and is easy to stow. Most tents use thin-strand *ripstop*, an extremely lightweight nylon woven in square grids that resists tears, or *taffeta*, which is a light, soft nylon. Some tents and almost all rain flies are made more waterproof and windproof by using a urethane coating on one side of the nylon.

Poles are usually aluminum, or in some cases, fiberglass or carbon. Aluminum is strong and less expensive.

Most tents are double walled and have a separate rain fly. The double-wall system allows the tent to be used without the rain fly in mild weather. The rain fly, usually waterproof urethane-coated nylon, sheds rain, enhances protection from the wind,

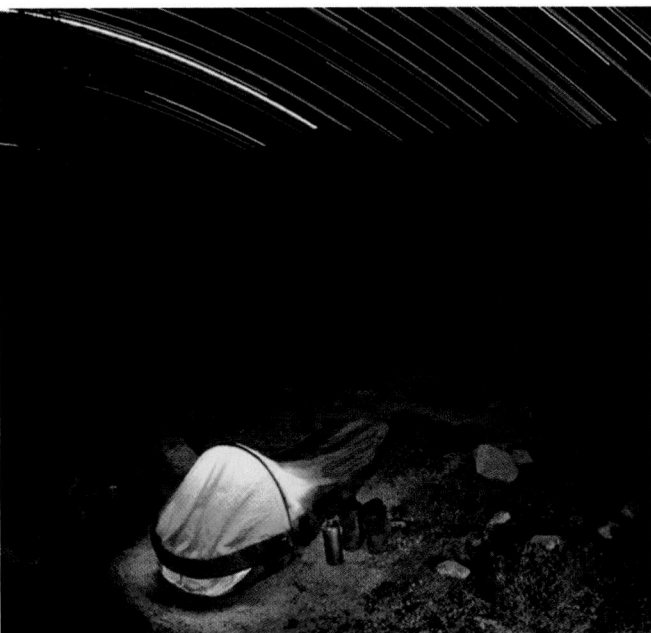

FIGURE 111-20 Bivouac camping under the stars. (*Copyright 2010, Outdoor Research Marketing.*)

and provides warmth because it traps a layer of air. The double-wall system allows the tent to "breathe" moisture through the tent and still accomplish weatherproofing with the second layer.

Certain three- or four-season tents are made with specialized fabrics in a single-wall construction without a separate rain fly. These do not breathe as well and are not as warm but are compact and light. They allow weatherproofing without the bulk and weight of two-layer tents. Ultralight mountaineers, backpackers, mountain bikers, and cyclists favor these when foul weather may be encountered, and when weight and space are at a premium and simplicity of setup is essential.

Shape and Size

Most wilderness tents are dome shaped. Compared with square or triangular tents, dome tents are lower profile, stronger in the wind and rain, easier to set up, lighter, and less bulky when packed. Ultralightweight tents (e.g., those used by ultralight backpackers and cyclists) are sometimes tunnel-shaped or hoop tents. They are set up with one or two hoops with guy lines and are usually not freestanding. A-frame tents are a more traditional style with a rectangular floor and a single center pole at each end. These tents are not freestanding but are very lightweight because they have the fewest poles. Large camping tents, 4 × 4 m (13.1 × 13.1 feet), with external poles are good for car-supported camping and expeditions but are too bulky and heavy for most other applications. Specialty tents, including plastic- and canvas-walled military or research tents, are used in extreme climates.

Tents are measured in square feet or the number of persons who will reasonably fit without backpacks or gear. A typical two- to three-person tent is approximately 2.3 to 4.2 m² (25 to 45 feet²). A typical four- to five-person shelter can be around 4.6 to 6.5 m² (50 to 70 feet²). Six- to eight-person shelters can be as large as 11.1 m² (120 feet²).

Bivouac Sack

A bivouac sack provides basic shelter. This one-person overbag provides protection from the elements in a very small package just large enough to encase a sleeping bag. Some have an aluminum pole that bends to form a hoop to keep the bivouac sac off the face when sleeping. Others are simple nylon bags that slide over the sleeping bag. These provide warmth, and with laminated waterproof coatings, can keep one fairly dry. They are especially useful for brief 1- or 2-day outings, for trips that require minimizing weight and bulk, and for mild-weather adventures. A bivouac sac is also a fairly lightweight option for an emergency shelter (Figures 111-21 to 111-23).

Tarps

Tarps and *wings* are floorless shelters that provide sun and rain protection, but little protection from the wind, insects, or cold, damp ground. These minimum shelters are excellent for ultralight backpacking; cycling in clear, warm weather; and for an emergency shelter. Some wings are freestanding, whereas others need to be tied to trees or vehicles with guy lines. Some can be supported by trekking poles (Figure 111-24). Used with depressions cut into snow, they can provide excellent protection in winter or alpine expeditions for cooking or sleeping (Figure 111-25).

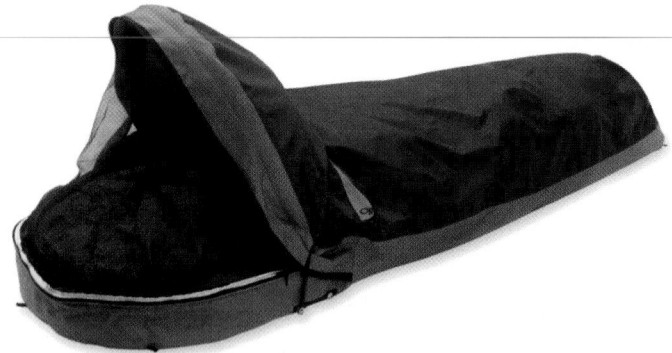

FIGURE 111-22 Outdoor Research Advanced Bivy—open. The Outdoor Research Advanced Bivy has a two-pole design to keep the material off the face and is an excellent lightweight option.

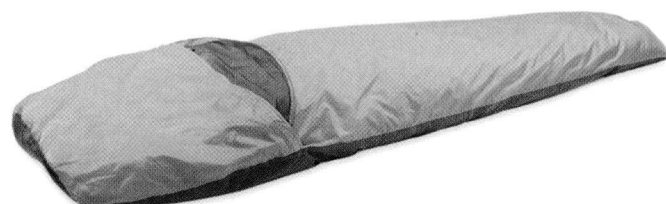

FIGURE 111-23 MSR AC-Bivy. Use a basic bivouac bag for a light-weight shelter in fair weather or as an emergency shelter for an unexpected night out.

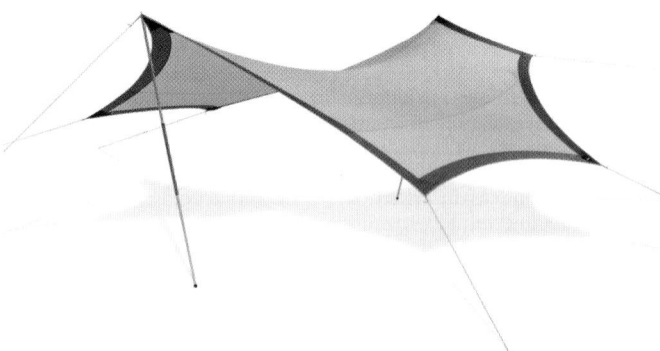

FIGURE 111-24 MSR Zing. Tarps can be used for shade and protection from rain and snow.

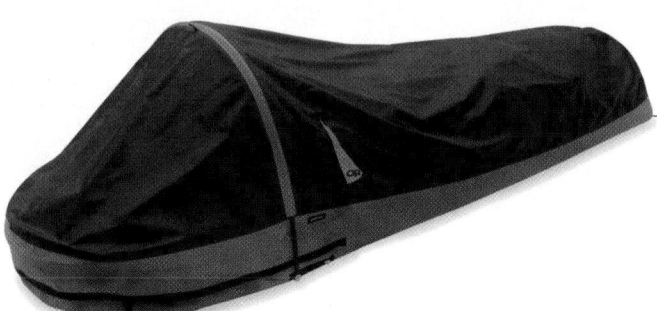

FIGURE 111-21 Outdoor Research Advanced Bivy—closed.

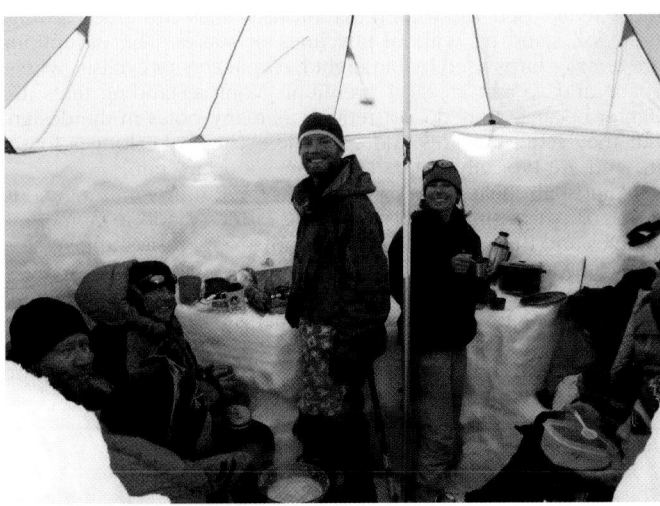

FIGURE 111-25 A snow kitchen. (*Courtesy Alaska Mountaineering School of Talkeetna; AMS Collection.*)

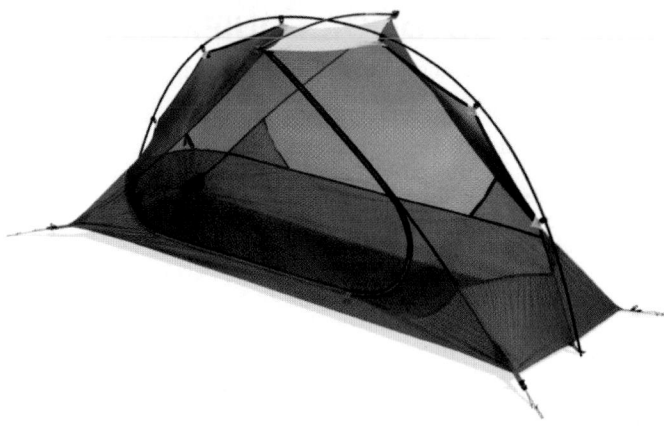

FIGURE 111-26 MSR Carbon Reflex 1 body. Lightweight summer tent with mesh panels.

Tents

Summer tents are usually all-mesh bug shelters or partial-mesh shelters with solid nylon panels at the apex to block the sun and provide shade (Figure 111-26).

Three-season tents are designed to withstand most weather conditions that occur outside of winter. They work well for all applications except mountaineering or severe wind and rain. Rain flies that extend to the ground are the most windproof and waterproof. Some less expensive tents have a rain fly that covers only the top one-third of the tent. Three-season tent sizes may range from one-person shelters to eight-person family tents.

Four-season tents are designed for mountain and winter use. Most have a full rain fly with a vestibule and minimize the use of mesh panels to conserve warmth. They are usually lower profile than are three-season tents, to minimize snow and wind effects, and are also usually constructed with four to six poles to maximize stability and handle loads of snow (Figure 111-27A). A four-season tent's main disadvantage is its bulk and weight. Most have internal guy points to further stabilize the tent in high winds and heavy snow loads. Some have air vents, because these tents do not breathe well.

Accessories

Many tents use accessories to improve function and versatility, as follows:

- Gear lofts and mesh pouches store clothing and equipment off the tent floor.
- Internal lash points can be used to rig clotheslines for drying wet clothing or to hang a flashlight.
- A footprint tarp protects the floor from rocks and dirt on the ground. This thin cloth keeps the tent dry.
- Mesh panels, mesh doors, and skylight panels work well for star gazing and ventilation and keep insects out of the tent.
- Large loops for stakes and guy lines secure the tent in wind and rain. Guy lines should be adjustable.
- Tent stakes help hold the tent on the ground and are sometimes necessary for nonfreestanding tents. These can be thin metal nails or hooks for dry, hard ground. In soft dirt, wide or large-diameter plastic stakes hold better. Long, wide stakes reach down into more compressed sand or snow. A stuff sack filled with snow, sand, or rocks, or "dead men" (stick/ski pole buried in the snow with line leading out) can be used to help secure a guy line (Figure 111-28). Skis are also helpful as "stakes" in snow.
- Many tents have a vestibule on the rain fly; this provides additional dry storage outside the tent (Figure 111-27B).
- Many tents have thicker, more durable material on the floor to protect from dirt and moisture.
- Some tents are "convertible," like the sleeping bags mentioned earlier. Weight and bulk can be adjusted depending on the weather conditions, length of outing, and terrain. For example,

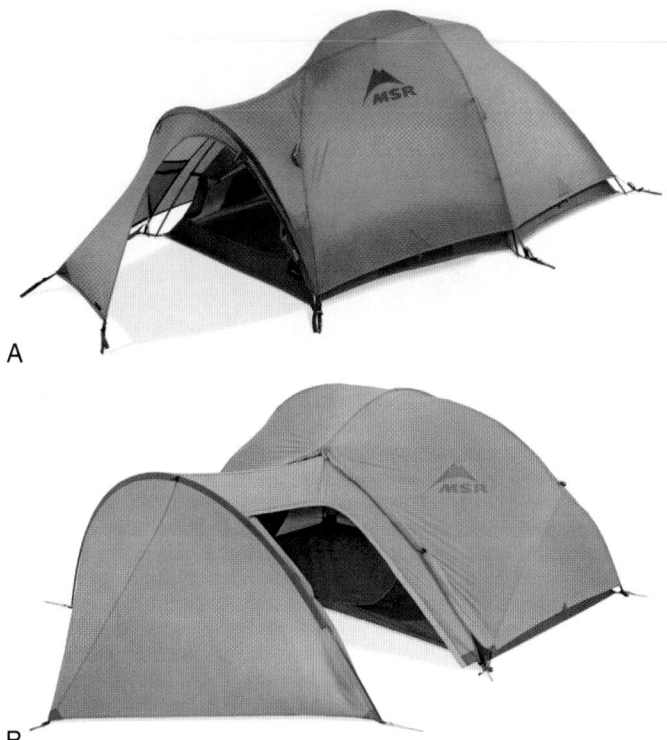

FIGURE 111-27 A, MSR Fury with fly. Standard four-season tent has a low profile with full-coverage fly and vestibule. **B,** MSR Gear Shed fly. Consider a large vestibule for extra space during inclement weather.

a four-season tent can be set up without one or two poles, or a vestibule can be detached. Some tents offer moderate wind and rain protection without the rain fly. Others allow the rain fly to be set up alone, to provide a simple floorless shelter (Figure 111-29).

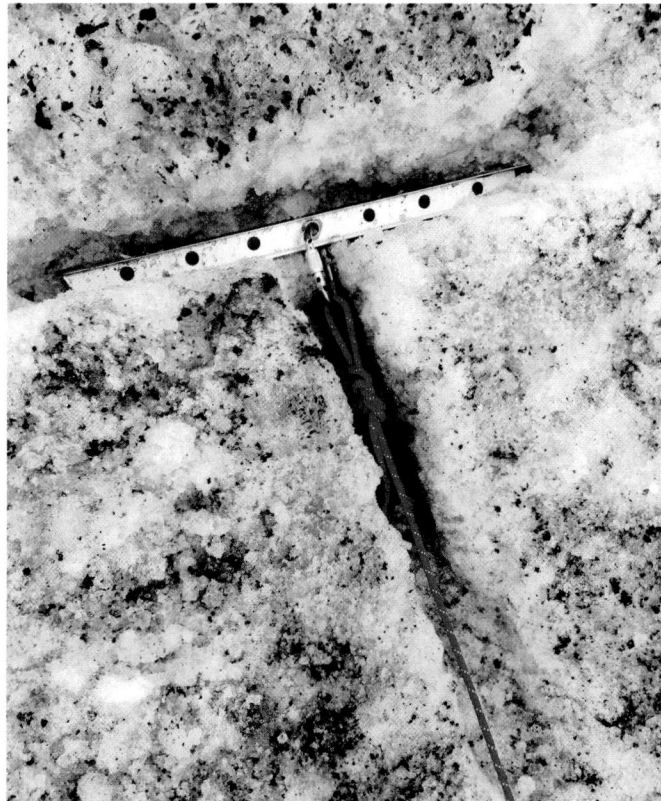

FIGURE 111-28 "Dead man" tent stake.

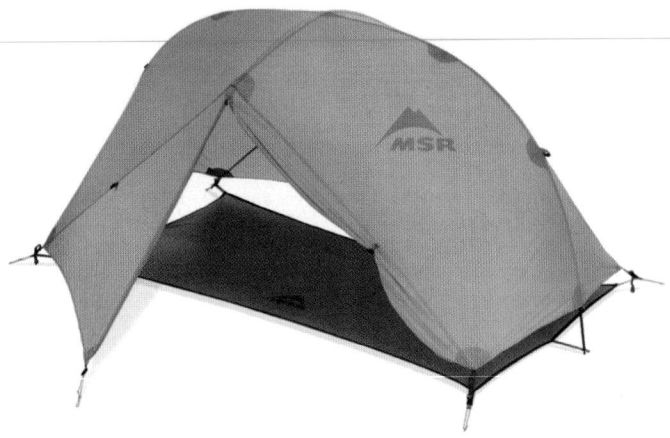

FIGURE 111-29 MSR Carbon Reflex two fly and footprint. To reduce weight during fair-weather camping, use a tent fly and footprint for shelter.

CARE OF OUTDOOR EQUIPMENT

Gear needs to be cleaned and inspected regularly. Replace worn or broken parts before beginning a trip. Carry spare parts and repair material (see Box 111-5). Make sure equipment, especially tents and sleeping bags, are dried thoroughly after use. Soft gear should never be stored in a compressed (stuffed) manner, because materials will break down more quickly. Tents will last longer if stored hung in a cool, dark place. Knives rust and tents mildew when stored damp.

Follow the manufacturer's recommendations on washing and cleaning. Some hardware can be cleaned in warm soapy water. Other equipment should only be rinsed with warm water. Equipment works better when it is clean and well lubricated.

Cooking utensils and pots should be washed with hot soapy water. If hot soapy water is unavailable, an alcohol-based cleanser may be used. Backcountry cooking is not the place to skimp on cleaning or hygiene.

SELECTED RESOURCES

Selected resources used in this text are available online at www.expertconsult.inkling.com.

CHAPTER 112
Native American Healing

KENNETH S. COHEN

KENNETH S. COHEN

Author's Note: A Word About Style
In writing about Native American healing, the third-person voice, common in scientific works, is generally considered neither appropriate nor ethical. It is personal experience and involvement that demonstrate to indigenous readers that the author is legitimate, has considered oral tradition as well as relevant literature, and is accountable to Native people and communities. It is an acknowledgment that the author is a human being rather than an "authority," and that what is known is always a mere raindrop compared to the immense ocean of the unknown. —KSC

The very concept of *Native American wilderness medicine* may seem redundant. Until the industrial age, all Native American medicine was learned, developed, and practiced in the wilderness. One might be of the mindset that the wisdom of ancient subsistence cultures has little relevance to the modern world. However, from an indigenous perspective, modern Americans are no less subsistence based (and therefore entirely dependent on the earth's resources) than were precontact (i.e., before 1492) Native Americans. As ecologist Gary Holtaus[33] explains, we are still a subsistence culture, although not a sustainable one. The Native American model of health, in which nature is the source of healing power, is as applicable today as at any time in the past.

Each of the thousands of precontact tribes of "Turtle Island," a common indigenous name for North America, had its strategies and tools for health, adaptation, and survival. Many of these are still used among the approximately 700 Native Nations that remain today. The methods reflect the variety of the North American landscape: The Yoeme of the Sonoran Desert recognize herbs that protect against heat and snakebite, whereas the Inupiaq in Alaska are more concerned with frostbite and mos-quito stings. Different remedies are found in the desert, plains, tundra, and mountains and near lakes, rivers, and seas. Similarly, the requirements and seasons for vision seeking, pilgrimage, and ceremony vary by latitude and longitude. In the Northern Plains, it is rare to engage in a fasting and prayer vigil before the first spring thunder. Certain Pacific Northwest peoples may seek spiritual power in the winter, because the rainy season is a good time to commune with the spirit of water.

With so much diversity, it is impossible to explore in depth the specifics of Native American wilderness medicine in a single chapter. These details are better gleaned from many excellent ethnographies, herbal texts,[19,20,27-29,31,38,49,51,53,65,69,80] and biographies of traditional healers,[4,9-11,34,37,41,42,48,79] as well as the few comprehensive surveys of Native healing ways.[5,17,47,74] This chapter introduces widely shared principles among Nations as well as the ethos on which Native American medicine is based, illustrating the applications of this worldview with clinical examples from various tribes and geographic regions. America's original holistic medicine can enhance the modern practice of integrative and wilderness medicine.

DEFINITIONS

NATIVE AMERICAN

Native Americans or American Indians are the indigenous peoples of North America. In Canada, it is also common to refer to the original peoples as *First Nations, aboriginal,* or *autochthones* (French). Native Hawaiians and indigenous Americans of Central and South America are not discussed, although they share many of the same principles and practices. Ultimately, there is no perfect or correct generalization for North America's original people, because the very concept of "Native American" was a political expediency when indigenous people sought unity in the face of common postcolonial challenges, including military, political, cultural, economic, social, and health. A morally acceptable term was also needed to substitute for the word *savages* and other demeaning labels or stereotypes common in postcontact discourse.

There is no single Native American or First Nations culture. There are more than 4.3 million indigenous Americans in the United States[57] and another 1.3 million in Canada,[66] which are divided into more than 1162 recognized Native governments: approximately 600 in Canada, 562 in the United States, and hundreds more in various stages of the recognition process.[60] Approximately 225 Native languages are spoken in the United States, and another 50 in Canada.[3,60] A far greater number of North American indigenous languages are extinct or are no longer spoken fluently. These languages are divided into 50 language families, many as different from each other as Romance (e.g., Italian) from Sino-Tibetan.

Old Hollywood movies and popular literature characterized as "New Age"[78] promote a particular type of generic Indian: in buckskins and feathered headdresses, speaking Tonto-like broken English, and frozen in popular imagination in western landscapes. Museum exhibits sometimes reinforce the impression that Native Americans are relics from the past rather than a people concerned about their future. Today's Native Americans wear business suits rather than buckskins, prize higher education, and generally identify themselves as Christian (i.e., approximately 85% in the southeastern United States). They are patriots who volunteer in the armed forces in higher percentages than any other ethnic minority. They live in houses and apartments, not in tipis.

Indigenous Americans live in two worlds: the culture of their ancestors and that of the modern United States and Canada. Health care choices are influenced by this duality. Although Native Americans are more likely to seek an allopathic physician than a traditional tribal healer, there remains widespread respect for many traditional remedies, such as prayers, herbal medicines, counseling, and ceremonies. Sometimes, ancient and modern healing methods are combined to create synergistic effects.[23,26] Prescription medicines *smudged* in sage smoke and prepared with prayer are believed to be more effective than other methods of administration. Counseling complements the sweat lodge for treatment of posttraumatic stress disorder.[12] Among diabetes patients, nutrient ratios are managed with a traditional native diet by substituting indigenous grains such as amaranth and wild rice for high-glycemic starches such as potatoes and bread. Native healers have always practiced "holistic" or "integrative" medicine. These terms take on more meaning as Native Americans find creative ways to combine the old and the new.

HEALTH

Like their Western counterparts, Native healers are concerned with relieving suffering, improving quality of life, and managing or curing disease. The World Health Organization's definition of health is congruent with that of many Native American healers: "Health is a state of complete physical, mental and social well-being and not merely the absence of disease or infirmity."[81] Native healers add to this definition two more elements: spiritual and environmental. Health becomes a state of balance characterized by physical, mental, social, spiritual, and environmental well-being. Implicit in this definition is a philosophy summarized by the saying, "All my relations" (or "relatives"). Whether recited in English or in a Native language (e.g., "Mitakuye Oyasin" in

Lakota), this phrase means that health is a state of connectedness in which stones, plants, animals, and people are recognized as family. A type of affirmation that may close a prayer, it is sometimes compared with the word *Amen,* but it means much more than that. *Amen,* which is Hebrew for "so be it," implies assent or approval, whereas *Mitakuye Oyasin* may be translated as "We are all children of the Great Spirit. May my words, prayer, song, and ceremonial actions be for the harmony and good of all."

"All my relations" is an expression of the recognition that family and community are essential elements of health. During precontact times, health and survival of a tribe depended on each person doing his or her part to the best of his or her ability. Indulging in shame, self-pity, acting-out behaviors, social withdrawal, or extravagance and excess consumption were not personal matters. What now would be considered "group therapy" might occur during a meeting or council that included one or more wise elders. Confidentiality was not an issue. Today, the value and importance of community remain, but psychological or psychiatric problems and the need for therapy are perceived as social stigma and cause for embarrassment. Confidentiality is an important matter, and patients will sometimes avoid or delay allopathic treatment until they can visit therapists or clinics far away, where office workers or other patients are less likely to recognize them.

TRADITIONAL HEALERS

Many Native healing methods, such as herbal medicine, massage, and music, are similar to complementary and alternative medicine (CAM) therapies. Traditional North American Indian healers are often willing to share these methods with the public and with health care colleagues through lectures, courses, articles, books, and more rarely, in collaborative research.[50] However, it is important to understand that when a technique is removed from its original context of culture, language, and geography, it may not be as effective. In addition, the Native American physician is expected to set an example of Native values by actually believing in the reality of spiritual forces. It is not enough to imitate a method such as blending an herbal tea.

Native American healers may be specialists or have broad expertise. Among some tribes, there are separate terms for herbalists, bonesetters, midwives, diagnosticians, ceremonial experts, and people known for their gifts in massage, counseling, dreaming, or prayer. Some healers are recognized as holy people, whose direct contact with transcendent realms gives them the intuition, knowledge, and power to adapt or create methods that best fit the needs of their patients. These healers are popularly called *medicine men, medicine women,* or *holy people.* Fools Crow[48] (Lakota) and Flora Jones[5,39] (Wintu) are examples of well-respected 20th-century medicine people. None of the English-language terms for indigenous healers is exact; these terms are often used indiscriminately in popular literature. A person described as a "medicine man" may be considered primarily an herbalist in his own tribe. An ethnographer may label a woman an "herbalist" who is in fact a medicine woman. In this chapter, the term "traditional healer" is used as a general category for all the various types of indigenous North American healers. Traditional healers may be male or female and young or old, although most are older than 50 years.

One becomes a traditional healer by any combination of an innate gift or talent; personal training, including ceremonial participation, vision seeking, fasting, or apprenticeship; and a ritual transfer of power from a previous healer. "Personal training," although primarily experiential, may include learning from texts (e.g., healing chants and practices transcribed by the Cherokee in their own language)[9] as well as from historic audio recordings and other media, including representations of healing practices in rock art or herbal remedies drawn on "pharmacopoeia sticks"[52] (Figure 112-1). "Apprenticeship" involves learning from the example, demonstration, mentorship, and wisdom shared by a teacher.

Any of the terms for traditional healers, especially *medicine man/woman,* are conferred by a community or group of Native people in recognition of years of wise and effective service. Although one may call oneself an "herbalist" or "traditional

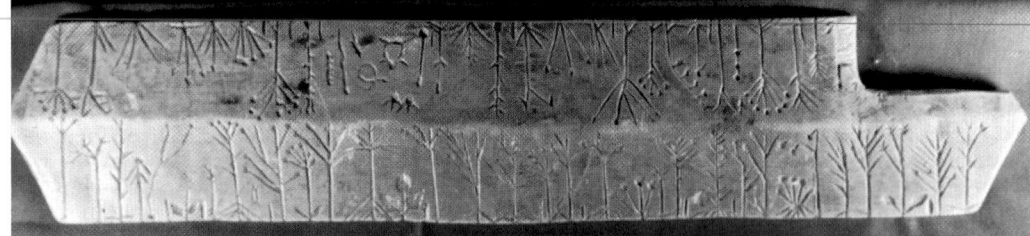

FIGURE 112-1 Nineteenth-century pharmacopoeia stick from the Museum of the Wisconsin Historical Society. *(Courtesy Daniel Moerman.)*

midwife," it is rare and considered egotistical to call oneself a "medicine person." In his book *Learning Journey on the Red Road,* Lakota medicine man Floyd Looks for Buffalo Hand calls himself a "spiritual interpreter."[45] As he once explained, "The only healer is the Great Spirit. I am only an interpreter" (personal communication, 1992). Most traditional healers have spent at least 7 to 10 years in rigorous training or apprenticeship before assuming their roles.

ELDER

The term *elder* occurs frequently in literature and discussions about Native American culture. Although this word may, at times, refer to a person's age, it more often means a keeper of ancient traditional wisdom. According to the Canadian Council of Elders, in the Algonquin Nation[1]:

An Elder is defined as someone who possesses spiritual leadership which is given by one's cultural and traditional knowledge. This knowledge is found in the teachings and responsibilities associated with sacred entities such as the Pipe, Wampum [sacred shell beads] belt, Drum and Medicine people. In addition to the spiritual recognition given by the Creator and the Spirit World, an elder is given the title and recognition as elder by other elders of his/her respective community and nation. Also one does not have to be a senior citizen to be an elder.

Various Indian Nations have their own definitions of the term *elder,* but the principles are similar. An elder passes along traditional values; he or she models, guides, and counsels people regarding how to live in a good way.

ETIOLOGY IN A WORLD OF "ALL MY RELATIONS"

In an interconnected and interdependent universe, it is impossible to posit a distinct cause for any disease. An infectious agent requires a vulnerable host, and the degree of vulnerability is affected by many factors, including genetics, environment, emotions, cognitive habits, diet, exercise, timing, and previous health history. Native Americans accept this biomedical model but believe that illness and trauma may also have hidden precipitating causes. For example, was the climbing accident a result of lack of technical skill, simple carelessness, or perhaps not paying attention to warnings from the spirit world in the form of omens or dreams (Figure 112-2)? Ethical and spiritual transgressions (e.g., a breach of taboo), such as disrespectful behavior in or toward nature, may also cause misfortune.

The powerful spirits of nature can be sources of curse or blessing. If one is in harmony with these spirits, even ordinarily dangerous or life-threatening events may cause little adverse effect. For example, a Cherokee medicine man deliberately entered a den of rattlesnakes and lived through 18 snakebites without medical treatment. This was a test issued by his mentor to see if the snake was indeed his helping spirit. If he lived, the answer was obvious. In another example, a young woman swimming near Daytona Beach, Florida, was stung multiple times by a box jellyfish that had wrapped around her leg. She suffered only a little discomfort, which she attributed to her connection with the local Seminole Indian culture and the nature and ocean spirits. Conversely, a person's negative attitude can immediately affect health. While participating in a sweat lodge ritual in Saskatchewan, Canada, a Native man vented anger about one of the other participants. Such a display is considered taboo

during a sweat, where there is a strong emphasis on the power of positive words. This man was the only one to suffer burns during the sweat, a phenomenon I had never before or since witnessed. (Although, as discussed later, even relatively safe therapies can become dangerous in the hands of unqualified practitioners.)

Considering common aspects of North American Indian culture, there are four general categories of pathogenesis: biomedical, environmental, psychological/psychosocial, and spiritual. Diseases may be caused by any combination of these factors.

BIOMEDICAL

The biomedical category includes all the etiologic factors recognized by modern medicine. Native American healers are part of the modern world and accept the scientific method as an

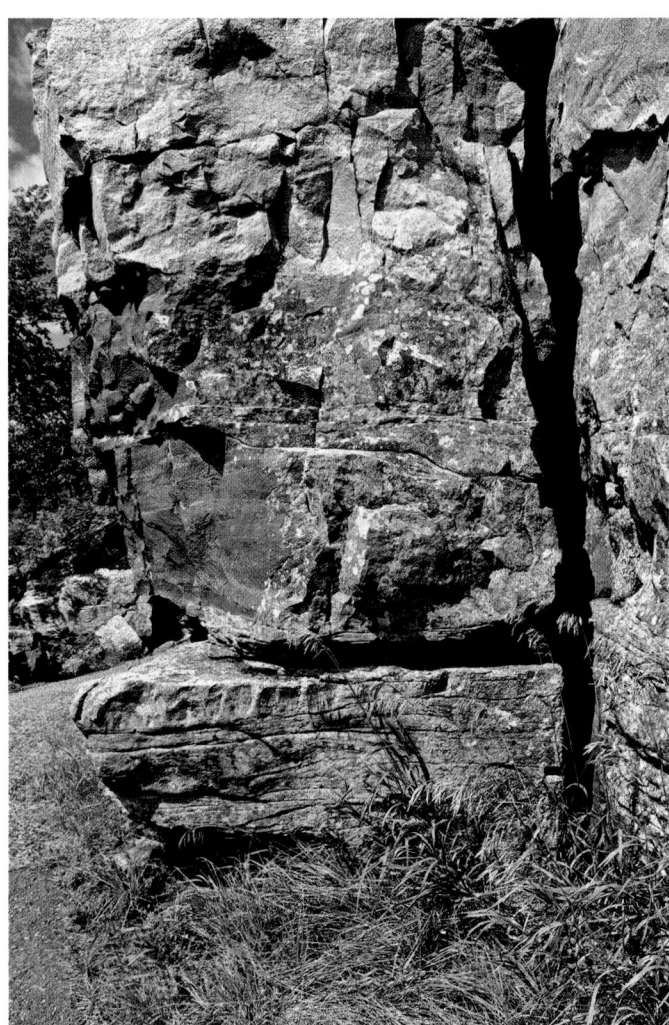

FIGURE 112-2 The Oracle Rock, a place for divination and insight, Pipestone National Monument, Minnesota. *(Photo by Ruth Hager—www.ruth-hager.artistwebsites.com.)*

important tool in the human search for truth. I have yet to meet a medicine man who would not go to a physician for diabetes management or for treatment of a bacterial infection. Diseases may certainly result from biochemical, metabolic, and mechanical imbalances; from viruses, bacteria, and parasites; from habits of posture and breathing; and from the influences of heredity and trauma. However, from the traditional healer's perspective, these are causal influences and cofactors rather than final explanations for disease. As one of my Native colleagues astutely commented, "Even germs have spirits." It is admirable that Western science can measure and predict the influence of microorganisms. On a psychological level, this satisfies the human need for certainty. However, for Native American healers, life falls outside the intellectual grid imposed by Western philosophies.

ENVIRONMENTAL

The term *environmental* refers to our connection with nature and nature's cycles as a major influence on health and well-being. In Plains Cree, one of the words for good health is "miyo-pimatisowin," literally "good" (*miyo*) and "alive" (*pimatisowin*). The term could be considered the Cree equivalent of "holistic health" and has a strong environmental component. Miyo-pimatisowin includes the exercise and endurance that are natural to anyone who spends a great deal of time outdoors, whether for subsistence activities or recreation. It connotes reliance on natural, unprocessed, local foods; the freedom to live in a way that honors one's land, people, and culture; and very importantly, a healthy environment for hunting, trapping, fishing, and foraging. Although only a small percentage of indigenous North Americans live by subsistence, there is nevertheless a commonly held philosophy that one cannot be healthy if the trout are unhealthy, the deer diseased, the water polluted, or the trees blighted.

Elders say that only one who spends time in nature will love nature; and only one who loves nature will protect her. Other things being equal, people who enjoy the outdoors are physically and psychologically healthier. "Nature-deficit disorder" has especially devastating effects on childhood development and soundness of adult decision making.[46] Nature, for Native people, is as important a role model as are parents or teachers. Animals remind people of essential values, such as courage, leadership, kinship, and harmony. To see fox or coyote pups frolicking reminds one of the important link between unstructured play and creativity, qualities sadly lacking in the world today. "Where do you like to play?" a third grader from San Diego was asked. "Inside," he replied, "because that's where the electric outlets are."[46] Children who play in nature are more resilient and better at reading and problem solving.

Wilderness, say indigenous people, is healing. The degree of healing power or influence may also vary, with some places having more or less, thus the customs of pilgrimage to and vision seeking at sacred sites (Figure 112-3). To spend more time in healing places is to enhance one's ability to resist and recover from disease. It is also the basis for recognizing healing herbs and connecting with their spirits, a necessity in Native herbal medicine.

PSYCHOLOGICAL/PSYCHOSOCIAL

The Cherokee traditional healer Rolling Thunder used to admonish, "Pollution begins in the mind" (Figure 112-4). Indeed, the reciprocal influence of mind and body, the core of today's psychoneuroimmunology, is well accepted in Native American medicine. "No evil sorcerer can do as much harm to you as you can do to yourself with negative thinking," the Samish traditional healer Johnny Moses once shared with me. Counseling, dream interpretation, and psychodrama (particularly the acting out of nighttime dreams) were common indigenous treatment modalities.[17,76] A positive attitude goes a long way toward enhancing the efficacy of any therapy or making such therapy unnecessary. Traditional healers are often experts at inducing the placebo effect.

Psychological and psychogenic diseases are of urgent concern to today's Native Americans.[18] Duran and Duran[23] have written insightfully about the prevalence of intergenerational post-traumatic stress disorder, resulting from the tragic history of

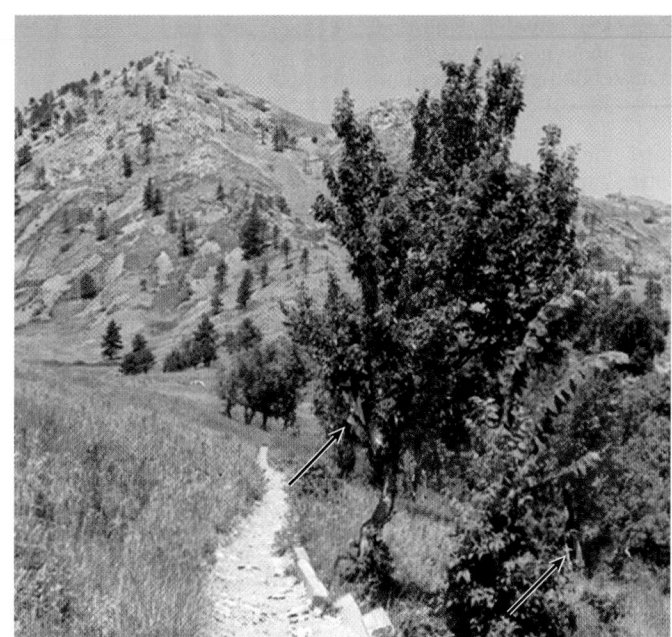

FIGURE 112-3 Bear Butte, South Dakota, holy place for the Lakota and many other tribes. Note the colored flags (prayer offerings) hanging from trees in the foreground.

Native peoples, their marginalization, the continuing challenges of racism, and the lasting effects of boarding school abuses and domestic violence. Some psychological problems are also the consequences of alcohol and drug abuse or birth defects, or associated with diseases such as diabetes and obesity. The breaking up of families and communities means that Native people now face problems on their own that would previously have been addressed by the group. Alienation and loneliness have replaced accountability and security. The programs most successful at treating psychological problems are integrative in nature, combining Western and indigenous therapies.[26,68]

In Native American medicine, major psychological influences on disease include sense of life purpose, degree of self-esteem, cognitive habits, and familial and social harmony.

Of these four, the first merits commentary. Native Americans believe that every person has a life purpose. To live a good life, one must prioritize discovering that purpose. This philosophy explains why dreams, and dream- or vision-quests, are so important in Native American culture. Equally important is to find the courage to live and express this purpose. A purpose not lived or a gift or talent that is kept locked up inside because of fear of failure, worry about disappointing others, and lack of self-esteem, is like stagnant water—a breeding ground for disease. We may become ill from our un-lived dreams just as we may heal by the

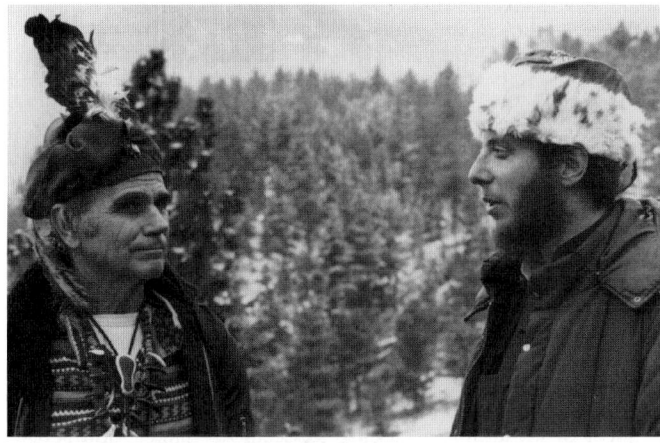

FIGURE 112-4 Rolling Thunder and the author, 1982.

dreams we live. To find and live one's purpose is to tell, with one's life, a good story. Many people lose joy in life or make and remake bad choices because they repeat to themselves a bad story. By contrast, good stories create meaning and purpose.

In 2004, I had the honor of presenting a talk about indigenous medicine to the Cree elders advisory council associated with a First Nations health center in Canada. As I was preparing, my adoptive Cree brother, Joseph, reminded me, "The elders will not listen if you give them information. They will pay attention if you present the information in the form of storytelling." One of the goals of the traditional healer is to hear and sense, often through intuition, the stories patients tell themselves, and then to help them "write" a better one. In counseling, raw information rarely heals.

SPIRITUAL

The term *spiritual* refers to the causes of illness that concern or originate in the spirit, soul, or transcendent realms. Unlike with popular Christianity, in Native American philosophy, spirit and soul may be attributes of stones, plants, and animals, not just people. Emotions are also spirits. Traditional Cree healers in Saskatchewan say that the spirits of hatred or shame may cause disease, just as the spirits of love and forgiveness can heal. However, spirit is not opposed to flesh. Aspects of the soul may be linked with the breath of life (*niya* in Lakota) or with the spirit or ghost that exists after the death of the body (*nagi* in Lakota). Spirit is an innate protecting force as well as a sacred power that may be gained by a person through sacrifice and contact with the divine (*sicun* in Lakota).[21] My Cree relatives distinguish between the appearance of the soul as a "ghost" (*tchi-pay*) while it remains on Earth and the soul (*at'-tshak*) that journeys to the spirit world.[24] The latter term, *at'-tshak,* is the root of the word for "star," which is *at'-tshakos.* The stars are the spirits of those who have passed on, and the trail they walk is the Milky Way. We can see that not only are spirit and matter not separate, but that the spiritual realm interpenetrates the ordinary. People can contact this other reality through prayer, ceremony, and waking or sleeping dreams.

Diseases always have a spiritual dimension. We are whole human beings, never divided, no matter how isolated parts look in a scan or under the microscope. In other words, whether the presenting symptoms suggest a predominantly biochemical, environmental, or psychosocial origin, a traditional healer also pays attention to spirit.

A person who is disconnected from his or her own soul or from the Great Spirit is only living a partial life and is more likely to become ill. Dreams are the royal road not only to the unconscious but also to the spirit world, and traffic goes both ways. In dreams, we contact spiritual realms, and these realms reach down to contact us. An effort to remember and interpret one's dreams by looking for clues to health and prevention of illness or misfortune is necessary for optimal health. Sometimes the traditional healer helps an unaware patient by searching for relevant information, both diagnostic and therapeutic, in the patient's dreams, or teaches methods to help the patient have and recall more meaningful dreams.

Contact with spirits may help prevent disease, but it can also cause disease. There is an ancient legend among the Cherokee and other Southeastern tribes that the spirits of animals caused disease as retribution for disrespectful hunting practices that now would be called "trophy hunting."[53] Illness results when people insult or mistreat animals, invade or destroy their habitat, or fail to show respect to animals while hunting or eating them. In *Crossing into Medicine Country*, Choctaw author David Carson[13] associates specific illnesses with various animals. If a person knows this connection, he or she may be able to relieve symptoms or cure disease by honoring the animal (e.g., with a feast among friends that is specifically intended to honor the animal) or by asking forgiveness from the offended animal spirit. As a sign of reconciliation, the animal may heal the illness directly or appear in a dream to offer advice.

Most of these animal-disease associations make good sense. For example, according to Carson's book, the millipede causes aching legs and lack of coordination. The moose may cause self-hatred, manifested as chain smoking, overeating, or destroying relationships without reason. Dog sickness is characterized by fever and delirium. Coyote sickness appears as obsession and addiction, including alcohol, drug, and sex addiction. It is no surprise that beavers may inflict constipation; one feels dammed up. Squirrels eat too much or too little. Turkeys swell with pride and may cause false pride, repressed anger, swollen glands, and cancer.

Spirits may be capricious, mischievous, or malevolent. For this reason, elders advise not contacting the realm of spirits unless one is in need, emotionally mature, or prepared and aided by a traditional healer. Sorcerers, popularly called *witches* by some Native tribes (although they are not to be confused with Western pagan Wicca traditions), can inflict harm by sending disease-causing spirits to their victims. Although many, if not most, of these phenomena are probably examples of the nocebo effect, negative intent may have concrete effects even if the victim does not believe in or is unaware of the "curse." Sorcerers may be hired by people to inflict harm and misfortune on other people, or they may be personally motivated to perform such criminal activities as a result of emotional imbalance (usually jealousy).[22,75]

There is also a traditional and widely held Native philosophy that negative actions eventually return to plague the perpetrator. Rolling Thunder taught that good deeds and bad deeds are both multiplied by seven to help or harm the person who performs them.[10] Tuscarora traditional healer Ted Williams[79] used to say that life is governed by natural and moral laws. To break these laws is the inner meaning of "breaking a taboo." To strike a child, disrespect an elder, pollute the earth, or to act with greed, malice, or egotism is to break the Creator's law. The result is illness in body, mind, or spirit.

ASSESSMENT AND DIAGNOSIS

Most healers base their diagnosis on intuition, sensitivity, and spiritual sight. A healer might sense or see that a patient's mind is clouded, soul fragmented, or body harboring an intrusive force or entity. He or she may dream or feel the spirit of a disease or early spiritual warning signs of cancer, heart disease, diabetes, or other conditions. Tactile clues during indigenous massage or noncontact energy healing (i.e., the hands held near the patient's body) are also important. The healer may feel heat (suggesting inflammation), cold (suggesting depletion), stagnation, pain, or other diagnostic sensations. Some traditional healers use therapeutic tools to refine their diagnoses. For example, a Kiowa colleague gave me what he called "an Indian x-ray machine," with instructions for its proper use: place a black cloth over the patient's body and then look, with the mind's eye, at the underlying tissues. Other healers may use beads to assess the gravity of an illness. For example, Cherokee healers turn black and white beads in the hands. If the black beads move more easily, the problem is serious; if the white beads move more easily, the meaning is good fortune and health. Clouds, patterns on stone or in flowing water, images seen while gazing at a quartz crystal, or the behavior of a campfire may become an indigenous Rorschach test with which the healer or patient reads the diagnosis and cure. The number of such possible tools is without limit.

Extrasensory phenomena are reported in association with traditional Native American diagnosis, reminding one of the out-of-body and clairvoyant skills of Edgar Cayce.[67] I know traditional healers who, when told of a physical trauma, travel psychically to the place of the occurrence to see it for themselves. They may find, at the site of an accident, a lost soul that needs to be retrieved. Other healers have "sympathy pains" starting hours or days before they see an unexpected client for the first time. I once experienced firsthand the work of an Ojibwe healer who specialized in diagnosing and treating from a distance. In 1989, she and I met during a conference in Ontario. Years earlier, septic arthritis had destroyed all the cartilage in both my hips. Noticing my disability, she offered to perform a healing on a specific day and time a few weeks later, after I returned to my home in Colorado. I did not remember the date I had scribbled in a small travel calendar. At the time, I was becoming increasingly skeptical because of the number of generally ineffective alternative healers who had tried to help me. I accepted my inability to climb stairs or to tie my shoelaces as an inconvenience with which I could live. However, one evening while sitting at my kitchen table, I felt a strange sensation, as though an electrically charged cloud surrounded me. I noticed that my hips, legs, and back had suddenly become comfortable. I bent forward and miraculously touched my toes. I then sat on the floor and crossed my legs, an impossible task both before and since. My range of motion was nearly normal. Of course, at this point, I remembered the meeting with the Ojibwe healer and, sure enough, this was the appointed evening. The change lasted for several hours. The next morning, when I woke up, I found that my previous level of disability had returned. For me, this healing remains a shining and encouraging example of the potential to heal and the power of indigenous medicine.

TREATMENT

In Native American healing, diagnosis and treatment are not rigidly divided and are often included in the same therapeutic session. This is true with ceremonial healing (e.g., the sweat lodge), with massage therapy, and especially with counseling. For example, ethnographers have noted the importance of dream interpretation and dream psychodrama among the Haudenosaunee.[76] Tribal members would act out ominous dreams to create more favorable outcomes and thus avoid misfortune. When telling the dream (i.e., diagnosis), the resolution (i.e., treatment) becomes obvious. Similarly, during counseling, the traditional healer listens to the patient and offers meaningful advice or spiritual therapies. My adoptive father, Andrew Naytowhow (Cree), a traditional healer, counseled people in prisons; he sometimes offered advice or "doctored" them with prayer and pipe ceremonies (Figure 112-5). Often, just talking about one's feelings was all the healing needed. He would also host "talking circles" among troubled youth. For a talking circle, after an opening prayer, each person speaks in turn, without interruption or commentary, sometimes followed by group discussion. I use counseling in my own traditional healing practice. After prayer and noncontact energy healing, one of my clients, a Native man in jail for assault, broke down in tears and admitted to me the tragic circumstances in his life that had led to his actions. This was an important step in his return to "the Good Red Road," the Native American path of a spiritual and ethical life.

Native American medicine is North America's original integrative medicine. Guided by a pragmatic philosophy of "use what works," traditional healers apply specific culture-bound methods of therapy, but may also combine or create entirely new treatment methods tailored to the needs of the patient. It is not unusual to bring insulin or an analgesic into a ceremony for

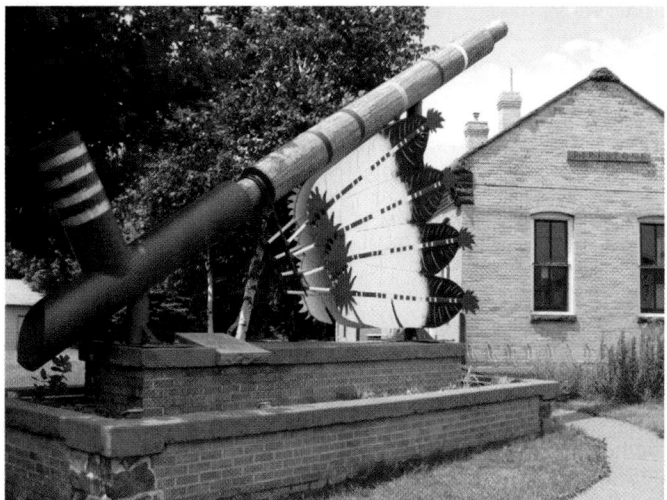

FIGURE 112-5 Giant replica of a Native American prayer pipe in Pipestone, Minnesota.

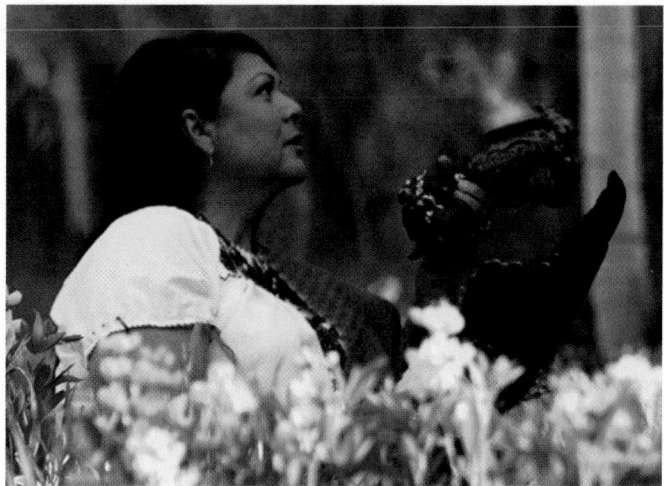

FIGURE 112-6 Griselda A. Sesma (Yoeme-Kumeyaay) offering sage smoke.

blessing and empowerment. Style of treatment may also vary according to the season, the availability of herbs, and spiritual directives received by the healer in the midst of therapy.

Because of these characteristics, Native American healing does not lend itself easily to replicable experiments. Despite the recognition of biochemical individuality, Western medicine promotes standard and uniform methods of therapy. By contrast, Native American medicine is adapted to the perceived or intuited needs of the patient. It is diverse, situational, and individualized.

Native American healing is also a holistic modality because, to borrow what has become a cliché, it seeks to treat the person rather than the disease. I remember a Navajo elder complaining that when he was in the hospital, he could not understand why the doctors seemed more interested in treating a piece of paper than in caring for him. They kept looking at the chart, but not at the patient himself.

The most common categories of Native therapeutics are smudging (i.e., cleansing with the smoke of a sacred plant [Figure 112-6]); prayer and chant; music; counseling; vision seeking, dreaming, and fasting; energy therapies; ceremonies; and herbs. These methods and their purposes are outlined in Table 112-1, an early version of which appeared in *Honoring the Medicine: The Essential Guide to Native American Healing.*[17] However, this is by no means an all-inclusive list.

An additional category not discussed here is Indian Christian healing. For the many Native Americans who identify themselves as Christian, the term *Native American healing* means methods of healing that are acceptable to their pastors and to their churches, such as the Catholic laying on of hands, revival meetings, and charismatic prayer groups. Some churches, such as the Native American Church[64] and the Indian Shaker Church in the Pacific Northwest,[59] integrate Christian symbolism with Native American songs and healing practices. Mexican Americans of Native or mixed background also blend indigenous and Christian elements in *curanderismo,* common throughout Central and South America, as well as in Arizona, Texas, Southern California, and wherever there are large Hispanic populations.[72] Although important culturally and socially, and reported to be effective for the treatment of many illnesses, Indian Christian healing is beyond the scope of this chapter.

CONTRAINDICATIONS

Like their allopathic colleagues, traditional healers are aware of contraindications that would make particular practices inadvisable. Some herbs may be dangerous during pregnancy, when administered with blood thinners, or for cancer patients, being toxic in incorrect dosages or having other negative effects. Similar precautions exist for other therapies, such as sweat lodges or prolonged fasts, which are inadvisable for hypertensive and diabetic patients, respectively. For these reasons, readers are advised

TABLE 112-1   Common Native American Therapeutic Methods

Method	Purpose
Smudging • Artemisia • Sage • Cedar • Sweetgrass • Juniper • Pine needles	Herbs burned to purify the healing space, healer, patient, helpers, and ritual objects; induce spiritual state of mind; increase awareness of both helpful and disease-causing forces; invite and offer respect to helping spirits.
Prayer and chant • Sacred expression • Communion • Invocation • Petition	Focus the mind on healing; engender positive, health-promoting values such as love, peace, acceptance, and trust; induce expanded and receptive state of consciousness in healer, patient, and helpers; commune with, invoke, empower, and express gratitude to sacred healing forces; increase patient self-esteem by helping him or her to feel worthy of divine help; attend gathering and administration of herbs or other medicines.
Music • Voice • Drum • Rattle • Flute • Whistle • Rasp • Clacker • Violin* • Bull-roarer	Same as for Prayer and chant, also: entrain consciousness and induce harmony and unity among healer, patient, and helpers; restore natural rhythms; unify with elements (e.g., flute: wind); accompaniment to any healing intervention, especially dance and ceremony.
Counseling • Talking things out • Advice of an elder or advisor • Storytelling • Dream and vision interpretation • Seeking guidance from nature • Healing imagery • Humor	Explore or clarify disease etiology and pathogenesis, including physical, behavioral, and spiritual components of disease; discover new sources of inner strength, confidence, and self-understanding; encourage positive behavioral changes, including strategies of coping with disease; strengthen family and community relations.
Vision seeking, dreaming, and fasting	Healer, patient, or both retrieve information, guidance, or solutions to problems or illness; attract and commune with helping spirits and spiritual power.
Energy therapies • Massage, sometimes with specific oils or herbal infusions • Laying on of hands • Indigenous acupuncture: thorns puncture therapeutic points • Noncontact treatment, including scooping harmful intrusive objects or forces • Blowing air, water, herbs, or teas on patient • Sucking disease from body • Stones, feathers, plants, earth, or pigments placed or brushed on or near the body	Aid healing of body, mind, and spirit; relieve pain; transmit healing intent, healing energy, and spiritual power.
Ceremony • Sweat lodge • Sacred pipe • Other tribal healing ceremonies (e.g., Diné sand painting, Salish winter spirit dances) • Ceremonies that belong to individual healers	Enact visions or instructions received from Spirit. Empower and provide a formal structure for healing methods; commune with natural and spiritual forces, the Great Spirit, or the spirit of the disease; induce positive and health-enhancing states of mind; affirm shared cultural identity and values.
Plant medicine (including seaweed) • Consumed (chewed, infused, fermented) • Poultices and salves • Rubbed, placed, brushed, or blown on patient • For bathing, smoking, or smudging • Other ritual uses	Enhance physical, mental, and spiritual balance; expand awareness of spiritual realms (e.g., dreaming/vision aid); combat specific physical or spiritual pathogens.

*The Apache violin or *tsii'edo'a'tl* ("wood that sings") is an ancient instrument that is played during some social songs, ceremonial songs, and healing rituals. The body of the instrument is made of the century plant, which is related to agave and common in Arizona.

not to try the formulas or methods described in this chapter without supervision of an expert practitioner.

Unfortunately, there are no statistical data that address the level of adverse effects of Native American medicine. One of the few reported cases is of a healthy 32-year-old Zuni woman who suffered a stroke from a left vertebral artery dissection after manipulation by a Native bonesetter. She was discharged from the hospital with warfarin anticoagulation therapy and improved quickly.[58] A glaring example of the dangers of Native therapies that are attempted by improperly trained individuals was in the widely publicized tragedy that occurred during a sweat lodge ceremony in Sedona, Arizona, on October 9, 2009, leaving three persons dead and 21 hospitalized. A traditional sweat lodge is a small, dome-like sauna covered by "breathable" blankets and hides, with room for 12 to 20 people. Participants have a chance to exit the lodge as needed or at prescribed times. In the Sedona sweat lodge, a monstrous 415-square-foot dome covered in plastic, approximately 60 people were trapped for 2 hours. Their leader, a non-Native motivational speaker, advised that they could survive their ordeal, but he was wrong.[15] There have been other, less dramatic examples of adverse effects, and many probably are not reported.

In all fairness, it seems likely that compared with allopathic interventions, the level of adverse effects in Native American healing is extremely low and certainly not greater than that attributable to Western or other culturally related medical practices.

AFTERCARE

Traditional healers, unless they have dual roles as physicians, psychotherapists, or other health care providers, generally do not follow up with phone calls or recommended appointments. Patients sometimes return to see healers, but it is their responsibility to request the visits. In addition, traditional healers rarely take notes or otherwise record encounters with their patients; there is a general disdain of note taking, photographing, or audio or video recording of healing interventions. Therefore, we know little about long-term results other than those obtained from anecdotal reports.

If recording occurred during diagnosis or treatment, it would be considered a distraction, dividing the mind and spirit of the healer and preventing full attention to the patient. Although few traditional healers today would claim that photographs or recorded words steal the soul or life force, a feeling remains that multimedia recording of sacred, ceremonial, and healing events is disrespectful to the powers that guide the healer. Recording creates a level of separation and abstraction, a step removed from what is happening in the moment; it freezes in time a passing phenomenon and is, in that respect, considered to be a false representation.

Given this caveat, there is nothing inherently wrong with documenting the effects of Native interventions after the therapeutic sessions and using this information to contribute to the literature on healing. As part of the continuing dialogue between indigenous and Western science, this is likely to occur more and more often.

PREVENTION

Native Americans today suffer from disproportionately high rates of diabetes, cancer, alcoholism, suicide, homicide, injuries, and tuberculosis. Conventional preventive medicine is well accepted, including behavioral and lifestyle changes, immunization, and education. Five hundred years ago, Native healers did not recognize prevention as a separate category of medicine: the elders with whom I have discussed this topic say that prevention was a result of living according to traditional values, including "a good heart and good mind" (a common expression), an emphasis on moderation, a caring family and community and feeling of belonging, and natural outdoor living in which organic food and exercise were facts of life. A clean environment, slower pace of life, and relatively low level of stress were also significant positive influences on health.

CLINICAL EXAMPLE: BACK PAIN

As an example of how these theories are applied clinically, consider the various tribal therapies for back pain, whether caused by congenital defect, stenosis, trauma (including strain, sprain, spasm, fracture, and various disk problems), arthritis, or as secondary to another condition such as renal cysts or cancer. Acute and chronic back pain were serious concerns among people whose survival depended on existence in the wilderness. Pain interferes with the ability to walk, run, climb, swim, defend, and practice subsistence activities such as hunting, planting, foraging, and fishing.

Herbal medicine is a common remedy for back pain. Salicin, the well-known analgesic in aspirin, was first listed in the U.S. Pharmacopoeia in 1882. It is found in all species of willow (*Salix*) and was a traditional pain remedy among many tribes. For example, the Blackfeet steeped willow twigs in boiling water for fever and pain. Alaskan Inupiat chewed on green willow bark specifically for back pain.[27] Alabama Indians applied a poultice made of the pulp of saw palmetto roots to a broken or injured back.[74] The Innu of Quebec and Baffin Island drank wintergreen root tea for back troubles of any kind. The Catawba from North and South Carolina crushed fresh horsemint leaves and steeped them in water. The tea was drunk every day to relieve back pain. They also used an arnica root wash for sprains and bruises.[14] The Kashaya Pomo of North Central California used a pepperwood leaf poultice for nerve pain. They also made a poultice from the root of cow parsnip (*Heracleum lanatum*), baking the root, mashing it, and placing it on the painful area under a rag, leaving it overnight.[29] Alaskan Aleut used a compress of heated cow parsnip leaves as a compress for muscle pain.[27] San Carlos Apache from Arizona made a dry poultice of greasewood (*Covillea tridentata*), heating the top of the plant and applying it directly to the painful area.[74] The creosote bush (*Larrea tridentata*), confusingly sometimes also called "greasewood," is used by many Arizona and Southern California tribes as a cure-all. Heated branches, twigs, or leaves are placed on the body to relieve pain. It is also common to treat pain with creosote steam or smoke.[20] Passamoquody herbalist Fredda Paul of Maine admires the healing properties of horsetail (*Equisetum arvense, Equisetum hyemale,* and *Equisetum sylvaticum*), also popularly called "shave grass." It is taken internally as a tea for aching or injured joints and ligaments and to help mend broken bones. Horsetail is rich in silica and may help build collagen.[40] As with other plants, it must be administered with care, because the silica may aggravate hemorrhoids, and the raw shoots contain toxic thiaminase. It is also inadvisable for persons with cardiovascular disease.

Calamus, a member of the sweet flag (*Acoraceae*) family, is an immensely popular herb among Native Americans. It commonly grows in swamps and near water in boreal forests and has a broad range of applications. The Cree of Montana, Alberta, and Saskatchewan call it *wacaskwatapih* ("muskrat root" or, more commonly, "rat root") and believe that muskrat meat is especially nourishing and spiritually potent because muskrats eat this healing root. Cree herbalists recommend chewing on the root to overcome fatigue during long hikes or strenuous activities. It is also applied for treatment of back pain. The fresh, or dried and ground, rhizome is chewed and used as a poultice for painful joints. The root may also be chopped and put in boiling water to make tea, which is then mixed with flour and applied as a hot paste over arthritic joints. The painful area is then wrapped with warm towels and left overnight.[49] The Muskogee Creek, who originally inhabited the region from Georgia to Alabama, use calamus tea in a similar manner, applying it within a hot compress to reduce inflammation and soothe sore joints and back pain. The Creek also use yarrow, another ubiquitous and popular plant, for painful or deep bruises from falls. The smashed leaves or a lukewarm tea made from the leaves are placed in a compress over the bruise. In a modern application, the leaves and flowers may also be soaked in isopropyl alcohol for 7 days to make an antiinflammatory liniment for joint pain and poor circulation.[19]

Cherokee and Hitchiti herbalist Tis Mal Crow[19] recommends a liniment made from Solomon's seal root (*Polygonatum biflorum*) for back pain, sprains, misaligned bones, and ruptured disks. The Tlingit and other Alaskan tribes make ointment or massage oil using skunk cabbage or devil's club (*Oplopanax horridus*) for joint and muscle pain.[32] Devil's club, sometimes called "Indian ginseng," is greatly admired among Northwest and Alaska Native peoples for its broad healing and spiritual qualities, and it is somewhat of a panacea[43] (Figure 112-7).

Massage is a universal remedy for pain. Native healing specialists called "bonesetters" are common among many tribes, from the Yurok of California to the Yoeme of Arizona. In addition to setting broken bones, many of them also practice massage or prescribe herbs that teach the bones how to mend. Traditional healers commonly practice laying on of hands, placing the hands

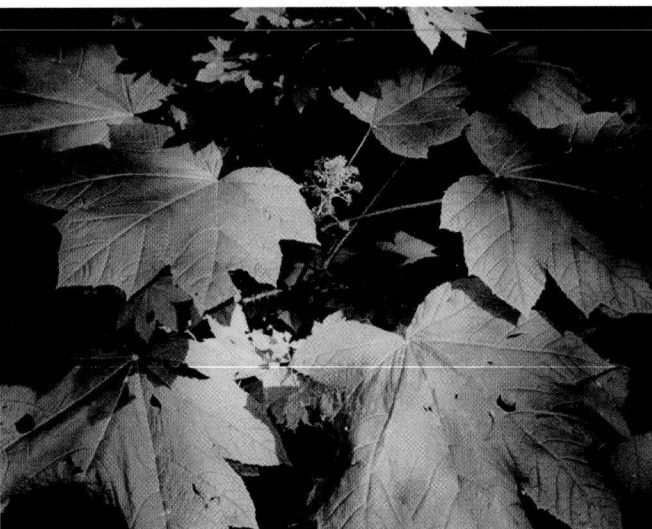

FIGURE 112-7 Devil's club, Sitka, Alaska.

on or near painful areas. In Washington State, practitioners of the Si.Si.Wiss "sacred breath" healing tradition may work on a patient with a combination of smudging (generally with cedar smoke), song, dance, prayer, candlelight, and healing gestures of the hands.[17,63] I have facilitated several Si.Si.Wiss healing ceremonies for patients with back pain. In one case, a 40-year-old white airline pilot joined a 2-hour healing ceremony without telling anyone about his diagnosis or symptoms. It was his first experience in a Native ceremony. A few years later, I met him by chance in a café, and he recounted an extraordinary story. He had been in a car accident 6 years earlier that had resulted in unremitting pain from three herniated disks: the third cervical and fourth and fifth lumbar vertebrae. The pain was significantly diminished the day after the ceremony; within 1 week, it was completely gone, and had never returned. A 60-year-old Comanche woman who had suffered from years of disk-related back pain asked me to "doctor" her. I smudged her with a mixture of artemisia and sweetgrass (*Hierochloe odorata*), waving the smoke over her body with a turkey feather fan. I then prayed to the Great Spirit for health and help while placing my palms directly on the painful area. I rested my palms there for about 10 minutes. The intervention closed with more prayers. Her pain was gone the next day and never returned.

As do modern massage therapists, Native healers use various oils to ease kneading and manipulation and to make the body more pliable. Oils were historically derived from animal fat, typically bear, bobcat, and raccoon.[74] The spirits of these animals were believed to contribute to the effectiveness of the massage. The power of massage could also be augmented by fanning the body with switches of cedar or other plants or by applying massage in a ceremonial or sanctified space such as a sweat lodge. Some traditional healers are especially efficacious because of the way they prepare themselves for healing. Cherokee healers warm their hands over an outdoor fire and then rub the painful area with circular motions of the palms.[74] Some healers imagine that they are becoming or communing with a dream helper, such as a badger, thunderbird (symbol of thunder, lightning, and life energy), or bear. In the minds of both healer and patient, it is perhaps the bear who "doctors" the patient and whose "paws" massage the painful area. The bear is one of the most common representations of healing among North American Indians. Because of the bear's winter hibernation, the bear is associated with sleeping, dreaming, and the intuitive insights that are considered essential to the practice of indigenous healing. Many tribes consider the bear an especially important teacher of herbal medicine. This may be a result of observing the bear's ability to self-medicate using plants in nature and knowing that humans, like bears, are the only North American mammals with a rotating forearm, giving them the manual dexterity to dig healing roots (Figure 112-8).

Back pain and spasms are often relieved by heat. This fact did not escape traditional healers, who recommended hot compresses, the heat of the sweat lodge, and bathing in hot springs. Rolling Thunder sometimes advised his patients to lie down on a "bed" of warm sand on the beach and consciously, meditatively allow the warmth to heal the back. Like the ancient Chinese, Native American healers for millennia have applied warmth to muscles, joints, or specific therapeutic points to relieve pain. In Chinese medicine, a small ball of moxa (mugwort) is burned at the end of the acupuncture needle to transmit heat and increase the therapeutic effect. Similarly, Cree Indians take a pinch of tinder fungus, found under the bark of birch trees, roll it into a matchstick shape, and burn it on the skin to treat arthritis.[49] Omaha Indians used stems of the shoestring plant in a similar fashion.[28] The Blackfoot sometimes inserted prickly pear or rose thorns into specific areas on the skin to relieve pain. These thorns may also have been heated by burning them. Historian Robert Beverley, Jr (1673-1722), reported that the Indians of Virginia fixed "a pain in any particular Joynt or Limb" by making a cone from soft or rotting wood in the knots in hickory or oak trees and burning it down to the skin over painful areas.[8] Most Native American languages have a word for life force or breath of life (*ni* in Lakota), similar to the Chinese concept of *qi*. It is logical to infer from this that indigenous acupuncture was not merely a counterirritant but rather an example of energy medicine.[35] However, counterirritants were not unknown. Many tribes, such as the Chehalis and Quileute of Washington, applied switches of stinging nettles to painful backs.[31]

Adolf Hungry Wolf[80] recounts a fascinating example of Blackfoot Indian "moxabustion" in his 1975 edition of *Teachings of Nature*. A Blackfoot elder told Hungry Wolf, "... a horse fell on me once. My knee really swelled up. My father told my mother to go get some thorns from a Rose bush, and he told her to bake them. ... He checked over my injured leg and he took one of the hot thorns and he pushed it in." His father inserted the thorns directly into the swollen area and then burned them down to the skin. He repeated the treatment later that same day. "This time the swelling went right down and I was able to walk. I guess that was a form of what they call, today, Acupuncture."[80]

Ceremonies may also be deemed effective against back pain, especially if the pain was caused by a negative or evil power, including anger, which may have lodged within the body; by offending an animal or natural phenomenon, such as the aurora borealis or lightning; by contact with the dead or ghosts; by lack of ceremonial preparations for military service or return from service; or by any other etiologic factor generally considered in the realm of spiritual.

There are no set rules regarding the frequency or overall length of Native healing therapies. An intervention lasting only a few hours or a day may bring a lasting cure. Navajo *sings*, which are ceremonies that may include baths, sand painting, and complex chants, may last 2, 5, or 9 nights. Some Native healers give the patient an herbal formula or ritual activity to perform for a set number of days, usually 4 or 7. Other healers may see

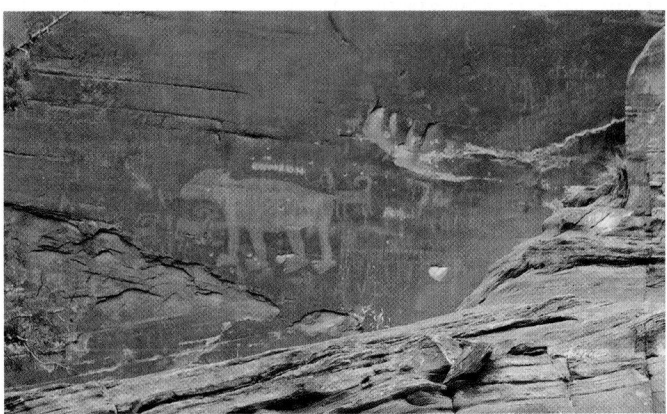

FIGURE 112-8 Life-size petroglyph of a bear near Moab, Utah.

their patients on a daily basis for 1 week or more. If the healer and his or her helpers have traveled a great distance, sometimes at considerable cost to the patient (who is expected to provide transportation costs, lodging, food, and a generous donation for services), the healer will work intensively to complete the treatment in as short a time as possible. A cure may require a commitment on the part of the patient to make lifelong behavioral changes or to perform ritual activities on a seasonal or yearly basis for a certain number of years. In contrast with the "fix-me" attitude that often accompanies allopathic medicine, patients receiving Native American healing treatments are expected to assume considerable responsibility for their own healing. Patients who comply with the healers' directives are much more likely to be cured.

Before leaving this brief survey of healing interventions for back pain, it is important to note that in precontact times, people who could not be cured or who lived with permanent disability were not rejected. Native patients among various tribes ingested datura (*Datura stramonium*) or peyote (*Lophophora williamsii*) to free the mind from pain and disability and to promote visions leading to a new sense of life purpose. I have heard from many elders that disability did not prevent one from living a useful life. On the contrary, a person who is weak in body is often pitied by the Creator and made especially strong in mind and spirit. These individuals find new ways to be of service.

THE CHALLENGES OF RESEARCH

Native American medicine is not found among the categories of CAM on the website of the National Center for Complementary and Alternative Medicine.[54] In various presentations and documents, I have advised officials from the National Institutes of Health that Native American medicine is too closely connected with political, economic, religious, and social issues to be considered a CAM method.[16,62] I was concerned that the benefits of research and control over its applications remain in the hands of the sovereign Native Nations to whom the healing methods belong. It would be a travesty for non-Native licensing or accreditation boards to create standards for or assume control over Native spirituality and culture.

The scientific analysis of Native American healing methods removed from their cultural context poses special challenges for creating standard conditions or replicable experiments. From an indigenous viewpoint, analyzing the chemistry and biologically active agents in plant medicines has limited value. To be effective, plants must be gathered by hand and not bought in a store or pharmacy. Native herbalists also pay attention to the time of day or season to dig roots or pick leaves and are careful to leave enough of a species for regrowth. The way an herbalist handles or prepares an herb (e.g., cutting, drying, mashing, crushing) may increase or decrease a plant's potency. For example, Mohegan herbalist Gladys Tantaquidgeon[69] states that many herbalists prefer to dry their medicines in the sun and crush them with a stone or wood mortar "to avoid contamination by metal."

Interventions vary according to the needs of the patient and intuition of the healer. The location is also considered an influence on treatment outcome. For example, an herbal medicine or massage received in a hogan, kiva, sweat lodge, or beautiful place in nature has a different effect than the same therapy applied in an office or hospital or studied in the laboratory. Songs and prayers may not be repeated, even when treating the same disease, and it is also possible that the powers they invoke are impossible to measure. A traditional healer would not wish to rule out the placebo effect, if it was a possibility. The presence of the healer, quality of relationship between healer and patient, and faith of the patient are powerful influences on treatment outcome. Levin[44] defines faith as "a confluence of belief, trust, and obedience in relation to God or the divine."

This does not mean that scientific research in this field is of no value. On the contrary, research can provide an alternative model for interpreting and appreciating healing phenomena.[50] Some prominent websites, including those of the American Cancer Society[2] and the University of California, San Diego Medical Center claim that the "[f]ormal research of the healing

ceremonies and traditions of Native Americans is almost nonexistent even though claims have been made regarding cures of a variety of ailments, including cancer."[73] This is not quite true. We have little data about Native American healing that has been conducted by traditional healers, especially in the context of their own communities or with members of their own tribes. At the same time, the major modalities applied by Native healers have been extensively researched and documented, including herbal medicine, music, touch, massage, and prayer. For example, in "Physical Fields and States of Consciousness," a 12-year research project conducted by the Menninger Clinic in Topeka, Kansas, scientists measured extraordinary surges in body potential, bioelectric fields, and brain-wave amplitude when various well-known healers, including some practitioners of Native American Medicine, attempted to emit healing energy, with or without an actual patient being present (Figures 112-9 and 112-10). At the same time, 600 control experiments with "regular" untrained participants produced no such phenomena.[30,70,71] Given the documented effects of drumming on brain waves and intuition, I believe that even stronger effects would have been evident if Native healers had used drums or other percussive instruments during these experiments.[36,55,56,61,77] However, this would have created movement artifacts, making data interpretation almost impossible. It is also likely that the sensory saturation common during Native rituals—olfactory (sage and cedar smoke), auditory (drumming), kinesthetic (dancing), and visual (masks and regalia)—causes synergistic neurophysiologic effects (e.g., blocking of pain signals).

Daniel Benor[7] has collected and analyzed hundreds of CAM and spiritual healing abstracts previously published in peer-reviewed journals. Many U.S. hospitals, particularly those serving

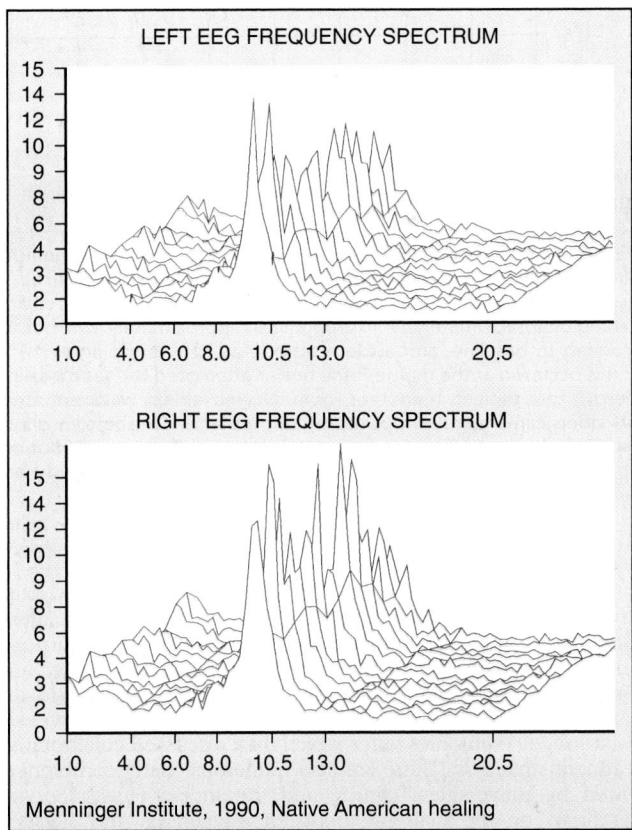

FIGURE 112-9 Left and right hemisphere electroencephalography (EEG) spectra from the Menninger Clinic, 1990. Subject practices Native American healing by mental focus on a distant patient, hidden from him in another office within the Menninger Clinic. Note coherence of upper (left) hemisphere with lower (right), peaking in the alpha range at approximately 10.5 Hz. This amplitude is unusually high, particularly for the right hemisphere.

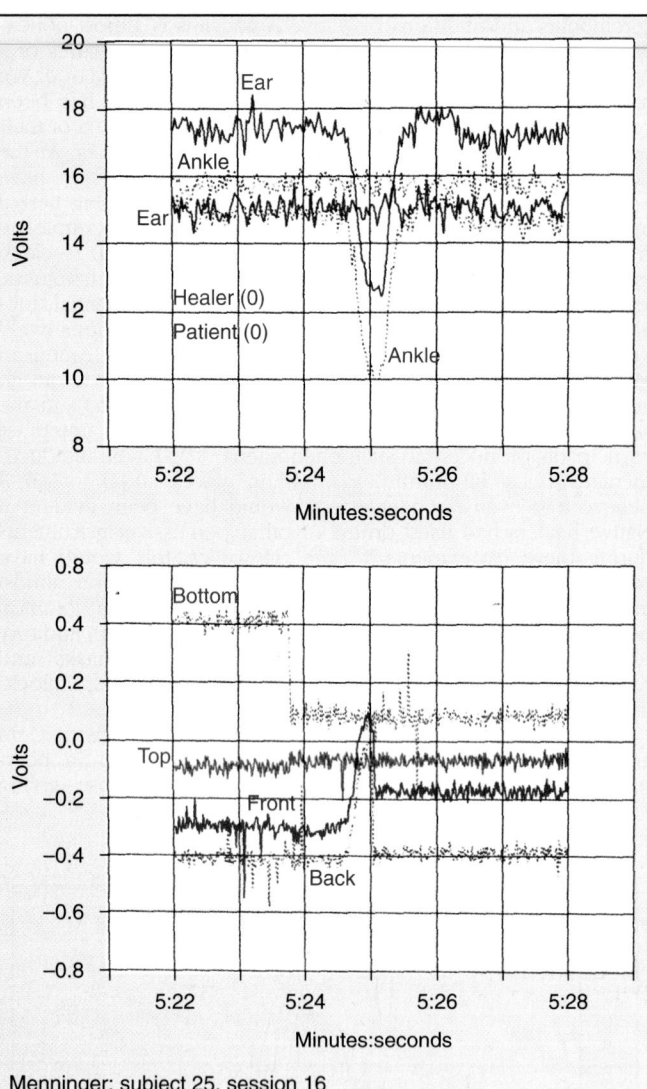

FIGURE 112-10 Anomalous changes in body potential, Menninger Clinic, 1990. Same subject (*healer*) and experimental session as in Figure 112-9. Upper graph shows the healer's baseline ear electrode reading of approximately 17 V, dropping to approximately 13 V before returning to baseline, and ankle electrode at 15 V dropping to 10 V. All this occurred at the moment the healer attempted to "send healing energy" to a patient in another room. No movement was permitted, and video cameras ruled out movement artifacts. The bottom graph displays voltage readings on four copper panels: bottom subflooring, top ceiling, front, and back. A significant spike in the front and back panels occurred in synchrony with the body potential surges.

Native patients or close to reservations, provide integrative health services that allow patients to be treated by traditional healers, often in special Indian treatment rooms reserved for that purpose. I have visited these facilities in New Mexico, Wyoming, and Washington. An administrator at one of these facilities told me that non-Indian physicians joined traditional healers in weekly sweat lodge ceremonies, after which they discussed collaborative treatment strategies. There are also numerous yearly conferences hosted by universities, clinics, and the Indian Health Service that focus on the dialogue between indigenous and Western medicine and the potential benefits of both research and clinical applications.

Returning to a theme from the beginning of this chapter, spending time in nature, whether camping, hiking, or on pilgrimage, has measurable effects on health. Louv[46] cites evidence for "nature-deficit disorder," linked with decreased creativity as well as cognitive and emotional difficulties in both adults and children. Becker and Seldon[6] explain the mechanism by which the earth's electromagnetic field influences healing and may program our biologic clocks and rhythms. Others have shown how rhythmic movement (e.g., healing and ceremonial dances) further encourages homeostasis. According to James R. Evans, Associate Professor of Psychology at the University of South Carolina (Columbia)[25]:

Some [researchers] perceive the human body as a collection of oscillating subsystems more or less in harmony with each other; the greater the harmony among the systems the less the "dis-ease," while the greater the dissonance the more severe the "dis-ease." According to some such views, internal order can be increased and hence the quality of the human "body symphony" enhanced by exposure to ordered stimuli such as certain music, poetry and rhythms of nature and/or by participation in rhythmic movement activities as diverse as dancing, jogging, and certain martial arts. One might guess that dancing to music under the stars on a beach would be highly conducive to reestablishment of internal order.

It is likely that positive health-enhancing entrainment may also occur between the healer and healed.[70,71] Through a process similar to what electrical engineers call "induction coupling," the information-carrying signals in one neural network produce similar signals in an adjacent biologic system. Of course, the opposite is also possible: an ill-prepared healer may resonate with the patient's disease or transmit his or her own disharmony.

The human race evolved in natural, not man-made, environments. As we become more familiar with these environments, we feel more fully human. The experience of belonging in nature—of being not stewards of the earth but rather, like a stone, a plant, or a fish in the sea, being a *part* of the earth's natural processes—is central to the practice and understanding of traditional healing. The healer draws on this connection to augment spiritual power. The wind, invoked through imagery and song, chases away pain; a healer-turned-wolf hunts for the scent of disease; a stone rubbed on the back strengthens bones. This creates a set of ever-changing variables probably impossible to measure.

In addition, it is important to consider that Native wilderness medicine today is different from that of the past. Modern lifestyles and habits create special challenges for a traditional healer. Many people, including Native Americans, are uncomfortable in the wilderness. Although people try to control it, when we are in nature, we are faced with a reality that is beyond our control and unpredictable. A fall or fracture in the forest may be doubly frightening; first because it happens in nature and second because it happens far from the security of a hospital. Alienation, helplessness, and fear exacerbate pain, impede healing, and may lead to panic. Thus, the very first task of the traditional healer is to communicate to the patient by word, deed, or symbol that the patient is safe and at home. The healer encourages the patient to accept and relax into a reality that, from a deeper perspective, has always been present.

REFERENCES

Complete references used in this text are available online at expertconsult.inkling.com.

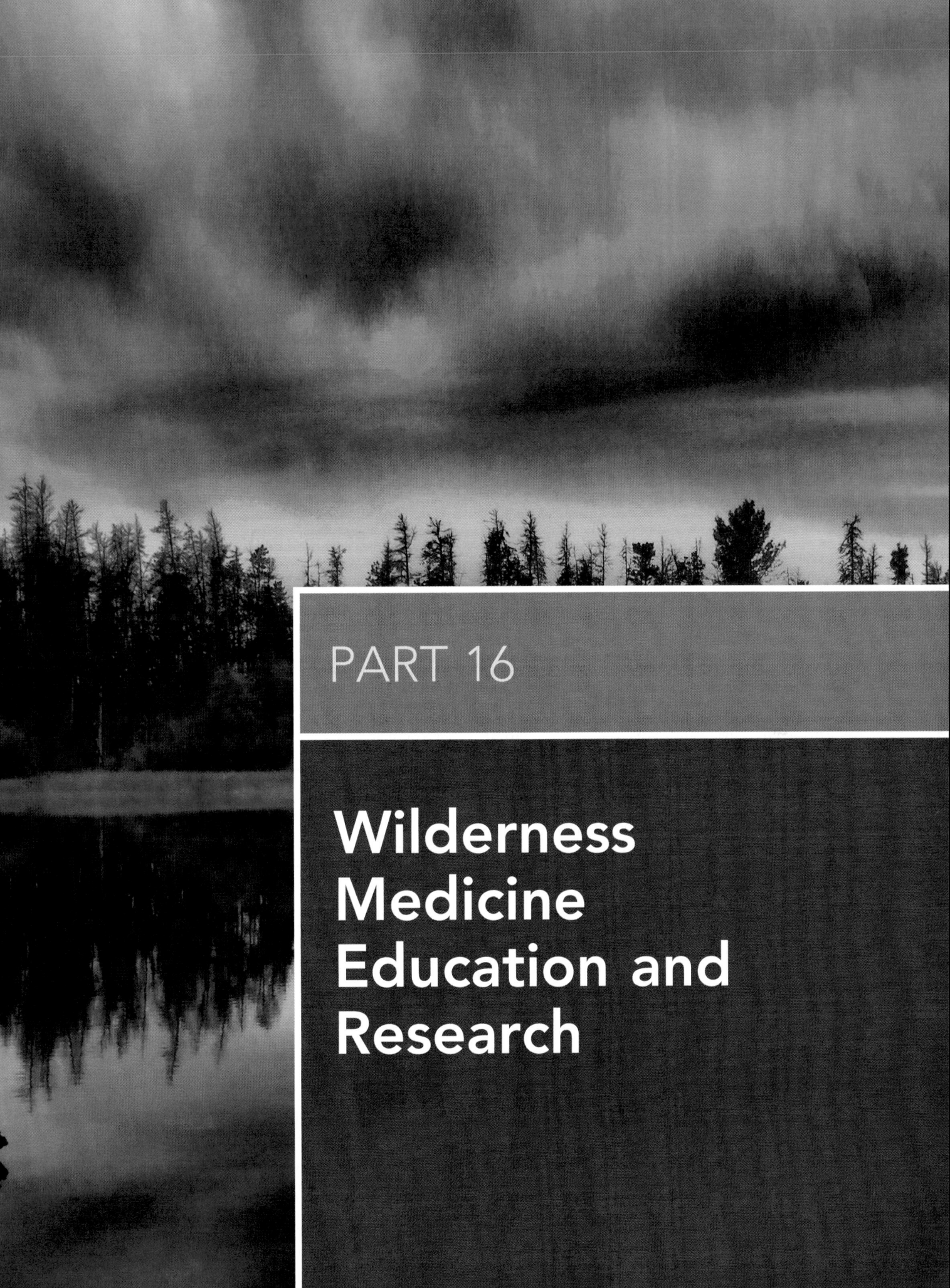

PART 16

Wilderness Medicine Education and Research

Whether the learner is an outdoor recreationalist or a physician specializing in one or more subdisciplines of wilderness medicine, wilderness medicine education has become increasingly popular and accessible. The features of wilderness medicine that make it attractive to an increasing number of people also present unique challenges to development of its educational programs. Training options and venues vary widely, from lecture sessions at conferences to fellowship programs lasting several years, and from first-aid courses for laypersons to semester-length programs combining wilderness, medical, and rescue curricula. The need for special attention to the learning process in the discipline of wilderness medicine has been recognized since the early 1990s; there are a growing number of collaborative efforts to define the core curriculum content and ensure the quality of the educational experience.[4,5,24,83] Work has been done at the individual program level to incorporate modern concepts of adult education in health care; however, little has been written about best practices and strategies for training wilderness medicine educators and designing training programs. There are no universally accepted standards for delivery of education or assessment of outcomes unique to this discipline.

The spectrum of learners in wilderness medicine is broad and diverse and closely mirrors the types of experiences to which the discipline applies. On one end of the spectrum are laypersons who seek to acquire knowledge on basic first aid, sometimes related to foreign travel, for reasons of safety or security. This group includes outdoors educators, guides, and outfitters who have not been medically trained. Next are persons seeking formal search and rescue medical training, including conventional emergency medical technician (EMT) and paramedic training tailored to the wilderness setting. The next level is represented by expeditionary advisors and multiple types of emergency care providers (e.g., EMTs, nurses, and physicians) who practice in isolated circumstances. Finally, there are technically oriented researchers and other professionals who seek topic- or environment-specific experience and fellowship with others who share their level of interest (Figure 113-1).

Early work by the Wilderness Medical Society (WMS) noted the differences between wilderness and urban prehospital emergency care.[120] These differences clearly illustrate what makes wilderness medicine education unique.

- Harsh environments greatly influence decisions on treatment and resourcing (Figure 113-2).
- There is a close link between basic survival needs and clinical care.
- Prolonged evacuation transport times of patients to definitive care are common.
- Uncommonly encountered injuries and clinical syndromes are seen because of exposure to extreme environments.
- Common illnesses and injuries require different approaches when complicated by austere circumstances.
- Advanced medical techniques may be required because of the nature of an injury or illness or prolonged transport times.
- Often, no immediate or reliable remote contact with a controlling physician in a definitive care setting is available.
- The need for improvisation of equipment and creative problem solving is typical.
- Expectations for successful management of a serious injury or illness are tempered by the circumstances.

- Standard urban protocols may be unrealistic or hazardous to caregivers.

Evolution of traditional models of adult education in health care has had a positive impact. These models incorporate widely varied teaching techniques that stimulate adults to learn difficult material at the deepest levels. Wilderness medicine challenges these models to deliver even more. The diverse nature of both teachers and learners adds another dimension. Traditional medical education tends to foster development of individualistic attitudes and may not produce practitioners who easily serve the needs of a group. However, successful management of situations that arise in the wilderness may hinge upon the ability of participants to serve as subordinate members of a team. Many wilderness medicine skills are not easy to learn and retain. They are technically difficult but also may need to be recalled immediately and applied accurately under adverse conditions with limited resources. Training often does not closely approximate the true impact of extreme surroundings on emergency or urgent care rendered in the wild.

As with any skill set, wilderness medicine techniques are best learned and maintained in the environments in which they will be applied. Wilderness medicine practitioners are typically action-oriented professionals who prefer to learn and practice their craft in the outdoors. Relying primarily on training in harsh environments may make it difficult to reliably deliver a high-quality learning experience that results in formation of lasting knowledge, however. In the field, absence of resources and presence of adverse conditions may limit the ability of advanced providers to use and maintain advanced skills. For example, physicians may well find themselves performing the same first aid, applying the same splints, and using the same hypothermia treatment as the lay provider, predominantly because resources are constrained (Figure 113-3).

This highlights the need to separate preparation and conditioning for the environment from education in order to facilitate the learning process.[4] Logistics and varying skill and physical conditioning levels of learners make it unreasonable to carry out full practical exercises for every wilderness medicine topic in every venue at which they are taught. As a result, most wilderness medicine programs combine traditional models of teaching (e.g., lecture format) with various types of experiential or event-based techniques.

Health care education generally serves independent groups that are homogeneous in their levels of education and learning experience. Groups such as nursing, medical, EMT, and physician assistant students have their own educational programs. Their professional preparation is generally addressed using subsets of educational techniques with little cross-pollination. Once a health care worker is fully certified in his or her field, the worker carries these differences forth as he or she becomes a learner and/or teacher in the continuing medical education/continuing education unit (CME/CEU) setting. It is from this educational melting pot that wilderness medicine draws its teachers.

In wilderness medicine, mixing groups (e.g., different specialties) of learners is inevitable. The groups represent different learning styles and all levels of health care certification and experience. In any given wilderness medicine educational program, one can find participants from most physician specialties seated next to EMTs of all levels and applications. Nursing vocations are well represented, as are PhD researchers, health care administrators, and laypeople with focused interests. Into this mix are thrown basic students from all health care vocations.

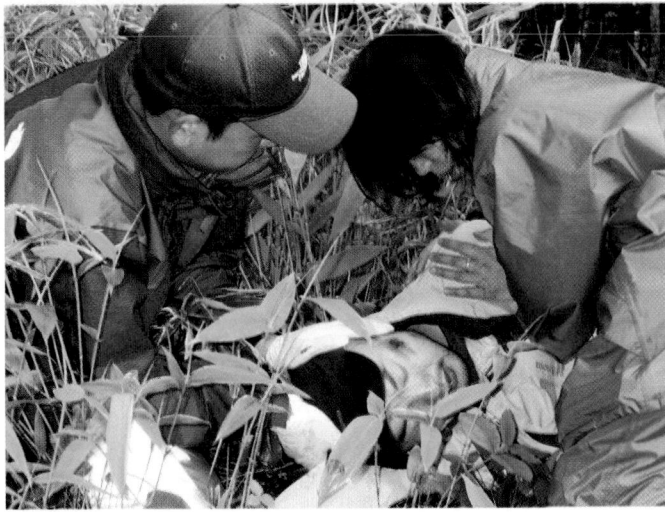

FIGURE 113-1 Wilderness medicine scenarios help learners of varied backgrounds function together in small teams. *(Courtesy Shana Tarter.)*

Finally, the growing international attention given to wilderness medicine as an academic discipline adds another factor. This mix of learners and blending of practical skills creates an interesting and often educationally enriching dynamic. In no other area of health care is the educational challenge at the same time so exciting and daunting.

Compounding the challenge of diverse learners are the varied educational backgrounds and teaching styles of the wilderness medicine educators. The process that prepares someone for a career as a leading academic pulmonary researcher produces different cognitive and practical skills than do mountaineering and scuba diving. The skill set required to effectively teach any of those highly technical wilderness medicine fields is different. The logistics of career management and available time make blending all desirable attributes and skills into the consummate wilderness medicine educator a rare event. This leads to a pool of educators whose teaching credentials might largely be derived from practical experience or notoriety rather than from having acquired specific training in planning and delivering adult education.

Instructors who provide wilderness medicine training should have a foundation in learning theory and skill at facilitating various elements of the learning process. It is unfortunate that although effective educators are instrumental in training practitioners, most practitioners are never formally trained as educators. Many persons who teach wilderness medicine do so because of their passion, but are without specific training or demonstrated competence as educators. The leap from providing patient care to teaching others to provide patient care can be significant.

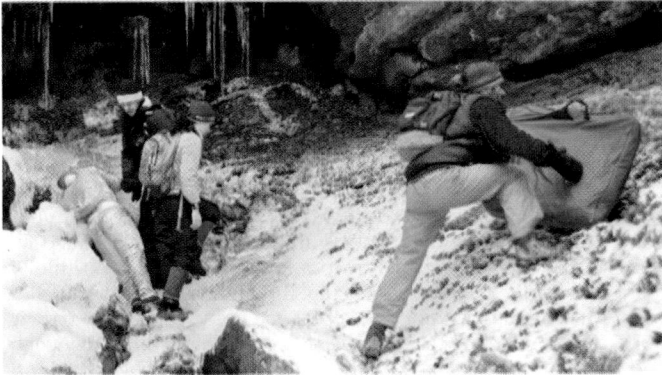

FIGURE 113-2 Wilderness medicine is a discipline practiced and learned in and around the extremes of environment. *(Courtesy Fred Baty.)*

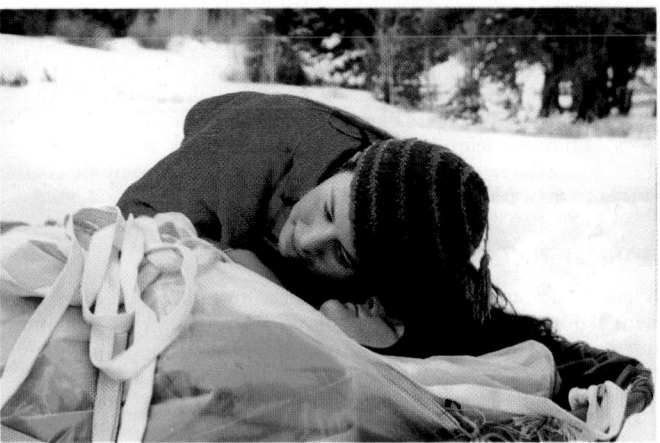

FIGURE 113-3 Wilderness medicine helps all providers focus on strong basic life support skills. *(Courtesy Melissa Gray.)*

Excellence in a clinical field does not necessarily translate to excellence as a clinical teacher.

One might presume that the high levels of education attained by individuals in these groups of learners would make the wilderness medicine educator's job easier. Except for the truly passive attendees to whom effective learning is less important than are the setting and experience, this proves not to be the case. Learners' expectations for receiving exciting, well-taught education are high, and they hold educators accountable. The well-prepared educator should have studied and understood the nature of a learner, just as an actor should be familiar with an audience.

Despite numerous adult education theories and the large amount of published work in this area, especially in disciplines of health care, there remains relatively little that specifically addresses wilderness medicine. Anecdotes, common sense, and the educational bias of the teacher are more common than hard evidence to support the preference of any education theory or its application over any other in this unique discipline. It is a general assumption that established techniques are of great use in wilderness medicine education. However, there remain two fundamental challenges. The first is determining which techniques work best for specific circumstances and how to apply them with specific types of learners. The second is preparing a cadre of wilderness medicine educators who are formally trained to understand the process and to make these applications work. Finally, as innovations, such as "digital health," accrue, wilderness medicine educators may find themselves among the first to determine their effectiveness.

PRINCIPLES OF ADULT LEARNING

There are important differences between the education of children and adults. These differences go far beyond the need for adults to be directive of their own learning and for children to be directed. Because of their general clientele, the details of the various learning theories may not be as important to wilderness medicine educators as an appreciation of some of their fundamental concepts. Although most wilderness medicine education is delivered to adult learners, the keen observer may note similarities to the education of school-age children. This speaks to the importance of attending to fundamental concepts. Much of the discipline is focused on acquiring skills meant to be used in emergency or urgent situations. These skills are most effectively taught by applying basic educational models.

Adult learning is generally predicated upon motivation. In the case of wilderness medicine, this might be personal enrichment, a professional opportunity, satisfying a job requirement, or an interesting continuing education experience. It may be that the learner is motivated by a previous experience for which the learner seeks validation of her or his actions or information that will allow the learner to perform more confidently in the future.

Regardless, the adult learner will generally present with a foundation of information and life experience that can at times be an impediment to assimilating new information. Adults tend to give greater credence to things they learned initially and are hesitant to reform their beliefs. Therefore, educators must create a safe opportunity for learners to explore their beliefs while coaching them toward a new understanding. Without developing this trust, students may remain resistant to learning.

BASIC PRINCIPLES

Some basic steadfast principles exist throughout modern academic thinking on adult education. The concept of proximity means that learning is enhanced and mastery achieved when new information or skills are used immediately. Classroom lectures in wilderness medicine are often necessary but are less effective with regard to proximity than are hands-on and small-group seminars.

Learners generally prefer educational approaches that focus on concepts and principles instead of fact-based information.[119] A concept derived from the teachings of Sir William Osler and known by nearly every classically trained physician holds that one should never spend time memorizing facts from a book at the expense of hands-on patient contact. This is why problem- and scenario-based learning has been incorporated into most modern health care education programs. The nuances of problem solving cannot easily be garnered from a book. Precious learning occurs at the bedside. Reading is important, but cannot replace education that takes place in "real life."

Learners respond favorably when they are able to participate in developing their own learning objectives.[119] The negotiation process between student and teacher that leads to properly established objectives builds relationships and trust that are at the foundation of the adult learning process. Participation by learners in goal setting facilitates ownership of the process and leads to higher levels of performance. Allowing this form of collaboration may seem counterintuitive to some, especially to educators used to teaching children, because they may use a more directive style of teaching.

Feedback to students may be the most important ingredient in solidifying learning and completing the education cycle.[119] To be effective, this should be direct, specific, and individualized to each learner. There are many reasons why this may not occur in health care education, ranging from the simple logistics of managing large classes to fear of retribution from students in the form of harsh evaluations if they feel they have been unduly criticized. However, these are not likely concerns in wilderness medicine education, because the typical program lends itself well to supporting a balanced learning experience. It also provides an opportunity to help students learn new study habits and improve skills performance. These habits transfer readily to learning other disciplines.

CONCEPTS, THEORIES, AND MODELS

There are numerous models to draw upon when developing an educational experience appropriate for the adult learner. One model seeks to balance the cognitive, emotional, and social needs of learners. Adult learners identify closely with the cognitive elements of learning, such as skills, knowledge, and understanding. To be more effective, the cognitive elements must be balanced with the emotional and social elements of the experience. Learner receptiveness is increased when the learning experience is enjoyable and respectful of diverse opinions. When the learner feels acknowledged, he or she will be more willing to participate, communicate, and cooperate. By balancing all three elements of an educational experience, the educator improves the opportunity for new learning to replace preconceptions.[56]

The Education Cycle

The notion that broad concepts of the process of learning can be applied as a cycle has been utilized in wilderness medicine education while planning a mountain medicine curriculum.[94] As depicted in Figure 113-4, the program director first makes an

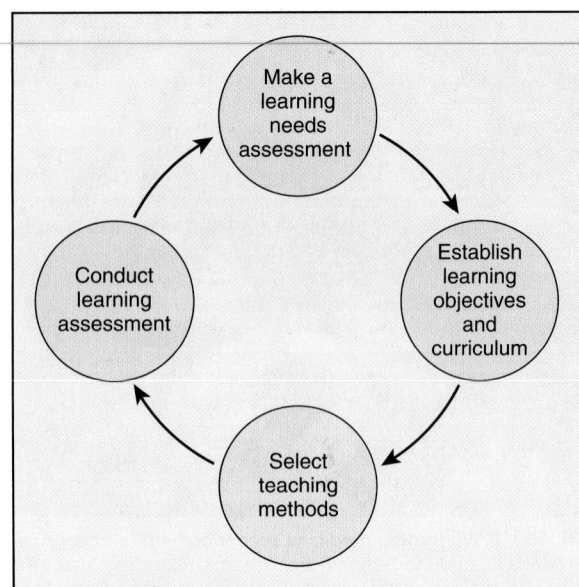

FIGURE 113-4 The education cycle.

assessment of the needs of the learners, getting to know the audience. Next is the often-underestimated task of establishing tailored and focused learning objectives. The educator then selects teaching methods and settings that best accomplish the objectives while meeting needs and expectations of the learners. Finally, after the experience, the educator makes an assessment to ascertain whether learning has occurred. This final step may be the most difficult and least attended. These elements will be addressed later in this chapter.

Experience-Based Learning

Kolb's model of learning is based on how individuals internalize and process learning experiences. Learners perform an action, referred to as a "concrete experience."[58] Then, they process the new information by "reflective observation." Next, they consider how the new information can be applied to their unique circumstances by using "abstract conceptualization." Having internalized the experience, they attempt it by "actively experimenting" with what they have learned to apply the knowledge and/or skills in new and unique ways. This model is reflected in several of the teaching and assessment techniques discussed later, especially those that address concrete skills.

Education and the Human Organism

Setting the conditions for learning can be conceptualized by using Maslow's famous explanation of how humans address fundamental needs.[74] Vella's work in popular education extends these ideas to the realm of education in the social context, but still deals with rudimentary human nature.[113,115]

Unmet physiologic needs, such as warmth and hunger, tend to impair learning because humans prioritize toward survival. Unfulfilled security needs, which Vella refers to as safety, distract from any process that does not pose such an immediate threat. In adult education, safety issues may be subtle.[113] Students who do not feel free to voice opinions or reveal a deficiency may be considered to lack a safe learning environment. Identification with a group of learners addresses the need for belonging that is used by organized team sports and the military. The need for self-esteem may be met by recognition for academic achievement in front of one's peers. Finally, the highest level of Maslow's concept, self-actualization, is represented by satisfied expectations on the part of the learner. By expanding these concepts and directly addressing each in the classic hierarchical fashion, an educator can remove many obstacles to learning during the planning phase of the educational experience. A learning event that accounts for them will have a high likelihood of success and have an impact on the student's life well beyond the experience.

Learner Sophistication

Another powerful tool available to teachers is identification of the level of understanding, or "sophistication," of the learner. Neal Whitman proposed four levels that learners traverse as they acquire new knowledge and skills. Correctly matching teaching methods to these will improve the overall experience by saving time, and increase the likelihood of fully meeting expectations.[119]

Most people begin the education journey at the level of being "unconsciously incompetent" and do not know enough about the material to know what they do not know. They become "consciously incompetent" as they gain appreciation for the amount and nature of the information they need to master. Next, they become "consciously competent," in that they know how to perform the skill or can use the information, but not yet with efficiency or at the level of mastery. The final stage, that of the teacher, is becoming "unconsciously competent." At this level, the learner becomes so practiced at the skill and the understanding is so well internalized that it can be performed to standard without consciously focusing on the process. The learner simply knows what to do.

Principles of Andragogy

There have been numerous efforts to roll learning theories together into a concise package of tools for health care education. To this end, the work of Malcolm Knowles is widely read and often cited by education academics. He put structure to the concept of helping adults learn and called it "andragogy." He suggested that through the principles of andragogy, adult learners are most successful when they are assisted in the process rather than directed through it unassisted.[55] Knowles made five basic assumptions about adult learners from which he derived his principles. They can be summarized as follows: (1) Adults tend to have internally and not externally focused motivations for learning; (2) the learning process should be related to solving real-life problems; (3) existing knowledge and experience greatly influence learning; (4) self-direction improves the learning experience; and (5) adults learn best with problem-based rather than subject-based methods. Knowles's seven principles of andragogy are summarized in Box 113-1.

Learner-Centered Education

Jane Vella has applied learning theory in unique ways to the social context across different cultures. She recognized that education lay at the heart of many social issues. The teacher's message is often lost in the delivery because of avoidable cross-cultural and interpersonal obstacles. She maintains that the key to adult learning is clear dialogue between the teacher and learner.[113,114] Educators too often fail to establish productive dialogue and hence select ineffective teaching approaches. Vella suggested that traditional hierarchical teacher-student roles be discouraged. Teachers should become facilitators. Barriers to dialogue are "addressed and eradicated." She offered to popular education a paradigm that places the learner at the center of the

---

BOX 113-2   Summary of Learner-Centered Principles

- Perform a learning needs assessment.
- Provide for learners' safety.
- Develop sound relationships to foster trust and encourage dialogue.
- Properly sequence learning tasks from simple to complex, and solo to groups.
- Provide opportunity for praxis—performing learning tasks and reflecting on the experience.
- Respect each learner's life, circumstances, autonomy, ideas, opinions, and time.
- Attend to ideas and feelings; link actions to them.
- Provide for immediate application of new skills and knowledge.
- Make dialogue more accessible by clarifying roles and reinforcing equity between teacher and learner.
- Use teamwork to enhance education.
- Engage learners directly by using small groups and an open exchange of ideas.
- Teachers and learners are accountable for what is learned. Learning must be tangible and observable.

---

educational universe. Her principles link theory to practical use in a way that enables learning in challenging circumstances. Vella's principles are summarized in Box 113-2.

Learning-Oriented Teaching Model

Cate and associates proposed their notion of a model of teaching based on concepts from educational psychology.[14] Their proposals are meant to influence all aspects of adult education, especially those of curriculum design, teaching techniques, and teacher assessment. An attractive feature is a method to "inventory" and match teaching and learning styles to improve outcomes. The authors build a model around what they identify as the "components of learning" and the "amount of guidance" that learners require to navigate the experience. Their premise is that, because education seeks to enable people to "function independently," the process should foster self-regulation of learning. In the model, learners mature from "externally guided" learning through "shared guidance" to self-guided or "internally guided" learning. This applies to both cognitive (what to learn) and affective (why to learn) components of learning.

Decision Making and Error

Wilderness medicine offers educators a controlled opportunity to help students look at how they make decisions and what traps or errors plague them in the process. By asking students to consider not only what decision they made, but also how they came to that decision, the educator can provide another tool to help develop the students' clinical reasoning skills. Able practitioners are expected to make appropriate decisions but commonly are not provided the tools to analyze their decision-making processes. Thus, they are less likely to be able to train others in the same skill.[17] Helping students recognize functional strategies and tools to avoid errors will create greater awareness for them in the future.

People make hundreds of decisions every day, most with little thought or consequence. These decisions may involve a small amount of research, or another opinion may be sought before making a choice. However, this sort of unstructured approach applied to wilderness medicine decision making can create problems for both caregivers and patients. Even small decisions, such as whether a treatment for wound infection appears to be efficacious, can have significant consequences if the infection becomes too difficult to manage in the wilderness and there is a missed opportunity for a simple evacuation. The distance from assistance and having to live with the consequences of a decision in an austere setting are important factors that inform wilderness medicine education.

In the wilderness, practitioners must make choices in environmentally challenging situations with incomplete information in the absence of external support or resources. Nevertheless,

---

BOX 113-1   Summary of Knowles' Principles of Andragogy

- The proper learning climate sets the stage for success.
- Adults prefer to actively participate in and contribute to planning for methods and curricula.
- Adults respond well to self-diagnosis of learning needs.
- Adults prefer to self-determine learning goals and objectives.
- Allow adults to identify their own resources for learning and formulate plans for their use.
- It is better to support adults while they implement their own learning strategies, rather than direct them through the process.
- Encourage reflective self-critique in the learning process.

there are predictable methods by which practitioners make decisions. The experience and ability to recognize patterns helps with perceptual decision making; protocols and analysis contribute to logical decision making. A skilled practitioner will engage all of these to a greater or lesser extent while making even a single decision, all the while remaining vigilant about potential errors and traps.

Experience is an important part of one's ability to recognize patterns and see similarities and differences between patients. The greater one's experience, the more one is able to develop a sense of typical and atypical presentations. Persons with limited experience may confuse experience with expertise, and even the experienced practitioner can make perceptual errors. Brains seek patterns. When a caregiver notices recognizable elements in a patient, it is possible to quickly anchor on a diagnosis that is not adjusted even when contradictory information becomes available.[36] Though objectivity is espoused, practitioners may seek evidence to support a conclusion rather than purposely trying to disprove it, which is known as confirmation bias. Decisions may be unduly biased by stress or emotion. Unconscious anxiety felt by the wilderness medicine provider when caring for a patient while thunderstorm clouds build, or the emotional connection to a recent patient with a similar presentation, can affect choices. Although a practitioner may have had significant experience managing a certain type of patient, if prior experience has all been in the controlled clinical setting, the stress of being in a remote setting may certainly influence decision making. How to manage this situation must somehow be taught to future wilderness medicine practitioners. Similar education missions are shared by the military, search and rescue professionals, ski patrollers, and expedition doctors.

To help sift through the overload of information that health care providers must manage, providers rely on heuristics or simple rules of thumb. For instance, if a patient has increased heart and respiratory rates and pale, cool, and clammy skin, a state of physiologic shock is suggested. Novice practitioners find heuristic shortcuts to diagnosis and treatment particularly useful when beginning to build a base of experience. However, heuristics can certainly be oversimplistic, situational, and sometimes incorrect. They can be applied quickly and might allow someone's initial thoughts and actions to focus in the right direction, but they carry the challenge of sometimes causing caregivers to cease thinking, investigating, and analyzing a given situation.

Another tool that is quite helpful is the protocol. One inherent challenge of providing wilderness medicine training to non–health care professionals is the inability for them to develop a solid patient care experience base prior to making challenging medical decisions in remote places. Even health care professionals may not be accustomed to making evacuation decisions. Protocols can help bridge the gap between training and experience. They also relieve the practitioner of relying on memory for many small details that can be easily looked up. Written guidelines covering the specifics of treatment, medication administration, and evacuation decisions help simplify complex situations. No set of protocols can cover every possible situation, but they can be a reasonable substitute for prompt access to expert opinion.

Finally, decisions can be made based on a studied analysis of the situation. In the clinical setting, this might involve using a variety of laboratory tests, as well as imaging and consultation. In the wilderness, the primary tool is patient assessment. Thorough, thoughtful, and careful assessment helps ensure that the provider makes rational decisions. Comprehensive assessment takes more time than does a general impression or applying a heuristic, but time is often available in the wilderness setting. The emphasis on ensuring that every patient receives a complete physical examination and determination of a full set of vital signs, and yields a thorough history, is one of the hallmarks of wilderness medicine training. When students take shortcuts through this process, a well-prepared educator will remind them that by doing so they are dangerously prone to making assumptions and denying themselves access to valuable information.

The strongest decision making balances the objectively observed with the subjectively perceived. It is important to

BOX 113-3 Kaufman's Principles to Guide Teaching Practice

- The learner should be an active contributor to the process.
- Learning should relate to understanding and solving real-life problems.
- Learners' knowledge and experience are critical and must be accounted for.
- Learners should have the opportunity to self-direct their learning.
- Learners should have ample opportunity to practice, self-assess, and receive constructive feedback.
- Learners should have frequent opportunities to reflect upon the learning process.
- Role models have a great impact on learning.

become mindful students and practitioners of the process. This self-awareness can help avoid consequential errors. Throughout the process, caregivers should prompt themselves to consider: What assumptions am I making? Am I missing or ignoring data that do not fit my pattern? What are the most likely and worst case scenarios? Have I considered alternative diagnoses? What emotions are influencing my thinking? Have I discussed my thinking with someone else? Have I sought input from my team? Have I used my protocols, checklists, and other resources? Can I step away from the situation to minimize my emotional connection and thereby create an objective space in which to think? After the situation is resolved, providers should reflect on each experience, assimilate learning, and seek feedback from others. If one cannot articulate how a decision was reached, one should strive to improve this skill.

Putting It All Together

Theories and models are meaningless without practical application. Direct extrapolation of ideas from theorists who have diverse backgrounds and agendas to the realm of wilderness medicine education is difficult. Kaufman reviewed several adult education theories in the context of health care education.[54] He examined them for key areas of commonality and offered simple principles to "guide" medical educators as they think about and plan educational experiences (Box 113-3). Wilderness medicine educators can easily adopt these.

EDUCATIONAL TECHNIQUES

There are a myriad of delivery techniques available to the modern medical educator. Although techniques have been extensively studied across many disciplines, the method of educating the medical learner in a way that results in consistently improved performance and outcomes exceeding other methods remains elusive. There is no single method that is effective for all types of learners in all settings. In wilderness medicine, this is compounded by the degree to which hands-on skills depend on a solid grasp of basic science combined with flexible application of clinical medicine.

Selection of the most effective methods depends largely on the setting and the expectations and needs of learners. The prudent curriculum designer avoids incorporating attractive methods of presentation designed to capture attention without substantively improving educational quality. Schweinfurth characterized the problem of finding the right mix of techniques when he described his use of interactive training among otolaryngology residents. He referenced comments from a focus group of trainees, discussing what he called "innovative learning strategies." He found that learners were hesitant to endorse innovative strategies, in order to avoid complex exercises that might compromise the limited time available to conduct didactic sessions. His learners found some attempts at innovation to be "too experimental" or a "waste of time."[101] The lesson should be that innovation, as an end in and of itself, may not serve the learner. Innovation that causes the learner to walk away with a sense of improvement can be considered successful.

Learning Strategies

Current literature on successful learning indicates that most students lack knowledge about helpful study strategies.[11] Traditional reliance on rereading material or repeated practice of a single skill, also known as massed practice, creates the illusion of knowledge. The familiarity that comes from reading material for the second or third time or the short-term improvement noted with repetition may be illusory and lead to overconfidence. Numerous studies show such short-term improvements do not last. Instead, learners need to build new study habits, which include self-testing, spacing and interleaving of material, and struggle. These strategies may feel less productive initially, but result in greater retention and application of knowledge.

Learners may engage in self-testing or retrieval practice by quizzing or being quizzed on previous material. Educators can facilitate this process through regular short quizzes, with scenarios requiring students to apply information learned at an earlier point. In-class exercises force students to recall information and compare and contrast it with similar information, and create structure for students to test each other. These strategies may create initial discomfort for the learner; however, the evidence is clear that learning will be deeper. When applied to clinical performance, both written testing and use of standardized patient experiences produced superior results on final written examinations compared with rereading and reviewing material. The students who trained with standardized patients performed better on final patient examinations than did those who trained solely by written testing.[62] This research underscores the important role that scenarios and simulation training play in wilderness medicine, as opposed to exclusive reliance on lectures and reading materials.

There is strong support for the concept of spacing or interleaving information by introducing new material before the individual has achieved mastery of the original content. The educator can apply spacing in the structure of skills practice. Rather than repeated practice of the same skill, consider multiple shorter practices throughout the educational experience. Students may gain initial experience with a specific skill and then later be asked to reproduce that skill in scenarios or other forms of practical assessment. This allows the student the opportunity to "forget" between experiences. The struggle to perform, sometimes called a desirable difficulty, strengthens the student's learning.[11] The educator can apply the concept of interleaving by consistently introducing new concepts and crafting scenarios that draw upon a mix of topics. Students may be challenged to consider solutions to problems they have yet to encounter. Using a scenario to introduce a new topic provides the opportunity for a student to apply problem-solving skills in the absence of preexisting knowledge. Even if the solution is initially incorrect, the student will demonstrate improved understanding when the topic is formally introduced.[11]

In addition to misperceptions about effective study strategies, most learners and educators still hold to the belief that receiving information in one's preferred individual learning style has a bearing on the quality of learning. The learning styles theory is well entrenched in education at all levels. There are myriad resources available to assess individual learning styles and prepare teachers to provide instruction for specific types of learners. Many learners will claim to know their preferred learning style and hold firmly to the belief that they will fail as learners unless provided instruction in a matching format. However, research does not uphold this belief. Learners misconstrue satisfaction with performance. What seems clear is the importance of matching the topic to the delivery method. When the instructional style is closely matched to the material, all learners perform better, regardless of their perceived learning style preference.[11,90]

Research also shows that learners who have the aptitude for building mental models out of general concepts, known as high-structure learners, are more capable of assimilating information than are low-structure learners, who rely on examples.[11] Educators can support high-structure learning by teaching in principles rather than absolutes. Students have a higher likelihood of successful problem solving when they can rely on decision-making principles or skills principles rather than single examples. For instance, teaching a student principles of a good wilderness splint (padded, not bulky, rigid, adjustable, digits accessible for assessment, joints above and below a fractured bone immobilized, bone above and below an injured joint immobilized) allows the student to problem solve with different materials regardless of the environment. Teaching the student to build one splint with specific tools may inadvertently restrict the student's ability to adapt when he or she is lacking those specific materials. The educator can facilitate the student's ability to recognize commonalities by highlighting and repeating patterns between topics. This will help the student to more quickly sift through information to improve the focus of the student's assessment and continue to enrich mental models as the knowledge base grows.

The adage "less is more" has a firm place in the world of education. Learners are frequently inundated with both volume and detail. Many are challenged to decode the underlying message buried in the mountain of information. Without understanding the fundamental and most critical concepts, it is unlikely that the recipient will apply information appropriately to solve a problem. Though the learner certainly bears some responsibility for this process, the educator must also be clear with the messaging. To this end, educators should consider applying a simple process to distill each topic into its fundamental essence before delivering the information (Box 113-4).

One approach is to teach a topic with three informative, yet simple, sentences. The sentences should reflect the underlying principles to be conveyed. This is a remarkably difficult activity until one practices and develops the skill. This exercise provides a valuable framework for lectures, practice sessions, and scenario debriefings. It also creates a structure for quizzing students to assess learning. It is easy to dismiss the idea of simplification as unsuitable to medical education. Yet, this seemingly rudimentary activity often highlights a lack of understanding of material on the part of the practitioner turned educator. Persons who excel at clinical education understand the power of making complex things simple. By modeling this with students, they provide an example of how students will ultimately communicate with patients.[99]

Lecture

Lecture is the most often used educational technique and is the default medium for most educators. This structured approach to information delivery feels familiar to both student and teacher. It offers several important advantages. Large amounts of information can be delivered in relatively short periods of time. Planning is generally easier for the lecture format. It requires little logistical support and only one teacher. It works well for highly technical information that the learner will most likely have to study again in order to internalize. Lectures can be easily enhanced with audiovisual aids. All of this adds up to a degree of efficiency that is highly attractive to the resource-limited educator. In one small but interesting study, Reed illustrated that, despite the availability of highly technical and resource-intensive teaching methods, a simple "low-cost, low-tech" lecture approach can offer rewards in terms of improved skill performance.[98]

The lecture technique has several equally important disadvantages. Learning is highly dependent on the delivery skill of the teacher. Because of the passive role played by the learner, many adults do not respond as well to this approach. It is generally

---

BOX 113-4 Example of Three-Sentence Class on Diabetes

Although diabetes is a complex disease process, the educator can practice simplifying information to help novice practitioners make decisions in remote settings.

1. Diabetes is a disease that affects the body's ability to process sugar.
2. Diabetics can become ill when they have too much or too little sugar.
3. If a known diabetic has a change in mental status, give sugar and evacuate.

BOX 113-5   Methods to Enhance a Lecture

- Clearly communicate the purpose of the lecture to learners.
- Be familiar with the culture, attitudes, expectations, professions, and experiences of learners.
- Pace the lecture; use the 12- to 20-minute rule for the span of attention. Break up the pace with discussions, a question-and-answer period, or group work.
- Personalize the presentation with examples.
- Speak from notes rather than complete scripts. Know the material!
- Use visual aids.
- Use critical incidents with which the learners are familiar to make teaching points and solidify learning.
- Leave with a question or challenge to encourage learners to explore further.
- Perform self-assessment through videos, learner evaluations, and other forms of appraisal.

---

accepted that levels of retention of material presented by pure lecture are lower than more active teaching techniques.[106] There is generally a limited opportunity for hands-on applications and practice. Thus, the usefulness of lectures is limited in some areas of wilderness medicine that are largely skills oriented. The more restricted the opportunity for student questioning and dialogue, the less effective becomes this technique. Students can often more effectively learn information to be presented by lecture by themselves, particularly when they are able to view the material in a supportive setting. Methods to enhance the lecture are listed in Box 113-5.

Length and depth of a lecture are dictated by both time limitations of the class and experience of the student group. They may also be influenced by expectations regarding prereading or study. Regardless, when planning a lecture for a wilderness medicine topic, teachers may find that using a simple five-section outline structure can be helpful. Beginning with the definition of the injury or illness, the teacher then provides background information relevant to the audience. For example, for the topic of cardiac chest pain, the wilderness first-aid student may only need to hear that "Chest pain can have many causes ranging from sore muscles to a heart attack. Two prominent causes are angina (heart pain) and heart attack (myocardial infarction)."

Learners may next be taught to recognize the condition. Typically, a description of signs and symptoms and supporting imagery works well for this purpose. Unless the goal is to teach clinical management of environmentally induced emergencies, one should consider how a condition can be realistically assessed in a wilderness setting rather than relying on information that will likely only be available in a traditional clinical setting. This can be followed by description and demonstration of wilderness treatments, accompanied by discussion of evacuation criteria for the injury or illness. It is helpful to distinguish between criteria for an evacuation (requiring medical care, but not an immediate threat to life or limb) and a rapid evacuation (threat to life or limb). The final step may be to consider relevant prevention strategies. This lecture flow will help students apply the information and make real-world decisions.

Although lecturing may feel like a straightforward skill, there are common pitfalls to be avoided. Instructors are responsible for creating a safe learning environment for students. Pertinent to lecturing, this is strongly associated with language choice. Profanity, judgmental descriptions of patients, use of only one gender pronoun, impatience with student questions, and inappropriate commentary generally undermine the educator's credibility and foster an environment where students are reluctant to ask questions. Rarely do instructors recognize when they are making off-putting comments, making self-awareness difficult. Another seemingly innocent tool that can be misapplied is the anecdote or story. The educator's intent may be to illustrate a teaching point. However, if learners perceive that the focus of the effort has become the teacher rather than the teaching, or if the story deviates from the message, it becomes a distraction.

The choice to include an anecdote or a story should be scrutinized with the same level of intentionality as is every other element of the teaching process.

Preparedness and familiarity with the topic are of critical importance. Memorization of material is minimally effective. The first few times that an instructor teaches a topic, some form of notes may be helpful for staying on task and tracking small details. Students will appreciate the use of notes if they support the flow of the lecture and the accuracy of its content; they will dislike the use of notes if they become a distraction, however. The lecturer is on a slippery slope if he or she reads the notes or slides to the class instead of engaging the class with eye contact and using audiovisual support tools primarily to enrich the lecture.

The desire to address the learning need at the moment or the fear of loss of credibility if the instructor is unable to answer a question can tempt the instructor to deliver incorrect or unhelpful information. Educators should be prepared to acknowledge the limitations of personal knowledge by answering "I don't know" to questions, with a commitment to follow up and obtain the answer for the student. This creates a sense of trust.

Time is an insidious factor that creeps into an instructor's vocabulary while teaching. Seemingly innocuous references to time can devalue the quality of the lecture. Phrases such as "We'll go quickly because we're running behind," "Let's skip the demo because I'm over time," "Take a quick 5-minute break," "Let's talk about that later so we can finish," or "Let's finish early so we can all get out of here" imply disorganization and poor time management on the part of the instructor and the instructor's assumption that the participants have little interest in learning. Students are in a course to learn and in many cases have paid for the privilege. An instructor owes it to students to provide as much education as possible in the allotted time window. An instructor's monologue about time and whether the class is ahead of or behind schedule should remain internal. Students are often oblivious to the small increments of time allotted to various topics. They tend to be concerned more with starting and ending the training day at the specified hours, and remaining true to the time allotted for breaks. By referencing time, students will become conscious of it. If the instructor does not reference time, the students will remain focused on the experience at hand and will not be influenced by instructor anxiety.

Finally, instructors must be attentive to all subtle nuances of professionalism. From attire to confidence with operation of the audiovisual equipment to management of the group, the instructor's educational competence will in part be judged by the little things done or not done.

Demonstration

It is challenging to take a skill that is commonplace and familiar and demonstrate it in a manner that is successfully reproducible at a high degree of quality by others. Educators are quickly enticed by the temptation to lapse into jargon-laced vocabulary and a presumption of knowledge and experience not appropriate for the audience. For example, by using technical terms or phrases such as "You all know how to tie a surgeon's knot," the educator may establish credibility or perhaps display prowess but in the process alienate learners who cannot tie the knot and now feel they are not welcomed into the elite circle of those who know how to tie it.

Demonstration of a skill(s) providing a particular type of care in a traditional clinical setting may not translate well to an effective presentation in a wilderness setting. Teachers must commit to the same high level, and perhaps more, of preparation when designing and practicing demonstrations as they do in crafting lecture notes and slides. Poorly executed, incomplete, or nonreproducible demonstrations that are visible by only a portion of the class are often the result of overestimating how familiar learners are with the skill. The goal of a demonstration is to create a final visual image for learners that serves as an enduring model.

To avoid demonstration pitfalls, the wilderness medicine educator can employ a few simple strategies. Although a frequent goal of wilderness medicine education is to train providers to improvise, the instructor should not improvise in order to complete a demonstration. Forethought when planning a demonstration may include such details as choosing individuals best suited to the task and making the teaching point, while also considering how best to be certain that the task can be successfully accomplished. When teaching how to turn (logroll) a patient as a single rescuer, one may select the largest individual in the group to serve as the patient in order to make the point that the skill is about mechanics and not strength, but also select a "rescuer" of sufficient strength to be able to turn the patient. If one is building a lower extremity splint, an individual with a fairly cylindrical leg may be chosen as the patient, rather than one with bulging thighs and skinny calves, to simplify splint construction. For an intravenous demonstration, one may select a student with easily located veins. Students will adapt their knowledge to real people and difficult situations, but the instructor's demonstration should be well performed and successful. Another factor is choosing the correct equipment. The instructor must ensure that demonstration gear is appropriately sized and in good working condition. For example, effectiveness of an otherwise good demonstration can be diminished by using a short sleeping bag to demonstrate a hypothermia wrap on a tall person. Considering the position of the demonstration patient and the instructor in relation to the class will maximize visibility and enhance learning. Students may be asked to leave their seats to come close and observe. They may find overuse of "pearls of wisdom" and discussion during the demonstration to be distracting. Minimizing distractions will focus students' attention on the skill being taught. The successful educator can often teach by showing without telling. Some skills lend themselves to a completely silent demonstration. Finally, practicing the demonstration in advance with the materials that will be used during the demonstration will avoid a cumbersome presentation in front of students and increase efficiency. Time is often limited, so the shorter the demonstration, the more time students will have to practice the skill, ask relevant questions, and receive answers.

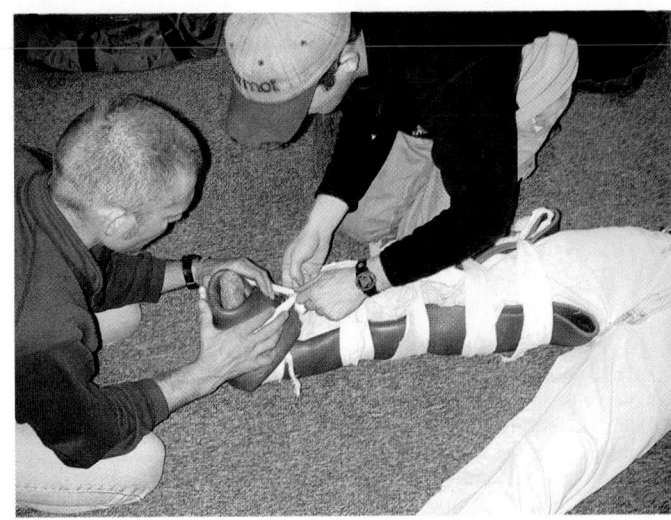

FIGURE 113-5 Practicing skills in a controlled environment builds confidence before learners apply the information in more challenging environments. *(Courtesy Gates Richards.)*

Skills Development Sessions

One attraction of wilderness medicine is its skills-rich content. Focus on improvisation provides ample opportunity for practicing techniques such as splint building, lifts and rolls, and wound closure. These practice sessions provide an opportunity for students to adapt and apply principles learned during lectures and demonstrations while receiving feedback and coaching. However, skills demonstrations notoriously have the opportunity to go astray if they are not carefully designed, planned, and performed.

Consideration should be given to appropriately matching the type of practice session to the topic. Some skills have a series of steps that should be practiced in sequence; certain assessments and cardiopulmonary resuscitation fall into this category. Some form of guided practice would be well suited for early practice with these topics. An instructor can lead a group in a step-by-step practice session, much like a square dance caller, to ensure that each student focuses on the task. Alternatively, students may guide each other through a series of steps using flow sheets or algorithms. As learners become more proficient with skills, they may become frustrated by this structure of practice, but it can be a helpful tool if it appears that learners are taking shortcuts in practice. The majority of skills-oriented learning tasks lend themselves to individual or small-group practice. If poorly managed, these opportunities can devolve into social time for students, who may see this as an opportunity to take care of unrelated needs. Inappropriately sized or poorly maintained equipment may force students to verbalize skills rather than practice them. To avoid this, establish strategies in advance to keep people focused on a task. Considerations include the group size, length of practice, types and operation of equipment, and practice outcomes. Teachers can facilitate the setup of instruction and transitions by dividing large groups into small practice groups, providing an ample supply of preapproved equipment, and briefing groups on what other materials they may use. Instructors should state the time limit for the session and indicate how many turns of practice of each particular skill

are expected for each student, and whether an instructor needs to assess the performance in some manner. Student performance during practice sessions often directly reflects the quality of demonstration provided to students. When watching students practice, it quickly becomes apparent when they fail to complete an element of the skill, usually because the instructor did not teach that element and, rather, finished the demonstration by verbalizing how the technique "should" be completed. The instructor must be present and engaged during practice sessions, which provide an excellent opportunity for individual evaluation and coaching (Figure 113-5).

Problem-Based Learning

A highly effective trend in health care education is using problem-based learning (PBL). PBL can take various forms, but generally learners are presented with a problem and guided through a structured discussion that leads to a preestablished solution. This learner-centered approach has proven popular among students and demonstrates comparable outcomes when compared with other, more traditional formats. An interesting aspect of PBL is that student-led experiences tend to be more highly favored among participants than those facilitated by faculty, yet the outcomes remain at least comparable in terms of satisfaction and examination scores.[41,104]

PBL offers great versatility to the curriculum planner. It can be used whether the focus is on acquiring pure fact-based knowledge or practical skills. It is most often applied in the small-group setting and therefore may pose logistics challenges in certain space- and resource-limited settings. It complements the strengths of small-group learning in that it reinforces communication and problem-solving skills, teamwork, individual responsibility for learning, and the need to share knowledge.[122] PBL tends to yield the best results when it is structured and forces learners to use critical thinking skills. It fosters the process of analysis, organized problem solving, and decision making, using group discussion to direct and reinforce learning. The general format for PBL is presented in Box 113-6.[7]

Case-Based Learning

Case-based learning is a subtype of PBL that is extremely useful in wilderness medicine education. It makes use of several powerful aspects of theory to solidify learning. This method improves outcomes over pure lecture for certain types of material. Many of the skills-oriented topics in wilderness medicine can be easily presented through scenarios and cases. The teacher can easily modify case scenarios to suit various learner levels, styles, and objectives. It can be modified for learning experiences in the field setting because, if properly planned, it requires minimal logistics support.

1. Presentation and evaluation of the problem
2. Generation of solutions to the problem (hypotheses)
3. Inquiry to review the hypothesis, including gathering information, such as laboratory tests and findings of a physical examination
4. Interview information
5. Application of the information gathered to the original problem
6. Review and synthesis of what has been learned and evaluation of the process

This technique motivates learners because it relates directly to the reasons for which they sought the experience. It offers an automatic sequence and information source for presentation, because cases flow in accordance with actual or simulated events. The teacher generally facilitates discussion and assists students with understanding and methods to organize information. Clinical problem-solving styles can easily be demonstrated.

Scenarios and Role-Play

Scenario-based, role-play training is quite familiar to most if not all prehospital emergency care educators. It maximizes many of the strengths of newer approaches to adult education because it guides self-motivated students through a process of "discovery" of the information.[70] The main role for teachers in this format is to facilitate, not direct, the learning process.[43] Being an expert in the clinical details of each case is less important than understanding how to apply PBL. This method is often scripted and makes use of actors, props, and moulage to simulate real-life situations. The logistics of carrying out this aggressive training technique may be prohibitive to some programs, but the investment is worth the effort in terms of retention of knowledge and improved outcomes shown by learners. Nearly all organizations that train prehospital wilderness medicine practitioners use some form of complex case- or scenario-based learning program. Role-play has benefits beyond the teaching and development of technical skills, notably including communication. Introduction of role-play as a training method may enhance the realism of technical skills training and lead to better patient-provider communication.[86]

Scenario- or simulation-based training is a popular choice for reinforcing assessment skills and providing opportunities for error in a low-risk environment. Learning will not occur simply by providing this type of experience, so whether using people in role-play or simulation mannequins for the scenario, it is crucial to design the experience with carefully crafted goals (Figure 113-6).

Role-play has benefits beyond teaching and learning technical skills. One recent randomized controlled trial confirmed the utility of using role-play when teaching communication skills. The authors of this study of medical students randomized to learn a skill with and without role-play concluded that, although there were no differences in technical performance between groups, introduction of role-play as a training method enhanced the realism of technical skills training and led to better patient-physician communication.[86]

Similar to practice sessions, scenario training should have established parameters that include time limits, an appropriate ratio of rescuers to patients, and allowable equipment. It should be both realistic and targeted to the audience. Because the topic is wilderness medicine, it follows that scenarios should teach, assess, and reinforce care delivered under austere and remote wilderness conditions. Although plane crashes and motor vehicle wrecks certainly occur during wilderness trips and are relevant for certain response entities, they do not represent the core of wilderness injuries and illnesses. Scenarios used early in an educational program should be straightforward and focus on reinforcing correct and consistent skill performance. This is generally accomplished by allowing only one or two rescuers per patient. As the education process progresses, scenarios can evolve in complexity and severity. Ending the program with a scenario celebrating the competent performance of basic skills sends students off with a memory they may find useful when they have to perform in the real world.

The following template is a helpful tool in developing successful scenarios. Note that the "story" is intentionally left as the final element. This focuses the developer on the goals of the experience and allows for the scenario to be used regardless of audience, location, or environmental challenges. By changing the story, the scenario can be made relevant to many audiences (Figure 113-7).

Scenario Template:
Three learning objectives or debriefing points
Ratio of rescuers to patients
Equipment needed
Time limit
Moulage (stage makeup for injuries) needed
Patient briefing, including the story, mechanism of injury or illness, injuries and associated symptoms, vital signs, acting cues, physical location boundaries

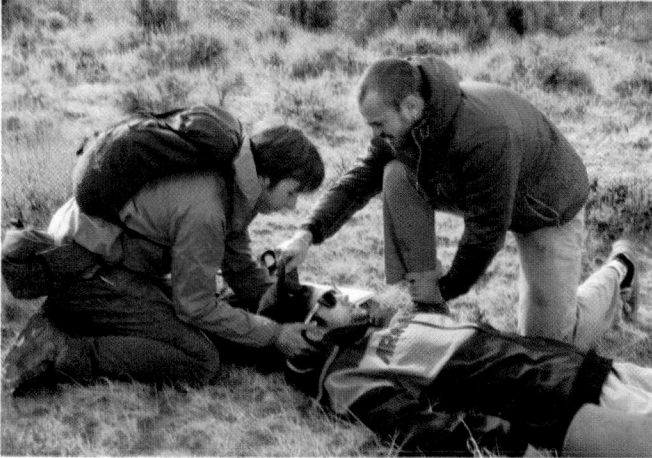

FIGURE 113-6 Role-play scenarios are an effective tool for reinforcing assessment skills and introducing decision making. *(Courtesy Marcio Paes Barreto.)*

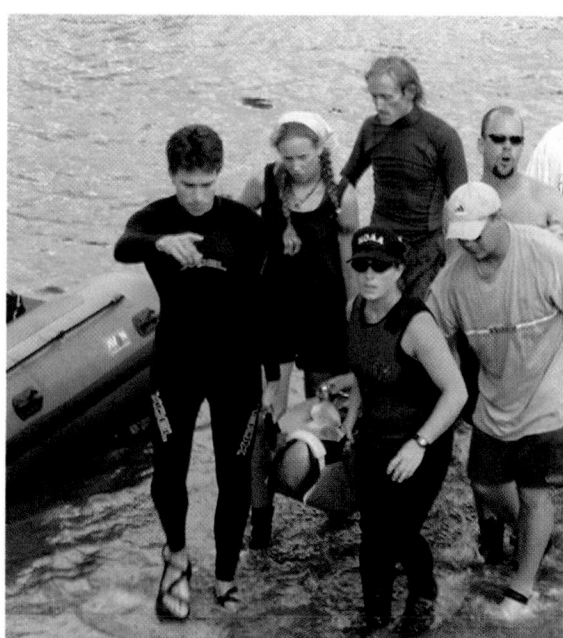

FIGURE 113-7 Wilderness medicine scenarios can be readily adapted to specific settings, such as marine operations. *(Courtesy Shana Tarter.)*

Rescuer briefing, including the story, location, time of day, resources, patient information, scenario goals or end point, performance expectations

Scenarios can be used to reinforce a previous topic or to introduce a new topic. It is simplest to set up many iterations of the same scenario, for example, five patients all with exactly the same condition and each rescue group manages the same situation. This facilitates simple, targeted debriefings. At times, it may be appropriate to set up a scenario to illustrate a differential diagnosis. For instance, some patients might exhibit a mild form of injury or illness, and others a severe form. In the debriefing, the instructor may highlight the differences and emphasize the implications for care. In multicasualty incident scenarios, each patient may have different injuries. Each level of variability adds preparation time, which runs the risk of taking away from student practice time.

Realism is a critical element of scenario-based training. Rescuers and patients should be coached to stay in their roles to create an emotional engagement with the experience. Patients may need a specific script to understand how to accurately portray learning objectives. Both underacting and overacting can be detrimental to the learning experience. Stage makeup, or moulage, can be incorporated to great effect. Having students play the roles of both rescuer and patient provides opportunity to gain experience applying new skills, as well as opportunity to provide feedback to others about those same skills (Figure 113-8).

Student safety is a priority. In scenarios, limiting the geographic distribution of students and ensuring there are adequate rescuers to manage each patient are ways to mitigate risk. Monitoring assessments, including the appropriateness of physical contact and language usage, are also important requirements.

Instructors or evaluators actively engage with the students during each scenario by watching their performance, correcting errors, and asking questions. When students are new to the skills, teaching and feedback are more directive. As they progress, students are prompted to consider their decision making or asked how their treatment meets or deviates from the key principles presented in a particular class.

It is common for students to see scenarios as problems that have a specific answer. After they believe they know the answer, they may cease their assessment and assume they are finished. The instructor can reinforce the importance of a complete assessment in a number of ways. Using moulage may help to create multiple injuries for students to find. If all major areas of the skin are visualized, discovering a simulated injury serves as a reward for a thorough physical examination. Scenarios may be designed with causal factors that can only be illuminated through a thorough interview and that are unlikely to be found early in the assessment. Simulated patients are told that rescuers must actually assess vitals each time; only after they are verbalized should any modifications be stated. Students can hold each other accountable for incomplete assessments.

Effective scenario debriefing is what helps solidify an experience into learning. Ultimately, a well-crafted debriefing session may illustrate the pitfalls of taking shortcuts to a diagnosis. As noted above, debriefing points should be the backbone of scenario construction. Two or three points of emphasis are generally appropriate for most scenarios. Considerations for debriefing points might include:

Does this patient need evacuation? Quickly or slowly? By what means?

Was this patient improving or deteriorating? How did you know?

Give a patient report as if you were making a cell phone call.

What principles did you apply in your treatment?

Was there a mechanism for a spinal injury?

What are your anticipated problems?

The debriefing should be structured and time efficient. A debriefing that is lengthy or generates multiple student questions may be indicative of poorly designed scenario outcomes or a scenario that was too complex.

Subject-Based Learning

The term *subject-based learning* (SBL) is a euphemism for traditional teacher-centered techniques of presenting information. The student in an SBL setting is the passive recipient of instruction rather than an active participant in the learning process. SBL methods typically present information on a broad topic in a format mainly based on lecturing. Health care curricula designed around SBL tend to be redundant, because broad topics may deal with the same or similar types of information. For example, a traditional first-year-of-medical-school, basic science curriculum will have a series of lectures on pharmacology, biochemistry, pathology, and microanatomy. Each will incorporate specific material on diabetes presented by different departments. The student may have to wait a year for a session focusing on diabetes that incorporates elements of pharmacology, biochemistry, pathology, and microanatomy.

Although SBL has a role, most health care educators have incorporated more learner-centered techniques, such as PBL, into their curricula. The main drawback of SBL is that by favoring efficient delivery and lengthy, complex curricula, it often fails to take advantage of features in adult learning theory that are known to lead to higher rates of retention and deeper learning.

Discussion

The technique of discussion is a versatile and highly effective teaching tool rooted in behavioral science. People learn better when information is presented in ways that challenge them to process it in more than one way. Although not as efficient as a lecture in terms of the quantity of information that can be delivered, it offers advantages to the wilderness medicine educator when teaching problem-solving skills and broad concepts that can be applied to many types of scenarios. Students more readily internalize material that they have to intellectually manipulate in various ways. The information is introduced, processed, and discussed. Students modify their own notions and then formulate solutions based on their new internal constructs of the problem. Learning is guided by the facilitator-teacher and reinforced by the students, all of whom are going through the same process and adopting a similar problem-solving skill set.

There are two basic modes of discussion-based learning.[60] The Socratic questioning method challenges students to identify the most important features of a specific problem and then reconstruct it using general principles that are the true focus of the discussion. Developmental discussion approaches the problem

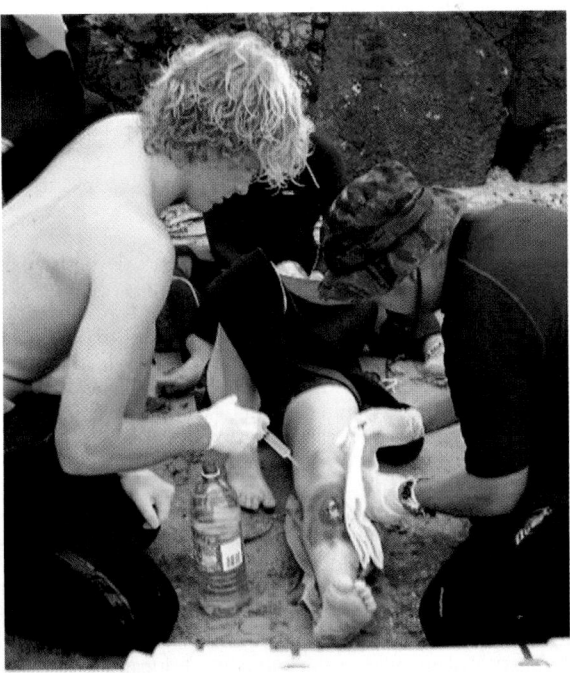

FIGURE 113-8 Moulage adds to the realism and the intensity of scenario-based training. *(Courtesy Shana Tarter.)*

in parts. It keeps all students focused on one part at a time and takes advantage of the group setting to ensure that teaching points are addressed.

Teacher-facilitators may highlight discussion with the powerful tools of analogy, discovery, and induction to stimulate learning and ensure retention.[22] The process of analogy illustrates concepts by asking students to use examples with which they are already familiar. The process of discovery leads students through a sequence of steps from the most basic to the more complex. This guides them to the final goal of deeper understanding of the principal learning objective. The process of induction asks students to take general lessons from specific examples or experiences, make comparisons, and draw new conclusions relevant to the learning objective. These three techniques can be applied in any setting that involves learner interaction with the teacher.

Small-Group Learning

Selection of a teaching method is highly influenced by the class size and quantity of information that must be learned. Large classes that must digest substantial amounts of information tend to push the faculty into selecting passive modes of teaching. The traditional CME conference at which hundreds of attendees review highly technical material is an example of this. Passive, lecture-based methods are not the most effective and often not the most efficient for all types of learning, especially in wilderness medicine. It is now widely accepted that skills-based learning presented in a small-group setting is a better way to teach practical skills.[64]

The problems inherent in teaching large groups can often be overcome by adopting a combined approach. In this strategy, the information is delivered in part to the entire group. Learners are then broken into small groups to conduct activities that allow them to discuss information, use information, and solidify learning. Within a small group, there is usually a more favorable teacher-to-learner ratio and greater self-direction of learning.

Wilderness medicine offers ample opportunity to use the combined approach or the pure small-group venue for teaching. Both rely upon the process and mechanics of group experiences. The simple act of breaking a large group into smaller groups does not constitute small-group teaching. This method requires the educator to possess skill and experience with group processes in order to avoid pitfalls that detract from learning. When done well, small-group learners take away solid lessons and the strong relationships that they had to build to learn them. However, if the teaching is done poorly, learners walk away dissatisfied with negative attitudes toward learning, the setting, and the discipline.

To understand group learning is to understand how individuals within the group interact. Bruce Tuckman's original concept of the developmental sequence of small groups should greatly influence how teachers plan and conduct these activities.[35,52,110,111] The general strategy for teachers is to become familiar with the stages, recognize their manifestations, and use a planned approach that gradually releases control of the teaching process to the group as members become more able to direct their own learning.

During the *forming stage,* group members get acquainted and become oriented to the setting. Student anxiety may hinder learning as interpersonal dynamics take shape. Students tend to adopt a passive mode of learning. They respond best during this stage to a more directive teaching style with clearly defined expectations and structured events.

During the *storming stage,* the group's identity begins to take shape among some members, while others continue to pursue individual goals over those of the group. Dissent may be voiced about leader- or teacher-directed tasks. Teachers should demonstrate strong but patient leadership to move through this stage without alienating group members. They should openly encourage support for group-generated goals.

During the *norming stage,* the group identity solidifies. Individual ownership of group goals and a greater affinity for teamwork are hallmarks. As they gain a sense of safety, members

who interact with other participants display genuineness. Leadership tasks should be directed to group members. Learning activities, such as role-play and case discussions, become most useful.

During the *performing stage,* the teacher acts only as a resource for the group, which has developed to a point of relative autonomy. The group is able to plan and conduct its own activities, as well as make self-assessments in an organized and productive fashion. Energy is spent on learning rather than on the interpersonal mechanics of the process.

The role of the teacher in a small-group setting should be oriented toward facilitation of learning rather than direct delivery of material. However, the teacher remains accountable and cannot take a completely hands-off approach and expect that objectives will be met. By attending to the details of process, the teacher ensures that the learners do not have to perform this task. The teacher creates the proper learning environment and keeps the process on track. Some common mistakes made by small-group "facilitators" include reverting to lecturing on the part of the teacher; a teacher who talks too much; students who do not participate unless prompted to do so or directly questioned; students who lack preparation for a session; students who are overbearing and domineering; and students who want to be provided with a quick and simple solution to a problem rather than engage in the process of group discovery.[49]

Despite not being part of the learner group, the teacher has great influence over the process and the outcomes. A poorly prepared teacher who ignores the internal dynamics of the group positions the experience for failure. Techniques available to avoid these problems include having agreed-upon rules for the conduct of sessions; having clearly stated tasks and objectives; using the rhetorical method of questioning to stimulate thinking; taking a lengthy pause after posing a question, allowing students to answer; not offering immediate solutions or guidance unless participants appear to be taking the wrong path; attending to body language and mannerisms of all participants, both when they are speaking and when they are listening; and addressing the entire group, rather than a single student, with mannerisms and eye contact.[49]

The general steps in preparing for and conducting small-group teaching are summarized in this way:

Establish the objectives or outcomes of the activity. What should the students be able to do?

Select the specific tasks and methods to achieve the desired outcomes (e.g., case presentation with discussion, or group project and presentation).

Choose appropriate facilitators and faculty.

Select and modify the environment and group size; make group assignments.

Prepare and coordinate for training support materials.

Familiarize oneself with the individuals and dynamics of the group; identify potential problems early.

Conduct the activity; modify techniques as required to address the unique needs of each group.

Assess learning; retrain as needed.

Assess methods, and modify them as needed for the next session or course.

Small-group learning is a rewarding and highly effective method of teaching. It requires preparation and experience. The characteristics of small-group learning make it the teaching method of choice for many wilderness medicine educational activities, especially when combined with techniques such as simulation, scenarios, and case presentations.

Distance Learning

Since the explosion of Internet-based applications has occurred, distance learning, traditionally provided via correspondence courses, has taken an entirely new direction. More people than ever find it possible to further their education without physically entering the classroom. Although web-based distance learning has found widespread application in many academic areas, it is a little-used tool in wilderness medicine education. It is not yet conducive to experiential education.

Recently, organizations have begun to offer hybrid wilderness medicine certification programs that include online prework and study paired with shorter-duration in-person training programs. This course model may be popular for students with limited availability away from their regular endeavors, but is not yet available on a large scale. Inadequate research exists to demonstrate whether students perform on par with those that spend a longer time immersed in in-person training.

The Internet offers many advantages for medical educators. Courses that are not offered as complete web-based packages can be supported by Internet applications such as email, distribution of materials, enrollment, needs assessments, and testing. To these can be added videoconferencing, discussion boards, live topic-specific chat rooms, and presentation of live events via video streaming. Nearly any software application that can be used on a home computer can be offered in some fashion over the Internet. With the advent of high-speed connectivity and constantly changing security programs, obstacles to efficiency and learner security have been minimized. Virtual learning environment software enables all of these applications to be managed efficiently while keeping the focus on the learner and not the technology.[45] The ability to hyperlink from any web page or digital document quickly brings an entire world of information to the learner.

For all of its attractiveness, the Internet is not a panacea for wilderness medicine education. There are two main disadvantages. First is the need for learners to possess sufficient computing power to allow rapid and efficient downloading and presentation of course materials. This is made worse when they travel to remote locations. It is worth recognizing that while online or hybrid learning may afford tremendous flexibility for students, it requires significant dedication to technology development, acquisition, oversight, and administrative support. Large organizations that offer this approach find it necessary to hire full-time support staff to provide a comprehensive and reliable product. Many wilderness medicine educators find it difficult to dedicate the resources necessary to bring it to full implementation. However, even small organizations find great usefulness in some applications.

For many wilderness medicine topics, passive approaches to learning, such as distance learning online, suffice to deliver information. It is up to the student to embrace the style and internalize the material. Basic science and clinical topics that can also be taught in a lecture format with audiovisual aids work well when presented online. However, much of the body of wilderness medicine knowledge, especially that dealing with the prehospital phase of care, is largely experiential and requires direct interaction with other people.

There are numerous ways that education can be delivered online. Broad categories include pure distance learning and the hybrid web-based course. In a completely web-based program, all course work, materials, sessions, and assessments are transmitted via the Internet; even assistance from teachers occurs by email or live message applications. This method is a true virtual learning experience. Alternatively, many organizations offer hybrid online courses in which students use Internet applications as an additional tool to complete portions of a course while they are also required to participate in periodic face-to-face sessions.

Many health care practitioners involve themselves in wilderness medicine because of the fellowship with other uniquely qualified and experienced professionals. As web-based applications become more widely used in wilderness medicine, educators will be increasingly challenged to ensure that learners do not feel isolated from their wilderness medicine peers and role models. The learner, not the technology, must remain at the center of the effort. Internet applications must be selected for how they enhance the learning experience, not merely for the sake of using a new technology.

Field Experiences

Medical schools and residencies have followed the lead of commercial wilderness prehospital emergency care (WPHEC) programs in moving learners out of the classroom and into the field.[70] Rotations and electives that include field training experiences of various lengths are now highly sought. These have the effect of maintaining high levels of student interest and satisfaction. They offer direct relevance and immediate application of newly learned skills. When coupled with an effective group process and feedback, the benefits of field training make this a powerful venue for skills-oriented education. These experiences are most often part of a curriculum that incorporates other techniques, such as lecturing and PBL, in a didactic setting (Figure 113-9).

Concerns include the safety and security of participants and liability issues for the sponsoring organization. The logistic support package can be expensive and complex. The quality of the experience is greatly influenced by uncontrollable factors, such as climate and weather. Proper screening and selection of participants are critical to success, especially in programs conducted in remote locations or physically demanding environments. Multiple techniques, such as scenarios and hands-on practical exercise, can be applied simultaneously to maximize the learning experience. Field training affords an opportunity to introduce nonmedical skills, such as leadership, wilderness survival, and land navigation.[70] This not only generates interest but also creates well-prepared learners and an overall lower level of risk.

OUTCOMES AND COMPETENCY-BASED EDUCATION

The notion that one should be able to demonstrate that a given intervention or technique will result in measurable, reproducible, and predictable outcomes is woven into the fabric of the scientific and business culture. Not surprisingly, in medicine, it is now taken for granted that recommended interventions are based on a body of evidence that shows improved reliability and safety. However, the seemingly fundamental ideas that data and evidence should drive educational program development and delivery and that programs should measure and be accountable for their outcomes (e.g., how their students perform) are relatively new to health care education. Successful programs determine specifically what they want their students to know or be able to demonstrate (competencies). They collect and assess data on the effectiveness of their teaching methods and then use that information to generate continual program improvements.

Over time, teaching programs across the spectrum of disciplines in health care education have adapted traditional teaching methods to a more modern approach using outcomes and competency-based principles. Most wilderness medicine programs have also adapted. For example, programs that offer

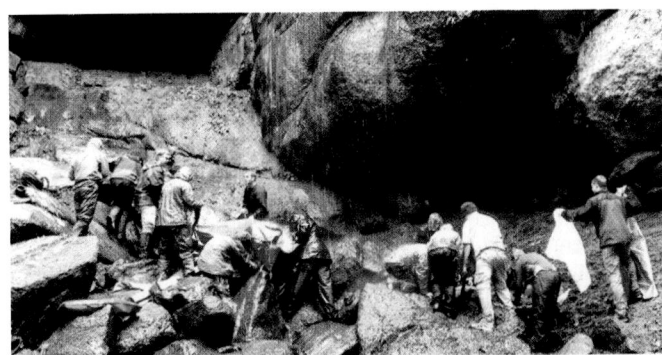

FIGURE 113-9 Learning conducted in the field under genuine conditions is a vital component of any comprehensive wilderness medicine course. This method enhances skills development for individuals and teams and facilitates several aspects of the 360-degree evaluation of learners. (*Courtesy Fred Baty.*)

medical school or graduate-level residency elective experiences that are approved by a parent academic institution may be required to demonstrate that curricula use measurable, competency-based objectives. Teaching methods and instruments used to evaluate learners who seek academic credit from parent institutions may be required to use competency-based formatting. Fortunately, most wilderness medicine educational programs incorporate fundamental concepts of adult education and have required only modest changes to curricula, training methods, and assessment tools. Many wilderness medicine programs do not require extensive modification with respect to outcomes-based education. Those that wish to satisfy specific compliance requirements generally use multiple and overlapping methods to assess learners and outcomes data to enable them to demonstrate continuous improvement in the educational program. Competency-based assessment tools are widely available on the Internet and can be modified for almost any wilderness medicine educational setting. When evaluating curricula and processes for competency-based improvements, programs may consider three areas: (1) Do learners achieve the established learning objectives? (2) Can the program demonstrate this with evidence? (3) How does the program demonstrate continuous improvement in its educational process?

ASSESSING LEARNERS' NEEDS

Performing proper assessment of the needs of students before designing a curriculum leads to a fulfilling experience for all. Jane Vella claims that this critical step is necessary to "truly honor the time investment of the learner and create the conditions for meaningful dialogue between learner and teacher."[113] People whose motivations for learning are ignored "quickly become bored and indifferent." They often walk away from the experience dissatisfied or without completing the program. A wilderness medicine course planner may query potential learners or other organizational stakeholders about their goals in attending an educational program. Organizations, such as camps and outdoor education programs, may be asked about the specific skills they want their staff members to master. Some examples of information the educational planner may wish to obtain:

1. Why do the students want to spend their valuable time learning this material?
2. What are the levels of training and vocation of the group?
3. Are any specific outcomes more important than others to the group?
4. What is the relevance of the wilderness medicine learning experience to them?
   - Job requirement
   - Prerequisite for another course
   - Enhancement of recreational activities
   - Preparation for emergencies
   - Acquiring knowledge for safer exotic travel
   - Sharing fellowship with other wilderness medicine practitioners
   - Creative diversion
   - Academic advancement

Learner-centered education principles tell us that the needs assessment should lead to modification of course content or structure to suit the individualized needs of the learner. To become fully invested, students should be able to shape to some degree what will be taught to them. Thorough, individualized modification of curriculum content based on a formal needs assessment is likely to be impractical for certain standardized certification experiences, such as wilderness first responder (WFR) courses. Detailed needs assessments are seldom completed for wilderness medicine CME conferences due to the wide variety of learner types and motivations. Advance study of students' expectations and reasons for attending allows for more focused and tailored instructional events. The needs assessment can be easily accomplished with a questionnaire delivered by postal or electronic mail, telephone contact, or a face-to-face interview. The actual format is not as important as the mere act of soliciting input from students. Allowing them to actively

dialogue about their learning will achieve buy-in. The curriculum design becomes overtly accountable to the students and results in much higher levels of internal motivation.

LEARNING OBJECTIVES

An area of wilderness medicine education that is often given cursory attention is that of providing well-constructed objectives for a course and for the individual learning activities contained therein. Most educators make an attempt, but well-written objectives are articulated too infrequently for the amount of education that is being delivered in the discipline.

Course objectives describe the overall purpose for students attending the course. They may include a job- or skill-related certification or simply enrichment skills and knowledge. They address what a participant should generally be able to do or know after completing the entire program. The objectives should be formalized, written, and distributed to anyone involved with curriculum design. They serve as a compass to guide all planning and design efforts. They also enable prospective participants to determine if the course is appropriate for them. For example, the objective of the wilderness first-aid course may be written as

"This course is intended to prepare the participant to perform basic first-aid procedures in locations where evacuations are primarily walk-outs or carry-outs with the assistance of local resources, and where local emergency medical services (EMS) access is expected in less than 8 hours. This is often in the context of short trips relatively close to assistance: day trips/camps, stationary wilderness camps, weekend family activities, and frontcountry outdoor recreation events."

Learning objectives are collections of words, pictures, or diagrams that tell others what the educator intends for learners to achieve.[64] Because they are designed for a specific activity or session, learning objectives should not be used as objectives or goals for an entire course. They are tailored to a single learning activity or a closely related group of activities; address preidentified needs and interests of the learner; are specific to levels and types of performance; are achievable, realistic, and time specific; and use verbs that specify behaviors that can easily be measured. When properly written, these objectives provide focus for individual instructors while preparing their offerings and guide selection of educational methods. Learning objectives establish outcomes rather than describe processes. The basic purpose of teaching is to facilitate learning in order to achieve measurable outcomes. A learning activity is a process designed to achieve a result. What students actually learn is the result and should be described in advance by objectives.[30]

A learning objective is constructed by describing an activity that elaborates specific knowledge or skills that a learner will be able to demonstrate following a successful learning activity. Well-written learning objectives are measured by written testing, observation, hands-on problem solving, or other methods of assessment. Words or phrases such as *know, think, appreciate, learn, comprehend, remember, perceive, understand, be aware of, be familiar with, have knowledge of,* and *grasp the significance of* are difficult to measure and are of little use when writing learning objectives in wilderness medicine. Examples of learning objectives that illustrate the concepts of being specific and measurable are as follows: The student will be able to …

…perform well during wilderness-setting role-play (not specific or measurable)

…carry an injured patient (specific; can be made more measurable)

…discriminate between edible and inedible wild plants (specific and measurable)

…feel more comfortable performing mass-casualty triage (neither specific nor measurable)

…express a point of view supported by valid evidence (specific and measurable)

Strong objectives, in addition to being performance based, specific, and measurable, are preceded by a condition statement to set the stage and aid with measurement specificity.[71] In writing objectives, answer the question: What should the participants be able to do and how well must they do it? Objectives must be

TABLE 113-1 Examples of Performance Verbs for Learning Objectives

Knowledge	Comprehension	Application	Analysis	Synthesis	Evaluation
Cite	Associate	Apply	Analyze	Arrange	Appraise
Count	Classify	Calculate	Appraise	Assemble	Assess
Define	Compare	Complete	Contrast	Collect	Choose
Draw	Compute	Demonstrate	Criticize	Compose	Critique
Identify	Contrast	Dramatize	Debate	Construct	Determine
Indicate	Describe	Employ	Detect	Create	Estimate
List	Differentiate	Examine	Diagram	Design	Evaluate
Name	Discuss	Illustrate	Differentiate	Detect	Judge
Point	Distinguish	Interpolate	Distinguish	Formulate	Measure
Read	Estimate	Interpret	Experiment	Generalize	Rank
Recite	Examine	Locate	Infer	Integrate	Rate
Recognize	Explain	Operate	Inspect	Manage	Recommend
Relate	Express	Order	Inventory	Organize	Revise
Repeat	Interpolate	Practice	Question	Plan	Score
Select	Interpret	Predict	Separate	Prepare	Select
State	Locate	Relate	Summarize	Produce	Test
Tabulate	Predict	Report		Propose	
Tell	Report	Restate			
Trace	Restate	Review			
Write	Review	Schedule			
	Translate	Sketch			
		Solve			
		Translate			
		Use			

clear and attainable. They are often constructed in an if ... then sequence to facilitate clarity. Focus on acquisition or reinforcement of a specific element of knowledge or skill.[30] Style options for constructing objectives include the following:

Given X materials and within Y minutes, the student will build a Z device strong enough to support 25 pounds.

At the completion of this teaching activity, participants will be able to ...

This last phrase is followed by a specific performance verb and the desired learning outcome. Examples of performance verbs are found in Table 113-1. The following is an example of a properly prepared set of objectives:

Aerospace Medicine Lecture: Fatigue, Desynchronosis, and Countermeasures

Time: 1200-1300

Speaker: Dr. Jane Doe

Lesson Objectives: At the conclusion of this activity the student will ...

Summarize the results of studies on the effects of fatigue on air crews.

Give examples of the deleterious effects of fatigue on human performance and the accident rate.

Define desynchronosis and give examples of applications of its understanding to aviation medical personnel.

Outline various countermeasures that are available, as well as some, such as melatonin, that are currently undergoing investigation.

ASSESSING LEARNING

The last step in the education cycle (see Figure 113-4) is making a formal assessment of whether or not learning has occurred.[94] There are several reasons for testing in wilderness medicine education beyond the obvious need to validate and certify students. Learning assessment can be a valuable extension of the learning process. Kromann observed that "testing as a final activity in an in-hospital resuscitation skills course for medical students increased learning outcomes compared with spending an equal amount of time in practice."[59] Students seldom come away from a properly conducted and reviewed examination without

having learned something. It can be said that this type of learning by assessment is the capstone of knowledge synthesis. Each examination completes the education cycle at a particular level and allows progression to the next with a higher degree of competence.

Learning assessments can be grouped for convenience into two general categories: formative and summative. Formative assessments are made before and throughout a course of instruction and have both learning and testing dimensions. Feedback after formative assessment is critical to shape additional learning. This type of assessment may take the form of a diagnostic examination to assess learners' needs and establish lesson objectives, or an intermediate examination to assess progress at a particular phase of training.

Summative assessments are generally used at the end of either a critical phase of training or course completion. This type of assessment is more often applied for certification and validation than as an extension of learning. Final course examinations and tests that lead to state or national certification in a vocation are examples of summative assessments.

TIMING OF EVALUATION

The learner uses feedback and information gained from formative evaluations to improve performance during the learning event or course. To be effective, formative evaluations must be provided to learners before the end of the training period. Although assessments rendered early in the training period allow more time for modifying performance, there may have been insufficient time for adequate and comprehensive assessment. Likewise, evaluation made later in the training period allows for more accurate and comprehensive assessment, but there may remain insufficient time for satisfactory remediation. Unless there are compelling reasons to render evaluations early (e.g., when questions of safety or impropriety arise), those provided to learners at the approximate midpoint of the training cycle tend to work well. These should be scheduled, anticipated by learners, and prepared and presented by faculty. Programs that use anonymous evaluation tools (e.g., at the end of a course) must collect and collate results from learners and faculty

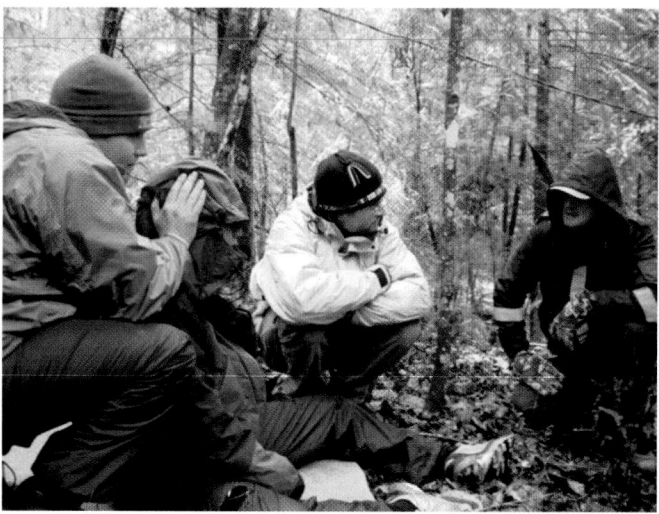

FIGURE 113-10 Timely and specific feedback is especially important in the types of hands-on, scenario-based training frequently conducted in wilderness medicine courses. *(Courtesy Fred Baty.)*

and analyze the results. This may decrease usefulness of the instrument by causing a separation of results from the actual training event.[19]

FEEDBACK

Regardless of which tools a program incorporates into the overall assessment system, dedicated opportunities for immediate feedback on performance must be used to ensure maximal learning. The basic goals of feedback are to improve student performance and to strengthen learning. Although formative and summative evaluations that take into account numerous individual events capture performance over a given period of time, immediate feedback is needed to give learners the opportunity to make adjustments based on their performance during specific events or very brief and focused training periods. Learners that are not provided this type of feedback will be left to rely on happenstance to succeed at course objectives (Figure 113-10).

Limited feedback may come in the form of corrections on written tests or other assignments. However, the bulk of this feedback is likely to be associated with performance on skills and in practical exercises or scenarios. Feedback is especially important in these types of hands-on, scenario-based clinical training events that are frequently conducted during wilderness medicine courses. Hands-on skill training requires concrete demonstration of proficiency and does not rely on an evaluator who makes presumptions of a learner's thought processes to make an assessment. Properly conducted feedback makes an immediate connection between outcomes of learner actions and expectations as established by goals and objectives. This solidifies learning in ways that are impossible with other evaluation tools. However, the benefit decreases rapidly as time increases from the event to delivery of feedback. Feedback is effective when it is given immediately after an event by a person who has observed the event.[19]

Instructors who know the learning objective for the lesson know what to look for in student performance. They are able to watch students practice a skill and use their observations to check whether students are performing correctly. This ongoing assessment and feedback helps in the coaching of skills and serves as a check on the effectiveness of the instruction.

Instructors must create an environment where high-quality objective feedback is both expected and normalized. Recipients should understand that feedback is specifically targeted at helping them improve their performance, rather than being a personal attack. Properly conducted objective feedback should be delivered verbally and focus on the individual's performance or actions, rather than on character or intent. In other words, feedback should focus on the performance, not the performer. Instructors may be reluctant to provide critical feedback for fear of hurting someone's feelings or setting up an environment of conflict, yet without good coaching, a student's skills will not improve. In one study of medical students, half received constructive feedback on a specific skill and the other half received only general compliments. The performance of students who received feedback improved, whereas the students who received only general compliments showed no change in skill level. The students who received compliments showed significantly higher satisfaction ratings.[12] Instructors must work to build learning environments where feedback and coaching both improve performance and create satisfaction.

The ability to craft specific messages can improve student receptiveness. For instance, when evaluating the quality of an improvised lower extremity splint, one may choose descriptive comments. Rather than using general qualitative statements such as "That splint is poor" or "That would never hold up in an evacuation," the teacher may provide specific feedback to help the student evaluate errors and correct them. One may use a more direct and interactive approach, such as "Recall that immobilizing the joint above and below the injury is an important principle of splinting. How might you alter your splint to improve immobilization of the knee?" This provides specific direction for improvement without the feeling of qualitative judgment.

A common pitfall of providing feedback is for the instructor to impose a particular personal preference or style onto a student's performance. One of the benefits of principle-based teaching is that there are many ways to achieve the same goal. The improvisational nature of wilderness medicine is among its most attractive features to new learners. Students may find creative ways to achieve the principles of a particular skill that do not resonate with the instructor. Students will feel undermined if the instructor habitually corrects an appropriate performance not for accuracy but for stylistic preference. The instructor can offer enrichment to the student, but suggestions about alternative solutions should be crafted so as not to denigrate the student's choices.

In addition to feedback related to cognitive knowledge and skills performance, wilderness medicine educators have the opportunity to observe students' performance in group settings and leadership roles. Educators can take the opportunity to help students develop in both of these areas. Although it may seem more challenging to provide feedback about team performance, the instructor can still objectify comments to provide growth for students. As with individual feedback, general qualitative statements such as "Your incomplete information caused the incident commander to make a poor decision" may result in suboptimal group learning. A more specific, interactive approach more appropriately addresses the learning situation, for example, "Your plan was to perform a complete patient assessment. What factors caused you not to finish your assessment? How might you avoid this in the future?"

THE 360-DEGREE EVALUATION

As part of the new focus on outcomes-based education, many training programs provide objectives-based assessments of learner performance. In addition, programs often incorporate an assessment system that receives input from multiple evaluators. This is also called a 360-degree evaluation system.

The 360-degree evaluation accepts contributions to the development of learners from all types of people in the general sphere of his or her influence. It offers training programs a process by which numerous and varied perspectives may be used to more accurately assess all aspects of performance. It is presumed that observations of learners made from different perspectives are more valid than are traditional, more narrowly focused assessments. The usefulness of 360-degree evaluations in specific wilderness medicine training programs has not been thoroughly evaluated; specific instruments relevant to these settings have not

- *Global assessment:* Faculty provide an overall, comprehensive evaluation.
- *Peer assessment:* Other learners at a similar level of training provide an evaluation.
- *Self-assessment:* Learner provides an assessment of his or her own performance.
- *Ancillary staff assessment:* Staff, administrative, or nursing personnel provide assessments.
- *Patient assessment:* Patients may be asked to provide comments or complete surveys.
- *Performance metrics:* Assessment of the performance is metrics based (e.g., productivity, test scores, chart reviews, quality data, timed events).

been proposed. However, 360-degree evaluations that are widely available and validated within graduate medical education can easily be modified and incorporated. Usefulness of this method of learner evaluation depends on factors such as length of the course, contact with participants not taking the course (e.g., role-players and patients), and types of events used as training tools (e.g., small-group field-training events). A 360-degree evaluation may be found to be more relevant for courses that are longer, with more varied types of learner interactions over time (Box 113-7).

ASSESSMENT DESIGN

Two key concepts that should be understood when designing learning assessment tools for wilderness medicine courses are reliability and validity. These are applied separately when discussing written and skills-oriented testing.[49,103] They are particularly relevant to WPHEC courses, such as WFR or WEMT, which rely heavily on skills-based testing.

A reliable testing instrument consistently measures the desired outcome, no matter how many times it is administered. A host of factors influence reliability. The length of time it takes to complete a test, characteristics of the examinees, logistical and administrative problems, and variation in examiner methods act to decrease the reliability of an examination and mask the learners' true level of competence. One cannot address the validity of an assessment tool until reliability is achieved.

A valid testing instrument is one that measures what it was designed to measure. Simply put, it reveals the actual level of learner competence. Apart from reliability problems, issues that negatively influence validity include cases and scenarios that are not directly relevant to the learning objectives, poorly structured or improperly selected test questions, testing stations that do not adequately examine the skills that were taught, and failure to seek an expert review of course content during the design phase. The measure of validity is done in terms of examination scores. Having removed obstacles to reliability and validity (see Evaluating the Assessment Tool, later), the educator may use scores to make a direct link from teaching methods to achieving learning objectives.

The two main approaches to learning assessment in health care that are pertinent to wilderness medicine are written and skills-based testing. Apprentice-style one-on-one teaching with feedback is useful in other areas of health care education, such as primary nursing programs and physician training courses, but is often impractical for wilderness medicine teaching activities.

Written assessments are still widely used in health care education despite the growing application and demonstrated usefulness of progressive teaching techniques, such as hands-on skills development and PBL. The questioning format of written assessment may take many forms, but all formats generally test a student's reasoning ability and accumulation of knowledge as opposed to practical application.

Schuwirth and van der Vleuten[100a] proposed a list of criteria to compare the advantages and disadvantages of various types of written test formats and questions: reliability and validity, educational impact (how students learn the material to prepare for examinations), cost-effectiveness (expense in terms of money and time), and acceptability (how both students and teachers view the examination's effectiveness and relevance). To account for these factors, the most preferred method of developing written examinations is to use several types of test questions in each instrument. The types of examination questions that may be considered include true or false, single-best-answer multiple-choice, multiple true or false, short-answer fill-in-the-blank, essay, case-based key feature, and extended matching.

Skills-based assessment is particularly relevant in wilderness medicine education. It is the mainstay of competency testing for most prehospital courses. The two general subtypes of skills-based assessment used in wilderness medicine are skills subset testing (sessions focused on a single skill or a few closely related skills) and case- or scenario-based skills stations. Basic learning theory tells us that this popular testing method should be highly effective in achieving objectives and delivering highly retained learning. This bears out in practical application. There are two important disadvantages of skills-based assessments. First, the logistic requirements necessary to conduct high-quality testing can be burdensome. Second, examiners require a high degree of skill with regard to the testing process and mechanics to ensure the reliability and validity of results. The general steps in conducting a skills-based learning assessment session are as follows:

Decide if the activity is for practice, formative (intermediate) assessment, or summative (end-of-course) assessment. Inform the learners.

Match learning objectives to scenarios and/or cases in the examination.

Select satisfactory examiners and role-players; conduct thorough briefings.

Obtain logistics support, and prepare the environment.

Thoroughly brief the learners.

Conduct the assessment; check progress; modify as required.

Conduct an initial assessment of the instrument.

Review results with learners.

Conduct a thorough assessment of the instrument with broader comparisons.

Feedback can be formalized and documented in evaluations of student performance. These learning tools are more common in longer programs than in short conference workshops or lay-person programs. Documenting student performance can consist of cognitive and practical test scoring. It may also expand beyond these objective measures to evaluations of the student's ability to lead and participate in groups, communicate, and perform in environments of uncertainty or adversity or the student's awareness of decision-making styles and techniques. These assessments flow from learning objectives. They should be based on assessment rubrics that can be communicated to the student to clarify standards for performance. These properly constructed rubrics can be effective tools for clarifying subjective assessments and expressing performance standards that may otherwise be difficult to comprehend.

For example, in addition to gaining wilderness medicine knowledge and skills, a program may have a learning objective that the students "effectively communicate patient information using the SOAP (subjective, objective, assessment, plan) format. The evaluation then includes the criteria of "verbal SOAP reports." The grading rubric is described in Table 113-2.

Another example would assess the following learning objective: Identify the decision-making technique used in a scenario. The evaluation criteria could be written as, "identifies the decision-making technique used in a scenario." The grading rubric is described in Table 113-3.

Evaluating the Assessment Tool

Educators must evaluate their learning assessment tools to ensure reliability and validity. Simple methods may be used. For written

TABLE 113-2 Feedback Tool A

Expert	Competent	Novice	Beginner
Speaks clearly; well organized; concise and complete verbal SOAP reports	Speaks clearly; missing some minor data; followed general format of verbal SOAP reports	Difficult to follow flow of information; missing key data points; inconsistent quality of verbal SOAP reports	Ineffective verbal communicator; used inappropriate language

assessments, a review of examination scores and comparing them to attendance is a good first step. It should come as no surprise that students who do not attend specific sessions would do poorly on test questions designed to assess learning on that topic. If this level of analysis points to attendance problems, then there are other issues in the course, such as objectives, content, and quality of instruction, that should be addressed before the quality of the examination.

The process of test item analysis correlates the number of examinees that missed a given question with overall test scores.[21] This can be done on two levels. The first is within the group that was being tested at a given course. The second is over a period of time among several groups that took the same examination. As with any internal assessment tool, the latter style leads to stronger conclusions but takes longer to complete. Internal pattern analysis of test scores can reveal that either the instruction was poor or the test question not well written. The basic principle is that if a large percentage of students received a high score on an examination but a similarly large percentage missed a particular test item, then either construction of the item or the teaching method is likely at fault. This technique loses power and specificity at lower overall examination scores among those that missed the item(s) in question.

Skills-based learning assessments can be evaluated for quality using similarly simple analytic tools.[21] The attendance comparison mentioned above is an obvious starting point when reviewing individual performance.

Mechanics or logistics of the testing setting that seem irrelevant to the actual demonstration of knowledge and skills may affect test scores. An examiner who did not attend precourse briefings and is not familiar with what was taught, or worse, with what is expected, poses a problem. This can be revealed by noting that a large percentage of examinees doing poorly at a given skill station despite doing well at other stations designed to test related skills. High-performing students that fail a particular station may be another warning sign. Testing stations that use role-playing with scenarios must account for the influence of the role-players. Poorly briefed actors that do not follow the script can make or break an otherwise competent learner.

Having made attendance comparisons and ruled out problems with the setting, examiners, and role-players, the problem if many students are doing poorly at a given skill station is most likely the quality of teaching. Retraining and retesting may be in order.

LIMITATIONS OF TRAINING

Training in all disciplines has limitations. It is impossible to supply an infinite amount of information to learners or to guarantee learning and retention of all material presented. Rather, the role of an effective training event is to provide a framework of knowledge for users to build upon through future experiences.

For example, there are some themes and goals common to nearly all wilderness medicine prehospital care courses. Graduates should be able to respond to wilderness emergencies, perform thorough assessments with only rudimentary tools, provide treatment using largely improvised equipment, function in challenging environmental conditions, and make decisions regarding treatment and evacuation. For some learners, this requires adapting existing knowledge to a new and sometimes poorly understood environment. For others, this training is the sum total of their medical experience. Regardless of students' experience and educational background or where they begin in this progression, and regardless of the length of the training event, there are assumed limitations to this educational medium.

CONTRIVED SITUATIONS

Medical education is plagued by the challenge of training new providers to recognize the typical, yet be prepared to manage the atypical. The newer the provider and shorter the length of training, the more likely it is that the education focuses on classic presentations. In the case of an introductory wilderness first-aid course for lay providers, the curriculum may focus solely on common wilderness medicine problems, leaving it to the caregiver to intuitively recognize when someone is seriously hurt or ill and requires additional care. The educator's job is to help students learn introductory concepts and assist them in recognizing patterns. As they gain additional education and experience, their ability to understand more complex concepts will evolve. If students are initially overwhelmed with too much detail, they will struggle to develop the framework on which to attach their future learning.

Simulations, scenarios, and case studies are useful tools to reinforce and apply learning. One of the helpful constructs of this type of experience is that the patient demonstrates a response to the provided treatment. As discussed above, scenarios have a time limit dictated by the structure and logistics of the setting. As a result, in order to illustrate a specific learning point, scenarios are often crafted with artificially accelerated patient responses or changes. For instance, in an effort to guide the caregivers toward a particular decision, the facilitator may instruct the patient to change his or her vital signs to indicate improvement or deterioration over the course of 10 minutes, whereas this change might more realistically occur over a longer time span. Students, especially those without extensive medical experience, may perceive that rapid change is typical and become confused when they do not see the same pattern in a real patient. It is also presumed that any given learner intervention will produce a notable outcome, either favorable or unfavorable, in the patient presentation. The educational risk is that the student may leave a class believing that the artificial construct of a scenario represents reality. A typical example is the notion that applying glucose paste to the gums of an unconscious patient

TABLE 113-3 Feedback Tool B

Expert	Competent	Novice	Beginner
Consistently identifies and can discuss the advantages and disadvantages of the decision-making tool used	Consistently identifies which decision-making tool is used	With coaching can identify which decision-making tool is used	Unaware or unable to identify which decision-making tool is used

for a few minutes (in a simulation) will return the patient to consciousness. Nevertheless, the positive reward of effective therapy likely remains the best teaching strategy. Consideration may also be given to including scenarios during which the patient does not improve or survive.

Some courses are specifically designed to teach rescue and evacuation skills, but most are concerned with managing the immediate needs of a patient. In the parlance of wilderness medicine, this is stated as "Assess and treat the patient, and then make an evacuation decision." The instructor will typically end a scenario at this point. In a true wilderness emergency, however, much of the hard work begins when the decision is made to evacuate the patient. Evacuation is often difficult, lengthy, and stressful for both the patient and rescuers. It is a challenge to prepare students of wilderness medicine to anticipate this hardship. They may be poorly equipped to handle the physical demands of the process, not familiar with providing long-term patient care, and not sufficiently resilient to endure the emotional challenges of a real evacuation. Without a frame of reference for remote places, students may harbor the conscious or subconscious illusion that evacuation is expedient and readily available by an external resource. To avoid this presumption, instructors should discuss methods of evacuation and emphasize that each choice must be tempered by an evaluation of the risks and benefits for the patient and the group. Scenarios may be crafted to reinforce the notion that self-evacuation by an injured individual may be the most reasonable choice. The faculty may design a scenario in which the group facilitates its own supported evacuation as a part of the exercise, so that the experience takes several hours or a day and requires that the group contend with the realities of long-term care for a patient (Figure 113-11).

Yet another limitation of training is artificial group cohesiveness. In general, participants in wilderness medicine education programs are eager to learn and value the experience of a conflict-free environment. Therefore, there is a general commitment to working together. Good educators create a structure that allows students to fill defined roles. In a real-world application, issues with leadership, teamwork, and communication may be far more challenging than the medical issues. Consideration should be given to including curriculum items that train wilderness medicine practitioners to fill leadership roles and to guide teams. Students should be expected to reflect on their experiences with group activities to better understand models and strategies of high-functioning teams.

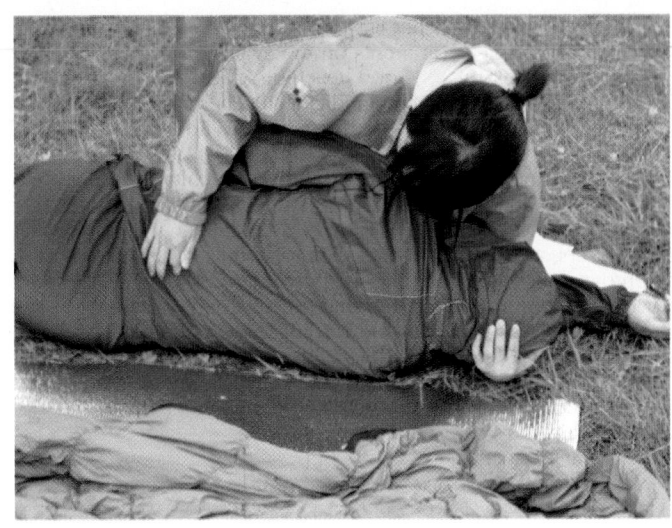

FIGURE 113-12 Wilderness medicine providers must learn to work independently and without the support of a larger team. *(Courtesy Shana Tarter.)*

Finally, although a wilderness medicine education program may create the opportunity to make hypothetical decisions, there is no aftermath. Real-world decisions have real consequences. Students of wilderness medicine must embrace the potential need to make autonomous decisions. In the clinical world, health care providers are accustomed to consulting with others with greater experience or expertise. In the remote setting, practitioners must be prepared for a lack of external communication and be ready to make decisions autonomously. Wilderness medicine courses can help prepare students for this eventuality by teaching and assessing decision-making skills. An experienced wilderness medicine faculty can guide students through a process of making difficult decisions and appropriately dealing with their uncertainty. There may be times when the influence of weather, terrain, darkness, and group dynamics alter the preferred medical decision. By providing opportunities for students to consider a multitude of factors in a given situation, the instructor creates the foundation that students will need to function in the demands of a remote environment (Figure 113-12).

TEACHING IN WILDERNESS MEDICINE
GOOD TEACHERS

What of the act of teaching in wilderness medicine? What is unique about the discipline compared with other areas of health care education that calls for wilderness medicine teachers to pay special attention to their delivery? As mentioned before, wilderness medicine instruction is often and understandably disconnected from the environment about which it informs. Teaching the fundamentals of altitude, depth, cold, or heat and their impact on the human condition requires that the initial knowledge base be largely acquired in a "safe" environment. The experiential phase that we presume solidifies learning for wilderness medicine practitioners often occurs in another setting at a different time, if it occurs at all. Therefore, to be effective, the material must be presented by faculty members that possess the ability to captivate and motivate learners. Paul Auerbach proclaimed, "The enthusiasm of the instructor is plainly apparent and can carry or lose the day. Regardless of the educational technique chosen, one must be 'into it' or the students will be soon flocking out of it."[4]

Just as wilderness medicine practitioners must draw from a solid base of knowledge to be creative when providing care in austere surroundings, wilderness medicine faculty must be familiar with and use all of the theory-based tools available to them to be successful, even in less-than-optimal teaching settings. Steve Donelan highlighted the issue by noting, "Instructors tend

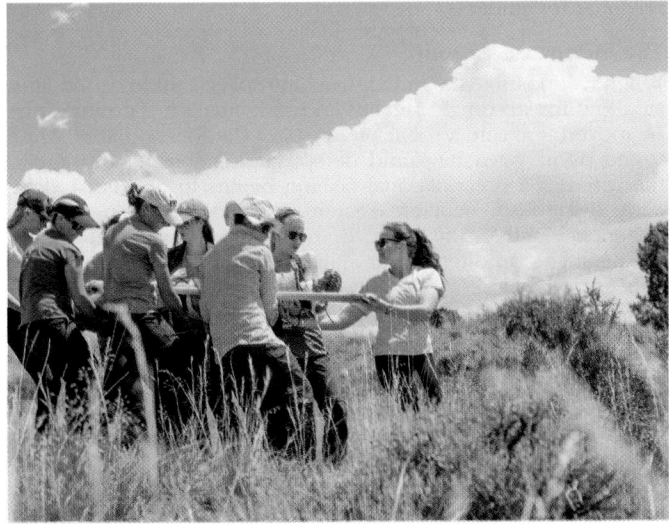

FIGURE 113-11 Extended scenarios help students experience the challenges of providing long-term care in a wilderness environment, including fatigue, hunger, stress, extremes of temperature, group conflict, and boredom. *(Courtesy Justin Alexandre.)*

to assume that if students stay awake and interested, pass the tests, and write nice comments on the evaluation forms, then the course is successful."[20] Good teaching does not just happen. Highly effective wilderness medicine teachers are as proficient with the teaching skill set as they are with the clinical "tools of the trade" in their unique area of expertise.

The credibility of wilderness medicine faculty is paramount. Beyond the obvious reasons for needing credibility as a teacher, most wilderness medicine learners are already well placed in their respective fields with years of educational experience. Moreover, it is not uncommon for wilderness medicine faculty to be addressing participants that are not only proficient at the topic in question but may be leading experts or researchers in that area. According to Auerbach, "If a teacher wishes to do more than read from a script, he or she must have some first-hand experience in the environment. Students are better than we imagine at rating our technical skills."[4]

For years, medical educators have studied the notion that the best clinical teachers all display a common set of characteristics. Numerous authors list qualities of good teachers based on learner surveys and outcomes assessments.[46,47,119] Some of these have special applicability to wilderness medicine education:

- Possess an excellent depth and breadth of knowledge about the topic(s)
- Are highly competent at the skill(s) being taught
- Are highly skilled at interpersonal interactions with learners
- Are enthusiastic about the role of teacher
- Possess good supervisory skills by providing appropriate feedback, timely and clear direction, and easy access to students for questions and guidance

THE EDUCATIONAL ENVIRONMENT

Hutchinson pointed out that "in adult learning theories, teaching is as much about setting the context and climate for learning as it is about imparting knowledge or sharing expertise."[45] Nearly everything that the teacher does influences a student's ability or willingness to learn. Wilderness medicine course planners that account for these factors enjoy a much higher likelihood of success than do those who simply present material with little accounting for process and environment. Two factors that can be influenced by providing the right environment are the motivation of learners and their perceptions of how relevant the material is to their lives. They derive their energy directly from the faculty and will respond in kind to the amount of effort that has gone into providing for the proper learning environment. They are quick to identify a poorly prepared program.

Motivating factors to consider when planning an educational experience include physical needs and comfort issues that may hinder learning, safety and security, group inclusion and identification, self-esteem (making learners feel important and relevant), and self-actualization through self-directed learning. This all leads to academic fulfillment resulting in a deeply ingrained understanding of the material. These mirror Maslow's well-known model for hierarchic needs satisfaction.

Tangible characteristics of the environment that affect learning seem insignificant to the overall goals of the course and are easily overlooked. If they are not properly accounted for in the course plan, learners may sense a lack of respect. The best-presented material by the most captivating, world-renowned teacher will not hold students' attention if students' primary motivational needs are not addressed. These include factors such as food and beverage availability; frequency of rest breaks; ambient lighting, noise, and temperature of the setting; lodging accommodations; access to telephone and Internet connections; access to public transportation and airports; and the availability of recreation during hours when training is not taking place.

Although it is impossible to solve every problem in any setting that is remote or exciting enough to host a wilderness medicine educational experience, problems should be addressed to the extent possible. Decisions should be made early about adequacy of the setting balanced against the need to conduct realistic training in or near the wilderness environment. Compromises may be

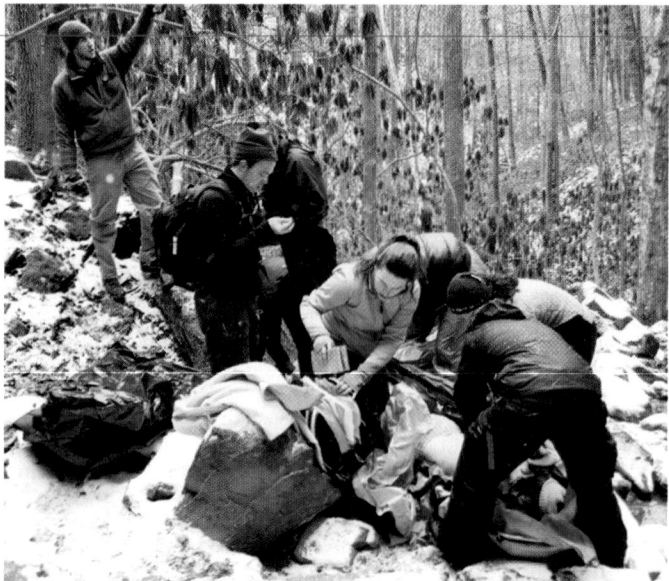

FIGURE 113-13 Successful realistic training in wilderness medicine strikes a balance between the competing demands for high-quality training on the one hand and the expense, safety, comfort, and distraction of learners on the other. *(Courtesy Fred Baty.)*

made that trade some degree of realism for comfort, and vice-versa. Potential problem areas should be made known to participants well in advance so that they may make choices about the importance of these factors and balance them against their own desire to receive the training (Figure 113-13).

THE CLASSROOM

In any given program, wilderness medicine educators will likely have both indoor and outdoor classroom settings available. Most courses will use both. Although these may seem interchangeable, assessment of their unique physical attributes will allow the educator to properly match the type of material being taught, expectations of learners, and course objectives with the most appropriate location. In either case, it is important to become familiar with the selected locations well in advance and to establish a transition plan that allows learners to smoothly flow from one to the other. Additionally, it is important to properly position amenities, such as restrooms, refreshments, and parking, to be a resource for students.

The Indoor Classroom

Whenever possible the indoor teaching space should be modified to allow for maximal visibility and participation. Furniture may be moved to create a semicircular space the focal point of which is the primary teaching and demonstration location. Arranging the room in a nontraditional fashion begins to engage students early and tends to generate excitement for the upcoming learning experience. When the space does not allow for a semicircular arrangement, an alternate arrangement, such as rows of tables and chairs angled in a chevron pattern, may suffice. This will preserve open floor space at the front of the room for demonstrations. If the number of participants is known, eliminate extra tables and chairs so that students fill all of the seating. This makes the classroom feel full and minimizes the effect of people sitting in the back row to avoid engagement. Because some practical sessions may occur in the indoor classroom, consideration should be given to preserving open floor space for this element of the class. Sometimes this can be accomplished without repeatedly moving the furniture. In small rooms, there may be the need to deconstruct and reconstruct seating arrangements regularly. It can be helpful to store equipment routinely used for outside scenarios near the classroom exit.

The Outdoor Classroom

The outdoor classroom can be an exciting and refreshing setting that adds a dimension to the experience not possible in a building. The location may be as simple as a small grassy area located between buildings, or a local park or wooded area. It could be as elaborate as a permanently constructed amphitheater-style teaching spot found commonly at summer camps. The instructor needs to assess the hazards associated with the outdoor space and actively manage the risks for and with the students. Is the space used by the local population for rest or recreation? Are there poisonous plants or aggressive insects, such as bees or hornets? Is the location too close to a busy road? A well-crafted scenario may be enough of a distraction that rescuers neglect to look for moving vehicles as they cross the street and approach the scene. Students who are not well prepared for the environment may struggle with rain, wind, cold, or heat in the outdoor classroom. The ambient noise may be such that effectively debriefing a practical experience outside may be frustrating. Finally, it is important to establish specific boundaries for the outdoor classroom that allow the instructor to monitor all students visually and to quickly intervene if necessary. This is especially critical for larger rescues or night rescues where patients may be widely dispersed. Consider bringing to the site a portable writing surface such as a dry-erase board or a butcher-block paper pad on a stand. This can be particularly helpful when debriefing students about a scenario, reinforcing principles, or providing instructions. In all cases, be careful to protect equipment in the outdoor classroom. Light gear blows away easily, notes left exposed can become saturated by rain, and stage makeup used in moulage for scenarios that is left in the sun will melt. Establish expectations for care of equipment with students ahead of time, so time is not spent chasing loose objects (Figures 113-14 and 113-15).

TRAINING AIDS

Equipment Considerations

An academic discipline such as wilderness medicine that studies and teaches the practical application of principles in harsh environments must rely heavily on hands-on, experiential learning. As such, educators and program organizers must anticipate the need to provide appropriate and adequate training equipment. It is reasonable to require students to bring appropriate personal equipment for self-care in the outdoors. However, it is not practical or efficient to require them to provide the equipment needed to learn a variety of new skills. With a large group, this means the program will need to provide a substantial amount of training gear. Planners will need to consider how many of each item will be required to ensure that the entire group of learners can practice a skill either simultaneously or in small groups of two to three persons. Examples of equipment include insulating pads,

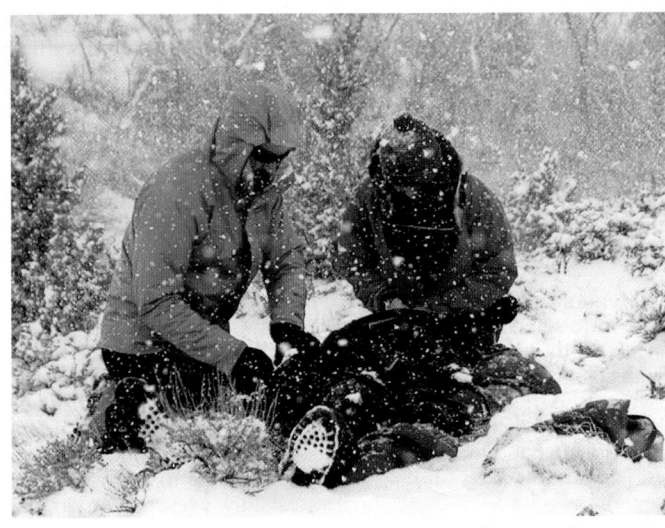

FIGURE 113-15 Challenging environmental conditions enhance the learning in wilderness medicine training and prepare students to function in a wide variety of situations. *(Courtesy Marcio Paes Barreto.)*

sleeping bags and tarps, bandaging and splinting material, athletic tape, extrication devices, old clothes, demonstration props such as EpiPen trainers, advanced airway trainers, suture kits, and gloves. If only a single example of a particular piece of equipment, such as a litter or portable ultrasound, is available, then the activity must be structured to allow for adequate hands-on time by all students. Finally, planners must establish well-defined and programmed processes for care, maintenance, transport, and storage of equipment.

Audio and Visual Aids

Audio and visual aids may take many forms, limited only by creativity of the teacher. The most basic may be a sand-covered stone upon which simple diagrams are drawn that communicate simple ideas and relationships. The most complex may be a multimedia presentation that incorporates diagrams, video, audio, and a computer or web-based interactive application to enhance learning by appealing to multiple senses. Despite the obvious advantages afforded by technology in preparing appealing and effective learning activities, pitfalls exist, largely related to the confusing or technically complex nature of the chosen technology.

The basic roles of visual aids are to illustrate the organization of a topic as it develops, to reinforce or highlight key material, and to provide an organizational "anchor" for the group that allows members to take notes, think, pose questions, and keep pace with the session.[23]

Examples of simple "low-tech" aids include terrain models, sand tables, dry-erase boards, paper charts, maps, and butcher-block flip charts. These offer significant advantages to wilderness medicine teachers because they are inexpensive and retain their usefulness in austere settings. The disadvantages of these dependable visual aids include the time required to prepare them, the fact that many are good for only a single use or topic, and their limited flexibility if changes occur in teaching objectives.

Technical audio and visual aids include overhead projectors, video machines, and computer or web-based software-driven and projected presentations. It is common for the modern lecturer to use a computer-based presentation program (e.g., PowerPoint, Keynote, Prezi). These tools make presentation and updating of visual images easy, help organize information, and facilitate presentations in large rooms and to large audiences. These all have the advantages of flexibility and appeal to multiple senses. If used properly and in the right setting, they enhance learning and provide a professional look to a degree that is unattainable with simple devices. However, they can seduce the educator to present entertainment instead of substance. They favor the use of bullet points instead of complete sentences. They

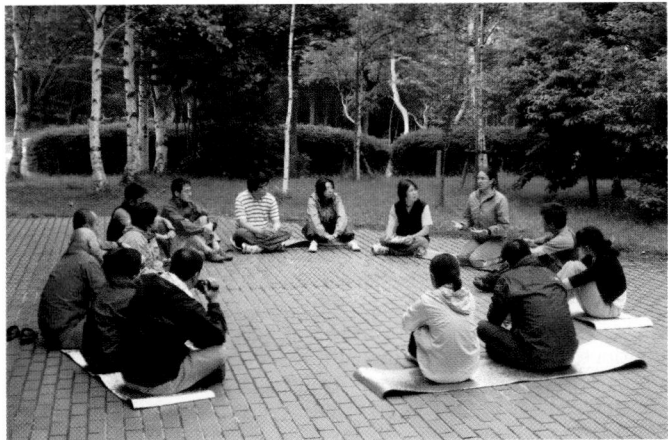

FIGURE 113-14 Wilderness medicine educators must be comfortable working in both indoor and outdoor classrooms. *(Courtesy Shana Tarter.)*

can lead the educator into the trap of showing a visual representation of something that, if demonstrated, would more effectively enhance learning. The tendency to darken a room for projection tends to dampen energy in the classroom. The inexperienced instructor may use the prefabricated visual resource as a crutch and default to reading the projected material. Class and conference participants are often oversaturated with computer-based presentations and appreciate the simple diagrams and personal engagement that comes when the educator uses a dry-erase board.

A mistake when preparing computer-based presentations is the tendency to want to use all of the "bells and whistles." There is a wide selection of graphics, animations, and interactive tools available to the educator who has even the most basic familiarity with standard software. The trick to preparing good presentations is to resist the temptation to use them. Anything that distracts learners from the main message of the graphic should be avoided. This includes sound effects, animated characters, moving text, and "wild and crazy" fonts. The best advice is to keep the presentations simple and personally test any presentation in the place where it will be used.

The obvious disadvantages of the high-tech methods to the wilderness medicine educator include expense and reliance upon additional technology, such as electricity, light bulbs, software, power cords, connectors, remote controls, computers, and, of course, Internet access. Not only must each teacher be comfortable with his or her subject, the teacher must know how to use computers and software packages and navigate the world-wide web. Many "high-powered" presentations have been aborted because of lack of a simple piece of equipment, an incompatible software program, Internet access difficulties, or a speaker who is not prepared to work with technologic devices.

Textbooks

Like any tool, textbooks are designed for specific purposes. It is important to address this issue before selecting a book to support an educational activity. The most important factor when selecting a textbook is to choose the right tool for the job. Some are intended to be encyclopedic and used mostly for reference. These tend to be larger and cover topics from a theoretical and evidence-based perspective. Although they act as good references and study resources, they may be unwieldy for use in wilderness medicine courses that focus on skills or are conducted in remote locations. They generally have greater application in the areas of wilderness medicine that cover theoretical and highly technical topics.

Some smaller textbooks are intended for use as summaries of larger works. These can even be condensed into quick-reference pocket versions. The disadvantage of these is the amount of information and important detail that is lost with each "condensation." They are seldom used as primary textbooks for courses; rather, they are adjuncts for rapid access to information already available elsewhere.

A third type of textbook is designed for use as a practical study guide. This type comes in various forms, but all appeal to the more practical areas of wilderness medicine that focus on prehospital care and acquisition of hands-on skills. Course planners may organize an entire curriculum around these highly flexible textbooks, or they may use certain sections to support an existing program of instruction.

Formats for modern textbooks include hard copy, electronic (CD-ROM) formats, and fully Internet-based formats. Publishers commonly integrate hard-copy textbooks with web-based tools that offer advanced features, such as updates, searches, and downloading of graphics and additional information.

Syllabus Material and Handouts

Students typically expect some form of syllabus to complement the learning experience. The main purpose of providing handouts is to supplement material provided in textbooks or presented in class. They are often used when faculty want to either summarize or reorganize information into a format that more closely matches the course's learning objectives. Handouts may be used to provide background information when more super-

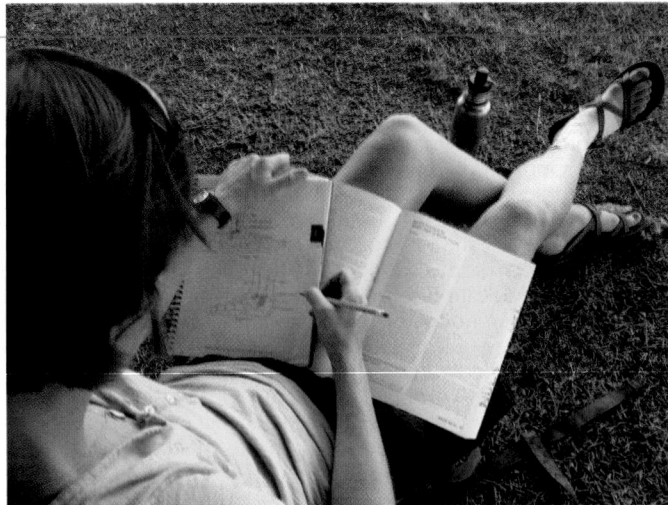

FIGURE 113-16 Wilderness medicine classes benefit from portable study materials that can be used by students, both in the classroom and during outside practice and scenarios. *(Courtesy Melissa Gray.)*

ficial treatments of material are offered in textbooks designed for skills-based or case-based learning. Other roles for handouts may be to provide a resource for conducting projects or self-examination and for updating information (e.g., clinical guidelines and procedural protocols) presented in published textbooks. Printed materials have the disadvantage of being less environmentally friendly and are likely to suffer the ill effects of harsh learning environments and daily wear and tear. However, they are portable, making them useful in programs with multiple training sites, practice sessions, and scenarios. Printed materials also tend to create less of a barrier between student and instructor than do digital computer-based materials (Figure 113-16).

Handouts that are meant for preclass preparation should be provided before the session. Those meant to recap or summarize may be best provided after the session to avoid distraction.[23] Some syllabus materials are meant to save students time in note taking by providing key points with spaces provided to fill in additional information. This serves the dual purpose of keeping students engaged and making them think about the information before summarizing it in their own words. This technique carries a risk that important information may be misquoted or missed entirely.

Handouts are sometimes intended for use as comprehensive study and preparation resources, much like a textbook. Settings where this may be most beneficial are resource-constricted courses held in remote locations that are not able to provide standard textbooks for all students to use.

A modern approach to the use of handouts is that of providing course materials in digital format, on a CD-ROM or thumb drive or in a web-based, downloadable version. Course planners must consider whether this serves the needs of the class. An instructor facing a room full of laptops cannot know whether students are focused on the material at hand or are distracted by activities unrelated to the class. This presents challenges to the wilderness medicine educator in that many activities are conducted at locations where the Internet is inaccessible and students may not want to bring computers. Some blend of digital and printed materials generally works well.

Whatever approach is used, a poorly prepared syllabus and support material detracts from learning as much as does a badly conducted session or inadequate teacher. No matter how well prepared and presented the learning activity, students will feel frustrated if they must navigate a disorganized, error-ridden syllabus.

Simulations

A thorough treatment of the history and perspectives of the use of simulation in medical education is offered by Gardner and

Raemer, whose description of the use of this educational tool in obstetrics and gynecology training remains relevant. They point out that among all the techniques available for transfer of medical skills and knowledge, "simulation is a practical and safe approach to the acquisition and maintenance of task-oriented and behavioral skills across the spectrum of medical specialties. It is a means to augment didactic instruction, providing an out-of-the-chair and hands-on experience in a safe environment without harming real patients."[37] The notion that nonhuman objects could be used to train medical practitioners is not new and is being used across many disciplines.[8,90,108,116]

Incorporation of computer- and Internet-based simulation technology across the spectrum of industries has been thoroughly adapted to health care education. Most medical schools and graduate medical education programs incorporate some form of simulation in their curricula.[9,37] Computer-based simulation technology has evolved to the point of offering virtual-world, individual- and team-based scenarios using preprogrammed patients to expand the breadth and depth of options available for medical education.[15,92,102] The potential for increased resources required to conduct this training and the associated expense are offset by expectations for increased quality of medical training and the improved outcomes that result (Figure 113-17).

Simulation technology is being used increasingly in medical training settings to enhance team training. As with any team-based vocation, medical teams that frequently practice their interactions are more effective and efficient. Teams that use simulation tools along with scenario-based role-play benefit greatly. This is particularly useful in first-responder and many other types of hands-on wilderness medicine training courses. Learning and reinforcement of basic teamwork principles are greatly facilitated by using scenario- and simulation-based training. These include leadership, followership, situational awareness, closed-loop communication, critical language, standardized responses, assertive communication, adaptive behaviors, workload management, and debriefing[44,87] (Figure 113-18).

Using simulation with computer-based mannequins and live patient role-play adds a dimension to skills-based training in

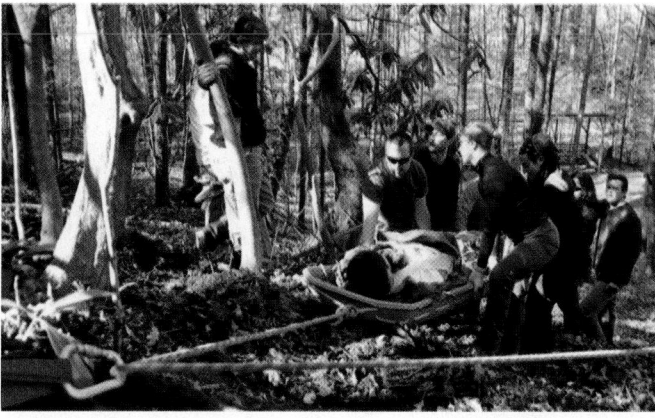

FIGURE 113-18 Medical simulation with scenario-based role-play training has become a vital tool in medical education to enhance team-based learning. *(Courtesy Fred Baty.)*

wilderness medicine not available with traditional teaching methods. Although this tool limits the quantity of information that can be covered and is resource intensive, it is a highly effective means of solidifying learning and conducting reliable and valid assessments of hands-on skills. Except for the important teaching paradigms of austerity, limited treatment resources, and improvisation, its use in wilderness medicine is fundamentally no different than how it is employed in other areas of health care education.

Important factors to consider when planning training using patient simulation are the setting, scene, acting, evaluation, and moulage.[73] The setting can be either indoors or outdoors so long as the proper clues are available to the learners. Highly realistic indoor settings call for elaborate surroundings and are often unnecessary. The basic function is to allow learners to quickly become familiar with the details of the scenario and make treatment and resource allocation decisions based on that information. Outdoor settings add more realism and use fewer resources but are subject to limitations imposed by weather and terrain. Even though prehospital courses in wilderness medicine orient their curricula toward anticipating, recognizing, and managing clinical syndromes using limited and often improvised equipment, using prefabricated and prepositioned props may make training more efficient and assessments more reliable.

The ability of learners to mentally immerse themselves in experiences using simulations seems to be directly related to the quality of the learning experience.[27] No matter the quality and high degree of fidelity of the simulation device used, the willingness of participants to "act the part" as though the situation were real for the duration of the training event facilitates the quality of their learning (Figure 113-19).

Managing the acting can be challenging. Much of what role-players will be asked to do will seem unnatural. Some persons will not have the personality or behavioral repertoire to make good role-players. This results in either overacting or underacting, both of which hinder learning and assessment. Thorough briefings about training goals and setting ground rules for role-players are crucial. Having role-players who are thoroughly familiar with the script ensures that training objectives are met and skills assessments remain reliable. Students within the group can be used for training and derive additional learning benefit from this experience. Outside role-players should generally be used as patients for skills testing. The variation in quality of role-players can be partly overcome by having experienced and thoroughly briefed faculty and examiners at each station.

When available, makeup devices enhance learning by adding a high degree of realism. Makeup may consist of inexpensive improvised items or costly, anatomically correct moulage kits designed specifically for this purpose. The overriding concern when improvising or selecting moulage is whether it enhances or detracts from achieving the learning objectives of the scenario.

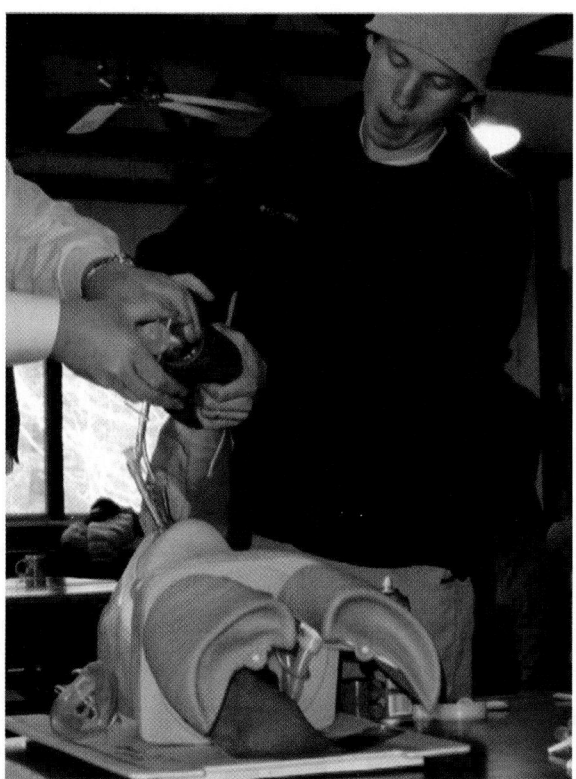

FIGURE 113-17 The use of simulation technology in wilderness medicine education often involves simple, low-technology models to enhance learning. *(Courtesy Fred Baty.)*

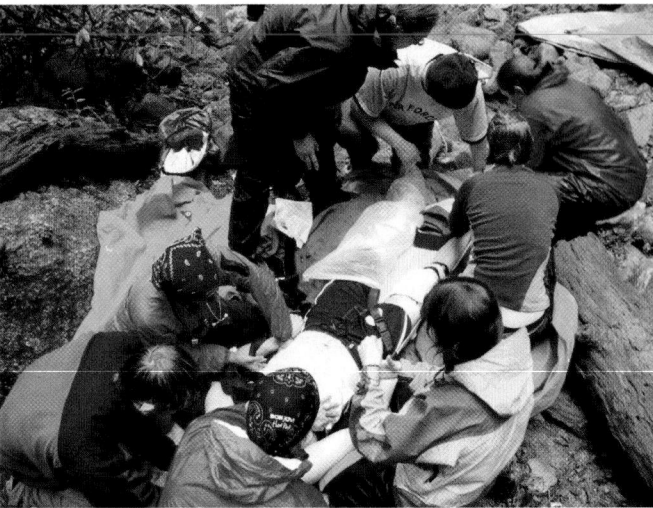

FIGURE 113-19 No matter the quality and high degree of realism provided by the equipment, the willingness of participants to "act the part" for the duration of the training event enhances the quality of learning.

If it directly supports the clinical syndrome being portrayed, then it is a good choice. If it does not, then it may confuse learners by causing them to make faulty assumptions. This has the overall effect of incorrect learning of material and leads to unreliable and invalid assessments (Figure 113-20).

Time spent in developing a fair and valid assessment process using patient simulation pays off. As previously mentioned, this is affected by many factors, such as quality and preparation of role-players and faculty, as well as environmental issues that are often beyond the control of the course director.

The notion of computer-simulated training dates back to the 1960s. Modern applications are taking the concept to a new level in the field of health care education. Patient simulation is particularly well suited for skills-oriented basic and advanced life support training in wilderness prehospital courses.[70] This tool

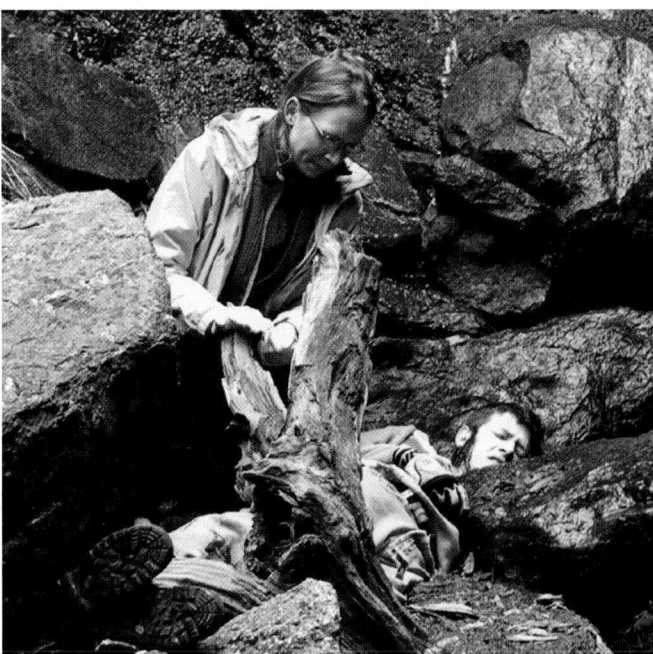

FIGURE 113-20 Simple moulage strategies can be combined with other inexpensive props to add realism to a clinical scenario. *(Courtesy Fred Baty.)*

merges computer technology with fundamental behavior-based adult learning principles to deliver effective teaching. Students are challenged and stimulated to high levels of performance. Information is delivered in a tangible, practical fashion with immediate reinforcement. Learners may repeat scenarios, make on-the-spot corrections of incorrect decisions, and see immediate results. Simulation at this level is more efficient than either problem- or scenario-based teaching, largely due to the high quality of feedback that learners receive when they observe the immediate consequences of their interventions.[70]

Some wilderness medicine training programs may be fortunate enough to have access to life-sized simulation mannequins that run algorithm-based software designed to deliver a response to anything the learner does or does not do. Software can be programmed to demonstrate any number of minor to life-threatening clinical presentations that are interpreted by the student as physiologic changes that would be expected in a real patient with a similar history and status. Interventions such as cardiopulmonary resuscitation, intravenous fluid administration, injectable medications, and endotracheal intubation can be delivered that, if performed properly and in the correct sequence, result in the expected clinical improvement. Information is delivered in a tangible, practical fashion with immediate reinforcement. Learners may repeat scenarios, make on-the-spot corrections of wrong decisions, and see immediate results. Simulation at this level is efficient due to the high quality of feedback that learners receive as they observe the immediate consequences of their interventions.[70] Certain mannequins of this type work well in the controlled indoor training setting with well-trained operators, but are not designed for use in an outdoor training environment.

An additional feature offered by this tool is assessment of learning. In relation to traditional forms of written testing, computer-based patient simulation using scenarios is one of the most effective learning assessment methods. To this already superb tool can be added computer-generated reports and video of the interaction that can be viewed individually or in groups, to reinforce teaching points and make corrections.

EVALUATION OF TEACHING

Assessment of the teaching process is an integral part of completing the education cycle. It is difficult to imagine how any course could flourish without a mechanism to self-evaluate and make periodic adjustments. This is part of what educators are accountable for when promising to deliver a product. Organizations that track, report, and maintain standards for awarding CME and CEU credit require this step to ensure that the quality of health care instruction is maintained at a high level. Evaluation is often viewed negatively by teaching staff. However, if done properly, it can take on a positive quality as a means to provide feedback. All curricula should evolve in ways that are responsive to students' needs. Formal self-evaluation requires a method to organize this process. The main purposes of course evaluation are as follows:[82]

Ensure that teaching is meeting students' needs.
Identify areas where teaching can be improved.
Facilitate allocation of faculty resources.
Provide feedback and encouragement for faculty.
Identify what is valued by educational organizations.
Facilitate curriculum development.

Course directors should look for correlations between results of course evaluations and academic testing. This requires well-constructed evaluation tools. Although a critique of the course should have no impact on whether or not students graduate, it must be treated like any other assessment to yield meaningful results. Several issues must be addressed when designing or selecting an effective evaluation instrument.

Method of Evaluation

There are three basic methods: individual interview, open discussion, and questionnaire and survey. Interview and discussion have limited roles in the overall, long-term process of improvement of most wilderness medicine courses, but have great usefulness in making short-term, on-the-spot adjustments. Questionnaires and surveys have the greatest applicability and will be discussed further.

Fairness and Confidentiality

All participants must be afforded the opportunity to evaluate the educational experience. Although it may not be feasible to make it mandatory, it should be highly encouraged. Questions should be constructed so that they do not unintentionally bias the results according to the responses of one group of learners (e.g., physicians versus EMTs). Most instruments are provided in a confidential fashion, whether or not names are provided on each questionnaire. The issue of anonymity has two schools of thought. One advocates anonymity to reduce the impact of bias and to make sure respondents feel free to offer an honest critique without fear of reprisal. The other requires students to provide their names but takes steps to guard against unintended disclosure and reprisal. This provides for responsible commentary and allows further clarification by individual students if needed. A reasonable compromise is to make it optional to provide names.

Usefulness of the Results

Like any other assessment, the ideal evaluation is reliable, valid, acceptable, and inexpensive.[82] Compromise in any of these areas will decrease usefulness of the instrument. A poorly designed or administered critique wastes valuable resources and time for both respondents and faculty. This lack of respect transforms the process into a meaningless exercise. The most important aspect to ensure that results will be useful is construction of the instrument (see later discussion). Another is to make students feel vested in the course so that thoughtful assessment has a purpose and comes naturally. This must be nurtured in the course design and should have already occurred before critique forms are handed out on the final day. Attend to the principle of proximity. For lengthy courses, ensure that there is time scheduled and reminders given each day to fill out critique forms for each session. A short, overall evaluation of the course can be done at the end. Students may be in a hurry to depart after academic activities are over and therefore rush through, or even omit, the evaluation process. A common technique to ensure that each student completes an evaluation is to require that he or she turns in a form before receiving a graduation or training certificate.

What to Evaluate

Participants may be queried about anything that is relevant to the conduct of the course. However, consideration must be given to the actual usefulness of the information and the time it takes to complete the form. At a minimum, students should be given the opportunity to rate and add additional commentary on the following components[21]:

Course design
Textbooks
Supplemental learning material (e.g., syllabus or handouts)
Audio and visual aids
Lecture and discussion sessions
Skills practice sessions
Scenarios, simulations, and practice examinations
Written examinations and quizzes
Instructors
The setting (e.g., administration, accommodations, and physical surroundings)

Format of the Evaluation Instrument

Selection of the proper format of the evaluation is critical. An improperly designed instrument with poorly worded questions may lead to meaningless results or faulty assumptions that lead to inappropriate modification of the course design. A valuable instrument is formed with respect for a student's time. Students will not fill it out properly if it is too lengthy or complicated. It should minimize the potential for error and confusion by reducing the amount of work and thought that goes into completing the form. Provide as much unique, identifying, course-related information as possible on the form. The fewer pages the better. One page is best. Instructions must be brief and clear.

A written commentary format gives immediate comprehensible feedback to the faculty that can be either positive or negative. However, it may be superficial and limited in scope. Comments may be difficult to translate into actionable information that leads to course improvements. Evaluations that use this method exclusively have limited reliability and validity.

The multiple-choice format facilitates tabulation and objective comparison. The choice of responses must be broad enough to avoid bias toward either end of the scale. In general, simple good-bad descriptors are less helpful than those that address the function and effectiveness of the item in question. Descriptive adjectives should be selected that match the component being evaluated. For example, adjectives describing helpfulness and effectiveness may be most appropriate when one is asking questions about class materials or procedures. A space for commentary should be provided after each question. Scaled forms on which the student must fill in a circle or cross off a number to rate the specific features of the course take less time to complete and are helpful in managing the results. A quick reminder about the nature of the item being rated may accompany these questions. Likert-type rating scales can be from 1 to 5, or 1 to 7, and may correspond to various forms of descriptors.

No matter what format is chosen, it is a good idea to leave room for several open-ended questions that address the most and least valuable portions of the course, as well as what improvements the respondent recommends. Responses to these tend to be highly contextual based on the background and personality of the student. However, multiple responses from a single class that focus on the same issue or several that are similar across multiple courses may indicate a need for change.

Providing the Results

Course directors should provide tabulated and summarized results of the evaluations to all faculty members. Both group and individual sessions with instructors may be beneficial to discuss the results and select process improvement strategies. Faculty members should see specific comments only about themselves and not those made about other instructors. There should also be some way to inform the students about the results of the evaluations and the resulting actions that were taken.

Evaluation of teaching is a critical component of the overall process of educating adults in any discipline. Learners and teachers at all levels expect this and sometimes look forward to it. With effort in planning and design work, the practice can become a very valuable tool for wilderness medicine educators.

PROGRAM AND CURRICULUM DEVELOPMENT

The notion continues to evolve that teaching in health care should be organized and standardized. How this is best accomplished remains to be determined. The uniqueness of wilderness medicine presents challenges while it affords educators opportunities for innovation in curriculum design. This applies equally to short certification-oriented courses, embedded curricula within longer programs of instruction, and limited CME/CEU programs.

In its most basic form, a curriculum is an expression of community values. To remain viable, it should reflect the current and changing values of the community it serves. Because students will ultimately return to the community to practice, this community of stakeholders should have a say in what they are taught. The educational topics should be directly relevant to their needs. This seems simple, but is an important underlying reason why curriculum design is often controversial in wilderness medicine. Who are the stakeholders? Apart from market dynamics, who gets to decide what should and should not be taught? To what standardizing body do wilderness medicine educators turn for guidance? Where is the evidence upon which to base judgments and decisions?

A growing body of literature seeks to refine what should be included in wilderness medicine education programs. Although there are taxonomies and lists of topics from which to draw, there exists no academic accreditation process or wilderness medicine oversight organization that ensures the relevance of these topics or that they are taught in a high-quality fashion. This allows for great variability in program content and delivery. The National Outdoor Leadership School's (NOLS) Wilderness Medicine Institute uses a triad of attributes: practicality, accuracy, and relevance, to help determine the curriculum content for its programs.

The formalized specialty practice of wilderness medicine is young. It has not yet experienced the scrutiny, peer-review, and standardization of techniques of other medical disciplines. The population of patients from which it can be determined whether a treatment is efficacious is small, which makes it challenging to perform certain types of research. Randomized controlled trials that study laypeople practicing first aid in the wilderness do not exist. NOLS extrapolates techniques from the urban clinical realm and applies them to the wilderness setting.

Absence of evidence-based standards combined with the culture of improvisation may lead the instructor to teach a technique, for example, how to use an improvised traction splint or advanced airway, which works well in the controlled classroom environment but fails in the field. Instructors must ask themselves whether anyone has successfully performed this technique outside the classroom or conference workshop. Often the answer is no, or at best, the sample size is small. In the absence of evidence or personal experience, seeking an anecdotal or a first-person account of the use of a technique helps reassure that what is taught will be effective when employed in the field.

The culture of medical education at the professional level values the accuracy and validity of information. Curriculum content that is evidence based relies upon established practice guidelines and informed expert opinion. By contrast, layperson first-aid training is often provided by well-intentioned but non-professional educators or practitioners who may unknowingly provide impractical practice advice and information that is poorly supported by the evidence.

RETENTION OF LEARNING

Despite increased availability of wilderness medicine education programs and establishment of wilderness medicine certification as the de facto standard for leading trips in the outdoors, there is a paucity of research related to wilderness medicine skills retention. There is a body of research in first-aid and basic life support education that documents rapid degradation of skills and knowledge.[2,6,48,63] In 2012, a targeted research study focused on graduates with no prior medical training or experience of a standardized 16-hour introductory wilderness first-aid course to evaluate knowledge and skills retention, as well as the students' perception of self-efficacy.[100]

The study evaluated knowledge retention, skills retention, and self-efficacy at 4, 8, and 12 months following training. The results demonstrated a few key findings that can help improve the design of wilderness medicine education programs. First and unsurprisingly, participants' skills deteriorated in as few as 4 months after their training experience and continued to deteriorate through the 12 months of the study. Most of the participants had no cause to practice their skills in any meaningful way after their course. Second, performance on a standardized, written knowledge assessment had little correlation to the quality of an individual's skill performance. This reinforces the need to dedicate ample time during wilderness medicine training to hands-on skills and application of knowledge through use of scenarios. First aid is largely a practical skill. Interestingly, an individual's confidence in the ability to perform as measured through the self-efficacy tool also lacked correlation with the ability to treat a simulated patient.

Wilderness medicine educators need to be aware of the limits of retention and design their curricula accordingly. Especially in layperson education, complex explanations and unnecessary detail will be forgotten, and even practiced skills will be quickly lost. A focus on simple, relevant, and practical skills, well-designed and well-coached practice, repetition of practice over time, and use of memory aids may be necessary to ensure competent performance in the field.

WILDERNESS MEDICINE INJURY AND ILLNESS DATA

Of everything that could be taught in a wilderness medicine course, how does the educator choose what is relevant to the audience? A good place to begin is to build an understanding of injury and illness patterns in the wilderness. Although wilderness medicine may be practiced in a variety of settings ranging from recreational camps to expeditions to disasters to remote medical clinics, incident data are relatively consistent. By using these data as the foundation for curriculum content, the educator will avoid developing material that may be overly influenced by anecdote or isolated experiences. Existing data can be roughly divided into data from outdoor adventure programs, remote clinical experiences, and wilderness EMS.

The NOLS Field Incident Database is the largest set of injury and illness reports from educational wilderness expeditions. It is currently in its 30th year, with more than 4 million person-days of experience and 14,000 incidents.[39,66,76] Over the last decade, the pace of research has increased, so there is a more substantial body of work that can inform practice and help focus training and decision-making tools. One can study incident data collected by youth groups, outdoor programs, park visitors, search and rescue teams, climbing programs, trekking organizations, and boating groups.[10,18,32,38,65,84,93,109,112,117] However, there remains a lack of credible incidence data from large segments of the outdoor recreation community, including college-based programs, scouting organizations, and many camps.

It is clear from examination of existing data that small wounds, sprains and strains, diarrhea, and flu-like illnesses make up most of the ailments faced by the outdoor leader, and that serious injury and illness are rare. When its incident database revealed these patterns, NOLS revised its WFR curriculum. Dramatic, unrealistic scenarios were deemphasized, and the focus moved toward developing the patient assessment skills needed to determine the need for and urgency of evacuation, and to address the prevention of wound infections, sprains and strains, diarrhea, and flu-like illnesses (Figure 113-21).

A glimpse of trends in wilderness EMS comes from looking at data from search and rescue teams, the National Park Service, and other state land management agencies. These data include both backcountry and frontcountry wilderness medicine, and reveal a set of serious injuries not seen in the outdoor education data. The data from search and rescue teams are weighted toward injury rather than illness, and, in addition to the expected orthopedic problems, there are deaths due to drowning. When one considers illness, there is a greater tendency for underlying medical issues to play a part in these data, especially at the

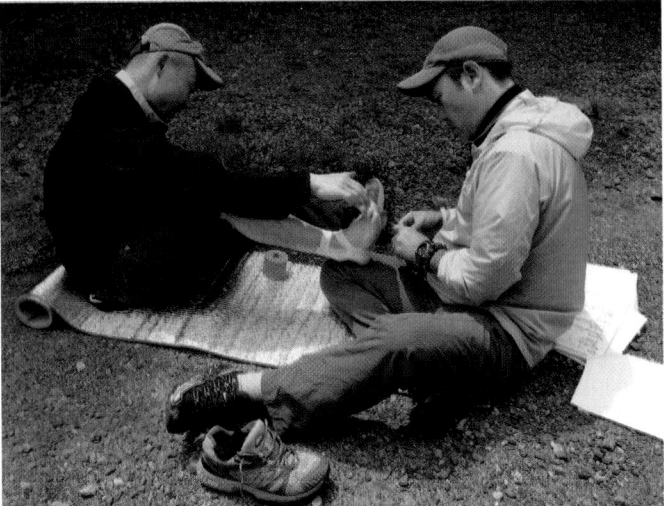

FIGURE 113-21 Basic skills, such as ankle taping, are important to include in wilderness medicine training. (*Courtesy Shana Tarter.*)

urban-wilderness interface. Cardiac emergencies are prominent; lung disease, diabetes, and the host of other illnesses in the general population also appear.[31,33,40,42,53,78,80,85,105]

Fortunately, the most common problems encountered in the field are not life threatening and can be identified as musculoskeletal, hygiene-related, and environmentally induced. Unfortunately, when a serious event occurs, field treatment is often limited by resources and evacuation is arduous or complicated.

From a course planning standpoint, one takes away important lessons from the growing knowledge of wilderness epidemiology. The first is the value of including prevention. The limits of practice in a wilderness context argue for a theme of prevention. Another lesson is that the strong presence of hygiene-related and communicable illnesses suggests the need for more attention to best practices in simple activities such as hand washing, cooking, and cleaning.[13,77]

The context of practice influences the content of the training program. Persons leading outdoor groups need to be prepared to manage overuse musculoskeletal injury and care for minor wounds with the goal of preventing infection. They need to know how to manage flu-like and gastrointestinal illnesses and how to recognize when a patient can stay in the field and when the patient needs to be assessed by a provider at a higher level of care. In addition, they need to be prepared to care for traumatic injury, including managing potential spine injuries (Figure 113-22).

The wilderness search and rescue provider is more likely to respond to serious injury or illness and needs to be able to adapt urban skills to the wilderness context; most importantly, the provider needs to have the judgment to know when an advanced skill is appropriate in the austere context, and the consequences of initiating an intervention that might need to be maintained for extended periods in austere conditions.

Persons evaluating and treating patients in a remote clinic setting need to be prepared for a broad scope of practice, especially what is common in the local environment. They need to understand what tools will be available and what will need to be improvised, the available inventory of medications and other therapies and how these might be resupplied, what to expect for evacuation and further care, and how to manage the long-term needs of their patients. The breadth of these learning needs challenges the educator to be thoughtful about including in their curriculum what will be practical and relevant for the student.

CONCEPTS AND MODELS

Prideaux described a curriculum as "existing at three basic levels: what is planned for the students, what is delivered to the students, and what the students experience." In practical application, a curriculum should be easily communicated to learners and educators, should be open to critique and modification, and should be easily implemented. More specifically, it should contain four elements: content, teaching and learning strategies, assessment processes, and teaching evaluation methods. The process of curriculum design attempts to form these elements into a tangible, usable device.[97]

Several models of health care curriculum design have been proposed. These evolved indirectly based on changing needs, values, and expectations of society. One that has emerged as being effective with great applicability to wilderness medicine is based on identifying, addressing, and assessing desired outcomes. This is appropriately referred to as "outcomes-based education." Although usually discussed in the context of clinical teaching settings, such as medical schools and residencies, the focus on outcomes is germane to wilderness medicine education. No matter how the details of a curriculum unfold in practice, keeping the focus on outcomes places the wilderness medicine learner at the center of the education cycle. The basic concept of this model requires that educators first decide what the students should know (outcomes), design a program of learning to allow them to achieve it, and then assess whether or not they achieved the desired results. The details of how educators make these determinations describe an elaborate and interesting process.

Numerous versions of curriculum design are used throughout the United States and Europe. Many have been reported in the wilderness medicine literature.[16,70,94-96,120] Steve Donelan has written extensively on the subject and offers detailed guidance.[21,25-29] Nearly all courses use a combination of techniques to deliver material to learners. A focus on outcomes is a common theme.

STEPS IN DESIGNING A CURRICULUM

The success or failure of any educational experience goes far beyond a title. Simply using a wilderness medicine label may initially attract enthusiasts. However, failing to deliver a rewarding learning experience that is rooted in fundamental educational concepts, that leverages the most modern technology when applicable and practicable, and that is clinically and practically useful in the field will send would-be attendees looking elsewhere for ways to spend their valuable time and money. The design of the curriculum lies at the heart of this issue. McGraw and Gluckman reported on the results of their efforts to bring wilderness medicine to undergraduate medical education at the University of Pennsylvania School of Medicine. A survey following the course indicated that a large number (40%) of respondents found the course to be the best experience they had undergone in medical school.[75] As Steve Donelan indicated in his commentary on their report, medical schools may have much to learn from these nontraditional courses, given the strength of their curricula and overall course design, quality of teaching, and relevance of the clinical information contained therein.[29a]

All aspects of curriculum design should be well thought out before resources are allocated. The general sequence starts with identification of the desired outcomes, or what the students should be able to do (including a learning needs assessment), addresses specific content (topics to be taught), selects teaching methods, develops learning assessment instruments, and, finally, constructs tools to evaluate the process.

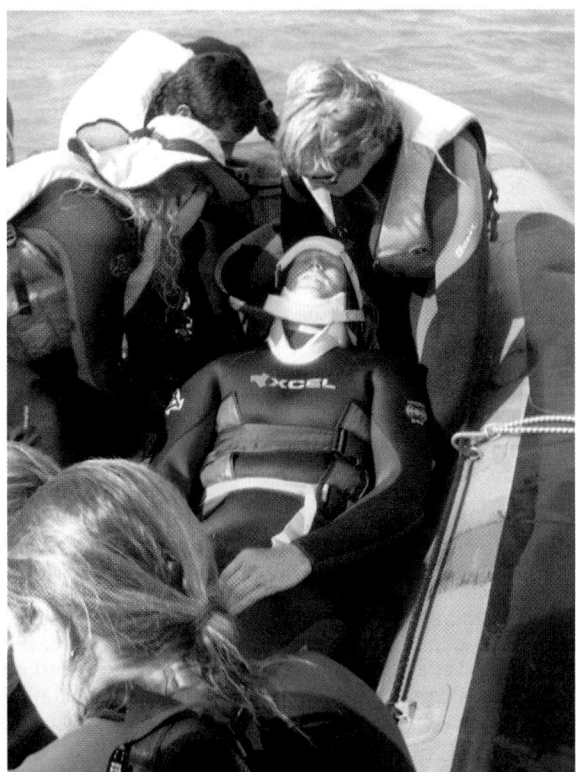

FIGURE 113-22 Management of spinal injuries in remote settings is a core topic in most wilderness medicine training events. *(Courtesy Shana Tarter.)*

Desired Outcomes

Outcomes are addressed on two levels: the overall course goals or objectives, and specific learning objectives for each session or activity. As discussed above, course goals describe the overall purpose for students attending the course. This may include a job- or skill-related certification or simply advancement of their general fund of knowledge. It addresses what they should be able to do or know after completing the entire program. All activities related to the formal curriculum should contribute in some way to these goals. This is similar to a large corporation that does institution-level analysis of its mission, vision, goals, and objectives. Any action resulting from this strategic planning that does not contribute in some way to the mission of the organization is at best distracting and possibly a hindrance. Individual learning objectives can be viewed in this context. Accomplishment of the course goals depends on them.

Two sources, or stakeholders, should be queried to determine outcomes at both levels. Potential learners may be asked using various methods (polling, focus groups, and questionnaires) what they think is important and what they would most like to learn. Organizations that hire or interface with potential graduates of the course may be asked for their input on what skills, knowledge, and qualities the graduates should possess. The goals and objectives should be formalized, written, and distributed to anyone involved with curriculum design. They serve as a compass to guide all planning and design efforts.

Determine the Content

After the course objectives are established, they are used as a basis to begin selecting major content divisions or sections. There is no "best" method of dividing the information, but it is generally agreed that sections should be easy to support with effective teaching and assessment methods based on sound learning theory (e.g., problem-based versus lecture-based courses, small-group discussion versus hands-on practical exercise). The organization of the original WMS WPHEC objectives suggests sections devoted to basic science, clinical science, EMS and evacuation procedures and equipment, field craft, and prevention. The major sections are further broken down into subsections or topics. The basic science section might be divided by topic-specific reviews of anatomic or physiologic systems. The field-craft section might be broken down into land navigation and wilderness survival. Land navigation may be further divided into sessions on map reading, compass use, celestial navigation, and use of global positioning system devices. It is this final level for which specific learning objectives are written. There are no absolutely right or wrong answers in selecting the specific content of a course. As long as the basic steps are followed, a suitable solution will reveal itself.

Select Teaching Methods

Methods for delivering the information should be selected after the course content has been established. Course planners should make use of several techniques and, if possible, vary them daily to maintain student interest. An entire day of hands-on practical exercise in frigid temperatures may detract as much from learning as a 10-hour day of back-to-back lectures. Intermixing the techniques by spending 2 hours outside and 2 hours indoors in small-group work, followed by 2 more hours outside, capped off with an hour or two of lecture at the end of the day, is an example of this type of variation. The only limits are the imagination of the course planners and simple logistics, such as moving or transporting learners and equipment between venues. Planners should make maximum use of the various forms of problem-based instruction and small-group work. Lectures should be limited to introductions and topics that absolutely do not lend themselves to the aforementioned techniques.

Of the steps in curriculum design, selection of teaching methods may be most influenced by the physical setting of the course. This includes the climate, terrain, and accommodations for teaching and lodging, as well as available support and equipment. The setting will sometimes be preestablished, forcing accommodations in curriculum design. At other times, the curriculum may contain flexible elements that will change as the features of the location change and unexpected opportunities arise.

Select Learning Assessment Instruments

Assessment of learning derives directly from the course objectives that are supported by the learning objectives. Written testing allows assessment of both. Some questions may be intended to evaluate knowledge of facts addressed by learning objectives from individual sessions. Others address the synthesis of information drawn from multiple sessions and in different sections. Written tests or quizzes can be used for formative assessment, whereas hands-on skills testing using scenarios and role-players may be used in practice, formative, and summative (end-of-course) roles. For some courses, skills-based assessments may be out of place, forcing planners to be skilled at constructing written examinations. The main concept in constructing assessment tools is to develop them based on well-written session and course objectives.

DEVELOPING THE COURSE EVALUATION

Evaluation of the course is the final step in the education cycle and curriculum design. Reserving this until last does not diminish its importance. Many highly effective examples of evaluation tools exist. Adhering to basic principles discussed earlier will lead to an effective instrument that informs continuous improvement and curriculum modification.

PLANNING FOR CONTINUING MEDICAL EDUCATION

Educational experiences intended to assist practitioners in maintaining currency, refreshing eroded skills and knowledge, or adding new skills and knowledge are vital to safety and viability across the spectrum of health care, including wilderness medicine. Despite the importance and use by all health care disciplines, there is a relatively small body of evidence beyond tradition, anecdote, and expert opinion to support use of any given educational technique or set of techniques over any another in planning and delivering CME.[89] Guidelines produced by some specialty-oriented professional organizations are based on evidence from the existing body of educational research. These attempt not only to elevate the effectiveness of CME but also to standardize training techniques within the discipline and inform the industry that has grown up to produce continuing education.[81] The body of literature on which these guidelines are based is not large and reflects the tremendous difficulty inherent in studying education in a way that is based on outcomes and that allows reliable cause-and-effect conclusions. It seems reasonable, however, to assert that continuing education for health care should adhere to fundamental principles of adult education. For example, augmenting a course based on a traditional lecture format by using multiple approaches for delivering information, such as multimedia presentations or interactive, small-group, case-based discussion, will enhance energy and improve learning. When practical to the setting, hands-on, practical exercises using scenario-based simulation is a preferable method to refresh, maintain, and learn new psychomotor skills.[1,57,89]

Development of programs designed to award credit for CME or CEU follows the same basic steps with respect to curriculum content. There are challenges unique to this type of activity that deserve special mention. The venue (setting) is more likely to affect the program of instruction, whether it is completely lecture based or uses a mix of teaching styles. Learners at CME/CEU events are more apt to form judgments about value based on the perceived quality of what they received balanced against how much they paid. Participants expect adequate physical space, facilities, accommodations, and amenities.

Many participants seek recreational diversion in addition to the learning experience. This must be addressed in the logistics planning and schedule. Holding an event at an attractive location with abundant recreational opportunities, and then cramming 50 hours of wonderful training into 4 days with no time for recreation will frustrate CME/CEU learners.

The selection process for faculty is often limited by the budget and availability of teachers. Although convention holds that only the most highly proficient and credentialed faculty should be selected, reality often forces a different approach. The search should begin early, because good teachers are highly sought after and have busy professional lives. Program chairs should attempt to obtain a commitment as early as possible and make a viable contingency plan for those that have to cancel or simply do not respond. The design of the program of instruction is closely linked to the selection of faculty for CME/CEU events. The notoriety of teachers often drives selection of their area of expertise as a subject in the curriculum. This also makes contingency planning all the more important when high-profile speakers need to cancel. Learners committed to a topic and speaker may feel slighted when the topic is not delivered or a substitute teacher appears.

After a program of instruction (curriculum) is set and faculty members are chosen, course materials are developed. Program chairs have two basic options to get this accomplished. They may establish the curriculum early, including learning objectives, and then ask faculty to develop and submit original material. This requires that faculty be given specific guidelines about how to prepare the materials, including the format and length. Standardization of presentation materials provides a professional appearance to the program that helps achieve buy-in from participants. The expertise, responsiveness, and quality of product vary greatly, so program chairs are wise to begin this process a year in advance. Another method is to provide prepared materials to the speakers in advance. They may or may not be allowed to make modifications depending on the desires of the program chair. This method has the advantage of being centrally controlled, dependable, and flexible when faculty members cancel. However, the workload of the program chair is increased because all materials must be developed, reviewed for accuracy and currency, and printed or otherwise reproduced.

Perhaps the most difficult part of conducting CME/CEU events is managing the administrative, business, and marketing tasks. These include contracting for venues, lodging and accommodations, speakers, printing, automation and training support, and materials. Developing marketing materials, such as flyers, brochures, and websites, requires skill with graphic design and layout and is usually beyond the expertise of most program chairs. A poorly designed brochure can kill an otherwise high-quality event. Arranging for CME/CEU credit, as well as the interface with the awarding organizations, poses a significant workload challenge. Course materials, including certificates, evaluation forms, syllabus, handouts, administrative guides, electronic storage media, and access to contracted wireless and on-line resources, must all be coordinated and produced. It is recommended that professional assistance be sought for these critical tasks at least 1 year in advance.

Using an organized approach to program and curriculum design that directly addresses objectives and follows the basic conventions discussed here will lead to successful outcomes, no matter the level of learner or type of activity.

PROFESSIONAL ORGANIZATIONS AND TRAINING PROGRAMS IN WILDERNESS MEDICINE

PROFESSIONAL SOCIETIES

Professional societies in the United States and elsewhere have guided establishment of academic standards in wilderness medicine education. These organizations typically sponsor CME events through large, sometimes international, meetings to further education, research, and international cooperation and sharing of knowledge. The WMS and the International Society for Mountain Medicine sponsor educational activities and publish their own peer-reviewed journals (*Wilderness and Environmental Medicine, High Altitude Medicine and Biology*). The WMS, for

BOX 113-8 Professional Societies Related to Wilderness Medicine

United States

Aerospace Medical Association	http://www.asma.org
American Alpine Club	americanalpineclub.org
American College of Emergency Physicians	acep.org
Appalachian Center for Wilderness Medicine	appwildmed.org
Divers Alert Network	diversalertnetwork.org
Institute for Altitude Medicine	altitudemedicine.org
International Society of Travel Medicine	istm.org
Mountain Rescue Association	mra.org
National Association for Search and Rescue	nasar.org
National Ski Patrol	nsp.org
Society for Academic Emergency Medicine	saem.org
Undersea and Hyperbaric Medical Society	uhms.org
Wilderness Medical Society	wms.org

Europe and Asia

Austrian Society for Mountain and High Altitude Medicine	alpinmedizin.org
German Society for Mountain and Expedition Medicine	bexmed.de
Himalayan Rescue Association Nepal	himalayanrescue.org
International Climbing and Mountaineering Federation	theuiaa.org
International Commission for Alpine Rescue	ikar-cisa.org
International Society for Mountain Medicine	ismm.org/
Japanese Society of Mountain Medicine	jsmmed.org/
Mountain Medicine Society of Nepal	mmsn.org.np/
Swiss Society for Mountain Medicine	mountainmedicine.ch

example, hosts CME events and offers fellowship recognition to members through its Academy of Wilderness Medicine. Several professional societies, including the American College of Emergency Physicians and the Society for Academic Emergency Medicine, possess wilderness medicine sections or interest groups. Other organizations, such as the Divers Alert Network and National Ski Patrol System, focus on specific content areas (Box 113-8).

CERTIFICATION PROGRAMS FOR OUTDOOR RECREATION AND EDUCATION

Wilderness medicine courses and certification programs exist in first aid, search and rescue, and other advanced topics for laypeople, first responders, physicians, and allied health professionals. In the past 20 years, these programs have proliferated. Growth of wilderness medicine education may be attributed to increasing accessibility of short-duration training for outdoor users, broadening scope of EMS response in nonurban or disaster settings, and the increase in training and certification requirements for outdoor leaders and guides. Although there presently is no consensus for an industry-wide, national standard for outdoor leader wilderness medicine training, the trend, influenced by leading groups in the field (e.g., the Wilderness Risk Managers Conference, accreditation organizations, insurance companies) or by land management permit requirements, is toward some form of certification in wilderness medicine. The Association for Experiential Education has program accreditation standards, which include a policy that wilderness programs enacted at least 4 to 6 hours from definitive care have at least one leader with WFR certification.[72] The American Camp Association requires the presence of persons who have completed, at a minimum, a 16-hour wilderness medicine course when access to EMS is more than 30 minutes.[3] NOLS requires WFR training for its field staff.[88] Outward Bound requires WFR training for the field staff if a program is more than 1 hour from definitive medical care[68] (Box 113-9).

In the 1970s, after decades of small-scale "mountain medicine" educational programs, modern wilderness medicine programs began in earnest. This occurred in tandem with growth of the outdoor education industry in order to meet the needs of trip leaders who needed more than urban-oriented first-aid courses.

In the early years of modern wilderness medicine programs, instructors, who were often outdoor enthusiasts interested in both wilderness and medicine, took what they had learned in urban-oriented, advanced first-aid or EMT courses and adapted

the curricula, based on experience and opinion, to fit their needs. Published research was sparse, and courses evolved based on experience, opinion, and available literature. Many of the credible textbooks of the time contained techniques, such as incision and suction for snakebite, that are now considered ineffective. Others included treatment recommendations that were beyond the scope of practice of a lay medical provider. At the time it was the best advice available.[34,67,121] In recent years, a group of providers of wilderness medicine courses have worked to define course content based on evidence and experience, resulting in publication of consensus statements on the Scope of Practice for both Wilderness First Aid (WFA) and WFR certifications.[50,51]

BOX 113-9 Wilderness Medicine Training Providers

Advanced Wilderness Life Support	awls.org
Adventure First Aid	adventurefirstaid.co.uk
Adventure Medic	theadventuremedic.com/courses/
Adventure Medical Consultants	lundycharters.com/maritime-and-wilderness-medicine/wilderness-first-responder
Aerie School of Backcountry Medicine	aeriemedicine.com/
All Aid First Aid	allaid.com.au/
American Red Cross	redcross.org/take-a-class/program-highlights/cpr-first-aid/wilderness-sports-pets #wilderness-remote-first-aid
American Safety and Health Institute	hsi.com/ashi/wildernessfirstaid/
Backcountry Medical Guides	backcountrymedicalguides.org/wilderness-first-responder/
Canadian Wilderness Medical Training	cwmt.ca/
Center for Wilderness Safety	wildsafe.com/
Coconino Community College	coconino.edu/list-of-course-descriptions/327-emergency-medical-services-ems
Desert Mountain Medicine	desertmountainmedicine.com/
Ecomed	ecomed.com.au/
Enviro-Tech International	etisurvival.com/wldmd.htm
Expedition Medicine	expeditionmedicine.co.uk
ExpedMed	expedmed.squarespace.com
First Lead	firstlead.com/
Foster Calm First Aid	fostercalm.com/
Front Range Institute of Safety	frisfirstaid.com
Great Smoky Mountains Institute	gsmit.org/wfr.html
Highlands Wilderness Training Institute	scotthembruff.wix.com/wildernesstraining#!wilderness-first-aid-training-courses/c8jf
International Wilderness Leadership School	iwls.com/courses/activity-2/first-aid-rescue
Longleaf Wilderness Medicine	longleafmedical.com/
Mountain Education and Development LLC	mountained.com/medical
Muir-Walker Medics Cooperative	uk.coop.muir-walker-medics-co-operative-limited
National Outdoor Leadership School Wilderness Medicine Institute	nols.edu/wmi
Outdoor Emergency Care	oectraining.com/courses
Pacific Alpine Institute	pacificalpineinstitute.com/coursedescriptions.html
Peak Emergency Response Training	peakemergencytraining.com
Remote 1st Response	remote1stresponse.com/
Remote First Aid Training Academy	remotefirstaid.com/courses
Remote Medical International	remotemedical.com/
Remote Rescue	remoterescuemed.com/
Rescue Dynamics	rescuedynamics.ca/emergency.htm
Rocky Mountain Adventure Medicine	adventuremed.ca
Sierra Rescue	sierrarescue.com/course-info/wilderness-first-aid-courses/
Sirius Wilderness Medicine	siriusmed.com/
Slipstream Wilderness First Aid Training	wildernessfirstaid.ca/
Stonehearth Open Learning Opportunities	soloschools.com/
University of Vermont	uvm.edu/cnhs/rems/
Wilderness Alert	wildernessalert.com/
Wilderness Emergency Care	wildernessemergencycare.com/
Wilderness Emergency Medical Services Institute	wemsi-international.org/
Wilderness First Aid	wfa.net/
Wilderness First Aid Australia	wildernessmedicine.com.au/
Wilderness First Aid Consultants	wfac.com.au/
Wilderness First Aid Course	sites.google.com/a/wildernessfirstaidcourse.org/wilderness-first-aid-course/home
Wilderness Medical Associates	wildmed.com/
Wilderness Medical Consultants	wildernessmedicalconsultants.ca/
Wilderness Medical Training	wildernessmedicaltraining.co.uk/
Wilderness Medicine	wilderness-medicine.com/
Wilderness Medicine Outfitters	wildernessmedicine.com/
Wilderness Medicine Training Center	wildmedcenter.com/
Wilderness Medicine of Utah	wmutah.org/
Wilderness Medicine Outfitters	wildernessmedicine.com/
Wilderness Medicine Training Center	wildmedcenter.com/
Wilderness Safety Consultants	wsc2.com/

TABLE 113-4 A Comparison of Wilderness First-Aid and Wilderness First-Responder Courses	
Wilderness First Aid (16 to 24 Hours)	**Wilderness First Responder (70 to 80 Hours)**
Wilderness first-aid courses are basic layperson first-aid programs. The curriculum focus is on performing a simple physical examination to identify obvious injuries or abnormalities; assessing signs, symptoms, and vital sign patterns; preventing medical problems anticipated by the activity and environment; treatment focused on stabilization of emergencies, initiation of specific and appropriate medical treatments (splints, wound care, spine injury management, managing environmental threats); and conservative decisions on the need for and urgency of evacuation. The wilderness first-aid curriculum neither includes such practices as administering medications other than epinephrine by autoinjector for anaphylaxis, nor does it include selective spine immobilization.	Wilderness first-responder courses are first-aid programs intended for nonmedical professionals who are acting as primary caregivers in a remote setting or as second rescuers for more highly trained persons. The scope of practice for a wilderness first responder is to prevent illnesses and injuries; identify illnesses and injuries; initiate reasonable and prudent field management; and identify red flag signs and symptoms necessitating evacuation for potentially life-threatening problems. The wilderness first responder is taught selective spine immobilization protocols and reduction of a selected set of joint dislocations.

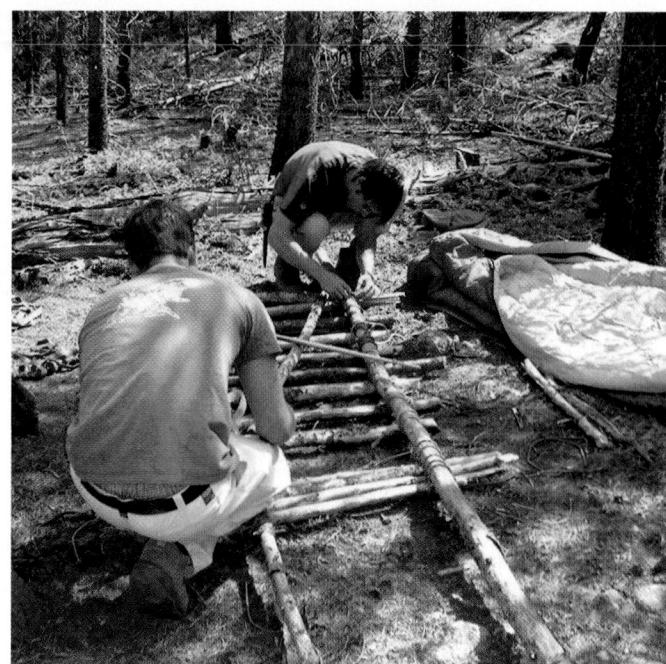

FIGURE 113-23 Wilderness medicine caregivers must develop skills to improvise equipment from the resources at hand. *(Courtesy Gates Richards.)*

Lay provider certification programs can be broadly divided into WFA (16 to 24 hours), Wilderness Advanced First Aid (32 to 40 hours), WFR (70 to 80 hours), and WEMT (150 to 200 hours). These programs are typically offered in a traditional classroom setting with access to out-of-doors practice space. They mix lectures with skills and scenarios. Successful completion of examinations results in certification lasting 2 to 3 years. Though the breadth and depth of topics covered in these courses vary, the courses share a foundation as defined in the WFA and WFR scope of practice documents (Table 113-4).

More recent developments include semester-long programs blending medicine, clinical experience, and rescue training. These programs average 12 weeks, include multiple certification opportunities, and offer undergraduate college credit. Some include international clinical experience; others focus on extended wilderness travel and technical rescue.

TRAINING FOR HEALTH CARE PROFESSIONALS

A similar series of certification programs exist for professionals. In addition to earning certifications, participants generally receive continuing education credits. These programs presume preexisting medical knowledge and focus on adapting existing understanding and experience to new contexts, as well as improvisation of equipment and materials (Figure 113-23).

Common certification programs include courses that add the wilderness medical skill set to urban EMT certification and advanced life support courses. The specific course and certification vary by provider. These courses typically range from 24 to 48 hours and carry a commensurate number of continuing education hours. Certification lasts 2 to 3 years. The courses are commonly classroom based, but may include outdoor experiences and perhaps an extended rescue experience. They provide a solid foundation for health care professionals looking to expand their sphere of practice, become involved with a local outdoor organization, or join a search and rescue team (Figure 113-24).

For individuals seeking deeper learning in wilderness medicine, there are more extended education programs. The WMS offers the Fellowship of the Academy of Wilderness Medicine. Successful completion of the education and experience requirements allows the WMS member to use the designation of FAWM to indicate this accomplishment.[118] The internationally recognized Diploma in Mountain Medicine includes intensive skills training focusing on the care of patients in technical mountain terrain.

MEDICAL SCHOOL, RESIDENCY, AND FELLOWSHIP OFFERINGS

Wilderness medicine training is gaining prominence within traditional medical education venues. Although it is historically closely aligned with emergency medicine, it can also be found as a component of family medicine, military medicine, and

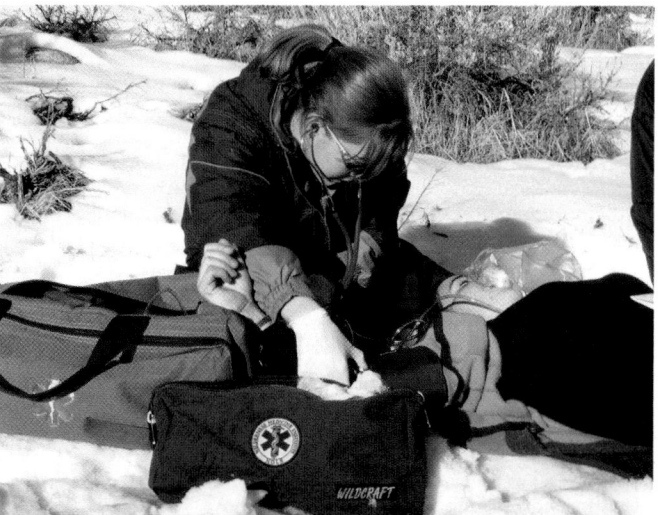

FIGURE 113-24 Specialty training courses help urban prehospital care providers adapt their knowledge to wilderness and austere environments. *(Courtesy Gates Richards.)*

BOX 113-10 Universities and Other Organizations Offering Electives in Wilderness Medicine for Medical Students

Belize Institute for Tropical and Wilderness Medicine	medschool.umaryland.edu/osr/training-belize.asp
Brown University	brown.edu/academics/medical/education/preclinical-electives/biol-6652
Cornell Medical College	cornellwm.org/
George Washington University	gwu.edu
Johns Hopkins University	hopkinsmedicine.org/emergencymedicine/residency/wilderness_medicine.html
Maine Medical Center	wildernessmedicineelective.com/
Marshall University	jcesom.marshall.edu/residents-fellows/programs/family-medicine/wilderness-medicine
NOLS and Harvard Affiliated Emergency Medicine Residency	nols.edu/wmi/courses/medicineinthewild.shtml
Saint Louis University	slu.edu/medicine/surgery/division-of-emergency-medicine/emergency-medicine -student-resources/medical-student-rotations
University of Arizona	medicine.arizona.edu/node/18288/wild-new-wilderness-medicine-program-ua-hones -patient-care-skills-austere-conditions/wild
University of California San Francisco, Fresno	fresno.ucsf.edu/undergrad/wilderness_medicine.html
University of Colorado	coloradowm.org/
University of Iowa	uiowa.edu/
University of Michigan	medicine.umich.edu/dept/emergency-medicine/education/other-programs/austere -environment-medicine
University of Nevada Las Vegas	medicine.nevada.edu/ome/electivesl; lasvegasemr.com/wilderness-medicine.html
University of New Mexico	unmmountainmed.com
University of South Alabama College of Medicine: Longleaf Wilderness Medicine	longleafmedical.com/medical-electives.html
University of South Carolina	emergencyresident.com/info_wilderness_medicine.php
University of Utah	awlsmedstudents.org/studentelective.html
University of Virginia	med.virginia.edu/emergency-medicine/education/medical-student-education/ wilderness-medicine
Wilderness Medical Associates, Canada	wildmed.com/wilderness-medical-courses/medical-professionals/wilderness-medical -elective
Wilderness Medical Society	wms.org/conferences/

disaster medicine. Wilderness medicine courses in medical schools and residencies have typically been formed by the efforts of an individual faculty member or students with personal interest in the topic. Until recently, little support existed for content consistency. However, within the past few years, there have been focused efforts to define core and elective topics for both student and resident electives and postresidency fellowships.

In 2014, there were at least 26 wilderness medicine electives for medical students and 12 for residents, more than three times the number in 2005. These electives typically last from 2 to 4 weeks and blend classroom learning with a wilderness experience. The emphasis of a given elective often closely parallels the interests of its medical director. Introduction of a wilderness experience creates an opportunity for instruction in general outdoor skills and preparedness. The results of an effort to achieve a consensus regarding core and elective elements was published in 2014.[61] Although this paper is largely based on expert opinion, it may help standardize the elective content for future programs. The growth of medical school electives in the past decade lends support to the notion that medical students value opportunities for education outside their traditional study topics. Wilderness experiential outings used as socialization events for an introduction to medical school further support the value of wilderness medicine education (Boxes 113-10 and 113-11).

More formalized effort is being put into standardizing content and recruitment and application processes for 1-year wilderness medicine fellowships. There exist at least 14 such fellowships, with more being developed. The American College of Emergency Physicians Wilderness Medicine Section established a task force to develop standardized content and a core curriculum for these fellowships and published the results of their 4-year project in 2014[69] (Box 113-12).

Beyond elective and fellowship opportunities, less formal structures exist for medical students and others to explore their interests. The WMS lists nearly 50 student interest groups on their website.[107] The Medical Wilderness Adventure Race (MedWAR; see Chapter 114) blends wilderness medicine skills with adventure-style racing and hosts events across the United States.[79] In addition, medical students can access the widely available certification training programs mentioned above.

CONTINUING MEDICAL EDUCATION CONFERENCES AND TRAVEL

An Internet search for wilderness medicine continuing medical education (CME) produces hundreds of results. The ability to combine required educational experiences with new and interesting content or possibly adventure travel draws professionals

BOX 113-11 Universities and Other Organizations Offering Electives in Wilderness Medicine for Residents

Belize Institute for Tropical and Wilderness Medicine	medschool.umaryland.edu/osr/training-belize.asp
Central Maine Medical Center	cmcfmrp.org/wimp-curriculum
Cornell Medical College	cornellwm.org/
George Washington University	gwu.edu
Johns Hopkins University	hopkinsmedicine.org/emergencymedicine/residency/wilderness_medicine.html
University of California San Francisco, Fresno	fresno.ucsf.edu/em/parkmedic/
University of Montana Wilderness Institute and Aerie School of Backcountry Medicine	umt.edu/wi/education
University of South Carolina	emergencyresident.com/info_wilderness_medicine.php

BOX 113-12   Universities and Other Organizations Offering Fellowships in Wilderness Medicine

Baystate Medical Center Wilderness Medicine Fellowship — baystatehealth.org/education-research/education/fellowships/wilderness-medicine

Eastern Virginia Medical School International and Wilderness Medicine Fellowship — evms.edu/education/centers_institutes_departments/emergency_medicine/fellowships/international_wilderness/

George Washington University Fellowship in Extreme Environmental Medicine — smhs.gwu.edu/emed/education-training/fellowships/environmental

Madigan Army Medical Center Austere and Wilderness Medicine Fellowship (Department of Defense only) — mamc.amedd.army.mil/education/graduate-medical-education/fellowships/austere-and-wilderness-medicine.aspx

Massachusetts General Hospital Wilderness Medicine Fellowship — massgeneral.org/education/fellowship.aspx?id=94

Medical College of Georgia at Augusta University Wilderness Medicine Fellowship — augusta.edu/mcg/em/ed/fellowships/wilderness/fellowship

Stanford University Wilderness Medicine Fellowship — emed.stanford.edu/specialized-programs/wilderness-medicine/fellowship/.html

State University of New York Upstate Medical University Wilderness and Expedition Medicine Fellowship — upstate.edu/emergency/education/fellowships/wilderness.php

University of California San Diego Wilderness Medicine Fellowship — healthsciences.ucsd.edu/som/emergency-med/education/fellowships/wilderness-medicine/Pages/default.aspx

University of California San Francisco, Fresno, Wilderness Medicine Fellowship — fresno.ucsf.edu/em/wilderness/

University of Colorado Wilderness Medicine Fellowship — coloradowm.org/

University of New Mexico Wilderness Medicine Fellowship — unmmountainmed.com

University of Utah Wilderness Medicine Fellowship — medicine.utah.edu/surgery/emergency_medicine/fellowships/wilderness_medicine

Yale School of Medicine Wilderness Medicine Fellowship — medicine.yale.edu/emergencymed/fellowships/

---

from many backgrounds. CME experiences provide an opportunity for individuals with similar interests to meet and engage. These experiences often draw well-known faculty with wilderness medicine research activities. The trend is for delivery of information through lectures or large-conference general sessions. Although this is a reasonable medium for conveying new knowledge and sharing research, it often lacks the opportunity for any form of practical application of the new material. Participants of CME events may still be ill-prepared to manage a situation that has been described to them but to which they have not been exposed in any tangible manner. Conference workshop sessions generally provide more opportunities for skills development, sometimes in a classroom, sometimes in the field. Participants should be encouraged to take advantage of these opportunities to develop confidence in functioning in remote environments.

Some CME programs include a travel component. This allows participants to practice skills in environments other than a classroom. The structure of these programs varies, with some offering day outings and others a more extended expedition experience. In either case, the participant is able to improve his or her wilderness travel knowledge in addition to gaining hands-on wilderness medicine experience.

REFERENCES

Complete references used in this text are available online at expertconsult.inkling.com.

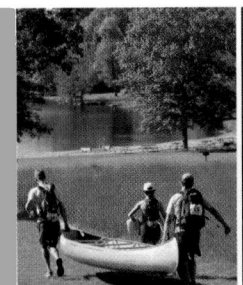

CHAPTER 114

MedWAR: Medical Wilderness Adventure Race

MICHAEL J. CAUDELL, DAVID J. LEDRICK, AND HILLARY R. IRONS

Simulations and scenarios are widely used for teaching in many professions, including wilderness medicine.[9] The last 10 years have seen a significant increase in the use of simulation, which has become an established part of graduate medical education. There is a growing body of literature on how best to use simulation equipment and instructional methods.[18,22,28,31,38] Simulation-based curricula have been developed to teach specific clinical skills, such as performing procedures, using teamwork, and making decisions, at all levels of medical training. Many resi-

dency programs have incorporated simulation as a formal part of a curriculum,[1,3,6,7,20,25,34,39] including educational programs for rural and wilderness medicine.[11,13,21,24,30] Both low-cost medical models[13,21,30] and highly realistic simulations[11] have been used for outdoor procedural skills and structured outdoor class settings such as advanced wilderness life support classes[11] and even the challenging and restricted space of an in-flight helicopter.[40]

Adventure racing, or the incorporation of multiple endurance disciplines into a single event, has roots that extend as far back

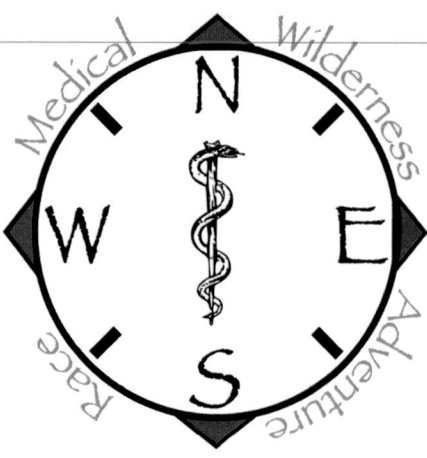

FIGURE 114-1 The MedWAR logo. *(Courtesy NAEAR and MedWAR.)*

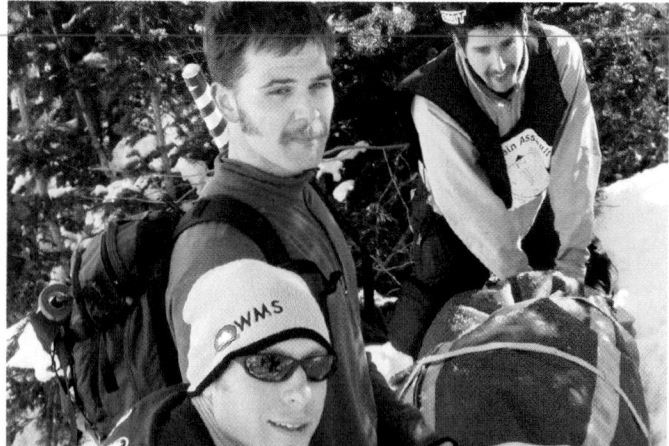

FIGURE 114-2 MedWAR Utah. *(Courtesy NAEAR and MedWAR.)*

as the Karrimor International Mountain Marathon in 1968. The Raid Gauloises was established in 1989 and is considered one of the first modern adventure races. The 1990s were a time of great expansion for adventure racing; the well-known Eco-challenge, produced in 1995, brought adventure racing to a wider audience and inspired other planners to establish races across the country. Adventure race distances range from shorter 2- to 6-hour events (sprint distance) to longer, 3- to 11-day events (expedition distance).[21] In 1998, the United States Adventure Racing Association (USARA) was founded to support the growing sport. Around this time, a number of faculty members from the Medical College of Georgia emergency medicine residency program took up the sport and provided inspiration for the Medical Wilderness Adventure Race (MedWAR) (Figure 114-1).

MedWAR MISSION STATEMENT

MedWAR combines wilderness medicine with adventure racing to teach and test wilderness medicine and survival skills (Box 114-1). Races are sprint distance events and typically cover 10 to 15 miles by foot, bike, boat, or skis. Teams may have three or four members, depending on the race, and may be composed of any combination of health care professionals, emergency personnel, students, and outdoor enthusiasts (Figure 114-2). There are no minimal knowledge or skill requirements and no divisions based on age, gender, or medical skill level. Teams must be self-sufficient and carry their own food and water throughout the race. They must also carry safety equipment and a medical kit. Part of the MedWAR challenge is deciding what to pack in the team's medical kit, just as would occur for an actual wilderness expedition.

THE HISTORY OF MedWAR

The first MedWAR was conceived in the fall of 2000, a few days after the founders competed in their first sprint distance adventure race. The idea became action when a group of medical students seeking a research project approached the Medical College of Georgia faculty and were offered the opportunity to help organize the inaugural event. In April 2001, 22 teams from eight states, along with teams from Canada and visiting students from Australia, spent the day learning wilderness medicine at

Wildwood Park near Augusta, Georgia. The original event included several hours of instruction, beginning in the morning. With no time limit, the last finishing teams struggled in at 2:00 AM the following morning. The event has been held in Georgia every spring since, although it has been relocated to a more rugged environment at Fort Gordon. In October 2002, the first event outside Georgia occurred at the Pinckney Recreation Area outside Ann Arbor, Michigan (Figure 114-3).

MedWAR caught on quickly. Many groups of motivated racers sought to bring the race closer to their homes. The first expansion race beyond the original Southeast Race in Georgia and the Midwest Race in Michigan was MedWAR North in Ontario, Canada, in 2003. MedWAR North was unique because it was the first winter race and included Nordic skiing, snowshoeing, and winter mountain biking. During its first year, the race was piggybacked onto a local adventure race, but soon thereafter MedWAR North broke away and held independent events. The MedWAR North racers take advantage of their winter setting by using scenarios with fallen ice climbers and victims of hypothermia, frostbite, and cold-water drowning. Displaying theatrical blood on snow makes for an impressive scene (Figure 114-4).

MedWAR North was the first race organized without the direct involvement of original Medical College of Georgia faculty members. The student organizers worked with the directors of the previous races, who offered advice on logistics, helped vet the scenarios, and assisted in writing questions. The students staged a successful and well-run event. The process, however, made it evident that a more formal mechanism should exist to assist future event organizers, coordinate race schedules, and advertise to participants.

BOX 114-1   MedWAR Mission Statement

To provide medical students, residents, health care professionals, and wilderness enthusiasts with a practical, interactive, and enjoyable curriculum for learning, applying, and evaluating emergency medical knowledge, skills, and techniques in a wilderness setting.

From MedWAR: medwar.org/mission.htm.

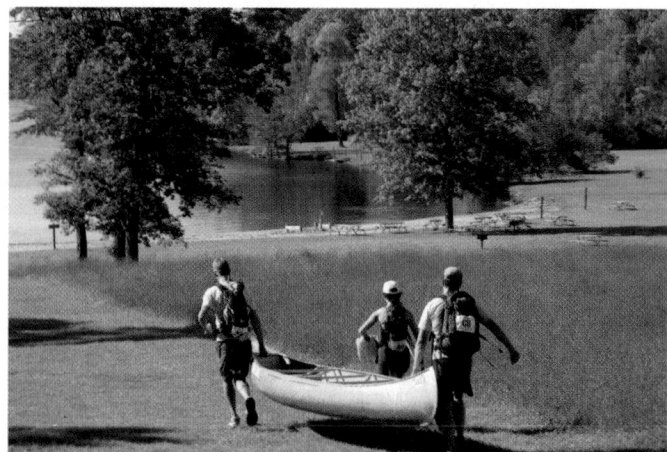

FIGURE 114-3 Midwest MedWAR in Pinkney, Michigan. Teamwork in action. *(Courtesy NAEAR and MedWAR.)*

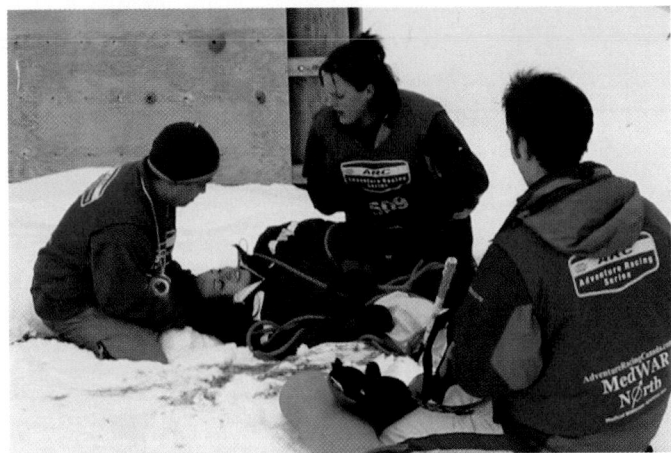

FIGURE 114-4 MedWAR North: a great moulage example. *(Courtesy NAEAR and MedWAR.)*

The first several MedWAR events were sanctioned by USARA, which helped with publicity and event insurance. It became clear that the educational mission of MedWAR meant it occupied a very small niche within USARA. In response, the organization North American Educational Adventure Racing (NAEAR) was created in 2003 to ensure that an event's educational focus would be upheld, regardless of the event format. In an effort to remain consistent, the published curriculum of potential medical issues for all events is the same, although different venues naturally lend themselves to different components. Through formation of a central organization, NAEAR has prevented competition among races in the same region, acted as a resource in writing and maintaining a question bank, and provided faculty oversight for the medical scenarios. NAEAR also offers advice on race organization and logistics and maintains a website for publicity and communication.

The Mid-Atlantic MedWAR began in spring 2006 in Virginia. The first race was held at Fort A.P. Hill with a course that heavily emphasized orienteering. The race has since been moved to Newport News Park, and the course has been changed to a multiloop one. It is now the third largest race held each year, with 35 to 40 teams.

The Northeast MedWAR was held in upstate New York for several years beginning in 2006; however, the original race organizers moved on, and so the race eventually lost support in the area.

MedWAR Utah came onto the scene in 2009 as the first global positioning system–based race. The race takes advantage of the altitude in Park City to simulate high-altitude illnesses and mountaineering injuries. An avalanche beacon is usually buried somewhere along the course.

In fall 2009, MedWAR Tennessee held its first race; races have opened in Pennsylvania and Southern California. Additional expansion races are in planning stages (Box 114-2).

BOX 114-2   Starting an Expansion Race

The rewards of starting a race are great, but it is not without a substantial amount of effort. New races are usually started by groups of interested medical students, residents, fellows, or attending physicians who have previously participated in an established race. Planning a new race takes approximately a year and requires a dedicated group of three to five core race directors and a pool of potential volunteers and racers. They are typically associated with a medical school or residency program, which brings in new ideas and new volunteers with each new class. If you are interested in starting a MedWAR expansion race, you can contact the sanctioning organization North American Educational Adventure Racing at naear@medwar.org.

THE MedWAR MODEL: HOW IT WORKS

MedWAR is an outdoor wilderness event; everything related to a MedWAR weekend pivots around this idea. MedWAR events are held around North America in all seasons; this means that every venue has a particular focus and feel, from the snowy north to the swamps of the southeast. The Midwest event is timed around the autumn changing of leaves, whereas the Utah event coincides with the Wilderness Medical Society's annual winter conference. The outdoor environment dictates everything from how the race will be planned to how competitors will need to prepare. Built-in safety margins and adaptability are crucial to MedWAR event planning; for example, at one venue, the temperature may be much colder and the water levels lower from year to year, and trails may need to be rerouted.

MedWAR is intended to be a safe event that allows each participant to step outside his or her level of comfort; however, it is not without risk. Line 1 of the liability waiver states "the only way to make this event entirely safe is to cancel it." For many competitors, MedWAR is an introduction to wilderness medicine and very often their first adventure race. Competitors are expected to prepare on their own for both the medical challenges and the time spent in the wilderness setting. The nature of adventure racing requires that teams be self-supported; therefore, they must carry adequate food and water for the duration of the event. Depending on the venue, racers may be out of sight of the competition and race staff for hours at a time, in a setting where it is possible to become lost. Race organizers, therefore, should inform competitors about the venue and how to communicate with the teams. Teams need to carry specific gear that would sustain them in the wilderness environment for a period of 24 hours in the event they were significantly delayed on the course. Mandatory gear for MedWAR typically includes a map and compass, a change of clothing, fire starting material, a space blanket, a light source, a whistle, and a water disinfection method. MedWAR courses must be planned with the novice in mind; directions must be more specific than might be the case in a typical adventure race and the trails and waterways used might need to be better established.

Learners at a MedWAR event receive little direct instruction prior to the race. Aside from course briefings and a basic review of water detoxification methods for safety reasons, participants learn through experience and self-preparation. The curriculum is published online prior to the event, and participants are asked to prepare for any of the challenges listed (Table 114-1). Learners are encouraged to carry and use references during the race. The intent of a MedWAR event is to offer competitors a chance to experiment, improvise, and apply principles that they have already learned.

Throughout the MedWAR event, teams encounter simulated wilderness medical emergencies. A team's response to a medical challenge is assessed through demonstration of specific criteria judged by experts to be "critical" to the management of a problem. The race presents several scenarios commonly seen in wilderness settings, and participants are asked to demonstrate their ability to recognize and manage a problem within a range of acceptable alternatives. Each team is allowed to have a unique solution, so long as it follows appropriate principles. In some cases critical actions must be performed in a specific order to be acceptable, such as ensuring scene safety prior to attempting rescue, or checking the neurovascular status of a limb before and after splinting. Some criteria must be met within a specific time to be considered complete, such as securing an airway within minutes of arrival on scene. Each scenario has its educational objectives built into the critical actions. The challenge of managing an unconscious patient who fell while crossing a stream may require that participants assess a scene for safety, perform an initial assessment, including airway and cervical spine protection, and then get the patient safely out of the water (Figure 114-5). There are multiple ways to accomplish each of these tasks, but the focus is on following management principles and demonstrating results. Task penalties are incurred for each missed critical action, thereby providing immediate educational feedback for

TABLE 114-1 MedWAR Curriculum

Type of Management	Specific Conditions Addressed
Musculoskeletal injury management	Strains and sprains
	Dislocations
	Fractures: splinting, traction
Soft tissue wound management	Lacerations
	Burns
	Punctures: with and without embedded objects
	Blisters
	Infection
	Frostbite or extremity immersion
	Animal bites
	Insect bites and stings
	Fishhook removal
Exposure injury and condition management	Hypothermia: full-body immersion
	Hyperthermia and heat stroke
	Altitude or mountain sickness
	Dehydration
	Hazardous materials exposure
	Poisonings
	Injections (animals, insects)
	Ingestions (foods, plants, liquids)
	Contaminated water or water disinfection
	Food or electrolyte deprivation
	Lightning and other weather conditions
	Drowning and river safety
	Fire issues: smoke inhalation, fire safety
	Avalanche safety and burial or rescue
	Crevasse extrication
Systemic injury and condition management	Shock
	Respiratory conditions and respiratory arrest (CPR)
	Cardiovascular conditions and cardiac arrest (CPR)
	Neurologic injuries and conditions
	Preexisting medical conditions (e.g., diabetes, sickle cell anemia)
	Diarrhea and fluid loss
General issues	Basic search and rescue
	Ethical issues in wilderness medicine
	Legal issues in wilderness medicine
	Scene assessment skills: multiple patients (wilderness triage)
	Patient assessment skills: multiple injuries
	Pediatric issues in wilderness medicine
	Orienteering
	Medical kit planning
	Expedition gear planning
	Communication issues
	Transition-to-hospital issues

From MedWAR: medwar.org/curriculum.htm.

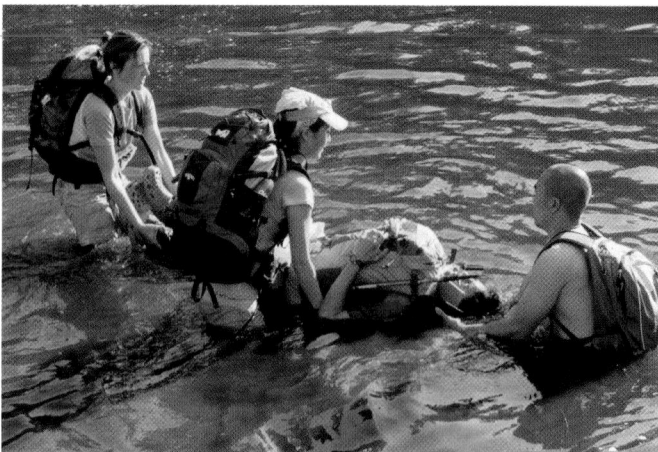

FIGURE 114-5 Southeast MedWAR: managing a cervical spine injury while safely moving a patient. *(Courtesy NAEAR and MedWAR.)*

climbing harnesses, may be provided by the race organizers. Teams might have to "earn" equipment by performing well in a scenario or providing a correct answer to a medical question. For instance, a syringe of "epinephrine" may be earned early in the race to be used later in an anaphylaxis scenario.

MedWAR is a competitive event, so the atmosphere at the starting and finishing lines is that of a race. However, its primary purpose, and what sets it apart from other races, is the goal of wilderness medicine education. Knowledge and competence are rewarded over speed. Using specific criteria grading supports an educational focus at each scenario. Failure to meet these criteria typically results in the team immediately performing a penalty on site, which serves the dual purpose of slowing the team down and reviewing the missed management principle. Time lost by performing a penalty is generally enough that a team moving slowly and using reference material will do better than a careless team that does not fully solve the problem. Performance bonuses are more difficult to execute at the practical stations due to difficulties with interrater reliability and the complexity of identifying multiple layers of management, but time bonuses may be earned by answering test questions. Questions worded in a typical board examination style, printed and laminated, are sometimes set on trees or stakes to mark the course, thus keeping competitors moving along the same path (Figure 114-6). In some instances, exhibits are used (Figure 114-7). Questions with passwords are also used as orienteering checkpoints or as optional time bonus points to extend the race for high-performing teams and to add a level of team strategy. At a typical MedWAR event,

participants' performances, a crucial portion of the education that participants gain during MedWAR. Well-trained volunteers are necessary to proctor multiple teams while maintaining the "race pace" atmosphere. Although the medical scenarios are simulated, it is necessary to create a believable scene that can be easily established and maintained by volunteers. Besides the cost of props, important considerations include the ability to transport equipment to scenario locations, having enough volunteers to staff scenarios, and having "victims" who agree to wear moulage. It is often more efficient and realistic to "injure" a team member than to have a volunteer actor. Most equipment is carried by teams as part of their required gear and medical kits. However, some safety equipment, such as personal flotation devices or

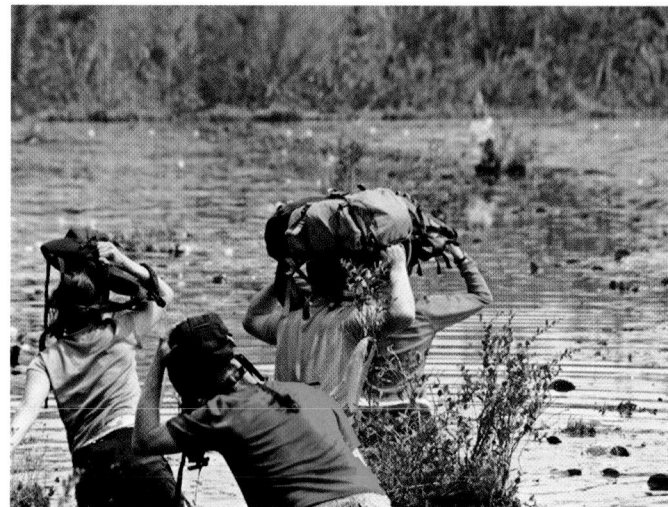

FIGURE 114-6 Southeast MedWAR: didactic questions keep racers on course. *(Courtesy NAEAR and MedWAR.)*

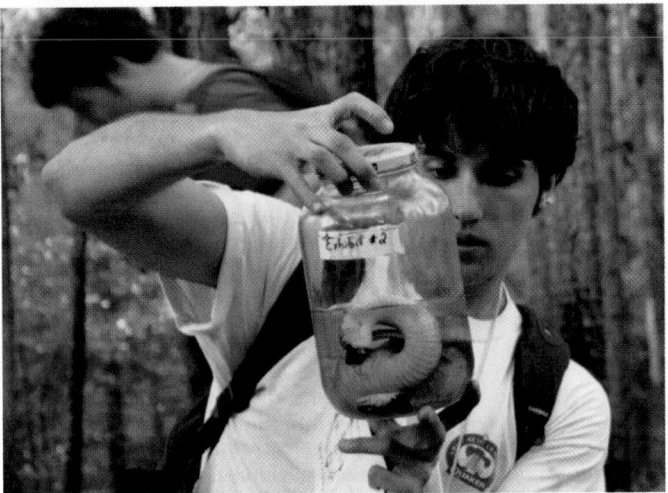

FIGURE 114-7 Snake identification at Southeast MedWAR: venomous or nonvenomous? *(Courtesy NAEAR and MedWAR.)*

each team moves along the course alone, usually out of sight of the other teams, with the winner unknown until all teams have finished and all didactic bonuses or penalties been tallied.

MedWAR planners have tried to make each event accessible to anyone willing to make the effort to participate. Anecdotally, MedWAR competitors tend to be medical students or residents with a better-than-average fitness level. Race directors have the challenge of creating an event difficult enough to be physically demanding for top competitors but within reach of novices. The Mid-Atlantic race has used two distinct courses to address this issue. Another difficulty in course design is creating a land navigation course for competitors with a wide range of experience in orienteering. Incorporating ropes or water challenges further tests the abilities of competitors and complicates event planning, but also significantly enriches the experience (Figure 114-8). When challenges requiring special skill, strength, balance, or tolerance of heights are incorporated, it is important that competitors are given an opportunity to complete the task with expert instruction and supervision, or to offer them an alternative challenge. On average, a top team can complete a well-planned course in half the time of a last-place team. A common way to extend the race for more competitive participants is to give them optional sections to complete for time bonuses. This section is usually a difficult orienteering challenge in which the team earns greater rewards according to the number of checkpoints they

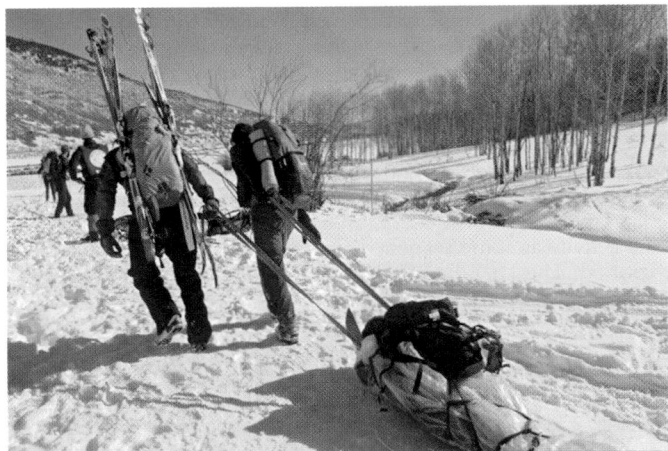

FIGURE 114-8 Southeast MedWAR: incorporating physical challenges enhances the race experience. *(Courtesy NAEAR and MedWAR.)*

visit. It is sometimes also necessary to reroute slower teams during the race for safety reasons due to time constraints.

The competition of a race environment enhances the educational value of a MedWAR event. This competitive aspect lends a sense of urgency similar to that of the stress of a survival situation with consequences for mistakes that make a difference in race outcome. Missing critical actions during a scenario may cause a significant delay or time penalty, and navigation errors may make the difference between finishing on the podium or in the middle of the pack. The place order of finishing gives competitors some measure of comparison with their peers. It also provides a forum for residents to challenge their attending physicians or wilderness medicine clubs from different schools.

There are many logistics challenges in creating a competitive event that sometimes involves upward of 100 participants. Planning the race begins with scouting the appropriate venue and creating a course that is challenging but also negotiable for most participants. Medical scenarios must be situated in areas accessible to volunteers and allow for transport of props and equipment. Rental of portable toilets and generators is sometimes necessary. Further problems include validating the medical scenarios and questions; obtaining permission to use land; securing race insurance; and having ready maps of the area, race T-shirts, and food for competitors and volunteers. Rental of boats, bikes, or ski equipment must be considered. On race day, competitors must be registered, have gear checked, receive race-specific instructions, be tracked on the course, be ushered through challenges without bottlenecks, be accounted for at the end of the race, and have their results accurately scored. After the race, the area needs to be cleaned, gear returned, results posted, and accounting done. In general, planning and executing a race is a 6- to 12-month process.

MedWAR RESEARCH

Although participating students sometimes view MedWAR as a competitive outdoor event with whimsical scenarios and dubious story lines, there has been an effort to maintain a high level of academic integrity in teaching wilderness medicine principles. There is validated research showing the educational value of simulation education. Several subsequent studies indicate that the scenario-based approach used by MedWAR has become an integral part of standard medical education.[1,3,6,7,20,25,34,39]

Initial publications were concept papers outlining the purpose and practicality of MedWAR.[12,14,17] Within 3 years of the first event, several hundred competitors, primarily medical students and residents from midwestern and southeastern U.S. states, had participated at a number of different venues. Each race maintained rigorous academic standards, realistic scenarios, and grading criteria that rewarded appropriate medical practice over speed. Although the agenda was not mandated, races tried to incorporate consistent lessons: a triage or mass casualty scenario, an airway problem, splinting, patient carry, wound care, and general wilderness survival skills. Didactic material was covered either by a written examination or questions posted throughout the race, allowing competitors to use whatever resources they carried, again rewarding a correct over a fast response (Figure 114-9).

While MedWAR was being refined, there was a push within medical education to emphasize simulation-based teaching as an effective way to educate students and residents. MedWAR is a simulation event that gives practitioners an opportunity to practice wilderness medicine skills in a safe environment. One commonly tested skill is the ability to obtain a surgical airway. A typical scenario requires a team to demonstrate noninvasive techniques first and then have the condition of the airway degenerate into a surgical emergency. This situation is an example of how a cost-effective model can be used to evaluate 30 to 40 teams (management instances) within a 2-hour period during a race. A model was created using styrofoam mannequin heads and tubing, materials easily obtained in a hardware store, and foam tape and ketchup packets (Figure 114-10). Based on the consensus opinion of experienced practitioners, this provided a convincing look and feel that were adequate for novice training.

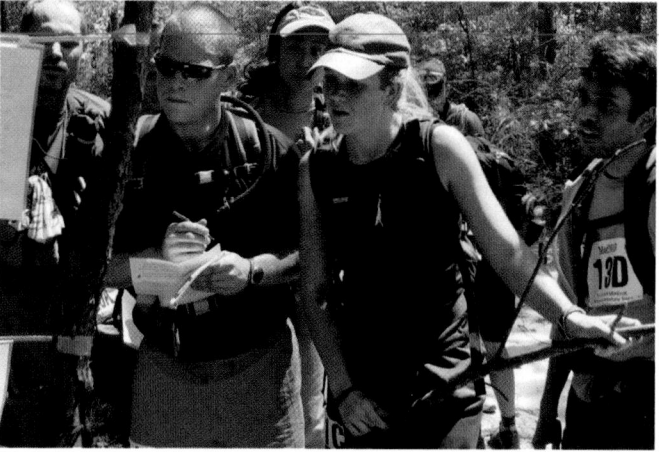

FIGURE 114-9 A correct response is more important than an erroneous fast response. *(Courtesy NAEAR and MedWAR.)*

The setup cost was $4.60, and the materials could be reused for approximately $0.65 per use.[2,13]

Based on formal participant feedback from surveys following multiple events, MedWAR was perceived as enjoyable and having educational value. In 2010, objective evidence was collected showing that participation improved medical performance and increased didactic knowledge. In one study, participants took a written test before and after the event.[16] Questions covered basic wilderness medicine topics; examination scores showed statisti-

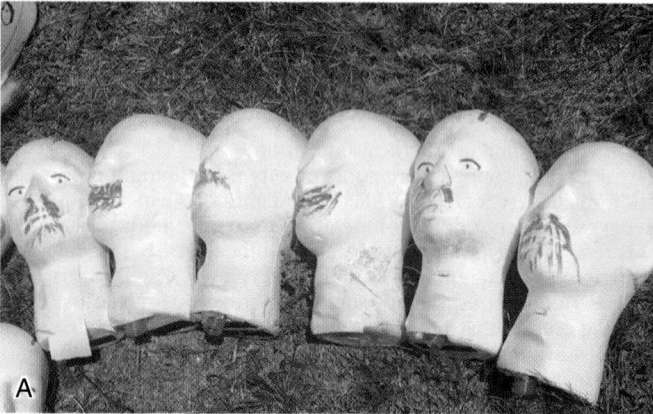

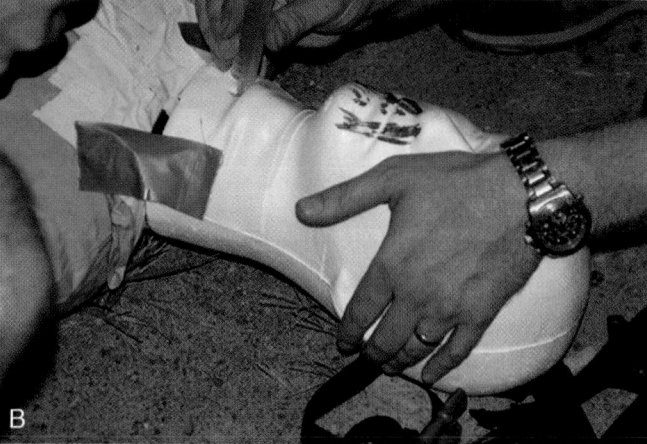

FIGURE 114-10 A and **B**, Midwest MedWAR: The clone army is an inexpensive reusable model for a surgical airway. *(Courtesy NAEAR and MedWAR.)*

cally significant improvement after the event, although pretest scores were high. A result more relevant to actual practice was demonstrated when participants were tested clinically.[24] A clinical scenario was created to test basic principles reinforced during a typical MedWAR event. The scenario contained 10 items considered to be critical actions, some of which had to be performed within a specified time to be considered complete. Actions were scored as "performed" or "not performed," and the scenario was timed from beginning to completion. A total of 34 teams were tested before the MedWAR event, and 31 teams completed a test after the event. The groups' pretest score was 71% of critical actions met (95% confidence interval [CI], 67.5% to 74.4%), and posttest score was 89.7% of critical actions met (95% CI, 86% to 93.3%). Mean improvement in postrace scenarios was 18.7% (n=31, 95% CI, 12.1% to 25.3%), with a significant paired two-tailed t-test (p < 0.001), showing that the race experience was effective in improving the number of postrace critical actions met.

As a form of standardized medical simulation, MedWAR events create an ideal setting to test an educational intervention. In 2012, two race organizers who were registered diagnostic medical sonographers wanted to evaluate novice providers' ability to learn from a brief on-line tutorial.[15] Few studies have examined the use of ultrasound (US) images to assist providers in making decisions about treatment and evacuation in wilderness settings. Participants in the 2012 Midwest MedWAR were asked to watch an on-line tutorial prior to the event. All participants received a unique log-in to allow accurate tracking of who watched the video. During the event, one medical challenge was presentation of US images of conditions that might be found in an austere setting and require interpretation. Of 72 study participants, 43 watched the training videos. Physicians (attending and resident) were significantly more likely to identify intraperitoneal fluid (89%) than were nonphysicians (64%), but the physician performance was not improved by watching the videos (89% vs 90%). Among the nonphysicians, those who watched the videos were significantly better at identifying intraperitoneal fluid (76% vs 47%). The results for identifying pneumothorax were similar but did not reach statistical significance. These findings suggest that for novice providers, an on-line training program followed by simulation testing provides a reasonable format for learning to interpret US images.

In 2012, the economic impact of a MedWAR event was assessed.[26] The demographics of MedWAR participants are more similar to those of a typically younger adventure race audience than to those of older, often better-funded physicians with a continuing medical education allowance. This economic study had value in estimating the impact of an event designed primarily for students. A survey of all volunteers and participants at the 2012 Midwest MedWAR was administered using questions modeled after a similar study. Most participants (44%) were receiving student loans; 39% had an annual income of between $20,000 and $60,000, with six participants reporting an income of over $80,000 annually. Participants traveled an average of 4.5 hours one way to come to the event, and 52 (58%) spent at least one night away from home, with nearly all camping in the host state park. Participants spent an average of $135 (range $20 to $385) on travel, food, and equipment independent of race entry fees and canoe rental. The registration cost was $135 per team of three. Each team was required to rent a canoe at a cost of $45. The estimated amount spent by a single participant on this event was $195, for a total of $20,475 for all 105 competitors. A dollar spent in a local economy translates into several dollars of total activity as some is spent, some saved, some taxed, and some exported. The spending multiplier formula is stated as

$$1/[\{1 - mpc * (1 - t)\} + mpm]$$

where *mpc* is the marginal propensity to consume, *t* is the income tax rate, and *mpm* is the marginal propensity to import. The local chamber of commerce placed the spending multiplier between 1.8 and 2.5 for this region, meaning that medical students, carpooling for half a day each way and camping during an adventure race, generated between $36,855 and $51,187 of economic benefit to the midwest region in this single weekend.

SIMULATIONS, SCENARIOS, AND EDUCATION IN MedWAR

Simulation-based curriculum studies have shown measurable benefits.[29] In a study by Ten Eyck, participating students demonstrated improvement in learning and greater satisfaction with a simulation-based curriculum than with group discussion.[35] Simulation has been shown to improve students' ability to manage medical emergencies[4] and demonstrate competence in procedural skills and theoretical knowledge.[10,32] Although a study by Lo and associates revealed no difference in performance of advanced cardiac life support after a 1-year interval, students demonstrated greater knowledge initially using highly realistic simulation training compared with traditional training, and student satisfaction was higher when highly realistic training was used.[19]

Staging a good simulation requires setting the scene, choosing actors, applying makeup or moulage, and undertaking an appropriate evaluation after the simulation.[5] Most scenes in MedWAR are realistic because events are held in austere environments (Figure 114-11). Some details are occasionally stipulated, including the altitude, environmental conditions, distance from help, and availability of communication.

Teamwork is an integral part of medicine, regardless of the setting. Use of scenarios for drills and training in multiple and various settings are widespread. Simulation and scenarios have been used to evaluate and improve team performance in health care.[27,33,37] When scenarios require active student participation, group dynamics play a prominent role. Scenario-based education is easier if group members know each other. For example, search and rescue teams of long-standing membership or firefighting teams that run drills, work, and live together usually function well in their team roles. In a wilderness medicine setting, group dynamics form and evolve while people are on an expedition or trek. In a wilderness medicine *education* setting, participants often do not know one another, in which case the group must grow and develop. In 1965, Bruce Tuckman proposed the following model of group development.[36]

- FORMING: Limited interactions between individuals due to a need for acceptance and fear of conflict.
- STORMING: Different individual ideas are presented and compete. Leaders begin to emerge.
- NORMING: Team begins to come together and work as a team.
- PERFORMING: This stage describes high-performance teams; they do not require external supervision.

MedWAR planners address the issues of group dynamics by formation of self-selected teams prior to an event, which usually places them at least into the "norming" stage of development,

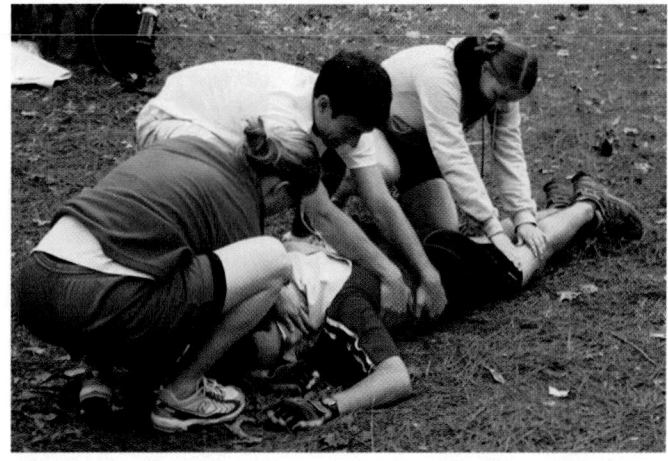

FIGURE 114-12 Group dynamics and teamwork are accelerated and solidified. *(Courtesy NAEAR and MedWAR.)*

and allows participants to focus on the tasks at hand rather than group dynamics and individual performances (Figure 114-12). The effectiveness of MedWAR simulations and scenarios may be enhanced by this preselection. The self-selection may allow a team member who is going to play a victim to let go of inhibitions and become a better actor.

Makeup and moulage may be difficult to provide when there are large numbers of race participants. However, many injuries and illnesses covered in the MedWAR curriculum (e.g., a fall with a head or cervical spine injury) do not require makeup. Efforts are made to make injuries look convincing, and appropriate props are also provided (Figure 114-13).

Medical equipment is an important part of the scenario performance. In MedWAR, each team is asked to bring the routine medical equipment they would take on an expedition to care for themselves or team members. The goal is for participants to

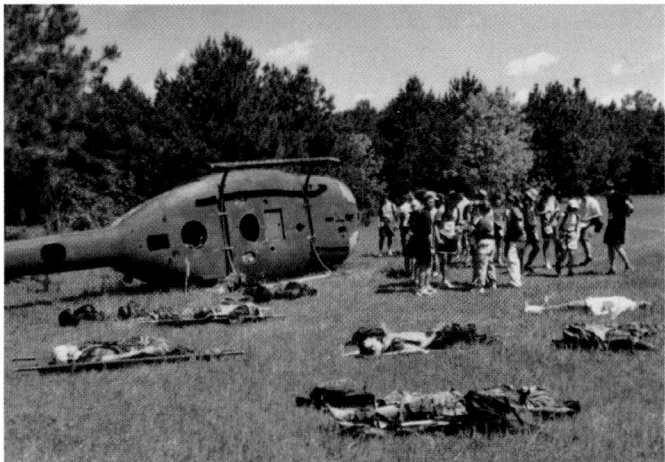

FIGURE 114-11 Southeast MedWAR: a simulated rescue helicopter crash. Participants had to care for the original patients that were being evacuated and then evaluate and treat victims of the simulated crash. *(Courtesy NAEAR and MedWAR.)*

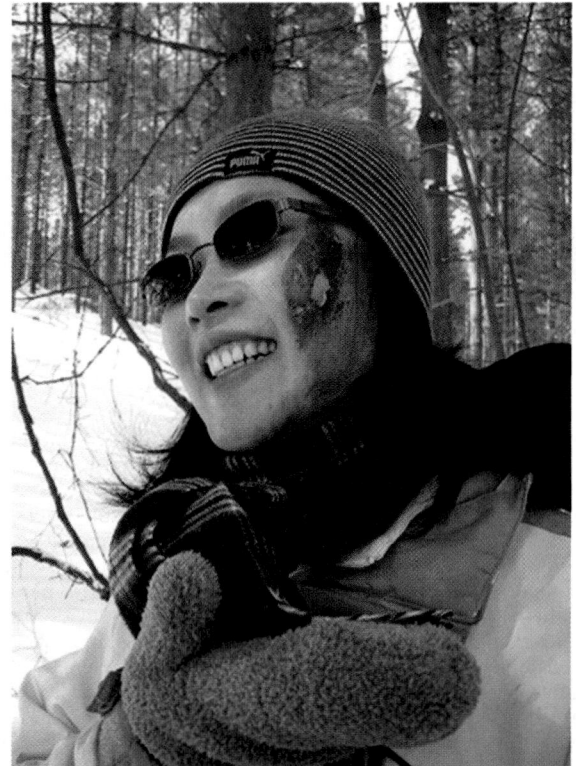

FIGURE 114-13 MedWAR North: another example of excellent moulage. *(Courtesy NAEAR and MedWAR.)*

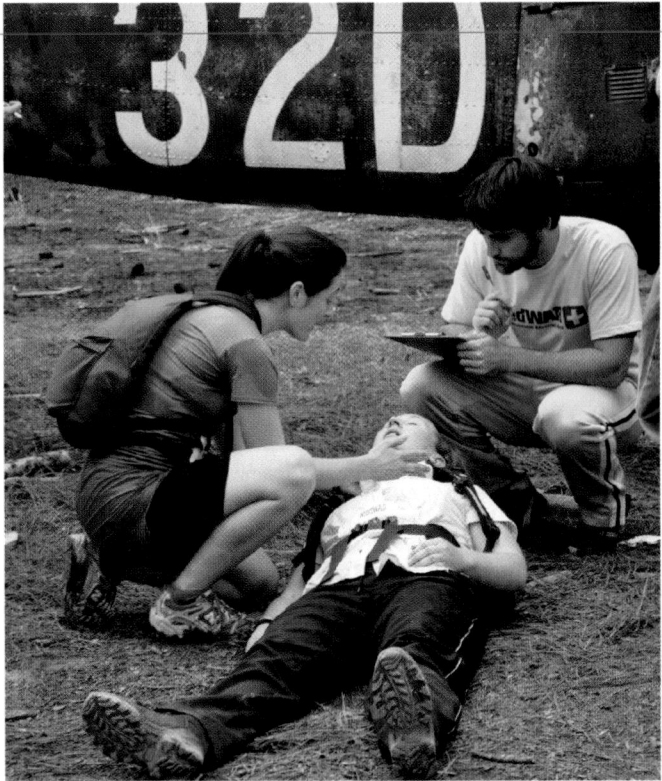

FIGURE 114-14 Southeast MedWAR: immediate feedback is given by well-trained proctors. *(Courtesy NAEAR and MedWAR.)*

noninvasive patient care action must be performed and not simply verbalized. Teams are expected to use the curriculum and anticipate what supplies they will need, thus providing their own material and equipment for each scenario. When possible, simulation equipment for invasive procedures is provided. Immediate feedback provides a memorable education event.

Stress is an important factor related to performance. Well-staged scenarios can be very stressful and emotionally powerful.[9] High-stress simulation training can help individuals learn to perform better in real-life stressful situations. Harvey and coworkers found that "in trainees, some aspects of performance and immediate recall appear to be impaired in complex clinical scenarios in which they exhibit elevated subjective and physiologic stress responses."[8] Highly realistic patient simulation produces significant stress. Müller and colleagues found that after 1 day of simulator training, the stress response as measured by salivary alpha-amylase was reduced. Clinical performance and nontechnical skills improved after 1 day of simulator training.[23] This intuitively correlates with many "inoculation" approaches to psychological stressors. The race aspect of MedWAR provides a sense of urgency similar to that of an urgent or emergent medical situation. The stress can be difficult to provide in other simulation settings where no time limitations or outside pressure exists.

CONCLUSION

MedWAR has been a highly successful program, incorporating wilderness medicine scenarios into an adventure race. This format provides a unique educational opportunity, accessible to many levels of health care providers and outdoor enthusiasts. MedWAR also provides a venue for innovative medical simulation models and for continuing medical education and simulation research.

learn to use the equipment they have, with some component of improvisation.

Using critical actions enables the MedWAR staff to provide quality evaluation and immediate feedback. Proctors are trained on how to evaluate each critical action (Figure 114-14). Each

REFERENCES

Complete references used in this text are available online at expertconsult.inkling.com.

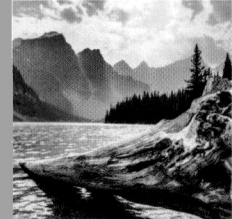

CHAPTER 115
Evidence-Based Wilderness Medicine

CHRISTOPHER R. CARPENTER AND BRENT E. RUOFF

In wilderness adventures, initial medical management must often be provided in austere settings that are quite unlike highly controlled research settings that occur in academic hospitals. Nonetheless, in order to optimize outcomes, medical providers who deliver health care in wilderness settings should be cognizant of contemporary research that best reflects the clinical scenarios they routinely confront in the wilderness. Wilderness medicine provides a unique compendium of knowledge as evidenced by an increasing number of publications addressing adventure-related illness or injury, ongoing research, and distinct journals committed to this body of expertise. Wilderness medicine is more than just another library of facts, however. It relies upon robust individuals with a sixth sense about concepts that work versus those that fail, based upon personal experiences in this environment.[6] Understanding the terminology, concepts, and resources that underlie research-based medical practice can simultaneously

ensure best-evidence "bedside" delivery and provide a framework for continuing to improve the science of wilderness medicine for future generations.[66] This chapter provides a roadmap for those who practice wilderness medicine to assimilate evidence-based medicine (EBM) principles into practice. It explores the roots and concepts underlying EBM and implementation science, explores common arguments against EBM, provides resources for wilderness medicine practitioners to employ EBM in heterogeneous settings, and highlights EBM using published wilderness medicine research.

WHAT EBM IS AND IS NOT

The term *evidence-based medicine* was coined in 1992 by Gordon Guyatt and the Evidence-Based Medicine Working Group as the overlap between clinician expertise, a patient's unique situation

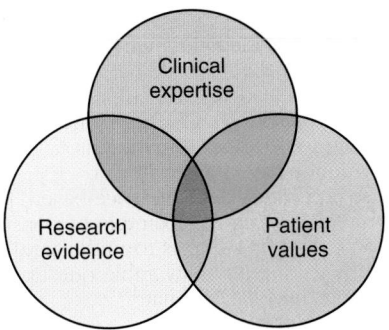

FIGURE 115-1 The EBM triad.

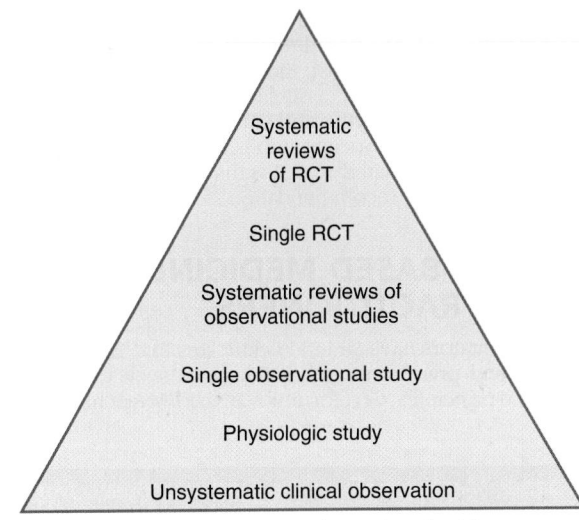

FIGURE 115-2 The EBM hierarchy of evidence.

and personal values, and research evidence (Figure 115-1).[21] Although graduate education, resident training, and postresidency practice improvement (continuing medical education) have espoused the virtues of research evidence since the Flexner report of the early 20th century, this definition and concept of EBM provided a new approach to incorporating clinical research into bedside practice. For example, the process of EBM provided a template to seek, find, appraise, and apply research findings to individual patients, as opposed to the passive dissemination of research that had been relied upon by investigators, journal authors, and educators in the decades following the Flexner medical revolution.[23] Through a series of peer-reviewed "how to use and appraise" manuscripts published in the *Journal of the American Medical Association* (JAMA),[27] EBM proponents supplied a toolbox for learners at all levels of training to use research evidence appropriate for their unique practice settings. This *JAMA* series is now available as a textbook entitled *User's Guide to the Medical Literature.*[28]

A growing body of evidence suggests that clinical experience alone is insufficient to ensure that patients receive contemporary, guideline-based medical care.[14] Half of the patients in the United States do not receive evidence-based management in primary care.[46] Information overload is a substantial proportion of the problem. For example, emergency medicine providers need to read 26 articles in the *Annals of Emergency Medicine* to find one manuscript that changes their practice.[49] Because there are over 4000 biomedical publications that appear every day in PubMed, it is hardly surprising that busy clinicians frequently overlook new innovations and updated guidelines.

EBM is one approach to help overloaded clinicians find, evaluate, and use clinical research in their practice, but it is not a panacea. Malcolm Gladwell's novel *Outliers* provides examples of many talented individuals in a variety of professions, with each expert sharing one key exposure: 10,000 hours of mentored training to master their domain.[23] Most clinicians lack a high-quality, mentored exposure to EBM during their medical training[11,37] and there is ample evidence that traditional CME is ineffective at altering professional practice or improving patient outcomes.[22] Because it is unlikely that clinicians working long hours with increasing patient volumes and paperwork burdens will have the luxury of Gladwell's 10,000-hour exposure, EBM critics portray the EBM construct of finding, appraising, and using clinical evidence as an unrealistic expectation.[29,59,64] Some of the arguments of EBM opponents are noted in Box 115-1.[64] However, these same critics offer no viable alternatives to EBM,[39,45] and a fiscally fragile and increasingly strained health care system demands adaptation to progress and a focus on moving beyond the status quo.

BOX 115-1 Problems Inherent to the Philosophy of Evidence-Based Medicine

EBM grading is detached from scientific reality.
EBM proceeds where logical positivism failed.
EBM reduces scientific methodology to a single step.
EBM confuses statistics with science.
EBM lacks evidence of efficacy; hence it is internally inconsistent.

THE EVIDENCE-BASED CLINICAL PRACTITIONER

Two key components of EBM are
1. Evidence alone is never enough.
2. Not all evidence is equally valid.

The first precept contends that there is an important and indispensable role for clinical expertise. Each clinician spends thousands of hours evaluating and contemplating myriad patient presentations and approaches to care. No textbook or journal manuscript will supplant this first-hand knowledge, which informs clinical intuition. In addition, patient priorities and values often trump clinical intuition and research evidence.

The second EBM precept refers to a hierarchy of research evidence. The hierarchy of evidence proposed by EBM leaders is depicted in Figure 115-2. In this hierarchical structure, systematic reviews and metaanalyses are considered the most accurate form of research evidence, followed by randomized controlled trials, metaanalyses of observational research, individual observational studies, case reports and case series, and bench research (e.g., physiologic studies), in order of the highest to lowest forms of clinical research evidence. The rationale for this hierarchy is that the highest forms of evidence are least likely to provide biased estimates of effect size, whether the research question is a therapy, diagnostic test, or prognostic factor. EBM proponents recognize that not every research question is amenable to a randomized controlled trial, so their emphasis is on ensuring the least biased estimate of effect size; hence the evidence hierarchy.

The evidence hierarchy can be illustrated using an example from wilderness medicine: frostbite. In 1978, Malhotra and colleagues used a rat model to assess the effect of bathwater temperature to treat frostbite.[44] Conclusions regarding the optimal water temperature were based on quantification of cold injury sustained on hind paws. On the EBM hierarchy of Figure 115-2, this physiologic study would represent a lower tier of evidence when extrapolated to humans.

In 2005, Twomey and associates evaluated tissue plasminogen activator (tPA) to treat severe frostbite. Twomey's experimental model assessed the lack of distal limb and digit perfusion using a technetium 99m (Tc-99m) bone scan. This case-control study used historical Tc-99m data from patients who ultimately required an amputation due to frostbite injury. Efficacy was evaluated by comparing the number of amputations in the patients treated with tPA with historical cohorts with amputations.[65] Compared with the Malhotra animal-model study, Twomey's data represent a higher level of evidence that is more applicable to human patients on whom this treatment would be applied. In other words, the case-control design is less likely to provide biased estimates of treatment efficacy than is the animal-based physiologic experiment, and can be applied to actual patients with more confidence, although case-control studies are far from definitive.

As described in detail in Chapter 9, significant evidence now exists to inform evidence-based rewarming and thawing of frost-bitten extremities in humans, including wound management, intervention timing, severity assessment, and pharmacologic interventions with thrombolytics and antiinflammatory medications. The Wilderness Medical Society published frostbite management guidelines in 2011, updated in 2014, that provide a level of evidence rating for each recommendation.[47,48]

EVIDENCE-BASED MEDICINE: EXPERTS VERSUS PRACTITIONERS

Some commentators have stratified clinicians into EBM experts or evidence-based practitioners.[25] EBM experts seek to understand existing EBM principles, develop innovative EBM teaching modules or measurement instruments, and disseminate these ideas within and around the House of Medicine. On the other hand, evidence-based practitioners are less interested in EBM as a teachable concept and more invested in applying research evidence using EBM at the patient-provider interface. Many resources exist for individuals seeking to become EBM experts.[32,61] The focus of this chapter is on evidence-based practitioners.

The stepwise approach for evidence-based practitioners is depicted in Box 115-2 using the example of nonsterile water for wound irrigation.[67] The first step is to understand what information is required by asking an answerable question. The question is formulated using the PICO format:[15]

P = patient population
I = intervention (therapy, diagnostic test, prognostic factor)
C = control group (if applicable)
O = outcomes of interest

BOX 115-2   An Example of the Evidence-Based Medicine Process

Step 1: Derive the PICO Question
PICO Question:
  Population: Patients with traumatic lacerations
  Intervention: Tap water (TW) irrigation
  Comparison: Sterile saline (SS) irrigation
  Outcome: Wound infection, pain scores, cosmetic appearance, cost

Step 2: Devise a Search Strategy and Find the Evidence
Use PubMed to conduct your initial search using a combination of the search terms "wound irrigation," "laceration," and "drinking water," but find no citations, so you next try the combination of search terms "wound irrigation," "laceration," and "tap water," which identifies 10 articles (see tinyurl.com/WoundWater2016).

Step 3: Select the Least Biased Clinical Research Using the Evidence Hierarchy (Figure 115-2).
A Multicentre Comparison of Tap Water Versus Sterile Saline for Wound Irrigation, Acad Emerg Med 14:404-410, 2007 (pmid.us/17456554).

Step 4: Appraise the Evidence Using the Appropriate Critical Appraisal Worksheet (in This Case, the Metaanalysis Critical Appraisal Form From the User's Guide to the Medical Literature—Table, Figure, and Page Numbers Refer to the Original Manuscript in *Academic Emergency Medicine*).

Guide	Comments
I. Are the results valid?	
A. Did experimental and control groups begin the study with a similar prognosis (answer the questions posed below)?	
1. Were patients randomized?	Yes. "Subjects were randomized to SS or TW irrigation by opening the next numbered study envelope for that institution." (p 405)
2. Was randomization concealed (blinded)?	No. Subjects and treating clinicians knew the allocation arms. For this particular question, blinding subjects and clinicians would be impractical, though not impossible. For example, one could use tap water bottled in saline bottles as a sham.
3. Were patients analyzed in the groups to which they were randomized?	No clear intention-to-treat analysis is stated, although Figure 1 (p 406) suggests analysis within treatment arms.
4. Were patients in the treatment and control groups similar with respect to known prognostic factors?	The anatomic distribution (Table 1, p 407) and wound mechanism/length/repair did not differ between the two groups. No details are provided on patient factors (age, gender, race, time-to-repair, follow-up proportion) by which to gauge patient-specific confounding variables.
B. Did experimental and control groups retain a similar prognosis after the study started (answer the questions posed below)?	
1. Were patients aware of group allocation.?	Yes
2. Were clinicians aware of group allocation?	Yes
3. Were outcome assessors aware of group allocation?	No. "Providers in the emergency department (ED) removing staples or sutures were blinded to the subject's allocation." (p 405)
4. Was follow-up complete?	71/715 subjects were lost to follow-up (35 SS, 36 TW). Of those who were followed, 54% returned to the ED and 46% were contacted by phone!
II. What are the results (answer the questions posed below)?	
1. How large was the treatment effect?	634/715 eligible subjects were enrolled and analyzed. Most of those not analyzed were lost to follow-up (71).
	The SS infection rate was 3.3% (11 subjects), and the TW infection rate was 4% (12 subjects; difference 0.7% with 95% CI = −2.2% to 3.6%). Only one infection required admission. All others were managed on outpatient basis.
	Based on a patient charge of $9.11 for SS irrigation supplies, 13.5/L of water for 2 minutes TW irrigation at $0.0011/L (cost per patient $.0.0015) and $0.60 per 3 feet of tubing for 36% of TW patients ($0.22 per patient) the authors extrapolate a savings of $65.6 million/year in the United States if TW is used in place of SS. This savings is based upon the worst case scenario 3.6% increased infection risk in TW all treated with Keflex.
2. How precise was the estimate of the treatment effect?	Narrow CI for infection rate. The upper margin of 3.6% would not dissuade most from using TW instead of SS.

BOX 115-2 An Example of the Evidence-Based Medicine Process—cont'd

Guide	Comments
III. How can I apply the results to patient care (answer the questions posed below)?	
1. Were the study patients similar to my patient?	Yes. ED patients presenting to academic medical centers with acute lacerations.
2. Were all clinically important outcomes considered?	No. The authors do not assess patient comfort or wound cosmetic appearance. Patient expectations may be an important, unmeasured impediment to routinely using TW rather than SS.
3. Are the likely treatment benefits worth the potential harm and costs?	Yes, TW appears to be equivalent to SS for acute traumatic laceration requiring emergency closure at a substantial cost savings.

Step 5: Summarize the Limitations of This Research and the Take-Home Message.

Limitations:
1. Unblinded (to patients and treating clinicians) convenience sampling. Because patients and clinicians were aware of allocation arm, bias (ascertainment bias, cointervention bias) is possible. In addition, convenience sampling could produce a selection bias.
2. Potential Hawthorne effect in the SS group because clinicians knew their patient outcomes were being monitored in a study setting. Did they irrigate longer, more carefully, or with greater volumes of saline than they otherwise would have?
3. Substantial lost to follow-up without any sensitivity analysis. Fortunately, equal numbers lost in SS and TW groups.
4. Nonvalidated telephone follow-up for 46% of those analyzed. Does anybody really think wound infection can be diagnosed over the phone as well as via face-to-face evaluation?
5. No statement of intention-to-treat analysis, although CONSORT diagram (Fig 1, p 406) suggests groups analyzed according to allocation assignment.
6. Underpowered study. Investigators calculated an a priori sample size of 1000 based upon a 10% infection rate. Doubling the observed 3.3% infection rate would recalculate a 1500-subject sample size. The current study only recruited 715 subjects (and only analyzed 634!), so they may have suffered a type I error (failed to detect a significant difference because of insufficient sample size).

Step 6: Determine Whether This Evidence Is Sufficient to Incorporate Into Your Practice.

Underpowered multicenter convenience sampling with substantial lost-to-follow-up and no sensitivity analysis suggests that TW may be equivalent to SS in uncomplicated traumatic lacerations requiring ED closure. If validated, these findings could simplify ED wound irrigation while saving $65.6 million/year in the United States alone.

SS, sterile saline; TW, tap water.

The PICO question is used to direct the search strategy that will acquire research evidence. Specific resources to find applicable evidence are discussed in the next section. Evidence-based practitioners prioritize evidence via the hierarchy of evidence (see Figure 115-2). The next step is to appraise the evidence. The User's Guide provides key questions for each type of research, including therapy, diagnosis, differential diagnosis, clinical decision rules, systematic reviews, harm, prognosis, and cost-effectiveness. Box 115-2 provides a real-life example of how evidence-based practitioners would use these principles to find the highest-quality research and then assess the risk of bias based upon the clinician's unique experience, patient population, and practice setting.

EVIDENCE-BASED MEDICINE RESOURCES FOR WILDERNESS MEDICINE PROVIDERS

A variety of free online resources exist to help physicians keep up to date on practice-changing or practice-enhancing research. Some of these resources are listed in Box 115-3. These products include synopses of journal club events across a variety of academic institutions. These often include reproducible PICO-based queries, critically appraised topics, associated podcasts, and social media feeds (e.g., Twitter and Facebook). Other resources, such as TheNNT.com, provide quantitative EBM reviews that may or may not be relevant to wilderness medicine but are searchable. In planning for a wilderness adventure, the content archived on these websites can be viewed as ready for educational sessions for wilderness providers to review.

In addition, free and unfiltered search engines exist for wilderness medicine providers with Internet access. PubMed (ncbi.nlm.nih.gov/pubmed) is commonly used and represents a medical librarian–archived resource made available by the National Library of Medicine. The PubMed website includes online tutorials to teach novice users how to optimize the search capability of this resource. As illustrated in Figure 115-3, PubMed Clinical Queries make up an extremely useful resource for clinicians to focus a search on therapy, prognosis, diagnostics, or clinical prediction guides.[1,41] Wilderness medicine providers can use Clinical Queries to quickly identify all of the research for a clinical question and then combine the findings with a search term such as "rural*" or "wilderness*" to isolate the most relevant studies for their setting (see Figure 115-3). PubMed also provides users with the capability to save search strategies and rerun them later. Some research indicates that physicians lack expertise in using PubMed and other search engines, so medical librarians are often quite helpful to enhance clinicians' capability to use these resources.[24,25] MEDLINE is another name for PubMed; OVID is a fee-based platform intended to add more user-friendly features to the PubMed search engine. Box 115-4 lists common terms used in evidence-based medicine; they may be helpful when doing searches.

Metaengines are electronic search products that simultaneously use medical terms to search PubMed, guidelines, textbooks, and other web-based resources. The TRIP database (tripdatabase.com/) is one prominent and free metaengine.[50] As demonstrated in Figure 115-4, TRIP provides the findings for a search

BOX 115-3 Free Evidence-Based Medicine Resources for Wilderness Medicine Providers

Search Engines
PubMed: ncbi.nlm.nih.gov/pubmed
TRIP: tripdatabase.com/

Journal Club Reviews
Eastern Virginia Medical School: emjournalclub.com/
Indiana University: http://emergency.medicine.iu.edu/research/ebm-journal-club/
Temple University: templeem.com/blog/
Washington University: http://emed.wustl.edu/education/EmergencyMedicineJournalClub

Quantitative Reviews
TheNNT.com: thennt.com/

Statistical Calculators
2×2 contingency table: statpages.org/ctab2x2.html
Posttest probability: dokterrutten.nl/collega/LRcalcul.html
Sample size calculator: http://homepage.stat.uiowa.edu/~rlenth/Power

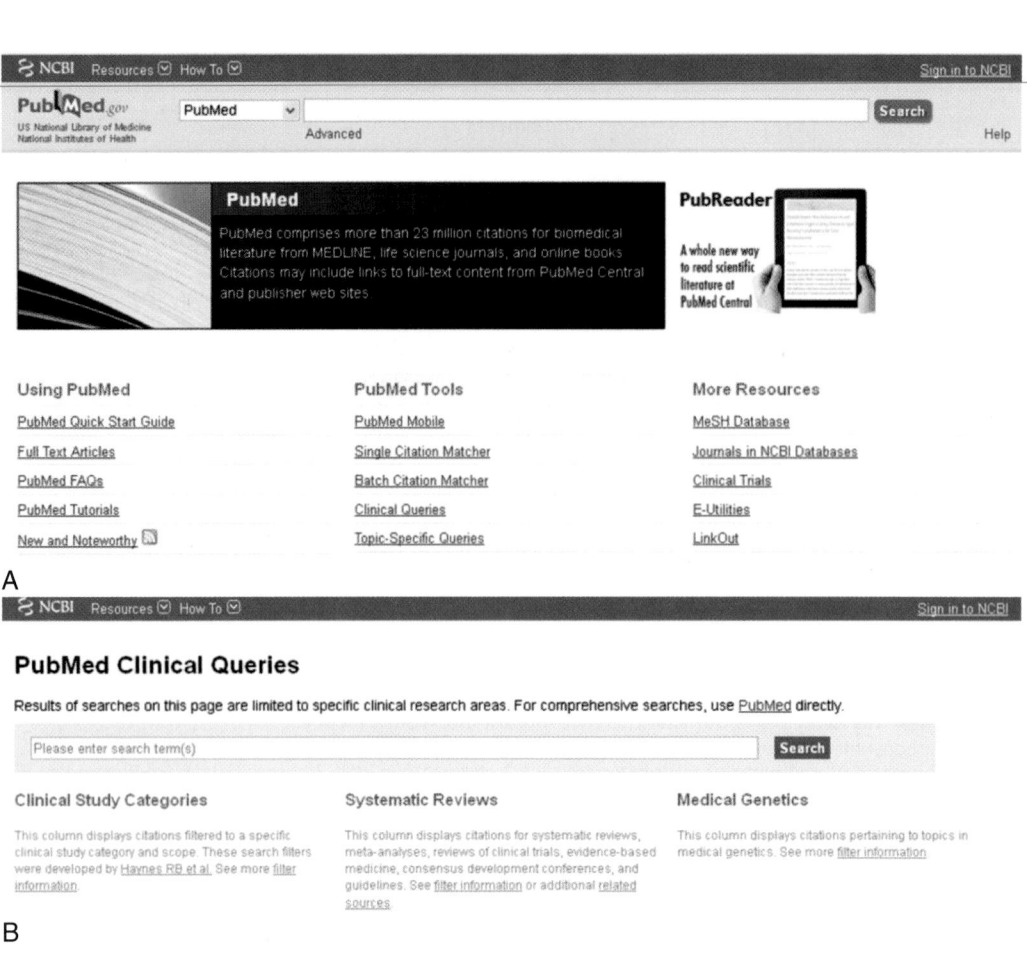

A

B

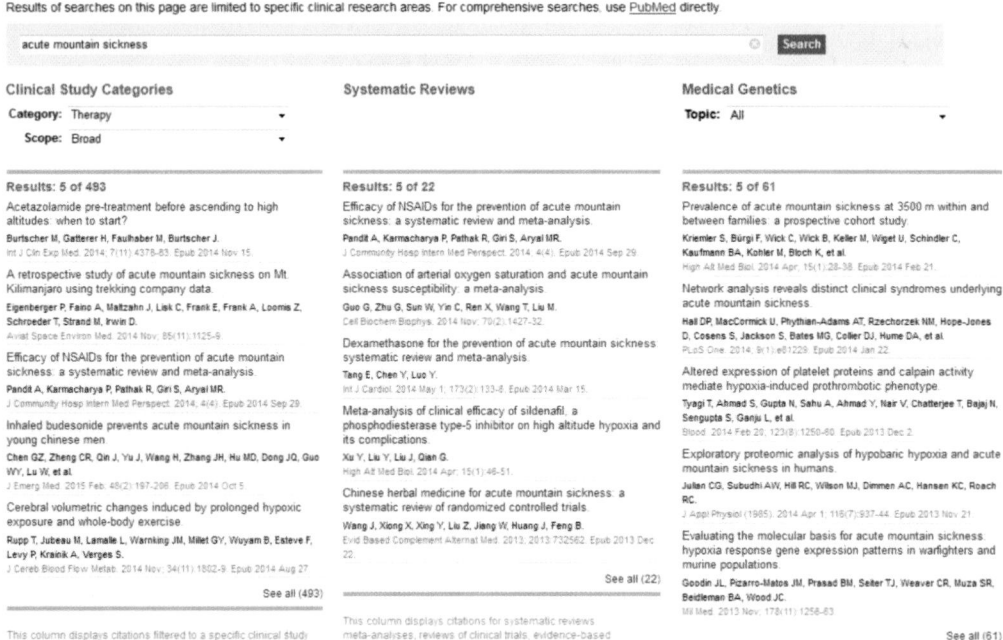

C

FIGURE 115-3 Free PubMed resources. **A,** Note PubMed QuickStart Guide and online tutorials, mobile applications, and clinical queries. Users can sign up for a National Center for Biotechnology Information (NCBI) account to save searches and receive email updates when relevant research is published based on established search strategies. **B,** Clinical Queries tab allows users to conduct broad or narrow searches for specific types of research. **C,** Sample Clinical Query of "acute mountain sickness" using the category "therapy" and "broad" scope. Other categories include etiology, prognosis, diagnosis, and clinical prediction guides. PubMed stratifies search results into clinical studies, systematic reviews, and medical genetics.

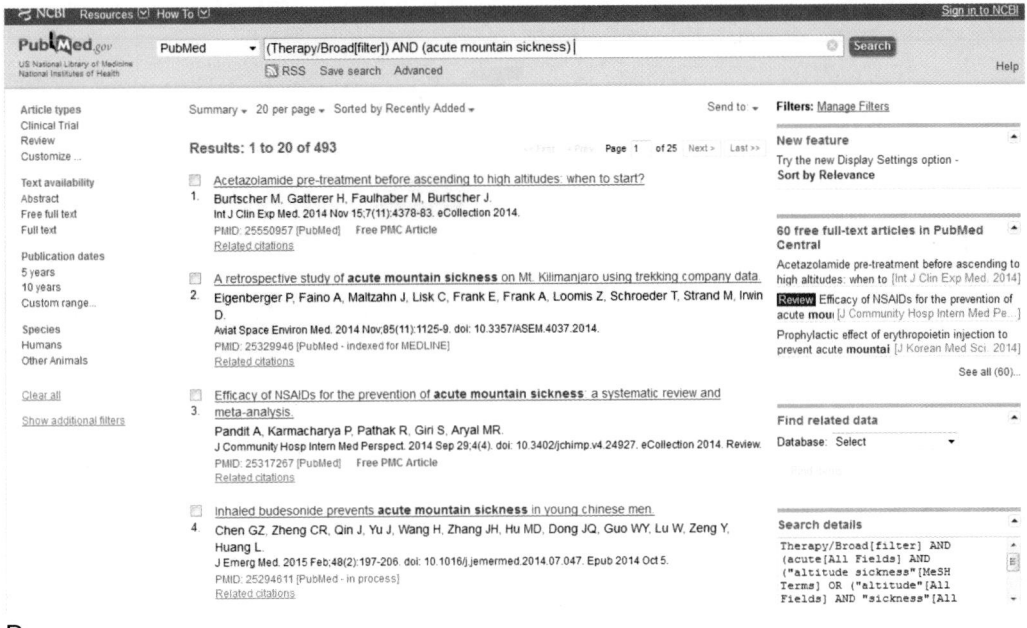

D

FIGURE 115-3, cont'd **D,** All of the PubMed citations under the Clinical Study category.

by listing the citations in the EBM hierarchy (see Figure 115-2). TRIP also allows users to save search strategies and can email users each month when new citations become available for a given search strategy or topic of interest.

Residency leaders in emergency medicine indicate that the primary skill set of EBM instructors ought to be the ability to identify secondary peer-reviewed resources for resident learners.[11] Secondary peer-reviewed literature is a snapshot synopsis of high-yield, practice-changing research with a critical appraisal already performed by a colleague in the field to which the research applies. Examples of secondary peer-reviewed resources include the journals *ACP Journal Club* and *Evidence-Based Medicine*.[30] The research summarized by secondary peer-reviewed journals undergoes a complicated process before reaching end-user bedside clinicians. In the case of *ACP Journal Club*, the McMaster Health Information Research Unit reviews 200 journals every month to identify higher-quality, minimally biased research methods. Once identified, these manuscripts are sent via email to at least three specialists in the applicable medical field(s), who rate the evidence for newsworthiness and likelihood of changing practice. The evidence that is rated by applicable medical specialties as both highly newsworthy and practice changing is then critically appraised with commentary by an EBM expert in that field. Wilderness medicine topics are included in these journals for conditions such as jellyfish stings[9] and tick bites,[51] but are

quite rare. Developing a similar product is an opportunity for wilderness medicine organizations and journals. Secondary peer-reviewed journals are not free, but many offer complimentary services to "push" the most compelling evidence to the medical specialists affected by the new research. For example, KT-Plus (plus.mcmaster.ca/kt/Default.aspx) can be accessed by anyone who signs up for this service.[31]

Although most textbooks represent authoritarian dictate, narrative review, or unsubstantiated opinion, several textbooks exist that use the EBM approach described above.[53,58] In addition, journals such as the *Annals of Emergency Medicine,*[52] *Academic Emergency Medicine,*[13] the *Canadian Journal of Emergency Medicine,* and the *Journal of Emergency Medicine*[68] now publish EBM series regularly. As EBM interest and expertise grow in wilderness medicine, similar series could be developed for relevant wilderness journals. The disadvantage of these textbooks' and journals' EBM series is that a large proportion of contemporary wilderness medical practice has little evidentiary basis, or even worse, available evidence is contradictory.[35]

Clinical guidelines are another resource for health care providers, but these are often viewed with skepticism for a variety of reasons.[10] Guidelines are often outdated and do not exist for many of the clinical situations faced on a daily basis. In the future, guidelines should become more applicable and transparent as the Grading of Recommendations Assessment Development and

---

BOX 115-4   Terms Used in Evidence-Based Medicine

Bias: deviation from the "truth" (i.e., the correct effect size) observed in the study as a result of the research design, conduct, or reporting.

Critical appraisal: the process of assessing the risk of bias and applicability to one's patient population and clinical setting when evaluating medical research manuscripts.

D&I/KT: dissemination and implementation/knowledge translation science, which is the approach of applying evidence in the clinical environment with consideration of pragmatic challenges, reproducibility, sustainability, unintended consequences, and costs.

EBM: evidence-based medicine, or the philosophical approach of seeking the overlap of patient circumstances/values, clinical expertise, and research evidence to yield optimal outcomes.

Effect size: the quantifiable impact that an intervention has upon an intended (or unintended) outcome or measure. In the case of a

therapy, the effect size is commonly expressed in terms of relative risk, absolute risk reduction, or number needed to treat and number needed to harm. On the other hand, in assessing a diagnostic test, the effect size is quantified using sensitivity, specificity, likelihood ratios, and receiver operator curve area under the curve. Understanding effect size empowers critical clinicians to (1) directly compare one intervention or test with another, and (2) communicate risk and benefit decisions with patients to facilitate shared decision making.

Metasearch engine: a software system that sends queries to several search engines or databases simultaneously.

Search engine: software system used to find evidence on the world-wide web.

Secondary peer-reviewed literature: journals or resources that provide critical appraisal and expert commentary about original research for other health care providers.

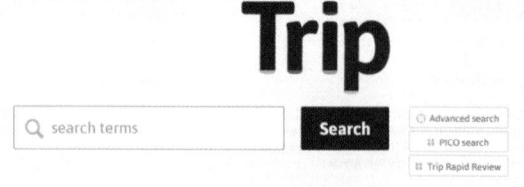

A

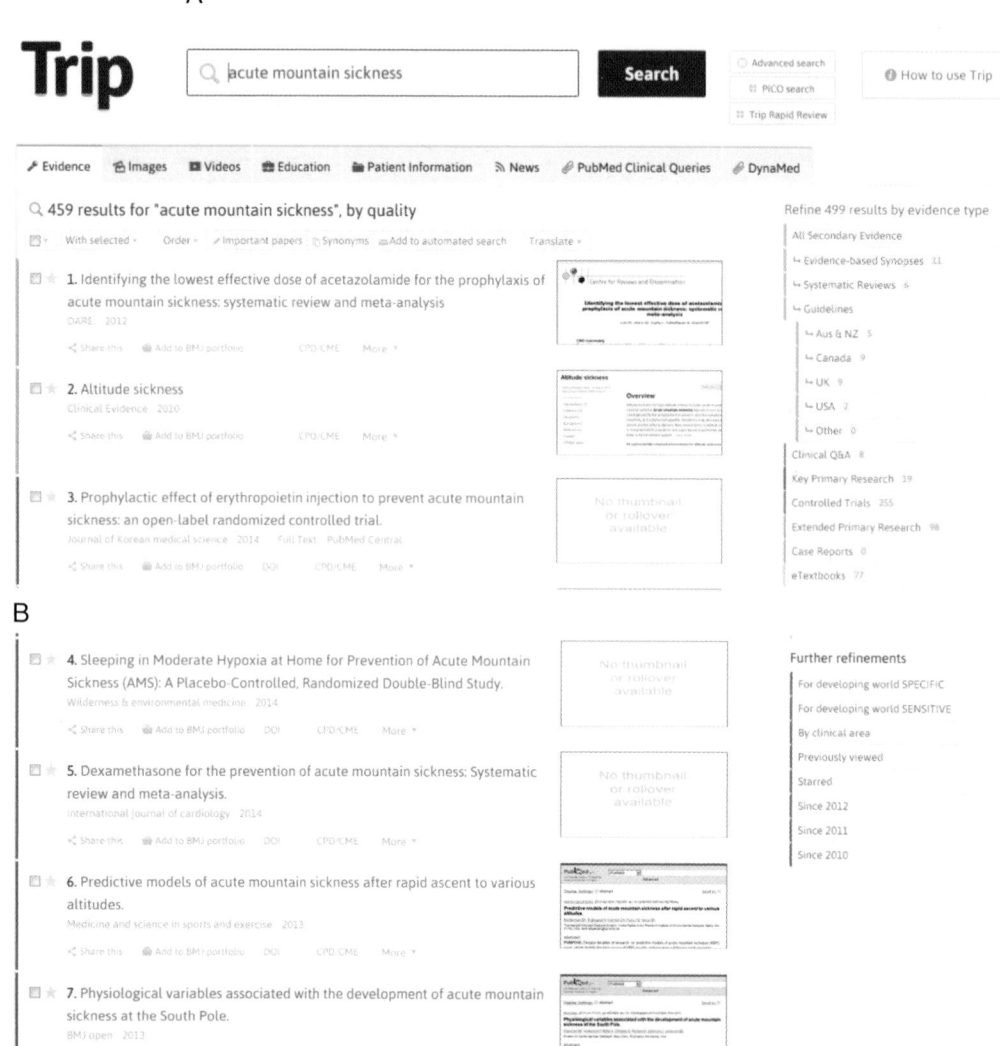

B

C

FIGURE 115-4 Free TRIP database resources. **A,** Enter search term. Note on the right that advanced and rapid search options are available, as is the possibility of constructing a PICO question upon which to base a search. **B,** TRIP search results for term *acute mountain sickness*. Note on the right that the results can be stratified by level of evidence using the hierarchy from Figure 115-2. Textbook chapters are included, and the findings most applicable to developing world settings can be identified with sensitive or specific filters. **C,** TRIP search results can also be stratified by "developing world" or "clinical area," as observed on the right of this screenshot.

FIGURE 115-4, cont'd D, Using the PICO function to refine the search. **E,** PICO-refined search results. See tabs at top with images, videos, educational materials, patient information, and news.

Recommendation (GRADE) criteria are used to develop them.[26] As the number of guidelines for core wilderness medicine issues expands, wilderness medicine providers will need to be part of the guideline development process to ensure that the recommendations are pragmatic and attainable for this environment.[42] Wilderness medicine guidelines are appearing with increasing frequency for frostbite,[48] hypothermia,[70] heat-related illness,[40] spine immobilization,[57] wound management,[56] acute altitude illness,[43] exercise-induced hyponatremia,[4] and lightning injuries,[16] among others.

MOVING BEYOND EVIDENCE-BASED MEDICINE: WHAT IS IMPLEMENTATION SCIENCE?

Once clinicians find and appraise the evidence, it is necessary to apply the new information when treating patients. The original descriptors of EBM acknowledged this portion of the process, but the complexities were oversimplified. Over the last 10 years, a new science has been developed to explore and promote the process of applying the evidence. In the United States this process is called dissemination and implementation (D&I) science, and in Canada it is called knowledge translation.[7,38]

Why is there the need for D&I research? In the past, investigators assumed that publication of new discoveries was a sufficient dissemination strategy to promote practice change in applicable clinical settings, but diffusion of innovations is more complex in medicine, public health, and policy making.[5,8] In fact, the delay between biomedical scientific discovery and widespread implementation usually extends beyond 10 years.[2,3,18,55] The 2001 Institute of Medicine report entitled "Crossing the Quality Chasm: A New Health System for the 21st Century" noted a "chasm" between medical advances and current medical care.[33] For example, McGlynn and colleagues examined 439 quality indicators in adult primary care patients from 12 U.S. cities and reported that only 55% routinely received recommended medical management.[46] The National Institutes of Health (NIH) recognized as early as 2000 that effective translational science would require a paradigm shift.[71] Many barriers exist between scientific discovery and clinical application, ranging from the level of the individual clinician to that of the health care system. These include clinical awareness in an era of information overload, balancing healthy skepticism with sufficient evidence of effectiveness, misaligned incentives for evidence uptake and care delivery, and an evolving understanding of D&I research methods. A conceptual leak is loss of clinically used information. These leaks at the provider-patient interface are depicted in Figure 115-5, along with specific examples driving each leak and solutions to slow the relative loss.[19] By understanding these factors, evidence-based practitioners can more efficiently introduce high-quality, practice-worthy research evidence into wilderness medicine.

The complexity of D&I is in the questions that remain unanswered by the EBM process, including

- How is the "best evidence" defined against the spectrum of research findings, particularly when there exists conflicting evidence?
- How is "best evidence" efficiently disseminated (publication, opinion leader)?
- What is the effective component of the intervention?
- Can this effective component be replicated with fidelity in one's setting? If adaptation is necessary, when is the modified intervention sufficiently dissimilar from the published intervention that it is a different intervention?
- What organizational culture is essential to facilitate local adoption?
- Is the intervention sustainable?
- What are the unintended consequences of the intervention?
- What are the financial and personnel costs to implement the intervention?

D&I science is distinct from the traditional understanding of scientific discovery. D&I researchers often engage in systems engineering and behavioral modification, a process that usually engages stakeholders beyond the clinical setting and includes administrative leadership, social services, case managers, home health care services, and policy makers. In addition, most professions have been developing D&I methods, but the disparate nomenclature across nonmedical and medical fields is confusing and limits penetration of similar concepts.[54] Using D&I principles to speed adoption of appropriate evidence in wilderness medicine settings is an emerging concept.

THE FUTURE OF EVIDENCE-BASED MEDICINE AND DISSEMINATION AND IMPLEMENTATION IN WILDERNESS MEDICINE

Since 1992, the process of EBM has continued to evolve and improve.[36] More recently, D&I developed as a necessary and distinct by-product of EBM. EBM and D&I each depend upon the other to be most useful for health care providers, as well as patients and society. EBM and D&I will continue to evolve. One important advance is development of a reliable and accurate instrument to identify practice-changing or practice-enhancing research pertinent to one specialty: the BEEM rater tool.[12,69] This instrument provides a validated method to filter the signal from the noise amongst the 4000+ biomedical publications that appear on PubMed every day, and can be important for busy clinicians who lack the time to find, appraise, and assimilate all of these data. In fact, most published research is not ready for widespread application.[34] Figure 115-6 provides an example of how the BEEM rater tool could be used as a filter for wilderness medicine practitioners to find high-quality (i.e., minimally biased), practice-worthy evidence applicable to this unique health care setting. These methods could be modified to identify wilderness medicine–ready research evidence primed for widespread dissemination by developing a network of wilderness medicine research literature raters.

Adult learning theory emphasizes the process of learning that is problem based and collaborative rather than didactic. A substantial body of evidence implies that the traditional conference-based didactic instructor-to-learner one-way information exchange is ineffective to ensure quality improvement in medicine.[17,22] Another ongoing development in the EBM world is use of social media to promote a "bottoms-up" approach to disseminating high-quality research evidence. For example, the podcast "Skeptics Guide to Emergency Medicine" provides brief synopses of BEEM rater

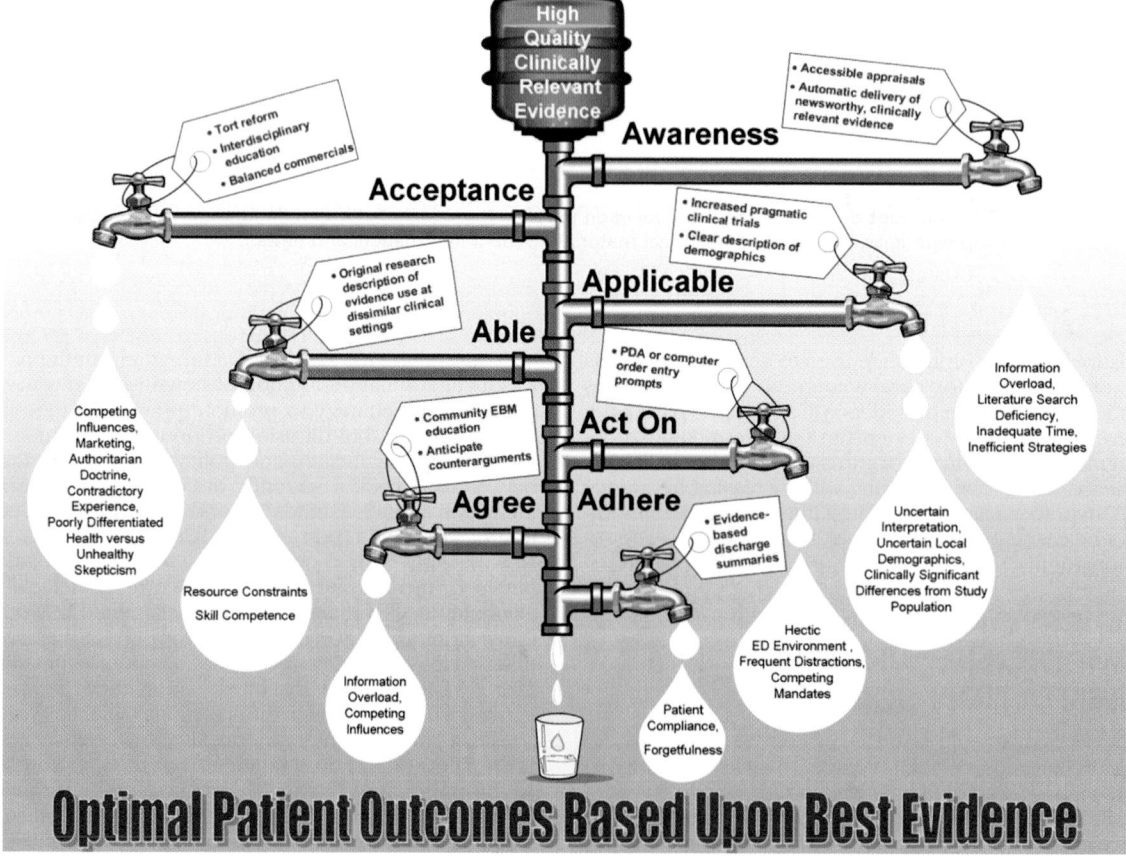

FIGURE 115-5 The knowledge translation pipeline. (*From Diner BM, Carpenter CR, O'Connell T, et al: Graduate medical education and Knowledge Translation: role models, information pipelines, and practice change thresholds. Acad Emerg Med 14(11):1008-1014, 2007.*)

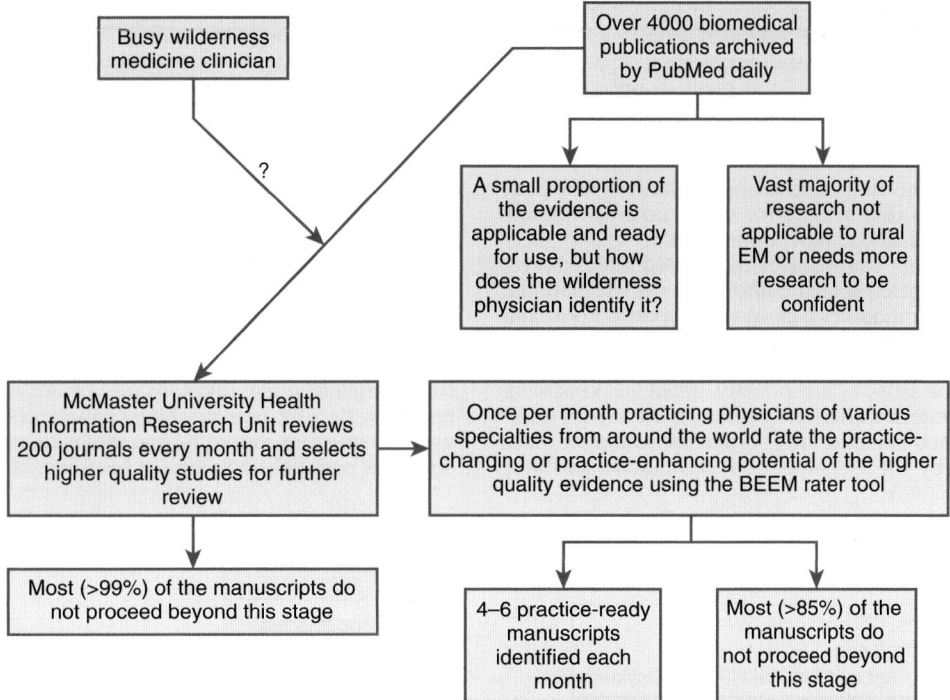

FIGURE 115-6 Potential application of the BEEM rater instrument.

tool–filtered evidence, targeting junior learners in an entertaining delivery mode using adult learning theory with the millennial audience in mind.[63] Other high-quality podcasts exist[20,60,62] and more could be developed for wilderness medicine aficionados.

CONCLUSION

Because of the austere environment in which wilderness injuries and illnesses occur, study of their prevention and acute treatment is quite challenging. Nonetheless, by using the principles of EBM, wilderness medicine providers can find, assess, and apply the most appropriate, least biased research to deci-

sion making in these scenarios. Furthermore, understanding the evolving concepts of implementation science provides wilderness medicine with a framework to move evidence to action and reduce unnecessary delays in translating evidence to wilderness care.

REFERENCES

Complete references used in this text are available online at expertconsult.inkling.com.

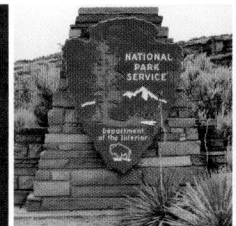

CHAPTER 116
National Park Service Medicine

SUSANNE J. SPANO

MISSION OF THE NATIONAL PARK SERVICE

The mission of the National Park Service (NPS) is to preserve natural and cultural resources for public enjoyment, education, and inspiration and to extend benefits of conservation throughout the United States and the world for future generations.[57] The mission is one century old. The NPS is responsible for both urban and wilderness areas. A brief history of national wild space conservation helps elucidate how emergency medical services (EMS) employed within the current park system have developed.

HISTORY OF THE NATIONAL PARK SERVICE

Although measures to preserve land for public use have been under way since the United States was founded, Congress did not create a unified federal agency to manage these areas until 1916.[7] In 1790, George Washington authorized for the first time that land should be reserved for the purpose of public enjoyment. This was in the District of Columbia, a planned city with a grand urban park system and parkways now known as the National Capital Parks.[14] In 1832, Congress created a precursor to modern national parks by setting aside four tracts of land surrounding Hot Springs, Arkansas, as the first federal reservation. This act was signed into law by President Andrew Jackson.[19]

President Lincoln used a federal land grant to preserve California's Yosemite Valley and the Mariposa Grove of Giant Sequoias. In 1864, these areas were ceded to the State of California to establish a state park.[49] In 1872, President Grant designated Yellowstone as the first national park. Because the park extended across borders of territories for which no governments existed, Yellowstone fell under federal jurisdiction.[15]

The next 44 years saw founding of the United States Forest Service, introduction of presidential authority to declare national monuments under the Antiquities Act under Theodore Roosevelt (1906), and founding of more than 39 national parks and monuments. Woodrow Wilson signed the National Park Service Organic Act in the summer of 1916.[54] The primary initial responsibility of the NPS was to protect wilderness resources. In 1933, Franklin D. Roosevelt issued an executive order consolidating sites previously managed by the Department of Agriculture and War

Department within the NPS.[50] This order broadened the NPS mission to encompass the natural, historical, and cultural heritage of the United States in both urban and wilderness environments. The NPS currently administers 407 units, covering more than 84 million acres in 50 states, the District of Columbia, and U.S. territories.[10]

ORGANIZATION OF THE NATIONAL PARK SERVICE

The NPS is a bureau of the Department of the Interior, headquartered in the Washington Support Office in Washington, DC. The director of the NPS reports to the Secretary of the Interior, who in turn reports to the President of the United States. The NPS is organized into divisions (led by deputy chiefs) that oversee branches (led by branch chiefs). Awareness of the NPS organizational structure should inform interactions with the EMS leadership at a national, regional, or local level (Figure 116-1).[36]

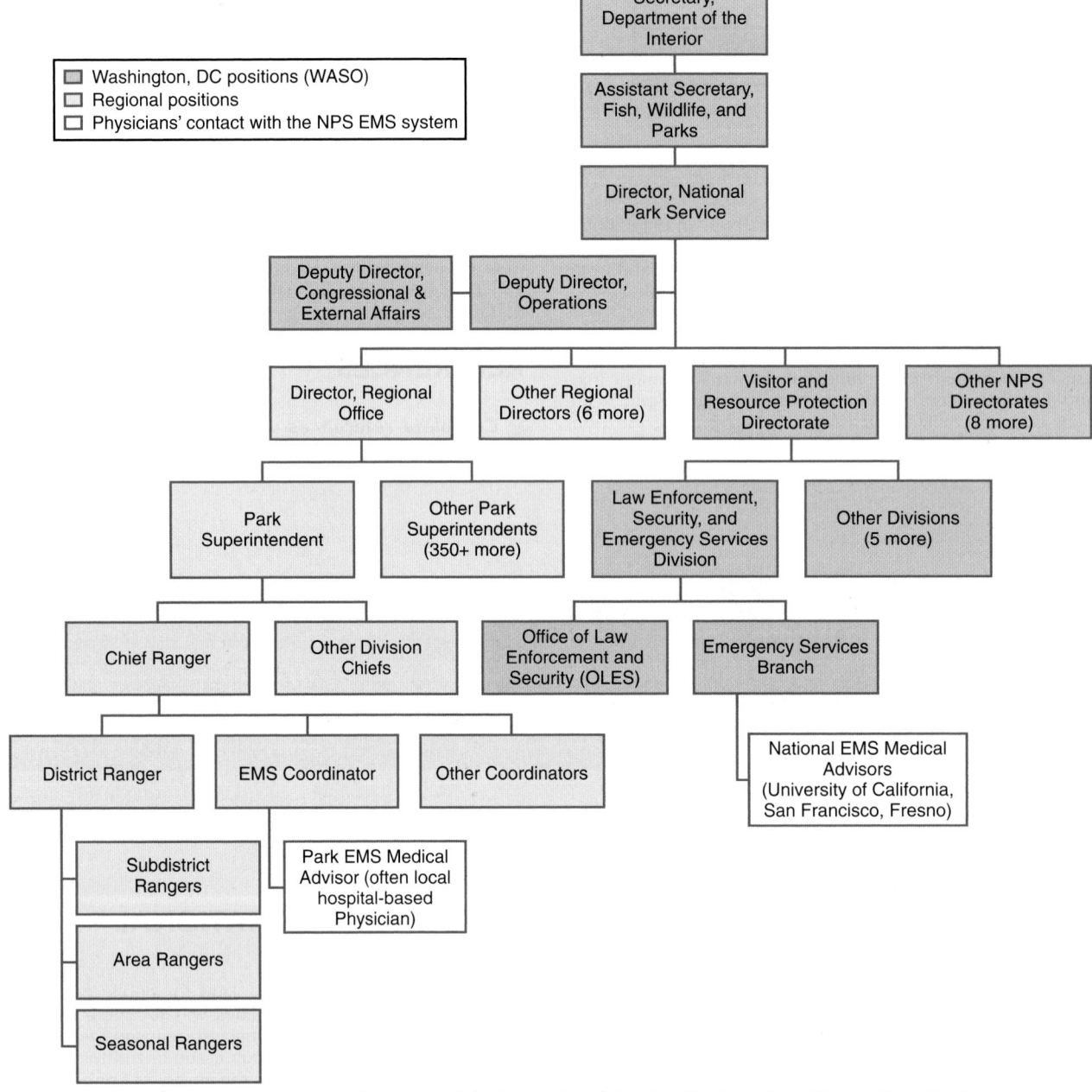

FIGURE 116-1 Organizational structure of the National Park Service. (Redrawn from National Park Service Organization Chart, National Park Service Reference Manual 51 Version 1.0, University of California San Francisco Fresno Emergency Medicine public website: fresno.ucsf.edu/em/parkmedic/lema.html.)

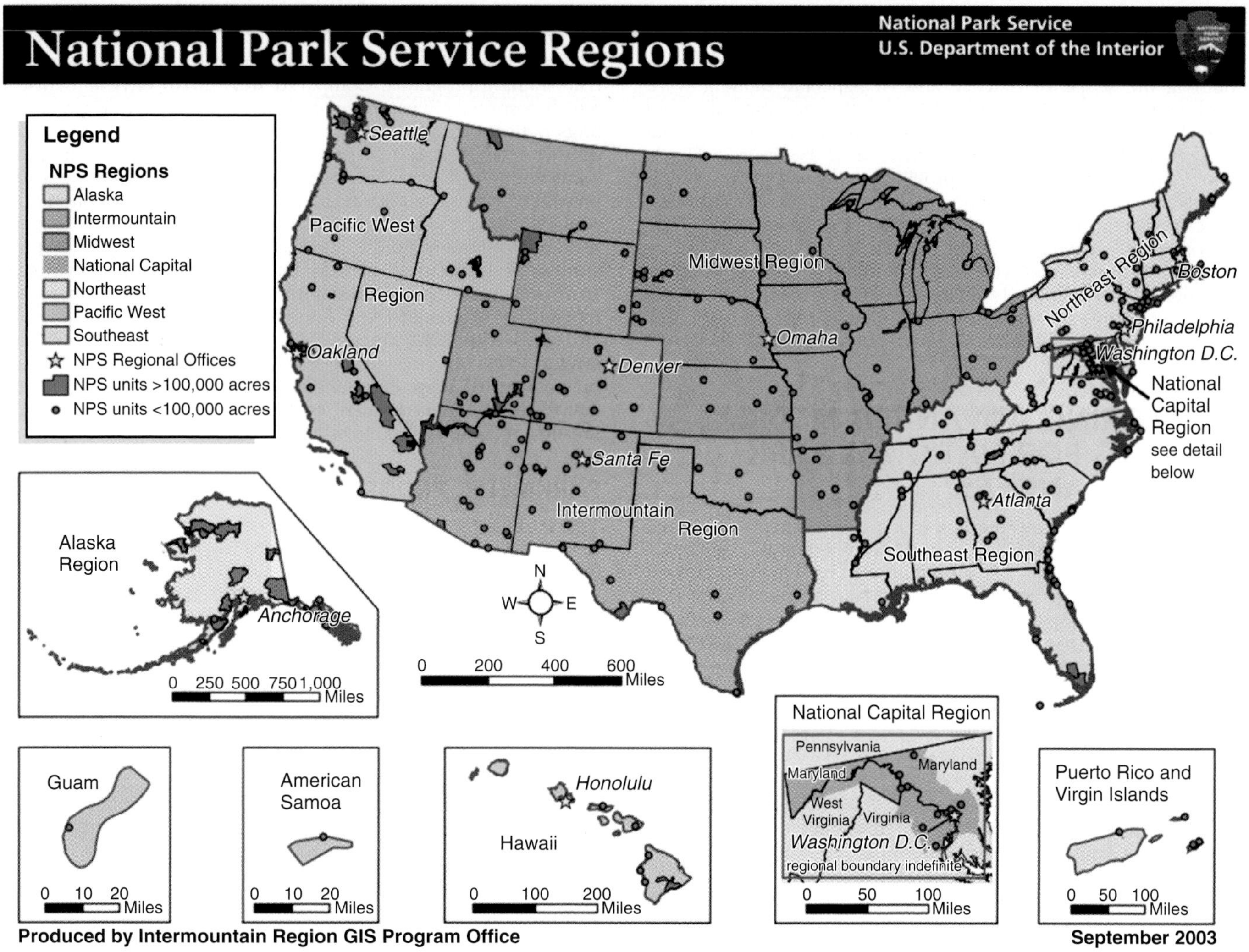

National Park Service Regions

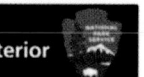

Legend

NPS Regions
- Alaska
- Intermountain
- Midwest
- National Capital
- Northeast
- Pacific West
- Southeast
- ☆ NPS Regional Offices
- ■ NPS units >100,000 acres
- • NPS units <100,000 acres

Alaska Region
Anchorage
0 250 500 750 1,000 Miles

Pacific West Region
Seattle
Oakland
Santa Fe
Intermountain Region
Denver
Midwest Region
Omaha
Northeast Region
Boston
Philadelphia
Washington D.C.
National Capital Region see detail below
Atlanta
Southeast Region

N W E S
0 200 400 600 Miles

Guam
0 10 20 Miles

American Samoa
0 10 20 Miles

Hawaii
Honolulu
0 100 200 Miles

National Capital Region
Pennsylvania
Maryland
Maryland
West Virginia
Virginia
Washington D.C.
regional boundary indefinite
0 50 100 Miles

Puerto Rico and Virgin Islands
0 50 100 Miles

Produced by Intermountain Region GIS Program Office   September 2003

FIGURE 116-2 The seven National Park Service Regions include Alaska, Intermountain, Midwest, Northeast, Pacific West, National Capital, and Southeast Regional Offices. *(From map produced by Intermountain Region Geographic Information Systems Program Office: nps.gov/gis/documents/nps_regions_11x8-5-new .pdf.)*

The deputy director of operations for the NPS oversees nine directorates (business services; cultural resources, partnerships, and science; information resources; interpretation, education, and volunteers; natural resource stewardship and science; park planning, facilities, and lands; partnerships and civic engagement; visitor and resource protection; and workforce and inclusion) and seven geographically based offices for regional management of the parklands (Figure 116-2).[25]

The NPS directorate responsible for delivery of emergency services is the Visitor and Resource Protection Directorate. This office's associate director is responsible for the policies and oversight of the NPS EMS. The directorate issues a reference and field manual *(Reference Manual-51 [RM-51])* that details NPS protocols, procedures, and medications allowed to be administered.[38] This directorate is also responsible for other operations (e.g., fire and aviation management; office of public health; wilderness stewardship, and law enforcement, security, and emergency services [LESES] division).[44]

The branch of Emergency Services is based within the LESES division of the Washington Support Office. The Branch Chief of Emergency Services is responsible for managing NPS EMS programs. The Branch Chief is assisted by the national EMS Medical Advisor and the regional EMS coordinators of the seven NPS regions. The national EMS medical advisor is the physician(s) contracted by the NPS to provide medical recommendations. Historically, this has been a member(s) of the core faculty in the Emergency Medicine Residency Program, University of California, San Francisco Fresno (UCSF Fresno).[31] Each

regional EMS coordinator inventories EMS data (e.g., certification levels of prehospital providers, regional centralized drug caches, medical supplies) within his or her service region.[29] Their recommendations (e.g., on system-wide quality improvements or adjustments in the appropriate prehospital scope of practice for the NPS EMS) are made to the Branch Chief of Emergency Services.

Day-to-day management and funding of EMS programs resides at the park level. Each park superintendent designates an EMS coordinator. This is often a ranger with additional responsibilities. A licensed physician serves as park EMS medical advisor (PEMS-MA).[29] The EMS coordinator and PEMS-MA are jointly responsible for park operational issues. This includes designating the requirements and scopes of practice for NPS EMS providers (e.g., emergency medical technician [EMT], paramedic). It also includes activities (i.e., routine training, continuing education, and quality improvement) intrinsic to any EMS system.[31] Each park's superintendent is ultimately responsible to ensure that a park EMS program is in compliance with the NPS Director's Order #51 (which outlines the policies and standards of the EMS program) and Reference Manual 51 (RM-51).

DIRECTOR'S ORDER #51

The Organic Act of 1916 delegated responsibility for the welfare of persons within parks to the NPS.[54] Within NPS-serviced recreational areas, emergency medical care is provided to approximately 13,000 of 279 million annual visitors.[5]

Rangers have been trained in first aid since the first park's inception. As visitation rose and incidents increased, levels of medical training have increased in step. In the 1970s, guidelines outlining the scope of practice and NPS-specific training were developed. In the 1980s and 1990s, a reference manual, field manual, and training programs were established under a National Emergency Medical Service Guideline.[29] In 2005, the NPS Director's Order #51 was issued and provided a detailed interpretation of policies, delegating specific authorities and responsibilities, and establishing the Parkmedic Program. The order reads: "The purpose of this Director's Order (DO) is to set forth NPS policy and a procedural framework for providing EMS. The policies, procedures, and standards in this document are to be implemented uniformly throughout the NPS inclusive of the U.S. Park Police. The details for implementation may be found in RM-51 and the EMS Field Manual."[29]

DEVELOPING ADVANCED MEDICAL TRAINING FOR NATIONAL PARK SERVICE RANGERS

The first formal advanced medical training for rangers was started by American mountaineer Dr. Thomas Hornbein at the University of Washington in 1968.[8] Dr. Hornbein and his climbing partner Willi Unsoeld were members of the first American expedition on Mt Everest in 1963, climbing via the treacherous West Ridge route.[20] As a former ranger in Mt Rainer National Park and practicing anesthesiologist, Dr. Hornbein developed a 110-hour curriculum covering emergency resuscitation and winter survival skills; it was taught in the park's off-season (January to April).

In the 1970s, EMS in the United States and the NPS developed rapidly. EMT certification programs became available throughout the country. In 1972, the first NPS EMT course (100 hours long) was taught at Camp Lejeune Marine Corps Base in North Carolina.[51] When Navy corpsmen returned from the Vietnam War, they brought remote first-aid skills from the battlefield to the backcountry; 23 rangers graduated with skills that included delivering a baby, reducing bony dislocations, establishing intravenous access, and administering medications.

The NPS Parkmedic Program developed in response to a 1976 accident, the Lost Soldier Cave Incident, in California. This Sequoia and Kings Canyon (SEKI) rescue of a spelunker with severe orthopedic injuries involved more than 18 persons, including a nurse, medical technician, volunteer climbers, four park rangers, and anesthesiologist (Dr. Harold Jakes), who served as an informal advisor to SEKI rangers.[8] The 22-hour rescue involved extrication of the immobilized victim through tight, twisting passageways and would not have been possible without pain medications administered by the registered nurse under direct physician orders from Dr. Jakes.

This experience highlighted the need for wilderness-specific EMS training programs. Compared with urban environments, in which responses were measured in minutes, in wilderness settings patients could be with rescuers for hours to days. In addition to a broad scope of practice (i.e., the ability to administer medications and provide lifesaving procedures), wilderness EMS providers needed authority to follow protocols to continue to provide care if medical control was unavailable due to exigencies such as equipment failure, electrical interference from lightning storms, or geographic barriers such as caves and canyons. In 1977, a new Parkmedic Program was adopted by the emergency medicine residents at UCSF Fresno based on training started by Dr. Jakes with SEKI rangers.[51] This program trained local park rangers to be prepared to meet NPS needs. The program focused on prehospital interventions and effective triage.[22] In 1978, the first formal "January Course" of the Parkmedic Program at UCSF Fresno graduated 20 rangers from Yosemite and SEKI.

PARKMEDIC PROGRAM

The Parkmedic certification course and the national NPS EMS medical advisors are based at the UCSF Fresno Medical Education Program.[45] The program develops and updates a range of national resources, including the RM-51[38]; *NPS First-Responder Field Manual* as an attachment to RM-51[33]; *NPS Medical Advisor Handbook*[31]; *NPS Paramedic Manual*[37]; *NPS Tactical EMS Protocols and Procedures Manual (RM-51T)*,[39] an online text for the Parkmedic training course: "Wilderness EMS, A Text for the NPS EMS Provider"[43]; and online training modules for tactical medicine, dislocation reductions, and epinephrine administration.[35] Current versions have restricted access for use within the NPS Servicewide for EMS operations, training, and continuing education requirements. Prior versions are available for public education through the UCSF Fresno emergency medicine website.

Certification and Authorization of Providers

NPS providers must demonstrate skills through a certifying body and be authorized to perform EMS within the national park unit to which they are assigned. The park EMS coordinator designates the scope of practice based on park and PEMS-MA recommendations. The National Registry of Emergency Medical Technicians (NREMT) oversees certification for levels other than basic training. Since 1970, the NREMT has administered a progressive process of EMS training, skills examination, and registration.[42] Six federal classifications (I to VI) are used to describe NPS prehospital care provider training levels.[40] Table 116-1 shows NPS EMS training levels and current recertification requirements.

TABLE 116-1	Emergency Medical Services Training Levels Available Within the National Park Service		
NPS Levels of EMS Training	**Description**	**Hours**	**Training Mandates**
Level I	CPR/AED provider: minimum level recommended for all NPS employees	10	Recertify every year
Level II	Basic first-aid provider: for those not normally involved in visitor contract duties but who may on occasion be confronted with having to provide initial medical care	8	Recertify every 3 years
Level III	Emergency medical responder (EMR): appropriate for fire suppression, search and rescue, and backcountry operations	50	Recertify every 2 years; 12-hour review course; 4-hour CPR refresher
Level IV	Emergency medical technician (EMT)	114	Recertify every 2 years; 24-hour BLS refresher course; 48-hours of CME
Level V	Advanced emergency medical technician (AEMT) *or* Parkmedic: requires current CPR certification and minimum of 1 year of EMT experience	340	Recertify every 2 years; 36-hour ALS refresher course; 36 hours of CME
Level VI	Paramedic: requires current CPR certification and current EMT certification	1000	Recertify every 2 years; 48-hour ALS refresher course; 24 hours of CME

AED, automated external defibrillator; ALS, advanced life support; BLS, basic life support; CME, continuing medical education; CPR, cardiopulmonary resuscitation; EMS, emergency medical service; NPS, National Park Service.
Adapted from National Park Service Training Mandates, edition 04/03/2003: nps.gov/training/mandated-training-list.doc.

BOX 116-1 Parkmedic Protocols

Adult Protocols
Abdominal pain
Allergic reactions
Altered mental status
Altitude illness
Altitude illness prophylaxis
Bites and stings
Burns
Cardiac arrest or dysrhythmias
Chest pain, cardiac
Childbirth
Dystonic reactions
Electrical and lightning
Frostbite
General medical illness

Heat illness
Hypothermia
Ingestions, poisoning
Respiratory distress
Scuba dive injury
Seizures
Shock without trauma
Submersion injury
Trauma (eye trauma, isolated extremity
    trauma, major trauma, trauma arrest)
Vaginal bleeding

Pediatric Protocols
Cardiac arrest or dysrhythmia
Medical illness or fever
Newborn resuscitation
Pediatric medical parameters
Trauma (major trauma, trauma arrest)

Adapted from National Park Service Reference Manual #51 version: 01/01/2015 (internal), University of California San Francisco Fresno Collaborative Learning Environment.

The first two levels, I (cardiopulmonary resuscitation [CPR]/automated external defibrillation [AED] provider) and II (basic first-aid provider), are not NREMT certified. NREMT certification covers the next four training levels: III (emergency medical responder [EMR]), IV (emergency medical technician [EMT]), V (advanced emergency medical technician [AEMT]), and VI (paramedic). Parkmedics are certified at level V, which allows a unique scope of practice not recognized by the NREMT skills examination.

Parkmedic (Level V) Scope of Practice

The Parkmedic scope of practice is unique to the federal NPS system. It is determined by the level of training, the federal protocols, and the provider's extended scope of practice endorsed by the administrator of each park within its jurisdiction.

Parkmedic Training

Parkmedic program training occurs nationally at the UCSF Fresno Center for Medical Education and Research. A biennial 6-week certification course or a 4-week Parkmedic refresher and recertification course is taught in alternating years.[45] Successful completion of didactics, skills performance, and procedure logs is required for graduation. Providers gain clinic skills by engaging in patient care in the affiliated level 1 trauma center emergency department, EMS ride-along activities, and simulated procedures employing high-fidelity models. Written and skills examinations are required for certification. Parkmedics are certified as AEMTs, but their scope of practice exceeds that of AEMTs in several areas.

Protocols for Parkmedics

The *NPS EMS Field Manual for Parkmedics* (RM-51) details symptom-based protocol management, procedural descriptions, and medication administration.[38] The Parkmedic's expanded scope of practice (beyond that of AEMTs) includes advanced airway management (e.g., supraglottic airway tube, endotracheal tube, endotracheal tube introducer), needle thoracostomy, Taser

dart removal, dislocation reductions, administration of additional intravenous medications, and a selective immobilization protocol that allows for decreased use of spinal motion restriction techniques.

NPS policy mandates that parks that will provide EMS at level IV or higher must implement the field manual standard protocols. This serves to ensure consistency of care and mitigates liability. NPS personnel transfer between parks during their careers. National protocols provide EMS uniformity despite transfers. Medical legal risks for physicians serving as medical advisors are also mitigated because standard protocols are nationally approved by the branch chief of emergency services and national medical advisor(s). Protocols are carefully vetted (sometimes at NPS EMS national conferences) before they are adopted. Ongoing feedback on current protocols from PEMS-MAs, rangers, and the Washington Support Office leadership is vital to modifying protocols as park needs change. In addition, a national NPS EMS advisory board composed of regional EMS coordinators, national medical advisors, and the branch chief of emergency services may convene to guide protocol revisions.

RM-51 protocols have two components: standing orders and base hospital communication failure orders. Standing orders have a stepwise structure. Step 1 is a reminder to assess a patient's airway, breathing, and circulation prior to any other steps. Step 2 highlights what pertinent findings should be sought in assessing patients within the protocol selected. Remaining standing orders systematically address field management of the presenting complaint. Communication failure orders (radio failure orders) outline procedures to follow if communication is lost between field and base hospital personnel, or when a radio connection cannot be established. These orders typically list procedural and/or medication administration recommendations relevant to the chosen protocol and can be enacted without a direct physician order. Box 116-1 lists RM-51 protocols.

All medications listed in the Parkmedic scope of practice are described in the RM-51 drug section (Box 116-2). Each medication description includes the scope of practice level (i.e.,

BOX 116-2 Medications Within the Scope of Practice for Parkmedics to Administer

Acetaminophen	Dexamethasone	Ipratropium
Acetazolamide	Dextrose 50%	Magnesium sulfate
Activated charcoal	Diltiazem	Midazolam
Adenosine	Diphenhydramine	Morphine sulfate
Albuterol	Dopamine	Naloxone
Amiodarone	Epinephrine	Nifedipine
Aspirin	Erythromycin ophthalmic	Nitroglycerine
Atropine sulfate	Fentanyl	Ondansetron
Bacitracin ointment	Glucagon	Oxytocin
Calcium gluconate	Glucose paste	Pralidoxime chloride
Cefazolin sodium	Hydromorphone	Sodium bicarbonate
	Ibuprofen	

Adapted from National Park Service Reference Manual #51 version: 01/01/2015 (internal), University of California San Francisco Fresno Collaborative Learning Environment.

EMT, Parkmedic, paramedic), medication class, mechanism of action, time to onset by route administered, duration of action, indications and contraindications, available formulations, age-appropriate dosing, additional notes, and cross-references to protocols that use the medication. An example is shown for acetaminophen (Figure 116-3).

RM-51 procedural protocols are formatted similarly (Box 116-3). For each procedure, absolute and relative indications and contraindications are listed. In addition, potential complications, equipment requirements, procedural steps, notes, and cross-references are presented. The scope of practice is the first line of the instructions. Some procedures (e.g., Gamow bag, King tube, nasogastric or orogastric tube) are listed as "per Local EMS Medical Advisor approved extended scope of practice" (i.e., the authority to determine the scope of practice resides within each park).

LOCAL CONTROL OF EXTENDED SCOPE OF PRACTICE

Decisions about which EMS training levels (I to VI) are to be deployed within an individual park are based on park needs, certifications of available rangers, and PEMS-MA recommendations.[31]

Acetaminophen (Tylenol)

Scope	EMT, Parkmedic, Paramedic.
Class	Antipyretic, analgesic.
Action	Elevates pain threshold and readjusts hypothalamic temperature-regulatory center.
Onset	PO/PR: 20 minutes.
Duration	4 hours.
Indications	Altitude illness. Febrile seizure. Fever. Mild pain.
Contraindications	Known hypersensitivity (rare).
Form	325 or 500 mg tablets. 160 mg/5 mL liquid.
Dosage	> 10–Adult: 1000 (975) mg PO every 4–6 hours. Do not exceed 4,000 mg in 24 hours. 0–10 yr: 15 mg/kg PO every 4–6 hours, max dose 1,000 mg. Do not exceed 4000 mg in 24 hours.
Notes	Small quantities of acetaminophen may be supplied to any person if requested for self-administration. The person should be offered an evaluation. A PCR does not need to be filled out if the person declines the evaluation and appears well. **REFERENCE PROCEDURE:** *When to Initiate a PCR (Patient Care Report/Run Sheet).* If the person appears acutely ill in your judgement, do your best to convince the person of the need for evaluation. A PCR shall be completed in this instance, even if the evaluation is declined. In general, acetaminophen and ibuprofen are interchangeable. The decision should be based on patient preference and contraindications.

Cross Reference

Procedures:	Protocols:	Drugs:
When to Initiate a PCR (Patient Care Report/Run Sheet)	Altitude Illness Bites and Stings Burns Childbirth Electrical and Lightning Injuries Eye Trauma Frostbite General Medical Illness – Adult Minor or Isolated Extremity Trauma Pediatric – Medical Illness/Fever Respiratory Distress Seizures Vaginal Bleeding	Ibuprofen (Motrin, Advil)

NPS EMS Field Manual
Version: 05/12

Drugs 3000-P

FIGURE 116-3 Standard formatting for medications approved for use in the current Parkmedic manual. *(Adapted from National Park Service Reference Manual 51 version 01/01/2015 [internal] University of California San Francisco Fresno Collaborative Learning Environment [UCSF CLE]. www.fresno.ucsf.edu/em/parkmedic/downloads/lemadocs/ParkmedicProtocol.pdf.)*

BOX 116-3 Procedures Within the Scope of Practice of Parkmedics

Automated external defibrillation	Fracture-dislocation	Oxygen administration
Base contact criteria	Gamow bag	Pelvic stabilization
Blood glucose determination	Intraosseous access	Rectal drug administration
Capnography	Intravenous access and intravenous fluid	Spine immobilization
Cardioversion defibrillation	administration	Standard reporting format
Continuous positive airway pressure	King tube	Transcutaneous pacing
Electronic control device dart removal	Mucosal atomizer device	Transtracheal jet insufflation
Endotracheal intubation	Multicasualty incident reporting format	Twelve-lead electrocardiogram
Endotracheal tube introducer	Nasogastric orogastric tube	When to initiate a patient care record
Epinephrine autoinjector	Needle thoracostomy	Wound care
Foreign body airway obstruction	Nerve agent antidote kit–Mark I	

Adapted from National Park Service Reference Manual #51 version: 01/01/2015 (internal), University of California San Francisco Fresno Collaborative Learning Environment.

NEEDS ASSESSMENT

RM-51 policies help parks perform evaluations of the EMS program at least every 3 years through the "needs assessment" process. Needs assessment is used to evaluate EMS (versus contemporary standards) and to match the local EMS program size to operational needs. The volume and types of calls, transport times, and local and regional available resources are taken into account. Each park's needs are individually judged. A small park near a metropolitan EMS catchment area (e.g., Adams National Historic Park, Massachusetts) may require only that providers have basic life support response certification. A large remote park with a high visitation rate (e.g., Yellowstone National Park) will need a more sophisticated program. A needs assessment process creates an EMS plan to guide each park's EMS program.

LEVEL OF EMS TRAINING OF NATIONAL PARK SERVICE PROVIDERS

Required EMS training levels (I to VI) depend on identified needs, park resources, and the number of cardiac event EMS responses. The EMS plan requires input from the PEMS-MA for parks providing level IV to VI services. A key distinction between level V and VI prehospital EMS care is paramedics' more sophisticated approach to cardiac emergencies (e.g., advanced training in rhythm interpretation and cardiac medication administration).

Many parks do not use level VI providers (paramedics). Those that do have paramedic services often contract with local EMS systems. Mutual aid agreements to provide paramedic coverage may be subcontracted (by season or to a specified area of the park with high visitor density) as part of a larger EMS system. Subcontracted medics are not NPS personnel. The EMS Plan for Lake Mead National Recreational Area (in Nevada and Arizona) includes seasonal level VI service through a regional EMS system. Parks rarely employ rangers to act exclusively as level VI EMS providers. Most EMS rangers are also federal law enforcement officers. Several large parks (e.g., Yosemite, Yellowstone, Grand Canyon, and Lake Mead) have dual-role rangers who act as both law enforcement officers and level VI medics. Parkmedic (level V) certification offers sufficiently advanced medical interventions without paramedic (level VI) cost and training requirements.

PARK EMS MEDICAL ADVISOR ROLE

EMS providers are not independent practitioners. RM-51 standing orders reviewed and signed by a PEMS-MA provide the legal basis for EMS providers to perform procedures and administer medications. An EMS provider's prehospital services are considered to be an extension of the licensed physician who has signed the RM-51 standing orders. Without standing orders, a level V to VI EMT is only authorized to operate under the skill level of a level IV EMT, regardless of prior medical training. Medical advisors may create park-specific standing orders not listed in RM-51. Park-specific orders must be approved by the EMS Field Manual Review Board prior to use. New protocols, procedures, or drugs may be approved for local level use or added to RM-51. Each medical advisor may restrict the range of RM-51 standing orders for use in the park without need for review by the Washington Support Office.

Medical Oversight

The PEMS-MA assumes responsibilities analogous to an urban EMS system's medical director. PEMS-MAs provide medical control, including policy review, protocol development and incident reviews; maintain quality assurance and continuous quality improvement (CQI) processes; and provide continuing education and access to larger annual training events. Park EMS plans that provide automated external defibrillator service or level IV to VI services are required to have a PEMS-MA. Parks with level III programs are encouraged to have a PEMS-MA.

Medical Control

Medical control is both offline and online. Online medical control allows direct communication between a physician and an EMS provider to make real-time recommendations during patient care. This ability is ideal for advanced life support care delivery or when prolonged field times are encountered. An example of the importance of online control (i.e., via radio) was seen when a Sequoia National Park Parkmedic received medical advice while caring for a solo climber with a femoral fracture on a ledge on 14,000-foot Mt Tyndall. During this 53-hour rescue, the Parkmedic administered intravenous fluids and pain medications overnight while awaiting a National Guard Blackhawk helicopter evacuation.[56] Medical control from a provider with a strong background in prehospital care delivery is preferred. Hospital-based emergency physicians often serve as PEMS-MAs. A base hospital emergency department physician with local EMS base hospital certification can provide 24-hour online medical control. EMS providers communicate with a dedicated physician or mobile intensive care nurses familiar with Parkmedic procedures and protocols. Standing orders (i.e., offline medical control or radio failure orders) can help guide advanced life support care if online medical control cannot be established. Offline medical control includes review of RM-51 standing orders.

QUALITY ASSURANCE AND CONTINUING QUALITY IMPROVEMENT

Quality assurance and continuous quality improvement (CQI) are separate processes to confirm delivery of appropriate care and identify means to improve future care. In quality assurance, the EMS coordinator, EMS supervisor, and, as needed, PEMS-MA regularly audit each provider's patient care records. Any cases judged to put a provider at risk of disciplinary action are reviewed by the PEMS-MA.[31] The NPS uses a single electronic format patient care record developed by emsCharts. This allows national-level CQI analysis.[51]

The CQI process is used to evaluate each park's program. It has retrospective, concurrent, and prospective components. Retrospective CQI personnel review electronic patient care records to evaluate trends in care across providers.[16] For example, within SEKI there are approximately 300 to 350 annual EMS contacts and approximately 10 patient contacts per each level IV or V provider. This allows specific feedback to individual providers and enables evaluation of cohort trends. The concurrent CQI process describes quality improvement when care is actually being delivered.[17] This may be performed by a supervisor (or person at the level of EMS coordinator) observing care of a patient. The prospective CQI process targets areas for future improvement using continuing education.[18] Through systematic chart review and direct observation, EMS providers can receive regular feedback to reinforce successful care delivery and identify skills that may be improved.

CONTINUING EDUCATION

Continuing education is mandated to maintain NREMT certification, address educational gaps identified by CQI processes, and provide opportunities for group trainings in critical, but infrequently used, clinical skills (e.g., endotracheal intubation, intraosseous line placement). Continuing education schedules should include monthly sessions with interspersed time-intensive skill refreshers and drills.

REFRESHER COURSES FOR NREMT RECERTIFICATION

The National Registry does not specifically recognize the Parkmedic level of training. Parkmedics certified prior to 2013 recertify at the EMT-intermediate (I-85) level. Parkmedics who were certified more recently recertify at the AEMT level. Requirements for a level V provider are 36 hours of documented continuing education sessions and completion of a 36-hour advanced life support refresher course (see Table 116-1). As previously noted, a 4-week Parkmedic refresher course is held at UCSF Fresno biennially. Urban EMS advanced life support refresher courses also satisfy this requirement. Because level IV EMT refresher courses are shorter (24 hours), they are often conducted within local parks.

CONTINUING EDUCATION SESSIONS

Monthly sessions fulfill continuing education requirements for NREMT recertification and prospective CQI program needs. CQI data–driven topics review recent cases to increase awareness of the EMS provider's responsibilities. Each park's PEMS-MA conducts continuing education sessions, which typically last 3 to 4 hours each. The medical advisor's handbook[31] recommends that each session include 1 hour each for didactics, procedural practice, and quality improvement, with time allotted for questions and answers. NPS continuing education sessions can be held indoors or in natural environments as guided by didactic goals (Figure 116-4). See Figure 116-5 for a sample continuing education schedule for Parkmedic and EMT-basic providers.

MULTICASUALTY INCIDENT DRILLS

Many parks perform multicasualty incident drills to teach EMS providers triage policies and practices using the incident command system. RM-51 includes multicasualty incident triage algorithms and procedure protocols with checklists, assigned roles, and explicit responsibilities for reference. RM-51 contains triage algorithms, including simple triage and rapid treatment (START) and a pediatric algorithm known as JumpSTART.[21,48] These algorithms have been widely used in the United States since the 1980s, although little published literature has examined their effectiveness.[4] Simulations using these drills (e.g., tabletop scenarios, elaborate high-fidelity exercises) are effective teaching tools (Figure 116-6). Participants should be guided to consider how each simulation could improve future prehospital care encounters. A post hoc review of an NPS backcountry lightning multicasualty incident (with multiple adult and pediatric victims) found that triage tags were not used (not part of helicopter rescue equipment) despite decades of annual high-fidelity scenario training exercises, including with a triage algorithm and tag use. Despite this, an improvised on-scene triage method, while not

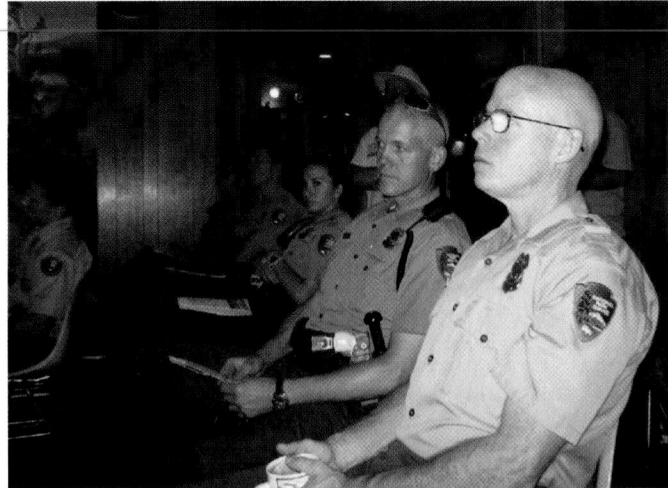

FIGURE 116-4 Sequoia and Kings Canyon National Park rangers participating in classroom-based continuing education. (*Courtesy Susanne J. Spano.*)

mirroring START/JumpSTART classifications, maintained rapid, appropriate evacuation priorities.[52] In addition to reviewing checklists and algorithms, drills should be designed to identify potential ways in which communications and care can be made more robust during future multicasualty incidents.

SPECIALIZED SUPPORT ASSETS

Specialized support services (e.g., air transport, technical rescue teams) are essential components to ensure that visitors are protected within the NPS. Specialized teams and equipment are available for local emergencies and nationwide deployment if required by a national crisis.

PERSONNEL AND NATIONAL RESPONSE

Each park ranger has multiple responsibilities within a park and must respond nationwide at the direction of the NPS director in event of an emergency.[3] Many full-time park rangers concurrently maintain training and certification in law enforcement, fire management, incident command system operations, search and rescue (SAR), and EMS. Additional training may be needed for some rangers in certain parks. Parks with large bodies of water may need rangers with scuba certification to maintain submerged cultural resources (e.g., Dry Tortugas National Park, Florida) and recover victims and wreckage from accidents (e.g., Isle Royale National Park, Michigan). Parks adjacent to international borders, or with large backcountry expanses, may benefit from tactical law enforcement teams, horse-mounted patrol rangers, and K9 units for law enforcement and lost person searches.

Park personnel may also request additional help from rescuers with technical rescue skills when a large response is needed. These technical rescuers can be found within the NPS or within community-based rescue organizations. In a request for mutual aid, park personnel may be temporarily reallocated to another park's jurisdiction when incident management requires such a move. Mutual aid responses enable a larger search effort than a single park could mount on its own. For example, the exhaustive search for veteran backcountry ranger Randy Morgenson in SEKI included 48 ground searchers, 4 helicopters, and 8 dog teams from park, military, and community SAR teams on just a single day.[2]

The NPS uses a 24/7 emergency incident communication center to report major incidents. The center (located in Shenandoah National Park, Virginia) expedites communications from field rangers to the director when a large coordinated response is needed.[30] The National Response Framework is the unified national response preplan for large-scale disasters and emergencies. NPS resources are a component of the National Response

Parkmedic CE Schedule 2008-2009

Meetings are at 9am. Two week schedule change notice can be given to Debbie Brenchley (EMS-C).

August 2008: Summer Break from CE

September 2008: Monday, September 29th
Topic: Chest Pain, Wounds, Eye injury, Lightning/Electrical
Procedures: Wound care, Combitube
Medications: Aspirin, Nitroglycerin, Neosporin Ophthalmic Ointment, Morphine
Resident Instructors: Drs. Schilling, Le, Kang

October 2008: Wednesday, October 8th
Topic: Allergic Reactions, Bites and Stings, Pediatrics
Procedures: Fracture dislocations, Epipen
Medications: Benadryl, Epinephrine, Morphine, Oxygen
Resident Instructors: Drs. Spano, Tsukamaki

November 2008: Monday, November 24th
Topic: Frostbite, Hypothermia, Burns, AMS
Procedures: Base Hospital Contact Criteria, Standard Reporting Format Accucheck
Medications: Bacitracin, Narcan, Glucose paste, Glucagon, Dextrose
Resident Instructors: Drs. Rubio, Urdanetta, Uranga

December 2008: Monday, December 9th
Topic: Abdominal pain, Cardiac Arrest, Childbirth
Procedures: AED, IV access, O_2 administration, Combitube, Delivery
Medications: Atropine, Epinephrine, Lidocaine, Bicarbonate, Oxytocin
Resident Instructors: Drs. Armenian, Caldwell, Eandi

January 2009: January Course

February 2009: Monday, February 23rd
Topic: Transport Decisions
Procedures: Intraosseous access, Rectal Drug administration, Transtracheal Jet Insufflation
Medications: Tylenol, Ibuprofen, Narcan, Glucose paste, Dextrose
Resident Instructors: Drs. Karaelias, Rodigin, Pham

March 2009: Monday, March 23rd
Topic: Ingestions / Poisoning / Seizures, Near Drowning
Procedures: Combitube, Epipen
Medications: Ipecac, Charcoal, Midazolam, Magnesium, Epinephrine
Resident Instructors: Drs. Ruegner, DeShields, Chacon-Lopez

April 2009: Monday, April 27th
Topic: GSW / booby traps, Trauma, Shock
Procedures: Fracture and dislocations, Dislocation reduction, Spine Immobilization, Needle thoracostomy
Medications: Ancef, Morphine, Reglan
Resident Instructors: Drs. James, Aggrewal, Hamilton

May 2009: Monday, May 25th
Topic: Altitude, Respiratory distress, Heat Illness
Procedures: Gamow bag
Medications: Nifedipine, Acetazolamide, Albuterol, Atrovent, Dexamethasone, Lasix
Resident Instructors: Drs. Schmitt, Chae, Kahwaji

June 2009: EMT REFRESHER

July 2009: MCI DRILL

FIGURE 116-5 Sample Parkmedic continuing education schedule for a park that has EMT and Parkmedic providers. *(Courtesy Susanne J. Spano and Ana Uranga.)*

Framework.[9] Preplan considerations include cataloguing qualified personnel, equipment, preexisting medical protocols, and communications plans that can operate between agencies and organizations at the local, state, or national level.

VOLUNTEERS-IN-PARKS PROGRAM

Former NPS Director George B. Hartzog, Jr., established the Volunteer-in-Parks (VIP) program in 1969, allowing the NPS to accept and use voluntary assistance from the public.[34] Anyone can be a VIP. Volunteer opportunities range from guiding interpretive programs to providing medical direction and emergency mountain rescue. Most PEMS-MAs are VIPs. Mountain rescue VIP positions are available in Denali National Park, Yosemite National Park, and Mt Rainier National Park.[6,11,26] VIPs are granted immunity from liability pursuant to the Federal Tort Claims Act.[55] If a negligence lawsuit is filed against a VIP, the United States is substituted as the defendant. VIP opportunities change often and can be found through the U.S. national volunteering site, through the NPS website, or by asking park personnel directly for information about them.[1,41] Volunteers are recognized for their efforts in donating more than 250 hours (free interagency pass), 500 hours (master volunteer ranger), and 4000 hours (presidential volunteer ranger) of service.[28] Volunteers have an enormous impact on the health and well-being of communities. According to the 2012 VIP report, 257,000 volunteers donated 6,784,971 hours, the equivalent of 3262 full-time employees.[32]

TECHNICAL RESCUES

Air operations and SAR teams are key specialized resources that complement an EMS plan. The NPS (e.g., Denali National Park, Alaska) uses advanced capabilities of fixed-wing and rotary aircraft and trained SAR technicians to save lives that might otherwise be lost.[8]

AIR OPERATIONS

The NPS has fixed-wing and rotary wing capabilities for carrying out park operations (i.e., EMS, law enforcement, and wildland fires management).[30] Given the prolonged transport times from remote national park locations to many level 1 trauma centers, parks may incorporate a neighboring EMS system's regional air ambulance services as part of their NPS EMS plan. Military aircraft can also be used for rescues because they typically have more robust operational abilities (e.g., can operate at higher altitudes, can carry heavier loads) than do civilian aircraft. In addition, military air operations are not subject to civilian flight restrictions (e.g., a ban on helicopter travel at night in mountainous terrain).[52] The U.S. Army National Guard and Reserve and U.S. Air Force Air National Guard units perform NPS rescues (e.g., Mt Denali, Mt Rainier, Yosemite, and Sequoia and Kings Canyon). Fire management is a large seasonal responsibility in larger western parks. Private helicopter services are often subcontracted (from May to October) for this purpose. In emergencies, these aircraft can be used to deliver personnel and supplies to remote areas of a park

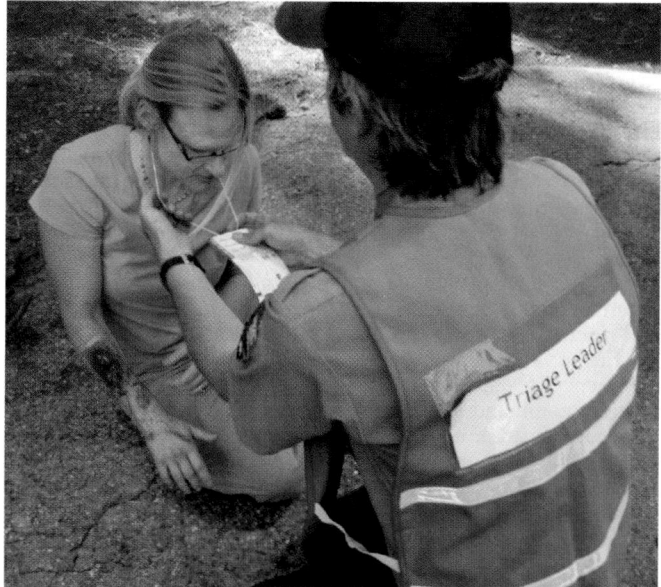

FIGURE 116-6 Multicasualty incident drill triage practice in Sequoia and Kings Canyon National Park. *(Courtesy Susanne J. Spano.)*

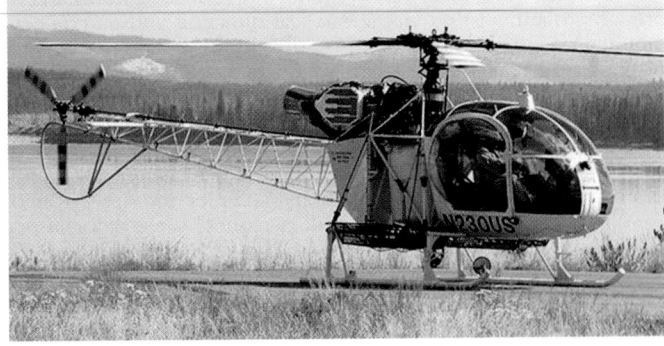

FIGURE 116-7 Wildland fire helicopter H 1109, a rental helicopter from Inyo National Forest (Aérospatiale SA 315B Lama, not litter capable) used in Sequoia and Kings Canyon National Park. These helicopters are not designed for medical rescues and do not accommodate supine patients, even in emergencies. *(Courtesy Jason Bauwens.)*

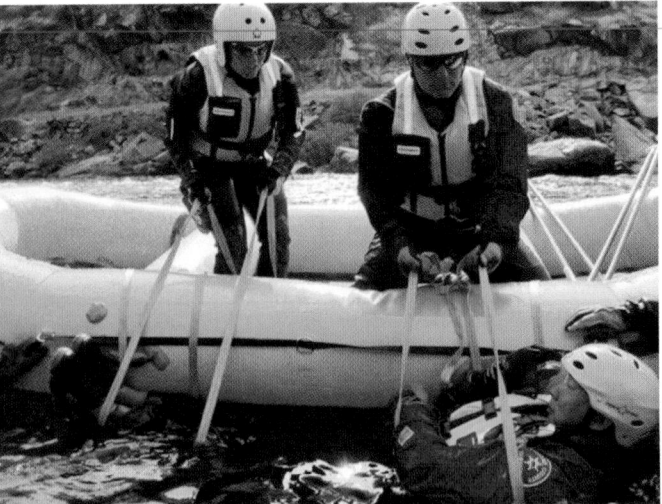

FIGURE 116-8 Swiftwater rescue training can include methods to safely transport an unresponsive victim in a paddleboat with minimal effort to the rescue crew. *(Courtesy Susanne J. Spano.)*

for rescue operations. They are not configured as an air ambulance and may not be able to accommodate a supine patient (Figure 116-7). The NPS also supports a fleet of fixed-wing and rotary wing aircraft in Grand Canyon, Death Valley, Lake Mead, Glen Canyon, and Big Bend National Parks, and throughout Alaska.[30]

The NPS branch chief of search and rescue, Ken Phillips, developed the National Search and Rescue Academy training manual on helicopter rescue. It includes sections on hoist rescues, helicopter rappelling, and helicopter short hauls.[46] Hoisting involves lifting a victim attached to a rescue hook via a hoist cable. Helicopter rappelling allows a rescuer to be inserted into a rescue location. Short hauls use fixed lines directly under helicopters to move a rescuer or victim. Short hauls entail prolonged rescuer and victim exposures to environmental conditions but decrease the need for the helicopter pilot to maintain prolonged hovering close to unforgiving terrain. They also increase the haul-load weight capacity because the load is situated directly under the helicopter, which minimizes lateral forces. Load-bearing equipment designed specifically for helicopter rescue use includes rescue bags, collapsible baskets, nets, seats, trail lines, straps, and harness systems. To safely implement helicopter rescue teams, careful training is essential. Flight operations involve inherent risks that may be fatal to air crews not well versed in helicopter techniques.[12]

SEARCH AND RESCUE TEAMS

National parks provide opportunities for citizens to hike, bike, swim, climb, and spelunk and to travel cross country within vast stretches of wilderness. This leads to the need for SAR capabilities. NPS has been at the forefront of SAR training in wilderness settings.[8] Anthologies describing prior NPS SAR events include a rescue on Yosemite's Half Dome in a lightning storm, the search for lost Sequoia ranger Randy Morgenson, and park-specific reviews of accidental deaths in the national parks since their inception.[2,12,13,24]

SAR teams typically employ several specialized units (e.g., mountaineering unit, jeep unit, mounted patrol or "posse" unit, and rescue dog unit with trained dog and handler teams) acting in concert to contribute to the overall rescue effort. All team members are trained in wilderness SAR management and the incident command system.

Mountaineer units are the most commonly deployed search teams in backcountry settings. An effective mountaineer team has members proficient in swiftwater rescue, high-angle rescue, and ground-searching methods. Swiftwater rescue training may use rope rescue systems, swimming techniques, and rescue aids to reach difficult areas and approach dangerous swiftwater environments during both day and night conditions[47] (Figure 116-8). High-angle rescue requires specific training (e.g., in common knots, principles of rope systems, rigging physics) and regular

practice in order to establish safe anchors, belay systems, mainline lifting systems, and victim extraction techniques[27] (Figure 116-9). Ground-searching tactics enable teams to locate lost persons who are alert and signaling for help, as well as unresponsive victims or subjects intentionally evading search efforts.[23] Methods include mantracking, hasty searching (i.e., techniques that are rapid and cursory), and grid searches (i.e., systematic and time consuming). Mantracking techniques using tracking tools, measurements, and a trained eye to identify signs of recent movement through an area and can reliably mark every step a subject makes. Expert teams can track a lost person crossing manmade features, such as a road or bridge.[53] Each of these specialized areas is based on simple principles, but all require diligent practice because skills may deteriorate over time. Certification courses allow opportunities for rescuers to refresh skills.

FUTURE DIRECTIONS

National park medicine is increasingly focused on the role of prevention. New rescue tactics, innovative medical technology, and ultralight and durable outdoor gear will undoubtedly affect how rescue teams and victims interact in wilderness settings, but

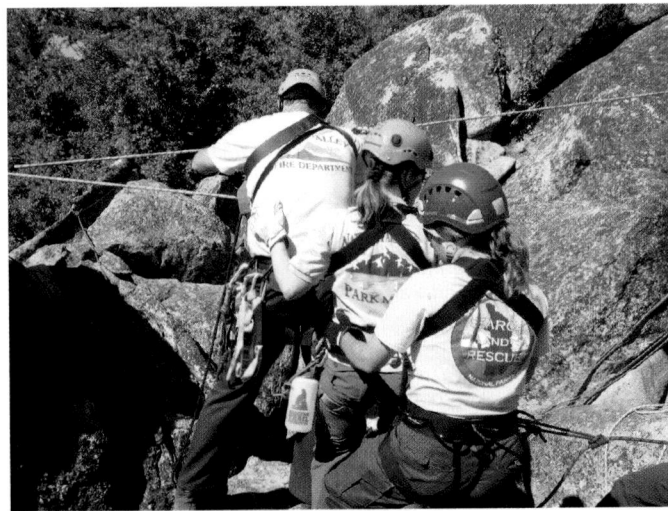

FIGURE 116-9 High-angle rescue training in Sequoia and Kings Canyon National Park. Training may involve multiagency events with Parkmedics, NPS search and rescue teams, and local fire rescue members who may be part of a future search and rescue effort. *(Courtesy Susanne J. Spano.)*

preventive measures are essential to sustaining public enjoyment of backcountry spaces. Educational public outreach already occurs in many national parks. Preventive SAR efforts are still in their infancy. It continues to be difficult to design and conduct research studies to measure whether costs and suffering are reduced by educational programs. Full conversion to a uniform electronic patient care record will allow the NPS EMS to identify trends in a way not previously possible. In the last decades, the NPS has developed an efficient prehospital response system to rapidly respond to accidents. The charge of future leaders within the NPS EMS community is to develop public education tools (e.g., educational outreach, statistical analysis) for accident prevention.

REFERENCES

Complete references used in this text are available online at expertconsult.inkling.com.

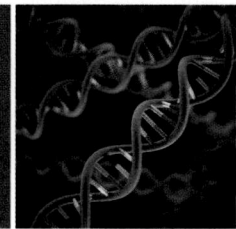

CHAPTER 117
Genomics in Wilderness Medicine

TATUM S. SIMONSON AND MARTIN J. MACINNIS

Human diseases involve disruptions in physiologic homeostasis. Genetic causes of disease are often explored by comparing cohorts of affected cases with unaffected controls or investigating inherited variations within families using linkage analysis. Diseases may be attributed to both genetic and environmental factors, and many (e.g., pulmonary hypertension, heart disease, cancer) are amenable to genetic research because they occur commonly with readily identifiable phenotypes. Similarly, some physical features (e.g., height or eye color) can be easily studied in a genetic context because they are common and stable over time.

Genetic studies on acute responses to environmental exposures (e.g., hypoxia, extremes of cold or heat, high levels of ultraviolet radiation) are more complicated. It may be difficult to standardize study conditions, identify proper "control" populations, and obtain appropriate sample sizes. Despite these limitations, genetic studies of wilderness-related diseases (based on individuals who have adapted to extreme conditions and those who have not) are currently under way. Many studies have focused on high-altitude adaptations, and others have explored responses to cold, ultraviolet radiation, and exercise.

GENETIC AND ENVIRONMENTAL INFLUENCES ON THE PHENOTYPE

According to the simplest explanation, *genetics* relates to the influence of the *genotype* (i.e., the sequence of the genome or a specific part of the genome) on the phenotype. A *phenotype* is the product of genetics and environment. The possible forms that a phenotype may take are called *traits* (Figure 117-1). Although the overwhelming majority of factors in the human genome are identical, numerous sites vary between individuals. These variable sites are referred to as *polymorphisms*. One category of variation is the *single nucleotide polymorphism* (SNP) or *single nucleotide variant* (SNV) (i.e., a single base pair that differs between individuals). Possible variants for a SNP/SNV are called *alleles* (or, more simply, genetic variants). Every human cell is diploid and so contains two copies of each *autosome*; therefore, each *locus* (position) in the genome has two alleles. These two alleles form the genotype at a particular locus (Figure 117-2). The genome guides the creation of proteins that carry out most biologic processes in our bodies. Alterations to the genome's nucleic acid sequence (e.g., alterations that influence structure, function, or expression of gene products, namely, proteins) can alter the phenotype.

If genetics describes the information in our genome, then *environment* refers to everything else. It may be easy to misconstrue environment to represent only our physical surroundings (i.e., altitude, cold, ultraviolet radiation); however, in the context of genetics, environment contains *all* of the external factors experienced by the organism (both abiotic and biotic). Genetics may be complex, but defining the effect of environment (in this broad context) on the phenotype is equally challenging. It is often the case that combined interactions between genetic and environmental factors ultimately create the variations in phenotypes.

Genetics is often used to explain the source of *variation* in phenotypes (i.e., to answer the question of whether individuals and populations are different because they differ genetically). To study the genetic basis of a phenotype in a population, that phenotype must vary (i.e., without phenotypic variation there are no phenotypic differences to explain).

Heritability is the ratio of genetic variance to total variance. Most genetic studies are interested in narrow-sense heritability (h^2), that is, the proportion of phenotypic variance attributable to *additive* genetic variance (i.e., variance from alleles whose contributions to the trait are independent of other alleles). This particular measure of heritability is used most often because it is related to the degree of resemblance between relatives.[246] The contribution of genetic and environmental variation to phenotypic variation is specific to the population under investigation. Even if genetic differences explain the majority of phenotypic variations in one population, environmental differences could explain the majority of phenotypic variations in another population.

As an example, imagine three human populations in which (1) everyone demonstrates an identical high tolerance of cold; (2) everyone demonstrates an identical low tolerance of cold; and (3) tolerance of cold is normally distributed (Figure 117-3). Genetics and environment unequivocally contribute to this phenotype. The question is whether *variation* in cold tolerance is due to genetic or environmental differences between individuals. The first two populations exhibit no variation. Whether genetic or environmental factors contribute more to a trait with nonexistent variation is moot. In contrast, there is considerable phenotypic variation in the third population. This population lends itself to the study of genetic versus environmental contributions to variation in cold tolerance. Variations in phenotype must exist for meaningful questions to be asked (e.g., Does a particular polymorphism explain the variation in cold tolerance, or do differences in diet explain the variation in cold tolerance?). Although

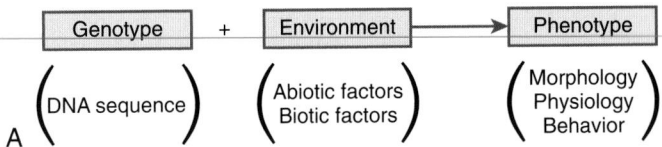

Phenotype	Qualitative traits	Quantitative traits
Eye color	Blue, green, brown, etc.	Density of pigment
Altitude tolerance	Low, moderate, high	Lake Louise Score
HIF1A gene expression	Increased, decreased	mRNA quantity
Enzyme activity	Increased, decreased	Enzyme activity

FIGURE 117-1 A, Relationship between genotype, environment, and phenotype. Subcategories are provided in parentheses below the boxes. **B,** Difference between a phenotype and a trait, and the difference between qualitative and quantitative traits. Note that a given phenotype can usually be examined in a qualitative or quantitative manner.

populations 1 and 2 are not very amenable to elucidating the role of genetic and environmental factors in isolation, they can be used to test hypotheses generated from studies performed in population 3. Alternatively, population 1 could be compared with population 2 to identify factors leading to their discrepant cold

tolerances (although differences in ancestry and other potential confounding factors would have to be considered before drawing firm conclusions). For more in-depth discussion of heritability, see the article by Visscher.[246]

ESTABLISHING THE GENETIC BASIS OF A TRAIT

Many studies take advantage of greater genetic similarity between relatives versus nonrelatives to determine if genetics contributes substantially to phenotypic variation. This relationship applies to families as well as larger populations. Comparisons are made using twins, closely related family members, and biogeographic groups (Figure 117-4). See Bouchard and colleagues[35] for a comprehensive discussion of quantitative genetics (Figure 117-5).

Monozygotic (MZ) twins are genetically identical, so phenotypic differences between MZ twins should be entirely due to environmental factors. In contrast, dizygotic (DZ) twins share only approximately 50% of their genomes (the same proportion that nontwin siblings share), and differences within pairs of DZ twins will be due to both genetic and environmental variation. *Twin studies* compare variation between MZ and DZ twin pairs. Greater resemblance within MZ pairs than DZ pairs indicates that genetic differences explain some of the variation. In contrast, similar resemblances within MZ and DZ pairs indicate that genetic differences explain very little of the variation. For more in-depth discussions of twin studies, see publications by Martin,[151] Boomsma,[30] and MacLeod.[148]

Twin studies can be difficult to conduct without large registries, but family studies can be used to gather evidence for a possible genetic basis of a phenotype. Family members are

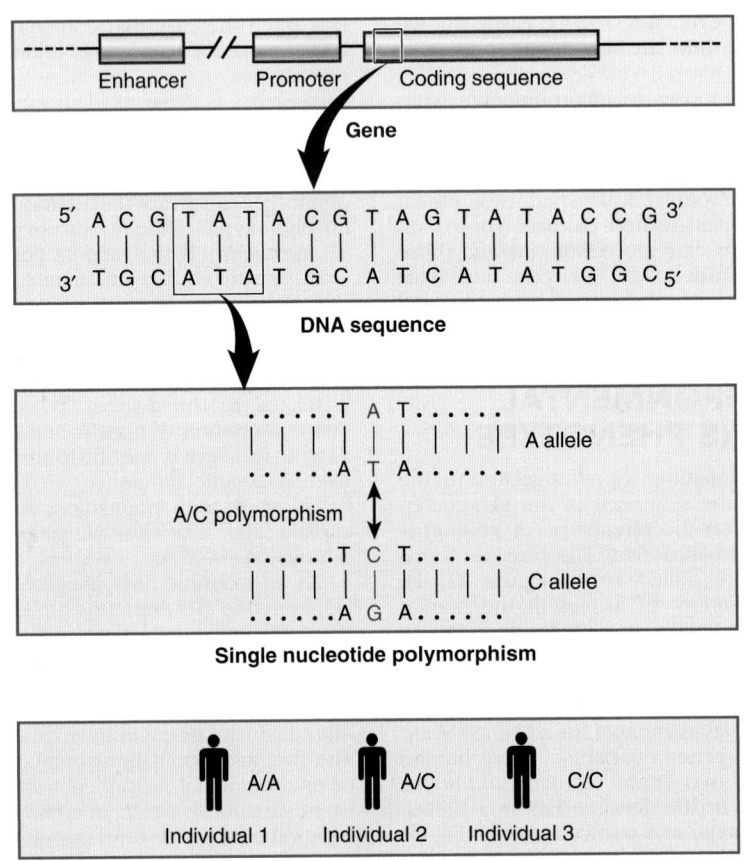

FIGURE 117-2 Schematic illustrating the hierarchy of genes, single nucleotide polymorphisms (SNPs), and alleles. Each individual's genome possesses the gene, but at the identified SNP, individuals possess two alleles (e.g., A or C), which may be the same (homozygous, A/A) or different (heterozygous, A/C).

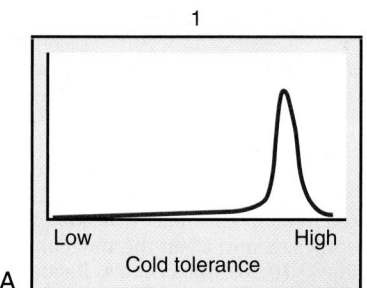
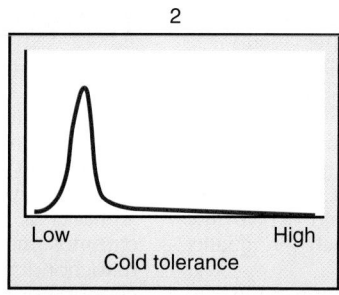
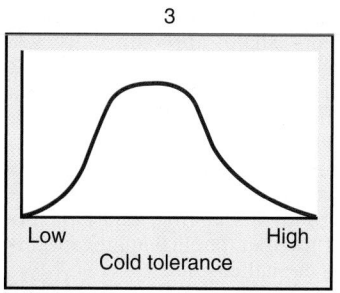

Population	Phenotypic variation	Within-population comparisons	Between-population comparison
1	Low	No	Yes
2	Low	No	Yes
3	High	Yes	Possible*

* Although between-population comparisons are possible with this population, they are not necessary, and a within-population design is preferred.

FIGURE 117-3 A, Three populations with different distributions of cold tolerance. Population 1 has uniformly high cold tolerance; population 2 has uniformly low cold tolerance; and population 3 has a normally distributed cold tolerance. **B,** Information related to potential within- and between-population studies that could be designed. Only population 3 is suitable for within-population comparisons, whereas populations 1 and 2 could be compared with each other but are not suitable for a within-population study of cold tolerance.

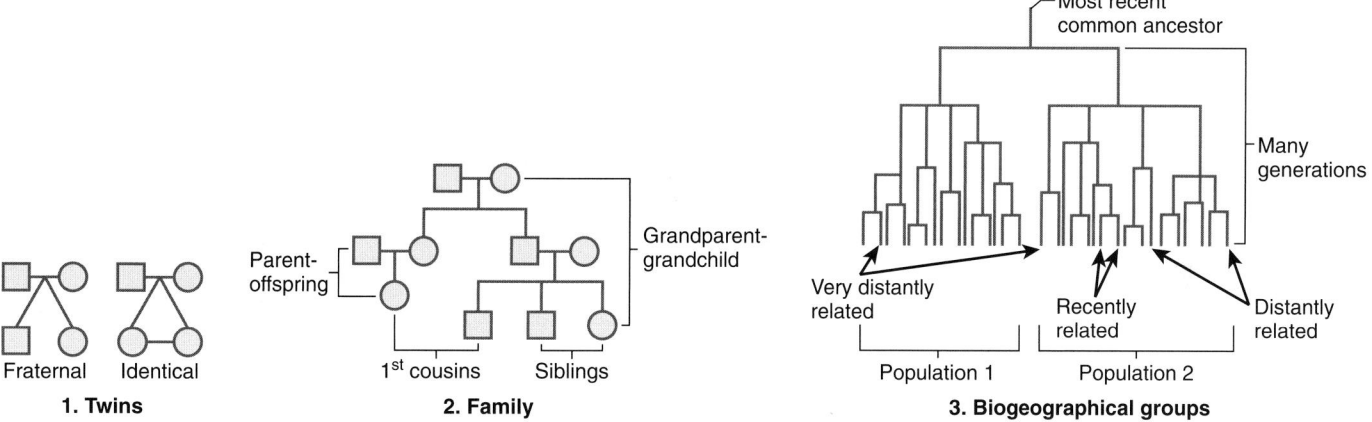

FIGURE 117-4 These schematics demonstrate the relatedness of fraternal and identical twins (1), family members (2), and distantly related populations (3). Pedigrees are not provided in biogeographical groups in order to illustrate the distant relationships that exist between any two populations.

In the early 1860s, Gregor Mendel hypothesized that "unit factors" controlled inheritance based on experiments in pea plants.

Scientists accepted the idea that genetic units were contained on chromosomes in the 1930s.

James Watson and Francis Crick reported the double helical structure of DNA in 1953.

Frederick Sanger developed the first rapid DNA sequencing technology in 1977.

Efforts to sequence the entire human genome gained momentum in the 1990s.

| 1860s | 1930s | 1940s | 1950s | 1960s | 1970s | 1980s | 1990s | 2000s |

Johann Friedrich Miescher succeeded in extracting pure nucleic acids from cells in the 1860s.

Experiments in bacteria and phage elucidated the chemical makeup of "unit factors" was deoxyribonuclease (DNA) in the 1940s.

In 1961, Marshal Nirenberg and colleagues discovered that DNA nucleotides are arranged in consecutive tri-nucleotide codes that comprise 20 amino acids.

In 1983, the locus of the first genetic disease (Huntington's disease) was mapped; the technique used to amplify DNA (polymerase chain reaction, PCR) was invented, leading to rapid analysis of DNA molecules.

In 2001, the draft sequence of the human genome was published; in 2005, HapMap provided haplotype map of the human genome.

FIGURE 117-5 Progress in genetics and genomics from the 1860s to the 2000s.

related to different extents (i.e., sibling-sibling and parent-offspring pairs share approximately 50% of their genomes; grandparent-grandchild and half-siblings, 25%; and first cousins, 12.5%). Statistical models using family data can be employed to determine the extent to which a phenotype is genetic.[31] If a trait is observed to aggregate in families (i.e., it is more common within a family than within the general population), this can be evidence that genetic variation contributes to the trait. Because shared environments among family members could explain the clustering of the trait, familial aggregation is relatively low-quality evidence for heritability.[151]

Members of a biogeographic group are often more similar to each other than to outsiders. Individuals within a population are assumed to be at least distantly related to each other, but more closely related to each other than to members of separate populations. As is the case with familial aggregation, a difference in a trait's prevalence across populations supports (but is not proof of) an influence of genetic variation. Shared environments can also explain the clustering of traits.

Studies establishing the genetic basis of a trait are typically pursued prior to molecular investigations. Researchers should have sufficient evidence to support the hypothesis that genetic differences contribute significantly to the phenotypic variation before they explore how genetic variants contribute to phenotypic variation.

If there is a genetic cause for phenotypic variation, at least one polymorphism will be associated with that phenotype (although the strength of this association may be small). If the phenotype has only two traits (e.g., case and control), the two alleles will be distributed unequally; one allele will be more common in cases and the other allele in controls. If we use the cold tolerance example above, we might find that the C allele of the C450T polymorphism is overrepresented in persons with a high cold tolerance. We would say that the C450T polymorphism is associated with the cold tolerance phenotype: the C allele associated with high cold tolerance (a trait), and the T allele associated with low cold tolerance (a trait). "Associated" is used because this type of study is not a true experiment (i.e., the genetic constitution of an individual is not manipulated). Methods used to identify associations are described in the following sections.

THE ERA OF GENOMICS

Recent advances in genomics have provided unprecedented insight into human variation and its role in disease susceptibility. The vast amount of the coded sequence in the human genome makes up more than 3.3 billion nucleotides of deoxyribonucleic acid (DNA) in the form of adenine (A), thymine (T), guanine (G), and cytosine (C) bases (see Figure 117-2). This genetic alphabet is organized within 22 linear *autosomes* and two sex chromosomes (allosomes; X and Y) in the nucleus and a circular mitochondrial genome (≈16,569 nucleotides) located in the mitochondria organelle of the cell. Nearly all cells (with the exception of mature red blood cells) have two copies of each autosome, two sex chromosomes, and several thousand copies of the mitochondrial genome.

A history of genetics and genomics in medicine is provided in Figure 117-5. First drafts of the human genome sequence, published in 2001, revealed that a relatively small number of genes (20,000 to 25,000) are encoded in our DNA, and many genes have functions similar to those of other organisms (e.g., worms and flies).[124,244] This knowledge supported the use of nonhuman animal models in experiments designed to test functional relevance of human genotype-phenotype relationships (Figure 117-6). Technologic advancements continue to facilitate sequencing efforts, providing extraordinary amounts of information from many human genomes and various other species.

Less than 2% of the human genome encodes proteins. The sequence of these protein-coding genes is transcribed through production of complementary messenger RNAs (mRNAs) and transported to the cytoplasm for translation into proteins based on three-nucleotide codons that represent 20 distinct amino acids. A cell's total collection of transcribed RNA (i.e., mRNA, tRNA, rRNA, and a wide range of nonprotein coding functional RNAs) is called the *transcriptome* (see Omics Revolution, later). A cell's total collection of proteins present at one time is called the *proteome* (Figure 117-7). The number of copies of a protein is highly variable between cell types. An abundant level (≈ 50,000 copies) of nearly 2000 proteins suggests general biochemical "housekeeping" activities in most cells. The transcriptome and proteome of a cell (i.e., which RNA and proteins are expressed and the quantity of each that is present at a given time) are

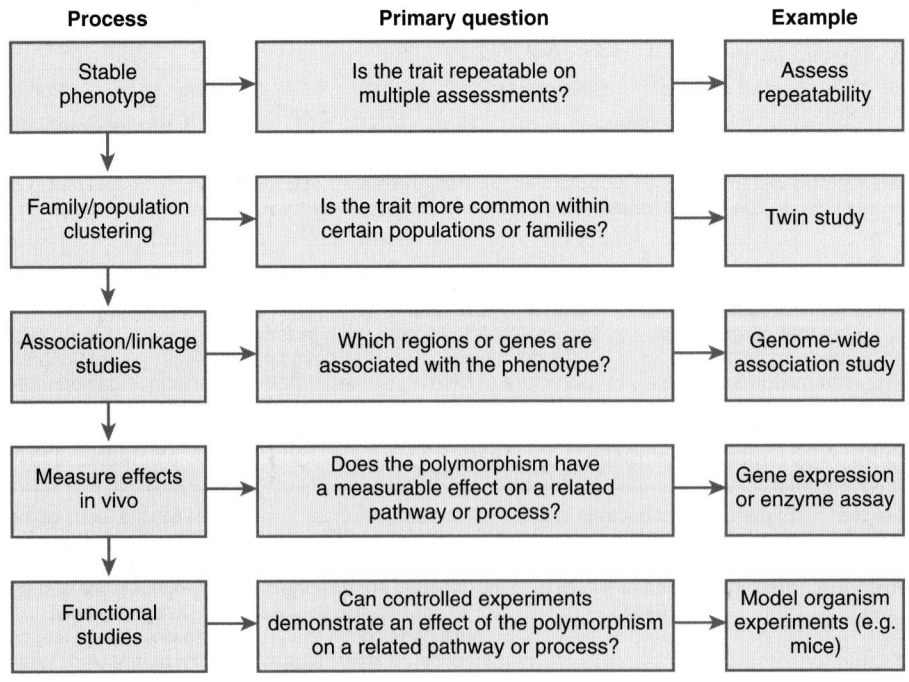

FIGURE 117-6 The typical process of determining whether variation in a particular phenotype is due to genetic variation. For each step in the process, the primary question posed at that step is provided, as well as an example of the type of analysis that would be performed.

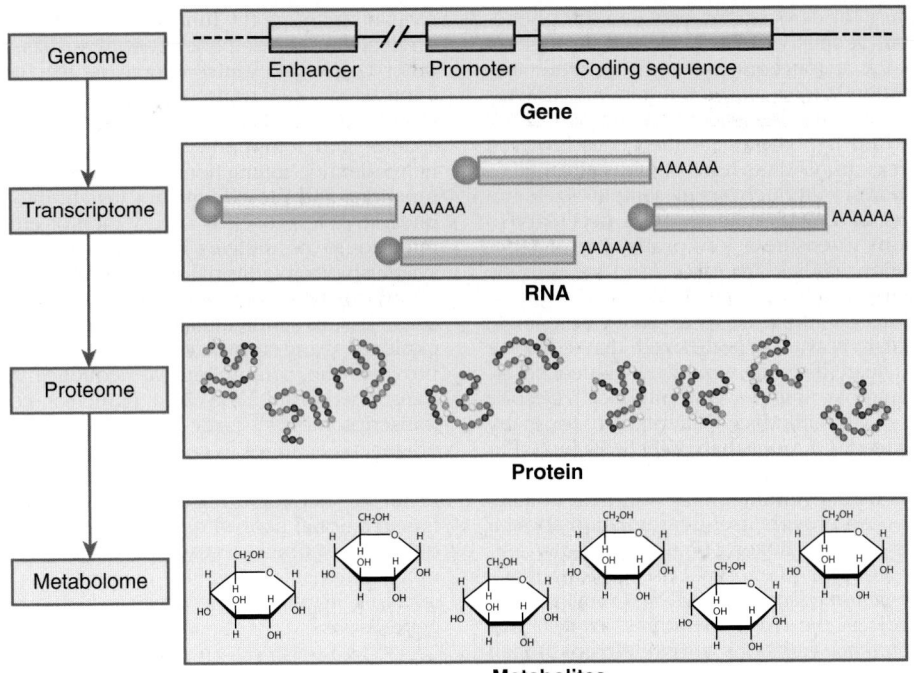

FIGURE 117-7 Hierarchy of the genome, transcriptome, proteome, and metabolome. The genome consists of genes and intervening sequences. The transcriptome consists of all RNA products transcribed from the genome. The proteome consists of all proteins produced from the transcriptome. The metabolome consists of all metabolites that accumulate in the cell, largely resulting from reactions and processes carried out by proteins. Note that the structure is hierarchical but that the lower levels can influence the upper levels. For example, metabolites could alter gene expression, which could modify the transcriptome, proteome, and metabolome.

determined by the genome in the context of the cell's development and the environment.

HUMAN GENETIC VARIATION

The International HapMap Project sequenced and catalogued SNPs in individuals of varying ethnic backgrounds so that common variations within human genomes could be studied. The initial SNP set included data from individuals of European, Yoruban African, Han Chinese, and Japanese descent.[107] The set was recently expanded to include individuals from more than 11 populations genotyped at more than 1.6 million SNP positions.[109] By showing that SNPs are generally inherited in large *haplotype* "blocks," this project granted insights into *linkage disequilibrium* in humans (i.e., by characterizing a small number of SNP signposts throughout the genome, insights into sequences of DNA are granted)[225] (Figure 117-8). Although the human genome contains more than 10 million common SNPs, characterization of only a subset (250,000 to 500,000) is required to "tag" the variation in human populations.[108]

Using low-cost, high-throughput genotyping methodologies, researchers can scan genomes of thousands of cases (i.e., individuals exhibiting a particular phenotype) and thousands of controls (i.e., individuals not exhibiting the phenotype of interest) to identify genomic regions associated with specific phenotypes. This method has been used to determine genetic links to various diseases (e.g., diabetes, psychiatric disorders, heart disease, and autoimmune disorders).

GENOME-WIDE ASSOCIATION STUDIES

The two primary study designs used to determine which genes and genetic variants are associated with a phenotype are *candidate-gene association studies*[55] and *genome-wide association studies* (GWASs).[97] In a candidate-gene association study, variants of a particular gene (i.e., the candidate) are chosen and tested for associations with a specific phenotype. For each individual, a phenotype is determined and a DNA sample is provided

for genotyping. One or more polymorphisms from the candidate gene are selected and tested for statistical association with the phenotype. Because candidate-gene association studies only examine a very small region of the genome (1 of ≈ 25,000 genes), successful candidate-gene studies require strong hypotheses to select the genes most likely related to the phenotype.

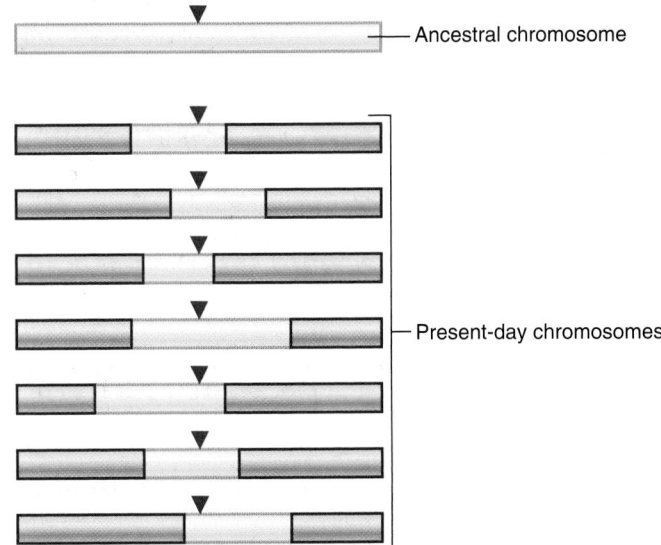

FIGURE 117-8 The mutation is indicated by a *red triangle*. Chromosomal stretches derived from the common ancestor of all mutant chromosomes are shown in *yellow*, and new stretches introduced by recombination are shown in *blue*. Markers that are physically close (that is, in the yellow regions of present-day chromosomes) tend to remain associated with the ancestral mutation, even as recombination limits the extent of the region of association over time. *(From Ardlie K, Kruglyak L, Seielstad M: Patterns of linkage disequilibrium in the human genome, Nat Rev Genet 3:299-309, 2002.)*

In contrast, GWASs test for associations between the phenotype and 100,000 or more genetic variants dispersed throughout the genome. This approach is conceptually similar to simultaneously performing association studies across the genome. GWASs have a greater chance of testing the genetic variant associated with the phenotype, and no hypotheses for the genes involved are required. For these reasons, GWASs have obvious advantages over candidate-gene studies. Although small sample sizes can limit the statistical power of GWAS analyses (it is necessary to make statistical corrections to ensure a low probability of false-positive results), replication studies are often used to examine the original GWAS findings.

In contrast to rare diseases attributed to a variant in a single gene (e.g., cystic fibrosis), it was hypothesized that complex common diseases (e.g., heart disease) would be influenced by genetic variation spread across multiple genomic loci.[76] Despite extensive research, data on the influence of heritability for many common diseases are limited. Of more than 3500 SNPs linked to common diseases or traits, most underlie only small effects (1.2 to 2 times the population risk).[96] Although they are small in magnitude, these associations can provide useful information about a condition or physiologic process (Boxes 117-1 and 117-2).

Efforts to identify genotype-phenotype associations have recently turned to *whole-genome sequence* analysis. Similar to the SNP-based HapMap project, the 1000 Genomes Project was designed to catalogue *sequence* variations across different human populations. The initial 1000 Genomes data set was collected from mother-father-child trios and unrelated individuals from four diverse human populations.[74] This data set enabled researchers to classify variants beyond common polymorphisms and SNVs by providing information about less frequent DNA polymorphisms (e.g., insertions, deletions, and structural variants). The collection contains whole-genome sequence data from approximately 2500 individuals representing 25 populations. As genome sequencing costs fall, efforts to complete whole-genome sequence and *exome* (protein-coding sequence) analysis are increasingly feasible for research purposes and to link genotypes to phenotypes.[12]

OMICS REVOLUTION

SNP association studies and comparative sequence analyses provide an unprecedented amount of information, but questions remain regarding the functional relevance of genetic variants. The original *omics* discipline, genomics, has provided a scaffold for other large-scale omics endeavors to characterize genome-wide expression (i.e., transcriptomics), protein properties (i.e., proteomics), and metabolic properties (i.e., metabolomics) in a spatial- and temporal-specific manner. These technologies can help identify interactions, regulatory networks, and molecular functions and provide greater insight into genome function. This integrative approach is one branch of emerging research efforts, referred to as *systems biology* (see nature.com/reviews/focus/systemsbiology/editorial/index.html for more information).

Information regarding variation in gene expression across cells, tissues, individuals, and populations is currently being explored using approaches such as *RNA-seq*.[252] This technology provides the comprehensive sequence of every RNA molecule transcribed from DNA in a particular cell population (i.e., the transcriptome)[162,179] and can also provide important insight into epigenetic changes in cells.[113] *Epigenetic analyses* reflect changes that occur in gene expression above (epi) the DNA level as a result of heterochromatin states (i.e., tightly packed, limited transcriptional access) or euchromatin states (i.e., lightly packed, often transcribed access) of DNA (Figure 117-9). Epigenetic modifications change in response to environmental cues,[80] resulting in phenotypic plasticity,[67] and may be inherited across generations.

FUNCTIONAL GENOMIC ELEMENTS

Evidence indicates that a vast array of functional genomic elements are harbored outside the approximately 1.5% of DNA that codes for proteins.[124] Comparative mammalian sequence alignments indicate that approximately 5% of the human genome is under evolutionary constraint, exhibiting levels of conservation across taxa that are far greater than the genome average, suggestive of important biologic functions.[135] Recent studies suggest even higher percentages of constraint (4% to 11%) if protein-coding regions are excluded.[138,253] Analyses of nonprotein coding regions of the genome reveal sequences that regulate gene expression (i.e., functional *enhancers, silencers,* and *insulators*) and sites at which DNA's transcription into RNA is initiated (i.e., *promoters*). Genomic segments that encode RNA transcripts that are not translated into proteins but play important functional

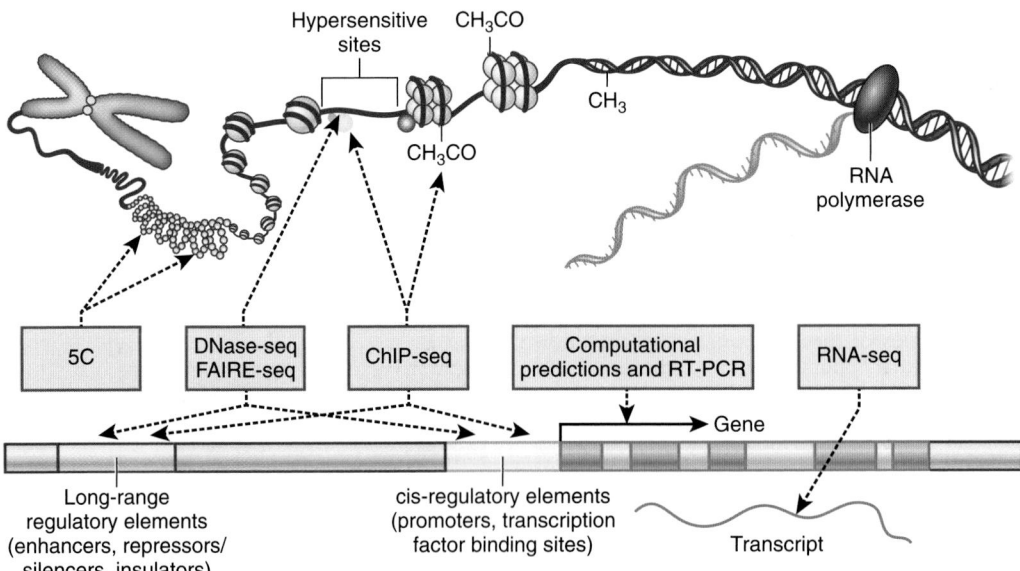

FIGURE 117-9 Diagram of ENCODE components. ENCODE aims to identify functional elements in the genome by annotating gene elements based on comparative genomics, bioinformatics, and comparative analyses. Regulatory elements are identified through assays that determine RNA sequence (indicative of gene expression), DNA hypersensitivity (open, eu-chromatin), DNA methylation, chromatin immunoprecipitation (ChIP), and ChIP-seq (to determine the sequence of protein-bound DNA elements). *(From Darryl Leja, National Human Genome Research Institute, and Ian Dunham, European Bioinformatics Institute: epigenomebrowser.org/encode.)*

BOX 117-1 Terms Used in Genomics

Term	Definition
Allele	One of two or more alternative forms of a gene that is found at the same place on a chromosome
Autosome	One of the 22 pairs of chromosomes not involved in the determination of sex
Candidate-gene association study	An approach that involves preselected genes or genetic variants of interest that are tested for relationships to phenotypes or disease states
Chromatin immunoprecipitation	Precipitation of a protein out of solution using an antibody specific to the chromatin mark of interest; this is used to assess interactions between proteins and DNA in the cell and provide information about gene regulation
Enhancer	A region of DNA to which activators (proteins that serve as transcription factors) bind and initiate transcription of a gene
Epigenetics	Reversible DNA or histone modifications that affect gene expression without altering the DNA sequence
Exome sequence	Protein coding portion of DNA sequence (< 2% in the human genome)
Genome	Complete genetic material of an organism; with respect to humans, the genome refers to the haploid set of chromosomes contained in the nucleus (the mitochondrial genome is considered separately)
Genome-wide association study	An approach that involves examination of genetic markers across the genomes of many people, with and without a particular phenotype or disease state, to test for relationships between genotype and phenotype
Genotype	Genetic constitution of an individual organism
Haplotype	A set of alleles found on the same chromosome that tend to be inherited together because of close proximity; alternatively, this definition can refer to one's genetic information at a set of polymorphisms on one chromosome that are not necessarily in strong linkage disequilibrium
Heritability	Proportion of observed differences on a trait among individuals of a population due to genetic differences; factors, including genetics, environment, and random chance, can all contribute to variation between individuals in their observable characteristics (in their phenotypes)
Insulator	A DNA element that, in order to regulate the enhancer influence of particular genes, blocks interaction between specific enhancers and promoters
Intronic sequence	Noncoding sequence removed from RNA through splicing
Linkage disequilibrium	A measure of the association (i.e., likelihood of coinheritance) of genetic variants (i.e., alleles) at different loci; when there is no association between genetic variants at different loci, they are in *linkage equilibrium*
Locus	Position of a gene or mutation on a chromosome
Methylome	All methylation modifications in the genome of a cell or population of cells (usually at a given point in time, under specific conditions)
MicroRNA	Small noncoding RNA molecule that functions in RNA silencing and posttranscriptional regulation of gene expression
Omics	Collective technologies used to explore roles, relationships, and actions of the various types of molecules that make up the cells of an organism; these technologies include genomics, ("the study of genes and their function" [Human Genome Project, 2003]), as well as transcriptomics and epigenomics, proteomics and metabolomics (entire sets of protein, metabolic factors), and others that are characterized under specific conditions.
Omics Reference genome	An assembly of nucleotide sequences used to represent the genome of a particular species; this sequence is used as a standardized platform to which genome data can be compared
Phenotype	Set of observable characteristics of an individual resulting from the interaction of its genotype with the environment
Phenotypic plasticity	Ability of one genotype to produce more than one phenotype when exposed to different environments
Polymorphism	A location (locus) in the genome that varies among members of a population; a polymorphism has two or more variants, and generally, the variant that is rarer must be present in ≥ 5% of the population or it is considered a mutation
Promoter	A region of DNA, upstream of the transcription start site, that initiates transcription of a particular gene
Proteome	The complete collection of proteins contained in a cell or a population of cells (usually at a given point in time, under specific conditions)
Quantitative trait loci	Genetic section of DNA that correlates with or is linked to variants associated with variation in a trait (a quantitative phenotype)
RNA-seq	Sequencing of all RNA transcripts in the cell, known as transcriptome profiling, determined using next-generation sequencing technologies
Selective sweep	Reduction or elimination of variation among the nucleotides in the neighboring DNA of a mutation as the result of recent and strong positive natural selection
Silencer	A region of DNA sequence to which proteins may bind and decrease gene expression
Single nucleotide polymorphism; (also known as single nucleotide variant)	DNA sequence variation occurring commonly within a population (e.g., 1%) in which a single nucleotide (A, T, C, or G) in the genome (or other shared sequence) differs between members of a biologic species or paired chromosomes
Systems biology	A biology-based interdisciplinary field of study that focuses on complex interactions within biologic systems, using a holistic approach (instead of traditional reductionism) to biologic and biomedical research
Transcriptome	Complete collection of RNA transcripts contained in a cell or a population of cells (usually at a given point in time, under specific conditions)
Twin studies	Methods used to assess genetic versus environmental contribution to traits; data from siblings and adoptees, from pedigree information, and from other aspects are commonly examined to determine the genetic role in development of a trait or behavior in twins
Whole-genome sequencing	A laboratory process that determines the complete DNA sequence of an organism's genome (also known as full-genome sequencing, complete-genome sequencing, and entire-genome sequencing)

BOX 117-2   Assessing the Quality of a Genome-Wide Association Study

1. Is the phenotype accurately and correctly defined?
2. Are potential confounding variables controlled between cases and controls?
3. Was the sample size appropriate?
4. Was the genotyping density appropriate?
5. Were the quality control steps sufficient?
6. Were previous associations replicated?
7. Were the statistical tests sufficiently stringent?
8. Was the result replicated in an independent population? Was the replication design sufficiently similar to the original study in terms of subject characteristics and phenotype?
9. Was the associated polymorphism demonstrated to have a functional role in the phenotype?

Attia J, Ioannidis JP, Thakkinstian A, et al: How to use an article about genetic association: C: what are the results and will they help me in caring for my patients? JAMA 301:304-308, 2009; Pearson TA, Manolio TA: How to interpret a genome-wide association study, JAMA 299:1335-1344, 2008.

roles (e.g., *microRNAs*, piRNAs, and structural and regulatory RNAs) have been extensively examined.[170,196]

The Encyclopedia of DNA Elements (ENCODE) Consortium suggests that most of the human genome contains DNA elements with biochemical relevance.[52] Extensive genome-wide expression analysis, initially completed in cell lines ranging from lymphoblastoid to primary liver cells, has provided candidate elements for future investigations of genome regulation. ENCODE analysis of RNA transcription helped identify epigenetic signatures of gene regulation (e.g., methyl marks on DNA [the *methylome*] and DNA hypersensitivity associated with decreased and increased transcription, respectively, and histone modifications associated with either repressive or activating transcriptional marks). Additional information regarding these regions is available at the ENCODE Data Coordination Center at the University of California Santa Cruz (UCSC) or on the UCSC Genome Browser (genome.ucsc.edu).

Many DNA variants associated with disease are identified within or near noncoding functional DNA elements. This provides important insight into the study of genetic variation and disease. Acute exposure to environmental wilderness conditions may initiate cellular, molecular, and, ultimately, physiologic compensations to such challenges. Understanding these responses will help advance our understanding of human disease, biology, and responses to environmental conditions.

TECHNOLOGIES FOR IDENTIFYING GENETIC VARIANTS AND THEIR ASSOCIATIONS WITH DISEASE

Various technologies may be employed to identify genetic variants and test for associations with disease. Genotyping or sequencing platforms allow for DNA and RNA sequence analyses, and various high-throughput methods may be used to detect epigenetic marks that influence gene expression and/or protein signatures and posttranslational modifications in cells or tissues. New genome-wide tools continue to improve accuracy and throughput, and investigators can select complementary approaches to address a wide range of research questions.

Microarrays based on hybridization techniques are used to assay large amounts of biologic material or simultaneously genotype multiple regions of the genome. Antibody arrays were among the first microarrays developed,[45] and "gene chips" followed in the 1990s.[208] Today, SNP hybridization microarrays can simultaneously genotype more than one million SNPs scattered throughout the genome. In these microarrays, chosen SNPs serve as reporters for a specific haplotype or DNA sequence. Precise DNA elements on the array are hybridized so that complementary sequencing of DNA or RNA can be performed under high-stringency conditions. This hybridization is detected and quantified by fluorophore-, silver-, or chemiluminescence-labeled targets. This technology is limited to specific markers, but has enabled progress (e.g., using GWASs and other genomic studies) by highlighting genetic patterns among individuals. In addition to DNA microarrays, various protein, peptide, and metabolism arrays are widely used for research.

In contrast to microarrays, *sequencing technologies* provide information across consecutive DNA or RNA sites in a targeted region or across the entire genome *(whole-genome sequencing)*. Next-generation sequencing technologies have revolutionized this effort through massively parallel sequencing.[220] The basic workflow requires library preparation (i.e., fragmenting and adding adapters to DNA that is then denatured and amplified). These fragments are sequenced and aligned with the *reference genome* (i.e., the nucleic acid sequence database that serves as the representative example of a species' genome).

Exome sequencing captures information from the protein-coding regions of the genome and has proved effective for identifying variants in rare Mendelian disease.[12] Knowledge of the protein-coding sequence has been applied to RNA sequencing for gene expression analysis (*RNA-seq* or whole-transcriptome sequencing). Additional efforts to categorize regulatory functions are achieved through *chromatin immunoprecipitation* (ChIP) followed by sequencing (ChIP-seq), and sequencing of methylated DNA (methyl-seq) (see Figure 117-9). In ChIP, interacting DNA-proteins (in chromatin) are cross-linked and sheared, and antibodies (targeted for specific proteins) precipitate a linked DNA-protein complex. The complex is then unlinked and the DNA purified for sequence analysis. ChIP is used to determine whether transcription factors and proteins (activating or repressive) are bound to a genomic region and so influence gene regulation and a phenotype of interest.

Sequencing technologies that are applied today have rapidly advanced since the 1980s (see Figure 117-6). Maxam-Gilbert (radiolabeled)[153] and Sanger (chain-termination)[205] sequencing preceded *de novo* sequencing of fragmented DNA. Shotgun sequencing, based upon fragmenting and then aligning genomic segments using overlapping regions, further improved output. Next-generation sequencing enabled parallel sequencing and simultaneous generation of millions of sequences. New methods (e.g., pyrosequencing, single molecule, Illumina/Solexa, SOLiD, Ion Torrent, nanoball, Heliscope, SMRT, nanopore, tunneling currents, and sequence by hybridization and mass spectrometry) are further advancing scientific techniques.[136]

Although such high-throughput technologies provide valuable insights, scientists need to determine the mechanism that enables gene variant(s) to *cause* a particular trait. These data can be obtained by testing mechanisms using genetically manipulated model organisms or cultured cells. For instance, demonstrating in a controlled experiment that a particular genetic variant decreases the rate of transcription of a gene or lowers the activity of the encoded enzyme provides good evidence that genetic association was causal.

GENETIC RESPONSES TO EXTREME ENVIRONMENTS

GENETICS AND ALTITUDE

Hypoxia and Acclimatization

High-altitude environments are physiologically stressful because of numerous abiotic factors (e.g., hypoxia, cold, heat, ultraviolet [UV] radiation, and wind). Although many stressors are easily mitigated (e.g., with warm clothing or sunscreen), the hypoxia of high-altitude environments cannot easily be avoided. Supplemental oxygen is expensive and difficult to carry; for these reasons, most humans at high altitude are constantly exposed to hypoxic stress.[256]

High-altitude hypoxia is due to hypobaria; ascent decreases barometric pressure and reduces partial pressure of oxygen.[256] High-altitude environments can be best simulated in chambers by decreasing the atmospheric pressure (i.e., hypobaric hypoxia) or the fraction of inspired oxygen (i.e., normobaric hypoxia). Although they are not equivalent, hypobaric hypoxia and normobaric hypoxia appear to elicit similar physiologic responses.[51,157,158,195]

Humans acclimatize to hypoxia through a series of physiologic responses (e.g., increased minute ventilation, bicarbonate diuresis, increased hemoglobin concentration).[14,17,206,219] Acclimatization to hypoxia increases oxygen availability and increases capacity for submaximal exercise.[69] Individual tolerance of acute and chronic hypoxia varies considerably.[145] Some individuals will develop acute altitude illnesses and others will remain healthy, despite traveling together and being exposed to the same hypoxic stress.[106] Similarly, only subsets of high-altitude natives and lifelong high-altitude residents develop chronic altitude illnesses.[199] Twin studies have demonstrated heritable control of ventilatory responses to hypoxia and hypercapnia and physiologic responses to hypoxic exercise (e.g., heart rate, oxygen saturation, and maximal oxygen uptake).[152] Additional evidence for individual responses to altitude comes from studies of altitude illness.

Altitude Illness

Altitude illness has acute and chronic presentations (Table 117-1). Acute altitude illness develops following a recent ascent to a new altitude (< 7 days, but most commonly at 1 to 4 days). The three major forms of acute altitude illness are acute mountain sickness (AMS), high-altitude cerebral edema (HACE), and high-altitude pulmonary edema (HAPE). Chronic altitude illnesses develop in

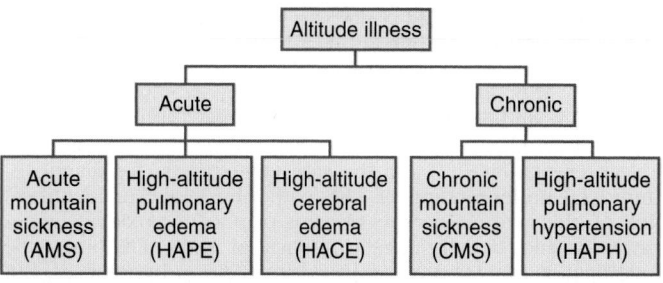

FIGURE 117-10 Altitude illnesses are either acute or chronic, depending on their typical time to onset.

humans following prolonged stays at high altitude (≥ 7 days, but more commonly several years). The most prominent chronic altitude illnesses are chronic mountain sickness (CMS) and high-altitude pulmonary hypertension (HAPH). Acute altitude illnesses are most likely to affect travelers to altitude; chronic altitude illnesses affect those who reside at altitude. Exceptions occur. Natives of high-altitude regions who travel to sea level can develop "reentry HAPE" on return to a high altitude,[104] and lowland residents can develop subacute mountain sickness (a condition similar to HAPH, characterized by right-heart failure) during a prolonged visit to high altitude[6] (Figure 117-10).

A brief review of high-altitude illnesses informs our discussion of genomics and personalized medicine. Please see Chapters 1 through 3 for a detailed review of altitude illness.

Acute Altitude Illnesses

Acute Mountain Sickness. Acute mountain sickness (AMS) is the most common form of altitude illness. It begins 6 to 10 hours after arrival at a higher altitude and resolves rapidly with descent.[70,85] Its prevalence depends on the altitude attained and the rate of ascent. AMS develops in normobaric and hypobaric hypoxia, but not in hypobaric normoxia,[195,197] suggesting that hypoxia (not hypobaria) is the primary precipitating factor for AMS.

The Lake Louise criteria define AMS as the presence of a headache (in the setting of a recent elevation change to > 2500 m), with at least one other symptom present (e.g., nausea, vomiting, dizziness, fatigue, or difficulty sleeping).[15] A Lake Louise score greater than or equal to 3 (with a headache) is diagnostic of AMS.

AMS symptoms are subjective and nonspecific and can mimic many other conditions (e.g., exhaustion, dehydration, alcohol hangover, and migraine).[18] Because symptoms are self-reported, the phenotype is subjective. Alternative questionnaires share similar flaws.[10,26,204,234,248,249] AMS likely results from hypoxia-induced cerebral perturbations,[106] and more research is needed to elucidate its physiologic basis.

Genetics of Acute Mountain Sickness. Differences in AMS susceptibility should encourage genetic study. The one twin study performed at altitude involved preverbal children, making generalizations to adults difficult.[267] A family history was not associated with AMS on an ascent to Mt Damavand, Iran (5671 m),[276] but AMS severity was correlated in brothers who ascended to Lake Gosainkunda, Nepal (4380 m).[143] Individuals of Tibetan ancestry seem less susceptible to AMS relative to other Asian populations (e.g., Han Chinese, Japanese).[133,263] Additional studies of twins, familial aggregation, family history, and biogeographic differences are needed.

Candidate-gene association studies have tested associations between AMS susceptibility and specific genetic variants.[147] None has identified a genetic variant with clinical utility. The angiotensin-converting enzyme (ACE) I/D polymorphism was originally associated with elite mountaineering performance; that is, relative to the general British population, elite climbers were more likely to carry the I allele, suggesting that these individuals had lower plasma ACE levels.[161] This is further supported by associations of the I/D polymorphism with arterial oxygen saturation in climbers ascending rapidly to 5000 m[259] and summit success on Mt Blanc, France.[241] Researchers hypothesized that

Altitude Illness	Advantages	Challenges and Considerations
Acute mountain sickness	Common Not fatal	Stability and repeatability Subjective diagnosis Ascent rate Altitude Timing of onset Susceptibility (age, gender) Comorbidities Many genes likely involved
High-altitude pulmonary edema	Objective diagnosis Stability and repeatability	Ascent rate Altitude Timing of onset Rare condition Rapidly fatal Susceptibility Comorbidities
High-altitude cerebral edema	Objective diagnosis Repeatability? Lasting signs of microhemorrhages	Stability and repeatability Ascent rate Altitude Timing of onset Rare condition Rapidly fatal Susceptibility Comorbidities
Chronic mountain sickness	Stable condition Objective diagnosis	Susceptibility (age, gender) Comorbidities Time at altitude Environmental factors
High-altitude pulmonary hypertension	Stable condition Objective diagnosis	Susceptibility (age, gender) Comorbidities Time at altitude

TABLE 117-1 Advantages, Challenges, and Considerations for Studies of Altitude Illness

this polymorphism could contribute to variation in AMS susceptibility (because susceptibility would hinder mountaineering). Several studies found that ACE polymorphisms were not associated with AMS at 3807 m, 4380 m, 4559 m, or 5895 m.[116]

Genetic studies of AMS susceptibility (see Table 117-1) have been hindered by AMS's unclear pathophysiology,[88,141] its variable presentation,[144,146] and the subjective criteria for diagnosis. Improved understanding of AMS pathophysiology or identification of objective biomarkers or signs of poor hypoxia acclimatization would benefit genetic studies of AMS. Genome-wide investigations might preclude need for *a priori* hypotheses, but more rigorous experimental designs and improved diagnoses will still be needed to strengthen genetic investigations into AMS susceptibility. If exposures (e.g., rate and final elevation of ascent) were standardized, results could more easily be compared across studies.

High-Altitude Cerebral Edema. High-altitude cerebral edema (HACE) is the rare, but potentially lethal, form of acute cerebral altitude illness defined by the presence of ataxia and/or altered mental status. It typically occurs at least 2 days after ascent to an altitude above 3000 m.[13] In the vast majority of cases, AMS precedes HACE.[85,86]

Magnetic resonance imaging studies of patients with HACE reveal vasogenic edema[87] and microhemorrhages in the corpus callosum,[60,115,210] indicating the blood-brain barrier has been disrupted. Without treatment or descent, HACE may within 24 hours progress to coma followed by death resulting from brain herniation.[13] Hemosiderin deposits (signs of brain microhemorrhages) remain in the brain of HACE survivors for decades.[210]

A HACE incidence of approximately 1% was reported in an early study.[84] A very large prospective study (> 14,000 high-altitude railway workers in China) reported a HACE incidence of 0.28%.[264]

Genetics of High-Altitude Cerebral Edema. The role of genetic variation in HACE susceptibility has not been investigated. No reports of individuals suffering repeated episodes of HACE or of familial aggregation of HACE have been published. Candidate-gene and genome-wide association studies have not been performed for HACE. Obtaining sufficient sample sizes to perform these studies would be advanced by the creation of a HACE database.

High-Altitude Pulmonary Edema. High-altitude pulmonary edema (HAPE) is the acute pulmonary manifestation of acute altitude illness and the leading cause of death due to acute illness. The onset of HAPE is generally 2 days after arrival at a new altitude (usually > 2500 m)[85,209] and is characterized by dyspnea at rest.[85,156,209] HAPE is a noncardiogenic form of pulmonary edema secondary to hypoxic pulmonary vasoconstriction as pulmonary arterial hypertension leads to stress failure of pulmonary capillaries and extravasation into alveolar spaces.[149,233] The HAPE incidence increases with ascent rate and altitude attained. Persons who are susceptible to HAPE demonstrate greater pulmonary artery pressure in response to normoxic exercise[82] and hypoxia (normobaric and hypobaric).[149] Persons susceptible to HAPE also have relatively lower level of exhaled nitric oxide.[41,63]

The risk of recurrence for HAPE is approximately 60% for persons who ascend to 4500 m in 2 days,[16] suggesting that a previous episode of HAPE is a strong risk factor for its redevelopment.

Genetics of High-Altitude Pulmonary Edema. HAPE is more amenable to research than is AMS or HACE. HAPE has demonstrable examination findings, which increases the certainty in diagnosis. HAPE is rare, but a subpopulation of susceptible individuals can be identified and studied prospectively with strong confidence in the quality of phenotypic data. HAPE field studies are still difficult because of its low incidence (and relatively longer time to onset) compared with AMS. Databases of individuals who have developed HAPE (as well as individuals who have traveled to high altitude but have not developed HAPE) are being created in an attempt to gather more information about the condition.[209]

HAPE family data include reports of HAPE susceptibility within siblings and within parent-offspring pairs.[68,105,140,212] Given that the incidence of HAPE is so low, reports of familial aggregation support a genetic cause (N.B., the potential effect of a shared environment cannot be ruled out). Biogeographic comparisons are not available for the incidence of HAPE.

Candidate genes investigated as markers of HAPE susceptibility are found in Table 117-2. A recent GWAS identified several candidate genes for HAPE susceptibility in Japanese individuals,[121] including a tissue inhibitor of metalloproteinase 3 (TIMP3), a gene whose product regulates the degradation of the extracellular matrix of lung tissue. Interaction of TIMP proteins and matrix metalloproteinases has been associated with various lung pathologies related to decreased structural integrity (e.g., edema, emphysema, fibrosis).[137] Based on the function of this gene and our current understanding of HAPE, this finding is intriguing. Intronic variants of the *EGLN1* gene have also been associated with HAPE in a population from India.[1] Research to confirm these results and to determine generalizability is needed.

Chronic Altitude Illnesses

Chronic Mountain Sickness. Chronic mountain sickness (CMS), or Monge's disease, is a condition that affects high-altitude natives and long-time residents of high altitude.[128] CMS generally develops after years of exposure to high altitude (i.e., ≥ 2500 m), gradually resolves with descent to lower altitudes, and can recur upon reascent to altitude.[128]

CMS is characterized by excessive erythrocytosis (females: hemoglobin ≥ 19 g/dL; males hemoglobin ≥ 21 g/dL). In addition, severe hypoxemia and pulmonary hypertension can occur.[128] Individuals with CMS can exhibit some symptoms similar to those of AMS (headache, dizziness, sleep disturbance, fatigue) in addition to dyspnea, tinnitus, alterations of memory, and bone or muscle pain.[126] Over time, pulmonary hypertension associated with CMS can cause right-heart failure (cor pulmonale) and congestive heart failure.[128]

Diagnosis of CMS requires exclusion of chronic pulmonary diseases or other chronic medical conditions that could cause severe hypoxemia.[128] A score is available to rate severity of CMS. Variables are rated on a scale of 0 to 3 and summed: breathlessness/palpitations, sleep disturbance, cyanosis, dilatation of veins, paresthesia, headache, tinnitus, and hemoglobin concentration.[128]

Only some highlanders develop CMS. Patients with CMS are hypoxic and may be hypercapnic due to relative hypoventilation.[127] In Andean patients with CMS, hypoxic ventilatory response is only modestly lower than that of healthy Andean highlanders,[127] suggesting that hypoxic ventilatory response is not the precipitating cause of CMS. Hypoventilation could result from erythrocytosis, because the hemodilution of patients with CMS increases ventilation[150,258]; however, whether or not erythrocytosis *causes* hypoventilation is unclear.[126] Limited increases in hemoglobin concentration counteract the effects of hypoxia by increasing oxygen-carrying capacity. Beyond a certain threshold, further increases in hemoglobin concentration increase blood viscosity and blood volume and become pathologic.[193,245] More research is needed to improve our understanding of the physiologic mechanisms leading to CMS.

The CMS prevalence varies widely between geographic locations and populations. There is a much higher prevalence of CMS in Andeans than in Tibetans despite both populations being native to regions of high altitude.[126,164] This difference is not due to location. The prevalence of CMS in Tibetan highlanders is approximately one quarter that of Han Chinese immigrants who inhabit the same region.[261] CMS has not been reported in Ethiopian highlanders.[126] The difference in incidence between Tibetans and Andeans could be the result of dissimilar physiology (e.g., higher alveolar ventilation and hypoxic ventilatory response and a lower hemoglobin concentration in Tibetans).[20,22,25,163]

Aging is associated with a greater prevalence of CMS: In one study, 27% of persons over 60 years, but only 7% of those between 20 and 29 years, had CMS.[129] Premenopausal females might be at lower risk for CMS.[125] A history of CMS, pulmonary dysfunction, hypopnea and sleep apnea, obesity, and exposure to environmental factors, such as air pollution and metals, could increase one's risk of developing CMS.[128]

TABLE 117-2 Candidate Genes Relevant to Wilderness Environment Phenotypes

Gene Symbol	Gene Name	Related Phenotype(s)	Protein Function*
ACE	Angiotensin I–converting enzyme	Responses to exercise training, exercise, performance, possibly AMS	Catalyzes conversion of angiotensin I to its physiologically active form, angiotensin II, which regulates blood pressure and fluid balance
ANP32D	Acidic (leucine-rich) nuclear phosphoprotein 32 family, member D	CMS	Tumor suppression
ARNT2	Aryl-hydrocarbon receptor nuclear translocator 2	Altitude adaptation	Under hypoxia, it forms a complex with HIF1alpha in the nucleus and binds to hypoxia response elements of oxygen-sensitive genes to increase transcription (i.e., a transcription factor)
BHLHE41	Basic helix-loop-helix family, member e41	Altitude adaptation	A transcription factor involved in the control of circadian rhythm and cell differentiation
CAMTA1	Calmodulin-binding transcription activator 1	Response to exercise training	Unclear
COL5A1	Collagen, type 5, alpha 1	Achilles tendinopathy	Alpha chain of a low-abundance fibrillar collagen
CREB1	cAMP-responsive element–binding protein 1	Response to exercise training	A transcription factor that binds to the cAMP-responsive element to induce expression
CYP19A1	Cytochrome P450, family 19, subfamily A, polypeptide 1	Physical activity	A monooxygenase that catalyzes the last steps of estrogen biosynthesis
CYP2C9	Cytochrome P450, family 2, subfamily C, polypeptide 9	Drug metabolism	Metabolizes many xenobiotics
CYP2C19	Cytochrome P450, family 2, subfamily C, polypeptide 19	Drug metabolism	Metabolizes many xenobiotics
CYP2D6	Cytochrome P450, family 2, subfamily D, polypeptide 6	Drug metabolism	Metabolizes as many as 25% of commonly prescribed drugs
CYP2E1	Cytochrome P450, family 2, subfamily E, polypeptide 1	Cold adaptation	A monooxygenase that catalyzes reactions involved in drug metabolism and the synthesis of cholesterol, steroids, and other lipids
CYP3A	Cytochrome P450, family 3, subfamily A	Salt homeostasis and hypertension	A monooxygenase that catalyzes reactions involved in drug metabolism and the synthesis of cholesterol, steroids, and other lipids
CYP3A4	Cytochrome P450, family 3, subfamily A, polypeptide 4	Drug metabolism	Metabolizes approximately 50% of commonly prescribed drugs
CYP3A5	Cytochrome P450, family 3, subfamily A, polypeptide 5	Drug metabolism	Metabolizes drugs as well as testosterone and progesterone
EDNRA	Endothelin receptor type A	Cold/hypoxia adaptation	Receptor for endothelin-1, a potent and long-lasting vasoconstrictor
EGLN1 (PHD2)	egl-9 family hypoxia-inducible factor 1	HAPE, altitude adaptation	Catalyzes hydroxylation of HIF1alpha protein to target the protein for degradation
EPAS1 (HIF2A)	Endothelial PAS domain protein 1	Altitude adaptation	A transcription factor that is regulated by oxygen tension
GUCY1A3	Guanylate cyclase 1, soluble, alpha 3	HAPH	Beta subunit of soluble guanylate cyclase, which catalyzes the conversion of GTP to 3′,5′-cyclic GMP and pyrophosphate
HBB	Hemoglobin, beta	Altitude adaptation (dogs)	A globin protein, which along with HBA, makes up the most common form of hemoglobin in adult humans, hemoglobin A
LEPR	Leptin receptor	Cold adaptation	A cytokine receptor for leptin that is involved in fat metabolism and lymphopoiesis
ME2	Malic enzyme 2, NAD(+)-dependent, mitochondrial	Cold adaptation	Catalyzes the oxidative decarboxylation of malate to pyruvate in the mitochondria [NAD(+)-dependent]
ME3	Malic enzyme 3, NADP(+)-dependent, mitochondrial	Cold adaptation	Catalyzes the oxidative decarboxylation of malate to pyruvate in the mitochondria [NADP(+)-dependent]
MICU1 (CBARA1)	Mitochondrial calcium uptake 1	Altitude adaptation	Regulates mitochondrial calcium uptake under basal conditions
NOS2	Nitric oxide synthase 2, inducible	Altitude adaptation	Synthesizes the signaling molecule nitric oxide
NOTCH1	Notch 1	Altitude adaptation	A transmembrane protein involved in developmental processes
PKLR	Pyruvate kinase, liver and red blood cell	Cold/hypoxia adaptation	Catalyzes the conversion of phosphoenolpyruvate to pyruvate and ATP (i.e., the rate-determining step of glycolysis)
PPARA	Peroxisome proliferator-activated receptor alpha	Altitude adaptation	A steroid hormone receptor that regulates lipid metabolism (i.e., a transcription factor)

Continued

TABLE 117-2 Candidate Genes Relevant to Wilderness Environment Phenotypes—cont'd

Gene Symbol	Gene Name	Related Phenotype(s)	Protein Function*
PPARG	Peroxisome proliferator-activated receptor gamma	Cold/hypoxia adaptation	A steroid hormone receptor that regulates adipocyte differentiation, as well as fatty acid storage and glucose metabolism (i.e., a transcription factor)
PRKAA1	Protein kinase, AMP-activated, alpha 1 catalytic subunit	Altitude adaptation	Catalytic subunit of AMP-activated protein kinase (AMPK), a cellular energy sensor that regulates key metabolic processes through phosphorylation
RGS18	Regulator of G-protein signaling 18	Response to exercise training	Attenuates the signal from G-proteins by increasing the activity of GTPase (increasing the conversion of GTP to GDP)
RYR2	Ryanodine receptor 2 (cardiac)	Response to exercise training	A receptor that when bound by calcium, releases calcium from the sarcoplasmic reticulum of cardiac muscle, triggering muscle contraction
SENP1	SUMO1/sentrin-specific peptidase 1	CMS	A cysteine peptidase that degrades members of the small ubiquitin-like modifier (SUMO) protein family
SGIP1	SH3-domain GRB2-like (endophilin) interacting protein 1	Physical activity	An endocytic protein that affects energy homeostasis
THRB	Thyroid hormone receptor, beta	Altitude adaptation	A nuclear hormone receptor for triiodothyronine (i.e., a transcription factor)
TIMP3	Metallopeptidase inhibitor 3	HAPE	Inhibits metalloproteinases, which degrade the extracellular matrix
TPMT	Thiopurine S-methyltransferase	Drug metabolism	Metabolizes thiopurine drugs
UCP3	Uncoupling protein 3	Cold adaptation	A skeletal muscle mitochondrial uncoupling protein that allows anions and protons to move between the inner and outer mitochondrial membranes (i.e., proton leak); ATP synthesis is separated from oxidative phosphorylation, with energy dissipated as heat
VAV3	Vav 3 guanine nucleotide exchange factor 1	Altitude adaptation	A guanine nucleotide exchange factor for Rho family GTPases; it is involved in angiogenesis
VKORC1	Vitamin K epoxide reductase complex, subunit 1	Drug metabolism	Reduces vitamin K 2,3-epoxide to its enzymatically activated form, which is essential for blood clotting

AMP, adenosine monophosphate; AMS, acute mountain sickness; ATP, adenosine triphosphate; cAMP, cyclic adenosine monophosphate; CMS, chronic mountain sickness; GDP, guanosine diphosphate; GMP, guanosine monophosphate; GTP, guanosine triphosphate; HAPE, high-altitude pulmonary edema; HAPH, high-altitude pulmonary hypertension; HIF, hypoxia-inducible factor; NAD, nicotinamide adenine dinucleotide; NADP, nicotinamide adenine dinucleotide phosphate.

Genetics of Chronic Mountain Sickness. Variation in CMS susceptibility across biogeographic groups is consistent with a genetic basis. A report of familial aggregation of CMS[192] led the way to recent candidate-gene and genomics investigations. Several candidate-gene association studies have been performed. Because they are limited by small sample size, they do not provide compelling evidence to link a specific gene or genetic variant to CMS susceptibility. A whole-genome sequencing study identified several genomic regions with haplotype patterns and frequencies consistent with the occurrence of selective sweeps.[274] These results are discussed in the next section on adaptation. In cultured fibroblasts, genes from a region containing SENP1 and ANP32D had greater expression in the CMS-derived cells. Similarly, decreasing expression of these genes increased the survival of flies exposed to hypoxia. SENP1 regulates erythropoiesis, so relative upregulation of this gene could have negative consequences for high-altitude dwellers (i.e., erythrocytosis).[49,270] ANP32D is an oncogene, but its putative role in the pathophysiology of CMS is unclear.

Cole and associates reported differences in the frequency of SENP1 genotypes (rs7963934) between cases and controls in two independent cohorts.[50] In the same cohorts, the previously associated ANP32D SNP (rs72644851) was not associated with CMS. Because the two variants are in strong linkage disequilibrium, the authors suggested that the two original associations could represent one selection signal. Whether the same genes influence susceptibility to CMS in other populations is unknown.

High-Altitude Pulmonary Hypertension. High-altitude pulmonary hypertension (HAPH) (i.e., chronic mountain sickness of the vascular type, high-altitude heart disease, or subacute mountain sickness) is a chronic form of altitude illness character-ized by excessive pulmonary artery pressure.[128] HAPH manifests following prolonged stays at altitudes above 2500 m. It can afflict high-altitude natives and lifelong residents of high altitude.[128]

HAPH is characterized by exaggerated pulmonary vasoconstriction, elevated pulmonary artery pressure (mean pulmonary artery pressures > 30 mm Hg and systolic pulmonary arterial pressures > 50 mm Hg), pulmonary vasculature remodeling, right ventricular hypertrophy, and congestive right-heart failure.[130] Excessive erythrocytosis may be present. HAPH can occur independent of CMS.[175]

In response to hypoxia, pulmonary vasculature constricts, elevating pulmonary artery pressure and pulmonary vascular resistance. With chronic hypoxia and increased pressure, pulmonary vessels remodel. In pulmonary arterial smooth muscle cells, calcium channels are upregulated and potassium channels are downregulated, leading to increased proliferation and vasoconstriction.[254] These vascular changes further increase vascular tone and increase thickness of the pulmonary vascular wall. The resulting elevated pulmonary vascular resistance augments right-heart afterload, which eventually leads to the right-heart failure associated with HAPH.[130]

HAPH prevalence increases in males and with increasing age.[131] In a group of Kyrgyz highlanders, 23% of males and 6% of females had electrocardiographic signs of cor pulmonale.[2]

Genetics of High-Altitude Pulmonary Hypertension. Familial aggregation for high-altitude heart disease (i.e., HAPH) was reported in three families living in the Qinghai region of China,[134] suggesting that HAPH susceptibility could be due to genetic variation or a shared environment. Tibetans generally have less pulmonary hypertension than do Andeans, which is consistent with genetic influence.[81]

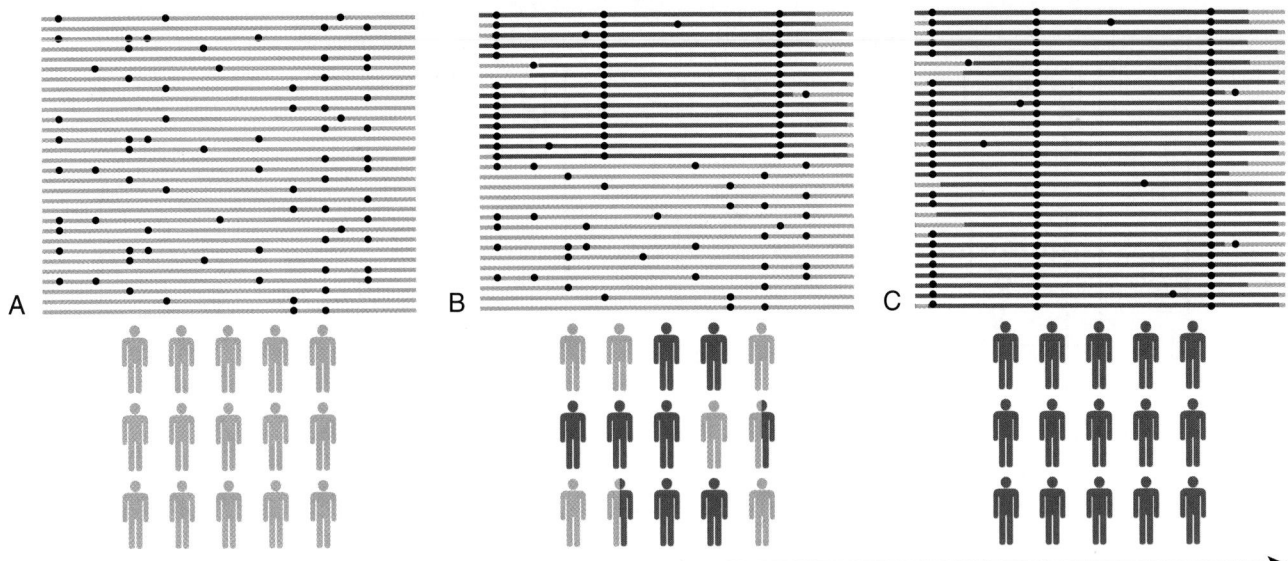

A selective sweep over hundreds of generations

FIGURE 117-11 Progression of a selective sweep in genomes sampled from a population across many generations. **A,** Neutrally evolving chromosomal regions aligned for 15 individuals. Patterns in **B** and **C** represent chromosomal regions indicative of partial and complete selective sweeps, respectively. Statistics are used to identify patterns of haplotype homozygosity, exhibited as decreased variation around an adaptive variant, within a single population or between populations. *(Modified from Simonson TS: Altitude adaptation: a glimpse through various lenses, High Alt Med Biol 16:125-137, 2015.)*

HAPH genetic analyses to date have focused on only a few candidate genes, and variants statistically associated with HAPH have not been replicated. A recent exome sequencing study of Kyrgyz highlanders with and without pulmonary hypertension identified GUCY1A3 (guanylate cyclase 1, soluble, alpha) as a candidate gene for HAPH susceptibility.[81] A rare missense mutation of the *GUCY1A3* gene was identified, and follow-up experiments revealed that the polymorphism under investigation altered activity of the soluble guanylyl cyclase (sGC) enzyme, which helps regulate pulmonary vascular homeostasis.[257] The authors hypothesized that the *GUCY1A3* variant protects against HAPH by enhancing sensitivity to nitric oxide. These findings highlight the importance of rare as well as common genetic variants involved in a phenotype.

High-Altitude Adaptation

Three continental populations have lived at high altitudes for hundreds of years. Ancestors of modern-day highlanders likely harbored beneficial variants in their genome sequences that have been selected over time.[23,27,29,224] Adaptive gene copies passed down over many generations create a pattern of variation distinct from neutrally inherited loci in the genome. The consequence of this process, called a *selective sweep*, may be detected by examining the variation of linked genetic markers *(haplotypes)*. These analyses highlight important genetic signals in genomic data from as few as 30 individuals, a stark contrast to the thousands of subjects often required to identify possible genetic contributions in GWASs[178] (Figure 117-11). Regions that exhibit an adaptive signal are expected to contain functional variants favored by selection and are therefore valuable candidates for detecting genotype-phenotype associations. In contrast, populations whose genomes do not face strong selective pressure for a particular trait typically exhibit a random pattern of genomic variation and may have many variants that contribute small effects to neutrally evolving phenotypes.

Tibetan, Andean, and Ethiopian populations have inhabited high-altitude regions for hundreds of generations, a long enough time for natural selection to occur. Physiologic and genomic analyses in these groups suggest distinct evolutionary paths[19] (Figure 117-12).

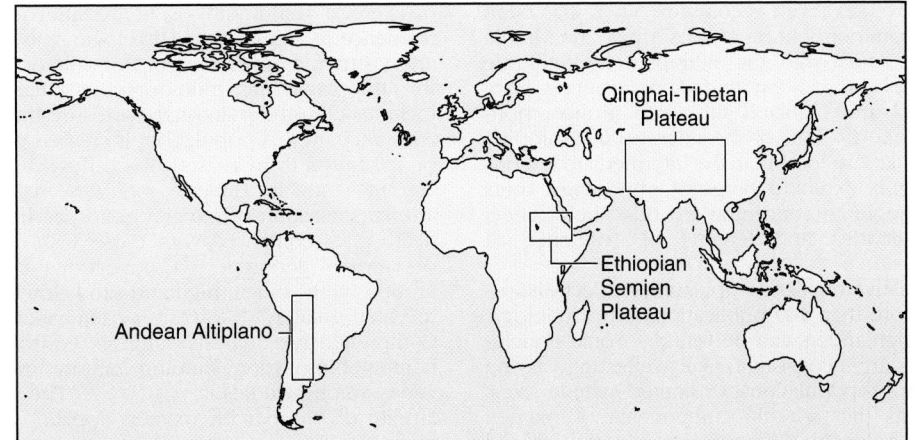

FIGURE 117-12 Map of high-altitude regions where data for evolutionary studies of adaptation have been collected. *(Modified from Simonson TS: Altitude adaptation: a glimpse through various lenses, High Alt Med Biol 16:125-137, 2015.)*

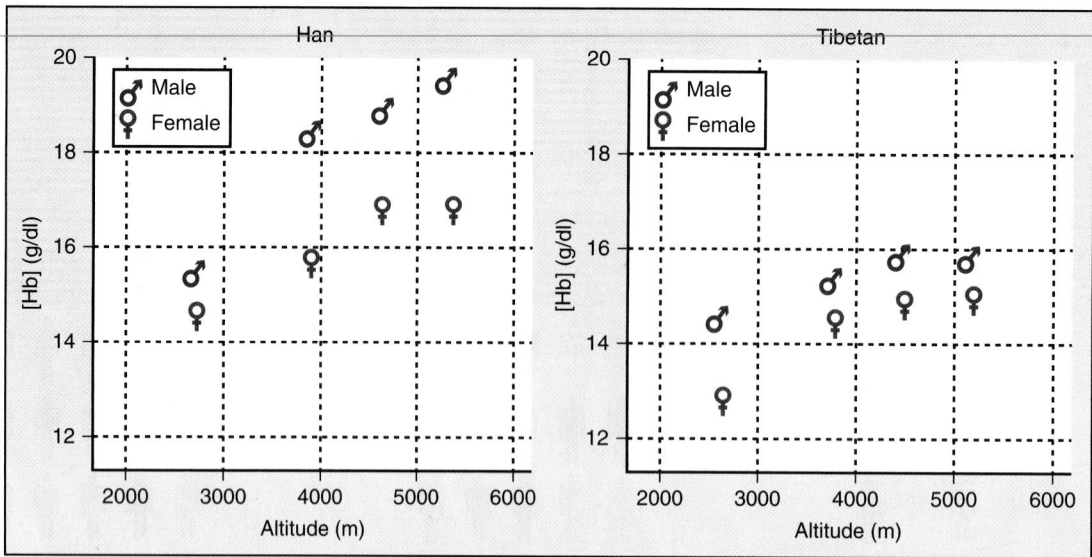

FIGURE 117-13 Hemoglobin concentration in Han Chinese and Tibetan males and females at various altitudes. *(From Gilbert-Kawai ET, Milledge JS, Grocott MPW, Martin DS: King of the mountains: Tibetan and Sherpa physiological adaptations for life at high altitude, Physiology 29:388-402, 2014.)*

The largest high-altitude region continuously inhabited by human populations is the Qinghai-Tibetan Plateau. Some regions of the plateau have been inhabited for up to 25,000 years,[5,187,273] and genetic relationships between ancestors of present-day Tibetan and Sherpa groups date to approximately 30,000 years ago.[112] The adaptive *EPAS1* gene segment identified in Tibetans is most similar to the sequence in an archaic Denisovan, suggesting introgression into the Tibetan gene pool approximately 40,000 years ago.[103] Archeologic findings indicate that areas in the northeast region of the plateau were more recently occupied (5000 years ago).[47] Considering the plateau's vast area (nearly 100 million square miles), it is not surprising that various groups (e.g., Amdo, Kham, and Ü-Tsang Tibetans) exhibit distinct population structures and vary in terms of adaptive signals.[224,265]

Archaeologic findings indicate that humans established residence in the Andean highlands shortly after inhabiting South America approximately 12,000 to 14,000 years ago, with subsequent migrations to and from neighboring coastal environments.[189] European admixture in the 17th and 20th centuries contributed to the genetic pool of present-day Aymara and Quechua populations. In various Andean populations, genetic variants from populations that have historically lived in lowland areas underlie aspects of their physiology (e.g., the capacity for exercise at altitude).[64]

In Ethiopia, the demographic history of various groups (i.e., Amhara, Oromo, and Tigray) that inhabit intermediate to high altitudes (> 1800 m above sea level) is complex. There has been substantial gene flow from northern regions of Africa, the Middle East, and sub-Saharan Africa into the Ethiopian high-altitude population gene pool.[215] In addition to factors resulting from mixing among lowland and highland Ethiopian groups, non-African components make up 50% of the ancestry in Ethiopian populations.[171] Subpopulations located in the intermediate regions and highlands of Ethiopia exhibit a range of physiologic traits (e.g., variations in hemoglobin concentration) that likely reflect distinct population histories and lengths of residence at altitude.

Traits exhibited by native highland populations reflect distinct evolutionary paths.[19] More than 100 publications on physiologic adaptations in native highlanders can be found.[77] Some conclusions from these studies are inconsistent, likely reflecting varying methodologies, varying subpopulations, or limited sample sizes. The consensus suggests that specific components of oxygen transport play unique roles in different continental highland populations.[19,20,28,77,166,177]

Hemoglobin concentration is generally elevated in sojourners after a couple of weeks at high altitude. Hemoglobin levels in Tibetans increase much less than in lowlanders examined at high altitudes (e.g., Han Chinese)[262] (Figure 117-13). Individuals of Tibetan and Amhara highland Ethiopian ancestry living above 4000 m may exhibit hemoglobin levels comparable to those in lowlanders at sea level.[19,207] Andean high-altitude populations exhibit an average of a few grams per deciliter more hemoglobin than is exhibited by Tibetans.[22] Low hemoglobin levels in Tibetans and the Amhara are associated with adaptive genetic loci (discussed below). The physiologic significance is unknown. It is not clear if elevated hemoglobin is the primary or secondary consequence of adaptive changes in the oxygen transport system[223,228] (Figure 117-14).

An important variable in oxygen transport is ventilatory sensitivity to hypoxia. Hypoxic ventilatory response measures the increase in minute ventilation in response to the decreased arterial partial pressures of oxygen. Tibetan hypoxic ventilatory response values are similar to those of unacclimatized lowlanders, and Andeans exhibit a lower response comparable to that of acclimatized lowlanders.[20,25,54] Tibetans have greater lung, residual, and tidal volumes, greater total lung and vital capacities, and greater diffusing capacity than do Han Chinese lowlanders.[61,117,232] Hypoxic pulmonary vasoconstriction directs pulmonary blood flow to better-oxygenated portions of the lung. Hypoxic pulmonary vasoconstriction is increased in many lowlanders at altitude,[174] resulting in pulmonary hypertension. Tibetans have muted hypoxic pulmonary vasoconstriction during rest or exercise at altitude[81] or after examination following extended residence at sea level.[176] Histologic study of Andean pulmonary artery structure gives evidence of pulmonary hypertension.[7,94,95,242] In Ethiopians, the pulmonary vascular response to hypoxia includes elevated pulmonary pressure but not increased vascular resistance. In this population, increased pulmonary pressure may be attributed to increased blood flow.[99]

One study in Tibetans indicates that mothers with a high–arterial saturation of oxygen genotype have decreased offspring death rates compared with those with a low–arterial saturation of oxygen genotype.[24] Comparisons of Tibetan and Sherpa groups with other highland and lowland populations have revealed greater,[40,48] lower,[21] or equivalent[120] oxygen saturations. Comprehensive analysis suggests equivalent saturations.[255] The hemoglobin-oxygen binding affinity in highland populations varies among studies.[11,165,167,203,223,235] The resting, in vivo, binding affinity of blood with oxygen appears higher in Andeans and highest in Tibetan groups.[11,223]

Compared with lowland Han Chinese at high altitude, Tibetan and Sherpa populations exhibit elevated heart rates,[185,186,232,260] greater stroke volume and cardiac output,[48,73,260] and less right

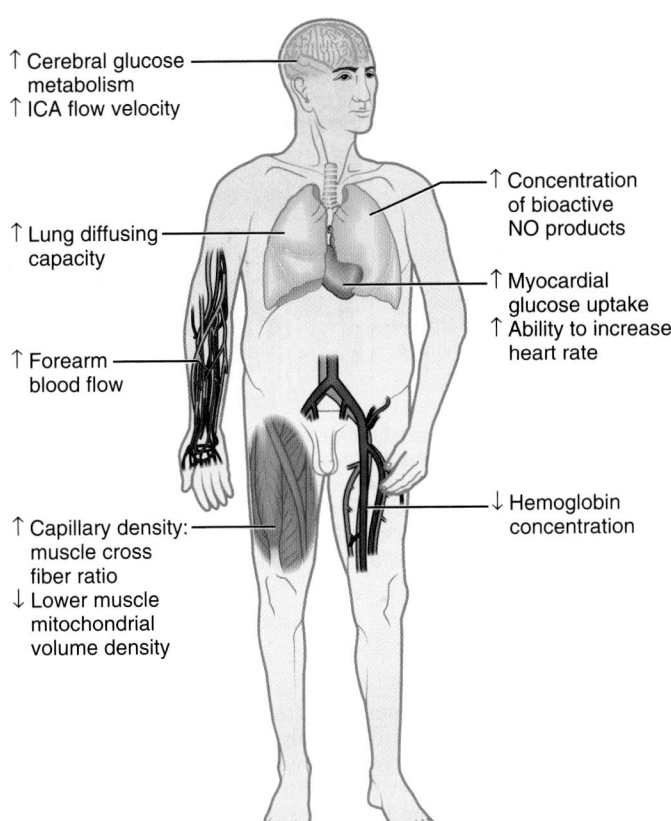

↑ Cerebral glucose metabolism
↑ ICA flow velocity

↑ Lung diffusing capacity

↑ Forearm blood flow

↑ Capillary density: muscle cross fiber ratio
↓ Lower muscle mitochondrial volume density

↑ Concentration of bioactive NO products

↑ Myocardial glucose uptake
↑ Ability to increase heart rate

↓ Hemoglobin concentration

FIGURE 117-14 Summary of physiologic differences described in Tibetan and Sherpa individuals, as compared with lowlanders. *(From Gilbert-Kawai ET, Milledge JS, Grocott MPW, Martin DS: King of the mountains: Tibetan and Sherpa physiological adaptations for life at high altitude,* Physiology *29:388-402, 2014.)*

heart hypertrophy.[89] Compared with lowlanders at altitude, Sherpa exhibit smaller left ventricular size.[227] Cardiac metabolism studies in Tibetans and Sherpas suggest a shift toward glucose metabolism (decreasing oxygen demand), possibly due to decreased energy reserve.[100] In Sherpas examined at low altitude, the myocardial phosphocreatine–to–adenosine triphosphate ratio is half that of lowlanders, but is not further depressed following administration of a hypoxic gas mixture. This suggests a metabolic optimization for cardiac hypoxic conditions.[98] In lowlanders acutely exposed to hypoxia, downregulation of beta-adrenergic receptors decreases sympathetic nervous system stimulation. In Tibetans, greater vagal dominance at high and low altitude has been reported.[275]

In the brain, improved autoregulation and increased oxygen delivery have been hypothesized to be beneficial at altitude. At extreme altitudes, Sherpas compared with lowlanders demonstrate decreased psychoneurologic symptoms and less mild cortical atrophy and/or periventricular high-intensity signal areas in the white matter.[71] Tibetans and Sherpas have a greater internal carotid artery blood flow velocity,[101] which may increase oxygen delivery. At high altitude, positron emission tomography scans of glucose metabolism in Sherpas and lowlanders are comparable, suggesting that reduced cerebral metabolism does not occur in Sherpas. A reduction is observed in Andean populations.[98]

Compared with lowland groups, native Tibetan and Andean highlanders exhibit greater birth weights.[164] The mean decline in lowlander birth weight is typically 100 g per 1000 m of altitude.[166] Increased uteroplacental oxygen delivery is attributed to increased common iliac blood flow into uterine arteries, with greater placental volumes and less uterine growth retardation. Compared with all other groups, Tibetans generally have lower rates of prenatal and postnatal death, premature birth, hypertension, and preeclampsia.[164,240,271]

Are physiologic differences in populations exposed to high altitude due to distinct evolutionary trajectories or to different temporal snapshots of a shared, consistent evolutionary process? Given that multiple adaptive traits and genetic factors have been described, it is likely that each evolutionary course is distinct.

No reports have specifically examined unfavorable outcomes in populations well adapted to altitude that descend to low altitude. Tibetan males born and raised at altitude that moved to sea level exhibited an average hemoglobin concentration significantly lower than that of sea-level Han Chinese at the same altitude (14.2 g/dL ± 0.9 g/dL vs 15.3 g/dL ± 1.2 g/dL, respectively).[176] This sea-level Tibetan cohort exhibits blunted pulmonary vascular responses to acute and sustained hypoxia, and at the cellular level demonstrates lower expression of certain genes regulated by hypoxia-inducible factor (HIF). These changes could have implications for oxygen signaling and processing, including the potential for metabolic inflexibility.[72]

Genetics of Altitude Adaptation. Permanent residents at altitudes more than 2500 m above sea level who exhibit adaptations to hypoxia have been most extensively studied in terms of altitude genomics. These groups provide a "natural experiment" in which genetic approaches can be used to uncover the causes of adaptive variation,[19] increase our understanding of the adaptive process, and help elucidate the causes of disease.

Efforts to identify adaptive genetic factors have included a candidate-gene approach, where single genes are sequenced and tested for associations with a trait of interest. This proved successful in identifying hemoglobin variants underling oxygen-binding affinity in high-altitude deer mice[230,231] and hummingbirds.[184]

Genome-wide signatures of selection have been identified using high-throughput genotyping technologies. These genomic regions are typically highlighted by dramatic differences in allele frequencies at particular loci or long continuous stretches of linkage disequilibrium, as a pattern of extended linkage disequilibrium is characteristic of a selective sweep (see Figure 117-11).

HIF is likely involved in altitude adaptation (Figure 117-15). HIF transcription factors are heterodimers, composed of a constitutively expressed HIF-1 beta (β) subunit and three labile alpha subunits (HIF-1α, HIF-2α, HIF-3α), that, under normal oxygen tensions, are targeted for degradation. In low-oxygen conditions (hypoxia), HIFs escape degradation and bind to a core DNA sequence within hypoxia response elements. HIFs recruit coactivators and increase transcription of hypoxia-responsive genes.

The alternative fates of HIF

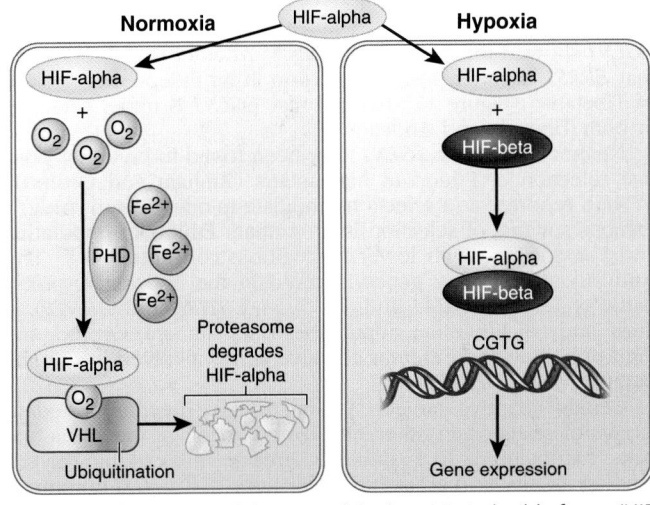

FIGURE 117-15 General diagram of the hypoxia-inducible factor (HIF) pathway. PHD, Prolyl hydroxylase; VHL, von Hippel-Lindau. *(From Petousi N, Robbins PA: Human adaptation to the hypoxia of high altitude: the Tibetan paradigm from the pregenomic to the postgenomic era.* J Appl Physiology *116:875-884, 2014.)*

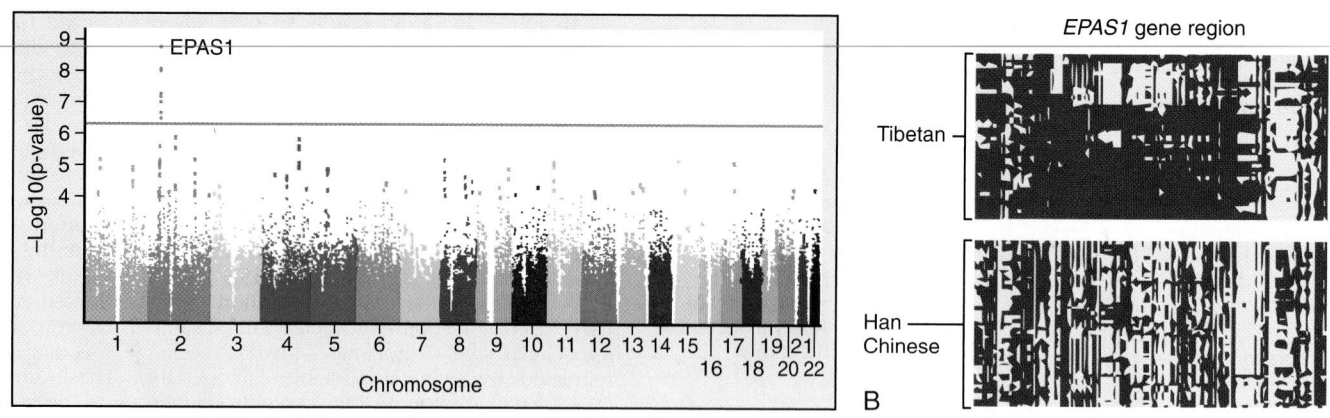

FIGURE 117-16 A, Results of a genome-wide allelic differentiation scan in Tibetans (chromosomes shown on the x-axis; significance, shown as −log10 of p value, on the y-axis). SNPs in the *EPAS1* gene region exhibit the most significant signal. **B,** Haplotype patterns in Tibetan (*top*) and Han Chinese (*bottom*) chromosomes in the genomic segment containing the *EPAS1* gene. (**A** from Beall CM, Cavalleri GL, Deng L, et al: Natural selection on EPAS1 (HIF2 alpha) associated with low hemoglobin concentration in Tibetan highlanders, Proc Natl Acad Sci USA 107:11459-11464, 2010; **B** from Simonson TS, Yang Y, Huff CD, et al: Genetic evidence for high-altitude adaptation in Tibet, Science 329:72-75, 2010.)

This facilitates acclimatization and adaptation to hypoxia by improving oxygen delivery and stimulating anaerobic glycolysis to compensate for insufficient oxidative phosphorylation. There are hundreds of known HIF target genes with established roles in developmental and physiologic processes (e.g., metabolism, proliferation and survival, iron and erythropoiesis, and vascular biology). These genes have been implicated in various disease states, including myocardial ischemia, stroke, different types of cancer, and pulmonary hypertension.[191,214]

Some of the strongest human adaptive signals have been identified in the genomes of native highland populations. A genome-wide scan of Andeans using a high-density SNP genotyping platform showed that thousands of SNPs were differentiated between Andean Quechuas residing at high altitude and nearby lowland populations.[29] This analysis focused on SNPs near HIF pathway genes. Thirty-six genes appeared to be under selection.

A study of Tibetans examined genome-wide patterns of SNPs and identified candidate genes within regions of the genome exhibiting a selective sweep.[224] Several of these genes intersected with an *a priori* list of functional candidates (e.g., *EGLN1*, *EPAS1*, and *PPARA*) in the HIF pathway. An analysis based on sequences from only protein-coding regions of the genome (i.e., the exome) identified 30 candidate genes in Tibetans of which *EPAS1* and *EGLN1* showed the strongest signals.[268] Another study confirmed that *EPAS1* is under positive selection in an independent cohort of Tibetans[23] (Figure 117-16) and that *EGLN1* is under selection in both Tibetans and Andeans.[27]

Neither *EPAS1* nor *EGLN1* have been found to be under positive selection in Ethiopian highlanders (Amhara and Oromo).[4] *PPARA*, reported as a selection candidate in one Tibetan study,[224] exhibits a signal of selection in an Amhara Ethiopian population and is associated with lower hemoglobin concentration.[207] This study identified other genes involved in the hypoxia response pathway (e.g., *CBARA1* and *VAV3*, and *THRB* and *ARNT2*). A third study of Ethiopian populations (i.e., Amhara, Oromo, and Tigray) highlighted different adaptive genes involved in the HIF pathway (e.g., *BHLHE41*).[102]

Certain adaptive targets in humans have been reported as targets of selection in other species.[222] Variants at the alpha and beta hemoglobin loci underlie greater hemoglobin-oxygen binding affinity in high-altitude deer mice[168,229,230] and hummingbirds in South America.[184] Adaptive signals at *EPAS1* and *HBB* have been identified in domesticated dogs at altitude.[66,79,251] Yak share an adaptive selection signal with Tibetans at the *ADAM17* locus.[188] In *Drosophila*, genes in the Notch pathway are top candidates of adaptation, and decreased expression of two

neighboring candidate genes, *SENP1* and *ANP32D*, originally identified through comparative analysis of Andeans with and without CMS, exhibit increased survival when exposed to hypoxia.[274] Gene expression at these two genes was also increased in fibroblasts derived from individuals with CMS compared with those without CMS[274] (Figure 117-17).

Some adaptive candidate genes appear unique to particular subpopulations within a geographic region. This may be due to (1) false-positive signals, possibly as a result of demographic history, (2) substructure among major groups, and/or (3) different analytic methods employed by various investigators,[265] including the selection of comparative populations.[102] Efforts to account for such differences in future studies and standardize methods will help elucidate adaptive genetic signals shared between groups, and help establish genetic causes for physiologic differences between native highland populations.

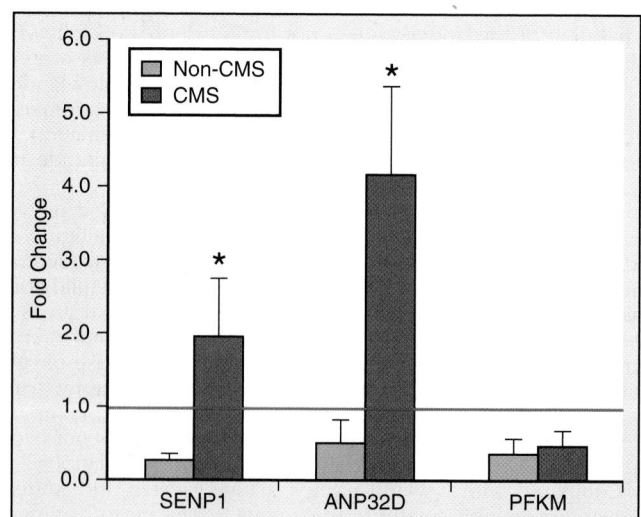

FIGURE 117-17 *SENP1* and *ANP32D* are both upregulated under hypoxia conditions in fibroblasts derived from subjects with chronic mountain sickness (*CMS*) compared with persons without the disorder (*green line* represents normoxia controls). (From Zhou D, Udpa N, Ronen R, et al: Whole-genome sequencing uncovers the genetic basis of chronic mountain sickness in Andean highlanders, Am J Hum Genet 93:452-462, 2013.)

GENETIC INFLUENCES ON ADAPTATION TO TEMPERATURE AND ULTRAVIOLET RADIATION

As human populations migrated throughout the past 100,000 years, they encountered diverse environments. These variables (e.g., altitude, as described in the previous sections, temperatures, ultraviolet (UV) light exposure, and food sources) may have contributed to phenotypes observed among human populations. Given that some traits are observed as gradients, both genetic contributions and phenotypic plasticity (as a result of genetic or epigenetic underpinnings) likely underlie these differences.

Major environmental components vary across geographic ranges (e.g., temperature and humidity). Body mass and frame are noted as distinct among geographically diverse human populations. People of northern compared with equatorial latitudes have shorter distal-to-proximal limb ratios.[118,198] It is hypothesized that elongated bodies more effectively dissipate heat than do more spherical forms. Similarly, Arctic populations exhibit increased basal metabolic rate compared with non-Arctic populations.[132]

Differences in UV exposure and melanin production correlate with geographic location. In northern latitudes, where damaging effects of UV exposure are relatively limited, lighter skin pigmentation is adaptive. Less melanin encourages sufficient UV penetration of the skin to allow for vitamin D production needed for calcium regulation and bone growth.[46,110]

Associations between SNPs and metabolic genes have been identified in polar ecoregion populations.[90] Genes involved in oxidative metabolism (ME2 and ME3), respiratory rate and body mass index (LEPR), cold resistance (UCP3), lipid oxidation, and brown adipose or nonshivering thermogenesis also harbor SNPs with extreme allele frequency differences or haplotype structures indicative of selection, suggesting a genetic underpinning to cold adaptation.[90,92] Evidence for climate adaptation (across nine climate variables) is provided in the Hancock and colleagues article of 2011.[91] SNPs associated with skin color, immunity and UV radiation, immunity and infection, and cancer pathways were also identified.[91]

Additional metabolic candidates of adaptation have been reported. Analyses of candidate genes from 52 worldwide populations suggest that variants in CYP3A are related to salt homeostasis and hypertension.[238,269] Various metabolic pathway genes appear as top candidates in Tibetan highlanders and neighboring or recent migrant Mongolian populations (e.g., EPAS1, PKLR, CYP2E1, EDNRA, PPARG). It is unclear if these signals reflect specific or integrated responses to environmental conditions (e.g., cold temperature in addition to hypoxia).[266]

GENETIC INFLUENCES ON EXERTION IN THE WILDERNESS

Many wilderness pursuits require increased levels of exertion for which a person may engage in a training regimen. Understanding individual variations in cardiovascular fitness and responses to exercise training is relevant to outdoor enthusiasts. Similarly, preventing exercise-related injuries and illnesses is especially important in remote and austere settings. Exercise genomics studies focus on explaining variations in cardiovascular fitness or exercise performance.[93]

PHYSIOLOGY OF EXERCISE

Exercise requires integration of many systems (e.g., cardiovascular, muscular, and respiratory systems). During exercise, muscle contractions require energy in the form of adenosine triphosphate (ATP), and production of ATP in the mitochondria requires oxygen. As exercise intensity increases, demand for ATP and for oxygen increases.

Total oxygen delivery, the amount of oxygen transported by the cardiovascular system each minute, is the product of the cardiac output (heart rate × stroke volume) and the arterial oxygen content. Cardiac output increases with exercise intensity. Arterial oxygen content remains relatively constant during exercise. To oxygenate blood and remove carbon dioxide, ventilation increases with exercise intensity. The peripheral vasculature contracts, redirecting blood to where it is most needed (i.e., exercising muscles) and away from where it is not needed (i.e., splanchnic region). With training, cardiac output is increased and greater ventilation rates can be achieved, increasing work rates.

The maximum volume of oxygen that can be taken up and used by the body is known as VO₂max. The theoretical upper limit for oxygen use is determined by cardiac output and oxygen extraction (i.e., the fraction of oxygen that can be extracted from blood). The VO₂max is determined by having subjects perform incremental exercise tests until they become exhausted. Cardiac output is a major factor in determining VO₂max, and is influenced by training status.[202] Changes in oxygen extraction occur with training, but these changes explain less of the change in VO₂max than do central adaptations.[201]

Physiologic factors influencing exercise performance include body morphology, endurance, strength, and power.[83] Each sport requires a different combination of these parameters. In addition, psychologic factors, training, and nutrition influence exercise performance.

EXERCISE GENOMICS

Exercise genomics studies first must determine the phenotype of interest. Studies may take a reductionist approach and measure a phenotype at the biochemical level or an applied approach and measure performance for a particular sport. Training heavily influences a person's physiology and performance. An elite athlete will have spent years training and practicing for a specific sport; this is likely the reason why training responsiveness is favored over exercise performance in genomics studies.[32,190] These factors must be considered when designing studies. For most exercise-related phenotypes, there is abundant variation among individuals. Twin and family studies indicate that genes may be associated with these phenotypes.

Human Variation and Studies Relating Genes to Performance

There is tremendous interindividual variation for exercise-related traits. Elite male endurance athletes (e.g., runners, cyclists, cross-country skiers) can have VO₂max values of 75 mL/kg/min or more and cardiac outputs of approximately 30 to 40 L/min.[56,65] VO₂max and cardiac output of elite female endurance athletes are lower but still high (e.g., ≥ 65 mL/kg/min and ≈ 25 L/min).[56,250] In young, trained men and women, VO₂max and cardiac output values are approximately 60 and 50 mL/kg/min and 25 and 20 L/min, respectively.[169] In comparison, untrained, recreationally active males might have VO₂max and cardiac output of approximately 45 mL/kg/min and 20 L/min, whereas females in this category have values of approximately 35 mL/kg/min and 15 L/min.[169] Improvements in VO₂max and individual traits in response to training are also highly variable.[9,34,247]

Other parameters related to exercise performance also vary (e.g., the proportion of type I muscle fibers in the vastus lateralis, height, and body mass index).[43] Given that the main factors underlying exercise performance (e.g., endurance, muscular strength, body composition, and height) are heritable and influenced by the environment (e.g., training and nutrition), it is not surprising that human exercise performance varies widely. The difficulty is in separating which of these phenotypic variations is attributable to genetic differences and which to environmental differences. We will discuss studies employing genomics-level techniques or studies that have been robustly replicated. The reader is directed to previous reviews for a more in-depth review of exercise genomics.[139]

Baseline Fitness

Family and Twin Studies. Family and twin studies have investigated the extent to which genetic differences explain variations in individual fitness levels. VO₂max is a heritable trait.[32] Heritability of baseline VO₂max was estimated to be approximately 50% in sedentary individuals.[34] Other exercise-related traits that are significantly heritable are the submaximal exercise work capacity and VO₂, ventilatory threshold, heart dimensions and mass, cardiovascular responses to exercise, muscular strength and endurance, flexibility and strength, fatigue resistance, neuromuscular performance, and body composition.[173,226] In addition to these physiologic parameters, the tendency of a person to participate in sports and leisure time physical activity has been reported to be heritable.[57]

Genetics of Exercise Capacity. Few genomics studies have attempted to determine which genes are associated with a baseline variation in exercise capacity. Several genome-wide linkage analyses have identified chromosomal regions associated with fatigue resistance,[237] exercise participation,[58] and physical activity levels.[42,221] These studies support a genetic basis for physical activity (and inactivity) but only identify regions of interest that harbor many genes. A GWAS to identify the specific genetic variants associated with variation in leisure time physical activity identified five such genes.[58] Two of these genes (*CYP19A1* in a Dutch sample; *LEPR* in an American sample) were replicated. A third gene (*SGIP1*) was not replicated but had a plausible physiologic role in exercise behavior. *SGIP1* and *LEPR* are expressed in the hypothalamus and are thought to regulate energy homeostasis. These studies suggest that genetic differences influence levels of physical activity in humans, even if individual genes have only modest effects.[119]

TRAINING RESPONSIVENESS

Due to differences in human activity levels and nutrition (i.e., environmental factors), it is difficult to investigate the role genetics plays in baseline fitness. More insight is likely gained by comparing individual responses with standardized exercise programs. These studies often use a within-subject design: subjects train for a set period of time and comparisons are made between pretraining and posttraining measurements. Genetic studies attempt to identify interactions between the genotype and training response.

Family and Twin Studies

The influence of heritability on responses to training has been studied. Increases in VO₂max following a standardized aerobic training protocol had a heritability of approximately 50% (coincidentally similar to the heritability for the baseline VO₂max).[33] Other responses to aerobic training found to be significantly heritable include cardiovascular responses to exercise, flexibility and strength, skeletal muscle enzyme activities, blood lipid concentrations, and glucose homeostasis.[37]

Genetics of Training Responsiveness

An early genomics study of training responsiveness used gene expression data in combination with genotype data.[239] The authors inferred that differential gene expression reflected underlying genetic variation in those genes. As such, associations between gene expression and the training response would indicate associations between the change in VO₂max and SNPs in those genes. The authors identified 11 SNPs that accounted for 23% of the variation in VO₂max trainability in the HERITAGE cohort. An independent GWAS performed on this same cohort identified a set of 21 SNPs, explaining 49% of the variation in VO₂max trainability (e.g., *CAMTA1*, *RGS18*, *RYR2*), or essentially all of the genetic variation in this trait[33] (Figure 117-18). None of the SNPs overlapped between the two studies, though 4 of 11 SNPs identified were close to significance (i.e., p < 0.008) in the GWAS. The study by Bouchard and associates[36] was recently supplemented with an integrative pathway analysis to discover specific pathways related to VO₂max trainability (e.g., protein kinase signaling, calcium signaling, immune responses, lipid metabolism, and cellular energetics).[75]

Nine SNPs associated with submaximal heart rate response to exercise training have been identified.[5] These SNPs explained the full heritability of the heart rate response to training (≈ 34%).[5]

These studies have limitations. In the HERITAGE family study, only sedentary individuals were tested, and the training protocol consisted of moderate-intensity continuous training and lasted 20 weeks. It is unclear whether the same genes would explain variation in training responses if subjects had a higher level of baseline fitness, performed other modes of training (i.e., high-intensity interval training), or trained for different durations.[32]

ATHLETIC PERFORMANCE

Another approach to identify genes involved in fitness is to compare athletes and nonathletes. Subjects are selected based on their success in organized sports. Given the paucity of successful international athletes, it can be difficult to obtain large sample sizes. Selecting appropriate controls is also difficult because athletic status is likely influenced by many environmental factors.

Family and Twin Studies

Athletic status was 66% heritable in a group of British female twins, suggesting that genetic variation could explain some of the differential success in organized sports.[59] Given that numerous exercise-related traits and responses to exercise training are

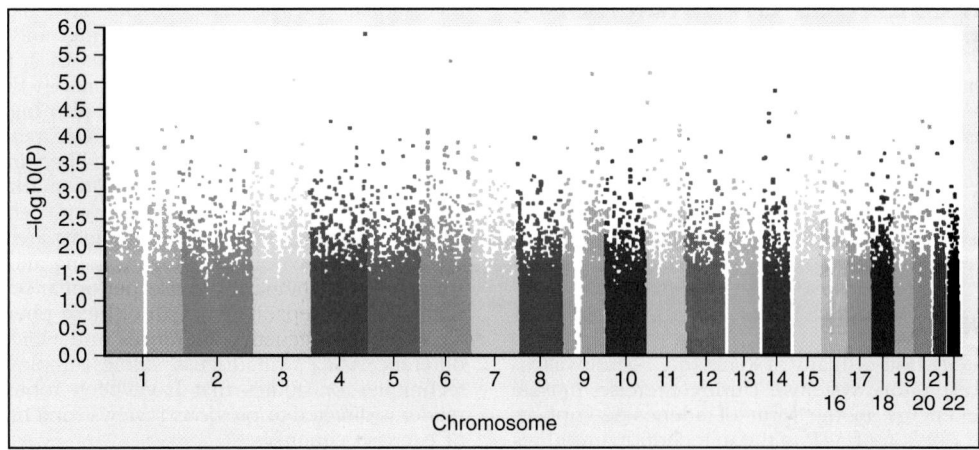

FIGURE 117-18 Results of a genome-wide association study (GWAS) for VO₂ response to exercise training in Caucasian individuals (chromosomes shown on the x-axis; significance, shown as –log10 of p value, on the y-axis). *(From Bouchard C, Sarzynski MA, Rice TK, et al: Genomic predictors of the maximal O₂ uptake response to standardized exercise training programs, J Appl Physiol 110:1160-1170, 2011.)*

heritable, it is reasonable to hypothesize that overall athletic ability is also a heritable trait.

Genetics of Athletic Performance

There are no published GWASs for athletic performance. In a recent review, Pitsiladis[181] references three abstracts presented in 2012 related to genomics in sprinting performance, suggesting that genomics data for elite athletic performance might be available soon. The same review also points out a number of existing cohorts that would be amenable to GWASs. Although genome-wide techniques have not been applied to this area of exercise science, a plethora of candidate-gene association studies have investigated the influence of specific genes on athletic success. The *ACE* gene will be discussed briefly as an example.

The *ACE* gene was the first one to be associated with human performance.[161] As previously noted, the II genotype is overrepresented in elite mountaineers relative to the general British population. In an independent sample of the same study, subjects with the II genotype demonstrated a greater training response to resistance exercise than did subjects with ID or DD genotypes. In most follow-up studies, the II genotype is associated with endurance performance,[83] except in elite Ethiopian[8] or Kenyan[213] runners. It is likely that one or more variant(s) in the *ACE* gene contribute to endurance performance but are not absolute indicators of potential athletic success. *ACTN3* is another gene often studied.[83]

SUSCEPTIBILITY TO INJURIES AND ILLNESSES RELATED TO EXERCISE

Understanding the variation in susceptibility to sports-related injuries and illnesses (e.g., concussions, exercise-induced asthma, and ligament injuries) is relevant to athletes, coaches, and physicians. Future genomics studies may inform clinical medical practice.

Achilles tendinopathy has been the subject of numerous candidate-gene association studies. Tendons are fibrous connective tissues composed largely of various collagen types and connect muscle to bone. Tendon injuries are among the most common (30% to 50%) sports injuries.[111] Both the soleus and gastrocnemius attach to the calcaneus via the Achilles tendon. Because these muscles are the major plantarflexors, large forces are placed on the Achilles tendon during weight-bearing exercise. Of sports injuries, 6% to 18% involve the Achilles tendon, and lifetime prevalence for Achilles tendon injury was estimated to be 6% in controls and approximately 50% in former competitive middle- and long-distance runners.[123]

Genetics of Achilles Tendon Injuries

Early reports suggested that blood type (i.e., encoded by the ABO locus located at 9q34) was associated with susceptibility to Achilles tendon injuries.[114,122] This locus is also the site of a more plausible physiologic association with tendon injuries, the alpha 1 type V collagen (*COL5A1*) gene. Follow-up studies have found that variants of this gene were associated with Achilles tendon pathology in South African and Australian populations.[160,217] Several other genes have been tested for association with Achilles tendon injury susceptibility: *TNC*,[159] *COL1A1*,[183] *COL12A1*,[216] *COL14A1*,[216] *TGFB1*,[182] *GDF5*,[182] and *IL1B, IL1RN*, and *IL6*.[218] Despite numerous investigations, insufficient evidence supports clinical utility (i.e., ability to suggest preventive measures or guide the prognosis) for these genetic biomarkers.[211] Identifying genes associated with tendinopathy may help provide insight into tendon pathophysiology.

GENETICS IN DIAGNOSTIC TESTS, TREATMENTS, AND PREVENTIVE MEASURES

PERSONALIZED MEDICINE

Advancements in genomics provide a greater understanding of how interindividual differences relate to disease predisposition and drug responses. Personalized medicine aims to tailor prevention and treatment to an individual's biologic profile. Genome sequencing (from blood or saliva) may be used to test for genetic contributions to disease or disease risk. Gene expression and other omic data can contribute to understanding an individual's risk of disease or response to environmental conditions.

PREDICTIVE MEDICINE

Predictive medicine works to assess probability of disease prior to its onset to minimize the impact on an individual. This effort uses information about an individual's environmental exposures and genetic makeup in association with proteomic and metabolomic biologic markers. Biologic markers may indicate early evidence of disease. Using DNA arrays or sequencing technologies, genetic risk loci can be detected years before disease onset.

Genetic testing may be recommended at different life stages. Prenatal testing, used to identify diseases or conditions in a fetus or embryo, is available to couples with an increased risk of genetic or chromosomal disorders. Tests may be minimally invasive (e.g., ultrasonography, maternal serum analyses, and maternal DNA tests) or may require invasive measures (e.g., needle aspiration for chorionic villus sampling of the placenta). Newborn screening is used to identify genetic disorders that require early treatment. In the United States, all newborns are tested for phenylketonuria and congenital hypothyroidism. Predictive risk testing (e.g., for breast cancer) uses genetic tests and a review of environmental factors to stratify the risk of disease. Diagnostic testing is used to confirm or specify the diagnosis of a particular disease. Carrier genetic testing determines whether one or both parents have a genetic variant that, if present as two copies, results in disease (e.g., cystic fibrosis). Preconception testing may be carried out on sperm and eggs to determine the risk of diseases and specific traits in offspring.

Direct-to-consumer genetic testing kits are available without physician authorization. Predictive approaches are based on probabilities, and are not able to determine with complete certainty that a disease will occur. In the absence of professional input, individuals may misinterpret genetic results.

Pharmacogenomics

Genetic variants influence individual drug responses. In different patients, a drug might have salutary effects, damaging effects, or no effects. Using analyses of multiple genes and epigenetic profiles, pharmacogenomics characterizes how acquired or inherited genetic variations contribute to function, absorption, distribution, metabolism, and elimination of a particular drug.

Rather than using a "one-size-fits-all" approach, pharmacogenomics uses an individual's genomic information to ensure that a medication dose has the greatest degree of effectiveness with minimal adverse effects. In the United States, millions of adverse drug reactions occur, leading to 100,000 deaths each year.[62] Many reactions are secondary to underlying genetic variants, typically found in a small proportion of the population.

Genes associated with pharmacogenomics are classified as pharmacodynamic or pharmacokinetic. *Pharmacodynamic genes* encode protein targets of drugs. These targets are often cell surface receptors, enzymes, or nuclear hormone receptors that modulate normal biologic function (e.g., agonists or antagonists). Genetic variation can alter properties (e.g., chemical or structural qualities) between a drug and its target protein. *Pharmacokinetic genes* encode proteins that influence availability of a drug (i.e., its absorption, distribution, metabolism, or elimination). Due to individual genetic variation, drugs that are processed in the body may be eliminated too quickly or slowly, with potentially deadly results.

As in GWASs, pharmacogenomic responses may be analyzed in a case-control (binary) or quantitative (dose) context. Individuals who exhibit an adverse response (e.g., myopathy after statin treatment) may be genotyped to look for associations. People with particular variants may want to consider alternative treatments based on predicted outcomes.

Pharmacogenomic testing of individuals for clinical care is not common practice. Data to provide molecular information about specific drugs and genes are publicly available (e.g., the Stanford University Pharmacogenomics Knowledge Base [PharmGKC]), but the data should not be used to make definitive decisions. Pharmacogenomic variants indicate the likelihood of a drug's being effective (e.g., a drug may be 90% effective if homozygous for a particular allele, 50% if heterozygous or homozygous for the alternate allele). SNPs in *quantitative trait loci* may explain some proportion of variation in a drug-metabolism trait, and may be used in predictive models of a drug response.

Genes associated with variance in drug metabolism and response include cytochrome P450s (CYP), the vitamin K epoxide reductase complex subunit 1 (*VKORC1*), and thiopurine methyl-transferase (*TPMT*). Of the 57 CYP-family genes, *CYP2D6, CYP2C19, CYP2C9, CYP3A4,* and *CYP3A5* account for the metabolism of approximately 80% of currently available prescription drugs.[272] *VKORC1* underlies the pharmacodynamics of the anticoagulant warfarin[236] because warfarin inhibits the *VKORC1* gene product, and *TPMT* is an enzyme associated with metabolic pathways that involve codeine, clopidogrel, tamoxifen, and warfarin.[53]

PERSONALIZED GENOMIC WILDERNESS MEDICINE

Adoption of personalized genomic approaches has limitations, including the uncertainty of clinical applications of associated genetic variants, expense, insufficient expertise to carry out and analyze genomic tests, and ethical questions raised by personalized medicine. This is true for conditions associated with wilderness travel.

Which Genes Should We Test?

Lack of clinical utility is the greatest impediment to using genomic medicine for conditions associated with wilderness travel. Given present knowledge, screening individuals for genetic variants is unlikely to improve patient care. For instance, although variants of the *TIMP3* gene were associated with susceptibility to HAPE in a Japanese population,[121] the association must be independently replicated to ensure validity before the information can be used for screening.

Susceptibility to many environmental stressors is likely complex; the interaction of multiple genetic variants and environmental factors determines one's susceptibility. A single genetic variant is likely to have only a small independent effect on an individual's susceptibility to an environmental condition (e.g., altitude, temperature, UV light) and is unlikely to alter clinical outcomes.

Genetic variants associated with the response to exercise training are better established. Genetic testing is being offered to provide insights into the training responsiveness of individuals,[38,200] as a means of identifying talent in younger athletes,[39,44,194] and as a way of determining susceptibility to sports injuries.[78,83,243]

Is the Test Worth It?

Individuals should not pursue genomic testing for the wilderness conditions discussed above. Even if a disease's genetic cause has been well characterized, testing for most benign conditions, especially those that can be easily avoided (i.e., susceptibility to AMS, which can be prevented by gradual ascent), is unlikely to influence outcomes.

Testing for genetic susceptibility to life-threatening conditions (e.g., HAPE or HACE) could provide greater benefit, but is unlikely to replace universal recommendations of gradual ascent.[142] In rare instances, individuals identified as susceptible to severe AMS, HAPE, or HACE could be excused from high-risk scenarios when proper acclimatization is not possible (e.g., in military efforts or search and rescue deployment).

Who Is Going to Interpret the Genomics Data?

Implementing individual genomic results into medical practice would require a full suite of knowledgeable health care professionals (i.e., physicians, nurses, pharmacists, genetic counselors) to recommend tests, answer questions, and interpret data. Many physicians do not have the necessary training in genomics and are not ready to deliver personalized medicine.[154] Although genetic counselors are trained to perform this role, there are not enough providers to absorb the burden of expanded personalized medicine.[154]

What Are the Ethical Concerns Surrounding Genomic Medicine?

The ethics of genomic medicine are still developing.[155,180] Sequencing an individual's genome provides more information than the average layperson (and perhaps even the best contemporary scientist) can fully appreciate. In addition to information about disease susceptibility and pharmaceutical effectiveness, an individual's genetic sequence contains information (e.g., ancestry, paternity, maternity, disease susceptibility) that many individuals might not want to know or want others to know.

Personalized medicine can identify treatments that are most likely to be successful, ineffective, or potentially detrimental but are likely more costly. Guarding against breaches of confidentiality and genetic discrimination will be constant concerns.

MOVING FORWARD

More than 2000 years ago, Hippocrates stated, "It's far more important to know what person the disease has, than what disease the person has." What is new in personalized medicine is the potential for genomics (and other omics-based technologies) to intimately describe molecular differences among individuals to personalize suitable treatments. With these tools, "what person the disease has" implies that a specific, molecular meaning can be determined.

Although adopting genomic medicine in the clinic will not be easy, this work is already informing medical care. Pearson and Manolio[172] state, "The primary use for GWA studies for the foreseeable future is likely to be in investigation of biologic pathways of disease causation and normal health and development." Genomics (and other omics-based research) can offer great insight into pathophysiologic processes, and can lead to better treatment, even if this treatment is not personalized. Omics technologies are already improving our understanding of high-altitude adaptation, chronic altitude illness, and HAPE. These processes and conditions likely will be further elucidated through the use of various omics-based methods.

Given the difficulties associated with investigating conditions most relevant to wilderness medicine, application of genomic medicine to this field will take time. Higher-quality genomics studies are needed to elucidate genetic variants associated with each condition. Answering whether genomic testing adds sufficient new data (beyond known risk factors) to justify the costs of screening will follow. A better understanding of the physiologic mechanisms underpinning each condition is necessary. Omics-based research can help provide this information.

REFERENCES

Complete references used in this text are available online at expertconsult.inkling.com.

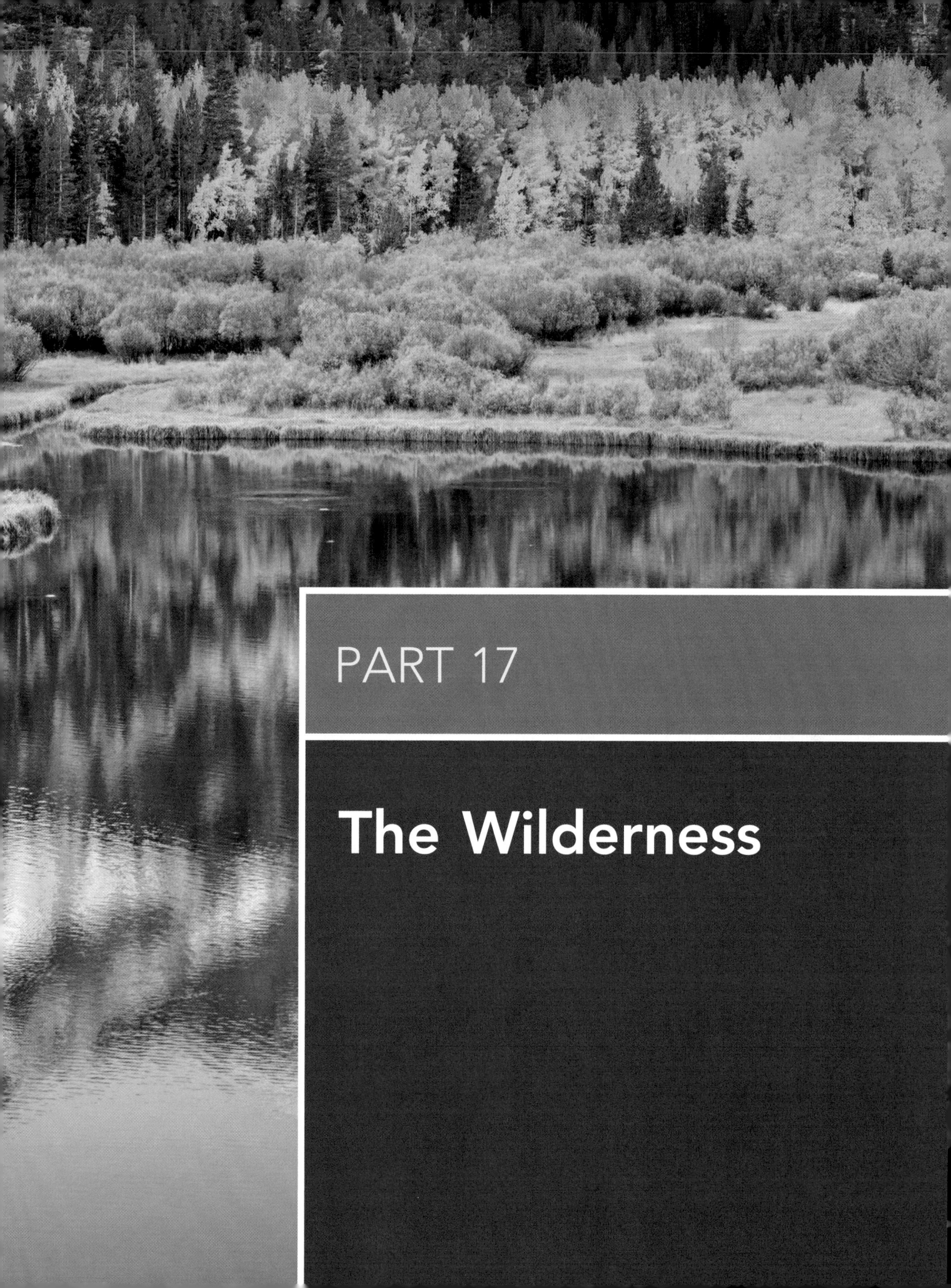

PART 17

The Wilderness

The year 2014 marked the 50th anniversary of the Wilderness Act of 1964. Public celebrations of the Wilderness Act were held across the United States to focus on the success of the National Wilderness Preservation System (NWPS). In 2014 the NWPS included more than 796 management units and had 110 million acres of publicly owned lands managed by the four federal land management agencies (Forest Service, National Park Service, Bureau of Land Management, Fish and Wildlife Service).

"Wilderness" is a word that carries various connotations and denotations among different people and cultures. Often, wilderness suggests a special place with human appeal or aversion that invokes an associated emotional, psychological, and mental state because of the natural and undeveloped characteristics of the area, whether real or perceived. Humans have a deep historical and cultural connection with "wild nature" because we have been shaped through human evolution by it, and in turn, we have modified it. Whether a person has a direct experience with wilderness, views wilderness in art and photography, or reads about the adventures of others in wilderness, the human reaction is complex and forms the basis for experiences and both conscious and subconscious memories.

In the United States and several other countries around the world, the term *wilderness* is associated with a legal definition for places that are legislatively protected.[10] The places selected and designated for protection follow certain general guidelines, and this political process is influenced by very strong and diverse groups of stakeholders and the general public. The management objectives for these areas include a variety of values, from preservation of the ecologic conditions and processes to human use and enjoyment (Figure 118-1). Although there is widespread public support for wilderness, there are divergent and polarized viewpoints on how to define wilderness, ranging from extreme protectionists who believe that humans have no place in wilderness to the utilitarian interests that hold that wilderness is a setting for economic development for recreation and tourism activities.

Although there are a variety of definitions, the United States has a legal definition of wilderness, even if somewhat vague, that is the basis for the creation of the NWPS. The purpose of this chapter is to outline the legal designation, management, and preservation of wilderness areas in the United States.[5]

HISTORICAL DEVELOPMENT OF THE WILDERNESS CONCEPT

The term *wilderness* historically was used to describe places that were untamed and not under control of humans, whereas *civilization* was the place of human control.[5,12] Areas of civilization that were cultivated and heavily influenced by human activities often bordered or were surrounded by areas that had minimal human influence. As world population has grown and more land area has come under human influence, wilderness has been lost to the point that it is now scarce in many areas of the world.

There are few places that are not now, or have not been at one time, under human control, habitation, cultivation, or influence. A gradient of human influence and impact exists from urban centers and rural areas to some wild country (e.g., wilderness) that has little or no human influence (Figure 118-2). The so-called human footprint on the world is large and expanding rapidly with population growth, road building, food production, power generation, industrialization, and human habitation. Some identifiable "last of the wild places" exist on each continent and might continue to do so with careful conservation of resources and protection worldwide of some remaining representative or remnant areas of each ecologic community type.[14]

In the United States, older adults have commented on the change in the landscape and extent of development in the country during their lifetime. The early history of the United States during European immigration was one of cultivating and taming the wild places and taking dominion over the land for human habitation. Wilderness was seen as a place for exploration and primitive travel, and most of the population often feared and avoided it. As the amount of land with wild conditions began to diminish, it was more appreciated as a change from cities and civilization. The public's interest in wild places evolved as these areas became scarce. Special places were first set aside as National Parks, such as Yellowstone, Yosemite, and the Grand Tetons. These areas were at first seen as park destinations for development of recreation and tourism, rather than as preserves.

The early interest in wilderness began with employees in the federal land-managing agencies, such as the U.S. Forest Service and U.S. National Park Service. After World War II, a greater public interest began to emerge to save areas for wilderness character. The emerging concern to save certain places by designating them for protection as wilderness was partly the result of interest in recreation experiences, coupled with a growing concern about rapid industrialization and population growth transforming the landscape through human activities. The U.S. population was more than 300 million by 2010.

Some would argue that few places in the world are "wilderness" in the strictest sense of the word. Thus, the more common use of the term *wilderness* is in relation to our perception of areas that are little known or predominantly under the influence of natural processes and forces. Although the term had been commonly applied to any large, remote area with natural characteristics, conditions, and processes, by 1964 it gained a new legal definition that was applied to federally owned land areas designated as wilderness by congressional action in the United States.

WILDERNESS LEGISLATION AND POLICY IN THE UNITED STATES

The U.S. Forest Service and U.S. National Park Service did not begin to set agency policies to protect primitive and roadless areas from development until the 1920s. During the following decades, roadless area inventories and administrative designations of wilderness occurred with increasing public interest. As recreational use and interest in these lands increased, professionals in the agencies and the public raised concerns that the administrative regulation (1) allowed too many development activities, such as mining, grazing, motorized access, and water resource development; (2) shifted boundaries or removed designation to permit resource development; (3) promulgated different regulations and management in different areas; and (4) had neither a distinct policy for wilderness preservation nor a national system with coordinated management.

The concept gradually evolved that legislative protection was needed to create a more permanent and coordinated national

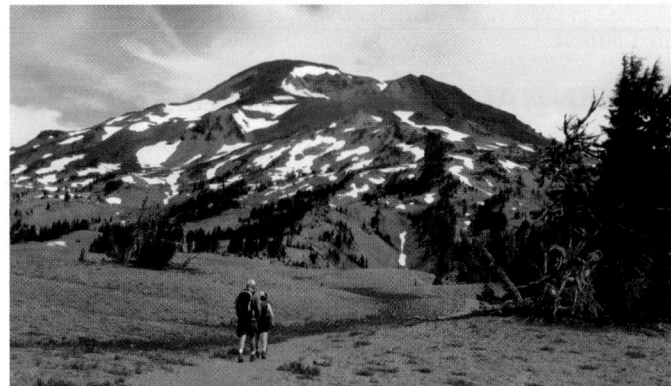

FIGURE 118-1 Day hikers en route to a summit attempt on snow-capped South Sister Mountain (3158 m [10,358 feet]) in the Three Sisters Wilderness, a 286,708-acre area managed by the U.S. Forest Service in west-central Oregon. *(Courtesy Chad P. Dawson.)*

system for wilderness preservation and management. From 1956 to 1964, more than 50 versions of a wilderness bill were introduced in the U.S. Congress, heavily debated, supported, and challenged by different interest groups. Political compromises were deemed necessary to have a wilderness bill finally passed into legislation, and so certain human activities were permitted in some areas, even though they would be nonconforming with the intent of the wilderness legislation.[5,15] These activities included mining, grazing, aircraft landings, and water resources development.

In 1964 the U.S. Congress passed The Wilderness Act (U.S. Public Law 88-577).[18] This legislation created the NWPS and was heralded by the environmental community and the general public as one of the most important pieces of conservation legislation in U.S. history.[15] A historian of wilderness policy and legislation, Scott[16] commented that "before there was a Wilderness Act, wilderness was, at best, an afterthought. Only the U.S. Forest Service had actually delineated wilderness areas, propelled by visionaries within its own ranks."

The Wilderness Act[18] defines a broad statement of policy for designating wilderness under the Act and recognizes the need to set aside significant natural areas for present and future generations because of the rapid loss of such resources, as follows:

In order to assure that an increasing population, accompanied by expanding settlement and growing mechanization, does not occupy and modify all areas within the United States and its possessions, leaving no lands designated for preservation and protection in their natural condition, it is hereby declared to be the policy of the Congress to secure for the American people of present and future generations the benefits of an enduring resource of wilderness. For this purpose there is hereby established a National Wilderness Preservation System to be composed of federally owned areas designated by Congress as "wilderness areas," and these shall be administered for the use and enjoyment of the American people in such manner as will leave them unimpaired for future use and enjoyment as wilderness, and so as to provide for the protection of these areas, the preservation of their wilderness character, and for the gathering and dissemination of information regarding their use and enjoyment as wilderness. (U.S. Public Law 88-577, section 2a)

This paragraph is referred to by land management agencies as the "guiding management intent" because it specifically refers to human "use and enjoyment," provided the areas were "unimpaired" and that management would ensure "preservation of their wilderness character."

Section 2c of The Wilderness Act[18] includes an important and often-quoted definition of wilderness that has led to much controversy and debate because although it is poetic in form, it has left room for interpretation, especially during legal hearings and court cases in the 50 years since its passage:

A wilderness, in contrast with those areas where man and his own works dominate the landscape, is hereby recognized as an area where the earth and its community of life are untrammeled by man, where man himself is a visitor who does not remain. An area of wilderness is further defined to mean … an area of undeveloped Federal land retaining its primeval character and influence, without permanent improvements or human habitation, which is protected and managed so as to preserve its natural conditions and which (1) generally appears to have been affected primarily by the forces of nature, with the imprint of man's work substantially unnoticeable; (2) has outstanding opportunities for solitude or a primitive and unconfined type of recreation; (3) has at least five thousand acres of land or is of sufficient size as to make practicable its preservation and use in an unimpaired condition; and (4) may also contain ecological, geological, or other features of scientific, educational, scenic, or historical value. (U.S. Public Law 88-577, section 2c)

The definition emphasizes that wilderness is in contrast to civilization, human influences, and habitation. The definition is an ideal that is tempered by four conditions to make it practical and applicable in a world that has historic human activities and impacts that may no longer be noticeable to visitors.

One of the conditions refers to "outstanding opportunities for solitude or a primitive and unconfined type of recreation." This phrase is often referred to as the "guiding principle for recreation and visitor management." A careful reading of the definition of wilderness makes it clear that preservation is the overall principle and reason for designating an area "wilderness." Certain types and amounts of recreation are permitted, provided the area is "protected and managed so as to preserve its natural conditions." This is an important principle to keep in mind when discussing recreation use and management (Figure 118-3), especially when it relates to primitive facilities and trails, backcountry travel, recreational equipment (e.g., removable climbing gear, backpacking stoves), and management interventions.

The use of helicopters and other motorized equipment during search and rescue operations is often regarded as a necessary exception to the natural preservation principle of wilderness, with the humanistic and legal rationale being that human health and safety should take precedence. However, the extent and frequency of search and rescue operations have led to such an intrusion in high-use mountain areas that "outstanding opportunities for solitude" are being diminished. Balancing human interest in risk-taking activities, such as helicopter drop-offs for high-altitude skiing or multiday high-wall rock climbing, with human self-preservation instincts for those injured or needing rescue will remain a controversial subject in wilderness management.

Creation of the NWPS with the Wilderness Act in 1964 was just the beginning of legislative designations. By 2014, more than 170 different laws were passed by the U.S. Congress designating new areas or adding acreage to existing areas.[5] In addition to the Wilderness Act, subsequent legislation over 50 years has clarified congressional intent to protect and manage the wildest remaining U.S. lands as wilderness and has expanded the NWPS. It is difficult to identify any natural resource issue—or any issue—for

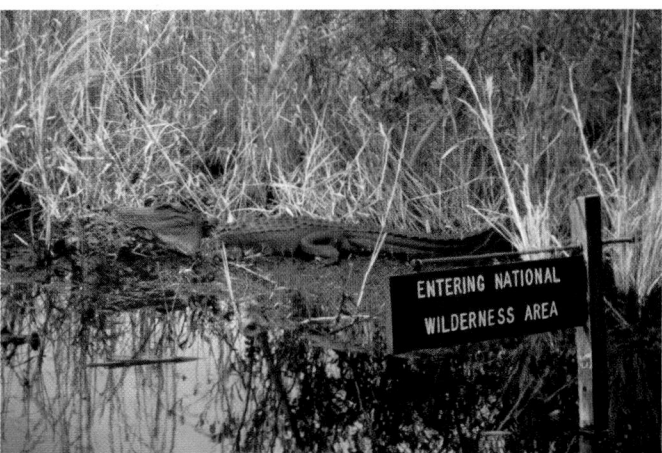

FIGURE 118-2 Wildlife is both an attraction and a danger to visitors in the Okefenokee Wilderness, a 353,981-acre wildlife refuge swamp and wilderness area managed by the U.S. Fish and Wildlife Service in southern Georgia. *(Courtesy Chad P. Dawson and Brian Dawson.)*

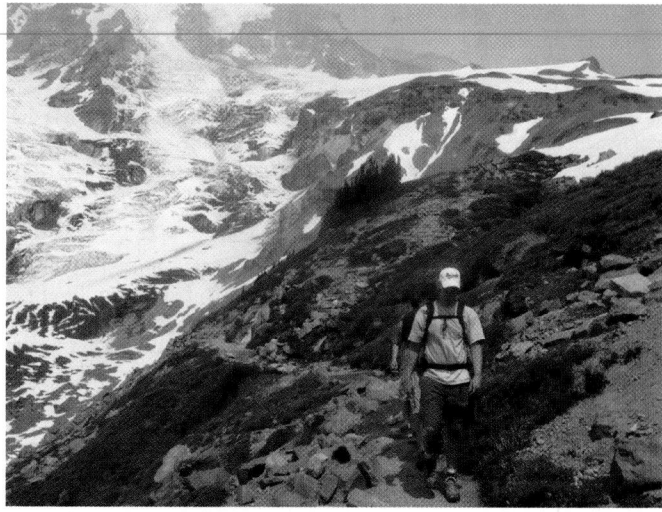

FIGURE 118-3 Tourists often test their snow-climbing skills on the easily accessible snowfields above Paradise in the Mt Rainier Wilderness (4393 m [14,410 feet]), a 228,480-acre wilderness area managed by the U.S. National Park Service in western Washington. *(Courtesy Chad P. Dawson.)*

which Congress has so consistently and so often confirmed its intent as it has with wilderness. The initial designation of 9.1 million acres of wilderness was followed by congressional designations in most of the years between 1964 and 2014 to add additional acres and units to the NWPS. The largest single increase was addition of approximately 56 million acres in Alaska under the Alaska National Interest Lands Conservation Act of 1980 (Public Law 96-487).

Many proposals for additional units and acreage are still being brought before the U.S. Congress and its committees. Several authors and organizations have predicted that more acreage will be added to the NWPS in coming decades, but estimates of those additions vary widely.[5,15] Scott[16] observed that, "however much wilderness Americans may choose to designate through their elected representatives, future generations are likely to judge that we preserved too little, rather than too much."

WILDERNESS STEWARDSHIP PHILOSOPHY

Some management of wilderness resources and experiences is necessary as visitor use increases and surrounding land management and use affect the wilderness area. The idea that we need management in an area that was intended to be free of the influences of modern human activities may appear paradoxical. However, wilderness stewardship is the management of human uses of wilderness and internal and external influences on wilderness to protect and preserve an area's solitude and naturalness, including natural processes and conditions. We highlight the following wilderness stewardship philosophy for managers:

Wilderness management should not mold nature to suit people. Rather, it should manage human use and influences so as not to alter natural processes. Managers should do only what is necessary to meet wilderness objectives and use only the minimum tools, regulations, and enforcement required to meet those objectives. In wilderness, people adapt to nature, to naturalness and solitude, and that is the source of human benefits from wilderness experience as well as the ecological and non-use benefits.

This stewardship philosophy is based on the wilderness legislation and is balanced between two often-debated ends of a continuum. At one end of the continuum is wilderness for its own sake with protection of the naturalness foremost, and at the other end is wilderness primarily for human use and enjoyment. The stewardship philosophy favors natural integrity of the wilderness ecosystems, with some accommodation for primitive styles of recreation and the opportunity for solitude. The long-term results are that the natural forces and processes that shaped and

formed the American wilderness will be evident in the wilderness that current stewards leave for future generations.

POTENTIAL THREATS TO WILDERNESS

Designating an area as wilderness is only the first step and must be followed by stewardship to maintain those areas that represent all that is left of many ecosystems, as well as natural landscapes that have not been cultivated, mined, developed, urbanized, or otherwise heavily altered by human activities. Numerous types of internal and external conditions, influences, and changes threaten wilderness resources and values, now and in the future.[9] Three examples of categories of threats are summarized here to highlight the concern about the future sustainability of wilderness conditions and processes.

Wilderness areas in many states are increasingly isolated fragments or remnants of historic ecosystems. As the surrounding landscape becomes more developed and inhabited, wilderness areas become ecologic islands that can continue with various processes, provided they are large enough or are not disconnected from other natural areas. This concern is most pronounced in the eastern United States, with its smaller wilderness areas, but the threat is felt throughout the country as the natural landscape is replaced by human influences, habitation, and manipulation.

Exotic and non-native species of plants and animals are invading wilderness and are direct threats to naturalness and wildness. Efforts to control and manipulate these invasive species can have additional impacts on wilderness conditions that are also undesirable. Invasive plant species, such as knapweed, cheatgrass, and purple loosestrife, can rapidly change an ecosystem and fundamentally alter its historic patterns and conditions for native plant and animal species.

Increasing commercial and public recreation use of wilderness and efforts to control its impacts are serious threats to wilderness resources and values. High visitor use has obvious impacts that can be identified, but what may not be as easily observed are changes to opportunities for solitude and the impacts of regulations and enforcement on social conditions. Regulation takes away some of the freedom of choice and spontaneity to explore that many visitors associate with wilderness experiences.

Nineteen categories of internal and external threats have been identified as change agents that affect wilderness conditions and values[5]:

1. Fragmentation and isolation of wilderness areas as ecologic islands
2. Impacts on threatened and endangered species
3. Increasing commercial and public recreation use
4. Permitted livestock grazing
5. Invasion of exotic and non-native species
6. Administrative access, facilities, and intrusive management
7. Adjacent land management and use
8. Private and public land inholdings within wilderness
9. Established mining claims
10. Wildland fire suppression activities
11. Reduced air quality
12. Reconstruction and maintenance of water projects and reduced water quality
13. Advanced communication and navigation technology that reduces solitude
14. Motorized and mechanical equipment trespass and legal use
15. Aircraft noise and airspace reservations
16. Urbanization and encroaching development
17. Global climate change
18. Legislation designating new wilderness areas with compromised wilderness conditions
19. Lack of political and financial support for wilderness protection and management

The concern is that few of these threats will diminish, and most are projected to increase in the coming decades. Land managers will need to monitor these potential threats to prepare management plans and activities to steward designated wilderness areas and minimize, mitigate, or remove the threats. The responsibilities at the national level for these wilderness

TABLE 118-1 Number of Designated U.S. Wilderness Management Units Under Agency Management and Their Acreage by 2014

U.S. Agency	Wilderness Units	Acres	Percentage of Total
Bureau of Land Management	222	8,736,087	8
Fish and Wildlife Service	71	20,702,488	19
Forest Service	442	36,385,240	33
National Park Service	61	43,932,843	40
TOTAL	796	109,756,658	100

From http://www.wilderness.net.

planning and management activities are primarily under the jurisdiction of four federal agencies.

WILDERNESS MANAGEMENT AGENCIES IN THE UNITED STATES

The NWPS included more than 796 units managed by four federal agencies and totaled 110 million acres of publicly owned lands by 2014 (Table 118-1). The four federal agencies administering the NWPS are the U.S. National Park Service (NPS), U.S. Bureau of Land Management (BLM), U.S. Fish and Wildlife Service (FWS) in the Department of Interior, and U.S. Forest Service (FS) in the Department of Agriculture. The NPS has the greatest total area of wilderness at 43.9 million acres and the fewest units for a federal agency; the largest area in the NWPS, Wrangell–St. Elias Wilderness (>9 million acres) in Alaska, is under NPS management. The FS has the largest number of wilderness units to manage and approximately one-third of the total NWPS acreage. The FWS manages 19% of the NWPS area, including the smallest unit in the system, 5-acre Pelican Island Wilderness in Florida. The BLM has significant acreage in some of the desert ecosystems of the west and manages many smaller units in its 8% of the NWPS.

The four federal land-managing agencies have promulgated regulations based on the wilderness legislation and have developed policy and management documents to steward the lands under their jurisdiction. In addition, the process of evaluating additional lands and managing them for potential inclusion in the NWPS continues for all four agencies. Although the NWPS is a national system operating under the same legislation, each agency has developed its own procedures and organizational approach to accomplishing the task of protecting the "enduring resource of wilderness," based on each agency's administrative mission and structure. Some of the different approaches to visitor and resource management can be confusing to visitors who do not have appreciation or understanding that the overall mission of each agency is different. For example, the FWS has a wildlife management mission that incorporates a national wildlife refuge system.

DISTRIBUTION OF WILDERNESS IN THE UNITED STATES

The 110-million-acre NWPS represents just over 4.5% of the U.S. land area, in contrast to the more than 6% of total acreage in urban and suburban land area or more than 20% of the total in agricultural cropland.[9] The NWPS is an attempt to designate wilderness areas that would represent the different geographic regions and ecosystems of the United States. The representation of ecosystems is not complete (<50% of types are represented), and it is more effective for some arid lands and mountain ecosystems of the west than for coastal lowlands, grasslands, and eastern hardwood forests.[9]

Forty-four of the states have federally designated wilderness, ranging from a 77-acre island wilderness area in Ohio to more than 57 million acres in the state of Alaska. The six states without federally designated wilderness are in the midwestern or northeastern United States. When the number of acres of designated wilderness in each state or region is compared with the total land area and total population, the pattern is an uneven distribution favoring the western United States.[5] Less than 5% of the NWPS is located in the eastern United States, where more than one-half of the population resides on over 40% of the U.S. land area. The Pacific and mountain regions of the western United States have approximately 22% of the population and more than 95% of the NWPS. The greatest disparity is that Alaska has more than one-half of the land area of the NWPS and less than 1% of the U.S. population.

Whereas the NWPS is based on the Wilderness Act of 1964 and federal land ownership, there are also 12 states that have designated state wilderness programs or areas on state-owned lands since the 1970s.[13] Most notable are 22 New York State wilderness areas (1.2 million acres in the Adirondack and Catskill Forest Preserves) and five Alaska state wilderness areas (1.1 million acres). The 12 states with wilderness programs or areas protect more than 3.2 million acres.[13] These areas are managed by the state land-managing agencies and are not part of the NWPS. Many states have legislation and management programs modeled after the federal Wilderness Act.

The NWPS is extensive and complex geographically and is often difficult for visitors to locate because it is generally shown on agency maps only as part of overall public land holdings. For example, the Boundary Waters Canoe Area Wilderness in Minnesota is part of the Superior National Forest. A helpful source to see the geographic distribution and location of the units in the NWPS is available at http://www.wilderness.net and is provided by the Wilderness Institute at the University of Montana's College of Forestry and Conservation, Arthur Carhart National Wilderness Training Center, and Aldo Leopold Wilderness Research Institute. This website also links to the managing federal agency, the wilderness area's legislative history, and visitor information sources.

WILDERNESS VALUES AND PUBLIC PERCEPTIONS

The American public is strongly supportive of wilderness designation and the NWPS.[1,3,4] Scott[16] reported a summary of seven different surveys in the United States from 1999 through 2002 that showed 48% to 81% of respondents supported designating more wilderness land in the United States into the NWPS. Our observations on the relationship between public visitors to wilderness areas and the values they hold for its protection indicate that the striking trend over time is for a broad base of support across American society and intense commitment from a subset to fight for wilderness protection[5]:

Although wilderness means something different to everyone, four central themes have consistently emerged: experiential, the direct value of the wilderness experience; the value of wilderness as a scientific resource and environmental baseline; the symbolic and spiritual values of wilderness to the nation and the world; and the value of wilderness as a commodity or place that generates direct and indirect economic benefits.

National surveys in 1994 and 2000 reported that more than 50% of the public indicated that 12 of 13 wilderness values were very or extremely important to them[4] (Table 118-2). These surveys showed a trend to increase the percentage for all 13 values, indicating a higher level of value.[3,4] The nonuse values tended to dominate the higher average value scores (scale ranged from "not important" to "extremely important"), with the highest value for protecting water quality and air quality. Strong support for the value of income from tourism related to industry use on wilderness lands tended to be reported by less than 30% of the respondents. Western U.S. residents were somewhat more often aware of the NWPS than were easterners (60% vs. 56%); conversely, eastern more often than western residents (53% vs. 48%) reported there was not enough land in the NWPS. Metropolitan

TABLE 118-2 Percentage of Americans (>16 Years of Age) Indicating a Response of "Very or Extremely Important" for 13 Wilderness Values

Wilderness Value	Percentage
Protecting water quality	93.1
Protecting air quality	92.3
Protection of wildlife habitat	87.8
For future generations	87.0
Protection for endangered species	82.7
Preserving ecosystems	80.0
Future option to visit	75.1
Just knowing it exists	74.6
Scenic beauty	74.0
Recreational opportunities	64.9
For scientific study	57.5
Providing spiritual inspiration	56.5
Income for tourism industry	29.7

From Cordell HK, Tarrant MA, Green GT: Is the public viewpoint of wilderness shifting? *Int J Wilderness* 9:27, 2003, with permission.

and urban more often than rural residents (54% vs. 44%) reported there was not enough land in the NWPS.[4]

WILDERNESS VISITORS

The diversity of wilderness visitors ranges from those who take short walks and view scenery and wildlife in an hour to multiday backpackers, week-long backcountry hunters with pack animals, and mountain climbers on expeditions. The growth in recreation demand and increasing popularity of many forms of recreation in wilderness are the result of U.S. population growth and a general upward trend in participation in many activities, on all types of sites, in the United States[1] on public or private lands. Although backcountry and wilderness use is distributed across the full geographic and sociodemographic spectrum, an identifiable 8.6% of the U.S. population has been labeled as "backcountry actives" by one researcher because of their 2.5 times or greater above-average participation in such activities as backpacking, wilderness visits, cross-country skiing, and day hiking.[1]

Studies at high-use federal agency sites of visitor use of wilderness in the mid-1990s estimated that more than 14 million visitors went to the wilderness per year. Public surveys of the general population in recent years estimated that visitation was closer to 40 million per year.[2] Most estimates of future growth suggest that wilderness use will continue to increase 2% to 4% per year, and that participation will continue across a wide range of activities.[1,2]

Recreation enthusiasts spending 7 or more days in wilderness or primitive areas per year are a growing market segment that includes participation in strenuous physical activities on a regular basis.[1] Improvements in and availability of high-technology gear permit travel in all types of weather conditions and terrain, so that regular use across the entire landscape makes it more difficult to manage use in general, as well as more challenging to conduct search and rescue operations. Risk-taking, exploring, and adventure activities are increasingly prevalent because of media exposure, easier access to sites, more available high-technology gear, more opportunities for initiation into activities, and more training and skill-building opportunities. There is some concern that communication equipment such as satellite cell phones and navigational equipment, such as handheld Global Positioning System (GPS) units, may contribute to the impression that a person could call for help more readily and therefore take greater risks than their skills otherwise would warrant.

One of the ways that people are initiated into wilderness use and gain training in primitive travel and living is through participation in Wilderness Experience Programs (WEPs). The number of WEP organizations and their clientele have grown rapidly in the United States in the past two decades.[7] Wilderness land managers recognize WEPs as a significant user group with a focus on programs in wilderness and primitive areas as one of their defining characteristics.[6]

The most prevalent three types of WEPs are (1) educational programs where the wilderness ecosystem is the focus of instruction, research, and field trips; (2) personal growth and development, where wilderness is the setting and metaphor for everyday life, with insights achieved from challenging activities and reflection; and (3) therapy and healing, where wilderness is the setting to seek restored normal functioning and a healthy balance through primitive living and traveling.[6,7] Although the healing aspects of a natural environment[8] and wilderness areas are well documented, the inherent risks of traveling in remote areas must be recognized through risk management assessment and contingency planning,[17] especially for human health and safety.

DISTRIBUTION OF WILDERNESS VISITOR USE

Visitor use is very unevenly distributed in geographic space and across time. Each wilderness has popular access points because of easy highway access from urban centers, information in guidebooks, word-of-mouth information dissemination, and many other factors. There is often congestion in visitor use at these access sites and crowding along popular trails and at campsites and destinations (e.g., lakes and ponds, scenic overlooks, historic sites). Many wilderness areas have these types of heavy-use access sites; conversely, each area also has places with very low or no use for a variety of reasons. This variation in visitation means that not every acre of wilderness or the associated experience has the potential to be experientially unique. Therefore, a continuum of solitude and naturalness exists across wilderness.

Some of the extreme variations in visitation are caused by seasonality and opportunity for use. Each area has a favored season for a given type of activity. Even though most hiking and camping activities occur during late spring through early fall, some areas have other peak-use times because of weather and opportunities present. For example, spring fishing and whitewater boating may occur in the same area, whereas fall hunting and backpacking during fall foliage may be followed by cross-country skiing and winter camping. Cooler weather in desert areas may bring visitors in nonsummer months (Figure 118-4). Warmer months in alpine areas may bring large numbers of visitors. Weekend and weekday variations are normal fluctuations resulting from work schedules.

Other variation patterns in visitation are caused by geographic location in the United States and proximity to urban population centers. The majority of use in each wilderness area comes from

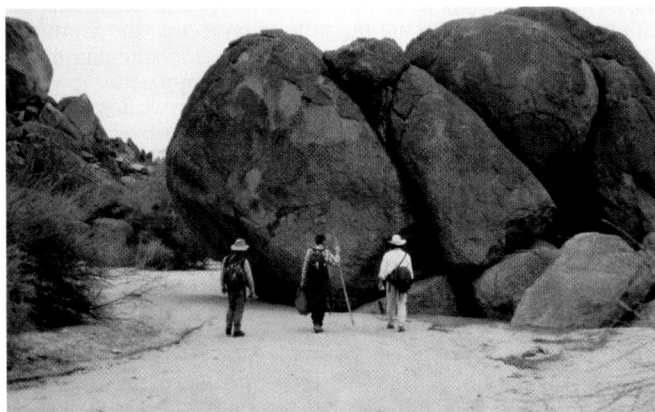

FIGURE 118-4 The lower Sonoran Desert in the North Maricopa Mountain Wilderness is a scenic and difficult place to access. Visitors may not understand the dangers of heat and dehydration in this 63,020-acre wilderness area managed by the U.S. Bureau of Land Management in southern Arizona, where temperatures commonly exceed 100° F (37.7° C). *(Courtesy Chad P. Dawson.)*

the surrounding region and states, regardless of whether one considers the urban-proximate White Mountain National Forest wilderness in New Hampshire or the Bob Marshall Wilderness in Montana. However, there is considerable long-distance travel and higher visitation to some of the larger and more popular wilderness areas that have unique opportunities and features. Every wilderness area has a great variation in the number of people at any given time and place. Although such variation in visitation is natural, the impacts may be difficult to manage, leading managers to use more direct and heavier-handed management techniques to reduce the negative consequences to resources and other users.

WILDERNESS MANAGEMENT PRINCIPLES

The guiding principles for managing wilderness areas[5] revolve around the idea that wilderness needs to be managed as a pristine extreme in the landscape (>4% of U.S. land area) to maintain the distinctive qualities that define and separate wilderness from other land uses (>95% of U.S. land area). Wilderness is managed from the biologically centered perspective. Environmental integrity and primeval conditions of wilderness are the basis for any human enjoyment, values, and benefits.

Managing wilderness as an *ecosystem* and not as a separate set of resource types (e.g., water, forests, wildlife) focuses managers on a more comprehensive perspective on the protected area. Most wilderness areas represent the remnants of ecosystems or entire ecosystems and, as such, need to be protected for present and future generations if they are to be available for humans to experience and enjoy. In addition, it is imperative that human uses and influences be managed to preserve wilderness conditions and characteristics, because without such stewardship, these remaining areas would lose their unique value in the U.S. landscape.

If wilderness is to be managed to maintain or improve wilderness conditions and not allow degradation on sites or across the area, it is essential to understand the carrying capacity of the area to sustain recreational use. One of the major components in managing wilderness recreational use is to manage use in favor of recreation and human activities that depend on wilderness conditions to achieve their goals, while not degrading wilderness conditions. In other words, there are other places to have various recreational experiences that do not require wilderness conditions. Thus, only those activities that require such conditions should be allowed in wilderness, and only as much as the area can sustain while maintaining its wilderness conditions and processes.

One of the implications of such a management philosophy is that wilderness is not primarily a place for recreational use, although it is permitted as long as it does not impinge on the capacity of the area to maintain its wilderness conditions and processes. All management activities, including search and rescue operations, should have as light an impact on the wilderness and user experience as possible. This is sometimes referred to as the "minimum tool or regulation" that achieves management objectives for the area and maintains the highest levels of naturalness and solitude. Examples are using hand tools instead of gas-powered tools in wilderness maintenance activities, using educational materials in place of direct trip management, and using minimal directional trail signs and not mileage markers.

Section 4c of The Wilderness Act provides for the administrative use of vehicles, such as aircraft and motorized equipment, when it is considered the minimum necessary for certain operations such as search and rescue (SAR). In the case of emergency situations, the use of aircraft, helicopters, and other motorized transport during SAR operations is often thought of as necessary for human health and safety. In some places, however, the extent and frequency of SAR operations have become an intrusion affecting both the environment (e.g., wildlife behavior) and the human experience of solitude. Balancing the need for effective and rapid SAR operations with impacts on the wilderness resources and experiences will be an increasingly controversial subject in wilderness management. Determining the level of SAR operations and activities that is effective with a minimal impact on wilderness resources and experiences is an ideal goal that needs further attention and study. For example, in nonemergency SAR operations, the minimum may be determined to be nonmotorized access using humans on foot to search or to carry out a victim with minor trauma.

WILDERNESS PRESERVATION AS A NATIONAL AND INTERNATIONAL MOVEMENT

The number of and membership in organizations involved in promoting wilderness designations, stewardship, information, and education have grown dramatically over the last 50 years. Organizations can be found at international, national, state, and local levels.

The U.S. legislative model has influenced some forms of international wilderness protection,[11] although variation in level and type of protection is complex and based on the cultural and legislative history in each country. The concept of wilderness is universal, but the national legislative approach used in the United States has been widely adopted by other countries, such as Canada, Australia, Finland, Russia, and South Africa.[11] There are dozens of international organizations that one can join to help protect wilderness. Some examples include the WILD Foundation (http://www.wild.org), Conservation International (http://www.conservation.org), and IUCN—The World Conservation Union (http://www.iucn.org). Many countries have strong public support for wilderness and related organizations that promote wilderness designation and stewardship.

As previously discussed, wilderness protection and management of federal lands in the United States is under jurisdiction of the NPS, BLM, FS, and WFS, each of which has policy and operational information that is important for visitors to understand. This information is available at agency websites but is easy to obtain through websites (e.g., http://www.wilderness.net) that allow access from a geographic map that in turn brings the viewer to useful information, ranging from the designating legislation to the managing agency and local-level contact offices for that wilderness unit. Obtaining local contact information and some general visitor management information makes wilderness visitation more enjoyable and improves the pretrip planning process, including compliance with local regulations.

Wilderness stewardship organizations in the United States include many that have been involved in wilderness issues for decades. Only a few examples are listed here: The Wilderness Society (http://www.wilderness.org), Sierra Club (http://www.sierraclub.org), American Wilderness Coalition (http://www.americanwilderness.org), Campaign for America's Wilderness (http://www.leaveitwild.org), Wilderness Watch (http://www.wildernesswatch.org), National Wildlife Federation (http://www.nwf.org), National Audubon Society (http://www.audubon.org), and the Izaak Walton League (http://www.iwla.org).

Wilderness preservation is a national and international movement comprising grass roots and membership organizations interested in protection and stewardship of dwindling wild areas. Although the concept and values of wilderness are supported by the general population of the United States and many other countries, it is the continued support and work of many people and organizations that stimulate the legislative and administrative branches of government to continue their efforts to maintain parts of the United States "wild" for present and future generations. The reader is encouraged to become part of that wilderness preservation movement. For a comprehensive resource, the reader is referred to Dawson and Hendee.[5]

REFERENCES

Complete references used in this text are available online at expertconsult.inkling.com.

Three miles southwest of the Kremlin, not far from Moscow's Olympic Stadium, lies the Novodevichiy Cemetery, one of the most celebrated burying places in Russia. Amid ornate memorials to former leaders such as Gromyko* and Khrushchev,[†] who were out of favor at the times of their deaths, and to giants of the arts, such as Chekhov[‡] and Shostakovich,[§] stands a white marble pedestal carrying the sculpted head of Vladimir Illich Vernadsky (1863-1945). Little known in the West, Vernadsky was a prescient observer of the emerging role of humans as makers of the global environment. It was he who first announced that we are living at a time when the power of mankind to change Earth now rivals that of geologic processes.[5] In the past, students of natural history could regard the human life span as a mere blink of a cosmic eye that witnessed little environmental change. At present, we are faced with the prospect that the planet may be fundamentally transformed by humans, perhaps within a few decades, but more probably over the next one or two generations.

This situation has not come about all at once, or equally everywhere. On a global scale, it has gradually built up over centuries, although the local manifestations of increased human agency sometimes have been masked by other processes. For example, conversion of "natural" ecosystems to "managed" ecosystems is a dominant feature on the global scale, but in some parts of the world, especially the United States and Western Europe, managed ecosystems are also being abandoned.

Such is the case in New Jersey, where hilltop 19th-century farmlands have largely reverted to regrowth forests.[21] The complications of environmental change might best be appreciated with the aid of a time machine, such as the one envisioned by H. G. Wells in 1895. Imagine, for a moment, being in a mature pine forest in southern New England. What might be observed as the machine slips into the past at this location? The surrounding landscape comes clearly into view. The pine trees shrink slowly down into youth as the years wind back, because most of today's pines trace their origin to abandonment of farmlands at or near the turn of the century. The pines disappear entirely in the late 19th century and are replaced by shrubs and eventually by grasses. By the mid-1800s, the local vicinity is completely open and appears as a shifting mosaic of agricultural crops and pasture, rotated in time and space. This is the high tide of farming in New England. Thereafter, the sequence goes into reverse. By the 18th century, trees begin to return, connecting the remnant patches of presettlement vegetation. Gradually, the forest closes in, and traces of human presence fade. Little breaks the monotony, apart from occasional fires started by lightning or native Americans clearing seasonal cultivation patches, or major windstorms that topple weaker trees. As the 16th century approaches, the landscape is essentially similar from decade to decade.

The time traveler's dominant impression is one of change. The preceding sequence of changes has been documented by many analysts of the New England landscape.[25] The sequence might be different elsewhere but is no less dynamic. Sometimes the changes are sudden and dramatic, and sometimes they are slow and imperceptible. Sometimes they are "natural" (e.g., storms), and sometimes they are caused by humans (e.g., forest clearance). For the bulk of human history, natural changes have seemed to dominate, although in fact people have been major shapers of the environment for millennia.[13,47,76] A casual observer of the New England landscape might conclude that the well-wooded 21st century scene is more "natural" than the cleared fields of the 1850s. However, today's scene is just as much a product of human choices as that of the 19th century, although different in composition and appearance.

In any event, deciding whether human or natural factors are responsible for a given environmental change is often difficult; these factors operate interdependently (Figure 119-1). It is widely believed that people have reached a critical threshold as environmental modifiers; they are able to equal or surpass the effects of nature. Humans have already significantly modified about half the Earth's land surface; portentous human-forced changes are becoming manifest in the entire biosphere. We can now speak of a human "transformation" of the global environment.[19,31,77]

This chapter addresses environmental change and its human dimensions, with special attention to implications created by the environment for the wilderness and wilderness medicine. What types of changes are likely to occur? How will they affect the natural environment, especially wilderness areas? What will be the consequences for society in general and for medical practitioners in particular? Can anything be done to improve our chances of successfully negotiating this impending time of dislocation and discontinuity?[48]

ISSUES OF ENVIRONMENTAL CHANGE

In recent years, a number of environmental change issues have come to prominence. These include climate change, stratospheric ozone depletion, erosion of biodiversity, population growth, and burgeoning pollution. These issues affect all environments, from urban centers to remote wilderness areas, and are examined on a variety of scales in this discussion. Although each issue is characterized by different expressions of change, all are interconnected. Local changes can aggregate to produce global effects, and global changes have many different disaggregated local effects.[77] In recognition of increasing human prominence, the present era of Earth's history is becoming known as the *Anthropocene*.[15,19] Current investigations of human-forced biogeochemical systems increasingly go beyond the separate issues previously noted, to adopt an integrated (holistic) perspective that spans the natural and social sciences.[25,31]

CLIMATE CHANGE

Weather is the state of the atmosphere at any specific time. *Climate* is the average weather pattern at a particular location. Weather and climate are usually described by such measures as temperature, precipitation, pressure, humidity, and wind speed and direction. In most parts of the world, these measures have been recorded for less than a century, so the actual historical record of direct observations is relatively brief compared with the human tenure of Earth. However, scientists are often able to extend the historical record by constructing synthetic climate data from other evidence, such as tree rings, fossils, concentrations of plankton in ocean sediments, pollen in sedimentary rocks, and isotopes of carbon and oxygen in rocks and glacial ice. For

---

*Andrei Gromyko (1909-1989); long time Foreign Minister of the USSR (1957-1985).

[†]Nikita Khrushchev (1894-1971); First Secretary Communist Party of the Soviet Union, 1953-1964.

[‡]Anton Pavlovich Chekhov (1860-1904); Russian novelist, short-story writer, essayist, and memoirist.

[§]Dmitri Dmitriyevich Shostakovich (1906-1975); Russian composer and one of the most celebrated composers of the 20th century.

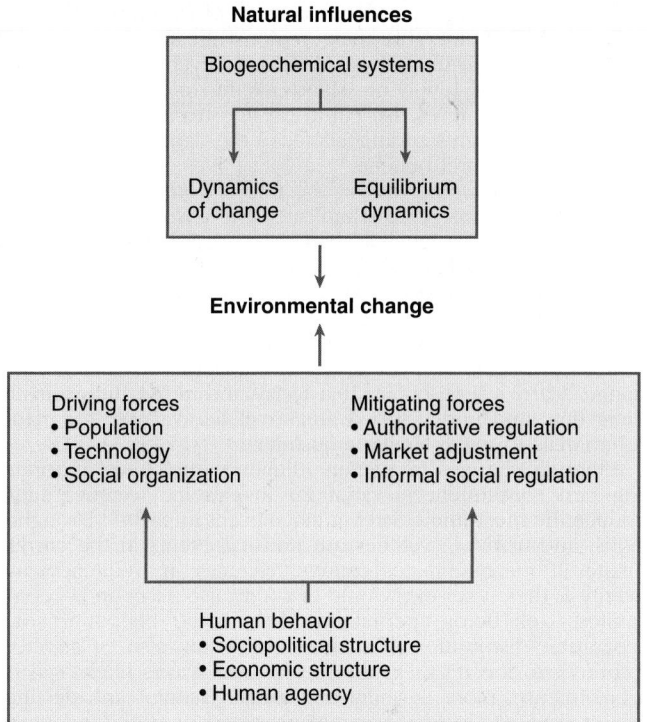

Natural influences

FIGURE 119-1 Human and natural forces for environmental change. *(Modified from Kates RW, Turner BL II, Clark WC: The great transformation. In Turner BL II, editor:* The earth as transformed by human action, *Cambridge, UK, 1990, Cambridge University Press.)*

example, narrow intervals between annual growth rings in trees and thin layers of organic material in lake sediments usually indicate cold, dry conditions. Clues such as these permit investigators to open a window on past climates.

Figure 119-2 illustrates trends in average global temperature during the past 10,000 years. Note that the global temperature has been in flux throughout this period. Not only has weather varied in relation to long-term average conditions, but the averages themselves have changed over time. For example, during the most recent ice age (about 10,000 years ago), average global temperatures were approximately 6°C (42.8°F) cooler than at present.[29] In other words, a massive environmental change (the

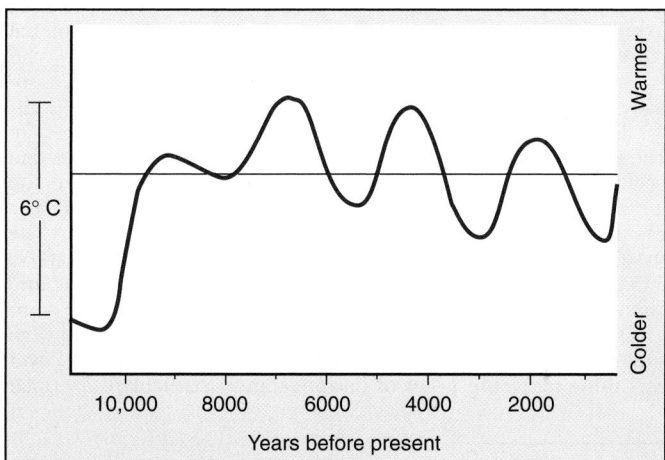

FIGURE 119-2 Variations of mean global temperature during the past 10,000 years. Horizontal line represents present global average temperature. *(Modified from Henderson-Sellers A, Robinson PJ:* Contemporary climatology, *New York, 1991, Wiley.)*

Wisconsin ice age) was connected with a relatively small climatic change. It is worthwhile remembering that regional changes in climate may or may not parallel global changes. For example, between 2600 and 2700 years ago—around the time of Socrates and Confucius—North America was colder and wetter than was the continental average since the end of the Wisconsin glaciation, whereas conditions in Europe were warmer and drier. Fortunately, the climate has remained within a range that sustains life for most of Earth's history, and the changes have occurred at very slow rates over thousands to millions of years.

Despite recent controversies regarding the accuracy of some climate science, a strong consensus exists among atmospheric scientists that global temperatures will rise significantly in coming decades.[41,70] One indicator of this trend is the fact that " … during 2014, the average temperature across global land and ocean surfaces was … the highest among all 135 years in the 1880-2014 record, surpassing the previous records of 2005 and 2010."[57] Although the global climate system is enormously complex, two factors point toward warming. First, it is known that certain greenhouse gases warm the atmosphere by trapping short-wave radiation reflected from the earth's surface when it is heated by solar radiation. Second, atmospheric concentrations of these gases, which include carbon dioxide (CO_2), methane, and nitrous oxide, are steadily increasing. Normally, the materials in greenhouse gases pass through long biogeochemical cycles between natural sources and natural sinks. For example, sulfur enters the atmosphere as sulfur dioxide from volcanic eruptions and washes back to the oceans in the form of mildly acidic rainfall, the constituents of which are later incorporated into bottom sediments. Human activities can increase source loads (e.g., emissions) and reduce the absorptive capacities of natural sinks. In the case of CO_2, the greenhouse gas that has raised the most environmental concern, both processes are at work simultaneously. Emissions of CO_2 have been increasing as energy-hungry societies burn petroleum hydrocarbons, coal, and wood. At the same time, forests that usually absorb huge amounts of atmospheric CO_2 continue to be cleared, although at rates less than that predicted in recent decades.[20]

Atmospheric scientists have estimated how climate might change as greenhouse gases accumulate. For this purpose, they rely heavily on *general circulation models* (GCMs) that mathematically simulate the global climate system. The chemistry and physics of climate are complex, and the models, although increasingly sophisticated, are still imperfect. Their accuracy is constrained both by the limits of current knowledge about the dynamics of the atmosphere and by the computational power of the most advanced supercomputers. They are also hedged with other limitations. For example, the present generation of GCMs is too coarse to provide more than a broad-gauge portrayal of atmospheric conditions in a lattice of 150- to 200-km-wide (90- to 120-mile-wide) regions over the earth's surface. The models are able to project some climate variables (e.g., temperature) with a high degree of accuracy, but there is lower confidence in their ability to predict other variables (e.g., precipitation). GCMs do not reveal storm systems that bring most of the weather to middle and high latitudes or smaller-scale features, such as hurricanes, tornadoes, and other extreme local winds. They also do not incorporate the role of clouds as reflectors and absorbers of energy. The models do not satisfactorily account for all the CO_2 believed to have been liberated into the atmosphere through human activities. Nonetheless, many scientists have considerable confidence in the accuracy of GCMs because of their relative success in replicating present and past climates.

The Intergovernmental Panel on Climate Change (IPCC), a large joint United Nations–World Meteorological Organization committee of leading Earth scientists, won the Nobel Peace Prize in 2007 for its work synthesizing existing research on climate change. It has completed five comprehensive assessments of the state of scientific knowledge and reached sobering conclusions. The most recent assessment (2014) concluded that there is now "unequivocal" evidence that global average temperatures are increasing and projected to rise by 1.5° to 2.0°C (by 2100, under most scenarios). Similarly, there is likely to be increasing disparity between wet and dry seasons and between wet and dry regions, as well as a continuing rise in global sea level at an accelerating rate.[36,75] Although the IPCC estimates embody a consensus about global warming, the level of agreement declines as researchers attempt to forecast the resulting impacts, especially at regional and local levels. An enhanced greenhouse effect would have a greater effect on global climate than would temperature alone. Solar radiation provides the energy that drives the climate system. The effects of a warmer atmosphere could produce a cascade of changes in many climate variables.[14] For example, precipitation and evaporation would also likely increase, especially over high latitudes, but with strong regional variations elsewhere. Increasingly accurate climate projections for regional patterns of climate change have been developed.[12,23] We will soon know a great deal more about regional patterns of climate change, because a large number of studies that combine GCM data and other indicators of climate are being conducted.[2]

The GCMs generally indicate that lower latitudes and lower elevations will be less affected by anticipated climate changes than will upper latitudes and higher elevations.[12] However, climate change impact simulations paint no simple pictures. For example, temperature changes in the tropics may be relatively small, but their effects on insects could be more deleterious than in higher latitudes, where insects are typically more heat tolerant.[18] Most likely, a mosaic of regional and local changes with varying impacts will occur along a spectrum from strongly positive to strongly negative, depending on how, when, and where they occur[25] (Table 119-1). For example, some tropical islands, particularly in the Indian Ocean, are likely to experience heavy precipitation combined with more frequent severe storms and rising sea levels. Other islands, such as those in the Caribbean, are also likely to see increasing sea levels, but may experience a decline in summer rainfall. The net impacts of such changes are difficult to assess, but the experiences of Indian Ocean islands

and coastlines during the massive tsunami of December 26, 2004, show just how vulnerable these regions already are to natural disasters. For the Andamans, Maldives, Seychelles, and other heavily populated low-lying islands of the Indo-Pacific Ocean, the results of sea level rise could be disastrous, whereas other places, such as high-standing islands of the Caribbean, could see offsetting agricultural benefits.[60]

More than any other factor, the rate of climate change is of concern to humans. GCMs indicate that absolute changes in temperature will be smaller than those that have occurred at other times during Earth's history. However, anticipated climate changes would still occur at a rate and magnitude that are unprecedented in human experience. Whereas past changes usually occurred slowly enough for plants and animals to adapt or migrate, examples exist of mass extinctions following rapid change. Many scientists fear that today and in the future, insufficient time and undeveloped areas will be available for plants and animals to make similar adjustments.

Although changes in average climate would have important long-term consequences, variations in extreme weather might produce the most immediate and significant impacts.[36] Droughts, floods, and tropical cyclones are unusual events in the current climate. If mean climates change, changes in frequency and severity of these extremes would probably also occur and become manifest well before permanent shifts could be confirmed.[28] Geographic distribution of such events would also be affected. According to the IPCC, in the future, heat waves likely will be "more intense, more frequent and longer lasting," and declines in frost days and cold waves are projected over all land areas. The frequency of extreme precipitation events would also likely increase everywhere.[35] There would be increased incidence of drought and water shortages. This may also have profound impacts for the local environment, particularly in locations where the local flora and fauna may not be adapted to prolonged dry periods. Sea level rise is likely to increase on all coasts, except in a few locations where land uplift negates its impacts. This is likely to lead to increased erosion and coastal flooding, increasing pressures on sensitive coastal environments, such as dunes and mangroves. Changes in both minimum and maximum temperatures experiences, particularly in the high latitudes and upload areas, are likely to have important impacts on the ability of some plant species to survive. In other areas, these changes may have a positive impact on some species because of increased length of the growing season.

Overall, the impacts of global climate change for wilderness areas will be complex and varied, influenced by a variety of local and regional factors as well as by global trends. As a result, natural hazards would likely pose increased risks to society. Moreover, exposure and vulnerability to extreme events would probably be exacerbated, because populations at risk might respond to the new conditions on the basis of outdated information and assumptions.[51] We might find that our previous experience prepared us to "fight the last war" rather than the current one.

STRATOSPHERIC OZONE DEPLETION

The stratosphere is a distinct layer of the upper atmosphere that occurs between 14.5 and 56 km (9 and 35 miles) above the ground. It contains significant concentrations of ozone (O_3), a gas that is formed when solar radiation splits oxygen atoms.* The stratospheric ozone layer absorbs most of the ultraviolet (UV) radiation from space that would otherwise damage plant and animal species.

During the 1970s and 1980s, researchers discovered that stratospheric ozone was being depleted, and that the ozone layer was thinning to the point of disappearance, particularly in polar

TABLE 119-1 Effects of Global Climate Change on Different Regions

Region	Climate Change Effects	Level
Africa	Water stress	High
	Food shortages	Very high
	Mosquito-borne and waterborne diseases	Very high
Europe	River and coast flooding	Medium
	Water stress	High
	Heat waves and air pollution	High
Asia	Flood damage	High
	Extreme heat deaths	Very high
	Drought-related malnutrition	Medium
Australasia	Coral reef and species loss	High
	Coastal flooding	Medium
North America	Wildfire destruction	Very high
	Heat wave deaths	High
	Extreme rainstorm damage	High
Latin America	Water stress in semiarid areas	Very high
	Urban flooding caused by extreme rainfall	Very high
	Decreased food production	Very high
Polar regions	Risk from permafrost, snow, and ice changes	High
	Food insecurity; unsafe drinking water	Very high
Small islands	Property losses caused by rising seas	High
	Loss of coastal land	Very high
Oceans	Decline in low-latitude fish catches	Medium
	Biodiversity loss from damaged corals	Very high
	Erosion and sedimentation of coasts	High

Modified from Climate change 2014: Impacts, adaptation, and vulnerability. In Field CB, Barros VR, Dokken DJ, et al (eds). Contribution of Working Group II to the Fifth Assessment Report of the Intergovernmental Panel on Climate Change. Cambridge: Cambridge University Press, United Kingdom.

*Ozone also accumulates near ground level as a byproduct of the photochemical modification of exhaust gases from automobiles and other sources of pollution. Concentrations of this type of ozone are sometimes reported in local news media, but the ground-level "ozone problem" should not be confused with the stratospheric one.

regions.[27,49] Chlorofluorocarbons (CFCs) were held to be at fault. For decades, these synthetic compounds had been manufactured in large quantities, mainly for use as aerosol propellants and refrigerants. Once CFCs escape into the atmosphere, they remain stable until reaching the stratosphere, where they decompose under the action of UV radiation. Chlorine atoms are released and bond with ozone atoms, breaking them down into oxygen and other products. As a result, the ozone shield is weakened or removed.

If the ozone layer is sufficiently depleted, intensity of UV radiation that reaches the earth's surface could be significantly increased. This could have deleterious consequences for human populations and plant and animal species. For humans, increased incidence of skin cancer, cataracts, and immune system suppression are three recognized effects of high UV exposure. Although humans might take precautions to protect themselves against UV radiation, such as reducing time spent outdoors or adding sunblock, sunglasses, and clothes, nonhuman species may not be able to make the necessary adaptations. Serious disruptions of human and agricultural systems are possible.

During their winter seasons, the Antarctic[61] and to a lesser extent the Arctic[46,73] have experienced elevated levels of UV radiation. "Ozone holes" have been clearly traced to CFCs. An international agreement, the Montreal Protocol, was reached to phase out CFC use by 1996. Much progress has been made toward that goal, but these compounds are still being produced in some developing countries, and the substitute chemicals that were introduced elsewhere may also contribute to global warming.[42] Chlorine atoms are extremely long-lived in the stratosphere, persisting perhaps for 100 to 200 years. There will continue to be some potential for additional ozone depletion in the decades to come.

EROSION OF BIODIVERSITY (See Chapter 120)

Loss of species or the habitats that support them is a controversial and potentially serious global problem that comes under the heading "erosion of biodiversity." Biodiversity is not an agent of change as are greenhouse gas buildup and ozone depletion. Rather, it is an index against which environmental changes can be assessed.[72] As with climate change and ozone depletion, biodiversity has a global to local range of dimensions.[34] Two aspects of biodiversity of great importance are numbers and interconnections of species.

Estimates of the number of existing species range widely because the state of knowledge about the planet's biologic resources is both uneven and incomplete.[74] It is estimated that the earth hosts between 5 and 15 million species. About 1.75 million of these have been named.[44] Higher-order mammals and birds in temperate ecosystems are well documented, but insects, worms, and microscopic life-forms in tropical regions are much less known. In the United States, approximately 100,000 species are recognized, but only about one-fifth of these have been surveyed to date.[74]

Paleobiologic research indicates that the number and type of species have varied greatly over time. New species evolve through adaptive genetic mutations, while others perish because of competitive pressures of natural selection. Emergence and disappearance rates depend on the speed and direction of environmental change and the ability of species to adjust. What is most troubling about the recent record is the disappearance of so many species. "Between 1600 and 1994, at least 484 species of animals and 654 species of plants (mostly vertebrates and flowering plants) became extinct. During this period, the rate of extinction in groups such as birds and mammals also increased dramatically. Nearly three times as many species of birds and mammals became extinct between 1810 and 1994 (112 species) as were lost between 1600 and 1810 (38 species)."[64] Plant losses are presumed to have been much greater. On some oceanic islands, such as Hawaii, disappearance of native animal species is almost total. Of 269 extinct Hawaiian species, most were either invertebrates (135 species) or plants (105 species). A majority of the rest are birds (15 species) and land snails (11 species).[74] Commercial forestry and fishing have proved particularly injuri-

ous to biodiversity because they simultaneously harvest desirable species and destroy undesirable species.[33] Agriculture and animal husbandry also contribute to species extinctions, especially by modifying habitats that support biota. Particular concerns have been expressed about threats to tropical forests and near extinction of certain marine species such as the northern cod, blue whale, and leatherback turtle. However, the problem is general in scope and may be most important for the "noncelebrity" species that do not elicit much human compassion.

It is estimated that approximately 32% of all U.S. species are now under serious pressure, sometimes to the point of threatened extinction (Tables 119-2 and 119-3).[74] However, the picture varies widely among particular groups of species (Table 119-4). Inhabitants of freshwater ecosystems, such as shellfish, crustaceans, amphibians, and fish, are much more likely to be in danger than are flowering plants, conifers, mammals, and birds.

TABLE 119-2 Percentage of U.S. Species at Risk

Status	%
Extinct	1.0
Critically imperiled	6.5
Imperiled	8.8
Vulnerable	15.4
Secure	69.3

Modified from Stein BA, Flack SR: Conservation priorities: The state of U.S. plants and animals, *Environment* 39:6, 1997.

TABLE 119-3 U.S. Species Groups at Risk

	Extinct	Imperiled	Vulnerable	Secure
Freshwater mussels	16.4	39.7	11.8	32.1
Crayfish	17.3	32.8	0.9	49.0
Amphibians	14.0	23.9	2.5	59.6
Freshwater fish	14.1	22.0	2.6	61.3
Flowering plants	16.6	15.8	0.9	66.7
Conifers	12.2	14.0	0.0	73.8
Ferns	11.9	8.9	0.7	78.5
Tiger beetles	13.6	6.3	0.0	80.1
Dragonflies	10.4	7.6	0.4	81.6
Reptiles	11.9	6.1	0.0	82.0
Butterflies	12.3	4.0	0.5	83.2
Mammals	9.1	7.2	0.2	83.5
Birds	5.4	5.8	3.3	85.5

Modified from Stein BA, Flack SR: Conservation priorities: The state of U.S. plants and animals, *Environment* 39:6, 1997.

TABLE 119-4 Species Threatened With Extinction: a Global Picture

Status	Numbers
Extinct	801
Extinct in the wild	63
Critically endangered	3947
Endangered	5766
Vulnerable	10,104
Near threatened	4467
Data deficient	10,497
Least concern	27,837
Other	255
Total species assessed	63,837

From 2012 IUCN *Red List of Threatened Species*. http://www.conservation.org/NewsRoom/pressreleases/Pages/Securing-the-web-of-life-31-Percent-of-Species-Threatened-with-Extinction.aspx. Accessed February 9, 2015.

Likewise, on the U.S. mainland, loss of biodiversity is more acute in Sunbelt states and east of the Mississippi River than in states of the northern Great Plains and the northern Rocky Mountains.

For many people, protection of threatened species is a moral imperative. For others, it is a luxury. Quite apart from moral issues, the rising rate of species extinction has practical implications. For example, loss of the planet's genetic stock hampers the search for wild strains of domestic crops that are resistant to pests and diseases that plague high-yield domestic varieties. The so-called Green Revolution that has helped to alleviate world hunger in recent decades owes much of its success to introduction of resistant wild genetic strains into commercial agriculture.

Biodiversity is also important for stability of global ecosystems. For example, the extent to which entire species can be eliminated from an ecosystem before it collapses is unknown. Likewise, the extent to which some nominally "wild" species may thrive under human management, while others succumb, is hotly debated.[24] Most ecologists believe that ecosystems containing a wide diversity of organisms are more resilient to change than are those with few species. Regardless of the degree of resilience, biodiversity and environmental change may be connected by negative feedback relationships. Environmental change may lead to loss of biodiversity that in turn produces lowered resistance to pressures for further change.

Despite intuitive, theoretical, and case study arguments in favor of preserving biodiversity, it has been difficult to agree on standardized measures of biodiversity or its loss. Deforestation of South American rain forests is a case in point. The Amazon Basin is one of the world's premier wilderness regions and is regarded as Earth's most important source of biodiversity. Perhaps impelled by dramatic and widely publicized reports of forest clearances by ranchers, homesteading farmers, and mineral firms in Brazil during the late 1980s, levels of international concern about loss of biodiversity in Amazonia have been high. As in most developing countries, however, comprehensive and reliable data on Brazilian deforestation are difficult to secure and interpret.[70,88]

Given the foregoing uncertainties, it is difficult to predict future rates of loss of biodiversity. The best available estimates suggest that about 3.5% of current bird species will likely become extinct by the year 2050, together with most large marine predators and much of species richness of freshwater ecosystems.[37]

POPULATION GROWTH

Human population is frequently cited as one of the primary driving forces behind contemporary environmental change. Beginning with the Reverend Thomas Malthus (1766-1834), many have argued that rising populations must eventually deplete resources and degrade environments, with potentially catastrophic consequences for the biosphere and the human populations who depend on it, because the earth is, for practical purposes, a closed system.[40] In the absence of interplanetary space travel on a scale impossible at present to destinations that are now unknown and perhaps nonexistent, Earth is our only home. This does not mean that it will be impossible for our

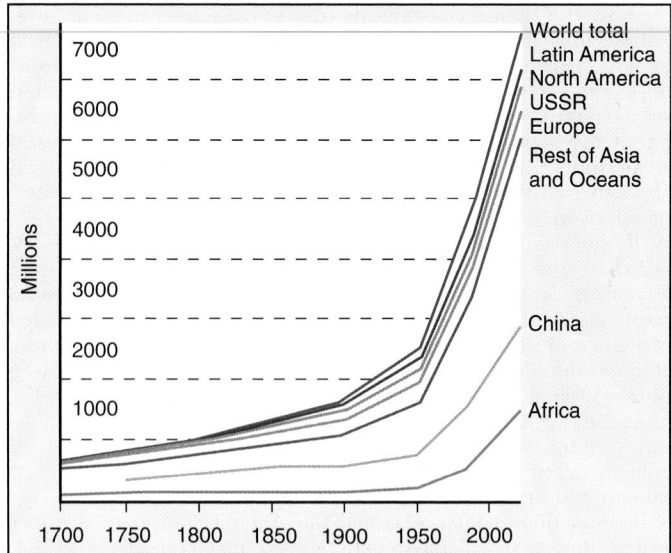

FIGURE 119-3 Global population (1700-2020). *(Modified from Demeny P: Population. In Turner BL II, editor:* The earth as transformed by human action, *Cambridge, UK, 1990, Cambridge University Press.)*

planet to hold additional human populations. The record of the past four centuries demonstrates that global carrying capacity is highly elastic up to some, as yet unreached, limit.[10] Leaving aside the argument that human ingenuity can make possible the support for larger populations indefinitely, clearly from the perspective of burdens on the physical environment, how people live is more important than the number of people. All other factors being equal, more affluent societies place heavier burdens on the physical environment than do poorer ones. For example, per-capita consumption of energy in the United States is more than 15 times higher than that in India.[65]

The global population has undergone unprecedented growth in the past several centuries (Figure 119-3). By 1800, Earth's population was approximately 1 billion. By 1920 it was approaching 2 billion. Three billion was reached by 1960, and the present number is more than 7 billion. The United Nations estimates that 9 to 11 billion people will be on Earth by 2050. Most of the new growth is likely to occur in developing countries of Asia, Africa, and Latin America (Table 119-5). The recent experience of China suggests that the process of development can itself perpetuate or increase historic rates of population growth, at least until economic conditions improve significantly.

Composition of future populations is an increasing concern of governments and individuals. In places such as Japan and Eastern Europe, natural increase is now well below the rate necessary to replace existing populations, whereas in the United States, increasing numbers are maintained largely by immigration. As a result, the fraction of national human populations older than

TABLE 119-5	Average Annual Percentage Rates of Population Increase							
	1700-1750	1750-1800	1800-1850	1850-1900	1900-1950	1950-1985	1985-2020	2014
Africa	0.0	0.0	0.1	0.4	1.0	2.6	2.7	2.5
Asia	0.3	0.5	0.5	0.3	0.8	2.1	1.4	1.1
Europe	0.3	0.6	0.7	0.7	0.6	0.6	0.1	0.0
Russia	0.3	0.7	1.0	1.0	0.7	1.2	0.6	−0.03
North America	0.8	1.0	3.2	2.6	1.2	1.3	0.6	0.4
Latin America	0.8	0.5	1.2	1.6	1.6	2.6	1.6	1.2
Oceania	—	—	—	—	1.6	1.9	1.2	1.1
World total	0.25	0.44	0.55	0.54	0.84	1.88	1.45	1.14

From Demeny P: Population. In Turner BL II, editor: *The earth as transformed by human action*, Cambridge, UK, 1990, Cambridge University Press. With additional information supplied by the author.

65 years is growing rapidly in the developed world. Meanwhile, increasing expertise in genetic manipulation holds out the prospect of significantly longer life span for populations who can afford the scientific research and medical care that will make this possible. Some segments of the world's population will become increasingly healthier and older, while others may remain caught in a cycle of brief, sickness-prone lives followed by early deaths.

Apart from the staggering societal impacts that such a change would produce, the implications for wilderness are considerable. For those who can be assured of longer lives, the quality of life experience, including the quality of their environments, may become of great importance. Wilderness areas would be among the most cherished places, and decisions about their future all the more portentous. Among developing countries, a different future might emerge, perhaps dominated by intense pressure to convert all available resources into support for survival. Although such scenarios are not difficult to envision, they carry a danger of indulging in stereotypic dichotomizations that ignore possibilities for a range of more nuanced outcomes.

The greatest uncertainties about future populations pertain to rates of migration and composition of families.[11] Rates of migration are shaped by many factors, including the extent to which the negative consequences of environmental change may lead to population displacement. If current patterns of migration continue, the majority of migrants will settle in large countries such as the United States, India, Pakistan, France, and Germany, where depending on their internal destinations, they may add to the burden of users on existing wilderness areas.

POLLUTION

Unwanted byproducts of production and consumption that exceed the absorptive capacity of the environment are known as *pollution*. Pollution comes in many forms, including solid physical materials, liquid chemical compounds, and energy (e.g., thermal pollution). Some pollutants (e.g., certain isotopes of plutonium) are highly toxic even in small amounts. Many materials that are beneficial in small amounts can be deleterious in large quantities. For example, phosphorus is a nutrient that limits biologic productivity in coastal and marine ecosystems. Small amounts of phosphorus can increase algal growth at the bottom of marine food chains. However, when large amounts of phosphorus-rich runoff from fertilizers or septic systems enter these environments, the entire population of algae can begin a period of explosive growth ("bloom"). Extensive blooms can produce "red tides" or "brown tides."[9] This occurs when algae prevent light from penetrating coastal waters and decomposition of dead algae consumes dissolved oxygen. Large fish kills are a frequent result.

The preferences of people for quick and convenient disposal of pollutants into available environmental sinks (e.g., soil, streams, groundwater, oceans, atmosphere) have sometimes been validated by incomplete science. For decades, in the United States and elsewhere, scientists advised policy makers that "the solution to pollution is dilution." As a result, physical and chemical wastes have been released into environments that had finite capacities for absorbing them. Once the absorptive capacities were reached, a variety of serious problems occurred. These included biologically "dead" rivers (e.g., Cleveland's Cuyahoga River), lakes (e.g., Lake Erie), and seas (e.g., sewage sludge dumping ground in the New York Bight off the coasts of New Jersey and Long Island). Although some of these conditions can be reversed, the remediation processes are slow, costly, contentious, and often incomplete. A growing body of evidence suggests that the aggregate effect of pollution may be jeopardizing functions of fundamental Earth systems. Buildup of atmospheric CO_2 is an excellent example of this concept.

Despite a large volume of evidence, effects of pollutants on receiving environments are not fully known.[13] This is partly because of lack of scientific knowledge about the normal (unpolluted) functioning of some environments, such as deep oceans and tropical forests. The volume and variety of materials released into the environment and their interactions complicate the study of effects of any single pollutant. Sometimes the effects of pollutants are subtle, long delayed, and far removed from the point of origin, making it difficult to connect causes and consequences. Occasionally, experts disagree about evidence of pollution impacts collected in the field and acquired from laboratory experiments. Even the impacts of well-studied events, such as the *Exxon Valdez* tanker grounding, are in dispute.[6,56] Nonetheless, there is broad consensus that the absorptive capacity of receiving media is not inexhaustible, and that pollution is a growing world problem pushing society against the limits of environmental resilience.

IMPACTS OF ENVIRONMENTAL CHANGE ON WILDERNESS AREAS

The task of assessing environmental change impacts in wilderness areas poses particularly difficult challenges to researchers. To begin with, the term *wilderness* is rarely used by scientists. For example, readers of the voluminous reports of the IPCC[36] might search in vain for references to wilderness impacts. Instead, there are comments about the effects of climate fluctuations on specific types of ecosystems, land covers, or land uses, such as forests or nature reserves, some of which may be defined as "wildernesses" by different interest groups.[53] Lack of references to wilderness in the scientific literature can be explained by emergence of a widely shared conviction among scientists that no part of the world is now truly "natural." As one prominent ecologist put it, "Overall, any clear dichotomy between pristine ecosystems and human-altered areas that may have existed in the past has vanished."[80] In other words, our environments are arranged on a continuum from intensely human-constructed places, such as cities, to places where the human presence is small, intermittent, or nonexistent, such as wilderness areas. Most places show evidence of both human and natural influences.

If scientists shy away from the term *wilderness*, the same cannot be said of political leaders and the general public. Unfortunately, in this larger arena, there is little agreement about meanings of wilderness, because some of them are rooted in religious views about the perfectibility of the earth.

In addition, people in different countries often interpret *wilderness* in different ways. "Naturalness" and "remoteness" are two frequently mentioned wilderness attributes, but measures of both can be highly subjective. Depending on the definition adopted, a wilderness area might include some of the world's most biologically productive ecosystems (e.g., tropical rain forests of Brazilian Amazon Basin) together with some of its least productive (e.g., Sahara desert), as well as some that have been thoroughly transformed by human activities (e.g., so-called urban wilderness areas like Portland, Oregon's Forest Park). Some analysts have attempted to cut through this Gordian knot by equating wilderness with "uninhabited areas" or "roadless places," but neither of these indicators is comprehensive in scope when it comes to accounting for all the places that humans perceive as "wild." Using the criterion of human intrusion, all of Antarctica might qualify as wilderness, for by most measures it is one of the least human-impacted places on Earth. However, very few of the specially protected areas that have been established in Antarctica were designated because of their wilderness values; although aesthetics and wilderness characteristics are among the main criteria for designating these protected areas, historic sites of human activity are much more protected.[32] In other words, in Antarctica, the rarity value of human impacts outranks the importance of more or less pristine wilderness.

In view of the potential for confusion that exists in discussions of wilderness, it is worthwhile to address some of the philosophic and evolutionary backgrounds of the term.[53]

The concept of wilderness can be found in several of the world's earliest cultures,[63] but formulation of a powerful philosophic and political movement that espouses the value of unaltered natural areas did not occur in the United States until the 19th and early 20th centuries.[67] Although the wilderness movement subsequently diffused elsewhere, widespread public concern for preservation of wild lands remains a characteristically American preoccupation,[69] perhaps because the contrast between

TABLE 119-6 Global Crop Land Changes (1700-1990) in 1000 ha

Region	1700	1750	1800	1850	1900	1950	1990
United States and Canada	3077	6606	15,009	170,444	199,413	235,327	232,771
Central and South America	15,348	15,333	16,602	18,980	31,950	79,024	149,456
Europe	67,292	73,315	79,878	87,028	106,734	143,983	139,129
Asia and Russia	135,514	179,054	239,826	324,859	424,820	603,186	698,279
Oceania	2147	3500	5788	9659	16,291	27,750	53,063
Japan	1425	1458	1492	1527	2119	4720	4596
World	265,631	321,302	401,611	537,060	813,425	1,229,985	1,477,600

From History Base of the Global Environment, HYDE. http://arch.rivm.nl/env/int/hyde/.
ha, Hectares (1000 hectares = 10,000,000 m²).

juxtaposed human-dominated landscapes and ostensibly "natural" ones is so apparent in the United States (e.g., California's Central Valley and Sierra Nevada mountains; Florida's Everglades and Gold Coast). Despite the volume of public debate about wilderness, the concept itself remains poorly defined, even in the United States.*

Most analysts recognize that *wilderness* refers to places that have one or all of three characteristics: (1) few or no permanent resident human populations, (2) unmanaged biogeochemical systems, and (3) no significant modification by modern technology. Places that meet these criteria might include deep oceans, high mountains, deserts, circumpolar lands, certain oceanic islands, coastal fringes, most areas of active vulcanicity, and some of the world's great forests (e.g., taiga, tropical rain forests).[†]

These three criteria are best regarded as necessary but not sufficient to identify an area as wilderness. Spatial dimensions must also be taken into account. An acre of wetland surrounded by shopping malls would not be considered wilderness, even if it is in biologically pristine condition. As a rule of thumb we have adopted, a wilderness usually encompasses at least several square miles.

If applied to the United States, the previous criteria would identify a great diversity of environments. Most would be marginal lands and waters beyond the boundaries of areas that are permanently settled, and perhaps without prospects for human occupancy or use in the long term. Some protected areas within the ecumene (inhabited lands) might also qualify as wilderness because they are administered as such. Most protected areas, however, such as national parks, national forests, and national recreational areas, would probably not meet all three major wilderness criteria because they are often subject to intensive management of residual plant and animal populations, as well as frequent human visits.[28]

CONVERSION OF WILDERNESS

In many parts of the world, the frontiers of wilderness areas are being pushed back as land is converted to managed uses. Economic growth and population increases are the ultimate driving forces of this conversion at the global scale. At local and regional levels, a variety of conversion processes are apparent. These include resource extraction industries (e.g., mining, forestry),

agriculture, animal husbandry, tourism, and commercial and residential uses. These processes are not confined to land. They also affect freshwater and shallow-water marine environments. Tourism exerts pressure on coral reefs in Belize, Kenya, and many other countries.

Most land conversion is driven by demands for additional cropland. The highest levels of land conversion are found in developing countries with rapidly growing populations. By comparison, land formerly devoted to crops is reverting to an uncultivated state in much of Europe, North America, and Japan (Table 119-6). Most of the world's prime agricultural lands have been brought under cultivation, so attention has turned to other terrains that are spatially and agriculturally marginal.[3] These are often wilderness areas. For example, during the past six decades, many formerly unpopulated parts of Sumatra and Borneo have been settled by government-sponsored "transmigrants" from the heavily populated Indonesian island of Java.

Land conversion may fragment existing wilderness areas by dividing them into smaller blocks. This process is well advanced in the Amazon rain forest of Brazil, where new, long-distance, government-built roads bring settlers.[50] As a result, ecologic "islands" are created that may not be sustainable. Forest-edge environments replace deep-forest ones. The islands may be too small to retain the previous diversity of species. Governments often attempt to protect such islands by designating them as parks or wilderness areas, but this may be insufficient to prevent further changes. In any case, to be effectively protected, such places often require intensive management of ecosystems and visitors, which defeats the objective of designating them as wilderness. Moreover, management actions may ripple through the ecosystems in unforeseen ways, perhaps contributing to the long-term conversion process.

HUMAN PENETRATION OF WILDERNESS AREAS

The number of people visiting wilderness areas is on the rise. In the United States, approximately 70 million persons per year visited them in 2008. Increase in visitation rates is not confined to the United States. The deadly South Asian tsunami of December 26, 2004, was notable in part for the number of foreign tourists included among the estimated 300,000 dead. Citizens of 44 different countries from outside the region became victims because they were vacationing in resorts located on exposed islands and remote coasts. Many such places were in or near wilderness areas. Among other issues, this "global" disaster highlights the increasing spread and penetration of humans into formerly remote places.

People have not figured prominently in conventional definitions of wilderness, but wilderness areas often contain significant human populations. Many of the remaining habitats of endangered tropical species survive because they are located in places far removed from the pressures of modern society. However, this does not mean that these areas are devoid of people. For example, the Bonobo chimpanzees of the central Congo and the rhinoceri and tigers of Assam are sheltered by thick forests that also are home to humans numbering in the hundreds of thousands to millions. Sometimes, the remoteness of these places has

---

*The definition included in the Wilderness Act (1964) is typically vague: " … an area where the Earth and its community of life are untrammeled by man, where man himself is a visitor who does not remain." For practical purposes "roadless areas" are often used as an indicator of wilderness in North America. Even in a well-researched region such as North America, exhaustive inventories of the species present in wilderness areas are generally lacking; at the global level, only the approximate distribution of wilderness areas has been mapped.

[†]How should formerly developed areas that have reverted to unmanaged states be classified? Many such areas can be found in Western Europe and North America (e.g., Adirondack Mountains of New York). Often, radical differences exist between predevelopment conditions and reverted conditions. For the purposes of this discussion, such areas are considered wilderness.

made them havens for dissident political movements and sites of civil conflicts that have had devastating effects on indigenous plants and animals. As advocates of international programs to mitigate the effects of climate change have observed, anti-deforestation programs will not be successful if they fail to gain the support of wilderness-resident human populations.[30,66]

Wilderness areas may be degraded without being converted to other uses. This usually occurs in one of three ways: direct impacts from increasing human presence, indirect effects of conventional industrial technologies in adjacent areas, and global effects of innovative, powerful, and often high-risk technologies.

DIRECT IMPACTS

Few parts of the planet have remained unexplored by humans at ground level. Formerly remote areas are penetrated for a variety of reasons. Winter sports entrepreneurs are shifting attention to Europe's ecologically fragile High Alps, because snowfields at lower altitudes shrink under the forcing action of rising temperatures.[18] In Canada, James Bay has been altered by a huge hydro-power scheme, and extraction of bitumen from the Athabasca Oil Sands is having profound impacts on local environments and ecosystems.[43] Gold prospecting has intruded into the innermost recesses of Amazonia and Angola. Philippine coral reefs are subject to cyanide poisoning in pursuit of aquarium fish.[17]

Penetration of wilderness is facilitated by modern industrial technologies, especially transportation technologies. For example, road building encourages invasion of wilderness areas for recreation, resource extraction, and other purposes. The roads themselves have environmental impacts ranging from vegetation clearance to drainage impedance, but their roles as conduits of change are even more significant. They bring new people, exotic materials, and different lifestyles to remote places. Similar inroads are made by boats and aircraft and their support facilities.

Because economic gain is an important incentive for wilderness penetration, recreational and esthetic needs also increase visitation. Hunting and fishing have long attracted visitors to wilderness areas, such as the Boundary Waters Canoe Area of northern Minnesota. Such pursuits are reinforced by "ecotourism." Increasing numbers of people want to visit remote areas to appreciate pristine beauty. For many people who formerly might have sought out Yellowstone National Park and the Grand Canyon, the destinations of choice include such places as Antarctica, the high Himalayas, Amazonia, and even Siberia. For many persons, the more remote the destination, the more attractive it is. Since most ecotourists want to visit the wilderness for only brief periods, they are whisked in and out by the most modern transportation technologies.

Visits from ecotourists can change wilderness environments. Seemingly insignificant impacts that are repeated can eventually become major problems. In the Masai Mara Reserve of Kenya's Serengeti Plains, the savanna ecosystem has been altered by photographic safaris. Safari camps require open campfires; fuel wood is scavenged from fallen trees that would otherwise provide important ecologic niches for local plants and animals. Climbing expeditions on Mt Everest have reported large volumes of garbage left by earlier expeditions. Decomposition is slow in the dry mountain air. Scarring of scientific sites in Antarctica by discarded refuse and vehicle tracks is well known. The Galápagos Islands, the one-time archetypical wilderness of Charles Darwin, are succumbing to the effects of their popularity with ecotourists. Geographers from the United States have assisted the government of Ecuador in carrying-capacity studies that form the basis for land-use regulations and other development controls to limit further degradation of these internationally valued sites.

INDIRECT IMPACTS

One of the most potent indirect impacts on wilderness areas follows introduction (inadvertent or intentional) of non-native species. Negative impacts have been demonstrated in the United States countless times, such as after the introduction of English sparrows, Asian gypsy moths, and Africanized "killer" bees. Everglades National Park in Florida is now one of the best places to

find imported Burmese pythons living in the wild.[22] In Glacier National Park, pack trips within the park were curtailed because horses were introducing exotic species of grasses picked up from stable feed and passed through the digestive tract within their feces.

The problems of small islands and introduced species are legendary. Guam's experience with the brown tree snake is a good example. These snakes are native to New Guinea, but several managed to travel to Guam on airplanes in 1962. They thrived in the absence of native snakes or predators. Now Guam has as many as 30,000 brown tree snakes per square mile, and they have devastated native bird species. These snakes are beginning to show up in the Hawaiian Islands, where conditions are also favorable for colonization. Although efforts to intercept the snakes are being increased, the potential outcome is discouraging.

HIGH-RISK TECHNOLOGIES

Technologic risks are increasingly familiar threats to modern industrial society. Such risks are usually perceived as limited to accidents in urban industrial zones such as Bhopal, India, where more than 3000 people died following accidental release of methylisocyanate gas in 1984. However, some technologies have the potential to affect very large areas at great distances from their point of origin, up to and including the entire global environment. For example, the *Deepwater Horizon* explosion and subsequent oil spill in the Gulf of Mexico produced widespread impacts across a range of marine ecosystems, including deepwater corals.[82] Increasing oil and gas exploration presents a variety of risks to wilderness areas.

Biotechnology exemplifies some of these powerful, high-risk technologies. Through genetic engineering, new organisms are being created, primarily for agricultural purposes. Nuclear technologies also carry environmental change potential. For decades after World War II, a massive nuclear war between the United States and Soviet Union was a serious possibility. This would have brought catastrophic changes to the earth as a whole.[62] Many military nuclear facilities were located in remote areas. With the end of the Cold War, this threat has diminished, but regional nuclear conflicts among lesser powers are still possible. The risks of accidents involving nuclear weapons remain a threat to some wilderness areas. Nuclear bombs have been lost at sea; improperly managed nuclear wastes have exploded in the Ural Mountains and elsewhere; and military nuclear wastes are buried on small Pacific islands, often within reach of rising sea levels. Environmental contamination around nuclear weapon–manufacturing plants in the United States has been reported, and nuclear submarine propulsion systems have been discarded into the Arctic Ocean north of Russia.

Civilian uses of nuclear technologies pose risks to wilderness areas. Accidents such as the explosion and fire at the Chernobyl nuclear power station and the meltdown at Fukushima, Japan, triggered by the combined effects of an earthquake and tsunami, had global repercussions. Deposition of highly radioactive fallout in Arctic areas of Scandinavia demonstrates that no wilderness is immune from the effects of major nuclear accidents. Proposed placement of a repository for high-level nuclear waste in Yucca Mountain in the middle of semiarid Nevada provides another example of the connection between high-risk technologies and wilderness areas.

CONSEQUENCES OF ENVIRONMENTAL CHANGE

Research on global environmental change continues to reveal an ever-greater number of connections between human and natural systems. Linkages among species in a given ecosystem, among different ecosystems, and among global biogeochemical systems have been described. Providing details about all vulnerable systems is not possible, but the range of interconnections can be illustrated by two examples: Canadian wilderness use and coral reefs.

Scientists have recently explored the likely impacts of environmental changes on users of wilderness areas in northern Canada. In one case, rising temperatures and increased precipitation were judged likely to pose few problems for rafters and canoeists on the Mackenzie River, but accompanying forest fires were seen as much greater threats. Farther north on Bathurst Island, the likelihood of increased winter snowfall, combined with larger summer insect populations, seemed likely to stress the existing large caribou herds to a point where hunting might have to be curtailed. Throughout the region, a shift from consumptive uses (e.g., hunting) of wilderness lands to nonconsumptive uses (e.g., scenic tourism) is a potential outcome.[8] Elsewhere in the Arctic, there might be serious effects on resident and visitor populations. For example[2]:

Indigenous people, dependent on climate conditions that support specific vegetation like forage for cattle and tundra climate commercial crops will need to change their lifestyle and adapt to suit the new environment. These changes in lifestyle would have long-term implications in all aspects including health. It is projected that although health conditions from frostbites and hypothermia would decrease with the reduction of cold stress in the region, heat-related diseases would become more common. Indirectly changes due to adjustments of dietary practices and weather conditions would change bacterial and viral proliferations that would result in specific health effects.

Coral reefs provide a second illustration of environmental change effects. Such reefs are among the most prized of wilderness ecosystems. Major reefs such as the Great Barrier Reef of Australia and the reefs off Belize are national and international treasures. Coral reefs cover only 0.17% of the ocean floor, an area approximately the size of Texas.[68,81] However, the importance of such reefs far exceeds their physical extent. Their biologic diversity is second only to that of tropical forests, and their productivity is among the highest in the world. They protect adjacent lands from wave action, nourish valuable fish populations, and generate millions of dollars in tourist revenues.

When subject to physical or chemical stress, coral "bleaches," losing color because of biochemical changes. Such stresses may be caused by fluctuations in sea level, temperature, or salinity and by pollution. Although reefs sometimes recover, bleaching often leads to death of the coral organisms and decomposition or disintegration of the reefs. In 1987, marine scientists began to notice high levels of coral bleaching and mortality off Puerto Rico. A worldwide pattern of severe coral bleaching began to emerge. Some scientists interpreted the problem as a harbinger of global warming, but it is unclear that this is the case. Nonetheless, coral reefs are vulnerable to temperature changes and sea level increases, so the threat of future damage is considerable. The best estimate is that sea level may rise an average of 1 m (3.3 feet) by 2100. Healthy reefs can grow upward by as much as 10 cm (4 inches) per decade, which may allow some reefs to adjust to rising sea level. However, if reefs are unhealthy, as the evidence of bleaching suggests, the rate of inundation may well exceed coral's ability to keep pace.[71]

Among the stresses that afflict coral reefs are coral mining for cement, dredging for navigation, coral collection for aquariums, and disruption by divers and commercial fishing. Many places also experience significant biochemical effects from coastal pollution and sediment or pollution runoff from land.

Loss of coral reefs is already significant. Estimates suggest that 5% to 10% of the world's living reefs have been destroyed by human activities. An additional 60% are thought to be at risk over the next 20 to 40 years.[85] The consequences for society are potentially enormous. Physical protection of coastlines could be drastically reduced. Locally, rich fisheries of coral islands could be diminished to the impoverished levels that typify deep oceans. Prized tourist attractions would disappear along with the revenues they generate. Opportunities for recovery of medicinal products (e.g., kainic acid) from reef organisms could be lost. Finally, the genetic resources of the planet could be further eroded. These are just some of the consequences of environmental change for one type of wilderness area. Similar, perhaps larger, effects may occur elsewhere.

ENVIRONMENTAL CHANGE AND MEDICAL EMERGENCIES

The causes and characteristics of many medical emergencies, and perhaps also the appropriate responses, are directly and indirectly connected with the environment in which they occur. This text contains many examples of medical challenges that are posed by environments in general and wilderness environments in particular. In some cases, an environmental agent (e.g., reptile bite, altitude sickness, wild animal attack) causes a medical emergency. In others, the environment affects the treatment of problems that are not environmentally created (e.g., wilderness trauma and surgical emergencies, hunting injuries, wilderness medical liability). In many cases, the environment serves as both agent and context. Inasmuch as the process of environmental change is global in scope, it probably will also affect wilderness medicine. A number of examples follow.

Increasing human penetration of wilderness areas by hikers, hunters, skiers, climbers, white-water boaters, and others is steadily driving up the number and cost of wilderness emergencies. For example, the U.S. National Park Service (NPS) spent $5.2 million on 2876 rescues in the United States in 2012.[79] NPS personnel, the U.S. military, and volunteers may be exposed to high risk when called on to retrieve inexperienced and underequipped parties. Given the rising cost of such operations, it has been proposed that individuals who participate in risky adventures should post rescue bonds before departing into the wilderness. California enacted a law that permits local authorities to charge persons who were aided up to $12,000 for each rescue performed by public agencies.[45] Similar laws exist in Hawaii, Idaho, Oregon, and New Hampshire. The combination of increasing populations and projected changes in environmental conditions can only add to future costs and difficulties of search and rescue in wilderness areas.

As settlement advances into wilderness areas, new patterns of disease are likely to emerge. For example, African land conversion from unmanaged wetlands to irrigated agriculture may spread the range of schistosomiasis and other waterborne diseases that are associated with drainage canals. Likewise, more people may be exposed to virulent diseases that are characteristic of wilderness ecosystems. Conversion of tropical forest in Africa may increase exposure to malaria carried by mosquitoes, onchocerciasis (river blindness) carried by Simulium flies, and trypanosomiasis (sleeping sickness) carried by tsetse flies.[4]

Pollutants often migrate into wilderness areas ahead of people. Air pollution is particularly mobile. Higher smokestacks are a common means of diluting airborne pollutants, but they also allow these materials to disperse more widely. Trees and lakes in New York State's Adirondack Mountains have been affected by acid rains transported from the Ohio Valley, and once clear vistas in the Grand Canyon have been obscured by smoke from a distant coal-fired power plant. The growing severity of winter haze in the Arctic is a problem.[73] Although the Arctic is a remote area, increasing haze has been observed there for almost a century. This smog consists of many different industrial pollutants that originate far to the south in industrial areas, especially the heavy manufacturing industries of Russia. Intense cold is the most obvious environmental health hazard in the Arctic, but buildup of industrial air pollutants may also have significant health effects, both directly on the body and indirectly through uptake by food sources from the Arctic environment.

The effect of weather on human mortality has long been a focus of biometeorologic research.[41] Box 119-1 lists a range of medical conditions that are weather related. For example, well-established linkages exist between high summer temperatures and human mortality, especially among elderly people. Although "global warming" need not mean that all parts of the earth will experience significantly elevated temperatures, some researchers are convinced that summer heat waves are likely to become more extreme, leading to increased mortality from this cause.[39]

The medical effects of UV radiation are known. Further erosion of the stratospheric ozone layer will undoubtedly increase the incidence of cataracts, skin cancers, and immune system

BOX 119-1 Causes of Death Considered to Be Weather Related

Active rheumatic fever
Adverse effects of medicinal agents
Cerebrovascular disease
Complications of medical care
Complications of pregnancy and childbirth
Contusion and crushing of intact skin surface
Diseases of the arteries, arterioles, and capillaries
Diseases of the blood and blood-forming organs
Diseases of the digestive system
Disease of the musculoskeletal system and connective tissue
Diseases of the nervous system and sense organs
Diseases of the skin and subcutaneous tissue
Diseases of the veins and lymphatics
Effects of foreign body entering through orifice
Endocrine, nutritional, and metabolic diseases
Fractures of the skull, spine, trunk, and limbs
Hypertensive disease
Influenza
Injury to nerves and spinal cord
Intracranial injury
Ischemic heart disease
Neoplasms: benign and malignant
Superficial injury
Toxic effects of substances of chiefly nonmedical sources

Modified from Kalkstein LS, Davis RE: Weather and human mortality: An evaluation of demographic and interregional responses in the United States, *Ann Assoc Am Geogr* 79:44, 1989.

diseases. Reduction of biodiversity threatens to reduce availability of natural materials that have medicinal value. Ethnobotanists are currently working with traditional shamans in Amazonia to catalog medicinal properties of plants in tropical forests. Marine species are also an important source of new medicines. Their decline will impair new drug discovery.

The "ozone hole" is a dramatic example of the expanding capacity of humans to modify the biosphere. Usually the process is inadvertent, and wilderness areas are not singled out for attention. Sometimes, however, the very remoteness and isolation of wilderness areas encourage dramatic environmental changes. Such was the case in northwest Alaska in 1962 when the U.S. government buried 15,000 pounds of radioactive soil at Point Hope.[55] The project was conducted by the U.S. Geological Survey acting in conjunction with the Atomic Energy Commission. The intent was to study effects of Arctic environments on radioactive isotopes. However, the burial was illegal; no public hearings were held, no markers were erected, and high-level wastes instead of low-level wastes were included. When the land was returned to the Inupiat (Eskimos) in 1971, they were not informed about the buried soils. They now attribute current elevated cancer rates to living and hunting for many years in a contaminated area. Government officials reject this view. The Point Hope case is not an isolated example. There is significant evidence that metropolitan governments have often tended to regard wilderness peripheries and their populations as dispensable when issues of national security and the welfare of metropolitan residents are at stake.[16]

COMPLEXITY AND UNCERTAINTY

Although we have ample reason to be concerned about environmental changes that lie ahead for wilderness areas, the subject is hedged with complexity and uncertainty. The potential for change exists, but it is difficult to be certain how fast and how far such changes will proceed. The following two cases illustrate some of the dimensions of complexity and uncertainty.

The north (Na Pali) coast of the Hawaiian island of Kauai is representative of wilderness areas that are particularly vulnerable to climate change. It is one of the most remote and beautiful places in Hawaii, accessible only on foot, from the ocean, or by air, weather permitting. The potential for increased rainfall, storminess, and sea level rise could radically alter this wilderness. For example, increased rainfall on Kauai's massive central peak, Mt Waialeale ("the wettest place on Earth"), would make for difficult hiking on steep Na Pali access trails that are already subject to erosion and landslides. The few available campsites near beaches may be eliminated by rising sea level. Sea caves that can be entered only by small, inflatable powerboats during calm conditions may become inaccessible. Flash floods in Na Pali streams may erode archeological sites, and increased moisture in the air would add to the mistiness that is now only an occasional feature of the area. Offshore waters host migrating whales that can be seen from the coast, but increased soil erosion might add to sediment loads and discourage the presence of these majestic mammals.

As the Na Pali coast becomes increasingly hazardous to visitors on foot, larger numbers may try to enter by helicopter, with more high technology–dependent visitors and fewer low technology–dependent ones. Health and safety emergencies may increase, or the mix of emergencies may change. The skies over Na Pali are already crowded with noisy aircraft. Crashes and deaths would likely increase. Leptospirosis from Na Pali streams may become more frequent. The bacteria were introduced from Southeast Asia in imported rats and pigs. In 1989, the Hawaiian Islands reported 66 cases of leptospirosis, with two resulting deaths.[54] Despite the potential for problems, no one can yet say with certainty which, if any, of these changes will occur. Still, we see strong indications that the Na Pali coast will not remain in its present state.

A second case that illustrates the complex interplay of environmental linkages and the potential for problems is provided by the highlands of Papua New Guinea.[1] Since the sweet potato was introduced to this area in the 1500s, it has become a staple crop for residents of remote mountain valleys. Sweet potatoes are susceptible to frost damage and tend to deplete mountain soils. In response to these constraints, villagers have developed specialized social and agricultural adjustments, including the practice of "mounding" and a complex system of resource exchanges between residents of higher elevations and lower elevations. Global warming might reduce the frost hazard, but increased precipitation or increased UV radiation could also threaten crop survival. At present, we have no way of confirming the extent and severity of possible changes. Clearly, however, a delicately balanced system of human ecology such as this would not remain unaffected by climate changes of the type anticipated in the next decades.

WHAT MIGHT BE DONE ABOUT LIMITING ENVIRONMENTAL CHANGE?

We have suggested that change is a dominant, perhaps "normal," feature of the world's landscapes and environments. What is different about the present era of environmental change is the extent to which it is directly attributable to human decisions and actions. It seems unlikely that people will do nothing if the anticipated changes are perceived as threatening, especially if they are also perceived as caused by humans. However, it is unlikely that responses to environmental change will be motivated solely by concern about environmental hazards, including medical emergencies in wilderness areas. Recognition is growing worldwide that improved environmental quality is an appropriate goal for all countries, not just developed ones. Therefore, public policies toward the environment will seek both to mitigate risks such as those connected with environmental emergencies and to secure rewards by safeguarding and enhancing valued resources, such as wilderness areas.

CHANGES IN ENVIRONMENTAL SCIENCE AND POLICY MAKING

This chapter initially appeared in the third edition of *Wilderness Medicine* (1995). It was written after the 1992 United Nations Conference on Environment and Development (UNCED) prompted creation of several landmark institutional instruments intended to guide governments and peoples toward economically and environmentally sustainable futures. Since then, the pace of international cooperation in support of these goals has greatly accelerated. By 2012, with the exception of a half-dozen developing countries and (notably) the United States, all of the world's nations had signed at least 10 of the 14 most prominent international governance agreements aimed at managing threats to environmental sustainability.*[78] Wilderness does not feature specifically in any of these agreements as a legal designation, but the roles of wild fauna and wild flora as indicators and maintainers of healthy environments loom large in several.

The picture is somewhat different at the level of national governments. Many countries have set aside wilderness areas and possess wilderness management systems, but these have typically evolved in piecemeal fashion and exhibit complex governance arrangements that imperfectly straddle jurisdictions of different agencies and organizations with differing agendas. Institutional complexity is the norm even in such places as New Zealand and Iceland, where wilderness has high cultural significance and enormous economic salience.[59,87] In the United States, the federal government has an explicit commitment to maintenance and protection of wilderness areas that is expressed in different policies among four major federal agencies, almost 200 separate wilderness-related laws, and thousands of guidance documents that govern wilderness management arrangements in different locations.[83]

The U.S. National Wilderness Preservation System (NWPS) includes 796 areas totaling 110 million acres in 44 states and Puerto Rico;[84] the separate Wild and Scenic Rivers System includes 12,598 miles of 203 rivers in 38 states and Puerto Rico.[52] The purpose of these designations is to protect relevant areas against significant modification by humans.[†] Most of the designated wilderness acreage is in Alaska (60%), and the bulk of the remainder in the 11 westernmost coterminous states (see Chapter 118). Typically, a wilderness area is embedded within and surrounded by other types of public land, such as national forests, national parks, or fish and wildlife reserves. Many types of human uses and activities permitted in the surrounding lands have spillover effects on the wilderness areas. Wilderness management is usually in the hands of the same agencies that administer the surrounding public lands and has frequently been a neglected stepchild of those agencies. Moreover, recent research has disclosed that the boundaries of wilderness areas are often poorly suited to permit survival of many species they contain. Especially in the case of migratory animals or those with large territorial ranges, what happens to them outside the wilderness is just as important as what happens within. Therefore, it makes little sense to restrict efforts for limiting environmental change solely to wilderness areas. Such efforts usually need to be applied to the private lands and waters that interdigitate with federally managed wilderness and nonwilderness areas.

Holistic management principles and tools that can be applied across governmental boundaries between and within countries are increasingly in demand. Some of these are available, but more are needed. For example, Environmental Impact Statements are decision support tools intended to provide holistic integrative assessments of proposed development actions with potentially undesirable effects on human environments, including wilderness areas.[7] Newer forms of holistic planning and management instruments (e.g., Health Impact Assessments) might take into account contributions of wilderness areas to human well-being that have previously been overlooked or undervalued.[58]

Although national and international government initiatives may have grabbed the headlines, adoption of international norms for private business practices has grown apace during the past 20 years. During the past two decades, the International Standards Organization has issued more than 230,000 compliance certificates to firms that met tighter environmental performance specifications.[78] Most of these focus on broad classes of environmental impact; they have positive indirect effects on wilderness areas and natural systems that sustain them.

Nongovernmental organizations (NGOs) have played key roles in fostering increased awareness of deleterious environmental changes and the growing human contribution to them. The IPCC's leadership of international efforts to apply scientific knowledge to the redress of unwanted climate changes is only the tip of a much larger iceberg founded on enhanced involvement of laypersons and local communities in decision making about environmental governance. This is made possible by modern electronic information and communication technologies (e.g., handheld computers, smartphones, Internet, social media, cloud sourcing, participatory mapping using geographic information science). These have ushered in a new era of volunteered geographic information that provides opportunities for increased use of lay knowledge in expert decision making and co-production of wilderness management systems previously a domain of experts.[26] Widespread availability of Global Positioning System (GPS) devices has reduced some of the uncertainties of wilderness navigation and, especially when coupled with satellite phones and other communications devices, affected the sense of remoteness formerly a signal characteristic of human experiences in the wilderness.

New environmental interest groups are joining the fray, including several connected with medicine, health, and human well-being. For example, the American Medical Association formed an Environmental Health Task Force charged with studying harmful environmental issues such as waste disposal and ozone depletion. In addition, the National Association of Physicians for the Environment was established in April 1992 to educate physicians about environmental hazards to human health and to develop recommendations for policy makers. In 2009, the World Health Professionals Alliance, a body that brings together representatives of national nursing, dentistry, pharmacy, and medicine associations across the globe, issued a statement on combating the effects of climate change that contained recommendations for changes in professional and public policies.[86]

Traditional conceptions of wilderness have emphasized the value of nature in a pristine condition—a condition that must be protected and preserved against human modifications. As argued here, such a view does not square with the vast bulk of scientific knowledge that recognizes the pervasiveness of past human impacts on natural systems and looks toward future environments that are even more completely human dominated. Such recognition implies that science and society might both consider restoration of degraded environments as well as preservation of minimally disturbed ones. *Restoration ecology* has become a new growth area in the environmental sciences and a new tool for environmental managers.[38] The implications for wilderness areas of such a shift are considerable. On the one hand, a restored watershed is not the same as one that has never been allowed to deteriorate, and a hand-reared endangered species is not the same as one that survives without direct human help. On the other hand, it is possible that environments might be restored to states that are functionally equivalent to wilderness. This raises fascinating but as yet unanswered questions. Would the availability of human-constructed alternatives to natural areas mean a slackening in political pressures to preserve "authentic" wilderness? Would "synthetic wildernesses" contain suites of medical risks similar to other types of wilderness? Current debates about the wisdom of changing existing wilderness protection statutes to accommodate climate change adaptation measures, which might involve more active human intervention in those places, are representative of the issues in play.

Looking across the range of environmental change issues and responses, new institutions and philosophies of human-nature relations are emerging and being linked to a broad range of

---

*Basel Convention, Cartagena Convention, Convention on Biological Diversity, Convention on International Trade in Endangered Species of Wild Fauna and Flora, Convention on Migratory Species, World Heritage Convention, Kyoto Protocol, Secretariat for the Vienna Convention and for the Montreal Protocol, Ramsar Convention, Rotterdam Convention, Stockholm Convention, Convention to Combat Desertification, Convention on the Law of the Sea, Framework Convention on Climate Change.

†http://www.fs.fed.us/recreation/programs/cda/wilderness.shtml.

public concerns. Issues of environmental change are seen as intertwined with issues of economics and security. The principle of diversity in natural systems, which imparts resilience in the face of stress, is being replicated in social systems. This is a hopeful sign at a time when environmental changes are unprecedented in rate and magnitude.

REFERENCES

> **Complete references used in this text are available online at expertconsult.inkling.com.**

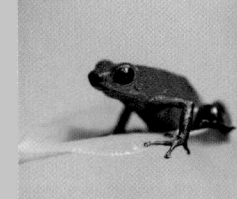

CHAPTER 120
Biodiversity and Human Health

RICHARD S. SALKOWE

Biodiversity is defined as the variety of all life-forms that inhabit Earth. From the earliest prokaryotic microorganisms that resided on this planet approximately 3.5 billion years ago to the megafauna that presently roam the vast plains of the Serengeti (Figure 120-1), this diversity of life is a result of competitive and cooperative relationships among species that have resulted in a delicate balance of natural processes that are essential to maintenance of human health. More than a century ago, the famous naturalist and preservationist John Muir stated, "Whenever we try to pick out anything by itself, we find it hitched to everything else in the universe." He was referring to inherent interrelationships that exist among the physical and biologic components of our environment. These relationships result in diverse ecosystems that serve to filter air, purify water, protect us from hazards, and provide essential food resources. What has become alarmingly evident is that the present rate of ecosystem destruction, species extinction, and loss of genetic variety on planet Earth is associated with a concurrent increase in prevalence of invasive species, severity of damage associated with natural disasters, and spread of infectious disease. Biodiversity is in a state of crisis, and the balance of nature that is critical to our sustainable existence is at risk.

Loss of species diversity is occurring at a rate that is 1000 to 10,000 times greater than the natural background rate.[36] This has an insidious effect on planetary and individual well-being. The effects are seen in the compromise of coastal estuaries that serve as natural waste filters and barriers to storm surges. The consequences are evident in bleached coral reefs that provide habitats for fish species and in clearing of tropical rain forests that serve as carbon sinks and provide oxygen for the environment.

In 1992 at the United Nations Earth Summit in Rio de Janeiro, 150 government leaders agreed to sustainable conservation of biologic diversity for preservation of planetary health. This agreement, adopted as the "Convention on Biodiversity," defined biologic diversity as "the variability among living organisms from all sources including, inter alia, terrestrial, marine and other aquatic ecosystems and the ecological complexes of which they are part; this includes diversity within species, between species and of ecosystems."[7] The United Nations Educational, Scientific, and Cultural Organization, in recognizing that biodiversity is the "basis for human existence," declared 2010 to be the International Year of Biodiversity in an attempt to increase awareness of the importance of biodiversity to human well-being.

UNDERSTANDING THE ETIOLOGY OF THE BIODIVERSITY CRISIS

> *What is man without the beasts? If the beasts were gone, men would die from great loneliness of spirit, for whatever happens to the beasts also happens to man. All things*

are connected. Whatever befalls the earth befalls the children of the earth.
> —*Chief Seattle of the Suquamish, 1854*

Chief Seattle's words are emblematic of the historic sentiments of people who were directly involved with the land for sustenance and shelter. Early civilizations revolved around small communal hunter-gatherer societies. These societies had integral dependence on interaction with nature. They were in constant contact with natural resources and depended on basic respect for the rhythms of nature to maintain societal sustainability. Native American Indians of the Eastern Cherokee Nation developed these ideals into a harmony ethic of noncompetitive and reciprocal symbiotic relations with nature and their fellow man[11] (see Chapter 112).

Successful hunter-gatherer societies gradually increased in population. Additional demand for food resources coincided with discovery of plant cultivation technology, leading to agrarian civilizations and additional needs pertaining to land ownership and permanent settlements. Agrarian culture and resultant success of permanent settlements eventually led to development of cities, states, and empires. The industrial revolution took hold as a result of advances in scientific discovery and need for greater productivity to meet the demands of a burgeoning populace. Civilization's advances gradually moved individuals further and further away from the necessity of physical contact with the natural world. Intermediaries with nature, such as farmers, fishers, and merchants, satisfied the sustenance needs of city dwellers. It is not coincidental that environmental degradation and biodiversity loss secondary to the byproducts of industrialization occurred without apparent knowledge in a society so seemingly independent of nature. It became easy to ignore an unknown and intangible threat, namely, biodiversity loss. Robert Ornstein and Paul Ehrlich[23] hypothesize that humans are affected by a lack of natural selection for response to slowly developing threats such as biodiversity loss. They explain this factor as follows[23]:

Hundreds of thousands or millions of years ago, our ancestors' survival depended in large part on the ability to respond quickly to threats that were immediate, personal, palpable: threats like the sudden crack of a branch as it is about to give way or the roar of a flash flood racing down a narrow valley. Threats like the darkening of the entrance of a cavern as a giant cave bear enters. Threats like lightning, threats like a thrown spear. Those are not threats generated by complex technological devices accumulated over decades by unknown people half a world away. Those are not threats like the slow atmospheric buildup of carbon dioxide from auto exhausts, power plants and deforestation; not threats like the gradual depletion of the ozone layer. Thus, the human mind evolved to register short-term changes from moment to moment, day to day, and season to season, and to overlook the backdrop against which those take place.

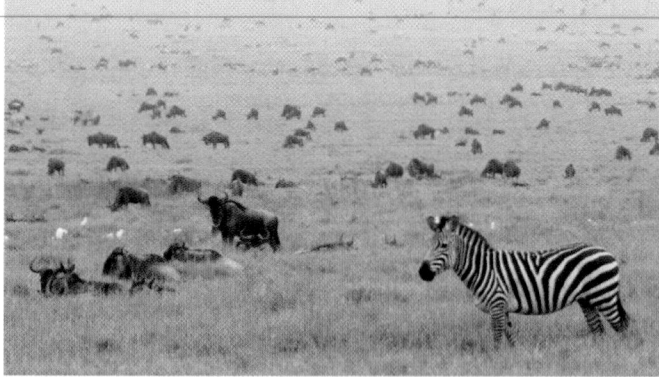

FIGURE 120-1 Zebra in the Serengeti during wildebeest migration. (*Courtesy David Dennis, cc-by-sa-2.0.*)

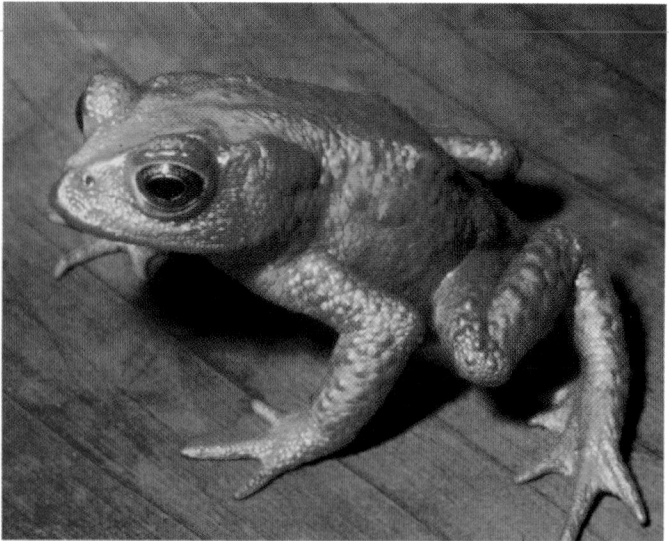

FIGURE 120-3 Monteverde golden toad. (*Courtesy U.S. Fish and Wildlife Service. Public domain.*)

The insidious processes of planetary degradation have reached a crisis phase. The miracle of the combustion engine and invention of plastics have become the potential bane of our existence, as shown by the consequences of injudicious burning of fossil fuels and discovery of toxic byproducts, such as dioxin and bisphenol A. Loss of biodiversity represents a unique challenge that demands an agenda for action. It is difficult enough to effectively communicate the risks associated with known technologic hazards, such as lead, mercury, and greenhouse gases. Convincing the public of the adverse consequences of the extinction of the dusky seaside sparrow (Figure 120-2) or the Montverde golden toad (Figure 120-3) represents an even greater challenge. Loss of these flagship species is a story that must be told, because the sparrow's demise is a tale of the health-related dangers of dichlorodiphenyltrichloroethane (DDT) and mismanagement of marshland in the United States. In this regard, extinction of a seemingly inconsequential avian species serves as an indicator of the ecologic dangers associated with pesticide exposure and loss of the water filtration and hazard protection services that marshlands provide to protect human health in coastal areas.

The Monteverde golden toad succumbed to a multitude of pressures associated with invasive species introduced by tourists and aquatic chytrid fungal infections that are theorized to be correlated with El Niño–induced climate change in the toad's former home range of Costa Rica. Loss of this particular species is indicative of the threat that amphibians face worldwide. A recent study revealed that 32% of the 6000 species of amphibians under analysis were threatened and 43% were in decline.[25] The potential medicinal value of chemical compounds that have been extracted from amphibians is evident in the 200 psychoactive alkaloids that have been extracted from the skin of frogs and toads.[1] Some of these compounds have been used in medical research pertaining to nerve and muscle disorders. The alkaloid known as *epibatidine,* which is synthesized from skin of the phantasmal poison frog, is being tested as a nonaddictive and nonsedating analgesic that exhibits 200 times the potency of morphine.[1] Bufogenin and bufotoxin, substances that have been extracted from parotid glands of toads from the same *Bufo* genus as the extinct Monteverde golden toad, exhibit adrenal and cardiovascular effects in humans.[1]

Further investigation of the adverse sequelae of biodiversity loss, as evidenced by ecosystem degradation, species decline, and loss of genetic diversity, provides additional validation of the corollary threat to human health.

THREATENED ECOSYSTEMS

Ecosystems represent abiotic and biotic components of an environment. Variation in ecosystems, from arid deserts of the South American Atacama to Siberian subarctic taiga forests, is determined by climatic and geologic characteristics of the respective regions. Mineral components of soil and nitrogen-fixing capacities of soil microbes; salinity, turbidity, and other hydrologic aspects of the respective environment; and the variety of flora and fauna that inhabit a region create a syncretic balance that is sustainable in a healthy ecosystem. Speciation within these respective biomes and ecosystems has developed over millions of years, as chronicled by successes and failures of living organisms that did (or did not) establish sustainable niches in a vast array of seemingly hospitable and inhospitable locales.

Ecosystems provide a multitude of features that are essential to human well-being. Food resources, fresh water, sediment retention, nutrient cycling, disease regulation, erosion control, air quality, and climate change depend on healthy ecosystems.[18] Human activities, ranging from land-use patterns associated with increased urbanization to clear-cutting of rain forest for agricultural purpose, have degraded the quality of ecosystems worldwide. The British ecologist, Norman Myers, developed the concept of "biodiversity hotspots" to identify areas of the planet with a high number of endemic species under extreme threats

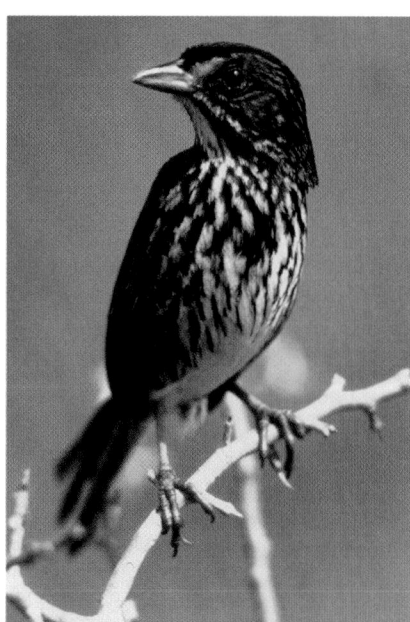

FIGURE 120-2 Dusky seaside sparrow. (*Courtesy U.S. Fish and Wildlife Service. Public domain.*)

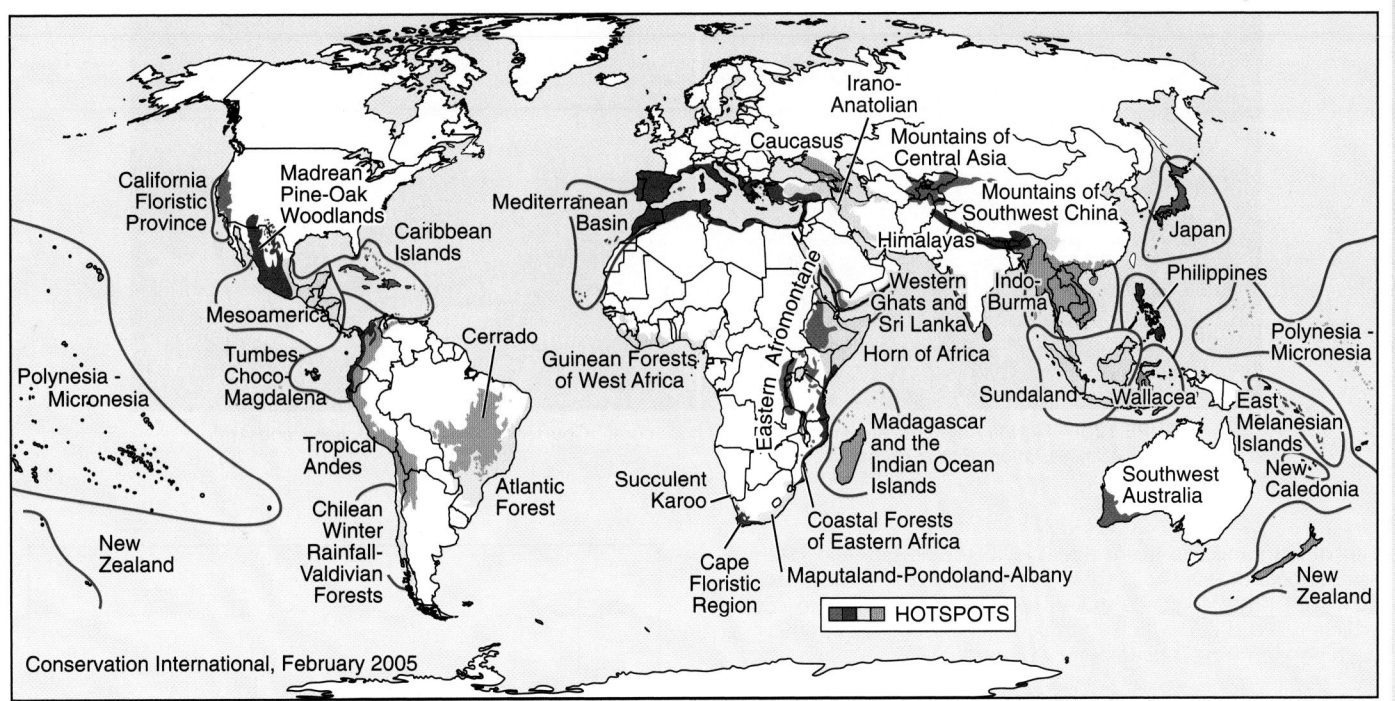

FIGURE 120-4 "Biodiversity hotspot" map. *(With permission from Conservation International.)*

to their ecosystems, as evidenced by loss of at least 70% of the natural vegetation.[6] Conservation International[6] states that "over 50 percent of the world's plant species and 42 percent of all terrestrial vertebrate species are endemic to the 34 biodiversity hotspots" (Figure 120-4).

Tropical rain forests exemplify the human health risks associated with ecosystem compromise. These biomes provide habitats for more than one-half of all plant and animal species in the world. Prior studies have counted 100 to 300 species in a 1-hectare area in South America. Approximately 25% of all pharmaceutical agents are estimated to contain compounds that are found in tropical rain forest plants.[2] The United Nations estimates that 13 million hectares of tropical forest are destroyed each year for logging and agricultural land clearing.[10] In South America, Mexico, and Guyana, rain forests have been cleared for cattle grazing, soybean farming, logging, and gold mining (Figure 120-5). Less than 1% of all tropical rain forest species have been evaluated for pharmacologic benefit. Degradation of this essential ecosystem has human health consequences that range from loss of potential lifesaving medicines to alterations in climate associated with carbon sequestration by forest trees and burning of forest land.

Mangrove estuaries and wetland sloughs represent another class of threatened ecosystems. Land development, agriculture, and aquaculture pursuits have led to loss of at least 35% of this ecosystem worldwide.[32] Considered to be one of the planet's most productive ecosystems, wetlands are referred to as "nature's kidneys," because they filter sediments and pollutants and regulate water flow. Mangroves act as a natural buffer to prevent coastal erosion and provide essential habitat for crustaceans, fish, and several other species. Runoff from excessive amounts of nitrogen- and phosphorus-based fertilizers used in monoculture farming leads to eutrophication of coastal forests and increased mortality of mangrove species as a result of root damage (Figure 120-6).

Coral reefs support more than 4000 species of fish and are home to approximately 25% of all marine species. In addition, reefs provide important breakwater protection for coastal areas during tropical storms. Scientists estimate more than 50% of the world's coral reefs face potential destruction by the year 2030.

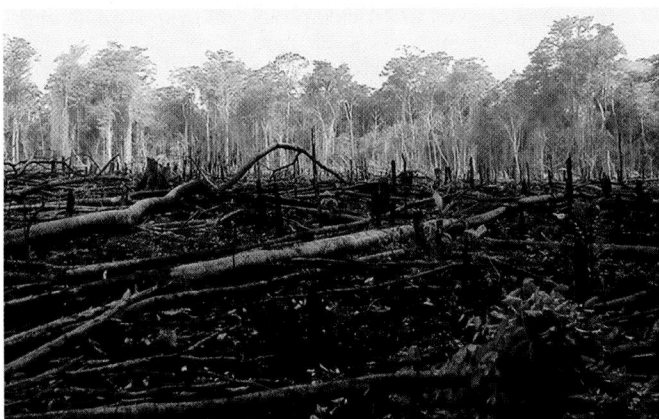

FIGURE 120-5 Tropical rain forest destruction in Mexico. *(Courtesy Azari Nicks. Public domain.)*

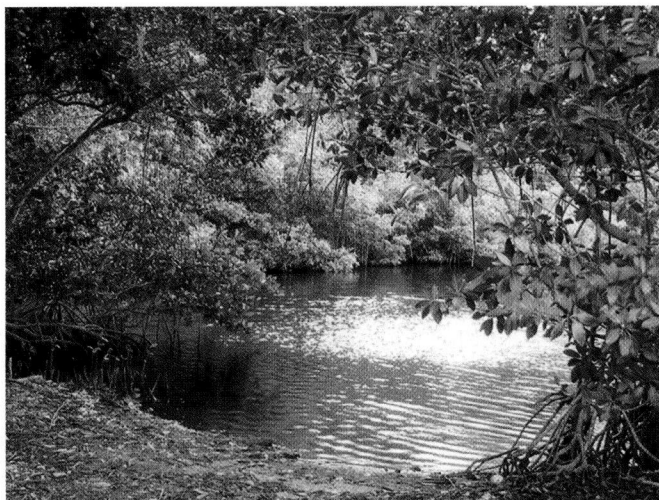

FIGURE 120-6 Everglades National Park mangrove tidal estuary. *(Courtesy Moni2. Public domain.)*

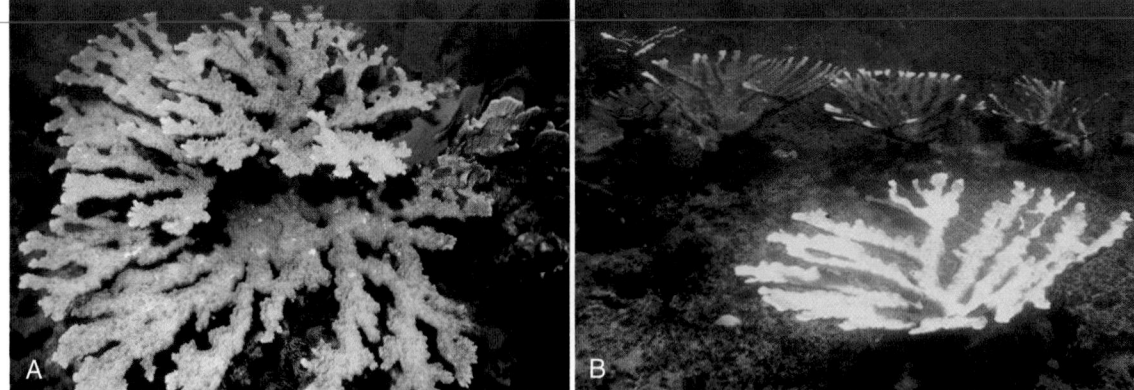

FIGURE 120-7 Florida Keys critically endangered elkhorn coral. *(Courtesy the National Oceanic and Atmospheric Administration. Public domain.)*

Global warming is a major threat to this important ecosystem; a sea temperature rise of 1° to 2°C (1.8° to 3.6°F) has been associated with physiologic stress and immune compromise to corals, which leave them with subsequent increased susceptibility to bacterial and fungal pathogens[3] (Figure 120-7).

SPECIES DECLINE

Species decline is another form of biodiversity loss. Variety of species in an ecosystem is critical to sustainability of the respective habitat. Excluding bacteria and viruses, approximately 1.5 million species have been taxonomically identified, and approximately 10 million species are believed to exist on Earth.[5] The 2008 *Living Planet Report* indicates that, between 1970 and 2005, the earth's wildlife populations declined by a third.[37] The International Union for Conservation of Nature has estimated that in 2010, 22% of all vertebrates, 34% of all invertebrates, 70% of all plants, and 50% of all fungi and protists were listed as critically endangered, endangered, or vulnerable species. Species that are considered threatened worldwide include 30% of all amphibians, 21% of mammals, and 86% of mosses.[16] Species are disappearing at the alarming rate of 1000 to 10,000 times the natural background rate of 1 to 10 species per year. E. O. Wilson, "the father of biodiversity," estimates the current extinction rate is 137 species per day in tropical rain forests alone[36] (Figure 120-8).

Invertebrate species, which represent approximately 76% of all life-forms, are experiencing a significant rate of extinction. Dam construction, water pollution, and deforestation have challenged the capacity of several invertebrate species to retain a foothold in ecosystems worldwide. A keystone species in the Antarctic ecosystem, the Antarctic krill, is indicative of the threats that face invertebrate species (Figure 120-9). Krill are an important food source for whales, seals, squid, penguins, and fish. In addition, these small crustaceans act as an essential component of the ocean's capacity to sequester carbon. Recession of the Antarctic ice pack and acidification of ocean waters associated with carbon dioxide emissions and global warming are challenges to vitality of the Antarctic krill.

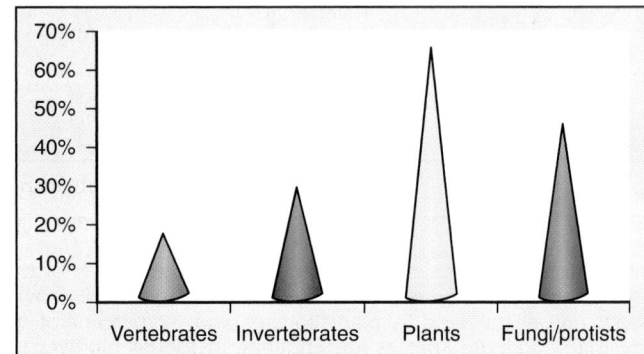

FIGURE 120-8 Extinction rate per millennium.

LOSS OF GENETIC DIVERSITY

Some analysts believe that the greatest threat to human welfare comes from losses of genetic diversity within species.[35] Farmers and pastoralists have used selective planting and breeding techniques for centuries to increase crop yield and product output. With the advent of techniques to genetically engineer crops for resistance to variations in climate and susceptibility to disease and pests, biodiversity of the gene pool has drastically altered. In 1970, the United States lost 15% of its Midwest corn crop as a result of a fungus that the genetically modified crop was unable to resist. By 2007, an estimated 73% of the U.S. corn crop was genetically modified or engineered. Uniformity of plant crops has led to pesticide-tolerant species. There is continuous need for further engineering of crops to resist pests and climatic influences, which were previously tolerable because of the capacity for a diverse gene pool to provide protection from adverse influences through the processes of natural selection. Although humans have dramatically increased crop yields, this has occurred at the risk of increased susceptibility to unanticipated pathogens

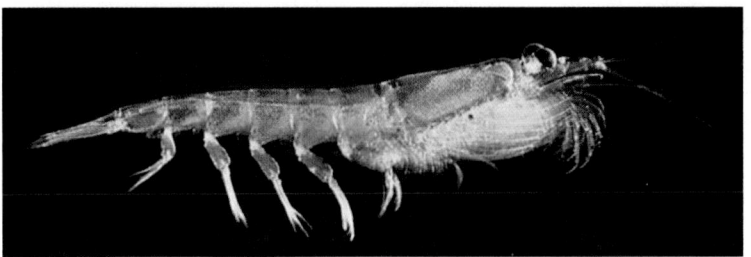

FIGURE 120-9 Antarctic krill. *(Courtesy Uwe Kils, Creative Commons, Share Alike 3.0.)*

and environmental extremes as a result of loss of indigenous strains that were well adapted to local ecosystems.[35]

Fragmentation of habitats caused by urbanization and deforestation has prevented species from interbreeding because of the loss of historic migration corridors, leading to genetic bottlenecks. Species ranging from the grizzly bear in the Central Canadian Rockies to the Florida panther in the Everglades face dangers associated with increased susceptibility to disease and genetic mutation caused by inbreeding of small populations. Loss of vitality in these species affects predator-prey relationships and ultimately contributes to spread of human pathogens (e.g., *Borrelia burgdorferi*, the causative agent of Lyme disease).

Genetic uniformity among honeybees has resulted in problems with reproduction and disease. A condition known as *colony collapse disorder* has led to an alarming die-off among honeybee colonies. This is a significant concern to beekeepers, who have witnessed decline of 30% to 90% of their hives in some parts of the United States. The disorder has been associated with lack of genetic diversity in managed beehives. The potential effect on apple, peach, soybean, and other honeybee-dependent crops could be devastating if these keystone pollinators continue to decline in number.

INVASIVE SPECIES

Introduction of species that are not indigenous to a particular ecosystem has become a global threat to biodiversity. This has posed a historic challenge to human health. The spread of disease to susceptible native populations led, in part, to the downfall of Mesoamerican civilizations as far back as the 16th century. Some alien species were intentionally introduced with intent to improve the local environment without awareness of possible negative repercussions. Africanized bees were imported to improve honeybee productivity in tropical regions of South America. Nile perch were introduced in an attempt to control aquatic weeds, and Brazilian pepper was planted as an attractive ornamental. In each case, lack of species competition in the introduced community allowed the invasive species to overwhelm the native species, with deleterious consequences for the entire ecosystem.

Zebra and quagga mussels are native to the Black and Caspian seas and are believed to have been inadvertently introduced to the Great Lakes region of the United States by emptying of ballast water from transatlantic commercial ships. Prolific female zebra and quagga mussels can produce up to 1 million eggs per year. These mollusks are clogging intake pipes that supply municipal water in Great Lakes cities. Both native mussel populations and freshwater ecosystems are threatened by these invasive species (Figure 120-10). In Florida, 10 of the 16 native bromeliad plant species are listed as threatened or endangered. The Mexican bromeliad weevil, inadvertently introduced by means of infested imported plants, represents a serious challenge to these vulner-

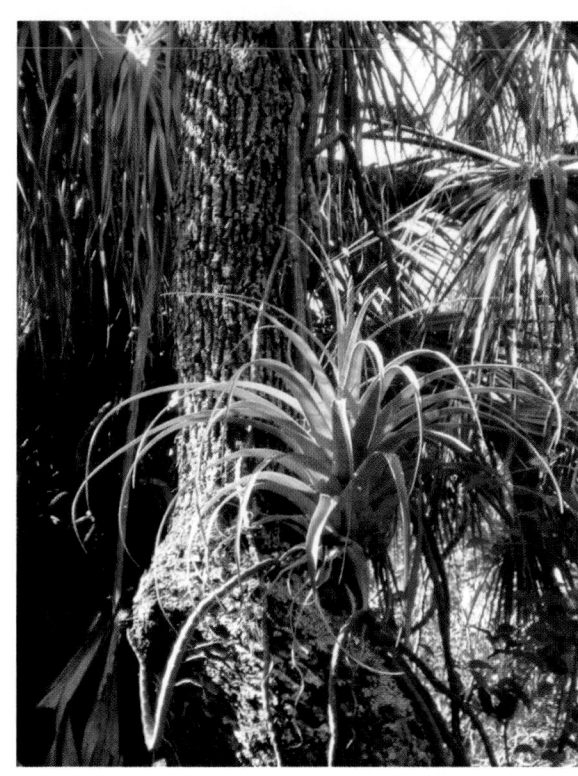

FIGURE 120-11 Florida bromeliad. *(Courtesy Richard Salkowe.)*

able plants. Extracts from bromeliads of the *Tillandsia* genus exhibit analgesic and antiviral properties (Figure 120-11). The danger of invasive species predation is exemplified by the risk of extinction of potentially beneficial bromeliad species. Exotic species, such as Burmese and African Rock pythons, invaded the Florida Everglades after pet owners released their animals into the wild. It is estimated that the Everglades are infested with a population of more than 10,000 of these snakes. Pythons compete with native species for food and habitat resources and represent a threat to several endangered species in the region (Figure 120-12). Approximately 50,000 species of introduced plants, animals, and microbes cause more than $120 billion in annual damages and control costs in the United States.

PUBLIC HEALTH CONCERNS

"More than any other biodiversity-related issue, effects on human health may make saving biodiversity an important societal goal."[35]

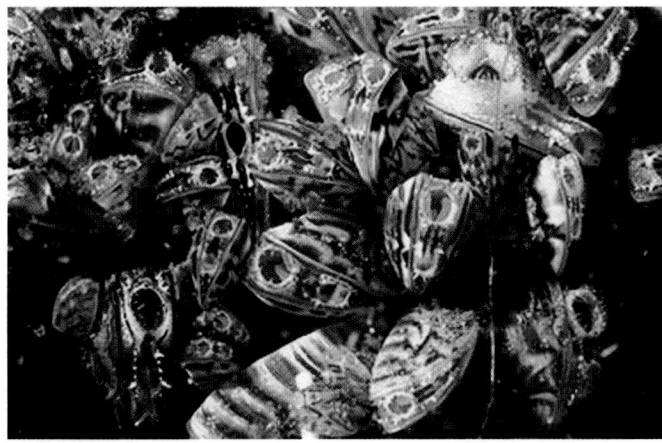

FIGURE 120-10 Zebra mussels. *(Courtesy GerardM, Creative Commons, Share Alike 3.0.)*

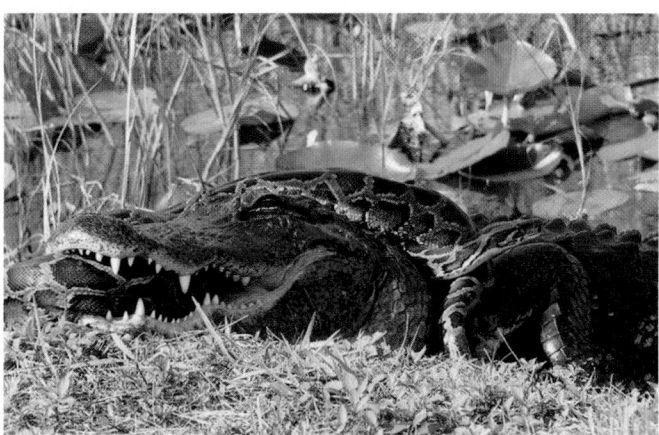

FIGURE 120-12 Burmese python and American alligator. *(Courtesy Lori Oberhofer, National Park Service.)*

The Wilderness Medical Society has defined five areas that relate biodiversity loss to public health concerns:
1. Altered epidemiology of diseases
2. Loss of biologic raw materials
3. Loss of models for medical research
4. Threatened food production
5. Threatened water resources

ALTERED EPIDEMIOLOGY OF DISEASES

Degraded ecosystems lose capacity to resist the challenges of disease and pestilence. The roles of invasive species, climate change, genetic uniformity, and altered predator-prey relationships have been previously highlighted with respect to relationships between biodiversity loss and disease epidemiology. Lyme disease exemplifies the ability for pathogens to spread in environments where an altered habitat disrupts normal relationships between predators and prey. Spread of *B. burgdorferi* has been enhanced by increased prevalence of the disease-carrying tick vector *Ixodes scapularis*. Altered habitats associated with urban sprawl and altered predator-prey relationships have allowed a burgeoning population of competent disease reservoirs in white-footed mice and deer that the female ticks use for blood meals before egg laying.

Nutrient runoff from fertilization and animal waste has become a significant concern with respect to biodiversity loss caused by eutrophication of nutrient-laden waters, with subsequent formation of harmful algal blooms (Figure 120-13). The Mississippi Dead Zone is an area where algal blooms have formed as a result of nitrogen and phosphorus runoff from fertilized cornfields in the U.S. Midwest. Decaying algal blooms lead to proliferation of oxygen-dependent bacteria. Resultant hypoxic waters, with 90% depletion in oxygen level, threaten vitality of the shrimp industry in the Gulf of Mexico. In addition, areas of high algal growth and warm water serve as ideal reservoirs for pathogens such as *Vibrio cholerae*. For areas in which hypoxic conditions are insufficient to affect productivity of copepod species, algal blooms are associated with a greater number of cholera-carrying copepods. Naturally occurring hydrocarbon-consuming bacteria have been active in clearing the remaining oil in the Gulf of Mexico after the 2010 *Deepwater Horizon* spill. These oil-related bacterial blooms are associated with 35% depletion in oxygen levels. The adverse effect on oxygen-dependent ocean species in the region remains under investigation.

LOSS OF BIOLOGIC RAW MATERIALS

Natural environments provide a vast pharmacologic potential: 57% of the 150 top prescription drugs sold in the United States in 1993 are in some way linked to natural products.[35] The World

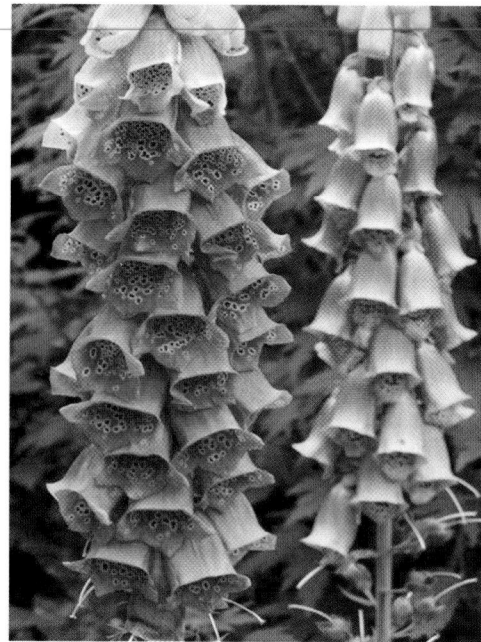

FIGURE 120-14 Foxglove flowers. *(Courtesy Jensflorian, Creative Commons Share Alike 3.0; and BerndH, Creative Commons Share Alike 2.5.)*

Health Organization (WHO) estimates that plant medicines account for more than $60 billion in worldwide sales. Revenue from chemotherapeutic drugs derived from the plant species *Taxus baccata* was $2.3 billion in 2000.[35] Many prescription medications are derived from plant products. The foxglove plant *Digitalis purpurea* is the source of digitalis. Deadly nightshade *Atropa belladonna* is the original plant source for atropine (Figure 120-14). Taxol is derived from bark of the threatened Pacific yew tree *Taxus brevifolia*. The Madagascar rosy periwinkle *Catharanthus roseus* is the source of vincristine and vinblastine[35] (Figure 120-15).

LOSS OF MODELS FOR MEDICAL RESEARCH

Species decline is associated with loss of biologic models that may help to understand human physiology and disease. Ancrod, a defibrinogenating agent derived from venom of the Malaysian pit viper, is being investigated as a treatment for acute ischemic stroke. Understanding the renin-angiotensin system evolved

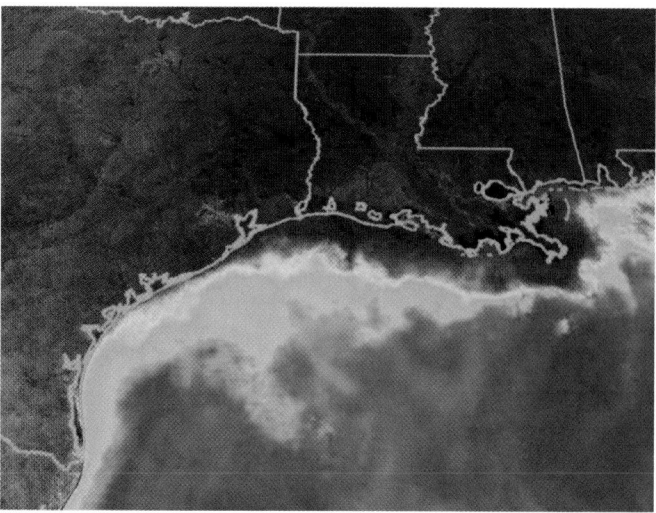

FIGURE 120-13 Mississippi Dead Zone. *(Courtesy National Aeronautics and Space Administration. Public domain.)*

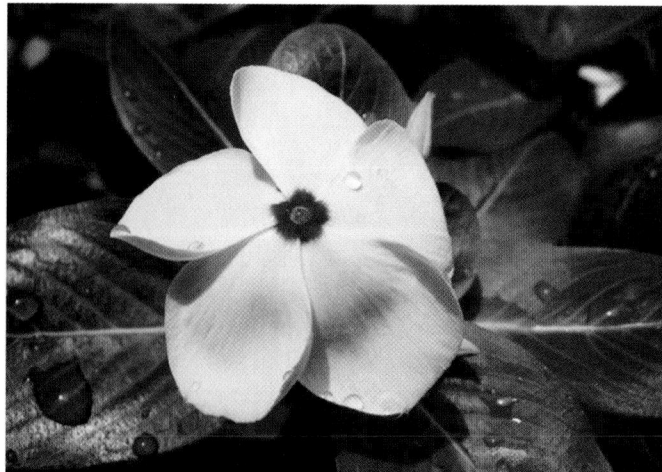

FIGURE 120-15 Madagascar rosy periwinkle. *(Courtesy titanium22, cc-by-sa-2.0.)*

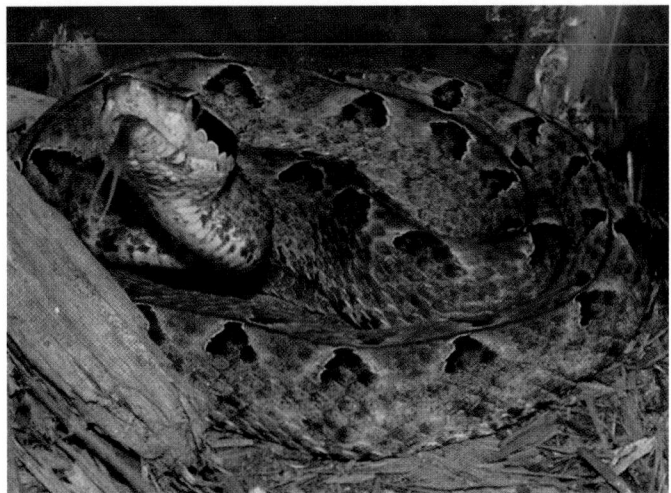

FIGURE 120-16 Malaysian pit viper. *(Courtesy Al Coritz, Creative Commons, Share Alike 3.0.)*

from study of South American pit viper venom that contains angiotensin-converting enzyme (ACE) factors. This led to development of synthetic ACE inhibitors[35] (Figure 120-16). The Gila monster of the southwestern United States is a venomous lizard that produces a glucagon-like peptide in its saliva (Figure 120-17). The synthetic version of this protein is the incretin mimetic, exenatide.

THREATENED FOOD PRODUCTION

At present, 15 crop plants provide 90% of the world's food-energy intake. High levels of monoculture farming and fertilizer use, in conjunction with genetic engineering of crops, have increased yield and resistance to pests and disease-causing organisms. However, loss of naturally acquired immunity to the full range of deleterious environmental factors that have affected our food crops is a concern. High-yielding varieties of genetically modified crops rely on heavy inputs of water, fertilizer, and pesticides. More than 900 pests now resist more than one pesticide. Pesticides also kill the natural enemies of pests, permitting an especially large explosion of those pests.[35]

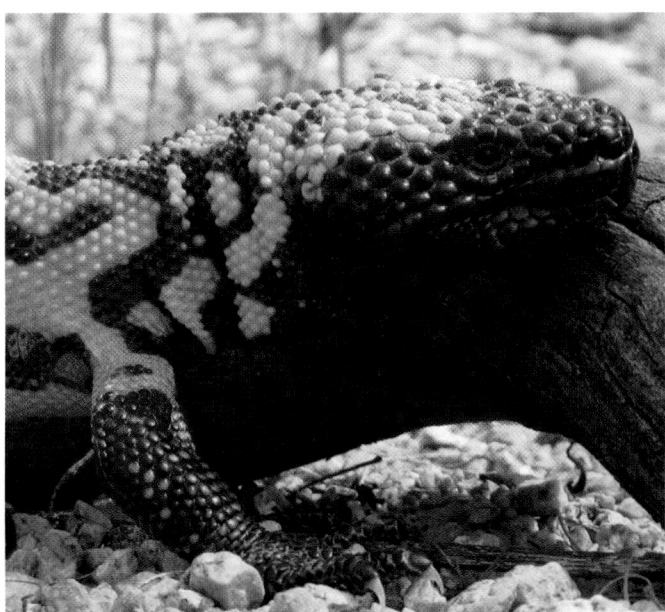

FIGURE 120-17 Gila monster. *(Courtesy Jeff Servoss, U.S. Fish and Wildlife Service.)*

Use of chemical dispersants as part of the containment response to the 2010 *Deepwater Horizon* oil spill disaster in the Gulf of Mexico has potential long-term deleterious effects on the region's ocean, coastal, and estuarine ecosystems. The Gulf of Mexico produces 25% to 30% of the annual seafood harvested in the United States, including 59% of the oyster production and 75% of the wild shrimp catch.[30] Scientists at the Dauphin Island Sea Lab, the state of Alabama's marine science education and research laboratory, are investigating the role of the coastal region's biodiversity in mitigating the adverse consequences of the event. The biopsychosocial impact on human health associated with any significant loss of biodiversity in this region extends from economic hardship to potential illness caused by environmental contaminants in the food chain.

THREATENED WATER RESOURCES

Water pollution from pesticides and industrial byproducts containing polychlorinated biphenyls (PCBs), bisphenol A, and phthalates has been associated with compounds that interfere with the function of endocrine hormones, resulting in developmental abnormalities and altered reproductive capacity. Alligator populations in Lake Apopka, Florida, have been in decline; nitrate-related endocrine disrupters may be the cause of observed abnormalities in sexual development.[14] The potential for endocrine disrupters to affect human health has been recognized, although there is no confirmatory evidence that these pollutants have definitively altered human reproductive function.[26]

CASE STUDY

The combined effects of ecosystem degradation and species decline as a risk to human health have raised concerns about one of the great river systems of the world. The Colorado River basin is considered the lifeline of the southwest. More than 20 million people depend on the Lake Powell portion of the river system for water and electricity. Lake Powell was formed between 1963 and 1980, when Glen Canyon slowly filled with backflow from the Colorado River after completion of the Glen Canyon Dam. This massive project was a component of the U.S. Bureau of Reclamation's plan to provide water and electricity to the growing population of the southwestern United States. The Glen Canyon and Colorado River ecosystem had previously developed over the course of 5 million years. However, during the span of 17 short years, it was drastically altered by the dam project. Examining this situation provides a window into the consequences of such an endeavor with respect to biodiversity and human health. Extinct and threatened native species in this region serve as indicators of ecosystem disruption and raise concerns pertaining to sustainability of a drastically altered natural environment.

"The native fish of the Colorado River system make up one of the most unusual assemblages of fish specially adapted to their environment found anywhere in the world."[29] The unique combination of geologic, hydrologic, and climatic factors that were found in the predam Colorado River basin led to natural-selection processes resulting in peculiar morphologic and behavioral characteristics in the native fish. Adaptations of the fish to extreme and severe river conditions include large streamlined bodies, large fins, and thick skin.[20] Larger fish of the Colorado River live an exceptionally long time and have depressed skulls with large predorsal humps and small eyes.[19] Niche partitioning for available resources led to development of structural variations within the fish native to this region, such as razorback sucker fish with "protrusible mouths and special gill rakers for sieving plankton or detritus."[19] Some of the native fish fauna have existed for 20 million years.[20] Speciation in this region was associated with demands placed on the aquatic biota. The native warm-water fish adapted to the "challenges of living in a highly variable environment subject to seasonal extremes of flow and water temperature, short term flow changes from local storm events, and highly turbid conditions"[29] associated with high-volume sediment transport. The previously mentioned unique morphologic features were most likely adaptations to the high-flow,

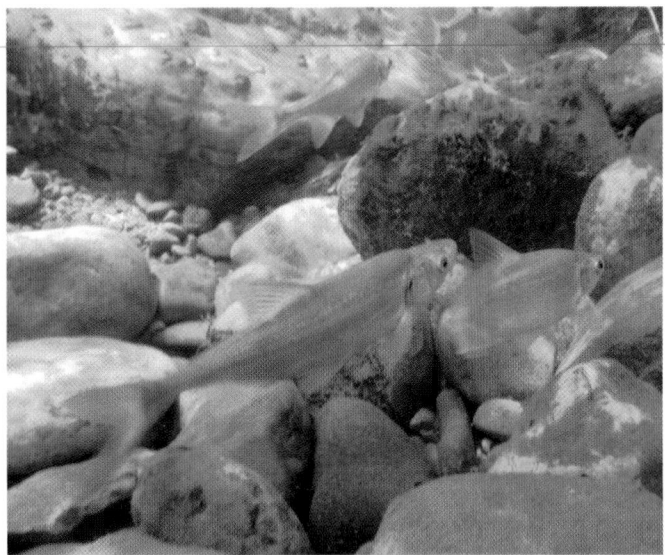

FIGURE 120-18 Humpback chub. *(Courtesy Melissa Trammell, National Park Service. Public domain.)*

sediment-laden waters of the Colorado River ecosystem. There are eight species of native fish in Glen and Grand Canyons, and six are endemic to the area: humpback chub (endemic); razorback sucker (endemic); Colorado squawfish (endemic); bonytail chub (endemic); roundtail chub (nonendemic); flannelmouth sucker (endemic); bluehead sucker (endemic); and speckled dace (nonendemic).[19] Four of the native fish are federally listed endangered species: humpback chub, razorback sucker, Colorado squawfish, and bonytail chub (Figure 120-18). Three of the native fish species are believed to be extirpated from the Glen and Grand Canyons: Colorado squawfish, bonytail chub, and roundtail chub.[29] Three native fish species retain relatively stable populations in the region: flannelmouth sucker, bluehead sucker, and speckled dace. The flannelmouth sucker is listed as a federal endangered species candidate and is protected in Arizona as a result of concerns regarding species decline.

Minckley[19] and Smith[28] have classified the native fish species of the Grand Canyon as dietary generalists. However, Minckley,[19] in reference to his earlier work, "characterized trophic relations in the native fish species based on qualitative and quantitative differences in selected foods and spatial segregation in feeding. Adult squawfish were piscivorous (fish eating). Flannelmouth suckers fed on insects and other benthic (bottom dwelling) animals. Bluehead suckers were adapted for scraping algae. Razorback suckers fed on detritus and plankton. Humpback chubs, speckled dace, and bonytail chub tend to be insectivores; although speckled dace have exhibited facultative omnivorous behavior." Classification of the native fish of this region as dietary generalists is tempered by empirical evidence of specialized structures and feeding behaviors that developed in response to specific demands of the river environment in this region.

"Before completion of the Glen Canyon Dam, the Colorado River was thought to be largely heterotrophic with little primary production in the sediment laden water."[4] Schmidt and colleagues[24] made note of the "allochthonous pre dam aquatic system," which refers to limited primary production of algae and existence of nutrient resources transported downstream by the river flow. This is confirmed by dietary habits of the native species, because the only fish (i.e., bluehead sucker) that used primary-producing algae as a food source was also able to sustain itself on other food sources. The predominant primary producer in the Glen Canyon and Grand Canyon aquatic ecosystem is the filamentous green algae *Cladophora*. The turbid sediment-laden waters of the Colorado River prevented sufficient penetration of sunlight to create an ideal environment for primary producers. Webb and colleagues[34] note that "the green alga *Cladophora glomerata* was present but not abundant in the river" before

completion of the Glen Canyon Dam. As a result of the limited algal resources, the native fish were dependent on carbon-based nutrients that were transported by river current. This process was contingent on scour of upstream flood-level algal remnants, diatoms, invertebrates, insects, fish, and plant debris from native riparian vegetation (e.g., willow, cottonwood).

A survey of Glen Canyon in 1958, before building the Glen Canyon Dam, revealed 17 species of fish, including 10 non-native types.[19] Intrusion of non-native fish is a significant factor in the demise of the native fishery. "Remarkable numbers of non-native fishes have been intentionally and inadvertently stocked into the Colorado River."[19] At least 20 species of non-native fish were planted in Utah before 1900.[27] Additional non-native fish were added for sport fishing, vegetation control, and as bait for the sport fishery. Minckley[19] states that "non-native fish have invaded essentially every habitat." Accidental introduction of gizzard shad during a 1998 largemouth bass stocking in Morgan Lake in New Mexico led to presence of this species in Lake Powell. This non-native shad species, also known as *stink shad,* may provide a food resource for the Lake Powell non-native striped bass fishery. However, there is significant concern that potential downstream spread of gizzard shad below the dam will compromise the food supply for the remaining native fish because of resource competition. Resultant competitive and predatory exclusion by non-native species, including channel catfish, trout, and voracious sunfish, has had a deleterious effect on native fish species. It is evident that even before development of the Glen Canyon Dam, there was significant pressure on native fish resources. The dam compounded the challenge to extant native fish.

A seasonal warm-water body with intermittent periods of inundation by floodwaters was immediately transformed into a constant cold-water river (i.e., 10°C [50°F])[21] with diurnal variations in flow and limited controlled flooding caused by opening the dam locks. The backwater and eddy habitats of native fish were compromised with respect to flood-induced habitat management, and the previously mentioned carbon-based debris-dependent ecosystem had been transformed. Clear discharge from the dam was established as a result of retention of sediment in the newly established Lake Powell. This provides for increased penetration of sunlight and significant increase in the primary-producing algal life-form *Cladophora*. Detritus and carbon-based debris flow were affected by the comparatively limited alteration in flow rate after the dam and the limited scour of higher-altitude vegetation that occurred from predam floods ranging from 2330 to 6230 m³/sec.[33]

The Glen Canyon Dam has created a compromise in the historic food supply, shelter, and thermal gradient conducive to spawning for the native fishery. Combined with predation and competition from non-native species, these adverse factors have led to the previously mentioned extirpation of three native species and "endangered" listing of two of the five remaining species. Valdez[31] summarized that as a result of the Glen Canyon Dam, several native fish species in this area are susceptible to "major threats from flow depletion, altered water chemistry, flooded habitat from reservoirs, introduced parasites and diseases, competition and predation from introduced non-native fish."

Introduced species have fared better in the postdam environment. Cold, clear outflow from the Glen Canyon Dam provides excellent conditions for growth of *Cladophora*, which is a food source for the freshwater scud *Gammarus lacustris*. Scud, annelids, and midge species are the primary dietary choices for rainbow trout in the area below Glen Canyon Dam. "The Lee's Ferry water below Glen Canyon Dam holds an estimated 50,000 trout over six inches long (17,000 over 12 inches) per mile in over 15 miles of water, according to the Arizona Game and Fish Department."[9] Daily change in water-flow release associated with electrical demand creates ideal feeding conditions for trout. When water levels drop significantly, millions of scuds become stranded on exposed gravel bars lining the banks. After 2 days of drying in the hot Arizona sun, the desiccated scuds are flushed into the current when the water rises again. As the dried shells float downstream, live fish go on a binge.[9] Although this carbon-based detritus would seem ideal for native fish accustomed to allochthonous food resources, cold-water temperature in the area between the dam and Lee's Ferry is not a conducive habitat or spawning ground for the native fishery. This leaves the abundant scour resource for the prime benefit of the cold-tolerant trout species.

The dam resulted in artificial creation of a prime non-native fish habitat in Lake Powell and the Grand Canyon. However, there is evidence that this is subject to a limited time period. "Lake Powell, an artificial reservoir on the Colorado Plateau, is beginning to suffer from high selenium levels in its sediments."[13] Two independent studies of largemouth bass from Lake Powell report that selenium concentrations in the fish greatly exceed national averages. This abnormally high selenium concentration in fish reflects the high concentration in the reservoir[8] and is a result of the dam blockage of normal downstream sediment transport. A growing body of literature continues to document extensive contamination of aquatic environments with selenium and the adverse effects in aquatic organisms.[15] Regardless of sediment toxicity, accumulation of a sediment load equal to 100 million tons per year is projected to potentially block the river outlet valves within 100 years.[12] The downstream trout fishery depends on a continued clear river-outlet discharge.

Creation of the dam has resulted in a variety of ecologic impacts regarding fishery resources. The native fish are the most vulnerable as a result of the effects of environmental pollutants, species competition, habitat modification, and gradual accumulation of sediment load in Lake Powell. There are continued efforts to ameliorate the effects of the dam on the native fishery while preserving the economically productive introduced sport fishery. The intractable nature of this environmental balancing act is firmly entrenched in the policy disputes associated with river management in this region. The inevitable fact is that choices and options will become progressively limited as the sediment load in Lake Powell eventually renders the dam ineffective for any economic or ecologic purpose consistent with present or historic use patterns. In addition, evaporative water losses in Lake Powell and potential diminished levels of stream flow associated with climate change could place the 20 million people who depend on this area for water and electricity at extreme risk.

The challenge to biodiversity in Lake Powell and the Colorado River basin is a challenge to human health. Biophysical alteration of a natural environment after construction of the Glen Canyon Dam has resulted in an unsustainable artificial ecosystem doomed to extinction under the pressures of sediment load and accumulation of arsenic, lead, selenium, boron, and mercury from upstream runoff sources. Resultant exposure to environmental contaminants and loss of water, electric, and economic resources will potentially create psychological and physiologic hardships for inhabitants of this region.

CONCLUSION

Lisa Newton[22] defines *sustainability* as activity that "can be maintained profitably and indefinitely without degrading the systems on which it depends." She suggests that no practice will be regarded as sustainable unless it can be continued without degrading the environment that nurtures it though the seventh generation from its initiation. It is evident that our historic land-use practices have led to ecosystem degradation, species decline, and loss of genetic diversity. The consequences of these actions are foreboding for human health and planetary well-being as we are exposed to emergent and resurgent infectious diseases and our food and water resources are placed at potential risk.

When referring to an ecologic conscience, Aldo Leopold[17] stated:

Obligations have no meaning without conscience, and the problem we face is the extension of the social conscience from people to land. Land ethic, then, reflects the existence of an ecological conscience, and this in turn reflects a conviction of individual responsibility for the health of the land. Health is the capacity of the land for self-renewal. Conservation is our effort to understand and preserve this capacity.

Those of us with an interest in wilderness medicine have a unique opportunity to serve as stewards of the environment and of our patients' well-being by increasing our understanding of the importance of biodiversity with respect to human health.

REFERENCES

Complete references used in this text are available online at expertconsult.inkling.com.

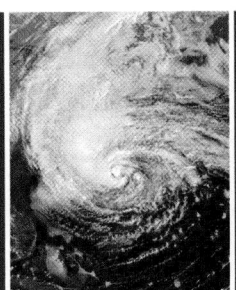

CHAPTER 121
Health Implications of Environmental Change

CAROLYN SIERRA MEYER AND JAY LEMERY

For 11,700 years, Earth's natural processes and related systems have remained relatively stable. For example, weather patterns, nutrient cycles, freshwater repositories, biodiverse forests, and prairie systems have nurtured growth of human societies. It is increasingly recognized that human actions modify these processes. Since the middle of the 19th century, human impact has accelerated, and it now threatens resilience of the planet. Humans burn fossil fuels, fertilize depleted soil, and irrigate deserts. The cumulative impact of environmental stressors directly afflicts humans by causing changing patterns of disease. Climate change and loss of biodiversity, among other impacts, threaten the quality and quantity of human life. Earth's planetary processes have global thresholds, or "tipping points"; crossing these boundaries may lead to changes that are not hospitable for human social structure or even survival. For example, there are limits to food production. Agricultural crops and livestock have physiologic limitations in certain thermal and water stress situations. Staple crops, such as maize, rice, wheat, and soybeans, grow only within the range of 40° C (104° F) to 45° C (113° F).[58] There are thresholds of global warming beyond which current agricultural practices will no longer be able to support large human civilizations. The global risk to food security will become alarmingly great if an increase occurs in global mean temperature of 4° C (7.2° F) to 6° C (10.8° F) or more.[56] Therefore, impacts of suboptimal nutrition and malnourishment may become severe as planetary temperature rises.

The wilderness medicine practitioner has a dual mandate to promote both patient wellness and a healthy environment. This chapter serves as a primer for understanding growing threats to human health caused by a changing environment. It addresses human-imposed impact on Earth's natural environmental processes and the effects on human health.

CLIMATE CHANGE

There is overwhelming scientific consensus that anthropogenic climate change is accelerating[23] (see Chapter 119). The Intergovernmental Panel on Climate Change (IPCC) is the leading international body for assessment of climate change. In 1988, the United Nations Environment Programme and the World Meteorological Organization established the IPCC to provide the world with a clear scientific view on the current state of knowledge regarding climate change and the potential environmental and socioeconomic impacts. Thousands of scientists worldwide contribute on a voluntary basis to these quadrennial reports. The thresholds for data to be included in the IPCC surpass that of contemporary peer-reviewed journals, and the science encompassed is considered to be of exceedingly high quality. The IPCC 2014 Synthesis Report states that anthropogenic "greenhouse" gases—atmospheric concentrations of carbon dioxide, methane, and nitrous oxide—have exponentially increased beyond historical cyclic variations measured over the past 800,000 years. Their effects are believed to be the dominant cause of the observed warming since the middle of the 20th century.[44] High levels of these greenhouse gases are linked to increases in intensity, frequency, and duration of heat waves,[48] melting of the Greenland and Antarctic ice sheets,[54] and increases in precipitation extremes, including heavy rainfall in some regions and drought in others.

VULNERABLE POPULATIONS

Climate variability and change do not affect all people equally. The vulnerable populations, whether measured in socioeconomic or demographic (e.g., extremes of age) terms, will bear a disproportionate burden of climate-related health effects.[27] Working Group II of the IPCC finds that regions of Africa with poor governance, tenuous public health and health care systems, and food and water insecurity will suffer the most from global climate change.[50] Factors that increase vulnerability include inadequate or no mosquito protection and limited to no access to health care facilities. Intense heat waves will increase mortality and morbidity in elderly people and persons with preexisting medical comorbidities. Increases in heavy rainfall and temperature will increase the risk of diarrheal diseases, dengue, and malaria, with the effects of these compounded by poor public health infrastructure. Increases in floods and droughts will exacerbate rural poverty in parts of Asia through negative impacts on certain crops, such as rice, resulting in increases in food prices with associated effects on nutrition.

Vulnerability is multifactorial, and data have clarified the etiology of climate exposure. Geographic location influences deterioration of health caused by climate change. Warming most affects persons who work outdoors in hot temperatures at the limits of thermal tolerance.[25] Populations in proximity to the present limits of the range of transmission of vector-borne diseases are most vulnerable to changes attributed to rising temperatures.[31] Communities situated on low-lying coral atolls experience the health impacts of soil salination, flooding, and freshwater reservoir contamination because of sea level rise.[41]

Age and gender are factors in the loss of health caused by climate change. Children and elderly persons are at increased risk for climate-related injuries and illnesses. Children are more physiologically susceptible to the destructive effects of malaria, diarrhea, and poor nutrition, all of which show increases from climate change.[35] Elderly people have a limited ability to respond to physiologic stressors, such as heat and air pollution, because they often have preexisting health conditions.[17] They also find it difficult to avoid the hazards and destruction of floods, heat

waves, and other extreme natural events because they tend to be less agile and less aware than are younger adults.

According to the World Health Organization (WHO), worldwide mortality from natural disasters, including droughts, floods, and storms, is higher among women than men.[60] Pregnant women in particular are at increased risk because they are more vulnerable to extreme heat, malaria, food-borne infections, and influenza.

Financially poor populations are at increased risk of loss of health caused by climate change. Mortality risk associated with tropical cyclones from 1970 to 2009 showed dependence on three major factors: storm intensity, quality of governance, and poverty level.[47] A study on the impacts of flooding in Bangladesh found that as average income and number of income sources increased, household risk was reduced. Poorer households took preventive action less often, were more severely affected by flooding, and received less assistance after the flooding than wealthier households.[7]

Indigenous peoples, populations of small island developing states, and resource-poor urban communities in developed countries, including the United States, are also particularly vulnerable to negative health impacts from climate change.[50]

DIRECT IMPACTS OF CLIMATE CHANGE ON HUMAN HEALTH

HEAT-RELATED HEALTH IMPACTS

Global warming is a relative misnomer. Although the past few years have been the warmest on record, some of the coldest and stormiest winter weather has occurred in the northeastern United States.[40] Climate denialists purport this to be evidence of conflicting data as to whether or not the earth is warming. A more accurate phrase would be *global energizing,* because as indeed we are consistently measuring the warmest years on record, the effects are not equally distributed in time or space. Local weather and temperature remain highly variable.

A *heat wave* is a prolonged period of excessively hot weather, beyond the normal seasonal temperature for a particular region. The association between hot days and increased morbidity and mortality is well established.[21] In Australia between 1968 and 2010, the ratio of summer-to-winter deaths increased in association with rising annual average temperatures.[6] Studies based on hospital admissions or emergency medical presentations during heat waves report increases in temperature-related morbidity, attributed to such conditions as cardiovascular, respiratory, and kidney diseases.[39] A Harvard School of Public Health study followed a U.S. cohort older than 65 with chronic disease from 1985 to 2006 and demonstrated reduced survival associated with greater variability of temperature. Dramatic short-term fluctuations in temperature variability have been shown to increase the risk of mortality.[65] Again highlighting vulnerability in socioeconomic groups, access to ventilation and the presence or absence of air conditioning contribute to the effects of high temperatures on humans. The 2003 Northern European heat wave contributed to more than 12,000 deaths in Paris alone, the vast majority being elderly persons of the lower socioeconomic neighborhoods without climate controls or preexisting knowledge of such unprecedented extreme weather.

The "urban heat island" effect is another well-documented result of heat waves in urban settings. Poorer neighborhoods without open parks or shaded areas have a significantly higher temperature change compared to average temperature than more affluent neighborhoods.[18] Health risks during heat extremes are greater in people who are physically active. Climate change especially impacts the health of manual laborers and persons who pursue outdoor recreation.[24]

FLOODS AND STORMS

Climate energizing through warming impacts frequency and severity of many weather events, including precipitation, drought, and cyclones. One such mechanism occurs when warmer ambient

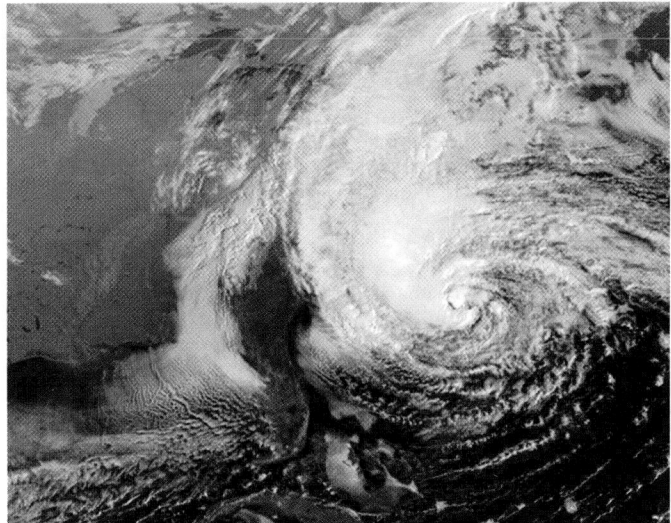

FIGURE 121-1 NOAA's GOES-13 satellite captured this visible image of the massive Hurricane Sandy on October 28, 2012, at 1302 UTC (9:02 AM EDT). *(Courtesy National Oceanic and Atmospheric Administration [NOAA].)*

temperatures increase evaporation, leading to higher absolute humidity. When more water is carried as vapor in the atmosphere, rain is less frequent, but rainstorms become more intense because the amount of water is greater in the storm clouds (Figure 121-1). Most climate models predict longer periods of drought interspersed with more intense rain events.

Floods are the most common extreme weather event. They affect and kill more people than any other form of natural disaster. The Center for Research on the Epidemiology of Disasters collects yearly data and reports that in 2011, six of the 10 largest natural disasters were flood events; 112 million people were affected and 3140 deaths were directly attributed to flooding.[19] Conservative estimates for health impact caused by storms and flooding suggest that 2.8 billion people were affected between 1980 and 2009, with more than 500,000 deaths. Worldwide, the frequency of river flooding has increased and caused greater economic losses because more population and property are present in flood plains. Flooding and storms cause death and disease through drowning, traumatic injury, hypothermia, and increased transmission of infectious disease. Flooding often causes groundwater contamination with feces, dead livestock, and chemicals leached from industrial facilities. Diarrheal disease, leptospirosis, insect vector–borne diseases, and cholera all increase in prevalence during and directly after flood events.[53]

Flooding has long-term implications on mental health. In one example involving a 2007 flood in Wales, United Kingdom, the prevalence of mental health symptoms, such as psychological distress, anxiety, and depression, was two to five times higher among individuals who reported flooding in their homes than among nonflooded individuals.[45]

HEALTH EFFECTS MEDIATED THROUGH NATURAL SYSTEMS

Global warming indirectly impacts human health through environmental and ecosystem changes. These changes include shifts caused by warmer conditions in territories and ranges of disease-carrying mosquitoes and ticks, more waterborne diseases, and increased precipitation and runoff.

VECTOR-BORNE DISEASES

Anthropogenic climate change impacts the burden of vector-borne diseases. A major determinant of the endemic range of vector-borne diseases is seasonal temperature. As the climate

warms, fewer pathogens languish in the cold, so the distribution of certain diseases expands. Mosquitoes and ticks primarily transmit vector-borne infectious diseases, such as malaria and dengue. Warmer temperatures increase metabolic rates of mosquitoes and ticks, affecting their nutritional requirements and increasing the drive to feed more frequently. Transmission potential of pathogens increases accordingly. Global warming directly affects survivability of pathogens and indirectly affects the vectors and reservoirs that harbor pathogens.[5]

Malaria (see Chapter 40)

Malaria is mainly caused by one of five parasites: *Plasmodium falciparum*, *P. vivax*, *P. malariae*, *P. ovale*, and *P. knowlesi*. Anopheline mosquitoes transmit the parasites. In 2013, there were an estimated 283 million cases of and 584,000 deaths from malaria worldwide, mostly among children younger than 5 years.[62] Increases in average planetary temperature and associated increases in precipitation likely favor malaria transmission. Warmer conditions will prolong malaria seasons and allow mosquito migration to higher latitudes, infecting populations not traditionally at risk. In 2014, researchers were shocked to discover malaria in Alaskan birds for the first time, as well as a recrudescence in southern Italy for the first time in 50 years.[30,52]

With increased average daily temperatures, areas previously below the lower limit of the range of viability for survival of the pathogens show increased transmission. However, the increase is not linear.[43] Even modest warming may drive increases in malaria transmission if conditions are otherwise suitable.[1]

Other Viral Diseases (see Chapter 39)

The incidence of dengue viral disease ("fever") has grown dramatically in recent decades. WHO currently estimates that there may be 50 to 100 million dengue infections worldwide every year. An estimated 500,000 people with severe dengue require hospitalization each year, many of whom are children. Approximately 2.5% of affected persons expire.[63] *Aedes aegypti* and *Aedes albopictus* mosquitoes transmit the virus to humans through bites during feeding periods. These mosquitoes are climate sensitive. Over the last few decades, climate conditions in certain areas have become more suitable for *A. albopictus* mosquitoes. A new serotype of dengue affecting a previously nonimmunized population was identified in Portugal in 2012.[2] This was in part attributed to climate change, according to the IPPC Fourth Assessment Report (AR4), because of an increase in the percentage of days per year with favorable temperature for disease transmission.[22] In 2013, new dengue cases occurred in Florida and the Yunnan province of China, two regions where it had not previously been observed; one report showed that the distribution of *A. albopictus* is highly correlated with annual temperature and precipitation.[64] Another study demonstrated that dengue incidence increased in Guangzhou, China, in association with temperature, humidity, and rainfall, and that wind velocity is inversely associated with rate of disease.[32]

Both typhoons and droughts affect vector populations and increase the incidence of infections. Typhoons bring extreme rainfall, high humidity, and water pooling, generating new mosquito breeding sites. Drought causes increases in rates of disease if households store water in containers that provide suitable mosquito breeding sites.

Other Vector-Borne Diseases

Hard ticks of the family Ixodidae transmit tick-borne encephalitis virus to humans. Europe and Asia have temperate regions where the disease is endemic, and climate change has resulted in expansion of Ixodidae tick territory and prolonged the season during which the ticks transmit disease.[5] During the 1970s, tick-borne encephalitis became more prevalent in central and eastern Europe. As reported in a study describing the Czech Republic, warm spring temperatures between 1970 and 2008 encouraged transmission of the tick-borne encephalitis virus. The transmission season lengthened, and disease spread to higher altitudes.[26]

Europe, Canada, and the United States are home to ticks infected with *Borrelia burgdorferi*, which causes Lyme disease. Many studies have shown associations between tick-borne diseases and climate. In North America, based on active and passive surveillance data, there is good evidence of northward expansion of the distribution of the *Ixodes scapularis* tick vector by 2060.[42]

This list correlating increased disease risk to expected climate change is extensive and a formidable challenge to public health. For instance, hantavirus causes rates of infection correlated to increases in temperature, precipitation, and relative humidity.[28] Plague has been linked to seasonal and internal variability in climate.[33] Other vector-borne diseases linked to climate variability include chikungunya fever, transmitted by the same mosquitoes (*A. aegypti* and *A. albopictus*) that transmit dengue virus; Japanese encephalitis, transmitted by *Culex tritaeniorhynchus* mosquitoes; and Rift Valley fever, transmitted by both *Aedes* and *Culex* mosquitoes.

WATERBORNE DISEASE

Anthropogenic climate change increases exposure to climate-sensitive waterborne pathogens. Warmer climate and increased severity and frequency of storms will result in a more sustainable habitat for pathogens and greater opportunity for mixing contaminated water sources with drinking water and agriculture. Most of these pathogens are introduced to the water by human and animal feces, which is directly related to poor sanitation and exacerbated by extreme precipitation and flooding, because latrines for human and animal waste often become comingled.

Most acute exposures to waterborne pathogens result in symptoms of gastroenteritis. These illnesses are generally self-limited, with the majority of symptoms lasting less than 1 week. However, some, such as cholera, can be devastating. Chronic exposure to waterborne pathogens carries long-term health consequences. Children are particularly at risk, because each episode of illness may jeopardize healthy growth by reducing caloric uptake and nutrient absorption. This problem is most profound with severe diarrheal diseases such as typhoid and dysentery, which progress from diarrhea to systemic syndromes with high rates of death.

CLIMATE CHANGE AS A THREAT MULTIPLIER

Every wilderness medicine practitioner should understand not only the direct causality of climate change on human health, but also the indirect effects. Undernutrition, mental illness, occupational health effects, food insecurity, and increases in violence and conflict may not be primarily caused by climate change, but all will be made worse by its consequences.[9]

MENTAL HEALTH

The American Psychological Association recently released a report on the broad psychological effects of climate change.[14] Psychological stress derives from both abrupt changes experienced during natural disasters and more gradual changes in the local environment. Natural disasters cause severe psychological trauma through personal injury, loss of family and friends, and loss of personal property or livelihood.[37] People who have recently experienced an acute trauma have high levels of distress and anxiety and may report panic attacks, difficulty sleeping, low motivation, and obsessive behavior.[12] This may lead to more long-term psychopathology, such as posttraumatic stress disorder (PTSD) or major depressive disorder. PTSD has been extensively documented in survivors of the urban flood from Hurricane Katrina and is linked to higher levels of substance abuse, depression, anxiety, and suicide. Disaster events produce strains on social relationships and may lead to forced migration, which is a devastating stressor because families and friends are separated and lose their systems of social support and access to primary health care.

More gradual effects of climate change, such as prolonged droughts and increases in mean temperature, also negatively affect mental health. Increases in average temperature are associ-ated with increased use of emergency mental health services, and warmer weather conditions increase the stress on people who already suffer from mental illness, exacerbating their disease and overwhelming their coping ability.[59] Even for people without mental illness, climate change is an additional source of stress and can affect some people deeply, causing feelings of loss, helplessness, and frustration because of inability to prevent the foreseen changes and their disastrous effects.[36]

NUTRITION

The effects of climate change on human nutrition are complex. Agricultural production, food prices, access to food, and human disease all impact nutrition and are expected to be affected by climate change. Extreme weather events, such as floods, droughts, and heat waves, exacerbate food insecurity. The IPCC concludes that climate change will have a substantial negative impact on per-capita calorie availability. Climate change will negatively impact childhood nutrition, particularly stunting of growth, and increase child deaths in developing countries.[22] Crop yield gains from warmer weather in the fields of Russia and Canada will not make up for loss of productivity in the global south, and the net result will be reduced quantity and quality of food harvested.[4] In most tropical regions, climate effects on crop yields are significant. For each degree above 30° C (86° F), African maize yields decrease by 1% under normal rain conditions and by 1.7% under drought conditions.[29] A study in Africa and South Asia revealed an 8% average yield reduction in crops of wheat, maize, sorghum, and millet as temperature increased and rainfall patterns changed.[58a]

VIOLENCE AND CONFLICT

Populations that are affected by violence and with weak civil institutions and poor governance are particularly vulnerable to the health impacts of climate change. The insecurity and full-scale natural disasters brought on by extreme weather events cause societal deterioration through exacerbation of existing or creation of new poverty situations. This adds to social strife and may escalate regional conflicts in parts of the world with little domestic capacity for resilience or adaptive response to a climate stressor.[16]

BIODIVERSITY LOSS

Destruction of species and mismanagement of natural ecosystems worldwide destabilizes the physical environment, increases vulnerability to the spread of human infectious disease, and promotes proliferation of pathogens that can affect the food supply and natural resources on which human health and well-being depend. Consider the vulnerability of agricultural monocultures. Pathogens spread more easily, and epidemics tend to be more severe, when the host plants (or animals) are more genetically homogeneous and crowded. Outbreaks of disease, insect infestations, and climatic anomalies pose a greater threat to monospecies ecosystems than to diverse ones, causing widespread crop and animal failures, undermining food security, and accelerating spread of diseases to human populations.

Biodiversity can be viewed in two ways, both of which are shrinking. *Genetic diversity* is diversity of genes within a species and functions as an information bank that determines the potential for life to evolve and adapt as the environment changes. Genetic diversity is difficult to measure on a global level, so as of now, global data do not exist for phylogenetic species variability. Species naturally go extinct at a rate of one to five species per year. Anthropogenic changes to ecosystems have increased the baseline extinction rate. The planet now loses species at a dramatically increased rate of 1000 to 10,000 species per year.[11]

Functional diversity concerns the behavior and effects of organisms in communities and ecosystems. Functional traits make up functional diversity. Functional traits are measurable aspects of an organism that reflect what it does and how it interacts with other organisms and its environment (e.g., size, diet, behavior). Functional groups are a set of species showing either similar responses to the environment or similar effects on major ecosystem processes. Functional diversity refers to the abundance of functional groups. For example, compare a section of tide pool that contains three different species of barnacle, and another section that has a starfish, sea grass, and an anemone. Each has three different species. However, the second section of tide pool has more functional diversity because each species interacts with the other organisms and the environment differently, and it also has different effect(s) on the ecosystem. Functional diversity allows for a resilient ecosystem, in this example, one that can withstand pathogens, invasive species, and extreme weather events and can provide continuous ecosystem services (e.g., clean water) for other sea life to thrive.

Some of the greatest pharmaceutical discoveries have come from nature. These include antiinflammatory, chemotherapeutic, antibiotic, and thrombolytic drugs. Our ecosystems are the raw materials for future discoveries in pharmaceuticals and biotechnology. The continued loss of biodiversity, to quote John Dingell, is "akin to burning the library without ever having read its books."[8a]

THREATS TO ECOSYSTEM SERVICES

Deforestation

Deforestation not only changes the climate, but also has direct effects on human health. As forest habitats are cleared for agriculture and urban development, human-wildlife interaction and conflict grow. Deforestation decreases the habitat available for wildlife species and can fragment these habitats into smaller patches separated by agricultural activities and human populations, thereby further promoting unhealthy interactions among pathogens, vectors, and hosts. This has been linked to expansion of "bush meat" consumption, which may have played a key role in emergence of both Ebola and human immunodeficiency virus (HIV) types 1 and 2 in Africa[46] (Figure 121-2).

This land system change likewise coincides with an upsurge in several infectious diseases, including Lyme disease, leishmaniasis, and malaria. With Lyme disease, aggressive land-use changes in the forests of North America have decreased the numbers of small-mammal predators because of habitat fragmentation. The probability that a deer tick will become infected with the *Borrelia* bacteria depends on the density of white-footed mice. As the density of white-footed mice increases because of fewer small-mammal predators, the infection rate of humans with Lyme disease increases accordingly.[8]

Deforestation also causes increases in noninfectious health risks to humans. Mercury is naturally found in rain forest soils

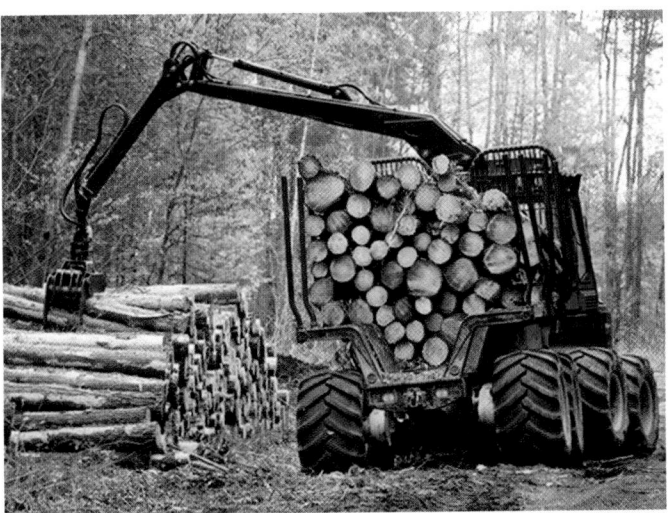

FIGURE 121-2 Deforestation may have played a role in the devastating Ebola virus outbreak. While cutting away swaths of African forest, loggers may have also been inadvertently creating convenient and unexpected pathways for the virus to spread. (*Courtesy* Inhabitat.com.)

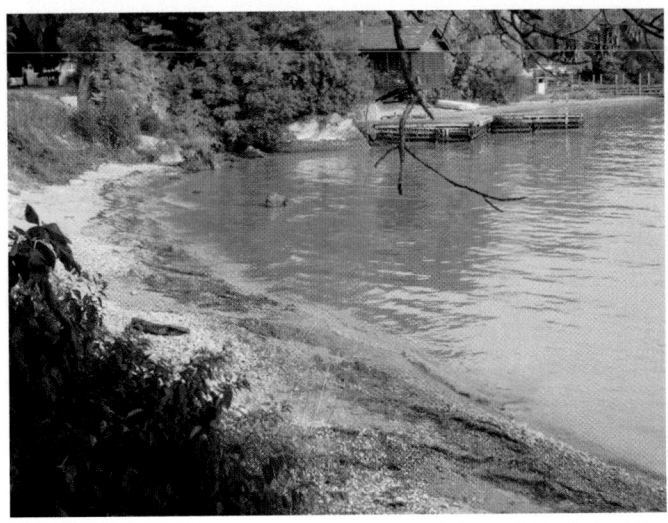

FIGURE 121-3 Harmful algal bloom, Kelley's Island, Ohio, Lake Erie, September 2009. (*Courtesy National Oceanic and Atmospheric Administration, Great Lakes Environmental Research Laboratory.*)

and is used to extract gold from riverbeds. Soil erosion after deforestation and gold mining adds significant mercury loads to rivers. The mercury collects in fish, making them hazardous to eat. Mercury suppresses the human immune system and is toxic to humans in very small amounts.

Lastly, land system change is implicated in mental health disruptions, such as a loss of personal identity and stress. Land-use changes causes a sense of loss called *solastalgia*, which is the experience of negatively perceived change to a home environment. As traditional landscapes where people live are irrevocably changed, people experience stress and negative emotions. Solastalgia is characterized by a sense of desolation and loss that is similar to the nostalgia experienced by people who are forced to migrate from their home environment. However, solastalgia relates to slow changes in the local environment.[14]

Nutrient Cycles

Nutrient cycles are natural processes in which chemical elements, such as nitrogen, phosphorus, and potassium, are continuously cycled among air, water, soil, and organisms. The ratios between elements in the environment are sensitive, so that perturbations impact biodiversity and can have downstream effects on human health. Fertilizer and fossil fuels have the greatest anthropogenic impact on phosphorus and nitrogen cycles, because these are the mainstay ingredients of chemical fertilizers used to replenish nutrients in agricultural lands. Fertilizer proliferation in nearly all parts of the world has resulted in cropland seep-off into watersheds that supply freshwater systems and ultimately the oceans. Freshwater nutrient inputs to the coastal oceans now exceed preindustrial fluxes by 10- to 15-fold in many parts of North America, Europe, and Asia.[3] The cumulative effect of concentrated pollution from different sources is known as "non–point source pollution" and is used to describe effects of watershed areas collecting agricultural pollutants in wetlands or other bodies of water.

Overconsumption of nitrogen compounds can directly affect human health. Nitrates in drinking water play a causative role in methemoglobinemia, or "blue baby syndrome," and are linked to reproductive problems and several cancers. Such nutrient loading into fresh and marine waters can also cause *eutrophication,* a complex process whereby excessive development of certain types of algae disturb aquatic ecosystems, which then become a threat to animal and human health (Figure 121-3). These *harmful algal blooms* (HABs) are the common link between algal blooms, red tides, green tides, fish kills, inedible shellfish, and blue algae. At their height, HABs can release dangerous hepatotoxins, neurotoxins, and dermatotoxins because of cyanobacteria overproliferation. People can be exposed to these

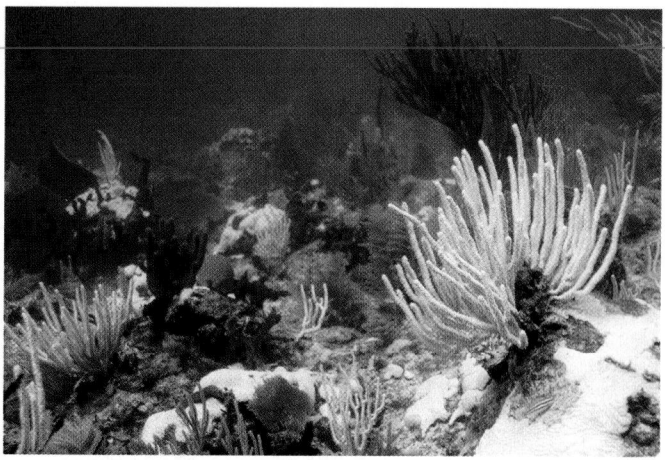

FIGURE 121-4 Most coral reefs exhibit very low annual accretion, with net carbonate production almost balanced against carbonate export, bioerosion, and dissolution. By reducing the growth rate, ocean acidification shifts the balance in favor of net carbonate loss. *(Courtesy National Oceanic and Atmospheric Administration, Coral Health and Monitoring Program.)*

toxins through consumption of contaminated drinking water or seafood, direct contact with contaminated water, and inhalation of aerosols.[61]

When algae die, they decompose, and the nutrients contained in that organic matter are converted into inorganic forms by microorganisms. This decomposition process consumes oxygen, which reduces the concentration of dissolved oxygen for healthy organisms in the ecosystem, and can instigate an anoxia-caused reduction in biodiversity.

Ocean Acidification

The IPCC Fifth Assessment Report (AR5) describes proliferation of planetary greenhouse gases over the past 150 years. By far the majority of this carbon dioxide (CO_2) is retained in the oceans. CO_2 retention in ocean waters influences carbonate chemistry, resulting in acidification (Figure 121-4). Marine organisms are particularly sensitive because aragonite, a form of calcium carbonate created by many marine organisms, dissolves in an acidic environment. This is thought to play a major role in the demise of coral reef biodiversity seen throughout the world in recent decades.[57] This affects many commercial sectors, including tourism and seafood aquaculture.[51] Ocean acidification has also been linked to less resilient coastal ecosystems in the face of extreme weather, nutrient pollution, and overfishing.[51]

FRESHWATER USE

Reduction in water availability for human uses can lead to decreases in health. About 36% of the global population lives in water-scarce regions, resulting in decreased population hygiene and concomitant increase in disease, because households, medical clinics, restaurants, and public places of convenience and hygiene are forced to use minimal water for cleaning. In the United States, the Environmental Protection Agency (EPA) has cited that areas in 36 states face water shortages. When water is scarce, people are forced to rely on drinking water sources that might not be safe. For example, in California in 2012-2013, the water quality in drought-stricken areas was found to have violated federal standards more than 1000 times. An estimated 38 million persons were exposed to contaminants such as arsenic, nitrates, radioactive minerals, and perchlorates (chemicals used in rocket fuel and explosives).[10]

About 70% of the available global freshwater supply is used to irrigate crops, much of which is used to feed livestock. As living standards improve in the developing world, meat consumption has increased, further putting pressure on available freshwater resources.[34]

New challenges to water quality have recently arisen. In the United States, emergence of chlorine-resistant pathogens, chemical contamination of water sources, aging water purification and transportation infrastructure, increased recreational water contamination, nontraditional water exposures (e.g., cooling towers at nuclear power plants), and increasing water reuse threaten public health.[13] Most municipal sanitation systems are designed to handle tons of human waste and toxic chemicals daily, yet worldwide have rarely kept pace with tremendous urban expansion. Many urban sewage networks operate at the margins of capacity and are subject to stress by even the most innocuous rainstorms. This is compounded by the fact that most urban areas do not absorb rainwater consistently, and absorb even less as arable land is put to other uses. A summer rain shower in a city can provide enough stress to allow dangerous runoff of untreated excrement and toxic material, often contaminating local water sources and public areas.

ATMOSPHERIC AEROSOL LOADING

Atmospheric aerosols, also known as particulate matter, are solid or liquid particles suspended in air, with diameters of approximately 0.002 to 100 µm. Primary atmospheric aerosols are particulates emitted directly into the atmosphere from volcanoes, sea spray, forest fires, dust storms, and vegetation in the form of pollen. Secondary atmospheric aerosols are particulates formed in the atmosphere by gas-to-particle conversion, including fossil fuel combustion, power plants, and industrial release of sulfates, nitrates, and some organic products. Atmospheric particulate matter impacts the climate and adversely affects human health, associated with approximately 7.2 million deaths per year from exacerbations of asthma, bronchitis, chronic obstructive pulmonary disease, and acute coronary syndromes.

Aerosol particles vary greatly in size, source, chemical composition, amount and distribution in space and time, and durability in the atmosphere. The smaller and lighter a particle, the longer it will remain in the air. Coarse particles are larger and heavier and are generated by industrial processes that involve crushing or grinding (e.g., construction, farming, mining). Fine particles originate from combustion sources and are formed by gaseous precursors. The size of the particle determines the risk to health. Particles that are 2 to 3 µm in size tend to deposit deeply in the terminal bronchioles and alveoli, whereas larger particles tend to deposit in upper (larger) bronchi, causing different symptoms and disease patterns. The upper bronchi are the part of the respiratory tract that has less interface with the blood supply, so symptoms mostly reflect lung inflammation and are manifested by cough, shortness of breath, and airway spasm or asthma-like symptoms. Smaller particles are especially toxic because they can reach the terminal bronchioles and even as deep as the alveoli, where they can enter the blood supply and travel to the rest of the body. The International Agency for Research on Cancer and WHO designate airborne particulates a group 1 carcinogen. Because of their unfiltered, deep penetration into the lungs and bloodstream, these particulates cause permanent DNA mutations, heart attacks, and premature deaths. In 2013, the European Study of Cohorts for Air Pollution Effects (ESCAPE) trial, a prospective cohort study involving 312,944 people in nine European countries, showed that no safe level exists for particulates, and that for every increase of 10 µg/m³ in particulate matter, the lung cancer rate increases by 22%.[49] Symptoms caused by acute exposure to atmospheric aerosols include shortness of breath, cough, and worsened asthma.

Dangerous atmospheric aerosols include pollen released from vegetation. Allergic diseases are common. In the United States alone, approximately 50 million Americans suffer from allergic conditions in response to airborne particulate allergens, including itchy eyes, rashes, rhinorrhea, cough, shortness of breath, bronchitis, and asthma.[38] Climate change and associated increases in land temperatures and CO_2 concentrations are drivers of plant metabolism and pollen production, as well as increased fungal growth and spore release. Increases in air temperature cause earlier flowering of prairie tall grass.[55] Increasing concentrations of grass pollen lead to more frequent ambulance calls because of asthma exacerbations.[20]

CHEMICAL POLLUTION

Chemical pollution refers to new substances, new forms of existing substances, and modified life-forms that have potential for unwanted effects. Anthropogenic introduction of novel entities causes concern when these entities exhibit persistence, have mobility across widespread distributions, and impact vital Earth system processes or subsystems.[57] Of special concern are new types of engineered materials, as well as naturally occurring elements, such as heavy metals that are mobilized by human activities. Release of chlorofluorocarbons into the atmosphere is an example of a synthetic chemical previously thought to be harmless that had unexpected impacts on the ozone layer. More than 100,000 substances exist in global commerce, and if one includes nanomaterials and plastic polymers that degrade to microplastics, the list is longer. Plastic microbeads, used as an exfoliant in certain bath products and cleansers, have been identified recently as a significant pollutant of the Great Lakes. According to a study released by the 5 Gyres Institute, parts of the shore around the lakes have 466,000 particles per square kilometer, with an average of 43,000 particles per square kilometer. Most of these plastic particles are meant to wash down the drain and are less than 1 mm in size.

Water stress worldwide forces people to turn to contaminated sources, increasing their exposure to toxic substances. Water contaminated with lead leached from pipes causes lead toxicity. Lead toxicity results in nervous system damage and developmental delays in children, as well as kidney damage and anemia. Waterborne arsenic exposure usually occurs through natural sources, although environmental contaminants occur from industrial processes associated with mining, metal refining, and timber treatment. Symptoms of arsenic exposure develop over 5 to 20 years and include skin discoloration and thickening (hyperkeratosis); cancers of the skin, bladder, kidneys, and lungs; and diseases of the blood vessels of the legs and feet. The EPA monitors the water supply for a number of synthetic and volatile organic contaminants (e.g., benzene, toluene) and inorganic contaminants (e.g., arsenic, copper) that pose potential threats to human health.

Extensive use of pesticides worldwide poses a great threat to human health. California is one of the few states collecting pesticide data. Between 1991 and 2000, almost 2 billion pounds of pesticides were used in that state alone. An estimated 1.2 billion pounds are used across the United States each year. Persons most at risk for injury are those who have regular, close exposure to pesticides. This includes agricultural workers and, to a lesser extent, populations who live close to farmland. Exposure to pesticides occurs through direct handling, agricultural runoff, and residue on food products. Organophosphates are the most frequently used pesticide and can affect the neurologic system. Toxicity manifests as loss of muscle control, salivation, defecation, bradycardia, and increased bronchial secretions.

Herbicides pose threats to human health. 2,4-D is one of the most widely used herbicides worldwide and is most often used on home lawns, rangeland, and pasture. Human cells that are exposed to 2,4-D undergo genetic damage. This herbicide has been linked to decreased sperm counts in exposed men.[15]

As the amount of chemicals in our environment increases to quantities that are impossible to monitor or study, it may be prudent to consider precautionary and preventive actions to mitigate the unknown risks of pollution. Strategies include further shifting the burden of proof of safety from the consumer to the producer, as well as developing "green chemistry" strategies focused on risk reduction.

REFERENCES

Complete references used in this text are available online at expertconsult.inkling.com.

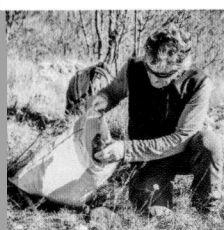

CHAPTER 122
Sustainability: Leave No Trace

NANCY V. RODWAY

"Sustainability has to be nonideological in order to be, well, sustainable.[4]" According to Tee L. Guidotti, sustainability is a culture, not an ideology, and will only succeed in that light. "The essence of sustainability is optimization of maximization of economic, social, and environmental benefits and operations performance across generations.[4]" The word implies preservation and respect for the future of Earth's resources and the health of its inhabitants. These concepts must become societal values rather than manipulable political agendas. Success in sustainability might be best achieved by technology rather than changes in human behavior, similar to engineering occupational exposure risk out of the workplace, rather than expecting worker compliance with personal protective equipment. Economic, social, and environmental sustainability must be driven by public opinion and supported by innovative technology. Public policy perhaps then will follow.

SUSTAINABILITY IN THE WILDERNESS

Decades ago, the Boy Scouts of America and Leave No Trace organization understood sustainability in the wilderness. The wilderness is not paved, and it is often delicate and easily damaged, sometimes permanently, by the human footprint. Fortunately, sustainability has long been applied to the wilderness. The Leave No Trace Center for Outdoor Ethics, located in Boulder, Colorado, is an educational, nonprofit organization dedicated to responsible enjoyment and active stewardship of the outdoors by all people worldwide. The principles of Leave No Trace (LNT) reflect a sense of stewardship and passion for the world and guide our passage, especially in untamed places.

SEVEN PRINCIPLES OF STEWARDSHIP

Seven guidelines are the official principles of Leave No Trace, Inc., and are copyrighted by the center. This copyrighted information has been reprinted with permission from the Leave No Trace Center for Outdoor Ethics (www.LNT.org):

1. Plan Ahead and Prepare
2. Travel and Camp on Durable Surfaces
3. Dispose of Waste Properly
4. Leave What You Find
5. Minimize Campfire Impacts

6. Respect Wildlife
7. Be Considerate of Other Visitors

Plan Ahead and Prepare

Before departing for an expedition, trip, or even a hike, research the environs and become familiar with the regulations for use. Acquire permits if needed. Plan party size accordingly, and limit size or split the group if necessary to minimize impact. Hike and camp separately if necessary. Avoid high-use times on popular trails, or do not travel at all if poor conditions, such as when a trail is muddy, would cause significant adverse impact. Use proper gear, such as a camp stove, and plan meals ahead to minimize waste. Repackage food before departure in reusable containers or plastic bags that can be easily packed out. Register at the trailhead or with the ranger, and be responsible and aware of personal and party limitations to minimize the chance of rescue. Use a map and compass to eliminate the need for rock cairns or markings on the trail that can mar the landscape for other travelers.

Travel and Camp on Durable Surfaces

Wherever traveling and camping, move on surfaces that are resistant to impact. These include rocky outcroppings, sand, gravel, dry grasses, snow, and water. Stay on well-traveled trails and hike in the center of the trail in single file. Do not shortcut. When boating, launch the craft from a durable area and camp at least 60 m (200 feet, 70 adult steps) from the waterfront. Good campsites, whether in the mountains, beach, desert, or plains, are found, not made. When campsites are not apparent and the area is pristine, try to disperse the impact rather than camp in a tight group.

Dispose of Waste Properly

For human waste, use outhouses where available. If necessary to use a cat-hole, dig it 6 to 8 inches (15 to 20 cm) deep, and choose a site far from water sources. Pack out toilet paper. Don't burn it. Disguise the hole as much as possible. Pack out feminine hygiene products, because they decompose slowly. Treat pet waste as human waste. Urine is generally environmentally tolerated, but nevertheless, urinate far from camps and trails. Aim to urinate on rocks or bare ground to discourage animals from eating tasty and salty urine-soaked foliage. On the water, a portable toilet has become standard practice and may be required by law. With regard to waste from cooking, attempt to plan meals to minimize leftovers that are tempting for wildlife and therefore potentially dangerous. Clean pots with hot water and a scant amount of soap, and scatter the dishwater, after it has been strained to remove food particles, at least 60 m (200 feet) from any water source.

Leave What You Find

Artifacts are often protected by law; leave them where they are found. Do not collect rocks or other portables. Take caution to avoid transporting plant species from one location to another on pack animals, on boots, or in tire treads.

Minimize Campfire Impacts

Avoid campfires unless they are essential for comfort or food preparation. If a campfire is unavoidable, use a fire ring and gather sticks and branches that have fallen on the ground. Do not cut down plants for fuel. Campfires on the beach are a little different; dig a shallow depression in the sand or gravel along the shoreline and, once the fire is cool, scatter the ashes and refill the depression.

Respect Wildlife

Observe wildlife from a safe distance, and do not approach them if you are not an expert. Do not feed wildlife. Avoid wildlife outright during mating season, nesting season, and when they are rearing young. When traveling with pets, keep them under control.

Be Considerate of Other Visitors

Be considerate of other visitors, natives, and native lands. Yield to other users on the trail and, when encountering pack animals, step to the downhill side of the trail. Avoid loud talk, music, and other cacophony.

SUSTAINABILITY IN SPECIAL ENVIRONS

The Mountains

Climbers, when traveling horizontally, can apply many of the aforementioned principles. Approach the route on an established trail, using a trail guide to minimize impact. Once vertical, certain caveats become more task and environ specific. Use only removable protection and as little chalk as possible. Avoid "scrubbing" or "gardening" the route, removing vegetation only when necessary for safety reasons. Do not climb near archeologically sensitive sites or animal habitats such as bird nests.

Toileting can be tricky. Urinating is generally not a problem, but defecating can be gravitationally and environmentally troublesome. In the past, it was allowable to drop waste in a paper bag over the edge of the rock. That is no longer acceptable for obvious reasons. In a pinch, feces can be smeared on the rocks (away from the route), but the preferred method is to pack waste out in a "poop tube," which is a piece of PVC pipe with a screw top that can be attached to the outside of a pack or haul sack, then emptied at the end of a climb or trip. Purchase a 30- to 60-cm (1- to 2-foot, depending on duration of your trip) length of PVC pipe approximately 10 cm (4 inches) in diameter and threaded on one end. Tightly glue a cap on the unthreaded end using PVC cement, and fit a threaded cap on the other end. Fashion a loop out of duct tape or other lashing to attach the screw cap to the piping to prevent it from becoming lost. The loop will also accommodate a carabiner to allow attachment to the outside of a pack. Defecate into small brown paper bags, add cat litter, place the bag into the tube, and then deposit the collection into a vault toilet or dumping station at the end of the trip. Do not flush the paper bags.[9]

Snow

Traveling and camping in the winter are difficult for humans and stressful for wildlife stressed by scarce food supplies. Avoid skiing or camping near game trails or in areas with obvious animal activity, to limit pressure on hungry animals. Campfires are not recommended, given the dearth of accessible firewood and temptation to harvest green wood fuel. When camping, make every effort to "fluff up" the trampled snow for the benefits of subsequent visitors, and do not leave visible "yellow snow" near well-traveled areas. Digging a cat-hole in the snow when winter camping is tempting, but simply leaves the frozen trophy to thaw on the exposed ground in the spring. Pack out all waste.[9]

Water

Waterways are often overused and are shared by recreational and nonrecreational users on motorized and nonmotorized crafts. In addition, water sports enthusiasts have varying levels of respect for scenic rivers, oceans, lakes, and delicate riparian environments. Some users litter beaches with trash. To limit impact in coastal environments, travelers should recreate within the intertidal zone because it is the most durable. Whenever possible, conduct all beach activities in this zone. Camp in an established campsite above the high-tide line of the intertidal zone, and tread on durable surfaces such as trails or rock. If fires are permitted and driftwood is available, build a campfire, if necessary, below high tide. Urinate below the high-tide line away from fellow campers and tidal pools. Use a cat-hole above the high-tide line or pack feces out if the environment is especially fragile. Launch and land watercraft on sand or gravel, avoiding dirt and vegetation. When on the water, do not approach marine wildlife; give all marine animals at least a 90-m (100-yard) berth. Do not dump waste into waterways.[9]

On rivers and freshwater, much of the aforementioned applies. Camp, where possible, in the river's floodplain. Bury human waste in a cat-hole at least 60 m (200 feet) from shore, or pack it out. For large groups such as rafting parties, consider a toilet tank or other latrine.[9]

Tundra

Tundra, the treeless vast soil of polar regions, is visited and traveled most often in the summer, the season when it is most vulnerable. During summer, the surface of tundra thaws to the depth of the permafrost, making it mushy. The thaw is the time when plants and burrowing animal life are most active in this layer. Trampling on summer tundra can be very destructive. When the thin layer of ground cover plants is destroyed, crystals in the underlying permafrost can melt because of increased sun exposure. This is called *thermokarsting* and can leave permanent scars, such as footprints and tire treads. Hiking and camping on durable surfaces are critical. If trails are not available, travel on shallow streambeds or snow, or, as a last resort, walk on tundra grasses rather than on lichen beds. Do not hike single file. For waste disposal, do not dig a cat-hole. Rather, smear feces on a rock or pack them out. Campfires are inappropriate.[9]

Alpine tundra, as opposed to the arctic type, occurs above tree line and has a short growing season (similar to arctic tundra) but has no permafrost. It is delicate but cannot undergo thermokarsting because of the absence of permafrost. This alpine landscape is home to a handful of hearty species of vegetation and adapted mammals. When traveling through alpine tundra, stay on the trail, because damage caused by shortcutting in this fragile environment can remain for several hundred years. Camping is generally discouraged because of the risk of lightning strike at this altitude, as well as soil sensitivity. If camping becomes necessary, try to use an established site or camp on a durable surface, such as rock, snow, or mineral soil. Avoid campfires. Tether trash and camping items to avoid their being blown away by high winds. With regard to human waste, many popular alpine destinations now require that visitors pack it out. However, a patient hiker can descend below tree line to dig a cat-hole if desperate.[9]

The Desert

Many desert soils are covered with a dark cryptobiotic crust, or *biocrust,* composed of cyanobacteria, algae, mosses, and lichen held together by organic materials. These crusts often cover a majority of the desert floor and help to stabilize the soil, fix nitrogen, and retain moisture. If disturbed, biocrusts may not regenerate for a century or more. In the desert, therefore, travelers must remain on designated trails to minimize damage to the biocrust or walk on durable surfaces, such as slickrock, gravel, or sand washes. Camp on durable surfaces or established campsites. Avoid campfires in this dry, treeless environment. Water is limited, so pack plenty. Wandering off the trail in search of water is detrimental for the soil and for thirsty desert creatures. Do not use precious water sources for bathing, because soaps and body oils contaminate the environment. In the desert, cat-holes are the preferred method for waste disposal, but keep them 60 m (200 feet) from any water source, because feces decompose slowly in arid climates.

SUSTAINABILITY AND THE HUMAN FOOTPRINT

According to the World Wildlife Fund, in the 21st century, humankind's footprint exceeds the earth's regenerative capacity by 30%.[5] Wildlife populations have declined by one-third over the last 35 years, and humans are consuming resources at a rate that far exceeds natural regenerative capacity. Biodiversity has declined as species have been overexploited. In 2005, the single largest human footprint was carbon in the form of carbon dioxide (CO_2) from combustion of fossil fuels; ambient CO_2 has grown more than 10-fold since 1961. At the present rate, humankind will need two planets to maintain the present level of consumption by the year 2030.[5] Two generations ago, humankind was an ecologic creditor. At present, two-thirds of our species live in countries that consume more natural resources than exist within their national borders. Therefore, these countries must depend on nations, often Third World countries, with fewer environmental restrictions for resources.

The earth provides food, water, material goods, and fuel. These resources have present economic value. Less salient and less marketable services include nutrient recycling, soil formation, pollination, pest control, and water purification, as well as the aesthetic, spiritual, and recreational provisions of the earth. Some natural resources with market value (e.g., fossil fuels) have been regulated, whereas others (e.g., the atmosphere) have been undervalued or regarded as a common good and therefore have had little to no market oversight, leading to exploitation and overuse. *Sustainability* is the science of managing humankind's footprint on Earth to achieve a balance between what humans use and what the earth can replenish.

ENERGY

The world is powered by fossil fuels that release CO_2 when burned. CO_2 is naturally present in the atmosphere as a trace component; it is released as a product of respiration by plants and animals and in small amounts from volcanoes and geysers. It is one of the greenhouse gases, which serve to keep the earth warm by absorbing and emitting infrared radiation. Without greenhouse gases, the earth would be much colder. The three main greenhouse gases—CO_2, methane (CO_4), and nitrous oxide (N_2O)—affect the atmosphere as functions of their chemistry and rate of decay. Methane, released by fossil fuel combustion, waste dumps, rice paddies, and livestock, accounts for 14.3% of greenhouse gas emissions but is greater than 20 times more effective at trapping heat than is CO_2. Nitrous oxide from fertilizers and industrial processes accounts for only 7.9% of emissions but is about 300 times more effective at trapping heat, ton per ton, than is CO_2.[16] In 1750, before industrialization, atmospheric CO_2 concentration was approximately 280 parts per million (ppm). By 2005, it had reached 379 ppm; the rate of increase from 1995 to 2005 was the highest in recorded history. More CO_2 in the atmosphere generally means more greenhouse gases and a warmer planet. CO_2 is the greatest contributor to global warming, accounting for 43% to 56% of all greenhouse gases, depending on the reference. The single largest contributor to atmospheric CO_2 is consumption of fossil fuels (e.g., coal, oil, natural gas) for energy in transportation, industry, and forestry.[16]

Oil is the most carbon-dense fossil fuel. Natural gas (methane) is the "cleanest" of the carbon-based fuels, because it has more hydrogen atoms per carbon molecule. For each unit of energy, methane produces 52.6 kg (117 lb) of emitted CO_2, compared with 73.8 kg (164 lb) released by burning oil. To achieve a similar amount of heat, one would need almost three times more weight of wood, which would release 88 kg (195 lb) of CO_2. Coal burns the dirtiest, producing 103 kg (227 lb) of CO_2 to achieve the same unit of energy.[3] Although some of these fuels are used primarily and directly for energy, such as in natural-gas stoves, fossil fuels are also burned in power plants to create electricity. Various sources of fuels are combusted or otherwise converted into heat to generate steam, which spins turbines that produce electricity. Electricity then enters the "grid," a large network of power lines, power stations, and transmission subsystems, to be distributed to homes and businesses (Box 122-1).

Worldwide, a majority of the electricity produced comes from coal. Coal combustion is the largest contributor to CO_2 worldwide, but its production and use damage more than just the atmosphere. Coal is extracted by underground, open-surface pit, and "mountaintop" mining. In mountaintop mining, mountaintop debris is deposited in the adjacent valley, destroying vegetation, soil, habitats, and the landscape aesthetics. Acid, along with heavy metals such as mercury, selenium, and arsenic, from this debris seeps into waterways and groundwater. Coal combustion is the largest source of human-made mercury pollution. Acid rain is produced by burning high-sulfur coal.[3]

Power stations can use any type of fuel (uranium, solar energy, biomass, oil, or methane) to power turbines to generate electricity, or the turbines can be turned directly by water and wind power. Although oil and natural gas burn cleaner than does coal, renewable sources of fuel can turn turbines and create electricity, so once the infrastructure is in place, the fuel is essentially free. According to the International Energy Agency, an intergovernmental energy policy advisor founded in the oil crisis of 1974 and located in France, renewable energy sources currently have the technologic potential to supply almost 20 times the current global energy demand, but presently account for no more than 17% of global energy consumption.[7] Biomass and hydropower provide less than 15% of global energy need, whereas wind and solar power fuel provide approximately 2%.

BOX 122-1   The Grid

Turbines that generate electricity from coal, natural gas, biomass, nuclear, wind, and solar power plants must distribute that power from the generating facility to end users. Many power plants are not located close to population centers, so they must transmit electricity via overhead (and occasionally underground) high-voltage transmission lines to substations closer to cities for voltage step-down and further distribution. Energy storage at the substations is inefficient, so electricity is best distributed in real time. A sophisticated system of controls is therefore necessary to ensure that electric generation matches demand. If supply and demand are mismatched, electricity generation and distribution can become overloaded, causing a blackout. To prevent this, generating and distributing stations are all interconnected in a "grid" or "power grid" to allow for redundancy in the system, creating a series of transmission triangles rather than a branching hub. These individual triangles are then connected regionally and nationally. The grid allows for generally uninterrupted electricity delivery through periods of high and low demand and high and low power generation, as can occur with intermittent renewable fuel sources. Finally, the miles of transmission lines of the grid act to pool and store electricity from various sources, both renewable and nonrenewable.

The network nature of the grid is ripe for computer management to improve efficiency. A "smart grid" delivers electricity from suppliers to consumers controlled by two-way digital technology. Such a system could alert the consumer, via smart meter devices such as a glowing orb, to high-use periods, giving direct feedback to limit electricity use during expensive peak demand periods. Alternatively, the system could automatically turn off selected high-demand appliances during peak periods, which can be cost and carbon saving, turning them back on as demand lessens. A smart grid can charge an electric vehicle at night, a time of low electricity demand. Renewable energy sources will need a smarter grid. As the world converts to renewable energy, which is mostly intermittent power, a smart system will be necessary to limit demand during peak periods. Some of this can be accomplished by pricing energy as a function of demand and allowing market forces to work.

A "home grid" extends some of these capabilities into the home to allow the individual homeowner to cut electricity cost and the individual's global footprint. Alternatively, individual homes can generate their own electricity "off the grid" or sell surplus to the grid. Many municipalities, regions, and countries already have established a smart or "smarter" grid.

RENEWABLE ENERGY

Renewable energies are essential contributors to the global energy menu and have the potential to reduce reliance on fossil fuel and to mitigate greenhouse gases, thereby lessening humans' ecologic footprint. Regions of the world differ in the types of renewable energy used, but overall, hydropower is the global renewable energy source of choice for electricity, and biomass for energy production.

BIOMASS

Biomass is an advanced form of photosynthetic solar power and a promising renewable replacement for fossil fuels in power plants. The energy generation is a relatively simple chemical process. Biomass is mashed and fermented with yeast to make ethanol. Ethanol is then burned for fuel. Initially, food crops such as corn were regarded as ideal biomass fuel options. However, the fossil fuel demands of industrial agriculture negated the benefits of decreased emissions. Corn was replaced by nonfood sources of biomass when the economic and social impacts of using food for fuel became obvious. Many sources of renewable (and sustainable) biocellulose work as sources of biomass. These include grasses (especially *Miscanthus* [elephant grass]), waste paper, corn silage, and bagasse waste from sugar cane production. One acre of sugar cane produces 2500 L (650 gal) of fuel; 1 acre of corn produces 1500 L (400 gal); and 1 acre of *Miscanthus* grass produces 4750 L (1250 gal). Soybeans can be used to make 174 L (46 gal) of biodiesel. Oil palms can be converted into 2300 L (610 gal) of biodiesel per acre.[3]

WIND POWER

Wind power, like biomass, is a form of solar energy, because atmospheric temperature differentials from the sun create wind. It is so abundant that it could fuel the entire planet five times over, and it is the fastest-growing renewable energy source. Wind power has the advantage of being rapidly installed, aesthetic, and scalable to the needs of the locale. An average windmill can generate enough electricity to power 400 average American homes; a smaller windmill 11 to 43 m (35 to 140 feet) tall can pay for itself after 6 years. The United States, Germany, and Spain generate the most electricity from wind power; however, India and China may soon surpass these countries because of their current investments in wind farms. England boasts the largest offshore wind farm in the North Sea, where winds are strong and reliable.[3]

A typical windmill stands 50 to 100 m (160 to 325 feet) tall and has blades that range from 27 to 45 m (90 to 150 feet) in length, making construction and transportation a challenge, especially for offshore wind farms. Wind farms are regarded as hazardous for birds. In reality, cats kill 3000 birds for every one struck by a windmill, and tall buildings flatten 19,000 birds for every windmill kill.[3] Despite this relative safety, engineers are perfecting sensors to halt windmill operation when birds are nearby. The largest drawback to wind power is its intermittency; power isn't generated if the wind doesn't blow.

SOLAR POWER

The sun radiates enough energy, were it to be captured properly to the earth in 1 hour, to power the entire planet for a year. Solar energy is the most common form used by persons trying to "live off the grid." Capturing solar power can be challenging because it is limited by clouds and darkness of night and is intermittent. Technically speaking, there are two mechanisms to harness solar energy. Solar rays on a large scale can be focused by curved mirrors to heat liquids that turn turbines in power plants. Alternatively, and usually on a smaller scale, photovoltaic cells convert sunlight directly into energy using semiconductor devices. Photovoltaic cells consist of a thin layer of silicon atoms that release free electrons when exposed to solar energy. They work in the presence of intermittent sunlight and can be deployed in small clusters or in large arrays. Free electrons flow out of the photovoltaic cell as electric current, which is converted to alternating current by an inverter for use in residential homes and other applications.

Solar power can also be harnessed in a passive manner by intelligent design of residential and commercial buildings. Orientation of the building can take advantage of winter sun and minimize summer glare. The roof can be colored to reflect or absorb intense heat and can serve as a solar water heater. Building materials, such as stone, can be chosen to absorb heat, whereas proper ventilation can circulate both cool and warm air to limit the use of fossil fuels.

GEOTHERMAL ENERGY

Geothermal energy has enough potential stored energy to satisfy the world's needs many times over, according to the United Nations World Energy Assessment Report.[15] Geothermal energy creates virtually no CO_2 emissions and is not intermittent, an advantage over other renewable sources. Geothermal activity is greatest where the tectonic plates meet, such as the Ring of Fire surrounding the Pacific Ocean. In addition, there are other naturally occurring hot spots where magma has found its way to the surface and created springs and geysers. Both these natural formations can serve as direct sources of hydrothermal energy, where natural steam is used to turn turbines. There is, however, the potential for geothermal energy in unsuspected locations. In many areas, rock below the ground surface is hot but dry. If rock temperature exceeds 149° C (300° F) and this bedrock is close enough to the surface to be cost-efficient, water can be injected into the ground in an Enhanced Geothermal System, and the resultant steam used to generate electricity. For personal consumption, a homeowner can install a geothermal heat pump to reduce the cost of heating and cooling a building. A hole is drilled 12 to 60 m (40 to 200 feet) below the surface, where the earth's temperature is a stable 16° C (60° F). A loop of copper pipes is installed, through which refrigerant pumped from the house circulates in the loop, exchanging heat from the home with the earth. In the summer, warm air in the home is absorbed by the refrigerant, then circulates underground to bring cool air back to the surface. The process is reversed in winter.

NUCLEAR ENERGY

Nuclear power, which generates heat through a controlled fission chain reaction using uranium, is an option to reduce carbon emissions. Uranium is the heaviest naturally occurring compound, containing 92 protons. When split, energy is released and the free neutrons collide with nearby uranium atoms, splitting them as well. "Control rods" of cadmium or other elements absorb some of the neutrons, limiting and controlling the reaction. The generated heat boils water into steam that turns an electric turbine. One pound of uranium contains as much energy as 3 million lb of coal.[3]

The United States is the current leader in nuclear power, with 100 active nuclear reactors, followed by France with 58 and Japan with 48. Nuclear engineers are aging and academic programs closing. The cost of building and maintaining a nuclear power plant has skyrocketed, and new reactors worldwide remain unfinished. According to the United National World Energy Assessment, 17% of global electricity production comes from nuclear power, behind coal (38.3%) and gas (18.1%).[15]

Nuclear energy has fallen out of public favor because of concerns about the consequences of long-term storage of radioactive waste, the public's hesitation to have this waste stored in its "backyard," and safety concerns after the accidents at Three Mile Island in 1979 (United States), Chernobyl in 1986 (USSR/Russia), and Fukushima Daiichi in 2011 (Japan). According to the U.S. Nuclear Regulatory Commission (NRC) and the International Atomic Energy Association (IAEA), the accident at Chernobyl released more than 100 times the radiation released by the two atomic bombs dropped by the United States on Japan in 1945 in World War II.[3]

Radiation is a natural phenomenon. Humans emit radiation from potassium-40 in the body and are exposed to naturally occurring radiation from elements and rocks (e.g., granite). Most living things are able to genetically withstand a certain amount of radiation. Radioactive waste, however, contains a number of radioisotopes that emit ionizing radiation that can be harmful to humans and the environment. Nuclear fuel, nuclear weapons, and health care industries produce nuclear waste. Waste generated by hospitals, such as contaminated towels, filters, and rags, is generally low-level waste that can be incinerated and buried in landfills, which poses insignificant long-term risk. Iodine-131, used in diagnosis and treatment of thyroid conditions, has a half-life of 8 days and is essentially gone from the body and environment in approximately 3 months. Plutonium-239, used for nuclear power and weapons, has a half-life of more than 24,000 years. Such high-level waste originates from spent reactor fuel and waste materials from reprocessing spent fuel rods. High-level waste is thermally hot and highly radioactive and remains so for many years. This waste is generally stored above ground or underwater for 3 to 5 years to allow it to cool before definitive disposal. The waste is contained, then relocated and disposed in a permanent, dry geologic site, far from human contact, with the surrounding rock providing a natural radiation barrier. Once filled, the disposal site is closed and sealed. Geologic disposal, regarded as the safest solution to radioactive waste, obviates the need for long-term storage facility maintenance and lessens the risk of terrorist acquisition. Despite the impressive safety record in the nuclear waste storage and disposal industry, public concern and opposition continue. Public opinion supports

long-term storage, which is a security risk, rather than permanent disposal.

The International Atomic Energy Agency (IAEA), headquartered in Vienna, Austria, was created in 1957 as an independent, intergovernmental, and science-based organization in the United Nations family. The IAEA publishes safety standards for transport and storage of radioactive waste and also maintains a databank, the Energy and Environment Data Reference Bank, which is a compilation of country-specific energy and environment-related indicators, such as CO_2 emissions per capita and overall energy statistics (http://www.iaea.org/inisnkm/nkm/aws/eedrb/). In 2005, the IAEA was the recipient of the Nobel Peace Prize for its efforts at ensuring that nuclear energy is used for peaceful purposes.

SUSTAINABLE LIVING

Renewable energy choices and decreased dependence on fossil fuels are the core of environmental sustainability; however, simple lifestyle changes can also lessen the individual human footprint. In the 2009 book, *Our Choice*, Al Gore reveals the CO_2 excesses of the Western diet.[3] Industrial agriculture uses 10 calories of energy from fossil fuel to produce 1 calorie of food, which does not include fuel burned to transport grain, meat, vegetables, and fruit. In the livestock industry, 3.18 kg (7 lb) of plant protein and 23,000 L (6000 gal) of water are required to produce 0.45 kg (1 lb) of beef. In addition, large livestock operations, such as those in Canada and California, release significant amounts of methane, a potent greenhouse gas, into the atmosphere. Natural gas, required for production of nitrogen fertilizer for industrial agriculture, releases 4.6 tons of CO_2 for every ton of fertilizer manufactured.[3] Nitrogen excess degrades the carbon content of soil as hungry soil bacteria consume fertilizer and release CO_2. Residual fertilizer enters the waterways, triggering robust algal blooms that starve water of oxygen, kill fish, and leave a dead zone. Cane sugar, another Western staple, is water intensive, requiring 1500 L (400 gal) of freshwater to produce 1 kg (2.2 lb) of sugar. Food choices can be more "sustainable" and carbon neutral if humans consume less meat, more fruits and vegetables, and purchase foodstuffs from local sources to minimize fuel used in transportation. Gardening is a green alternative, especially if natural fertilizers (manure or garden spoilage) are used.

Clothing choices can be sustainable. Cotton production, similar to beef and sugar, has a large water footprint, requiring 2900 L (800 gal) of water to produce one cotton shirt.[5]

SUSTAINABLE HOSPITALS

According to the U.S. Department of Energy, hospitals are among the most energy-intensive facilities, producing 2.5 times the CO_2 emissions of commercial office buildings and releasing more than 13.5 kg (30 lb) of CO_2 emissions per square foot.[17] Besides consuming large amounts of energy, hospitals use toxic elements and chemicals for diagnosis, treatment, and decontamination, potentially threatening health of the environment, patients, visitors, and health care workers. The 21st century has seen an emphasis on sustainable and healthy health care with such initiatives as the Global Health Security Initiative (GHSI; http://www.ghsi.ca/), Health Care Without Harm (www.noharm.org), Practice Greenhealth (www.practicegreenhealth.org), and The Center for Health Design (www.healthdesign.org). The focus of these initiatives is to improve architectural design to improve energy efficiency and to eliminate waste, improve management of medical waste, eliminate mercury in hospitals, and provide sustainable and organic options in hospital cafeterias. In addition, green hospitals are using environment-friendly cleaning products and more eco-friendly building practices, which can improve working conditions for employees and improve air quality for patients and visitors.

Medical waste is an environmental challenge. The vast majority of medical waste is incinerated, releasing CO_2, mercury, and dioxins, among other byproducts. Because paper waste makes up about one-half of hospital waste, many hospitals are replacing paper surgical gowns with reusable ones and medical charts with electronic medical records. Sharps containers can be reused, saving money and oil. There are biodegradable bedpans made of recycled phone books and beeswax.

SUSTAINABLE TRAVEL

Traveling in a carbon-neutral or carbon-friendly fashion seems straightforward. One should walk or bicycle when possible and use public transportation, such as a train or bus, where available, favoring trains for short trips and buses for long distances. Air travel is the most carbon intense, with short flights emitting more carbon per traveler per mile than do longer ones; nonstop flights are easier on travelers and the environment. The eco-conscious traveler can purchase a carbon offset to neutralize environmental impact. Using an online carbon calculator, a traveler pays a fee, based on calculated carbon emissions, to a service organization that typically plants trees, captures methane, or builds a windmill to offset the CO_2 emitted. The growing popularity of this practice has created Internet scams, so the carbon-offset industry is striving for transparency and legitimacy. Trusted carbon-offset sellers include Terrapass, which has a simple carbon footprint calculator and carbon gift certificates; Native Energy; and the Climate Trust, which is focused on eco-friendly businesses. The Gold Standard (www.cdmgoldstandard.org), a nonprofit organization under Swiss law that operates a certification program for carbon credits, is supported by multiple nongovernmental organizations (NGOs), World Wildlife Fund International, Greenpeace International, and others. It is regarded as the international certifying body for premium-quality carbon credits.

Critics of the concept of purchasing carbon offsets believe that the presence of an "easy carbon out" only encourages carbon use when we should be preventing its release. In addition, how can the purchaser ensure that the tree was planted and survived, and/or that the project funded by the carbon offsets was not previously scheduled? The Gold Standard and critics discourage reliance on tree planting for many reasons, including difficulty with verification.

HYDRAULIC FRACTURING

Hydraulic fracturing, or fracking, is an issue that cannot be ignored in any discussion of sustainability. Fracking is a method for extraction of oil or natural gas from tight formations of shale or other rock located thousands of feet underground (Figure 122-1). It has made the United States one of the world's leading producers of natural gas and has contributed to declining natural-gas prices.[14] Natural gas is regarded as a cleaner "bridge fuel" between the carbon-heavy fossil fuels of coal and oil and the carbon-neutral renewable energy sources such as wind power. When burned, natural gas emits less CO_2 per unit of energy than when oil or coal is burned. However, if the gas is leaked directly into the atmosphere, methane (natural gas) is 86 times more potent than CO_2 over a period of 20 years. The global-warming impact of methane falls to 34 over a period of 100 years because methane has a life span of only 12.4 years in the atmosphere, much shorter than that of CO_2.[18]

Natural gas, or methane, can be found in pockets and loose rock formations such as sandstone, where it is easily accessed by conventional drilling methods. Unfortunately, conventional oil and gas reservoirs in the United States have long ago been pumped dry. Newer technologies with horizontal drilling methods can extract natural gas from tight rock formations, such as shale, where methane is less accessible. Rock formations amenable to fracking exist throughout the world. However, one of the largest shale gas formations is the Marcellus shale region that underlies Ohio, Pennsylvania, New York, Maryland, Virginia, and West Virginia in the United States. Fracking, the newer unconventional horizontal drilling method, accesses reservoirs previously inaccessible or too expensive to drill. In this process, a vertical well is drilled into the rock formation many hundreds to thousands of feet underground, generally far below the water table. Once

the vertical drill reaches the shale or other rock, it is then directed horizontally for thousands of feet, along the horizontal length of the targeted rock formation. The vertical portion of the well is cased with a steel lining to prevent groundwater contamination. The horizontal portion of the wellbore is lined with perforated piping. The well is then "fracked." A mixture of large amounts of water, chemicals, and sand is injected under high pressure into the well, creating fractures in the shale that are propped open by the injected sand. Fracked wells typically produce oil and gas for 3 years.[14] Along with marketable fuels, fracked wells produce wastewater that contains some of the injected chemicals, dissolved clays, salts, heavy metals, and radioactive substances. Once a fracked well becomes economically unproductive, it is "capped" to prevent leakage of methane into the atmosphere.[14]

WATER POLLUTION

Unconventional drilling requires millions of gallons of water to frack a well and creates millions of gallons of wastewater for disposal, a serious concern when fracking occurs in water-starved areas.[14] Even if water is abundant, such as in the Marcellus shale region, wastewater produced from fracking can contaminate groundwater and surface water. The chemical toxicity of wastewater is often unknown because drilling companies protect the identity of chemicals used in fracking as a "trade secret" despite that dangerous and carcinogenic chemicals such as toluene, benzene, and xylene have been identified.[2] In Ohio, the state passed a bill that, in the event of an emergent medical exposure, physicians can acquire proprietary information regarding chemicals used in fracking; however, the physician must keep the identity of the chemical confidential.[13] The radioactivity of fracking wastewater limits disposal options; the safest method is injection into deep injection wells. Transportation of water to the disposal site is risky because truck traffic can be hazardous.[11] Wastewater from fracking can also be reused on site but more often is placed in lined temporary holding pits created locally until permanent disposal is available. Occasionally, wastewater is transported to specialized water treatment facilities because regional septic wastewater treatment plants cannot accommodate radioactive wastewater.[14] In one instance, tributaries of the Ohio River were contaminated with barium, strontium, and bromides when wastewater was treated at a municipal treatment plant.[6] In West Virginia, wastewater is legally sprayed on local roads or grounds. All these disposal methods are vulnerable to leakage and have the potential for subversion. Cases of groundwater contamination have been documented in Ohio and Pennsylvania.[14] Surface water contamination, through accident or subversion, has the potential to poison fish, wildlife, and local livestock; these contaminated animals can potentially enter the food chain.[14] Methane from fracked wells can contaminate local drinking water, although the gas itself poses a significantly greater risk to the atmosphere. Methane-contaminated water is not hazardous to drink but poses a risk of combustion. A study of private wells near fracking sites showed that 75% of wells within 1 km (0.6 mile) of hydraulic fracturing sites in the Marcellus shale in Pennsylvania were contaminated with methane isotopically identical to the fracked gas.[6]

The true extent of contamination of surface and groundwater by fracking wastewater is unknown. The Energy Policy Act of 2005 created a loophole that exempted the oil and gas extraction industry from the National Environmental Policy Act, and thus fracking companies are not legally obligated to consider environmental impacts of oil and gas extraction. This loophole also exempts the fracking industry from most provisions of the Safe Drinking Water Act of 1974. As a result, much of the fracking industry goes unregulated. The work of regulating hydraulic fracturing has fallen to the states and localities, with disparate results. Water quality data before drilling are often unavailable, because fracking companies are not required to perform these tests, making the causation of water contamination difficult. When proof of water contamination is attributable to fracking, legal proceedings and settlements often include confidentiality

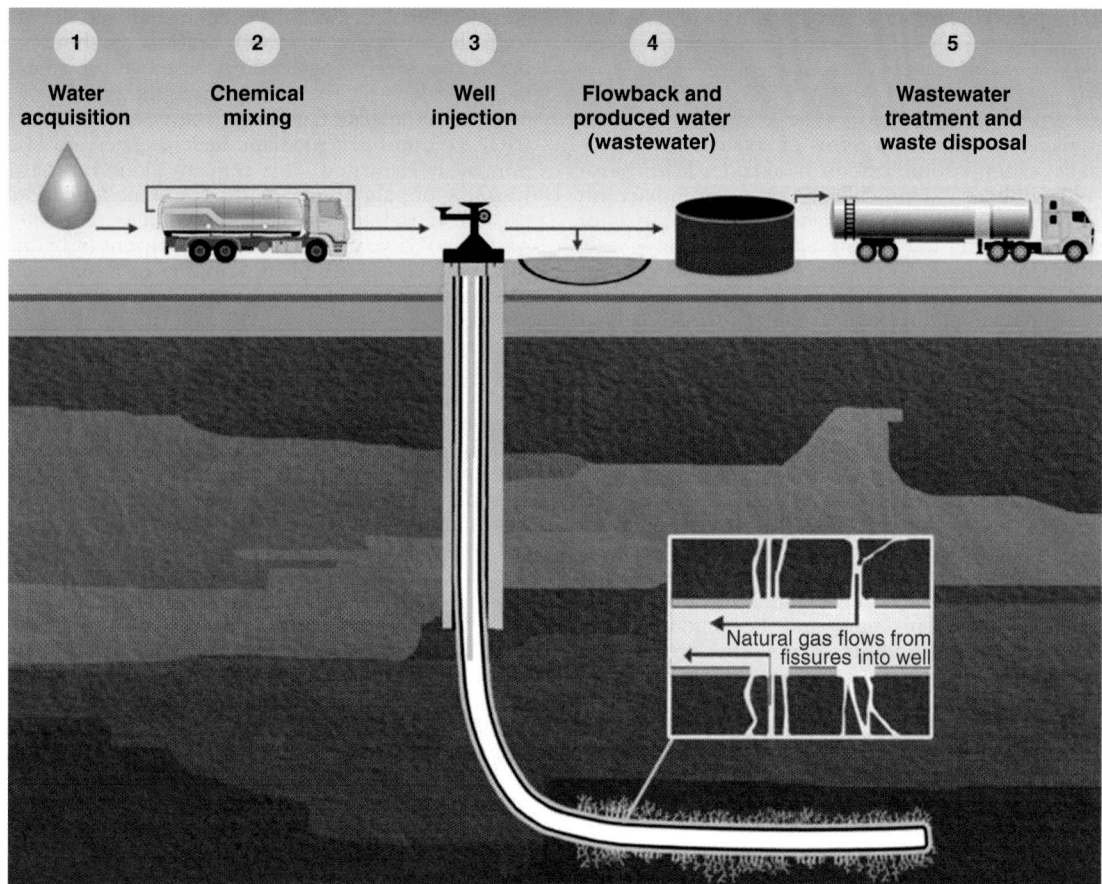

FIGURE 122-1 Stage 1: Water Acquisition[1]

Large volumes of water are withdrawn from groundwater[2] and surface water[3] resources to be used in the hydraulic fracturing process.

Potential Impacts on Drinking Water Resources

Change in the quantity of water available for drinking

Change in drinking water quality

Stage 2: Chemical Mixing

Once delivered to the well site, the acquired water is combined with chemical additives[4] and proppant[5] to make the hydraulic fracturing fluid.

Potential Impacts on Drinking Water Resources

Release to surface and groundwater through on-site spills and leaks

Stage 3: Well Injection

Pressurized hydraulic fracturing fluid is injected into the well, creating cracks in the geologic formation that allow oil or gas to escape through the well to be collected at the surface.

Potential Impacts on Drinking Water Resources

Release of hydraulic fracturing fluids to groundwater caused by inadequate well construction or operation

Movement of hydraulic fracturing fluids from the target formation to drinking water aquifers through local human-made or natural features (e.g., abandoned wells, existing faults)

Movement into drinking water aquifers of natural substances found underground, such as metals or radioactive materials, which are mobilized during hydraulic fracturing activities

Stage 4: Flowback[6] and Produced Water[7] (Hydraulic Fracturing Wastewaters)

When pressure in the well is released, hydraulic fracturing fluid, formation water, and natural gas begin to flow back up the well. This combination of fluids, containing hydraulic fracturing chemical additives and naturally occurring substances, must be stored on-site, typically in tanks or pits, before treatment, recycling, or disposal.

Potential Impacts on Drinking Water Resources

Release to surface water or groundwater through spills or leakage from on-site storage

Stage 5: Wastewater Treatment and Waste Disposal

Wastewater is dealt with in one of several ways, including, but not limited to, disposal by underground injection, treatment followed by disposal to surface water bodies, or recycling (with or without treatment) for use in future hydraulic fracturing operations.

Potential Impacts on Drinking Water Resources

Contaminants reaching drinking water caused by surface water discharge and inadequate treatment of wastewater

Byproducts formed at drinking water treatment facilities by reaction of hydraulic fracturing contaminants with disinfectants

[1]Recently, some companies have begun recycling wastewater from previous hydraulic fracturing activities, rather than acquiring water from ground or surface resources.

[2]Groundwater is the supply of freshwater found beneath the earth's surface, usually in aquifers, which supply wells and springs. It provides a major source of drinking water.

[3]Surface water resources include any water naturally open to the atmosphere, such as rivers, lakes, reservoirs, ponds, streams, impoundments, seas, and estuaries. It provides a major source of drinking water.

[4]Chemical additives are used for a variety of purposes (see examples in Table 4, p. 29, of the hydraulic fracturing Study Plan). A list of publicly known chemical additives found in hydraulic fracturing fluids is provided in Appendix E, Table E1, of the hydraulic fracturing Study Plan.

[5]Proppant is a granular substance such as sand that is used to keep the underground cracks open once the hydraulic fracturing fluid is withdrawn.

[6]Flowback.

[7]Produced water.

(Courtesy U.S. Environmental Protection Agency (EPA). http://www2.epa.gov/hfstudy/hydraulic-fracturing-water-cycle.)

AIR QUALITY

Air quality is typically measured in terms of six "criteria pollutants"—particulate matter, ozone, carbon monoxide, lead, nitrogen oxides, and sulfur dioxide—chosen for their impact on human cardiorespiratory health and carcinogenicity. In areas of fracking, particularly during the drilling and completion phase, particulate matter and ozone levels are increased because of truck traffic and emissions from drilling.[14] In addition, volatile hydrocarbons from fracking fluids, such as benzene, toluene, and xylene, are released into the air, causing at least noxious odors.[2] Toxic air pollutants near fracking sites in Texas have included formaldehyde, chloroform, and carbon tetrachloride.[1] Objective data on air pollution from fracking are limited because drilling sites are restricted with only remote data ("fence studies") available. A 2013 report from the Office of the Inspector General of the United States concluded: "Limited data from direct measurements, poor quality emission factors, and incomplete NEI [National Emissions Inventory] data hamper EPA's ability to assess air quality impacts from oil and gas production activities. With limited data, human health risks are uncertain, states may design incorrect or ineffective emission control strategies, and the EPA's decisions about regulating this industry may be misinformed."[14]

SEISMIC ACTIVITY

Hydraulic fracturing, the particular process of initially injecting the chemicals/sand/water into a well to fracture the rock formation, causes small earthquakes, generally undetectable at the surface.[14] Disposal of wastewater into deep injection wells is associated with more significant seismic activity. The largest earthquake caused by deep water injection, rated at 5.7 magnitude, occurred in November 2011 in Oklahoma.[14] Improvements in well site-selection can mitigate this risk, particularly when fracking is considered in earthquake-prone areas, such as near fault lines.

SAND MINING

Hydraulic fracturing accounts for 41% of all the silica sand used in the United States, triggering a silica sand surface strip-mining boom, especially in the upper Midwest.[14] The sudden expansion of silica strip mining creates an environmental concern as silica dust is harmful to workers at mines, workers at well sites, and residents living near fracked wells. In 2012, the National Institute for Occupational Safety and Health (NIOSH) issued a hazard alert for workers at fracking sites after discovering elevated levels of silica in the air near many wells.[12] Silicosis is a pulmonary disease caused by inhaling silica dust that can have a latency period of more than 10 years.

GLOBAL WARMING

Combustion of methane releases less CO_2 into the atmosphere per energy generated than combustion of other fossil fuels, such as oil or coal. Although less carbon friendly than renewable energy sources, methane is regarded as the most environmentally safe fossil fuel. However, if methane gas is leaked directly into the atmosphere before burning, it is very damaging. One molecule of methane creates an atmospheric global-warming footprint that is 86 times greater than one molecule of CO_2.[18] Using present practices, a fracked well typically releases 3.6% to 7.9% of "fugitive methane" into the atmosphere. A Cornell study of the carbon footprint of shale gas used for consumer heat generation estimated that, with the 3.6% to 7.9% rate of fugitive methane, a fracked well creates a larger CO_2 footprint than does an oil well, with a 1.7% to 6% methane leak, over a 20-year period.[6] When methane is burned for electricity, excluding the consumer component, the CO_2 footprint produced by shale gas is somewhat better because of the efficiency of gas power plants over coal power plants, but methane is still more damaging to the atmosphere than coal or oil. The longer the estimated time, the smaller is the difference, because methane remains in the atmosphere for a shorter period than CO_2 but is a much more potent greenhouse gas. According to the Cornell study, shale gas creates a larger estimated carbon footprint in timescales of less than about 50 years.[6] The National Oceanic and Atmospheric Administration (NOAA) found that methane leakage rates are even higher than previously estimated. This concern alone can hasten the global-warming tipping point (the point in time when interventions can no longer stabilize the global-warming process) to within the next 15 to 35 years.[2] The carbon footprint of hydraulic fracturing can be easily mitigated by trapping or flaring fugitive methane; present U.S. federal regulatory requirements do not mandate this.[14]

NATIONAL PARKS IN THE UNITED STATES

Drilling for methane and oil has already occurred in 12 national parks and threatens the borders of many others, especially parks that are atop shale formations.[10] The surface footprint of a fracking drilling well site, approximately 2.5 acres, is much larger than conventional wells to allow room for chemical storage tanks, holding pits, and roads for heavy truck traffic.[10,14] The sheer size of the footprint has great potential to fragment habitats and impact native wildlife species within and around a national park.[10] This can potentially affect biodiversity and stability of plant and animal species, and alter migration patterns and grazing habitats. Flaring of methane gas from fracked wells near and within national parks, although good for the atmosphere, causes significant light obscuration in lands that were previous nighttime viewing destinations, such as the Theodore Roosevelt National Park in North Dakota.[10] Noise pollution from fracking is disruptive to visitors. Water extraction for drilling can impact the amount and quality of water in rivers coursing through national parks, in addition to concerns about fracking wastewater. Visitors heading east from Glacier National Park encounter a sign warning against poisonous gases from fracking operations.[10]

CONCLUSION

The shale gas boom has created a market where the United States will rapidly become a net exporter of natural gas.[2] However, the typical boom-and-bust cycles of energy extraction have historically created abandoned oil and gas wells and abandoned coal mines. These leave taxpayers with cleanup bills and are an environmental risk until the sites are remediated.[12] Although most states in the United States have small bonding requirements for well plugging (some as low as $100 per well), few states have established policies that require drillers to have bonds, trust funds, or insurance policies to cover well reclamation once the well has lost its profitability.[12] These funds would cover restoration of the environment, compensation of victims for damage to property and health, provision of alternate sources of water if needed, and full restoration of damaged public infrastructure (e.g., road damage from heavy truck traffic). With such low bonding rates, the oil and gas industry has little incentive to reclaim sites. Between 2001 and 2008, 127 mines in West Virginia and 227 mines in Pennsylvania were abandoned and the posted bonds forfeited; this may increase as falling fuel prices financially pressure drilling companies.[12]

The National Resources Defense Council opposes expanding fracking without additional safeguards to protect human health and the environment.[11] The U.S. Environmental Protection Agency (EPA) is now working on a comprehensive study of the environmental impacts of hydraulic fracturing. Objective scientific data regarding the environmental safety of unconventional drilling are difficult to find. Legal settlements for groundwater contamination of private wells often include confidentiality agreements. Academic studies have been sponsored by the fracking industry without appropriate attribution, coined "frackademia."[14] Policy makers and regulators are subjected to financial and environmental pressures from both corporate lobbyists in favor of fracking and voters and landowners strongly opposed to fracking. Direct measurement of air and water quality data at and around fracking well sites is regularly restricted to "fence studies" where the

agreements, limiting public discourse and availability of objective data.

fracked site is known, but the industry does not routinely reveal the location of fracking sites, wastewater pits, or injection wells. The overall paucity of objective environmental data regarding the impact of hydraulic fracturing on human and environmental health has created a biased informational landscape, impairing public debate as well as policy formation. Geisinger Health Systems, sitting atop the Marcellus shale in Pennsylvania, is presently conducting a comprehensive epidemiologic survey on the health implications of fracking using 2.6 million available electronic health records.[2]

However, the present informational vacuum cannot adequately predict the short-term and long-term impacts of fracking. In a 2013 review of the impact of fracking on public health, Finkel and Hays[2] summarize the data: "no sound epidemiologic study has been done" to quantify fracking's impact on human and environmental health. They conclude, "Natural gas has been in shale formations for millions of years; it isn't going anywhere."

THE CHALLENGE

A mere two generations ago, humankind was an ecologic creditor, using fewer natural resources than were generated by the planet. By 2010, fueled by population growth and individual consumption, we have amassed environmental debt. We must learn to live within our ecologic means. Each country has a measurable ecologic footprint equivalent to the sum of all the land and water required to support its consumption and absorb its waste. According to the 2008 *Living Planet Report,* this global sum exceeded the planet's available supply in the 1980s, and by 2005, demand was 30% greater than was biocapacity.[5] The United States and China have the largest individual footprints, with each country consuming 21% of the planet's biocapacity. Much of China's footprint is caused by its large population. India is a distant third at 7%. These three countries have among the highest natural biocapacities in the world but are now in ecologic debt. Many developed countries have ecologic footprints that far exceed their biocapacity and increasingly depend on the remaining creditor countries for resources.

Scientists cannot accurately predict precisely when the earth will reach an ecologic "point of no return." According to the World Wildlife Fund and the *Living Planet Report* of 2005, we have the technology to return the earth to biostability by controlling population, limiting individual consumerism, and decreasing the amount of resource use and waste production.

Global population in 2015 was more than 7,291,000,000 (http://www.worldometers.info/). A nation's ecologic footprint is a function of its population, natural resources used, and waste produced. Lowest-income countries have had the greatest increases in population. Increases in middle-income population and consumerism have led to the highest per-person footprint, accounting for 39% of the total per-capita footprint. High-income countries account for 36% of the footprint, primarily from increases in per-person carbon footprint rather than increases in population.[5] To achieve sustainability, lower-income nations would benefit from family-planning services, education, and empowerment of women regarding childbearing choices. In middle- and high-income countries, family planning may be helpful; however, renewable energy sources and investment in resource-efficient cities are also important. In addition, material consumerism in richer countries, along with the accompanying electronic waste, has reached unprecedented levels. A culture of nonmaterial personal rewards could help ease this particular ecologic stress.

The largest gap between biocapacity and ecologic footprint is caused by energy consumption. Energy production from burning fossil fuels accounts for 45% of the global ecologic footprint.[5] Energy in all forms is a global issue. Its unfettered production, distribution, and use are unsustainable. The energy status quo is a threat not only to the environment but also to social equity and national security. Energy externalities are not only environmental (acid rain, global warming, radiation exposure) but social (black lung disease, asthma exacerbation, malignancies). External costs vary by energy source, being greatest for coal, followed by oil, and then by renewable energy sources.[15] The "free market," which has neglected these long-term costs in the past, can include them, pricing energy as a function of energy's total cost, rather than its subsidized cost. This may encourage consumers to purchase greener products and use renewable energy sources. A multifaceted approach to sustainability in the home and workplace, on the road, and in the wilderness, along with significant political will, is needed, because no single approach is adequate to sustain the earth and democratize energy for all people.

Renewable energies, including biomass, hydropower, wind, solar and geothermal, account for a few percent of the total global energy market because of technologic reasons and a disabling policy environment that subsidizes fossil fuel–based energy. Leadership to advance innovation in energy may come from Third World countries with less entrenched infrastructures. Once the infrastructure is in place, renewable fuel is essentially free. "Success" in the future will be measured in financial, social, and environmental terms. The addition of "environmental success" to our cultural lexicon will require leadership, sense of urgency, and global effort.

REFERENCES AND SELECTED RESOURCES

Complete references and selected resources used in this text are available online at expertconsult .inkling.com.

OCEAN STATISTICS

The ocean may be defined as the vast body of saline water that occupies the depressions of the earth's surface. More than 97% of the water on or near the earth's surface is contained in the ocean; less than 3% is held in land ice, groundwater, and all the freshwater lakes and rivers.

Traditionally, we have divided the ocean into artificial compartments called *oceans* and *seas* by using the boundaries of continents and imaginary lines such as the equator. In fact, the ocean has few dependable natural divisions and is only one great mass of water. The Pacific and Atlantic Oceans and the Mediterranean and Baltic Seas, so named for our convenience, are in reality only temporary features of a single world ocean. In this chapter, I refer to the ocean as a single entity, with subtly different characteristics at different locations but with very few natural partitions. Such a view emphasizes the interdependence of the ocean with land, life, water, atmospheric and oceanic circulation, and natural and human-made environments.

Earth's ocean exists because of a fortuitous combination of circumstances. Our planet's orbit is roughly circular around a relatively stable star. Earth is large enough to hold an atmosphere, but not so large that its gravity would overwhelm. Its neighborhood is tranquil—supernovae have not seared its surface with ionizing radiation. Our planet generates enough warmth to recycle its interior and generate the raw materials of atmosphere and ocean, but is not so hot that lava fills vast lowlands or roasts complex molecules. Best of all, our distance from the Sun allows the earth's abundant surface water to exist in the liquid state. Ours is a clement ocean world; surely *Oceanus* would be a better name for our watery home.

The ocean moderates temperature and dramatically influences weather. The ocean borders most of the planet's largest cities. It is a primary shipping and transportation route that provides much of our food. From its floor is pumped more than one-third the world's supply of petroleum and natural gas. The dry land on which almost all of human history has unfolded is hardly visible from space, because nearly three-quarters of the planet is covered by water.

BRIEF APPRECIATION OF THE OCEAN'S HISTORY AND MODERN OCEAN TOOLS

The ocean did not prevent the spread of humanity. By the time European explorers set out to "discover" the world, native peoples met them at almost every landfall. Ocean transportation offers people the benefits of mobility and greater access to food supplies. Any coastal culture skilled at raft building or small-boat navigation would have economic and nutritional advantages over less-skilled competitors. Thus, from the earliest period of human history, understanding and appreciating the ocean and its life-forms benefited those people patient enough to learn.

Systematic application of marine science began at the Library of Alexandria in Egypt. Founded during the third century BC at the behest of Alexander the Great, the library and adjacent museum could be considered the first university in the world.

When any ship entered the harbor, the books (actually, scrolls) it contained were by law removed and copied; the copies were returned to the owner and the originals kept for the library. Caravans arriving by land were also searched. Manuscripts describing the Mediterranean coast were of great interest, and traders quickly realized the competitive benefit of this information.

The second librarian at Alexandria (from 235 to 192 BC) was the Greek astronomer, philosopher, and poet Eratosthenes of Cyrene. This remarkable man was the first to calculate the circumference of the earth using geometry. The Greek Pythagoreans had realized that Earth was spherical by the sixth century BC, but Eratosthenes was the first to estimate its true size.

Scientific oceanography began with the departure of *HMS Challenger* from Plymouth, England, in 1872. Conceived by Wyville Thomson, a professor of natural history at Scotland's University of Edinburgh, and his Canadian-born student, John Murray, *HMS Challenger*'s 4-year cruise was the first research expedition devoted completely to marine science, and it also holds the record as the longest such voyage. Other scientific expeditions had been launched previously, such as the voyages of Captain James Cook, RN, and the United States Exploring Expedition under Charles Wilkes, but these were hybrid military and scientific undertakings. The *HMS Challenger* voyage is notable for being the first purely scientific oceanographic endeavor. Stimulated by their own curiosity and with the inspiration of Charles Darwin's voyage in *HMS Beagle*, Thomson and Murray convinced the Royal Society and British government to provide a Royal Navy ship and trained crew for a prolonged and arduous voyage of exploration across the oceans of the world. They coined a word for their enterprise: *oceanography*. Although the term literally implies only marking or charting, it has come to refer to the science of the ocean.

The demands of scientific oceanography have become greater than the capability of any single voyage. Modern oceanography depends on an interlocking suite of terrestrial and space-based sensors. Among the most interesting are the radar altimeters borne by *TOPEX/Poseidon/Jason*, as the project is known, a train of satellites orbiting 1336 km (830.2 miles) above Earth in a pattern that allows coverage of 95% of the ice-free ocean every 10 days. Experiments that are occurring as part of this 5-year program include sensing water vapor over the ocean, determining the precise location of ocean currents, and determining wind speed and direction. The most revolutionary devices are the satellites' *TOPography Experiment,* which use radar positioning devices to allow researchers to determine position to within 1 cm (0.4 inch) of Earth's center. Computers can then determine the height of the sea surface with unprecedented accuracy.

Disregarding waves, tides, and currents, researchers have found the ocean surface can vary from the ideal smooth (ellipsoid) shape by as much as 200 m (656 feet). The reason is that the pull of gravity varies across Earth's surface depending on the nearness or farness of massive parts of the earth. An undersea mountain or ridge "pulls" water toward it from the sides, forming a mound of water over itself. For example, a typical undersea volcano with a height of 2000 m (6562 feet) above the seabed and a radius of 20 km (12.4 miles) would produce a 2-m (6.6-feet) rise in the ocean surface. This mound cannot be seen with the unaided eye because the slope of the surface is very gradual. The large features of the seabed are amazingly and accurately reproduced in the subtle standing irregularities of the sea surface. Hundreds of previously unknown features have been discovered using the data provided by this project.

Small robot submersibles were much in the news during the *Deepwater Horizon* oil spill in the Gulf of Mexico in 2010. These nimble devices can manipulate valves, lift and reposition equipment, and act as remote sets of eyes for decision-makers. Scientists use them to probe submerged geologic features, examine shipwrecks, and measure water.

Perhaps the most imaginative new technology being incorporated into submersibles is *telepresence,* the extension of a person's senses by remote manipulators. A scientist might wear a helmet containing small stereo television screens and earphones, and place his hands in special gloves equipped with tactile feedback units. Movements of his head and hands would be duplicated by a robot on the seafloor, and sensations "felt" by the robot would be relayed back to the scientist through the TVs, earphones, and gloves. He or she would thus have the sensation of being on the seafloor and could take samples, manipulate tools, or just look around. Other researchers could watch or participate at distant locations via a high-speed data link.

Personal investigation is still an important option. As amazing as are robots, satellites, and multibeam systems, sometimes there is no substitute for actually *seeing*—focusing a well-trained set of eyes on the ocean floor.

The most difficult problem is to reach extreme depths, but amazingly, scientists have visited the bottom of the deepest ocean basin. On 23 January 1960, U.S. Navy lieutenant Don Walsh and Dr. Jacques Piccard descended to a depth of 11,022 m (6.85 miles) into the Challenger Deep, an area of the Mariana Trench discovered in 1951 by the British oceanographic research vessel *Challenger II.* The vehicle used in the descent was *Trieste,* a deep-diving submersible designed like a blimp with a very strong and thick (and cramped) steel crew sphere suspended below. A blimp uses helium gas for buoyancy, but a gas would be compressed by water pressure; so gasoline, which is relatively incompressible, was used to provide lift. The trip was repeated by film director James Cameron in 2012 in a vehicle of different design.

We have come a long way since the 1960s. *Alvin,* the best-known and oldest of the deep-diving manned submarines now in operation, has made more than 4500 dives since its commissioning in 1964. Recently refurbished and certified to even greater depths, *Alvin* will continue to explore the Mid-Atlantic Ridge and other seabed features of interest to geologists and biologists. *Alvin*'s abilities have been surpassed by a new class of manned vehicles, the most capable of which are Japan's *Shinkai* 6500 and China's *Jaiolong.* These submarines can reach depths greater than 7000 m (22,966 feet).

WATER CHARACTERISTICS

Water is so familiar and abundant that we do not always appreciate its unusual characteristics. Two major concepts are reviewed here. The first is the influence of water on global temperatures. Liquid water's thermal characteristics prevent broad swings of temperature during day and night and, through a longer span, during winter and summer. Heat is stored in the ocean during the day and released at night. A much greater amount of heat is stored through the summer and given off during the winter. Liquid water has an important thermostatic balancing effect—an oceanless Earth would be much colder in winter and much hotter in summer than the moderate climates we experience. The second concept is the influence of density on ocean structure. Ocean structure and large-scale movement depend on changes in the density of seawater, with this density dependent on temperature and salt content.

Perhaps the most important physical properties of water are related to its behavior as it absorbs or loses heat. Water's unusual thermal characteristics prevent wide temperature variation from day to night and from winter to summer, permit vast amounts of heat to flow from equatorial to polar regions, and power Earth's great storms, wind waves, and ocean currents.

Heat and temperature are related concepts but are not the same. *Heat* is energy produced by random vibration of atoms or molecules. On average, water molecules in hot water vibrate more rapidly than do water molecules in cold water. Heat is a measure of how many molecules are vibrating and how rapidly they are vibrating. *Temperature* records only how rapidly the molecules of a substance are vibrating. Temperature is an object's response to the input (or removal) of heat. The amount of heat required to bring a substance to a certain temperature varies with the nature of that substance.

Heat capacity is a measure of the heat required to raise the temperature of 1 gram of a substance by 1°C. Different substances have different heat capacities, and not all substances respond to identical inputs of heat by rising in temperature the same number of degrees (Table 123-1). Heat capacity is measured in calories per gram per degree centigrade.

Because of the great strength and large number of the hydrogen bonds between water molecules, more heat energy must be added to speed up molecular movement and raise water's temperature than would be necessary in a substance held together by weaker bonds. Liquid water's heat capacity is therefore among the highest of all known substances. This means that water can absorb (or release) large amounts of heat while changing relatively little in temperature.

The uniqueness of water becomes even more apparent when one considers the effect of temperature change on water's density. Most substances become denser as they become colder. Pure water generally becomes denser as heat is removed and its temperature falls, but water's density behaves in an unexpected way as its temperature approaches the freezing point. As the water continues to cool, its framework of hydrogen bonds becomes more rigid; this causes the liquid to expand slightly because the molecules are held slightly farther apart. Water becomes slightly less dense as cooling continues, until 0°C (32°F) is reached; this is the point at which water begins to freeze and change state by crystallizing into ice. At this point, the density of the water decreases abruptly. Ice is therefore lighter than an equal volume of water. Ice increases in density as it becomes colder than 0°C; however, no matter how cold it becomes, ice never reaches the density of liquid water. Because it is less dense than water, ice "freezes over" as a floating layer instead of "freezing under" as do the solid forms of virtually all other liquids.

Progressive transition from liquid water to ice crystals requires continued removal of heat energy; the change in state does not occur instantly throughout the mass when the cooling water reaches 0°C (32°F). Removal of heat does not stop when some of the water in the freezing water mass reaches the freezing point, but the decline in temperature stops. Although heat continues to be removed, the water will not become colder until the water mass has changed state from liquid (water) to solid (ice). Heat may therefore be removed from water when it is changing state (i.e., when it is freezing) without the water dropping in

TABLE 123-1	Heat Capacity of Common Substances*
Substance	**Heat Capacity† in Calories/gram/°C**
Silver	0.06
Granite/sand	0.20
Aluminum	0.22
Alcohol (ethyl)	0.30
Gasoline	0.50
Acetone	0.51
Ice (not freezing or thawing)	0.51
Pure liquid water	1.00
Ammonia (liquid)	1.13

*Heat capacity is a measure of the heat required to raise the temperature of 1 gram of a substance by 1°C.
†Different substances have different heat capacities. Note how little heat is required to raise the temperature of 1 gram of silver by 1°C. Of all common substances, only liquid ammonia has a higher heat capacity than liquid water.

temperature. Indeed, continued removal of heat is what makes the change in state possible. Heat is released as hydrogen bonds form to make ice, and that heat must be removed to allow more ice to form. This heat is called the *latent* heat of fusion (from the Latin *latere,* meaning "to be hidden").

The implications of this odd thermal behavior are striking. More than 18,000 km³ (11,185 miles³) of polar ice that covers as many as 20 million km² (12.4 million miles²) of surface thaws and refreezes in the southern hemisphere each year; this is an area of ocean larger than South America. The annual change in sea ice cover is less in the Arctic, averaging about 5 million km² (3.1 million miles²). Incoming solar heat melts ice in the local polar summer, but the ocean's temperature does not change. The situation reverses during the winter: the water freezes, and again the temperature does not change. Models suggest that without this thermostatic effect—or if ice "froze under" rather than "froze over"—Earth would be a much different planet, perhaps roiled by near-transonic winds peaking about 1 month after the equinoxes at equatorial latitudes.

The total quantity or concentration of dissolved inorganic solids in water is its *salinity.* The ocean's salinity varies from about 3.3% to 3.7% by mass, depending on such factors as evaporation, precipitation, and freshwater runoff from the continents. However, the average salinity is usually given as 3.5%. Most of the dissolved solids in seawater are salts that have been separated into ions. Sodium (Na^+) and chloride (Cl^-) are the most abundant of these ions.

The many ions present in seawater react with each other and with water molecules in complex ways to modify the physical properties of pure water:

- The heat capacity of water decreases with increasing salinity. In other words, less heat is necessary to raise the temperature of seawater than is required to raise the temperature of freshwater by the same amount.
- Dissolved salts disrupt the webwork of hydrogen bonding in water. As salinity increases, the freezing point of water becomes lower; the salts act as a form of antifreeze. Sea ice therefore forms at a lower temperature than does ice in freshwater lakes.
- Because dissolved salts tend to attract water molecules, seawater evaporates more slowly than does freshwater. Swimmers usually notice that freshwater evaporates quickly and completely from their skin, but seawater lingers.
- *Osmotic pressure,* which is the pressure exerted on a biologic membrane when the salinity of the environment is different from that within cells, rises with increasing salinity. This is a key factor related to the transport of water into and out of cells.

These four properties, which vary with the quantity of solutes dissolved in water, are called water's *colligative* properties (Latin *colligatus,* "to bind together"). Because colligative properties are the properties of solutions, the more concentrated (saline) the solute, the more important these properties become. Because it is not a solution, pure water has no colligative properties.

Because about 3.5% of seawater consists of dissolved substances, boiling away 100 kg of seawater theoretically produces a residue with a mass of 3.5 kg. Because variations of 0.1% are significant, however, oceanographers prefer to use the parts-per-thousand notation (‰) rather than percent (%, parts-per-hundred notation) when discussing these materials. The seven ions listed below oxygen and hydrogen in Table 123-2 make up more than 99% of this residual material; sodium and chloride make up 85% of the total. When seawater evaporates, its ionic components combine in many different ways to form table salt, Epsom salts, and other mineral salts.

Seawater also contains minor constituents. The ocean is sort of an "Earth tea"; almost every element present in Earth's crust and atmosphere is also present in the oceans, although sometimes in extremely small amounts. Only 14 elements have concentrations in seawater of more than 1 part per million. Elements present in amounts less than 0.001‰ (1 part per million) are known as *trace elements.*

Remembering the effectiveness of water as a solvent, one might think that the ocean's saltiness has resulted from the ability

TABLE 123-2 Major Constituents of Seawater at 34.4‰ Salinity

Constituent	Concentration in Parts per Thousand (‰) or Grams per Kilogram (g/kg)	Percent by Mass
Water Itself		
Oxygen	857.8	85.8
Hydrogen	107.2	10.7
Most Abundant Ions		
Chloride (Cl^-)	18.980	1.9
Sodium (Na^+)	10.556	1.1
Sulfate (SO_4^{2-})	2.649	0.3
Magnesium (Mg^{2+})	1.272	0.1
Calcium (Ca^{2+})	0.400	0.04
Potassium (K^+)	0.380	0.04
Bicarbonate (HCO_3^-)	0.140	0.01
Total	999.377 g/kg	99.99%

of rain, groundwater, or crashing surf to dissolve crustal rock. Much of the sea's dissolved material originated in that way, but is crustal rock the source of all the ocean's solutes? An easy way to find out would be to investigate the composition of salts in river water and compare this to that of the ocean as a whole. If crustal rock is the only source, the salts in the ocean should be like those of concentrated river water; however, they are not. River water is usually a dilute solution of bicarbonate and calcium ions, whereas the principal ions in seawater are sodium and chloride. The magnesium content of seawater would be higher if seawater were simply concentrated river water. The proportions of salts in isolated salty inland lakes (e.g., Utah's Great Salt Lake, the Dead Sea) are much different from the proportions of salts in the ocean. Thus, weathering and erosion of crustal rock cannot be the only source of sea salts.

The components of ocean water with proportions that are not accounted for by the weathering of surface rocks are called *excess volatiles.* The sources of these excess volatiles are Earth's deeper layers. The upper mantle appears to contain more of the substances found in seawater (including the water itself) than are found in surface rocks, and their proportions are about the same as found in the ocean. Convection currents slowly churn Earth's mantle, causing the movement of tectonic plates. Because of this activity, some deeply trapped volatile substances escape to the exterior, outgassing through volcanoes and rift vents. These excess volatiles include carbon dioxide (CO_2), chlorine, sulfur, hydrogen, fluorine, nitrogen, and water vapor. This material, along with residue from surface weathering, accounts for the chemical constituents of today's ocean.

Some of the ocean's solutes are hybrids of the two processes of weathering and outgassing. Table salt (sodium chloride) is an example of this. Sodium ions come from the weathering of crustal rocks, whereas chloride ions come from the mantle by way of volcanic vents and outgassing from midocean rifts. As for the lower-than-expected quantity of magnesium and sulfate ions in the ocean, research at a spreading center east of the Galápagos Islands suggests that the chemical composition of seawater percolating through midocean rifts is altered by contact with fresh crust. The water that circulates through new ocean floor at these sites is stripped of magnesium as well as of a few other elements. The magnesium seems to be incorporated into mineral deposits, but calcium is added as hot water dissolves adjacent rocks.

Recent research has shown that temperature and density gradients inside seamounts also drive great quantities of water into close association with hot geologic bits. The ocean contains about 15,000 seamounts, and the volume of seawater circulated through them may exceed the amounts associated with ridges. Astonishingly, all the water in the ocean is thought to cycle through the seabed at rift zones every 1 to 2 million years.

OCEAN STRUCTURE

Heat combines with salinity to define ocean structure. A liter of seawater weighs between 2% and 3% more than a liter of pure water because of the solids (often called *salts*) dissolved in seawater. The density of seawater is thus between 1.020 and 1.030 g/cm³ compared with 1.000 g/cm³ for pure water at the same temperature. Cold, salty water is denser than warm, less salty water. Seawater's density increases with increasing salinity, increasing pressure, and decreasing temperature. Figure 123-1 shows the relationship between temperature, salinity, and density. Note that two samples of water can have the same density at different combinations of temperature and salinity.

Much of the ocean is divided into three density zones: the surface zone, pycnocline, and deep zone. The *surface zone,* or mixed layer, is the upper layer of ocean. Temperature and salinity are relatively constant with depth in the surface zone because of the action of waves and currents. The surface zone consists of water in contact with the atmosphere and exposed to sunlight; it contains the ocean's least dense water and accounts for only about 2% of total ocean volume. This layer typically extends to a depth of about 150 m (500 feet), but depending on local conditions, may reach a depth of 1000 m (3300 feet) or may be absent entirely.

The *pycnocline* (Greek *pyknos,* "strong," and Latin *clinare,* "to slope" or "to lean") is a zone in which density increases with increasing depth. This zone isolates surface water from the denser layer below. The pycnocline contains about 18% of all ocean water.

The *deep zone* lies below the pycnocline at depths of more than about 1000 m (3300 feet) in midlatitudes (40 degrees south to 40 degrees north). There is little additional change in water density with increasing depth through this zone. This deep zone contains about 80% of all ocean water.

The pycnocline's rapid density increase with depth is mainly the result of a decrease in water temperature. The surface zone is well mixed, with little decrease in temperature with depth. In the next layer, temperature drops rapidly with depth. Beneath it lies the deep zone of cold, stable water. The middle layer, the zone in which temperature changes rapidly with depth, is called the *thermocline.* Falling temperature is the major contributor to the formation of the pycnocline.

Thermoclines are not identical in form in all areas or latitudes. Surface temperature is proportional to available sunlight. More solar energy is available in the tropics than in the polar regions, so the water there is warmer. The ocean's sunlit upper layer is thicker in the tropics, both because the solar angle there is more nearly vertical and because water in the open tropical ocean contains fewer suspended particles and is therefore clearer than

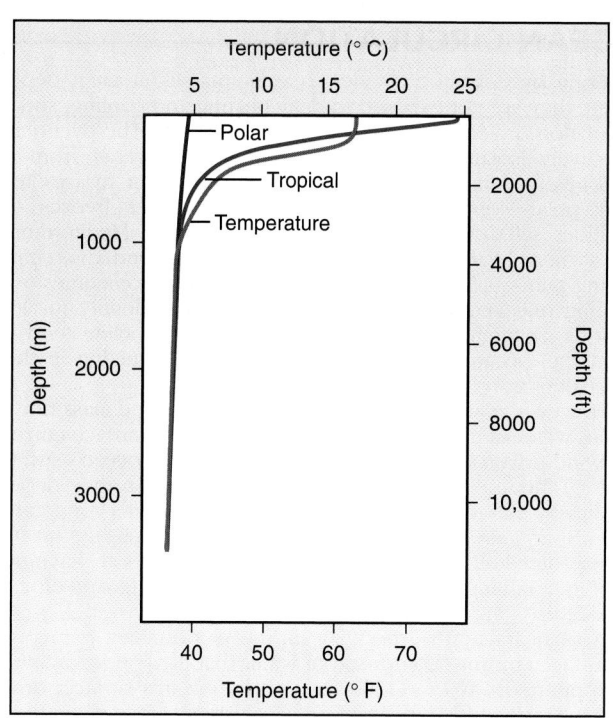

FIGURE 123-2 Typical temperature profiles at polar, tropical, and middle (temperate) latitudes. Note that polar waters lack a thermocline.

water in open temperate or polar regions. Because the ocean is heated to a greater depth, the tropical thermocline is deeper and much more pronounced than thermoclines at higher latitudes. The transition to the colder, denser water below is more abrupt in the tropics than at high latitudes.

Polar waters, which receive relatively little solar warmth, are not stratified by temperature and generally lack a thermocline because surface water in the polar regions is almost as cold as water at great depths.

Figure 123-2 contrasts polar, tropical, and temperate thermal profiles, showing that the thermocline is primarily a mid- and low-latitude phenomenon. Thermocline depth and intensity vary with season, local conditions (e.g., storms), currents, and many other factors.

The vertical movement of large volumes of water from the surface to great depths (and vice versa) is possible only where surface-water density is similar to deep-water density. The great difference in temperature—and therefore density—between surface water and deep water in the tropics makes the water column very stable and prevents an exchange of surface and deep water. This stability is maintained even though the surface of the tropical ocean is in constant horizontal motion, churned by tropical cyclones and stirred by currents.

Vertical movement of water in the northern polar ocean is also limited. There, however, the stratification is caused largely by a salinity difference between surface water and water at great depths. The surface of the Arctic Ocean receives a large volume of freshwater runoff from Siberian and Canadian rivers. Continental masses block the formation of large currents, and the landlocked northern ocean communicates sluggishly with other ocean areas, so the surface water tends not to mix with deeper water or to flow to lower latitudes.

By contrast, the southern polar ocean is only weakly stratified. The cold temperature of southern ocean surface water closely matches that of deep water, so no thermocline divides surface water from deep water (see Figure 123-2). The absence of confining continental margins and mixing at the boundaries of the Antarctic Circumpolar Current minimize salinity differences. Turbulence and weak stratification encourage a huge volume of deep-water upwelling, which contributes to high surface nutrient levels and high biologic productivity.

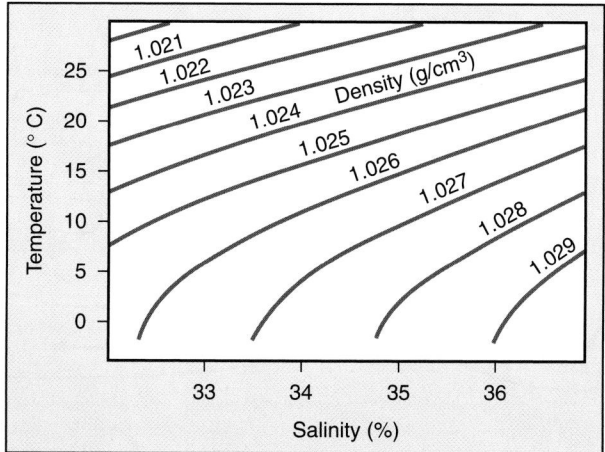

FIGURE 123-1 The complex relationships between temperature, salinity, and density of seawater. Note that two samples of water can have the same density at different combinations of temperature and salinity.

OCEAN CIRCULATION

Layering by density traps dense water masses at great depths, where they are not exposed to daily heating and cooling, surface circulation driven by winds and storms, or light. The pycnocline effectively isolates 80% of the world ocean's water from the 20% involved in surface circulation. Dense water masses form near polar continental shelves (as cold water freezes and excludes salt) or in enclosed areas such as the Mediterranean Sea (where evaporation exceeds precipitation and river input, raising salinity). These heavy-water masses sink, sometimes overlapping one another and often retaining their identity for long periods. Separate water masses below the pycnocline tend not to merge, because little energy is available for mixing in these quiet depths.

However, water does circulate in the ocean. The mass flow of ocean water in currents occurs in two forms: (1) surface currents are wind-driven movements of water at or near the ocean's surface; and (2) thermohaline currents (so named because they depend on density differences caused by variations in water's temperature and salinity) are the slow, deep currents that affect the vast bulk of seawater beneath the pycnocline (see later). Both have very important influences on Earth's temperature, climate, and biologic productivity, and will change as Earth's climate varies.

A small fraction of the water in the world ocean is involved in surface currents, comprised of water that flows horizontally in the uppermost 400 m (1300 feet) of the ocean's surface, driven mainly by wind friction. Most surface currents move water above the pycnocline.

The primary force responsible for surface currents is wind. Surface winds form global patterns within latitude bands. Most of Earth's surface wind energy is concentrated in each hemisphere's trade winds (i.e., easterlies) and westerlies. Waves on the sea surface transfer some of the energy from the moving air to the water using friction. This tug of wind on the ocean surface begins a mass flow of water, and the water flowing beneath the wind forms a surface current.

Because of the Coriolis effect, northern hemisphere surface currents flow to the right and southern hemisphere currents flow to the left of the wind direction. Continents and basin topography often block continuous flow and help deflect the moving water into a circular pattern, clockwise in the northern hemisphere and counterclockwise in the southern hemisphere. This flow around the periphery of an ocean basin is called a *gyre* (Greek *gyros,* "a circle").

There are six great current circuits in the world ocean, two in the northern hemisphere and four in the southern hemisphere. Five are geostrophic gyres, gyres that flow around the periphery of an ocean basin: the North Atlantic gyre, South Atlantic gyre, North Pacific gyre, South Pacific gyre, and Indian Ocean gyre. Although it is a closed circuit, the sixth and largest current is technically not a gyre because it does not flow around the periphery of an ocean basin. The West Wind Drift, or Antarctic Circumpolar Current, as this exception is called, flows endlessly eastward around Antarctica, driven by powerful, nearly ceaseless westerly winds. This greatest of all the surface ocean currents is never deflected by a continent. Figure 123-3 shows the major surface currents of the world ocean.

Assisted by the winds, surface currents distribute tropical heat worldwide. Warm water flows to higher latitudes, transfers heat to the air and cools, moves back to low latitudes, and absorbs heat again; the cycle then repeats. The greatest amount of heat transfer occurs at midlatitudes, where about 10^{15} calories of heat are transferred each second; this is 1 million times as much power as is consumed by the entire world's human population in the same length of time.

This combination of water flow and heat transfer from and to water influences climate and weather in several ways. For example, during the winter, Edinburgh, Dublin, and London are bathed in eastward-moving air only recently in contact with the

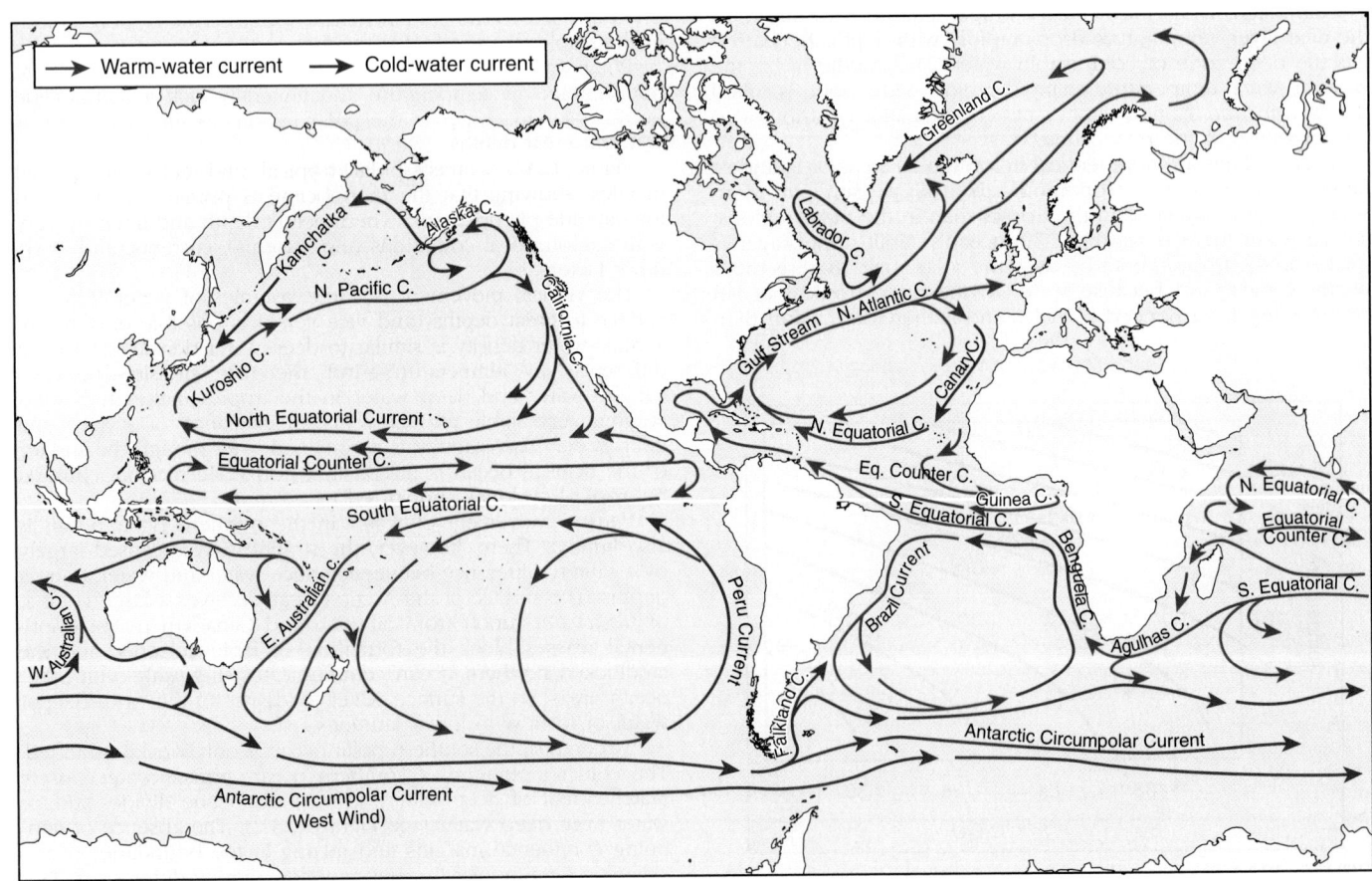

FIGURE 123-3 A chart showing the names and usual directions of the world ocean's major surface currents. The powerful western boundary currents flow along the western boundaries of ocean basins in both hemispheres.

relatively warm North Atlantic Current. Scotland, Ireland, and England have a maritime climate. These places are warmed in part by the energy of tropical sunlight transported to high latitudes by the Gulf Stream.

At lower latitudes on an ocean's eastern boundary the situation is often reversed. Mark Twain supposedly said that the coldest winter he ever spent was a summer in San Francisco. Summer months in that West Coast city are cool, foggy, and mild. Alternatively, Washington, DC—on nearly the same line of latitude as San Francisco but on the western boundary of an ocean basin—is known for its all-but-intolerable August heat and humidity. The California Current, carrying cold water from the north, comes close to the coast at San Francisco. Air normally flows clockwise in summer around an offshore zone of high atmospheric pressure. Wind approaching the California coast loses heat to the cold sea and comes ashore to chill San Francisco. Summer air often flows around a similar high off the East Coast (i.e., the Bermuda High). Therefore, winds that approach Washington, DC, blow from the south and east. Heat and moisture from the Gulf Stream contribute to the capital's oppressive summers. Alternatively, during the winter, Washington, DC, is colder than San Francisco, because westerly winds approaching Washington, DC, are chilled by the cold continent over which they cross.

Surface currents affect the uppermost layer of the world ocean (i.e., about 10% of its volume), but horizontal and vertical currents also exist below the pycnocline in the ocean's deeper waters. Because density is largely a function of water temperature and salinity, the movement of water as a result of differences in density is called *thermohaline circulation* (Greek *therme*, "heat," and *halos*, "salt"). The entire ocean is involved in slow thermohaline circulation, a process responsible for the large-scale vertical movement of ocean water and circulation of the global ocean as a whole.

Formation and downwelling of deep water occurs in the polar regions. Antarctic Bottom Water, the most distinctive of the deep-water masses, is characterized by salinity of 34.65‰, temperature of $-0.5°C$ (30°F), and density of $1.0279 g/cm^3$. This water is noted for its extreme density (it is the densest in the world ocean), the great amount of it produced near Antarctic coasts, and its ability to migrate north along the seafloor.

Most Antarctic Bottom Water forms near the Antarctic coast south of South America during winter. Salt is concentrated in pockets between crystals of pure water and then squeezed out of the freezing mass to form a frigid brine. Between 20 and 50 million m^3 of this brine form every second. The water's great density causes it to sink toward the continental shelf, where it mixes with nearly equal parts of water from the southern Antarctic Circumpolar Current.

The mixture settles along the edge of Antarctica's continental shelf, descends along the slope, and spreads along the deep-sea bed, creeping north in slow sheets. Antarctic Bottom Water flows many times more slowly than the water in surface currents: in the Pacific, it may take 1000 years for this water to reach the equator; 600 years later, it may be as far away as the Aleutian Islands at 50 degrees N latitude. Antarctic Bottom Water also flows into the Atlantic Ocean basin, where it flows north at a faster rate than in the Pacific. Antarctic Bottom Water has been identified as high as 40 degrees N latitude on the Atlantic floor, a journey that will have taken some 750 years to complete.

Similar water masses form in the North Atlantic and even at the Gibraltar outlet of the Mediterranean Sea. However, none is as dense as Antarctic Bottom Water. Oxygen is delivered to organisms in the deepest ocean basins by these slowly creeping water masses.

The great quantities of dense water sinking at polar ocean basin edges must be offset by equal quantities of water rising elsewhere. Figure 123-4 shows an idealized model of thermohaline flow.

Note that water sinks relatively rapidly in a small area where the ocean is very cold, but rises much more gradually across a very large area in the warmer temperate and tropical zones. It then slowly returns poleward near the surface to repeat the cycle. The continual diffuse upwelling of deep water maintains the

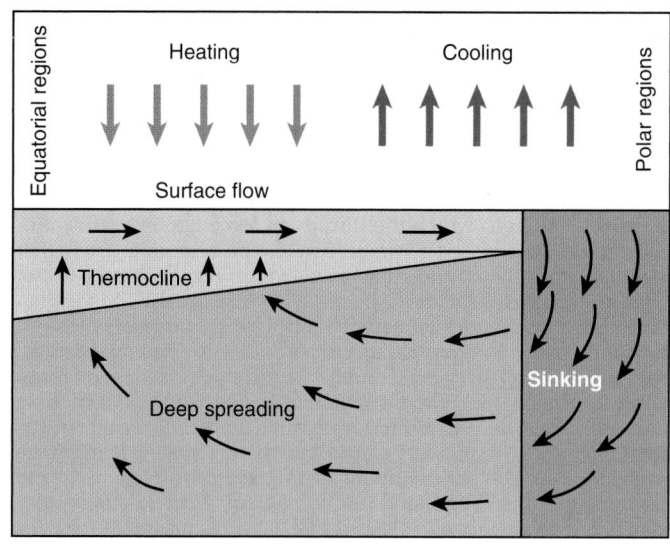

FIGURE 123-4 The classic model of a pure thermohaline circulation, caused by heating in lower latitudes and cooling in higher latitudes. Note that the low- and mid-latitude thermocline is "held up" by continuous replacement from below.

existence of the permanent thermocline found everywhere at low latitudes and midlatitudes. This slow, upward movement is estimated to be about 1 cm (0.4 inch) per day over most of the ocean. If this rise were to stop, downward movement of heat would cause the thermocline to descend and would reduce its steepness. In a sense, the thermocline is "held up" by the continual, slow, upward movement of water.

OCEAN MOVEMENT: WAVES, TIDES, AND TSUNAMIS

Wind waves, ocean tides, and tsunamis are expressions of energy moving across the ocean surface. Waves are disturbances caused by the movement of energy from a source through a medium (i.e., solid, liquid, or gas). As the energy of the disturbance travels, the medium through which it passes moves in specific ways. Sometimes this movement is visible as crests or ridges in the medium. The traveling crests produce the appearance of movement we see in a wave. In an ocean wave, a ribbon of energy is moving at the speed of the wave, but water is not. In a sense, the wave is an illusion.

Picture a resting seagull as it bobs on the wavy ocean surface far from shore. The gull moves in circles: up and forward as the tops of the waves move to its position, down and backward as the tops move past. Each circle is equal in diameter to the wave's height. Energy in waves flows past the resting bird, but the gull and its patch of water move only a very short distance forward in each up-and-forward, down-and-back wave cycle. The water on which the bird rests does not move continuously across the sea surface, as is suggested by the wave illusion. To clarify the important idea of wave as illusion, imagine yourself at a sports stadium where spectators are doing "the wave." Your role in wave propagation is simple: you stand up and sit down in precise synchronization with your neighbors. Although you move only a few feet vertically, the wave of which you were a part circles the arena at high speed. You and all the other participants stay in place, but the wave moves faster than anyone can run.

Transfer of energy from water particle to water particle in these circular paths or orbits transmits wave energy across the ocean surface and causes the waveform to move. This type of wave is known as an *orbital wave*; it is a wave in which particles of the medium (water) move in closed circles as the wave passes. Orbital ocean waves occur at the boundary between two fluid media (i.e., air and water) and between layers of water of different densities. Because the waveform moves forward, these waves are a type of progressive wave.

The progressive wave that moved the gull was probably caused by wind. Other forces can generate much greater progressive waves in which water molecules move through much larger circular or elliptical orbits. Some of these waves are so large that they do not appear to us as waves at all, but rather as the slow sloshing of water in a harbor or bay, as dangerous flooding surges of water, or as rhythmic and predictable ocean tides.

Ocean waves are classified by the disturbing force that creates them, the extent to which the disturbing force continues to influence the waves after they are formed, the restoring force that tries to flatten them, and their wavelength. (Wave height is not often used for classification, because it varies greatly depending on water depth, interference between waves, and other factors.)

Wind blowing across the ocean surface provides the disturbing force for *capillary waves* and *wind waves*. Arrival of a storm surge or seismic sea wave in an enclosed harbor or bay, or a sudden change in atmospheric pressure, is the disturbing force for the resonant rocking of water known as a *seiche*. Landslides, volcanic eruptions, and faulting of the seafloor associated with earthquakes are the disturbing forces for *seismic sea waves*, which are also known as *tsunamis*. The disturbing forces for tides are changes in the magnitude and direction of gravitational forces among Earth, Moon, and Sun in combination with Earth's rotation.

A wave that is formed and then propagates across the sea surface without the further influence of the force that formed it is known as a *free wave*. When wind waves move away from the storm that created them, or when the storm ceases, they continue without the injection of additional wind energy. Likewise, tsunamis—waves caused by submerged landslides or earthquakes—continue to move across the ocean surface long after the landslide or earthquake has stopped moving.

By contrast, a *forced wave* is maintained by its disturbing force. Tides are forced waves that depend on the gravitational attraction of the moon and sun.

Restoring force is the dominant force that returns the water surface to flatness after a wave has formed in it. If the restoring force of a wave were quickly and fully successful, a disturbed sea surface would immediately become smooth, and the energy of the embryo wave would be dissipated as heat. However, that is not what happens. Waves continue after they form because the restoring force overcompensates and causes oscillation. The situation is analogous to a weight bobbing at the bottom of a very flexible spring, constantly moving up and down past its normal resting point.

The restoring force for very small water waves (i.e., those with wavelengths of <1.73 cm [0.68 inch]) is *cohesion,* the property that enables individual water molecules to stick to each other by means of hydrogen bonds. The same force that makes tea creep up on the sides of a teacup tugs the tiny wave troughs and crests toward flatness.

All waves with wavelengths of more than 1.73 cm (0.68 inch) depend mostly on gravity to provide the restoring force. Gravity pulls the crests downward, but inertia of the water causes the crests to overshoot and become troughs. The repetitive nature of this movement, like the spring weight moving up and down, gives rise to the circular orbits of individual water molecules in an ocean wave. These larger waves are called *gravity waves*. Because the circular motion of water molecules in a wave is nearly free of friction, gravity waves can travel across thousands

of miles of ocean surface without disappearing, eventually breaking on a distant shore.

Wavelength is an important measure of wave size. Table 123-3 lists the causes and typical wavelengths of capillary waves, wind waves, seiches, seismic sea waves, and tides.

Most characteristics of ocean waves depend on the relationship between their wavelength and water depth. Wavelength determines the size of the orbits of water molecules within a wave, but water depth determines the shape of the orbits. The paths of water molecules in a wind wave are circular only when the wave is traveling in deep water. A wave cannot "feel" the bottom when it moves through water deeper than half its wavelength because too little wave energy is contained in the small circles below that depth. Waves moving through water deeper than half their wavelengths are known as *deep-water waves*. A wave has no way of "knowing" how deep the water is, only that it is in water deeper than about half its wavelength. For example, a wind wave with a 20-m (66-feet) wavelength will act as a deep-water wave if it is passing through water deeper than 10 m (33 feet).

The situation is different for wind-generated waves close to shore. The orbits of water molecules in waves moving through shallow water are flattened by proximity of the bottom. Water just above the seafloor cannot move in a circular path, only forward and backward. Waves in water shallower than 0.05 their original wavelength are known as *shallow-water waves*. For example, a wave with a 20-m (66-feet) wavelength will act as a shallow-water wave if the water is less than 1 m (3.3 feet) deep.

Transitional waves travel through water deeper than 0.05 their original wavelength but shallower than one-half their original wavelength. For the previously discussed example, this would be water between 1 m (3.3 feet) and 10 m (33 feet) deep.

Of the five wave types listed in Table 123-3, only capillary waves and wind waves can be deep-water waves. To understand why, remember that most of the ocean floor is deeper than 125 m (400 feet), one-half the wavelength of very large wind waves. The wavelengths of the larger waves are much longer; the wavelength of seismic sea waves usually exceeds 100 km (62 miles). No ocean is 50 km (31 miles) deep, so seiches, seismic sea waves, and tides are forever in water that to them is shallow or transitional in depth. Their huge orbit circles flatten against a distant bottom that is always less than one-half a wavelength away.

In general, the longer the wavelength, the faster the wave energy will move through the water. For deep-water waves this relationship is shown in the formula:

$$C = L/T$$

where *C* represents speed (celerity), *L* is wavelength, and *T* is time or period in seconds.

The speed of all ocean waves is controlled by gravity, wavelength, and water depth. The speed of a deep-water wave may also be approximated by the formula:

$$C = \sqrt{gL}/2\pi$$

where *g* is acceleration due to gravity, which is 9.8 m/sec². Because *g* and π (3.14) are constants,

$$C = 1.251\sqrt{L}$$

TABLE 123-3	Disturbing Forces, Wavelengths, and Restoring Forces of Ocean Waves		
Wave Type	**Disturbing Force**	**Typical Wavelength**	**Restoring Force**
Capillary wave	Usually wind	Up to 1.73 cm (0.68 inch)	Cohesion of water molecules
Wine wave	Wind over ocean	60-150 m (200-500 feet)	Gravity
Seiche	Change in atmospheric pressure, storm surge, or tsunami	Large and variable; a function of ocean basin size	Gravity
Seismic sea wave (tsunami)	Faulting of seafloor, volcanic eruption, or landslide	200 km (125 miles)	Gravity
Tide	Gravitational attraction or rotation of Earth	Half of Earth's circumference	Gravity

where C is measured in m/sec and L in meters. Note in both instances that wave speed is proportional to wavelength.

Wavelength is difficult to determine at sea, but period is comparatively easy to find. For example, an observer simply times the movement of waves past the bow of a stopped ship. If the period (T) is known, speed (S) can be calculated from the relationship:

$$C \text{ (in m/sec)} = gT/2\pi$$
$$= 9.8 \text{ m/sec}^2 \times T \text{ (in sec)}/2 \times (3.14)$$
$$= 1.56T$$

where g is acceleration caused by gravity.

The speed of shallow-water waves is described by the equation:

$$C = \sqrt{gd} \text{ or } C = 3.1\sqrt{d}$$

where C is speed in m/sec, g is acceleration from gravity (9.8 m/sec^2), and d is the depth of the water in meters. The period of a wave remains unchanged regardless of the depth of water through which it is moving. However, as deep-water waves enter the shallows and touch bottom, their speed is reduced and their crests "bunch up," so their wavelengths shorten.

Comparing deep-water wind waves with shallow-water seismic sea waves is like comparing apples with oranges, but the following paragraphs demonstrate the general relationship between wavelength and wave speed: the longer the wavelength, the greater the speed. Remember that energy (not the water mass itself) is moving through the water at the astonishing speed of 760 km/hour (472.2 miles/hr) in seismic sea waves; this is the same speed as a jet airliner.

Long-wavelength, shallow-water progressive waves caused by rapid displacement of ocean water are called *tsunamis;* this is a descriptive Japanese term combining *tsu,* "harbor," with *nami,* "wave." Tsunamis that are caused by the sudden, vertical movement of Earth along fault lines (i.e., the same forces that cause earthquakes) are properly called *seismic sea waves.* Tsunamis can also be caused by landslides, icebergs falling from glaciers, volcanic eruptions, asteroid impacts, and other direct displacements of the water surface. Note that all seismic sea waves are tsunamis, but not all tsunamis are seismic sea waves.

Displacement of surface water by small seismic fractures causes "small" tsunamis. Although less energy is released by landslides than by most seismic fractures, the resulting sea waves are still very destructive for people or structures near their point of origin. This is especially true if the wave is formed within a confined area.

Seismic sea waves originate on the seafloor when Earth movement along fault lines displaces seawater. When the seismic sea wave in the Indian Ocean occurred on December 26, 2004, it ruptured along a submerged fault line, lifting the sea surface as much as 10 m (33 feet). Gravity pulled the crest downward, but the momentum of the water caused the crest to overshoot and become a trough. The oscillating ocean surface generated progressive waves that radiated from the epicenter in all directions. Waves would also have formed if the fault movement were downward. In that case, a depression in the water surface would have propagated outward as a trough; the trough would have been followed by smaller crests and troughs caused by surface oscillation.

It seems strange to refer to tsunamis—with wavelengths of up to 200 km (124.3 miles)—as shallow-water waves. However, one-half their wavelengths would be 100 km (62.1 miles), and even the deepest ocean trenches do not exceed 11 km (6.8 miles) in depth. Therefore, these immense waves never find themselves in water deeper than one-half their wavelengths. As with any shallow-water wave, seismic sea waves are affected by the contour of the bottom and are usually refracted, sometimes in unexpected ways. Detailed analysis of the 2004 event showed that the midocean ridges acted as topographic waveguides. These shallow-water waves were in constant contact with the seabed and appear to have followed the Southwest Indian Ridge below the southern tip of Africa to the Mid-Atlantic Ridge.

We are familiar with the steepness of a wind wave and the short period of a few seconds between its crests. Tsunamis are much different. After a tsunami is generated, its steepness (i.e., ratio of height to wavelength) is extremely low. This lack of steepness, in combination with the wave's very long period (i.e., 5 to 20 minutes), enables it to pass unnoticed beneath ships at sea. A ship on the open ocean that encounters a tsunami with a 16-minute period would rise slowly and imperceptibly for about 8 minutes, to a crest only 0.3 to 0.6 m (1 to 2 feet) above average sea level; it would then ease into the following trough 8 minutes later. With all the wind waves around, such a movement would not be noticed.

However, as the tsunami crest approaches shore, the situation changes rapidly and often dramatically. The period of the wave remains constant, its velocity drops, and the wave height greatly increases. As the crest arrives at the coast, observers would see water surge ashore in the same way as a very high and fast tide. In confined coastal waters relatively close to their points of origin, tsunamis can reach a height of 30 m (100 feet). The wave is a fast, onrushing flood of water and not the huge, plunging breaker of popular movies and folklore. Tsunamis can be catastrophic even if the wave crests are not that high; imagine a smaller wave inundating a flat, low-lying coast. The combination of wave height and "run up" (i.e., the distance the waves move ashore) determines a tsunami's lethality.

The wave energy spreads through an enlarging circumference as a tsunami expands from its point of origin. People onshore near the generating shock have reason to be concerned because the energy will not have dissipated much. Because of its low elevation and proximity to the earthquake epicenter, the Indonesian city of Banda Aceh was essentially demolished during the December 2004 event.

The same seismic sea wave reached the coast of India about 3 hours later. By this time, the wave circumference was enormous and its energy more dispersed. Even so, successive waves surged onto Sri Lankan, Indian, and African beaches at regular intervals for more than 2 hours.

Note that the destruction was not caused by one wave, but by a series of waves spaced at regular intervals. Some energy from the main tsunami wave was distributed into smaller waves ahead of or behind the main wave as it moved. If the epicenter of the displacement responsible for a tsunami is far away, sea level at shore will rise and fall as these waves arrive. The interval between crests (i.e., the wave period) is usually about 15 minutes. Coastal residents far from a tsunami's origin can be lulled into thinking the waves are over; they return to the coastline only to be injured or killed by the next crest. This behavior contributed to the enormous loss of life around the Indian Ocean.

Destructive tsunamis strike somewhere in the world an average of once each year. An earthquake along the Peru-Chile Trench on May 22, 1960, killed more than 4000 people; the associated tsunami reached Japan, 14,500 km (9010 miles) away, killing 180 people and causing $50 million in structural damage. Los Angeles and San Diego harbors in California were badly disrupted by seiches excited by the tsunami.

The catastrophic seismic sea wave that struck northern Japan on 11 March 2011 was the result of a rupture along a submerged fault that lifted the sea surface as much as 6 m (20 feet) in places. Gravity pulled the crest downward, but the momentum of the water caused the crest to overshoot and become a trough. The oscillating ocean surface generated progressive waves that radiated from the epicenter in all directions. Because of its low elevation and proximity to the earthquake epicenter, parts of the Miyagi and Iwate prefectures were inundated by the March 2011 wave. The Sendai region, adjacent to the epicenter, suffered the greatest damage. More than 20,000 people were killed or declared missing in the surrounding area. Nuclear power plants in the area were seriously damaged and leaked radioactive substances into air, land, and ocean. The economic loss will almost certainly amount to about 3% of a year's production by the world's third-largest economy, more than US$310 billion.

Modern tsunami warning systems depend on seabed seismometers and submerged devices and satellites that watch the shape of the sea surface.

CONDITIONS FOR OCEANIC LIFE

Marine organisms depend on the ocean's chemical composition and physical characteristics for life support. Any aspect of the physical environment that affects living organisms is called a *physical factor*. Living in the ocean often has advantages over living on land; for example, physical conditions in the sea are usually milder and less variable than physical conditions on land. The most important physical factors for marine organisms are light, temperature, dissolved nutrients, salinity, dissolved gases, acid-base balance, and hydrostatic pressure.

These physical factors work in concert to provide the physical environment for oceanic life. Additional biologic factors (i.e., biologically generated aspects of the environment) also affect living organisms. These biologic factors include diffusion, osmosis, active transport, and surface-to-volume ratio.

Too much or little of a single factor can adversely affect the function of an organism. Such a factor is called a *limiting factor*, a physical or biologic necessity with a presence that, in inappropriate amounts, limits the normal action of the organism. For example, in an ocean area where everything is perfect for photosynthesis (i.e., warmth, nutrients, adequate CO_2) except for light, no photosynthesis would occur, because light is the limiting factor. If light was present but nitrates absent, nitrate nutrients would be the limiting factor.

Marine organisms are often subject to great pressure from the constant weight of water above them, but hydrostatic pressure presents very little difficulty for them. In fact, the situation in the ocean is parallel to that on land. Land animals live in air pressurized by the weight of the atmosphere above them (i.e., $1 kg/cm^2$).

Pressures inside and outside an organism are essentially the same, both in the ocean and at the bottom of the atmosphere. Thus, marine organisms do not require heavy shells to keep from being crushed by hydrostatic pressure. Great pressure has chemical effects: gases become more soluble at high pressure, some enzymes are inactivated, and metabolic rates for a given temperature tend to be slightly higher. However, these effects are felt only at great depth. Unless marine organisms have gas-filled spaces in their bodies (e.g., lungs, swim bladders), a moderate change in pressure has little effect.

All cells of every organism are enclosed by membranes, which are essentially complex films through which a few select substances can move. A cell's membranes are greatly affected by salinity of the surrounding water.

Salinity of seawater can vary in places as a result of rainfall, evaporation, runoff of water and salts from land, and other factors. Surface salinity varies most, with lows of 6% or less along the coast of the inner Baltic Sea in early summer, to year-around highs exceeding 40% in the Red Sea. Salinity is less variable with increasing depth, with the ocean typically becoming slightly saltier with depth.

Change in salinity can physically damage cell membranes, and concentrated salts can alter protein structures. Salinity can affect the specific gravity and density of seawater and therefore buoyancy of an organism. Salinity is also important because it can cause water to enter or leave a cell through the membrane, changing the cell's overall water balance. Seawater is nearly identical in salinity to the interior of all but the most advanced forms of marine life, so maintaining salt balance—and therefore water balance—is easy for most marine species.

Almost all marine organisms require dissolved gases, particularly CO_2 and oxygen, to stay alive. Oxygen does not easily dissolve in water, and as a result, about 100 times as much gaseous oxygen exists in the atmosphere as in the ocean. However, CO_2, which is essential to primary productivity, is much more soluble and reactive in seawater than is oxygen (Table 123-4).

Although up to 1000 times as much CO_2 as oxygen can dissolve in water, normal values at the ocean surface average around 50 mL/L for CO_2 and approximately 6 mL/L for oxygen. At present, the ocean holds about 60 times as much CO_2 as the atmosphere. Because of this abundance, marine plants almost never run out of CO_2.

TABLE 123-4 The Solubility of Gases in Seawater Decreases as Temperature Rises*

Temperature	Solubility (mL/L at Atmospheric Pressure and Salinity of 33‰)		
	Nitrogen	Oxygen	Carbon Dioxide
0°C (32°F)	14.47	8.14	8700.0
10°C (50°F)	11.59	6.42	8030.0
20°C (68°F)	9.65	5.26	7350.0
30°C (86°F)	8.26	4.41	6600.0

Modified from Walton-Smith FG: *CRC handbook of the marine sciences.* Cleveland, Ohio, 1974, CRC Press.
*Note that the data shown represent values at saturation.

Deep water tends to contain more CO_2 than does surface water. Why should this be? Table 123-4 shows the relationship between water temperature and its ability to dissolve gases; note that colder water contains more gas at saturation. You may recall that the deepest and most dense seawater masses are formed at the surface in the cold polar regions, and more CO_2 can dissolve in that low-temperature environment. The dense water sinks, taking its large load of CO_2 to the bottom, and the pressure at depth helps keep it in solution. CO_2 also builds in deep water because only heterotrophs (animals) live and metabolize there, and because CO_2 is produced as decomposers consume falling organic matter. No photosynthetic primary producers are present in the dark depths to use this excess CO_2, because there is not enough sunlight for photosynthesis to occur.

Rapid photosynthesis at the surface lowers CO_2 concentrations and increases the quantity of dissolved oxygen. Oxygen is least plentiful just below the limit of photosynthesis because of respiration by many small animals at middle depths.

Low oxygen levels can sometimes be a problem at the ocean surface. Plants produce more oxygen than they use, but they produce it only during daylight hours. The continuing respiration of plants at night will sometimes remove much of the oxygen from the surrounding water. In extreme cases, this oxygen depletion may lead to the death of the plants and animals in the area, a phenomenon most noticeable in enclosed coastal waters during spring and fall plankton blooms.

The greatest variability in levels of dissolved gas is found at the surface near shore. Less dramatic changes occur in the open sea.

Ocean temperature varies with depth and latitude. The average temperature of the world ocean is only a few degrees above freezing. Warmer water is found only in the lighted surface zones of the temperate and tropical ocean and in deep, warm, chemosynthetic communities. Although temperature ranges of the ocean are considerable, they are much narrower than comparable ranges on land.

What are the implications of the ocean's temperature for living things? The rate at which chemical reactions occur in an organism largely depends on the molecular vibration known as *heat*. Because agitation brings reactants together, warmer temperatures increase the rate at which chemical reactions occur. Thus, an organism's metabolic rate increases with temperature. The metabolic rate approximately doubles with each temperature rise of 10°C (18°F). The interior temperature of an organism is directly related to the rate at which it moves, reacts, and lives.

The great majority of marine organisms are ectothermic, which means that they have an internal temperature that stays very close to that of their surroundings. A few complex animals (e.g., mammals, birds, some of the larger and faster fishes) are endothermic; they have a stable, high internal temperature.

In general, the warmer the environment of an ectotherm within its tolerance range, the more rapidly its metabolic processes will proceed. Tropical fish in a heated aquarium eat more food and require more oxygen than goldfish of the same size living in an unheated but otherwise identical aquarium. Tropical fish generally grow faster, have a faster heartbeat, reproduce more rapidly, swim more swiftly, and live shorter lives. The

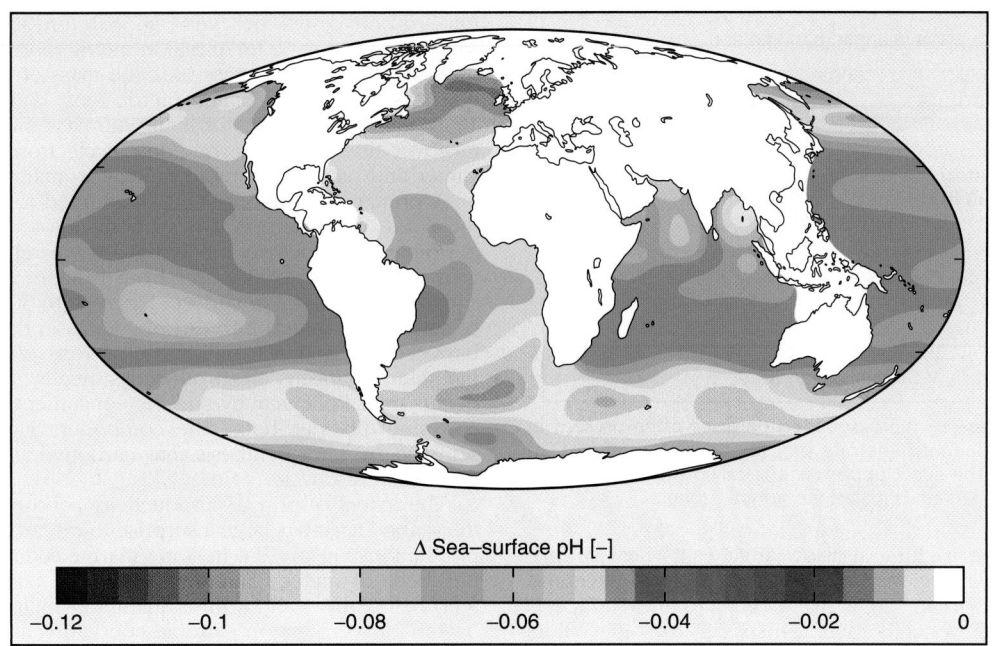

FIGURE 123-5 The ocean is becoming more acidic as it absorbs additional carbon dioxide from the atmosphere. A less alkaline environment will make it more difficult for organisms to build hard structures containing calcium (e.g., shells, coral). The chart shows changes in sea surface pH between the 1700s and the late 1990s.

upper limit of temperature that an ectotherm can tolerate is often not much higher than its optimum temperature. The lower limit is usually more forgiving because molecules are merely slowed.

Compared with ectotherms, endotherms can tolerate a tremendous range of external temperatures (e.g., a whale migrating from polar waters to the tropics, an emperor penguin incubating an egg at −51°C [−60°F]). However, their internal temperatures vary only slightly. Sophisticated thermal-regulation mechanisms make it possible for endotherms to live in a variety of habitats, but they pay a price. Their high metabolic rates make proportionally high demands on food supply and gas transport, but the benefit of having a biochemistry fine-tuned to a single efficient temperature is worth the regulatory difficulties involved.

Another physical condition that affects ocean life is the acid-base balance of seawater. The complex chemistry of Earth's life-forms depends on precisely shaped enzymes, which are large protein molecules that accelerate the rate of chemical reactions. When strong acids or bases distort the shapes of these vital enzymes, the chemical reactions they govern may not function normally.

Seawater's average pH is about 8. The dissolved substances in seawater act to buffer pH changes, preventing broad swings of pH when acids or bases are introduced. The normal pH range of seawater is much less variable than that of soil, and terrestrial organisms are sometimes limited by the presence of harsh alkali soils that damage cell components.

Although seawater remains slightly alkaline, it is subject to some variation. When dissolved in water, some CO_2 becomes carbonic acid. In areas of rapid plant growth, pH will rise because the plants use CO_2 for photosynthesis. Because temperatures are generally warmer at the surface, less CO_2 can dissolve. Surface pH in warm, productive water is usually around 8.5.

At middle depths and in deep water, more CO_2 may be present. Its source is animal and bacterial respiration. With cold temperatures, high pressure, and no photosynthetic plants to remove it, this CO_2 will lower the pH of water and make it more acid with increasing depth. Thus, deep, cold seawater below 4500 m (14,764 feet) has a pH around 7.5. This lower pH can dissolve calcium-containing marine sediments. A drop to pH 7 can occur at the deep ocean floor when bottom bacteria consume oxygen and produce hydrogen sulfide.

Concentrations of CO_2 are rising in the atmosphere. Much, perhaps most, of this increase comes from burning fossil fuels to support human industry and economic growth. Some researchers

believe that this rapid increase in CO_2 could overwhelm the carbonate buffer system in surface waters and cause surface oceanic pH to drop. Even slightly more acidic seawater would interfere with formation of calcareous materials, such as coral skeletons, plankton tests, and some other hard parts of marine organisms. Figure 123-5 shows recent changes in oceanic pH.

MARINE PRIMARY PRODUCTIVITY

Primary productivity involves synthesis of organic materials from inorganic substances by photosynthesis or chemosynthesis. Primary productivity is expressed in grams of carbon bound into organic material per square meter of ocean surface area per year: $gC/m^2/yr$. The immediate organic material produced is the carbohydrate glucose, and dissolved CO_2 provides carbon for the glucose.

A *nutrient* is a compound required for an organism to produce organic matter. Some nutrients help form the structural parts of organisms, some make up the chemicals that directly manipulate energy, and some have other functions. A few of these necessary nutrients are always present in seawater, but most are not readily available.

The main inorganic nutrients required for primary productivity include nitrogen (as nitrate) and phosphorus (as phosphate). As any gardener knows, plants require fertilizer, mainly nitrates and phosphates, to grow. Ocean gardeners have more trouble raising crops than do their terrestrial counterparts, because the most fertile ocean water contains only about 0.0001 of the available nitrogen of topsoil. Phosphorus is even more scarce in the ocean, but fortunately, living things need less of it, because they have only about 1 atom of phosphorus for every 16 atoms of nitrogen.

Nitrogen and phosphorus are often depleted by autotrophs during times of high productivity and rapid reproduction. Also in short supply during rapid growth are dissolved silicates (used for shells and other hard parts) and trace elements such as iron and copper (used in enzymes, vitamins, and other large molecules). Marine plants must recycle these nutrients.

On land, most photosynthesis proceeds at or just above ground level. However, seawater, unlike soil, is relatively transparent, which allows photosynthesis to proceed for some distance below the ocean surface. At the same time, incoming sunlight must run a gauntlet of difficulties before it can be absorbed by chlorophyll in marine autotrophs.

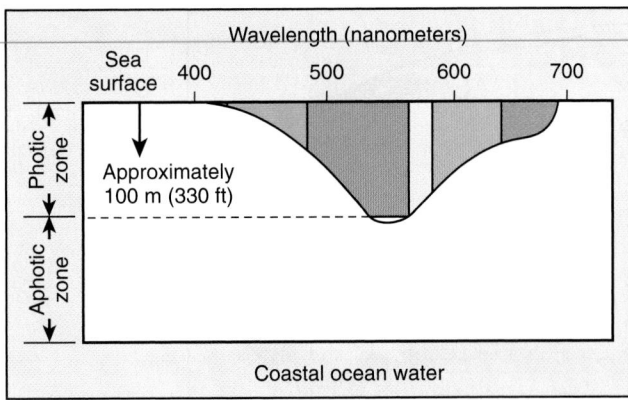

FIGURE 123-6 Because of the suspended particles often present in coastal waters, light cannot penetrate very far; approximately 100 m (330 feet) is typical. The sunlit upper zone is called the *photic zone,* and the dark ocean beneath is called the *aphotic zone.*

Most sunlight approaching at a low angle (e.g., near sunrise or sunset, in the polar regions) reflects off the water surface and does not enter the ocean. Light that penetrates the surface is selectively absorbed; water is more transparent to some colors of light than to others. In clear water, blue light penetrates to the greatest depth, whereas red light is absorbed near the surface. Light energy absorbed by water turns to heat.

The number and characteristics of particles in the water also limit the depth to which light penetrates. These particles—which may include suspended sediments, dust-like bits of once-living tissue, or the organisms themselves—scatter and absorb light. High concentrations of particles quickly absorb most blue and ultraviolet light. This absorption, in combination with the reflection of green light by chlorophyll within the producers, changes the color of productive coastal waters to green.

How far down does light penetrate? Figure 123-6 shows the depths reached by light of various wavelengths (i.e., colors) in the ocean. The *photic zone* is the uppermost layer of seawater lit by the sun. Because of the abundant small organisms and light-scattering particles, the photic zone near the coasts usually extends to about 100 m (330 feet), and in midlatitude waters it reaches down to about 150 m (500 feet). In clear tropical waters in the open ocean, instruments much more sensitive than human eyes have detected light at much greater depths; the present record is 590 m (1935 feet) in the tropical Pacific. The *aphotic zone,* the permanently dark layer of seawater beneath the photic zone, extends below the sunlit surface to the seabed. The vast bulk of the ocean is never brightened by sunlight.

Photosynthesis proceeds slowly at low light levels. Most of the biologic productivity of the ocean occurs in the upper part of the photic zone called the *euphotic zone* (Greek *eu,* "good"). This is the zone in which marine autotrophs can capture enough sunlight energy for plant primary production by photosynthesis to exceed the loss of carbohydrates by respiration. Although it is difficult to generalize about the ocean as a whole, the euphotic zone typically extends to a depth of approximately 70 m (230 feet) in the midlatitudes (as averaged over an entire year). The upper productive layer of ocean is a very thin skin indeed; the water within this zone amounts to less than 1% of world ocean volume, yet almost all marine life depends on this fine, illuminated band.

Phytoplankton, which are minute drifting photosynthetic organisms, produce between 90% and 96% of the surface ocean's carbohydrates. Seaweeds, which are larger marine photosynthesizers, contribute only 2% to 5% of the ocean's primary productivity. Chemosynthetic organisms probably account for 2% to 5% of the total primary productivity in the water column. Although estimates vary widely, recent studies suggest that total ocean productivity ranges from 75 to 150 gC/m²/yr. For comparison, a well-tended alfalfa field produces about 1600 gC/m²/yr.

How does marine productivity compare with terrestrial productivity? Recent research suggests the global net productivity in marine ecosystems is 35 to 50 billion metric tons of carbon bound into carbohydrates per year; global terrestrial productivity is roughly similar at 50 to 70 billion metric tons per year. However, the total producer biomass (i.e., the mass of living tissue) in the ocean is only 1 to 2 billion metric tons, compared with 600 to 1000 billion metric tons of living biomass on land. As the rapid turnover time indicates, nutrients cycle from producer to consumer and back much more quickly in marine ecosystems.

A primary producer's mass is assumed to be about 10 times the mass of the carbon it has bound into carbohydrates. Thus, a primary productivity of 100 gC/m²/yr represents the yearly growth of about 1000 grams from primary producers for each square meter of ocean surface. Since 35 to 50 billion metric tons of carbon are bound into carbohydrates in the ocean each year, between 350 and 500 billion metric tons of marine plants and plantlike organisms are produced annually. Each year, the producers' metabolic activity and the consumers that graze on them consume this vast bulk. The component atoms are then reassembled by photosynthesis into carbohydrates in a continuous solar-powered cycle.

The extent of primary productivity by chemosynthesis within the seabed itself has been a surprise to researchers. High bacterial populations are present in some marine sediments to a depth of hundreds of meters. Samples have been taken at 842 m (2762 feet) below the seafloor in sediments 14 million years old. These bacteria are thriving in extreme conditions at these depths; they have high diversity and are well adapted to life in the subsurface. In fact, a single gram of rock may harbor 10 million bacteria.

These specialized organisms are usually called *extremophiles,* because they are capable of life under extreme conditions (Figure 123-7). Bacteria and similar organisms known as *archaea* have been found in fractured rocks more than 3 km (1.8 miles) below the surface of Africa at the same depth. As with bacteria, a single gram of rock may harbor 10 million archaea. Specialized organisms have been seen in hot oil reservoirs below the North Sea and the North Slope of Alaska (where they cause oil to "sour") and in volcanic rock 1220 m (4000 feet) below the surface of the island of Hawaii. Bacterial biomass in sediments and solid rock

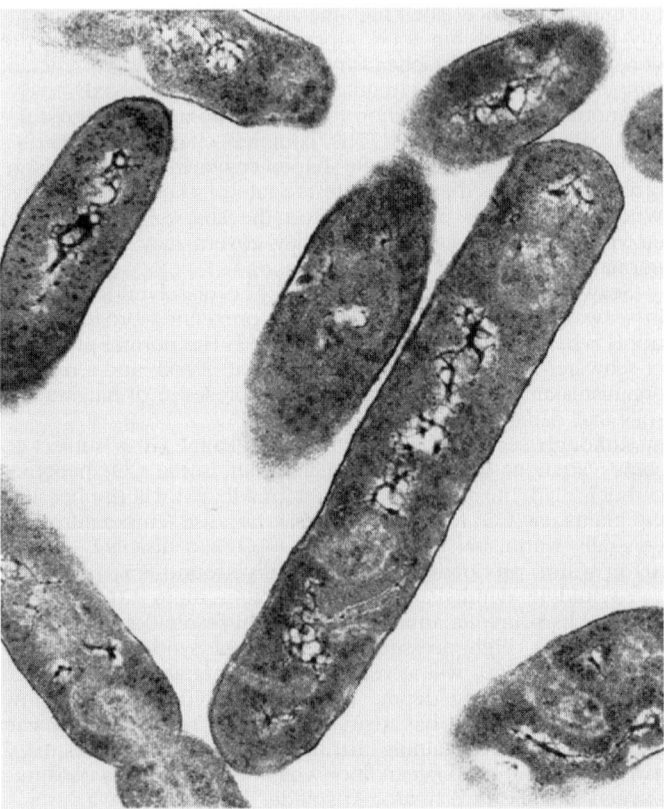

© 2007 Thomson Higher Education

FIGURE 123-7 Deep-living chemosynthetic bacteria cultured from the minute spaces between mineral crystals in solid rock.

may represent at least 10% of the total known Earth surface biomass (although more than a few biologists believe this estimate to be low by at least an order of magnitude). Some of these organisms can tolerate the extreme temperatures found at hydrothermal vents.

Photosynthetic and chemosynthetic organisms can be called either *primary producers* or *autotrophs,* because they make their own food. The bodies of autotrophs are rich sources of chemical energy for any organisms capable of consuming them. *Heterotrophs* are organisms such as animals that must consume food from other organisms because they are unable to synthesize their own food molecules. Some heterotrophs consume autotrophs, and some consume other heterotrophs.

We can label organisms by their positions in a "who eats whom" feeding hierarchy called a *trophic pyramid.* The primary producers at the bottom of a trophic pyramid are mostly chlorophyll-containing photosynthesizers. The animal heterotrophs that eat them are called *primary consumers* or *herbivores;* the animals that eat these primary consumers are called *secondary consumers,* and so on, to the *top consumer* or *top carnivore.*

The mass of consumers becomes smaller as energy flows toward the top of the pyramid. In other words, there are many small primary producers at the base and very few large top consumers at the apex. Only about 10% of the energy from the organisms consumed is stored in the consumers as flesh, so each level is about one-tenth the mass of the level directly below. The rest of the energy is lost as waste heat as organisms live and work to maintain themselves.

Pyramid constructs can lead to the misconception that one type of fish eats only one other type of fish (and so on). Real communities are more accurately described as *food webs;* these are groups of organisms linked by complex feeding relationships in which the flow of energy can be followed from primary producers through consumers. Organisms in a food web almost always have some choices of food species.

IMPORTANT PLANKTONIC AUTOTROPHS

Autotrophic plankton that generate glucose by photosynthesis are generally called *phytoplankton* (Greek *phyton,* "plant"). A huge and nearly invisible mass of phytoplankton drifts within the euphotic zone, which is the productive sunlit surface layer of the world ocean. Although the water within the euphotic zone amounts to less than 2% of world ocean volume, most pelagic marine life depends on this fine, illuminated band.

There are at least eight major types of phytoplankton, the most prominent being the diatoms and dinoflagellates. As noted earlier, recent research suggests that very small producers, most of which are forms of cyanobacteria and archaea, may be responsible for much more oceanic primary productivity than are their larger and better-known counterparts.

Apart from cyanobacteria, the most productive photosynthetic organisms in the plankton are the diatoms. *Diatoms* evolved comparatively recently and began to dominate phytoplanktonic productivity during the Cretaceous Period, about 100 million years ago. Their abundance and photosynthetic efficiency increased the proportion of free oxygen in Earth's atmosphere. More than 5600 species of diatoms are known to exist. The larger species are barely visible to the unaided eye. Most are round, but some are elongated, branched, or triangular (Figure 123-8).

For more effective light absorption, *chlorophyll,* which is the main photosynthetic pigment, is accompanied in diatoms by accessory pigments. These yellow or brown pigments give most diatoms a yellow-green or tan appearance. Diatoms store energy as fatty acids and oils, which are compounds that are lighter than their equivalent volume of water and assist with flotation. Buoyancy is a potential problem for diatoms because the weight of their heavy silica frustule seems at odds with their need to stay near the sunlit ocean surface. Oil floats, glass sinks, and a balanced amount of both reduces cell density and lightens the load. Not all diatoms, however, need to float. Many nonplanktonic species lie on shallow bottoms, where light and nutrients are

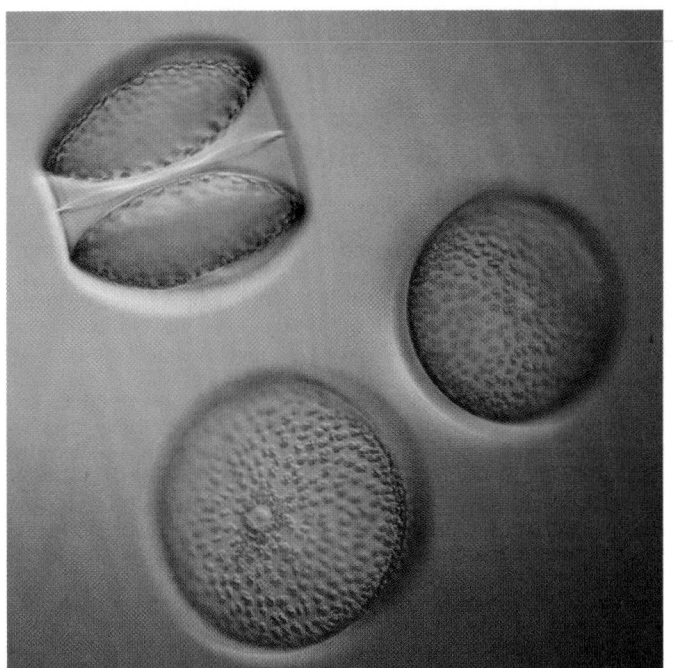

FIGURE 123-8 Diatoms of the genus *Coscinodiscus.* One is shown reproducing.

able to support photosynthesis. These benthic species are almost always elongated (pennate) in shape.

Like diatoms, *dinoflagellates* are single-celled autotrophs (Figure 123-9). Dinoflagellates are not as productive as diatoms, and they appear to have evolved much earlier. A few species live within the tissues of other organisms (e.g., the zooxanthellae of coral animals), but the majority of dinoflagellates live free in the water. Most have two whip-like flagella in channels grooved in their protective outer cell wall of cellulose. One flagellum drives the organism forward, whereas the other causes it to rotate in the water; thus the name, derived from the Greek word *dino,* meaning "whirling," and the Latin *flagellum,* "whip." These flagella allow dinoflagellates to adjust their orientation and vertical position to make the best photosynthetic use of available light or to move vertically in the water column to obtain nutrients.

Dinoflagellates are widely distributed, solitary organisms that reproduce by simple fission; they rarely form colonies. During reproduction, the cellulose covering that surrounds most species splits, and the single cell divides in half. Each daughter cell subsequently replaces the missing portion of covering. Under favorable conditions, the organisms can reproduce once a day, growing in number but not in size.

Some species of dinoflagellates can become so numerous that the water turns rusty red because light is reflecting from the accessory pigments within each cell. These species are usually responsible for the phenomenon referred to as a *red tide,* or

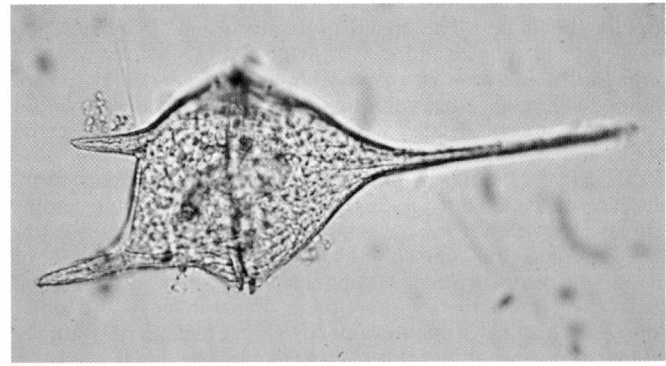

FIGURE 123-9 A dinoflagellate of the genus *Ceratium. (Courtesy Tom Garrison.)*

more generally, as a *harmful algal bloom* (HAB). During times of such rapid growth, which is usually in the spring, the concentration of microscopic planktonic organisms may briefly reach 6 to 8 million per liter.

HARMFUL ALGAL BLOOMS

An HAB occurs when high concentrations of phytoplankton adversely affect the physiology of nearby organisms. HABs do not always turn water red, and the organisms that cause them are not always visible. A number of factors are thought to contribute to HABs, including warm surface temperature, reduced salinity, optimal nutrient and light conditions, and a mechanism (e.g., gentle onshore winds) that physically concentrates the dinoflagellates.

Although the dinoflagellates responsible for most red tides are comparatively simple organisms, some have the ability to synthesize potent toxins as byproducts of metabolism. Among the most effective poisons known, these toxins may affect nearby marine life if ingested, or may even indirectly poison humans through the food chain. Some of the toxins are similar in chemical structure to the muscle relaxant curare, but much more potent (see Chapter 77).

The number and severity of HABs appear to be increasing. Perhaps this is not surprising; coastal waters receive industrial, agricultural, and domestic wastes, rich in nitrogen and other plant nutrients that stimulate algal growth. In addition, the long-distance transport of algal species in the ballast water of cargo vessels can introduce alien species into coastal waters, where they may thrive in the absence of the organisms that naturally consume them. Australia has recently issued strict guidelines for discharging ballast in the country's ports.

BIOGEOCHEMICAL CYCLES

The atoms and small molecules that make up the biochemicals—and thus the bodies—of organisms move between the living and nonliving realms in biogeochemical cycles. Living organisms are supported and sustained by huge, nonliving chemical reserves, and there is large-scale transport of elements between the reserves and the organisms themselves. Sometimes the environment contains enough of a required element to sustain life; sometimes the element is in short supply and is thus limiting. The tropical and temperate ocean is usually highly stratified, with a warm, less dense layer of water (the mixed zone) separated from the cold, dense, deep zone by a strong pycnocline. In the surface mixed layer, the atoms and small molecules that make up the bodies of organisms may cycle rapidly for a time among predators, prey, scavengers, and decomposers. When these organisms die, their bodies can sink below the sunlit upper sea and pycnocline to become isolated from the rapid biologic activity of the surface. Regions of upwelling are critical to returning these substances to the surface, if only for a short reprieve, before their eventual incorporation into deep sediments, from which only the very slow progress of tectonic cycles will liberate them.

As you read about the biogeochemical cycles described later in this chapter, remember that the elements and small molecules forming the tissues of an organism are always on the move. They may cycle rapidly in and out of living things, or they may be trapped in Earth for vast spans of time. However, the nature of the cycles dictates what will live where, which creatures will be successful, and ultimately, what will be the composition of the ocean and atmosphere.

The largest biogeochemical cycle is the global carbon cycle. Because of its ability to form long chains to which other atoms can attach, carbon is the basic building block of all life on Earth. Carbon enters the atmosphere as CO_2 through respiration of living organisms, volcanic eruptions that release carbon from rocks deep in Earth's crust, burning of fossil fuels, and other sources. When levels of atmospheric CO_2 are high, Earth's surface temperature rises as a result of the greenhouse effect.

Large and small plants and plantlike organisms capture sunlight and use this energy to incorporate, or fix, CO_2 into organic molecules. Some of these molecules are used as food, and some become structural components. When an animal eats a plant or plantlike organism, the carbon can do one of the following: (1) be incorporated into the animal's body for growth; (2) be respired by the animal (i.e., taken apart to harvest the energy); or (3) be excreted back into the seawater as what is called *dissolved organic carbon* (DOC). Typically, about 45% of the carbon from an ingested plant is used for growth, 45% is used for respiration, and 10% is lost as DOC. The end product of respiration is CO_2, a gas eventually lost to the atmosphere. Most of the DOC is rapidly used by bacteria, which are in turn eaten by protozoa, which are eaten by zooplankton, which are then eaten by fish; this is called the *microbial loop*. Eventually, the organisms (or at least their hard parts, containing calcium carbonate) sink below the mixed layer and begin the long fall toward the seabed. Most of the carbon in this calcium carbonate is turned into CO_2 by bacteria long before it hits the bottom, but a small percentage (<1%) reaches the sediments and is buried. The carbonate sediments can be uplifted over geologic time and weathered so that the carbon is eventually returned to the biologically active upper sea.

Because of the large amount of CO_2 available in the ocean, and because CO_2 from the atmosphere dissolves readily in seawater, marine organisms almost never suffer from a deficit of available carbon. For life in the sea, the critical bottlenecks lie elsewhere, mainly in the nitrogen, phosphorus, and iron cycles.

Nitrogen is a critical component of proteins, chlorophyll, and nucleic acids. Like carbon, nitrogen may be found in the bodies of organisms, as a dissolved gas, and as dissolved organic matter known as *dissolved organic nitrogen*.

One might think nitrogen would be abundantly available in the ocean, because nitrogen accounts for 48% of the dissolved gas in seawater by volume. However, most organisms cannot use free nitrogen in the atmosphere and ocean directly. It must first be bound with oxygen or hydrogen, or *fixed*, to usable chemical forms by specialized organisms, usually bacteria or cyanobacteria. Thus, oceanic regions are frequently nitrogen limited; growth of plants and plantlike organisms is often held back by lack of available nitrogen.

Forms of nitrogen available for uptake by living things are ammonium and nitrate, an ion formed by oxidation of ammonium and nitrite. Nitrate runoff from soil is an especially rich source of this often limiting nutrient, which explains why coastal water tends to support greater plankton populations than does oceanic water. Nitrogen is assimilated by small plants and plantlike organisms and then recycled as animals excrete ammonium and urea. These reduced forms of nitrogen are then oxidized back into nitrate, through nitrite, by nitrifying bacteria. In the deep ocean, most nitrogen is in the form of nitrate. In anoxic sediments and certain low-oxygen regions of the ocean, denitrifying bacteria use nitrate in respiration and convert nitrate back to nitrite and nitrogen gas, which is lost to the atmosphere. The other major loss occurs when nitrogen-containing organisms and debris are buried in ocean sediments.

Iron is used in minute quantities in the reactions of photosynthesis, in certain enzymes crucial to nitrogen fixation, and in the structure of proteins. Other essential trace metals, such as zinc, copper, and manganese, are also used by organisms in small quantities, primarily in enzymes. Although in absolute terms, organisms require only tiny quantities of iron, the concentration of iron in seawater relative to the concentration of nutrients, such as nitrogen and phosphorus, can sometimes be so low that phytoplankton growth is limited by the availability of iron. Although iron is one of the most abundant elements in Earth's crust, it is nearly insoluble in oxygenated seawater, and the little dissolved iron that is present is highly reactive, sticks to falling particles, and sinks to the bottom of the water column.

In general, the biogeochemical cycles of the trace metals follow the pattern of uptake and recycling in the surface ocean and regeneration, sometimes over long periods of time, at depth. However, much remains to be learned about the interactions between living organisms and trace metals. Iron and other trace metals exist in many chemical forms in seawater. Discovering what these forms are, how transformation between forms occurs, and availability of different forms to marine organisms are major foci of current research in trace metal biochemistry.

MARINE ENVIRONMENTAL ISSUES

Human demand has exceeded Earth's ability to regenerate resources since at least the early 1980s. Since 1961, human demand on Earth's organisms and raw materials has more than doubled and now exceeds Earth's natural replacement capacity by at least 20%. Our present rate of consumption is clearly unsustainable. The ocean's great volume and relentless motion dissipate and distribute natural and synthetic substances. For this reason, humans have long used the sea as a dump for wastes. The ocean's ability to absorb is not inexhaustible, however, and the ocean is being severely affected by human activity.

A *pollutant* causes damage by interfering directly or indirectly with the mechanical or biochemical processes of an organism. Many pollutants are harmful to human health. Some pollution-induced changes may be instantly lethal; other changes may weaken an organism over weeks or months, alter the dynamics of the population of which it is a part, or gradually unbalance the entire community.

An organism's response to a particular pollutant depends on its sensitivity to the combination of *quantity* and *toxicity* of that pollutant. Some pollutants are toxic to organisms in tiny concentrations. For example, photosynthetic ability of some species of diatoms is diminished when chlorinated hydrocarbon compounds are present in parts-per-trillion quantities. Other pollutants may seem harmless, as when fertilizers flowing from agricultural land stimulate plant growth in estuaries. However, these pollutants may be hazardous to certain organisms but not others. For example, crude oil interferes with the delicate feeding structures of zooplankton and coats the feathers of birds, but simultaneously serves as a feast for certain bacteria.

Pollutants also vary in their *persistence*; some reside in the environment for thousands of years, whereas others last only minutes. Pollutants may break down into harmless substances spontaneously or through physical processes (e.g., shattering of large molecules by sunlight). Sometimes pollutants are removed from the environment through biologic activity. For example, some marine organisms escape permanent damage by metabolizing hazardous substances to harmless ones. Indeed, many pollutants are ultimately biodegradable; that is, they can be broken down by natural processes into simpler compounds. However, many pollutants resist attack by water, air, sunlight, or living organisms, because the synthetic compounds of which they are composed resemble nothing in nature.

Determining the ways in which pollutants are changing the ocean and the atmosphere is often difficult for researchers. Environmental impact cannot always be predicted or explained. As a result, marine scientists vary widely in their opinions about what pollutants are doing to the ocean and atmosphere and what to do about it. Environmental issues are frequently emotional, and media reports tend to sensationalize short-term incidents (e.g., oil spills) rather than more serious, long-term problems (e.g., climate change, effects of long-lived chlorinated hydrocarbon compounds). Figure 123-10 summarizes sources of marine pollution.

OIL POLLUTION

Public perception equates marine pollution with oil spills. Oil is a natural part of the marine environment. Oil seeps have been leaking large quantities of oil into the sea for millions of years; indeed, natural seeps are the largest source of oil in the ocean. The amount of oil entering the sea has increased in recent years, however, because of our growing dependence on marine transportation for petroleum products, offshore drilling, nearshore refining, and street runoff carrying waste oil from automobiles.

The world's accelerating thirst for oil is currently running at about 3800 L *per second*, slightly more than half of which is transported to market in large tankers. In the 1990s, approximately 1.3 million metric tons of oil entered the world ocean

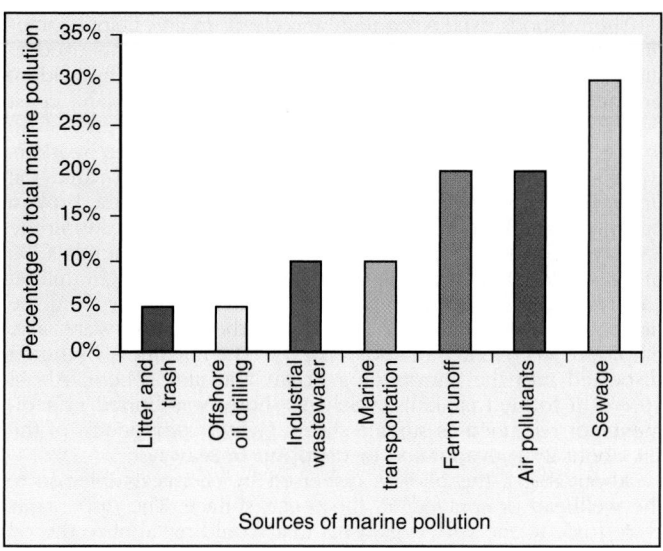

FIGURE 123-10 Sources of marine pollution. *(Data from Garrison, T: Oceanography: An invitation to marine science, 8th ed, Independence, Ky, 2013, Cengage Learning.)*

each year. Natural seeps accounted for almost half this annual input, or 600,000 metric tons. About 8% of the total was associated with marine transportation. Some of this oil was not spilled in well-publicized tanker accidents but was released during loading, discharging, and flushing of tanker ships. Between 150,000 and 450,000 marine birds are believed to be killed each year by oil released from tankers.

Much more oil reaches the ocean in runoff from city streets, or as waste oil dumped down drains, poured into dirt, or hidden in trash destined for a landfill. Each year, more than 900 million liters (about 240 million gallons) of used motor oil—about eight times the volume of the 2010 Gulf of Mexico spill—finds its way to the sea. This used oil is much more toxic than crude oil because it has developed carcinogenic and metallic components from the heat and pressure within internal combustion engines. Not all hydrocarbon pollution is "wet." Aromatic compounds released when crude oil evaporates eventually find their way back into the ocean.

Spills of *crude* oil are generally larger in volume and more frequent than spills of refined oil. Most components of crude oil do not dissolve easily in water, but those that do can harm the delicate juvenile forms of marine organisms, even in minute concentrations. The remaining insoluble components form sticky layers on the surface that prevent free diffusion of gases, clog feeding structures in adult organisms, kill larvae, and decrease sunlight available for photosynthesis. Crude oil is ultimately biodegradable. Although crude oil spills look terrible and generate great media attention, most forms of marine life in an area recover from the effects of a moderate spill within about 5 years.

Spills of *refined* oil, especially near shore where marine life is abundant, can be more disruptive for longer periods. The refining process removes and breaks up the heavier components of crude oil and concentrates the remaining lighter, more biologically active ones. Components added to oil during the refining process also make it more toxic. Spills of refined oil are of growing concern because the amount of refined oil transported to the United States rose dramatically through the 1980s and 1990s.

The volatile components of any oil spill eventually evaporate into the air, leaving the heavier tars behind. Wave action causes the tar to form into balls of varying sizes. Some of the tar balls fall to the bottom, where they may be assimilated by bottom organisms or incorporated into sediments. Bacteria eventually decompose these spheres, but the process may take years to complete, especially in cold polar waters. This oil residue, especially if derived from refined oil, can have long-lasting effects on seafloor communities.

The methods used to contain and clean up an oil spill sometimes cause more damage than the oil itself. Detergents used to disperse oil are especially harmful to living things. An accident on the *Deepwater Horizon* oil platform off the Louisiana coast on 20 April 2010 resulted in the largest accidental release of oil in the history of the U.S. petroleum industry. Eleven workers were killed, 17 injured, and the rig itself failed and sank. Oil under high geologic pressure shot from the stump of the broken drill pipe. The best estimate of the total release of oil during the 85 days required to plug the well is 4.9 million barrels (206 million gallons) of crude oil, of which 800,000 barrels (33 million gallons, about 16%) were captured by direct recovery from the drill head. Skimming and burning at the surface were also employed, recovering an additional 8%. The remainder of the oil dispersed into the surrounding ocean and atmosphere. About 26% of it formed tar balls, washed ashore, was buried in sediments, or remained as surface sheen. Lighter components of the oil, about 25%, evaporated or dissolved in seawater.

About 8% of the oil was dispersed by chemicals injected at the wellhead or sprayed on the ocean surface. The dispersants were toxic to the very organisms that would metabolize the oil naturally. A vast amount of dispersant, mostly the chemical Corexit, was deployed; estimates suggest that 2 million gallons were sprayed over the water or injected directly into the gushing wellhead on the seafloor. When mixed with the dispersant, oil that would normally float was able to linger far below the surface and affect fishes and bottom-dwelling organisms. Research continues, but it has been suggested the dispersed oil was more likely to be toxic than the crude oil by itself.

The best way to deal with oil pollution is to prevent it from happening. Tanker design is being modified to limit the amount of oil intentionally released in transport. Oil companies limit new tanker construction to stronger, double-hull designs, and platforms to contain redundant fail-safe components. During the past decade, improved production technology and safety training of personnel have significantly reduced both blowouts and daily operational spills. Currently, accidental spills from platforms represent about 1% of petroleum discharged in North American waters and about 3% worldwide.

PLASTIC WASTE

Plastic waste is another serious and growing problem. Approximately 134 million metric tons of plastic are produced each year, of which 10% ends up in the ocean. Americans use more plastic per person than any other nationality. Americans generate about 31 million metric tons of plastic waste, about 120 kg (264 lb) per person, each year. They consume an average of 167 plastic bottles of water per person per year—about 25 million per hour!

Slightly more than 4% of world oil production goes into the manufacture of plastics.

The attributes that make plastic items useful to consumers—durability and stability—make them a problem in marine environments. Scientists estimate that certain forms of synthetic materials, such as plastic six-pack holders, will not completely decompose for 400 years. Although oil spills receive more attention as a potential environmental threat, plastic is a much more serious danger. Oil is harmful, but plastic does not biodegrade.

The problem is not confined to the coasts. The North Pacific subtropical gyre covers a large area of the Pacific where the water slowly circulates in a clockwise direction. Winds are light. The currents tend to move any floating material into the low-energy center of the gyre. There are few islands on which this floating material can beach, so it remains in the gyre. This area, about the size of Texas, has been dubbed the "Eastern Pacific Garbage Patch." A smaller, western Pacific equivalent has formed midway between San Francisco and Hawaii; another lies off the U.S. East Coast. One researcher estimates the weight of the debris trapped in gyres to be about 3 million metric tons, comparable to 1 year's deposition at Los Angeles's largest landfill.

Hundreds of marine mammals and thousands of seabirds die each year after ingesting or being caught in plastic debris. Sea turtles mistake plastic bags for jellyfish prey and die from intestinal blockages. Seals and sea lions starve after becoming entangled in nets or muzzled by six-pack rings. The same rings strangle fish and seabirds. About one-quarter million Laysan albatross chicks die each year when their parents feed them bits of plastic instead of food (see Figure 123-10).

Plankton productivity is adversely affected by plastics. Sunlight, wave action, and mechanical abrasion break plastic into ever smaller particles. This microfine plastic debris tends to attract oily toxic residues such as polychlorinated biphenyls, dioxin, brominated flame retardants, and other noxious organic chemicals. In the middle of the Pacific Ocean, 1 million times the amount of toxins are concentrated on the plastic debris and plastic particles (e.g., microbeads used in mildly abrasive skin cleaners) than are estimated to reside in ambient sea water. The microscopic plastic particles outweighed zooplankton by six times in water taken from the North Pacific subtropical gyre. Filter-feeding zooplankton mistake plastic particles for food, and the attendant synthetic chemicals may be interfering with aspects of phytoplankton physiology.

Not all plastic floats. About 70% of discarded plastic sinks to the ocean bottom. In the North Sea, Dutch scientists have counted 110 pieces of litter for every square kilometer of seabed, or about 600,000 metric tons in the North Sea alone. These plastics can smother benthic life-forms.

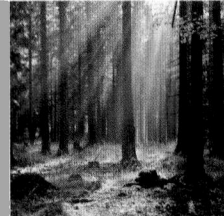

CHAPTER 124
Brief Introduction to Forestry

DONALD L. GREBNER AND PETE BETTINGER

Although forests have provided material, safety, and welfare for thousands of years, only in the last 100 years have humans begun to manage forests carefully. Early humans used forests as a source of shelter and products to sustain primitive communities. More recently, humans have used forests to develop modern economies. For most of human history, humans have only minimally impacted forested resources, largely because of low and widely dispersed population densities. More recently, human populations have expanded dramatically, leading to increased interactions between people and forested landscapes.

When the first European colonists arrived at the eastern seaboard of North America, settlers could only marvel at the immensity of the forested landscape.[6] For centuries, it seemed as if this resource had no limit and could never be depleted. Humans entered the forest and extracted material to build houses, hunted game to provide food, and used wood to support smelting of iron ore.[8] Settlers converted forested lands to develop agricultural fields to produce crops, which were used to feed themselves and expand communities. A culture of sustainability was not inherent.

Forested landscapes may pose risks to people as they travel in and around them. These landscapes can be flat or steep, wet or dry, and densely vegetative or sparsely covered. Types of birds, mammals, insects, reptiles and amphibians, and fish found in forests vary depending on latitude, elevation, and physiographic features. Size and shape of water bodies found within forested landscapes vary greatly, from small ponds to large lakes, and from seasonal streams that only flow at certain times of the year to swift rivers carrying melted-snow water from mountainous peaks. The landscapes vary depending on location, which can be extremely important in case of medical emergencies and search and rescue operations. Landowners and land managers who care for these landscapes can have important impacts on risks assumed by visitors. Small, private forest landowners, as well as larger industrial landowners, typically have easy access to their properties. However, in certain areas, particularly in the eastern part of North America, access to these lands is often restricted. State, province, and county governments that control public forests typically allow unimpeded access, as do national forests and parks. Many privately owned forested areas in Scandinavia allow free public access. Larger forests in less densely populated and remote areas often have poorer access characteristics (e.g., roads may not be well maintained), which can pose critical challenges to search and rescue teams as well as to medical evacuation.

DEFINITIONS

FORESTRY

Forestry involves management of forests to meet economic, ecologic, or social goals. Early references to the term *Forstwesen*, which is similar to "forestry," can be traced to Europe in the early to mid-19th century, in association with publications such as the *Swiss Forestry Journal* (now called *Schweizerische Zeitschrift fur Forstwesen*). Forestry as a profession began in Europe during the Middle Ages, when royalty was interested in controlling which persons hunted wildlife on crown lands.[2] In Germany, exclusive hunting rights in forests were provided to nobility from the ninth through the 18th centuries.[5] Given humankind's long-term use of forests to locate food, it was an important task for foresters to conserve a sufficient supply of animals for their countries' inhabitants (in particular their nobles) to hunt. At present, perceptions of forests are much different. In some countries (e.g., Scotland), forestry practice outcomes are now among the lowest environmental concerns of local societies (i.e., when compared to treatment of human waste or nuclear technology), but forest practices remain important social concerns with respect to climate change.[4]

In Europe, the transition from managing forests as wildlife habitat to timber production preceded that within the United States. This transition did not begin in the United States until the middle to later 1800s. Early European settlers viewed the North American forested landscape as endless and placed little emphasis on resource management. Attention focused on resource extraction, as was pursued with nonrenewable resources (e.g., coal, petroleum). Early American foresters trained in Europe, such as Bernhard Fernow (Prussia) and Gifford Pinchot (France), led the way in developing the profession of forestry in the United States. Pinchot was instrumental in founding the Society of American Foresters (SAF).

The Dictionary of Forestry (http://dictionary of forestry.org) of the SAF defines *forestry* as "the profession embracing the science, art, and practice of creating, managing, using, and conserving forests and associated resources for human benefit and in a sustainable manner to meet desired goals, needs, and values."[3] This definition has changed over time, becoming more complex with increased recognition of the benefits, not previously

considered, that forests provide to individuals as well as to human society.

During the late 1800s and early 1900s, there were growing concerns about excessive harvesting of trees from forested landscapes. This contributed to development of scientific forestry as well as efforts to establish a national park system that focused on protection of "wild" forested landscapes. These events led to debate over whether public forests should be "conserved" and managed for human needs, or whether they should be "preserved" and managed to minimize human interaction with their innate resources. Advocates of the "conservation" perspective included Pinchot, and advocates of the "preservation" perspective included John Muir. Debate over management of forests is ongoing. Whether forest are managed or preserved can have significant implications for structure and health of a forested landscape, as well as for how people interact with the forest.

For much of the 1900s, forestry schools taught students such skills as how to manage a forest, focusing on extraction of wood, how to reforest cutover areas, and how to implement fire protection strategies. During the early phases of the forestry profession's development, American society was largely agrarian in nature. Since that time, more than 85% of the U.S. population now resides in an urban environment. This dramatic change in U.S. demographics has important implications for how people view forests and forested landscapes. These changes have also impacted how foresters and other natural resource professionals manage forested landscapes and ecosystems, for what are often competing uses.

FOREST

What defines a forest can vary depending on standards set by societies, as well as the perspective of individuals or organizations tasked with managing them. For some, any area that contains trees can be viewed as a forest. For others, a stand of trees at the north end of their cornfield is simply considered a woodlot, not a forest. The size of a forest can play a critical role in shaping one's perspective on what is or is not a forested landscape. Some forests can be 100 acres, about 40 hectares (ha), whereas others can be 100,000 acres (~40,470 ha) or even as large as a 1 million acres (~404,700 ha). The SAF dictionary defines a forest as "an ecosystem characterized by a more or less dense and extensive tree cover, often consisting of stands varying in characteristics such as species composition, structure, age class, and associated process, and commonly including meadows, streams, fish and wildlife."[3]

The U.S. Forest Service[7] uses a different definition, as found in its Forest Inventory and Analysis (FIA) program:

Land that is at least 10 percent stocked with trees of any size, or that formerly had such tree cover and is not currently developed for a nonforest use. The minimum area for classification of forest land is one acre. The components that make up forest land and all noncommercial forest land.

This definition is consistent with that used by the Food and Agriculture Organization (FAO) of the United Nations[1]:

Land with tree crown cover (or equivalent stocking level) of more than 10 percent and area of more than 0.5 hectares (ha). The trees should be able to reach a minimum height of 5 meters (m) at maturity *in situ*. May consist either of closed forest formations where trees of various stories and undergrowth cover a high proportion of the ground; or open forest formations with a continuous vegetation cover in which tree crown cover exceeds 10 percent. Young natural stands and all plantations established for forestry purposes which have yet to reach a crown density of 10 percent or tree height of 5 m are included under forest, as are areas normally forming part of the forest area which are temporarily unstocked as a result of human intervention or natural causes but which are expected to revert to forest.

The FAO definition is similar to others but is more specific. Forests are basically areas with a number of trees that vary in size and shape. They can include other features (e.g., bodies of water, meadows, open areas) and can accommodate wildlife, insects, and fish. In many cases, humans live there.

A forest's classification as *wilderness* depends on remoteness of a forested area, size of forested area, and presence (or lack of) human structures as well as the presence (or lack of) human activity. Typically, wilderness areas are those where forests are not actively managed. A wilderness can be situated in a forested landscape, but not all wilderness areas are forested areas. Wilderness areas are managed from a "preservationist" perspective, which allows virtually no human interference in ecologic processes occurring on those properties. The SAF forestry dictionary refers to the Wilderness Act of 1964 in its definition of a wilderness area[3]: "A wilderness, in contrast with those areas where man and his works dominate the landscape, is hereby recognized as an area where the earth and its community of life are untrammeled by man, where man himself is a visitor who does not remain."

In the United States, a wilderness area is an area that the U.S. Congress has designated as such, regardless of the land's past use. The Sleeping Bear Dunes is a great example of a recently designated wilderness area. Located along Lake Michigan, the dunes are places where people have often recreated. Others, such as the Sipsey Wilderness Area located within the Bankhead National Forest in northwestern Alabama, are largely devoid of human structures except around their boundaries. The Sipsey Wilderness Area contains one remnant road that is being slowly reclaimed by nature as time passes, and the area hosts a wide collection of diverse plant and animal species, beautiful rock formations, waterfalls, and pristine river ways. It is also a popular hiking and camping destination.

Key differences between wilderness and nonwilderness areas center on the amount of human activity and whether human presence is transitory. Regardless of a forest's official designation, wilderness and nonwilderness forests both have the same attributes. All forests have a distinctive vertical structure of vegetation dominated by trees. In mature forests, trees dominate the *overstory,* the uppermost portion of the forest. This canopy section can be home to different types of wildlife, including birds and insects, as well as mammals such as flying squirrels. Beneath the canopy layer are three other layers of forest. The next level down from the canopy, the *midstory,* comprises trees that are either more shade tolerant or suppressed by the overstory canopy. These trees are shade tolerant and live and grow in lower levels of sunlight. Trees that are shade intolerant require more sunlight and are more likely to be found in the canopy layer. The next layer is called the *understory,* or *shrub layer,* and includes smaller trees as well as shrubs. Not all forests have this layer. Forests with extensive shrub layers can be difficult to navigate. In some parts of the United States, landowners may burn their properties because it makes it easier for them to travel through the forest. Below the shrub layer are found the *herbaceous layer* and *grass layer,* which are located just above the soil. These lower layers provide food and cover to numerous wildlife species. Their presence can depend on sufficient levels of sunlight reaching the forest floor. Not all forest structures are alive. Dead trees, known as "snags," may be standing in the midstory or overstory, and downed logs may be lying on the ground.

Trees and Rainfall

Types of tree species are an important aspect of forests. Which tree species exist in a forest depends not only on region of the world, but also on latitude and other physiographic and climatic factors (e.g., elevation, average local rainfall, average seasonal temperatures). A forest in Maine may be composed of species such as balsam fir (*Abies balsamea*), white spruce (*Picea glauca*), red maple (*Acer rubrum*), sugar maple (*Acer saccharum*), quaking aspen (*Populus tremuloides*), white (paper) birch (*Betula papyrifera*), and American beech (*Fagus grandifolia*). As one moves further south, changes in average annual temperatures prohibit many of these species from being found at lower latitudes or elevations. In Mississippi, a common tree species is loblolly pine (*Pinus taeda*). It can be found throughout the southern United States, but as one moves further north, loblolly pine becomes less common because it is susceptible to damage caused by ice storms.

Rainfall is a crucial factor in determining structure and species composition of a forest. In general, the eastern United States receives more rainfall than does the western part, except along the Pacific Coast. Areas west of the Rocky Mountains (e.g., northern California to Washington) are typically wetter than the eastern sides of the Cascade or Sierra Nevada Ranges. Redwood (*Sequoia sempervirens*) trees in northern California need sea fog for optimal growth, whereas ponderosa pines (*Pinus ponderosa*) are generally found much farther inland and often east of the Cascade or Sierra Nevada Ranges and can thrive in much drier climates.

Factors affecting forest type and structure are important for a variety of reasons. First, abundance of different types of species can impact what can be used for human consumption. Different tree species have different useful properties to humans, animals, and insects. The forest structure can affect who enters the forest and why they would do so. Drier forests tend to possess fewer trees that are more widely spaced. This landscape can be more prone to fire. In addition, drier forests provide fewer opportunities for finding water, which would be important to hikers and campers.

Where substrate (soil) conditions are favorable, and where seeds or seedlings (if planted) are provided, forests will become established. The establishment phase can occur after a natural disaster or following human activity. Many conifers are shade-intolerant trees. Full sunlight (e.g., large openings) may be required to successfully reestablish coniferous forests. Shade-tolerant trees may not require full sunlight for successful reestablishment. If left unattended, forests progress through stages of "succession." In the last stage of forest succession, the *climax stage,* the forest ecosystem perpetuates itself indefinitely through minor changes in forest structure, including individual tree mortality and regrowth of trees in the resulting gaps created. Currently, the climax stage of forests is often not attained because of human intervention.

TYPES OF FORESTS

Forests naturally occur in areas that are conducive to tree growth and are influenced by factors such as latitude, elevation, soil condition, and precipitation. Different environments lead to very different types of forests. The three major forest biomes found around the world are the boreal, temperate, and tropical. Each contains ecosystems with similar climatic characteristics. Boreal and temperate biomes contain forests with trees that become dormant in the winter. Tropical biome contains forests that have a year-long growing cycle.

Boreal forests are found in higher latitudes (e.g., Canada and Russia in northern hemisphere) and mainly contain conifers such as spruces and firs (Figure 124-1). Growing season is generally short, and forests can be located on relatively dry sites (e.g., western Alberta) or wet sites (peat bogs). *Montane* (i.e., high-elevation forests) can be found in the boreal biome or in temperate and tropical biomes. These forests also typically contain conifers; a good example is the dry coniferous forests of the Rocky Mountain range in the intermountain western United States (Figure 124-2). For these forests, elevation influences the amount of precipitation available for trees to grow.

Temperate deciduous forests contain oaks, maples, hickories, and much broader variety of broad-leaved trees that are typically found in the Appalachian Mountains and northeastern part of the United States (Figure 124-3), as well as vast areas of northern Europe. Temperate coniferous forests contain pines or firs; a good example of these are the pine forests along the southeastern U.S. Coastal Plain (Figure 124-4). Between these two forest types and across the eastern U.S. and northern Europe are mixed temperate coniferous and deciduous forests. In the U.S. Pacific Northwest, temperate rain forests contain fir and hemlock trees (Figure 124-5). Precipitation patterns influenced by the Pacific Ocean result in high annual rainfall amounts, and tree growth in this type of forest can be substantial. Throughout California and southern Europe, forests grow in climates that typically have wet winters and long, dry summers. These are often characterized as woodlands, chaparral, or Mediterranean forests (Figure 124-6).

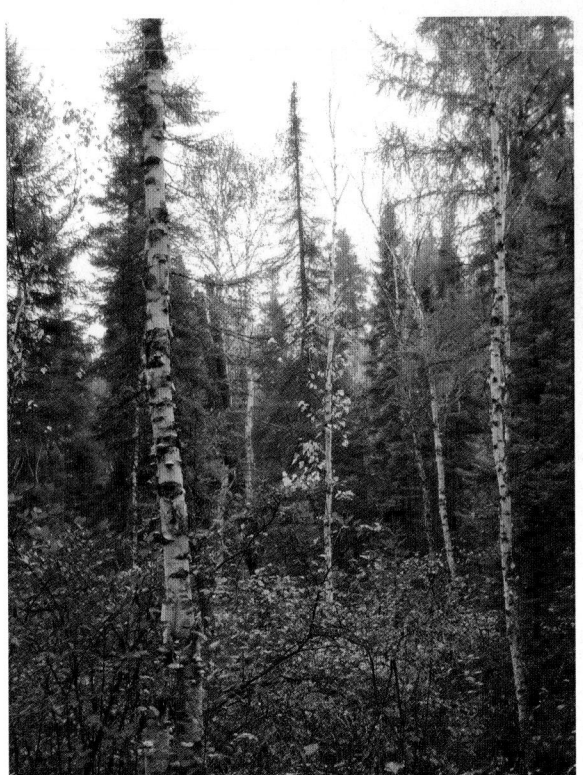

FIGURE 124-1 Boreal forest, northern Minnesota. *(Courtesy Steven Katovich, USDA Forest Service. www.Bugwood.org.)*

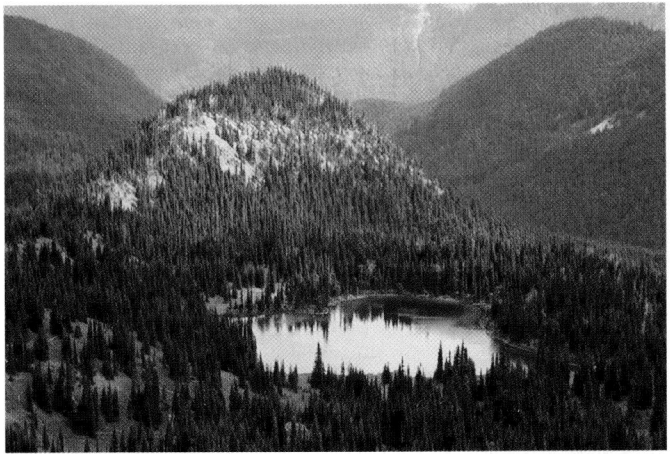

FIGURE 124-2. Montane forest. *(Photo from Wikimedia Commons; courtesy Walter Siegmund.* https://commons.wikimedia.org/wiki/File:Clover_Lake_8556.JPG; *licensing agreement:* https://creativecommons.org/licenses/by-sa/3.0/deed.en.)

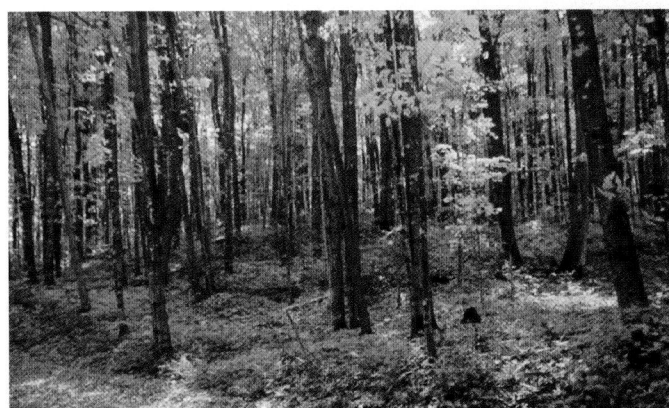

FIGURE 124-3 Temperate deciduous forest, northern United States. *(Courtesy Joseph O'Brien, USDA Forest Service. www.Bugwood.org.)*

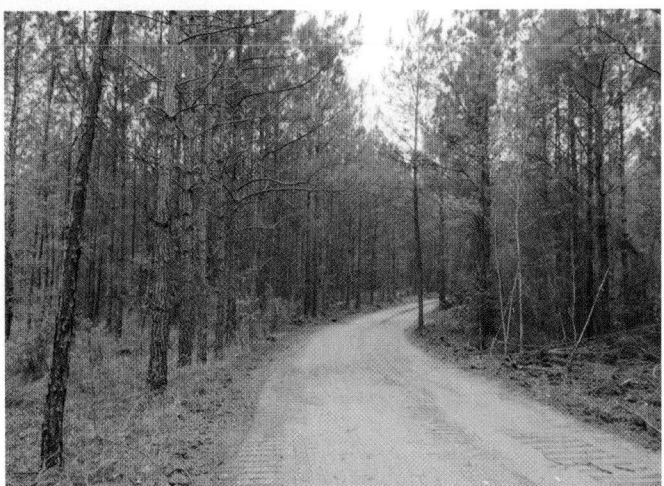

FIGURE 124-4 Temperate pine forest, south Georgia. *(Courtesy Chuck Bargeron, University of Georgia. www.Bugwood.org.)*

Tropical deciduous forests can be found along the east coast of South America and the east coast of India, among other locations. Tropical rain forests are located throughout the Amazon Basin and Central America (Figure 124-7). Precipitation occurs nearly year-round in these forests. Monsoon tropical forests are somewhat different and involve a prolonged dry season and short rainy season. Cloud forests have a consistent low-level cloud cover at the tree canopy level (Figure 124-8). Examples of these can be found in Hawaii and Central America.

The gradient between forests and prairies or deserts can contain savannah forests (Figure 124-9). These areas are often grassy and contain sparse amounts of trees. Examples are the xeric scrublands of the intermountain western United States and subtropical deserts.

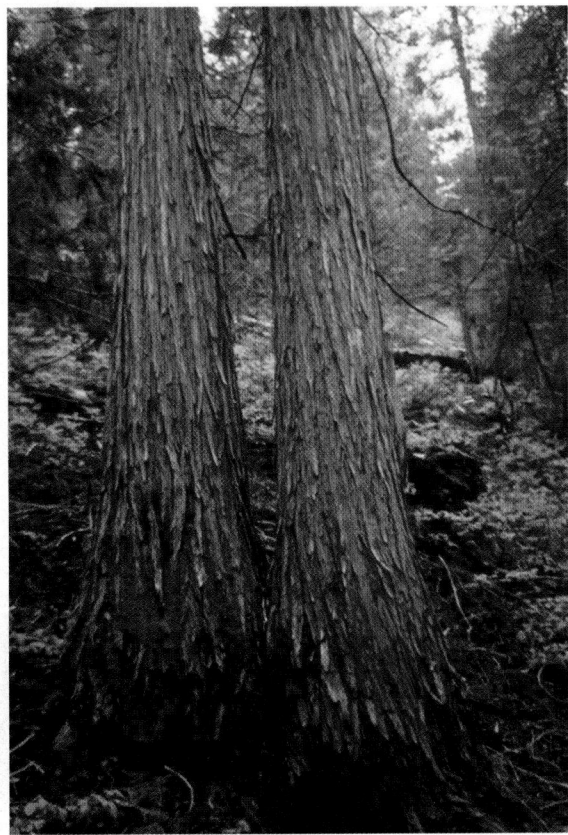

FIGURE 124-5 Temperate rain forest, Alaska. *(Courtesy Dave Powell, USDA Forest Service, retired. www.Bugwood.org.)*

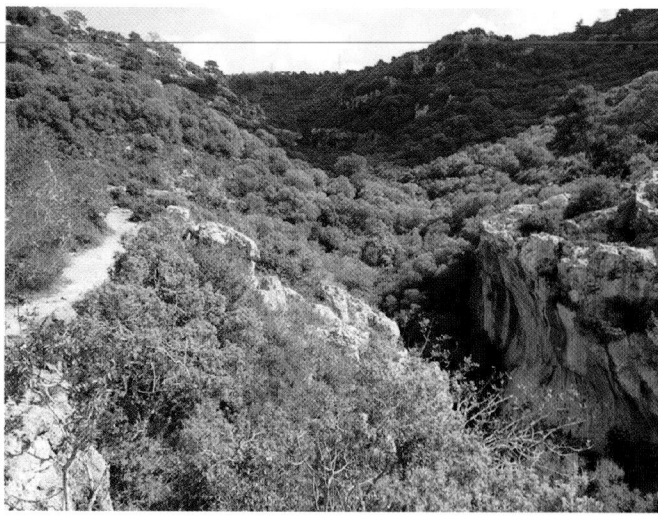

FIGURE 124-6 Mediterranean forests. *(Photo from Wikimedia Commons; courtesy Ramessos.* https://commons.wikimedia.org/wiki/File:KleineSchweizIsrael.jpg; *licensing agreement:* https://creativecommons.org/licenses/by-sa/3.0/deed.en.)

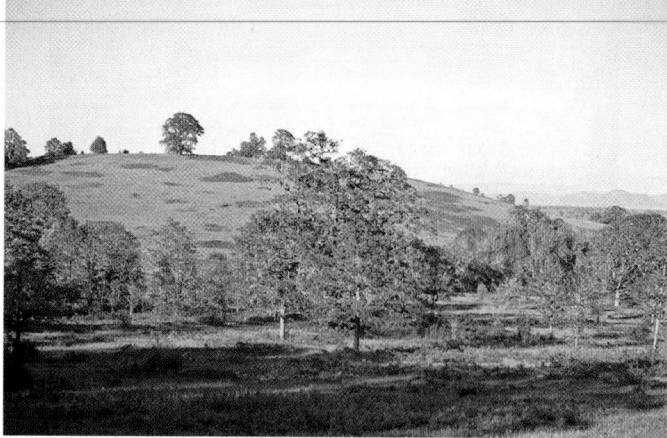

FIGURE 124-9 Savannah forests. *(Photo from Wikimedia Commons; courtesy Gentry George, US Fish and Wildlife Service.* https://commons.wikimedia.org/wiki/File:Bald_top_oak_savannah.jpg; *licensing agreement: public domain.)*

IMPORTANCE OF FORESTS TO PEOPLE

Forests provide services to people and their communities. What people desire from forests can change over time depending on the changes in technology. During the early development of human society, forests provided wood used to cook food as well as to generate warmth. Wood was used to create tools to create weapons for hunting and self-defense. Early human societies depended heavily on hunting and gathering foodstuffs from the forest. This can still be seen in modern times in remote areas of the world where indigenous peoples are found. Forests in both early and modern human societies have played an important role in spiritual and religious practices. Many people prefer a particular forest area that, when visited, provides a sense of calm and peace.

Many types of products or commodities come from forests.[2] For example, "wood products" can be considered to be solid wood, pulp and paper, composites and engineered woods, chemicals, and non–timber-based products. Solid-wood products include items such as boards, beams, posts, fuel wood, charcoal, piles, posts, furniture, barrels, kegs, casks, musical instruments, sailing masts, tool handles, weapons, ice hockey sticks, gun stocks, flooring, canoes, bowls, utensils, pencils, chests, and knickknacks.

Paper production began in China almost 2000 years ago. The process has evolved over time so that now a wide variety of pulp and paper products are produced. Common products include writing and copying paper, printing paper, books, magazines, newspapers, post-it (or sticky) notes, calendars, envelopes, maps, business cards, holiday cards, photographic paper, and wrapping paper. Wood pulp is often used for creating napkins, newspapers, magazines, books, maps, toilet tissue, diapers, and paper towels. Other paper-based products include the corrugated cardboard containers widely used as packaging.

Composites and engineered products are created from small pieces of wood that are arranged and glued together to create a resource with a specific, desired property. A well-known composite and engineered product is plywood, which is made from peeled layers of wood that are overlaid with each other and glued together. Particleboard is another composite-based product made from chips, sawdust, and shavings. Oriented strand board is made from wood wafers, and newer products (e.g., decking, seating, and in some cases sidewalks) are currently made from combining wood fibers and plastic polymers to create wood-plastic composites.

Forests provide chemicals and residues. Some common chemicals that have been created include creosote (a wood preservative), acetone (a solvent), and acetic acid (used to make wood glue). Other chemicals produced include formic acid, butyric acid, propionic acid, methanol, turpentine, and various other oils and acids. Naval stores were typically extracted from specific tree

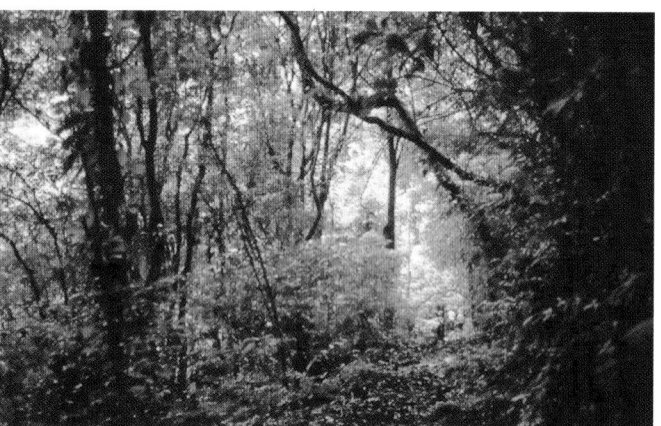

FIGURE 124-7 Tropical rain forest, Honduras. *(Courtesy Howard F. Schwartz, Colorado State University.* www.Bugwood.org.)

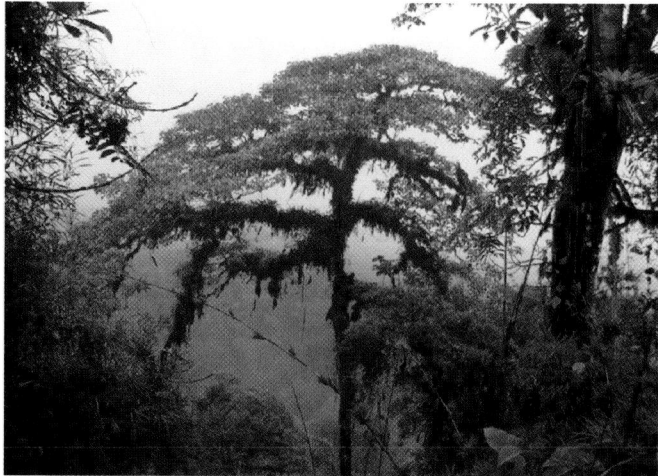

FIGURE 124-8 Cloud forest, Ecuador. *(Courtesy Paul Bolstad, University of Minnesota,* www.Bugwood.org.)

species, such as pines, to provide resin, pitch, and tar for ship-yards. In addition, lye is created by leaching potash from deciduous tree species and can be used in making soap.

Although wood-based products derived from forest resources are extremely important, many non–timber-based products provide spiritual, medicinal, food-based, or recreational value to humans and society. In certain U.S. areas, people enjoy extracting sap from (tapping) maple and birch trees to create syrups. In Europe, mushroom picking is a common forest-based activity. Some people collect medicinal plants, such as yarrow (*Achillea millefolium*), wild ginger (*Asarum canadense*), mayapple (*Podophyllum peltatum*), ginseng (*Panax quinquefolius*), witch hazel (*Hamamelis virginiana*), and sarsaparilla (*Smilax regelli*).

Wildlife habitat is an important nontimber forest product. Wildlife habitats are environments where vertebrates and invertebrates procreate and obtain shelter, food, and water. Many landowners view wildlife habitat as important because it can provide conditions favorable for supporting preferred species. Encouraging wildlife habit may promote better hunting, animal- and bird-watching opportunities, and protection of endangered species. Recreation is an important nontimber benefit. In forested landscapes, this usually refers to activities such as camping, hiking, backpacking, mountain biking, canoeing, fishing, hunting, bird watching, rock climbing, zip lining, and spelunking. Another important nontimber product is provision of water from forested ecosystems.

HUMAN INTERACTION WITH FORESTS

Foresters or natural-resource professionals interact with the forest in different ways, depending on the management objectives for a forested landscape. One of the most common objectives for managing a forested landscape is to maximize a financial return. This typically entails extraction of biologic material from the landscape. This objective is achieved through extraction or harvesting of trees to be sold to various types of forest products manufacturing facilities. The harvesting system employed depends on type of topography, forest access, and type(s) of tree species. Areas that are flat typically employ harvesting systems that use feller-bunchers to harvest trees (Figure 124-10) and then skidders to drag the trees to a landing area close to an access road. In steeper terrain, it is common to see loggers using chainsaws for felling trees and in the western United States, employing cable logging systems (Figure 124-11). These systems use a tower and cables to drag logs up to the roadside for placement on trucks.

People visit forests for recreational purposes. Hunting is a common activity. Although considered a recreational sport in many areas, foresters consider hunting an important tool for managing wildlife populations. The decline of natural predators, such as wolves (*Canis lupus*), cougars (*Puma concolor*), and bears in many areas, as well as changes in vegetative communities helps promote expansion of white-tailed deer (*Odocoileus*

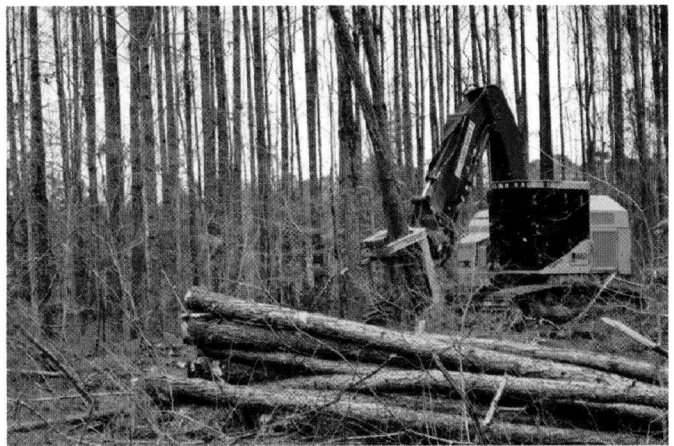

FIGURE 124-10 Feller-buncher. *(Photo courtesy USDA Forest Service. www.Bugwood.org.)*

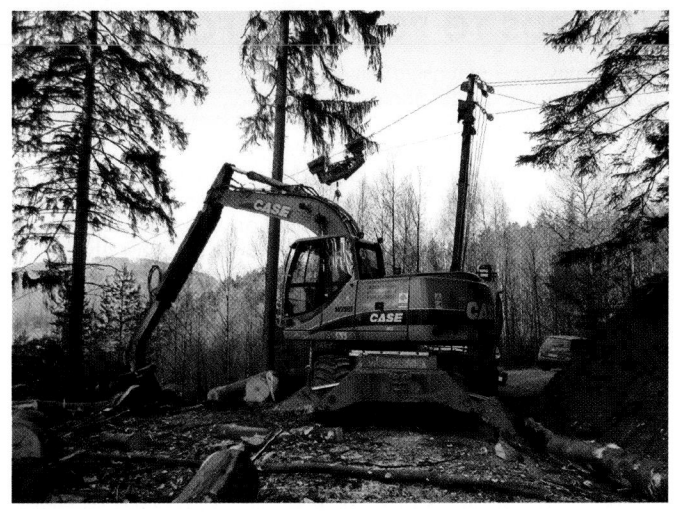

FIGURE 124-11 High-lead cable logging system with loader in the foreground, tower and carriage in background. *(Courtesy Donald L. Grebner, Mississippi State University.)*

virginianus) and elk (*Cervus canadensis*) populations. On smaller forested properties, one may find hunting camps in remote locations. In the United States, large landowners, such as real estate investment trusts (REITS), forest products companies, and timber investment management organizations (TIMOS), often lease large portions of their lands to hunt clubs to generate additional revenues, as well as recruit people to monitor activities on forested properties. Game wardens, who typically are state employees, are responsible for monitoring hunting activities on state lands.

As we noted, recreation activities situated in forests include day hiking, backpacking, camping, rock climbing, mountain biking, skiing, spelunking, bird watching, and mushroom and berry picking. Topography can dictate the types of potential activities. For example, mountainous areas are popular for rock climbers, spelunkers, skiers, backpackers, and campers. Time of year can be equally important. Mushroom and berry pickers forage in the woods during growing seasons (summer months). Bird watchers depend on location and time of year and on species linked to those landscapes. Especially in state or national forests, natural-resource professionals actively promote these recreational opportunities.

Foresters measure various natural resources throughout the year. Successful forest management requires considerable data. Foresters identify living plant species, location, and size and density (heights and diameters). They measure amount of dead vegetation, both standing as snags and as the volume of dead trees lying on the forest floor. Foresters measure these conditions over time to evaluate forest growth and health. Foresters conduct field surveys to measure density and populations of wildlife. These animals may include common white-tailed deer or endangered and threatened species, such as the American bald eagle (*Haliaeetus leucocephalus*) or red-cockaded woodpecker (*Leuconotopicus borealis*). Natural-resource professionals and other scientists often monitor water quality in remote rivers and streams and in lakes and ponds.

Forest fires, whether wildfires started by lightning strikes or arson or planned prescribed fires, are of special interest to foresters. When wildfires are found in remote locations, firefighters known as "smoke jumpers" will parachute into "hot spots" in an attempt to put out a fire quickly before it spreads. If they are unsuccessful, large numbers of people may be employed to build firebreaks around burning areas to control a fire's spread. Aircraft equipped to carry water or fire-retardant chemicals may be used to extinguish fire or suppress a fire. Wildfires can be greatly influenced by the amount of dry vegetation on the forest floor, topography, and general weather conditions. Prescribed fires employ many of the same personnel and equipment but are typically planned events for which firebreaks and other safeguards are put in place before the fire is started.

HAZARDS TO PEOPLE IN FORESTS

People may face extensive hazards in forested landscapes. Both natural-resource professionals and laypersons can become disoriented and lost, especially in forests with dense understory and overstory levels. Misdirection can lead to panic and feelings of being lost, which can lead to poor decision making and injuries. Foresters are trained to use a compass, and many carry Global Positioning System (GPS) instrumentation and cellular phones with GPS capabilities. However, these tools may not always be available or may fail. Nonprofessionals venturing into the forest may not have these tools but may possess a cell phone with GPS tracking capability.

Forests pose risk for injuries incurred by falling or by being hit by falling objects. Risks are increased when traveling off trail or on uneven terrain where it is difficult to see hidden holes covered by vegetation. Walking on top of downed trees is particularly hazardous. Falls can result in both blunt trauma (i.e., against the ground or tree) and penetrating trauma (i.e., impalements on broken stems or branches) that can be fatal. Travelers in the forest may be exposed to falling rocks and debris upslope and falling branches and trees under canopies. Falling branches that are loosened from a tree's crown through wind events are called "widow makers." Foresters can be injured or killed by falling dead trees or snags, especially while evaluating their suitability for wildlife habitat. Additional hazards include hypothermia, hyperthermia, and exposure to flash floods.

Traveling through uneven topography can be physically stressful and pose hazards. Difficulty of traveling through a forest is influenced by the number of live trees, composition of the understory, and density of fallen tree branches. Managers of recreation facilities typically develop trails to reduce the impact of these impediments and to provide higher-quality experiences for people wanting to walk through forests. In undeveloped forests, considerable exertion may be required to navigate through a forest, particularly in areas with steep or uneven topography. Field foresters are therefore typically required to be in good physical condition.

Forests also pose risk of exposure to infectious diseases. In North America, these include giardiasis, West Nile virus disease, Rocky Mountain spotted fever, rabies, and Lyme disease. Insects, mammals, and reptiles may pose hazards. Bee stings can be life threatening. Animal bites can produce lacerations and infections. Large animals, such as deer, moose (*Alcesalces*), or mountain goats (*Oreamnos americanus*), may attack a person if threatened. Their size, horns, and hooves may lead to fatal blunt and penetrating trauma. It is prudent to use care when stepping over logs or other woody debris in uneven terrain to avoid bites and envenomation. Toxic plants pose hazards. In North America, the most common toxic plant is poison ivy (*Toxicodendron radicans*).

Forest management operations (e.g., tree harvesting, road building, invasive insect and plant control) pose unique hazards. Heavy machinery can crush a person's limb or body; chainsaws and axes can cause puncture wounds and severe lacerations. Vehicles can roll over on steep slopes. Someone may be struck because of standing in the path of a falling tree. Where harvesting operations use overhead cable systems for dragging logs up steep terrain, cables can snap under high tension, and logs can also slip from their harnesses (chokers) and crush persons. Heavy equipment is a hazard during road construction. Also invasive insect and plant control operations also pose hazards because of the extensive use of chemicals.

Forest fires are extremely hazardous to foresters and others working, living, or recreating in forested areas (see Chapter 14). Firefighters use heavy equipment and chainsaws to create firebreaks, which are critical to slowing progression of or containing a fire. Hilly terrain and changes in wind patterns pose threats to firefighters, who may become trapped by rapidly advancing fires. Firefighters can employ "back fires" initiated upwind of a human-made or natural firebreak that burn available fuel back to the wildfire and thus widen the firebreak.

REFERENCES

Complete references used in this text are available online at expertconsult.inkling.com.

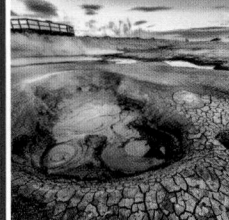

CHAPTER 125
Brief Introduction to Earth Sciences

WAYNE D. RANNEY

The planet Earth is a rocky sphere covered in a rich veneer of life. Even without its biologic life, however, Earth could still be considered alive because of the way that it creates heat in its interior. Although sometimes overlooked or even taken for granted, this heat engine creates a multitude of tangible effects on Earth's surface, including earthquakes and volcanoes felt and witnessed by all living beings. Escape of heat from the earth's interior drives the motions of the continents (which move at about the rate our fingernails grow) to create the mountains and ocean basins that cover the globe. Formation of these uplifted and down-warped features on Earth's surface determines circulation patterns in the world's oceans, which in turn redistributes warm water heated in the tropics toward the more temperate and polar regions. These ocean circulation patterns work in conjunction with feedback from various orbital phenomena, including the sun and the inclination of Earth's spin axis, to drive our planet's climate system. Tropical forests, arid and sandy deserts, temperate growing regions, and polar ice caps are all the result of this system. All life on Earth is affected by this multitude of inputs, which originate from the simple starting point that the earth generates its own heat and can be considered "alive" on the inside. The moon, as well as some other planetary bodies, is not alive in this sense. This chapter explores some of the products of existence on a living planet. Civilization and all life-forms respond to, and are affected by, the sometimes dramatic effects that are felt and experienced on planet Earth.

EARTH'S ORIGIN

Recent advances in astronomical measurements have allowed for consensus on the age, origin, and life cycle of the universe and its component parts. These observations into deep space reveal that the Big Bang occurred about 13.8 billion years ago (it is possible at this time to observe outward to about 380,000 years after the Big Bang). Considering the antiquity of the age of the universe, it could be said that our relatively "average" solar system is *only* about one-third of this age, or about 4.566 billion years old.

Our sun and its solar system formed as did many other common stars, from a *nebula* (Latin for "cloud"), which is composed of the scattered remains of previously existing stars (Figure 125-1). Stars have a life cycle from birth to death that begins in nebulae (Figure 125-2). As the far-flung material begins to collapse inward and coalesce, it swirls into a *protostar* that is surrounded by a disk of gas and dust. The gas and dust particles begin to adhere to one another and eventually grow into *protoplanets*. It is believed that only 1 million years elapsed from the initial collapse of a nebula to the birth of our protostar and the protoplanets. Then, for about 50 to 100 million years, these protoplanets collided with various neighbors to create the *planetesimals*. During this time, a large planetesimal hit Earth with a glancing blow to create the moon. Planetesimals in turn collided to form the planets we know today. The solar system is about halfway through its life cycle. About 5 billion years from now, the sun will have used up its inheritance of hydrogen fuel and begin to die, first becoming a red giant, and then exploding into the surrounding region to become the interstellar dust and gas that will eventually collapse into future stars. The cycle will begin anew.

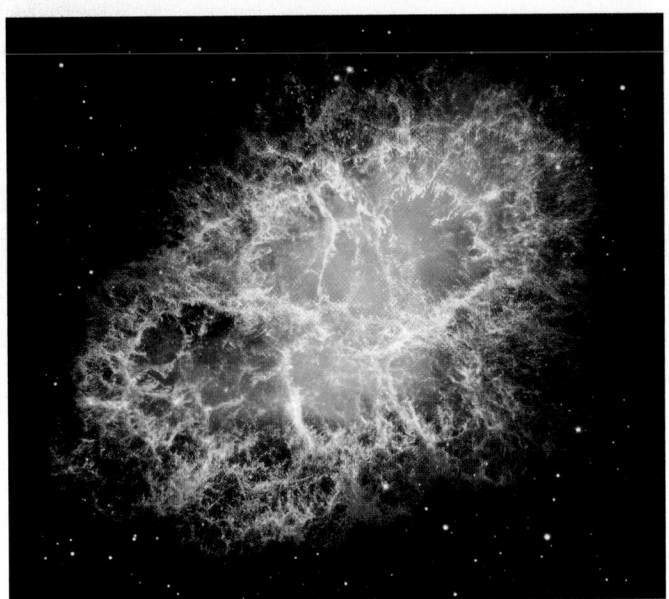

FIGURE 125-1 The Crab Nebula is an example of the material that once made up a solar system. The light from this nebula reached Earth in the year 1054, but it is 6500 light-years from Earth, meaning that it exploded about 7500 years ago.

EARTH'S INTERIOR STRUCTURE

To the geologist, Earth can be considered "alive" because of the way in which it generates its own heat, causing its interior to roil and convulse and its surface to be subjected to constant motion and change. Physical expressions of this living nature are the many earthquakes and volcanoes that shake our existence on this restless planet. The moon is an example of a "dead" planet in that it does not generate its own heat and thus does not presently have active volcanoes or tectonic earthquakes. Our planet extends from its core to the outer reaches of the atmosphere (the atmosphere can be considered a part of the layered Earth). The planet is technically an oblong spheroid, meaning that it bulges slightly at the equator and is squashed minimally at the poles. It has a radius of nearly 6400 km (4000 miles) and is layered into concentric shells with the heaviest, densest layers at the center and the least dense on the outside. The contrast in density between these layers is the result of differences in the composition of each layer and increasing pressure toward the center. In composition from the center outward, our rocky Earth contains

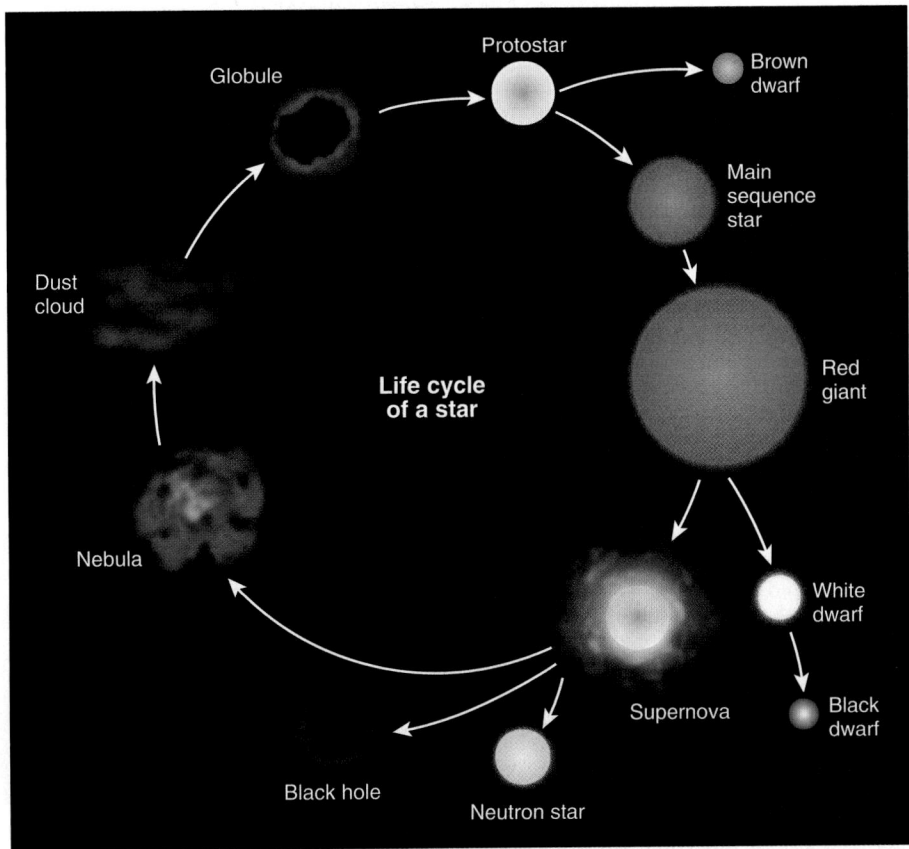

FIGURE 125-2 Life cycle of a typical star, such as our sun.

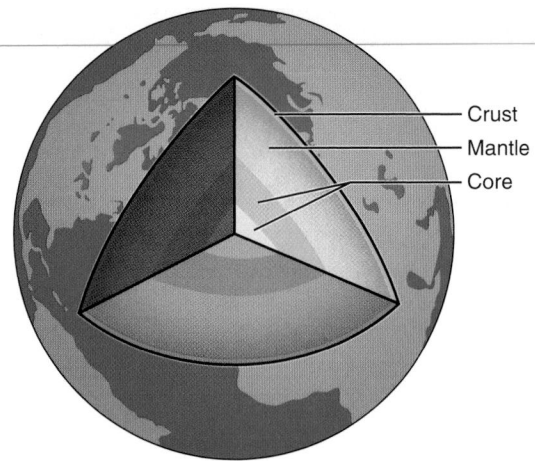

FIGURE 125-3 Earth's concentric layers consist of the core (both inner solid and outer liquid), mantle, and crust.

the core, mantle, and crust. A second scheme differentiates the earth's interior based on the variable properties that the rocks exhibit pertaining to their depth and pressure. These layers do not correspond precisely to the compositional layers just mentioned and are known as the asthenosphere and lithosphere, which together correspond only to the upper few hundred miles of the earth's interior (Figure 125-3).

EARTH'S COMPOSITION

The *core* is the densest part of the earth and was created when the heaviest components of the planet "sank" inward during its formation. It consists of two parts, a solid inner core and liquid outer core, both composed of iron, nickel, and sulfur. No one has ever sampled the core; its density and temperature are too great to access, among many other physical limitations. Its composition is determined in two ways: from the makeup of metallic meteorites whose chemistry mimics that of the earth's interior, and from the way earthquake waves propagate through the earth's interior. Even though both parts of the core exist at essentially the same temperature (4000° to 7000° C [7232° to 12,632° F]), the inner core is solid because of the extreme pressure on it. The area near the core-mantle boundary contains pockets of radioactive elements, which undergo fission and create the earth's internal heat. Uneven distribution of these radioactive pockets drives convection and movement of the mantle and ultimately, the earth's living mobility, and gives rise to its magnetic field.

Surrounding the core is the *mantle*, a layer not quite as thick as the core but comprising almost 80% of Earth's volume. It is composed of iron- and magnesium-silicate minerals, which often combine with other elements, such as aluminum, iron, calcium, sodium, magnesium, and potassium. This chemistry makes it only about one-third as dense as the core. No one has sampled the mantle, but in some instances, fragments have been carried to the earth's surface by volcanic eruptions or, rarely, when mantle material is scraped up onto the earth's surface by plate tectonic processes (see next section). Even though it is solid, the mantle "flows" slowly on the currents of heat that are generated at the core-mantle boundary. All solid material, even rock, can flow when subjected to enough heat and pressure.

The outermost, rocky layer of the earth is the *crust*. We live on the crust and interact with aspects of it every day, from copper in our cell phones, to aluminum and steel in our cars, to salt on the dinner table. This relatively thin layer is proportionally equal to that of the skin of a peach or an apple. In fact, a peach may be a perfectly proportional analog to Earth, with its central pit mimicking the core, its juicy flesh representing the mantle, and its thin skin as the crust (Figure 125-4). Two types of crust exist on Earth. Ocean crust underlies most of the ocean basins and is relatively dense (3.3 times as dense as water) but relatively thin, at only 5 to 10 km (3 to 6 miles) thick. These properties cause ocean crust to have a low average elevation of about 5 km (3

miles) below sea level and therefore be covered with seawater. There are a few places where strands of the ocean crust have been forcibly shoved up onto the continents, leaving samples that are easily obtained. Modern technology now allows us to sample the ocean floor. The average composition of ocean crust is very close to that of basalt rock.

Continental crust underlies all the continents and is less dense (2.7 times as dense as water) than ocean crust but on average is much thicker, at about 30 to 80 km (20 to 50 miles) thick. It therefore stands higher on Earth's surface than the ocean crust. The average composition of continental crust is very close to that of granite rock. Because continental crust is less dense than ocean crust, the continents essentially "float" on the mantle, which is why they rise above sea level to form land. The outermost edges of most continents are sometimes inundated with seawater. These fringes of the continents are called *continental shelves* and may extend out to sea up to 225 km (140 miles). The geologic record provides abundant evidence that these shelves have often been more extensive in the past than at present, forming what are known as *epicontinental seas* ("upon the continent"). This partially explains why areas far from the sea today sometimes expose marine rocks on land (Figure 125-5).

Examination of how rocks behave in the upper part of the earth's interior reveals two layers: the *asthenosphere* (meaning "without strength" or "weak layer") and the *lithosphere* ("rocky" or "rigid layer"). The asthenosphere is slightly more than 320 km (200 miles) thick and is found up to 100 km (60 miles) below the lithosphere. It exhibits temperatures close to the melting temperature of rock (about 1600° C [2900° F]) and thus consists of mushy, plastic-like rock containing pockets of molten material. Therefore, the asthenosphere behaves as a ductile (bends without breaking) material and is structurally weak. Its weak, ductile properties impair the velocity of earthquake waves; in fact, this is how the asthenosphere was first recognized. It is sandwiched between stronger, more rigid layers above and below and provides the medium on which Earth's tectonic plates "float." The asthenosphere can be viewed as a yielding cushion upon which the continents drift (Figure 125-6).

The lithosphere has the properties of a rigid, brittle medium. It is formed from the entire crust and very uppermost part of the mantle, which is cool enough at this level to be brittle. The lithosphere is 1 to 60 miles thick (1.6 to 100 km), is relatively strong, and floats on the ductile asthenosphere. The brittle nature of the lithosphere causes it to behave like a broken eggshell, and thus it is broken into a series of tectonic plates (from the Greek *tectos*, "to build"). Heat generated near the core-mantle boundary is what drives slow convection of the mantle, which ultimately allows the brittle lithosphere to move across the face of the earth and fracture into plates. The lithosphere can be viewed as pieces of Styrofoam drifting in a swimming pool, with water currents generated beneath them by activation of the filter system. The

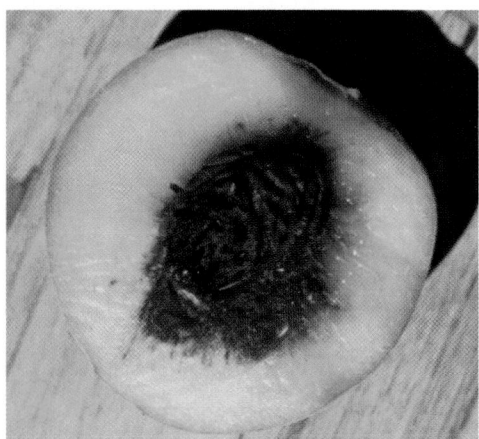

FIGURE 125-4 Various layers inside a peach may serve as a convenient analog to Earth's interior, with the peach pit representing the core, the flesh representing the mantle, and the thin skin of the peach representing Earth's crust. (*Photo by Wayne Ranney.*)

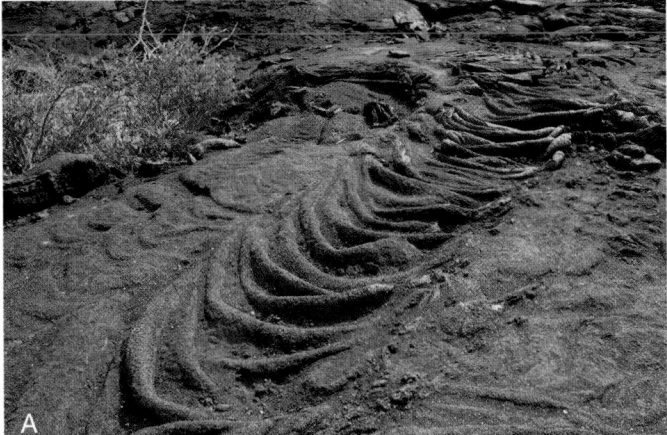

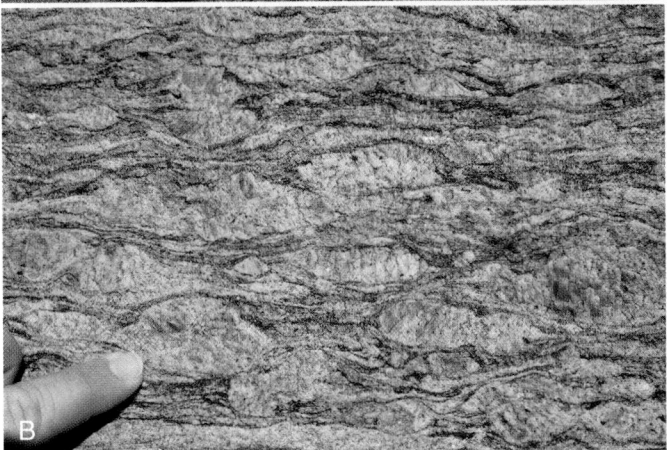

FIGURE 125-5 The two types of earth crust are exemplified by two rock types: **A,** basalt lava flow on the Galápagos Islands, and **B,** granite outcrop in Rio de Janeiro. *(Photos by Wayne Ranney.)*

process of plate tectonics drives most landscape-forming processes and is the overriding theory that has shaped much geologic thought in the past 50 years.

THE BRITTLE, RESTLESS CRUST: PLATE TECTONICS

The branch of geology that studies movements of the earth's lithosphere is called *plate tectonics.* Based on an enormous amount of evidence, geologists developed this theory in the 1960s. It holds that the lithosphere, the outermost rigid layer of the earth, is divided into separate sections called *plates,* which move in response to convection of the mantle, itself a byproduct of radioactive decay in the earth's interior. Plate tectonic processes build up mountains and down-warp basins. This facilitates erosion of mountains, which delivers sediment to the basins. Most geologic concepts are related to plate tectonics (Figure 125-7 and Box 125-1).

A considerable amount of tectonic activity occurs along the plate boundaries, or margins. Earthquakes and volcanoes are concentrated along these narrow boundaries, which run in an arcuate pattern across the earth's surface, like the stitches of a baseball (Figure 125-8). Three major types of plate boundaries are recognized on Earth: (1) *divergent margins,* where plates separate and new ocean crust is formed; (2) *convergent margins,* where one plate crashes into another and is sometimes consumed or destroyed in subduction; and (3) *transform* or *strike-slip margins,* where plates slide past one another and where crust is generally not created or destroyed.

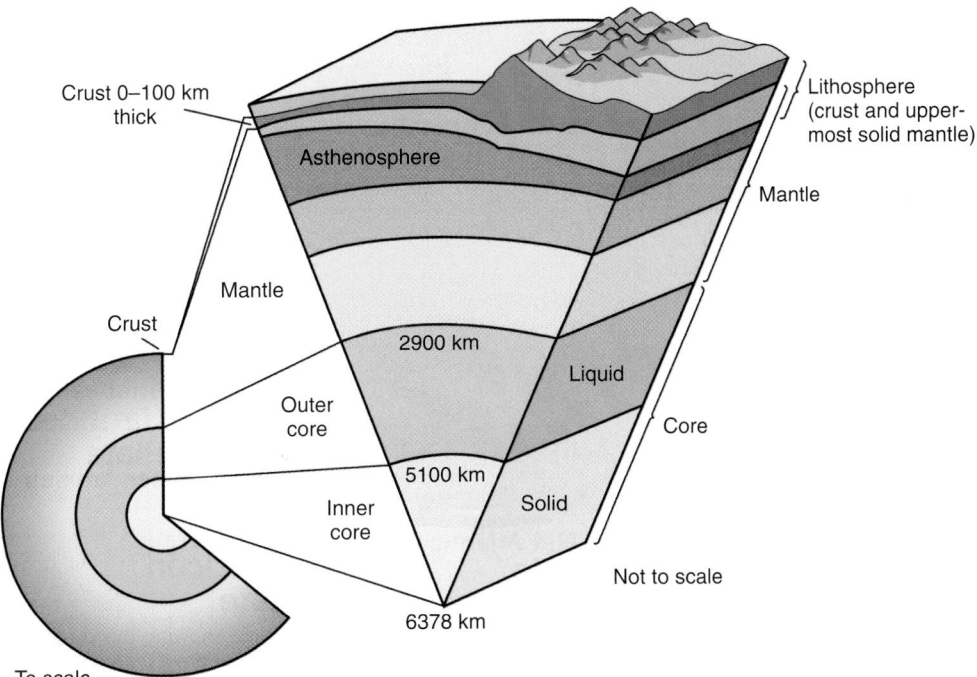

FIGURE 125-6 The lithosphere is composed of the crust and rigid part of the upper mantle. The aesthenosphere lies below it and is the ductile portion of the mantle. *(From* http://upload.wikimedia.org/wikipedia/commons/thumb/8/8a/Earth-cutaway-schematic-english.svg/2000px-Earth-cutaway-schematic-english.svg.png.*)*

DIVERGENT PLATE MARGINS

Also known as *spreading centers,* divergent plate margins are places where plates move away from one another. They are sinuous but lengthy traces that reveal where heat is escaping from the earth's interior. Portions of the upper mantle melt here and force their way into the overlying crust, causing it to separate. As the older crust is pushed away, lava takes its place and solidifies into a rock type called basalt. This process produces long, sinuous chains of submarine mountains called *midocean ridges.* Evidence for this slow, ongoing process comes from the increasing age of ocean crust away from the midocean ridges, alternating bands of magnetism that run parallel to these spreading centers, and mirror images of these phenomena produced on either side of the spreading centers. In fact, the observation of alternating bands of magnetism in ocean crust first led to the concept of seafloor spreading. Basalt contains appreciable amounts of iron, and when it is extruded on the ocean floor, preserves a record of the earth's changing magnetic field. Because the earth's magnetic poles occasionally switch from north to south, and vice versa, an alternating magnetic signature is progressively recorded in ocean crust at spreading centers. This pattern of alternating magnetism is identical on either side of the ridge, showing how the crust has spread apart. Midocean ridges occur in all the world's major oceans (Figure 125-9).

CONVERGENT PLATE MARGINS

When new crust is formed at midocean ridges, something must be destroyed on the opposing edge of the plate (unless the earth is growing larger, an idea for which there is no evidence). Zones where crustal plates move together and are often destroyed are called *convergent plate margins.* They occur variably between two oceanic plates (as in the Japan, Philippines, or Aleutian island chains), two continental plates (as in the Himalayan chain, where the Indian plate is colliding with the Eurasian plate), or between an ocean and a continent, such as the western edge of South America. The South American example provides a typical series of events. As lithospheric plates converge, the oceanic crust that is being pushed from behind at the spreading center (and tending to be denser and cooler) sinks beneath the lighter, continental crust in a process called *subduction.* As the ocean plate is subducted, usually at an angle of 35 to 60 degrees, it is pushed into the earth, where portions of it melt after achieving a depth of about 100 km (60 miles), although parts of the descending slab can reach depths of 640 km (400 miles) before melting entirely. Pockets of molten material then rise buoyantly through the continental crust, creating slightly curved chains of volcanoes called *volcanic arcs* (Figure 125-10). These arcs typically erupt through overthickened crust, formed by the convergence of two plates. Oceanic trenches form offshore, where the ocean crust slides beneath the continental edge and can be quite deep. Plate boundaries where two continents collide are also the site of convergence but generally do not produce volcanism. This is because when two pieces of continental crust meet, they are equally buoyant to preclude subduction. Thus, no melting occurs in continent-to-continent convergence. Great mountain ranges such as the Himalayas are thrust upward in these settings, resulting in continental rocks becoming greatly deformed and folded.

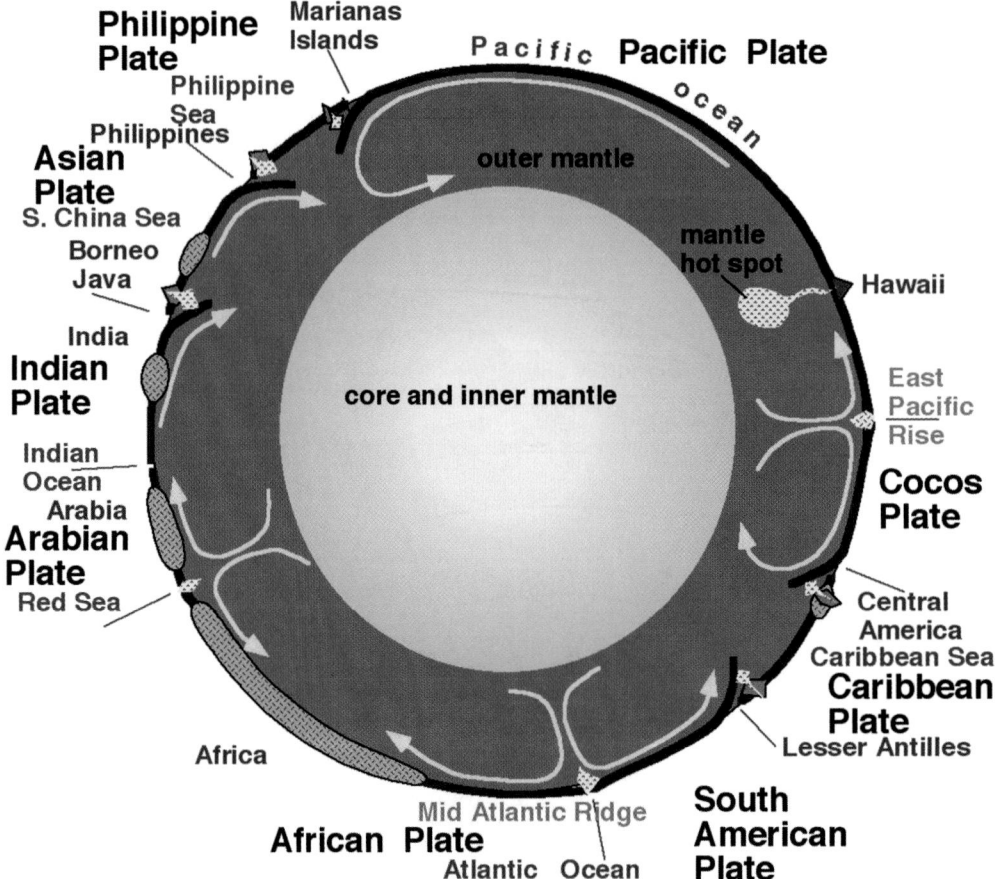

FIGURE 125-7 Cross section through Earth at about 10 degrees north latitude showing the components of plate tectonic theory. The *yellow arrows* show convection cells in the mantle that drive the surface motion of the earth's plates. Continental crust is depicted in *pinkish color* with ocean crust as a *solid dark line.* The plate boundaries are shown with *thin red lines* pointing to the crust. Major tectonic features are named and labeled as plates in *black,* oceans in *purple,* arcs and continental crust in *dark green,* and midocean ridges in *orange.* All thicknesses depicted are exaggerated and not to scale. *(Courtesy Ron Blakey.)*

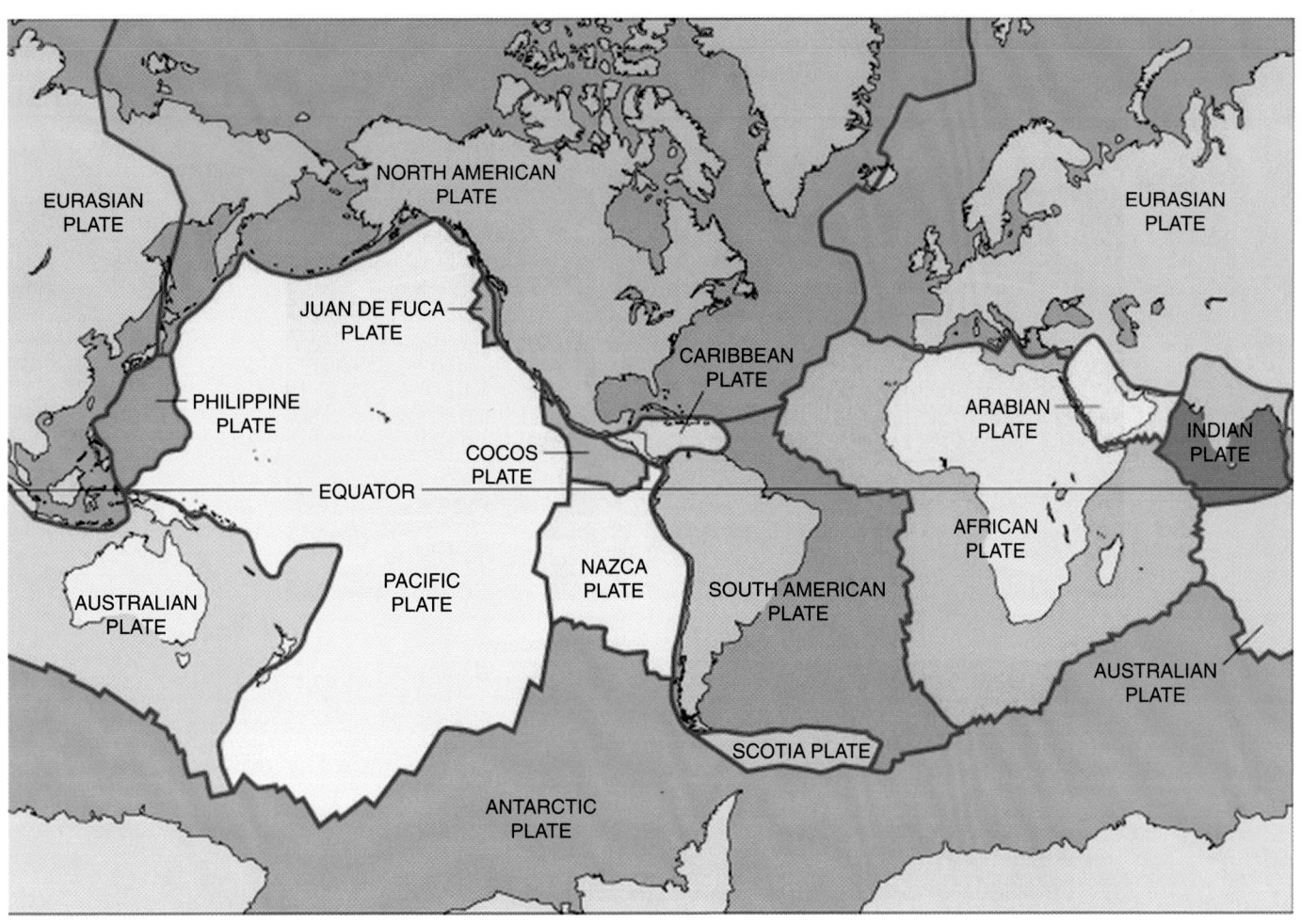

FIGURE 125-8 Map of the earth showing its major plates. *Lighter* shade of any color shows the continental portion of the plate, while *darker* color shows the oceanic component of the same plate. Fifteen of the largest plates are labeled here, with dozens of smaller plates not shown. *(From the United States Geological Survey.* http://pubs.usgs.gov/gip/dynamic/slabs.html. *Accessed February 9, 2016.)*

STRIKE-SLIP OR TRANSFORM PLATE MARGINS

Some plates slide horizontally past one another in such a way that little or no creation or destruction of crust occurs. Such boundaries are called strike-slip or transform margins because the plate motions transform the offset laterally. Few volcanoes occur in these tectonic settings because there is no subduction and consequent melting of the crust. Earthquakes, however, are quite abundant and tend to be rather destructive as the two rigid plates grind past one another. The San Andreas Fault in California and the Alpine Fault in New Zealand are the most famous examples of such plate boundaries. Earthquakes, therefore, are the result of breaking of brittle lithosphere. When this solid rock is subjected to stress, it sends off shock waves that generate earthquakes. Most earthquakes occur along the earth's plate boundaries, but it is also possible to have intraplate earthquakes, such as the famous New Madrid, Missouri, quakes of 1811-1812 or the Virginia earthquake of August 23, 2011. Plotting major earthquake epicenters over time clearly delineates the location of the plate boundaries. Shallow earthquakes tend to occur along all plate boundaries, whereas intermediate and deep earthquakes occur only in subduction zones along convergent margins. Shallow earthquakes are defined as those occurring down to 60 km (40 miles); intermediate, between 60 and 320 km (40 and 200 miles); and deep, 320 to 640 km (200 to 400 miles). Below this depth, the mantle is ductile and rocks do not break.

Mountains, the most obvious result of the uplift generated by Earth's tectonic system, are formed in many ways. Almost all mountain ranges are located near present or ancient plate boundaries. The Appalachian chain formed near an ancient plate boundary, and the Andes formed on a modern margin.

Mountains at convergent margins are the result of plates pushing rock together, which thickens the crust either by squeezing it or by forcing some sections to override other sections (*thrusting*). Volcanoes can form mountains as molten material accumulates on the surface and cools into rock. Mountains are also created at divergent plate boundaries because upwelling heat initially swells the earth's crust before it rifts apart; the flow of hot material expands the crust upward, and piles of volcanic material are added to its top.

A less obvious but no less important result of tectonism is formation of tectonic or sedimentary basins. These form in conjunction with mountain uplift but are often overlooked by non-geologists because they do not form the rugged, spectacular scenery of a mountain range. Sedimentary basins, however, are corollaries of the same tectonic story. As plates converge, they unevenly warp the crust into both mountains and basins. Consider the way a throw rug is variably warped as it is pushed along a hardwood floor into a wall. You can see both humps (mountains) and depressions (basins) that form on the rug's surface. In tectonic settings, rocks are eroded off the mountains and transported by rivers and wind into the basins. These basins preserve most of the earth's sedimentary deposits, which reveal details about Earth's prior environments, climate, and life. It is the workings of plate tectonics that allows this clear view into the ancient past.

TECTONIC ORIGIN OF ROCKS

Pervasiveness of plate tectonics on Earth creates the conditions necessary to form the many different types of rocks found on our planet. These rocks constitute the record of Earth's history.

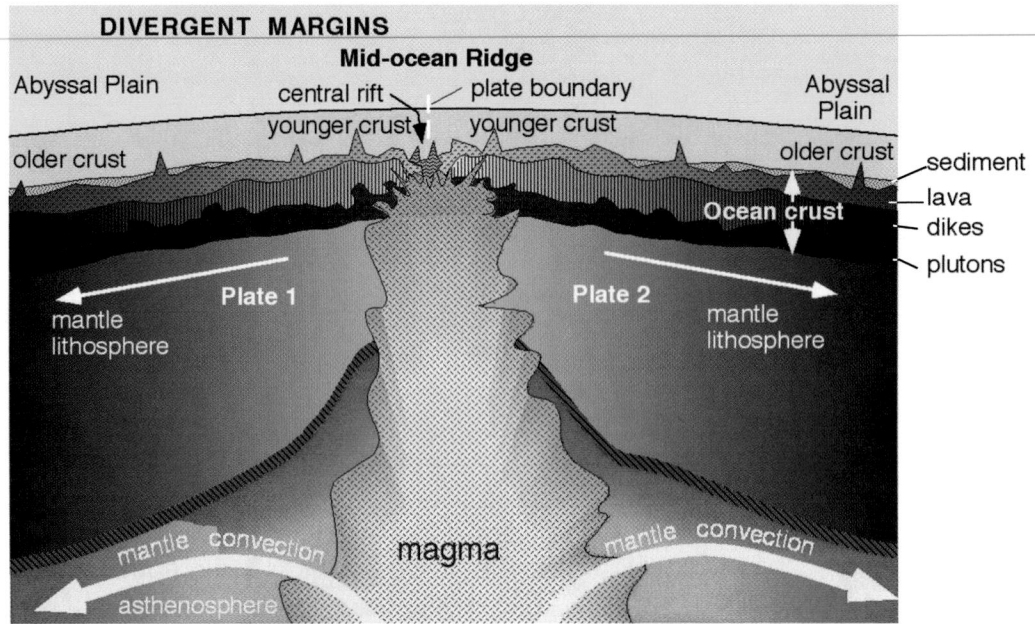

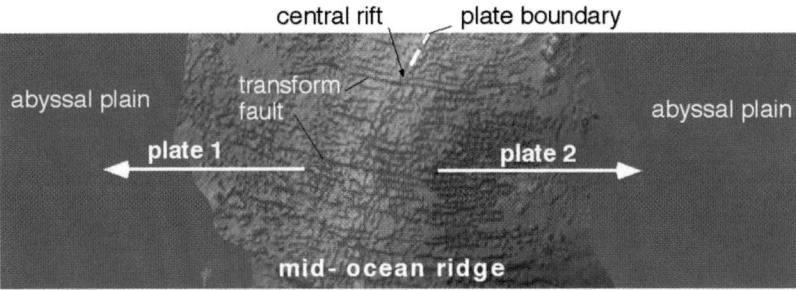

FIGURE 125-9 Cross section through a typical midocean ridge or divergent plate margin. Note how magma rises through the lithosphere and is erupted onto the ocean floor, creating new ocean crust. *(Courtesy Ron Blakey.)*

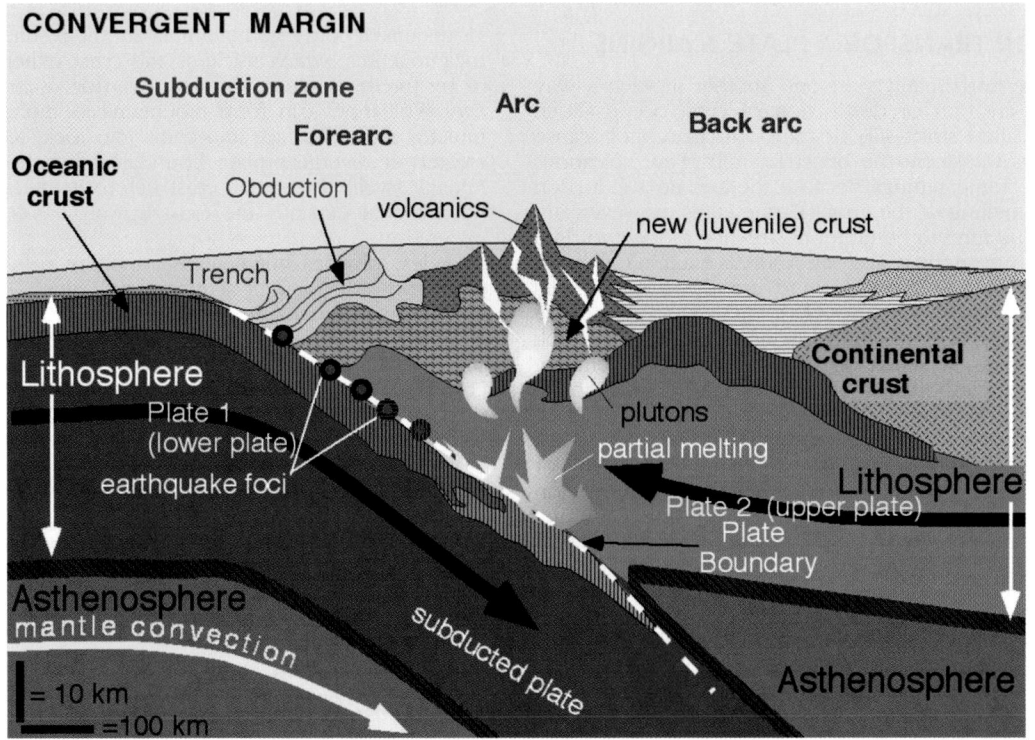

FIGURE 125-10 Convergent margins form where oceanic crust is subducted beneath the edge of a continent (or between two continents or the edge of another ocean plate). Although some material may be scraped off near the top *(obduction)*, most descends beneath the continent because ocean crust is cooler and denser than continental crust. Melting of the subducted plate at depth of about 100 km (60 miles) creates magma that erupts into the crumpled edge of the continent to create a volcanic arc. The Andes Mountains in South America are a good example of this type of plate margin. *(Courtesy Ron Blakey.)*

ROCK CYCLE

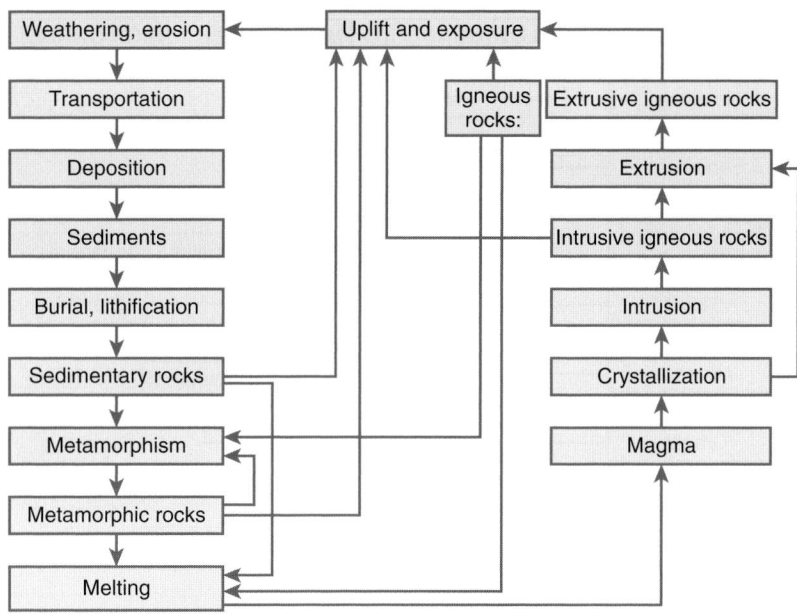

FIGURE 125-11 Typical rock cycle showing the relationship among the three classes of rocks. Follow the "Uplift and exposure" box (top, center) counterclockwise for the simplest cycle, noting only that rocks can take "shortcuts" at any stage within the circle.

Most people are familiar with the three main types of rocks: igneous, metamorphic, and sedimentary, but many may not be aware of the close relationship these rocks have with tectonic processes (Figure 125-11). Igneous and metamorphic rocks, which contain groupings of one or more mineral crystals, are the so-called crystalline rocks. They form from heat and except for volcanic rocks, within the earth. Sedimentary rocks contain a record of Earth's surface and form from broken bits of other rocks (including other sedimentary rocks), precipitation of solutions, or compaction of shells.

Igneous Rocks

Igneous comes from the Latin word meaning "to ignite" ("burning" or "fiery"). Igneous rocks are born of heat. When the earth's crust or upper mantle is subjected to extreme heat, melting occurs and molten magma is formed. Therefore, all igneous rocks originate initially as magma. Some of this magma may remain deep within the crust, where it cools slowly to form solid rock (e.g., granite). Such rocks take a long time to form, which allows for growth of large crystals as the magma cools and solidifies. Such igneous rocks are called *intrusive* or *plutonic* (after Pluto, the Roman god of the underworld). They contain coarse-grained crystals that are easily seen without magnification. Large bodies of plutonic rock are called *plutons* or *batholiths*; small bodies less than 259 km² (100 miles²) are called *stocks* (Figure 125-12).

Some magma makes its way to the surface in liquid form and flows out rather gently, or it is blasted out violently onto Earth's surface. This igneous material cools relatively quickly, and crystals often do not have time to form. If crystals form, they are very fine-grained and are not usually visible without magnification. Basalt lava flows or rhyolite ash beds are examples of *extrusive* or *volcanic* rocks (after Vulcan, the Roman god of the forge).

Volcanoes are simply mountains composed of piles of volcanic material—cinders, lava, and ash—erupted from a central vent. Volcanoes are classified according to their shape or the processes that form them. *Shield volcanoes* form from piles of extremely fluid basalt lava that flows and cools far from the vent; they tend to be broad at the base with a very low profile, reflecting the low viscosity of the lava. *Cinder cones* (or *scoria cones*) are formed from small droplets of molten rock that erupt into the air and cool as pea-sized particles in a steep pile around the vent. Cinder cones tend to be the smallest volcanoes, at about 300 m (1000 feet) in height. *Composite volcanoes* or *stratovolcanoes* are formed from alternating layers of andesite lava flows and ash. These form some of the largest, most symmetric, and dangerous mountain peaks on Earth: Mt St Helens, Mt Fuji, and Mt Pinatubo are examples. These types of volcanoes yield huge amounts of ash. When this material travels to distant basins, it can become preserved within sedimentary layers. These ash beds are readily dated and allow geologists to date strata, which otherwise could

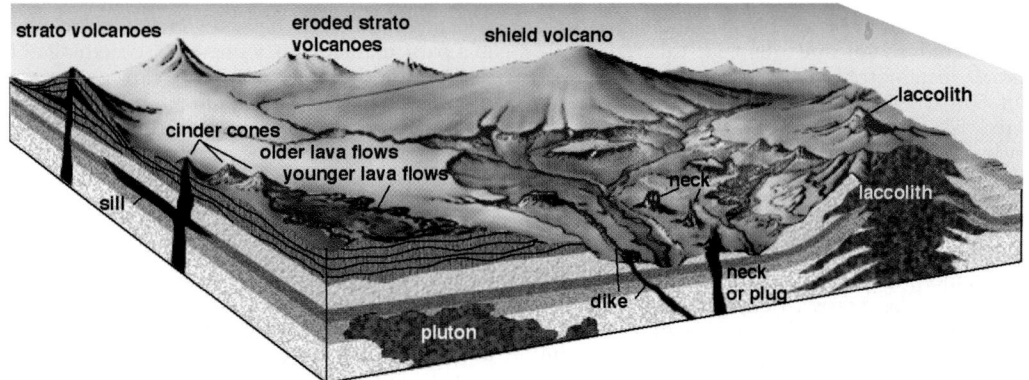

FIGURE 125-12 Hypothetical landscape, showing many of the igneous landforms that can be found on Earth. *(Courtesy Ron Blakey.)*

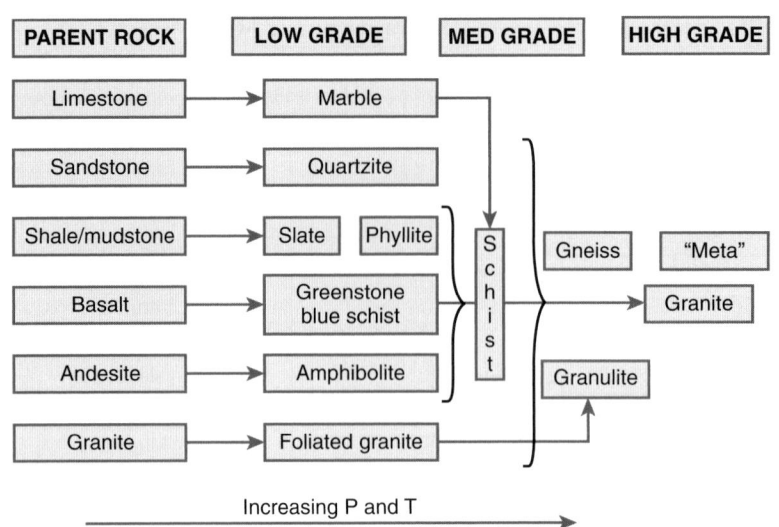

FIGURE 125-13 Protolith or parent rocks and their metamorphic equivalents, with increasing grade of metamorphism shown *left* to *right*.

not be dated directly. *Dome volcanoes,* the last type of volcanic edifice, form from very viscous magma that resists flow away from the vent.

Volcanoes have the potential to cause much destruction. Lava flows pose an obvious hazard, but more serious are volcanic explosions and their associated gases, hot dust (ash), and mud-flows triggered by melting ice and snow. The more destruction and death associated with volcanic eruptions, the more they are reported. However, many significant eruptions in unpopulated areas go virtually unreported and unnoticed.

Metamorphic Rocks

Rocks formed by heat and pressure, regardless of their original makeup, are called metamorphic rocks. The word *metamorphic* means "changed form." These rocks have been altered considerably since their original incarnation. Heat and pressure applied by tectonic processes (with perhaps associated magmatism) can cause a significant change in the appearance of a rock, such that an entirely new rock is formed. These changes include formation of entirely new minerals, recrystallization of old minerals (usually with an increase in crystal size), or alignment, banding, or segregation of differently colored minerals. Some common metamorphic rocks are slate, marble, quartzite, schist, and gneiss. Each of these has an original rock type, or *protolith,* from which it formed. The protoliths can often be determined by the overall chemistry and texture of a metamorphic rock and may help in determining the ancient setting of the prealtered rocks (Figure 125-13).

There is a relative increase in metamorphic grade as rocks become subjected to increasing temperatures and pressures. *Low-grade* metamorphic rocks begin to form between 200° and 300°C (392° and 572°F). Examples of these are phyllite and slate (both different grades of altered shale) and quartzite (altered sandstone). *Medium-grade* metamorphism begins at 300°C (572°F) and ends at about 500°C (932°F). These rocks include schist (increasingly altered shale), marble (from limestone), and amphibolite (from basalt). *High-grade* metamorphism begins at about 500°C [932°F]) and includes gneiss (extremely altered shale or granite) and migmatite (tectonically deformed and cooked granite). At about 950°C (1742°F), rocks begin to melt, and the igneous environment begins.

Through time, metamorphic rocks find their way back to the surface in tectonic uplifts, where erosion exposes them to view. Awareness of all these rock-forming processes is useful in deciphering the seemingly unconnected parts of Earth's history. The metamorphic grade in a rock allows us to know the specific conditions that existed during its creation. Certain minerals can grow only within a narrow range of temperatures and pressures, and geologists use the known depths where those conditions are

present today to infer the ancient depth of the rocks when they were created. The chemistry of the rock can suggest a protolith, which can divulge the specific sedimentary environment of the rock before its burial and metamorphism. This may provide a clue to its tectonic setting just before the mountain-building event that changed it. Taken together, all this information might reveal a sensible sequence of tectonic events in which a rock originated in a sedimentary basin, only to become involved in a convergent mountain-building event that folded, buried, and altered the rock deep within the earth.

The beauty of the plate tectonic concept and of modern geologic thought is that discreet bits of evidence scattered across the globe allow us to know the sequential evolution of our planet, if only we can recognize the evidence. Before the birth of this concept, metamorphic rocks could only be described in stone-faced prose and dry classification schemes that were simply organized around their texture. Attempts were made to interpret how the rocks might have originated, but there was no single, fundamental concept that could show a link between the seemingly unrelated aspects of a rock's metamorphic grade, its sedimentary protolith, or how it was uplifted and exposed. A plate tectonic view has allowed us to see how the transitions in Earth's history have been actualized. Many of the details are still being determined, but scientists continue to unravel Earth's history at an astounding rate.

DYNAMICS OF SEDIMENTATION AND SEDIMENTARY ROCKS

Sedimentary rocks are the most important surface rocks in reconstructing the details of past events. If sedimentary rocks are found in a particular area, they preserve something of the surface history that occurred there. We usually can recognize parts of that past, because all modern environments also existed in the past. Geologists are like detectives who arrive at a crime scene long after the fact. In much the same way that 20-year-old fingerprints can pinpoint the person who left the scene of a crime, ordinary sandstone, limestone, and mudstone record the specific environments that once covered an area, even if that area is now completely changed. Sediments accumulate in layers called *strata* to form sedimentary rocks. Because strata form under surface conditions, they reflect the extent and nature of the environments in which they formed. This allows geologists to reconstruct the ancient landscapes that once existed on Earth. *Clasts* (broken grains or particles) in sedimentary rocks tell us about the parent rocks from which they were derived. Clasts can also tell us about the conditions of weathering, erosion, and the transportation history of the grains. Fossils in sedimentary rocks reflect specific ecologic and

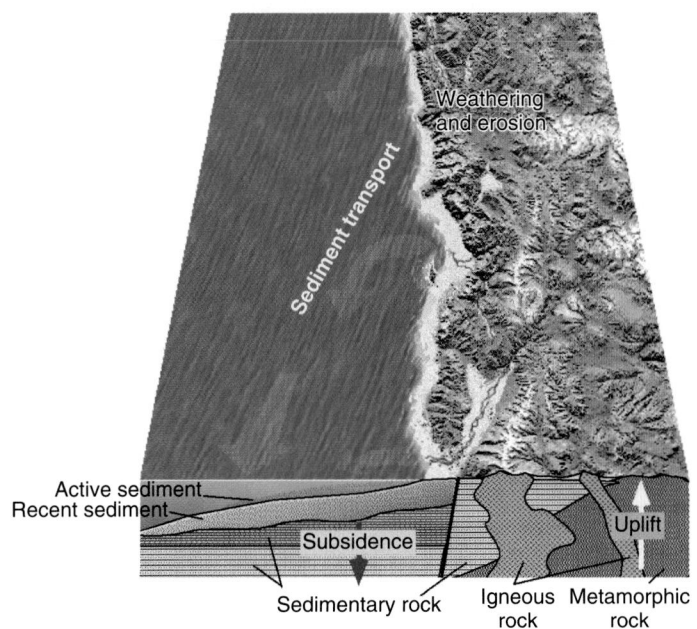

FIGURE 125-14 Sedimentary cycle, in which rocks of any type are uplifted, weathered, eroded, and transported to a depositional basin. Subsidence in the basin creates the space where the sediment becomes buried and lithified. *(Courtesy Ron Blakey.)*

environmental conditions at the site of deposition. *Evaporite rocks* such as halite and gypsum tell us about the chemistry of waters, as well as the climate during deposition. Organic material also reflects the extent of the fecundity of the biosphere.

Ironically, sedimentation begins with weathering and erosion. Any type of rock exposed on Earth's surface eventually breaks down as it is subjected to vagaries of the atmosphere or hydrosphere. Eventually, these clasts are transported downwind or downstream and come to rest in a basin. Formation of sedimentary rocks involves initial weathering (physical or chemical) and erosion of preexisting rocks, transportation of the broken pieces to other areas as sediment, and its ultimate deposition as a layer of new sediment. These steps can be presented graphically in a *sedimentary cycle*. Factors such as the tectonic setting, climate, rock types in the source area, and distance to the sea affect the sedimentary cycle (Figure 125-14).

Weathering is the breakdown and change of rocks at or near the earth's surface. Many rocks are formed under heat and pressure within the earth, where there are relatively low amounts of water. Conversely, the surface of the earth has lower temperatures and pressures but large amounts of water. These opposed conditions tend to cause minerals to change either by physical breakdown of the rock or by chemical alteration. Physical weathering is decrease in the size of clasts from larger pieces to smaller ones. Freeze-and-thaw processes in rock cavities split off chunks of rock and are a good example of physical weathering. Chemical alteration in composition of the parent material is an illustration of chemical weathering. For example, feldspar, a common mineral in granite, interacts chemically with rain and groundwater to form clay minerals. This process results in a new substance with totally different properties than the parent mineral. Chemical weathering results in release of dissolved ions, such as calcium, iron, and silica, into the surface water and/or groundwater. These ions are carried by surface water to the sea and become the source of dissolved sea salts. They are carried by groundwater through rocks and often become the cementing agents for loose sediment (e.g., turning sand into sandstone).

Erosion is the process that removes weathered bits of rock and carries them to a new site. It is accomplished by moving water, blowing wind, soil creep, or flowing glacial ice. Erosion by running water forms the canyons and gullies that are so prevalent on our planet. The force of running water removes loose particles and is the method by which canyons are lengthened, deepened, and widened. Each new flood carries away more material to increase the size of the canyon. Meanwhile, weathering loosens

more material, and the process continues. Erosion by running water is by far the most important aspect of this process. Wind erosion is much less important with respect to the amount of material moved but can affect weakly cemented rocks when they are buffeted by other particles traveling with the wind. The most efficient erosion is that accomplished by glacial ice. Glaciers form when more snow is deposited in winter than melts in spring and summer. This must occur for a number of successive years for major glaciers or ice fields to form. As ice accumulates and thickens, it flows downhill and has a tremendous capacity to erode soil and even solid rock. Ice is a major factor in sculpting some landscapes, especially in mountainous areas.

Numerous factors affect the rate and type of erosion that occurs across the landscape. Climate determines the distribution and amount of precipitation and thus the pace of erosion. Arid landscapes tend to be more angular in appearance than humid landscapes because erosion is concentrated along river courses, even if those channels are usually dry. Intervening areas (mesas and plateaus) between the major rivers have much slower rates of erosion in this dry environment and thus stand tall relative to the deep canyons. Humid areas, such as Brazil or the eastern seaboard of North America, experience considerable chemical weathering, and the intervening areas between rivers tend to "round off" at about the same rate as the rivers dissect. Elevation and *relief* (the elevation difference between the highest and lowest points in a given area) are other important factors and determine the potential energy of running water and how far the water drops to attain *base level*, defined as the final destination of a stream, usually a lake or the ocean, which is the ultimate base level. Steep-gradient rivers tend to both deepen and lengthen their channels. If a river has a steep gradient to base level, erosion will be facilitated.

Bedrock type can determine the ultimate shapes we see on landscapes. Harder rocks, such as granite or limestone, tend to produce steep-walled canyons, whereas softer rocks such as shale or mudstone typically yield broader valleys. The geologic age of a landscape (how long the area has been subjected to the current conditions of weathering and erosion) determines the overall appearance of a landscape. Relatively young landscapes tend to be more rugged and angular in appearance and to have the greatest relief. Older landscapes tend to have more rounded slopes and hills and to be mostly low-lying with broad, open river valleys.

Many areas undergo erosion as *mass movement*. Mass movement involves pulses or relatively short spurts of activity where large amounts of material move downslope. The type of mass movement is related to the type of material being moved by erosion and amount of water associated with the process. Mudflows involve large amounts of water and relatively fine material, such as soil and mud. Rockfalls involve little water and large amounts of loose rock. *Slumps* are sudden slippage, usually of water-saturated soil or rock, and *creep* involves movement of water-saturated soil and rock by means of numerous small pulses of short duration. Mass movement causes billions of dollars of damage worldwide on an annual basis. Roads, buildings, and other cultural features can be destroyed rapidly, often without warning.

The products of erosion are usually transported by water, wind, or ice and then deposited (Figure 125-15). These deposits include gravel, sand, and mud (technically a mixture of clay and silt particles), precipitates (material that changes from solution to solid in bodies of water), and organic deposits (material formed from living organisms). Common precipitates include halite (common salt), gypsum, potash, and some limestones. Common organic deposits include most limestones, coals, and phosphates.

Sedimentary rocks can be dated by several different methods, including *fossils,* the remains of organisms that lived during deposition. Because life has changed constantly throughout geologic time, fossils can be used to date sedimentary rocks in a relative way. They do not tell us "how many millions of years ago," but rather "what came first" and "what came later." Fossils that are widespread laterally but that lived for only a short time make excellent *index fossils*, used to correlate widely separated rock units. Presence of datable grains and volcanic ash beds allows absolute dating that can tell us "how many millions of years ago." Dating of clasts, such as zircon, must be used with

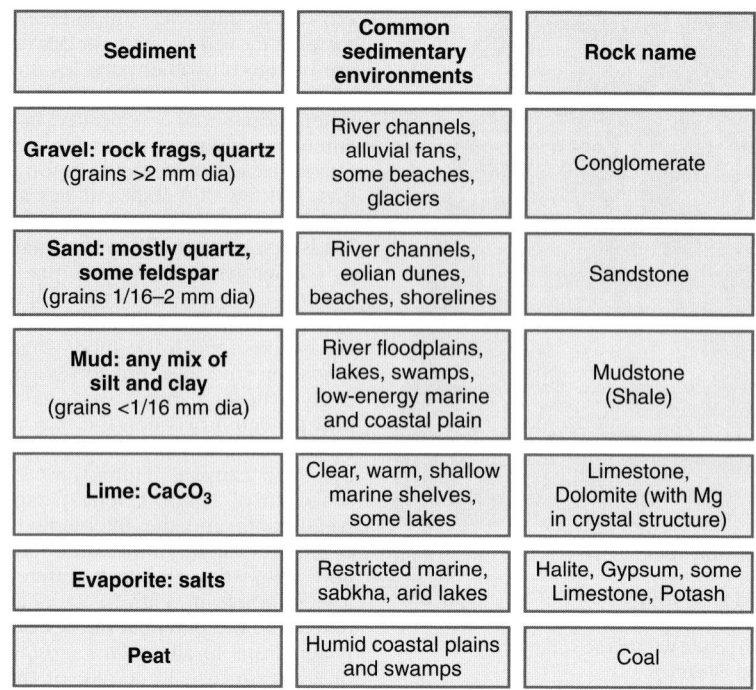

FIGURE 125-15 Sediment types with their equivalent rock names and the environments in which they form.

care, because the grains provide only the age of the parent rock, not the age of the sedimentary deposit. Using this method, geologists may only be able to tell a strata's maximum age. Volcanic ash beds are an important dating method for sedimentary strata. Ash deposits originate from eruptions far away and are carried by the wind to become trapped in the deposits of a sedimentary basin. Their presence in strata can be cryptic and difficult for an untrained eye to detect, but once found, provide useful dating tools and yield increasingly reliable dates. Taken together, use of fossils and datable materials has allowed global correlation of strata.

PRESENT-DAY GEOLOGY AS A KEY TO UNDERSTANDING THE PAST

The concept of using the present to understand the past is an invaluable tool to the geologist. This concept is called *uniformitarianism* and widely applied in the field of historical geology. For example, one can study the processes and subsequent deposits associated with the flooding of a major modern-day river. As floodwaters recede, they leave behind newly deposited sediment, and geologists may trench through the sand, mud, and debris to observe what is preserved. They will look to see how the grains of sand are arranged, what sizes they are, and how they all "stack up" when viewed comprehensively. Geologists are interested in a sediment's *texture* and the *sedimentary structures* it contains. The texture and structure of these modern flood deposits (which have first-person accounts that verify how they originated) can be used to help recognize ancient flood deposits whose origins were not directly observed. In this way, flood events that happened many millions of years ago can be documented, showing how a present reality becomes a key to understanding the past. Because the same rigorous observations are performed on other types of deposits, such as sand dunes in the Sahara, deltas in India, and beaches in eastern North America, a body of knowledge exists that helps to interpret and differentiate the various types of deposits, regardless of their antiquity.

This ability to "read the rocks" has only evolved in the last 250 years. Before that, people saw oddly located fossils and lacked the geologic framework to make sense of how seashells came to rest in the mountains. Before development of geologic

thought, they could not know that rocks contained a sequential record of Earth history. Modern geologic concepts began with the Age of Enlightenment at the end of 18th century and have progressed such that it is now possible to reconstruct major portions of Earth's past, even though there were no humans present to witness it. Several assumptions need to be accepted, however, most importantly that the processes acting on the earth today are similar to those that have acted in the past. The evidence, critically reviewed by thousands of scientists, is overwhelming that the earth behaves today much as it has in the past.

HOW ROCKS ARE DATED

Many nonscientists express skepticism when presented with ideas regarding the staggering antiquity of Earth. They wonder, "How can it be known?" that events happened hundreds of millions or billions of years ago. Certain physical properties of some common elements allow scientists to discover how long ago rocks formed or events occurred. It involves radioactive decay from a parent product into a daughter product. These naturally occurring decay series happen at a known and constant rate. One example is radiocarbon decay. Organisms such as animals and plants absorb carbon-14 (^{14}C) from the atmosphere. When their living functions cease, they stop absorbing ^{14}C, which is radioactive and begins to decay to ^{12}C. The half-life of ^{14}C is 5730 years (±40 years), meaning that after that amount of time, half the ^{14}C has decayed to ^{12}C. This radiocarbon method is good for dating organic matter less than about 62,000 years old. After that, there is insufficient residual ^{14}C to obtain a ratio.

Therefore, other decay series must be used to date older materials. Some common decay series used to date rocks are uranium-235 to lead-207 (half-life, 700 million years); uranium-238 to lead-206 (half-life, 4.5 billion years); potassium-40 to argon-40 (half-life, 1.3 billion years); and rubidium-87 to strontium-87 (half-life, 50 billion years).

GEOLOGIC TIME

The concept of geologic time, or *deep time*, exposes humans, who are used to much smaller time frames, to vast numbers of years. One million years is difficult to comprehend even to the geologist, yet represents only a fraction of Earth's history. An analogy may help. Medium-sized sand grains, the common building block of many sedimentary rocks and widespread in modern sand dunes and beaches, are approximately 10 mm ($\frac{1}{25}$ inch) in diameter. Although 25 sand grains laid side by side in a line is only 2.5 cm (1 inch), 1 billion sand grains would stretch over more than 1015 km (630 miles). Astonishingly slow geologic rates, such as the movement of the earth's plates, can accomplish amazing feats in a relatively short geologic time span. For example, with an average rate of plate motion at about 2.5 cm (1 inch) per year, the Atlantic Ocean has widened another 14 m (44 feet) since Christopher Columbus sailed from Spain to the New World in 1492. In just 100 million years, widening of the Atlantic has proceeded more than 1900 km (1200 miles) (Figure 125-16).

THE GRAND CANYON: AN EXAMPLE OF EARTH SCIENCE AT WORK

INTRODUCTION AND PHYSICAL SETTING

The Grand Canyon is one of Earth's most iconic landscapes (Figure 125-17). It provides an exceptional window into the workings of planet Earth and serves to highlight the basic concepts presented in this chapter. Grand Canyon National Park offers a host of colorful viewpoints from the rim that present visitors a platform from which to view a spectacular display of Earth history. Numerous trails leave the rim to provide access to the Colorado River, offering an exciting white-water ride through the length of the canyon. Almost everyone who visits the canyon is immediately impressed with its immense size, rugged and colorful topography, and stunning skies and changeable weather.

The Colorado River and its tributaries have likely carved the Grand Canyon in only the last 5 to 6 Ma (*mega-annum,* or million years ago), but neither the exact age nor the specific processes that acted to create it are resolved. The river flows through the canyon for 450 km (277 miles), but nowhere can the canyon be viewed in its entirety from the ground. On average, the canyon measures about 16 km (10 miles) wide, with an extreme width of 29 km (18 miles). It is more than 1.6 km (1 mile) deep in most places, with about 4170 km³ (1000 miles³) of rock having been removed by erosion. Much of this material now resides in the area of the Gulf of California, where the Colorado River ends its 2333-km (1450-mile) journey to the sea.

The canyon is located entirely within the state of Arizona and on the southwestern edge of the Colorado Plateau, one of 26 geographic provinces described within the boundaries of the United States. Because of its extreme relief and longitudinal profile, the canyon is home to 1750 species of plants (more than any other National Park in the country), 373 species of birds, 47 reptile species, and 34 species of mammals. Its archaeological record extends back at least 4500 years and is based on radiocarbon-dated willow-stick figurines found in caves. The record may extend back 12,000 years or more, to the time when people first arrived in the Americas, but based only on a single projectile point, found on the canyon's South Rim.

Persons of European descent first saw the canyon in 1540, when native guides led members of the Coronado Expedition to the canyon's edge. These explorers were not impressed, and the canyon was not truly appreciated by humans until the first geologist visited in 1858. From that time onward, people have come to the Grand Canyon to experience its sublime grandeur and spectacular vistas. Today, it is visited by almost 5.5 million people a year, with more than 40% coming from outside the United States.

CREATING THE ROCKS: 2 BILLION YEARS OF EARTH HISTORY

Basement Rocks

The geologic story at Grand Canyon National Park begins about 1840 Ma, when other *terranes* collided with North America and became attached to it (a *terrane* is a discreet portion of the crust containing related rocks with a shared geologic history) (Figure 125-18). This collision compressed the rocks and both raised mountains on the surface and folded them to great depths within the crust, altering them to medium- to high-grade metamorphic rocks. Garnet minerals within rocks exposed today reveal burial depths of up to about 25 km (15 miles) with temperatures of 750°C (1382°F). They are now formally described as the Grand Canyon Metamorphic Suite, but historically are known as Vishnu Schist.

At even greater depths, the same rocks were melted and then rose buoyantly into the still-deforming metamorphic assemblage. These rocks were intruded as light-colored granitic dikes and plutons between about 1710 and 1660 Ma. They have been formally classified as the Zoroaster Plutonic Complex, but are historically known as the Zoroaster Granite. The resulting assemblage of igneous and metamorphic rocks records the dynamic changes that added crust to the North American continent over a 180-million-year period.

The entire assemblage of metamorphic and igneous rocks is informally referred to as the "Vishnu basement" (Figure 125-19). Mica minerals within the schist record how the overlying 21 km (13 miles) of rock was eroded away between 1350 and 1254 Ma. As erosion continued through time, the confining pressures were gradually lessened, and the rocks below rose isostatically. This is how rocks once found at 21 km (13 miles) down were brought back to the earth's surface. A generally flat-lying erosion surface was ultimately worn down to near sea level.

Grand Canyon Supergroup

Following this period of erosion, during which the Vishnu basement rocks were planed to near sea level, sediments began to be deposited on top of them around 1250 Ma. These rocks belong to the Grand Canyon Supergroup, a package of mostly sedimentary rocks containing nine formations that is more than 3800 m (12,500 feet) thick. The lower part of the Supergroup records deposition in offshore (limestone), nearshore (shale), and continental (sandstone) environments. A volcanic period with eruptive lava flows and forceful intrusions ended deposition about 1100 Ma.

The upper part of the Supergroup was preceded by an interval of erosion lasting up to 400 million years, and the rocks in this package were laid down in shallow marine and nearshore settings. Few rocks of this age (between 780 and 740 Ma) are known on Earth. The Grand Canyon Supergroup contains an important record of the diversification of single-celled life and the appearance of heterotrophic life—organisms that gain their nutrition from other organisms rather than exclusively through photosynthesis.

The Grand Canyon Supergroup is found in only about 10% of the canyon and always as isolated, fault-bounded, and tilted blocks. The preserved blocks represent areas that were downfaulted low into the ancient crust, allowing them to escape subsequent erosion. Blocks that were faulted higher were eroded away completely between 650 and 540 Ma. Some lithologies in the Supergroup were particularly resistant to erosion and stood as cliffs on the ancient landscape. These cliffs were preserved beneath the next package of rocks (Figure 125-20).

Paleozoic Rocks

A 1200-m (4000-foot) section of flat-lying Paleozoic strata makes up the upper four-fifths of the walls of Grand Canyon, composing the easily recognizable, stratified profile of the canyon (Figure 125-21). These rocks record deposition over a 255-million-year period spanning the length of the Paleozoic Era. There are 14 separate formations that make up this stack of rocks, each with a distinctive story to tell about the environments that once existed there (Figure 125-22).

Cambrian-age rocks include the Tapeats Sandstone, Bright Angel Shale, and Muav Limestone. This three-part assemblage exposes a continental-to-marine sequence that records the gradual onlap (about 30 million years) of the sea onto the continental margin (Figure 125-23). A hiatus of no less than 135 million years separates the Muav Limestone from the Devonian-age Temple Butte Limestone. This rock unit is only exposed in

GEOLOGIC TIME SCALE

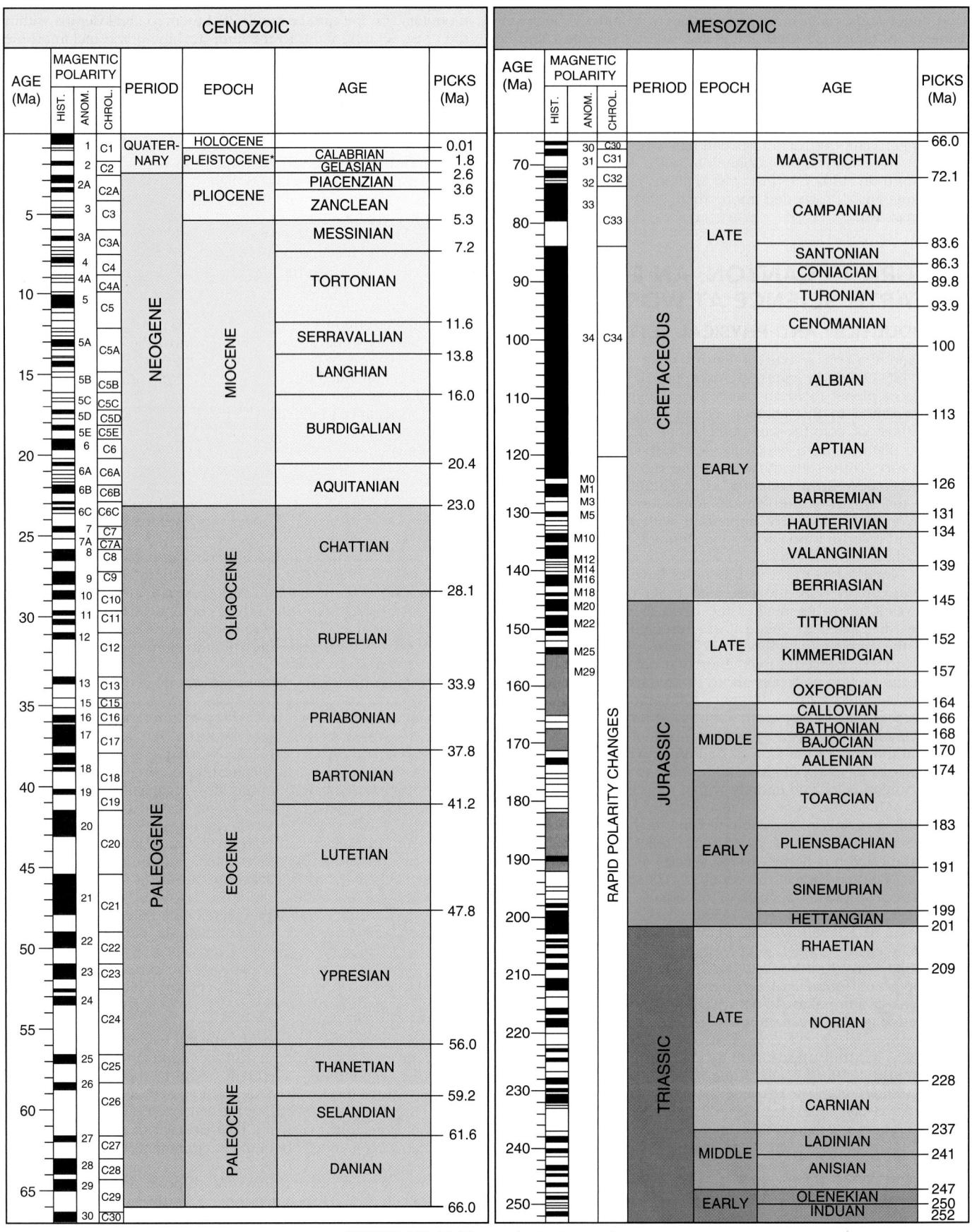

FIGURE 125-16 The geologic time scale.

GEOLOGIC TIME SCALE continued

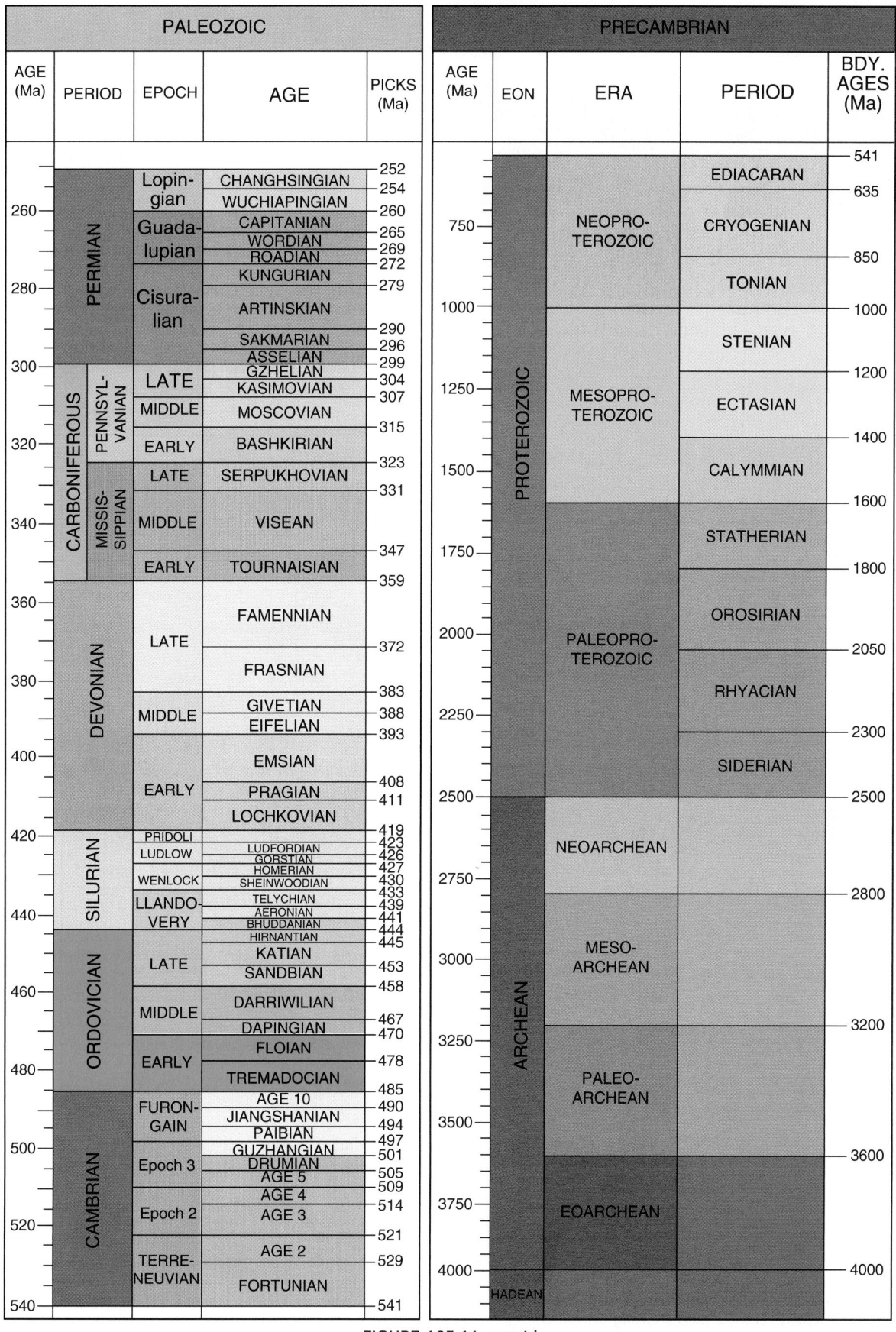

PALEOZOIC				
AGE (Ma)	PERIOD	EPOCH	AGE	PICKS (Ma)
260	PERMIAN	Lopin-gian	CHANGHSINGIAN	252
			WUCHAPINGIAN	254
		Guada-lupian	CAPITANIAN	260
			WORDIAN	265
			ROADIAN	269
280		Cisura-lian	KUNGURIAN	272
			ARTINSKIAN	279
			SAKMARIAN	290
300			ASSELIAN	296
	CARBONIFEROUS	PENNSYL-VANIAN	LATE	GZHELIAN	299
				KASIMOVIAN	304
		MIDDLE	MOSCOVIAN	307
320		EARLY	BASHKIRIAN	315
		MISSIS-SIPPIAN	LATE	SERPUKHOVIAN	323
					331
340		MIDDLE	VISEAN	
		EARLY	TOURNAISIAN	347
360	DEVONIAN	LATE	FAMENNIAN	359
380			FRASNIAN	372
		MIDDLE	GIVETIAN	383
			EIFELIAN	388
400		EARLY	EMSIAN	393
			PRAGIAN	408
			LOCHKOVIAN	411
420	SILURIAN	PRIDOLI		419
		LUDLOW	LUDFORDIAN	423
			GORSTIAN	426
		WENLOCK	HOMERIAN	427
			SHEINWOODIAN	430
		LLANDO-VERY	TELYCHIAN	433
440			AERONIAN	439
			BHUDDANIAN	441
			HIRNANTIAN	444
	ORDOVICIAN	LATE	KATIAN	445
			SANDBIAN	453
460		MIDDLE	DARRIWILIAN	458
			DAPINGIAN	467
		EARLY	FLOIAN	470
480			TREMADOCIAN	478
	CAMBRIAN	FURON-GAIN	AGE 10	485
			JIANGSHANIAN	490
			PAIBIAN	494
500		Epoch 3	GUZHANGIAN	497
			DRUMIAN	501
			AGE 5	505
		Epoch 2	AGE 4	509
			AGE 3	514
520			AGE 2	521
		TERRE-NEUVIAN		529
540			FORTUNIAN	541

PRECAMBRIAN			
AGE (Ma)	EON	ERA	PERIOD	BDY. AGES (Ma)
	PROTEROZOIC	NEOPRO-TEROZOIC	EDIACARAN	541
750			CRYOGENIAN	635
			TONIAN	850
1000		MESOPRO-TEROZOIC	STENIAN	1000
1250			ECTASIAN	1200
1500			CALYMMIAN	1400
		PALEOPRO-TEROZOIC	STATHERIAN	1600
1750			OROSIRIAN	1800
2000			RHYACIAN	2050
2250			SIDERIAN	2300
2500	ARCHEAN	NEOARCHEAN		2500
2750				2800
3000		MESO-ARCHEAN		
3250				3200
3500		PALEO-ARCHEAN		3600
3750		EOARCHEAN		
4000	HADEAN			4000

FIGURE 125-16, cont'd

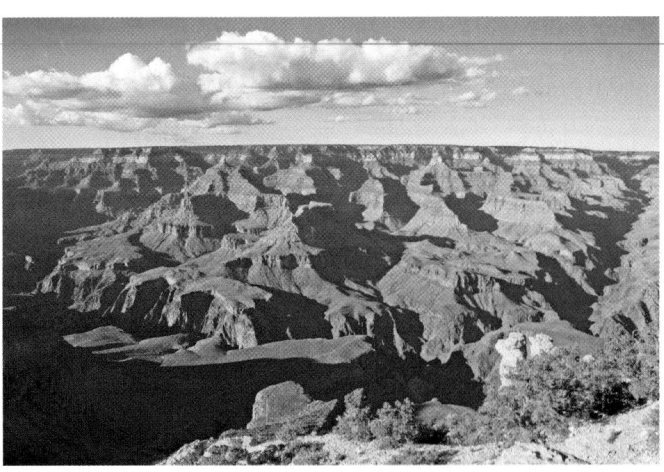

FIGURE 125-17 The Grand Canyon of the Colorado River in Arizona is perhaps our planet's best monument to geologic time, sedimentation, and erosion. *(Photo by Wayne Ranney.)*

discontinuous channels in eastern Grand Canyon that thicken and converge into a 120-m-thick (400-foot-thick) continuous deposit in the western canyon.

Overlying the Temple Butte Limestone is the Redwall Limestone, a Carboniferous-age massive cliff-former located midway up the canyon walls. The deposit is 150 m (500 ft) thick and formed in an open marine setting that contains abundant crinoid, bryozoan, brachiopod, and coral fossils (Figure 125-24). The Tapeats to Redwall section of rocks reflects the passive margin (continental shelf) conditions that existed in western North America during the early Paleozoic, after the opening of the proto–Pacific Ocean.

Upper Carboniferous to Permian rocks known as the Supai Group document the gradual replacement of marine environments to more continental conditions during the late Paleozoic. The Supai rocks are interpreted in ascending order as nearshore, coastal floodplain, and eolian (wind-derived) deposits. Some vertebrate trackways have been found. The overlying brick-red Hermit Formation consists of sandstone, mudstone, and pebble conglomerate. It formed on a broad coastal plain in mostly fluvial (river) and eolian settings.

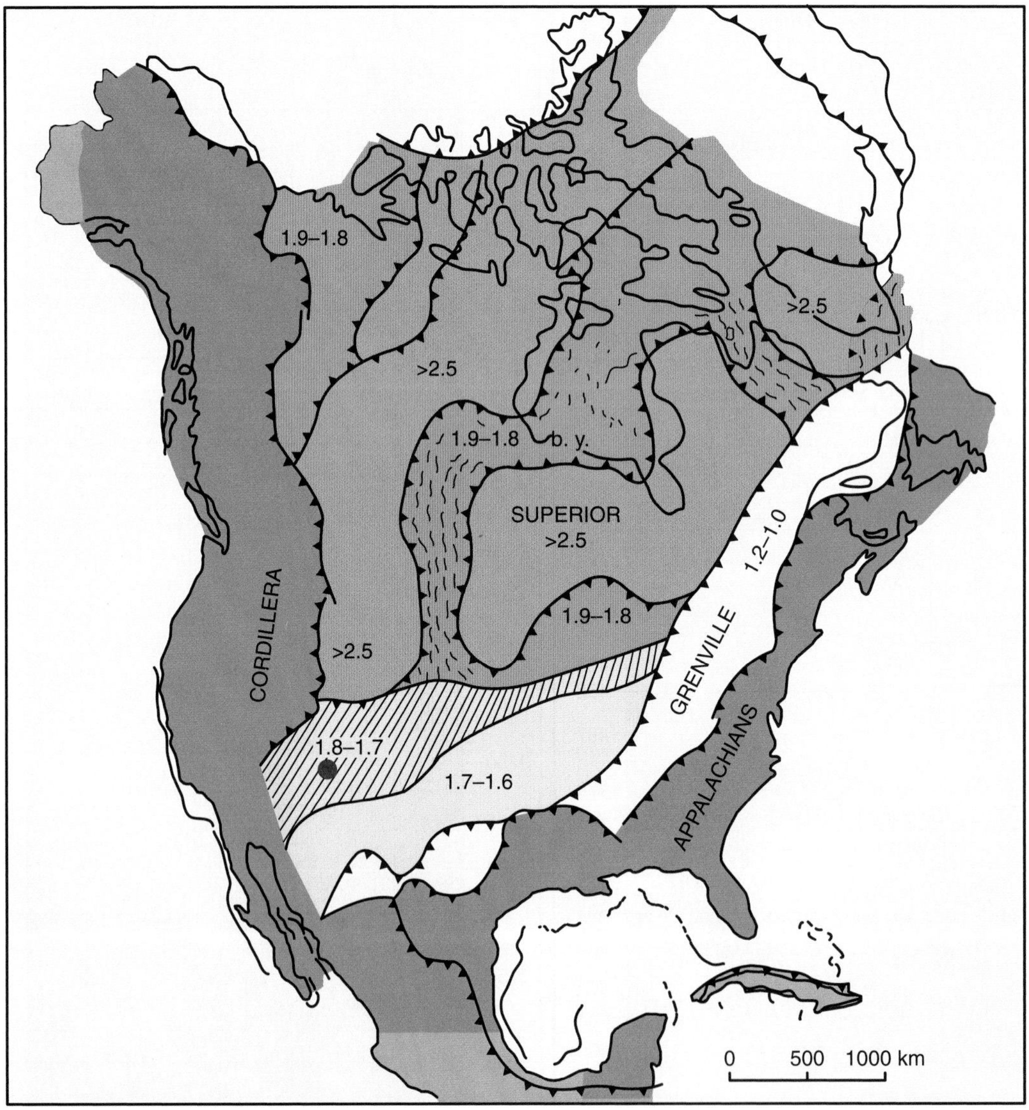

FIGURE 125-18 Map showing incremental growth of the North American continent. The oldest parts of the crust, formed more than 2500 million years ago (Ma), are labeled in *orange*; crust between 1900 and 1800 Ma, in *green*; 1800 to 1600 Ma, in *yellow*; and less than 300 Ma, in *blue*. The Vishnu rocks in the Grand Canyon are part of a terrane that arrived about 1750 to 1680 Ma. Red dot indicates approximate location of the Grand Canyon.

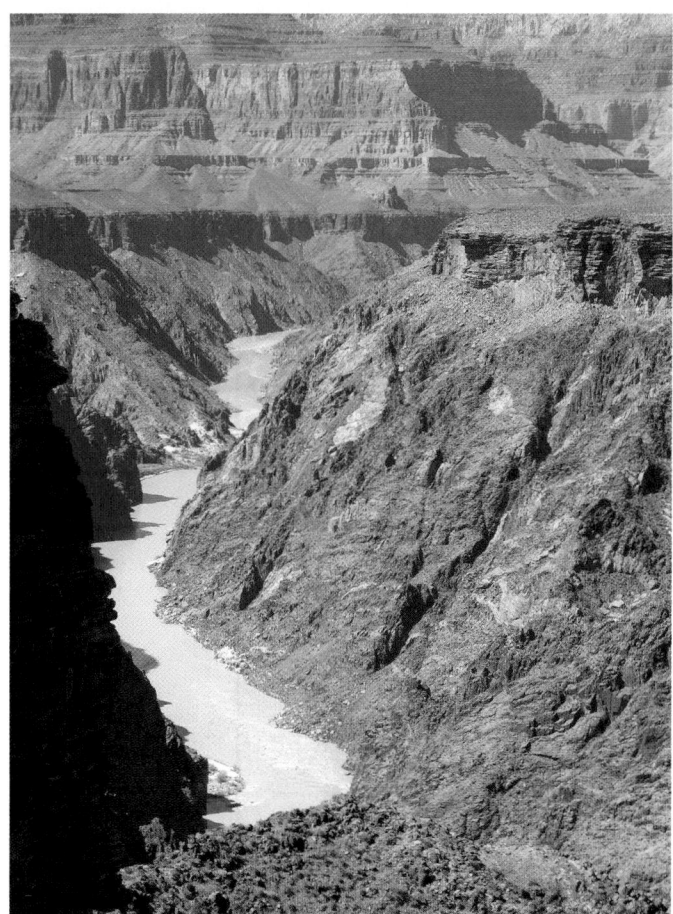

FIGURE 125-19 Spectacular view of the Vishnu basement rocks in the Inner Gorge of the Grand Canyon. *(Photo by Wayne Ranney.)*

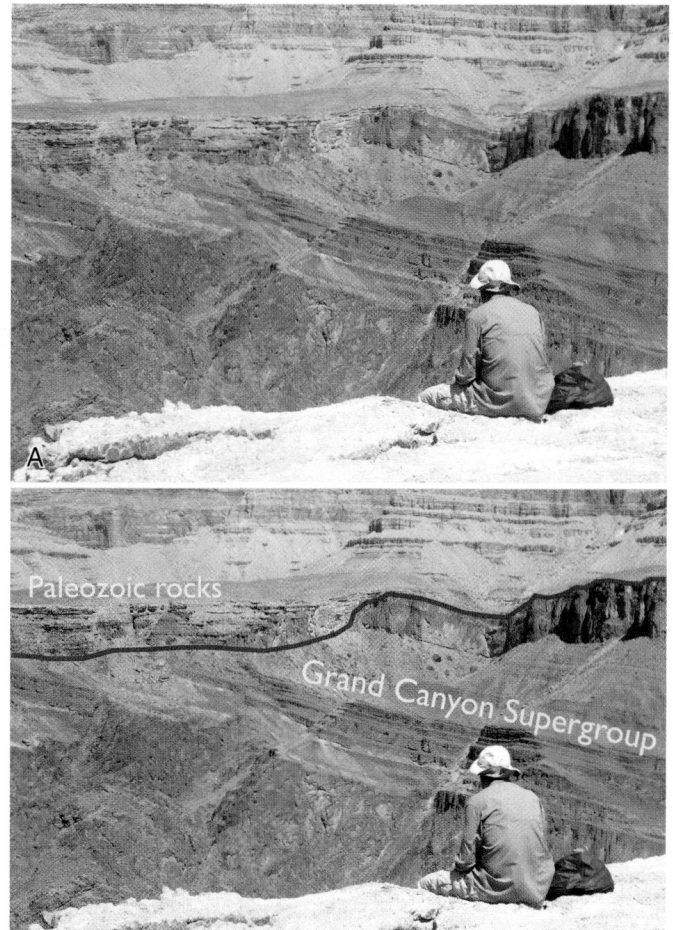

FIGURE 125-20 **A,** The Grand Canyon Supergroup, originally more than 3658 m (12,000 feet) thick, is found in only about 10% of the Grand Canyon and is tilted everywhere when seen. **B,** The *red line* shows the eroded top surface of the Supergroup, with a resistant cliff standing in the center of the photo. The younger, flat-lying Paleozoic layers *(top)* ultimately buried the Supergroup rocks. *(Photo by Wayne Ranney.)*

The next deposit is the Coconino Sandstone, a pale-yellow unit that is 100 m (330 feet) thick and forms sheer cliffs everywhere within the canyon. It originated in an arid, inland dune environment similar to the modern desert in the Sahara (Figure 125-25). Some layers contain numerous and well-preserved reptile trackways. The overlying Toroweap Formation is often overlooked in Grand Canyon because it forms slopes of easily eroded siltstone and gypsum that are covered in trees. It was deposited along the shore of a sea that encroached from the west. Capping the Grand Canyon and completing the entire Paleozoic section is the Kaibab Limestone. It represents a final transgression of the late Paleozoic sea into the area. Numerous chert horizons (a microcrystalline form of silica that often precipitates from seawater) help to solidify the Kaibab and make it the durable rock that "holds up" the strata in the canyon.

Mesozoic Rocks

A voluminous stack of Mesozoic-age rocks once covered the Grand Canyon area, but erosion has removed most of them. These rocks were once on the order of 1500 to 3000 m (5000 to 10,000 feet) thick and can be found in Zion and Bryce Canyon National Parks to the north, on the Navajo Indian Reservation to the east, and near Las Vegas, Nevada, to the west. Because the Grand Canyon lies between the three areas, it is logical to assume the rocks were once here as well, before erosion stripped them away.

Cenozoic Rocks

Rocks of Cenozoic age are relatively scarce at the Grand Canyon, because this was a time of regional uplift and erosion. Some river gravels are preserved that may indicate a time when the Grand Canyon began to form, no earlier than about 70 Ma. More recent volcanic rocks are located in the western Grand Canyon, where basalt lava, ranging in age from 830,000 to 1000 years, erupted

along a 16-km (10-mile) stretch of the Colorado River. Numerous flows and cones are found perched above and within the canyon walls, with one remnant having traveled 135 km (84 miles) down the river channel, while others are perched up to 330 m (1100 feet) high. Up to 17 lava dams blocked the Colorado River, and

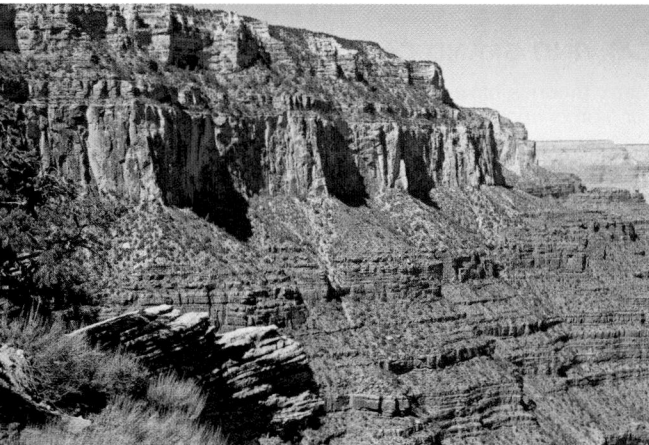

FIGURE 125-21 Paleozoic rocks were deposited in the Grand Canyon from 525 to 270 Ma and form the upper four-fifths of the canyon walls. *(Photo by Wayne Ranney.)*

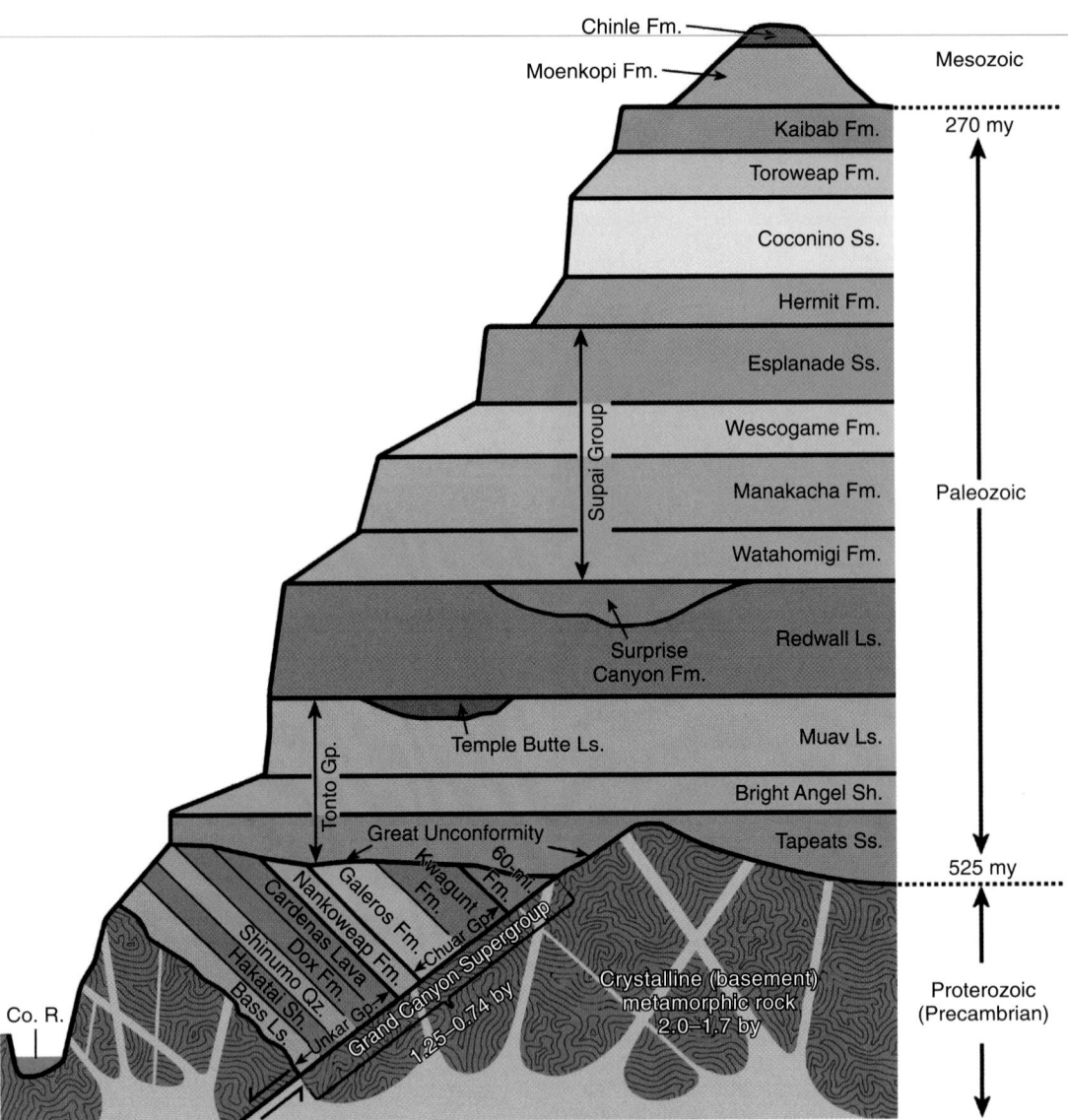

FIGURE 125-22 Rock column for the Grand Canyon.

on at least five occasions, huge outburst floods were the result of catastrophic failure of these dams. Deposits from these outburst floods are found 45 to 200 m (150 to 650 feet) above the modern channel, with clast sizes up to 30 m (100 feet) in diameter.

CARVING GRAND CANYON

Many theories have been proposed for how the Colorado River (or some ancestor to it) actually carved the Grand Canyon. Despite extensive research, some important details about its formation have escaped full detection. However, a broad outline is known, and future research will likely elucidate more of the story. This much is known: the Colorado River and its tributaries excavated this great space; it could not have happened before about 70 Ma; and it is likely that much of what we see today has formed in just the last 5 or 6 million years.

For approximately 455 million years, the Grand Canyon region was situated near, and many times below, sea level, thus precluding the presence of a deep canyon. A fantastic 4.8-km-thick (3-mile-thick) section of stratified rocks reveal this long-lived nearshore setting, a time when the rocks in Grand Canyon were formed. Beginning about 70 million years ago, the region was uplifted as the Farallon Plate was subducted beneath western North America. This event, known as the *Laramide orogeny* (an orogeny is a mountain-building event), uplifted a broad section

of the continent from southern Arizona to the Rocky Mountains. A range of mountains southwest of the Grand Canyon, called the Mogollon Highlands, caused the first rivers to run from the southern mountains to the northeast, exactly opposite the direction of the modern Colorado River. This drainage lasted until at least 25 million years ago (Figure 125-26).

It is currently under debate if portions of the Grand Canyon could have been cut by this early northeast drainage system. Modern laboratory techniques are being used to tease more information out of Grand Canyon's stubborn rocks, but to date have yielded conflicting data. One group of researchers proposes that by about 70 Ma, some portions of the canyon were cut to within 100 m (330 feet) of its current depth, whereas another group says that only one of five subsections of the canyon was carved at this early date.

Geologists "lose sight" of the river and canyon for about 20 million years, because a period of erosion or perhaps even nondeposition ensued. This certainly was the time of drainage reversal, whereby the old northeast-directed system gave way to the current southwest-flowing river. Deposits at the mouth of the Grand Canyon that are between 16 and 6 million years old show that the modern river might not have been flowing here before about 5 or 6 million years ago. This is why the majority of geologists think that the river (and thus the canyon) could be no older than this age. However, some alternative scenarios have been proposed that can explain why no Colorado River sediment

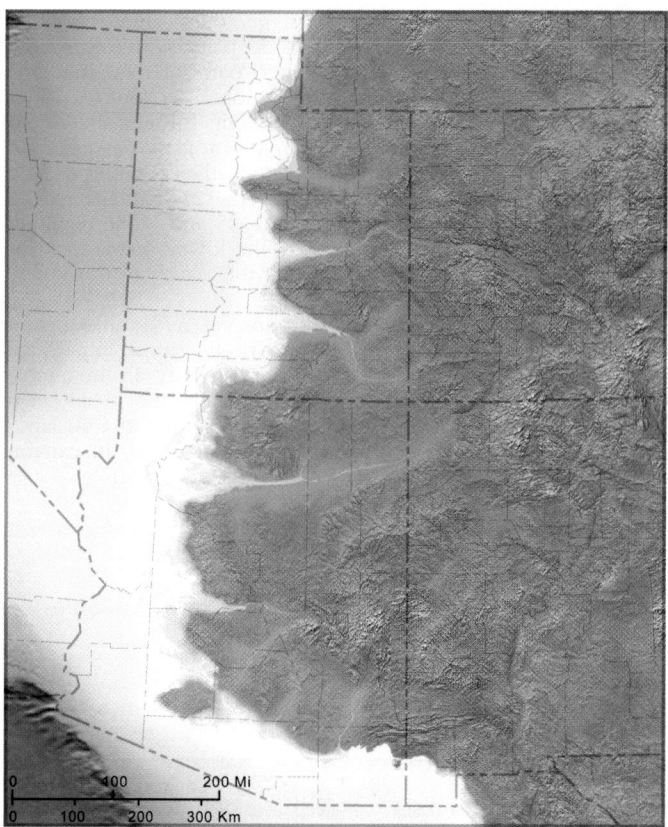

FIGURE 125-23 Paleogeographic view of the Four Corner states during deposition of the Tapeats Sandstone 525 Ma. The map reflects a time before land plants evolved; thus the land area (*right*) is shown as *brown*. (*From Blakey R, Ranney W. Ancient landscapes of the Colorado Plateau, 2008, Grand Canyon Association.*)

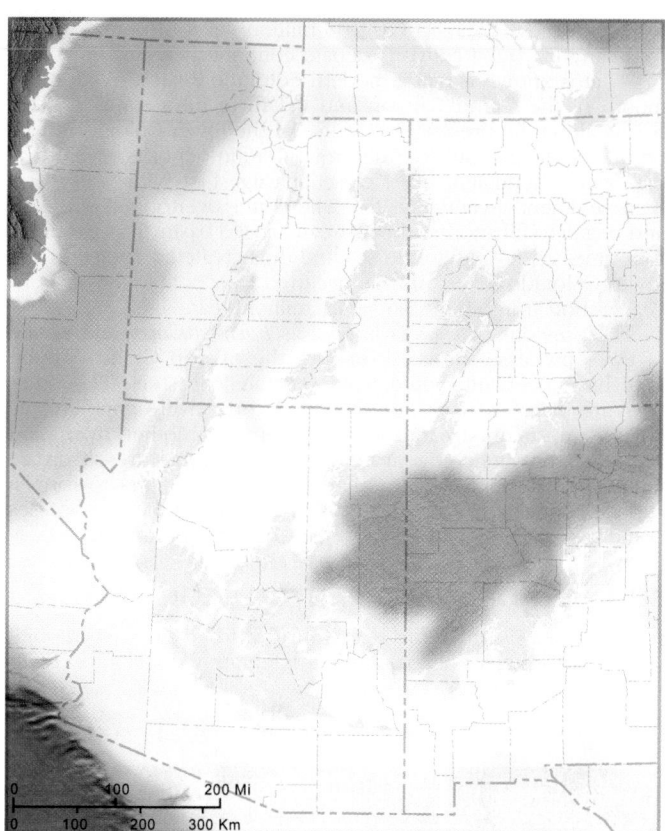

FIGURE 125-24 The Redwall Sea covered much of the American Southwest about 340 Ma.

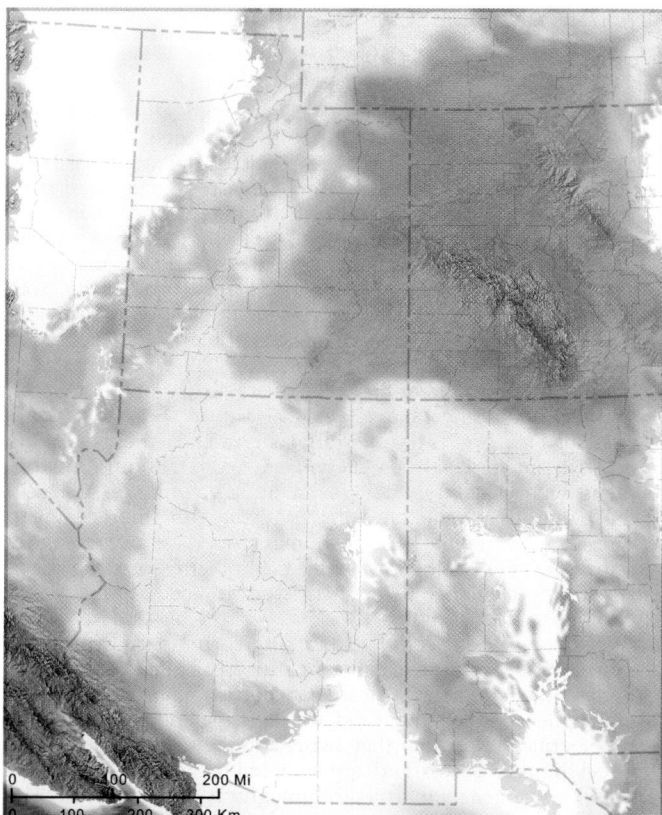

FIGURE 125-25 The Coconino Sandstone reveals the presence of a Sahara-like desert in the Grand Canyon area about 275 Ma.

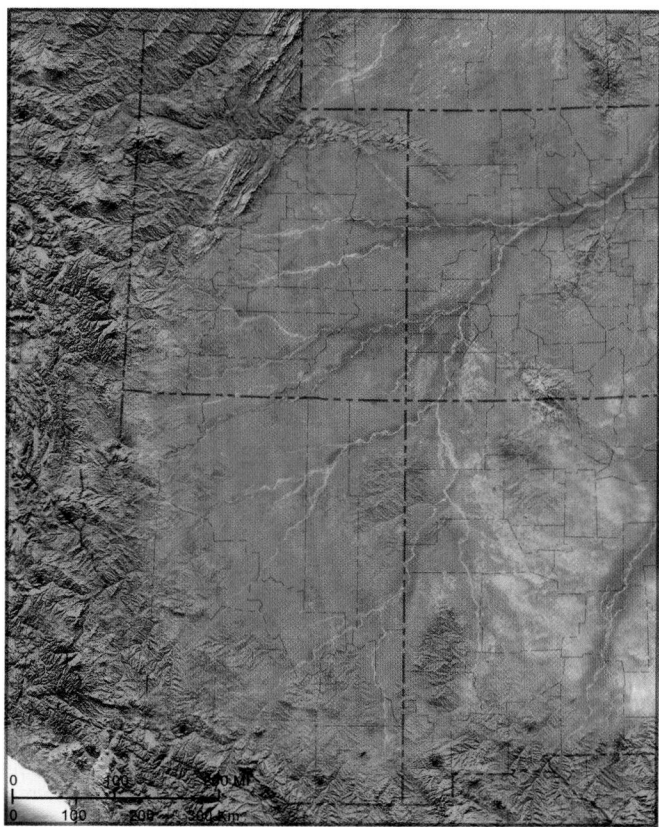

FIGURE 125-26 When the sea finally left the Grand Canyon region for the last time, an initial river system developed from the Mogollon Highlands (*bottom*) to the northeast. This is opposite to the direction of the modern river system and lasted for at least 45 million years.

resides in these deposits (16 to 6 million years old), and so the "old canyon/young canyon" debate continues.

What is known is that a modern Colorado River arrived at the mouth of the Grand Canyon and began to fill a series of lake basins along the present-day course of the lower Colorado River on its way to the Gulf of California. Certain deposits reveal that the river sequentially filled closed basins, first with water and then sediment. Eventually, the lake water overtopped a divide and began to fill another downstream closed basin. This occurred four times on its way to the sea and thus created a course of the lower Colorado River. All this occurred over a 1- to 1.5-million-year period from about 5.6 to 4.1 million years ago.

The previous process is known as *basin spillover* and is one of three processes invoked for how the river in Grand Canyon may have been integrated from separate ancestors. The other two are *headward erosion,* whereby one river lengthens its channel upstream to intersect and capture another river, and *karst collapse*, whereby groundwater establishes a subsurface connection through caverns that ultimately collapses to form a surface connection. Any one, two, or all three of these processes could explain the Colorado River in the Grand Canyon.

SUMMARY OF GRAND CANYON GEOLOGY

A picture that is emerging is that headward erosion, basin spillover, and/or karst collapse helped integrate the Colorado River and create the Grand Canyon. Most geologists agree that the canyon we see today is the result of deep incision within only the last 5 to 6 million years. However, parts of this "modern" canyon may overprint or incorporate some sections of older canyons. A broad outline of the major events forming the Grand Canyon is now possible: (1) the Laramide orogeny produced an initial river system with drainage to the northeast, with possible early segments of Grand Canyon carved; (2) drainage in the region became disrupted between about 25 and 6 Ma, resulting in few deposits; and (3) integration of the lower Colorado River by basin spillover created an outlet to the sea from the Rocky Mountains.

The Grand Canyon continues to inspire as a unique and remarkable landform. It remains one of the most impressive outdoor laboratories for the study of Earth history. In the almost 160 years that it has been studied scientifically, much has been learned about fluvial processes acting on an uplifted, arid landscape. Over time, and with improved dating methods, the canyon will continued to reveal more of its secrets.

SELECTED RESOURCES

Selected resources used in this text are available online at expertconsult.inkling.com.

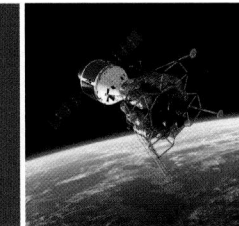

CHAPTER 126

Space Medicine: The Next Frontier

THOMAS H. MARSHBURN, RICHARD W. COLE, AND REBECCA S. BLUE

Humans are at the threshold of a phase of exploration equal in significance to any yet undertaken by the species. Having developed technology that enables escape from the gravitational forces that hold us to the earth's surface, human space programs have demonstrated that we can survive, function, and perform complex tasks in continuous microgravity. The past century has witnessed humans piloting spacecraft through launches, landings, rendezvous, and dockings in Earth orbit; constructing complex vehicles and habitats that allow long-term occupancy; and expanding human presence in the Solar System beyond the limits of Earth's atmosphere.

An international coalition of space programs from the United States, Russia, Europe, Canada, and Japan continuously inhabit low Earth orbit. We have collectively experienced more than 15 years of human presence aboard the International Space Station (ISS), the largest space vehicle ever assembled, with a module length of 50.9 m (167 feet) and a habitable volume of about 906.14 m^3 (32,000 feet^3) (Figure 126-1). More recently, China has joined the roster of spacefaring nations, launching five-crewed missions since 2003 and maintaining the Tiangong-1 space station in low Earth orbit for visiting crews since 2012.

With increasing human experience in space, the field of space medicine continues to mature and advance, improving understanding of the unique threats spaceflight poses to human health and developing a foundation of medical diagnosis and treatment techniques specific to spaceflight-related concerns. While drawing heavily from many medical and surgical specialties, aerospace medicine is a unique field of study and medical practice. It addresses the challenges of maintaining long-term human health and performance in the face of the following four fundamental threats:

1. *Microgravity.* Astronauts travel in craft with sufficient energy to attain a free-fall state in perpetuity, no longer encumbered by Earth's gravity gradient. The resultant unloading of body fluids and tissues has profound effects on human physiology and health and can have an impact on timing and mechanism of recovery from injury and illness. Further, the microgravity environment alters the ability to deliver medical care.

2. *Radiation.* The farther humans travel into space, away from the protective shroud of Earth's geomagnetosphere, the more they are exposed to greater intensities of highly ionizing radiation, pervasive throughout the universe. This type of radiation has the potential to inflict immediate injury and long-term harm to human health.

3. *Psychological effects of isolation.* Living in space entails living in close quarters with few crewmates in a dangerous environment, with visual and tactile surroundings quite dissimilar to those found in daily life on Earth, and an unprecedented disconnect from the rest of humankind. The psychological impact of this unique combination of stressors can be a significant challenge to human performance during space exploration.

4. *The spacecraft environment.* To survive in space, astronauts must rely entirely on small, enclosed, Earth-like ecosystems aboard their vehicles. These systems maintain a breathable atmosphere, water and food supply, hygiene methods, and other critical elements that, when disrupted, can negatively affect human health and are vulnerable to any insults that could endanger their structural integrity.

Despite these challenges, access to space may soon increase exponentially. Spacefaring nations are expanding their reach toward the goals of habitation on the lunar surface, interplanetary

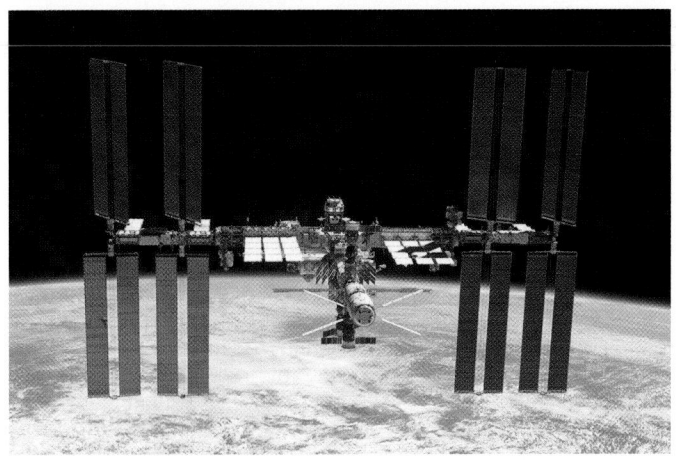

FIGURE 126-1 The International Space Station (ISS), a National Research Laboratory currently orbiting the earth approximately 250 nautical miles above Earth's surface. Assembled by five partner agencies, the ISS has been continuously manned since November 2000.

travel to Mars, and commercial spaceflight offered to the general population. Acknowledging this rapid expansion of spaceflight and the unique role of space as the ultimate wilderness environment, this chapter summarizes the distinctive environmental factors experienced by astronauts; describes the clinically relevant physiologic and psychological effects of space travel, particularly as related to human function and adaptation in space; and provides an understanding of the medical practice of modern flight surgeons and astronaut physicians. We further explore gaps in current clinical understanding with respect to the knowledge we must gain to reduce barriers to longer and more expansive space travel in the future.

THE SPACEFLIGHT ENVIRONMENT

The spaceflight environment is complex and variable. In general, space is uninhabitable to humans and fraught with dangers that would rapidly prove fatal without the protection afforded by a vehicle with intrinsic life support systems. Major challenges of the spaceflight environment include pressure (specifically, lack of pressure), thermal concerns, gaseous factors (e.g., availability of oxygen, concentrations of carbon monoxide and carbon dioxide), presence of onboard hazardous materials (e.g., coolants, propellants, other contaminants), and risk of fire.

PRESSURE

The human body requires a certain amount of ambient pressure to sustain life. Humans exposed to vacuum conditions, as exist outside of Earth's atmosphere, would experience a number of physiologic insults, including decompression illness, hypoxia and impeded gas exchange, and ebullism (the evolution of body fluids to gas); each of these insults can rapidly lead to physiologic dysfunction and death. Integrity of life support systems, particularly in providing the livable pressure atmosphere, is a major determinant of human survival in spaceflight.

Spaceflight Decompression Risks

Decompression is a serious concern during spaceflight and can occur either intentionally or from a contingency event, such as collision, structural failure, or human error. Intentional decompressions occur in normal flight operations, usually to support spacewalks, or extravehicular activities (EVAs). Astronauts performing EVAs do so in spacesuits that operate at pressures lower than the common sea level cabin pressure of 14.7 pounds per square inch absolute (psia), typically between 4 and 6 psia depending on the suit, using 100% oxygen (O_2) as a breathing gas. To prevent evolution of tissue nitrogen bubbles during decompression to these lower pressures, ISS astronauts perform an O_2 prebreathe session to afford nitrogen washout, followed

by a staged decompression within the airlock to final suit pressure. The usual EVA sortie lasts for about 6 hours, after which crews can fairly rapidly recompress back to station sea level pressure. Although such intentional depressurizations can cause injury, including decompression sickness (DCS), such events are rare. In fact, the only recorded DCS events in spaceflight occurred with planned cabin depressurization during launch of a Gemini spacecraft from sea level to an in-flight operating pressure of 5 psia, when a crewmember experienced sharp pain in one knee. The same astronaut experienced similar pain when he later launched in an Apollo spacecraft.[89]

Contingency depressurization is of greater concern than are planned decompression protocols with respect to likelihood of crew injury. The most likely events leading to contingency depressurization are collision with other vehicles, as occurred between the Russian Mir station and an uncrewed cargo vessel in 1997, and hypervelocity orbital debris impact. Whereas vehicle collision can be avoided with engineering and human factor practices, orbital debris is a much less controlled hazard. As human presence in space has increased, so has the risk of orbital debris impacts. Any component of derelict spacecraft, including abandoned stages, decomposing satellites, or even minute debris such as paint particles, can pose a risk to other space vehicles. While orbital debris pieces larger than 10 cm (4 inches) in diameter can be carefully tracked and avoided by means of ground-based radar, smaller pieces are difficult to track and can be highly damaging because of the speeds at which they travel. The highest-risk objects are 1 to 10 cm in (0.4 to 4 inches) diameter, large enough to be seen by ground radar but not tracked and avoided, and still able to transmit highly damaging force to spacecraft. The force imparted by collision with even a small debris particle is surprisingly large because of the velocity of the object and kinetic energy being proportional to the square of this velocity. For example, a 1 cm^2 (0.15 $inch^2$) piece of aluminum weighing 3 g (0.0066 lb) and traveling at orbital velocity of approximately 8 km/sec (17.89 miles/hr) in low Earth orbit would deliver 96,000 J of force on impact. The effects of orbital debris impacts depend on velocity of the debris, angle of impact, and the object mass, as well as sensitivity of the surface that is hit. A small, glancing blow may not cause significant damage to a heavily reinforced portion of a space vehicle, but it could cause catastrophic damage to a solar panel. Unfortunately, impacts are now a feature of space travel, with numerous reports of impact craters found on space vehicles, one of the largest being 3.8 mm (0.15 inch), on the window of Soyuz T-9 in 1983.[170]

The longer a vehicle stays in orbit, the greater its exposure to some manner of debris, and the more important it is to ensure that shielding is effective. The ISS has the most robust shielding ever flown and routinely performs maneuvers to adjust the orbit of the entire station to avoid collision with orbital debris; even so, small debris impacts do occur. For this reason, protocols are in place to prepare astronauts for a contingency decompression after debris strike or vehicle collision. In a decompression event, sensors would alarm at a pressure differential of greater than 1.0 psi/hr or a total pressure decrease of 0.4 psi. Crews are trained to respond by first ensuring individual access to supplemental O_2 and a clear route to an escape vehicle, then detecting and isolating the leak or, in worst-case scenarios, abandoning the station to return to Earth.

Decompression-Related Injuries

Decompression-related injuries in spaceflight are expected to be similar to those seen in other dysbaric events, such as rapid pressure changes during scuba diving or rapid decompression of an aircraft at altitude. Sequelae can include hypoxia from reduced partial pressure of oxygen (Po_2), barotrauma events (e.g., pneumothorax, gastrointestinal barotrauma), musculoskeletal decompression symptoms (e.g., joint pain), neurologic sequelae of DCS, and arterial gas embolism (clinical manifestations are discussed in Chapters 71 and 72). DCS is avoided during nominal decompression procedures for EVA through a combination of prebreathing 100% O_2 and staged crew decompression to facilitate nitrogen washout (Figure 126-2). One recently adopted adjunct

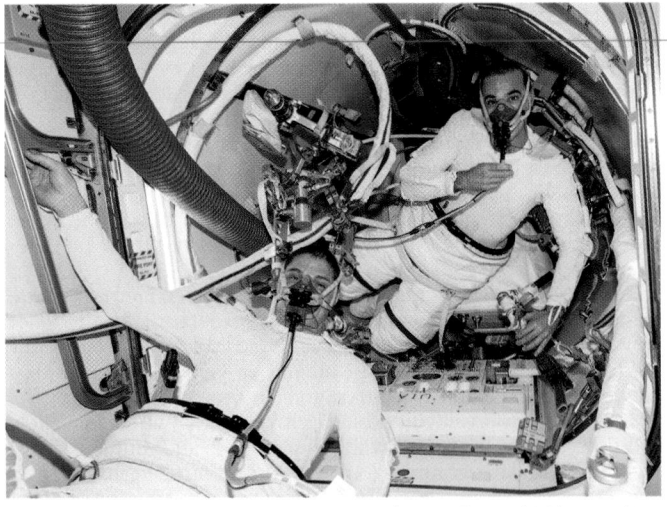

FIGURE 126-2 Astronauts Rick Mastracchio (*right*) and Mike Hopkins in preparation for a spacewalk in the ISS airlock, breathing 100% oxygen while donning their spacesuits as part of a protocol to reduce the risk of decompression sickness. Note the white cooling and ventilation undergarments that crews wear inside their spacesuits to regulate body temperature.

is addition of a light-exercise protocol; extensive research has evaluated exercise as a means of accelerating nitrogen washout during reduced-pressure O_2 prebreathe sessions.[36] Another option is to lengthen the O_2 prebreathe, then decompress directly to suit pressure, although this may imply logistical overhead of more in-suit time before decompression.

Accidental DCS events during a controlled decompression could occur; most would be expected to be treatable by returning to sea level pressure and continuing to breathe 100% O_2.[126] Decompression injury could also be treated on orbit by using an EVA suit as a pressure chamber. At standard sea level atmospheric pressure inside the ISS, the suit with the affected crewmember inside can be further pressurized with 100% O_2 to attain 22 psia. Although this is not as effective as a hyperbaric chamber and a standard hyperbaric protocol, the increased pressure may offer some benefit for acute DCS injuries, although isolation of the affected crewmember in a suit would limit other examination and interventional opportunities.[73] Further, limitations of on-orbit medical capability renders treatment of most of the more severe decompression-related conditions listed practically untenable, and evacuation and return to Earth may be necessary.

With the most catastrophic events, exposure to true vacuum conditions is also possible. If crewmembers are exposed to ambient pressure of less than 1 psia, ebullism occurs in addition to the classic DCS, hypoxia, and barotrauma insults. *Ebullism* is spontaneous evolution of water in tissues from a liquid to gaseous state at ambient pressures of less than 47 mm Hg (~0.9 psia), where the boiling point of water is less than or equal to the homeostatic temperature of the human body.[165] In *ebullism syndrome,* multiple insults occur, including anoxia, trapped-gas expansion and formation of nitrogen and water vapor bubbles, and rapid body fluid loss.[165] With an explosive decompression to vacuum conditions, crewmembers would be rapidly rendered unconscious, generally in less than 10 seconds. Even if astronauts were wearing supplemental O_2, the ambient pressure would be too low to allow for effective pulmonary gas exchange. Within 30 seconds of exposure, severe neurologic hypoxic sequelae would occur, leading ultimately to brain death as a result of hypoxia or ischemic insult from bubble formation within the vasculature. Bubbles can also form within thoracic organs, including the heart, and impede intrathoracic circulation, compounding ischemic insult. Circulatory arrest would rapidly follow.

However, very short exposures to complete vacuum are survivable. In 1966, a spacesuit technician was exposed during a test to near-vacuum conditions for 30 seconds in an altitude chamber after his suit umbilical accidentally disconnected from its pressurized O_2 supply. The technician lost consciousness in 12 to 15 seconds,[197] although was later able to report noting a fizzing sensation on his tongue from sublimation of saliva. He regained consciousness seconds after rapid repressurization and surprisingly, suffered no sequelae (LeBlanc J: Personal communication, 2015). An individual exposed to 22,555 m (74,000 feet) equivalent altitude for approximately 3 minutes in another vacuum chamber accident suffered pulmonary barotrauma and massive pulmonary and neurologic sequelae of DCS, with eventual clinical resolution after hyperbaric and prolonged medical treatment.[120] Protocols have been developed and published for treatment of ebullism syndrome based on successful rehabilitation of these individuals and continuous advancement of supportive medical care.[165] Aside from rapid recompression to cabin atmosphere, few options exist for ebullism treatment on orbit. Unless exposure is isolated to a single crewmember and ambient pressure could be rapidly restored, or exposure occurs during a rapid descent to normal atmosphere during reentry, ebullism injury in a spacecraft vehicle would likely prove rapidly fatal.

In-Flight Decompression Events

Despite careful debris tracking and avoidance and extensive crew training on the risks and mitigations of loss of cabin pressure, significant decompressions have occurred during human spaceflight. In 1997, the Russian Spektr module was damaged and depressurized by a collision with an uncrewed Progress resupply ship during an attempted docking with the Mir space station. In this case, the crew quickly sealed the hatch to the leaking Spektr, preventing further depressurization in the remaining modules of the space station and avoiding crew injury.

A more catastrophic loss of pressure occurred in 1971 when a pressure-equalization valve failed during reentry in the Soyuz 11 spacecraft at an altitude of 168 km (105 miles). The three cosmonauts aboard the Soyuz (Georgi Dobrovolskiy, Vladislav Volkov, and Victor Patsayev) rapidly lost consciousness during the decompression, and it is believed they had suffered fatal injuries within 1 minute of exposure. Preliminary autopsy results reportedly revealed intracerebral and pulmonary hemorrhage as a result of the approximately 10-minute exposure to near-vacuum conditions.[205]

Given the potential for catastrophic outcomes of decompression-related events in spaceflight, prevention of any loss of cabin pressure will remain of the utmost importance in vehicle design, trajectory and orbital maneuvering, and crewmember training.

OXYGEN

Directly related to the atmospheric pressure of a space vehicle cabin is the amount of O_2 available. Decreases in ambient pressure lead to resultant decreases in the partial pressure of O_2 available for gas exchange, which can lead to hypoxic symptoms despite compensatory pulmonary and cardiac responses. All current crewed vehicles, including the ISS and all its resupply craft, are nominally pressurized to 14.7 psia with a dual-gas system at near-terrestrial composition (21% O_2 and 79% nitrogen). However, astronauts are occasionally exposed intentionally to lower ambient pressures, most often during EVA. Lower spacesuit pressures are useful for many reasons, particularly for manipulating suit components such as gloves, improving mobility, and reducing the physical strain of activity within the suits. However, in addition to the risk of DCS, the lower pressure of a spacesuit does expose astronauts to the potential for hypoxia from reduced PO_2. Given these lower pressures and the simplicity of a single-gas system, suits are operated at 100% O_2.

Given the risk of vehicular depressurization or disruption of the internal gas environment from equipment malfunction, spacecraft are rigorously monitored for O_2 levels, and an insidious decrease in PO_2 would likely be detected by automatic sensing systems before symptomatically affecting the crew. Similarly, the EVA suit environment is carefully monitored for pressure and levels of O_2 and carbon dioxide. Any slight disruption of the internal suit environment would prompt rapid termination of an

EVA and return to the safety of the vehicle. Disruption of the cabin environment would prompt the crew to seek individual supplemental O_2 equipment to mitigate hypoxia until the problem is addressed, or in the worst-case scenario, the vehicle is abandoned.

The aerospace medicine practitioner must remain hypervigilant for hypoxic signs and symptoms because of the potential for exposure of entire astronaut crews to hypoxic conditions. At an ambient pressure of 10 psi (equivalent-pressure altitude, 3408 m [10,000 feet]), PO_2 drops to 109 mm Hg (~2 psi), and intra-alveolar concentrations of O_2 approach 60 mm Hg (~1.16 psi).[79] Decompression of the cabin atmosphere from 14.7 to 10 psia or lower would prompt physiologic compensatory responses to hypoxia in most individuals. Immediate responses are identical to those in patients at high altitude: hyperventilation and tachycardia to increase tissue O_2 delivery. Crewmembers may report more obvious evidence, such as ear popping, if decompression is rapid. However, hypoxic conditions secondary to dysfunction of gas-mixing systems may not be accompanied by a pressure differential, and the only signs or symptoms of a hypoxic environment may be vague and poorly defined feelings of fatigue, malaise, apprehension, paresthesias, visual changes, and nausea. Because none of the immediate symptoms of acute hypoxia can be considered pathognomonic, clinicians must remain vigilant for any crewmember complaints that may suggest an insidious hypoxic event and thus the need for O_2 replenishment or supplementation.

CARBON DIOXIDE

On Earth, production of carbon dioxide (CO_2) as a normal byproduct of ventilation is physiologically insignificant, because the gas is rapidly dispersed into the atmosphere and CO_2 concentration remains quite low, at an average of 0.23 mm Hg (.004 psi, or 0.03%). However, in a closed spacecraft environment, CO_2 would rapidly build up without effective atmospheric scrubbers. Therefore, cabins must be designed not only to provide the O_2 that a crew requires, but also to remove the CO_2 that the crew produces. Cabin scrubbers, typically adsorbents such as lithium hydroxide or zeolite, accomplish this task by chemically removing CO_2 from the cabin atmosphere. However, components of CO_2 removal systems have a limited lifetime, making it impractical to maintain CO_2 continuously at terrestrial levels. Furthermore, without effective airflow, localized concentrations of CO_2 can exist in microgravity, particularly around a stationary crewmember's face. For this reason, forced convection is established by using cabin fans in an attempt to ensure effective cabin airflow and avoid stagnant gas concentrations. Because structural elements may disturb airflow, astronauts are often exposed to elevated levels of CO_2, particularly in less ventilated areas or more populated spaces within the cabin, where individuals and their CO_2 byproducts tend to congregate and accumulate.

It was previously believed that physiologic effects of elevated CO_2 would be recognized only at levels of greater than 12 mm Hg (0.2 psi, or 1.5% CO_2). However, more recent evidence suggests that alterations in mood can occur at levels as low 0.5% CO_2 (4 mm Hg, 0.07 psi).[130] Headache is the most common initial complaint of CO_2 toxicity in space and has been reported at levels of less than 5 mm Hg of CO_2 in the cabin atmosphere. Because CO_2 is known to be a potent vasodilator that can increase cerebral blood flow and therefore possibly affect intracranial pressure (ICP), elevated CO_2 is also a possible contributor to suspected ICP increases on long-duration missions. This phenomenon is discussed later.

In a standard developed from terrestrial data and in concert with U.S. Occupational Safety and Health Administration (OSHA) and National Institute for Occupational Safety and Health (NIOSH) recommendations published in the 1980s, the average 24-hour CO_2 levels aboard the ISS were initially allowed to climb up to 7.6 mm Hg (0.14 psi).[101] This limit was later lowered to 5.3 mm Hg (0.1 psi) after several individuals onboard reported CO_2-related symptoms at the 7.6 mm Hg level; the decrease was further supported by new ground-based information from the early 1990s that suggested elevated CO_2 could lead to secondary

effects, including discomfort and decreased exercise tolerability.[242] However, astronauts continued to report symptoms even at the 5.3 mm Hg level. Crew symptomatology includes headache, fatigue, and self-reports of decreased work efficiency. Although there is significant interindividual variability, the frequency of symptoms resulted in the CO_2 threshold being lowered again in 2013, to 4.0 mm Hg (0.07 psi, or 0.5%).

New data continue to accumulate. In general, CO_2 levels below 2.3 mm Hg (0.04 psi, or 0.3%) seem to cause few crew symptoms, but levels as low as 2.3 to 2.7 mm Hg (0.04 to 0.05 psi, or 0.3 to 0.35%) can result in complaints of headache or feelings of "full-headedness" and decreases in crew work efficiency. Currently, CO_2 levels are generally maintained below 3.0 mm Hg (0.06 psi, or 0.4%) to minimize symptoms, with allowable excursions above this limit for periods less than 24 hours.

TEMPERATURE

The touch temperature of external spacecraft objects in low Earth orbit can range from approximately −100°C to +130°C (−148°F to +266°F) between shaded and sunlit sides of the vehicle (Figure 126-3). These extremes require active thermal control and insulation of crewed vehicles to ensure temperature management within habitable ranges for crewmembers. On the ISS, the crew controls the temperature to a typical range of 21° to 22°C (69.8° to 71.6°F), a "shirtsleeve" environment. However, this is a greater challenge than it appears because in the space environment, convection (transfer of heat through air or fluid currents) does not naturally occur; as a result, heated objects tend to stay warm, and cold objects tend to stay cold. Temperature variations in space are primarily determined by radiation; only objects receiving direct or reflected sunlight become warmed, and objects that fall into shadow rapidly cool to the low temperature extremes.

These temperature variations become apparent to a spacewalker during EVA. Despite a spacesuit's insulation, electric glove heaters, and manual temperature controls, the surface temperatures of a spacecraft are noticeable. Spacesuit gloves are designed to protect human skin from incidental contact with the ISS external surface temperatures, but they function best in touch temperatures ranging from −115°C to +115°C (−175°F to +239°F). Therefore, contact with surfaces receiving direct sunlight may be too hot for suit gloves to mitigate the heat delivered to an astronaut's hand. Likewise, prolonged contact with metal surfaces entirely encased in shadow can result in numbness despite the

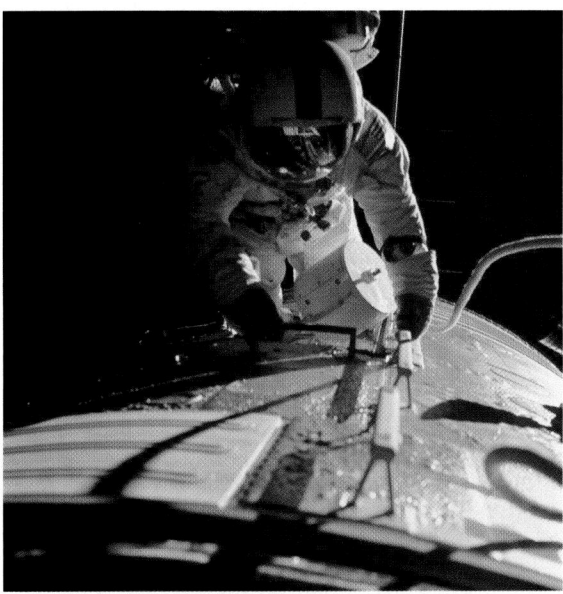

FIGURE 126-3 Astronaut Ron Evans performing a spacewalk during the transit of the Apollo 17 spacecraft from the moon back to Earth. *(Courtesy NASA.)*

use of glove heaters or, worse, might lead to significant injury. During one ground chamber test, a shaded object in a vacuum became so cold as to cause a frostbite injury from instrument handling through suit gloves. Should such an injury occur during spaceflight, limited medical capabilities could lead to permanent damage.

Thermal conduction from structural contact is not the only thermal concern for an astronaut during EVA. Work outside the spacecraft can be very demanding. Even the simplest tasks require exquisite control of a human-suit complex with considerable mass in the microgravity environment. As a result, astronauts can and do overheat during rigorous EVA activities. The human body cools through many mechanisms, but the most rapid and effective method of body heat loss is through vasodilation and convection through blood flow to the skin surface and transfer of heat to the environment. Due to the lack of natural convection in spaceflight, an overheated astronaut may experience significant delay in body cooling, leading to heat stress, fatigue, and other sequelae of heat illness. During EVA, astronauts wear cooling undergarments that circulate cooled water over the astronaut's skin, allowing convective heat transfer from the body to the cooling garment. Even with this mitigation in place, crewmembers must take care to ensure that they are allowing themselves sufficient time to cool down after particularly demanding activity, such as EVA or even daily exercise activity in the cabin, and remain vigilant for evidence of thermal stress. Some evidence suggests that body heat dissipation after long-duration flight remains impaired after landing, such that astronauts must remain wary of heat stress even after they return to Earth.[64]

Within the cabin, the environment can reach temperature extremes that challenge the crew's health. On the Mir space station, failures of the cooling and electrical systems in 1997 led to internal station temperatures of greater than $40°C$ ($104°F$).[198] After the Apollo 13 command module lost power, temperatures as low as $3°C$ ($37.4°F$) were recorded in the cabin.[18] In another example, in 1985, a Soyuz crew was launched to reclaim and repair the Salyut-7 space station, which had experienced a power failure earlier that year. The electrical systems had been nonfunctional for months before the rescue mission, and the cosmonauts who boarded the derelict station entered one of the most extreme environments encountered in spaceflight. Wearing winter coats, hats, and gloves, the crew worked in subfreezing temperatures, estimated at $−10°C$ ($14°F$), to repair the station successfully.

CARBON MONOXIDE

Carbon monoxide (CO) formed from the catabolism of hemoglobin is another metabolite that can normally accumulate in spacecraft, at a rate of 32 mg per crewmember per day.[206] Most sources agree that CO levels below 70 parts per million (ppm) would not often cause symptoms; however, in the enclosed environment of a spacecraft, levels could rise rapidly if removal systems failed, and pockets of poorly circulated air may result in areas of higher CO concentration, as occurs with CO_2 buildup. The rate of CO accumulation would depend on the size of the spacecraft and efficiency of the CO removal mechanisms. For example, if CO is not actively removed, CO levels could rise to about 20 ppm in 20 days with three crewmembers in a habitable volume of 100 m^3 (3500 $feet^3$).[101] Current spacecraft utilize catalytic oxidizers for CO removal; under normal circumstances, CO accumulation is generally not a significant concern. However, CO release as a byproduct of fire is a greater risk, as discussed later.

PROPELLANTS AND COOLANTS

Accidental release of onboard propellants and coolants could pose a significant risk to astronauts. The most common propellants used in spaceflight, nitrogen tetroxide as an oxidizer and monomethyl hydrazine as fuel, are extremely hazardous. To mitigate the risk to crewmembers, these compounds are usually contained in tanks located outside the habitable volume of the vehicle (Figure 126-4). Unfortunately, leaks occur. During the Apollo-Soyuz mission in 1975, the three-member U.S. crew was exposed to 250 ppm of nitrogen tetroxide for about 5 minutes

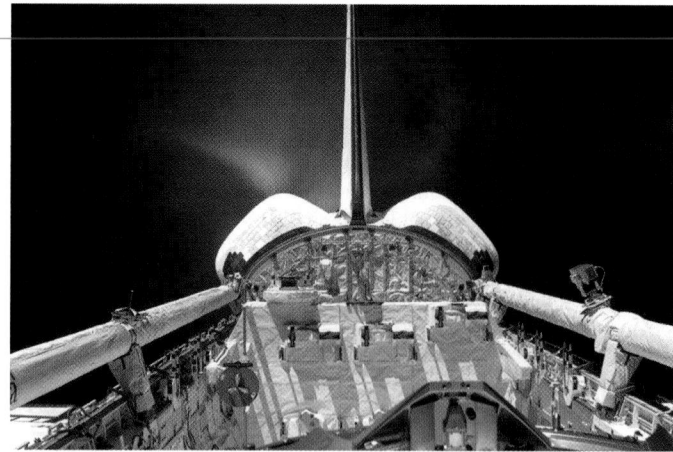

FIGURE 126-4 Emissions visible from the Space Shuttle's orbital maneuvering system during an orbital correction. Once in orbit, nitrogen tetroxide and monomethyl hydrazine are often used to provide thrust to spacecraft.

during reentry, when a valve misconfiguration allowed the gas to enter the crew cabin. Nitrogen tetroxide decomposes into nitric acid on contact with mucous membranes and is a potent irritant, causing damage to mucosal membranes and lung tissue. The crewmembers began to suffer from a burning sensation in their eyes, throats, and lungs immediately after exposure and developed significant pulmonary edema shortly after landing, requiring hospitalization and observation. Fortunately, all three crewmembers recovered completely.[51,199]

Hydrazine can be similarly irritating to mucous membranes. Significant exposure can also lead to nervous system injury, causing seizures, coma, and eventually death. Furthermore, hydrazine can cause damage to other major organs, including liver, spleen, and thyroid. Exposure to hydrazine would be of great concern during prelaunch fueling or a postlanding fuel dump. Typically, vehicles dump unused fuel shortly before or after landing; this could pose a concern to a crewmember or ground-recovery worker who might be exposed. Halocarbons are another class of potential contaminants, particularly because they are used inside the crew cabin as cleaning agents, coolants, and fire suppressants. Concentrations above 1% are known to cause cardiac irritation that can lead to dysrhythmias; these levels have not been seen in spacecraft.[101] Ethylene glycol, used in the internal cooling system of the Apollo spacecraft and Mir space station, leaked into the cabin atmosphere during a Mir mission in 1997, causing ocular and respiratory irritation in the crew. Fortunately, inhaled ethylene glycol does not pose the high risk of systemic toxicity seen with oral ingestion,[101] and the crew experienced no systemic effects.

The ISS uses liquid ammonia, pressurized in coolant lines that run outside the station, to transfer heat to space. When leaked, ammonia forms snow-like crystals near the point of leakage. During EVA, when working on these lines, astronauts may be exposed to crystallized ammonia and carry the compound on their suits into the cabin, contaminating the internal atmosphere of the airlock. If a crewmember were to come in direct contact with ammonia, exposure as low as 20 ppm would be immediately noticeable and irritating to the eyes and mucous membranes, and inhalations of 150 ppm could cause inflammation of the upper airway. Higher levels of exposure can cause tracheobronchial burns, pulmonary edema, and even death.[241] Given the risks associated with ammonia exposure, several steps are taken to prevent contaminating the internal atmosphere of the ISS after EVA. Exposing a suit to sunlight during EVA, a technique known as a "bake-out," can accelerate sublimation of any ammonia contamination. Bake-outs are required before airlock ingress any time suit contamination is suspected. In addition, colorimetric testing kits reside in the airlock to detect the presence of residual ammonia in the air after repressurization. If contamination is discovered, multiple atmosphere purges and repressurizations of the airlock may be required to dump contaminants fully before returning the crew into the habitable volume of the ISS.

FIRE

Fires are quite possible onboard spacecraft; three occurred during the Space Shuttle program from electrical arcing and combustion of wiring insulation or electrical components. Fires within the closed volume of a spacecraft can be dangerous, not only because of the flames but also because toxic pyrolytic products, such as hydrogen chloride, hydrogen cyanide, and CO, are released into the habitable volume. The Space Shuttle events produced minor combustion products easily scrubbed from the atmosphere, but more significant fires have occurred. In 1997, a fire broke out aboard the Mir space station when a solid-fuel O_2 generator (frequently used at that time to add O_2 to the environment) malfunctioned, leading to an uncontrolled and intense flame. The flames caused damage to station panels and internal structures and released thick clouds of smoke into the cabin before the crewmembers were able to extinguish the fire. This event almost led to evacuation of the station and highlighted the dangers of an uncontrolled flame in the cabin. During a separate event aboard the Mir station, paper filters inside an overheated catalytic oxidizer ignited, releasing a significant amount of CO, with measured levels as high as 400 ppm. At least one crewmember reported headache and nausea from that exposure.[101]

To minimize the risk of fire, O_2 levels are kept at the nominal constituent level of 21%. Materials onboard the ISS are carefully selected whenever possible to be flame retardant and to minimize toxic off-gassing. An example is minimizing plastics that off-gas high levels of cyanide. Care is taken to ensure that crewmembers always have immediate and unhindered access to nearby supplemental O_2 stores and fire suppressants, with a clear path to the escape vehicles. If a fire occurs and is controllable, clearance of pyrolytic contaminants is achieved with airflow and filtering. Combustion products typically absorb quickly into water vapor; thus, condensers in air-conditioning systems can assist in removing these compounds. Lastly, the crew has access to colorimetric sensors for real-time detection of atmospheric contaminants and to ensure that the air has been adequately purified.

WATER

Historically, such as during the Mercury and Gemini missions, water for drinking and hygiene has been provided to crews from storage tanks or from water generated as a byproduct of the electrochemical combination of hydrogen and O_2 in fuel cells, as occurred on the Apollo spacecraft and the Space Shuttle. At present, the ISS Water Recovery System (WRS) recycles potable water from urine, cabin humidity condensate, and spacesuit wastewater. Water from the ISS WRS is also fed into an oxygen generation assembly that produces O_2 and hydrogen through electrolysis. The O_2 created is released into the cabin atmosphere; the remaining hydrogen is combined with CO_2 in a separate system, which can then produce more water for consumption. This highly efficient generation of water reduces the weight of stowed water and consumables that must be launched and delivered to the ISS to support the nominal six-person crew; weight savings have been reported as high as 6804 kg (15,000 lb) per year.

Water contamination can be a significant risk on spacecraft. Waterborne microbes can be transported into spacecraft water systems from terrestrial sources or from crewmembers and crew activities. Potable water is chemically disinfected before crew consumption through a variety of mechanisms. Russian water stores are purified using silver biocide, and U.S. systems typically use iodination. However, use of iodine raises a concern for thyroid dysfunction. To mitigate this risk, a resin filter is used to remove iodine just before water consumption.[160] Despite disinfection efforts, water contamination occurs. *Burkholderia cepacia* and *Staphylococcus aureus* were the most frequently identified organisms in Space Shuttle and ISS water sources.[100,188] Although *B. cepacia* has fairly low virulence, *S. aureus* contamination is a concern because food cooked in *S. aureus*–contaminated water

could cause food poisoning. Water spilled aboard spacecraft, if allowed to accumulate, can support microbial life. On the Mir station, condensate accumulations found behind panels after a prolonged period of water system leaks contained stable microbial colonies of algae, bacteria, ciliates, and protozoa.[198,180] No illness has been attributed to microbial contamination in spacecraft water, but prevention of biofilm growth on water system hardware is critical because of the risk and difficulty associated with handling caustic cleaning liquids in microgravity.

Chemical contamination of water systems can occur. As mentioned, the ISS uses condensate recovery and recycling to potable water; atmospheric contaminants could accumulate in condensate and contaminate drinking water. For this reason, certain chemicals, such as isopropyl alcohol, are not used aboard the ISS. In addition, water storage and filtering systems can themselves add contaminants; for example, an early iteration of the iodine removal system led to an accidental ingestion of significant levels of trialkylamines caused by resin leaching. In this case, preflight radiation sterilization of the resin accidentally caused chemical breakdown of the resin material and production of the contaminating byproduct, which leached into the water during filtration.[17]

DUST, PARTICULATES, AND OTHER CONTAMINANTS

Dust and particulates can affect a spacecraft's habitability in the weightless environment, particularly because such particulates, in the absence of gravity, do not settle on surfaces. Flakes of skin, clothing lint, food particles, and particulates from experiments are often found in samples of analyzed spacecraft air. Of particular concern are particles larger than 100 μm, which are the particle sizes most often associated with airborne microorganisms.[100,24] Ventilation systems aboard contemporary vehicles tend to be robust, relying on high-efficiency particulate arrestance (HEPA) filters to maintain a clean environment. In more confined spaces, such as an astronaut's private quarters, crewmembers can often recognize visible levels of particulate matter, particularly skin flakes. Known as *scurf,* skin flakes are released throughout long-duration spaceflight, particularly from skin surfaces that are not used in a microgravity environment, such as calluses and thickened soles on the feet. Another common source of particulate contamination is the lithium hydroxide (LiOH) compound used in CO_2 removal systems. In spacecraft such as the Space Shuttle or Soyuz, which lack the space and power for regenerative CO_2 removal systems, LiOH cartridges are used and replaced frequently, and small LiOH particles are often released during the exchange. Inhalation of LiOH dust can cause self-limited respiratory irritation.[101]

Crews are specifically trained to remove themselves from releases of "noncontainable" particulate flurries and don surgical masks and goggles if returning to work in the area. Also, the risk of particulate contaminant in any newly arriving vehicle is increased; settled tools, screws, and dust from recent manufacturing and stowage operations on Earth can escape detection until they begin to float in microgravity. For this reason, crewmembers wear surgical masks and safety goggles during the first entry into most newly docked cargo vehicles.

Human spaceflight experience to date has revealed other contaminants that can be expected to build up in the closed ecosystem of spacecraft, most often caused by off-gassing of materials. Formaldehyde, halocarbons in hardware cleaning agents, and trace organic compounds are frequently found in air samples in spacecraft, suggesting the need for continued occupational surveillance of air pollutants during long-duration flight.[101] Space station maintenance operations require close proximity of crewmembers to other exotic compounds, including cadmium and nickel (used as anticorrosives in fluid lines) and urea, sulfuric acid, and trivalent chromium (found in waste management systems). Microgravity permits unexpected and ubiquitous sources of exposure; fluids can be free floating, adherent to walls, or hidden behind panels. Thus, accidental contact or even inhalation may be more likely than on Earth, particularly in the close quarters of a spacecraft.

Other environmental considerations will arise with future planetary missions. Close contact with alien soils and dust will be inevitable, so aerospace medicine practitioners will need to anticipate potential hazards from dust that is carried into habitats for study or as a contaminant on space suits and tools. Apollo astronauts reported significant dust contamination of the vehicle cabin after lunar excursions, even noting that the dust seemed to somewhat aerosolize in the low lunar gravity and led to unavoidable inhalation of the particles. In ground studies of animal models, pulmonary inflammation, thickening of alveolar septa, fibrosis, and granulomas have all been demonstrated after lunar dust exposure, although no Apollo astronaut is known to have had such sequelae.[127] Concerns over dust contamination of cabins have led scientists and engineers to develop alternative methods to transfer a surface-walking astronaut into a vehicle, such as "docking" a spacesuit to the vehicle wall and climbing out of the suit into the vehicle, thereby avoiding bringing the dusty suit inside. Creative methods to mitigate particulate exposures will be increasingly important as renewed lunar and then interplanetary travel is realized.

THE RADIATION ENVIRONMENT

Space radiation consists of multiple particle and electromagnetic wave types with a broad spectrum of energies. The solar wind, a continuous efflux of stellar material from the sun and made up primarily of electrons and protons, bathes Earth's magnetic field. Solar particle events, which are jets of high-energy protons and other atomic species, including helium nuclei (alpha particles), also periodically erupt into interplanetary space, occasionally striking the earth and the orbital environment. Galactic cosmic rays (GCR), likely arising from distant supernovas and traveling at relativistic speeds, also contribute to this radiation milieu.

The most common range of orbital altitudes for crewed vehicles is between 240 and 480 km (150 and 300 miles). The ISS orbits between 328 and 432 km (205 and 270 miles) above the surface of the earth. While crews in low Earth orbit (LEO) receive substantially higher radiation doses than occur with terrestrial exposures, the crews still reside well within the Earth's geomagnetosphere (GMS), which deflects much of the solar wind and GCR. The inner and outer Van Allen belts, layered torus-shaped fields of electrons and protons encircling the earth along geomagnetic field lines, represent a further radiation risk to orbiting astronauts (Figure 126-5). The lower margin of the Van Allen belts is closer to Earth above the South Atlantic, because of the offset between Earth's center of mass and its rotational axis, creating a region known as the South Atlantic Anomaly (SAA), where radiation levels are much higher even in LEO. Spaceflight crews in LEO spend only a small fraction (~10%) of travel time traversing the SAA, but incur the majority of their total mission radiation dose there.[192] In addition, captured particles travel along Earth's magnetic field lines and gather closer to Earth's surface at the magnetic poles, creating a region of denser particle concentrations at higher latitudes. Thus, the highest LEO radiation exposures are incurred in polar orbits, where a vehicle travels north to south around the earth, and in orbits that pass through the SAA.

The space radiation environment varies temporally as well as spatially; solar wind intensity and flare frequency wax and wane over an 11-year solar cycle. While increased activity near the peak of the cycle, known as *solar max,* injects more solar electrons and protons into the GMS and increases the radiation burden from these lower-energy particles, it simultaneously expands the solar magnetic field, which better deflects the more highly energetic GCR and lowers the overall radiation dose.[45] Another source of space radiation arises from collisions between GCR and the spacecraft hull, which produce showers of secondary particles. The radiation dose that a crew traveling in LEO can expect to receive therefore largely depends on orbital altitude and inclination, timing of the mission relative to the solar cycle, and the potential for secondary particle creation. Much more distant travel, such as missions to the moon and farther destinations, requires leaving the earth's GMS and exposing crews to the full brunt of solar and GCR, increasing exposure rates to GCR as much as threefold over lower orbital altitudes.[45] *Solar particle events* (SPEs) associated with solar flares, unimpeded by Earth's GMS, may represent the most potent radiation event for a crew traveling outside LEO.

Current spacecraft aluminum hulls provide some protection to crews from space radiation,[192] although the secondary generation of particles from GCR and aluminum collisions adds to the radiation environment inside of the spacecraft. Proton-dense hydrogenated materials, such as water or polyethylene, are excellent absorbers of ionizing radiation and have been considered for use as linings of "safe haven" compartments within interplanetary spacecraft, where the crew could camp for the hours to days required for an SPE to pass.[57] Kevlar can be used for micrometeoroid protection; it demonstrates shielding effectiveness against heavy ions of approximately 80% that of water.[144] However, shielding capability is limited by the weight of effective materials, which may become prohibitive for larger vehicles designed to travel greater distances from Earth. For longer and more distant missions, the most effective means of decreasing exposures would be by limiting transit time through interplanetary space. Electromagnetic or nuclear propulsion engines that provide substantially more thrust over current chemical rocket engines could significantly shorten travel duration through interplanetary space, but this capability depends on advances in rocket propulsion technology.[57]

Radiation Health Effects

Significant ionizing radiation exposure can result in biologic tissue damage and an array of adverse health events on two time scales. Acute radiation effects include burns, vomiting, hemorrhage, and even death, whereas chronic effects include increased mutagenicity, accelerated senescence, and chromosomal alterations causing carcinogenesis and genomic instability.[91] Although the short-term effects largely result from single doses of radiation, long-term issues arise with repetitive and cumulative dosages.

Correlating terrestrial exposures with doses spaceflight crews could experience is problematic because terrestrial exposures consist largely of single-particle types with limited energy spectra, whereas space radiation is a mix of multiparticle species with much higher energies, as well as electromagnetic wave radiation.[56] Because little is known about the biologic effects of many of these exotic particle types, the range of uncertainty in dose calculations can be high. It is expected, however, that acute clinical effects seen with high-dose terrestrial radiation exposure, including nausea, vomiting, fatigue, alterations to blood cell production, and even death, could also occur with high-dose acute space radiation exposures.[94,111] Similarly, long-term effects, such as mutagenesis, are expected to be similar to prolonged

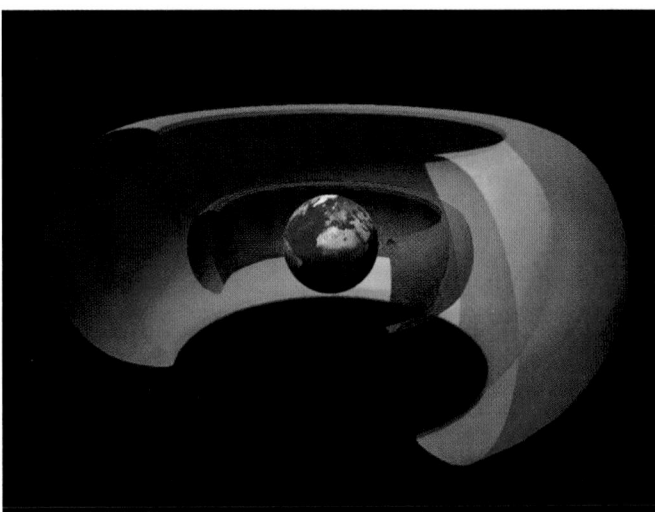

FIGURE 126-5 Artist's rendition of the Van Allen belts, consisting of solar protons and electrons that are trapped by Earth's magnetic field. *(Courtesy NASA.)*

accumulation of radiation dosages. In addition, single-cell studies have demonstrated that damage from a single high-energy atomic particle can propagate into long-term effects, such as mutagenesis from chromosomal aberrations caused by a single impacting particle.[65] Other evidence suggests that space radiation may have tissue-specific effects on the ocular lens, bone turnover, and the nervous and cardiovascular systems, in addition to the mutagenic risk.

The health effects of human radiation exposure are commonly measured in sieverts (Sv). For context, an acquired dose of 1 Sv carries with it a 5.5% increased chance of eventually developing cancer. Terrestrial background radiation doses vary with region, but a person living in the U.S. generally receives a dose of approximately 0.0066 millisievert (mSv)/day. In LEO, the typical dose is about 75 times higher, about 0.5 mSv/day.[192] Crewmembers may receive higher exposures, closer to 1 mSv/day, during EVA, simply because of the lack of spacecraft shielding.[192] A crewmember on board the ISS for 6 months is exposed to radiation dosage still well below acute terrestrial dose exposure limits that would drive a measurable increase in cancer incidence.[142] Higher exposures would be expected, of course, with more distant or interplanetary travel. However, little is known about the biologic effects of exposure to high-energy heavy particles associated with unshielded GCR, so making health impact predictions for deep-space missions is difficult.

Cancer risk aside, the only measured pathophysiologic effect in astronauts from radiation exposure is a consistent increase in lymphocyte chromosomal aberrations after long-duration flight, relative to before flight.[72] However, an insufficient population has traveled in space, and insufficient time has passed since the beginning of human spaceflight, to detect an increase in cancer incidence in the astronaut population (Van Baalen M: Personal communication, 2015). Data on doses to astronaut crews have been accumulating since the early days of spaceflight. Crewmembers carry dosimeters on their person throughout their mission, including during EVAs. Other dosimeters are distributed throughout the interior of the ISS to develop spatial and temporal radiation maps of the living quarters. These passive dosimeters can be read and analyzed only after landing; however, a tissue equivalent proportional counter (TEPC) located on board the ISS can be read in real time for particle event monitoring. Other active dosimeters and space weather satellites are available to determine real-time changes in dose in case of unexpected SPEs. This suite of devices significantly adds to the data available to improve the collective knowledge of radiation characteristics in LEO.

Monitoring and Risk Reduction

Because no OSHA limit exists for spaceflight and terrestrial guidelines are too restrictive, the U.S. National Aeronautics and Space Administration (NASA) has sought external guidance from the National Council on Radiation Protection and Measurements (NCRP) and the National Radiation Council (NRC) in determining an acceptable radiation exposure risk level for astronauts, and to recommend means to quantify and mitigate these risks. The NCRP stated that human spaceflight should be conducted while keeping radiation exposure risk "as low as reasonably achievable" (ALARA). Currently, the limit set for astronauts in LEO is a 3% increased incidence (95% confidence interval) of fatal cancer above the background incidence in the normal terrestrial population.[46] Risk reduction currently is largely accomplished through mission planning. Orbital altitude and inclination, mission duration, and timing with the solar cycle can be incorporated into flight planning to reduce exposure. These flight-profile characteristics are largely fixed for operations aboard the ISS, although a few mission parameters can be adjusted to reduce dose. For example, timing spacewalks to occur during orbits that do not transit the SAA can reduce an astronaut's unshielded exposure to elevated radiation levels. Flight rules have been developed to guide a rapid response to acute radiation events (e.g., SPEs) by terminating an EVA, reorienting the ISS, or directing the crew to cease working and move to a safe haven in a more heavily shielded part of the station.

Limiting an individual astronaut's time in space is the other means of risk reduction currently practiced. Before assignment of astronauts to a mission, the total radiation burden predicted for that mission is combined with each astronaut's radiation history from previous occupational, medical, and spaceflight exposures.[111] An individual's gender and age at first spaceflight are major determinants of susceptibility to mutagenicity from space radiation, because women and younger individuals are more susceptible to effects from identical dosages than men or older individuals.[46] These factors are also incorporated into an astronaut's risk calculation.

MISSION CONSIDERATIONS

Spaceflight missions vary in time, trajectory, and intent. However, a number of physiologic phenomena are usually experienced during the various phases of flight, including the preflight period, launch, time spent in microgravity, reentry, and landing. These events, as well as strategies to minimize unwanted effects, are described next, specifically with an introduction to the signs and symptoms experienced by the astronaut or witnessed by the aerospace physician.

PREFLIGHT

Space programs usually institute a period of quarantine for about 2 weeks before launch, primarily to prevent infectious illness from affecting the launching crew. A comprehensive quarantine program creates a controlled environment that raises awareness among workforce and family members to limit their contact with the crew and enables a medical screening process for visitors. Children younger than 14 years, who are less able to recognize their own infectious disease symptoms and are more likely to be carriers, constitute the greatest threat of infecting the crew.

A quarantine period has other benefits as well. The final weeks before a spaceflight can be an intensely active time for the astronaut, often requiring last-minute academic preparation and contacts with family, friends, trainers, and program managers. Sequestering the crew in a controlled environment can assist in limiting distractions and enables establishment of a well-balanced work-rest schedule. Furthermore, missions to orbiting destinations, such as the ISS, may require launches at any time of the day to synchronize the trajectories of the launching and destination spacecraft. A controlled lighting environment in a quarantine facility can assist sleep-shifting the crew to help ensure optimal wakefulness at launch. Finally, since crewed spacecraft have very small interiors with primitive waste and hygiene systems, astronauts occasionally desire liquid diets or enemas just before launch, to minimize the need for defecation in the first days of flight, which an adequate quarantine facility and staff can facilitate.

Regardless of precautions taken, an aerospace physician may see a number of physiologic alterations in a crew preparing to launch. Astronauts are often sleep-deprived on the day of launch, if not from the academic workload of preparation for the flight or an extended circadian shift, then certainly from the emotional excitement of anticipating their flight. Wary of inadvertent injury, prelaunch astronauts may limit their exercise intensity and thus may not be at their peak physical condition. They may also be slightly dehydrated, having reduced their oral intake to limit the need for urination or defecation in the first hours of their mission.

LAUNCH

To reach Earth orbit using current chemical propulsion rockets, astronauts nominally undergo acceleration forces of three to four times that of gravity (+3 to 4 G) for approximately 8 to 9 minutes. This acceleration occurs in peaks and valleys to balance human and structural tolerance and fuel and engine performance, eventually attaining a target orbital velocity of approximately 28,000 km/hr (17,500 miles/hr) for the altitudes usually occupied by orbiting spacecraft. While acceleration loads on the order of several Gs may be endured by humans, the human body is particularly vulnerable to excess acceleration in the head-to-toe

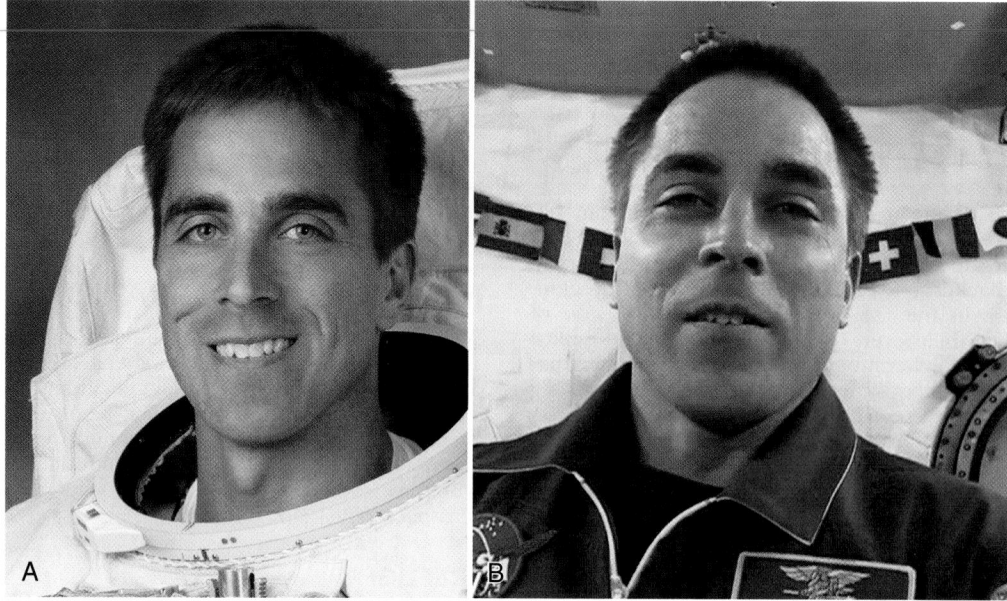

FIGURE 126-6 The facial "puffiness" common among astronauts in space is attributed to headward fluid shifts in microgravity, as demonstrated clearly in these preflight and in-flight images of astronaut Chris Cassidy during his 6-month mission aboard the ISS as a member of Expeditions 35 and 36 in 2013.

direction (+Gz). +Gz acceleration results in blood pooling in the lower extremities, which can overcome the cardiovascular system's ability to provide adequate blood flow to the brain and possibly lead to G-induced loss of consciousness. Given these necessary acceleration loads, most spacecraft position crewmembers in a recumbent posture such that the major accelerations of rocket ascent are taken in the more favorable chest-to-back direction (+Gx).

As crews assume a recumbent position in the vehicle on the pad before launch, a cephalad intravascular fluid shift occurs, as it would in any individual in such a position, and the resultant central volume increase triggers atrial and carotid stretch receptors to activate a baroreceptor-mediated decrease in cardiac output and, eventually, inhibition of antidiuretic hormone (ADH) production, ultimately resulting in diuresis. This effect can be dramatic; in studies during the Space Shuttle era, measurements of central venous pressure (CVP) at the cardiac atrium obtained from indwelling venous catheters in three astronauts showed a rise from a standing-position pressure of 5 to 6 cm H_2O to 10 to 12 cm H_2O after the astronauts took their seats before launch.[20]

During launch, crewmembers experience multiple vibroacoustic and acceleration stimuli. The noise and vibrational motion inside the spacecraft, although dramatic, are largely dampened by the crewmember's seat, spacesuit, and helmet, so that astronauts are able to hear radio-voiced commands, speak, monitor instruments, and write on a kneeboard. The overlying sustained 3 to 4 +Gx acceleration to orbital velocity is clearly noticeable, however, in the sensation of heaviness in the limbs and anterior-to-posterior chest pressure. The CVP at this time increases up to 15 to 17 cm H_2O[20] (Video 126-1).

EFFECTS OF MICROGRAVITY

The human cardiovascular system evolved with venous valves and neuroendocrine responses to ensure adequate cerebral blood flow while standing upright under Earth's gravitational influence. Likewise, inner ear otolith organs determine head and body position and sense motion relative to a gravitational field. These physiologic mechanisms remain active when the spacecraft attains LEO, the rocket engines shut down, and the spacecraft begins its free-fall trajectory. Precisely at this moment of engine cutoff, the influence of gravity on the human body vanishes. The astronaut can sense a rapid, remarkable cephalad shift of their intravascular fluid volume, unweighting of limbs, and lifting of intraperitoneal organs, not unlike what one feels in the first few seconds of free-fall on Earth. Crewmembers immediately perceive pressure at the base of the skull and a sense of levitation from the seat as they rise against the pressure of seat restraints. The vestibulo-ocular reflex, which integrates sensed gravitational cues from otolith organs with eye movement and visual input of perceived spatial position, is now essentially uncoupled. Without sensed gravity to help establish a local vertical, crewmembers may feel as if they are hanging upside down, and any head movement can induce a sensation of tumbling.

In these first minutes in orbit, the astronaut may experience sinus congestion, similar to what may be felt with a slight head-down posture on Earth, manifesting in some as a headache. Facial edema, particularly in areas of loose skin such as the eyelids, and an increase in conjunctival injection are often soon visually apparent (Figure 126-6). In fact, forehead soft tissue thickness measured in microgravity with ultrasound showed a 9% increase after several weeks of spaceflight, relative to measurements obtained on Earth.[155] Reductions in leg circumference can be noted after only a few hours in microgravity, and jugular venous distention is also often discernible. Remarkably, CVP decreases to 0 to 3 cm H_2O on arrival into microgravity,[20] unlike the CVP rise associated with the recumbent position on Earth. Decrease in CVP may be caused by a number of mechanisms, including decreased intrathoracic pressure, decreased external cardiac constraint, diuresis, and intravascular volume depletion,[63] as discussed in detail later.

Human physiologic adaptation to weightlessness continues over days and weeks of life in space, as microgravity induces changes in fluid volume and body morphology, and neural and hormonal regulation ensues. These changes can be detected in both short-duration flights of 18 days or less and long-duration flights of 1 month or more. Experience with long-duration flight has led to recognition that these physiologic changes ultimately result in a newly adapted, weightless state of the human organism, a condition explored further in this chapter.

Space Adaptation Syndrome

Motion sickness is one of the most prominent symptom complexes affecting astronauts on entry into microgravity and may occur within minutes of engine shutdown. Conventionally named space adaptation syndrome (SAS), space motion sickness consists of headache, nausea, vomiting, malaise, loss of appetite, and occasionally disorientation. SAS is common and has been studied extensively in attempts to predict susceptibility and determine prophylaxis and treatment measures. The cause of SAS is believed to be a mismatch between movement of the visual surround and neurovestibular stimulation, with headward fluid shifts as a possible contributor. This discordance between visual and neurovestibular inputs is often provoked by head motions and can be attributed to the microgravitational lifting of otoliths away from sensory hair cells in the vestibular labyrinth of the inner ear. As the head moves, the human body expects a resultant activation of the inner ear hair cells by otolithic movement; in microgravity, floating otoliths fail to activate the hair cells, leading to this mismatch and the sequelae of SAS. It has been postulated that cephalad fluid shifts may result in increased intracranial pressure that alters the responses of vestibular receptors, further contributing to the syndrome.[90] Confining launch restraints and the small internal volume of early Mercury, Gemini, and Soyuz spacecraft likely prevented freedom of movement sufficient to elicit symptoms of SAS; thus, the syndrome was not appreciated until the Apollo program. As many as 60% to 80% of all astronauts are affected by some degree of SAS, although the vast majority of cases resolve within 48 hours. Rare cases have been known to persist for up to 14 days before resolution of symptoms.[90] Incidence is decreased for repeat flyers, suggesting either some degree of retained adaptation or use of cognitive strategies to mitigate provocative movements.

Most crewmembers are able to perform operational tasks despite symptoms; early in the Space Shuttle program, only 13% were unable to complete their scheduled work in the first hours of flight because of SAS.[48] Some suggest that adrenergic stimulation from the excitement of the first minutes in space can suppress symptoms.[47] Limiting head movement can also minimize symptoms, but this is often difficult with the required work and occasional unintentional tumbling early in flight before controlled motions are mastered in microgravity.

Thornton and Bonato[227] review the differences between terrestrial and SAS-related motion sickness. Of particular interest is the different character of emesis in space. SAS-induced emesis may be described as "wet burps," which may reflect the lack of a distinct gastric air-fluid level in microgravity. SAS emesis can also occur without prodrome and with rapid onset. Containing small amounts of vomitus in the microgravity environment is relatively simple with readily accessible gauze-lined emesis bags, which take advantage of the predominance of surface tension forces to wick and trap fluids.

Unfortunately, there are few training-related means of reducing the incidence of SAS. Preflight exposure to cross-coupled angular acceleration stimuli, such as off-axis rotating chairs, have been unsuccessful in preventing SAS.[77] Likewise, bouts of aerobatic and parabolic flight during preflight training have not reduced the incidence of SAS in the astronaut population.[93] Preflight adaptation training by exposing crews to novel gravito-inertial surrounds and stimulations in the laboratory has shown some success in reducing motion sickness during parabolic flight and simulator exposure[29,71] but has not been shown to be successful for SAS prophylaxis.

Pharmaceutical agents remain the most effective treatment for SAS.[47,103] Metoclopramide, scopolamine (oral and transdermal), promethazine (oral, rectal, and intramuscular), and meclizine have all been used as SAS pharmacologic countermeasures. Intramuscular promethazine was the preferred in-flight medication to combat SAS during most Space Shuttle missions and was routinely given before sleep so the sedative side effect would not affect operational performance.[103] Because the onset of SAS occurs shortly after orbital insertion, prophylactic medications are also frequently taken before launch. Dextroamphetamine can be added to promethazine or scopolamine oral preparations to counteract associated drowsiness and sedation, with the added benefit of further antiemetic properties. Of all the medications used to treat SAS at clinically useful doses, ground-based studies showed that meclizine seems to have the least influence on cognitive function, and meclizine taken 12 to 14 hours preflight and repeated 2 hours before launch has recently become the prophylactic pharmacologic countermeasure of choice among U.S. crewmembers to prevent SAS symptoms.[183]

Currently, ISS mission planners allow 48 hours for an adaptation period for SAS resolution before scheduling heavy operational work or mission-critical activities such as spacewalks. SAS is now accepted as an unavoidable consequence of the first few days of microgravity adaptation; work schedule planning and medications to alleviate symptoms are the main means of preventing further mission impact.

POSTFLIGHT

Eventually, humans acclimate to a new functional normal during their time in microgravity, but this transformation results in deconditioning of some physiologic systems required for basic performance on Earth. Returning astronauts may suffer from neurovestibular balance disorders, cardiovascular deconditioning, bone loss, and muscle atrophy. The postflight state is influenced by duration of flight, in-flight countermeasure activities (e.g., exercise), nutritional state, and individual variability. With dedicated countermeasure performance, many long-duration spaceflight crews have demonstrated the ability to function independently immediately after return to Earth, being able to stand, ambulate, and perform light work at the landing site. Others will require significant assistance because of symptomatic orthostasis and disruption of balance. Discussions later in this chapter summarize the physical findings the aerospace practitioner can expect to see in crewmembers immediately on their landing after a long-duration flight.

PHYSIOLOGIC CONCERNS OF SPACEFLIGHT

The following sections delineate many common medical findings in humans after spaceflight, focusing specifically on various physiologic systems and microgravity sequelae. Expression of many of these symptoms is proportional to the duration of flight; longer periods in weightlessness result in more extreme physiologic adaptations. As with many extreme environmental scenarios, the human body adapts, often remarkably, to tolerate and even thrive in the microgravity environment.

CARDIOVASCULAR ISSUES

Headward fluid shifts, tissue unloading, and an almost complete lack of postural or ambulation loading drive the majority of changes in the cardiovascular system in weightlessness. This nullified hydrostatic and hypokinetic state, different from recumbency or even head-down positioning on Earth,[176] is unique in human experience. The cardiovascular system seems to function well with these changes, but the adaptation process has not been completely characterized, and its long-term systemic and end-organ effects have not been fully identified or completely understood.

As previously mentioned, on cessation of acceleration forces at the moment of main engine cutoff, the astronaut's intravascular fluid redistributes cephalad. Unweighting of tissue structures induces thoracic expansion, which is believed to increase venous compliance, allowing thoracic venous accommodation of the onrush of blood volume (up to 2 L) from the lower extremities and splanchnic vascular beds into the thorax.[20,228] The CVP decrease previously noted is accompanied by cardiac accommodation of the increased fluid load, evidenced by increased venous return, enlarged cardiac chamber volumes, and significant increase in cardiac output.[232] This indicates that despite decreased CVP, a central transmural venous pressure increase occurs in microgravity,[63] most likely caused by decreases in pleural and lung parenchymal pressures and release of pericardial constraint.[84,235] Thus, fluid shifts from the lower to the upper body increase the pressures across the cardiac chamber walls and thus increase cardiac preload. Frank-Starling–induced elevations in stroke volume and cardiac output follow, with cardiac output increases of 15% to 22% maintained 1 week into flight[175] and for up to 40% after 3 months of microgravity.[173] The presence of jugular venous distention in some crewmembers in microgravity despite a reduction in CVP is not completely understood but clearly shows that this clinical sign cannot be relied on as an indicator of right-sided heart dysfunction in the space-adapted individual in the same way as it would be in a terrestrial patient.

Monitoring of blood pressure (BP) and heart rate (HR) in long-duration astronauts on the ISS has shown either no change[95] or decreases of 10 mm Hg or less in mean or diastolic arterial pressures[9,173] compared with preflight recumbent or ambulatory conditions, indicating a drop in peripheral vascular resistance (PVR) to accommodate the increase in cardiac output previously noted.[173] However, unlike in recumbency on Earth, circulating noradrenaline and sympathetic nerve activity remain high in microgravity,[58,59] so this decrease in PVR must be controlled by mechanisms other than a baroreflex-induced decrease in sympathetic nervous activity.[173,174]

Investigations since the Apollo program have established that reduction in intravascular fluid volume stabilizes at approximately a 15% decrease from preflight in approximately 5 days.[4] As a response to the increase in central vascular volume, immediate diuresis would be expected, but this has not been observed in space. Instead, total body water is preserved.[132] This finding suggests that Starling forces induce fluid shifts from intravascular into interstitial and intracellular compartments,[132,176] resulting in a novel cardiovascular euvolemic state in microgravity. Hemoconcentration resulting from this decrease in intravascular water is believed to trigger a process, termed *neocytolysis*, in which newly released red blood cells (RBCs) are selectively removed from the circulation to reestablish a normal hematocrit.[6] Loss of young, larger RBCs results in overall RBC mass reduction that stabilizes at 10% to 15% loss by 1 week into flight.[5] Although astronauts seem to function well in space after these trends stabilize, the adapted state may be inadequate to maintain a normal cardiovascular response to standing in normal Earth gravity on return from spaceflight. Much research has been devoted to this issue of orthostatic intolerance after landing.

As noted earlier, return of gravity can pool blood in the lower body and lead to orthostatic intolerance during and initially after landing. As many as 20% of astronauts after short-duration flight and up to 80% after long-duration flight[161] experience postflight presyncopal symptoms, with a somewhat higher incidence among female astronauts.[233] Low PVR, hypovolemia, and blunted adrenergic response are considered to contribute to this phenomenon.[141]

Lower-body negative pressure (LBNP) techniques, in which the legs and lower torso are inserted into a small vacuum chamber and exposed to a reduced pressure (usually 1 psi below ambient), were used on orbit during the Skylab and Space Shuttle programs as a tool to simulate the orthostatic stress of landing (Figure 126-7). A series of investigations found that a 5-hour session of in-flight LBNP, in combination with hypertonic saline ingestion, maintained HR and systolic BP similar to the preflight response to orthostatic stress.[32] LBNP is considered a possible

peripheral neurovascular stimulant that may help prepare crews for return to Earth and resultant hydrostatic stress, but its benefit was found to extinguish within 2 days, leaving astronauts just as susceptible to orthostasis after that period. Given the significant amount of time required to use LBNP as a prelanding countermeasure and the extinguishing benefits, LBNP is not used by U.S. astronauts,[31] although the Russian program has continued to use LBNP exposure for its cosmonauts in the few weeks before return to Earth.

Other means of reducing postflight orthostatic intolerance have been adopted. An inflatable lower-body antigravity (anti-G) suit was used during Space Shuttle launch and landing to prevent blood from pooling in the lower body during +Gz (head-to-toe) acceleration exposures. This was particularly relevant to Space Shuttle crewmembers who were returned from short-duration flight in an upright seated position, rather than in the recumbent position in U.S. and Russian capsules. Arterial pressure was higher in astronauts who inflated their anti-G suit during acceleration exposure than in those who did not inflate them.[184] In addition, a liquid cooling garment was worn inside later Space Shuttle reentry suits to reduce thermal stress and allow astronauts to regulate their individual body temperature, which improved overall tolerance of the physiologic stresses of reentry. Use of this liquid cooling garment, in combination with the anti-G suit, resulted in a significantly lower average HR than in astronauts who did not use either countermeasure.[184] In the Russian space program, Soyuz crewmembers currently wear an elastic compression garment during reentry and on the days immediately after landing, to provide venous compression and improve cardiac return from the extremities. A graded compression garment has also been developed to apply progressive pressures from the feet to the abdomen for use after long-duration and exploration missions; it has been shown to prevent tachycardia and to increase total peripheral resistance when standing after short-duration spaceflight.[216]

Crewmembers return to Earth relatively dehydrated compared to the terrestrial norm. "Prehydration," or fluid loading, with oral water and salt in the hours before return to Earth is another effective countermeasure against orthostasis.[21] Alfrey and colleagues[5] described a 27% decline in stroke volume and 14% drop in cardiac output in astronauts who did not fluid load before reentry. Effective fluid loading countermeasures have been demonstrated to help prevent this reduction of stroke volume and cardiac output.

By 2 weeks into a long-duration mission, aerobic capacity has been shown to decrease by 17% from preflight values. Although it can trend toward preflight values with sufficient exercise, aerobic capacity can decrease again to 15% to 22% below preflight baseline after landing.[141,164] With a supervised physical rehabilitation program, aerobic capacity returns to preflight levels by 30 days after landing.[164] Considerable variability exists between crewmembers in alterations of aerobic capacity during and after flight, apparently related to intensity of aerobic exercise while in orbit.[164] Intense exercise countermeasures during flight can effectively prevent postflight aerobic deconditioning. Even with in-flight exercise, diminished aerobic capacity can be expected both during flight and in the first weeks after landing from long-duration flight, most likely as a result of intravascular volume losses, which can take several days to return to normal, and from dilutional anemia that results from the intravascular fluid replenishment, recovery from which can take weeks.[211]

Dysrhythmias

Since the beginning of human space exploration, there has been concern about increased risk of dysrhythmias in microgravity. One instance of paroxysmal supraventricular tachycardia resulted in early termination of a Russian space station mission,[171] and another episode was implicated in termination of a Russian spacewalk.[83]

Short-duration spaceflight has not been shown to predispose crews to clinically significant dysrhythmias,[196,82] although rates of clinically benign ectopy can increase during physiologically demanding activity, such as spacewalks.[83] Preliminary results of Holter monitoring of astronauts on long-duration missions aboard

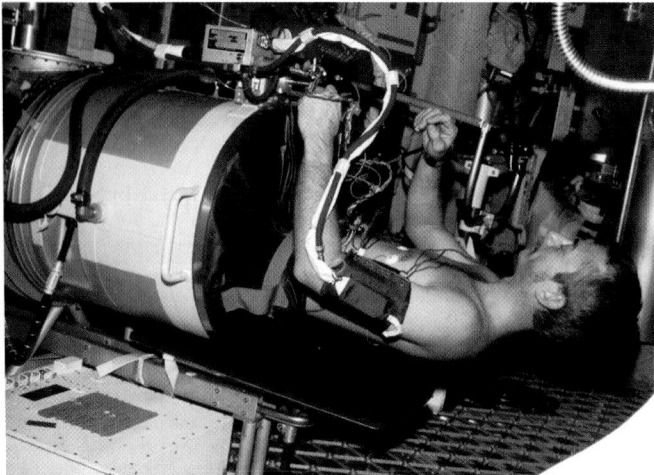

FIGURE 126-7 Astronaut Owen Garriott using the lower-body negative pressure (LBNP) device in an experimental protocol aboard the Skylab Space Station during the Skylab 3 mission in 1973.

the ISS indicate no evidence of clinically significant electrocardiographic abnormalities[88] (Levine B: Personal communication, 2013), suggesting that spaceflight conditions do not cause an increase in ventricular dysrhythmia risk. In-flight ECG monitoring is currently performed in the U.S. program only during exercise testing and spacewalks, as an objective measure of activity level during these events.

Cardiovascular Fitness

The potential for cardiac atrophy from lack of physical demand in microgravity has been a concern. Decreases in cardiac mass measured with magnetic resonance imaging (MRI) in astronauts after short-duration spaceflight and in terrestrial bed-rested subjects[185] suggested that significant cardiac atrophy could occur after 1 week or more of exposure to microgravity. However, rapid recovery of left ventricular (LV) mass to preflight values, detected in crewmembers after 4 days of short-duration flight, suggests that LV mass changes can be explained by dehydration or microgravity-induced fluid shifts alone.[223]

Reduction in postflight aerobic fitness has been noted since the Gemini program, with decreases in peak O_2 consumption ($\dot{V}O_2$max) of up to 22% relative to preflight values.[30,141] Generally, crewmembers experience a 15% to 20% decrease in $\dot{V}O_2$max over the first month of flight, which can improve over several months with adequate access to in-flight aerobic exercise, approaching preflight levels in some individuals. However, postflight $\dot{V}O_2$max usually remains below preflight levels; after a 6-month mission, average $\dot{V}O_2$max significantly decreased to 10% to 15% below preflight values.[66,164]

Aerobic exercise aboard the ISS is provided by using a cycle ergometer and a treadmill with a load-bearing harness (Figure 126-8 and Video 126-2). Thirty minutes of aerobic exercise with protocols that generate O_2 consumption at 75% of a crewmem-

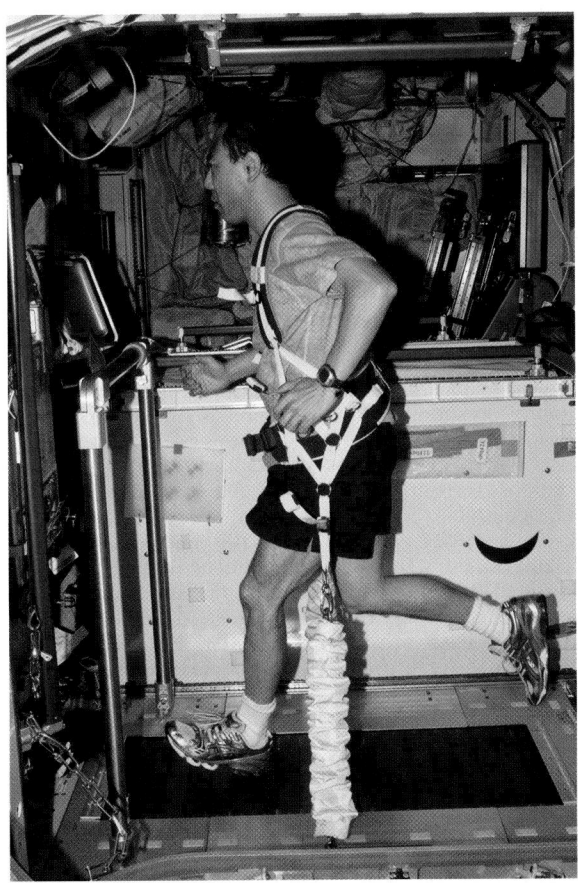

FIGURE 126-8 Astronaut Satoshi Furukawa using the T2, a vibration-isolated treadmill used extensively for exercise aboard the ISS. Note the white loading harness and bungees that pull the astronaut onto the treadmill with a force equivalent to up to 80% of the astronaut's body weight.

ber's $\dot{V}O_2$max are scheduled 6 days per week on the ISS. Participation in robust aerobic exercise during spaceflight has also been increasingly recognized as a mitigator of postflight orthostasis after even short-duration exposure to microgravity.[137]

Monitoring and Treatment

Screening potential spaceflight crewmembers for cardiac disease is the most effective means of preventing cardiac issues from having an impact on space missions. Hypertension, cardiac structural abnormalities, evidence of inflammation of the myocardium or pericardium, cardiac tumors, and symptomatic atherosclerotic disease are considered disqualifying for selection as a career astronaut. Tachydysrhythmias and conduction defects can be disqualifying, depending on symptoms, persistence, and associated underlying conditions. Catheterizations are not routinely used because of cost and risk considerations, but a coronary artery calcium score (CACS) determined by electron-beam computed tomography (CT) scanning, in conjunction with a Framingham risk evaluation, is currently used to stratify astronauts into low-, medium-, or high-risk categories.

After selection, a program of exercise, nutrition counseling, and annual monitoring is followed to detect, prevent, and delay progression of atherosclerotic disease in susceptible individuals. Members of the astronaut corps are generally fit, but for some astronauts, age alone constitutes an independent risk factor; average age in the astronaut corps was 44 years for women and 45 years for men in 2002.[84] When disease resulting in flight disqualification is identified in an active astronaut, definitive treatment can be appropriate in select cases and can result in return-to-flight status. For example, radioablation of ectopic foci and accessory conductive tracts has been performed in astronauts diagnosed with new-onset atrial fibrillation and resulted in successful subsequent spaceflights. In addition, detecting early stages and progression of atherosclerotic disease has been a major component of an astronaut's annual physical examination. Risk can be decreased by reducing low-density lipoprotein (LDL) to less than 100 mg/dL by means of diet and medications and by increasing $\dot{V}O_2$max as determined by exercise stress testing. While hypertension is considered disqualifying on selection, single-agent antihypertension control can be instituted in an already-qualified astronaut. Risk of a life-threatening cardiac event during a mission still exists because no prevention program will be perfectly sensitive to detecting and mitigating cardiac disease.

Future Research

The extent to which redistribution of fluid within body compartments during spaceflight affects long-term human health is unknown. It has become apparent that fluid shifts and tissue unweighting in microgravity impose a profound change on cardiovascular, neuroendocrine, musculoskeletal, and hematologic systems. There is further evidence for effects even at the cellular level, in size, contour, shape, and distribution of renal microtubules and changes in mechanotransduction of various cell types.[172] A recently discovered phenomenon, known as visual impairment and intracranial pressure, may result from the unique vascular response to the fluid shifts and tissue compression changes associated with microgravity. Likewise, we are only just beginning to understand the effects of ionizing radiation on vascular viability and rate of cardiovascular aging. Investigations are currently underway to detect evidence of insidious radiation damage to blood vessels that can manifest as intimal thickening, changes in vascular reactivity, or increases in O_2 radicals in blood or urine.[10]

VISUAL IMPAIRMENT/INTRACRANIAL PRESSURE SYNDROME

Concerns related to the effects of long-duration spaceflight on human vision have been expressed for decades. Some crewmembers have historically reported minor changes in visual acuity during or after spaceflight, with symptoms often resolving after return to Earth. Prolonged vision changes that required more significant or chronic corrections have been largely attributed to age-related presbyopia. However, toward the end of the Space Shuttle era, a postflight funduscopic examination and fluorescein angiography of a visually affected long-duration ISS crewmember identified findings that could not be attributed to presbyopia alone.[2] Subsequent medical surveillance since this seminal case has included more detailed eye examinations and advanced imaging technologies to further characterize these findings, including pre- and postflight imaging, regular visual acuity and field testing during flight, ultrasonography of the globe and optic nerve, and similar detailed examinations throughout the pre-, in-, and postflight periods. Findings show that a significant proportion of astronauts exhibit combinations of hyperopic shifts, optic disc edema, posterior globe flattening, optic nerve sheath distention, nerve fiber layer thickening, choroidal folds, cotton-wool spots, and elevated postflight cerebrospinal fluid (CSF) pressure, with variable expression of any given finding.[146]

This constellation of findings was noted to have similarities with idiopathic intracranial hypertension (IIH, formerly "pseudotumor cerebri"), which raised concern for the potential of increased intracranial pressure (ICP) secondary to microgravity exposure leading to ocular and visual alterations.[125] Previous evidence from Russian cosmonauts serving aboard the Mir station suggested that ICP elevation may result from long-duration spaceflight, as indicated by postflight optic disc edema.[166] Intracranial hypertension was thus rapidly identified as a possible causative factor for these ocular structural findings, and a provisional name of *visual impairment/intracranial pressure* (VIIP) was coined to denote this variable yet prevalent phenomenon. Interestingly, not all affected astronauts expressed persistent visual symptoms; some cases resolved on return to Earth, whereas other cases retained visual acuity changes or mild elevations of ICP for months to years after landing.[2,146] Because of this variability and the potential for significant disability given the wide range of ocular and neuroanatomic findings, VIIP has become recognized as one of the top health risks of human spaceflight, and substantial resources have been allocated to study the phenomenon.

The etiology of VIIP is unclear, although elevated ICP is thought to be a significant contributor. ICP elevations likely occur secondary to a number of possible factors. The cephalic fluid shift caused by microgravity is thought to cause cerebral venous congestion leading to increased ICP. Intense resistive exercise performed to prevent bone and muscle loss is capable of causing intermittent but potent spikes in intraabdominal and intrathoracic pressures; these intermittent Valsalva-like events may have a smaller but additive effect on ICP.[154] Insufficiency of internal jugular venous valves has been proposed as a factor predisposing to ICP elevation for some groups of terrestrial patients[53,169] and might play a role in ICP alterations in the astronaut population. Elevated concentrations of CO_2 in the vehicle atmosphere may be another contributing factor, because CO_2 is known to cause cerebral vasodilation and subsequently ICP elevation. As previously described, permissible CO_2 concentrations have undergone scrutiny over the years because symptoms suggestive of CO_2 toxicity have been reported at lower concentrations. One investigation also suggests that exposure to chronically elevated CO_2 level during flight may lead to the impaired cerebrovascular CO_2 reactivity seen after landing from long-duration missions.[244] The duration of spaceflight may affect cerebral autoregulation. Cerebral autoregulation in response to LBNP was preserved 2 weeks into short-duration spaceflight[98] and after long-duration flight,[244] but cerebrovascular sensitivity to CO_2 after long-duration spaceflight showed significant reduction in cerebral blood flow response relative to before flight.[244] Increased dietary sodium has also been suggested as a contributor to ICP elevation, precipitating a substantial reduction in allowable sodium levels in the ISS diet.[128] Also considered is the interplay of CSF production and ICP in space. Recently returned astronauts with significant posterior globe flattening had, on average, 70% increased CSF production relative to preflight values, as measured by MRI,[124] suggesting a more nuanced contribution to ICP increases than that caused by venous congestion alone.

Although these clinical and imaging data suggest ICP elevation as a likely contributor for VIIP development,[146,125,124] actual in-flight ICP remains speculative. Ultrasound measurements of optic nerve sheath diameter and globe dimensions show changes that suggest in-flight rise of ICP, but data are not conclusive. Postflight lumbar punctures have been performed on a few affected individuals and showed normal to mildly increased opening pressures.[146] Ocular findings have been out of proportion to these ICP values, but the timing of the lumbar puncture (performed when the busy postflight schedule allowed) may have missed elevations that had since normalized. In-flight lumbar puncture in microgravity has not been performed for many reasons, including sterility concerns and operational risks; even if single ICP values could be obtained from in-flight lumbar puncture, there is no guarantee that measurements would be representative of the ICP during an entire flight duration. Options exist for continuous ICP measurement over several months and involve parenchymal or subdural implantable devices, but these methods carry an additional set of risks.

Fluid shift contribution to increased ICP has been demonstrated in several animal and human spaceflight analog studies. An immediate increase in ICP was seen in rats during analog testing using vacuum drop tests,[78] and a rhesus monkey flown on a Russian biosatellite showed increased ICP within minutes of arriving in microgravity.[229] Elevated human ICP has likewise been seen immediately on head-down tilt,[131] and a recent study showed ICP to be higher both in the supine position and during parabolic flight relative to the upright seated position.[131] Given the inability to "sit" or "stand" in space, the time-averaged ICP in microgravity may be higher than on Earth, where humans spend most of the day upright.

Clinical signs and symptoms of VIIP syndrome vary widely among affected individuals. Interestingly, alterations of ocular anatomy are more likely to occur in the right eye.[146] Female astronauts have presented thus far with milder signs and symptoms than have males,[13] and thus far there have been no reported cases of frank optic disc edema in female astronauts. This gender difference may be related to differences in vascular compliance; overall, male astronauts with VIIP findings have been older than their nonaffected counterparts. Age might contribute to decreased vascular compliance. Affected crewmembers have shown alterations of their folate and vitamin B_{12} one-carbon metabolism pathway, suggesting this trait may predispose a subset of astronauts to developing VIIP.[245] A spectrum of expression of VIIP-related findings suggests biologic variability between individual responses to spaceflight and warrants determination of potential risk factors. A case study of a repeat long-duration astronaut indicated that previous spaceflight experience with ocular abnormalities may be a predictor for developing VIIP findings during a subsequent mission, and repeat flight may have a cumulative effect on the VIIP process.[145]

Medical management of VIIP syndrome is multifactorial, with the goal of preserving vision by managing increased ICP, reducing dietary sodium, avoiding medications or exposures that might increase ICP, and judicious use of medications to lower CSF production. Terrestrially, ICP may be lowered with carbonic anhydrase inhibitors to protect optic nerve function. Although this drug class may have utility in VIIP patients, it could worsen VIIP manifestations by lowering intraocular pressure out of proportion to ICP and thus increase the pressure differential experienced by orbital structures. Corticosteroids may be used in addition to acetazolamide in patients with severe papilledema, although concerns surround the potential for rebound of elevated ICP after cessation. Although not routinely used in terrestrial clinical populations with increased ICP, omeprazole may be considered for treatment of VIIP findings because it is known to decrease CSF production in animal models.[102,143] Medical evacuation from space would be considered in extreme cases, such as impeding retinal compromise or new onset of neurologic findings such as diplopia.

MUSCULOSKELETAL ISSUES

Life and work during a space mission generally demands little from the postural muscles and load-bearing skeleton of the human body. Prolonged, unmitigated exposures to microgravity can therefore result in significant muscle atrophy and bone loss in an otherwise healthy astronaut. Even with regularly scheduled resistive and aerobic exercise, whole-body dual-energy x-ray absorptiometry (DEXA) scans of astronauts returning from long-duration flight in both the Russian and the U.S. space program have shown site-specific areal bone mineral density (aBMD) loss rates of 1% per month in the spine and 1.5% per month at the hip,[129] rates higher than those seen in postmenopausal women.[167,194] A review of the first 23 missions to the ISS showed that, although no astronaut had postflight aBMD values commensurate with osteoporosis, several astronauts evaluated had statistically significant aBMD decrements in the lumbar spine and/or hip (femoral trochanter, femoral neck, or total hip), with some showing aBMD decreases greater than 10% in both areas.[136,179] Recovery to preflight levels of aBMD after return to Earth from the standard 6-month mission in microgravity can take up to 1 year, and 3 years in some cases.[204,207] Removing gravitational compression and postural muscle tension on the human skeleton seems to be the cause of these losses, with studies providing evidence for upregulation of osteoclastic activity in space that outstrips the normally balancing effects of osteoblasts.[225]

Likewise, significant muscle atrophy and functional declines have been measured in the lower back, hips, and lower limbs of individuals after missions longer than 6 weeks. If atrophy is unmitigated, its magnitude appears to correlate with flight duration, associated with a shift of muscle fiber type from slow type I to fast type II phenotypes.[61,76] Muscle volume losses of 4% in the psoas and 17% in the gastrocnemius, as measured by MRI,[134] as well as loss of knee flexion and extension isokinetic torque of 31% and 27%, respectively,[138] have also been observed after long-duration missions.

Atrophy of bone and muscle, which limit function on return to Earth's gravitational environment, can affect in-flight performance. Typical workday activities in space place little demand on the musculoskeletal system, but translating (moving) massive objects across modules, using tools to maintain station systems, and operating mechanisms such as hatches require in-flight maintenance of strength and endurance. Crewmembers must learn to balance any pushing or pulling force with a counterforce in their work, often by the use of postural muscles to brace themselves against a structure. EVAs in particular demand significantly more strength and endurance than usual mission activities, particularly in the upper extremities. For example, two crewmembers conducting a Salyut spacewalk after almost 2 months in space had difficulty opening their hatch and reentering the station airlock.[170] After this event, the Russian program established an upper-body exercise regimen and arm ergometry test that cosmonauts must now pass before EVA.

Various resistive exercise devices have been employed on spacecraft in an attempt to minimize microgravity-induced bone and muscle losses. Sufficiently high loads to the musculoskeletal system, applied through a series of exercises that focus on postural muscle groups and load-bearing skeletal sites, are essential. In one study, a device capable of generating 300 lb-equivalent loads used for 1 hour a day in a variable exercise regimen, including squats, dead lifts, and heel raises, neither prevented loss of muscle mass or decreases in force or power,[76,230] nor preserved bone.[179] A more recent device, launched to the ISS in 2008, uses adjustable piston-driven vacuum cylinders and an inertial flywheel to simulate the constant mass and inertia of free weights on Earth. The Advanced Resistive Exercise Device (ARED) delivers loads ranging from 20 to 600 lb equivalent, and its daily use on board during 6-month missions has demonstrated the capability to reduce aBMD loss significantly in the pelvis, hip, and trochanter, as well as preserve lean tissue mass[210,212] (Video 126-3).

Preservation of bone and muscle also depends on adequate energy intake and vitamin D supplementation.[212] The required daily exercise during a space mission may place a greater metabolic demand on the human body than working and living on Earth. Absence of ultraviolet light exposure during spaceflight in conjunction with decreased vitamin D intake can significantly reduce body vitamin D stores, further adding to bone loss. Stein

and colleagues[215] demonstrated that astronauts on short-duration Space Shuttle flights averaged a negative energy balance while in space, consuming only 70% of predicted caloric requirements, likely because of food palatability and compressed schedules that limit time for food preparation. Crews are more likely to attain the recommended caloric and mineral intake with present-day menus and their wider variety of food choices, along with readily available vitamin D supplementation.

The bisphosphonate drug alendronate has also been evaluated during spaceflight as a potential pharmacologic adjunct to exercise in preventing bone loss. In a recent study, exercise in addition to alendronate attenuated all indices of bone loss, including aBMD, trabecular alterations, serum markers of bone turnover, and urinary calcium excretion.[135] Because alendronate was evaluated during the time ARED use became routine, the degree of aBMD preservation attributable to the drug alone cannot be ascertained at this time.[179]

Given the benefits of exercise in maintaining musculoskeletal health, exercise hardware systems will continue to be a critical component of future spacecraft. However, exercise hardware development is not without its challenges. One of the most important issues in providing effective exercise countermeasures is the need for vibration isolation of any exercise equipment from its vehicle interface to avoid unwanted mechanical stress on spacecraft structure. Efforts are underway to develop more compact systems that can work within the smaller spacecraft interiors expected for exploration-class spaceflights, and that demonstrate greater reliability for these missions where resupply is impractical, yet still provide musculoskeletal stresses similar to a 1-G environment. Investigations are also underway to develop resistive exercise protocols that require less crew time but maintain bone and muscle fitness, by incorporating more explosive movements of the large muscles of posture and locomotion. Still to be determined are the long-term effects, if any, of radiation on bone remodeling from the higher radiation doses that accrue with flights outside Earth's GMS.[239]

The long-term health effects of microgravity-induced bone loss are unknown, particularly when considered in combination with expected age-related losses. Quantitative CT used to evaluate volumetric BMD in astronauts shows slower recovery rates in the more metabolically active trabecular compartment of bone in astronauts after long-duration flight, despite preservation of aBMD (measured by DEXA), suggesting that bone remodels itself with altered architecture during microgravity exposure.[129,158] It is unclear how this alteration affects fracture risk, or whether it reduces age of onset or characteristics of age-related osteoporosis.[179,207]

PSYCHIATRIC AND BEHAVIORAL HEALTH

Most astronauts find months of life and work in space to be an enriching experience, but there are many stressors inherent to spaceflight that can threaten psychological health of spaceflight crews. Identifying and reducing these stressors are essential to mission success, particularly for deep-space exploration. Significant effort is put toward maintaining behavioral and psychiatric health, supporting crew cohesion and productive crew-ground interactions, and working with ground control teams to minimize crew overwork and circadian dyssynchrony (asynchrony).

Some negative stressors inherent to spaceflight are common to analog environments, including remote polar or subsea stations. Studies of populations deployed to these environments are useful in helping define risks to behavioral and mental health for astronauts who experience similar conditions, and in evaluating methods and products to mitigate these risks. Stressors inherent in both spaceflight and analog missions include confinement, stimulus reduction, social crowding, workload responsibilities, and potential for unhealthy crew social dynamics.[92,182] Another similarity is physical separation of deployed teams from their nuclear social networks, during preparation and for duration of the mission itself. A spaceflight of 6 months is the culmination of 1.5 to 2.5 years of training that includes frequent travel to international training centers. Family crises and world events, completely unrelated to the mission, can affect crews; one cosmonaut withdrew from ground communication for several days on receiving news of a family member's death during a long-duration flight.[35]

Other stressors are found only in spaceflight. Microgravity is both a source of immense fascination for the crew and a complicating element in planning and executing most daily activities. At the same time, the microgravity environment initiates a process of physiologic adaptation with unknown changes in sleep demand and cognitive effort needed to perform several or complex tasks.[92] Other characteristics of the typical spacecraft environment include continuous cabin fan noise, dim lighting conditions, altered circadian cues (including 16 day-night cycles per workday in orbit), variations in air contaminants, and high levels of ionizing radiation exposure.

The spaceflight experience also carries unique positive characteristics, including the qualities of life in microgravity, awareness of membership in an elite group,[221] and, perhaps most important, the visual impact of Earth as seen from orbit[96] (Figure 126-9). Even so, behavioral or psychological challenges can arise during flight. A review of Space Shuttle postmission debriefs conducted from 1981 to 1989 found a total of 34 comments regarding behavioral symptoms, most often anxiety and annoyance;[16] symptoms of stress, tension, mood elevation, and depression were also mentioned in a subsequent review.[208] Crews on Russian and U.S. long-duration missions have shown signs and symptoms associated with negative intracrew interactions, a tendency toward detachment from ground-support teams, symptoms of depression, irritation, boredom, and both overwork and underwork.[37,114]

Psychosocial aspects unique to a long-duration crew aboard the ISS include its small size, with typically only three to six members, its international makeup, and the high levels of education and motivation in each of its members. In addition, the crew in LEO is in near-continuous communication with ground specialists, allowing mission control centers to constantly supervise work activity on board, which can at times undermine crew autonomy or increase workload (Figure 126-10).

Given the demanding schedule and operational requirements of spaceflight activities, disruptions of sleep and sleep quality are known to occur during both short- and long-duration missions. Crews are often required to shift their own circadian rhythms, particularly before dynamic events such as launch, landing, and docking of newly arriving spacecraft. Since 1990, astronauts have undergone scheduled exposures to bright light during preflight quarantine to induce circadian shifts as needed to accommodate launch times or in-flight shift work.[218,238] Sleep-shift protocols that delay, rather than advance, the circadian rhythm are practiced aboard the ISS as needed before major dynamic operations, because most individuals find that delaying their circadian cycle

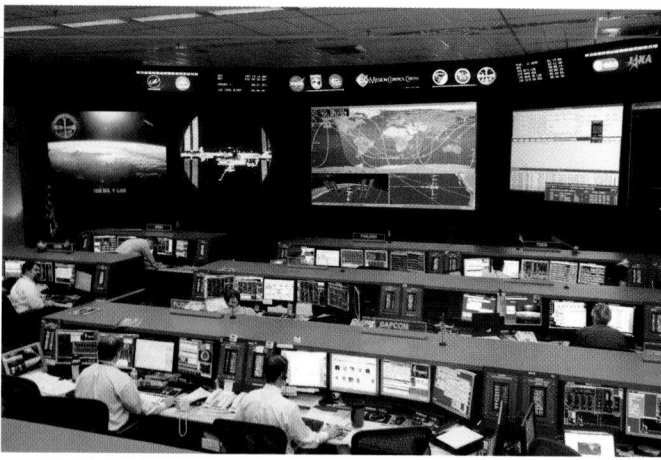

FIGURE 126-10 Mission Control at the Johnson Space Center in Houston. Flight directors lead a team of engineers and scientists to monitor the ISS and work with the in-flight crew to successfully complete space missions. *(Courtesy NASA.)*

(in other words, going to bed later than usual) is more tolerable than a phase advance (going to bed earlier than normal). "Slam-shifting," a sudden shift in the sleep/wake cycle for one-time critical operations, is sometimes practiced. One study identified that as many as 13% of flight days were spent in slam-shifted cycles.[123] These disruptions of sleep cycles can add to social or operational pressures and further precipitate crew irritation or stress.

Dedicated efforts are made to reduce the psychological stressors of spaceflight. Selection of astronauts is in part based on their demonstration of qualities suitable for work in the spacecraft environment, including strong teamwork and coping skills, high level of motivation, competency, self-discipline and sensitivity, and history of good social relationships.[181,208] After selection, annual psychiatric and psychological interviews are conducted to confirm fitness for duty. Once astronauts are assigned to a mission, a dedicated behavioral health and performance program provides active support to crewmembers and their families. This focuses on behavioral health, fostering positive crew and family interactions, while monitoring and mitigating disruptions to sleep and circadian rhythms.[15,209] During a mission, astronauts speak privately every 2 weeks with the same psychiatric and psychology professionals with whom they trained before flight. In addition, crewmembers are able to use e-mail and connect to private calls or videoconferences with their families. These are some of the many advantages of near-Earth spaceflights that are capable of real-time voice and video communication.

As with any deployed team, optimizing crew workload is a common challenge on ISS missions. This includes managing the risk of performance being compromised by extended duty days, irregular work schedules, and high workload.[149] In LEO, managing work/rest schedules requires satisfying research and maintenance requirements, planning sleep shifts, and accommodating off-duty time. Preestablished scheduling guidelines include methods of increasing crew autonomy and establishing "payback," utilizing increased time off for more efficient operational activities; this provides a means of managing workload during periods with an accelerated operational tempo. Psychiatrists and psychologists have also derived flight rules defining appropriate sleep-shifting schedules both to prevent accumulation of fatigue and to shift the crew's circadian nadir away from times when they must perform critical activities, such as robotic operations. Sleep aids are available in onboard medical kits to support circadian shifting.[62,190] Symptoms of depression, if detected through crew medical conferences, are generally treated with conservative measures that may include focusing on ensuring adequate rest in the schedule and providing positive feedback to the crew.[62] Antidepressants are available in the space medical supply for severe or prolonged symptoms, but their use has not been required to date. Similarly, antipsychotic and anxiolytic

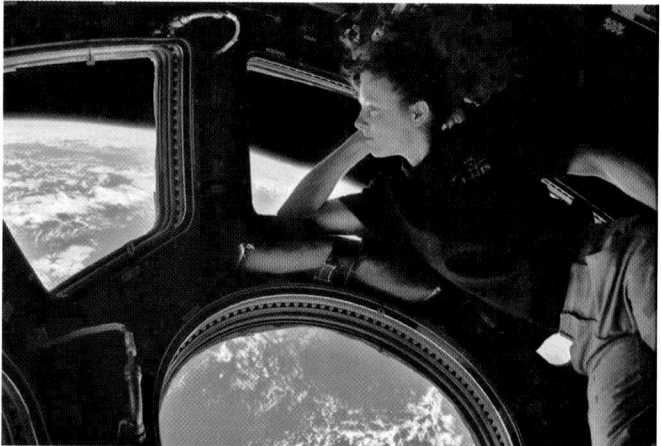

FIGURE 126-9 Astronaut Tracy Caldwell-Dyson takes a break from work aboard the ISS to view Earth through the largest windows ever constructed for spacecraft. The view of Earth from space is often cited as one of the most enjoyable aspects of spaceflight.

medications are available, but have yet to be needed during spaceflight.[62]

In the future, crews of missions beyond Earth orbit will experience a level of isolation unique in human existence. The distances involved will prevent real-time communications with any terrestrial social network; the round-trip journey for a signal from Earth to the Martian surface could take 45 minutes. The view of Earth, one of the most pleasing aspects of today's missions, will not be present for much of the time during these expeditionary flights. In anticipation of these challenges, current research focuses on further defining personality traits and personal skills that, according to our long-duration experience to date, would be desirable characteristics for future expeditionary crews. Our experience continues to provide lessons in the value of increasing crew autonomy and in ensuring adequate sleep and work/rest balance. Self-assessment tools are being developed to assist remote crews in prevention, assessment, and management of sleep disruption, fatigue, and psychosocial problems.[27] The lessons learned in continued human missions to LEO will be invaluable in designing for the psychological challenges of the longer expeditionary missions of the future.

DERMATOLOGY AND HYGIENE

After a few days in microgravity on orbit, the normal skin desquamation process becomes a fascinating spectacle. In fact, an astronaut recently returned from a long-duration mission can be identified by both the lack of calluses on the foot sole and the addition of a corn on the foot dorsum, formed after months in flight by repeated abrasion of wedging the feet under handrails for positional stability.

Understanding underlying physiologic changes in human skin is largely subjective. Crewmembers often describe delayed healing time for small cuts and abrasions, but this has not been objectively documented. One experiment found delayed epidermal cellular proliferation and loss of elasticity in one crewmember during flight compared with after flight. Coarser skinfolds in magnified images showed changes similar to those in aging skin, and results suggest slowing of epidermal cell turnover from the basal layer to the stratum corneum during flight.[231] The effects of ionizing radiation, immune changes, or microgravity are unclear with respect to these findings.

As discussed earlier, water is a precious commodity during spaceflight. Because of the microgravity challenges of containing free-floating water and detergents, there are no running water showers or handwashing stations in current spacecraft. Personal hygiene consists of using an array of moistened wipes, dry wipes, and towels. Without laundering available, crews simply wear the same clothing on a rotation schedule and discard their clothing after a certain duration of use (every 2 weeks on the ISS). While this might suggest that the ISS would be a rather pungent environment, body odor is generally minimal: clothes remain generally clean because of lack of terrestrial dirt, and in microgravity, without body weight pressing down on socks or underwear, clothes generally "hover" around the body and can remain surprisingly clean despite normal perspiration. Even so, it is worth noting that contact dermatitis, folliculitis, and fungal infections have occurred on long-duration missions. Whether this level of hygiene predisposes astronauts to superficial skin infection is not clear.

Skin trauma is one of the most common injuries reported by astronauts during spaceflight.[202] Although generally minor, skin injuries can affect crewmembers on an almost daily basis. Constant handling of rough materials, such as Nomex fabric or Velcro, will abrade a crewmember's hands and fingers. Minor cuts are common because the hands are so frequently used for mobilization and stabilization. Primary irritant contact dermatitis is also common; EVAs, exercise tests, and scientific payloads require repeated application of electrocardiographic electrodes, the usual cause of this condition. Other dermatologic conditions include tinea pedis and cruris infections.[80]

Skin trauma from working in a spacesuit deserves special attention. A pressurized suit glove acts as a rigid, jointed shell, and pressure points on the hands and elsewhere are common during and after spacewalks.[202,219] This pressure has been known to cause bruising of hand extensor tendons and digital neuropraxia. Strong, continuous fingertip pressure in the suit glove is desired by spacewalkers to enhance tactility throughout arm range of motion; however, this pressure typically causes trauma to the nail bed matrix. Protective measures, such as applied synthetic enamels or cyanoacrylate adhesives, have been tried with variable success. The moist environment of the glove after hours of continuous work and perspiration can contribute to fungal growth, so that onychomycosis may have to be treated in the compromised nail bed.[219]

With the absence of atmospheric filtering, excessive ultraviolet (UV) radiation exposure is another risk inherent to spaceflight. Although most windows aboard spacecraft have coatings to prevent transmission of UV radiation, some are uncoated to fulfill science requirements in Earth and astronomy observations. Skin exposed to solar nonionizing radiation transmitted through non–UV-protected windows can sustain first- and second-degree burns within seconds. As a result, even momentary exposure to light through these windows is avoided.

In-flight treatment for dermatologic problems includes topical corticosteroids and antibiotics, using terrestrial treatment regimens in consultation with ground medical support. Photography is perhaps the most useful diagnostic tool for dermatologic conditions, particularly to assist ground specialists in diagnosing persistent cases.

TRAUMA

Minor trauma, such as contusions, abrasions, and superficial cuts, particularly to the hands as previously noted, is a common occurrence during spaceflight.[202] Activities most often associated with these injuries include interfacing with exercise machines, stowage operations, and translation about the spacecraft. Work in space occasionally requires moving massive objects such as experiment racks, so that more serious crush injuries, particularly to the hands, are possible because of an object's inertial mass. Scalp lacerations, while uncommon, are possible as well from accidental collision against spacecraft structure during crew locomotion, particularly early in a mission before crewmembers have developed their skills in microgravity. Soft tissue trauma also frequently occurs from prolonged work inside the rigid confines of the pressurized spacesuit, which can cause contusions of the hands and feet.

The hardware available to repair lacerations on orbit is similar to that found in the terrestrial clinic or wilderness medical kit. A limited variety of nylon and polypropylene sutures, curved needles, hemostats, forceps, iris scissors, cyanoacrylate tissue adhesive, staples, and bandages are available on board. The main challenge in repairing a wound in space, however, is in setting up the worksite and stabilizing hardware. Maintaining sterile technique is more difficult without the organizing assistance of gravity: Velcro, bungees, magnetic strips, and tape are most often used for this purpose. Wound irrigation is necessary, particularly because of the increased airborne particulate burden inside spacecraft, but irrigation can be challenging in microgravity. Towels or loose-weave gauze can capture fluids effectively in space (but may require some planning).[22]

In vitro studies have shown variable results with respect to integrity of the healed wound in space; abnormal cellular migration and collagen formation, as well as increased inflammation, have been observed.[189] Likewise, aerospace practitioners and astronauts have subjectively noted increased rates of wound infection of up to 50%.[159] The greater challenge with more serious wounds may be to balance complexity of repair with in-flight medical capability and degree of disability if definitive treatment is not rendered in flight. Considerations include limited capability of the medical kit and skill level of the medical officer, who may not be a physician and is likely to have had only a few hours of training. In these situations, photographic documentation and conferences with ground specialists may be essential.

Inertial loads from impacts and sudden motion can be significant, given the speeds crewmembers can attain in translating through the relatively large volume of the ISS and the torque that can be imparted to a single hand or foot acting as a pivot to stabilize the entire mass of the body (Video 126-4). Foot restraints are used throughout the ISS, both inside and outside the spacecraft. Although essential to stabilize oneself for close work, foot restraints can allow transfer of torsional stress, for example, to the knee if only one foot is constrained. Minor knee injuries, such as ligamentous sprains, have occurred. No fractures have occurred in space, but accidental entrapment of a finger or foot between panels or handrails during translation could result in hand or foot fractures. One phalangeal dislocation occurred on Skylab by such a mechanism; fortunately, one of the other crewmembers happened to be a physician and was able to perform rapid relocation of the digit.[38]

Back pain is also a common complaint among crewmembers. In a review by Kerstman and colleagues,[117] back pain was shown to affect 52% of U.S. astronauts during spaceflight. Onset typically occurs on the first flight day, usually resolving by the second day. The pain has features of musculoskeletal or myofascial origin, is typically located in the lumbar region, and is most often mild. Radicular symptoms can also arise, with lancinating pain and patchy anesthesia over the lower extremities. Spinal column lengthening likely contributes to in-flight back pain as a natural consequence of body gravitational unloading.[117,200] One study demonstrated that crewmembers can expect to "grow" 2 to 6 cm (0.8 to 2.36 inches) above their terrestrial preflight height during even short-duration missions, demonstrating significant spinal elongation in microgravity and resultant strain on spinal nerves.[19,220] In general, back pain is alleviated by donning the treadmill harness to impart a compressive load on the spine,[117] or more often by pulling the knees to the chest in a fetal position and stretching the lumbar musculature. Some crewmembers use a strap behind the back and around the knees to maintain this fetal position during sleep.

Herniated nucleus pulposus (HNP) is increasingly recognized as a postflight injury among astronauts, after both short- and long-duration missions.[110] The incidence of both cervical and lumbar HNP is four times higher in astronauts than in terrestrial cohorts in the 12 months after landing.[110] Although the mechanism of this increased incidence is unknown, persistent spinal elongation in microgravity, with intermittent compression from using a harness for treadmill exercise or from loading while performing squats on the ARED, may predispose an astronaut to annulus stress that manifests as postflight herniation.[117] To protect themselves from vertebral disk injuries, astronauts limit heavy load lifting or overaggressive return to nominal exercise regimens for at least 2 weeks after landing.

Shoulder injury constitutes another prominent musculoskeletal risk for astronauts. Spacewalk training in particular is known to be associated with shoulder rotator cuff injuries.[219] Astronauts spend at least 72 hours overall in the spacesuit in an underwater simulated weightless environment before a mission, working continuously for 5 to 6 hours at a time. Training for and executing spacewalks in the U.S. program generally involves repetitive, sustained shoulder joint stress, pulling and pushing the mass of the body and the 250-lb spacesuit during translation. Since the spacesuit is designed around a hard upper-torso component, rotator cuff impingement against the arm opening can occur with arm abduction, flexion, and external rotation (Video 126-5). Rotator cuff tendon strains, subacromial bursitis, and labral tears, usually of the superior labral anterior-to-posterior (SLAP) variety, are relatively common and occur more frequently in astronauts training for and performing EVA[200] (Scheuring R: Personal communication, 2015). In-flight acute shoulder injury is rare but has occurred during the process of spacesuit doffing and during Apollo lunar surface operations after using a drilling tool on the lunar surface.[14]

One of the periods of greatest risk of musculoskeletal injury for astronauts is the preflight period. An injury during this time can have significant impact on the upcoming mission or even prevent an astronaut from flying. In one review of an 8-year span during Space Shuttle operations, astronauts sustained ligamentous sprains and fractures during preflight athletic activity and flight training that resulted in 28 orthopedic surgical procedures during this period. Knee injuries accounted for the majority of the surgical conditions, and running, skiing, and basketball were most frequently associated with injuries.[104] Restricting and monitoring athletic activity, along with improved awareness of the risk of preflight injury, are necessary to prevent impacts of such injuries on space missions.

For finger, wrist, and ankle strains during flight, current spaceflight medical kits contain compression bandages and splinting devices similar to those found in a wilderness medical kit. Cold packs are available, although refrigeration in spacecraft is primarily used to support research and will not likely be available on deep-space exploration missions because of weight and power restrictions. It is not known how bone callous integrity and formation rate in response to a fracture would be affected by microgravity, although investigations in simulated microgravity indicate the potential for alterations to the fracture healing process.[178] A graded loading protocol, such as on the treadmill using an adjustable loading harness, would likely need to be devised for rehabilitation and functional recovery.

For shoulder injuries, in-flight evaluation of soft tissue structures using ultrasound has been performed in space,[60] and nonsteroidal antiinflammatory drugs (NSAIDs) are generally used by crewmembers for exacerbations of a chronic problem in flight. Efforts are currently focused on preflight prevention and early detection and intervention for musculoskeletal and traumatic injuries, in particular shoulder injuries associated with EVA training in water immersion. This includes a consistent exercise regimen to help protect the shoulder through a rotator-strengthening and scapular stabilization program. Still, surgical intervention is often required. Sports medicine specialists are assisting in development of a new spacesuit, which will include new torso/upper arm configurations to allow more freedom of shoulder and upper arm movement and minimize the risk of shoulder injury.

IMMUNOLOGY

Radiation exposure, altered sleep cycles, noise, isolation, allergens, and other terrestrial factors are known immunologic stressors experienced during spaceflight. In addition, microgravity itself directly or indirectly alters the human immune system and may disturb its performance and response to host or environmental pathogens.[40,163,226] Dysregulation of the immune system may increase the risk of contracting infectious diseases during spaceflight. Astronauts and cosmonauts aboard the Mir space station experienced a number of infectious disease events, including conjunctivitis, upper respiratory infections,[156] otitis media/externa, pharyngitis, urinary tract infections, and skin infections. Severe infections or those not responding to antimicrobials may require medical evacuation from LEO. In 1985, one Soviet cosmonaut developed prostatitis while on board the Salyut-7 space station and was medically evacuated after his condition did not improve.[112] Even with all these incidents, no increased incidence of infectious disease has been attributable to spaceflight factors, relative to terrestrial experience.

Alterations of blood hematologic components have been documented in crewmembers and persist for the duration of ISS flights. Decreased resistance to viruses is suggested by cytokine shifts observed in humans and animals during spaceflight. Of note, microgravity alters production of the interferon class of cytokines, reducing the quantity of available defenders to combat invading viruses.[140,214] Furthermore, antiinflammatory cytokines in mice[12] and astronauts[42] have been shown to increase in microgravity; this could weaken the inflammatory response needed to combat immunologic insults. Leukocyte cell distribution shifts have also been observed after spaceflight. Granulocyte percentages from peripheral blood have been shown to increase (although this change is likely caused by demargination with the stress of landing) and lymphocytes to decrease after landing, whereas monocytes remain relatively unchanged when measured after short-duration flights.[43] In multiple studies, T-cell function has been shown to be impaired in both short- and long-duration spaceflight.[41,81,121] The extent of immunologic alterations and amount of time needed to return to baseline after flight depend on the flight duration and accompanying stress levels.[69] Stress hormone elevation during spaceflight may also play a role.

It is uncertain whether allergic or hypersensitivity reactions that have occurred in space result from these immune system changes. Basophil granulocytes contain histamine and have an important role in human allergic response, and the increased granulocyte percentage seen in spaceflight may worsen allergic symptoms. Cosmonauts have demonstrated hypersensitivity to several substances during long-duration spaceflights.[69] Likewise, NASA astronauts have reported numerous atypical allergies and prolonged rashes while on board the ISS. There have been 3.29 cases of skin rashes per person-year of U.S. spaceflight,[97] a rate significantly greater than the incidence of skin rashes in the general terrestrial population (0.044 case/person-year),[118] although the terrestrial data may be limited because these data represent only individuals who sought medical attention for skin complaints.

The risk of infectious disease reflects a balance among host defense strength, host exposure, and the pathogen's capability to evade the host defense. There is some evidence that pathogen virulence is influenced by microgravity-induced alterations in pathogen mechanotransduction. For example, *Salmonella* has been shown to increase in virulence during spaceflight.[172] Larger particulates, such as sloughed skin, offer microorganisms a unique harbor in microgravity. While terrestrial gravity causes these particulates to settle, spaceflight gives free-floating particulates enhanced potential for inhalation, resulting in direct contact with an astronaut's ocular, nasal, and respiratory mucous membranes. Cramped conditions in small vehicles may also lead to transfer of microorganisms between crewmembers.[186,187] Fortunately, geographic isolation of a crew in space from the terrestrial population allows introduction of a new contagious process only when a new crewmember arrives, and virulent pathogens are generally hindered from hitchhiking to space by a strict, immediately preflight quarantine process.

Even with these precautions, in at least one instance, a recently arrived Space Shuttle astronaut disseminated an upper respiratory infection throughout the ISS and Space Shuttle crews. Furthermore, the quarantine process cannot be effective against reactivation of latent viruses. An average of 65% of asymptomatic ISS astronauts reactivated latent varicella-zoster virus, and 82% shed Epstein-Barr virus during their mission.[37,162] It is unknown whether microgravity-induced alterations render immune cells less able to defend against growth of cancer cells induced by the increased radiation exposure outside Earth's atmosphere.

Prevention is the primary space medicine countermeasure against immune disorders. Acquired immunity is enhanced with preflight immunizations against specific disease processes, such as influenza and herpes zoster. Routine sampling of ISS air, water, and surfaces is used to gauge potential pathogenic challenges to crewmembers' host defense systems. Monitoring and early intervention through station cleaning also prevent biofilm propagation across spacecraft surfaces, which could otherwise result in unhygienic conditions during spaceflight. Modern spacecraft engineered with efficient ventilation systems, adequate air filters, microbial limits on launching space vehicles, and strict quarantine before launch help prevent occurrence or transfer of infectious illness in space.

For onboard treatment, ISS medical kits contain standard topical, oral, and injectable medications to combat active infections and hypersensitivity reactions. Ground-based flight surgeons assist crews in selection of a medical regimen and evaluate treatment progression.

Future immune countermeasures may include nutritional supplements. Cervantes and Hong[28] suggested that astronauts may be able to maintain a healthy microbiome by supplementing a well-managed diet with probiotic therapies. Immunotherapies, such as recombinant cytokines, monoclonal antibodies and immunoconjugates, immunomodulators, activated immunocytes, and gene therapy, are other countermeasures that could someday be tailored for spaceflight.

Infectious disease, viral reactivation, hypersensitivity, and increased risk of cancers are the principal immunologic concerns during spaceflight. Immunologically impaired crew health could

result in poorly executed tasks, early mission termination, or at worst, loss of crew life. Even a minor illness can result in substantial mission costs, particularly if illness forces an evacuation and early mission termination. Fortunately, the incidence of infectious disease remains low.

UROLOGY

Renal stone formation, urinary retention, and urinary tract infections (UTIs) are the most prevalent genitourinary disorders in spaceflight.[113] Specific stresses associated with spaceflight elevate the risk of urinary problems during flight and in the pre- and postflight periods and contribute to formation of renal stones. Decreased urine output from reduced plasma volume or fluid restriction is known to lead to increased urinary solute concentrations. Fluid restriction can result from limited access to water during launch and landing operations, during spacewalks, and during the compressed timeline of on-orbit operations. Intentional fluid restriction may be practiced by some astronauts to avoid use of primitive hygiene systems (e.g., simple absorbency garments) during launch and spacewalks. Increases in urinary calcium and phosphate from leaching of bone, secondary to skeletal unloading in microgravity, and increased dietary salt contribute to an elevated risk of forming urinary calculi.[236,237]

Kidney stones can be incapacitating and risk crew health, safety, and mission success. The one reported case of a symptomatic renal stone in spaceflight involved a Russian cosmonaut who experienced severe lower abdominal pain that spontaneously resolved, barely preventing an emergency deorbit.[133] The postflight period may also carry increased risk of kidney stones. Some NASA astronauts experienced kidney stones during the 12 months following their spaceflight. These kidney stones might have developed during spaceflight, or the postflight period may continue to increase the risk of kidney stone formation.

American astronauts are screened for the presence of renal stones with ultrasound imaging both at selection and again on assignment to a long-duration mission, and their stone formation risk is evaluated through measurement of stone risk parameters (urinary analytes, pH, urine volume, and supersaturation of calcium oxalate, calcium phosphate, and uric acid).[112] In an effort to prevent stone formation, astronauts are encouraged to ensure adequate oral intake of water, sufficient to maintain urine output of 2 L/day.[112] In addition, the ISS food system is undergoing reformulation to decrease the sodium content of food items, potentially changing the urinary biochemistry environment to make it less conducive to stone development.

During spaceflight, should symptoms suggestive of acute ureterolithiasis arise, remote guided ultrasound imaging can be used to localize and measure ureteral stone size or to detect the presence of obstruction or alternate diagnoses. Urinalysis using standard reagent sticks can be performed in flight; the presence of blood may assist with diagnosis. For confirmed cases, in-flight kidney stone treatment would mirror standard terrestrial symptomatic care. Tamsulosin, ketorolac, morphine, ondansetron, promethazine, and intravenous (IV) rehydration are available in the current ISS medical kit. Medical evacuation may be required depending on the astronaut's condition, ultrasound characteristics, and associated complications, such as concomitant urinary infection or inability to manage nausea and emesis.

Urinary retention has occurred during both short- and long-duration spaceflight. Intentional voiding delay, possibly because astronauts may prefer not to use absorbent pads during launch, landing, and EVA, may contribute to this incidence. In the close quarters of spacecraft, psychosocial ("shy" bladder) influences may be a contributor because there is often limited privacy for bathroom activities. In addition, anticholinergic and sympathomimetic side effects of medications used during spaceflight (e.g., promethazine, pseudoephedrine) are likely a predominant influence on the frequency of urinary retention. Lastly, absence of gravity may be a separate, unique contribution to urinary retention in spaceflight.[217]

Terrestrially, urinary retention is almost exclusively seen in older men secondary to prostatic hypertrophy; in spaceflight, women represent a larger percentage of this incidence. Most spaceflight cases of urinary retention have occurred in the first 30 days of space missions, implicating SAS (and thus antiemetic medication use and dehydration) as a causative factor. Urinary retention during a mission can generally be treated successfully with a variety of urinary catheters (straight or indwelling) available from the current ISS medical kit. Ultrasound evaluation of bladder urine volume to determine the need for catheterization has been shown to reduce the rate of this procedure terrestrially, reducing bladder or ureteral irritation and nosocomial UTIs; this may be a useful adjunct in spaceflight.[108]

Cystourethritis has occurred during both short- and long-duration spaceflight. Stepaniak and colleagues[217] reported two cases associated with bladder catheterization during shuttle flights. Urinary infection has also been described in one returning Apollo astronaut,[14,112] and one Russian medical evacuation resulted from a case of septic UTI/prostatitis during a long-duration space mission.[112] Currently, in-flight UTI diagnosis is limited to symptoms and simple urinalysis; urine cultures cannot be obtained, and UTIs must be treated empirically. Onboard antibiotic stores are limited, and even a single case of UTI can significantly deplete resources.

GYNECOLOGY AND REPRODUCTIVE ISSUES

Women comprise about 10% of the more than 500 individuals who have flown into space on short- or long-duration missions and have participated in most aspects of spaceflight activity. The flight experience of female astronauts has not revealed any obvious difference in incidence of gynecologic disorders in space or after landing, compared with the terrestrial population.[105,113] However, a 2014 review of the life sciences literature on physiologic adaptation to spaceflight highlights the lack of spaceflight data pertaining to reproductive physiology.[153]

Medical screening criteria for women are the same as for men, with the exception of breast and reproductive system evaluations. Maintenance of women's health before spaceflight follows the same practice as does terrestrial clinical medicine, with the addition of pelvic and abdominal ultrasound examinations every 5 years. On assignment of a female astronaut to a long-duration flight, repeat pelvic ultrasound is required to detect uterine or ovarian abnormalities that may have arisen since the astronaut's selection. During flight, menstrual suppression has been practiced by about one-half of female U.S. astronauts, including use of levonorgestrel implants and oral contraceptives.[99,105] For astronauts who choose to continue menstruating during their mission, standard sanitary products are available, and control and disposal of blood and blood products present no greater challenge in microgravity than do other routine hygiene activities. Although microgravity seems to have no effect on menstrual cycling,[105] the overall picture of spaceflight effects on the hypothalamic-pituitary-ovarian cycle has yet to be fully explored. Microgravity poses a greater challenge for women to maintain hygiene after urination. Toilet designs use controlled airflow in place of gravity to collect and contain urine, and each female astronaut uses a custom-made funnel to interface with the perineum. Surface tension causes urine to collect in the vaginal orifice or remain in the distal urethra in some women, making postvoid drying more difficult. Although this phenomenon is described as a relatively minor annoyance,[105] care must be taken to prevent UTI.

Preventing bone loss during a long-duration spaceflight is of particular interest given the existing risk of bone mineral density loss in postmenopausal women. Fortunately, there appear to be no gender differences in musculoskeletal response to microgravity or in the efficacy of in-flight impact and resistive exercise in preventing bone loss.[210] Adherence to the in-flight fitness regimen, estrogen replacement for postmenopausal astronauts,[39,50] and particular attention to adequate dietary calcium and vitamin D supplementation are necessary to help mitigate potentially additive osteoporotic influences. Bisphosphonates have been shown to be effective as an adjunct to in-flight exercise[135] and are also offered to postmenopausal astronauts to help protect the skeleton in microgravity.

The cardiovascular response to spaceflight shows gender differences. In stand tests conducted after Space Shuttle missions, women had a significantly higher incidence of presyncope than did men, likely from gender differences in cardiovascular response to orthostatic stress. Men tend to respond with a greater increase in PVR, whereas women respond with a greater increase in HR.[68] Recent improvements in maintaining cardiovascular and musculoskeletal fitness during long-duration missions seem to be reducing the incidence of postflight orthostatic intolerance for both men and women.

Radiation exposures are expected to put women at greater risk than men to long-term health. For all ages, ionizing radiation exposure limits for female astronauts are lower than for their male counterparts. The additional cancer risk for the breast and ovaries, the higher lung cancer risk from radiation in women, and other gender-related differences in natural cancer incidence contribute to an overall higher risk of cancer for women exposed to space radiation.[168] Likewise, the longer female life expectancy allows more time for any postflight carcinogenesis to arise.[75] Organ dose equivalents are a few percent higher for women because of their smaller body mass shielding. Female astronauts are therefore at a greater risk of exceeding their career limits for radiation than men are for an equivalent radiation exposure.[45]

Pregnancy is contraindicated for most astronaut training activities and is disqualifying for spaceflight. Flying time in high-performance jets is limited to no later than the first trimester of pregnancy (although most women choose not to fly at all during pregnancy) because of the concern for exposure to high-acceleration forces with potential ejection, possibility of accidental cockpit decompression, hypoxia, and similar risks. Other training risks include rapid pressure changes with standard spacesuit training in vacuum chambers, which includes exposure to 100% O_2, hypercarbia, and depressurization deltas as great as 10 psi from ambient. These and other exposure risks, such as the risks of increased radiation on a developing fetus, require deferral of spaceflight training and flight itself for the pregnant astronaut. Additionally, abnormalities have been demonstrated in neonatal mammals exposed to microgravity during their fetal development, with observable detriments to function of the neurovestibular system.[195]

Spaceflight is not known to affect postflight female fertility. No differences in rates of conception or spontaneous abortion have been detected in female astronauts compared with age-matched controls. Because many female astronauts choose to delay their first pregnancy until completion of selection, training, and their first spaceflight, they often require assisted reproductive technology due to advanced maternal age. Success rates for both natural pregnancy and assisted reproduction in these women are similar to those of nonastronaut cohorts of the same age.[105] For long-duration missions, preflight cryopreservation of embryos or oocytes may be desired, because of the risk in delaying a pregnancy after years of flight and training and the risk of ionizing radiation exposure to reproductive organs.

OPHTHALMOLOGY

Ophthalmologic issues have historically been the predominant reason for disqualification from astronaut selection.[109] Visual acuity, stereopsis, color vision, intraocular pressure (IOP), the fundus, and visual fields[150] are all evaluated in the selection physical examination. However, acuity standards for selection have relaxed since the beginning of the U.S. space program. Currently, visual correction with laser-assisted in situ keratomileusis (LASIK) or photorefractive keratectomy (PRK) is acceptable.[74] Visual correction is common during spaceflight; approximately 80% of U.S. astronauts wear some form of correction. Contact lenses are often worn, and one astronaut has also flown in space with bilateral intraocular lens replacements, demonstrating no instability or visual defects.[147]

The spaceflight environment can be particularly hazardous to the eyes. Microgravity increases the risk of ocular injury from free-floating objects, and increased particulate burden in cabin air raises the incidence of foreign body contamination. Cephalad fluid shifting also contributes to elevated IOP early in flight,[54]

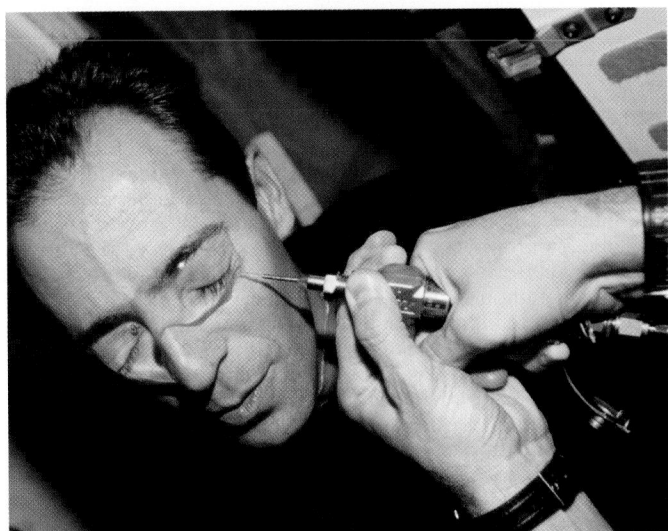

FIGURE 126-11 Astronaut Jean-Francois Clervoy demonstrates an effective spaceflight technique for removing foreign bodies from the eye using potable water. In microgravity, the water forms a dome that bathes the eyes and can in most cases remove offending particulates.

likely from engorgement of the choroid,[148] and is probably a component of the spectrum of physiologic changes that affect visual acuity, retinal vascular diameter, and the optic nerve, the constellation of findings known as the VIIP syndrome (see Visual Impairment/Intracranial Pressure Syndrome, earlier).

Minor ocular injuries resulting in limited, self-resolving ocular irritation are a daily fact of life in space. Crewmembers often find their work or mealtime halted for a few moments to remove a foreign body from the eye or to flush out mild irritants (Figure 126-11). As previously noted, certain activities, particularly entry into a newly arrived spacecraft and packing operations, pose a particular risk for corneal abrasions from atmospheric debris. Crews are required to wear safety glasses during initial entry into newly arrived cargo vehicles, because dust, lint, or metallic debris can easily escape detection during ground cleaning operations and find its way into the open cabin space on arrival to microgravity. The momentum of free-floating particles on impact with the cornea is generally insufficient to embed a foreign body; however, larger free-floating objects, such as tools or writing pens, particularly if tethered to the worksite or crewmember and hovering near the face during work, can pose a risk of eye injury. Corneal abrasions from larger free-floating objects, requiring ocular examination and antibiotic ointment, have occurred several times during flight and usually resolve in 24 to 36 hours. Elastic straps can be particularly hazardous because of the significant potential energy that can be released when they are stretched and snapped back into place. In one crewmember, failure of an exercise cord with elastic snap-back caused traumatic iridocyclitis with photophobia and a decrease in visual acuity in the affected eye, resolving 10 days after the initial injury.

Greater particulate contamination in spacecraft air and difficulty maintaining appropriate hygiene in microgravity without running water likely create increased microbial load to the eye. Sterile infiltrative keratitis has occurred during missions, diagnosed after flight upon discovery of corneal infiltrative scarring. Erythromycin ointment and ciprofloxacin 0.3% solution are available in space medical kits; however, even these medications pose challenges in the microgravity environment. In the absence of gravity, liquid ophthalmologic medications must be placed directly onto the eye so that surface tension can wick the solution onto the conjunctival surface. Therefore, contamination of the dropper tip is likely, and some wasted dropper fluid is expected. Ophthalmologic ointments are preferred for use in space;[74] otherwise, extra liquid preparations are provided to compensate for waste and contamination.

Work aboard the ISS at times requires proximity to caustic materials, such as the sulfuric acid used to treat urine before recycling it into potable water, or lithium hydroxide, a common particulate in CO_2 removal systems. Eye protection is mandatory for procedures involving these systems. If an ocular toxic exposure occurs that requires copious irrigation, an eyewash station using potable water and modified swim goggles can flush potable water across each eye at a rate of 1 L/min[203] (Figure 126-12).

For more complex and serious ocular injuries, communication with the ground is essential. Still images are valuable for ground evaluation of injury severity. Ultrasound is useful in visualizing injuries and can be immediately streamed to the ground to facilitate real-time guidance and diagnostic assistance. Comprehensive ocular examinations using B-mode ultrasonography and Doppler with remote guidance are regularly performed as part of a periodic in-flight ocular examination.[33] Optical coherence tomography, currently aboard the ISS, can also be used to measure the size and depth of corneal foreign bodies, abrasions, and ulcers.

Radiation poses an ophthalmologic risk during spaceflight. Window coatings protect astronauts from the intense solar UV radiation found outside Earth's atmosphere, but as noted earlier, some windows are uncoated to allow transmission of the full electromagnetic spectrum for scientific observations. Exposure of the eye to radiation transmitted through these windows has occurred and quickly results in UV keratitis.[133] "Light flashes," noted by crewmembers in a darkened compartment or when the eyes are closed, occur when energetic particles hit the retina[70] and are reminders of the ionizing radiation environment in space. The GCR component of space radiation has been found to be associated with increased risk of cataracts,[44] although a subsequent 5-year NASA study of lens opacities in astronauts showed no increase in cataract progression with subsequent flight exposure.[34] These findings are relevant to the long-term ophthalmologic health of pilots participating in high-altitude sorties as well

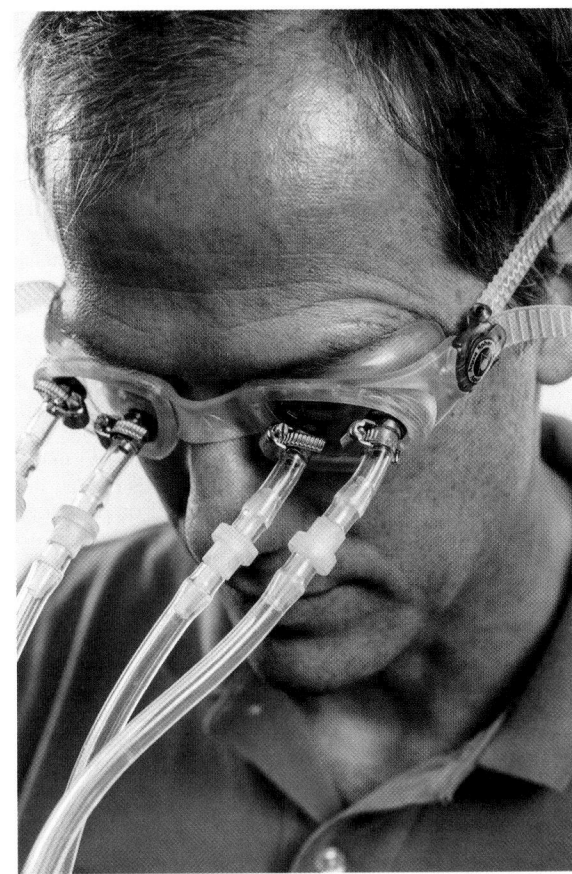

FIGURE 126-12 The emergency eyewash system, demonstrated here by astronaut Tom Marshburn during training. The system can flush the eyes with copious amounts of potable water to remove chemical contaminants, capturing the waste water in a plastic waste bag (not shown).

as of astronauts, particularly those who will crew vehicles traveling beyond LEO on extended exploration missions.[111]

OTOLARYNGOLOGY

Microgravity, cephalic fluid shifts, pressure and PO_2 differentials, and noise exposure are all components of spaceflight that can affect otolaryngologic structures. Nasal congestion is a common occurrence during spaceflight. Mucosal swelling associated with cephalic fluid shifts is believed to be the major contributor to congestion symptoms; pharyngeal mucosal hyperemia has been noted in the normal physical examination in space.[87] Although the cephalic fluid shift can increase the thickness of soft tissue structures above the clavicles, in microgravity there is no posterior displacement of the tongue, soft palate, uvula, or epiglottis, as occurs with the supine position terrestrially. Snoring and signs of obstructive apnea were reduced relative to pre- and postflight measurements and were almost eliminated during in-flight sleep studies conducted on the Space Shuttle,[52] perhaps a welcome finding given that living in close quarters is a common characteristic of life aboard spacecraft.

Nasal congestion can wax and wane in severity during a mission. Symptoms seem to vary depending partly on adequacy of air ventilation in the spacecraft interior, suggesting an allergic component to congestive episodes. Blockage of air ventilation filters has been associated with increased congestion among the crew, and symptom improvement has been noted after filter cleaning.[157] Although symptoms associated with upper respiratory infection (URI) are rare during spaceflight since the establishment of preflight quarantine, they remain the most common otolaryngologic complaint.[3] URI symptoms can be particularly troublesome when compounded with nominal nasopharyngeal congestion. Of note, rhinorrhea is not often seen in space because of the lack of gravity-assisted drainage of nasopharyngeal secretions; this may also exacerbate congestion. Intranasal oxymetazoline, cromolyn, mometasone, and oral antihistamines are available in the onboard medical kits.

Upper respiratory congestion is of particular concern during procedures that require cabin or spacesuit atmospheric pressure changes. Atmospheric pressure in the Space Shuttle and the U.S. airlock on the ISS is decreased during preparations for EVA as part of a DCS prevention protocol. Within the airlock, pressure in the U.S. and Russian spacesuit is reduced from the normal 14.7 psia to 4.2 to 5.8 psia, to allow sufficient flexibility of limbs and hands as the airlock pressure drops for hatch opening into the vacuum of space. Repressurization after an EVA has led to sinus pressure discomfort from blockage of sinus ostia or eustachian tubes in some congested astronauts. EVA crewmembers use yawning, swallowing, and jaw movement to help maintain patency of the eustachian tubes. Valsalva maneuver, if needed, must be done by compressing the nares against a foam block on the inside of the helmet, since EVA crewmembers are unable to access their face with their hands when fully suited. After an EVA, swollen mucosal blockage can again cause problems, and EVA astronauts have reported pain from barotitis media. Prophylactic nasal decongestants (oxymetazoline and/or pseudoephedrine) may be used before EVA as a preventive measure, and symptomatic crewmembers can pause the airlock pressurization process to allow equalization of inner ear pressure when necessary. URIs can exacerbate any of these symptoms, so astronauts with URI symptoms are not allowed to perform EVAs.

Delayed barotitis, also called O_2 otitis, can occur during aviation training or after an EVA as a result of breathing pure O_2. In this condition, O_2 is absorbed in the middle-ear mucosa for up to 24 hours after low-pressure exposure. This absorption creates enough negative middle-ear pressure to cause discomfort if active equilibrium is not initiated. Most often, astronauts report delayed barotitis symptoms after a sleeping period when they are not sufficiently awake to perform these equilibration maneuvers.

Otitis externa is occasionally seen with use of earplugs on orbit. If required, antimicrobial ear drops must be administered by inserting a wick or by allowing the dropper tip to touch the external canal skin such that the surface tension allows the drops to adhere to the skin. Dry cabin air and cephalic fluid shifts are believed to predispose crews to epistaxis, another common otolaryngologic malady that occurs during spaceflight.[3] Anterior nasal bleeds can occur spontaneously or after nose blowing, and crewmembers are trained to apply direct external nasal pressure at the onset of epistaxis. If bleeding continues, oxymetazoline, silver nitrate, and lidocaine with epinephrine are available in the ISS medical kit. Posterior epistaxis has not occurred in space, although nasal packing and Foley catheters are available to tamponade a posterior bleed. Sulfamethoxazole-trimethoprim is available as prophylaxis against infection from nasal packing.

Astronauts are exposed to a wide range of vibroacoustic energy throughout a mission, so hearing protection is another aspect of spaceflight preventive care. Astronauts are exposed to significant noise from rocket engines during a launch phase, and high sound pressure levels also occur on board space vehicles in orbit. The main contributors to noise in the orbital phase of flight are internal to the spacecraft and include exercise hardware, experiment payloads, ventilation fans, and pumps. Astronauts living aboard space stations experience less noise than exists in many industrial workplaces, but because they live and work continuously in the same environment for 6 months or more, progressive hearing loss from occupational noise exposure is considered a risk of long-duration spaceflight. Also at risk are speech intelligibility, sleep, and detection of alarms. Space station hardware degradation and refurbishment and the constant addition of new experiment payloads result in a dynamic acoustic environment, which necessitates occupational hearing surveillance for crewmembers and monitoring of the spacecraft sound environment for long-duration missions. Onboard hearing assessments, acoustic dosimeters, and pre- and postflight audiometry are all utilized for hearing surveillance and to identify the need for improved hearing protection. Hearing-protective devices that have been used in spaceflight include foam earplugs, custom-made earplugs, passive headsets, and active noise reduction headsets. Rather than personal hearing protection, however, engineering controls are the preferred means of protecting crews from excessive noise levels.

DENTAL CONCERNS

Dental problems requiring urgent or emergency care pose significant risk in the space environment. Although no specific aspect of spaceflight presents a unique risk for dental issues, the freedom of multidirectional movement possible in spacecraft (and therefore inadvertent impacts between an astronaut and vehicle component) and the tendency for crewmembers to hold small tools or other items in their teeth while using their hands for movement control can increase the risk of tooth fracture. Launch vibrations have been known to dislodge dental crowns, and airlock operations place astronauts at risk for barodontalgia. Apical abscesses, usually from undiagnosed dental caries, can lead to significant and even debilitating pain.

Proper preflight monitoring and dental care are paramount for limiting the risk of mission impact caused by dental problems. Astronaut oral care is focused on prevention. Crewmember dental examinations and prophylaxis are required annually after selection and 1 to 3 months before launch, so that any issues identified can be remedied. During flight, the dental kit includes a dental mirror, explorer, spoon evacuator, and elevator. Dental extraction forceps and anesthetic are also available for intractable tooth pain. Carpules for anesthetic injection are prefilled with bupivacaine for ease of preparation in microgravity. Before launch, crewmembers learn simplified examination techniques and simple dental procedures, including temporary filling application, crown cementation, and dental injections.

GASTROINTESTINAL ISSUES

Once SAS symptoms have resolved, gastrointestinal (GI) function seems to readily adapt to microgravity (see Space Adaptation Syndrome, earlier). However, some mild GI symptoms often arise during space missions. Constipation is a common GI complaint among spaceflight crews early in flight; although the cause is unknown, some degree of decreased gastric motility is likely present in flight.[86,191] Onboard medical kits include fiber supplements and bisacodyl to be used as needed, and constipation usually self-resolves within 1 week of arrival in microgravity.[157] Reflux symptoms are also common and are usually associated with ingestion of a large meal or large bolus of fluid; symptomatic treatments are available to crewmembers as needed.

Because GI diagnostic and surgical capabilities aboard spacecraft are extremely limited, preflight GI abnormalities are identified and addressed before flight. Screening colonoscopy, endoscopy, and abdominal ultrasonographic examinations are performed on astronaut candidates at selection. Abnormalities, such as the presence of gallstones, biliary sludge, or evidence of inflammation in the gallbladder or pancreas, discovered in the intervening period between selection and assignment to a flight, would require aggressive treatment or surgical resolution and a sufficient recovery period before medical approval would be given to return to training or flight. Management of abdominal pain of unknown etiology has generated much discussion among aerospace practitioners and surgical specialists.[11,24] Acute surgical abdomen, such as suspected appendicitis or cholecystitis, is a significant concern. It may be possible to perform some degree of diagnostic imaging for such conditions using the onboard ultrasound, but true suspicion of these conditions would likely result in early termination of the mission and return to Earth. Before evacuation, the mainstay of treatment would be antibiotic control of the infection with the goal of walling off an abscess to prevent rupture until return to Earth for definitive treatment. IV access capability, parenteral fluids, antibiotics, and pain control are available on board, along with sufficient hardware to attempt percutaneous drainage of an abdominal abscess under remote guidance and ultrasonic visualization.[119]

Prophylactic appendectomies or cholecystectomies are performed by some sponsoring agencies before Antarctic and other long-duration deployments. These have not been instituted to date in the U.S. space program,[26] however, in part because of the increased risk of small bowel obstruction from adhesions. The risk of an acute abdomen has been considered sufficiently low given the prescreening mandated before flight, and because the average age of the astronaut corps is higher than the age of peak incidence for appendicitis.[7] This practice may be reconsidered because improvements in laparoscopic technique decrease the terrestrial surgical risk to an otherwise healthy astronaut in training, and as space missions extend deeper into space,[11] an emergency return to Earth becomes less tenable.

NEUROLOGY

The human nervous system undergoes a rapid adaptive process in microgravity and again on return to Earth. Neurovestibular changes, oculomotor function (e.g., eye-hand coordination, gaze tracking), alterations in sensory perception, changes in proprioception, and cognitive effects (e.g., three-dimensional visual perception, mental spatial representation), must all take place for an astronaut to function effectively in microgravity.[193] In microgravity, the influence of otolith inputs on central nervous system (CNS) sensory integration seems to decrease,[115,116,177] resulting in a central prioritization of retinal information over vestibular inputs.[67] At the same time, semicircular canal inputs seem to be unaffected.[115,116] Degradation of proprioception[115,116,177] and remembered limb position,[234] loss of orientation without visual cues,[85] and decrements in visuomotor tracking[122] and dual-task performance[151] have been detected during in-flight investigations.

Given these profound and rapid CNS alterations, it is not surprising that neurovestibular complaints are the most common neurology-associated issues that arise during spaceflight, and their severity seems to be correlated with flight duration.[243] Neurovestibular symptoms are often reported with motion sickness early in flight, contributing to the diagnosis of SAS (described earlier). Symptoms similar to those of SAS, collectively termed *entry adaptation syndrome,* often occur in crewmembers immediately on return to Earth. In addition, astronauts have demonstrated marked ataxia, poor hand-eye control, and neurovestibular confusion with any rapid motion in the early postlanding period. In-flight exercise is increasingly recognized as providing some mitigation of postflight neurovestibular ataxia.[8] A dedicated rehabilitation regimen in the first few weeks after return to Earth is intended to return crewmembers to their preflight fitness levels and to reduce the risk of injury as they assume activities of daily life on Earth. Exercises are tailored to one's individual neurovestibular state, with increasingly challenging exercises that promote multisensory integration.[243] The rehabilitation period also allows the clinician to observe the return of neuromotor function during the readaptation process.

Regarding specific neurologic complaints, headaches occur fairly frequently in flight; up to two-thirds of astronauts have reported at least one headache during their mission, even when they had not suffered from headaches on Earth. Headaches occurring early in flight are likely associated with fluid shifts, SAS, or caffeine withdrawal. The etiology of headaches after the first days of a mission are not as easily discernible, although elevated CO_2 levels have been suggested as an inciting factor in some crewmembers.[130] Cerebral venous hypertension has been postulated as well and may be caused by venous insufficiency similar to that suspected with acute mountain sickness or in patients with idiopathic intracranial hypertension.[240] In-flight medical kits contain acetaminophen and NSAIDs; these medications can be used as needed for headache.

Objective measures of crew performance rarely show decrements aside from those related to fatigue. Crewmembers often note a need for increased focus to prevent mistakes early in flight; fatigue, sensory overload, and other nonspecific stressors likely contribute to this effect, making any specific effects caused by microgravity difficult to extract.[152] CO_2 may be a contributor in some cases; some crewmembers have reported that only after CO_2 levels were reduced for operational reasons did they notice greater mental clarity and ease in performing their daily tasks.[130] Space radiation damage to the CNS is increasingly recognized as a potential risk to astronauts on extended-duration missions beyond LEO. Rodents exposed to heavy ion radiation have shown CNS pathology similar to that seen with aging, including CNS atrophy[222] and decreases in cell division with alterations in behavior.[224]

ONBOARD MEDICAL CAPABILITY

In-flight medical capability has expanded to keep up with the growing demands associated with increasingly complex mission profiles. The current makeup and function of the ISS Health Maintenance System (HMS) distinctly express the aggregate experience of space physiology and space medicine, coupled with operational and technologic advances of recent decades. Similar to wilderness medical supplies, the contents of the HMS are based on predictions of most likely medical threats and the medical expertise of the in-flight crew, and must be reasonable in terms of weight, volume, safety, and compliance with vehicle requirements. In addition to general limitations on mass and volume, constraints exist for certain types of equipment, such as alcohol-containing products (because of their volatility and contamination of condensate reclamation systems) and radiographic equipment (because of power use and electromagnetic interference). Shelf life stability is also a critical factor that must be considered due to cost of launch and resupply logistics.

All ISS crews are trained to respond autonomously to emergency medical conditions, such as anaphylaxis, choking, and cardiopulmonary arrest. Because of significant preflight training time limitations, this training is procedure focused, has a very narrow scope, and is limited to lifesaving functions. ISS crewmembers are typically not physicians, and training for select crew medical officers (CMOs) is limited to less than 40 hours in the 15 months before launch. Computer-based "just-in-time" instructional and ground-based physician coaching are available before medical procedures are performed in orbit.

MEDICAL KITS

Medical supplies that are unique to individual astronauts are flown in a personal ISS Medical Accessory Kit (IMAK). These items could include personal medical devices such as shoe orthotics (for use with treadmill exercise), contact lenses and eye care accessories, and medications used to treat chronic conditions. This kit is launched with the crewmember and is also used to deliver resupply items to the various ISS medical kit packs.

The ISS onboard HMS is a collection of consumable and durable equipment used to monitor crew health as well as respond to illnesses and injuries. ISS medical kits are collections of primarily consumable goods, separated into nine different notebook-like packs, ideal for viewing all contents at a glance and for quick transport to a worksite. The packs are color coded, items are individually restrained, and packs are organized in functional groups according to medical problem, frequency of use, or resupply efficiency. The most frequently used medications are stowed separately for easier access.

Kit contents vary according to their intent and function. Over-the-counter and prescription medications are available; many of the medications are designed for astronaut use at their own discretion, with notification of the ground physician for awareness and resupply needs. Diagnostic equipment, including hemodynamic monitors, otoscopes, and ophthalmoscopes, are also readily available to the crew. Less common and injectable medications, dental cements, urinary catheterization equipment, and wound care equipment are stored separately; crewmembers are required to notify ground physicians when using such equipment. Lastly, there is a separately contained Emergency Medical Treatment Pack with advanced life support consumables, including a bag-valve-mask, intraosseous access kit, and injectable medications for treatment of anaphylaxis and cardiopulmonary arrest. Sufficient supplies, as well as an automated external defibrillator (AED), are available to progress through two rounds of assessment and medication delivery for basic life support and advanced cardiac life support algorithms. There is also a rigid plastic platform, fixed to the cabin deck, with integrated restraint straps to stabilize a patient for medical procedures and transport, similar to a medical backboard. It also provides electrical isolation to protect the CMO(s) and space station avionics during defibrillation (Figure 126-13).

Using injectable medications or fluid rehydration poses challenges unique to the microgravity environment. Although modified off-the-shelf bags of normal saline are available on the ISS, medical officers must ensure adequate air/water separation before injection, generating angular acceleration by spinning the IV bag and driving fluid to the outside of the spin radius. A similar technique must be employed with syringes to minimize infusion of air into IV lines or during intramuscular injections.

DIAGNOSTIC IMAGING

Onboard imaging equipment is limited to ultrasound technique. The ISS ultrasound unit is a lightweight, modified commercial device that is primarily used to support scientific research. A phased-array probe and a curvilinear probe are available for

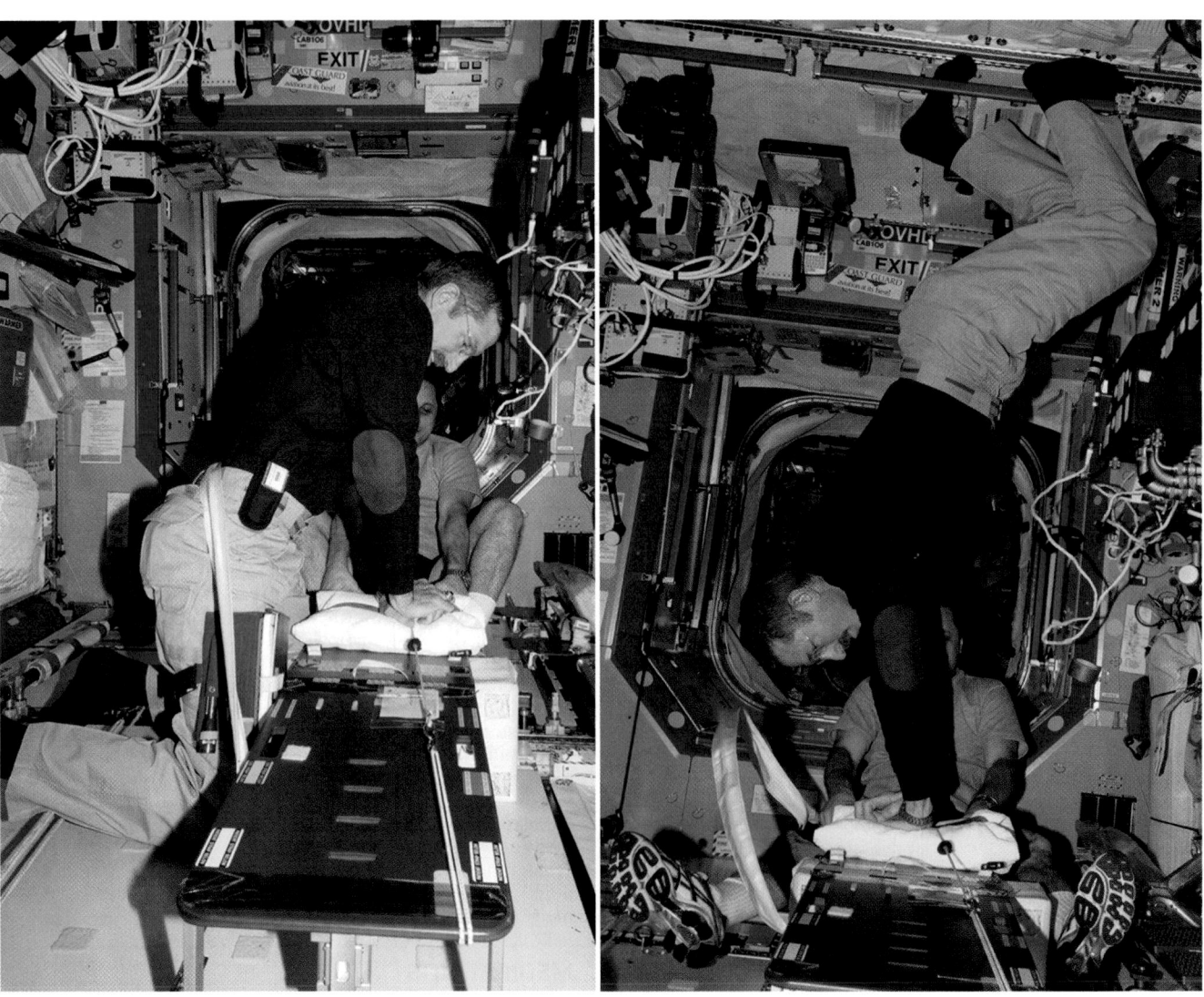

FIGURE 126-13 Astronaut Dan Burbank demonstrates two methods for performing chest compressions during refresher medical training aboard the ISS. The table shown provides patient restraint, a rigid platform for medical interventions as shown here, and electrical isolation from a patient requiring defibrillation.

abdominal, cardiac, thoracic, and transcranial Doppler imaging. High-frequency probes (linear and curvilinear) are available for imaging more superficial structures, such as blood vessels, muscles, and bones. The crew routinely uses ultrasound to perform occupational surveillance of ocular structures, usually guided in real time by imaging experts and ground investigators. Also, the ultrasound and remote guiders are available in the event of a medical contingency to assist with diagnosis and treatment.

Absence of gravity offers both challenges and advantages to ultrasound imaging (Video 126-6). The patient, operator, and hardware must be physically restrained in congruent positions during the exam, typically by using foot restraints. Imaging joints under stress (i.e., valgus/varus) can unintentionally reposition the entire patient rather than the joint alone; occasionally, additional operators, restraints, or ingenuity are needed to ensure patient stability.

Most astronauts undergo preflight photography training. Given the need for photographic documentation of so many aspects of a human spaceflight, high-quality camera equipment is easy to find aboard most spacecraft. Ground-based physicians use downlinked still and video imagery to evaluate skin and mucous membranes, urine reagent stick results, the tympanic membrane, and other visual targets in symptomatic astronauts. Tympanic membrane images obtained with a commercially available otoscope are an important part of the medical examination before and after a spacewalk. Corneal abrasions can also be photo-documented with a high-quality digital camera.

FUTURE CAPABILITIES

Enhanced diagnostic capability that can operate under the constraints of minimal size, weight, power requirements, and complexity will be desired for future generations of spaceflight medical kits. Near-infrared spectroscopy for noninvasive blood chemistry analysis[213] has been investigated for use in spaceflight. Enhancement of surgical care capabilities may entail the ultimate challenge in significantly expanding medical capabilities, because this involves balancing risk and capability against the specific aspects of a spaceflight scenario, such as remoteness, duration, and crew size. Clearly, the significant overhead associated with a terrestrial standard of surgical care, including extensive perioperative imaging, nursing care, delivery of anesthesia, sterility maintenance, and postoperative care,[11] makes application of a terrestrial surgical standard unobtainable in the spacecraft environment. Even so, ideas regarding future surgical capabilities currently drive an integrated assessment of spacecraft design, acceptable medical risk, and requirements for preflight preventive procedures. Evaluations of standard surgical preparation and technique in parabolic flight[23,25] have been performed, highlighting the challenges in maintaining hardware restraint and sterility in microgravity. Interventional radiologic techniques have likewise been considered as a means of further reducing the weight and complexity of hardware required to perform minimally invasive repair in space.[139] The need for a physician in long-duration deep-space missions seems likely, and this physician should have a skill set that includes percutaneous venous access for hydration and medication delivery, ultrasound for diagnosis and procedure guidance, proficiency in treating ophthalmologic and genitourinary problems, and sufficient surgical skills to treat dental problems and repair soft tissue trauma.

SUMMARY AND FUTURE CONSIDERATIONS

Much has been learned in the past 50 years to enable habitation of space, and humans have demonstrated a remarkable ability to adapt, both physiologically and behaviorally, to extended stays in low Earth orbit. Still, much work remains to be done to understand this new frontier, to reduce the risk that the inherent dangers of the spaceflight environment will affect human health, and to maximize human effectiveness. We are still only beginning to understand the space-normal human and time course of each body system as it adapts to microgravity, and how best to arrest

processes that trend toward a state that is injurious on return to normal gravity. Although current countermeasures seem to protect the musculoskeletal and cardiovascular systems from the hypokinesis associated with microgravity, we are still unclear on the mechanical integrity of trabecular bone formed in space, and whether a permanent state of increased fracture exists. The pathologic mechanisms and long-term outcomes of VIIP syndrome, the most recently recognized microgravity-induced syndrome, are largely unknown, and knowledge gaps remain regarding individual susceptibility and effective mitigation strategies. The International Space Station, operating in a high-ionizing-radiation environment, offers a platform to better understand effects of a unique radiation population on cells and human physiology. As more astronauts fly, we will better understand the permanency of microgravity- and radiation-induced effects, as well as gender differences in these physiologic changes.

Regarding medical care delivery, knowledge is lacking about the pharmacodynamics, pharmacokinetics, and bioavailability of drugs in the setting of microgravity, particularly given the confounders of body fluid shifts, radiation effects on wound healing, immunosuppression, and lack of sterile capabilities in orbit.[49,55] There is still much to understand about minimizing risk through diagnostic evaluation of individuals during astronaut selection and improved preflight health maintenance programs, as well as determining which medical conditions should truly be considered risky or disqualifying for spaceflight. Commercial access to space will broaden the flying population and include a wider distribution of age and underlying medical conditions. This will improve our understanding of human limits to the stressors of launch, landing, and exposure to microgravity, expanding our collective knowledge of the human body in space.[1,106,107]

The health and function of humans in space will always be intimately tied to the engineering systems that propel and sustain crews, so that the medical risk for missions outside low Earth orbit will largely depend on the capabilities of future spacecraft. While crews will remain dependent on adequacy of rocket and spacecraft integrity to deliver them safely to and from space, advances in propulsion could have the greatest overall effect on medical risk by reducing transit times and therefore minimizing human exposure to ionizing radiation and microgravity. Improved shielding of spacecraft may be necessary to protect crews from the continual background radiation and intermittent solar particle events. As popular media have identified, exposure to the microgravity environment could be further reduced with artificial gravity generation through radial acceleration of rotating vehicles, although this approach carries significant engineering challenges.

As distance from Earth increases, so does the ability to resupply dwindling medical and life support equipment, such that more robust environmental control systems, exercise hardware, better food storage, and improved onboard medical capability will be necessary. Crewmembers will be less able to interact effectively with Earth-based experts and their nuclear social groups. Destinations for longer missions are likely to include the moon, an asteroid, or Mars, where extravehicular activities (spacewalks) are likely to be conducted, and next-generation spacesuits should incorporate ergonomic improvements that cause less injury, particularly to the shoulders, and better accommodate both genders and a wider variety of body types. Neurovestibular compromise on arrival into a new fractional-gravity gradient is still a concern, and methods for adapting crewmembers to gravity gradients will need to be considered. Spacecraft intended for deep-space missions, for the foreseeable future, will be small in size, and onboard medical systems will need to be designed to fit within these limits. The medical system will compete with other components essential to human survival, such as adequate water supply, power to run environmental control systems, and sufficient fuel to reach the destination with a margin for safety. Minimizing the weight and volume of medical hardware, reducing the number of consumable components, or perhaps including components that can be easily manufactured onboard through three-dimensional printing, will be desirable. There will be significant pressure to simplify medical delivery in space.

Our continued experience with long-duration flights will likely uncover other unexpected long-term effects of adaptation to microgravity and contribute further to the basic knowledge of human physiology. Spaceflight programs will continue to be both the recipients of and the contributors to advances in disease detection and health maintenance and to a better understanding of human disease as a whole.

ACKNOWLEDGMENTS

The authors wish to express thanks to the following individuals who provided expert guidance in the writing of this chapter: Dr. Michael Barratt, Dr. Peter Norsk, Dr. Yael Barr, Dr. Jean Sibonga, Dr. Mary Van Baalen, Dr. Gary Beven, Dr. Al Holland, Dr. Richard Scheuring, Dr. John Clark, Robert Pietrzyk, Dr. Brian Crucian, Dr. Richard Jennings, Dr. Serena Aunon, Dr. Richard Danielson, Dr. Robert Gibson, Malinda Hailey, Dr. Ashot Sargsyan, Dr. Mary Wear, Sara Mason, and Jennifer McDonald, as well as the Longitudinal Study of Astronaut Health.

REFERENCES

Complete references used in this text are available online at expertconsult.inkling.com.

Drug Stability in the Wilderness

BEAU A. BRIESE AND MILLICENT M. BRIESE

ENVIRONMENTAL FACTORS INFLUENCING DRUG STABILITY

The main environmental factors affecting drug stability are temperature, light, and humidity. In addition, additives included with a medication can preserve or, under certain conditions, diminish a drug's efficacy during long-term storage.

Extreme temperatures and light can cause medications to spontaneously decompose, reassemble, or react with air, contaminants, or a drug's otherwise inactive ingredients. Exposure to high humidity can decrease a drug's rate of dissolution, the bottleneck step in bioavailability of drugs taken by mouth. Common additives, such as bicarbonate or D5W, and dilution can drastically reduce robustness and durability of some medications in extreme environments. Knowing a medication's anticipated rate of breakdown indicates how to titrate the dosage during extended periods in the field and how often to resupply. The most accurate understanding of the robustness of a medication's efficacy in the wilderness stems from evidence-based research.

Manufacturers generally recommend little variation in storage temperatures. Brief excursions into temperatures below the minimum or beyond the maximum recommended temperatures for a given drug are often acceptable, so long as two conditions are met: (1) the drug is not exposed to a maximum temperature constituting excessive heat for a period longer than 24 hours and (2) the mean kinetic temperature (MKT), or average temperature, for the drug remains at or below the maximum temperature of its ideal range.[25] These less commonly known rules for excursions ease medical fieldwork related to wilderness emergency situations of short duration by minimizing the amount of artificial cooling absolutely necessary in the field, depending on the drugs involved.

Being mindful of the season for which one estimates the MKT enables one to anticipate conditions that risk degrading drug potency and composition. Monthly MKTs were recorded for an emergency medical services (EMS) vehicle in South Africa that was not equipped with an electrical cooling system.[21] For the 12-month study period, the MKT was 24.7°C (76.5°F), just under the 25°C (77°F) limit for drugs needing controlled room temperature storage. However, the 6-month period between the Southern Hemisphere's warmer months of October through March had an excessive MKT of 27°C (80°F).

Helm and colleagues evaluated how season affected storage temperatures in unpowered containers in prehospital EMS vehicles that included a helicopter, ambulance, and physician car in southern Germany.[12] Despite the temperate climate, storage temperature exceeded 25°C (77°F) 33% to 45% of time in summer, and was less than 0°C (32°F) 19% of the time in winter.

In another study, epinephrine kept primarily at room temperature but exposed to extreme heat for 8 hours per day had impaired drug durability following dilution. Exposure to 5°C (41°F) did not cause epinephrine (1:1000 or 1:10,000 concentration) degradation at 4, 8, and 12 weeks. At 70°C (158°F), no 1:1000 epinephrine was lost, but only 36% of 1:10,000 epineph-

rine remained at 12 weeks.[11] Similarly, 7 days of constant exposure to 65°C (149°F) caused no depletion of 1:1000 epinephrine but complete destruction of 1:10,000 epinephrine.[5] Degraded 1:10,000 epinephrine is less effective in clinical use. Compared with controls stored at room temperature, at least 30% more (by volume) 1:10000 epinephrine exposed cyclically to 70°C for 8 or 12 weeks was required to achieve the same physiologic effect.[11]

The effect of dry desert heat on drug stability has also been studied. Valenzuela and associates studied degradation of 23 prehospital drugs stored in an unventilated drug box in a metal storage shed in arid Tucson, Arizona during the dry desert heat of summer.[26] The drugs included aminophylline, atropine, bretylium tosylate, calcium chloride, dexamethasone, dextrose, diazepam, diphenhydramine, dopamine hydrochloride, epinephrine, furosemide, isoetharine, isoproterenol, lidocaine, metoprolol tartrate, morphine sulfate, naloxone, nifedipine, nitroglycerin tablets, phenobarbital, sodium bicarbonate, thiamine, and verapamil. This 4-week study exposed the drugs to temperatures that ranged from 28° to 39°C (82° to 102°F). By the end of the study, only isoproterenol, epinephrine, and nifedipine exhibited noteworthy chemical changes. Isoproterenol was 11% less potent. Although the epinephrine itself remained unaffected, the pH of its storage solution degraded, creating a more acidic solution. As with epinephrine, nifedipine remained stable, but its delivery vehicle was compromised. The nifedipine capsules melted.

In the temperate climate of Los Angeles County in southern California, Gill and colleagues evaluated how exceeding the recommended MKT in advanced life support paramedic vehicles affected drug concentrations.[10] The 45-day study measured temperature and drug concentrations of atropine, epinephrine, and lidocaine in 15 different geographic locations, including one laboratory control, an inland airport, a harbor, six high desert neighborhoods, and six inland suburbs. The manufacturers of all three drugs recommended storage at 20° to 25°C (68° to 77°F), with temperatures not to exceed 40°C (104°F) for periods of more than 24 hours. The authors' findings indicate that atropine, epinephrine, and lidocaine can withstand an MKT of up to 29°C (84°F) for up to 45 days without degradation. The study also concluded that those drugs could tolerate spikes up to 52°C (125°F) for a cumulative time of up to 13 hours (795 minutes) without degradation.

Drugs can withstand only so much heat and cold before they begin to lose potency. Gammon and colleagues tested stability of 23 prehospital drugs thermally cycled between 12-hour periods at −6°C (21°F) and 54°C (129°F) for 1 month.[9] The drugs included adenosine, albuterol, amiodarone, atropine, diltiazem, dopamine, epinephrine, etomidate, haloperidol, heparin, hydralazine, ipratropium, labetalol, lidocaine, naloxone, nitroglycerin, ondansetron, oxytocin, procainamide, succinylcholine, terbutaline, thiamine, and vasopressin. Eight drugs degraded to less than 90% potency: diltiazem, dopamine, haloperidol, ipratropium, lidocaine, naloxone, nitroglycerin, and succinylcholine.

Mathijssen and associates examined antibiotics stored at constant temperatures ranging from −80°C to 37°C (−112° to 99°F) for up to 1 year.[16] Antibacterial activity of linezolid and clindamycin pills and solution was unchanged. However, efficacy of oxacillin and cefazolin diminished when stored at 37°C (99°F) for 1 month or at 20°C for 6 months. Activity of vancomycin became substandard when stored at 37°C (99°F) for 6 months.

EXPIRATION DATES AND SHELF LIFE

The United States Pharmacopeia (USP) requires manufacturers to list a drug's shelf life as the time during which a drug's potency (or concentration of active product) is guaranteed to be 90% to 110% of its listed potency (or concentration).[25] Expiration dates are based on the shelf life of a drug under ideal, manufacturer-suggested conditions of temperature, humidity, light exposure, and packaging integrity. When stored in environments that do not correlate with those listed by the manufacturer, the printed expiration date no longer indicates whether a drug is potent. For this reason, multiple studies have evaluated the rate and extent of degradation and loss of potency for numerous drugs under various circumstances.

Tropical climates pose difficulty for drugs susceptible to heat and humidity. One concern is that drugs from one climate may not be optimized for use in another environment. Risha and colleagues evaluated two primary markers of potency, namely drug content and bioavailability, for ciprofloxacin and diclofenac tablets in Tanzania by exposing the drugs to the following conditions: temperature of 40° ± 2°C (104° ± 4°F) and 75% ± 5% relative humidity.[20] Drug content and bioavailability were tested at the beginning of the study and again at 3 and 6 months for eight formulations of ciprofloxacin from Belgium and India, and for four formulations of diclofenac sodium from Belgium, India, Malaysia, and Cyprus. All formulations of both drugs complied with the USP required level of 90% to 110% of labeled drug content during the entire span of the study. Oral bioavailability remained within required levels for all formulations of ciprofloxacin, because all formulations complied with ciprofloxacin's dissolution regulations, dissolving 80% or more of the drug within 30 minutes. However, dissolution levels were substandard for two of the four diclofenac formulations. Those from Camden (Malaysia) and Remedica (Cyprus) failed to dissolve during the full course of the dissolution test. This indicates that although a drug may be active, stable, and of proper concentration, it still may be inaccessible after ingestion if, because of environmental exposures, it can no longer dissolve. Drug potency and dissolution should be tested regularly, because the robustness of a drug in more extreme environments may vary between manufacturers, formulations, and batches.

Maintaining drug integrity requires quality control in all steps of the process, from manufacturing through storage to delivery. In preparing for an expedition, be mindful that drugs purchased in certain locations may be less potent and durable than those purchased elsewhere. Twagirumukiza and associates studied 16 formulations of the medications atenolol, captopril, hydrochlorothiazide, methyldopa, and propranolol, 10 purchased from Rwandan pharmacies and 6 reference formulations purchased in Belgium or France.[24] All drug formulations were labeled with expiration dates indicating that at least 2 years of shelf life remained. Of the 10 formulations purchased in Rwanda, 2 exhibited substandard percentages of content on initial receipt. After 6 months, 7 of the 10 medications purchased in Rwanda had less than 90% of their original content, and 6 had impaired dissolution profiles. This indicated both reduced content and diminished bioavailability of the remaining medication.

PACKAGING

Where drugs are stored significantly influences their stability and safety. Packaging can shield drugs from environmental assaults, but only when conditions optimize the packaging's performance. For example, glass or plastic syringes containing medication, such as epinephrine, for immediate use may develop hairline cracks when frozen, leading to leakage and compromising stability and sterility of the remaining drug.

Independent of environmental conditions, packaging can negatively influence a drug's stability by leaching chemicals into drugs, absorbing drugs, and reacting with medications. These effects may reduce efficacy of stored medications and increase potential for their toxicity. Polyvinylchloride (PVC) is known to contain toxic compounds that may seep into drugs in trace amounts; the most infamous is the carcinogen diethylhexyl phthalate, which represents 30% to 80% of the weight of medical bags and intravenous (IV) tubing that contain PVC.[22] Medications can also be absorbed by the PVC itself. Alternative packaging materials, such as polypropylene and polyethylene, have demonstrated lower risk for absorption than does PVC for medications such as nitroglycerin and diazepam.[23] Over extended periods, glass containers can deposit reactive alkali decomposition materials into drugs. Leaching, absorption, and reactivity of packaging made of glass, PVC, polypropylene, and polyethylene have not been studied for most medications.

Although packaging may protect a drug from environmental extremes and degradation, packaging might degrade the drug, reducing its bioavailability. For example, blister packs of atenolol from Alpharma maintain bioavailability after 28 days at temperatures of 40°C (104°F) and humidity levels of 75%, but blister packs of atenolol from CP Pharmaceuticals do not, even though both versions of atenolol, when not stored in blister packs, are equally robust in some similar environmental conditions.[7]

Hoye and colleagues evaluated efficacy of hydrofluoroalkane (HFA) inhalation aerosols commonly used in albuterol metered-dose inhalers (MDIs) for proficiency in drug delivery at high temperatures.[13] The study included (1) a 185-day evaluation of albuterol (Proventil) HFA and albuterol (Ventolin) HFA MDIs stored in extreme temperatures but tested at room temperature and (2) evaluation of the performance of the MDIs when actuated at 4°, 22°, 47° and 60°C (39°, 72°, 117°, and 140°F). In the first portion of the study, inhaler frames warped and canisters had a minor increase in rates of propellant leakage, but showed integrity for the size of emitted particles and the dose per actuation. Proper drug delivery was unaffected by storage at temperatures ranging from −3° to 88°C (26° to 190°F). The second portion of the study concluded that the amount of drug successfully delivered decreased as the temperature at the time of delivery increased. The dose per actuation was more drastically reduced for the Proventil HFA MDI, for which 15% less albuterol was dispersed at 60°C (140°F) than at 4°C (39°F); the Ventolin HFA MDI exhibited only an 8% decrease. It is therefore recommended that propellant-based drug delivery systems be sprayed in conditions as close as possible to the manufacturer's storage parameters.

It is not always possible to keep drugs in the original packaging. Drugs stored outside of the manufacturer's container might exhibit significantly altered shelf lives. Rawas-Qalaji and associates evaluated the effects of the duration of humidity and sunlight on the stability of 0.3 mg of 1 mg/mL epinephrine transferred to unsealed syringes stored at high temperatures.[19] Their study examined four standardized storage environments at a constant 38°C (100.4°F): darkness with low (15%) humidity, darkness with high (95%) humidity, sunlight with low (15%) humidity, and sunlight with high (95%) humidity. Results suggest that presence or absence of sunlight did not affect injectable epinephrine. On the other hand, low humidity accelerated decomposition. Syringes placed into low humidity decreased to 90% potency by the end of the second month, and drastically dropped to 60%, 55%, and 39% potency at the end of months three, four, and five, respectively. Syringes placed into high humidity statistically fared better. Their epinephrine reduced to 90% potency by the end of the third month and dropped below regulation limits, falling to 83% and 82% in months four and five, respectively. Humidity is protective of repackaged epinephrine solution.

Repackaged lidocaine solution is stable over a moderate range of temperatures. In one study, lidocaine placed into 2-mL Tubex cartridges (20 mg/mL) and lidocaine diluted with 5% dextrose in plastic infusion bags (4 mg/mL) remained potent and stable for 3 months at room temperature; the latter also remained stable for 3 months under refrigeration at 4°C (39°F).[14]

Storage of drug mixtures can cause loss of potency and bioavailability that worsens with time. One percent lidocaine buffered with bicarbonate at a pH range of 7.38 to 7.41 remained effective for up to 1 week, decreasing in potency by approximately 10%, the lowest acceptable loss of potency, after 1 week of storage.[2] Avoid storing pills of different drugs in the same container, because interactions in storage can reduce dissolution rates, as occurs when atenolol is costored with some formulations of generic aspirin.[7]

Other forms of drug costorage are extremely stable. Implantable infusion systems are helping previously impaired individuals return to the outdoors. Mixtures of bupivacaine and clonidine with either morphine or hydromorphone have been shown to remain stable in implantable infusion systems at 37°C (99°F) for 90 days.[3]

For small pill storage, be aware that some pill containers appear to maintain pill integrity more than do others. One study demonstrated that Medidose pill packs maintained atenolol's bioavailability more effectively than did either blister packs or refillable pill containers at 25°C (77°F), but the converse was true at 40°C (104°F) and 75% humidity.[7] Place such pill packs in a water-sealed, light-tight container not containing PVC. Brands such as SealLine, Seattle Sports, Dry Pak, and Sea to Summit offer bags that meet these requirements.

STERILITY

Some drugs must be mixed with buffer or saline solutions prior to use. When preparing these solutions, caution should be taken to ensure sterile formulation. Brief exposures of less than 4 hours to air do not appear to compromise sterility. Carrasco and colleagues evaluated stability and sterility of saline infusion solutions.[18] Solutions of 0.9% saline in their original containers were transferred to polyethylene bottles or PVC bags, each equipped with a 1.5-μm bacterial filter, air intake, and nonextendable three-way valve with protected caps. These solutions were placed in various mobile intensive care units in urban portions of western Andalusia, and tested for sterility after 24, 48, and 72 hours. Bacterial colonization was found within 1.7% of the 8028 cultures tested from 672 solution units. Only two cultures contained clinically relevant concentrations greater than 5 colony-forming units per milliliter. No significant difference existed between sterility of saline infusion solutions used immediately and those repackaged up to 72 hours prior to use.

STORAGE

The site selected to store medications affects drugs' stability either by shielding drugs from extremes of environment or by increasing the chance that medications will be exposed to those extremes.

Air conditioning and refrigeration, humidifiers and desiccants, and light control can create a stable environment for medications. Short of an ongoing energy source to power climate-controlled storage, all storage systems eventually fail in one or more ways to protect medication from ambient environmental conditions. Furthermore, storage systems can actively damage drugs. For example, storage containers can prolong exposure to high temperatures if they are overinsulated in heated environments, or can create an environment that is too arid when air conditioning is used, destabilizing drugs such as some formulations of epinephrine.

Vehicular storage is convenient in many wilderness and tactical settings. It offers a mobile source of medications and potential power supply for artificial cooling.

McMullan and associates evaluated the potency of midazolam, diazepam, and lorazepam, stored in the air-conditioned cabs of four EMS vehicles in two EMS systems in the southwestern United States.[17] After 120 days of being exposed to an MKT of 32°C (90°F), only the minimal acceptable potency of 90% (95% confidence interval [CI]: 85% to 95%) of lorazepam remained at 90 days. At 120 days, the concentration was below the acceptable level of potency at 86% (95% CI: 81% to 92%).

Air ambulances expose the drugs they carry to extremes that are similar to those of ground ambulances. Madden and associ-

ates evaluated ambient and internal temperatures of nylon drug bags carried on EMS helicopters in Texas.[15] Temperatures within the nylon bags failed to comply with the USP recommendations for room temperature of 15° to 30°C (59° to 86°F) on 49% of winter days, 62% of winter nights, 56% of summer days, and 27% of summer nights.

Other cooling and heating methods include ice packs and chemical heat or cold packs. Given the density of water, ice packs are heavy; chemical packs are expensive, given the vast quantities needed in most circumstances.

Nonelectric "coolers" sometimes heat their contents and generally should not be relied on for drug storage. Vehicle windows and the sides of some coolers passively transform solar into thermal energy, acting as solar cookers. Although these storage units might be effective in resisting rising temperatures, when overheated they maintain high temperatures well after the heat of the day. Nonelectric "cooler" insulation neither cooks nor heats, but provides a temporary buffer to temperature change. It lacks capacity for maintaining any temperature for more than a period of minutes to hours; the duration is determined by the specific insulator. An exception to this is the Cambodian Cooler Box, a 24-L chamber of thin galvanized iron covered by cotton sack cloth connected to a top dish holding 9 L of water.[4] At an MKT of 27°C (81°F) in Cambodian drug storerooms, the cooler box reduced the percentage of hours at more than 30°C (86°F) from 4.5% outside the box to 0.1% in the box.

Electrical systems cool more consistently do than nonpowered systems. The Koolatron P9 Traveler III Cooler runs on 12-volt car adapters, weighs 3 kg (7 lb), stores 7 L, and cools to 11°C to 22°C (20°F to 40°F) below the ambient temperature. Its durability is inconsistent. Dison and M-Cool manufacture portable insulin cases that provide 0.1 to 0.2 L of storage, weigh 0.5 to 1.5 kg (1 to 3 lb), last 8 to 24 hours with batteries, and can take AV or AC power. Insulin cases with portable solar systems weighing less than (7 kg) (15 lb) are available from Goal Zero and Instapark.

DuBois studied the temperature of nonelectrically and electrically cooled drug storage boxes on ground EMS vehicles in the Sonoran Desert of California when outside temperatures were 29° to 38°C (84° to 100°F).[8] Temperatures in nonelectrically cooled compartments were often as hot, and occasionally up to 6°C (10°F) hotter than, was ambient air temperature. While the vehicles were immobile, the temperature in electrically cooled compartments remained at approximately 27°C (81°F) when set at 25°C (77°F) to 38°C (100°F). However, when the vehicles were mobile, the temperature in those same compartments occasionally increased to up to 41°C (106°F), exceeding the ambient temperature and manufacturer's maximum suggested storage temperature by 12°C (22°F) for 16 of 17 drugs stored in these EMS vehicles. This indicates the vulnerability to high temperatures of even electrically cooled mobile systems.

All modalities risk uneven temperatures for multiple drugs stored in the same compartment.

DRUGS FOR A BASIC FIELD KIT

A basic field medical kit includes the following types of medications:
Analgesic
Antianaphylactic and antiallergy
Antibiotic
Antiemetic
Antiepileptic
Antipyretic
Sterile fluid (for IV use)

HOW TO READ THE DRUG LIST

The following list summarizes stable conditions for drugs most likely to be included in field or tactical medical kits.[1,6] The list offers options for similar types of drugs, depending on the particular requirements of the users.

Certain terms are used for brevity's sake. *Room temperature* is defined as 15° to 30°C (59° to 86°F). *Controlled room temperature* is defined as 20° to 25°C (68° to 77°F). *Excessive heat* is defined as a temperature exceeding 40°C (104°F).

In the United States, availability of medications is subject to regulations of the Food and Drug Administration and Drug Enforcement Agency (DEA). The following labels note drug availability in the United States: OTC (over-the-counter), Rx (prescription required), DEA Schedule (S II, S III, or S IV indicating drugs with abuse potential, with S II having the greatest abuse potential and S IV the least), or NA (not available).

Packaging and inert compounds used with a medication may vary, especially for generic drugs. In all cases, information from the manufacturer should supplement the guide below.

Deviation from the manufacturer's recommendations is the decision of the treating medical professional and not recommended by the authors of this Appendix. Medications are generally listed by their generic names. Mention of trade names does not imply endorsement.

DRUG LIST

ACETAMINOPHEN CAPSULES, TABLETS, ORAL SOLUTION, AND SUPPOSITORIES (OTC)

Store capsules, tablets, and the oral solution at a controlled room temperature. Most are fairly stable in light, moisture, and heat, but high humidity should be avoided for gel-coated capsules. High humidity and light should be avoided for oral-dissolving and chewable tablets. Excessive heat (≥ 40°C [104°F]) should be avoided for extended-release tablets. Solid forms of acetaminophen remain stable for 3 years and liquid forms remain stable for 2 years from the date of manufacture. Store suppositories at 8° to 25°C (46° to 77°F).

ACETAMINOPHEN WITH CODEINE TABLETS AND ORAL SOLUTION (S III)

Store tablets and the solution in light-resistant containers at a controlled room temperature.

ACETAMINOPHEN WITH HYDROCODONE TABLETS AND ORAL SOLUTION (S II)

Store tablets and the solution in light-resistant containers at a controlled room temperature.

ACETAZOLAMIDE TABLETS, EXTENDED-RELEASE CAPSULES, ORAL SOLUTION, AND INJECTION (RX)

Store tablets and extended-release capsules at a controlled room temperature. Brief excursions to 15° to 30°C (59° to 86°F) are permitted for tablets. Dry powder for the injection solution should be stored in an unopened vial at a controlled room temperature. Powder reconstituted with 5 mL sterile water is stable for 12 hours at room temperature, and is stable for 3 days if refrigerated at 2° to 8°C (36° to 46°F).

An extemporaneous formulation can be prepared in three ways:

To prepare a solution of acetazolamide 50 mg/mL, crush 20 acetazolamide 250-mg tablets in 25 mL glycerin or distilled water. Add flavored syrup or 2:1 simple syrup or flavored syrup to bring the total volume to 100 mL. Shake well before use. This solution should be stored under refrigeration and is stable for 1 week.

To prepare a solution of acetazolamide 5 mg/mL, crush two acetazolamide 250-mg tablets in 7 mL polyethylene glycol 400, 53 mL propylene glycol, 15 mL 70% sorbitol solution, 15 mL 85% sucrose solution, 1 mL sweet syrup, 0.5 mL ethanol, and 8 mL of 0.1M citrate to achieve a total volume of 100 mL.

The solution can be prepared in a concentration of acetazolamide 25 mg/mL by crushing 10 acetazolamide 250-mg tablets in 50 mL Ora-Sweet and 50 mL Ora-Plus. Store the solution in an opaque container at room temperature. This solution remains stable for 60 days.

ACETIC ACID OTIC SOLUTION (OTC)

Store the solution in an airtight, light-resistant container at room temperature. Protect from heat.

ALBUTEROL TABLETS, SYRUP, AND INHALED FORMULATION (RX)

Store tablets at 2° to 25°C (36° to 77°F). Store extended-release tablets at 15° to 30°C (59° to 86°F). Store syrup at 2° to 30°C (36° to 86°F). Store capsules for inhalation at room temperature.

For the inhalation route, be certain that albuterol is at room temperature prior to use. For the nebulization route, store albuterol solution for inhalation 0.083% (Proventil), 0.5% (Ventolin), and 0.42% or 0.21% (Accuneb) at 2° to 25°C (36° to 77°F). Accuneb nebulized solution must be used within 1 week after removal from the foil pouch. In the pouch, Ventolin Nebules inhalation solution can be stored at 2° to 8°C (36° to 46°F) for up to 6 months and remains stable at room temperature for 14 days.

Store albuterol aerosol inhalers containing chlorofluorocarbon propellants at room temperature. Store albuterol sulfate aerosol inhalers containing hydrofluoroalkane (HFA) propellants out of direct sunlight at 15° to 25°C (59° to 77°F). To avoid bursting, do not exceed 49°C (120°F). Do not puncture or incinerate. If infrequently used, Ventolin HFA is stable for 6 months from removal from the pouch. Store Ventolin HFA canisters with the mouthpiece down. If frequent nebulization is required, 200 mcg/mL of albuterol sulfate inhalation solution in normal saline remains stable for 7 days at room temperature or under refrigeration when placed in polyvinyl chloride or polyolefin bags, polypropylene syringes and tubes, or borosilicate glass tubes.

ALOE VERA GEL, OINTMENT, AND LAXATIVES (OTC)

Store gel, ointment, and laxatives away from excessive heat and prolonged strong direct light.

AMIODARONE TABLETS, ORAL SOLUTION, INHALANTS, AND INJECTIONS (RX)

Store tablets in a light-resistant container at a controlled room temperature. An extemporaneous 5 mcg/mL formulation can be created by crushing five amiodarone 200-mg tablets into a 200-mL solution of 1:1 of Ora-Plus to Ora-Sweet or Ora-Sweet SF. Solution stored in a glass or plastic bottle under refrigeration remains stable for 91 days. The solution remains stable at room temperature for 6 weeks. Shake before use. Store conventional amiodarone ampules at a controlled room temperature. Ampules may be briefly removed for use at temperatures of 15° to 30°C (59° to 86°F). Protect all injection solutions from light and excessive heat. Do not freeze.

ANTACIDS (OTC)

Store aluminum hydroxide and magnesium hydroxide (often called milk of magnesia) products in tightly sealed containers at a controlled room temperature. Store calcium carbonate conventional tablets at 15° to 30°C (59° to 86°F). Store calcium carbonate chewable tablets below 25°C (77°F). Protect all products from light, moisture, and excessive heat. Do not freeze.

ASPIRIN TABLETS, ORAL SOLUTION, AND SUPPOSITORIES (OTC)

Store tablets and solution in tightly sealed, light-resistant containers at room temperature. Protect from moisture. Store suppositories in the original sealed wrapper at 2° to 15°C (35° to 59°F). Do not freeze. Protect from light, moisture, and excessive heat. Discard aspirin if a strong vinegar odor is present, because potency may be significantly decreased.

ATENOLOL TABLETS (RX)

Store tablets in light-resistant containers at a controlled room temperature.

ATROPINE INJECTION AND OPHTHALMIC SOLUTION (RX)

Store ophthalmic and injection solutions in light-resistant containers at room temperature. In order to prevent contamination, do not touch the applicator tip directly to the eyes or skin. Atropine sulfate 1 mg/mL injection solutions in Tubex (0.5-mL and 1-mL) packaging have been shown to remain stable for 3 months. Atropine methyl nitrate 10 mg/mL solutions have been shown to remain stable for 6 months. Inspect the solution prior to administration for the presence of particulate matter, cloudiness, or discoloration, and discard if present. Do not freeze.

AZITHROMYCIN TABLETS, ORAL SOLUTION, INJECTION, AND OPHTHALMIC SOLUTIONS (RX)

Store tablets at room temperature. Store dry powder for reconstitution below 30°C (86°C). After reconstitution, store suspension at 5° to 30°C (41° to 86°F) and discard after use. After reconstitution, store extended-release solution at a controlled room temperature and use at room temperature. Do not refrigerate or freeze. The solution remains stable for 12 hours. Shake oral azithromycin suspension before use and do not take simultaneously with antacids containing aluminum or magnesium. The injection solution remains stable for 24 hours if stored at 30°C (86°F), or for 7 days if stored under refrigeration below 5°C (41' F). Store ophthalmic solution in an unopened bottle under refrigeration at 2° to 8°C (36° to 46°F), and at 2° to 25°C (36° to 77°F) once opened. The solution remains stable for 14 days.

BACITRACIN TOPICAL FORMULATION (OTC)

Store the aqueous topical formulation at 2° to 8°C (36° to 46°F) for up to 1 week. Store the nonaqueous topical formulation at room temperature for 3 days, and for longer periods if stored in an anhydrous base, such as lanolin and paraffin.

BISMUTH SUBSALICYLATE TABLETS AND ORAL SOLUTION (OTC)

Store tablets and suspension in tightly sealed containers at room temperature. Protect from direct light and excessive heat. Do not freeze the suspension.

BRETYLIUM TOSYLATE (RX)

Store at a controlled room temperature.

BUPIVACAINE INJECTION (RX)

Store the injection solution at a controlled room temperature. Protect solutions containing epinephrine from light. Bupivacaine hydrochloride 1.25 mg/mL in 0.9% sodium chloride injection solution in disposable polypropylene syringes is stable for 32 days at 3° to 23°C (37° to 73°F).

BUTORPHANOL TARTRATE NASAL SPRAY AND IM AND IV INJECTIONS (S IV)

Store nasal spray at room temperature. Store the injection solution in the original container at 20° to 25°C (68° to 77°F). Protect from light. Discard if discoloration occurs or particulate matter forms in injection solution.

CALCIUM CHLORIDE, CALCIUM GLUCEPTATE, AND CALCIUM GLUCONATE INJECTION (RX)

Store injection solutions of calcium chloride, calcium gluceptate, and calcium gluconate at room temperature. Sterile solutions of calcium in water are indefinitely stable.

CALENDULA TOPICAL FORMULATION (OTC)

Protect from heat, moisture, and direct light.

CEFTRIAXONE INJECTION (RX)

Store dry powder for solution preparation in a light-resistant container at or below 25°C (77°F). Dry powder for injection solutions should not be combined with diluents containing calcium, such as Ringer's or Hartmann's solution, because there will be particulate formulation. After constitution, intramuscular (IM) solutions in water or normal saline remain stable for 2 days at 25°C (77°F) and for 10 days refrigerated at 4°C (39°F) in a concentration of 100 mg/mL; however, at a concentration of 250 mg/mL, such solutions remain stable for only 24 hours at 25°C (77°F) and 3 days refrigerated at 4°C (39°F). IV solutions at concentrations of 10, 20, and 40 mg/mL remain stable for 2 days at 25°C (77°F) and for 10 days refrigerated at 4°C (39°F). Do not refrigerate injection solutions that contain 5% dextrose and 0.9% or 0.45% sodium chloride diluent solutions. IV solutions of ceftriaxone that contain 5% dextrose and 0.9% sodium chloride solution can be frozen at −20°C (−4°F) in PVC or polyolefin containers and remain stable for 26 weeks. Thaw at room temperature before use, and discard any unused, thawed solution.

CEPHALEXIN CAPSULES, TABLETS, AND ORAL SOLUTION (RX)

Store capsules at room temperature. The suspension is stable for 14 days under refrigeration.

CHARCOAL, ACTIVATED (OTC)

Store activated charcoal in an airtight container. Sealed aqueous suspensions are stable for 1 year.

CIPROFLOXACIN TABLETS, CAPSULES, ORAL SOLUTION, INJECTION, OPHTHALMIC SOLUTION, AND OTIC SOLUTIONS (RX)

Store tablets below 30°C (86°F). Store extended-release tablets at 25°C (77°F). Brief excursions are permitted at room temperature. Store microcapsules and diluent for oral suspensions below 25°C (77°F). Do not freeze. After reconstitution, the solution should be stored below 30°C (86°F); it remains stable for 14 days. Store the ophthalmic solution in original vials at 2° to 25°C (36° to 77°F). Protect from light and excessive heat. Do not freeze tablets or oral and ophthalmic solutions. Store the otic solution in a light-resistant container at room temperature of 15° to 25°C (59° to 77°F).

CROTALIDAE ANTIVENOM (RX)

Store vials at 2° to 8°C (36° to 46°F). Do not freeze. Use within 4 hours of reconstitution.

CYCLOPENTOLATE HYDROCHLORIDE OPHTHALMIC SOLUTION (RX)

Store ophthalmic solution in the original container at room temperature. Use only if the sealing neckband on the container is intact.

DABIGATRAN TABLETS (RX)

Store in a tightly sealed container at 25°C (77°F). Brief excursions are permitted at room temperature. Protect from moisture. Once the container has been opened, use within 4 months.

DEET (N,N-DIETHYL-META-TOLUAMIDE, DIETHYLTOLUAMIDE)–CONTAINING INSECT REPELLENT (OTC)

Store the repellent below 49°C (120°F). Store away from heat and flame.

DERMABOND (2-OCTYL CYANOACRYLATE) TOPICAL SKIN ADHESIVE (RX)

Store the adhesive below 30°C (86°F). Discard if the package is open or has been tampered with. Discard the excess after use because the adhesive hardens on exposure to air. Protect from moisture and direct heat.

DEXAMETHASONE TABLETS AND ORAL, INJECTION, IMPLANTATION, INTRAVITREAL, AND OPHTHALMIC SOLUTIONS (RX)

Store tablets in a light-resistant container at a controlled room temperature. Protect from moisture. Store the oral solution in the original bottle and only dispense with the supplied calibrated dropper at a controlled room temperature. Once opened, the oral solution remains stable for 90 days. Discard if precipitation forms. Store the implantation, intravitreal, and ophthalmic solutions at room temperature. Extemporaneous formulations remain stable for 91 days.

DEXTROAMPHETAMINE TABLETS, CAPSULES, AND ORAL SOLUTION (S II)

Store non–extended-release capsules and tablets at room temperature. Store extended-release capsules and tablets at a controlled room temperature. Store the elixir in an airtight, light-resistant container at room temperature.

DEXTROSE ORAL SOLUTION (OTC) AND INJECTION (RX)

Store oral solution in a well-filled, airtight container. For injection, do not exceed 25°C (77°F). Do not freeze or expose to extreme heat. Discard if cloudy prior to use and discard any unused portions once open.

DIAZEPAM TABLETS, ORAL SOLUTION, SUPPOSITORIES, AND INJECTION (S IV)

Store tablets, oral solution, and suppositories at room temperature. Protect from light, heat, and moisture. Do not freeze the oral solution. Suppositories are stable for 8 months at 40°C (104°F) and can withstand at least three freeze-thaw cycles. Brief excursions are permitted to room temperature. Store the injection solution at a controlled room temperature. Do not refrigerate.

DIGOXIN TABLETS AND INJECTION (RX)

Store at a controlled room temperature. Brief excursions are permitted to room temperature. Protect from light. Protect tablets from moisture.

DILTIAZEM TABLETS, ORAL SOLUTION, AND INJECTION (RX)

Store tablets at 25°C (77°F). Brief excursions are permitted to 15° to 30°C (59° to 86°F). Avoid excess humidity. An extemporaneous formulation of a 1-mg/mL solution can be prepared using 250 mg diltiazem (2.5 mL of diltiazem hydrochloride stock solution) combined with dextrose, fructose, mannitol, sorbitol, or sucrose to a volume of 250 mL. A solution of 12-mg/mL diltiazem can be prepared by crushing 16 tablets of 90-mg diltiazem in 10 mL of 1:1 mixtures of Ora-Plus with either Ora-Sweet or Ora-Sweet SF or in 1:4 mixtures of flavored syrup with simple syrup and then bringing the solution to a total volume of 120 mL. Protect from light.

DIPHENHYDRAMINE TABLETS, ORAL SOLUTION (OTC), AND INJECTION (RX)

Store at a controlled room temperature in a light-resistant container. Do not freeze oral and injection solutions.

DOMEBORO (ACETIC ACID AND ALUMINUM ACETATE) OTIC SOLUTIONS (OTC)

Store otic solutions in a tightly sealed container at either room temperature or under refrigeration. Protect from direct light, heat, and moisture. Do not freeze.

DOPAMINE HYDROCHLORIDE INJECTION (RX)

Store the injection in a light-resistant container. Discard if the injection has yellow-brown discoloration or if pH outside of the 4.0 to 6.4 range is detected, because these are indications of decomposition. Dopamine 6.4 mg/mL in 5% dextrose injection is stable at a controlled room temperature for up to 24 hours in ambient humidity and in the presence of light.

DOXYCYCLINE CAPSULES, TABLETS, ORAL SOLUTION, AND INJECTION (RX)

Store capsules and tablets in light-resistant containers at room temperature. Store doxycycline hyclate delayed-release tablets in light-resistant containers at a controlled room temperature. Brief excursions are permitted at room temperature. Store lyophilized powder in a light-resistant container at a controlled room temperature. Refrigerate in a light-resistant container immediately after reconstitution, or dilute the injection solution to 0.1 to 1 mg/mL within 12 hours after reconstitution, where it will remain stable for up to 48 hours at 25°C (77°F) and 72 hours at 4°C (39°F). Avoid direct sunlight during storage and infusion. Infusions of doxycycline made with lactated Ringer's or 5% dextrose in lactated Ringer's diluents must be used within 6 hours of reconstitution to ensure stability. Solutions of 10 mg/mL doxycycline in sterile water can be frozen and stored at −20°C (−4°F) and remain stable for up to 8 weeks. Avoid excess heat after thawing and discard any unused thawed solution.

EDOXABAN TABLETS (RX)

Store at a controlled room temperature. Brief excursions are permitted at room temperature.

EMLA (LIDOCAINE/PRILOCAINE) TOPICAL FORMULATION (RX)

Store EMLA at room temperature. Do not freeze. Discoloration does not necessarily indicate lack of stability. Precipitate indicates that the solution is not stable.

EPINEPHRINE INJECTION AND TOPICAL, INHALED, AND INTRANASAL FORMULATIONS (RX)

Store injection ampules at 5° to 25°C (41° to 77°F). Do not freeze. Injection ampules stored at 38°C (100°F) will last less than 3 months at low humidity (15%) and less than 4 months at high humidity (85%). An extemporaneous formulation of a topical anesthetic solution can be prepared with 2.25 mg/mL of racemic epinephrine hydrochloride, 40 mg/mL of lidocaine hydrochloride, 5 mg/mL of tetracaine hydrochloride, and 0.63 mg/mL of sodium metabisulfite. Store this topical solution in a light-resistant container at 18°C (64°F) for no more than 4 weeks, and at 4°C (39.2°F) for up to 26 weeks. Store the epinephrine inhaler at a controlled room temperature. Do not exceed 49°C (120°F). Do not puncture or incinerate the inhaler. Store the intranasal solution in a light-resistant container at 15° to 25°C (59° to 77°F). Do not freeze.

ERYTHROMYCIN TABLETS, ORAL SOLUTION, AND TOPICAL OINTMENT (RX)

Store tablets and oral solution at less than 30°C (86°F). Reconstituted granules must be used within 10 days. Reconstituted erythromycin ethyl succinate solution must be used within 14 days if kept at room temperature. Reconstituted EryPed solution should be stored at less than 25°C (77°F) and used within 35 days. Refrigeration of the suspension is encouraged for the best taste. Optimal stability is maintained at pH above 6.0, with significant decomposition at or below pH of 4.0. Store the topical ointment at less than 27°C (81°F).

FAMOTIDINE TABLETS (OTC) AND INJECTION (RX)

Store regular and chewable tablets at a controlled room temperature. Brief excursions for chewable tablets to room temperature are permitted. Protect from moisture. Store injection vials in a light-resistant container at 2° to 8°C (36° to 46°F).

FENTANYL ORAL LOZENGES, SUBLINGUAL TABLETS, SUBLINGUAL SPRAY, BUCCAL FILM, INJECTION, AND INTRANASAL FORMULATION (RX)

Store oral lozenges, sublingual tablets, sublingual spray, and buccal film at a controlled room temperature. Brief excursions to room temperature are permitted. Protect from moisture. Do not freeze. Store the injection solution in a light-resistant container at a controlled room temperature. Store the intranasal canister in a light-resistant container at 2°C to 25°C (36°F to 77°F).

FLUOCINOLONE ACETONIDE TOPICAL OINTMENT, OTIC SOLUTION, AND SHAMPOO (RX)

Store topical cream, ointment, and shampoo at room temperature. Do not freeze. Store the otic solution at a controlled room temperature.

FURAZOLIDONE TABLETS AND SOLUTION (NA)

Store tablets and liquid in light-resistant containers. Tablets can be crushed and administered with a spoonful of corn syrup. Exposure to strong light may cause darkening.

FUROSEMIDE TABLETS, SOLUTION, AND INJECTION (RX)

Store tablets and solution in light-resistant containers at 25°C (77°F). Brief excursions are permitted to 15° to 30°C (59° to 86°F). Protect from moisture. Store the injection solution in a light-resistant container at room temperature. Discard all types of furosemide if discoloration occurs.

GLUCAGON INJECTION (RX)

Store dry powder in a light-resistant container at a controlled room temperature. Do not freeze. Powder remains stable for 24 months. Use the injection solution immediately after reconstitution and discard unused portions.

HALOPERIDOL TABLETS AND INJECTION (RX)

Store tablets in a tightly closed, light-resistant container at a controlled room temperature. Store the injection solution in a light-resistant container at room temperature. Do not freeze.

HYDROCORTISONE TABLETS, SOLUTION, INJECTION, AND TOPICAL CREAM (RX)

Store tablets, oral solution, injection, and topical cream at room temperature in the original container. Protect from light, moisture, and heat. Do not freeze the oral solution or injections.

HYDROMORPHONE TABLETS, SOLUTION, SUPPOSITORIES, AND INJECTION (S II)

Store tablets, solution, suppositories, and injectables in light-resistant containers at a controlled room temperature. Excursions are permitted to 15° to 30°C (59° to 86°F). Slight yellow discoloration of the injection liquid does not affect potency.

IBUPROFEN TABLETS AND SOLUTION (OTC)

Store the tablets at a controlled room temperature and the solution at room temperature.

INSULIN (REGULAR) INJECTION AND INHALED FORMULATION (RX)

Store the subcutaneous and IV injections in a light-resistant container refrigerated at 2° to 8°C (36° to 46°F). Do not freeze. Store the open vials at room temperature for up to 31 days. Store inhalers refrigerated at 2° to 8°C (36° to 46°F). Store at room temperature for up to 10 days. Discard unused cartridges from an open blister pack strip after 3 days.

INTRAVENOUS SOLUTIONS (D$_5$W, NS, LR, D$_5$NS, AND OTHER ADMIXTURES)

Store solutions below 90°C (194°F) and preferably at room temperature for ease of use. Pure sodium chloride and lactated Ringer's solutions at concentrations used in medicine are unlikely to show precipitation at 0°C (32°F), or if frozen for 3 months.

ISOPROTERENOL HYDROCHLORIDE INHALANT AND INJECTION (RX)

Store the inhalation solution and injection in light-resistant containers at room temperature. The injection is stable indefinitely in normal saline. Avoid excessive heat. Discard inhalation or injection solution if pink or brown discoloration or precipitation occurs. Store isoproterenol (5 mg/L) in 5% dextrose in water at room temperature. This solution remains stable for 24 hours.

IVERMECTIN TABLETS (RX)

Store below 30°C (86°F).

KALETRA (LOPINAVIR/RITONAVIR) TABLETS (RX)

Store tablets at a controlled room temperature. Brief excursions are permitted at room temperature. Once the tablet container is opened or tablets are exposed to high humidity, tablets remain stable for up to 2 weeks.

KETOCONAZOLE TABLETS, SHAMPOO, FOAM, AND GEL (RX)

Store tablets in light-resistant containers at a controlled room temperature. Protect from heat and moisture. Store the shampoo in a light-resistant container below 25°C (77°F). Store the foam in a light-resistant container at a controlled room temperature. Do not refrigerate. Avoid direct light. Store the foam at a controlled room temperature with excursions permitted to room temperature.

Store drops in a tightly sealed container below 30°C (86°F).

LACOSAMIDE TABLETS, ORAL SOLUTION, AND INJECTION (RX)

Store at a controlled room temperature. Brief excursions are permitted at room temperature. The oral solution remains stable for up to 7 weeks after the bottle has been opened. Do not freeze. Once the injection is diluted, store at room temperature for up to 4 hours.

LACRISERT (HYDROXYPROPYL METHYLCELLULOSE) OPHTHALMIC SOLUTION (RX)

Store drops in a tightly sealed container below 30°C (86°F).

LEMON GRASS (CYMBOGOGON) CITRONELLA OIL TOPICAL FORMULATION (OTC)

Store at room temperature. Protect from heat, moisture, and direct light.

LEVETIRACETAM TABLETS, ORAL SOLUTION, AND INJECTION (RX)

Store immediate-release tablets, extended-release tablets, and oral solution at 25°C (77°F). Brief excursions are permitted at room temperature. The injection diluted in solution in a polyvinyl chloride bag is stable for at least 24 hours. Discard the unused portion of the vial after opening.

LEVOFLOXACIN TABLETS, SOLUTION, INJECTION, AND OPHTHALMIC FORMULATION (RX)

Store tablets at 15° to 30°C (59° to 86°F). Store the oral solution at 25°C (77°F). Brief excursions are permitted at 15° to 30°C (59° to 86°F). The injection solution remains stable for 72 hours if stored at or below 25°C (77°F). Injection solution can be diluted in plastic or glass containers, and then frozen at −20°C (−4°F), where it remains stable for up to 6 months. Thaw slowly (no hot water baths or microwaves) at 25°C (77°F) or under refrigeration at 8°C (46°F). Use immediately after thawing. Do not refreeze. Store flexible containers of premixed solutions in a light-resistant container at or below 25°C (77°F). Avoid excessive heat and do not freeze. Store levofloxacin 0.5% and 1.5% ophthalmic solutions at 15° to 25°C (59° to 77°F).

LIDOCAINE INJECTION AND TOPICAL, INTRADERMAL, AND OPHTHALMIC SOLUTIONS (RX)

Store injection solution in a light-resistant container at room temperature. Do not freeze. Do not reuse "one-time-use" injection bottles, because they lack methylparaben preservative. Store the topical gel and jelly at a controlled room temperature. Store the viscous topical preparation, topical patches, and intradermal powder in sealed original packaging at room temperature at 15° to 30°C (59° to 86°F).

LIDOCAINE/EPINEPHRINE/TETRACAINE (LET) TOPICAL SOLUTION (RX)

Store solution in a light-resistant container. The solution remains stable at 18°C (64°F) for 4 weeks, and at 4°C (39°F) for 26 weeks.

LINDANE (GAMMA-HEXACHLOROCYCLOHEXANE) LOTION AND SHAMPOO (RX)

Store lotion and shampoo at a controlled room temperature.

LOPERAMIDE HYDROCHLORIDE CAPSULES (OTC)

Store capsules at 15° to 25°C (59° to 77°F). Placing the contents of 10 of the 2-mg capsules in hard fat, such as suet, leaf lard, or fatback lard, and rolling into shape can also create rectal suppositories of 20 mg loperamide.

LORAZEPAM TABLETS, ORAL SOLUTION, AND INJECTION (S IV)

Store tablets in a tightly sealed container at a controlled room temperature. Store oral solution at 2° to 8°C (36° to 46°F). Discard an opened bottle after 90 days. Store IM and IV solutions in light-resistant containers at 2° to 8°C (36° to 46°F).

MALARONE (ATOVAQUONE/PROGUANIL) TABLETS (RX)

Store in a light-resistant container at a controlled room temperature. Brief excursions to room temperature are permitted.

MANNITOL INJECTION (RX)

Store vials of mannitol solution and powder for reconstitution at a controlled room temperature. Discard the unused portion of the solution. Concentrations of 15% or more may crystallize when exposed to lower temperatures. To resolubilize crystals, place the vial in a heated water bath at 60° to 80°C (140° to 176°F) and shake occasionally. Using a microwave is not recommended, because the vial is likely to explode. Cool to room temperature before use. Do not heat the solution if a white flocculent precipitate forms after contact with PVC, because crystals will re-form rapidly.

MEBENDAZOLE TABLETS (RX)

Store at 15° to 25°C (59° to 77°F).

MEPERIDINE HYDROCHLORIDE TABLETS, ORAL SOLUTION, AND INJECTION (S II)

Store tablets and the oral solution at a controlled room temperature. Brief excursions are permitted to 15° to 30°C (59° to 86°F). Store the injection solution in a light-resistant container at a controlled room temperature.

METOPROLOL TABLETS, ORAL SOLUTION, AND INJECTION (RX)

Store tablets at a controlled room temperature. Brief excursions are permitted to room temperature. An extemporaneous oral suspension solution can be created by combining 12 crushed 100-mg metoprolol tablets with a small amount of Ora-Sweet, Ora-Sweet SF, or Ora-Plus and bringing the volume to 120 mL with water. The suspension remains stable for 60 days under refrigeration. Shake well before use. Store the injection ampules in tight, light-resistant, moisture-free containers at a controlled room temperature.

METRONIDAZOLE CAPSULES, TABLETS, AND INJECTION (RX)

Store capsules at 15° to 25°C (59° to 77°F). Store extended-release tablets at a controlled room temperature. Brief excursions are permitted to room temperature. Store the injection solution in a light-resistant container at room temperature.

MIDAZOLAM ORAL SOLUTION AND INJECTION (S IV)

Store oral solution at a controlled room temperature. Brief excursions are permitted to 15° to 30°C (59° to 86°F). Store injection solution at a controlled room temperature. The injection solution may be stored for at least 28 days at 3° to 25°C (37° to 77°F).

MODAFINIL TABLETS (S IV)

Store tablets at a controlled room temperature.

MORPHINE SULFATE TABLETS, EPIDURAL SUSPENSION, AND INJECTION (S II)

Store tablets in light-resistant containers at a controlled room temperature. Excursions are permitted to room temperature.

Store the epidural extended-release suspension under refrigeration at 2° to 8°C (36° to 46°F). Do not freeze. Unopened vials remain stable for 30 days at a controlled room temperature. Do not return vials to the refrigerator once they have been stored at room temperature. Solution withdrawn from the vial can be stored at room temperature for up to 4 hours prior to administration. After that, all withdrawn solution should be discarded.

Store injection solution in the original carton at a controlled room temperature. Brief excursions are permitted to 15° to 30°C (59° to 86°F). Do not freeze. Discard any unused solution.

Pain cocktails containing preservatives without alcohol or chloroform water will remain stable for 3 weeks after compounding.

MOXIFLOXACIN TABLETS, ORAL SOLUTION, INJECTION, AND OPHTHALMIC ROUTE (RX)

Store tablets and injection solution at a controlled room temperature. Brief excursions are permitted to 15° to 30°C (59° to 86°F). Do not refrigerate injection solution because precipitate forms. Extemporaneous oral suspension can be formed to create 60 mL of 20 mg/mL moxifloxacin hydrochloride by combining three crushed 400-mg tablets with 30 mL of Ora-Plus, Ora-Sweet, or Ora-Sweet SF. When stored in a light-resistant amber plastic bottle, oral suspension remains stable for 90 days if stored at 23° to 25°C (73° to 77°F). Store 0.5% moxifloxacin ophthalmic solution at 2° to 25°C (36° to 77' F).

MUPIROCIN TOPICAL FORMULATION (RX)

Store cream and ointment at a controlled room temperature. Do not freeze cream.

NALBUPHINE HYDROCHLORIDE INJECTION (RX)

Store injection solution in a light-resistant container at a controlled room temperature.

NALOXONE HYDROCHLORIDE INJECTION (RX)

Store injection solution ampules and vials in original containers at a controlled room temperature. Use infusion solutions within 24 hours of opening. For Evzio, store between 15° and 25°C (59° and 77°F). Brief excursions are permitted to 4° to 40°C (39° to 104°F).

NEOSPORIN OINTMENT (OTC)

Store ointment in the original container with the cap tightly sealed at room temperature. Protect from light, moisture, and heat.

NIFEDIPINE CAPSULES, TABLETS, ORAL SOLUTION, AND INJECTION (RX)

Store capsules in a light-resistant container at 15° to 22° (59° to 77°F). Store tablets in a light-resistant container below 30°C (86°F). An extemporaneous formulation of an oral solution can be made by combining five nifedipine 10-mg tablets and soaking them in a small amount of 1% hypromellose for 5 minutes and then bringing the total volume to 50 mL with 1% hypromellose. Package the 1-mg/mL extemporaneous suspension in single-dose syringes stored in opaque black plastic bags. Solution remains stable for 28 days at 6° or 22°C (43° or 72°F).

Store injection solution in a light-resistant container below 25°C (77°F). Because the infusion is extremely light sensitive, the solution retains its potency for 1 hour in daylight and 6 hours in artificial light. Do not remove the vial from the container until immediately before use.

NITROGLYCERIN CAPSULES, SUBLINGUAL TABLETS AND SPRAYS, INJECTION, PATCHES, AND TOPICAL FORMULATION (RX)

Store capsules at room temperature. Store sublingual tablets and sprays at a controlled room temperature. Protect tablets from moisture. Sprays may have brief excursions to room temperature. Store concentrated nitroglycerin for injection solution in a light-resistant container at room temperature. Injection solutions in polyolefin containers can be stored at room temperature for at least 24 hours. Premixed nitroglycerin in either normal saline or 5% dextrose can be stored for 48 hours at room temperature and 7 days under refrigeration. The extemporaneous formulation of solutions with a concentration of 0.035 to 1 mg/mL in glass containers remains stable for 70 days at room temperature and 6 months under refrigeration. Store transdermal patches at room temperature. Store topical ointment at a controlled room temperature.

NORFLOXACIN TABLETS, ORAL SOLUTION, AND OPHTHALMIC SOLUTION (RX)

Store tablets at a controlled room temperature in tightly sealed containers. Brief excursions to room temperature are permitted. Extemporaneous oral solution can be created by crushing three 400-mg tablets into a small amount of Ora-Plus and flavored syrup to taste and bringing the total volume to 60 mL to create a 20-mg/mL solution. Under experimental conditions, the suspension remains stable (containing ≥ 93% norfloxacin) for at least 56 days at a temperature of 23° to 25°C (73.4° to 77°F) or under refrigeration at 3° to 5°C (37.4° to 41°F). Store the ophthalmic solution at room temperature.

OFLOXACIN TABLETS, INJECTION, OPHTHALMIC SOLUTION, AND OTIC SOLUTION (RX)

Store tablets in a tightly sealed container below 30°C (86°F). Store single-use vials and premixed bottles of injection solution in light-resistant containers at room temperature. Brief exposure to temperatures up to 40°C (104°F) are permitted. Do not freeze. In diluted concentrations between 0.4 and 4 mg/mL and stored in a glass or plastic container, solution remains stable for 14 days under refrigeration at 5°C (41°F), or for 6 months frozen at −20°C (−4°F). Solution will remain stable for up to 14 days under refrigeration at 2° to 8°C (36° to 46°F) after thawing. Do not use hot water or a microwave oven for rapid thawing. Store ophthalmic and otic solutions at 15° to 25°C (59° to 77°F).

PENICILLIN G PROCAINE INJECTION (RX)

Store at 2° to 8°C (36° to 46°F). Avoid freezing. Injection is stable for 7 days at 25°C (77°F) and 1 day at 40°C (104°F). Wycillin remains stable for 6 months if stored at room temperature.

PENICILLIN GK AND G SODIUM INJECTION (RX)

Store penicillin GK vials at a controlled room temperature. Once they have been diluted, refrigerate for up to 7 days. Once prepared, penicillin G solutions remain stable and free from allergenic components for 24 hours at room temperature or under refrigeration. At a concentration of 40 million units/L, more than 90% potency was retained for 1 month for penicillin GK, and for 39 days for penicillin G when stored in PVC containers at −20°C (−4°F), and for 70 days for penicillin G under refrigeration.

PHENOBARBITAL TABLETS, SOLUTION, AND IM AND IV INJECTIONS (S IV)

Store tablets, oral solution, and IM and IV injection solutions in tightly sealed light-resistant containers at a controlled room temperature. Protect oral solution and tablets from moisture. Slight discoloration is allowable. Discard the solution if there is more discoloration or any precipitation.

PHENYLEPHRINE INJECTION AND OPHTHALMIC SOLUTION (RX) AND NASAL SPRAY (OTC)

Store injection solution in a light-resistant container at a controlled room temperature. Brief excursions to room temperature are permitted. Once it has been diluted, the solution is stable for 4 hours at room temperature and 24 hours if refrigerated. Store nasal spray in light-resistant containers at room temperature. Refrigerate ophthalmic solution. Discard all forms of phenylephrine if brown discoloration occurs or a precipitate forms.

PHENYTOIN CAPSULES, TABLETS, ORAL SOLUTION, AND INJECTION (RX)

Store capsules, tablets, and oral solution at a controlled room temperature. Keep extended-release tablets and oral solution in a light-resistant container. Do not freeze oral solution. Store phenytoin sodium injection solution at a controlled room temperature. The solution is usable while clear or faintly yellow. Discard if the solution becomes hazy or if a precipitate forms and persists at room temperature. Because phenytoin is more stable in saline than in dextrose, use or discard phenytoin in 5% dextrose solution within 2 hours of mixing.

POLYSPORIN OINTMENT (RX)

Store at room temperature. Do not freeze.

POTASSIUM PERMANGANATE ASTRINGENT SOLUTION (OTC)

Store solution in a tightly sealed container at 15° to 30°C (59° to 86°F).

POVIDONE-IODINE SOLUTION (OTC)

Store solution at a controlled room temperature. Brief excursions are permitted to 15° to 30°C (59° to 86°F).

PREDNISONE TABLETS AND ORAL SOLUTION (RX)

Store tablets and oral solution at a controlled room temperature. Brief excursions to room temperature are permitted. Extemporaneous formulations should be stored at room temperature or under refrigeration, and will remain stable for 1 to 2 months.

PROCHLORPERAZINE CAPSULES, TABLETS, ORAL SOLUTION, AND INJECTION (RX)

Store capsules, tablets, and solution in tightly closed light-resistant containers at room temperature. Slight yellow discoloration is acceptable. Discard if more discoloration develops. If preparing an IV admixture, use it immediately or dissolve the prochlorperazine in a dextrose solution and store under refrigeration in a light-resistant container. Prochlorperazine 5 mg/mL or 10 mg/2 mL retained 100% potency when it was stored at room temperature in Tubex containers for 3 months.

PROMETHAZINE CAPSULES, TABLETS, SOLUTION, INJECTION, AND SUPPOSITORIES (RX)

Store capsules, tablets, and oral and injection solutions in a light-resistant container at a controlled room temperature. Light pink discoloration of white promethazine tablets does not indicate a significant loss of potency. Discard the solution if color or precipitate develops. Refrigerate suppositories. Suppositories remain stable at room temperature for 2 weeks, and under refrigeration for weeks.

PSEUDOEPHEDRINE AND PSEUDOEPHEDRINE/ TRIPROLIDINE CAPSULES AND TABLETS (OTC)

Store capsules and tablets in light-resistant containers at 15° to 25°C (59° to 77°F). Protect them from moisture.

RIVAROXABAN TABLET (RX)

Store at 25°C (77°F). Brief excursions are permitted to room temperature.

ROCURONIUM INJECTION (RX)

Store at 2° to 8°C (36° to 46°F). Do not freeze. Injection solutions can be stored at a controlled room temperature for 60 days. Open vials should be used within 30 days.

SILDENAFIL TABLETS (RX)

Store tablets at a controlled room temperature. Brief excursions are permitted to room temperature.

SIMETHICONE CAPSULES, TABLETS, DROPS, AND ULTRASOUND SUSPENSION (OTC)

Store capsules, tablets, and drops in a light-resistant container below 40°C (104°F), and preferably at room temperature. Do not freeze.

SODIUM BICARBONATE TABLETS, INJECTION, AND SUPPOSITORIES (RX)

Store tablets at room temperature. Do not refrigerate. Store injection solution at a controlled room temperature in an airtight container to stop the solution from changing to sodium carbonate. Brief exposure to 40°C (104°F) does not affect stability or potency.

SODIUM SULFACETAMIDE TABLETS, CREAM, LOTION, OINTMENT, AND OPHTHALMIC ROUTE (RX)

Store tablets and cream in light-resistant containers at 15° to 30°C (59° to 86°F). Do not freeze vaginal cream. Store 10% sulfacetamide topical lotion and ointment at room temperature. The lotion will remain stable for 4 months. Do not freeze. Store ophthalmic solution in a light-resistant container at 8° to 15°C (46° to 59°F). Discard if it becomes darkened.

SUCCINYLCHOLINE INJECTION (RX)

Store at 2° to 8°C (36° to 46°F). The injection solution is stable at a controlled room temperature for 14 days. Once it has been diluted, discard within 24 hours.

TEMAZEPAM CAPSULES (S IV)

Store capsules in light-resistant containers below 30°C (86°F). Protect from moisture.

TETANUS TOXOID, TETANUS TOXOID/ DIPHTHERIA/ACELLULAR PERTUSSIS, AND HYPERIMMUNE TETANUS GLOBULIN VACCINE SOLUTIONS (RX)

Store vaccine solutions at 2° to 8°C (36° to 46°F). Do not freeze. The solutions are stable for 72 hours at a controlled room temperature.

TETRACAINE HYDROCHLORIDE OPHTHALMIC SOLUTION (RX)

Store ampules in light-resistant containers at 2° to 8°C (35.6° to 46.4°F) to prevent oxidation and crystallization. Tetracaine hydrochloride remains stable for 3 days at room temperature, and retains the original manufacturer's expiration date if returned to refrigeration. For topical "LET" solution information, see the Lidocaine/Epinephrine/Tetracaine entry.

TETRACYCLINE CAPSULES, TABLETS, ORAL SOLUTION, INJECTION, AND TOPICAL OINTMENT (RX)

Store capsules, tablets, oral solution, and topical ointment in light-resistant containers at room temperature. Reconstituted solutions are stable for 12 hours, and tetracycline hydrochloride is stable in 5% dextrose and water for 6 hours. Do not use outdated products, because they may cause proximal renal tubular acidosis and Fanconi's syndrome.

TOLNAFTATE TOPICAL ANTIFUNGAL SOLUTION (OTC)

Store topical solution at room temperature. Solidification may occur at lower temperatures, but the solution reliquefies easily when warmed.

TRIAZOLAM TABLETS (S IV)

Store tablets at a controlled room temperature.

TRIMETHOPRIM/SULFAMETHOXAZOLE (80 MG/400 MG) TABLETS, ORAL SOLUTION, AND INJECTION (RX)

Store tablets, oral solution, and unopened injection vials at a controlled room temperature. Protect tablets from moisture. Store the oral solution in a light-resistant container. Injection solution, including 80 mg trimethoprim in 100 mL D_5W, is stable for 4 hours, but will last longer if it is more dilute. Vials drawn into a polypropylene syringe will remain stable for 60 hours. Do not refrigerate. Do not inject intramuscularly. Discard if cloudiness or precipitation develops.

TRUVADA (EMTRICITABINE/TENOFOVIR) TABLETS (RX)

Store in a tightly closed container at 25°C (77°F). Brief excursions are permitted at room temperature.

VERAPAMIL HYDROCHLORIDE CAPSULES, TABLETS, AND INJECTION SOLUTION (RX)

Store verapamil sustained-release and all immediate-release tablets in a light-resistant container at 15° to 25°C (59° to 77°F). Immediate-release tablets remain stable for 3 years. Protect all tablets and capsules from moisture. An extemporaneous oral suspension of 50 mg/mL verapamil can be created from 20 of the 80-mg verapamil tablets in a 1:1 mixture of Ora-Plus with Ora-Sweet, Ora-Sweet SF, or flavored syrup mixture (1:4 concentrated flavoring to simple syrup). When stored in light-resistant amber polyethylene terephthalate bottles, the solution retains 91% potency for 60 days at 25°C (77°F) or under refrigeration at 5°C (41°F).

Store verapamil hydrochloride powder and premixed vials in a light-resistant container at room temperature. Protect from moisture. Discard unused portions of the injection solution.

WARFARIN TABLETS (RX)

Store in a light-resistant container at room temperature. Protect from moisture.

ZINC SALTS (OTC)

Store zinc salts in an airtight, nonmetallic container. An extemporaneous formulation of an oral solution can be made up for zinc sulfate by combining 22 g of zinc sulfate powder with 250 mL of flavored syrup and bringing the total volume to 500 mL with purified water. The solution of 10 mg/mL zinc remains stable for 60 days under refrigeration, or for 12 months after addition of a paraben concentrate for a final zinc concentration of 0.5%.

ZOLPIDEM TABLETS, SUBLINGUAL TABLETS, AND SPRAY (S IV)

Store sublingual, immediate-release, and extended-release tablets and oral spray in a light-resistant container at a controlled room temperature. Protect from light and moisture. Brief excursions are permitted to temperatures of 15° to 30°C (59° to 86°F). Do not freeze.

REFERENCES

Complete references used in this text are available online at expertconsult.inkling.com.

Index

Page numbers followed by "*f*" indicate figures, "*t*" indicate tables, and "*b*" indicate boxes.